Contents

For a more detailed Table of Contents, see page xiii.

ASM Handbook®

Volume 21
Composites

Prepared under the direction of the
ASM International Handbook Committee

Daniel B. Miracle and Steven L. Donaldson, Volume Chairs

Scott D. Henry, Project Editor
Charles Moosbrugger, Technical Editor
Gayle J. Anton, Editorial Assistant
Bonnie R. Sanders, Manager of Production
Nancy Hrivnak and Carol Terman, Copy Editors
Jill Kinson, Production Editor
Kathryn Muldoon, Production Assistant
William W. Scott, Jr., Director of Technical Publications

Editorial Assistance
Jill Brown
Kelly Ferjutz
Edward J. Kubel, Jr.
Heather Lampman
Elizabeth Marquard
Beverly Musgrove
Mary Jane Riddlebaugh
Juli Williamson

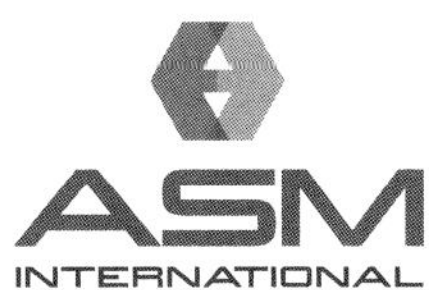

Materials Park, Ohio 44073-0002
www.asminternational.org

First printing, December 2001
Second printing, May 2002
Third printing, January 2005
Fourth printing, March 2006
Fifth printing, June 2007
Sixth printing, October 2008
Seventh printing, January 2012
Eighth printing, July 2017

Comments, criticisms, and suggestions are invited, and should be forwarded to ASM International.

Library of Congress Cataloging-in-Publication Data

ASM International

ASM Handbook
Includes bibliographical references and indexes
Contents: v.1. Properties and selection—irons, steels, and high-performance alloys—v.2. Properties and selection—nonferrous alloys and special-purpose materials—[etc.]—v.23. Materials for medical devices

1. Metals—Handbooks, manuals, etc. 2. Metal-work—Handbooks, manuals, etc. I. ASM International. Handbook Committee. II. Metals Handbook.
TA459.M43 1990 620.1'6 90-115
SAN: 204-7586

ISBN-13: 978-0-87170-703-1
ISBN-10: 0-87170-703-9

ASM International®
Materials Park, OH 44073-0002
www.asminternational.org

Printed in the United States of America

Foreword

ASM International is proud to offer *Composites* as Volume 21 of the *ASM Handbook*. The nominal basis for this volume was the *Engineered Materials Handbook,* Volume 1, published in 1987. However, this new edition is, to a large degree, a brand new volume. New or greatly expanded coverage is provided, in particular, in the Sections on constituent materials, analysis and design, and processing. New sections have been added to address the important topics of maintenance, repair, and recycling. Coverage of polymer-matrix composites has been enhanced to address the latest materials advances and new application areas. Coverage of metal-matrix and ceramic-matrix composites has been revamped and greatly expanded to reflect the increasing industrial importance of these materials.

With the release of this new edition of the *Composites* volume, it seems like a natural transition for it to become part of the *ASM Handbook* series. The *Metals Handbook* series was renamed the *ASM Handbook* in the mid-1990s to reflect the increasingly interrelated nature of materials and manufacturing technologies. Since that time the *ASM Handbook* has incorporated increasing amounts of information about nonmetallic materials in each new and revised volume. ASM expects that other volumes in the *Engineered Materials Handbook* will become part of the *ASM Handbook* when they are revised.

Creating the new edition of this monumental reference work was a daunting task. We extend thanks and congratulations on behalf of ASM International to the Volume Chairs, Dan Miracle and Steve Donaldson, and the Volume's 13 Section Chairs for the outstanding job they have done in developing the outline for the revision and guiding its development. Our gratitude is also due to the over 300 international experts from industry, academia, and research who contributed as authors and reviewers to this edition. In addition, we express our appreciation to the ASM International editorial and production staff for their dedicated efforts in preparing this volume for publication.

Aziz I. Asphahani
President
ASM International

Michael J. DeHaemer
Managing Director
ASM International

Policy on Units of Measure

By a resolution of its Board of Trustees, ASM International has adopted the practice of publishing data in both metric and customary U.S. units of measure. In preparing this Handbook, the editors have attempted to present data in metric units based primarily on Système International d'Unités (SI), with secondary mention of the corresponding values in customary U.S. units. The decision to use SI as the primary system of units was based on the aforementioned resolution of the Board of Trustees and the widespread use of metric units throughout the world.

For the most part, numerical engineering data in the text and in tables are presented in SI-based units with the customary U.S. equivalents in parentheses (text) or adjoining columns (tables). For example, pressure, stress, and strength are shown both in SI units, which are pascals (Pa) with a suitable prefix, and in customary U.S. units, which are pounds per square inch (psi). To save space, large values of psi have been converted to kips per square inch (ksi), where 1 ksi = 1000 psi. The metric tonne (kg $\times$ 10^3) has sometimes been shown in megagrams (Mg). Some strictly scientific data are presented in SI units only.

To clarify some illustrations, only one set of units is presented on artwork. References in the accompanying text to data in the illustrations are presented in both SI-based and customary U.S. units. On graphs and charts, grids corresponding to SI-based units usually appear along the left and bottom edges. Where appropriate, corresponding customary U.S. units appear along the top and right edges.

Data pertaining to a specification published by a specification-writing group may be given in only the units used in that specification or in dual units, depending on the nature of the data. For example, the typical yield strength of steel sheet made to a specification written in customary U.S. units would be presented in dual units, but the sheet thickness specified in that specification might be presented only in inches.

Data obtained according to standardized test methods for which the standard recommends a particular system of units are presented in the units of that system. Wherever feasible, equivalent units are also presented. Some statistical data may also be presented in only the original units used in the analysis.

Conversions and rounding have been done in accordance with IEEE/ASTM SI-10, with attention given to the number of significant digits in the original data. For example, an annealing temperature of 1570 °F contains three significant digits. In this case, the equivalent temperature would be given as 855 °C; the exact conversion to 854.44 °C would not be appropriate. For an invariant physical phenomenon that occurs at a precise temperature (such as the melting of pure silver), it would be appropriate to report the temperature as 961.93 °C or 1763.5 °F. In some instances (especially in tables and data compilations), temperature values in °C and °F are alternatives rather than conversions.

The policy of units of measure in this Handbook contains several exceptions to strict conformance to IEEE/ASTM SI-10; in each instance, the exception has been made in an effort to improve the clarity of the Handbook. The most notable exception is the use of g/cm^3 rather than kg/m^3 as the unit of measure for density (mass per unit volume).

SI practice requires that only one virgule (diagonal) appear in units formed by combination of several basic units. Therefore, all of the units preceding the virgule are in the numerator and all units following the virgule are in the denominator of the expression; no parentheses are required to prevent ambiguity.

Preface

It should be apparent with just a quick glance through this Volume that a great deal of technical progress has been made since the first edition was published in 1987 (as *Engineered Materials Handbook*, Volume 1). Much of the earlier promise of high performance organic-matrix composites (OMCs) has been fulfilled. These materials are now the preferred design solution for an expansive scope of applications. Earlier concerns related to high cost and marginal manufacturability have been satisfactorily addressed through high volume and innovative design and manufacturing, including extensive use of unitized design and construction. A clear example of the success in these areas is illustrated by the growing use of high-performance composites in the commodity applications of civil infrastructure. Nonetheless, cost and manufacturability continue to be areas of vigorous development and hold hope for significant future advancements, along with the development of composite materials with higher specific properties, higher operating temperatures, and improved supportability. One can expect to see broad advances in innovative structural concepts and certification methods in the future.

The progress in metal-matrix composites (MMCs) has been equally remarkable. Although only marginal coverage was warranted in the first edition, MMCs now represent a significant material option in the international marketplace. The world market for MMCs was over 2.5 million kg (5.5 million pounds) in 1999, and an annual growth rate of over 17% has been projected for the next several years. Significant applications are in service in the aeronautical, aerospace, ground transportation, thermal management/electronic packaging, and recreation industries. The ability to offer significant improvements in structural efficiency and to excel in several other functional areas, including thermal management and wear, and to utilize existing metalworking infrastructure have aided this progress. Continued future extension into both new and existing markets is expected.

While ceramic-matrix composite (CMC) technology is still largely centered in the research and development phase, significant advancements have been made. Some commercial applications now exist, and strategies for growing market insertion are being pursued. The traditional motivation of structural performance and environmental resistance at the highest application temperatures continue to provide incentive for development. Recent important research accomplishments provide growing optimism that significant aeropropulsion structural applications will be fielded in the coming decade.

The primary objective of *ASM Handbook*, Volume 21, *Composites* is to provide a comprehensive, practical, and reliable source of technical knowledge, engineering data, and supporting information for composite materials. Coverage of OMCs and MMCs is provided in a balanced fashion that reflects the maturity of each material class. Given the current status of CMC materials, less coverage is provided, but it, too, is focused in areas of current industrial importance. This Handbook is intended to be a resource volume for nonspecialists who are interested in gaining a practical working knowledge of the capabilities and applications of composite materials. Thus, coverage emphasizes well-qualified information for materials that can be produced in quantities and product forms of engineering significance. This Volume is not intended to be a presentation of fundamental research activities, although it certainly provides an important reference for scientists engaged in the development of new composite materials. The full range of information of importance to the practical technologist is provided in this Volume, including topics of constituent materials; engineering mechanics, design, and analysis; manufacturing processes; post–processing and assembly; quality control; testing and certification; properties and performance; product reliability, maintainability, and repair; failure analysis; recycling and disposal; and applications.

This new edition builds on the success of the version published as Volume 1 of the *Engineered Materials Handbook*. Information on OMCs has been updated to reflect advancements in this technology field, including improvements in low cost manufacturing technologies and significantly expanded applications in areas such as infrastructure. Progress in MMCs has been particularly dramatic since the previous edition, and new information on these materials provides an up-to-date comprehensive guide to MMC processing, properties, applications, and technology. CMCs also have entered service in limited applications since the previous edition, and the coverage of these materials reflects this progress. These three classes of composites are covered in each Section of the Volume as appropriate to provide a unified view of these engineered materials and to reduce redundancies in the previous edition.

We would like to offer our personal, heartfelt appreciation to the Section Chairpersons, article authors, reviewers, and ASM staff for sharing both their expertise and extensive efforts for this project.

Daniel B. Miracle
Steven L. Donaldson
Air Force Research Laboratory

Officers and Trustees of ASM International (2000–2001)

Members of the ASM Handbook Comittee (2000–2001)

Previous Chairs of the ASM Handbook Comittee

Authors and Contributors

R.C. Adams
Lockheed Martin Aeronautical Systems

Suresh Advani
University of Delaware

David E. Alman
U.S. Department of Energy

Finn Roger Andressen
Reichhold AS

Keith B. Armstrong
Consultant

B. Tomas Åström
IFP SICOMP AB

Amit Bandyopadhyay
Washington State University

Yoseph Bar-Cohen
Jet Propulsion Laboratory

Robert J. Basso
Century Design Inc.

Mark Battley
Industrial Research Limited

Joseph J. Beaman, Jr.
University of Texas at Austin

John H. Belk
The Boeing Company

Tia Benson Tolle
Air Force Research Laboratory

Barry J. Berenberg
Caldera Composites

John Bootle
XC Associates Inc.

Chris Boshers
Composite Materials Characterization Inc.

Richard H. Bossi
The Boeing Company

David L. Bourell
University of Texas at Austin

Dennis Bowles
Northrop Grumman Corporation

Jack Boyd
CyTech Fiberite Inc.

Maureen A. Boyle
Hexcel Corporation

Shari Bugaj
FiberCote Industries Inc.

Frank Burzesi
XC Associates Inc.

Flake C. Campbell
The Boeing Company

Karl K. Chang
DuPont

K.K. Chawla
University of Alabama

N. Chawla
Arizona State University

Eric Chesmar
United Airlines

Richard J. Chester
Aeronautical and Maritime Research Laboratory

S. Christensen
The Boeing Company

William F. Cole II
United Airlines

Bruce Crawford
Deakin University

George Dallas
TA Instruments

Joseph R. Davis
Davis & Associates

J.A. DiCarlo
NASA Glenn Research Center

Cynthia Powell Doğan
U.S. Department of Energy

Roderick Don
University of Delaware

Steven L. Donaldson
Air Force Research Laboratory

Louis C. Dorworth
Abaris Training Resources Inc.

Richard Downs-Honey
High Modulus New Zealand Limited

T.E. Drake
Lockheed Martin Aerospace

Lawrence T. Drzal
Michigan State University

G. Ehnert
Menzolit-Fibron GmbH

D. Emahiser
GKN Aerospace

Roger W. Engelbart
The Boeing Company

Don O. Evans
Cincinnati Machine

Richard E. Fields
Lockheed Martin Missiles and Fire Control

Lynda Fiorini
XC Associates Inc.

Gerald Flanagan
Materials Sciences Corporation

Mark S. Forte
Air Force Research Laboratory

Marvin Foston
Lockheed Martin Aeronautical Systems

Luther M. Gammon
The Boeing Company

C.P. Gardiner
Defence Science & Technology Organisation, Australia

Nicholas J. Gianaris
Visteon Corporation

Ian Gibson
The University of Hong Kong

Lawrence A. Gintert
Concurrent Technologies Corporation

Jonathan Goering
Albany International Techniweave Inc.

John W. Goodman
Material Technologies Inc.

J.H. Gosse
The Boeing Company

Michael N. Grimshaw
Cincinnati Machine

Olivier Guillermin
Vistagy Inc.

H. Thomas Hahn
Air Force Office of Scientific Research

Paul Hakes
High Modulus New Zealand Limited

William C. Harrigan
MMC Engineering Inc.

L.J. Hart-Smith
The Boeing Company

Brian S. Hayes
University of Washington

Dirk Heider
University of Delaware

Edmund G. Henneke II
Virginia Polytechnic Institute and State University

John M. Henshaw
University of Tulsa

G. Aaron Henson III
Design Alternatives Inc.

Rikard B. Heslehurst
Australian Defence Force Academy

Arlen Hoebergen
Centre of Lightweight Structures TUD-TNO

Leslie A. Hoeckelman
The Boeing Company

Michael J. Hoke
Abaris Training Resources Inc.

J. Anders Holmberg
SICOMP AB

K. Hörsting
Menzolit-Fibron GmbH

Warren H. Hunt, Jr.
Aluminum Consultants Group Inc.

Michael G. Jenkins
University of Washington

L. Kahn
Georgia Institute of Technology

Vistasp M. Karbhari
University of California, San Diego

Kristen M. Kearns
Air Force Research Laboratory

Shrikant N. Khot
University of Delaware

Jeffrey J. Kilwin
The Boeing Company

Jim Kindinger
Hexcel Corporation

Donald A. Klosterman
University of Dayton

Frank K. Ko
Drexel University

Greg Kress
Delta Air Lines

Lawrence F. Kuberski
Fischer U.S.A.

R. Kühfusz
Menzolit-Fibron GmbH

Joseph M. Kunze
Triton Systems

Joe Lautner
Gerber Technology Inc.

Richard D. Lawson
The Boeing Company

David Lewis III
Naval Research Laboratory

Hong Li
PPG Industries Inc.

R. Liebold
Menzolit-Fibron GmbH

Shyh-Shiuh Lih
Jet Propulsion Laboratory

Jim R. Logsdon
EMF Corporation

Peter W. Lorraine
General Electric Company

Bhaskar S. Majumdar
New Mexico Institute of Mining and Technology

Ajit K. Mal
University of California, Los Angeles

Cary J. Martin
Hexcel Corporation

Jeffrey D. Martin
Martin Pultrusion Group

James J. Mazza
Air Force Research Laboratory

John E. McCarty
Composite Structures Consulting

Douglas A. McCarville
The Boeing Company

Colin McCullough
3M Company

Lee McKague
Composites-Consulting Inc.

James McKnight
The Boeing Company

J. Lowrie McLarty

Carol Meyers
Materials Sciences Corporation

Andrew Mills
Cranfield University

Daniel B. Miracle
Air Force Research Laboratory

Stephen C. Mitchell
General Electric Aircraft Engines

John E. Moalli
Exponent Failure Analysis Associates

Robert Moore
Northrop Grumman Corporation

A.P. Mouritz
RMIT University

John Moylan
Delsen Testing Laboratories

Thomas Munns
ARINC

John D. Neuner
Hexcel Corporation

Steven R. Nutt
University of Southern California

T. Kevin O'Brien
U.S. Army Research Laboratory

Michael J. Paleen
The Boeing Company

Awadh B. Pandey
Pratt & Whitney

Robert T. Parker
The Boeing Company

Tim Pepper
Ashland Chemical Company

Stanley T. Peters
Process Research

Charles W. Peterson
Azdel bv

Daniel R. Petrak

J. Gary Pruett
Hitco Carbon Composites

Shahid P. Qureshi
Georgia-Pacific Resins Inc.

Naveen Rastogi
Visteon Chassis Systems

Suraj P. Rawal
Lockheed Martin Astronautics

Scott Reeve
National Composite Center

Susan Robitaille
YLA Inc.

Carl Rousseau
Bell Helicopter

Paul A. Roy
Vantage Associates Inc.

C.D. Rudd
University of Nottingham

Daniel R. Ruffner
The Boeing Company

A.J. Russell
Dockyard Laboratory Pacific, DRDC

John D. Russell
Air Force Research Laboratory

Adam J. Sawicki
The Boeing Company

Henry A. Schaefer
The Boeing Company

Jeffrey R. Schaff
United Technologies Research Center

Hans-Wolfgang Schröder
EADS Deutschland GmbH

Mel M. Schwartz
Sikorsky Aircraft (retired)

Daniel A. Scola
University of Connecticut

Tito T. Serafini

Steven M. Shepard
Thermal Wave Imaging, Inc.

M. Singh
QSS Group Inc.
NASA Glenn Research Center

Raj N. Singh
University of Cincinnati

Cory A. Smith
DWA Aluminum Composites

E. Murat Sozer
KOC University

Horst Stenzenberger
Technochemie GmbH

Rich Stover
Lockheed Martin Aeronautics

Patricia L. Stumpff
Hartzell Propeller Inc.

Joseph E. Sumerak
Creative Pultrusions Inc.

Kirk Tackitt
U.S. Army Research Laboratory

E.T. Thostenson
University of Delaware

R.S. Trask
DERA Farnborough

J. Tucker
Southern Research Institute

Rebecca Ufkes
Ufkes Engineering

Barry P. Van West
The Boeing Company

Anthony J. Vizzini
University of Maryland

Frederick T. Wallenberger
PPG Industries Inc.

Paul J. Walsh
Zoltek Corporation

Stephen Ward
SW Composites

Jeff L. Ware
Lockheed Martin Aeronautics

James C. Watson
PPG Industries Inc.

David Weiss
Eck Industries Inc.

Mark Wilhelm
The Boeing Company

D.M. Wilson
3M Company

Rod Wishart
Integrated Technologies Inc. (Intec)

Mike R. Woodward
Lockheed Martin Aeronautics

Richard P. Wool
University of Delaware

H.M. Yun
NASA Glenn Research Center

F.W. Zok
University of California, Santa Barbara

A. Zureick
Georgia Institute of Technology

Carl Zweben
Composites Consultant

Reviewers

John W. Aaron
The Boeing Company

R.C. Adams
Lockheed Martin Aeronautical Systems

John C. Adelmann
Sikorsky Aircraft

Suresh Advani
University of Delaware

Suphal P. Agrawal
Northrop Grumman Corporation

Klaus Ahlborn
Mitras Composites Systems

Bob Allanson
GKN Westland Aerospace

David P. Anderson
University of Dayton Research Institute

Donald A. Anderson
The Boeing Company

Douglas L. Armstrong
Fiber Innovations Inc.

Keith B. Armstrong
Consultant

B. Tomas Åström
IFP SICOMP AS

Mohan Aswani

Mark Battley
Industrial Research Limited, New Zealand

Behzad Bavarian
California State University, Northridge

Matthew R. Begley
University of Connecticut

Arie Ben-Dov
Israel Aircraft Industry

Tia Benson Tolle
Air Force Research Laboratory

Albert Bertram
Naval Surface Weapons Center

Edward Bernardon
Vistagy Inc.

R.T. Bhatt
NASA Glenn Research Center

Greg Black
Northrop Grumman Corporation

Tom Blankenship
The Boeing Company

George A. Blann
Buehler Ltd.

Ben R. Bognar
BP Amoco Chemicals

Gregg R. Bogucki
The Boeing Company

Raymond Bohlmann
The Boeing Company

Collin Bohn
The Boeing Company

Chris Boshers
Composite Materials Characterization Inc.

Dennis Bowles
Northrop Grumman Corporation

Alfonso Branca
Top Glass s.p.a.

Mike Brun
General Electric

Doug Brunner
Lockheed Martin

Bruce L. Burton
Huntsman Corporation

Mark Bush
University of Western Australia

Rick Callis
Hexcel Corporation

Flake C. Campbell
The Boeing Company

Gene Camponeschi
NSWCCD

Jay Carpenter
Creative Tooling

Mark T. Carroll
Lockheed Martin Aeronautics

Patrick E. Cassidy
Southwest Texas State University

Gilbert B. Chapman II
DaimlerChrysler Corporation

K.K. Chawla
University of Alabama

N. Chawla
Arizona State University

Judy Chen
The Boeing Company

Richard J. Chester
Aeronautical and Maritime Research Laboratory

Mark Chris
Bell Helicopter Textron

Stan Chichanoski
Steinerfilm Inc.

Bruce Choate
Northrop Grumman Corporation

Linda L. Clements
C & C Technologies

Todd Coburn
Adroit Engineering

William F. Cole II
United Airlines

Doug Condel

John Cooney

Bruce Cox
DaimlerChrysler Corporation

Jim Criss
Lockheed Martin Aeronautics

Alan Crosky
University of New South Wales

Maxwell Davis

J.G. Dean
Lockheed Martin

Thomas J. Dearlove
General Motors Corporation

Leen Deurloo
Adzel bv

Herve Deve
3M Company

José Manuel Luna Díaz
EADS-CASA Airbus

George DiBari
International Nickel

Jack Dini
Consultant

John Dion
BAE Systems

Alan Dobyns
Sikorsky Aircraft

Jim Door
Duke Engineering

Louis C. Dorworth
Abaris Training Resources Inc.

Timothy E. Easler
COI Ceramics Inc.

Jim Epperson

Jay Fiebig
Warner Robins Air Logistics Center

Richard E. Fields
Lockheed Martin Missiles and Fire Control

Lynda Fiorini
XC Associates Inc.

John Fish
Lockheed Martin Aeronautics Company

Gerald Flanagan
Materials Sciences Corporation

Marvin Foston
Lockheed Martin Aeronautical Systems

Rob Fredell
U.S. Air Force Academy

David H. Fry
The Boeing Company

H. GangaRao
West Virginia University

Samuel P. Garbo
Sikorsky Aircraft

Slade Gardner
Lockheed Martin Aeronautics

C.P. Gardiner
Defence Science and Technology Organisation

Rikard Gebart
Luleå University of Technology

Gerald A. Gegel

Guy M. Genin
Washington University

Dipankar K. Ghosh
Vanderplaats R&D Inc.

Nicholas J. Gianaris
Visteon Corporation

A.G. Gibson
University of Newcastle upon Tyne

John W. Goodman
Materials Technologies Inc.

Peter Grant
The Boeing Company

Stephen A. Green
Sikorsky Aircraft

John Griffith
The Boeing Company

John Gruss
The Boeing Company

John W. Halloran
University of Michigan

Gail Hahn
The Boeing Company

William C. Harrigan
MMC Engineering Inc.

Neil M. Hawkins
University of Illinois

Randy Hay
Air Force Research Laboratory

Paul Hergenrother
NASA Langley Research Center

Mike Hinton
DERA Farnborough

Michael J. Hoke
Abaris Training Resources Inc.

Richard C. Holzwarth
Air Force Research Laboratory

DeWayne Howell
CompositeTek

Kuang-Ting Hsiao
University of Delaware

Donald Hunston
National Institute of Standards and Technology

Warren H. Hunt, Jr.
Aluminum Consultants Group Inc.

Frances Hurwitz
NASA Glenn Research Center

John W. Hutchinson
Harvard University

William Jandeska

Dave Jarmon
United Technologies

Michael G. Jenkins
University of Washington

Paul D. Jero
Air Force Research Laboratory

Richard A. Jeryan
Ford Motor Company

Eric Johnson
Virginia Polytechnic Institute and State University

Robert M. Jones
Virginia Polytechnic Institute and State University

Ronald J. Kander
Virginia Polytechnic Institute and State University

Vistasp M. Karbhari
University of California, San Diego

Allan Kaye
BAE Systems

Ronald J. Kerans
Air Force Research Laboratory

Hamid Kia

Christopher J. Kirschling
Reichold Chemicals Inc.

James Klett
Oak Ridge National Laboratory

Eric S. Knudsen
Fiberline Composites A/S

Greg Kress
Delta Air Lines

Raymond B. Krieger, Jr.
Cytec-Fiberite Inc.

Arun Kumar
Seal Laboratories

Murray Kuperman
United Airlines (retired)

Jeremy Leggoe
Texas Tech University

Bradley A. Lerch
NASA Glenn Research Center

James Leslie
ACPT Inc.

Chris Levan
BP Amoco Carbon Fibers

Stanley Levine
NASA Glenn Research Center

John Lewandowski
Case Western Reserve University

Jian Li
The Boeing Company

Denny Liles
BGF Industries Inc.

Mike Lindsey
Lockheed Martin

Steve Loud
Composites Worldwide Inc.

David Maas
Flightware

Tönu Malm
Metallvägen

John F. Mandell
Montana State University

Rod Martin
Materials Engineering Research Laboratory

Frederick J. McGarry
Massachusetts Institute of Technology

Lee McKague
Composites-Consulting Inc.

Stewart E. McKinzy
TWA Inc.

Aram Mekjian
Mektek Composites Inc.

Greg Mellema
Abaris Training Resources Inc.

James D. Miller
Cool Polymers

Robert J. Miller
Pratt & Whitney

Andrew Mills
Cranfield University

Daniel B. Miracle
Air Force Research Laboratory

Jack Mitrey
Ashland Chemicals

Peter Mitschang
Institute für Verbundwerkstoffe GmbH

Dale Moore
Naval Air Systems

A.P. Mouritz
RMIT University

Alvin Nakagawa
Northrup Grumman Corporation

James Newell

Theodore Nicholas
Air Force Research Laboratory

T. Kevin O'Brien
U.S. Army Research Laboratory

Mark Occhionero
Ceramic Process Systems

Tim A. Osswald
University of Wisconsin

Steve Owens
Lockheed Martin

Ron Parkinson
Nickel Development Institute

Steven Peake
Cytec-Fiberite Inc.

John Peters
A&P Technology

Bruce Pfund
Special Projects LLC

Fred Policelli
FPI Composites Engineering

Richard D. Pistole

Kevin Potter
University of Bristol

(Paul) Mack Puckett

Naveen Rastogi
Visteon Chassis Systems

Suraj P. Rawal
Lockheed Martin Astronautics

James Reeder
NASA Langley Research Center

David L. Rose
Polese Company

Tom Rose

Carl Rousseau
Bell Helicopter

Roger Rowell

C.D. Rudd
University of Nottingham

Daniel R. Ruffner
The Boeing Company

John Russell
Air Force Research Laboratory

Adam J. Sawicki
The Boeing Company

Robert E. Schafrik
GE Aircraft Engines

Warren C. Schimpf
Advanced Fiber Technology

John R. Schlup
Kansas State University

Daniel A. Scola
University of Connecticut

Mark Shea
The Boeing Company

Bill Schweinberg
Warner Robins Air Logistics Center

R. Ajit Shenoi
University of Southampton

Robert L. Sierakowski
Air Force Research Laboratory

Raymond J. Sinatra
Rolls Royce Corporation

J.P. Singh
Argonne National Laboratory

Lawrence H. Sobel
Northrop Grumman Corporation (retired)

Jonathan E. Spowart
UES Incorporated

David A. Steenkamer
Ford Motor Company

W. Kent Stewart
Bell Helicopter Textron

Bob Stratton

Brent Strong
Brigham Young University

Brent Stucker
University of Rhode Island

Patricia L. Stumpff
Hartzell Propeller Inc.

Susan Sun
Kansas State University

Jerry Sundsrud
3M Company

John Taylor
Borden Chemical

Roland Thevenin
Airbus

L. Scott Thiebert
Air Force Research Laboratory

Rodney Thomson
CRC for Advanced Composites
Structures Ltd.

Katie E.G. Thorp
Air Force Research Laboratory

Richard E. Tressler
Pennsylvania State University

Francois Trochu
Ecole Polytechnique de Montreal

Willem van Dreumel
Ten Cate Advanced Composites bv

Richard Van Luven
Northrup Grumman Corporation

Barry P. Van West
The Boeing Company

James Vaughan
University of Mississippi

Albert A. Vicario
Alliant Techsystems Inc.

Anthony J. Vizzini
University of Maryland

Shawn Walsh
Army Research Laboratory

Steve Wanthal
The Boeing Company

Stephen Ward
SW Composites

Charles R. Watson
Pratt & Whitney

Kevin Waymack
The Boeing Company

David Weiss
Eck Industries Inc.

Dan White
dmc^2 Electronic Components Corporation

Mary Ann White
Alliant Techsystems Inc.

Paul D. Wienhold
Johns Hopkins University

J.L. Willet
USDA/ARS/NCAUR

Martin Williams
ADI Limited

Mark Wilhelm
The Boeing Company

D.J. Williamson
The Boeing Company

Dale W. Wilson
Johns Hopkins University

David Wilson
3M Company

Warren W. Wolf
Owens Corning

Ernest Wolff
PMIC

Hugh Yap
Aerocell Inc.

Chun Zhang
Florida State University

Contents

Introduction to Composites

Chairpersons: Daniel B. Miracle and Steven L. Donaldson, Air Force Research Laboratory

---

Introduction to Composites

Daniel B. Miracle and Steven L. Donaldson, Air Force Research Laboratory

A COMPOSITE MATERIAL is a macroscopic combination of two or more distinct materials, having a recognizable interface between them. Composites are used not only for their structural properties, but also for electrical, thermal, tribological, and environmental applications. Modern composite materials are usually optimized to achieve a particular balance of properties for a given range of applications. Given the vast range of materials that may be considered as composites and the broad range of uses for which composite materials may be designed, it is difficult to agree upon a single, simple, and useful definition. However, as a common practical definition, composite materials may be restricted to emphasize those materials that contain a continuous matrix constituent that binds together and provides form to an array of a stronger, stiffer reinforcement constituent. The resulting composite material has a balance of structural properties that is superior to either constituent material alone. The improved structural properties generally result from a load-sharing mechanism. Although composites optimized for other functional properties (besides high structural efficiency) could be produced from completely different constituent combinations than fit this structural definition, it has been found that composites developed for structural applications also provide attractive performance in these other functional areas as well. As a result, this simple definition for structural composites provides a useful definition for most current functional composites.

Thus, composites typically have a fiber or particle phase that is stiffer and stronger than the continuous matrix phase. Many types of reinforcements also often have good thermal and electrical conductivity, a coefficient of thermal expansion (CTE) that is less than the matrix, and/or good wear resistance. There are, however, exceptions that may still be considered composites, such as rubber-modified polymers, where the discontinuous phase is more compliant and more ductile than the polymer, resulting in improved toughness. Similarly, steel wires have been used to reinforce gray cast iron in truck and trailer brake drums.

Composites are commonly classified at two distinct levels. The first level of classification is usually made with respect to the matrix constituent. The major composite classes include organic-matrix composites (OMCs), metal-matrix composites (MMCs), and ceramic-matrix composites (CMCs). The term "organic-matrix composite" is generally assumed to include two classes of composites: polymer-matrix composites (PMCs) and carbon-matrix composites (commonly referred to as carbon-carbon composites). Carbon-matrix composites are typically formed from PMCs by including the extra steps of carbonizing and densifying the original polymer matrix. In the research and development community, intermetallic-matrix composites (IMCs) are sometimes listed as a classification that is distinct from MMCs. However, significant commercial applications of IMCs do not yet exist, and in a practical sense these materials do not provide a radically different set of properties relative to MMCs. In each of these systems, the matrix is typically a continuous phase throughout the component.

The second level of classification refers to the reinforcement form—particulate reinforcements, whisker reinforcements, continuous fiber laminated composites, and woven composites (braided and knitted fiber architectures are included in this category), as depicted in Fig. 1 (Ref 1). In order to provide a useful increase in properties, there generally must be a substantial volume fraction ($\sim$10% or more) of the reinforcement. A reinforcement is considered to be a "particle" if all of its dimensions are roughly equal. Thus, particulate-reinforced composites include those reinforced by spheres, rods, flakes, and many other shapes of roughly equal axes. Whisker reinforcements, with an aspect ratio typically between approximately 20 to 100, are often considered together with particulates in MMCs. Together, these are classified as "discontinuous" reinforcements, because the reinforcing phase is discontinuous for the lower volume fractions typically used in MMCs. There are also materials, usually polymers, that contain particles that extend rather than reinforce the material. These are generally referred to as "filled" systems. Because filler particles are included for the purpose of cost reduction rather than reinforcement, these composites are not generally considered to be particulate composites. Nonetheless, in some cases the filler will also reinforce the matrix material. The same may be true for particles added for nonstructural purposes, such as fire resistance, control of shrinkage, and increased thermal or electrical conductivity.

Continuous fiber-reinforced composites contain reinforcements having lengths much greater than their cross-sectional dimensions. Such a composite is considered to be a discontinuous fiber or short fiber composite if its properties vary with fiber length. On the other hand, when the length of the fiber is such that any further increase in length does not, for example, further increase the elastic modulus or strength of the composite, the composite is considered to be continuous fiber reinforced. Most continuous fiber (or continuous filament) composites, in fact, contain fibers that are comparable in length to the overall dimensions of the composite part. As shown in Fig. 1, each layer or "ply" of a continuous fiber composite typically has a specific fiber orientation direction. These layers can be stacked such that each layer has a specified fiber orientation, thereby giving the entire laminated stack ("laminate") highly tailorable overall properties. Complicating the definition of a composite as having both continuous and discontinuous phases is the fact that in a laminated composite, neither of these phases may be regarded as truly continuous in three dimensions. Many applications require isotropy in a plane, and this is achieved by controlling the fiber orientation within a laminated composite. Hybrid organic-metal laminates are also used, where, for exam-

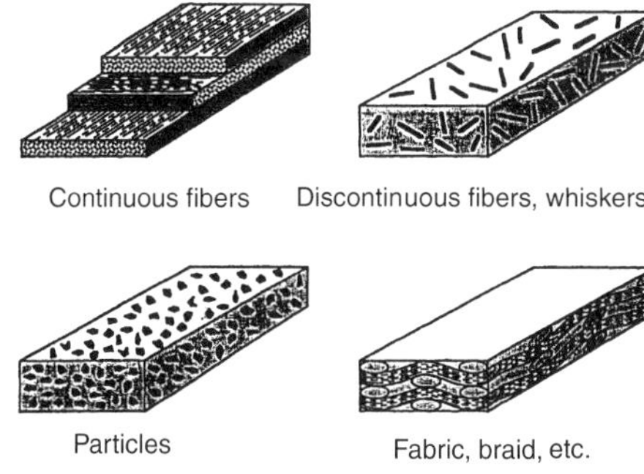

Fig. 1 Common forms of fiber reinforcement. In general, the reinforcements can be straight continuous fibers, discontinuous or chopped fibers, particles or flakes, or continuous fibers that are woven, braided, or knitted. Source: Ref 1

ple, layers of glass/epoxy are combined with aluminum alloy sheets. These laminates provide improved wear, impact and blast resistance, and fire resistance.

The final category of fiber architecture is that formed by weaving, braiding, or knitting the fiber bundles or "tows" to create interlocking fibers that often have orientations slightly or fully in an orientation orthogonal to the primary structural plane. This approach is taken for a variety of reasons, including the ability to have structural, thermal, or electrical properties in the third or "out-of-plane" dimension. Another often-cited reason for using these architectures is that the "unwetted" or dry fiber preforms (fibers before any matrix is added) are easier to handle, lower in cost, and conform to highly curved shapes more readily than the highly aligned, continuous fiber form.

In addition to these general categories, it is possible to create fiber architectures that are combinations of two or more of these categories. For example, it is possible to create laminated structures of both knitted fabric and continuous fiber layers. The design flexibility offered by composites is truly infinite!

A Brief History of Composite Materials

Organic-matrix composites, or OMCs, originated through efforts in the aerospace community during World War II to produce materials with specific strength and stiffness values that were significantly higher than existing structural materials. In addition, existing aerospace structural alloys, such as those based on aluminum, were subject to corrosion and fatigue damage, and OMCs provided an approach to overcome these issues. By the end of the war, glass-fiber-reinforced plastics had been used successfully in filament-wound rocket motors and demonstrated in various other prototype structural aircraft applications. These materials were put into broader use in the 1950s and provided important improvements in structural response and corrosion resistance. Commercial applications in consumer sporting equipment in the 1960s provided a larger market, which improved design and production capabilities, established consumer familiarity and confidence, and lowered costs.

Defense spending during the Cold War ensured sufficient resources for research and development of new, high-technology materials, and a market for their application. The significant number of new military aircraft, and the large numbers of systems ordered, provided an ideal environment for the development and insertion of high-performance OMCs. The energy crisis during the 1970s provided a significant incentive for the introduction of OMCs into commercial aircraft, and the successful experience in military aircraft was an important factor in their acceptance in the commercial industry. Dramatic improvements in structural efficiency became possible during this period, through the introduction of high-performance carbon fibers. Improved manufacturing capabilities and design methodologies provided the background for significant increases in OMC use for military and commercial aircraft and spacecraft structures.

Over the past 30 years, OMCs have won an increasing mass fraction of aircraft and spacecraft structures. This is demonstrated by the fact that the vintage 1970s application of OMCs to fighter aircraft was typically confined to tailskins and other secondary or "noncritical" flight structures. For example, only 2% of the F-15 E/F was comprised of OMCs. During the subsequent years, significant government and private investments were made toward research, development, fabrication, testing, and flight service demonstration of composite materials and structures. Parallel programs were also ongoing for the use of composites in military and civilian land and naval vehicles. For example, the development of fiberglass structures for boats and other marine applications was extremely successful and now accounts for a significant portion of composite production volume. During these years, confidence in using composite materials increased dramatically. This was also a period of great innovation in manufacturing, assembly, and repair method development.

The advantages demonstrated by composites, in addition to high stiffness, high strength, and low density, include corrosion resistance, long fatigue lives, tailorable properties (including thermal expansion, critical to satellite structures), and the ability to form complex shapes. (This advantage was demonstrated in the ability to create "low observable," or stealth, structures for military systems.) An example of recent OMC application is the next-generation U.S. tactical fighter aircraft, the F-22. Over 24% of the F-22 structure is OMCs. The B-2 bomber, shown in Fig. 2, is constructed using an even higher percentage of composites, as are current helicopter and vertical lift designs. For example, the tilt-rotor V-22 Osprey is over 41% composite materials. The upper-use temperature of PMCs has also increased dramatically: early epoxies were considered useable (for extended periods) up to 121 °C (250 °F). Current generation polymers, such as bismaleimides, have increased that limit to around 204 °C (400 °F), and the use of polyimide-matrix composites has extended the range to 288 °C (550 °F).

Once considered premium materials only to be used if their high costs could be justified by increased performance, OMCs can now often "buy their way onto" new applications. This is

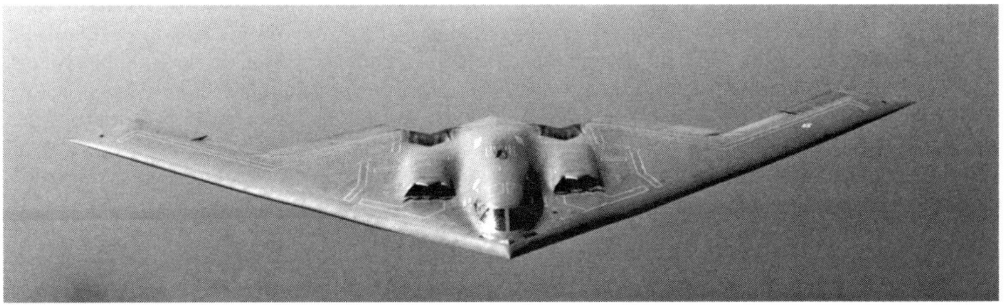

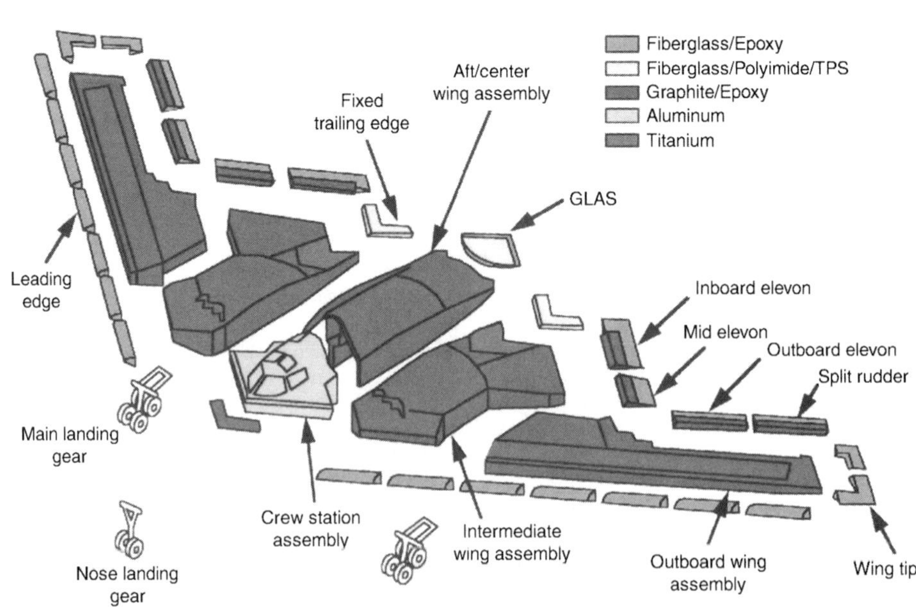

Fig. 2 The U. S. Air Force B-2 advanced "stealth" bomber, which is constructed to a large extent of advanced composite materials

due not only to a dramatic drop in materials costs, but also in advances in the ability to fabricate large, complex parts requiring far less hand labor to manually assemble. A recent example of this is the addition of large composite structures in the tail and landing gear pods on the C-17 cargo aircraft. Clearly, the applications, technology, confidence, and other considerations of high-performance OMCs have expanded dramatically since the 1980s. Perhaps the most dramatic example of this is the growing use of high-performance OMCs in the commodity market of infrastructure.

Metal-Matrix Composites. The first focused efforts to develop MMCs originated in the 1950s and early 1960s. The principal motivation was to dramatically extend the structural efficiency of metallic materials while retaining their advantages, including high chemical inertness, high shear strength, and good property retention at high temperatures. Early work on sintered aluminum powder was a precursor to discontinuously reinforced MMCs. The development of high-strength monofilaments—first boron and then silicon carbide (SiC)—enabled significant efforts on fiber-reinforced MMCs throughout the 1960s and early 1970s. Issues associated with processing, fiber damage, and fiber-matrix interactions were established and overcome to produce useful materials. Although these were very expensive and had marginal reproducibility, important applications were established, including 243 structural components on the space shuttle orbiters. Recession in the early 1970s produced significant research and development funding cuts, leading to an end of this phase of MMC discovery and development.

In the late 1970s, efforts were renewed on discontinuously reinforced MMCs using SiC whisker reinforcements. The high cost of the whiskers (Ref 2) and difficulty in avoiding whisker damage during consolidation led to the concept of particulate reinforcements (Ref 3). The resulting materials provided nearly equivalent strength and stiffness, but with much lower cost and easier processing. A renaissance in both discontinuous and fiber-reinforced MMCs continued through the 1980s. Major efforts included particle-reinforced, whisker-reinforced, and tow-based MMCs of aluminum, magnesium, iron, and copper for applications in the automotive, thermal management, tribology, and aerospace industries. In addition, monofilament-reinforced titanium MMCs were developed for high-temperature aeronautical systems, including structures for high-mach airframes and critical rotating components for advanced gas turbine engines. Significant improvements in performance and materials quality were matched by an increasing number of mostly small businesses that specialized in the production of MMC components for target markets. One by one, MMC applications entered service during this timeframe. However, these successful insertions were not often widely advertised, and so the full impact of MMC technology was not widely appreciated.

In the early 1990s, a U.S. Air Force Title III program provided a significant investment to establish an MMC technology base for the aerospace industry in the United States. This program produced several landmark military and commercial aerospace applications of discontinuously reinforced aluminum (DRA), which are described in some detail in the Section "Applications and Experience" in this Volume. In addition to these dramatic successes, new MMC insertions in the ground transportation, industrial, and thermal management/electronic packaging industries far exceeded the growth in the aerospace industry. Thus, the insertion of new materials in military and commercial aircraft has actually lagged behind the industrial sector, reversing the trend of earlier years for the insertion of new materials. The MMC market for thermal management and electronic packaging alone was five times larger than the aerospace market in 1999, and this gap is expected to increase in the coming five years, due to aggressive growth in the ground transportation and thermal management markets (Ref 4).

Ceramic-Matrix Composites. Ceramic-matrix composite development has continued to focus on achieving useful structural and environmental properties at the highest operating temperatures. The high risk associated with this task foreshadows the relatively small number of commercial products. However, development of CMCs for other uses has also been pursued, and significant commercial products now exist. These are described in the article "Applications of Ceramic-Matrix Composites" in this Volume.

General Use Considerations

General Characteristics. First and foremost, composites are engineered materials that have been designed to provide significantly higher specific stiffness and specific strength (stiffness or strength divided by material density)—that is, higher structural efficiency—relative to previously available structural materials. In composite materials, strength and stiffness are provided by the high-strength, high-modulus reinforcements. The actual magnitude in composite strength and stiffness can be controlled over a significant range by controlling the volume fraction of reinforcements and by selecting reinforcements with the desired levels of strength and stiffness. In fiber-reinforced composites, the strength and stiffness may be further controlled by specifying the fiber orientation. The highest levels of properties are achieved when all fibers are aligned along the primary loading direction within the composite. However, this simultaneously produces a material with the lowest specific properties for loads perpendicular to the fiber direction. These highly anisotropic properties must be considered in the use of the material. Of course, various laminate architectures can be produced to provide isotropy within a plane, and this is often done with OMCs.

Figure 3 shows the specific strength and specific stiffness of a wide range of engineering structural materials. The highest structural efficiency is obtained with graphite-fiber uniaxially reinforced epoxy matrix (graphite 0° in Fig. 3), and this provides part of the motivation for the widespread use of these materials. However, this material also provides the lowest structural effi-

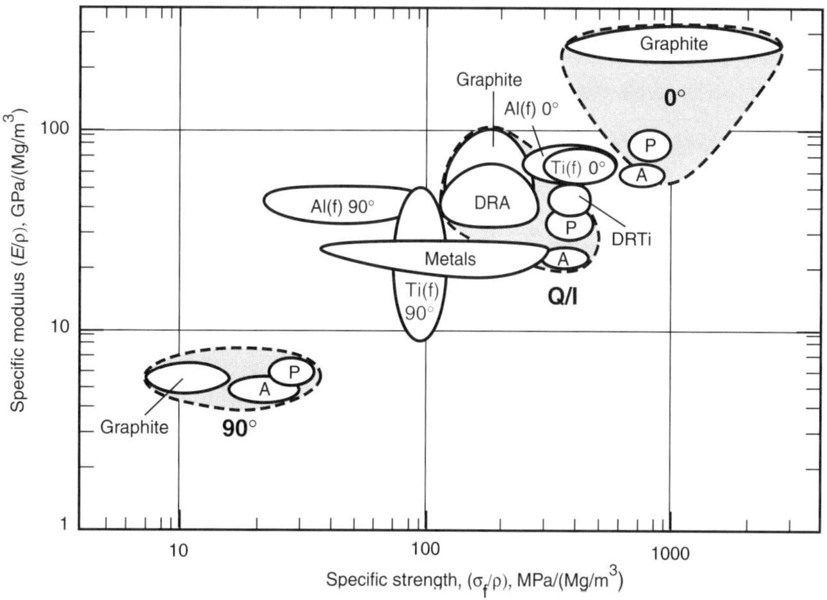

Fig. 3 Materials selection chart depicting normalized strength and stiffness characteristics for various materials systems. Note the high amount of anisotropy (or directional dependence) in composite materials, which can be exploited to create extremely lightweight structures. DRA, discontinuously reinforced aluminum; DRTi; discontinously reinforced titanium; Q/I, quasi-isotropic; P, polyacrylonitrile PAN fibers; A, aramid fibers

ciency for loads that are normal to the fiber axis (graphite 90°). There are two common approaches for dealing with the low properties in the off-axis condition. The first is to use the axially reinforced material in components with largely axial loading, so that the off-axis stresses on the composite are minimal, and the material is used most efficiently. The second approach is to cross-ply the reinforcement so that some fraction of the fibers are aligned along the off-axis loads. Both approaches are fully successful and have been used extensively, thereby overcoming the poor transverse properties of OMCs. A great deal of flexibility exists in the lay-up of a composite, so that the fraction of fibers in any given direction can be tailored in proportion to the load that must be supported. In-plane isotropy is required in some applications, so a quasi-isotropic (Q/I) graphite/epoxy laminate is produced. This is most often accomplished by orienting the laminating plies at equal numbers of 0°, 90°, +45°, and –45° plies, although there are other stacking sequences that will result in in-plane isotropy. The specific stiffness of quasi-isotropic laminated OMCs is significantly higher than structural metals. The highest specific strength of these materials is superior to all common structural metals, with the exception of a few specialty β–titanium alloys and ultrahigh-strength steels.

Fiber-reinforced metals provide axial and transverse properties that fall between the extremes of the axial and transverse graphite/epoxy OMCs. However, the technology base for fiber-reinforced MMCs is less mature. Processing difficulties currently limit the ability to form complex shapes for SiC monofilament-reinforced titanium alloys. Further, cross-plied architectures have not been successfully demonstrated in any commercial fiber-reinforced MMC. While the high cost of constituent materials dramatically limits the appeal of MMCs reinforced with monofilaments, aluminum alloys reinforced with a tow-based alumina reinforcement are commercially available and can be significantly cheaper than graphite/epoxy OMCs. As a result, these are finding applications in industries that are typically very cost-sensitive. Fiber-reinforced MMCs are now entering applications in limited areas where the metallike behavior is important, including high bearing strength, good wear resistance, high electrical conductivity, and elevated temperature operation. Some of these applications are discussed in the Section "Applications and Experience" in this Volume.

Particle-reinforced metals provide essentially isotropic properties that are in the same general range as graphite/epoxy quasi-isotropic material (Fig. 3). Discontinuously reinforced aluminum is currently by far the most widely used MMC. For reinforcement volume fractions of ≤25%, DRA has structural efficiency that overlaps that of quasi-isotropic OMCs and has good fracture toughness and ductility, so that a number of important structural applications have been established. (See the articles "Aeronautical Applications of Metal-Matrix Composites" and "Automotive Applications of Metal-Matrix Composites" in this Volume.) The fracture properties for higher volume fractions are lower, but these materials are used widely for wear-resistant applications and for thermal management and electronic packaging. The relatively low cost and ease of manufacturing makes DRA an affordable material where high structural efficiency is required. Discontinuously reinforced titanium (DRTi) is less mature than DRA, but already has several important applications established, including intake and exhaust valves in production automobile engines. (See the article "Automotive Applications of Metal-Matrix Composites" in this Volume.) Current DRTi materials have reinforcement volume fractions of ≤20%, and significant improvements are expected for higher reinforcement volume fractions. Current DRTi materials provide a balance of specific strength and specific stiffness that is superior to that of any isotropic engineering material, including quasi-isotropic OMCs.

Almost all high-strength/high-stiffness materials fail because of the propagation of flaws. A fiber of such a material is inherently stronger than the bulk form, because the size of a flaw is limited by the small diameter of the fiber. In addition, if equal volumes of fibrous and bulk material are compared, it is found that even if a flaw does produce failure in a fiber, it will not propagate to fail the entire assemblage of fibers, as would happen in the bulk material. When this material is also lightweight, there is a tremendous potential advantage in specific strength and/or specific stiffness over conventional materials. These desirable fiber properties can be converted to practical application when the fibers are embedded in a matrix that binds them together, transfers load to and between the fibers, and protects them from environments and handling. In addition, fiber-reinforced composites are ideally suited to anisotropic loading situations where weight is critical. The high strengths and moduli of these composites can be tailored to the high load direction(s), with little material wasted on needless reinforcement.

To be useful for structures, materials must offer more than just strength and stiffness. Damage tolerance, fatigue resistance, environmental resistance, and other secondary properties are also required so that the composite can perform its primary structural function. Additional functional properties for which a composite may be developed include high thermal or electrical conductivity (or conversely, electrical and/or thermal insulation), good wear resistance, controlled CTE, and/or environmental resistance. Although composites with significantly different constituents can be conceived to optimize any of these functional properties, the typical organic and metallic composite systems described previously provide a useful range of these functional properties. Specifically, in addition to high strength and stiffness, the reinforcements commonly used in OMCs and MMCs generally have low CTE, high hardness, good electrical and thermal conductivity, and good chemical inertness. As a result, the structural composites in common use can also be tailored to provide other useful functional properties with only minor alterations. The balance of properties obtained in these composites typically cannot be obtained in any other monolithic material. Examples of these functional applications are provided in the Section "Applications and Experience" in this Volume.

Materials Selection and Use. The selection of an optimal material for an intended application is a difficult and multidisciplinary task that requires careful understanding and analysis of a great many variables. The simple introductory comments given previously regarding the two primary figures of merit for structural applications provide a useful starting point for bounding this multivariable problem, but do not address the difficulty associated when trade-offs between competing characteristics must be made. The information and approaches required to help with these decisions are covered in some detail throughout this Volume, so the purpose of this brief introduction is to outline broad considerations and approaches that may help to quickly bound the problem to a tractable and well-defined set of issues.

As a starting point, the application requirements and constraints must be clearly understood. This allows definition of the primary design criteria. An approach for comparing the response across the full range of candidate materials for carefully selected relevant pairs of figures of merit to achieve these primary design criteria has recently been provided (Ref 5). To support this approach, graphical representation of a vast amount of materials properties has been undertaken and completed—these are often commonly referred to as "Ashby plots." Figure 3 provides a simple example of such a representation, because specific stiffness and specific strength are the figures of merit to resist an axial deflection or to support a given load, respectively, at minimum mass. Pairwise comparisons of figures of merit for many other design objectives provide a flexible and complete methodology for quickly bounding a difficult materials selection problem. Additional information on the use of Ashby plots is provided in the article "Material Selection Charts" in *Materials Selection and Design,* Volume 20 of *ASM Handbook.*

As explicitly engineered materials, composites in actual use integrate materials specification and component design. For example, the number and orientation of plies is typically explicitly considered during the design of components produced from OMCs. By tailoring the local architecture to the component geometry and anticipated stresses, the designer is able to take best advantage of the materials properties and to produce the component at a minimum mass. In fact, the relatively high raw material cost and high lay-up cost of OMCs has led to a highly unitized approach to design and manufacturing. This has dramatically reduced the cost of manufacture by reducing material waste and by eliminating high labor costs associated with extra manufacturing and joining steps. Fewer parts also lead to reduced inventory and overhead costs. The high structural efficiency and tailorability of OMCs has enabled this important integration in design and materials specification, and this unitized design and manufacturing approach has largely offset the high perceived costs of high-performance OMCs. While similar approaches cannot currently be achieved with fiber-reinforced MMCs, the concept of selective reinforcement in regions of high stress has been considered and is likely to find application in the near future.

Technology Overview

With some few exceptions, only "high-performance" composites are considered in this Volume. These are composites that have superior performance compared to conventional structural metals. Thus, the focus for OMCs is on continuous fiber-reinforced composites, although the principles are often applicable to other types of composites as well. Continuous fiber-reinforced composites are generally referred to as simply fiber-reinforced composites, and in some cases, as merely fiber composites or composites. Composites with organic (resin) matrices are emphasized throughout this Volume, because these OMCs are by far the most commonly used structural composites. Nonetheless, MMCs are now an established technology with strong impact and growing applications, and so MMCs are discussed explicitly throughout this Volume. Only very limited discussion of CMCs is provided in this Volume.

The following is an introduction to composite materials constituents, product forms, and fabrications processes. The purpose is to provide a simple overview that may serve as a point of departure for the nonspecialist. More detailed information is provided on each of these topics elsewhere in this Volume.

Reinforcements

The principal purpose of the reinforcement is to provide superior levels of strength and stiffness to the composite. In a continuous fiber-reinforced composite, the fibers provide virtually all of the strength and stiffness. Even in particle-reinforced composites, significant improvements are obtained. For example, the addition of 20% SiC to 6061 aluminum provides an increase in strength of over 50% and an increase in stiffness of over 40%. As mentioned earlier, typical reinforcing materials (graphite, glass, SiC, alumina) may also provide thermal and electrical conductivity, controlled thermal expansion, and wear resistance in addition to structural properties.

By far the most widely used reinforcement form in high-performance OMCs are fiber tows. These typically consist of thousands of fine filaments arranged in a single bundle. A fiber tow can be handled as a single unit and so can be wrapped or woven using commercial equipment. Fiber tows also have important applications in MMCs and CMCs. Fiber monofilaments are used in OMCs, MMCs, and CMCs; they consist of a single fiber with a diameter generally ≥100 μm (4 mils). In MMCs, particulates and chopped fibers are the most commonly used reinforcement morphology, and these are also applied in OMCs. Whiskers and platelets are used to a lesser degree in OMCs and MMCs.

Glass Fibers. Initial scientific and engineering understanding of fiber-reinforced organic-matrix composites was based on studies of glass-fiber-reinforced composites. Both continuous and discontinuous glass-fiber-reinforced composites have found extensive application, ranging from nonstructural, low-performance uses, such as panels in aircraft and appliances, to such high-performance applications as rocket motor cases and pressure vessels. The reasons for the widespread use of glass fibers in composites, both in the past and in the present, include competitive price, availability, good handleability, ease of processing, high strength, and other acceptable properties. Furthermore, the advent of highly efficient silane coupling agents, which are very compatible with either polyester or epoxy matrices, provided a strong and much-needed boost in property translation and in environmental durability.

The glass fiber most commonly used is known as E-glass, a glass fiber having a useful balance of mechanical, chemical, and electrical properties at very moderate cost. Typical strength and stiffness levels for the individual filaments are about 3450 MPa (500 ksi) tensile strength and 75.8 GPa (11×10^6 psi) Young's modulus. Higher-performance, higher-cost S-2 glass fibers have properties of 4830 MPa (700 ksi) tensile strength and a modulus of 96.5 GPa (14×10^6 psi). For specialized applications, such as ablatives, thermal barriers, antenna windows, and radomes, high-silica and quartz fibers are also used.

Boron fibers were the first high-performance monofilament reinforcement available for use in advanced composites. Developed and first marketed in the early 1960s, these high-strength, high-modulus fibers found application in composite structural components on the U.S. Air Force F-15 and the U.S. Navy F-14 aircraft. Because these aircraft are still in service and the high costs of changeover are unacceptable, boron fibers are still being used today, even though carbon fibers are now available with equivalent or better properties at a significantly lower price. Boron-epoxy composites have been used in the sporting goods industry, and boron fibers have been used in MMCs because of their excellent mechanical properties, thermal stability, and reduced reactivity with the matrix (compared to carbon fibers). Boron fibers are produced as a rather large monofilament fiber or "wire" (100 to 200 μm, or 4 to 8 mils, diameter) by chemical vapor deposition (CVD) of boron onto a tungsten or pyrolyzed carbon substrate. The resulting fibers have excellent strength (3450 MPa, or 500 ksi) and stiffness (400 GPa, or 58×10^6 psi). Because of their large fiber diameters, they form composites having extremely high compressive strengths. However, because both the precursor gases and the manufacturing process are inherently expensive, boron fibers cannot be expected to compete with carbon fibers on the basis of cost alone. The use of boron fibers has seen somewhat of a resurgence lately in the use of composite patch repairs of crack damage in aluminum aircraft structure.

Carbon Fibers. Although the search for high-performance reinforcing fibers was highly successful, the early limited demand outside the military aerospace industry did not permit the cost reductions that would have resulted from more extensive use. As a result, widespread industrial applications for the variety of new materials progressed very slowly in all but specialty applications where higher costs could be justified. Factors that changed this situation were the extensive use of carbon-fiber-reinforced composites in recreational equipment and the increased cost of energy in the early 1970s. The promise of commercial quantities of carbon-fiber materials from a number of sources at attractive prices created a resurgence of interest in advanced composites in the general aerospace industry. Currently, carbon fibers are the best known and most widely used reinforcing fibers in advanced composites. Although there are many reasons for this situation, two factors predominate. First, the manufacturing technology for carbon fibers, although complex, is more amenable to large-scale production than are those of many of the other advanced fibers. Second, carbon fibers have very useful engineering properties that, for the most part, can be readily translated into usable composite physical and mechanical properties.

Carbon fibers are available from a number of domestic and foreign manufacturers in a wide range of forms having an even wider range of mechanical properties. The earliest commercially available carbon fibers were produced by thermal decomposition of rayon precursor materials. The process involved highly controlled steps of heat treatment and tension to form the appropriately ordered carbon structure. Rayon has been largely supplanted as a precursor by polyacrylonitrile (PAN). Polyacrylonitrile precursors produce much more economical fibers because the carbon yield is higher and because PAN-based fibers do not intrinsically require a final high-temperature "graphitization" step.

Polyacrylonitrile-based fibers having intermediate-modulus values of about 240 to 310 GPa (35 to 45×10^6 psi), combined with strengths ranging from 3515 to 6380 MPa (510 to 925 ksi), are now commercially available. Because carbon fibers display linear stress-strain behavior to failure, the increase in strength also means an increase in the elongation-to-failure. The commercial fibers thus display elongations of up to 2.2%, which means that they exceed the strain capabilities of conventional organic matrices. The diameter of carbon fibers typically ranges from 8 to 10 μm (0.3 to 0.4 mils). Polyacrylonitrile-based fibers are available in various "tow sizes," meaning the number of carbon fibers per bundle. Currently, tow sizes range from low (1000 fibers per tow) at high cost ($40 to $70 per pound) to very high tow counts (hundreds of thousands of fibers per tow) for less than $10 per pound.

Carbon fibers are also manufactured from pitch precursor for specialty applications. Pitch-fiber properties typically include high modulus and thermal conductivity, as might be required on satellite structures. Modulus values in commercially available fibers range up to 825 GPa (120×10^6 psi).

Aramid Fibers. Aramid is a generic term for a class of aromatic polyamide fibers introduced commercially during the early 1960s. These high-performance fibers are all variations of poly para-phenyleneterephthalamide. A broad range of properties are available. Kevlar 149 (DuPont), for example, has a tensile modulus of 180 GPa (26×10^6 psi) and tensile strength of 3450 MPa (500 ksi). The more commonly used Kevlar 49 (DuPont) has a tensile modulus of 131 GPa (19 $\times 10_6$ psi) and a tensile strength of 3620 MPa (525) ksi).

Aramid fiber is unusual in that it is technically a thermoplastic polymer (like nylon), but rather than melting when heated, it decomposes before reaching its projected melting temperature. With polymerization, it forms rigid, rodlike molecules that cannot be drawn from a melt, as textile fiber molecules can, but must instead be spun from a liquid crystalline solution in sulfuric acid. The polymerization and manufacturing processes for aramid fibers are complex and exacting and involve many aggressive chemical species.

The high strength of aramid fiber, combined with a fiber modulus considerably higher than S-glass, gave it early application in filament-wound rocket motor cases, gas pressure vessels, and lightly loaded secondary structures on fixed-wing commercial aircraft and helicopters. The fiber shows linear tensile stress-strain behavior to failure, but unlike inorganic fibers, is surprisingly damage tolerant. However, it also displays far lower strength in compression than carbon and other inorganic fibers and relatively poor adhesion to matrix resins. Moisture uptake may also need to be considered. Nevertheless, because of properties such as its high specific strength, low density, and toughness, significant markets exist.

Other Organic Fibers. Another common category of fibers are ultrahigh-molecular-weight polyethylene fibers, such as Spectra from AlliedSignal Inc. The modulus of Spectra can range up to 113 GPa (16×10^6 psi), with tensile strengths up to 3250 MPa (470 ksi). These fibers have high chemical, impact, and moisture resistance, as well as low density, good vibration damping, and low dielectric constant. Major applications include ballistic armor, radomes, boats, and other recreational products.

Silicon Carbide Monofilaments. Silicon carbide monofilaments have been developed for reinforcements in MMCs based on aluminum and titanium alloy matrices and for CMCs. Fibers that are now commercially available are all produced by CVD of fine-grained β-SiC, which is deposited on either a tungsten or a carbon filament core. Each of the fibers also uses a carbon-based coating to improve fiber strength by healing surface defects, to improve handleability, and to protect the fiber from interaction with the metal matrix during consolidation and use. The monofilaments range in diameter from 100 to 142 μm (4 to 5.6 mils). The CTE for all of the SiC monofilaments is 4.5×10^{-6}/°C, (2.5×10^{-6}/°F) and the density is 3.0 g/cm^3 (0.11 lb/in.^{3}) for fibers with a carbon core and 3.4 g/cm^3 (0.12 lb/in.^{3}) for fibers deposited on tungsten. There are currently three manufacturers of SiC monofilament.

Textron Systems markets the venerable SCS-6 monofilament, which has been used longer than any other SiC monofilament. It is deposited on a carbon core by a two-pass process, which produces a distinct change in grain size at the fiber midradius. A multilayer carbon-based coating consists of an intentional gradation in silicon content to enhance the coating effectiveness. The overall fiber diameter is 142 μm (5.6 mils). The minimum specified average properties are 3450 MPa (500 ksi) strength and 345 GPa (50×10^6 psi) stiffness. The typical average properties are 4300 MPa (625 ksi) strength and 390 GPa (56×10^6 psi) stiffness. There is a great deal of data and experience behind this fiber, which has been produced by the same process since 1983. Process improvements have led to the Textron Systems Ultra SCS fiber. While the carbon core, fiber coating, and fiber diameter are identical to the SCS-6, the SiC possesses a finer grain size that is uniform across the fiber diameter. The minimum average specified properties are 5860 MPa (850 ksi) strength and 360 GPa (52×10^6 psi) stiffness. The typical average values obtained are 6550 MPa (950 ksi) strength and 415 GPa (60×10^6 psi) stiffness.

Two SiC monofilaments are available from the Atlantic Research Corporation (Gainesville, VA). Trimarc-1 is 127 μm (5 mils) in diameter on a tungsten core, with a multilayer carbon coating 4 to 5 μm (0.16 to 0.20 mils) thick. The typical mean fiber strength is 3550 MPa (515 ksi), and the modulus is 420 GPa (61×10^6 psi). Trimarc-2 is deposited on a carbon core and is 142 μm (5.6 mils) in diameter. The typical strength is 3790 MPa (550 ksi), and the typical modulus is 400 to 414 GPa (58 to 60×10^6 psi). The Sigma SiC monofilament is produced by QinetiQ, formerly the Defence Evaluation and Research Agency (DERA), in the United Kingdom. The DERA Sigma 1140+ fiber is 100 μm (4 mils) in diameter, is produced on a tungsten core, and has a carbon coating about 5 μm (0.2 mils) thick. The typical strength is between 3400 to 3500 MPa (490 to 510 ksi), and the modulus is 380 GPa (55×10^6 psi).

Alumina-Fiber Reinforcements. A number of alumina (Al_2O_3) fibers have been developed and used for MMCs and CMCs, including ceramic tows and monofilaments. At present, production MMCs only use alumina tows. The most commonly used material is the Nextel 610 fiber produced by 3M (St. Paul, MN). This is ≥99% α–alumina and has a density of 3.96 g/cm^3. Tows are available that contain from 400 to 2550 filaments per tow. The mean filament diameter is 10 to 12 μm (0.4 to 0.5 mils). The typical fiber properties are 2930 MPa (425 ksi) strength and 373 GPa (54×10^6 psi) modulus. The CTE is 7.9×10^{-6}/°C.

Particulate reinforcements in MMCs typically use abrasive-grade ceramic grit. This provides a ready commercial source, and the high volumes associated with the abrasives industry help maintain a low cost. Silicon carbide, alumina, and boron carbide (B_4C) are most often used. Titanium carbide (TiC) is also used for iron and titanium alloy matrices. While TiB is used as a reinforcement in discontinuously reinforced titanium alloys, this reinforcement is typically obtained by in situ reaction with TiB_2. Silicon carbide offers the best strength and stiffness for aluminum matrices, but is slightly more expensive than alumina. "Green" SiC offers better strength and thermal conductivity relative to "black" SiC, and so is used where these properties are important. Typical grit sizes used are between F-600 (mean grit size between 8.3 to10.3 μm, or 0.33 to 0.41 mils) and F-1200 (mean grit size between 2.5 to 3.5 μm, or 0.11 to 0.14 mils). Alumina is slightly cheaper than SiC, and so is attractive where cost is critical, such as in the automotive sector. Alumina is slightly more dense than SiC and has a higher CTE. Alumina is chemically more stable than SiC in molten aluminum, and so is frequently used in cast DRA. Silicon carbide particulates are still used for cast MMCs, and silicon is added as an alloying addition to reduce the reactivity with the molten metal.

Matrices

The purpose of the matrix is to bind the reinforcements together by virtue of its cohesive and adhesive characteristics, to transfer load to and between reinforcements, and to protect the reinforcements from environments and handling. The matrix also provides a solid form to the composite, which aids handling during manufacture and is typically required in a finished part. This is particularly necessary in discontinuously reinforced composites, because the reinforcements are not of sufficient length to provide a handleable form. Because the reinforcements are typically stronger and stiffer, the matrix is often the "weak link" in the composite, from a structural perspective. As a continuous phase, the matrix therefore controls the transverse properties, interlaminar strength, and elevated-temperature strength of the composite. However, the matrix allows the strength of the reinforcements to be used to their full potential by providing effective load transfer from external forces to the reinforcement. The matrix holds reinforcing fibers in the proper orientation and position so that they can carry the intended loads and distributes the loads more or less evenly among the reinforcements. Further, the matrix provides a vital inelastic response so that stress concentrations are reduced dramatically and internal stresses are redistributed from broken reinforcements. In organic matrices, this inelastic response is often obtained by microcracking; in metals, plastic deformation yields the needed compliance. Debonding, often properly considered as an interfacial phenomenon, is an important mechanism that adds to load redistribution and blunting of stress concentrations. A broad overview of important matrices is provided subsequently.

Organic matrices for commercial applications include polyester and vinyl ester resins; epoxy resins are used for some "high-end" applications.

Polyester and vinyl ester resins are the most widely used of all matrix materials. They are used mainly in commercial, industrial, and transportation applications, including chemically resistant piping and reactors, truck cabs and bodies, appliances, bathtubs and showers, and automobile hoods, decks, and doors. The very large number of resin formulations, curing agents, fillers, and other components provides a tremendous range of possible properties.

The development of highly effective silane coupling agents for glass fibers allowed the fabrication of glass-fiber-reinforced polyester and vinyl ester composites that have excellent mechanical properties and acceptable environmental durability. These enhanced characteristics have been the major factors in the widespread use of these composites today.

The problems of attaining adequate adhesion to carbon and aramid fibers have discouraged the development of applications for polyester or vinyl ester composites that use these fibers. Although there are applications of high-performance fiberglass composites in military and aerospace structures, the relatively poor properties of advanced composites of polyester and vinyl ester resins when used with other fibers, combined with the comparatively large cure shrinkage of these resins, have generally restricted such composites to lower-performance applications.

Other Resins. When property requirements justify the additional costs, epoxies and other resins, as discussed subsequently, are used in commercial applications, including high-performance sporting goods (such as tennis rackets and fishing rods), piping for chemical processing plants, and printed circuit boards.

Organic matrices for aerospace applications include epoxy, bismaleimide, and polyimide resins. Various other thermoset and thermoplastic resins are in development or use for specific applications.

Epoxy resins are presently used far more than all other matrices in advanced composite materials for structural aerospace applications. Although epoxies are sensitive to moisture in both their cured and uncured states, they are generally superior to polyesters in resisting moisture and other environmental influences and offer lower cure shrinkage and better mechanical properties. Even though the elongation-to-failure of most cured epoxies is relatively low, for many applications epoxies provide an almost unbeatable combination of handling characteristics, processing flexibility, composite mechanical properties, and acceptable cost. Modified "toughened" epoxy resin formulations (typically via the addition of thermoplastic or rubber additives) have improved elongation capabilities. In addition, a substantial database exists for epoxy resins, because both the U.S. Air Force and the U.S. Navy have been flying aircraft with epoxy-matrix structural components since 1972, and the in-service experience with these components has been very satisfactory.

Moisture absorption decreases the glass transition temperature (T_g) of an epoxy resin. Because a significant loss of epoxy properties occurs at the T_g, the T_g in most cases describes the upper-use temperature limit of the composite. To avoid subjecting the resins to temperatures equal to or higher than this so-called wet T_g (the wet T_g is the T_g measured after the polymer matrix has been exposed to a specified humid environment and allowed to absorb moisture until it reaches equilibrium), epoxy resins are presently limited to a maximum service temperature of about 120 °C (250 °F) for highly loaded, long-term applications and even lower temperatures (80 to 105 °C, or 180 to 220 °F) for toughened epoxy resins. Although this limit is conservative for some applications, its imposition has generally avoided serious thermal-performance difficulties. Considerable effort continues to be expended to develop epoxy resins that will perform satisfactorily at higher temperatures when wet. However, progress in increasing the 120 °C (250 °F) limit has been slow.

Bismaleimide resins (BMI) possess many of the same desirable features as do epoxies, such as fair handleability, relative ease of processing, and excellent composite properties. They are superior to epoxies in maximum hot/wet use temperature, extending the safe in-service temperature to 177 to 230 °C (350 to 450 °F). They are available from a number of suppliers. Unfortunately, BMIs also tend to display the same deficiencies (or worse) as do epoxies: they have an even lower elongation-to-failure and are quite brittle. Damage tolerance is generally comparable to commercial aerospace epoxy resins. Progress has been made to formulate BMIs with improved toughness properties.

Polyimide resins are available with a maximum hot/wet in-service temperature of 232 °C (450 °F) and above (up to 370 °C, or 700 °F, for single use short periods). Unlike the previously mentioned resins, these cure by a condensation reaction that releases volatiles during cure. This poses a problem, because the released volatiles produce voids in the resulting composite. Substantial effort has been made to reduce this problem, and there are currently several polyimide resins in which the final cure occurs by an addition reaction that does not release volatiles. These resins will produce good-quality, low-void-content composite parts. Unfortunately, like BMIs, polyimides are quite brittle.

Other Thermosetting Resins. The attempt to produce improved thermosetting resins is ongoing, with major efforts focusing on hot/wet performance and/or impact resistance of epoxies, BMIs, and polyimides. Other resins are constantly in development, and some are in commercial use for specialized applications. Phenolic resins, for example, have been used for years in applications requiring very high heat resistance and excellent char and ablative performance. These resins also have good dielectric properties, combined with dimensional and thermal stability. Unfortunately, they also cure by a condensation reaction, giving off water as a by-product and producing a voidy laminate. However, they also produce low smoke and less toxic by-products upon combustion and are therefore often used in such applications as aircraft interior panels where combustion requirements justify the lower properties. Cyanate esters are also used as matrix materials. Their low-moisture-absorption characteristics and superior electrical properties allow them to see applications in satellite structures, radomes, antennas, and electronic components.

Thermoplastic Resins. The dual goal of improving both hot/wet properties and impact resistance of composite matrices has led to the development, and limited use, of high-temperature thermoplastic resin matrices. These materials are very different from the commodity thermoplastics (such as polyethylene, polyvinyl chloride, and polystyrene) that are commonly used as plastic bags, plastic piping, and plastic tableware. The commodity thermoplastics exhibit very little resistance to elevated temperatures; the high-performance thermoplastics exhibit resistance that can be superior to that of epoxy.

Thermoplastic-matrix materials are tougher and offer the potential of improved hot/wet resistance and long-term room-temperature storage. Because of their high strains-to-failure, they also are the only matrices currently available that allow, at least theoretically, the new intermediate-modulus, high-strength (and strain) carbon fibers to use their full strain potential in the composite. Thermoplastics are generally considered to be *semicrystalline* (meaning the atoms in the polymer chains arrange themselves in regular arrays to some degree) or *amorphous* (meaning there is no local order to the molecular chains). These materials include such resins as polyether etherketone, polyphenylene sulfide, polyetherimide (all of which are intended to maintain thermoplastic character in the final composite), and others, such as polyamideimide, which is originally molded as a thermoplastic but is then post-cured in the final composite to produce partial thermosetting characteristics (and thus improved subsequent temperature resistance). Thermoplastic matrices do not absorb any significant amount of water, but organic solvent resistance is an area of concern for the noncrystalline thermoplastics.

Metal and Ceramic Matrices. Unlike their organic counterparts, the metal alloy matrix in MMCs provides an important contribution to the strength of the composite. This results not only from the higher strength of metal alloys relative to organic resins typically used as matrices, but also from the fact that most MMCs currently have discontinuous reinforcements and a much higher matrix volume fraction. Metal-matrix composites are currently in service using matrices based on alloys of aluminum, titanium, iron, cobalt, copper, silver, and beryllium. Copper, silver, and beryllium MMCs are mostly used for thermal management and electrical contacts; iron MMCs are used for industrial wear-resistant applications, such as rollers and tool dies; and titanium MMCs are used primarily for automotive, aerospace, and recreational products. Cobalt MMCs (cemented carbides, or cermets) are included here as an MMC, although not all agree upon this classification, while oxide-dispersion-strengthened nickel is explicitly excluded, because strengthening in these alloys occurs by a dislocation mechanism rather than a load-sharing mechanism. By far the most widely produced MMCs are based on aluminum alloy matrices, and these are in current use for automotive and rail ground transportation, thermal management and electronic packaging, aerospace, and recreational applications.

A wide range of cast and wrought aluminum alloys are used as matrices in aluminum MMCs. A standard nomenclature, American National Standards Institute (ANSI) H35.5-1997, has been established for aluminum MMCs: 2009/SiC/15p-T4. The first four digits (or three digits for cast alloys) are the Aluminum Association alloy designation, which specifies the matrix alloy composition. This is followed by the reinforcement composition and the reinforcement volume fraction (in volume percent). A single letter signifies the reinforcement morphology ("p" is particle, "w" is whisker, and "f" is fiber). The standard Aluminum Association temper designation is used at the end of the MMC designation, as appropriate.

The most widely used MMC casting alloys are based on aluminum-silicon, which are used to produce foundry ingots. The high-silicon aluminum alloys improve castability and minimize chemical interaction with the SiC reinforcements during melting. Common matrix alloy compositions are based on aluminum casting alloys such as 359, 360, and 380. The modifications generally include higher silicon and sometimes higher magnesium or manganese or lower copper (Ref 6). Infiltration casting also often uses aluminum-silicon alloys, such as A356, and this is common for materials used in thermal management. However, wrought alloy compositions, including common 2*xxx* and 6*xxx* alloys, can also be used for infiltration casting. For pressureless casting, the matrix composition is carefully controlled to provide the desired reactions and microstructures. Silicon is typically at 10% (by weight), and 1% Mg (by weight) is also critical.

Cast billets or blooms for subsequent thermomechanical processing often use wrought matrix alloys containing magnesium, such as 2024 and 6061. Billet obtained by powder metallurgy also uses conventional wrought alloy compositions, or may use modified alloys that have been optimized for use in an MMC matrix. Two examples are 6091, which is a modified 6061 alloy, and 6092, which is a modification of 6013. Often, the modification involves a small reduction in the concentration of alloy additions used for grain refinement, because the reinforcing particulates restrict grain growth. Also, a maximum level is specified for oxygen to ensure that the powder does not introduce a large fraction of oxide particles.

Metal-matrix composites of copper, beryllium, and silver are used primarily for their excellent electrical and thermal properties, and reinforcements are added for control of thermal expansion or improved wear resistance. The matrix is usually the pure element to retain the excellent thermal or electrical properties. Typical reinforcements, such as molybdenum in copper and silver, tungsten and tungsten carbide in copper, and beryllium oxide in beryllium, are insoluble in the matrix.

Titanium MMCs use conventional wrought alloy matrices when the reinforcement is continuous. For current applications, Ti-6Al-2Sn-4Zr-2Mo (Ti-6242) is used. (See the article "Aeronautical Applications of Metal-Matrix Composites" in this Volume.) Other commercial alloys, such as Ti-6Al-4V and Timetal 21S, have been used extensively in development and component demonstrations. A number of alloys have been used in research and development of DRTi. The largest commercial application of DRTi by far is for automotive intake and exhaust valves. The intake valve uses Ti–6Al–4V as the matrix, but the exhaust valve requires a high-temperature matrix alloy. The composition used is Ti-6.5Al-4.6Sn-4.6Zr-1.0Mo-1Nb-0.3Si (Ref 7, 8).

Ceramic-matrix composites currently in use generally use SiC or inhibited carbon as the matrix. The role of the matrix is to provide the required wear and abrasion resistance, or to protect the fiber from oxidation and damage.

Material Forms

Composite materials are generally available in a range of raw product forms. These forms provide a standardized unit for cost-effective production and are a convenient input for manufacturing processes. Further, standardizing the raw product form allows better control over constituent composition and distribution. A brief discussion of the raw product forms used most often in composite manufacture is provided subsequently.

Organic-Matrix Composites. Continuous reinforcing fibers are available in many product forms, ranging from monofilaments (for fibers such as boron and SiC) to multifilament fiber bundles, and from unidirectional ribbons to single-layer fabrics and multilayer fabric mats. The organic matrices are generally mixed from the individual components if the matrix is a thermoset, or are available as sheet, powders, or pellets if the matrix is a thermoplastic. The reinforcing fibers and matrix resins may be combined into many different nonfinal material or product forms that are designed for subsequent use with specific fabrication processes. In the case of continuous fibers, these combinations of unidirectional fiber ribbons, tows, or woven fabrics with resin and formed into broad sheets are called prepregs. (In some cases, the fiber tows are impregnated with resin and wound back on spools, still as tows, to form "towpregs.") At this stage, prepregs/towpregs are still largely uncured.

Using prepregs rather than in-line impregnation of the fibers during the final composite fabrication process can offer significant advantages. Prepregs can have very precisely controlled fiber-resin ratios, highly controlled tack and drape (in the case of thermoset matrices), controlled resin flow during the cure process, and, in some processes, better control of fiber angle and placement. Prepreg materials can be produced and stored, normally under refrigeration for thermosetting matrices, and then used in processes ranging from hand lay-up to highly automated filament winding, tape laying, or tow placement. Processes such as pultrusion and braiding can also use prepreg forms instead of in-line resin impregnation. While the latter may be lower in initial cost, it may be prohibitive for some resin systems (such as thermoplastics), and parameters such as fiber-resin ratio may not be as easily controlled, as is the case with a prepreg.

Discontinuous fiber-reinforced product forms include sheet molding compounds, bulk molding compounds, injection molding compounds, and dry preforms fabricated for use in resin infusion processes. Many other forms of reinforcement exist, primarily in fiberglass materials. Both continuous and discontinuous mats, with and without binder materials, are available. Of course, composites reinforced primarily with discontinuous fibers have lower mechanical properties than those with continuous fibers. This is because all of the loads in discontinuous fiber composites must be carried by the matrix in shear from fiber length to fiber length (shear lag). In addition, fiber volume in discontinuous fiber composites is normally quite a bit lower than is typical in continuous fiber composites.

Composite materials are very often used as facesheets and combined with core materials to form sandwich structures. Common forms for core materials are foams (open and closed cell), honeycomb (often made from fiberglass, aramid, or aluminum) whereby the longitudinal axes of the cells are perpendicular to the primary plane of the structural sandwich, and foam-filled honeycomb. Sandwich structures have extremely high structural bending stiffness, which is exploited in bending- and buckling- critical applications.

Metal-Matrix Composites. The largest supplier of MMC primary product forms is Alcan Engineered Cast Products (formerly Duralcan USA). Billet and blooms for wrought processing and foundry ingots for remelting are produced by a patented casting process. Batches of 6.8 metric tons are melted, and the ceramic particles are suspended in the melt by a high-energy mixing process. The molten MMC is then cast into bloom, billet, or ingot. These material forms are then provided to customers who apply secondary forming operations, such as extrusion, forging, rolling, or remelting and casting.

The aerospace industry relies upon MMC billet produced by a powder metallurgy process. The primary process, performed by DWA Aluminum Composites, mixes matrix and reinforcing powder in a high-shear mixer, then outgases and consolidates the powder into billet. Billet sizes over 360 kg (800 lb) are typical, and billets up to 450 kg (1000 lb) are available.

A major portion of the MMC market relies upon components produced in near-net shape processes other than recasting of foundry ingot. The most commonly used processes are infiltration casting and squeeze casting. In both cases, carefully produced porous ceramic preforms are required. Infiltration preforms of ceramic particulates are produced by either a slurry-casting approach, by powder pressing, or by injection molding. These preforms provide a uniform distribution of the reinforcement and a controlled porosity for infiltration. In addition, the preform provides adequate "green strength" to resist the pressures that are sometimes applied during infiltration. Another important near-net shape process is a proprietary in situ casting technique used by DMC^2 Electronic Components (formerly Lanxide Electronic Components). As the MMC is formed in situ during solidification, special MMC foundry ingot or preforms are not required.

Wire and tape product forms of continuously reinforced aluminum MMCs are now commercially available. The MMC has a reinforcement volume fraction of approximately 55% alumina (Nextel 610). The wire is by far the most common form. A variety of diameters is available, but 2.6 mm (0.10 in.) is the median diameter. These are produced by a patented process by 3M.

Fabrication Processes

Organic-Matrix Composites. A host of processes exist for the fabrication of OMC components. Fiber-reinforced composites used in most high-performance applications are laminated with unidirectional (or fabric) layers at discrete angles to one another (such as in plywood), thereby allowing for highly tailored directional stiffness and strength properties. A variety of fiber-placement processes are available to achieve this desired combination of orientations. Two common processes are lay-up (by hand or machine) and filament winding/tow placement. With lay-up, material that is in prepreg or dry fiber form (dry fibers contain no resin, so this form typically consists of knitted, braided, or woven layers) is cut and laid up, layer by layer, to produce a laminate of the desired number of plies and associated ply orientations. In filament winding/tow placement, a fiber bundle or ribbon is impregnated with resin and wound upon a mandrel to produce a shape: with filament winding it is often a simple geometry, such as a tube or pressure vessel; with tow placement the shapes can often be more complex. As mentioned before, filament winding/tow placement may use wet liquid resin or prepreg.

Composite fiber-placement fabrication procedures can be labor intensive, so most major composite component fabricators are developing and/or using automatic fabrication equipment. Such equipment is often used for composite components that have a relatively large area and reasonable production rate. Two methods predominate. One involves laying up the plies with tape. Large tape-laying machines are computer controlled, include gantry robot systems, and are equipped with a specially designed tape-dispensing head. Another method involves the cutout of entire plies from unidirectional broad goods using laser, waterjet, or reciprocating-knife cutters. Cutout ply patterns are transferred to a tool and laid up by hand or automatic equipment with specially designed pick-up and lay-down heads. Laser-generated guidelines can be projected onto a part to indicate the location of the next part to be placed.

If the fiber-placement process involved the use of "dry" fibers, the next step in the process is to infuse this dry fiber preform with liquid resin. One of the most basic processes to do this is called resin transfer molding (RTM). In the RTM process, the dry fiber preform is first placed in an open matched mold. The mold is closed and resin is injected into ports in the mold. Excess air is forced out other vents in the mold. In vacuum-assisted resin transfer molding, vacuum can be applied to the vent ports to assist in drawing the resin into the fiber preform and removing any trapped air. There are many variations of the resin infusion process. For example, for cost reduction, molds can contain a single-sided hard tool side, where the opposite side of the tool can just be a simple, flexible vacuum bag. Other variations contain an air gap or high permeability layers over the planform surface of the part, to allow the liquid resin to flow quickly over and "above" the surface, before the slower process of diffusing through the preform (hence, using this method, the liquid has only to diffuse through the preform thickness, not across the part width direction as in RTM). In one variation of this process (liquid compression molding), once the resin has flowed through the air gap over the preform, the tool can be further closed creating additional pressure to force the resin into the preform. Probably the oldest of all methods of resin infusion is "wet lay-up," in which the fibers, typically textiles, are dipped in the resin (or the resin squeegeed into the textile layer) and the wet layer is placed on a single-sided mold.

The fiber placement (and resin infusion, if appropriate) process is followed by some type of cure process to harden (cross link) the polymer-matrix resin. For a low-cure-temperature or two-part mix thermoset matrix, this may simply involve holding the part at room temperature until cure completion. However, for applications involving elevated-temperature service or for thermoplastics, there must be an elevated-temperature cure. Filament-wound parts may be cured at elevated temperature in an open oven; in some cases, consolidation and surface finish may be improved by applying an external female mold or vacuum bag. Lay-ups are most commonly consolidated by applying both heat and pressure in an autoclave, but they may also be molded, pressed, or vacuum bag cured. (For example, in the RTM process, the molds themselves may be heated.)

There are also special fabrication processes, such as pultrusion, that combine fiber placement, consolidation, and elevated-temperature cure in one continuous operation. The pultrusion process is a low-cost, high-volume method to produce long parts with constant (or nearly constant) cross section containing fibers aligned predominantly along the longitudinal axis of the part. The pultrusion process is a continous "line" process, whereby fiber tows are mechanically gripped and pulled from their spools, through a resin bath, then through a heated die containing the desired cross section of the part. Another common industrial process is compression molding, typically whereby flat sheets of preimpregnated fibers are placed in an open heated mold. The mold halves are subsequently closed and the resin then cured to final shape.

To select the best composite fabrication process, the designer generally chooses the process that will provide an acceptable-quality component for the lowest cost. In evaluating cost and quality, however, tooling cost, production rate, materials cost, desired part finish, and many other factors must be considered. Only after all the pertinent factors have been weighed can the fabrication method (or the material) be selected.

Metal-Matrix Composites. Nearly twice the volume of MMCs are produced by casting and other liquid routes compared to solid-state fabrication, and this gap is expected to widen in coming years. This is lead by automotive applications, such as engine block cylinder liners and brake components, and in the thermal management industry. By a great margin, aluminum MMCs are the most commonly cast materials. A wide variety of techniques are now commercially established, including pour casting, infiltration casting, and in situ processing.

Casting typically begins with a foundry ingot material, as described previously. Upon remelting, the molten composite must be well stirred to keep the reinforcements well distributed. Both SiC and alumina reinforcements have a density slightly higher than aluminum alloys, and so tend to settle. Settling is avoided with boron carbide reinforcements in aluminum alloys, because the densities are nearly identical, but the higher cost of these reinforcements has restricted their use in high-volume applications. In cast aluminum MMCs using SiC reinforcements, the liquid metal temperature must be kept below about 730 °C (1346 °F) to avoid the formation of aluminum carbide, Al_3C_4. Due to the higher viscosity of the MMC, this process is typically used for reinforcement volume fractions of ≤20%. The Alcan material has been successfully cast using a number of standard techniques, including green sand, bonded sand, permanent mold, plaster mold, investment, lost foam, and centrifugal casting (Ref 6). Small but important modifications are sometimes required for MMC casting. For example, the design of gating systems must specifically take account of the higher melt viscosity, so that air entrapment is avoided. With proper design, excellent results have been obtained.

Pressure casting of MMCs has been used commercially since the early 1980s. In this process (often called "squeeze casting"), a porous ceramic preform is introduced into a permanent mold cavity. A fixed volume of molten metal alloy is introduced and is rapidly pressed into the ceramic preform by a mechanical force. After solidification, the part is ejected from the mold, and the process is repeated. Because the process is very rapid, it is well suited for high volumes, such as those represented by the automotive industry. Another feature leading to good cost-effectiveness is the reusability of the permanent mold. A notable example of squeeze-cast components are the selectively reinforced MMC pistons introduced by Toyota Motor Manufacturing in 1983 as the first commercial MMC application in the automotive industry. Production rates of over 100,000 per month have been achieved (Ref 4).

A number of approaches are used for the production of components via infiltration casting. The primary difference between these techniques is in the amount of gas pressure applied to force the molten metal into the porous ceramic preform. Typical gas pressures range from 5.5 MPa (800 psi) to 10.3 MPa (1500 psi). The hydrostatic pressure and moderate rates of pressurization eliminate the need for high-strength tooling and minimize the possibility of damaging the preform as the molten metal is infiltrated. The mold is not permanent, but five to ten parts can typically be produced from a single mold before replacement. While excellent results can be obtained, a pressure chamber with adequate volume and heating capability is required. This process is well suited to aerospace components, where high quality and low or moderate production volumes are required, or to electronic packaging, where the small component size allows up to several hundred parts to be made in a single run.

A pressureless process is used to produce MMCs by infiltrating a porous, nonreactive ceramic preform. The aluminum alloy contains magnesium, and the infiltration is conducted in a nitrogen atmosphere. The magnesium reacts with the nitrogen gas to form Mg_3N_2, which enables spontaneous infiltration of the ceramic preform. As the molten aluminum is drawn into the preform, the Mg_3N_2 is reduced to form aluminum nitride, and the magnesium is released into solid solution (Ref 6).

The fabrication processes established for the metalworking industry, such as extrusion, forging, and rolling, are typically used for particle-reinforced MMCs with only small modifications. Extrusion of MMCs is used extensively: in the automotive industry (for example, driveshafts for trucks and the Chevrolet Corvette), for aerospace components (such as the fan exit guide vane of Pratt and Whitney 4*xxx* series gas turbine engines), and recreation products (such as bicycle frame tubing). Extrusion billet up to 51 cm (20 in.) in diameter has been commercially extruded. Some commercially produced components represent significant geometrical complexity. Excellent dimensional tolerances and surface finish can be achieved in the as-extruded product. Hard-face extrusion die coatings are often used to extend die life.

Commercial MMC components are also produced by rolling and forging. Rolled MMC product includes plate and sheet. Plate is used for applications such as clutch plates, thermal management input material, and fuel access doors in the aerospace industry. Sheet is used primarily for aerospace components, and material over 76 cm (30 in.) has been produced. Rolling preforms are produced by both casting and powder metallurgy processes. Forging of MMCs is used for fatigue-critical applications, such as helicopter rotor blade sleeves. A cylindrical extrusion preform is blocker-forged and then closed-die forged to the final shape. Excellent dimensional tolerances are maintained. Forging is being developed for automotive connecting rods. The microstructural refinement provided by the forging process improves the fatigue response, which is a critical requirement for this application.

The processes described previously are those most extensively used for existing applications. Many other fabrication processes are being used or have been established for MMCs, including spray forming, drawing, piercing, and ring rolling.

Machining and finishing operations for MMCs are similar to those used for metals. By far the greatest experience exists for aluminum MMCs. Standard mills, lathes, and computer numerical control machines can be used, as long as the cutting parameters are properly selected. Because of the strong, hard, ceramic reinforcements in MMCs, significant tool wear results when using simple high-speed steel tools and even carbide tools. However, economies of machining identical to that obtained with conventional tooling can be achieved in MMCs using polycrystalline diamond (PCD) on a unit-operation basis. Tool wear is reduced and surface quality improved for more aggressive cuts and higher speeds, improving the overall speed of machining. Experience at Alcan has shown that coarse-grained PCD (15 to 40 μm, or 0.6 to 1.6 mils) provides the best overall performance and cost-effectiveness (Ref 4). In some cases, operations in MMCs provide superior results compared to unreinforced metals.

Applications

The purpose of this brief introduction is to provide broad insights and unifying themes regarding the diverse applications of composite materials. An overview of OMC use is highlighted. The dramatic progress in the technology and application of MMCs is discussed, and the current status of CMC applications is provided. Because of their recent maturity to the point of becoming a robust commercial technology, the subsequent section on MMC applications is somewhat expanded in this introduction. Detailed information relating to the application of composite materials over a broad range of categories is provided in the Section "Applications and Experience" in this Volume.

Organic-Matrix Composite Applications

Based on their high-performance properties, reduced-cost manufacturing methods, and the higher level of confidence among users, the use of OMC materials has expanded greatly since the mid-1980s. These applications are well documented in the "Applications and Experience" Section of this Volume, as well as in other sources (Ref 7). High-performance composites were borne of the need for extremely high-performance aircraft structures during the days of the Cold War. The military aerospace markets still constitute a major user of the higher-end performance materials. For example, the B-2 bomber, F-22 fighter, Joint Strike Fighter, F-18E/F aircraft, Eurofighter, Gripen aircraft, and Rafale aircraft in production, on the books, or in prototype form are all constructed using high percentages of OMCs. Current-production helicopters are now largely composite. On the commercial side, OMCs constitute a significant portion of the new large Boeing 777 and planned Airbus jumbo A380, which reportedly will contain the first carbon fiber wing center secton in a large commercial aircraft, in addition to extensive, OMC use in tail surfaces, bulkheads, and fuselage keel and floor beams), as well as intermediate-sized transport aircraft and business jets, and they are prevalent in many small commercial and homebuilt aircraft. Space applications for OMCs have flourished, from satellite structures (where low CTE, in addition to low weight, is a major advantage of OMCs) to the use of OMCs in booster fairings, shrouds, and tanks. The maturity of high-temperature OMC structures has afforded the use of OMCs in many engine applications for both air and space vehicles.

The sports and recreation market continues to be one of the primary consumers of composite raw materials. Golf clubs, bicycles, snowboards, water skis, tennis rackets, hockey sticks, and so on— the list of consumer products now produced using OMCs is extensive and commonplace. On the marine side, the consumer use of fiberglass OMCs in low- to high-end boats is the norm. Military ships have seen several applications of OMCs, primarily topside structures and minesweepers. Carbon-fiber composites can be seen in high-performance engine-powered, sail-powered, and human-powered racing boats.

A potentially huge market exists for composite materials in the upgrading of the infrastructure needs. For example, 31% of the highway bridges in the United States are categorized as structurally deficient. To address this, many activities are underway at national, state, and local levels to use composites to repair and, in some cases, replace deficient bridges. Figure 4 shows an example of an all-fiberglass bridge being installed in Butler County, Ohio. This bridge is fully instrumented to detect structural performance loss. At the time of this writing, the bridge has almost four years of service with, almost no maintenance required. Composites have also been used for seismic enhancement of existing highways and bridges.

Land vehicles have also benefited greatly from the application of OMCs. Military armored vehicles have been demonstrated that offer ballistic protection of their occupants in addition to light weight. The demand for energy-efficient and low-maintenance vehicles has spurred composites use in advanced automobile, truck, bus, and train commercial products. Production parts include everything from small linkage assemblies to very large exterior structural panels.

Rounding out the OMC application discussion are a host of products. For example, the medical industry has applied OMCs to products ranging from implanted orthopedic devices to x-ray tables and lightweight assistance devices. (An example is shown in Fig. 5). Industrial applications include electronic housings, large rollers, tanks, robotic arms, and so on. Spoolable piping for oil wells allows deeper wells due to the increased strength and reduced "hang weight" of composite tubular products. In short, the development and use of OMCs were initially spurred by early investments based on military need, and, based on those successes, have now dramatically taken off in the private sector, based solely on their commercial merits.

Metal-Matrix Composite Applications

In 1999, the MMC world market amounted to over 2.5×10^6 kg (2500 metric tons). While this is hardly remarkable relative to production volumes of more historical structural materials, it certainly illustrates that MMCs are no longer a marginal technology and have passed the threshold into a self-sufficient materials technology. This is also clearly demonstrated by the number of functions and the wide range of applications that are satisfied by MMCs. In this subsection, instructive selected applications are briefly presented in each of the major existing markets to illustrate the breadth and impact of current applications and to highlight application trends. This introduction is by no means exhaustive, and more detailed information is provided in the Section "Applications and Experience" and in other information sources cited in this Volume. Some of the subsequent information was taken from a recent market analysis of MMCs (Ref 4).

Ground Transportation/Automotive. The ground transportation industry (automotive and rail) accounted for 62% of the total MMC world market by volume in 1999. However, the high production rates and imperative emphasis on low cost resulted in a surprisingly low total market share by value—only 7%! By far the single most prevalent composite used in this sector is DRA. The most common application strategy is to displace components made of cast iron or steel, maximizing weight reductions. However, replacement of steel based simply on reduced weight is clearly an inadequate motivation for the use of DRA; otherwise most of an automobile structure would be displaced. Therefore, components are targeted where other benefits besides simple weight reduction are possible, so that the additional cost of insertion can be justified. Selected applications that illustrate the additional benefits obtained by the use of MMCs are provided subsequently.

A selectively reinforced piston head was introduced by Toyota Motor Manufacturing in 1983. Produced by squeeze casting, this was a reasonably low-cost and high-rate production process. The reinforcements provided improved wear resistance and lower thermal conductivity, so that more of the heat generated by the combustion gases was available for producing work. Further, the MMC provided a lower CTE than unreinforced aluminum, so that tighter tolerances and hence, higher pressure and better performance were obtained. Squeeze-cast piston liners have been used in the Honda Prelude since

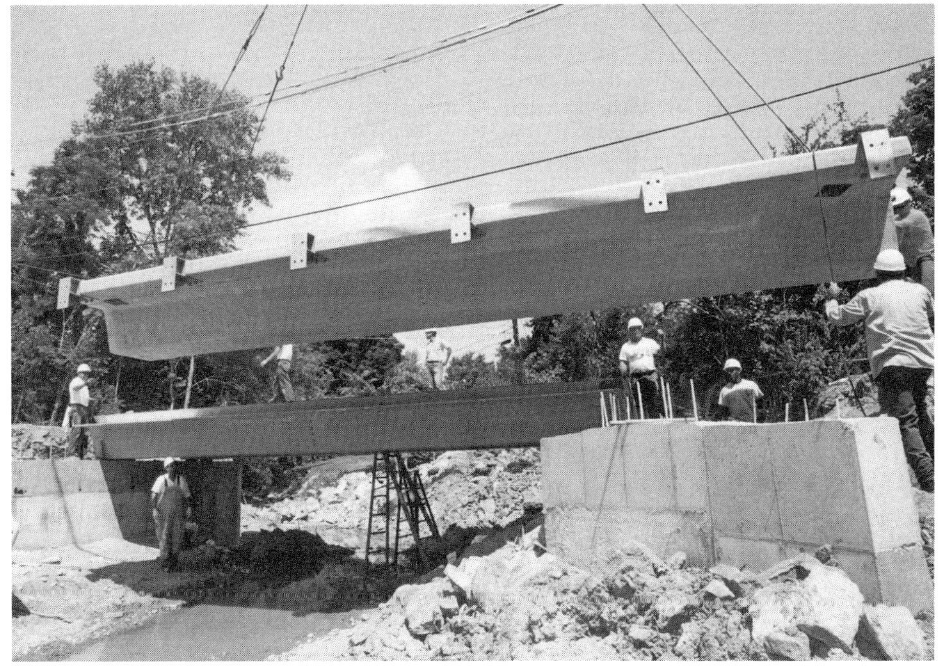

Fig. 4 All-composite bridge in Butler County, Ohio. Factory-constructed primarily using glass fiber, the bridge was trucked to the site and installed in less than one day.

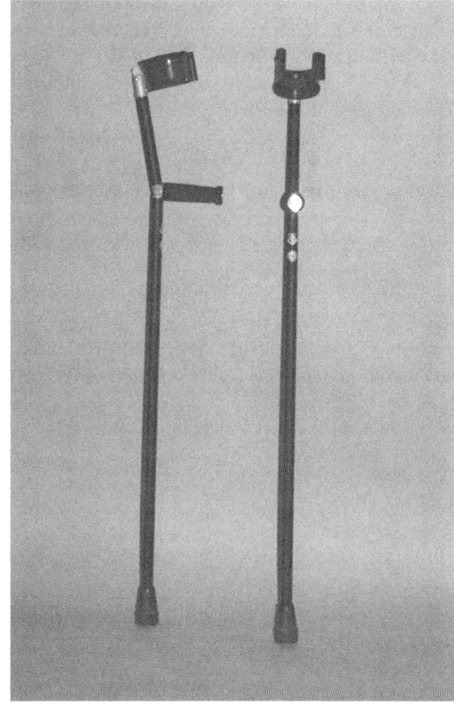

Fig. 5 Carbon/epoxy composite crutch. This crutch is stronger than its aluminum counterpart yet weighs 50% less, is quieter, and is more aesthetically pleasing.

1990, displacing cast iron inserts (Fig. 6). In a novel manufacturing process, the engine block casting and piston liner preform infiltration are performed simultaneously, eliminating the cost of assembly associated with the cast iron inserts. More importantly, the MMC liners provided improved wear resistance, so that the overall liner thickness could be reduced. This yielded an increase in engine displacement, so that more horsepower is obtained from the same overall powerplant weight and volume. Finally, the thermal conductivity of the MMC is much higher than the cast iron liner, so that the operating temperature is decreased, resulting in extended engine life.

Automotive driveshafts represent a component application motivated primarily by structural properties. Driveshaft design is limited by rotational instability, which is controlled by the specific stiffness of the driveshaft material. The higher specific stiffness of DRA relative to steel or aluminum allows a longer driveshaft of a given diameter. This is important in trucks and large passenger cars, where two-piece metal driveshafts are often used. Replacement with DRA allows a single-piece driveshaft. Not only is significant weight saved as a result of material substitution, but elimination of the central support for the two-piece unit provides additional weight savings. Finally, MMC driveshafts require less counterweight mass compared to steel. In all, as much as 9 kg (20 lb) have been saved by this application. Metal-matrix composite driveshafts were first introduced in the Chevrolet S-10 and GMC Sonoma in 1996, and have been used in the Chevrolet Corvette beginning in 1997. In 1999, Ford Motor Company introduced MMC driveshafts in the "Police Interceptor" version of the Crown Victoria.

Other significant MMC components include automotive and rail brake components, DRA snow tire studs, and DRTi automotive intake and exhaust valves in the Toyota Altezza. Additional information is provided in the article "Automotive Applications of Metal-Matrix Composites" in this Volume.

Thermal Management and Electronic Packaging. Materials for thermal management and electronic packaging requre high thermal conductivity to dissipate large, localized heat loads, and a controlled CTE to minimize thermal stresses with semiconductor and ceramic baseplate materials. Previous preferred materials include Kovar, an Fe-Ni-Co alloy with 17% Co, and copper MMCs reinforced with molybdenum or tungsten to lower the CTE. Copper-MMCs reinforced with graphite or diamond have been developed, but are less frequently used. A beryllium/beryllium oxide MMC is sometimes used where weight is most critical, but cost and health concerns limit this application. Aluminum MMCs with 55 to 70% SiC are now widely used for thermal management applications.

Aluminum MMCs, such as DRA, provide better performance (higher thermal conductivity) relative to previous preferred materials. For example, DRA has a thermal conductivity that is nearly ten times higher than Kovar and up to 20% higher than copper-molybdenum and copper-tungsten MMCs. Discontinuously reinforced aluminum provides a dramatic weight reduction, 65 to 80% relative to copper-molybdenum and copper-tungsten, providing an important functional benefit for aerospace components and a significant commercial advantage for portable electronics, such as laptop computers and cellular telephones. Finally, processing innovations yield significant cost reductions for DRA components. Net shape processing reduces machining, which is difficult and costly for Kovar and copper MMCs reinforced with molybdenum or tungsten, and enables integration of the infiltration step with bonding to ceramic baseplate and incorporation of wire feed-throughs, resulting in fewer processing steps. Together, these provide cost savings of up to 65%.

Unlike the automotive market, MMCs for the electronic packaging sector are high value-added. Although this is the second-largest MMC market in terms of volume (26.5%), it is by far the largest in terms of value (66%) (Ref 4). Current applications of MMCs include radio frequency packaging for microwave transmitters in commercial low-earth orbit communications satellites (Fig. 7) and for power semiconductors in geosynchronous earth orbit. Metal-matrix composites are also used as power semiconductor baseplates for electric motor controllers and for power conversion in cell phone ground station transmitting towers. Finally, MMCs are being more widely used as thermal management materials for commercial flip-chip packaging of computer chips. Additional details are provided in the article "Thermal Management and Electronic Packaging Applications" in this Volume.

Aerospace. Several DRA applications emerged in the early 1990s as a result of defense investment in the United States. The ventral fin on the F-16 aircraft was experiencing a high incidence of failure as a result of unanticipated turbulence. Of the several materials and design options considered, DRA sheet was chosen as the best overall alternative. The higher specific strength and stiffness, good supportability, and affordability were considerations in the final selection of DRA. As a result of the successful experience with DRA in this application, the F-16 project office selected DRA to solve a cracking problem of the fuselage at the corners of fuel access doors. Again, the mechanical properties of DRA and retention of the same form, fit, and function led to the selection of DRA as the final solution. Discontinuously reinforced aluminum was also qualified and entered service in a commercial gas turbine application (fan exit guide vanes) as a result of this program. Discontinuously reinforced aluminum double-hollow extrusions replaced solid graphite/epoxy to resolve an issue with poor erosion and ballistic impact response. Discontinuously reinforced aluminum also resulted in a cost savings to the manufacturer of well over $100 million.

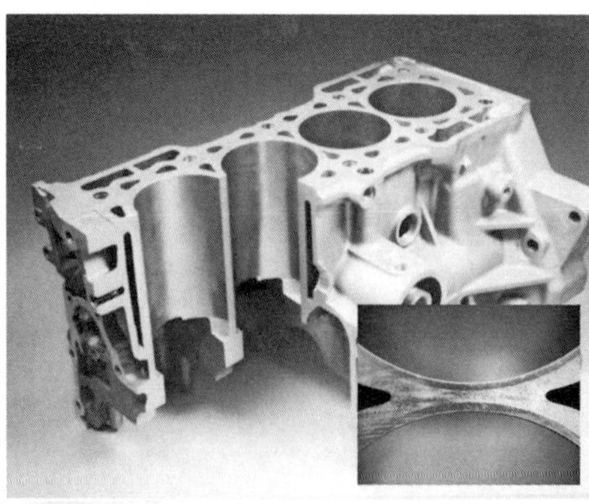

Fig. 6 Cutaway section of the Honda Prelude 2000 cc cast aluminum engine block with integral MMC piston liners. A cross section of the MMC liners is shown in the inset. These piston liners have been in production since 1990.

Continuously reinforced titanium-matrix composites (TMCs) are bill of material for nozzle actuator piston rods for the Pratt and Whitney F119 engine in the F-22. Specific strength and specific stiffness, along with good fatigue response at a maximum operating temperature of 450 °C (850 °F), are the requirements. The hollow TMC rod replaced a solid rod of precipitation-hardened stainless steel and has resulted in a direct weight savings of 3.4 kg (7.5 lb) per aircraft. This is the first aerospace application of TMC materials. Following the successful specification of TMCs for this part, TMCs are now specified for nozzle actuator links in the General Electric F110 engine for the F-16 aircraft. Additional details for each of these applications are provided in the Section "Applications and Experience" in this Volume.

Industrial, Recreational, and Infrastructure. Metal-matrix composites are used for a range of applications in these sectors, including DRA for bicycle frames and iron-based MMCs reinforced with TiC (Ferro-TiC, Alloy Technology International, Inc.) for wear-resistant tool and die coatings and industrial rollers. A continuously reinforced aluminum MMC produced by 3M is being used in high-performance automotive applications and has completed certification testing for overhead power transmission conductors (Ref 4). Steel cable is typically used as the core for "high-tension" power conductors. The steel bears the weight of the aluminum conduc-

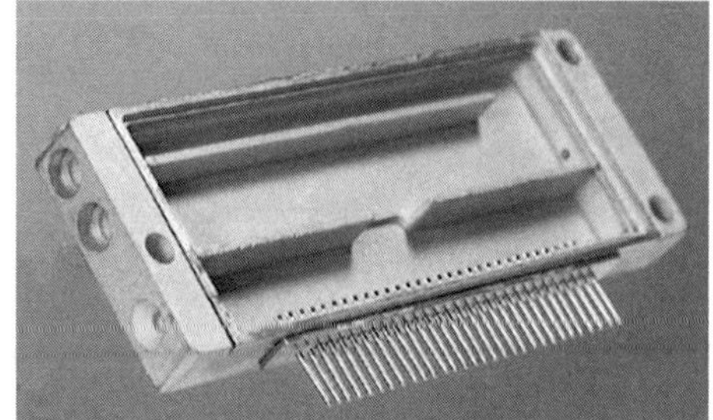

Fig. 7 An AlSiC radio frequency microwave packaging used in commercial low-earth orbit communications satellites. Courtesy of General Electric Company

tor, but carries little of the current, due to a low electrical conductivity (only one-eighth that of aluminum). Depending on the specifics of the transmission installation, the conductor can heat to temperatures in excess of 200 °C (400 °F) during peak use. In regions of the world such as Japan, the conductors can operate above 200 °C (400 °F) under continuous use and as high as 240 °C (460 °F) or more during peak loads. Sagging due to thermal expansion is an issue. The important properties for conductor cores are specific strength, electrical conductivity, CTE, high-temperature capabilities, and cost. Increased demand for electricity and the impact of deregulation requires utility companies to consider means for increasing the ampacity (i.e., the maximum current flow in the line). Higher ampacity produces higher conductor temperatures, resulting in line sagging that requires significant tower modifications to maintain needed line clearance. Tower construction is the major cost associated with new or increased power transmission and includes considerations such as purchasing right of way, satisfying environmental impacts, and design and construction costs. The ability to avoid the costs associated with tower construction provides the opportunity for new conductor materials. The aluminum MMC conductor provides the strength of steel cable at less than half the density. More importantly, the MMC conductor carries four times more current than steel and has a CTE one-half that of steel. Although the aluminum MMC conductor is more expensive than conventional conductors on a unit-length basis, the ampacity gains are significant, with projected increases of 200 to 300% with no tower modifications required. Thus, at a system level, the use of MMC conductors may provide an attractive cost savings. A cross section of a conductor with an aluminum MMC core is shown in Fig. 8.

An aluminum MMC reinforced with boron carbide particulates is now being used for nuclear waste storage casks. The casks must meet stringent requirements for both transportation and long-term storage. The MMC is used as a liner for a carbon-steel outer container. The required neutron-absorbing capabilities are provided by the B_{10} isotope in boron carbide. Each cask uses 2.3 tonnes (2.5 tons) of aluminum-boron carbide MMC, and the first cask was delivered in 2000.

Summary. A number of insights are available regarding the application of MMCs discussed previously. The initial motivation for the application of MMCs typically comes from improved performance, such as lighter weight from better specific structural properties, improved thermal conductivity, or better wear resistance. In addition, pressures imposed by legislative, economic, or environmental concerns often play an important role. Examples include legislated financial penalties for failure to comply with corporate average fuel economy requirements for lighter, more fuel-efficient automobiles, regulatory requirements for nuclear storage, and environmental impact from the construction of towers for new overhead power conductors. Of course in every case, cost is a primary selection criterion. Although MMCs are almost always more expensive on a per-pound basis relative to the material displaced, an overall cost reduction is often a result of several considerations. Novel or simplified processing reduces costs and can eliminate steps, resulting in a cheaper component. Life cycle considerations (reduced repair frequency, higher reliability, longer life) further enhance the cost comparison. Finally, system-level benefits are sometimes obtained, such as increased engine displacement for MMC cylinder liners or reduced tolerances for MMC pistons, which further extend the payoff. The multifunctionality offered by MMCs greatly aids in obtaining these additional benefits.

The first successful entry of MMCs into a system is the most difficult. This reflects the lack of designer familiarity with MMCs. However, additional applications often follow the first use, as designer familiarity and confidence grows. These follow-on applications may be within the same system or company, but can also be from a competitor. Examples include the fuel access doors, which followed the ventral fin for the F-16, and specification of DRA driveshafts in Chevrolet trucks, followed by use in the Chevrolet Corvette, and then insertion in the Ford Crown Victoria.

Unlike the paradigm during the Cold War era, the first applications of MMCs have, by and large, come from the commercial sector. Both high-volume/low-cost and low-volume/high value-added technologies have been successfully pursued for MMCs. This has provided the incentive for establishing the technology base for further expansion.

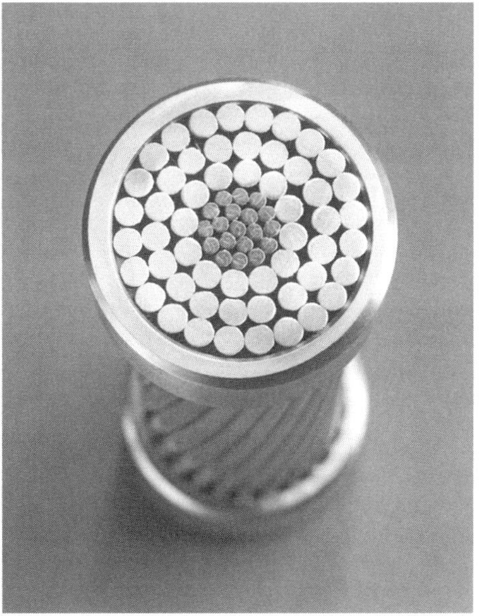

Fig. 8 Cross section of an electrical conductor for power transmission. The core consists of 19 individual wires made from a continuously reinforced aluminum MMC produced by 3M. The MMC core supports the load for the 54 aluminum wires and also carries a significant current, unlike competing steel cores. Courtesy of 3M

Ceramic-Matrix Composite Applications

Ceramic-matrix composites have successfully entered service as exhaust nozzle flaps and seals in the F414 engine, now used in the Navy F-18 E/F (Fig. 9). The exhaust temperature of the F414 is over 80 °C (145 °F) higher than for the F404 engine used in the previous version of the F-18. As a result, the metal flaps and seals were failing in tens of hours. The CMC parts consist of a Nicalon (Dow Corning Corp.) fiber with an inhibited carbon matrix. A thick SiC overcoat and glaze provide protection from oxidation. There are 12 flaps and 12 seals per engine, and the seals are attached to metal backing plates with metal rivets and a zirconia overcoat. The seals are subjected to the highest temperatures, and the flaps must support the largest mechanical loads. Further, the flaps must survive a high thermal gradient, and the CMC is subjected to rubbing with the back face of the seal. Insertion of the CMC flaps and seals has produced a weight savings of nearly 1 kg (2 lb) per engine relative to the metal parts. Because this mass is at the very back of the aircraft, additional weight savings can be obtained by removing ballast to shift the center of gravity of the aircraft. The CMC flaps have a useful life that is at least double the design requirement of 500 hours.

Ceramic-matrix composites are now also commercially available as brake rotors for automobiles. Short carbon fibers and carbon powder are pressed and sintered into a porous green compact, which is then easily machined to shape. This part is then reheated and infiltrated with molten silicon, which reacts with the carbon to form SiC. The resulting disc is 50% lighter than conventional discs, yielding a 20 kg (44 lb) weight saving in the Porsche 911 Turbo. Since the rotor weight is unsprung, improved handling also results. The wear rate is half that of con-

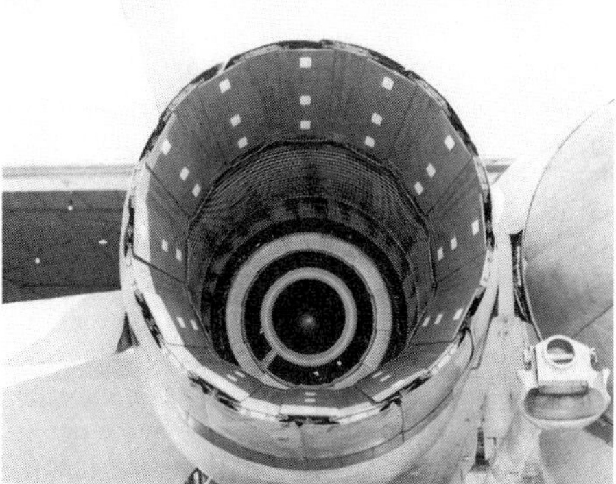

Fig. 9 Exhaust nozzle of an F414 engine on an F-18 E/F aircraft, showing the twelve sets of CMC flaps and seals. The white areas on the seals are a zirconia overcoat for mechanical fasteners. Over an order-of-magnitude increase in life has been obtained with the CMC flaps and seals.

ventional metal rotors, and a service life of 300,000 km (185,000 miles) is reported. The new Porsche braking system uses an MMC brake pad. Ceramic-matrix composite brake rotors have also been demonstrated for the Inter-City Express high-speed trains in Germany, where a total weight savings of 5.5 metric tons is obtained per trainset.

View of the Future

A conservative view has been taken in this Volume, which emphasizes current technologies and known applications. Growth in the volume, applications, value, and impact of composites technologies is expected as a result of the natural growth of many of the existing applications. Infrastructure applications of OMCs and both automotive and thermal management components for MMCs typify this expected growth. However, there are also many composites applications in new uses and representing new technologies that are now on the verge of certification. In addition, robust research and development over the coming years is expected to provide entirely new composite materials options, opening up entirely new markets. In the closing part of this article, the prognosis for each of these possibilities is briefly discussed.

Organic-Matrix Composites. Without a doubt, military requirements fueled investments in the development of advanced composites from the 1940s through the end of the Cold War (around 1990). Since that time, however, Department of Defense requirements for advanced composites have begun to represent only a small portion of the total amount of OMCs used by all markets combined. As discussed previously, the rise in the use of OMCs in transportation, recreation, infrastructure, and industrial applications is fully expected to continue to increase. Current active research areas provide some insight into OMC technologies that will mature to practical application in both the short and long term. These future directions can be broken down into three areas: materials and processing advances, advances in structural concepts, and progress in design and certification.

Development of polymers that can withstand sustained use in realistic service environments of both moisture and high temperatures (exceeding 370 °C, or 700 °F) is expected to allow for the increased use of PMCs in hot structural areas. Current research into nanophase reinforcements, essentially third-phase reinforcements, has already shown some progress on this front. Processing of OMCs is also evolving. For example, research into the use of electron beam curing shows promise of being able to cure large structures less expensively than by using traditional autoclaves. In terms of advanced structural concepts, the highly anisotropic nature of OMCs has only begun to be exploited. Current structures often appear similar to traditional isotropic metallic ones (for example, orthogonal rib/stringer designs), in which OMCs are used primarily for their light weight and high stiffness and strength. To fully use the high-fiber properties, unconventional three-dimensional structural architectures are being explored. In addition, research into "multifunctional" materials and structures is being pursued. Examples include structures that serve thermal management, self- or external assessment, self-repair, and self-actuation functions. (An example of this would be the use of active embedded layers for vibration damping in helicopter rotor blades.)

The current aerospace structural design process relies on a "building-block" approach. This approach has served the military well, as is evidenced by the large weight savings provided by OMCs, while the number of structural failures has been negligible. However, this approach requires, for example, large statistical databases of materials properties to be established early in the structural design cycle. This leaves little flexibility for large, real-time changes in the structure to optimize design and minimize cost. As the fidelity, validation, and integration of analytical models (micromechanical through structural) increases, ultimately it is believed that structures can be designed and "tested" almost entirely analytically. This would dramatically shorten the design cycle and allow for the exploration of vast numbers of design concepts, all at very low cost. The expensive experimental testing, although probably always required to some extent, will be dramatically reduced.

Metal-Matrix Composites. For MMCs, a conservative annual market growth rate of between 15 to 20% has been projected through 2004 (Ref 4). This will be led by the ground transportation industry (automotive and rail), and in the high value-added thermal management and electronic packaging sector. Additional applications are expected to result from increased experience and confidence in MMCs, based on prior use and on natural market growth. The growth in the automotive and rail industry is expected from increasing pressure for light weight, fuel economy, and reliability. In the thermal management and electronic packaging industry, increased MMC use will result from the dramatic growth in this industry for new networking and wireless communications installations. The largest market by far, and the largest projected growth, is for DRA, which is expected to double in production volume between 1999 and 2004 (Ref 4).

This growth is anticipated from existing technologies and applications. However, significant new applications and markets are being pursued vigorously for MMC technologies that are now on the verge of widespread acceptance. A notable example is the relatively low-cost continuously reinforced aluminum MMC produced by 3M. Significant progress has been achieved in the last two years toward the acceptance of this material for overhead power transmission conductors (high tension wires), as briefly discussed previously. This application, if successful, will represent a dramatic increase in the worldwide MMC market and may be nearly equal to the entire annual volume of the ground transportation market. The simple, flexible material form (wire and tape) is amenable to use in a wide range of other applications. The uniaxial configuration is ideal for hoop and tube or rod configurations, and it can easily be used as an insert for selective reinforcement of components. Many potential applications are currently being pursued, including flywheel containment, high-speed electric motors, and high-performance automotive components. A novel process using the tape preform is being pursued to produce large cryogen tanks for rocket propulsion, paving the way for building large structures from a simple-to-manufacture material form.

In the farther term, technology innovations leading to new and significantly improved MMC materials can be expected as a result of the robust international activity in MMC research and development. Two examples are DRA for elevated-temperature use and aerospace-grade DRTi. Titanium alloys are specified in many applications, especially aerospace, where the use temperature exceeds the current limit for aluminum alloys, about 150 °C (300 °F). The titanium is more expensive, more difficult to machine, and heavier, yet is required to support the use temperature. A modest increase in use temperature, to about 200 °C (400 °F), will provide the opportunity to replace many aerospace components currently made of titanium with an aluminum material. Discontinuously reinforced titanium shows very attractive structural properties (Fig. 3) and is currently used commercially in automotive valves for the Toyota Altezza (Ref 9). However, the approaches taken to ensure that cost goals were met are incompatible with aerospace requirements. Research and development of DRTi for aerospace applications show that this MMC has the potential of exceeding the structural efficiency of all metallic materials, and of cross-plied graphite/epoxy. While initial volumes are not expected to be large, the promise afforded by this material and other advanced MMC technologies makes the future bright for MMCs.

ACKNOWLEDGMENTS

Portions of this article have been adapted from T.J. Reinhart and L.L. Clements, Introduction to Composites, *Composites,* Volume 1, *Engineered Materials Handbook,* ASM International, 1987, p 27–34.

REFERENCES

1. Carl Zweben, Composite Materials and Mechanical Design, *Mechanical Engineer's Handbook*, 2nd ed., Myer Kutz, Ed., John Wiley & Sons, Inc., New York, 1998.
2. A.P. Divecha, S.G. Fishman, and S.D. Karmarkar, Silicon Carbide Reinforced Aluminum—A Formable Composite, *JOM*, Vol 33 (No. 9), 1981, p 12–17

3. S.G. Fishman, Office of Naval Research, private communication, 1997
4. M.N. Rittner, "Metal Matrix Composites in the 21st Century: Markets and Opportunities," Report GB-108R, Business Communications Co., Inc., Norwalk, CT, 2000
5. M.F. Ashby, *Materials Selection in Mechanical Design,* Pergamon Press, Oxford, U.K., 1992
6. J.R. Davis, Ed., *Metals Handbook Desk Edition,* 2nd ed., ASM International, 1998, p 674–680
7. *High Performance Composites Source Book 2001,* Ray Publishing, www.hpcomposites.com
8. T. Saito, A Cost-Effective P/M Titanium Matrix Composite for Automobile Use, *Adv. Perform. Mater.* Vol 2, 1995, p 121–144
9. F.H. Froes and R.H. Jones, *Light Met. Age,* Vol 57 (No. 1, 2), 1999, p 117–121

Constituent Materials

Chairperson: Steven R. Nutt, University of Southern California

Introduction to Constituent Materials

Steven R. Nutt, University of Southern California

THIS SECTION describes the major matrix resins and reinforcing fibers used in composite materials, as well as some of the intermediate material forms available for composite fabrication. The Section begins with articles that provide coverage of the various fibers and matrices used in composites, including their structure, chemistry, and properties.

Constituent Material Forms

For the engineer, knowledge of the constituent material properties and understanding of the origins of those properties is important for the task of defining a composite structure for a particular application. This knowledge is needed to understand how that structure will respond to an imposed load or stimulus under a set of conditions. Often, fiber properties are the most important with respect to composite performance, as in the properties of tensile strength and stiffness of a unidirectional composite in the fiber direction. However, other aspects of composite performance depend more strongly on matrix properties, such as the maximum upper-use temperature and interlaminar shear properties. In other cases, the fiber and matrix sometimes contribute to the composite response in direct proportion to their respective volume fractions (e.g., composite dielectric constant and moisture absorption). And finally, there are countless documented examples where performance is determined by the (complex) interaction between the fibers and the matrix, a topic discussed in the article "Interfaces and Interphases."

Fortunately for the composites engineer, a wide variety of high-performance fibers and resins are commercially available, affording unprecedented flexibility and latitude in structural design. The most commonly used constituent materials include fibers of glass, carbon, and aramid, followed by various high-temperature ceramics. In addition, a host of polymeric resins are used, as well as metallic alloys and even ceramics. However, the constituent materials continue to evolve, as evidenced by the recent introduction of carbon nanotubes and nanofibers, as well as new varieties of carbon fiber and high-temperature ceramic fibers. On the matrix side, resins continue to improve through modified formulations and the introduction of fillers, such as silicate-based nanoclay particles (added to produce nanocomposites) and toughening agents, both of which result in enhanced performance.

Fibers. A general introduction to and comparison of the most significant fiber types is provided in the article "Introduction to Reinforcing Fibers." At the time of publication, the most widely used, economical reinforcement in polymer-matrix composites is E-glass fiber. When higher stiffness and strength are required, carbon fibers and aramid fibers are employed. There are a wide variety of carbon fibers, differing primarily in the degree of graphitization, which affects modulus and strength, and the number of fibers per tow. Recent years have seen the price of certain types of carbon fiber plummet to the \$10/kg (\$5/lb) range, opening the door to a wide variety of commercial/industrial applications that were previously cost-prohibitive. Ceramic fibers based on alumina, alumina-silica, and silicon carbide are used to reinforce metallic alloys and ceramics, and in some cases, to reinforce polymers where unique physical properties are required, such as low dielectric constants or infrared transparency. Improvements to fiber performance and reductions in fiber cost will greatly change the way in which composites are used, and expand the use of composites beyond aerospace and sporting goods and into other sectors of industry.

Matrix Materials. The polymer matrix resins considered in this Section include both thermosetting and thermoplastic types, with emphasis on the former because they account for more than 80% of all matrices in reinforced plastics and essentially all matrices used in advanced composites. The most widely used thermosetting resins are the polyesters, which are most often combined with E-glass. This combination accounts for the bulk of the fiber-reinforced plastics (FRP) market. Polyesters offer a combination of low cost, versatility in many processes, and reasonably good property performance unmatched by any other resin type. The most common orthophthalic types and the premium isophthalic types, bisphenol A fumarate, chloendic, and vinyl ester, are discussed in this Section.

For more demanding structural uses, epoxy resins are the preferred candidates. Although the amount of epoxies used in reinforced plastics is small in comparison to the volume of polyester used, epoxy use dominates the more demanding aircraft/aerospace structural applications. Epoxy resins are of particular interest to structural engineers because they provide a unique balance of chemical and mechanical properties combined with extreme processing versatility. Epoxy resin performance is highly dependent on the formulation, which includes the base resin, curatives, and the modifiers. A practical introduction to these basic formulary components and epoxy-resin selection is provided in this Section.

Several high-temperature polymeric matrices are also covered, including cyanate ester, polyimide, and bismaleimide resins. These tend to be more expensive resin systems, and are employed in applications where the high-temperature performance justifies the additional cost. Cyanate esters, or polycyanurates, bridge the gap in thermal performance between engineering epoxy resins and high-temperature polyimides. Polyimide resins are used when optimum thermal stability at high temperature is required. Although polyimides may be thermosetting or thermoplastic, most composite applications use the thermosetting types, which are fully covered in this Section. The addition-type bismaleimide (BMI) resins are also covered in this Section.

The use of high-performance thermoplastics as matrices in continuous fiber reinforced composites is currently an area characterized by very low use but very high interest. This Section addresses continuous fiber reinforced thermoplastics. The focus is on materials suitable for fabrication of structural laminates such as might be used for aerospace.

The Section also includes articles that address metallic, ceramic, and carbon matrices, including the distinct advantages and limitations of these materials.

Intermediate Material Forms. Also covered in this Section are some of the intermediate material forms available for composite fabrication. These are often used as components that are joined with other components and assembled into a structure, and/or as ways of arranging and controlling the fiber architecture. Examples include sandwich core materials, fabrics and preforms, fiber mats, and braids. While the coverage is not comprehensive, the articles offer the engineer a shopping list that complements the Sections in this Volume that focus on design, manufacturing, and material properties. A key advantage of working with composite materials is the opportunity to integrate material properties, design, and manufacturing technique so that the end product—a completed structure—is optimized from both a performance and an economics standpoint.

Selection Factors

The individual articles within this Section are written to give an understanding of the composite raw materials available today and how they are processed. Because there is a great deal of flexibility in the manufacture of composite material forms, engineers and designers are encouraged to be creative when selecting a particular material form. If a particular form fits a particular design and manufacturing technique but is not listed here, engineers and designers are encouraged to ask for what they want.

Most of the forms listed are the result of such requests. For example, the tow sizes available for glass and carbon fibers resulted from particular needs. In the first case, large bundles of glass were needed to feed choppers to make sheet molding compounds. After the request was made and the potential market was found to be significant, large multiple-strand bundles in center-pull packages were developed. In the case of carbon fibers, the need for woven fabrics to form complex shapes brought a request for smaller tows. The resulting 1000, 3000, and 6000 (1, 3, and 6K) filament tows are now used to produce woven goods. More recently, the need for lower-cost carbon fiber for commercial/industrial applications led to the availability of much larger tows (48K to >200K). Similar examples can be cited for prepreg tape width, resin content, and thickness. Thus, constituent raw material forms can be adjusted to meet evolving requirements.

An all-important factor in material selection is cost, an area where composites historically have not fared well. However, recent declines in carbon fiber prices, coupled with improvements in low-cost manufacturing methods and continued demand for high structural efficiencies have begun to change the reputation of composites. As composites begin to compete with traditional low-cost materials, material cost will continue to be an important factor. Some guidelines to keep in mind are:

- *Fiber:* the greater the number of filaments per tow, the lower the cost
- *Resin:* the lower the performance temperature, the lower the cost
- *Prepreg:* the wider the product (tape or fabric), the lower the cost

The proper selection of constituent materials and material form to fit the structural application and the process design is critical to the success of the endeavor. Adding performance almost always adds cost, and cost savings generally begin with material selection.

Introduction to Reinforcing Fibers

Frederick T. Wallenberger, PPG Industries, Inc.

REINFORCING FIBERS are a key component of polymer-matrix composites (PMCs), ceramic-matrix composites (CMCs), and metal-matrix composites (MMCs). They impart high strength and stiffness to the matrix material that they modify, and in addition, may offer other valuable properties such as low dielectric constant, high temperature resistance, or high creep resistance. Depending on the design requirements, it is possible to select an appropriate composite-reinforcing fiber to manufacture a commercial composite part having high value-in-use. The composite will achieve the desired property values for a specific or generic application at a reasonable cost, even though the cost of the fibers themselves may appear high (Ref 1).

Overview

Composite-reinforcing fibers can be categorized by chemical composition, structural morphology, and commercial function. Natural fibers such as kenaf or jute are derived from plants and are used almost exclusively in PMCs. Oxide glass fibers (Ref 2) are derived from a mixture of oxides; silica, or quartz, fibers are from a single oxide. They are amorphous and primarily used to reinforce thermoplastic and thermoset PMCs. Aramid fibers (Ref 3) are crystalline polymer fibers and mostly used to reinforce PMCs. Carbon fibers (Ref 3) are based on ordered planar structures; they are primarily used to reinforce PMCs. Ceramic fibers are polycrystalline. Oxide ceramic (e.g., silica-alumina and pure alumina) fibers and nonoxide ceramic (e.g., silicon carbide) fibers (Ref 4) are used to reinforce CMCs and MMCs (Ref 5).

Value-in-Use. In a PMC, the primary function of a reinforcing fiber is to increase the strength and stiffness of a matrix material so that the resulting part can satisfy the design requirements or replace an existing part at equal strength, stiffness, and lower weight. In a CMC, the primary function of a reinforcing fiber is to facilitate the use of a given part at the highest possible ultimate-use temperature, offer superior fracture toughness, and prevent premature brittle failure. In a MMC, the primary function of a reinforcing fiber is to sustain the ultimate-use temperature of the part by preventing ductile failure. The value-in-use of a selected reinforcing fiber, whether based on a single property or on a combination of selected properties, depends on its cost as indexed to that property or combination of properties (Ref 1).

Specific Modulus and Specific Strength. Polymeric-matrix composite reinforcing fibers have adequate strength and yield adequate composite strength. Their value-in-use, therefore, depends mostly on their stiffness or elastic modulus (GPa). In transportation, aircraft, and aerospace applications, value-in-use additionally depends on their density, g/cm^3 (lb/in.^{3}), and therefore on the specific modulus. Specific properties are material properties divided by the density of the material. Specific modulus and specific strength are commonly expressed in units of length, for example, 10^6 meter (Mm). (Units of modulus or strength over density are also used. In SI units, this is Mpa · m^3/Mg. See the article "Material Property Charts" in *Materials Selection and Design,* Volume 20 of *ASM Handbook,* for example. The design engineer is cautioned to observe the units when comparing specific property data from multiple sources.) The specific modulus of PMC reinforcing fibers ranges from 25 to 437 Mm (Table 1, Fig. 1), thus facilitating the design of composites with vastly different part stiffness at equal weight, or with vastly lower part weight at equal stiffness.

Fiber Toughness. Toughness is the ability of a material to absorb work, which is proportional to the area under the stress-strain curve. It is the actual work per unit volume or unit mass that is required to rupture the material, so it is a measure of impact damage resistance. Some PMCs require high toughness. Amorphous reinforcing

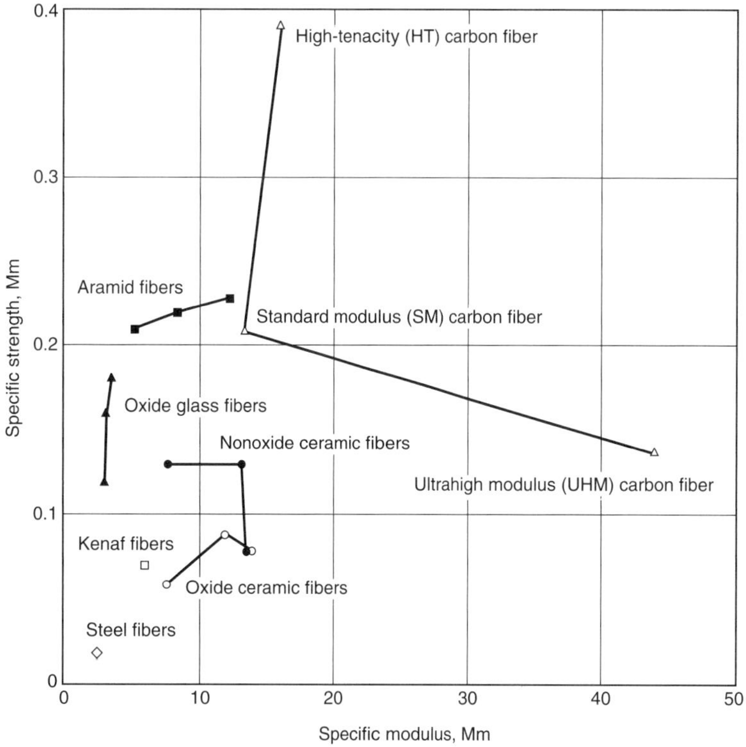

Fig. 1 Specific properties of selected reinforcing fibers

fibers, such as E-glass, S-glass, and single-crystal sapphire fibers, have high elongation at break and offer high fiber and composite toughness. Carbon fibers are typically more brittle, having lower elongation at break, and thus have lower fiber and composite toughness. Fracture toughness is the measure for damage resistance of CMCs (Ref 6).

Ultimate-Use Temperature. CMC and MMC reinforcing fibers, in contrast to PMC reinforcing fibers, have low to moderate stiffness or moduli (Fig. 1). Their function is not to stiffen an already stiff ceramic part, but to prevent brittle failure and to facilitate its use at the highest possible ultimate-use temperature of 1000 to 1400 °C (1830 to 2550 °F).

Nonmechanical Properties. Depending upon their chemical composition, PMC reinforcing fibers can offer additional value-in-use, due to their nonmechanical properties, such as electrical properties ranging from high conductivity to superior insulation. They can lower vibration transmission and thus provide quieter parts. The life cycle cost can be a greater value due to the extended life of the composite resulting from its corrosion resistance.

PMC Reinforcing Fibers

The following overview of PMC reinforcing fibers focuses on the cost-considered value-in-use of specific modulus and ultimate-use temperature of selected fibers in four fiber categories: natural fibers, oxide glass fibers, aramid fibers, and carbon and graphite fibers (Table 1 and Fig. 1). The individual reinforcing fibers in each category were deliberately selected to represent those commercial products that have the highest, midpoint, and lowest values, respectively, of specific modulus and of ultimate-use temperature.

Natural Plant Fibers. Kenaf, sisal, hemp, and jute are finding commercial use in automotive PMCs, where they offer adequate performance in interior composite applications (Ref 6) at a lower cost than that of comparable composites from incumbent reinforcing fibers. The density

Table 1(a) Comparative properties and costs of selected high-performance reinforcing fibers for polymer-matrix composites

Trade name	Generic name	Manufacturer	Composition	Ref	Density		Elastic modulus		Tensile strength		Specific modulus(a)	Specific strength(a)	Break elongation	Coefficient of thermal expansion		Fiber diameter		Ultimate-use temperature		Estimated unit cost(b)	
					g/cm^3	lb/in.^{3}	GPa	10^6 psi	MPa	ksi	Mm	Mm	%	10^{-6}/K	10^{-6}/°F	μm	10^{-6} in.	°C	°F	$/kg	$/lb
Natural fibers																					
...	Kenaf	Kafus	63% cellulose	6	1.52	0.0549	90	13.0	1000	145	6.0	0.067	2	...	...	...	...	<150	<300	0.5–1	0.45–2.20
Oxide glass fibers																					
...	E-glass	Owens-Corning, PPG, Vetrotex	Borosilicate	1, 2	2.54	0.0918	76–79	11.0–11.5	3100–3800	450–550	3.1–3.2	0.124–0.153	4.8	5	2.78	5–20	200–800	500	930	1.5–4	0.68–1.81
...	S-glass	Owens-Corning, Vetrotex, Nittobo	Mg/Al silicate	1, 3	2.48	0.0896	88–91	12.7–13.2	4400	638	3.6–3.7	0.181	5.7	2.9	1.61	5–10	200–900	750	1380	10–13	4.54–5.90
Astro-quartz	Quartz	Vetrotex	Silica 90.999%	1, 3	2.15	0.0777	69	10.0	3400	493	3.3	0.161	5	0.5	0.28	9	350	1050	1920	260	118
Aramid fibers																					
Technora T-200	LM	Teijin	Poly p-phenylene-terephthalamide	1, 3	1.39	0.0502	70	10.2	3000	435	5.1	0.220	4.4	...	...	12	472	160	320	20	9
Twaron	IM	Akzo	Poly p-phenylene-terephthalamide	1, 3	1.45	0.0524	121	17.6	3100	450	8.5	0.218	2	–3.5	–1.94	12	472	160	320	...	...
Kevlar 149	HM	DuPont	Poly p-phenylene-terephthalamide	1, 3	1.47	0.0531	179	26.0	3500	508	12.4	0.243	2	–2	–1.11	12	472	160	320	...	...

LM, low modulus; IM, intermediate modulus; HM, high modulus. (a) Calculated from actual strength and modulus data tabulated in Ref 3. (b) U.S. dollars.

Table 1(b) Comparative properties and costs of selected high-performance reinforcing fibers for ceramic-matrix and metal-matrix composites

Trade name	Generic name	Manufacturer	Composition	Ref	Density		Elastic modulus		Tensile strength		Specific modulus	Specific strength	Break elongation	Coefficient of thermal expansion		Fiber diameter		Ultimate-use temperature		Estimated unit cost(a)	
					g/cm^3	lb/in.^{3}	GPa	10^6 psi	MPa	ksi	Mm	Mm	%	10^{-6}/K	10^{-6}/°F	μm	10^{-6} in.	°C	°F	$/kg	$/lb
Metal fibers																					
Brunsmet	...	Brunswick Corp.	Austenitic steel	8	7.9	0.2854	197	28.6	1450	210	2.54	0.0187	...	8.5	4.72	12	472	1100	2010	...	...
Carbon and graphite fibers																					
Panex	SM	Zoltek	Carbon	1, 3	1.74	0.0629	228	33.1	3600	522	13.4	0.211	1.5	...	...	8	320	500	930	20	9
Torayca T1000	HT	Toray	Carbon	1, 3	1.82	0.0658	294	42.3	7100	1030	16.5	0.398	2.4	...	...	7	280	500	930	...	...
Thornel K-110X	UHM	BP Amoco	Carbon	1, 3	2.18	0.0788	966	140.0	3100	450	45.2	0.145	0.3	–1.5	–0.83	10	394	500	930	...	...
Oxide ceramic fibers																					
Nextel 610	...	3M	>99% alumina	1, 4	3.88	0.1402	373	54.1	2900	421	9.80	0.076	0.80	7.9	4.39	14	551	950	1740	594(b)	270(b)
Nextel 720	...	3M	85% alumina	1, 4	3.4	0.1228	260	37.7	2100	305	7.80	0.063	0.81	6	3.33	12	472	1050	1920	550(b)	250(b)
Saphikon	...	Saphikon	α-sapphire	1, 4	3.96	0.1431	470	68.2	3500	508	12.1	0.090	2.0	9	5	125	4921	<1400	<2550	66,000(b)	30,000(b)
Non-oxide ceramic fibers																					
Tyranno LM	...	Ube	9.8% O, 1.0% Zr	1, 4	2.48	0.0896	192	27.8	3300	479	7.90	0.136	2.2	3.5	1.94	11	433	<1200	<2190	...	...
...	SCS-6	Textron	SiC on C core	1, 4	3	0.1084	390	56.6	4000	580	13.3	0.136	...	4.6	2.56	140	5512	<1400	<2550	5,500(b)	2,500(b)
Hi-Nicalon-S	...	Nippon Carbon	99.8% SiC, 0.2% O	1, 4	3.1	0.112	420	60.9	2600	377	13.8	0.086	0.7	3.5	1.94	12	472	<1400	<2550	6,900(b)	3,136(b)

SM, standard modulus, HT, high tenacity; UHM, ultrahigh modulus. (a) U.S. dollars. (b) Ref 4

of kenaf fibers is 1.52 g/cm^3 (0.0549 lb/in.^{3}) (Table 1, Fig. 1) and its specific modulus of 6.0 Mm is therefore higher than that of commercial low modulus aramid fibers (5.1 Mm). Sustained use of fibers is possible at temperatures below 150 °C (300 °F).

Oxide Glass Fibers. Three types of oxide glass fiber are used as reinforcements for composites: silicate E-glass, silicate S-glass, and ultrapure silica fibers. E-glass is commercially available as a boron-containing and a boron-free variant. Owens Corning, PPG, and Vetrotex sell boron-containing E-glass. Owens Corning also sells boron-free E-glass under the trade name Advantex. S-glass is the predominant version of a group of high-strength fibers, which is sold by Owens Corning. Other high-strength fibers are R-glass, which is sold by Vetrotex, and Te-glass, which is sold by Nitto Boseki. Ultrapure silica fibers are also known as quartz fibers, despite the fact that they are amorphous and do not therefore exhibit the otherwise typical hexagonal crystal structure of quartz. An ultrapure silica fiber is sold by Vetrotex under the trade name Astroquartz.

The density of these three glass fibers increases from 2.15 g/cm^3 (0.0777 lb/in.^{3}) for silica glass fibers to 2.54 g/cm^3 (0.0918 lb/in.^{3}) for E-glass. The specific modulus, as reflected in Table 1 and Fig. 1, increases from 3.1 Mm for E-glass to 3.6 Mm for S-glass. This is an important property for transportation and aircraft composites. The ultimate-use temperature ranges from 500 °C (930 °F) for E-glass to 1050 °C (1920 °F) for silica/quartz glass fibers.

Aramid Fibers. Three grades of aramid fibers are known: low modulus (LM), intermediate modulus (IM), and high modulus (HM) fibers. The LM fiber is sold by Teijin under the trade name Technora T-200, the IM fiber is sold by Akzo under the trade name Twaron, and the HM fiber is sold by DuPont under the trade name Kevlar 140. The specific density increases from 1.39g/cm^3 (0.0502 lb/in.^{3}) for the LM fiber to 1.47 g/cm^3 (0.0531 lb/in.^{3}) for the HM fiber. Strength increases from 3.0 GPa (435 ksi) for the LM fiber to 3.5 GPa (510 ksi) for the HM fiber. Modulus increases from 70 GPa (10 $\times$ 10^6 psi) for the LM fiber to 179 GPa (26 $\times$ 10^6 psi) for the HM fiber. The specific modulus increases from 5.1 Mm for the LM fiber to 12.4 Mm for the HM fiber. The specific modulus of aramid fibers is an important property for aircraft composites. It is higher than that of the family of oxide glass fibers but lower than that of the family of carbon fibers. The temperature at which sustained use of aramid fibers is possible is about 160 °C (320 °F) (Ref 7).

Carbon and Graphite Fibers. Five grades of carbon fibers are known (Ref 3): standard modulus (SM), ultrahigh modulus (UHM), high modulus (HM), high tenacity-high strength (HT) or intermediate modulus (IM), and low modulus (LM) fibers. The LM fibers are fibrous carbons used as gland packing, furnace insulation, and as reinforcement to provide toughness. Three examples were selected for this overview. They represent the extreme values of strength and modulus within the wide range of fiber properties that are commercially available today. In order of increasing specific modulus, they are SM, HT, and UHM fibers. The SM fiber is sold by Zoltek under the trade name Panex, the HT fiber is sold by Toray under the trade name Torayca T1000, and the UHM fiber is sold by BP Amoco under the trade name Thornel K-100X.

The density of carbon fibers increases from 1.74 g/cm^3 (0.0629 lb/in.^{3}) for the HT fiber to 2.18 g/cm^3 (0.0788 lb/in.^{3}) for the UHM fiber. High-tenacity carbon fibers have the highest strength (7.1 GPa, or 1030 ksi) and specific strength (0.398 Mm) of any known reinforcing fiber. Ultrahigh modulus carbon fibers have the highest modulus (966 GPa, or 140 $\times$ 10^6 psi) and specific modulus (45.2 Mm) of any known reinforcing fiber. The ultrahigh specific modulus is an important property for aircraft and aerospace composites. Carbon fibers are electrically conductive. The temperature at which sustained use of carbon fibers is possible in oxidative environments is about 500 °C (930 °F).

CMC and MMC Reinforcing Fibers

This overview of CMC and MMC reinforcing fibers focuses primarily on the cost-considered value-in-use of the ultimate-use temperature of selected fibers in three fiber categories: metal fibers or wires, oxide ceramic fibers, and non-oxide ceramic fibers. The individual reinforcing fibers in each category were deliberately selected to represent those commercial products that have the highest, midpoint, and lowest values of specific modulus and ultimate-use temperature, respectively.

Metal Fibers or Wires. Steel, tungsten, beryllium, and other metal fibers are used (Ref 8). Due to their relatively high densities, their specific moduli are low and their reinforcing value is limited. They do offer high ultimate-use temperatures. Beryllium is a useful but toxic fiber. Steel fibers offer the lowest specific modulus (and value-in-use) among all known composite reinforcing fibers. The Brunswick Corporation sells a steel fiber under the trade name Brunsmet, as well as other metal fibers.

Oxide Ceramic Fibers. Increasing demand for fibers with a much higher ultimate-use temperature than that of oxide glass fibers has resulted in two families of ceramic fibers: oxide ceramics and non-oxide ceramics. These fibers are used in CMCs and MMCs. The 3M Company sells polycrystalline alumina and silica-alumina fibers under the trade name Nextel 610 and Nextel 720, respectively, and Saphikon sells a single-crystal alumina (sapphire) fiber under the trade name Saphikon.

The density of oxide ceramic fibers increases from 3.40 g/cm^3 (0.123 lb/in.^{3}) for Nextel 720, a polycrystalline fiber containing 85% alumina and 15% silica, to 3.96 g/cm^3 (0.143 lb/in.^{3}) for Saphikon, a single-crystal sapphire fiber containing 100% α-alumina. Because of the high density of these fibers, their specific strength (0.063–0.090 Mm) is lower than those of carbon, aramid, non-oxide ceramic, and oxide glass fibers. It is comparable to that of steel and natural fibers. The specific modulus of ceramic oxide fibers, which increases from 7.80 Mm for Nextel 720 fibers to 12.1 Mm for sapphire fibers, is intermediate between that of carbon and aramid fibers. The temperature at which sustained use of these oxide ceramic fibers is possible is about 1200 °C (2200 °F).

Non-oxide Ceramic Fibers. Non-oxide and oxide ceramic reinforcing fibers have different properties and are aimed at different applications (Ref 4). Non-oxide fibers include polycrystalline silicon carbide and silicon nitride fibers. Ube sells a silicon carbide fiber that contains 9.8% O and 1.0% Zr under the trade name Tyranno LM. Textron sells a sheath/core fiber with a silicon carbide sheath and a carbon core under the designation SCS-6. Nippon Carbon sells a near-stoichiometric silicon carbide fiber under the trade name Hi-Nicalon-S. The properties of these fibers are shown in Table 1 and Fig. 1.

The density of silicon carbide fibers increases from 2.48 g/cm^3 (0.0896 lb/in.^{3}) for Tyranno ZM to 3.10 g/cm^3 (0.112 lb/in.^{3}) for Hi-Nicalon-S fibers. The specific modulus increases from 7.90 Mm for Tyranno ZM to 13.8 Mm for Hi-Nicalon-S fibers. It is comparable to that of oxide ceramic fibers. The highest temperature at which sustained use of SCS-6 and of Hi-Nicalon-S is possible is about 1400 °C (2550 °F).

Summary and Conclusions

Composite reinforcing fibers have high value-in-use in a wide range of commercial applications. Commercial glass fibers have high value-in-use in low-cost, high-volume, commodity PMCs where they offer satisfactory reinforcement at a fiber price ranging from \$1.50/kg for first-quality products to \$4.25/kg for multiaxial glass reinforcements. Commercial aramid, carbon, oxide ceramic and non-oxide ceramic reinforcing fibers have high value in high-cost, low-volume applications where the cost ranges from \$20/kg for LM aramid and SM carbon fibers to \$6,900/kg for Hi-Nicalon-S silicon carbide fibers. Commercial sapphire fibers have high value-in-use in extremely costly specialty applications where they offer otherwise unattainable reinforcing properties at \$66,000/kg.

REFERENCES

1. F.T. Wallenberger, *Advanced Inorganic Fibers—Processes, Structures, Properties, Applications,* Kluwer Academic Publishers, Dordrecht, the Netherlands, 1999
2. T.F. Starr, *Glass-Fibre Dictionary and Data-*

book, 2nd ed., Chapman & Hall, London, 1997

3. T.F. Starr, *Carbon and High Performance Fibres,* Directory and Databook, 6th ed., Chapman & Hall, London, 1995
4. National Materials Advisory Board Committee, D.W. Johnson, Chair, "Ceramic Fibers and Coatings," National Research Council, Publication NMAB-494, National Academic Press, Washington, D. C., 1998
5. V.I. Kostikov, *Fibre Science and Technology,* Chapman & Hall, London, 1995
6. A. Kelly, *Concise Encyclopedia of Composite Materials,* Revised ed., R.W. Cahn and M.B. Beaver, Ed., Pergamon, Elsevier Science Ltd., Oxford, 1994
7. A.R. Bunsell, *Fibre Reinforcements for Composite Materials,* Elsevier, Oxford, 1988
8. J.V. Milewski and H.S. Katz, *Handbook of Reinforcements for Plastics,* Van Nostrand Reinhold Company, New York, 1987

Glass Fibers

Frederick T. Wallenberger, James C. Watson, and Hong Li, PPG Industries, Inc.

GLASS FIBERS are among the most versatile industrial materials known today. They are readily produced from raw materials, which are available in virtually unlimited supply (Ref 1). All glass fibers described in this article are derived from compositions containing silica. They exhibit useful bulk properties such as hardness, transparency, resistance to chemical attack, stability, and inertness, as well as desirable fiber properties such as strength, flexibility, and stiffness (Ref 2). Glass fibers are used in the manufacture of structural composites, printed circuit boards and a wide range of special-purpose products (Ref 3).

Fiber Forming Processes. Glass melts are made by fusing (co-melting) silica with minerals, which contain the oxides needed to form a given composition. The molten mass is rapidly cooled to prevent crystallization and formed into glass fibers by a process also known as fiberization.

Nearly all continuous glass fibers are made by a direct draw process and formed by extruding molten glass through a platinum alloy bushing that may contain up to several thousand individual orifices, each being 0.793 to 3.175 mm (0.0312 to 0.125 in.) in diameter (Ref 1). While still highly viscous, the resulting fibers are rapidly drawn to a fine diameter and solidify. Typical fiber diameters range from 3 to 20 μm (118 to 787 μin.). Individual filaments are combined into multifilament strands, which are pulled by mechanical winders at velocities of up to 61 m/s (200 ft/s) and wound onto tubes or forming packages. This is the only process that is described in detail subsequently in the present article.

The marble melt process can be used to form special-purpose, for example, high-strength fibers. In this process, the raw materials are melted, and solid glass marbles, usually 2 to 3 cm (0.8 to 1.2 in.) in diameter, are formed from the melt. The marbles are remelted (at the same or at a different location) and formed into glass fibers. Glass fibers can also be down drawn from the surface of solid preforms. Although this is the only process used for manufacturing optical fibers, which are not discussed in this Volume, it is a specialty process for manufacturing structural glass fibers such as silica or quartz glass fibers. These and other specialty processes are highlighted wherever appropriate but not discussed in full. Additional details about fiber forming are provided in the section "Glass Melting and Fiber Forming" in this article.

Sizes and Binders. Glass filaments are highly abrasive to each other (Ref 4). "Size" coatings or binders are therefore applied before the strand is gathered to minimize degradation of filament strength that would otherwise be caused by filament-to-filament abrasion. Binders provide lubrication, protection, and/or coupling. The size may be temporary, as in the form of a starch-oil emulsion that is subsequently removed by heating and replaced with a glass-to-resin coupling agent known as a finish. On the other hand, the size may be a compatible treatment that performs several necessary functions during the subsequent forming operation and which, during impregnation, acts as a coupling agent to the resin being reinforced.

Glass Fiber Types

Glass fibers fall into two categories, low-cost general-purpose fibers and premium special-purpose fibers. Over 90% of all glass fibers are general-purpose products. These fibers are known by the designation E-glass and are subject to ASTM specifications (Ref 5). The remaining glass fibers are premium special-purpose products. Many, like E-glass, have letter designations implying special properties (Ref 6). Some have tradenames, but not all are subject to ASTM specifications. Specifically:

Letter designation	Property or characteristic
E, electrical	Low electrical conductivity
S, strength	High strength
C, chemical	High chemical durability
M, modulus	High stiffness
A, alkali	High alkali or soda lime glass
D, dielectric	Low dielectric constant

Table 1 gives compositions and Table 2 gives physical and mechanical properties of commercial glass fibers.

General-purpose glass fibers (E-glass variants) are discussed in the following section of this article, which provides an in-depth discussion of compositions, melt properties, fiber properties (Ref 12), methods of manufacture, and significant product types. An in-depth discussion of composite applications can be found in other articles in this Volume.

Glass fibers and fabrics are used in ever increasing varieties for a wide range of applications (Ref 13). A data book is available (Ref 14) that covers all commercially available E-glass fibers, whether employed for reinforcement, filtration, insulation, or other applications. It lists all manufacturers, their sales offices, agents, subsidiaries, and affiliates, complete with addresses, and telephone and fax numbers. And it tabulates key properties and relevant supply details of all E-glass fiber grades, that are available in the market today.

Special-Purpose Glass Fibers. S-glass, D-glass, A-glass, ECR-glass, ultrapure silica fibers, hollow fibers, and trilobal fibers are special-purpose glass fibers. Selected special-purpose glass fibers are discussed in the subsequent section of this article. That section reviews compositions, manufacture, properties, and applications to an extent commensurate with their commercial use (Ref 15).

A companion data book (Ref 16) is available that covers all commercially available high-strength glass fibers including S-glass and, all silica or quartz glass fibers, including Astroquartz and Quartzel. It also lists a wide range of woven fabrics, that are commercially available in the market of today, ranging from S-glass/aramid, S-glass/carbon, silica/aramid, and silica/carbon yarns to silica/boron yarns. In addition, it covers all commercially available carbon, ceramic, boron, and high-temperature polymer fibers and yarns. This data book also lists all yarn counts, fabric constructions, fabric weights, and commercial sources.

ASTM Test Methods. ASTM has published standard test methods for glass density (Ref 17), alternating current loss characteristics and dielectric constant (Ref 18), direct current conductance of insulating materials (Ref 19), dielectric breakdown voltage and dielectric strength (Ref 20), softening point of glass (Ref 21), annealing point and strain point of glass by fiber elongation (Ref 22), annealing point and strain point of glass by beam bending (Ref 23), viscosity (Ref 24), liquidus temperature (Ref 25), and coeffi-

Table 1 Compositions of commercial glass fibers

Fiber	Ref	Composition, wt% SiO_2	B_2O_3	Al_2O_3	CaO	MgO	ZnO	TiO_2	Zr_2O_3	Na_2O	K_2O	Li_2O	Fe_2O_3	F_2
General-purpose fibers														
Boron-containing E-glass	1, 2	52–56	4–6	12–15	21–23	0.4–4	. . .	0.2–0.5	. . .	0–1	Trace	. . .	0.2–0.4	0.2–0.7
Boron-free E-glass	7	59.0	. . .	12.1	22.6	3.4	. . .	1.5	. . .	0.9	. . .	. . .	0.2	. . .
	8	60.1	. . .	13.2	22.1	3.1	. . .	0.5	. . .	0.6	0.2	. . .	0.2	0.1
Special-purpose fibers														
ECR-glass	1, 2	58.2	. . .	11.6	21.7	2.0	2.9	2.5	. . .	1.0	0.2	. . .	0.1	Trace
D-glass	1, 2	74.5	22.0	0.3	0.5	. . .	. . .	. . .	. . .	1.0	<1.3	. . .	. . .	. . .
	2	55.7	26.5	13.7	2.8	1.0	. . .	. . .	. . .	0.1	0.1	0.1	. . .	. . .
S-, R-, and Te-glass	1, 2	60–65.5	. . .	23–25	0–9	6–11	. . .	. . .	0–1	0–0.1	. . .	. . .	0–0.1	. . .
Silica/quartz	1, 2	99.9999	. . .	. . .	. . .	. . .	. . .	. . .	. . .	. . .	. . .	. . .	. . .	. . .

cient of linear thermal expansion of plastics (Ref 26).

Some fiber properties (Ref 4), such as tensile strength, modulus, and chemical durability, are measured on the fibers directly. Other properties, such as relative permittivity, dissipation factor, dielectric strength, volume/surface resistivities, and thermal expansion, are measured on glass that has been formed into a bulk patty or block sample and annealed (heat treated) to relieve forming stresses. Properties such as density and refractive index are measured on both fibers and bulk samples, in annealed or unannealed form.

General-Purpose Glass Fibers

Types. Two generic types of E-glass (Ref 6) are known in the market today. The incumbent E-glass contains 5 to 6 wt% of boron oxide. Stringent environmental regulations require the addition of costly emission abatement systems to eliminate boron from the off-gases of boron-containing melts. Alternatively, the use of environmentally friendly boron-free E-glass is required. These melts do not contain, and therefore do not emit, boron into the environment during processing. As a result, a boron-free E-glass product was recently introduced into the market by Fiberglas (Owens Corning Corp., Toledo, OH) under the trademark Advantex.

Commercial boron-containing E-glass comes in two variants. One commercial variant is derived from the quaternary SiO_2-Al_2O_3-CaO-MgO (Ref 2, 4, 6, 27), and the other is derived from the ternary SiO_2-Al_2O_3-CaO phase diagram (Ref 2, 4, 6, 28). Commercial E-glasses in the ternary SiO_2-Al_2O_3-CaO system contain a small amount (<0.6 wt%) of MgO that is not deliberately added but obtained as by-product (or tramp) from other ingredients. On the other hand, commercially available boron-free E-glass is derived from the quaternary SiO_2-Al_2O_3-CaO-MgO phase diagram (Ref 2, 7, 8, 29).

ASTM standards for E-glass (Ref 5) cover all three commercial E-glass variants, distinguishing E-glasses by end use. Compositions containing 5 to 10 wt% by weight of boron oxide are certified for printed circuit board and aerospace applications. Compositions containing 0 to 10 wt% by weight of boron oxide are certified for general applications. According to these standards, E-glass compositions for either type of application may also contain 0 to 2 wt% alkali oxide and 0 to 1 wt% fluoride. The more recent boron-free E-glass variants may also be fluorine-free.

Oxide Compositions. E-glasses of any type are general-purpose fibers because they offer useful strength at low cost. Table 1 presents the oxide components and their ranges for the two types of E-glass fibers that are currently being produced and used in composites. A range is given for each with regard to its oxide components because each manufacturer, and even different manufacturing plants of the same company, may use slightly different compositions for

Table 2 Physical and mechanical properties of commercial glass fibers

Fiber	Log 3 forming temperature(a), °C	Log 3 forming temperature(a), °F	Liquidus temperature, °C	Liquidus temperature, °F	Softening temperature, °C	Softening temperature, °F	Annealing temperature, °C	Annealing temperature, °F	Straining temperature, °C	Straining temperature, °F	Bulk density, annealed glass, g/cm^3
General-purpose fibers											
Boron-containing E-glass	1160–1196	2120–2185	1065–1077	1950–1970	830–860	1525–1580	657	1215	616	1140	2.54–2.55
Boron-free E-glass	1260	2300	1200	2190	916	1680	736	1355	691	1275	2.62
Special-purpose fibers											
ECR-glass	1213	2215	1159	2120	880	1615	728	1342	691	1275	2.66–2.68
D-glass	. . .	. . .	. . .	. . .	770	1420	. . .	. . .	475	885	2.16
S-glass	1565	2850	1500	2730	1056	1935	. . .	. . .	760	1400	2.48–2.49
Silica/quartz	>2300	>4170	1670	3038	. . .	. . .	. . .	. . .	. . .	. . .	2.15

Fiber	Coefficient of linear expansion, 10^{-6}/°C	Specific heat, cal/g/°C	Dielectric constant at room temperature and 1 MHz	Dielectric strength, kV/cm	Volume resistivity at room temperature $\log_{10}$ (Ω cm)	Refractive index (bulk)	Weight loss in 24 h in 10% H_2SO_4, %	Tensile strength at 23 °C (73 °F), MPa	Tensile strength at 23 °C (73 °F), ksi	Young's modulus, GPa	Young's modulus, 10^6 psi	Filament elongation at break, %
General-purpose fibers												
Boron-containing E-glass	4.9–6.0	0.192	5.86–6.6	103	22.7–28.6	1.547	~41	3100–3800	450–551	76–78	11.0–11.3	4.5–4.9
Boron-free E-glass	6.0	. . .	7.0	102	28.1	1.560	~6	3100–3800	450–551	80–81	11.6–11.7	4.6
Special-purpose fibers												
ECR-glass	5.9	. . .	. . .	. . .	. . .	1.576	5	3100–3800	450–551	80–81	11.6–11.7	4.5–4.9
D-glass	3.1	0.175	3.56–3.62	. . .	. . .	1.47	. . .	2410	349	. . .	. . .	. . .
S-glass	2.9	0.176	4.53–4.6	130	. . .	1.523	. . .	4380–4590	635–666	88–91	12.8–13.2	5.4–5.8
Silica/quartz	0.54	. . .	3.78	. . .	. . .	1.4585	. . .	3400	493	69	10.0	5

(a) The log 3 forming temperature is the temperature of a melt at a reference viscosity of 100 Pa · s (1000 P). Source: Ref 2, 7–10, 11

the same glass. These variations result mainly from differences in the available glass batch (raw materials). Tight control is maintained within a given production facility to optimize compositional consistency and maximize production efficiencies.

As shown in Table 1, commercial, boron-containing E-glass compositions (Ref 1, 2, 4, 6, 12, 24) differ substantially from boron-free E-glass compositions. The silica content for commercial boron-containing E-glasses ranges from 52 to 56 wt% by weight, and for commercial boron-free E-glasses from 59 to 61 wt%. The alumina content generally ranges from 12 to 15 wt% for these boron-containing E-glasses and from 12 to 13.5 wt% for these boron-free E-glasses. The calcia content ranges from 21 to 23 wt% for these commercial boron-containing E-glasses and from 22 to 23 wt% for these boron-free E-glasses.

For commercial, boron-containing, ternary or quaternary E-glasses, the magnesia content ranges from 0.4 wt% (tramp only) to greater amounts if magnesia (dolomite) is deliberately added. For commercial boron-free E-glasses, it ranges from 3.1 to 3.4 wt% (see Table 1). The boron oxide content ranges from 5 to 6% for commercial boron-containing E-glasses, and it is zero for boron-free E-glasses. The titania content ranges from 0.4 to 0.6 wt% for commercial boron-containing E-glasses. For boron-free E-glasses, it ranges from 0.5 wt% (Ref 8) to 1.5 wt% (Ref 7) (see also Table 1).

Environmentally friendly E-glass melts are boron-free and fluorine-free. However, the log 3 fiber forming or fiberization temperature (T_F) of boron-free E-glass melts may be as much as 100 to 110 °C (180 to 200 °F) higher than that of boron-containing E-glass melts (Fig. 1). The log 3 forming temperature is the temperature of a melt at a reference viscosity of 100 Pa · s (1000 P). In addition, the softening point of boron-free E-glass is 60 to 90 °C (110 to 160 °F) higher also than that of a boron-containing E-glass. The higher process temperature requires more process energy, but the higher softening point facilitates higher use temperatures.

Melt Properties. According to Table 2, the log 3 forming temperature, T_F, of boron-containing E-glasses ranges from 1140 to 1185 °C (2085 to 2165 °F). The liquidus temperature (T_L) is the temperature below which solid (crystals) will form. It ranges form 1050 to 1064 °C (1920 to 1945 °F). The difference between forming and liquidus temperature (ΔT) ranges from 81 to 90 °C (146 to 162 °F). In contrast, the log 3 fiber forming temperature of boron-free E-glasses ranges from 1250 to 1264 °C (2280 to 2307 °F), the liquidus temperature from 1146 to 1180 °C (2095 to 2155 °F), and the difference between forming and liquidus temperature (ΔT) from 86 to 104 °C (155 to 187 °F) (Ref 7–10). Finally, the softening point of boron-containing E-glasses ranges from 830 to 860 °C (1525 to 1580 °F); that of boron-free E-glasses is about 916 °C (1680 °F).

Mechanical Properties. Table 2 also compares the mechanical properties of the boron-free and boron-containing E-glasses. Elastic modulus (or fiber stiffness) of boron-free E-glasses is about 5% higher than that of boron-containing E-glasses, while pristine, virgin, or single-filament tensile strength is said to be about the same for both types of E-glasses when both are tested at room temperature (Ref 8, 9).

Physical Properties. In addition, Table 2 compares the physical properties of the boron-free and boron-containing E-glasses. Most importantly, the corrosion resistance of boron-free E-glasses was found to be seven times higher than that of boron-containing E-glasses when tested at room temperature for 24 h in 10% sulfuric acid. It approaches that of ECR glass fibers (Ref 9, 10).

Boron-free E-glasses have a slightly higher density (2.62 g/cm^3) than boron-containing E-glasses (2.55 g/cm^3), but the density of both fibers is lower than that of ECR glass (2.66 to 2.68 g/cm^3), a corrosion-resistant special-purpose fiber. Boron-free E-glasses have a higher refractive index and linear expansion coefficient than boron-containing E-glass fibers. The refractive index of both E-glasses is lower than that of ECR glass. The linear expansion coefficient of ECR glass fibers is midway between that of the two E-glasses.

Boron-free E-glasses have a slightly higher dielectric constant (7.0) than boron-containing E-glasses (5.9 to 6.6) when measured at room temperature and at a frequency of 1 MHz. As a result, boron-containing, but not boron-free, E-glass fibers are needed for electronic circuit boards and aerospace applications. On the other hand, boron-free and boron-containing E-glass fibers are used in structural composites where the dielectric constant is of no concern. Composite and laminate uses of all glass fibers are discussed in other articles in this Volume.

Special-Purpose Glass Fibers

Types. Special-purpose fibers, which are of commercial significance in the market today, include glass fibers with high corrosion resistance (ECR-glass), high strength (S-, R-, and Te-glass), with low dielectric constants (D-glass), high strength fibers, and pure silica or quartz fibers, which can be used at ultrahigh temperatures. These fibers will be discussed in the following paragraphs. Others special-purpose fibers include A-glass, C-glass, hollow fibers, bicomponent fibers, and trilobal fibers. These special-purpose glass fibers have recently been reviewed in detail (Ref 2).

ECR-Glass. The corrosion resistance of glass fibers is determined by their chemical structure. It has already been noted in the preceding section on general-purpose glass fibers that boron-free E-glass fibers derived from the quaternary SiO_2-Al_2O_3-CaO-MgO phase diagram have higher acid resistance than E-glass fibers that are derived from the ternary SiO_2-Al_2O_3-CaO phase diagram but have high boron levels. The ECR glass fibers offer enhanced long-term acid resistance and short-term alkali resistance (Ref 27).

The addition of high levels of ZnO and TiO_2 to the boron-free quaternary E-glass system further enhances the corrosion resistance of the resulting ECR glass fibers while at the same time reducing the log 3 forming temperature. The product and process advantage are obtained at a cost penalty. About 2% ZnO and two additional percent TiO_2 are required, and both materials are known to be costly batch ingredients.

S-Glass, R-Glass, and Te-Glass. The tensile strength of glass fibers is determined by the structure connectivity of the silicate network, notably, by the absence of alkali oxides, which are not readily integrated into the structure. The structure of boron oxide, though being a part of the network, is weaker than that of silicon oxide, and therefore, boron oxide serves as a flux. Several high-strength glass fibers are known, including S-glass, Te-glass, and R-glass (Ref 2). All offer 10 to 15% higher strength than E-glass at room temperature, but their real value is their ability to withstand higher in-use temperatures than E-glass. These fibers are used in military applications. Stringent quality-control procedures are necessary to meet military specifications.

S-glass and Te-glass are derivatives of the ternary SiO_2-Al_2O_3-CaO system. R-glass is a derivative of the quaternary SiO_2-Al_2O_3-CaO-MgO system. S-glass and S-2 glass fibers, a product variant, have the same glass composition (Ref 2) but different coatings. While internal structural uniformity (high strength) is achieved with these boron-free and alkali-free compositions, their forming temperatures are higher than that of E-glass. Attainment of high in-use temperatures is a definite product advantage, but

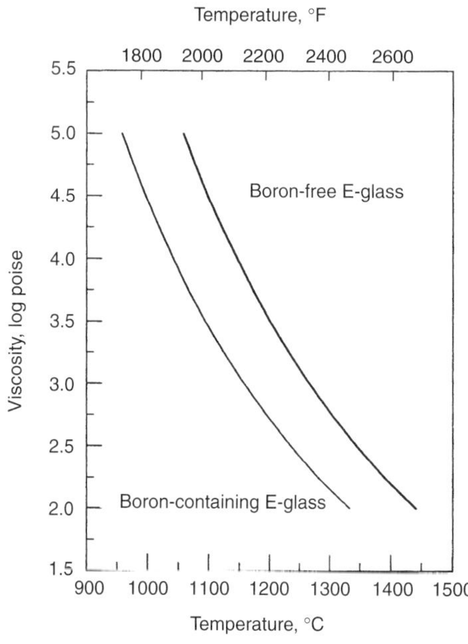

Fig. 1 Viscosity of boron-free and boron-containing E-glass

higher melt temperatures, more process energy, and more costly bushing alloys are required.

Silica/Quartz Fibers. Glass fibers with increasing SiO_2 levels can be used in applications requiring increasingly high in-use temperatures. High-silica fibers (95% SiO_2) are amorphous glass fibers. They are obtained by acid leaching of borosilicate E-glass fabrics, which are, in turn, used as insulation blankets at temperatures up to 1040 °C (1900 °F). Pure silica fibers (99% SiO_2) are made by dry spinning from aqueous water-glass solutions. They are known by the tradename "Silfa" and mostly are used as yarns, for example, for wire insulation at temperatures up to 1090 °C (1990 °F). For details see Ref 2. They are not used in composite applications and are therefore not shown in Table 2.

Ultrapure silica glass fibers or quartz fibers (99.99% SiO_2), which are down-drawn from preforms (Ref 2) in a containerless process, are also amorphous, despite the fact that the trivial name "quartz" or trade names Quartzel and Astroquartz would imply the presence of the hexagonal crystal structure of quartz. Ultrapure silica (quartz) fibers combine superior high-temperature resistance with superior transparency to ultraviolet (UV) and longer wavelength radiation. For example, in a composite radome on the nose of an aircraft, they protect delicate radar equipment from flying objects, lightning and static discharge (Ref 30). The purest of all commercial silica glass or quartz fibers (99.999% SiO_2) are obtained by dry-spinning of a reagent grade tetraethylorthosilicate sol-gel (Ref 2).

All ultrapure silica glass or quartz fibers are used in yarn and in composite applications and are, therefore, shown in Table 2. Ultrapure and pure silica yarns and fabrics can be used at temperatures up to 1090 °C (1990 °F), high silica fabrics at up to 1040 °C (1900 °F), and S-glass, Te-glass, and R-glass yarns and fabrics at up to 815 °C (1500 °F) (for process and product details see Ref 2).

D-Glass. The electrical properties of glass fibers are determined by their volume resistivity, surface conductivity, dielectric constant and loss tangent (Ref 2). E-glass with its relatively high dielectric constant is the major reinforcing fiber for printed circuit board (PCB) laminates in the market today, but miniaturization drives the industry toward specialty fibers with lower dielectric constants and lower dielectric loss tangents.

Several low D-glass variants are known. All have very high B_2O_3 levels (20 to 26%) and, therefore, much lower dielectric constants than E-glass (4.10 to 3.56 versus 6.86 to 7.00). Those D-glass variants having low dielectric loss tangents as well (Ref 8) are said to offer the highest value in-use when used to reinforce PCB laminates. Because of their high cost, however, any D-glass version will remain a low volume specialty fiber. The very high boron-oxide levels, which are needed and in part emitted from the melt, may require an entirely different specialty process (see Ref 2 for details).

For very different reasons, ultrapure silica fibers, hollow E-glass fibers, S-glass, and other high-temperature fibers have lower dielectric constants than solid E-glass. They, too, can and are being used to reinforce printed circuit board (PCB) laminates. However, silica fibers have a low modulus and are, therefore, less effective as reinforcing fibers. Hollow fibers, although initially effective because of their low dielectric constant, lose their dielectric properties if moisture can seep into the laminate structure.

Glass Melting and Fiber Forming

A glass is an amorphous solid obtained by cooling a melt (i.e., liquid phase) sufficiently fast that crystallization (devitrification) cannot occur. When the melt is cooled slowly, crystallization can occur at the liquidus temperature, T_L, where crystals and melt are in equilibrium, or below. Glass fibers are therefore obtained at high cooling rates. Chemically, a glass consists of a silica network. Other oxides facilitate melting, homogenizing, removal of gaseous inclusions, and fiber formation at optimum temperatures. This section addresses the generic glass-melting and fiber-forming process, including the viscosity versus temperature profile that is required for general-purpose E-glass glass fibers and, more specifically, for E-glass fibers containing 5 to 6% boron oxide (see Ref 1 for details).

Depending on fiber diameter, optimum fiber formation is achieved with melts having a viscosity ranging from log 2.5 to log 3 P. The generic melting and forming process that is required for boron-free E-glass is the same as that required for boron-containing E-glass, but the viscosity/temperature profile differs. The relative forming temperatures can be deduced from the Fulcher curves shown in Fig. 1. They will be proportionately higher for boron-free E-glass at equal melt viscosities between log 2.5 to log 3.0 P. This section does not address the glass melting and fiber forming processes required for the special-purpose glass fibers, that is, ECR-glass, S-glass, ultrapure silica fibers, and D-glass (see Ref 2).

Batch Mixing and Melting. The glass melting process begins with the weighing and blending of selected raw materials. In modern fiberglass plants, this process is highly automated, with computerized weighing units and enclosed material transport systems. The individual components are weighed and delivered to a blending station where the batch ingredients are thoroughly mixed before being transported to the furnace.

Fiberglass furnaces generally are divided into three distinct sections (Fig. 2). Batch is delivered into the furnace section for melting, removal of gaseous inclusions, and homogenization. Then, the molten glass flows into the refiner section, where the temperature of the glass is lowered from 1370 °C (2500 °F) to about 1260 °C (2300 °F). The molten glass next goes to the forehearth section located directly above the fiber-forming stations. The temperatures throughout this process are prescribed by the viscosity characteristics of the particular glass. In addition, the physical layout of the furnace can vary widely, depending on the space constraints of the plant.

Fiberizing and Sizing. The conversion of molten glass in the forehearth into continuous glass fibers is basically an attenuation process (Fig. 3). The molten glass flows through a platinum-rhodium alloy bushing with a large number of holes or tips (400 to 8000, in typical production). The bushing is heated electrically, and the heat is controlled very precisely to maintain a constant glass viscosity. The fibers are drawn down and cooled rapidly as they exit the bushing.

A sizing is then applied to the surface of the fibers by passing them over an applicator that continually rotates through the sizing bath to maintain a thin film through which the glass filaments pass. It is this step, in addition to the original glass composition, which primarily differentiates one fiberglass product from another.

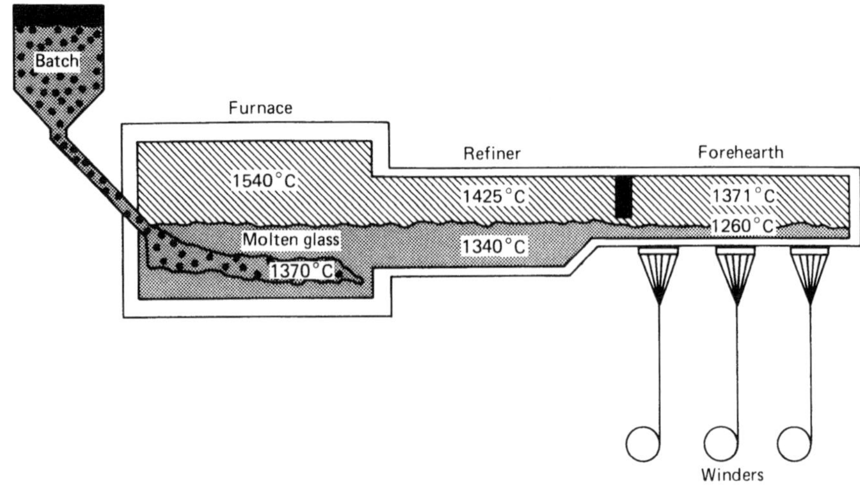

Fig. 2 Furnace for glass melting

The components of the sizing impart strand integrity, lubricity, resin compatibility, and adhesion properties to the final product, thus tailoring the fiber properties to the specific end-use requirements. After applying the sizing, the filaments are gathered into a strand before approaching the take-up device. If small bundles of filaments (split strands) are needed, multiple gathering devices (often called shoes) are used.

Fiber Diameters. The attenuation rate, and therefore the final filament diameter, is controlled by the take-up device. Fiber diameter is also affected by bushing temperature, glass viscosity, and the pressure head over the bushing. The most widely used take-up device is the forming winder, which employs a rotating collet and a traverse mechanism to distribute the strand in a random manner as the forming package grows in diameter. This facilitates strand removal from the package in subsequent processing steps, such as roving or chopping. The forming packages are dried and transferred to the specific fabrication area for conversion into the finished fiberglass roving, mat, chopped strand, or other product.

In recent years, processes have been developed to produce finished roving or chopped products directly during forming, thus leading to the term *direct draw roving* or *direct chopped strand*. Special winders and choppers designed to perform in the wet-forming environment are used in these cases (Fig. 4).

Yarn Nomenclature. It is standard practice in the fiberglass industry to refer to a specific filament diameter by a specific alphabet designation, as listed in Table 3. Fine fibers, which are used in textile applications, range from D through G. One reason for using fine fibers is to provide enough flexibility to the yarn to enable it to be processed in high-speed twisting and weaving operations. Conventional plastics reinforcement, however, uses filament diameters that range from G to T.

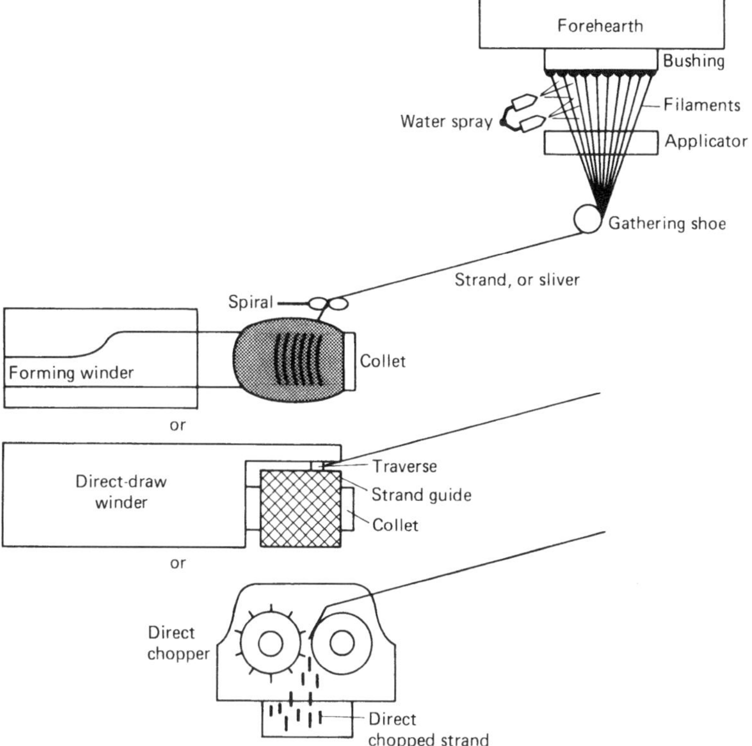

Fig. 3 Fiberglass forming process

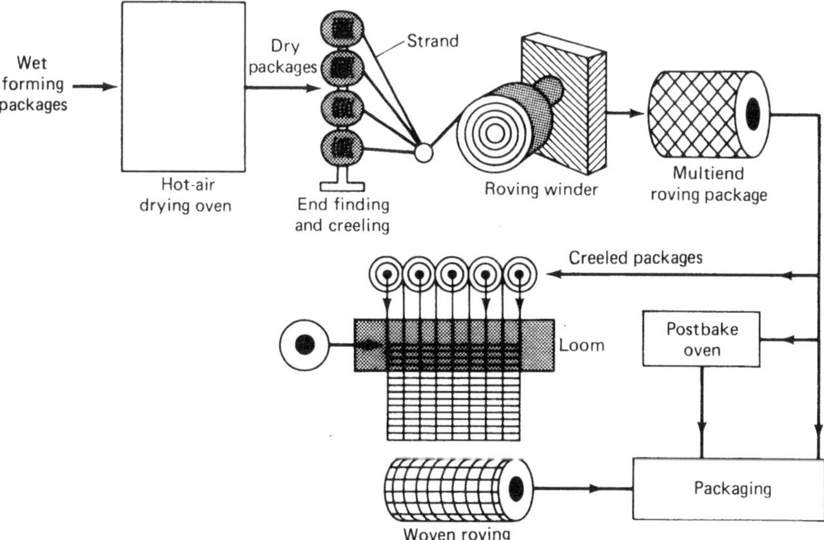

Fig. 4 Multiend roving process production

Important Commercial Products

Once the continuous glass fibers have been produced they must be converted into a suitable product form for their intended composite application. The major finished forms for E-glass fibers are continuous roving, woven roving, fiberglass mat, chopped strand, and yarns for textile applications.

Fiberglass roving is produced by collecting a bundle of strands into a single large strand, which is wound into a stable, cylindrical package. This is called a multiend roving process. The process begins by placing a number of oven-dried forming packages into a creel. The ends are then gathered together under tension and collected on a precision roving winder that has a constant traverse-to-winding ratio, and is called the waywind. This ratio has a significant effect on package stability, strand characteristics, and ease of payout in subsequent operations. The yield (meter per kilogram, or yard per pound) of the finished roving is determined by the number of input ends and the yield of the input strand or sliver. Final package weight and dimensions can be made to vary widely, depending upon the required end-use. Figure 4 shows the entire process.

Rovings are used in many applications. When used in a spray-up fabrication process, the roving is chopped with an air-powered gun that propels the chopped-glass strands to a mold while simultaneously applying resin and catalyst in the compact ratio. This process is commonly used for bath tubs, shower stalls, and many marine applications. In another important process, the production of sheet molding compound (SMC), the roving is chopped onto a bed of formulated polyester resin and compacted into a sheet, which thickens with time. This sheet is then placed in a press and molded into parts. Many fiber-reinforced plastic (FRP) automotive body panels are made by this process.

Filament winding and pultrusion are processes that use single-end rovings in continuous form. Applications include pipes, tanks, leaf springs, and many other structural composites. In these processes the roving is passed through a liquid resin bath and then shaped into a part by winding the resin-impregnated roving onto a mandrel or by pulling it through a heated die. Because of a property called *catenary* (the presence of some strands that have a tendency to sag within a bundle of strands), multiend rovings sometimes do not process efficiently. Catenary is caused by uneven tension in the roving process that results in poor strand integrity.

While providing desirable entanglement for transverse strength in pultrusion, the looser ends in the roving may eventually cause loops and breakouts in close-tolerance orifices, making reinforced plastics processing difficult. Consequently, the process of direct forming single-end rovings was developed by using very large bushings and a precision winder specially designed to operate in the severe forming environment. No subsequent step other than drying is required. Single-end rovings have become the preferred product for many filament-winding and pultrusion applications.

Woven roving is produced by weaving fiberglass rovings into a fabric form. This yields a coarse product that is used in many hand lay-up and panel molding processes to produce FRPs. Many weave configurations are available, depending on the requirements of the laminate. Plain or twill weaves provide strength in both directions, while a unidirectionally stitched or knitted fabric provides strength primarily in one dimension. Many novel fabrics are currently available, including biaxial, double-bias, and triaxial weaves for special applications.

Fiberglass mats may be produced as either continuous- or chopped-strand mats. A chopped-strand mat is formed by randomly depositing chopped fibers onto a belt or chain and binding them with a chemical binder, usually a thermoplastic resin with a styrene solubility ranging from low to high, depending on the application. For example, hand lay-up processes used to moderate corrosion-resistant liners or boat hulls require high solubility, whereas closed-mold processes such as cold press or compression molding require low solubility to prevent washing in the mold during curing.

Table 3 Filament diameter nomenclature

Alphabet	Filament diameter, μm	Filament diameter, 10^{-4} in.
AA	0.8–1.2	0.3–0.5
A	1.2–2.5	0.5–1.0
B	2.5–3.8	1.0–1.5
C	3.8–5.0	1.5–2.0
D	5.0–6.4	2.0–2.5
E	6.4–7.6	2.5–3.0
F	7.6–9.0	3.0–3.5
G	9.0–10.2	3.5–4.0
H	10.2–11.4	4.0–4.5
J	11.4–12.7	4.5–5.0
K	12.7–14.0	5.0–5.5
L	14.0–15.2	5.5–6.0
M	15.2–16.5	6.0–6.5
N	16.5 17.8	6.5 7.0
P	17.8–19.0	7.0–7.5
Q	19.0–20.3	7.5–8.0
R	20.3–21.6	8.0–8.5
S	21.6–22.9	8.5–9.0
T	22.9–24.1	9.0–9.5
U	24.1–25.4	9.5–10

Continuous-strand mat is formed in a similar manner but without chopping, and, usually, less binder is required because of increased mechanical entanglement, which provides some inherent integrity. Continuous-strand mat may be used in closed mold processes and as a supplemental product in unidirectional processes such as pultrusion, where some transverse strength is required. A number of specialty mats are also produced. Surfacing veil made with C-glass is used to make corrosion-resistant liners for pipes and tanks. Surfacing veils made from other glass compositions are used to provide a smooth finished surface in some applications. Glass tissue is used in some vinyl flooring products.

Combinations of a mat and woven roving have been developed for specific products in recent years. In many lay-up processes the laminate is constructed from alternate layers of fiberglass mat and woven roving. Fiberglass producers thus began to provide products that make this process more efficient. The appropriate weights of fiberglass mat (usually chopped-strand mat) and woven roving are either bound together with a chemical binder or mechanically knit or stitched together. This product can then be used as a significant labor saver by the fabricators.

Chopped strand products are produced by two major processes. In the first process, dried forming packages are used as a glass source. A number of strand ends are fed into a chopper, which chops them into the correct length, typically 3.2 to 12.7 mm ($\frac{1}{8}$ to $\frac{1}{2}$ in.). The product is then screened to remove fuzz and contamination and boxed for shipment (Fig. 5). The second process, used in recent years to produce many chopped-strand products, is the direct-chop process. In this process, large bushings are used in forming, and the strands are chopped in a wet state directly after sizing is applied. The wet, chopped strands are then transported to an area where they are dried, screened, and packaged. The direct-chop process has provided the industry with a wide variety of chopped reinforcements for compounding with resins.

Chopped glass is widely used as a reinforcement in the injection molding industry. The glass and resin may be dry blended or extrusion compounded in a preliminary step before molding, or the glass may be fed directly into the molding machine with the plastic resin. Hundreds of different parts for many applications are made in this manner. Chopped glass may also be used as a reinforcement in some thermosetting applications, such as bulk molding compounds.

Milled fibers are prepared by hammer milling chopped or sawed continuous strand glass fibers, followed by chemically sizing for some specific applications and by screening to length. Fiber lengths typically vary from particulates to screen opening dimensions for the reported nominal length (0.79 to 6.4 mm, or $\frac{1}{32}$ to $\frac{1}{4}$ in.). As such, milled fibers have a relatively low aspect ratio (length to diameter). They provide some increased stiffness and dimensional stability to plastics but minimal strength. Their use is primarily in phenolics, reaction-injection molded urethanes, fluorocarbons, and potting compounds.

Fiberglass paper is the reinforcing element for fiberglass roofing shingles. Chopped strands of 25 to 50 mm (1 to 2 in.) length are usually used in making fiberglass paper or a thin fiberglass mat. In this process, chopped fibers are dispersed in water to form a dilute solution. The fiberglass strands filamentize during the mixing and dispersion process. The solution is pumped onto a continuously moving chain, where most of the water is removed by vacuum, leaving behind a uniformly distributed, thin fiberglass mat. A binding resin is added on-line, followed by drying and curing, to form the fiberglass paper. This paper is then combined with the appropriate resin system to form roofing shingles.

Textile yarns are fine-fiber strands of yarn from the forming operation that are air dried on the forming tubes to provide sufficient integrity to undergo a twisting operation. Twist provides additional integrity to yarn before it is subjected to the weaving process, a typical twist consisting

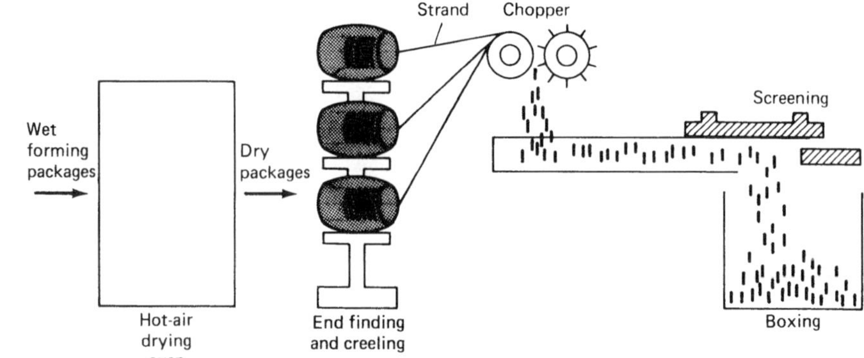

Fig. 5 Chopped-strand production

of up to one turn per inch. The twisting operation is shown in Fig 6. In many instances, heavier yarns are needed for the weaving operation. This is normally accomplished by twisting together two or more single strands, followed by a plying operation. Plying essentially involves retwisting the twisted strands in the opposite direction from the original twist. The two types of twist normally used are known as S and Z, which indicate the direction in which the twisting is done. Usually, two or more strands twisted together with an S twist are plied with a Z twist in order to give a balanced yarn. Thus, the yarn properties, such as strength, bundle diameter, and yield, can be manipulated by the twisting and plying operations.

The yarn nomenclature for fiberglass yarns consists of both letters of the alphabet and numbers. For instance, in ECG 75 2/4:

- The first letter specifies the glass composition, in this case, E-glass.
- The second letter specifies the filament type (staple, continuous, texturized) (in the case, of ECG 75 2/4, continuous).
- The third letter specifies the filament diameter (in this case, G).
- The next series of numbers represents the basic strand yield in terms of $\frac{1}{100}$ th of the yield (in this case, 75 means 7500 yd/lb).
- The fraction represents the number of strands twisted together (numerator) to form a single end and the number of such ends plied together (denominator) to form the final yarn. In the above case, 2/4 means two basic strands are twisted together to form a single end, and four such ends are plied together (usually in the opposite direction) to form the final yarn.

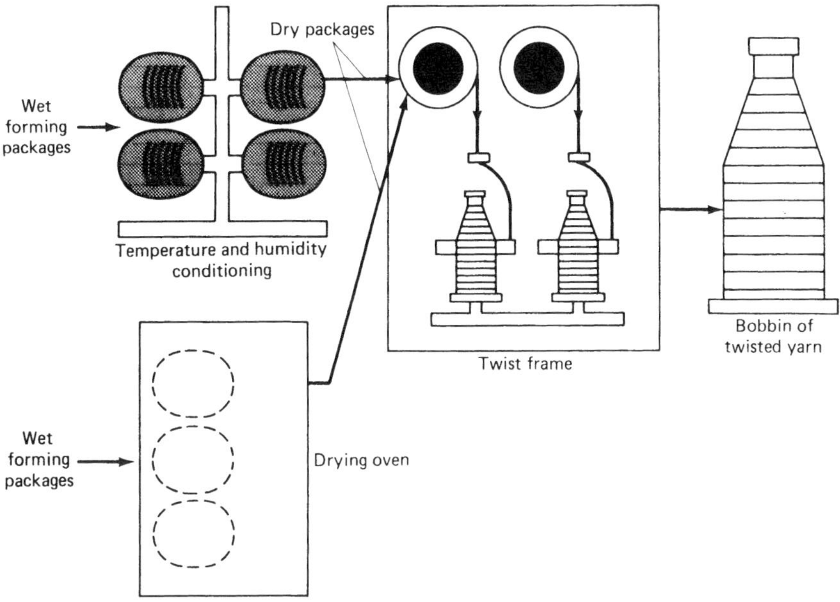

Fig. 6 Twisting

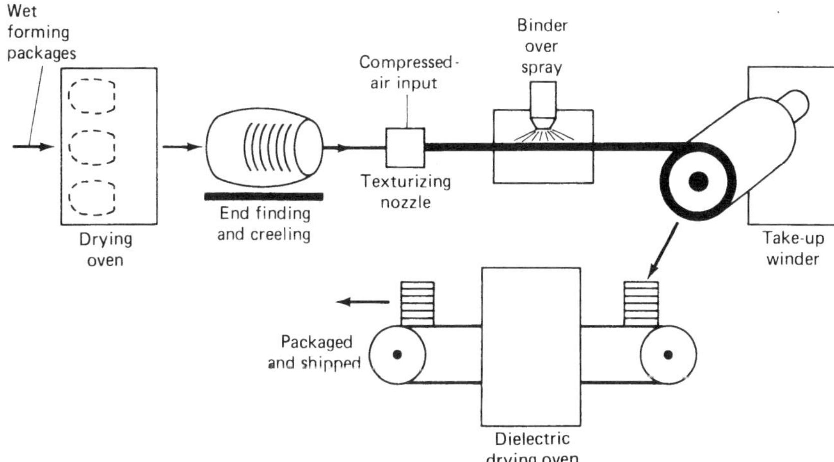

Fig. 7 Texturizing

The product brochures from various weavers as well as to Ref 4 should be consulted for details on commercially available fabrics. The *Glass-Fibre Dictionary and Databook* (Ref 14) should be consulted for even greater detail and/or for a summary of all commercially available yarns.

Fiberglass Fabric. Fiberglass yarns are converted to fabric form by conventional weaving operations. Looms of various kinds are used in the industry, but the air jet loom is the most popular. The major characteristics of a fabric include its style or weave pattern, fabric count, and the construction of warp yarn and fill yarn. Together, these characteristics determine fabric properties such as drapability and performance in the final composite. The fabric count identifies the number of warp and fill yarns per inch. Warp yarns run parallel to the machine direction, and fill yarns are perpendicular.

There are basically four weave patterns: plain, basket, twill, and satin. Plain weave is the simplest form, in which one warp yarn interlaces over and under one fill yarn. Basket weave has two or more warp yarns interlacing over and under two or more fill yarns. Twill weave has one or more warp yarns floating over at least two fill yarns. Satin weave (crowfoot) consists of one warp yarn interfacing over three and under one fill yarn to give an irregular pattern in the fabric. The eight-harness satin weave is a special case, in which one warp yarn interlaces over seven and under one fill yarn to give an irregular pattern. In fabricating a composite part, the satin weave gives the best conformity to complex contours, followed in descending order by twill, basket, and plain weaves.

Texturized Yarn. Texturizing is a process in which the textile yarn is subjected to an air jet that impinges on its surface to make the yarn "fluffy" (Fig. 7). The air jet causes the surface filaments to break at random, giving the yarn a bulkier appearance. The extent to which this occurs can be controlled by the velocity of the air jet and the yarn feed rate. The texturizing process allows the resin-to-glass ratio to be increased in the final composite. One of the major applications of texturized yarns is as an asbestos replacement.

Carded Glass Fibers. Carding is a process that makes a staple fiberglass yarn from continuous yarn. The continuous yarn is chopped into 38 to 50 mm (1.5 to 2.0 in.) lengths, and then aligned in one direction in a mat form. It is finally converted to a staple yarn. The yarn produced by this process can absorb much more resin than texturized yarn. Carded glass fibers are also used as an asbestos replacement in friction applications, such as automotive brake linings.

REFERENCES

1. K.L. Loewenstein, *The Manufacturing Technology of Continuous Glass Fibers*, 3rd revised ed., Elsevier, 1993
2. F.T. Wallenberger, Structural Silicate and Silica Glass Fibers, in *Advanced Inorganic*

Fibers Processes, Structures, Properties, Applications, F.T. Wallenberger, Ed., Kluwer Academic Publishers, 1999, p 129–168
3. F.T. Wallenberger, Melt Viscosity and Modulus of Bulk Glasses and Fibers: Challenges for the Next Decade, in *Present State and Future Prospects of Glass Science and Technology*, Proc. of the Norbert Kreidl Symposium (Triesenberg, Liechtenstein), 1994, p 63–78
4. D.M. Miller, Glass Fibers, *Composites*, Vol 1, *Engineered Materials Handbook*, ASM International, 1987, p 45–48
5. "Standard Specification for Glass Fiber Strands", D 578-98, *Annual Book of ASTM Standards*, ASTM
6. P.K. Gupta, Glass Fibers for Composite Materials, *Fibre Reinforcements for Composite Materials*, A.R. Bunsell, Ed., Elsevier Publishers, 1988, p 19–72
7. J.F. Sproull, Fiber Glass Composition, U.S. Patent 4,542,106, 17 Sept 1985
8. W.L. Eastes, D.A. Hofman, and J.W. Wingert, Boron-Free Glass Fibers, U.S. Patent 5,789,329, 4 Aug 1998
9. "Advantex Glass Fiber, A New Era in Composites Technology—Systems Thinking", Product Bulletin, Owens Corning, 1998
10. F. Rossi and G. Williams, A New Era in Glass Fiber Composites, Proc., 28th AVK Conf. (Baden-Baden, Germany), 1-2 Oct 1997, p 1–10
11. O.V. Mazurin, M.V. Streltsina and T.P. Shvaiko-Shvaikovskaya, Viscosity of Silica, *Handbook of Glass Data*, Part A, Elsevier, 1983, p 75
12. P.F. Aubourg and W.W. Wolf, "Glass Fibers-Glass Composition Research," presented at Glass Division Meeting (Grossinger, NY), American Ceramic Society, Oct 1984
13. J.C. Watson and N. Raghupathi, Glass Fibers, in *Composites*, Vol 1, *Engineered Materials Handbook*, ASM International, 1987, p 107–111
14. T.F. Starr, *Glass-Fibre Dictionary and Databook*, 2nd ed., Chapman & Hall, 1997
15. W.W. Wolf and S.L. Mikesell, Glass Fibers, *Encyclopedia of Materials Science and Engineering*, 1st Edition, 1986
16. F.T. Starr, *Carbon and High Performance Fibres, Directory and Databook*, ed. 6, Chapman & Hall, 1995
17. "Standard Test Method for Density of Glass by Buoyancy," C 693, *Annual Book of ASTM Standards*, ASTM
18. "Standard Test Methods for A-C Loss Characteristics and Permittivity (Dielectric Constant) of Solid Electrical Insulating Materials," D 150, *Annual Book of ASTM Standards*, ASTM
19. "Standard Test Methods for D-C Resistance or Conductance of Insulating Materials," D 257, *Annual Book of ASTM Standards*, ASTM
20. "Standard Test Method for Dielectric Breakdown Voltage and Dielectric Strength of Solid Electrical Insulating Materials at Commercial Power Frequencies," D 149, *Annual Book of ASTM Standards*, ASTM
21. "Standard Test Method for Softening Point of Glass," C 338, *Annual Book of ASTM Standards*, ASTM
22. "Standard Test Method for Annealing Point and Strain Point of Glass by Fiber Elongation," C 336, *Annual Book of ASTM Standards*, ASTM
23. "Standard Test Method for Annealing Point and Strain Point of Glass by Beam Bending," C 598, *Annual Book of ASTM Standards*, ASTM
24. "Standard Practice for Measuring Viscosity of Glass Above the Softening Point," C965, *Annual Book of ASTM Standards*, ASTM
25. "Standard Practices for Measurement of Liquidus Temperature of Glass by the Gradient Furnace Method," C829, *Annual Book of ASTM Standards*, ASTM
26. "Standard Test Method for Coefficient of Linear Thermal Expansion of Plastics," D 696, *Annual Book of ASTM Standards*, ASTM
27. J.F. Dockum, Jr., Fiberglass, in *Handbook of Reinforcement for Plastics*, J.V. Milewski and H.S. Katz, Ed., Van Nostrand Reinhold Company, New York, 1987, p 233–286
28. R.A. Schoenlaub, "Glass Compositions," U.S. Patent 2,334,961, 5 Dec, 1940
29. R.L. Tiede and F.V. Tooley, "Glass Composition," U.S. Patent 2,571,074, 23 Nov, 1948
30. L.L. Clements, Composite Radomes Protect and Perform, *High Performance Composite*, September/October 2000, p 44–47

Carbon Fibers

Paul J. Walsh, Zoltek Corporation

CARBON FIBERS, after a 40 year period of development and use in specialized applications, are now on the brink of broad commercialization. Their use is growing rapidly, fueled by significant price reductions during the 1990s and increasing availability. Changes in the performance/price ratio have resulted in the increased penetration of composites into applications formerly held by metals and has enabled their use in other applications previously not possible with existing materials. Additionally, market conditions increasingly favor designs for commercial products that are lighter, stronger, faster, and more fuel efficient—designs that are possible with carbon fibers. No longer relegated to aerospace, carbon fiber composites are now being adopted in fields such as automotive, civil infrastructure, offshore oil, and paper production.

History

The earliest commercial use of carbon fibers is often attributed to Thomas Edison's carbonization of cotton and bamboo fibers for incandescent lamp filaments (Ref 1). However, practical commercial use of carbon fibers for reinforcement applications began in the late 1950s with the pursuit of improved ablative materials for rockets (Ref 2). Union Carbide marketed a carbonized rayon based fabric in the early 1960s (Ref 3). DuPont's work with "black Orlon" in the late 1950s showed that acrylics could be thermally stabilized, while Shindo in Japan and Watt et al. in the United Kingdom demonstrated that, by using tension through the carbonization process, high mechanical properties could be realized (Ref 4).

Activity increased rapidly during the 1960s and 1970s to improve the performance/price ratio of carbon fibers. Much of this effort focused on evaluation of various precursors, since carbon fiber can be made from almost anything that yields a quality char upon pyrolysis. Donnet and Bansal (Ref 5) present a good overview of various researchers' efforts to evaluate different precursors, including PAN (polyacrylonitrile), pitch, rayon, phenol, lignin, imides, amides, vinyl polymers, and various naturally occurring cellulosic materials.

Overall carbon fiber demand grew to approximately 1000 metric tons by 1980, fueled primarily by the aerospace industry, with the sporting goods industry taking some excess capacity and off-specification fiber. Polyacrylonitrile-based carbon fiber usage had exceeded all other precursors at that time. This was a surprise to some, since the anticipation in the late 1970s had been that the significantly lower raw material price and higher char yield of pitch would result in the winning combination. However, higher processing costs are required to make a spinnable pitch, so better overall properties for PAN fibers resulted in their dominance. Rayon was relegated to third place, despite having a lower raw material cost, because inferior properties and a low char yield (20 to 25%) after carbonization made for a higher overall cost. Properties can be improved by stress graphitization at high temperatures, but this increases cost further, making the fiber even less desirable. Rayon is still used today for insulating and ablative applications but not for structural applications.

By the mid-1990s, a new cost-effective, PAN-based carbon fiber made from a modified textile precursor was being aggressively promoted by companies like Zoltek and Fortafil for commercial applications. In 1995, one manufacturer announced the goal of reaching a price level of $5/lb ($11/kg) by the year 2000, which brought alot of attention to and greatly accelerated application development (Ref 6). An overall trend of improved performance/price ratio for both pitch and PAN fiber manufacturers has sustained this growth.

Carbon fiber demand has grown to an estimated 16×10^6 kg (35×10^6 lb) per year (Ref 7). Usage in 1997 was estimated at 30% aerospace, 30% sporting goods, and 30% commercial/industrial applications, with the industrial applications poised for the greatest growth (Ref 8).

Manufacture of Carbon Fibers

Precursor sources used, in order of volume, are PAN, pitch, and rayon. Although the specific processing details for each precursor is different, all follow a basic sequence involving spinning, stabilization, carbonization, and application of a finish or sizing to facilitate handling, as shown in Fig. 1. Discontinuous carbon fiber whiskers are also now produced in a batch process from

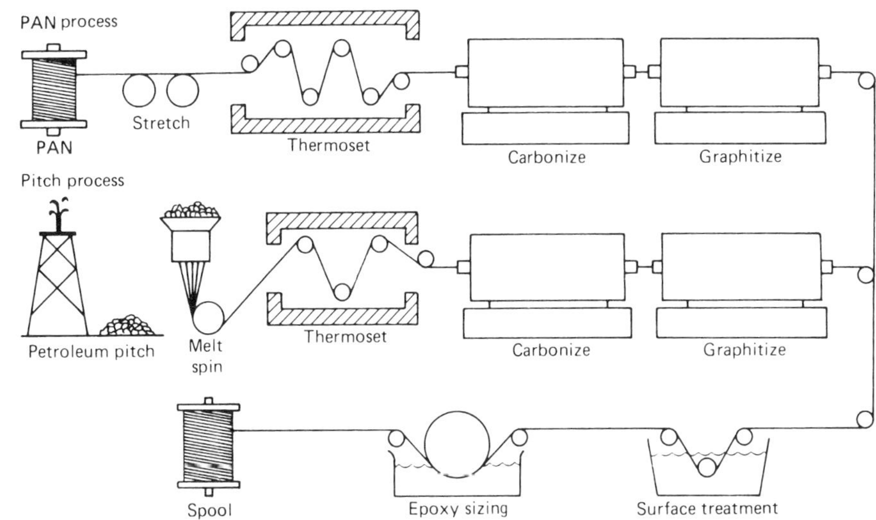

Fig. 1 The processing sequence for polyacrylonitrile (PAN) and mesophase-pitch-based precursor fibers shows the similarities for the two processes. Highly oriented polymer chains are obtained in PAN by hot stretching, while high orientation in pitch is a natural consequence of the mesophase (liquid crystalline) order.

hydrocarbon gases using a vapor-liquid-solid growth mechanism.

PAN-based Carbon Fibers. The majority of all carbon fibers used today are made from PAN precursor, which is a form of acrylic fiber. Precursor manufacture is accomplished by spinning the PAN polymer into filaments using variants of standard textile fiber manufacturing processes. The PAN fibers are white in color, with a density of approximately 1.17 g/cm^3 (0.042 lb/in^3) and a molecular structure comprised of oriented, long chain molecules. Stabilization involves stretching and heating the PAN fibers to approximately 200 to 300 °C (390 to 570 °F) in an oxygen-containing atmosphere to further orient and then crosslink the molecules, such that they can survive higher-temperature pyrolysis without decomposing. Stretching after spinning and during stabilization helps develop the highly oriented molecular structure that allows development of a high tensile modulus and improved tensile strength upon subsequent heat treatment.

Carbonization of standard and intermediate modulus fiber typically involves pyrolyzing the fibers to temperatures ranging from 1000 to 1500 °C (1800 to 2700 °F) in an inert atmosphere, typically to a 95% carbon content. An additional high heat treatment step is included just after carbonization for some very high-modulus fibers. During carbonization, the fibers shrink in diameter and lose approximately 50% in weight. Restraint on longitudinal shrinkage helps develop additional molecular orientation, further increasing mechanical properties.

After carbonization, the fibers may be run through a surface treatment step designed to clean and attach functional groups to the fiber surface, which increases bond strength with matrix resins. Most manufacturers use an electrolytic oxidation process that creates carboxyl, carbonyl, and hydroxyl groups on the surface for enhanced bonding. A sizing or finish is then applied to minimize handling damage during spooling and enhance bonding with matrix resins. The fiber is then spooled.

Today, there is differentiation among manufacturers between those who use a modified textile-type PAN precursor and those who use an aerospace-type precursor. The textile-type precursor is made on a very large scale in modified-acrylic textile fiber plants in tows or rovings consisting of >200,000 filaments. The tows are then split down into smaller bundles (approximately 48,000 filaments) after carbonization for spooling. Aerospace precursor is made in smaller specialty plants and processed in 3000 (3K) to 12K filament tows that can be assembled into 24K or larger tows after carbonization. Manufacturing cost is lower for the textile-type precursor, due to higher line throughputs, larger economies-of-scale, and less handling of smaller tow bundles. This type fiber is more targeted for industrial applications. The aerospace-type precursor, because it is processed in smaller tow sizes, is less fuzzy and available in the small tow sizes favored by the aerospace industry, for whom it was originally developed. Physical properties can be similar for both types.

Pitch-Based Fibers. Pitch is a complex mixture of aromatic hydrocarbons and can be made from petroleum, coal tar, asphalt, or PVC (Ref 9). Starting raw material selection is important to the final fiber properties. Pitches must be processed through a pre-treatment step to obtain the desired viscosity and molecular weight in preparation for making high-performance carbon fibers. The pre-processed pitch contains "mesophase", a term for a disk-like liquid crystal phase (Ref 10) that develops regions of long-term ordered molecules favorable to manufacture of high-performance fibers. Without this step, the result is an isotropic carbon fiber with low strength and low modulus of less than 50 GPa (7×10^6 psi) (Ref 11). Process details of the final composition and method of spinning mesophase pitch are generally held secret by the manufacturers.

Once spun, the stabilization, carbonization, surface treatment, application of sizing, and spooling of pitch-based fibers follows a sequence similar to the manufacture of PAN-based fibers, as shown in Fig. 1. Actual process parameters, such as temperatures, ramp rates, and time at temperature for stretch and stabilization, are different for pitch than for PAN. Gas species evolved during pyrolysis and their onset of evolution are very different for PAN and pitch. The response to heat treatment is also greater for mesophase-pitch-based fibers at higher temperatures, a consequence of their more ordered starting molecular structure. For example, a mesophase-pitch-derived fiber processed to the same temperature as a PAN fiber will exhibit higher density and thermal and electrical conductivity, all else being equal.

Other Precursors. Rayon is processed in similar fashion to PAN, as shown in Fig. 1; the difference is the actual process parameters used.

Carbon fiber "whiskers" can be formed from gas-phase pyrolysis via catalyzed cracking of hydrocarbon gases like methane. One process involves growth of a thin carbon tube of 10 to 50 nm from a submicron iron particle in a hydrocarbon-rich atmosphere, followed by a secondary process of thickening the tube by chemical vapor deposition of carbon on the surface (Ref 12). Others have discussed similar processes, some capable of longer length fibers (Ref 13). Although only discontinuous fibers are fabricated, they have unique properties approaching those of single crystal graphite in some cases.

Available Formats for Fibers. Commercially available carbon fibers are produced by a multitude of manufacturers with a wide range of properties and tow sizes. Carbon fibers are available in many of the same formats as glass fiber. These formats include continuous filament-spooled fiber, milled fiber, chopped fiber, woven fabrics, felts, veils, and chopped fiber mattes. Most fiber today is spooled, and then processed into other formats in secondary operations. The size of the carbon fiber tow bundle can range from 1000 filaments (1K) to more than 200K. Generally, aerospace carbon fibers are available in bundles of 3K, 6K, 12K, and 24K filaments, while most commercial-grade fibers are available in 48K or larger filament counts. Composite fabrication equipment, such as filament winders and weaving machines, must be adapted to handle the larger cross section of commercial grade fiber.

Properties and Characteristics of Carbon Fibers

Composites made from carbon fiber are five times stronger than grade 1020 steel for structural parts, yet are still five times lighter. In comparison to 6061 aluminum, carbon fiber composites are seven times stronger and two times stiffer, yet 1.5 times lighter. Carbon fiber composites have fatigue properties superior to all known metals, and, when coupled with the proper resins, carbon fiber composites are one of the most corrosion resistant materials available. Certain mesophase-pitch-based carbon fibers possess thermal conductivity three times greater than copper. The electrical conductivity of PAN and pitch-based carbon fibers is used to dissipate static electricity in a wide variety of computer-related products. They do not melt or soften with heat, allowing them to be used in such high temperature applications as rocket nozzles and aircraft brakes. In fact, their strength actually increases with temperature in non-oxidizing atmospheres. These unique properties are the result of the fiber microstructure, in both the axial and transverse directions.

Axial Structure. Envision a single carbon filament as a long cylinder with a diameter of approximately 7 μm. Packed within this cylinder are tiny undulating ribbon-like crystallites which are intertwined and oriented more or less parallel to the axis of the cylinder (Ref 14–16). The length and straightness of these crystallite "ribbons" determines the modulus of the fiber. A model of the axial structure of a PAN-based carbon fiber is shown in Fig. 2.

On a finer scale, each ribbon-like crystallite is comprised of multiple wrinkled layers. Each layer is made of carbon atoms arranged like chicken wire in a hexagonal structure characteristic of graphite, called a graphene plane. Strong covalent C-C bonds within the layer plane give the potential for high strength and stiffness. Weak van der Waals bonding between the layer planes gives rise to poor shear resistance, but also allows thermal and electrical conductivity. Loose electrons and thermal energy in the form of phonons take advantage of the weak bonding between layer planes and use the inter-plane space as a corridor to travel. The width of the ribbons, the number of graphene layers comprising their thickness, and the length of the ribbons help determine the electrical and thermal characteristics of the carbon fiber, as well as contribute to fiber modulus. Typically, larger and more oriented graphene planes result in higher thermal and electrical conductivity.

Improving the orientation of the microstructure can also increase filament tensile modulus, thermal conductivity, electrical conductivity, and density. This can be accomplished by plastic deformation (for example, stretching the fiber) and/or heat treatment. Figure 3 shows x-ray diffraction results relating heat treatment temperature to the degree of preferred orientation of the microstructure (Ref 17, 18). The degree of preferred orientation represents the average angle at which the crystallites lie relative to the fiber axis; a zero degree angle means that the crystallites are perfectly aligned with the fiber axis. Transmission electron microscopy shows that the ribbons undulate, such that their amplitude is greater than their wavelength. Any reported measurement of preferred orientation is therefore only an average. The data clearly shows improved orientation with increasing heat treatment temperature. Figure 3 also shows that for heat treatment temperatures above 1600 °C (2900 °F) the mesophase pitch-based fiber will orient more than the PAN fiber, a result of larger crystallite sizes that PAN precursors are not able to achieve. The relationship between preferred orientation of the microstructure and modulus is illustrated in Fig. 4. Increased orientation results in increased fiber modulus, as expected.

Increases in fiber tensile modulus can also be obtained by stretching the fiber during stabilization and carbonization. In this case, mechanical rather than thermal energy provides the impetus for molecular realignment.

Transverse Structure. While axial orientation determines modulus, fiber strength is determined by the number and size of flaws and by the transverse and axial orientation. A variety of transverse textures are possible (Ref 19), including a common one described as "onion skin". In this structure, the graphene layer planes at the fiber surface align like the layers of an onion. In the center core region of the fiber, the layers are randomly oriented. Most of the microstructural pores and flaws are found in either the transition from the skin to the random core region, or in the core region; flaws resulting from damage induced during precursor or carbon fiber processing are observed on the surface. Some pitch fibers have very large graphene layers in a flat orientation reminiscent of the old Pan-Am Airlines insignia. Some of the ultra-high modulus fibers >900 GPa (130 $\times 10^6$ psi) have a radial structure like the spokes of a wheel.

Unlike the axial structure, the radial structure of the carbon filament depends upon precursor type and processing (Ref 20–24).

Flaw size and flaw density reduce the strength of a carbon fiber. However, because the fiber is bundled with thousands or millions of other fibers in a composite, the strength is an average effect. Fiber manufacturers control the strength of the overall fiber bundle through rigorous process control.

Effect of Structure on Properties. Fibers made from PAN precursors generally exhibit higher tensile and compressive strength, higher strain at failure, and lower modulus as compared to mesophase-pitch-based fibers. The structure of PAN-based carbon fibers leads to a good balance in properties and is responsible for their dominance in structural applications. Relatively good layer alignment and small crystallite stack heights minimize interlayer shear failure, which improves compressive strengths while maintaining good tensile strength (Ref 25). A model of a 400 GPa (58 $\times$ 10^6 psi) PAN-based carbon fiber is shown in Fig. 5 (Ref 26).

PAN fibers used to be categorized into standard modulus, intermediate, and high modulus. New offerings by fiber producers have blurred these categories somewhat. The differences between the three categories for fibers made from a particular precursor are due to combinations of mechanical stretching, heat treatment, and/or precursor spinning. Distinctions are also made between aerospace and commercial-grade carbon fibers. The difference relates to the type of precursor used; commercial grades use a lower cost, modified textile-type PAN. Polyacrylonitrile chemistry is similar between the two, and differences relate more to processing. Generalized properties for PAN-based fibers are presented in Table 1.

Larger crystallite size and greater orientation of mesophase-pitch-based fibers give them superior modulus, thermal conductivity, and lower thermal expansion characteristics as compared to PAN-based fibers. Satellite applications make extensive use of pitch-based fibers and take advantage of all three properties. Table 2 lists general properties of mesophase-pitch-based fibers.

One of the most beneficial properties of all carbon fibers is their superior fatigue resistance in composites. Unlike glass or aramid fibers, carbon fibers do not suffer from stress rupture, and demonstrate complete elastic recovery upon unloading (Ref 27–29). Creep is not observed in carbon fibers at temperatures below 2200 °C (3990 °F) (Ref 30).

The carbon content of low-modulus carbon fibers is less than 99%, largely because of retained nitrogen (Ref 31). Increasing carbon contents

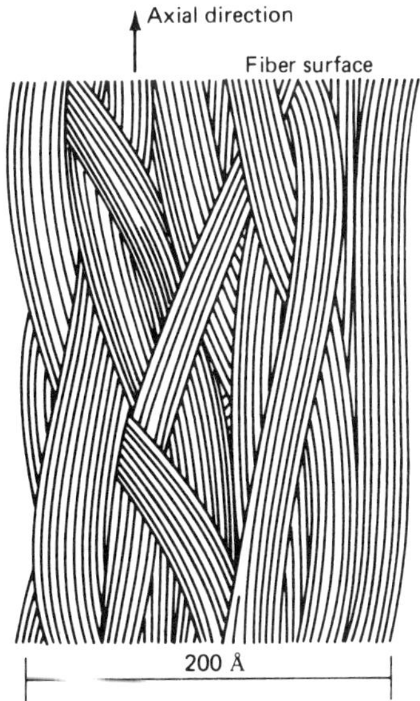

Fig. 2 The undulating ribbon structure of the graphene layers for a PAN-based carbon fiber with a 400 GPa (600 $\times$ 10^6 psi) modulus. The ribbons at the surface have lower amplitude than in the core. There are about 20 graphene layers in the ribbons in the core and about 30 near the surface.

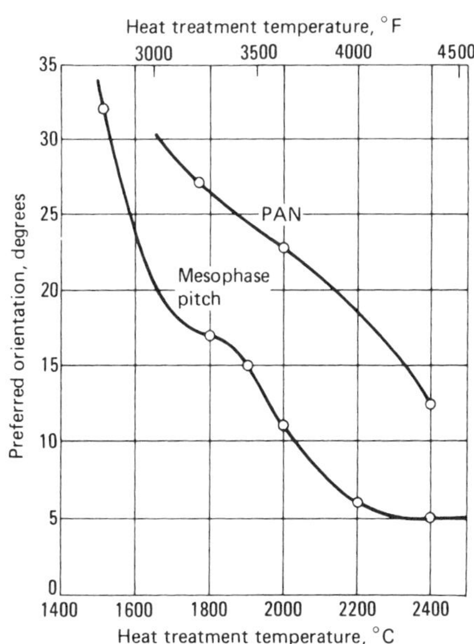

Fig. 3 The preferred orientation of the graphene planes is determined by the heat treatment temperature and the precursor type. Source: Ref 14, 18

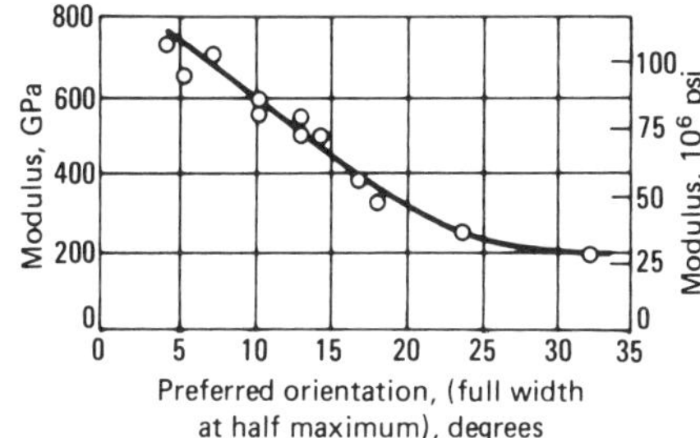

Fig. 4 The modulus of a carbon fiber is determined by the preferred orientation, microstructure, and elastic constants. The relationship between modulus and preferred orientation for a pitch-based carbon fiber is shown.

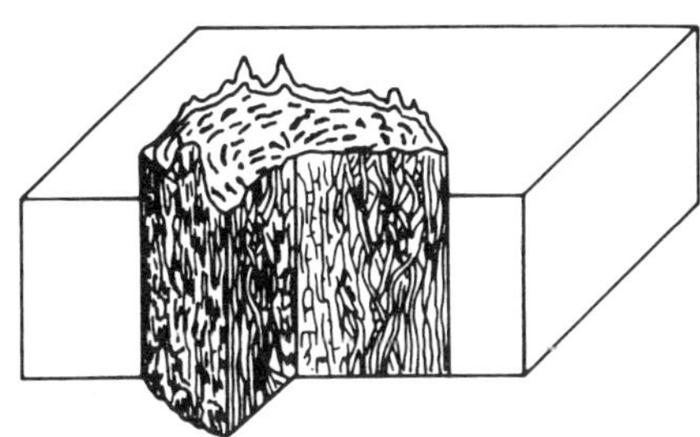

Fig. 5 A 400-GPa (60 $\times$ 10^6 psi) modulus PAN-based fiber. Source: Ref 26

Table 1 Properties of PAN-based carbon fibers

Property	Commercial, standard modulus	Aerospace		
		Standard modulus	Intermediate modulus	High modulus
Tensile modulus, GPa (10^6 psi)	228 (33)	220–241 (32–35)	290–297 (42–43)	345–448 (50–65)
Tensile strength, MPa (ksi)	380 (550)	3450–4830 (500–700)	3450–6200 (600–900)	3450–5520 (600–800)
Elongation at break, %	1.6	1.5–2.2	1.3–2.0	0.7–1.0
Electrical resistivity, μΩ · cm	1650	1650	1450	900
Thermal conductivity, W/m · K (Btu/ft · h · °F)	20 (11.6)	20 (11.6)	20 (11.6)	50–80 (29–46)
Coefficient of thermal expansion, axial direction, 10^{-6} K	–0.4	–0.4	–0.55	–0.75
Density, g/cm^3 (lb/in.^{3})	1.8 (0.065)	1.8 (0.065)	1.8 (0.065)	1.9 (0.069)
Carbon content, %	95	95	95	+99
Filament diameter, μm	6–8	6–8	5–6	5–8
Manufacturers	Zoltek, Fortafil, SGL	BPAmoco, Hexcel, Mitsubishi Rayon, Toho, Toray, Tenax, Soficar, Formosa		

and densities are achieved through higher heat treatment temperature, which removes nitrogen and provides greater crystalline perfection.

Electrical and thermal conductivity also increase with increasing crystalline perfection and purity (Ref 32). The electrical conductivity of carbon fibers must be taken into account when processing, since free-floating fibers can short out electrical equipment. Dust-proof, gasketed NEMA 12 enclosures (as specified by the National Electrical Manufacturers Association) are recommended for electrical cabinets, as are covers over electrical outlets (Ref 33).

Room temperature coefficients of thermal expansion (CTE) in the axial direction are slightly negative for low modulus carbon fibers, and grow increasingly negative for the higher modulus fibers. At temperatures above 700 °C (1290 °F), the axial CTE of all fibers turns positive (Ref 34). Composite designers are able to couple the negative CTE of high modulus fibers with appropriate matrix materials to make composites with a CTE of zero over limited temperature ranges.

Interfacial Bonding. Resins and molten metals do not easily wet carbon fibers, due to the relatively inert, non-polar fiber surface. Glass fibers depend upon coupling agents to chemically bond with resins; carbon fibers never achieve strong bonds. Instead, carbon fiber depends upon a combination of mechanical and weak chemical bonding with the matrix material. Surface treatments used by carbon fiber manufacturers populate the fiber surface with active chemical groups such as hydroxyls, carboxyls, and carbonyls (Ref 35). These form bridges between the fiber and resin, and depend upon the number of bonds rather than the strength of the bonds to achieve a strong interface.

Reactivity with Other Compounds. As an inorganic material, carbon fibers are not affected by moisture, atmosphere, solvents, bases, and weak acids at room temperature (Ref 36). However, oxidation becomes a problem at elevated temperatures. For low-modulus PAN-based fibers and high-modulus PAN- or pitch-based fibers, the threshold for oxidation for extended operating times is 350 °C (660 °F) or 450 °C (840 °F), respectively (Ref 37). Impurities tend to catalyze oxidation at these low temperatures and somewhat improved oxidation resistance can be expected with higher-purity fibers (Ref 38).

Typical Applications of Carbon Fibers

Carbon fiber usage is growing in a variety of applications, including aerospace, sporting goods, and a variety of commercial/industrial applications. Growth is fastest in the commercial/industrial applications. In many instances, carbon composites have displaced metal parts, despite being more expensive on a direct-replacement purchased cost basis. Where successful, carbon composites have lowered total system costs through reduced maintenance, faster processing speeds, and improved reliability. Many new uses under development are enabling, meaning applications that were not practical with metal or other materials are now possible with carbon composites.

Aerospace. Perhaps nowhere is the need to save weight greater than in the aerospace industry. Early growth of the carbon fiber industry was driven almost exclusively by the desire for higher performance aircraft made possible with carbon fiber composites. Today, carbon fiber is used on aircraft for primary and secondary structures. Use is growing, having already established a strong track record in primary structures on military aircraft. All of these applications use carbon fiber for its high specific strength and specific stiffness. Fiber formats used include prepreg for layup processes and fabrics for resin transfer molding and similar processes.

Satellites incorporate very high modulus pitch-based carbon fibers, partly for the high stiffness-to-weight ratios and partly for their negative axial coefficient of thermal expansion.

Sporting Goods. Golf club shafts are presently the largest sporting goods application for carbon fibers. Lighter weight and higher stiffness shafts, made possible with carbon fiber, allow club manufacturers to place more weight in the clubhead, which increases club head speed for improved distance. Most golf shaft manufacturing today is done with unidirectional prepregged sheets of carbon fiber in a roll wrapping operation. Some shafts are filament wound.

Carbon fiber fishing rods are favored by fisherman for their lightweight and sensitive touch. The rods are manufactured via a roll-wrapping process similar to golf shafts, using unidirectional prepreg. Most racquets for tennis, racquetball, and squash are made from prepregged carbon fiber that is sheeted, wrapped around a bladder, and cured. Carbon composite arrows are fabricated by either of two processes: pultrusion or roll wrapping. Skis and bicycle components tend to use fabrics made from carbon fiber.

Commercial and Industrial Applications. Large volumes of milled and chopped carbon fiber are used to impart static dissipating properties to trays for processing semiconductors, and for computer printer and copier machine parts. Parts are injection molded from thermoplastics that have been pre-blended with carbon fiber in a compounding extruder. The carbon fiber is used for its electrical conductivity and ability to

Table 2 Properties of mesophase pitch-based carbon fibers

Property	Low modulus	High modulus	Ultra-high modulus
Tensile modulus, GPa (10^6 psi)	170–241 (25–35)	380–620 (55–90)	690–965 (100–140)
Tensile strength, MPa (ksi)	1380–3100 (200–450)	1900–2750 (275–400)	2410 (350)
Elongation at break, %	0.9	0.5	0.4–0.27
Electrical resistivity, μΩ · cm	1300	900	220–130
Thermal conductivity, W/m · K (Btu/ft · h · °F)	. . .	. . .	400–1100 (230–635)
Coefficient of thermal expansion in axial direction, 10^{-6} K	. . .	–0.9	–1.6
Density, g/cm^3 (lb/in.^{3})	1.9 (0.069)	2.0 (0.072)	2.2 (0.079)
Carbon content, %	+97	+99	+99
Filament diameter, μm	11	11	10
Manufacturers	BPAmoco, Mitsubishi Kasei		BPAmoco

provide lightweight reinforcement to thermoplastics.

Carbon fiber drive shafts and couplings have replaced steel shafts for cooling towers and many other torque-transmitting applications. Properties that favor carbon composites include corrosion resistance, light weight, and high stiffness, which reduces vibration. Filament winding processes are used to fabricate the shafts and incorporate fiber into various angles tailored for the torque and vibrational characteristics required of the application.

The desire for faster processing in the papermaking and film casting industry has encouraged growth of carbon composite rollers, which spin faster and have less deflection than steel rollers. Roller diameters up to one meter are now routinely fabricated with carbon fibers on automated filament winding machines.

Speed and precision are also drivers for weaving machine components, such as rapiers, that are made from pultruded carbon composite shapes.

Injection of liquids into oil wells to stimulate production is currently being performed with spoolable carbon composite pipe. The pipe is made in a continuous process whereby a thermoplastic liner is pulled through multiple sets of rotating creels containing carbon fiber spools. The fiber is wetted with resin and wrapped onto the liner, which serves as the mandrel. The tube is cured in-line, and spooled at the other end. Although spoolable carbon composite pipe is more expensive than spoolable steel pipe, its usage is increasing because of superior fatigue performance, which results in improved reliability. Stress corrosion during unspooling and respooling is responsible for premature failure of steel spoolable pipe.

Depletion of shallow water oil fields and the move into deeper water has raised oil company interest in carbon composites. Development programs are underway to moor large oil platforms to the ocean bottom via tethers constructed from pultruded carbon fiber rods. Carbon fiber tethers are the leading contender for use in water depths beyond 1500 m (5000 ft); this shift is based on its lightweight and high stiffness, which minimize the natural frequency of the platform due to wave motion. Steel tethers used in shallower depths are impractical in deeper water, because they cannot support their own weight hanging from the platform.

Pultrusion companies that are eyeing the tether application are also pursuing carbon composite tendons for pre- and poststressing of precast concrete. Unlike glass fiber, carbon composite rods are inert to alkaline attack and corrosion and satisfy the increased useful life requirement imposed by many municipalities for infrastructure projects. Another pultrusion application, carbon composite rebar, is being developed for use along the waterfront to combat the high costs of corrosion induced structural damage.

Seismic retrofitting of bridge columns and walls has been extensively performed in Japan with sheets of carbon fiber "wallpaper" or fabrics that are saturated with resin and applied to the concrete structure. The high stiffness of the carbon minimizes movement of the concrete and the inertness to corrosion insures long term protection.

The electrical properties of carbon fiber and the ability to configure the material into a semipermeable membrane with defined mass transport properties make carbon the material of choice as the electrode in polymer electrolyte fuel cells to power next generation engines.

Anticipated Developments in Carbon Fibers

Much of the effort expended for carbon fibers today is directed at cost reduction. It appears that the prospects for cost reduction have stimulated interest in many new applications. Certainly, as prices come down, opportunities for new applications grow.

Future funding and technology development for carbon fibers will most likely be directed towards application development, a trend experienced in the glass fiber industry. Areas of opportunity include lowering cost and improving speed of manufacturing processes.

Education and familiarity with composite materials are increasing, but are still well below that of metals. We can expect the demand for carbon fibers to grow in large steps as more engineers learn how to design with carbon fibers.

Property standardization is another expected trend. Glass fiber is easy for a designer to design with, since E-glass and S-glass are standards by which many suppliers produce. Carbon fiber suppliers have many grades to choose from, with little commonality among producers. As large applications for carbon fiber develop, customers will demand standardization among carbon fiber producers.

REFERENCES

1. T. Edison, U.S. Patent 223,898, 1880
2. R. Bacon and M.M. Tang, Carbonization of Cellulose Fibers I, *Carbon*, Vol 2, 1964, p 211
3. R. Bacon and C.T. Moses, *High-Performance Polymers—Their Origin and Development*, R.B. Seymour and G.S. Kirshenbaum, Ed., Elseveir, 1986, p 341
4. W. Schimpf, Advanced Fiber Technologies, personal communication, 2000
5. J.B. Donnet and R.C. Bansal, *Carbon Fibers*, 2nd ed., Marcel Dekker, 1990
6. "Zoltek Corporation 1994 Annual Report," St. Louis, 1995
7. Zoltek Corporation, unpublished data, 2000
8. K. Shariq, E. Anderson, and M. Yamaki, "Carbon Fibers," Chemical Economics Handbook Market Research Report, SRI International, Menlo Park, CA, July 1999
9. J.B. Donnet and R.C. Bansal, *Carbon Fibers*, 2nd ed., Marcel Dekker, 1990, p 55
10. J.D. Brooks and G.H. Taylor, The Formation of Graphitizing Carbons from the Liquid Phase, *Carbon,* Vol 3, 1965, p 185–193
11. R.P. Krock, D. Carolos, and D.C. Boyer, Versatility of Short Pitch-Based Carbon Fibers in Cost Efficient Composites, *42nd Conf. of Composites Institute*, SPI, Feb 1987
12. A. Oberlin, M. Endo, and T. Koyama, Filamentous Growth of Carbon Through Benzene Decomposition, *J. Cryst. Growth*, Vol 32, 1976, p 335
13. G.G. Tibbetts, *Carbon Fiber Filaments and Composites*, J.L. Figueiredo et al. Ed., Kluwer Academic Publishers, 1990, p 73–94
14. G.D. D'Abate and R.J. Diefendorf, The Effect of Heat on the Structure and Properties of Mesophase Precursor Carbon Fibers, *Proc. of the 17th Biennial Conf. on Carbon*, American Carbon Society, 1985, p 390
15. R. Perret and W. Ruland, The Microstructure of PAN-Based Carbon Fibers, *J. Appl. Crystallogr.*, Vol 3, 1970, p 525
16. S.C. Bennett and D.J. Johnson, Structural Characterization of a High Modulus Carbon Fibre by High-Resolution Electron Microscopy and Electron Diffraction, *Carbon*, Vol 14, 1976, p 177
17. G.D. D'Abate and R.J. Diefendorf, The Effect of Heat on the Structure and Properties of Mesopause Precursor Carbon Fibers, *Proc. of the 17th Biennial Conf. on Carbon*, American Carbon Society, 1985
18. C.W. LeMaistre and R.J. Diefendorf, The Origin of Structure in Carbonized PAN Fibers, *SAMPE Q.*, Vol 4, 1973, p 1
19. D.D. Edie and E.G. Soner, *Carbon-Carbon Materials and Composites*, J.D. Buckley and D.D. Edie, Ed., Noyes Publications, 1993, p 50
20. C.W. LeMaistre and R.J. Diefendorf, The Origin of Structure in Carbonized PAN Fibers, *SAMPE Q.*, Vol 4, 1973
21. R.J. Diefendorf and E.W. Tokarsky, "The Relationships of Structure to Properties in Graphite Fibers, Part I," AFML-TR-72-133, Air Force Materials Laboratory, 1971
22. R.J. Diefendorf and E.W. Tokarsky, "The Relationships of Structure to Properties in Graphite Fibers, Part II," AFML-TR-72-133, Air Force Materials Laboratory, 1973
23. R.J. Diefendorf and E.W. Tokarsky, "The Relationships of Structure to Properties in Graphite Fibers, Part III," AFML-TR-72-133, Air Force Materials Laboratory, 1975
24. R.J. Diefendorf and E.W. Tokarsky, "The Relationships of Structure to Properties in Graphite Fibers, Part IV," AFML-TR-72-133, Air Force Materials Laboratory, 1975
25. L. Singer, "Overview of Carbon Fiber Technology," *Material Technology Center Newsletter*, Southern Illinois Univ. at Carbondale, Spring 1994
26. E.W. Tokarsky and R.J. Diefendorf, High Performance Carbon Fibers, *Polym. Eng. Sci.,* Vol 15 (No. 3), 1975, p 150
27. R.J. Diefendorf, Clemson University, unpublished data

28. J. Awerback and H.T. Hahn, "Fatigue and Proof Testing of Unidirectional Graphite/ Epoxy Composites," Fatigue of Filamentary Composite Materials, *STP 636, Am. Soc. for Testing and Materials*, 1977, p 248
29. T.T. Chiao, C.C. Chiao, and R.J. Sherry, Lifetimes of Fiber composites Under Sustained Tensile Loading, *Proceedings of the 1977 Int. Conf. on Fracture Mechanics and Technology*, 1977
30. L.A. Feldman, High Temperature Creep Effects in Carbon Yarns and Composites, *Proceedings of the 17th Biennial Conference on Carbon,* American Carbon Society, 1985, p 393
31. R.J. Diefendorf, Carbon/Graphite Fibers, *Composites*, Vol 1, Engineered Materials Handbook, ASM International, 1987, p 51
32. A.A. Bright and L.S. Singer, Electronic and Structural Characteristics of Carbon Fibers from Mesophase Pitch, *Proceedings of the 13th Biennial Conference on Carbon*, American Carbon Society, 1977, p 100
33. Zoltek Corporation, technical bulletin, St. Louis, MO, 1999
34. R. J. Diefendorf, Carbon/Graphite Fibers, Composites, Vol 1, Engineered Materials Handbook, ASM International, 1987, p 52
35. W. Schimpf, Advanced Fiber Technologies, person communication, 2000
36. N.C.W. Judd, The Chemical Resistance of Carbon Fibers and a Carbon Fibre/Polyester Composite, *Proceedings of the First Int. Conf. on Carbon Fibers*, Plastics Institute, 1971, p 258
37. D.W. McKee and V.J. Memeault, Surface Properties of Carbon Fibers, *Chemistry and Physics of Carbon*, Vol 17, Marcel Dekker, 1981, p 1
38. D.W. McKee and V.J. Memeault, Surface Properties of Carbon Fibers, *Chemistry and Physics of Carbon*, Vol 17, Marcel Dekker, 1981, p 1

Aramid Fibers

Karl K. Chang, E.I. Du Pont de Nemours & Company, Inc.

ARAMID FIBERS held the distinction of having the highest strength-to-weight ratio of any commercially available reinforcement fiber at the time of their first commercial introduction in the early 1970s. The earliest aramid fibers, produced by E.I. Du Pont de Nemours & Company, Inc., under the tradename of Kevlar, were initially targeted at reinforcement of tires and plastics. The characteristics of light weight, high strength, and high toughness have led to the development of applications in composites, ballistics, tires, ropes, cables, asbestos replacement, and protective apparel. Since those early days other para-aramid fibers have been developed, including Twaron by Accordis BV, Technora by Teijin, Ltd, and improved variations of Kevlar fibers.

H_2N–C₆H₄–NH_2 + Cl–C(=O)–C₆H₄–C(=O)–Cl →

Para-phenylene diamine | Terephthaloyl chloride

Poly para-phenyleneterephthalamide (PPD-T)

Fig. 1 Chemical structure of para-aramid

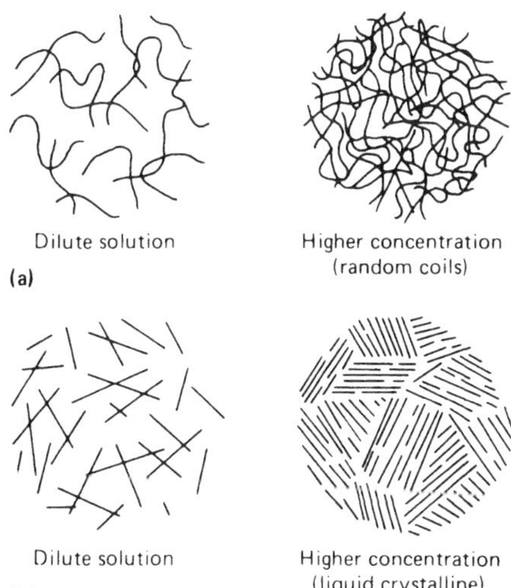

Fig. 2 Polymer states in solution. (a) Flexible molecules. (b) Rigid molecules

Fiber Manufacturing

The chemical composition of Kevlar aramid fiber is poly para-phenyleneterephthalamide. This fiber, also known as PPD-T, is made from the condensation reaction of paraphenylene diamine and terephthaloyl chloride (Fig. 1). The aromatic ring structure contributes high thermal stability, while the para configuration leads to stiff, rigid molecules that contribute high strength and high modulus.

Para-aramid fibers belong to a class of materials known as liquid crystalline polymers. Because these polymers are very rigid and rodlike, in solution they can aggregate to form ordered domains in parallel arrays (Ref 1). This is shown in Fig. 2 and contrasted to more conventional, flexible polymers, which in solution can bend and entangle, forming random coils.

When PPD-T solutions (in concentrated sulfuric acid solvent) are extruded through a spinneret and drawn through an air gap during fiber manufacture, the liquid crystalline domains can orient and align in the direction of flow (Ref 2–5), as shown in Fig. 3. With PPD-T, there is an exceptional degree of alignment of long, straight polymer chains parallel to the fiber axis. This structure, which has been analyzed and characterized extensively (Ref 6–9), is anisotropic and gives higher strength and modulus in the fiber longitudinal direction than in the radial direction. It is also fibrillar, as shown in Fig. 4, which has a profound effect on fiber properties and failure mechanisms. Subsequent high-temperature processing under tension can further increase the orientation of the crystalline structure and result in higher fiber modulus.

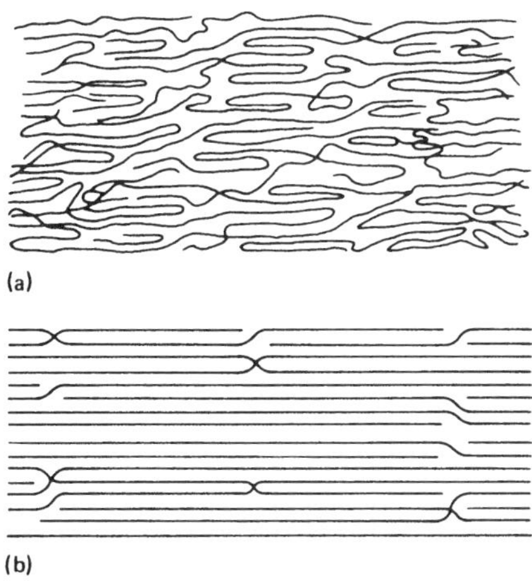

Fig. 3 Polymer chain orientation. (a) Conventional organic, characterized by chain folds, misalignment, and crystalline and amorphous regions. (b) Para-aramid, characterized by long, straight chains without folds, parallel to the fiber axis, crystalline

Fiber Forms and Applications

The major fiber forms are continuous filament yarns, rovings, and woven fabrics, and discontinuous staple and spun yarns, fabrics, and pulp.

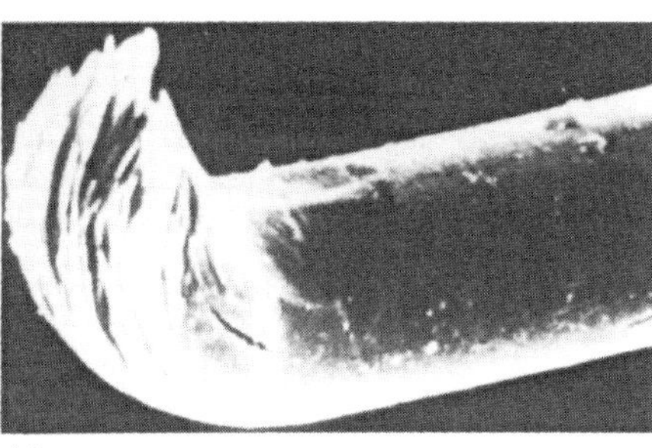

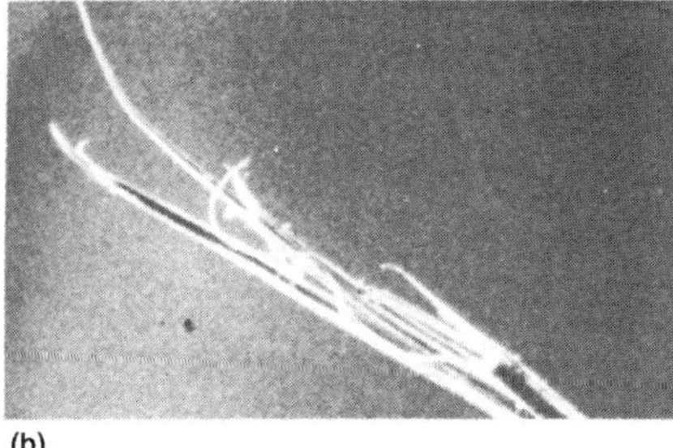

Fig. 4 Fibrillar structure of Kevlar aramid fibers. (a) Loop break. (b) Tensile failure

Table 1 Kevlar 49 yarn and roving sizes

Denier	Yield m/kg	Yield yd/lb	Number of filaments
55	163,636	81,175	25
195	46,155	22,895	134
380	23,684	11,749	267
720	12,500	6,200	490
1,140	7,895	3,916	768
1,420	6,388	3,144	1,000
1,860	4,877	2,400	1,000
2,160	4,225	2,097	1,000
2,450	3,673	1,822	1,333
2,840	3,169	1,572	1,333
4,560	1,973	980	3,072
5,680	1,585	786	2,666
7,100	1,268	630	5,000
8,520	1,056	524	3,999

Aramid is also available as textured yarn, needle-punched felts, spunlaced sheets, and wet-laid papers.

Yarns and Rovings. Kevlar 49 is a high-modulus aramid fiber that is available in 11 yarn sizes and four roving sizes, as shown in Table 1. Yarns are multifilament products that are spun directly during fiber manufacture and range from a very fine, 25-filament yarn to 1333-filament yarns. Rovings are produced by combining ends of yarns in a process similar to that used to produce glass fibers. For example, four ends of 1140-denier yarn are combined to make 4560-denier roving. Denier, a textile unit of linear density, is the weight in grams of 9000 m of yarn or roving (1 denier = 1.111×10^{-7} kg/m). Table 2 lists the yarn and roving sizes of Kevlar 29, which has a lower tensile modulus than Kevlar 49 and is used extensively in ballistic armor, asbestos replacement, and certain composites when greater damage tolerance is desired. Kevlar 149, with a tensile modulus 25 to 40% higher than Kevlar 49, is available as 1420-denier yarn.

Because aramid yarns and rovings are relatively flexible and nonbrittle, they can be processed in most conventional textile operations, such as twisting, weaving, knitting, carding, and felting. Yarns and rovings are used in the filament winding, prepreg tape, and pultrusion processes. Applications include missile cases, pressure vessels, sporting goods, cables, and tension members.

Table 2 Kevlar 29 yarn and roving sizes

Denier	Yield m/kg	Yield yd/lb	Number of filaments
200	45,000	22,320	134
400	22,500	11,160	267
600	15,000	7,440	400
720	12,500	6,200	500
840	10,714	5,314	560
850	10,588	5,252	560
900	10,000	4,960	500
1,000	9,000	4,464	666
1,500	6,000	2,976	1,000
2,250	4,000	1,984	1,000
3,000	3,000	1,488	1,333
15,000	600	298	10,000

Fabrics and Woven Rovings. Conventional woven fabric is the principal aramid form used in composites. Of the wide range of fabric weights and constructions available, those most commonly used are identified in Table 3 (Ref 10). Many of these aramid fabrics of Kevlar were designed and constructed to be the volume equivalent to the same style number of fiberglass fabric. Generally, fabrics made of a very fine size of aramid yarn are thin, lightweight, and relatively costly, and they are used when ultralight weight, thinness, and surface smoothness are critical. Fabrics are available from weavers worldwide. Plain, basket, crowfoot, and satin weave patterns are available. Generally, crowfoot and satin weaves are recommended when a high degree of mold conformability is required. Heavy, woven roving fabrics are also available and are used in marine applications where hand lay-up is appropriate and for hard ballistic fabrics. Unidirectional fabrics are used when maximum properties are desired in one direction. Applications for high-modulus aramid fabrics include commercial aircraft and helicopter secondary composite parts, particularly facings of honeycomb sandwich constructions, boat hulls, electrical and electronic parts, ballistic systems, and coated fabrics.

Textured aramid can be processed through a high-velocity air jet to attain filament loops in the continuous filament yarn. This produces a bulkier yarn that has more air space between the filaments and a drier, less slick, tactile characteristic. The yarn is used in asbestos replacement to give the composite a higher resin-to-aramid ratio and in protective apparel to achieve superior textile aesthetics.

Although continuous filament forms dominate composite applications, the use of aramid in discontinuous or short fiber forms is rapidly increasing. One reason for the increase is that the inherent toughness and fibrillar nature of aramid allows the creation of fiber forms not readily available with other reinforcing fibers.

Staple and Spun Yarns. Staple or short aramid fiber is available in crimped or uncrimped form in lengths ranging from 6.4 to 100 mm (0.25–4.0 in.). Crimped versions that are 25 mm (1.0 in.) or longer are used to make spun yarns on conventional cotton, woolen, or worsted system equipment. Spun yarns formed in this way are not as strong or as stiff as continuous aramid filament yarns, but are bulkier, pick up more resin, and have tactile characteristics similar to cotton or wool. They are used in asbestos replacement (for example, clutch facings) and as sewing thread. The shorter aramid fibers, crimped and uncrimped, are used to reinforce thermoset, thermoplastic, and elastomeric resins. Applications include automotive and truck brake and clutch linings, gaskets, electrical parts, and wear-resistant thermoplastic parts. Selection of a crimped or uncrimped form usually depends on the resin-fiber mixing method or on equipment used for the specific application. Special mixing methods and equipment are usually necessary to achieve uniform dispersion of the aramid fiber.

Fabrics and Felts. Woven and knit fabrics made from aramid spun yarns are available. They are used in asbestos replacement and in protective apparel because of their resistance to cutting, puncture, abrasion, or thermal exposure. Aramid staple is also processed into needle-punched felts, which are used in asbestos replacement, ballistic armor, and marine laminates.

Pulp. Kevlar is available in a unique short fiber form known as pulp (Fig. 5). It is a very short fiber (2–4 mm, or 0.08–0.16 in.) with many attached fibrils. These fibrils are complex in that

Table 3 Kevlar 49 fabric and woven roving specifications

Style No.	Weave	Basis weight g/m²	Basis weight oz/yd²	Fabric construction ends/cm	Fabric construction ends/in.	Yarn denier	Fabric thickness mm	Fabric thickness 10^{-3} in.
Light weight								
166(a)	Plain	30.6	0.9	37 × 37	94 × 94	55	0.04	1.5
199(a)	Plain	61.13	1.8	24 × 24	60 × 60	55	0.05	2
120	Plain	61.1	1.8	13 × 13	34 × 34	195	0.11	4.5
220	Plain	74.7	2.2	9 × 9	22 × 22	380	0.11	4.5
Medium weight								
181	Eight-hardness satin	169.8	5.0	20 × 20	50 × 50	380	0.23	9
281	Plain	169.8	5.0	7 × 7	17 × 17	1140	0.25	10
285	Crowfoot	169.8	5.0	7 × 7	17 × 17	1140	0.25	10
328	Plain	230.9	6.8	7 × 7	17 × 17	1420	0.33	13
355	Crowfoot	239.9	6.8	7 × 7	17 × 17	1420	0.30	12
500	Plain	169.8	5.0	5 × 5	13 × 13	1420	0.28	11
Unidirectional								
143	Crowfoot	190.2	5.6	39 × 8	100 × 20	380 × 195	0.25	10
243	Crowfoot	227.5	6.7	15 × 7	38 × 18	1140 × 380	0.33	13
Woven roving								
1050	4 × 4 basket	356.6	10.5	11 × 11	28 × 28	1420	0.46	18
1033	8 × 8 basket	509.4	15.0	16 × 16	40 × 40	1420	0.66	26
1350	4 × 4 basket	458.5	13.5	10 × 9	26 × 22	2130	0.64	25

(a) Only available on special order; custom fabric will be woven to specifications.

they are curled, branched, and often ribbonlike. They are a direct result of the inherent fibrillar structure of this fiber. The large surface area (40 times standard fiber) and high aspect ratio of the fibrils (greater than 100) can provide very efficient reinforcement. In general, pulp is more easily mixed into resin formulations than is staple fiber and is now used extensively in replacing asbestos in gaskets, friction products, sealants, caulks, and coatings (Ref 11, 12).

Spunlaced Sheets. Aramid staple fibers can be processed into lightweight, nonwoven sheet structures. One of the available forms is spunlaced sheet, in which webs of staple fibers are entangled by high-pressure water jets. No binder resin is used. These sheets are low-density (0.008–0.16 g/cm^3), lightweight (0.02–0.07 kg/m^2, or 0.5–2.0 oz/yd^2) structures that are very drapable and readily impregnated. Applications include surfacing veil, printed circuit boards, and fire-blocking layers in aircraft seating.

Papers. The dominant aramid paper used in advanced composites in honeycomb sandwich constructions is made from Nomex aramid fiber (Ref 13). It is chemically related to Kevlar, but its tenacity and modulus are considerably lower and are more like those of conventional textile fibers. A range of Nomex papers in varying thicknesses and weights are available. Honeycomb cores of Nomex are also available; densities range from 0.24 to 0.14 g/cm^3 (Ref 14).

Fig. 5 Aramid pulp

Aramid chopped fibers and pulp can be processed into wet-laid papers on conventional fourdrinier machines. Applications include asbestos replacement, such as in gasketing and automatic transmissions. Straight, uncrimped fibers can be used to maximize stiffness and mechanical properties of the wet-laid papers. These thin, lightweight papers are readily impregnated and can be cost competitive with expensive, lightweight, thin, continuous filament fabrics. Composites that use these papers are being developed for printed circuit boards, aerospace, and industrial applications (Ref 15). Proprietary papers based on para-aramid floc and meta-aramid fibrids are also available.

Materials Properties

Key representative properties of para-aramid fibers are given in Table 4. Kevlar 49 is the dominant form used today in structural composites because of its higher modulus. Kevlar 29 is used in composites when higher toughness, damage tolerance, or ballistic stopping performance is desired. An ultrahigh-modulus fiber, Kevlar 149, is also available.

Tensile modulus of para-aramid fibers is a function of the molecular orientation. As a spun fiber, Kevlar 29 has a modulus of 62 GPa (9 × 10^6 psi). In composite form, it has a modulus (83 GPa, or 12 × 10^6 psi) that is slightly higher than that of E-glass (69 GPa, or 10 × 10^6 psi). Heat treatment under tension increases crystalline orientation, and the resulting fiber, Kevlar 49, has a modulus of 131 GPa (19 × 10^6 psi). Kevlar 149 has an even higher modulus (179 GPa, or 26 × 10^6 psi) and is available on special order. This modulus approaches the theoretical maximum predicted for para-aramid fibers (Ref 18).

The tensile strength of para-aramid fiber is in the range of 3.6 to 4.1 GPa (0.525–0.600 × 10^6 psi). This is more than twice the strength of conventional organic fibers such as nylon 66 and is 50% greater than the strength of E-glass roving. It is believed that tensile failure initiates at fibril ends and propagates via shear failure between the fibrils.

Tensile Properties in Hot/Wet Conditions. High-modulus para-aramid yarns show a linear decrease of both tensile strength and modulus when tested at elevated temperatures in air (Fig. 6). More than 80% of these properties are retained at 180 °C (355 °F). Figure 7 shows retention of room-temperature yarn strength after long exposures at elevated temperatures. More than 80% of strength is retained after 81 h at 200 °C (390 °F).

At room temperature, the effect of moisture on tensile properties is <5%. At elevated tem-

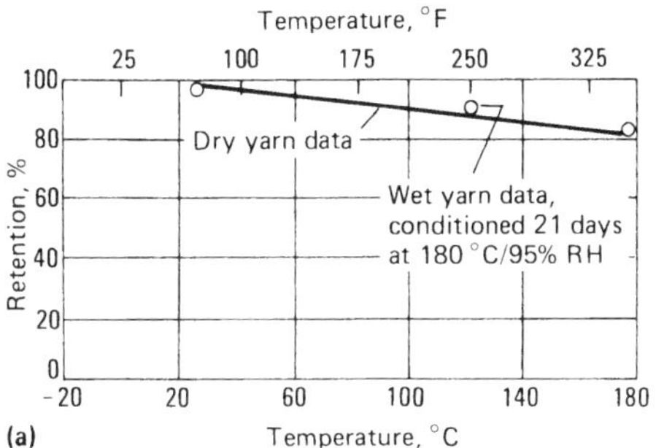

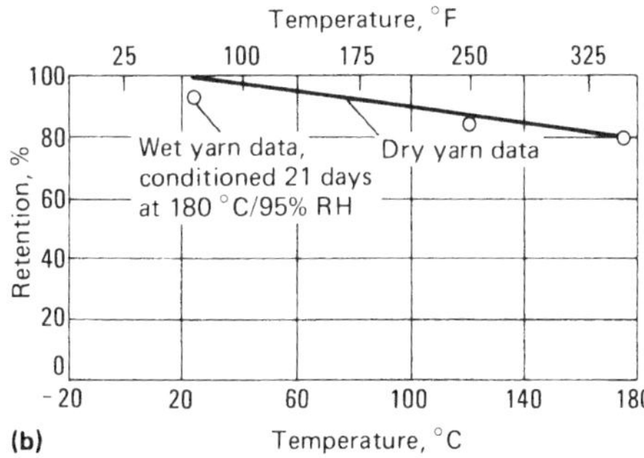

Fig. 6 Effect of temperature on tensile strength and modulus of dry and wet Kevlar 49 aramid yarn. (a) Tensile strength. (b) Tensile modulus

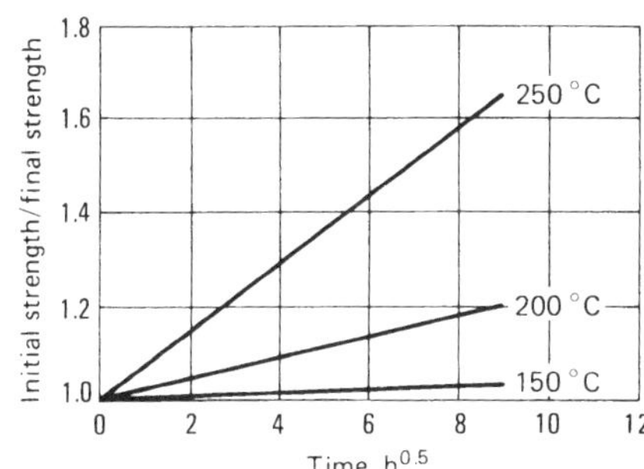

Fig. 7 Room-temperature tensile strength retention after air aging of Kevlar 49 aramid yarn at various temperatures

Table 4 Properties of para-aramid fibers

Material	Density, g/cm^3	Filament diameter		Tensile modulus(a)		Tensile strength(a)		Tensile elongation, %	Available yarn count, No. filaments
		μm	μin.	GPa	10^6 psi	GPa	10^6 psi		
Kevlar 29 (high toughness)	1.44	12	470	83	12	3.6 2.8(b)	0.525 0.400(b)	4.0	134 10,000
Kevlar 49 (high modulus)	1.44	12	470	131	19	3.6–4.1	0.525–0.600	2.8	25–5,000
Kevlar 149 (ultrahigh modulus)	1.47	12	470	179	26	3.4	0.500	2.0	1,000

(a) ASTM D 2343, impregnated strand (Ref 16). (b) ASTM D 885, unimpregnated strand (Ref 17).

perature, the effect of moisture appears to be reversible: yarn conditioned for 21 days at 180 °C (355 °F)/95% relative humidity tested at high temperature had essentially the same behavior as dry yarn (Fig. 6). Tests of yarn while immersed in hot water suggest a loss of 10% due to the water alone (Ref 19–20).

Creep and Fatigue. Para-aramid is resistant to dynamic and static fatigue (Fig. 8 and 9). Creep rate is low and similar to that of fiberglass, but unlike glass, para-aramid is less susceptible to creep rupture (Ref 21).

Compressive Properties. Although para-aramid fiber responds elastically in tension, it exhibits nonlinear, ductile behavior under compression. At a compression strain of 0.3 to 0.5%, a yield is observed (Fig. 10). This corresponds to the formation of structural defects known as kink bands (Fig. 11), which are related to compressive buckling of para-aramid molecules. As a result of this compression behavior, the use of para-aramid fibers in applications that are subject to high strain compressive or flexural loads is limited. The compressive buckling characteristics have also led to developments of crashworthy structures that rely on the fail-safe behavior of aramid composites under sustained high compressive loads (Ref 23).

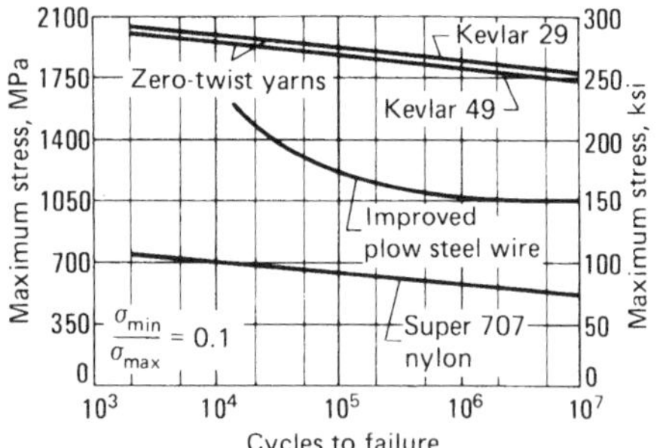

Fig. 8 Comparative tension-tension fatigue for yarns and wire

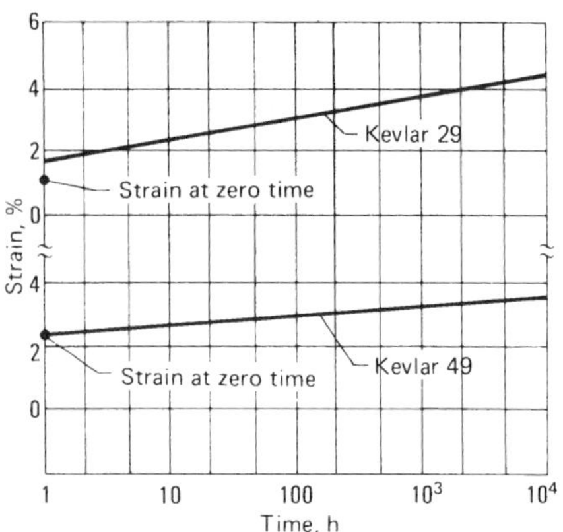

Fig. 9 Creep of Kevlar 29 and Kevlar 49 aramid yarns at 50% of ultimate strength

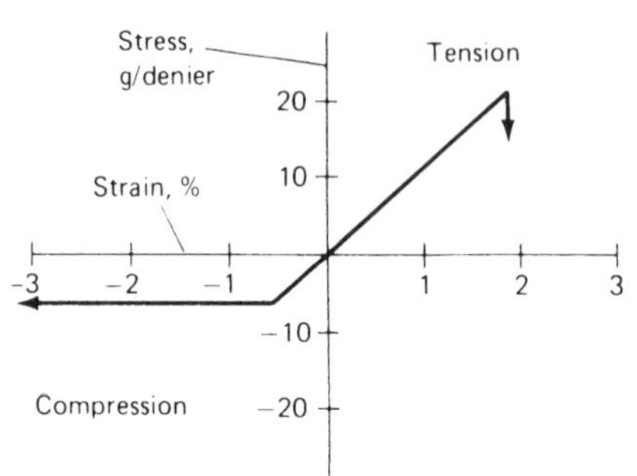

Fig. 10 Para-aramid stress-strain behavior in tension and compression

Toughness. Para-aramid fiber is noted for its toughness and general damage tolerance characteristics (Ref 24). In part, this is related directly to conventional tensile toughness, or the area under the stress-strain curve. Toughness is also related to composite impact resistance and ballistic stopping power (Ref 25, 26). The para-aramid fibrillar structure and compressive behavior contribute to composites that are less notch sensitive (Ref 27) and that fail in a ductile, nonbrittle, or noncatastrophic manner, as opposed to glass and carbon (Ref 28).

Thermal Properties. The aromatic chemical structure of para-aramid imparts a high degree of thermal stability (Fig. 12). Fibers from PPD-T do not have a literal melting point or a glass transition temperature (T_g) (estimated at ≥375 °C, or 710 °F), as normally observed with other synthetic polymers. They decompose in air at 425 °C (800 °F) and are inherently flame resistant (limiting oxygen index of 0.29). They have utility over a broad temperature range of about –200 to 200 °C (–330 to 390 °F), but are not generally used long term at temperatures above 150 °C (300 °F) because of oxidation (Fig. 7). Para-aramid fiber has a slightly negative longitudinal coefficient of thermal expansion of -2×10^{-6}/K and a positive transverse expansion of 60×10^{-6}/K.

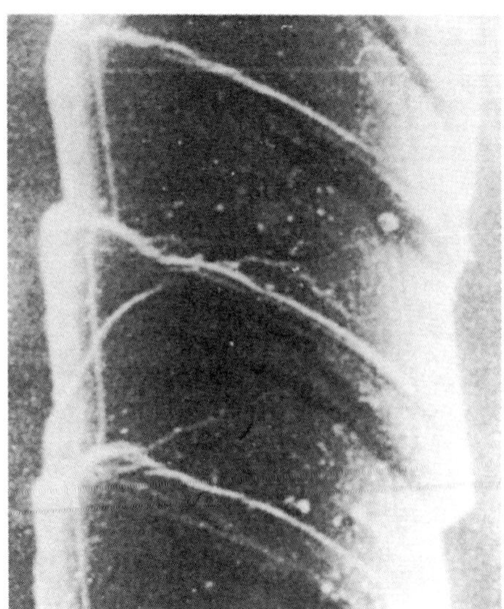

Fig. 11 Kink bands from severe compression. Source: Ref 22

Para-aramid fiber has a low thermal conductivity that varies by about an order of magnitude in the longitudinal versus transverse direction. Heat of combustion is about 35 MJ/kg (15000 Btu/lb). The specific heat versus temperature is shown in Fig. 13.

Electrical and Optical Properties. Para-aramid is an electrical insulator. Its dielectric constant of ~4.0, measured at 10^6 Hz, is lower than that of fiberglass and about the same as that of quartz. The index of refraction of para-aramid fiber is 2.0 parallel to the fiber axis and 1.6 perpendicular to the fiber axis. E-glass is 1.55 in both directions.

Environmental Behavior. Para-aramid fiber has an equilibrium moisture content that is determined by the relative humidity, as shown in Fig. 14. At 60% RH, equilibrium moisture of Kevlar 49 is about 4%. Kevlar 149 has a corresponding value of about 1.5%. Physically, the diameter of an aramid filament changes by 0.5% with a corresponding 1% change in fiber moisture content.

Para-aramid fiber can be chemically degraded by strong acids and bases. It is resistant to most other solvents and chemicals (Ref 6). Ultraviolet radiation also can degrade para-aramid. The degree of degradation depends on material thick-

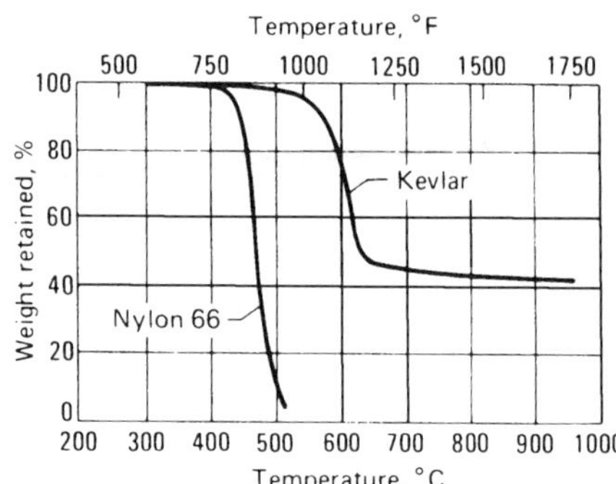

Fig. 12 Thermal stability; thermogravimetric analysis done at 20 °C (70 °F)/min in nitrogen

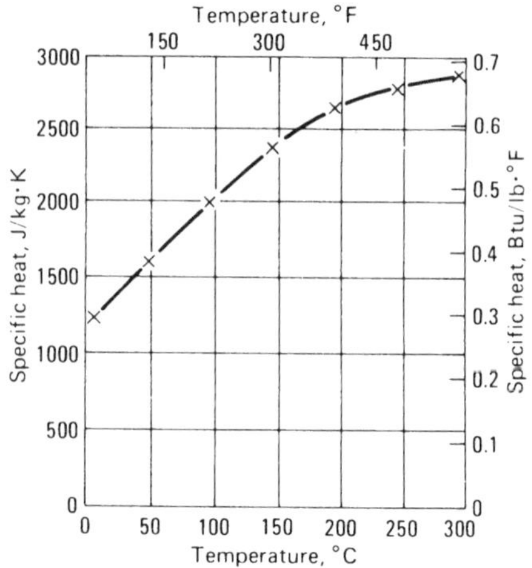

Fig. 13 Effect of temperature on the specific heat of Kevlar 49 aramid

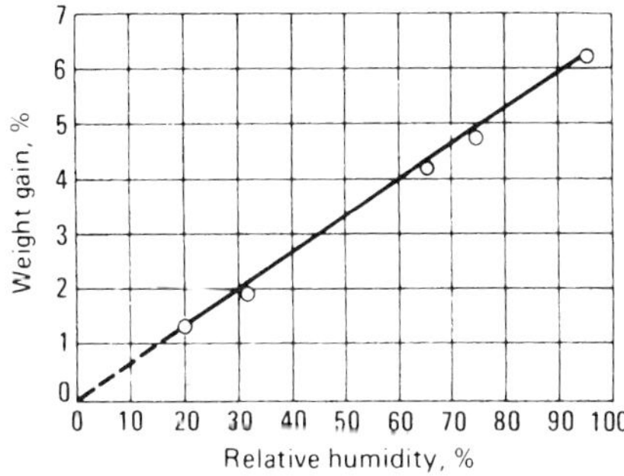

Fig. 14 Equilibrium moisture content versus relative humidity for Kevlar 49 at room temperature

ness because para-aramid is self-screening. In polymeric composites, strength loss of para-aramid has not been observed (Ref 29).

Para-aramid is resistant to electron radiation, as shown in Table 5. Vacuum outgassing has been performed on para-aramid yarn that had been predried at 125 °C (257 °F) for 24 h under a vacuum of 1.3×10^{-4} Pa (10^{-6} torr). With a colorless deposit of 0.02 wt% micro volatile condensible materials (VCM), there was a 2.28% weight loss.

Future Developments

The most promising new market opportunity for composite materials today is infrastructure. Composite solutions for repair and strengthening of bridges and buildings can be considerably less expensive and faster than conventional steel and reinforced concrete. Major earthquakes in California, Japan, and Italy since 1994 have accelerated the adoption of composite materials in infrastructure applications. Aramid systems were developed and commercialized in Japan for seismic retrofit of railway and highway bridge columns after the Kobe earthquake in 1995. In addition to structural properties, the damage tolerance and impact-resistant properties of aramid fibers also make them the fiber of choice for strengthening bridge supports to resist vehicular impact and for strengthening masonry walls to resist blast loads (Ref 30).

Table 5 Effect of electron radiation on Kevlar 49

Using resonant transformer and filament wrapped in aluminum foil over dry ice, conditions of exposure were 1 Mrad every 13.4 s, 0.5 mA, 2 MV, and 30 cm (10 in.) distance.

	Single-filament properties				
	Tenacity		Tensile modulus		
Mrad exposure	MPa	ksi	GPa	10^6 psi	Elongation, %
0	2860	415	128	18.6	2.4
100	2940	426	130	18.8	2.4
200	3010	436	133	19.3	2.5

REFERENCES

1. P.J. Flory, Molecular Theory of Liquid Crystals, in *Advances in Polymer Science,* Vol 59, Springer-Verlag, 1984, p 1–36
2. P.W. Morgan, *Macromolecules,* Vol 10, 1977, p 1381
3. S.L. Kwolek, P.W. Morgan, J.R. Schaefgen, and L.W. Gulrich, *Macromolecules,* Vol 10, 1977, p 1390
4. H. Blades, U.S. Patent 3,767,756, 1973
5. H.M. Caesars, *Chem. Fibers Int.,* April, 2000, p 161–164
6. H.H. Yang, *Kevlar Aramid Fiber,* John Wiley & Sons, 1993
7. D. Tanner, J.A. Fitzgerald, W.F. Knoff, and J.J. Pigliacampi, "Aramid Fiber Structure/Property Relationships and Their Applications to Industrial Materials," Paper presented at Japan Fiber Society Meeting, Aug 1985
8. M.G. Northolt, *Eur. Polym. J.,* Vol 10, 1974, p 799
9. V. Gabara, High Performance Fibres 1: Aramid Fibres, *Synthetic Fibre Materials,* H. Brody, Ed., Longman Scientific and Technical, Essex, England, 1994, Chapter 9
10. *Kevlar 49 Data Manual,* E.I. Du Pont de Nemours & Co., Inc., May 1986
11. "Kevlar and Nomex Specialty Additives for Enhanced Performance," E.I. Du Pont de Nemours & Co., Inc., Oct 1998
12. "Kevlar Brand Pulp in Adhesives, Sealants, Coatings and Fiber Reinforced Plastics," E.I. Du Pont de Nemours & Co., Inc., March 1999
13. "Nomex Brand Paper Type 412 Properties and Performance," E.I. Du Pont de Nemours & Co., Inc.
14. H.Y. Loken, Tradeoffs in Honeycomb Cored Designs, *Aircraft Eng.,* Dec 1988
15. M.P. Zussman and D.J. Powell, Nonwoven Aramid—A Cost Effective Surface Mount Laminate Reinforcement, *J. Surface Mount Technol.,* Oct 1992
16. "Standard Test Method for Tensile Properties of Glass Fiber Strands, Yarns, and Rovings Used in Reinforced Plastics," D 2343, *Annual Book of ASTM Standards,* ASTM
17. "Standard Methods of Testing Tire Cords, Tire Cord Fabrics, and Industrial Filament Yarns Made from Man-Made Organic-Base Fibers," D 885, *Annual Book of ASTM Standards,* ASTM
18. E.E. Magat, *Philos. Trans. R. Soc., (London) A,* Vol 294 (No. 463), 1980
19. W.S. Smith, Environmental Effects on Aramid Composites, *Proc. Society of Plastics Engineers Conference,* Dec 1979
20. N.J. Abbott et al., "Some Mechanical Properties of Kevlar and Other Heat Resistant, Nonflammable Fibers, Yarns and Fabrics," AFML-TR-74-65, Part III, Air Force Materials Laboratory, March 1975
21. P.G. Riewald et al., Strength and Durability Characteristics of Ropes and Cables from Kevlar Aramid Fibers, *Oceans '77 Conference Record,* Third Combined Conference, Marine Technology Society and Institute of Electrical and Electronics Engineers, Oct 1977
22. M.G. Dobb, D.J. Johnson, and B.P. Saville, *Polymer,* Vol 22 (No. 7), 1981, p 960
23. J.D. Cronkhite, Design of Helicopter Composite Structures for Crashworthiness, Technical Symposium V, *Design and Use of Kevlar Aramid Fiber in Composite Structures,* E.I. Du Pont de Nemours & Co., Inc., April 1984
24. M.W. Wardle, Designing Composite Structure for Toughness, Technical Symposium V, *Design and Use of Kevlar Aramid Fiber in Composite Structures,* E.I. Du Pont de Nemours & Co., Inc., April 1984
25. M.W. Wardle and E.W. Tokarsky, Drop Wings Testing of Laminates Reinforced with Kevlar Aramid Fibers, E-Glass and Graphite, *Composites Technology Review,* ASTM, 1983
26. L.H. Miner, "Fragmentation Resistance of Aramid Fabrics and Their Composites," paper presented at Symposium on Vulnerability and Survivability (San Diego, CA), March 1985
27. C. Zweben, Fracture of Kevlar 49, E-Glass and Graphite Composites, paper presented at ASTM Symposium on Fracture Mechanics of Composites, ASTM, Sept 1974
28. M.W. Wardle, Aramid Fiber Reinforced Plastics—Properties, *Comprehensive Composite Materials,* Vol 2, A. Kelly and C. Zweben, Ed., Elsevier Science, 2000, p 200–229
29. R.H. Stone, "Flight Service Evaluation of Kevlar 49/Epoxy Composite Panels in Wide Body Commercial Transport Aircraft," Contractor Report 159231, National Aeronautics and Space Administration, March 1980
30. J.R. Cuninghame and B. Sadka, Fibre Reinforced Plastic Strengthening of Bridge Supports to Resist Vehicle Impact, *Proc. 20th International SAMPE Europe Conference,* M.A. Erath, Ed., Society for the Advancement of Material and Process Engineering, April 1999, p 391–403

Ceramic Fibers

D.M. Wilson, 3M Specialty Fibers & Composites
J.A. DiCarlo and H.M. Yun, NASA Glenn Research Center

CONTINUOUS-LENGTH CERAMIC FIBERS are commercially available in two general classes for the reinforcement of ceramic-matrix composites (CMC): (1) oxide fibers, based on the alumina-silica (Al_2O_3-SiO_2) system and on α-alumina (α-Al_2O_3), and (2) nonoxide fibers, based primarily on β-phase silicon carbide (SiC). These fibers are typically produced with small diameter (<20 μm) and in polycrystalline form with small grain size (<1 μm). When compared to single-crystal fibers or whiskers of the same compositions, the polycrystalline fibers are easier to handle and offer significantly lower production costs, but reduced creep resistance and temperature capability. Thermostructural capability is degraded further with the presence of amorphous or creep-enhancing second phases in the grain boundaries. Nevertheless, a variety of oxide and nonoxide polycrystalline-ceramic fibers exist today with sufficient crystallinity, purity, and performance capability to reinforce metal- and ceramic-matrix composites that can compete with metallic alloys at low and high temperatures. Literature reviews detail the process methods, properties, and applications for numerous ceramic-fiber types that have been developed since the 1970s (Ref 1–5). However, only certain types have reached the stage in which they have been used to reinforce different CMC systems with composite-property databases available in the open literature. For the sake of brevity, this article focuses only on these commercial types because they have demonstrated their general applicability as CMC reinforcement.

Fiber Production

The most common approach for producing polycrystalline-ceramic fibers is by spinning and heat treating chemically derived precursors. For oxide fibers, sol-gel processing is used. The sol-gel process uses chemical **sol**utions or colloidal suspensions, which are shaped into fibers, then **gel**led (usually by drying) and heat treated to convert the gelled precursor to ceramic. In the case of fibers based on SiC and silicon nitride, fibers are spun from organometallic "preceramic" polymer precursors, followed by cross-linking (curing) and heat treatment steps to convert the fibers to ceramic materials (Ref 5). The use of chemical precursor technology allows the commercial preparation of ceramic fibers with properties not accessible by traditional fiber-forming technology, such as spinning of molten glasses. A key characteristic of ceramic fibers is their ultrafine microstructure, with grain sizes sometimes in the nanometer range. Fine grains are required for good tensile strength (>2000 MPa, or 300 ksi), but can be detrimental to creep resistance (Ref 6). The precursor processes also allow fiber production in the form of continuous-length multifilament tows or rovings, which are typically coated with a thin polymer-based sizing and then supplied to customers on spools. These sized tows are flexible and easily handled so that they can be woven or braided into fabrics, tapes, sleeves, and other complex shapes. Most small-diameter fiber manufacturers also supply fibers in fabric form since composite-fabrication processes generally require an initial step of fabric stacking and near-net shaping into final product forms. Continuous-length monofilaments of single-crystal Al_2O_3 and polycrystalline SiC with diameters >50 μm are also commercially available. Although employed to reinforce both metal and ceramic composites, they are limited in their flexibility, shapeability, and affordability, and thus are considered here mainly for property comparison.

Composite Applications

Applications for oxide-based fibers take advantage of their oxidation resistance, moderate temperature capability (to 1100 °C, or 2000 °F), chemical stability, and relatively low cost. Many oxide-fiber CMC do not require interfacial fiber coatings or composite overcoatings for debonding; instead, composite toughness is generated by crack deflection in porous oxide matrices. This provides an additional cost benefit, but may limit temperature capability in order to avoid matrix sintering. Although displaying a lower toughness to surface flaws and surface coatings, oxide-based fibers are preferred over nonoxide reinforcements in corrosive environments such as in waste incineration, hot gas filtration, certain heat exchanger applications, and metal-matrix composites (especially aluminum). In addition, oxide fibers have major commercial uses in high-temperature thermal insulation applications requiring flexible, lightweight, and oxidation-resistant continuous fibers, such as sleeves for pipes and electrical cables, high-temperature shielding, belts, blankets, and gasket seals. The cost of most small-diameter oxide fibers ($200–1000/kg) is higher than that of glass and carbon fibers, but lower than that of SiC fibers ($1,000–13,000/kg).

Applications for nonoxide SiC-based fibers typically center on CMC for high-temperature structural applications (>1100 °C, or 2000 °F), where lower creep and grain-growth rates in comparison to oxide fibers allow better dimensional stability and strength retention under the combined conditions of temperature and stress. The SiC-based fibers can also provide greater thermal and electrical conductivity, higher as-produced strength, and lower density. However, under oxygen-containing environmental conditions, the exposed surfaces of silicon-based fibers will degrade slowly due to silica growth and surface recession. However, silica is among the most protective of scales, so that, in a general sense, SiC has very good oxidation resistance. It follows then that SiC-based fibers are generally preferred for CMC applications that require both long-term structural service under environmental conditions that minimally expose the fibers to oxygen, and upper-use temperatures higher than possible with oxide/oxide CMC and state of the art metallic superalloys. Minimal oxygen exposure is typically achieved by incorporating the fibers in dense protective matrices of similar composition and thermal expansion, such as in SiC/SiC composites. Extensive developmental efforts are underway to use these SiC/SiC CMC in land- and aero-based gas turbine engines for hot-section components that require service for thousands of hours under combustion gas environments.

Properties of Commercial Fibers

Commercial oxide fibers can be divided into two compositional classes: (1) alumina-silica fibers, that is, those consisting of a mixture of transition alumina and amorphous silica, and (2) alumina fibers consisting primarily of α-Al_2O_3. As indicated in Table 1, these two classes contain a variety of fiber types from different manufacturers, with substantially different as-produced microstructures and properties. In general, the alumina-silica fiber types display lower strength, modulus, thermal expansion, and density than the fibers based on α-Al_2O_3. The higher strength and modulus plus the superior thermochemical stability of the more crystalline α-Al_2O_3 fibers make them the preferred oxide candidates for the reinforcement of metal- and ceramic-matrix composites. However, the moderate strength and lower stiffness of the alumina-silica fibers allow better strain to failure and flexibility, both very important properties for the use of textile-grade fibers in thermal insulation applications.

In the alumina-silica fibers, alumina is present as transition aluminas (η-Al_2O_3 or γ-Al_2O_3). Because transition aluminas have very fine grain size (10–100 nm), these fibers have good strength. Commercial alumina-silica fibers contain SiO_2 to preserve the submicrometer transition alumina microstructure and therefore fiber strength and flexibility for extended periods above 1100 °C (2000 °F). However, SiO_2 remains as an amorphous glassy phase; this can compromise chemical stability and creep properties at high temperature. Above 1200 °C (2200 °F), alumina-silica fibers will crystallize over time to form either mullite ($3Al_2O_3 \cdot 2SiO_2$) or α-Al_2O_3, which commonly results in large grains and low fiber strength. Nextel 440 ceramic oxide fibers, which contain 2 wt% B_2O_3, do not degrade during the crystallization to mullite. B_2O_3 promotes the formation of fine-grained mullite via a $9Al_2O_3 \cdot 2B_2O_3$ intermediate phase. However, B_2O_3 increases fiber creep rate and can also increase reactivity and therefore strength degradation with certain matrices.

In comparison to fibers containing transition aluminas and amorphous silica, fibers containing crystalline α-Al_2O_3 are more resistant to shrinkage at high temperatures caused by crystallization and sintering and can have higher creep resistance under load at high temperatures. The chemical stability of α-Al_2O_3 fibers reduces reactivity with oxide matrices, providing much higher strength in porous matrix composites. Nextel 720 fiber, although it contains 15 wt% SiO_2, can be considered to be based on α-Al_2O_3 because it contains greater than 50 vol% of α-Al_2O_3. Thus it has a much higher modulus, chemical stability, and creep resistance compared with the alumina-silica fibers discussed previously. Saphikon, which is a melt-grown single-crystal Al_2O_3 monofilament, has the highest as-produced strength (3500 MPa, or 500 ksi) and does not creep until well above 1400 °C (2600 °F). However, unlike polycrystalline fibers, the strength of Saphikon fiber decreases substantially at moderate temperatures (e.g., below 500 °C, or 900 °F) due to environmentally assisted slow crack growth. For applications with thermal gradients, one disadvantage of the α-Al_2O_3 fibers is their high thermal expansion and low thermal conductivity (<5 W/m · K), which can result in high thermal stresses.

Commercial Nonoxide (SiC-Based) Fibers. Table 2 lists some key technical details related to the microstructure and properties of a variety of SiC-based fiber types of interest for CMC reinforcement. These types range from fibers with very high percentages of oxygen and excess carbon, such as Nicalon and Tyranno Lox M, to the near-stoichiometric (atomic C/Si $\approx$ 1) fibers, such as Sylramic. These large compositional differences not only impact chemical and thermostructural properties, but also result in a large variation in electrical properties (Ref 5). Because of their high production costs and need to be protected from oxidizing environments, SiC-based fibers have yet to reach the market status enjoyed by oxide fibers, which also have applications outside of structural composites (e.g., high-temperature thermal insulation). For sake of completeness, Table 2 also includes some nonoxide carbon-based fibers that also have been used for CMC reinforcement. Typically the carbon fibers are very low in cost and display the best intrinsic behavior of all fiber types, particularly regarding intrinsic thermal stability, creep resistance, and as-produced tensile strength. However, under oxidizing conditions, the exposed surfaces of carbon fibers quickly convert to gas at temperatures as low as 400 °C (750 °F). Thus these fiber types have only been considered for CMC that are well protected from oxidizing service conditions by matrices and/or external composite coatings and that are required to experience these conditions for relatively short times. Ceramic composites such as C/SiC are typically targeted for high-temperature applications of short duration in oxygen, such as brake pads and structural components in advanced space-propulsion systems.

The primary process methods used to produce SiC-based fibers with small (<20 μm) and large (>50 μm) diameters are polymer pyrolysis and chemical vapor deposition (CVD), respectively. For the polymer route, precursor fibers typically based on polycarbosilane are spun into multifilament tows, which are then cured and pyrolzed to form strong fibers at process temperatures up to ~1200 °C (2200 °F). This maximum process temperature is dictated by the fact that during the early fiber production steps, a small amount of oxygen can be unwontedly introduced into the fiber microstructure. This results in oxide-based impurity phases that, in the presence of carbon and carbides, tend to decompose into gases that leave the fiber above 1200 °C (2200 °F), thereby creating porosity and less than optimal fiber tensile strength (Ref 5). Because it is often desirable to fabricate and use CMC for long times above 1200 °C (2200 °F), advanced process methods that limit the oxide phases have recently been developed. In one method, the oxygen pickup is reduced, for example, by curing under electron irradiation (Hi-Nicalon and Hi-Nicalon-S). In another method, any oxide-based impurities are allowed to decompose at higher temperatures, and then the remaining SiC grains are sintered into strong fibers that are dense, oxygen-free, and nearly stoichiometric. For example, to form the Tyranno SA and Sylramic fiber types, aluminum and boron sintering aids are introduced,

Table 1 Commercial oxide fiber types for CMC reinforcement

Tradename	Manufacturer	Composition(a), wt%	Avg. grain size, nm	Density, g/cm^3	Avg. diameter, μm	Filaments per tow	Current cost (<5 kg), $/kg	Avg. RT tensile strength		RT tensile modulus		Thermal expansion, ppm/°C (to 1000 °C)
								MPa	ksi	GPa	10^6 psi	
Alumina-silica based												
Altex	Sumitomo	85 A + 15 S	25	3.3	15	500/1000	330–550	2000	290	210	30	7.9
Alcen	Nitivy	70 A + 30 S (80 + 20, 60 + 40)	. . .	3.1	10–7	1000	. . .	2000	290	170	25	. . .
Nextel 312	3M	62 A + 24 S + 14 B_2O_3	<50	2.7	10–12	420/780	190–230	1700	250	150	22	3
Nextel 440	3M	70 A + 28 S + 2 B_2O_3	<50	3.05	10–12	420/780	380–490	2000	290	190	28	5.3
Nextel 550	3M	73 A + 27 S	<50	3.03	10–12	420/780	475–730	2000	290	193	28	5.3
α-alumina based												
Almax	Mitsui Mining	99.5 A	600	3.6	10	1000	815	1800	260	330	48	8.8
Nextel 610	3M	>99 A	100	3.9	12	420/780/2600	330–660	3100	450	373	54	7.9
Nextel 650	3M	89 A + 10 ZrO_2 + 1 Y_2O_3	100	4.1	11	780	400–660	2500	360	358	52	8.0
Nextel 720	3M	85 A + 15 S	100–500	3.4	12	420/780	440–1010	2100	300	260	38	6.0
Saphikon	Saphikon	100 A	Single crystal	3.98	125	Mono-filament	50,000	3500	510	460	67	9

RT, room temperature. (a) A, alumina; S, silica

Table 2 Commercial nonoxide fiber types for CMC reinforcement

Tradename	Manufacturer	Composition, wt%	Avg. grain size, nm	Density, g/cm^3	Avg. diameter, μm	Filaments per tow	Current cost (<5 kg), $/kg	Avg. RT tensile strength		RT tensile modulus		RT axial thermal conductivity, W/m · k	Thermal expansion, ppm/°C (to 1000 °C)
								MPa	ksi	GPa	10^6 psi		
Silicon-carbide based (pure stoichiometric SiC: Si = 70 wt%, C = 30 wt%)													
Nicalon, NL200	Nippon Carbon	56 Si + 32 C + 12 O	5	2.55	14	500	~2000	3000	440	220	32	3	3.2
Hi-Nicalon	Nippon Carbon	62 Si + 37 C + 0.5 O	10	2.74	14	500	8000	2800	410	270	39	8	3.5
Hi-Nicalon type S	Nippon Carbon	69 Si + 31 C + 0.2 O	100	3.05	12	500	13,000	~2500	360	400–420	58–61	18	...
Tyranno Lox M	Ube Industries	55 Si + 32 C + 10 O + 2.0 Ti	1	2.48	11	400/800	1500/1000	3300	480	187	27	1.5	3.1
Tyranno ZMI	Ube Industries	57 Si + 35 C + 7.6 O + 1.0 Zr	2	2.48	11	400/800	1600/1000	3300	480	200	29	2.5	...
Tyranno SA 1-3	Ube Industries	68 Si + 32 C + 0.6 Al	200	3.02	10–7.5	800/1600	~5000	2800	410	375	54	65	...
Sylramic	Dow Corning	67 Si + 29 C + 0.8 O + 2.3 B + 0.4 N + 2.1 Ti	100	3.05	10	800	10,000	3200	460	~400	~58	46	5.4
Sylramic-iBN	Dow Corning, NASA	Sylramic + in situ BN surface (~100 nm thick)	>100	3.05	10	800	>10,000	3200	460	~400	~58	>46	5.4
SCS-6-9	Textron Specialty Materials	70 Si + 30 C + trace Si + C on ~30 μm C core	~100 by ~10	~3	140–70	Monofilament	~9000	~3500	510	390–350	57–51	~70	4.6
Ultra SCS	Textron Specialty Materials	70 Si + 30 C + trace Si + C on ~30 μm C core	~100 by ~10	~3	140	Monofilament	~9000	~6000	870	390	56	~70	4.6
Carbon-based													
T300	Amoco	92 C + 8 N	~2	1.76	7	1000 to 12,000	250–100	3700	540	231	34	8.5	–0.6
IM7	Hercules (Hexcel)	>99 C, trace N	~2	1.77	5	6000/12,000	70–50	5300	770	275	40	6.0	–0.2
UHM	Hercules (Hexcel)	>99 C, trace N	~2	1.87	4.5	3000/12,000	350–100	3500	510	440	64	110	–0.5
P120	Amoco	>99 C	~80	2.17	10	2000	1900	2400	350	830	120	640	–1.45
K321	Mitsubishi Kasei	>99 C, trace N	...	1.90	10	1000 to 12,000	...	2000	290	176	26	...	...

RT, room temperature

respectively, into the fibers prior to pyrolysis in order to facilitate fiber densification during excursions to process temperatures greater than 1700 °C (3100 °F). In comparison to the pyrolyzed fibers, the final sintered fibers usually contain larger grains that are beneficial for improved fiber creep resistance and thermal conductivity. For the Sylramic fiber, creep and oxidation resistance are further improved when the boron sintering aids are reduced by a postprocess thermal treatment to form the Sylramic-iBN fiber that contains a thin in situ BN coating on the fiber surface (Ref 7).

Stoichiometric SiC fibers with high strength, thermal conductivity, and creep resistance can also be produced by the CVD route, which typically uses methyl-trichlorosilane to vapor deposit fine columnar-grained (~100 nm long) SiC onto a small-diameter (~30 μm) continuous-length carbon monofilament (Ref 1). Chemical vapor deposited-SiC fibers on small-diameter (~13 μm) tungsten monofilaments are also commercially available, but due to high-temperature reactions between the SiC and tungsten, these fibers are more suitable as reinforcement of metal-matrix composites for low- and intermediate-temperature applications. Although the CVD-SiC fibers have displayed very high strengths (~6000 MPa, or 900 ksi, for the Ultra SCS fiber), the final fibers are monofilaments with diameters greater than 50 μm. Laboratory attempts have been made to reduce their diameters and to produce multifilament tows, but issues exist concerning finding substrate filaments with the proper composition and diameter, methods for spreading these filaments during deposition to avoid fiber-to-fiber welding, and low-cost gas precursors for the CVD-SiC.

Fibers for High-Temperature CMC Applications

With increasing temperature, ceramic fiber properties such as elastic modulus and thermal conductivity decrease slowly in a monotonic manner, so that the room-temperature values for these properties in Tables 1 and 2 represent, in a relative manner, how these fiber types differ across a wide temperature range. Fiber strength follows the same trend of a slow monotonic decrease with temperature up to about 800 and 1000 °C (1500 and 1800 °F) for polycrystalline oxide and SiC-based fibers, respectively. However, above these temperatures, factors such as composition, grain size, impurity content, and prior thermostructural history have a significant impact on rate of fiber strength degradation with time and temperature. This strength behavior is typical of the time-dependent fracture of monolithic ceramics in which as-produced flaws grow slowly in size (slow crack growth) at elevated temperatures; whereas creep mechanisms aid in the more rapid growth of the same flaws or in the nucleation and growth of new microcracks and cavities at higher temperatures. Currently, pure and stoichiometric SiC fiber types with grain sizes of ~0.2 μm provide the best combination of low- and high-temperature tensile strength (Ref 6).

To better understand fiber thermostructural capability over a long time period, one can exam-

Table 3 1000 h upper-use temperatures for oxide-based ceramic fibers as estimated from single fiber creep-rupture results in air

Fiber	Fiber stress, 100 MPa (15 ksi)				Fiber stress, 500 MPa (75 ksi)			
	1% creep		Fiber fracture(a)		1% creep		Fiber fracture(a)	
	°C	°F	°C	°F	°C	°F	°C	°F
Alumina-silica types								
Nextel 312	...	...	750	1400	...	...	650	1200
Altex, Nextel 550	...	...	950	1750	800	1450	850	1550
α-alumina types								
Almax	900	1650	950	1750	NA	NA	800	1450
Nextel 610	950	1750	950	1750	850	1550	850	1550
Nextel 650	...	...	1000	1800	NA	NA	900	1650
Nextel 720	...	...	1100	2000	NA	NA	1000	1800
Saphikon	...	...	>1400	>2550	NA	NA	1250	2300

(a) For 25 mm (1 in.) gage length. Source: Ref 6–9

Table 4 1000 h upper-use temperatures for SiC-based ceramic fibers

Estimated from single fiber creep-rupture results in air and argon atmospheres

		Fiber stress, 100 MPa (15 ksi)				Fiber stress, 500 MPa (75 ksi)			
		1% creep		Fiber fracture(a)		1% creep		Fiber fracture(a)	
Fiber	Atmosphere	°C	°F	°C	°F	°C	°F	°C	°F
Nonstoichiometric types									
Tyranno Lox M	Air	1100	2000	1250	2300	<1000	<1800	1100	2000
Tyranno ZMI, Nicalon	Air	1150	2100	1300	2400	1000	1800	1100	2000
	Argon	1150	2100	1250	2300	1000	1800	1100	2000
Hi-Nicalon	Air	1300	2400	1350	2500	1150	2100	1200	2200
	Argon	1300	2400	1300	2400	1150	2100	1150	2100
Near-stoichiometric types									
Tyranno SA	Air	1350	2500	>1400	>2600	1150	2100	1150	2100
	Argon	1300	2400	1400	2600	NA	NA	1150	2100
Hi-Nicalon type S	Air	...	...	>1400	>2600	NA	NA	1150	2100
	Argon	NA	NA	1400	2600	NA	NA	1150	2100
Sylramic	Air	NA	NA	1350	2500	NA	NA	1150	2100
	Argon	NA	NA	1250	2300	NA	NA	1150	2100
Sylramic-iBN	Air	...	...	>1400	>2600	NA	NA	1300	2400
	Argon	NA	NA	1300	2400	NA	NA	1150	2100
Ultra SCS	Air	...	...	...	...	1350	2500	>1400	>2600

(a) For ~25 mm (1 in.) gage length. Source: Ref 6–9

ine literature data that show the effects of temperature, time, stress, and environment on the creep and fracture behavior of various fiber types of CMC interest (Ref 7–11). In general, the maximum temperature/time/stress capability of the more creep-prone fibers is limited by the fiber tendency to display excessive creep strains (>1%) before fracture. On the other hand, the temperature/time/stress capability of the more creep-resistant fibers is limited by fiber fracture at low creep strains (<1%), the values of which are often dependent on the environment. These limitations are illustrated in Tables 3 and 4, which show the approximate upper-use temperatures of some commercial oxide and SiC fibers, respectively, as determined from simple stress-rupture measurements on single fibers. These upper-use temperatures were determined by using the available data for fiber creep and fracture time versus stress and temperature, and the assumption that the maximum temperature-limiting condition occurred either when the fiber creep strain exceeded 1% in 1000 hours or when the fiber fractured in 1000 hours. Fiber stresses of 100 and 500 MPa (15 and 70 ksi) were assumed, which are typical of the range of stresses experienced by fibers within structural CMC. A "not applicable" (NA) notation in the tables indicates that the more creep-resistant fibers fractured before reaching a creep strain of 1%. Figure 1 compares the estimated 1000 h upper-use temperatures for all the ceramic fibers based on single fiber fracture as measured at 500 MPa (70 ksi) in air.

For the oxide fibers tested in air, Table 3 shows Nextel 312 has the lowest thermostructural capability due to its high content of noncrystalline phases. The maximum capability of the Altex and Nextel 550 fibers, both alumina-silica fibers, and the α-Al_2O_3 Nextel 610 and Almax fibers are similar; while Nextel 650 fiber and Nextel 720 fiber display the best thermostructural capability of all the commercially available polycrystalline types. Nextel 650 fiber, which contains yttria-stabilized zirconia as a second phase, benefits primarily from the Y^{3+} dopant, which has been shown to slow diffusion and creep in Al_2O_3 (Ref 12, 13). Nextel 720 fiber, on the other hand, benefits from a high content of mullite, a highly creep-resistant oxide compound, and from a unique crystalline structure of interpenetrating phases that reduces creep by grain boundary sliding (Ref 14). The highest-performing oxide fiber is the Saphikon single crystal fiber, which has no measurable creep in the *c*-axis orientation below 1400 °C (2600 °F), but suffers from high-temperature diffusion-controlled crack growth (Ref 9).

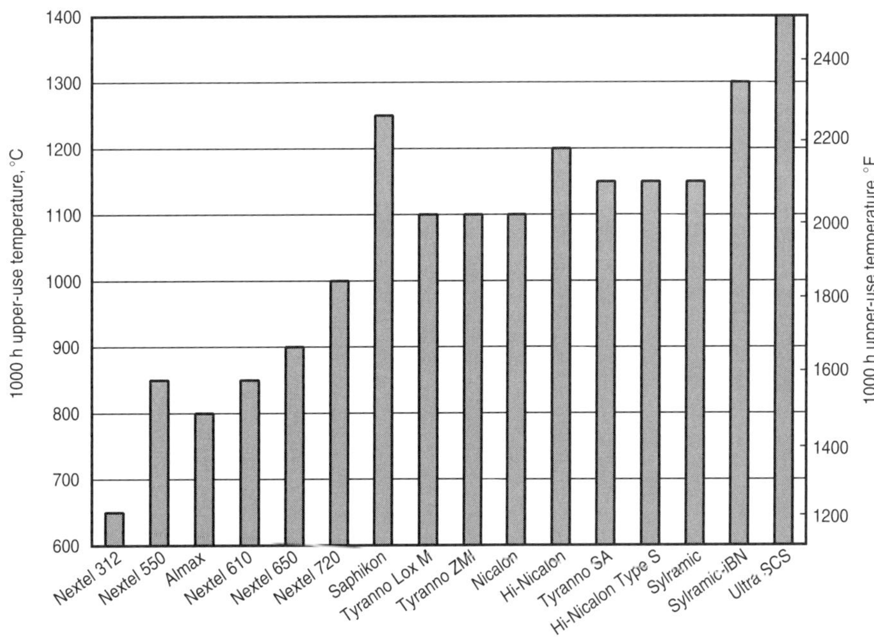

Fig. 1 Estimated 1000 h upper-use temperatures for small- and large-diameter ceramic fibers based on the fracture of single fibers measured at 500 MPa (70 ksi) in air at 25 mm (1 in.) gage length

Table 4 shows the approximate upper-use temperatures for commercial SiC fibers as determined from single fiber testing up to 1400 °C (2600 °F) under air and argon environments. These upper-use temperatures, when compared to those of Table 3, clearly indicate the greater thermostructural capability of the SiC fibers over the oxide-based fibers (see also Fig. 1). Although the stoichiometric and purer SiC fiber types display the best capability, some of these fiber types display better behavior in air than argon, with the Sylramic fiber types showing the largest difference. The improved capability in air can be attributed in part to a measurable reduction in intrinsic creep rate for some fiber types (Ref 7), and in part to the formation of a thin silica layer on the fiber surface. This layer minimizes vaporization of thermally unstable phases and, by blunting surface flaws, increases the creep-rupture strain of all fiber types by ~100%. For CMC service under oxidizing conditions, this environmental effect can be important, because air may be the effective fiber environment if the CMC matrix is cracked and inert gas the environment if the matrix is uncracked. Another important observation from Tables 3 and 4 and Fig. 1 is that the fracture-limited upper-use temperatures of the more creep-resistant fibers are not measurably better than those of their more creep-prone counterpart fibers; for example, compare Nextel 650 versus Nextel 610, Hi-Nicalon type S versus Hi-Nicalon, and Tyranno SA versus Tyranno Lox M.

Future Directions

Because of their low atomic diffusion and high thermal conductivity, pure stoichiometric

SiC fibers are the preferred reinforcement for CMC products that are required to operate for long times at temperatures greater than state of the art metal alloys (>1100 °C, or 2000 °F). While reduction in production costs and improvement in high-temperature thermal conductivity and fracture life are high-priority developmental issues for future SiC-based fibers, another important issue is improvement of the fiber surfaces against oxygen attack. In this area, possibilities exist for the development of oxidation-resistant fiber coatings that are deposited on tows after fiber processing, or better yet in terms of cost reduction, are formed in situ during fiber production or service. Some of the developmental fibers, such as the Hi-Nicalon-type fibers coated with CVD-BN from Nippon Carbon (Ref 15) and the in situ BN-coated fibers from the University of Florida (Ref 16) and Bayer Company (Ref 17), are moving in these directions. These coating approaches should also be beneficial for reducing fiber abrasion and strength degradation during the complex weaving and braiding processes typically needed for some CMC products.

Although the creep resistance of oxide fibers is inferior to SiC-based fibers, recently developed oxide fibers have demonstrated adequate creep resistance for use in structural composites up to 1100 °C (2000 °F). Further increases in temperature capability are possible. The use of dopants (e.g., Y^{3+} in Nextel 650 fibers) has been shown to provide a promising route to improved high-temperature capability in oxide fibers. Another fertile area for research is the development of fine-grained, fully crystalline fibers of creep-resistant multicomponent oxides such as yttrium-aluminum-garnet (YAG) and mullite. Both YAG and mullite fibers have been developed at several laboratories (Ref 8, 18) and have exhibited even better creep resistance than Nextel 720 fibers. The advantages of environmental stability and low cost will continue to provide incentive for further improvements in high-temperature properties of oxide fibers.

REFERENCES

1. *Composites,* Vol 1, *Engineered Materials Handbook*, ASM International, 1987, p 58–65
2. J.A. DiCarlo and S. Dutta, Continuous Ceramic Fibers for Ceramic Composites, *Handbook On Continuous Fiber Reinforced Ceramic Matrix Composites,* R. Lehman, S. El-Rahaiby, and J. Wachtman, Jr., Ed., CIAC, Purdue University, West Lafayette, Indiana, 1995, p 137–183
3. "Ceramic Fibers and Coatings," National Materials Advisory Board, Publication NMAB-494, National Academy Press, Washington, D.C., 1998
4. A.R. Bunsell and M.H. Berger, *Fine Ceramic Fibers*, Marcel Dekker, New York, 1999
5. H. Ichikawa and T. Ishikawa, Silicon Carbide Fibers (Organometallic Pyrolysis), *Comprehensive Composite Materials*, Vol 1, A. Kelly, C. Zweben, and T. Chou, Ed., Elsevier Science Ltd., Oxford, England, 2000, p 107–145
6. J.A. DiCarlo and H.M. Yun, Microstructural Factors Affecting Creep-Rupture Failure of Ceramic Fibers and Composites, *Ceramic Transactions,* Vol 99, 1998, p 119–134
7. H.M. Yun and J.A. DiCarlo, Comparison of the Tensile, Creep, and Rupture Strength Properties of Stoichiometric SiC Fibers, *Cer. Eng. Sci. Proc.,* Vol 20 (No. 3), 1999, p 259–272
8. R.E. Tressler and J.A. DiCarlo, High Temperature Mechanical Properties of Advanced Ceramic Fibers, *Proceedings of HT-CMC-1*, R. Naslain, J. Lamon, and D. Doumeingts, Ed., Woodland Publishing, Ltd., Cambridge, England, 1993, p 33–49
9. R.E. Tressler and J.A. DiCarlo, Creep and Rupture of Advanced Ceramic Reinforcements, *Proceedings of HT-CMC-2*, *Ceramic Transactions,* Vol 57, 1995, p 141–155
10. H.M. Yun and J.A. DiCarlo, Time/Temperature Dependent Tensile Strength of SiC and Al_2O_3-Based Fibers, *Ceramic Transactions,* Vol 74, 1996, p 17–26
11. H.M. Yun, NASA Glenn Research Center, Creep-Rupture Behavior of Tyranno SiC Fibers, private communication, 1997
12. D.M. Wilson and L.R. Visser, Nextel™ 650 Ceramic Oxide Fiber: New Alumina-Based Fiber for High Temperature Composite Reinforcement, *Cer. Eng. Sci. Proc.,* Vol 21 (No. 4), 2000, p 363–373
13. J. Bruley, J. Cho, H.M. Chan, M.P. Harmer, and J.M. Rickman, Scanning Transmission Electron Microscopy Analysis of Grain Boundaries in Creep-Resistant Yttrium-And Lanthanum-Doped Alumina Microstructures, *J. Am. Ceram. Soc.,* Vol 82, 1999, p 2865–2870
14. D.M. Wilson, S.L. Lieder, and D.C. Lueneburg, Microstructure and High Temperature Properties of Nextel 720 Fibers, *Cer. Eng. Sci. Proc.,* Vol 16 (No. 5), 1995, p 1005–1014
15. H. Ichikawa, Nippon Carbon Company, private communication, 2000
16. M.D. Sacks and J.J. Brennan, Silicon Fibers with Boron Nitride Coatings, *Cer. Eng. Sci. Proc.,* Vol 21 (No. 4), 2000, p 275–281
17. P. Baldus, M. Jansen, and D. Sporn, Ceramic Fibers for Matrix Composites in High-Temperature Engine Applications, *Science,* Vol 285, 1999, p 699–703
18. M.H. Lewis, A. Tye, E.G. Butler, and P.A. Doleman, Oxide CMCs: Interphase Synthesis and Novel Fibre Development, *J. Europ. Ceram. Soc.,* Vol 20, 2000, p 639–644

Discontinuous Reinforcements for Metal-Matrix Composites

Cory A. Smith, DWA Aluminum Composites

DISCONTINUOUSLY REINFORCED METAL-MATRIX COMPOSITES (DRMMCs) are commonly used today in many aerospace and industrial applications. They offer a wide range of attractive material properties, both mechanical and physical, that cannot be achieved using conventional engineering alloys. These enhanced materials properties are the direct result of the interaction between the metallic matrix and the reinforcement. This article focuses on the production of particulate reinforcements used in DRMMC materials systems, their physical and materials properties, and the particle shape and overall morphology.

Reinforcement Roles

In a DRMMC materials system, the reinforcement strengthens the metal matrix both extrinsically, by load transfer to the ceramic reinforcement, and intrinsically, by increasing dislocation density (Ref 1). The interaction between the particulate reinforcement and the metallic matrix is the basis for the enhanced physical and materials properties associated with DRMMC materials systems. Composite materials properties can be tailored to meet specific engineering requirements by selecting a particular reinforcement and varying the amount added to the metal matrix. In this fashion, the physical and mechanical properties of the composite materials system can be controlled with some independence. Increasing the reinforcement volume in a composite system increases mechanical properties, such as elastic modulus, ultimate strength, and yield strength, while reducing the thermal expansion and, in some cases, the density of the composite system. Unfortunately materials properties such as ductility and fracture toughness typically decrease with increasing reinforcement volume.

The increase in both the elastic modulus and strength (ultimate and yield) is believed to be due to the difference in thermal expansion between the ceramic reinforcement particles and the metallic matrix during processing. During the production of these composites, both the reinforcement and matrix are heated to processing temperature, brought to thermomechanical equilibrium, and then allowed to cool. The thermal contraction of the metallic matrix during cooldown is typically much greater than that of the reinforcement, which leads to a geometric mismatch. At the ceramic-metal interface, this geometrical disparity creates mismatch strains that are relieved by the generation of dislocations in the matrix originating from sharp features on the ceramic reinforcement.

Discontinuously reinforced metal-matrix composite materials systems are commonly used in applications that require high specific materials properties, enhanced fatigue resistance, improved wear resistance, controlled expansion, or the ability to absorb neutron radiation (boron carbide). Additionally, DRMMC may be designed to yield a materials system that offers multiple roles. Some examples of multiple roles are DRMMC materials systems that offer high strength and fatigue resistance for aerospace and mechanical applications, thermal management coupled with expansion control for space-borne applications, moderate strength and neutron absorption capabilities for nuclear applications, high strength and wear resistance for heavy equipment applications, and impact/energy dissipation for armor applications. The correct selection of reinforcement is very important in yielding desired resultant materials properties. An improper reinforcement selection may lead to less-than-desirable composite materials properties, difficulty in fabrication of end product, and high cost.

DRMMC Reinforcements

The most common DRMMC materials systems used for current aerospace structural applications are silicon carbide (SiC) and boron carbide (B_4C) particulate reinforcement in an aluminum alloy matrix. Aluminum oxide particles are a lower-cost alternative most commonly used for casting applications. Titanium carbide is being investigated for high-temperature applications. Table 1 lists the mechanical and physical properties of various ceramic reinforcements commonly used in the manufacture of modern DRMMC materials systems. Table 2 lists the characteristics for commonly used reinforcements.

Silicon Carbide. Discontinuously reinforced metal-matrix composite materials systems based on SiC are the most commonly used and most mature at this time. The benefits of using SiC as reinforcement are improved stiffness, strength, thermal conductivity, wear resistance, fatigue resistance, and reduced thermal expansion. Additionally, SiC reinforcements are typically low-cost and are relatively low-density. Figure 1 shows the size distributions for commonly used SiC grits ranging from F1500 to F360. The "F" nomenclature is defined by Federation of the European Producers of Abrasives (FEPA) standards, which govern abrasive grit-size distributions in Europe.

The production of SiC was first reported by Berzelius in 1810 and again in 1821. It was later rediscovered during various electrothermal ex-

Table 1 Mechanical and physical properties of various ceramic particulate reinforcements commonly used in the manufacture of modern discontinuously reinforced metal-matrix composites

Ceramic	Density, g/cm^3	Elastic modulus		Knoop hardness	Compressive strength		Thermal conductivity		Coefficient of thermal expansion		Specific thermal conductivity, $W \cdot m^2/kg \cdot K$
		GPa	10^6 psi		MPa	ksi	$W/m \cdot K$	$Btu \cdot ft/h \cdot ft^2 \cdot °F$	$10^{-6}/K$	$10^{-6}/°F$	
SiC	3.21	430	62.4	2480	2800	406.1	132	76.6	3.4	6.1	41.1
B_4C	2.52	450	65.3	2800	3000	435.1	29	16.8	5.0	9.0	11.5
Al_2O_3	3.92	350	50.8	2000	2500	362.6	32.6	18.9	6.8	12.2	8.3
TiC	4.93	345	50.0	2150	2500	362.6	20.5	11.9	7.4	13.3	4.2

periments by Despretz in 1849 and Marsden in 1881. However, Acheson was the first to recognize its potential industrial importance. Acheson applied electric current through a mixture of powdered coke and clay and found that the carbon electrode was covered in hard, shiny crystals. Acheson later discovered that these crystals had much better abrasive properties than the emery powder that was in general use at the time.

Table 2 Characteristics of commonly used reinforcements

Relative size	FEPA grit size	Particle diameter (d_{50}), μm (μin.)	Advantages	Limitations
Particulate reinforcements				
Fine	F1500	1.7 (68)	Greatest strength and stiffness contribution	Tendency to agglomerate
	F800	6.5 (260)	Highest fatigue resistance	Blending difficulty (powder/casting)
			Lowest resultant coefficient of thermal expansion	Lowered ductility
				High cost
				Segregation during casting common
Medium	F600	9.3 (370)	Excellent balance between properties (elevated strength and good ductility) and ease of manufacturing	Necessary for high-volume reinforcement systems
	F360	22.8 (9120)		Good balance between properties and raw material costs
				Good balance between manufacturing ease and resultant ductility
Coarse	F12	1700 (0.068 in.)	Good wear resistance	Lowest benefit to resultant properties
			High ductility and ease of manufacturing	
			Great for armor applications	
Whisker reinforcements				
Fine (submicron)	...	...	Highest resultant properties in the fiber direction	Highly anisotropic resultant properties
Coarse	...	...		Greatly affected by damage (fracture) during processing
				High cost
				Difficult to process
Spheres and low-aspect-ratio shapes				
Fine (micron range) glass microspheres	...	...	Greatly lowers density	...
Coarse (inch range) aluminum oxide or zirconium oxide	...	...	Good for wear resistance and armor applications	...

FEPA, Federation of the European Producers of Abrasives

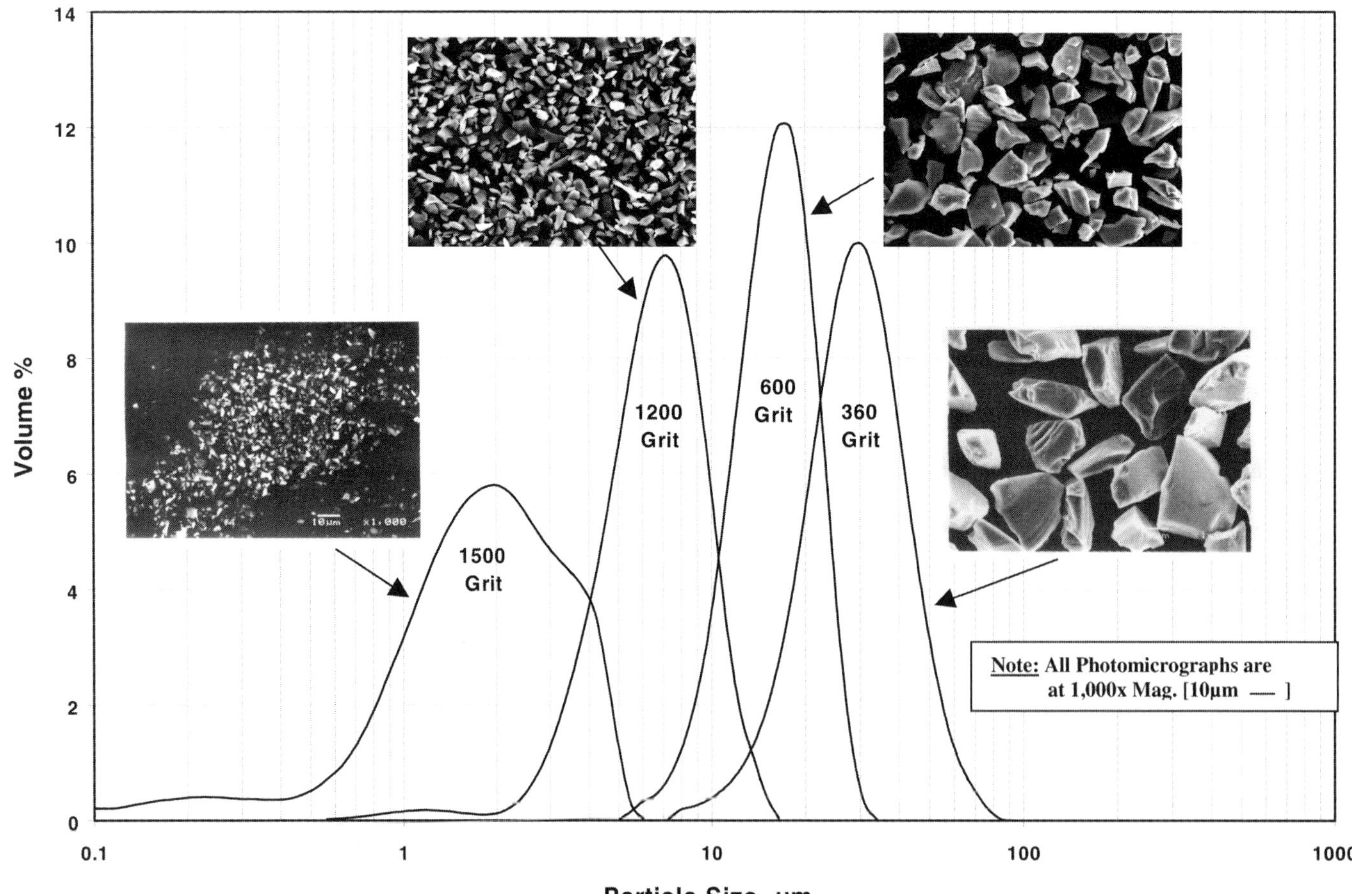

Fig. 1 Variation in particle size distribution and morphology as a function of grit size for F1500, F1200, F600, and F360 grit SiC powders

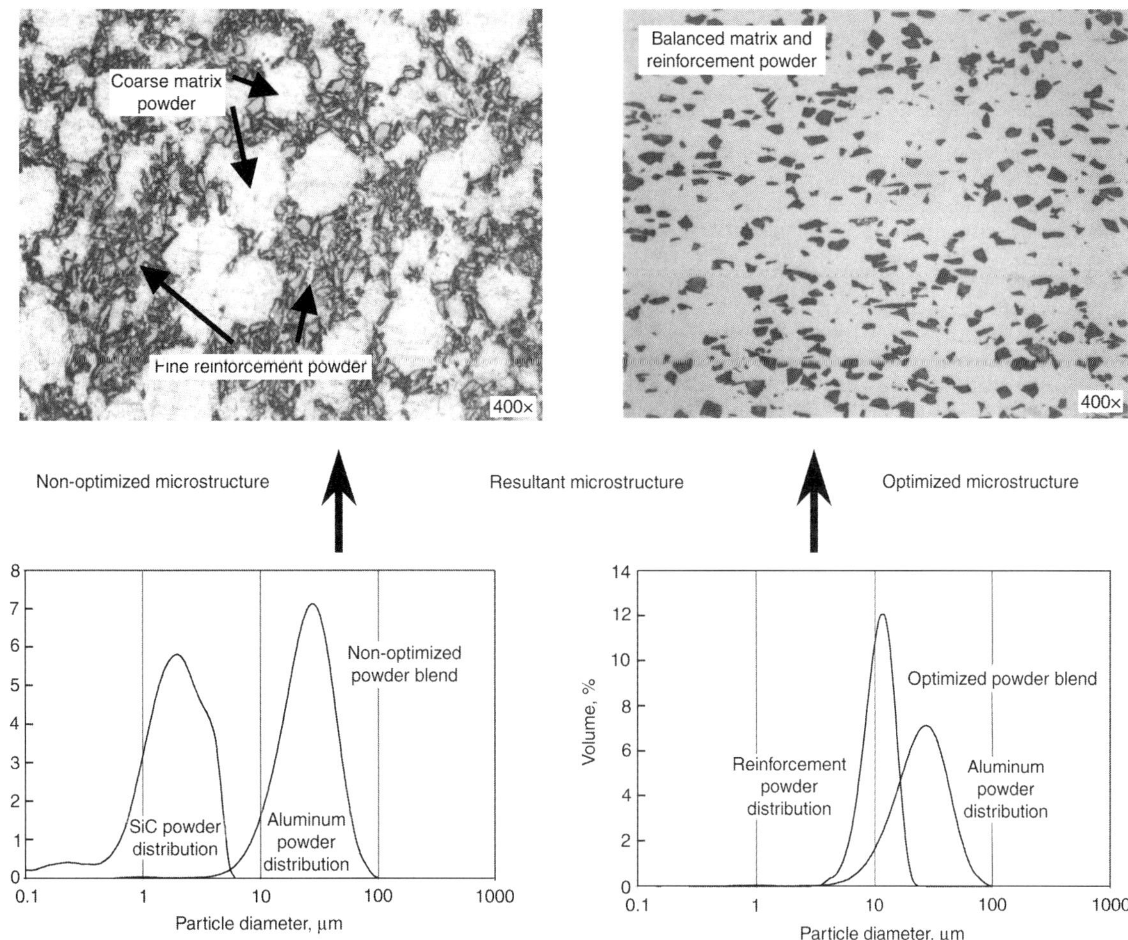

Fig. 2 Effect of microstructure optimization for 20 vol% SiC discontinuously reinforced aluminum metal-matrix composites

As a result, he founded the Carborundum Company in 1891 for the production of SiC. An important development in the production of SiC in resistance furnaces came in 1972 to 1974, when Elektroschmelzwerk Kempten (ESK) developed a furnace that collected reaction-produced gases and used them for energy production and, in doing so, contributed to environmental protection (Ref 2).

Silicon carbide is produced industrially from silicon dioxide and carbon, which reacts as follows:

$$SiO_2 + 3C \rightarrow SiO + 2CO \quad \text{(Eq 1)}$$

The reaction is strongly endothermic, with the enthalpy change, $\Delta H = 618.5$ kJ/mol (4.28 kW · h/kg) (Ref 3). The reaction takes place in several stages:

$$SiO_2 + C \rightarrow SiO + CO \quad \text{(Eq 2)}$$

The initiation reaction follows Eq 2 and is thermodynamically possible above 1700 °C (3100 °F), beginning when the SiO_2 melts. The next stages are:

$$SiO + C \rightarrow Si + CO \quad \text{(Eq 3)}$$

$$Si + CO \rightarrow SiC \quad \text{(Eq 4)}$$

The SiC is formed as an encrustation on the carbon grains, ultimately causing the reaction to cease. The SiC then further reacts:

$$SiC + 2SiO \rightarrow 3SiO + CO \quad \text{(Eq 5)}$$

$$SiC + SiO \leftrightarrow 2Si(g) + CO \quad \text{(Eq 6)}$$

where Eq 6 is the equilibrium reaction and is mainly responsible for the formation of large SiC crystals. The yield and quality of the SiC are seriously affected by any impurities present in the raw materials. Therefore, high-purity raw materials must be used.

Particle size and shape are important factors in determining materials properties. Fatigue strength is greatly improved with the use of fine particles, and the uniform distribution of reinforcement is improved by matching the size of the reinforcement to the size of the matrix particles. Figure 2 illustrates the benefit to uniformity of particle distribution of selecting the proper reinforcement size for the matrix powder being used. Figure 3 summarizes the effect of

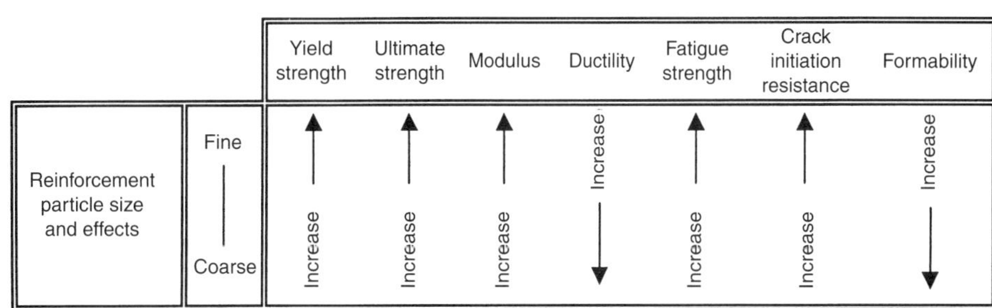

Fig. 3 Materials properties and formability as a function of reinforcement particle size

variation in particle size on several composite properties.

The shape of a particle is characterized by its aspect ratio, the ratio of its longest to shortest linear dimension. Most ceramic reinforcement particles have a low aspect ratio, being blocky with sharp edges. They are easy to produce by simple milling and therefore comparatively inexpensive, yielding composites with approximately isotropic properties. Whiskers and platelets are particles with higher aspect ratios. Figure 4 shows a high-aspect-ratio SiC particle. Although they are typically more expensive and harder to work with than the blocky particles, high-aspect-ratio particles are used when anisotropic properties are desired, concentrating the benefits of the reinforcement into a limited direction.

Boron carbide is a commonly used reinforcement when low composite density is important, when low reactivity with the matrix is needed, and when neutron absorption is required. Figure 5 shows the morphology for B_4C particulates at 1000× (Fig. 5a) and at 5000× (Fig. 5b). When anisotropic composite properties are necessary, B_4C whiskers are used (Fig. 6). This form is expensive and rarely used. Some naturally occurring boron atoms (B^{10}) have a high neutron-absorption cross-section area. Consequently, B_4C, having four boron atoms per structural unit, is an important reinforcement for use in nuclear containment applications. Boron carbide is more inert in the presence of aluminum at high temperatures than is SiC. Its nonreactivity makes it more suitable for applications involving welding or casting.

The large-scale production of B_4C is based on the carbothermic reaction of boric acid:

$$2B_2O_3 + 7C \rightarrow B_4C + 6CO \qquad \text{(Eq 7)}$$

The reaction is strongly endothermic, producing 1812 kJ/mol (9.1 kW · h/kg), and is usually carried out at 1500 to 2500 °C (2700 to 4500 °F) in an electric furnace, as in the case of SiC. The starting mixture is an intimate mixture of boric acid and carbon (petroleum coke or graphite). Large quantities of carbon monoxide (2.3 m^3/kg) are generated, and boron can be lost to evaporation of boric acid at high temperatures. In an electrothermic process used by ESK, the product is cooled and the unreacted outer-zone material is removed to leave a fused coarse-grained B_4C of high purity. This B_4C is obtained in the form of regular blocks, which are broken up and milled to produce the B_4C grain size appropriate for final use. Additionally, B_4C of high purity is produced by other methods. These include the magnesiothermic reaction of magnesium and boric acid in the presence of carbon:

$$2B_2O_3 + 6Mg + C \rightarrow B_4C + 6MgO \qquad \text{(Eq 8)}$$

synthesis from elements:

$$(4 + x)B + C \rightarrow B_{4+x}C + C \qquad \text{(Eq 9)}$$

the reduction of boron trichloride by hydrogen in the presence of carbon:

$$4BCl_3 + 6H_2 + C \rightarrow B_4C + 12HCl \qquad \text{(Eq 10)}$$

and by chemical vapor deposition:

$$4BCl_3(BBr_2) + CH_4 \rightarrow B_4C + 12HCl(Br) \qquad \text{(Eq 11)}$$

The B_4C whiskers shown in Fig. 6 were produced by chemical vapor deposition.

Aluminum oxide particulate is another ceramic powder commonly used in reinforcement of DRMMC materials systems. The resultant benefits are not as great as some of the previously mentioned reinforcements, that is, SiC and B_4C. Aluminum oxide (Al_2O_3) reinforcement

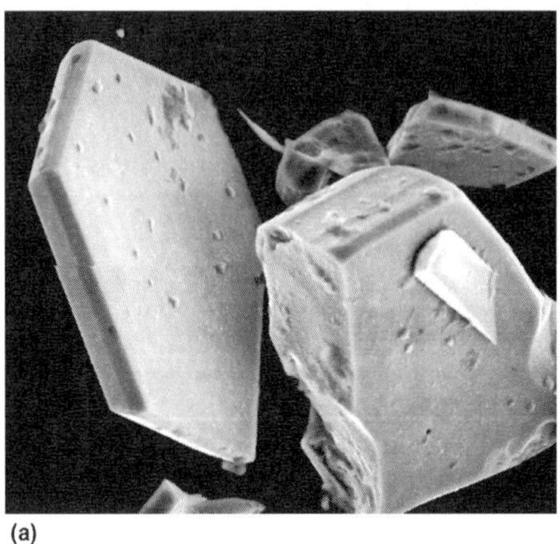

(a)

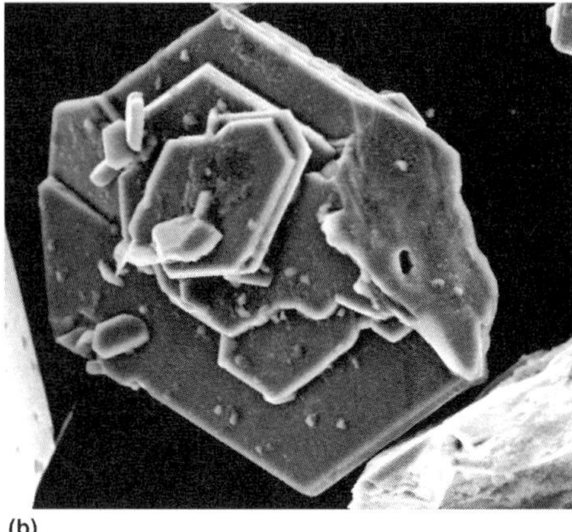

(b)

Fig. 4 Silicon carbide platelet reinforcement showing the basal plane morphology in the β phase. 1000×

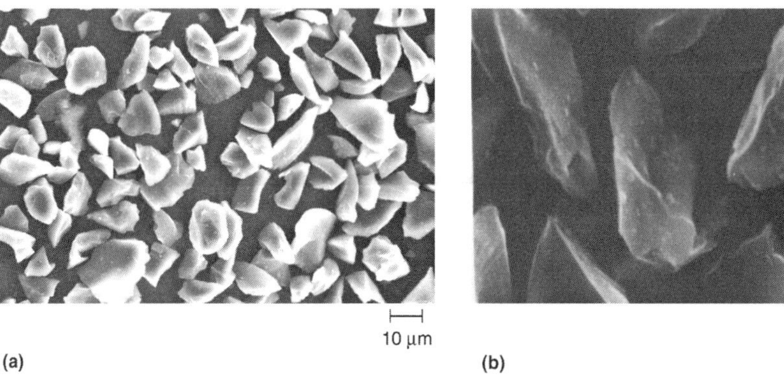

Fig. 5 Inherent morphology of B_4C particulate. (a) 1000×. (b) 5000×

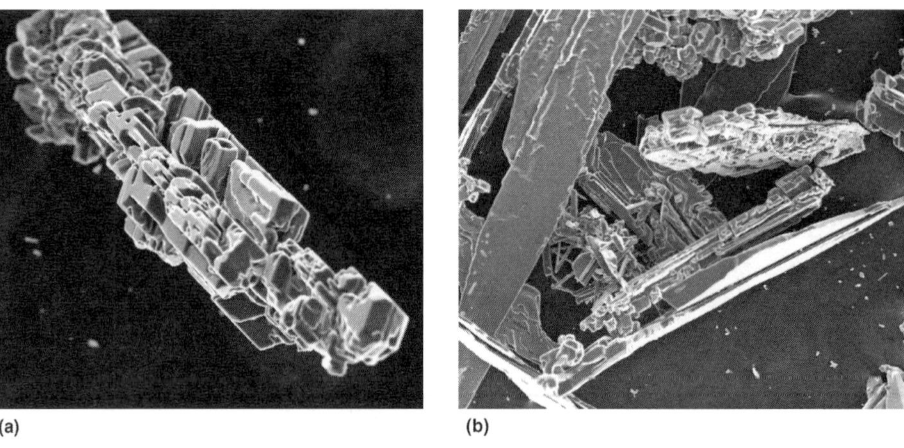

Fig. 6 Boron carbide whisker reinforcement, showing polycrystalline microstructure for different whisker morphologies. (a) 200×. (b) 100×

powders possess very low reactivity in molten metal baths (casting) and are relativity low-cost. The resultant composite properties, such as stiffness, strength, and fracture toughness, are not as high as those of either the SiC or B_4C reinforcement. However, the low reactivity and low cost make this reinforcement very attractive for the production of cast metal-matrix composites (MMCs) that require moderate strengths and stiffness improvements while retaining good wear resistance.

Titanium carbide (TiC) is not a widely used ceramic reinforcement powder. However, its inherent high-temperature stability is attractive for use in elevated-temperature applications, where high strength, stiffness, and creep resistance are required. This reinforcement is used primarily in titanium- and nickel-base alloy MMC materials systems that require stability at very high temperatures (up to 1100 °C, or 2000 °F). In these applications, all previously discussed reinforcements would rapidly react into brittle intermetallics, leading to less-than-desirable MMC properties. The use of this reinforcement comes at a price: TiC is very dense when compared to SiC, B_4C, and Al_2O_3 and, as a result, tends to be used only when very demanding high-temperature composites are necessary. The tensile strength of 20 vol% TiC in a matrix of nickel-base 718 alloy has been shown by DWA Aluminum Composites to be greatly improved over that of the monolithic 718 alloy between temperatures of 650 and 1100 °C (1200 and 2000 °F). It is also believed by current investigators to provide enhanced creep resistance. Iron-base materials systems reinforced with TiC are the best candidates for extrusion dies, where extremely high strength and wear resistance are necessary at elevated temperatures, such as extrusion of DRMMC materials systems.

Reinforcement Chemistry

When designing DRMMC materials systems, care must be taken to distinguish between the bulk chemistry and the surface chemistry of the reinforcement. The bulk chemistry describes the crystalline interior and controls the overall resultant materials properties. Typically, higher-purity ceramic powder yields higher composite performance, usually with higher raw material costs. In the case of surface chemistry, the composite designer must consider the contribution of incidental elemental additions to the overall DRMMC system. For example, SiC powders typically possess both silicon dioxide (SiO_2) and elemental silicon (Si) on their surfaces. If the concentration of these two species is high enough, the targeted DRMMCs chemistry may exceed alloy composition limits. Boron carbide reinforcements are affected in the same manner with contributions of free carbon, boron, and boric acid. The same is true for most available ceramic reinforcements widely used today.

ACKNOWLEDGMENTS

The author wishes to thank Behzad Bavarian, California State University, Northridge, Roman Kurth, ESK-SiC GmbH, and Tim Loftin, DWA Aluminum Composites.

REFERENCES

1. R.W. Hertzberg, *Deformation and Fracture Mechanics of Engineering Materials,* 3rd ed., John Wiley & Sons, 1989
2. K. Liethschmidt, ESK GmbH, Werk Grefrath, Frechen, Federal Republic of Germany, Ullmann's Encyclopedia of Industrial Chemicals, Vol A 23, VCH Publishers, 1993
3. JANAF Thermochemical Tables, 2nd ed., National Standard Reference Data Series, National Bureau of Standards, June 1971

Continuous Fiber Reinforcements for Metal-Matrix Composites

Colin McCullough, 3M Company, Electrical Products Division

FOR THE REINFORCEMENT of metal-matrix composites (MMCs), four general classes of materials are commercially available: oxide fibers based primarily on alumina and alumina-silica systems, nonoxide systems based on silicon carbide, boron fibers, and carbon fibers. Two general fiber forms are available: tow-based fibers that are typically small diameter (<20 μm) multifilament rovings or tows and monofilaments that are generally large diameter. The final choice of fiber for any composite system is governed not only by performance aspects, but also by the compatibility of the fiber with the matrix metal, the composite fabrication process, the handling character of the fiber and the mechanical requirements of the fiber/matrix interface. Note that metal fibers such as steel and tungsten are also used for reinforcing metals, but that in this article the topic is limited to nonmetallic fibers.

Composite applications take advantage of various properties of the fiber. The most common are high tensile strength, high tensile modulus, low coefficient of thermal expansion, and low density. The four general classes of fibers are discussed in the sections that follow.

Aluminum Oxide Fibers

Today the most common approach for producing polycrystalline tow-based ceramic fibers is by spinning and heat treating chemically derived precursors, which in the case of oxide fibers are sol-gel precursors. The use of chemical precursor technology allows the commercial preparation of ceramic fibers with properties not accessible by traditional fiber-forming technology, such as spinning of molten glasses. Traditional slurry processing methods can also be used to spin fibers (Almax, FP). A key characteristic of ceramic fibers is their ultrafine microstructure with grain sizes sometimes in the nanometer range. Fine grains are required for good tensile strength (>2 GPa, or 290 ksi). These processes also allow fiber production in the form of continuous-length multifilament tows or rovings, which are typically coated with a thin polymer-based sizing and then supplied to customers on spools. These sized tows are flexible and easily handled so that they can be woven or braided into fabrics, tapes, sleeves, and other complex shapes. Most small-diameter fiber manufacturers also supply fibers in fabric form. Further discussion of these tow-based alumina fibers can be found in the article "Ceramic Fibers" in this Volume.

Monofilament alumina is available as a 125 μm diam single-crystal fiber, which is grown directly from the molten oxide (Ref 1). This fiber has been studied for reinforcing some of the intermetallic-matrix composites such as titanium aluminides and nickel aluminides (Ref 1).

Key properties of commercially available fibers are listed in Table 1. Tow-based alumina fibers are used extensively for aluminum alloy reinforcement, and while generally nonreactive with molten aluminum there is the danger of a degrading reaction with alloying elements in some aluminum alloys (e.g., those containing magnesium) (Ref 2). These fibers are used principally where low density, high tensile and compression strengths, and high stiffness are desired in the composite. Additionally, good off-axis properties result from the strong bonding between aluminum and alumina, and the chemical stability of the fiber aids in producing good elevated-temperature properties (Ref 3).

Silicon Carbide Fibers

For fibers based on silicon carbide (SiC), the most common approach for producing polycrystalline tow-based ceramic fibers is by spinning and heat treating chemically derived precursors based on polymer precursors. As with the alumina-based tow materials, fine grain sizes are produced that promote high strength, and the ability to make multifilament rovings permits woven, braided, and fabric fiber forms. The multifilament form of SiC has been used to reinforce aluminum alloys (Ref 4). Further discussion of these tow-based fibers can be found in the article "Ceramic Fibers" in this Volume.

There are also commercially available forms of monofilament SiC. These are made using a continuous chemical deposition process in which a mixture of hydrogen and chlorinated alkyl silanes are reacted at the surface of a heated substrate wire. The substrate (fiber core) can be either tungsten or a spun carbon filament (see Table 2). The bulk fiber then consists of fine-grained β-SiC. Key properties are listed in Table 1. These fibers are used principally to reinforce titanium alloys where the low density, high tensile strength, high stiffness, and elevated-temperature capability offer the potential of great weight savings in high-speed-rotating jet-engine structures. However, to promote good load sharing between fibers in the composite and thus a high tensile strength, a low-strength, lubricious fiber coating is needed to create a "weakly bonded" interface system and additionally to act as a protective diffusion barrier. Table 2 summarizes the coatings for the SiC monofilaments.

Boron Fibers

Boron fibers are made using chemical vapor deposition. A fine tungsten wire provides a substrate, and boron trichloride gas is the boron source. Continuous production provides for boron filaments of 100 and 140 μm diameter. Key properties are listed in Table 1. Boron fibers have been used principally in reinforcing aluminum alloys where low density, high tensile and compression strengths, and high stiffness result. The bare fiber may be used with solid-state composite forming, but with liquid processing routes the fiber needs to be coated with either B_4C or SiC in order to eliminate reaction with the fiber and the accompanying loss of fiber properties. More expansive coverage of these fibers is provided in the article "Ceramic Fibers" in this Volume.

Carbon Fibers

Two classes of carbon fiber, polyacrylonitrile (PAN) and pitch-based fibers, derive quite dif-

Table 1 Commercial fibers for reinforcement of metal-matrix composites

Tradename (manufacturer)	Composition	Average grain size, nm	Density, g/cm^3	Average diameter, μm	Tow count	Current cost, (<5 kg), \$/kg	Average tensile strength at room temperature		Tensile modulus at room temperature		Axial thermal conductivity at room temperature, W/m · K	Thermal expansion, ppm/°C (to 1000 °C)
							GPa	ksi	GPa	10^6 psi		
Alumina-silica-based fibers												
Altex (Sumitomo)	85% Al_2O_3 + 15% SiO_2	25	3.3	15	500, 1000	330–550	2.0	290	210	30	...	7.9
Nextel 312 (3M)	62% Al_2O_3 + 24% SiO_2 + 14% B_2O_3	<500	2.7	10–12	420, 780	90–230	1.7	247	150	22	...	3
Nextel 440 (3M)	70% Al_2O_3 + 28% SiO_2 + 2% B_2O_3	<500	3.05	10–12	420, 780	380–490	2.0	290	190	28	...	5.3
α-alumina-based fibers												
Almax (Mitsui Mining)	99.5% Al_2O_3	600	3.6	10	1,000	815	1.8	260	330	48	...	8.8
Nextel 610 (3M)	>99% Al_2O_3	100	3.9	12	420, 780, 2600	330–660	3.1	450	373	54	...	7.9
Saphikon (Saphikon)	100% Al_2O_3	Single	3.98	125	Monofilament	50,000	3.5	507	460	67	...	9
Boron-based fibers												
Boron (Textron Specialty Materials)	Boron	2	2.57 2.50	100 140	Monofilament	700	3.6	522	400	58	...	4.5
SiC-based fibers												
Nicalon, NL200 (Nippon Carbon)	Si-C-O, 10 O	2	2.55	14	500	2,000	3.0	435	220	32	3	3.2
Hi-Nicalon (Nippon Carbon)	SiC, 30 C, 0.5 O	4	2.74	14	500	8,000	2.8	406	270	39	8	3.5
Hi-Nicalon-S (Nippon Carbon)	SiC, 0.2 O	20	3.05	13	500	13,000	2.5	363	400–420	58–61	18	...
Tyranno Lox M (Ube Industries)	Si-Ti-C-O, 10 O, 2 Ti	1	2.48	11	400, 800	1,500/1,000	3.3	479	187	27		3.1
Tyranno SA 1-3 (Ube Industries)	SiC, 0.3 O, <2 Al	100 to >200	3.02	10–7.5	800, 1,600	5000	2.8	406	375	54	65	...
Sylramic (Dow Corning)	SiC, 3 TiB_2, 2 B	150	3.05	10	800	10,000	3.2	464	400	58	46	5.4
SCS-6, SCS-9 (Textron Specialty Materials)	SiC, trace Si/trace C	100 × 10	3.0 2.8	140	Monofilament	9,000	3.5	507	380 290	55 42	70	4.6
Ultra SCS (Textron Specialty Materials)	SiC, trace Si/trace C	100 × 10	3.0	140	Monofilament	9,000	6.2	900	410	59	70	4.6
Trimarc (Atlantic Research Corp.)	SiC, trace Si/trace C	...	3.3	125	Monofilament	...	3.5	507	425	62	...	...
Sigma 1140, 1240 (DERA)	SiC, trace Si/trace C	...	3.4	100	Monofilament	...	3.5	507	400	58	...	...
Carbon-based fibers												
T300 (Amoco)	92 C, 8 N	2	1.76	7	1,000–12,000	250–100	3.65	529,250	231	34	8.5	–0.6
IM7 (Hercules/ Hexcel)	C, trace N	Same	1.77	5	6,000, 12,000	70–50	5.30	768,500	275	40	6.0	–0.2
UHM (Hercules/ Hexcel)	C, trace N	Same	1.87	4.5	3,000, 12,000	350–100	3.45	500,250	440	64	110	–0.5
P120 (Amoco)	99^+% C	80	2.17	10	2,000	1,900	2.41	349,450	830	120	640	–1.45

ferent structures and properties: the PAN being higher strength, lower modulus with little graphitization of the fiber surface, and the pitch being moderate strength, high modulus with greater levels of surface graphitization. The article "Carbon Fibers" discusses the characteristics of carbon fibers in more detail. Key properties of some carbon fibers are shown in Table 1. The combination of high strength, modulus, low coefficient of thermal expansion, low density, and low cost seemingly make them a desirable choice to reinforce metals. However, structural carbon fibers are still not widely used in MMCs, for example, aluminum and magnesium alloys, despite much research and development activity. Several technical issues remain to be solved, including: the reactivity during composite processing, the reactivity at elevated temperatures, the oxidation resistance of the fiber at elevated temperatures, the corrosion resistance due to the inherent galvanic coupling between carbon and the metal matrix (aluminum or magnesium), and the corrosion resistance related to the leaching of any fiber-matrix reaction products (e.g., aluminum carbide) (Ref 5–8).

Carbon fibers have also been used to reinforce copper for thermal-management applications, but the difficulties encountered relate to both the poor bond strength and high wetting angle between carbon and copper, necessitating the use of coatings or reactive elements to increase the bond strength. Generally, the low bond strength between carbon fibers and any of the common metals (aluminum, magnesium, copper) is a difficulty because poor off-axis properties result. In aluminum the pitch fibers appear to be less reactive, but their handling characteristics (high modulus, brittle) make fabrication a more difficult task. Additionally, the high-modulus fibers also have a high thermal conductivity, which makes them attractive for use in combined structural/thermal-management applications.

Future Outlook

Future developments in fibers for MMCs are intimately tied up with the successful commercialization of MMCs in general. The properties and performance of the fibers are already good, and wider commercial use of MMCs would help drive the price down by increasing the demand for volume. Technical activity is needed in addressing the interface behavior for system-specific applications and would include both mechanical behavior and chemical stability. This

Table 2 Coating schemes for SiC monofilament fibers

Fiber	Diameter, μm	Fiber core	Fiber coating
SCS-6	140	33 μm carbon core	3 μm carbon layer + graded C-Si layer
Ultra SCS	140	33 μm carbon core	3 μm carbon layer + graded C-Si layer
Trimarc	125	12.5 μm W + C layer	3 μm carbon layer + $(H\text{-}S\text{-}H)^2$ layer
Sigma 1140+	100	14 μm tungsten core	3–5 μm carbon layer
Sigma 1240	100	14 μm tungsten core	1 μm carbon layer + TiB_x layer

can include surface chemistry of the fiber, fiber coatings, and so on.

REFERENCES

1. K.S. Kumar and G. Bao, Intermetallic-Matrix Composites: An Overview, *Compos. Sci. Technol.*, Vol 52, 1994, p 127–150
2. C. McCullough, P. Galuska, and S.R. Pittman, Criteria for Matrix Selection in Continuous Fiber Aluminum Matrix Composites, *Design Fundamentals of High Temperature Composites, Intermetallics, and Metal-Ceramic Systems*, R.Y. Lin, Y.A. Chang, R.G. Reddy, and C.T. Liu, Ed., TMS, 1995, p 15–28
3. H.E. Deve and C. McCullough, Continuous-Fiber Reinforced Al Composites: A New Generation, *J. Met.*, Vol 47 (No. 7), 1995, p 33–37
4. S. Yamada, S. Towata, and H. Ikuno, Mechanical Properties of Aluminum Alloys Reinforced with Continuous Fibers and Dispersoids, *Cast Reinforced Metal Composites*, ASM International, S.G. Fishman and A.K. Dhingra, Ed., 1985, p 109–114
5. M. De Sanctis, S. Pelletier, Y. Bienvenu, and M. Guigon, On the Formation of Interfacial Carbides in a Carbon Fibre-Reinforced Aluminum Composite, *Carbon*, Vol 32 (No. 5), 1994, p 925–930
6. R.S. Bushby and D. Scott, Evaluation of Aluminum-Copper Alloy Reinforced with Pitch-Based Carbon Fibres, *Compos. Sci. Technol.*, Vol 57, 1997, p 119–128
7. I.H. Khan, The Effect of Thermal Exposure on the Mechanical Properties of Aluminum-Graphite Composites, *Metall. Trans. A*, Vol 7A, 1976, p 1281–1289
8. B. Wielage and A. Dorner, Corrosion Studies on Aluminum Reinforced with Uncoated and Coated Carbon Fibers, *Compos. Sci. Technol.*, Vol 59, 1999, p 1239–1245

Fabrics and Preforms

WOVEN MATERIALS, in laminate form, are currently displacing more traditional structural forms primarily because of the availability of fibers (such as carbon and aramid) whose enhanced mechanical properties in composite form surpass the property values of corresponding hardware in aluminum or steel on a strength-to-weight basis.

Woven broad goods, considered to be intermediate forms, present these fibers in a more convenient format for the design engineer, resin coater, and hardware fabricator. The many variations of properties made possible by combining different yarns and weaves allow the structural engineer a wide range of laminate properties. The designer should understand the operation of weaving hardware and textile design details in order to select the best fabric style.

This article describes the types of fabrics and preforms that are used in the manufacture of advanced composites and related selection, design, manufacturing, and performance considerations.

Unidirectional and Two-Directional Fabrics

The fabric pattern, often called the construction, is an *x*, *y* coordinate system. The *y*-axis represents warp yarns and is the long axis of the fabric roll (typically 30 to 150 m, or 100 to 500 ft). The *x*-axis is the fill direction, that is, the roll width (typically 910 to 3050 mm, or 36 to 120 in.). Basic fabric weaves are few in number, but combinations of different types and sizes of yarns with different warp/fill counts allow for hundreds of variations.

The most common weave construction used for everything from cotton shirts to fiberglass stadium canopies is the plain weave, shown in Fig. 1. The essential construction requires only four weaving yarns: two warp and two fill. This basic unit is called the pattern repeat. Plain weave, which is the most highly interlaced, is therefore the tightest of the basic fabric designs and most resistant to in-plane shear movement. Basket weave, a variation of plain weave, has warp and fill yarns that are paired: two up and two down. The satin weaves represent a family of constructions with a minimum of interlacing. In these, the weft yarns periodically skip, or float, over several warp yarns, as shown in Fig. 2. The satin weave repeat is x yarns long and the float length is $x - 1$ yarns; that is, there is only one interlacing point per pattern repeat per yarn. The floating yarns that are not being woven into the fabric create considerable looseness or suppleness. The satin weave produces a construction with low resistance to shear distortion and is thus easily molded (draped) over compound curves, such as an aircraft wingroot area. This is one reason that satin weaves are preferred for many aerospace applications. Satin weaves can be produced as standard four-, five-, or eight-harness forms. As the number of harnesses increases, so do the float lengths and the degree of looseness and sleaziness, making the fabric more difficult to control during handling operations. Textile fabrics generally exhibit greater tensile strength in plain weaves. This distinction fades in the composites field.

The ultimate laminate mechanical properties are obtained from unidirectional-style fabric (Fig. 3), where the carrier properties essentially vanish in the laminate form. The higher the yarn interlacing (for a given-size yarns), the fewer the number of yarns that can be woven per unit length. The necessary separation between yarns reduces the number that can be packed together. This is the reason for the higher yarn count (yarns/in.) that is possible in unidirectional material and its better physical properties. Unidirectional material has the most "unbalanced" weave and is usually reserved for special applications involving hardware with axial symmetry (such as a carbon-fiber-reinforced shuttle motor case) fabricated using a tape-wrapping operation.

A weave construction known as locking leno (Fig. 4), which is used only in special areas of the fabric, such as the selvage, is woven on a shuttleless loom. The gripping action of the intertwining leno yarns anchors or locks the open selvage edges produced on rapier looms. The leno weave helps prevent selvage unraveling during subsequent handling operations, but is unsatisfactory for obtaining good laminate physical properties. However, it has found applications where a very open (but stable) weave is desired.

The textile designer is concerned with only a few fabric parameters: type of fiber, type of yarn, weave style, yarn count, and areal weight. Standard methods for measuring such parameters are well documented in Ref 1.

The verification of quality is an important aspect of the aerospace materials business. Quality is usually governed by military specification as part of the purchasing requirements. Typical quality defects, such as missing or broken warp or fill yarns, fabric misorientation (pucker), and misweaves in the pattern due to equipment failure or foreign material on the fabric, are documented in Ref 1 and 2.

Weave construction is the realm of the textile engineer, but fabric mechanical properties and how they translate into the laminate are concerns of the composite design engineer. Maximum directional properties for the minimum material (thickness) are attained with unidirectional-style material. The more usual goal of balanced properties requires two-directional styles. The fiber obviously dominates those properties carried by the fabric into a structural composite.

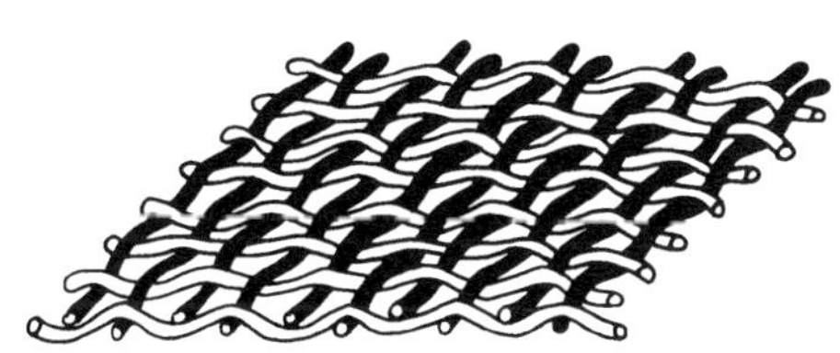

Fig. 1 Plain weave, yarn interlacing

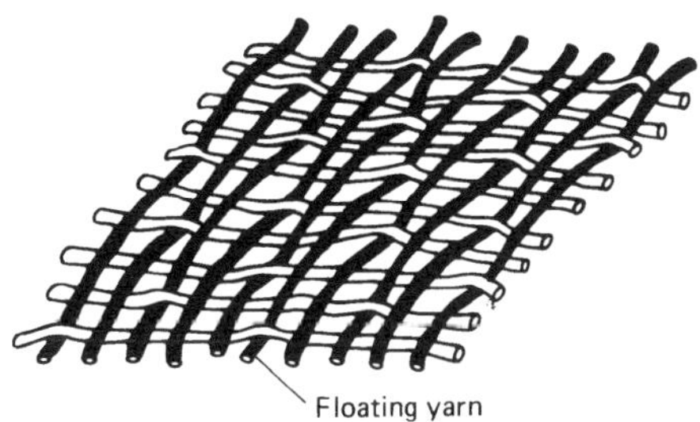

Fig. 2 Five-harness satin weave, interlacing

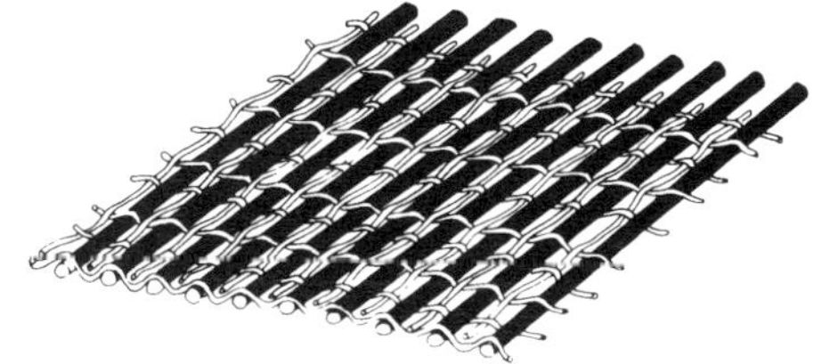

Fig. 3 Unidirectional weave

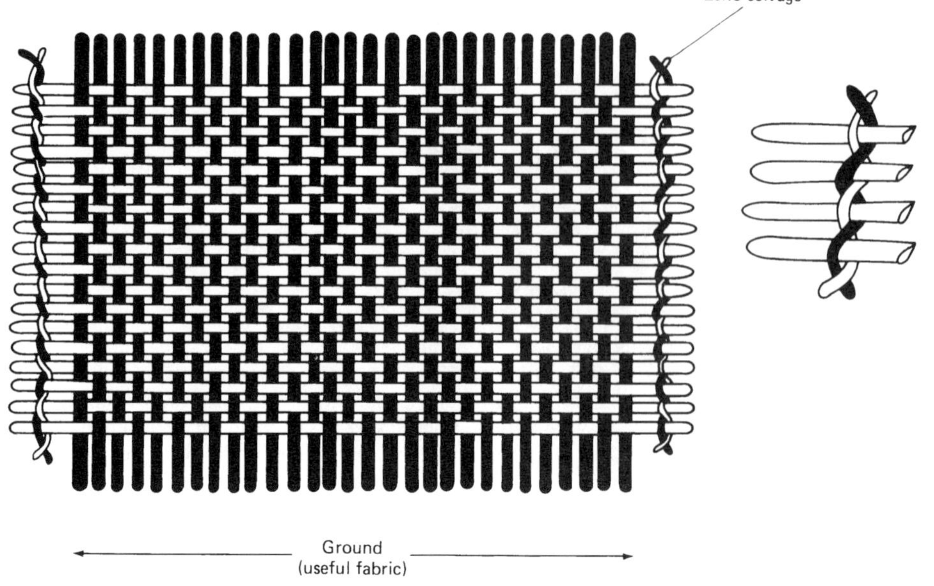

Fig. 4 Full-width plain weave with leno selvage

The fiberglass industry has these well-established fabric styles and categories:

Fabric weight	Areal wt, kg/m^2 (oz/yd^2)	Thickness, μm (mil)
Light	0.10–0.35 (3–10)	25–125 (1–5)
Intermediate	0.35–0.70 (10–20)	125–250 (5–10)
Heavy	0.50–1.0 (15–30)	250–500 (10–20)

The newer carbon and aramid fiber industries are somewhat oriented to custom design, but as the aerospace market matures, a few fabric constructions may become standards. Table 1 provides a sampling of styles that have found uses, along with corresponding order-of-magnitude epoxy resin composite properties.

The following data illustrate the relative market importance of various aerospace textile intermediate forms:

Woven	90+%
Filament winding	5%
Braided	<1%
Knit	<1%
Prepregs	(a)

(a) Depends on prepreg manufacture and its market segment/product line

Hybrid Fabrics

Hybrid fabrics are those woven from several different types of fibers, in contrast to fabrics woven from a single type of fiber. Table 2 shows typical properties of one hybrid graphite/aramid fabric. Combining fiber reinforcements allows the designer considerable flexibility. Among the reasons for the hybridization of graphite composites are (1) adding another fiber to a predominantly graphite composite in order to overcome the inherent disadvantages of graphite, (2) adding graphite fibers to a predominantly nongraphite composite or structure in order to take advantage of the benefits of graphite, and (3) producing a lower-cost structure. Normally, the impact resistance of graphite fiber composites can be improved by adding high-strength fibers with a greater strain-to-failure ratio than graphite. Several energy-absorbing mechanisms that have been proposed include interlacing resin layers to absorb energy and using fillers to stop cracks. Table 3 shows typical hybrid graphite/aramid and graphite/glass impact properties.

Graphite hybrid composites can be fabricated using conventional techniques and can be combined with boron, glass, aramid fibers, or metals in a laminated structure. Hybrids usually have the same matrix and can be fabricated by the cocuring process.

Multidirectionally Reinforced Fabrics

With the emergence of carbon-carbon composites and the resultant increased use of composite materials for high-temperature aerospace applications, the anisotropic nature of two-directionally oriented fabric presented a design problem: Although mechanical properties were satisfactory in the two directions containing reinforcement fabric, the mechanical properties in the third direction were matrix dominated and typically more than an order of magnitude less than in the reinforced direction. This problem was especially critical in applications involving high thermal stresses, such as carbon-carbon composite ballistic reentry nose tips and solid rocket throats. The obvious solution was to add fiber reinforcement in the third direction, and additional directions when necessary, to provide composite materials with isotropism approaching that of metals.

Early work in multidirectional reinforcement, preformed in the late 1960s, emphasized the development of geometric principles for a variety of fiber orientations, ranging from orthogonal, three-directional to eleven-directional reinforcement.

By the mid 1970s, it became apparent that the high cost of hand-assembled preforms (a preshaped fibrous reinforcement) would severely limit the application of multidirectionally reinforced composites to a very few aerospace applications. As a result, development activities began to de-emphasize the more complicated reinforcement geometries and concentrate on three-directional reinforcements, seeking to nar-

Table 1 Typical fabric styles and composite properties

Weave	Yarns/in., warp × fill	Weight kg/m^2	Weight oz/yd^2	Thickness at 25 kPa (3.4 psi) mm	Thickness at 25 kPa (3.4 psi) in.
Typical fabric weaves					
Eight-harness satin	24 × 23	0.370	10.9	0.46	0.018
Eight-harness satin	24 × 23	0.370	10.9	0.48	0.019
Plain	12½ × 12½	0.190	5.6	0.30	0.012
Five-harness satin	24 × 24	0.125	3.7	0.20	0.008
CFS	24 × 12	0.20	6.0	0.23	0.009
Plain	11½ × 11½	0.19	5.7	0.25	0.010
Five-harness satin	11 × 11	0.370	10.9	0.50	0.020
Plain	8 × 8	0.525	15.5	0.81	0.032
Eight-harness satin	10½ × 10½	0.755	22.2	1.0	0.040
Plain	10 × 10	0.345	10.2	0.48	0.019
8HS	21 × 21	0.393	11.6	0.38	0.015

Property	Value
Typical composite properties (balanced weave)	
Tensile strength, MPa (ksi)	620–690 (90–100)
Tensile modulus, GPa (10^6 psi)	69–76 (10–11)
Flexural strength, MPa (ksi)	690–900 (100–130)
Flexural modulus, GPa (10^6 psi)	62–69 (9–10)
Compressive strength, MPa (ksi)	620–690 (90–100)
Compressive modulus, GPa (10^6 psi)	62–69 (9–10)
Short beam shear strength, kPa (psi)	55–69 (8–10)
Specific gravity	1.6

Table 2 Properties of graphite, aramid, and hybrid fabric composites compared to 0°/90° laminates made from unidirectional layers (data normalized to 65 vol% fiber)

Ratio of aramid to graphite fiber	Tensile modulus, 0°/90°		Tensile modulus, fabric		Fabric efficiency, %	Tensile strength, 0°/90°		Tensile strength, fabric		Fabric efficiency, %	Compressive strength, 0°/90°		Compressive strength, fabric		Fabric efficiency, %
	GPa	10^6 psi	GPa	10^6 psi		MPa	ksi	MPa	ksi		MPa	ksi	MPa	ksi	
100/0	36.5	5.29	35.8	5.19	98	579	84.0	544	78.9	94	165	23.9	152	22.0	92
50/50	55.1	7.99	48.2	6.99	87	572	83.0	400	58.0	70	407	59.0	227	32.9	56
25/75	69.6	10.1	57.2	8.30	82	661	95.9	434	62.9	66	641	93.0	317	45.0	49
0/100	72.3	10.5	59.9	8.69	83	730	105	434	62.9	59	965	140	558	80.9	58

Source: Ref 3

row the program scope and to optimize the three-directional configuration for specific applications, such as reentry nose tips and solid rocket motor throats. This optimization included fiber selection, heat treatment variations, and wave balance.

With the scope of multidirectional reinforcement development this reduced, it became possible to design and fabricate semiautomated equipment to reduce preform costs while increasing quality by eliminating the human error potential associated with hand assembly. As a result of these activities, semiautomated weavers were developed by the late 1970s and used to produce propulsion hardware for strategic weapon systems. At the present time, fully automated computer-controlled three-directional weavers are operational.

Reinforcement Materials

There are few limits on the composition of reinforcement fibers that can be woven into three-dimensional preforms; if a material can be made into a fiber, it can probably be woven into some type of three-directional preform. Fibers that have been woven into three-directional preforms include carbon-graphite, glass, silica, alumina, aluminosilicates, silicon carbide, cotton, and aramid. When design requirements necessitate, it is possible to weave a three-directional preform with a combination of fibers, as illustrated by the silica/carbon cylinder in Fig. 5.

Generally, the only limitation to fiber selection is the combination of brittle fibers and small yarn bend radii, the latter being caused by either weave geometry or the yarn delivery system of the automated weaving machine. This is particularly true of carbon and graphite fibers, which account for about 90% of all three-directional woven preforms. High-modulus graphite fiber is particularly prone to fracture during preform construction.

Table 3 Impact resistance of hybrid composites

Hybrid composite(a), wt%	Izod impact strength, unnotched	
	J/m	ft · lbf/in.
Graphite, 100%	1495	28
Graphite, 75%; aramid, 25%	1815	34
Graphite, 50%; aramid, 50%	2349	44
Aramid, 100%	2562	48
Graphite, 100%	1495	28
Graphite, 75%; glass, 25%	2349	44
Graphite, 50%; glass, 50%	2989	56
Glass, 100%	3843	72

(a) With epoxy matrix. Source: Ref 4

Weave Geometry

There are more than 20 varieties of multidirectionally reinforced preforms. Only the three variations of three-directional preforms that are most widely used and best characterized are described here, however.

Polar weave three-directional preforms have reinforcement yarns in the circumferential, radial, and axial (longitudinal) directions, as shown in Fig. 6. Preforms of this geometry normally contain 50 vol% fibers that can be introduced equally in the three directions. Some variation in relative yarn distribution can be accomplished when a specific application requires unbalanced properties. For example, if high-hoop tensile strength is required, additional fibers can be added in the circumferential direction, at some sacrifice of radial and longitudinal properties.

Although originally developed as 305 to 510 mm diam (12 to 20 in. diam) thick-walled cylinders, polar weave three-directional preforms are presently fabricated in a number of body-of-revolution shapes, including cylinders, cylinders/cones, and convergent/divergent sections. When nonaxisymmetric shapes are needed, such as leading edges or conic/rectangular transitions, a two-step process is used. First, preform of appropriate geometry is woven. Next, the preform is placed in a metal die, deformed into the required shape, and impregnated with a suitable resinous material to ensure geometric stability during the remainder of the densification process, as shown in Fig. 7. It may or may not be necessary to slit the preform before deformation; although the leading-edge example in Fig. 7 required slitting, a simpler deformation from conic to conic/rectangular would not.

Present size limitations for three-directional polar weave cylindrical preforms are an approximate maximum of 210 cm (84 in.) in diameter and 130 cm (50 in.) in length. Wall thicknesses vary from 6.4 to 200 mm (0.25 to 8 in.). Inside diameters are limited to 75 mm (3 in.) because of space requirements for the weaving mechanism.

Although yarn spacing is not discussed in specific quantitative terms because of the large number of variables, some general observations are appropriate. In a polar weave three-directional preform, the angular spacing of the radial fibers

Fig. 5 Cylinder showing the combined use of silica and carbon fibers

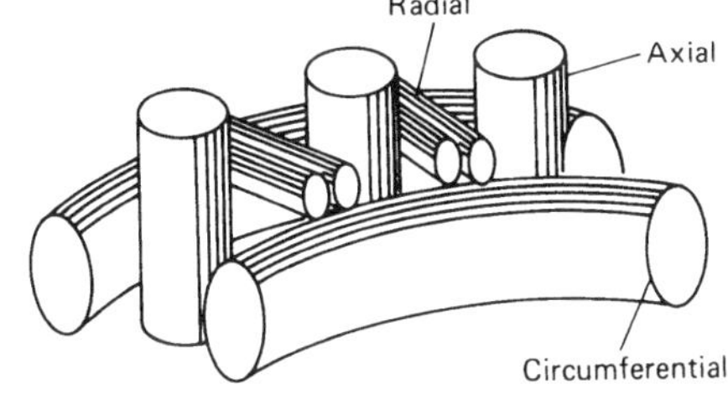

Fig. 6 Geometry of 3-D polar weave preform

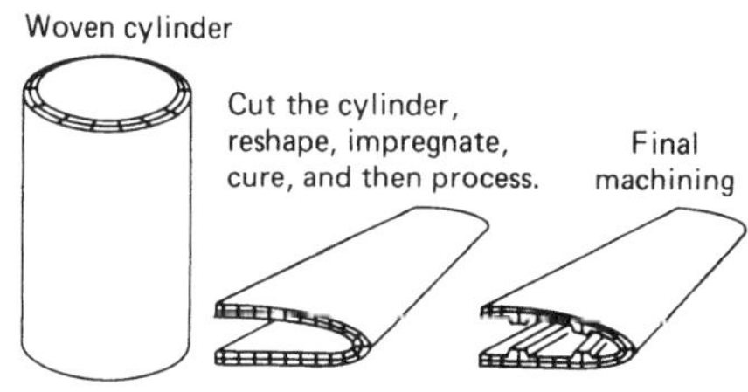

Fig. 7 Deformation of three-dimensional cylindrical preform to form a leading edge

is a critical factor. The number and diameter of the radial yarn bundles remain constant as they move from the inside diameter to the outside diameter of the part, forming a pie-shaped "corridor" of increasing width. The volume percentage of radial fibers is therefore lower at the outside diameter than at the inside diameter. To account for this and to maintain a uniform fiber volume throughout the preform, the fiber bundle size of both the circumferential and longitudinal yarns is increased.

Orthogonal weave three-directional preforms have reinforcement yarns arranged in an orthogonal (Cartesian) geometry, with all yarns intersecting at 90° angles, as shown in Fig. 8. Typical yarn content varies from 45 to 55%, similar to that of a polar weave preform. These fibers can be introduced uniformly in each of the three directions to provide isotropic properties or in unbalanced amounts when design considerations require anisotropic properties. Unlike polar weave preforms, they are rarely woven to near-net configuration. Instead, they are woven as blocks, and parts are machined to the requisite size and shape.

In regard to yarn spacing, it is worth noting that orthogonally woven three-directional preforms generally have a much finer unit cell size than their polar weave counterparts, resulting in superior mechanical properties and erosion resistance after densification into a composite.

Angle interlock, also known as warp interlock is a multilayered fabric in which the warp yarns travel from one surface of the fabric to the other, holding together up to eight layers of fabric, thus creating a thick, two-directional fabric, as shown in Fig. 9(a). When higher in-plane strength is needed, additional stuffer yarns can be added to create a quasi three-directional fabric, as shown in Fig. 9(b).

Although angle interlock fabric is economical to produce on commercially available weaving equipment, its use has been limited. Because it is unavailable in closed shapes, its use when closed cones/cylinders are required necessitates the use of joints and their attendant plane of weakness.

Stitched fabric and needled felt can be marginally included in a summary of three-directional preforms and fabrics. Although both materials have reinforcement fibers in all three directions, the amount of fiber in the cross-ply direction is frequently such a small fraction of the total fiber volume that the cross-ply mechanical properties are only slightly better than the matrix dominated properties of two-directional materials.

Prepreg Resins

Fibers that are preimpregnated with matrix resin in the uncured state are known as prepregs. Either continuous- or chopped-fiber prepregs are supplied to a part fabricator to the laminated or molded. The laid-up part is then subjected to heat and pressure to cure (chemically react) the resin. Prepreg has become an article of commerce because it frees the end user from having to develop resin formulations and impregnate fiber. The composite material can be bought with resin content, resin type, and fiber type already made to order. Handling characteristics such as curing time and temperature can be controlled to precise levels to meet user requirements. Prepregs can be divided into at least two classes: those suitable for high-preformance applications (including aerospace applications) and those to be used in lower-performance molding compounds. Aerospace applications demand high-performance, high-quality composites and moldings. The lower-performance applications use sheet molding prepregs for automotive components and appliance housings. The two general classes differ widely in composition, handling, part manufacture, and use.

Prepreg Resins for High-Performance Applications

The reinforcement in prepregs supplied for aerospace application is typically carbon fiber. The high strength and stiffness of carbon, coupled with its low density, result in composites with higher performance/weight ratio than is possible in either metals or composites using glass fiber. The prepreg consists of resin-impregnated fiber in either uniaxial or woven form.

The part fabricator requires a prepreg with tack, drape, and a certain tack life and out time. Tack is the tendency of two plies or layers to adhere sufficiently to allow laying-up of complex parts yet allow a clean strip-back if layers are applied incorrectly. Too low an adhesion level will allow layers to slip, while too aggressive a level will not allow repositioning. Drape is the ability of the prepreg to bend and conform to mold curvature. Tack life refers to the amount of time that the prepreg can be at room temperature and still retain enough tack for lay-up. Out time is the total amount of time that the prepreg can be left at room temperature before curing and still make a good part. Fabricators must consider all of these handling characteristics, in addition to the cured properties generated by certain resin and fiber combinations.

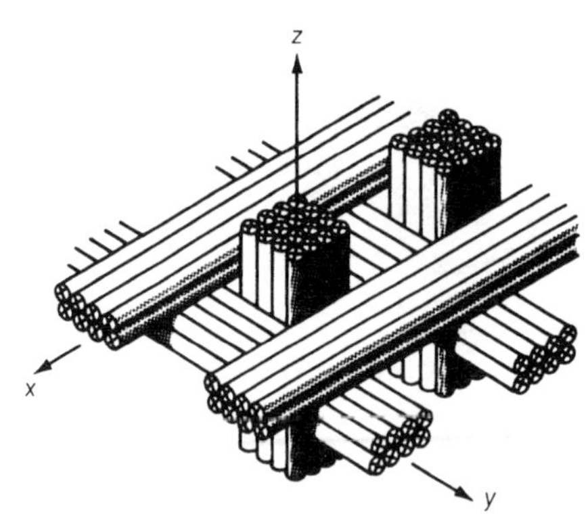

Fig. 8 Geometry of three-dimensional orthogonal weave preform

Epoxy Resins. A resin chemistry that satisfies both manufacturing and composite property requirements is based on epoxy resins with a latent curative system. The cure system will be slow, at room temperature, to prevent reactions that reduce tack, drape, and out time, but sufficiently rapid at elevated temperatures to permit reasonably short curing times. Even the most latent systems in use do not completely eliminate room-temperature reaction. After the fiber is impregnated with resin, it is stored and shipped at low temperatures. The material is allowed to warm to room temperatures for lay-up. Typically, a one-year storage life at –20 °C (0 °F) is provided.

The epoxide group is well known and is a mature technology (Ref 5–7). A wide range of epoxy-containing ingredients are available, as well as a wide range of curing agents and catalysts. Resins with different viscosities, amounts of reactive groups, and structures are available. Additives that change the uncured resin viscosity, reduce brittleness, or impart some other property are available. Aromatic backbones and high functionality give a strong high-temperature, highly cross-linked matrix that is usually brittle. Aliphatic epoxies and low functionality usually result in matrices with higher elongation, lower temperature capability, and higher toughness. The primary resin for aerospace application is *N,N,N′,N′*-tetraglycidyl-4,4′-methylenebisbenzenamine. When reacted with the appropriate curative, it yields a hard resin with temperature capabilities of about 190 to 205 °C (375 to 400 °F).

Curatives. The epoxide group can react chemically with other molecules to form a three-dimensional network. This chemical reaction changes the liquid resin into a load-bearing solid. Curing agent scan include amines, anhydrides, acids, and many others. Two commonly used

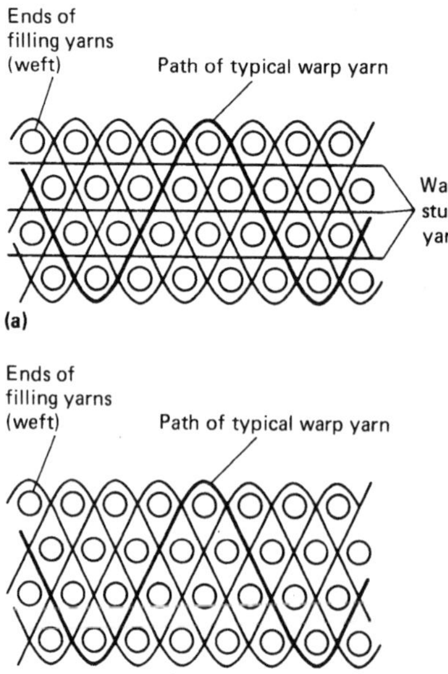

Fig. 9 Geometry of angle-interlock fabric (a) with and (b) without added stuffer yarns

amine curatives for prepreg resins are 4,4′-diaminodiphenylsulfone and dicyandiamide. Other curatives are too reactive with the epoxies at low and room temperatures, resulting in an unacceptable reduction of storage and use life. Dicyandiamide appears to decompose at elevated temperatures of 145 to 154 °C (290 to 310 °F) to yield other nitrogen-containing species, which cause the curing reaction to occur. The curative 4,4′-diaminodiphenylsulfone may or may not completely dissolve in the epoxy resins. Insolubility contributes to its latent curing behavior. Curatives are usually mixed with epoxy content on a 1-to-1 chemical basis. In the calculation of amounts, each hydrogen of the amine group is considered to react with one epoxy group. The actual mix ratio may be varied to optimize desired properties.

Catalysts are used to accelerate the latent curatives in order to achieve a complete cure in a shorter time. Boron trifluoride (BF_3) can be rendered latent by complexing with nitrogen-containing compounds, such as monoethylamine. Other amines can be used to adjust latency.

The types of amines and epoxies used for prepregs react slowly at room temperature, and elevated temperatures are needed for complete cure and attainment of ultimate properties. However, as a general rule, the temperature-use capability of the cured resin is slightly above the actual curing temperature. Therefore, a room-temperature system will operate at room temperature within a range; a formulation cured at 175 °C (350 °F) will perform at or somewhat above that temperature.

The actual mixture of epoxy resin or resins, curative, and catalyst that is formulated and blended is designed to meet end-use, prepregging, handling, and storage requirements. Low-viscosity resin components are used to reduce overall viscosity and aid in prepreg manufacture and flow during curing. Aromatic epoxies that differ in epoxy functionality are used to vary the cross-link density. Highly cross-linked aromatic resins used in aerospace prepregs make a very strong composite that is nonetheless brittle; flexibilizers or tougheners may be added to decrease brittleness. The amount of type of epoxy resins is varied to maximize desired composite properties as well as improve processing and handling characteristics.

Cure cycles for resin formulations are determined empirically. A given cure cycle may have several hold steps on the temperature rise to the maximum cure temperature. Hold steps at a given temperature allow resin flow to ensure a void-free part. They also prevent runaway temperature increases caused by rapid rates of reaction and cross-linking. The programmed heat-up cycle allows reactive groups to be consumed at a rate that permits removal of the heat of reaction. Subsequent heating to a higher temperature (and higher polymerization rate) is safe, because the amount of reactive material has been reduced. Conversely, hold steps can build viscosity through a reaction that reduces resin flow when the temperature is increased. Cure cycles recommended by the prepreg supplier are designed for specific composite thicknesses and resin formulations. Significant departures from customary lay-ups and cure schedules should be reviewed for safety as well as for achievement of ultimate properties.

Another epoxy application for prepregs is in circuit boards. Glass is used for this application because carbon fiber is electrically conductive. The combination of glass and epoxy resin yields good electrical properties, in addition to good temperature capabilities and ease of epoxy chemistry processing.

High-temperature epoxy resins have maximum continuous-use temperature of 205 to 230 °C (400 to 450 °F). Temperature spikes up to 290 °C (550 °F) can be tolerated by some formulations based on epoxy novolacs. The amine-cured epoxy resins are also affected by water. Because of the hydroxyl groups generated during cure, water is absorbed readily and acts like a plasticizer. Water exposure can reduce the operating temperature by 56 °C (100 °F). Although much effort has been spent to synthesize polymers that possess adequate thermal and water resistance, very few have proved to be economically feasible. However, two chemical approaches appear able to solve the problem: addition polyimides and condensation polyimides (Ref 8).

Addition polyimides are based on the reaction of bismaleimide molecules with aromatic amines or dienes. These systems possess temperature capabilities in excess of 260 °C (500 °F). Addition polyimides are similar to epoxies in that no volatiles are released by the polymerization reaction. In order to achieve the high-temperature properties, autoclave cures at 175 °C (350 °F) are followed by postcures at 315 to 340 °C (600 to 650 °F) in a free-standing oven. The primary drawback to addition polyimides is their extreme brittleness, which can be compensated for, somewhat, but usually at the loss of temperature capability or water resistance.

Condensation polyimides have temperature capabilities exceeding 315 °C (600 °F) and are not as brittle as the addition polyimides. A polyimide solution of in situ polymerization of monomer reactants consists of a mixture of monomers dissolved in solvent. The monomers are latent, as in the case of prepreg epoxy resins, but react at high temperatures. The presence of solvent, as well as the liberation of volatiles during polymerization, can create voids in the cured parts. The cure cycle and devolatilization are critical for producing high-quality parts.

Glass-phenolic and carbon-phenolic prepregs are used in specialty flame-resistant and ablative applications (Ref 9, 10), including aircraft interior panels and exit cones for rocket motors. Phenolic resins have excellent heat resistance, but their drawbacks include brittleness and the need for press curing at high pressures to suppress volatiles generated during the cross-linking reaction.

More detailed information is provided in the articles "Epoxy Resins," "Bismaleimide Resins," and "Phenolic Resins"in this Volume.

Prepreg Resins for Lower-Performance Applications

Sheet molding compounds (SMCs), used in applications where the high performance and high cost of carbon prepregs are not justified, consist of continuous or chopped fibers and a polyester or vinyl ester resin. The formulation includes inorganic filler, thixotrope, catalyst, release gent, and pigments. Processing conditions usually are 1 to 3 min in a press at 90 to 150 °C (200 to 300 °F).

Sheet molding compound is manufactured by calendaring a strip that contains the fiber and resin. Because of the latent nature of the catalyst, molding compounds can be stored and shipped at ambient temperature.

The two types of resin families that are used—polyester and vinyl ester—are similar in chemistry. A typical polyester resin is formed by the reaction of glycols and dibasic acids and anhydrides. Other unsaturated compounds, such as styrene, are added to cross-link and act as a diluent. Curing is accomplished by peroxide-initiated free-radial polymerization.

Vinyl ester resins are manufactured by reacting unsaturated carboxylic acids and epoxies.

As in the case of polyesters, styrene or vinyl toluene is used as a diluent for processing and chemical reactions. Vinyl esters are tougher, shrink less, and are more resistant to chemical attack than polyesters.

For both families, the composition of the resin affects the physical properties of a final part. The type of chemical backbone and diluent will allow weather resistance, chemical resistance, impact properties, and flow during processing to be tailored to fit the application. The curing time and storage life is altered by the amount and type of catalyst, accelerator, and inhibitors

Additional information about SMCs in provided in the article "Molding Compounds" in this Volume.

Woven Fabric Prepregs

Woven fabric prepregs are one of the most widely used fiber-reinforced resin forms. Fabrics typically offer flexibility in fabrication technique, but a higher cost than other prepreg forms. The designer must consider these and other factors before selecting a prepreg form for structural application. Information about fabric types and weave patterns is provided in the section "Unidirectional and Two-Directional Fabrics" in this article.

Fabrics can be prepregged using either a hot-melt or a solvent-coating process. The hot-melt process uses a machine similar to that used for fabricating unidirectional tape. Resin can be applied to the fabric either by using prefilmed substrate paper, a "knife over roll," or a similar coating mechanism. Solvent coating is typically accomplished by immersing the fabric into a bath containing 20 to 50% of a solvent and resin

Table 4 Fiber bundle dimensions

Material	Yield/tow m/kg	Yield/tow yd/lb	Filament size μm	Filament size μin.
Graphite (1000 to 12,000 filaments per tow)	300–1200	150–600	5–10	200–390
Fiberglass (2450–12,240 filaments per tow)	490–2400	245–1200	4–13	160–510
Aramid (800–3200 filaments per tow)	2000–7850	980–3900	12	470

mixture and then drying the fabric in a one-pass or multipass former coater. The two techniques generate different characteristics in the prepreg:

Hot melt

- Less drape and lower tack, due to higher resin viscosity, which in turn is due to lack of residual solvent in the prepreg
- Better hot/wet mechanical properties, less flow, and longer gel time, due to the absence of volatiles
- Higher cost, due to slower process speed and higher resin scrappage

Solvent coating

- Better drape, due to lower resin viscosity and, usually, higher tack
- Residual solvent of 1 to 2%, which incurs longer gel time, higher flow, and lower hot/wet mechanical properties
- Lower cost, due to increased process speed and reduced resin waste.

Fabrication Techniques. Woven fabric prepregs can be darted to conform to convoluted shapes of low-stressed items. Darting is the practice of slitting the prepregs at locations where folds would normally occur in a lay-up; the excess material at those locations is removed completely, and the remaining edges butted together. As an alternative, the prepreg can be slit where a crease would normally form, and the excess material can overlap, provided that it is wrinkle free. When the former method is used, an additional ply may be required to compensate for the weak butt joints in the lay-up. Darting is not recommended for highly stressed, lightweight construction; on those occasions, prepregs should be cut in predetermined patterns such that joints in successive plies do not coincide. Overlapping joints must be deliberately placed and joint widths must be controlled. Usually, patterns for precutting the prepregs allow for 13 mm (0.5 in.) overlaps on the lay-up.

When woven fabric reinforcements are laid up on convoluted shapes, weave patterns become distorted and the fiber directions change. Orientations of 0°, ±60° or 0°, ±45°, 90° are used to compensate for undetermined deficiencies. These plying sequences provide reinforcements for laminate plane quasi-isotropic properties. However, ply alignments of heavily draped lay-ups of fabric-reinforced prepregs are difficult to control. Colored tracer fibers, woven into the fabrics, simplify the lay-up and inspection of the composite.

Structural composites that are required to resist loads must be designed to obtain reproducible properties. Their shapes should permit the plies to be oriented in predetermined directions. Whether the lay-up is produced manually or is automated, the principles behind the lay-up techniques are similar. When the structural shapes permit, the most reproducible properties are developed by laying up plies that are cut to size and then applied to transfer films. These transfer films, or polyester film templates, are indexed to specified ply locations and orientations with respect to the mold. Plies that are laid up on templates are transferred to molds without additional distortion; after the plies are laid up and transferred, the templates are removed.

Anisotropies of a fabric-reinforced prepreg in one ply are corrected with equal but opposite anisotropy in adjacent plies. The symmetry achieved by making these corrections is important to avoid distortions in the cured laminates Other corrections are sometimes made by cross-plying compensating misalignments to attain orthotropy (Ref 11).

Unidirectional Tape Prepregs

Prepreg tapes of continuous-fiber reinforcement in uncured matrix resin are one of the most widely used forms of composite materials for structural applications. Tapes offer the designer advantages in the areas of economics and translation of fiber properties. Prepreg tape is a collimated series of fiber-reinforcing tows impregnated with a matrix resin. Before tape is manufactured from fiber, the fiber is usually found in a spooled form with widely varying tow size, weight per unit length (denier), and filament size, as shown in Table 4.

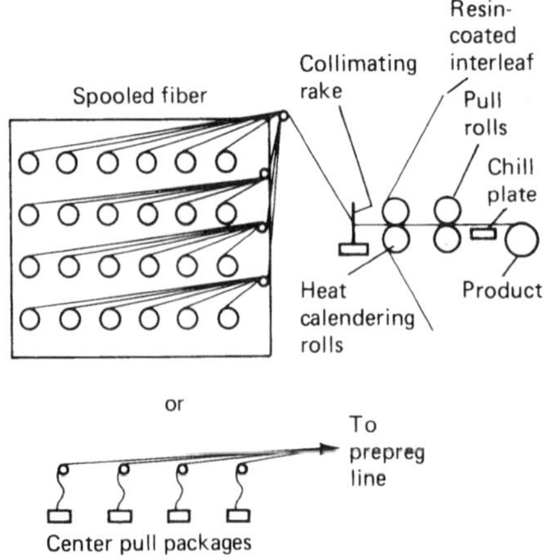

Fig. 10 Typical prepreg machine

Tape Manufacture and Product Forms

The fiber is typically converted into a prepreg by bringing a number of spooled tows into a collimated form, as shown in Fig. 10. The prepregging operation consists of heating a matrix resin to obtain low viscosity and creating a well-dispersed fiber-resin mass. The amount of fiber is controlled by the number of tows brought into the prepreg line, and the resin can be cast onto the substrate paper either on the prepreg line or in a separate filming operation to obtain the desired fiber-resin ratio. The prepreg is calendered to obtain a uniform thickeness and to close fiber gaps before being wound on a core. Substrate paper is ordinarily left between layers of tape. The paper can be any releasing film, but is typically a calendered paper coated with a nontransferable, cured silicone coating. Figure 11 shows a typical spool of graphite-epoxy prepreg tape, which is available in a wide variety of widths, thicknesses, and package sizes.

Using narrow (75 mm, or 3 in.) prepreg tape usually results in a minimal material loss of 7 to 10%. Narrow tape is ideally suited for a very expensive material, such as boron-epoxy. However, using narrow tape increases labor costs, which must be balanced against material costs.

Tape Properties

Reinforcement fibers by their nature are anisotropic (reinforcing primarily in one direction). Consequently, unidirectional tapes reinforce primarily in the 0° direction of the reinforcing fibers. Other structural properties also vary depending on fiber direction.

Tapes offer the best translation of fiber properties because the fibers are not crimped or distorted as in fabric prepregs. Significant differences exist between tape and fabric mechanical properties. Figures 12 and 13 show typical tensile property translation differences between tape and fabric prepregs.

Properties such as tack, flow, gel time, and drape are critical to proper selection of material form.

Tack should be adequate to allow the prepreg to adhere to prepared molding surfaces or preceding plies for a lay-up, but light enough to part

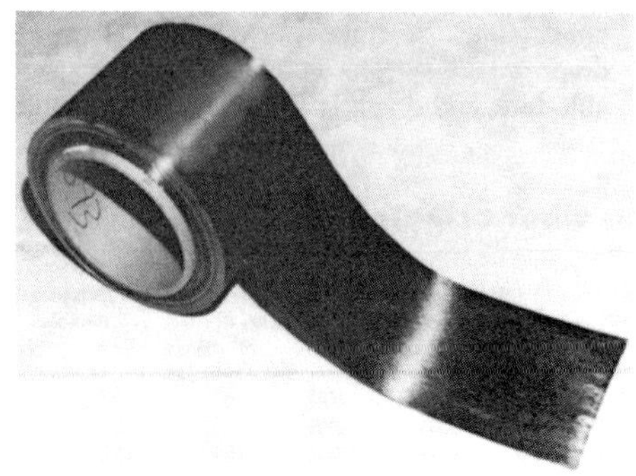

Fig. 11 Spool of graphite-epoxy tape

from the backing film without loss of resin. Tack qualities can be specified to require the prepreg to remain adhered to the backing until a predetermined force is applied to peel it off.

Prepregs with excessive tack generally are difficult to handle without disrupting resin distribution and fiber orientation or causing a roping (fiber bundling) of the reinforcements. Constituents are not reproducible because undetermined amounts of resin are removed when the release film or backing is separated from prepreg. In general, all the disadvantages of wet lay-up systems are inherent to overly tacky prepregs.

Prepregs with no tack are either excessively advanced, have exceeded their normal storage life, or are inherently low in tack. Such materials cannot attain adequate cured properties and should be discarded. Exceptions are silicones and some polyimides, which can only be prepared with no tack. Lay-ups with these materials are limited to those situations where lower mechanical properties can be tolerated in exchange for improved heat resistance or electrical properties. A lack of tack in thermoplastic prepregs does not interfere with their consolidation, provided that they can be heated to the melting point of the polymer during processing.

Flow is the measure of the amount of resin squeezed from specimen as it cures (under heat and pressure) between press platens. Flow measurement indicates the capability of the resin to fuse successive plies in a laminate and to bleed out volatiles and reaction gases. Flow can be an indicator of prepreg age or advancement. It is often desirable to optimize resin content and viscosity to attain adequate flows. In some cases, prepreg flow can be controlled by adding thickening or thixotropic additives to the resin.

Gel time, the measure of the time a specimen remains between heated platens until the resin gels or reaches a very high viscosity stage (Ref 11), can be an indicator of the degree of prepreg advancement. The useful life of prepregs is limited by the amount of staging or advancement. Most prepregs are formulated to attain a useful life of ten days or more at standard conditions. Life can be prolonged by cold storage, but each time the prepreg is brought to thermal equilibrium at lay-up room temperatures, useful life is shortened. Gel time measurements are used as quality control verifications (Ref 11).

Drape is the measure of the formability of a material around contours, which is critical to fabrication costs. Tape drapability is typically measured by the ability of a prepreg to be formed around a small-radius rod. The pass/fail criterion for drape is the ability to undergo this forming without incurring fiber damage. This measurement translates to the ability of fabrication personnel to form the prepreg to complex tools. Of the physical properties mentioned, drape is one property where tapes differ from other prepreg forms. Tapes are typically less drapable than fabric forms of prepreg, and this difference must be considered when specifying a prepreg form for manufacture.

It is essential that prepregs for structural applications be staged to desirable tack and drape qualities. The combination of manageable tack and drape is sometimes best attained from woven satin fabric-reinforced prepregs. Cross-plied or multiplied prepregs are sometimes used to provide transverse strengths for lay-ups of broad goods. The term "broad goods" refers to wide prepreg tape (>305 mm, or 12 in.) that consists of one or more plies of tape oriented at 0° or off-axis to each other.

Multidirectional Tape Prepregs

When a number of tape plies are laminated at several orientations, the strength of the composite increases in the transverse direction. As the number of oriented plies is increased, the isotropic strength is approached asymptotically.

Multidirectional tapes can be manufactured with multiple plies of unidirectional tape oriented to the designer's choice. These tapes are available in the same widths and package sizes as unidirectional tape, with varying thickness. Up to four or five plies of tape, with each ply typically being 0.125 mm (0.005 in.), can be plied together in various orientations to yield a multidirectionally reinforcing tape. Figure 14 depicts the difference between unidirectional and multidirectional tapes.

By using a preplied quasi-isotropic prepreg, the fabricator can avoid a substantial lay-up cost. However, preplied prepregs are typically more costly than unidirectional prepregs because of the additional work necessary to ply the tape.

Multioriented prepreg performance can be accurately predicted from test data that have been generated on these configurations. Tables 5 and 6 show typical mechanical property data for these lay-ups compared with other structural materials.

Cross-plied tapes offer controlled anisotropy, that is, properties can be varied and modified in selected directions, but these tapes are generally more expensive than unidirectional tapes because of the additional manufacturing steps. This disadvantage is often overcome, however, by the cost savings from using a preplied tape in part lay-up.

Properties are controlled by the number of plies of tape oriented in critical directions. Figures 15 and 16 show typical changes in tensile properties and when ply orientation is changed.

Tape Manufacturing Processes

Tape manufacturing processes fall into three major categories: hand lay-up, machine-cut patterns that are laid up by hand, and automatic machine lay-up.

Hand Lay-Up. Historically, tapes have primarily been used in hand lay-up applications in which the operator cuts lengths of tape (usually 305 mm, or 12 in.) and places them on the tool surface in the desired ply orientation. Although this method uses one of the lower-cost forms of reinforcement and has a low facility investment, it results in a high material scrap rate, fabrication time/cost, and operator-to-operator part variability. The scrap factor on this type of operation can exceed 50%, depending on part complexity and size.

Auxiliary processing aids should be used extensively to expedite the lay-up operation and to use molds and tools more efficiently. It is customary to presize the laid-up ply before it is applied to the mold. Usually, an auxiliary backing is fixed in position on the lay-up tool, which is sometimes equipped with vacuum ports to anchor the backings. Plies are oriented to within ±1° using tape-laying heads, or manually, using straight edges, drafting machine dividing heads (Ref 4) or ruled lines on the table (Ref 4).

Indexes or polyester film templates also can be used to reduce the lay-up times on molds. The presized plies are first laid up and oriented on the templates. When the mold is available for the lay-up, the plies are positioned on them and transferred. Positioning is achieved by using the

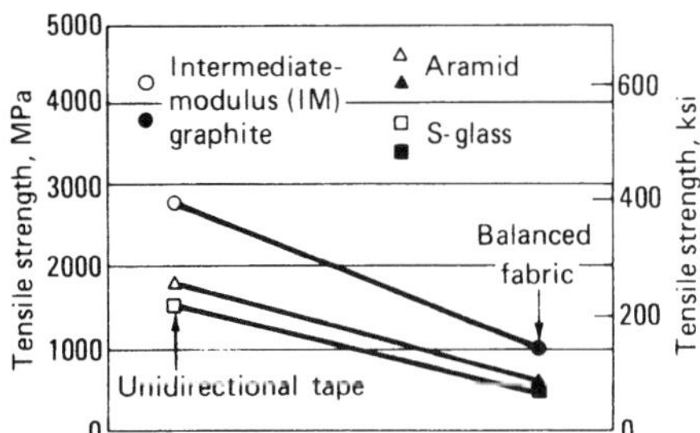

Fig. 12 Tensile strength comparison—fiber-epoxy tape versus fabric

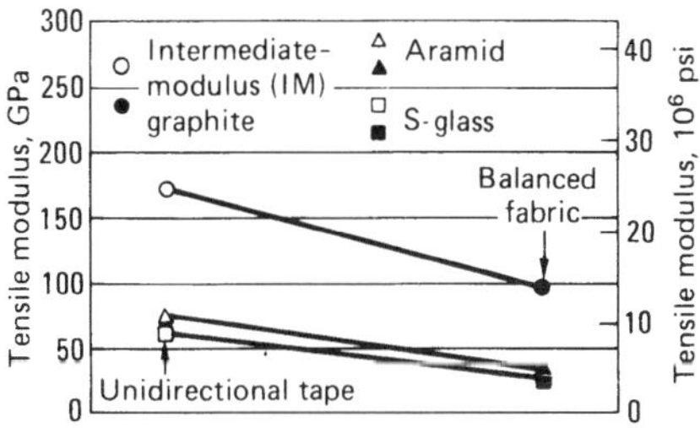

Fig. 13 Tensile modulus comparison—fiber-epoxy tape versus fabric

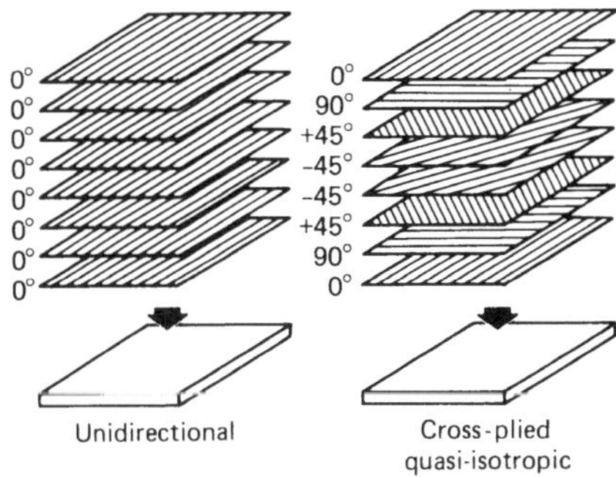

Fig. 14 Unidirectional versus quasi-isotropic lay-ups

references used for indexing. Reference posts for the templates are sometimes located on the mold; corresponding holes in the templates fit exactly over the posts. In some cases, the templates are shaped so that they fit only one way in the mold. The plies are rubbed out from the templates onto the mold, the mold is removed, the bleeder systems are laid up, and the assemblies are bagged and cured.

Machine-Cut Patterns. More advanced technology uses machine-cut patterns that are then laid up by hand. This method of manufacture involves a higher facility cost but increases part fabrication output and reduces operator error in lay-up. The right-sized pattern can be automatically cut in one or more ply thicknesses using wider tapes of up to 1500 mm (60 in.), which are potentially more economical to fabricate.

The cut is normally done on a pattern-cutting table, where up to eight plies of material are laid up. Various templates are located on top of the lay-up, and the most economical arrangement is determined by matching templates. The patterns are then cut and stored until required. Cutting of plies can be done by laser, water jet, or high-speed blades. The machine-cut method is often used in modern composites shops and is best suited for broad goods and wide tapes. A typical cutting machine is shown in Fig. 17.

Automatic Machine Lay-Up. Numerically controlled automatic tape-laying machines, especially in the aerospace industry, are now programmed to lay down plies of tape in the quasi-isotropic patterns required by most design applications. In addition to being able to lay down a part in a short time and with reduced scrappage, robotics also lend consistency to lay-down pressures and ply-to-ply separations. These advantages are rapidly causing the aerospace industry to switch from hand lay-up operations. Automatic tape layers are evolving from being able to handle only limited tape widths and simple tool contours to being able to fabricate large, heavily contoured parts. Additional information is provided in the article "Automated Tape Laying" in this Volume.

Table 5 Comparative strength/weight versus material form

Material(a)	Strength, 0°, MPa	Strength, 0°, ksi	Strength, 0°/±45°/90°, MPa	Strength, 0°/±45°/90°, ksi	Density, g/cm^3	Strength/density, 0°, 10^6 cm	Strength/density, 0°, 10^6 in.	Strength/density, 0°/±45°/90°, 10^6 cm	Strength/density, 0°/±45°/90°, 10^6 in.
Graphite									
High-strength, low modulus	2.2	0.32	0.73	0.11	1.55	14.3	5.63	4.8	1.9
High-strength, intermediate modulus	2.4	0.35	0.80	0.12	1.52	...	...	...	...
Low-strength, high modulus	1.2	0.17	0.43	0.06	1.63	15.1	5.94	2.7	1.1
S-glass	1.8	0.26	0.76	0.11	1.99	9.2	3.6	3.9	1.5
E-glass	0.82	0.12	0.52	0.075	1.99	4.2	1.7	2.7	1.1
Aramid	1.5	0.22	0.39	0.057	1.36	10.9	4.29	2.9	1.1
Aluminum	...	0.41	0.059	...	2.77	...	1.5	0.59	...
Steel	...	2.1	0.30	...	8.00	...	2.6	1.0	...

(a) In epoxy-resin matrix

Table 6 Comparative stiffness/weight versus material form

Material(a)	Stiffness, 0°, MPa	Stiffness, 0°, ksi	Stiffness, 0°/±45°/90°, MPa	Stiffness, 0°/±45°/90°, ksi	Density, g/cm^3	Stiffness/density, 0°, 10^6 cm	Stiffness/density, 0°, 10^6 in.	Stiffness/density, 0°/±45°/90°, 10^6 cm	Stiffness/density, 0°/±45°/90°, 10^6 in.
Graphite									
High-strength, low modulus	0.15	0.022	0.046	0.0067	1.55	0.98	0.39	0.30	0.12
High-strength, intermediate modulus	0.17	0.025	0.065	0.0094	1.52	1.14	0.45	0.43	0.17
Low-strength, high modulus	0.20	0.029	0.052	0.0075	1.63	1.25	0.49	0.33	0.13
S-glass	0.055	0.0080	0.0025	0.0036	1.99	0.28	0.11	0.13	0.051
E-glass	0.041	0.0059	0.018	0.0026	1.99	0.21	0.083	0.09	0.035
Aramid	0.073	0.011	0.025	0.0026	1.36	0.59	0.23	0.19	0.075
Aluminum	...	0.069	0.010	...	2.77	...	0.25	0.098	...
Steel	...	0.19	0.028	...	8.00	...	0.24	0.094	...

(a) In epoxy-resin matrix

Prepreg Tow

Another form of prepreg is a towpreg, which is either a single tow or a strand of fiber that has been impregnated with matrix resin. The impregnated fiber is typically wound on a cardboard core before being packaged for shipment. Because a towpreg is potentially the lowest-cost form or prepreg, it is of significant interest to designers. It also lends itself to potentially low-cost manufacturing schemes, such as filament winding. Towpreg is being considered by filament winders as a way to combine the advantages of low-cost part manufacture and high-performance matrix resins. The fibers that are typically used are shown in Table 7.

Manufacture. Most towpregs are converted in a solvent-coating process (Fig. 18) in which base resin is first dissolved in a mix containing 20 to 50% solvent and resin. The dry fiber is then routed through the solvent-resin mix and dried in a tower consisting of one or more heated zones. Resin content is controlled either by using metering rolls after impregnation or by adjusting the solvent-resin ratio. This drying step reduces volatiles and advances the resin so that the towpreg will not adhere to itself during unspooling in part manufacture. Towpregs can also be manufactured in a hot-melt operation by filming resin on substrate paper, impregnating strands be-

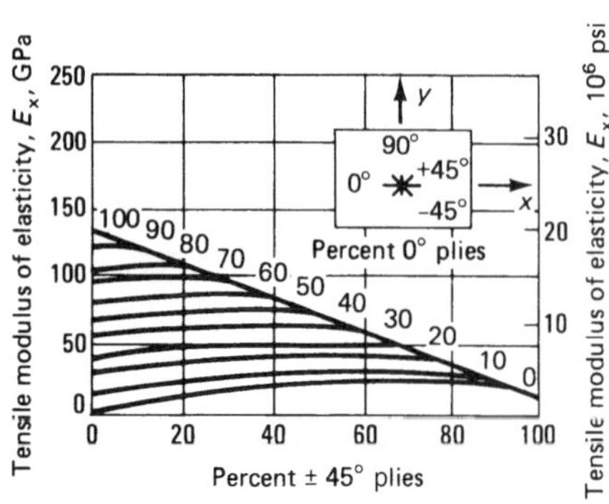

Fig. 15 Tensile modulus of elasticity of carbon-epoxy laminates at room temperature

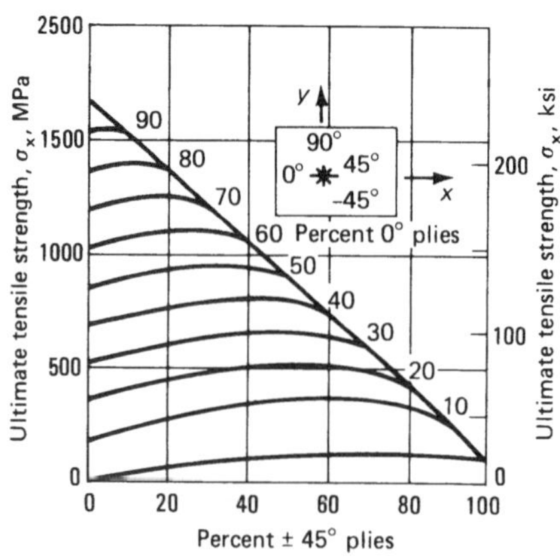

Fig. 16 Ultimate tensile strength of carbon-epoxy laminates at room temperature

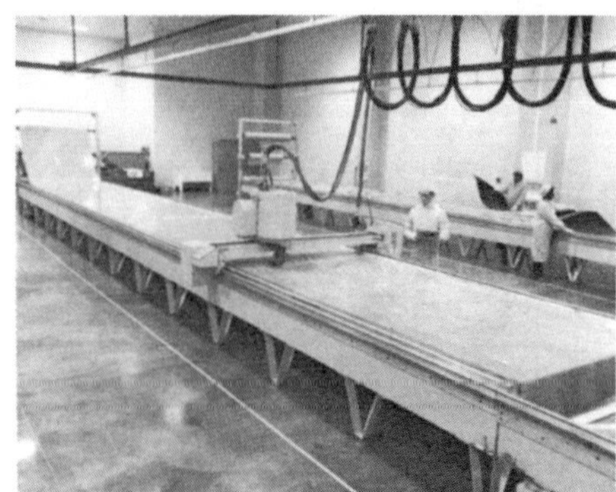

Fig. 17 Gerber cutting machine

Table 7 Fiber tow characteristics

Before impregnation

	Yield/tow		Filament size	
Material	m/kg	yd/lb	μm	μin.
Graphite (1000–12,000 filaments/tow)	300–1200	150–600	5–10	200–390
Fiberglass (2450–12,240 filaments/tow)	490–2400	245–1200	4–13	160–510
Aramid (800–3200 filaments/tow)	2000–7850	980–3900	12	470

Table 8 Towpreg form parameters

Parameter	Typical range
Strand weight per length, g/m (lb/yd)	0.74–1.48 (0.00150–0.0030)
Resin content, %	28–45
Tow width, cm (in.)	0.16–0.64 (0.06–0.25)
Package size, kg (lb)	0.25–4.5 (0.5–10)

tween two layers of filmed paper, and then advancing the resin to an intermediate point between freshly mixed and cured (B-staging) on a prepreg line. However, this tends to result in a higher-cost towpreg.

Forms. Table 8 shows typical form parameters that a manufacturing shop might specify. A designer must evaluate the size and complexity of the part being designed before selecting material parameters. Resin content will determine part mechanical performance and thickness by determining fiber volume, assuming that little or no resin is lost in the curing process. Tow width, which is important in establishing ply thickness and gap coverage, can be modified during laydown. Package size can be important to manufacturing personnel, especially when more than one spool is used in the manufacturing process. In such cases, manufacturing personnel often try to match the sizes of spools that are used in order to minimize spool doffs (changes) and splices in the manufactured part.

To determine the mechanical properties of a towpreg, it can be tested by a single-strand type of test or by winding tows on a drum to specified thicknesses and then laying up laminates from this wind. Mechanical properties of towpregs are comparable to those of tapes, if they are cured under autoclave conditions. Filament-sound structures that are not autoclave cured will typically have higher void contents than autoclave-cured parts.

Applications. The two basic uses for towpregs are as a filler in hard-to-form areas and in joints of structural components such as I-beams (Fig. 19) and as a replacement for low-performance filament-winding resins in filament-winding operations. Using a towpreg as a filler material in areas where tape or fabric prepregs will not lay down involves hand lay-up.

Most of the development in towpreg technology has been in the area of winding, particularly using a graphite-epoxy towpreg. The six-axis winding machine (Fig. 20) unspools the towpreg bundles and collimates them into a band of prepregs before laying down a unified band. The band of prepreg can be laid into complex cylindrical or nongeodesic forms, as shown in Fig. 21. This technology has the potential of making significant inroads into complex low-cost aerospace-grade part manufacture and may revolutionize the amount of composites and types of techniques used in aircraft fuselage manufacture. Additional information on towpreg is provided in the article "Filament Winding" in this Volume.

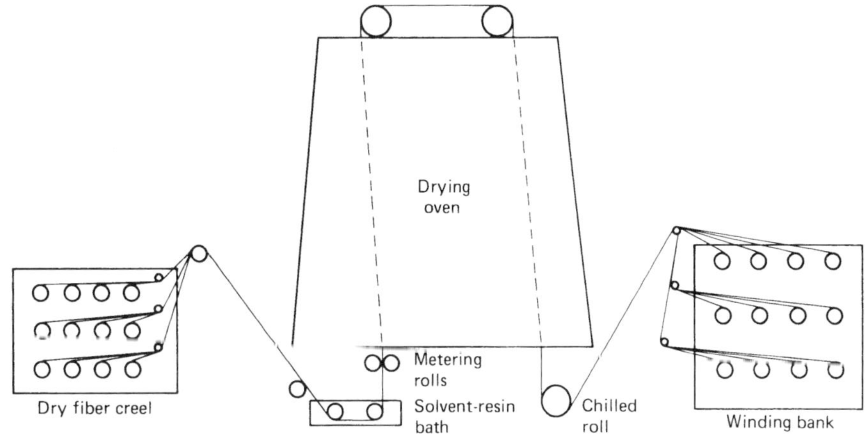

Fig. 18 Typical towpreg manufacturing process

ACKNOWLEDGMENTS

The information in this article is largely taken from the following articles in *Composites,* Volume 1, *Engineered Materials Handbook,* ASM International, 1987:

- W.D. Cumming, Unidirectional and Two-Directional Fabrics, p 125–128
- F.S. Dominguez, Unidirectional Tape Prepregs, p 143–145

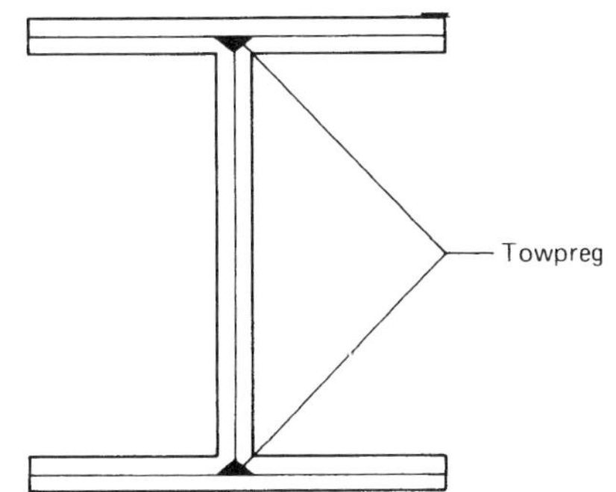

Fig. 19 Towpreg used a filler in an I-beam

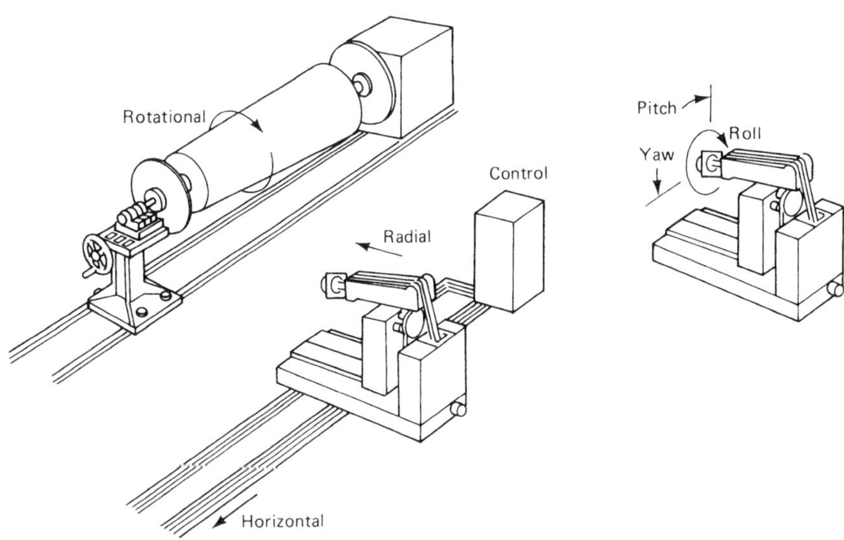

Fig. 20 Six-axis winding machine

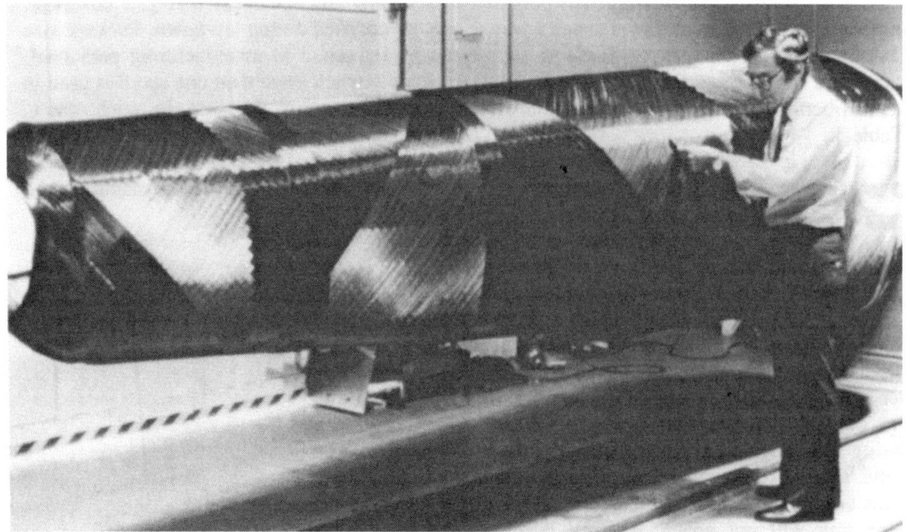

Fig. 21 Complex structure wound with towpreg on six-axis winding machine

- F.S. Dominguez, Multidirectional Tape Prepregs, p 146–147
- F.S. Dominguez, Prepreg Tow, p 151–152
- F.S. Dominguez, Woven Fabric Prepregs, p 148–150
- F.P. Magin III, Multidirectionally Reinforced Fabrics and Preforms, p 129–131
- W.T. McCarvill, Prepreg Resins, p 139–142

REFERENCES

1. *Textiles*, Vol 7.01 and 7.02, *Annual Book of ASTM Standards*
2. "Textile Test Methods," Federal Specification 191a, 1978
3. C. Zweben and J.C. Norman, "Kevlar" 49/ "Thornel" 300 Hybrid Fabric Composites for Aerospace Applications, *SAMPE Q.*, July 1976
4. G. Lubin, *Handbook of Composites*, Van Nostrand Reinhold, 1982
5. H. Lee and K. Neville, *Handbook of Epoxy Resins*, McGraw-Hill, 1967
6. L.S. Penn and T.T. Chiao, Epoxy Resins, *Handbook of Composites*, G. Lubin, Ed., Van Nostrand Reinhold, 1982 p 57–88
7. P.F. Bruins, *Epoxy Resin Technology*, Wiley-Interscience, 1968
8. K.L. Mittal, Ed., *Polyimides*, Vol 1, Plenum, 1984
9. A. Knop and L.A. Pilato, *Phenolic Resins*, Springer-Verlag, 1985
10. K.L. Forsdyke, G. Lawrence, R.M. Mayer, and I. Patter, The Use of Phenolic Resins for Load Bearing Structures, *Engineering with Composites*, Society for the Advancement of Material and Process Engineering, 1983
11. B.D. Agarwol and L.J. Broutman, *Analysis and Performance of Fiber Composites*, John Wiley & Sons, 1980

SELECTED REFERENCES

- F.K. Ko and G.-W. Du, Processing of Textile Preforms, *Advanced Composites Manufacturing*, T.G. Gutowski, Ed., John Wiley & Sons, 1997, p 157–205
- M.M. Schwartz, *Composite Materials*, Vol 2, *Processing, Fabrication, and Applications*, Prentice Hall, 1997, p 114–125

Braiding

Frank K. Ko, Drexel University

BRAIDING is a textile process that is known for its simplicity and versatility. Braided structures are unique in their high level of conformability, torsional stability, and damage resistance. Many intricate materials placement techniques can be transferred to and modified for composite prepreg fabrication processes. The extension of two-dimensional braiding to three-dimensional braiding has opened up new opportunities in the near-net shape manufacturing of damage-tolerant structural composites.

In the braiding process, two or more systems of yarns are intertwined in the bias direction to form an integrated structure. Braided material differs from woven and knitted fabrics in the method of yarn introduction into the fabric and in the manner by which the yarns are interlaced. Braided, woven, and knitted fabric are compared in Table 1 and Fig. 1.

Braiding has many similarities to filament winding (see the article "Filament Winding" in this Volume). Dry or prepreg yarns, tapes, or tow can be braided over a rotating and removable form or mandrel in a controlled manner to assume various shapes, fiber orientations, and fiber volume fractions. Although braiding cannot achieve as high a fiber volume fraction as filament winding, braids can assume more complex shapes (sharper curvatures) than filament-wound preforms. The interlaced nature of braids also provides a higher level of structural integrity, which is essential for ease of handling, joining, and damage resistance. While it is easier to provide hoop (90°) reinforcement by filament winding, longitudinal (0°) reinforcement can be introduced more readily in a triaxial braiding process. In a study performed by McDonnell Douglas Corporation, it was found in one instance that braided composites can be produced at 56% of the cost of filament-wound composites, because of the labor savings in assembly and the simplification of design (Ref 1). By using the three-dimensional braiding process, not only can the intralaminar failure of filament-wound or tape laid-up composites be prevented, but the low interlaminar properties of the laminated composites can also be prevented. A comprehensive treatment of braiding that does not directly relate to composites is provided in Ref 2.

Because of its knot-tying origins, braiding is perhaps one of the oldest textile technologies known to man. From the Kara-Kumi, an Oriental braid for ornamental purposes, to heavy-duty ropes, braids have long been used in many specialized applications. Their modern applications include sutures and high-pressure hose reinforcement. In short, braids have been used wherever a high level of torsional stability, flexibility, and abrasion resistance are required. On the other hand, because of their lack of width and relatively low productivity (due to machine capacity), braids have not gained as widespread use in the textile industry as have woven, knitted, and nonwoven fabrics.

As a result of the relatively low use of braids as a textile and clothing material, publications related to braiding are limited. Braids were considered a crafting art in the 1930s (Ref 3); one of the earliest treatments of braids as an engineering structure appeared in an article by W.J. Hamburger in the 1940s (Ref 4) in which the geometric factors related to the performance of braids were examined. The first comprehensive discussion of the formation, geometry, and tensile properties of tubular braids was given by D. Brunnschweiler (Ref 5, 6) in the 1950s. From the machinery and processing point of view, an informative book was written by W.A. Douglass (Ref 7) in the early 1960s. Relating processing parameters to the structure of braids, two articles (Ref 8, 9) reflect the sophistication of the development of braiding technology in Germany. A beautifully illustrated review on the historical development of braiding and its applications and manufacture was published by Ciba-Geigy Corporation (Ref 10). Serious consideration of braids as engineering materials did not occur until the later part of the 1970s, when researchers from McDonnell Douglas described the use of braids for composite preforms (Ref 11) to reduce the cost of producing structural shapes. About the same time, the first published article on the structural mechanics of tubular braids by S.L. Phoenix appeared (Ref 12), as well as an extended treatment by C.W. Evans of braids and braiding for a pressure hose, which is a flexible composite (Ref 13).

Since the 1980s, most of the published information on braids has been related to composites (Ref 1, 11, 14, 15). A large concentration of articles on three-dimensional braiding has been appearing in the literature. Addressing the delamination problem in state-of-the-art composites and demonstrating the possibility of near-net shape manufacturing, the articles on three-dimensional braiding can be categorized into the areas of applications (Ref 16), processing science and structural geometry (Ref 17), structural analysis (Ref 18), and property characterization (Ref 19). As indicated in this brief review of the literature, braids have gained popularity in the composite industry because of the technological needs of structural composites for the inherent uniqueness of braided structures, as well as the recent progress in hardware and software development for braiding processes. At this point, two-dimensional and three-dimensional triaxial braids are more developed and widely applied than complex three-dimensional braids.

Coupled with the fully integrated nature and the unique capability for near-net shape manufacturing, the current trend in braiding technology is to expand to large-diameter braiding; develop more sophisticated techniques for braiding over complex-shaped mandrels, multidirectional braiding, or near-net shapes; and the extensive use of computer-aided design and manufacturing.

This article describes basic terminology, braiding classifications, and the formation, structure, and properties of the braided structures, with specific attention to composites.

Table 1 A comparison of fabric formation techniques

Parameter	Braiding	Weaving	Knitting
Basic direction of yarn introduction	One (machine direction)	Two (0°/90°) (warp and fill)	One (0° or 90°) (warp or fill)
Basic formation technique	Intertwining (position displacement)	Interlacing (by selective insertion of 90° yarns into 0° yarn system)	Interlooping (by drawing loops of yarns over previous loops)

Braiding Classifications

One of the most attractive features of braiding is its simplicity. A typical braiding machine (Fig. 2) essentially consists of a track plate, spool carrier, former, and a take-up device. In some cases, a reversing ring is used to ensure uniform tension on the braiding yarns. The resulting braid geometry is defined by the braiding angle, θ, which is half the angle of the interlacing between yarn systems, with respect to the braiding (or machine) direction. The tightness of the braided structure is reflected in the frequency of interlacings. The distance between interlacing points is known as pick spacing. The width, or diameter, of the braid (flat or tubular) is represented as *d*.

Table 2 Braiding classifications

Parameter	Biaxial	Triaxial	Multiaxial
Dimension of braid	Two-dimensional	Three-dimensional	Three-dimensional
Shaping	Formed shape	Formed shape	Net shape
Direction of braiding	Horizontal	Vertical	Inverted vertical
Construction of braid	1/1	2/2	3/3
Control mechanism for carrier motion	Positive	Positive	Jacquard
Braiding type	Circular	Flat	Jacquard, special

The track plate supports the carriers, which travel along the path of the tracks. The movement of the carriers can be provided by devices such as horn gears, which propel the carriers around in a maypole fashion. The carriers are devices that carry the yarn packages around the tracks and control the tension of the braiding yarns. At the point of braiding, a former is often used to control the dimension and shape of the braid. The braid is then delivered through the take-up roll at a predetermined rate. If the number of carriers and take-up speed are properly selected, the orientation of the yarn (braiding angle) and the diameter of the braid can be controlled. The direction of braiding is an area of flexibility, because it can be horizontal, vertical from bottom to top, or inverted.

When longitudinal reinforcement is required, a third system of yarns can be inserted between the braiding yarns to produce a triaxial braid with 0° ± θ° fiber orientation. If there is a need for structures having a greater thickness than that produced as a single braid, additional layers (plies) of fabric can be braided over each other to produce the required thickness. For a higher level of through-thickness reinforcement, multiple-track braiding, pin braiding, or three-dimensional braiding can be used to fabricate structures in an integrated manner. The movement of the carriers can follow a serpentine track pattern or orthogonal track pattern by means of a positive guiding mechanism and/or Jacquard-controlled mechanism (lace braiding). Jacquard braiding uses a mechanism that enables connected groups of yarns to braid different patterns simultaneously. Various criteria and braiding classifications are shown in Table 2. For simplicity, and to be consistent with the literature in the composite community, the dimensions of braided structures are used as the criteria for categorizing braiding. Specifically, a braided structure having two braiding-yarn systems with or without a third laid-in yarn is considered two-dimensional braiding. When three or more systems of braiding yarns are involved to form an integrally braided structure, it is known as three-dimensional braiding.

Two-Dimensional Braiding

The equipment for two-dimensional braiding is well established worldwide, but especially in West Germany. One of the oldest braiding machine manufacturers in the United States is Mossberg Industries (also known by its former

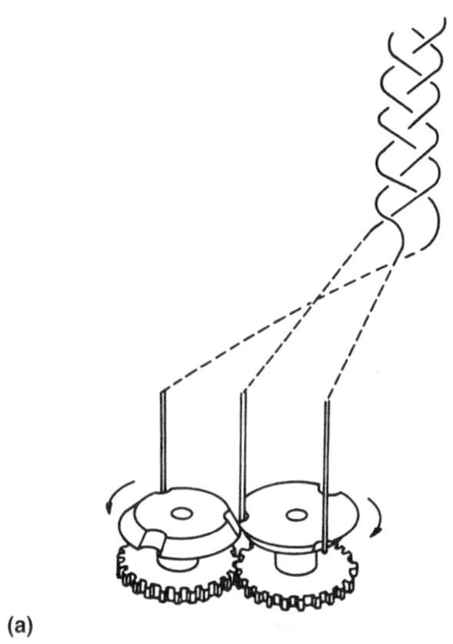

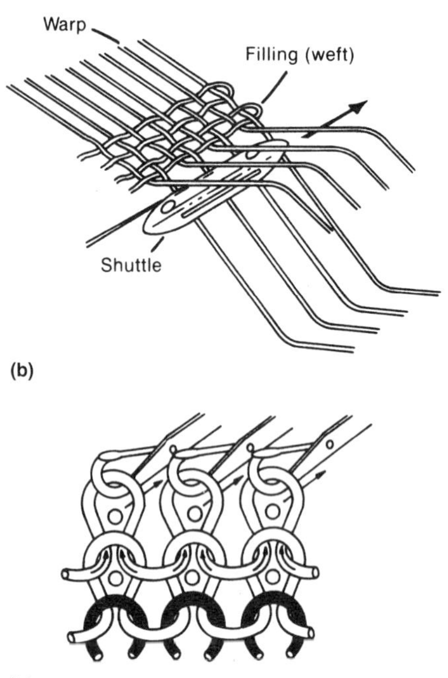

Fig. 1 Fabric techniques. (a) Braided. (b) Woven. (c) Knitted

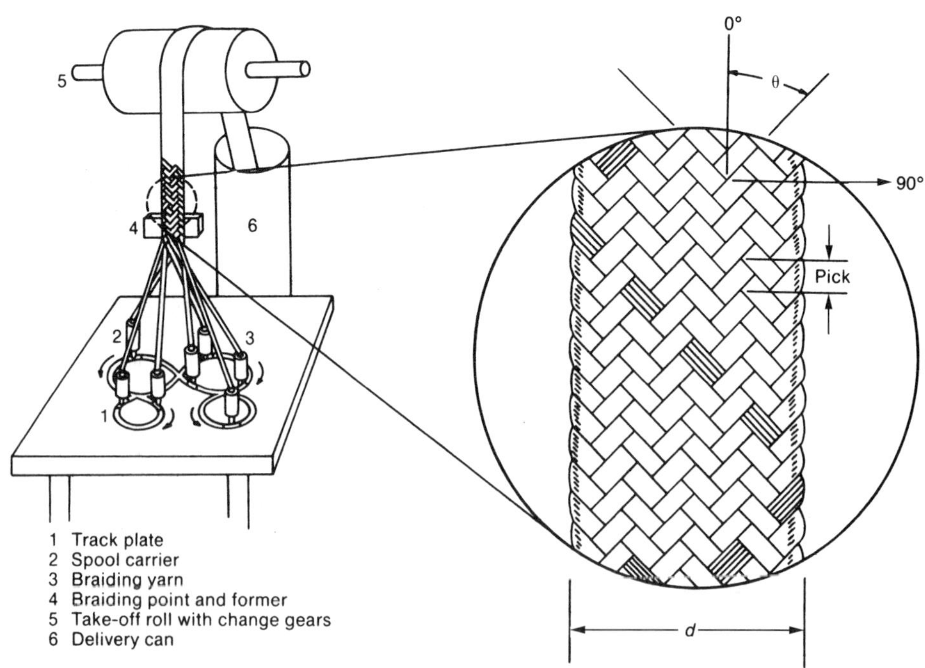

Fig. 2 Flat braider and braid

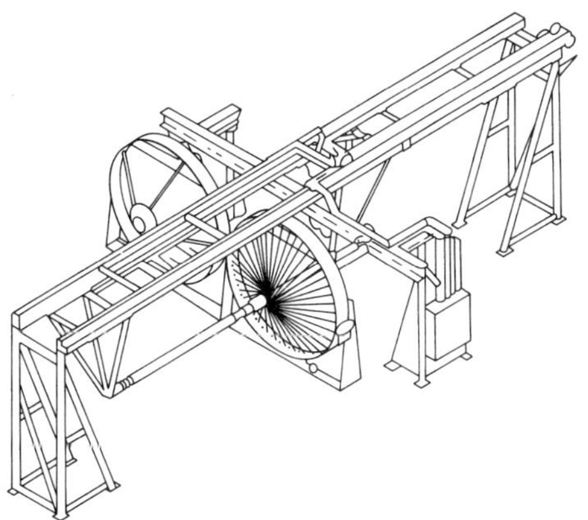

Fig. 3 Braiding machine, 144-carrier model

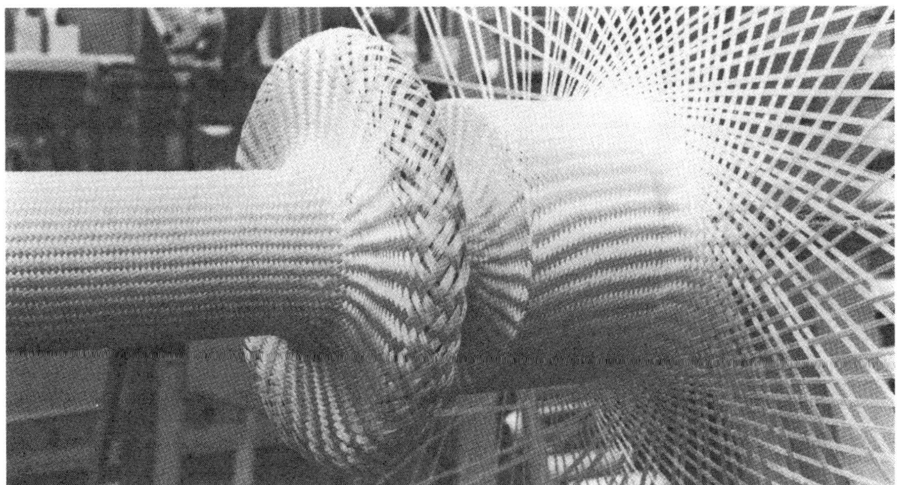

Fig. 4 Formation of fiberglass preform for composite coupling shaft

name, New England Butt, and now called Wardwell Braiding Machine Company), which manufactures braiders ranging from three-carrier to 144-carrier models. There are a number of braid manufacturers actively producing braided preforms and/or developing braided composites. A sample list of these companies is given in Table 3. A wide range of applications has been reported by these companies, including medical, recreational, military, and aerospace uses, as defined in Table 4.

Table 3 U.S. braid manufacturers

A & P Technology, Inc.	Kentucky
Albany International Research	Massachusetts
Amatex	Pennsylvania
Atlantic Research	Virginia
Fabric Development	Pennsylvania
Fiber Concepts	Pennsylvania
Fiber Innovations	Massachusetts
Fiber Materials	Maine
Newport Composites	California
Polygon	Indiana
Techniweave	New Hampshire
U.S. Composites	New York

Table 4 Applications of braided fabrics and composites

Aircraft fuselage frames	Net shape rigid armor
Aircraft interiors	Personal armor
Aircraft propellers	Pressure vessels
Artificial limbs, tendons, bone	Racing canoes
Automotive parts	Racing cars (structural panels)
Boats	Racing sculls and catamarans
Boat masts	Radar dishes
Bridge components	Radomes
Chemical containers	Record brushes
Drive shafts	Robot arms and fingers
Elbow fittings	Rocket launcher
Fishing rods	Rocket motor casing
Frame of airplane seats	Rolling ferel drum
Glider	Rotor blades
Glider airplanes	Satellite frames
Golf clubs	Ski poles
Hang-glider frames	Skis
Hockey and ice hockey sticks	Space struts
Jet engine ducts	Spar and blades
Jet engine spinner	Sport cars
Lightweight bridge structures	Squash rackets
Lightweight submersibles	Stiffened panels
Machine parts	Stocks for high jumping
Military equipment	Surfboats
Model aircraft	Tennis rackets
	Wind generator propellers and D-spars
	X-ray tables

Figure 3 illustrates a 144-carrier horizontal braider that is capable of biaxial or triaxial braiding. The versatility of braiding for forming complex structural shapes is illustrated in Fig. 4, which shows a fiberglass preform for a composite coupling shaft being formed in the Fibrous Materials Research Laboratory at Drexel University, using a 144-carrier braiding machine. Using a similar braiding machine, a racing car chassis has also been fabricated (Fig. 5) by that laboratory.

Governing Equations. The mechanical behavior of a composite depends upon fiber orientation, fiber properties, fiber volume fraction, and matrix properties. To conduct an intelligent design and selection process for using braids in composites, an understanding of fiber volume fraction and geometry as a function of processing parameters is necessary. The fiber volume fraction is related to the machine in terms of the number of yarns and the orientation of those yarns. The fiber geometry is related to the machine by orientation of the fibers and final shape.

Braided fabrics can be produced in flat or tubular form by intertwining three or more yarn systems together. The bias interlacing nature of the braided fabrics makes them highly conformable, shear resistant, and tolerant to impact damage. Triaxial braiding can be produced by introducing 0° yarns, as shown in Fig. 6, to enhance reinforcement in the 0° direction.

Multilayer fabrics can be formed by simply braiding back and forth or overbraiding in the same direction to build up the thickness of the structure. Each layer can be biaxial or triaxial. The fiber type and braid angle can be varied as needed.

Because of the highly conformable nature of braided structures, braiding has undergone a great deal of development in recent years (Ref 18). The formation of shape and fiber architecture is illustrated in Fig. 7, which depicts the process of braiding over an axisymmetric shape of revolution according to instructions generated through a process kinematic model. The governing equations for the model and the input parameters summarized in Tables 5 and 6 (Ref 20) form the basis for a computer-controlled braiding process.

Geometric parameters include distribution of braiding angles, yarn volume fraction, and fabric-covering factor along the mandrel length. Processing variables include profiles of the braiding and mandrel advance speeds versus

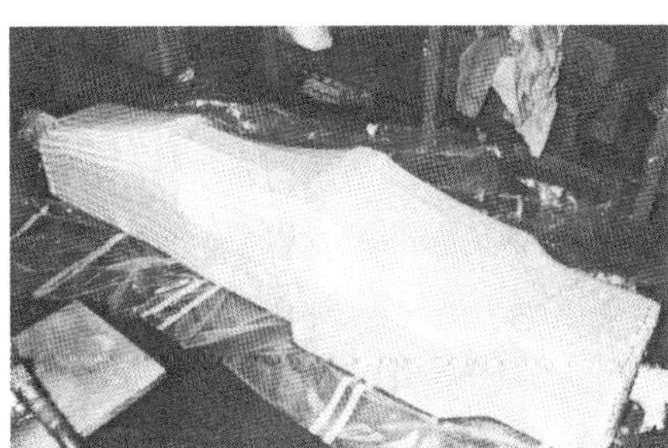

Fig. 5 Braided fiberglass car chassis

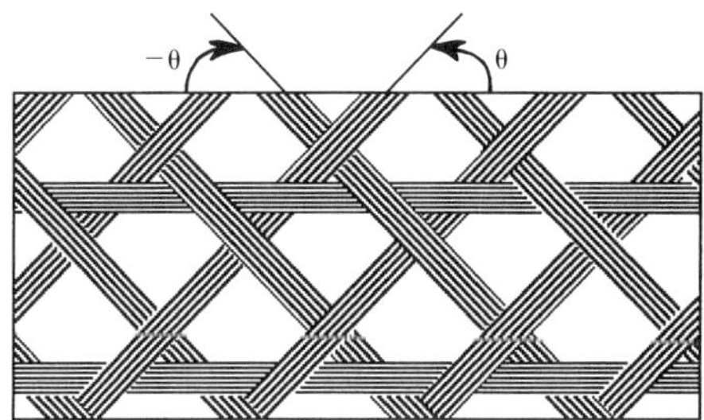

Fig. 6 Structure of triaxial braid

processing time. The equations in Table 6 give the relationship between geometric parameters and processing variables, describe current machine status (braid length and convergence length), and provide process limits due to yarn jamming.

Braiding angle can range from 5° in almost parallel yarn braid to approximately 85° in a hoop yarn braid. However, because of geometric limitations of yarn jamming, the braiding angle that can be achieved for a particular braided fabric, as defined in Table 6, depends on the following parameters: number of carriers, N_c, braiding yarn width, w_y, mandrel radius, R_m, and half-cone angle, γ, of the mandrel.

When the mandrel has a cylindrical shape, that is, $\gamma = 0$, the fiber volume fraction (V_f) of the biaxial braid becomes:

$$V_f = \frac{\kappa \supseteq w_y \supseteq N_c}{4 \supseteq \pi \supseteq R_m \supseteq \cos\theta} \qquad \text{(Eq 1)}$$

where κ is the fiber packing fraction, w_y is the yarn width, N_c is the number of braiding carriers, R_m is the radius of mandrel, and θ is the orientation angle of yarns. We define the braid tightness factor, η, as the ratio of the total width of either $+\theta$ or $-\theta$ yarns to the mandrel perimeter, namely:

$$\eta = \frac{w_y \supseteq N_c}{4 \supseteq \pi \supseteq R_m} (0 < \eta \leq 1) \qquad \text{(Eq 2)}$$

which must be maintained within the range of 0 to 1 to avoid yarn jamming. Combining Eq 1 and 2, the fiber volume fraction is expressed as:

$$V_f = \kappa \frac{\eta}{\cos\theta} \qquad \text{(Eq 3)}$$

Figure 8 shows the process window for the fiber volume fraction versus the braid angle at various levels of fabric tightness factor, based on Eq 3. The fiber packing fraction again is assumed to be 0.8. As can be seen, for a given fabric tightness factor, the fiber volume fraction increases with an increase in the braid angle, until the yarn jamming point is reached. In designing braided preforms, their fiber volume fraction and fiber orientation angles are usually determined from the composite properties desired. To achieve the requirement for the desired fiber volume fraction and orientation angle, it is only necessary to select a specific fabric tightness factor (either by changing the braiding carrier numbers, the width of braiding yarns, or a combination of the two) as defined by Eq 3.

Three-Dimensional Braiding

Three-dimensional braiding technology is an extension of two-dimensional braiding technology, in which the fabric is constructed by the intertwining or orthogonal interlacing of yarns to form an integral structure through position displacement.

A unique feature of three-dimensional braids is their ability to provide through-the-thickness reinforcement of composites as well as their ready adaptability to the fabrication of a wide range of complex shapes ranging from solid rods to I-beams to thick-walled rocket nozzles.

Three-dimensional braids have been produced on traditional maypole machines for ropes and packings in solid, circular, or square cross sections. The yarn carrier movement is activated in a restricted fashion by horn gears. A three-dimensional cylindrical braiding machine of this form was introduced by Albany International Corporation, with some modification that the yarn carriers do not move through all the layers (Ref 21). Three-dimensional braiding processes without using the horn gears, including track and column (Ref 22) and two-step (Ref 23), have been developed since the late 1960s in the search for multidirectional reinforced composites for aerospace applications. The track and column method is concentrated upon for analysis.

A generalized schematic of a three-dimensional braiding process is shown in Fig. 9. Axial yarns, if present in a particular braid, are fed directly into the structure from packages located below the track plate. Braiding yarns are fed from bobbins mounted on carriers that move on the track plate. The pattern produced by the motion of the braiders relative to each other and the axial yarns establishes the type of braid being formed, as well as the microstructure.

Track and column braiding is the most popular process in manufacturing of three-dimensional braided preforms. The mechanism of these braiding methods differs from the traditional horn gear method only in the way the carriers

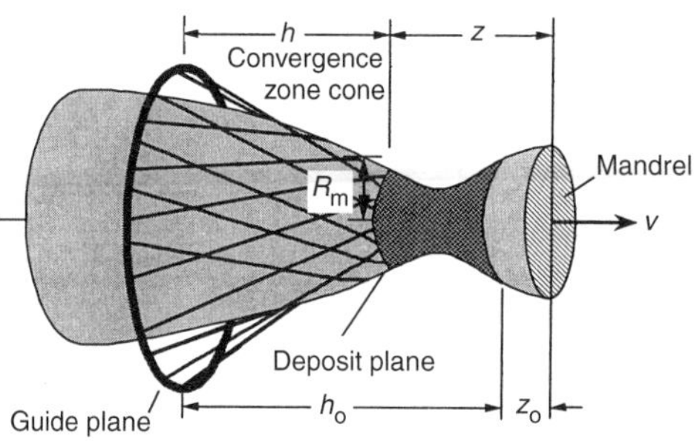

Fig. 7 Braid formation over mandrel. For definition of variables see Table 5.

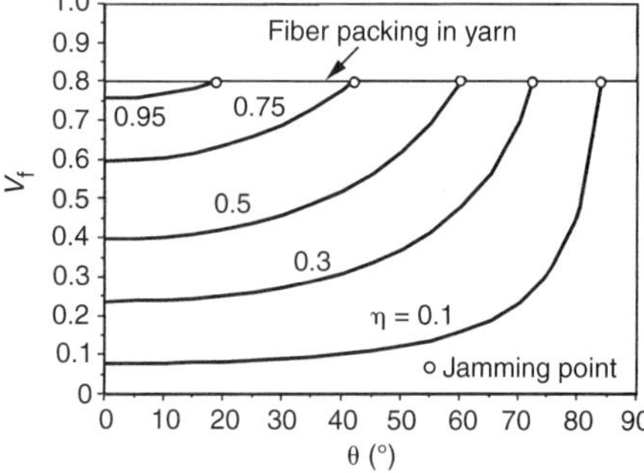

Fig. 8 Process window of fiber volume fraction for two-dimensional braid

Table 5 Key inputs and outputs for computer-controlled braiding

Inputs	
Constants	
Guide radius	R_g
Number of carriers	N_c
Yarn width	w_y
Mandrel shape	$R_{m(z)}$
Initial conditions	
Convergence zone length	h_o
Starting deposit location	z_o
Key inputs/outputs	
Local braid angle	$\theta(z)$
Local yarn volume fraction	$V_{y(z)}$
Machine speed profiles	$v(t)$, $\omega(t)$
Auxiliary outputs	
Convergence zone length	$h(t)$
Local cone half-angle	$\gamma(z)$
Velocity of braid formation	$\frac{dz(t)}{dt}$

Table 6 Governing equations for computer-controlled braiding

Convergence length	$v(t) = \frac{dh(t)}{dt} + \frac{R_{m(z)} \supseteq \omega(t) \supseteq h(t)}{R_g \sqrt{1 - \left[\frac{R_{m(z)}}{R_g} + \frac{h(t)}{R_g} \tan\gamma(z)\right]^2}}$
Braid angle	$\theta(z) = \tan^{-1}\left[\frac{R_g}{h(t)} \cos\gamma(z) \sqrt{1 - \left[\frac{R_{m(z)}}{R_g} + \frac{h(t)}{R_g} \tan\gamma(z)\right]^2}\right]$
Fiber volume fraction	$V_{f(z)} = \frac{\kappa \supseteq w_y \supseteq \sin\gamma(z)}{2 \supseteq R_{m(z)} \supseteq \cos\theta(z) \supseteq \sin\left[\frac{2 \supseteq \pi \supseteq \sin\gamma(z)}{N_c}\right]}$
Yarn jamming criterion	$\theta_{max(z)} = \cos^{-1}\left[\frac{w_y \supseteq \sin\gamma(z)}{2 \supseteq R_m \supseteq \sin\left[\frac{2 \supseteq \pi \supseteq \sin\gamma(z)}{N_c}\right]}\right]$

are displaced to create the final braid geometry. Instead of moving in a continuous maypole fashion, as in the solid braider, these three-dimensional braiding methods invariably move the carriers in a sequential, discrete manner. Figure 10(a) shows a basic loom setup in a rectangular configuration. The carriers are arranged in tracks and columns to form the required shape, and additional carriers are added to the outside of the array in alternating locations. Four steps of motion are imposed to the tracks and columns during a complete braiding machine cycle, resulting in the alternate X- and Y-displacement of yarn carriers, as shown in Fig. 10 (b)–(e). Since the track and column both move one carrier displacement in each step, the braiding pattern is referred to as 1 × 1. Similar to the solid braid, the 0° axial reinforcements can also be added to the track and column braid as desired. The formation of shapes, such as T-beam and I-beam, is accomplished by the proper positioning of the carriers and the joining of various rectangular groups through selected carrier movements.

The assumptions made in the geometric analysis of three-dimensional braids given by Du and Ko (Ref 24) are as follows: no axial yarns; rectangular loom with 1 × 1 braiding pattern; braider yarns have circular cross sections, same linear density, and constant fiber packing fraction; yarn tensions are high enough to ensure a noncrimp yarn path; and the braid is mostly compacted so that each yarn is in contact with all its neighboring yarns. In other words, the braid is always under the jamming condition.

Figure 11(a) shows the unit cell identified from the analysis. The unit cell consists of four partial yarns being cut by six planes. Clearly, there does not exist such a unit cell that only consists of four complete yarns. The dimensions of the unit cell are $\frac{1}{2} h_{x'}$ in x'-direction, $\frac{1}{2} h_{y'}$ in y'-direction, and $\frac{1}{2} h_z$ in the z-direction (braid length), where $h_{x'}$ and $h_{y'}$ can be calculated from the yarn diameter, d, its orientation angle, α, and the fabric tightness factor, η. The dimension h_z is actually the pitch length of braid formed in a complete machine cycle (four steps). This length is one of the key parameters in controlling the fabric microstructures. The cross sections of the unit cell at $\frac{1}{2} h_z$, $\frac{3}{8} h_z$, $\frac{1}{4} h_z$, $\frac{1}{8} h_z$, and 0 are shown in Fig. 11(b)–(f), respectively. As can be seen, each unit cell cross section consists of four half-oval cross sections of yarn. The fiber volume fraction can then be derived based on this observation.

The braid has the tightest structure when each yarn is in contact with all its neighboring yarns, in other words, the yarns are jammed against each other. At the jamming condition, fiber volume fraction, V_f, can be derived from the geometric relationship:

$$V_f = \frac{\pi}{2}\kappa\frac{\cos\theta}{1+\cos^2\theta} \quad \text{(Eq 4)}$$

where κ is the fiber packing fraction (fiber-to-yarn area ratio) and θ is the angle of braider yarn to braid axis (yarn orientation angle). Due to the bulky fiber and nonlinear crimp nature, it is difficult to fabricate the braid with tightest structure. In practice, the yarn orientation angle (braiding angle) is determined from the yarn diameter and braid pitch length. The fiber volume fraction is controlled by the braiding angle and the braid tightness factor. The governing equations are (Ref 25):

$$\theta = \sin^{-1}\sqrt{\frac{8}{(h_z/d)^2+4}} \quad (h_z \geq 2d) \quad \text{(Eq 5)}$$

$$V_f = \frac{\kappa\eta}{\cos\theta} \leq \frac{\pi}{2}\kappa\frac{\cos\theta}{1+\cos^2\theta} \quad \text{(Eq 6)}$$

where d is the yarn diameter, h_z is the pitch length of braid formed in a machine cycle (four braiding steps), and η is the fabric tightness factor. The tightness factor is within the range of 0 to $\pi/4$ and must be so selected that the required fiber volume fraction is achieved and also that the over-jamming condition is avoided.

Figure 12 shows the V_f-θ relationship prior to and at the jamming condition, based on the governing equations. The fiber packing fraction, κ, is assumed as 0.785. As can be seen, there are three regions of fiber volume fraction. The upper region cannot be achieved due to the impossible fiber packing in a yarn bundle. Jamming occurs when the highest braiding angle is reached for a given fabric tightness factor, η. The nonshaded region is the working window for a variety of V_f-θ combinations. Clearly, for a given fabric tightness, the higher braiding angle gives higher fiber volume fraction, and for a fixed braiding

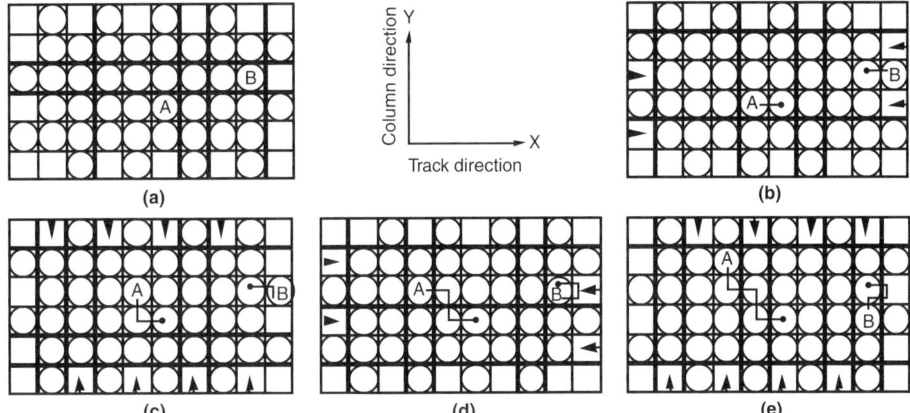

Fig. 10 Formation of a rectangular three-dimensional track and column braid, using 4 tracks, 8 columns, and 1 × 1 braiding pattern

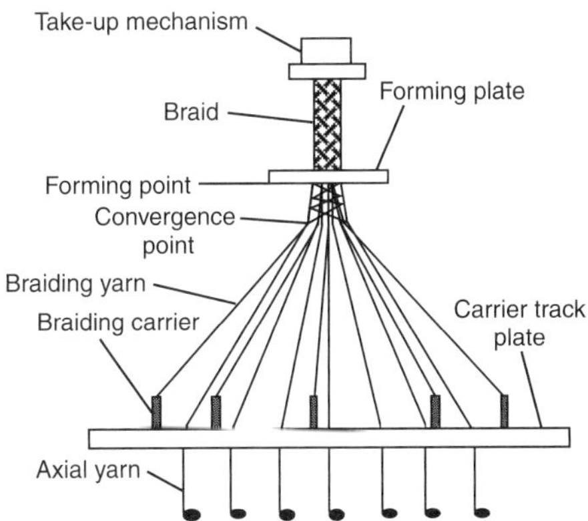

Fig. 9 Schematic of a generalized three-dimensional braider

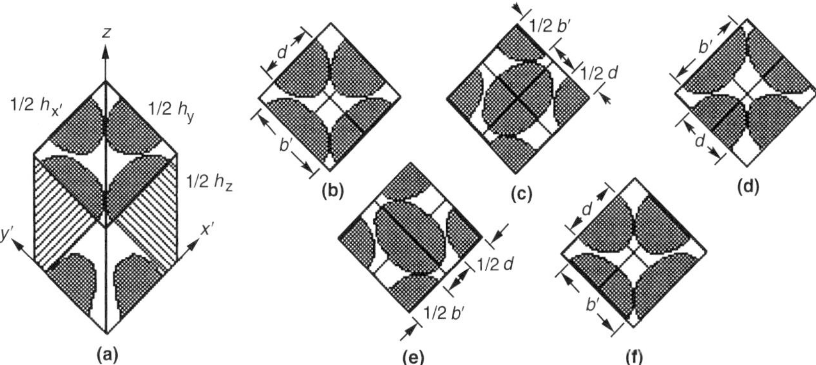

Fig. 11 Unit cell geometry of three-dimensional braid. (a) Unit cell. (b) Unit cell cross section at $z = \frac{1}{2} h_z$. (c) Unit cell cross section at $z = \frac{3}{8} h_z$. (d) Unit cell cross section at $z = \frac{1}{4} h_z$. (e) Unit cell cross section at $z = \frac{1}{8} h_z$. (f) Unit cell cross section at $z = 0$.

angle, the fiber volume fraction is greater at higher tightness factors.

Properties of Braided Composites

The properties of braided composites are not as well characterized as those for unidirectional tape or woven ply laid-up laminated composites. For two-dimensional braided composites, most of the studies have been on tubular braids. For three-dimensional braid, a database is beginning to be accumulated in academia and government laboratories. In addition to the near-net shape formability, the most outstanding properties noted for two-dimensional and three-dimensional braid composites are their damage tolerance and their ability to limit impact damage area.

Two-Dimensional Braid Composites. In a study by D.E. Flinchbaugh (Ref 26) on tubular braided S-2 fiberglass-epoxy composites, it was reported that the tensile strength of the braided composites is comparable to that of mild steel at a much lower density. Table 7 summarizes these results. The composite had a density of 1.66 g/cm^3 and a fiber volume fraction of 75%.

The properties of triaxial braided graphite-epoxy composites was demonstrated by T. Tsiang et al. (Ref 27). As shown in Table 8, the hoop modulus was quite sensitive to the braiding angle. In the longitudinal direction, because of the 0° yarn introduced in the triaxial braiding process, the modulus was less sensitive to the braiding angle. It was also shown that the addition of longitudinal yarns can address the concern for the lack of compressive resistance in braids.

In another study by D. Brookstein and T. Tsiang (Ref 28), it was demonstrated, as shown in Fig. 13, that the capability for the formation of holes in the braiding process revealed the superiority of open hole and pin hole strength over that of machined holes.

Three-Dimensional Braid Composites. Since 1983, an intensive effort has been devoted to studying three-dimensional braid composites. Mostly funded by the government, a rather extensive database is being generated in U.S. government laboratories (with the majority in the Naval labs) and in academia (Drexel University and the University of Delaware). The preforms used in these studies are primarily supplied by Drexel University and Atlantic Research Corporation. Although research work on three-dimensional braid composites has been carried out on polymer, metal, and ceramic-matrix composites as well as on carbon-carbon composites, the largest database by far is in polymeric-matrix composites. Therefore, for illustration purposes, only their properties are described subsequently.

General Mechanical Properties. The most comprehensive mechanical characterization of three-dimensional braid composite properties to date has been carried out by A.B. Macander et al. (Ref 29). In this study, the effect of cut-edge bundle size and braid construction were examined through tensile, compressive, flexural, and shear tests. It was found that the test specimens were sensitive to cut edges. As shown in Table 9, the tensile strength of a graphite-epoxy (T300/5208) composite was reduced by approximately

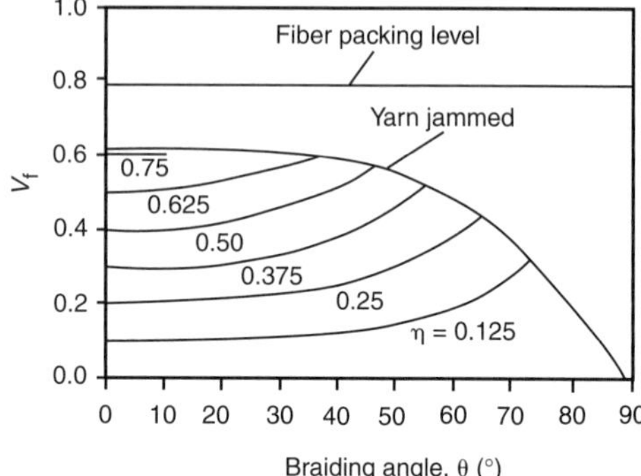

Fig. 12 Relationship of fiber volume fraction to braiding angle for various fiber tightness factors (η)

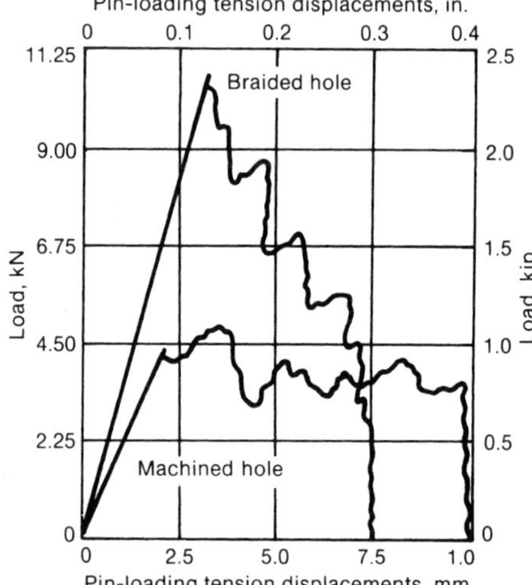

Fig. 13 Strengths of braided holes and machined holes

Table 7 Properties of two-dimensional braided S-2 fiberglass-epoxy composites

	Tensile strength				Compressive strength					
	Hoop		Long		Hoop		Long		In-plane shear	
Braid angle, degree	MPa	ksi	MPa	ksi	MPa	ksi	MPa	ksi	MPa	ksi
89	1320	192	21	3	700	102	220	32	55	8
86.75	1250	182	83	12	380	55	100	14	75	11
82.50	1030	149	...	...	330	48	...	...	...	...
78	730	106	...	...	275	40	...	...	...	...

Table 8 Properties of triaxial braided graphite-epoxy composites

		E_{LT}		E_{LC}		E_{HT}				
Braid angle, degree	V_f, %	GPa	10^6 psi	GPa	10^6 psi	GPa	10^6 psi	ν_{LHT}	ν_{LHC}	ν_{HLT}
45	33.8	61.4	8.9	62.7	9.1	6.8	0.98	0.56	0.64	0.044
63	29.3	49.0	7.1	49.6	7.2	15.2	2.20	0.43	0.45	0.088
80	56.3	...	...	52.4	7.6	43.6	6.32	...	0.13	0.110

V_f, fiber volume; *E*, modulus of elasticity; ν, Poisson's ratio

Table 9 Three-dimensional braided graphite-epoxy composite property data

1 × 1.3 × 1 and 1 × 1 × 11-braid patterns with uncut and cut edges. Fiber volume (V_f), 68%

	Fiber type and braid pattern					
Property(a)	T300(b), 1 × 1 (uncut)	T300, 1 × 1 (cut)	T300, 3 × 1 (uncut)	T300, 3 × 1 (cut)	T300, 1 × 1 × ½ fixed (uncut)	T300, 1 × 1 × ½ fixed (cut)
Tensile strength, MPa (ksi)	665.6 (96.5)	228.7 (33.2)	970.5 (140.8)	363.7 (52.7)	790.6 (114.7)	405.7 (68.9)
Elastic modulus, GPa (10^6 psi)	97.8 (14.2)	50.5 (7.3)	126.4 (18.3)	76.4 (11.1)	117.4 (17.0)	82.4 (12.0)
Compressive strength, MPa (ksi)	...	179.5 (26.0	...	226.4 (32.8)	...	385.4 (55.9)
Compressive modulus, GPa (10^6 psi)	...	38.7 (5.6)	...	56.6 (8.2)	...	80.8 (11.7)
Flexural strength, MPa (ksi)	813.5 (118.0)	465.2 (67.5)	647.2 (93.9)	508.1 (73.3)	816.0 (118.3)	632.7 (91.8)
Flexural modulus, GPa (10^6 psi)	77.5 (11.2)	34.1 (4.9)	85.4 (12.4)	54.9 (8.0)	86.4 (12.5)	60.8 (8.8)
Poisson's ratio	0.875	1.36	0.566	0.806	0.986	0.667
Apparent fiber angle	±20°	±20°	±12°	±12°	±15°	±12°

(a) Tension and compression specimens were tabbed at grip ends. (b) T300 graphite yarn, 30,000 tow

Table 10 Three-dimensional braided graphite-epoxy composite properties as a function of braid pattern

Uncut specimens, 25.4 mm (1 in.) wide including comparative data for a laminated fabric composite. Tensile specimens were tabbed with 1.6 mm ($\frac{1}{16}$ in.) thick, 25.4 mm (1 in.) × 63.5 mm ($2\frac{1}{2}$ in.) glass-reinforced plastic tapered tabs at grip ends. Celion 6K and 12K specimens had cut edges for the short-beam shear tests only.

	Fiber type and braid pattern						
Property	AS-4, 3K 1 × 1	AS-4, 6K 1 × 1	Celion, 6K 1 × 1	AS-4, 12K 1 × 1	Celion, 12K 1 × 1	T300, 30K 1 × 1	T300, Eight harness satin fabric
V_f, %	68	68	56	68	68	68	65
Tensile strength, MPa (ksi)	736.8 (106.8)	841.4 (122.0)	857.7 (124.4)	1067.2 (154.790)	1219.8 (176.910)	655.6 (96.530)	517.1 (75.000)
Elastic modulus, GPa (10^6 psi)	83.5 (12.1)	119.3 (17.3)	87.8 (12.7)	114.7 (16.6)	113.1 (16.4)	97.8 (14.2)	73.8 (10.7)
Short-beam shear, MPa (ksi)	114.8 (16.6)	126.0 (18.2)	71.4 (10.3)	121.4 (17.600)	71.4 (10.350)	...	69.0 (10.000)
Poisson's ratio	0.945	1.051	0.968	0.980	0.874	0.875	0.045
Flexural strength, MPa (ksi)	885.3 (128.4)	739.8 (107.3)	...	1063.3 (154.210)	...	813.5 (117.990)	689.5 (100.000)
Flexural modulus, GPa (10^6 psi)	84.5 (12.3)	95.2 (13.8)	...	1385.2 (20.1)	...	77.5 (11.2)	65.5 (9.5)
Apparent fiber angle	±19°	±15°	±15°	±13°	±17.5°	±20°	0°

60%. When longitudinal yarns (0°) were added, the strength reduction was less than 50%. Accordingly, care should be exercised in the preparation of braided composites to ensure that the yarns on the surfaces are not destroyed. In the same table, one can also see the effect of braid construction and thus, the resulting surface fiber orientation. From a 1 × 1 construction to a 3 × 1 construction, the surface fiber orientation was reduced from 20° to 12°, which resulted in an increase in tensile strength from 665.6 MPa (96.5 ksi) to 970.5 MPa (140.8 ksi).

In Table 10, the effect of yarn bundle size is illustrated. It was found that the tensile strength and modulus of the three-dimensional braid composites tend to increase as fiber bundle size increases. This is apparently related to the dependence of fiber orientation on yarn bundle size. A larger yarn bundle size produced lower crimp (fiber angles) and thus higher strength and modulus. From both Tables 9 and 10, one will notice that although the strength and modulus of the braided composites were significantly higher than those of the 0°/90° woven laminates, the Poisson's ratio (or specific Poisson's ratio) of the braided composites were exceedingly high, from 0.67 to 1.36. To address the instability characteristics in the transverse direction, it was found in the Drexel University laboratory that by adding 10 vol% transverse (90°) yarns, the Poisson's ratio of the braided composites can be reduced to 0.27 at a reduction of strength and modulus from 1250 MPa (180 ksi) and 100 GPa (15 × 10^6 psi) to 10 MPa (155 ksi) and 90 GPa (13 × 10^6 psi), respectively.

Damage Tolerance. The first indication of the damage tolerance capability of the three-dimensional braid composites was observed by L.W. Gause and J. Alper (Ref 30). In the drill hole test performed on three-dimensional braided Celion 12K/3501 (BASF Corporation), composites and quasi-isotropic composites, it was found that the braided composites were quite insensitive to the drill hole (retaining over 90% of the strength). In the case of the quasi-isotropic composites, a 50% reduction in strength was observed. In the same study, it was also found that although the braided composites did not increase the damage threshold, they did successfully limit the extent of impact damage of graphite-epoxy, compared to that of conventional laminated constructions. Similar observations were also made by F. Ko and D. Hartman on glass-epoxy composites (Ref 31) as well as on carbon-polyetheretherketone (PEEK) composites (Ref 32). The three-dimensional braid glass-epoxy required significantly higher levels of energy to initiate and propagate damage than did the laminated composites under drop weight impact test. In the study of three-dimensional braid commingled Celion 3K-PEEK thermoplastic composites, it was found, as shown in Fig. 14, that the compression-after-impact-strength of the three-dimensional composites was less sensitive than for the state-of-the-art, unidirectional tape laid-up graphite-PEEK composites. The most drastic difference, however, was the impact damage area of the three-dimensional braid composite, compared to that of the laminated composites. As shown in Fig. 15, an order of magnitude lower damage area was attained with the braided composites, compared to the laminated composites.

Properties of Three-Dimensional Braid Composite I-Beams. To illustrate the design flexibil-

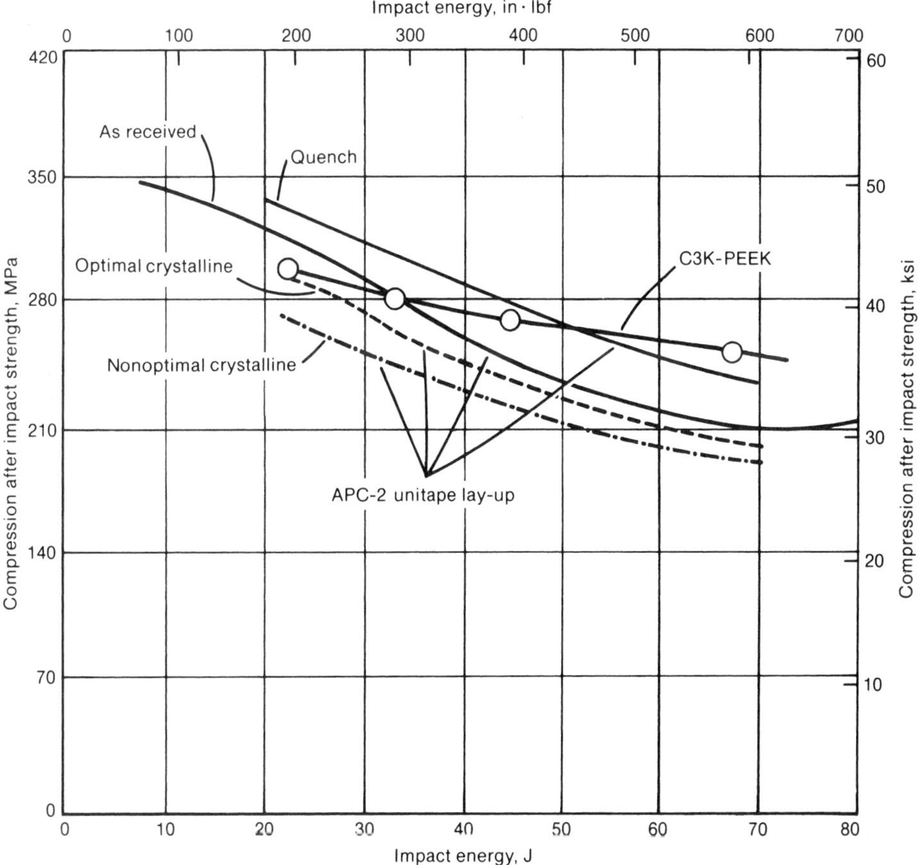

Fig. 14 Effect of impact energy level on compression after impact strength for three-dimensional braid comingled and laminated carbon-PEEK composites

Table 11 Properties of three-dimensional braid glass-polyester I-beams

	I-beam 1	I-beam 2	I-beam 3
Geometry	Braid	Braid/lay-in	Braid/lay-in
Fiber	Glass	Glass/glass	Glass/carbon
Fiber volume, %	50	60	65
Length, mm (in.)	452 (17.8)	460 (18.1)	447 (17.6)
Test span, mm (in.)	305 (12.0)	305 (12.0)	305 (12.0)
Width, mm (in.)	31 (1.2)	31 (1.2)	32 (1.25)
Height, mm (in.)	32 (1.25)	33 (1.3)	33 (1.3)
Tensile modulus, GPa (10^6 psi)	18.34 (2.66)	30.54 (4.43)	44.82 (6.5)
Compressive modulus, GPa (10^6 psi)	21.10 (3.1)	30.54 (4.43)	68.26 (9.9)
Flexural strength, MPa (ksi)	150.5 (21.8)	237.9 (34.50)	292.0 (42.3)
Compressive modulus, GPa (10^6 psi)	20.62 (3.0)	29.44 (4.27)	68.67 (9.96)
Compressive strength, MPa (ksi)	145.1 (21.0)	176.4 (25.58)	175.9 (25.51)

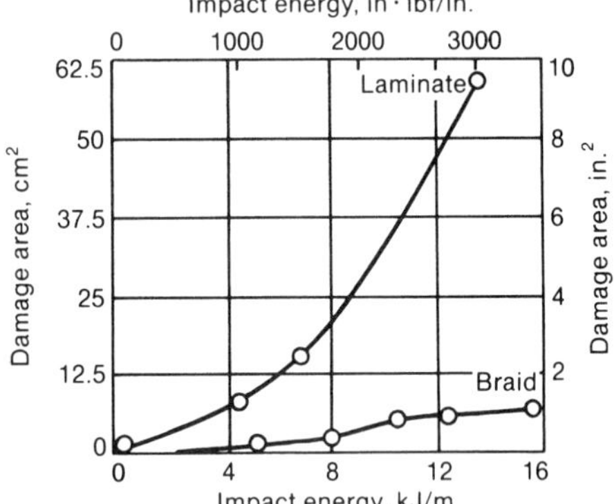

Fig. 15 Effect of impact energy on damage area of three-dimensional braid comingled and laminated carbon-PEEK composites

ity and the structural properties of the three-dimensional braid net-shape composite, a study was carried out by S.S. Yau, T.W. Chu, and F.K. Ko on three-dimensional braided E-glass-polyester I-beams (Ref 33). It was demonstrated that mechanical properties of the net-shape composites can be tailored by the strategic placement of materials in the braiding process. For instance, in Table 11, it can be seen that the addition of longitudinal glass yarns in the flanges of the I-beam led to a more than 50% increase in tensile and compressive moduli. Instead of fiberglass, the addition of unidirectional carbon yarns in the flanges of the I-beam produced as much as a three-fold increase in compressive resistance. Furthermore, the delamination failure found in laminated composites was not observed in any of the I-beams as a result of the high degree of through-thickness strength in the three-dimensional braided composites.

REFERENCES

1. L.R. Sanders, Braiding—A Mechanical Means of Composite Fabrication, *SAMPE Q.*, 1977, p 38–44
2. F.K. Ko, *Atkins and Pearce Handbook of Industrial Braids,* 1988
3. C.A. Belash, Braiding and Knotting for Amateurs, *The Beacon Handicraft Series,* The Beacon Press, 1936
4. W.J. Hamburger, Effect of Yarn Elongations on Parachute Fabric Strength, *Rayon Textile Monthly,* March and May, 1942
5. D. Brunnschweiler, Braids and Braiding, *J. Textile Ind.,* Vol 44, 1953, p 666
6. D. Brunnschweiler, The Structure and Tensile Properties of Braids, *J. Textile Ind.,* Vol 45, T55-87, 1954
7. W.A. Douglass, *Braiding and Braiding Machinery,* Centrex Publishing, 1964
8. F. Goseberg, The Construction of Braided Goods, *Band-und Flechtindustrie,* No. 2, 1969, p 65–72

9 F. Goseberg, "Textile Technology-Machine Braids," training material instructional aid, All Textile Employers Association, 1981

10. W. Weber, The Calculation of Round Braid, *Band-und Flechtindustrie,* No. 1, Part 1, 1969, p 17–31; No. 3, Part 11, 1969, p 109–119
11. R.J. Post, Braiding Composites—Adapting the Process for the Mass Production of Aerospace Components, *Proc. 22nd National SAMPE Symposium and Exhibition,* Society for the Advancement of Material and Process Engineering, 1977, p 486–503
12. S.L. Phoenix, Mechanical Response of a Tubular Braided Cable with Elastic Core, *Textile Res. J.,* 1977, p 81–91
13. C.W. Evans, *Hose Technology,* 2nd ed., Applied Science, 1979
14. J.B. Carter, "Fabrication Techniques of Tubular Structures from Braided Preimpregnated Rovings," Paper EM85-100, presented at Composites in Manufacturing 4, Society of Mechanical Engineers, 1985
15. B.D. Haggard and D.E Flinchbaughy, "Braided Structures for Launchers and Rocket Motor Cases," paper presented at JANNAF S and MBS/CMCS Subcommittee Meeting, MDAC/Titusville, Nov 1984
16. R.A. Florentine, Magnaswirl's Integrally Woven Marine Propeller—The Magnaweave Process Extended to Circular Parts, *Proc. 38th Annual Conf.,* Society of the Plastics Industry, Feb 1981
17. F.K. Ko and C.M. Pastore, "Structure and Properties of an Integrated 3-D Fabric for Structural Composites," Special Technical Testing Publication 864, American Society for Testing and Materials, 1985, p 428–439
18. A. Majidi, J.M. Yang, and T.W. Chou, Mechanical Behavior of Three Dimensional Woven Fiber Composites, in *Proceedings of the International Conference on Composite Materials* V, 1985
19. C. Croon, Braided Fabrics: Properties and Applications, *19th National SAMPE Symposium,* Society for the Advancement of Material and Process Engineering, March 1984
20. G.W. Du, P. Popper, and T.W. Chou, Process Model of Circular Braiding for Complex-Shaped Preform Manufacturing, *Proc. Symposium on Processing of Polymers and Polymeric Composites,* American Society of Mechanical Engineers (Dallas, Texas), 25–30 Nov 1990
21. D.S. Brookstein, Interlocked Fiber Architecture: Braided and Woven, *Proc. 35th Int. SAMPE Symposium,* Vol 35, Society for the Advancement of Material and Process Engineering, 1990, p 746–756
22. R.T. Brown, G.A. Patterson, and D.M. Carper, Performance of 3-D Braided Composite Structures, *Proc. Third Structural Textile Symposium* (Drexel University, Philadelphia, PA), 1988
23. P. Popper and R. McConnell, R. 1987. A New 3-D Braid for Integrated Parts Manufacturing and Improved Delamination Resistance—The 2-Step Method, *32nd International SAMPE Symposium and Exhibition*, Society for the Advancement of Material and Process Engineering, 1987, p 92–103
24. G.W. Du and F.K. Ko, Unit Cell Geometry of 3-D Braided Structure, *Proc. ASC Sixth Technical Conference,* 6–9 Oct 1991 (Albany, NY), American Society for Composites
25. G.W. Du and F.K. Ko, Geometric Modeling of 3-D Braided Preforms for Composites, *Proc. 5th Textile Structural Composites Symposium,* 4–6 Dec 1991 (Drexel University, Philadelphia, PA)
26. D.E. Flinchbaugh, "Braided Composite Structures," paper presented at the Composites Material Conference, Aug 1985 (Dover)
27. T. Tsiang, D. Brookstein, and J. Dent, Mechanical Characterization of Braided Graphite/Epoxy Cylinders, *Proc. 29th National SAMPE Symposium,* Society for the Advancement of Material and Process Engineering, 1984, p 880
28. D. Brookstein and T. Tsiang, Load-Deformation Behavior of Composite Cylinders with Integrally Formed Braided and Machined Holes, *J. Compos. Mater.,* Vol 19, 1985, p 477
29. A.B. Macander, R.M. Crane, and E.T. Camponeschi, Fabrication and Mechanical Properties of Multidimensionally (X-D) Braided Composite Materials, *Composite Materials: Testing and Design (Seventh Conference),* STP 893, J.M. Whitney, Ed., American So-

ciety for Testing and Materials, 1986, p 422–443

30. L.W. Gause and J. Alper, "Mechanical Characterization of Magnaweave Braided Composites," paper presented at the Mechanics of Composites Review, Oct 1983, Air Force Materials Laboratory
31. F. Ko and D. Hartman, Impact Behavior of 2-D and 3-D Glass/Epoxy Composites, *SAMPE J.,* July/Aug 1986, p 26–29
32. F.K. Ko, H. Chu, and E. Ying, Damage Tolerance of 3-D Braided Intermingled Carbon/PEEK Composites, *Advanced Composites: The Latest Developments*, Proceedings of the Second Conference on Advanced Composites, ASM International, 1986, p 75–88
33. S.S. Yau, T.W. Chu, and F.K. Ko, Flexural and Axial Compressive Failures of Three Dimensionally Braided Composite I-Beams, Composites, Vol 17 (No. 3), July 1986

Epoxy Resins

Maureen A. Boyle, Cary J. Martin, and John D. Neuner, Hexcel Corporation

THE FIRST PRODUCTION OF EPOXY RESINS occurred simultaneously in Europe and in the United States in the late 1930s and early 1940s. Credit is most often attributed to Pierre Castan of Switzerland and S.O. Greenlee of the United States who investigated the reaction of bisphenol-A with epichlorohydrin. The families of epoxy resins that they commercialized were first used as casting compounds and coatings. The same resins are now commodity materials that provide the basis for most epoxy formulations (Ref 1–3).

Epoxy resins are a class of thermoset materials used extensively in structural and specialty composite applications because they offer a unique combination of properties that are unattainable with other thermoset resins. Available in a wide variety of physical forms from low-viscosity liquid to high-melting solids, they are amenable to a wide range of processes and applications. Epoxies offer high strength, low shrinkage, excellent adhesion to various substrates, effective electrical insulation, chemical and solvent resistance, low cost, and low toxicity. They are easily cured without evolution of volatiles or by-products by a broad range of chemical specie. Epoxy resins are also chemically compatible with most substrates and tend to wet surfaces easily, making them especially well suited to composites applications.

Epoxy resins are routinely used as adhesives, coatings, encapsulates, casting materials, potting compounds, and binders. Some of their most interesting applications are found in the aerospace and recreational industries where resins and fibers are combined to produce complex composite structures. Epoxy technologies satisfy a variety of nonmetallic composite designs in commercial and military aerospace applications, including flooring panels, ducting, vertical and horizontal stabilizers, wings, and even the fuselage. This same chemistry, developed for aerospace applications, is now being used to produce lightweight bicycle frames, golf clubs, snowboards, racing cars, and musical instruments.

To support these applications, epoxy resins are formulated to generate specific physical and mechanical properties. The designers of these systems must balance the limitations of the raw materials and the chemistry with the practical needs of the part fabricator. While the simplest formulations may combine a single epoxy resin with a curative, more-complex recipes will include multiple epoxy resins, modifiers for toughness or flexibility or flame/smoke suppression, inert fillers for flow control or coloration, and a curative package that drives specific reactions at specified times.

When selecting a thermoset resin, consideration is usually given to tensile strength, modulus and strain, compression strength and modulus, notch sensitivity, impact resistance, heat deflection temperature or glass transition temperature (T_g), flammability, durability in service, material availability, ease of processing, and price. Epoxy resins are of particular interest to structural engineers because they provide a unique balance of chemical and mechanical properties combined with extreme processing versatility. In all cases, thermoset resins may be tailored to some degree to satisfy particular requirements, so formulation and processing information are often maintained as trade secrets.

The three basic elements of an epoxy resin formulation that must be understood when selecting a thermoset system are the base resin, curatives, and the modifiers. When formulating an epoxy resin for a particular use, it is necessary to know what each of these components contributes to the physical and mechanical performance of the part during and after fabrication. The subsequent sections may be used as a practical introduction to formulary components and epoxy resin selection.

Base Resins

The term "epoxy resin" describes a broad class of thermosetting polymers in which the primary cross linking occurs through the reaction of an epoxide group. In general, an epoxy resin can be thought of as a molecule containing a three-membered ring, consisting of one oxygen atom and two carbon atoms (Fig. 1).

While the presence of this functional group defines a molecule as an epoxide, the molecular base to which it is attached can vary widely, yielding various classes of epoxy resins. The commercial success of epoxies is due in part to the diversity of molecular structures that can be produced using similar chemical processes. In combination with judicious selection of a curing agent and appropriate modifiers, epoxy resins can be specifically tailored to fit a broad range of applications.

It is important to understand basic production techniques in order to appreciate the available resins and how they differ from each other. Epoxy resins are produced from base molecules containing an unsaturated carbon-carbon bond. There are two processes that can be used to convert this double bond into an oxirane ring: dehydrohalogenation of a halohydrin intermediate and direct peracid epoxidation. While both processes are used to produce commercial epoxy resins, the halohydrin route is more common and is used to produce a wider variety of materials (Ref 4).

The most important raw material used in epoxy resin production is epichlorohydrin, which, with the exception of the cycloaliphatic resins, is used as a precursor for nearly every commercially available epoxy resin.

Catesonics and Defining Characteristics. Epoxy resins used in commercial composite applications can be loosely categorized as those suitable for structural or high-temperature applications, and those best suited to nonstructural or low-temperature applications. A primary indicator of service or use temperature of a polymeric composite is the glass transition temperature (T_g). The T_g is the temperature below which a polymer exists in the glassy state where only vibrational motion is present, whereas above this temperature, individual molecular segments are able to move relative to each other in what is termed the "rubbery state." The modulus of a material above its T_g is typically several orders of magnitude lower than its value below the T_g, so this becomes an important consideration when selecting an epoxy resin. The T_g is also strongly affected by the presence of absorbed moisture or solvents. Thus, exposure to moisture or solvents must also be taken into account when

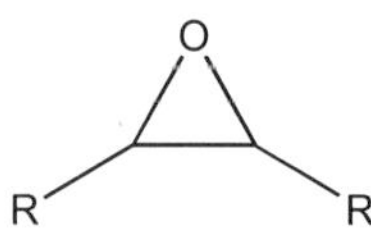

Fig. 1 Basic chemical structure of epoxy group

selecting or designing resins for particular applications.

The glass transition temperature of a cured epoxy resin is dependent upon the molecular structure that develops in the matrix during cure, which is driven by characteristics such as cross-link density, stiffness of the polymer backbone, and intermolecular interactions. It is generally agreed, however, that cured resin formulations suitable for elevated temperature applications are largely determined by cross-link density. The T_g is therefore closely related to cure temperature and will change as the cure temperature changes, so a resin system cured at a low temperature will have a lower T_g than the same system cured at a higher temperature. Every system, however, will have an ultimate T_g determined by its formulation that cannot be enhanced by an increase in cure temperature. In most cured epoxy resins, T_g will lag cure temperature by 10 to 20 °C (20 to 35 °F). It is important to remember that the molecular structure and other characteristics of the cured product are equally dependent on the base resin, the curing agent, and modifiers employed in the formulation.

In addition to service temperature, there are many other physical and chemical differences between the commercially available epoxy resins that dictate both their ultimate use and how they are processed. Primary physical differences between uncured epoxy resins products within a family are material form and viscosity at room temperature, which can range from very thin liquids to solids. Application or processing guidelines often dictate what viscosity or form is required. For example, a solid or semisolid candidate is inappropriate in a wet lay-up application where low viscosity at room temperature is required. As processing capabilities are developed or modified, new material forms become available. The most commonly used resins can be purchased as powders, liquids, solutions produced from various solvents, and, in some cases, as aqueous emulsions.

Another key characteristic that determines resin suitability for use is the epoxy equivalent weight (EEW), which can be defined as the weight of the resin per epoxide group. The equivalent weight of a polymer is used to calculate the stoichiometric ratio between the epoxy and curing agent in order to optimize the cured properties. Dividing the molecular weight of a resin by the number of epoxide groups per molecule can approximate the equivalent weight of a resin. In practice, this estimate will be low as most available resins consist of distribution of molecular weights rather than the single idealized structure. Therefore, epoxy resin vendors routinely determine the EEW of each production lot experimentally as part of their quality control protocols.

Elevated-temperature base resins are those that cure to yield somewhat inflexible molecular structures. Rigidity can be built into the cured matrix in several ways: through the incorporation of aromatic groups, an increase in the number of reactive sites (epoxy groups) per molecule, or a reduction of the distance between reactive sites. The three primary classes of epoxies used in composite applications are phenolic glycidyl ethers, aromatic glycidyl amines, and cycloaliphatics.

Phenolic glycidyl ethers are formed by the condensation reaction between epichlorohydrin and a phenol group. Within this class, the structure of the phenol-containing molecule and the number of phenol groups per molecule distinguish different types of resins.

The first commercial epoxy resin in this class, the diglycidyl ether of bisphenol-A (DGEBA), remains the most widely used today. The structure of pure DGEBA is shown in Fig. 2. Various grades of material are available from multiple suppliers, some of which are summarized in Table 1. The primary distinction between these grades is their viscosity, which can range from 5 to 14 Pa · s (5,000 to 14,000 cP) at 25 °C (77 °F). As equivalent weight increases so does viscosity. Viscosity is ultimately dependent on the molecular weight distribution, with lower molecular weight or purer materials having a lower viscosity and a higher tendency to crystallize upon storage.

Modifying the ratio of epichlorohydrin to bisphenol-A during production can generate high molecular weight resin variants. This growth in molecular weight increases the viscosity, resulting in resins that are solid at room temperature. Higher molecular weight analogs are used to adjust resin viscosity and tack at the expense of lower glass transition temperatures. Small increases in fracture toughness may also be observed as cross-link density decreases.

A variation on this theme is seen in the hydrogenated bisphenol-A epoxy resins. In this process, the epoxy resin is first formed from epichlorohydrin and bisphenol-A. Next, the aromatic benzene ring is converted to cyclohexane, producing a cycloaliphatic material. This results in a low-viscosity, moderately reactive resin with a structure analogous to the DGEBA-types.

An important variant is the epoxy resin produced from tetrabromo bisphenol-A. These bro-

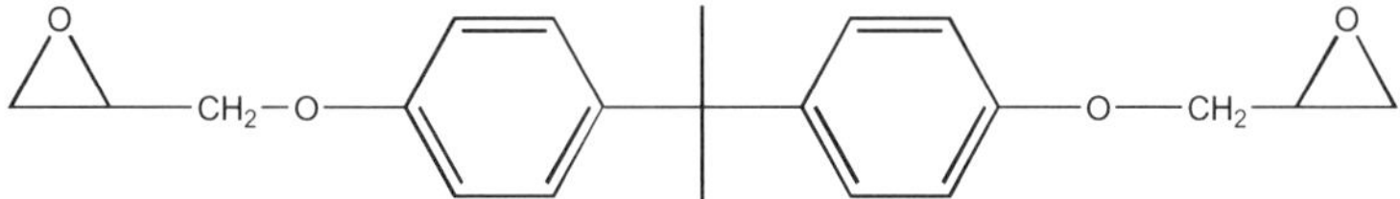

Fig. 2 Chemical structure of diglycidyl ether of bisphenol-A

Table 1 Epoxy resins

Chemical class	Form	Functionality(a)	Equivalent weight(b)	Viscosity at 25 °C (77 °F)		Trade name (supplier)
				Pa · s	cP	
Diglycidyl ether of bisphenol-A	Liquid	2	174–200	5–20	5,000–20,000	Epon 825, 828 (Shell) GY 2600, 6004, 6005, 6008, 6010, 6020 (Vantico) DER 330, 331, 332 (Dow) Epiclon 840, 850 (DIC)
	Solid	2	>500	...	...	Epon 1001, 1002, 1004, 1007, 1009 (Shell) GT 6063, 6084, 6097 (Vantico) DER 661, 662 (Dow) Epiclon 1050, 2050, 3050, 4050, 7050 (DIC)
Diglycidyl ether of bisphenol-F	Liquid	2	165–190	2–7	2,000–7,000	Epon 862 (Shell) GY 281, 282, 285 (Vantico) DER 354, 354LV (Dow) Epiclon 830, 835 (DIC)
Phenol novolac	Semisolid	2.2–3.6	170–210	varies	varies	EPN 1138, 1139, 1179, 1180 (Vantico) DEN 431, 438 (DOW) N-738, 740, 770 (DIC)
Cresol novolac	Semisolid	2.7–5.4	200–245	varies	varies	ECN 1273, 1280, 1285, 1299, 9511 (Vantico) N-660, 665, 667, 670, 673, 680, 690, 695 (DIC)
Bisphenol-A novolac	Semisolid-solid	...	...	...	...	SU 2.5, 3, 8 (Shell)
Dicyclopentadiene novolac	Solid	...	210–280	...	...	Tactix 556 (Vantico) HP-7200 (DIC)
Triglycidyl ether of trisphenol-methane	Solid	3	150–170	...	...	Tactix 742 (Vantico)
Triglycidyl p-aminophenol	Liquid	3	95–115	0.55–5	550–5,000	MY 0500, 0510 (Vantico) ELM-100 (Sumitomo)
Tetraglycidyl methylene dianiline	Liquid-semisolid	4	109–134	...	...	MY 720, 721, 9512, 9612, 9634, 9655, 9663 (Vantico) Epiclon 430 (DIC) ELM-434 (Sumitomo)
3,4 epoxycyclohexylmethyl-3,4-epoxycyclohexane carboxylate	Liquid	2	131–143	0.25–0.45	250–450	CY 179 MA (Vantico) UVR-6105, 6110 (Union Carbide)

(a) Number of reactive sites per molecule. (b) Weight of resin per unit epoxide.

minated resins are used to impart flame retardancy into the final product and are commonly used in electrical applications. Multiple forms are available with various bromine contents and molecular weight ranges. This category of resins ranges from nearly pure diglycidyl ether of tetrabromo bisphenol-A to high molecular weight analogs similar to those available with the standard bisphenol-A resins.

Another type of phenolic epoxy resin is the diglycidyl ether of bisphenol-F. This material has a lower viscosity than most DGEBA resins and is commonly used to reduce mix viscosity while limiting reductions in glass transition temperature. Moderate improvements in chemical resistance are seen when bis-F resins are used in place of bis-A resins. Unlike the bisphenol-A-based resins, high molecular weight versions are not readily available (Ref 5).

Phenol and cresol novolacs are another two types of aromatic glycidyl ethers (Fig. 3). These resins are manufactured in a two-step process. Combining either phenol or cresol with formaldehyde produces a polyphenol that is subsequently reacted with epichlorohydrin to generate the epoxy. High epoxy resin functionality and high cured T_g characterize these resins and differentiate them from the difunctional bisphenol-A/F resins. The phenol novolacs are high-viscosity liquids while cresol novolacs are typically solids at room temperature. They are of general interest because excellent temperature performance can be achieved at a relatively modest cost.

Other important epoxy novolacs include bisphenol-A novolacs and novolacs containing dicyclopentadiene. Bisphenol-A novolacs achieve excellent high-temperature performance. Dicyclopentadiene novolacs impart increased moisture resistance to a resin (Ref 6).

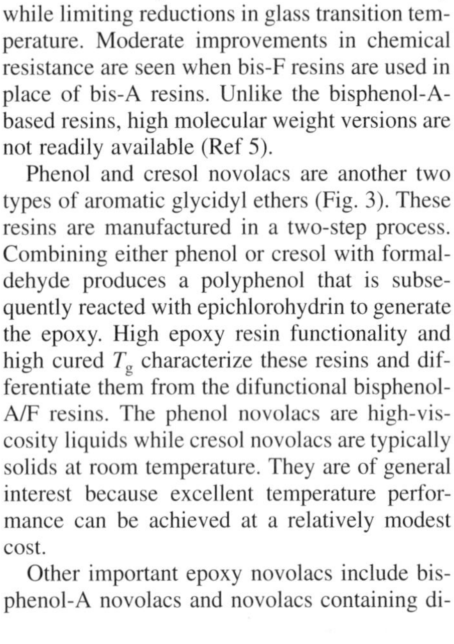

Glycidyl amines are formed by reacting epichlorohydrin with an amine, with aromatic amines being preferred for high-temperature applications. The most important resin in this class, tetraglycidyl methylene dianiline (TGMDA), is shown in Fig. 4.

This resin is used extensively in advanced composites for aerospace applications due to its excellent high- temperature properties. In general, these resins are more costly than either the difunctional bisphenols or the various novolacs. Advantages of TGMDA resins include excellent mechanical properties and high glass transition temperatures. Glycidyl amines are high-viscosity liquids or semisolids at room temperature. As with the DGEBA resins, a variety of grades are available, again dependent upon purity, molecular weight, and particle size.

Another glycidyl amine, triglycidyl p-aminophenol (TGPAP), consists of three epoxy groups attached to a single benzene ring. This resin exhibits exceptionally low viscosity at room temperature, from 0.5 to 5.0 Pa · s (500 to 5000 cP). The mechanical properties and glass transition temperatures approach those obtained with the tetrafunctional resins. Because of its low viscosity, TGPAP resins are commonly blended with other epoxies to modify the flow or tack of the formulated system without loss of T_g. The primary disadvantage is cost, which can be 6 to 8 times that of commodity bis-A resins.

Other commercial glycidyl amines include diglycidyl aniline and tetraglycidyl meta-xylene diamine. The primary advantage of these resins is their low room-temperature viscosity, which makes them useful for applications requiring very high resin flow, such as filament winding or liquid molding.

Cycloaliphatics are differentiated from other epoxies by containing an epoxy group that is internal to the ring structure rather than external or pendant (Fig. 5). Very low viscosity (0.25–0.45 Pa · s, or 250–450 cP, at 25 °C, or 77 °F) and relatively high thermal-mechanical performance (for an aliphatic resin) characterize this class of materials. The high T_gs possible with cycloaliphatics are primarily due to the difference in structure formed upon cross-linking. The cross-link formed upon curing is attached directly to the cyclic backbone structure. While this cyclic structure is aliphatic and therefore more flexible than the aromatic materials described previously, the distance between cross-links is reduced. While many materials have been described in the literature, as of 2000, only a few are available on the open market (Ref 7, 8). It may be important to note that unlike bis-A epoxies, cycloaliphatic epoxies react very slowly with some amines at room temperature.

Other resins. A wide variety of other epoxy resins are available, including epoxidized oils and specialty, low-volume or experimental high-performance resins. These materials are conceptually similar to those discussed previously.

A list of commonly used epoxy resins and their suppliers may be found in Table 1.

Epoxy Resin Curatives

Epoxy resins will react with a large number of chemical species called curatives or hardeners. (Other terms often used, sometimes incorrectly, are catalysts and accelerators.) The most commonly used chemical classes of curatives are amines, amine derivatives, and anhydrides. Other classes of curing agents are mentioned briefly at the end of this section. Those seeking a more comprehensive guide to epoxy resin curatives should refer to one of several books on the subject (Ref 9, 10).

When selecting resin-curative combinations, the application or end use defines the resin characteristics that must be built into a particular system. Epoxy resins can be formulated in an infinite number of ways to manipulate characteristics such as system stability, cure kinetics, physical form, T_g, mechanical performance, and chemical resistance. Cure times can range from seconds to days, with some heat-activated systems being latent for months to years at room temperature. The uncured formulated resin can be solid, rubbery or liquid, tacky or dry, and can cure at temperatures from 5 to 260 °C (40–500 °F). The cured product can be soft and pliable or rigid and glassy, with glass transition temperatures ranging from below room temperature to 260 °C (500 °F) and tensile elongations from 1% to over 100%. The following sections are meant to give a quick overview of commercially available curatives as of 2001. The materials have been separated into the general categories of room-temperature cure, room- or elevated-temperature cure, elevated-temperature cure, and miscellaneous curatives. In some cases, a single curative or class of curatives may fit in more than

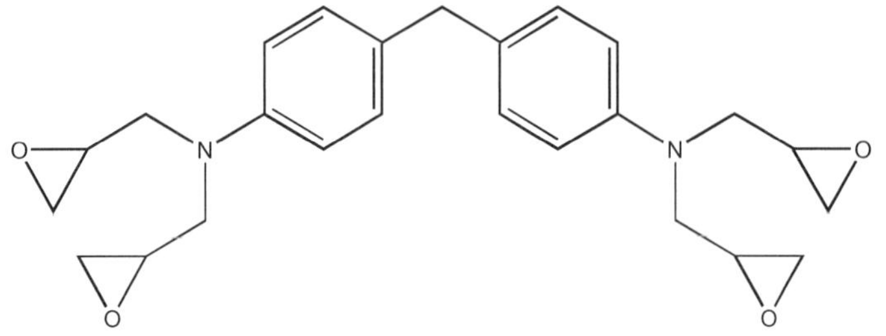

Fig. 3 Chemical structure of phenol novolac. A cresol novolac contains a methyl group on each benzene ring

Fig. 4 Chemical structure of tetraglycidyl methylene dianiline (TGMDA)

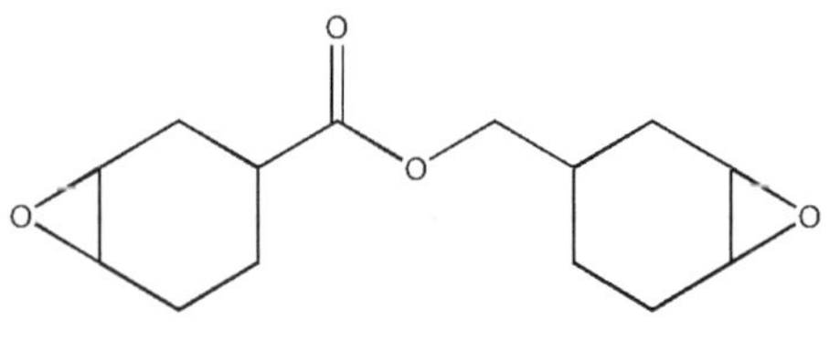

Fig. 5 Chemical structure of a typical cycloaliphatic epoxy resin

one of these categories, however, no effort has been made to identify where classifications overlap.

Room temperature curing agents include aliphatic amines, polyamides, and amidoamines.

Aliphatic amines are the curatives most often paired with epoxy resins. When the functionality and cure mechanism of each component is understood, these materials are used in stoichiometric amounts, though mix ratios are more often determined experimentally and curative levels recommended in units of phr (parts curative per 100 parts bis-A epoxy). The reaction mechanisms of epoxy resin with primary, secondary and tertiary amines are illustrated in Fig. 6. Primary and secondary amines proceed as addition reactions where one nitrogen-hydrogen group reacts with one epoxy group. Reaction with tertiary amines results from the unshared electron pair on the nitrogen. Since there are no secondary hydroxyl groups generated, the resin may be said to homopolymerize. Numerous combinations are available since the various epoxy structures available may contain one, two, three, or more reactive sites and the amine can contain multiple nitrogen-hydrogen groups. Both the number and the distance between reactive groups affect material performance. The distance between reactive groups can vary, with few, widely spaced sites yielding soft and very flexible products while frequent, short separations yield hard and brittle products (Ref 12).

Commonly used primary amines are diethylene triamine (DETA), triethylene tetramine (TETA), tetraethlylenepentamine (TEPA), and N-aminoethyl-piperazine (N-AEP). Even though these amines will cure at room temperature, T_g and subsequent-use temperature are often improved by an elevated-temperature cure or postcure. The enhanced T_g of these baked materials however, will always be 10 to 20 °C (20 to 35 °F) below cure temperature.

The reactivity of some primary amines allows them to cure under adverse conditions where the substrate and surrounding environment may be cold and damp. Primary amines are highly exothermic and may be adducted with epoxy resins, ethylene, or propylene oxides to render curatives with higher viscosity, less reactivity, and less toxicity than the pure amines. Amine basicity must be carefully controlled in applications where workers come into contact with uncured materials.

Other aliphatic amines sometimes used as epoxy curatives are meta-xylenediamine (MXDA) and the polymeric form of MXDA, which are available as liquids. These curatives contain an aromatic ring but react as aliphatic amines, which gives them cured properties closer to that of the aromatic amines.

Polyetheramines, also known by the trade name Jeffamine (Texaco Inc.), are an interesting class of curative that are available as difunctional or trifunctional liquids with low viscosity and vapor pressure. These materials contain primary amines located on secondary carbons, which gives them relatively long pot lives due to the methyl groups adjacent to the nitrogen. They can be accelerated with nonyl phenol or proprietary compounds available from Huntsman Chemical. Low shrinkage, good clarity, and high toughness or flexibility characterize the cured products. When cured with a standard bis-A epoxy, tensile elongation can vary from 2 to over 100% with tensile strengths from 7 to 70 MPa (1 to 10 ksi) (Ref 13).

Tertiary amines (Lewis bases) react by catalytic anionic polymerization (Fig. 7) (Ref 14). The reactivity of tertiary amines varies widely as the electron density around the nitrogen changes. The composition and location of hydrocarbon groups on the amine will affect the electron density. Homopolymerization results in higher glass transition temperatures, better chemical resistance, and a more brittle product than a resin that has cured through an addition reaction. They may be used as sole curatives at a level of approximately 1 to 6 phr or as accelerators for other curing agents, such as polyamides, amidoamines or anhydrides. Examples of tertiary amines are pyridine, triethylamine, and 2,4,6-tris(dimethylaminomethyl)phenol (Ref 15).

Cycloaliphatic amines are characterized by having at least one amino group attached directly to a saturated ring. Examples are isophoronediamine (IPDA) and methylene-di(cyclohexylamine) (PACM). In their unmodified state, they harden under ambient conditions but require heat to attain full cure. They can be modified to cure quickly under cold, damp conditions (at temperatures as low as 0–5 °C) and yield less blush, higher T_g, and toughness than aliphatic amines; therefore, these materials are often used in industrial applications, such as floor coatings, mortars, and grouts.

Polyamides, like polyamines, are classified as primary, secondary, or tertiary depending on the substituents on the amide group (Fig. 8). They are condensation products of polyamines and dimer acids or fatty acids. In general, polyamides are less reactive than most polyamines, therefore, they are often modified or adducted in order to increase ambient reactivity, decrease viscosity, and increase compatibility with epoxy resins. They offer excellent adhesion, low toxicity, and good toughness but tend to be somewhat dark in color, which may limit their application. Polyamides are often used for coatings, adhesives, and sealants.

Amidoamines (which are sometimes classified as amides or amide/imidazolines by their vendors) contain both amide and amine groups (Fig. 9). They are reaction products of monobasic carboxylic acids (usually the acids derived from C_{16}–C_{19} fats and oils) and aliphatic polyamines. Those materials containing the imidazoline group (a five-membered ring structure) may exhibit more rigidity in the cured backbone result-

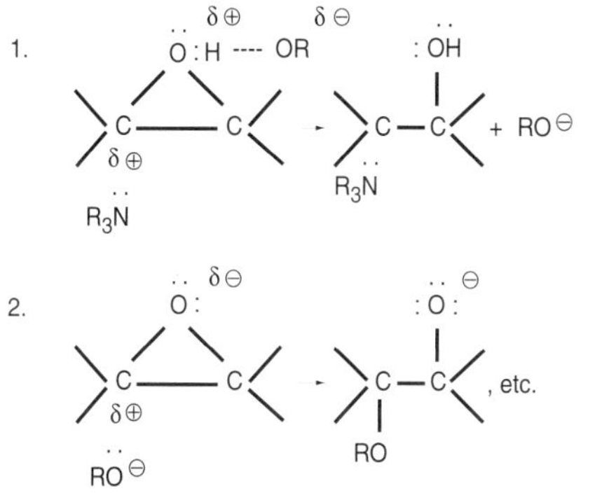

Fig. 7 Epoxy/tertiary amine (Lewis base) reaction mechanism

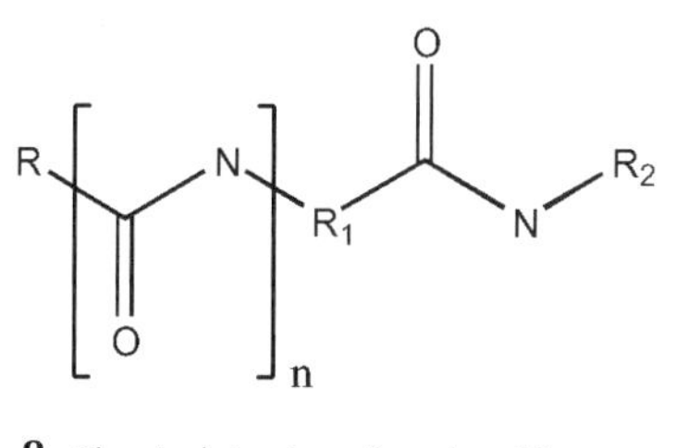

Fig. 8 Chemical structure of a polyamide

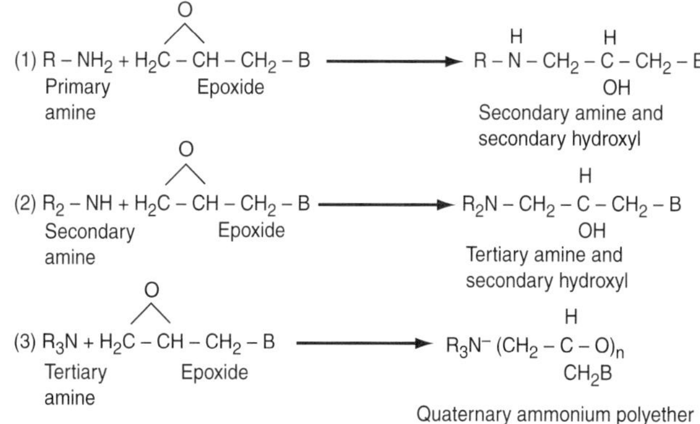

Fig. 6 Epoxy/amine reactions. (1) The primary amine group reacts with the epoxide group to provide secondary amine groups. (2) The secondary amine groups further react with the epoxide groups and generate tertiary amine groups. In both instances the hydroxyl groups are formed, which are believed to catalyze the amine-epoxide reaction. (3) The teriary amine group exerts a catalytic effect and causes the epoxide group to self-polymerize to form a polyether. Source: Ref 11

ing in a higher T_g. Amidoamines are low-viscosity amber liquids that have very long pot lives and afford good toughness, flexibility, and adhesion, particularly to concrete. They are used when low volatility and minimal skin irritation are desired. This class of curative also tends to yield better moisture resistance than aliphatic polyamines. Both polyamides and amidoamines may be only marginally compatible with epoxy resins, which means that they must be very thoroughly mixed before use. When stirred, the epoxy-curative may need to partially react before they become fully compatible with each other (Ref 16, 17).

Selection Factors. Cycloaliphatic amines, polyamides, and amidoamines can be used at a wide range of stoichiometric ratios to generate the desired handling or cured properties. Although both an amine value (functionality of the amine) and equivalent weight are available from the vendor, these curatives are generally compounded following recommended use levels given in units of phr. Glass transition temperatures vary between 5 and 55 °C (40 and 130 °F) after cure at room temperature and may be increased substantially with elevated temperature or postcure. Tensile strengths range between 21 and 59 MPa (3 and 8.5 ksi) and elongations between 3% and 8.5% (Ref 16).

Aliphatic amines, their adducts, and derivatives are available from a number of companies who offer a profusion of products (Table 2). The sheer number of options may seem confusing to the formulator, so it becomes important to note that a number of vendors have unique designations or trade names for what are basically the same product. Selection may hinge on purity, form, packaging, availability, or price. Many other products are proprietary adducts and mixtures that may contain accelerators and coreactants, such as free-aliphatic amines, benzyl alcohol, nonyl phenol, phenol, and salicylic acid. It is also important to understand that multiple formulations using different curing agents and different epoxies may yield the same cured properties but differ in the other parameters, such as mix viscosity, pot life, cure time, or appearance. Uses can range from electronics and encapsulation to thermosetting adhesives, flooring grouts, and trowel coatings. A general performance comparison of the major aliphatic amine types, which represent the bulk of room-temperature curatives, can be found in Fig. 10 (Ref 16).

Room or Elevated Temperature Curing Agents. Unlike the amines and amides discussed earlier, the following two classes of curatives, BF_3 complexes and imidazoles, contain variants that may be cured safely at room temperature and at elevated temperature. Instead of pot lives of minutes to hours, these compounds may be modified to remain latent at room temperature for periods ranging from hours to days. They are often used as accelerators in conjunction with other epoxy curatives.

Boron trifluoride-amine complexes (Lewis acids) cure epoxy resins by catalytic cationic polymerization. The mechanism is shown in Fig. 11 (Ref 18). Pure boron trifluoride (BF_3) reacts with standard bis-A epoxy in seconds, so room-temperature stability is built into the molecule by adducting BF_3 with various amines. These curatives, most of which are proprietary, may be stabilized by the addition of excess amine, which also reduces the elevated-temperature reactivity. The complexes are available as liquids that vary in latency, activation temperature, and cured properties. Systems can be formulated to cure in hours at room temperature or they may be designed as stable at room temperature and require elevated-temperature cures. Boron trifluoride complexes are used to generate resin castings and coatings with T_gs of up to 200 °C (390 °F). As with amine cures, the product T_g will usually lag behind the cure temperature by approximately 20 °C (36 °F).

With standard epoxy resins the cure reaction is rapidly triggered and highly dependent on temperature, so elevated-temperature cures can be long and often occur in a step-wise manner to prevent uncontrollable exotherms that can degrade physical properties, making a part unusable. One of the benefits of this class of curative is that they are used at relatively low levels (4–17 parts to 100 parts epoxy) (Ref 19).

Substituted imidazoles are a unique class of curatives that find applications in electronic, structural adhesive, automotive, and aerospace composites. They are generally employed as accelerators for the reaction between epoxies and other curatives but can also be highly effective as sole curing agents. They are one of the most efficient of the Lewis bases, initiating anionic

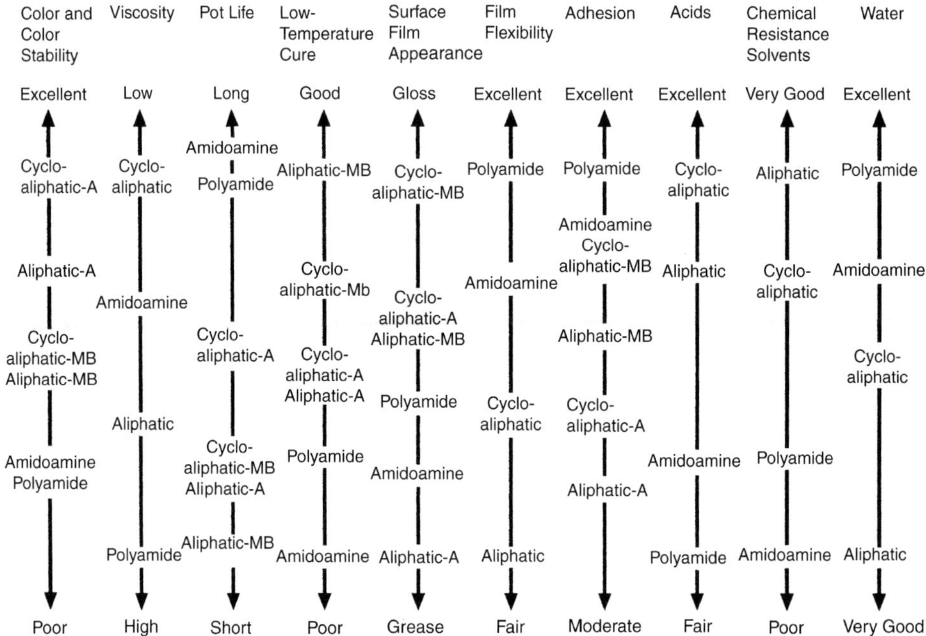

Fig. 10 Comparison of some amine curative classes. A, adduct-type curative; MB, Mannich base-type curative

Fig. 9 Chemical structure of an amidoamine

Fig. 11 Epoxy/Lewis acid reaction mechanism

homopolymerization of the epoxy resin at very low loadings (<8 phr). Imidazole curatives are tailored by substitution with organic groups on the ring, chemically blocking active amine hydrogen on the ring, and by salt formation with ring nitrogen. These modifications result in molecules that are rendered latent through steric hindrance or insolubility in room-temperature epoxy resin. Imidazole cures are characterized by high glass transition temperatures (which usually exceed the cure temperature), room-temperature latency that ranges from several hours to 6 months, and rapid cure beyond the activation temperature. Initial cures are generally 1.5 to 2 h at 80 to 100 °C (175 to 210 °F) while postcures range from 2 to 4 h at 150 to 200 °C (300 to 390 °F). The chemical resistance of the cured product is similar to that achieved with aromatic amines, and T_gs can exceed 200 °C (390 °F). Imidazoles are also used as accelerators in anhydride cures (Ref 20).

Elevated Temperature Curatives include aromatic amines and anhydrides.

Aromatic amines are generally fine-powder curatives that are blended or melted into epoxy resin. Some of the products mentioned subsequently will also be available as supercooled liquids or eutectic blends to facilitate mixing at room temperature. The aromatics tend to be more expensive than the aliphatic amines and fewer variants are available. An aromatic amine has the nitrogen of the nitrogen-hydrogen group directly bound to an aromatic ring. The aromatic amines are used in high-performance composites and generally require high- temperature cures to yield superior T_gs and greater chemical resistance than the same epoxy resins cured with aliphatic amines. The reaction of aromatic amines with epoxy resins follows the same mechanisms seen in Fig. 6. The reaction is slower due to lower nucleophilicity and steric factors, so formulated systems can show extended room-temperature out times. Although not as toxic as aliphatic amines, most aromatic amines are considered to be skin sensitizers or irritants and must be handled with the proper precautions.

One of the first aromatic amines used in industry, 4,4′-diaminodiphenyl methane (represented as DADM, MDA, or DDM in the literature), exhibits one of the best balances of properties available from a curative; however, it is currently used infrequently since it has been identified as a suspected carcinogen. The toxic nature of MDA has impeded the introduction of new aromatic amines with related structures because they too would be suspected carcinogens. The alkyl-substituted versions of this molecule, such as methylene-bis(dimethylaniline) and methylene-bis(diisopropylaniline) (MPDA), are less toxic and are commercially available. The phenylenediamines follow the same pattern, with the alkyl-substituted derivatives such as diethyltoluenediamine being significantly less toxic than the base molecule. When the methylene group of MDA is replaced with a sulfone, the result is diaminodiphenylsulfone (DDS), which is well known and widely used in the aerospace industry. When cured with bis-A epoxy, DDS will yield higher T_g, tensile modulus, and elongation than either MDA or MPDA. In addition, DDS tends to be more latent at room temperature.

Anhydrides are another major class of epoxy curing agents (Fig. 12) (Ref 21), that are available in a variety of physical forms from various suppliers. Most of the products in use in epoxy-composite applications are low- viscosity liquids or moderate-viscosity eutectic blends; nonetheless, some solid anhydrides are also available. The reaction mechanism between an anhydride curing agent and epoxy resin is complex, because three competing reactions take place. The anhydride reacts with the epoxy hydroxyls to form half-esters. The half-ester containing the free carboxyl group is then available to react with an epoxide ring, which generates another hydroxyl. The newly formed hydroxyl can react with another anhydride or, in the presence of free acid, it can react with another epoxy to form an ether linkage.

Formulating with anhydrides requires some experimentation because the desired ratio of anhydride to epoxy can vary widely depending on materials selected, the concentration of hydroxyl groups in the formulation, and the presence of an accelerator. Anhydrides are usually used at between 0.4 to 1.1 equivalents to the epoxy. As with amine curatives, the equivalent weight is defined as the molecular weight divided by the number of functional sites (in this case, anhydride groups) on the molecule. In general, the reaction of epoxy resin with anhydride is more sluggish than with aliphatic amines or amides, with lengthy cure and postcure profiles being required to generate desired properties. Primary cure occurs between 80 to 150° C (175–300 °F) with postcures ranging to 200° C (3900 °F). Accelerators, usually tertiary amines or imidazoles, are used in the range of 0.5 to 3.0% to catalyze the epoxy anhydride reaction and speed up the cure. Representative anhydrides are methyl tetrahydro- phthalic anhydride, nadic methyl anhydride, and methyl hexahydro-phthalic anhydride. Some commonly used accelerators are dimethylaminomethylphenol, benzyl-dimethylamine, phenylimidazole, and ethylmethylimidazole.

Anhydrides are selected as curatives when low viscosity, noncritical mix ratios, low potential for skin irritation, and long pot life are desired. As cured resins they can yield high T_gs, excellent electrical properties, low shrinkage, and retention of physical and electrical properties above the T_g. Polyanhydrides can offer excellent toughness and thermal shock resistance. Saturated liquid anhydrides offer excellent color, ultraviolet stability, and moisture resistance. Unsaturated anhydrides offer low cost and very low viscosity. The disadvantages of using an anhydride curative are moisture sensitivity (where the anhydride reacts with atmospheric moisture to hydrolyze into the corresponding diacids), brittleness (when unmodified), and only general formulation recommendations from vendors (experimentation is often required to achieve desired performance). Uses are casting, potting, encapsulation, and filament winding. It is noteworthy that cycloaliphatic epoxies are also cured with anhydrides in the presence of an accelerator (Ref 22).

Miscellaneous Curing Agents. Dicyandiamide (generally referred to as "dicy") is widely used as an epoxy curative in composite applications where room-temperature stability is desired and rapid elevated- temperature cure is attractive. It may be employed as a sole curing agent but most often finds use paired with sub-

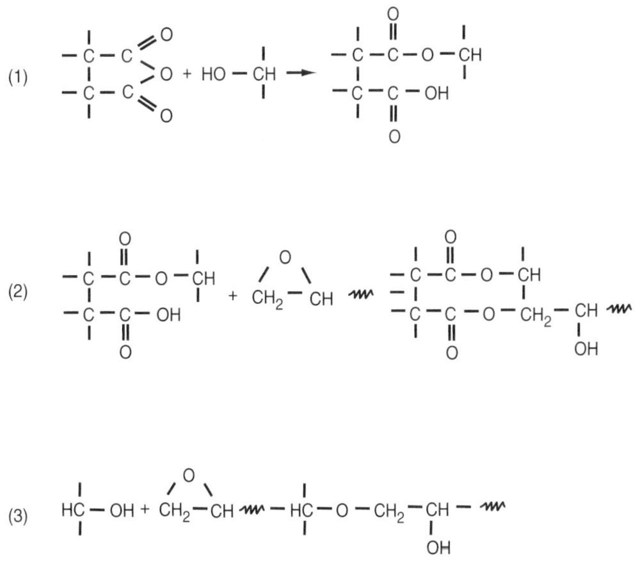

Fig. 12 Epoxy/anhydride reaction mechanism. (1) The opening of the anhydride ring with an alcoholic hydroxyl to form the monoester. (2) Subsequent to (1), the nascent carboxylic groups react with the epoxide to give an ester linkage. (3) The epoxide groups react with nascent or existing hydroxyl groups, catalyzed by the acid, producing an ether linkage.

stituted ureas, substituted imidazoles, or as a cure accelerator for aromatic amines. Dicy is a fine white powder available in a variety of particle size distributions. Particle size distribution may significantly affect resin cost and reactivity as well as cured-product properties, so care should be taken in the selection of the appropriate grade. Dicy tends to be insoluble in epoxy at room temperature, and the reaction doesn't initiate until solubility is achieved (between 80 and 90 °C, or 175 and 195 °F, in most epoxy resins). During cure it decomposes, allowing all four nitrogen atoms to react; therefore, one molecule of dicy can react with six or seven epoxy groups (Ref 23). When used alone, full cure is attained in approximately two hours at temperatures between 145 and 175 °C (295 and 345 °F). When combined with substituted ureas (like monuron or diuron), cures take place at 120 to 175 °C (250–345 °F) over a period of minutes to hours, depending on curative concentrations. The combination of dicy with a substituted imidazole can cure epoxy at temperatures down to about 100 °C (210 °F) with cure time dependent on concentration and temperature selection. In most formulations, dicy is used at a level of 3–7 phr with an optional 2–4 parts of accelerator.

Polysulfides, thiols, or mercaptans (which are terminated with the S-H group) historically have not been used as sole epoxy curatives because these end groups are not acidic enough to thoroughly cure the resin. They have been used as reactive modifiers to increase the toughness or flexibility. Relatively new accelerated compounds are available that cure in seconds at temperatures as low as –40 °C (–40 °F). The cure mechanism is shown in Fig. 13. These curatives are used in adhesive applications where rapid cure is required and the sulfur odor of the curative doesn't prohibit use. Common applications are industrial road marker adhesives and commercial patch kits (Ref 24).

Alternate Cure Methods. One of the newer trends in the composites industry is to look at cutting production costs and decreasing cycle times by using radiation-curable resin systems (Ref 25, 26). Radiation sources are ultraviolet (UV), infrared (IR), or electron beam (EB). These methods of cure use radiation to physically or chemically change organic materials, forming cross-linked polymer networks. Historic applications are in the coatings, electronics, printing, and adhesives industries where only a thin film of resin is being cured or dried. Some benefits of radiation cures are energy efficiency, rapid cure times measured in seconds, dimensional stability, pollution abatement as solvent is eliminated from the process, low exotherm potential that permits the use of temperature-sensitive substrates, and no cure until source exposure. Disadvantages are large capital expense, difficulty in penetrating thick parts, and the sensitivity of the reaction mechanism to impurities. There are also limitations due to raw material availability and cost.

Epoxy acrylates can be cationically cured with aryl-sulfonium salt photoinitiators. Polyols are often added to the formulation for flexibilizing or cross-linking. Amines cannot be used in epoxy acrylate systems because they deactivate the sulfonium salts.

Standard cycloaliphatic and bis-A epoxies can be homopolymerized by exposure to radiation; however, cure times will be greater than those obtained with the epoxy acrylates, and the fundamental work to understand curing mechanisms has not been completed.

A higher-energy nonthermal curing method uses EB radiation. Initial equipment cost is very high because parts must be irradiated within a shielded room, but cures are very rapid and high volumes are realized with little overall energy. While there is some temperature increase in the part during cure, it is minor, so inexpensive tooling materials may be considered (including wood). Like UV curing systems, most nonamine-containing epoxies can be used and the initiators are similar. Cure shrinkage is lower than with traditional hardeners, so this is an attractive option for parts with tight dimensional tolerances. Although EB curing of composites is relatively new and work still needs to be done to commercialize the process, preliminary results suggest that the thermal and mechanical properties of these systems may eventually meet most requirements for high-performance applications.

A list of some commonly used curatives and their suppliers may be found in Table 2.

Modifiers

The third major category of epoxy formulation constituents is modifiers. They are used to provide specific physical and mechanical performance in both the uncured and cured resin. General categories of modifiers include rubbers, thermoplastics, diluents, flame retardants, fillers, and pigments and dyes. In this discussion, examples are limited to a few types per category. It is important to note that while some materials offer multiple desirable characteristics, others demand trade-offs in processing or final product performance that must be carefully considered. Table 3 gives some examples of frequently used modifiers, with suppliers. Complete and updated lists may be found in a variety of publications including *Thomas Register* and *Modern Plastics Encyclopedia*.

Rubber Additives. Rubbers are used to increase flexibility, fatigue resistance, crack resistance, and energy absorption (toughness) in epoxy resins and can be separated into two categories, reactive or nonreactive. These polymers may be employed as liquid, solid, or particulate components in a formulation.

The concepts of resin and composite toughness are complex and may be somewhat ambiguous because definitions vary depending on audience and applications discussed. To simplify, toughness is defined as an increase in the stress or energy needed to reach an identified failure point. The definition of failure point is linked to the specific application and will vary as part design and materials selection changes.

Fracture mechanisms involved in toughening epoxy composites with rubbers have been widely investigated. Publications by Kinloch and Young (Ref 27), Yee and Pearson (Ref 28, 29), and Bascom and Huntsdon (Ref 30) discuss the subject in great detail. Toughening is principally due to plastic deformation of the matrix and rubber particle at the crack tip. In rubber-modified resin systems, this deformation is achieved through crazing, shear band formation, particle cavitation, bridging, and voiding for stress relaxation at a crack tip.

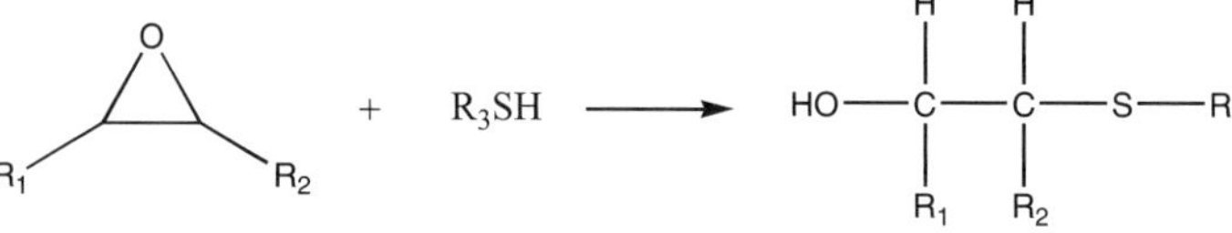

Fig. 13 Epoxy-thiol reaction

Table 2 Epoxy curatives

Curative class	Suppliers
DETA, TETA, TEPA, IPDA	Air Products, Dow Chemical
Aliphatic amine adducts	Air Products, Ajinomoto, Dow, Emerson & Cuming, Henkel, Hoechst-Celanese, Hüls America, Polychem, Reichold Chemical, Rhone-Poulenc, Shell, Vantico
Tertiary amines (Lewis bases)	Air Products, Henkel, Lindau, Lonza, Reichold Chemicals, Vantico
Cycloaliphatic amines	Air Products, Reichold Chemical, Rhone-Poulenc, Vantico
Polyamides	Air Products, Dow, Henkel, Reichold Chemical, Rhone-Poulenc, Shell, Vantico
Amidoamines	Air Products, Henkel, Hoechst-Celanese, Reichold Chemical, Rhone-Poulenc, Shell, Vantico
Aromatic amines	Air Products, BASF, Buffalo Color, CVC Specialty Chemicals, Dow Chemical, Rhone-Poulenc, Shell
Anhydrides	Dow, Humprey Chemical, Lindau Chemicals, Leepoxy Plastics, Lonza, Oxychem, Milliken Chemicals, Reichold Chemicals, Vantico
BF_3–amine complexes	Air Products, Leepoxy Plastics
Dicyandiamide	Air Products, CVC Specialty Chemicals, SKW, Vantico
Substituted ureas	Air Products, CVC Specialty Chemicals, SKW, Vantico
Thiols	Henkel
Ultraviolet cure initiators	Union Camp

The liquid rubbers most often used in epoxy composites are carboxyl-terminated butadiene acrylonitrile copolymers, or CTBNs. CTBNs are miscible with most epoxy resins, so they can easily be added to formulations with only modest increases in room-temperature resin viscosity. These long-chain polymers have terminal carboxyl groups that may be reacted with epoxy to decrease cross-link density and increase tensile elongation. Once the rubber becomes an integral part of the matrix however, decreases in strength, modulus, and T_g are unavoidable. In order to moderate the negative impact of rubber addition in the cured part, the candidate rubber must be carefully selected and blended into the epoxy formulation (usually at levels below 30 phr) so that during cure it phases out of solution to form discrete domains within the epoxy matrix. This phenomenon is referred to as in situ particle formation. It is believed that cure kinetics and cure temperature play a critical role in determining final particle size and morphology, which in turn affects part performance (Ref 31).

Solid acrylonitrile-butadiene rubbers have higher molecular weights than the liquid rubbers. Loadings are generally low due to a rapid increase in resin viscosity as rubber content increases. They can be dissolved directly into the epoxy or addition can be facilitated with a solvent that is later removed. In all cases, the rubber must phase out of solution during cure in order to effectively toughen the resin without sacrificing modulus and thermal performance.

The acrylonitrile content of the rubber is an important consideration when choosing a rubber modifier. As the nitrile content of a rubber increases, solubility increases and eventual particle size in the cured matrix decreases. While a variety of rubbers are effective tougheners in DGEBA, rubbers with high-acrylonitrile content are generally used with the more polar novolac epoxies. Unreactive rubbers are not generally used in epoxy composite applications because they tend to have the drawbacks of both rubbers and thermoplastics.

Preformed rubber particles are occasionally used in composites when both the particle size distribution and the volume fraction of particles in the cured resin need to be closely controlled. If they are totally insoluble in the matrix, a formulation can contain high loadings without the rapid increase in viscosity present with high-molecular-weight soluble polymers. To be effective as tougheners, the surface of the particle needs to react with or adhere well to the matrix. The benefit of using preformed particles is that they generate a consistent matrix morphology that is independent of cure conditions. However, the particles may be expensive, difficult to disperse in the base resin, and their presence may make processing more challenging (Ref 32, 33).

Thermoplastic Additives. Thermoplastics (TPs) are used much like rubbers to increase the fracture toughness of epoxy resins. They may be dissolved into the formulation or added as a particulate. Only relatively low-molecular-weight TPs can be dissolved in epoxy resin, and not all TPs are compatible with epoxy, so options are limited when selecting a toughener of this type. Thermoplastics commonly used in epoxy composites are phenoxy, polyether block amides, polyvinyl butyral, polyvinyl formal, polysulfone, polyethersulfone, polyimide, polyetherimide, and nylon.

The ability to toughen epoxy resins with both rubbers and TPs is closely related to the cross-link density of the thermoset matrix. Thermoplastics differ from rubbers in that they are more effective tougheners in highly cross-linked matrices because phase separation will occur at lower concentrations as matrix rigidity increases (Ref 34). As with rubbers, the morphology of the cured resin will impact the effectiveness of the additive. Unlike rubbers, TPs do not tend to adversely affect T_g and modulus. If used in very small amounts the TP may remain dissolved in the epoxy matrix to form an interpenetrating network, however, when used in concentrations high enough to positively affect measures of toughness, the TP will phase out during cure to form discrete plastic domains (Ref 35). Most TPs have limited use as components in epoxy formulations because the viscosity of the resin increases dramatically with only moderate loadings of TP. The effectiveness of the TP-rich domains in the cured part may also be limited by the relatively poor interface between them and the matrix. Other potential drawbacks when using high loadings of TP are an increase in solvent sensitivity and decreases in resistance to creep and fatigue.

Epoxy Diluents. There are a number of resins that are used as diluents in epoxy composites. In most cases these are very low-viscosity reactive monofunctional epoxies, although there are a few difunctional resin diluents available. While monofunctional resins such as butyl glycidyl ether, phenyl glycidyl ether, and cresyl glycidyl ether are effective in reducing viscosity, their use will result in a reduction of thermal and mechanical properties. As a rule, the lower-molecular-weight compounds are most effective as diluents but they also tend to be volatile and are often irritants, therefore, they must be used in controlled environments. The higher-molecular-weight materials are less toxic and impact other properties less, but they are generally used at higher loadings since they are not as effective at reducing viscosity. In order to address this trade-off, several epoxy manufacturers supply blends of high-volume resins preblended with diluent to alleviate the need for the user to handle them. As with other types of additives, the formulator selects a particular diluent to balance physical needs with thermal-mechanical performance.

Flame Retardants. Flame retardants (FRs) can be added to epoxy resins as a filler, or the matrix can be built to incorporate FR characteristics. Generally, the more carbon and hydrogen in a polymer system, the more flammable it is. The presence of halogens and char-forming aromatics in the epoxy-curative based resin decrease flammability. FR modifiers operate through the three mechanisms that govern the pyrolysis and combustion of polymers; the condensed phase, the vapor phase, and physical inhibition (Ref 36, 37). Fillers such as alumina trihydrate ($Al(OH)_3$) and magnesium hydroxide ($Mg(OH)_2$) are effective in inhibiting combus-

Table 3 Epoxy resin modifiers

Class	Type	Form	Supplier
Rubbers	CTBN	Liquid-reactive	B.F. Goodrich, Zeon
		Solid-reactive	B.F. Goodrich, Zeon
		Particulate	Zeon
Thermoplastics	Phenoxy	Pellets and powders	Phenoxy Specialties
	Polyether block amide	Pellets and powders	Atochem America
	Polyvinyl butyral	Pellets and powders	DuPont, Solutia, Tomen
	Polyvinyl formal	Pellets and powders	Tomen
	Polysulfone	Pellets and powders	Amoco, BASF
	Polyether sulfone	Pellets and powders	Amoco, BASF, Sumitomo
	Polyimide	Pellets and powders	Ciba, DuPont, Mitsui
	Polyetherimide	Pellets and powders	GE Plastics
	Polyamide	Pellets and powders	Creanova, DuPont
Diluents	Monofunctional and difunctional	Liquid	CVC, Shell, Vantico
Flame retardants	Brominated reactive	Liquid, resin, solid	Akzo Nobel, Ameribrom, Great Lakes
	Aluminum trihydrate	Powders	Alcan, Amspec, Franklin Ind., Harwick
	MgOH	Powders	Harwick, Lonza, Morton
	Antimony oxide	Powders	Amspec, Great Lakes, Laurel Ind.
	Phosphates	Liquids and powders	Albright & Wilson, Clariant, Harwick, Solutia
Fillers	Carbon black	Powder	Cabot, DJ Enterprises, Degussa, Ashland
	Glass beads	. . .	Cataphote Inc., Ferro, Potters Industries
	Fumed silica	Flocculent	Cabot, Degussa
	Microballoons	Inorganic	3M, Dow Corning, Mitsubishi, PQ Corp.
		Organic	Dow, PQ Corp., Union Carbide, Zeolite
	Fibers, whiskers	. . .	Alcoa, Amoco, Intercorp Zinc, Nyco,
	Clays	. . .	ECC Int., J.M. Huber - Eng. Materials, U.S. Silica
	Talc	. . .	Luzenac America, Specialty Minerals Inc.
Pigments and dyes	Organics and inorganics	Powders and pastes	Americhem, Colorco, Engelhard, Ferro, Lily

CTBN, carboxyl-terminated butadiene acrylonitrile

tion by undergoing endothermic decomposition and liberating water into the gaseous state during combustion. The oxides produced may also form an insulating barrier that prevents oxygen from reaching the unconsumed polymer. Unfortunately, they must be used at loadings of 30 to 40% by weight, which prohibits their use in many composite applications. Chlorinated or brominated epoxy resins and curing agents may be combined with antimony, phosphorous, or boron compounds to lower flammability of epoxy composites. These compounds work in the gas phase to liberate free radicals trapping ·H and ·OH, thereby blocking the chain reactions that contribute to decomposition. They also work in the condensed phase to catalyze reactions that form nonvolatile products and char. One standard approach to formulating a flame-retardant cured epoxy resin employs the use of brominated epoxy resin (approximately 10–15% Br content by weight) combined with antimony trioxide powder at levels of 5 to 10% by weight. The synergistic effects of combining halogens with metal-oxides have been researched extensively. Currently there is a trend to minimize the use of halogens because they have a negative environmental impact and they produce highly toxic and corrosive hydrogen-halide gases during combustion.

Unreactive Fillers. Fillers are used in epoxy resins as extenders, reinforcements, and to impart specific physical characteristics such as low density, low flow, shrinkage reduction, and thermal or electrical conductivity. The types of fillers used vary widely but can generally be categorized as minerals, metals, glass, fibers, carbon, and miscellaneous organics. Physically, they can be used in a variety of forms including powders, pulps, flakes, flocks, spheres, microballoons, short fibers, and whiskers. When compounding filled systems, variables to take into consideration are the volume fraction of the filler, particle characteristics (size, shape, surface area, and particle size distribution), filler aspect ratio, the strength and modulus of the filler, adhesion of the filler to the resin, the viscosity of the base resin, and the toughness of the base resin (Ref 38, 39). The specialty applications and extensive product lines of fillers used in epoxy composite materials prohibit detailed discussion in this article, however, the following generalities should be considered when selecting fillers.

The maximum loading possible in epoxy resin is generally about 50% by volume in low-viscosity resins and may be significantly less when working with complex systems of high-initial viscosity. Other factors to take into account during processing are aggregate formation and particle wetting. Particles may be treated with interfacial agents to aid wetting by the matrix, and care must be taken to make sure particle distribution is uniform and aggregates are dispersed. Final resin viscosity must be low enough to allow air or volatile removal from the resin before or during cure in order to minimize void formation. In general, increasing filler content increases the modulus and compressive strength of the resin. In most cases, the strength of the filler directly affects the strength of the composite. It is important to note that when weak or brittle fillers such as microballoons are used, the filler may increase the overall toughness of the resin by acting as an energy dissipating "defect" in the matrix (Ref 40). To a certain extent, particle size and shape are independent of modulus as long as the volume fraction remains constant. Shape and size become important during processing or when particle packing or particle orientation affects the isotropy of the part. Increasing filler-aspect ratio increases the resistance to crack propagation, but it also rapidly increases resin viscosity, decreasing the amount of filler that can be used (Ref 41).

Pigments and Dyes. Epoxy resins may be colored using a wide variety of pigments and dyes, both organic and inorganic. Pigments are insoluble particles dispersed in a resin, whereas dyes are soluble organic molecules. Dyes are generally not suitable for epoxy composite applications due to temperature limitations. If they are to be used, care should be taken to identify materials that are compatible with target systems and remain inert in them. The large number of colorant manufacturers and the wide range of color compounds make it possible to color match epoxy products to customer specifications. A resin or prepreg vendor that offers color matching will maintain a large inventory of pigments that are blended to obtain target shades and hues.

It is important to evaluate the color of a particular resin-reinforcement combination only after it has gone all the way through final processing and cure steps. Most epoxy resins have color of their own that must be taken into account, and presence of a second phase will affect final part appearance. Changes in resin morphology or cure temperature will affect the color and clarity of the part. Other factors affecting part appearance are resin content, filler, fiber, and fabric type. Pigments compatible with epoxy resins are available as powders, slurries, or pastes. Predispersed pigments are desirable, as dispersion of powders can be difficult without the right equipment. Powders may be available in a number of grades that reflect ranges in particle size distribution (Ref 42).

Additional additives occasionally found in epoxy resins are flexibilizers, plasticizers, liquid and resinous extenders, antioxidants, light stabilizers, internal mold releases, and antifoams. It is important to note that there are a number of suppliers for each of these modifiers and that the vendors may be extremely helpful in selecting candidate materials for the less-experienced formulator.

Epoxy Resin Model Formulations

The following examples of epoxy resin formulations illustrate how raw materials are combined to tailor a formulation to a specific application. It should be noted that these examples are intended for illustrative purposes only. Raw materials vendors should be contacted to recommend mix ratios and safe handling practices. The potential hazards associated with mixing and curing these resin formulations are not addressed in this article. The formulator or manufacturer must make an independent assessment of process safety for each material before it is used.

These model systems are typical of epoxy resin formulations used in composite applications. In each case, an attempt has been made to identify practical considerations that must be addressed by the potential user. The examples include a room-temperature-curing wet lay-up system (Ref 43), a room-temperature-curing paste adhesive (Ref 44), a toughened elevated-temperature-curing film adhesive (Ref 45), and a high-performance elevated-temperature-cure aerospace prepreg resin (Ref 46).

Example 1: Room-Temperature-Curing Wet Lay-Up System. The key characteristics of a room-temperature-curing wet lay-up system (Table 4) are low viscosity, adequate pot life, and reactivity. Both the epoxy (part A) and the amine (part B) are liquids that may be blended easily at room temperature (mix viscosity 1560 cps). The part B is generally added to the part A as it is stirred. Additives may be premixed into either the A or the B or they may be included as part of the mixing procedure. Regardless of how the system is modified, the finished resin must have a low-enough final viscosity to thoroughly penetrate the target reinforcement or thoroughly wet the surface to be coated. In the example presented, the formulated resin can be applied to a fibrous reinforcement (usually glass fabric or mat) shortly after mixing and then placed on a mold and cured at room temperature. Care should be taken to introduce as little air as possible into the resin during mixing to minimize voids in the finished part.

Some room-temperature-curing systems will require 10 to 20 minutes of mixing to fully blend the curative with the resin. If mixing is not adequate, the part may cure with a tacky surface.

Table 4 Composition of a room-temperature-cure wet lay-up system

Component	Content, wt%
Diglycidyl ether of bisphenol-A	62.3
Ancamine 2143	37.7

Source: Ref 43

Table 5 Cured resin properties of wet lay-up model system

Property	Value
Glass transition temperature (T_g), °C (°F)	51 (123)
Heat distortion temperature, °C (°F)	49 (120)
Tensile strength, MPa (ksi)	51 (7.45)
Tensile modulus, MPa (ksi)	2979 (432)
Tensile elongation, %	2.8
Hardness, Shore D	81

Source: Ref 43

Since these systems are highly reactive at room temperature, they should be mixed in small quantities and used as soon as possible to prevent premature gellation or destructive exotherm. Room-temperature-curing resins tend to be mass sensitive, so large quantities of compounded resin need to be moving at all times to facilitate heat transfer and prevent hot spots from developing. The introduction of fillers will also dissipate heat to reduce the chance of destructive exotherm and increase gel time (working life). To avoid the dangers inherent in mixing large masses, there are a number of chambered mixing devices available that will continually mix and dispense small quantities of resin. A 150 g mass of this model system at 25 °C (77 °F) will gel in 42 minutes, yet has a thin-film set time of seven hours. If the ambient temperature is increased, the set time will decrease; conversely at 4 °C (40 °F), the thin-film set time increases to 21 hours. Properties obtained after a cure of seven days at 25 °C (77 °F) can be found in Table 5.

Example 2: Room-Temperature-Curing Paste Adhesive. The resin is produced (Table 6) by blending the Hycar 1300x16 (B.F. Goodrich) with Ancamide 400 (Air Products Polymers, LP) to create a viscous liquid (part B). This mixture is then added to the epoxy resin (part A) while stirring to form a high-viscosity adhesive. Note that if the viscosity of A differs significantly from that of B, the resin becomes difficult to mix, so it is not uncommon to find modifiers predissolved or predispersed in both the A and the B.

Like Example 1, this resin system is reactive at room-temperature, therefore it should be mixed in small quantities and used immediately. The inclusion of a Hycar liquid rubber in the formulation yields the high toughness required for an adhesive and increases the viscosity so that the adhesive will stay where it is put. Hycar 1300x16 is an amine-terminated acrylonitrile-butadiene copolymer that decreases tensile strength and modulus while greatly increasing the elongation to failure and toughness of the cured product. Ancamide 400 promotes room-temperature cure and reduces the resin viscosity. The properties obtained after curing 14 days at ambient temperature are found in Table 7. Like most room-temperature-cured systems, strength will increase with time or if the part is heated above room-temperature.

Example 3: Elevated-Temperature-Cure Film Adhesive. This system (Table 8) is intended for parts that can be bonded (cured) at elevated temperatures. Like the paste adhesive, the film adhesive achieves toughening through incorporation of a liquid rubber, Hycar 1300x9 (B.F. Goodrich), which is a carboxyl-terminated acrylonitrile-butadiene copolymer with acrylonitrile content of 18%. In addition to the rubber, toughness is obtained by the reaction of bisphenol-A with the epoxy to increase the molecular weight between reactive sites, thus decreasing cross-link density. Unlike the two previous resins, this example includes 11.5% MY9512 (Vantico Inc.), a tetra-functional epoxy which increases T_g, providing temperature resistance at the expense of toughness. Triphenylphosphine is used to catalyze both the reaction between the epoxy and carboxylic acid groups on the rubber and the epoxy-bisphenol-A reaction. The curative package is dicy/diuron; dicy is the curative and diuron the accelerator.

The resin is made by first reacting the rubber and the phenol with the epoxies at elevated-temperature. The viscosity of the base resin will increase substantially as the reactions take place. The mix is then cooled and the curatives are dispersed into the resin. Although the curatives are stable at room-temperature, care must be taken to make sure that the resin is well below reaction initiation temperature when they are added to the other components, or uncontrollable exotherm may occur. It is important to remember that even latent systems may exotherm when heated, so the resin should always be stirred when at elevated temperatures and should be maintained at as low a temperature as possible until it is used. The use of a rubber decreases the T_g, whereas the addition of the multifunctional epoxy increases it, illustrating how the components of a formulation are balanced to yield desired properties. The system is cured at 180 °C (355 °F) for two hours to yield the properties found in Table 9.

Some critical considerations when developing or selecting a film adhesive are:

- *Room-temperature resin viscosity:* Film adhesives, depending on use, may need to be dry and tack-free or very tacky. The substitution of solid or liquid bis-A epoxy for the Epon 828 in this example will allow the tack to be tailored. In almost all instances, a film adhesive must be flexible enough at room temperature so that it does not crack or break when used. The application of a scrim cloth or other support will substantially increase the robustness of the adhesive.
- *Resin rheology:* At cure temperature, the adhesive must flow enough to wet the surface and develop a suitable bond line, but not so much that it runs out of the bond area.
- *Adhesive strength:* The type or the amount of toughener used in a formulation must be balanced against resin T_g because the incorporation of a toughener will tend to lower T_g.
- *Porosity:* The presence of gaseous or fugitive components in the adhesive film may result in significant void formation in the bond line, thereby decreasing the strength of the bond. Adhesives are often degassed before filming in order to eliminate residual gases and air bubbles from the product.

Example 4: A Typical High-Performance Aerospace Resin. This formulation (Table 10) is produced by dissolving the crystalline curative (DDS) into hot epoxy resin (MY9512) at 125 °C (255 °F). Care should be taken to monitor the resin at all times while it is being heated. It should be noted that the system may exotherm with prolonged heating at this processing temperature. The resin is then usually applied to a fibrous reinforcement to make prepreg. Prepreg is the term used to describe the fiber-resin combination. While this resin is relatively brittle, excellent elevated-temperature performance is obtained by the combination of the tetrafunctional epoxy with DDS. This is evidenced by the mechanical properties shown in Table 11.

Table 6 Composition of an ambient-curing paste adhesive

Component	Content, wt%
Diglycidyl ether of bisphenol-A	56.6
Ancamide 400	26.4
Hycar 1300x16	17.0

Source: Ref 44

Table 7 Cured properties of a paste adhesive after 14 days at ambient temperature

Property	Value
Tensile strength, MPa (ksi)	33.3 (4.833)
Tensile modulus, MPa (ksi)	1220 (117)
Tensile elongation, %	12
Hardness, Shore D	77
Heat distortion temperature, °C (°F)	60 (140)
Izod notch impact strength, J/m (ft · lbf/in.)	56.5 (1.06)

Source: Ref 44

Table 8 Formulation of a high-temperature film adhesive

Component	Content, wt%
Epon 828	57.3
MY9512	11.5
Bisphenol-A	8.0
Hycar 1300x9	15.4
Dicyandiamide	5.3
Diuron	2.2
Triphenylphosphine	0.3

Source: Ref 45

Table 9 Cured properties of a high-temperature film adhesive cured two hours at 180 °C (355 °F)

Property	Value
Glass transition temperature (T_g), °C (°F)	157 (315)
Single lap shear strength at ambient temperature, MPa (ksi)	18.0 (2.61)
Interlaminar fracture toughness, J/m^2 (in. · lbf/in.^{2})	
G_{Ic}	800 (4.6)
G_{IIc}	2250 (12.9)

Source: Ref 45

Table 10 Composition of a high-performance aerospace resin

Component	Content, wt%
MY720	69.4
4,4′-DDS	30.6

Source: Ref 46

Some critical considerations when developing or selecting an aerospace grade resin are:

- *Room-temperature resin viscosity:* Aerospace-grade composite materials are often used to build large parts with complex contours so, once again, tack is a key product characteristic, with most tack-life requirements ranging from one to three weeks. How the part is fabricated (by hand or using special equipment) will dictate the specific tack needed. The substitution of higher- or lower-viscosity MY9512 variants in this example would allow the tack to be tailored. In almost all instances, both overall tack life and tack stability over that period of time are desired.
- *Resin rheology:* At cure temperature, the resin must flow enough to thoroughly wet the reinforcement, allow consolidation, and provide a pathway for trapped air and volatiles to escape. Insufficient flow can result in a cured part that is improperly consolidated, contains voids, and exhibits surface roughness. Too much flow can result in resin starvation, which also leads to parts with internal voids and external roughness.
- *Thermal-mechanical properties:* The final part application will dictate whether or not a basic epoxy resin system needs to be modified. This model system, as written, generates a strong, high-modulus part with a high T_g. It can easily be modified to provide a number of different characteristics. For examples, adhesive strength can be attained by incorporation of rubber, toughness by adding thermoplastics or rubbers, and hot/wet properties can be improved by the addition of a dicyclopentadiene novolac resin.

Safety

Epoxy resins and their associated products may be safely handled if care is taken to follow all recommendations made by materials suppliers. Product data sheets and technical service experts are usually available to aid in product selection. Vendors will always recommend processes for compounding, fabrication, and curing of composite parts. There are a number of publications that outline the environmental, safety, and health considerations related to the use of epoxy composite materials. It is important to understand that some epoxy resin systems and composite operations will require much more stringent controls than others, due to the specific chemicals and processes being used (Ref 47, 48).

General guidelines include but are not limited to:

- Read and understand all product literature and Material Safety Data Sheets (MSDSs) before exposing yourself or your workplace to any chemical. The MSDS will list all hazards associated with the product, including hazardous ingredients, exposure limits, exposure routes, health risks, effects of short and long term exposure, personal protection information, reactivity data, fire and explosion data, spill or leak procedures, special precautions, first aid procedures, and regulatory data. The MSDS will also include physical data about the material, including vapor pressure, vapor density, melting and boiling point, solubility in water, and specific gravity. Material Safety Data Sheets are required for all hazardous materials sold or transported in the United States and Europe.
- Work with uncured epoxy resins in areas with adequate ventilation. In some cases, this may require an enclosed area with a high rate of air exchange to minimize exposure through inhalation as well as irritation to the eyes, skin, and mucous membranes.
- Conventional personal protective equipment including barrier creams, gloves, respirators, and safety glasses should always be worn. Depending on work conditions, disposable or dedicated clothing should be provided in the workplace and washed routinely. Skin sensitization (contact dermatitis) and respiratory sensitization may occur when adequate industrial hygiene practices are not employed.
- Always follow manufacturer's directions carefully, especially with regard to mass of resin used, mixing procedure, and curing operations. Epoxy resins react exothermically and the heat generated may, if uncontrolled, cause fires or explosions.

Future Trends

Epoxy resins have been successfully used in composite applications since the 1960s. It is fair to say that this market has matured, as evidenced by the following facts. First, consumption of epoxy resins in composite applications has largely stagnated. From 1971 to 1984, use in the United States increased fourfold, from 21 to 86.8 million pounds, with most of this growth occurring in the late 1970s. Through the next decade, usage was essentially constant at approximately 83.7 million pounds in 1993. Second, of the three major U.S. producers of epoxy resins (Shell Chemical, Dow, and Ciba-Geigy), two (Shell and Ciba) have either sold or announced the sale of their epoxy resin businesses. The third, Dow, has concentrated away from the high-performance multifunctional resins and toward difunctional liquid resins, which compose the largest overall market segment. Finally, many of the specialty epoxy resins and curatives introduced since the 1980s have been withdrawn from the market and are no longer available. In the aerospace arena, industry consolidation has been reflected downstream by the intermediaries who manufacture formulated epoxy resin products as well as in the aerospace manufacturers themselves. This trend is driven by an overall industry emphasis on lower cost rather than improved performance. The introduction of epoxy composite materials into non-traditional markets continues but will not significantly affect the overall business until material and conversion costs can compete with those of commodity thermoplastics.

Given the maturity of the market and the technology, it's difficult to generalize with regard to future needs and research. It is clear, however, that the most serious barrier to the introduction of new chemistries is raw materials cost. Many of the specialty materials introduced since the mid-1980s (and later withdrawn from the market) were unsuccessful because the technological advantages they offered did not offset their high costs. Basic bisphenol-A epoxies are available on the order of \$1–3/lb., with high-end multifunctionals ranging from \$8–20/lb. To survive in this climate, new epoxy resin raw materials need to offer technical and/or handling advantages *and* be priced competitively. Without price competitiveness, it is unlikely that new raw materials, regardless of technical advantage, will be successfully employed in future composite programs. Additional factors that impede the introduction of new raw materials are decreases in the price of carbon fiber, which is now approaching the cost of the resins, improvements in strength and chemical resistance of glass fibers, and efficiencies in manufacturing methods.

A second barrier to the development of new epoxy resins and modifiers is the cost and time required in getting them approved for use. Before a new material can be sold commercially in a country, it must be registered by governmental agencies under regulations such as the Toxic Substances Control Act in the United States and the European Inventory of Existing Commercial Chemical Substances in the European Union. Registration requires a significant and expensive evaluation of the toxicological risks associated with a new substance. Unfortunately, the developers of new materials often find themselves in a no-win position. They cannot justify the expense of testing and registering a new material without a clearly identified market. Their customers, in turn, are reluctant to develop applications based on these new materials when long-term availability is not confirmed.

Beyond the requirement that any new developments be price competitive with existing technologies, several possibilities for future development exist. These include significant cost reduction for standard high-performance resin components, user-friendly materials, recyclable material forms, and processing operations that enable the displacement of conventional epoxy

Table 11 Cured properties of a high-performance aerospace resin

Property	At ambient temperature	At 150 °C (302 °F)
Tensile strength, MPa (ksi)	58.3 (8.45)	44.5 (6.46)
Tensile modulus, MPa (ksi)	3723 (540)	3723 (540)
Tensile elongation, %	1.8	1.9
Glass transition temperature (T_g), °C (°F)	177 (350)	. . .
Heat distortion temperature, °C (°F)	238 (460)	. . .
Charpy impact strength, unnotched, J (ft · lbf)	7.7 (5.7)	. . .

Source: Ref 46

materials. Some general trends within the aerospace market are toward lower-cost materials forms and lower-cost processing methods. Nonaerospace applications are achieving cost- cutting targets by using large tow carbon fibers to reduce fiber cost, low-temperature-rapid cures to reduce processing cycles, and preformed reinforcements to reduce hand work. Both markets are evaluating materials that increase the design flexibility. These include a single resin available in multiple materials forms, thin tapes, alternate lay-up techniques such as tape and tow placement, and high-modulus carbon fibers.

REFERENCES

1. H. Lee and K. Neville, *Handbook of Epoxy Resins*, McGraw-Hill, 1967
2. S.H. Goodman, *Handbook of Thermoset Plastics*, Noyes, 1986, p 133–182
3. J.A. Brydson, *Plastics Materials*, Iliffe Books Ltd./D. Van Nostrand Co., 1966, p 451–483
4. H. Lee and K. Neville, *Handbook of Epoxy Resins*, McGraw-Hill, 1967, Chap. 2 and 3
5. "Chemical Resistance Guide for Protective Coatings," Technical Bulletin SC:2298-95, Shell Chemical Company, 1995
6. "Tactix 556 Datasheet," Vantico
7. S.P. Qureshi (Amoco), U.S. Patent 4,686,250, Aug 1987
8. "Cyracyre Cycloaliphatic Epoxides," Technical Bulletin UC-958B, Union Carbide
9. H. Lee and K. Neville, *Handbook of Epoxy Resins*, McGraw-Hill, 1967
10. C. May, *Epoxy Resins Chemistry and Technology*, Marcel Dekker Inc., 1988
11. "Epoxy Resin Curing Agents, Comparative Performance Properties," Henkel Technical Bulletin, 1998
12. H. Lee and K. Neville, *Handbook of Epoxy Resins*, McGraw-Hill, 1967, p 7–2
13. Jeffamine Polyoxypropyleneamine Curing Agents for Epoxy Resins, Texaco Chemical Company 102-0812, 1992
14. H. Lee and K. Neville, *Handbook of Epoxy Resins*, McGraw-Hill, 1967, p 5-4
15. H. Lee and K. Neville, *Handbook of Epoxy Resins*, McGraw-Hill, 1967, p 5-4–5-12
16. "Epoxy Curing Agents and Diluents," Technical Bulletin 125-9613, Air Products, 1996
17. H. Lee and K. Neville, *Handbook of Epoxy Resins*, McGraw-Hill, 1967, p 10-3–10-4
18. M. Goosey, M. Roth, T. Kainmuller, and W. Seiz, Epoxy Resins and Their Formulation, *Plastics for Electronics,* Academic Publishers, 1999, p 103
19. H. Lee and K. Neville, *Handbook of Epoxy Resins*, McGraw-Hill, 1967, p 5-13–5-16, 11-4–11-8
20. "Epoxy Curing Agents and Diluents," Technical Bulletin 125-9613, Air Products, 1996
21. "Formulating with Dow Epoxy Resin," Technical Bulletin No. 296-346-1289, Dow Chemical, 1996, p 23
22. P.S. Rhodes, "*Advances in* Anhydride Epoxy *Systems*," 23rd International SAMPE Technical Conference, 1991
23. "Dyhard Epoxy Resin Hardeners," Technical Bulletin D-8223 Trostberg, SKW Trostberg, p 6
24. S.H. Goodman, *Handbook of Thermoset Plastics*, Noyes, 1986, p 157
25. C. Eberle, C. Janke, L. Klett, and G. Wrenn, "Radiation Curing of Composites Tutorial," Oak Ridge National Laboratory, 4 April 1999
26. D. Howell, "1999 Electron Beam Curing of Composites-Workshop Proceedings," Oak Ridge, TN, 20-21 April 1999
27. A.J. Kinloch and R.J. Young, *Fracture Behavior of Polymers*, Elsevier, 1983
28. A.F. Yee and R.A. Pearson, "Toughening Mechanisms in Elastomer Modified Epoxy Resins," NASA Contractor Report 3718, 1983
29. A.F. Yee and R.A. Pearson, "Toughening Mechanisms in Elastomer Modified Epoxy Resins, Part 2," *NASA Contractor Report 3852*, 1984
30. W.D. Bascom and D.L. Huntsdon, International Conference of Toughening Plastics, 22.1, London, 1978
31. Henry S.-Y. Hsich, Morphology and Properties Control on Rubber-Epoxy Alloy Systems, *Polym. Eng Sci.,* Vol 30 (No. 9), May 1990, p 493-510
32. B.L. Burton and J.L. Bertram, Design of Tough Epoxy Thermosets, *Polymer Toughening*, Marcel Dekker Inc., 1996, p 339–379
33. B.S. Hayes, J.C. Seferis, E. Anderson and J. Angal, Novel Elastomeric Modification of Epoxy/Carbon Fiber Composite Systems, *J. Adv. Mater.* Vol 28 (No. 4), 1997, p 20–25
34. M. Stängle, V. Altstädt, H. Tesch, and T. Weber, Thermoplastic Toughening of 180 °C Curable Epoxy Matrix Composites – a Fundamental Study, *Advanced Materials: Cost Effectiveness, Quality Control, Health and Environment, Proc. of the 12th Int. European SAMPE*, May 1991, Elsevier, p 33–42
35. S. Horiuchi, A.C. Street, T. Ougizawa, and T. Kitano, Fracture Toughness and Morphology Study of Ternary Blends of Epoxy, Poly(Ether Sulfone) and Acrylonitrile-Butadiene Rubber, *Polymer,* Vol 35 (No. 24), 1994, p 5283–5292
36. M. Lewin, Flame Retardant Mechanisms, *Conf. Proc.: Recent Advances: Flame Retardant Polymer Materials,* Business Communications Co., 1990
37. E.D. Weil, R.H. Hansen, and N. Patel, Fire and Polymers: Hazards, Identification and Prevention, *ACS Symposium Series*, 0097-6156; 425, 1990, p 97–108
38. I.S. Miles and S. Rostami, *Multicomponent Polymer Systems*, Longman/Wiley, 1992, p 207–268
39. H.S. Katz and J.V. Milewski, *Handbook of Fillers and Reinforcements*, Van Nostrand Reinhold, 1978
40. R. Bagheri and R.A. Pearson, Role of Particle Cavitation in Rubber-Toughened Epoxies: II. Inter-Particle Distance, *Polymer*, Vol 41, 2000, p 269–276
41. A.C. Roulin-Moloney, W.J. Cantwell, and H.H. Kausch, Parameters Determining the Strength and Toughness of Particulate-Filled Epoxy Resins, *Polym.Compos.*, Vol 8 (No. 5), 1987, p 314–323
42. S. Gordon, *Modern Plastics Encyclopedia*, 1991, p 167–170
43. Air Products Data Sheet for Anchamine 2143
44. B.F. Goodrich Technical Bulletin
45. J.H. Klug and J.C. Seferis, J.E. Green, S. Beckwith, and A.B. Strong, Ed., Model Epoxy Adhesive Systems: Influence of Prereaction Methods, *29th International SAMPE Technical Conference,* 1997, p 449–461
46. "Araldite MY720 Data Sheet," Vantico Specialty Chemicals
47. H.-P. Chu, Environmental, Safety, and Health Considerations–Composite Materials in the Aerospace Industry, *NASA Conference Publication 3289,* 1994
48. *Safe Handling of Advanced Composite Materials,* 3rd ed., SACMA, 1996

Polyester Resins

Tim Pepper, Ashland Chemical Company

UNSATURATED POLYESTER (UPE) RESIN is used for a wide variety of industrial and consumer applications. In fact, more than 0.8 billion kg (1.7 billion lb) was consumed in the United States in 1999. This consumption can be split into two major categories of applications: reinforced and nonreinforced. In reinforced applications, resin and reinforcement, such as fiberglass, are used together to produce a composite with improved physical properties. Typical reinforced applications are boats, cars, shower stalls, building panels, and corrosion-resistant tanks and pipes. Nonfiber reinforced applications generally have a mineral "filler" incorporated into the composite for property modification. Some typical nonfiber reinforced applications are sinks, bowling balls, and coatings. Polyester resin composites are cost effective because they require minimal setup costs and the physical properties can be tailored to specific applications. Another advantage of polyester resin composites is that they can be cured in a variety of ways without altering the physical properties of the finished part. Consequently, polyester resin composites compete favorably in custom markets.

Polyester Resin Chemistry

Polyesters are macromolecules that are prepared by the condensation polymerization of difunctional acids or anhydrides with difunctional alcohols or epoxy resins. Unsaturated polyester resins, commonly referred to as "polyester resins," are the group of polyesters in which the acid component part of the ester is partially composed of fumaric acid, a 1,2-ethylenically unsaturated material. Maleic anhydride is the predominant source of this fumarate. Maleic anhydride is incorporated into the polyester backbone and then isomerized to provide fumarate esters (commonly referred to as unsaturated polyesters). In most cases, the polymer is dissolved in styrene to provide a solution that will typically have a viscosity in the range of 0.2 to 2 Pa · s (200–2000 cP). Other reactive vinyl monomers, such as vinyl toluene, diallyl phthalate, or methyl methacrylate may be used to obtain specific properties. The resin viscosity is tailored for specific fabrication processes in which the resin is ultimately "cured" via a free-radical process. A final formulation may include resin, inorganic filler, fiberglass reinforcement, and a free-radical initiator, such as an organic peroxide. This final formulation is formed against a mold prior to the cross-linking reaction between the unsaturated polymer and the unsaturated monomer. The "curing" is a cross-linking chain reaction, converting the low-viscosity solution into a three-dimensional thermoset plastic (Ref 1). This is referred to as the cure. Terminology has developed to distinguish between various types of UPEs.

General-purpose resins are a group of resins generally used because of their low cost. While processing parameters can affect this, the cost of the raw materials tends to limit the type of unsaturated polyesters selected. The resins used in this area are commonly referred to as PET, DCPD, and ortho resins. While PET (polyethylene terephthalic) resin and orthophthalic anhydride are sources of low-cost saturated acids, DCPD (dicyclopentadiene) is typically coupled with maleic anhydride during an initial step, prior to both the isomerization and the condensation polymerization. Dicyclopentadiene improves the solubility of the polyester resin in styrene. As one drives toward lower-cost resins, solubility in styrene is a serious concern. Dicyclopentadiene offers a low-cost solution. Due to government regulations aimed at minimizing styrene emissions in open molding, a subset of general-purpose resins, "low-styrene" resins, has been developed. These resins tend to have a higher dependency on DCPD and are cooked to a lower molecular weight. This allows less styrene to be used to achieve the desired viscosity, and performance generally suffers.

Isophthalic resins are based on isophthalic acid and maleic anhydride. The incorporation of isophthalic acid creates a high-molecular-weight resin with good chemical and thermal resistance and good mechanical properties. The use of nonpolar glycols contributes to improved aqueous resistance, which is required to protect the fiberglass.

Bisphenol A (BPA) fumarate resins are prepared by the reaction of propoxylated BPA with fumaric acid. The result is a relatively nonpolar polyester with a reduced number of ester linkages. The reduced number of ester linkages contributes to excellent corrosion resistance. Bisphenol A fumarates were once the workhorse of the corrosion-resistant composite industry. In recent years, they have been replaced by isophthalic resins for mildly corrosive applications and bisphenol A epoxy based vinyl esters in more aggressive environments. Currently, BPA fumarates are used almost exclusively in applications requiring exceptional corrosion resistance to caustic environments.

Chlorendic resins are prepared using either chlorendic anhydride or chlorendic (HET) acid (Ref 2) reacted with maleic anhydride. Composites made from these resins have excellent chemical resistance and some fire retardancy because of the presence of chlorine. Chlorendic resins are used in applications requiring exceptional resistance to acidic or oxidizing environments. In many of these environments, metals are attacked quite aggressively, while chlorendic resin composites generally perform much better.

Vinyl ester resin is the common name for a series of unsaturated resins that are prepared by the reaction of a monofunctional unsaturated acid, typically methacrylic acid, with an epoxy resin. The epoxy resin is "end-capped" with an unsaturated ester to form the vinyl ester resin. The resulting polymer, which contains unsaturated sites only in the terminal positions, is mixed with an unsaturated monomer, generally styrene. At this point, the appearance, handling properties, and curing characteristics of vinyl ester resins are the same as conventional polyester resins. However, the corrosion resistance and mechanical properties of vinyl ester composites are much improved over standard polyester resin

Table 1 ASTM test methods for characterizing mechanical properties of polyester resins

Properties	ASTM Test Method
Tensile strength, modulus, and % elongation	D 638
Flexural strength and modulus	D 790
Compressive strength, modulus, and % compression on break	D695
Izod impact	D256
Heat distortion	D 648
Barcol hardness	D 2583

Table 2 Mechanical properties of clear-cast (unreinforced) polyester resins

Material	Barcol hardness	Tensile strength		Tensile modulus		Elongation, %	Flexural strength		Flexural modulus		Compressive strength		Heat-deflection temperature	
		MPa	ksi	GPa	10^6 psi		MPa	ksi	GPa	10^6 psi	MPa	ksi	°C	°F
Orthophthalic	...	55	8	3.45	0.50	2.1	80	12	3.45	0.50	...	...	80	175
Isophthalic	40	75	11	3.38	0.49	3.3	130	19	3.59	0.52	120	17	90	195
BPA fumarate	34	40	6	2.83	0.41	1.4	110	16	3.38	0.49	100	15	130	265
Chlorendic	40	20	3	3.38	0.49	...	120	17	3.93	0.57	100	15	140	285
Vinyl ester	35	80	12	3.59	0.52	4.0	140	20	3.72	0.54	...	...	100	212

Table 3 Mechanical properties of fiberglass-polyester resin composites (glass content, 40 wt%)

Material	Barcol hardness	Tensile strength		Tensile modulus		Elongation, %	Flexural strength		Flexural modulus		Compressive strength		Izod impact	
		MPa	ksi	GPa	10^6 psi		MPa	ksi	GPa	10^6 psi	MPa	ksi	J/mm	ft · lbf/in.
Orthophthalic	...	150	22	5.5	0.8	1.7	220	32	6.9	1.0	...	...	...	...
Isophthalic	45	190	28	11.7	1.7	2.0	240	35	7.6	1.1	210	30	0.57	10.7
BPA fumarate	40	120	18	11.0	1.6	1.2	160	23	9.0	1.3	180	26	0.64	12
Chlorendic	40	140	20	9.7	1.4	1.4	190	28	9.7	1.4	120	18	0.37	7
Vinyl ester	...	160	23	11.0	1.6	...	220	32	9.0	1.3	210	30	...	...

composites. These improved properties have enabled vinyl ester resins to become the workhorse of the polyester custom corrosion industry. However, the properties of vinyl ester resins are not as easily tailored to a specific application as are standard unsaturated polyester resins. This combined with the use of higher-cost raw materials has somewhat limited the ability of vinyl ester resins to penetrate the unsaturated polyester resin market.

Within each of these five resin classifications, specific polyesters can be formulated by varying the starting materials. Specific properties such as flexibility, thermal properties, fire retardancy, and hydrophobicity can be altered (Ref 3) by varying the type of dihydric alcohol/epoxy resin used or by varying the fumaric/saturated acid ratio.

Low-profile additives (LPAs) are a class of saturated resins that are used for dimensional stability. Although these materials are not UPEs, they play a very important role in the use of UPEs. One of the problems associated with the use of UPEs is that they shrink volumetrically about 6 to 8% upon curing. This creates challenges in fabricating a high-quality surface and/or maintaining the dimensional stability of a part. Low-profile additives offer a unique solution to this problem when processing at elevated temperatures. Addition of an LPA to a UPE formulation reduces or eliminates shrinkage. Some formulations using LPAs can actually have expansion greater than the original mold or form size. Since the LPA does not chemically react with the UPE or styrene, care should be taken in determining the type and amount of LPA used.

Mechanical Properties

Mechanical properties are often the critical factor in selecting a polyester resin for a specific application. Table 1 lists the common test methods of the American Society for Testing and Materials (ASTM) that are used to characterize the mechanical properties of polyester resin composites.

While the physical properties of polyester composites are predominately controlled by reinforcement, the physical properties of the polyester resin do affect the durability and thermal performance. Representative examples of clear-cast polyester resin data are shown in Table 2. It should be noted that within each class of resins, modifications are made to the polymer. These modifications effectively trade off thermal performance for increased toughness (Table 2). Table 2 highlights the differences among the classes of polyesters. Isophthalic resins tend to show higher tensile and flexural properties than orthophthalic resins. This may be because isophthalics usually form more linear, higher-molecular-weight polymers than orthophthalics. In contrast, the BPA fumarate and chlorendic resins are formulated for service in aggressive corrosive conditions and consequently are much more rigid. This results in clear castings that are brittle and have low tensile elongation and strength. The vinyl ester, because of its bisphenol diepoxide content, exhibits excellent tensile and flexural properties as well as high elongation.

In this article, it is impossible to discuss thoroughly the effects that dihydric alcohols, acids, levels of unsaturation, monomer types and amounts, and cure temperatures have on mechanical properties; however, Ref 4 provides an excellent review. In general, increasing the chain length of the dihydric alcohol increases the flexibility of the cross-linked resin. The same occurs with saturated acids. Aromatic groups, in either the dihydric alcohol or acid component, increase stiffness and hardness.

Using a reinforcing fiber to produce a polyester composite dramatically improves both the tensile and flexural properties. Table 3 lists the same five samples as Table 2; however, Table 3 shows the mechanical properties of the fiberglass reinforced polyester resin composites. In Tables 4 and 5, the properties obtained were dependent on the amount and type of glass fiber used. The last two entries in Table 5 show the influence of fiberglass orientation. Both contained 70 wt% glass fiber, but the unidirectional composite showed much higher tensile properties and flexural modulus when tested in the glass fiber di-

Table 4 Effect of glass content on mechanical properties of fiberglass reinforced polyester composites

Material	Glass content, wt%	Flexural strength		Flexural modulus		Tensile strength		Tensile modulus		Compressive strength	
		MPa	ksi	GPa	10^6 psi	MPa	ksi	GPa	10^6 psi	MPa	ksi
Orthophthalic	30	170	25	5.5	0.80	140	20	4.8	0.70	...	...
	40	220	32	6.9	1.00	150	22	5.5	0.80	...	...
Isophthalic	30	190	28	5.5	0.80	150	22	8.27	1.20	...	...
	40	240	35	7.58	1.10	190	28	11.7	1.70	210	30
BPA fumarate	25	120	17	5.1	0.74	80	12	7.58	1.10	170	24
	35	150	22	8.27	1.20	100	14	10.3	1.50	170	24
	40	160	23	8.96	1.30	120	18	11.0	1.60	180	26
Chlorendic	24	120	17	5.9	0.85	80	11	7.58	1.10	140	21
	34	160	23	6.89	1.00	120	18	9.65	1.40	120	18
	40	190	28	9.65	1.40	140	20	9.65	1.40	120	18
Vinyl ester	25	110	16	5.4	0.79	86.2	12.5	6.96	1.01	180	26.5
	35	260	37.3	9.52	1.38	153.4	22.25	10.8	1.56	230	34
	40	220	32	8.89	1.29	160	23	11.0	1.59	210	30

Table 5 Effect of glass type and amount on mechanical properties of fiberglass reinforced polyester composites

Type of glass fiber reinforcement	Glass content, wt%	Density, g/cm^3	Tensile strength, MPa	Tensile strength, ksi	Tensile modulus, GPa	Tensile modulus, 10^6 psi	Elongation, %	Flexural strength, MPa	Flexural strength, ksi	Flexural modulus, GPa	Flexural modulus, 10^6 psi	Compressive strength, MPa	Compressive strength, ksi
Neat cured resin	0	1.22	59	8.6	5.40	0.783	2.0	88	12.8	3.90	0.565	156	22.6
Chopped-strand mat	30	1.50	117	17.0	10.80	1.566	3.5	197	28.6	9.784	1.419	147	21.3
	50	1.70	288	41.8	16.70	2.422	3.5	197	28.6	14.49	2.102	160	23.2
Roving fabric	60	1.76	314	45.5	19.50	2.828	3.6	317	46.0	15.00	2.175	192	27.8
Woven glass fabric	70	1.88	331	48.0	25.86	3.750	3.4	403	58.4	17.38	2.520	280	40.6
Unidirectional roving fabric	70	1.96	611	88.6	32.54	4.720	2.8	403	58.4	29.44	4.270	216	31.3

Source: Ref 1

Table 6 Comparative properties of fiberglass reinforced polyester composites and various metals

Material	Glass content, wt%	Density, g/cm^3	Flexural strength, MPa	Flexural strength, ksi	Flexural modulus, GPa	Flexural modulus, 10^6 psi	Tensile strength, MPa	Tensile strength, ksi	Tensile modulus, GPa	Tensile modulus, 10^6 psi
Unidirectional glass roving, rod and bar	70	2.0	690	100	40	6	690	100	40	6
Unidirectional glass roving, sheet	50	1.6	205	30	15	2	140	20	12	1.8
Chopped-strand mat	30	1.5–1.7	110–190	16–28	6.9–8.3	1.0–1.2	60–120	9–18	6–12	0.8–1.8
Aluminum sheet	...	2.8	140	20	70	10	40–190	6–27	70	10
Stainless steel	...	8.0	210–240	30–35	190	28	210–240	30–35	190	28
Low-carbon steel	...	8.0	190	28	210	30	200–230	29–33	210	30

Material	Elongation, %	Compressive strength, MPa	Compressive strength, ksi	Impact strength, J/mm	Impact strength, ft · lbf/in.	Thermal conductivity, W/m · K	Thermal conductivity, Btu · in./h · ft^2 · °F	Specific heat, kJ/kg · K	Specific heat, Btu/lb · °F	Coefficient of thermal expansion, 10^{-6}/K
Unidirectional glass roving, rod and bar	1.5	410	60	2.6	49	0.70	5	1.0	0.24	5
Unidirectional glass roving, sheet	1.5	140	20	0.96	18	0.60	4	1.2	0.28	9
Chopped-strand mat	1–1.2	100–170	15–25	0.2–0.64	4–12	0.20–0.25	1.2–1.6	1.3–1.4	0.31–0.34	20–35
Aluminum sheet	30–40	...	...	...	...	120–130	810–1620	0.92–0.96	0.22–0.23	20–25
Stainless steel	40–50	210	30	0.45–0.59	8.5–11	14–25	96–185	0.50	0.12	15–20
Low-carbon steel	38–50	190	28	...	...	35–65	260–460	0.42–0.46	0.10–0.11	10–15

rection. The properties of unidirectional composites are even more anisotropic than typical polyester laminates. Mechanical properties measured transverse to the glass direction will approach those observed for clear castings. The pultrusion or filament-winding process commercially produces polyester composites employing unidirectional reinforcements. They can be used in structural applications where strength or stiffness is required in only one direction. In Table 6, physical properties of fiberglass reinforced polyester resin composites are compared to those of various metals.

As mentioned earlier, different types of reinforcement affect mechanical properties. While E-glass is the most commonly used reinforcement in polyester resins, S-glass, aramid, and carbon fibers can also be used. Table 7 compares a variety of reinforcements in both orthophthalic polyester and vinyl ester resins. While the tensile strength of the orthophthalic polyester was much improved with aramid, no such improvement was seen with the vinyl ester.

Inorganic fillers are commonly used in polyester resin composites. While they do improve stiffness, as shown by an increase in modulus (see Table 8), they have little effect on other strength characteristics. They are used primarily to reduce cost.

As expected, mechanical properties at elevated temperatures vary significantly among the general classifications of polyester resins (Fig. 1). The extreme rigidity and high glass transition temperature (T_g), of BPA fumarate and chlorendic polyesters result in high flexural strength retention up to 120 °C (250 °F). Vinyl esters also show performance advantages over isophthalic polyesters in fatigue studies (Fig. 2, Ref 5). The advantage of vinyl ester was evident at elevated temperatures (Ref 6). At 105 °C (220 °F), vinyl ester and isophthalic polyester composites (60% glass) were cycled to a stress level of 60 to 70 MPa (9–10 ksi). After 200,000 cycles, the drop in flexural modulus was only 5% for the vinyl ester, compared to 12% for the isophthalic polyester. The thermal performance of vinyl esters, combined with their excellent mechanical properties and toughness, explains why they are often chosen for structural resin composites.

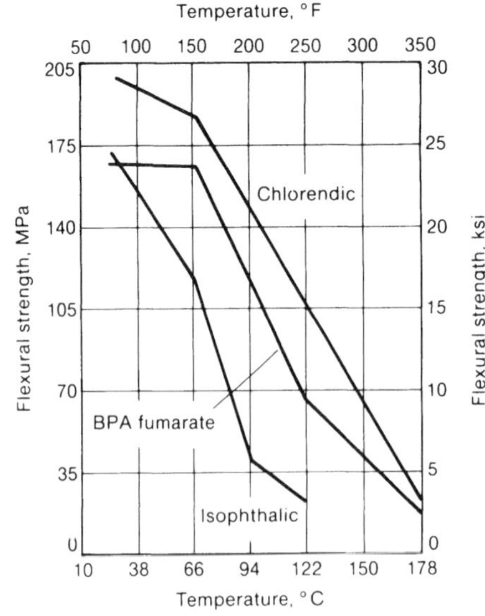

Fig. 1 Flexural strength versus temperature, glass-polyester composites of 40% glass

Thermal and Oxidative Stability

Polyester resins are commonly used in elevated-temperature applications, especially in the electrical and corrosion-resistance areas. At temperatures above 150 °C (302 °F), the polymer begins to slowly dissociate chemically. The temperature at which this decomposition occurs depends on the structure of the polyester used. Regardless of the polymer composition, at temperatures near 300 °C (570 °F), the cured polyester resin will undergo spontaneous decom-

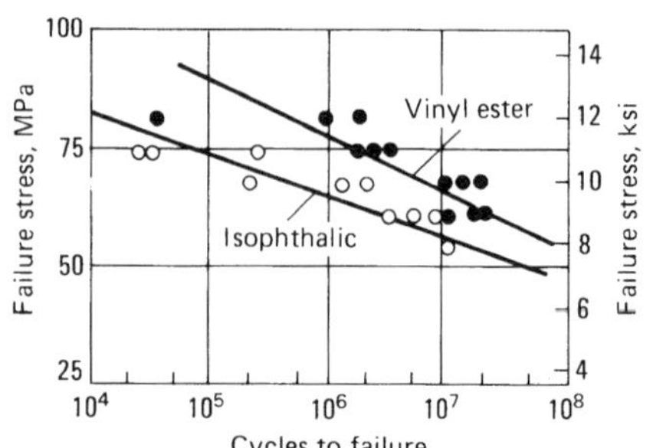

Fig. 2 Flexural fatigue strength

Table 7 Effect of reinforcement on mechanical properties of polyester-matrix composites

Material	Tensile strength, MPa	Tensile strength, ksi	Tensile modulus, GPa	Tensile modulus, 10^6 psi	Elongation, %
E-glass-ortho polyester					
Ambient temperature	157	22.8	11.0	1.59	1.7
50 °C (125 °F)	148	21.5	8.41	1.22	2.4
65 °C (150 °F)	140	20.3	7.31	1.06	2.6
S-glass-ortho polyester					
Ambient temperature	159	23.0	10.3	1.49	1.9
50 °C (125 °F)	165	24.0	8.55	1.24	2.6
65 °C (150 °F)	157	22.8	7.38	1.07	2.6
Aramid-ortho polyester					
Ambient temperature	212	30.7	12.5	1.82	2.0
50 °C (125 °F)	208	30.2	11.5	1.67	2.1
65 °C (150 °F)	200	29.0	9.52	1.38	2.4
E-glass-vinyl ester					
Ambient temperature	206	29.9	12.6	1.83	2.1
50 °C (125 °F)	192	27.9	11.4	1.66	2.2
65 °C (150 °F)	201	29.2	11.6	1.68	2.4
S-glass-vinyl ester					
Ambient temperature	198	28.7	11.4	1.66	2.2
50 °C (125 °F)	172	25.0	9.6	1.39	2.3
65 °C (150 °F)	199	28.8	10.3	1.49	2.5
Aramid-vinyl ester					
Ambient temperature	189	27.4	12.1	1.76	1.8
50 °C (125 °F)	221	32.0	11.7	1.70	2.2
65 °C (150 °F)	218	31.6	11.7	1.69	2.2

position. This is characteristic of vinyl polymers and is caused by their depolymerization to form monomeric species.

Among polyesters, high-molecular-weight UPEs and epoxy vinyl esters show better stability above 150 °C (302 °F) than low-molecular-weight UPEs. High-molecular-weight isophthalic, PET, DCPD, and BPA fumarate resins, when formulated properly, can perform very well in thermal applications (Fig. 3). In thermal stability, nonhalogenated resins outperform halogenated resins. While some chlorinated resins have respectable thermal stability, brominated resins universally have poor thermal stability with aromatic bromides performing somewhat better than aliphatic bromides. Low-styrene (general-purpose) resins also exhibit poor thermal stability. The same is true for orthophthalic resins, as they tend to be low-molecular-weight resins. In spite of their poor thermal stability, orthophthalic resins perform well in moderate- to low-temperature applications and are often

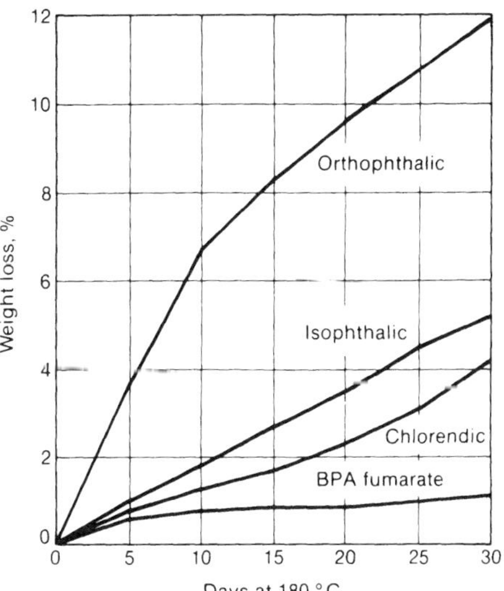

Fig. 3 Thermal stability of glass-polyester composites at 180 °C (355 °F)

preferred in such applications because of their low cost.

Monomer type also plays an important role in the thermal stability of a polyester resin. For example, a polyester resin in vinyl toluene shows superior thermal stability when compared to the same resin in styrene. This is attributed to the strong copolymer bonds formed with the fumarate unsaturation. Even after aging at 200 °C (390 °F), an isophthalic resin in vinyl toluene has better flexural strength retention than an isophthalic resin in styrene (Fig. 4). While vinyl toluene versions of an isophthalic polyester and a BPA fumarate showed comparable performance at 200 °C (390 °F), the BPA fumarate had much better flexural strength retention at 220 °C (430 °F) (Fig. 5) and 240 °C (465 °F) (Fig. 6).

Chemical Resistance

Polyester resins have been used for many years in applications requiring resistance to chemical attack. Parts made from UPEs have corrosion-resistant properties that complement most metals. As an environment increases in polarity, it becomes less aggressive toward parts made from UPEs. Numerous applications for corrosion-resistant tanks, pipes, ducts, and liners can be found in the chemical process and pulp and paper industries. Resin selection depends on

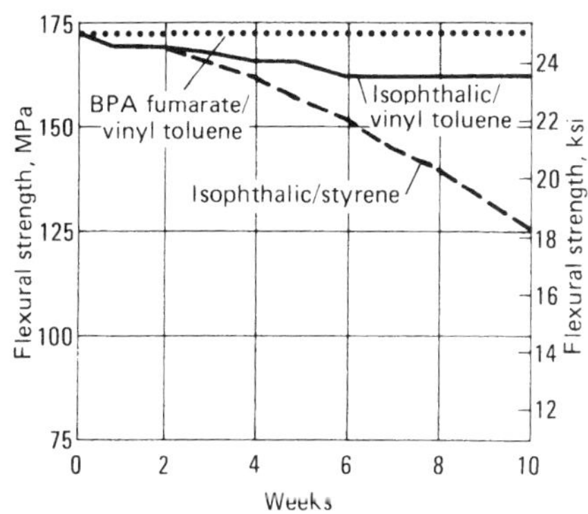

Fig. 4 Flexural strength retention of glass-polyester composite when aged at 200 °C (390 °F), tested at room temperature

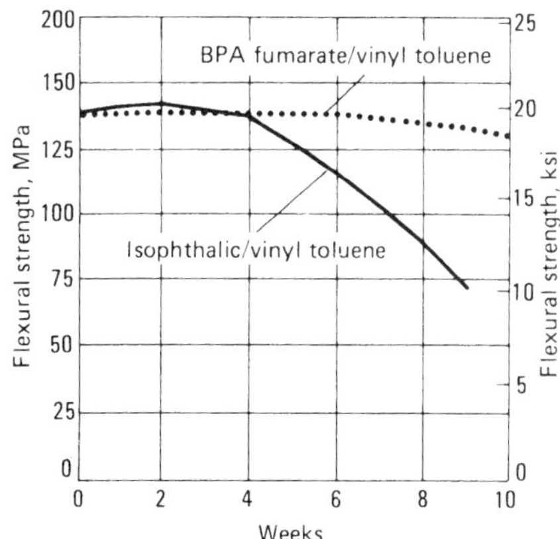

Fig. 5 Flexural strength retention of glass-polyester composite when aged at 220 °C (430 °F), tested at room temperature

the specific chemical environment to be contained. Table 9 shows how four different classes of polyester resin perform in several environments. Isophthalic resins perform well in both mild aqueous and mild organic environments. Generally, they are the most economic resin choice. Vinyl ester resins are typically used in more aggressive environments. A properly selected vinyl ester resin will perform well in many applications. When the environment becomes more aggressive, premium polyesters are preferred. Premium polyester resins offer improved corrosion resistance for specific applications. Chlorendic resins are chosen for strong acid and oxidizing environments, especially at elevated temperatures, while BPA fumarate resins are better in caustic environments. Using glass fiber

Table 8 Effect of filler and glass fiber reinforcement on mechanical properties of polyester resins

Reinforcement material	Flexural strength, MPa	Flexural strength, ksi	Flexural modulus, GPa	Flexural modulus, 10^6 psi	Tensile strength, MPa	Tensile strength, ksi	Tensile modulus, GPa	Tensile modulus, 10^6 psi	Elongation, %	Barcol hardness	Heat deflection temperature(a), °C	Heat deflection temperature(a), °F
Neat resin casting (A material)	129	18.7	3.60	0.522	70.0	10.1	3.50	0.507	3.0	30	58	135
80 pph A; 20 pph $CaCO_3$ (B material)	109	15.8	4.30	0.623	52	7.5	5.60	0.812	1.26	45	67	150
74 pph B; 26 pph 2.5 cm long chopped strand (C material)	183	26.5	6.10	0.884	116	16.8	9.694	1.406	1.72	45	>260	>500

pph, parts per hundred. (a) For 250 μm (10 mil) deflection at 1.82 MPa (0.264 ksi). Source: Ref 1

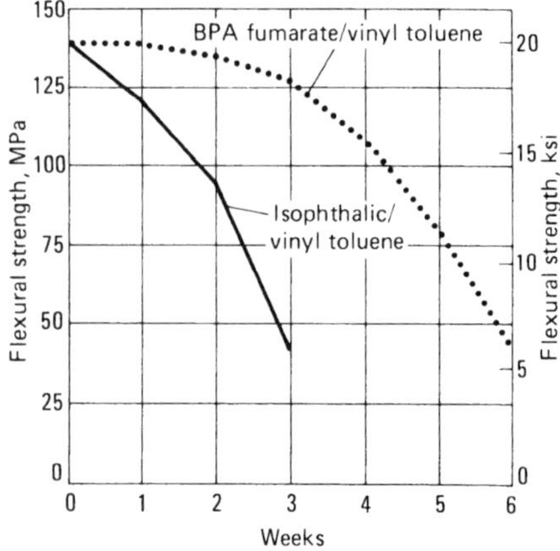

Fig. 6 Flexural strength retention of glass-polyester composite when aged at 240 °C (465 °F), tested at room temperature

Table 9 Corrosion resistance of glass fiber polyester resin composites

Resin	75% H_2SO_4 80 °C (175 °F)	15% NaOH 65 °C (150 °F)	5.25% NaOCl 65 °C (150 °F)	Xylene Ambient	Deionized water 100 °C (212 °F)	Seawater 80 °C (180 °F)
Isophthalic	–	–	–	+	–	–
Chlorendic	+	–	–	+	+	+
BPA fumarate	–	+	–	+	–	+
Vinyl ester	–	–	+	–	–	+

Table 10 Effect of methyl methacrylate on the gloss retention of weathered polyester panels

Components	Panel number 1	2	3	4	5
Polyester, %	75	75	60	60	60
Methyl methacrylate, %	25	. . .	20	10	0
Styrene, %	0	25	20	30	40
Gloss retention, %	5.2	48	83.5	56.5	11.8

Source: Ref 8

Table 11 Electrical properties of glass-polyester composites

Volume resistivity, 50% relative humidity, Ω · m	10^{10}–10^{12}
Dielectric strength, kV/mm (kV/in.)	
Short-time, 3.2 mm (⅛ in.)	13.6–16.5 (345–420)
Step-by-step, 3.2 mm (⅛ in.) increments	10.8–15.4 (275–390)
Dielectric constant	
60 Hz	5.3–7.3
1 kHz	4.68
1 MHz	5.2–6.4
Dissipation factor	
60 Hz	0.011–0.041
1 MHz	0.008–0.022
Arc resistance	120–200

does not improve the corrosion resistance of polyester resins and, in some cases, actually reduces performance. This is especially true in hydrofluoric acid or strong caustic environments where the chemicals actually attack and dissolve glass. In this and other special cases, reinforcing materials, such as carbon fibers, may be preferred (Ref 7).

Ultraviolet (UV) Resistance

Polyester resins are used in many outdoor applications. They can survive exposure to the elements for periods exceeding 30 years, although some discoloration and loss of strength will occur. The onset of surface degradation is marked by a yellow discoloration that becomes progressively darker as erosion and surface stress crazing occur. In translucent systems, this UV radiation causes yellowing of the composite as a whole, although the color is usually more intense on the surface. The negative effects of UV exposure can be effectively eliminated with the addition of UV stabilizers to the outermost resin layer. Monomer selection also affects UV stability. Styrene and other aromatic vinyl monomer derivatives are more susceptible to oxidative degradation and are usually supplemented with more resistant acrylate or methacrylate monomers. Of the acrylate monomers, methyl methacrylate (MMA) is the most common. When MMA is copolymerized with styrene, the cured polyesters have superior durability, color retention, and resistance to fiber erosion (Ref 8).

The improved UV resistance with MMA is evident in Table 10, which compares four polyester resins composed of identical polymers and four different monomer systems. These resins were used to prepare glass fiber reinforced panels that were exposed to outdoor weathering for five years. The gloss retention for styrene/MMA monomer blends was much greater than for either monomer alone. The refractive index of MMA is also lower than that of styrene, allowing the formulation of polyester resins with a refractive index matched to the glass fibers. This, combined with improved UV resistance, has resulted in the use of MMA polyesters to fabricate glass reinforced transparent building panels that can be used in greenhouses, skylights, and other applications. Using UV-absorbing chemical additives, such as the substituted benzophenones or benzotriazoles, can further reduce the effect of radiation.

Electrical Properties

Most organic polymers have medium to excellent electrical properties. Wide ranges of thermoset and thermoplastic materials are used in the

Table 12 Electrical properties of isophthalic polyester 3.2 mm (⅛ in.) laminates with various fillers

Filler	Dielectric strength short time, kV/mm	Dielectric strength short time, kV/in.	Volume resistivity, 10^{-13} Ω · m	Dielectric constant, 1 MHz	Dissipation factor, 1 MHz	Dielectric constant, 1 kHz	Dissipation factor, 1 kHz	Dielectric constant, 60 Hz	Dissipation factor, 60 Hz	Arc resistance Avg	Arc resistance Max	Arc resistance Min	Track resistance, V	Dielectric breakdown short time, kV	Dielectric breakdown step-by-step, kV
Calcium carbonate	15.0	380	7.8	4.10	0.007	4.18	0.005	4.19	0.003	157	181	140	840	58	61
Gypsum $CaSO_4$	14.4	365	2.1	3.69	0.011	4.04	0.023	4.19	0.027	153	184	141	840	70	55
Aluminum trihydrate	15.4	390	2.6	3.67	0.009	3.81	0.010	3.89	0.011	183.5	184	183	860	67	51
Clay	14.4	365	6.4	4.08	0.018	4.61	0.040	5.10	0.057	182.5	183	182	840	59	57

Note: Isophthalic polyester resin based on a vinyl toluene monomer

Table 13 Electrical properties of BPA fumarate polyester 3.2 mm (⅛ in.) laminates with various fillers

Filler	Dielectric strength short time, kV/mm	Dielectric strength short time, kV/in.	Volume resistivity, 10^{-13} Ω · m	Dielectric constant, 1 MHz	Dissipation factor, 1 MHz	Dielectric constant, 1 kHz	Dissipation factor, 1 kHz	Dielectric constant, 60 Hz	Dissipation factor, 60 Hz	Arc resistance Avg	Arc resistance Max	Arc resistance Min	Track resistance, V	Dielectric breakdown short time, kV	Dielectric breakdown step-by-step, kV
Calcium carbonate	6.1	155	1.6	3.94	0.005	4.00	0.004	4.03	0.004	140	143	133	840	58	52
Gypsum $CaSO_4$	5.9	150	3.3	3.72	0.009	4.03	0.024	4.24	0.029	144	151	137	820	50	40
Aluminum trihydrate	11.8	300	3.3	3.64	0.008	3.81	0.015	3.93	0.025	182	184	181	820	55	52
Clay	12.6	320	3.5	4.08	0.023	4.68	0.043	5.11	0.053	183	184	181	840	61	43

Note: BPA fumarate polyester resin based on a vinyl toluene monomer electrical and electronics industries. Applications in which polyester resins have been used include the insulation of motor windings, encapsulation of electrical components, fabrication of printed circuit boards, high-voltage standoff insulators, switch boxes, and miscellaneous equipment for high-voltage line work. Typical electrical properties of polyester resins are shown in Table 11. Tables 12 and 13 show specific data on an isophthalic polyester and a BPA fumarate as well as the influence of filler type.

Because many electrical applications require performance at elevated temperatures, polyester resin composites must have good thermal stability. Thermal stability and electrical performance at elevated temperatures are directly related, as can be seen by comparing the retention of dielectric strength at 200 °C (390 °F), shown in Fig. 7, with the retention of flexural strength at 200 °C (390 °F), shown in Fig. 4. As with flexural strength, a vinyl-toluene-based polyester outperforms a styrene-based polyester. At temperatures above 200 °C (390 °F), vinyl-toluene-based BPA fumarates outperform vinyl-toluene-based isophthalic polyesters (Fig. 8, 9).

Large electrical equipment, such as high-voltage motors or generators, often operate at elevated temperatures. In such applications, the electrical property of greatest concern is the dissipation factor, especially the dissipation factor versus the temperature. Polyester resins can be formulated for a low dissipation factor at elevated temperatures (Fig. 10). They are used as electrical varnishes at continuous-use temperatures up to 180 °C (355 °F).

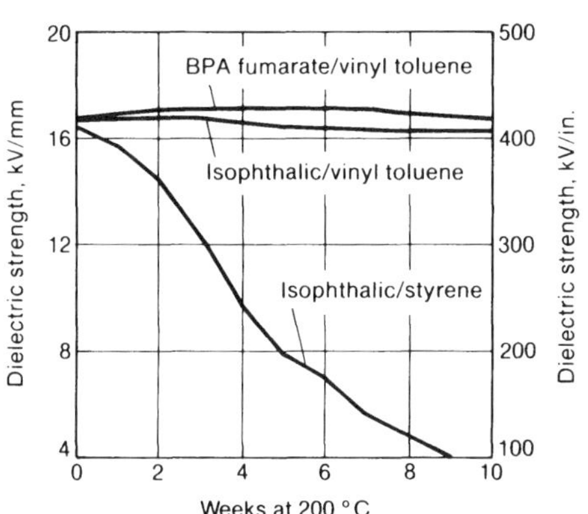

Fig. 7 Dielectric strength retention of glass-polyester composite when aged at 200 °C (390 °F), tested at room temperature

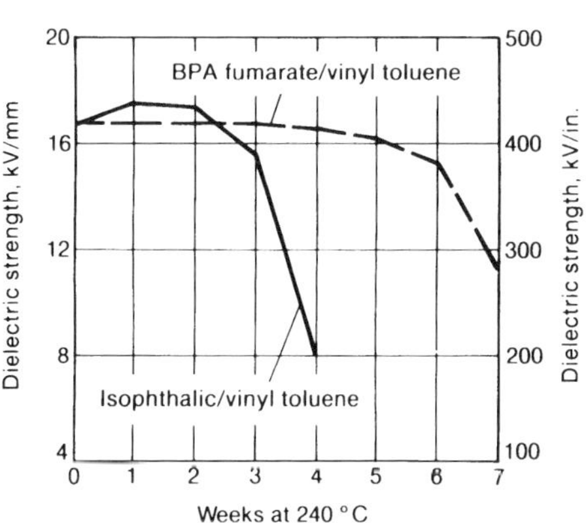

Fig. 9 Dielectric strength retention of glass-polyester composite when aged at 240 °C (465 °F), tested at room temperature

Flame-Retardant Polyester Resins

All organic materials, including polyesters, will burn in the presence of a flame. In many applications, polyester resins are required to have some degree of resistance to burning. This can be accomplished by using either a filler or a specially formulated flame-retardant polyester resin, depending on the degree of resistance required. The addition of filler is the more economical route to achieving flame retardancy in parts made from UPEs. However, the addition of filler increases weight and compromises tensile properties.

Incorporating halogen into a polyester resin is an effective way of improving flame retardance. This can be accomplished using a halogenated dibasic acid, such as chlorendic anhydride or tetrabromophthalic anhydride, or a halogenated dihydric alcohol, such as dibromoneopentyl glycol or tetrabromobisphenol A. At equivalent concentrations, bromine is much more effective than chlorine. Additives such as antimony oxides and ferrous oxide act as synergists with halogenated polyesters and improve their flame-retardancy properties (Ref 9).

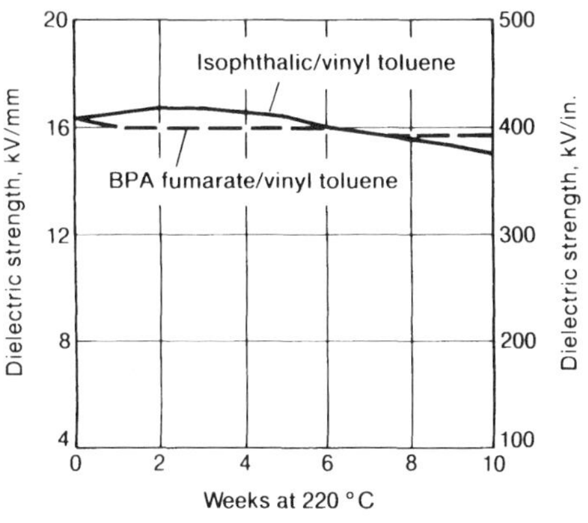

Fig. 8 Dielectric strength retention of glass-polyester composite when aged at 220 °C (430 °F), tested at room temperature

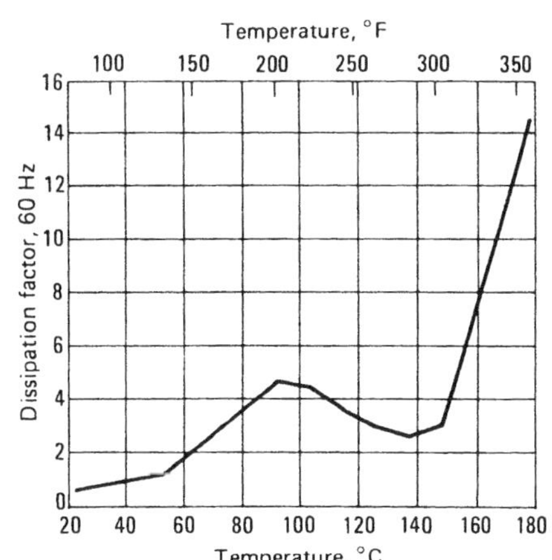

Fig. 10 Isophthalic polyester at 2.4 kV/mm (60 kV/in.)

Burning rate and smoke generation are measured using the Steiner Tunnel Test (ASTM E 84). In this test, a gas burner is placed at one end of a 53 cm by 7.6 m (21 in. by 25 ft) section. The distance the flame travels and the amount of smoke generated are measured (by the obscuration of a photoelectric beam). These are compared to two standards: red oak board, which is given a rating of 100 for flame spread and smoke generation, and asbestos cement, which is given a rating of 0 for both flame spread and smoke generation. Smoke generation is also measured with an NBS smoke chamber, which uses a photoelectric cell to measure smoke buildup in a closed chamber. The sample is burned either with or without a direct flame. When NBS smoke chamber testing is used, it is often common to use ASTM E 162, Flame Spread Index, to measure this variable.

Table 14 compares the performance of several resins using the above-mentioned fire and smoke tests. In each of these tests, the halogenated resin clearly outperforms the orthophthalic resin. Ferrous oxide also reduces smoke generation in the NBS chamber when compared to antimony oxide.

Table 15 compares various filled and unfilled polyester resin composites. The improvement of an orthophthalic resin by the incorporation of alumina trihydrate (ATH) is dramatic, the flame spread is reduced from 350 to 64. However, halogenated resins reach this level of performance

Table 14 Performance of selected polyester composites in fire tests

Material or test	System I	System II	System III
Material			
Resin	100(a)	100(b)	100(c)
Alumina trihydrate	100	100	100
Antimony oxide	...	57	...
Ferrous oxide	...	...	5
Test method and property			
ASTM E 162			
Flame spread index	75	7	7
ASTM E 84			
Flame spread	120	23	25
Smoke emission	608	270	268
NBS chamber: flaming mode			
Maximum density	203	433	264
90 s density	2.5	18	11
240 s density	162	245	128
NBS chamber: nonflaming mode			
Maximum density	481	400	350
90 s density	1	1	5
240 s density	16	45	50

(a) Orthophthalic resin. (b) HET acid resin A, 26% Cl. (c) HET acid resin B, 26% Cl. Source: Ref 10

Table 15 Flame spread and smoke emission characteristics of unfilled and filled polyester systems

Glass reinforced laminates 3.2 mm (1/8 in.) thick, containing 30% glass, tested in accordance with ASTM E 84

Component or property	System formulation and property value									
	100(a)	100(b)	100(b)	100(c)	100(d)	100(d)	100(e)	100(e)	100(f)	100(f)
Unfilled system										
Antimony oxide	...	...	5	...	...	5	...	5	...	5
Flame spread	350	60	25	...	60	15	67	20	69	18
Smoke emission	1100	780	450	...	747	731	980	1043	837	838
Filled system										
Alumina trihydrate, phr	100	100	100	100	100	100	100	100	100	100
Antimony oxide	...	5	...	...	5	...	5	...	5	...
Ferrous oxide	...	...	5	5	...	5	...	5	...	5
Flame spread	120	23	20	25	10	25	18	10	10	12
Smoke emission	608	270	242	168	364	260	450	400	761	620

(a) Orthophthalic resin. (b) HET acid resin A, 26% Cl. (c) HET acid resin B, 26% Cl. (d) Dibromotetrahydrophthalic resin, 18% Br. (e) Dibromoneopentyl glycol resin, 18% Br. (f) Tetrabromophthalic resin, 18% Br. Source: Adapted from Ref 10

without the incorporation of any filler. Halogenated resins with a synergist show only a slight reduction in flame spread when ATH is added, but smoke emission is greatly reduced. When comparing brominated and chlorinated resins, 26% Cl gave comparable flame and smoke results as 18% Br.

ACKNOWLEDGMENT

This revised article is largely built around the original article "Polyester Resins" by Charles D. Dudgeon, Ashland Chemical Company, from *Composites,* Vol 1 of the *Engineered Materials Handbook.*

REFERENCES

1. M. Grayson and D. Eckroth, Ed., *Encyclopedia of Chemical Technology,* 3rd ed., Vol 18, John Wiley & Sons, 1982, p 575
2. P. Robitschek and C.T. Bean, Flame Resistant Polyesters from Hexochlorocyclopentadiene, *Ind. Eng. Chem.,* Vol 46, 1954, p 1628
3. E.N. Doyle, *The Development and Use of Polyester Products,* McGraw-Hill, 1969, p 258
4. H.V. Boenig, *Unsaturated Polyesters: Structure and Properties,* Elsevier, 1964
5. B. Das, H.S. Loveless, and S.J. Morris, Effects of Structural Resins and Chopped Fiber Lengths on the Mechanical and Surface Properties of SMC Composites, *36th Annual Conference of the Reinforced Plastics Composites Institute,* The Society of the Plastics Industry, 1981
6. P.K. Mallick, Fatigue Characteristics of High Glass Content SMC Materials, *37th Annual Technical Conference,* Society of Plastics Engineers, 1979, p 589
7. H.S. Kliger and E.R. Barker, A Comparative Study of the Corrosion Resistance of Carbon and Glass Fibers, *39th Annual Conference of the Reinforced Plastics/Composites Institute,* The Society of the Plastics Industry, 1984
8. A.L. Smith and J.R. Lowry, Long Term Durability of Acrylic Polyesters versus 100% Acrylic Resins in Glass Reinforced Constructions, *15th Annual Conference of the Reinforced Plastics/Composites Institute,* The Society of the Plastics Industry, 1960
9. E. Dorfman, W.T. Schwartz, Jr., and R.R. Hindersinn, "Fire-Retardant Unsaturated Polyesters," U.S. Patent 4,013,815, 1977
10. J.E. Selley and P.W. Vaccarella, Controlling Flammability and Smoke Emissions in Reinforced Polyesters, *Plast. Eng.,* Vol 35, 1979, p 43

Bismaleimide Resins

BISMALEIMIDE (BMI) RESINS are a relatively young class of thermosetting polymers that are gaining acceptance by industry because they combine a number of unique features including excellent physical property retention at elevated temperatures and in wet environments, almost constant electrical properties over a wide range of temperatures, and nonflammability properties. Bismaleimides have become a leading class of thermosetting polyimides. Their excellent processibility and balance of thermal, mechanical, and electrical properties have made them popular in advanced composites and electronics.

Composites of the BMI class are used on some of the most important and complex, high-performance applications ranging from military programs such as the U.S. Air Force's F-22 to Formula-1 race cars. The most important attribute of BMIs is the highest service temperature capability of an addition-cure matrix resin combined with epoxy-like autoclave processing. The BMI matrix composites provide the highest composite mechanical properties available through 177 °C (350 °F)/wet with damage tolerance equivalent to the best epoxies. Certain BMIs are capable of extended service at 230 to 290 °C (450 to 550 °F), approaching the performance of PMR-15 (see the article "Polyimide Resins" in this Volume). BMIs also are suitable for resin transfer molding (RTM) processing. This article first discusses BMI chemistry and then describes the use of BMI in composites. An analysis of the current applications illustrates how the advantages of BMIs have been exploited and perhaps suggests how these advantages might be extended to other applications.

BMI Resin Chemistry

Horst Stenzenberger, Technochemie GmbH, Germany

Bismaleimides are best defined as low molecular weight, at least difunctional monomers or prepolymers, or mixtures thereof, that carry maleimide terminations (Fig. 1). Such maleimide end groups can undergo homopolymerization and a wide range of copolymerizations to form a highly cross-linked network. These cure reactions can be effected by the application of heat and, if required, in the presence of a suitable catalyst.

The first patent for cross-linked resins obtained through the homopolymerization or copolymerization of BMI was granted to Rhone Poulenc, France in 1968 (Ref 1), followed by a series of patents related to poly(amino BMIs) (Ref 2), which were synthesized from BMIs and aromatic diamine. Following the initial patent disclosures, numerous chemical modifications have been carried out and mixtures formulated to improve processibility and cured resin properties. Melt-processible BMI systems specifically designed for fiber reinforced applications are described in a patent granted to Technochemie in 1974 (Ref 3). The approach of blending selected BMI monomers and further formulating them with reactive diluents or comonomers provided formulated resins that are equivalent in processing to the conventional 177 °C (350 °F) service epoxy resins. The breakthrough with respect to application as tacky autoclavable prepreg was achieved through a divinylbenzene modified BMI system (Ref 4) that was used to build the delta wings of the General Dynamics F16XL demonstrator combat aircraft (Ref 5) and parts of the McDonnell Douglas AV8-B vertical takeoff aircraft (Ref 6).

The principal concern with BMI resins has been their inherent brittleness owing to their high cross-link density. Ciba Geigy, however, demonstrated that BMI and o,o′-diallylbisphenol A (DABA) copolymers are much tougher than high-temperature epoxies (Ref 7). The BMI/DABA copolymers were patented in Switzerland in 1975, but the significance of the invention, that is, their toughness, was not recognized before toughness became an issue to the aerospace industry. Experience has taught that a useful BMI-resin comprises both a BMI part and a comonomer part.

Bismaleimide Building Blocks

A standard synthesis of N,N′-arylene BMI (Fig. 2) involves the chemical dehydration of N,N′-arylene bismaleamic acid with acetic anhydride in the presence of a catalyst (sodium acetate) at temperatures below 80 °C (175 °F) (Ref 8). The yield of the pure recrystallized BMI is usually 65 to 75%. Various byproducts, such as isoimides and acetanilides, are responsible for the relatively low yield of pure BMI. Almost every aromatic diamine can be converted to the corresponding BMI. However, the most widely used building block is 4,4′-bismaleimidodiphenylmethane, because the precursor diamine is readily available and inexpensive. Bismaleimides based on aromatic diamines are crystalline substances with high melting points. For reasons of processibility, BMIs with low melting points are the preferred building blocks for composite resins. The BMI-building blocks primarily used

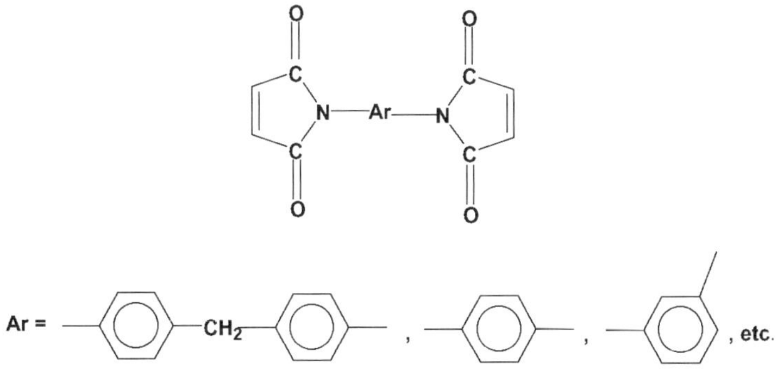

Fig. 1 General structure of bismaleimide resin

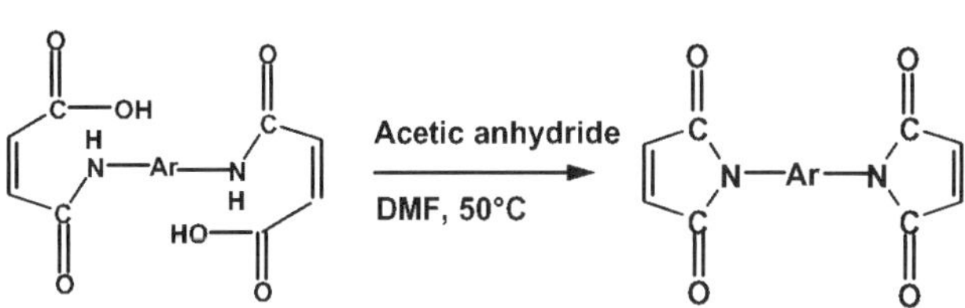

Fig. 2 The synthesis of bismaleimide from bismaleamic acid. DMF, dimethyl formamide

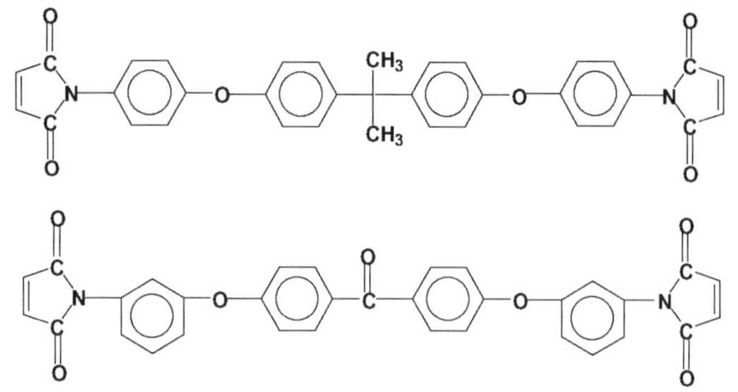

Fig. 3 Bismaleimide of polyaromatic diamines

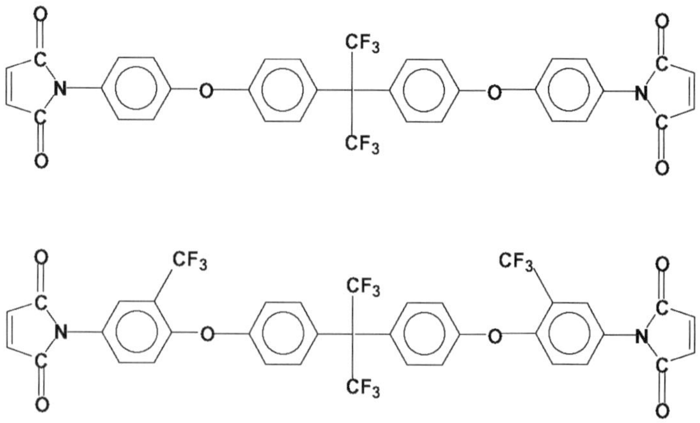

Fig. 4 Fluorine containing bismaleimides

in commercial BMI resins are 4,4′-bismaleimidodiphenylmethane, 2,4-bismaleimidotoluene, 1,3-bismaleimidobenzene, and sometimes, aliphatic BMIs based on n- or iso-alkanes.

Because of the toxicity problems associated with methylene dianiline (MDA) (4,4′-diaminodiphenylmethane), the BMI precursor and other diamines with only one or two aromatic rings, polyaromatic diamines, and BMIs based on them are of increasing interest. In the past, it was almost impossible to introduce novel BMI building blocks with increased molecular weight because of the processing problems associated with the high melting points and high melt viscosities. With the new processing techniques, such as powder prepregging and blending with reactive diluents such as DABA, such limitations could be partly overcome. Examples of polyaromatic BMIs are provided in Fig. 3.

The most important property of a BMI is its ability to undergo a temperature-induced polymerization. The maleimide double bond is highly activated owing to the adjacent carbonyl groups of the maleimide ring. Therefore, heating the BMI above its melting point effects polymerization. The cure exotherm peak temperature taken from a dynamic differential scanning calorimetry (DSC) scan is used to characterize the reactivity of individual BMIs. The reactivity is influenced by the chemical nature of the residue between the maleimide terminations and by the molar mass between the reactive maleimide groups. Normally, electron-donating groups such as alkyl groups reduce the BMI reactivity, provided they are present in the phenyl ring that carries the maleimide group. On the other hand, electron-attracting groups such as SO_2, carbonyl, and so on, have the opposite effect. Increasing the molecular weight between cross links (Mc) generally provides a more latent system owing to steric effects.

In their early days, the most important application for BMI resins was multilayer printed circuit boards. In this area, resins with low dielectric constants are required. Hitachi Research Laboratory, Japan recently reported the thermal and dielectric properties of fluorine-containing BMIs (Ref 9). The chemical structures of two fluorinated BMIs investigated are provided in Fig. 4.

Bismaleimides and maleimide-terminated prepolymers have been considered for systems with improved fire, smoke, and toxicity properties. For such applications, phosphorous-containing BMIs are of interest because they provide high limiting-oxygen index (LOI) values.

Besides the fact that synthesizing new BMI building blocks and investigating their application potential are still desired, the BMI building block is not the final resin product. Although building blocks usually make up 50 to 75 wt% of the resin, other ingredients—such as comonomers, reactive diluents, processing additives, elastomers, and catalysts—are combined with BMI to obtain a product suitable for the application considered. The application areas for BMI resins are reinforced composites for printed circuit boards (with glass fabric), structural laminates (with glass, carbon, and aramid fibers), and moldings (with short fibers and particulate fillers).

Bismaleimide Resin Systems

In order to fulfill the processing requirements, BMI building blocks have to be formulated into products that enable their use as highly concentrated solutions, powders, or hot melts. An early attempt in BMI modification with respect to achieving a meltable, noncrystalline resin was made by blending a complex mixture of BMIs and crystallization inhibitor (Ref 10). The resin (Compimide 353), although it is not a formulated product, shows a very low melting transition and a low viscosity at 110 °C (230 °F). This specific resin system can be further formulated with a wide range of vinyl and/or allyl compounds to provide prepreg resins that are tacky at room temperature and suitable for low-pressure autoclave molding.

The divinylbenzene approach to modify BMI into a hot-melt prepreg system was followed by U.S. Polymeric/British Petroleum (now Cytec Fiberite) (Ref 11). The resin system, known in the industry under the trade name V378A, was the first BMI formulation used in primary aircraft application. Although the resin is relatively brittle in comparison with epoxy resin, it provides outstanding high-temperature mechanical properties in both dry and wet environments. V378A prepreg can be cured under standard low autoclave pressure of 700 kPa (7 bars) and temperatures similar to current 177 °C (350 °F) curing epoxy systems. However, postcure temperatures of 245 to 260 °C (475 to 500 °F) are required to maximize elevated-temperature strength retention.

Polyaminobismaleimides. The reaction of a BMI with a functional nucleophile (diamine, aminophenol, aminobenzhydrazide, etc.) via the Michael addition reaction converts a BMI building block into a polymer. The nonstoichiometric reaction of an aromatic diamine with a BMI converts the BMI into a polyaminobismaleimide as shown in Fig. 5.

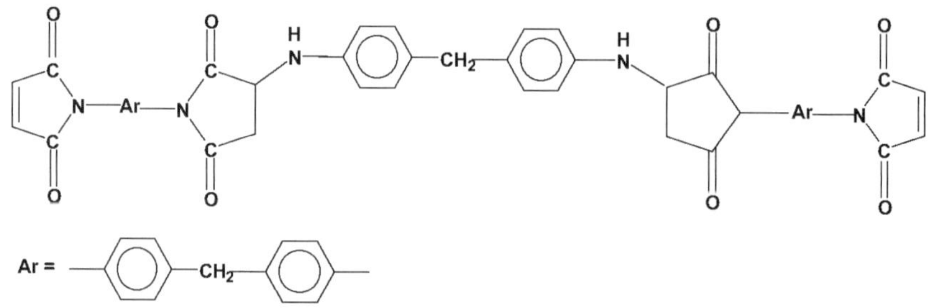

Fig. 5 Bismaleimide/MDA Michael addition product

The reaction product of 4,4′-bismaleimidodiphenylmethane and 4,4′-diaminodiphenylmethane, known as Kerimide 601, is prepolymerized to such an extent that the resulting prepolymer is soluble in aprotic solvents such as N-methylpyrrolidone, dimethylformamide, and the like, and therefore can be processed via solution techniques to prepreg. Kerimide 601 was mainly used in glass fabric laminates for electrical applications and became the industry standard for polyimide-based printed circuit boards. Recently the resin has been taken off the market because of the high free methylene dianiline (MDA) content in the product. The MDA is a suspected carcinogen.

Another approach to processible BMI resin via a Michael addition chain extension is the reaction of BMI, or a low-melting mixture of BMIs, with aminobenzoic hydrazide to provide a resin that is soluble in various solvents, such as acetone, methylene chloride, and dimethylformamide (DMF) (Ref 12). The idealized chemical structure for a 2:1 BMI-aminobenzhydrazide resin is provided in Fig. 6.

Two resin systems based on this chemical concept are commercially available from Technochemie (now a subsidiary of Laporte PLC) under the name Compimide 183 (solid resin with no solvent) and Compimide 1206-R55 (resin solution in DMF) for use in printed circuit boards. Typical properties of Compimide 1206 printed circuit laminates are provided in Table 1.

The BMI/amine Michael adduct resins may be further modified and blended with other thermosets or reactive diluents to achieve either specific end-use properties or processibility. Epoxy resins are very suitable for the modification of BMI/primary amine adducts, because the secondary amine functionality in the aspartimide structure is a curative for the epoxy group.

A modified BMI-epoxy resin system has been developed and introduced by Shell Chemical Company. The system is a highly reactive blend of a BMI, Compimide 1206 R55, and Epon resin 1151, a polyfunctional epoxy resin (Ref 13). In this polyimide resin, no free MDA is present. This is an important feature because MDA has been identified as an animal carcinogen and a possible human carcinogen. The resin system has been fully evaluated for use in multilayer printed circuit boards (Ref 14). Catalysts such as methylimidazole or phenylimidazole are recommended for processing and for adjusting the processing window. The properties of two BMI-epoxy electrical laminates are provided in Table 2.

The Compimide 1206/Epon 1151 BMI/epoxy concept is particularly interesting because the ratios of BMI and epoxy resin may be varied widely to possibly tailor the thermal and electrical properties.

Bismaleimide/Bis(Allylphenol) Resins. The copolymerization of a BMI with DABA is a resin concept that has been widely accepted by the industry because BMI-DABA blends are tacky solids at room temperature and therefore provide all the desired properties in prepregs, such as drape and tack, similar to epoxies. Crystalline BMI can easily be blended with DABA, which is a high-viscosity fluid at room temperature. On heating, BMI-DABA blends copolymerize via complex ENE and Diels Alder reactions as outlined in Fig. 7.

Reportedly, DABA is an attractive comonomer for BMIs because the corresponding copolymer is tough and temperature resistant (Ref 15). Toughness, however, is a function of the BMI-DABA ratio employed in the resin mix. In one study, optimized toughness properties were achieved when BMI and DABA were employed at a close to 2:1 molar ratio (Ref 16), as can be seen from Table 3.

Diallylbisphenol is commercially available under the trade name Matrimide 5292 from Ciba Geigy. Other comonomers of the o-allylphenol type have been synthesized and copolymerized with BMI (Ref 17). Bis(3allyl-4-hydroxyphenyl)-p-diisopropylbenzene, in particular, provided even better toughness properties than the BMI-DABA system.

Table 1 Properties of BMI (Compimide 1206) printed circuit laminates

Property	Value
Dielectric constant at 1 MHz	4.6–4.7
Dielectric loss constant at 1 MHz	0.01
Dielectric strength, V/μm	29.5
Volume resistivity, Ω · cm	10^{15}
Water absorption(a), %	<1
Heat stability at 287 °C (550 °F), s	>60
Thermal expansion coefficient, 10^{-6}/°C	
x, *y* directions	14–16
z direction	36–38
Flammability in comparison with UL 94	
3 mm (0.12 in.) laminate	V-0
1.5 mm (0.06 in.) laminate	V-1

Compimide 1206 is equivalent to Compimide 183. Properties measured using 1.0–1.5 mm (0.04–0.06 in.) glass fabric laminates. (a) After postcure at 210 °C (410 °F)

Table 2 Properties of BMI-epoxy electrical laminates

Property	Value for laminate composition (BMI/epoxy) of 70/30	50/50
Flexural strength at 23 °C (73 °F), MPa (ksi)	462 (67)	441 (64)
Flexural modulus at 23 °C (73 °F), GPa (10^6 psi)	22 (3.2)	21 (3.0)
Dielectric constant at 23 °C (73 °F)	4.32	4.48
Dissipation factor at 23 °C (73 °F)	0.0083	0.0098
Dielectric strength, V/μm	30	31
Volume resistivity, Ω · cm	2.1×10^{16}	1.9×10^{16}
Surface resistivity, Ω · cm	3.8×10^{16}	$>1.9 \times 10^{16}$
Flammability, UL-94	V-0	V 0
Methylene chloride, mg uptake	1.1	1.7
Water absorption, wt%		
103 kPa steam, 1 h	0.28	0.31
Boiling, 24 h	1.32	1.24

BMI resin is Compimide 1206. Epoxy is Epon 1151.

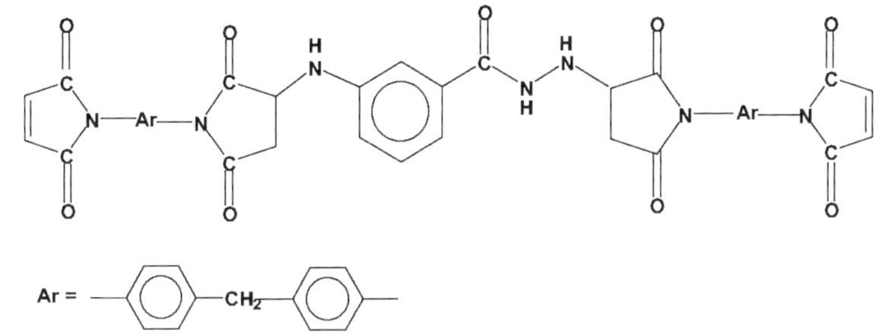

Fig. 6 Michael addition product of BMI-aminobenzhydrazide

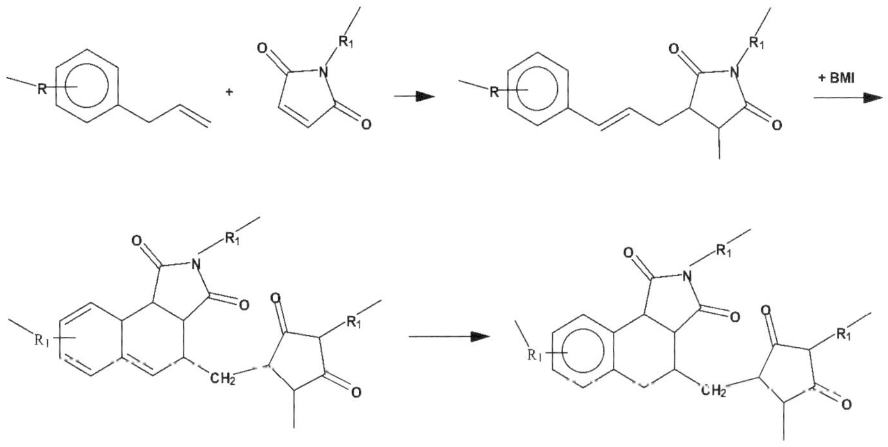

Fig. 7 Copolymerization of BMI with DABA

Bismaleimide Resins via Diels-Alder Reaction. The Diels-Alder reaction can also be employed to obtain thermosetting polyimides. If BMI (the bisdienophile) and the bisdiene react nonstoichiometrically, with BMI in excess, a prepolymer carrying maleimide terminations is formed as an intermediate, which can then be cross-linked to yield a temperature-resistant network.

A new Diels-Alder comonomer for BMI is bis(o-propenylphenoxy) benzophenone. This comonomer is commercially available from Technochemie under the trade name Compimide TM123. It is of particular interest because the BMI/bis(o-propenylphenoxy)benzophenone copolymers are very temperature resistant. The synthesis involves a straightforward nucleophilic halogen displacement reaction. The o-allylphenol reacts with 4,4′-difluorobenzophenone at 160 °C (320 °F) in N-methylpyrrolidone as a solvent in the presence of potassium carbonate as a catalyst. The alkaline reaction conditions are responsible for the o-allyl → o-propenyl isomerization (Ref 18).

The bis(o-propenylphenoxy)benzophenone, Compimide TM123, is commercially available from Technochemie, Germany. It is a low-melting, low-viscosity material that can easily be melt blended with BMI and then cured at temperatures of 170 to 230 °C (340 to 445 °F). The BMI/Compimide TM123 copolymer resin is attractive because of its extremely high temperature stability. It shows a better thermal oxidative stability than all other commercially available BMI systems. The copolymerization chemistry of BMI/propenylphenyl resins is provided in Fig. 8.

Continuing Development of BMI Resin Systems. The target in BMI resin technology for composite applications is to improve properties such as toughness and thermal stability and at the same time reduce moisture absorption. BMI comonomers influence such properties significantly. The DABA concept is favored when high toughness properties are desired. Compimide TM123 [bis(o-propenylphenoxy) benzophenone] on the other hand provides systems with excellent thermal oxidative stability. Figure 9 shows the weight retention versus aging time at 275 °C (525 °F) for up to 1000 h of a BMI-DABA system versus two BMI-Compimide TM123 resins. It is obvious that the Compimide TM123 neat resin is by far superior to the BMI-DABA resin.

Another important property of BMI-comonomer blends is processibility. Processibility includes working viscosity and cure kinetics or reactivity. A comparative study of the relative reactivity of alkenyl-functionalized modifiers for BMI was recently published (Ref 19). Differential scanning calorimetry measurements suggest that propenyl-functionalized aromatic comonomers do react more readily than the allylic analogues. For a series of recently synthesized bis[3-(2-propenylphenoxy) phthalimides], it could be demonstrated that these are by far more reactive than their allylphenoxy analogs (Ref 20). Therefore allylphenoxy comonomers are to be favored when processibility is desired. However, the thermal oxidative stability is superior for the propenylphenoxy reactive diluents and comonomers.

The key to improved BMI systems is the properties of the comonomer employed for the BMI resin. The BMI itself is limited to a very few chemical structures; 4,4′-bismaleimidodiphenylmethane represents the most important one because it is readily available and relatively inexpensive.

Research in the area of improved BMI resin systems is still ongoing. Technochemie has synthesized propenyl-group-functionalized poly(arylen ether ketone) high polymers and could demonstrate that these are excellent tougheners for BMIs; however, these systems suffer from high glass-transition temperatures and poor processibility (Ref 21). Many other chemical concepts to modified BMI systems have been published (Ref 22), but only a few combine all the desired properties for advanced fiber composites.

Table 3 Properties of BMI/DABA copolymers

	BMI/DABA molar ratio			
Property	**1.2/1**	**1.5/1**	**2/1**	**3/1**
Flexural strength, MPa (ksi)	186 (27.0)	188 (27.3)	174 (25.2)	131 (19.0)
Flexural modulus, GPa (10^6 psi)	4.02 (0.58)	3.94 (0.57)	4.05 (0.59)	4.14 (0.60)
Deflection at breaking, %	7.78	7.30	5.53	3.50
Fracture toughness				
Plane-strain (K_{Ic}), MPa $\sqrt{m}$ (ksi $\sqrt{in.}$)	0.97 (0.88)	0.86 (0.78)	0.80 (0.73)	0.64 (0.58)
Interlaminar (G_{Ic}), J/m^2 (in. · lbf/in.^{2})	197 (1.10)	158 (0.88)	133 (0.74)	83 (0.46)
Glass transition temperatures (T_g), °C (°F)	279 (534)	282 (540)	288 (550)	288 (550)

BMI resin is compimide 353A; curing conditions: 175 °C (350 °F)/3 h + 230 °C (445 °F)/4 h

Fig. 8 Copolymerization chemistry of BMI-propenylphenyl resins

BMI Composites

Jack Boyd, Cytec Fiberite Inc.

Most advanced composite parts in the aerospace industry use epoxy resins. Epoxies have earned wide acceptance because of their excellent mechanical properties, extended service temperature range, and ease of part manufacture. However, many applications require service temperatures higher than the capability of epoxies. Some BMI composites are being selected for those applications, because they are capable of higher temperature use than epoxies, yet possess epoxy-like processing. Through this avenue, BMI composites are gaining important applications and acceptance.

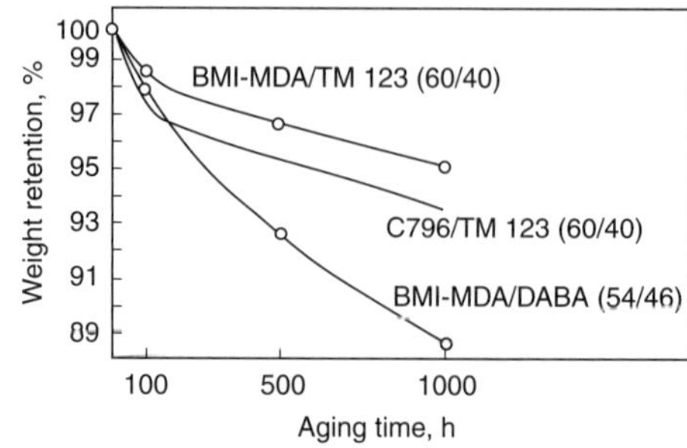

Fig. 9 Thermo-oxidative stability of BMI-comonomer systems (DABA versus Compimide TM123). Aging temperature, 275 °C (525 °F)

The first BMI composites, developed in the early 1980s, possessed excellent mechanical properties in the 150 to 230 °C (300 to 450 °F) temperature range, but exhibited low damage tolerance. Research to improve BMI damage tolerance resulted in the development of a resin (Cycom 5250-4, Cytec Fiberite Inc.) with improved damage tolerance and excellent mechanical properties. The 5250-4 is being used as a matrix resin for composites that serve as the primary construction material for the F-22 Raptor, which is the first large-scale production use of BMI composites.

Mechanical Properties

Compression Strength. Fiber-dominated properties such as tensile strength are similar for most composites. Properties such as damage tolerance and compression at elevated temperatures differentiate matrix resins. The industry has not as yet established a standard measurement of composite service temperature. However, service temperature is often defined as the temperature when the open-hole compression (OHC) strength of moisture-saturated, quasi-isotropic specimens is equal to 205 MPa (30 ksi). The 5250-4 composite OHC strength is 240 MPa (35 ksi) at 177 °C (350 °F)/wet, indicating a service temperature capability of at least 177 °C (350 °F) (Table 4).

The aerospace industry is using a number of medium-toughness epoxies (MTEs) as the baseline for new applications. For example, the MTE, Cycom 977-3/IM-7, was selected for the F-18E/F program. The MTEs possess a good balance of high mechanical properties, good damage tolerance, and the highest OHC strengths for epoxy based composites. The OHC strength of 5250-4 composites equals or exceeds the values of Cycom 977-3.

Damage Tolerance. The aerospace industry has determined through experience that high compression properties are more important than damage tolerance in many applications. However, most designs still have damage tolerance requirements. For designs that do not require the highest level of damage tolerance, the medium-toughness epoxies are being selected. The compression after impact (CAI) strength of a leading MTE, 977-3/G40-800, is 180 to 200 MPa (26 to 29 ksi) after impact of 6.7 J/mm (1500 in. · lbf/in.). The 5250-4 matrix provides a similar level of damage tolerance, 185 to 200 MPa (27 to 29 ksi) (Table 4, Fig. 10). Some designs require the highest level of damage tolerance. Table 4 and Fig. 10 also compare a high-toughness epoxy (HTE), Cycom 5276-1/G40-800, with 5250-4 and 977-3 composites. While the 5276-1 composite has the highest CAI strength (at >305 MPa, or 44 ksi), it also has the lowest OHC strength (248 MPa, or 36 ksi) at 80 °C (180 °F)/wet.

Bismaleimide composites are not limited to the medium toughness level. They can be formulated to provide the highest levels of toughness. Cycom 5280 provides CAI values >305 MPa (44 ksi) while maintaining the same high service temperature of the 5250-4 system (Fig. 10). This CAI value equals that of the high-toughness, 5276-1 epoxy composite. As a historical comparison, a first-generation epoxy is also shown in Fig. 10 with the CAI and OHC lower than the MTE or BMI. The improvements exhibited by the BMIs and epoxies are the result of the research conducted over the last 15 years to provide composites to the aerospace industry with superior capability.

Composite Applications

Recent applications show that BMI composites offer:

- Mechanical properties higher than those of epoxies at elevated temperature resulting in either lower weight or increased safety margins
- Epoxy-like processing using standard autoclave cure processes
- Installed cost similar to epoxy parts

F-22 Raptor Fighter Jet. The F-22 will be the frontline fighter for the U.S. Air Force in the twenty-first century. This program was the most sought-after composite application in the 1980s, and the high strength and high service temperature of the 5250-4 BMI system led designers to use it on half of the composite parts. The F-22 airframe is 24% composite, 39% Ti, 16% Al, 6% steel, and 15% other materials. Cycom 5250-4/IM-7, BMI, accounts for about 50% of the composite weight with the balance epoxy. The epoxy prepreg is the medium-toughness Cycom 977-3/IM-7. Product forms are unidirectional tape and fabric and fiberglass fabric. The BMI adhesive is FM 2550, which is used to fabricate complex sandwich structures.

The BMI wings, which give the F-22 a modified delta shape, are particularly noteworthy. The wings are designed for extended supersonic

Table 4 Typical mechanical properties of 5250-4 and leading epoxies

Property	5250-4/IM-7 BMI(a)	977-3/G40-800 MTE(b)	5276-1/G40-800 HTE(c)
Tensile properties at RT			
Strength, MPa (ksi)	2827 (410)	2758 (400)	2827 (410)
Modulus, GPa (10^6 psi)	161 (23.4)	163 (23.7)	164 (23.8)
0° compression strength, MPa (ksi)			
Room temperature (RT)	1689 (245)	1689 (245)	1586 (230)
80 °C (180 °F)/wet	1586 (230)	1448 (210)	1310 (190)
Open-hole compression strength, MPa (ksi)			
RT	324 (47)	325 (47)	310 (45)
80 °C (180 °F)/wet	283 (41)	283 (41)	248 (36)
120 °C (250 °F)/wet	262 (38)	262 (38)	193 (28)
175 °C (350 °F)/wet	241 (35)	. . .	. . .
Compression after impact strength (6.7 J/mm, or 1500 in. · lb/in.), MPa (ksi)	185–200 (27–29)	180–200 (26–29)	303–324 (44–47)
Glass transition temperature (T_g)(d), °C (°F)			
Dry	280 (540)	210 (410)	180 (360)
Wet	210 (410)	165 (325)	145 (290)

BMI, bismaleimide; MTE, medium-toughness epoxy; HTE, high-toughness epoxy. IM-7 and G40-800 carbon fibers provide nearly identical mechanical properties (tensile strength, 5516 MPa, or 800 ksi; modulus of elasticity, 290 GPa, or 42 × 10^6 psi). Fiber areal weight, 145 g/m^2; resin content, 34%. (a) Cure cycle for 5250-4: 175 °C (350 °F)/6 h cure plus 225 °C (440 °F)/6 h postcure. (b) Cure cycle for 977-3: 180 °C (355 °F)/6 h. (c) Cure cycle for 5276: 175 °C (350 °F)/2 h. (d) Dynamic mechanical analysis (DMA) storage modulus using tangent intercept method

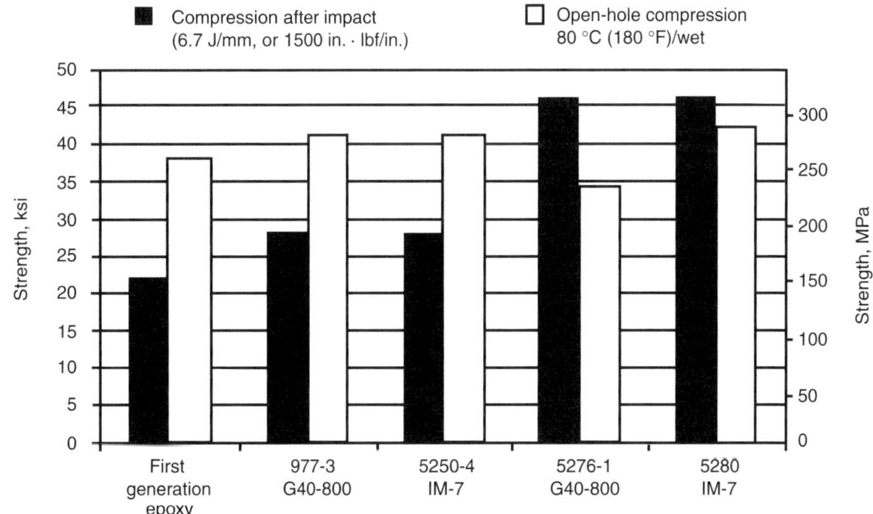

Fig. 10 Mechanical property comparison of BMI and epoxy composites

cruising at Mach 1.5 and for withstanding extremely "high G" maneuvers. The wings are large, flat structures and are, therefore, where composites can be most efficiently exploited to save weight. The wing materials are 35% composite, 42% Ti, and 23% Al and other materials. Each triangular-shaped wing measures 4.9 m (16 ft) (side of body) by 5.5 m (18 ft) (leading edge) and weighs about 900 kg (2000 lb). Each wing contains about 320 kg (700 lb) of composites, the majority of which is 5250-4/IM-7 BMI composite. The understructure is composed of titanium and composite spars. Each wing contains approximately 7000 holes to attach the composite skins to the titanium and composite understructure. This is the reason why high open-hole compression strength is vital.

C-17 Aft Flap Hinge Fairing Structure. The C-17 is the U.S. Air Force heavy-lift aircraft. The 5250-4 composites are used to build the aft flap hinge fairing structure that is attached to the trailing edges, four per wing, of the C-17 wings. Each measures about 1.5 m (5 ft) long, 0.6 m (2 ft) high, and 0.3 m (1 ft) wide. They are constructed by Aerostructures Hamble at its Southampton, United Kingdom facility. Figure 11 shows the four fairings installed on the wings.

The original fairing design was epoxy composite. A detailed analysis, however, indicated that the fairing would experience engine exhaust during routine operation, calling for an actual service requirement of 200 °C (390 °F). Therefore, the part design was switched to BMI because that is the only matrix resin with the required use temperature and with epoxy-like processing. A schematic of the fairing is shown in Fig. 12. All of the structure is built with BMI except for the forward bulkheads and lower access cover, which are built with epoxy composite. A 5250-4/T650-35 fabric is used for the BMI structures. All of the panels are monolithic, about 9 plies (365 g/m^2 fiber areal weight), with the exception of the side covers and lower tray, which are constructed with 2 to 3 plies of BMI fabric over glass phenolic honeycomb core. The skin is bonded to the core using FM 2550 BMI adhesive.

The hinge-fairing program shows that BMI composites have reached the maturity of epoxy composites in terms of availability, producibility, and ease of design, thus providing the capability of rapid scale-up. The C-17 was the first application to use BMI to accommodate engine exhaust impingement. Exhaust can heat a part beyond the capability of epoxies. In such situations, BMI composite is an alternate candidate to metal.

Thrust Reverser Structures (Ref 23). Engine components are an application where the elevated temperature capability of BMI composites can be fully exploited. The 5250-4 composites and 2550 adhesive are used in two major thrust reverser applications. One of these is the inner fixed cowl structure for the Pratt & Whitney 4168 engine built by Middle River Aircraft Systems for use on the Airbus Model A330. The inner cowl of the thrust reverser is stationary and surrounds the hot engine core. It provides the primary attachments of the thrust reverser to the engine, access to engine components, and inlets for airflow for various engine or aircraft systems. Figure 13 shows a schematic of the 5250-4/T650-35, one-piece inner core cowl. The structure is approximately 2.7 m (9 ft) long and 3.0 m (10 ft) in cross section. The composite part integrates many of the individual components of a metal part. It saves about 16 kg (35 lb) weight compared to a metal structure.

The inner core cowl consists of a precured outer skin, local precured reinforcing doublers, aluminum honeycomb core, and a precured inner skin. Because the forward section of the inner cowl is part of the sound-suppression system for the engine, this portion has perforated BMI outer skin with the aft portion having a solid BMI outer skin. Now in service, this structure provides excellent performance with no unanticipated in-service problems.

Helicopter Tail Boom (Ref 24). Bell Helicopter Textron (BHT) has developed a BMI composite tail boom for its Model 412/212 helicopters to replace the existing metal tail boom. The tail boom will be exposed to hot engine exhaust during routine use, as well as a corrosive and fatigue environment. 5250-4 composite and 2550 adhesive were selected for this application based on their high-temperature performance, outstanding mechanical properties, and extensive use history.

The tail boom features and requirements are monocoque boom section, integral vertical fin, support of the tail rotor, drive system, and support of the synchronized elevator. Typically, composite parts cost more to manufacture than metal. Bell Helicopter Textron was able to over-

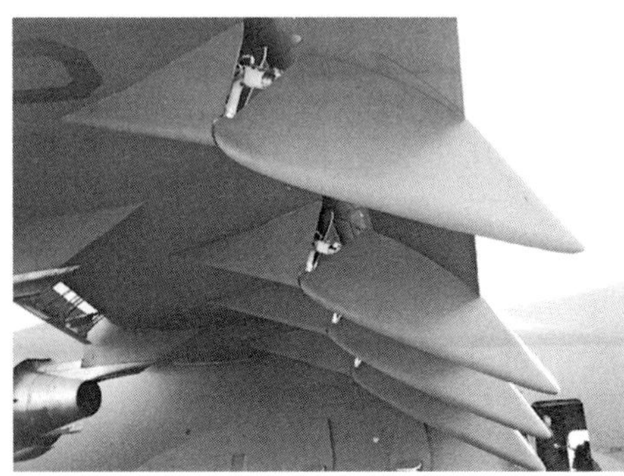

Fig. 11 C-17 aft flap fairings

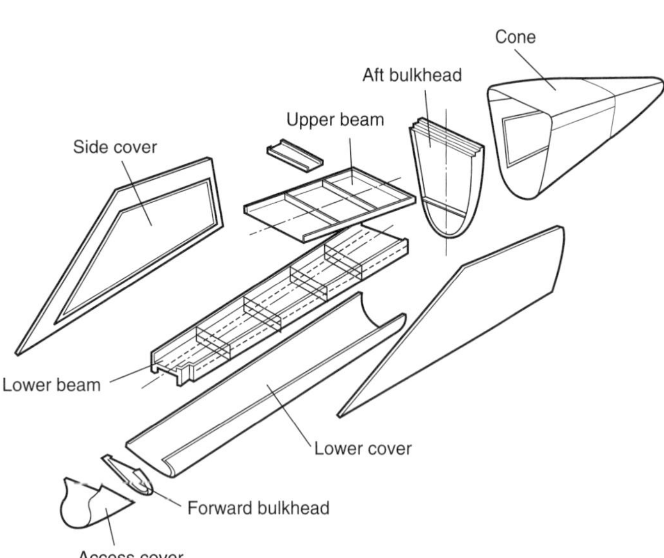

Fig. 12 Schematic of aft flap hinge fairing structure

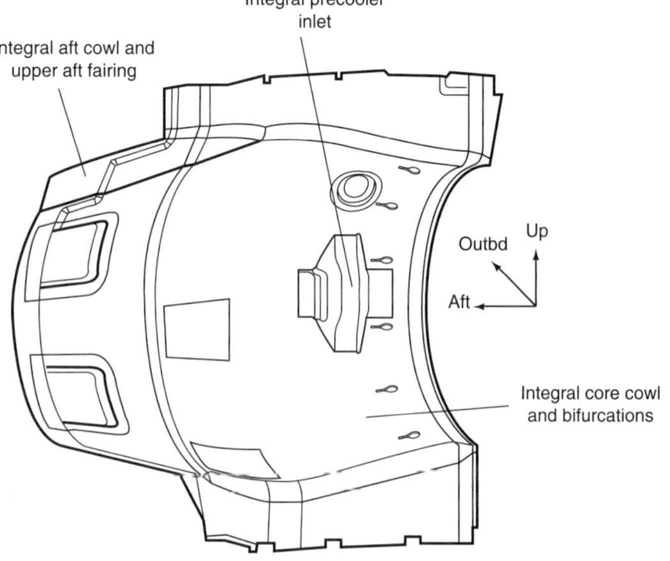

Fig. 13 One-piece inner cowl for Pratt & Whitney 4168 made from BMI composite (Cycom 5250-4)

come this potential difficulty by designing the tail boom for low-cost manufacture. The primary objective in designing for producibility is to achieve low recurring costs, which translates into minimizing the number of parts, reducing the lay-up cycle and assembly process times. The 6.4 m (21 ft) long tail boom is a bonded assembly comprising a four-piece skin construction extending the full length, with internal substructure composing only 17 components and no mechanical fasteners (Fig. 14).

The BMI tail boom will also save money in service compared to the metal tail boom. Its lower weight will reduce fuel costs and increase range, while the inherent composite corrosion and fatigue resistance will minimize maintenance. This application shows that BMI composites, if designed for producibility, can be cost competitive with metal structures.

Formula 1 Race Cars. Formula 1 racing is highly competitive. Designers will use any material that provides improved performance over metal parts. Composites of BMI have found extensive and increasing use on race cars. They are applied to structures in hot areas of engines and transmissions and in and around exhaust systems and areas where exhaust impinges a structure.

Resin Transfer Molding

Resin transfer molding (RTM) is finding increasing use because it can reduce composite manufacturing cost. Final assembly is one of the most costly aspects of composite part manufacture. Composites molded with a vacuum bag, single-mold surface typically have dimensional variation part to part. During assembly, shims and reinforcement parts are used to accommodate that variation. The technology of RTM is capable of making parts with tight dimensional tolerances because all dimensions are defined by the mold. Processing by RTM can be efficient to make complex parts where many different shapes and contours are brought together, requiring tight tolerances.

The 5250-4 prepreg resin provides composites with excellent properties and the capability of operating in high-temperature environments. A derivative, Cycom 5250-4RTM (Ref 25), makes an outstanding RTM resin. This resin has been selected for a wide variety of RTM applications. The largest use is on the F-22, which is one of the first production aircraft taking advantage of RTM. A further advantage of 5250-4RTM is that the 5250-4 composite database is transferable. 5250-4RTM is one component and homogenous. The resin is used by heating and injecting into the mold. The RTM process requires low viscosity for several hours. 5250-4RTM has less than 10 P viscosity for over 4 h (Fig. 15), which meets the requirements of any process.

The RTM process is used to manufacture over 400 F-22 parts. One challenging application is the sine wave spars. Initially, standard prepreg was used, but fiber distortion was encountered due to the complexity of the spar shape. The RTM process solved this and other fabrication problems, while reducing manufacturing cost by 20%. The tight dimensional tolerances provided by the RTM process decreased by half the number of reinforcement parts needed for installing the spars in the wings. The F-22 5250-4RTM applications demonstrate the capability of manufacturing complex parts.

Table 5 Properties of BMI 5250-4 composites with and without postcure

Cure cycle	Open-hole compression 80 °C (180 °F)/wet MPa	ksi	Open-hole compression 120 °C (250 °F)/wet MPa	ksi	Compression after impact (6.7 J/mm, or 1500 in. · lbf/in.) MPa	ksi	Glass-transition temperature (T_g) °C	°F
Standard cycle: 175 °C (350 °F)/6 h plus 225 °C (440 °F)/6 h	283	41	262	38	186–200	27–29	282	540
205 °C (400 °F)/2 h	290	42	. . .	. . .	193	28	251	484
190 °C (375 °F)/6 h	290	42	262	38	193	28	247	477

5250-4 reinforced with IM-7 was used in all tests. Postcure not required for service below 150 °C (300 °F)

Cure and Post Cure Requirements

One factor that limits wider BMI use is that BMIs require higher cure temperatures than used for epoxies. Tests in this section show that for applications not requiring the highest T_g, the cure temperature can be reduced to 190 °C (375 °F) with no trade-off in mechanical properties (Ref 26). Most civil aerospace applications use 80 °C (180 °F)/wet as the design condition. The 80 °C (180 °F)/wet open-hole compression (OHC) strength is the same whether 5250-4 is cured at 190 °C (375 °F)/6 h or 205 °C (400 °F)/2 h with no postcure or cure using the standard cure followed by postcure (Table 5). The 120 °C (250 °F)/wet OHC is also the same, regardless of cure condition, as was the damage tolerance. The only difference is T_g. The T_g is lower at the lower temperature cures. However, this level of T_g is adequate for uses below about 150 °C (300 °F).

Elevated-Temperature Applications

The 5250-4 matrix can be used at 230 °C (450 °F), but the service life is about 2500 h due to oxidative weight loss. PMR-15, an industry standard condensation polyimide, has higher temperature capability and is usually selected for ap-

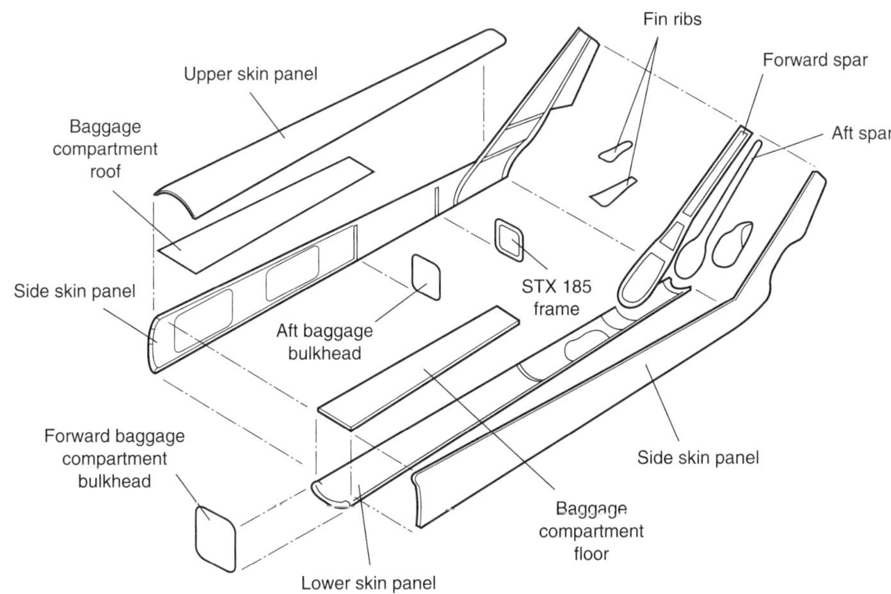

Fig. 14 Bell Helicopter Model 412 tail boom made from BMI composite (Cycom 5250-4)

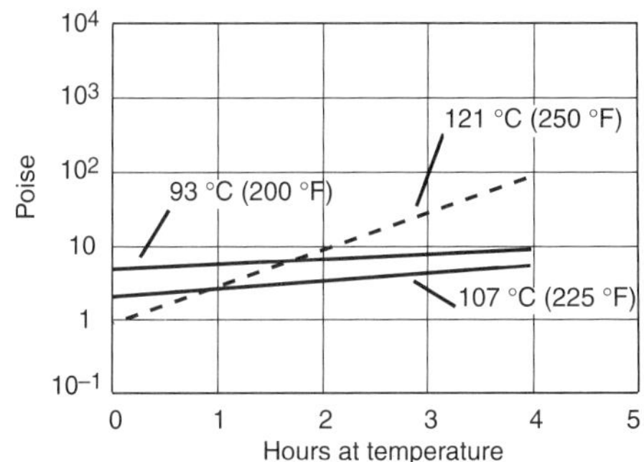

Fig. 15 Viscosity and pot life of BMI resin 5250-4RTM

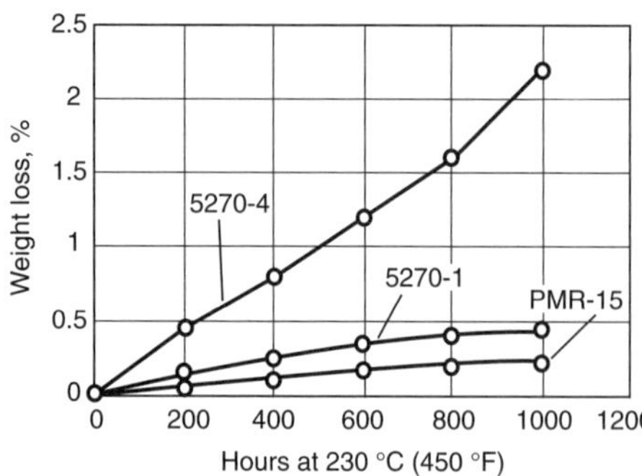

Fig. 16 High-temperature performance of BMI composites versus PMR-15 composites. Reinforcing fiber, T650-35

plications at 230 °C (450 °F) and above. However, PMR-15 has processing disadvantages. It cures by a condensation reaction, and volatiles are formed. The bagging, tooling, and cure cycle must be designed to allow volatile removal in order to consolidate parts. PMR-15 can be RTM processed, but the technique has limitations due to the volatiles formed. Therefore, there existed a need for a BMI that approached the performance of PRM-15 without the processing disadvantages. The 5270-1 matrix was developed to have the highest temperature capability of a BMI resin (Ref 27). There are no volatiles released during cure so 5270-1 processes like an epoxy and can be RTM processed using standard techniques.

High Temperature Aging Comparison. Composites held at elevated temperature are slowly oxidized and lose weight. One of the most critical tests for elevated temperature applications is how well the composite resists weight loss at the service temperature. The industry typically uses side-by-side, isothermal aging for accelerated weight loss testing. Figure 16 shows comparisons of 5270-1, PMR-15, and 5250-4 at 230 °C (450 °F). The composite of 5270-1 loses much less weight than 5250-4 composite. It loses only twice as much weight as PMR-15. Similar results are obtained in 260 °C(500 °F) aging where 5270-1 composite loses only twice as much weight as PMR-15.

Since volatiles are not formed during cure, 5270-1 resin can also be processed by standard RTM methods for resins without volatile components. The 5270-1 system can be considered a potential replacement for PMR-15 in current applications, and the first choice candidate when an application requires high service temperature.

Conclusions

New matrix resin classes are accepted by the aerospace composite industry only when they offer significant advantages over epoxy-based systems. The BMI composites offer the advantages of higher temperature capability with epoxy-like processing. Bismaleimide has successfully made the transition from experimental composites in the early 1980s to application on some of the most important aircraft programs. The wide variety of applications shows that BMI composites can be manufactured into an extensive array of parts. The BMI composites now include systems with high damage tolerance, RTM capability, and thermal stability approaching that of PMR-15. Bismaleimide resins offer the widest service range of any matrix resin class and excellent mechanical properties.

REFERENCES

1. F. Grundschober and J. Sambeth, U.S. Patent 3,380,964, 1968
2. M. Bargain, A. Combat, and P. Grosjean, British Patent Specification 1,190,718, 1968
3. H. Stenzenberger, U.S. Patent 3,966,864, 1974
4. S. Street, 25th National SAMPE Symposium, 1980, p 366
5. L. McKague, 28th National SAMPE Symposium, 1983, p 640
6. B.L. Riley, 2nd International Conf. on Fibre Reinforced Composites, Proc., University of Liverpool, U.K., 1986, p 153
7. S. Zahir and A. Renner, Swiss Patent Application 7988, 1975
8. H.N. Cole and W.F. Gruber, U.S. Patent 3,127,414, 1964
9. A. Nagai, A. Takahashi, M. Suzuki, and A. Mukoh, *Appl. Polym. Sci.*, Vol 44, 1992, p 159
10. H. Stenzenberger, *J. Appl. Polym. Sci.*, Vol 22, 1973, p 77
11. S. Street, U.S. Patent 4,351,932, 1982; U.S. Patent 4,454,283, 1984
12. H. Stenzenberger, U.S. Patent 4,211,861, 1980
13. A. Pigneri, E.C. Galgoci, R.J. Jackson, and G.E. Young, 1st International SAMPE Electronics Conf., 1987, p 657
14. M.J. Davis and T.R. Sense, IPC Fall Meeting, Chicago, 1987
15. J. King, M. Chaudhari, and S. Zahir, 29th National SAMPE Symposium, 1984, p 392
16. H. Stenzenberger and P. König, *High Perf. Polym.*, Vol 1 (No. 3), 1989, p 239
17. H. Stenzenberger and P. König, *High Perf. Polym.*, Vol 1 (No. 2), 1989, p 133
18. H. Stenzenberger et al., 32nd International SAMPE Symposium, 1987, p 44
19. J.M. Barton, I. Hamerton, R.J. Jones, and J.C. Stedman, *Polym. Bul.*, Vol 27, 1991, p 163
20. H. Stenzenberger and P. König, *High Perf. Polym.*, Vol 3, 1991, p 41
21. H. Stenzenberger and P. König, *High Perf. Polym.*, Vol 5, 1993, p 123
22. H. Stenzenberger, Addition Polyimides in 117 Advances in Polymer Science, *High Perf. Polym.*, P.M. Hergenrother, Ed., 1994
23. 9th DOD/NASA/FAA Conf. on Fibrous Composites and Structural Design, November, 1991
24. With permission from Bell Helicopter Textron Inc.
25. A. Taylor, *SAMPE J.*, Vol 36, 2000, p 17–24
26. D. Lavery and J. Boyd, *Proc. of the 40th International SAMPE Symposium and Exhibition*, 1995, p 632
27. J. Boyd and A. Kuo, *Proc. of the 39th International SAMPE Symposium and Exhibition*, 1994, p 588

Polyimide Resins

Daniel A. Scola, University of Connecticut

POLYIMIDE MATERIALS can be categorized by their temperature capabilities into those with an upper limit of 230 °C (450 °F) for extended time periods, and those capable of extended use up to 315 °C (600 °F). Bismaleimides, phenylethynyl-containing polyimides, and some condensation polyimides such as Avimid-K3 belong in the former category, while those materials such as PMR-15, LARC-TPI, Avimid-N and BPDA/TFMB belong in the latter. In terms of chemistry, there are two general types of commercial polyimides: thermoplastic polyimides, derived from a condensation reaction between anhydrides or anhydride derivatives and diamines, and cross-linked polyimides, derived from an addition reaction between unsaturated groups of a preformed imide monomer or oligomer. The imide monomers or oligomers are also derived from the typical condensation reaction to form the imide group, but polymer formation stems from the addition reaction. For completeness, the chemistry of both types and process conditions to fabricate articles are described in this article. Bismaleimides are not reviewed in this article. (See the article "Bismaleimide Resins" in this Volume.)

Properties and Applications

The specific advantages and disadvantages of two types of polyimides are summarized in Table 1. These are generalized conclusions regarding each type, because there are exceptions, which depend on chemical structure.

The condensation polyimides, which are linear long-chain thermoplastic polymers, have high melt viscosity, thereby requiring high pressures and temperatures for neat resin molding or composite processing. However, the highly aromatic nature of these systems coupled with flexible groups, such as ether, hexofluorosopropylidene, or methylene within the backbone structure, yields materials with good toughness, excellent thermal and thermooxidative stability, and moderate to high glass transition temperatures (T_g).

The addition-type polyimides, derived from preformed oligomers, undergo thermal cross linking or chain extension to form a thermoset. The oligomer molecular weight controls the processability, the degree of cross linking or chain extension, and the T_g. However, because no volatiles are released during processing, and the oligomers have a melt or softening region where the viscosity is relatively low near the temperature region where the addition reaction occurs, moderate to low pressure is required during processing to consolidate the part being fabricated.

Polyimides are finding wide applications because of their unusual properties. The polyimides derived from aromatic dianhydrides and aromatic diamines containing stable flexible units in the backbone exhibit:

- High thermal and thermo-oxidative stability up to 400 °C (750 °F)
- Excellent mechanical properties, both at room temperature and elevated temperatures
- Film- and fiber-forming ability
- Excellent adhesive properties, both at room temperature and elevated temperature
- Nonflammability—will not support combustion

Fluorine-containing polyimides exhibit the properties listed previously, as well as low dielectric constant. Polyimides containing func-

Table 1 General attributes of condensation (thermoplastic) and addition-type (cross-linked) polyimides

Polyimide type	Advantages	Disadvantages
Condensation (thermoplastic)	Thermoplastic (reprocessability)	Poor processability
	Moderate to high glass transition temperatures (T_g)	Volatiles released in processing
	Toughness	High pressure required in processing
	Excellent thermal and thermo-oxidative stability	
Addition-type (cross-linked)	Processability	Limited reprocessability
	Cross linked	Brittle
	High T_g	Poor thermal and thermo-oxidative stability
	No volatiles in processing	
	Low pressure required in processing	

Table 2 Applications of polyimides by industry

Industry	Applications
Electronics	Flexible circuits
	Flexible connectors
	Chip carriers
	Tape automated bonding
	High-density interconnect applications
	Photosensitive polyimides
Aircraft	Wire insulation
	Motor windings
	Electrical switches
	Structural adhesives
	Structural composites
	Foam insulation
	Bushings
	Baffles
	Flanged bearings
	Thrust washers
	Thrust discs
	Seal rings
Automobile	Electrical switches
Medical	Pacemakers
	Eye lens implants
Machining	Abrasive cutting wheels
Gas purification	Membranes
Aerospace	Rockets
	Spacecraft (composite, adhesives, coatings)
Military applications	Composites, adhesives, coatings
Manufacturing	Discs in compressor valve systems

Table 3 Applications of high-temperature polyimide composites in aircraft engines

Sector	Applications
Military engines	Stator vanes
	Shrouds (fan section)
	External nozzle flaps
	Bushings
	Bearings
	Intermediate cases
	Augmenter ducts
	Fan ducts
	Nose cones
Commercial engines	Core cowls (nacelles)
	Union rings (variable vane actuation system)
	Stator vanes (low-pressure compressor)
	Externals gear box housing and support structures
	Washers
	Bushings
	Bearings

tional or pendant groups in the backbone of the aromatic dianhydride or/and diamine exhibit some of the properties listed previously, as well as selective gas permeability.

Since the mid-1980s, the application areas for high-temperature polyimides have continually grown. This is because of the ability to vary the polymer structure, thereby tailoring the properties for specific applications. Polyimide products are used in a variety of applications, such as coatings, adhesives, composite matrices, fibers, films, foams, moldings, membrane, liquid crystalline displays, and insulation. A list of general application areas by industry is given in Table 2. Specific applications of high-temperature polyimides for aircraft are listed in Table 3. Clearly,

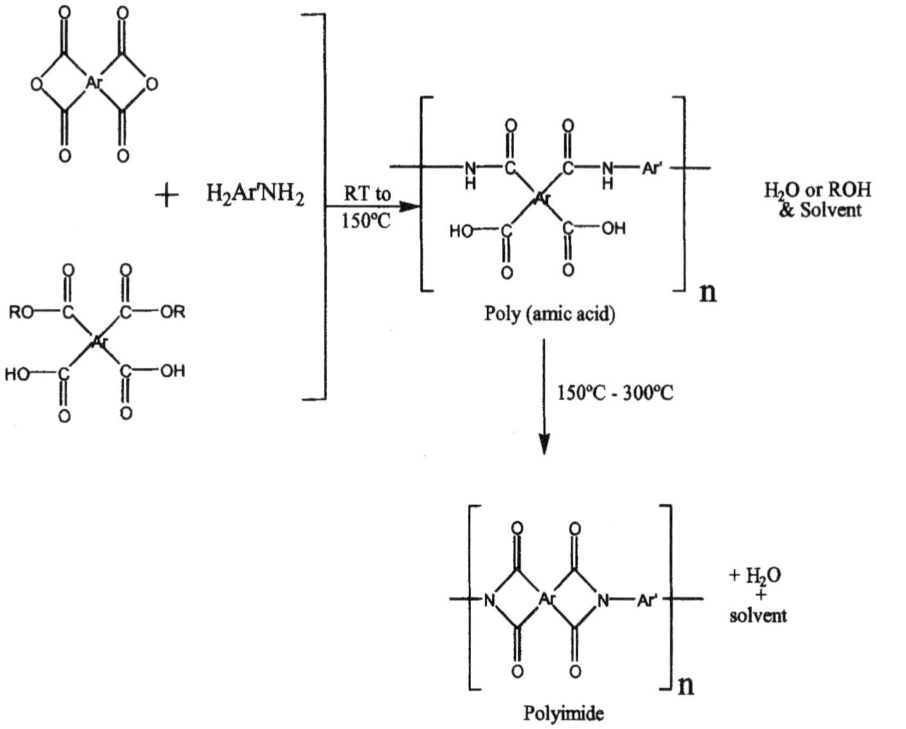

Fig. 1 General reaction for condensation polyimides. Solvents can be NMP, DMF, or m-cresol diglyme.

Table 4 Commercial polyimide materials

Developer/source	Material	Supplier
DuPont	Kapton film	DuPont
	Vespel parts	DuPont
DuPont Tribon	Vespel composites	DuPont Tribon Composites
DuPont Electronics/Hitachi Chemical	Pyralin series (solution)	HD Microsystems
DuPont/Cytec Fiberite	Avimid-N (prepreg, powder)	Cytec Fiberite
	Avimid-K3 (prepreg, powder)	Cytec Fiberite
	Avimid-K3B (prepreg, powder)	Cytec Fiberite
	Avimid-R (prepreg, powder)	Cytec Fiberite
	Avimid-RB (prepreg, powder)	Cytec Fiberite
	Avimid-K3A (prepreg, powder)	Cytec Fiberite
BF Goodrich Aerospace	Superimide 800 (solution)	Goodrich Aerospace
Monsanto/IST (Japan)	Skybond 700 series	IST
Monsanto/IST (Japan)/Cytec Fiberite	Skybond 700 series (prepreg)	Cytec Fiberite, Hexcel, YLA, Inc.
Mitsui Chemical	Aurum (all forms)	Mitsui Chemical
BP Amoco	Ultradel (solution)	BP Amoco
	Torlon (pellets)	BP Amoco
General Electric	Ultem (pellets)	General Electric
TRW/U.S. Air Force	AFR 700B (solution, powder)	Imitec, Inc., Eikos, Inc., Daychem Labs, Inc., SP Systems, Hy Comp, Inc.
TRW/U.S. Air Force/Cytec Fiberite	AFR 700B (prepreg)	Cytec Fiberite, SP Systems
National Aeronautics and Space Administration (NASA) Glenn Research Center	PMR-15 (solution, powder)	Imitec, Inc., Eikos, Inc., Daychem Labs, Inc., Hy Comp, Inc.
	PMR-15 (prepreg)	Cytec Fiberite, YLA, Inc.
	PMR-II-50 (solution, powder)	Imitec, Inc., Eikos, Inc., Daychem Labs, Inc., Hy Comp, Inc.
	PMR-II-50 (prepreg)	Cytec Fiberite, YLA, Inc.
	Modified PMR-15 (solution, powder)	Imitec, Inc., Eikos, Inc., Daychem Labs, Inc., Hy Comp, Inc.
NASA Langley Research Center/ Cytec Fiberite	PETI-5 (solution, powder)	Imitec, Inc.
	PETI-5 (prepreg)	Cytec Fiberite
	LARC RP-46 (prepreg)	Cytec Fiberite, YLA, Inc.
NASA Langley Research Center	LARC RP-46 (solution, powder)	Imitec, Inc., Eikos, Inc., Daychem Labs, Inc., Hy Comp, Inc.
	LARC-SI (solution, powder)	Imitec, Inc., Eikos, Inc.
Imitec, Inc.	Imitec 772 (solution, powder)	Imitec, Inc.
	Imitec 927 (solution, powder)	Imitec, Inc.

Table 5 Developmental high-temperature polyimide resins

Designation	Monomer components	Ref
BPDA/TFMB	BPDA/TFMB	1, 2, 3, 4
3F-PI	3FDA/$ArNH_2$	5–8
36F-PI	6FDA/3FDA/$ArNH_2$	5–8
8F-PI	8FDA/$ArNH_2$	9
Ar-3FD	ArDA/3FDAM	10–12
PTPEI	PEPA/BPDA/3,4′-ODA/ APB/DPEB	13, 14
PPEI	PA/BPDA/3,4′-ODA/ APB/DPEB	13, 14
PE Ultem 3000	BPADA/*m*-PDA/PEPA	15
2,2′,3,3′-BPDA/ $ArNH_2$	BPDA/$ArNH_2$	16
BTDA/TPER	BTDA/TPER	17
BPDA/TPER	BPDA/TPER	18
ARDA/DABTF	ArDA/3.5-DABTF	19
PMMDA/$ArNH_2$	PDMDA/$ArNH_2$	20
PMR-15 replacement	BTDA/3,3′DDS/NE	21
	BTDA/BAPP/NE	22
	BTDA/BAX/NE	23, 24
	BTDA/DMBZ/NE	25, 26
	BTDA/BABN/NE	23, 27
	BTDA/BPAP/NE	23, 27
	BTDA/BISP/NE	28
	BTDA/1,2,4- OBABTF/NE	29
	BTDA/3,5-DABTF/NE	29
	BTDA/MC's/NE	29
	BTDA/TAB/NE	30, 31
	BTDA/APB/NE	31
	BNDA/$ArNH_2$/NE	27, 30, 32
	PBDA/$ArNH_2$/NE	27, 30, 32
	ArDA/TMBZ/NE	23, 31, 33
	3FDA/$ArNH_2$/NE	34, 35

PTPEI, pendant, terminal phenylethynyl imide oligomer; PPEI, pendant phenylethynyl imide oligomer; 3FDA, 4,4′-(2,2,2-trifluoro-1-phenylethylidene) diphthalic anhydride or dimethyl ester; PEPA, 4- phenylethynylphthalic anhydride; BPDA, 3,3′,4,4′-biphenyl-tetracarboxylic dianhydride or dimethyl ester; 3,4′-ODA, 3,4′-oxydianiline; DPEB, 3,5-diamino-4′-phenylethynyl benzophenone; p-PDA, para-phenylenediamine; 6FDA, 4,4′-(1,1,1,3,3,3-hexafloroisopropylidene) diphthalic anhydride or dimethyl ester; 8FDA, 4,4′-(2,2,2-trifluoro-1-pentafluorophenylethylidene) dipthalic anhydride; BTDA, 3,3′-4,4′-benzophenone tetracarboxylic acid dianhydride or dimethyl ester; TFMB, 2,2′-trifluoromethyl biphenylene diamine or 2,2′-bis(trifluoromethyl)benzidene; BisP, 1,3-bis (4′-aminophenylisopropylidene) benzene; BAX, 1,4-bis (4′-amino benzyl) benzene; DMBZ, 2,2′-dimethylbenzidine; BNDA, 4,4-bis (1,1-binapthyl-2-oxy, 1,1′-binepthyl-2,2′-oxy) dipthalic anhydride or dimethyl ester; BAPP, 2,2-bis (4-aminophenoxyphenyl) propane; ArDA, aromatic dianhydrides; 3FDAM, 4,4′-(2,2,2,-trifluoro-1-phenylethylidene) diphenyl diamine; NE, dimethyl ester of 5-norbornene 1,2-dicarboxylic acid; PBDA, 4,4′-(1,1′-biphenyl-2-oxy) diphthalic anhydride or dimethyl ester; APB, 1,3-(4,4′-aminophenoxy) benzene; $ArNH_z$, aromatic diamines; TAB, 1,3,5-tris (4-aminophenoxy) benzene; BPADA, 2,2′-bis(phenoxy isopropylidene) 4,4′-diphthalic anydride or Bisphenol A-4,4′-diphthalic anhydride; TPER, 1,3-bis (4-aminophenoxy) benzene; MC's, 1,3 and 1,4 bis (aminobenzyl and aminobenzoyl) benzenes; 1,2,4-OBABTF, 4,4′-oxybis (3-trifluoromethyl) benzamine; 3,5,-DABTF, 3,5-diaminobenzotrifluoride; PDMDA, 3,3′-bis (3,4-dicarboxyphenoxy) diphenylmethane dianhydride; TMBZ, 2,2′,6,6′-tetramethylbenzidine; 2,2′,-BPDA, 2,2′,3,3′,-biphenyltetracarboxylic dianhydride or dimethylester; PE, phenylethynyl end-capped; PPQ, polyphenylquinoxaline (solution sample from H. Hergemrother, NASA Langley Research Center); IP-600, ethynyl end-capped imide oligomer (no longer commercially available); L-20, BTDA/4-BDAF 4,4′-(p-aminophenoxyphenyl-hexafluoroisopropylidene); L-30, BTDA/4-BDAF 4,4′-(p-aminophenoxyphenyl-hexafluoroisopropylidene); Sixef-44, 6FDA/6FDAM, 2,2-(4-aminophenyl)-hexafluoroisopropylidene); PBI, polybenzimidazole

Table 6 Thermal properties of polyimides

Material	Glass transition temperature (T_g)		Cure temperature		Postcure temperature		Postcure time, h	T_g after postcure		Approximate upper-use temperature	
	°C	°F	°C	°F	°C	°F		°C	°F	°C	°F
Thermoplastic polyimides											
Avimid-N (Ref 36–39)	371	700	350	660	416	780	8	407	760	316	600
Avimid-K (Ref 40–42)	250	480	316	600	...	...	...	...	...	225	437
Avimid-K3A (Ref 40–42)	222	430	316	600	...	...	...	...	...	225	437
Avimid-K3B (Ref 40–42)	235	460	316	600	...	...	...	...	...	225	437
LARC-TPI (Ref 43)	265	510	340	640	...	...	...	...	...	300	572
3F-PI (Ref 5–8)	371	700	370	700	416	780	8	410	770	316	600
36F-PI (Ref 5–8)	371	700	365	690	416	780	8	405	760	316	600
LARC-SI (Ref 44)	251	480	300	570	...	...	...	...	...	230	446
Ultem 1000 (Ref 45)	210	410	200	390	...	...	...	...	...	267	510
Skybond 700 Series (Ref 46)	330	630	330	630	...	...	...	...	...	316	600
Aurum New TPI (Ref 47)	250	480	300	570	...	...	...	...	...	260	550
BPDA/TFMB (Ref 1–4)											
From solution cure	290	550	200	390	...	...	...	...	...	316	600
Solid state cure	340	640	350	660	...	...	...	...	...	316	600
Kapton H (Ref 48)	360	680	400	750	...	...	...	...	...	316	600
Pyralin PI 2525 (Ref 49)	320	610	400	750	...	...	...	...	...	316	600
Pyralin PI 2610 (Ref 49)	400	750	350	660	...	...	...	...	...	316	600
Pyralin PI 2540 (Ref 49)	360	680	350	660	...	...	...	...	...	225	527
BP Amoco Ultradel 4212 (Ref 50)	295	560	350	660	...	...	...	...	...	...	...
Vespel SP-I (Ref 51)	360	680	400	750	...	...	...	...	...	287	549
Torlon 4203 (Ref 52)	267	510	350	660	...	...	...	...	...	225	437
2,2′,3,3′-BPDA-4,4′-ODA (Ref 16)	319	610	280	540	...	...	...	...	...	300	572
BTDA/TPER (Ref 17)	210	410	300	570	...	...	...	...	...	250	482
BPDA/TPER (Ref 18)	230	450	300	570	...	...	...	...	...	250	482
PDMDA/ArNH2(4,4′-MDA) (Ref 20)	210	410	300	570	...	...	...	...	...	250	482
Cross-linked polyimides											
Avimid-R (Ref 53,54)	310	590	360	680	...	...	...	...	...	250	528
Avimid-RB (Ref 55)	348	660	360	680	...	...	...	...	...	250	528
PMR-15 (Ref 56–60)	340	640	316	600	370	700	8	395	740	316	600
LARC RP-46 (Ref 61, 62)	280	540	316	600	370	700	8	395	740	300	572
AFR 700B (Ref 63–65)	370	700	390	730	416	780	8	455	850	316	600
Superimide 800 (Ref 66)	300	570	316	600	316–400	600–750	32	385	730	316	600
PETI-5 (Ref 13, 14)	270	520	370	700	...	...	...	...	...	250	482
PMR-II-30 (Ref 67–69)	350	660	316	600	370	700	24	390	730	316	600
VCAP-II-50 (Ref 70)	311	590	316	600	343	650	126	362	680	275	527
BTDA/DMBz/NE (Ref 25, 26)	433	810	316	600	316	600	8	420	790	275	527
PE Ultem 3000 (Ref 15)	230	450	370	700	...	...	...	...	...	250	482
3FDA/p-PDA/NE (Ref 35)	310	590	371	700	370	700	20	385	730	316	600

the range of applications for the polyimides is a good indication of the ability to modify molecular structure for specific properties. Hundreds of research polyimide materials have been synthesized over the years, but only a few are commercially available at the present time. However, many research polyimides are available from specialty chemical houses. A partial list of available polyimides and their sources is shown in Tables 4 and 5.

The glass transition temperatures and upper temperature capabilities of the two types of polyimides are listed in Table 6. The thermal properties of the polyimides depend on the presence of flexible units, such as ether, isopropylidene, methylene, hexafluoroisopropylidene, and carbonyl in the backbone of the polymer chain, or bulky side groups pendant to the backbone structure. These groups can also affect solubility. Disruption of regularity by the copolymerization of two dianhydrides with two diamines also affects solubility.

An important consideration in the selection of a polyimide for a composite application is resin toughness. An interesting correlation of resin toughness versus estimated cost is shown in Table 7. The polyether imide (PEI) Ultem has the most favorable toughness/cost correlation. As with all polyimides, this property must be balanced between other properties, such as processability, T_g, temperature capability, and mechanical properties.

A summary of the thermo-oxidative stability of several polyimides at 316 °C (600 °F) and 371 °C (700 °F) is given in Tables 8, 9, and 10. The data clearly show that the fluorinated aromatic polyimides possess the highest thermo-oxidative stability.

Table 7 Relationship of resin toughness to cost

Resin type	Interlaminar fracture toughness (G_{Ic}) at 23 °C (73 °F)		Approximate cost		Toughness per unit cost(a)
	J/m^2	ft · lbf/ft^2	\$/kg	\$/lb	
PETI-5	4800	330	230	500	2
Avimid-K3B	1400	100	45	100	31
Avimid-N	2500	170	180	400	14
PMR 15	300	20	30–40	70–90	8–10
AFR 700B(b)	2500?	170?	180	400	14
BMI	330	20	70	150	5
Ultem (PEI)	~5000	~340	3	6	1667

(a) Interlaminar fracture toughness (G_{Ic}) in J/m^2 divided by cost in \$/kg. (b) Toughness value listed with a question mark in source. Source: Ref 71

A comparison of common physical and mechanical properties of polyimides is provided in Table 11.

Chemistry of Condensation-Type Polyimides

These materials, discovered in 1908 by T.M. Bogert and R.R. Renshaw (Ref 75) and made practical by W.M. Edwards and I.M. Robertson

(Ref 76), are derived from polyamic acids by either chemical or thermal treatment over a temperature range from room temperature to 370 °C (700 °F). The polyamic acids are produced by a series of step growth reactions at room temperature from a dianhydride or dianhydride derivative and a diamine. The general reaction for polyimide formation is illustrated in Fig. 1. The structures of several commercially available thermoplastic polyimides are shown in Fig. 2.

Synthesis (General). Thermoplastic polyimides are prepared in dimethylacetamide (DMAC) or N-methyl pyrrolidinone (NMP) by dissolving the appropriate diamine in the solvent at room temperature under nitrogen. The dianhydride is added as a solid or a slurry in the solvent while stirring over a period of one-half hour. The reaction is allowed to continue from 6 to 24 h while stirring under ambient conditions, depending on the relative reactivities of the diamines and dianhydride. The polyamide acid solution thus produced can be sampled for determination of intrinsic viscosity or analyzed by gel permeation chromatography (GPC) for molecular weight or analyzed by other methods as required. The polyamide acid solution can be used to prepare polyamide acid or polyimide powder, thin films, supported adhesive tape, and to impregnate unidirectional carbon fiber, carbon cloth, or other fiber/cloth substrate.

Alternatively, thermoplastic polyimides can also be prepared by dissolving the dialkyl ester (methyl, ethyl, or isopropyl) of the dianhydride in ethanol at room temperature, followed by the addition of the aromatic diamine. This polyimide precursor solution can also be used to prepare powder, thin films, supported adhesive tape, and impregnated carbon fiber, carbon cloth, or other fiber/cloth substrate. The polyamide acid can be converted to the polyimide by thermal methods or by chemical methods, described subsequently.

Processing of Polyamide Acid Precursor Solution to Polyimide. The polyamide acid solution can be converted thermally in solution to the polyimide by: the addition of a sufficient quantity of toluene or o-xylene, followed by azeotropic distillation of water in a Dean-Stark trap overnight; by refluxing the polyamide acid solution containing 1 to 2 wt% isoquinoline catalyst (based on solvent) for 6 h; or by the addition of ten-fold excess of acetic anhydride with pyridine or triethylamine catalyst at a 4 to 1 weight ratio, followed by heating at 100 °C (210 °F) for 3 h.

The polyamic acid solution can also be prepared in m-cresol solvent instead of DMAC or NMP at room temperature and converted to the polyimide by refluxing at 200 °C (390 °F) with or without a catalyst (1 to 2 wt% isoquinoline based on m-cresol) for 4 h. The polyimide powder is isolated as described in the following paragraphs.

NMP or DMAC polyamic acid solution is added while stirring vigorously to a methanol/water (50:50) solution. The precipitated polyamic acid powder is filtered and washed again in methanol and water, then dried at 125 °C for 24 h in a vacuum, or at 200 °C (390 °F) for 4 h in vacuum. The polyamic acid powder is converted to polyimide in an oven at 150 °C (300 °F) for 1 h + 250 °C (480 °F) for 1 h + 275 °C (525 °F) for 1 h.

Alcohol solutions of the diester and diamine composition are concentrated to a solvent-free polyamic acid powder in a vacuum oven at 60 °C (140 °F) for 2 h. The polyamic acid powder is converted thermally to polyimide powder at 150 °C (300 °F) for 1 h + 250 °C (480 °F) for 2 h + 275 °C (525 °F) for 1 h.

Preparation of Polyimide Films from Thermoplastic Polyamic Acid Precursors. Centrifuged NMP or DMAC solutions of the polyamic acids are cast on a clean glass plate and heated

Table 8 Thermo-oxidative stability of high-temperature polymers at 316 °C (600 °F) (air flow, 100 cm^3/min, or 6 $in.^3$/min)

		Weight loss, %, after indicated number of hours					
Polymer	Cure and postcure	91	408	1079	2000	2927	4122
Avimid-N	(a)	0.8	1.3	2.4	4.2	5.8	10.7
p-PPQ	(b)	0.7	2.9	12.1	...	51.1	74.9
PMR-15	(c)	2.3	5.7	13.4	3.4	55.4	84.9
IP-600	(d)	1.8	8.2	19.8	...	68.5	89.2
LARC-TPI	(e)	6.8	12.1	19.9	...	46.5	82.2
L-20	(f)	1.9	6.6	21.3	...	72.8	100
L-30	(f)	1.5	5.8	20.9	...	86.1	100
PBI	(g)	0.4	11.5	40.8	...	100	...
Sixef 44	(h)	...	1.0	2.1	...	5.3	...
PMR-II-30	(i)	...	2.9	7.7	14	20.9	28.0
PMR-II-50	(i)	...	2.4	4.3	9.0	10.8	15.0
3F-PI	(j)	...	...	4.0	9.8	13.0	...
36F-PI	(j)	...	...	3.0	5.0	...	...
AFR 700B	(k)	...	...	...	30.0	...	...

See Table 5 for abbreviations and definitions. (a) 316 °C (600 °F)/1 h + 340 °C (645 °F)/4 h. (b) 325 °C (615 °F)/1 h + 360 °C (680 °F)/4 h. (c) 316 °C (600 °F)/1 h + 316 °C (600 °F)/16 h. (d) 316 °C (600 °F) 2 h + 375 °C (705 °F)/4 h. (e) 316 °C (600 °F)/1 h + 340 °C (645 °F)/4 h. (f) 335 °C/1 h + 360 °C (680 °F)/2 h. (g) Sample obtained from Celanese Corp. as a 50 mm (2 in.) diam × 6 mm (1/4 in.) thick disk. (h) Sample obtained from Hoechst-Celanese (6FDA/6FDAM). (i) 316 °C (600 °F)/1 h + 343 °C (650 °F)/2 h + 371 °C (700 °F)/26 h. (j) 316 °C (600 °F)/1 h + 370 °C/24 h and 416 °C (780 °F)/8 h. Source: Ref 7, 8, 60, 72

Table 9 Thermo-oxidative stability of polyimides at 370 °C (700 °F), 1 atm (air-circulating oven)

		Weight loss, %, after indicated number of hours(a)				
Resin system	Cure and postcure	25 h	100 h	200 h	300 h	400 h
Avimid-N	(b)	1.10	3.1	4.8	8.0	...
6F-PDA-1, Avimid-N(control)	(b)	1.15	3.3	...	...	11.8(f)
3F-PDA (3F-PI)	(b)	1.10	4.0	...	...	71.0(f)
Sixef 44	(b)	...	5.0	8.0	10.0	...
PMR-II-30	(c)	2.5	5.9	18 (264 h)	8.0(e)	...
PMR-II-50	(c)	...	4.5	11.0 (264 h)	5.5(e)	28.7
PMR-15	(d)	5.7	17.1	...	18.2(e)	...
AFR 700B	(b)	1.57	6.4	...	...	...
36F-PI	(b)	0.64	1.8	...	...	...

See Table 5 for abbreviations and definitions. (a) Source: Ref 7, 8, 60, 72, except where noted. (b) Cure and postcure for Avimid-N, 6F-PDA-1, 3F-PDA, 36F-PI, Sixef 44, and AFR 700B: 316 °C (600 °F)/1 h + 371 °C (700 °F)/24 h + 416 °C (780 °F)/8 h. (c) Cure and postcure for PMR-II-30 and PMR-II-50: 316 °C (600 °F)/1 h + 343 °C (650 °F)/2 h + 371 °C (700 °F)/26 h. (d) Cure and postcure for PMR-15: 316 °C (600 °F)/17 h + 371 °C (700 °F)/24 h. (e) Source: Ref 73. (f) Source: Ref 74. PMR-II-50 postcured 371 °C (700 °F)/18 h. 6F-PDA and 3F-PDA postcured 371 °C (700 °F)/8 h. Phthalic anhydride end-capped (aging conditions, not stated). Source: Ref 7, 8, 60, 72, 73, 74

Table 10 Thermo-oxidative stability of polyimides at 371 °C (700 °F), 4 atm (air flow, 100 cm^3/min, or 6 $in.^3$/min)

		Weight loss, %, after indicated number of hours				
Resin system	Cure and postcure	10 h	25 h	50 h	75 h	100 h
Avimid-N	(a)	1.61	2.30	4.26	6.10	10.5
6 F-PDA (control)	(a)	1.12	2.54	5.07	7.65	12.2
3 F-PDA	(a)	1.20	2.66	5.71	8.50	12.1
PMR-II-30	(b)	...	4.19	7.55	...	15.1
PMR-II-50	(b)	...	3.41	6.60	...	...
PMR-15	(c)	...	6.60	...	...	25.2
AFR 700B	(a)	...	4.28	8.83	13.4	18.8
36F-PDA	(a)	...	1.57	3.40	6.0	9.1

See Table 5 for abbreviations and definitions. (a) Cure and postcure for Avimid-N, 6F-PDA, 3F-PDA, 36F-PDA, AFR 700B: 316 °C (600 °F)/1 h + 370 °C (700 °F)/24 h + 416 °C (780 °F)/8 h. (b) Cure and postcure for PMR-II-30 and PMR-II-50: 316 °C (600 °F)/1 h + 343 °C (650 °F)/2 h + 371 °C (700 °F)/26 h. (c) Cure and postcure for PMR-15: 316 °C (600 °F)/17 h + 371 °C (700 °F)/24 h. Source: Ref 8, 72

at 80 °C (175 °F) in a vacuum for 1 h. The tack-free film is then cured at 100 °C (210 °F), 200 °C (390 °F), and 300 °C (570 °F) for 1 h at each temperature. The film is removed from the glass surface by immersion into warm water. Alternatively, an alcohol solution of the polyamic acid precursor is centrifuged, and then the solution is cast on a clean glass plate using a doctor blade. The film solution is placed in a chamber under flowing nitrogen at room temperature for 4 h to become a tack-free film, and cured according to the schedule described previously.

Chemistry of Addition-Type Polyimides

General structures of several types of addition-type polyimides are shown in Fig. 3. Specific structures of the more common materials are shown in Fig. 4. Generally, these materials are low-molecular-weight imide oligomers containing unsaturated end caps, capable of forming an addition-type reaction. In some cases, these unsaturated groups can also be located as pendant groups in the backbone of the oligomer unit.

Phenylethynyl-Containing Imide Oligomers

Since 1985, considerable efforts have been made in the area of phenylethynyl-containing imide oligomers, where the phenylethynyl group can be located at chain ends (Ref 77–83), pendant to the main chain (Ref 84, 85), as well as pendant and terminal (Ref 13, 14, 86–90) to the main chain, shown schematically in Fig. 5. Of the many phenylethynyl end-capped and pendant imide oligomer structures investigated, the phenylethynyl (PE) end-capped imide oligomer, known as PETI-5 (Ref 81) and having a calculated molecular weight of 5000 g/mol, has been extensively characterized as an adhesive (Ref 13, 14, 91–93) and as a composite-matrix resin (Ref 13, 14, 94–96). This material offered the best combination of properties of the oligomers investigated.

The PE end groups are thermally and chemically stable at the conditions necessary to form the imide oligomers. The imide oligomers undergo thermal cure at 370 °C (700 °F) without volatile evolution, to provide polyimides with an excellent combination of thermal stability, mechanical strength, adhesion, and toughness (Ref 13, 14, 81).

The basic chemistry of the PE series of imide oligomers is illustrated by the two reaction schemes (Fig. 5 and 6). The PE end-capped imide oligomers to produce the PETI series of polyimides are shown in Fig. 6. Oligomers containing PE groups pendant to the oligomeric chain end-capped with phthalic anhydride (labeled PPEI) and oligomers with pendant and terminal PE groups (labeled PTPEI) are shown in Fig. 7.

Preparation of Phenylethynyl-Containing Imide Oligomers (Ref 13, 14, 81). The PE end-capped oligomers are prepared from the reactants 3,3′,4, 4′-biphenyltetracarboxylic acid anhydride (BPDA), 3,4′-oxydianiline (3,4′-ODA) and 1,3-bis (3-aminophenoxy) benzene (APB), and 4-phenylethynylphthalic anhydride (PEPA). 3,5-diamino-4-phenylethynyl benzo-

Table 11 Physical and mechanical properties of polyimides

Material	Density, g/cm^3	Tensile strength		Tensile modulus		Flexural strength		Flexural modulus	
		MPa	ksi	GPa	10^6 psi	MPa	ksi	GPa	10^6 psi
Avimid-N (Ref 36–39)	1.40	110	16.0	4.1	0.60	...	...	...	...
Avimid-K3 (Ref 40–42)	1.31	102	15.0	3.6	0.52	...	...	...	...
Avimid-K3A (Ref 40–42)	1.35	83	12.0	3.3	0.49	...	...	...	...
Avimid-K3B (Ref 40–42)	1.34	93	13.4	3.4	0.49	...	...	...	...
Avimid-R (Ref 53, 54)	...	117	16.9	3.6	0.52	...	...	...	...
Avimid-RB (Ref 55)	...	86	12.5	3.8	0.55	...	...	...	...
PMR-15 (Ref 56–59)	1.32	38.6	5.6	3.9	0.57	176	25.5	4.0	0.58
Skybond 701 (Ref 46)	1.35	69	10.0	4.1	0.60	...	...	...	...
Ultem 1000 (Ref 45)	1.27	104	15.2	3.0	0.43	145	21	3.4	0.48
Torlon 4203 (Ref 52)	1.38	186	27.0	4.4	0.64	211	30.7	4.5	0.66
LARC- SI (Ref 44)	1.37	141	19.6	4.0	0.58	...	...	...	...
LARC-TPI (film) (Ref 43)	1.40	166	24.0	3.6	0.51	...	...	...	...
Kapton H film (Ref 48)	1.42	173	25.0	3.0	0.43	...	...	...	...
Vespel SP-1 (Ref 49)	1.34	72	10.5	...	...	83	12.0	3.2	0.45
Pyralin film PI 2610 (Ref 49)	1.40	352	52	8.4	1.22	...	...	...	...
Pyralin PI 2540 (Ref 49)	1.42	104	15.3	1.3	0.20	...	...	...	...
Pyralin PI 2525 (Ref 49)	1.45	113	13.5	2.5	0.36	...	...	...	...
Aurum (new TPI) (Ref 47)	1.33	96	13.4	...	...	138	20.0	3.0	0.43
Super Imide 800 (Ref 66)	1.41	...	...	...	...	...	...	...	...
AFR 700B (Ref 64, 65)	1.41	94	13.1	4.7	0.69	...	...	...	...

Material	Izod impact strength, notched		Strain-to-failure, %	Glass transition temperature (T_g)		Interlaminar fracture toughness (G_{Ic})	
	J/m	ft · lbf/in.		°C	°F	J/m^2	in. · lbf/in.^{2}
Avimid-N (Ref 36–39)	42.7	0.8	6.0	340	644	2400	13.4
Avimid-K-3 (Ref 40–42)	...	...	14	250	482	1400	9.3
Avimid-K3A (Ref 40–42)	...	...	...	222	432	1400	9.3
Avimid-K3B (Ref 40–42)	...	...	4.4	237	459	1400	9.3
Avimid-R (Ref 53, 54)	...	...	3.3	310	590	...	...
Avimid-RB (Ref 55)	...	...	2.4	349	660	...	...
Skybond 701 (Ref 46)	53.4	1.0	1.0	330	626	...	...
PMR-15 (Ref 53, 56–59)	53.4	1.0	1.5	340	644	280	1.57
Ultem 1000 (Ref 45)	53.4	1.0	60	210	426	...	...
Torlon 4203 (Ref 52)	133.5	2.5	20	267	512	3900	21.9
Kapton H film (Ref 48)	23	0.43	7.5	360	680	~2000	~11.6
Vespel SP-1 (Ref 51)	...	...	7.5	>360	>680	~2000	~11.6
Pyralin PI 2610 (Ref 49)	...	...	40	>400	>754	~2000	~11.6
Pyralin PI 2540 (Ref 49)	...	...	40	360	680	...	...
Pyralin PI 2525 (Ref 49)	...	...	15	320	608	...	...
Aurum (new TPI) (Ref 47)	91	1.7	90	250	482	...	...
LARC-SI (Ref 44)	...	...	7.2	248	479	4200	28
LARC-TPI film (Ref 43)	21.4	0.40	8.5	259	498	...	...
Super Imide 800 (Ref 66)	...	...	...	388	730	...	...
AFR 700B (Ref 64, 65)	...	...	...	370	698	...	...

Table 12 Physical properties of phenylethynyl end-capped imide oligomers (PETIs) of various molecular weights

Calculated molecular weight ($\bar{M}_n$) g/mol	ηinh(a), dL/g	Melting temperature (T_m)		Initial (uncured) T_g(b)		T_g (cured)(c)		Imide minimum melt viscosity, Pa · s, at indicated temperature
		°C	°F	°C	°F	°C	°F	
1250	0.15	320	610	170	340	288	550	500 (335 °C, or 635 °F)
2500	0.20	330	630	210	410	277	530	9000 (371 °C, or 700 °F)
5000	0.27	357	675	210	410	270	520	100,000 (371 °C, or 700 °F)

(a) Inherent viscosity (in deciliters per gram) determined on 0.5% (w/v) NMP solution of the amide acid at 25 °C (77 °F). (b) Determined on powdered sample by differential scanning calorimetry at a heating rate of 20 °C/min (36 °F/min). (c) Determined on powdered sample cured in a sealed aluminum pan for 1 h at 371 °C (700 °F). Source: Ref 13

Table 13 Properties of phenylethynyl end-capped polyimides

Calculated molecular weight ($\bar{M}_n$) g/mol	Fracture toughness				Unoriented tensile properties at 23 °C (73 °F)					Tensile shear strength			
	K_{Ic}		G_{Ic}		Strength		Modulus		Elongation	At room temperature		At 177 °C (350 °F)	
	MPa $\sqrt{m}$	ksi $\sqrt{in.}$	J/m^2	ft · lbf/ft^2	MPa	ksi	GPa	10^6 psi	break, %	MPa	ksi	MPa	ksi
1250(a)		...	...	...	...	...	...	...	...	36.6	5.3	31.7	4.6
2500(b)	3.9	3.5	426(a)	29(a)	...	...	...	...	...	...	...	...	...
2500(a)	3.7	3.4	3878	266	151.7	22.0	3.5	0.51	14	1462	212	37.2	5.4
5000(a)	3.9	3.5	4295	294	129.6	18.8	3.1	0.45	32	48.3	7.0	37.9	5.5

(a) Molding cured for 1 h at 371 °C (700 °F). (b) Molding cured for 1 h 350 °C (660 °F). Source: Ref 13

phenone (DPEB) and phthalic anhydride (PA) were added to place PE randomly (pendant) along the oligomeric chain. PEPA and DPEB are added together to form PE terminal to and along the backbone of the oligomeric chain.

The PE oligomers are prepared by dissolving the appropriate diamines 3,4′-ODA, APB, and, in some cases, DPEB in N-methyl pyrrolidinone or dimethylactamide at room temperature under nitrogen. The dianhydride (BPDA) and end-cappers (PEPA or PA, as required) are added in one portion as a slurry in NMP to the stirred diamines. The solids concentration is subsequently adjusted to 25 to 35% (w/w) with additional solvents. A mild exotherm is observed during the first few minutes of the reaction. The solution is stirred for about 24 h at room temperature under nitrogen. Aliquots are removed to determine the inherent viscosity and for GPC analysis to assess molecular weight and molecular weight distribution, or other properties as desired.

The polyamic acid/NMP or DMAC solution is used to prepare thin films, supported adhesive tape, and impregnated unidirectional carbon fiber, carbon cloth, or other fiber/cloth substrate, and cured as described subsequently for film, powder, or composites. The amide acid oligomer is converted to the imide oligomer by adding sufficient toluene or o-xylene to the solution, followed by azeotropic distillation of water in a Dean-Stark trap overnight in nitrogen. The imide oligomers typically precipitate during this imidization process. The pale yellow powder is isolated by adding the reaction mixture to water, filtering, and washing with water and then methanol. It is dried at 200 °C (390 °F) in air to constant weight. This yellow imide oligomer powder can be used to mold polyimide specimens.

Cross-linked Phenylethynyl-Containing Polyimides (Ref 13, 14, 81). Final cure of phenylethynyl-containing imide oligomers occurs about 370 °C (700 °F) over a 1 to 2 h period. The mechanism of the cure process is not completely understood, but it is believed that the major cure reaction is the ethynyl-to-ethynyl reaction to form double bonds or polyene structures (chain extension) (Fig. 8) (Ref 97–99).

Fabrication of Molded Phenylethynyl Polyimide Specimens. Powdered imide oligomers are compression molded in a stainless steel mold under 345 kPa (50 psi) pressure by heating to 370 °C (700 °F) for 1 to 2 h (Ref 13, 14).

Preparation of Phenylethynyl-Containing Polyimide Film (Ref 13, 14). Phenylethynyl-containing oligomeric amide acids in NMP or DMAC (20 to 35 wt%) are centrifuged; the decantate is doctored onto a clean plate glass surface and dried to a tack-free surface in 80 °C (175 °F) in a vacuum for 4 h or at 80 °C (175 °F) in an oven in nitrogen for 24 h. The films on glass are imidized by heating at 100, 225, 300, and 370 °C (210, 435, 570, and 700 °F) for 1 h at each temperature. The film is removed by immersion in warm water.

Constituent Properties of Phenylethynyl-Containing Polyimides (Ref 13, 14). The effect of molecular weight of PETI oligomers and cured polymer on inherent viscosity, T_g, and imide minimum melt viscosity is shown in Table 12. As expected, the inherent viscosities and T_gs for uncured oligomer and imide minimum melt viscosity increase with molecular weight. The T_gs of the cured oligomer are higher for the

Table 14 Physical properties of phenylethynyl-containing imide oligomers and polyimides

Oligomer	ηinh(a), dL/g	Melting temperature T_m, °C	Melting temperature T_m, °F	Glass transition temperature (T_g)(b), Initial, °C	Initial, °F	Cured(c), °C	Cured(c), °F	Imide minimum melt viscosity, Pa · s, at 371 °C (700 °F)
PETI-5(d)	0.27	286	547	210	410	270	518	100,000
PPEI(d)	0.31	. . .	. . .	209	408	279	534	600,000
PTPEI(d)	0.32	282	540	231	448	313	595	1,150,000

(a) Inherent viscosity (in deciliters per gram) determined on 0.5% (w/v) NMP solution of the amide acid at 25 °C (77 °F). (b) Determined on powdered sample by differential scanning calorimetry at heating rate of 20 °C/min (36 °F/min). (c) Determined on powdered sample cured in a sealed aluminum pan for 1 h at 371 °C (700 °F). (d) Molecular weight ($\bar{M}_n$) 5000 g/mol. Source: Ref 14

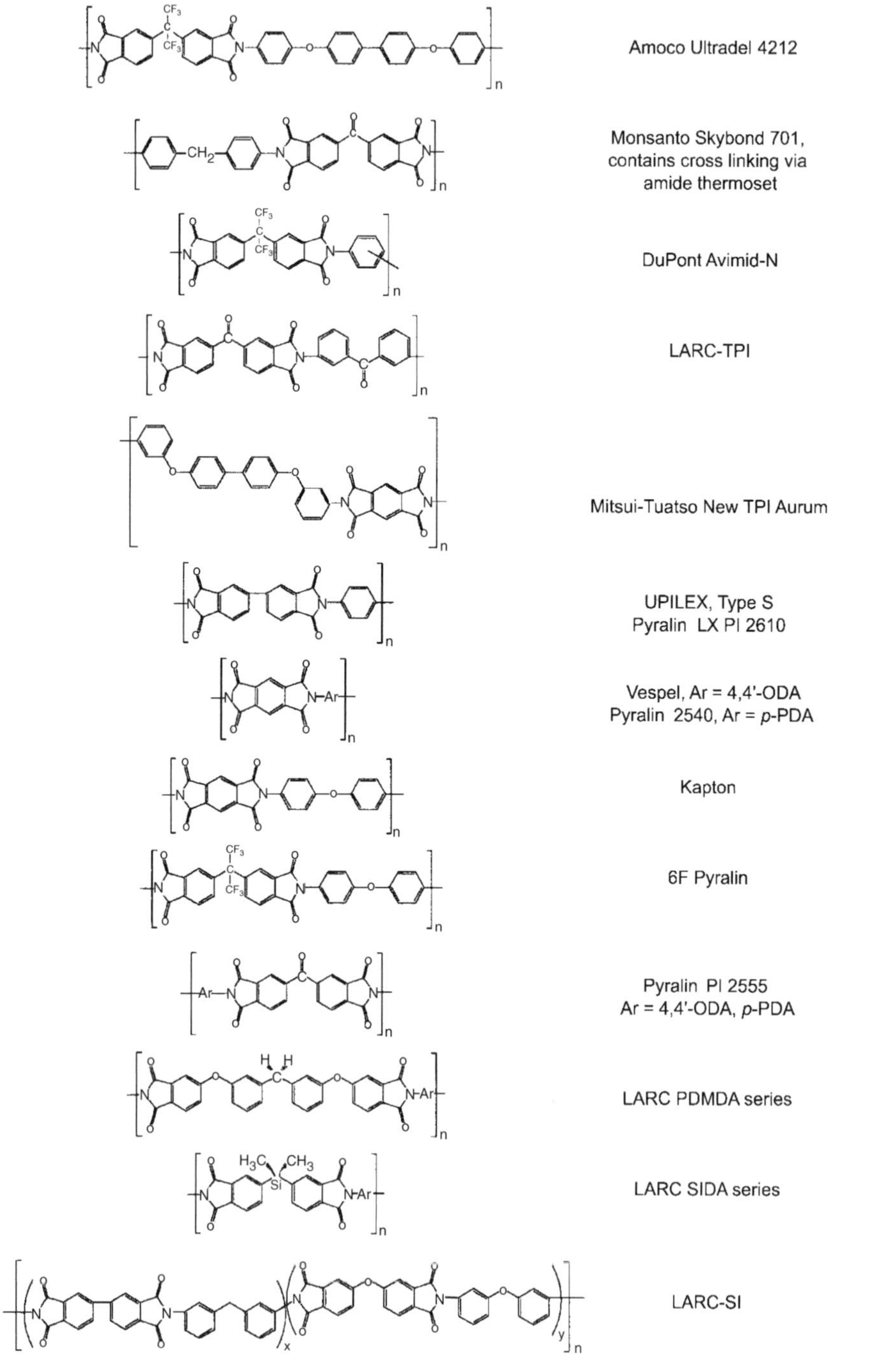

Amoco Ultradel 4212
Monsanto Skybond 701, contains cross linking via amide thermoset
DuPont Avimid-N
LARC-TPI
Mitsui-Tuatso New TPI Aurum
UPILEX, Type S
Pyralin LX PI 2610
Vespel, Ar = 4,4′-ODA
Pyralin 2540, Ar = *p*-PDA
Kapton
6F Pyralin
Pyralin PI 2555
Ar = 4,4′-ODA, *p*-PDA
LARC PDMDA series
LARC SIDA series
LARC-SI

Fig. 2 Structures of selected commercially available condensation polyimide resins

lower-molecular-weight oligomer, presumably due to higher cross-link density. The tensile properties, neat resin fracture, and adhesive properties of the various PETIs are shown in Table 13. The PE end-capped material with calculated molecular weight 5000 g/mol, PETI-5, was selected for extensive evaluation in composites.

The properties of cured phenylethynyl-containing polymers, comparing terminal (PETI-5), pendant (PPEI), and pendant/terminal (PTPEI) each with a calculated molecular weight of 5000 g/mol, are shown in Tables 14 and 15. PETI-5 has the lowest cured T_g and also the lowest melt viscosity, as expected. The best material, from a processing view, is PETI-5. The tensile properties of unoriented thin films of these same polymers are shown in Table 15. As expected, the PPEI (pendant) and PTPEI (pendant/terminal) polymers demonstrate the best tensile properties at 175 °C (350 °F).

Nadic End-Capped Polyimides

Nadic end-capped polyimides, also called reverse Diels-Alder polyimides (Ref 100, 101) and represented by PMR-15 and RP-46, not only undergo the amidation and imidization reactions to form a low-molecular-weight oligomer typical of condensation polyimides, but also undergo an irreversible Diels-Alder reaction leading to a high-molecular-weight cross-linked polyimide. Processing of this resin is further complicated by isomerization of the endo-nadic end-capped imide oligomer to the exo-isomer (Ref 102, 103). These latter two reactions distinguish the RDA addition-type polyimides from the condensation polyimides.

The first process step is amide formation, which occurs between room temperature and 150 °C (300 °F) (Fig. 9). In the second step, imidization occurs over a temperature range of 150 to ≥250 °C (300 to ≥480 °F). Simultaneously, in the temperature range of 175 to 260 °C (350 to 500 °F), isomerization of the endo-isomer to the exo-isomer occurs (Fig. 10) (Ref 102, 103). Finally, in the fourth step, an irreversible Diels-Alder reaction of the endo/exo-oligomers occurs, yielding the reactive intermediates cyclopentadiene and bismaleimide oligomers (Fig. 11). These recombine to form a stable cross-linked polyimide. The critical steps in the processing of this polyimide are the removal of residual by-products due to the imidization reaction and the removal of low-molecular-weight components formed during the various process steps.

It should be noted that the cross-linking mechanism for PMR-15 and other related addition polyimides, such as RP-46 and PN-modified PMR polyimide, remains controversial. There are at least three mechanisms that have been proposed in the literature (Ref 104–109). The cross-linking mechanism of PMR-15 described in this article represents just one of these mechanisms.

LARC RP46. LARC RP46 polyimide was developed (Ref 61) as an alternative to PMR-15, because the diamine in PMR-15,4,4′-methylenedianiline (4,4′-MDA) is carcinogenic. LARC RP46 substitutes 3,4′-oxydianiline (3,4′-ODA) for 4,4′-MDA to form a nontoxic nadic, end-capped PMR system, although the mutagenic and carcinogenic effects of this material are unknown. This material has essentially equivalent mechanical property characteristics to PMR-15 in graphite composites, but constituent properties of the neat resin have not been reported. The chemistry of this material is similar to that for PMR-15.

Other Addition-Type Polyimides. There are several other nadic end-capped polyimides similar to PMR-15, but different in the monomer composition and stoichiometry. However, the chemistry of these materials is similar.

PMR-II-30 and PMR-II-50 are examples. The molecular structures are shown in Fig. 4. AFR 700B and Superimide 800 are end-capped with nadic groups on one end of the oligomer chain. These materials differ from PMR-15 in composition and end-cap stoichiometry, and therefore the cross-linking mechanism is more complex than in PMR-15. The structures of these materials are also shown in Fig. 4. In addition to the nadic end-capped materials, the vinyl end-capped PMRs are also available. The ends of this imide oligomer are bonded to vinyl groups. This material cross links by a simple vinyl addition to give a saturated hydrocarbon cross-linked structure. The structure of this material is shown in Fig. 4.

Table 15 Tensile properties of phenylethynyl-containing polyimides

Oligomer	Test temperature, °C	Test temperature, °F	Strength, MPa	Strength, ksi	Elastic modulus, GPa	Elastic modulus, 10^6 psi	Elongation at break, %
PETI-5(a)	23	73	129.6	18.8	3.1	0.45	32
	177	350	84.1	12.2	2.3	0.33	83
PPEI(a)	23	73	117.2	17.0	3.9	0.57	7
	177	350	64.1	9.3	2.6	0.38	9
PTPEI(a)	23	73	139.3	20.2	3.4	0.49	10
	177	350	78.6	11.4	2.2	0.32	9

(a) Molecular weight ($\bar{M}_n$), 5000 g/mol. Source: Ref 14

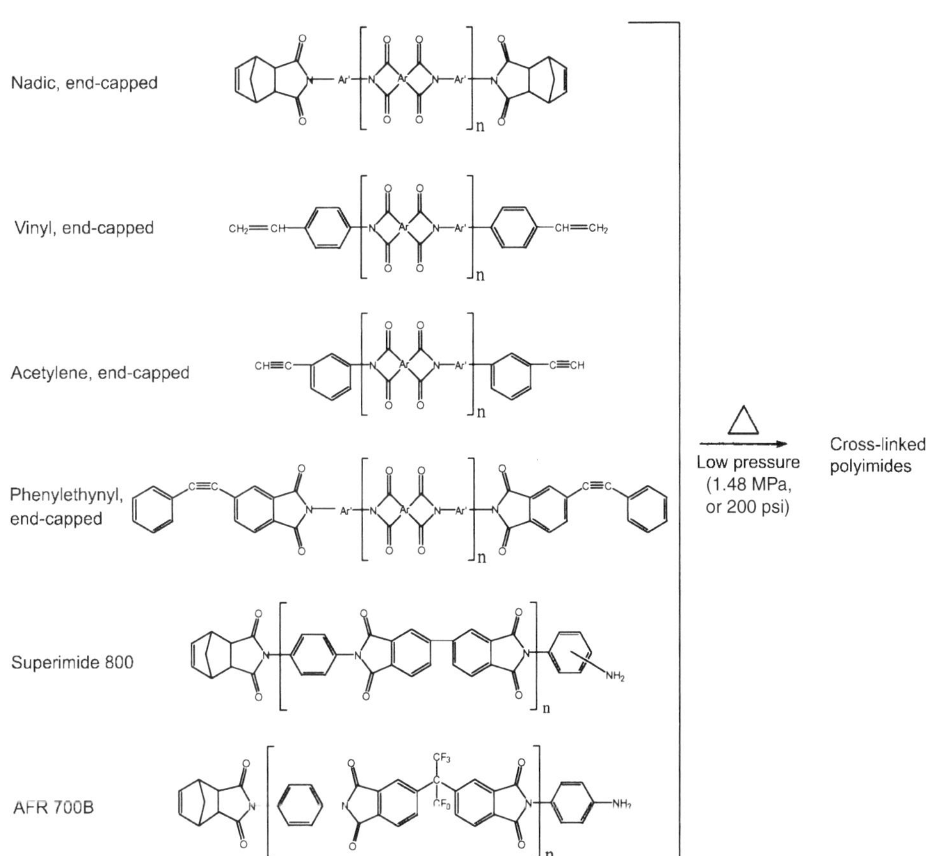

Fig. 3 General structures of addition-type polyimides

Preparation of Nadic End-Capped Amic Acid Oligomer Resin Solutions

PMR-15 Polyimide. The prepolymer composition of this material consists of three monomers: monomethyl ester of 5-norbornene-2, 3-dicarboxylic acid; dimethyl ester of 3,3′, 4,4′-benzophenone tetracarboxylic acid, and 4,4′-methylene dianiline, in the mole ratio of 2:2.087:3.087 (Ref 100, 101). These monomers undergo a reaction to yield PMR-15 polyimide (Fig. 9).

The idealized structure of the imide oligomer resulting from thermal treatment of this monomer mixture (free of solvent), as well as the molecular weight of each segment of the oligomer, is shown in Fig. 12. The theoretical empirical formula for this oligomer, where $n = 2.087$, is $C_{93.61}H_{59.392}N_{6.174}O_{14.435}$, yielding a molecular weight of 1501.56. Dimethyl ester of 5-norbornene 1,2-dicarboxylic acid (13.285 g, 0.0677 mol) is added to a methanol solution of benzophenone tetracarboxylic acid dimethyl ester (BTDE) (60 wt%) (27.296 g, 0.0766 mol), while stirring at room temperature. The diamine (4,4′-MDA, 20.460 g, 0.10319 mol) is then added to the ester solution. The solution is stirred at room temperature until the diamine dissolves. This resin solution can be used to impregnate glass, carbon, or other cloth materials, as well as to impregnate fiber tows to form unidirectional fiber/resin tape. The resin solution can be used to form films or resin powder.

Preparation of Resin Powder and Resin Discs. The PMR-15 resin solution is allowed to concentrate at room temperature to a viscous oil. The solution is dried at 60 °C (140 °F) in vacuum for 2 h to a solid foam. The foam is ground to a powder and thermally treated at 125 °C (255 °F) for 1 h and 200 °C (390 °F) for 1 h and 250 °C (480 °F) for 1.5 h to form an imidized oligomer. Resin discs are fabricated by placing the imidized powder (about 5.0 g) in a 25 mm (1 in.) diam stainless steel mold. The mold is placed in a preheated press (150 °C, or 300 °F). The temperature is raised to 200 °C (390 °F) at 5 °C/min at contact pressure, then a pressure of 28 MPa (4000 psi) is applied at temperature and held for 10 minutes. The temperature is raised to 250 °C (480 °F) at 2 °C (3.5 °F)/min, 4000 psi, held for 10 minutes, and then the pressure is released and reapplied. The temperature is raised to 315 °C (600 °F) at 2 °C/min, 4000 psi, and held for 1 h. The mold is cooled to 275 °C (525 °F) and the pressure is released. The resin disc is removed and postcured at 315 °C (600 °F) for 16 h in the free state or at a higher temperature to increase the glass transition temperature and thermo-oxidative stability. Greater stability is generated when the material is postcured at 370 °C (700 °F) for 24 h.

Preparation of Adhesive Film. The PMR-15 resin solution, prepared as described previously, is brushed onto glass scrim cloth, and the solvent is allowed to evaporate to produce a tacky film. The process is repeated until sufficient resin is deposited on the scrim cloth to give a finished adhesive bond thickness of about 0.13 mm (0.005 in.).

Preparation of Adhesive Bond Specimens. The impregnated glass scrim cloth is cut to the

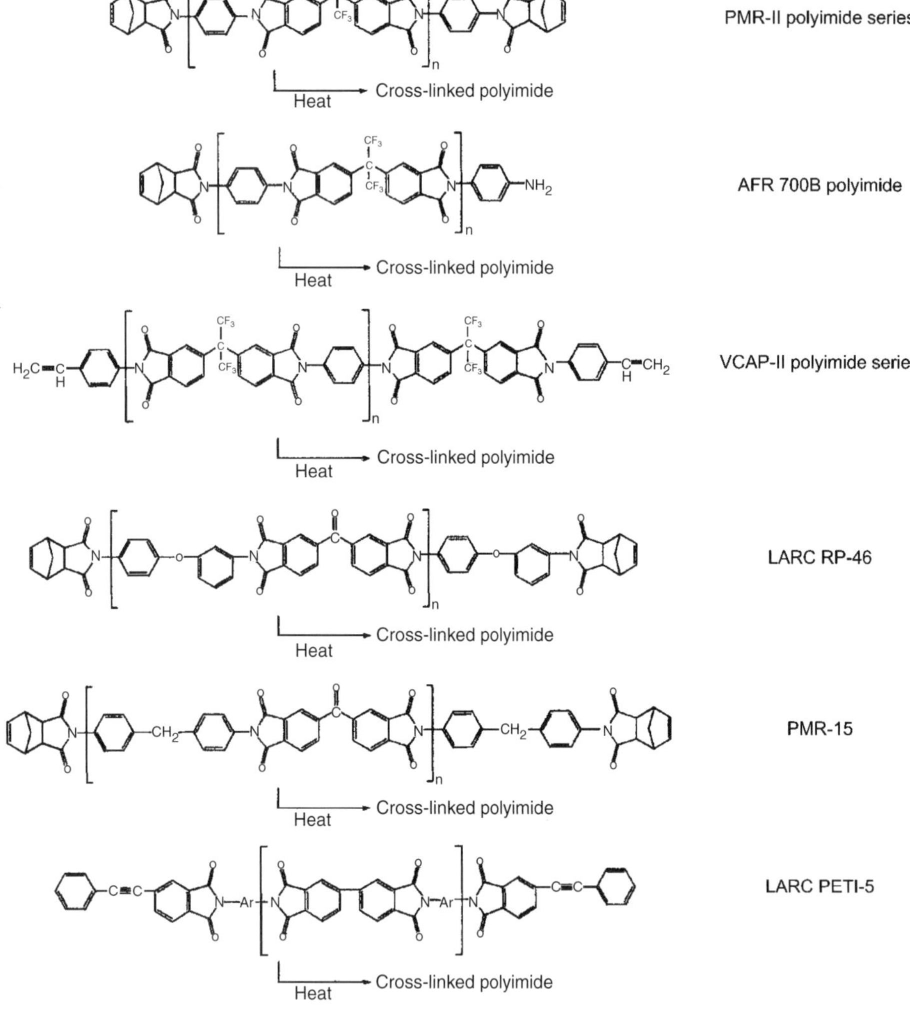

Fig. 4 Structures of selected addition-type polyimides (thermosets)

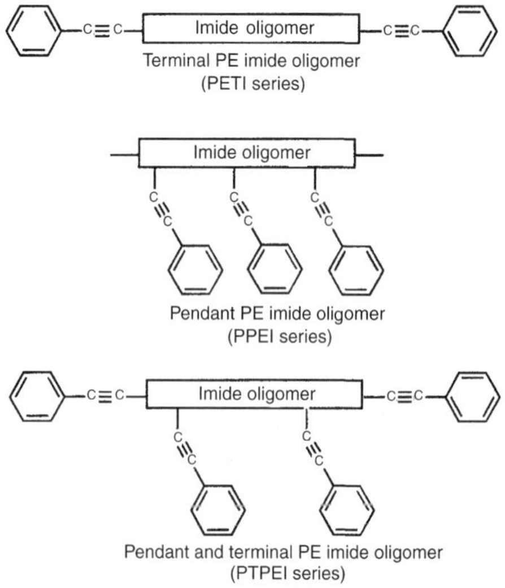

Imide oligomer
Terminal PE imide oligomer (PETI series)
Imide oligomer
Pendant PE imide oligomer (PPEI series)
Imide oligomer
Pendant and terminal PE imide oligomer (PTPEI series)

Fig. 5 Schematic of phenylethynyl-containing imide oligomers. Source: Ref 14

dimensions required for bonding. The cut adhesive scrim cloth is placed on one of the surface-treated specimens to be bonded. The other part of the specimen to be bonded is placed on the adhesive specimen. The bond specimen is placed in a specially designed tool to maintain dimensions of the bonded area. It is placed in a vacuum bag or autoclave, the temperature is raised to 275 °C (525 °F) at 2 °C/min, pressure is applied (700 kPa, or 100 psi), and then the temperature is raised to 315 °C (600 °F) at 100 psi and held for 1 h under these conditions.

Preparation of Films. The PMR-15 resin solution is filtered, the solution is doctored onto a clean plate glass surface, and dried to a tack-free surface at 80 °C (175 °F) in a vacuum. The film is then cured at 150 °C (300 °F) for 1h + 200 °C (390 °F) for 1 h + 250 °C (480 °F) for 1 h + 275 °C (525 °F) for 1 h + 316 °C (600 °F) for 1 h. The film is removed by immersion in warm water.

Constituent Properties of PMR-15

PMR-15 is extremely resistant to most organic solvents, including aliphatic hydrocarbons, ether, ketones, aromatic hydrocarbons, and chlorinated aliphatic and aromatic hydrocarbons. It is hydrolyzed in strong acids and strong bases, including aqueous hydrazine solutions, at elevated temperatures. The constituent materials properties are listed in Table 16.

Current State of the Art

In terms of commercial availability, the polyimides listed in Table 4 define the current technology. The polyimide materials listed in these tables have application as matrices for composite adhesive coating materials, film-forming materials, and electronic materials. The polyimide materials used to make these components are available as solutions, pellets, powder, adhesives films, impregnated unidirectional fiber tape or cloth, and as freestanding films. Specific polyimides are available in solution for applications in electronic applications. Most of these materials are identified only by specific company designations and not by chemical composition. The processing characteristics for each type of polyimide and their applications have been described previously.

Outlook

Improvement in polyimide processability is essential for the ability to manufacture polyimide parts, such as composites, at costs competitive to other metal parts. In order to improve processability, a reduction in the melt viscosity of the polyimide material is an absolute necessity. For the long-chain high-molecular-weight, highly aromatic thermoplastic materials, such as Avimid-N, LARC-TPI, or BPDA/TFMB, this is not readily possible. Low-molecular-weight end-capped oligomers are potential candidates for the development of polyimide oligomers for improved processability. The phenylethynyl end-capped imide oligomers appear to hold considerable promise, because low viscosity versions of the phenylethynyl end-capped imide oligomers have already been developed and are being tested (Ref 89, 111). Research efforts to replace 4,4′-methylene dianiline (4,4′-MDA) in PMR-15 with a nonmutagenic and noncarcinogenic diamine will continue both from the health viewpoint and for process improvements (Ref 112). NASA Glenn Research Center is the lead organization behind this research effort (Ref 23, 27, 32). Therefore, the approach toward developing

Table 16 Constituent properties of PMR-15 polyimide

Property	PMR-15 polyimide
Density, g/cm^3	1.32(a)
Glass transition temperature (T_g), °C (°F)	
After 16 h at 316 °C (600 °F)	340 (662)(a)
After 1 h at 316 °C (600 °F)	320 (680)
Morphology	Amorphous, cross-linked
Tensile strength (dry) at room temperature, MPa (ksi)	8.6 (5.6)(b)
Tensile modulus (dry) at room temperature, GPa (10^6 psi)	39 (0.57)
Tensile strain-to-failure, %	1.1
Flexural strength (dry), MPa (ksi)	
At room temperature	176 (25.5)(c)
At 288 °C (550 °F)	73 (10.7)(c)
At 316 °C (600 °F)	72 (10.4)(c)
At 343 °C (650 °F)	52 (7.6)(c)
Flexural modulus (dry), GPa (10^6 psi)	
At room temperature	4.0 (0.58)(c)
At 288 °C (550 °F)	2.3 (0.34)(c)
At 316 °C (600 °F)	1.9 (0.27)(c)
At 343 °C (650 °F)	1.8 (0.26)(c)
Fracture toughness	
K_{Ic}, MPa $\sqrt{m}$ (ksi $\sqrt{in.}$)	1110 (1010)(d)
	648 (590)(e)
G_{Ic}, J/m^2 (ft · lbf/in.^{2})	280 (1.6)(d)
	94 (0.52)(e)
Izod impact strength, notched, J/m (ft · lbf/in.)	53.37 (1.0)
Equilibrium moisture absorption(e) at 95% relative humidity and 71 °C (160 °F), wt%	4.2
Weight loss, %, at 288 °C (550 °F) in flowing air (100 cm^3/min, or 6 in.^{3}/min)(f)	
After 1000 h	0.3
After 2000 h	0.8
After 3000 h	2.0
Coefficient of thermal expansion(e), 10^6 K	14

(a) Ref 60. (b) Ref 56. (c) Ref 58. (d) Ref 59. (e) Ref 57. (f) Ref 110

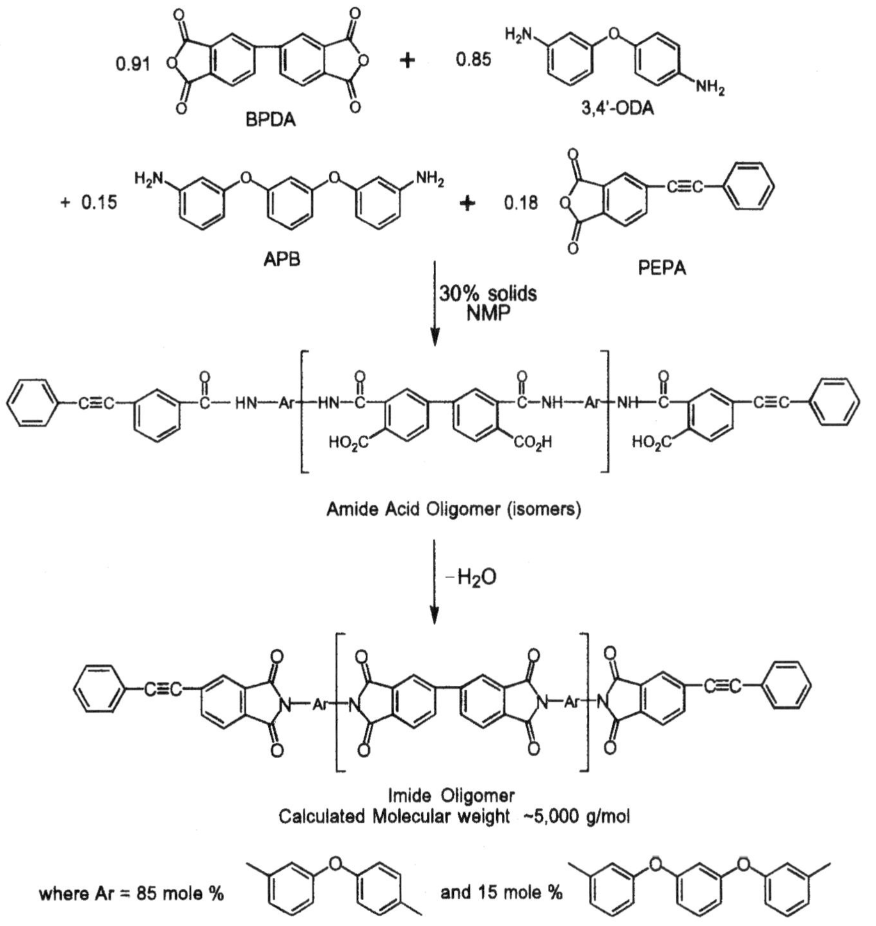

Fig. 6 Phenylethynyl end-capped imide oligomers. Source: Ref 13

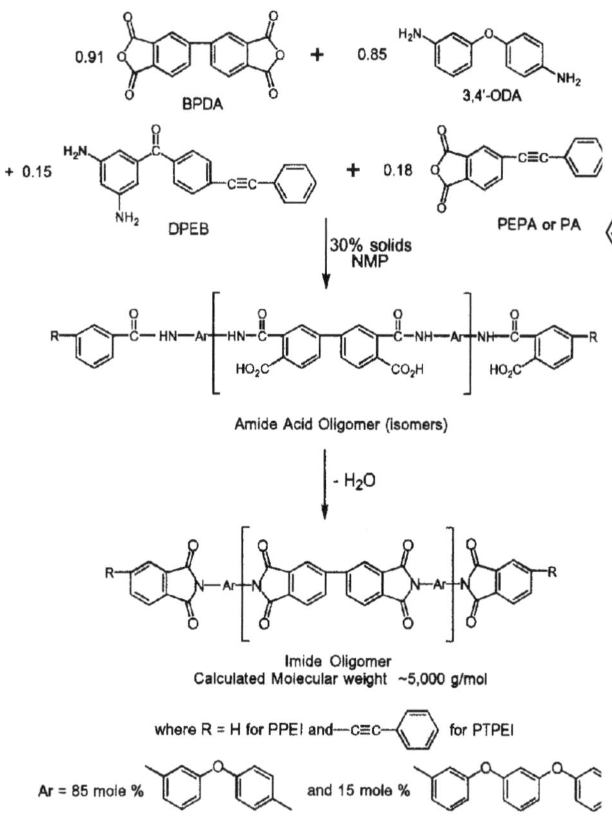

Fig. 7 Phenylethynyl terminal and pendant imide oligomers. Source: Ref 13

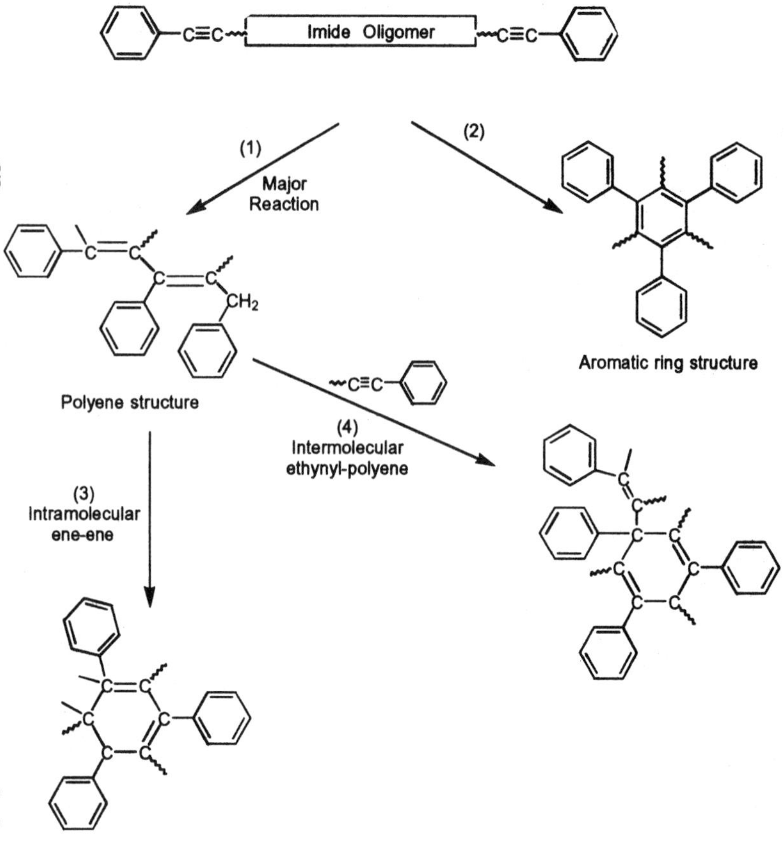

Fig. 8 Proposed phenylethynyl curing process. Source: Ref 97

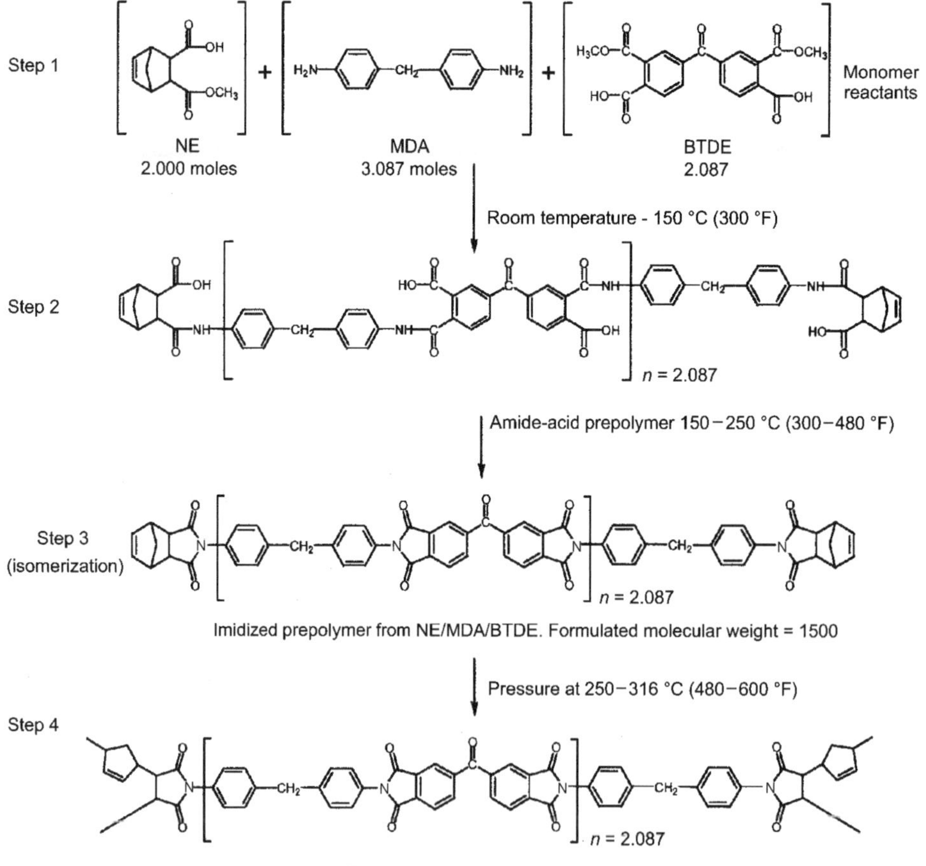

Fig. 9 General reaction scheme for PMR-15 reverse Diels-Alder polyimide. NE, monomethyl ester of nadic anhydride; MDA, 4,4′-methylene dianiline; BTDE, diethyl ester of 3,3′,4,4′-benzophenone tetracarboxylic acid dianhydride. Source: Ref 100, 101

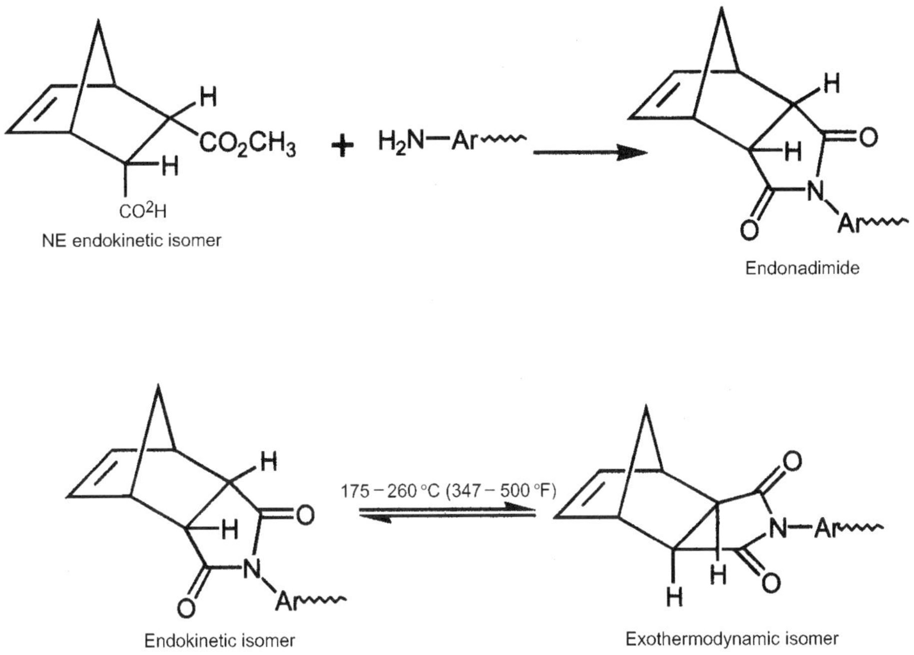

Fig. 10 Isomerization during PMR-15 polymerization. Source: Ref 102, 103

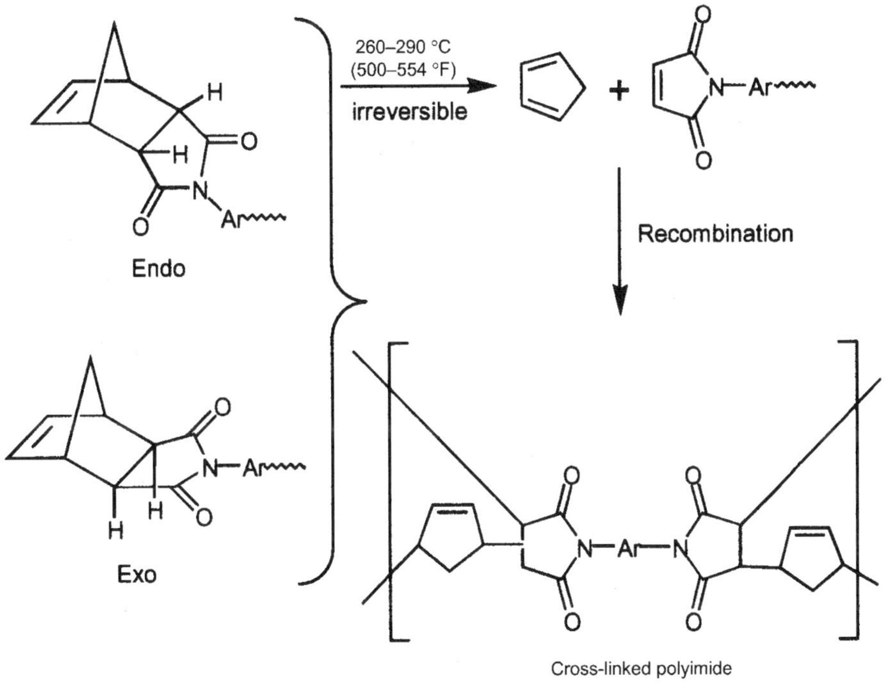

Fig. 11 Reverse Diels-Alder reaction during cure. Source: Ref 104–109

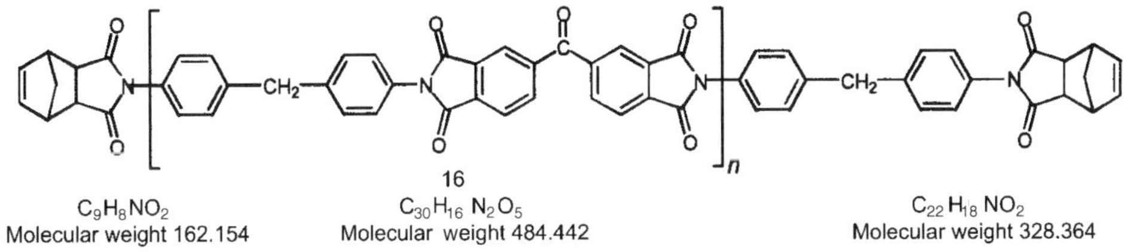

Fig. 12 Idealized PMR-15 structure

polyimides with improved processability without undue sacrifice of other desirable properties can be summarized as follows:

- Control of molecular weight
- Blends of low-molecular-weight, low-melting, low-viscosity, reactive phenylethynyl viscosity modifiers with phenylethynyl end-capped oligomers
- Blends of star-shaped, branched, and linear oligomers
- Design of monomers and oligomers with structured features to increase bulkiness, free volume, and prevent interchain interactions
- Change of bonding in the aromatic rings from para to a mixture of para and meta.

There is always the need to lower the dielectric constant of polyimides for application in the electronic and microelectronics industries. Several important publications deal with the influence of fluorine on the dielectric constant (Ref 9, 113–117). A novel approach for reducing the dielectric constant of polyimides is the formation of nanofoam polyimides (Ref 118, 119). Basically, this approach replaces polyimide polymer with air, which has a dielectric constant of 1.00.

In addition to processing, research efforts will continue to improve thermo-oxidative stability (Ref 9, 120), improve selectivity of gas separation membranes (Ref 121–125), develop proton exchange membranes (Ref 126, 127) for fuel cell applications, improve solubility (Ref 16, 128–131) for coatings, and improve optical properties (Ref 132–138) such as optical anisotropy (Ref 132) for liquid crystal displays. Photosensitive polyimides as photo resists for use in the field of microelectronics is of continued interest (Ref 139). The newest areas of polyimide research involve the development of nanostructured silica-polyimides (Ref 140, 141) and polyimide foam for structural and insulation applications (Ref 142, 143) for use over a temperature range of –250 to 250 °C (–420 to 480 °F).

REFERENCES

1. F.W. Harris, S.L.C. Hsu, and C.C. Tso, Synthesis and Characterization of Polyimides Based on 2,2′ Bis (Trifluoromethyl)-4,4′-Diaminobiphenyl, *Polym. Prepr.*, Vol 31 (No. 5), 1990, p 342
2. S.Z.D. Cheng, F.E. Arnold, Jr., A. Zhang, S.L.C. Hsu, and F.W. Harris, Organosoluble, Segmented Rigid-Rod Polyimide Film: Structure Formation, *Macromolecules*, Vol 24, 1991, p 5856–5862
3. M. Eashoo, D. Shen, Z. Wu, C.J. Lee, F.W. Harris, and Z.D. Cheng, High Performance Aromatic Polyimide Fibers: Thermal Mechanical and Dynamic Properties, *Polymer* Vol 34 (No. 15), 1993, p 3209–3215
4. J.C. Coburn, P.D. Soper, and B.C. Auman, Relaxation Behavior of Polyimides Based on 2,2′-Disubstituted Benzidines, *Macromolecules*, Vol 28, 1995, p 3253–3260
5. D.A. Scola, High Temperature Fluorinated

Polyimides, U.S. Patent 4,742,152, 3 May 1988
6. D.A. Scola, Fluorinated Condensation Copolyimides, U.S. Patent 5,298,600, 29 March 1994
7. D.A. Scola, Synthesis and Thermo-Oxidative Stability of [1,4-Phenylene-4,4′-(2,2,2-Trifluoro-Phenyl Ethylidene) Bisphthalimide] and Other Fluorinated Polyimides, *J. Polym. Sci A, Polym. Chem.*, Vol 31, 1993, p 1997–2008
8. D.A. Scola and M. Wai, The Thermo-Oxidative Stability of Fluorinated Polyimides and Polyimide/Graphite Composites at 371 °C, *J. Appl. Polym. Sci.*, Vol 52, 1994, p 421–429
9. E. Vaccaro and D.A. Scola, Novel Fluorinated Polyimides, *Proc. High Temple Workshop XX*, 24–27 Jan 2000 (San Diego, CA), U.S. Department of Defense and National Aeronautic and Space Administration
10. G.R. Husk, P.E. Cassidy, and K.L. Gebert, Synthesis and Characterization of a Series of Polyimides Derived from 4,4′(2,2,2-Trifluoro-1-Trifluoromethyl) Ethylidene] Bis [1,3-Isopbenzofurandione], *Macromolecules*, Vol 21, 1988, p 1234–1238
11. C.A. Arnold, J.D. Summers, and J.E. McGrath, Syntheses and Physical Behavior of Siloxane Modified Polyimides, *Polym. Eng. & Sci.*, Vol 29 (No. 20), 1989, p 1413–1418
12. M.E. Rogers, H. Grubbs, A. Brennan, D. Rogriques, G.L. Wilkes, and J.E. McGrath, Very High T_g, Fully Cyclized, Soluble Polyimides, *Advances in Polyimide Science and Technology, Proc. Fourth International Conference on Polyimides*, 30 Oct to 1 Nov 1991, (sponsored by the Society of Plastics Engineers), C. Feger, M.M. Khojasteh, and N.S. Htoo, Ed., Technomic, Lancaster, PA, p 33–40
13. P.M. Hergenrother, J.W. Connell, and J.G. Smith, Jr., Phenylethynyl Containing Imide Oligomers, *Polymer*, Vol 41, 2000, p 5073–5081
14. J.G. Smith, Jr., J.W. Connell, and P.M. Hergenrother, The Effect of Phenylethynyl Terminated Imide Oligomer Molecular Weight on the Properties of Composites, *J. Compos. Mater.*, Vol 34, (No. 7), 2000, p 614–627
15. J.E. McGrath, B. Tan, V. Vasuderan, G.W. Meyer, A.C. Loos, and T. Bullions, Syntheses and Characterization of High Performance Thermosetting Polyimides for Structural Adhesives and Composite Matrix Systems, paper presented at 28th International SAMPE Technical Conf., 4–7 Nov 1996, Society for the Advancement of Material and Process Engineering, 1996, p 29–38
16. Y. Tang, W. Huang, J. Luo, and M. Ding, Syntheses and Properties of Aromatic Polyimides Derived from 2,2′,3,3′-Biphenyltetracarboxylic Dianhydride, *J. Polym. Sci., Polym. Chem.*, Vol 37, 1999, p 1425–1433
17. V. Ratta, A. Ayambem, J.E. McGrath, and G.L. Wilkes, Crystallization and Multiple Melting Behavior of a New Semicrystalline Polyimide Based on 1,3-Bis (4-Amino Phenoxy) Benzene (TPER) and 3,3′,4,4′-Benzophenonetetracarboxylic Dianhydride (BTDA), American Chemical Society, *Polymeric Materials Science and Engineering (PMSE) Abstracts*, Vol 81, 1999, p 303–304
18. S. Srinivas, F.E. Caputo, M. Graham, S. Gardner, R.M. Davis, J.E. McGrath, and G.L. Wilkes, Semicrystalline Polyimides Based on Controlled Molecular Weight Phthalimide End-Capped, *Macromolecules*, Vol 30, 1977, p 1012–1022
19. M.K. Gerber, J.R. Pratt, A.K. St.Clair, and T.L. St.Clair, Polyimides Prepared from 3,5-Diaminobenzotrifluoride, *Polym. Prepr.*, Vol 31 (No. 1), 1990, p 340–341
20. H.G. Boston, A.K. St. Clair, and J.R. Pratt, Polyimides derived from a Methylene-Bridged Dianhydride, *J. Appl. Polym. Sci.*, Vol 46, 1992, p 243–258
21. D.A. Scola, 3,3′-DDS-PMR-16-5, A Non-Toxic Form of PMR-15, *Proc. High Temple Workshop X*, 29 Jan–1 Feb 1990, U.S. Department of Defense and National Aeronautic and Space Administration
22. R. Vannucci, Non-MDA PMR Polyimides, *Proc. High Temple Workshop XV*, 16–19 Jan 1995, U.S. Department of Defense and National Aeronautic and Space Administration
23. M. Meador, High Temperature Polymers and Composites for Aeropropulsion, *Proc. High Temple Workshop XVII*, 10–13 Feb 1997, U.S. Department of Defense and National Aeronautic and Space Administration
24. R. Gray, Resin Transfer Molding of High Temperature Composites, *Proc. High Temple Workshop XVIII*, 20–22 Jan 1998, U.S. Department of Defense and National Aeronautic and Space Administration
25. K.C. Chuang, J.E. Waters, and D.H. Green, A High T_g Thermosetting Polyimide, paper presented at 42nd International SAMPE Symposium and Exhibit, Society for the Advancement of Material and Process Engineering, 1997, p 1283–1290
26. K.C. Chuang, J.D. Kinder, D.L. Hull, D.B. McConville, and W.J. Joungs, Rigid-Rod Polyimides Based on Noncoplanar 4,4′-Biphenylenediamines: A Review of Polymer Properties vs. Configuration of Diamines, *Macromolecules*, Vol 30 (No. 23), 1997, p 7183–7190
27. M. Meador, R.K. Eby, C.A. Gariepy, B.N. Nguyen, D. Hubbard, and J. Williams, Processable Polyimides, *Proc. High Temple Workshop XIX*, 1999, U.S. Department of Defense and National Aeronautic and Space Administration
28. R. Gray, E. Collins, and L. Livingston, Resin Transfer Molding of High Temperature Composites, *Proc. High Temple Workshop XIX*, 1–4 Feb 1999, U.S. Department of Defense and National Aeronautic and Space Administration
29. R. Vannucci, P. Delvigs, and R. Gray, Non-Toxic PMR-Type Polyimides, *Proc. High Temple Workshop XVIII*, 20–22 Jan 1998, U.S. Department of Defense and National Aeronautic and Space Administration
30. J. Sutter, A Review of NASA Advanced High Temperature Engine Materials Technology Program (HiTEMP) in Polymer Matrix Composites, *Proc. High Temple Workshop XVII*, 10–13 Feb 1997, U.S. Department of Defense and National Aeronautic and Space Administration
31. B.N. Nguyen, R.K. Eby, and M. Meador, Development of Processable PMR-Type Polyimides with Star Branched Structures, *Proc. High Temple Workshop XX*, 24–27 Jan 2000, U.S. Department of Defense and National Aeronautic and Space Administration
32. C.A. Gariepy, R.K. Eby, and M.A. Meador, An Approach to Processable Polyimides, *Proc. High Temple Workshop XX*, 24–27 Jan 2000, U.S. Department of Defense and National Aeronautic and Space Administration
33. K.C. Chuang and J.D. Kinder, Polyimides Based on 2,2′,6,6′-Tetramethylbenzidine, *High Perform. Polym.*, Vol 7 (No. 1), 1995, p 81–92
34. D.A. Scola, High Temperature Fluorinated Polymers, U.S. Patent 4,801,682, 31 Jan 1989
35. A.J. Hu, J.Y. Hao, T. He, and S.Y. Yang, Synthesis and Characterization of High-Temperature Fluorinated-Containing PMR Polyimides, *Macromolecules*, Vol 32, 1999, p 8046–8051
36. F.E. Rogers, Polyamide-acids and Polyimides from Hexafluoroisopropylidene Bridged Diamine, U.S. Patent 3,356,648, 5 Dec 1967
37. D.G. Coe, Diaryl Fluoro Compounds, U.S. Patent, 3,310,573, 21 March 1967
38. H.H. Gibbs and C.V. Breder, High Temperature Laminating Resins Base on Melt Fusible Polyimides, *Advances in Chemistry*, American Chemical Society Symposium Series 142, *Copolymers, Polyblends and Composite*, 1975, p 442–457
39. "Avimid N Composite Materials," Data Sheet H-16044, DuPont
40. R.C. Boyce, T.P, Gannett, H.H. Gibbs, and H.R. Wedgewood, Processing, Properties and Applications of K-Polymer Composite Materials Based on Avimid K-111 Prepregs, paper presented at 32nd Annual SAMPE Symposium and Exhibition, Society for the Advancement of Material and Process Engineering, 1987, p 169–184
41. A.R. Wedgewood, Melt Processable Polyimides For High Performance Applications, paper presented at 24th International

SAMPE Technical Conference, Society for the Advancement of Material and Process Engineering, 1992, p T385–T398
42. "Processing Characteristics of Avimid K Composite Materials," Data Sheet H-14473, DuPont, April 1989
43. Mitsui Toatsu Chemical, Inc., data sheet
44. "High-Performance Polyimide LARC-TPI," NASA Langley Research Center, data sheet
45. "Ultem 1000," Data Sheet VLT-301B, General Electric Co.
46. "IST," Technical Data Bulletin 50421, Monsanto, Springfield, MA, also private communication
47. "Auvum," Data Sheet Series A-00 through E-00, Mitsui Toatsu Chemicals, Inc.
48. "DuPont Kapton," Data Sheet E-72087, DuPont, Jan 1985
49. "LX-Series—Product Information and Process Guidelines," H.D. Micro Systems (an enterprise of Hitachi Chemical and DuPont Electronics), data sheet, Dec 1997
50. Bulletin UL-P3e, R1197, BP Amoco
51. "DuPont Vespel," Brochure 216129B, DuPont, April 1994; also DuPont Engineered Parts Group, brochure
52. "Torlon 4203," commercial data sheet, Amoco Chemical Corporation, July 1974
53. R.J. Boyce and J.P. Gannett Avimid R: A New High Temperature Polyimide Matrix Composite, *Proc. High Temple Workshop*, 16–19 Jan 1995, U.S. Department of Defense and National Aeronautic and Space Administration
54. J.M. Sonnett, R.J. Boyce, and J.P Gannett, Avimid R: A New High Temperature Organic Matrix Composite, *HiTEMP Conf. Proc.*, Oct 1994 (Cleveland, OH), NASA Lewis Research Center
55. S. Peak, J. Pratte, and R.J. Boyce, Avimid RB High Temperature Non-MDA Polyimide Composite Prepreg System, paper presented at 44th International SAMPE Symposium and Exhibit, Society for the Advancement of Material and Process Engineering, 1999, p 96–102
56. P.J. Canvana and W.F. Winters, " PMR-15 Polyimide/Graphite Composite Fan Blade," NASA CR-135113, National Aeronautic and Space Administration, Feb 1976
57. "PMR-15," Data Sheet F670, Hexcel Corporation, April 1986
58. "PMR-15," Data Sheet PI-2337, Ferro Composite Division (now Cytec Fiberite)
59. D.A. Scola and D.J. Parker, Fracture Toughness of Bismaleimide and Other Resins, *Proc. 43rd Annual Technical Conference and Exhibition*, Society of Plastics Engineers, *Antec '85*, Vol 31, 1986, p 399–400
60. D.A. Scola and J.H. Vontell, High Temperature Polyimides, Chemistry and Properties, *Polym. Compos.,* Vol 9 (No. 6), 1988, p 443–452
61. R.H. Pater, LARC-RP46, A New 700 °F Matrix Resin Having Attractive Overall Properties, *Proc. High Temple Workshop XII*, 27–30 Jan 1992, U.S. Department of Defense and National Aeronautic and Space Administration
62. Y. Xiao, X.D. Sun, C.D. Simone, and D.A. Scola, Cure and Postcure of RP-46, a Nadic End-Capped Polyimide and a Bisnadimide Model Compound, *High Perform. Polym.*, to be submitted 2001
63. T.T. Serafini, P.G. Cheng, K.K. Ueda, and W.F. Wright, Improved High Temperature Resistant Matrix Resins, 22nd International SAMPE Technical Conference, Society for the Advancement of Material and Process Engineering, 1990, p 94–107
64. J.D. Russell, and J.L. Kardos, Crosslinking Characterization of a Polyimide, AFR 700B, *Polym. Compos.*, Vol 18 (No. 5), 1997, p 595–612
65. B.P. Rice and K. Johnson, AFR700B: An Overview, *HiTEMP Review 1993*, NASA Conference Publication 19117, 25–27 Oct 1993
66. S. Prybla, Super Imide 800, *Proc. High Temple Workshop XVI*, 29 Jan to Feb 1996, U.S. Department of Defense and National Aeronautic and Space Administration; also M. Dyer, BF Goodrich Aerospace, personal communication
67. T.T. Serafini, R.D. Vannucci, and W.B. Alston, "Second Generation PMR Polyimides," NASA TMX-71894, 1976
68. R.D. Vannucci and D. Cifani, 7000F Properties of Autoclave Cured PMR-II Composites, paper presented at 20th International SAMPE Technical Conference, Society for the Advancement of Material and Process Engineering, 1988, p 562–575
69. D.A. Scola, J.H. Vontell, and J.P. Pinto, *A Comparison of the Thermo-Oxidative Stability of PMR-II Type and PMR-15 Polyimides in Graphite Composites*, Vol XXXVI, Society of Plastics Engineers, 1990, p 1300–1301
70. K.C. Chuang, R.D. Vannucci, I. Anasari, L.L. Cerny, and D.A. Scheiman, High Flow Addition Curing Polyimides, *J. Polym. Sci. A, Polym. Chem.*, Vol 32, 1994, p 1341–1350
71. R.J. Morgan, E.E. Shin, J. Zhou, J. Lincoln, and B. Rozenberg, Current Durability Issues on High Temperature Polymers Matrix Composites for Aero-Space Applications, *Proc. High Temple Workshop XIX*, 1–4 Feb 1999, U.S. Department of Defense and National Aeronautic and Space Administration
72. D.A. Scola, Polyimides for 370 °C Applications, *Proc. Fourth Interdisiplinary Symposium on Recent Advances in Polyimides and Other High Performance Polymers*, 18–21 Jan 1993, American Chemical Society
73. R.D. Vannucci, PMR Polyimide Compositions for Improved Performance at 371 °C , *SAMPE Q.*, Vol 19 (No. 1), 1987, p 31–36
74. M.J. Turk, A.S. Ansari, W.B. Alston, G.S. Gahn, A.A. Frimer, and D.A. Scheiman, Evaluation of the Thermal Oxidative Stability of Polyimides via TGA Techniques, *J. Polym. Sci. A, Polym. Chem.*, Vol 37, 1999, p 3942–3956
75. T.M. Bogert and R.R. Renshaw, *ACS Symposium Series 132*, C.A. May, Ed., Vol 30, American Chemical Society, 1980, p 1140
76. W.M. Edwards and I.M. Robertson, U.S. Patent 2,710,853, 1955
77. F.W. Harris, K. Sridhar, and S. Das, Polyimide Oligomers Terminated with Thermally-Polymerizable Groups, *Polym. Prepr.*, Vol 25 (No. 1), 1984, p 110–111
78. F.W. Harris, A. Pamidimukkala, R. Gupta, S. Das, T. Wu, and G. Mock, Syntheses and Characterization of Reactive End-Capped Polyimide Oligomers, *J. Macromol. Sci.-Chem.,* A21 (No. 8, 9), 1984, p 1117–1135
79. C.W. Paul, R.A. Schultz, and S.P. Fenelli, Polyimides End-Capped with Diaryl Substituted Acetylene: Composites, Molding Material, Adhesives, Electronics, U.S. Patent 5,138,028,11 Aug 1992; also C. Feger, M.M. Khoyastech, and M.S. Htoo, Ed., *Advances in Polyimide Science and Technology*, Technomic Publishing Co., Inc., 1993, p 220–244
80. P.M. Hergenrother, R.G. Bryant, B.J. Jensen, and S.J. Havens, Phenyl Ethynyl-Terminated Imide Oligomers and Polymers Therefrom, *J. Polym. Sci. A, Polym. Chem.*, Vol 32, 1994, p 3061–3067
81. P.M. Hergenrother and J.W. Smith, Jr., Chemistry and Properties of Imide Oligomer End-Capped with Phenylethynylphthalic Anhydrides, *Polymer*, Vol 35 (No. 22), 1994, p 4857–4864
82. J.A. Johnston, F.M. Li, F.W. Harris, and T. Takekoshi, Synthesis and Characterization of Imide Oligomers End-Capped with 4-(Phenylethynyl) Phthalic Anhydrides, *Polymer*, Vol 35, 1994, p 4865–4873
83. G.W. Meyer, T.E. Glass, H.J. Grubbs, and J.E. McGrath, Syntheses and Characterization of Polyimides End-Capped with Phenylethynylphthalic Anhydride, *J. Polym. Sci. A, Polym. Chem.*, Vol 33, 1995, p 2141–2149
84. B.J. Jensen, P.M. Hergenrother, and G. Nuokogu, Polyimides with Pendant Ethynyl Groups, *Polymer*, Vol 34 (No. 3), 1993, p 630–635
85. J.W. Connell, J.G. Smith, Jr., and P.M. Hergenrother, Properties of Imide Oligomers Containing Pendant Phenylethynyl Groups, *High Perform. Polym.*, Vol 9, 1997, p 309–321
86. J.G. Smith, Jr., J.W. Connell, and P.M. Hergenrother, Imide Oligomers Containing Pendant and Terminal Phenylethynyl Groups, *Polymer*, Vol 38 (No. 18), 1997, p 4657–4665
87. J.W. Connell, J.G. Smith, Jr., and P.M. Hergenrother, Adhesive and Composite

Properties of Cured Imide Oligomers Containing Pendant and Terminal Phenylethynyl Groups, paper presented at 29th International SAMPE Technical Conference, Society for the Advancement of Material and Process Engineering, 1997, p 317–331

88. J.W. Connell, J.G. Smith, Jr., and P.M. Hergenrother, Imide Oligomers Containing Pendant and Terminal Phenylethynyl Groups II, *High Perform. Polym.*, Vol 10, 1998, p 273–283
89. J.G. Smith, Jr. and J.W. Connell, Chemistry and Properties of Imide Oligomers from Phenylethynyl Containing Diamines, *High Perform. Polym.*, Vol 12, 2000, p 213–223
90. P.M. Hergenrother, R.G. Bryant, B.J. Jensen, J.G. Smith, Jr., and S.F. Wilkinson, Chemistry and Properties of Phenylethynyl Terminate Imide Oligomers and their Cured Polymers, paper presented at International SAMPE Symposium and Exhibition, Society for the Advancement of Material and Process Engineering, 1994, p 961–968
91. B.J. Jensen, R.G. Bryant, and P.M. Hergenrother, Adhesive Properties of Cured Phenylethynyl- Terminated Oligomers, *J. Adhes.*, Vol 54 (No. 1–4), 1995, p 57–66
92. R.J. Cano and B.J. Jensen, Effect of Molecular Weight on Processing and Adhesive Properties of the Phenylethynyl-Terminated Polyimide LARC—PETI-5, *J. Adhes.*, Vol 60, 1996, p 113–123
93. T. Hou, B.J. Jensen, and P.M. Hergenrother, Processing and Properties of IM7/PETI Composites, *J. Compos. Mater.*, Vol 30 (No. 1), 1996, p 109–122
94. P.M. Hergenrother and M.L. Rommel, Mechanical Properties of a Reactive End-Capped Polyimide Based Composite from Polyamic Acid, paper presented at 41st International SAMPE Symposium and Exhibition, Society for the Advancement of Material and Process Engineering, 1996, p 1061–1072
95. M. Rommel, L. Konopka, and P.M. Hergenrother, Composite Properties of Cured Phenylethynyl Containing Imide Oligomers, paper presented at 28th International SAMPE Technical Conference, Society for the Advancement of Material and Process Engineering, 1996, p 14–28
96. J.W. Connell, J.G. Smith, P.M. Hergenrother, and M.L. Rommel, Neat Resin, Adhesive and Composite Properties of Reactive Additive/PETI-5 Blends, *High Perform. Polym.*, Vol 12 (No. 2), 2000, p 323–333
97. X. Fang, X.-Q. Xie, C.D. Simone, M.P. Stevens, and D.A. Scola, A Solid State ^{13}C NMR Study of the Cure of ^{13}C-Labeled Phenylethynyl End-Capped Polyimides, *Macromolecules*, Vol 33, 2000, p 1671–1681
98. C.C. Roberts, J.M. Apple, and G.E. Wnek, Curing Chemistry of Phenylethynyl-Terminated Imide Oligomers: Synthesis of ^{13}C-Labeled Oligomers and Solid-State NMR Studies, *J. Polym. Sci. A, Polym. Chem.*, Vol 38, 2000, p 3486–3497
99. T.V. Holland, T.E. Glass, and J.E. McGrath, Investigation of the Thermal Curing Chemistry of the Phenylethynyl Groups Using a Model Arylether Imide, *Polymer*, Vol 41, 2000, p 4965–4990
100. H.R. Lubowitz, "Polyimide Polymers," U.S. Patent 3,528,590, 15 Sept 1970
101. T.T. Serafini, P. Delvigs, and G.R. Lightsey, Thermally Stable Solutions of Monomeric Reactants, *J. Appl. Polym. Sci.*, Vol 16 (No. 4), 1972, p 905–916; also U.S. Patent 3,765,149, July 1973
102. P.R. Young and A.C. Chang, Characterization of Geometric Isomers of Norbornene End-Capped Imides, *J. Heterocylic Chem.*, Vol 20, 1983, p 177–182
103. D.A. Scola and J.H. Vontell, Some Chemical Characteristics of the Reverse-Diels-Alder (RDA) Polyimide, PMR-15, *Proc. Second International Conference on Polyimides: Chemistry, Characterization, and Applications*, Society of Plastics Engineers, Inc., 1985, p 247–252
104. M.A. Meador, J.C. Johnston, and P.J. Cavano, Elucidation of the Cross-Link Structure of Nadic End-Capped Polyimides Using NMR of ^{13}C-Labeled Polymers," *Macromolecules*, Vol 30, 1997, p 515–519
105. A.C. Wong and W.M. Ritchey, Nuclear Magnetic Resonance of Study of Norbornene End-Capped Polyimides I, Polymerization of N-Phenylnadimide, *Macromolecules*, Vol 14, 1981, p 825–831
106. Y. Liu, X.D. Sun, X.-Q. Xie, and D.A. Scola, Kinetics of the Crosslinking Reaction of a Bisnadimide Model Compound in Thermal and Microwave Cure Processes, *J. Polym. Sci. A: Polym. Chem.*, Vol 36, 1998, p 2653–2665
107. H.R. Lubowitz, New Thermosetting Resins For Composites, *ACS Div. Org. Coatings Plast. Chem. Pap.*, Vol 31 (No.1), American Chemical Society, 1971, p 560–568
108. E.A. Burns, R.J. Jones, R.W. Vaughn, and W.P. Kendrick, "Nadimide," CR-72633 12-16, NASA, 1970
109. T.T. Serafini, P. Delvigs, and G.R. Lightsey, Thermally Stable Solutions of Monomeric Reactants, *J. Appl. Polym. Sci.*, Vol 16, 1972, p 905–915
110. D.A. Scola, Thermo-Oxidative Stability and Moisture Absorption Behavior of Glass- and Graphite Fiber-Reinforced PMR-Polyimide Composites, paper presented at 22nd National Symposium and Exhibition, Society for the Advancement of Material and Process Engineering, 1977, p 238–252
111. C. Simone and D.A. Scola, "Novel Fluorinated Polyimides" *Proc. Fluoro Polymer 2000*, American Chemical Society, 15–18 Oct 2000
112. B. Nguyen, R.K. Eby, and M.A. Meador, High Temperature PMR-Type Polyimides with Branched Structure: Syntheses and Characterization, *Polym. Prepr.*, Vol 41 (No. 1), 2000, p 225–226
113. A.E. Feiring, B.C. Auman, and E.R. Wenchoba, Syntheses and Properties of Fluorinated Polyimides from Novel 2,2′-Bis (Fluoroalkoxy) Benzidenes, *Macromolecules*, Vol 26 (No. 11), 1993, p 2779–2784
114. G. Hougham, G. Tesero, and J. Shaw, Syntheses and Properties of Highly Fluorinated Polyimides, *Macromolecules*, Vol 27 (No. 13), 1994, p 3642–3649
115. B.C. Auman, Fluorinated Low Thermal Expansion Coefficient Polyimides for Interlayer Dielectric Applications: Thermal Stability, Refractive Index and High Temperature Molecules Measurements, *Mater. Res. Soc. Proc.*, Vol 381, 1995, p 19
116. J.O. Simpson and A.K. St. Clair, "Fundamental Insight on Developing Low Dielectric Constant Polyimides," *Thin Solid Films*, 1997, p 308–309
117. S. Hermciuc, E. Hamciuc, I. Sava, I. Diaconu, and M. Bruma, New Fluorinated Poly (Imide-Ether-Amide)s, *High Perform. Polym.*, Vol 12, 2000, p 205–276
118. J.L. Hedrick and Y. Charlier, High Temperature Polyimide Nanofoams, *Polym. Prepr.*, Vol 35 (No. 1), 1994, p 245–346
119. J.L. Hedrick, K.R. Carter, R. Ritcher, R.D. Miller, T.P. Russell, V. Flores, D. Meccereyes, and P.H. Jerome, Polyimide Nanofoams from Alphatic Polyester-Based Copolymers, *Chem. Mater.*, Vol 10 (No. 1), 1998, p 39–49
120. S. Tamai, W. Yamashita, and A. Yamaguchi, Thermo-Oxidatively Stable Polyimides and Their Chemical Structures, *J. Polym. Sci. A, Polym. Chem.*, Vol 36, 1998, p 1717–1723
121. I.C. Kim, J.H. Kim, K.H. Lee, and T.M. Tak, Preparation of Soluble Polyimides and Ultrafiltration Membrane Performances, *J. Appl. Polym. Sci.*, Vol 75, 2000, p 1–9
122. G.A. Polotskaya, V.P. Sklizkova, N.D. Kozhurnikova, G.K. Elyashevich, and V.V. Kudryavtsev, Formation and Analysis of a Polyimide Layer in Composite Membranes, *J. Polym. Sci.*, Vol 75, 2000, p 1026–1032
123. S.B. Mkasks, R.V. Bhingarkar, M.B. Sabne, R. Mercier, and S.P. Vernekar, Synthesis and Characterization of End-Capped Polyimides and Their Gas Permeability Properties, *J. Appl. Polym. Sci.*, Vol 77 (No. 3), 2000, p 627–635
124. J.H. Kim, B.-J. Chang, S.-B. Lee, and S.Y. Kim, Incorporation of Fluorinated Side Groups into Polyimide Membranes on Their Pervaporation Properties, *J. Membr. Sci.*, Vol 169 (No. 2), 2000, p 185–196
125. J. Fang, H. Kita, and K. Okamoto, Hyperbranched Polyimides for Gas Separation Applications I, Syntheses and Character-

ization, *Macromolecules*, Vol 33 (No. 13), 2000, p 4639–4660

126. C.J. Wang, W. Harrison, J. Mecham, R. Formato, R. Kovan, P. Osenar, and J.E. McGrath, Synthesis of Sulfonated Poly (Arylene Ether Sulfones) via Direct Polymerization, *Polym. Prepr.* Vol 41 (No. 1), 2000, p 237–2381
127. Y. Zhang, M. Litt, R.F. Savinell, J.S. Wainright, and J. Vandramini, Molecular Design of Polyimides Toward High Proton Conducting Meterials, *Polym. Prepr.*, Vol 41 (No. 2), 2000, p 1651–1562
128. C.S. Wang and T.S. Leu, Soluble Polyimides Containing Napthalene Structure, *Polym. Prepr.* Vol 41 (No. 2), 2000, p 1205–1206
129. T.L. Grubb, K.L. Ulery, T.J. Smith, G.L. Tullos, H. Yagci, L.J. Mathia, and M. Langsam, Highly Soluble Polyimides from Sterically Hindered Diamines, *Polymer*, Vol 40, 1999, p 4279–4288
130. I.C. Kim and J.M. Tak, Synthesis and Characterization of Soluble Random Coplyimides, *J. Appl. Polym. Sci.*, Vol 74, 1999, p 272–277
131. C.-P. Yang and H.-W. Yang, Preparation and Characterization of Organosoluble Copolyimides Based on a Pair of Commercial Aromatic Dianhydride and One Aromatic Diamine, 1,4-Bis (4-Aminophenoxy)-2-Tert-Butybenzene Series, *J. Appl. Polym. Sci.*, Vol 75 (No. 1), 2000, p 87–95
132. S.Z.D. Cheng, F. Li, E.P. Savitsks, and F.W. Harris, Molecular Design of Aromatic Polyimide Films, as Uniaxial Negative Birefrigent Optical Compensators in Liquid Crystal Displays, *TRIP*, Vol 5 (No. 2), Feb 1997, p 51–58
133. B. Li, T. He, and M. Ding, Correlation Between Chain Conformation and Optical Anisotropy of Thin Films of an Organo-Soluble Polyimide, *Polymer*, Vol 38 (No. 26), 1997, p 6413–6416
134. S. Akimoto, M. Jikei, and M.-A. Kakimoto, A Novel Photosensitive Polyimide: A Polyimide Containing the Hydroxy Triphenylamine Structure with Diazonaphthoquinone, *High Perform. Polym.*, Vol 21 (No. 11), 2000, p 177–184
135. L. Bes, A. Rosseau, B. Bouterin, R. Mercier, B. Sillion, and E. Joussaere, Synthesis and Characterization of Aromatic Polyimides Bearing Nonlinear Optical Chromophores, *High Perform. Polym.*, Vol 12 (No. 1), 2000, p 169–176
136. M.H. Davey, V.Y. Lee, L.-M. Wu, C.R. Moylan, W. Volksen, A. Knoesen, R.D. Miller, and T.J. Marks, Ultra High Temperature Polymers for Second-Order Nonlinear Optics, Synthesis and Properties of Robust, Processable, Chromophere-Embedded Polyimides, *Chem. Mater.*, Vol 12 (No. 6), 2000, p 1679–1693
137. H.Y. Woo, H.-K. Shim, K.-S. Lee, M.-Y. Jeong, and T.-K. Lim, An Alternate Synthetic Approach For Soluble Non-Linear Optical Polyimides, *Chem. Mater.*, Vol 11 (No. 2), 1999, p 218–226
138. K. Han, W.-H. Jang, and T.-H. Rhee, Syntheses of Fluorinated Polyimide and Their Application of Passive Optical Waveguides, *J. Appl. Polym. Sci.*, Vol 72 (No. 10), 2000, p 2172–2177
139. M. Berrada, F. Carriere, B. Coutin, P. Monjol, H. Sekiguchi, and R. Mercier, Novel Negative-Type Soluble Photosensitive Polyimides: Synthesis and Characterization, *Chem. Mater.*, Vol 8 (No. 5), 1996, p 1029–1034
140. Y. Chen and J.O. Iroh, Synthesis and Characterization of Polyimide/Silica Hybrid Composites, *Chem. Mater.,* Vol 11, 1999, p 1218–1222
141. S.J. Hobsen and K.J. Shea, Bridged Bisimide Polysilsequioxane Xerogels: New Hybrid Organic-Inorganic Materials, *Chem. Mater*., Vol 9, 1997, p 616–623
142. E.S. Weiser, J.F. Johnson, T.L. St. Clair, Y. Echigo, H. Kaneshiro, and B.W. Grimsley, Polyimide Foams for Aerospace Vehicles, *High Perform. Polym.*, Vol 12, 2000, p 1–12
143. V.E. Yudin, J.U. Otaigbe, and V.N. Artemiera, Processing and Properties of a New High Temperature Lightweight Composites Based on Foam Polyimide Binder, *Polym. Comp.*, Vol 20 (No. 3), 1999, p 337–345

Phenolic Resins

Shahid P. Qureshi, Georgia-Pacific Resins, Inc.

PHENOLICS are thermosetting resins produced by the reaction of phenol or substituted phenol with an aldehyde, usually formaldehyde, in the presence of a catalyst (Ref 1). Phenolic resin composites offer superior fire resistance, excellent high-temperature performance, long-term durability, and resistance to hydrocarbon and chlorinated solvents. This article describes the chemistry of phenolic resins, reviews their characteristics and properties for various composites manufacturing processes, and discusses some representative applications.

Phenolic Resin Chemistry

In the reaction of the phenol with the aldehyde, the catalyst used and the ratio of formaldehyde to phenol determines the type of resin produced. Phenolic resins based on an acid catalyst and formaldehyde-to-phenol (F/P) molar ratio of less than 0.9 to 1 are called novolacs, and those prepared from an alkaline catalyst and an F/P molar ratio of greater than 0.9:1 are known as resoles. Oxalic and sulfuric acids are used to synthesize novolacs. Aliphatic amines or hydroxides of ammonium, sodium, lithium, potassium, barium, and calcium are used to produce resoles. For both novolacs and resoles, 37–52% formaldehyde solution in water (methylene glycol, $CH_2(OH)_2$ is commonly used.

For novolac synthesis, the initial reaction is the formation of a carbonium ion by the action of the acid catalyst on the methylene glycol; this ion then reacts with phenol to produce methylolphenol:

$$HO\text{-}CH_2\text{-}OH + H^+ \rightarrow HO\text{-}CH_2^+ + H_2O$$

methylene glycol, acid, carbonium ion, water

$$HO{-}CH_2^{\oplus} + \text{phenol} \longrightarrow \text{methylol phenol} + H^{\oplus}$$

carbonium ion, phenol, methylol phenol, acid

In an acidic medium, the methylol group is extremely unstable and will react immediately with an additional phenol or methylolated phenol to produced novolac:

$$\text{methylol phenol} + \text{phenol} \longrightarrow \text{diphenyl methane} + H_2O$$

methylol phenol, phenol, diphenyl methane, water

Diphenyl methane is the novolac with the lowest molecular weight. Novolacs are thermoplastic resins and require a coreactant hexamethylenetetramine (HEXA) to become thermosetting resins. The reaction requires heat.

Synthesis of base-catalyzed resole proceeds via addition of formaldehyde to phenol to produce hydroxymethyl phenols:

$$C_6H_5OH + NaOH \longrightarrow C_6H_5O^- + Na^+ + H_2O$$

phenol, caustic, phenolic anion

This phenolic anion then reacts with the hydrated formaldehyde (methylene glycol) to produce a methylolphenol:

$$\text{phenolic anion} + HO{-}CH_2{-}OH \longrightarrow \text{ortho methylol phenol} + OH^{\ominus}$$

phenolic anion, methylene glycol, ortho methylol phenol, alkali

trimethylol phenol

Resoles contain various orthomethylol and para methylol groups, free phenol, free formaldehyde, water, and/or solvent. Resoles do not require an external catalyst and undergo self-polymerization under heat with evolution of water. The versatility of phenolic resins in a broad spectrum of market areas requires the production of novolac and resole resins in a variety of physical states, such as powder, hot melt, solvent-based, or aqueous solution resins.

Novolac powders with HEXA are commonly used in molding compounds with chopped glass and carbon fibers. Other applications include the binder in brake linings, grinding wheels, foundry molds, and general molding compounds. In more recently developed composite applications, novolac/HEXA are not used because they do not meet processing and cure requirements of composite fabrication processes.

Phenolic resole resins are commonly used in manufacturing of fiber reinforced composites. The use of phenolic resins in glass and carbon fiber composites is growing, primarily due to their low flame spread, low smoke generation, and low smoke toxicity properties (Ref 2, 3), which are achieved without the use of mineral fillers or fire retardant additives (Fig. 1 and Tables 1 and 2). In some specialty applications, the demand is increasing for high-temperature phenolics. If properly formulated and cured, phenolics perform much like high-temperature polyimides (Ref 4). Phenolics also provide excellent chemical resistance, to such compounds as chlorinated and hydrocarbon solvents (Ref 5). Interestingly, with all these superior properties, phenolics are relatively inexpensive.

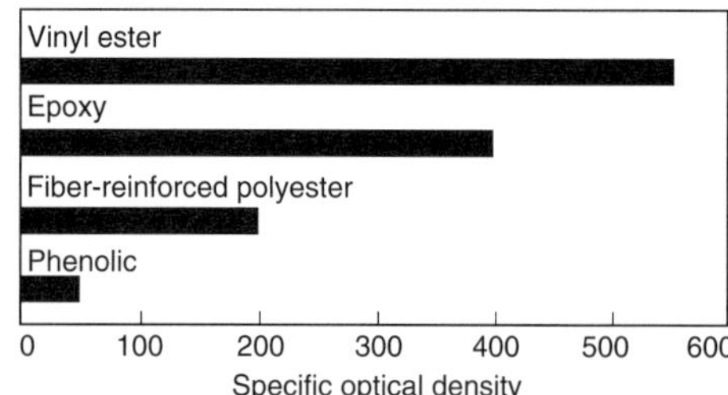

Fig. 1 Smoke optical density (ASTM E 662) comparison of selected resins

Table 1 Flame spread index and smoke density comparison of thermosetting resins (ASTM E 84 tunnel test)

Resin	Flame spread index	Smoke density
Phenolic	10	10
Halogenated polyester	15	600–800
Halogenated vinyl ester	45	600–800
Methacrylate vinyl ester with 150 phr aluminum trihydrate	20	40

phr, parts per hundred parts resin

In the 1980s, the Federal Aviation Administration tightened aerospace fire specifications for smoke and heat release tests. The purpose was to increase the evacuation time for passengers in airplane fires to exit safely. Glass and carbon fiber composites made with phenolic resins met these severe fire specifications. Today, phenolic composites are the material of choice for walls, ceilings, and floors of aircraft interiors (Ref 6). Since 1990, the use of phenolic resins has been gradually increasing for nonaerospace applications, which include mass transit, construction, marine, mine ducting, and offshore structures (Ref 7–13). These areas traditionally used other resins, such as polyesters, vinyl esters, and epoxies. These resins are being replaced with phenolics for specific applications with stringent fire resistance requirements.

To participate in the growing market, phenolic resin manufacturers have responded to the current and future market needs and have tailored the resin chemistry for the following state-of-the-art fabrication processes: solution/hot-melt process, pultrusion, vacuum infusion, filament winding, sheet molding, and hand lay-up (Ref 5, 13–15). Typical viscosity and cure characteristics of phenolic resins for these processes are summarized in Table 3.

Further details on fabrication processes, phenolic technology, and recent applications for phenolic composites are detailed below.

Phenolic Prepregs

The solution process involves impregnation of unidirectional fiber, woven fabric, or nonwoven fabric with phenolic resin having viscosity from 0.3–1.0 Pa · s (300–1000 cP) at 25 °C (77 °F) with 40–75% solids. Methanol, ethanol, isopropanol, and ketones are common solvents. For the solution process, the substrate is passed through a resin-containing bath and then into a heated vertical or horizontal tower for removal of solvent and water and B-staging. Process parameters are adjusted to achieve desired combination of flow, resin content, tack, and volatiles. The treated material, called *prepreg*, is rolled for storage and shipping. Phenolic prepregs offer significantly longer storage life than epoxy prepregs due to the nature of the phenolic chemistry. Prepregs are cured under heat (120–175 °C, or 250–350 °F) and pressure (345–3450 kPa, or 50–500 psi) to prepare laminates. Manufacturers of phenolic prepregs are Cytec-Fiberite, M.C. Gill, Hexcel, J.D. Lincoln, Lewcott Corporation, and Aerocell.

Conventional applications of solution-based thermal cured phenolic composites are in ballistic components. Typical properties are summarized in Table 4 (Ref 5). The composites are prepared with unmodified resin (Borden SC1008, GP 445D05) and polyvinyl butyral and with woven fabric of aramid, S-glass, or ultra-high molecular weight polyethylene. The composites are used in helmets, land vehicles, and military aircraft. Other traditional applications of solution prepreg include a carbon-carbon composite. The phenolic/carbon fiber prepreg is cured and carbonized to achieve carbon-carbon composite (Ref 16). These composites are used when high temperature performance is critical; current applications include rocket motors, aerospace engine components, aircraft brakes, and racing car brakes.

Table 2 Pittsburgh smoke toxicity test results for selected resins

Material	LC_{50}(a), g
Phenolic	86.5
Unsaturated polyester	34.0
Halogenated polyester	9.1
Epoxy	23.0
Polyvinyl chloride	8–30

(a) LC_{50} indicates the mass of material required to cause smoke concentration that is fatal to 50% of test animals after 30 minutes of exposure when burned at 822 °C (1510 °F). Lower values indicate greater toxicity.

Phenolic Honeycomb

Phenolic prepregs based on carbon, aramid, or glass fibers are used as face sheets on Nomex honeycomb to construct sandwich panels for aerospace applications such as cargo liners, walls, galleys, ceilings, and floors. The sandwich panel structure is selected due to its high strength-to-weight ratio. For densification, Nomex honeycomb is also treated with either solvent or waterborne phenolic resole resins (Ref 17). There is no alternate resin that meets the adhesion, low flammability, and processing requirements of Nomex honeycomb. For aerospace honeycomb applications, the honeycomb phenolic resin should meet requirements, such as those specified in MIL-R-9299C (now cancelled). This specification calls for the extensive evaluation of mechanical properties at room temperature and at 260 °C (500 °F). Several commercial resins, such as SC1008 (Borden) and GP 5236, GP 445D05, and GP 307T35 (Georgia-Pacific), have achieved the requirements outlined in this specification. Compressive, tensile, and flexural properties of phenolic/glass laminates (containing at least 14 plies) meet MIL-R-9299C specification requirements and are similar to those reported for epoxy and polyester composites (Ref 18–19). Sandwich panels based on Nomex honeycomb, prepreg face sheets, and Tedlar (polyvinyl fluoride) decorative film have been used for ceilings and side walls of aircraft interiors (Boeing 8-222 specification).

The honeycomb manufacturing process is shown in Fig. 2. An aramid paper is used to manufacture untreated honeycomb. The honeycomb is coated with multiple layers of phenolic resin for densification of the honeycomb core. By using face sheets of phenolic composite for epoxy composites with a honeycomb core, the highest strength-to-weight and stiffness-to-weight ratios for many configurations can be obtained. Key aerospace requirements for the panels are low heat release, low smoke, and high peel strength (adhesion of cured prepreg to Nomex). For aircraft interiors, strength and flammability requirements continue to increase, and modified phenolics that achieve higher peel strength and maintain the flammability behavior of phenolics have been developed (Ref 6).

The following two prepreg products are commercially available: SP-2400 (Ref 6), which was developed for Boeing 8-226 specification, and Bakelite epoxy-modified phenolic (Ref 20–21), which is used for floors of the Airbus 340. Three Boeing specifications are summarized in Table 5.

The sandwich panels are also used in California's Bay Area Rapid Transit (BART) subway cars. Until 1979, BART passenger subway cars had relatively lenient flame spread and smoke specification requirements. A fire broke out onboard a BART subway train in the Transbay

Table 3 Phenolic resins for composites

Composites manufacturing process	Resin type (solvent)(a)	Viscosity at 25 °C (77 °F) Pa · s	cP	Catalyst	Cure temperature °C	°F
Filament winding	PF (water)	0.5–2.0	500–2,000	Acid	65–95	150–200
	PRF (water/alcohol)	0.5–2.0	500–2,000	Formaldehyde	25–65	75–150
Hand lay-up	PF (water)	0.5–2.0	500–2,000	Acid	25–80	75–180
Pultrusion	PF (water)	2.0–10.0	2,000–10,000	Base	165–245	325–475
	PRF (water/alcohol)	2.0–10.0	2,000–10,000	Formaldehyde	165–245	325–475
Sheet molding and bulk molding	PF (water)	1.0–2.0	1,000–2,000	Base	150–175	300–350
Solution	PF (water/alcohol)	0.3–1.0	300–1,000	Base/neutral	120–175	250–350
Hot melt	PF (water)	50–100	50,000–100,000	Base/neutral	120–175	250–350
Honeycomb	PF (water/alcohol)	0.5–1.0	500–1,000	Base/neutral	120–175	250–350

(a) PF, phenol formaldehyde; PRF, phenol resorcinal formaldehyde

Table 4 Properties of phenolic prepreg resins and composites

Property	Value
Flexural strength (ASTM D 790), MPa (ksi)	620–690 (90–100)
Flexural modulus (ASTM D 790), GPa (10^6 psi)	28–31 (4.0–4.5)
Tensile strength (ASTM D 638), MPa (ksi)	415–485 (60–70)
Compressive strength (ASTM D 695), MPa (ksi)	485–620 (70–90)
OSU heat release (ASTM E 906)	
At 2 min, kW · min/m^2	15
At peak, kW/m^2	30
NBS maximum smoke density (ASTM F 814)	15 (max)

Composite: 14-ply, 7781 glass, 30–32% resin, cured at 175 °C (350 °F) for 1 h at 1380 kPa (200 psi). Source: Ref 5 and 18

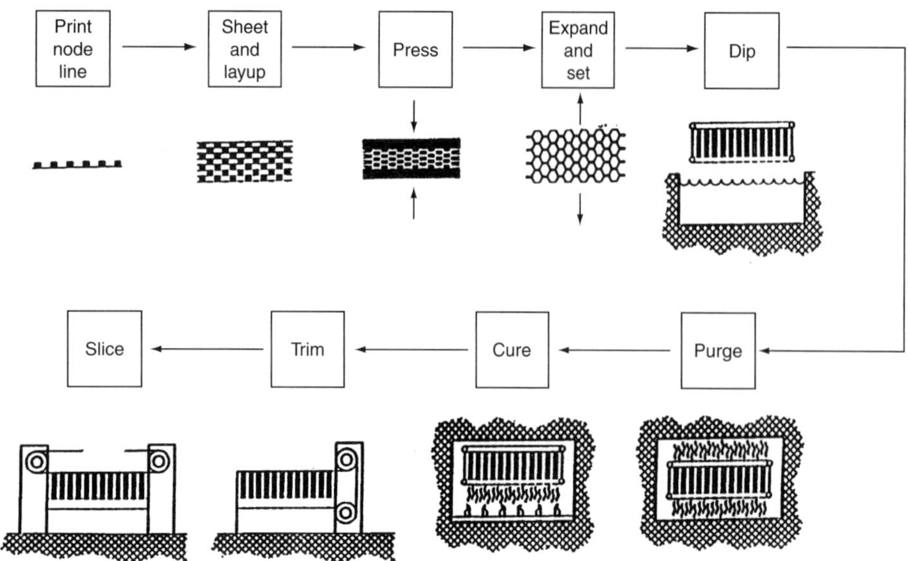

Fig. 2 Honeycomb manufacturing process

Table 5 Boeing phenolic prepreg specification requirements for aircraft interior structures

Property	Sandwich panels and laminates (BMS 8-226)	Crushed core glass fiber (BMS 8-222)	Crushed core graphite fiber (BMS 8-274)
NBS maximum smoke density at 4 min	20 max	20 max	20 max
OSU heat release			
At 2 min, kW · min/m^2	30–65	65	30–65
At peak, kW/m^2	45–65	65	45–65
Peel strength in 76 mm (3 in.) width, N/m (lbf/in.)	1750 (10)	1050–1750 (6–10)	875–1225 (5–7)
Flexural strength, MPa (ksi)	61–138 (8.8–20.0)	83–110 (12.0–16.0)	124–143 (18.0–20.7)

Tunnel, killing a fireman and injuring 46 passengers. As a result of this tragedy, the California Public Utility Commission ordered BART to use phenolic composites for ceilings, sidewalls, and endwalls (Ref 22).

Phenolic Pultrusion

Pultrusion is a cost-effective process that provides composites on a continuous basis. Fibers are pulled through a resin bath and then through the heated die. At the end of the die, sufficiently cured and rigid composite is pulled and cut to desired length. The most commonly used resins are unsaturated polyesters and vinyl esters with peroxide catalysts; these composites are useful in marine applications, power transmission, and construction. Phenolic resole resins are used to manufacture pultruded composites when low flammability is needed. Thermal-cured (without an external catalyst) and formaldehyde-cured resorcinol resins have been successfully converted to pultruded composites. Phenolic resins with viscosity of 2–10 Pa · s (2,000–10,000 cP) and 68 to 75% solids have been processed through the pultrusion equipment (Ref 10, 13, 23). The viscosity range desired for the process is achieved through residual water, phenol monomer, and/or ethanol. Due to low viscosity, fillers (clay, zinc borate, and/or aluminum trihydrate) at the 10 to 20% level can be used to obtain a smooth surface. Compared to polyesters, phenolic pultruded parts contain higher fiber volume (due to solvent loss and to counteract the inherent brittleness of phenolics); however, the mechanical properties are similar (Ref 10). Mechanical properties of phenolic and polyester pultruded composites are compared in Table 6 (Ref 10).

In the phenolic pultrusion process, Strongwell has conducted extensive research and has manufactured phenolic grating for offshore oil platforms. The grating can withstand direct flame contact without major structural damage. Also, it has low thermal conductivity and the strength of steel grating at a lighter weight than steel. Phenolic grating can withstand 1.75 times the load of equivalent steel grating. This combination of properties was not available with alternate organic matrix materials. Therefore, phenolic grating has replaced steel grating at several offshore oil platforms.

For these first commercial applications of phenolic grating, glass fiber and mold release suppliers have developed phenolic-compatible mat, roving, and mold release chemicals. Phenolic resins from Georgia-Pacific and Borden Chemical have been qualified (Ref 14, 23) for the grating applications. Research work continues (Ref 23–25) to improve the strength and toughness of phenolic pultruded composites to extend their applications into structural areas such as walkways, decking for tunnels/mass transit, and automotive, aircraft, and marine structures. To extend into structural applications, toughened phenolic resin technology is needed. The market requirements are faster line speeds and at least 20% higher strength than the first-generation products. In this area, the line speed has been improved from 25–76 cm/min (10–30 in./min) (Ref 25), and a 20% improvement in strength has been achieved (Table 7).

Table 6 Properties of glass-fiber-reinforced phenolic and polyester pultruded composites

Property	Phenolic	Polyester
Tensile strength, MPa (ksi)	310 (45)	483 (70)
Flexural strength, MPa (ksi)	359 (52)	607 (88)
Compressive strength, MPa (ksi)	352 (51)	310 (45)

Source: Ref 10

Table 7 Properties of catalyzed phenolic pultruded composites

Property	Latent base catalyst, phr(b) 0	5	10
Line speed, cm/min (in./min)	76 (30)	76 (30)	76 (30)
Glass-transition temperature (T_g), max(a), °C (°F)	308 (586)	326 (619)	335 (635)
Flexural strength, MPa (ksi)	403 (58.5)	417 (60.5)	481 (69.8)
Flexural modulus, GPa (10^6 psi)	14.8 (2.14)	16.1 (2.33)	16.5 (2.39)
Short beam shear strength, MPa (ksi)	24.8 (3.6)	25.5 (3.7)	29.0 (4.2)

Pultruded bar, 64 × 3 mm (2.5 × 1/8 in.). Pultrusion temperature conditions: zone 1, 205 °C (400 °F); zone 2, 230 °C (450 °F); zone 3, 245 °C (475 °F). Fiber roving, Johns Manville 507AA-13; mat, CertainTeed Uniflo U528. (a) As determined by dynamic mechanical analysis (DMA) loss modulus. (b) phr, parts per hundred parts resin

Phenolic Filament Winding

Filament winding of phenolics has been well established in the industry. Phenol-formaldehyde resins with an acid catalyst and resorcinol resins with paraformaldehyde catalyst are currently used. The process of filament winding with phenolic systems is little different in principle from winding with other systems such as vinyl esters, polyesters, and epoxies. The processing requirements include the following:

- Resin viscosity of 0.5–2.0 Pa · s (500–2000 cP)
- Pot life for resin/catalyst mixture must be greater than 30 min
- Gel time at 80 °C (180 °F) must be 90–150 s
- Cure temperature must be 65–95 °C (150–200 °F)

Resin manufacturers have developed latent acids for filament winding phenolic resin (Ref 13, 26–28). The latent catalyst gives pot lives equal to those of polyester mixes, while maintaining the cure speed required by fabricators. After a 50–80 °C (120–180 °F) cure, filament-wound pipes give adequate strength and dimensional stability and glass-transition temperatures (T_g) from 95–150 °C (200–300 °F). If a higher T_g is needed, the pipes are removed from the mandrel and then post-cured for T_g improvement. Table 8 shows the T_g development with cure of a filament-wound pipe (Ref 29).

Due to superior fire resistance, phenol-formaldehyde-based filament-wound composites are currently being used for ventilation ducting in mining and tunneling. Applications include such projects as the Channel Tunnel and the Thames Water London Ring Main. The pipes are used in mining to carry methane. Besides being fire safe, they are extremely light to handle (approximately a quarter of the weight of steel), and the installation rates are up to six times faster than those for the equivalent steel pipe. Phenol-resorcinol-formaldehyde resins have been used since the 1980s in Factory Mutual clean room ducting applications (Fig. 3) (Ref 30–31).

Filament wound phenolic composites are being used for offshore oil platform water piping systems. The state-of-the-art technology is based on a filament wound epoxy resin system. To meet the severe fire requirements, the epoxy pipes required a thick layer of intumescent coating. To eliminate this labor intensive and costly procedure, Ameron Fiberglass Pipe Group developed phenolic pipes that have passed the fire and high-temperature tests without the intumescent coating. The filament-wound pipe, based on a polysiloxane-modified phenolic system, demonstrated higher mechanical properties and improved weathering resistance than the pipes without the siloxane modification (Ref 32). The piping system (pipes, joints, and adhesives) under jet fire certification must withstand 5 minutes of exposure in dry state, followed by 15 minutes of exposure, filled with flowing water at 1000 kPa (10 bar) pressure. The piping system will not only survive a fire, but will also deliver pressurized water where it is needed at the critical times.

For protection of damaged utility and transmission poles, PoleCare Industries, a subsidiary of Chemical Specialties, Inc., has wrapped the poles with latent-acid-cured phenolic resin and glass fabric composites. This approach is more cost-effective than replacing the pole, due to the complexity of the system supported by the pole. Repaired phenolic-wrapped poles perform better than new ones. The composite wrap increases strength, and the fire resistance is an advantage for farming areas, where fields are burned off, and in regions such as California, where wildfires are a continual threat. The long-term durability of the phenolic-wrapped pole is currently being monitored by nondestructive tests. After five years in the field, the wrapped poles show no apparent degradation in performance or durability (Ref 5).

Phenolic Sheet Molding Compounds

The use of phenolics for sheet molding compounds (SMC) has been researched since the 1980s (Ref 33). The technology challenge was to match resin viscosity, handling, and cure properties of the polyester SMC to avoid any special processing and equipment adjustments for fabricators and end users. Both acid-catalyzed and base-catalyzed phenolics have been investigated. An acid-catalyzed system is not acceptable due to corrosion of the existing polyester molds. For SMC processes, resin requirements are low viscosity (greater than 1.5 Pa · s, or 1500 cP, at 25 °C, or 77 °F), high solids (less than 75%), and minimal levels of monomers (phenol, formaldehyde) and solvents (water, alcohol). A typical SMC composition is shown in Table 9. The SMC product is aged/matured to achieve desired release and flow for molding. The maturation time depends on the level and type of catalysts. Recently, latent-based catalysts were found effective in reducing the maturation time without any reduction in shelf life of the matured SMC.

Quantum Composites has commercialized nonacid phenolic SMC products for specific aircraft and military applications. In the aerospace industry, phenolic SMC products have been successfully produced by Kaiser Compositek since 1993 as air scoops in inner fan duct for aircraft engine structures. Phenolic SMC was chosen because of the ease of molding to the required shape with light.

Recently, a chopped carbon fiber/phenolic SMC product, Enduron 4685 by Fiberite, was used to manufacture the base and cover of the IBM Think Pad 701 (Ref 34). Key attributes of

Table 8 Flexural properties and glass-transition temperatures for filament-wound pipes

Property	Polyester	Latent acid cured phenolic
Resin content, %	43.1	38.7
Flexural strength, MPa (ksi)	460 (66.7)	386 (56.0)
Flexural modulus, GPa (10^6 psi)	10.5 (1.53)	15.9 (2.3)
Glass-transition temperature (T_g), °C (°F)	120 (250)	120 (250)
After postcure(a)	130 (270)	155 (310)
After postcure(b)	135 (275)	205 (400)
After postcure(c)	140 (280)	230 (450)

(a) 30 min at 150 °C (300 °F). (b) 30 min at 150 °C (300 °F) + 30 min at 175 °C (350 °F). (c) 30 min at 150 °C (300 °F) + 30 min at 175 °C (350 °F) + 30 min at 205 °C (400 °F)

Table 9 Typical composition of a phenolic sheet molding compound

Material	Content, parts by weight
Phenolic resin (GP 652D58)	100.0
Base catalyst (GP 012G23)	2.0
Calcium oxide	1.5
Clay	60.0
Chopped glass fiber	60.0
Release agent	1.0

Typical cure, 150–205 °C (300–400 °F) for 2–5 min

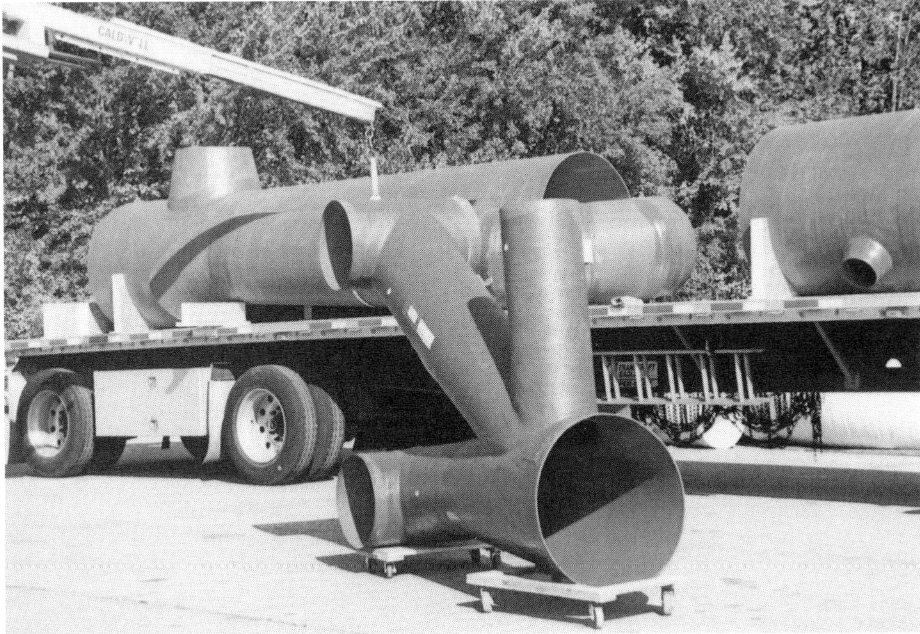

Fig. 3 Factory Mutual filament-wound phenolic ducting. Courtesy of Composites USA

Table 10 Properties of phenolic and polyester hand lay-up composites

Property	Phenolic	Polyester
Flexural strength, MPa (ksi)	225 (32.6)	235 (34.1)
Flexural modulus, GPa (10^6 psi)	12.4 (1.8)	9.7 (1.4)

carbon fiber/phenolic SMC are high thermal resistance (since newer computers generate more heat) and a very low shrinkage value.

Phenolics for Hand Lay-Up

The hand lay-up or wet lay-up process is widely used for making composites with chopped strand mat and polyester resins. Resin requirements are a viscosity of 0.5–2.0 Pa · s (500–2000 cP), 10–60 min pot life for resin/catalyst mixture, and 60–80 °C (140–175 °F) cure temperature. Due to the market demand, phenolic technology was advanced to achieve polyester-like processing, mechanical properties (Table 10), pot life, and cure speed.

Waterborne phenolic resole resins with sulfonic acid and phosphate ester catalyst are used for hand lay-up processes. The latent phosphate ester (Ref 27) or phosphonic acid (Ref 28), in conjunction with p-toluene sulfonic acid, was effective in meeting pot life and cure speed requirements of the hand lay-up process. Due to the condensation cure and solvent loss, phenolic laminates are more porous than polyester laminates. This shortcoming is addressed using a phenolic-based surface coat. A thixotropic phenolic-based surface paste is available. The paste is brushed or sprayed on the mold and allowed to partially cure before the glass is applied and the hand lay-up process is completed. The surface paste-coated panels are then subjected to the desired paint color. This is a three-step process, compared to the two-step process of lay-up and gel coating for polyester laminates; fabricators have requested a pigmentable phenolic-compatible gel coat to eliminate the painting step. Recently, acrylic gel coats that show good adhesion to the phenolic composite substrate have been introduced. Developmental work continues to meet the needs of the mass transit industry with phenolics.

In Europe, hand lay-up phenolic composites have been used in mass transit since 1988, after a fire broke out at the King's Cross Station, which killed thirty-one people and injured several hundred others. In response to this tragedy, the British government established a Code of Practice (BS 6853) that includes flame spread and smoke limitations for composites used in underground railways. Phenolic composites from Georgia-Pacific and Borden Cellobond products are the only composites that meet the code requirement (Ref 22). Most of the underground railways in France and the Scandinavian countries have followed the specifications of the United Kingdom and switched to phenolic composites.

For mass transit applications in the United States, the current flame spread index requirements (less than 35, per ASTM E 162) and smoke emission specifications (smoke density at 4 min less than 200) for passenger rail vehicles can be met with fiber-reinforced polyesters and vinyl esters. However, with an increasing awareness for reducing fire hazards and improving passenger safety, the United States may follow the example of Britain. If the smoke specification requirement is reduced to less than 20, the use of phenolics will be required (Ref 35).

Recently, phenolic hand lay-up, latent-acid-cure technology has been used to manufacture large (1.8 by 5.4 m, or 6 by 18 ft) panels for constructing composite homes. American Structural Composites (Reno, NV) demonstrated the advantages of phenolic composite homes compared with homes built with traditional construction materials. The phenolic panels eliminate the possibility of termite damage and provide better fire safety and easier construction (Ref 36).

Conclusions

In the 1990s, phenolic resin technology advanced to meet the processing requirements of state-of-the-art composites fabrication processes. Phenolic resin composites offer superior fire resistance, excellent high-temperature performance, long-term durability, and resistance in hydrocarbon and chlorinated solvents. These benefits are available at no additional cost, compared to other thermosetting resins. Mechanical properties of the composite depend on the fabrication process, resin content, and fiber configuration. Fire safety attributes are less sensitive to these variables; they are more a function of the resin/fiber ratio. In recent years, the technology improvements in phenolic resins include the development of low-emission resins, latent acids for desired pot life/cure temperature, and modifiers for higher strength. Application of phenolic composites continues to increase where fire safety is a primary requirement.

REFERENCES

1. A. Gardziella, L.A. Pilato, and A. Knop, *Phenolic Resins Chemistry, Applications, Standardization, Safety and Ecology,* Springer-Verlag, 1999
2. T.H. Dailey, Jr. and J. Shuff, "Phenolic Resins Enhance Public Safety by Reducing Smoke, Fire and Toxicity in Composites," paper presented at the 46th Annual Conf., Composites Institute, 18–21 Feb 1991, Society of the Plastics Industry Inc.
3. U. Sorathia, T. Dapp, and C. Beck, *Fire Performance of Composites, Mater. Eng.,* Sept 1992, p 10
4. "High Temperature Graphite Phenolic Composites," NASA Tech Briefs MFS 28795, Technical Support Package, George C. Marshall Space Flight Center, 1994
5. A. Mekjian and S.P. Qureshi, "Phenolic Resins Technology," paper presented at the Composites Fabricator Association Annual Convention, 18–21 Oct 1995
6. H. Gupta and M. McCabe, "Advanced Phenolic Systems for Aircraft Interior," paper presented at the FAA International Conf. for the Promotion of Advanced Fire Resistant Aircraft Interior Materials (Atlantic City, NJ), 9–11 Feb 1993
7. K.L. Forsdyke, "Phenolic Matrix Resins: The Way to Safer Reinforced Plastics," paper presented at the 46th Annual Conf., Composite Institute, 18–21 Feb 1991, Society of the Plastics Industry Inc.
8. S.F. Trevor, "Fire Hard Composites," tutorial seminar presented at the 40th SAMPE Symposium, 8–11 May 1995
9. A. Mekjian, "Phenolic RTM: A Boon to Mass Transit," paper presented at the 49th Annual Conf.: Session 2-B, Composite Institute, Society of the Plastics Industry Inc., 1994
10. S.P. Qureshi, "High Performance Phenolic Pultrusion Resin," paper presented at the 51st Annual Conf., Composites Institute, Society of the Plastics Industry Inc., 1996
11. J.L. Folker and R.S. Friedrich, High Performance Modified-Phenolic Piping System, *Proc. International Composites Expo '97* (Nashville, TN), Session 22A, 1998
12. K. Namaguchi, "Phenolic Composites in Japan," a database of the American Chemical Society, paper presented at the 54th Annual Conf., Composites Institute, Society of Plastics Industry Inc., 1999
13. J.G. Taylor, Phenolic Resin Systems for Pultrusion, Filament Winding and Other Composite Fabrication Methods, *44th International SAMPE Symposium,* Society for the Advancement of Material and Process Engineering, 23–27 May 1999, p 1123
14. "Dura Grid Phenolic Grating," product bulletin, Strongwell, Bristol, VA, 1996
15. G. Walton, Manufacturers Tackle Phenolic Processing Challenges, *High-Perform. Compos.,* Jan/Feb 1998
16. D.L. Schmidt, K.E. Davidson, and L.S. Theibert, *SAMPE J.,* Vol 32 (No. 4), 1996 p 44
17. S.P. Qureshi and R.A. McDonald, Low Emission, Water-Borne Phenolics for Prepregs and Honeycomb Applications, *37th International SAMPE Tech. Conf.,* Vol 39, Society for the Advancement of Material and Process Engineering, 1994, p 1023
18. S.P. Qureshi, "Fire Resistance and Mechanical Properties for Phenolic Prepregs," paper presented at the FAA International Conf. (Atlantic City, NJ), 9–11 Feb 1993
19. G. Lubin, *Handbook of Composites,* Van Nostrand Reinhold Company, New York, NY, 1982, p 146, 154
20. A. Butcher, L.A. Pilato and M.W. Klett, En-

vironmentally and User Friendly Phenolic Resin for Pultrusion, *International SAMPE Tech. Conf.,* Vol 29, Society for the Advancement of Material and Process Engineering, 1997, p 635
21. K. Jellinek, B. Meier, and J. Zehrfeld, Bakelite Patent EP 0242512, 1987
22. C. King and J.R. Zingaro, "Phenolic Composites in the Aircraft Industry and the Necessary Transition to the Mass Transit Rail Industry," paper presented at the 51st Annual Conf., Composites Institute, Society of the Plastics Industry Inc., 1996
23. J.F. Mayfield and J.G. Taylor, "Advanced Phenolic Pultruded Grating for Fire Retardant Applications," *31st International SAMPE Tech. Conf.,* 26–30 Oct 1999, Society for the Advancement of Material and Process Engineering, p 142
24. H.-D. Wu, M.-S. Lee, Y.-D. Wu, Y.-F. Su, and C.-C. Ma, "Pultruded Fiber-Reinforced Polyurethane-Toughened Phenolic Resin," *J. Appl. Polym. Sci.,* Vol 62, 1996, p 227–234
25. Product Brochure GP652D79/GP012G23 Pultrusion System, Georgia-Pacific, 2001
26. "Toughened Phenolic Resins for Pultrusion Applications," Georgia-Pacific Resins, Inc., unpublished results, Dec 2000
27. Process for Hardening Phenolic Resins, Patent EP 0539098, 1 July 1998
28. Thermosetting Phenolic Resin Composition, U.S. Patent 864,003, Jan 1999
29. S.P. Qureshi, Recent Developments in Phenolic Resins Technology and Composites Applications, *31st International SAMPE Tech. Conf.,* 26–30 Oct 1999, Society for the Advancement of Material and Process Engineering, p 150
30. "Factory Mutual Approved Products for Clean Room Ducting Applications," ATS Products, Richmond, California
31. U.S. Patent 5,202,189, 13 April 1993
32. Phenolic Resin Compositions with Improved Impact Resistance, U.S. Patent 5,736,619, 7 April 1998
33. M. Gupta and D.W. Hoch, Phenolic Sheer Molding Compounds, *31st International SAMPE Symposium,* 1986, Society for the Advancement of Material and Process Engineering, p 1486
34. K. Fisher, Fabricating with Chopped Carbon Composites, *High-Perform. Compos.,* Vol 5 (No. 1), 1997, p 23
35. "The Mass Transit Market Place," The Society of the Plastics Industry, Winter 1996
36. D.O. Carlson, Automated Fiberglass Composite Wall Panel Plant is Developing Housing's Future, *Automated Builder,* Feb 2000, p 8

Cyanate Ester Resins

Susan Robitaille, YLA Inc.

CYANATE ESTER (CE) RESINS are a family of high-temperature thermosetting resins—more accurately named polycyanurates—that bridge the gap in thermal performance between engineering epoxy and high-temperature polyimides. In addition to their outstanding thermal performance, CE resins have several desirable characteristics that justify their higher cost in many applications. They possess a unique balance of properties and are particularly notable for their low dielectric constant and dielectric loss, low moisture absorption, low shrinkage, and low outgassing characteristics. Despite their relatively high cost they have found wide applications in electronics, printed circuit boards, satellite and aerospace structural composites, and low-dielectric and radar applications. They can be formulated for use as high-performance adhesives, syntactic foams, honeycomb, and fiber-reinforced composites and are often found in blends with other thermosetting resins such as epoxy, bismaleimide, and engineering thermoplastics (Ref 1).

E. Grigat (Ref 2) first successfully synthesized aryl cyanate monomers in the early 1960s, and in 1963, a process was developed to produce the monomers commercially. In the 1970s, the first patents for CE resins were awarded to Bayer AG and Mobay. These patents focused primarily on their use in printed circuit boards (PCBs), using a bisphenol A-based prepolymer. In the late 1970s, patents were licensed to Mitsubishi Gas Chemical and Celanese. Mitsubishi marketed a CE and bismaleimide blend under the name BT resin. Both blended and 100% CE resins systems were initially targeted into the PCB industry. In the 1980s, Hi-Tech Polymers, formerly Celanese, was instrumental in the commercial development of CE resin technology by producing and characterizing a wide array of different polymer backbones with CE functionality. Dave Shimp and Steve Ising of Hi-Tech Polymers are noted for their great contribution to the applications and development of CE polymers during this period (Ref 1–3).

By the mid 1980s, work was proceeding on the development of commercial CE and CE/epoxy blends for aerospace and PCB applications. This work was undertaken because of keen interest in improving the hot/wet performance of composites for both structural composites and electronic applications. Cyanate esters were selected for development because of their excellent low moisture-absorbing characteristics and high mechanical and thermal performance. But, due to their high cost and lack of a comprehensive database, they did not penetrate into the large commercial aircraft and structural composite industry. They did, however, find acceptance for dimensionally critical applications in space structures where weight-to-stiffness trade-offs allow higher materials costs. Lower-cost CE resins and CE blends with epoxy and with bismaleimide were eventually developed and entered the electronics industry; these lower-cost resins and blends currently account for approximately 80% of CE use. Estimated CE resin use in 1999 was approximately 400,000 lb (Ref 4).

Cyanate Ester Chemistry

Cyanate ester resins are available as low-melt crystalline powder, liquid, and semisolid difunctional monomers and prepolymers of various molecular weights. Higher molecular weight resins are also available as solid flake or in solution. Prepolymers are formed by controlling the cyclotrimerization of monomers in an inert atmosphere, then thermally quenching the resin when it approaches the desired molecular weight.

The most widely used method for commercial production of CE resins is the low-temperature reaction of a cyanogen halide, such as cyanogen chloride, with alcohol or phenol in the presence of a tertiary amine. The low reaction temperatures are desirable in order to reduce the formation of the undesirable by-product diethylcyanamide, a volatile contaminant. It is also important to fully react the phenol during the synthesis, because free, unreacted phenol will catalyze the cyclotrimerization reaction, and significantly reduce shelf life of the resin, and increase the potential for an uncontrollable exothermic reaction during heating.

Due to the extreme hazard of handling and manufacturing with cyanogen halides, there are few companies in the world that are capable of producing commercial quantities of CE resins. As of 2001, Mitsubishi Gas Chemical, Lonza, and Vantico are the main suppliers of CE monomers and prepolymers.

Optionally, cyanogen bromide can be used instead of cyanogen chloride. Because it is a solid, it is easier to handle safely; however, it is more likely to form diethylcyanamide by reacting more aggressively with the tertiary amine. This can be avoided by substituting potassium or sodium hydroxide for the amine or by using alcoholates directly (Ref 1).

Commercially, CE resins are available in monomer and prepolymer forms with several different backbone structures. The general structure of CE resins is a bisphenol, aromatic, or cycloaliphatic backbone with generally two or more ring-forming cyanate functional groups (–O–C≡N–). The differences in backbone and the substituent pendent groups result in a variety of structure/property relationships. Table 1 describes the available physical forms of the monomers or prepolymers, their approximate cost, and the applications for each of the resin types. Materials suppliers formulate these basic components into proprietary systems by combining different CE resins or blending them with other thermosets or thermoplastics, or by adding catalysts, fillers, and flow and toughness modifiers. Cure, or conversion to a thermoset, occurs by cyclotrimerization of three functional groups to produce a triazine ring. The cured polymer forms a three-dimensional cross-linked network consisting of triazine rings linked to the backbone structure through ether groups. Figure 1 depicts the reaction from monomer to prepolymer to thermoset network. The resulting cured matrix has several interesting characteristics. In most cases, this type of linkage provides greater flexibility and higher strain to failure of the cured polymer than multifunctional, unmodified epoxies and bismaleimide resins (Ref 3, 5).

The selection of catalyst is important to the curing process of CE resins. Studies performed by D. Shimp et al. show that cure rates can vary depending on the type, addition level, and whether or not a reaction accelerator is used. The most common type of catalysts are chelates and carboxylate salts of transition metals. The metals act as coordination catalysts and complex with the –OCN groups, bringing three reactive groups together to form the triazine ring structure. The reaction does not evolve any volatiles. The transition metal used to catalyze the polymerization does not play an important role in the final properties of the fully cured polymer. This means that the same triazine ring structure will be produced, regardless of the type of transition metal selected; however, it does directly affect its percent conversion and cure rate at specific temperatures, which in turn affect the glass transition temperature (T_g) and the thermal oxidative and hydrolytic stability of the cured system.

Cyanate ester resins are autocatalytic at temperatures above 200 °C (390 °F) and can be cured without catalyst. Their heat of reaction is higher than epoxy resins, which can be problematic if attempting fast cure cycles of thick laminates or compounding large masses of polymer at elevated temperatures. The heat of reaction for the OCN groups are approximately 105 kJ/mole compared to 50 to 58 kJ/mole for epoxy systems. Cyanate ester resins are also sensitive to contaminants and impurities, especially phenols, transition metals, amines, Lewis acids, alcohols, and water, which will all increase the reaction rate (Ref 1, 6).

Properties and Characteristics

Many of the beneficial characteristics of CE resins contrast with those of epoxies and are directly related to the chemical structure of the resin. The most attractive attributes of CE chemistry evolve from the cured matrix structure. While there are differences in performance depending on the backbone structure and formulation, all forms contain a notably low concentration of dipoles and hydroxyl groups in the cured structure. They can also have a moderate cross-link density and high free volume. These

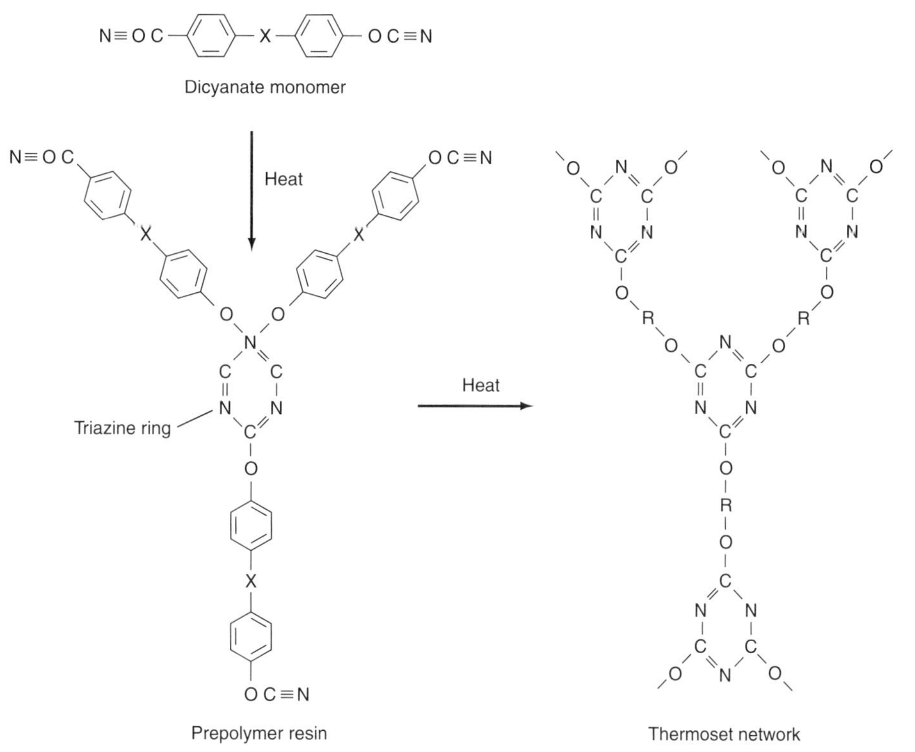

Dicyanate monomer

Heat

Triazine ring

Heat

Prepolymer resin

Thermoset network

Fig. 1 Cure of cyanate resins by cyclotrimerization of cyanate ester monomer and prepolymer

Table 1 Available forms of cyanate ester resins

Form	Structure	Physical state	Cost $/kg	Cost $/lb	Applications
XU366, 378	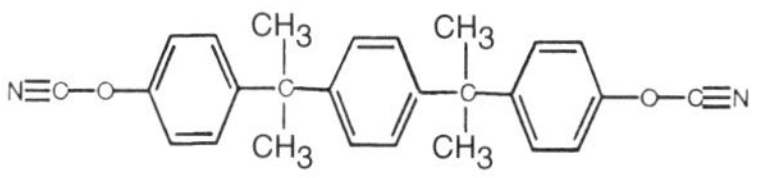	Viscous liquid, amorphous semisolid	29–34	65–75	Telecommunication satellites, radomes, adhesives (120 °C, or 250 °F, cure)
Bisphenol A dicyanate	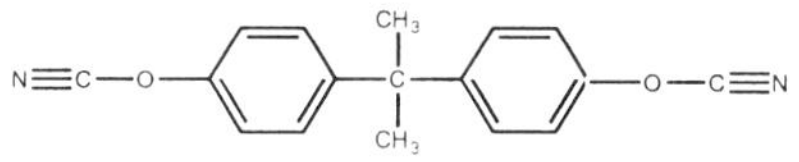	Crystal powder, viscous liquids, solid flake, solution	9–14	20–30	Radomes, multilayer high-speed printed circuit boards, solvent for thermoplastics
Ortho methyl dicyanate	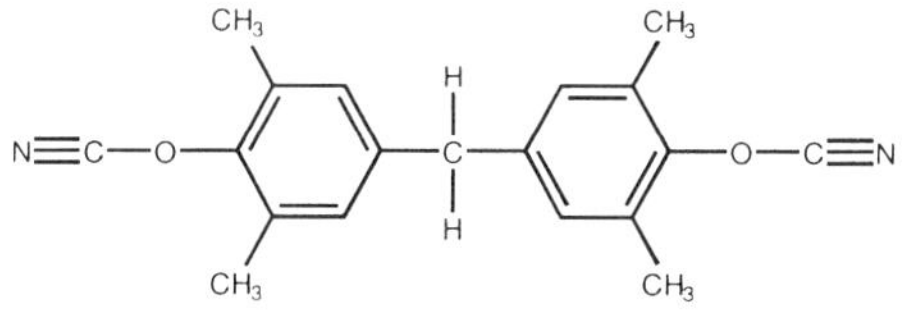	Crystal powder, semisolid, amorphous solid	11–14	25–30	Radomes, primary structures, flexible circuitry, high-speed printed circuit boards, adhesives
L-10 monomes	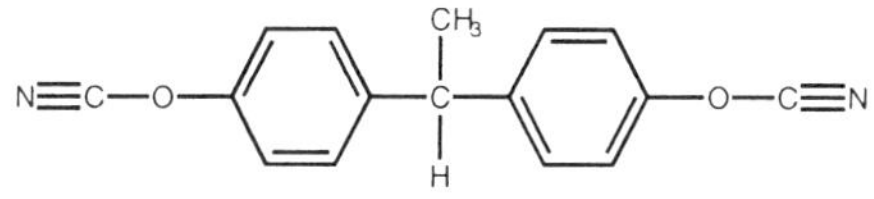	Low viscosity liquid or crystal	36–45	80–100	Radomes, satellites, syntactic foams, primary structures, solvent for thermoplastics
XU7187 dicyclopentadiene	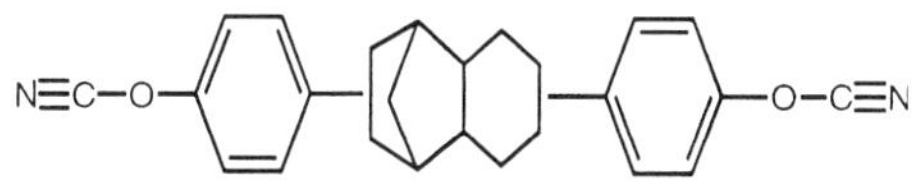	Semisolid amorphous (0.7L is core shell rubber toughened)	36–50	80–110	Telecommunications or satellites, primary structures, structural syntactic cores, radomes, adhesives
Phenol triazine PT-30, 60	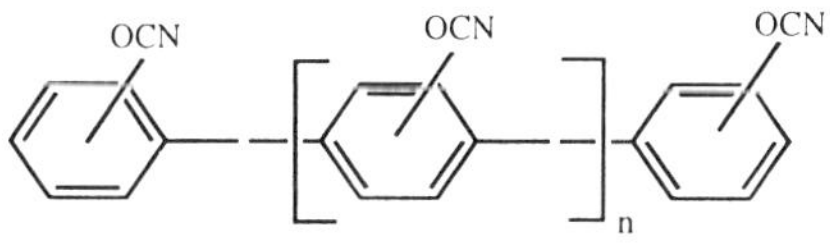	Viscous liquid or semisolid amorphous	27–34	60–75	High-temperature applications: wet winding, carbon-carbon, ablatives

Data courtesy of Vantico, formerly Ciba Giegy

result in lower moisture absorption, higher diffusivity, low cure shrinkage, low coefficient of thermal expansion (CTE), and low dielectric constant and dielectric loss when compared with epoxy and bismaleimide (BMI) systems. These attributes are particularly attractive for stable structures, PCBs, and radar and low dielectric applications. Figure 2 is a graph of moisture absorption of CE neat resins (RS-3) and an epoxy (3501-6), both cured at 180 °C (360 °F). The cured resins were conditioned at 100% relative humidity and 25 °C (77 °F) for more than 1000 days. The moisture absorption behavior comparison between the CE and epoxy resins shows that the CE reaches moisture equilibrium quickly and at much lower total absorption level. This is also reflected in the overall lower coefficient of moisture expansion of CE resins when compared to epoxies.

The resin modulus and toughness characteristics depend, in part, on the backbone structure and cross-link density of the polymer. For satellite structures, improved toughness and elongation to failure result in fewer microcracks due to thermal cycling and a more stable structure. Figure 3 compares microcracking of several CE and epoxy resins, all of which are space-qualified systems. The laminates were made using XN-70A, a 690 GPa (100×10^6 psi) modulus pitch fiber at 60% fiber volume. The CE systems produced fewer microcracks overall after 2000 cycles, with the microcrack density increasing rapidly from zero to 500 cycles and then stabilizing. The exception to this stabilization is the lower-temperature curing epoxy system (130 °C, or 270 °F) that appears to continue microcracking after 2000 cycles.

Cyanate ester can be toughened by the same mechanisms used for epoxy resins, with the expected change in the balance of modulus, T_g, and strain to failure. The ability to modify and toughen CE-based resins makes them appropriate for adhesives and toughened composite applications. One prepolymer system available from Vantico, XU71787 0.07l, incorporates a proprietary submicron core shell rubber particle. It is very efficient in improving the fracture toughness (K_{Ic}) of the matrix at low concentrations without significantly reducing the T_g of the resin. A comparison of mechanical and physical properties of cured neat resins used to formulate matrix systems is found in Table 2. All resins were cured at 175 °C (350 °F) and postcured to

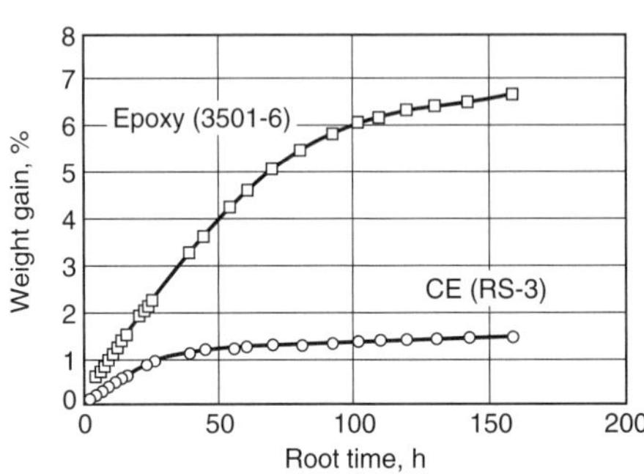

Fig. 2 Moisture absorption of 180 °C (360 °F) cured epoxy and CE neat resins at 100% relative humidity and 25 °C (77 °F) for more than 1000 days

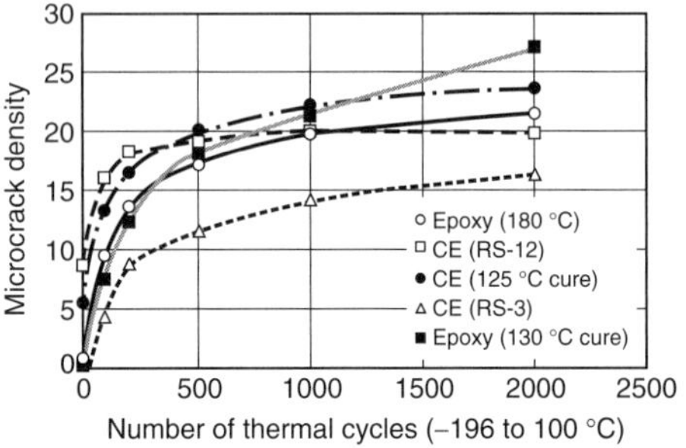

Fig. 3 Comparison of microcracking behavior of cyanate ester and epoxy laminates (reinforced with graphite fiber XN70A, modulus >690 GPa, or 100×10^6 psi). Source: Nippon Graphite Fiber Corporation

Table 2 Mechanical and physical properties of cyanate ester resins

Property(a)	Bisphenol A dicyanate	Ortho methyl dicyanate	Arocy L10	XU366, XU378	Phenol triazine	XU71787 0.2L	XU7178 0.7L CSR
Mechanical properties							
Tensile strength, MPa (ksi)	88 (13)	73 (11)	87 (13)	76 (11)	48 (7)	70 (10)	...
Tensile modulus, GPa (10^6 psi)	3.17 (0.5)	2.97 (0.4)	2.90 (0.4)	3.16 (0.5)	3.11 (0.5)	3.2 (0.5)	...
Elongation to break, %	3.2	2.5	3.8	3.5	1.9	2.7	...
Flexural strength, MPa (ksi)	174 (25)	161 (23)	162 (23)	119 (17)	79 (11)	124 (18)	102 (15)
Flexural modulus, GPa (10^6 psi)	3.11 (0.5)	2.9 (0.4)	2.9 (0.4)	3.31 (0.5)	3.59 (0.5)	3.31 (0.5)	2.36 (0.3)
Flexural elongation to break, %	7.7	6.6	8.0	3.7	2.1	4.0	7.5
Strain energy release rate (G_{Ic}), J/m^2	140	175	190	210	60	70	490
Thermal properties							
Glass transition temperature (T_g) (DMA), °C (°F)	289 (552)	252 (486)	258 (496)	182 (360)	320 (608)	265 (509)	254 (489)
Coefficient of thermal expansion (TGA), 10^{-6}/°C (10^{-6}/°F)	64 (36)	71 (39)	64 (36)	70 (39)	62 (34)	66 (37)	66 (37)
Coefficient of moisture expansion, 10^{-6}/%M	...	...	...	...	...	1250	1250
Onset of degradation (TGA), °C (°F)	411 (772)	403 (757)	408 (766)	390 (734)	412 (774)	405 (761)	...
Char yield in nitrogen (N_2) atmosphere (TGA), %	41	48	43	39	62	32	...
Flammability, UL-94							
1st ignition, s	33	20	1	>50	14	>50	...
2nd ignition, s	23	14	>50	...	7	...	...
Hygrothermal and chemical properties							
Water absorbed at saturation, 100 °C (210 °F), %	2.5	1.3	2.4	0.6	3.8	1.2	...
Onset of hydrolysis at 100 kPa (1 bar) steam and 120 °C (250 °F), h	200	>600	NA	NA	NA	>600	...
Weight loss onset in NaOH solution at 50 °C (120 °F), days	9	>70	NA	28	NA	10	...
Electrical properties							
Dielectric constant							
At 1 GHz, dry	2.79	2.67	2.85	2.53	2.97	2.76	...
At 1 MHz, dry	2.91	2.75–2.8	2.98	2.64–2.8	3.08	2.80	2.9
At 1 MHz, wet	3.32	3.13	3.39	2.90	NA	3.22	...
Dissipation factor							
At 1 GHz, dry	0.006	0.005	0.006	0.002	0.007	0.005	0.005
At 1 MHz, dry	0.005	0.002	0.005	0.001	0.006	0.002	...
At 1 MHz, wet	0.015	0.010	0.016	0.004	NA	0.011	...
Other characteristics							
Density at 25 °C (77 °F), g/cm^3	1.21	1.17	1.23	1.14	1.24	1.19	1.18
Supplier	Vantico, Mitsubishi Chemical	Vantico	Vantico	Vantico	Vantico, Lonza	Vantico	Vantico

(a) DMA, dynamic mechanical analysis; TGA, thermogravimetric analysis

>95% conversion. This table shows the differences in the commercially available resins. Additional data are available from the materials suppliers (Ref 3, 7, 8).

Processing

Cyanate ester resins have prepreg processing requirements similar to epoxy and BMI resins and are prepregged using traditional hot-melt and solution-coating processes. The preferred method of incorporating reinforcements is by hot-melt or other solvent-free processing due to possible contamination by water when using solvent-coating processes. For the PCB prepregs, solvent impregnation is used because of better production efficiencies for solution coating large volume, low-flow systems.

Cyanate esters also have composite processing characteristics similar to epoxy resins. They are available as hot-melt prepregs, tow preg, wet-winding resins, molding compounds, resin transfer molding (RTM) resins, adhesive systems, and syntactic core materials. They can be consolidated using autoclave, vacuum bag, press, pultrusion, RTM, Seemans composite resin injection molding process, or vacuum-assisted resin transfer molding methods.

Curing of CE resins and prepregs is generally performed at elevated temperatures. Low-temperature cures are possible but will result in a system with significantly shorter out times as well as overall low cyanate conversions, <80%, without postcuring. Low conversions of OCN groups can cause poor hydrolytic chemical stability, low T_g, brittleness, and higher dielectric properties. Postcuring should be considered if optimal properties are required, especially at elevated service temperatures. In order to achieve adequate conversions of the OCN reactive groups and useable room temperature out times, most resin systems are formulated to cure at temperatures between 120 and 180 °C (250 and 360 °F). It is recommended that CE resins be postcured to 235 to 315 °C (455 to 600 °F) for structural service temperatures at or above 180 °C (360 °F).

For structural laminates, a chelated metal catalyst, such as cobalt or copper, is typically used. Other catalysts used to cure CE resins include zinc, manganese, and iron. Metal chelates will give longer pot life than metal carboxylates, and the addition of active hydrogen compounds, such as nonyl phenol, acts as co-catalysts and solvents for the metal coordination catalyst. They play an important role in percent conversion at temperature, resulting in longer pot life. For practical reasons, some metal catalysts should be avoided because, in the presence of moisture, they can promote hydrolysis of the OCN groups to form carbamates. The formation of carbamates reduces the ultimate T_g and thermal stability of the resin and can lead to delamination at elevated temperatures, due to the decomposition of carbamate structure to CO_2 gas and an amine group. Metal catalysts that promote the formation of carbamates are tin, lead, antimony, and titanium, and, to a lesser extent, zinc (Ref 6, 9, 10).

The formation of carbamates in CE resins is one of the few disadvantages of CE resins when compared to BMI or epoxies. It is generally accepted that, for most high-performance composites, exposure to moisture contamination during the cure must be controlled. In the case of CE, the most predominant contamination problem by far occurs when the resins are exposed to moisture during the cure process. Carbamate contamination of CE systems due to the reaction with moisture in structural composites has been noted since the early 1990s, when the first structural parts were fabricated for space structures using low CTE composite tooling. Shimp et al. have characterized the reaction (Ref 3). The general reaction for the formation of carbamate is shown in Fig. 4.

Carbamate formation can occur when moisture is able to diffuse into the laminate or adhesive and react with the polymer system during the cure process. This problem is most noticeable on structures that are cured against undried composite tools, with moisture-laden bagging materials, fibers, foam, or honeycomb cores. The formation of the carbamate group proceeds by hydrolysis of the OCN functional group to form a carbamate. With additional heating above 150 °C (300 °F), the carbamate group decomposes and forms an amine and carbon dioxide. The carbon dioxide gas can cause blistering and delamination, as noted by Shimp and Ising (Ref 7) in early postcured Kevlar (DuPont) laminates. The amount of carbamate formed is also dependent on the catalyst used in the formulation; zinc catalysts promoted the carbamate formation more than copper or cobalt. During thermal decomposition of the carbamate into carbon dioxide and amine, it is possible for unreacted OCN groups to react with the amine and form a more stable linear polymer structure, or isourea (Ref 1, 3, 9).

Moisture contamination problems do not always result in blistering or delamination. For composites cured against undried composite tooling, the problem generally is restricted to the tool surface of the laminate. In severe cases it can be detected as a rough, friable surface on laminates. If the formation and/or decomposition of the carbamate structure has occurred, the surface of the laminate will be soluble in a ketone such as acetone or methyl ethyl ketone. Depending on the cure conditions, Fourier transform infrared examination of the extract can detect the carbonyl peak at around 1750 cm^{-1}. This can be misleading; if the carbamate has decomposed fully due to elevated cure temperatures and is no longer present, only a much stronger-than-normal NH stretch peak around 3500 cm^{-1} may be detected. A characteristic change of the cured cyanate, if carbamates have been formed, is a decrease in the T_g of the resin.

In order to alleviate the risk of moisture forming carbamates during cure, some easy precautions and techniques can be used. These include predrying and dry storage of composite tools, drying and outgassing of foam cores, drying fabrics, and modifying the cure cycle to remove moisture from the materials before the cure reaction begins. Even changes in the vacuum bag lay-up, for instance, allowing a good path for trapped moisture to be removed from the vacuum bag and keeping the part under an active vacuum throughout the cure, have been found to be useful in minimizing the problem. The reaction of water and CEs proceeds very slowly at room temperature and is generally not a problem as long as good materials storage practices are used. This should include the use of heat-sealable aluminum-coated Mil bags, storage with desiccant, and avoiding long-term or repeated moisture contamination.

Another useful tool to determine the potential presence of carbamates and their decomposition on suspect parts is detailed electron spectroscopy for chemical analysis (ESCA), which is used for determining elemental and chemical bond information for elements that have atomic numbers greater than helium. This method can be used to determine the existence of carbamate groups (seen as carbonyl –C = O) or the amine and subsequent isourea structure formed from carbamate decomposition. ESCA will also detect other potential surface contaminates, such as silicone and fluorine (Ref 11).

Properties For Selected Applications

Space Applications. The ability to save weight by replacing heavier metal structures with composites has been a common thread for justifying the use of more-expensive composites for the last twenty-five years, especially for space applications. Depending on the launch platform used, it is estimated that each pound of weight removed from the structure at launch saves between \$5,000 and \$30,000. Epoxy and BMI resins were the first systems to be used for satellite composite structures, but problems soon became apparent with these systems. Matrix microcracking during thermal cycling with unmodified systems reduced structural stiffness and caused instability. Rubber-toughened resin systems did not hold up to radiation exposure, losing strength, stiffness, and thermal performance. Epoxy and BMI resins absorbed moisture while being stored prior to launch and, in the vacuum

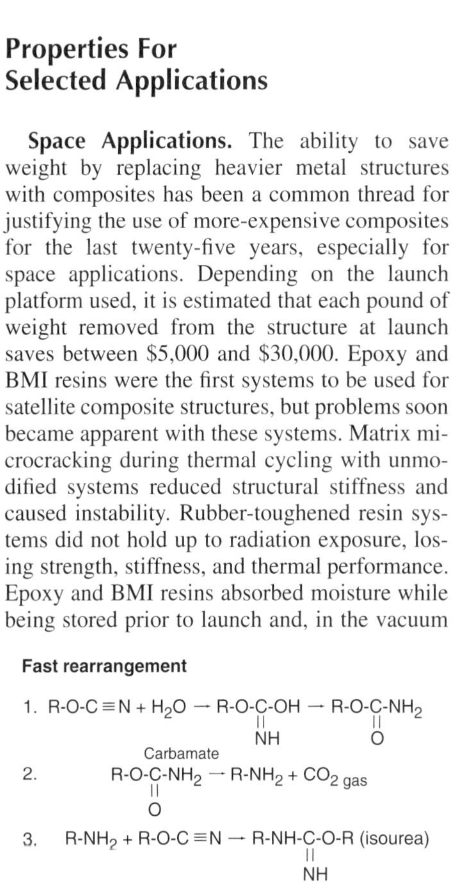

Fast rearrangement

1. R-O-C≡N + H_2O → R-O-C(=NH)-OH → R-O-C(=O)-NH_2

Carbamate

2. R-O-C(=O)-NH_2 → R-NH_2 + CO_2 gas

3. R-NH_2 + R-O-C≡N → R-NH-C(=NH)-O-R (isourea)

Fig. 4 Reaction of cyanate ester and water, formation and decomposition of carbamate, reaction of amine with OCN group. Source: Ref 3

of space, outgassed absorbed moisture, resulting in structural instability as the matrix changed dimensionally and degraded thermal performance. Outgassing also produced condensation of moisture on sensitive reflectors, mirrors, and optics, reducing signals or making them inoperable.

The characteristics that make CE resins a more-suitable choice for space structures and ultimately led to their wide acceptance were their low outgassing, good cryogenic temperature performance, low cure shrinkage, low microcracking from thermal cycling, good radiation resistance (Ref 11, 12), and low coefficient of moisture absorption, low CTE, and low density. Table 3 shows typical laminate performance of 180 °C (360 °F) cured CE prepreg resin systems on carbon, graphite, Kevlar, and quartz fibers. The values are averages of commercially available 100% CE prepreg systems that are qualified for satellite and radome applications.

Combining the CE resins with ultrahigh modulus pitch and polyacrilonitrile (PAN) fibers (modulus >517 GPa, or 75 × 10^6 psi) allows the design and fabrication of near-zero CTE composite structures of unparalleled stiffness and stability. Control of CTE is of special interest for space applications such as antennas, reflectors, optical benches, signal devices, feed horn, mux cavities, arrays, and mirrors. It allows the fabricator to build structures that are dimensionally stable during thermal cycling in the space environment from –160 to 180 °C (–250 to 350 °F), allowing improved signal and focal accuracy.

Radomes. Advancements in radar systems, microwave communications, and targeting and tracking electronics using higher frequencies and energy levels has contributed to more-demanding conditions for electromagnetic windows. The frequency ranges required by these systems are between 600 MHz and 100 GHz. Some of the advanced, high-powered systems require materials that are not only transparent to the electromagnetic signal, but can perform at the elevated temperatures that can be produced as the signal passes through the structure. The placement of radomes as primary structure on advanced aircraft requires that they perform well both structurally and electromagnetically. Because of the excellent mechanical properties and very low dielectric properties of cyanate ester, thinner, lightweight structural radomes can be produced, reducing signal loss over a wide frequency range. Their low moisture absorption also provides consistent signal performance.

Reinforcements for these structures are typically glass, quartz, Kevlar, or Spectra polyethylene fibers. Syntactic core materials and lightweight molding compounds can be produced easily using CE resins, and, by adding modifiers and fillers, the dielectric properties can be tuned to specific dielectric constant and loss tangent values. In addition to the contribution CE resins make to low dielectric applications in radomes, they are also suitable for radar-absorbing structures. By combining several layers of material, each with different radar absorbing, transmitting, and canceling properties, the radar signature of a structure can be significantly reduced (Ref 13).

Printed Circuit Boards. The largest application for CE resins is in the electronics industry. In many of the most-demanding applications, CE resins have replaced epoxy novolac systems. The primary reasons are their high T_g (>220 °C or 430 °F), low dielectric properties, very low chloride levels, low moisture absorption, and their ability to be formulated to meet UL 94 flammability requirements. The greatest use in the electronics industry is in multilayer circuit boards and mulitchip modules, which account for 70 to 80% of CE resin usage.

The demand for higher processing speeds and higher frequency capability requires the use of materials with very low dielectric loss properties. The large volume use of CE resins requires formulations that are capable of high-speed prepreg and laminating techniques. Prepreg used for PCB applications is often produced using the solution-coating process and is catalyzed for fast laminating cycles, which increase the throughput of the PCB product. Many PCB cyanate ester formulations are modified with epoxy, BMI, and thermoplastic blends and provide superior bonding to copper foils and higher glass transition properties when compared to FR-4 epoxy laminates (Ref 13).

Cyanate ester resins are compatible at high loading levels with many inorganic fillers, particles, flakes, nanofillers, glass and ceramic balloons, and fibers and can be combined with high-conductivity (>900 W/m · K) fillers and fibers

Table 3 Composite properties of 180 °C (360 °F) cyanate ester prepreg systems

		Unidirectional prepregs				Other fabric-reinforced composites		
Property	ASTM test method	CE/M46J	CE/M55J	CE/XN-70A	CE/K13D2U	Fabric 120 CE/Kevlar	Fabric 4581 CE/quartz	Fabric 1K PW CE/T300
Tensile properties at 0°								
Tensile strength, MPa (ksi)	D 3039	2048 (297)	2000 (290)	1669 (242)	1786 (259)	586 (85)	689 (100)	834 (121)
Modulus of elasticity, GPa (10^6 psi)	D 3039	234 (34)	327 (47)	427 (62)	578 (84)	35 (5)	26 (4)	67 (10)
Poisson's ratio	D 3039	0.31	...	0.32	...	...	...	...
Ultimate strain, %	D 3039	...	...	0.38	...	...	...	...
Tensile properties at 90°								
Tensile strength, MPa (ksi)	D 3039	43.6 (6.3)	33 (5)	45 (7)	16.5 (2.4)	...	...	107 (16)
Modulus of elasticity, GPa (10^6 psi)	D 3039	6.5 (0.9)	6.5 (0.9)	6.8 (1.0)	4.1 (0.6)	...	...	42 (6)
Poisson's ratio	D 3039	0.0040	...	0.004	...	...	...	...
Compressive properties at 0°								
Compressive strength, MPa (ksi)	D 695 MOD	1179 (171)	834 (121)	334 (48)	315 (46)	279 (40)	538 (78)	814 (118)
Compressive modulus, GPa (10^6 psi)	D 695 MOD	220 (32)	301 (44)	423 (61)	557 (81)	33.6 (4.9)	25.5 (3.7)	61.0 (8.8)
Compressive properties at 90°								
Compressive strength, MPa (ksi)	D 695 MOD	234 (34)	...	...	...	...	...	...
Compressive modulus, GPa (10^6 psi)	D 695 MOD	6.89 (1.0)	...	...	...	...	...	...
Short beam shear, MPa (ksi)	D 2344	72 (10)	74 (11)	80 (12)	40 (6)	35 (5)	68.9 (10.0)	76 (11)
In-plane shear strength, MPa (ksi)	D 3518	84 (12)	90 (13)	58.6 (8.5)	29 (4)	...	...	138 (20)
In-plane shear modulus, GPa (10^6 psi)	D 3518	3.8 (0.6)	4.8 (0.7)	4.4 (0.6)	4.7 (0.7)	...	...	4.8 (0.7)
Flexural strength, MPa (ksi)	D 790	1324 (192)	1206 (175)	586 (85)	571 (83)	415 (60)	897 (130)	1020 (148)
Flexural modulus, GPa (10^6 psi)	D 790	226 (33)	297 (43)	317 (46)	508 (74)	34 (5)	48 (7)	62 (9)
Dielectric constant at 8 GHz	...	...	...	...	...	3.0–3.1	3.20	...
Dielectric loss at 8 GHz	...	...	...	...	...	0.004–0.006	0.001–0.005	...
Coefficient of moisture expansion in a 0°/90° laminate, 10^{-6}/%M	...	...	...	63/1064	4/1701	...	...	130
Thermal conductivity at room temperature, W/m · K								
0° longitudinal	(a)	4.60	54.00	172	448	...	...	...
0° transverse	(a)	0.70	1.80	5.8	...	...	...	...
Coefficient of thermal expansion in a quasi-isotropic laminate (60% V_f), 10^{-6}/°C (10^{-6}/°F)	(a)	0.03 (0.06)	–0.02 (–0.03)	–0.26 (–0.46)	...	...	...	...
Coefficient of thermal expansion in the through-thickness direction, 10^{-6}/°C (10^{-6}/°F)	...	...	...	8.48 (15.27)	...	...	...	...

Results normalized to 60% fiber volume fraction (V_f). Average of available data for 180 °C (360 °F) cure systems, not to be used for design. (a) Precision Measurements Instruments Corp. test method

to produce molded heat sinks for thermal management applications.

Outlook

Cyanate ester resins offer excellent benefits when compared to other thermoset resins. Currently, the use of CE resins in composites has been restricted by their high cost. New developments for CE resins are focused on lower-cost solutions for synthesizing the resins, resin blends, and copolymers and fully understanding the cure mechanism to allow lower cure temperatures with high conversions. Additionally, work is being pursued to identify modifications for lower moisture absorption, lower coefficient of moisture expansion, and improved dielectric properties. Throughout the development of new CE resins, one area that continues to be investigated is changes in backbone chemistry. This work is ongoing, by functionalizing different polymer backbones with cyanate functional groups and characterizing the subsequent properties, enabling new uses or improvements in CE properties.

In the electronics industry, the performance requirements of PCBs are continually increasing, and rapid advancement is being made on the performance limits of the epoxy resins. Ultimately, CE resins will become the materials choice for this market, but their potential will be limited by their high cost. It is essential that economical manufacturing methods and raw materials supplies be developed. Lowering the cost of CE resins in order to meet the demand and cost constraint of the electronic market will not only lead to CE resins expanding into more electronic components, but will aid in their acceptance into large aerospace and commercial markets.

REFERENCES

1. A.W. Snow, The Synthesis, Manufacture and Characterization of Cyanate Ester Monomers, *Chemistry and Technology of Cyanate Ester Resins*, Hamerton, 1994
2. E. Grigat and R. Putter, German Patent 1,195,764, 1963
3. D.A. Shimp, J.R. Christenson, and S.J. Ising, "Cyanate Ester Resins—Chemistry, Properties and Applications," Technical Bulletin, Ciba, Ardsley, NY, 1991
4. B. Woo, Vantico, personal correspondence, Oct 2000
5. R.J. Zaldivar, "Chemical Characterization of Polycyanurate Resins," Aerospace Technical Report 96-(8290)-1, Aerospace Corporation, 1996
6. J.P. Pascault, J. Galy, and F. Mechin, Additives and Modifiers for Cyanate Ester Resins, *Chemistry and Technology of Cyanate Ester Resins*, Hamerton, 1994
7. D.A. Shimp and S.J. Ising, *35th International SAMPE Symposium*, 2–5 April 1990, p 1045–1056
8. H. Sue, I. Garcia-Meitin, and D.M. Pickleman, Toughening Concept In Rubber-Modified High Performance Epoxies, *Elastomer Handbook,* 1993, p 661–699
9. D.A. Shimp, *32nd International SAMPE Symposium,* 1987, p 1063–1072
10. Hi-Tek Polymers Inc., U.S. Patent 4,847,233, 1989
11. S. Robitaille and M. Saba, Designing High Performance Stiffened Structures, ImechE Seminar, 2000, p 1–11
12. A. Tavlet, A. Fontaine, and H. Schonbacher, Compilation of Radiation Test Data, CERN, 1998
13. D.A. Shimp, Technology Driven Applications for Cyanate Ester Resins, *Chemistry and Technology of Cyanate Ester Resins*, Hamerton, 1994, p 282–327

Thermoplastic Resins

Lee McKague, Composites-Consulting, Inc.

THERMOPLASTICS have attractive mechanical properties for many supersonic aircraft requirements and for most commercial aircraft requirements. They also offer dimensional stability and attractive dielectric characteristics. Good flame-retardant and wear-resistant characteristics also are common. Table 1 qualitatively compares current-generation thermoplastics and thermosets.

This article addresses thermoplastic resins used as matrix materials for continuous fiber reinforced composites. The focus is on materials suitable for fabrication of structural laminates such as might be used for aerospace applications. Chopped fiber reinforced molding systems are not discussed. High-temperature polymers suitable only for manufacture of small parts, such as washers and bushings, also are not included. Secondary attention is paid to materials whose elevated-temperature properties limit their applications to sporting goods or other low-service-temperature products.

Background

First-Generation Resins. Thermoplastic resins for structural composites began to receive serious attention in the 1980s. This resulted because composite structures made with first-generation thermosetting resins were easily damaged by low-velocity impacts, such as from a dropped wrench. Some fighter aircraft structures were being delaminated by such impacts. Alarmingly, a delamination could be formed without leaving visual evidence on the impacted surface. Worse yet, subsequent structural loads could cause enlargement of the delamination.

Previous decades had focused on high performance, that is, low structural weight. In the 1980s, new attention was placed on achieving an acceptable level of damage tolerance and durability. Significant investigations were launched to devise test methods to characterize damage tolerance and durability (Ref 1–7) and to establish threshold requirements. The favored method of evaluating damage tolerance of a composite has evolved to be testing for compression strength of a laminate after it sustains an impact of 6.67 J/mm (1500 in. · lbf/in.). This test has been conducted per Suppliers of Advanced Composite Materials Association (SACMA) method SRM 2R-94. Although SACMA is no longer an active organization, testing companies in the United States still use the test method. An alternate procedure is National Aeronautics and Space Administration (NASA) 1142-B11.

Searches were initiated for tougher materials, and thermoplastic polymers were identified as a candidate option. They were perceived as inherently tough and resistant to damage from low-velocity impacts. Significant programs were funded by the U.S. Air Force, the U.S. Navy, and NASA.

Thrusts from Department of Defense (DoD) and NASA programs spurred research by various companies. Altogether, these efforts sought to identify suitable thermoplastic resins, to develop composite products, to learn how to fabricate aircraft components, and to characterize resulting performance. Because needs were centered first on improving composite performance in fighter aircraft, thermoplastics were sought that also could yield attractive elevated-temperature properties.

Fighter platforms evolving during the 1980s typically were designed to perform at speeds up to Mach 2.0 to 2.2. At these speeds, aerodynamic friction can cause adiabatic and stagnation heating of aircraft skins to temperatures of 132 to 171 °C (270–340 °F). An acceptable material would have to have good retention of mechanical properties at these temperatures, as well as being resistant to impact damage at ambient temperatures.

Most of the many distinct thermoplastic polymers have found commodity applications that typically have modest service temperature requirements. Less than a dozen polymers have been considered for engineering applications at higher temperatures, such as are required for many aerospace structural composites. The restrictive factor has been the relationship of processing to elevated-temperature properties.

Many polymers may have a glass transition temperature (T_g) or melting temperature (T_m) that seems high. However, the stiffness and mechanical performance of thermoplastics progressively diminish as these points are approached. To have good properties at temperatures of 132 °C (270 °F) or higher, the T_g or T_m must be well above the intended use temperature. Yet, only above T_g or near melting do

Table 1 Qualitative comparison of current thermoplastics and thermosets

Characteristic	Thermoplastics	Thermosets
Tensile properties	Excellent	Excellent
Stiffness properties	Excellent	Excellent
Compression properties	Good	Excellent
Compression strength after impact	Good to excellent	Fair to excellent
Bolted joint properties	Fair	Good
Fatigue resistance	Good	Excellent
Damage tolerance	Excellent	Fair to excellent
Durability	Excellent	Good to excellent
Maintainability	Fair to poor	Good
Service temperature	Good	Good
Dielectric properties	Good to excellent	Fair to good
Environmental weakness	None, or hydraulic fluid	Moisture
NBS smoke test performance	Good to excellent	Fair to good
Processing temperatures, °C (°F)	343–427 (650–800)	121–315 (250–600)
Processing pressure, MPa (psi)	1.38–2.07 (200–300)	0.59–0.69 (85–100)
Lay-up characteristics	Dry, boardy, difficult	Tack, drape, easy
Debulking, fusing, or heat tacking	Every ply if part is not flat	Typically every 3 or more plies
In-process joining options	Co-fusion	Co-cure, Co-bond
Postprocess joining options	Fastening, bonding, fusion	Fastening, bonding
Manufacturing scrap rates	Low	Low
Ease of prepregging	Fair to poor	Good to excellent
Volatile-free prepreg	Excellent	Excellent
Prepreg shelf life and out time	Excellent	Good
Health/safety	Excellent	Excellent

thermoplastics become soft enough for the mechanical forming or shaping required for manufacturing parts.

Based on the author's experience, an approximate rule of thumb is that polymer softness sufficient for part processing must occur 180 °C (325 °F) or more above the intended maximum structural use temperature. Adequate composite stiffness at the intended use temperature results from this margin. Another desirable result is resistance to creep when elevated-temperature design loads are applied. Restated, this rule of thumb means that component manufacturing operations have been required to occur well above 315 °C (600 °F).

These high temperatures, together with the typical lack of tack of thermoplastic prepregs, have required processing techniques that are significantly different from those used for thermosetting composites. One low-cost technique has been lay-up and heat consolidation of a flat laminate, followed by thermoforming to the required part shape (Ref 8). Both consolidation and thermoforming might be done in a press.

Depending on size or shape of contoured parts, another technique has involved heat tacking of each ply during lay-up. This compensates for lack of tack that otherwise would allow plies to slip off the contoured tool. It also better enables thickness tailoring of the laminate. Such lay-up usually is followed by autoclave consolidation.

Autoclave process parameters for consolidation can involve compacting at pressures of 1.38 to 2.07 MPa (200–300 psi) and temperatures as high as 343 to 382 °C (650–720 °F). At such autoclave conditions, preparation for processing is much more difficult. Ancillary materials for vacuum bagging must possess high-temperature resistance; bagging films such as Kapton or Upilex are required. In addition, bagging must be done more carefully. One of the highest-temperature tough thermoplastics is polyether etherketone (PEEK). Autoclave processing of PEEK is done at a nominal temperature of 380 °C (715 °F), and the process cycle is long because of autoclave heat-up and cool-down times.

Altogether, these factors have meant higher cost. In the early 1990s, such cost disadvantages caused some companies to stop marketing certain thermoplastic composites. Development of new, innovative approaches has been required to combat high costs.

Second-Generation Resins. As previously noted, durability and damage tolerance requirements created a drive toward increased application of thermoplastics. However, the emerging market threat of thermoplastics spurred development of a second, tougher generation of thermosetting resins. As illustrated in Fig. 1, these tougher thermosetting resins improved by a factor of 1.3 in compression strength after impact (CSAI). Open-hole compression strength (OHCS), another critical design property, also improved. However, by comparison composites made with polyetherimide (PEI) and PEEK had CSAI values more than twice as high as the first-generation graphite/epoxies, also illustrated in Fig. 1.

Meanwhile, the military was pressed by timing requirements for new programs, such as the F-22 and the F-18E&F. Based on many tests and evaluations, it was concluded that improvements provided by second-generation thermosets would satisfy mission requirements. Although thermoplastics still required extensive development of processing methods, these thermosets processed the same as—and even better than—first-generation thermosets. This led emerging military programs to use materials such as IM7/977-3 graphite/epoxy and IM7/5250-4 graphite/BMI (Ref 9). As a consequence of these factors, applications of thermoplastic composites to military aircraft during the 1990s were quite limited.

Third-Generation Resins. Recently, a third generation of thermosets has achieved CSAI and OHCS values that approach those of PEI and PEEK, also shown in Fig. 1. Based on military experience, some members of this later generation of thermosets appear likely to meet most durability and damage-tolerance requirements while preserving much of the lower-cost processing options generally offered by thermosets. Despite this potential rivalry, thermoplastics are gaining applications as their advantageous characteristics become better known and as new, cost-effective processing methods evolve.

One such significant application of thermoplastics is to commercial aircraft, which do not sustain supersonic flight temperatures. Here, the demand for excellent damage tolerance and durability dominated decisions. Consequently, resins that would be marginal or unacceptable in many military aircraft applications could easily meet many commercial aircraft performance requirements.

In addition to impact resistance, thermoplastics offer excellent abrasion resistance. They exhibit attractive dielectric properties, and these properties are not significantly shifted by moisture absorption. In most cases, high-temperature thermoplastic composites also have excellent environmental and solvent resistance.

Thermoplastic composites have promised these and other advantages. Capturing these advantages has been slow, due in part to reduced military spending on aircraft. In the commercial sector, significant recent progress has been made in understanding where and how to use thermoplastic composites and how to reduce the costs of structures. For some thermoplastic resins, manufacturing approaches have been developed that yield very favorable processing costs. Perhaps more significantly, they open up component assembly options that enable large total-cost savings. As a result, commercial applications of thermoplastics have blossomed.

Categories and Characteristics

Thermoplastic materials are divided into categories based on fundamental differences in morphology. These morphologies are described as crystalline, semicrystalline, and amorphous.

Semicrystalline materials have domains of highly ordered molecular structure (crystallites)

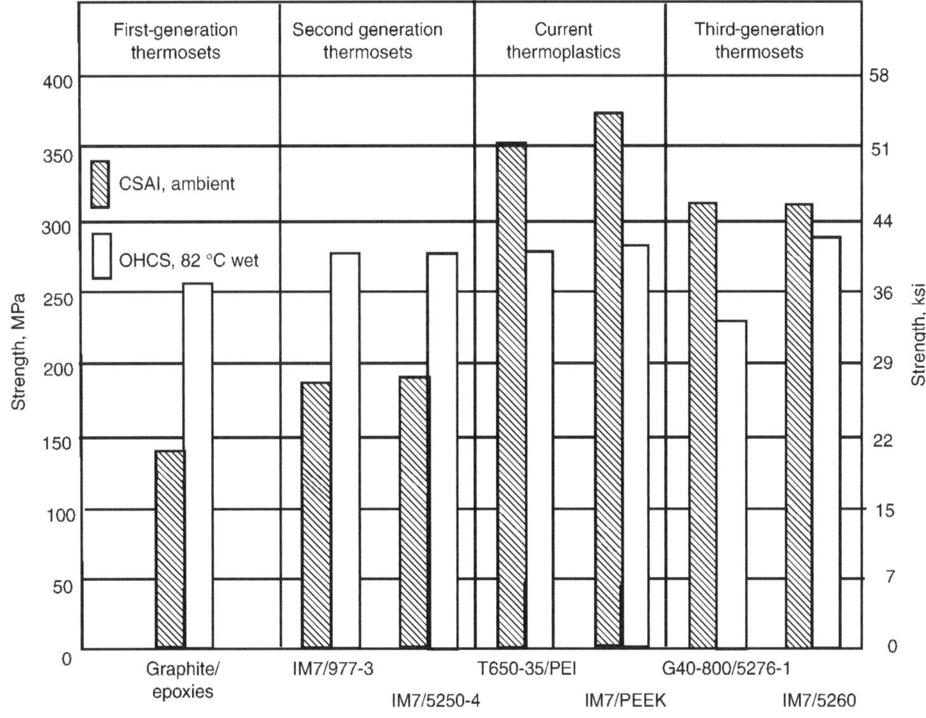

Fig. 1 Compression properties of thermosets and thermoplastics. Source: Ref 9 and manufacturer data (PEI, Hexcel Corp.; PEEK, Cytec Fiberite)

having well-defined melting points. Crystalline development is a thermodynamic and transport phenomena controlled by balance in mobility and free energy of molecules. Cooling rate can influence crystalline content and distribution (Ref 10).

The effects of crystallinity are similar to cross linking in that resin stiffness and solvent resistance increase with increasing crystalline content (Ref 11). Above the T_g softening occurs more gradually in crystalline materials than in amorphous materials and progresses toward a melting point that is characterized by a sudden change to an apparent liquid state. In this respect, crystallinity is quite different from cross linking, where the material thermally degrades without entering a liquid state.

Semicrystalline materials typically exhibit very good chemical resistance. Unlike thermoset composites, a great degree of useful strength and stiffness may remain well above the T_g of these thermoplastic composites.

Amorphous, high-temperature resins have randomly ordered molecular structures and do not exhibit a sharp melting point. Instead, they soften gradually with rising temperature. Amorphous resins lose their strength quickly above their T_g, even when reinforced with continuous fibers. Physical aging effects, creep behavior, and sensitivity to fatigue also are more pronounced.

At the beginning of 2000, only a few thermoplastic polymers have emerged to dominate the aerospace field. These high-temperature polymers are PEEK, PEI, polyphenylene sulfide (PPS), and polyetherketone ketone (PEKK). Although PEKK exhibits excellent properties, its applications have progressed at a slower rate.

Chemical structures of these and some mid-temperature-range thermoplastic materials are illustrated in Fig. 2. Table 2 compares T_g, processing temperature range, and morphology for several polymers.

Of these polymers, PEEK has become one of the most widely known and used materials. Through work toward a variety of aerospace requirements, such as the F-22 fighter aircraft, mechanical properties have been well characterized (Ref 13). Effects of various environmental agents—including solvents, acids, hydraulic fluids, and fuels—have been assessed with favorable results. Other materials that have been well characterized are PPS and PEI, reinforced with either glass or carbon fibers (Ref 14–16). Some of these properties are presented and discussed in the section "Properties" in this article.

Product Forms

Thermoplastic composite materials are available in a variety of forms, as are thermosetting composites. There are significant differences, however. Perhaps one of the most significant differences is that fabric reinforced thermoplastic prepreg typically have been sold in discontinuous sheet form rather than in roll form. Usual size has been 107 by 366 cm (48 by 120 in.). Also, fabric forms often have been sold as consolidated laminates involving some number of plies with either standard or custom ply orientations.

Unidirectional prepreg has been sold in roll form, but with a maximum roll width only one-fourth to one-fifth that typical of thermosetting prepreg. The standard width has been 30.5 cm (12 in.), but almost any more narrow width has been available. Slit tape and single tow forms have become commonly available.

For various reasons, not all combinations of thermoplastic resin/reinforcement are actively marketed. It is common to find PEEK applied to unidirectional material but not to fabric material. Polyetherimide and PPS, on the other hand, are more commonly marketed with fabric forms.

Impregnation

The operations used to combine thermoplastic resins with fine-diameter reinforcing fibers are both a science and an art. They are the domain of companies whose business is manufacture and marketing of prepreg or semipreg materials.

Semipreg is the term often used with thermoplastic materials because the resin may be more nearly a coating rather than an impregnation. This is more typical with fabric reinforcements than with unidirectional reinforcements.

No particular attempt is made here to distinguish between prepreg and semipreg for any particular material combination. In any case, material suppliers typically regard the exact method and set of parameters used for a particular resin/fiber combination to be proprietary. Discussion here, then, is merely for the purpose of providing

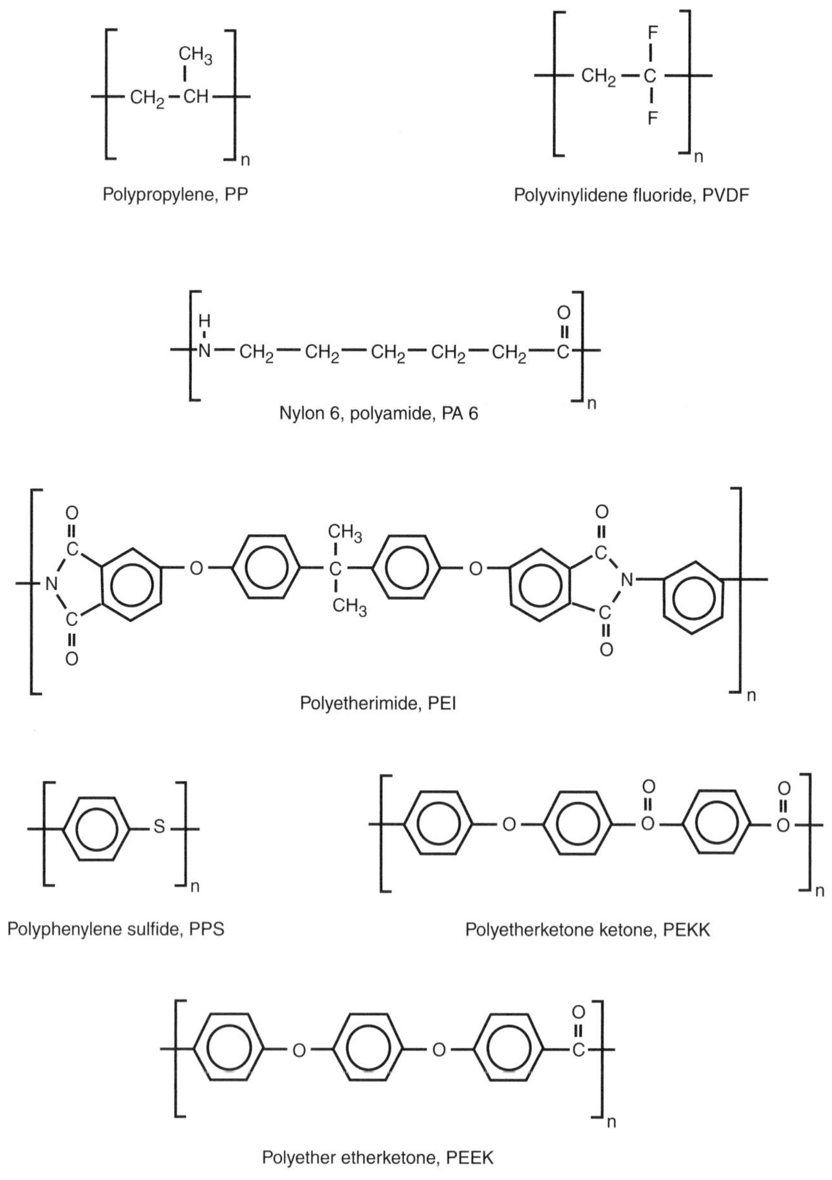

Fig. 2 Chemical structures of mid- and high-temperature thermoplastics

a general introduction to the operations and issues associated with the production and use of thermoplastic-matrix composites.

As indicated in Table 1, impregnation with thermoplastic resins is much more difficult than with thermosetting resins because thermoplastics generally are much more viscous. Increasing temperature lowers the viscosity, but in some polymers decomposition can result before very low viscosity is realized.

Many thermoplastics are insoluble by most organic solvents, or their properties are significantly degraded by attempts to thin them using solvents. The consequence is that thorough impregnation can be extremely difficult. Some polymers, however, are readily soluble in select organic solvents. This enables fairly conventional solvent impregnation and is a method that has been used for PEI composites.

Four strategies have been advanced to deal with impregnation difficulties. Two strategies involve heat plus mechanical methods, and the other two involve delivering the thermoplastic in a form that enables intermixing with the reinforcing fibers prior to melting of the resin.

One of the mechanical methods is based on the fact that the viscoelastic behavior of thermoplastics is non-Newtonian (Ref 17). As a result, it is possible to achieve a significant reduction in viscosity through shear thinning. This type of approach could be considered for a viscous polymer that was insoluble in any environmentally acceptable solvent. It is believed that this method is not widely used.

The second, more common mechanical method involves stacking a film layer over fabric. The resin film is heated above the melt or softening temperature and forced into the fabric with pressure, such as from a press platen.

One of the intermixing strategies involves drawing or spinning the resin into fibers that then are commingled with the reinforcing fibers (Ref 18). The resinous fibers of this mixed fiber bundle are then melted or softened. If commingling is adequately achieved, then effective impregnation is achieved. The process to form the thermoplastic fibers represents an added cost, but in volume this can be a very small cost.

The second intermixing strategy involves combining powdered resin with the reinforcing fibers. Electrostatic attraction methods are used in a fluidized bed process to apply the powder coating. The polymer then is melted to form the prepreg (Ref 19, 20). Sometimes the material may be sold prior to resin melting, so that the drapable, no-tack material achieves its actual impregnation after part lay-up—during the part consolidation step. Mechanically producing powders with very small particle sizes represents an added cost that can be larger than the cost of drawing the polymer into fibers. However, the net cost of combining the polymer and fibers can be less than for solvent impregnation (Ref 21). For some polymers, an alternate strategy involves precipitation from reactors, but sizes tend to be quite a bit larger than for mechanically formed powders.

Processing

Lay-up of thermoplastic composite panels and parts is conceptually similar to lay-up with thermosetting composites in that plies are cut to shape and applied ply by ply. Beyond this similarity, however, the processes are quite different. The difference is driven by the typical lack of tack inherent in most thermoplastic prepregs.

For parts of certain size having contour, the first ply may be held to the tool by tape at the corners or by some other suitable method. Then, each subsequent ply must be heat tacked to the one below it. The heat-tacking process is analogous to a spot-welding process. A standard soldering iron with a blunt-shaped tip is applied with light pressure after heating the tip to a suitable temperature that is well above the T_g of the resin. For some thermoplastics the tip may be heated to as much as 500 °C (932 °F). This causes local melting and fusion of the resin to the ply below.

Fiber placement processes can be used to create a part using slit tape or tow prepreg. The entire surface of the slit tape or tow is heated as it is being laid, fusing it to the layer below. If the part is a body of revolution, then the process is similar to filament winding (see the article "Filament Winding" in this Volume). If the part is more nearly planar, then special care in the design of the part, tooling, and process may be necessary. As the laminate is built up, out-of-plane forces sufficient to cause warping or bowing away from the tool may result from nonsymmetry of the plies, and microcracking of the matrix also might result. In such a case, it may be necessary to create a part that is not optimum from a structural standpoint, but that approximates pairwise symmetry during the lay-up to total laminate thickness.

The fiber-placement process may provide adequate in situ consolidation, but for other lay-up methods it generally will be necessary to consolidate laminates after lay-up is complete. If the part is flat or nearly so, consolidation can occur either in a press or an autoclave. Press consolidation is somewhat easier, but in many production shops, press sizes are smaller than autoclave sizes.

Forming. As mentioned in the discussion of material forms, a common fabric reinforced product form is consolidated sheet, analogous to plywood except that it can be thermoformed whereas plywood cannot. From such sheets, patterns are cut that are subsequently formed to the required shape of the intended part. Figure 3 illustrates this method for multipart fabrication of rib stiffeners.

Several processes are used to create part shapes with consolidated sheet material. Typically, these processes are analogous to sheet metal forming, drawing, and bending operations. The processes include roll forming, mold or die forming, and diaphragm forming.

Assembly of elements or parts into a component can be accomplished without the need to drill holes and install fasteners. Although such conventional assembly can be employed, it is the unique ability of thermoplastics to undergo postforming remelting and fusion that can be especially attractive.

Fusion bonding enables structural components to be assembled without use of mechanical fasteners. All of the components to be joined can be heated and fused together. This can be accomplished with externally applied heating methods,

Table 2 Characteristics of mid- and high-temperature thermoplastics

Polymer	Glass transition temperature (T_g)		Melting point		HDTUL(a)		Processing temperature		Type of morphology
	°C	°F	°C	°F	°C	°F	°C	°F	
Polypropylene (PP)	−4	25	170	338	99	210	191–224	375–435	Crystalline
Polyvinylidene fluoride (PVDF)	−10	−50	171	340	149	300	232–246	450–475	Crystalline
Acrylic, polymethyl methacrylate (PMMA)	100	212	...	...	86	187	199–246	390–475	Amorphous
Nylon 6 polyamide (PA6)	60	140	216	420	177	350	246–274	475–525	Crystalline
Nylon 12 (PA12)	46	115	178	352	138	280	200–240	392–464	Crystalline
Polyphenylene sulfide (PPS)	88	190	285	545	181	358	329–343	625–650	Crystalline
Polyetherimide (PEI)	218	424	...	...	210	410	316–360	600–680	Amorphous
Polyether etherketone (PEEK)	143	290	345	653	171	340	382–399	720–750	Crystalline
Polyetherketone ketone (PEKK)	156	313	310	590	...	...	327–360	620–680	Crystalline

(a) Heat-deflection temperature under load, 455 kPa (66 psi). Sources: Ref 12, Applied Fiber Systems, Cytec Fiberite Advanced Composites, Ten Cate Advanced Composites, www.plasticsusa.com

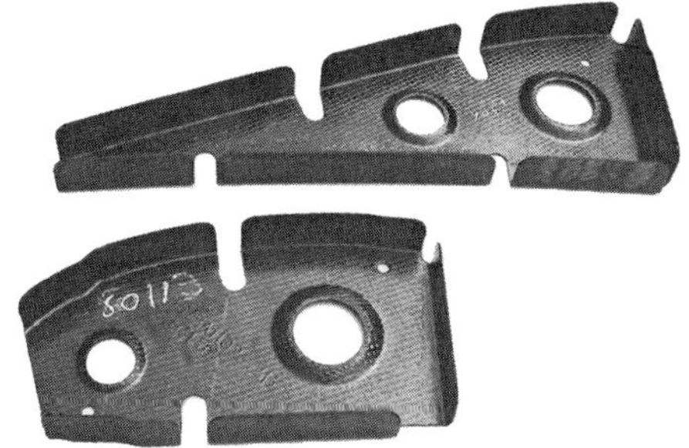

Fig. 3 Dornier 328 landing flap ribs, thermoformed from pattern blanks. Courtesy of Ten Cate Advanced Composites bv

by resistance heating of screens or wires placed at the interfaces, or by induction heating involving the reinforcing fibers. All of these methods can produce excellent adhesion. However, if the entire part details are heated to fusion, special tooling may be required to prevent dimensional distortions. If the resin is in the semicrystalline state, a higher temperature will be required for fusion bonding than if the resin is in the amorphous state.

A similar, but different, approach is to place a lower-melting thermoplastic film between the faying surfaces, such as a film of PEI between two PEEK-matrix parts (Ref 22). All of the elements or parts can be heated together with contact pressure applied to the bond areas, and with less rigorous tooling requirements. Polyetherimide and PEEK are uniquely miscible, helping make the resulting interface quite strong.

Process Temperature Effects. For many thermoplastics, high-temperature properties and resistance to environmental fluids result from achieving the semicrystalline state. Once the semicrystalline state is achieved, those regions of the material exhibit a higher melting point than the adjacent, amorphous-state material. In addition, it has been found that crystallinity and crystalline morphology influence fracture toughness of carbon/PEEK (Ref 23).

Fiber diameter may affect PEEK morphology. The smaller, 5 μm IM6 fibers exhibit better fracture toughness than the larger 7 μm AS4 fibers. However, differences in total energy under the stress-strain curves may cause much of this (Ref 24). Since IM7 fibers are similar in diameter and properties to IM6 fibers, similar effects can be expected.

Some influence over the extent of crystallinity is achieved by controlling the rate of cooling from the melt phase. Polyether etherketone has a characteristic limit of about 30% conversion to the semicrystalline state. Faster cooling can reduce the extent of crystallinity. While an increased level of crystallinity improves solvent resistance and strength, it also creates a more brittle material. A slow cooling rate of 1 °C/min results in a 40% reduction in fracture toughness of AS4/PEEK compared with fast cooling at 50 °C/min (Ref 24). For most parts this is good news with respect to processing because faster cooling means shorter cycle time. However, it also suggests that a very thick PEEK laminate might have properties that vary through the thickness.

Process temperatures, as well as cooling rates, have a significant influence on final morphology and the resulting properties. In carbon/thermoplastic polyimide composites, processing at temperatures above T_g caused reduction in and even irreversible loss of crystallizability (Ref 25). This same kind of behavior has also been reported for carbon/PEEK (Ref 10).

From this information it is clear that processing parameters, fiber size, and possibly fiber surface characteristics interact in the establishment of crystallinity. Together, these findings suggest that there is much yet to be determined about reinforcement, processing, and property interrelationships in thermoplastic composites.

Costs

Much has been said about the cost benefits of manufacturing thermoplastic composite parts; however, a more important consideration is matching the right material and process to the application. Thermoplastics, if not properly targeted and processed, can be much more expensive than thermosets. However, when properly targeted and processed, thermoplastics can offer extremely attractive cost benefits.

An example of missing the mark in touting thermoplastics has been the focus on not needing refrigerated storage or of not having out-life limitations. Although these are genuine benefits, they offer trivial cost savings against costs in an efficiently run thermoset manufacturing shop. Savings from eliminating refrigerated storage can quickly and easily be overwhelmed by significant losses in other areas.

One such area of potential cost liability is in lay-up. Throughout the history of composites, the largest recurring labor-cost contributor has been putting the composite material into the shape of the intended part. Basically, 40 to 60% of the total finished-part cost is involved in this portion of part fabrication. Ply-by-ply lay-up on a contoured tool is a time-consuming process step. This is true when one is using thermoset material that has ideal tack qualities. When using thermoplastic material that has no tack, heat tacking of each ply easily can double or triple lay-up time.

Lay-up costs can be turned from liability to advantage by lay-up and consolidation of flat laminates, followed by thermoforming to the desired part shape. Flat laminate lay-up is quick and does not require ply-by-ply heat tacking. For small parts, the laminate can be large enough so that multiple copies of the required pattern blank can be cut from it after consolidation, as is illustrated by Fig. 3. To a significant degree, the labor involved in lay-up of material for one part provides laid-up material for other parts as well. Current methods and strategies, however, tend to limit such approaches to constant thickness laminates. Without internal part ply-drops, the inherent benefit from tailorability of composites is missed. Also, the shape of the part, together with elongation that might occur perpendicular to the fibers, must be geometrically compatible with a starting blank that is flat. Appreciable elongation parallel to the fibers does not occur.

Another strategy for conquering lay-up costs is to employ computer-controlled tape or tow placement machines. A heating device located at the roll nip, the place where the slit tape or tow meets the surface of the part being built, causes melting of the thermoplastic to a degree sufficient to achieve tacking and in situ compaction.

Although no rigorous cost-analysis studies are known to be publicly available at the time of this writing, it can be assumed that thermoplastics will benefit from automated placement methods as do thermosetting materials. A number of studies have shown that total manufacturing costs can be reduced 20 to 35% by use of automated material-placement machines. With thermoplastics, though, total savings from hot tape lay-up will be larger than with thermosets because compaction occurs during lay-up, and autoclave cure is not required.

Generally, production volumes must be substantial to effectively amortize the cost of automated placement equipment. Cost of such equipment can range from approximately $2 million to $7 million (U.S. dollars), depending on the size of the equipment required and the sophistication needed for process control. Most machines currently cost closer to the high end of this cost band.

Processing parts in an autoclave is another way to spend more money than would be required with thermoset composites. The high softening and melt temperatures involved with structural thermoplastics, and the higher consolidation pressures needed for compaction combine to require a more expensive autoclave and to complicate the recurring autoclave processing. Choices of vacuum-bagging materials are limited to more expensive products, and the reliability of sealing and survival is severely challenged.

Consequently, if one autoclaves an element or structure that will be joined to another element or structure by mechanical fastening, then there is more likely to be a cost disadvantage in using thermoplastics. In such a case, one would want to justify the material selection on the basis of some unique property or structural benefit. Thermosets have made great strides since the initial thrust toward thermoplastics, and some now offer most of the benefits available from thermoplastics.

If, however, the element or structure will be joined to another thermoplastic structure by fusion bonding, then the liability of having made the element or structure in an autoclave will be negated. In this case, the polymer in the elements or structures melts and joins them together in the same way that the plies in a laminate are fused and bonded together. Assembly of structural elements by mechanical fastening is time consuming and expensive. Usually it is more expensive than lay-up of the part. Fusion bonding, by comparison, is very cost effective and can enable a large reduction in total component costs.

In fact, the opportunity to unitize structural details, whether through autoclave processing or some other approach to manufacturing, is extremely significant (Ref 26). In Europe, Dassault Aviation, Eurocopter, and Aerospatiale are actively pursuing the use of thermoplastics for fabrication of unitized fuselage structure (Ref 27). This development involves automated fiber placement of PEEK tape, together with in-process fusion of skin and understructure details. An approach of this nature can yield extremely attractive cost advantages and damage resistance.

Of course, the thermoset community also is pressing toward the advantages of structural un-

Table 3 Properties of glass fiber reinforced thermoplastic-matrix composites (7781-8HS E-glass reinforcement)

Properties	Polyetherimide(a)	Polyphenylene sulfone(a)	Polyetherketone ketone(b)
Specific gravity, g/cm^3	1.91	1.93	1.79
Tensile strength, MPa (ksi)			
Warp	484 (70)	324 (47)	300 (44)
Weft	445 (65)	306 (44)	296 (43)
Tensile modulus, GPa (10^6 psi)			
Warp	26 (3.8)	23 (3.3)	23 (3.3)
Weft	24 (3.5)	22 (3.2)	21 (3.0)
Compression strength, MPa (ksi)			
Warp	727 (105)	526 (76)	317 (46)
Weft	676 (98)	378 (55)	283 (41)
Compression modulus, GPa (10^6 psi)			
Warp	29 (4.2)	27 (3.9)	21 (3.0)
Weft	27 (3.9)	26 (3.8)	20 (2.9)
Flexural strength, MPa (ksi)			
Warp	669 (97)	489 (71)	413 (60)
Weft	585 (85)	452 (66)	393 (57)
Flexural modulus, GPa (10^6 psi)			
Warp	28 (4.1)	24 (3.5)	19 (2.8)
Weft	25 (3.6)	21 (3.0)	18 (2.6)

Sources: (a) Ten Cate Advanced Composites bv. (b) Cytec Fiberite Advanced Composites

itization. It now is feasible, and practical, to achieve with thermosets any assembly that might be pursued with thermoplastics. With care in the design approach, the result can be even lower in cost than with thermoplastics.

Properties

The thermoplastic resins discussed in this article can each be combined with a number of different fibers and fabrics. Glass and carbon fibers are the most prevalent choices.

Table 3 contains typical property values for polymers combined with 7781 style E-glass fabric. Polyether etherketone is not represented in this group, because its high performance and its comparatively difficult, high-temperature processing make it unattractive to combine with glass fabric. It has been used, however, with unidirectional S2 glass; Table 4 compares PEEK and PEKK properties for unidirectional S2 glass reinforcement.

Table 5 compares design properties of PEEK, PEKK, and PEI reinforced with unidirectional carbon fiber reinforcements. Polyetherimide and PPS resins have been extensively characterized with carbon fabrics. Table 6 contains typical property values for PEI and for PPS combined with both 5HS and plain-weave carbon fabrics (Ref 14–16). Neither PEEK nor PEKK appear to have been well characterized with carbon fabrics, that is, with respect to design properties.

Environmental resistance of thermoplastics generally is quite good. Depending on the grade of the material, PEI may be much less resistant than PPS or PEEK. The most commonly used grade of PEI is Ultem 1000, which is soluble in chlorinated solvents such as methylene chloride and chloroform. In the late 1980s methylene chloride was being used by the Air Force as a paint stripper, so it was a significant detriment to consideration of PEI for military aircraft. Such use of methylene chloride has been discontinued.

Hydraulic fluid (Skydrol) also has been found to attack PEI. As a result, use of Ultem 1000 is confined to the interior of commercial aircraft such as Airbus A3XX. Another grade of PEI, Ultem D5000, is fairly inert with respect to hydraulic fluid. At this time, use of this grade has not become prevalent. Table 7 qualitatively compares the effects of various environmental agents on PEI (Ultem 1000), PPS, PEKK, and PEEK.

As indicated in Table 7, thermoplastics generally have excellent resistance to degradation effects from water, either immersed or from high humidity. They also have very good dielectric properties, making them useful for radomes. Thermoset materials are hygroscopic, and absorbed moisture causes a gradual shift in dielectric behavior, degrading performance.

Table 8 summarizes representative thermal properties of various thermoplastic composites.

Applications

Work to apply thermoplastic composites to commercial aircraft has been underway since the early 1990s. An early application was the main landing gear door of the Fokker 50 aircraft (Ref 28, 29). Certification of this structure was completed in March 1998.

Thermoplastic composites are gaining recognition for their toughness and for attributes that can enable recurring cost savings. A wide variety of applications have been made that range from tertiary and secondary structures to primary structures that required Federal Aviation Administration (FAA) certification. An example of primary structure is the pressure floor panels of the Gulfstream V aircraft, which received certification in December 1996 (Ref 30).

To date, applications of thermoplastic composites have ranged from small, simple, structural details such as ribs or spars up to relatively large, unitized structures. Table 9 lists some of the applications that have been made. This list is intended to convey a sense of potential use and is not inclusive of all current applications of thermoplastics. In gathering this list it appears that the lower processing temperature, lower material cost, and amorphous character of PEI favor processing it into parts more so than the semicrystalline PPS or the higher-temperature PEEK.

Figure 4 illustrates the fixed wing leading edge assemblies of the Airbus A340-500/600. This is one of the largest thermoplastic structures made for aircraft exteriors. It is a cost-saving ap-

Table 4 Properties of glass reinforced thermoplastic-matrix composites (unidirectional S2-glass tape reinforcement)

Properties	PEEK	PEKK
0° tensile strength, MPa (ksi)	1170 (170)	1675 (243)
0° tensile modulus, GPa (10^6 psi)	55 (8.0)	52 (7.5)
0° compression strength, MPa (ksi)	1100 (160)	1220 (177)
0° compression modulus, GPa (10^6 psi)	55 (8.0)	. . .

Fiber volume = 60–61%. Source: Cytec Fiberite

Table 5 Properties of carbon fiber reinforced thermoplastic-matrix composites (unidirectional carbon fiber tape reinforcement)

Properties	AS4/PEKK(a)	T650-35/PEI(b)	AS4/PEEK(a)	IM7/PEEK(a)
Fiber volume, %	60	58	61	61
0° tensile strength, MPa (ksi)	1965 (285)	2050 (297)	2070 (300)	2896 (420)
0° tensile modulus, GPa (10^6 psi)	127 (18.4)	139 (20.2)	138 (20.0)	169 (24.5)
0° compression strength, MPa (ksi)	1068 (155)	1720 (249)	1283 (186)	1206 (175)
0° compression modulus, GPa (10^6 psi)	121 (17.6)	133.5 (19.4)	124 (18.0)	. . .
0° flexural strength, MPa (ksi)	1930 (280)	1630 (236)	2000 (290)	2084 (302)
0° flexural modulus, GPa (10^6 psi)	128 (18.6)	123.4 (17.9)	124 (18.0)	157 (22.8)
±45 in-plane shear strength, MPa (ksi)	131 (19.0)	91 (13.2)	186 (27.0)	179 (26.0)
±45 in-plane shear modulus, GPa (10^6 psi)	6.8 (0.99)	5.0 (0.73)	5.7 (0.83)	5.5 (0.80)
Open-hole tension strength, MPa (ksi)	335 (48.6)	. . .	386 (56.0)	476 (69.0)
Open-hole compression strength, MPa (ksi)	325 (47.1)	321 (46.6)	324 (47.0)	324 (47.0)
Compression strength after impact, MPa (ksi)	274 (39.7)	352 (51.1)	338 (49.0)	370 (53.7)
$(0_2, \pm 45)_{2s}$ tensile strength, MPa (ksi)	. . .	1200 (174)	. . .	. . .
$(0_2, \pm 45)_{2s}$ tensile modulus, GPa (10^6 psi)	. . .	78.0 (11.3)	. . .	. . .
$(0_2, \pm 45)_{2s}$ compression strength, MPa (ksi)	. . .	1070 (155)	. . .	. . .
Short-beam shear strength, MPa (ksi)	98 (14.2)	101 (14.7)	. . .	. . .

Sources: (a) Cytec Fiberite Advanced Composites. (b) Hexcel Composites

plication representing the structural unitization potential enabled by the melt fusion characteristics of thermoplastics. Outer shell and rib stiffeners are fused together without use of mechanical fasteners.

As mentioned in the previous section, thermoplastics can maintain excellent dielectric properties during service because of their low moisture absorption. This stability has led recently to application of PEKK reinforced with 7781 style quartz fabric for radomes (Ref 31). Figure 5 illustrates a PEKK radome on the Air Force RC-135 aircraft.

Future Directions

It is clear that elevated-temperature structural performance requires a material with a high T_g or melt temperature. However, it also is clear that process temperatures required for high-temperature systems, such as PEEK, inhibit component manufacturing. This has been a retarding force that has slowed the progress of thermoplastics toward the wide acceptance and use in production applications that thermosets have enjoyed. Boardiness and lack of tack of the prepreg materials have made lay-up difficult and expensive. Because of such qualities it has not been possible to use thermoplastics in the same manner as thermosets. New strategies have been necessary, and this need has slowed progress and acceptance.

High nonrecurring costs for elevated-temperature manufacturing equipment, and high recurring costs for elevated-temperature manufacturing operations are detriments. Pursuit is questionable, then, of even higher temperature thermoplastics because of the potential for further negative impacts on equipment costs and recurring manufacturing costs. In the foreseeable future, therefore, principal work is likely to center on currently applied materials.

Based on these factors, conjecture about future development involving existing materials leads toward development of more cost-effective manufacturing methods. If thermoplastic composites are approached with the same perspective as for thermoset composites, thermoplastics usually will fail to deliver competitive costs. Hence, new design and manufacturing strategies will be required.

Heretofore, thermoplastic prepreg manufacturing limitations with fabrics have led to production of plywood-sized sheets. This has led to creation of plywoodlike laminates, sold to part

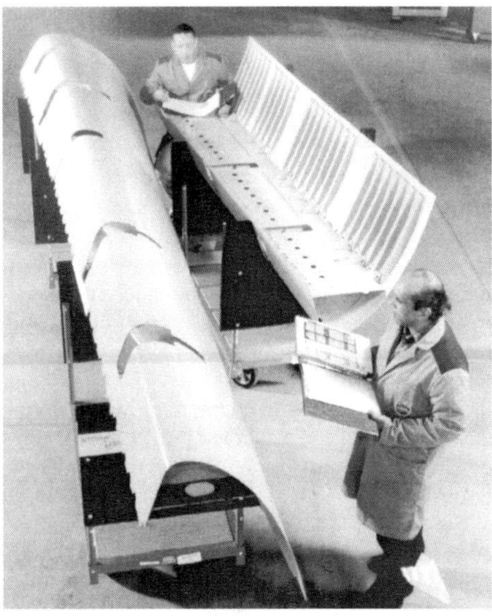

Fig. 4 Airbus A340-500/600 unitized, fixed-wing, leading edge (J-nose) assemblies. Courtesy of Fokker Aerostructures

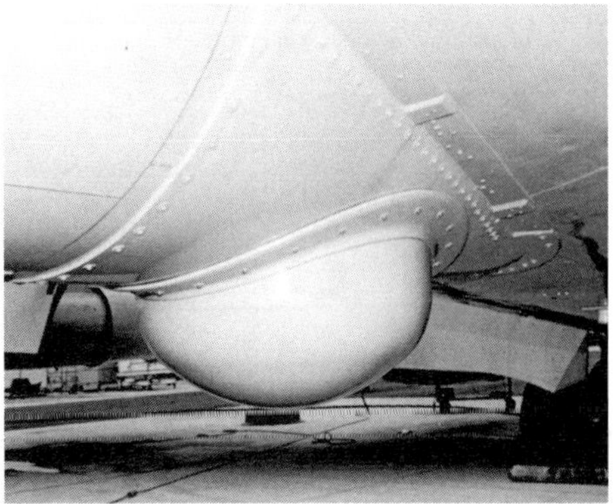

Fig. 5 Quartz/PEKK radome on RC-135 aircraft. Courtesy of Raytheon Systems Co.

Table 6 Properties of carbon fabric reinforced thermoplastic-matrix composites (T300J-3K carbon fabric reinforcement) versus unreinforced thermoplastics

Properties	5HS/PEI	5HS/PPS	Plain PEI	Plain PPS
Tensile strength, MPa (ksi)				
Warp	656 (95)	592 (86)	670 (97)	670 (97)
Weft	673 (98)	725 (105)	626 (91)	569 (83)
Tensile modulus, GPa (10^6 psi)				
Warp	56 (8.1)	54 (7.8)	59 (8.6)	56 (8.1)
Weft	58 (8.3)	54 (7.8)	56 (8.1)	54 (7.8)
Compression strength, MPa (ksi)				
Warp	750 (109)	589 (85)	632 (92)	606 (88)
Weft	754 (109)	513 (74)	642 (93)	459 (67)
Compression modulus, GPa (10^6 psi)				
Warp	52 (7.5)	55 (8.0)	53 (7.7)	52 (7.5)
Weft	52 (7.5)	52 (7.5)	52 (7.5)	51 (7.4)
Flexural strength, MPa (ksi)				
Warp	870 (126)	854 (124)	809 (117)	750 (109)
Weft	793 (115)	842 (122)	769 (112)	750 (109)
Flexural modulus, GPa (10^6 psi)				
Warp	50 (7.3)	52 (7.6)	47 (6.8)	47 (6.8)
Weft	44 (6.4)	50 (7.2)	46 (6.7)	51 (7.3)
In-plane shear strength, MPa (ksi)	118 (17.1)	110 (16.0)	125 (18.1)	100 (14.5)
In-plane shear modulus, GPa (10^6 psi)	3.4 (0.49)	4.2 (0.60)	3.4 (0.49)	3.9 (0.57)
Open-hole tensile strength, MPa (ksi)	270 (39.2)	274 (39.7)	261 (37.9)	261 (37.9)
Open-hole compression strength, MPa (ksi)	268 (38.9)	259 (37.6)	275 (39.9)	239 (34.7)
Bearing strength at yield, MPa (ksi)	...	391 (56.7)	...	352 (51.1)
Bearing strength, ultimate, MPa (ksi)	...	738 (107)	...	652 (94.6)

Fiber volume 50%. Source: Ten Cate Advanced Composites bv

Table 7 Environmental resistance of selected thermoplastic resins

Environmental agent	PEI(a)	PPS(a)	PEKK(b)	PEEK(b)
Water or humidity	Good	Excellent	Excellent	Excellent
JP-4, JP-5 fuels	Excellent	Excellent	Excellent	Excellent
Hydraulic fluid (Skydrol)	Very poor	Excellent	Excellent	Excellent
Methylene chloride	Poor	Good	Excellent	Good
Methyethylketone	Poor	Excellent	Excellent	Excellent
Ethylene glycol	Good	Excellent	Excellent	Excellent

Note: PEI is Ultem 1000 Grade. Sources: (a) Ten Cate Advanced Composites bv. (b) Cytec Fiberite Advanced Composites

Table 8 Thermal characteristics of carbon reinforced thermoplastics

Properties	T300/PEI(a)	AS4/PEEK(b)	AS4/PEKK(b)
Density, g/cm^3 (lb/in.^{3})	1.51 (0.055)	1.61 (0.058)	1.58 (0.057)
Specific heat, J/kg · °C (Btu/lb · °F)	1264 (0.302)	1100 (0.263)	860 (0.205)
Thermal conductivity			
Parallel to fibers, W/m · K (Btu · in./h · ft^2 · °F)	4.46 (30.9)	4.92 (34.1)	...
Perpendicular to fibers, W/m · K (Btu · in./h · ft^2 · °F)	0.43 (2.98)	0.61 (4.23)	0.41 (2.84)
Coefficient of thermal expansion			
Parallel to fibers, 10^{-7}/°C (10^{-7}/°F)	...	2.80 (5.04)	3.00 (5.40)
Perpendicular to fibers, 10^{-5}/°C (10^{-5}/°F)	3.10 (5.58)	3.00 (5.40)	4.40 (7.92)

Standard modulus (227.5 GPa, or 33 × 10^6 psi) carbon fibers. Sources: (a) Ten Cate Advanced Composites bv. (b) Cytec Fiberite Advanced Composites

fabricators. This has robbed designers of one of the most valuable aspects of composites: tailorability that involves internal buildups or ply-drops to reinforce selected regions of a part that will be most highly loaded. Some parts (relatively few) can be made effectively with constant thickness.

Whether at the prepregger or at the part fabricator's facility, there will need to be more effective means to lay-up tailored laminates. This need most likely will result in new forms of lay-up equipment. One form might be equipment that creates the equivalent of warp-knit materials such as are evolving with thermosets. Here, sheet material would be produced that incorporate ±45 orientations along with the traditional 0/90 orientations.

Another means to improve tailorability is toward less labor-intensive methods of laying up small components. These would be components that are not candidates for fiber placement and whose shape and performance requirements are not compatible with thermoforming of sheet material. This might lead to development and use of a flexible cobot, that is, a robot that is integrated into human operations—controlled by human operators and coordinated with their activities. After an operator has positioned a ply, such a device might help by forcefully holding the ply in place against a contoured tool while heating to fuse or spot tack it to the ply below.

An additional, obvious manufacturing endeavor is further improvement in fiber-placement machines and processes, moderation of capital equipment costs, and generalization of the kinds of components for which fiber placement is advantageous. The dynamics of in situ consolidation will need to be modeled and better understood.

Still another obvious effort is toward increased unitization of structures. An emerging example is Dassault's hot tape lay-up and fusion of thermoplastic skin over thermoplastic stiffeners. Melt fusion processing provides a means to eliminate the high costs of drilling and countersinking holes and of buying and installing fasteners.

Pursuit of approaches to increase the "pull-off" capability of a melt-fused member can be expected. Success in this might enable wider spacing of stiffeners, improving structural efficiency and further reducing costs.

Conjecture about the future also leads to development of new applications. The author suggests that use of thermoplastic composites may expand toward cryogenic applications, particularly for cryogenic tanks. Factors that may lead in this direction are: (1) some thermoplastic composites may be resistant to microcracking effects from cryogenic exposures (Ref 32), and (2) hot-head fiber placement or winding methods may enable more cost-effective manufacture of such tanks (Ref 33, 34).

The latter factor also may favor extending applications into a variety of additional parts that are bodies of revolution. Such parts might be used *as* bodies of revolution, such as fuselage structure, or, two or more pieces might be cut out of such a body to serve such functions as leading edges, fairings, and cowlings.

Table 9 Applications of various polymers

Polymer	Applications
Polyetherketone ketone	RC-135 parabolic and blade radomes
Polyether etherketone	Airbus A320 vertical stabilizer brackets EH 101 helicopter floor F-117 rudder assembly F-22 weapons bay doors F-22 access covers OH-58D helicopter horizontal stabilizer Rafale engine tunnels
Polyphenylene sulfide	Airbus A330-200 rudder nose ribs Airbus A340 aileron ribs Airbus A340-500/600 fixed-wing leading-edge assemblies Airbus A340-500/600 inboard wing access panels Airbus A340-500/600 keel beam connecting angles Airbus A340-500/600 keel beam ribs Airbus A340-500/600 pylon panels Fokker 50 main landing gear door
Polyetherimide	737 smoke detector pans 737/757 galleys 747 stowage bins 767 aircraft acoustical tile 767 and other Boeing aircraft brackets Airbus A320 bulk cargo floor sandwich structural panels Airbus A330-340 lower wing fairings A3XX main stair case (developmental) Beluga heavy-duty entrance floor panels Dornier 328 landing flap ribs Dornier 328 ice protection plates Fokker 50 ice protection plates Fokker 50 trailing-edge wing shroud skins Fokker 70/100 structural floor panels Galleys on most commercial aircraft models Gulfstream G-V structural floor panels Gulfstream IV and V rudder ribs Gulfstream IV and V rudder trailing edges LearJet air steps M829E3 SABOT

ACKNOWLEDGMENT

Several individuals and companies have provided vital information that has been used for figures and to shape and populate the data tables in this article. Although a lot of information is available on the Internet, no "one-stop" information source has been found. Also, no Internet site currently offers "cutting-edge" information. Consequently, the following companies and individuals are gratefully acknowledged:

- Steve Peake and James Pratte, Cytec Fiberite, Havre de Grace, MD
- W.H. "Skip" Face, Ten Cate Advanced Composites bv, Fountain Valley, CA
- Willem H.M. van Dreumel, Ten Cate Advanced Composites bv, Nijverdal, The Netherlands
- Bob Buyny, Hexcel Corp., Dublin, CA
- Tim Greene, Applied Fiber Systems, Clearwater, FL
- Slade Gardner, Lockheed Martin Aeronautics Co., Fort Worth, TX
- Gerald Heard, Raytheon Systems Co., Greenville, TX

REFERENCES

1. J.G. Williams, T.K. O'Brien, and A.J. Chapman III, Conference Publication 2321, National Aeronautics and Space Administration, 1984
2. S. Oken and J.J. Hoggatt, AFWAL-TR-803023, Air Force Wright Aeronautical Laboratories, 1980
3. M.G. Maximovich, Development and Applications of Continuous Graphite Reinforced Thermoplastic Advanced Composites, *19th National SAMPE Symposium*, Vol 19, Society for the Advancement of Material and Process Engineering, 1974, p 262–281
4. E.J. Stober, J.C. Seferis, and J.D. Keenan, *Polymer*, Vol 25, 1984, p 1845
5. P.E. McMahon and L. Ying, Contractor Report 3607, National Aeronautics and Space Administration, 1982
6. G.R. Griffiths et al., *SAMPE J.*, Vol 20 (No. 32), 1984
7. "Standard Tests for Toughened Resin Composites," Reference Publication, rev. ed., National Aeronautics and Space Administration, 1983, p 1092
8. T.P. Kueterman, Advanced Manufacturing of Thermoplastic Composites, *ASM Conf. Proc., Advanced Composites*, 2–4 Dec 1985, American Society for Metals, p 147–153
9. J. Boyd, Bismaleimide Composites Come of Age: BMI Science and Applications, *SAMPE J.*, Vol 35 (No. 6), Nov/Dec 1999, p 13–22
10. H.-H. Kausch and R. Legras, Ed., *Advanced Thermoplastic Composites Characterization and Processing*, Hanser Publishers, 1993, p 113
11. S.L. Rosen, *Fundamental Principles of Polymeric Materials*, John Wiley & Sons, 1993, p 84
12. *Engineering Plastics,* Vol 2, *Engineered Materials Handbook,* ASM International, 1988
13. *Thermoplastic Composite Materials Handbook,* Cytec Fiberite, Havre de Grace, MD
14. "Results of the Qualification Test Program of CETEX Carbon Fabric (CD0286) Reinforced PPS (HC/C)," Report 5906.11, Ten Cate Advanced Composites, Nijverdal, The Netherlands, 12 June 1998
15. "Results of the Qualification Test Program of CETEX Carbon Fabric (CD0206) Reinforced PPS (HC/C)," Report 5906.30, Ten Cate Advanced Composites, Nijverdal, The Netherlands, 22 June 1998

16. "E Glass Fabric Reinforced Polyetherimide," CETEX Product Information, GI 0303 (SS 0303/8463), Ten Cate Advanced Composites, Nijverdal, The Netherlands
17. N.G. McCrum et al., *Principles of Polymer Engineering*, Oxford University Press, 1988, p 272–274
18. S.H. Olsen, Manufacturing with Commingled Yarn, Fabrics, and Powder Prepreg Thermoplastic Composite Materials, *SAMPE J.*, Vol 26, 1990, p 31–36
19. J. Muzzy et al., Electrostatic Prepregging of Thermoplastic Matrices, *Proc. 34th International SAMPE Symposium*, Society for the Advancement of Material and Process Engineering, 1989, p 1940–1951
20. "Tow Flex Product Guide," Applied Fiber Systems, Clearwater, FL
21. E. Werner, Powder-Based Prepreg Fabric: What, How, Why?, *Proc. 42nd International SAMPE Symposium*, Vol 42, Society for the Advancement of Material and Process Engineering, 1997, p 706–719
22. S. Zelenak et al., The Performance of Carbon Fiber Reinforced PEEK Subassemblies Joined Using a Dual Resin Bonding Approach, *Proc. 37th International SAMPE Symposium*, Society for the Advancement of Material and Process Engineering, 1992, p 1346–1356
23. T.Q. Li et al., Dependence of the Fracture Toughness of Thermoplastics Composite Laminates on Interfacial Interaction, *Compos. Sci. Technol.*, Vol 60 (No. 3), 2000, p 465–476
24. H.-H. Kausch and R. Legras, Ed., *Advanced Thermoplastic Composites Characterization and Processing,* Hanser Publications, 1993, p 173–191
25. A.P. Deshpande and J.C. Seferis, Crystallizability in a Model High-Performance Thermoplastic-Matrix Composite, *J. Thermoplast. Compos. Mater.*, Vol 12 (No. 6), 1999, p 498–514
26. J.G. Hutchins, "Operational Durability of Thermoplastic Composites in Primary Aircraft Structure," 52nd Annual Forum, American Helicopter Society (Washington, D.C.), 4–6 June 1996
27. S. Maison et al., Technical Developments in Thermoplastic Composite Fuselages, *19th SAMPE Europe/JEC International Conference* (Paris), 22–24 April 1998, Society for the Advancement of Material and Process Engineering, p 3–15
28. W. Schijve, Fokker 50 Thermoplastic Main Landing Gear Door: Design and Justification, *Proc. 38th International SAMPE Symposium,* Society for the Advancement of Material and Process Engineering, 1993, p 259–269
29. A.R. Offringa, Fokker 50 Main Landing Gear Door: Thermoplastic Processing, *Proc. 38th International SAMPE Symposium,* Society for the Advancement of Material and Process Engineering, 1993, p 270–281
30. Company information brochure, Fokker Aerostructures, Papendrecht, The Netherlands
31. "Thermoplastic Aircraft Radome Forming Process Offers High Volume, Low Cost," Success Story from the Air Force Research Laboratory, posted at www.ml.afrl.af.mil/successes/1999/ss99-98295.html
32. S.J. Rios and R. Arrowood, Impact Damage in E-Glass/Polypropylene Compared to E-Glass Thermoset Laminates, *Proc. 44th International SAMPE Symposium*, SAMPE '99, 23–27 May 1999, Society for the Advancement of Material and Process Engineering, p 1768–1779
33. R.J. Langone et al., Continued Development of Automated, in situ Processing for Thermoplastic Composite Structures and Components, *Proc. 42nd International SAMPE Symposium*, 4–8 May 1997, Society for the Advancement of Material and Process Engineering, p 56–64
34. O. Christen et al., Thermoplastic Winding with Direct Impregnation: Cost-Effective Production of Pressure Cylinders, *Kunst. Plast. Europe*, Vol 89 (No. 4), 1999, p 18–19

Molding Compounds

MOLDING COMPOUNDS are plastic materials in varying stages of pellets or granulation that consist of resin, filler, pigments, reinforcement, plasticizers, and other ingredients ready for use in a molding operation. This article describes sheet molding compounds, bulk molding compounds, and injection molding compounds. Additional information about the resins and reinforcements used in these materials is provided in other articles in this Section. Detailed information on processing is provided in the Section "Manufacturing Processes" in this Volume.

Sheet Molding Compounds

Sheet molding compound (SMC) refers to both a material and a process for producing glass-fiber-reinforced polyester resin items. The material is typically composed of a filled, thermosetting resin and a chopped or continuous strand reinforcement of glass fiber. The uncomplicated SMC processing machine (Fig. 1) produces molding compound in sheet form that is not unlike that of rolled steel. The size of the machine is designated by the width of the sheet it produces. Machine manufacturers generally offer a range of sizes from 0.6 to 1.5 m (2 to 5 ft), the most common being 1.2 m (4 ft).

The process starts in the paste reservoir (below the chopper in Fig. 1), which meters a specified amount of resin filler paste onto a plastic carrier film. The paste consists of several ingredients, which can be changed to fit the particular needs of specific processing conditions and applications. The carrier film passes under a chopper, which cuts glass roving into 25 mm (1 in.) lengths. After the glass falls to the resin bed, another carrier film with another layer of paste is added on top, sandwiching the glass between the two layers.

When the paste is first mixed and put in the SMC machine, it has the consistency of pancake batter. After maturation, when the thickening agents have had the opportunity to react, the material attains the consistency of heavy putty or caulking compound. Once matured, all carrier film is removed, the SMC material is cut into charges, and the charges are placed in matched metal die molds made of machined steel. A high-tonnage hydraulic press then applies molding pressure. The application of heat and pressure causes the SMC to flow to all areas of the mold. Heat from the mold, normally 150 °C (300 °F), also activates the catalyst in the material, and cure or cross linking takes place. The part is then removed from the mold.

A number of advantages can be credited to the SMC compression molding process:

- High-volume production
- Excellent part reproducibility
- Low labor requirement per unit produced
- Minimum material scrap
- Excellent design flexibility (from simple to very complex shapes)
- Parts consolidation
- Weight reduction

Material Components

With an unsaturated polyester resin system as its base, the resin paste incorporates other materials for desirable processing and molding characteristics and optimal physical and mechanical properties. Glass-fiber reinforcements improve the performance of polyester by upgrading mechanical strength, impact resistance, stiffness, and dimensional stability. Other additives are catalysts, fillers, thickeners, mold release agents, pigments, thermoplastic polymers, polyethylene powders, flame retardants, and ultraviolet absorbers, all of which are mixed by the SMC manufacturer to exact proportions for specific resin paste formulations. Some ingredients, such as release agents and thermoplastic syrups, can be added by the resin supplier. As described below, each additive provides important properties to the SMC, either during the processing and molding steps or in the finished parts. Additional information on additives provided in Ref 1.

The catalyst initiates the chemical reaction (copolymerization) of the unsaturated polyester and monomer ingredients from a liquid to a solid state. This is the primary purpose of a catalyst. Heat from the mold causes the catalyst to decompose, which activates the monomer and polyester to form cross-linked thermosetting polymers.

Catalysts are only a small part of an SMC resin formulation. Generally, the addition of 0.3 to 1.5 wt% of catalytic agents will adequately promote the cross-linking reaction. Organic peroxides are the principal catalysts used for SMC

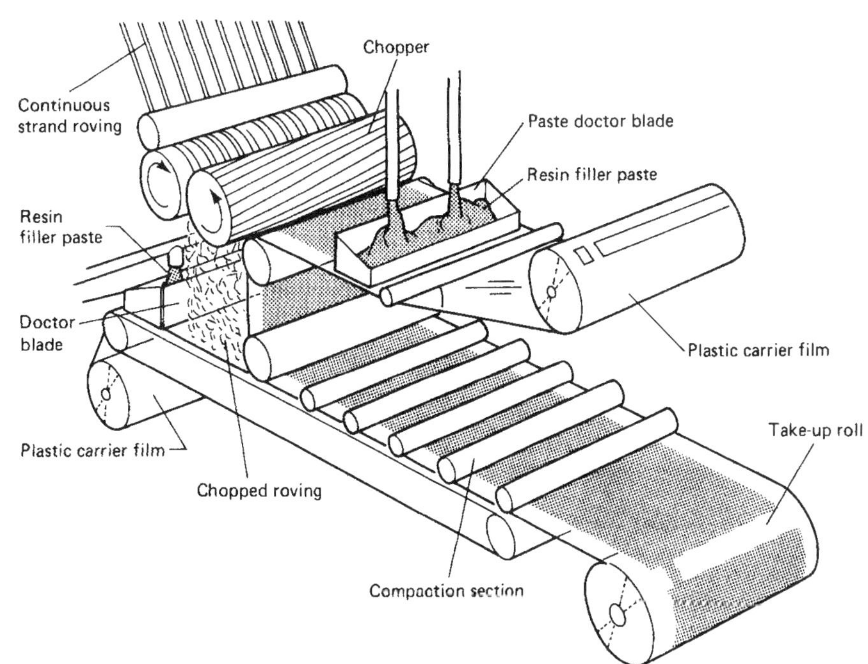

Fig. 1 Sheet molding compound processing machine

resin pastes. The temperature at which the curing process is to be carried out usually determines the selection of a catalyst. For any given catalyst-resin system there is an optimal temperature at which peroxide decomposition initiates the monomer-resin polymerization process. Since SMC is usually molded at temperatures of 132 to 165 °C (270 to 330 °F), catalysts that are the most effective as polymerization initiators over this temperature range are the ones used most often.

Fillers enhance the appearance of molded parts, promote flow of the glass reinforcement during the molding cycle, and reduce the overall cost of the compound. Commonly used fillers include calcium carbonate, hydrated alumina, and clay. Calcium carbonates are readily available and can be added to polyester resin in large amounts, while still maintaining a processable paste. They assist in reducing shrinkage of the molded parts and in distributing glass reinforcement for better strength uniformity. Hydrated alumina fillers are incorporated in SMC formulations to provide flame retardancy while maintaining good electrical properties. They are used in most electrical and appliance applications and in some construction applications where material requirements call for specific Underwriters' Laboratories (UL) standards established for flame spread, burning, and smoke density. Kaolin clays are sometimes combined with calcium carbonates or hydrated aluminas. When they represent 10 to 20% of the total filler weight, the clays serve to control paste viscosity, promote flow, and improve resistance to cracking in molded parts.

Thickeners include calcium and magnesium oxides and hydroxides. They initiate the reaction that transforms the mixture of SMC ingredients into a handleable, reproducible molding material. Usually 1 to 3% of the SMC resin formulation is thickener. It is the final ingredient added to the resin mix, and it begins the chemical thickening process immediately.

The thickening reaction must:

- Be slow enough to allow wet-out and impregnation of the glass reinforcement
- Be fast enough to allow the handling required by molding operations, as soon as possible after the impregnation step, in order to keep storage inventories low
- Give a viscosity at molding temperatures that is low enough to permit sufficient flow to fill out the mold at reasonable molding pressures
- Give a viscosity at molding temperatures that is high enough to carry the glass reinforcement along with the resin paste as it flows into the mold
- Level off in the moldable range to give a long shelf life

A typical thickening curve is shown in Fig. 2.

Release agents are common components of SMC formulations. They are selected on the basis of their melting points being just below that of the molding temperature. In theory, the release agent at the molding compound-mold surface interface melts upon contact and forms a barrier against adhesion.

Commonly used internal release agents include zinc stearate, calcium stearate, and stearic acid. Zinc stearate has a melting point of 133 °C (272 °F) and can be used at molding temperatures up to 155 °C (310 °F). Calcium stearate, with a higher melting point of 150 °C (302 °F) can be used at molding temperatures up to 165 °C (330 °F). Stearic acid should be used only if molding temperatures are below 127 °C (260 °F).

Mold release agents must be used at the lowest concentration possible to do an adequate job, which normally is a concentration less than 2 wt% of the total compound. Excessive amounts can reduce mechanical strength, cause objectionable cosmetic appearance on the molded part surface, and affect paint and/or bond adhesion characteristics.

Pigments are supplied as either dry powders or paste dispersions. Two advantages of paste dispersion pigments are that there are fewer agglomerates in the SMC resin paste and that they can be added at lower concentrations than dry powders. Pigment concentration generally is 1 to 5 wt% of the resin paste. Pigments can affect the cure time and shelf life stability of SMC systems and may accelerate or inhibit the reactivity of the catalyst-resin system. Thus, preevaluation of the reactivity of a specific pigment is essential.

Thermoplastic polymers are combined with polyester resins to achieve low polymerization shrinkage for many SMC applications. Shrinkage is primarily controlled by varying the polyester/thermoplastic ratio. It is possible to attain near-zero shrinkage in molded parts when thermoplastic polymers are added to polyester resins at concentrations of 40 wt% of the total resin system.

There are a number of thermoplastic additives that are compatible with polyester resins developed for SMC low-shrink and low-profile systems. Among those in use are acrylics, polyvinyl acetate, styrene copolymers, polyvinyl chloride (PVC), PVC copolymers, cellulose acetate butyrate, polycaprolactones, thermoplastic polyester, and polyethylene powder.

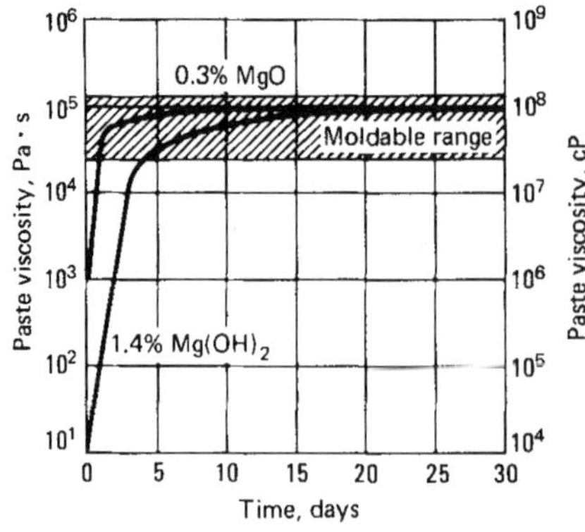

Fig. 2 SMC paste thickening curve

Flame Retardants. As a filler, hydrated alumina compounds normally satisfy most UL requirements, but more stringent flammability classifications necessitate the use of flame-retardant additives. These additives are used in conjunction with hydrated alumina fillers and halogenated polyester resins to provide maximum retardancy performance. Flame-retardant additives recommended for SMC are antimony trioxides, tris (2,3,-dibromopropyl) phosphates, chlorinated paraffins, and zinc borates. Two of these additives are often combined at 1-to-1. ratios to offer more selective properties. About 3 to 5% of the SMC formulation consists of these additives.

Ultraviolet (UV) absorbers can be added to SMC resin blends when the molded parts need to withstand extended exposure to sunlight. Generally, SMC resins are stabilized with approximately 0.1 to 0.25% of UV absorber of the benzotriazole or benzophenone type.

Physical Properties

The typical SMC properties shown in Table 1 represent a broad range of data on composites having 15 to 30% glass reinforcements. Many of these properties were tested on specific SMC formulations to better define their suitability for various end-product applications. Standard test methods, developed by ASTM and others, were used. Mechanical properties were obtained on both dry (as-molded) and wet (2 h submersion in boiling water) test specimens. Additional properties normally reported on dry specimens include Izod impact (notched and unnotched), Barcol hardness, water absorption, and heat distortion.

It should be noted that most standardized laboratory tests are, at best, a simplification or approximation of what may happen to a finished part in use. The shape and dimensions of the test specimens and the procedure by which they are molded practically never duplicate those of any end product.

Table 1 Typical mechanical properties for sheet molding compounds with 15 to 30 wt% glass fiber

Tensile modulus, GPa (10^6 psi)	11–17 (1.6–2.5)
Tensile strength, MPa (ksi)	55–138 (8–20)
Elongation at failure, %	0.3–1.5
Compressive strength, MPa (ksi)	103–206 (15–30)
Flexural modulus, GPa (10^6 psi)	96–138 (1.4–2.0)
Izod impact strength, notched, J/m (ft · lbf/in.)	430–1176 (8–22)
Dielectric strength, kV/cm (V/mil)	120–160 (300–400)
Heat distortion temperature, °C (°F)	150–205 (300–400)
Thermal conductivity, W/m · K (Btu · in./h · ft^2 · °F)	0.19–0.25 (1.3–1.7)
UL flammability class, V	945
Rockwell hardness number	H50–H112
Specific gravity	1.7–2.1
Density, g/cm^3	1.7–2.1
Coefficient of thermal expansion, 10^{-6}/K	15–22

Mixing Techniques for SMC Resin Pastes

The three types of resin paste mixing techniques for an SMC operation are batch, batch/continuous, and continuous.

Batch mixing is an economical method adequate for preparing small amounts of resin paste for short production runs or for evaluating an experimental formulation. All raw materials can be mixed in a single mixing unit. The disadvantages are:

- Material efficiencies are low (generally considered to be 85% or less); the resin paste often becomes too thick for good wet-out of the glass.
- Batch-to-batch variations of the resin paste can lead to SMC inconsistencies.
- Additional manpower is required to make the paste and deliver it to the SMC machine.

The SMC supplier generally can justify a more automated resin-mixing system if large quantities of material are to be produced.

Batch/continuous mixing has these primary advantages over the batch system:

- More reproducible resin paste thickening
- Higher material efficiencies
- Less manpower

This mixing technique normally employs two tanks, A and B, one for holding the thickenable resin bath mix (A) and the other for holding the thickener material or component in a nonthickenable resin mix (B). A metering pump or cylinder is used to proportion each side of the paste system and simultaneously pump the paste through a static or dynamic mixer to the paste doctor (metering) blades. Batch mixing equipment for each paste side is still required in this system, but the combined A and B resin paste delivered to the machine has marked improvement in reproducibility.

Continuous mixing eliminates a separate resin paste mixing facility, which is its biggest advantage over the batch/continuous mixing system. Predetermined amounts of the liquid ingredients are individually pumped into a continuous mixer. The dry ingredients can be preblended or fed individually by automatic-metering equipment into the same continuous mixer. The amount of thickened resin paste in the continuous mixer can be kept to a minimum level for delivery to the SMC machine. Better control of the resin mix is accomplished, because reproducible pumping and metering rates are used. The continuous-mixing system also provides higher material efficiencies than either the batch or batch/continuous system. A change of resin formulation of the normal clean-up operation wastes only a small amount of material. Only the head of the mixer requires cleaning (flushing) with a suitable solvent, whereas in the batch/continuous system, all lines must be flushed, which involves more cleaning time and greater material waste. Water jacketing of the continuous-mixing head in an automatic system offers temperature control, thereby maintaining a more reproducible resin paste. The temperature of the resin mix is critical in viscosity control, with 32 °C (90 °F) at the time the thickening ingredient is added considered optimal. The continuous-mixing system (Fig. 3) is best for long runs. The length of set-up time makes short runs of various formulations impractical.

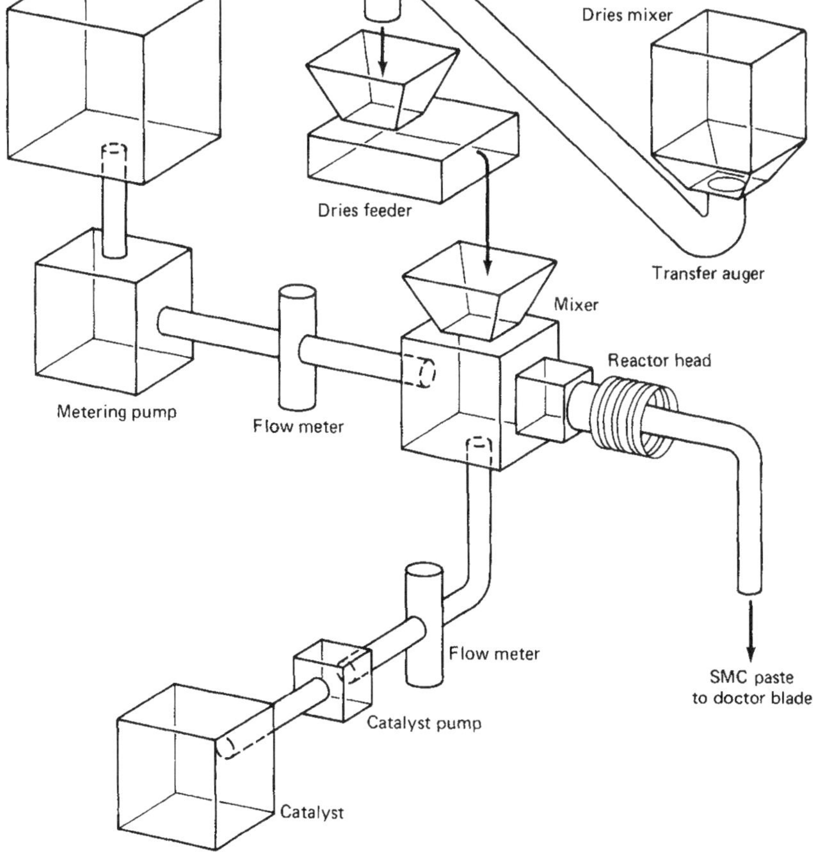

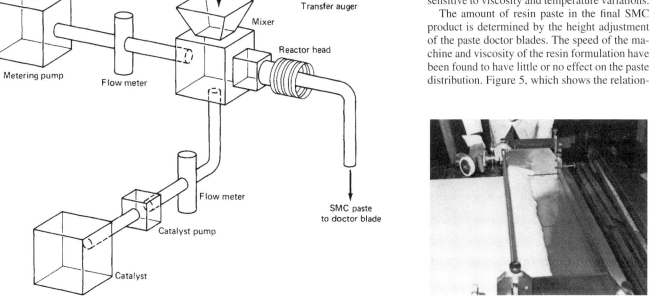

Fig. 3 Continuous SMC paste mixing system

SMC Machines

The two most common types of SMC machines are the continuous-belt and the beltless machines. Each type has unique design features, although the functional operations of both are very similar (see Fig. 1). Both types can handle chopped roving or chopped and continuous strand mat glass reinforcements.

Paste Metering. There are two adjustable paste doctor blades (Fig. 4) on the SMC continuous-belt machine, which meter a predetermined thickness of resin paste onto upper and lower carrier films of (usually untreated) polyethylene that is 0.05 mm (0.002 in.) thick. Paste doctor blades are adjustable for both product width and thickness. They are rigid blades positioned vertically to the belt and are beveled to a fine edge on the side of the belt away from the paste flow. The bevel makes the metering of the paste less sensitive to viscosity and temperature variations.

The amount of resin paste in the final SMC product is determined by the height adjustment of the paste doctor blades. The speed of the machine and viscosity of the resin formulation have been found to have little or no effect on the paste distribution. Figure 5, which shows the relation-

Fig. 4 Adjustable paste metering blades

ship of paste weight to paste doctor blade settings, is representative of the settings for each of the two paste doctor blades when a typical SMC resin paste formulation (1.5 to 1 filler ratio) is used.

Compaction. After the materials are brought together, they go through a compaction section to help push the resin paste through the glass to ensure wet-out of the glass. The two designs commonly used for compaction sections are serrated steel rollers and a chain belt.

Serrated Steel Rollers. This type of compaction system consists of three series of serrated steel rollers. The first series initiates the wet-out process, the second more intimately compacts the partially wet-out sheet, and the third completes the wet-out. There are a number of roller designs that do an adequate job of compacting the glass-resin sheet, but one particularly popular design uses grooved, spiral-cut roller flutes to force the resin paste into the glass pack with some lateral movement. Usually the rollers are pneumatically adjustable so that they can be set for maximum pressures (equal at each end) without causing shifting of the fibers or buildup of resin paste.

Chain Belt. New machines can be equipped with one or two dual wire mesh belt compaction modules. The two-dual module unit supports the sheet of SMC on both sides with a flexible wire mesh as it follows a sinusoidal path through the unit. The two modules have different mesh sizes in order to increase the range of materials that can be compounded, with the upstream module having a coarser mesh than the downstream module. The reasoning behind this is that a coarse mesh forces the resin paste to the center of the glass layer, and the fine mesh spreads the paste evenly through the layers. The compaction modules can also impart an oscillating motion to the movement of the upper belt to aid wet-out.

Take-up. SMC production machines are normally equipped with a dual turret take-up system for continuous operation, although festooning into 1350 to 1800 kg (3000 to 4000 lb) boxes is becoming more popular. The speed of the turrets is controlled by a weighted dancer roll that automatically adjusts to the correct tension as the SMC roll diameter increases. Electronic devices can be used to provide torque control on the wind-up mandrel.

When a full roll of SMC is ready, the sheet is cut and transferred to the second wind-up turret. The full roll is taped to prevent unwinding, and a vapor barrier sleeve is applied. The sleeve film can be any material, such as aluminum foil or monomer resistant film, that can contain the styrene monomer in the SMC and prevent UV light or moisture contamination. SMC rolls may vary in weight, but for shelf life stability and/or shipping in cardboard boxes, a weight of about 450 kg (1000 lb) per roll is considered the maximum. Sheet molding compound rolls for in-house storage and subsequent molding are suspended on racks that are mounted on wheels or designed for transporting by forklift vehicles.

Maturation Room Environments. A common practice among SMC processors is to condition their products in a temperature-controlled environment, known as a maturation room, to provide a uniform, reproducible viscosity for sheet molding. Maturation rooms are usually maintained at temperatures in the range of 29 to 32 °C (85 to 90 °F). Storage times may vary from 1 to 7 days, depending on the resin formulations. Maturation of most SMC formulations requires approximately 3 days.

Output and Feed Requirements. A single SMC machine can satisfy the material requirements of many molding presses. At 100% efficiency and continuous operation, one 1.2 m (4 ft) SMC machine can produce 11×10^9 g (25×10^6 lb) of molding compound per year.

Bulk Molding Compounds

Bulk molding compounds, or fiber-reinforced thermoset molding compounds, represent the original engineering plastic materials. Phenolic molding compounds reinforced with cellulose fibers were developed by L. Baekeland early in the twentieth century. Fiberglass reinforcement and polyester, melamine, and epoxy resin systems extended the range of thermoset material capabilities. More recent developments of carbon and aramid fibers and of polyimide and silicone matrices offer further enhancements of the engineering properties that are available in thermoset molding compounds.

Thermoset materials reinforced with long fibers offer excellent engineering properties in a moldable material. Bulk molding compounds can be molded into a variety of complex shapes by methods that can be readily automated for high-volume production. At the same time, their engineering properties can approach those attainable with continuous fiber-reinforced composites.

Formulation

There is a general similarity in the many formulations of bulk molding compounds. However, because of the wide variety of reinforcements, thermoset resins, and additives available, a multitude of compounds can be tailored for a variety of uses. Most compounds consist of:

- Resin matrix, with the necessary hardeners, catalysts, and plasticizers to make a moldable composition capable of curing
- Fiber reinforcement
- Additives, such as colorants, lubricants for mold release, and others for special properties, such as flame retardancy, dimensional stability, and crack resistance

Processing

Just as there are many formulations, there are many ways to compound and process the requisite raw materials into a bulk molding compound. These methods influence the final physical properties. Minimizing damage to the fiber reinforcement during processing is a key factor in maintaining optimal-strength properties.

Compound Preparation. One of the most common processing methods is the use of the sigma blade mixer. With this method, fiber reinforcement is charged to the mixer in prechopped form. Resin matrices are added in liquid form, such as polyester resins dissolved in styrene, or a varnish solution of resin (such as a phenolic) dissolved in methanol. With polyester bulk molding compound, the material is ready to mold when it is discharged from the mixer. With material made from a varnish, the solvent has to be volatilized and the resin advanced to a moldable viscosity.

Other methods of manufacture are used to obtain a longer chop length or a higher loading of reinforcement. One method is to pull reinforcement from a roving form through a dip tank of resin varnish, evaporate the solvent, and chop to length. Prepreg fabric can also be diced or chopped, with fabric used as the reinforcement. The resultant fabric is in a macerated form.

Molding Methods. Bulk molding compounds are processed by compression, transfer, and injection molding. Compression molding is used for large parts and wherever strength is critical to a molded part. This molding method causes the least amount of damage to reinforcing fibers, and in some cases, the orientation of the fibers can be predetermined.

A particular use of transfer molding is to mold inserts into the part, by prepositioning them in the mold prior to the transfer operation. Transfer molding is also used to ensure accurate dimensions in the end part and reduce cleanup of molded flash.

Injection molding is capable of the highest degree of automation and lowest processing cost. Special techniques are needed to feed the bulky materials into the injection machine. This process is not widely used for bulk molding compounds because of the poor flow characteristics of many compounds.

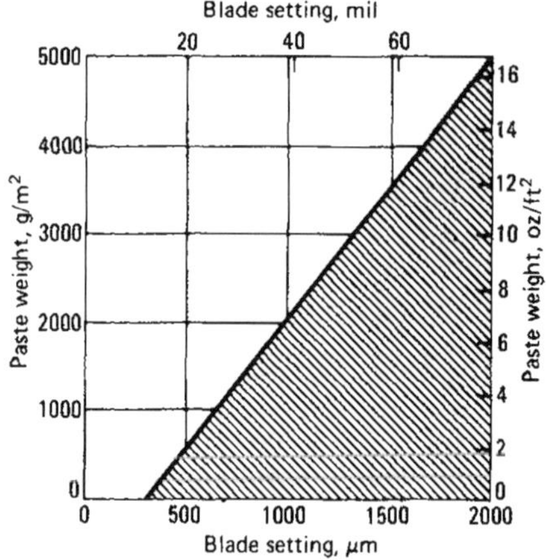

Fig. 5 Paste metering blade setting versus resin paste weight for typical SMC formulation

Properties A discussion of the effects of fiber type and length and matrix type on thermoset bulk molding compounds follows.

Effect of Fiber Type. The translation of fiber properties to bulk molding compounds that use the same matrix, fiber length, and percentage of fiber but different types of fiberglass, carbon, and aramid fibers, is shown in Table 2. Specific gravity, as might be expected, translates well with the fiber properties. Tensile and flexural strengths, and flexural modulus especially, also closely follow fiber properties. However, compressive strength properties show a distinct pattern of higher values produced by fiberglass reinforcement, followed by polyacrylonitrile-(PAN-) based carbon-fiber materials. Aramid-fiber compounds have lower compressive-strength values. PAN-based carbon fibers, being brittle, demonstrate the lowest Izod impact strength. Glass fibers have higher elongation values than aramid fibers, but are notch sensitive. The toughness of aramid fibers is demonstrated by their higher impact values; the difficulty encountered in cutting aramid fibers is demonstrated by this property.

Effect of Fiber Length. Generally, the longer the fiber reinforcement, the higher the physical properties. Typical lengths range from 3.2 to 50 mm (⅛ to 2 in.), with 3.2 mm (⅛ in.), 6.4 mm (¼ in.), and 12.7 mm (½ in.) predominating. The tensile, flexural, and particularly the impact strength properties show great improvement with increasing fiber length. Modulus values also show improvement with increasing length, but to a lesser degree than strength values.

The values for strength and modulus properties listed in Table 3 were obtained from compression molded test specimens. Partial orientation of the fiber reinforcement is obtained by mold geometry and resin flow. Orientation of the fiber reinforcement can be used with long fiber-reinforced bulk molding compounds to enhance performance in molded parts.

Effect of Matrix. Epoxy is used whenever the best structural performance is required, and polyimide is used when higher temperature performance is a criterion. Phenolics are used for their good heat-resistant and flame-retardant properties. Polyester is used in electrical applications that require high arc track resistance. Silicone does not offer good structural properties, but is used in applications where temperatures requiring continuous exposure up to 300 °C (570 °F) are needed.

The comparison in Table 4 of properties of bulk molding compounds reinforced with 12.7 mm (1/2 in.) chopped fiberglass measured at room temperature shows that an epoxy matrix yields the best structural properties. Polyimide and phenolics are close in their performance at room temperature. The slight advantage of polyimide improves with increasing temperature. Polyester offers good performance in electrical applications. Silicones, although unimpressive at room temperature, maintain their mechanical properties at temperatures up to 300 °C (570 °F).

Injection Molding Compounds

Injection molding compounds are thermoplastic or thermosetting materials and their composites, which are specifically formulated for the injection molding process. This process requires

Table 2 Properties of composite materials molded from bulk molding compounds

Material			Typical values													
				Fiber		Tensile strength		Flexural strength		Flexural modulus		Compressive strength		Impact strength	
Fiber type	Fiber product code	Resin type	Specific gravity, g/cm^3	wt%	vol%	MPa	ksi	MPa	ksi	GPa	10^6 psi	MPa	ksi	J/mm	ft · lbf/in.
Fiberglass	Type E	Epoxy	1.88	63	46	190	27	470	68	28	4.1	290	42	1.6	30
Fiberglass	Type S-2	Epoxy	1.85	63	46	210	30	430	62	30	4.3	260	38	1.7	32
PAN-based carbon	High-strength	Epoxy	1.48	58	49	140	20	330	48	38	5.5	190	28	0.55	10
PAN-based carbon	High- modulus	Epoxy	1.51	58	48	170	25	340	50	55	8.0	210	30	0.70	13
Aramid	Kevlar 49	Epoxy	1.34	53	49	160	23	290	42	21	3.0	150	22	1.8	34
Aramid	Kevlar 29	Epoxy	1.33	53	49	110	16	270	39	19	2.8	130	19	2.1	40

Table 3 Effect of chop length on properties of compression molded composite materials

Material					Typical values												
			Chop length			Fiber		Tensile strength		Flexural strength		Flexural modulus		Compressive strength		Impact strength	
Fiber type	Fiber product code	Resin type	mm	in.	Specific gravity, g/cm^3	wt%	vol%	MPa	ksi	MPa	ksi	GPa	10^6 psi	MPa	ksi	J/mm	ft · lbf/in.
Fiberglass	Type E	Epoxy	6.4	¼	1.88	63	46	120	17	270	39	25	3.6	190	27	0.75	14
Fiberglass	Type E	Epoxy	12.7	1.2	1.88	63	46	190	27	470	68	28	4.1	290	42	1.6	30
Fiberglass	Type E	Epoxy	31.8	1¼	1.88	63	46	310	45	760	110	32	4.6	290	42	2.8	53
Fiberglass	Type E	Phenolic	12.7	½	1.78	56	34	110	16	240	35	21	3.0	240	35	1.1	20
Fiberglass	Type E	Phenolic	25.4	1	1.78	56	34	120	18	280	40	24	3.5	260	37	1.6	30
Fiberglass	Type E	Polyimide	6.4	¼	1.90	63	47	100	15	250	36	19	2.8	230	34	0.04	7
Fiberglass	Type E	Polyimide	12.7	½	1.95	63	47	140	21	260	37	21	3.1	220	32	1.2	22
PAN-based carbon	High-strength	Epoxy	12.7	½	1.48	53	49	140	20	330	48	38	5.5	190	28	0.55	10
PAN-based carbon	High-strength	Epoxy	50.8	2	1.44	53	49	160	23	470	68	38	5.5	220	32	1.0	18

Table 4 Effect of resin matrices on properties of composite materials produced from bulk molding compounds

Material			Typical values													
				Fiber		Tensile strength		Flexural strength		Flexural modulus		Compressive strength		Impact strength	
Fiber type	Fiber product code	Resin type	Specific gravity, g/cm^3	wt%	vol%	MPa	ksi	MPa	ksi	GPa	10^6 psi	MPa	ksi	J/mm	ft · lbf/in.
Fiberglass	Type E	Epoxy	1.88	63	46	190	27	470	68	28	4.1	290	42	1.6	30
Fiberglass	Type E	Polyimide	1.95	63	47	140	21	260	37	21	3.1	220	32	1.2	22
Fiberglass	Type E	Phenolic	1.78	56	34	110	16	240	35	21	3.0	340	35	1.1	20
Fiberglass	Type E	Polyester	1.98	55	39	80	12	170	25	17	2.5	180	26	0.8	15
Fiberglass	Type E	Silicone	2.02	46	34	30	4	70	10	14	2.0	80	11	0.25	5

materials capable of being fed into a molding machine, transported to accumulate pressure, injected through channels, and made to flow into a small opening in the mold. The process may cause major changes in both the physical and chemical properties of the molding compound. Because of their resistance to flow, neither high-molecular-weight resins nor long reinforcing fibers, or flakes, can be effectively manipulated through the molding process. Consequently, parts produced from molding compounds represent a compromise between optimal physical properties and the essential ability to flow under pressure. This compromise is offset by the ability to produce three-dimensional products with holes, ribs, and bosses, often without secondary operations or direct labor.

While the flow process has the potential to physically change the molding compound, these changes are not always negative. Improved homogeneity, better reinforcement wetting, and higher physical properties may be achieved if the response of the molding compound to the injection process conditions is well understood. Where this understanding is absent, reinforcements may be broken, and polymers may be either degraded or prematurely cured. This article focuses on enhancing the general understanding of the forces that these compounds encounter in the injection molding process, rather than on the thousands of commercially available molding compounds. Table 5 itemizes the more common thermoplastic and thermosetting molding compounds and indicates where, within the four subprocesses of injection molding, specific formulations demand special care or attention.

The injection process (Fig. 6) may be divided into four specific zones in which the molding compound properties may be changed. These zones, which correspond to the four injection molding subprocesses, are:

- Feeding the molding compound into the molding machine
- Transporting and melting the compound, while developing pressure
- Injecting the molding compound through runners and gates
- Flowing the molding compound material into the mold cavity

Within each of these areas, several forces may combine to affect one molding compound in a manner entirely different from the way they affect another. The uniformity of a thermoplastic may be improved by the combination of shearing forces and heat, while the fibrous reinforcement of a thermoset molding compound may be broken, or the polymers may be prematurely cured. An extremely high shear rate may be beneficial to an unfilled polymer blend or alloy, but similar conditions might cause another molding compound to flow unevenly.

Plastic resins obtained directly from a chemical reaction rarely exhibit the properties that are essential to meet the flow requirements for feeding into injection machines. Therefore, a separate compounding operation is used to convert the form of a resin while also introducing the stabilizers, lubricants, reinforcements, filters, and even the pigments that will constitute the final injection molding compound formulation. During this operation, the molding compound resin may be exposed to heat, shearing forces, and ambient moisture. Most "virgin" molding compounds carry a history of these events. The nominal molecular weight distribution, length of the reinforcement (if one is used), and moisture content may vary as a result.

In most cases, the chemical effects are slight and would require precision analytical instruments to detect. It is wise, however, to monitor the consistency of the average molecular weight of the "as received" molding compound, using ASTM D 1238 (Ref 2), ASTM D 3123 (Ref 3), or gel-permeation chromatography.

Because fiber length may be dramatically reduced during compounding (Ref 4) some compounders of glass- or carbon-fiber composites coat the strands of fibers with coupling agents or molten/fluid ingredients and chop them into pellets of the desired length to ensure a specific fiber length in the "after compounding" product.

Moisture will usually interfere with thermoset curing reactions. Compounding, unless done in

Table 5 Common thermoplastic and thermoset molding compounds

		Potential subprocess problem areas			
Base polymer	Principal applications	Feeding	Transporting	Injecting	Flowing
Thermoplastics					
ABS	Furniture, cabinets, containers, trim	(b)	(h)(i)	(k)(l)(n)(o)	(q)
Acetal	Clock gears, miniature engineered parts	(b)	(f)(h)(i)(j)	(o)	(p)(s)
Acrylic	Automobile light lenses, plastic glazing	(b)	(h)(i)	(k)(l)(n)(o)	(q)
Cellulose	Esters trim, moldings, screwdrivers	(b)	(h)(i)	(k)(l)(n)(o)	(q)(r)
Polycarbonate	Auto bumpers, traffic lights, lenses	(b)(c)	(f)(h)(i)(j)	(k)(l)(n)(o)	(q)
Polyester	Appliance parts, pump and electrical housings	(b)(c)	(h)(i)(j)	(o)	(p)(s)
Polyethylene	Houseware, food storage, dunnage	(b)	(i)	(o)	(p)
Fluoroplastics	Corrosion/solvent-resistant parts	(b)(c)	(f)(i)(g)	(k)(l)(n)(o)	(q)
Polyimide	Aerospace items, electrical insulators	(b)(c)	(h)(i)(j)	(k)(l)(n)(o)	(q)
Ionomer	Bumper rub strips, golf ball covers	(b)	(h)(i)	(k)(l)(n)(o)	(p)
Nylon	Auto parts, bearing retainers, appliances	(b)(c)	(h)(i)(j)	(o)	(p)(s)
Polyphenylene oxide and alloys	Auto instrument panels	(b)	(h)(i)(j)	(k)(l)(n)(o)	(q)(r)
Polypropylene	Battery cases, auto parts, containers	(b)	(h)(i)	(o)	(p)(s)
Polystyrene	Toys, advertising displays, picture frames	(b)	(h)(i)	(k)(l)(n)(o)	(q)
Polysulphone	Camera cases, aircraft parts, connectors	(b)(c)	(h)(i)(j)	(k)(l)(n)(o)	(q)
Polyvinyl chloride	Soft steering wheels, trim items	(b)	(f)(h)(i)(j)	(k)(l)(n)(o)	(q)(r)
Thermosets					
Alkyd	Switches, motor housings, pot/pan handles	(a)(b)	(g)(h)(i)(j)	(k)(l)(m)(n)(o)	(q)(r)(s)(t)
Allyl	Electrical connectors, circuit boards	(a)(b)	(g)(h)(i)(j)	(k)(l)(m)(n)(o)	(q)(r)(s)(t)
Epoxy	Electrical insulators, electronic cases	(b)(e)	(g)(h)(i)(j)	(k)(l)(m)(n)(o)	(q)(r)(s)(t)
Polyester	Automotive structural parts	(d)(e)	(g)(i)(j)	(k)(l)(m)(n)(o)	(p)(q)(r)(s)(t)
Polyimide	Aircraft components, aerospace parts	(a)(d)(e)	(g)(h)(i)(j)	(k)(l)(m)(n)(o)	(p)(q)(r)(s)(t)
Melamine	Dinnerware, microwave cookward	(b)	(g)(h)(i)(j)	(k)(l)(m)(n)(o)	(q)(r)(s)(t)
Phenolic	Distributor caps, plastic ash trays	(a)(b)	(g)(h)(i)(j)	(k)(l)(m)(n)(o)	(q)(r)(s)(t)
Urethane	Automotive body panels, bumpers	(a)(d)(e)	(g)(i)	(l)(m)(o)	(q)(r)(t)
Vinyl ester	Composite car/truck springs, wheels	(b)(d)(e)	(g)(i)(j)	(k)(l)(m)(n)(o)	(p)(q)(r)(s)(t)

(a) Moisture may chemically react to degrade the polymer base. (b) Drying is recommended to avoid splay in molded product. (c) Drying is essential to prevent molecular weight attrition. (d) Drying may volatilize monomers essential to the curing reaction. (e) Fiber reinforcement breakage may occur during force feeding. (f) Overheating may cause explosive depolymerization. (g) Overheating may cause premature curing of (thermoset) compound. (h) Venting is recommended to remove volatiles and reduce splay. (j) Overheating may produce chemical changes in the base polymer. (k) Fast injection of the molding compound can lead to serious overheating. (l) Filled or reinforced compounds will exhibit much higher viscosity. (m) Open runners required because material can cure in closed channels. (n) Melt fracture may occur with high injection speed. (0) Fiber-filler orientation will occur if molding compound is reinforced. (p) Major sink marks may develop if part sections are thick, not uniform. (q) Weak knitlines may develop if compound packing pressure is low. (r) Large mold vents recommended to allow volatiles to escape. (s) Hot molds required to promote cure, crystalline growth. (t) Curing reaction may produce peak exotherm, leading to degradation.

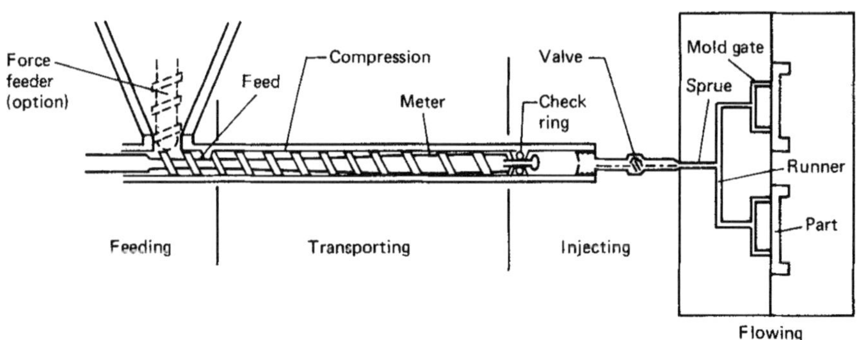

Fig. 6 The tortuous path of injection molding compounds

controlled environments, may introduce extreme moisture content variations between the extremes of dry winter periods and humid summer days. Thermoplastic molding compounds are often produced as extruded strands and quenched in water. The moisture content of thermoplastics produced in this manner may vary, based on the efficiency of the compounder's driers and the moisture-sealing effectiveness of the shipping containers. Thermoplastic molding compounds should be dried before feeding. At the very least, moisture can affect surface quality, cause steam erosion of the mold, or interfere with the curing reaction. At worst, moisture can actually interfere with polymerization, and hence diminish the molecular weight of certain condensation thermoplastics, such as nylon, polycarbonate, or polyester, or consume vital cross-linking sites in thermoset compounds, such as urethanes. Hopper driers and routine quality assurance tests are usually all that is required to ensure that compounding has not already changed the chemistry of the plastic.

Feeding thermoplastic, thermoset, or composite molding compounds is greatly facilitated when they are in the form of dry, free-flowing pellets. However, if this is not the case, the feeding process may cause variations in both the base polymer and any reinforcements. Typically, the molder will elect to integrate some or all of the compounding operations into the feeding and transport processes. The injection of liquid pigments, cointroduction of glass fibers and thermoplastic pellets, and building of a bulk molding compound at the press are examples of this dual-process integration. While economically feasible, compounding integration during the molding process should not be attempted without a solid understanding of the underlying effects on a molding compound.

Molding compounds that are sticky, rubbery, or powdery present feeding problems that often require specialized prefeeders. Force-feeding units may be employed, although the potential improvement in mixing may be outweighed by fiber-length attrition in reinforced molding compounds. There are mechanical auger-feeder devices and so-called strap feeders that are designed to introduce a ribbon of molding compound (usually rubber) directly into the feed throat of the injection molding machine. Auxiliary feeders generally add no heat to the molding compound.

Transporting the molding compound forward from the feed section to the injection section often provides high shearing forces, heat, and extensive mixing, which can be good or bad depending on the polymer. In normal processing of thermosets, the transport zone is designed only to densify the molding compound by removing entrapped gases. For thermoplastics, the densification process requires heat. A pressure gradient, required to degas both thermoplastics and thermosets, is produced by use of variable flight depth (tapered) screws to provide pumping, compression, decompression, and mixing functions. The design of these screws will vary greatly from thermoplastic to thermoset, from crystalline to amorphous polymers, and from inherently solid to potentially volatile materials (see Fig. 7). The description of an injection molding screw is complex and involves two key factors: the length and the compression ratio.

Short screws are recommended for heat-sensitive thermosetting injection molding compounds. Longer screws are needed for thermoplastic molding compounds that must be both compressed and melted. The compression ratio is determined by dividing the "open volume" in the feed zone of the screw by the volume at the end of the screw. Thermoplastic molding compounds require compression ratios in the range of 2.0 to 3.0 or more. Thermoset molding compounds rarely require compression ratios above 1.5. Exactly how the compression is achieved is also of great importance to the ultimate properties of the molding compound. A heat-sensitive thermoset should not be compressed quickly during the transport process, because reinforcing fiber lengths will be broken and/or excessive heat will be created. Similarly, a thermoplastic molding compound should not be compressed quickly, unless the intent is to create a hot spot of extremely high work energy. The specification of the screw profile of the injection molding machine is just as vital as the specification of its compression ratio and length.

Thermoplastic molding compounds must be gradually melted, compressed, degassed (if volatile), sheared (if crystalline and amorphous), and accumulated before injection. This must be accomplished with minimal thermal gradient, at the lowest possible temperature, and with minimal heat history. Otherwise, the part cooling time will be extended, part shrinkage may vary, and the potential for polymer degradation may be increased, although degradation is not always the result. Reinforced thermoplastic molding compounds of improved strength may be obtained if sufficient time is allowed for the polymer to wet the reinforcement surface (Ref 5). The proper compression ratio for an injection molding screw will be slightly greater than the bulk density of the as-received molding compound divided by the density of the molten metal (melt).

Crystalline thermoplastics, such as acetal, nylon, polypropylene, and polyester, should be processed with screws containing a meter zone (no further compression) at the end of the profile. The meter zone is really a high shear zone where the crystalline regions can be more effectively melted or fluxed. Amorphous thermoplastics, such as acrylonitrile-butadiene-styrene, styrene, polycarbonate, and acrylic, require little, if any, meter zone (Ref 6), because it would create useless shear and heat that could reduce molecular weight, which in turn could reduce impact strength.

Volatile materials must be removed from any molding compound to prevent either internal voids or splay (a fanlike surface defect near the gate) on the part. With thermoplastic molding compounds, a two-stage "vented" screw may be employed, as shown in Fig. 7. Only thermally stable molding compounds can safely employ two-stage injection molding screws. The orderly transport of molding compound is interrupted where the second screw stage begins. Thermally unstable molding compounds may accumulate, and the increased residence of time and heat will degrade them at this vent point. Attaching a vacuum pump to this vent point will further reduce the volatile content of the molding compound.

Thermoset molding compounds are rarely vented, because their formulations usually include a proportion of potentially volatile, low-molecular-weight monomers that are needed later in the molding process to cross link the resin. Venting could seriously deplete these vital ingredients. The objective of the transport process in the injection molding of thermosets is to preserve both the physical and chemical integrity of the compound, while providing mixing and densification. Low compression ratios are required to prevent the reduction of reinforcing fiber length and to avoid the mechanical heat. Any hot spots could prematurely initiate the curing reaction. For this reason, it is standard operating procedure to cool the barrel of an injection mold-

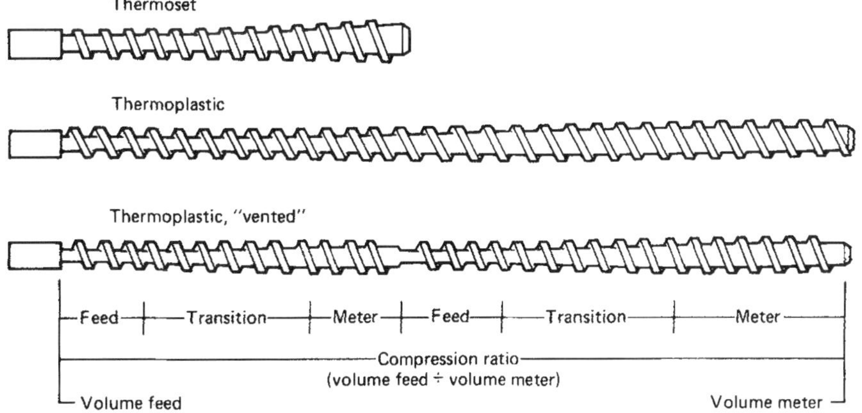

Fig. 7 Injection molding compound screws

ing machine that is used for thermosets, whereas the barrel is always heated for use with thermoplastics.

In either thermoplastic or thermoset injection molding, the end of the transport process is the accumulation of a volumetrically predetermined amount (shot) of compound, under pressure, somewhere in front of the screw. In some thermoplastic molding techniques, such as molding of structural foam, this shot is held in an accumulator. Normally, however, the shot is accumulated between the end of the screw and the end of the barrel. The screw must be allowed to slide back out of the barrel, under some controlled back pressure, to allow for this accumulation. In the subsequent injection subprocess, the travel of the screw is reversed, because the shot is forced forward.

A check ring, ball check, or some other mechanical valve must be placed at the tip of the screw to prevent the molding compound from flowing back down the screw during the subsequent injection. The resistance to flow through these devices can be so difficult that the polymer and any reinforcement will be degraded. The development of the free-flow check ring concept minimizes this difficulty (Ref 7). Another mechanical device, the nozzle valve, is needed to contain the molding compound within the barrel of the injection machine as the shot is being accumulated. As with the check ring, nozzle valves can be areas of extremely high shear, work energy, and heat. In some cases, nozzle valves can be eliminated by assuming that the tail end of the prior shot acts as a mechanical plug. This is effective only if the back pressure is low and the viscosity of the molding compound is high. Otherwise, the nozzle will "drool" after the molded part is removed.

Injecting thermoset molding compounds is done directly into the mold cavity through a single hole known as a sprue. The potential thermal instability of thermoset molding compounds usually precludes the use of "close" manifold systems used to support multicavity thermoplastic injection molding. When molding thermoplastics, however, the molding compounds will flow from the sprue into a system of "runners" leading to the gate of the mold. Injection pressures of up to 100 MPa (15 ksi) are employed to cause the molding compound to flow, although higher pressures are available on special injection machines equipped with boosters. The compound must flow if the mold is to be filled, and molding compounds are formulated specifically for this moment. If the flow is inadequate under the available conditions, an internal lubricant or processing aid may be used by the molding compound formulators to ensure that the molding compound flows smoothly without melt fracture or jetting (Ref 8), that is, the formation of disorderly ropelike patterns.

Jetting can occur as a result of fill rate in materials without these additives; it is a process phenomenon rather than a material condition. As the molding compound is injected from the nozzle through the sprue and then forward toward the mold, the narrowness of the runners exerts high shearing forces. In some cases, the presence of additional shear is beneficial, because it lowers the apparent viscosity in those molding compounds that exhibit shear thinning. Under these high-shear conditions, fibrous and flake reinforcements will align parallel to the runner walls. Random orientation will become flow orientation. As the compound reaches the entrance, or gate, of the mold, it will begin to flow into the cavity unless there is a gate valve restriction. Gate valves may be used in thermoplastic molding compound applications to avoid the scrap loss associated with the runner system. In some cases, however, these restrictions may create conditions of high shear and heat.

Flowing from the gate into the mold cavity proceeds as in the runner system. If the molding compound is reinforced and the gates are smaller than the fiber lengths, the reinforcements will break (Ref 5). If the formulator, compounder, and molder have all done their jobs, the molding compound should flow in an even front, or curtain. Experimenting with short shots, shown in Fig. 8, is a valuable analytical tool. Successively increasing the size of a short shot should produce a progressively more complete product with good surface finish. The presence of splay, bubbles, pits, or roughness indicates that something is wrong in the preceding feed, transport, and injection subprocesses. There are two notable exceptions to this rule. Rib sink, or a reverse vein appearance over a rib, is normal in a short shot. The molding compound has not been "packed out." If the molding compound is a structural foam, the front will not be smooth, as in a properly delivered unfoamed short shot, because under the tremendous injection pressure it will tend to explode into the unpressurized mold.

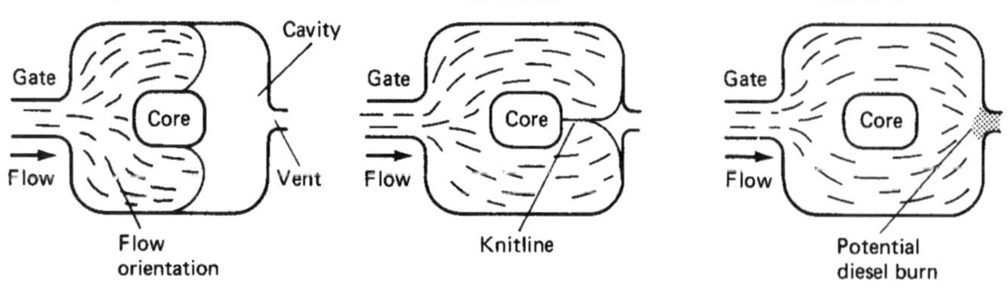

Fig. 8 Flowing molding compounds into molds

In order to inject the molding compound into a mold, the air within the mold must be adequately vented. Usually this is accomplished by determining the last area to be filled and providing a narrow vent slot from this point to the outside edge of the mold. When the mold fills to a point that is inaccessible to the parting line plane, an undersized ejector pin or flatsided pin may be used. If either of these actions is not taken or if the vents clog with processing oils or volatile additives, the force of injection may locally ignite the molding compound. Known as diesel burn, the ignition is caused by compressing the combustible oxygen in the mold. The molding compound within a burn area is chemically destroyed, and adjacent areas also may be affected.

Knitlines occur in any part that is molded in a cavity with more than one gate, or in any part where the molding compound is forced to flow around a pin or core. In cases of high shear stress, reinforcements such as talc, mica, and glass may physically protrude from the molding compound front. If knitlines are formed under these conditions, they will have greatly reduced strength. Although knitlines may be nearly invisible to the eye, they are areas of very high stress, fiber orientation, and potential weakness. To maximize the strength of a knitline, it is necessary to arrange the mold gating such that the melt fronts join before the completion of the shot. The molding compound fronts may thereby "scuff" together with sufficient force to achieve a higher-strength knit.

At the end of the flow process, the mold cavity will be filled. Depending upon whether the molding compound is thermoplastic or thermoset, it will begin to cool or cure. The cold molds used for crystalline thermoplastics must be held above the minimum crystalline growth temperature of the molding compound. Crystallinity initiators and so-called nucleated resins accelerate the rate of crystal growth but generally do not effectively lower the minimum crystal growth temperature. When thermoplastics crystallize, they shrink. If the mold is too cold to permit crystallization, the molded part will crystallize at some later time/temperature schedule, which may cause warpage or distortion. Thermoset molding compounds must cure. To initiate their chemical cross-linking reactions, it is necessary to heat the mold above the initiation temperature of the curing reaction. Once initiated, thermoset reactions liberate exothermic heat. At its peak, the heat produced in this manner may raise the molded temperature above the polymer degradation threshold. Thick thermoset molding compound products may present extreme difficulties both in the ability to uniformly initiate the curing process and, once initiated, to control the heat generated during the curing process.

ACKNOWLEDGMENTS

This article has been adapted from the following articles in *Composites,* Volume 1, *Engineered*

Materials Handbook, ASM International, 1987:

- J.J. McCluskey and F.W. Doherty, Sheet Molding Compounds, p 157–160
- W.G. Colclough, Jr. and D.P. Dalenberg, Bulk Molding Compounds, p 161–163
- F.J. Meyer, Injection Molding Compounds, p 164–167

REFERENCES

1. General Additives for Plastics and Elastomers, *Engineered Materials Handbook Desk Edition*, ASM International, 1995, p 287–291
2. "Standard Test Method for Flow Rates of Thermoplastics by Extrusion Plastometer," D 1238, *Annual Book of ASTM Standards,* ASTM
3. "Standard Test Method for Spiral Flow of Low-Pressure Thermosetting Molding Compounds," D 3123, *Annual Book of ASTM Standards,* ASTM
4. R.A. Schweizer, "Glass Fiber Length Degradation in Thermoplastics Processing," Paper presented at the 36th Annual Conference, Reinforced Plastics/Composites Institute, 1981
5. S. Newman and F.J. Meyer, Mica Composites of Improved Strength, *Polym. Compos.* Vol I (No. 1), Sept 1980, p 37
6. Zero Meter Screws, *Plast. World,* March 1982, p 34
7. A.J. Keeney, "Free Flow Check Ring and Zero Metering Screw," Paper presented at the 37th Annual Conference, Reinforced Plastics/Composites Institute, 1982
8. K. Oda, et al., Jetting Phenomena in Injection Mold Filling, *Polym. Eng. Sci.,* Vol 16 (No. 8), Aug 1976, p 585

SELECTED REFERENCES

- *Handbook of Reinforced Plastics*, Reinhold, 1978
- G. Lubin, Ed., *Handbook of Composites,* Van Nostrand Reinhold, 1982
- H.G. Kia, *Sheet Molding Compound Materials: Science & Technology,* Hanser Gardner, 1993
- R.B. Seymour, *Reinforced Plastics: Properties and Applications,* ASM International, 1991

Metallic Matrices

Awadh B. Pandey, Pratt & Whitney

METALLIC MATRICES are essential constituents for fabrication of metal-matrix composites (MMCs). Research and development on MMCs have increased considerably in the last decade due to their improved modulus, strength, wear resistance, thermal resistance, and fatigue resistance—and improved consistency in properties and performance in general—compared to the unreinforced matrix alloys. The concept of MMCs is based on using the best characteristics of two different materials, such as ductility and toughness of metallic matrices and the modulus and strength of ceramic reinforcements, to make a material with superior properties compared to the unreinforced metals. The reinforcements are added extrinsically or formed internally by chemical reaction. The properties of MMCs depend on the properties of matrix material, reinforcements, and the matrix-reinforcement interface. While a variety of matrix materials has been used for making MMCs, the major emphasis has been on the development of lighter MMCs using aluminum and titanium alloys, due to the significant potential of improvement in the thrust-to-weight ratio for the aerospace, space, and automotive engines.

The reinforcements are either in the form of continuous fibers or discontinuous reinforcements, such as chopped fibers, whiskers, particulates, or platelets. Metal-matrix composites can contain either continuous or discontinuous or a combination of both these reinforcements. The main advantage of discontinuously reinforced composites over continuous ones is that they can be fabricated using processing techniques similar to those commonly used for unreinforced matrix materials, which makes them more cost-effective. In addition, discontinuously reinforced composites have relatively more isotropic properties than continuously reinforced composites, due to the lower aspect ratio and more random orientation of the reinforcements.

The use of MMCs as ventral fins on F-16 aircraft and as fan exit guide vanes in commercial aerospace engines has attracted the attention of several researchers in the recent past. The life of the ventral fin has been increased significantly by the use of discontinuously reinforced aluminum (DRA). The role of matrix properties becomes more important in discontinuously reinforced composites compared to the continuous composite, due to a difference in the strengthening mechanisms for both these systems. The strength of continuously reinforced composites is mainly determined by the ability of load transfer from the matrix to the continuous fiber. Thus, the properties of fiber and the matrix-fiber interface become more important than the matrix property itself. This is evident in room temperature properties. For higher temperature, the role of matrix material becomes more important, because the high-temperature properties are controlled by diffusion in the matrix alloys. In discontinuously reinforced composites, the matrix material has a crucial role, because the strength of discontinuous composite depends on many other mechanisms in addition to the load transfer to the reinforcements. The other mechanisms responsible for strengthening in the discontinuous composites are the finer grain size, finer subgrain size, increased dislocation density, increased kinetics for precipitation hardening, and some degree of Orowan strengthening. The mechanical properties of discontinuously reinforced composites are dominated by the behavior of matrix alloys.

The choice of matrix material depends mainly on the strength, temperature, density, and cost requirements for the intended applications. For example, titanium appears to be an obvious candidate for very high-strength and moderate-temperature applications. However, aluminum may compete with titanium on the basis of specific properties, because of its significantly lower density, even though the strength and temperature capability of aluminum is lower than that of titanium. Also, the lower cost of aluminum compared to titanium provides an additional benefit for aluminum. Other factors, such as ductility, fracture toughness, and fatigue resistance, become more important once a particular metal is selected.

One of the most important factors is the compatibility of the matrix material with the reinforcement. Compatibility in this case means that there is no undesirable chemical reaction at the interface of the matrix and reinforcement. This reaction can sometimes lead to the formation of intermetallic compounds at the interface that may have the deleterious effect of transferring load to the reinforcements. Also, the reaction products may act as sites for crack nucleation.

The maximum mechanical property benefits MMCs often provide due to the presence of reinforcement are increased modulus, strength, and fatigue strength. However, the ductility and fracture toughness of MMCs are known to be inferior to those of the unreinforced matrix alloys, because the ductility and toughness of most ceramic reinforcements are very low. These properties are very important for any load-bearing structural applications. Therefore, it is apparent that the matrix alloys having higher ductility and fracture toughness are desirable for MMC applications.

Research in the area of aluminum-matrix composites has been concentrated mainly toward development of DRA composite, because of the ease of processing. Pure metal is usually not considered as a matrix material for MMCs, because the properties of pure metals are not attractive. Three classes of aluminum alloys have been chosen in the past for fabrication of MMCs:

- Wrought commercial aluminum alloys, such as 6061, 2124, and 7075, and cast aluminum alloys, such as aluminum-silicon and aluminum-magnesium
- The lighter aluminum-lithium alloys, such as 8090
- High-temperature aluminum alloys, such as aluminum-iron- and aluminum-scandium-base alloys

Most of the earlier studies have focused on understanding of the composite behavior rather than developing newer aluminum alloys. Work on developing a newer matrix alloy suitable for MMCs has focused on the modification of existing aluminum alloy compositions. Among these three alloy systems, maximum efforts have been put into developing MMCs with commercially available aluminum alloys (Ref 1, 2). These alloys were selected for MMCs because they offer good properties, are well understood, and are commercially available. While aluminum-lithium has considerable potential in terms of lowering density and improving modulus, only a few studies are available with regard to MMCs (Ref 3, 4). This may be partly related to the fact that aluminum-lithium itself is in the early development stage. Because commercially available aluminum alloys cannot be used at higher temperatures, the high-temperature aluminum alloys based on Al-Fe-V-Si and aluminum-scandium have been used to improve the high-temperature capability of MMCs. While significant potential exists for developing a newer aluminum alloy with improved properties for a wide range of temperatures, limited studies are available in this area (Ref 5–7).

Titanium-matrix composites with continuous fibers have received considerable attention in the past for improving strength and modulus of titanium alloys at ambient and high temperatures (Ref 8–10). Initially the efforts were concentrated on Ti-6Al-4V, which is the workhorse titanium alloy, with major emphasis on understanding the interfacial behavior. The studies were also focused on evaluating fiber strength, because the strengthening in the composite depends on the strength of the fiber and the quality of the interface. The understanding of interface characteristics is very important, because the transverse strength of continuous fiber composite is usually inferior. Different types of fibers were used to manufacture titanium composites with different fiber strengths. Subsequently, considerable studies have been conducted to exploit ordered intermetallics Ti_3Al and TiAl (γ), which offer improved high-temperature properties for MMCs applications. These ordered intermetallics have excellent high-temperature strengths, but lower room-temperature ductility. More recently, significant interest has been generated on discontinuously reinforced titanium (DRTi) composite to take advantage of isotropic properties. While both ingot and powder metallurgy (P/M) routes have been used, more emphasis was on the powder technique to reduce reaction between the matrix and reinforcement and also to provide more uniform distribution of reinforcement.

Aluminum Alloys

Aluminum alloys can be categorized in three different classes: commercial aluminum alloys, low-density and high-modulus alloys, and high-temperature alloys. The details of these alloys are given subsequently.

Commercial Aluminum Alloys

Commercial aluminum alloys can be classified in the following categories:

- *Wrought heat treatable alloys,* such as Al-Mg-Si (6000), Al-Cu-Mg (2000), and Al-Zn-Mg (7000), which require heat treatment to develop high strength through precipitation hardening. These alloys offer a wide range of strength and ductility. They have been used extensively in aerospace and other structural applications and have also been used for MMC development.
- *Wrought non-heat-treatable alloys,* such as aluminum-magnesium and aluminum-manganese, which provide strengthening through solid solution and dislocation structure introduced by cold work. The strengths of these alloys are not suitable for aerospace applications. These alloys have found applications in the automotive industries. These alloy systems have found limited use in MMC fabrications, due to their lower strengths.
- *Casting alloys,* which are based principally on the aluminum-silicon, aluminum-copper and aluminum-magnesium alloy systems. These alloys usually have a medium level of strength and ductility and are used in applications with complicated component geometries. Casting alloys have been used extensively for MMC applications.

Wrought heat treatable aluminum alloys are the most common alloys in the aluminum family. Among the three common series of alloys, 6000, 2000, and 7000, Al-Mg-Si (6000-series) alloys are very attractive for MMCs due to their high ductility and toughness, although strengths of this series are lower than the other two series. Table 1 lists the compositions and tensile properties of some selected 6000-series alloys. The Al-Mg-Si alloys are widely used in medium-strength applications due to their very good ductility, weldability, corrosion resistance, and immunity to stress-corrosion cracking. Magnesium and silicon are added in the 6000 series either in balanced amounts to form quasi-binary Al-Mg_2Si or with an excess of silicon needed to form Mg_2Si precipitate. Alloy 6061 is one of the most common alloys in the 6000 series, which has balanced compositions of magnesium and silicon. This also contains 0.2% Cr, which provides improved corrosion resistance. While the presence of excess silicon improves age hardening response, it may reduce the ductility and cause intergranular embrittlement, due to segregation of excess silicon to grain boundaries. This alloy also contains titanium for controlling recrystallization, because most of the aluminum alloys usually contain chromium, manganese, zirconium, or titanium for grain refinement purpose. Alloy 6092 (Al-1.0Mg-0.6Si-0.85Cu-0.15Ti-0.3Fe), a modification of 6061 alloy, is a P/M alloy developed by DWA Composites, Inc. (Ref 11). The ventral fin and the fan exit guide vane were manufactured using a wrought powder metallurgy 6092/SiC/17.5p composite. The 6000-series alloys are suitable for MMC applications requiring medium strength and high ductility.

The 2000-series alloys have been used in several aerospace applications, due to their higher strengths compared to the 6000-series alloys. Table 1 shows the properties of some common 2000-series alloys used for aerospace and also for MMC applications. This series of alloys contain copper and magnesium to provide precipitation strengthening through formation of metastable precipitate of S′ (Al_2CuMg) for higher-magnesium-containing alloys and precipitation of θ′ (Al_2Cu) for higher copper-to-magnesium ratio alloys upon heat treatment. They also contain some other elements, such as chromium, zirconium, manganese, or titanium, to control the grain size. Alloy 2124, a purer version of 2024, is the most common alloy with lower amounts of iron and silicon contents. Iron and silicon are usually present in all the aluminum alloys as impurities. These elements can have a detrimental effect on ductility and fracture toughness of aluminum alloys. The toughness of 2124 alloy is improved significantly by reducing the iron and silicon content in the alloy (Ref 12). It is almost always desired to keep the amount of iron and silicon as low as possible in most of the aluminum alloys to preserve ductility and toughness, because these elements form large intermetallic particles, which can cause the nucleation of voids by debonding or cracking. This concern is particularly important for MMC applications, because the ductility and toughness of MMCs are lower than those of the matrix alloys due to the presence of the reinforcements.

Other 2000-series alloys that are of interest are 2014, 2219, and 2618. These alloys have been used for slightly higher-temperature applications. The higher copper-to-magnesium ratio provides improved properties at elevated temperatures, due to formation of θ′ (Al_2Cu) precipitate. Alloys 2014 and 2219 have high copper-to-magnesium ratios (Table 1). On the other

Table 1 Typical tensile properties and fracture toughness of selected heat treatable aluminum alloys

			Yield strength in 0.2%		Ultimate tensile strength			Fracture toughness (K_{Ic})	
Alloy	Composition	Temper	MPa	ksi	MPa	ksi	Elongation, %	MPa $\sqrt{m}$	ksi $\sqrt{in.}$
6061	Al-1Mg-0.6Si-0.25Cu-0.19Cr-0.1Ti-0.7Fe	T6	275	39.9	310	45.0	12	27	25
6063	Al-0.7Mg-0.4Si-0.1Cu-0.1Cr-0.1Ti-0.35Fe	T6	215	31.2	240	34.8	12	...	...
2014	Al-4.5Cu-0.5Mg-0.26Mn-0.7Fe-0.8Si	T6	410	59.5	480	69.6	13	31	28
2024	Al-4.3Cu-1.5Mg-0.6Mn-0.5Fe-0.5Si	T8	450	65.3	480	69.6	6	26	24
2124	Al-3.9Cu-1.5Mg-0.6Mn-0.3Fe-0.2Si	T8	440	63.8	490	71.1	8	32	29
2618	Al-2.3Cu-1.6Mg-1Ni-1.1Fe-0.15Fe-0.15Si	T61	330	47.9	435	63.1	10	...	...
2219	Al-6.3Cu-0.02Mg-0.3Mn-0.3Fe-0.2Si-0.1Zr	T87	315	45.7	475	68.9	10	36	33
7075	Al-5.6Zn-2.5Mg-1.6Cu-0.23Cr-0.2Ti	T73	430	62.4	500	72.5	13	32	29
7050	Al-6Zn-2.3Mg-2.3Cu-0.11Zr-0.15Fe-0.12Si	T7	510	74.0	550	79.8	11	33	30
7090(a)	Al-8Zn-2.5Mg-0.95Cu-1.45Co-0.15Fe-0.12Si	T7	580	84.1	620	89.9	9	26	24
7091(a)	Al-6.5Zn-2.5Mg-1.45Cu-0.4Co-0.15Fe-0.12Si	T7	545	79.0	590	85.6	11	46	42
CW67(a)	Al-9Zn-2.5Mg-1.5Cu-0.14Zr-0.1Ni	T7	580	84.1	614	89.1	12	43	39

(a) Alloys prepared by powder metallurgy processing

hand, 2618 contains additional elements, such as manganese, iron, and nickel with low diffusivity, which provides improved strengthening at elevated temperatures due to the formation of thermally stable dispersoids, such as Al_6Mn, Al_3Fe, Al_3Ni, and Al_9FeNi, respectively. Alloy 2219 is being used in cryogenic liquid tank for space application due to its higher strength and fracture toughness at cryogenic temperatures. In addition, 2219 has good creep strength at elevated temperatures. While 2014, 2219, and 2618 can be used at slightly higher temperatures compared to the conventional aluminum alloys, they cannot be used above 150 to 170 °C (300 to 340 °F). A modified version of 2219 with composition Al-6.3Cu-0.45Mg-0.3Ag-0.3Mn-0.15Zr is very attractive for MMC applications. The role of silver is to promote uniform precipitation of Ω-phase as very thin plates on {111} matrix planes, as shown in Fig. 1 (Ref 12). This Ω-phase has close relationship with θ (Al_2Cu), which forms as equilibrium precipitate. The Ω-phase is stable up to 200 °C (390 °F). The room-temperature strength and creep strength of this alloy are superior to that of 2219 alloy. The yield strength of this silver-containing alloy is 520 MPa (75 ksi) in the T6 condition, compared to 390 MPa (57 ksi) for 2219 alloy. The 2000-series alloys exhibit superior fatigue resistance compared to the 7000-series alloys, as shown by the fatigue crack growth rate (*da/dN*) versus the stress-intensity factor range (ΔK) in Fig. 2 (Ref 13). The higher threshold stress intensity and lower rate of crack growth in the 2000 series may be attributed to the higher ductility of 2000-series alloys compared to 7000 alloys.

The 7000-series alloys have received special attention in aerospace industries, because they provide the highest strength among all aluminum alloys. Table 1 shows the composition and properties of some common 7000 alloys. This series of alloys contain zinc and magnesium to provide precipitation hardening through formation of η′ (Zn_2Mg) phase. The role of copper is to improve stress-corrosion cracking resistance of these alloys. In addition, small amounts of chromium, zirconium, titanium, or manganese are also present for controlling recrystallization. The presence of zirconium also provides improved strength and toughness and reduced quench sensitivity of the alloys, in addition to the grain-size control. Alloy 7075, the most common alloy in this series, provides a good combination of strength, ductility, and toughness. The 7000-series alloys exhibit inferior stress-corrosion cracking resistance in the peak-aged condition; therefore, these alloys are used mostly in the T73 condition. The T73 condition is a duplex aging treatment employing higher-temperature aging (170 °C, or 340 °F) followed by peak aging at 120 °C (250 °F). Strength in the T73 condition is reduced, compared to the peak-aged condition.

Significant advances have taken place in the development of newer 7000 alloys such as 7090, 7091, and CW 67, using a P/M approach in order to improve the strength, toughness, and stress-corrosion cracking resistance by using the benefits of rapid solidification. This approach uses rapidly solidified powder produced by gas atomization, followed by compaction and extrusion of the powder. As shown in Table 1, the properties of all the P/M alloys are improved significantly over ingot metallurgy 7075 alloy. These alloys contain cobalt, nickel, or zirconium, which form very fine dispersoids of Al_9Co_2, Al_3Ni, and Al_3Zr, respectively, depending on the composition. These dispersoids effectively pin the grain boundaries, providing considerable strengthening through Hall-Petch relation. The grain size of P/M alloys is much finer than that of the ingot-based alloys (as shown in Fig. 3), which helps in achieving improved strengthening. The CW 67 has the best combination of strength and toughness, indicating significant potential for MMC applications to derive maximum benefit from matrix properties. As evident from Table 2, the strength of DRA depends significantly on the strength of the matrix alloy for a fixed volume fraction of reinforcement (Ref 14). These DRA materials are made by P/M approach to provide a uniform distribution of reinforcement particles in the matrix. Powder metallurgy is a preferred approach for making DRA today, because this can provide higher strength, ductility, and toughness than that of cast DRA materials. The strength of DRA containing 7091 alloy is higher than that of DRA containing 6061 and 2124, indicating that the 7000 alloys are more attractive for high-strength applications. It should also be noted that the effect of matrix alloys on the properties of DRA is more pronounced than that of volume fraction of reinforcement. The effect of matrix heat treatment on the properties of a powder metallurgy 7093/15 vol% SiC discontinuously reinforced aluminum is shown in Table 3 (Ref 15,16). The yield strength of this DRA material is very high (640 MPa, or 93 ksi) in the peak-aged condition. This table also indicates that the strength, ductility, and fracture toughness of DRA depend significantly on the heat treatment.

Wrought non-heat-treatable aluminum alloys include manganese and magnesium where

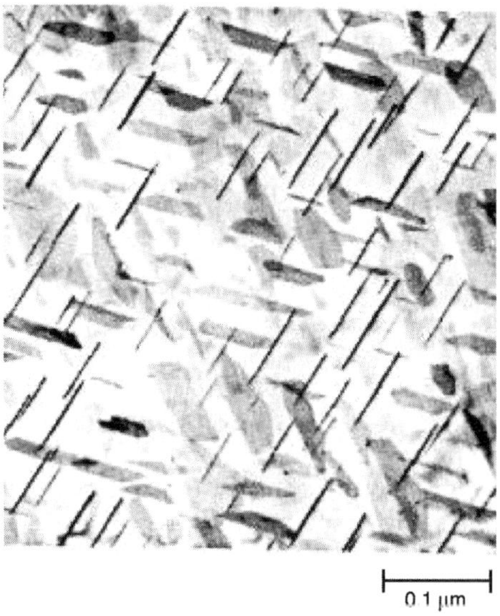

0.1 μm

Fig. 1 Transmission electron microscopy microstructure showing Ω–phase precipitated on the {111} planes in an Al-Cu-Mg-Ag alloy. ΔK_{th}, change in threshold stress-intensity factor. Source: Ref 12. Courtesy of R.J. Chester

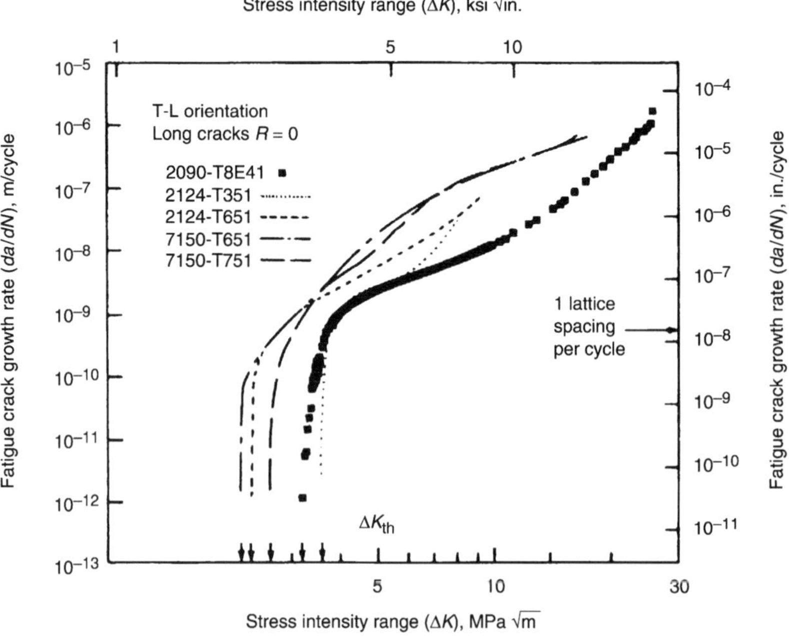

Fig. 2 Variation of fatigue crack growth rate (*da/dN*) versus stress-intensity factor range (ΔK) for various aluminum alloys, showing higher crack growth resistance for aluminum-lithium alloy. ΔK_{th}, change in threshold stress-intensity factor. Stress ratio (R) is 0. T-L is transverse or longitudinal. Source: Ref 13

strengthening is derived from solid-solution and strain hardening. Strain hardening is associated with the increase in dislocation density from cold deformation. Table 4 shows the tensile properties of some selected non-heat-treatable alloys. As can be noted from the table, the strengths of these alloys are lower than heat treatable aluminum alloys, because precipitation hardening cannot be imparted in these alloys. The ductility of these alloys in the strain-hardened condition (H) is not very high, due to increased dislocation density present in this material. Because magnesium is known to be a good solid-solution strengthener, the strength of higher-magnesium-content alloys, such as 5456, is superior to aluminum-manganese-based alloys. It also suggests that the strength of aluminum-magnesium alloys increases with magnesium content. These alloys have not been used much for MMC applications, due to their lower strengths. The solid-solution strengthening alone is not sufficient to provide required strengthening. A combination of solid-solution and dispersion hardening in the presence of fine dispersoid particles may provide sufficient strengthening. In addition, P/M would be required for making these alloys, because more magnesium can be taken into solution by extending the solid solubility by rapid solidification, and also, fine dispersoids can be formed.

Cast Aluminum Alloys

Cast aluminum alloys consist of two groups: one with copper and the other with silicon. Alloys with silicon as the major alloying addition are the most important ones, because silicon imparts high fluidity by the presence of a larger volume of aluminum-silicon eutectic. The eutectic is formed between aluminum solid solution and silicon, with about 12.7% Si content. The eutectic is composed of individual cells within which the silicon particles appear to be interconnected. Table 5 shows the tensile properties of some selected cast aluminum alloys. The strength and ductility of aluminum-copper alloys, especially 201, are very attractive. However, the castability of aluminum-copper is not as good as aluminum-silicon alloys, due to the greater tendency for hot tearing and hot shortness in aluminum-copper alloys. Hypoeutectic and hypereutectic aluminum-silicon alloys are commercially available; hypoeutectic is more common, because these alloys can provide slightly higher ductility. Finer eutectic via rapid cooling is preferred to impart more ductility in the alloys. The refinement of eutectic can also be achieved by small additions of sodium or strontium. Figure 4 shows the microstructures of Al-12 wt% Si in the unmodified and modified conditions. Finer microstructures in aluminum-silicon alloys result from sodium additions, because sodium depresses the eutectic temperature by almost 12 °C (22 °F) and thereby reduces the potency of nucleating sites for the eutectic phase, silicon. The fracture toughness of modified aluminum-silicon alloys improves significantly over unmodified alloy, due to the finer structure of the former alloy.

Aluminum-silicon alloys have been used extensively for making MMCs via various casting techniques. Unlike P/M in casting there is a reaction between molten aluminum alloys and the reinforcements, particularly with SiC forming the deleterious product Al_4C_3 at the interface. The reaction between aluminum and SiC can be

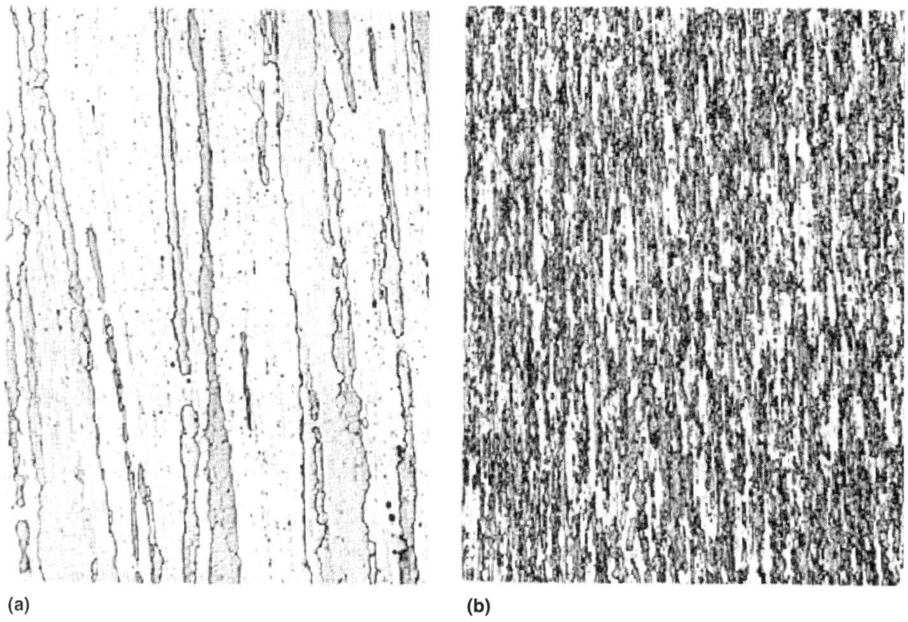

Fig. 3 Microstructures of 7000-series aluminum alloy in the (a) cast and (b) P/M conditions, showing finer grain size for P/M alloy. Source: Ref 12

Table 2 Effect of matrix strength on the tensile properties of powder metallurgy DRA materials

Alloy	SiC content, vol%	Modulus, GPa	Modulus, 10^6 psi	Yield strength, MPa	Yield strength, ksi	Ultimate tensile strength, MPa	Ultimate tensile strength, ksi	Elongation, %
6061 (wrought)	...	68.9	10.0	275.8	40.0	310.3	45.0	12
6061	20	103.4	15.0	413.7	60.0	496.4	72.0	5.5
6061	30	120.7	17.5	434.3	63.0	551.6	80.0	3
2124 (wrought)	...	71	10.3	420.6	61.0	455.1	66.0	9
2124	20	103.4	15.0	400	58.0	551	79.9	7
2124	30	120.7	17.5	441.3	64.0	593	86.0	4.5
7091 (wrought)	...	72.4	10.5	537.8	78.0	586.1	85.0	10
7091	20	103.4	15.0	620.6	90.0	724	105.0	4.5
7091	30	127.6	18.5	675.7	98.0	765.3	111.0	2

Table 3 Influence of heat treatment on the tensile properties and fracture toughness of powder metallurgy DRA composite (7093/15 vol% SiC)

Heat treatment(a)	Young's modulus, GPa	Young's modulus, 10^6 psi	Yield strength in 0.2%, MPa	Yield strength in 0.2%, ksi	Ultimate tensile strength, MPa	Ultimate tensile strength, ksi	Elongation, %	Fracture toughness (K_{Ic})(b), MPa $\sqrt{m}$	Fracture toughness (K_{Ic})(b), ksi $\sqrt{in.}$
Solution treated	91.0	13.2	430	62.4	577	83.7	8.0	25.4	23.1
Underaged	89.9	13.0	503	73.0	629	91.2	5.9	19.0	17.3
Peak aged	95.6	13.9	642	93.1	694	100.7	1.8	15.7(c)	14.3(c)
Overaged 1	91.5	13.3	591	85.7	642	93.1	2.4	19.6(c)	17.8(c)
Overaged 2	93.0	13.5	447	64.8	514	74.5	7.0	22.1	20.1
Overaged 3	89.2	12.9	369	53.5	451	65.4	7.6	25.3	23.0
Solution treated + 5% deformation	91.9	13.3	507	73.5	592	85.9	5.4	19.6	17.8

(a) Solution treated: 490 °C (915 °F)/4 h + water quenched (WQ). Underaged: 490 °C (915 °F)/4 h + WQ + 120 °C (255 °F)/25 min. Peak aged: 490 °C (915 °F)/4 h + WQ + 120 °C (255 °F)/24 h + air cooled (AC). Overaged 1: 490 °C (915 °F)/4 h + WQ + 120 °C (255 °F)/24 h + AC + 150 °C (300 °F)/8 h + AC. Overaged 2: 490 °C (915 °F)/4 h + WQ + 120 °C (255 °F)/24 h + AC + 170 °C (340 °F)/36 h + AC. Overaged 3: 490 °C (915 °F)/4 h + WQ + 120 °C (255 °F)/24 h + AC + 170 °C (340 °F)/97 h + AC. (b) K_{Ic} values were obtained from valid J_{Ic} data. (c) Fracture toughness values are based on the maximum load, because the specimens failed following elastic loading.

written as (Ref 17):

$$Al\ (l) + 3SiC\ (s) = Al_4C_3\ (s) + 3Si \quad \text{(Eq 1)}$$

where Si represents silicon in solution of aluminum. The stepwise reaction leading to the formation of Al_4C_3 can be given by

$$SiC\ (s) = Si + C \quad \text{(Eq 2)}$$

$$3C + 4Al\ (l) = Al_4C_3\ (s) \quad \text{(Eq 3)}$$

The previous equations show that SiC has to go into solution in order to form Al_4C_3 by reaction with aluminum from the matrix. One of the factors that controls the extent to which SiC would go into solution is the activity of silicon in aluminum. If the activity of silicon in the alloy were sufficiently high, then the dissolution of SiC would be reduced significantly. Therefore, aluminum-silicon alloys with silicon contents over 8 to 9 wt% are required to avoid reaction with SiC. Alloys without sufficient silicon cannot be used for making MMCs with SiC reinforcement in casting. However, non-silicon-containing alloys can be used with Al_2O_3, TiB_2, and B_4C for making MMCs. Alloys containing magnesium react with Al_2O_3, forming $MgAl_2O_4$ (spinel) at the interface. The spinel is not detrimental to the properties of MMCs. Therefore, it is important to select matrix alloys and reinforcements in such a way that the formation of detrimental reaction products is prevented.

There is a continued interest in the development of cast DRA, with the objective of achieving good strength, ductility, and fracture toughness at lower cost. Alcan has conducted a considerable amount of work on DRA materials with two alloy systems: aluminum-silicon alloys with SiC as the reinforcement and 2014 alloy with Al_2O_3 as the reinforcement (Ref 2). Silicon carbide and Al_2O_3 reinforcements are both slightly denser than the matrix alloys, so particulate settling is an issue that requires attention. Alcan has used a proprietary stirring process for wetting and dispersion of reinforcements in the melt and has produced composite material with good properties. The advantage with this technique is that reinforcement contents up to 30 vol% can be added easily.

MMCC Inc. and Triton Systems Inc. have been involved in pressure infiltration casting (PIC) of DRA. MMCC Inc. has used an aluminum-silicon alloy and 2014 alloy as matrices, whereas Triton Systems Inc. has used 2219 as a matrix for DRA applications. Aluminum-silicon alloys have been used with SiC, and 2014 has been used with Al_2O_3 reinforcements. As mentioned previously, 2219 has good strength and toughness at cryogenic temperatures suitable for space applications. The PIC process requires a high-quality preform for infiltration. Although reasonably high strengths can be achieved using the PIC process, the ductility is very low (less than 1%), as shown in Table 6. This is partly because of the very high volume fraction (40 to 60%) of reinforcements present in the DRA materials produced using the PIC process. Brake calipers for potential automotive application have been made by MMCC Inc. using the PIC process. Current technology is not able to produce high quality preforms with reinforcement volume fractions below about 40%, thus limiting material produced by the PIC process.

Lanxide Corporation has patented techniques known as Primex and Primex Cast, which have been used to make DRA materials via pressureless infiltration at a lower cost compared to PIC processes. These techniques are based on the unique capability to infiltrate ceramic reinforcements with molten aluminum without application of pressure or vacuum. To produce DRA

Table 4 Typical tensile properties of selected non-heat-treatable aluminum alloys

Alloy	Composition	Temper	Yield strength in 0.2%, MPa	Yield strength in 0.2%, ksi	Ultimate tensile strength, MPa	Ultimate tensile strength, ksi	Elongation, %
1100	Al-0.12Cu-0.1Zn-1Si + Fe (CP Al)	O	35	5.1	90	13.1	35
		H18	150	21.8	165	23.9	5
3003	Al-1.2Mn-0.12Cu-0.7Fe-0.6Si	O	25	3.6	110	16.0	30
		H18	185	26.8	195	28.3	7
3004	Al-1.25Mn-1.1Mg-0.25Zn-0.7Fe-0.3Si	O	70	10.2	180	26.1	20
		H38	250	36.3	280	40.6	5
5052	Al-2.5Mg-0.25Cr-0.4Fe-0.25Si	O	90	13.1	195	28.3	25
		H38	255	37.0	270	39.2	7
5456	Al-5.1Mg-0.25Zn-0.75Mn-0.12Cr-0.2Ti	O	160	23.2	310	45.0	24
		H24	280	40.6	370	53.7	12
5083	Al-4.5Mg-0.7Mn-0.25Zn-0.Cr-0.15Ti	O	115	16.7	260	37.7	22
		H34	255	37.0	325	47.1	10

Table 5 Typical tensile properties of selected cast aluminum alloys

Alloy	Composition	Temper	Yield strength in 0.2%, MPa	Yield strength in 0.2%, ksi	Ultimate tensile strength, MPa	Ultimate tensile strength, ksi	Elongation, %
201	Al-4.6Cu-0.35Mg-0.35Mn-0.2Ti	T6	345	50.0	415	60.2	5
213	Al-7.0Cu-2Si-2.5Zn-0.6Mn-0.1Mg	T533	185	26.8	220	31.9	0.5
355	Al-5Si-0.5Mg-0.5Mn-1.2Cu-0.35Zn-0.25Ti	T6	235	34.1	280	40.6	1
356	Al-7.0Si-0.25Cu-0.3Mg-0.35Mn-0.35Zn-0.25Ti-0.6Fe	T6	205	29.7	230	33.4	4
357	Al-7.0Si-0.55Mg-0.12Ti-0.055Be	T6	221	32.1	283	41.0	3
360	Al-9.5Si-0.6Fe-0.35Mn-0.15Mg-0.5Ni-0.5Zn	T6	265	38.4	310	45.0	1
413	Al-12Si-2Fe-1Cu-0.5Ni-0.5Zn-0.35Mn	F1	140	20.3	265	38.4	2
518	Al-8Mg-1.8Fe-0.35Mn-0.25Cu	F1	130	18.9	260	37.7	10

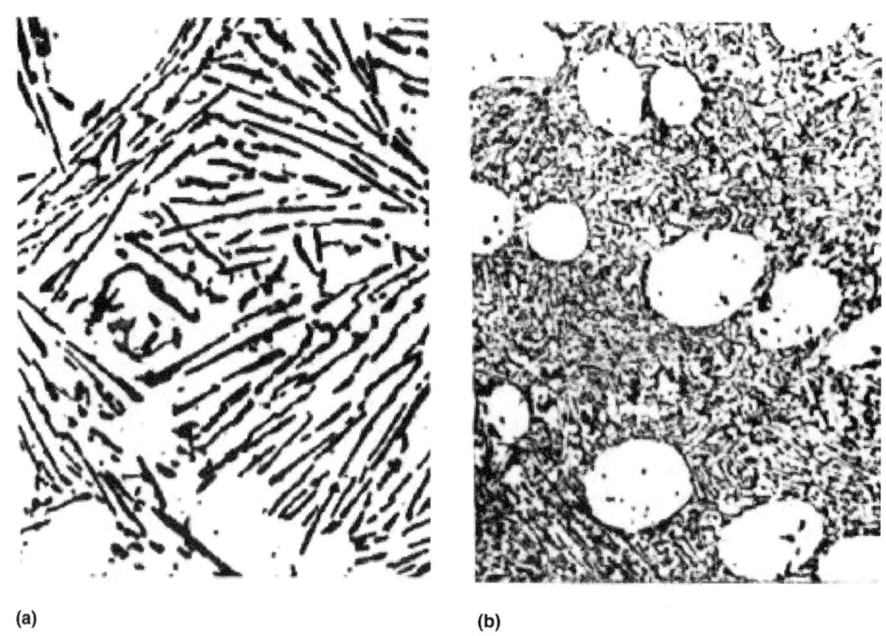

Fig. 4 Microstructures of aluminum-silicon alloy in the (a) unmodified and (b) modified conditions. Source: Ref 12. Courtesy of J.A. Cheng

Table 6 Typical tensile properties and fracture toughness of cast DRA materials

Alloy	Reinforcement	Temper	Young's modulus GPa	Young's modulus 10^6 psi	Yield strength MPa	Yield strength ksi	Ultimate tensile strength MPa	Ultimate tensile strength ksi	Elongation, %	Fracture toughness MPa $\sqrt{m}$	Fracture toughness ksi $\sqrt{in.}$	Reference
2219	40 vol% SiC	T4	...	...	276	40.0	345	50.0	0.8	...	...	Triton
Al-Si	40–55 vol% SiC	T6	180–200	26.1–29.0	...	...	300–500	43.5–72.5	...	10–25	9.1–22.8	MMCC
Al-Cu-Mg	40–55 vol% Al_2O_3	T6	170–190	24.7–27.6	...	...	300–500	43.5–72.6	...	15–30	13.7–27.3	MMCC
Al-10Si-1Mg	20 vol% SiC	T6	108	15.7	334	48.4	353	51.2	0.52	15.8	14.4	MSE
Al-10Si-1Mg	30 vol% SiC	T6	125	18.1	...	...	371	53.8	0.4	14.7	13.4	MSE
Al-10Si-1Mg	40 vol% SiC	T6	147	21.3	270	39.2	370	53.7	0.4	...	...	MSE
Al-7Mg	60 vol% Al_2O_3	...	202	29.3	441	64.0	454	65.8	0.5	15.1	13.7	MSE

References are Triton Systems Inc., MMCC Inc., and MSE Materials Inc.

materials, magnesium is added to the alloy and the infiltration is carried out in a nitrogenous atmosphere at a temperature above the melting point of the aluminum alloy. Using this technique, reasonably good properties in DRA have been obtained, as shown in Table 6. The brake discs made out of cast DRA using the Primex pressureless infiltration technique have been used successfully on all four wheels of the Lotus Elise. Several other automotive components for potential applications have been made from cast DRA using the pressureless infiltration technique.

Low-Density, High-Modulus Alloys

Lithium is a unique alloying element for aluminum because it reduces density and improves the modulus of the aluminum alloy considerably. It has high solid solubility (4 wt% at 610 °C, or 1120 °F) in aluminum and responds to age hardening, due to precipitation of an ordered, metastable phase $\delta'(Al_3Li)$ that is coherent and has small misfit with the matrix (Fig. 5). Due to these characteristics, aluminum-lithium alloys have attracted considerable attention in the past for the development of new-generation low-density, high-modulus alloys for aerospace and space structures. Specifically, aluminum-lithium alloys have been considered for cryogenic propellant tank applications.

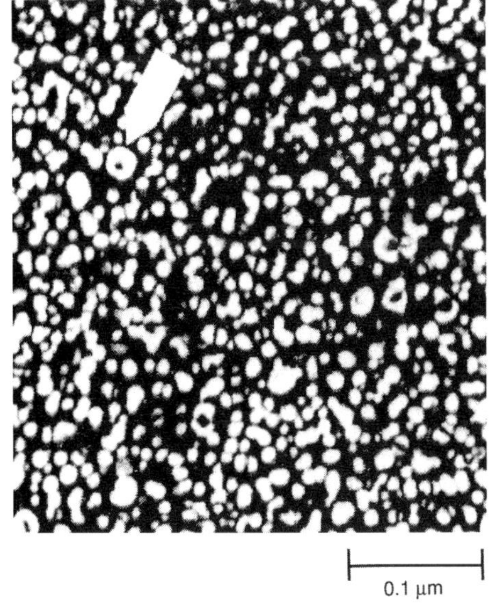

Fig. 5 Transmission electron microscopy microstructure showing δ′ precipitate in an Al-Li-Mg-Zr alloy. Source: Ref 12. Courtesy of D.J. Lloyd

Binary aluminum-lithium alloys suffer from low ductility and fracture toughness, due to severe strain localization resulting from the shearing of coherent δ′ precipitates by moving dislocations. Therefore, significant work has been done to develop ternary and quaternary alloys with dispersoids capable of dispersing dislocations more homogeneously. Table 7 lists the compositions and properties for some selected aluminum-lithium-based alloys. There are two categories of aluminum-lithium-based alloys: modified aluminum-copper alloys (such as Weldalite, Martin Marietta Corporation) that have small lithium additions to enhance strength and alloys (such as 8090 and 2091) with higher lithium contents to maximize density reduction. The quaternary alloys based on Al-Li-Cu-Mg (such as 8090) are the most common, due to a good combination of strength, ductility, and toughness. The Al-Li-Cu-Mg alloys are strengthened by three types of precipitates: δ′ (Al_3Li), T1 (Al_2CuLi), and S′ (Al_2CuMg). Most of the aluminum-lithium alloys contain a small amount of zirconium, similar to other aluminum alloys. The role of zirconium here is twofold: Al_3Zr controls recrystallization and grain growth, and Al_3Zr particles have similar $L1_2$ structure as δ′ substituting to the Al_3Li precipitate forming $Al_3(Li_xZr_{1-x})$ (Ref 18). The presence of zirconium improves strength and toughness in aluminum-lithium based alloys.

The 2090 alloy containing Al-Li-Cu is hardened by δ′ and the hexagonal T1 phase (Al_2CuLi) that forms as thin plates on {111} planes. Plates of θ′ (Al_2Cu) may also be present in this alloy. Because nucleation of T1 and θ′ are difficult, cold working is required prior to aging to promote uniform precipitation on dislocations (T8 condition). The 2091, 8090, and 8091 alloys contain S′ precipitate, which is resistant to shearing by dislocations, promoting more homogeneous deformation. These alloys provide improved precipitation in the T8 condition. Figure 2 indicates that aluminum-lithium alloy has superior crack growth resistance to 2000- and 7000-series alloys. The Russian alloy 1421 (Al-Li-Mg-Sc-Zr) also shows good strength and ductility (Table 7). These alloys—which have good mechanical properties and are light, weldable, and corrosion resistant—are used for fuel tanks, fuselage stringers, cockpits, and other aircraft parts. The Weldalite, with a small addition of silver in the Al-Li-Cu-Mg-Zr alloy, has very high strength (700 MPa, or 100 ksi), good weldability (Ref 19), and was developed by Martin Marietta Corporation.

While some of the aluminum-lithium alloys show a very good combination of strength, ductility, and toughness in addition to lower density and higher modulus, the use of aluminum-lithium alloys has been very limited as matrices for DRA applications (Ref 3, 4). This is mainly due to the fact that that P/M version of aluminum-lithium is not attractive because of severe oxidation of aluminum-lithium powder, and these alloys cannot be used easily for making cast DRA with SiC.

High-Temperature Aluminum Alloys

The commercial aluminum alloys and aluminum-lithium alloys cannot be used at tempera-

Table 7 Typical tensile properties of selected lithium-containing aluminum alloys

Alloy	Composition	Temper	Yield strength in 0.2% MPa	Yield strength in 0.2% ksi	Ultimate tensile strength MPa	Ultimate tensile strength ksi	Elongation, %	Fracture toughness (K_{Ic}) MPa $\sqrt{m}$	Fracture toughness (K_{Ic}) ksi $\sqrt{in.}$
2091	Al-2Li-2.1Cu-1.5Mg-0.1Zr	T8X (UA)	370	53.7	460	66.7	15	40	36
		T851	475	68.9	525	76.1	9	25	23
8090	Al-2.4Li-1.3Cu-0.9Mg-0.16Zr	T81(UA)	360	52.2	445	64.5	11	45	41
		T6	400	58.0	470	68.2	6	35	32
		T851	455	66.0	510	74.0	7	30	27
2090	Al-2.3Li-2.7Cu-0.3Mg-0.5Zr	T83	510	74.0	565	81.9	5	...	...
8091	Al-2.6Li-2Cu-0.85Mg-0.16Zr	T851	515	74.7	555	80.5	6	22	20
1421	Al-5Mg-2Li-0.2Mn-0.2Sc-0.15Zr	T8	330	47.9	470	68.2	10	65	59
Weldalite 049	Al-6.3Cu-1.3Li-0.4Mg-0.4Ag-0.18Zr	T8	725	105.1	797	115.6	9.8	...	...

UA, underaged

tures above 150 °C (300 °F), due to rapid coarsening of strengthening precipitates and loss of mechanical properties in these alloys and loss of mechanical properties. There is an increasing demand for high-temperature aluminum alloys for aerospace and space applications to substitute for titanium alloys at temperatures up to 315 °C (600 °F) (Ref 20–24). A considerable amount of work was done in the 1990s to develop high-temperature alloys via a rapid solidification process (Ref 5–7). However, the use of these alloys for MMCs has been limited, mainly due to lower ductility and fracture toughness of these alloys. Also, processing of MMCs with high-temperature alloys as matrices requires careful control of temperature during processing to prevent coarsening of dispersoids.

Aluminum-scandium-based alloys provide a unique opportunity for developing improved ambient- and high-temperature properties. Scandium is known to be a potent strengthener in aluminum alloys (Ref 25). While aluminum-scandium alloys have potential for making MMCs using casting techniques, studies on MMCs do not exist. The higher-scandium-containing aluminum alloys have been investigated for MMC applications using P/M technique (Ref 26, 27). The aluminum-scandium-based alloys have the potential to provide a new class of MMCs, due to the balanced strength, ductility, and toughness in this system.

Another class of aluminum alloys that has attracted the attention of researchers in the recent past is the amorphous aluminum alloys for elevated-temperature applications (Ref 28–30). While significant research on amorphous structure has been carried out in the past, the present emphasis is toward development of bulk amorphous structure in alloys using conventional processing techniques. Recently, a large initiative in the area of amorphous alloys has been started by the Defense Advanced Research Projects Agency in the United States. Although these alloys have not been used as matrices in MMCs, they may be used in the future, with further advancement in understanding.

Titanium Alloys

Titanium alloys are very attractive for MMC applications, due to their higher strength and temperature capability compared to aluminum alloys. Despite significant potential for discontinuously reinforced titanium MMCs in various applications, much less emphasis has been given for development of this class of materials until recently. A significant amount of work has been carried out for developing continuously reinforced MMCs to derive substantial strengthening and stiffening at ambient and elevated temperatures (Ref 8–10). While Ti-6Al-4V and Ti-15V-3Cr-3Sn-3Al have been used commonly for MMC applications, other alloys, such as titanium aluminides, were also considered with specific objectives. The alloy Ti-6Al-4V is the most common alloy in the titanium family and has been used in many applications.

The alloying in titanium largely depends on the ability of elements to stabilize either the low-temperature α- or high-temperature β-phase, which is related to the number of bonding electrons (Ref 31). Alloying elements with electron-to-atom ratios of less than four stabilize the α-phase, and elements with electron-to-atom ratios greater than four stabilize the β-phase in titanium. Elements with a ratio of four are neutral. All of the transition elements stabilize the β-phase in titanium, except some rare earth elements. Also, titanium has a high solubility for most of the elements, except a few rare earth elements. The phase diagram of titanium can be categorized as α- and β-stabilizers. The α–stabilizers are the elements that provide complete solubility, with a peritectic reaction such as titanium-oxygen and titanium-nitrogen, and those that have limited α-stability, with a peritectoid reaction into β plus a compound, such as titanium-boron, titanium-carbon, and titanium-aluminum. The β-stabilizers consist of two categories: β-isomorphous and β-eutectoid. In the β-isomorphous systems, an extra β-solubility range exists with only a restricted α-solubility range, such as titanium-molybdenum, titanium-tantalum, and titanium-vanadium. In the β-eutectoid systems, for example, titanium-chromium and titanium-copper, the β-phase has a limited solubility range and decomposes into α and a compound. It is customary to classify titanium alloys into three main groups, designated as α, α + β, and β.

The alloys Ti-6Al-4V and Ti-15V-3Cr-3Sn-3Al have been used with SCS-6 silicon carbide monofilament reinforcements for MMC applications with reasonable success (Ref 32). These alloys have good ductility at room temperature, which helps achieve rule-of-mixture tensile properties in MMCs. The need for materials that possess superior specific strength and specific modulus at high temperatures has focused attention on a different class of alloys, titanium aluminides. There has been considerable interest in niobium-rich Ti_3Al alloys for continuous fiber-reinforced MMC applications, due to the presence of an orthorhombic (O) phase based on the compound Ti_3AlNb. This O-phase was first found in a Ti-25Al-12.5 Nb (at.%) alloy. The O-phase is similar in nature to α2 (Ti_3Al, DO_{19} structure), however it differs in the lattice arrangement of niobium with respect to titanium. The O-phase has been identified in titanium alloys containing 20 to 30 at.% Al and 11 to 30 at.% Nb, and such alloys are known as O-alloys. Orthorhombic alloys such as Ti-22Al-23Nb (at.%) have good creep resistance, tensile strength, ductility, and thermomechanical fatigue behavior (Ref 33). Improvements in properties such as tensile strength and toughness also have been observed in Ti-25Al-17Nb (at.%) alloy (Ref 34). Because of the attractive combination of room-temperature ductility and elevated-temperature strength, O-alloys have been considered as matrix alloys for continuously reinforced MMCs. Additional advantages of O-based alloys are reduced reaction with SiC fibers and improved environmental resistance compared to most other titanium aluminide alloys. The matrix alloy plays a key role on the properties of continuously reinforced titanium MMCs (Ref 8).

Table 8 shows the tensile properties of an O-alloy in different heat treatment conditions (Ref 35). The table indicates that the strength of the Ti-25Al-17Nb (at.%) alloy is very high and ductility is low after supertransus treatments, whereas for subtransus treatments, it shows much higher ductility with not much reduction in strength. Ductility for subtransus heat treatment ranges from 7 to 14%, which is excellent for MMC matrices. The higher ductility of this alloy helped in efficient use of fiber strength during longitudinal loading of MMCs, as shown by the properties of SiC fiber-reinforced orthorhombic MMCs in Table 9 (Ref 35). The table also includes the properties of the monolithic O-alloy

Table 8 Effect of heat treatment on room-temperature properties of Ti-25Al-17Nb alloy sheet

Heat treatment(a)	α2 phase, vol%	β2 phase, vol%	O phase, vol%	Yield strength		Ultimate tensile strength		Elongation, %
				MPa	ksi	MPa	ksi	
Supertransus treatment								
1190 °C (2175 °F)/0.25 h + AQ	...	...	...	...	...	1154	167.4	1.2
Subtransus treatments								
As-rolled	64.1	35.9	0	681	98.8	775	112.4	10.7
925 °C (1700 °F)/24 h + FC	76.4	23.6	0	617	89.5	840	121.8	12.3
1050 °C (1920 °F)/1 h + WQ + 850 °C (1560 °F)/2 h + WQ	57.5	23.9	18.6	691	100.2	906	131.4	14
1050 °C (1920 °F)/1 h + CC + 850 °C (1560 °F)/2 h + FC	53.4	25.8	20.8	564	81.8	805	116.8	10.7
1075 °C (1970 °F)/1 h + CC + 850 °C (1560 °F)/24 h + FC	43.3	13	43.7	587	85.1	780	113.1	9.5
1100 °C (2010 °F)/1 h + CC + 850 °C (1560 °F)/2 h + FC	17.9	19.7	61.8	569	82.5	748	108.5	7
1125 °C (2060 °F)/1 h + CC + 850 °C (1560 °F)/2 h + FC	17.1	18.9	64	547	79.3	785	113.9	10.2

(a) AQ, air quenched; FC, furnace cooled; WQ, water quenched; CC, control cooled at 28 °C (50 °F)/min

to provide a comparison with MMCs. In the case of a $[0]_4$ MMC, heat treatment has significantly improved the ultimate tensile strength (UTS) and ductility; whereas in the case of $[90]_4$, the heat treatment did not produce as significant improvement in the UTS and ductility. It is known that fiber-matrix debonding under transverse loading can produce a high stress concentration around the fibers. Such stresses can initiate matrix cracks, which can rapidly grow to failure if the fracture toughness of the matrix is low. The low ductility observed for $[90]_4$ MMCs is related to the low toughness of the titanium aluminide matrix. When the matrix possesses sufficient toughness, as in the case of SCS-6/Ti-15V-3Cr-3Al-3Sn metal-matrix composites, room-temperature ductility of about 1.4% was observed (Ref 36). Table 9 also includes the data for single-ply niobium-coated SCS-fiber-based MMCs in the transverse loading condition that show some improvement in the UTS and ductility.

Significant residual stresses brought about by the mismatch in coefficient of thermal expansion (CTE) between the fiber and the matrix, in combination with limited matrix ductility has caused a major concern with regard to the thermal cycling capability of the titanium aluminide composite system. In earlier studies, chemical interactions in the interfacial region led to the formation of a β-depleted zone, within which cracks often formed from thermal stresses. However, subsequent studies on matrix alloys with higher levels of niobium, from 22 to 27 at.%, showed that the β-depleted zone was eliminated. In fact, a β-enriched zone in the interfacial region led to significantly improved properties under thermal cycling conditions. Studies of MMCs based on other intermetallics with limited ductility, such as titanium aluminide alloys, further emphasize the importance of matching the matrix and fiber CTEs. Significant damage is often observed in TiAl/SiC metal-matrix composites, while $TiAl/Al_2O_3$ metal-matrix composites exhibit far less damage as a result of a much closer match in CTE between the matrix and the reinforcement.

The progress made in the development of fiber-reinforced titanium MMCs since the 1980s is underscored by the successful military applications now in use (see the article "Aeronautical Applications of Metal-Matrix Composites" in this Volume). While many of the matrix-related issues for O-matrix alloys were adequately addressed in the 1990s, expanded applications of fiber-reinforced titanium MMCs await the development of more-reliable composite processing and lower-cost reinforcements.

Discontinuously reinforced titanium composites have received significant attention in the recent past, with the aim of developing materials having a good combination of strength, ductility, fatigue resistance, and fracture toughness. The major benefit of DRTi over continuous fiber MMCs is that relatively more isotropic properties can be achieved in DRTi. Discontinuously reinforced titanium can be processed using conventional techniques. Due to the reaction between SiC and titanium alloys, SiC is not a preferred reinforcement for titanium alloys. Particles of TiB and TiC have been considered commonly as reinforcements for making DRTi, due to their attractive properties, including compatibility with the matrix alloys. Titanium diboride (TiB_2) is not thermally stable in conventional titanium alloys and therefore, cannot be used as a stable reinforcement. However, TiB_2 can be used to make TiB reinforcement dispersed in titanium alloys by conversion at higher temperatures. While casting can be used to make DRTi (Ref 37), more emphasis has been given to the P/M approach to achieve improved properties through controlled microstructure in the material.

A significant amount of work has been done in Japan (Ref 38–40) to develop DRTi for automotive applications. An elemental powder approach using titanium sponge fines was used to reduce the cost of MMCs. This approach also provided a high degree of freedom in the selection of alloy compositions suitable for processing. The processing approach consists of mixing elemental powder of the desired composition, compacting by using cold isostatic pressing (CIP), and then sintering at high temperature in vacuum. This process eliminated the use of hot isostatic pressing (HIP), thereby reducing the cost of the composite. In order to develop an alloy suitable for elemental blending, many alloys were considered for MMC evaluation using elemental powder blending, including Ti-6Al-4V (Ref 38). Boron powder was used to produce TiB by reaction with titanium during high-temperature sintering of the powder. Except for gamma alloy, where TiB_2 is the stable compound, TiB in the form of plates or needles was found to be a stable reinforcement in α, α-β, and β alloys. A clean interface at TiB/Ti was observed in these MMCs.

The effect of matrix alloys such as α, α-β, and β on the modulus of DRTi is shown in Fig. 6. The modulus value depends on the type of matrix alloys. The aluminum-rich alpha alloy shows the highest modulus for a given TiB fraction, indicating the potential of this alloy for high-modulus applications. Figure 7 shows the comparison of yield strength and creep deflection of the as-sintered DRTi with different matrix alloys. The wrought alloy IMI 834 and 21-4N steel are also used in the plots for comparison purposes. The yield strength of MMC with Ti-Al-Sn-Zr-Nb-Mo-Si is the highest at 800 °C (1470 °F). The creep resistance of this MMC is also better than MMCs with other titanium alloys, except gamma-based MMCs. These plots indicate that by careful selection of a matrix alloy, one can design DRTi with superior thermal resistance relative to typical heat-resistant steel (Ref 38).

In order to make MMCs suitable for hot working, a new β-alloy, Ti-4.3Fe-7.Mo-1.4Al-1.4V, has been developed that is compatible with the elemental blending approach (Ref 38). Figure 8 compares hot workability of the developed β-matrix MMC and Ti-6Al-4V-based MMC. The data for commercial medium-carbon steel is also included for a comparison. The β-matrix MMC shows better hot workability than both Ti-6Al-4V-based MMC and medium-carbon steel. This suggests that β-matrix MMC can be processed

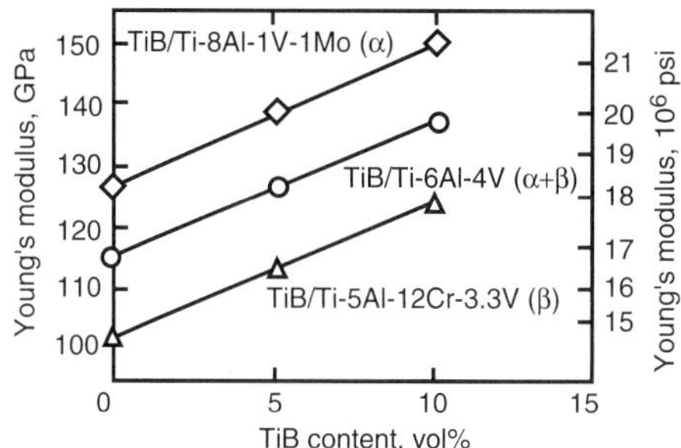

Fig. 6 Effect of matrix alloy on the Young's modulus of DRTi material, showing higher modulus for the composite with alpha alloy. Courtesy of T. Saito, Toyota Corp.

Table 9 Effect of heat treatment on tensile properties for Ti-25Al-17Nb matrix alloy and SCS-6/Ti-25Al-17Nb

Heat treatment	α2, vol%	β2, vol%	O, vol%	Young's modulus, GPa	Young's modulus, 10^6 psi	Yield strength, MPa	Yield strength, ksi	Ultimate tensile strength, MPa	Ultimate tensile strength, ksi	Elongation, %
Matrix alloy										
As-processed	74.8	16.3	8.9	97.3	14.1	781	113.3	801	116.2	1.09
1050 °C (1920 °F)/1 h + CC + 850 °C (1560 °F)/2 h + FC	64.1	19.2	16.7	88.2	12.8	670	97.2	759	110.1	4
$[0]_4$ SCS-6/Ti-25Al-17Nb										
As-processed	80	11.5	8.5	192.6	27.9	...	...	1367	198.3	0.86
1050 °C (1920 °F)/1 h + CC + 850 °C (1560 °F)/2 h + FC	68.5	12	19.5	170.3	24.7	...	...	1579	229.0	1.15
$[90]_4$ SCS-6/Ti-25Al-17Nb										
As-processed	80	11.5	8.5	145	21.0	...	...	256	37.1	0.2
1050 °C (1920 °F)/1 h + CC + 850 °C (1560 °F)/2 h + FC	68.5	12	19.5	114.2	16.6	...	...	250	36.3	0.23
[90] NbSCS-6/Ti-25Al-17Nb										
As-processed	53.3	15.6	31.1	118	17.1	...	...	397	57.6	0.4

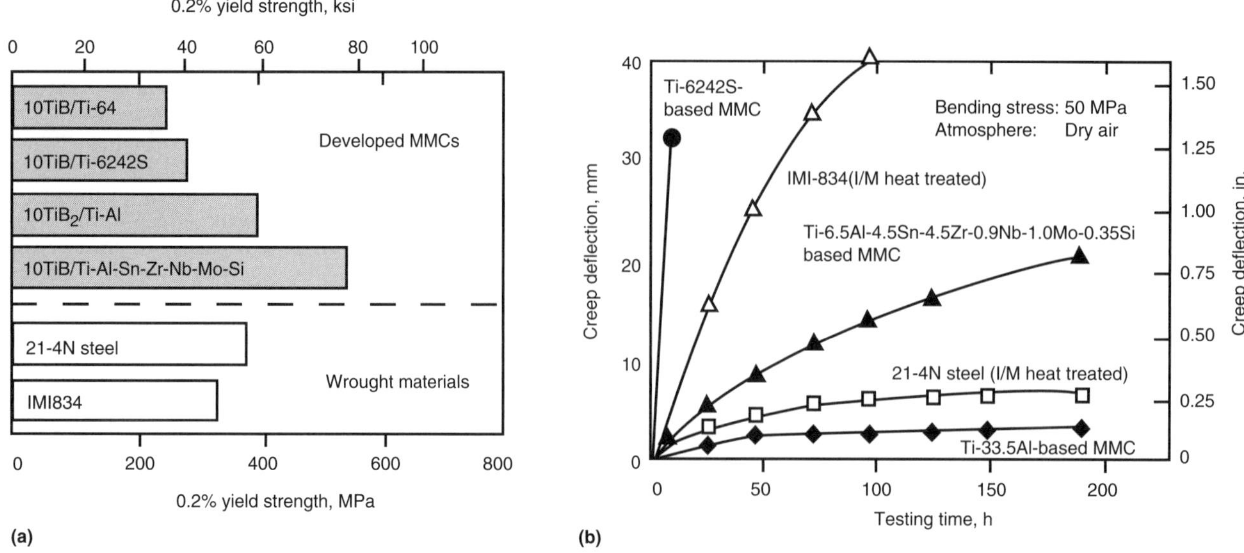

Fig. 7 Effect of matrix alloys on (a) strength and (b) creep of titanium composite at 800 °C (1470 °F). I/M, ingot metallurgy. Courtesy of T. Saito, Toyota Corp.

successfully using a high-temperature forging operation. Figure 9 shows the tensile properties of the β-matrix MMC in the sinter-swaged and annealed condition. Compared with the as-sintered Ti-6Al-4V-based MMC, the β-matrix MMC shows significantly higher strength and ductility. This suggests that the β-Ti-4.3Fe-7.0Mo-1.4Al-1.4V alloy is a very effective matrix alloy for MMC applications The high performance was achieved from cheap sponge fine powder using CIP and sintering processes only. The material yield was as high as 100% allowing postprocessing after sintering to a minimum level. Metal-matrix composites of Ti-6Al-4V/TiB are being used for intake valves, and a high-temperature Ti-Al-Zr-Sn-Nb-Mo-Si/TiB metal-matrix composite is being used for exhaust valves in the Altezza car made by Toyota Motor Manufacturing (Ref 39, 40). Over 500,000 valves have been produced, with no failures, underscoring the maturity of this technology in the automotive market. Additional details of this application are provided in the article "Automotive Applications of Metal-Matrix Composites" in this Volume.

Alloy Ti-6Al-4V has been used with TiC reinforcement to make MMC using a cold and hot isostatic pressing (CHIP) process developed by Dynamet Technology Inc. (Ref 41). The CHIP process consists of CIP of blended elemental matrix alloy powders and reinforcement particles, followed by vacuum sintering and HIP to provide completely densified products with near-net shape. The MMC developed using the CHIP process is commercially known as CermetTi-X, where "X" denotes the volume fraction of reinforcement. CermetTi-10 consists of Ti-6Al-4V with 10 vol% of TiC particles. The Young's modulus of CermetTi-10 is significantly improved over Ti-6Al-4V from room temperature to 650 °C (1200 °F). The room-temperature yield and tensile strengths are retained up to higher temperatures. Ductility of the MMC is lower than that of the matrix alloy at all temperatures. However, the difference between the MMC and matrix alloy ductility gets smaller at higher temperature (650 °C, or 1200 °F). The creep stress rupture property of the MMC is higher by an order of magnitude relative to the matrix alloy at 540 °C (1000 °F). The fracture toughness of the MMC is reasonably high, 28 MPa $\sqrt{m}$ (25 ksi $\sqrt{in.}$), even though the ductility is low. The fatigue properties of the MMC are comparable to those of the cast Ti-6Al-4V alloy. The improvements in high-temperature strength and modulus of the MMC increase the use-temperature limit relative to unreinforced Ti-6Al-4V by approximately 110 °C (200 °F). Prototype parts made using CermetTi MMC include domed rocket cases, missile fins, and aircraft engine component preforms (Ref 43).

While casting has also been used in many studies (Ref 37–38), rapid solidification can provide improved properties, due to the finer and uniform distribution of reinforcement in the matrix (Ref 42, 43). Fine dispersions of borides and carbides in the powder have been produced by inert gas atomization. The rapidly solidified powder was consolidated using HIP and/or extrusion. Discontinuously reinforced titanium with Ti-6Al-4V/TiB, Ti-6Al-4V/TiC, and Ti-6Al-4V/TiB + TiC were produced using this technique. A significant improvement in properties was observed in DRTi containing TiB reinforcements (Ref 43), compared to the Ti-6Al-4V matrix. Most of these studies concentrated on developing MMCs using different processing techniques with Ti-6Al-4V alloy as a matrix. Little effort has been put into developing newer matrix alloys for DRTi applications.

Conclusions

Both DRA and DRTi are well-established materials with significant commercial markets. Generally, the matrix alloys are based upon alloys developed for use as monolithic materials. Small modifications in chemistry and processing have provided alloy characteristics more suitable for a matrix alloy, while simultaneously producing notable improvements in materials performance. Additional evolution in discontinuously

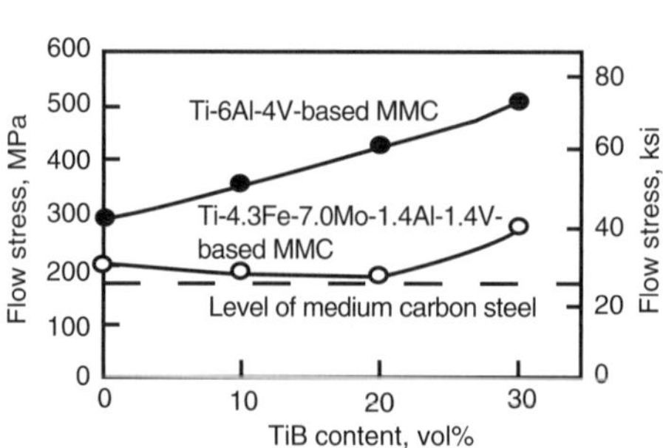

Fig. 8 Influence of matrix alloy on the hot workability of titanium composites. Strain rate, 10^{-2} s^{-1}. Test temperature, 973 K. Courtesy of T. Saito, Toyota Corp.

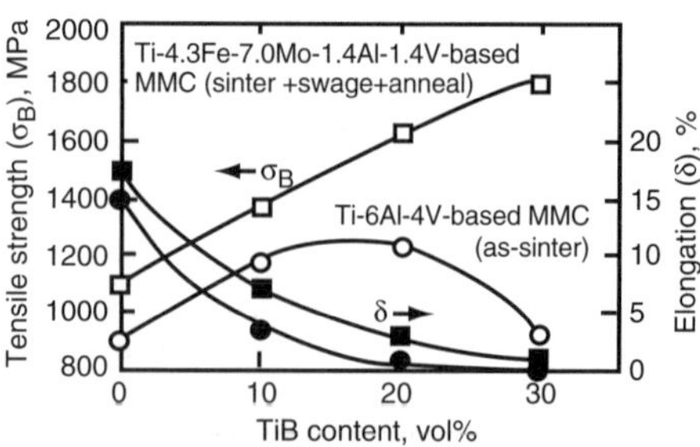

Fig. 9 Comparison of strength of titanium composites with different matrices, suggesting much higher strength for the composite with beta-matrix alloys. Courtesy of T. Saito, Toyota Corp.

reinforced MMCs may be achieved by further matrix alloy development.

There is a significant potential of DRA and DRTi materials for several applications. Future work should be directed in the following areas in order to widen the existing applications of discontinuously reinforced aluminum and titanium composites:

- Improvement in the ductility and fracture toughness of DRA materials by developing more fracture-resistant matrix alloys
- Improvement in the high-temperature capability of DRA materials through development of newer heat-resistant matrix alloys
- Improvement in the fracture properties of DRTi through better understanding of processing effects and failure mechanisms in matrix alloys

REFERENCES

1. D.L. McDanels, *Metall. Trans. A*, Vol 16, 1985, p 1105
2. D.J. Lloyd, *Int. Mater. Rev.*, Vol 39, 1994, p 1
3. D. Webster, *Metall. Trans. A*, Vol 13, 1982, p 1511
4. P. Poza and J. Llorca, *Metall. Trans. A*, Vol 30, 1999, p 845
5. D.J. Skinner, in *Dispersion Strengthened Aluminum Alloys*, Y.-W. Kim and W.M. Griffith, Ed., *TMS Annual Meeting*, Jan 1988 (Arizona), p 181
6. Y.-W. Kim, in *Dispersion Strengthened Aluminum Alloys*, Y.-W. Kim and W.M. Griffith, Ed., *TMS Annual Meeting*, Jan 1988 (Arizona), January 1988, p 157
7. I.G. Palmer, M.P. Thomas, and G.J. Marshall, in *Dispersion Strengthened Aluminum Alloys*, Y.-W. Kim and W.M. Griffith, *TMS Annual Meeting*, Jan 1988 (Arizona), p 217
8. D.B. Miracle, B.S. Majumdar, S. Krishnamurthy, and M. Waterbury, in *Metal Matrix Composites, Proc. Ninth Int. Conf. on Composite Materials*, A. Miravete, Ed., Woodhead Publishing Ltd., 1993, p 610
9. F.H. Froes, D. Elon, and H.R. Bomberger, "Titanium Technology: Present Status and Future Trends," Titanium Development Association, 1985
10. H.A. Lipsitt, in *High Temperature Ordered Intermetallic Alloys*, C.C. Roch, C.T. Liu, and N.S. Stoloff, Ed., Materials Research Society, 1985, p 351
11. M. van den Bergh, DWA Composites, Inc., private communication, 1996
12. I.J. Polmear, *Light Alloys: Metallurgy of the Light Metals*, Halsted Press, Great Britain, 1996
13. E.A. Starke, Jr. and W.E. Quist, New Light Alloys, *AGARD Conf. Proc. No. 444*, Advisory Group For Aerospace Research and Development (NATO), Oct 1988 (Netherland), p 4
14. W.C. Harrigan, *Discontinuous Silicon Fiber MMC$_s$ Composites*, Vol 1, *Engineered Materials Handbook*, ASM International, 1987, p 889
15. A.B. Pandey, B.S. Majumdar, and D.B. Miracle, *Metall. Trans. A*, Vol 29, 1998, p 1237
16. A.B. Pandey, B.S. Majumdar, and D.B. Miracle, *Metall. Trans. A*, Vol 31, 2001, p 921
17. G. Selvaduray, R. Rickman, D. Quinn, D. Richard, and D. Rowland, in *Interfaces in Metal-Ceramics Composites*, R.Y. Lin, R.J. Arsenault, G.P. Martins, and S.G. Fishman, Ed., *TMS Annual Meeting*, Feb 1990 (Anaheim, CA), p 271
18. F.W. Gayle and J.B. Vander Sande, *Rapidly Solidified Powder Aluminum Alloys*, ASTM STP 890, M.E. Fine and E.A. Starke, Jr., Ed., ASTM, 1986, p 137
19. W.E. Quist and G.H. Narayan, Aluminum-Lithium Alloys, *Aluminum Alloys—Contemporary Research and Applications*, A.K. Vasudevan and R.D. Doherty, Ed., Academic Press, Inc., Boston, 1989, p 219
20. C.M. Adam and R.E. Lewis, Rapidly Solidified Crystalline Alloys, S.K. Das, B.H. Kear, and C.M. Adam, Ed., *Proc. TMS/AIME Meeting*, May 1985 (New Jersey), p 157
21. K.S. Chan, Dispersion Strengthened Aluminum Alloys, Y.-W. Kim and W.M. Griffith, Ed., *TMS Annual Meeting*, Jan 1988 (Arizona), p 283
22. E. Bouchand, L. Kubin, and H. Octor, *Metall. Trans. A*, Vol 22, 1991, p 1021
23. M.S. Zedalis and M.E. Fine, *Metall. Trans A*, Vol 17, 1986, p 2187
24. W.E. Frazier and M.J. Koczak, Dispersion Strengthened Aluminum Alloys, Y.-W. Kim and W.M. Griffith, Ed., *TMS Annual Meeting*, Jan 1988 (Arizona), p 573
25. L.S. Toropova, D.G. Eskin, M.L. Kharakterova, and T.V. Dobatkina, in *Advanced Aluminum Alloys Containing Scandium: Structure and Properties*, Gordan and Breach Science Publishers, Moscow, Russia
26. A.B. Pandey, K.L. Kendig, and D.B. Miracle, "Discontinuously Reinforced Aluminum for Elevated Temperature Applications," presented at *TMS Annual Meeting*, Feb 2001 (New Orleans)
27. R. Unal and K.U. Kainer, *Powder Metall.*, Vol 41, 1998, p 119
28. Y. Kawamura, A. Inoue, K. Sasamori, and T. Masumoto, *Scr. Metall.*, Vol 29, 1993, p 275
29. K. Ohtera, A. Inoue, and T. Masumoto, *First International Conf. Processing Materials for Properties*, H. Henen and T. Oki, Ed., The Minerals, Metals and Materials Society, 1993, p 713
30. A. Inoue and H. Kimura, *Mater. Sci. Eng.*, Vol A286, 2000, p 1
31. F.H. Froes, Y.-W. Kim, and F. Hehmann, *J. Met.*, Aug 1987, p 14
32. P.R. Smith, F.H. Froes, and J.T. Cammett, in *Mechanical Behavior of Metal Matrix Composites*, J.E. Hack and M.F. Amateau, Ed., TMS-AIME, Warrendale, Pa, 1983, p 143
33. D. Banerjee, in *Intermetallic Compounds: Principles and Practice*, J.H. Westbrook and R.L. Fleischer, Ed., John Wiley & Sons Ltd., New York, NY, Vol 2, 1994, p 91
34. S. Krishnamurthy, P.R. Smith, and D.B. Miracle, *Scr. Metall.*, Vol 31, 1994, p 653
35. C.J. Boehlert, B.S. Majumdra, S. Krishnamurthy, and D.B. Miracle, *Mater. Trans. A*, Vol 28A, 1997, p 309
36. B.S. Majumdar and G.M. Newaz, *Phil. Mag.*, Vol 66, 1992, p 187
37. J.A. Philliber, F.-C. Dary, F.W. Zok, and C.G. Levi, "Cast Metal Matrix Composites: Processing, Properties and Applications," *TMS Fall Meeting*, Oct 1996 (Cincinnati, OH)
38. T. Saito, *Adv. Perform. Mater.*, Vol 2, 1995, p 121
39. T. Yamaguchi, H. Morishita, S. Iwase, S. Yamada, T. Furuta, and T. Saito, "Development of P/M Titanium Engine Valves," SAE Technical Paper 2000-01-0905, Society of Automotive Engineers International, 2000
40. F.H. Froes and R.H. Jones, *14th International Titanium Application Conf. and Exhibition*, Oct 1998 (Monte Carlo, Monaco)
41. S. Abkowitz and P. Weihrauch, *Adv. Mater. Process.*, Vol 7, 1989, p 31
42. C.Y. Yolton and J.H. Moll, Crucible Materials Corporation, private communication, 1999
43. Z. Fan, A.P. Miodownik, L. Chandrashekaran, and M. Ward-Close, *J. Mater. Sci.*, Vol 29, 1994, p 1127

Ceramic Matrices

Daniel R. Petrak

FIBER-REINFORCED CERAMIC-MATRIX COMPOSITES (CMCs) have received a great deal of interest since the 1980s for their potential as high-temperature structural materials. This new class of composites has been the subject of many research programs aimed at ultimately producing components for turbine engines for aerospace and power generation and components for space applications and a variety of industrial uses. Currently, these materials are considered to be expensive relative to available alternatives. Progress on development of design methods and evaluation of full-scale components has been slow. This may be due to the wide variety of chemistries for both matrices and reinforcements and also the process methods used for fabrication. Other factors limiting CMCs use are cost and the poor oxidation resistance of interfacial coatings. This discussion is directed at the matrices for the composites; therefore, attention is focused on the process methods and matrix chemistries. Issues related to reinforcements and interfaces are discussed in other articles in this Volume. In general, the processes of interest include:

- Pressure-assisted glass-matrix densification
- Chemical vapor infiltration (CVI)
- Melt infiltration (MI)
- Polymer infiltration and pyrolysis (PIP)
- Sol-gel processing

In essence, all of the previously mentioned methods involve use of a ceramic, preceramic, or metal phase as a fluid or vapor phase reactant to form the matrix. Each processing technique and specific matrix chemistry types of interest are discussed subsequently. Emphasis is placed on microstructural features that influence ultimate composite properties.

Pressure-Assisted Densification

Some of the first successful efforts to produce tough ceramic-matrix composites involved hot pressing of glass or glass ceramics (Ref 1, 2). This work was done with graphite fibers (various vendors), large-filament SiC fibers (Textron Specialty Materials), and ceramic grade (CG) Nicalon fibers (Nippon Carbon Co.). The composites were prepared by slurry coating the fibers with glass frit. Layers or plies of fiber were stacked in a graphite die and then heated under pressure to consolidate the composite above the fusion point of the glass. Typically, the matrices produced in these studies had low porosity and were impermeable to liquids.

The use of glass-ceramic matrices such as $MgO-Al_2O_3-SiO_2$ systems produced crystallized matrices that could be tailored to control matrix thermal expansion and therefore, control the differential stress between the matrix and the fiber. Perhaps most importantly, these studies permitted an understanding of the role of fiber-matrix interfacial layers to be developed. Although many of these composites have useful properties, they are inherently expensive, because the process is size- and shape-limited.

Chemical Vapor Infiltration

Chemical vapor deposition has been recognized as an important process to produce solid materials. It has been used to produce materials for semiconductors and also for structural ceramics (Ref 3). Chemical vapor deposition methods have been useful in producing all of the individual components of ceramic-matrix composites, that is, fibers, interface coatings, and matrices. The term CVI has been used to refer to the process for deposition of interphase and matrix in fiber-reinforced composites. Although the CVI process has been used to produce many carbides, nitrides, borides, and oxides, its use to prepare SiC is most widely known (Ref 4, 5, 6).

Silicon carbide CVI matrices are often produced by heating methyltrichlorosilane or dichlorosilane and hydrogen to a temperature of 900 to 1100 °C (1600 to 2000 °F) at a pressure of 10 to 100 kPa (1.5 to 15 psi). These deposition conditions permit the use of reinforcements such as graphite, crystalline SiC, Si-C-O fibers (such as CG Nicalon), and Si-C-O-Ti fibers (such as Tyranno, Ube Industries Inc., New York, NY).

The SiC phase produced by this method is beta-SiC. Depending upon the actual deposition time, temperature, and other variables, CVI deposition tends to close off matrix pores. Machining the surface of the composite can open the pores to permit additional matrix densification. Depending upon the thickness of the composite, that process can be repeated until the desired density and porosity are achieved. The CVI process is normally considered complete when the overall porosity is 10 to 15%. Most CVI materials are prepared under isothermal and isobaric conditions. However, thermal gradients and pressure gradients can be used to minimize porosity and to manufacture certain geometrical shapes more efficiently.

The typical microstructure of two-dimensional fabric laminates produced by the CVI process is characterized by dense matrix regions near the fibers tows and by rather coarse pores (10 to 200 μm) in the regions between plies or within the tows (Fig. 1). The SiC-matrix phase is essentially continuous but does not necessarily protect the fibers and the fiber-matrix interface coating from the environment. The ability of the SiC matrix to protect the interface coating is often dependent on the thickness of the coating, its chemistry, and actual environmental conditions. Porosity and matrix stress cracking will allow the ingress of oxygen, which will degrade the interface coating.

Melt Infiltration

The MI method to produce ceramic composites involves producing a reaction-bonded SiC-Si matrix by infiltrating a porous SiC preform with silicon metal. An excellent review of this process and material was given by Corman et al. (Ref 7, 8). The MI technology has evolved over more than 30 years and is covered by a number of patents. Early versions of the technology were called "Silcomp" (General Electric Co.). Silcomp is prepared by infiltrating molten silicon into a porous preform containing carbon in a fibrous form.

More recent versions of the technology include the use of SiC fibers with a BN-based interface coating. Preforms of the coated fiber can be prepared by laminating with a carbon-producing resin or by using CVI methods to produce a porous preform, followed by slurry casting SiC particles into the open porosity of the preform. Densification of the porous preform is accomplished by silicon infiltration. The infiltration step is done in vacuum, at a temperature above the melting point of the silicon alloy. This process results in a nearly fully dense composite. Figures 2 and 3 show examples of MI composites from General Electric Company.

Figure 2 is a micrograph of an MI composite prepared from Hi-Nicalon fiber and the tow-winding method to prepare a tape, followed by laminating with a resin. The resin is then pyrolyzed to produce carbon in the preform, followed by silicon infiltration to yield a low-porosity SiC-Si matrix. Figure 3 shows a similar structure, but with Sylramic SiC fiber from Dow Corning, Midland, MI. The preform in Fig. 3 was made from two-dimensional cloth and was prepared by using a CVI method, followed by slurry casting and silicon melt infiltration. The "white" phase in Fig. 2 and 3 is silicon metal; the dark rings around the fibers are interface coatings.

The SiC-Si MI matrix nearly matches the thermal expansion of the high-temperature SiC fibers. It is also a higher thermal conductivity material than the CVI SiC matrix due to its low porosity and the presence of silicon. The MI matrix, along with improved interface coatings and environmental barrier coatings, makes the MI matrix composites candidates for high-temperature structural applications, such as components for power-generating turbines.

Polymer Infiltration and Pyrolysis

The PIP method for producing ceramic matrices makes use of preceramic polymers to form the composite shapes and also to densify the composite matrix. A number of preceramic polymers were developed in the 1970s and 1980s that led to the fabrication of silicon-based fibers and other ceramic applications. Those polymers included polycarbosilanes, polysilanes, polysilazanes, and polysiloxanes. The early efforts to fabricate CMCs by the PIP method (Ref 9) were only marginally successful, because as they were made before the role of interface coatings was known. For that reason, they most often resulted in low strength and brittle materials. That work did, however, suggest lower-cost routes for producing large and complex parts with ceramic composites. In addition to the autoclave molding or compression molding methods discussed subsequently, other techniques, such as filament winding, injection molding, and pultrusion, can be used to manufacture CMCs by the PIP method.

Later, with the availability of carbon-coated CG Nicalon fiber and then commercial sources of BN coatings on Nicalon and higher-temperature fibers, a number of PIP-based CMCs were promoted (Ref 10–16). Basically, all of the PIP composites were prepared by variants of the methods shown in Fig. 4. The process steps through the polymer cure step are essentially the same as for the preparation of organic-matrix composites. The matrix precursors are often ceramic powder-filled preceramic polymers, mixed by ball milling to make a slurry. The slurry is used to infiltrate the space between the interface-coated fibers in a woven fabric or tape. If solvent is used, it is removed by evaporation. The prepreg is then ready for laminating in a press or autoclave. The stack of prepreg layers is heated under moderate pressure to debulk and then cure the laminate. After the cured part is trimmed and inspected, the composite is converted to a ceramic by heating in a nonreactive atmosphere to pyrolyze the matrix. Pyrolysis removes volatiles such as hydrogen, methane, and sometimes ammonia from the polymer, leaving a ceramic char. Different polymers produce different char chemistries. They include Si-C-O, Si-N-C, and SiC or Si_3N_4 under different conditions of atmosphere and temperature. Depending upon char yield (percentage of original weight of polymer retained after pyrolysis), the char density, and the

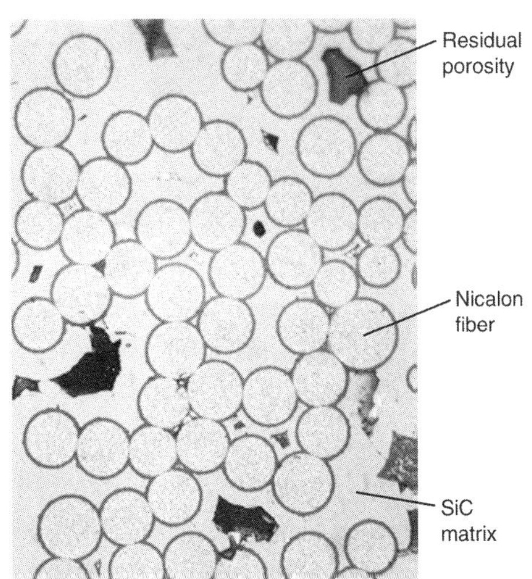

Fig. 1 Typical microstructure of a fabric laminate produced by the chemical vapor infiltration process. The micrograph shows fibers in only one direction in one tow.

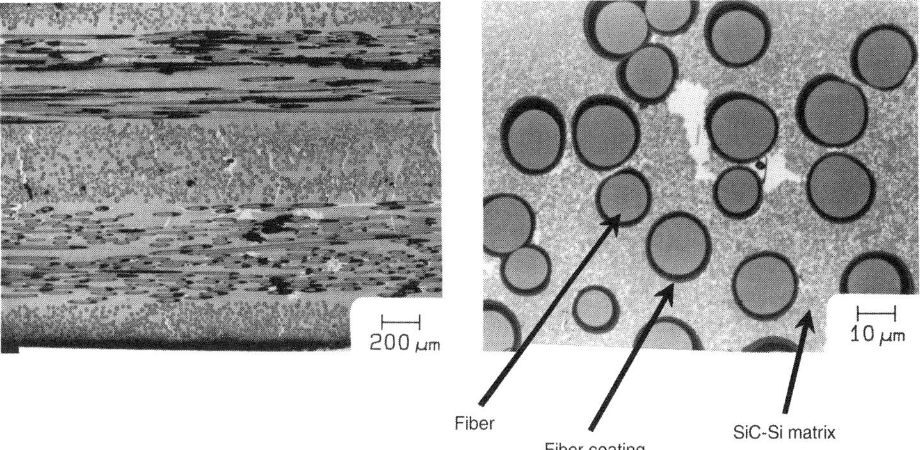

Fig. 2 Micrographs of a melt infiltrated composite prepared from Hi-Nicalon fiber and the tow-winding method to create a tape that is then laminated with a resin. The resin is pyrolyzed to produce carbon in the preform. The silicon infiltration is then done to produce a low-porosity SiC-Si matrix.

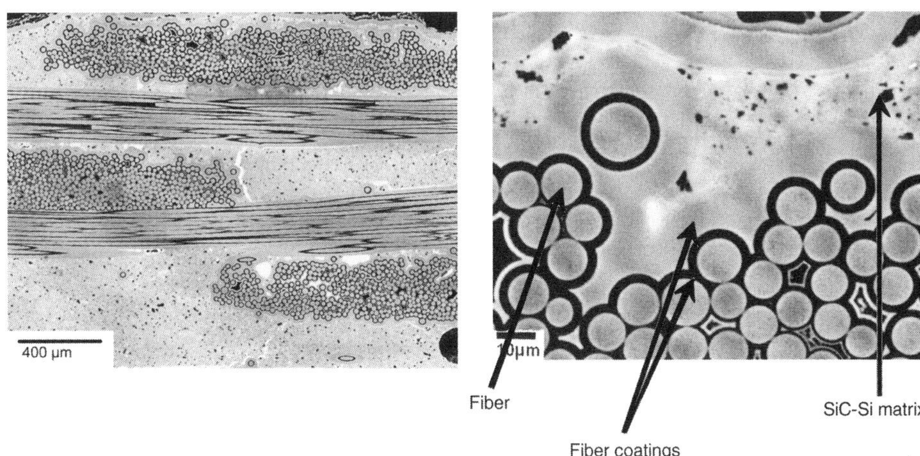

Fig. 3 Micrographs of a melt infiltrated composite reinforced with Sylramic SiC fiber. The preform was made from two-dimensional cloth and was prepared by using a CVI method, followed by slurry casting and silicon melt infiltration.

amount of powder filler used in the matrix, porosity will be created in the matrix. The level of that porosity can be up to 35% of the volume of the composite.

If the porosity left in the composite is higher than desired, the polymer used to prepare the prepreg can be used to reinfiltrate the pores, followed by pyrolysis to form additional matrix. This procedure of reinfiltrating the porosity and heating to a pyrolysis temperature can be repeated until the porosity is reduced to an acceptable level. As few as 4 and as many as 15 or 16 pyrolysis cycles are typically required to complete the process. Fully processed PIP composites can have as little as 3 to 5% open porosity, although total porosity is usually approximately 10%.

Figure 5 shows a microstructure of a CG Nicalon fiber composite prepared with a polysilazane-derived matrix (Ref 17). The matrix includes a Si_3N_4 powder filler. The measured open porosity in the composite was less than 5%. Inspection of the micrograph shows that cracks occur in the matrix during the first pyrolysis, and that most of the porosity generated by those cracks has been filled with matrix from subsequent reinfiltrations. Although the PIP composites tend to have some residual open porosity, the formulation of the polysilazane-derived matrix described previously retains good tensile and fatigue properties at 1100 °C (2000 °F) in air for hundreds of hours. That effect occurs because surface oxidation seals porosity to protect the interface and the fiber.

Silicon-based polymer-derived matrices typically produce amorphous silicon containing glasses when pyrolyzed at temperatures at which CG Nicalon fiber is stable, that is, less than 1200 °C (2200 °F). The use of higher-temperature fibers, such as Hi-Nicalon, Hi-Nicalon S, and Sylramic SiC, permits higher-temperature processing. It is possible to produce crystalline SiC and Si_3N_4 by heating to appropriate temperatures. Depending on the level of oxygen in the char, crystalline phases can be produced in the 1400 to 1600 °C (2550 to 2900 °F) temperature range. However, the volume char yield of the polymer will decrease to levels of less than 20% in some cases, due to the higher density of crystalline phases. The specific gravity of amorphous chars ranges from 2.2 to 2.5, whereas the specific gravity of crystalline SiC is 3.2.

Although many PIP composites have nonoxide chemistries, Szweda et al. (Ref 18) from General Electric Company have used silicon-based preceramic polymers to produce oxide matrices. This permits the polymer to provide the same shape-forming advantages of known organic-matrix composites technologies, similar to the nonoxide precursor capabilities. By processing in air, the SiO_2-containing matrix chemistries can be produced. According to Szweda et al., the processing can be done from 600 °C (1100 °F) to as high as 1400 °C (2550 °F) to produce various solid reactions with ceramic filler particles to form lathlike grains in the matrix. This type of structure minimizes matrix shrinkage and preserves porosity in the matrix to avoid the bonding of matrix to fibers. Fibers useful in producing this type of composite must be stable in the processing and use environment, typically air. Examples include sapphire filaments and weavable oxide tows. One advantage of this process is that only one high-temperature process step is required to make a composite. However, reinfiltration with the polymer can be done to tailor the amount and nature of the porosity.

Sol-Gel Processing

Sol-gel processing (Ref 19) has been used to prepare many oxide compositions in the form of powders, fibers, coatings, and ceramic matrices in CMCs. Sol-gel processing is a chemical solution method to produce ceramic oxides. Two methods are normally used: metal salts or alkoxide precursors. An example of a metal salt is ZrOCl, and an example of an alkoxide precursor is tetraethylorthosilicate. Alkoxides are often preferred, because higher yields and better purity can be achieved with their use.

Combinations of a sol along with solid ceramic powders are often used to prepare a matrix precursor. The sol can act as a carrier and also the binder for the powder in forming a prepreg with the ceramic reinforcing fiber. Once a composite is formed from the preform, the sol can be gelled to make the composite rigid. The composite fabrication process can be filament winding, laminating of two-dimensional prepreg, or injection molding of two- or three-dimensional

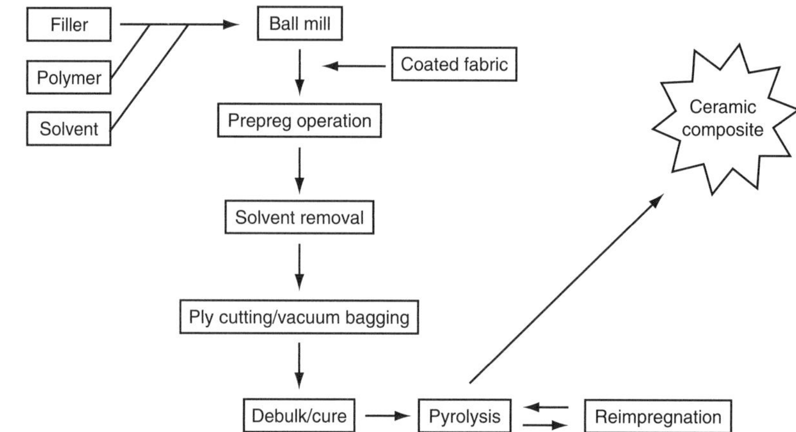

Fig. 4 Polymer infiltration process

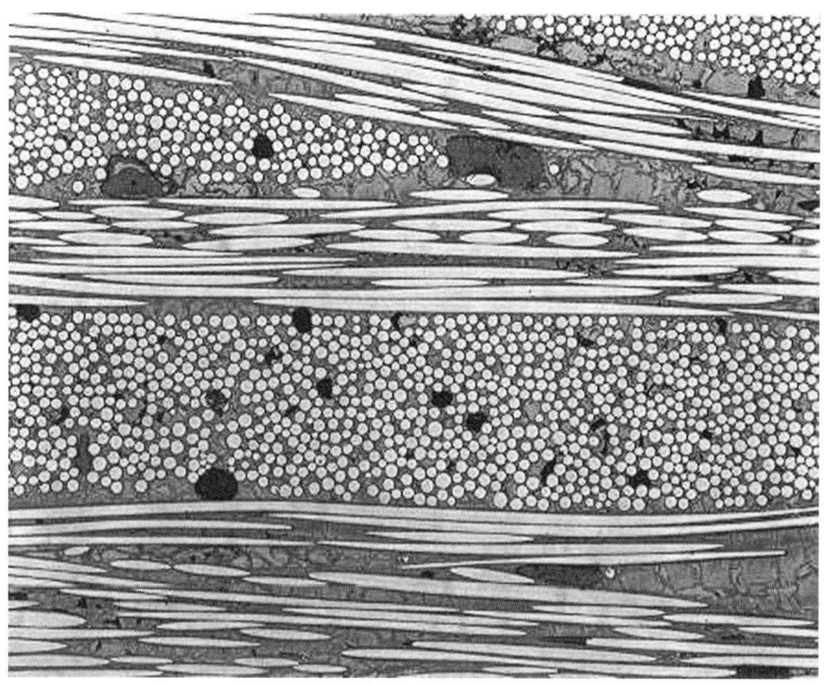

Fig. 5 Microstructure of a CG Nicalon fiber composite prepared from a polysilazane-derived matrix

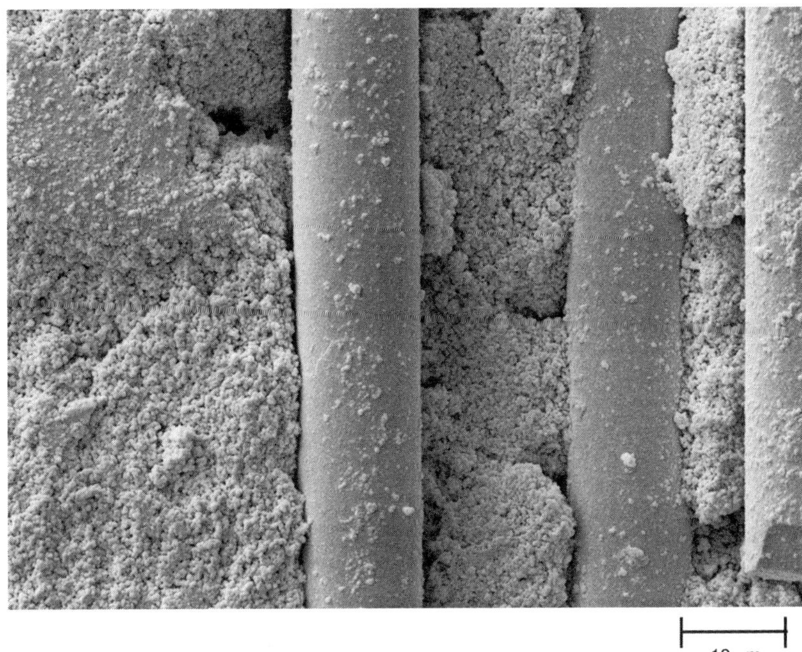

Fig. 6 Micrograph of a sol-gel-derived Nextel 610 fiber-reinforced aluminum-oxide-matrix composite. Courtesy of John Paretti, COI Ceramics Inc.

preforms. Gelling of the sol often can be done by heating, by slight drying, or by a chemical reaction such as exposure to ammonia.

The use of reactive and/or inert filler particles is often very important to reduce matrix shrinkage and cracking during drying and conversion to the final ceramic-matrix chemistry and structure. The typical sol-gel-derived ceramic matrix contains 25 to 40% open porosity after heating to a final process temperature and is of low strength. There are two approaches to selecting the level of desired porosity in these matrices. If the reinforcing fiber does not have an interface coating, then a moderately high level of porosity is generally required to control fiber-to-interface bonding. However, high levels of matrix porosity also typically correspond to low interlaminar strength properties. The introduction of oxidatively stable interface coatings on oxide reinforcements has been studied (Ref 20). Interface coatings, such as $LaPO_4$, are being developed to permit the use of higher-density matrices that should lead to better matrix-dominated properties, higher thermal conductivity, and better erosion resistance.

Figure 6 is a micrograph of a sol-gel-derived Nextel 610 (3M Corporation, St. Paul, MN) fiber-reinforced aluminum-oxide-matrix composite. The composite has nominally 30% porosity and was produced using a two-dimensional cloth lay-up method. The material exhibits a tensile strength of 190 MPa (28 ksi) and an interlaminar shear strength of 11.3 MPa (1.6 ksi).

REFERENCES

1. J. Aveston, G.A. Cooper, and A. Kelly, *Proc. Conf. on Properties of Fibers and Composites*, IPC Science and Technology Press, Guildford, 1971
2. K.M. Prewo, J.J. Brennan, and G.K. Layden, Fiber Reinforced Glasses and Glass Ceramics for High Performance Applications, *Am. Ceram. Soc. Bull.*, Vol 65 (No. 2), 1986, p 305–313
3. F.S. Galasso, *Chemical Vapor Deposited Materials*, CRC Press, 1991
4. L.R. Newkirk, R.E. Riley, H. Sheinberg, F.A. Valencia, and T.C. Wallace, Preparation of Titanium Diboride and Boron Carbide Composite Bodies, *Proc. Conf. Chemical Vapor Deposition*, 14–19 Oct 1979 (Los Angeles, CA), The Electrochemical Society, 1979
5. D.P. Stinton, A.J. Caputo, and R.A. Lowden, Synthesis of Fiber-Reinforced SiC Composites by Chemical Vapor Deposition, *Am. Ceram. Soc. Bull.*, Vol 65 (No. 2), 1986, p 347–350
6. R. Naslain, Two-Dimensional SiC/SiC Composites Processed According to the Isobaric-Isothermal Chemical Vapor Infiltration Gas Phase Route, *J. Alloy. Comp.*, Vol 188 (No. 1992), p 42–48
7. G.S. Corman, K.L. Luthra, and M.K. Brun, Silicon Melt Infiltrated Ceramic Composites—Process and Properties, *Progress in Ceramic Gas Turbine Development*, M.K. Ferber, M. van Rhoode, and D.W. Richerson, Ed., ASME Press, 2001
8. G.S. Corman, M.K. Brun, and K.L. Luthra, "SiC Fiber Reinforced SiC-Si Matrix Composites Prepared by Melt Infiltration (MI) for Gas Turbine Applications," presented at International Gas Turbine and Aeroengine Congress and Exhibition, 7–10 June 1999, (Indianapolis, IN)
9. F. Chi and G. Stark, Fiber Reinforced Glass Matrix Composites, U.S. Patent 4,460,639, Dow Corning, July 1984
10. S.T. Schwab et al., "Infiltration/Pyrolysis Processing of SiC Fiber-Reinforced Si_3N_4 Composites," NASA-CP 3175, Part 2, 1992, p 721–738
11. Ceramic Fiber-Reinforced Silicon Carboxide Composite, U.S. Patent 5,464,594, Allied Signal, Nov 1995
12. S.T. Gonczy and P.D. Dubois, Flexural Properties of a 2D Blackglas Nicalon Composite as a Function of Processing and Porosity, *Proc. Materials Challenge: Diversity and Future*, Vol 40-I (Covina, CA), Society for the Advancement of Material and Process Engineering, 1995, p 446–456
13. S.T. Gonczy, E.P. Butler, N.R. Khasgiwale, L. Tsakalakos, W.R. Cannon, and S.C. Danforth, Blackglas-Nicalon Composites with CVD Boron Nitride Fiber Interface Coatings, *Ceramic Engineer and Science Proc. 19th Conf. on Composites and Advanced Ceramics*, 9–12 Jan 1995 (Cocoa Beach, FL), Vol 16 (No. 4), p 433
14. D.R. Petrak, Polymer Derived Ceramics, *Ceramics and Glasses, Engineered Materials Handbook*, Vol 4, ASM International, 1991, p 223–226
15. T.E. Easler, D.R. Petrak, and A. Szweda, Sylramic Ceramic-Matrix Composites Processing and Properties, *Ceram. Trans.*, Vol 96, 1999, p 113–122
16. R. Jones, A. Szweda, and D. Petrak, Polymer Derived Ceramic Matrix Composites, *Compos.: Part A*, Vol 30, 1999, p 569–575
17. D. Petrak, G. Stark, and G. Zank, Method for Making Ceramic Matrix Composites, U.S. Patent 5,707,471, Dow Corning, Jan 1998
18. Fiber Reinforced Ceramic Matrix Composite Member, U.S. Patent, 5,488,017, General Electric, Jan 1996
19. C.X. Campbell, S.K. El-Rahaiby, and D.W. Freitag, "Processing and Affordability of Ceramic Matrix Composites," Ceramics Information Analysis Center report, Contract DLA900-90-D-0304, 4 Oct 1995
20. P. Morgan and D. Marshall, Fibrous Composites Including Monazites and Xenotimes, U.S. Patent 5,665,463, Rockwell International, Sept 1997

Carbon Matrices

James Gary Pruett, Hitco Carbon Composites

APPLICATIONS involving very high temperature or highly corrosive environments often have requirements that exceed the capabilities of plastic or epoxy matrix composites. Even metal matrices frequently are unable to meet the requirements of the applications. Carbon, which is often included in a discussion of ceramic materials, can sometimes mimic the properties of ceramic matrix composites, but the wide range of processing options and final matrix properties justifies the separation of this material into its own category of matrix materials.

Pure Carbon Forms

Graphite and Diamond. Elemental carbon owes its variety and versatility to the nearly equivalent energy between its two primary forms: (1) diamond, where carbon atoms bond equally to four other carbon atoms, and (2) graphite, where carbon atoms bond equally to three other carbon atoms and weakly to many other carbon atoms. The diamond structure (Fig. 1b) extends uniformly in all three directions to form a very hard crystalline material. The graphite structure (Fig. 1a) is normally pictured as a planar assembly of atoms arranged in hexagonal patterns, much like "chicken" wire. Multiple planes of the basic sheet structure are stacked in a regular pattern, such that alternating planes are exactly matched and aligned. Both the diamond and graphite structures create long-range interconnectivity (theoretically infinite crystal lattices), resulting in large macroscopic crystals in nature (diamonds and natural graphite flakes).

The net thermodynamic energy required to transform between diamond and graphite is very small (less than one kilocalorie per mole, with graphite the more stable), yet diamond is very stable even at elevated temperatures. The stability is due to a large energy barrier necessary to convert between the two. The energy barrier is associated with a concerted simultaneous change in bonding of many atoms and the resulting large atomic displacements required. Very high temperatures and pressures are necessary to overcome the barrier. This explains why natural diamonds are found deep in ancient volcano pipes and why synthetic diamond production requires specialized ultrahigh pressure, high-temperature reactor systems.

Since the 1980s, additional methods of making artificial diamonds have been developed that do not require such high temperatures and pressures. With precise control of the gas mixtures, diamond films have been grown with an ordinary acetylene torch. Plasma torches, microwave discharges, and hot filament reactors have also been used with success, as described by Bachman (Ref 1). These approaches avoid the energy barrier between graphite and diamond by constructing the diamond material a few carbon atoms at a time from a carbon-containing gas such as methane or acetylene, rather than trying to transform a bulk graphite form.

The combination of nearness in energy and propensity for large interconnectivity gives rise to many intermediate mixed structures between diamond and graphite that are also metastable. On the graphite end of this spectrum are near-graphites, which exhibit long-range order in a given plane of carbon atoms (so-called graphene sheets), but whose planes are stacked somewhat randomly and exhibit a range of angles of in-plane rotation between adjacent sheets. Moving toward more disorder, the graphene sheets can be contorted, split, twisted, and reconnected with a resulting high level of defects and void structures. The logical end to this sequence would be a totally random and very hard, glassy network of carbon atoms with an amorphous morphology. As these amorphous structures contain more three-dimensional diamondlike structures, the material begins to resemble a diamond lattice.

These intermediate structures have wide property ranges that are exploited in carbon matrix composites. They are all highly metastable, especially the glassy forms, and, for all practical purposes, are stable and useful over wide temperature ranges. Under normally accessed temperatures and pressures, the graphite form is the most stable.

Fullerenes and Nanotubes. A third "new" form of carbon recently discovered, the fullerenes, is qualitatively different from the traditional forms of carbon. The fullerenes are actually molecular forms of pure carbon. The connectivity between the atoms is "closed," in that all bonds are satisfied within a short distance. For example, C_{60} is a stable carbon molecule whose structure was worked out by Kroto, Curl, and Smalley (Ref 2) to be that of a soccer ball (mixture of hexagons and pentagons of carbon atoms connected in a closed structure). This is also the structure presented by Buckminster Fuller's geodesic dome, from which the common name of the material is derived. If additional six-carbon atom rings are added around the circumference of C_{60}, it becomes cigar shaped and, eventually, a closed-end tube, referred to as single wall nanotubes.

All of these new forms of carbon should be thought of as molecular forms of carbon that

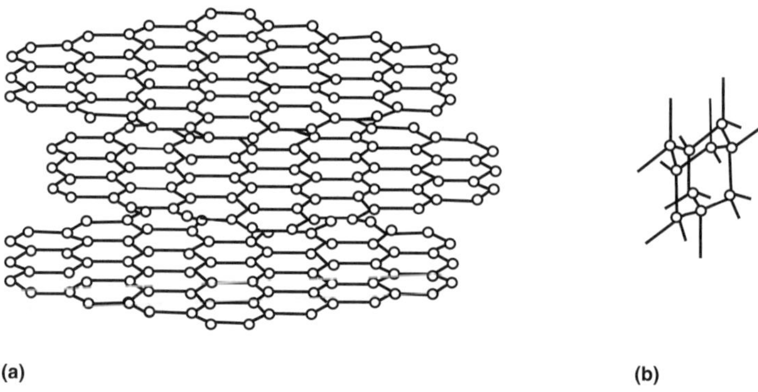

Fig. 1 Primary forms of elemental carbon. (a) Graphite structure with extended sheets of hexagonal units. (b) Diamond structure with each carbon atom having four equivalent bonds in an interconnected network

condense into various phases. For example, crystals of C_{60} have been separated and examined by x-ray diffraction, and "condensed" ropes of single wall nanotubes are the most commonly observed structures of nanotubes in the laboratory. These carbons are less metastable than the graphite or diamond forms, due primarily to the higher energy related to the carbon pentagons. As a result they tend to convert to graphitic or glassy forms of carbon when heated to moderately high temperatures. As a molecular form of pure carbon, there are some potential advantages of this material as a matrix precursor, if not as the actual matrix. Since there is no other element present except carbon, it could have a unique role as a zero-mass loss precursor to other forms of carbon. Laboratory examples of composites made by using some of these materials began to emerge in the late 1990s.

The commercial importance of each of these forms as matrix materials varies widely. A graphitic carbon matrix is a desired goal for composites whose primary function is heat transfer. Large quantities of aircraft brake materials are made with the specification of having a highly ordered graphite structure in the matrix. The graphite structure is also desirable when a better resistance to oxidation at high temperature is advantageous. These matrices are readily made either by choosing the right conditions for pyrocarbon deposition, or by using highly graphitic pitch-precursor materials for liquid impregnation. For purely structural applications, a less-graphitic and more-glassy carbon matrix material is often used, which requires less high-temperature processing. Diamond as a matrix material is not commercially available due to the difficulty of achieving the diamond structure within the bulk of a composite. The new fullerene materials have been used in the laboratory as matrix materials and matrix precursors, but suffer from the high cost and low availability of the starting materials.

Matrix Formation Methods

General Considerations. Carbon, since it does not melt or flow even at quite high temperatures, must be introduced into a matrix in a precarbon or presolid form, similar to any refractory matrix material. Inclusion in a matrix can be done in a variety of ways. The earliest method employed was by the introduction of a precarbon liquid followed by solidification and carbonization of the carbon precursor. Later, the matrix was formed by the introduction of a carbon-containing gas into a hot porous part, with subsequent chemical decomposition of the gas to elemental solid carbon within the porous part. In the case of liquid infiltration, the liquid flow properties can also be used to introduce finely divided solid carbon or modifying materials into the matrix as fillers or modifiers for a variety of end-use properties. The whole process can be catalyzed or uncatalyzed, and it can be aided with a variety of energy-enhanced processes such as plasmas or electrical discharges.

Table 1 illustrates the variety of carbon types and the corresponding general methods used to create them or incorporate them into a matrix of a composite.

Liquid Precursors. Liquid precursors are generally one of three types: thermoplastic (viscosity decreasing with temperature), thermosetting (transforming to nonfluid state at increased temperature), and evaporative or solvent carriers (disappearing entirely during later processing).

Thermoplastic varieties are relatively easy to process to a noncarbon composite state, but present significant challenges to convert to pure carbon. Their thermoplastic behavior requires that they either be confined within the object by external means, or be chemically treated (stabilized) prior to heating to carbonization temperatures. Petroleum- or coal-based pitch materials are a good example of this type. Most pitches are solids at room temperature. They can be dissolved in a volatile solvent or heated to reduce their viscosity to the point that they can infiltrate a porous object or preform. Since the pitch material melts prior to carbonization, the object to be filled must be held within a closed container that, at the fluid temperature of the pitch, subjects the object to complete immersion in the fluid. The fluid can enter the porous part by capillary action or by using external pressure. As the material continues to be heated, the pitch will begin to solidify through condensation reactions, a process that releases gaseous products. Unless held at high pressure, these gaseous products tend to cause the pitch fluid to foam, displacing pitch from the preform. Prior to reaching the foaming reaction, the pitch material can be exposed to an oxidizing environment at an elevated temperature over a period of time. This treatment induces an oxidative cross-linking among the constituents of the pitch, causing it to permanently harden. Further increase in temperature causes decomposition to form solid carbon, but no fluid phase occurs and the carbon is retained in the object. The net result is that a process using this type of carbon precursor requires the steps of fluidization (by heat or solvent), infiltration, confinement and stabilization, final carbonization, and removal of the object from waste-carbonized precursor. Other thermoplastic forms can be treated similarly.

Thermosetting Fluids. At an elevated temperature and without the introduction of additional materials, thermosetting fluids possess the property of curing to a solid that will not melt at a higher temperature. Some of these materials cure with an exothermic reaction that releases water. Others cure without the release of any volatile materials. From a fabrication process perspective, this is a very useful behavior because reinforcing material can be preimpregnated with the precursor material, compression and heat molded, and cured to a near-net shape in one step. The resulting near-net shape part can then be carbonized and further processed to finish the composite structure with no further fixtures or confinement. This process is at least the first step in the fabrication of a large number of aircraft brake materials made of carbon matrix composites.

Evaporative Precursors. Some more-recently developed methods use a carrier fluid, which is evaporated prior to carbonization, to carry powdered materials into the reinforcement structure; the powders themselves have no or much-reduced fluidity even at very high temperatures. In this technique, a solids-loaded carrier fluid is introduced to the reinforcement through a preimpregnation process or by multiple soaking and evaporation steps. The purpose is to obtain a very high carbon content in the matrix prior to carbonization. Subsequent carbonization then results in a high carbon yield within the composite while reducing the number of processing cycles. Variations of this technique have long been used with standard precursor fluids to introduce fillers into the composite. Either pure carbon (carbon black or advanced pitch-derived carbon particles) or active fillers, such as boron-containing compounds or silicon carbide, can be added for the purpose of modifying the performance properties of the composite.

Processing Characteristics and Properties. All liquid precursor methods for producing a carbon matrix suffer from one problem: the precursor materials always have a lower carbon content per unit volume than does the desired carbon matrix. Therefore, there is always a reduction in volume of the precursor when going to the final matrix. In addition, most of the liquid precursor materials lose some of their carbon content and all of their noncarbon content during the carbonization process. The most commonly used phenolic heat-set resins, for example, lose up to 50% of their mass when being carbonized. This mass loss also produces waste products in the process that must be handled carefully as potential health risks (polyaromatic and phenolic species). This mass and volume loss results in a fully dense, precarbonized composite that becomes porous and weak after carbonization. This situation is

Table 1 Carbon forms and methods used to incorporate them into a composite matrix

Carbon form	Liquid	Particulate	Pyrolytic	Catalyzed	Enhanced
Graphite	X	X	X	X	
Turbostratic graphite	X	X	X		
Glassy carbon	X	X	X		
Diamond		X			X
Fullerene	X			X	
Nanotube		X		X	

X, applicable method

usually remedied by multiple reimpregnation and carbonization steps, reaching a diminishing return at around 5 to 10% porosity. As a result, a high premium is placed on carbon yield in the process. Poor carbon yields are obtained from polyesters and epoxides (<20%). Useful yields are obtained from epoxy-novalac, furan, and phenol formaldehyde resins (>50%). Some difficult-to-obtain materials, such as polyphenylene, have been shown to give over 80% carbon yields. Pitch materials, when processed at high pressure, can give yields in the 80% range. In general, the more aromatic structure in the precursor, the higher the carbon yield. Carbon yield can be increased by selection of precursor, by use of fillers, or by carrying out the carbonization at high pressure to inhibit the loss of volatile carbon species during carbonization. The high pressure impregnation and carbonization method was developed specifically to overcome this mass loss issue in pitch materials.

The matrix shrinkage of liquid precursors can have a profound effect on the composite properties as well. Carbon and noncarbon loss during carbonization is often a source of damage in the structure, especially during the early stages when there are no passages for the material to escape. When the evolved species collect in isolated voids and exert pressures that exceed the local material strength, larger voids can open and create damaged regions (primarily delaminations). During later stages when a network of connected cracks has developed, this danger is largely over. As a result, careful attention is often paid to the carbonization process temperature versus time profile to avoid these dangers in manufacturing.

The nature, location, and size of the shrinkage cracks is also a subtle but important issue in the processing of these matrix materials. If the crack structure is to be used as the conduit for later infiltration steps, it is important to have a structure that is compatible with the next processing step. When a region of resin surrounded by reinforcement begins to shrink, stress occurs in any direction that the reinforcement is constrained and unable to move with the shrinking matrix. When the stress extends to the area of lowest material strength, a crack opens in that area to relieve the stress. As the material continues to shrink, stress builds up again until another weak area is found, thereby creating a new crack or extending the size of an old crack. While some of the shrinkage can occur as net dimensional shrinkage of the composite, the fiber or other reinforcement often holds the part shrinkage to a small value, resulting in substantial porosity within the part. The shrinkage can result in either a few large cracks or a large number of smaller cracks within the part. This behavior is often dictated by a combination of resin strength at various stages during carbonization, stress induced by shrinkage at those stages, and the interfacial strength between the carbonizing matrix precursor and the reinforcing network.

For example, in traditional two-dimensional fabric composites, it is relatively easy for the part to shrink in a direction perpendicular to the fabric planes. There are no fibers oriented in that direction to maintain the dimensional stability of the article. Stress buildup in the direction normal to the plane is rare, and few, if any, cracks are found in that direction in the composite. In the two orthogonal directions, however, the composite dimensions are constrained, and quite large stresses build up during matrix shrinkage. Two general cases can occur, as illustrated in Fig. 2. If the reinforcement-matrix interface is strong, the stress will build up until the material strength of the matrix itself is matched, causing a crack to occur within the matrix material. For a strong matrix material, this most often results in the formation of a few large cracks within the composite structure. These appear as ribbonlike cracks when viewing the fiber bundle cross section (Fig. 2a). These cracks are often nearly equally spaced, indicating a classic stress field in one direction that results in cracks at even intervals. The second case (Fig. 2b) is if the matrix-reinforcement interface is very weak, or if the matrix itself has little strength. In this case, cracks begin to occur at very low stress levels, and the final structure has many very fine cracks with few large cracks. A fine-cracking structure is usually obtained when there is a very weak surface bonding between the matrix and the reinforcement or any fillers present. This creates a large number of weak crack sites during matrix shrinkage.

Chemical Vapor Infiltration. Pyrolytic carbon deposition from hydrocarbon gases has been known and used for many years. The process was first developed to provide carbon overcoats on nuclear fuel pellets. Relatively early in the development of carbon matrix composites, the method was adapted to infiltrate a porous preform with pyrolytic carbon. In this process a porous carbon or other refractory material reinforcing structure is placed inside a closed furnace vessel and heated in the presence of a carbon-containing gas, usually natural gas. The process is normally run at a reduced pressure, about 20 mbar (2 kPa), and with sufficient hydrocarbon gas flow to reduce residence time in the furnace to less than a few seconds. This type of process is referred to as isothermal chemical vapor infiltration (CVI). Hydrogen gas is often added as a side reaction moderator. The temperature is usually between 800 and 1100 °C (1470 and 2010 °F) in order to slow the deposition rate down such that deposition occurs throughout the part rather than just at the surface. The process is a very complex multi-step reaction in which the initial gas components decompose to more reactive gases, while all the time diffusing into the porous parts and converting to solid carbon as it contacts surfaces. It is not surprising then that variations in both chemistry and deposition rate can and do occur in large furnaces where the diffusion length of the gas is much smaller than the furnace during the transit time through the furnace. A large part of the commercial success of this process is due to the artful control of such variables.

The highly complex nature of the process has led to some misunderstanding of the limitations of the isothermal CVI. The presence of the gas phase side reactions that leads to ever-increasing reactivity of the molecules produced gives rise to furnace limitation effects on the kind of processing that can be done. If the gas flow is too low and residence time is too long in the furnace,

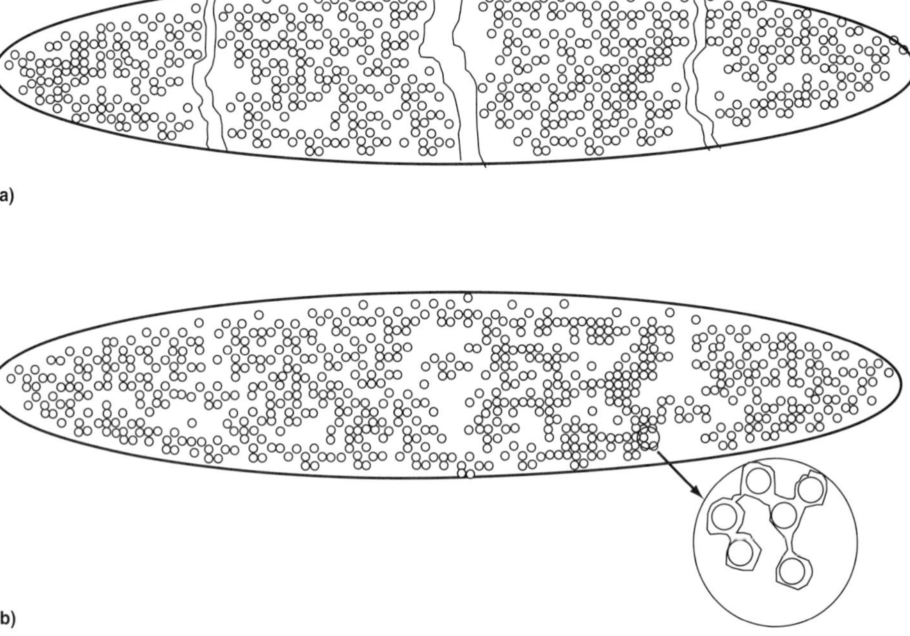

Fig. 2 Effects of shrinkage. (a) Shrinkage cracks in matrix carbon when matrix is strongly bonded to reinforcement. (b) Debonding and shrinkage in matrix when matrix is weakly bonded to reinforcement

reactive species build up that eventually (and non-linearly) lead to soot formation. Long before soot is formed, species are generated that are so reactive they deposit carbon on the first surface they encounter, leading to surface coatings on the parts and necessitating costly and time-consuming unloading and machining. Such sooting also is most apparent in regions of restricted flow within a furnace. These same species, if generated within the pores of the part, are rapidly depleted due to the high surface area-volume ratio within the part, contributing to the desired internal deposition but never advancing to the sooting stage. This soaking up of soot-forming precursors leads to the observation that soot plumes are usually associated with regions of the furnace away from reacting parts. The surface coating is often blamed on the intrinsic limitations of isothermal CVI as being an "outside-in" process. In reality, the reactivity of the initial species introduced into the furnace is low enough that such limitations are not realized. In small furnaces where it is easy to avoid side reactions, successful infiltration of parts can proceed at many times the speed of the process practiced in large furnaces. A recent series of demonstrations and measurements by Huttinger (Ref 3) clarifies this process and has the potential of modernizing the isothermal CVI process practice, or at least clarifying most of the issues in its commercial use. Huttinger has even demonstrated that proper attention to the issues of this complex process can actually succeed in adding carbon to the matrix from the inside-out rather than the reverse.

In other efforts to overcome the issues of isothermal CVI processing, two other vapor deposition concepts have been developed. One method, which was developed to overcome the diffusional mass transport limitations, is known as forced flow CVI. In this process, the part to be infiltrated is fixtured in such a way that gases flowing in the reactor are forced to move through the part by pressure gradients, rather than being limited to diffusion due to concentration gradients. This process has indeed been demonstrated to allow much faster infiltration times. Its commercial acceptance is probably limited by the prior installation of an ample amount of isothermal CVI capacity, and by the fact that in large production, it is often impractical to arrange the fixtures and gas flow patterns to accommodate multiple parts and complex part geometries.

Another method that has been developed is known as thermal gradient CVI. In this process a thermal gradient is developed across the object to be infiltrated, such that the reaction proceeds slowly on the outside of the part that is relatively cool while proceeding rapidly on the inside of the part where it is hot. In some examples, the gradient is obtained by natural radiative cooling of the hot exterior of the parts exposed to cold reactor walls, and in other examples by the boiling of a hydrocarbon source liquid in contact with the outside surfaces of the part. As the reaction proceeds, the hot zone migrates to the outside, resulting in very high filling efficiencies in notably short periods of time. This method, while very successful, also suffers in some commercial applications where complex part geometries are not amenable to this type of processing. In addition, this method suffers from the consideration that the thermal gradient requires considerable power per unit being processed, resulting in high power costs to establish a large volume production based on the technique.

For all of the CVI processing options, there are two very significant advantages of CVI processing over liquid precursor processing. First, when infiltration is complete, the matrix is all carbon with no processing shrinkage to damage the composite. Second, the type of pyrocarbon in the matrix can be tailored to range from highly graphitic to very isotropic.

Since all CVI processing is a surface deposition rather than a volume deposition process, carbon is deposited layer by layer until the pore is either inaccessible through a closed neck, or it is completely filled. As long as the pores being filled are small in size, this layer-by-layer process is economical and relatively fast. Typical surface thickness growth rates in commercial isothermal CVI processing are on the order of 0.02 μm per hour, requiring about 50 hours of processing time to fill all pores below 2 μm in diameter. Larger pores are clearly an important issue, and successful commercial applications of isothermal CVI have paid close attention to the pore size distribution in the parts to be infiltrated. When preceded by a liquid infiltration step, the issues associated with crack size during carbonization are of clear importance. The resulting relatively crack-free composite structures tend to be of the highest strength class of composites using the same reinforcements.

Pyrocarbon has been known for many years to be produced in a wide range of microstructures. Some rough processing maps have been produced to indicate the types of conditions necessary to create the different carbon types. In general, slower deposition rates using precursor species that contain acetylenic, if not aromatic, bond units tend to give more graphitic structures. Such pyrocarbons can have as-grown densities above 2.0 g/cm^3 and can be converted to nearly pure graphite at reasonably achievable temperatures. On the other hand, using either high deposition rates or precursor species with little or no aromatic content can lead to pyrocarbons that have densities below 1.4 g/cm^3, almost no graphitic character, and unresponsiveness to heat treatment. The desired type of carbon can therefore be controlled to fit the performance requirements of the final composite.

Matrix Contribution to Composite Properties

All carbon matrix forms exhibit the characteristic thermal and chemical stability of carbon, but they do not all result in the same final properties of the composite. Although composite properties are often dominated by the reinforcement properties, some properties, such as interlaminar shear and interlaminar tensile, are matrix dominated. In addition, properties such as thermal and electrical conductivity can be strongly affected by the matrix material type. Even the more traditional structural properties are affected by the density and/or porosity of the composite, which are almost entirely due to the matrix or to the process of forming the matrix. Finally, some performance properties of composites, such as friction coefficient and wear in brakes and clutches, are such complex functions of the composite constituents that the matrix material and its processing can never be disregarded.

High thermal and electrical conductivity are best obtained by having as high a graphitic content in the matrix as possible. This is moderated by the fact that both electrical and thermal conductivity of graphite are highly anisotropic, so the alignment of the graphitic planes in the final composite is as important as the presence of the graphite itself, if thermal conductivity is desired in a particular direction. If the composite is produced using isothermal CVI or related techniques, the graphitic planes usually align with the surface they are grown on. Thus, if a fiber reinforcement is used, the direction of highest thermal conductivity is aligned along the fiber direction. Liquid impregnation processing has less of a templating effect on the graphitic plane orientation in the matrix, so the matrix contribution is more uniform in direction, but is less dramatic in any one direction.

The effects of crack size and porosity on the strength of the material is well established, so to minimize these effects, careful attention must be paid to the matrix and the process of making it. Since part density is such an easy property to measure and is directly correlated with part porosity for a composite of a given structure, density is often used as a property to correlate with strength. Caution should be exercised, however, since such a wide range of matrix densities can be realized that a fully dense, near-zero porosity part of high strength could be made with a density below that of a weak and still-porous composite.

Alteration of Properties by Heat Treatment. Since graphite is the most stable form of carbon under normal conditions, nongraphitic forms of carbon can be converted to more graphitic forms by applying heat to the composite after matrix formation. In cases where the object will be used at very high temperature, the preheating of the composite is also beneficial for stabilizing the properties during use. As mentioned previously, the transformation of the metastable forms of carbon to graphite requires a high temperature to overcome barriers to the transformation. For the wide variety of imperfections that are possible in a nongraphitic carbon, it is not surprising that some of those imperfections would become annealed at lower temperatures, while others would require very high temperatures. A great deal of differentiation in carbon materials comes from whether they can be heat treated to achieve graphitic character, and the temperature required to achieve that character. For easily heat-treated materials (mesophase pitch-derived carbon and anisotropic pyrocarbons), it may only be necessary to heat to temperatures of 1930 to 2200 °C (3500 to 4000 °F), while other materials (isotropic pitch-derived carbons, isotropic pyrocarbons, and phenolic resin chars) may require up to 2760 °C (5000 °F) to achieve the same structure. Some materials resist becoming graphite at even those extreme conditions.

Future Directions and Needs

Future changes in the practice of carbon matrix composites most likely will be driven by the cost requirements necessary to transform the material from a military and aerospace specialty to a commercially viable substitute for monolithic graphites or specialty metals and coatings. Lower-cost production methods are required, which primarily means continuous, hands-off processing and more sophisticated control of process variables. On the materials side, low cost, ultrahigh-yield carbon precursors are required. It will also be helpful when a balance is struck between the performance required and the level of processing of the composite. Many of the new rapid densification techniques being developed will need to find a new market-pull application. This will allow them to move around the momentum established by the brakes market for carbon matrix composites, which has driven and frozen the technology due to long qualification times and incorporation of the technology into a vertically integrated manufacturing process.

REFERENCES

1. P.K. Bachman, *Ullman's Encyclopaedia of Industrial Chemistry,* Vol A26, 1996, p 720–725
2. H.W. Kroto, J.R. Heath, S.C. O'Brien, R.F. Curl, and R.E. Smalley, *Nature (London),* Vol 318, 1984, p 162–163
3. W. Benzinger and J.J. Huttinger, *Carbon,* Vol 37 (No. 6), 1999, p 941

SELECTED REFERENCES

- Timothy D. Burchell, Ed., *Carbon Materials for Advanced Technologies*, Pergamon, 1999
- G. Savage, *Carbon-Carbon Composites*, Chapman and Hall, 1992
- C.R. Thomas, Ed., *Essentials of Carbon-Carbon Composites*, Royal Society of Chemistry, 1993

Interfaces and Interphases

Lawrence T. Drzal, Michigan State University

FIBER-MATRIX ADHESION is a variable to be optimized in order to get the best properties and performance in composite materials. The contemporary view of adhesion rests on an *interphase* model in which not only the actual chemical and physical interactions between fiber and matrix are considered, but also the structure and properties of both the fiber and the matrix in the region near the interface. While not a "phase" in the true sense of the word (that is, an identifiable volume with uniform properties), the term has come to be used to describe a region of finite dimensions where the local properties vary from those of the bulk phases. Although our understanding of this interphase is far from complete, the studies completed to date provide some insight into selection of surface treatments and finishes for certain classes of fiber and matrix constituents. An optimal design methodology starts with the specification of the fiber and matrix from a structural consideration. Once the constituents are selected, the focus is on the creation of a beneficial fiber-matrix interphase. This interphase region where the fiber and matrix interact has to be designed for both processing and performance. Although no quantitative models are available for interphase optimization, various thermodynamic and materials science principles coupled with a growing body of experimental data allow us to understand the interphase as well as to qualitatively design the interphase. The tools available for analysis and design include selection of surface treatments for surface structural and chemical modification; the use of surface finishes and/or sizes to ensure thorough wetting and protection of the fiber; creation of interphases with desirable stiffness, toughness, and failure modes; and quantitative and qualitative characterization tests for measuring fiber-matrix adhesion levels compatible with the structural environment and constituent materials.

Interface and Interphase

A composite material is the combination of any two or more constituents, one of which has superior mechanical properties but is in a difficult-to-use form (e.g., fiber, powder, etc.). This superior constituent is usually the reinforcement, while the other constituent (the matrix) serves as the medium in which the reinforcement is dispersed and serves to transmit external loads from reinforcing fiber to fiber. The resultant composite is a material whose properties are close to those of the reinforcement constituent, but in a form that can be easily fabricated into a structural component. Included in this definition of the reinforcing materials are particulate, fiber, flake, and sheet reinforcements. Matrices may be ceramic, metallic, polymeric, and cementitious.

Interface. Since their inception, composite materials behavior has been predicated on the use of structure-property relationships accounting for the fiber and matrix constituents. Factors such as constituent composition, physical morphology, and geometrical arrangement have been incorporated in models that can predict composite mechanical behavior. Since the 1980s, however, the realization that "acceptable" properties of the interface between reinforcement and matrix are necessary for coupling of the reinforcement to the matrix and behavior that agrees with the structure-property models, for example, rule-of-mixtures. An optimized interface is necessary for the composite to achieve maximum static and dynamic mechanical properties and environmental resistance. Indeed, interfacial adhesion between fiber and matrix is based on empirical methods for optimization in most commercial composites marketed today. In optimized commercial materials, the interface functions as an efficient transmitter of forces between fiber and matrix. As such, as long as the interface is intact, composite materials behavior can be adequately described by models that assume ideal adhesion between fiber and matrix and consider the interface to be a two-dimensional boundary.

Interphase. Fiber-matrix adhesion is viewed as a necessary criterion for achieving acceptable composite properties. The patent literature contains numerous chemical formulations, processes, and procedures designed to increase fiber-matrix adhesion levels so that acceptable composite mechanical properties could be achieved. As our understanding of the relationship of fiber-matrix adhesion to composite mechanical properties has increased (Ref 1), it has become apparent that adhesion not only is necessary, but also, if properly designed, can enhance the composite mechanical properties and performance. Although our quantitative understanding of the fiber-matrix interface and the mechanisms of adhesion is not completely developed at this time, it is possible to optimize the fiber-matrix interphase in much the same manner as composite design methodologies are optimized. The key to success in this endeavor is using the concept of a fiber-matrix interphase as a framework upon which to build this methodology. For the illustration of the concept of "interphase," comments will be directed to and examples will be selected from polymeric matrix composites.

Research since 1990 has expanded the concept of the fiber-matrix interface, which exists as a two-dimensional boundary, into that of a fiber-matrix *interphase* that exists in three dimensions (Ref 2). The complexity of this interphase can best be illustrated with the use of a schematic model, which allows the many different characteristics of this region to be enumerated, as shown in Fig. 1.

By definition, the interphase exists from some point in the fiber where the local properties begin to change from the fiber bulk properties, through the actual fiber-matrix interface, into the matrix where the local properties again equal the bulk properties. Within this region, various components of known and unknown effect on the interphase can be identified. For example, the fiber may have morphological variations near the fiber surface, which are not present in the bulk of the fiber. The surface area of the fiber can be much greater than its geometrical value, because of pores, pits, or cracks present on the surface. The atomic and molecular composition of the fiber surface can be quite different from the bulk of the fiber. Surface treatments can add surface chemical groups or remove the original surface, giving rise to a chemically and structurally different region. Exposure to air before composite processing can result in the adsorption of chemical species, which may alter or eliminate certain beneficial surface reactivity. These adsorbed materials may also desorb at the elevated temperatures seen in composite fabrication and be a source of volatiles, which, if not removed, can be the origin for voids that disrupt the interface. The thermodynamic surface energy of the fiber is a result of these factors. A necessary condition for acceptable interfacial interaction between the reinforcement and the matrix is determined by its surface free energy and that of the matrix. Usually this means that the surface energy of the reinforcement must be greater than that of the matrix.

Once the fiber surface and matrix come into contact, both chemical and physical bonds can form at the interface. Surface chemical groups can react with chemical groups in the matrix, forming chemical bonds. Van der Waals attractive forces, hydrogen bonds, and electrostatic bonds can also form, depending on the system. The number and type of each strongly influence the interaction (i.e., adhesion) between fiber and matrix. The structure and properties of the matrix in the interphase can also be influenced by proximity to the fiber surface. The presence of the reinforcement and its chemical and physical nature can alter the local morphology of the matrix in the interphase region. Unreacted matrix components and impurities can diffuse to the interphase region, altering the local structure and interfering with intimate contact between fiber and matrix or producing a material with little useful mechanical properties.

Each of these phenomena can vary in magnitude and can occur simultaneously in the interphase region. Depending on the materials system, the interphase itself can be composed of any or all of these components and can extend in thickness from a few to a few thousand nanometers. Furthermore, each interphase is formed during composite processing and, therefore, may not be in its equilibrium configuration as a result of processing constraints. The structure of this region can have profound effects on the performance of the composite in terms of its mechanical strength and chemical and thermal durability. The exact composition and properties of this region must be understood if accurate predictive models of interphase behavior are to be developed and integrated into a model of composite performance. Sufficient knowledge of the interphase and its effect on fiber-matrix adhesion and composite mechanical performance has been achieved so that the fiber-matrix interphase can be engineered through the use of fiber surface treatments, coupling agents, and sizings in a rational manner to optimize composite performance. Even though it is not yet possible to either quantify or predict the formation of this "interphase" from first principles, it can serve as a framework on which the interactions between composite constituents can be studied and the interphase can be designed in an optimal manner.

Interphase Thermodynamics

One of the keys to obtaining effective composite properties is ensuring thorough infiltration of the fiber tow by the matrix. This infiltration process is limited by the interfacial thermodynamics. Wettability of the fiber by the matrix is taken as a necessary prerequisite for the formation of any composite material (Ref 3). Often, microscopic examination of the fracture surfaces of composite materials shows bare reinforcement surfaces, and/or the presence of voids is taken as an indication that "good wetting" has not occurred. Frequently, poor off-axis mechanical properties are attributed to less-than-ideal fiber-matrix adhesion that is related to poor wetting. There is a linkage between fiber surface chemistry, matrix surface free energy, thermodynamic wetting of the fiber by the matrix, and adhesion of the matrix to the fiber. The generation of adhesion during composite processing is a dynamic event that can be affected by processing conditions and that ultimately can affect composite properties.

Thermodynamics provides an excellent framework upon which to study the surface of the fiber and matrix and to quantify the interactions that can occur when they are brought together. For small-molecule liquids where the time constants for the rearrangement of molecules is short, *equilibrium thermodynamic relationships* are available that describe the interactions between the solid surface and the liquid phase and can be used to understand and predict polymer-matrix interaction with the reinforcing fiber (Ref 4). Although care must be taken when applying these relationships to polymer systems, because the viscosity and kinetics may prevent equilibrium from being attained in the composite fabrication time frame, thermodynamics does provide a useful framework upon which to understand fiber-matrix interactions.

Surface Energy. An atom or molecule on the surface of a liquid or a solid has a net force acting on it, pulling it toward the interior of that phase. The manifestation of this force is commonly called the surface tension (also called "surface energy"). In a liquid where the rearrangement of molecules takes place on the microsecond scale, the surface tension can be observed creating a "skin" on the liquid. Liquids that are composed of molecules that exert dispersion forces alone (e.g., hexane) have low values of surface tension, and liquids with a highly polar nature (e.g., water) have large values of the surface tension. Solids have a surface free energy also, but because the atoms in the surface cannot rearrange spontaneously as in a liquid, its surface appears to be unaffected by any disturbance.

Contact Angle. When a liquid having a surface tension γ_{LV} is placed on a solid surface with surface tension γ_{SV}, the liquid will spontaneously form a droplet or spread out into a film (Fig. 2). If a droplet is formed, a relationship between the solid surface tension and the liquid surface tension can be derived, if the surface tensions are considered to be vectors acting at the edge of the drop. The surface free energy of the solid-liquid interface is labeled γ_{SL} and the equilibrium can be expressed as:

$$\gamma_{SV} = \gamma_{SL} + \gamma_{LV} \cos\theta$$

where θ is the angle formed by the drop surface with the solid surface, measured through the liquid. Various established physical-chemical methods are available for measuring the surface

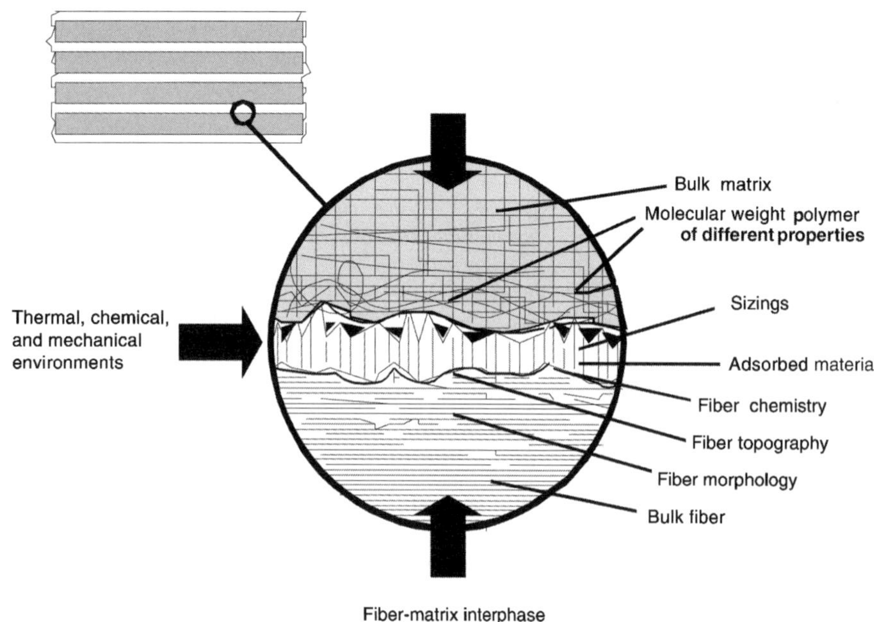

Fig. 1 Schematic diagram of the fiber-matrix interphase and some of the factors that contribute to its formation. Source: Ref 2

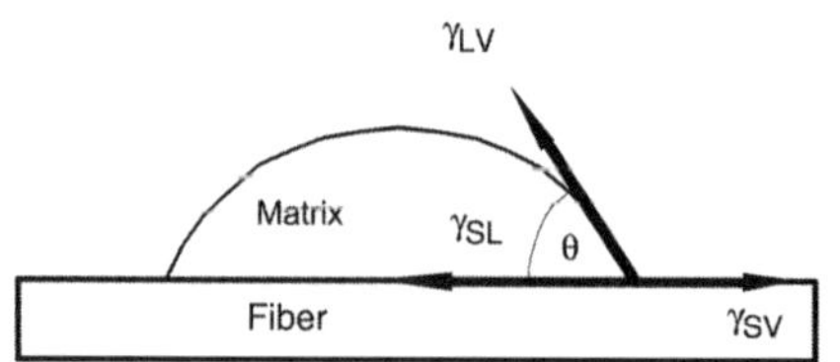

Fig. 2 Schematic diagram of the contact angle and its surface free energy (tension) components

tension of a liquid. Optical methods and gravimetric methods are available for measuring the angle that the droplet makes with the solid surface. Neither the solid surface tension nor the solid-liquid interfacial tension can be measured directly, but the difference between the two is the product of the cosine of the contact angle and the liquid surface tension.

Liquids that form contact angles greater than 90° are called "nonwetting." Liquids that form a contact angle less than 90° are termed "wetting." If the liquid does not form a droplet, that is, the contact angle is 0°, the liquid is said to be "spreading," and the relationship does not hold.

The equilibrium is expressed by an inequality where:

$$\gamma_{sv} - \gamma_{SL} \geq \gamma_{LV}$$

because as the liquid flows, it is decreasing the solid-vapor interface. Closer inspection of this relationship leads to the conclusion that for all cases of wetting and spreading, the surface tension of the wetting liquid must be greater than the solid surface tension.

Work of Adhesion. A term frequently used is "work of adhesion" (W_a), which gives an expression for the thermodynamic work necessary to create a solid-vapor surface and a liquid-vapor surface by:

$$W_a = \gamma_{LV} + \gamma_{SV} - \gamma_{SL}$$

pulling apart the solid-liquid interface. By substituting the equilibrium expression for the droplet forming the contact angle, the work of adhesion is given by:

$$W_a = \gamma_{LV}(1 + \cos\theta)$$

This expression is a thermodynamic work and as such, is a reversible equilibrium value. Likewise, it is not to be confused with the work of disrupting an adhesively bonded interface between reinforcing fiber and matrix that includes many substantial energy-absorbing and dissipative processes. This thermodynamic expression actually states that the maximum value of the work of adhesion occurs when the contact angle is equal to zero, and the work of adhesion is twice the surface tension of the liquid.

Solid Surface Energy. Although these expressions apply to equilibrium situations, they can be used to understand the wetting process in a polymer-reinforcement system as well. Zisman used these concepts to identify a critical solid surface tension for polymers. He noted that if the cosine of the contact angle were plotted against the contacting liquid surface tension, a straight line would result that intersected the 0° line at some value of the surface tension. By testing a variety of polymer surfaces, he found that there was a characteristic value for γ_O, which was an intrinsic characteristic of the solid. If a liquid had a surface tension greater than γ_O, the liquid would form a droplet on the surface, and if it was less, it would spread on the surface. This concept reinforced the rule that for spreading to occur, the surface tension of the liquid had to be less than that of the solid.

Kaelble (Ref 5) built upon some earlier work of Fowkes and proposed that the surface tension, or more properly, the surface free energy, of a liquid or a solid is composed of dispersion interactions and higher order ones, such as polar interactions. If liquids with known dispersion and polar components of their surface free energy were used as contacting fluids with solid surfaces, the polar and dispersive components of the solid could be determined. This resulted in an expression for the work of adhesion that was related to the contact angle and the liquid surface free energy, which could be measured directly through the following expression, where the surface tensions refer to the dispersive (D) and polar (P) components of the solid (SV) and liquid (LV) phases.

A plot of the left-hand side of this equation versus the ratio of the square roots of the polar-to-dispersive ratios of the contacting liquids results in a straight line whose slope and intercept determine the dispersive and polar component of the surface free energy of the solid:

$$\frac{\gamma_{LV}(1+\cos\theta)}{2\gamma_{LV}^{D^{1/2}}} = \gamma_{SV}^{D^{1/2}} + \gamma_{SV}^{P^{1/2}} \frac{\gamma_{LV}^{P^{1/2}}}{\gamma_{LV}^{D^{1/2}}}$$

Recently, an alternative to the polar-dispersive approach has been developed in which the surface free energy is divided into a dispersive component in a manner similar to the Kaelble formulation, but the polar component is replaced by acid and base components (Ref 6). This acid-base model has a more solid theoretical foundation and is gaining wider acceptance.

Wetting and Wicking. Although the discussions on wettability have focused on the thermodynamics between the fiber surface and the matrix, real composite systems are very large assemblies of small-diameter fibers. A key to creating good composite properties is infiltration of the matrix into this fiber assembly, or tow, during the processing steps. The small interstices in the tow can create very large capillary forces that aid in the wetting process. This capillary force is commonly characterized as a pressure drop, due to the surface tension acting in the small capillaries. A relation quantifying this driving force for infiltration is:

$$\Delta P = \Delta\rho g h = \frac{\gamma_{LV} - \cos\theta}{2r}$$

where the height of the rise, h, of a liquid of density, ρ, is directly related to the liquid surface tension, γ_{LV}, the cosine of the contact angle, θ, and inversely related to the radius, r, of the capillary, and where g is the gravitational constant. The contact angle controls the capillary forces, because at $\theta = 90°$, the capillary force vanishes, and at $\theta > 90°$, infiltration is prevented.

As stated earlier, the thermodynamic analysis of wetting and capillarity is true for equilibrium conditions. Thermoplastic polymer melts or thermoset polymer mixtures are high-viscosity fluids that may never reach true thermodynamic equilibrium during the processing of a composite. Yet the condition predicted by the analysis is valid. That is, the surface tension of the fiber must be greater than that of the matrix. A properly designed interphase should employ surface chemical treatments, finishes, and/or sizings to minimize the contact angle between matrix and reinforcement and to gain the most assistance from capillary forces during composite processing. This will ensure displacement of any moisture and assist the transport of voids from the composite during processing.

Surface Modification Strategies

Because wetting is a necessary prerequisite for optimal processing, thermodynamics tells us that the surface free energy of the matrix should be less than the surface free energy of the solid. Most polymers have low values of surface free energy (tension), that is, 20 to 45 mJ/m^2, which decrease slightly with increasing temperature. Solids, on the other hand, can have surface energies that vary over orders of magnitude if they are in the pristine state. Solid surfaces that have been exposed to the ambient environment want to minimize their surface free energy and, therefore, adsorb material or grow oxides to lower their surface free energy. In some cases, this "native" surface can have a surface free energy lower than that of the polymer matrix. In order to increase the solid surface free energy, surface treatments, finishes, and sizings have been developed to enhance the wettability of a solid surface.

Surface Treatments. The term "surface treatment" usually refers to a chemical treatment that imparts an altered surface chemistry to a material, primarily in the outermost layer, increases the surface energy, and/or creates beneficial microtopographical features without a deliberate coating of the surface. These treatments can be applied from the gas or liquid phase, be acidic or basic, or involve bombardment of the surface with radiation of various types. In most cases, effective surface treatments also remove surface material, that is, etch the surface to some degree. From a composite processing viewpoint, the use of a surface treatment is desirable to promote wettability and intimate contact between the fiber and the matrix.

Surface Finishes. The term "surface finish" is usually applied to describe coatings applied to reinforcement surfaces after or in conjunction with surface treatments. In many commercial examples for thermoset-matrix composites, finishes are the base resin component of the matrix applied from solvent solution or water emulsion to the reinforcement surface without any curing agent, to thicknesses of about 100 nm. The purpose is to protect the reinforcement surface during handling operations. Most reinforcements are very "flaw sensitive," and even the slightest contact with another hard surface can introduce critical-sized flaws that reduce strength. The 100 nm surface finish layer prevents actual contact between reinforcing entities. Finishes can be used with any reinforcement and have been developed primarily by the textile industry to aid in keeping fiber tows together during the textile steps that are sometimes required in composites manufacture. They find the widest use with carbon- and polymeric-reinforcing fibers. Another use for surface finishes is to protect the surface chemistry from environmental attack or contamination of the surface and consequent reduction in the surface free energy. Because the finish is an unpolymerized layer, exposure to the matrix or essentially the same composition during processing allows the finish to be solubilized and removed from the fiber surface.

From a processing viewpoint, finishes are very helpful in assisting and ensuring that the wetting and infiltration steps are complete. Well-designed surface finishes promote infiltration, disbursement, and wetting of individual reinforcements by their presence. Because the finishes are placed on the reinforcements from solution (both organic solvent and water-based), retention of solvent and volatilization during the early portion of the processing cycle is a potential problem. The high surface area of the fibers, their small size, and their large volume make the generation of voids a potential problem. If the composition of the finish is susceptible to chemical aging during long-term ambient storage, its solubility may be reduced to the point where it becomes confined to the fiber-matrix interface and is detrimental to both processing and adhesion.

Surface Sizings. In the composites industry, the term "sizing" has come to mean any surface coating applied to a reinforcement to protect it from damage during processing, aid in processing, or improve the mechanical properties of the composite. Surface sizings are similar physically to surface finishes, that is, they are applied to the fibers in thicknesses of approximately 0.1 μm, but differ in their chemical composition. They are almost always used with glass fibers and sometimes used with other reinforcements. Surface treatments are sometimes confused with sizings, especially in carbon-fiber reinforcement technology (Ref 7). The distinction between sizing and surface treatment is fairly clear in the case of carbon fibers, but is less clear in the case of boron fibers that are treated chemically to form a boron carbide or boron nitride coating (Ref 8). A useful definition is that a sizing is a deliberate coating of the reinforcement, which may incidentally react chemically with the surface; a surface treatment is a deliberate chemical modification of the reinforcement, which may incidentally result in the formation of a coating. Other terms used synonymously for sizing include finishing agent, which comes from the textile industry and refers to fiber coatings that render flexibility, drape, and special features, such as fire retardance, to fabrics. This term still finds use in fibrous composite nomenclature, especially for woven glass or carbon-fiber products. Sometimes sizing is referred to as a coupling agent when it is designed to enhance composite mechanical properties or durability.

Typical sizings solutions (Ref 9) contain a silane coupling agent or combinations of coupling agents, as well as other ingredients, such as film formers, antistatic agents, and lubricants. Sizings are applied to glass fibers from solution immediately at the point of glass manufacture. They are formulated to protect the glass-fiber surface from corrosive attack by water from the ambient environment. The silanes are hydrolyzed and react with glass-fiber surface hydroxyls to form very stable siloxane bonds. The remaining ingredients in the sizings systems are there to protect the glass surface from mechanical damage and to promote infiltration by the matrix. Titanate and zirconate chemistries are also used in addition to silane chemistries.

Sizings designed to protect the reinforcement during processing must coat the surface uniformly. For this reason, polymers that are widely used in the coating industry because of their good film-forming ability (Ref 10) are also used as sizing agents. Typical examples are starch and starch derivatives, the vinyl polymers, and the phenoxys. The choice is dictated by a number of considerations: compatibility with the matrix polymer, the level of protection required (for example, weaving is more severe on continuous fibers than prepregging of unidirectional tape), pliability or drape of the sized tow or cloth (for example, a stiff, "boardy" fabric is difficult to process), and cost. Sizings are usually applied at a level of 1.0 wt% or less, making it necessary to remove and dispose of large volumes of solvent. Environmental pollution and cost considerations mandate that the sizing be applied from aqueous media, which requires that it be soluble in water or able to be applied as a water-based emulsion.

Ideally, a sizing should be chemically compatible with the matrix polymer and should not adversely affect the mechanical properties of the interphase between reinforcement and matrix. If these requirements cannot be met, the sizing may be removed by washing or heating before processing the reinforcement into the final composite form. However, these manipulations usually either damage the fiber or leave residues that may prevent good bonding between reinforcement and matrix. Nevertheless these fugitive sizings are still used, especially for woven reinforcements.

There are a variety of film-forming polymers that are compatible with the more widely used polyester and epoxy-matrix resins. However, there are very few sizings that can be used with the newer high-temperature matrix polymers, such as the bismaleimides and polyimides, or with the tough thermoplastic matrices, such as polyphenylene sulfide or polyether etherketone. One approach to developing sizing for these newer matrix materials is to use the polymers themselves as the sizing. However, they usually do not have the wetting and spreading behavior necessary to form a uniform coating. Developing sizings for these new matrix polymers, especially for carbon-fiber-reinforced composites, is essential in order to realize their full potential.

Sizing systems are usually proprietary, and the manufacturer's recommendations must be followed, especially the storage conditions. Sizing systems are reactive, and the chemical reactions that can occur during long-term storage can make the sizing insoluble and/or lower in surface free energy, resulting in poor infiltration and wetting. Sizings are an essential factor in fibrous composites technology. They are critical in composites manufacturing and can have both negative and positive effects on composites properties. A sizing may adversely affect the mechanical properties of the composite. For example, a sizing that holds the filaments in a bundle so that the strand (tow) can be chopped for discontinuous fiber composites hinders later efforts to disperse the fibers during injection molding or extrusion.

As stated earlier, in commercial practice, the silanes are often applied with a film-forming polymer. Presumably, the coating polymer becomes entangled in the silane network along with the matrix polymer. The composition of this complex interphase is critical to understanding the moisture durability of composite materials. The possible interpenetration formation of silane and epoxy molecules is a subject of recent study (Ref 11).

Surface Modification Examples

Adhesion between fiber and matrix and its modification for composite structural applications must start with consideration of the stresses that the structural element will experience in its operational environment. In addition, the thermal and chemical (i.e, moisture) environments must be specified. This in turn dictates the fiber and matrix constituents to be used in the composite. The interphase will change depending on the matrix (e.g., thermoset or thermoplastic) as well as the reinforcing fiber (e.g., glass, carbon, or polymeric). Each constituent has different but related requirements for the interphase from both a processing and performance perspective.

Glass Fibers. For example, in glass fibers, the native fiber surface is mainly an inorganic oxide. This surface quickly adsorbs water that creates a hydroxylated surface. If exposure to moisture is continued, the adsorption of water corrodes the fiber surface, creating critical-sized flaws that reduce fiber strength. This corrosion process can vary in intensity, depending on the glass-fiber composition. In all cases, however, the glass surface must be protected from the chemical attack of water. Organofunctional silanes, titanates, and/or zirconates (Ref 12) are produced for this purpose and have been shown to be very effective in reducing or eliminating corrosive attack of the glass surface (Ref 6).

The silanes readily form three-dimensional polysiloxane networks through hydrolysis and condensation of the alkoxy groups. This polymerization is acid-base catalyzed, and the silanes are frequently applied from acid solution. It has been demonstrated experimentally (Ref 13) that these silanes form a polymeric network on solid substrates that, as in the case of glass, has an occasional chemical attachment to the surface. It has been suggested that this is a relatively open network that is easily penetrated by the molecules of the matrix polymer (Ref 14), so that an entanglement of the polymer networks is formed in the interphase region between matrix and reinforcement. This polymer network formation does not, in itself, explain how the silanes protect the boundary from attack by water. It does, however, present a more realistic picture of the adsorbed silane film. However, despite all the studies of silanes on glass (and other) surfaces, the mechanisms involved in their protection of the glass-polymer interface are not well understood.

Most commercial glass-fiber treatments are formulated sizes, which contain a silane or similar molecule, but are blended in a solution with a film-former, antistatic agent, lubricant, or other ingredients in a proprietary formulation. These sizes are applied to the fiber surface in thicknesses of about 0.1 μm. The formulation is empirically designed to be compatible with the matrix used with the glass fiber. In addition to providing corrosion protection to the fiber, the sizing surface treatments provide protection for the fiber surface during handling operations to prevent surface damage, ensure compatibility with the matrix, and aid in the infiltration of the matrix into the fiber tows during processing.

Carbon Fibers. Carbon fibers do not have a reactive surface in the same sense as glass fibers. The basal plane of graphite that forms the majority of the carbon-fiber surface is very stable and unreactive. However, the edges and corners of these planes and of the resulting crystallites are the sites at which chemical reactions can take place. The percentage of reactive edge area varies directly with the fiber modulus and the precursor polymeric fiber. For the intermediate-modulus fibers used in the largest number of applications, only 20% of the fiber surface contains surface chemical groups (mostly oxygen) that can be reacted with other molecules under most conditions (Ref 15). Attempts to increase the surface functional group content usually result in a loss of fiber strength, because the oxidation of carbon fibers invariably creates flaws that are greater than the critical size. Surface chemical treatments used to treat carbon-fiber surfaces also etch away the native fiber surface formed during the carbonization and graphitization of the fiber. This in itself creates a surface that can withstand much higher shear loadings and therefore, is largely responsible for the increase in adhesion seen with chemical surface treatments (Ref 16). Attempts at elucidating the amount of chemical reaction between fiber surface and matrix have shown that only a few percent of these groups react with the matrix (Ref 17). Surface "finishes" are commonly used with surface chemical treatments for carbon fibers. These finishes are much simpler than sizings for glass fibers. Finishes are usually a matrix component applied from solvent to the fiber surface to create a layer about 0.1 μm in thickness. Because the composition is the same as the matrix, wetting and impregnation of the fiber tow is enhanced, the carbon-fiber surface is protected from damage during handling, the fiber chemical reactivity is protected until processing, and the tow can be used with textile processing equipment with a minimum of difficulty (Ref 6).

Polymeric Fibers. Reinforcing fibers made from polymers have surfaces that are low in energy and require some surface treatment to enhance their wettability. The polymeric-fiber surface is, for the most part, unreactive, and the use of coupling agents is generally not effective. Finishes can be used, but are viewed as "processing aids" that enhance the impregnation and infiltration of the tow. Polymeric-fiber surfaces are not as sensitive to abrasion as the surfaces of glass or carbon fibers, and the use of a finish does not add to its protection. Likewise, corrosion is not an issue with polymers, and the absorption of moisture is generally small. The application of a finish could reduce moisture pickup, however. Chemical treatments, corona treatments, radio frequency discharge, microwave plasma, and so on are all used to alter the native polymeric-reinforcing-fiber surface. The resulting reported enhancement in adhesion is almost invariably due to removal of low-energy contaminants from the fiber surface coupled with the addition of surface chemical species that improve the wettability. Indeed, it has been shown that in the case of aramid fibers (and probably for all highly oriented polymeric-reinforcing fibers), the upper limit in fiber-matrix adhesion is related to the intrinsic interfibrillar strength of the fiber itself in its surface layer (Ref 18).

Fiber-Matrix Adhesion Measurements

The effectiveness of a fiber surface modification approach ultimately must be evaluated based on its relationship to fiber-matrix adhesion and the composite mechanical properties. There have been several techniques developed to measure fiber-matrix adhesion levels and the effect of the surface modification on the effective properties of composites. These methods can broadly be classified into three separate categories: direct methods, indirect methods, and composite lamina methods. The *direct* methods include the fiber pullout method, the single-fiber fragmentation method, the embedded fiber compression method, and the microindentation method. The *indirect* methods for fiber-matrix adhesion testing include the variable curvature method, the slice compression test, the ball compression test, dynamic mechanical analysis, and voltage contrast x-ray spectroscopy. The *composite* lamina methods include the 90° transverse flexural and tensile tests, three- and four-point shear, ±45° and edge delamination tests, the short beam shear test method, and the mode I and mode II fracture tests.

It should be pointed out that while the indirect methods provide a qualitative method of ranking the adhesion between fiber and matrix, and the composite lamina test methods actually measure fiber-matrix interface-sensitive composite properties, the direct methods not only provide a measure of fiber-matrix adhesion, but can also provide information about fiber-matrix failure mode and a method to measure the energy involved in fracture of the fiber-matrix interface. This last parameter is important in relating fiber-matrix adhesion to composite toughness.

Direct Methods. The direct methods of characterizing the fiber-matrix adhesion and the interphase have relied on the use of single-fiber-matrix test methods for measuring adhesion and failure modes. The first technique proposed was the fiber pullout method (Ref 19), which was developed in the early stages of composites research when the fibers were much larger and easier to handle than they are today. There have been variations in the experimental details pertaining to the fabrication of the test coupon and to the execution of this test, mainly in the matrix portion, but overall, the procedures to fabricate samples, the experimental protocols, and the data analysis remain the same. In the pullout version, the fiber is pulled out of the matrix, which can be a block of resin, a disc, or a droplet. The use of very small droplets reduces the difficulties in preparing thin discs of resin and can reduce the variability in exit geometry (Ref 20). These advantages have made this test very popular since the 1990s. In this test, the load and displacements are monitored continuously, and upon fiber pullout, the load registered at complete debonding of the fiber from the matrix is converted into interfacial shear strength. The advantage of this method is that it allows testing of brittle and/or opaque matrices.

Another popular method is the embedded single-fiber fragmentation test. Here, a single fiber is totally encapsulated in the polymeric matrix that has been formed into a tensile dogbone-shaped coupon, which in turn is loaded in tension. An interfacial shear stress transfer mechanism is relied upon to transfer tensile forces to the encapsulated fiber through the interphase from the polymeric matrix (Ref 21, 22). The fiber tensile strength, σ_f, is exceeded, and the fiber fractures inside the matrix tensile coupon. This process is repeated, producing shorter and shorter fragments until the remaining fragment lengths are no longer sufficient in size to produce further fracture through this stress transfer mechanism. A simple shear-lag analysis is applied to analyze the experimental data based on the length of the resulting fiber fragments, the fiber diameter, and the fiber tensile strength, in order to calculate the interfacial shear strength.

Another method proposed in the 1960s by Outwater and Murphy (Ref 23) uses a single fiber aligned axially in a rectangular prism of matrix. A small hole is drilled in the center of the specimen through the fiber. The prism is placed under a compressive load, and the propagation of an interfacial crack is followed with increasing load. The mode II fracture toughness of the interface can be calculated from this data based on the strain in the resin (ε_r), the tensile modulus of the fiber (E_f), the frictional shear stress (τ), the length of the interfacial crack (x), and the fiber diameter (a).

An in situ microindentation measurement technique has also been proposed for measuring the fiber interfacial shear strength (Ref 24). It involves the preparation of a polished cut surface of a composite in which the fibers are oriented perpendicular to the surface. A small hemispherical indenter is placed on an individual fiber, and the force and displacements are monitored to the point at which the fiber detaches from the matrix.

Indirect Methods. The indirect methods for fiber-matrix-adhesion-level measurement include the variable curvature method, the slice compression test, the ball compression test, the fiber-bundle pullout test, the use of dynamic-mechanical thermal analysis, and voltage contrast x-ray photoelectron spectroscopy (VCXPS).

Narkis et al. (Ref 25) proposed the use of a single-fiber specimen in which the fiber is embedded along the centerline in the neutral plane of a uniform cross-sectional beam. The beam is placed in nonuniform bending according to an elliptical bending geometry with the aid of a template. This causes the shear stress to build up from one end of the fiber according to the gradient of curvature of the specimen. Careful observation of the fiber in the specimen allows location of the point at which the fiber fails as a result of a maximum shear stress criterion. The stress along the fiber is calculated as a function of the matrix tensile modulus, the beam width, the first moment of transformed cross-sectional area, and constants from the equation of the ellipse. Some of the advantages of this technique are that a single fiber or fiber tow can be used, the results do not depend on fiber strength, and sample preparation is relatively easy. Some of the disadvantages are that the debond front is not so easy to detect, and the results are sensitive to the location of the single-fiber layer within the cross section of the coupon.

The slice compression test has been applied to polymer-matrix composites, even though it was developed to probe the interface in ceramic-matrix composites (Ref 26). A thin slice sample of unidirectional composite is produced with the cut surface perpendicular to the fiber axis. The surfaces are cut and polished to be parallel to each other and perpendicular to the fibers. The thin slice is loaded in compression in the fiber axis direction with two plates. One of the plates is made of a very hard material, such as silicon nitride, and the other of a soft material, for example, pure aluminum that can deform as the fibers are compressed into it. The thickness of the slice must be controlled to allow the fibers to debond without failing in compression as well as to allow them to slide inside through the matrix. The depth of the fiber indentation into the plate can be related to the interfacial shear strength (Ref 27).

Carman et al. (Ref 28) developed a test called the mesoindentation test that used a hard, spherical ball indenter to apply a compressive force to a surface of the composite perpendicular to the fiber axis. The indenter was much larger than the diameter of a single fiber; therefore, when the ball was forced into the end of the composite, it made a permanent depression in the material. From the size of the depression and the force-deflection curve, they calculated a mean hardness pressure as a function of strain in the coupon. Qualitative differences have been reported in tests conducted on carbon-fiber-epoxy composites where the fiber-matrix adhesion had been varied systematically.

The fiber bundle pullout method (Gopal et al., Ref 29) is similar to the single-fiber pullout method except that instead of using a single fiber, a bundle of fibers is used. A coupon is fabricated in which a bundle of fibers or a lamina of unidirectional fibers is cast in a block of matrix. Transverse notches are cut into the coupon near the end of the fiber bundle. The coupon is loaded in tension with the load applied parallel to the fiber axes. The load versus displacement curve can be monitored and the debonding point detected. In a similar manner to the way data are reduced for the single-fiber pullout test, the interfacial shear strength between the bundle of fibers and matrix can be calculated.

Ko et al. (Ref 30) examined a carbon-fiber-epoxy system in which the interfacial properties have been varied by the use of dynamic mechanical analysis. They report a change in the tan δ-peak attributable to changes in the fiber-matrix adhesion. Chua (Ref 31) also measured a shift in the loss factor for glass-polyester systems that corresponded to changes in the condition of the fiber-matrix interphase. Perret et al. (Ref 32) measured both the loss factor and the change in the shear modulus with increasing displacement and detected a change in composite properties with a change in the fiber-matrix adhesion. Yuhas et al. (Ref 33) have used ultrasonic wave attenuation to establish correlations with short beam shear data. This method was useful for poorly bonded systems, but was not sensitive to well-bonded interfaces. Wu used localized heating coupled with acoustic emission events to detect interfacial debonding (Ref 34).

Laser Raman spectroscopy can be applied to the fiber-matrix interface in order to determine the actual stresses that exist at the interface. Laser Raman spectroscopy is a visible light spectroscopy that relies on the inelastic scattering of visible light photons from a surface. Certain chemical groups in a material or on a surface can scatter incident radiation at characteristic frequencies. Tuinstra and Koening (Ref 35) showed that certain characteristic frequencies in the Raman active bands of graphite and other fibers are sensitive to the level of applied stress or strain. There is a measurable shift in the characteristic frequency that is proportional to the applied strain. A small (1 μm) spot generated by a laser beam can be scanned along a fiber surface and provide the Raman information, which can be converted to the local stresses in the fiber. A transparent matrix incorporating fibers having a Raman active band (e.g., aramid, high-modulus graphite) can be analyzed with this method (Ref 36).

A recent method for determining information about fiber-matrix adhesion is a technique identified as VCXPS (Ref 37). This method relies on the VCXPS characterization of the fracture surface of high volume fraction fiber composites. A unidirectional coupon is fractured in an opening mode to produce a fracture surface. This fracture surface containing fibers and polymer is placed inside of an x-ray photoelectron spectroscopy spectrometer for analysis. X-ray photons are directed at the surface, causing the emission of photoelectrons. These electrons are collected and analyzed for quantity and energy, which contains useful information about the atomic composition of the surface as well as the molecular environment of the atoms on the surface. During the process of photoelectron emission, nonconducting (insulating) samples will acquire a charge and cause peaks to shift from their neutral position. This happens in nonconductive materials such as polymers, but does not happen in conducting materials such as carbon fibers. As a result, the carbon peak begins to split into two peaks as charge builds up on the surface. One carbon peak, due to the conductive carbon fiber, stays at the neutral position while the other portion, due to the polymer, shifts, depending on the magnitude of the charge on the surface. The height and width of the peaks and the shift in energy are related to the content of the conducting carbon fiber and nonconductive polymer remaining on the fracture surface. As a result, the ratio of the two carbon peaks is a qualitative indicator of the degree of adhesion. For example, if the ratio of the nonconductive carbon peak to the conductive carbon peak is large, the fracture surface contains a large amount of nonconductive polymer and very little conductive carbon fiber. This can be interpreted as being due to good adhesion between the fibers in the matrix, causing failure to occur in the weaker polymer matrix between fibers. On the other hand, if the ratio of the nonconductive carbon peak to the conductive carbon peak is small, many bare carbon fibers are exposed on the fracture surface, indicating poor adhesion between the fiber and the matrix. In cases where the same carbon fibers are used with various polymeric matrices, a semiquantitative relationship between this parameter and fiber-matrix adhesion has been developed.

Composite Laminate Tests. Composite laminate tests are often used to measure fiber-matrix adhesion, but none of these tests measures interfacial properties alone. The obvious tests to be conducted are those in which the fiber-matrix interface dominates the results, such as shear properties. Numerous techniques have been developed for measuring shear properties in fiber-reinforced composite laminates. The most commonly used test methods for in-plane shear characterization are the $[\pm 45]_S$ tension test (Ref 38) and the Iosipescu test (Ref 39). To determine the interlaminar shear strength, the short beam shear test (Ref 40) is more frequently used. In all these cases, standard protocols exist for preparing the samples, conducting the tests, reporting the data, and analyzing the results. These include ASTM and Automotive Composites Consortium standards. A careful experimental study has been published relating differences in fiber-matrix adhesion to these tests (Ref 41).

Issues in the Use of Adhesion Test Methods. Overall, the use of any of the direct, indirect, or composite lamina tests in the hands of a skilled experimenter can provide a consistent way of ranking fiber-matrix adhesion regardless of the method chosen. However, one should be aware that there are various issues related to the use of these tests that limit their applicability. One issue is the identification of the appropriate parameter for characterizing the fiber-matrix interface. All of the direct and indirect tests have been developed with the goal of measuring the fiber-matrix interfacial shear strength. However, several of these tests are really fracture tests and are more properly used if the interfacial fracture energy is calculated. On the other hand, interfacial fracture energy is rarely used to evaluate or measure fiber-matrix adhesion or to design composite materials. Another factor that must be considered is the preparation of the samples. The single-fiber tests are very sensitive to the careful preparation of samples and the careful selection of fibers for testing within those samples. Testing conditions are likewise very important. While normally one would conduct any of these tests at reasonably slow strain rates, in microtesting, the strain rates used are only nominally slow. These strain rates become extraordinarily high when taking into account the small dimensions of the distances over which these tests are conducted. There is also evidence that in dealing with viscoelastic polymer composites, creep effects can be important and must be considered. Finally, the data analysis methods associated with these techniques rely on the assumption of a value for the modulus of the matrix near the fiber surface for reduction of the test results into a usable parameter, whether it is strength or energy. The literature contains numerous references indicating that the structure of the polymer near the fiber surface can be quite different from the bulk polymer. Indeed, the modulus in some cases can be quite a bit lower or higher than the bulk matrix, depending on the system investigated (Ref 42). At the present time, there is no accurate method for measuring the interface modulus that may exist in dimensions of a few tens to a few hundreds of nanometers from the fiber surface. Until such a quantitative measurement is available, it is not possible to accurately relate interfacial tests, whether single fiber or microscopic, to composite properties.

Interphase Processing

Implicit in the preceding discussion has been the assumption that the fiber-matrix interphase has attained its final equilibrium state. This may not always be true, however. The desire for reducing costs and increasing production speeds is leading to development of alternatives to conventional convective thermal processing methods (e.g., reaction injection molding, microwave processing, radio frequency processing, ultraviolet light processing, electron beam processing) and fast-reacting polymerization chemistries (e.g., urethane, vinyl ester, cationic, etc.), resulting in gelation or consolidation times of minutes or seconds. The fiber-matrix interphase may not reach an equilibrium state under these constraints, especially in systems that rely on the use of fiber finishes and sizings. Research in this area is underway and will eventually lead to time-dependent models for interphase formation, but in the interim, the role of processing must be considered in any fiber-matrix interfacial research or design.

Interphase Effects on Fiber-Matrix Adhesion

An optimal interphase must be designed with the materials, the process, and the final operational environment of the composite in mind. The choice of surface treatment, finish, or size will depend, to a large extent, on the reinforcing element in the composite as well as the polymeric matrix. Surface treatments should be selected to remove the native surface and leave behind one that is rich in surface functionality to promote thermodynamic wetting. The concept of chemical bonding at the interphase should not be used exclusively in selecting a surface treatment.

The application of surface finishes should be considered for all brittle reinforcements as both a protector of the mechanical strength of the reinforcement as well as an aid in enhancing the infiltration and wetting of the reinforcement during the composite processing steps. The surface free energy and solubility of the finish in the matrix should be considered to ensure optimal processability. The choice of an organic solvent or water-based carrier for the deposition of the finish will be determined by the processing conditions. Water requires temperatures in excess of 100 °C (210 °F) for complete removal. This must be accomplished at the low-viscosity stage to allow for water migration out of the composite. Organic solvents offer a wide range of processing temperatures, but may be an environmental concern.

The use of a sizing system incorporating silanes (or titanates or zirconates) is a requirement for glass-fiber systems to ensure that the glass-fiber surface is protected from corrosion. At the same time, the silane functionality must be chosen to ensure chemical compatibility with the matrix.

For the treated, finished, or sized systems, close attention must be paid to the level of adhesion generated as well as the interfacial failure mode at the point of fiber fracture. The operational environment of the composite will dictate the level of adhesion and the desirable failure mode. In most cases, an optimum in interfacial properties will be desired.

If the interphase is considered to have some finite size, it plays a role in the mechanical performance of the composite. At a minimal level, the interphase structure is responsible for the level of adhesion that ensures continuity in the transfer of forces from fiber to matrix, allowing the composite to function as one mechanical entity. The interphase also acts as a failure site when a fiber fails. Either interfacial or matrix failure can result. It is tempting to extrapolate that high levels of adhesion are the most desirable condition for the composite, and that a high degree of chemical bonding is the best way to achieve this condition. This is not the case, and there is a practical limit to the adhesion level that can be produced in any fiber-matrix system.

If a stress analysis is conducted on a single isolated fiber in the matrix, an expression for the local shear stress similar to one attributable to Cox (Ref 43) can be derived. Closer inspection of the terms shows that there are fiber-dependent terms, geometric terms related to the fiber geometry and position, and matrix-dependent terms. If the interphase is considered to exist as a component of the composite near the fiber surface, its mechanical properties limit the degree of adhesion. In a study (Ref 44) where single-fiber methods were used to measure fiber-matrix adhesion, a dependence on the interphase shear modulus was found in composites fabricated from identical fibers and with identical matrix chemistries in which the distance between cross links was systematically varied and therefore produced matrices with identical chemistries but with different mechanical properties. Figure 3 shows that the adhesion varied as the product of the square root of the matrix shear modulus. This indicates that when fiber surface treatments affect the resulting structure of the polymer in the interphase, when the surface finishes produce an interphase different in modulus from the bulk, or when the surface sizings create an interphase with a modulus different from the bulk matrix, it is the interphase properties and not the bulk properties that determine the level of adhesion. In a similar manner, the fracture properties of the composite are controlled by the interphase structure and properties.

Interphase and Fiber-Matrix Adhesion Effects on Composite Mechanical Properties

There are numerous examples of published studies in which correlations between the interphase, fiber-matrix adhesion, and composite mechanical properties for different combinations of reinforcing fiber and matrix and fiber-matrix adhesion have been made. The carbon-fiber-epoxy systems have been studied extensively. As an example, results from one recently published study is used for illustration purposes here (Ref 45).

Consider a carbon-fiber-epoxy system consisting of one carbon fiber with three different surface treatments combined with a low-temperature, amine-cured epoxy. Unidirectional composite prepregs were fabricated at 67% fiber volume fraction from one type of carbon fiber whose surface has been modified in three different ways to produce three distinct levels of adhesion and two different failure modes. The mechanical characterization tests were conducted according to ASTM protocols.

The "A"- type carbon fibers used in this study are produced by high-temperature inert gas graphitization of polyacrylonitrile fiber. The AU-4 fibers are "as-received," that is, removed from the heat treatment ovens without any further surface treatment. The AS-4 fibers are surface treated with an electrochemical oxidation step that optimizes the adhesion to epoxy matrices, and the AS-4C fibers are coated with a 100 to 200 nm layer of epoxy applied from an organic solvent directly onto the surface-treated AS-4 fibers. The surface chemical and topographical features of these reinforcing fibers have been characterized using a variety of techniques (Ref 46–48). The adhesion of these carbon fibers to the epoxy matrix has been quantified through single-fiber fragmentation tests. The results are shown in Fig. 4.

The adhesion has changed significantly with surface treatment. Compared to the untreated AU-4 fiber, the surface treatment (AS-4) has increased the interfacial shear strength 100%. Application of the fiber sizing (AS-4C) has produced another 25% increase. It is important to note that along with the increase in adhesion is a change in failure mode. Failure of the "as-received" AU-4 interface is through the outer layer of the carbon fiber, while pure interfacial failure takes place in the AS-4 as a result of the surface treatment, indicating that the fiber surface treatment not only adds reactive chemical groups, but also removes the initial defect-laden surface and leaves behind a structurally sound surface that is capable of sustaining high mechanical loads without failure. Both factors are responsible for the improvement in adhesion. The surface-treated carbon fibers are coated with 100 nm of an epoxy resin without any curing agent (AS-4C). The mechanism by which this surface finish increases the level of fiber-matrix adhesion is that the finish layer interacts with the bulk matrix and causes a local change in properties in the fiber-matrix interphase. The modulus of the in situ epoxy-rich finish layer has been shown to increase over that of the bulk matrix, but the material also becomes more brittle. This can readily be seen in a comparison of the composite fracture surfaces of the A-4/epoxy composites where only the adhesion and interphase have been altered, as shown in Fig. 5. Notice the fractured, brittle-appearing surface on the AS-4C samples that have the stiff and brittle fiber sizing.

The results obtained for on-axis properties, off-axis properties, and interlaminar fracture toughness present compelling evidence for the effect of the interphase on fiber-matrix adhesion and composite mechanical properties. The on-axis properties (such as longitudinal tensile, compressive, and flexural properties) are dominated by fiber properties, whereas the off-axis properties (such as transverse tensile and flexural, in-plane and interlaminar shear) and interlaminar fracture toughness are dominated by matrix and interfacial properties. The sensitivity of composite properties to fiber-matrix adhesion will be governed by how matrix and fibers are connected and how the applied load is transferred and distributed in composite. For example, in the case of longitudinal tension, the matrix and fibers are connected through fiber-matrix interface in parallel, and most of the applied load is borne by fibers. Therefore, as far as the mechanism of load distribution is concerned, the fiber-matrix adhesion should not be expected to play a dominant role in the longitudinal tensile behavior as long as there is some level of adhesion. If fiber-matrix adhesion is very low, stress transfer at points of fiber fracture will be inadequate, causing the growth of flaws which reduce strength. Changes in the failure modes resulting from the change in fiber-matrix adhesion may have an effect on the longitudinal tensile strength. On the other hand, in the case of transverse tension, the matrix and fibers are connected through the fiber-matrix interface in series, and all the three components, that is, fiber, matrix, and interface/interphase, carry equal load. In such a case, the fiber-matrix adhesion should be expected to have a dominant effect on the composite properties.

Composite On-Axis Properties. Figure 6 compares the longitudinal compressive and longitudinal tensile strength properties of the three composite systems. The longitudinal tensile and compressive moduli are insensitive to fiber-matrix adhesion, because in on-axis specimens, fiber and matrix are connected through the interface in parallel. The applied load is carried by the longitudinal fibers. The role of interface (and matrix) is limited to transferring stress from highly stressed fibers to the neighboring fibers carrying relatively low stress, so as to result in a uniform stress distribution in the composite.

The average longitudinal tensile strengths (σ_{11}^{f}) of the three composite materials increase with increasing fiber-matrix adhesion for the low (AU-4) and intermediate (AS-4) values. However, when the fiber-matrix adhesion is increased to the highest level (AS-4C), the strength does not increase. Analysis of the failure modes of the tensile coupons indicates that tensile strength increases with increasing interfacial shear strength only as long as the failure is primarily interfacial. However, if the interfacial strength is too weak, the composite fails prematurely, because of cumulative weakening of the material. On the other hand, when interfacial bond strength is very large, the failure mode changes from interfacial to matrix, and the composite behaves like a brittle material, that is, it becomes "notch-sensitive." Thus, excessive fiber-matrix bond strength may

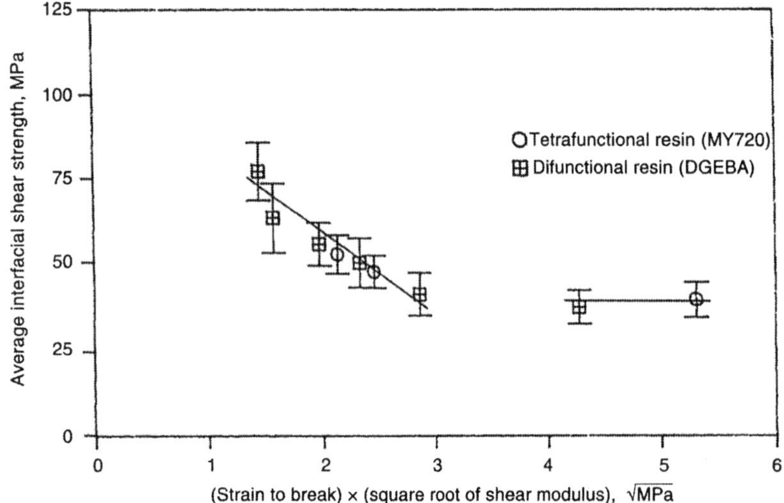

Fig. 3 Fiber-matrix adhesion dependence on interphase and matrix properties. Source: Ref 44

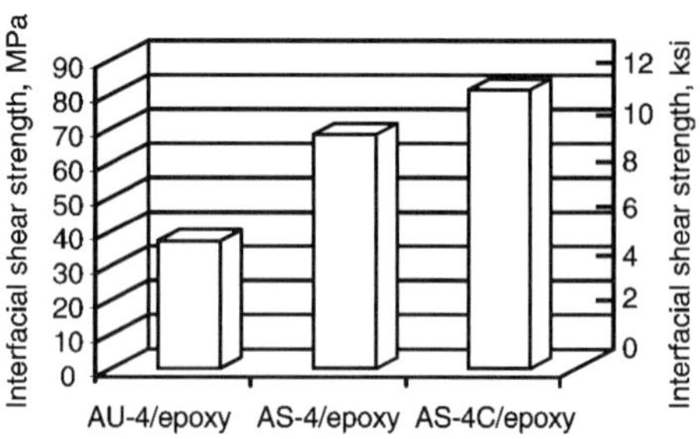

Fig. 4 The adhesion of the A-4 carbon fibers to the epoxy matrix, as quantified through single-fiber fragmentation tests. The fiber-matrix adhesion increases in the order AU-4 > AS-4 > AS-4C. AU-4 has the lowest level of adhesion and fails by a frictional debonding mode; AS-4 has an intermediate level of adhesion and fails by an interfacial crack growth mode; AS-4C has the highest level of adhesion and fails by a matrix-cracking mode perpendicular to the fiber axis. Source: Ref 45

have a detrimental effect on the longitudinal tensile strength of the composite.

There is an increasing trend toward greater composite compressive strength, with increasing fiber-matrix adhesion as well. The increase in the compressive strength corresponding to the increase in the fiber-matrix adhesion from the low (AU-4) to the intermediate (AS-4) value and then the subsequent more rapid increase in the strength at the highest (AS-4C) value suggests that both the improved shear strength between fiber and matrix coupled with the presence of the high-modulus, brittle interphase around the graphite fibers contribute to the greater compressive strength of these composites. The fibers surrounded by matrix material in unidirectional composites subjected to compressive load are like beam columns that are laterally supported on an elastic foundation. The integrity of fiber-matrix interface will determine the effectiveness of the surrounding elastic foundation, which will, in turn, affect the compressive properties of a unidirectional composite. In the composites having the poorest value of fiber-matrix adhesion, the fibers in the delaminated regions are easily separated from the matrix, resulting in global delamination buckling under in-plane compressive loading. In the composites with the intermediate values of fiber-matrix adhesion, delamination is contained only near the specimen edges. Local interfacial failure, however, does take place, and in such a case, the fiber columns may locally behave like beam columns, resting in matrix tunnels. With increasing applied load, local microbuckling may start in this fiber column and propagate in the adjacent fiber columns, resulting in final failure of the specimen. In the AS-4C/epoxy composites where the interlaminar shear strength (ISS) is the highest, the delamination, interfacial failure, and transverse tensile failure due to Poisson's effect are prevented by the strong fiber-matrix adhesion. In addition, the high-modulus, strong interphase around carbon fibers in AS-4C/epoxy composites provides strong lateral support to the graphite-fiber columns. Thus, the fibers can be compressively loaded to their maximum capacity.

Composite Off-Axis Properties. A comparison between transverse flexural, tensile, and short beam shear strength is shown in Fig. 7. There is a significant difference between transverse flexural and transverse tensile strengths. Not only is the transverse flexural strength more sensitive to changes in fiber-matrix adhesion, it is much higher than the transverse tensile strength. The higher values and higher sensitivity of the transverse flexural strength compared to the transverse tensile strength can be explained by the nonuniformity of stress in the three-point flexure test.

In the case of short beam shear strength, increasing composite shear strength is measured with the intermediate level of adhesion, but levels off or slightly decreases for the composite with the highest level of adhesion. This is also explained earlier by the different failure mode produced by the samples with the highest level of adhesion. The short beam shear specimens fail prematurely under matrix-failure-dominated conditions encountered with the AS-4C specimen.

Composite Fracture Properties. A comparison between the mode I and mode II interlaminar fracture toughness (G_{Ic} and G_{IIc}) for the three material systems is shown in Fig. 8. The dominant micromechanical event responsible for the increased mode I fracture toughness of AS-4C/epoxy compared to that of the AS-4/epoxy is increased matrix deformation resulting from the improved fiber-matrix adhesion. Although the AS-4C fibers are surrounded by the low fracture toughness interphase, the gain in the composite fracture toughness from the improved adhesion is larger than the loss resulting from the brittle interphase. Thus, even in the composite system having highly cross-linked, brittle epoxy system, the interfacial strength must be increased to a sufficiently high level in order to maximize the composite interlaminar fracture toughness.

This observation suggests that resin fracture toughness is fully transferred to the composite. In addition, there are several other toughening mechanisms that are present in composite but are absent in the bulk resin specimen. For example, in a composite, if the interfacial shear strength is stronger than the matrix strength, the crack

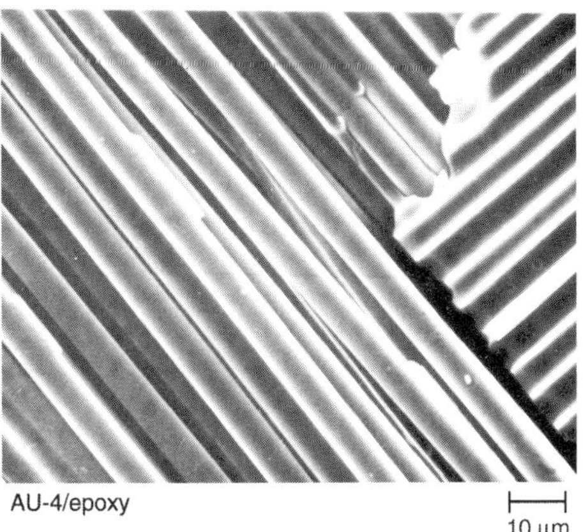

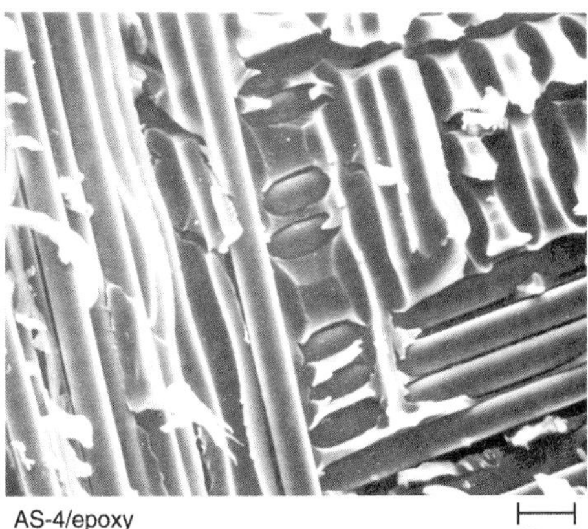

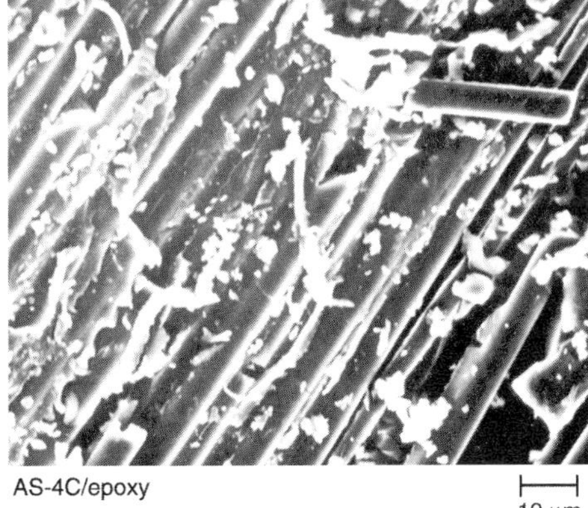

Fig. 5 Fracture surface of A-4/epoxy $[\pm45]_{3S}$ composites, illustrating the different nature of the failure mode and interphase properties. The fiber-matrix adhesion decreases in the order AS-4C > AS-4 > AU-4. AU-4 and AS-4 exhibit interfacial failure modes; AS-4C fails in a matrix-dominated mode. The presence of the fiber sizing on the AS-4C fiber has created a brittle interphase. Source: Ref 45

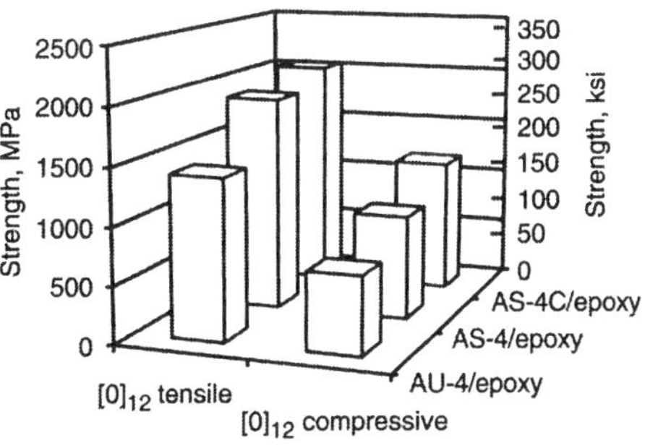

Fig. 6 Comparison between the tensile and compressive properties of the three types of $[0]_{12}$ A-4 carbon-fiber-epoxy composites. The modulus values are similar in both the loading modes. The compression test yields much smaller strength than tensile strength. Also, the compressive strength is more sensitive than the tensile strength to fiber-matrix adhesion. The fiber-matrix adhesion decreases in the order AS-4C > AS-4 > AU-4. AU-4 and AS-4 exhibit interfacial failure modes; AS-4C fails in a matrix-dominated mode. Source: Ref 45

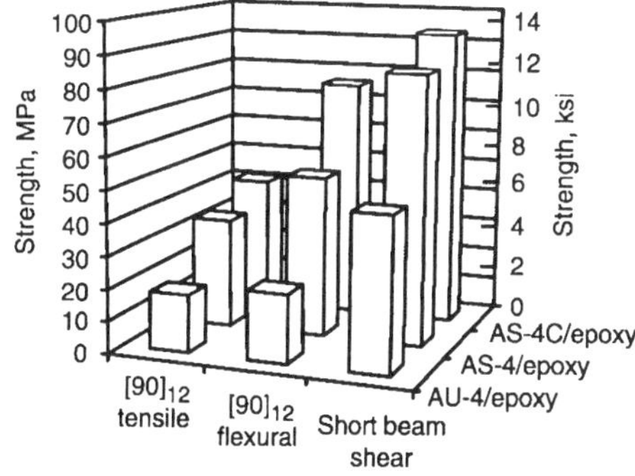

Fig. 7 Comparison between the transverse tensile and flexural properties for $[90]_{12}$ and the short beam shear strength of A-4 carbon-fiber-epoxy composites. The flexural strength is much higher than the tensile strength. The interlaminar shear strength and transverse tensile and flexural strengths all show the same trends. The fiber-matrix adhesion decreases in the order AS-4C > AS-4 > AU-4. AU-4 and AS-4 exhibit interfacial failure modes; AS-4C fails in a matrix-dominated mode. Source: Ref 45

will prefer to go through the weaker resin rather than breaking the stronger fibers. However, because of intermingling of fibers (resulting from high consolidation pressures during processing) and very small thickness between the plies (of the order of one fiber diameter), there is no plane containing only resin. In such a situation, the crack must always go around fibers, creating a much larger fracture surface area. Moreover, the resistance to crack growth will be increased by the misaligned fibers that may lie in the path of the advancing crack. All these mechanisms contribute to the composite fracture toughness. It has been suggested that the contribution of each of these toughening mechanisms to the composite fracture toughness will be highest for an optimal thickness of the resin-rich region (Ref 49).

In correlating the effect of fiber-matrix adhesion on G_{IIc} and the observed failure modes, it is shown that by improving the adhesion, the primary failure mode changes from interfacial failure to the matrix failure. The work required to cause matrix fracture is significantly larger than that to cause the failure of the interface having low ISS. When the fiber-matrix adhesion is strong, several energy-absorbing phenomena, such as matrix deformation, matrix cracking, fiber pullout, interfacial failure, and so on, take place. As a result, the G_{IIc} of the composites shows significant improvement when fiber-matrix adhesion is increased. At a certain level when the interfacial strength approaches the matrix strength, the additional increase in the ISS may not yield much improvement in the fracture toughness of the composite. The similarities in the fracture surface morphologies of the AS-4/epoxy and AS-4C/epoxy suggest that almost the full potential of the interface has already been realized in the AS-4/epoxy composites. Therefore, the percentage increase in the G_{IIc} corresponding to the increase in the ISS from the medium to the highest levels is much smaller than that corresponding to the increase in the ISS from the low to the medium levels. The brittle matrix failure that was believed to be due to the presence of the brittle interphase around the AS-4C fibers also may have canceled part of the gain in the G_{IIc} resulting from the increase in fiber-matrix adhesion.

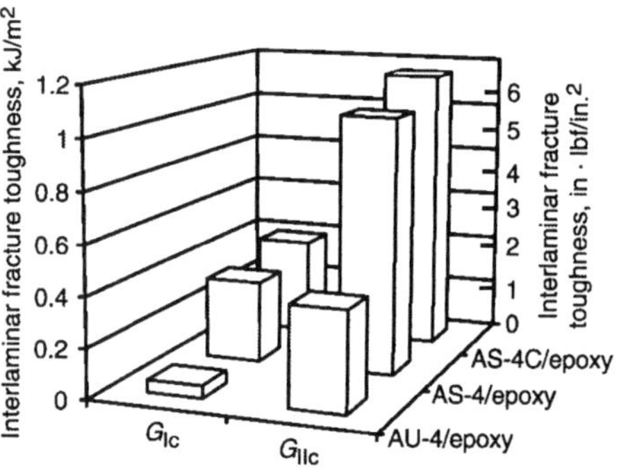

Fig. 8 Comparison between the mode I and mode II fracture toughness of the three composite materials. The mode II fracture toughness is about three times higher than the mode I fracture toughness. The fiber-matrix adhesion decreases in the order AS-4C > AS-4 > AU-4. AU-4 and AS-4 exhibit interfacial failure modes; AS-4C fails in a matrix-dominated mode. Source: Ref 45

Comparison between results from the single-fiber and composite tests indicates that two key parameters must be obtained from single-fiber tests in order to explain composite property data. They are the level of adhesion and the failure mode, that is, interfacial or matrix. Fiber-matrix adhesion and the "interphase" affect composite properties in different ways, depending on the state of stress and failure mode created at the fiber-matrix interphase.

Conclusions

The fiber-matrix interphase structure exists and can be the major factor in controlling fiber-matrix adhesion and can strongly influence the resulting composite properties. Although many studies have been conducted with the goal of deriving structure-property relationships for fiber-matrix interphases in composite systems, little analytical success has been achieved. As our understanding of the chemistry, physical properties, and morphology of the interphase increases, predictive relationships between the interphase, fiber-matrix adhesion, and composite mechanical properties can be expected to develop. In the future, microengineering of the fiber-matrix interphase will be used to optimize the properties and performance of composites materials.

REFERENCES

1. R. Yosomiya, Y. Morimoto, A. Nakajima, Y. Ikada and T. Suzuki, *Adhesion and Bonding in Composites,* Marcel Dekker, Inc., New York, 1990
2. L.T. Drzal, *Advances in Polymer Science II*, Vol 75 K. Dusek, Ed., Springer-Verlag, 1985
3. W.D. Bascom and L.T. Drzal, "The Surface Properties of Carbon Fibers and Their Adhesion to Organic Polymers," NASA Technical Report 4084, July 1987
4. A.W. Adamson, *Physical Chemistry of Surfaces*, 5th ed., Wiley Interscience, 1990
5. D.H. Kaelble, *Physical Chemistry of Adhesion*, Wiley Interscience, 1971
6. E.A. Plueddemann, *Silane Coupling Agents*, Plenum Press, New York, 1982
7. J.B. Donnet and R.C. Bansal, *Carbon Fibers*, Marcel Dekker, 1985
8. M. Basche, "Interfacial Stability of Silicon Carbide Coated Boron Filament Reinforced Metals," *Interfaces in Composites*, STP 452, American Society for Testing Materials, 1968, p 130
9. E.P. Plueddeman, Interfaces in Polymer Matrix Composites, *Composite Materials*, Vol 6, L.J. Broutman and R.H. Krock, Ed., Academic Press, 1975
10. R.R. Meyers and J.S. Long, Ed., *Film Forming Compositions, Parts I and II*, Marcel Dekker, 1968
11. K. Hoh, H. Ishida, and J.L. Koenig, The Diffusion of Epoxy Resin into a Silane Coupling Agent Interphase, *Composite Interfaces*, H. Ishida and J.L. Koenig, Ed., Elsevier, 1986, p 251
12. S.J. Monte, G. Sugarman, and D.J. Seeman, "Titanate Coupling Agents—Current Applications," paper presented at Rubber Division Meeting, May 1977, American Chemical Society, p 40
13. W.D. Bascom, Structure of Silane Adhesion Promoter Films on Glass and Metal Surfaces, *Macromolecules*, Vol 5, 1972, p 792
14. H. Ishida and Y. Suzuki, Hydrolysis and Condensation of Aminosilane Coupling Agents in High Concentration Aqueous Solutions: A Simulation of Silane Interphase, *Composite Interfaces*, H. Ishida and J.L. Koenig, Ed., North-Holland, 1986
15. G. Hammer and L.T. Drzal, *Appl. Surf. Sci.*, Vol 4, 1980, p 340–355
16. L.T. Drzal, M. Rich, and P. Lloyd, *J. Adhes.*, Vol 16, 1983, p 1–30
17. K.J. Hook, R.K. Agrawal, and L.T. Drzal, *J. Adhes.*, Vol 32,1990, p 157–170
18. J. Kalantar and L.T. Drzal, *J. Mater. Sci.*, Vol 25, 1990, p 4194–4202
19. L.J. Broutman, "Measurement of the Fiber-Polymer Matrix Interfacial Strength," *Interfaces in Composites*, STP 452, American Society for Testing and Materials, 1969, p 27–41
20. B. Miller, P. Muri, and L. Rebenfeld, A Microbond Method for Detremination of the Shear Strength of a Fiber/Resin Interface, *Compos. Sci. Technol.*, Vol 28, 1987, p 17–32
21. A. Kelly and W.R. Tyson, Tensile Properties of Fiber-Reinforced Metals: Copper/Tungsten and Copper/Molybdenum, *J. Mech. Phys. Solids*, Vol 13, 1965, p 329–350
22. L.T. Drzal, M.J. Rich, J.D. Camping, and W.J. Park, "Interfacial Shear Strength and Failure Mechanisms in Graphite Fiber Composites," Paper 30-C, 35th Annual Technical Conf., Reinforced Plastics/Composites Institute, The Society of the Plastics Industry, 1980
23. J.O. Outwater and M.C. Murphy, The Influences of Environment and Glass Finishes on the Fracture Energy of Glass-Epoxy Joints, Paper 16-D, *Proc. 24th Annual Technical Conf.*, The Society of the Plastics Industry, 1969
24. J.F. Mandell, J.-H Chen, and F.J. McGarry, "A Microdebonding Test for In-Situ Fiber-Matrix Bond and Moisture Effects," Research Report R80-1, Department of Materials Science and Engineering, Massachusetts Institute of Technology, Feb 1980
25. M. Narkis, E.J.H. Chen, and R.B. Pipes, Review of Methods for Characterization of Interfacial Fiber-Matrix Interactions, *Polym. Compos.*, Vol 9(No.4), Aug 1988, p 245–251

26. D.G. Brandon and E.R. Fuller, Jr., *Ceram. Eng. Soc. Proc.*, Vol 10, 1989, p 871
27. N. Shafry, D.G. Brandon, and M. Terasaki, *Euro-Ceramics*, Vol 3, 1989, p 453–457
28. G.P. Carman, J.J. Lesko, K.L. Reifsnider and D.J. Dillard, *J. Comp. Mater.*, Vol 27, 1993, p 303–329
29. P. Gopal, L.R. Dharani, N. Subramanian, and F.D. Blum, *J. Mater. Sci.*, Vol. 29, 1994, p 1185–1190
30. Y.S. Ko, W.C. Forsman, and T.S. Dziemianowicz, Carbon Fiber-Reinforced Composites: Effect of Fiber Surface on Polymer Properties, *Polym. Eng. Sci.*, Vol 22, Sept 1982, p 805–814
31. P.S. Chua, Characterization of the Interfacial Adhesion Using Tan Delta, *SAMPE Q.*, Vol 18 (No. 3), April 1987, p 10–15
32. P. Perret, J.F. Gerard, and B. Chabert, A New Method to Study the Fiber-Matrix Interface in Unidirectional Composites: Application for Carbon Fiber-Epoxy Composites, *Polym. Test.*, Vol 7, 1987, p 405–418
33. D.E. Yuhas, B.P. Dolgin, C.L. Vorres, H. Nguyen, and A. Schriver, Ultrasonic Methods for Characterization of Interfacial Adhesion in Spectra Composites, *Interfaces in Polymer, Ceramic and Metal Matrix Composites*, H. Ishida, Ed., Elsevier, 1988, p 595–609
34. W.L. Wu, "Thermal Technique for Determining the Interface and/or Interply Strength in Polymeric Composites," National Institute of Standards and Technology, Polymers Division Preprint, 1989
35. T. Tuinstra and J.L. Koening, *J. Compos. Mater.*, Vol 4, 1970, p 492–400
36. J.-K. Kim and Y.-W Mai, *Engineered Interfaces in Fiber Reinforced Composites*, Elsevier Science Ltd., London, 1998, p 21–24
37. J.D. Miller, W.C. Harris, and G.W. Zajac, *Surf. Interface Anal.*, Vol 20, 1993, p 977–983
38. P.H. Petit, "A Simplified Method of Determining the In-plane Shear Stress-Strain Response of Unidirectional Composites," STP 460, American Society for Testing and Materials, 1969, p 63
39. D.E. Walrath and D.F. Adams, Analysis of the Stress State in an Iosipescu Shear Test Specimen, Department Report UWME-DR-301-102-1, Composite Materials Research Group, Department of Mechanical Engineering, University of Wyoming, Laramie, June 1983
40. J.M. Whitney, I.M. Daniel, and R.B. Pipes, "Experimental Mechnaics of Fiber Reinforced Composite Materials," Monograph 4, Society for Experimental Stress Analysis, 1982
41. L.T. Drzal and M.S. Madhukar, *J. Mater. Sci.*, Vol 28, 1993, p 569–610
42. X. Dirand, E. Hilaire, E. Lafontaine, B. Mortaigne, and M. Nardin, *Composites*, Vol 25, 1994, p 645–652
43. H.L. Cox, Br. *J. Appl. Phys.*, Vol 3, 1952, p 122
44. V. Rao and L.T. Drzal, *Polym. Compos.*, Vol 12, 1991, p 48–58
45. L.T. Drzal and M. Madhukar, Fiber-Matrix Adhesion and Its Relationship to Composite Mechanical Properties, *J. Mater. Sci.*, Vol 28, 1993, p 569–610
46. L.T. Drzal and M.J. Rich, "Effect of Graphite Fiber-Epoxy Adhesion on Composite Fracture Behavior," *Research Advances in Composites in the United States and Japan*, ASTM STP 864, ASTM, 1985, p 16–26
47. L.T. Drzal, Composite Interphase Characterization, *SAMPE J.*, Vol 19, 1983, p 7–13
48. L.T. Drzal, M.J. Rich, M.F. Koenig, and P.F. Lloyd, Adhesion of Graphite Fibers to Epoxy Matrices II. The Effect of Fiber Finish, *J. Adhes.*, Vol 16, 1983, p 133–152
49. W.L. Bradley and R.N. Cohen, "Matrix Deformation and Fracture in Graphite-Reinforced Epoxies," *Delamination and Debonding of Materials*, ASTM STP 876, W.S. Johnson, Ed., ASTM, 1985, p 389–410

SELECTED REFERENCES

- W.J. Feast and H.S. Munro, *Polymer Surfaces and Interfaces*, John Wiley, 1987
- Y.A. Gorbatkina, *Adhesive Strength of Fibre-Polymer Systems*, Ellis Horwood Ltd., London, 1992
- R.A.L. Jones and R.W. Richards, *Polymers at Surfaces and Interfaces*, Cambridge University Press, 1999
- J.-K. Kim and Y.-W. Mai, *Engineered Interfaces in Fiber Reinforced Composites*, Elsevier Science Ltd., London, 1998
- A.J. Kinloch, *Adhesion and Adhesives, Science and Technology*, Chapman and Hall, 1987
- Y.S. Lipatov, *Polymer Reinforcement*, ChemTec Publishing, Toronto, 1995
- J.V. Milewski and H.S. Katz, *Handbook of Reinforcements for Plastics*, Van Nostrand Reinhold, 1987
- P.S. Theocaris, *The Mesophase Concept in Composites*, Springer-Verlag, New York, 1987
- R. Wool, *Polymer Interfaces, Structure and Strength*, Hanser Gardner, Cincinnati, 1995
- S. Wu, *Polymer Interface and Adhesion*, Marcel Dekker, New York, 1982
- R. Yosomiya, K. Morimoto, A. Nakajima, U. Ikada, and T. Suzuki, *Adhesion and Bonding in Composites*, Marcel Dekker, 1990

Lightweight Structural Cores

Jim Kindinger, Hexcel Composites

LIGHTWEIGHT STRUCTURAL CORES were first used on aircraft in the 1940s to reduce weight and increase payload and flight distance. They were incorporated into the aircraft design to replace the heavier conventional sheet and stringer or beam support approach, and their incorporation into sandwich panels has been a basic structural concept in the aerospace industry since the 1950s. In 2000, virtually every commercial and military aircraft depends on the integrity and reliability offered by lightweight structural cores. Current lightweight structural cores are classified into three primary types: honeycomb, balsa, and foam. There are numerous substrate materials within the honeycomb and foam categories. Lightweight structural cores can have a density as small as 16 kg/m^3 (1 lb/ft^3).

Honeycomb

Four primary manufacturing methods are used to produce honeycomb:

- Adhesive bonding and expansion
- Corrugation and adhesive bonding
- Corrugation and braze welding
- Extrusion

The most common manufacturing method for honeycomb is adhesive bonding and expansion. Honeycomb substrates are bonded using heat-curable epoxy-based adhesives. Corrugation is a slower method and typically is used to manufacture higher-density honeycombs, which are either adhesive bonded or braze welded. Adhesive bonding is less expensive than braze welding. Braze welding is used only with steel and specialty metal honeycomb materials, which are usually used in high-temperature applications. The extrusion process is used with ceramic honeycomb and a few thermoplastic honeycombs.

Honeycomb Cell Technology. The honeycomb industry has its own terminology to define the various aspects of honeycomb core (Fig. 1). The bonded portion of a honeycomb cell is called the node, while the single-sheet portion is called a free cell wall. Cell size is measured between two parallel sides of the hexagonal cell. Honeycomb is available in cell sizes ranging from 1.6 to 35 mm (0.062–1.375 in.); most common sizes are 3, 5, 6, 9, 13, and 25 mm (0.125, 0.1875, 0.25, 0.375, 0.5, 0.75, and 1 in.). Honeycomb densities range from 16 to 880 kg/m^3 (1–55 lb/ft^3). When specifying honeycomb, the user needs to stipulate the material, cell configuration, cell size, and density.

Cell Configuration. Honeycomb is available in a variety of cell configurations; the most appropriate configuration depends on application requirements. Available honeycomb cell configurations include:

- Hexagonal
- Reinforced hexagonal
- Overexpanded (OX)
- Square
- Flex-Core
- Double Flex-Core
- Spirally wrapped (Tube-Core)
- Cross-Core
- Circular (tubular core)

Flex-Core, Tube-Core, and Cross-Core are trademarks of Hexcel Corporation (San Francisco, CA).

Figure 2 illustrates various honeycomb cell configurations; the most common is hexagonal. A hexagon is one of nature's most efficient shapes for providing structural support. A reinforcement layer can be incorporated in the cellular structure along the nodes in the ribbon direction (reinforced hexagonal configuration) to increase mechanical properties. An OX cell configuration is a hexagonal honeycomb overexpanded in the width (W), or transverse direction. This configuration approaches a rectangular shape, which is preferred when the core needs to be curved or formed around one axis. The OX cell increases shear properties in the W direction and decreases length (L), or longitudinal shear properties compared with hexagonal honeycomb. Making the node very narrow relative to the length of a free cell wall results in a square cell configuration, which provides nearly equal shear strength and modulus in the L and W directions. A Flex-Core or double-Flex-Core cell configuration is ideal when necessary to form parts having compound curvatures. A Tube-Core spirally wrapped cylinder or a cross-core cell configuration is used in applications requiring specific energy absorption. Cross-Core provides energy absorption strength in multiple directions. A circular cell configuration is available for some solvent-bonded thermoplastic honeycombs. In addition to the above cell configurations for structural applications, a very small square cell configuration is available for use in catalytic-converter and heating, ventilation, and air conditioning (HVAC) applications.

Kraft paper	Specialty metals
Thermoplastics	Titanium
Polyurethane	Nickel-base alloys
Polypropylene	Hastelloy
Others	Inconel
Aluminum	Waspaloy
Alloy 5052	René
Alloy 5056	Cobalt-base alloys
Alloy 3003	Haynes
Alloy 3104	Aramid fibers
Carbon steel	Nomex
Stainless steel	Korex
300 series	Kevlar
Precipitation hardenable (PH)	Fiberglass
	Carbon
	Ceramic

Various corrosion-resistant coatings are available for aluminum and steel honeycomb. The most common corrosion-resistant coatings are chromate based and phosphoric acid anodization based. Phosphoric acid anodization provides enhanced honeycomb-to-facing bond strength in sandwich panel construction and enhanced protection in hot/wet and salt environments. Cell wall thicknesses for aluminum, steel, and specialty metal honeycombs range from 0.002 to

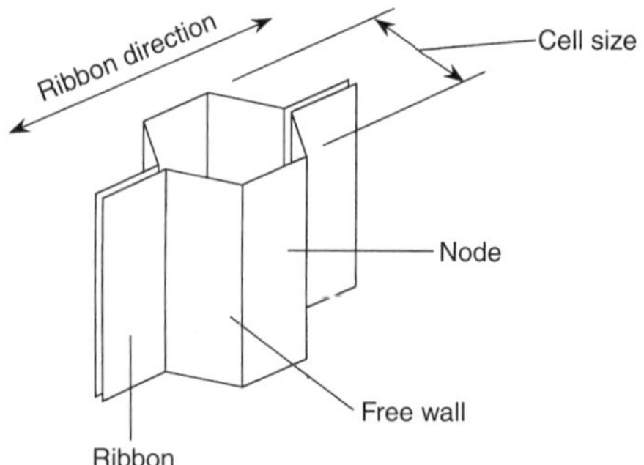

Fig. 1 Honeycomb cell terminology

0.15 mm (0.0009–0.006 in.). Metallic honeycomb cell walls are available either perforated or nonperforated.

In addition to the substrate, some of the nonmetallic honeycombs are reinforced with resin, which increases density and mechanical properties. Honeycomb substrate materials that can be strengthened with the addition of resin include kraft paper, aramids, fiberglass, and carbon. Resins used to reinforce nonmetallic honeycombs are phenolic, polyimide, and epoxy.

Phenolic resin is by far the most common due to its adherence, fire resistance, and relatively low cost. Polyimide resin is much more expensive than phenolic resin, but provides high-temperature resistance and low dielectric properties. Epoxy resin, also relatively expensive, is used in specialty applications, such as satellites.

Each honeycomb material provides certain properties and has specific benefits. Selection of the proper honeycomb material for a given application is a trade-off between properties and cost. General attributes of honeycomb materials are:

- *Kraft paper:* Relatively low strength, good insulating properties, available in large quantities, lowest cost
- *Thermoplastics:* Good insulating properties, good energy absorption and/or redirection, smooth cell walls, moisture and chemical resistance, environmentally compatible, aesthetically pleasing, relatively low cost
- *Aluminum:* Best strength-to-weight ratio and energy absorption, good heat transfer properties; electromagnetic shielding properties; smooth, thinnest cell walls; machinable; relatively low cost
- *Steel:* Strong, good heat transfer properties, electromagnetic shielding properties, heat resistance
- *Specialty metals:* Relatively high strength-to-weight ratio, good heat transfer properties, chemical resistance, heat resistance to very high temperatures
- *Aramid fiber:* Flammability resistance, fire retardance, good insulating properties, low dielectric properties, good formability
- *Fiberglass:* Tailorable shear properties by lay-up, low dielectric properties, good insulating properties, good formability
- *Carbon:* Good dimensional stability and retention, high-temperature property retention, high stiffness, very low coefficient of thermal expansion, tailorable thermal conductivity, relatively high shear modulus, very expensive
- *Ceramic:* Heat resistance to very high temperatures, good insulating properties, available in very small cell sizes, very expensive

Properties. Most honeycombs are anisotropic; that is, properties are directional. Honeycomb L, W, and T orientation is shown in Fig. 3. The highest compressive and tensile strength of honeycomb is in the T direction; other directions are substantially weaker. Honeycomb provides shear strength in the L and W directions. For the hexagonal-cell configuration, the shear strength and modulus are greatest in the L direction. The shear strength is nearly equivalent in the L and W directions in both the rectangular and the square cell configurations. The Cross-Core cell configuration is designed to have good structural properties in two directions. The most important strength properties used to quantify honeycomb are:

Hexagonal; Reinforced hexagonal; Overexpanded (OX) core; Flex-Core; Double Flex-Core; Tube-Core; Cross-Core; Square

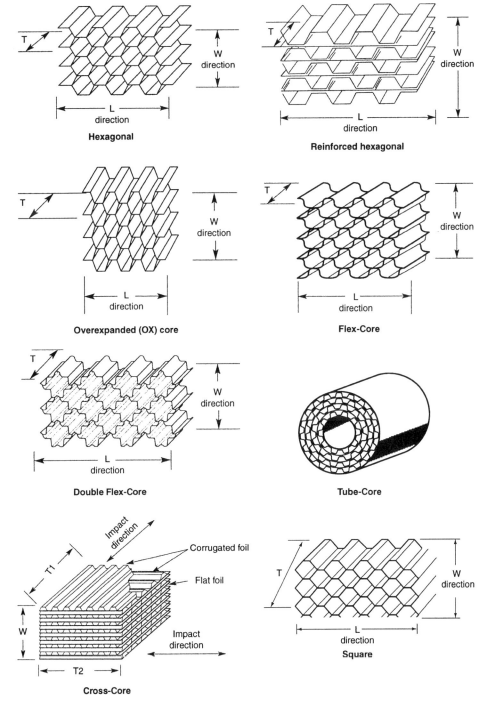

Fig. 2 Honeycomb cell configurations. L, length; T, thickness, W, width

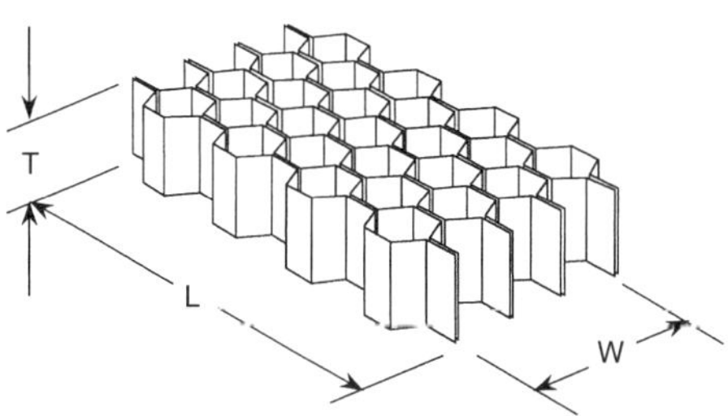

Fig. 3 Honeycomb orientation: L (length or ribbon), W (width), and T (thickness) directions

- Compressive strength, either as bare core or stabilized with facings
- Compressive modulus, measured as stabilized with facings
- Crush strength, for energy absorption applications
- Shear strength and modulus in the L and W directions

Figure 4 shows a typical load-deflection curve for honeycomb.

Balsa

Balsa is a natural wood product with elongated closed cells; it is available in a variety of grades that correlate to the structural, cosmetic, and physical characteristics. The density of balsa (96–288 kg/m^3, or 6–18 lb/ft^3) is less than one-half of the density of conventional wood products (480–720 kg/m^3, or 30–45 lb/ft^3). However, balsa has a considerably higher density than the other types of structural cores. Balsa is not available in densities less than 96 kg/m^3 (6 lb/ft^3).

Foam

The mechanical properties of foams are typically isotropic. A variety of foams can be used as core including:

- Polystyrene (better known as styrofoam)
- Phenolic
- Polyurethane
- Polypropylene
- Polyvinyl chloride (PVC), under the tradenames Divinycell, Klegecell, and Airex
- Polymethacrylimide, under the tradename Rohacell

Polystyrene foam is the least expensive, but has relatively low mechanical properties. It is commonly used for disposable packaging. Phenolic foam has very good fire-resistant properties and can have very low densities, but it has relatively low mechanical properties. Polyurethane foam is relatively inexpensive and is used primarily in automotive applications, requiring moderate structural properties. Polypropylene foam is used primarily in automotive applications requiring more demanding structural properties. Polyvinyl chloride (PVC) foam is used primarily in the marine industry for pleasure craft. Polymethacrylimide foam is much more expensive than the other types of foams, but has greater mechanical properties and is used primarily in aerospace and recreation product applications.

Specifying Structural Core

Determining which structural core type to use requires knowing the relevant application requirements. Factors to consider include:

- Materials
- Size
- Density
- Mechanical properties
- Environmental compatibility
- Formability
- Durability
- Thermal behavior
- Cost versus performance

The various attributes of honeycomb, balsa, and foam are compared in Table 1. A relative cost/performance comparison is shown in Fig. 5. Aluminum honeycomb offers the optimal cost/performance characteristics.

Sandwich Structures

In many applications, lightweight structural cores are used in a sandwich panel. The primary

Table 1 Comparison of selected properties and attributes for lightweight structural core materials

Property or attribute	Honeycomb	Balsa	Foam
Density (typical), kg/m^3 (lb/ft^3)	Expanded: 32–192 (2–12) Corrugated: 160–880 (10–55)	96–288 (6–18)	32–288 (2–18)
Moisture resistance	Excellent	Fair	Excellent
Chemical resistance	Fair to excellent	Fair to very good	Fair to very good
Flammability resistance	Excellent	Poor	Fair to excellent
High-temperature resistance	Adhesive bonded: to 177 °C (350 °F) Braze welded: to between 370 and 815 °C (700 and 1500 °F) depending on material	To at least 95 °C (200 °F)	Typically to 80 °C (180 °F); varies by type, but mechanical properties decrease significantly at higher temperatures
Strength and stiffness	Excellent	Excellent	Fair
Energy absorption and crush strength	Constant crush strength value	Not used for energy absorption	Increasing stress with increasing strain
Impact resistance	Fair to excellent	Very good	Fair to poor
Fatigue strength	Good to excellent	Very good	Fair to poor
Abrasion resistance	Good integrity	Fair	Friable
Acoustic attenuation	Yes	Yes	Yes
Formability	Various cell configurations for different shapes	Must cut (e.g., scoring), or use joined strips	Requires molds or scoring
Cost	Inexpensive (kraft paper) to very expensive (carbon)	Moderate	Very inexpensive (polystyrene) to expensive (polymethacrylimide)

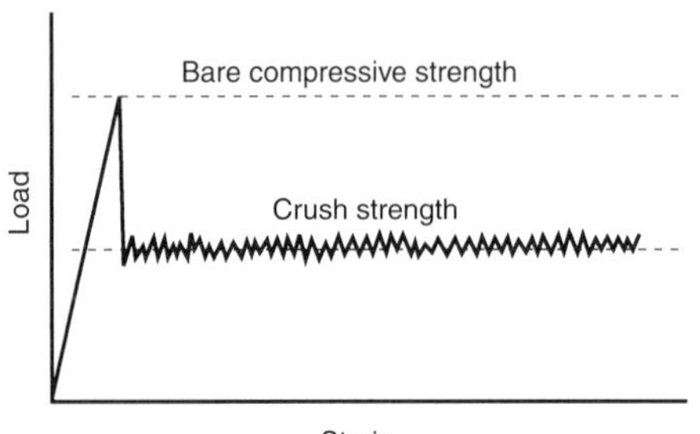

Fig. 4 Typical load-deflection curve for honeycomb

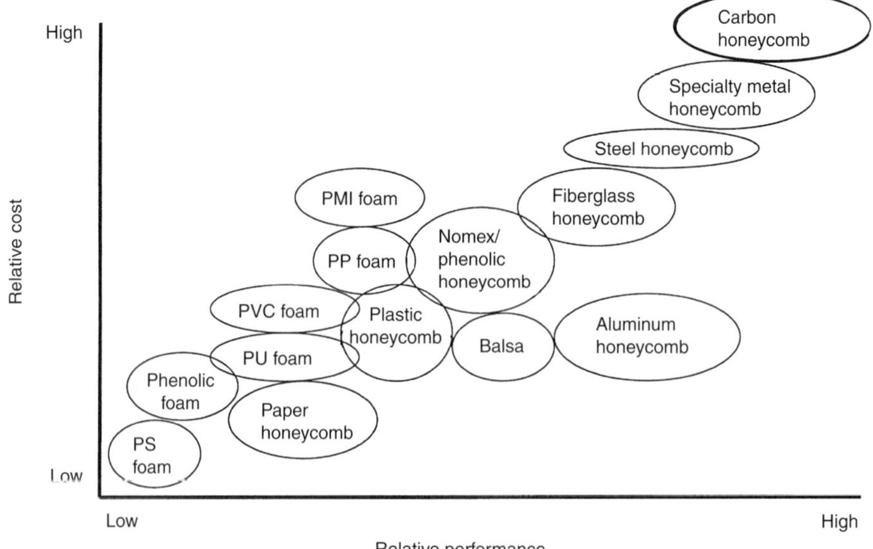

Fig. 5 Cost versus performance of various lightweight structural cores. PMI, polymethacrylimide; PP, polypropylene; PVC, polyvinyl chloride; PU, polyurethane; PS, polystyrene

advantages of a sandwich panel design are weight savings and increased stiffness compared with alternative designs.

A typical sandwich consists of two thin, high-strength facings bonded to a thick, lightweight core. Each component by itself is relatively weak and flexible, but when combined in a sandwich panel they produce a structure that is stiff, strong, and lightweight. Common facing materials for sandwich panels include aluminum, steel, fiberglass, kraft paper, wood, carbon, nonwovens, and prepregs.

Sandwich Concept. The basic concept of a sandwich panel is that the facings carry the bending loads and the honeycomb core carries the shear loads. In most cases the facing stresses are uniformly distributed. The honeycomb core offers no resistance to bending. In other words, the bending modulus, E', of the core is assumed to be zero. This assumption leads to a uniform shear stress throughout the core thickness.

Deflection, in all structures, consists of two components: bending deflection and shear deformation. In nonsandwich structures, such as steel plate, the shear deformation often is negligible and therefore is neglected. In a sandwich structure, on the other hand, the shear deformation can be significant. In most cases it accounts for about 1% of the bending deflection, although it can be much greater for thick panels or short spans. A typical sandwich panel, formed by adhesive bonding thin skins to a honeycomb core, is shown in Fig. 6.

The honeycomb concept produces extremely stiff and strong structures at minimum weight. Table 2 is a generic example of honeycomb effectiveness: a 0.81 mm (0.032 in.) thick piece of aluminum is compared to two sandwiches made by halving the aluminum into two facings and bonding honeycomb core between them. In bending, the thickest of the two sandwich panels is 37 times stiffer and more than 9 times stronger than the aluminum sheet, with a weight increase of only 6%.

Benefits of sandwich panels containing lightweight structural cores instead of alternative designs include:

- High strength-to-weight ratio
- Impact and damage resistance
- High rigidity (stiffness)-to-weight ratio
- Fatigue resistance
- Durability
- Tailorable heat transfer and insulation properties
- Fire resistance with tailored self-extinguishing and low-smoke properties
- Ability to include fasteners and attachments

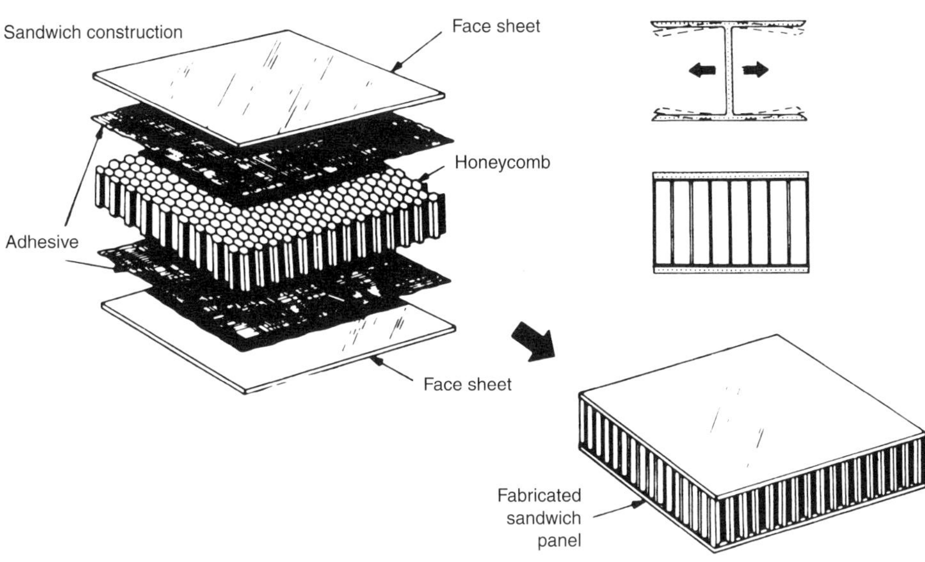

Fig. 6 Honeycomb sandwich panel components

Table 2 Honeycomb sandwich panel structural efficiency

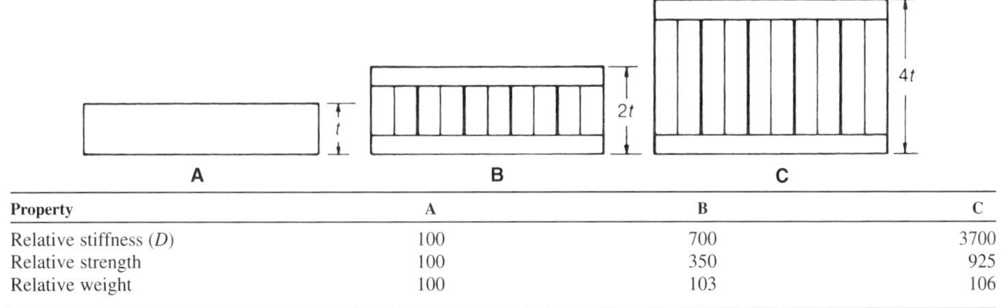

Property	A	B	C
Relative stiffness (D)	100	700	3700
Relative strength	100	350	925
Relative weight	100	103	106

SELECTED REFERENCES

- "Bonded Honeycomb Sandwich Construction," Hexcel TSB 124, Hexcel Composites
- J. Corden, Honeycomb Structure, *Composites,* Vol 1, *Engineered Materials Handbook,* ASM International, 1986
- Hexcel Cross-Core data sheet, Hexcel Composites
- J. Kindinger, "HexWeb Honeycomb Attributes and Properties," Hexcel Composites, 1999
- J. Kindinger, "Honeycomb Sandwich Panels," Hexcel Composites, 1999

Bio-Based Resins and Natural Fibers

Richard P. Wool and Shrikant N. Khot, University of Delaware

ADVANCES in genetic engineering, natural fiber development, and composite science offer significant opportunities for new, improved materials from renewable resources, which can be biodegradable and/or recyclable with enhanced support for global sustainability. Newly developed soy-based plastics and adhesive materials are being evaluated and tested by end-users and converters for high-volume applications in agricultural equipment (Fig. 1), automotive components (car and truck parts), civil infrastructure (bridges and highway components), marine structures (pipes and offshore equipment), rail infrastructure (carriages, box cars, and grain hoppers), and the construction industry (formaldehyde-free particle board, ceilings, engineered lumber). This article describes the synthesis, manufacturing, and properties of both the neat soy-based resins and the glass, flax, and hemp composites.

Bio-Based Resins

Polymers and polymeric composites are derived from petroleum reserves, and as the number of applications of polymeric materials continues to increase, an alternative source of these materials becomes more important. Since 1996, a broad range of chemical routes to use natural triglyceride oils as a basis for polymers, adhesives, and composite materials has been developed (Ref 1–3). These materials have economical and environmental advantages over petroleum-based materials, making them an attractive alternative. Natural oils, which can be derived from both plant and animal sources, are abundantly found in all parts of the world, making them an ideal alternative chemical feedstock. These oils are predominantly made up of triglyceride molecules, which have the 3-armed star structure shown in Fig. 2. Triglycerides are composed of three fatty acids joined at a glycerol juncture. Most common oils contain fatty acids that vary from 14 to 22 carbons in length, with 0 to 3 double bonds per fatty acid. In Table 1, the fatty-acid distributions of several common oils are shown (Ref 4). There are more exotic oils, which are composed of fatty acids with other types of functionalities, such as epoxies, hydroxyls, cyclic groups, and furanoid groups (Ref 5). Due to the many different fatty acids present, it is apparent that on a molecular level, these oils are composed of many different types of triglycerides with numerous levels of unsaturation. With newly developed genetic engineering techniques, the variation in unsaturation can be controlled in plants such as soybean, flax, and corn.

Besides their application in the foods industry, triglyceride oils have been used quite extensively to produce coatings, inks, plasticizers, lubricants, and other agrochemicals (Ref 6–12). Within the polymer field, the application of these oils to toughen polymer materials has been investigated. There has been an extensive amount of work in their use to produce interpenetrating

Table 1 Fatty-acid distribution in various plant oils

Fatty acid	C:DB(a)	Canola	Corn	Cottonseed	Linseed	Olive	Palm	Rapeseed	Soybean	High oleic(b)
Myristic	14:0	0.1	0.1	0.7	0.0	0.0	1.0	0.1	0.1	0.0
Myristoleic	14:1	0.0	0.0	0.0	0.0	0.0	0.0	0.0	0.0	0.0
Palmitic	16:0	4.1	10.9	21.6	5.5	13.7	44.4	3.0	11.0	6.4
Palmitoleic	16:1	0.3	0.2	0.6	0.0	1.2	0.2	0.2	0.1	0.1
Margaric	17:0	0.1	0.1	0.1	0.0	0.0	0.1	0.0	0.0	0.0
Margaroleic	17:1	0.0	0.0	0.1	0.0	0.0	0.0	0.0	0.0	0.0
Stearic	18:0	1.8	2.0	2.6	3.5	2.5	4.1	1.0	4.0	3.1
Oleic	18:1	60.9	25.4	18.6	19.1	71.1	39.3	13.2	23.4	82.6
Linoleic	18:2	21.0	59.6	54.4	15.3	10.0	10.0	13.2	53.2	2.3
Linolenic	18:3	8.8	1.2	0.7	56.6	0.6	0.4	9.0	7.8	3.7
Arachidic	20:0	0.7	0.4	0.3	0.0	0.9	0.3	0.5	0.3	0.2
Gadoleic	20:1	1.0	0.0	0.0	0.0	0.0	0.0	9.0	0.0	0.4
Eicosadienoic	20:2	0.0	0.0	0.0	0.0	0.0	0.0	0.7	0.0	0.0
Behenic	22:0	0.3	0.1	0.2	0.0	0.0	0.1	0.5	0.1	0.3
Erucic	22:1	0.7	0.0	0.0	0.0	0.0	0.0	49.2	0.0	0.1
Lignoceric	24:0	0.2	0.0	0.0	0.0	0.0	0.0	1.2	0.0	0.0
Average number of double bonds per triglyceride		3.9	4.5	3.9	6.6	2.8	1.8	3.8	4.6	3.0

(a) C, number of carbons; DB, number of double bonds. (b) Genetically engineered high oleic-acid-content soybean oil (DuPont)

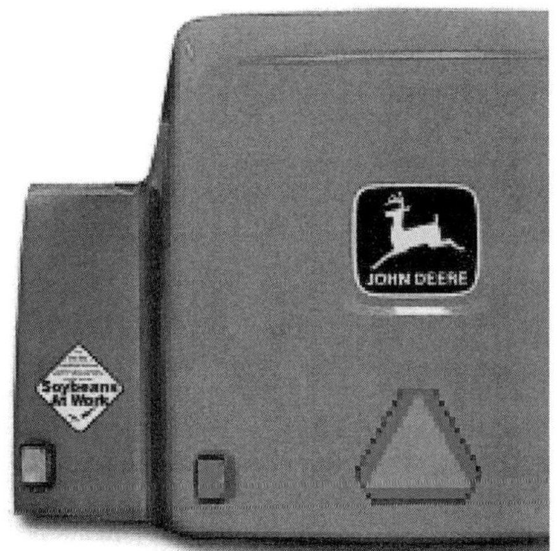

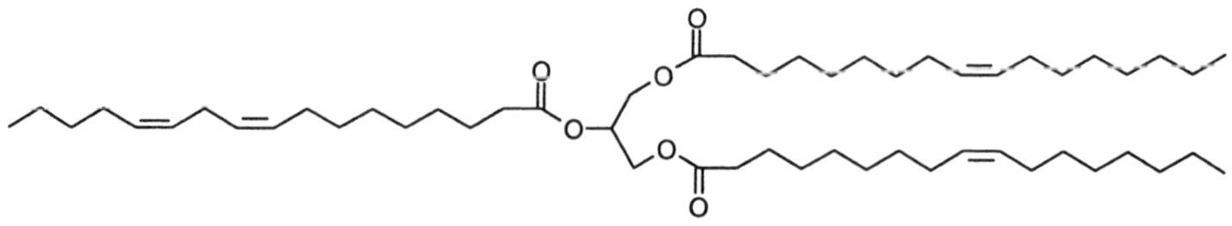

Fig. 1 Harvester part manufactured using soybean-oil-based polymer resin

Fig. 2 Triglyceride molecule, the major component of natural oils

networks (IPNs), which has been reviewed by Barrett and coworkers (Ref 13). It was found that IPNs formed by triglycerides could increase the toughness and fracture resistance in conventional thermoset polymers. For example, Qureshi and coworkers developed an IPN consisting of cross-linked polystyrene and an epoxidized linseed-oil elastomer (Ref 14). Similarly, Devia and coworkers produced IPNs with cross-linked polystyrene and castor-oil elastomers (Ref 15–17). Many other efforts have been made to use various types of triglycerides as tougheners in the polymer field (Ref 18–21).

Recently, there has been renewed interest in developing polymers predominantly based on triglyceride-derived monomers. Such materials do not depend on triglycerides as additives within the material, but rather as major components in the polymer matrix. Li and coworkers have examined using fish, soybean, and tung oil as comonomers in producing rigid plastic materials (Ref 22–25). Using these oils in their natural form and in conjugated forms, thermoset polymers were formed by cationic polymerization with other monomers, such as styrene, divinyl benzene, and cyclopentadiene. Similarly, work in the authors' laboratory at the University of Delaware since 1996 has developed several methods for producing polymers from triglycerides.

Synthetic Pathways for Triglyceride-Based Monomers. The triglyceride contains many active sites amenable to chemical reactions. These are the double bond, the allylic carbons, the ester group, and the carbon alpha to the ester group. These active sites can be used to introduce polymerizable groups on the triglyceride using the same synthetic techniques that have been applied in the synthesis of petroleum-based polymers. The key step is to reach a high level of molecular weight and cross-link density, as well as to incorporate chemical groups that are known to impart stiffness in a polymer network (e.g., aromatic or cyclic structures). Several synthetic pathways have been found to accomplish this, as illustrated in Fig. 3 (Ref 3). In structures 5, 6, 7, 8, and 11, the double bonds of the triglyceride are used to functionalize the triglyceride with polymerizable chemical groups. From the natural triglyceride, it is possible to attach maleinates (5) (Ref 7, 12) or convert the unsaturation to epoxies (7) (Ref 26–28) or hydroxyl functionalities (8) (Ref 29, 30). Such transformations make the triglyceride capable of reaction via ring-opening or polycondensation polymerization. These particular chemical pathways are also accessible via natural epoxy- and hydroxyl-functional triglycerides, as demonstrated by past work (Ref 13, 15–17). It is also possible to attach vinyl functionalities to the epoxy- and hydroxyl-functional triglycerides. Reaction of the epoxy-functional triglyceride with acrylic acid incorporates acrylates onto the triglyceride (6), while reaction of the hydroxylated triglyceride with maleic anhydride incorporates maleate half-esters and esters onto the triglyceride (11). These monomers can then be blended with a reactive diluent, similar to most conventional vinyl-ester resins, and cured by free-radical polymerization.

The second method for synthesizing monomers from triglycerides is to reduce the triglyceride to monoglycerides through a glycerolysis (3A) reaction or an amidation reaction (2, 3B) (Ref 31–36). Monoglycerides have found much use in the field of surface coatings, commonly referred to as alkyd resins, due to their low cost and versatility (Ref 32). In those applications, the double bonds of the monoglyceride are reacted to form the coating. However, monoglycerides are also able to react through the hydroxyl groups via polycondensation reactions with a comonomer, such as a diacid, epoxy, or anhydride. Alternatively, maleate half-esters can be attached to these monoglycerides (9), allowing them to polymerize via free-radical polymerization.

The third method is to functionalize the unsaturation sites as well as reduce the triglyceride into monoglycerides. This can be accomplished by glycerolysis of an unsaturated triglyceride, followed by hydroxylation (4), or by glycerolysis of a hydroxy-functional triglyceride. The resulting monomer can then be reacted with maleic anhydride, forming a monomer capable of polymerization by free-radical polymerization (10).

These bio-based monomers, when used as a major component of a molding resin, exhibit properties comparable to conventional polymers and composites, and these properties are presented. Additionally, their use as a matrix in synthetic- and natural-fiber-reinforced composites is presented

Acrylated epoxidized soybean oils (AESO) (Fig. 4) are synthesized from the reaction of acrylic acid with epoxidized triglycerides. Epoxidized triglycerides can be found in natural oils, such as vernonia plant oil, or can be synthesized from more common unsaturated oils, such as soybean oil or linseed oil, by a standard epoxidation reaction (Ref 37). The natural epoxy oil, vernonia oil, has an epoxy functionality of 2.8 epoxy rings per triglyceride (Ref 14). Epoxidized soybean oil is commercially available (e.g., Vikoflex 7170, Atofina Chemicals Inc.) and is generally sold with a functionality of 4.1 to 4.6 epoxy rings per triglyceride, which can be identified via proton nuclear magnetic resonance (^{1}H-NMR) (Ref 19, 38). Epoxidized linseed oil is also commercially available (Vikoflex 7190, Elf Atochem Inc.) when higher epoxy content is required. Predominantly, these oils are used as an alternative plasticizer in polyvinyl chloride in place of phthalates (Ref 39–41). However, research has been done to explore their use as a toughening agent (Ref 19–21, 42, 43). With the addition of acrylates, the triglyceride can be reacted via addition polymerization. Acrylated epoxidized soybean oil has been used extensively in the area of surface coatings and is commercially manufactured in forms such as Ebecryl 860 (UCB Chemicals Co.) (Ref 8, 44, 45). Urethane and amine derivatives of AESO have also been developed for coating and ink applications (Ref 9, 10, 46).

The reaction of acrylic acid with epoxidized soybean oil occurs through a substitution reaction and has been found to have first-order dependence with respect to epoxy concentration and second-order dependence with respect to acrylic acid concentration (Ref 47). However, epoxidized oleic methyl ester has been found to

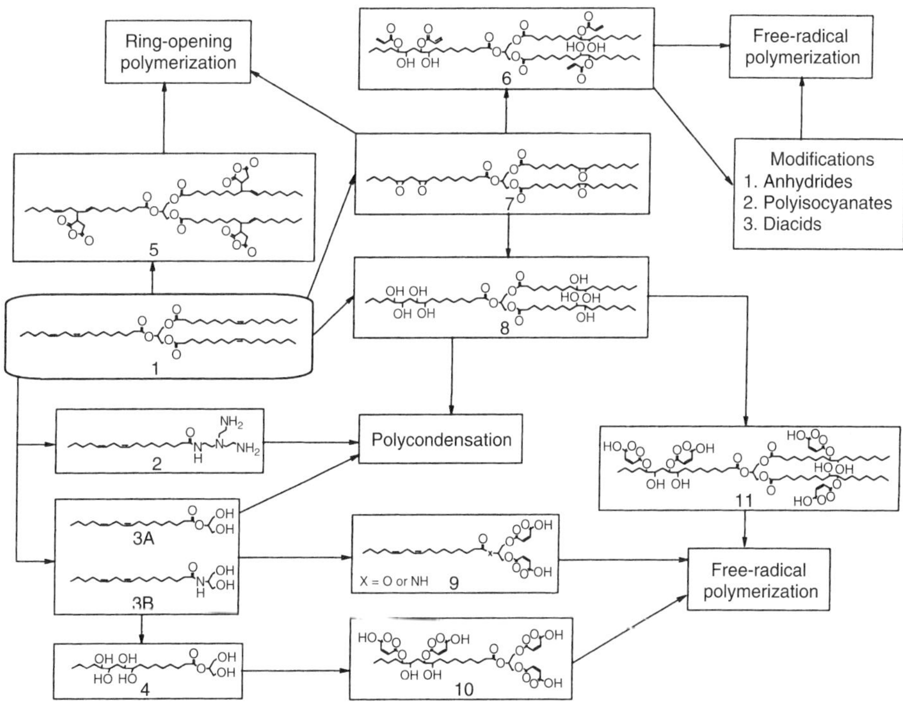

Fig. 3 Chemical pathways leading to polymers from triglyceride molecules. See text for discussion. Source: Ref 1, 3

display second-order dependence on both epoxy and acrylic acid concentrations (Ref 48). Although the reaction of epoxidized soybean oil with acrylic acid is partially acid catalyzed by the acrylic acid, the use of additional catalysts is common. Tertiary amines, such as N,N-dimethyl aniline, triethylamine, and 1,4-diazabicyclo[2.2.2]octane, are commonly used (Ref 38, 49). Additionally, organometallic catalysts have been developed that are more selective, reducing the amount of epoxy homopolymerization (Ref 50, 51).

Acrylated epoxidized soybean oil can be blended with a reactive diluent, such as styrene, to improve its processability and control the polymer properties to reach a range acceptable for structural applications. By varying the amount of styrene, it is possible to produce polymers with different moduli and glass transition temperatures. Changing the molecular weight or functionality of the acrylated triglyceride can also modify the polymer properties. Consequently, a range of properties and therefore, applications, can be found. After the acrylation reaction, the triglyceride contains both residual amounts of unreacted epoxy rings as well as newly formed hydroxyl groups, both of which can be used to further modify the triglyceride by reaction with a number of chemical species, such as diacids, diamines, anhydrides, and isocyanates. The approach presented here is to oligomerize the triglycerides with reagents that have chemical structures conducive to stiffening the polymer, such as cyclic or aromatic groups. Reaction of the AESO with cyclohexane dicarboxylic anhydride (CDCA) forms oligomers, increasing the entanglement density and introducing stiff cyclic rings to the structure. Reaction of the AESO with maleic acid also forms oligomers as well as introduces more double bonds. While it is desirable to maximize the conversion of hydroxyls or epoxies, at high levels of conversion the viscosity increases dramatically. Eventually, this can lead to gelation, so careful monitoring of the reaction must be conducted. After oligomerization, the modified AESO resin can be blended with styrene and cured in the same manner as the unmodified AESO resin.

Maleinized soyoil monoglyceride (SOMG/MA) (Fig. 4) is synthesized from the triglyceride oil in two steps (Ref 33). The first step is a standard glycerolysis reaction to break the triglycerides into monoglycerides. This reaction involves a breakdown of the triglycerides by reaction with glycerol, which has been reviewed in detail by Sonntag (Ref 31). The product is generally a mixture of mono- and diglycerides. To aid in the conversion, excess glycerol can be used. Additionally, the reaction can be run in solvent or in the presence of an emulsifier catalyst (Ref 34). Once the reaction is completed, it is possible to separate a portion of the unreacted glycerol by rapidly cooling the product (Ref 33). However, the presence of glycerol is not detrimental to the end polymer, because it can be reacted with maleic anhydride in the same manner as the monoglycerides and incorporated into the end-polymer network.

The maleinization of the SOMG mixture at temperatures below 100 °C (210 °F) produces monoglycerides, diglycerides, and glycerol maleate half-esters. This reaction makes no attempt to produce a polyester, and the half-ester formation is expected to proceed at low temperatures in the presence of either acid or base catalysts without any by-products. A good indication of the success of this reaction is to follow the signal intensity ratio of maleate vinyl protons to fatty-acid vinyl protons (N_M/N_{FA}) in the ^{1}H-NMR spectrum. The use of 2-methylimidazole and triphenyl antimony as catalysts has been shown to be successful when conducting the reaction at temperatures of 80 to 100 °C (175 to 210 °F) with a 3 to 2 weight ratio of glycerides to maleic anhydride (N_M/N_{FA} = 0.85) (Ref 33, 52). Once these maleates have been added, the monoglycerides can react via addition polymerization. Since maleates are relatively unreactive to each other, the addition of styrene increases the polymerization conversion as well as imparts rigidity to the matrix.

To increase the glass transition temperature (T_g) and modulus of the SOMG/MA polymer for higher performance, more rigid diols can be added during the maleinization reaction. Such diols are neopentyl glycol (NPG) and bisphenol A (BPA), which are known to produce rigid segments in polymer chains. While their addition to the maleinization mixture will reduce the renewable resource content of the final resin, they should result in higher T_g values for the end polymer. The synthesis of maleate half-esters of organic polyols, including NPG and BPA, and the cross linking of the resulting maleate half-esters with a vinyl monomer, such as styrene, have been reported in two patents (Ref 53, 54). The literature is replete with examples of unsaturated polyesters prepared from NPG and maleic anhydride with some other polyols and diacids (Ref 55–58). However, the copolymers of NPG and BPA bis-maleate half-esters with SOMG maleate half-esters is new.

Maleinized hydroxylated oil (HO/MA), as shown in Fig. 4, is synthesized in a manner similar to both the AESO monomer and the SOMG/MA monomer. The double bonds of the triglyceride are converted to hydroxyl groups, which are then used to attach maleates similar to the SOMG/MA synthesis. As can be seen in Fig. 3, there are two routes to synthesize the hydroxylated triglyceride. The first path is through an epoxidized intermediate. By reacting the epoxidized triglyceride with an acid, the epoxies can be easily converted to hydroxyl groups (Ref 29, 59). Alternatively, the hydroxylated oil can be synthesized directly from the unsaturated oil in a manner similar to that described by Swern and coworkers (Ref 30). After hydroxylation, the oil can be reacted with maleic anhydride to functionalize the triglyceride with maleate half-esters. A molar ratio of 4 to 1 anhydride to triglyceride was used in all cases, and the reaction catalyzed with N,N- dimethylbenzylamine. Once the maleinization reaction is finished, the monomer resin can be blended with styrene, similar to the other resins presented here.

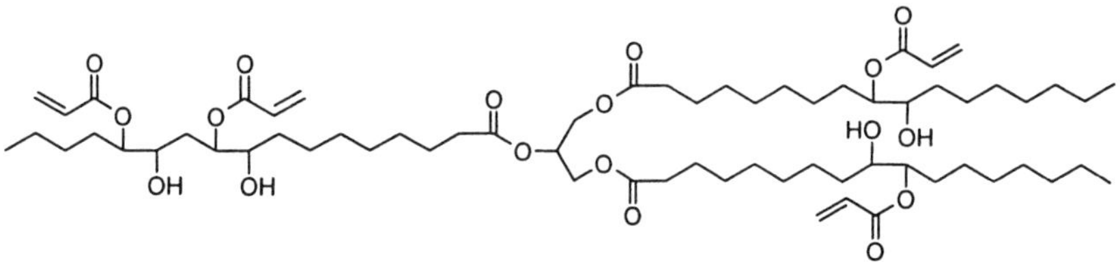

Acrylated epoxidized soybean oil (AESO)

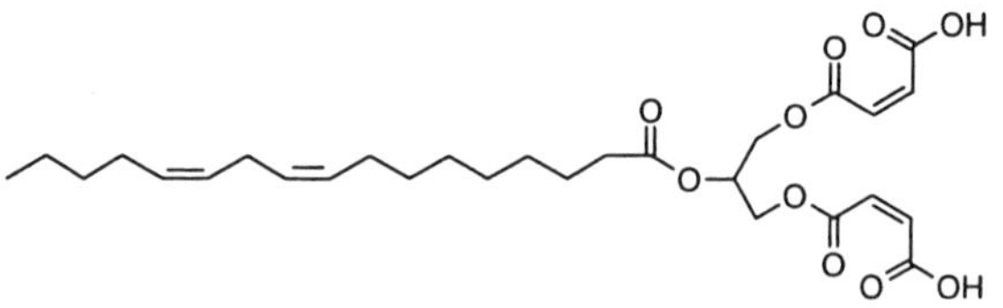

Maleinated soybean oil monoglyceride (SOMG/MA)

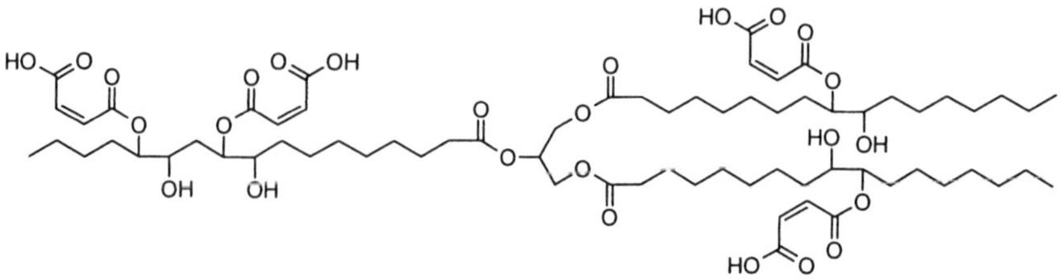

Maleinated hydroxylated soybean oil (HSO/MA)

Fig. 4 Triglyceride-based monomers

Neat Resin Properties

AESO Polymer Properties. The pure AESO polymer exhibits a tensile modulus of approximately 440 MPa (64 ksi). At a styrene content of 40 wt%, the modulus increases significantly to 1.6 GPa (232 ksi), almost a fourfold increase. In this region, the dependence on composition appears to be fairly linear. The ultimate tensile strengths of these materials also show linear behavior. The pure AESO exhibits a strength of approximately 6 MPa (0.9 ksi), while the polymers with 40 wt% styrene show much higher strengths of approximately 21 MPa (3.0 ksi). The dynamic mechanical analysis (three-point bending geometry) indicates that even at temperatures as low as –130 °C (–200 °F), these polymers have not reached a characteristic glassy plateau. All compositions exhibit moduli on the order of 4 GPa (580 ksi), but have not reached a plateau. At higher temperatures in the rubber behavior region, the compositions show moduli inversely proportional to the amount of styrene present. According to rubber elasticity theory (Ref 60), the lower-styrene-content polymers have a higher cross-link density, as observed in Fig. 5.

The dynamic mechanical properties of the AESO polymers modified by CDCA and maleic acid were found to be better than the unmodified polymers. The storage modulus (E') of the unmodified AESO resin at room temperature is 1.3 GPa (189 ksi), while the CDCA modification increases E' to 1.6 GPa (232 ksi). The maleic acid modification provides the most improvement, raising the E' to 1.9 GPa (276 ksi). The glass transition temperature, as indicated by the peak in tan δ (the ratio of the loss modulus, E'', to the storage modulus, E'), does not show any large increase from the anhydride modification. However, the maleic acid modification shifts the tan δ peak by almost 40 °C (72 °F), showing a peak at 105 °C (220 °F). The increased broadness of the peak can be attributed to increased cross-link density.

The previous dynamic mechanical behavior is a combination of two factors, cross-link density and plasticization. As the amount of AESO is increased, the number of multifunctional monomers also increases. Therefore, the overall cross-link density is expected to be greater with increasing amounts of AESO, as supported by the high-temperature moduli shown in Fig. 5. Increasing the cross-link density has been found to slow the transition in E' from glassy to rubbery behavior. Additionally, the tan δ peak broadens and decreases in height (Ref 61). The other factor in the dynamic mechanical behavior, plasticization, is due to the molecular nature of the triglyceride. The starting soybean oil contains fatty acids that are completely saturated and cannot be functionalized with acrylates. Therefore, these fatty acids act in the same manner as a plasticizer, introducing free volume and enabling the network to deform more easily. The addition of even small amounts of plasticizer to polymers has been known to drastically broaden the transition from glassy to rubbery behavior and reduce the overall modulus (Ref 61).

This plasticizer effect presents an issue that may be inherent to all-natural triglyceride-based polymers that use the double bonds to add functional groups. However, with advances in genetic engineering capabilities, it may be possible to reduce this trend by reducing the amount of saturated fatty acids present, thus sharpening the glass-rubber transition. This issue is addressed later in the properties of HO/MA polymers produced from genetically engineered high-oleic-content oil and synthetic triolein oil. The existence of some saturated fatty acids, though, can contribute to improved toughness and ballistic impact resistance (Ref 62).

SOMG/MA Polymer Properties. The tan δ peak for the SOMG/MA polymer occurs at around 133 °C (271 °F), and the polymer has an E' value of approximately 0.92 GPa (133 ksi) at room temperature. The T_g of this polymer is lower due to the broad molecular weight distribution of the SOMG maleates. The distribution of soyoil monoglyceride monomaleates, monoglyceride bismaleates, diglyceride monomaleates, and glycerol trismaleates has been confirmed by mass spectral analysis, which has been reported in a previous publication (Ref 63). Additionally, the molecular structure of the monomer is such that the fatty acid "tail" is not incorporated into the network, introducing additional free volume. The tensile tests performed on the copolymers of SOMG maleates with styrene showed a tensile strength of 29.4 MPa (4.26 ksi) and a tensile modulus of 0.84 GPa (122 ksi).

SOMG/NPG Maleates (SOMG/NPG/MA) Polymer Properties. The dynamic mechanical analysis of SOMG/NPG/MA polymers showed a tan δ peak at approximately 145 °C (293 °F) and an E' value of 2 GPa (290 ksi) at room temperature. The 12 °C (22 °F) increase in the T_g and the considerable increase in the modulus of the copolymers of SOMG/NPG maleates with styrene compared to that of the SOMG maleates can be attributed to the replacement of the flexible fatty-acid chains by the rigid methyl groups of NPG. The overall dynamic mechanical behavior of the SOMG/NPG/MA polymer was very similar to that of the SOMG/MA. However, despite the higher T_g and modulus, there remained a broad glass transition. The tensile strength of the SOMG/NPG/MA polymer was found to be 15.6 MPa (2.26 ksi), whereas the tensile modulus was found to be 1.49 GPa (216 ksi).

Maleinized pure NPG polymerized with styrene (NPG/MA) has been prepared in work by E. Can et al. (Ref 64) to compare its properties with the SOMG/NPG/MA polymer. Dynamic mechanical analysis of the NPG/MA showed a tan δ peak at around 103 °C (217 °F) and an E' value around 2.27 GPa (329 ksi) at 35 °C (95 °F). The high T_g value observed for the SOMG/NPG/MA system (~145 °C) must be a synergetic effect of both the NPG and SOMG together, because the T_g value observed for the NPG/MA system (~103 °C, or ~217 °F) is much lower. This is probably due to the incorporation of the fatty-acid unsaturation into the polymer in the SOMG/NPG/MA system. The comparatively higher E' value observed for the NPG maleates, on the other hand, explains the increase in the E' observed for the SOMG/NPG/MA system compared to that of the SOMG/MA system. The decrease in tensile strength of the SOMG/NPG/MA system compared to that of SOMG/MA might be attributed to a broader molecular weight distribution of this system compared to that of the SOMG maleates.

SOMG/BPA Maleates (SOMG/BPA/MA) Polymer Properties. The dynamic mechanical analysis of this polymer showed a tan δ peak at around 131 °C (239 °F) and an E' value of 1.34 GPa (194 ksi) at 35 °C (95 °F). The introduction of the rigid benzene ring on the polymer backbone made a considerable increase on the modulus of the final polymer, compared to that of the SOMG maleates. The T_g of this polymer, however, was not very different from that of the SOMG maleates (133 °C, or 271 °F). This has been attributed to a lower yield in the maleinization of the BPA, as determined from ^{1}H-NMR data (Ref 52). Like the SOMG/NPG/MA polymer, the SOMG/BPA/MA displayed the characteristic gradual glass transition.

HO/MA Dynamic Mechanical Polymer Properties. The dynamic mechanical properties of the HO/MA polymers were found to be better than those of the AESO polymers. Little variation was seen between the polymers made from the different oils. At room temperature, the storage moduli for all of the oils existed between 1.45 and 1.55 GPa (210 and 225 ksi), showing no dependence on saturation level. The dynamic mechanical behavior was very similar between the different oils, with the typical behavior shown in Fig. 6. The maximum in tan δ ranged from 107 to 116 °C (225 to 241 °F), which are all substantially higher than the AESO-based resin. These properties are fairly close to those shown by conventional petroleum-based polymers. However, the distinctive triglyceride behavior still exists, in that the glass transitions are

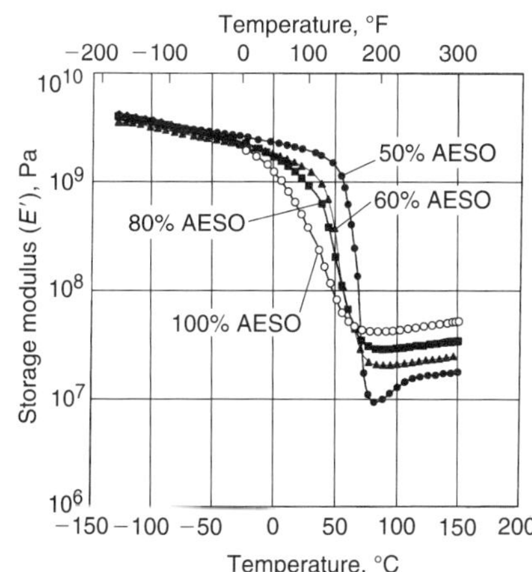

Fig. 5 Storage modulus (E') of AESO-styrene copolymer as a function of temperature

extremely broad, and even at room temperature, the materials are not completely in a glassy state. Again, this is probably due to the saturated fatty acids of the triglycerides acting as a plasticizer. As shown in Fig. 7, the behavior is linear, suggesting that if higher levels of functionality are reached, the properties should improve accordingly. However, it is expected that past a certain extent of maleate functionality, the property dependence will plateau. Work is currently being pursued to test the limits of this behavior.

It was previously stated that the broadness in the glass transition might be inherent to all triglyceride-based polymers. However, work with genetically engineered oil and synthetic oil has shown that it is possible to reduce this characteristic (Ref 65). The genetically engineered high-oleic soybean oil has an average triglyceride functionality of three double bonds/triglyceride and the fatty-acid distribution shown in Table 1. The maleinized form of this oil had a maleate functionality of two maleates/triglyceride. The properties of polymers from this material were compared to polymers from triolein oil, which is monodisperse, consisting only of oleic fatty-acid esters (18 carbons long, one double bond). The maleinized triolein oil had a maleate functionality of 2.1 maleates/triglyceride. Thus, the only difference between the two oils is the fatty-acid distribution of the high-oleic oil versus the monodisperse triolein oil. It was found that the T_g of these two polymers does not seem to differ much, judging from either their tan δ peak or the inflection in the E', but the broadness of the transitions do differ: the triolein polymer has a sharper E' transition from the glassy region to the rubbery region. This was evident also in the tan δ peak, which has a higher peak height. However, the transition is not yet as sharp as petroleum-based polymers. This is probably due to the triolein monomer having a functionality of only two maleates/triglyceride. Consequently, there is still a plasticizer effect present. However, this effect may be reduced by controlling the reaction conditions to reach higher conversions.

Triglyceride-Based Composite Materials

Four types of triglycerides typically make up a composite resin system: sizing, matrix, rubber toughening, and material modification. For natural fibers, or unsized glass or carbon, about 1% of the system consists of the sizing molecules. These have groups that allow them to bond both to the surface as well as to the matrix. A strong fiber-matrix interface bond is critical for high-strength composites. The ability to apply the sizing in situ offers considerable savings of time and cost, especially for all-natural composites that are intended to be low-cost. The chemical modification on the sizing is chosen with respect to specific interactions on the natural-fiber surface. The matrix consists of the dominant phase binding the fibers together in the composite, and it can be selected with respect to required material properties (hydrophilicity, biodegradability, flammability, dielectric, etc.). The rubber-generating molecules (5 to 20%) can be made in situ or synthesized separately, depending on the manufacturing conditions. The rubber particles, when used at the optimal concentration, impart considerable impact resistance to both the neat resin and the composite. Other triglycerides are chemically modified to tailor the optical, thermal, electrical, and mechanical properties of the composite.

All of the resins presented here are suitable for use as a matrix in a composite material. Their low viscosity and method of curing make them ideal candidates for use in conventional resin transfer molding (RTM) processes. Most polymer-matrix composites are made by embedding strong fibers, such as carbon, aramid, glass, or natural fibers, in a polymer matrix. The high strength and modulus of the embedded fibers impart strength and rigidity to the material that surpass that of the neat polymer (Ref 66).

Natural-Fiber Reinforcements. While most composite materials use synthetic fibers such as carbon or glass, in recent years, natural fibers have attracted the attention of the composite community as a potential reinforcement, due to the high cost of synthetic fibers. These natural fibers are based on cellulose and offer advantages of biodegradability, low density, nonabrasive nature, and low cost.

Depending on their origin, natural fibers can be grouped into seed, bast, leaf, and fruit qualities. Bast- and leaf-quality fibers are the most commonly used in composite applications. Examples of bast fibers include hemp, jute, flax, ramie, and kenaf. Leaf fibers include sisal and banana leaf fibers. Properties for these fibers include excellent tensile strength and modulus, high durability, low bulk density, good moldability, and recyclability. These natural fibers have an advantage over glass fibers in that they are less expensive, are abundantly available from renewable resources, and have a high specific strength. While high-performance carbon fibers remain superior to natural fibers in high-end applications, natural fibers have comparable properties to glass fibers in high-volume applications (Ref 67). The properties of flax, jute, sisal, and hemp fibers are shown in Table 2 and compared to the commonly used E-glass fiber (Ref 68). The most notable natural fiber is the flax fiber, which has a modulus higher than that of E-glass. Flax is also less dense, thereby producing a lighter composite with good mechanical properties.

Numerous studies on the properties of natural-fiber composites have appeared in the literature. These studies have considered a range of natural fibers, including jute (Ref 69–73), banana (Ref 74), agave (Ref 74), hemp (Ref 74, 75), flax (Ref 75–77), bamboo (Ref 78), pineapple (Ref 79), and rubber wood (Ref 80). For certain applications, the mechanical properties of natural-fiber composites, such as those made from flax or hemp fiber, are not sufficient due to the low strength of these fibers. However, combining natural fibers with stronger synthetic fibers, such as glass, could offer an optimal balance between performance and cost. These "hybrid" composites (discussed in a later section), which use two different types of fiber, have been examined in such forms as jute/glass hybrids with epoxy- and polyester-matrix materials (Ref 81, 82).

In all of the previous work, the natural fibers were combined with petroleum-derived matrix resins. The resins presented here offer the unique potential of combining natural fibers with resins based on natural, renewable resources. The properties of glass-reinforced composite materials made from the AESO and HSO/MA resins, as well as all-natural fiber-composite materials reinforced by flax and hemp fibers, are presented here (Ref 83). Additionally, the properties of hy-

Table 2 Properties of natural and E-glass fibers

Fiber	Density, g/cm^3	Tensile modulus		Tensile strength	
		GPa	ksi	MPa	ksi
Flax	1.50	100	14,500	1100	160
Jute	1.45	2.5–13	360–1885	460–530	67–77
Sisal	1.45	9.4–15.8	1363–2292	570–640	83–93
Hemp	1.48	...	...	690	100
E-glass	2.54	76	11,022	1500	218

Source: Ref 68

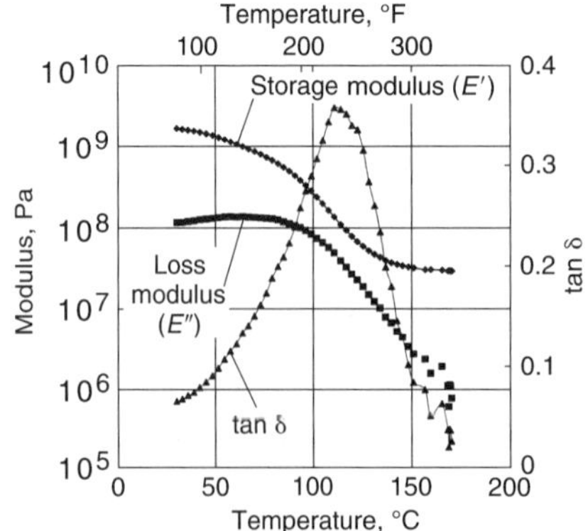

Fig. 6 Representative dynamic mechanical behavior for HO/MA polymers

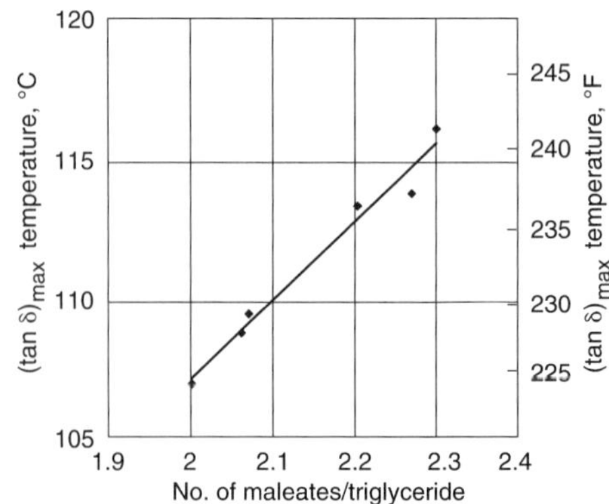

Fig. 7 Peak in tan δ as a function of maleate functionality

Table 3 Tensile and compressive properties of glass-fiber reinforced AESO-based polymer and Dow PC100 vinyl-ester polymer

Polymer	Testing direction	Tensile strength		Tensile modulus		Compressive strength		Compressive modulus	
		MPa	ksi	GPa	10^6 psi	MPa	ksi	GPa	10^6 psi
AESO	0°	463	67.2	24.8	3.60	303	43.9	24.8	3.60
Dow PC100	0°	458	66.5	23.8	3.45	421	61.1	23.4	3.39
AESO	90°	322	46.7	20.7	3.00	181	26.3	20.7	3.00
Dow PC100	90°	324	47.0	17.6	2.55	339	49.2	17.9	2.60

brid composites manufactured from AESO-based resins reinforced with flax and glass fibers are reviewed (Ref 84).

AESO and HSO/MA Glass-Fiber Composites

The properties of the glass-fiber reinforced AESO composites made by RTM are shown in Table 3 (Ref 3). The tensile strength, tensile modulus, and compressive modulus are similar to the properties of the commercial vinyl-ester resin, Dow PC100 (Dow Chemical Co.). The only shortcoming is the compressive strength of the AESO resin, which can be attributed to the lower strength of the AESO neat polymer. However, according to dynamic mechanical analysis, the AESO composite still displayed a T_g close to that of the neat polymer at approximately 80 °C (175 °F). This is much lower than the T_g of the vinyl-ester polymer, which was found to be about 128 °C (262 °F). Figure 8 shows a commercial composite part that was made with soy-based resins and glass fibers by RTM. The agricultural equipment part in Fig. 1 was manufactured similarly.

The HSO/MA composite properties were found to be even more successful at replicating the properties of a vinyl-ester composite, as shown in Table 4. The flexural modulus and compressive strength for the HSO/MA composite were of the same magnitude as the vinyl-ester composite, while the flexural strength was found to be slightly lower. Additionally, the T_g of the HSO/MA composite was found to be approximately 128 °C (262 °F), which equals that found for the vinyl-ester composite.

These results indicate that although the properties of the neat soyoil-based polymers are less than those of the vinyl-ester polymers, the composite material properties with the same fiber and resin content are very similar. In tensile deformation, the fiber reinforcement is able to support the majority of the load, leading to an acceptable modulus and strength. The area in which improvement is needed is in compression deformation, where the polymer bears the majority of the stress.

Table 4 Flexural and compressive properties of HSO/MA-based polymer and Dow 411C50 vinyl-ester polymer

Polymer	Flexural modulus		Flexural strength		Compressive strength	
	GPa	10^6 psi	MPa	ksi	MPa	ksi
HSO/MA	34.5	5.00	669	97	200	29
Dow DK 411C50	35.8	5.19	813	118	290	42

Natural-Fiber Composites

The use of natural fibers with the natural-oil resins described herein promises to give economical, potentially biodegradable or recyclable engineering materials with a high level of vegetable-based raw materials. Such materials have a low market cost and are attractive with respect to global sustainability. As the composite industry becomes more environmentally responsible, resins such as these should find increasing commercial use. Excellent inexpensive composites were made using natural fibers, such as hemp, straw, flax, jute, and wood. It has been found that the soy-based resins have a strong affinity for natural fibers and form an excellent fiber-matrix interface, as determined by scanning electron microscope analysis of fractured composites. Other abundantly available natural products, such as lignin and starch, can make substantial contributions to the composite properties by acting as toughening agents, increasing adhesion between matrix, fillers, and fibers, modifying the biodegradability, improving the antistatic properties, and acting as reinforcement fillers.

The use of natural fibers as a reinforcing fiber or filler in composites has received a lot of attention, as recently reviewed by Williams et al. (Ref 83) and Mohanty et al. (Ref 85). The fibers possess certain properties that make them an attractive alternative to glass fibers. These properties include high specific strength and modulus, low density, low cost, and easy recyclability. The fibers are also safer to handle than glass fibers. Glass fibers produce glass particles that can damage the lungs if inhaled during handling. Natural fibers have been used as reinforcements in both thermoplastics and thermosets. However, the combination of hydrophilic lignocellulosic fibers with hydrophobic resins has led to compatibility problems at the interface. The interface between the matrix and the fibers is very crucial in determining the mechanical properties in composites, and researchers have focused on studying ways to improve the fiber-matrix interface. This problem is often addressed through the use of sizing agents within the composite.

Sizing agents are specifically designed to have chemical functionalities to adhere to both the reinforcing fibers and the polymer matrix. Typically, the sizing agent concentration is of the order of 1 to 2 wt% and provides stronger bonding between the fibers and the matrix, which is essential to the manufacture of high-performance composite materials. Some of the soy-based resins presented here can be used as sizing agents for the natural fibers, with the selection of the correct functional groups. For example, hydrophilic hydroxylated oils that have been maleinized can bond to the fiber as well as the matrix, strengthening the interface.

The low density of natural fibers makes them an attractive alternative to glass fibers in certain applications. The automotive industry is cur-

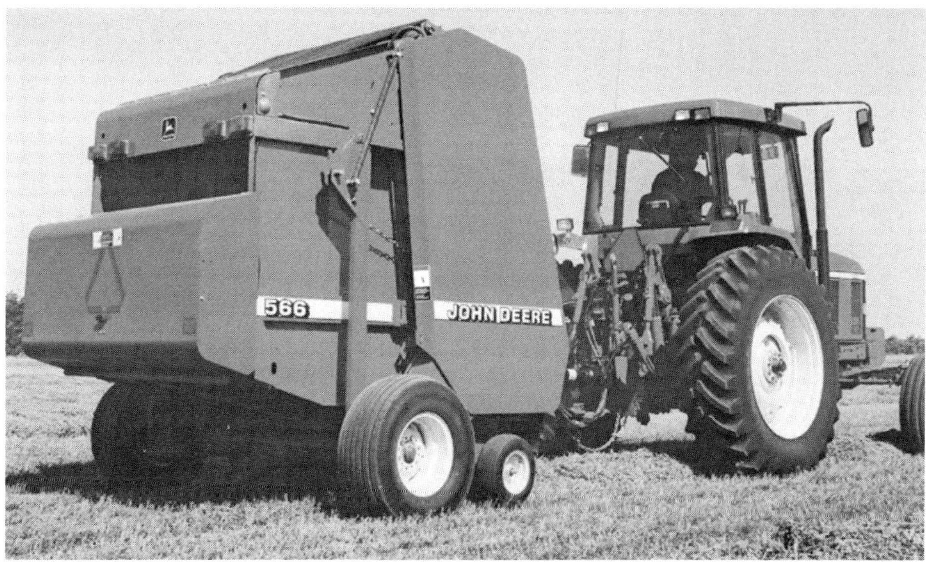

Fig. 8 Round hay bailer. The 2.5 × 1 m (8 × 3 ft) panel containing the name "John Deere" was made from a soy-based resin. Courtesy of John Deere, Moline Illinois

rently using this to their advantage in the battle to reduce the weight of vehicles in order to improve fuel efficiency. The German automotive industry has been a leader in this trend, and several U.S. companies are exploring their use. Parcel shelves, door panels, instrument panels, arm- and headrests, and seat shells can all be made using natural fibers. The construction and furniture industry is also embracing the use of these composites. Superior particle- and fiberboard can be manufactured using natural fibers as reinforcement or fillers in a polymeric matrix. The panel-type composites produced have properties that are comparable to that for wood. The most common resin used to bond the lignocellulosic fibers together is urea formaldehyde. Phenol and melamine formaldehyde are also used as adhesives. The possibility of more stringent regulation of resins containing formaldehyde and the need to reduce the dependence on petroleum products has lead to the search for alternative adhesives for particle- and fiberboards. The use of a plant-triglyceride-based resin as an adhesive in particleboard production is an interesting possibility that is currently being investigated. The farm machinery industry is another industry that provides an attractive application for these materials. It provides a good marketing point for farm machinery producers to use products made by their customers in their products. Combining the natural fibers with plant-triglyceride-based resins produces a very attractive low-cost composite with much potential in this industry. In the future, the greatest impact of natural fibers with bio-based resins may be seen as a wood lumber substitute.

Flax Composites. Flax comes from the stem of the flax plant of the species *Linum usitatissimum*. The flax plant provides linseed oil from the seeds and fibers from the stem. Fibers obtained from the stem of the plant are known as bast fibers. The fiber can be processed to produce linen fabric, which happens to be one of the first plant fibers used by man for making textile. The same fibers obtained from the stem can be used as reinforcement in composite applications. Flax is readily available in North America and Europe. Canada is the world's leader in the production and export of flax, growing 2.1 million acres in 1997. However, only 15% of these acres are being used in industrial pulping of fine paper. Clearly, there is a huge source of untapped flax fibers available for use in composite applications. In the United States, 146,000 acres of flaxseed was planted in 1997, producing 2.17 million bushels (55,143 metric tons) of flax. Most of the flax in the United States is grown in Minnesota, North Dakota, and South Dakota.

The tensile strength of the AESO/flax-fiber composite was found to have a maximum value of 30 MPa (4.4 ksi) at 34% fiber content, which is comparable to the tensile strength of the AESO neat resin (~30 MPa). The flexural strength showed a similar trend, exhibiting a maximum value at approximately 34% fiber content. The flexural moduli of these materials behaved similarly, showing a maximum at 34% fiber content. However, the tensile moduli showed an increase with fiber content, as shown in Fig. 9. Other researchers have noticed this optimization phenomena in strength, which has been explained in terms of increasing fiber-fiber interactions as the fiber content increases (Ref 67). This reduces the level of fiber-matrix interaction, thereby weakening the composite. Percolation theory has also been used to explain this effect (Ref 62).

The tensile or flexural fracture stress, σ, of composites with natural fibers can be determined by the vector percolation model of fracture (Ref 86):

$$\sigma \sim \left[E(\phi)(1-\phi/\phi_c)\right]^{1/2}$$

where $E(\phi)$ is the composite modulus as a function of fiber volume fraction, ϕ, and ϕ_c is a critical fiber fraction. This assumes that natural fibers have defects distributed along their length whose concentration is proportional to ϕ. At a critical concentration $\phi = \phi_c$, the latter equation predicts that the composite becomes fragile. Since the composite stiffness $E(\phi)$ is typically an increasing function of ϕ, as shown in Fig. 9, this relation predicts that in the linear approximation for $E(\phi)$, σ will attain a maximum at some ϕ^* value. From the work of Williams et al. (Ref 83), $\phi^* \approx 35\%$, such that we expect $\phi_c \approx 70\%$. Elimination of such defects via sizing design, internal repair, and healing processes would substantially increase the tensile properties of natural-fiber composites.

Hemp Composites. Hemp fibers are obtained from the bast fibers of the plant *Cannabis sativa*. The fiber has received much negative publicity due to its close relation to marijuana. Both plants are identical in appearance, but differ in their level of tetrahydrocanabinol (THC). Tetrahydrocanabinol is the chemical responsible for giving marijuana its psychoactive properties. Industrial hemp fibers contain less than 0.5% THC, whereas marijuana has anywhere from 3 to 15% THC. The hemp plant is native to China, but by 1750 had become the largest agricultural crop in the world, with extensive use as cloth, canvas, rope, and oil. The 1937 Marijuana Tax Act lead to the demise of industrial hemp as an agricultural crop in the United States. At the time, the government had no way of telling the plants apart. Both plants ended up being regulated under the same law, and by 1958, the government had stopped granting licenses to grow hemp. However, the hemp industry is making a strong comeback. Hemp is a very versatile fabric and can be used in many different products. It has found use in textile, home furnishing, paper, construction, and automotive industry.

Composites made of 20 wt% hemp fiber (supplied by Hempcore of England) were found to display tensile strength of 35 MPa (5.1 ksi) and modulus of 4.4 GPa (638 ksi). The mechanical properties of the all-natural composites are comparable to the properties shown by wood. For example, a typical hardwood has a tensile modulus of about 10 GPa (1450 ksi), with a fracture stress of about 30 MPa (4.4 ksi) when the stress is exerted parallel to the fiber axis and about 3 MPa (0.4 ksi) when the stress is exerted normal to the fiber-grain axis. The considerable advantage of the all-natural composites is that the unidirectional high properties of wood can be obtained in all directions for the randomly oriented fiber composite. In addition, the ease of manufacturing complex shapes via normal composite liquid molding operations provides a significant cost as well as ease-of-fabrication advantage for these materials. In countries such as China, the depletion of forests to supply wood for the housing industry is strongly discouraged, and the natural-fiber composites would make an excellent substitute for construction lumber.

Hybrid composites were manufactured using glass (E-glass woven fiber) and Durafiber grade 2 flax fibers (Cargill Limited Inc.) in an AESO-based polymer (Ref 84). These were manufactured in symmetric and asymmetric manners by RTM. In the symmetric hybrid composites (G/F/G), a layer of flax fiber (F) was sandwiched in between two layers of glass fiber (G). The asymmetric composites (G/G/F) were produced by uniformly arranging the flax fibers at the bottom of the mold in a random mat and then placing the two layers of woven glass fabric on top. The AESO resin was then injected with vacuum assist into the mold and cured. The tensile modulus, tensile strength, and compressive strength of hybrid composites for different glass/flax ratios and composite constructions are shown in Table 5. As can be expected, these properties all increase with increasing glass-fiber content. The 100% flax-fiber-reinforced materials show a tensile strength and modulus of 26.1 ± 1.7 MPa (3.8 ± 0.2 ksi) and 1.9 ± 0.1 GPa (275 ± 15 ksi), respectively, while the 100% glass-fiber-reinforced materials show tensile strength and modulus of 128.8 ± 1.1 MPa (18.7 ± 0.16 ksi) and 5.2 ± 0.1 GPa (754 ± 15 ksi), respectively. As shown in Table 6, the asymmetric composites have tensile moduli very similar to the moduli of the symmetric composites. However, the tensile and compressive strengths of the asymmetric composites were noticeably less than the symmetric composites. This is due to the different

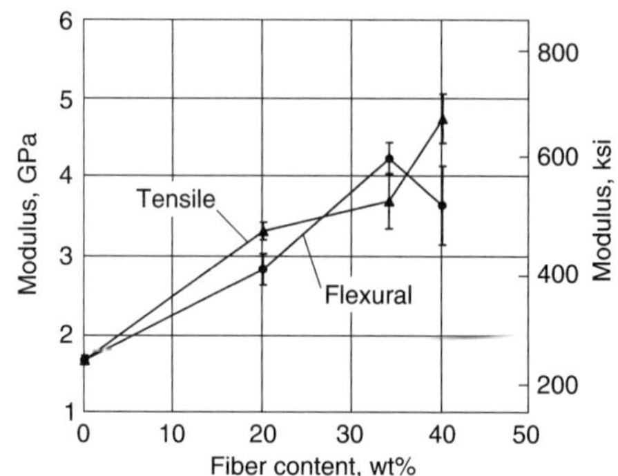

Fig. 9 Modulus dependence on composition for flax (Durafiber-grade 2)-reinforced AESO polymer

modes of failure exhibited by the two types of composites. The symmetric composites undergo tensile failure at the peak load while the asymmetric composites fail by shear delamination at the glass/flax interface due to the difference in the tensile moduli of the two fiber types.

The flexural properties of the glass/flax hybrid composites are shown in Table 7. The flexural modulus and strength for the glass-fiber composite are much higher than those for the flax-fiber composite due to the higher modulus and strength of glass fibers. The 100% flax-reinforced composites display a flexural strength and modulus of 61.0 ± 3.4 MPa (8.8 ± 0.5 ksi) and 3.8 ± 0.2 GPa (551 ± 29 ksi), respectively. The 100% glass-fiber-reinforced composites have a flexural strength and modulus of 205.5 ± 4.5 MPa (29.8 ± 0.65 ksi) and 9.0 ± 0.2 GPa (1305 ± 29 ksi), respectively. Additionally, there is an obvious anisotropy in the behavior of the asymmetric composites, depending on the surface that bears the load. The maximum flexural strengths were obtained when the flax surface was the surface bearing the exerted load or impact. In such an orientation, the glass fibers bear a tensile load during the bending of the sample.

The impact energy of the hybrid composites ranged from 13.3 ± 0.3 to 28.7 ± 1.2 J (9.8 ± 0.2 to 21.2 ± 0.9 ft · lbf). The maximum impact energy absorbed (28.7 ± 1.2 J, or 21.2 ± 0.9 ft · lbf) was shown by the asymmetric 40/60 glass/flax ratio composite when the flax surface was the load-bearing face. The energy absorption by the symmetric hybrid composites seems to be only marginally higher than that of the 100% glass-fiber composite, a difference made even more insignificant considering the standard deviations. Thus, to reduce cost and weight, flax could be used in place of glass as the outer laminates in composites subjected to impact. The transverse impact is the most common in-service loading mode in composites. In structural applications it could be an impact from a dropped tool; in aircraft applications it could be an impact from a bird; and in aerospace applications it could be an impact from space debris.

Ballistic Impact Resistance of Soy Resin Composites

High-performance polymer composites based on aramid fibers, S-glass fibers, and more recently, gel-spun polyethylene fibers are widely used in applications demanding protection from ballistic impact. These applications include personal armor and armor for equipment. The armor is designed with respect to the threat level, that is, anticipated projectiles, type of ammunition and weapons, velocity of projectiles, and so on. For very high-velocity protection, an armor with a ceramic front plate and a polymer composite backing is selected. For personal protection where the weight of the armor is an important issue, fibers with a low density, such as aramid and gel-spun polyethylene, are commonly used. For equipment protection, on the other hand, S-glass fibers are used.

The ballistic impact of composites is measured in terms of the *V*50 parameter, which is defined as the velocity, *V*, at which the probability of complete penetration of the target by the projectile is 50%. This involves firing a minimum of six shots at the target, such that three are complete penetrations and three are partial penetrations. The *V*50 is then given by the average of the six strike velocities. In the current study, ballistic impact resistance was determined on S-glass fiber-reinforced soy-based resin panels (305 × 305 × 19 mm, or 12 × 12 × 0.75 in.). The panels were made by the Seeman composite resin infusion molding process (SCRIMP) method at room temperature and cured at 110 °C (230 °F) for 60 min. The composite consisted of 28 woven S-glass fabric layers. The composite was found to have a *V*50 of about 550 m/s (1,800 ft/s) using 50 caliber (13.5 g) blunt-nosed fragment-simulating projectiles. This ballistic impact resistance is at least comparable to, if not better than, epoxy- and vinyl-ester-based composites. The composites were found to absorb the kinetic energy of the impacting projectiles by tensile failure of fibers, fiber pull-out, delamination, and shear between different layers in the composite.

When 19 mm (0.75 in.) thick ceramic tiles (Coors alumina, CoorsTec) were placed on the soy-based composite, the ballistic impact *V*50 resistance improved to 950 m/s (3,100 ft/s) for 20 mm (53.75 g) projectiles. The role of a ceramic frontface backed by a polymer composite backplate is to spread the impact energy over a larger area. The hard ceramic plate also deforms and blunts the projectile. On ballistic impact, the ceramic is shattered and it spreads the impact over a much larger area. The delocalized energy is then absorbed by the polymer-composite backplate. This increases the amount of energy absorbed and therefore improves the ballistic performance. The enhanced impact resistance of soy-based composites is also attributed to both the low-temperature beta relaxation (similar to polycarbonate), which occurs by virtue of the floppy nature of the triglyceride, coupled with the excellent frictional energy dissipation, which the resin-fiber interface generates during impact.

Biodegradable Composites

Most of the plant-oil-based composite resins described in this article were found to be nonbiodegradable, as required for the traditional long-life applications, but some, such as the ami-

Table 5 Tensile and compression properties of symmetric glass/flax hybrid composites

	Weight fractions		Tensile modulus		Tensile strength		Compressive strength	
Glass/flax ratio	Glass	Flax	GPa	ksi	MPa	ksi	MPa	ksi
100/0	0.35	0.00	5.2 ± 0.1	754 ± 15	128.8 ± 1.1	18.7 ± 0.16	89.8 ± 3.2	13.0 ± 0.46
80/20	0.25	0.06	3.5 ± 0.1	508 ± 15	123.3 ± 1.2	17.9 ± 0.17	71.6 ± 2.6	10.4 ± 0.38
60/40	0.23	0.16	3.2 ± 0.1	464 ± 15	109.1 ± 1.0	15.8 ± 0.15	62.3 ± 3.1	9.0 ± 0.45
40/60	0.16	0.24	2.9 ± 0.2	420 ± 29	82.6 ± 1.4	12.0 ± 0.20	33.6 ± 0.8	4.9 ± 0.12
0/100	0.00	0.31	1.9 ± 0.1	275 ± 15	26.1 ± 1.7	3.8 ± 0.25	18.5 ± 2.4	2.7 ± 0.35

Table 6 Tensile and compression properties of asymmetric glass/flax hybrid composites

	Weight fractions		Tensile modulus		Tensile strength		Compressive strength	
Glass/flax ratio	Glass	Flax	GPa	ksi	MPa	ksi	MPa	ksi
80/20	0.25	0.06	3.4 ± 0.1	493 ± 15	111.7 ± 2.1	16.2 ± 0.30	65.3 ± 4.8	9.5 ± 0.70
60/40	0.24	0.16	3.1 ± 0.1	450 ± 15	90.6 ± 2.4	13.1 ± 0.35	46.2 ± 0.6	6.7 ± 0.09
40/60	0.16	0.25	2.7 ± 0.3	392 ± 44	68.9 ± 2.1	10.0 ± 0.30	30.1 ± 2.2	4.3 ± 0.32

Table 7 Flexural properties and energy absorption on impact of glass/flax hybrid composites

Glass/flax ratio	Weight fractions		Composite construction	Loading/impact face	Flexural modulus		Flexural strength		Energy absorbed	
	Glass	Flax			GPa	ksi	MPa	ksi	J	ft · lbf
100/0	0.35	0.00	...	...	9.0 ± 0.2	1305 ± 29	205.5 ± 4.5	29.8 ± 0.65	16.5 ± 0.2	12.2 ± 0.1
80/20	0.25	0.06	Symmetric	...	6.9 ± 0.2	1001 ± 29	130.3 ± 3.0	18.9 ± 0.44	17.7 ± 1.9	13.0 ± 1.4
	0.25	0.06	Asymmetric	Glass	6.3 ± 0.3	914 ± 44	87.8 ± 3.9	12.7 ± 0.57	13.3 ± 0.3	9.8 ± 0.2
	0.25	0.06	Asymmetric	Flax	5.0 ± 0.1	725 ± 15	189.0 ± 8.5	27.4 ± 1.23	25.8 ± 1.1	19.0 ± 0.8
60/40	0.23	0.16	Symmetric	...	6.0 ± 0.2	870 ± 29	115.3 ± 2.5	16.7 ± 0.36	18.0 ± 0.3	13.3 ± 0.2
	0.24	0.16	Asymmetric	Glass	4.0 ± 0.3	580 ± 44	80.1 ± 0.7	11.6 ± 0.10	14.7 ± 0.3	10.8 ±
	0.24	0.16	Asymmetric	Flax	4.7 ± 0.3	682 ± 44	146.9 ± 5.5	21.3 ± 0.80	27.6 ± 2.6	20.3 ± 1.9
40/60	0.16	0.24	Symmetric	...	5.8 ± 0.5	841 ± 73	83.3 ± 5.4	12.1 ± 0.78	18.5 ± 0.2	13.6 ± 0.1
	0.16	0.25	Asymmetric	Glass	3.8 ± 0.1	551 ± 15	73.2 ± 7.5	10.6 ± 1.09	15.1 ± 0.3	11.1 ± 0.2
	0.16	0.25	Asymmetric	Flax	3.3 ± 0.4	479 ± 58	111.1 ± 9.5	16.1 ± 1.38	28.7 ± 1.2	21.2 ± 0.9
0/100	0.00	0.31	...	...	3.8 ± 0.2	551 ± 29	61.0 ± 3.4	8.8 ± 0.49	1.4 ± 0.2	1.0 ± 0.1

dated monoglyceride, were found to be biodegradable (as determined by weight loss in soil burial tests), as might be expected for materials made with triglycerides. The biodegradable composites could be useful in applications where the biodegradability is an important component of the materials performance in aquatic and terrestrial environments, or in municipal solid waste management where composting and landfill reclamation are considered to be important. Compostable packaging and products that are disposed in the environment would particularly benefit from the new soy-based materials. The variety of biodegradable thermoplastics resins, natural fibers, and their biocomposite properties have recently been reviewed by Mohanty et al. (Ref 85). The four mechanisms of degradation of composites (biodegradation, microorganism degradation, photo degradation, and chemical degradation) and the kinetics of biodegradation of starch-based composites have also been examined (Ref 85).

Conclusions

Triglyceride oils derived from plants have been used to synthesize several different monomers for use in structural applications. These monomers have been found to form polymers with a wide range of properties. Composite materials have been manufactured using these resins and have produced a variety of durable and strong materials. Besides glass fibers, natural fibers such as flax and hemp were used. The properties exhibited by both the natural- and synthetic-fiber-reinforced composites can be combined through the production of hybrid composites. These materials combine the low cost of natural fibers with the high performance of synthetic fibers. Their properties lie between those displayed by the all-glass and all-natural composites. Characterization of the polymer properties also presents opportunities for improvement through genetic engineering technology.

This area of research sets a foundation from which completely new materials can be produced with novel properties. Work is continuing to optimize the properties of these materials and understand the fundamental issues that affect them. In this manner, more renewable resources can be used to meet the material demands of many industries.

REFERENCES

1. S.N. Khot, J.J. La Scala, E. Can, S.S. Morye, G.R. Palmese, S.H. Kusefoglu, and R.P. Wool, *J. Appl. Polym. Sci.*, 2001, in press
2. R.P. Wool, *Chemtech,* Vol 29, 1999, p 44
3. R.P. Wool, S.H. Kusefoglu, G.R. Palmese, R. Zhao, and S.N. Khot, U.S. Patent 6,121,398, 2000
4. K. Liu, *Soybeans: Chemistry, Technology, and Utilization,* Chapman and Hall, New York, 1997
5. F. Gunstone, *Fatty Acid and Lipid Chemistry,* Blackie Academic and Professional, New York, 1996
6. A. Cunningham and A. Yapp, U.S. Patent, 3,827,993, 1974
7. G.W. Bussell, U.S. Patent, 3,855,163, 1974
8. L.E. Hodakowski, C.L. Osborn, and E.B. Harris, U.S. Patent 4,119,640, 1975
9. D.J. Trecker, G.W. Borden, and O.W. Smith, U.S. Patent 3,979,270, 1976
10. D.J. Trecker, G.W. Borden, and O.W. Smith, U.S. Patent 3,931,075, 1976
11. D.K. Salunkhe, J.K. Chavan, R.N. Adsule, and S.S. Kadam, *World Oilseeds: Chemistry, Technology, and Utilization,* Van Nostrand Reinhold, New York, 1992
12. C.G. Force and F.S. Starr, U.S. Patent 4,740,367, 1988
13. L.W. Barrett, L.H. Sperling, and C.J. Murphy, *J. Am. Oil Chem. Soc.,* Vol 70, 1993, p 523
14. S. Qureshi, J.A. Manson, L.H. Sperling, and C.J. Murphy, *Proc. American Chemical Society* (New York), 1983
15. N. Devia, J.A. Manson, L.H. Sperling, and A. Conde, *Polym. Eng. Sci.,* Vol 19, 1979, p 878
16. N. Devia, J.A. Manson, L.H. Sperling, and A. Conde, *Polym. Eng. Sci.,* Vol 19, 1979, p 869
17. N. Devia, J.A. Manson, L.H. Sperling, and A. Conde, *Macromolecules,* Vol 12, 1979, p 360
18. L.H. Sperling, C.E. Carraher, S.P. Qureshi, J.A. Manson, and L.W. Barrett, *Polymers from Biotechnology,* Plenum Press, New York, 1991
19. A.M. Fernandez, C.J. Murphy, M.T. DeCosta, J.A. Manson, and L.H. Sperling, *Proc. American Chemical Society* (New York), 1983
20. I. Frischinger and S. Dirlikov, *Polym. Commun.,* Vol 32, 1991, p 536
21. J. Rosch and R. Mulhaupt, *Polym. Bull.,* Vol 31, 1993, p 679
22. F. Li, R.C. Larock, and J.U. Otaigbe, *Polymer,* Vol 41, 2000, p 4849
23. F. Li and R.C. Larock, *J. Appl. Polym. Sci.,* Vol 78, 2000, p 1044
24. F. Li and R.C. Larock, *J. Polym. Sci. B, Polym. Phys.,* Vol 38, 2000, p 2721
25. F. Li, D.W. Marks, R.C. Larock, and J.U. Otaigbe, *Polymer,* Vol 41, 2000, p 7925
26. A. Meffert and H. Kluth, Denmark Patent 4,886,893, 1989
27. B. Rangarajan, A. Havey, E.A. Grulke, and P.D. Culnan, *J. Am. Oil Chem. Soc.,* Vol 72, 1995, p 1161
28. F.A. Zaher, M.H. El-Malla, and M.M. El-Hefnawy, *J. Am. Oil Chem. Soc.,* Vol 66, 1989, p 698
29. A. Friedman, S.B. Polovsky, J.P. Pavlichko, and L.S. Moral, U.S. Patent 5,576,027, 1996
30. D. Swern, G.N. Billen, T.W. Findley, and J.T. Scanlan, *J. Am. Chem. Soc.,* Vol 67, 1945, p 1786
31. N.O.V. Sonntag, *J. Am. Oil Chem. Soc.,* Vol 59, 1982, p 795
32. D.H. Solomon, *The Chemistry of Organic Film Formers,* Wiley, New York, 1967
33. E. Can, master's thesis, Bogazici University, 1999
34. D. Swern, *Bailey's Industrial Oil and Fat Products,* Wiley, New York, 1979
35. M. Hellsten, I. Harwigsson, and C. Brink, U.S. Patent 5,911,236, 1999
36. F.W. Cain, A.J. Kuin, P.A. Cynthia, and P.T. Quinlan, U.S. Patent 5,912,042, 1995
37. K. Eckwert, L. Jeromin, A. Meffert, E. Peukert, and B. Gutsche, U.S. Patent 4,647,678, 1987
38. S.N. Khot, master's thesis, University of Delaware, 1998
39. J. Wypych, *Polyvinyl Chloride Stabilization,* Elsevier, Amsterdam, 1986
40. J.K. Sears and J.R. Darby, *The Technology of Plasticizers,* Wiley, New York, 1982
41. K.D. Carlson and S.P. Chang, *J. Am. Oil Chem. Soc.,* Vol 62, 1985, p 934
42. I. Frischinger and S. Dirlikov, in *Interpenetrating Polymer Networks, Advances in Chemistry Series,* L.H. Sperling, D. Kempner, and L. Utracki, Ed., American Chemical Society, Vol 239, 1994, p 517
43. R. Raghavachar, R.J. Letasi, P.V. Kola, Z. Chen, and J.L. Massingill, *J. Am. Oil Chem. Soc.,* Vol 76, 1999, p 511
44. R.M. Pashley, T.J. Senden, R.A. Morris, J.T. Guthrie, and W.D. He, U.S. Patent 5,360,880, 1994
45. W.R. Likavec and C.R. Bradley, U.S. Patent 5,866,628, 1999
46. G.W. Bordon, O.W. Smith, and D.J. Trecker, U.S. Patent 4,025,477, 1974
47. J.J. La Scala, S.P. Bunker, and R.P. Wool, *J. Am. Oil Chem. Soc.,* in preparation
48. S.P. Bunker, master's thesis, University of Delaware, 2000
49. T.-J. Chu and D.-Y. Niou, *J. Chin. Inst. Chem. Eng.,* Vol 20, 1989, p 1
50. A.T. Betts, U.S. Patent 3,867,354, 1975
51. E.L. Mitch and S.L. Kaplan, *Proc. 33rd Annual Society of Plastics Engineers Technical Conference* (Atlanta, GA), 1975
52. E. Can, S. Kusefoglu, and R.P. Wool, *J. Appl. Polym. Sci.,* Vol 81, 2001, p 69
53. H.C. Gardner and R.J. Cotter, European Patent 20,945, 1981
54. P. Thomas and J. Mayer, U.S. Patent 3,784,586, 1974
55. S.H. Lee, T.W. Park, and S.O. Lee, *Polymer (Korea),* Vol 23, 1999, p 493
56. H. Shione and J. Yamada, Japanese Patent 11,147,222, 1999
57. H. Hasegawa, Japanese Patent 11,240,014, 1999
58. L.K. Johnson and W.T. Sade, *J. Coatings Tech.,* Vol 65, 1993, p 19
59. T.W.G. Solomons, *Organic Chemistry,* Wiley, New York, 1992
60. P.J. Flory, *Principles of Polymer Chemistry,* Cornell University, Ithaca, New York, 1975
61. L.E. Nielsen and R.F. Landel, *Mechanical*

Properties of Polymers and Composites, Marcel Dekker, New York, 1994
62. R.P. Wool and S.N. Khot, *Proc. Advanced Composites at the University of New South Wales ACUN-2* (Sydney, Australia), 2000
63. S.H. Kusefoglu, R.P. Wool, and E. Can, *J. Appl. Polym. Sci.,* in preparation
64. E. Can, S.H. Kusefoglu, and R.P. Wool, *J. Appl. Polym. Sci.,* 2001, in press
65. J.J. La Scala and R.P. Wool, *J. Amer. Oil Chem. Soc.,* 2001, in press
66. N.G. McCrum, C.P. Buckley, and C.B. Bucknall, *Principles of Polymer Engineering,* Oxford University Press, New York, 1997
67. L.U. Devi, S.S. Bhagawan, and S. Thomas, *J. Appl. Polym. Sci.,* Vol 64, 1997, p 1739
68. A.K. Bledzki, S. Reihmane, and J. Gassan, *J. Appl. Polym. Sci.,* Vol 59, 1996, p 1329
69. A.K. Saha, S. Das, D. Bhatta, and B.C. Mitra, *J. Appl. Polym. Sci.,* Vol 71, 1999, p 1505
70. P. Ghosh and P.K. Ganguly, *Plast., Rubber Compos. Process. Appl.,* Vol 20, 1993, p 171
71. J. Gassan and A.K. Bledzki, *Polym. Compos.,* Vol 18, 1997, p 179
72. T.M. Gowda, A.C.B. Naidu, and C. Rajput, *Compos. Part A: Appl. Sci. Manuf.,* Vol 30, 1999, p 277
73. R.J.A. Shalash, S.M. Khayat, and E.A. Sarah, *J. Pet. Res.,* Vol 8, 1989, p 215
74. S. Mishra and J.B. Naik, *J. Appl. Polym. Sci.,* Vol 68, 1998, p 1417
75. T. Czvikovszky, H. Hargitai, I. Racz, and G. Csukat, Beam Interactions with Materials and Atoms, *Nucl. Instrum. Methods Phys. Res. B,* Vol 151 (No. 1–4), May 1999, p 190–195
76. P.R. Hornsby, E. Hinrichsen, and K. Tarverdi, *J. Mater. Sci.,* Vol 32, 1997, p 443
77. K.P. Mieck, R. Luetzkendorf, and T. Reussmann, *Polym. Compos.,* Vol 17, 1996, p 873
78. X. Chen, Q. Guo, and Y. Mi, *J. Appl. Polym. Sci.,* Vol 69, 1998, p 1891
79. J. George, M.S. Sreekala, S. Thomas, S.S. Bhagawan, and N.R. Neelakantan, *J. Reinf. Plast. Compos.,* Vol 17, 1998, p 651
80. H.D. Rozman, B.K. Kon, A. Abusamah, R.N. Kumar, and Z.A.M. Ishak, *J. Appl. Polym. Sci.,* Vol 69, 1998, p 1993
81. R.M. Kishore, M.K. Shridhar, and R.M.V.G.K. Rao, *J. Mater. Sci. Lett.,* Vol 2, 1983, p 99
82. A.N. Shah and S.C. Lakkad, *Fibre Sci. Technol.,* Vol 15, 1981, p 41
83. G.I. Williams and R.P. Wool, *J. Appl. Compos.,* Vol 7 (No. 5), 2000, p 421
84. S.S. Morye and R.P. Wool, *Polym. Compos.,* in press
85. A.K. Mohanty, M. Misra, and G. Hinrichsen, *Macromol. Mater. Eng.,* Vol 276, 2000, p 1
86. R.P. Wool, *Polymer Interfaces: Structure and Strength,* Hanser Gardner, Munich, 1995

Engineering Mechanics, Analysis, and Design

Chairperson: Scott Reeve, National Composite Center

Introduction to Engineering Mechanics, Analysis, and Design

Scott Reeve, National Composite Center

COMPOSITE MATERIALS offer amazing opportunities for delivering structures that are optimized to meet design requirements. The flexibility to tailor a design for each application also means that design and analysis for composites are more complex than for traditional materials. Full utilization of the advantages of composite materials requires an understanding of the mechanics at multiple levels, the analytical approaches and tools, and the methodologies employed in the design process. This Section of the Volume introduces many of the engineering approaches used in composite industry. The Section is comprised of three general areas: mechanics, analysis, and design.

Mechanics

The mechanics area addresses composites at two levels: micromechanics and macromechanics. The article "Micromechanics" provides an understanding of the behavior of the fiber and resin constituents and how their combination affects higher level composite behavior. Micromechanics played a significant role in the formative years of composites development. Micromechanics has limitations in predicting higher level lamina properties, so many current approaches use macromechanics (addressed in the article "Macromechanics Analysis of Laminate Properties"). As composite analysis continues to expand, refinements in micromechanics and fracture mechanics will enable the full capability of composites to be modeled and exploited.

Analysis

Macromechanics uses the ply level as the building block for analyzing composite laminate behavior. Lamination theory is used to accurately predict laminate properties. These analysis methods address:

- Stress-strain relationship for membrane and bending response
- Thermal and moisture effects
- Inelastic behavior
- Strength and failure
- Interlaminar stresses

The article "Hygrothermal Behavior" illustrates the importance of considering thermal and moisture effects. The article "Characterizing Strength from a Structural Design Perspective" concerns analyzing the strength of composites, critical to predicting failure of any laminate. Successful use of two-dimensional composites requires an understanding of interlaminar stresses, and fracture mechanics offers a promising method for this need (see the article "Fracture Mechanics of Composite Delamination"). Composites provide excellent damping properties and are much less sensitive to fatigue degradation than metals. Two articles, "Damping Properties" and "Fatigue and Life Prediction," address these topics.

Structural analysis is the next level beyond laminate analysis. It addresses loadings and geometries that occur when the composite laminates are used in functional structure. The structural analysis topics discussed in this Volume include:

- Bolted and bonded joints
- Stability
- Damage tolerance
- Out-of-plane effects
- Sandwich structure

"Bolted and Bonded Joints" discusses considerations necessary to integrate all composite parts in the overall product. The stress concentrations associated with the load transfer at joints are one of the most important areas that must be analyzed. "Instability Considerations" addresses buckling analyses specially formulated for orthotropic materials and laminates. The article "Damage Tolerance" addresses the use of empirical and analytical methods for assessing the damage tolerance of composite laminates and structures. Design guidelines and lessons learned for damage tolerance have been accumulated in three decades of composite applications. As the advantages of composites in integrated structures are exploited, the complex configurations often result in out-of-plane loads on the laminate shells and integrated parts. Analyses of the out-of-plane effects are needed to ensure satisfactory performances, as discussed in the article "Out-of-Plane Analysis." Sandwich structures continue to be widely used as weight-efficient designs to carry bending and pressure loads. "Analysis of Sandwich Structures" discusses design and analysis along with unique aspects when using composite facesheets.

The orthotropic nature of composites along with the complexity of integrated structures necessitates the use of numerical analysis to fully determine the loads, stresses, and strains that occur in the composite structure. The capabilities of numerical analyses to address the unique issues of composite structures has greatly increased in the past years, and the article "Finite Element Analysis" addresses current methods, limitations, and uses. The article "Computer Programs" reviews current state-of-the-art software that is available and easily used on personal computers. The software programs analyze all levels of composites, from micromechanics to macromechanics to structure.

The final article on analysis, "Testing and Analysis Correlation," addresses the importance of correlating test results and analytical data. Tests results inspire improvements to the scope and accuracy of analysis methods. Validated analysis methods that correctly predict test failure modes and strengths can confidently be used to reduce the quantity of tests (and costs) necessary to substantiate the use of composites in structures.

Design

The third general area in this Section addresses design. The first article, "Design Criteria," describes the types of criteria that must be considered when applying composite materials. The next article, "Design Allowables," explains the procedures involved in generating design allowables. Establishing design values is a critical foundation for beginning the design and analysis process. The ability to design complex and integrated composite structures has been greatly enhanced by the availability of computer aided design (CAD), described in "Computer-Aided Design and Manufacturing." The exponential growth of computing power and software packages provides the designer with tools to quickly and accurately develop composite designs. The CAD packages are now integrated with downstream manufacturing functions. This integration of design, tooling, and manufacturing, discussed in "Design, Tooling, and Manufacturing Interaction," is very important to the successful and cost-efficient application of composites.

In the design and analysis of practical composites structures, one factor that must not be overlooked is cost, discussed in "Cost Analysis." Future growth of composite applications is dependent on the design of cost-effective parts. Affordability has become much more important, even in high-performance aircraft. The article on cost analysis emphasizes this issue and discusses the development of cost models to assist the designer. Another tool to reduce the overall cost of composite development is discussed in the article "Rapid Prototyping." Low-cost methods of prototyping parts provides quick feedback to improve designs and identify manufacturing issues early in the design process. The composite industry has developed a collective body of knowledge that provides guidelines and lessons learned for using composite materials (see the article "Design Guidelines"). These assist both new and experienced users in all aspects of composite material selection, design, analysis, and manufacturing. The guidelines are especially beneficial for topics in which analysis methods have not been fully developed and designers must rely on empirical results and experience.

The final two articles, "Engineering Mechanics, Analysis, and Design of Metal-Matrix Composites" and "Fracture Analysis of Fiber-Reinforced Ceramic-Matrix Composites," address the unique aspects that must be considered when using metal-matrix and ceramic-matrix composites.

Micromechanics

WITH INCREASING USE of high-strength and high-stiffness fibers in materials designed to yield a desired set of properties, new interest has arisen in the relationships between the mechanical and physical properties of composites and those of their constituents. A study of the property relationships facilitates analysis of the performance of structures using these heterogeneous materials and provides guidelines for the development of improved materials.

The entire design process has been greatly affected by inclusion of the material design phase in the structural design process. In the preliminary design, the materials considered will usually include many that are still experimental, for which property data are not available. Thus, preliminary material selection may be based on analytically predicted properties. The analytical methods used are the result of studies of the relationship between the effective properties of composites and their constituents (studies that, although not actually conducted at a microscopic level, are frequently described by the term micromechanics). When the relationships between the overall or average response of a composite and the properties of its constituents are understood, the nonhomogeneous composite can be represented by an effective homogeneous (and, usually, anisotropic) material. The properties of this homogeneous material are the effective properties of the composite; that is, they are the properties that give the average values of the state variables in the composite. When the effective properties of a unidirectional composite have been determined, the material may be viewed as a homogeneous anisotropic material for many aspects of the design process. The evaluation of these effective properties is the major topic of this article.

Physical Properties of Fiber Composites: General Concepts

A unidirectional fiber composite (UDC) consists of aligned continuous fibers that are embedded in a matrix (Fig. 1). Fibers currently used are glass, carbon, graphite, and boron; typical matrices are polymeric, such as epoxy, and light metallic, primarily aluminum alloys. The physical properties of a UDC as measured by means of laboratory specimens are called effective properties. A typical specimen is a flat coupon containing many fibers. The effective physical properties are functions of both fiber and matrix physical properties, of their volume fractions, and perhaps also of statistical parameters associated with fiber distribution. The fibers usually have circular cross sections with little variability of diameters. A UDC is clearly anisotropic, because properties in the fiber direction are different from properties transverse to the fibers. The effective properties that are considered herein include elasticity, thermal expansion coefficients, moisture swelling coefficients, static and dynamic viscoelastic properties, conductivity, and moisture diffusivity.

Traditionally, material properties have been obtained experimentally and have been compiled in handbooks. Such an approach is not practical for fiber composites because of their large variety. There are many kinds of carbon and graphite fibers with different anisotropic properties, and there are many kinds of matrix materials with different properties (Ref 1). There also are different environmental effects on those matrix properties. Because experimental determination of all the effective anisotropic properties of interest is impossible, analytical procedures must be developed (on the basis of fiber and matrix properties, volume fractions, and perhaps fiber distribution) to determine those properties. The task of experimentation is to check the validity of the analytical procedures. Thus, the properties are determined from the point of view of structural mechanics, not of materials science. Indeed, composite materials are complicated structures, not materials in the classical sense.

A variety of analytical methods that may be used to determine various properties of a UDC are described in the following sections. Details of derivations may be found in Ref 2 and 3. Reference 4 is also helpful.

Elastic Properties

The elastic properties of a material are a measure of its stiffness and are used to determine the deformations produced by loads. In a UDC, the stiffness is provided by the fibers; the matrix prevents lateral deflection of the fibers. An illustration may be obtained by comparing a bundle of stiff fibers with a UDC containing the same amount of fibers embedded in a polymeric matrix. If the stiffness of the polymer is neglected, the bundle and the UDC will have the same stiffness for a tensile load; in this case, the bundle functions like a rope. However, if compressive load is applied to the bundle in the fiber direction, the bundle will buckle at once; its stiffness for this load is zero. This is in contrast to the UDC, which has the same stiffness for compressive and tensile loads, because the matrix prevents fiber buckling until high values of load are applied. Similarly, the bundle has no transverse tensile stiffness, because the fibers will separate at once. This again will be prevented in the UDC by the matrix.

The elastic properties of a UDC are functions of the elastic properties of fibers and matrix and of their relative volumes in the composite material. Clearly, the stiffness in the fiber direction is much greater than the stiffness transverse to the fibers. If a load is applied in the fiber direction, it is carried primarily by the fibers, which deform very little and constrain the matrix to small deformation. On the other hand, in the direction normal to the fibers, the matrix is a continuous load-carrying structure and the fibers move with the deforming matrix, not significantly impeding deformation. Therefore, the stiffness in the direction transverse to the fibers is much less than the stiffness in the fiber direction, making the material highly anisotropic.

For engineering purposes, it is necessary to determine Young's modulus in the fiber direction (large), Young's modulus transverse to the fibers

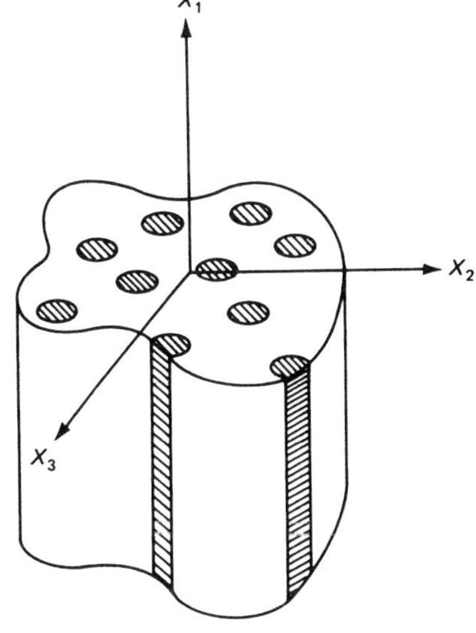

Fig. 1 Unidirectional fiber-reinforced composite

(small), shear modulus along the fibers, and shear modulus in the plane transverse to the fibers, as well as various Poisson's ratios. This can be done in terms of simple analytical expressions.

Elastic properties of homogeneous materials are defined by relations between homogeneous (constant) stress and strain. Because of the various symmetries, there are 21 independent elastic moduli or compliances in the most general case.

The fundamental property of a fiber composite or any other composite material is statistical homogeneity. This implies that the properties of a sufficiently large sample element containing many fibers are the same as those of the entire specimen. Because the fibers are usually randomly placed, there is no preferred direction in the transverse x_2x_3 plane, which implies that the UDC is statistically transversely isotropic.

Experimental determination of the properties of homogeneous materials is based on induction of homogeneous states of stress and strain in suitable specimens. The mathematical interpretation is the application of suitable boundary conditions in terms of tractions of displacements that produce homogenous states of stress and strain, or so-called homogeneous boundary conditions. Examples are simple tension, pure shear, and hydrostatic loading. An experimenter would naturally think to apply the same homogeneous boundary conditions to composite specimens. In this case, however, the states of stress and strain in the specimen are no longer homogeneous but highly complex. The variations of stress and strain on any plane through the composite material are random; nothing specific distinguishes the variation on one plane from that on another. Such stress and strain fields are called statistically homogeneous. They consist essentially of constant averages with superimposed random noise and are produced in geometrically statistically homogeneous specimens subjected to homogeneous boundary conditions. Consequently, effective elastic properties are defined by relations between average stress and average strain.

A typical transverse section of a UDC shows random fiber placement; hence, the material is statistically transversely isotropic. Its effective elastic stress-strain relations have the form:

$$\begin{aligned}\bar{\sigma}_{11} &= n^*\bar{\varepsilon}_{11} + \ell^*\bar{\varepsilon}_{22} + \ell^*\bar{\varepsilon}_{33}\\ \bar{\sigma}_{22} &= \ell^*\bar{\varepsilon}_{11} + (k^* + G_T^*)\bar{\varepsilon}_{22} + (k^* + G_T^*)\bar{\varepsilon}_{33}\\ \bar{\sigma}_{33} &= \ell^*\bar{\varepsilon}_{11} + (k^* + G_T^*)\bar{\varepsilon}_{22} + (k^* + G_T^*)\bar{\varepsilon}_{33}\end{aligned} \quad \text{(Eq 1a)}$$

$$\begin{aligned}\bar{\sigma}_{12} &= 2G_L^*\bar{\varepsilon}_{12}\\ \bar{\sigma}_{23} &= 2G_T^*\bar{\varepsilon}_{23}\\ \bar{\sigma}_{13} &= 2G_L^*\bar{\varepsilon}_{13}\end{aligned} \quad \text{(Eq 1b)}$$

with inverse

$$\begin{aligned}\bar{\varepsilon}_{11} &= \frac{\bar{\sigma}_{11}}{E_L^*} - \frac{\nu_L^*}{E_L^*}\bar{\sigma}_{22} - \frac{\nu_L^*}{E_L^*}\bar{\sigma}_{33}\\ \bar{\varepsilon}_{22} &= -\frac{\nu_L^*}{E_L^*}\bar{\sigma}_{11} + \frac{\bar{\sigma}_{22}}{E_T^*} - \frac{\nu_T^*}{E_T^*}\bar{\sigma}_{33}\\ \bar{\varepsilon}_{22} &= -\frac{\nu_L^*}{E_L^*}\bar{\sigma}_{11} - \frac{\nu_T^*}{E_T^*}\bar{\sigma}_{22} + \frac{\bar{\sigma}_{33}}{E_T^*}\end{aligned} \quad \text{(Eq 1c)}$$

where * denotes effective property relating values of state property, n^* is C_{11}^*, ℓ^* is C_{12}^* (refer to Eq 12), E_L^* is the longitudinal Young's modulus in fiber direction, ν_L^* is the associated longitudinal Poisson's ratio, E_T^* is the transverse Young's modulus, normal to fibers ν_T^* is the associated transverse Poisson's ratio (in transverse plane), G_T^* is the transverse shear modulus, G_L^* is the longitudinal shear modulus, and k^* is the transverse bulk modulus. Figure 2 illustrates the loadings associated with these properties. The Poisson's ratio, ν_L^*, is an abbreviated notation for ν_{LT}^*, which defines the transverse strain due to a stress E^*_L in the fiber (L or 1) direction. Similarly, the Poisson's ratio ν_T^* is an abbreviated notation for ν_{TT}^*, which defines strain in transverse direction 3 due to stress E_T in transverse direction 2, or vice versa. There is also a Poisson's ratio ν_{TL}^*, which defines strain in the longitudinal direction due to stress E^*_T in the transverse direction, but it is seldom used and does not enter into the stress-strain relations presented here. Its value is given by $\nu_{TL}^* = \nu_{LT}^* E_T^* / E_L^*$. All of these Poisson's ratios are illustrated in Fig. 2.

The longitudinal shear modulus G_L^* is an abbreviation for $G_{LT}^* = G_{TL}^*$, which is associated with shear acting on perpendicular longitudinal and transverse planes. Similarly, the transverse shear modulus G_T^* is an abbreviation for G_{TT}^*, associated with shear or transverse perpendicular planes.

The effective modulus k^* is obtained by subjecting a specimen to the average state of strain:

$$\bar{\varepsilon}_{22} = \bar{\varepsilon}_{33}$$

All others vanish, in which case it follows that:

$$(\bar{\sigma}_{22} + \bar{\sigma}_{33}) = 2k^*(\bar{\varepsilon}_{22} + \bar{\varepsilon}_{33})$$

Unlike the other properties listed, k^* is of little engineering significance but is of considerable analytical importance.

Only five of the properties in Eq 1 are independent. The most important interrelations of properties are:

$$n^* = E_L^* + 4k^*\nu_L^{*2} \quad \text{(Eq 2a)}$$

$$\ell^* = 2k^*\nu_L^* \quad \text{(Eq 2b)}$$

$$4/E_T^* = 1/G_T^* + 1/k^* + 4\nu_L^{*2}/E_L^* \quad \text{(Eq 2c)}$$

$$2/(1-\nu_T^*) = 1 + k^*/(1 + 4k^*\nu_L^{*2}/E_L^*)G_T^* \quad \text{(Eq 2d)}$$

$$G_T^* = E_T^*/2(1+\nu_T^*) \quad \text{(Eq 2e)}$$

Computation of effective elastic moduli is a difficult problem in elasticity theory. It is first necessary to assume a suitable arrangement of fibers and thus a geometrical model of UDC. Suitable homogeneous boundary conditions are then applied to fiber-reinforced specimens. For example, to compute k^*, it is convenient to apply displacement boundary conditions for which there is not external longitudinal deformation and for which the plane deformation in the transverse plane is isotropic, preserving the shape of the cross section. To find the associated average stress, however, it is necessary to determine in detail the elastic displacement fields in matrix and fibers. These displacements must satisfy the differential equation of elasticity theory in matrix and fibers, the displacement and traction continuity conditions at fiber-matrix interfaces, and the external boundary conditions. Once these displacements are known, the strain fields are computed by differentiation, the stress fields are found from the local Hooke's laws, and then the stress average, which is necessarily proportional to the strain average, is computed. Then, $2k^*$ is the coefficient of proportionality.

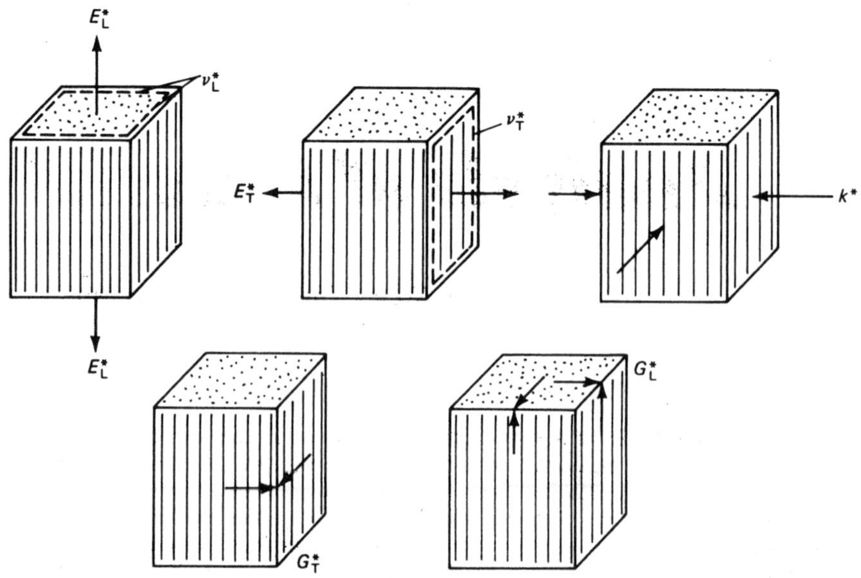

Fig. 2 Basic loadings associated with effective elastic properties. Symbols are defined in text.

In view of the difficulty of the problem, only a few simple models permit exact analysis. One kind of model is periodic arrays of identical circular fibers, for example, square and hexagonal periodic arrays (Fig. 3). These models are analyzed by numerical finite-difference or finite-element procedures. It is necessary in each case to identify a suitable repeating element of the fiber composite and to express its boundary conditions on the basis of symmetry requirements in terms of the external boundary conditions (see, for example, Ref 2). The hexagonal array was apparently analyzed first in Ref 5 and the square array in Ref 6. It should, however, be noted that the square array is not a suitable model for most UDC analyses because it is tetragonal but not transversely isotropic. Further discussion on periodic arrays is available in Ref 7.

The only existing model that permits exact analytical determination of effective elastic moduli is the composite cylinder assemblage (CCA), introduced in Ref 8. To construct the model, one might imagine a collection of composite cylinders, each consisting of a circular fiber core and a concentric matrix shell. The sizes of outer radii b_n of the cylinders may be chosen at will. The size of fiber core radii a_n is restricted by the requirement that in each cylinder the ratio a_n/b_n be the same, which also implies that matrix and fiber volume fractions are the same in each composite cylinder. It may be shown that for various loadings of interest, each composite cylinder behaves as some equivalent homogeneous cylinder. A hypothetical homogeneous cylindrical specimen is assigned these equivalent properties and is progressively filled out with composite cylinders. Because the radii of the cylinders can be arbitrarily small, the remaining volume can be made arbitrarily small. In the limit, the properties of the assemblage converge to the properties of one composite cylinder. The construction of CCA is shown in Fig. 4. A desirable feature of the model is the randomness of fiber placement; an undesirable feature is the large variation of fiber sizes. It will be shown, however, that the latter is not of serious concern.

Analysis of the CCA gives closed-form results for the effective properties k^*, E_L^*, ν_L^*, n^*, ℓ^*, and G_L^* and close bounds for the properties G_T^*, E_T^*, and ν_T^*. Such results are listed below for isotropic fibers, with the necessary modifications for transversely isotropic fibers. Details of derivation are given in Ref 2 and 9.

$$k^* = \frac{K_m(K_f+G_m)V_m + K_f(K_m+G_m)V_f}{(K_f+G_m)V_m + (K_m+G_m)V_f} = K_m + \frac{V_f}{1/(K_f-K_m)+V_m/(K_m+G_m)} \qquad \text{(Eq 3)}$$

$$E_L^* = E_m V_m + E_f V_f + \frac{4(\nu_f-\nu_m)^2 V_m V_f}{V_m/K_f + V_f/K_m + 1/G_m} \cong E_m V_m + E_f V_f \qquad \text{(Eq 4)}$$

where K_m and K_f are the bulk moduli of elasticity of matrix and fiber, and V_m and V_f are the volume fractions of matrix and fiber. The last is an excellent approximation for all UCDs.

$$\nu_L^* = \nu_m V_m + \nu_f V_f + \frac{(\nu_f-\nu_m)(1/K_m - 1/K_f)V_m V_f}{V_m/K_f + V_f/K_m + 1/G_m} \qquad \text{(Eq 5)}$$

$$G_L^* = G_m\left[\frac{G_m V_m + G_f(1+V_f)}{G_m(1+V_f)+G_f V_m}\right] = G_m + \frac{V_f}{1/(G_f-G_m)+V_m/2G_m} \qquad \text{(Eq 6)}$$

As indicated previously, the result for G_T^* is a pair of bounds on the actual value. One or the other of these bounds is recommended, depending on the ratios of the constituent properties (to compute the resulting E_T^* and ν_T^* Eq 2c and 2d are used). When $G_f > G_m$ and $K_f > K_m$, the upper bound is recommended:

$$G_{T(+)}^* \sim G_T^* = G_m\left[1+\frac{(1+\beta_m)V_f}{\rho-\left[1+3\beta_m^2 V_m^2/(\alpha V_f^3+1)\right]V_f}\right] \qquad \text{(Eq 7)}$$

where

$$\alpha = \frac{\beta_m - \gamma\beta_f}{1+\gamma\beta_f} \qquad \rho = \frac{\gamma+\beta_m}{\gamma-1}$$

$$\beta_m = \frac{1}{3-4\nu_m} \qquad \beta_f = \frac{1}{3-4\nu_f}$$

$$\gamma = \frac{G_f}{G_m}$$

When $G_f < G_m$ and $K_f < K_m$, the lower bound is recommended:

$$G_{T(-)}^* \sim G_T^* = G_m\left[1+\frac{(1+\beta_m)V_f}{\rho-\left[1+\beta_m^2 V_m^2/(\alpha V_f^3-\beta_m)\right]V_f}\right] \qquad \text{(Eq 8)}$$

The result (Eq 8) is of interest for metal matrix composites consisting of carbon and graphite fibers in an aluminum matrix because in that case, the elastic properties G_m and K_m of the matrix are larger than the G_{Tf} and K_f of the fibers. Note that K_m in Eq 3 is the isotropic plane-strain bulk modulus.

For transversely isotropic fibers, there are the following modifications (Ref 2, 9):

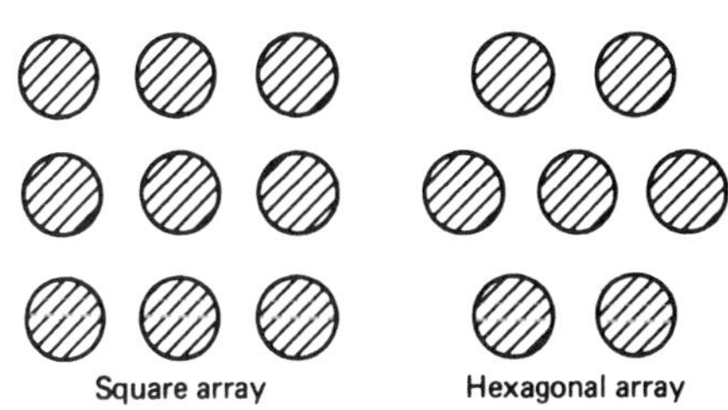

Fig. 3 Models of fiber arrays for numerical computation of properties

For k^* $\quad k_f$ is the fiber transverse bulk modulus

For E_L^*, ν_L^* $\quad E_f = E_{Lf}$, $\nu_f = \nu_{Lf}$, k_f as above (Modification 1)

For G_L^* $\quad G_f = G_{Lf}$

For G_T^* $\quad G_f = G_{Tf}$, $\beta_f = k_f/(k_f+2G_{Tf})$

A rational approximate evaluation of G_T^* of the CCA model is developed (Ref 3) by assuming that any composite cylinder behaves as if it were embedded in the effective medium with effective shear modulus G_T^*.

Numerical analysis of the effective elastic properties of the hexagonal-array model reveals that their values are extremely close to those predicted by the CCA model, as given by the preceding equations. The simple analytical results given here predict effective elastic properties with sufficient engineering accuracy. They are of considerable practical importance for two main reasons. They permit easy determination of effective properties for a variety of matrix properties, fiber properties, and volume fractions, and they constitute the only approach known today for experimental determination of carbon fiber properties.

With respect to the first reason, it is to be noted that the variety of matrix properties to be considered arises not only from the choice of different materials but also, and perhaps more importantly, from environmental changes of properties of a specified matrix. Significant examples are property changes due to temperature, moisture absorption, fatigue damage accumulation, and radiation. Thus, environmental changes of composite stiffness can be determined by measurement of environmental matrix stiffness changes and computation of such changes for the composite. This avoids a great deal of expensive experimentation.

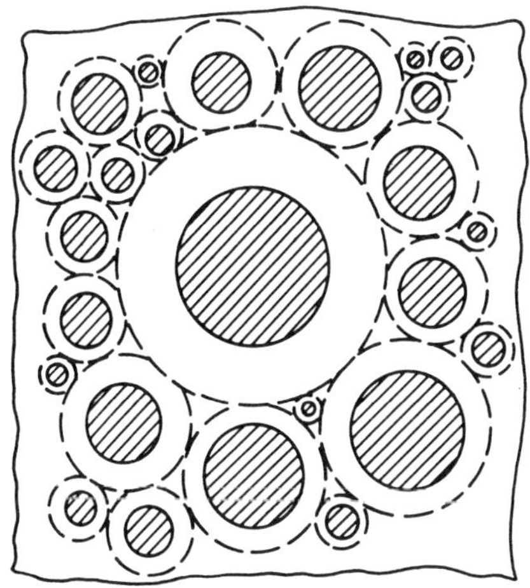

Fig. 4 Composite cylinder assemblage (CCA)

With respect to the second reason, it should be recalled that a carbon or graphite fiber has five independent elastic properties (Eq 2a to 2e) and that its diameter is of the order of 0.01 mm (0.0004 in.). It is thus impossible to measure directly the elastic properties except for E_L in the fiber direction. A remaining alternative is to measure the elastic modulus of the matrix and the five effective elastic moduli of the composite and then to compute the five fiber elastic properties from Eq 3 to 7 with Modification 1. The current standard method for doing this is to prepare a flat UDC specimen and measure the effective elastic properties by ultrasonic wave propagation. The principle of the method is to measure various wave velocities in various directions relative to the fiber direction. Because wave velocities are defined in terms of elastic moduli and density, their measurement determines the elastic moduli. Table 1 lists the anisotropic elastic properties of a carbon fiber having an axial modulus of 350 GPa (50×10^6 psi). Its properties were determined in this fashion by using carbon-epoxy specimens. The fiber properties obtained were then used to compute the elastic properties of a UDC consisting of an aluminum matrix and the carbon fiber. Also shown is the comparison between measured and computed composite elastic properties, based on the results (Eq 3 to 6, Eq 8) of Ref 10. The agreement is excellent.

The foregoing results are of sufficient accuracy and reliability to provide a predictive tool for evaluation of effective elastic properties of fiber composites. Various approximate treatments given in the literature are at least as complex and are less reliable than those presented here. Attempts have also been made to devise empirical or semiempirical equations for effective elastic properties, but in view of the complexity of the problem, this is not a helpful approach.

For purposes of laminate analysis, it is important to consider the plane-stress version of the effective stress-strain relations. Let x_3 be the normal to the plane of a thin, unidirectionally reinforced lamina. The plane-stress condition is defined by:

$$\bar{\sigma}_{33} = \bar{\sigma}_{13} = \bar{\sigma}_{23} = 0 \qquad \text{(Eq 9)}$$

Then, from Eq 1:

$$\begin{aligned} \bar{\varepsilon}_{11} &= \frac{\bar{\sigma}_{11}}{E_L^*} - \frac{\nu_L^*}{E_L^*}\bar{\sigma}_{22} \\ \bar{\varepsilon}_{22} &= -\frac{\nu_L^*}{E_L^*}\bar{\sigma}_{11} + \frac{\bar{\sigma}_{22}}{E_T^*} \\ 2\bar{\varepsilon}_{12} &= \frac{\bar{\sigma}_{12}}{G_L^*} \end{aligned} \qquad \text{(Eq 10)}$$

The inversion of Eq 10 is:

$$\begin{aligned} \bar{\sigma}_{11} &= C_{11}^*\bar{\varepsilon}_{11} + C_{12}^*\bar{\varepsilon} \\ \bar{\sigma}_{22} &= C_{12}^*\bar{\varepsilon}_{11} + C_{22}^*\bar{\varepsilon}_{22} \\ \bar{\sigma}_{12} &= 2G_L^*\bar{\varepsilon}_{12} \end{aligned} \qquad \text{(Eq 11)}$$

where

$$\begin{aligned} C_{11}^* &= \frac{E_L^*}{1 - \nu_L^{*2} E_T^* / E_L^*} \\ C_{12}^* &= \frac{\nu_L^* E_T^*}{1 - \nu_L^{*2} E_T^* / E_L^*} \\ C_{22}^* &= \frac{E_T^*}{1 - \nu_L^{*2} E_T^* / E_L^*} \end{aligned} \qquad \text{(Eq 12)}$$

The value of ν_L^* for polymeric matrix composites at the usual 60 vol% of fiber is of the order of 0.25, while the ratio E_T^* / E_L^* is of the order of 0.1 to 0.2. Consequently, the denominator is usually practically equal to unity; hence, the approximation:

$$\begin{aligned} C_{11}^* &\cong E_L^* \\ C_{12}^* &\cong \nu_L^* E_T^* \\ C_{22}^* &\cong E_T^* \end{aligned} \qquad \text{(Eq 13)}$$

Thermal Expansion and Moisture Swelling

The elastic behavior of composite material discussed in the previous section was concerned with deformations produced by stresses, thus by loads. Deformations are also produced by temperature changes and absorption of moisture, thus by environmental changes. The two phenomena are similar and therefore discussed together. A change of temperature in a free body produces thermal strains, while moisture absorption produces swelling strains. The relevant physical parameters to quantify these phenomena are coefficients of thermal expansion (CTEs) and coefficients of swelling.

Fibers have significantly smaller CTEs than do polymeric matrices. The CTE of glass fibers is 5.0×10^{-6}/K while a typical epoxy value is 54×10^{-6}/K. Carbon and graphite fibers are anisotropic in thermal expansion. The CTEs in the fiber direction are usually extremely small, either positive or negative, of the order of 0.9×10^{-6}/K. It follows that a UDC will have very small CTEs in the fiber direction because the fibers will restrain matrix expansion. On the other hand, transverse CTEs will be much larger because the fibers move with the expanding matrix and thus provide less restraint to matrix expansion.

These phenomena are of considerable practical importance, particularly for laminates made of unidirectionally reinforced layers. When such a laminate is heated, the free expansion of any layer is prevented by the adjacent laminae because the fiber directions in all layers are different. This causes internal stresses that could be considerable. To compute these stresses, it is necessary to know the CTEs of the layers. Procedures to determine the CTEs in terms of elastic properties and the CTEs of component fibers and matrix are discussed in this section.

A physically similar situation arises in moisture swelling. Polymers absorb moisture in a wet environment and consequently swell. When this swelling is restrained, stresses are produced. If a UDC is placed in a wet environment, the matrix absorbs moisture but, with the exception of aramid, the fibers do not. Therefore, the fibers restrain—literally prevent—swelling in the fiber direction but not in the direction transverse to the fibers. Thus, the UDC is highly anistropic with respect to moisture swelling.

When a laminate absorbs moisture, the same phenomenon occurs as with heating. Because free swelling of the layers cannot take place, internal stresses develop, which can be computed if the UDC coefficients of swelling are known. Procedures for computing those coefficients are also discussed in this section.

The CTEs of homogeneous solids are defined by the strains produced by unit change of temperature in bodies that are free of load and thus free of stress. The main engineering importance of thermal expansion is in the stresses produced when temperature changes occur under conditions of constraint and free expansion is prevented.

The CTEs of a composite are defined by the average strains produced by unit temperature change. In this case, however, free thermal expansion cannot take place on the microscale, because the difference in constituent CTEs will

Table 1 Comparison of experimental and analytical results for elastic properties of a graphite-aluminum composite

Property	Value
Graphite fiber (T50)	
Young's modulus, GPa (10^6 psi)	
Longitudinal (E_L)	388 (56.3)
Transverse (E_T)	7.17 (1.04)
Bulk modulus (K), GPa (10^6 psi)	7.03 (1.02)
Shear modulus, GPa (10^6 psi)	
Transverse (G_T)	2.41 (0.350)
Longitudinal (G_L)	6.79 (0.985)
Poisson's ratio	
Longitudinal (ν_L)	0.23
Transverse (ν_T)	0.486
Matrix (aluminum 201)	
Young's modulus (E), GPa (10^6 psi)	71.0 (10.3)
Shear modulus (G), GPa (10^6)	26.7 (3.87)
Poisson's ratio (ν)	0.33
Composite (30% T50, 70% Al)	
Young's modulus, GPa (10^6 psi)	
Longitudinal (E_L^*)	
Experimental	160 (23.2)
Analytical	166 (24.1)
Transverse (E_T^*)	
Experimental	29.6 (4.30)
Analytical	32.0 (4.64)
Shear modulus, GPa (10^6 psi)	
Transverse (G_T^*)	
Experimental	10.3 (1.50)
Analytical	10.4 (1.51)
Longitudinal (G_L^*)	
Experimental	18.5 (2.69)
Analytical	18.6 (2.70)
Poisson's ratio, transverse (ν_T^*)	
Experimental	0.43
Analytical	0.41

produce microstresses when the temperature changes. Thus, failure of a composite material can be caused by changes in temperature. The CTEs of a UDC are indispensable for stress analysis of laminates subjected to temperature changes.

Consider a free cylindrical specimen of a UDC under uniform temperature change, ΔT, implying that the boundary temperature T is changed $T + \Delta T$. When a composite body is subjected to uniform boundary temperature, the temperature will also be uniform throughout the constituents. On the other hand, the stresses and strains in the phases are nonuniform and complex. The stress-strain relations of Eq 1 in the presence of temperature change then assume the form:

$$\begin{aligned}\bar{\varepsilon}_{11} &= \frac{\bar{\sigma}_{11}}{E_L^*} - \frac{\nu_L^*}{E_L^*}\bar{\sigma}_{22} - \frac{\nu_L^*}{E_L^*}\bar{\sigma}_{33} + \alpha_L^*\Delta T \\ \bar{\varepsilon}_{22} &= -\frac{\nu_L^*}{E_L^*}\bar{\sigma}_{11} + \frac{\bar{\sigma}_{22}}{E_T^*} - \frac{\nu_T^*}{E_T^*}\bar{\sigma}_{33} + \alpha_T^*\Delta T \\ \bar{\varepsilon}_{33} &= -\frac{\nu_L^*}{E_L^*}\bar{\sigma}_{11} - \frac{\nu_T^*}{E_T^*}\bar{\sigma}_{22} + \frac{\bar{\sigma}_{33}}{E_T^*} + \alpha_T^*\Delta T\end{aligned} \quad \text{(Eq 14)}$$

where α_L^* is the effective axial expansion coefficient, and α_T^* is the effective transverse expansion coefficient.

This definition would indicate that to compute α_{ij}^*, it would be necessary to compute the detailed strain fields in the two phases of a composite subjected to uniform temperature rise. Fortunately, however, this is not necessary; it has been found (Ref 11) that there is a unique mathematical relation between the effective CTEs and the effective elastic properties of a two-phase composite (for the general relations, see Ref 2 and 12). The present discussion is confined to specific cases of interest for a UDC. When fibers and matrix are isotropic:

$$\begin{aligned}\alpha_L^* &= \alpha_m + \frac{\alpha_f - \alpha_m}{1/K_f - 1/K_m}\left[\frac{3(1-2\nu_L^*)}{E_L^*} - \frac{1}{K_m}\right] \\ \alpha_T^* &= \alpha_m + \frac{\alpha_f - \alpha_m}{1/K_f - 1/K_m}\left[\frac{3}{2k^*} - \frac{3(1-2\nu_L^*)\nu_L^*}{E_L^*} - \frac{1}{K_m}\right]\end{aligned} \quad \text{(Eq 15)}$$

where α_m and α_f are the matrix and fiber isotropic expansion coefficients, K_m and K_f are the matrix and fiber three-dimensional bulk modulus, and E_L^*, ν_L^*, and k^* are the effective axial Young's modulus, axial Poisson's ratio, and transverse bulk modulus. These equations are suitable for glass-epoxy and boron-epoxy or boron-aluminum composites. They have also been derived in Ref 13 and 14.

For carbon and graphite fibers, it is necessary to consider the case of transversely isotropic fibers whose elastic and thermal expansion behavior is characterized by five independent elastic constants and two independent thermal expansion coefficients. This complicates the results considerably (Ref 7, 9):

$$\begin{aligned}\alpha_L^* &= \alpha_m + (\alpha_{Lf} - \alpha_m)\left[P_{11}(S_{11}^* - S_{11}) + 2P_{12}(S_{12}^* - S_{12})\right] + 2(\alpha_{Tf} - \alpha_m) \\ &\quad \left[P_{12}(S_{11}^* - S_{11}) + (P_{22} + P_{23})(S_{12}^* - S_{12})\right] \\ \alpha_T^* &= \alpha_m + (\alpha_{Lf} - \alpha_m)\left\{P_{11}(S_{12}^* - S_{12}) + P_{12}\left[S_{22}^* + S_{23}^* - (S_{22} + S_{23})\right]\right\} \\ &\quad + 2(\alpha_{Tf} - \alpha_m)\left\{P_{12}(S_{12}^* - S_{12}) + \tfrac{1}{2}(P_{22} + P_{23})\left[S_{22}^* + S_{23}^* - (S_{22} + S_{23})\right]\right\}\end{aligned} \quad \text{(Eq 16)}$$

where

$$P_{11} = (\Delta S_{22} + \Delta S_{23})/D$$

$$P_{12} = -\Delta S_{12}/D$$

$$P_{22} + P_{23} = \Delta S_{11}/D$$

$$D = \Delta S_{11}(\Delta S_{22} + \Delta S_{23}) - 2\Delta S_{12}^2$$

$$\Delta S_{11} = 1/E_{Lf} - S_{11}$$

$$\Delta S_{12} = -\nu_{Lf}/E_{Lf} - S_{12}$$

$$\Delta S_{22} + \Delta S_{23} = \tfrac{1}{2}(1/k_f + 4\nu_{Lf}^2/E_{Lf}) - (S_{22} + S_{23})$$

$$S_{11} = 1/E_m$$

$$S_{12} = -\nu_m/E_m$$

$$S_{22} + S_{23} = (1 - \nu_m)/E_m$$

$$S_{11}^* = 1/E_L^*$$

$$S_{12}^* = -\nu_L^*/E_L^*$$

and

$$S_{22}^* + S_{23}^* = \tfrac{1}{2}(1/k^* + 4\nu_L^{*2}/E_L^*)$$

Frequently, fiber and matrix CTEs are functions of temperature. It is not difficult to show that Eq 15 and 16 remain valid for temperature-dependent properties if elastic properties are taken at final temperature and CTEs are taken as secant values between that temperature and the stress-free temperature.

To evaluate the CTEs from Eq 15 or Eq 16, it is necessary to know the effective elastic properties k^*, E_L^*, and ν_L^*. These may be taken as the values predicted by the CCA model as given by Eq 3, 4, and 5 with Modification 1 when the fibers are transversely isotropic. Comparison of the values thus obtained with a numerical analysis performed for a hexagonal array of carbon fibers (with an axial modulus of 210 GPa) in epoxy (Ref 15) shows that the results obtained are numerically indistinguishable.

The CTEs of carbon and graphite fibers can be measured directly only in the fiber direction, thus obtaining α_L. Direct measurement of transverse α_T is not possible because of the minute fiber diameters. Again, the only possible way to evaluate α_T is to measure α_L^* and α_T^* experimentally for a specified composite and then compute α_T from Eq 16. If the equations are written in the form:

$$\begin{aligned}\alpha_L^* &= \alpha_m + (\alpha_{Lf} - \alpha_m)a_{11} + (\alpha_{Tf} - \alpha_m)a_{12} \\ \alpha_T^* &= \alpha_m + (\alpha_{Lf} - \alpha_m)a_{21} + (\alpha_{Tf} - \alpha_m)a_{22}\end{aligned} \quad \text{(Eq 17)}$$

it follows that:

$$\begin{aligned}\alpha_{Lf} &= \alpha_m + \frac{(\alpha_L^* - \alpha_m)a_{22} - (\alpha_T^* - \alpha_m)a_{12}}{a_{11}a_{22} - a_{12}a_{21}} \\ \alpha_{Tf} &= \alpha_m + \frac{(\alpha_T^* - \alpha_m)a_{11} - (\alpha_L^* - \alpha_m)a_{21}}{a_{11}a_{22} - a_{12}a_{21}}\end{aligned} \quad \text{(Eq 18)}$$

Figure 5 shows typical plots of the effective CTEs of graphite-epoxy. For 0.50 fiber volume fraction, the axial expansion coefficient, α_L^*, is practically equal to that of the fibers. Because many carbon and graphite fibers have small negative axial expansion coefficients, many composites with such fibers have small negative or practically vanishing axial expansion coefficients. It is also interesting that for small fiber volume fractions, the transverse CTE becomes larger than the matrix CTE, which is the maximum constituent CTE.

With respect to deformation due to moisture, when a body that absorbs moisture is placed in a wet environment, moisture will diffuse through the external boundary. The internal moisture concentration, C, is defined by the mass of moisture accumulated per unit volume and is initially a function of space and time. Ultimately, the moisture concentration will stabilize and become time independent. The time-dependent stage is called the transient stage, and the ultimate time-independent stage is called the stationary stage. There is a complete mathematical analogy between the equations describing heat conduction and moisture diffusion, in both the transient and stationary stages. Thus, in the latter stage, the concentration C satisfies the Laplace equation.

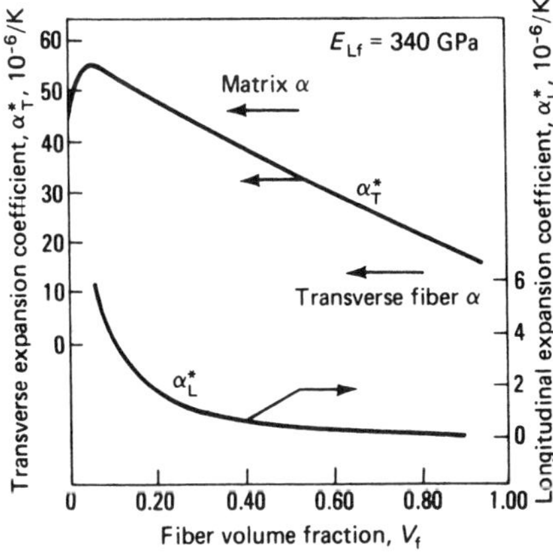

Fig. 5 Effect of fiber volume fraction on thermal expansion for representative carbon-epoxy composite

When a composite with a polymeric matrix is placed in a wet environment, the matrix will begin to absorb moisture. However, the moisture absorption of most fibers used in practice is negligible. Aramid fibers alone do absorb significant amounts of moisture when exposed to high humidity. The total moisture absorbed by an aramid-epoxy composite, however, may not be substantially greater than that absorbed by other epoxy composites.

In most composites, the fibers act as barriers to moisture diffusion, analogous to perfect insulators in heat conduction, After sufficient time has elapsed, the matrix will be in an equilibrium moisture state with uniform concentration on the boundary. After a long time in this stage, the moisture concentration throughout the matrix will also be uniform, and thus the same as the boundary concentration. It is customary to define the specific moisture concentration, c, by:

$$c = C/\rho \qquad \text{(Eq 19)}$$

Thus, c is the mass of moisture per unit mass, a nondimensional number. The swelling strains due to moisture are functions of c and, to a first approximation, are given by:

$$\varepsilon_{ij} = \beta_{ij} c \qquad \text{(Eq 20)}$$

where β_{ij} are the swelling coefficients.

If there are also mechanical stresses and strains, the swelling strains are superimposed on the latter, which is exactly analogous to the thermoelastic stress-strain relations of an isotropic material where β replaces the CTE and c replaces the temperature. The swelling coefficients of most fibers are zero since their moisture absorption is negligible. (Aramid fiber swelling coefficients are unknown.) It follows that moisture swelling of a UDC is mathematically analogous to thermal expansion of such a composite with vanishing fiber expansion coefficients. Therefore, all of the results previously given for thermal expansion can be transcribed to moisture swelling. The effective swelling coefficients, β^*_{ij}, are defined by the average strains produced in a free sample subjected to uniform unit change of specific moisture concentration in the matrix. Thus, these coefficients follow directly from the equations for CTEs.

Other aspects of moisture absorption and transient and steady state are discussed in Ref 16 and 17, which also contain survey articles on this subject.

With respect to the important question of simultaneous moisture swelling and temperature rise, often called hygrothermal behavior, the simplest approach is to assume that thermal expansion strains and moisture swelling strains can be superimposed. Thus, for a free specimen:

$$\bar{\varepsilon}_{11} = \alpha^*_L \Delta T + \beta^*_L c$$
$$\bar{\varepsilon}_{22} = \bar{\varepsilon}_{33} = \alpha^*_T \Delta T + \beta^*_T c \qquad \text{(Eq 21)}$$

In this situation, the matrix elastic properties in Eq 15 and 16 may be functions of the end temperature and the equilibrium moisture concentration, c; this dependence must be known in order to evaluate α^*_L, α^*_T, β^*_L, and β^*_T in Eq 21.

Viscoelastic Properties

All polymers exhibit time dependence. This manifests itself by the increase with time of deformations under constant load, which is called creep, and, conversely, by the decrease with time of stresses under deformation constraints, which is called relaxation. Another important effect of time dependence is the damping of vibrations due to energy dissipation in the polymeric matrix. The significance of all these phenomena increases with rise in temperature.

The effects described are of considerable engineering importance for fiber-reinforced composite structures, because stresses and deformations determined on the basis of elastic analysis may change considerably with time because of polymeric matrix time dependence. Vibration damping is a beneficial effect that is of particular significance for the higher vibration modes, which often become negligible because of damping.

The simplest description of time dependence is linear viscoelasticity. Viscoelastic behavior of polymers manifests itself primarily in shear and is negligible for isotropic stress and strain. This implies the elastic stress-strain relation:

$$\sigma_{11} + \sigma_{22} + \sigma_{33} = 3K(\varepsilon_{11} + \varepsilon_{22} + \varepsilon_{33}) \qquad \text{(Eq 22)}$$

where K, the three-dimensional bulk modulus, remains valid for polymers. When a polymeric specimen is subjected to shear strain ε_{12}, which does not vary with time, the stress needed to maintain this shear strain is given by:

$$\sigma_{12}(t) = 2G(t)\varepsilon^0_{12} \qquad \text{(Eq 23)}$$

where $G(t)$ is defined as the shear relaxation modulus. When a specimen is subjected to shear stress σ^0_{12} constant in time, the resulting shear strain is given by:

$$\varepsilon_{12}(t) = \tfrac{1}{2} g(t)\sigma^0_{12} \qquad \text{(Eq 24)}$$

and $g(t)$ is defined as the shear creep compliance.

Typical variations of relaxation modulus and creep compliance with time are shown in Fig. 6. These material properties change significantly with temperature. The relaxation modulus decreases, and the creep compliance increases. This implies that stiffness decreases with temperature. The initial values of these properties at time-zero (at the beginning of deformation) are denoted $G(0)$ and $g(0)$ and are the elastic properties of the matrix. Note that $G(0)\, g(0) = 1$. If the applied shear strain is an arbitrary function of time, commencing at time zero, Eq 23 is replaced by:

$$\sigma_{12}(t) = 2G(t)\sigma_{12}(0) + 2\int_0^t G(t-t')\frac{d\varepsilon_{12}}{dt'}dt' \qquad \text{(Eq 25)}$$

Similarly, for applied shear stress, which is a function of time, Eq 24 is replaced by:

$$\varepsilon_{12}(t) = \tfrac{1}{2} g(t)\sigma_{12}(0) + \tfrac{1}{2}\int_0^t g(t-t')\frac{d\sigma_{12}}{dt'}dt' \qquad \text{(Eq 26)}$$

The viscoelastic counterpart of the Young's modulus is obtained by subjecting a cylindrical specimen to axial strain ε constant in space and time. Then:

$$\sigma_{11}(t) = E(t)\varepsilon^0_{11} \qquad \text{(Eq 27)}$$

and $E(t)$ is the Young's relaxation modulus. If the specimen is subjected to axial stress σ^0_{11} constant in space and time, then:

$$\varepsilon_{11}(t) = e(t)\sigma^0_{11} \qquad \text{(Eq 28)}$$

and $e(t)$ is the Young's creep compliance (Fig. 6).

Obviously $E(t)$ is related to K and $G(t)$, and $e(t)$ is related to k and $g(t)$. The relations are not simple (Ref 18). To write the viscoelastic stress-strain relations for general states of three-dimensional stress and strain, it is customary to separate stress and strain into isotropic (or hydrostatic) and deviatoric parts. Thus:

$$\sigma_{ij} = \sigma\delta_{ij} + S_{ij} \qquad \sigma = \tfrac{1}{3}(\sigma_{11} + \sigma_{22} + \sigma_{33})$$
$$\varepsilon_{ij} = \varepsilon\delta_{ij} + e_{ij}$$
$$\varepsilon = \tfrac{1}{3}(\varepsilon_{11} + \varepsilon_{22} + \varepsilon_{33}) \qquad \text{(Eq 29)}$$

where ij represents range indices varying from 1 to 3. Then:

$$\sigma(t) = 3K\varepsilon(t)$$
$$S_{ij}(t) = 2G(t)e_{ij}(0) + 2\int_o^t G(t-t')\frac{\partial e_{ij}}{\partial t'}dt'$$
$$e_{ij}(t) = \tfrac{1}{2} g(t)s_{ij}(0) + \frac{1}{2}\int_o^t g(t-t')\frac{\partial s_{ij}}{\partial t'}dt' \qquad \text{(Eq 30)}$$

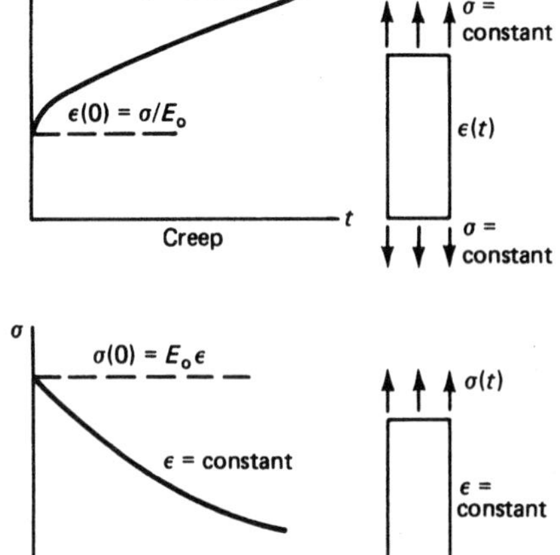

Fig. 6 Viscoelasticity as shown by the creep and stress relaxation behavior over time

where S_{ij} represents the deviatoric stress components.

The problem is to evaluate the effective viscoelastic properties of a UDC in terms of polymeric matrix viscoelastic properties and the elastic properties of the fibers. (It is assumed that the fibers themselves do not experience any time-dependent effect.) This problem has been resolved in general fashion in Ref 19 and 20, which show that the Laplace transforms of the effective relaxation moduli and creep compliances of a composite can be written in terms of expressions for effective elastic moduli in which elastic matrix properties are replaced by Laplace transforms of viscoelastic matrix properties. The main difficulty is the inversion of these Laplace transforms into the time domain. Details and applications of such procedures are given in Ref 2. Only some simple illustrative cases are presented here.

Detailed analysis shows that the viscoelastic effect in a UDC is significant only for axial shear, transverse shear, and transverse uniaxial stress. For any of average strains $\bar{\varepsilon}_{22}, \bar{\varepsilon}_{23}$, and $\bar{\varepsilon}_{12}$ constant in time, thus stress relaxation, the time-dependent stress responses will be, respectively:

$$\begin{aligned} \bar{\sigma}_{22}(t) &= E_T^*(t)\bar{\varepsilon}_{22} \\ \bar{\sigma}_{23}(t) &= 2G_T^*(t)\bar{\varepsilon}_{23} \\ \bar{\sigma}_{12}(t) &= 2G_L^*(t)\bar{\varepsilon}_{12} \end{aligned} \quad \text{(Eq 31)}$$

For any of stresses $\bar{\sigma}_{22}$, $\bar{\sigma}_{23}$, and $\bar{\sigma}_{12}$ constant in time, thus creep deformation, the time-dependent strain responses will be, respectively:

$$\begin{aligned} \bar{\varepsilon}_{22}(t) &= e_T^*(t)\bar{\sigma}_{22} \\ \bar{\varepsilon}_{23}(t) &= \tfrac{1}{2}g_T^*(t)\bar{\sigma}_{23} \\ \bar{\varepsilon}_{12}(t) &= \tfrac{1}{2}g_L^*(t)\bar{\sigma}_{12} \end{aligned} \quad \text{(Eq 32)}$$

where the material properties in Eq 31 are effective relaxation moduli and the properties in Eq 32 are associated effective creep functions. All other effective properties may be considered elastic. This implies in particular that if a fiber composite is subjected to stress $\bar{\sigma}_{11}(t)$ in the fiber direction, then:

$$\begin{aligned} \bar{\sigma}_{11}(t) &\cong E_L^*\bar{\varepsilon}_{11}(t) \\ \varepsilon_{22}(t) &= \bar{\varepsilon}_{33}(t) \sim -\nu_L^*\bar{\varepsilon}_{11}(t) \end{aligned} \quad \text{(Eq 33)}$$

where E_L^* and ν_L^* are the elastic results (Eq 4 and 5) with matrix properties taken as initial (elastic) matrix properties. Similar considerations apply to the relaxation modulus k^*.

The simplest case of the viscoelastic properties entering into Eq 31 and 32 is the relaxation modulus $G_L^*(t)$ and its associated creep compliance, $g_L^*(t)$. A simple result has been obtained for fibers that are infinitely more rigid than the matrix (Ref 2). In this case, the elastic result (Eq 6) reduces to:

$$G_L^* = G_m \frac{1+V_f}{1-V_f}$$

For a viscoelastic matrix, the corresponding results are:

$$\begin{aligned} G_L^*(t) &= G_m(t)\frac{1+V_f}{1-V_f} \\ g_L^*(t) &= g_m(t)\frac{1-V_f}{1+V_f} \end{aligned} \quad \text{(Eq 34)}$$

This result is an acceptable approximation for glass fibers in a polymeric matrix and an excellent approximation for boron fibers in a polymeric matrix. However, it is not applicable to carbon or graphite fibers in a polymeric matrix, since the axial shear modulus of these fibers is not large enough in relation to the matrix shear modulus to justify rigid-fiber approximation. In this case, it is necessary to use the correspondence principle previously mentioned. Laplace transform inversion can be carried out by representing the matrix in terms of a viscoelastic spring-dashpot model (see Ref 2 and 19). The situation for transverse shear is more complicated and involves complicated Laplace transform inversion (Ref 20).

All polymeric matrix viscoelastic properties, such as creep and relaxation functions, are significantly temperature dependent. If this temperature dependence is known, all of the results given in this section can be obtained for the temperature of interest by introducing into the results matrix properties at that temperature.

At elevated temperatures, the viscoelastic behavior of the polymeric matrix may become nonlinear. In this event, the UDC will also be nonlinearly viscoelastic and all the results given are not valid. The problem of analytical determination of nonlinear properties is, of course, much more difficult than the linear problem. Some results are given in Ref 21.

Conduction and Moisture Diffusion

The conductivity of a UDC implies both thermal and electrical conductivity. Because all of the conductivity problems are governed by the similar equations, the results obtained also apply to dielectric and magnetic properties and to steady-state moisture diffusion. The various equivalent physical quantities in these different areas are listed in Table 2. The language of thermal conductivity will be used in the following discussion.

Let $T(x)$ be a steady-state temperature field in a homogeneous body. The temperature gradient is given by:

$$H_i = \frac{\partial T}{-\partial x_i} \quad \text{(Eq 35)}$$

and the heat flux vector by:

$$D_i = \mu_{ij}H_j \quad \text{(Eq 36)}$$

where μ_{ij} is the conductivity tensor. The inverse of Eq 36 is:

$$H_i = \xi_{ij}D_j \quad \text{(Eq 37)}$$

where ξ_{ij} is the resistivity tensor. In an isotropic material:

$$\begin{aligned} D_i &= \mu H_i \\ H_i &= \xi D_i \\ \xi &= 1/\mu \end{aligned} \quad \text{(Eq 38)}$$

For a transversely isotropic material, such as carbon and graphite fibers with x_1, the axis of transverse isotropy (fiber axis):

$$\begin{aligned} D_1 &= \mu_L H_1 \\ D_2 &= \mu_T H_2 \\ D_3 &= \mu_T H_3 \end{aligned} \quad \text{(Eq 39)}$$

where μ_L is longitudinal conductivity and μ_T is transverse conductivity.

A simple, common example is heat conduction through a slab whose faces are maintained at different temperatures, T and $T + \Delta T$. Then:

$$\begin{aligned} H_1 &= -\frac{\Delta T}{h} \\ D_1 &= \mu_{11}H_1 \end{aligned}$$

where h is the slab thickness and μ_{11} is the conductivity coefficient normal to the faces of the slab.

Because a UDC is statistically transversely isotropic, it has two different effective conductivities, μ_L^* in the fiber direction and μ_T^* transverse to the fibers. The effective constituent relations are analogous to Eq 39:

Table 2 Equivalent physical quantities

Physical subject	T	$H = -\Delta T$	D	μ_{ij}	ξ_{ij}
Thermal conduction	Temperature	Temperature gradient	Heat flux	Heat conductivities	Resistivities
Electric conduction	Electric potential	Electric field intensity	Current density	Electric conductivities	Resistivities
Electrostatics	Electric potential	Electric field intensity	Electric induction, electric displacement	Dielectric constants, permittivities	
Magnetostatics	Magnetic potential	Magnetic field intensity	Magnetic induction	Magnetic permeabilities	
Moisture diffusion	Concentration	Moisture gradient	Moisture flux	Diffusivities	

$$\overline{D}_1 = \mu_L^* \overline{H}_1$$
$$\overline{D}_2 = \mu_T^* \overline{H}_2 \quad \text{(Eq 40)}$$
$$\overline{D}_3 = \mu_T^* \overline{H}_3$$

where overbars denote averages over the representative volume element (RVE).

It can be shown (Ref 2) that for isotropic matrix and fibers, the axial conductivity μ_L^* is given by:

$$\mu_L^* = \mu_m V_m + \mu_f V_f \quad \text{(Eq 41)}$$

and for transversely isotropic fibers:

$$\mu_L^* = \mu_m V_m + \mu_{Lf} V_f \quad \text{(Eq 42)}$$

where μ_{Lf} is the longitudinal conductivity of the fibers. The results (Eq 41 and 42) are valid for any fiber distribution and any fiber cross section.

The problem of transverse conductivity is mathematically analogous to the problem of longitudinal shearing (Ref 2). It follows that all results for the effective longitudinal shear modulus, G_L^*, can be interpreted as results for transverse effective conductivity, μ_T^*. In particular, for the CCA model:

$$\mu_T^* = \mu_m \left[\frac{\mu_m V_m + \mu_f (1 + V_f)}{\mu_m (1 + V_f) + \mu_f V_m} \right] = \mu_m + \frac{V_f}{1/(\mu_f - \mu_m) + V_m / 2V_m} \quad \text{(Eq 43)}$$

These results are for isotropic fibers. For carbon and graphite fibers, μ_f should be replaced by the transverse conductivity of the fibers, μ_{Tf} (Ref 9).

As in the elastic case, there is reason to believe that Eq 43 represents with great accuracy all cases of circular fibers that are randomly distributed and are not in contact. The reason, again, is the numerical coincidence of hexagonal-array numerical analysis results with the number predicted by Eq 43.

To interpret the results for moisture diffusion, the quantity μ_m is interpreted as the diffusivity of the matrix. Because moisture absorption of fibers is negligible, μ_f is set equal to zero. The results are then:

$$\mu_L^* = \mu_m V_m$$
$$\mu_T^* = \mu_m \frac{V_m}{1 + V_f} \quad \text{(Eq 44)}$$

that leads to the interesting relation:

$$\mu_L^* / \mu_T^* = 1 + V_f \quad \text{(Eq 45)}$$

ACKNOWLEDGEMENT

This article is adapted from B.W. Rosen and Z. Hashin, Analysis of Material Properties, *Composites,* Volume 1, *Engineered Materials Handbook,* ASM International, 1987, p 185–205. ASM International thanks Gerald V. Flanagan, Materials Sciences Corporation for helping with this adaptation.

REFERENCES

1. R.J. Palmer, "Investigation of the Effect of Resin Material on Impact Damage to Graphite/Epoxy Composites," NASA CR-165677, National Aeronautics and Space Administration, March 1981
2. Z. Hashin, "Theory of Fiber Reinforced Materials," NASA CR-1974, National Aeronautics and Space Administration, 1972
3. R.M. Christensen, *Mechanics of Composite Materials,* Wiley-Interscience, 1979
4. R. Hill, Theory of Mechanical Properties of Fiber Strengthened Materials, I, Elastic Behavior, *J. Mech. Phys. Solids,* Vol 12, 1964, p 199–212
5. G. Pickett, AFML TR-65-220, 1965; also, Elastic Moduli of Fiber Reinforced Plastic Composites, *Fundamental Aspects of Fiber Reinforced Plastic Composites,* R.T. Schwartz and H.S. Schwart, Ed., Wiley-Interscience, 1968, p 13–27
6. D.F. Adams, D.R. Doner, and R.L. Thomas, AFML TR-67-96, 1967. Also *J. Compos. Mater.,* Vol 1, 1967, p 4–17, p 152–165
7. G.P. Sendeckyj, Elastic Behavior of Composites, *Mechanics of Composite Materials,* Vol II, G.P. Sendeckyj, Ed., Academic Press, 1974
8. Z. Hashin and B.W. Rosen, The Elastic Moduli of Fiber Reinforced Materials, *J. Appl. Mech.,* Vol 31, 1964, p 223–232
9. Z. Hashin, Analysis of Properties of Fiber Composites With Anistropic Constituents. *J. Appl. Mech.,* Vol 46, 1979, p 543–550
10. G.V. Blessing and W.L. Elban, Aluminum Matrix Composite Elasticity Measured Ultrasonically, *J. Appl. Mech.,* Vol 48, 1981, p 965–966
11. V.M. Levin, On the Coefficients of Thermal Expansion of Heterogeneous Materials, *Mechanics of Solids,* Vol 2, 1967, p 58–61
12. B.W. Rosen and Z. Hashin, Effective Thermal Expansion Coefficients and Specific Heats of Composite Materials, *Int. J. Eng. Sci.,* Vol 8, 1970, p 157–173
13. R.A. Schapery, Thermal Expansion Coefficients of Composite Materials Based on Energy Principles, *J. Compos. Mater.,* Vol 2, 1968, p 380ff
14. B.W. Rosen, "Thermal Expansion Coefficients of Composite Materials," Ph.D. thesis, University of Pennsylvania, 1968
15. T. Ishikawa, K. Koyama, and S. Kobayashi, Thermal Expansion Coefficients of Unidirectional Composites, *J. Compos. Mater.,* Vol 12, 1978, p 153–168
16. G.S. Springer, Environmental Effects on Epoxy Matrix Composites, *Fifth Conference on Composite Materials: Testing and Design,* STP 674, S.W. Tsai, Ed., American Society for Testing and Materials, 1979, p 291–311
17. S.W. Tsai and H.T. Hahn, *Introduction to Composite Materials,* Technomic, 1980
18. R.M. Christensen, *Theory of Viscoelasticity,* Academic Press, 1971
19. Z. Hashin, Viscoelastic Behavior of Heterogeneous Media, *J. Appl. Mech.,* Vol 32, 1965, p 630–636
20. Z. Hashin, Viscoelastic Fiber Reinforced Materials, *AIAA J.,* Vol 4, 1966, p 1411–1417
21. R.A. Schapery, Viscoelastic Behavior of Composites, *Mechanics of Composite Materials,* Vol II, G.P. Sendeckyj, Ed., Academic Press, 1974

Macromechanics Analysis of Laminate Properties

THE PROPERTIES of unidirectional composite (UDC) materials are quite different from those of conventional, metallic materials. The primary difference, from an analytical viewpoint, results from the material anisotropy. The UDC materials typically have exceptional properties in the direction of the reinforcing fibers but poor to mediocre properties perpendicular (transverse) to the fibers. Thus, with the exception of one-dimensionally loaded members (for example, truss members), UDC materials would be expected to perform poorly compared to conventional materials. The problem then is how to obtain maximum advantage from the exceptional fiber directional properties while minimizing the effects of the low transverse properties. One obvious solution is to use the approach taken in the manufacture of plywood.

Plywood consists of layers, or plies, of wood bonded together, with the wood grain in each ply oriented perpendicular to the adjacent plies. With this orientation of the plies of wood, the lesser properties of the wood perpendicular to the grain are augmented by the superior properties in the direction of the wood grain. At the same time, however, the superior properties in the grain direction cannot be fully utilized because of the perpendicular plies.

The bonding of individual UDC plies is used to form laminates. The plies, or laminae, are oriented such that the effective properties of the laminate match the loading environment. Laminate effective material properties are tailored to meet performance requirements through the use of lamination theory.

Lamination theory can be considered a form of structural analysis but can also be used when a structural material is being designed. This adds another level of effort to the design process but allows the structural material to be tailored to match the loadings. Thus, if a 2-to-1 biaxial loading environment is prescribed, the structural laminate can be designed for a 2-to-1 strength. The amount of material is thereby minimized in a way that is not possible with conventional materials.

This article first presents a treatment of UDC stress-strain relations in the forms appropriate for analysis of thin plies of material. The analysis is then developed for an assemblage of plies (laminate), and finally the stress-strain relations for a thin, laminated plate are developed for the case of plate membrane forces and bending moments.

For purposes of structural analysis, it is desirable to represent a laminate by a set of effective stiffnesses, just as a homogeneous plate is defined by its extensional and bending stiffnesses. Accordingly, the calculation of these laminate mechanical properties is defined and illustrated in this article. Also, the analysis is expanded to include treatment of laminate expansion resulting from temperature and moisture changes.

Next, calculations of temperature and moisture distributions through the thickness of a laminate are discussed. With this information and the definition of applied loads or deformations, the stresses in each ply can be calculated. Procedures for doing this are presented.

The sections just described deal with what may be classified as the nondestructive response of the laminate to external load and environment. The next sections address laminate failure resulting from static, cyclic, and impact loading conditions. The final section describes intra- and interlaminar cracking behavior.

Lamina Stress-Strain Relations

A laminate is composed of unidirectionally reinforced laminae oriented in various directions. The elastic stress-strain relations of the lamina are expressed in this article in matrix form using a different notation for elastic properties. With x_1 in the fiber direction, x_2 transverse to the fibers in the plane of the lamina, and x_3 normal to the plane of the lamina, these material properties define the lamina properties:

$$\begin{aligned} E_1 &= E_L^* & \nu_{12} &= \nu_L^* \\ E_2 &= E_3 = E_T^* & \nu_{23} &= \nu_T^* \\ G_{12} &= G_L^* & G_{23} &= G_T^* \end{aligned} \qquad \text{(Eq 1)}$$

where E represents Young's modulus of elasticity, ν is Poisson's ratio, G is shear modulus, L is longitudinal, T is transverse, and * represents the effective properties.

Furthermore, the laminae, at this point, are treated as effective, homogeneous, transversely isotropic materials, and the strains are written without overbars. Thus,

$$\begin{Bmatrix} \varepsilon_{11} \\ \varepsilon_{22} \\ \varepsilon_{33} \\ 2\varepsilon_{23} \\ 2\varepsilon_{13} \\ 2\varepsilon_{12} \end{Bmatrix} = \begin{bmatrix} \frac{1}{E_1} & \frac{-\nu_{12}}{E_1} & \frac{-\nu_{12}}{E_1} & 0 & 0 & 0 \\ \frac{-\nu_{12}}{E_1} & \frac{1}{E_2} & \frac{-\nu_{23}}{E_2} & 0 & 0 & 0 \\ \frac{-\nu_{12}}{E_1} & \frac{-\nu_{23}}{E_2} & \frac{1}{E_2} & 0 & 0 & 0 \\ 0 & 0 & 0 & \frac{1}{G_{23}} & 0 & 0 \\ 0 & 0 & 0 & 0 & \frac{1}{G_{12}} & 0 \\ 0 & 0 & 0 & 0 & 0 & \frac{1}{G_{12}} \end{bmatrix} \begin{Bmatrix} \sigma_{11} \\ \sigma_{22} \\ \sigma_{33} \\ \sigma_{23} \\ \sigma_{13} \\ \sigma_{12} \end{Bmatrix} \qquad \text{(Eq 2)}$$

where ε is strain and σ is stress. Account has been taken of the symmetry relations:

$$\frac{\nu_{21}}{E_2} = \frac{\nu_{12}}{E_1} = \frac{\nu_{31}}{E_3} = \frac{\nu_{13}}{E_1}\quad \frac{\nu_{23}}{E_2} = \frac{\nu_{32}}{E_3}$$

It has been common practice in the analysis of laminates to use engineering shear strains rather than tensor shear strains. Thus, the factor of 2 has been introduced into the stress-strain relations of Eq 2.

The most important state of stress in a lamina is plane, that is:

$$\sigma_{13} = \sigma_{23} = \sigma_{33} = 0 \qquad \text{(Eq 3)}$$

because it occurs for both in-plane loading and bending at a sufficient distance from the laminate edges. In this case, Eq 2 reduces to:

$$\begin{Bmatrix} \varepsilon_{11} \\ \varepsilon_{22} \\ 2\varepsilon_{12} \end{Bmatrix} = \begin{bmatrix} \frac{1}{E_1} & \frac{-\nu_{12}}{E_1} & 0 \\ \frac{-\nu_{12}}{E_1} & \frac{1}{E_2} & 0 \\ 0 & 0 & \frac{1}{G_{12}} \end{bmatrix} \begin{Bmatrix} \sigma_{11} \\ \sigma_{22} \\ \sigma_{12} \end{Bmatrix} \qquad \text{(Eq 4)}$$

which may be written:

$$\{\varepsilon_\ell\} = [S]\{\sigma_\ell\}$$

where ℓ identifies lamina coordinates, and $[S]$, the compliance matrix, relates the stress and strain components in the principal material directions.

The three relations in Eq 4 relate the in-plane strain components to the three in-plane stress components. For this plane stress state, the three additional strains can be found to be:

$$\varepsilon_{23} = \varepsilon_{13} = 0$$

$$\varepsilon_{33} = -\sigma_{11}\frac{\nu_{13}}{E_1} - \sigma_{22}\frac{\nu_{23}}{E_2}$$

and thus the complete state of stress and strain is determined.

The relations in Eq 4 can be inverted to yield:

$$\{\sigma_\ell\} = [S]^{-1}\{\varepsilon_\ell\} \qquad \text{(Eq 5)}$$

or

$$\{\sigma_\ell\} = [Q]\{\varepsilon_\ell\}$$

where the matrix $[Q]$ is defined as the inverse of the compliance matrix and is known as the reduced lamina stiffness matrix. Its terms can be shown to be given by:

$$[Q] = \begin{bmatrix} Q_{11} & Q_{12} & 0 \\ Q_{12} & Q_{22} & 0 \\ 0 & 0 & Q_{66} \end{bmatrix}$$

$$Q_{11} = \frac{E_1}{E_1 - \nu_{12}^2 \dfrac{E_2}{E_1}}$$

$$Q_{22} = \frac{E_2}{E_1 - \nu_{12}^2 \dfrac{E_2}{E_1}} \qquad \text{(Eq 6)}$$

$$Q_{12} = \frac{\nu_{12} E_2}{E_1 - \nu_{12}^2 \dfrac{E_2}{E_1}}$$

$$Q_{66} = G_{12}$$

The notation used for the $[Q]$ matrix follows from the simplified engineering representation of the fourth-rank stiffness tensor. Each pair of subscripts of the stiffness components is replaced by a single subscript according to the scheme:

11 → 1 22 → 2 33 → 3
23 → 4 31 → 5 12 → 6

The reduced stiffness and compliance matrices, Eq 6 and 4, relate stresses and strains in the principal material directions of the material. To define the material response in directions other than these material coordinates, transformation relations must be developed for the material stiffnesses.

In Fig. 1, two sets of coordinate systems are shown. The 1-2 coordinate system corresponds to the principal material directions for a lamina, while the x-y coordinates are arbitrary and are related to the 1-2 coordinates through a rotation about the axis out of the plane of the figure. The angle, θ, is defined as the rotation from the arbitrary x-y system to the material 1-2 system (θ is positive for a counterclockwise rotation).

The transformation of stresses from the 1-2 system to the x-y system follows the rules for transformation of tensor components. Thus:

$$\begin{Bmatrix} \sigma_{xx} \\ \sigma_{yy} \\ \sigma_{xy} \end{Bmatrix} = \begin{bmatrix} m^2 & n^2 & -2mn \\ n^2 & m^2 & 2mn \\ mn & -mn & m^2 - n^2 \end{bmatrix} \begin{Bmatrix} \sigma_{11} \\ \sigma_{22} \\ \sigma_{12} \end{Bmatrix} \qquad \text{(Eq 7)}$$

or

$$\{\sigma_x\} = [\theta]\{\sigma_\ell\}$$

where $m = \cos\theta$ and $n = \sin\theta$. In these relations, the subscript x is used to refer to the laminate coordinate system.

The same transformation matrix $[\theta]$ can also be used for the tensor strain components. However, since the engineering shear strains have been used, a different transformation matrix is required. Thus:

$$\begin{Bmatrix} \varepsilon_{xx} \\ \varepsilon_{yy} \\ 2\varepsilon_{xy} \end{Bmatrix} = \begin{bmatrix} m^2 & n^2 & -mn \\ n^2 & m^2 & mn \\ 2mn & -2mn & m^2 - n^2 \end{bmatrix} \begin{Bmatrix} \varepsilon_{11} \\ \varepsilon_{22} \\ 2\varepsilon_{12} \end{Bmatrix} \qquad \text{(Eq 8)}$$

or

$$\{\varepsilon_x\} = [\psi]\{\varepsilon_\ell\}$$

where $[\psi]$ is now the transformation matrix.

Given the transformations for stress and strain to arbitrary coordinate systems, the relations between stress and strain in the laminate system can be determined. Substituting Eq 7 and 8 into Eq 5 yields:

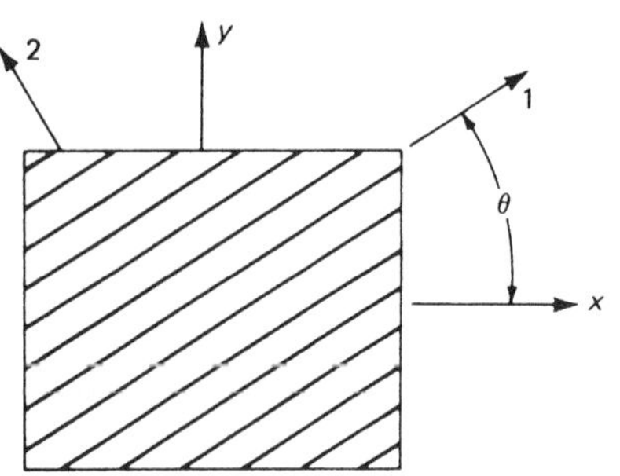

Fig. 1 Coordinate systems; 1, 2, principal material coordinates; x, y, laminate or arbitrary coordinates

$$\{\sigma_x\} = [\bar{Q}]\{\varepsilon_x\} \qquad \text{(Eq 9)}$$

The reduced-stiffness matrix, $[\bar{Q}]$, relates the stress and strain components in the laminate coordinate system. Here:

$$[\bar{Q}] = [\theta][Q][\psi]^{-1} \qquad \text{(Eq 10)}$$

The terms within $[\bar{Q}]$ are defined by the appropriate matrix multiplication to be:

$$\bar{Q}_{11} = Q_{11}m^4 + Q_{22}n^4 + 2m^2n^2(Q_{12} + 2Q_{66})$$
$$\bar{Q}_{12} = m^2n^2(Q_{11} + Q_{22} - 4Q_{66}) + (m^4 + n^4)Q_{12}$$
$$\bar{Q}_{16} = [Q_{11}m^2 - Q_{22}n^2 - (Q_{12} + 2Q_{66})(m^2 - n^2)]mn$$
$$\bar{Q}_{22} = Q_{11}n^4 + Q_{22}m^4 + 2m^2n^2(Q_{12} + 2Q_{66})$$
$$\bar{Q}_{26} = [Q_{11}n^2 - Q_{22}m^2 + (Q_{12} + 2Q_{66})(m^2 - n^2)]mn$$
$$\bar{Q}_{66} = (Q_{11} + Q_{22} - 2Q_{12})m^2n^2 + Q_{66}(m^2 - n^2)^2$$
$$\bar{Q}_{21} = \bar{Q}_{12}$$
$$\bar{Q}_{61} = \bar{Q}_{16}\bar{Q}_{62} = \bar{Q}_{26} \qquad \text{(Eq 11)}$$

where the subscript 6 has been retained in keeping with the discussion following Eq 6. Thus:

$$[\bar{Q}] = \begin{bmatrix} \bar{Q}_{11} & \bar{Q}_{12} & \bar{Q}_{16} \\ \bar{Q}_{21} & \bar{Q}_{22} & \bar{Q}_{26} \\ \bar{Q}_{16} & \bar{Q}_{26} & \bar{Q}_{66} \end{bmatrix} \qquad \text{(Eq 12)}$$

A feature of the $[\bar{Q}]$ matrix that is immediately noticed as being dissimilar to previous constitutive relations is that $[\bar{Q}]$ is fully populated. The additional terms that have appeared in $[\bar{Q}]$, namely, $\bar{Q}_{16}$ and $\bar{Q}_{26}$, relate shear strains to extensional loading and vice versa. This effect of a shear strain resulting from an extensional stress is shown in Fig. 2.

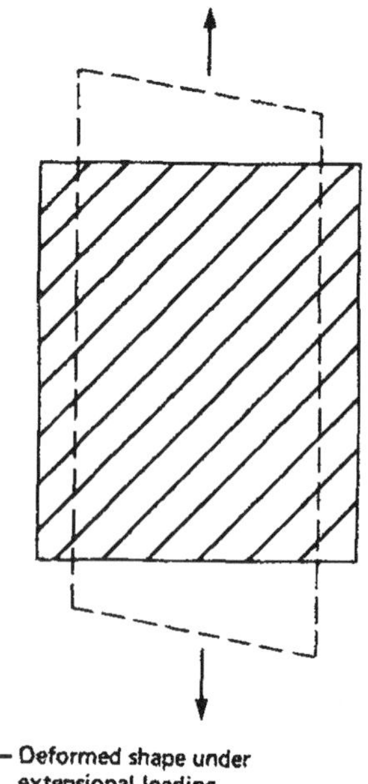

Fig. 2 Extensional-shear coupling

Referring to Eq 11, each of the extensional-shear coupling terms can be seen to contain a sine-cosine multiplier term. Obviously, if either sin θ or cos θ is zero, the extensional-shear coupling terms are zero. For the product sin θ cos θ to be zero, the angle θ must be 0° or 90°. Physically, this means that the fibers are either parallel or perpendicular to the loading direction. For this case, extensional shear coupling does not occur in an orthotropic material, because the loadings are in the principal material directions (Eq 4).

The procedure used to develop the transformed stiffness matrix can also be used to find a transformed compliance matrix. Thus:

$$\{\varepsilon_\ell\}=[S]\{\sigma_\ell\}$$
$$\{\varepsilon_x\}=[\psi][S][\theta]^{-1}\{\sigma_x\} \qquad \text{(Eq 13)}$$
$$\{\varepsilon_x\}=\left[\bar{S}\right]\{\sigma_x\}$$

The relations between the terms in $[\bar{S}]$ and $[S]$ are developed by a procedure identical to that for the relations between $[\bar{Q}]$ and $[Q]$.

With the stress-strain relations now defined in the laminate coordinate system, lamina stiffnesses can also be defined in this system. Thus, expanding the last of Eq 13 yields:

$$\begin{Bmatrix}\varepsilon_{xx}\\ \varepsilon_{yy}\\ 2\varepsilon_{xy}\end{Bmatrix}=\begin{bmatrix}\bar{S}_{11} & \bar{S}_{12} & \bar{S}_{16}\\ \bar{S}_{21} & \bar{S}_{22} & \bar{S}_{26}\\ \bar{S}_{16} & \bar{S}_{26} & \bar{S}_{66}\end{bmatrix}\begin{Bmatrix}\sigma_{xx}\\ \sigma_{yy}\\ \sigma_{xy}\end{Bmatrix}$$

The engineering constants for the material can be defined by specifying the conditions for an experiment. Thus, the ratio $\sigma_{xx}/\varepsilon_{xx}$, for $\sigma_{yy} = \sigma_{xy} = 0$, is the Young's modulus in the x direction. For this same stress state, $-\varepsilon_{yy}/\varepsilon_{xx}$ is Poisson's ratio. In this way, the lamina stiffnesses in the coordinate system of Eq 13 are found to be:

$$E_x=\frac{1}{\bar{S}_{11}}$$
$$E_y=\frac{1}{\bar{S}_{22}}$$
$$G_{xy}=\frac{1}{\bar{S}_{66}} \qquad \text{(Eq 14)}$$
$$\nu_{xy}=-\frac{\bar{S}_{21}}{\bar{S}_{11}}=-\frac{\bar{S}_{12}}{\bar{S}_{11}}$$

It is sometimes desirable to obtain elastic constants directly from the reduced stiffnesses, $[\bar{Q}]$, by utilizing Eq 9. In the general case where the $\bar{Q}_{ij}$ matrix is fully populated, this can be accomplished by using Eq 14 and the solution for $\bar{S}_{ij}$ as functions of $\bar{Q}_{ij}$ obtained from the inverse relationship of the two matrices. Another approach is to evaluate extensional properties for the case of zero shear strain, $\varepsilon_{xy} = 0$, as opposed to the previous case of zero shear stress, $\sigma_{xy} = 0$. For single stress states and zero shear strain it is found that, in terms of the transformed stiffness matrix terms (Eq 12), the elastic constants are:

$$E_x=\bar{Q}_{11}-\frac{\bar{Q}_{12}^2}{\bar{Q}_{22}}$$
$$E_y=\bar{Q}_{22}-\frac{\bar{Q}_{12}^2}{\bar{Q}_{11}} \qquad \text{(Eq 15)}$$
$$\nu_{xy}=\frac{\bar{Q}_{12}}{\bar{Q}_{22}}=\frac{\bar{Q}_{21}}{\bar{Q}_{22}}$$

Also:

$$G_{xy}=\bar{Q}_{66}$$

Referring to the terms in the $[\bar{Q}]$ matrix (Eq 11) and the stiffness relations (Eq 15), it can be seen that, in general, the elastic constants in an arbitrary coordinate system are functions of all of the elastic constants in the principal material directions as well as the angle of rotation.

The variation of elastic modulus E_x with angle of rotation is shown in Fig. 3 for a typical graphite-epoxy material. For demonstration purposes, two different shear moduli have been used in generating the figure. The differences between the two curves demonstrate the effect of the principal material shear modulus on the transformed extensional stiffness. The two curves are identical at θ = 0° and θ = 90°. This is to be expected, because at these angles, the extensional stiffness, E_x, is simply E_1 or E_2. Between the two end points, substantial differences exist. For the smaller shear modulus, from approximately 50° to just less than 90°, the extensional stiffness is less than the E_2 value. This is a most interesting result, indicating that for these angles, the material stiffness is governed more strongly by the principal material shear modulus than by the transverse extensional stiffness.

The curves of Fig. 3 can also be used to determine the modulus E_y, simply by reversing the angle scale. Thus, the values shown at 0° correspond to E_y at 90° and the values at 90° correspond to E_y at 0°.

With the transformed stress-strain relations, it is now possible to develop an analysis for an assemblage of plies, that is, a laminate.

Lamination Theory

The development of procedures to evaluate stresses and deformations of laminates is crucially dependent on the fact that the thickness of laminates is so much smaller than the in-plane dimensions. Typical thickness values for individual plies range between 0.15 and 0.25 mm (0.005 and 0.010 in.). Consequently, aerospace laminates using from 8 to 50 plies are generally still thin plates and therefore can be analyzed on the basis of the usual simplifications of thin-plate theory.

Analysis of isotropic thin plates is an old, established field in which in-plane loading and bending are usually analyzed separately. The former is described by plane stress elastic theory, and the latter is described by classical plate-bending theory. This separation is possible because the two loadings are uncoupled; when both occur, the result is given by superposition. In the case of anisotropic laminates, in-plane loading and bending are generally coupled and must be treated together. It is only for symmetric laminae stacking sequences that uncoupling occurs. Consequently, lamination theory will be developed first for the general case, and simplifications will then be introduced.

The classical assumptions of thin-plate theory are:

- The thickness of the plate is much smaller than the in-plane dimensions.
- The strains in the deformed plate are small compared to unity.
- Normals to the undeformed plate surface remain normal to the deformed plate surface.
- Vertical deflection does not vary through the thickness.
- Stress normal to the plate surface is negligible.

On the basis of the second, third, and fourth assumptions, the displacement field in the plate, u, can be expressed as:

$$u_z=u_z^0(x,y)$$
$$u_x=u_x^0(x,y)-z\frac{\partial u_z}{\partial x} \qquad \text{(Eq 16)}$$
$$u_y=u_y^0(x,y)-z\frac{\partial u_z}{\partial y}$$

with the x-y-z coordinate system defined as in Fig. 4. These relations (Eq 16) indicate that the in-plane displacements consist of a midsurface displacement, designated by the superscript 0, plus a linear variation through the thickness. The

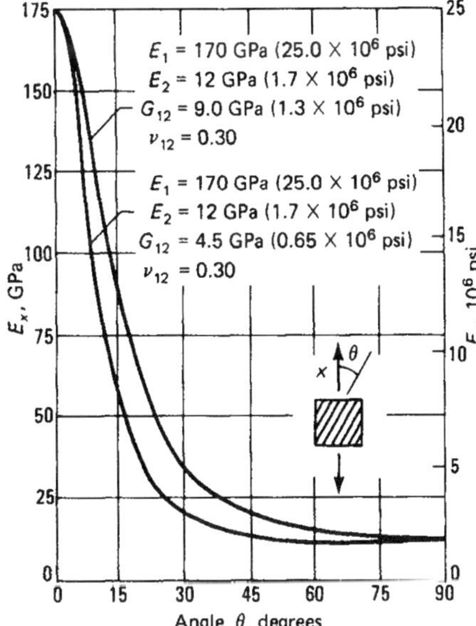

Fig. 3 Variation of E_x with angle of rotation and G_{12} for typical graphite-epoxy materials

two partial derivatives are simply bending rotations of the midsurface. The use of the fourth assumption prescribes that u_z not vary through the thickness. The z coordinate is measured from the midsurface of the plate. This is a natural convention for a laminate that is symmetrically stacked with reference to the midsurface but an arbitrary one when this is not the case.

The linear strain displacement relations are:

$$\varepsilon_{xx} = \frac{\partial u_x}{\partial x}$$
$$\varepsilon_{yy} = \frac{\partial u_y}{\partial y} \qquad \text{(Eq 17)}$$
$$\varepsilon_{xy} = \frac{1}{2}\left(\frac{\partial u_x}{\partial y} + \frac{\partial u_y}{\partial x}\right)$$

Performing the required partial differentiations yields:

$$\varepsilon_{xx} = \varepsilon^0_{xx} + z\kappa_{xx}$$
$$\varepsilon_{yy} = \varepsilon^0_{yy} + z\kappa_{yy} \qquad \text{(Eq 18)}$$
$$2\varepsilon_{xy} = 2\varepsilon^0_{xy} + 2z\kappa_{xy}$$

or

$$\{\varepsilon_x\} = \{\varepsilon^0\} + z\{\kappa\}$$

where

$$\{\varepsilon^0\} = \begin{Bmatrix} \dfrac{\partial u^0_x}{\partial x} \\ \dfrac{\partial u^o_y}{\partial_y} \\ \left(\dfrac{\partial y^o_x}{\partial y} + \dfrac{\partial u^0_y}{\partial x}\right) \end{Bmatrix} \qquad \text{(Eq 19)}$$

and

$$\{\kappa\} \equiv \begin{Bmatrix} \kappa_{xx} \\ \kappa_{yy} \\ 2\kappa_{xy} \end{Bmatrix} = \begin{Bmatrix} -\dfrac{\partial^2 u_z}{\partial x^2} \\ -\dfrac{\partial^2 u_z}{\partial y^2} \\ -2\dfrac{\partial^2 u_z}{\partial x \partial y} \end{Bmatrix} \qquad \text{(Eq 20)}$$

Thus, the strain at any point in the plate is defined as the sum of a midsurface strain, $\{\varepsilon^0\}$, and a curvature, $\{\kappa\}$, multiplied by the distance from the midsurface.

For convenience, as is usual in plate theory, stress and moment resultants will be used rather than stresses for the remainder of the development (Fig. 5). The stress resultants, N, are defined as:

$$\{N\} = \begin{Bmatrix} N_{xx} \\ N_{yy} \\ N_{xy} \end{Bmatrix} = \int_{-h}^{h} \{\sigma_x\} dz \qquad \text{(Eq 21)}$$

and the moment resultants, M, are defined as:

$$\{M\} = \begin{Bmatrix} M_{xx} \\ M_{yy} \\ M_{xy} \end{Bmatrix} = \int_{-h}^{h} \{\sigma_x\} z dz \qquad \text{(Eq 22)}$$

where the integrations are carried out over the plate thickness, $2h$.

Noting Eq 9 and 18, relations between the stress and moment resultants and the midplane strains and curvatures can be written as:

$$\{N\} = \int_{-h}^{h} \{\sigma_x\} dz = \int_{-h}^{h} \left[\bar{Q}\right](\{\varepsilon^0\} + z\{\kappa\}) dz \qquad \text{(Eq 23)}$$

$$\{M\} = \int_{-h}^{h} \{\sigma_x\} z dz = \int_{-h}^{h} \left[\bar{Q}\right](\{\varepsilon^0\} + z\{\kappa\}) z dz \qquad \text{(Eq 24)}$$

Since the transformed lamina stiffness matrices are constant within each lamina and the midplane strains and curvatures are constant with respect to the z coordinate, the integrals in Eq 23 and 24 can be replaced by summations, Σ, over the total number of plies.

Introducing three matrices equivalent to the needed summations, the relations can be written as:

$$\{N\} = [A]\{\varepsilon^0\} + [B]\{\kappa\}$$

$$\{M\} = [B]\{\varepsilon^0\} + [D]\{\kappa\}$$

or

$$\begin{Bmatrix} N \\ \hline M \end{Bmatrix} = \begin{bmatrix} A & B \\ B & D \end{bmatrix} \begin{Bmatrix} \varepsilon^0 \\ \hline \kappa \end{Bmatrix} \qquad \text{(Eq 25)}$$

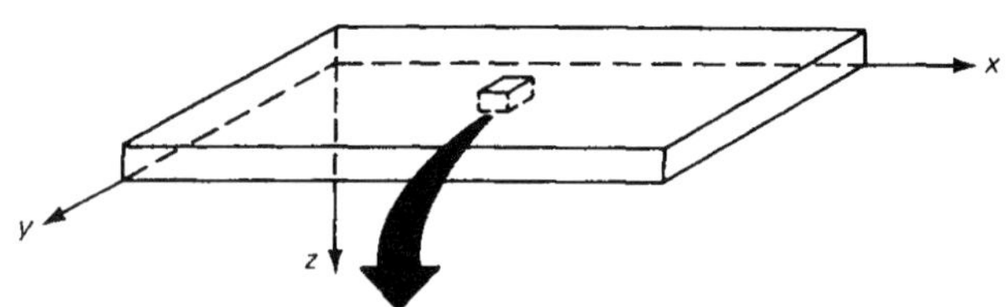

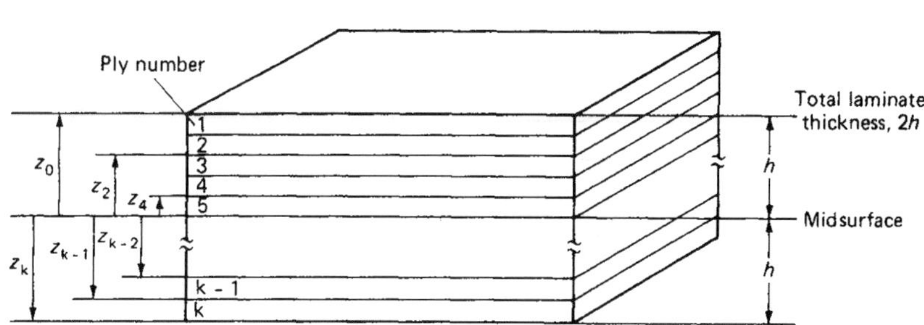

Fig. 4 Laminate construction

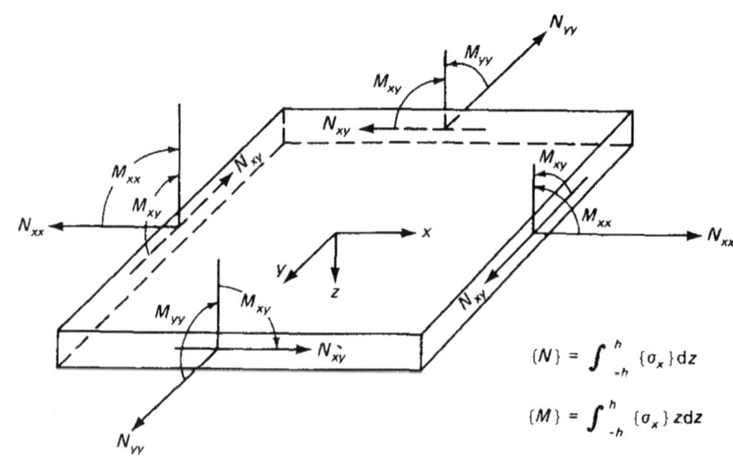

Fig. 5 Stress and moment resultants

where the stiffness matrix is composed of the following 3 by 3 matrices:

$$[A]=\sum_{i=1}^{K}\left[\bar{Q}\right]^{i}(z_i - z_{i-1})$$
$$[B]=\frac{1}{2}\sum_{i=1}^{K}\left[\bar{Q}\right]^{i}(z_i^2 - z_{i-1}^2) \qquad \text{(Eq 26)}$$
$$[D]=\frac{1}{3}\sum_{i=1}^{K}\left[\bar{Q}\right]^{i}(z_i^3 - z_{i-1}^3)$$

where K is the total number of plies, z_i is defined as in Fig. 4, and superscript i denotes a property of the ith ply. Note that $z_i - z_{i-1}$ is equal to the ply thickness. Here the reduced lamina stiffnesses for the ith ply are found from Eq 11 using the principal ply properties and orientation angle of each ply in turn. Thus, the constitutive relations for a laminate in terms of stress and moment resultants have been developed.

In examining the relations (Eq 25), the first interesting feature revealed is a coupling between bending and extension. The $[B]$ matrices relate stress resultants to bending curvatures and moment resultants to midplane strains. Thus, for a general laminate, the application of a stress resultant produces curvatures, and application of a bending moment produces extensional strain. The feature is known as bending-extensional coupling.

In typical structural laminates, bending-extensional coupling is eliminated by proper specification of the stacking sequence. Stacking sequence refers to the order in which the various plies are put together. From the relations for computing the $[B]$ matrix (Eq 26), it can be seen that if the plies are arranged in an even z function (symmetric about the midplane), the $[B]$ matrix is eliminated. Thus, if the laminate is designed with identically oriented plies at equal distances from the midsurface, bending-extensional coupling is eliminated.

Other forms of coupling are inherent in the relations (Eq 25). To examine these couplings, it is necessary to evaluate individual terms in the $[A]$, $[B]$, and $[D]$ matrices. The most general form of these matrices, combined as in Eq 25, is:

$$\begin{bmatrix} A_{11} & A_{12} & A_{16} & B_{11} & B_{12} & B_{16} \\ A_{21} & A_{22} & A_{26} & B_{21} & B_{22} & B_{26} \\ A_{16} & A_{26} & A_{66} & B_{16} & B_{26} & B_{66} \\ B_{11} & B_{12} & B_{16} & D_{11} & D_{12} & D_{16} \\ B_{21} & B_{22} & B_{26} & D_{21} & D_{22} & D_{26} \\ B_{16} & B_{26} & B_{66} & D_{16} & D_{26} & D_{66} \end{bmatrix}$$

In general, the $[A]$, $[B]$, and $[D]$ matrices are fully populated. Thus, there is coupling between membrane extension and membrane shear (A_{16}, A_{26}) and between bending and twisting (D_{16}, D_{26}). Both of these forms of coupling can be eliminated by judicious ply orientation and stacking sequence selection, but in some cases this selection may be impractical. Extensional-shear coupling can be eliminated by specifying a balanced construction. Balance indicates that for every $+\theta$ ply, there is a $-\theta$ ply. These plies do not have to be adjacent to satisfy this requirement.

When bending-twisting coupling is undesirable, it can be eliminated, but only by using a unidirectional or cross-ply construction. Unidirectional construction implies that all layers have the same orientation, which is aligned with the loading direction. A cross-ply laminate has plies oriented at 0° and 90° only, again oriented with the loading direction. It is also possible to limit the effect of bending-twisting coupling by other means. If a symmetric laminate is constructed with many plies, and plies with the same angular orientation are not grouped together, the magnitude of the D_{16} and D_{26} terms will be reduced with respect to the other terms in the $[D]$ matrix. Thus, while the bending-twisting coupling is not eliminated, its effect is reduced. In certain applications, such coupling may be desirable.

Laminate Properties

The previous section presented the development of the relations between midsurface strains and curvatures and membrane stress and moment resultants. The elastic stiffnesses in these relationships are functions of the ply elastic constants and the ply orientations and arrangement or stacking sequence. In the present section, these results will be used to calculate plate bending and extensional stiffnesses suitable for use in structural analysis. The effects of orientation variables on plate properties are also discussed.

For practical structures it is necessary to understand not only the mechanical loading conditions but also the effects of temperature changes on laminate behavior. Thus, the thermal expansion characteristics of laminates will be presented. Further, for polymeric matrix composites, high moisture content has been found to cause dimensional changes. This effect is treated in this section to define effective swelling coefficients.

In general, as shown previously, laminates exhibit coupling between bending and extension. Elimination of this coupling was shown to be possible through the specification of midplane symmetric construction. This leads to a natural division of laminates into symmetric and nonsymmetric categories.

Before these two laminate categories are discussed, typical laminate notation is described. A shorthand notation has been devised and is in common use. The basis for the notation comes from the fact that structural laminates typically have repeating groups of plies and pairs of plies at $+\theta$ and $-\theta$ angles. Using these groupings, the laminate construction

[0°/0°/45°/–45°/90°90°/–45°45°0°0°]

can be specified as:

[45°/– 45°/0°/0°/90°/0°/0°/– 45°/45°]

The numerical subscript indicates the number of adjacent identical plies. Adjacent balanced angle plies are lumped together, and the subscript s indicates that the pattern is repeated in reverse order, forming a symmetric laminate. A multiplier subscript is also used to denote multiple groups of plies. Thus, the laminate

[45°/–45°/0°/0°/45°/–45°/0°/0°/0°/0°/–45°/45°/0°/0°/–45°/45°]

is specified as:

$$\left[\pm 45°/0_2^{\circ}\right]_{2s}$$

When the central ply of a symmetric laminate is not repeated, this is denoted by an overbar. Thus the laminate

[45°/–45°/0°/0°/90°/0°/0°/–45°/45°]

is specified as:

$$\left[\pm 45°/0_2^{\circ}/\overline{90°}\right]_{s}$$

Additional conventions can be designated, but those shown here are usually sufficient.

Symmetric Laminates. Because a symmetric laminate does not exhibit coupling between extension and bending, the design of composites is considerably simplified because symmetric constructions behave somewhat similarly to conventional materials. Recalling Eq 25 and noting that for this case the $[B]$ matrix is zero, the relations can be rewritten as:

$$\begin{Bmatrix} N_{xx} \\ N_{yy} \\ N_{xy} \end{Bmatrix} = \begin{bmatrix} A_{11} & A_{12} & A_{16} \\ A_{12} & A_{22} & A_{26} \\ A_{16} & A_{26} & A_{66} \end{bmatrix} \begin{Bmatrix} \varepsilon_{xx}^0 \\ \varepsilon_{yy}^0 \\ 2\varepsilon_{xy}^0 \end{Bmatrix} \qquad \text{(Eq 27)}$$

and

$$\begin{Bmatrix} M_{xx} \\ M_{yy} \\ M_{xy} \end{Bmatrix} = \begin{bmatrix} D_{11} & D_{12} & D_{16} \\ D_{12} & D_{22} & D_{26} \\ D_{16} & D_{26} & D_{66} \end{bmatrix} \begin{Bmatrix} \kappa_{xx} \\ \kappa_{yy} \\ 2\kappa_{xy} \end{Bmatrix}$$

Since the extensional and bending behavior are uncoupled, effective laminate elastic constants can be readily determined. Inverting the stress resultant midplane strain relations yields:

$$\{\varepsilon^0\} = [A]^{-1}\{N\} = [a]\{N\}$$

$[a]$ is called the elastic compliance matrix from which the laminate elastic constants are seen to be:

$$E_x = \frac{1}{2ha_{11}} \quad G_{xy} = \frac{1}{2ha_{66}}$$
$$E_y = \frac{1}{2ha_{22}} \quad \nu_{xy} = -\frac{a_{12}}{a_{11}} \qquad \text{(Eq 28)}$$

where the divisor $2h$ corresponds to the laminate thickness.

Noting that the $[A]$ matrix consists of $[\bar{Q}]$ matrices from each layer in the laminate, it is obvious that the laminate elastic properties are functions of the angular orientation of the plies. This is illustrated in Fig. 6 for a typical high-modulus graphite-epoxy system. The lamina properties for this material are listed in Table 1. The laminae are oriented in $\pm\theta$ pairs in a symmetric, balanced construction, creating what is called an angle-ply laminate.

Figure 6 indicates a variation in extensional modulus similar to that shown for the off-axis unidirectional material (Fig. 3). The differences between an off-axis material and an angle-ply laminate are due to the effects of extensional-shear coupling. In an off-axis material, extensional loadings produce shear deformations as well as extensional deformations. In an angle-ply laminate, the shear deformations are eliminated through internal constraints. Since the shear strains are eliminated, the material exhibits higher effective stiffnesses.

Two other features are noteworthy in Fig. 6, namely, the variation of shear modulus and Poisson's ratio. The shear modulus is equal to the unidirectional value for $\theta = 0°$ and $\theta = 90°$; it rises sharply and reaches a maximum at $\theta = 45°$. The peak at 45° can be explained by noting that shear is equivalent to a combined state of equal tension and compression loads oriented at 45°. Thus, the shear loading on a $[\pm 45°]$ laminate is equivalent to tensile and compressive loading on a $[0°/90°]_s$ laminate. Effectively, the fibers are aligned with the loading; hence, the large shear stiffness.

An even more interesting effect is seen in the variation of Poisson's ratio. The peak value in this example is greater than 1.5. In an isotropic material, this would be impossible. In an orthotropic material, the isotropic restrictions do not hold, and a Poisson's ratio greater than one is valid and realistic. In fact, large Poisson's ratios are typical for laminates constructed of UDC materials with the plies oriented at approximately $\pm 30°$.

This effect can readily be explained by referring to Fig. 7, which shows two separate loadings on a $\pm 30°$ lamina. When a positive N_{xx} load is applied, the deformed shape contains a positive ε_{xx} and a negative ε_{xy}. In the $[\pm 30°]_s$ laminate, the shear strain is constrained by the presence of the –30° plies, causing an internal shear load, which eliminates the shear strain. The large Poisson's ratio is a result of this internal shear load. As shown in the second part of Fig. 7, a compressive N_{yy} load promotes a positive ε_{xy}. Because of material symmetries, the application of a positive N_{xy} would produce a compressive ε_{yy}. Therefore, the positive internal shear load required to constrain the shear strains developed by the positive N_{xx} in the first part of Fig. 7 produces a compressive ε_{yy}. Thus, the Poisson-induced strain is made up of two components: First, the applied tensile N_{xx} produces a compressive ε_{yy}, and, second, the induced positive N_{xy} produces a compressive ε_{yy}. Thus, the large Poisson's ratio is simply a function of extensional-shear coupling in the individual laminae.

Because of the infinite variability of the angular orientation of the individual laminae, presumably a laminate could be constructed having a stiffness which behaves isotropically in the plane of the laminate by using a large number of plies having small, equal differences in their orientation. It can be shown that a symmetric, quasi-isotropic laminate can also be constructed with as few as six plies, three plies above and three below the midplane. The simplest quasi-isotropic laminate is $[0°/\pm 60°]_s$. A general rule for describing a quasi-isotropic laminate states that the angles between plies are equal to π/N, where N is an integer greater than or equal to 3, and the number of plies at each orientation is identical, in a symmetric laminate. For plies of a given material, all such quasi-isotropic laminates will have the same elastic properties, regardless of the value of N.

As was stated, a quasi-isotropic laminate has in-plane stiffnesses which follow isotropic relationships. Thus:

$$E_x = E_y = E_\theta$$

where the subscript θ indicates any arbitrary angle. Additionally,

$$G_{xy} = \frac{E_x}{2(1 + \nu_{xy})}$$

There are two items which must be remembered with respect to quasi-isotropic laminates. First and foremost, only the elastic in-plane properties are isotropic; the strength properties, in general, will vary with direction. The second item is that two equal moduli, $E_x = E_y$, do not necessarily indicate quasi-isotropy. This second item is graphically demonstrated in Table 2 where three laminates each have identical E_x and E_y moduli.

The first two laminates in Table 2 are actually the same. If one rotates the $[0°/90°]_s$ laminate 45°, it is easily seen that it becomes a $[\pm 45°]_s$ laminate. Note that the extensional moduli of these laminates are not the same and that the shear modulus in each laminate is not related to the extensional moduli and Poisson's ratio. For these laminates, the π/N relation has not been satisfied and they are not quasi-isotropic.

The third laminate has plies oriented at 45° to each other, but there are not equal numbers of plies at each angle. This laminate is also not quasi-isotropic. This can be verified by computing a shear modulus using the isotropic relation.

The discussion of symmetric laminates has thus far centered on membrane behavior. It has been shown that symmetric laminates can be

Table 1 Properties of a high-modulus graphite-epoxy lamina

E_1 = 170 GPa (25.0 × 10^6 psi)
E_2 = 12 GPa (1.7 × 10^6 psi)
G_{12} = 4.5 GPa (0.65 × 10^6 psi)
ν_{12} = 0.30
ρ = 0.056
α_1 = –0.54 × 10^{-6}/K
α_2 = 35.1 × 10^{-6}/K
σ_L^{tu} = 758 MPa (110.0 ksi)
σ_T^{tu} = 28 MPa (4.0 ksi)
σ_L^{u} = 62 MPa (9.0 ksi)
σ_L^{cu} = 758 MPa (110.0 ksi)
σ_T^{cu} = 138 MPa (20.0 ksi)
V_f = 0.6

Note: Ply thickness, 0.13 mm (0.0052 in.)

Table 2 Elastic properties of laminates

	E_xE_y			G_{xy}	
	GPa	10^6 psi	ν_{xy}	GPa	10^6 psi
$[0°/90°]_s$	92.46	13.41	0.038	4.5	0.65
$[\pm 45°]_s$	16.4	2.38	0.829	44.5	6.46
$[0°/90°/+45°/–45°/90°/0°]_s$	75.64	10.97	0.213	17.9	2.59

Note: See Table 1 for lamina properties.

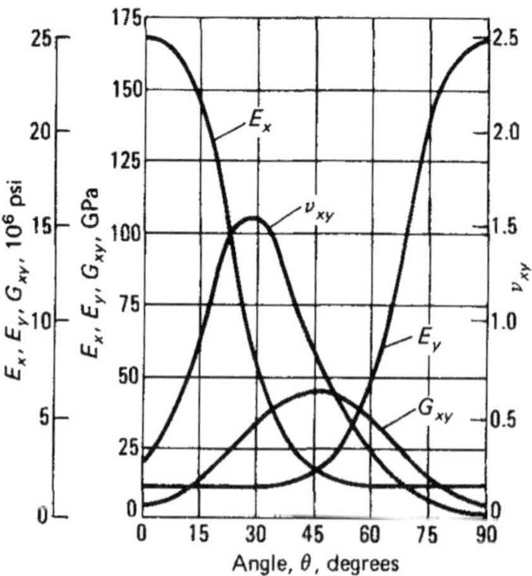

Fig. 6 Laminate elastic constants for high-modulus graphite-epoxy system, $[\pm\theta]_s$

Fig. 7 Extensional-shear coupling and Poisson's ratio

constructed that are very well behaved in the membrane sense. The bending behavior of symmetric laminates is considerably more complex, primarily due to the arrangement of the plies throughout the thickness of the laminate.

Unsymmetric Laminates. The use of laminates that are not midplane symmetric introduces some fundamental difficulties for the designer and analyst, the most important being how one defines the membrane and bending stiffnesses of such a material. Because this type of laminate bends when subjected to membrane loading, how is an extensional modulus defined? Conversely, since the material extends when subjected to a bending load, how is a bending stiffness defined?

Basically, there are two approaches to defining these elastic constants. A membrane stiffness can be derived either with zero curvatures or with zero bending moments, and a bending stiffness can be defined with either zero membrane strains or zero membrane forces. In both cases, the stiffness defined will be greater when the bending-extensional coupling is restrained. The nature of the problem can sometimes help the designer determine which approach to use.

In order to define stiffnesses of unsymmetric laminates with constrained bending-extensional coupling, it is necessary to use zero curvatures for extension and zero midplane strains for bending. Writing the full constitutive relations:

$$\begin{aligned}\{N\} &= [A]\{\varepsilon^0\} + [B]\{\kappa\} \\ \{M\} &= [B]\{\varepsilon^0\} + [D]\{\kappa\}\end{aligned} \qquad \text{(Eq 29)}$$

the extensional stiffness can be found by substituting $\kappa = 0$; thus:

$$\{N\} = [A]\{\varepsilon^0\} \qquad \text{(Eq 30)}$$

and bending stiffness can be found by substituting $\{\varepsilon^0\} = 0$.

$$\{M\} = [D]\{\kappa\} \qquad \text{(Eq 31)}$$

The relations shown in Eq 30 and 31 are identical to those used in symmetric laminates; therefore, the constrained stiffnesses are identical to those of symmetric laminates. However, moment resultants are required to develop the zero curvatures in Eq 30, and stress resultants are required to develop the zero midplane strains in Eq 31.

The moment resultants that are developed because of the prescribed zero curvatures can easily be determined. Solving Eq 30 for the resulting midplane strains yields:

$$\{\varepsilon^0\} = [A]^{-1}\{N\} \qquad \text{(Eq 32)}$$

Substituting these into Eq 29, while noting that the curvatures are zero, yields:

$$\{M\} = [B]\{\varepsilon^0\}$$

or

$$\{M\} = [B][A]^{-1}\{N\} \qquad \text{(Eq 33)}$$

Stress resultants developed because of curvature restraint can be found similarly. Thus:

$$\{\kappa\} = [D]^{-1}\{M\}$$

$$\{N\} = [B]\{\kappa\} \qquad \text{(Eq 34)}$$

or

$$\{N\} = [B][D]^{-1}\{\kappa\} \qquad \text{(Eq 35)}$$

Defining stiffnesses without constraining the bending-extensional coupling requires more effort. Referring to Eq 29, the extensional stiffnesses can be found by specifying that $\{M\} = 0$. Therefore:

$$\{0\} = [B]\{\varepsilon^0\} + [D]\{\kappa\} \qquad \text{(Eq 36)}$$

The curvatures can then be found to be:

$$\{\kappa\} = -[D]^{-1}[B]\{\varepsilon^0\} \qquad \text{(Eq 37)}$$

Substituting these into the first set of relations in Eq 29 yields:

$$\{N\} = [A]\{\varepsilon^0\} + [B](-[D]^{-1}[B]\{\varepsilon^0\}$$

or

$$\{N\} = ([A] - [B][D]^{-1}[B])\{\varepsilon^0\}$$

or

$$\{N\} = [A^*]\{\varepsilon^0\} \qquad \text{(Eq 38)}$$

The effective laminate extensional stiffnesses can now be found using the relations in Eq 28 and the effective stiffness matrix $[A^*]$.

An effective bending stiffness matrix can be determined similarly by specifying $\{N\} = 0$. Thus:

$$\{0\} = [A]\{\varepsilon^0\} + [B]\{\kappa\} \qquad \text{(Eq 39)}$$

Now the midplane strains are seen to be:

$$\{\varepsilon^0\} = -[A]^{-1}[B]\{\kappa\} \qquad \text{(Eq 40)}$$

and the second of relations in Eq 29 is rewritten as:

$$\{M\} = (-[B][A]^{-1}[B] + [D])\{\kappa\}$$

or

$$\{M\} = [D^*]\{\kappa\} \qquad \text{(Eq 41)}$$

yielding an effective bending stiffness matrix, $[D^*]$.

Thermal Expansion. As the use of composite materials becomes more common, they are subjected to mechanical and environmental loading conditions that are increasingly severe, and with the advent of high-temperature resin systems, the range of temperatures over which the composite system can be used has increased. Thus, it is necessary to understand the response of laminates to temperature and moisture, as well as to applied loads. Previously, laminate extensional and bending stiffnesses were determined; in this section, laminate conductivities and expansivities will be defined.

The presence of stresses induced by free thermal expansion is new to the designer and analyst of conventional materials. The mechanism that produces such stresses is qualitatively described in Fig. 8, which shows that free laminae and bonded laminae (laminate) expand differently. In the direction shown, the 0° plies will develop tensile stress, while the 90° ply will develop compressive stress because of the differences between the laminae and laminate thermal expansion coefficients. This effect is similar to heating a conventional material and providing constraints such that thermal expansion strains cannot develop.

To determine quantitatively the laminate thermal expansion coefficients and thermally induced stresses, it is necessary to begin at the ply level. The thermoelastic relations for strain in the principal material directions are:

$$\{\varepsilon_\ell\} = \{\varepsilon_\ell^M\} + \{\alpha_\ell\}\Delta T$$

or

$$\{\varepsilon_\ell\} = \{\varepsilon_\ell^M\} + \varepsilon_\ell^T \qquad \text{(Eq 42)}$$

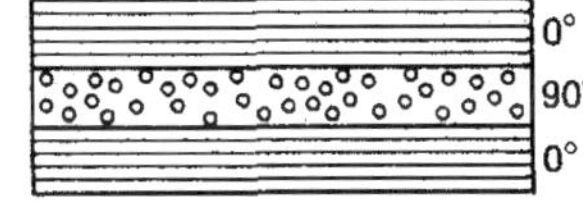

Heating of free laminae

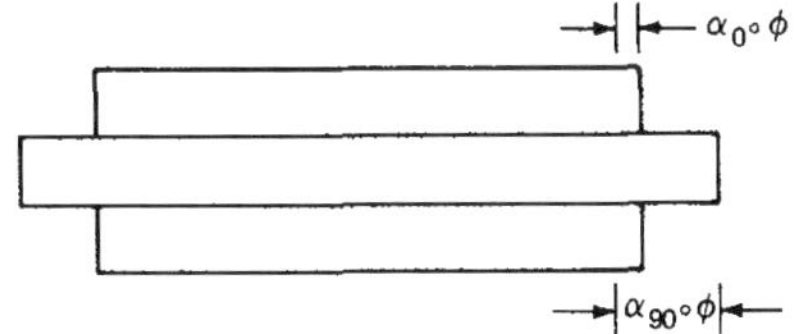

Heating of laminate

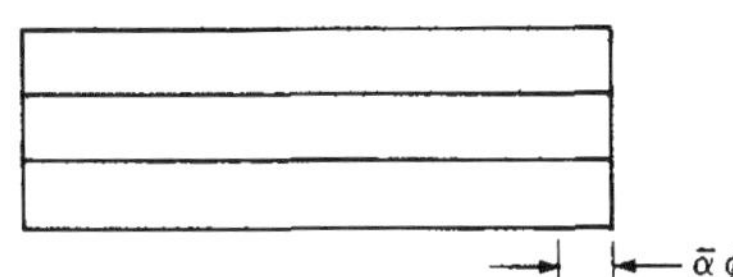

Fig. 8 Thermally induced loads

The vector $\{\alpha_\ell\}$ represents the free thermal expansion coefficients of a ply. The individual components are:

$$\{\alpha_\ell\} = \begin{Bmatrix} \alpha_1 \\ \alpha_2 \\ 0 \end{Bmatrix} \quad \text{(Eq 43)}$$

and ΔT represents a change in temperature. The thermal strains, $\{\alpha_\ell\}\Delta T$, are the lamina free thermal expansions. They produce no stress in an unconstrained lamina. The thermal expansion coefficients, α_1 and α_2, are the effective thermal expansion coefficients α_L^* and α_T^*, respectively, of the unidirectional composite.

Substituting for mechanical strain terms in Eq 42 and inverting, yields:

$$\{\sigma_\ell\} = [Q]\{\varepsilon_\ell\} - \{\Gamma_\ell\}\Delta T \quad \text{(Eq 44)}$$

where

$$\{\Gamma_\ell\} = [Q]\{\alpha_\ell\}$$

The components in the thermal stress coefficient vector, $\{\Gamma_\ell\}$, can be shown, by carrying out the indicated multiplication, to be:

$$\{\Gamma_\ell\} = \begin{Bmatrix} \dfrac{E_1\alpha_1 + \nu_{12}E_2\alpha_2}{\Delta} \\ \dfrac{E_2\alpha_2 + \nu_{12}E_1\alpha_1}{\Delta} \\ 0 \end{Bmatrix} \quad \text{(Eq 45)}$$

where

$$\Delta = 1 - \frac{E_2}{E_1}\nu_{12}^2$$

The vector $\{\Gamma_\ell\}\Delta T$ physically represents a correction to the stress vector, which results from the full constraint of the free thermal strains in a lamina.

Both the thermal expansion vector, $\{\alpha_\ell\}\Delta T$, and thermal stress vector, $\{\Gamma_\ell\}\Delta T$, can be transformed to an arbitrary coordinate system using the relations developed for stress and strain transformation (Eq 7 and 8).

With transformed thermal expansion and stress vectors, it is possible to develop thermoelastic laminate relations. Following directly the development of Eq 21 to 25, the membrane relations are:

$$\{N\} = [A]\{\varepsilon^0\} + [B]\{\kappa\} + \{N^T\} \quad \text{(Eq 46)}$$

where

$$\{N^T\} = -\int_{-h}^{h} \{\Gamma_x\}\Delta T \, dz \quad \text{(Eq 47)}$$

Similarly, the bending relations are

$$\{M\} = [B]\{\varepsilon^0\} + [D]\{\kappa\} + \{M^T\} \quad \text{(Eq 48)}$$

where

$$\{M^T\} = \int_{-h}^{h} \{\Gamma_x\}\Delta T \, z dz$$

The integral relations for the thermal stress resultant vector, $\{N^T\}$, and thermal moment resultant vector, $\{M^T\}$, can be evaluated only when the change in temperature variation through the thickness of the laminate is known. For uniform temperature change through the thickness, the term ΔT is constant and can be factored out of the integration, yielding:

$$\{N^T\} = \Delta T \sum_{i=1}^{K} \{\Gamma_x\}^i (z_i - z_{i-1})$$
$$\{M^T\} = \frac{1}{2}\Delta T \sum_{i=1}^{K} \{\Gamma_x\}^i (z_i^2 - z_{i-1}^2)$$

With the relations in Eq 46 and 48, it is possible to determine effective laminate coefficients of thermal expansion and thermal curvature. These quantities are the extension and curvature changes resulting from a uniform temperature distribution.

Noting that for free thermal effects $\{N\} = \{M\} = 0$, and defining a free thermal expansion vector as

$$\{\alpha_x\} = \{\varepsilon^0\}\frac{1}{\Delta T} \quad \text{(Eq 50)}$$

and a free thermal curvature vector as

$$\{\delta_x\} = \{\kappa\}\frac{1}{\Delta T} \quad \text{(Eq 51)}$$

the relations in Eq 46 and 48 can be solved. After suitable matrix manipulations, the following expressions for thermal expansion, $\{\alpha_x\}$, and thermal curvature, $\{\delta_x\}$, are found:

$$\{\alpha_x\} = \frac{1}{\Delta T}[L_1]^{-1}([B][D]^{-1}\{M^T\} - \{N^T\}) \quad \text{(Eq 52)}$$

$$\{\delta_x\} = \frac{1}{\Delta T}[L_2]^{-1}([B][A]^{-1}\{N^T\} - \{M^T\}) \quad \text{(Eq 53)}$$

where

$$[L_1] = [A] - [B][D]^{-1}[B]$$

$$[L_2] = [D] - [B][A]^{-1}[B]$$

The relations in Eq 52 and 53 are complicated expressions containing the $[A]$, $[B]$, and $[D]$ matrices. In many practical cases, the laminates of interest are symmetric, which simplifies the expressions considerably. For symmetric laminates, the bending-extensional coupling vanishes (that is, $[B] = 0$), and the relations are reduced to the form:

$$\{\alpha_x\} = -\frac{1}{\Delta T}[A]^{-1}\{N^T\}$$
$$\{\delta_x\} = -\frac{1}{\Delta T}[D]^{-1}\{M^T\} \quad \text{(Eq 54)}$$

Examination of the relations for $\{M^T\}$, Eq 49, shows that the symmetry that eliminates the $[B]$ matrix also eliminates the $\{M^T\}$ vector. Thus:

$$\{\delta_x\} = \{0\} \quad \text{(Eq 55)}$$

and no curvatures occur because of uniform temperature changes in symmetric laminates.

The variation of the longitudinal thermal expansion coefficient for a symmetric angle-ply laminate is shown in Fig. 9 to illustrate the effect of laminae orientation. At $\theta = 0°$, the term α_x is simply the axial lamina coefficient of thermal expansion; at $\theta = 90°$, α_x equals the lamina transverse thermal expansion coefficient. An interesting feature of the curve is the large negative value of α_x in the region of 30°. In Fig. 6, the value of Poisson's ratio also behaves peculiarly in the region around 30°. The odd variation of both the coefficient of thermal expansion and Poisson's ratio stems from the magnitude and sign of the shear-extensional coupling in the individual lamina.

Previously, classes of laminates were shown to have isotropic stiffnesses in the plane of the laminate. Similarly, laminates that are isotropic in thermal expansion within the plane of the laminate can be specified. The requirements for thermal expansion isotropy are considerably less restrictive than those for elastic constants. In fact, any laminate that has two identical, orthogonal

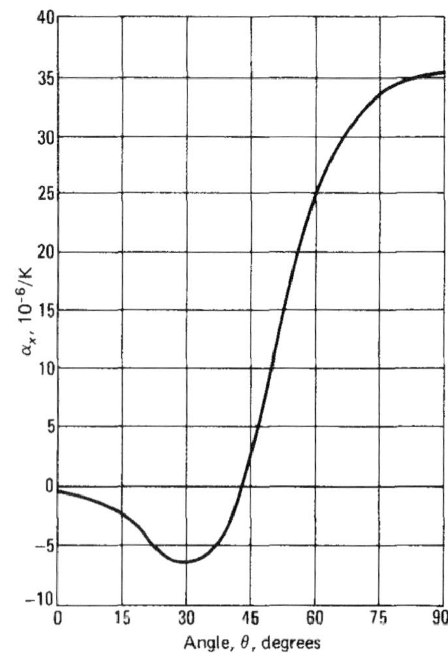

Fig. 9 Thermal expansion coefficients for high-modulus graphite-epoxy system, $[\pm\theta]_s$

thermal expansion coefficients and a zero-shear thermal expansion coefficient is isotropic in thermal expansion. Thus, $[0°/90°]_s$ and $[\pm 45°]_s$ laminates are isotropic in thermal expansion even though they are not quasi-isotropic for elastic stiffnesses.

Laminates that are isotropic in thermal expansion have thermal expansions of the form:

$$\{\alpha_x\} = \begin{Bmatrix} \alpha_x \\ \alpha_y \\ \alpha_{xy} \end{Bmatrix} = \begin{Bmatrix} \alpha^* \\ \alpha^* \\ 0 \end{Bmatrix} \quad \text{(Eq 56)}$$

where the term α^* can be shown to be a function of lamina properties only, as follows:

$$\alpha^* = \alpha_1 + \frac{(\alpha_2 - \alpha_1)(1 + \nu_{12})}{1 + 2\nu_{12} + \dfrac{E_1}{E_2}}$$

Thus, for a given ply material, all laminates that are isotropic in thermal expansion have identical expansion coefficients.

Moisture Expansion. Resin matrix composites are said to be hygroelastic when the matrix absorbs and desorbs moisture from and to the environment. The primary effect of moisture sorption is a volumetric change in the laminae. When a lamina absorbs moisture, it expands; when moisture is lost, the lamina contracts. Thus, the effect is similar to thermal expansion.

In a lamina, a free moisture expansion coefficient vector can be defined as:

$$\{\varepsilon_\ell\} = \{\beta_\ell\}\Delta M \quad \text{(Eq 57)}$$

where

$$\{\beta_\ell\} = \begin{Bmatrix} \beta_1 \\ \beta_2 \\ 0 \end{Bmatrix}$$

and ΔM is moisture change by weight. Noting that the relations in Eq 57 are identical to those of thermal expansion, with $\{\beta_\ell\}$ substituted for $\{\alpha_\ell\}$ and ΔM substituted for ΔT, it can easily be seen that all of the relations developed for thermal effects can be used for moisture effects, as long as the substitutions mentioned are performed.

The procedure required to determine moisture gains or losses are described in the section "Stresses Due to Temperature and Moisture" subsequently in this article. The analytical procedures detailed here allow for the prediction of moisture-induced stresses when the percent moisture change is known for the laminate. As with the thermoelastic analysis, only elastic effects have been treated.

Conductivity. The conductivity (thermal or moisture) of a laminate in the direction normal to the surface is equal to the transverse conductivity of a unidirectional fiber composite. This follows from the fact that normal conductivity for all plies is identical and unaffected by ply orientation.

The in-plane conductivities will be required for certain problems involving spatial variations of temperature and moisture. For a given uniform state of moisture in a laminate, the effective thermal conductivities in the x and y directions can be obtained by methods entirely analogous to those used previously for stiffnesses:

$$\mu_x = \frac{1}{2h}\sum_{i=1}^{K}(\mu_1 m^2 + \mu_2 n^2)t_{\text{ply}}^i \quad \text{(Eq 58)}$$

$$\mu_y = \frac{1}{2h}\sum_{i=1}^{K}(\mu_1 n^2 + \mu_2 m^2)t_{\text{ply}}^i \quad \text{(Eq 59)}$$

where μ_1 is the conductivity in the fiber direction, μ_2 is the conductivity transverse to the fibers, m is cos θ^i, n is sin θ^i, θ^i is the orientation of ply i, t_{ply} is the thickness of ply i, K is the total number of plies, and $2h$ is the laminate thickness. The results apply to symmetric as well as to asymmetric laminates. The results for moisture conductivity are identical.

Thermal and Hygroscopic Analysis

This section is concerned with the distribution of temperature and moisture through the thickness of a laminate. The mathematical descriptions of these two phenomena are identical, and the physical effects are similar. Some of these aspects have already been discussed.

A free lamina undergoes stress-free deformation due to temperature change or moisture

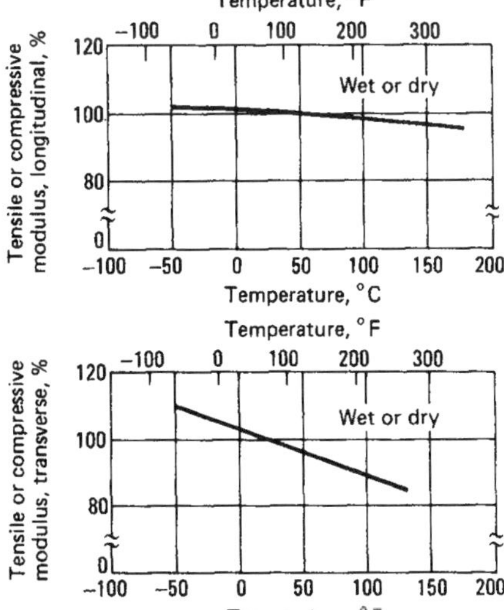

Fig. 10 Effects of moisture and temperature on lamina stiffness measured at room temperature

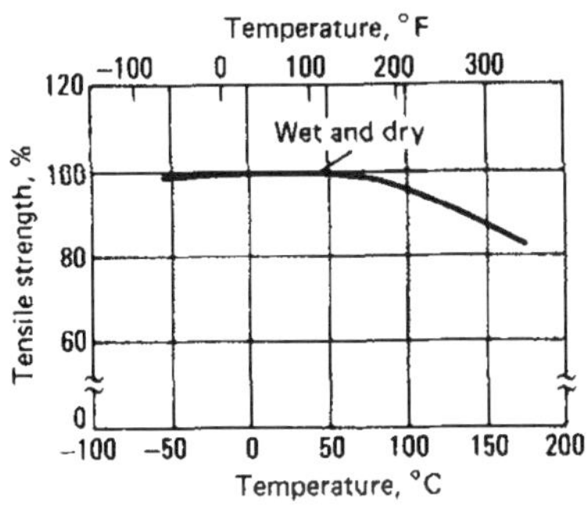

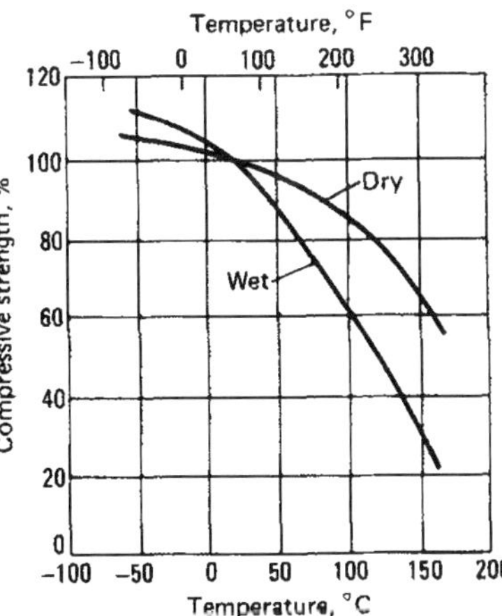

Fig. 11 Effects of moisture and temperature on lamina longitudinal strength, measured at room temperature

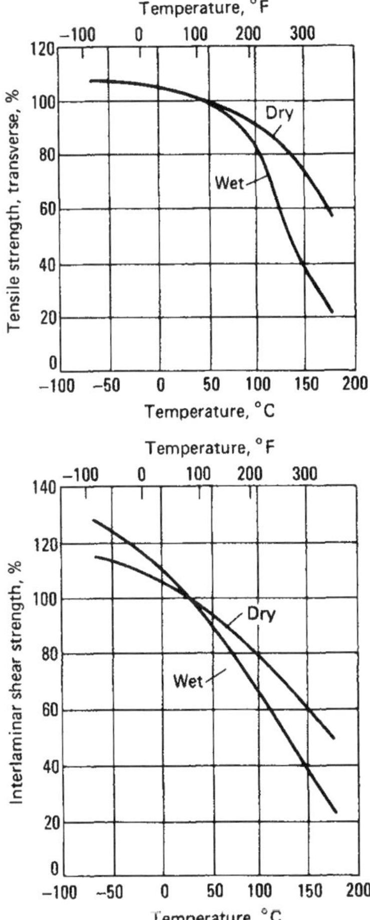

Fig. 12 Effects of moisture and temperature on lamina matrix-dominated strengths measured at room temperature

swelling. In a laminate, stress-free deformation is constrained by adjacent layers, producing internal stresses. In addition to the swelling-induced stresses, temperature and moisture content also affect the properties of the material. These effects are primarily related to matrix-dominated strength properties. Figure 10 (Ref 1) indicates that for the typical graphite-epoxy system, moisture has little or no effect on stiffness. Figures 11 and 12 (Ref 1) show a large variation in strength, with the exception of axial tension. In each of these figures, the presence of moisture is seen to decrease the elevated-temperature strengths of the material while neither detrimentally affecting nor increasing the lower-temperature strengths.

The principal strength-degrading effect is related to a change in the glass transition temperature of the matrix material. As moisture is absorbed, the temperature at which the matrix changes from a glassy state to a viscous state decreases. Thus, the elevated-temperature strength properties decrease with increasing moisture. Limited data suggest, however, that this process is reversible. When the moisture content of the composite is decreased, the glass transition temperature increases and the original strength properties return.

In Fig. 10, 11, and 12, the term *wet* indicates that the material is fully saturated. This condition corresponds to a state of equilibrium with the environment at which the relative humidity is nearly 100%. The equilibrium moisture content at full saturation for typical epoxy composite systems ranges from about 1.0 to 2.5% weight gain.

All of these considerations also apply in the case of temperature rise in the sense that the matrix and therefore the laminae lose stiffness and strength when the temperature rises. Therefore, this effect is primarily important for matrix-dominated properties.

The differential equation governing time-dependent moisture sorption of an orthotropic homogeneous material is given by:

$$D_1 \frac{\partial^2 c}{\partial x_1^2} + D_2 \frac{\partial^2 c}{\partial x_2^2} + D_3 \frac{\partial^2 c}{\partial x_3^2} = \frac{\partial c}{\partial t} \quad \text{(Eq 60)}$$

where t is time, x_1, x_2, x_3 are coordinates in principal material directions, c is the specific moisture concentration, and D_1, D_2, and D_3 are moisture diffusivity coefficients. Equation 60 is based on Fick's law of moisture diffusion and is entirely analogous to the equation governing time-dependent heat conduction, with temperature, φ, replacing concentration, c, and thermal conductivities, μ_1, μ_2, and μ_3 replacing the moisture diffusivities. For a transversely isotropic lamina, with x_1 in the fiber direction, x_2 in the transverse direction, and $x_3 = z$ in the direction normal to the lamina:

$$D_1 = D_L$$

$$D_2 = D_3 = D_T \quad \text{(Eq 61)}$$

These quantities are analogous to the thermal conductivities of a UDC.

An important special case is one-dimensional diffusion or conduction through the thickness of a lamina. In this case, Eq 60 reduces to:

$$D_T \frac{\partial^2 c}{\partial z^2} = \frac{\partial c}{\partial t} \quad \text{(Eq 62)}$$

This equation also applies to moisture diffusion or thermal conduction through a laminate, in the direction normal to its laminae planes, since all laminae are homogeneous in the z-direction with equal diffusion coefficients, $D_T = D_z$.

Equation 62 is applicable to the important problem of time-dependent moisture diffusion through a laminate where the two faces are in different moisture environments. After enough time has elapsed, the concentration settles down to a time-independent (so-called stationary) state. In this state, since c is no longer time-dependent, Eq 62 simplifies to:

$$\frac{d^2 c}{dz^2} = 0$$

Thus, c is a linear function of z, and if the laminate faces are in environments with constant saturation concentrations, c_1 and c_2, then:

$$c = \frac{1}{2}\left[(c_2 - c_1)z/h + c_2 + c_1\right] \quad \text{(Eq 63)}$$

where the laminate thickness is $2h$, and z originates in the middle surface. In the important case where $c_2 = c_1$, Eq 63 reduces to:

$$c = c_1 = \text{constant} \quad \text{(Eq 64)}$$

The foregoing discussion of moisture also applies to heat conduction.

Solutions to the time-dependent problem, Eq 62, are readily available, and considerable work has been performed in the area of moisture absorption (Ref 2). The most interesting feature of the solutions to Eq 62 relates to the magnitude of the coefficient D_z, which is a measure of the speed of moisture diffusion. In typical epoxy matrix systems, D is of the order of 645×10^{-8} mm^2/s (1×10^{-8} in.^{2}/s) to 645×10^{-10} mm^2/s (1×10^{-10} in.^{2}/s). The diffusion coefficient is sufficiently small that full saturation of a resin matrix composite may require months or years, even when subjected to 100% relative humidity.

The approach typically taken for design purposes is to assume a worst-case scenario. If the material is assumed to be fully saturated, reduced allowable strengths can be computed. This is a conservative approach, because typical service environments do not generate full saturation. It is used because it allows for inclusion of the effects of moisture in a relatively simple fashion. Design databases are growing and analytical methods are maturing, so that the worst-case combinations of environment factors can be considered for the specific materials and loading being studied. In the cases where moisture absorption is detrimental, full saturation can be assumed.

In the case of heat conduction, the time required to achieve the stationary state, the analogue of saturation, is extremely rapid. Thus, the transient time-dependent state is generally of little practical importance for laminates.

Laminate Stress Analysis

The physical properties defined in the section "Laminate Properties" in this article enable any laminate to be represented by an equivalent homogeneous anisotropic plate or shell element for the purpose of structural analysis. The results will be the definition of stress resultants, bending moments, temperature, and moisture at any point on the surface defining the plate. (Temperature and moisture distributions through the thickness of the plate will also be defined when they exist.) With this definition of the local values of the state variables, a laminate analysis is next performed to determine the state of stress in each lamina in order to assess margins for each critical design condition.

Stresses Due to Mechanical Loads. To determine stresses in the individual plies, the laminate midplane strain and curvature vectors must be used. Writing the laminate constitutive relations as:

$$\left\{\frac{N}{M}\right\} = \left[\begin{array}{c|c} A & B \\ \hline B & D \end{array}\right] \left\{\frac{\varepsilon^0}{\kappa}\right\} \quad \text{(Eq 65)}$$

shows that a simple inversion will yield the required relations for $\{\varepsilon^0\}$ and $\{\kappa\}$. Thus:

$$\left\{\frac{\varepsilon^0}{\kappa}\right\} = \left[\begin{array}{c|c} A & B \\ \hline B & D \end{array}\right]^{-1} \left\{\frac{N}{M}\right\} \quad \text{(Eq 66)}$$

Given the strain and curvature vectors, the total strain in the laminate can be written as:

$$\{\varepsilon_x\} = \{\varepsilon^0\} + z\{\kappa\} \quad \text{(Eq 67)}$$

The strains at any point through the laminate thickness are now given as the superposition of the midplane strains and the curvatures multiplied by the distance from the midplane. Thus, the strain field at the center of ply i in a laminate can be seen to be:

$$\{\varepsilon_x\}^i = \{\varepsilon^0\} + \frac{1}{2}\{\kappa\}(z^i + z^{i+1}) \quad \text{(Eq 68)}$$

where the term

$$\frac{1}{2}(z^i + z^{i+1})$$

corresponds to the distance from the midplane to the center of ply i. Curvature-induced strains at a point through the laminate thickness can be defined simply by specifying the distance to the point in question from the midplane.

The strains defined in Eq 68 correspond to the arbitrary laminate coordinate system. These strains can be transformed into the principal material coordinates for this ply by using transformations developed previously. Thus:

$$\{\varepsilon_\ell\}^i = \left[\theta^i\right]^{-1}\{\varepsilon_x\}^i \quad \text{(Eq 69)}$$

where the superscript i indicates which ply and therefore which angle of orientation is to be used. Because the orientations of the various plies may differ, it is necessary to use the transformation matrix corresponding to the proper ply orientation.

With the strains in the principal material coordinates defined, stresses in these same coordinates are written using the lamina reduced stiffness matrix (Eq 5). Thus:

$$\{\sigma_\ell\}^i = \left[Q^i\right]\{\varepsilon_\ell\}^i \quad \text{(Eq 70)}$$

Again, it is important that the stiffness matrix used correspond to the correct ply, as each ply may be of a different material.

The stresses in the principal material coordinates can be determined without the use of principal material strains. Using the strains defined in the laminate coordinates (Eq 68) and the transformed lamina stiffness matrix (Eq 9, 11, 12), stresses in the laminate coordination system are written as:

$$\{\sigma_x\}^i = \left[\bar{Q}^i\right]\{\varepsilon_x\}^i \quad \text{(Eq 71)}$$

and these stresses are then transformed to the principal material coordinates. Thus:

$$\{\sigma_\ell\}^i = \left[\theta^i\right]^{-1}\{\sigma_x\}^i \quad \text{(Eq 72)}$$

Reviewing these relations, it can be seen that for the case of symmetric laminates and membrane loading, the curvature vector is zero. This implies that the laminate coordinate strains are identical in each ply and equal to the midplane strains. The differing angular orientation of the various plies will promote different stress and strain fields in the principal material coordinates of each ply.

Stresses Due to Temperature and Moisture. When the equations for the thermoelastic response of composite laminates were developed, it was indicated that thermal loading in laminates can cause stresses within the plies even when the laminate is allowed to expand freely. The stresses are induced because of a mismatch in thermal expansion coefficients between plies oriented in different directions. Either the mechanical stresses of the preceding section or the thermomechanical stresses to be calculated in this section can be used to evaluate laminate strength.

To determine the magnitude of thermally induced stresses, the thermoelastic constitutive relations (Eq 46, 48) are required. Since free thermal effects require that $\{N\} = \{M\} = 0$, these relations are written as:

$$\begin{Bmatrix} 0 \\ 0 \end{Bmatrix} = \left[\begin{array}{c|c} A & B \\ \hline B & D \end{array}\right]\begin{Bmatrix} \varepsilon^0 \\ \kappa \end{Bmatrix} + \begin{Bmatrix} N^T \\ M^T \end{Bmatrix} \quad \text{(Eq 73)}$$

Inverting these relations yields the free thermal strain and curvature vectors for the laminate:

$$-\left[\begin{array}{c|c} A & B \\ \hline B & D \end{array}\right]^{-1}\begin{Bmatrix} N^T \\ M^T \end{Bmatrix}\begin{Bmatrix} \varepsilon^0 \\ \kappa \end{Bmatrix} \quad \text{(Eq 74)}$$

Proceeding as before, the strain field in any ply is written as:

$$\{\varepsilon_x\}^i = \{\varepsilon^0\} + z^i\{\kappa\} \quad \text{(Eq 75)}$$

Stresses in the laminate coordinates are written as:

$$\{\sigma_x\}^i = \left[\bar{Q}^i\right]\{\varepsilon_x\}^i - \{\Gamma_x\}^i\,\Delta T^i \quad \text{(Eq 76)}$$

which can then be transformed to the principal material coordinates. Thus:

$$\{\sigma_\ell\}^i = \left[\theta^i\right]^{-1}\{\sigma_x\}^i \quad \text{(Eq 77)}$$

As was shown for mechanically induced loadings, the stresses can be found in another fashion. Transforming the strains of Eq 75 directly yield

$$\{\varepsilon_\ell\}^i = \left[\theta^i\right]^{-1}\{\varepsilon_x\}^i \quad \text{(Eq 78)}$$

Recalling Eq 44, stresses in the principal material coordinates are written as:

$$\{\sigma_\ell\}^i = \left[Q^i\right]\{\varepsilon_\ell\}^i + \{\Gamma_\ell\}^i\,\Delta T^i \quad \text{(Eq 79)}$$

Some interesting physical interpretations can be obtained by restricting the discussion to uniform-temperature fields and symmetric laminates. In the presence of these restrictions, the coupling matrix, $[B]$, and the thermal moment resultant vector, $\{M^T\}$, vanish, and:

$$\{\varepsilon^0\} = \{\alpha_x\}\Delta T$$

and

$$\{\kappa\} = \{0\}$$

The strains in the laminate coordinates are identical in each ply. Thus:

$$\{\varepsilon_x\}^i = \{\varepsilon^0\} = \{\alpha_x\}\Delta T \quad \text{(Eq 80)}$$

For this case, it can be shown that:

$$\{\sigma_x\}^i = \left[\bar{Q}^i\right](\{\alpha\} - \{\alpha_x\}^i)\Delta T \quad \text{(Eq 81)}$$

These relations indicate that stresses induced by the free thermal expansion of a laminate are related to the differences between the laminate and the ply thermal expansion vectors. Thus, the stresses are proportional to the difference between the amount the ply would freely expand and the amount the laminate will allow it to expand.

A further simplification can be found if the laminate under investigation is isotropic in thermal expansion. It can be shown that if this class of laminates is subjected to a uniform temperature change, the stresses in the principal material coordinates are identical in every ply. The stress vector can be shown to be:

$$\{\sigma_\ell\} = \frac{E_{11}(\alpha_{22} - \alpha_{11})\Delta T}{1 + 2\nu_{12} + \dfrac{E_{11}}{E_{22}}}\begin{Bmatrix} 1 \\ -1 \\ 0 \end{Bmatrix} \quad \text{(Eq 82)}$$

where the transverse direction stress is equal and opposite to the fiber direction stress. This is important because unidirectional transverse material strengths are typically an order of magnitude lower than fiber direction strengths.

A similar development can be generated for moisture-induced stresses. All of the results of this section apply when the moisture swelling coefficients, $\{\beta_1\}$, are substituted for the thermal expansion coefficients, $\{\alpha_1\}$.

Netting Analysis. Another approach to the calculation of ply stresses is sometimes used for membrane loading of laminates. This procedure, called netting analysis, treats the laminate as a net; that is, all loads are carried in the fibers while the matrix material is present only to hold the geometric position of the fibers.

Since only the fibers are assumed to be loaded in this analytical model, stress-strain relations in the principal material directions can be written as:

$$\sigma_{11} = E_1\varepsilon_{11}$$

or

$$\varepsilon_{11} = \frac{1}{E_1}\sigma_{11} \quad \text{(Eq 83)}$$

and

$$E_2 = G_{12} = \sigma_{22} = \sigma_{12} = 0$$

The laminate stiffnesses predicted by means of a netting analysis will be smaller than those predicted using lamination theory, because of exclusion of the transverse and shear stiffnesses from the formulation. This effect is demonstrated in Table 3 for a quasi-isotropic laminate consisting of high-modulus graphite-epoxy. The stiffness properties predicted using a netting analysis are on the order of 10% smaller than those predicted using lamination theory. Experimental work has consistently shown that lamination theory predictions are more realistic.

Although the stiffness predictions using netting analyses are of limited value, such an analysis can be used as an approximation of the response of a composite in which the matrix has been damaged. In this sense it may be considered a worst-case analysis and is frequently used to predict ultimate strengths of composite laminates.

Interlaminar Stresses. The analytical procedures that have been developed in this article can be used to predict stresses within each lamina in a laminate. The stresses predicted are planar because of the assumed state of plane stress. There are cases for which the assumption of plane stress is not valid and a three-dimensional stress analysis is required.

An example of such a case exists at certain free edges in laminates where stress-free boundary conditions must be imposed. When the laminate in Fig. 13 is subjected to a membrane loading in the x direction, Poisson's ratio mismatches between the 0° plies and the $\pm 60°$ plies will introduce a stress in the y direction in each ply. Additionally, extensional-shear coupling effects will generate equal but opposite shear stresses in the 60° and –60° plies. In Fig. 13, all σ_y and σ_{xy} stresses must vanish at $y = \pm b$ to satisfy the stress-free boundary conditions. This cannot be accomplished with lamination theory; a three-dimensional analysis is required.

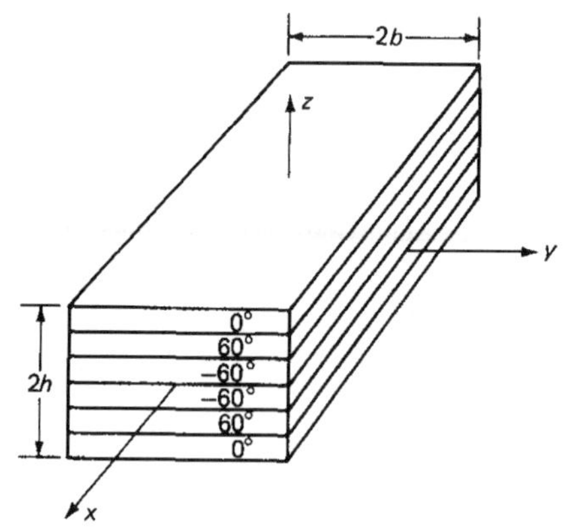

Fig. 13 Laminate construction (interlaminar stress example)

Using equilibrium and symmetry considerations, the other components of stress which arise at the free edge can be visualized. In Fig. 14, lamination theory stresses are shown for the uniaxial loading discussed previously; it can be seen that the laminate analysis satisfies equilibrium in the y direction but not the conditions at the free boundary. Thus, additional forces are required to satisfy the boundary conditions. For example, in the 0° plies, a compressive σ_y is predicted using lamination theory. This does not satisfy the boundary condition locally. A second, self-equilibrating set of edge stresses may be regarded as a superposed stress field that brings the lamination theory stresses to the necessary boundary values. Thus, an interlaminar shear stress, σ_{yz}, develops between the 0° and 60° plies. This introduces an x-moment disequilibrium even though the y-direction force equilibrium has been satisfied. To achieve x-moment equilibrium, a couple is needed. The required couple develops as an interlaminar normal stress distribution which, in Fig. 15, is seen to be compressive at $y = b$. For a couple to develop, the normal stress must change sign as the distance from the free edge increases.

In Fig. 16, a similar situation exists with respect to the in-plane shear stresses, σ_{xy}. At the free edge, $y = b$, these stresses must vanish. Therefore, the other component of interlaminar shear stress, σ_{xz}, develops, and the stress-free boundary conditions are satisfied. In each case it is seen that lamination theory satisfies strain compatibility and equilibrium, while the interlaminar stresses satisfy the stress-free boundary conditions.

The sign of the interlaminar normal stress at the free edge can be of great importance. As can be inferred from previous discussions, a large Poisson's ratio mismatch between plies produces large interlaminar normal stresses. If these stresses are tensile, the laminate may split between plies, or delaminate, under membrane loading. Obviously, if the laminate is designed such that expected loadings produce only compressive interlaminar normal stresses at the free edges, delamination will not occur.

The free-edge problem occurs wherever ply stresses must become zero to satisfy boundary conditions. Thus, any free edge, including holes, may introduce interlaminar stresses. The consequences of these stresses obviously need to be evaluated for structural applications, particularly where fatigue loadings are present. It can become extremely complex to provide quantitative analytical treatment of free-edge stresses in all but the most simple geometric shapes. In most cases, the possibility of delaminations due to the effects of free edge stresses is tested experimentally.

Nonlinear Stress Analysis. All of the preceding material in this article has related to laminae that behave in a linear elastic fashion. However, composites can behave in a nonlinear fashion because of such factors as internal damage or because of nonlinear stress-strain behavior of the polymeric matrix. Matrix nonlinearity (or microcracking) can result in laminae that have nonlinear stress-strain curves for transverse stress or axial shear stress. When this situation exists, the previously presented elastic laminate stress analysis must be replaced by a nonlinear analysis. A convenient procedure for doing this is found in Ref 3.

Table 3 Laminate elastic constants

Analysis	E_x GPa	E_x 10^6 psi	E_y GPa	E_y 10^6 psi	G_{xy} GPa	G_{xy} 10^6 psi	ν_{xy}
Lamination theory	64.9	9.42	64.9	9.42	24.5	3.55	0.325
Netting analysis	57.4	8.33	57.4	8.33	21.6	3.13	0.333

Note: Unit thickness: high-modulus graphite-epoxy

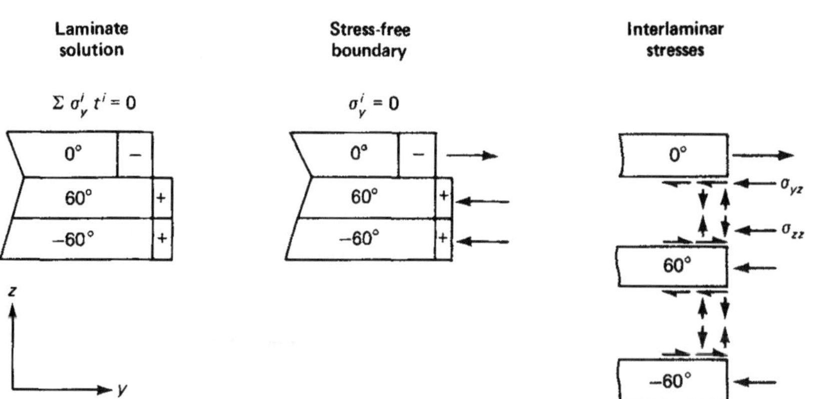

Fig. 14 Equilibrium and boundary conditions, y direction. t^i, thickness of ith ply

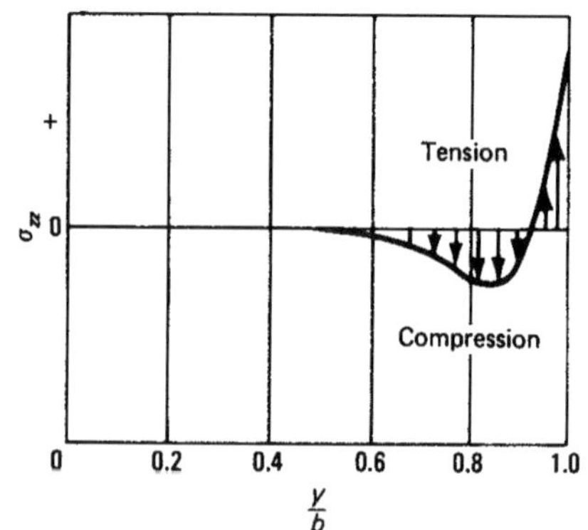

Fig. 15 Interlaminar normal stresses and moment equilibrium

This subject is of importance primarily for such specialized applications as dimensionally stable space structures. Hence, further treatment is beyond the scope of this article.

Strength and Failure

Methods for stress analysis of laminates subjected to mechanical loads, temperature changes, and moisture absorption are described in the previous section. The main reason for performing a stress analysis is to determine or assess the strength of a laminate. The problem is of primary practical significance, because design without knowledge of strength characteristics is impossible. Such information for laminates cannot be obtained on a purely experimental basis, because the number of candidate laminates is immense, and each of them is an anisotropic structural element. Thus, in each case it would be necessary to determine a set of strengths and to incorporate them into a failure criterion for a laminate under combined load. The situation is much more complex than for a UDC where the one-dimensional strengths can be obtained experimentally and only one failure criterion under combined stress is needed. In the present case, however, the one-dimensional strengths of a laminate are by themselves of great variety, because they depend on stacking sequence and layer orientations. To complicate matters further, both in-plane and bending loads must be considered.

This situation clearly requires analytical criteria for strengths of laminates, which, unfortunately, are not yet available. Consequently, the approaches and methods discussed will be both quantitative and qualitative.

The case of a perfect laminate, which does not contain defects of any kind, is considered first. When such a laminate is loaded in its plane, a simple stress distribution results, consisting of plane stress in each layer and a complex three-dimensional stress distribution at the edges that involves interlaminar normal and shear stress. Some of these stress components may become large at the edges; theoretically, they may become infinite. This at once indicates several modes of initial failure. Away from the edges, a laminate may fail either in what may be called a fiber mode, implying rupture or buckling of fibers, or in what may be called a matrix mode, implying longitudinal cracking parallel to the fibers. Since the state of stress is planar, there are no other failure modes. The advantage of the criteria to be developed for these modes is that they predict not only failure but also the mode. At the edges, the interlaminar stresses may produce delamination as the initial failure. The major difficulties of analytical strength definition are determining failures subsequent to the initial failure and providing a criterion for when these will produce ultimate failure of the laminate.

Initial Failure. For a laminate that is loaded by in-plane forces and/or bending moments, the stresses in the layers at a sufficient distance from the edges can be obtained by the methods developed in the previous section "Laminate Stress Analysis" in this article. If there is no external bending, if the membrane forces are constant along the edges, and if the laminate is balanced and symmetric, the stresses in the kth layer are constant and planar. With reference to the material axes of the laminae, fiber direction x_1 and transverse direction x_2, they are written σ_{11}^k, σ_{22}^k, and σ_{12}^k. Failure will occur when either one of the following failure criteria is satisfied:

Fiber mode

$$\left(\frac{\sigma_{11}^k}{\sigma_L^u}\right)^2 + \left(\frac{\sigma_{12}^k}{\tau_L^u}\right)^2 = 1$$

Matrix mode

$$\left(\frac{\sigma_{22}^k}{\sigma_L^u}\right)^2 + \left(\frac{\sigma_{12}^k}{\tau_L^u}\right)^2 = 1 \quad \text{(Eq 84)}$$

where σ_L^u is ultimate longitudinal stress and τ_L^u is ultimate longitudinal shear stress. It is necessary to distinguish between tensile (case a) and (case b) compressive normal stresses. Thus:

$$\sigma_L^u \begin{cases} \sigma_L^{tu} & \sigma_{11} > 0 \ \text{(a)} \\ \sigma_L^{cu} & \sigma_{11} < 0 \ \text{(b)} \end{cases} \quad \text{(Eq 85)}$$

$$\sigma_T^u \begin{cases} \sigma_T^{tu} & \sigma_{22} > 0 \ \text{(a)} \\ \sigma_T^{cu} & \sigma_{22} < 0 \ \text{(b)} \end{cases} \quad \text{(Eq 86)}$$

where σ_T^u is ultimate transverse stress, σ_L^{tu} and σ_T^{tu} are ultimate tensile stress, longitudinal and transverse; and σ_L^{cu} and σ_T^{cu} are ultimate compressive stress, longitudinal and transverse. Sometimes the simplistic maximum-stress criterion is used to assess the initiation of failure. For the *k*th lamina, the maximum-stress criterion assumes the form:

$$\begin{aligned} -\sigma_L^{cu} &\le \sigma_{11}^k \le \sigma_L^{tu} \\ -\sigma_T^{cu} &\le \sigma_{22}^k \le \sigma_T^{tu} \\ |\sigma_{12}|^k &\le \tau_L^u \end{aligned} \quad \text{(Eq 87)}$$

The maximum-stress criterion typically overestimates the strength of a lamina, because the interaction of stress components is neglected. Some stress interaction is obtained when the maximum-strain criterion is used. This involves replacing the stresses by ε_{11}, ε_{22}, and ε_{12} and replacing the ultimate stresses by the corresponding ultimate strains.

The failure criteria (Eq 84) must be used for each layer. The layer for which the criteria are satisfied by the lowest external load will define the load that produces the initial laminate failure, while also identifying the layer that fails and the nature of the failure (that is, fiber failure or cracking along fibers). This is called first-ply failure.

Bending occurs when there are external bending and/or twisting moments or when the laminate is not symmetric. In these cases, the stresses σ_{11}^k, σ_{22}^k, and σ_{12}^k in a layer are linear in x_3. Consequently, the stresses assume their maximum and minimum values at the layer interfaces; thus, the failure criteria (Eq 84) must be examined for each layer at these locations.

The situation is much more complicated for the edge stresses, where the state of stress is three-dimensional and must be obtained by numerical analysis in each case. The major problem is that there are edge stress singularities, that is, some interlaminar stresses become theoretically infinite. Numerical methods cannot uncover the nature of a singularity, but there are analytical treatments (Ref 4) that do this. The major problem is how to assess the implication for failure of such edge stress singularities, a problem as

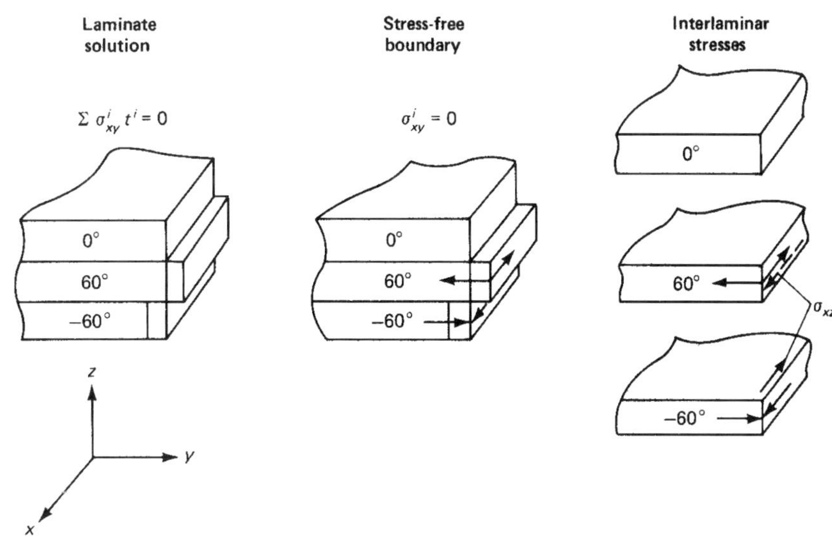

Fig. 16 Equilibrium and boundary conditions, *x* direction

yet unresolved. The situation is reminiscent of fracture mechanics in the sense that stresses at a crack tip are theoretically infinite, thus singular. Fracture mechanics copes with this difficulty in terms of a criterion for crack propagation that is based either on the amount of energy required to open a crack or, equivalently, on the value of the stress intensity factor. Similar considerations seem to apply for edge singularities, but the situation is much more complicated, since a crack initiating at the edge will propagate between anisotropic layers. It appears, therefore, that the problem of edge failure must be relegated to experimentation for the time being.

Subsequent Failures. In many cases, laminates have considerable strength remaining after first-ply failure; the difficult and important problem arises of analytically determining subsequent failures. As noted, this problem is far from resolved and an active area of research in composite materials. A simplistic, well known approach to this problem is as follows: when initial failure takes place, the failure may occur in the fiber or in the matrix mode. In the first case, the stiffness in the fiber direction, E_L, is reduced; in the second case, the elastic properties, E_T and G_L, are reduced. These elastic properties are not reduced to zero, because the initial failure produces cracks in the layer and the uncracked regions remain bonded to adjacent layers. Although a precise estimate of these stiffness reductions is not yet available, the simplest (but drastic) assumption is that E_L reduces to zero in the fiber mode and that E_T and G_L reduce to zero in the matrix mode. Since a laminate will usually not survive a fiber-mode failure, the progressive-failure cases of interest are initial and subsequent failures in the matrix mode. If it is assumed that, for failure of a lamina group in the matrix mode, E_T and G_L of that group can be set equal to zero, eventually the basic assumptions of netting analysis result. For netting analysis, the ultimate load is defined by the state at which E_T and G_L vanish in all laminae.

To demonstrate these effects, some specific examples of membrane loadings will be considered. The unidirectional lamina properties used in the examples are listed in Table 1.

The predicted load-strain response of a $(0°/\pm 45°)_s$ laminate subjected to three different membrane-loading environments is shown in Fig. 17, 18, and 19. For simplicity, failure analyses for these examples have been performed using the maximum-stress failure criterion.

The laminate loading in Fig. 17 consists of uniaxial tension in the direction of the 0° fibers, or the laminate x direction. The laminate response is seen to be linear to the load where the 0° fibers fail in axial tension. Because the failure mode is fiber breakage, no additional load-carrying capability exists.

In Fig. 18, the laminate loading consists of uniaxial tension perpendicular to the 0° fiber direction, or in the laminate y direction. The laminate response in this example is not linear to first fiber failure. Two distinct knees exist in the load-strain response. The first slope discontinuity corresponds to a transverse tensile failure in the 0° fibers. At this point, the lamina properties for the 0° plies are modified to account for the damage. Thus, for the 0° plies, the moduli E_2 and G_{12} are set to zero, and the laminate properties are reformulated.

Subjecting this damaged laminate to additional loading then yields transverse tensile failure in both the 45° and −45° plies, resulting in the second knee in the load-strain curve. When a new laminate is again formulated with all plies having moduli E_2 and G_{12} set to zero, additional loading produces fiber compressive mode failure in the 0° plies (followed immediately by fiber tensile mode failure in the 45° and −45° plies), which corresponds to the ultimate strength under N_{yy} loading.

The final membrane-loading state considered is an applied N_{xy} (Fig. 19). The response under this shear loading produces a single matrix-mode failure before ultimate or fiber-mode failure.

Examination of the three figures reveals major differences in laminate response under different loading states, simply because the ply stress states are very different from each other. This is apparent in Table 4, in which the states of stress in each ply of the laminate are listed at first-ply

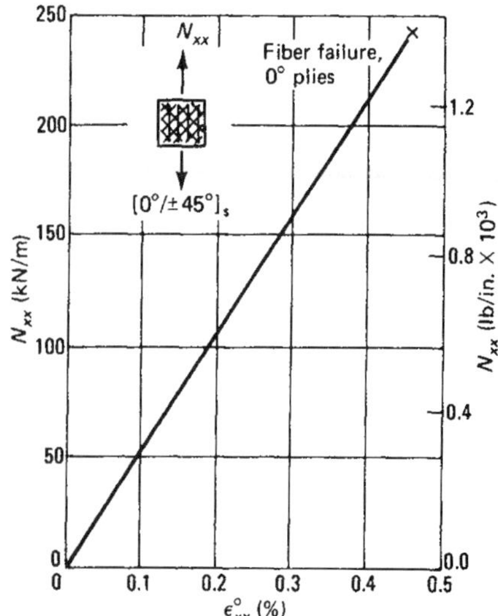

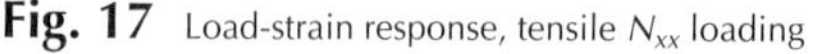

Fig. 17 Load-strain response, tensile N_{xx} loading

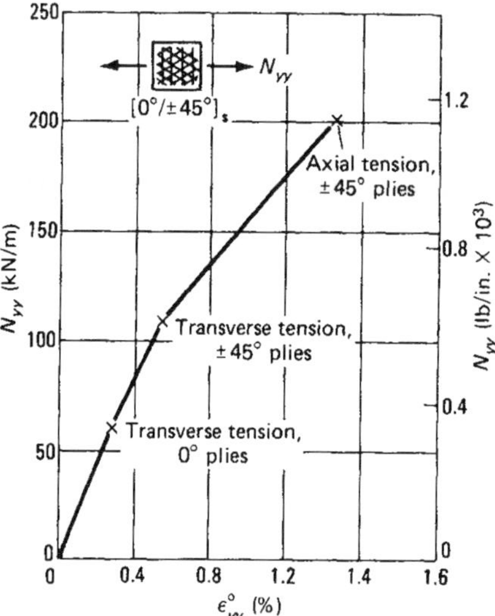

Fig. 18 Load-strain response, tensile N_{yy} loading

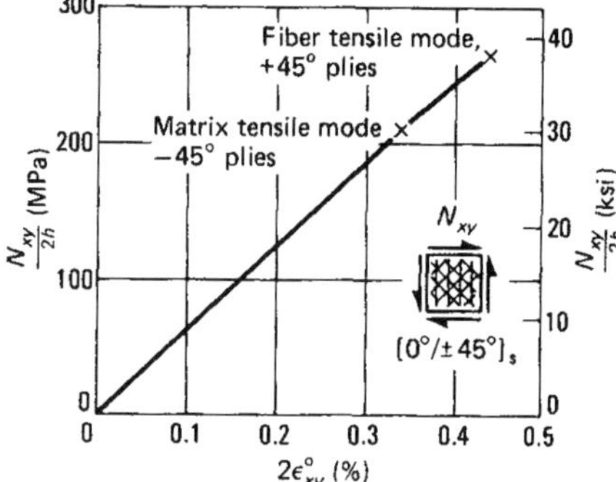

Fig. 19 Stress-strain response, N_{xy} loading

Table 4 Ply stresses at first-ply failure, $[0°/\pm 45°]_s$ laminate

	0° plies						45° plies						−45° plies					
	σ_1		σ_2		σ_{12}		σ_1		σ_2		σ_{12}		σ_1		σ_2		σ_{12}	
Loading, MPa (ksi)	MPa	ksi	MPa	ksi	MPa	ksi	MPa	ksi	MPa	ksi	MPa	ksi	MPa	ksi	MPa	ksi	MPa	ksi
$\frac{N_{xx}}{2h} = 308$ (44.7)	760	110.0(a)	−25	−3.6	0.0	0.0	88.3	12.8	7.58	1.10	−35.4	−5.14	88.3	12.8	7.58	1.10	35.4	5.14
$\frac{N_{yy}}{2h} = 75.2$ (10.9)	−140	−19.9	30	4.0(a)	0.0	0.0	150	22.4	13.4	1.95	15.4	2.23	154	22.4	13.4	1.95	−15.4	−2.23
$\frac{N_{xy}}{2h} = 208$ (30.2)	0.0	0.0	0.0	0.0	30.0	4.35	570	82.2	−28	−4.0	0.0	0.0	567	−82.3	28	4.0(a)	0.0	0.0

(a) Critical stress value

failure under the three membrane loadings applied. The stresses listed in Table 4 demonstrate that at the three different first-ply failure loads, different stress components in different plies are critical. When subjected to N_{xx} loading, the fiber-direction stress in the 0° plies reaches the lamina strength value first, hence promoting failure. The other ply stresses are not critical at this load. Under N_{yy} loading, the first stress component to reach the lamina strength is the transverse stress in the 0° plies. Shear loading produces a critical stress in the –45° plies in transverse tension. Thus, the critical stresses depend on loading direction.

The differences between first-ply failure and ultimate failure are shown in Fig. 20, in which the laminate failure surface for combined in-plane extensional stresses is shown for the laminate discussed above. The dashed curve defines the combination of applied laminate stresses for which the first-ply failure occurs in the matrix mode. The solid curve defines the combined laminate stress states, which result in failure of a ply in the fiber mode. Note that for most positive values of N_{yy}, a matrix-mode failure precedes the first fiber-mode failure. Conversely, for negative values of N_{yy}, the first-ply failure is always a fiber-mode failure. The large region between these two surfaces indicates the potentially limiting effect of low transverse and shear strengths of the individual plies and hence the limiting effect of the matrix properties.

The related failure surfaces for combined laminate membrane extensional and shear stress are presented in Fig. 21, which shows that for large membrane shear stresses, the first-ply failure is in the matrix mode. Again, the potential for performance improvement through changes in matrix properties appears to be worth considering.

The failure surfaces of Fig. 20 and 21 illustrate the importance of knowing the difference between the loads causing first-ply failure and ultimate failure. It is first necessary to determine whether there is additional load capacity in the laminate beyond the point of first-ply failure. A necessary condition for this is stability of the laminate (that is, it must be able to carry loads) after the loss of laminae stiffnesses associated with matrix-mode failure. For example, an angle-ply laminate ($\pm\theta$) experiencing matrix-mode failure when subjected to an axial load will be unable to carry that load. However, any laminate having fibers oriented in three or more directions can generally carry load after matrix-mode failure. An estimate of load-carrying capability can be obtained by using netting analysis.

In Table 5, laminate analysis predictions for first-ply failure strength and ultimate failure strength are shown, as well as netting analysis predictions for ultimate failure strength. In both the N_{yy} and N_{xy} loadings, the netting-analysis strength predictions are considerably larger than the first-ply failure laminate analysis predictions, indicating that considerable strength remains beyond first-ply failure. The netting analysis, however, predicts a lower strength than lamination theory for N_{xx} loadings, indicating that first-ply failure corresponds to ultimate failure. Because of the trends of the type indicated in Table 5, netting analysis can be a useful tool in composite strength predictions.

Strength. A conventional definition of material strength is the maximum static stress, or combination of stresses, that can be carried by the material. For example, in a simple uniaxial tensile test, strength is the highest stress achieved before the material breaks. In a metal, other points on the material stress-strain curve have also been found to be significant in considering the maximum stress to be applied to a material; for example, the proportional-limit stress and the material 0.2% offset yield stress are valuable measures of material strength. Similarly, in composites, several characteristic stress levels should be considered in the evaluation of strength. The primary stress levels of interest are the stress at which first-ply failure occurs and the maximum static stress (stress resultant divided by laminate thickness) that the laminate can carry.

In the calculation of first-ply failure, residual thermal stresses must be considered. Residual stresses are the ply stresses induced in a laminate as a result of fabrication processes. Typical resin matrix composites are formed under a combination of elevated temperature and pressure, which promotes matrix curing. When the laminate is subsequently cooled to room temperature, significant residual processing stresses develop. How to include these stresses in the failure analysis presents a problem. The rationale for including them is obvious: the stresses exist after processing and can therefore be expected to influence the occurrence of first-ply failure. However, there is also a rationale for not including them. Because all resin matrix materials exhibit viscoelastic, or time-dependent, effects, a significant portion of the residual processing stresses can be assumed to dissipate through stress relaxation. Additionally, the processing stresses may be reduced through the introduction of transverse matrix microcracking. A limited amount of cracking may occur without significantly affecting the laminate elastic properties. This problem is complicated by the difficulty of measuring the residual stresses in a laminate and of observing first-ply failure during a laminate test.

From an analytical point of view, when laminae properties are known, it is possible to cal-

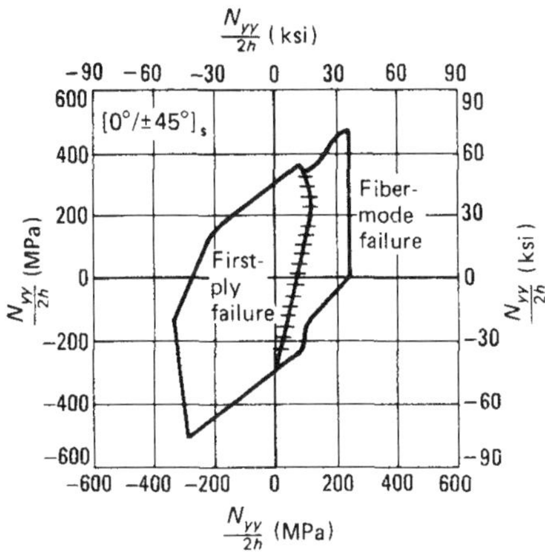

Fig. 20 Laminate failure surface for combined in-plane extensional stress states

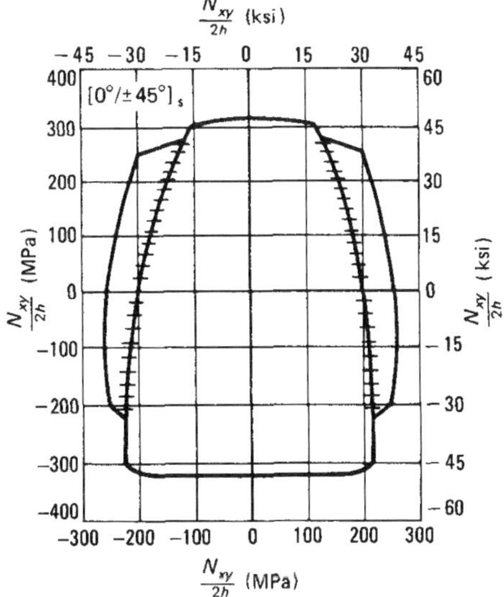

Fig. 21 Laminate failure surface for combined in-plane extensional and shear stress states

Table 5 Failure loads and modes, $[0°/\pm45°]_s$ laminate

	Laminate analysis						Netting analysis		
	First-ply failure load			Ultimate failure load			Ultimate load		
Loading type	MPa	ksi	Failure mode	MPa	ksi	Failure mode	MPa	ksi	Failure mode
$\frac{N_{xx}}{2h}$	308	44.7	Axial tension, 0° plies	308	44.7	Axial tension, 0° plies	250	36.5	Axial tension, 0° plies
$\frac{N_{yy}}{2h}$	75.2	10.9	Transverse tension, 0° plies	250	36.6	Axial tension, ±45° plies; axial compression, 0° plies	250	36.5	Axial tension, ±45° plies; axial compression, 0° plies
$\frac{N_{xy}}{2h}$	208	30.2	Transverse tension, –45° plies	270	38.7	Axial tension, 45° plies	250	36.5	Axial tension, 45° plies; axial compression, –45° plies

culate a laminate stress-strain curve (including or excluding residual thermal stress effects) and determine first-ply failure, subsequent ply failures, and maximum stress at failure. From an experimental point of view, it is possible to measure a laminate stress-strain curve and determine proportional-limit stress and maximum stress. The existence of these different characteristic stress levels in laminated composite materials must be recognized, just as both a yield stress and an ultimate stress are known to characterize metallic materials. These stress levels for composites, as for metals, must be used with different factors of safety. At present, the proper action seems to be to use analytical strength predictions (both first-ply failure and ultimate failure) in the preliminary design phase, and experimental strength values for final design.

When experimental strength data are used for laminates, the problem of combined loading conditions arises again. The difficulties of combined-load testing preclude the purely experimental approach; the uncertainties of failure mechanism cloud the choice of analytical interaction criteria. A reasonable approach appears to be represented by the following sequence: analytical calculation of ultimate strength via netting analysis, or any other straightforward method; use of the analytical result to define the shape of the interaction curve; use of experimental data for single-stress components to define amplitudes of the interaction curve; and confirmation via limited combined-stress testing for a condition of practical interest.

It is common practice in the aerospace industry to neglect the residual thermal stresses in the calculations of ply failure. Data to support this approach do not appear to be available. However, at the present time, damage tolerance requirements limit allowable strain levels in laminates to a range of 3000 to 4000 μm/m. This becomes the dominant design restriction and eliminates the need to resolve the effects of residual thermal stresses. As materials of improved impact resistance are developed, first-ply failure calculations will become more significant. It appears that thermal stresses should be included in first-ply failure calculations unless their omission were to create an improved degree of conservatism. Careful stress-strain testing of laminate coupons should be used to define design allowables.

Whichever stress values are used, design charts in the form of so-called carpet plots are of great value for the selection of the appropriate laminate. Figure 22 presents a representative plot of this type for the axial tensile strength of laminates having various proportions of plies oriented at 0°, ±45°, and 90°. Appropriate strength data suitable for preliminary design can be found for various materials in Ref 1 and 5.

Fracture. The presence in a structure of a hole or other discontinuity introduces local stress concentrations that, if high, can result in initial localized failure. In metals, a common consequence of these effects is the formation of a small crack at the region of stress concentration. When there is a combination of high stress intensity and low resistance of the metal to crack propagation, the result is failure due to cracking. This failure mechanism is generally termed fracture. The mathematical technology that has been developed to treat this problem uses fracture mechanics methods and is called structural-integrity technology (Ref 1).

For composite laminates, the problem is complicated by the heterogeneity of the material, both at the microscale level and on a layer-to-layer basis. The complexity of this problem is illustrated by the laminate analysis of a plate with a hole. In a symmetric, balanced laminate having a circular hole and subjected to in-plane axial tension, the plate may be regarded as an orthotropic plate whose properties are the effective laminate moduli defined in the section "Laminate Properties" in this article. Solutions for stress concentrations in such a plate are available (Ref 6). The stresses obtained from such a solution define local values of the stress resultants, which can be treated as the stress resultants applied to the actual laminate. In general, at any point in the plate this will define a combined loading with all three stress resultants being nonzero. Following the laminate stress analysis methods, the stress state in each ply can then be found, thereby defining the variation of ply stresses throughout the plate.

Sample results obtained by the above procedure are presented in Fig. 23. The tangential stress around the periphery of the hole is plotted. The solid line represents the stress from the orthotropic plate analysis, which is equivalent to the average value of the in-plane ply stresses. At the edge of the hole, these average tangential stresses are the only nonzero components of the stress resultants; elsewhere in the plate all three stress resultants generally will be nonzero. The dotted lines are the tangential stresses in the individual plies computed from laminate theory. In general, all the stress components in each ply will be nonzero, even at the edge of the hole. This is the same effect as treated in the discussion of interlaminar stress: The boundary conditions are satisfied in laminate analysis only by the average stresses.

In Fig. 23, the lamina stresses at the edge of the hole will not be correct, and interlaminar stresses will exist. These interlaminar shear stresses are shown in Fig. 24 at the various ply interfaces; the interlaminar normal stresses are shown in Fig. 25 at the midsurface interface. These interlaminar stresses are normalized with respect to the average applied stress. The magnitudes of these stresses are substantial.

Associated with the interlaminar stresses is a modification of the in-plane stress state in each ply. Thus, as described for the free-edge problem, the only nonzero in-plane stress component in each ply at the edge of the hole is the tangential stress, $\sigma_{\theta\theta}$. This combination of in-plane and interlaminar stresses varies strongly with the coordinate. The variation takes place near the hole, where the average in-plane stress components

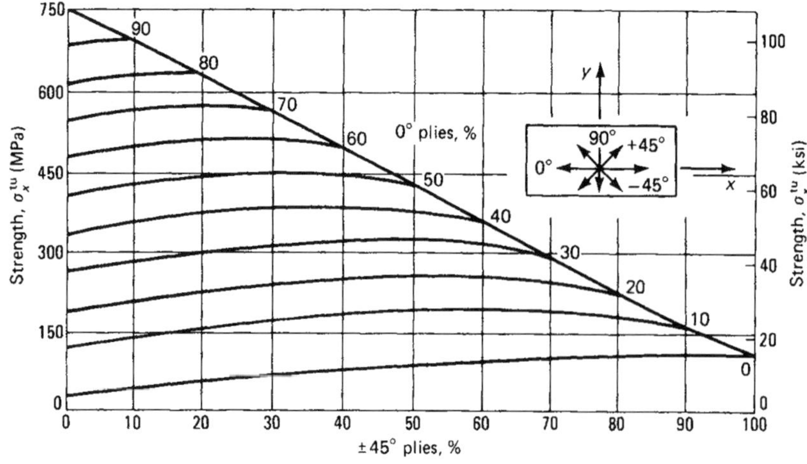

Fig. 22 Tensile strength of $[0°_i/\pm45°_j/90°_k]_s$ family of high-modulus graphite-epoxy laminates at room temperature

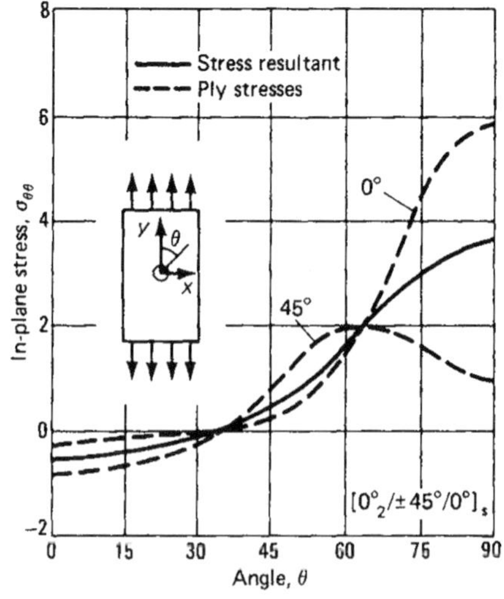

Fig. 23 Laminate theory calculations for stresses around a hole

are also varying. This complex state of stress can cause various failure mechanisms. Clearly, interlaminar disbonding is a possibility at various locations at or near the edge of the hole. Intraply matrix-mode failure in any ply is another possibility. At elevated stress levels, it is reasonable to expect diverse local matrix failures. This complex problem can be treated by the method described below.

Using the laminate properties methods, the effective in-plane laminate stiffnesses, E_x, E_y, and G_{xy}, may be calculated for any laminate. With these properties specified, a balanced symmetric laminate may be regarded, for purposes of structural stress analysis, as a homogeneous, orthotropic plate. Orthotropic elasticity theory may be used for evaluating stresses around a hole in such a plate (Ref 6). Examples of the resulting stress concentrations are shown in Fig. 26 for various carbon-epoxy laminates. The laminae orientation combinations influence both the magnitude and the shape of the stress variation in the vicinity of the hole. The high stresses at the edge of the hole may initiate fracture.

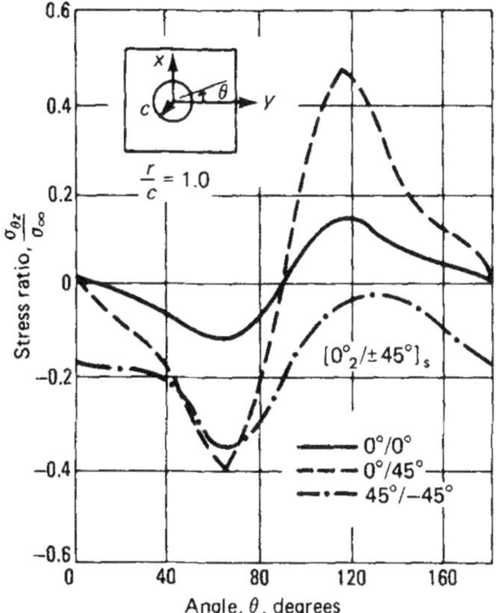

Fig. 24 Interlaminar shear stress at a hole

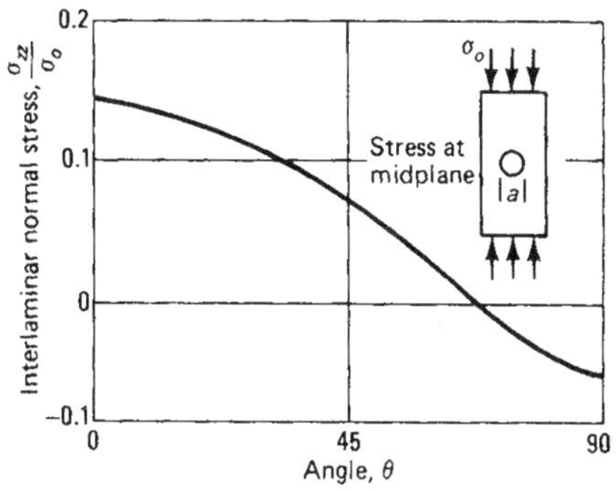

Fig. 25 Interlaminar normal stress at a hole

If the laminate fails as a brittle material, fracture will be initiated when the maximum tensile stress at the edge of the hole equals the strength of the unnotched material. In a tensile coupon with a hole, as in Fig. 26, the failure will occur at the minimum cross section and will initiate at the edge of the hole, where the stress concentration is at a maximum. The stress-concentration factor of interest is one that includes the finite-width effect, illustrated in Fig. 27 for an isotropic plate with a central, circular hole. Stress distributions are shown for various ratios of hole diameter, a, to plate width, W.

The basic stress-concentration factor for this problem is the ratio of the axial stress at the edge of the hole ($x = a/2$ and $y = 0$) to the applied axial stress, σ_∞. For small holes in an isotropic plate, this factor is equal to 3. For large hole sizes, the average stress at the minimum section, σ_n, is higher than the applied stress, σ_∞, and is given by the relation:

$$\sigma_n = \frac{\sigma_\infty}{\left(1 - \frac{a}{W}\right)} \quad \text{(Eq 88)}$$

The net section stress-concentration factor, K_n, is the ratio of the maximum stress to this average stress. Thus:

$$K_n = \frac{\left[\sigma\left(\frac{a}{2}, 0\right)\right] / \sigma_\infty}{1 - \frac{a}{W}} \quad \text{(Eq 89)}$$

Laminate fracture for the elastic-brittle case will occur at stress σ_{fr}, that is:

$$\sigma_{fr} = \frac{\sigma^{tu}}{K_n} \quad \text{(Eq 90)}$$

A material that fails in this fashion is called a notch-sensitive material. In contrast, a ductile material will yield locally, alleviating the stress-concentration effect. In the extreme, this will result in a uniform stress distribution at the net section, as shown in Fig. 28. For this case, failure will occur when the average net section stress equals the material strength, or:

$$\sigma_{fr} = \sigma^{tu}\left(1 - \frac{a}{W}\right) \quad \text{(Eq 91)}$$

A material that fails in this way is known as a notch-insensitive material. Practical laminates

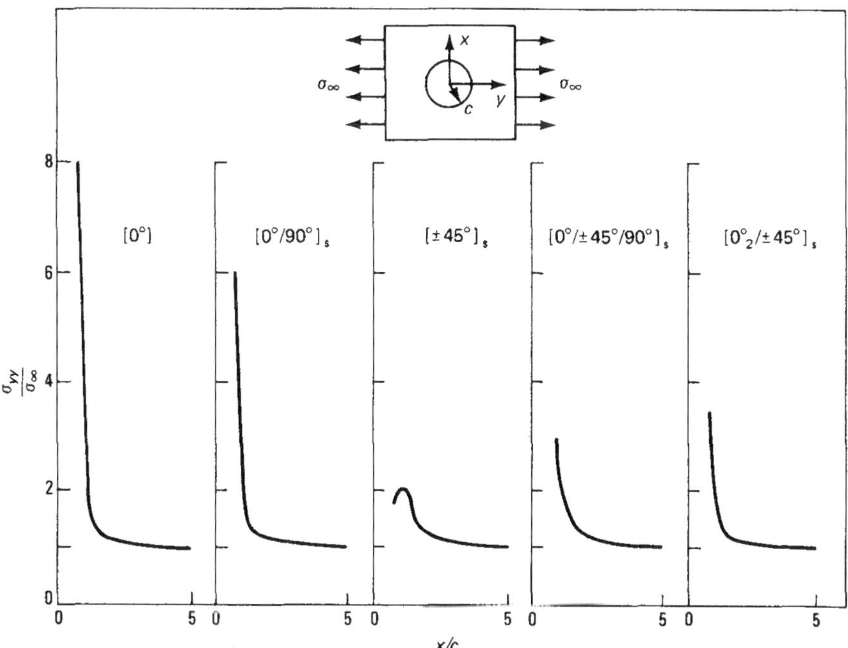

Fig. 26 Stress-concentration factors for a circular hole in a homogeneous, orthotropic, infinite plate

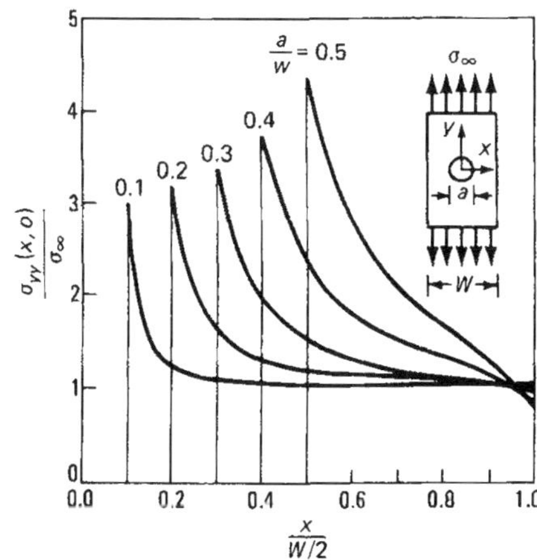

Fig. 27 Stress distribution around a hole in a finite-width plate

may be expected to fail in a fashion that is neither of these two extreme cases.

Various matrix damage effects are expected to occur at the maximum-stress locations. These localized damages reduce the material stiffness and diminish and spread the stress-concentration effects. As a result, although fracture will occur because of stress concentration, it can be expected to occur because of lesser stress-concentration factors than those calculated from orthotropic elastic stress analysis of the notched laminate. Semiempirical methods for evaluating this reduction in stress concentration have been proposed.

The point stress theory (Ref 7) proposes that the elastic-stress distribution curve (Fig. 26) be used but that the stress concentration be selected at a distance, d_0, from the edge of the hole. Thus, the numerator of Eq 89 should be evaluated at the point $x = a/2 + d_0$. The characteristic length d_0 must be evaluated experimentally. The average-stress theory (Ref 7) takes a similar approach by proposing that the elastic-stress distribution be averaged over a distance, a_0, to obtain the stress concentration. Thus:

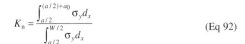

$$K_n = \frac{\int_{a/2}^{(a/2)+a0} \sigma_y d_x}{\int_{a/2}^{W/2} \sigma_y d_x} \quad \text{(Eq 92)}$$

Again, the characteristic dimension, a_0, must be found experimentally. The two approaches are illustrated in Fig. 29. For both methods, the resulting stress concentration is used in Eq 90 to define the fracture stress.

Representative results are plotted in Fig. 30 to illustrate the differences associated with the different types of material behavior. The ratio of strength of the plate with a hole, σ_{fr}, to that of an unnotched laminate, σ^{tu}, is plotted as a function of hole size. For the notch-insensitive material, this course clearly shows a linear decrease in failure stress with hole size due to the reduction in net cross-sectional area. The lower curve, for a notch-sensitive material, shows an immediate drop in strength with the introduction of even a small hole due to the local stress-concentration effect. The semiempirical theories (both have similar effects) show a rapid but more modest drop due to stress concentration. Experimental data for laminates support the use of either of the semiempirical theories for fracture of a laminate with a hole.

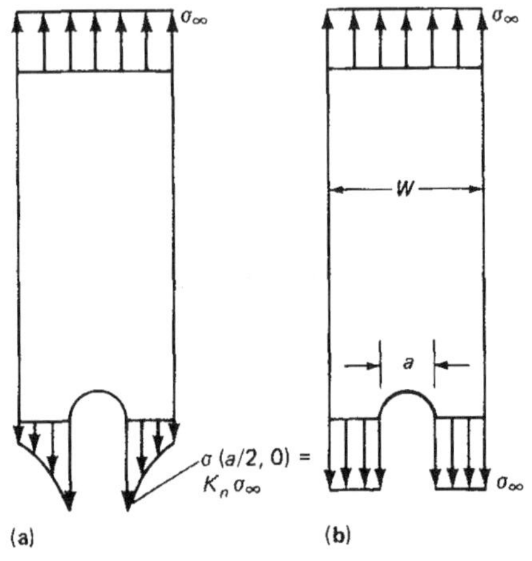

Fig. 28 Idealized limit cases for failure. (a) Notch-sensitive. (b) Notch-insensitive

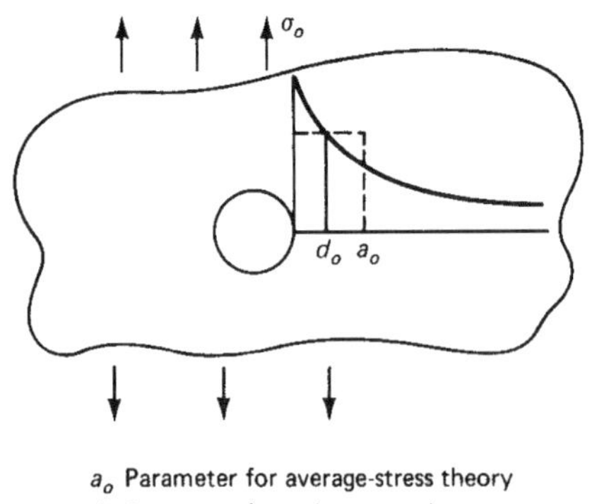

Fig. 29 Representation of characteristic dimensions for semiempirical fracture theories

Intra- and Interlaminar Cracking

The ply cracking and delamination discussed earlier may be analyzed using an energy method. This method basically integrates the laminate stress analysis and the concept of effective material flaws into the classical theory of fracture mechanics. The laminate stress analysis is used to determine three-dimensional state of stress in constituent plies. Elastic fracture mechanics criteria are used to describe the propagation behavior of matrix cracks. However, in order to render a rational prediction for matrix crack initiation, the concept of effective material flaws is first introduced.

In this concept, two basic types of effective flaws are postulated. First, for the unidirectional ply, there exists a known distribution of effective intralaminar flaws, lying in the ply thickness direction, as shown in Fig. 31(a). These flaws effect intralaminar cracking. Second, in each ply-to-ply interface, there exists a known distribution of effective interfacial flaws, lying parallel to the ply interface, as shown in Fig. 31(b).

At this point, the effective flaws remain a hypothetical quantity, though they are considered inherent properties of the basic ply material system. It is postulated that the presence of the effective flaws does not effect any change in the elastic constitutive properties of the ply. But, at some critical laminate loading, one (or more) of the flaws can be transformed into a matrix crack that is measurable at the phenomenological scale.

The condition governing the transformation from a particular effective flaw to a detectable matrix crack is provided by a criterion of the theory of brittle fracture (Ref 8). Because the size and the location of a particular flaw are known, it is possible to perform an elastic stress analysis by treating the flaw as a crack; the crack-tip stress intensity factor $K(a_0, \sigma_0)$ or the strain energy release rate $G(a_0, \sigma_0)$ can be calculated in terms of the initial crack (flaw) size, a_0, and the applied laminate load, σ_0. The condition for a_0 to propagate and to become detectable is given, for example, by:

$$G(a,\sigma_0) = G_c \quad \text{at } a = a_0 \quad \text{(Eq 93)}$$

where G_c is the material fracture toughness against the considered mode of matrix crack propagation. The stability of propagation is determined by the functional dependence of G on the crack size, a. Namely, if $dG/da > 0$ at $a = a_0$, the propagation is unstable; if $dG/da < 0$, the propagation is stable; that is, there is no crack growth.

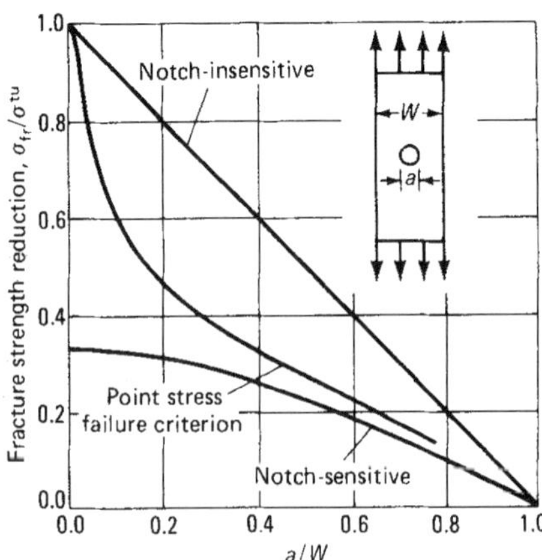

Fig. 30 Approximate-failure theories

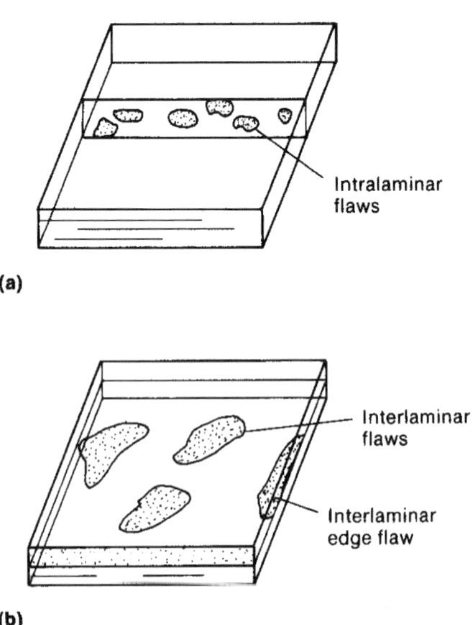

Fig. 31 View of (a) effective intralaminar flaws. (b) Effective interlaminar flaws

Interlaminar Cracking, Free-Edge Delamination

The energy approach outlined previously has been applied to analyze the initiation and propagation of free-edge delamination (Ref 9, 10). In order to illustrate the specific procedures involved in the energy analysis, let us consider the $[\pm 25°/90°]_s$ tension coupon. When this coupon is loaded in uniaxial tension ε_0, significant interlaminar stresses develop near the free edges. In fact, these interlaminar stresses are large enough to cause free-edge delamination as the first failure mode in the laminate. Of course, the question is at what critical ε_0 and in which ply interface will the delamination initiate. Also, the question of delamination stability must be answered.

Interface Flaw. To answer these questions, begin with the assumed distribution of interfacial (effective) flaws. Identify in each ply interface and along the laminate free edge the most dominant effective flaw having a uniformly elongated shape with a width a_0 (Fig. 31b). This interfacial flaw is capable of transforming into an interfacial crack as soon as the laminate stress field reaches the critical level.

Energy Release Rate Curve. Second, the most dominant edge flaw is treated as a crack of the same size, a_0, and the crack tip strain energy release rate $G(a_0, \varepsilon_0)$ is calculated.

The strain energy release rate, G, when calculated numerically, can be expressed in explicit terms of the crack size a, and the applied laminate strain, ε_0.

$$G(a, \varepsilon_0) = C_\varepsilon(a)\, 2t\varepsilon_0^2 \qquad \text{(Eq 94)}$$

where $C_\varepsilon(a)$ is a coefficient function explicitly depending on a but implicitly depending on the location of a ply interface, the ply stacking sequence of the laminate, and the ply elastic constants.

If the residual thermal stresses due to laminate curing are significant and their effects are to be included in the calculation of G, it then is necessary to define the laminate stress-free temperature, T_0. Usually, T_0 is approximately the same as the laminate curing temperature. Thus, at the ambient temperature, T, the laminate is exposed to a uniform thermal loading, $\Delta T = T - T_0$. In such a case, the strain energy release rate due to the combined loading of ε_0 and ΔT can be expressed as:

$$G(a, \varepsilon_0, \Delta T) = \left[\sqrt{C_\varepsilon}\, \varepsilon_0 - \sqrt{C_T}\, \Delta T\right]^2 (2t) \qquad \text{(Eq 95)}$$

where C_T is another coefficient function expressed in terms of a. Note that a minus sign associated with the ΔT term is only a convention, because the value of ΔT is always negative.

Figure 32 shows the computed strain energy release rate coefficient functions C_ε for interfacial cracking in the midplane (90°/90° interface) and the −25°/90° interface. Note that the computed C_ε curve for delamination in the midplane contains exclusively mode I energy, as it should, while the C_ε curve for delamination in the −25°/90° interface contains both mode I and mode III energies. The ratio of mode I energy to mode III energy in the latter case is about 0.8. Similarly, Fig. 33 shows the strain energy release rate coefficients C_T for delamination in each of the same two ply interfaces.

It is seen that the characteristics of all the energy curves are similar. Namely, the curve rises sharply from 0 at $a = 0$ and reaches a limiting value at $a = a_m$. The physical meaning of a_m is not exactly known. However, the free-edge effect may be interpreted as fully developed when a delamination reaches the size a_m. The size of a_m is approximately of the order of a couple of ply thicknesses for most laminate situations (Ref 10).

Determining the Exact Delaminating Interface. A comparison of magnitudes of the strain energy release rate curves for the $[\pm 25°/90°]_s$ laminate shown in Fig. 32 and 33 shows that edge delamination in the laminate midplane would release more strain energy than delamination in the −25°/90° interface. Whether the midplane (mode I) or the −25°/90° interface (mixed modes) will delaminate, however, is determined by the fracture criterion of Eq 93, for which the material fracture toughness G_c and the effective flaw size a_0 are yet to be specified.

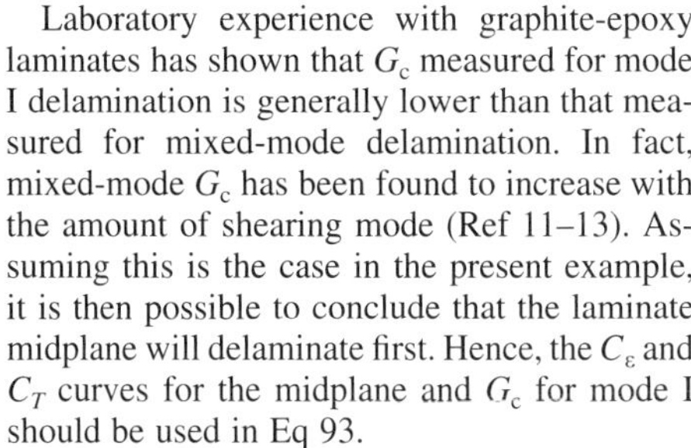

Laboratory experience with graphite-epoxy laminates has shown that G_c measured for mode I delamination is generally lower than that measured for mixed-mode delamination. In fact, mixed-mode G_c has been found to increase with the amount of shearing mode (Ref 11–13). Assuming this is the case in the present example, it is then possible to conclude that the laminate midplane will delaminate first. Hence, the C_ε and C_T curves for the midplane and G_c for mode I should be used in Eq 93.

Determining the Critical Laminate Strain. With the interface and mode of delamination identified, the last information needed in using Eq 93 is the size of a_0. Because a_0 is a hypothetical quantity, however, it is essentially a random variable. Yet, given the functional relationship $G(a)$ as expressed in Eq 94 or 95 and the values for ΔT and G_c, a one-to-one relationship between ε_0 and a can be obtained from Eq 93 (Fig. 34). If all the possible values of a_0 are represented by some probability function, $f(a_0)$, then there is a corresponding range of ε_0 values for which Eq 93 is satisfied. While the exact size, a_0, of the most dominant effective flaw is not known, the minimum critical ε_0, which is associated with all values of $a_0 > a_m$, can now be determined from Fig. 34.

As mentioned before, the value of a_m is on the order of one or two ply thicknesses, while the actual initial edge delamination observable at the macroscale is on the order of the laminate thickness. Hence, delamination onset can be predicted by the minimum critical strain associated with $a_0 > a_m$. Thus, from Eq 93 and in conjunction with Eq 95, the predicted minimum critical strain for initial delamination propagation is given by:

$$(\varepsilon_0)_{cr} = \frac{\left[\sqrt{(G_c/2t)} + \sqrt{C_T}\, \Delta T\right]}{\sqrt{C_\varepsilon}} \quad \text{at } a > a_m \qquad \text{(Eq 96)}$$

where the coefficients C_ε and C_T are taken from the calculated energy curves for the midplane.

To determine the propagation stability, the functional form of C_ε and C_T for all $a > a_m$ is examined. Accordingly, it is concluded that the stability behavior of free-edge delamination is

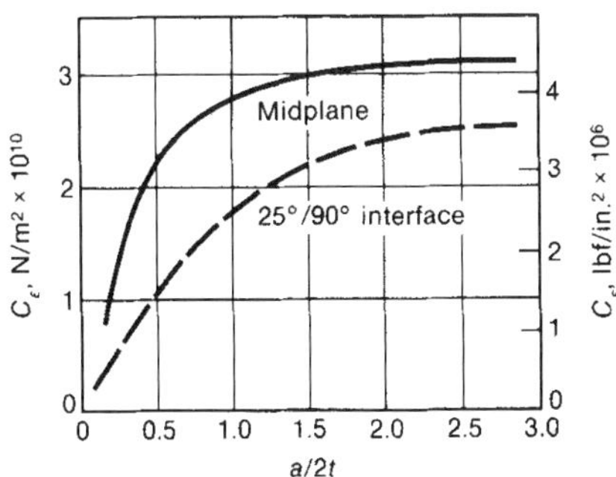

Fig. 32 Strain energy release rate coefficients, C_ε, for interfacial cracking in the 90°/90° and the −25°/90° interfaces of the $[\pm 25°/90°]_s$ laminate

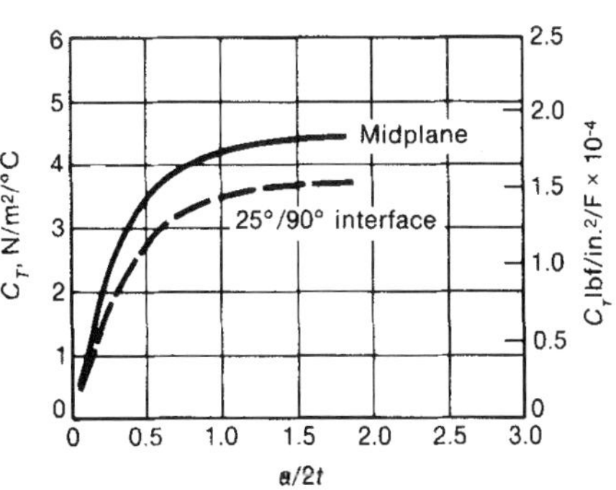

Fig. 33 Strain energy release rate coefficients, C_T, for interfacial cracking in the 90°/90° and the −25°/90° interfaces of the $[\pm 25°/90°]_s$ laminate

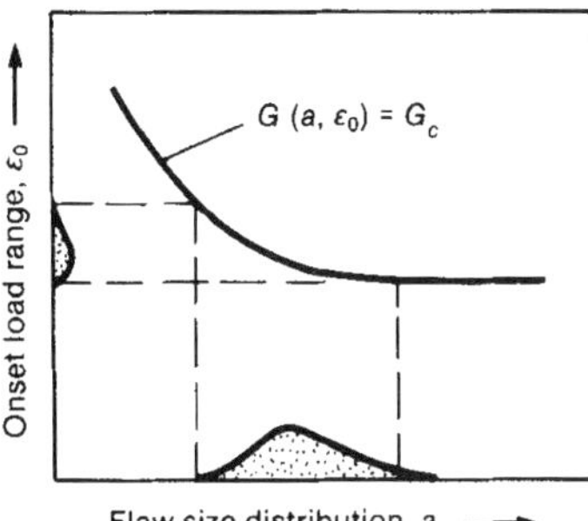

Fig. 34 Fracture relationship between the critical load range (ε_0) and the effective flaw size distribution $f(a)$

neutral. In reality, however, the propagation is generally stable, with the degree of stability depending on whether other modes of matrix cracking develop subsequent to delamination initiation.

Intralaminar Cracking, Transverse Cracks

The energy analysis procedures outlined above for the free-edge delamination problem have also been applied to simulate intralaminar cracking in laminates (Ref 14). Here, the $[0°/90°]_s$ graphite-epoxy tensile coupon serves as an example. As discussed earlier, free-edge effect is relatively unimportant when the coupon is under uniaxial tension. Hence, an analysis of transverse cracking in the 90° layer can be developed without regard to the influence of free-edge stresses.

Initiation and Growth Characteristics. At the macroscopic scale, the formation of a transverse crack is simply a sudden separation of the 90° layer. When this happens, it often gives off acoustic emissions. At the microscopic scale, however, the exact nature of the event is unclear. It may be postulated again that the crack is caused initially by the coalescence of those material microflaws that lie in the thickness direction in the 90° layer. The effect of this coalescence is represented by the propagation of an effective flaw (Fig. 31a) in the thickness direction. The crack, however, is unable to propagate through the 0° ply and is either arrested at or blunted to propagate along the 0°/90° interface. The latter then becomes a localized delamination. In either case, the propagation is not catastrophic. This allows an increase of the applied tension, which, in turn, can cause another transverse crack to form at another location. In this manner, a series of transverse cracks can be formed along the length of the coupon as a function of the tension loading.

Figure 35 shows a plot for the number of transverse cracks (per centimeter length) versus applied tension relationships, obtained by testing a family of $[0°/90°_n/0°]$ coupons ($n = 1, 2, 3, 4$) made of the T300/934 graphite-epoxy system (Ref 15). From the plot, it can be seen that for the $n = 1$ coupon, transverse cracking did not occur until the load had reached the critical level, causing fiber breaking in the 0° plies. For the other three coupons, however, each yielded a cumulative crack development curve that is characteristically distinct from the others. These results clearly indicate that the occurrence of any one particular crack in a given coupon is essentially probabilistic in nature but that the developmental character of the cumulative cracks as a whole seems to follow a rather deterministic rule.

Effective Flaws. Now, for the sake of simplicity, it may be assumed that the effective intralaminar flaws are one-dimensional, being oriented in the ply thickness direction, as shown in Fig. 36. The linear size of an individual flaw is denoted by $2a$, and its location is denoted by x. Then, for the unidirectional ply (thickness $2t$), the discrete random variables (a_i, $i = 1, M$) and (x_i, $i = 1, M$) characterize the size and the location distributions of the effective intralaminar flaws. At this point, the exact values for (a_i) and (x_i) are not known, but are assumed to be inherent ply properties. As such, these can be determined by some suitable experimental measurements to be discussed subsequently.

When two or more 90° plies are grouped together, such as in the $[0°/90°_n/0°]$ coupons with $n > 1$, the effective flaw size distribution in the grouped plies will be different from that of the single ply, although their spacing distribution may be assumed to be the same. Here, a volumetric rule (Ref 16) can be used to express the flaw size distribution, $(a_{i,n})$, in n-plies in terms of the flaw sizes, (a_i), of the single ply:

$$a_{i,n} = a_i(n)^{2/\alpha} \qquad \text{(Eq 97)}$$

where $i = 1, M$, and α is an arbitrary constant related to the distributional characteristics of (a_i) and the particular volumetric rule used in deriv-

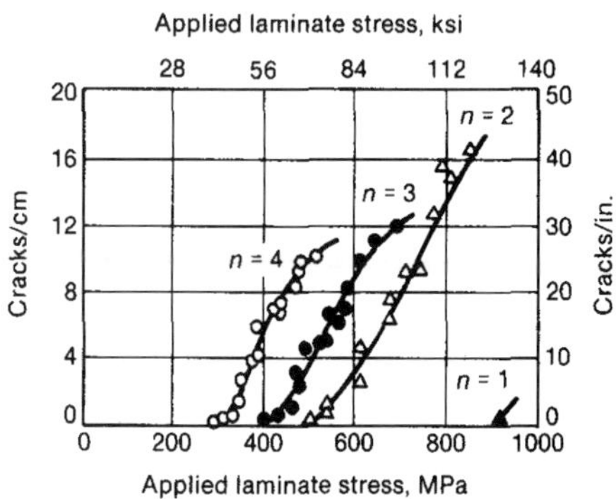

Fig. 35 Experimental crack density versus load plots for a family of T300-934 $[0°/90°_n/0°]$ laminates under uniaxial tension, 2 specimens each. $n = 1, 2, 3, 4$

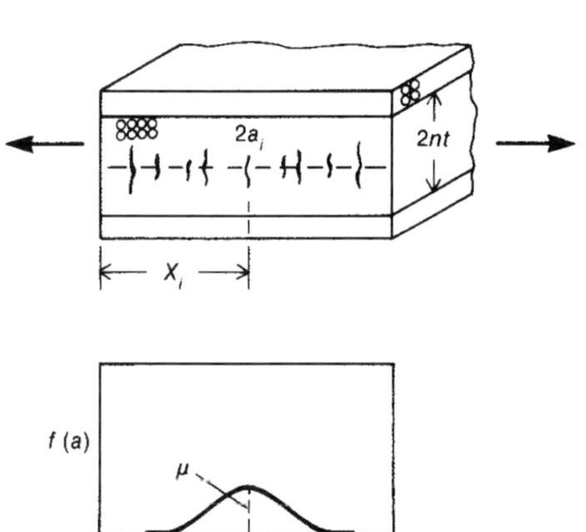

Fig. 36 Idealized effective intralaminar flaw distribution in the 90° layer

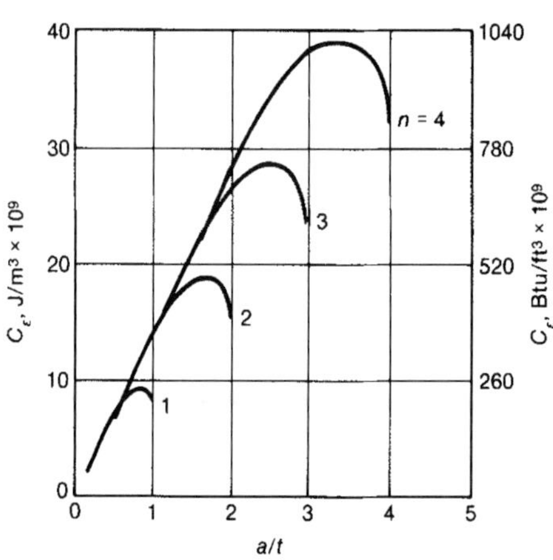

Fig. 37 Strain energy release rate coefficients, C_ε, for transverse cracking in $[0°/90°_n/0°]$ laminates, $n = 1, 2, 3, 4$

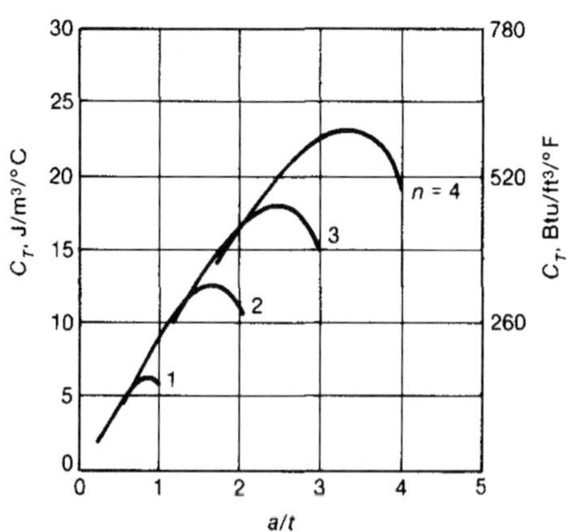

Fig. 38 Strain energy release rate coefficients, C_T, for transverse cracking in $[0°/90°_n/0°]$ laminates. $n = 1, 2, 3, 4$

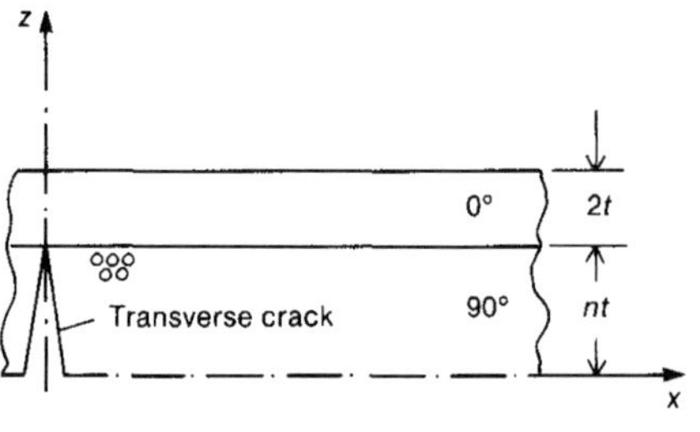

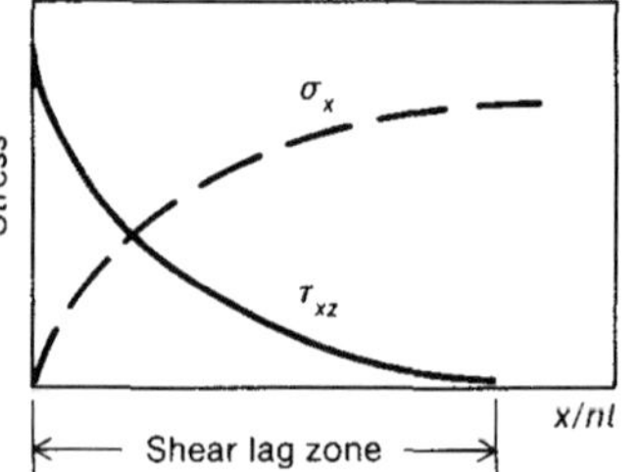

Fig. 39 Shear lag zone due to a transverse crack in the $[0°/90°]_s$ laminate

ing the relationship in Eq 97 (see, for example, Ref 16).

Onset of the First Crack. The $[0°/90°_n/0°]$ coupon is now considered under the applied tensile strain, ε_0, as shown in Fig. 36. Each of the flaws is capable of propagating into a transverse crack. The propagation of any one of the flaws, say the ith flaw a_i, is governed by Eq 93. There, the strain energy release rate $G(a_i, \varepsilon_0, \Delta T)$ associated with the ith flaw must first be calculated. In addition, the fracture toughness, G_c, must also be determined a priori. It is noted that for the present problem, transverse cracking is essentially in mode I. Hence, G_{Ic} should be determined first and then used in Eq 93.

The calculation of $G(a_i, \varepsilon_0, \Delta T)$ can be performed by finite-element procedures. The calculated G is then expressed in the form of Eq 95. Figures 37 and 38 show, respectively, the $C_\varepsilon(a)$ and $C_T(a)$ functions for $n = 1, 2, 3, 4$. Here, the unique character of the C_ε or C_T curves is worth noting. It is seen that both C_ε and C_T increase sharply from $a = 0$ to reach their respective maxima, $C_{\varepsilon,max}$ and $C_{T,max}$; these maxima occur at about three-fourths the thickness of the 90° layer. After this point, they both decrease toward the 0°/90° interface at $a = nt$. This behavior is consistent with the observed fact that transverse cracking can be initially unstable (that is, in giving off acoustic emissions) but is immediately arrested at the 0°/90° interfaces.

Now, for the first crack to form, let the largest of (a_i) be denoted by a_{max}. Then, the critical strain (ε_0) for the onset of the first crack is given by Eq 96 for $a = a_{max}$ and $G_c = G_{Tc}$.

Actually, because each (a_i) must be smaller than the half-thickness of the 90° layer, nt, and in all likelihood, a_{max} is only slightly less than nt, a minimum $(\varepsilon_0)_{cr}$ can be found by substituting $C_{\varepsilon,max}$ and $C_{T,max}$ in Eq 96.

Shear Lag Effect. Assume that the transverse crack is arrested at the 0°/90° interfaces. Then, the local tensile load formerly carried by the unbroken 90° layer is now transferred to the adjacent 0° plies. If the 0°/90° interface bonding is strong, a slip of the interface (delamination) is not possible. Then, a localized interlaminar shear stress τ_{xz} is developed near the transverse crack termini, as shown in Fig. 39. This interlaminar shear stress decays exponentially a small distance away from the transverse crack, and at the same time, the in situ tensile stress σ_x in the 90° layer regains its far-field strength. This local load transfer zone, known as the shear lag zone, is proportional to the thickness of the 90° layer, $2nt$. Hence, the thicker the 90° layer, the larger the shear lag zone. For the present problem, one side of the shear lag zone is about $12nt$.

If there is an effective flaw located near a transverse crack (Fig. 40), the flaw is under the influence of the shear lag casted by the transverse crack. The degree of influence depends on their relative distance, s. Specifically, if the size of this flaw is $2a$, and the associated strain energy release rate is $G(a, \varepsilon_0, \Delta T, s)$, then the shear lag effect on the strain energy release rate can be expressed by the factor, $R(s)$, defined by:

$$R(s) = \frac{G(a, \varepsilon_0, \Delta T, s)}{G(a, \varepsilon_0, \Delta T)} \qquad \text{(Eq 98)}$$

where $G(a,\varepsilon_0,\Delta T)$ is calculated without the influence of shear lag. It may be noted that the numerical range of $R(s)$ is between 0 and 1, as shown in Fig. 40.

If a flaw is situated between two consecutive cracks, then it is under the shear lag effect from both cracks. The associated strain energy release rate, G^*, is given by:

$$G^*(a,\varepsilon_0,\Delta T) = R(s_l)G(a,\varepsilon_0,\Delta T)R(s_r) \qquad \text{(Eq 99)}$$

where s_l and s_r are distances from the flaw to the left crack and the right crack, respectively.

Multiple Cracks. After the formation of the first crack from the largest flaw in (a_i), subsequent cracks can form from the remaining flaws at laminate strain appropriately higher than $(\varepsilon_0)_{tr}$. A Monte Carlo search routine is then commenced to determine the next flaw that yields the highest strain energy release rate G^*, with the shear lag effect casted by any existing crack or cracks included. The laminate strain corresponding to the next crack, which should be higher than $(\varepsilon_0)_{cr}$, is determined by using G in Eq 96.

Successive searches for the next most energetic flaws follow, and the entire load sequence of transverse cracks is simulated. In essence, this search procedure mimics the transverse cracking process as it would occur naturally.

Determining the Effective Flaw Distribution. The difficulty in the preceding simulation procedure lies in the fact that the effective flaws are hypothetical quantities and that they can only be determined indirectly at the macroscale. Appropriate experiments in which distributed intralaminar cracks occur must be devised.

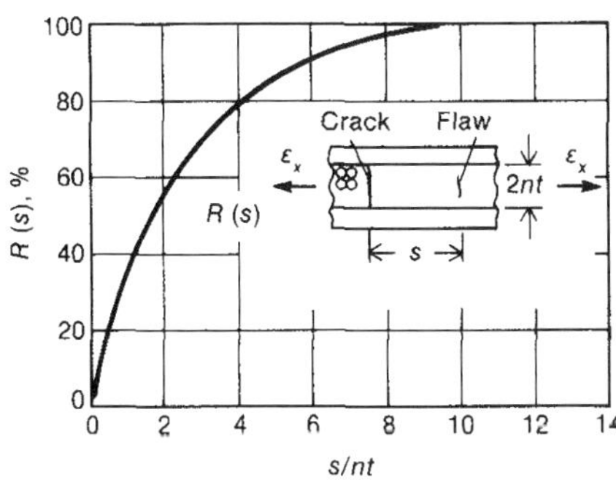

Fig. 40 Strain energy release rate retention factor, $R(s)$

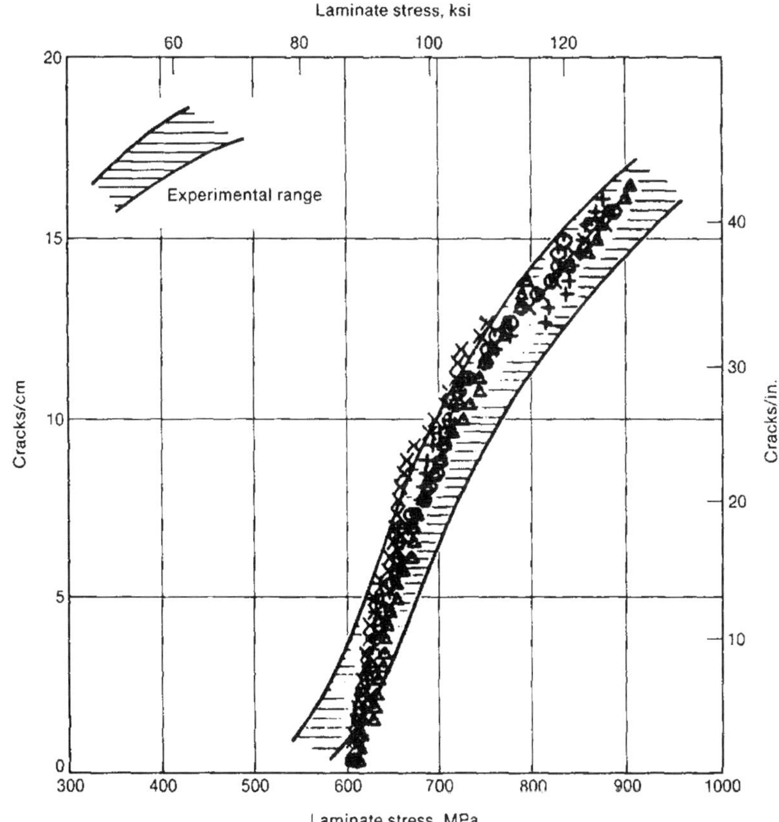

Fig. 41 Experimental (shaded) and simulated (points) transverse crack density versus laminate tension relations. Data from four $[0°_2/90°]_s$ coupons

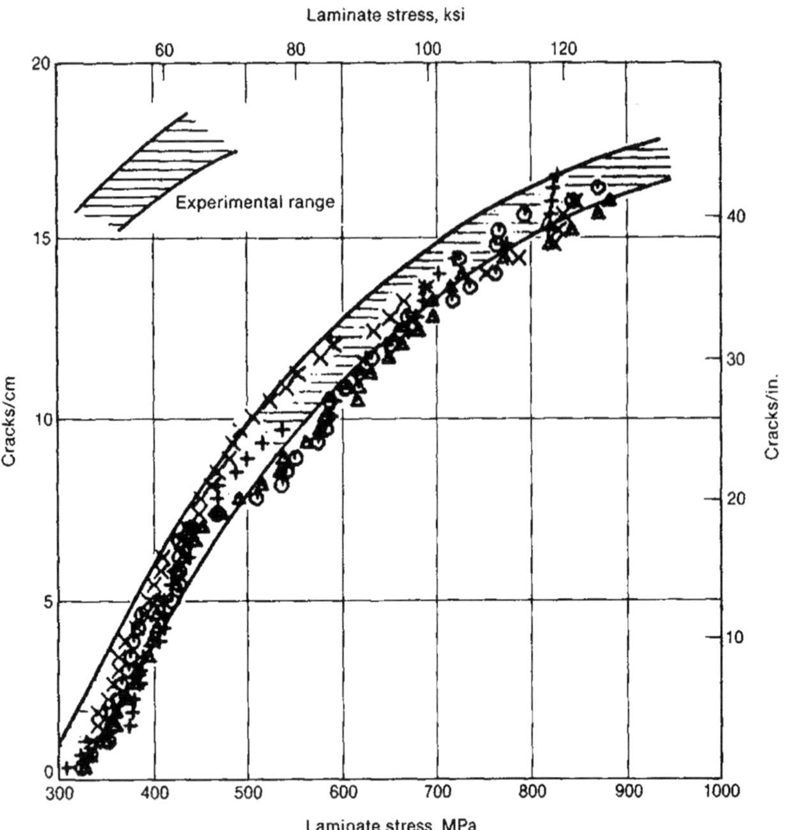

Fig. 42 Experimental (shaded) and simulated (points) transverse crack density versus laminate tension relations. Data from four $[0°_2/90°_2]_s$ coupons

In Ref 16, the effective flaw distribution in $[90°_2]$was determined by testing $[0°_2/90°]_s$ tension coupons. The shaded band in Fig. 41 was formed by test data obtained from four specimens, plotted in terms of crack density versus applied tension (average laminate stress). This band, statistically speaking, resembles a cumulative formation behavior of the transverse cracks as a function of the applied tension. The band possesses a certain position relative to the stress scale, a certain characteristic curvature, and an asymptotic value in the crack density scale.

This band is used to determine the flaw distribution in the $[90°_2]$ layer. To do so, a random number generation scheme is employed. First, the number of flaws, M, in a unit length of the 90° layer is assumed. Second, a set of M random values is generated in the interval of (0,1). These M random values are assigned to be (x_i), which are the locations of the flaws along the unit length of the 90° layer. Third, the sizes of the M flaws (a_i) are described by a Weibull cumulative function:

$$F(a) - 1 - \exp\left[\left(\frac{a}{\beta}\right)^{\alpha}\right] \quad \text{(Eq 100)}$$

with the parameters α and β so far being unknown.

A new set of M random values is again generated in the interval (0,1). These values are then assigned to (F_i), corresponding to the values of $F(a)$ at $a = a_i$. Thus, for appropriately assumed values of α and β, one determines from Eq 100 the flaw size a_i for each assigned value of F_i.

With the flaw distribution (sizes and locations) now characterized, though the values of α, β, and M are still assumed, a simulation of the transverse cracking process can be performed as outlined previously. The correct choices of α, β, and M must be ones that closely simulate the experimental band shown in Fig. 41. Generally, α primarily affects the curvature of the band, β shifts the band along the stress scale, and M determines the asymptotic value of the band on the crack density scale (Ref 16). Figure 41 shows the crack density development relations for four simulated specimens, along with a set of appropriately chosen α, β, and M values.

With α, β, and M chosen from the preceding experiment, flaw size distribution in any number of grouped 90° plies can be found using Eq 97. For example, the band in Fig. 42 represents the experimental results from four $[0°_2/90°_2]_s$ coupons, while the simulated results for four samples of the same coupons are shown by scattered dots. Figure 43 shows a similar comparison for four $[0°_2/90°_4]$ coupons. In both cases, the basic flaw distribution found from the $[0°_2/90°_2]_s$ coupons was used in conjunction with Eq 97 in the simulation.

Of course, the uniqueness of the determined flaw distribution in the basic ply cannot be proved. Specifically, the values of α, β, and M determined experimentally could assume different sets of values for the same set of experiments. This difficulty, it is felt, will remain as long as an exact analysis of the cracking mechanisms at the fiber-matrix scale is unavailable.

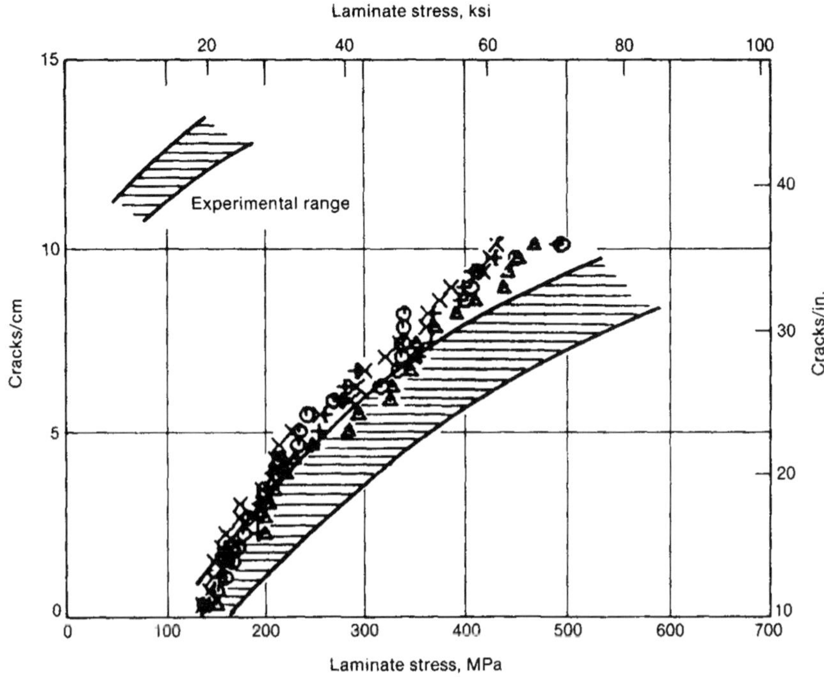

Fig. 43 Experimental (shaded) and simulated (points) transverse crack density versus laminate tension relations. Data from four $[0°_2/90°_4]_s$ coupons

ACKNOWLEDGMENTS

This article was adapted from the following articles in *Composites,* Volume 1, *Engineered Materials Handbook,* ASM International, 1987:

- E.A. Humphreys and B.W. Rosen, Properties Analysis of Laminates, p 218–235
- A.S.D. Wang, Strength, Failure, and Fatigue Analysis of Laminates, p 236–251

ASM International would like to thank H. Thomas Hahn, Air Force Office of Scientific Research for adapting the preceding articles for this edition.

REFERENCES

1. *Advanced Composites Design Guide,* 3rd ed., North American Rockwell Corporation, AFML F33615-71-C-1362, Air Force Materials Laboratory, Jan 1973
2. C. Shen and G.S. Springer, Moisture Absorption and Desorption of Composite Materials, *J. Compos. Mater.,* Vol 10, 1976, p 1
3. Z. Hashin, D. Bagchi, and B.W. Rosen, "Nonlinear Behavior of Fiber Composite Laminates," NASA CR-2313, National Aeronautics and Space Administration, April 1974
4. S.S. Wang and I. Choi, Boundary Layer Thermal Stresses in Angle-Ply Composite Laminates, *Modern Developments in Composite Materials and Structures,* J.R. Vinson, Ed., American Society of Mechanical Engineers, 1979, p 315–342
5. *Plastics for Aerospace Vehicles, Part I, Reinforced Plastics,* MIL-HDBK-17A, Department of Defense, Jan 1971
6. G.N. Savin, "Stress Distribution Around Holes," NASA TT-F-607, National Aeronautics and Space Administration, Nov 1970
7. J.M. Whitney and R.J. Nuismer, Stress Fracture Criteria for Laminated Composites Containing Stress Concentrations, *J. Compos. Mater.,* Vol 8, 1974, p 253–265
8. A.A. Griffith, The Phenomena of Rupture and Flow in Solids, *Phil. Trans. R. Soc.* (London) A, Vol 221, 1920, p 163–198
9. A.S.D. Wang and F.W. Crossman, Initiation and Growth of Transverse Cracks and Edge Delamination in Composite Laminates, Part 1, An Energy Method, *J. Compos. Mater.,* Vol 14, 1980, p 71–87
10. F.W. Crossman, W.J. Warren, A.S.D. Wang, and G.E. Law, Initiation and Growth of Transverse Cracks and Edge Delamination in Composite Laminates, Part 2, Experimental Correlation, *J. Compos. Mater.,* Vol 14, 1980, p 88–106
11. D.J. Wilkins, J.R. Eisenmann, R.A. Camin, W.S. Margolis, and R.A. Benson, Characterizing Delamination Growth in Graphite-Epoxy, *Damages in Composite Materials,* STP 775, American Society for Testing and Materials, 1982, p 168–183
12. A.S.D. Wang, N.N. Kishore, and W.W. Feng, On Mixed-Mode Fracture in Off-Axis Unidirectional Graphite-Epoxy Composites, *Progress in Science and Engineering of Composites,* Vol 1, Japan Society for Composite Materials, 1982, p 599–606
13. A.J. Russell and K.N. Street, Moisture and Temperature Effects on the Mixed-Mode Delamination Fracture of Unidirectional Graphite-Epoxy, *Delamination and Debonding of Materials,* STP 876, American Society for Testing and Materials, 1985, p 349–370
14. A.S.D. Wang, P.C. Chou, and S.C. Lei, A Stochastic Model for the Growth of Matrix Cracks in Composite Laminates, *J. Compos. Mater.,* Vol 18, 1984, p 239–254
15. F.W. Crossman and A.S.D. Wang, The Dependence of Transverse Cracking and Delamination on Ply Thickness in Graphite-Epoxy Laminates, *Damages in Composite Materials*, STP 775, American Society for Testing and Materials, 1982, p 118–139
16. S.C. Lei, "A Stochastic Model for the Damage Growth During the Transverse Cracking Process in Composite Laminates," Ph.D. thesis, Drexel University, 1986

Characterizing Strength from a Structural Design Perspective

L.J. Hart-Smith, J.H. Gosse, and S. Christensen, The Boeing Company

THIS ARTICLE presents a comprehendable and comprehensive physics-based approach for characterizing the strength of fiber-reinforced polymer composites. It begins with background information on the goals and attributes of this method The article then addresses the characterization of fiber failures in laminates, because these are at the highest strengths that can be attained and, therefore, are usually the design objective. An exception would be if the design goal is to maximize energy absorption, rather than static strength. The discussion proceeds to situations in which the matrix fails first, either by intent, by design error, or because of impact damage. The state of the modeling propagation and arrest of matrix damage follows.

Comparisons of this physics-based approach are then made to empirically based failure theories.

Background on Characterization

The mechanical properties of fiber-polymer composites can be characterized at a number of levels—at the constituent level, at the lamina level, and at the laminate level. The appropriate level at which to characterize a specific property varies with that property. Some cannot be characterized at any level higher than for the isolated constituent. Others cannot possibly be measured until the fibers have been embedded in the resin. The approach adopted here is to measure the properties at the most relevant level and, equally, to characterize them in the model at the highest level that does not lose the minimum level of physical definition that is needed. There is a conscious rejection of the common hypothesis that fiber-polymer composites need not be modeled with any greater precision than for a homogenized lamina that does not even differentiate between layers with fibers in one or two directions. However, equally, there is an acknowledgement that it is not possible to predict laminate strengths on the basis of the properties of dry fibers and bulk resin alone. What is presented here is the *least* complicated model that is simultaneously sufficiently comprehensive to cover the standard needs for the design of fibrous composite structures.

The basic analysis is performed at the customary unidirectional lamina level, for a number of reasons:

- A most-practical limitation is the need for compatibility with standard finite-element analysis codes, such as ANSYS, ABACUS, NASTRAN, and COSMOS. Even so, it is vital to incorporate strain magnification factors to differentiate, when necessary, between strains in the fibers, the matrix, and the laminae.
- It is also necessary to include all contributions to residual thermal stress, those that exist within isolated unidirectional laminae as well as those that are caused by laminating together plies of different fiber orientations. The former set are customarily referred to as *intralaminar* thermal stresses and the latter as *interlaminar* thermal stresses. The basic analysis is performed in terms of strains, rather than stresses, because the properties governing the strength of both the fibers and the matrix turn out to be simpler to express, and comprehend, that way.
- The unidirectional lamina is the lowest possible level at which certain phenomena can be characterized without misrepresenting the physics governing the behavior of structural laminates. Modeling a woven fabric layer as a single ply, for example, precludes all possibility of assessing matrix failures in that layer. In addition, modeling at the lamina strain level makes it possible to superimpose different possible failure mechanisms to identify the sequence in which they would occur. This capability is particularly important in the context of damage propagation.

It is most important to emphasize that all analyses presented here are physics based. None rely on curve fits to make up for incomplete understanding of the phenomena. It is likely that there are still more features of the behavior of fiber-polymer composites that have not been accounted for, because there may be further as-yet-unidentified properties awaiting discovery. In the event that such enlightenment does occur, in the future, there will be no need to revise any of the analyses that are governed by the properties that already are included. This is often not the case with even the best of empirical analyses.

The analyses are presented for unidirectional tape laminae, but apply equally to woven fabric layers when they have been properly decomposed into two equivalent orthogonal tape layers in the manner described in Ref 1. Backing out the equivalent "ply" properties ensures that the appropriate level of crimping in the fibers is accounted for. Since matrix-dominated transverse properties cannot be measured for bidirectional laminates, the transverse properties of unidirectional laminae are used. (Fiber crimping has no effect on these.)

Tools for the analyst who does not need to know everything about composites are also addressed, because there are some well-established and reliable approximate methods that cover a great number of design requirements. These include the maximum-strain model (Ref 2) for glass-fiber-reinforced plastics and the truncated maximum-strain model (Ref 3) for polymers reinforced by carbon fibers. At the constituent level, however, the representation of the individual fibers is the same. The difference shows up at the lamina level, because of the vastly different transverse stiffnesses of the two fibers, in comparison with the stiffness of the matrix. Further differences arise from the different fiber strains-to-failure in comparison with that of the matrix. These theories can be used quite safely by anyone who understands what they cannot do. They have only limited capacity in regard to matrix failures. One must either design laminates that are fiber-dominated for all loads the structure will experience, thereby avoiding matrix failures by precluding their occurrence until after the limit load has been reached, or one must use a more comprehensive theory that properly represents matrix failures if there is no simple design solution available. It should be noted that these particular empirical failure models are 100% mechanistic, so their capabilities and limitations are easily established. What must be avoided are those theories, usually referred to as interactive, in which the theories cannot possibly be related to physical phenomena, and for which, therefore, no bounds of applicability have ever been established.

Because the models presented here are more closely tied to more fundamental physical properties than is customary, the analysis methods are actually simpler than usual, because there is no need to compensate for effects that are present in the test coupons and structure, but not included in the analysis. In addition, the reliance on a mechanistic basis permits complete characterizations with fewer reference properties than have been needed in the past.

There have been a great number of composite failure models published elsewhere. Several are described in Ref 4. The authors are aware of these prior works, some of which are discussed here. However, most of them advocate different approaches, based on models for homogeneous anisotropic solids, that cannot characterize the behavior of the heterogeneous fiber-polymer composite laminates as fully as the methods discussed here.

There is a statistical variability to all of the materials properties discussed here. It is assumed that proper interpretation of the data is applied, using mean values for elastic constants and A- or B-allowables for strengths, depending on the application. However, it is necessary to add a warning that most of the variability perceived in the past has nothing to do with the properties in question, but is the result of inappropriate design of many of the standard test coupons, which is compounded by the difficulties in testing any brittle materials. Bonded tapered tabs where loads are introduced have been a chronic source of premature failure, peeling off the outermost plies of the coupon. The inherent variability in fiber and polymer properties is no greater than for typical metal alloys. Most of the time, only the highest test result in each set comes close to being valid, particularly when there is great scatter. Fortunately, the pedigree of the reference properties can be separated from the theories in which they are used.

The characterization of fiber failures in laminates is presented first. Then situations in which the matrix fails first either by intent, by design error, or because of impact damage follow. It is shown that the longitudinal compressive strength of embedded fibers can be limited by the ability of the matrix to support them. It is also affected by stacking sequence and by blocking of parallel plies. The new models have shown progress in also covering the propagation and arrest of matrix damage, followed by its possible spreading further at still higher loads or by catastrophic failure of the matrix, the fibers, or both. However, it is considered premature to claim that the tools have been developed to such a robust level for analysis of events subsequent to the initial structurally significant damage. In any event, the ability to tolerate further load application is very dependent on the application. It is far more likely to be permissible for structures subjected to only single monotonic loads than for structures like those in aircraft. In aircraft, many different loads can be applied in random order, and the strengths would become path-dependent, or worse, if the onset of significant structural damage were not defined as design ultimate strength in each case.

The Strength of Embedded Fibers under Arbitrary Biaxial Loads

There are three basic failure mechanisms by which fibers can fail, but only one of these, *shear*, can cover all possible states of combined stress (Ref 5). The other two, *brittle fracture* and *compressive instability*, are limited to specific domains on the strain plane and become local truncations superimposed on the primary shear failure envelope, which is shown in Fig. 1 for isotropic glass fibers and in Fig. 2 for orthotropic carbon fibers.

Maximum-Strain Failure Diagrams. For the reader unfamiliar with strain failure diagrams, important elements of it are detailed. A shear strain envelope for fibers is shown in Fig. 1. The longitudinal fiber strains, ε_L, are plotted horizontally, following the usual convention that positive strains are extensions and negative ones are compressive. ε_0 is the longitudinal strain at failure. Strains in the transverse direction, ε_T, are

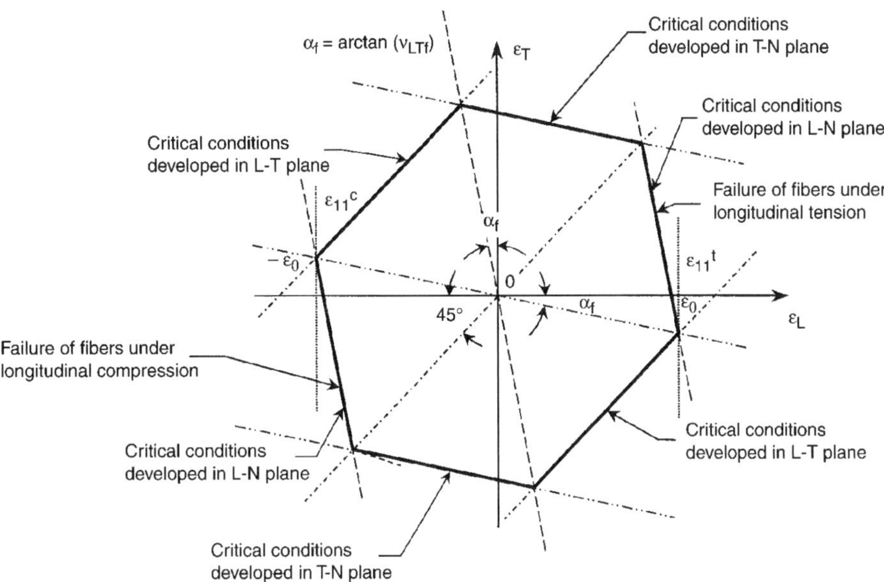

Fig. 1 The strength of glass fibers embedded in polymer matrices, in terms of fiber strains

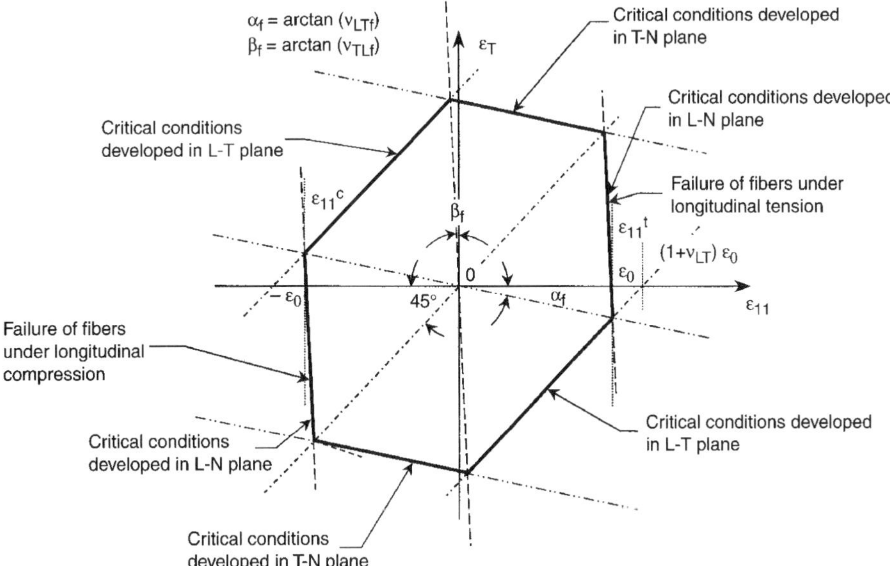

Fig. 2 The strength of carbon fibers embedded in polymer matrices, in terms of fiber strains

plotted vertically. The area within the irregular hexagon represents conditions of strain less than the failure criterion. The failure limits are represented by the hexagon itself. As noted in Fig. 1, the sides each represent a different set of critical conditions. N is the normal, perpendicular direction to the L-T plane, where L and T refer to the longitudinal and transverse in-plane direction relative to the fibers. The angle α_f is related to ν_{LTf} (the major Poisson's ratio of strain in the T-direction to the strain in the L-direction, caused by stress in the L-direction). In Fig. 2, the angle β_f is related to the minor Poisson's ratio, ν_{TLf} (the ratio of the strain in the L-direction to strain in the T-direction, due to stress in the T-direction).

Figure 1 shows the shear failure envelope for isotropic glass fibers, and Fig. 2 presents orthotropic carbon fibers. Only the major Poisson's ratio is involved for glass fibers, while two are needed for the carbon fibers.

Biaxial Strains. Figure 2 identifies the various planes, with respect to the fiber axes, that become critical with changes in the combination of biaxial strains. The same conditions pertain for glass fibers. It is significant that the uniaxial tensile and compressive fiber strengths *must be equal* according to this failure mechanism, thus $\varepsilon_{11}^t = \varepsilon_{11}^c$. This is why a fiber shear failure mechanism was proposed in Ref 6, because this equality had been observed for the carbon fibers of the day. However, there also needs to be provision for other failure mechanisms, because the equality is not true for high-strain carbon fibers, unless they are specially stabilized, and was probably never true for glass fibers. The shear failure mechanism is necessarily sensitive to transverse stresses acting on the fibers whenever the sign of those stresses is opposite to that acting along the length of the fiber.

Uniaxial Stress. Other failure mechanisms are sensitive to only the longitudinal stress in the fiber. One example is brittle fracture of glass fibers resulting from surface imperfections, such as those caused by attack by moisture. Another is failure of carbon fibers, initiating where defects were created in the original precursor from which the fibers were drawn. Both of these phenomena can be added to Fig. 1 and 2 in the form of constant stress cutoffs parallel to the nearly vertical lines therein. The measured longitudinal tensile strength of the fibers will reflect the lower of these two possibilities. It will not be possible to differentiate between the two without microscopic analysis. The reason why the older high-strength carbon fibers, like T-300, appear to be governed by shear failures is presumably that, in that case, the brittle fracture cutoff lies beyond the shear failure limit. These additional tensile cutoffs are combined with the basic shear failure envelope in Fig. 3.

Conservative Shear Strength Limits. The structural analyst may have little interest in knowing which failure mechanism governs tensile fiber strengths, particularly in the case of glass fibers. The engineers stressing carbon-fiber-reinforced laminates may have a little interest, because of the difficulty of locating what to them appears to be a 45° sloping cutoff in the second and fourth quadrants of their customary maximum-strain failure model. There are very few reliable data points with which to locate what is perceived as the shear failure envelope if the fibers fail by brittle fracture first. It has become customary in such cases to relocate the 45° sloping cutoffs to pass through the measured unidirectional tension strength, as shown in Fig. 4. Doing so is clearly conservative. However, new German test techniques (Ref 7) offer hope that reliable direct measurements of fiber shear failure may become possible. In their technique, a single layer of 45° fibers is wound around a carrier tube that is sufficiently strong and buckle-resistant that the strain at failure of embedded fibers subjected to nominally equal and opposite strains can be established. (Note that it is a little more complicated than this, of course. The transverse strain will be equal to the longitudinal strain only at the lamina level. There will be somewhat less transverse strain developed in the fibers themselves—very much less in the case of glass fibers. There may also be residual longitudinal compression applied to the fibers, par-

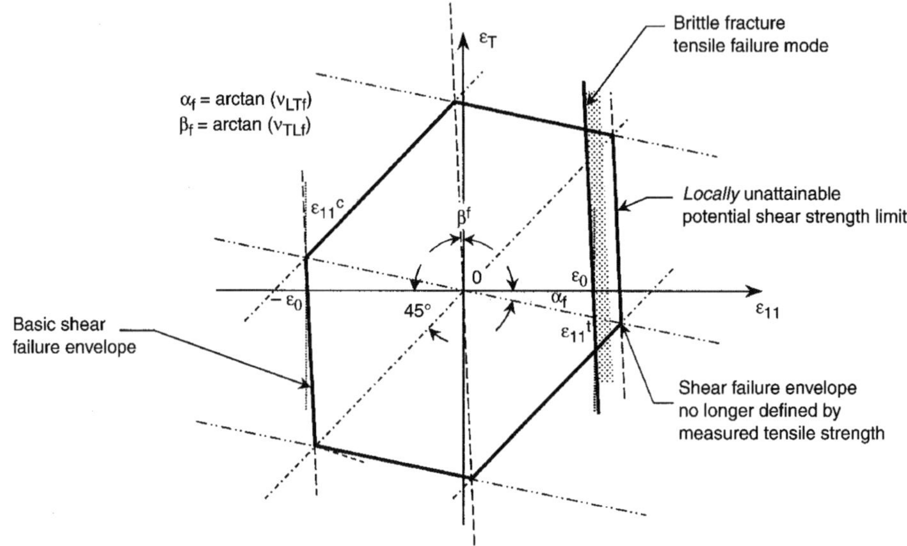

Fig. 3 Additional tensile strength limits for fibers embedded in polymer matrices. The shaded area is affected by the brittle fracture mechanisms.

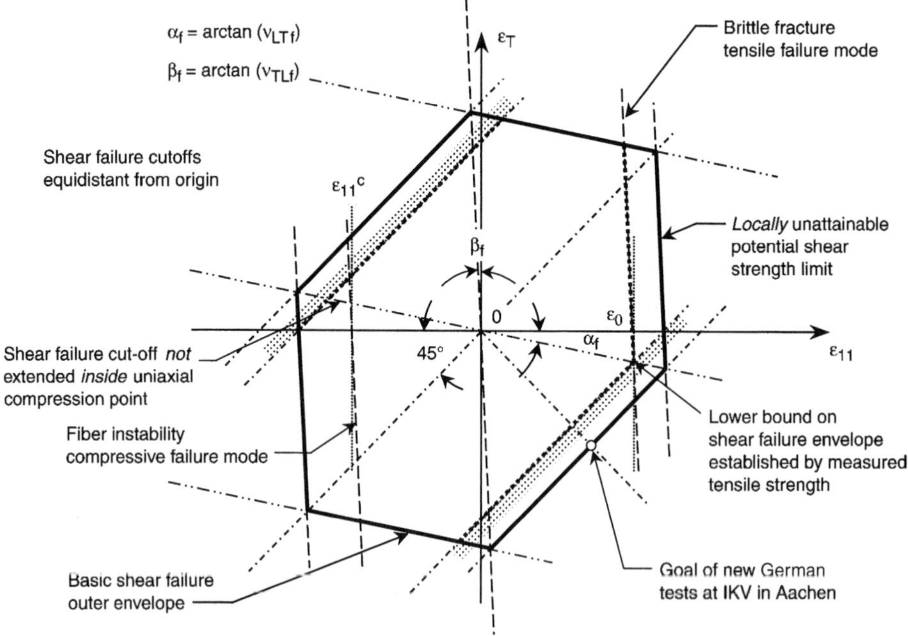

Fig. 4 Conservative establishment of shear strength limits for embedded fibers. Shear failures in the second and fourth quadrants have been relocated, as indicated by the gray bands.

ticularly in the case of carbon fibers, because of thermal dissimilarities between the fibers and the underlying carrier tube. Nevertheless, all of these effects can be compensated for by standard micromechanical analyses. This German technique is actually a major breakthrough, relying only on identifying the most suitable material for the carrier tube, to ensure that it does not fail first. It can obviously be extended to all biaxial states of strain, permitting systematic verifications of any proposed fiber failure envelope.)

Compressive Strength. The customary measured longitudinal compressive strengths (or strains-to-failure) of high-strain carbon fibers are clearly far less than those shown in Fig. 2. Only completely stabilized individual fibers have been shown to have such strengths and failure modes, as reported in Ref 8. Most of the time, the matrix in typical laminae or laminates is unable to stabilize the fibers sufficiently well to attain the shear failure strength. Various forms of instability can precede reaching the compression strength limits shown in Fig. 1 and 2. This process is actually quantified later in this article in the context of matrix failures. It will suffice here to say that this limit has been conventionally represented as an experimentally located constant strain line on the lamina strain plane, which is shown subsequently to be closely equivalent to a constant stress limit at the fiber level, parallel to the closest-to-vertical lines shown in Fig. 1 and 2 and closer to the origin. This has been a reliable empirical technique for structural design, provided that the designs are *restricted* to the laminates in which there are fibers in a sufficient number of directions, and in which extreme limits on blocking of parallel unidirectional plies discourages the incidence of serious failures in the matrix. The in situ compression strength of fibers is actually far more complicated at this level of physical reality, as is discussed later. It should be noted that the data analysts for MIL-HDBK-17 (Ref 9) are confirming that there does not seem to be a unique lamina compressive strength, the way there is for the equivalent tensile strength.

It should also be noted that the two 45° sloping lines in Fig. 1 and 2, and their derivatives, remain equidistant from the origin, even when the in situ longitudinal tensile and compressive strengths differ. In the absence of specific test data to precisely locate these portions of the fiber failure envelope, the correct (conservative) procedure is to locate both of them by the higher of the longitudinal tensile and compressive strengths.

The Strength of Embedded Fibers Characterized at the Lamina Level

The strain in the matrix parallel to the fibers must obviously be the same as in the fibers, except at free edges. However, this is not true in the transverse direction. Therefore, allowance must be made for the differences between transverse strain in the fiber, the matrix, and the lamina. Analyses for accomplishing these distinctions have been around for decades, but recognition of the need to employ them seems to have been appreciated only by some researchers and analysts focusing on mechanistic failure models. Reference 5 contains some simple approximate solutions for this problem, based on continuity of stress through the diameters of the aligned fibers. Because the factors so derived are in the form of ratios, the calculations are isolated from the added complication that there is variation in stress through the thickness of each lamina. The steps involved in these calculations are illustrated in Fig. 5, starting from the exactly 45° slope for the fibers and determining the corresponding slope for the lamina. The strain amplification factors, R_ε, depend slightly on the fiber array, K, and appreciably on the fiber volume fraction, V_f, so it is important to be consistent in the values used.

At the pure transverse tension case, in the absence of longitudinal stress, a typical amplification factor, R, between the transverse strain in the lamina and that in glass fibers is a little over 5, while that for carbon fibers is only about 1.5. Figure 5 displays this latter case. Because the Poisson's ratio for the lamina is about 50% higher than for the carbon fiber, the slope of the lamina-level failure envelope in the second and fourth quadrants is little affected by the distinction between transverse strains in the fiber and the lamina. For glass fibers, on the other hand, the slope is increased to almost 90°. Both of these seemingly contradictory slopes are based on the *same* fiber failure mechanism, shear between axes at ±45° to the longitudinal axis of the fibers, as explained in Ref 5. Note that the same kind of transverse strain amplification factors apply to all other states of biaxial stress, too. All of the nearly vertical lines become even more so, because $\beta << \beta_f$. This difference arises because of the expansion of transverse strains needed to fail the fibers, when expressed at the lamina rather than fiber level. The failure envelope for the glass-fiber lamina is expanded so much in the transverse direction that it is obvious that longitudinal fiber failures in any orthogonal (90°) plies would precede transverse failures in the fibers in the reference (0°) lamina, even if the matrix were strong enough to apply such stresses (which it is not).

Having explained the origin of the various facets of the embedded fiber failure envelope, by starting at the constituent level, it is appropriate to relate them to the more traditional establishment of these same facets at the lamina strain level. This is because the actual measurements on which the model is based are made at that level. Only the thermoelastic constants of the constituents are needed at that lower level for the strain amplification and residual thermal stress calculations. Historically, only two measurements have been made for fiber failures, one in longitudinal tension and the other in longitudinal compression. There is now hope that a third may

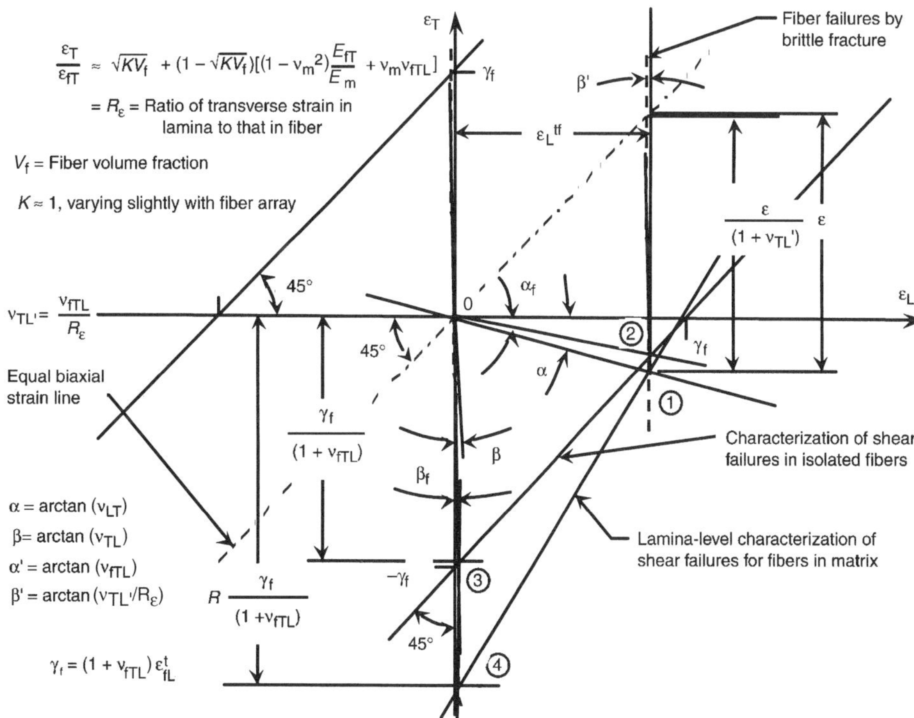

Fig. 5 Strain amplification factors between fiber- and lamina-level models for fibers embedded in polymer matrices. Circled numbers 1 through 4 indicate the sequence by which the points were located. γ_f is the fiber shear strain, E_{fT} is transverse modulus of elasticity of the fiber, and E_m is the modulus of elasticity of the matrix. Subscripts f, m, L, and T refer to fiber, matrix, longitudinal, and transverse, respectively.

be added, to locate the fiber shear cutoffs whenever they cannot be defined precisely by the higher of the longitudinal tension and compression states. The lamina-level measurements and the underlying constituent failure mechanisms are related in Fig. 6 for a typical carbon-fiber polymer lamina. The corresponding diagram for a glass-fiber-reinforced polymer lamina would be far taller, as in Fig. 7, and the 45° sloping lines in the glass-fiber reference plane would be almost vertical at the lamina level.

Actually, the *entire* outer failure envelope is defined by the shear failure mechanism within the fibers, but many people associate *only* the second and fourth quadrants with that mechanism, because they are thinking at the macro-, rather than micro-, level. Failure to add this cutoff, in those quadrants, to the commonly used maximum-strain failure criterion would have no effect on strengths predicted in the first and third quadrants, for any fibrous reinforcements, but would over-estimate the in-plane shear strengths for ±45° laminates, or sublaminates, for carbon fibers.

The nearly vertical lines in Fig. 6 in the first and third quadrants are so close to vertical that it is a reasonable approximation to simplify analyses by making them true "constant strain" lines at the lamina level, even though they originated as constant stress lines at the fiber level, as explained previously. This has been done in Fig. 7, which also shows how the lamina-level envelope for glass-fiber failures is expanded tremendously in the transverse (vertical) direction in comparison with the corresponding carbon-fiber envelope.

It is important to note how few fiber-dominated strength measurements are actually needed to employ this failure model—*three at the maximum*, with only two being used customarily, as shown in Fig. 7. The *entire* shear failure envelope is defined by a single strength measurement. The unidirectional tension and compression strengths are relatively easy to obtain, when they are different. This is provided that one pays attention to the many difficulties that have been encountered in the past and focuses only on the simpler test coupons that have been well validated in the process of explaining the premature failures with other coupons. The shear reference strength has been difficult to establish experimentally in the past, again because of the use of inappropriate test coupons. See the article "Lamina and Laminate Mechanical Testing" in this Volume. (Significantly, the present model is consistent with the best of these measurements, using the Douglas bonded tapered rail-shear test coupon described in Ref 10.) Most of the time, the measured strengths would undercut the measured uniaxial tension strength, which is impossible. It is shown in the subsequent section on matrix failures that even the embedded fiber compression strength can be dispensed with, in most cases. The highest possible compression strength cannot exceed the limit set by the shear failure mechanism, which is usually defined by the tension strength measurement, except for boron filaments, which are stronger in compression than in tension. Despite the great number of test coupons that are incapable of measuring these embedded fiber reference strengths, those that are reliable are extremely simple to perform, as described in Ref 1.

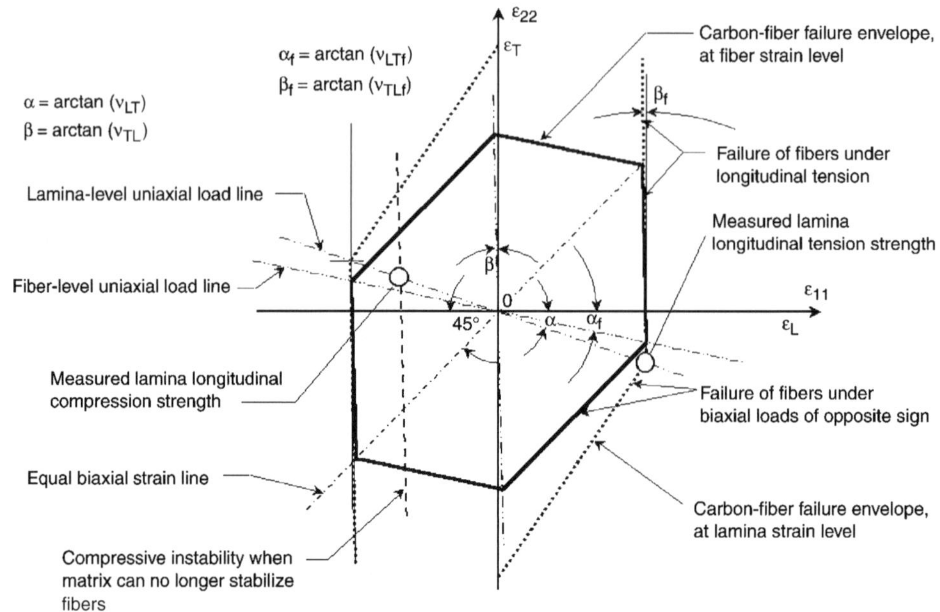

Fig. 6 Fiber failure envelopes at the constituent and lamina strain levels for carbon fibers in a polymer. Circles indicate lamina test data points.

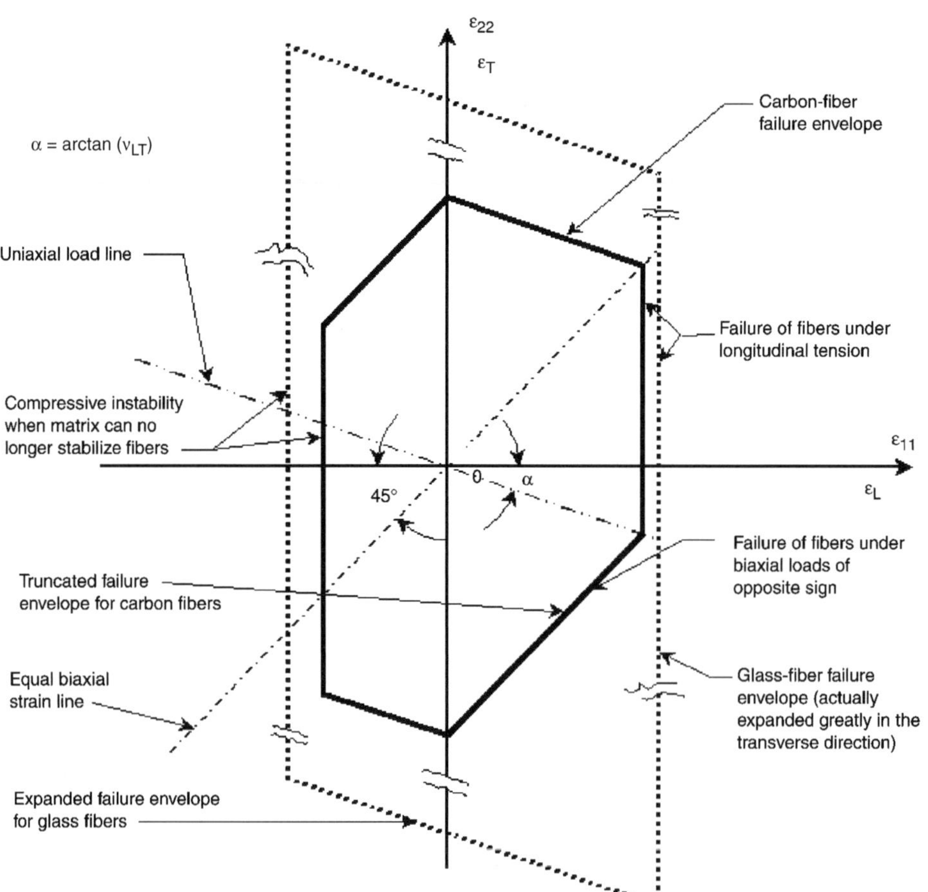

Fig. 7 Fiber failure envelopes at the lamina strain level for carbon and glass fibers. Glass-fiber envelope is not to scale, being actually much taller.

Strength Properties for Polymer Matrices Confined Between Fibers

Just as there are only three possible mechanisms of failure for glass and carbon fibers embedded in polymer matrices, there are only two possible mechanisms—and therefore only two physical properties—describing the *initiation* of failure in the constrained polymer. These are *dilation* and *distortion* (Ref 11). These two characteristics alone are universally applicable, because they are *intrinsic materials properties*. The *orientation* of the fracture surface is defined by the largest principal strain, but the strain itself is not an intrinsic property. Additional properties are needed to describe the propagation of damage, and they are introduced later.

Dilation. The parameter characterizing dilatational (volume increase) failure is the first strain invariant, J_1. This is simply the sum of the three principal strains, although, actually, it has the same value with respect to any triorthogonal coordinates. This invariant is defined as:

$$J_1 = \varepsilon_1 + \varepsilon_2 + \varepsilon_3 \qquad \text{(Eq 1)}$$

If the local volume of the matrix is increased sufficiently, failure will occur by cracking on a plane perpendicular to the highest principal strain. Because most fiber-polymer composites are cured at elevated temperatures, it is necessary to account for microlevel strains equivalent to the thermally induced residual thermal stresses in the matrix, because of the constraints from the fibers. The strains in Eq 1 are with respect to the stress-free state of the matrix.

If a sufficiently good transverse tension test is available for a unidirectional (90°) lamina, a superficial lower bound estimate for J_1 can easily be established from the simple formula:

$$J_1 \approx \varepsilon_T(1 - 2\nu_{TL}) \qquad \text{(Eq 2)}$$

in which L and T refer to the customary longitudinal (0°) and transverse (90°) directions of the fiber. The residual thermal stresses will increase this value. Because ν_{TL} is extremely small for unidirectional composite laminae, J_1 will be roughly on the order of the transverse strain-to-failure. However, there is more to the process of establishing the value of J_1 than this. It is well known that most attempts to measure ε_T can result in premature failures. The most consistently good results have been obtained by surrounding the block of 90° layers by surfacing plies of soft ±45° glass or carbon fabric. (It is recommended that the number of nested 90° plies be between 10 and 20.) It is then necessary to use the finite-element method or standard lamination theory to analytically compensate for the fact that the surfacing plies have different thermoelastic properties from the core of 90° plies, but the improvement in test results, often by as much as a factor of two, justifies this added work. In any event, it is also necessary to employ a micromechanical model (Fig. 8) to account for the strain amplifications between matrix and lamina, arising from their different mechanical and thermal properties of the fiber and polymer, so that the true state of strain is defined. There are five mechanical amplification factors that are multiplied by the five nodal mechanical tensor strain components, three for shear and two for the components normal to the fiber direction. The J_1 invariant is then always evaluated by Eq 1. At the observed load drop, corresponding to the initiation of transverse cracks within the 90° plies, the coupon should be analyzed at the interior of the laminate and not at the laminate free edge. The justification for this procedure can be found in Ref 11. The critical location is also traditionally found to be located at the interstices between the fibers, as is evident in Fig. 8. At that location, *all* strain components are typically positive, because of the customary residual thermal stresses. The radial strain in the matrix immediately adjacent to the fibers is typically negative, because of the same residual thermal stresses*. This has the effect of reducing J_1 there and making the interstices between the fibers more critical most of the time. It should also be noted that the highest contribution to J_1 often comes from the residual thermal stress parallel to the stiff fibers, an increment of strain that is overlooked in most analyses. The macrolevel strain in the matrix parallel to the fibers is obviously extremely limited. However, J_1 must be evaluated with respect to a stress-free condition for the matrix. For this reason, a second micromechanical model, such as that in Fig. 8, is prepared for thermal stresses alone. The six nodal thermal strain components are superimposed on the six micromechanical strain components. With both the nodal mechanical and thermal strain tensors properly modified for micromechanical effects, they can now be added together for all selected nodes. Nodal calculation of any quantity can now proceed.

It is sometimes necessary to differentiate between conditions at stress-free edges of laminates and in the middle of each lamina, where planes perpendicular to the fibers remain plane. Fig. 8 shows that there is a difference between the J_1 values at these two locations, so it is important to use the appropriate values. Figure 8 shows only one end of the model; the front face is actually a section cut through its middle. This process to establish the micromechanical amplification factors and thermal strains for superposition is done only once, at the time of incoming receiving inspections, and J_1 is treated just like any other effective universal property, such as the longitudinal tensile strain to failure, ε_0, or fiber failures in the lamina. The evaluation process for J_1 is influenced by the fiber volume fraction and by the temperature at which the tests are performed, but is valid for all fiber patterns. The approximation given in Eq 2 fails to account for some of the needed effects and is *not* a universal

*The authors have not yet examined the situation for room-temperature-curing laminating resins and therefore cannot predict *where* the highest strains will develop in the matrix in that case. Nevertheless, the procedure outlined above will lead to the correct property. It should also be noted that the value of J_1 will also change when the laminate is saturated with absorbed moisture, but more from the change in polymer properties than from any relief of thermal stresses due to "swelling." In any event, even if the swelling was able to completely nullify the residual thermal stresses, it would do so at *only one temperature*. Increments of intralaminar (and interlaminar) residual thermal stress would be reintroduced *every* time the operating temperature was changed. No justification has ever been provided for omitting consideration of *intra*laminar residual thermal stresses in the manner adopted by so many other authors, who have formulated their models at the macrolevel and thereby overlooked microlevel effects that influence the macrolevel behavior. Any chemical contraction of the resin should be a fixed quantity, independent of temperature, and should therefore be accounted for automatically in the estimate for J_1, because these effects would be present in the test specimen.

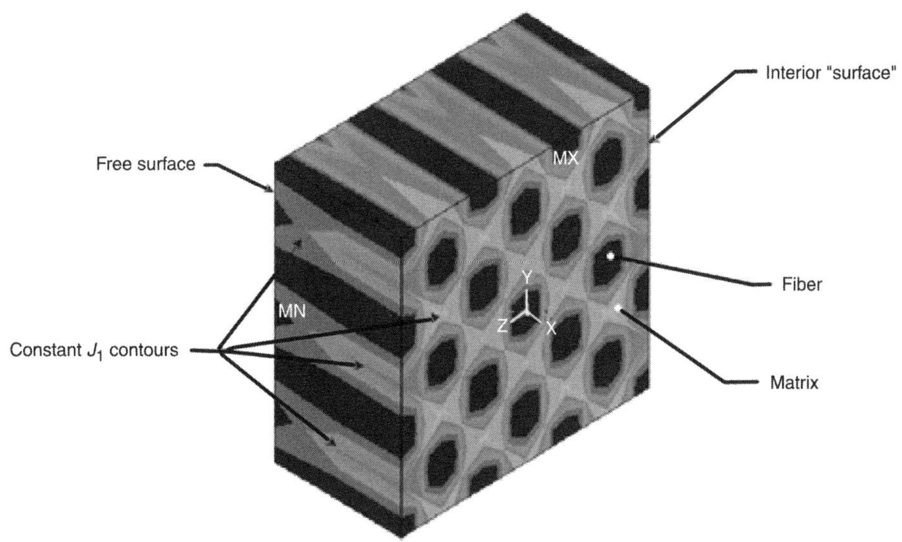

Fig. 8 Micromechanical model to relate lamina-level strains to constituent-level strains in unidirectional lamina. Shading represents contours of constant J_1, which is the sum of the three principal strains. Typically, radial strains in the matrix immediately adjacent to the fibers are negative, so J_1 is lower here and higher between the fibers. MX indicates where the strain in variant J_1 reaches its maximum value; MN identifies the minimum.

property. (As noted earlier, there are correct levels at which the properties should be established.)

It is very important that all the micromechanical models be prepared using standard, universally available computer codes, so that they can be reproduced by *any* user of these theories. Under these conditions, the preparation and use of these models is not at all difficult. Nevertheless, the number of fibers in the cross section and the length of the model must be such as to ensure that the model is long enough to exceed the load transfer distances between fibers and matrix. (This may be set at ten fiber diameters, if no specific data are available.)

Distortion. The other effective strength property of constrained polymers is a function of the second deviator of strain, or equivalent strain (also referred to as the von Mises shear strain). The equivalent strain is also an invariant, being defined as:

$$\varepsilon_{eqv} = \sqrt{[(\varepsilon_1' - \varepsilon_2')^2 + (\varepsilon_2' - \varepsilon_3')^2 + (\varepsilon_3' - \varepsilon_1')^2]/2} \quad \text{(Eq 3)}$$

in which the ε_i's are the *local* principal strains in the matrix, also including strains equivalent to the residual thermal stresses. Because all of the differences between strains in Eq 3 are shear strains, this invariant characterizes *distortion* of the polymer in the *absence* of any change in volume. A superficial estimate of the order of magnitude of the equivalent strain can be established from a pure in-plane shear load with respect to the L and T (1 and 2) axes. A shear strain of γ_{LT} is equivalent to equal-and-opposite longitudinal strains of $\gamma_{LT}/2$, so Eq 3 would predict that:

$$\varepsilon_{eqv} \approx \sqrt{\frac{3}{4}}\gamma_{LT} = 0.87\gamma_{LT} \quad \text{(Eq 4)}$$

However, this test is very difficult to perform reliably. A more accurate test from which to deduce the critical equivalent strain is by transverse compression, by an amount ε_{22}^c. In this case, the critical equivalent strain is approximated by the relation:

$$\varepsilon_{eqv} \approx \varepsilon_{22}^c \sqrt{[(1+\nu_{21})^2 + (1+\nu_{23})^2 + (\nu_{23} - \nu_{21})^2]/2} \approx \sqrt{\frac{13}{9}}\varepsilon_{22}^c \quad \text{(Eq 5)}$$

if we assume that $\nu_{21} \approx 0$ and $\nu_{23} \approx \frac{1}{3}$.

Equations 3 and 5 imply a relationship between γ_{LT} and ε_{22}^c on the order of:

$$\varepsilon_{22}^c \approx \gamma_{LT}/1.39 \quad \text{(Eq 6)}$$

We should *not*, therefore, expect these to be independent properties in the way they have been perceived in the past. They are *both* governed by the *same* failure mechanism.

As with the property J_1, the precise value of ε_{eqv} is a material property that needs to be established only once, using a micromechanical model to properly account for the differences between the lamina-level strains and those in the constituents. At the macrolevel, the residual thermal stresses cannot create distortions in the 1-2 and 1-3 planes, with respect to fibers in the 1-direction, away from free edges. However, between the fibers, such shear strains *can* exist in the 2-3 plane, because of the radial compressive stresses and hoop tension stresses around the fibers.

Figure 9 is a three-dimensional plot of these two matrix failure criteria, with the distortional condition portrayed by an infinitely long, circular cylinder and the dilatational condition shown as a flat plate cutoff, perpendicular to the axis of this cylinder, precluding the attainment of the distortional failures in the presence of quite small dilation (volume increase). A most important implication of this criterion is that the two modes of matrix failure do not interact. This is easy to understand, because distortion can occur in the absence of dilation, and vice versa. However, there are many different sets of strains that can equate to satisfying the critical distortion criterion. This criterion indicates that failure is not possible under equal triaxial compression.

A zero transverse stress ($\sigma_3 = 0$) section cut through the failure envelope in Fig. 9 is clearly consistent with the truncated ellipse failure model for constrained polymers reported by Sternstein et al. (Ref 12) and others (see inset in Fig. 9). However, it should be noted that zero transverse stress at the lamina level does not translate directly to the absence of this stress at the constituent level, because of the customary induced thermal stresses. The application of this matrix failure model has shown that the –45° sloping line for critical J_1 values in Fig. 9, at the constituent level, can look very different when expressed in terms of lamina strains, being almost rectangular for a 0°/90° laminate because of the high residual thermal stresses.

An interesting observation surfaced during a discussion on this theory with colleagues at the Defence Evaluation and Research Agency in England, concerning the randomness of fiber arrays. Given that studies by these authors and others have confirmed only a weak influence of the nature of regular fiber arrays (hexagonal, square, diamond, etc.), but a significant influence of fiber volume fraction, it would seem that the micromechanical models used for these analyses could have the number of fibers in the element adjusted to simulate the varying fiber spacing in real laminates.

The two properties J_1 and ε_{eqv} cover the initiation (rather than the progression) of matrix failure under all states of combined stress, including interlaminar and intralaminar residual thermal stresses induced by the thermal dissimilarity between the fiber and polymer materials. Both can be deduced reliably by quite simple tests, transverse tension and transverse compression of unidirectional laminae. These would need to be repeated for a range of temperatures, because all polymer properties are known to be sensitive to this as well as other environments. However, the presence of the fibers embedded in the polymer matrix can cause the initial matrix damage to be arrested. (Cracks parallel to the fibers in unidirectional laminae will spread catastrophically from initiation.) Additional effective ply strength properties are needed to characterize the progression of such damage. It should be obvious that matrix cracks are more likely to be arrested by laminates with fibers in multiple directions and in laminates in which the plies in the different directions are thoroughly interspersed rather than blocked or nested together.

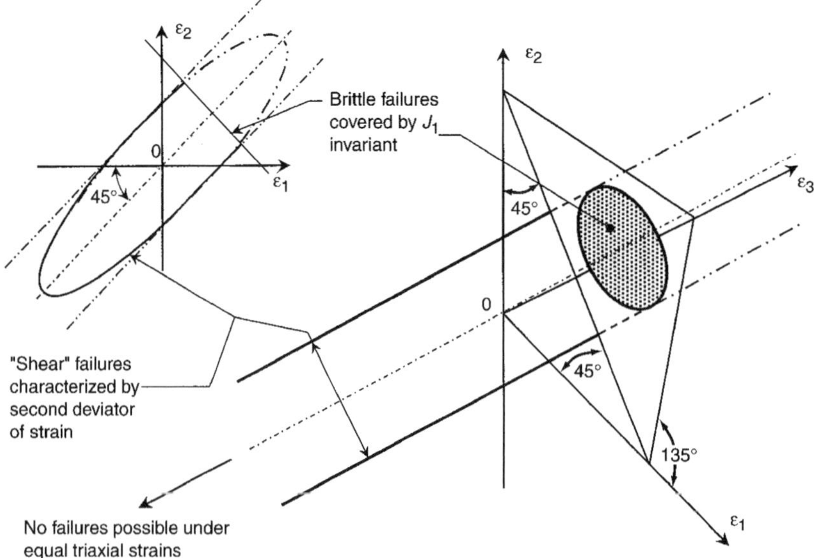

Fig. 9 Two-mechanism characterization of matrix failures in composite laminates. Distortion is shown at the long, circular cylinder and dilation as the flat plate cutoff perpendicular to the cylinder.

Effects of Combined Loading on Matrix Failure Envelope

Considerable progress has been made in applying the matrix failure model described previously to the classical interaction between in-plane shear and transverse tension and compression stresses acting on a unidirectional lamina, and no need has been found for any further properties or for any changes in J_1 and ε_{eqv}, which are the only properties involved in the initiation of matrix failures. Figure 10 shows German test data for biaxial loads of a unidirectional glass lamina in which the predictions have been fitted to only two points, the transverse strains to failure in tension and compression. The measured in-plane shear strain was not involved.

These results indicate that there is no opportunity for subsequent progressive damage if the initial failure is by dilation. However, it is clear that substantial subsequent damage can be tolerated before catastrophic failure occurs. The assessment shown for damage progression has been fitted to only *one* test point. The *same* value of the J_2 invariant is used for all of the other predictions. The damage-progression model was still under development when this article was prepared, so further details must await subsequent publications.

Characterization of Progressive Matrix Damage

Although the ability to reliably assess the onset of damage initiation within the polymeric matrix phase is important, the ultimate goal in failure analysis is usually to determine the ultimate failure loads of composite structures. (In some structures subjected to multiple loads in random order, the *onset* of damage may need to be *defined* as design ultimate strength.) Understanding damage initiation allows for the simulation of damage progression and ultimate failure.

Actual damage can involve transverse ply cracks, delaminations, fiber-matrix debonding, and fiber fracture. At present, it is important to track this damage explicitly. Recent efforts by the authors to simulate the presence of matrix damage (no fiber failure) through abstract means have been successful, but the methods are new and not yet developed to the level where they can be used in production environments.

Although the damage initiation mechanisms are not synergistic, it can be assumed that damage progression will involve both dilatational and distortional deformations. Equations 1 and 3 can be used to express J_2 (the second invariant of strain) as a function of both J_1 and γ, where J_2 is the sum of the products of the principal strains:

$$J_2 = \varepsilon_1'\varepsilon_2' + \varepsilon_1'\varepsilon_3' + \varepsilon_2'\varepsilon_3' = \frac{(J_1^2 - \gamma^2)}{3} \qquad \text{(Eq 7)}$$

The result is a critical arrest property, (J_2^a), that can be used to map matrix damage once matrix damage has been initiated without fiber failure. The arrest property, J_2^a, can be determined by analyzing an angle-ply laminate in tension with no grip-to-grip fiber support. At the onset of damage initiation (the onset of nonlinearity in the load-displacement curve), a one-inch wide laminate will instantly suffer damage across the width of the laminate. J_2^a is then numerically extracted from the center of the laminate at the damage initiation load. The damage arrest property is an effective intrinsic material property of the lamina. J_2^a is only valid when fiber failure does not occur, and it only identifies what elements should have their matrix-dependent moduli, E_2, E_3, G_{12}, G_{13}, and G_{23}, reduced. The final local analysis will have each ply represented by a single element (more if convergence through the laminate thickness has not been achieved). Expressing failure mechanisms as mathematical functions allows for each element to be checked against all currently understood failure mechanisms. Each mathematical function results in a number between 0, for complete degradation, to 1, for no degradation. The failure mechanism that results in the lowest fraction is used to reduce the matrix-dependent moduli for the element under assessment. Currently, five failure mechanisms have been documented mathematically and are given in Eq 8 to 12, where *rf* refers to reduction factor.

Reduction factor a is given as:

$$rfa = \frac{\varepsilon_{eqv}}{\gamma} \qquad \text{(Eq 8)}$$

It has been shown that the critical value of J_2^a is always a negative value. Inspection of Eq 7 indicates that for J_2^a to be negative, damage progression must be distortionally dominant. Therefore, the first failure mechanism, Eq 8, is simply the ratio of the critical value of γ, the equivalent strain, ε_{eqv}, divided by the element average value of γ for a given state of deformation. This failure mechanism would dominate in a laminate subject to in-plane tension.

Reduction Factor b. If a laminate is subject to out-of-plane deformation, transverse cracks may occur that could lead to delaminations. This failure mechanism is expressed mathematically as:

$$rfb = \frac{\gamma_{ip}}{\gamma} \qquad \text{(Eq 9)}$$

Here, γ_{ip} is the element value of γ where only the in-plane tensor strain components are included. γ is the element value of γ where the entire strain tensor is included. As out-of-plane behavior is reduced, Eq 9 approaches unity, and Eq 8 will govern moduli degradation.

Reduction Factors c and d. If the ply volume decreases and becomes negative, and the maximum principal strain is positive, then at some point, damage will initiate within the ply, but damage progression will be very different than when the ply volume is increasing. In this case, damage progression will be retarded. Another regime lies in between volume expansion and contraction. These two additional failure mechanisms are expressed mathematically in Eq 10 and 11:

$$rfc = \frac{(1 + rff)}{2} \qquad \text{(Eq 10)}$$

if $J_1 + J_{1crit} < 0$ *and* where $rff = \min(rfa, \ rfb)$.

$$rfd = \frac{(rfc + rff)}{2} \qquad \text{(Eq 11)}$$

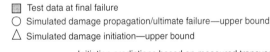

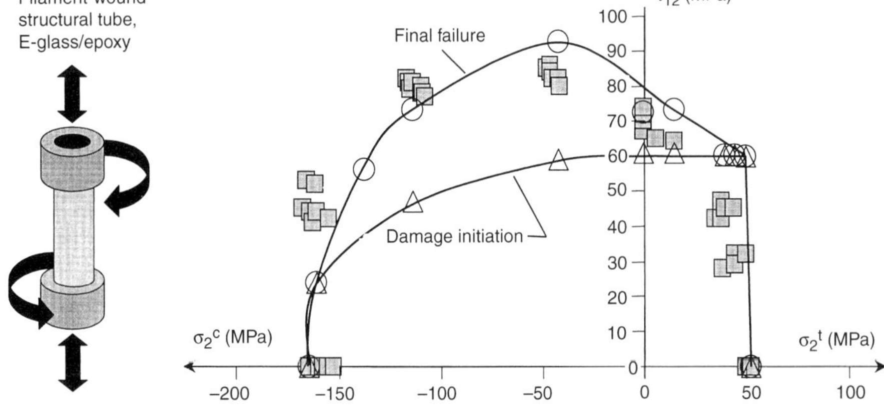

Fig. 10 Damage initiation, propagation, and ultimate failure of biaxially loaded E-glass/epoxy composite tubes. σ_2^t and σ_2^c are axial tension and compression. τ_{12} is in-plane shear stress.

if $J_1 < 0$ and $J_1 + J_{1crit} > 0$ and where again *rff* is defined as previously.

Reduction Factor e. Finally, if a deformed ply has longitudinally compressed fibers, then the ply modulus in the fiber direction is temporarily reduced by the smallest of Eq 8 to 11. This measure is temporary and only occurs for the current state of deformation. Damaged laminates suffering fiber compression may not fail catastrophically. As a result, strains may redistribute as a function of the reduced lateral support supplied by the damaged matrix. If the next state of deformation does not involve longitudinal fiber compression, and the fiber has not failed, then the modulus in the fiber direction is restored to its original value. This final failure mechanism is mathematically expressed as:

$$rfe = \min(rfa, rfb, rfc, rfd) \quad \text{(Eq 12)}$$

In all cases, if fiber failure has occurred, then all ply moduli are reduced to 0.001% of their original values. For a converged model, every ply within every element is assessed as previously stated, resulting in a simulation of matrix damage propagation that is tied to the current state of deformation. The resulting property-reduction methodology is therefore nonarbitrary and reflects a realistic simulation of damage and its effects on critical structural behavior.

Empirical Failure Envelopes for Multidirectional Laminates

The preceding physics-based failure envelopes are easily related to two reliable, widely used empirical failure envelopes. These are the maximum-strain model used so successfully by Puck and his disciples in Germany for glass-fiber-reinforced laminates (Ref 13) and the truncated maximum-strain failure model for carbon-fiber-reinforced laminates developed independently at several aircraft factories in the United States (Ref 3). Despite a common heritage at the constituent level, these materials are surprisingly different at the lamina level, because of the relative strains-to-failure. Glass fibers have such high strains-to-failure that it is common for structurally significant matrix failures to precede fiber failures by large margins. On the other hand, carbon fibers have such low strains-to-failure that it is quite easy to design laminates in which structurally significant matrix failures do not occur until long after limit loads have been attained or, in some cases, not until after the fibers have failed. Matrix damage from impacts is a separate issue and can clearly precede failures under the in-plane load to which structures are designed. In both cases, microcracks of no structural significance occur in the matrix, preceding any cracks that are important; in most cases, even virgin laminates are riddled with insignificant microcracks caused by residual thermal stresses.

Maximum-Strain Model. The consequence of these relative strains-to-failure is that Puck's roughly ellipsoidal failure envelope for glass-fiber-reinforced polymers is predominantly defined by matrix failures, under transverse loads and shear, truncated at the ends by fiber failure cutoffs, as shown in the simplified model characterized in Fig. 11. The reader is referred to the published works of Puck and his students for further details on this kind of analysis.

In contrast with his better-known contemporaries, Puck, in the 1960s, pointed all those who chose to follow him in the *right* direction, that the use of only mechanistic failure models was the path to follow. His progress was eventually limited by a decision to formulate his criteria at the homogenized lamina level, with no micromechanical considerations.

Because of his dissatisfaction with the models used in America, as far as the ability to predict real matrix failures was concerned, Hart-Smith had developed empirical models (for matrix failures), which he used until his collaboration with Gosse. These met with mixed success, but had always been recognized as incomplete. One failure mechanism, matrix failure under in-plane shear, could be coped with by use of secant moduli appropriate to the strains actually developed, as explained in Fig. 12.

The predictions from such a model are reasonably consistent with test data on laminates, but were always at odds with cracking failures

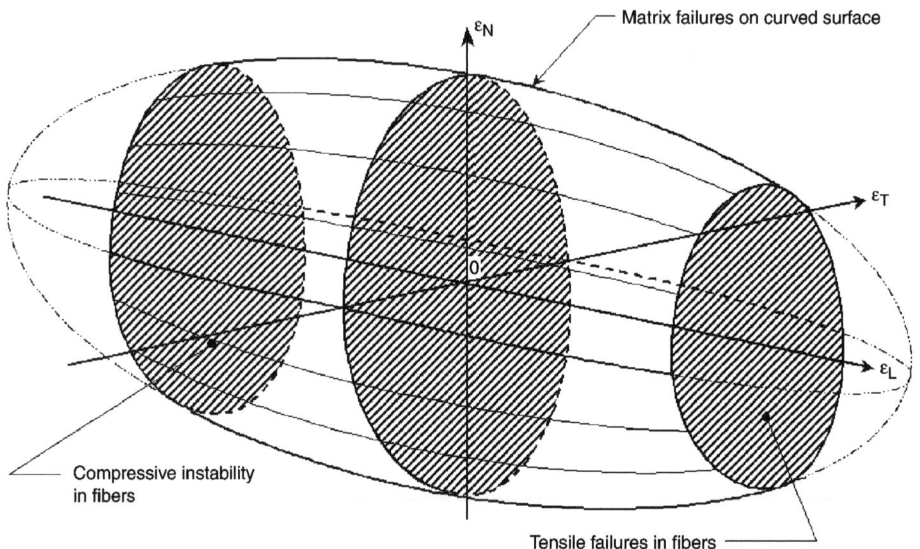

Fig. 11 Lamina-level failure model for glass-fiber-reinforced laminates

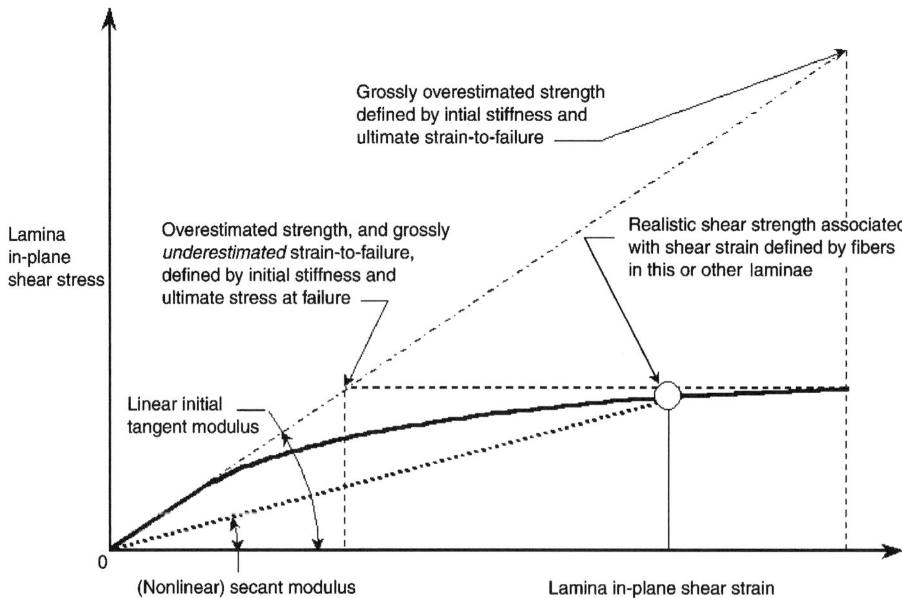

Fig. 12 Approximate modeling of in-plane shear deformation of matrix, at lamina level, in terms of secant moduli

in the matrix by transverse tension within each ply. It has long been clear that two unrelated mechanisms were involved, as indicated in Fig. 9. Hart-Smith's model for such cracking was a straight-line cutoff on the unidirectional lamina strain plane, but there was no basis for locating it. Recent calculations by Gosse have indicated that even the slope, parallel to the locus for a pure axial load in the fibers, was in need of improvement.

It is planned that Gosse's matrix failure criteria in Fig. 9 will, at some future date, be depicted in full for both unidirectional laminae and 0°/90° laminates. Preliminary calculations to this end have confirmed the existence of a straight-line (planar) cutoff for failures governed by the J_1 invariant, dominated by tensile σ_{22} stresses. Not surprisingly, they have also identified a curved surface for those matrix failures governed by the equivalent shear strain, γ_{crit}. Indeed, there is every expectation that the general form of Puck's failure model in Fig. 11 will be confirmed, except for the presence of a flat cutoff, rather than Puck's distorted ellipse, to cover the second failure mechanism. These exploratory calculations have necessitated a reappraisal of all prior matrix failure models. The planned new calculations at the lamina and laminate level will be coupled by failure criteria at the constituent level. There will be no way of progressing from lamina behavior to laminate behavior, as *has* been possible for fiber failures. The authors are therefore deferring any further recommendations about the use of approximate analyses for matrix failures until they have developed a more complete understanding. What can be anticipated, however, is that *complete* matrix failure initiation envelopes at the lamina and laminate levels will be defined by only two reference properties, just as they have been (and continue to be) for fiber failure envelopes.

Truncated Maximum-Strain Model. The truncated maximum strain failure envelope for a unidirectional carbon/epoxy lamina is shown in Fig. 13. It is customarily presented for orthogonal 0° and 90° plies to provide transverse strain limits that would otherwise be much further from the origin, as indicated in Fig. 6. The failure envelope is almost completely defined by fiber failures in the longitudinal-transverse plane, with vertical walls also defined by fiber failures, and an approximately horizontal roof defined by a constant matrix shear strain at failure. Exactly the same envelope is employed for both embedded and isolated laminae, even though there is a difference in regard to transverse tension loads, as noted previously. There is no separation between the onset of failure and catastrophic final destruction when there are no transverse fibers in adjacent plies to arrest the spread of any initial damage. Even so, for structures that can be subjected to varying combinations of biaxial loads in random order, it is necessary to *define* the onset of structurally significant matrix damage as design ultimate strength. Otherwise, it would be necessary to face the intractable problem of path-dependent strengths.

The longitudinal tension and compression strengths are defined by the simple relation:

$$\varepsilon_L^{\,c} \le \varepsilon_{11} \le \varepsilon_L^{\,t} \qquad \text{(Eq 13)}$$

The 45° sloping cutoffs are defined by:

$$|\varepsilon_{11} - \varepsilon_{22}| = (1 + \nu_{LT})\varepsilon_0 \qquad \text{(Eq 14)}$$

in which the longitudinal strain, ε_0, is the numerically greater of the tensile and compressive longitudinal strains-to-failure, $\varepsilon_L^{\,t}$ and $\varepsilon_L^{\,c}$, and ν_{LT} is the primary Poisson's ratio for the unidirectional lamina. Transverse strain limits are effectively defined by the failure under longitudinal tension or compression of other plies in the laminate, at different orientations. For laminates not containing plies in a sufficient number of directions to be fiber-dominated, it has become standard in the aircraft industry to apply transverse strain limits as if such fibers had been present, to limit the design matrix strains. These limits have customarily been defined to be the same as for the fiber longitudinal strains at failure, but it was learned during the preparation of Ref 15 that this was appropriate only for laminates in the 0°, ±45°, 90° family. In laminates with fibers in other directions, it was found that the arbitrary transverse cutoffs should be defined by:

$$|\varepsilon_{22}| = (1 + \nu_{LT})\varepsilon_0 - \nu_{LT}\varepsilon_{11} \qquad \text{(Eq 15)}$$

The matrix in-plane shear limits are set by horizontal plateaus parallel to the fiber reference plane:

$$|\gamma_{12}| \le \gamma_{LT} \qquad \text{(Eq 16)}$$

For laminates and laminae with fibers in only the 0° and 90° directions, there are no further matrix shear failure cutoffs in the approximate analyses. However, standard transformation equations should be used to convert the 0° and/or 90° shear failure plateau into the corresponding nonhorizontal planes for plies with fibers in other directions. For example, the corner truncations shown in the second and fourth quadrants of Fig. 13 would be supplemented by parallel cutoffs, further from the origin, for matrix shear failure cutoffs between fibers in the ±45° directions.

The same set of equations can be applied for glass-fiber-reinforced laminates by omitting Eq 10, as indicated in Fig. 7.

The failure envelope in Fig. 13 is totally noninteractive. However, this relies upon laminates in which the layers of fibers are triangulated so that they behave as structures rather than mechanisms, and in which parallel plies are not blocked together. If they were, failure could be caused by interlaminar stresses not addressed in the present analysis of potential matrix failures. Good design practice for multidirectional laminates calls for restrictions to no more than 0.25 mm (0.010 in.) of parallel fibers adjacent to a 90° change in fiber directions and no more than 0.50 mm (0.020 in.) of parallel fibers adjacent to a 45° change in fiber direction. The preferred fiber patterns shown in Fig. 14 place limits on the deviation from the quasi-isotropic pattern. These are particularly important for laminates with loaded bolt holes. Coarser limits on percentage of fibers in each direction are shown for minimum-gage, lightly loaded panels, because there are insufficient plies, in total, to create overloaded interfaces. Nevertheless, it is common

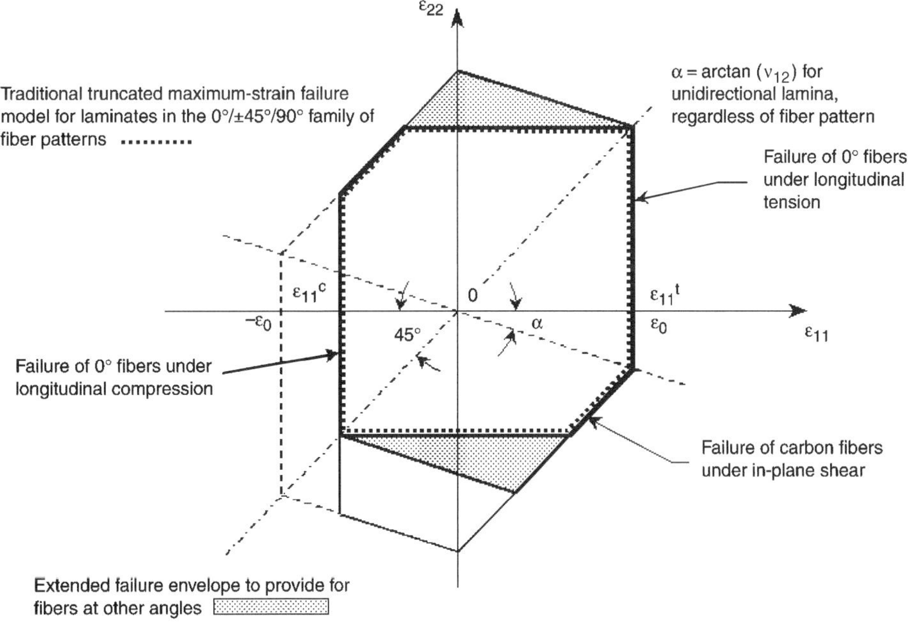

Fig. 13 Truncated maximum-strain failure envelope for carbon-fiber-reinforced polymers at the lamina and laminate strain levels

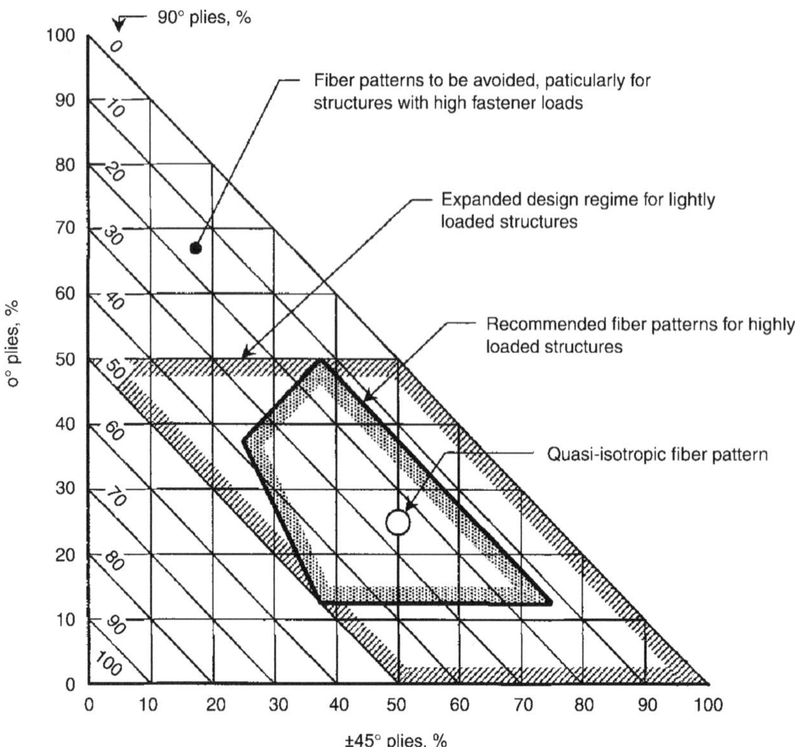

Fig. 14 Preferred fiber patterns for carbon-fiber-reinforced polymers

practice to include nearly quasi-isotropic reinforced edges, for bolt holes, surrounding minimum-gage facesheets (particularly when they are split into two even thinner layers on each side of sandwich cores.)

The truncated maximum-strain failure model was developed because, without it, the projected in-plane shear strengths for $\pm 45°$ carbon/epoxy laminates, according to the original (untruncated) maximum-strain model described in Ref 2, would be far too high in light of even the best test data.

Provided that they were used in such a way as not to violate physical reality, the approximate matrix properties in Eq 2, 4, and 5 could be employed without consideration of micromechanical effects as a *lower bound* set of properties for simplified analyses of some problems. The inclusion of intralaminar residual thermal stresses and an accounting of the greater strains in the matrix than in the lamina in the proper evaluation of these two properties would only increase their value. The authors recommend this approach only with caution, but it must be said that even this would be far more accurate than many established analysis procedures for predicting the strength of composite laminates.

Conclusions

The simple-to-comprehend physics-based failure criteria presented here for the embedded constituents of fiber-polymer composites provide the first *comprehensive* procedure for predicting the strength of composite laminates. Other than for calculating elastic stiffnesses for laminae and laminates, there is no such thing as a homogeneous composite material, only a composite of materials. It is vital to characterize the failure of the constituents separately and in a manner that includes all of the relevant macro- and microlevel stresses and strains. It has been found that strain-based models are the most appropriate formulations, for both fibers and polymer matrices. It is significant that each of the materials properties on which these analyses are based is independent of all others. All of these properties can be measured directly, although it is necessary to analytically compensate for the effects of residual thermal stresses, which cannot be measured, on the basis of measured properties for the fiber and matrix constituents. Even the simple lamina-level approximate analyses recorded here are fully mechanistic. Not one of the analyses relies on empirical curve fits through unexplained test data. It is no longer necessary to know the answer before it can be predicted.

REFERENCES

1. L.J. Hart-Smith, Backing Out Composite Lamina Strengths from Cross-Ply Testing, *Comprehensive Composite Materials*, A. Kelly and C. Zweben, Ed., Elsevier, London, 2000, p 149–161
2. M.E. Waddoups, Characterization and Design of Composite Materials, *Composite Materials Workshop*, S.W. Tsai, J.C. Halpin, and N.J. Pagano, Ed., Technomic, 1968, p 254–308
3. L.J. Hart-Smith, The Truncated Maximum-Strain Composite Failure Model, *Composites*, Vol 24 (No. 7), 1993, p 587–591
4. E.E. Gdoutis, K. Pilakoutas, and C.A. Rodopoulos, *Failure Analysis of Industrial Composite Materials*, McGraw-Hill, 2000, p 99–104
5. L.J. Hart-Smith, "The First Fair Dinkum Macro-Level Fibrous Composite Failure Criteria," McDonnell Douglas Paper MDC 97K0009, presented to 11th International Conference on Composite Materials, 14–18 July 1997 (Gold Coast, Australia); in Proc. Vol I, p I-52 to I-87
6. P.D. Ewins and R.T. Potter, Some Observations on the Nature of Fibre Reinforced Plastics and the Implications for Structural Design, *Philos. Trans. R. Soc. (London) A*, Vol 294, 1980, p 507–517
7. Meeting on composites at Institut für Kunstoffverarbeitung, IKV (Institute for Plastics Processing), Aachen, Germany, 5–8 Sept 2000, private communication
8. S. De Teresa, "Piezoresistivity and Failure of Carbon Filaments in Axial Compression," *Carbon*, Vol 29, 1991, p 397–409
9. MIL-HDBK-17-1E, *Composite Materials Handbook*, Vol 1, Department of Defense, Aug 1996
10. J.B. Black, Jr. and L.J. Hart-Smith, "The Douglas Bonded Tapered Rail-Shear Test Specimen for Fibrous Composite Laminates," Douglas Paper 7764, presented to 32nd International Society for the Advancement of Material and Process Engineering Symposium and Exhibition, 6–9 April 1987 (Anaheim, California); in Proc., p. 360–372
11. J.H. Gosse, S. Christensen, and L.J. Hart-Smith, "Strain Invariant Failure Criteria for Polymers as Binders for Composite Materials, Part 1: Damage Initiation," submitted for publication
12. S. Sternstein and L. Ongchin, Yield Criteria for Plastic Deformation of Glassy High Polymers in General Stress Fields, *Polym. Prepr.* Vol 10, 1969, p 1117–1124
13. A. Puck and W. Schneider, "On Failure Mechanisms and Failure Criteria of Filament-Wound Glass-Fiber/Resin Composites" presented at Conf. Research Projects in Reinforced Plastics, 20 March 1968 (London); published in *Plastics & Polymers*, Feb 1969, p 33–42
14. L.J. Hart-Smith, Predictions of a Generalized Maximum-Shear-Stress Failure Criterion for Certain Fibrous Composite Laminates, McDonnell Douglas Paper MDC 97K0011, *Compos. Sci. Technol.*, Vol 58 (No. 7), 1998, p 1179–1208

Fracture Mechanics of Composite Delamination

T. Kevin O'Brien, U.S. Army Research Laboratory

DELAMINATION, a separation of the fiber-reinforced layers that are stacked together to form laminates, is one of the most commonly observed failure modes in composite materials. The most common sources of delamination are the material and structural discontinuities that give rise to interlaminar stresses (Fig. 1). Delaminations occur at stress-free edges due to a mismatch in properties of the individual layers, at ply drops (both internal and external) where thickness must be reduced, and at regions subjected to out-of-plane loading, such as bending of curved beams. There are three fundamental failure modes, as shown in Fig. 2:

- *Mode I*: opening mode
- *Mode II*: in-plane shearing mode
- *Mode III*: tearing or scissoring shearing mode

Locally, delaminations typically form due to some combination of these fracture modes.

The interlaminar fracture toughness (IFT) is a measure of the ability of a material to resist delamination. For the most general cases, the strain energy release rate values for each mode (G_I, G_{II}, G_{III}) are calculated for the configuration and loading of interest. These values must be compared to the critical value, which has been determined from material characterization tests. The critical IFT value is determined from the same combination of fundamental modes to predict delamination onset and growth.

Delamination Characterization

Typical mixed-mode I and II delamination failure criterion is shown in Fig. 3. The IFT is determined as a critical value of the strain energy release rate, G_c, plotted as a function of the mixed-mode ratio, G_{II}/G, where $G = G_I + G_{II} + G_{III}$. The pure mode I opening case is stated as $G_{II}/G = 0$, and the pure mode II case is represented by $G_{II}/G = 1$. These properties are determined using test methods that are being evaluated and standardized by ASTM and other national standards organizations, as well as the International Standards Organization (ISO) (Ref 1). The pure mode I data are generated using a double-cantilever beam (DCB) test (Ref 2–4). The pure mode II data generally are generated using an end-notched flexure (ENF) test (Ref 5, 6). The mixed-mode I and II data are generated using a mixed-mode bending (MMB) test (Ref 7–9). As shown in Fig. 3, the apparent toughness generally increases monotonically between the pure opening mode I case and the pure shear mode II case. Furthermore, due to the complex micromechanisms involved, the scatter of test data is very large for the mode II case (Ref 10). The test specimens are shown in Fig. 4. For cases where a mode III fracture toughness is required,

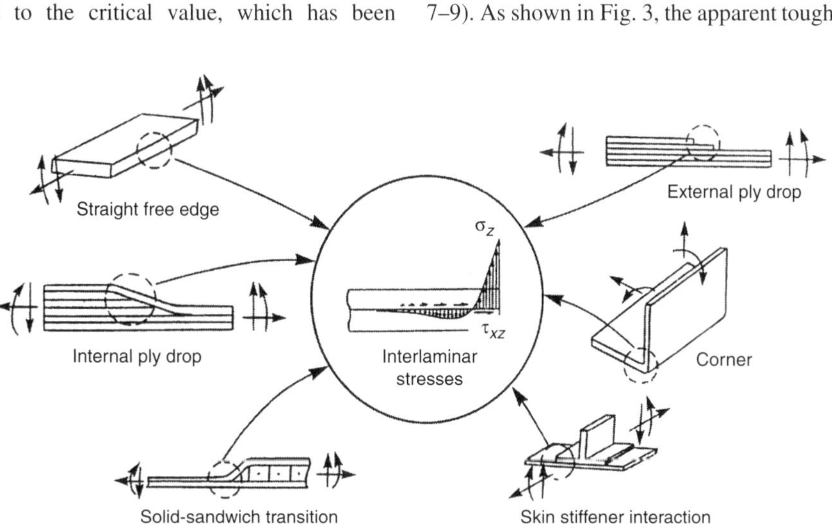

Fig. 1 Delamination sources at geometric and material discontinuities

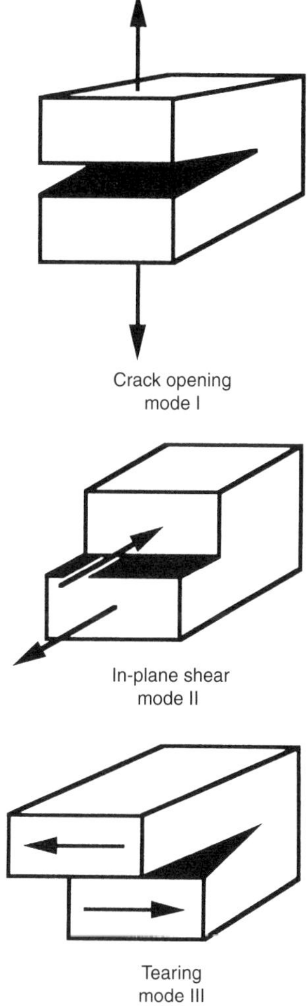

Fig. 2 Three basic modes of delamination fracture

the edge-cracked torsion (ECT) test is preferred (Ref 11, 12).

Because delaminations often form and grow under cyclic loads, a fatigue characterization is also desired. The classical Paris law for fatigue crack growth (which describes crack growth per load cycle as a function of the range in the stress-intensity factor) has often been generated (Ref 13–15); however, the exponents in these power laws are quite high compared to similar characterizations for metals. Hence, a no-growth threshold approach is often proposed instead (Ref 16–19). Furthermore, for mode I fatigue, fiber bridging typically develops in the unidirectional DCB specimens (Ref 1, 17). This fiber bridging can cause a growing crack to arrest artificially early, yielding a nonconservative threshold value (Fig. 5a). Therefore, as shown in Fig. 5(b), an alternate G versus N onset curve is typically generated to achieve a threshold characterization for delamination onset (Ref 17–20).

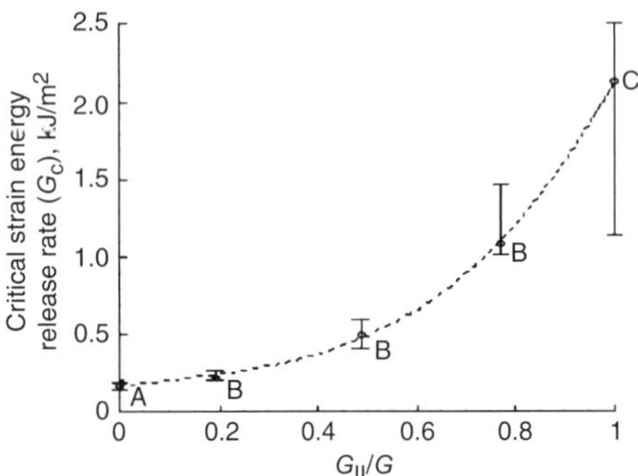

Fig. 3 Critical strain energy release rate, G_c, as a function of the mixed-mode ratio for graphite/epoxy IM7/E7T1-2. A, pure mode I; B, mixed mode I and mode II; C, pure mode II

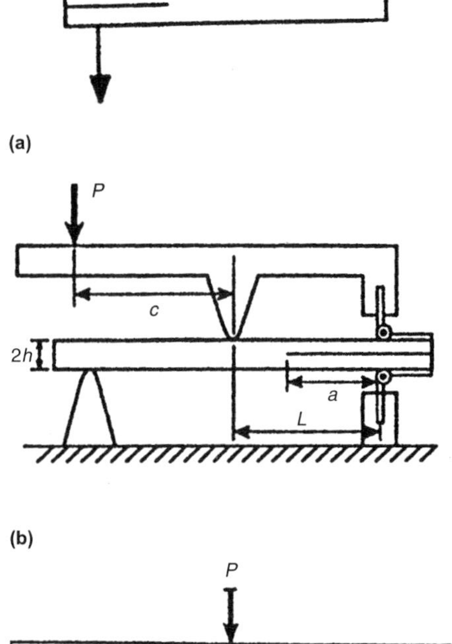

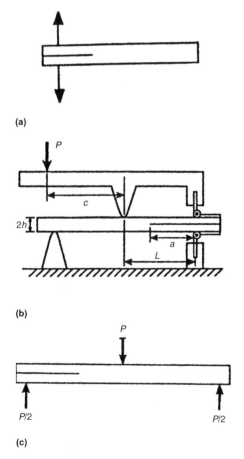

Fig. 4 Test specimens for determining G_c. (a) Mode I, double-cantilever beam (DCB). (b) Mixed mode I and mode II, mixed-mode bending (MMB). (c) Pure mode II, end notch flexure (ENF)

Delamination Analysis

As noted earlier, the strain energy release rate, G, associated with onset and growth, must be determined to predict delamination. Typically, a plot of the G components due to the three fundamental fracture modes (G_I, G_{II}, G_{III}) and the total $G = G_I + G_{II} + G_{III}$ are calculated as a function of delamination length, a, using the virtual crack closure technique (VCCT) in a finite element analysis (FEA) (Ref 21, 22). The VCCT technique, depicted in Fig. 6, utilizes the product of nodal forces and the difference in nodal displacements, to calculate the G components for each fracture mode. Alternate methods have also been proposed for calculating G (Ref 23–25). For predicting delamination onset in two-dimensional problems, the peak value of the G versus a distribution is compared to the mixed-mode fracture criterion of Fig. 3. The VCCT technique has also been extended to three-dimensional problems (Ref 26), including those involving delamination growth due to sublaminate instability in compression loaded laminates (Ref 27) and the three-dimensional effect in skin-stiffener pull-off delamination failure (Ref 28).

Delamination Prediction

Flexbeam Fatigue Life Prediction. Helicopter composite rotor hubs contain tapered flex-

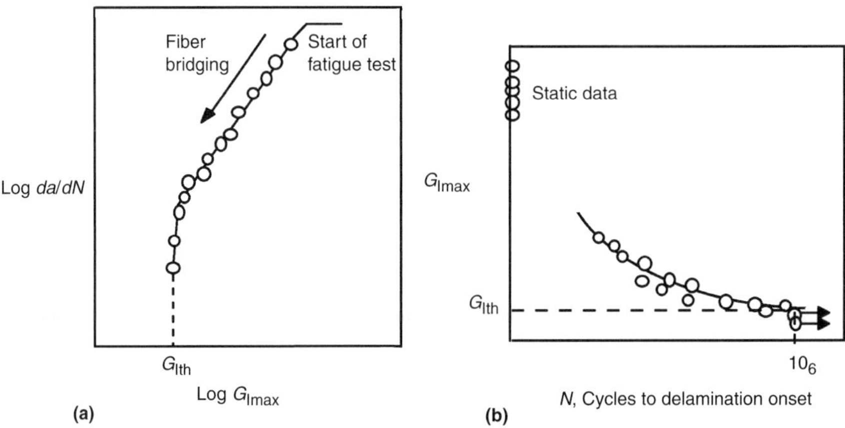

Fig. 5 Experimental techniques to obtain a strain energy release threshold, G, for delamination onset. (a) By delamination arrest. (b) By delamination onset

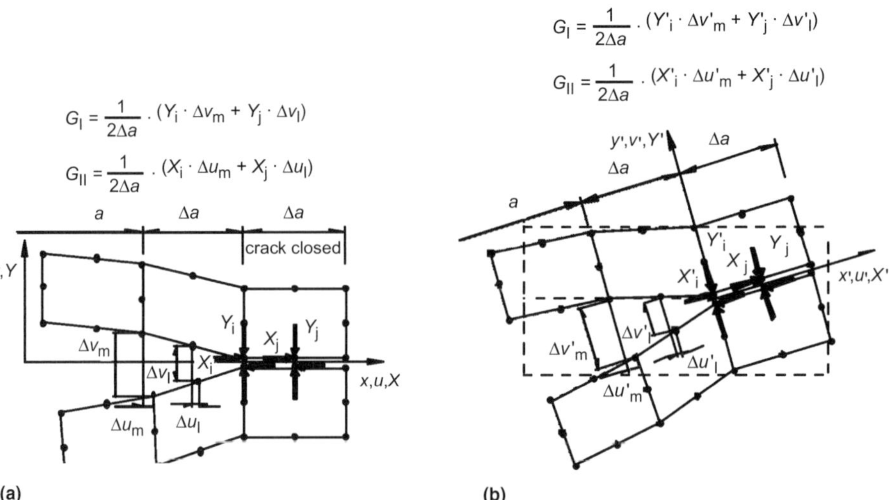

Fig. 6 Finite elements used for the virtual crack closure technique (VCCT). Eight-noded quadrilateral elements are used in (a) linear and (b) nonlinear analysis.

beams with large numbers of ply terminations, or *ply drops*, to taper the beam thickness. These ply drops may act as delamination initiation sites in the flexbeam under high combined tension and cyclic bending loads. Reference 29 describes how one-sixth sized flexbeams were tested (Fig. 7) and analyzed to determine the fatigue life, identified as onset of delamination. The ply drops of the flexbeams are detailed in Fig. 8. Fatigue delamination onset test data are plotted in Fig. 9. This characterization of the material is compared to the *G* distributions determined by FEA using VCCT, for the conditions shown in Fig. 10. The analysis results in the prediction of the onset of unstable delaminations from ply drops to characterize the fatigue life given in Fig. 11.

Skin/Stiffener Pull-Off Strength and Life. Figure 12 shows the prediction of pull-off loads that cause separation of the flange of a hat stiffener from the skin of a composite part. The pull-off loads associated with delamination onset were predicted by comparing *G* values calculated from FEA using VCCT to the mixed-mode delamination failure criteria in Fig. 3 and 4 (Ref 30).

Subsequent studies led to the development of the simple specimen for studying skin-stiffener debonding (Fig. 13), which consists of a skin bonded to a tapered flange laminate (Ref 31, 32). Most recently, a generalized fatigue methodology based on the approach used in Ref 29 was developed and used to predict the delamination onset life for skin-stiffener debonding under cyclic loading (Fig. 14) (Ref 33).

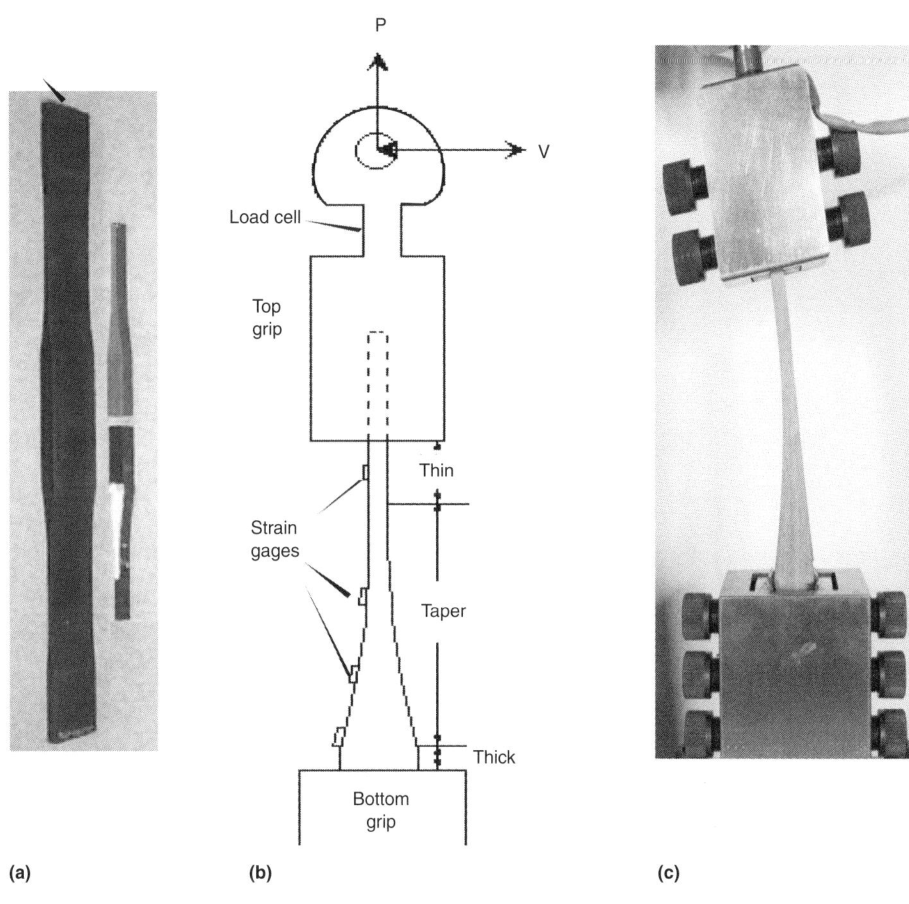

Fig. 7 Testing of helicopter composite rotor hub flexbeams in tension and bending. (a) Full beam and one-sixth size beam. (b) Drawing of one-sixth size section in test fixture. (c) Flexbeam specimen in the tension and bending test load frame

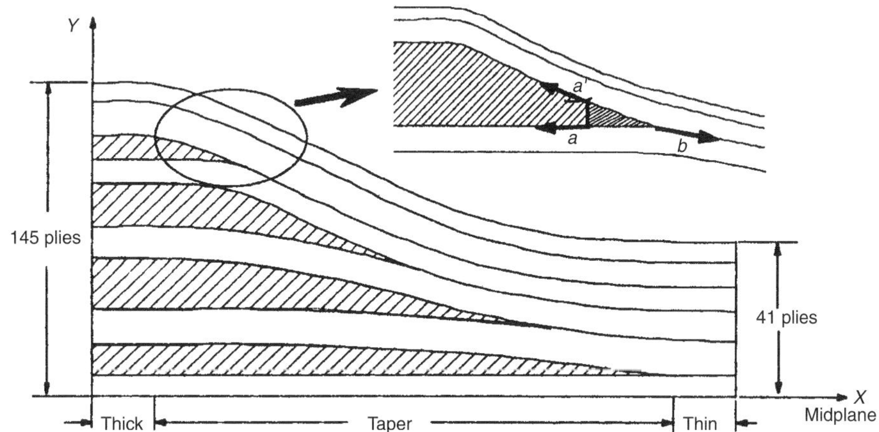

Fig. 8 Detail of flexbeam ply drops

REFERENCES

1. T.K. O'Brien, Interlaminar Fracture Toughness: The Long and Winding Road to Standardization, *Compos. B: Eng.*, Vol 29B, 1998, p 57–62
2. T.K. O'Brien and R.H. Martin, Round Robin Testing for Mode I Interlaminar Fracture Toughness of Composite Materials, *J. Compos. Technol. Res.*, Vol 15 (No. 4), 1993, p 269–281
3. "Standard Test Method for Mode I Interlaminar Fracture Toughness of Unidirectional Fiber-Reinforced Polymer Matrix Composites," D 5528-94a, *Annual Book of ASTM Standards,* ASTM, Vol 15.03, 1994, p 272–281
4. "Fibre-Reinforced Plastic Composites—Determination of Mode I Interlaminar Fracture Toughness, G_{Ic}, for Unidirectionally Reinforced Material," IS-15024, International Standards Organization, 2000
5. A.J. Russell, "Measurement of Mode II Interlaminar Fracture Energies," Materials DREP Report 82-0, Defence Research Establishment Pacific, 1982
6. R.H. Martin and B.D. Davidson, Mode II Fracture Toughness Evaluation Using a Four-Point Bend End Notched Flexure Test, *Plast. Rubber Compos.*, Vol 28 (No. 8), 1999, p 401–406
7. J.R. Reeder and J.H. Crews, Jr., The Mixed-Mode Bending Method for Delamination

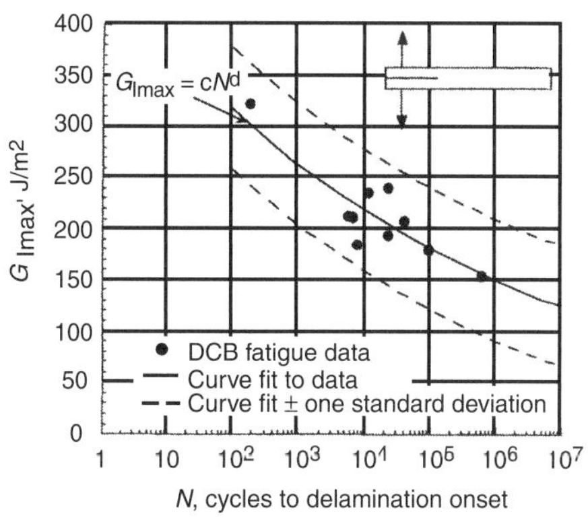

Fig. 9 Double cantilever beam (DCB) fatigue data of material delamination characterization

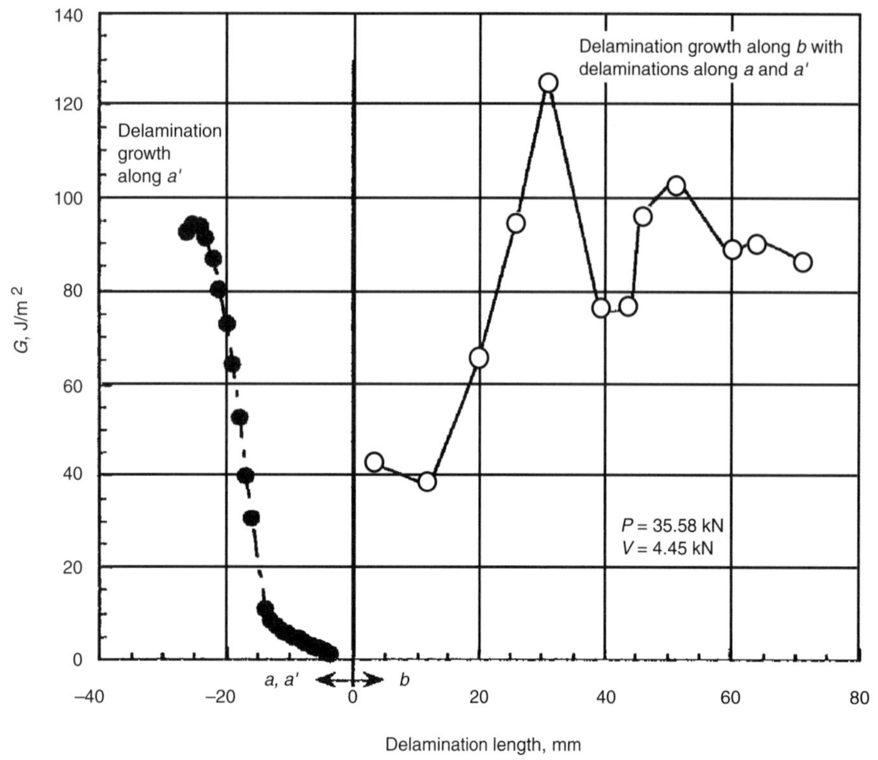

Fig. 10 Finite element analysis using VCCT to determine strain energy release. Delamination growth, a, a', and b; directions are shown in detail of Fig. 8.

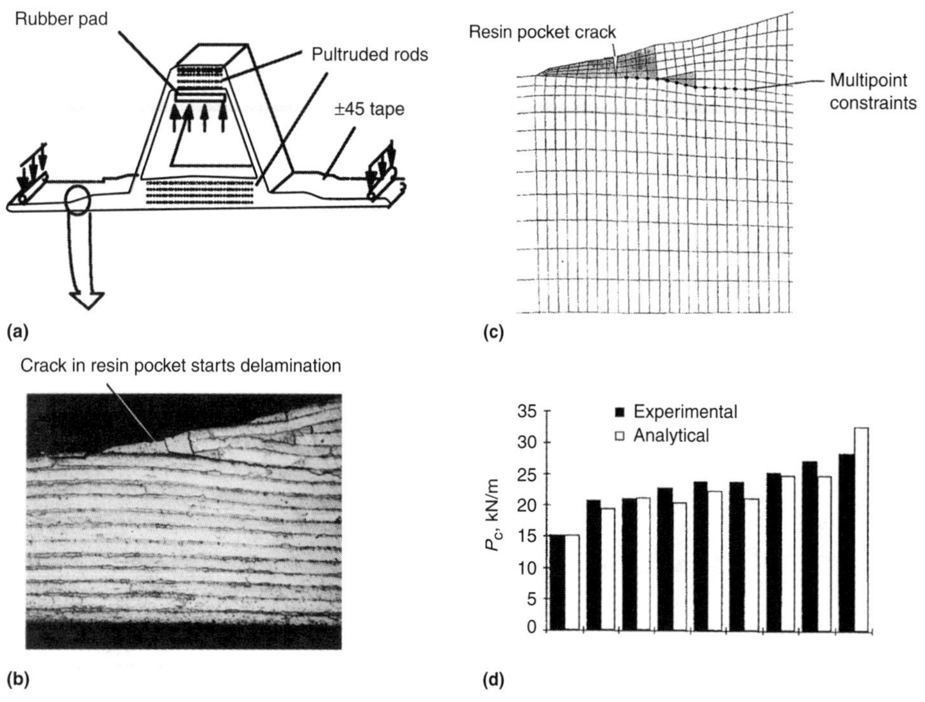

Fig. 12 Hat stiffener as part of composite skin. (a) Test configuration with loading indicated (b) Micrograph of flange tip region (c) FEA mesh used to model the flange tip region (d) Comparison of experimental and analytical results of the pull-out loads for individual specimens

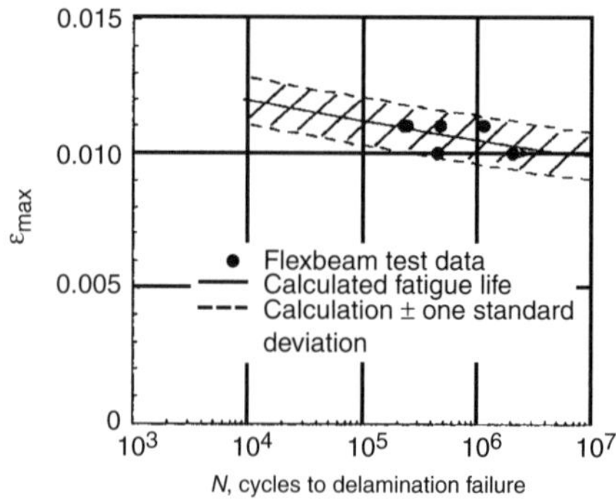

Fig. 11 Flexbeam life prediction

Testing, *AIAA Journal*, Vol 28 (No. 7), July 1990, p 1270–1276

8. J.R. Reeder and J.H. Crews, Jr., Redesign of the Mixed-Mode Bending Delamination Test to Reduce Nonlinear Effects, *J. Compos. Technol. Res.*, Vol 14, 1992, p 12–19
9. J.R. Reeder, Refinements to the Mixed-Mode Bending Test for Delamination Toughness, *Proc. American Society for Composites 15th Technical Conf.*, Technomic, Sept 2000, p 991–998
10. T.K. O'Brien, Composite Interlaminar Shear Fracture Toughness, G_{IIc}: Shear Measurement or Sheer Myth?, *Composite Materials: Fatigue and Fracture, Seventh Volume,* STP 1330, ASTM, 1998, p 3–18
11. S.M. Lee, An Edge Crack Torsion Method for Mode III Delamination Fracture Testing, *J. Compos. Technol. Res.*, Vol 15 (No. 3), fall 1993, p 193–201
12. J. Li, S.M. Lee, E.W. Lee, and T.K. O'Brien, Evaluation of the Edge Crack Torsion (ECT) Test for Mode III Interlaminar Fracture Toughness of Laminated Composites, *J. Compos. Technol. Res.,*Vol 19 (No. 3), July 1997, p 174–183
13. P.C. Paris and G.C. Sih, "Stress Analysis of Cracks," STP 381, *Fracture Toughness Testing and its Applications,* ASTM, June 1964, p 30–83
14. Y.J. Prel, P. Davies, M. Benzeggagh, and F.X. de Charentenay, "Mode I and Mode II Delamination of Thermosetting and Thermoplastic Composites," STP 1012, *Composite Materials: Fatigue and Fracture, Second Volume,* ASTM, April 1989, p 251–269
15. K. Kageyama, I. Kimpara, I. Ohsawa, M. Hojo, and S. Kabashima, "Mode I and Mode II Delamination Growth of Interlayer Toughened Carbon/Epoxy Composite System," STP 1230, *Composite Materials: Fatigue and Fracture, Fifth Volume,* ASTM, Oct 1995, p 19–37
16. T.K. O'Brien, "Towards a Damage Tolerance Philosophy for Composite Materials and Structures," STP 1059, *Composite Materials: Testing and Design, Ninth Volume,* ASTM, Feb 1990, p 7–33
17. R.H. Martin and G.B. Murri, "Characterization of Mode I and II Delamination Growth and Thresholds in AS4/PEEK Composites," STP 1059, *Composite Materials: Testing and Design, Ninth Volume,* ASTM, 1990, p 251–270
18. T.K. O'Brien, G.B. Murri, and S.A. Salpe-

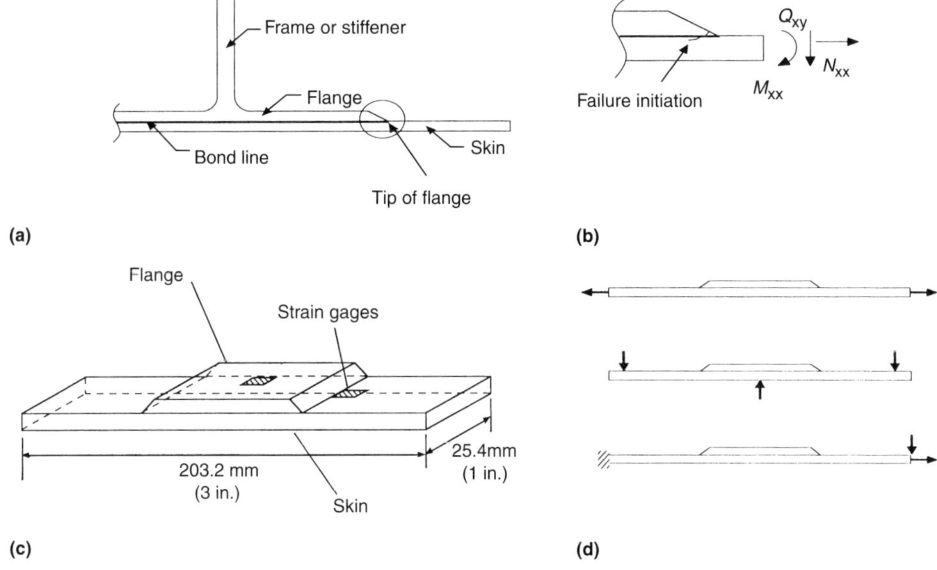

Fig. 13 Simplified test specimen for skin-stiffener debonding. (a) Cross section of composite part. (b) Detail of flange tip. (c) Simplified test specimen. (d) Loads applied to skin

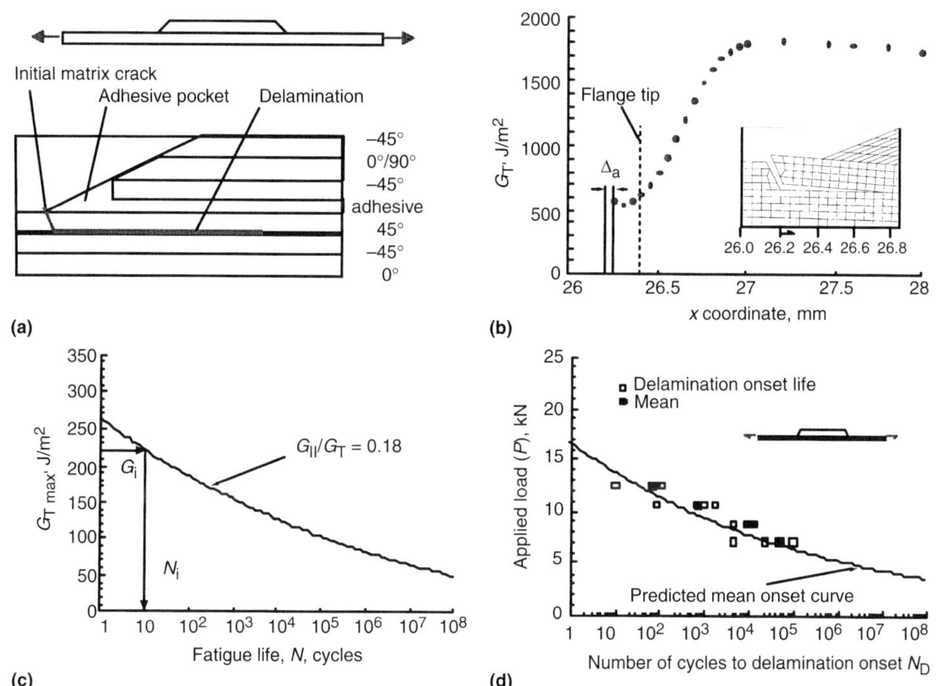

Fig. 14 Skin-stringer debonding fatigue life prediction methodology. (a) Detail of lamina with initial delamination. (b) FEA using VCCT analysis; initial delamination is modelled. (c) Characterization data. (d) Life prediction of the skin-stringer interface

kar, "Interlaminar Shear Fracture Toughness and Fatigue Thresholds for Composite Materials," STP 1012, *Composite Materials: Fatigue and Fracture, Second Volume,* ASTM, April 1989, p 222–250

19. G.B. Murri and R.H. Martin, "Effect of Initial Delamination on Mode I and Mode II Interlaminar Fracture Toughness and Fatigue Fracture Thresholds," STP 1156, *Composite Materials: Fatigue and Fracture, Fourth Volume,* ASTM, June 1993, p 239–256
20. "Standard Test Method for Mode I Fatigue Delamination Growth Onset of Unidirectional Fiber-Reinforced Polymer Matrix Composites," D6115-97, *Annual Book of ASTM Standards,* ASTM, Vol 15.03, 1997, p 338–343
21. E.F. Rybicki and M.F. Kanninen, A Finite Element Calculation of Stress Intensity Factors by a Modified Crack Closure Integral, *Eng. Fract. Mech.,* Vol 9 1977, p 931–938
22. I.S. Raju, Calculation Of Strain-Energy Release Rates With Higher Order And Singular Finite Elements, *Eng. Fract. Mech.,* Vol 28, 1987, p 251–274
23. G. Flanagan, A Sublaminate Analysis Method for Predicting Disbond and Delamination Loads in Composite Structures, *J. Reinf. Plast. Compos.*, Vol 12, 1993, p 876–887
24. B.D. Davidson, Analytical Determination of Mixed-Mode Energy Release Rates for Delamination Using a Crack Tip Element, *Fracture of Composites*, Vol 120–121, *Key Engineering Materials*, 1996, p 161–180
25. B.D. Davidson, H. Hu and R.A. Schapery, An Analytical Crack Tip Element for Layered Elastic Structures, *J. Appl. Mech.*, Vol 62, 1995, p 243–253
26. R. Krüger, M. König, and T. Schneider, Computation of Local Energy Release Rates Along Straight and Curved Delamination Fronts of Unidirectionally DCB and ENF Specimens, *Proc. 34th AIAA-SDM Conf.,* La Jolla, CA, 1993, p 1332–1342
27. J.D. Whitcomb, Three Dimensional Analysis of a Postbuckled Embedded Delamination, *J. Compos. Mater.,* Vol 23, Sept 1989, p 862–889
28. J. Li, "Three-Dimensional Effect in the Prediction of Flange Delamination in Composite Skin-Stringer Pull-Off Specimens," *Proc. of American Society for Composites 15th Technical Conf.,* 25–27 Sept 2000, p 983–990
29. G.B. Murri, T.K. O'Brien, and C.Q. Rousseau, Fatigue Life Methodology for Tapered Composite Flexbeam Laminates, *J. Am. Helicopt. Soc.,* Vol 43 (No. 2), April 1998, p 146–155
30. J. Li, T.K. O'Brien, and C.Q. Rousseau, Test and Analysis of Composite Hat Stringer Pull-off Test Specimens, *J. Am. Helicopt. Soc.,* Vol 42 (No. 4), Oct 1997, p 350–357
31. P.J. Minguet and T.K. O'Brien, Analysis of Test Methods for Characterizing Skin/Stringer Debonding Failures in Reinforced Composite Panels, STP 1274, *Composite Materials: Testing and Design, Twelfth Volume,* ASTM, Aug 1996, p 105–124
32. R. Krueger, M.K. Cvitkovich, T.K. O'Brien, and P.J. Minguet, Testing and Analysis of Composite Skin/Stringer Debonding Under Multi-Axial Loading, *J. Compos. Mater.*, Vol 34 (No. 15), 2000, p 1264–1300
33. K. Krueger, I.L. Paris, T.K. O'Brien, and P.J. Minguet, Fatigue Life Methodology for Bonded Composite Skin/Stringer Configurations, *Proc. American Society for Composites 15th Technical Conf.,* Technomic Publishers, Sept 2000, p 729–736

Hygrothermal Behavior

Daniel R. Ruffner, The Boeing Company

HYGROTHERMAL BEHAVIOR of cured composite materials relates to the combined and commonly synergistic effects of moisture absorption and temperature on various physical, chemical and mechanical properties. While effects for polymer-matrix composites can be substantial, thermosetting matrices are typically much more affected than thermoplastic matrices. Although hygrothermal effects should be irrelevant for metal- and ceramic-matrix composites, their responses as newer materials and as classes are still somewhat uncertain. This article concentrates on polymer-matrix composites and is limited to the effects of moisture absorption after an established cure of the material has been completed. Effects of moisture absorption on uncured prepreg or adhesive materials on the material properties after cure can also be present but are not covered in this article. The galvanic electrochemical mechanisms experienced by some carbon/bismaleimide composites also are not covered.

General Considerations in Assessing Hygrothermal Behavior

Moisture absorption for composite materials is primarily a diffusion process dependent on environmental conditions. As a result, time is an important factor in reproducing these effects. Since moisture absorption to saturation under typical field environmental conditions can take years, the ability to reproduce these effects in the lab in the more reasonable time frame of days or weeks is critical. Validating that the accelerated aging technique used has not changed the expected field degradation mechanisms and failure modes and their effects on the performance of the material then becomes a concern.

Since hygrothermal testing is accelerated aging designed to reproduce years of exposure in service, an understanding of the conditions of service is important. The same material may be adequate for worldwide environmental conditions in excess of 20 years but fail rapidly in an industrial application with steam exposure. For many aerospace applications a service life of 20 years has been used, but with life extension and aging aircraft programs already in effect, this lifespan should be carefully reconsidered. Since the use of composite materials has expanded, potential service lives have grown from just a few years for some sporting goods to 30 to 50 years anticipated for marine and civil applications such as bridge refurbishment.

While moisture exposure typically induces the greatest degradation for most composite materials, the effects on the material of other fluids and solvents must also be assessed, at least to a degree where it is clear that moisture is in fact the most critical factor. In aerospace, the exposure to solvents, fuels, and hydraulic and deicing fluids is (at least) screened for (typically), in addition to performing the hygrothermal studies described here.

Since this is fundamentally an accelerated aging process, there is a real concern about aging performed under conditions so extreme as to change the material state at the end of conditioning from that which would be expected in service. The intent is that after accelerated conditioning for a period of weeks, the state of the coupon or structure closely approximates the condition that would be expected after years of service. If this is not accomplished, the results may be useless, or, worse, misleading. The inferences from the results on what the long-term durability of the material will be must be clearly understood as a form of extrapolation, with the associated uncertainty. Even though each material combination must be treated individually, similar results on closely related materials that have undergone successful testing and field service are frequently used to validate results to some degree.

Several different goals are associated with work in hygrothermal behavior. One is to ensure that the worst-case environmental conditions are being represented when attempting to characterize or qualify a composite material for a specific application. Even if the only moisture conditions to be represented in testing are the two extremes, completely dry and completely saturated, creating data for both conditions for every property is burdensome and almost always unnecessary. The task is to ensure that hygrothermal effects are well represented for the material properties and conditions that will control the success of the application.

Some work is dedicated to greater understanding of the diffusion phenomena as experienced by composite materials, the factors associated, and the effects such as failure modes. Much of this work is of general benefit, even if the application is just characterization of specific materials for specific applications. If the moisture absorption weight gain data from the characterization is analyzed and seen to be normal Fickian diffusion (that is, diffusion that has the same magnitude in all directions), it can provide additional assurance about the stability of the material. While the discovery of non-Fickian diffusion does not necessarily present a problem, it can indicate phenomena such as the collection of moisture at the fiber/matrix interface or in voids. For some applications this may still be acceptable, but for other critical applications this could mean that the long-term durability of the composite material in its intended environment has not been ensured.

Absorbing moisture induces some degree of volumetric expansion, which can induce warping and other structure-performance effects similar to thermal expansion issues, in addition to the fundamental effects on the base properties of the material. While this is not commonly the most critical loading condition, it can be an issue and should be considered, as appropriate for the application.

A great deal of the uncertainty associated with hygrothermal effects is the range of differences present based on the combination of materials that make up the composite. Since the exact formulation of most commercially available composite materials is not public knowledge, making comparisons based on composition may not even be possible. Processing can also affect the hygrothermal response; for example, cure cycle differences result in changes in cure state and quality such as void volume. New processes should also be assessed, at least establishing the worst case condition for the current process for a given material. As a result of this sensitivity, some assessment of hygrothermal behavior must be made for every variant of a composite material. This sensitivity partially explains the wide range of literature values for seemingly identical materials.

As more substantial and critical composite structures have been fielded, the thickness of some is now greater than could conceivably be saturated with moisture, even under continuous worst case environmental exposure for the intended life of the structure. If modeling using the appropriate material parameters can establish this condition, then insisting on saturation for coupon and structural testing may be excessively conservative.

The worst case environmental condition is generally taken as 26 °C (79 °F) with 85% relative humidity and, as such, is used for many aerospace composite applications. The condition of the composite material after exposure to 20 years at 26 °C (79 °F) and 85% relative humidity is what is being attempted to be reproduced in the lab in one to two orders of magnitude less time. If exposure to conditions such as engine temperatures or other industrial environments is anticipated, then they may be more critical than the ambient environmental exposure.

Most composite structure is eventually assembled into larger structures, requiring either mechanical fasteners or adhesive bonding. The effects of moisture on mechanically fastened joints can be assessed in the same manner as other mechanical property tests. Adhesives used are subject to most of the same hygrothermal issues as discussed for composite materials, although glass transition temperature requirements may be less stringent.

Resins or Matrices

Since the majority of the moisture is typically absorbed by the resin, the type of resin used as a matrix can obviously have a substantial effect on the response of the composite. Epoxies are the most common thermosetting-matrix materials for aerospace, but moisture absorption and effects on properties can vary by an order of magnitude. Other thermosetting matrices include polyimides, polyester, and vinyl esters. High-performance thermoplastic matrices such as polyether etherketone (PEEK) are typically used for continuous fiber composites and have low moisture absorption properties, while others such as nylon used for discontinuous fiber composites exhibit fairly high moisture absorption.

Various materials are used to modify the base resin to improve properties such as toughness. These can be materials such as rubber, thermoplastic, or polyurethane and can substantially change the hygrothermal behavior with the same basic matrix and fiber. A variety of curing agents and catalysts are used, modifying the chemistry of the final matrix and its response.

Reinforcements

The type of reinforcement can substantially change the hygrothermal behavior. Carbon fibers are generally considered to be unaffected by most moisture conditions, and the interface between the fiber and resin is usually relatively stable. While the glass fiber itself is largely unaffected by moisture, surface effects can be substantial. Adhesion of the resin to the glass fiber is critical, and is affected by the sizes, finishes, and binders applied. The surface of the fiber can also be attacked. Aramid fibers are unusual in that they can absorb a higher weight percentage of moisture than the matrix and, as such, should be scrutinized as much as the resin. Hybrid forms, using, for example, carbon and glass reinforcements, should be evaluated individually and at least checked in the hybrid form.

The form of the reinforcement can have some influence on hygrothermal behavior. If the fiber/resin interface is compromised and moisture collects, then continuous fibers allow an easier path for progression than discontinuous fibers. In the same manner, unidirectional material may react slightly differently than fabric or braided forms, although some of this difference may be due to the different finishes applied. In the same manner, the stacking sequence can have some influence of the damage progression. Random mats or preforms that have a substantial quantity of binder applied can absorb more moisture.

The surface treatments, coupling agents, sizes, finishes and binders applied to the surface of fibers used to improve resin adhesion and handling can critically affect hygrothermal performance and should be carefully selected and documented.

Processing

Fabrication processing can affect the hygrothermal behavior of composites, primarily as a function of the resulting quality of the completed composite. Oven cures have become more common with cost considerations, but with only vacuum pressure for consolidation, void volume typically increases. Collection of liquid moisture in voids is a common reason for the appearance of non-Fickian diffusion from weight gain data. Resin content and fiber volume differences also change absolute weights, since the resin is typically the primary component absorbing moisture.

Regardless of the fabrication process, every thermosetting composite material undergoes some sort of time-and-temperature cure cycle profile where the chemical changes such as chain extension and crosslinking occur. The pressure applied during the cure cycle can be set aside for this discussion, for while the pressure applied during cure can result in physical changes such as consolidation or development of voids, for common composite-cure processes, it has a negligible effect on the chemical changes occurring during cure.

Since the cure cycle is where chemical changes are occurring, differences in cure cycles can result in differences in the chemical end-state for the resin matrix. While some nominal degree of variation in cure cycles is unavoidable and typically negligible, substantial differences can significantly influence many composite responses, including hygrothermal behavior. A simple case is the result of unreacted curing agent being trapped in the matrix. Since curing agents can be hygroscopic, small changes in the quantity of residual curing agent can result in relatively large differences in the amount of moisture absorbed by the resin. Other chemical changes in parameters such as molecular weight and cross-link density can also occur, with similar results.

The final dwell in a cure cycle is commonly 2 h at 120 to 180 °C (250 to 350 °F) for many epoxies. While there can be some effects from the time and temperature profile leading up to the final dwell, called path dependence, the profile usually becomes critical only with extreme deviations or specific materials. Many changes in composite performance can be attributed to changes in the final dwell time and temperature, including hygrothermal behavior such as moisture weight gain.

The percent weight gain of moisture as a function of cure-cycle final dwell time and temperature for a 120 °C (250 °F) curing glass/epoxy material can be seen in Fig. 1. This response surface shows that the material absorbs the most moisture with a cure cycle of about 110 °C (230 °F) for about an hour. This would be a strong indication of an undercure resulting from use of this dwell, although the material may still be acceptable for some applications. With relatively small increases in time and/or temperature for the final dwell, the moisture absorption can be substantially reduced. More dramatic reduction in moisture absorption with substantially higher time or temperature must be weighed against other chemical and mechanical changes that are also a function of cure, such as those seen in Fig. 2 for elevated-temperature wet compression strength.

Diffusion

Moisture absorption for composite materials is primarily a diffusion-based process. Diffusion

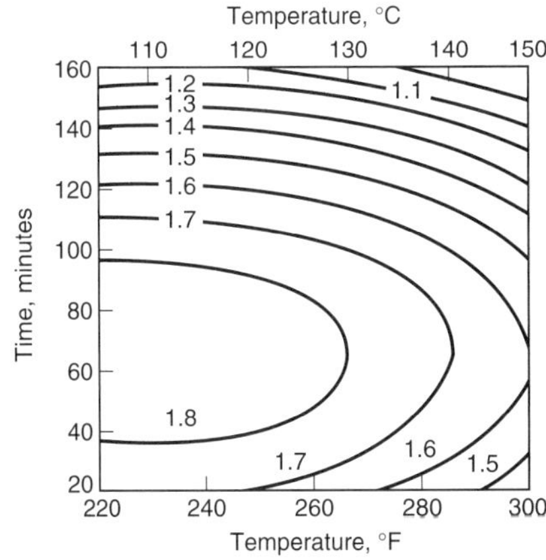

Fig. 1 Moisture absorption at saturation (weight percent) as a function of cure cycle final dwell time and temperature (120 °C, or 250 °F, cure glass/epoxy)

is classically described as Fickian. For some materials a time effect has been noted, and modified Fickian models have been proposed in response. Characterization of the diffusion-based process of moisture absorption has been the focus of a great deal of work. Some work is concerned with achieving saturation, typically a worst-case moisture exposure, for material characterization. When the moisture absorption, seen as weight gain, slows to a predetermined level, the coupon or part is ready for testing.

Even if the aim of a particular project is just to assure saturation of particular parts or coupons, a more basic understanding can assist in determining the time frame necessary to achieve the saturation desired and confirm assumptions made about the moisture absorption of the material. This ability becomes critical for thicker structure where saturation within the service life is not anticipated.

Two primary factors govern diffusion behavior: the rate at which the moisture is absorbed and the final saturation level achieved. The rate at which moisture absorption occurs is typically a function of the temperature to which the material is exposed, not the moisture level or relative humidity exposure. The saturation moisture absorption achieved after long exposure to the temperature and humidity condition is usually governed by the moisture level or relative humidity to which the material is exposed. Thus the temperature and moisture level work together to determine the rate and ultimate quantity of moisture absorbed by the material.

Many examples of composite materials demonstrating non-Fickian behavior have been reported in the literature. While this behavior may not exclude a material for a particular application, it frequently indicates non-diffusion processes of interest. The diffusion process describes the physical absorption of moisture in a material. If other processes occur in parallel, they can change the moisture absorption process and the associated weight gain. If only diffusion is assumed to be occurring, the weight gain profile could appear non-Fickian. An example of Fickian weight gain can be seen in Fig. 3, along with several non-Fickian profiles.

Since diffusion only covers the physical absorption of moisture, if the material has locations for liquid moisture to collect, a dual mechanism is in place. One common feature that allows the collection of liquid moisture in the laminate is voids or porosity. Another is failure of the bond between the fiber and resin, allowing collection of fluid at this interface. Chemical changes to the resin such as hydrolysis can also change the moisture absorption.

One frequent cause of non-Fickian behavior is use of a conditioning temperature near or exceeding the glass-transition temperature, T_g of the resin. Many resin and composite properties change substantially and sometimes unpredictably near or exceeding the T_g. Unless the composite is for some reason actually being considered for use in these conditions, the conditioning temperature should almost always be at least 10 to 15 °C (20 to 30 °F) below the T_g anticipated for the composite at the end of conditioning. Epoxies can lose 20 °C (35 °F) in T_g temperature for each 1% of moisture weight gain. The T_g may also be cure dependent, as seen in Fig. 4 for the cure final dwell time and temperature. Exceeding this T_g limit can result in substantially different mechanisms and failure modes and irreversible moisture absorption. Thus the appearance of non-Fickian behavior may actually be an indication of undesired initial or aged conditions for the composite and deserving of further investigation.

Hygrothermal Testing and Conditioning

Separate coupons are typically used to assess fundamental hygrothermal behavior. When they are conditioned alongside mechanical test coupons or even parts to assess moisture absorption, they are termed traveler coupons or travelers. To avoid the coupon configuration from affecting the observed behavior, the traveler should reflect the as-processed material for the other coupons or parts as closely as possible. If coupons are being used just to monitor moisture absorption to saturation, they should reflect the thickest portion of the coupons or parts. If diffusion through the thickness of the structure is anticipated as the primary mode, then the width and length of the coupon should be at least 10 times the thickness. For determination of fundamental hygrothermal properties, a range of coupon thicknesses may be used.

If there were no fiber or interface effects, then neat resin and composite results would be comparable. Since this is rarely completely true, composite samples should be used, although additional samples of neat resin can be used to further discern the nature of the moisture absorption and effects.

To achieve a reference dry state prior to conditioning so the full moisture absorption can be characterized, coupons are first dried until weight losses are negligible. It is critical that this drying- (and subsequent conditioning-) temperature exposure does not further the cure of the resin beyond what will be seen for the fielded structure. As a rule, the drying and conditioning temperature should be at least 10 to 15 °C (20 to 30 °F) below the maximum cure temperature used.

The drying can be performed in a desiccator with or without vacuum or in an oven with or without desiccant or vacuum to speed drying. Commonly 65 °C (150 °F) for at least 48 h is employed. If the traveller coupons are being used just to assure saturation, and have seen the same history as the mechanical coupons or parts they represent, the drying step is frequently omitted.

Exposure to 70 °C (160 °F) at 85 to 95% relative humidity for 30 to 60 days is an informal standard for aerospace application and is a good starting point for evaluation. Determining the conditions of saturation is important. As saturation is approached, the rate of moisture absorption decreases exponentially, and the additional moisture absorbed in reaching full saturation becomes insignificant. Several different metrics are

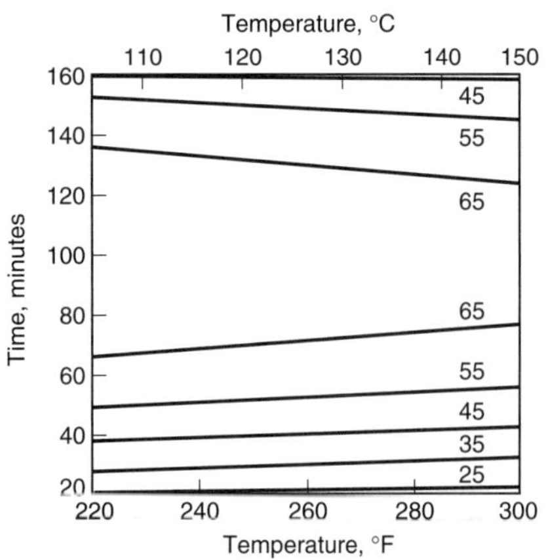

Fig. 2 Elevated temperature wet compression strength (ksi) as a function of cure cycle final dwell time and temperature (120 °C, or 250 °F, cure glass/epoxy)

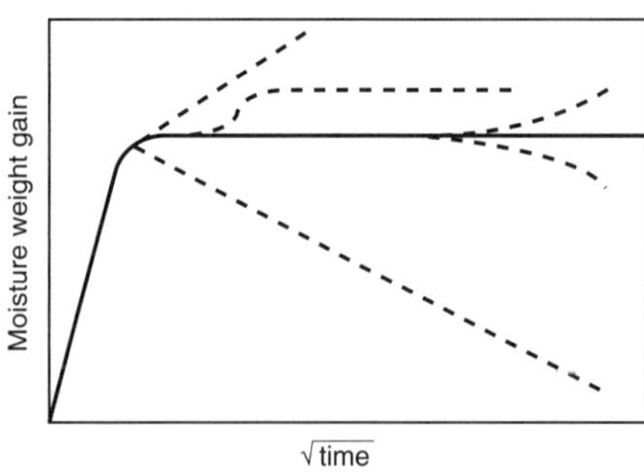

Fig. 3 Fickian (solid line) and common non-Fickian moisture weight gain profiles

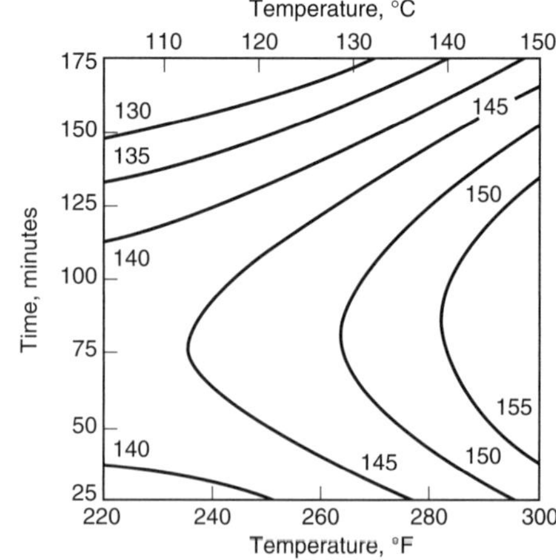

Fig. 4 Glass transition temperature (in degrees Celsius, as determined by differential scanning calorimetry) as a function of cure cycle final dwell time and temperature (120 °C, or 250 °F, cure glass/epoxy)

used, including three consecutive 24 h measurements, each of which represents less than 1 or 2% of the total weight gain. Typically at least three coupons are used, and the moisture loss during weight gain measurement is considered insignificant.

Frequently water immersion is used to speed the moisture absorption. While this may be appropriate, especially for receiving inspection functions, care must be taken to correlate moisture absorption in humid air to immersion. It is common for longer exposures to immersion to create degradation worse than that normally experienced in the field. Immersion in 30 °C (86 °F) water is used to simulate long-term exposures, while immersion from 90 °C (195 °F) to boiling is used for rapid conditioning, such as for receiving inspection of materials. Immersion temperatures of about 60 °C (140 °F) for 14 days or more have been used for conditioning of coupons before material-characterization mechanical testing.

Some have conditioned with exposure to steam up to 150 °C (300 °F), but unless this is representative of actual service, it typically induces excessively conservative degradation. For a given humidity level for most polymer matrices, there is an upper-limit temperature beyond which the degradation extent and mechanism change dramatically.

Coupons that can be fully dried after completion of saturation can provide additional insight on the degradation mechanism(s) at work. If the moisture-absorption weight gain can be completely reversed on drying, then only physical changes are indicated (although it is possible for leaching losses to match moisture weight gain from physically bound or chemically reacted water).

If it cannot be fully reversed, then chemical degradation such as through hydrolysis is indicated. Substantial chemical changes do not provide confidence in the long-term durability of the material or indicate excessively accelerated aging.

Mechanically loading or pressurizing coupons while they are being conditioned has shown to have some influence but is not commonly considered. Finally, "pulse" loading of the moisture has been performed to further accelerate conditioning to saturation. A higher temperature and/or pressure is used for the initial conditioning to encourage the more rapid absorption of moisture. The remainder of the conditioning is then performed at the standard condition. Validated moisture-absorption models can be especially useful when such complex hygrothermal histories are used for conditioning or to represent actual service conditions.

Nondestructive test methods such as pulse-echo ultrasonics have been used to gage the absorption of moisture. Correlation of laboratory results can then be used to gage the condition of the fielded structure. This can also be correlated with visually observable changes in the material, as well as fractographic examination such as that performed in a scanning electron microscope.

Degradation Mechanisms and Failure Modes

An understanding of the degradation mechanisms and failure modes is a critical part of using accelerated aging to predict long-term behavior of the material. Effects can be seen in the fiber, in the matrix, and at the interface or interphase between.

While hygrothermal degradation of the fiber itself is not common for most glass and carbon fiber reinforcement applications, it is characteristic for aramid fibers, which may absorb more moisture than the resin. Degradation of the resin can take several different forms. Physical changes such as plasticization are largely reversible. Chemical changes such as hydrolysis or chain scission are usually more severe and irreversible. Cracks, peeling, and other surface modifications can be experienced, as well as leaching of components such as unreacted curing agent.

The interface between the resin and fiber can be attacked, destroying the fiber bonding and allowing water to collect. Since the collection of liquid water is not a diffusion-based process, this can make the moisture weight gain appear non-Fickian. A distinct phase that has shared characteristics with the fiber bond and the resin can be created in the composite, which can experience different effects.

The ratio of reversible moisture weight loss by drying after saturation to total moisture weight absorption at saturation can be used as a rough measure of the ratio of reversible to irreversible mechanisms. This can be somewhat misleading if there are competing mechanisms, such as leaching of material for weight loss with permanent weight gain from moisture captured in a chemical degradation mechanism.

A final mechanism is the swelling and volumetric stress that can be developed with moisture absorption. While typically only a significant factor for relatively thick coupons and some parts, it can generally be treated analytically in the same manner as thermal- and cure- induced volumetric changes and stresses.

Properties

The effect of moisture absorption can be negligible or dominate the application of the material. Hygrothermal effects can range from damping characteristic improvements, strength degradations, and little change to moduli. If effects are present, lesser differences are usually seen on fiber-dominated properties versus resin-dominated properties. Exceptions occur when the interface between the fiber and resin is attacked, preventing load transfer.

Physical and chemical effects to the composite have already been discussed in some detail, so mechanical property effects are primarily discussed here. The effect of hygrothermal conditioning can be a function of not just the property but also a function of loading conditions and rates. Thermal spike and freeze/thaw cycles have been used as part of the conditioning process to represent field usage. Changes in toughening mechanisms can occur, leading to changes in failure modes from tough to brittle. Fatigue, creep and impact properties can also be adversely affected. In some cases, the variability of a particular property will be affected, with or without changes to the mean value. Many mechanical property effects will be highly correlated. In many cases, it is not necessary to exactly characterize the effect but only to establish that for this particular property, it is not a worst case condition.

A comparison of wet- and dry-test results for a glass/epoxy material can be seen in Fig. 5. For compression and shear, the moisture exposure induces some level of reduced strength regardless of temperature. For tensile strength, a reduction is seen at elevated temperature, but there is no effect at room temperature. At cold temperatures the dry condition appears to be more critical than the wet condition. As is frequently

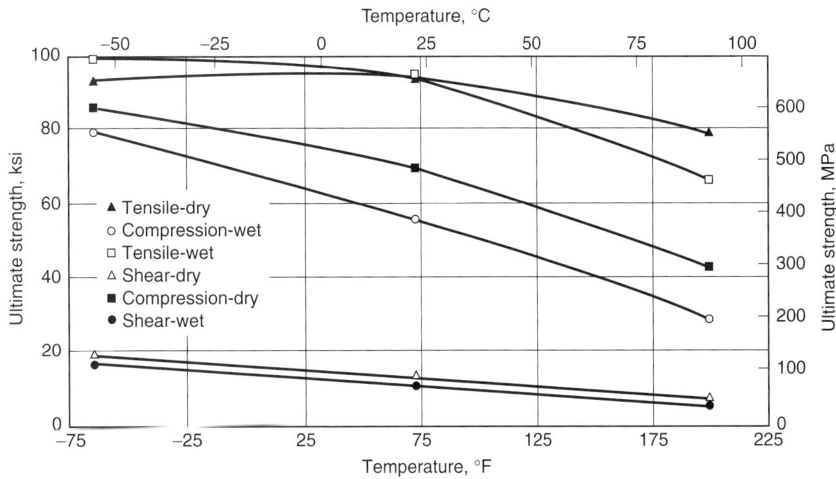

Fig. 5 Mechanical properties for dry and moisture saturated glass/epoxy material as a function of test temperature

seen for many materials and applications, hot/wet is the most critical condition for each of the properties shown.

There is an obvious test-temperature dependence on the extent of the hygrothermal effect. In addition, drying of the coupon during test can have a substantial effect on the results in a nonconservative manner. Unsteady-state temperature and moisture conditions are being experienced while the coupon is being heated to the test temperature. Weighing the coupons immediately after test and using a model to determine the actual moisture state at the time of failure can be useful.

SELECTED REFERENCES

- R.D. Adams, and M.M. Singh, The Dynamic Properties of Fibre-Reinforced Polymers Exposed to Hot, Wet Conditions, *Compos. Sci. Technol.*, Vol 56, 1996, p 977–997
- M. Akay, S. Kong Ah Mun, and A. Stanley, Influence of Moisture on the Thermal and Mechanical Properties of Autoclaved and Oven-Cured Kevlar-49/Epoxy Laminates, *Compos. Sci. Technol.*, Vol 57, 1997, p 565–571
- D.R. Askins, "Characterization of EA9396 Epoxy Resin for Composite Repair Application," WL-TR-92-4060, National Technical Information Service, Oct 1991
- L.E. Asp, The Effects of Moisture and Temperature on the Interlaminar Delamination Toughness of a Carbon/Epoxy Composite, *Compos. Sci. Technol.*, Vol 58, 1998, p 967–977
- S.E. Buck, D.W. Lischer, and Sia Nemat-Nasser, The Durability of E-Glass/Vinyl Ester Composite Materials Subjected to Environmental Conditioning and Sustained Loading, *J. Compos. Mater.*," Vol 32 (No. 9), 1998, p 874–892
- C. Cappelletti, A. Rivolta, and G. Zaffaroni, Environmental Effects on Mechanical Properties of Thick Composite Structural Elements, *J. Compos. Technol. Res.*, Vol 17 (No. 2), April 1995, p 107–114
- D. Choqueuse, P. Davies, F. Mazeas, and R. Baizeua, Aging of Composites in Water: Comparison of Five Materials in Terms of Absorption Kinetics and Evolution of Mechanical Properties, *High Temperature and Environmental Effects on Polymeric Composites*, Vol 2, ASTM STP 1302, T.S. Gates and A.H. Zureick, Ed., ASTM, 1997, p 73–96
- P.J.C. Chou, D. Ding, and W.H. Chen, Damping of Moisture-Absorbed Composite Rackets, *J. Reinf. Plast. Compos.*, Vol 19 (No. 11), 2000, p 848–862
- D.M. Cise, and R.S. Lakes, Moisture Ingression in Honeycomb Core Sandwich Panels: Directional Aspects, *J. Compos. Mater.*, Vol 31 (No. 22), 1997, p 2249–2263
- I. Ghorbel, and P. Spiteri, Durability of Closed-End Pressurized GRP Pipes under Hygrothermal Conditions, Part I: Monotonic Tests, *J. Compos. Mater.*, Vol 30 (No. 14), 1996, p 1562–1580
- I. Ghorbel, Durability of Closed-End Pressurized GRP Filament Wound Pipes under Hygrothermal Aging Conditions. Part II: Creep Tests, *J. Compos. Mater.*, Vol 30 (No. 14), 1996, p 1581–1595
- J.M. Hale, A.G. Gibson, and S.D. Speake, Tensile Strength Testing of GRP Pipes at Elevated Temperatures in Aggressive Offshore Environments, *J. Compos. Mater.*, Vol 32 (No. 10), 1998, p 969–986
- Y. Jayet, R. Gaertner, P. Guy, R. Vassoille, and D. Zellouf, Application of Ultrasonic Spectroscopy for Hydrolytic Damage Detection in GRFC: Correlations with Mechanical Tests and Microscopic Observations, *J. Compos. Mater.*, Vol 34 (No. 16), 2000, p 1356–1368
- M.L. Karasek, L.H. Strait, M.F. Amateau, and J.P. Runt, Effect of Temperature and Moisture on the Impact Behavior of Graphite/Epoxy Composites: Part I: Impact Energy Absorption, *J. Compos. Technol. Res.*, Vol 17 (No. 1), Jan 1995, p 3–10
- M.L Karasek, L.H. Strait, M.F. Amateau, and J.P. Runt, Effect of Temperature and Moisture on the Impact Behavior of Graphite/Epoxy Composites: Part II: Impact Damage, *J. Compos. Technol. Res.*, Vol 17 (No. 1), Jan 1995, p 11–16
- W.J. Liou, Effects of Moisture Content on the Creep Behavior of Nylon-6 Thermoplastic Composites, *J. Reinf. Plast. Compos.*, Vol 17 (No. 01), 1998, p 39–50
- Z.A. Mohd Ishak, U.S. Ishiaku, and J. Karger-Kocsis, Hygrothermal Aging and Fracture Behavior of Short-Glass-Fiber-Reinforced Rubber-Toughened Poly(butylene terephthalate) Composites, *Compos. Sci. Technol.*, Vol 60, 2000, p 803–815
- T. Morii, I. Nobuo, K. Kiyosumi, and H. Hamada, Weight-Change Analysis of the Interphase in Hygrothermally Aged FRP: Considerations of Debonding, *Compos. Sci. Technol.*, Vol 57, 1997, p 985–990
- A.K. Mukhopadhyay and R.L. Sierakowski, On the Thermoelastic and Hygrometric Response of Sandwich Beams with Laminate Facings and Honeycomb Cores, Part IV: A Dynamic Theory, *J. Compos. Mater.*, Vol 34 (No. 3), 2000, p 174–198
- A. Nakai, S. Ikegaki, H. Hamada, and N. Takeda, Degradation of Braided Composites in Hot Water, *Compos. Sci. Technol.*, Vol 60, 2000, p 325–331
- O.O. Ochoa and G.R. Ross, Hybrid Composites: Models and Tests for Environmental Aging, *J. Reinf. Plast. Compos.*, Vol 17 (No. 9), 1998, p 787–799
- H. Parvatareddy, A. Pasricha, D.A. Dillard, B. Holmes, and J.G. Dillard, High Temperature and Environmental Effects on the Durability of Ti-6Al-4V/FM5 Adhesive Bonded System, *High Temperature and Environmental Effects on Polymeric Composites,* Vol 2, ASTM STP 1302, T.S. Gates and A.H. Zureick, Ed., ASTM, 1997, p 149–174
- *Polymer Matrix Composites*, Vol 1 and 3, MIL-HDBK-17, DODSSP, Naval Publications and Forms Center, Philadelphia, PA
- B.A. Pratt, and W.L. Bradley, Effect of Moisture on the Interfacial Shear Strength: A Study Using the Single Fiber Fragmentation Test, *High Temperature and Environmental Effects on Polymeric Composites,* Vol 2, ASTM STP 1302, T.S. Gates and A.H. Zureick, Ed., ASTM, 1997, p 64–72
- L. Prian, R. Pollard, R. Shan, C.W. Mastropietro, T.R. Gentry, L.C. Bank, and A. Barkatt, Use of Thermogravimetric Analysis to Develop Accelerated Test Methods to Investigate Long-Term Environmental Effects on Fiber-Reinforced Plastics," *High Temperature and Environmental Effects on Polymeric Composites,* Vol 2, ASTM STP 1302, T.S. Gates and A.H. Zureick, Ed., ASTM, 1997, p 206–222
- S. Roy, Modeling of Anomalous Moisture Diffusion in Polymer Composites: A Finite Element Approach, *J. Compos. Mater.*, Vol 33 (No. 14), 1999, p 1318–1343
- T. Shimokawa, Y. Hamaguchi, and H. Katoh, Effect of Moisture Absorption on Hot/Wet Compressive Strength of T800H/PMR-15 Carbon/Polyimide, *J. Compos. Mater.*, Vol 33 (No. 18), 1999, p 1685–1697
- G.C. Sih, J.G. Michopoulos, and S.C. Chou, Ed., *Hygrothermoelasticity*, Martinus Nijhoff Publishers, Dordrecht, The Netherlands, 1986
- G.S. Springer Ed., *Environmental Effects on Composite Materials*, Technomic Publishing Co., Westport, CT, 1981
- G.S. Springer Ed., *Environmental Effects on Composite Materials,* Vol 2, Technomic Publishing Co. Inc., 1984
- S. Srihari, and R.M.V.G.K. Rao, Hygrothermal Characterization and Diffusion Studies on Carbon/Epoxy Composites, *J. Reinf. Plast. Compos.*, Vol 18 (No. 10), 1999, p 921–930
- S. Srihari and R.M.V.G.K. Rao, Hygrothermal Characterization and Diffusion Studies on Glass-Epoxy Composites, *J. Reinf. Plast. Compos.* Vol 18 (No. 10), 1999, p 942–953
- "Standard Practice for Conditioning Plastics for Testing," ASTM D 618, *ASTM Standards*, Vol 08.01, ASTM
- "Standard Test Method for Moisture Absorption Properties and Equilibrium Conditioning of Polymer Matrix Composite Materials," ASTM D 5229, *ASTM Standards*, Vol 15.03, ASTM
- M. Todo, T. Nakamura, and K. Takahashi, Effects of Moisture Absorption on the Dynamic Interlaminar Fracture Toughness of Carbon/Epoxy Composites, *J. Compos. Mater.*, Vol 34 (No. 8), 2000, p 630–648
- T.K. Tsotsis and S.M. Lee, Long-Term Durability of Carbon- and Glass-Epoxy Composite Materials in Wet Environments, *J.*

Reinf. Plast. Compos., Vol 16 (No. 17), 1997, p 1609–1621

- P.C. Upadhyay and J.S. Lyons, Effect of Hygrothermal Environment on the Bending of PMC Laminates under Large Deflection, *J. Reinf. Plast. Compos.*, Vol 19 (No. 06), 2000, p 465–491
- P.C. Upadhyay and J.S. Lyons, Hygrothermal Effect on the Large Deflection Bending of Asymmetric PMC Laminates, *J. Reinf. Plast. Compos.*, Vol 19 (No. 14), 2000, p 1094–1111
- M.R. VanLandingham, R.F. Eduljee, and J.W. Gillespie, Jr., The Effects of Moisture on the Material Properties and Behavior of Thermoplastic Polyimide Composites, *High Temperature and Environmental Effects on Polymeric Composites*, Vol 2, ASTM STP 1302, T.S. Gates and A.H. Zureick, Ed., ASTM, 1997, p 50–63
- E. Vauthier, J.C. Abry, T. Bailliez, and A. Chateauminois, Interactions Between Hygrothermal Aging and Fatigue Damage in Unidirectional Glass/Epoxy Composites, *Compos. Sci. Technol.*, Vol 58, 1998, p 687–692
- F.D. Wall, S.R. Taylor, and G.L. Cahen, The Simulation and Detection of Electrochemical Damage in BMI/Graphite Fiber Composites Using Electrochemical Impedance Spectroscopy, *High Temperature and Environmental Effects on Polymeric Composites*, ASTM STP 1174, C.E. Harris and T.S. Gates, Ed., ASTM, 1993, p 95–113
- J. Wang, D. Kelly, and W. Hillier, Finite Element Analysis of Temperature Induced Stresses and Deformations of Polymer Composite Components, *J. Compos. Mater.*, Vol 34 (No. 17), 2000, p 1456–1471
- H.L. Yeh and H.Y. Yeh, The Variation in Through-Thickness Hygrothermal Expansion Coefficients of Laminate Composites, *J. Compos. Mater.*, Vol 34 (No. 14), 2000, p 1200–1215
- G. Zaffaroni, Two-Dimensional Moisture Diffusion in Hybrid Composite Components, *High Temperature and Environmental Effects on Polymeric Composites*, Vol 2, ASTM STP 1302, T.S. Gates and A.H. Zureick, Ed., ASTM, 1997, p 97–109
- Y. Zhong and J. Zhou, Study of Thermal and Hygrothermal Behaviors of Glass/Vinyl Ester Composites, *J. Reinf. Plast. Compos.*, Vol 18 (No. 17), 1999, p 1619–1629
- J. Zhou and J.P. Lucas, The Effects of a Water Environment on Anomalous Absorption Behavior in Graphite/Epoxy Composites, *Compos. Sci. Technol.*, Vol 53, 1995, p 57–64

Fatigue and Life Prediction

Jeffrey R. Schaff, United Technologies Research Center

DURABILITY AND DAMAGE TOLERANCE are significant concerns for safety and product liability in the design of composite structures. This is particularly true for components that experience dynamic loading, such as rotorcraft blades, propellers, turbine blades, and so on. Although advancements have been made in composite life prediction methods, these methods are not sufficiently mature to predict the fatigue life of full-scale components with only coupon fatigue data. As a result, components are largely designed and certified through a series of tests that are supported by analysis. In practice, the cost and risk of designing and certifying a robust structure can be significantly reduced based on a building-block approach, where the design is validated in coupon and sub-component through full component testing. The building-block approach is discussed in the article "Overview of Testing and Certification" in this Volume. Simplifying analyses and guidelines are used in a supporting role to address fatigue in the design and development process in meeting specific durability and damage tolerance requirements.

Fatigue is defined as the degradation of the integrity of a material as a result of external conditions that vary with time. These external conditions are usually in the form of a fluctuating mechanical load and stress, but can also be in other forms, such as a thermally induced cyclic stress or cyclic exposure to moisture. The integrity of the material is commonly measured in terms of mechanical properties, such as stiffness and strength. The loss in stiffness of a material may create an instability in a structural component, and loss in strength is directly associated with the failure of a component. Such a failure can occur at a small fraction of the static strength of a material. In this sense, fatigue in composite materials is observed through accumulation of damage that initiates and progresses during cyclic loading and exposure to environment. The cyclic loading causes damage, reducing the strength until the material can no longer sustain even the service loading, that is, the load for which the material was designed.

In comparison with metals, advanced composites exhibit superior fatigue performance due to their high fatigue limit and resistance to corrosion. Fatigue damage in composite materials is very complex, due to several damage mechanisms occurring at many locations throughout a laminate. Damage is observed in a series of mechanisms, such as matrix cracking, fiber fracture, longitudinal cracking, crack coupling, and delamination growth. As a result of this damage, composite components generally do not fail due to a single, large macrocrack (as do metals), but rather fail due to a series of interdependent damage events.

In the design of composite structures for durability and damage tolerance, the primary concerns are out-of-plane failures, such as delamination, material degradation associated with environment, stability under compression loading, large degree of scatter in fatigue life, and bearing failure of joints. This article offers introductory discussion on fatigue damage process, methodologies assessing fatigue behavior, and life prediction models. For detailed discussions of fatigue and life prediction of composite materials, the reader is encouraged to refer to Ref 1 to 3.

Fatigue Damage

Knowledge of the individual damage mechanisms and their progression is key to understanding the fatigue behavior of composite materials. For illustration purposes, the damage mechanisms are introduced for a quasi-isotropic laminate under tension-compression fatigue loading. For a more detailed discussion of damage process, see Ref 1. Damage is defined by several localized mechanisms. Further complicating matters, these damage mechanisms are abundant, that is, they occur at many unpredictable locations throughout the laminate. There are five major damage mechanisms: matrix cracking, fiber breaking, crack coupling, delamination initiation, and delamination growth. Figure 1 illus-

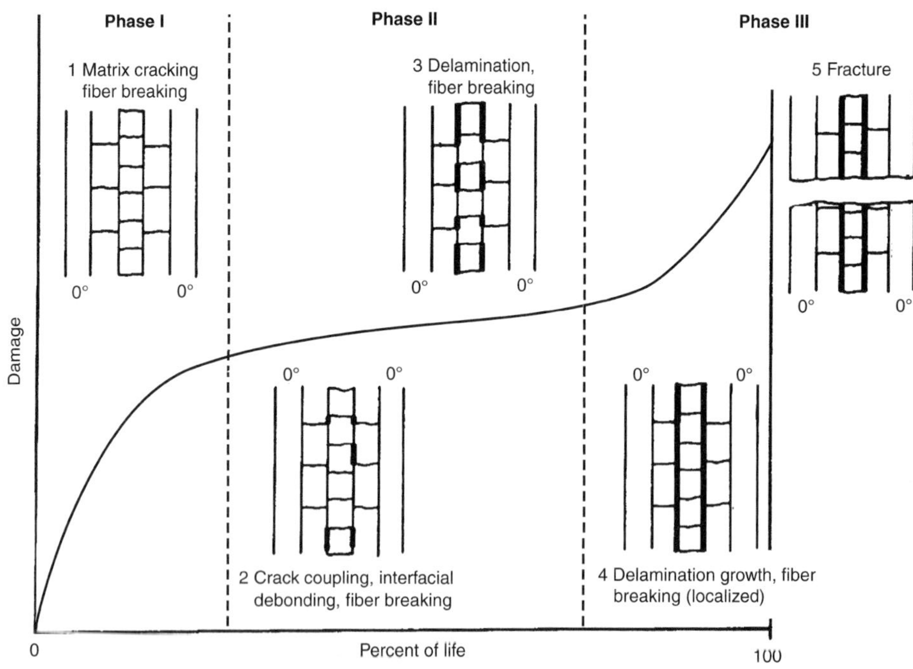

Fig. 1 Three phases of fatigue damage represented on a damage curve. Phase I, matrix cracking; Phase II, fiber fracture, crack coupling, and start of delamination; Phase III, delamination growth and final fracture. Five damage mechanisms are illustrated. Adapted from Reifsnider (Ref 1)

trates the damage state versus percent of life for the three phases of damage progression.

Phase I: Matrix Cracking. In the first phase, the damage consists primarily of matrix cracks. Overall, the damage in this phase is relatively small and occurs in the first 10 to 25% of life (Ref 4). The loss in stiffness is typically less than 10% of the original stiffness, and the strength loss is negligible. However, future damage events are strongly dependent on matrix cracking, which initiates during the first phase. Matrix cracks grow from flaw sites continuously distributed throughout the laminate. As the fatigue loads fluctuate, matrix cracks develop in the off-axis 45° and 90° plies. These matrix cracks are more likely to initiate under tensile loads and will occur first in the 90° plies. Figure 2 shows the crack pattern in a $[0°/90°/\pm45°]_s$. The matrix crack runs through the thickness of the 90° plies and terminates at the 0° plies. Measurement of matrix cracks in controlled fatigue experiments suggests the crack density reaches a saturation state that can be described by the ply thickness and material properties (Ref 5–7).

Phase II: Fiber Fracture, Crack Coupling, and Delamination Initiation. The second phase consists primarily of fiber fracture, local debonding, and delamination initiation, and occurs over the next 70 to 80% of the life of the laminate. Damage develops at a slower rate than in Phase I. As the load increases, stress concentrations develop at the intersection of the matrix cracks and the 0° fibers where these cracks are blunted. These stress concentrations cause fibers to fracture in the adjacent plies. Large tensile stresses located at the tip of the matrix cracks induce longitudinal cracks in the direction of the 0° fibers and perpendicular to the matrix cracks. This damage mechanism is called crack coupling and includes the combination of matrix cracks and longitudinal cracks. Crack coupling is illustrated in Fig. 3 using a cross-ply laminate that has been subjected to a fatigue loading. In this figure, transverse matrix cracks and longitudinal cracks are visible. In the later stages of Phase II, delamination initiation becomes the dominant damage mechanism. Strong interlaminar stresses develop at the intersection of matrix cracks and longitudinal cracks, creating a favorable situation for delamination initiation.

Phase III: Delamination Growth and Fracture. In the final phase of fatigue damage, internal stresses cause the damage mechanisms to increase in intensity. The longitudinal cracks grow, thereby isolating the 0° fibers. Also, the delaminations continue to grow between ply interfaces. Delaminations separate the main laminate into a series of sublaminates. In this phase, a rapid decay of stiffness has been experimentally observed (Ref 8). Eventually, the strength of the laminate is reduced enough to cause catastrophic failure. Note that compression fatigue loads may accelerate the delamination growth, due to buckling of the sublaminates.

Fatigue Methodologies

As with metals, there are two classical approaches for design and analysis of fatigue-loaded composite components: safe life and damage tolerance. The damage tolerance approach assumes that all engineering components contain flaws. These flaws are considered allowable if the defects, or defect growth, do not affect structural performance. Defect growth is predicted using empirical crack growth laws and linear elastic fracture mechanics (Ref 9). The safe life or fatigue life technique involves characterization of the total fatigue life to failure in terms of cyclic stress or strain range. In this technique, engineering components are designed for a certain life-based on empirical stress (or strain) versus life (*S-N*) curves and on cumulative damage growth laws (Ref 9). A variation of these approaches, sometimes referred to as enhanced safe life, characterizes *S-N* relationships where the test specimens purposely contain potential manufacturing defects and in-service damage. The best source of current practices on durability and damage tolerance is MIL-HDBK-17, Volume 3 (Ref 3).

Safe Life and *S-N* Relationships. The *S-N* curve was first implemented by Wohler in the 1860s to understand the effect of stress on the fatigue life of railroad axles. The *S-N* curve quantifies the relationships between fatigue life and applied stress amplitude. The curve is developed using constant stress amplitude fatigue tests at several stress levels. Each *S-N* curve represents one loading type, as defined by its stress ratio, $R = \sigma_{min}/\sigma_{max}$, where σ_{min} and σ_{max} are the minimum and maximum stress, respectively. In the safe life approach, the *S-N* relation is used in design to establish a maximum allowable stress (or strain) and/or to predict statistically based minimum fatigue life with a cumulative damage fatigue model. There are significant shortcomings of the safe life approach. First, the damage mechanisms and damage processes of Fig. 1 are combined into a single, phenomenological damage parameter. Furthermore, the structural composite produces a multiaxis stress state due to its anisotropy and multiaxis loading,

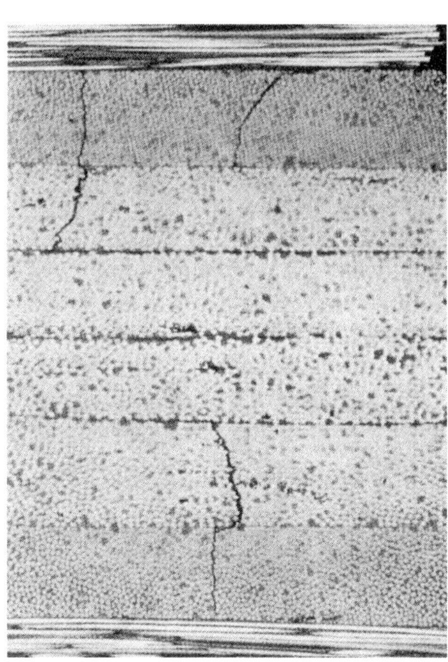

Fig. 2 Micrograph showing crack pattern in matrix of $[0°/90°/\pm45°]_s$ graphite/epoxy laminate under a static load of 483 MPa (70 ksi). Cracks in 90° plies have linked to those in +45° plies, but have not propagated to the 0° plies.

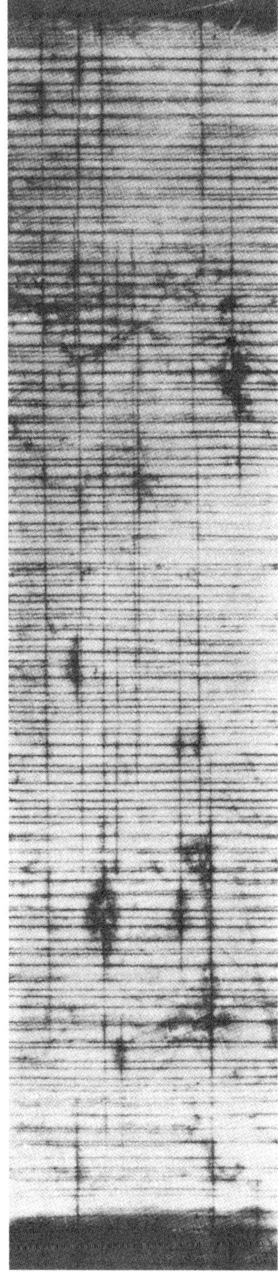

Fig. 3 Radiograph of graphite/epoxy laminate using image-enhancing penetrant to reveal transverse and longitudinal cracking and local delaminations

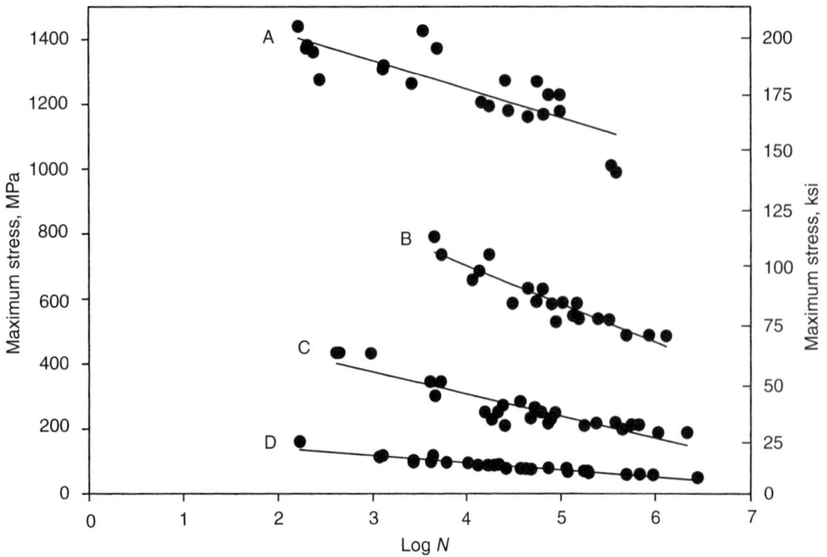

Fig. 4 *S-N* curves for T300/934 graphite/epoxy laminates. Log life in cycles, *N*, vs. maximum load. Loading is equal tension-compression, $R = -1.0$. Curves are A, unidirectional $[0°]_{16}$; B, cross-ply $[0°/90°]_{4s}$; C, quasi-isotropic $[0°/\pm45°/90°]_{2s}$; D, angle-ply $[\pm45°]_{4s}$. Adapted from Ref 10

whereas the *S-N* relationships are indicative of a simplified stress state, especially for unidirectional coupons. Thus, test results obtained from coupons cannot easily be directly applied to complex structures, due to differences in manufacturing, loading, environment, and damage states. However, even with these limitations, well-planned *S-N* experiments can be very useful for studying many variables in design.

A typical *S-N* curve is graphically represented in Fig. 4 for a series of T300/934 graphite/epoxy laminates under tension-compression loading. The influence of composite lay-up can be inferred from inspection of Fig. 4 by comparison of the fatigue behavior for unidirectional $[0]_{16}$, cross-ply $[0/90]_{4s}$, angle-ply $[\pm45°]_{4s}$, and quasi-isotropic $[0°/\pm45°/90°]_{2s}$ laminates. Although some correlation has been made between unidirectional fatigue behavior and that of multidirectional laminates, it is best to characterize laminates of interest rather than infer *S-N* curves from unidirectional data. This is in part due to the acceleration of damage associated with off-axis matrix cracking and crack coupling. Compared with metals, the curves of the composite offer relatively high fatigue threshold, and the slope is relatively low due to insensitivity of the graphite fiber to fatigue. For practical laminates, the slope of the *S-N* curve tends to increase, becoming less negative as the percentage of off-axis plies increases (Ref 11).

The effect of loading can be determined upon comparison of *S-N* curves for stress ratios, *R*, reflecting tension-tension, compression-compression, and tension-compression loading. Study of fatigue data consistently suggests that tension-compression loading is the most severe, followed by compression-compression and tension-tension (Ref 12–14). A master diagram is a graphical means of simultaneously presenting fatigue lives for many stress ratios. In a master diagram, the stress amplitude, $\sigma_{amp} = (\sigma_{max} - \sigma_{min})/2$, is plotted as the ordinate, and the mean stress, $\sigma_m = (\sigma_{max} + \sigma_{min})/2$, is plotted as the abscissa. Stress ratio is introduced through lines of constant stress ratio, R ($R = \sigma_{min}/\sigma_{max}$). These stress ratio lines have a slope of $(1-R)/(1+R)$ and radiate from the origin. These lines are separated into four distinct load types: tension-tension (T-T), tension-dominated tension-compression (T-C), compression-dominated tension-compression (C-T), and compression-compression (C-C). Figure 5 illustrates the master diagram for T300/5308 $[0°/45°/90°/-45°]_{2s}$ laminates.

For a case where the stress was cyclic and varied between 400 MPa (58 ksi) tension and compression, the mean stress is 0. The stress ratio (*R*) is –1. The family of all cases of cyclic load-

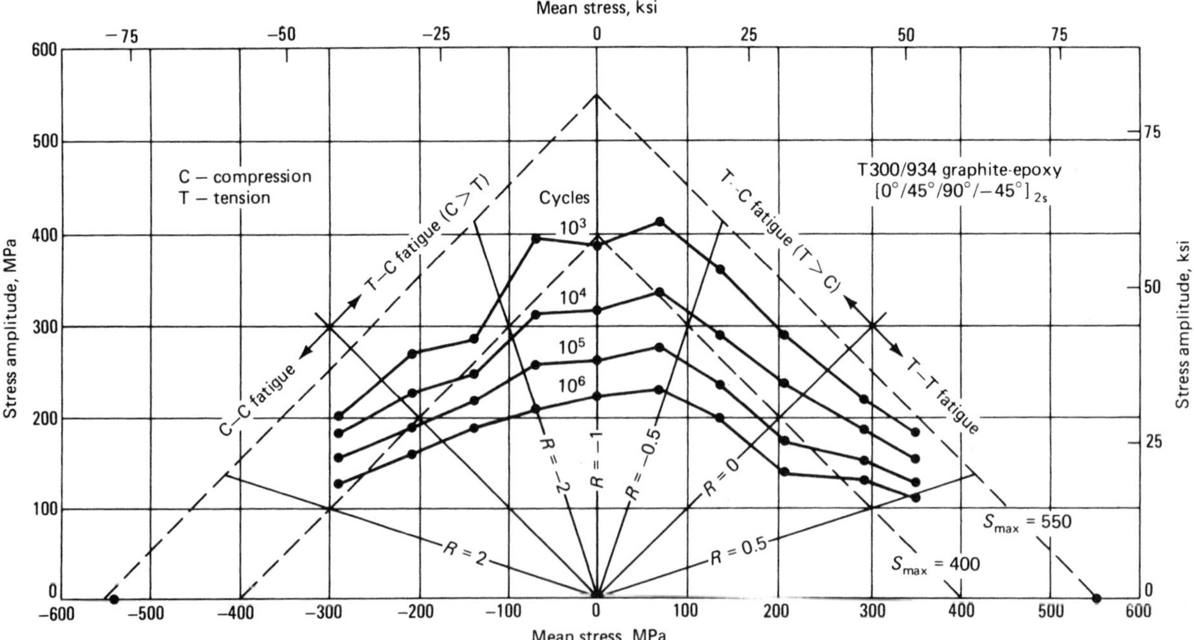

Fig. 5 Master diagram for $[0°/+45°/90°/-45°]_{2s}$, T300/5208 graphite/carbon quasi-isotropic laminate. Maximum stress, S_{max}, are dotted lines. Stress amplitude, $S_{amp} = (S_{max}-S_{min})/2$, vs. mean stress, $S_m = (S_{max} + S_{min})/2$. $R = S_{min}/S_{max}$

ing where the compression stress equals the tensile stress would fall on the vertical axis, where $R = -1$ and the mean stress would be 0. Cases where the tensile load is greater than the compressive load fall to the right of this line, as do pure tensile loads. More compressive loads and pure compressive loads fall to the left. Note the dotted lines indicating the maximum stress ($S_{max} = \sigma_{max}$) on the master diagram.

Recall that a primary concern in the fatigue of composites is delamination. However, the *S-N* data of Fig. 4 and 5 represent in-plane axial loading and provide little use in characterizing interlaminar failure. Thus, it is prudent to develop *S-N* relationships between interlaminar stresses and interlaminar failure. Experience has shown that three- or four-point short beam shear testing can be used to correlate cyclic interlaminar shear stress with delamination. The test method for noncyclic loads is discussed in "Out-of-Plane Analysis" in this Volume. This can be supplemented with interlaminar normal stress fatigue behavior if interlaminar tension stresses are expected. The axial tension-tension and short beam shear *S-N* curves are plotted in Fig. 6 for unidirectional graphite/epoxy laminates. ASTM D 3479 and D 2344 provide test practices for an axial tension-tension fatigue specimen and for a static strength by short beam shear specimen, respectively.

The fatigue data of Fig. 4 and 6 can be characterized by the following common expressions in semilog or power form, respectively:

$$S = A + B \log N \quad \text{(Eq 1)}$$

$$KS^{b}N = 1 \quad \text{(Eq 2)}$$

where *S* is the applied stress parameter; *N* is the fatigue life; *A* and *B* are parameters for Eq 1; and *K* and *b* are parameters for Eq 2. The *S-N* curves of Fig. 4 are reported in Table 1 in the form of Eq 1. "B" corresponds to the slope of the line and "A" corresponds to the y-intercept.

In developing *S-N* curves, the stress level, stress ratio, and environment should bound the anticipated in-service exposure. Typically, tests are performed at three to five stress levels for a given *R* ratio, where 6 to 10 replicates are preferred at each stress level to quantify the statistical variations of life. Furthermore, fatigue behavior should characterize both in-plane and out-of-plane failure modes.

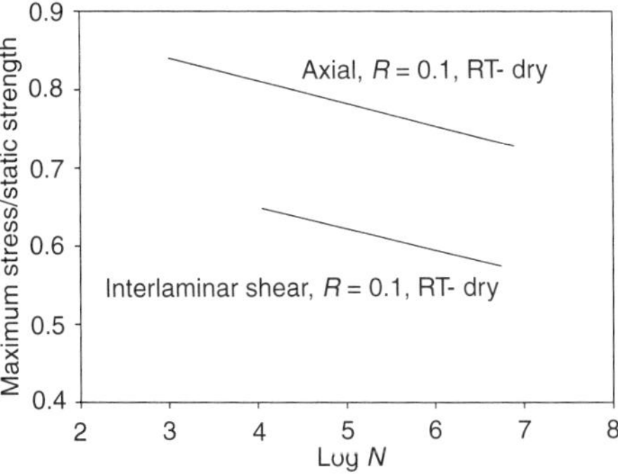

Fig. 6 *S-N* curves for 6350/AS unidirectional laminates. RT, room temperature (Ref 15)

Failure of composite specimens under identical conditions produces a high degree of scatter, in comparison with metals. Thus, statistical treatment of the fatigue data is of particular interest. The distribution of static strength and fatigue life can be described mathematically by a two-parameter Weibull function (Ref 16). A two-parameter Weibull density function is given by:

$$f(x) = \frac{\beta}{\alpha}\left(\frac{x}{\alpha}\right)^{\beta-1} \exp\left[-\left(\frac{x}{\alpha}\right)^{\beta}\right] \quad \text{(Eq 3)}$$

where α is the scale parameter and β is the shape parameter. The scale parameter, α, represents the location of the 63.2 percentile of the distribution. The Weibull parameters are determined to mathematically fit the experimentally determined distributions by well-established techniques, such as the maximum likelihood method (Ref 17). The shape parameter for composite materials is typically between 14 and 40 for static strength and between 1.4 and 4.0 for fatigue life. For comparison, shape parameter for commonly used metals is approximately 7.0, indicating a greater degree of scatter for composites. The same information can also be cast into another form, called a cumulative Weibull distribution function. This function is a cumulative sum of the density function and is given by:

$$F(x) = 1 - \exp\left[-\left(\frac{x}{\alpha}\right)^{\beta}\right] \quad \text{(Eq 4)}$$

where $F(x)$ is the probability that x exceeds α. Equations 3 and 4 describe the fatigue life distribution for a single loading. Given data at three stress levels for a given *R*-ratio, the *S-N* relations of Eq 1 and 2 can be expressed in terms of Weibull scale parameter by substituting $N = \alpha$. This provides a statistical representation of the *S-N* curve. Examples of Weibull fatigue life distributions are summarized in Table 2 for selected data reported in Ref 18.

Often the *S-N* curves are used in the design process to establish maximum stress (or strain) values called allowables. In fatigue these are established for both in-plane stresses as well as interlaminar stresses. An A- or B-basis allowable specifies a maximum allowable stress representing a probabilistic statement equal to 95% lower confidence bound that the probability of survival is at least 0.99 for *A*-basis or 0.90 for *B*-basis. The calculation of stress allowable is reported in Shyprykevich (Ref 19) and the MIL-HDBK-17. Additional sources of *S-N* fatigue data are listed in Table 3.

Damage Tolerance Approach. The damage tolerance approach has evolved from metals to composite applications within the aerospace industry among others. Damage tolerance is defined as the ability of a structure to sustain design loads in the presence of damage caused by fatigue, corrosion, environment, accidents, and other sources, until such damage is detected, through inspections or malfunctions, and repaired. This approach measures the safe operation of the structure through linkage of damage state, schedule inspections, likelihood of detection, and damage progression. Thus, damage tolerance is an integral part of fatigue and life prediction. Detailed discussion of this approach and analysis is provided in the articles "Damage Tolerance" and "Fracture Mechanics of Composite Delamination" in this Volume.

Table 1 *S-N* parameters for T300/934 laminates, *R* –1.0

Curve(a)	Laminate	A, MPa	B, MPa
A	Unidirectional	1597	–87.7
B	Cross-ply	1170	–117
C	Quasi-isotropic	578	–67.3
D	Angle-ply	186	–22.5

(a) See Fig. 4. Source: Ref 10

Table 2 Fatigue life distributions using Weibull function

Laminate	R	σ_{amp} MPa	σ_{amp} ksi	Log α	β
Glass/epoxy cross-ply	0.05	183	26.5	2.775	2.4
	0.05	160	23.2	3.453	4.2
	0.05	137	19.9	4.249	2.0
	0.05	115	16.7	5.342	1.7
Graphite/epoxy quasi-isotropic	0.1	179	26.0	5.968	1.3
	0.1	167	24.2	6.108	4.5
	0.1	159	23.1	6.591	1.8
	–1.0	344	49.9	4.434	1.7
	10	155	22.5	5.988	2.4
Graphite/epoxy angle-ply	0.1	82.7	12.0	4.214	3.7
	0.1	71.8	10.4	4.942	5.7
	0.1	54.9	7.96	6.061	6.0
	–1.0	109.7	15.91	4.740	7.1
	10	88.0	12.8	5.192	3.4

For selected data from Schoff and Davidson (Ref 18). *R* $\sigma_{min}/\sigma_{max}$; σ_{amp}, stress amplitude; Log α, log life; β, shape factor

Table 3 Summary of composite *S-N* fatigue data

Reference	Material	Comment
Kadi and Ellyin (Ref 12)	Glass/epoxy	Unidirectional *S-N* curves at several *R*-ratios
Rotem and Nelson (Ref 10)	Graphite/epoxy	Unidirectional and laminate *S-N* curves
Schutz and Gerharz (Ref 14)	Graphite/epoxy	Laminate *S-N* curves at several *R*-ratios and spectrum loading
Askins (Ref 20)	Graphite/epoxy	Unidirectional and laminate *S-N* curves
Badaliance and Dill (Ref 21)	Graphite/epoxy	Laminate *S-N* curves at several *R*-ratios and spectrum loading
Reifsnider and Jen (Ref 22)	Various	Unidirectional and laminate *S-N* curves
Dexter and Baker (Ref 23)	Graphite and aramid/epoxy	Short beam shear *S-N* curves with environmental effects
Ridley and Cropper (Ref 24)	Graphite/epoxy	Laminate *S-N* curves at several *R*-ratios and spectrum loading

In the damage tolerance approach, prediction of damage growth and future damage states is aided by composite fracture mechanics analysis. The dominant mechanism leading to failure in metals is crack growth. The *Paris law*, which is a primary tool to predict flaw growth in metals, relates the rate of growth of a macrocrack to the change in stress-intensity factor induced by the loading. The Paris law is written in the form:

$$\frac{da}{dN} = C(\Delta K)^m \quad \text{(Eq 5)}$$

where da/dN is the crack growth rate; C and m are empirical constants; and ΔK is the stress-intensity factor range. Recalling the complex damage states of Fig. 1, the damage of a composite is not well characterized as a single, dominant crack. In most composites there are many microcracks and delaminations. In some cases in which there is a dominant macrocrack or delamination, the Paris law may be used for an approximation of life to a defined crack size. In this case, the stress-intensity factor (ΔK) is replaced in Eq 5 by strain energy release rate (ΔG). In a similar manner, interlaminar fracture models can be used to determine if a delamination will initiate and grow from a flaw. For the special case where the dominant failure mechanism is delamination, interlaminar fracture methods based on strain energy release rate and virtual crack closure principles, as proposed by O'Brien (Ref 25) and summarized by Martin (Ref 26), have shown promise.

Regardless of which approach is taken, the damage tolerance requirements are ultimately satisfied in practice by testing full-scale components with engineered defects to a statistically based lifetime.

Delamination

Fatigue is generally not considered the limiting factor in design, due to high fatigue thresholds. This is particularly true for static structures. Consider airframe structures in aerospace applications, where the structure is designed to satisfy damage tolerance criteria, which results in low stress levels in these structures. It is generally accepted that fatigue does not represent a design constraint in these composite structures. The exceptions are structures that are subjected to high cycle fatigue or dynamic loading, components that are prone to delamination, or structures not designed for damage tolerance.

Delamination is a critical issue in fatigue and generally results from high interlaminar normal and shear stresses. Figure 7 shows structural elements in which high interlaminar stresses are common. Experience has shown these elements to be prone to delamination. These elements include free edges, termination of plies in taper regions, radius of stiffeners or channel sections, closeout regions of sandwich structures, and skin-stiffener attachments. Either by testing or analysis, the elements of Fig. 7 must be designed to limit the occurrence of delamination. Analysis consists of three-dimensional finite-element analysis (FEA) or specialized solutions for elements of Fig. 7. In particular, interlaminar normal stresses that result in an opening mode fracture should be minimized. In testing, the building-block approach is strongly recommended. A relatively large number of tests are performed at the coupon level to establish design allowables for different loading and environments. A smaller number of tests at the element and subcomponent level are required to demonstrate the reliability of the manufacturing and structural concept.

The work of Dexter and Baker (Ref 23) is perhaps the best reference on environmental effects on composite structures. In this work, the effect of moisture and aging was characterized in a ten-year study of laboratory coupons as well as a fifteen-year study of in-service flight exposure of helicopter structures.

Life Prediction Models

For purposes of this review, fatigue models for composite materials under cyclic loading are classified broadly as either *mechanistic* or *phenomenological*. In a mechanistic-based approach, the damage is modeled discretely, thus allowing direct prediction of initiation and growth of damage. For example, O'Brien (Ref 25) suggests the application of linear fracture mechanics and FEA to predict the initiation of delamination. These models are useful in damage tolerance assessments and are further discussed in the article "Fracture Mechanics of Composite Delamination" in this Section. Phenomenological fatigue methodologies, which generally define damage in terms of macroscopically measured properties such as strength or stiffness, are easily incorporated into existing design practices. These models are simply applied to multistress-level loading and are traditionally associated with safelife.

Palmgren-Miner Rule. Perhaps the most simple life prediction model is the Palmgren-Miner rule (Ref 27, 28):

$$\sum_{i=1}^{m} \frac{n_i}{N_i} = 1 \quad \text{(Eq 6)}$$

where m is the number of different stress levels; n_i is the number of stress cycles at level i; and N_i is the number of cycles to failure at the stress amplitude corresponding to level i. The fatigue life, N_i, is determined from the appropriate *S-N* curve. The Palmgren-Miner rule assumes that damage can be quantified as the ratio of the number of cycles at an applied stress amplitude divided by the fatigue life at that stress amplitude. In general, the Palmgren-Miner rule provides poor predictive capability for composite materials (Ref 18, 21).

Advanced Residual Strength Models. Advancements in life prediction have been largely in the development of stiffness- and strength-based fatigue models. Talreja (Ref 29) developed a continuum damage model relating stiffness to local damage states. Strength-based fatigue models applied to composite materials originated with the works of Halpin et al. (Ref 30) and were advanced by Yang and Du (Ref 31). These models were modified by Reifsnider et al. (Ref 32) and incorporated into MRLife, a composite analysis code that uses normalized strength relations for a given ply based on unidirectional static and fatigue properties. MRLife allows selection of failure criteria, strength degradation functions, and stiffness degradation functions. The strength-based residual strength model has shown good predictive capability for spectrum fatigue loading (Ref 18). It is considered as a good alternate life prediction model to the Palmgren-Miner rule.

Figure 8 presents the residual strength relation that is used by the model for constant amplitude fatigue. The solid line in the figure "tracks" the Weibull scale parameter for residual strength, that is, the 63.2 percentile of the strength distri-

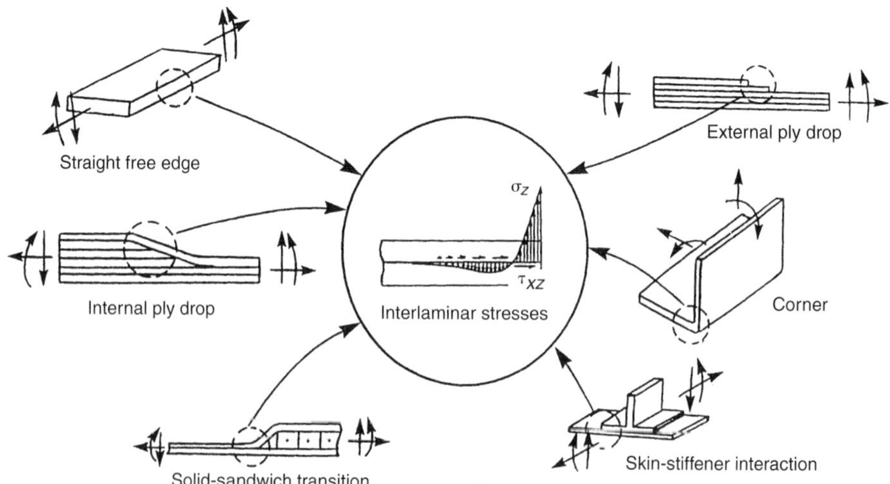

Fig. 7 Structural configurations with high interlaminar stresses. σ_z is tensile stress and τ_{xz} is shear stress.

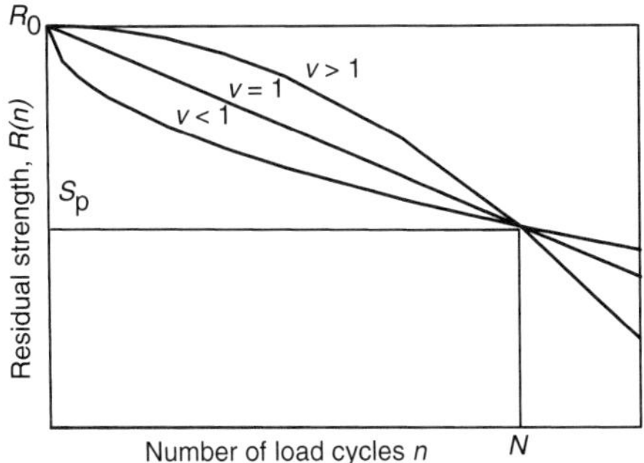

Fig. 8 Residual strength, $R(n)$, relation for constant amplitude loading. R_0 is the original static tensile or compressive strength; S_p is the peak stress magnitude; v is a strength degradation parameter.

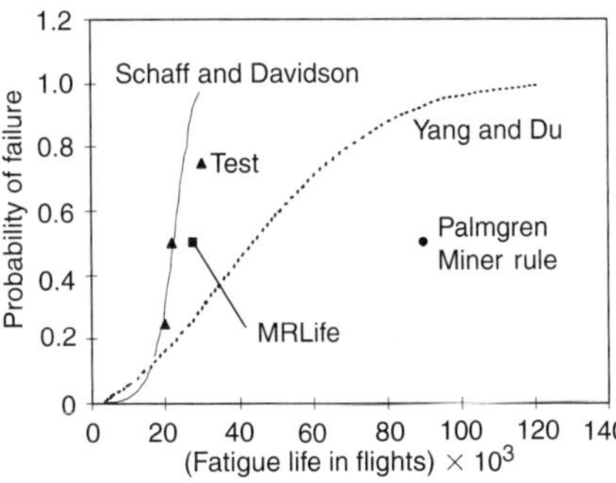

Fig. 9 Comparison of prediction and observed results for spectrum fatigue data of Schutz and Gerharz (Ref 14), Schaff and Davidson (Ref 18), Yang and Du (Ref 31), MRLife (Ref 32), and Palmgren-Miner rule (Ref 27, 28)

bution, as the scale parameter for strength decreases with increasing cycling. The equation of this line is given by:

$$R(n) = R_0 - (R_0 - S_p)\left(\frac{n}{N}\right)^v \quad \text{(Eq 7)}$$

where $R(n)$ is the residual strength scale parameter after n cycles; R_0 is the static strength scale parameter; S_p is the peak stress *magnitude* of the constant amplitude loading; N is the scale parameter for the fatigue life distribution; and v is the strength degradation parameter.

For constant amplitude loading with a positive mean stress, S_p is the maximum stress; for constant amplitude loading with a negative mean stress, S_p is the magnitude of the minimum stress. R_0 is the scale parameter for the distribution of static strength. The scale parameter for the fatigue life distribution, N, is found by an S-N curve or from a master diagram similar to Fig. 5. The strength degradation parameter, v, controls the overall shape of the residual strength relation. It is obtained by comparing the predicted and observed life distributions for constant amplitude fatigue loading. When $v >> 1$, "sudden death" behavior is simulated; when $v = 1$, a linear strength degradation is simulated; and when $v < 1$, the behavior of those laminates that experience an early, sudden loss in strength is simulated. The values of R_0, N, and v are dependent on laminate lay-up, materials system, geometry, and the type of loading (i.e., uniaxial, biaxial, shear, etc.). Therefore, model characterization tests must be performed for each variation. Initially, the strength distribution is equal to the static strength distribution. During fatigue loading, the entire distribution experiences a degradation in strength. As cycling continues and the mean strength degrades, the residual strength of the weaker structures will fall below the maximum applied stress, and failure will occur. The probability of failure during constant amplitude fatigue loading, that is, the probability that the residual strength is less than the peak stress, S_p, may also be expressed in the form of a Weibull distribution as:

$$P[\hat{R}(n) \le S_p] = 1 - \exp[-(S_p / R(n))^{B_f(n)}] \quad \text{(Eq 8)}$$

where $B_f^{(n)}$ is a yet-to-be-determined Weibull shape parameter for residual strength. Substituting the residual strength relation, Eq 7, into Eq 8 gives:

$$P[\hat{R}(n) \le S_p] = 1 - \exp \times \left[-\left(\frac{S_p}{R_0 - (R_0 - S_p)\left(\frac{n}{N}\right)^v}\right)^{B_f(n)}\right] \quad \text{(Eq 9)}$$

A review of the fatigue data in open literature indicates that strength data becomes increasingly scattered with increasing fatigue loading prior to static testing. In Eq 9, this is controlled by the Weibull shape parameter, B_f. Smaller values of B_f correspond to broader, more dispersed, distributions. In Eq 9, B_f is assumed to initially equal the static strength shape parameter, B_s, and to linearly degrade to the limiting value of the fatigue life shape parameter, B_l.

Life predictions by strength-based fatigue models are compared to experimental results reported by Schutz and Gerharz (Ref 14) for uniaxial loading of $[0_2°/\pm45°/0_2°/\pm45°/90°]_s$ graphite/epoxy test specimens. Comparisons are made for a loading spectrum simulating the stress history on upper wing skin at wing root of fighter aircraft. The load spectrum contains sixteen load levels and a peak compressive stress of 652.5 MPa (94.6 ksi). The models were characterized with fatigue life data at three stress ratios: –1.0, –1.66, and –5.0. Experimental and theoretical fatigue life results are shown in Fig. 9. The predictions demonstrate good correlation with experiment and better agreement than that of Yang and Du (Ref 31). The Palmgren-Miner rule was unconservative by factor of three in prediction of the mean fatigue life. Overall, strength-based fatigue models have shown better predictive ability for mean life than the Palmgren-Miner rule.

REFERENCES

1. R.L. Reifsnider, *Composite Materials Series: Fatigue of Composite Materials*, Vol 4, Elsevier Science Publishing Company, New York, 1991
2. R. Talreja, Fatigue of Fiber Composites, *Materials Science and Technology: Structure and Properties of Composites*, Vol 13, T.W. Chou, Ed., VCH Publishers, Weinheim, 1993
3. *Composite Materials*, Military Handbook 17, *Materials Usage Design and Analysis*, Vol 3, Department of Defense, Philadelphia, PA
4. W.W. Stinchcomb and C.E. Bakis, Fatigue Behaviour of Composite Laminates, *Composite Materials Series: Fatigue of Composites*, Vol 4, 1991, p 105–178
5. R.Y. Kim, Experimental Assessment of Static and Fatigue Damage of Graphite/Epoxy Laminates, *Advances in Composite Materials*, Vol 2, *Proc. Third International Conference on Composite Materials* (Paris), A.R. Bunsell, Ed., 1980
6. A.S.D. Wang and F.W. Crossman, Initiation and Growth of Transverse Cracks and Edge Delamination in Composite Laminates, Part I An Energy Method, *J. Compos. Mater.*, supplement, 1980
7. K.W. Garrett and J.E. Bailey, Multiple Transverse Cracking in Glass Fiber Epoxy Cross-Ply Laminates, *J. Mater. Sci.*, Vol 12, 1977
8. H.T. Hahn and R.Y. Kim, Fatigue Behavior of Composite Laminates, *J. Compos. Mater.*, Vol 10, 1976, p 156–180
9. S. Suresh, *Fatigue of Materials*, Cambridge University Press, New York, 1991
10. A. Rotem and H.G. Nelson, Residual Strength of Composite Laminates Subjected to Tensile-Compressive Fatigue Loading, *J. Compos. Technol. Res.*, Vol 12 (No. 2), 1990, p 76–84
11. J.M. Whitney, "Fatigue Characterization of Composite Materials," AFWAL-TR-79-4111, Air Force Materials Laboratory, 1979
12. E.H. Kadi and F. Ellyin, Effect of Stress Ratio on Fatigue of Unidirectional Glass Fiber/Epoxy Composite Laminates, *Composites*, Vol 25, 1994
13. I.R. Farrow, "Damage Accumulation and Degradation of Composite Laminates Under Aircraft Service Loading: Assessment and Prediction Vol I and II, Ph.D. thesis, Cranfield Institute of Technology, 1989
14. D. Schutz and J.J. Gerharz, Fatigue Strength of a Fibre-Reinforced Material, *Composites*, Vol 8 (No. 4), 1977, p 245–250
15. J.R. Schaff and A. Dobyns, "Fatigue Analysis of Helicopter Tail Rotor Spar," AIAA Report 98-1738, American Institute of Aeronautics and Astronautics - ASM Symposium (Long Beach), 1998
16. W. Weibull and G.W. Weibull, "New Aspects and Methods of Statistical Analysis of Test Data with Spatial Reference to the Normal, the Log Normal, and the Weibull Distributions," FOA Report D 20045 DB, Defense Research Institute, Stockholm, 1977
17. R. Talreja, "Estimation of Weibull Parameters for Composite Materials Strength and Fatigue Life Data," STP 723, American So-

ciety for Testing and Materials, 1981, p 297–311
18. J.R. Schaff and B.D. Davidson, A Life Prediction Methodology for Composite Structures, Part I: Constant Amplitude and Two Stress Level Fatigue Loading, and Part II: Spectrum Fatigue Loading, *J. Compos. Mater.*, Vol 31 (No. 2), 1997, p 128–181
19. P. Shyprykevich, The Role of Statistical Data Reduction in the Development of Design Allowables for Composites, *Test Methods and Design Allowables for Fibrous Composites*, Vol 2, American Society for Testing and Materials, Philadelphia, PA, 1989, p 111–135
20. D.R. Askins, "Development of Engineering Data on Advanced Composite Materials," AFWAL-TR-81-4172, Air Force Materials Laboratory, 1982
21. R. Badaliance and H.D. Dill, "Effects of Fighter Attack Spectrum on Composite Fatigue Life," AFWAL-TR-81-3001, Air Force Flight Dynamics Laboratory, 1981
22. K.L. Reifsnider and M.H.R. Jen, "Composite Flywheel Durability and Life, Part II: Long Term Materials Data," UCRL-15523-Pt.2, Lawrence Livermore Laboratory, 1982
23. H.B. Dexter and D.J. Baker, Flight Service Environmental Effects on Composite Materials and Structures, *Adv. Perform. Mater.*, Vol 1 (No. 1), F.H. Froes, Ed., 1994
24. G.S. Ridley and D.J. Cropper, "Fatigue and Damage Tolerance Design Data for Carbon Fibre Composites," Bae-MSM-R-GEN-0454, British Aerospace Public Limited Company, 1986.
25. T.K. O'Brien, "Towards a Damage Tolerance Philosophy for Composite Materials and Structures," ASTM STP 1059, *Composite Materials: Testing and Design*, Vol 9, S.P. Garbo, Ed., ASTM, 1990, p 7–33
26. R.H. Martin, Incorporating Interlaminar Fracture Mechanics into Design, *International Conf. Designing Cost-Effective Composites*, *ImechE Conf. Trans.*, Professional Eng. Publishing, London, 15–16 Sept 1998, p 83–92
27. M.A. Miner, Cumulative Damage in Fatigue, *J. Appl. Mech.*, Vol 12, 1945, p 159–164
28. A. Palmgren, Die Lebensdauer von Kugellagern, *Zeitschrift des Vereins Deutscher Ingenieure*, Vol 68, 1924, p 339–341
29. R. Talreja, A Continuum Mechanics Characterization of Damage in Composite Laminates, *Proc. R. Soc. (London), A*, 1985, p 399
30. J.C. Halpin, T.A. Johnson, and M.E. Waddoups, Kinetic Facture Models and Structural Reliability, *Int. J. Fract. Mech.*, 1972
31. J.N. Yang and S. Du, An Exploratory Study into the Fatigue of Composites under Spectrum Loading, *J. Compos. Mater.*, Vol 17, 1983, p 511–526
32. K.L. Reifsnider, S.W. Case, and Y.L. Xu, "MRLife: A Strength and Life Prediction Code for Laminated Composite Materials," Virginia Polytechnic Institute and State University, 1996

Damping Properties

VIBRATIONAL AND DAMPING CHARACTERISTICS OF composites are important in many applications, including ground-based and airborne vehicles, space structures, and sporting goods. In response to a transient or dynamic loading, structures can experience excessive vibrations that create high noise levels, stress fatigue failure, premature wear, operator discomfort, and unsafe operating conditions. An understanding of various theoretical and experimental aspects to vibration in composites is essential to the efforts to avoid or eliminate these potential problems.

In the past, the damping capacity of conventional engineering materials has not generally provided sufficient energy dissipation to limit resonant or near-resonant amplitudes of vibration. The position has been further aggravated by the development of high-strength alloys of aluminum and titanium, which generally have lower damping than those provided by their weaker counterparts. Conventional structures have many additional sources of energy dissipation, such as bolted and riveted joints, lubricated bearings, and so on. In space applications, because of the absence of a surrounding fluid or gas, aerodynamic damping is essentially zero, thus removing an important source of energy dissipation, especially in thin-sheet structures. However, when using composite materials, it is usually necessary to use adhesively bonded joints, because bolts and rivets tend to pull out. This seriously reduces structural damping, which makes material damping far more important. This situation can be alleviated in fiber-reinforced materials by making a suitable choice of components so that the damping derives essentially from the matrix and fiber-matrix interface. It is therefore more important to understand the mechanisms of damping in composites and to appreciate their significance than is the case for metallic materials.

The main sources of internal damping in a composite material arise from microplastic or viscoelastic phenomena associated with the matrix and from relative slipping at the interface between the matrix and from relative slipping at the interface between the matrix and the reinforcement. Thus, excluding the contribution from any cracks and debonds, the internal damping of the composite will be influenced by:

- The properties and relative proportions of matrix and reinforcement in the composite (the latter is usually represented by the volume fraction of the reinforcement, V_f)
- The size of the inclusions
- The orientation of the reinforcing material to the loading axis
- The surface treatment of the reinforcement

In addition, loading and environmental factors, such as amplitude, frequency, and temperature, may affect damping.

To cover the dynamic properties of all composite materials is beyond the limited scope of this article. Only those advanced composites used in stress-bearing situations in modern engineering are discussed. Unreinforced polymers are not covered here, except as a component of the composite, nor are composites with randomly oriented fibers, nor those containing nonfibrous reinforcements. The damping and moduli of short-fiber composites have been reviewed by S.A. Suarez et al. (Ref 1). Because modulus and damping are interrelated, both are considered.

The vibration properties of concern are the damping and the dynamic modulus, which are defined in Fig. 1. When subjected to a stress cycle, all materials show a nonsingular relationship between stress and strain. The modulus is given by the mean of the stress-strain loop. For most materials, there is little ambiguity in this definition, because the loop is almost indistinguishable from a straight line. The area, ΔU, of the loop represents the work done against "internal friction" and is the amount of energy dissipated during the cycle.

It can be seen from Fig. 1 that the maximum strain energy stored per unit volume in the cycle is $U = \sigma^2/2E = E_\varepsilon^2/2$. The specific damping capacity, Ψ, of the material is defined as:

$$\Psi = \frac{2\pi}{Q} = 2\delta = 2\pi\eta = 4\pi C = 2\pi\left(\frac{f_2 - f_1}{f_n}\right)_{3\text{dB}} \quad \text{(Eq 1)}$$

where Q is the quality (amplification) factor, δ is the logarithmic decrement, η is the loss factor, C is the proportion of critical damping, f_n is the natural frequency (Hz), and f_1 and f_2 are the half-power (3 dB) points.

Finally, it must be emphasized that just as there are many possible sources of energy dissipation in structures, most apparatuses for measuring damping need some method of applying the cyclic loads, measuring the dynamic response, and locating the specimen in some frame of reference. Many authors have not been sufficiently careful in making such measurements with metals and composites. Whereas thermoplastics often have substantial amounts of damping, structural metals and composites do not. It is therefore crucially important that any damping data used should be from an impeccable source. All things being equal, the lowest damping values quoted for a given material are likely to be the nearest to the truth. Not only should damping measurements be carefully made, but the apparatus must be purged of extraneous losses by calibrating it with some metal of very low damping properties (such as high-strength titanium or aluminum alloys).

Unidirectional Composites

The basic building block of layered composite structures is a single lamina of unidirectionally reinforced material. All the fibers are considered to be parallel and lying in the direction of the major axis of the specimen.

Longitudinal shear involves the twisting of a bar of an aligned composite. Thus, the longitudinal shear modulus of carbon-fiber-reinforced plastic (CFRP) or glass-fiber-reinforced plastic (GFRP) is principally a function of the matrix shear modulus, the fiber shear modulus, and the volume fraction of fibers. None of the existing micromechanics theories accurately fits the experimental data (Ref 2), but the numerical prediction of D.F. Adams and D.R. Doner (Ref 3)

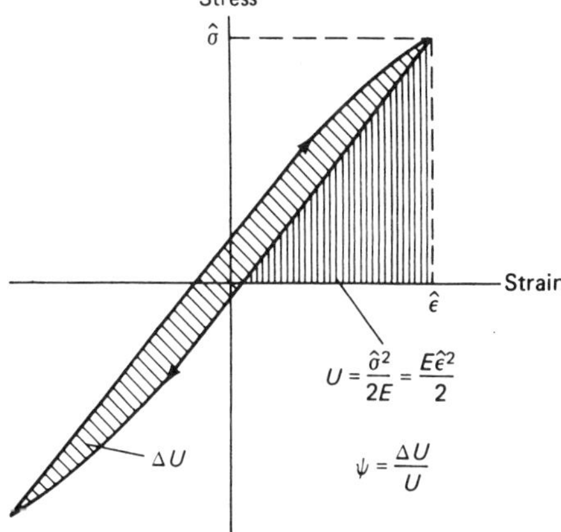

Fig. 1 Definition of specific damping capacity, Ψ. ΔU, energy dissipated per cycle; U, maximum stored energy

gives good agreement. From the type of curve shown in Fig. 2, it is possible to determine the fiber volume fraction, V_f, if the matrix shear modulus, G_m, is known, and vice versa.

For longitudinal shear loading, it can be shown that for viscoelastic materials (Ref 4):

$$\Psi_{LT} = \frac{\Psi_m(1-V_f)\{(G+1)^2 + V_f(G-1)^2\}}{[G(1+V_f)+1-V_f][G(1-V_f)+1+V_f]} \quad \text{(Eq 2)}$$

where f and m represent fiber and matrix, V_f is the fiber volume fraction, G is the ratio of the shear modulus of the fiber to that of the matrix, and Ψ is the specific damping capacity. For many fiber-matrix combinations, G is of the order of 10, which leads to a composite specific damping capacity that is not influenced very much by the fiber volume fraction. This relationship is shown in Fig. 3 for a typical carbon-fiber-reinforced composite, along with an alternative solution proposed by R.D. Adams and D.G.C. Bacon (Ref 2). To allow a comparison of these predictions with the variety of experimental data, the damping values have been nondimensionalized. To explain the lower damping measured in their torsional tests, R.D. Adams and D.G.C. Bacon cited effects that were due to fiber misalignment and dilatational strains in the materials that contribute little to the damping but add significantly to the stored strain energy. Thus, if the damping capacity or shear modulus of the matrix is known, it is possible to estimate the damping and shear modulus of a composite with a given volume fraction. Alternatively, by using curves such as those in Fig. 3, or the similar ones given by R.G. Ni and R.D. Adams (Ref 5), it is possible to estimate the properties of a composite with a given volume fraction if those at some other volume fraction are known.

Longitudinal Tension/Compression. The longitudinal Young's modulus, E_L, (the tensile modulus in the direction of the fibers in a unidirectional composite) is given by the rule of mixtures and is:

$$E_L = E_f V_f + E_m(1 - V_f)$$

where E_f and E_m are the fiber and matrix Young's moduli, and V_f is the fiber volume fraction. This rule is well obeyed experimentally, as shown in Fig. 4, and may be used as a check on any parameter, provided the others are known. This relationship was derived for normal axial loading (tension or compression), but also applies in flexure, provided that shear effects can be neglected. The scatter of the experimental results in Fig. 4 is mainly due to fiber misalignment, which is usually worse at low volume fractions. Other errors can be due to incorrect assessment of the volume fraction. It is also possible to predict the damping capacity of a unidirectional material when it is stressed in the fiber direction by using the rule of mixtures and assuming that all the energy dissipation occurs in the matrix. This gives the equation:

$$\Psi_L = \Psi_m(1 - V_f)\, E_m/E_L$$

where E is Young's modulus and L represents longitudinal tensile/compressive properties of the composite.

However, it is found that this expression considerably underestimates the measured value of Ψ_L, even when considerable effort has been made to eliminate extraneous losses (Fig. 5). Basically, there are several factors contributing to the discrepancy. First, the smaller the fiber diameter, the larger the surface area of fiber per unit volume. R.D. Adams and D.F. Short (Ref 6) showed that for 10, 20, 30, and 50 μm (390, 790, 1200, and 1950 μin.) diam glass fibers in polyester resin, there was a consistent increase in Ψ_L with reduction in fiber diameter. Second, the problem of misalignment is not insignificant, as is shown subsequently for angle-ply composites. Third, any structural imperfections, such as cracks and debonds, lead to interfacial rubbing and, hence, to additional losses. Finally, the unidirectional lamina is very often loaded in flexure rather than uniform in-plane tension or compression. Thus, although the effect of shear is negligible in stiffness measurements, this is less true for damping because shear damping is essen-

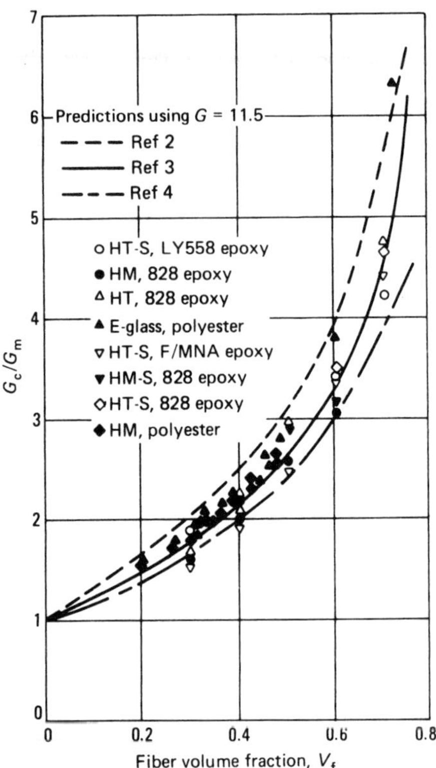

Fig. 2 Variation of reduced composite longitudinal shear modulus (G_{LT}/G_m) with fiber volume fraction (V_f)

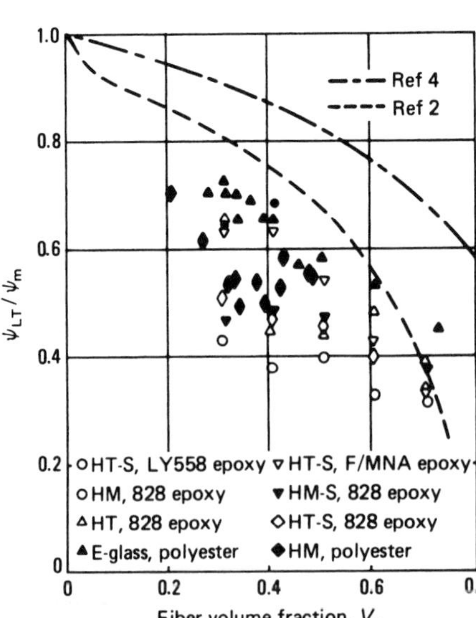

Fig. 3 Variation of the ratio of longitudinal shear damping (Ψ_{LT}) to the matrix damping (Ψ_m) with volume fraction (V_f)

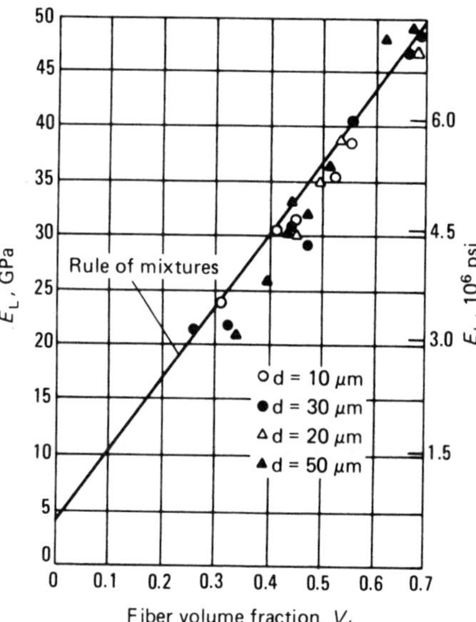

Fig. 4 Longitudinal Young's modulus (E_L) against fiber volume fraction (V_f) for different glass fibers

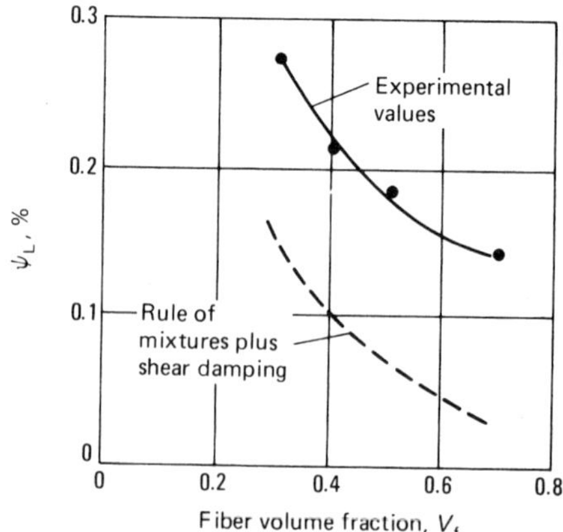

Fig. 5 Variation of flexural damping (Ψ_L) with fiber volume fraction (V_f) for HT-S carbon fiber in epoxy resin

tially that of the matrix, and Ψ_{LT} is of the order of 50 to 100 times larger than Ψ_L.

Although only a small percentage of the energy is stored in shear, it can make a substantial contribution to the total predicted value of damping. Figure 6 shows that as the aspect ratio of a beam was reduced from 90 to 50, the shear damping contribution was increased. Further, by subtracting the shear damping from the experimental values, the effect of aspect ratio is essentially eliminated.

The difference remaining between the rule of mixtures prediction and the "experimental minus shear" values was mainly due to the combination of misalignment internal flaws, and fiber diameter. It has been suggested that the discrepancy can be explained by the composite being modeled such that it considers damping of the fibers. Unfortunately, this is unlikely to be a realistic solution because the damping of the fibers is extremely small. R.D. Adams (Ref 7) has directly measured the longitudinal shear damping of a variety of single carbon fibers and found values of the order of 0.13% specific damping capacity. This gives a loss factor of the order of 2×10^{-4}. In tension/compression, the graphite microfibrils that make up the carbon-fiber structure will be preferentially stressed in their strong direction, with much less interfacial slipping than might occur in torsion. Thus, the longitudinal damping (tension/compression) ought to be at least an order of magnitude lower than that measured in torsion, giving a loss factor of approximately 2×10^{-5}. There is, therefore, no way in which damping of this level can reasonably be used to explain the discrepancies in the micromechanic models. On the other hand, it is known that aramid fibers possess quite high damping levels, even in tension/compression, and might therefore offer an exception to the previous generalization.

Transverse Tension/Compression. In the transverse direction, damping is, as in shear, very heavily matrix-dependent. Again, there is no reliable micromechanics theory for predicting Ψ_L. Experiments covering a wide variety of fibers, from E-glass to high-modulus carbon, showed that transverse damping is largely independent of both fiber type and surface treatment. Volume fraction, like longitudinal shear, does have a significant effect on Ψ_L. Some experimental results to illustrate this point are given in Fig. 7. Figure 8 shows the transverse Young's modulus, E_T, which, like G_{LT} (Fig. 2), is seen to increase markedly with volume fraction. The theoretical curve is based on the expression proposed by S.W. Tsai and H.T. Halpin (Ref 8), and the values are for a glass composite for which it has been assumed that the longitudinal and transverse moduli of the glass fibers are identical (that is, the fiber is isotropic). This cannot be assumed for carbon fibers, which are highly anisotropic.

General Comments on the Simple Loading of Laminae. While the various micromechanics theories, including those proposed by S. Chang and C.W. Bert (Ref 9), are sufficiently accurate for predicting moduli, they are generally poor at predicting damping. This is because the various theories do not contain some of the important factors (such as microcracks, misalignment, and surface area) that contribute to the damping of unidirectional materials while having little effect on the moduli. Without the development of some very complex models, it is unlikely that the situation can be changed in the near future. The only safe feature is that, with the possible exception of aramid fibers, there is essentially no damping in the fibers themselves.

R.G. Ni and R.D. Adams (Ref 5) used a combination of micromechanics and experimental results to produce a series of predictive curves for the variation of the unidirectional moduli and damping values with fiber volume fraction. They also showed the importance of using the correct volume fraction for this basic data. Thus, when predictions of the damping for laminated plates are being made, it is important to know the volume fraction of both the plates and the unidirectional material used in making the prediction. Guides were given for converting data, and an example showed the errors that can occur if the corrected data are not used. It is suggested that the Ni and Adams approach is far more suitable in practical terms than trying to evolve increasingly complex micromechanics models. A further practical point is that it is difficult to make representative pure resin (matrix) specimens, the results of which are necessary for any micromechanics prediction. This is because the resins used for making preimpregnated fiber sheets or tapes (prepregs) contain volatiles that are difficult to remove from the bulk without creating bubbles or causing other chemical changes in the cured blocks.

Off-Axis Loading. When the specimen axis, and thus the direction of loading, is at an angle, θ, to the fiber direction in a unidirectional composite, an off-axis situation exists.

R.D. Adams and D.G.C. Bacon (Ref 10) derived closed-form expressions for the damping, Ψ_θ, of a unidirectional beam with fibers at an angle to that of the specimen axis. Figure 9 shows the theoretical and experimental values of Ψ_θ for a CFRP beam, together with the separate theoretical contributions from stresses in the L, T, and LT directions. Figure 9 also shows the separate contributions from direct stresses in the direction of the fibers Ψ_L, transverse to the fibers Ψ_T, and in shear, Ψ_{LT}. The theoretical prediction and experimental measurements of the variation of Young's modulus, E_θ, with angle, are also shown in Fig. 9. Excellent agreement between theory and experiment is shown for both modulus and damping.

R.D. Adams and D.G.C. Bacon showed that, for a carbon composite in which $E_L >> G_{LT}$, $E_L >> E_{LT}$, $\Psi_L << \Psi_T$, and $\Psi_L << \Psi_{LT}$, then to

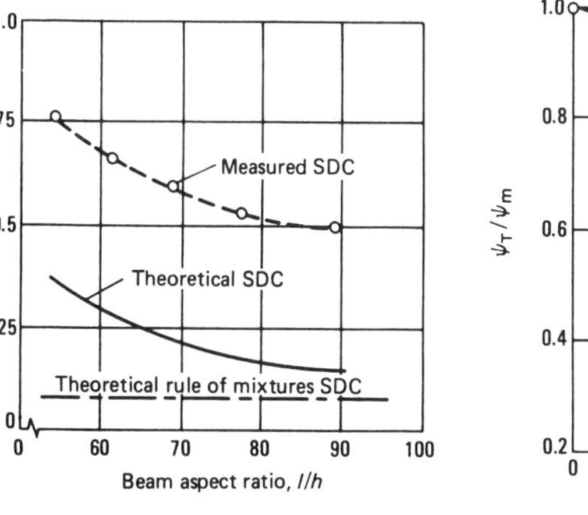

Fig. 6 Variation of flexural damping (Ψ_L) with aspect ratio l/h (l, length; h, thickness) for high-modulus carbon fiber in DX209 epoxy resin V_f = 0.5. SDC, shear damping contribution

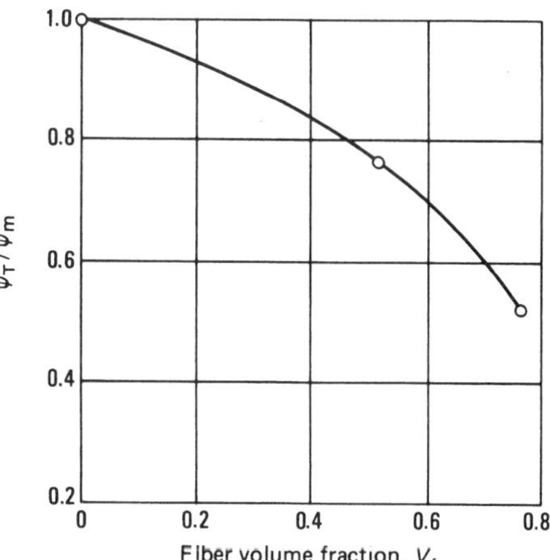

Fig. 7 Variation of ratio of transverse damping (Ψ_T) to matrix damping (Ψ_m) with fiber volume fraction (V_f). Results from GFRP specimens in flexure

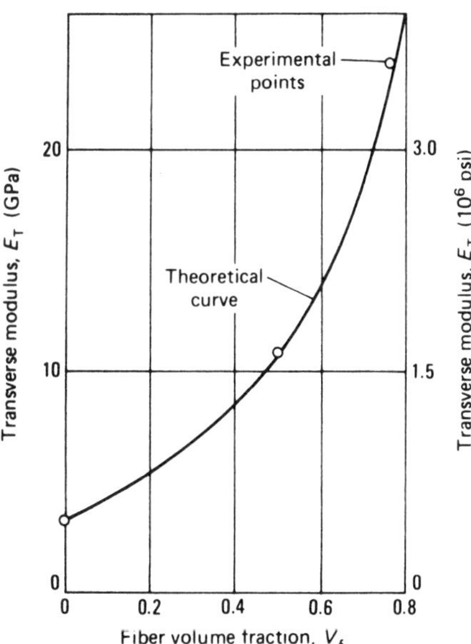

Fig. 8 Variation of the transverse modulus (E_T) with fiber volume fraction (V_f) of GFRP in flexure. E_{fT} = 70 GPa (10×10^6 psi). E_m = 3.21 GPa (0.466×10^6 psi)

a very good approximation over the range $5° < \theta < 90°$:

$$\Psi_\theta = \frac{1}{S_{11}}\left[\frac{\psi_T}{E_T}\sin^4\theta + \frac{\psi_{LT}}{G_{LT}}\sin^2\theta\cos^2\theta\right]$$

where S_{11} is the compliance in the direction of the specimen axis.

Beams Cut From Laminated Plates

In practice, structures made from composites contain a series of layers of unidirectional fibers such that each layer has some predetermined orientation with respect to the defined dimensions of the structure (Fig. 10). The orientations and transverse dispositions of the fibers depend on the loads to be carried (strength) and the deflections that can be tolerated (stiffness). For any arrangement of layers, it is now possible to predict not only structural strength and stiffness, but also inherent damping. Laminated plate theory is used to evaluate the contributions to damping made by each layer. Beams are a special case of plates, but are often treated separately because the theory of vibrating beams is much easier than that of plates. In an article of this length, the theory can only be outlined. A fuller treatment is given by R.G. Ni and R.D. Adams (Ref 11).

The constitutive equation relating stresses, σ, and strains, ε, in the kth lamina is (using standard notation for composites):

$$\begin{bmatrix}\sigma_1\\ \sigma_2\\ \sigma_6\end{bmatrix}_k = \begin{bmatrix}Q_{11} & Q_{12} & Q_{16}\\ Q_{12} & Q_{22} & Q_{26}\\ Q_{16} & Q_{26} & Q_{66}\end{bmatrix}_k \begin{bmatrix}\varepsilon_1\\ \varepsilon_2\\ \varepsilon_6\end{bmatrix}_k$$

where the values Q_{ij}^k are the stiffness matrix components in the specimen system of axes 1, 2, 3 of the kth lamina, and are obtained from the values in the axes related to the fiber direction x, y, z by using the appropriate geometric transformation. For a beam specimen, the stresses σ_2 and σ_6 (transverse and interlaminar shear) can generally be neglected in comparison with σ_1 although M.M. Wallace and C.W. Bert cite cases where this may not always be so (Ref 12).

With the appropriate geometric transformation, these stresses can be converted from the specimen axes to the fiber directions. It is then possible to calculate the stresses in the fiber direction σ_x (that is, σ_L), normal to it σ_y (that is, σ_T), and the shear components σ_{xy} (that is, σ_{LT}). The total energy stored in the x (or L) direction, Z_L, for example, can then be calculated, and the energy dissipation in this layer and in this direction can then be given by:

$$\Delta Z_L = \Psi_L \cdot Z_L$$

For the beam, the overall specific damping capacity, Ψ_{ov}, is then given by the total energy dissipated divided by the total energy stored:

$$\Psi_{ov} = \frac{\Sigma\Delta Z}{\Sigma Z} = \frac{\psi_L Z_L + \psi_T Z_T + \psi_{LT} Z_{LT}}{Z_L + Z_T + Z_{LT}} \qquad \text{(Eq 3)}$$

If the elastic moduli and damping coefficients are known for the unidirectional material, it is possible to calculate the overall damping of a beam. R.G. Ni and R.D. Adams (Ref 11) gave the theory for generally laminated beams and obtained excellent agreement with the measured results.

Whereas specimens with all the layers at θ will twist as they are bent, the twisting can be restrained internally by using several layers at $\pm\theta$. The damping contributions can again be assessed, and the measured values accounted for (Ref 10, 11). Figure 11 shows theoretical predictions and experimental measurements for the modulus and damping of a series of CFRP beams made with ten layers of high-modulus carbon fibers in epoxy resin, alternately at $\pm\theta$. Note that the modulus is higher than that of the off-axis specimens because of the internal restraint, while the damping is generally lower.

More generally, laminated composites, as shown in Fig. 10, are commonly used in practice. Fortunately, the same method as that just described can be used to predict damping. Figure 12 shows the excellent agreement between theory and experiment for the variation of damping (and stiffness) with θ of a symmetrical, high-modulus, graphite-fiber-reinforced epoxy plate. Beam specimens were cut at angles from –90° to +90° relative to the fiber direction in the outer layer of this (0°, –60°, +60°)$_s$ plate.

Laminated Plates

Fiber-reinforced plates of various shapes and different boundary conditions (free, clamped, and hinged) commonly occur in practice. Designers need to be able to predict the stiffness parameters and damping values of such plates for conditions such as aeroelasticity, acoustic fatigue, and so on. Much attention has been devoted to stiffness predictions, but very little to damping. The objective here is to develop a suitable mathematical model that can be used to predict the damping values of plates laminated from fibers of various types at various orientations. Such is the mathematical complexity of the equation of motion of plates (even those made

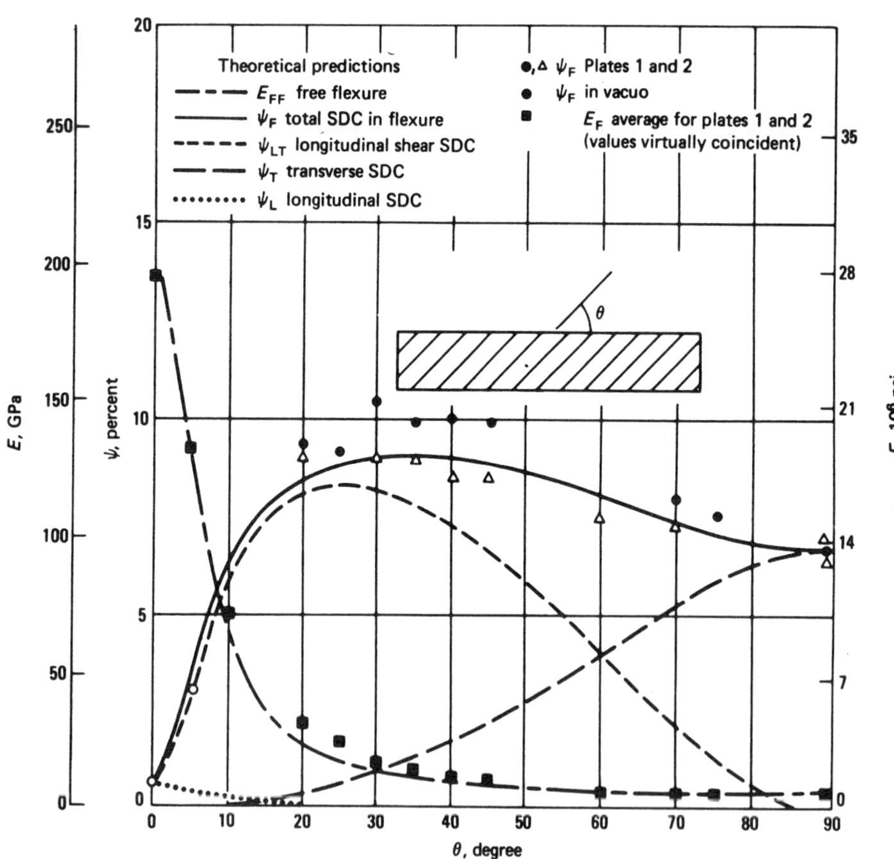

Fig. 9 Variation of flexural Young's modulus (E) and Damping (Ψ) with fiber orientation (θ) for high-modulus carbon fiber in DX209 epoxy resin. $V_f = 0.5$

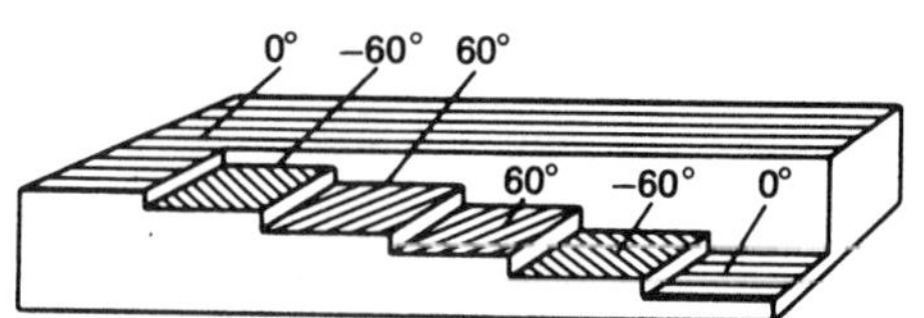

Fig. 10 Lamina stacking arrangement for (0°, –60°, 60°)$_s$ laminate. The suffix s indicates symmetry of stacking about the midplane.

from isotropic materials) that closed-form solutions exist only for special cases, such as hinged (simply supported) rectangular plates and circular plates (involving Bessel functions). The solution is therefore best obtained using finite-element techniques, which can readily accommodate different shapes, thicknesses, and boundary conditions. Some examples are given by P. Cawley and R.D. Adams (Ref 13).

All the plates discussed here are midplane symmetric, which eliminates bending-stretching coupling. It is, however, possible to include this effect in the analysis if asymmetrical laminates are used.

The first ten modes of vibration of a typical plate can be adequately described by using a coarse finite-element mesh with six elements per side (6 × 6 = 36 elements for a rectangular plate). The essence of the technique is first to determine the values of strain energy stored because of the stresses relative to the fiber axes of each layer of each element. Use of modulus parameters determined from unidirectional bars makes it possible to determine the total energy stored in each layer of each element. These are then summed through the thickness to give the energy stored in each element (related to the strains and the mean elasticity matrix for the element). It is then possible to use standard finite-element programs and avoid the mathematical complication of working in terms of the standard plate equations. This approach provides the stiffness of the plate, the maximum strain energy, U, stored in any given mode of vibration, the natural frequencies, and the mode shape. The energy dissipated in an element of unit width and length situated in the kth layer can also now be determined. This is done by transforming the stresses and strains to the fiber directions and using the damping properties of 0° bars. The energy dissipated in the element in the kth layer is integrated over the whole area of the plate, and contributions of each layer are summed to give ΔU, the total energy dissipated in the plate. The overall specific damping capacity, Ψ_{ov}, is then given by $\Psi_{ov} = \Delta U/U$. Alternatively, the damping can first be summed through the thickness of the damped element to give a damped element stiffness matrix. This can then be treated by standard finite element techniques (Ref 14).

It is useful to express in the mathematical terms the technique described previously. The maximum strain energy, U, is obtained as for an undamped system as follows:

$$U = \frac{1}{2}\int_v \{\varepsilon_{ij}\}^T\{\sigma_{ij}\}dV \qquad \text{(Eq 4)}$$

where ε_{ij} and σ_{ij} are the strains and stresses related to the fiber direction, and V refers to the volume.

This equation may be reduced to a standard form as:

$$U = \tfrac{1}{2}\{\delta\}^T[K]\{\delta\} \qquad \text{(Eq 5)}$$

where $\{\delta\}$ is the nodal point displacement matrix. Here, five degrees of freedom for each nodal point and eight nodal points for each element are used, and $[K]$ is the stiffness matrix. In the evaluation of the maximum strain energy, U, the Young's modulus of 0° and 90° unidirectional fiber-reinforced beams, E_L, E_T, and the shear modulus of a 0° unidirectional rod, G_{LT}, are used, Now:

$$\Delta U = \int_v \delta(\Delta U)dV \qquad \text{(Eq 6)}$$

where $\delta(\Delta U)$ is the energy dissipated in each element, and is defined as:

$$\delta(\Delta U) = \delta(\Delta U_1) + \delta(\Delta U_2) + \delta(\Delta U_{23}) + \delta(\Delta U_{13}) + \delta(\Delta U_{12})$$

$$\delta(\Delta U_1) = \tfrac{1}{2}\Psi_L\varepsilon_{11}\sigma_{11} \quad \delta(\Delta U_2) = \tfrac{1}{2}\Psi_T\varepsilon_{22}\sigma_{22}$$

and

$$\delta(\Delta U_{23}) = \tfrac{1}{2}\Psi_{TT}\varepsilon_{23}\sigma_{23}$$

$$\delta(\Delta U_{13}) = \tfrac{1}{2}\Psi_{LT}\,\varepsilon_{13}\,\sigma_{13}$$

$$\delta(\Delta U_{12}) = \tfrac{1}{2}\Psi_{LT}\,\varepsilon_{12}\,\sigma_{12}$$

where subscript 1 denotes the fiber direction, while 2 and 3 denote the two directions transverse to the direction of the fibers, and Ψ_L, Ψ_T, and Ψ_{LT} are the associated damping capacities that are also obtained from tests on unidirectional beams.

We may now reduce Eq 7 to matrix form as:

$$\Delta U = \tfrac{1}{2}\int_v \{\varepsilon_{ij}\}^T[\Psi]\{\sigma_{ij}\}dV \qquad \text{(Eq 7)}$$

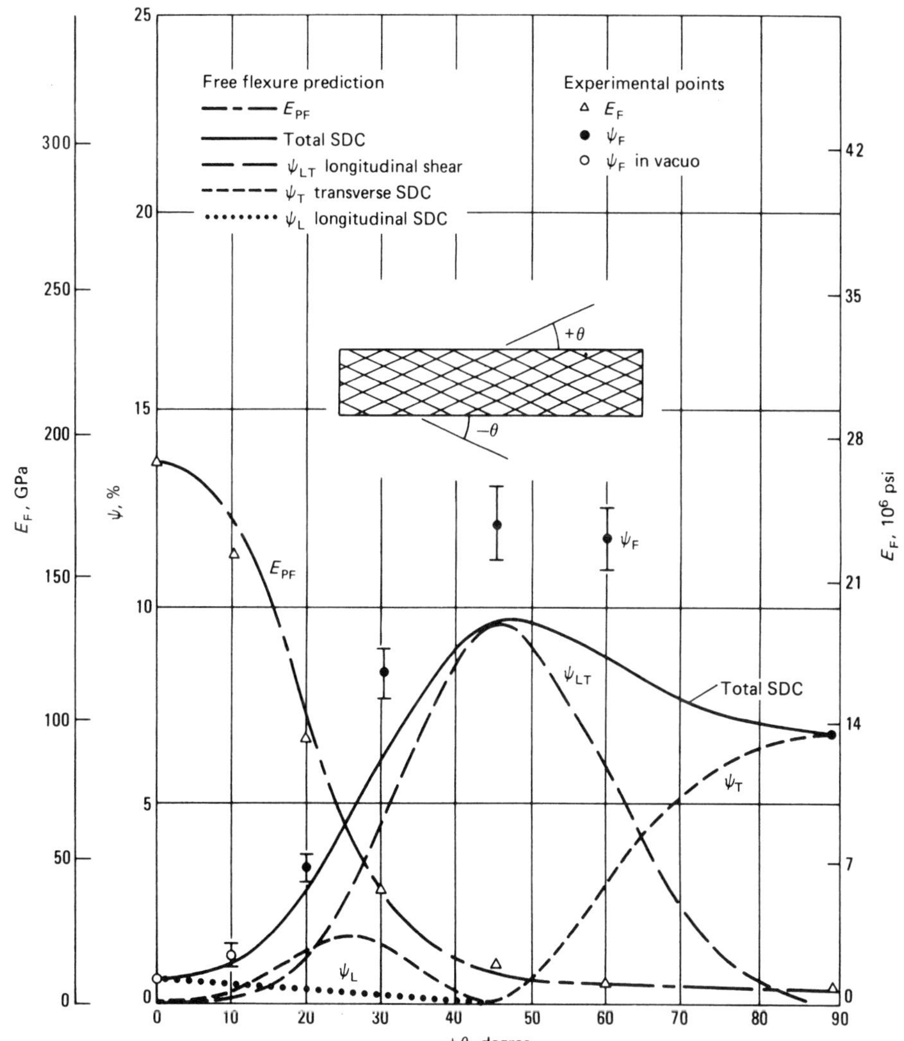

Fig. 11 Variation of flexural Young's modulus (E_f) and damping (Ψ) with ply angle ±θ for high-modulus carbon fiber in DX209 epoxy resin. V_f = 0.5

where:

$$[\Psi]=\begin{bmatrix} \psi_L & 0 & 0 & 0 & 0 \\ 0 & \psi_T & 0 & 0 & 0 \\ 0 & 0 & \psi_{TT} & 0 & 0 \\ 0 & 0 & 0 & \psi_{LT} & 0 \\ 0 & 0 & 0 & 0 & \psi_{LT} \end{bmatrix}$$

Using the same method as with Eq 4, Eq 7 may be reduced to:

$$\Delta_U = \tfrac{1}{2}\{\delta\}^T[K_d]\{\delta\} \qquad \text{(Eq 8)}$$

where $\{\delta\}$ is the same matrix as in Eq 4 and was obtained from the finite-element results. The stiffness matrix of the damped system is $[K_d]$, and it may be evaluated separately. D.X. Lin, R.G. Ni, and R.D. Adams described this method in much more detail (Ref 14).

Some results are given for theoretical predictions and experimental measurements on several plates made from glass or high-modulus carbon fibers in DX210 epoxy resin. The plates were made of 8 or 12 layers of preimpregnated fiber to give different laminate orientations; details of the plates used are given in Table 1. The material properties used in the theoretical prediction are given in Table 2. All the values in this table were established either by using beam specimens cut from a unidirectional plate (longitudinal and transverse damping and Young's moduli) or cylindrical specimens (for measuring the shear modulus and damping in torsion). It should be noted that the value of the torsional damping of a bar with fibers at 90° to the axis, Ψ_{23}, is not important in the prediction, because changing it from 6% to 15% gave no significant difference to the overall theoretical results. In the prediction, Ψ_{23} is taken as the same value as Ψ_{12}, which is the value of torsional damping of a unidirectional rod in longitudinal shear. Because of variations in the fiber volume fraction of the plates, the material properties used in the theoretical prediction were each corrected from a standard set given for 50 vol%, using the method of R.G. Ni and R.D. Adams (Ref 11). The plates were vibrated in the free-free condition (with all the edges freely supported). Although hinged or clamped edges can be readily incorporated into the finite element model, they are not easy to reproduce in an experiment. Figures 13 and 14 show, for the first six free-free modes, the theoretical prediction and experimental results of CFRP plates for various fiber orientations. On the whole, there is good agreement between the predicted and measured values. Mode 6 in plate 3 could not be obtained experimentally because the input energy from the transient technique used for measuring the frequency and damping (Ref 15) was insufficient. Figures 15 and 16 give

Table 1 Plate data

Plate number	Material	No. of layers	Density, g/cm³	V_f	Ply orientation
1	CFRP(a)	8	1.446	0.342	$(0°, 90°, 0°, 90°)_s$(b)
2	CFRP	12	1.636	0.618	$(0°, -60°, 60°, 0°, -60°, 60°)_s$
3	GFRP	8	1.813	0.451	$(0°, 90°, 0°, 90°)_s$
4	GFRP	12	2.003	0.592	$(0°, -60°, 60°, 0°, -60°, 60°)_s$

(a) Using high-modulus carbon fiber. (b) *s* represents midplane symmetric.

Table 2 Moduli and damping values for materials used in the plates

	E_L		E_T		G_{LT}						
Material	GPa	10^6 psi	GPa	10^6 psi	GPa	10^6 psi	ψ_L, %	ψ_T, %	ψ_{LT}, %	ν_1,ν_2	V_f
HMS-DX210(a)	172.1	30.0	7.20	1.04	3.76	0.55	0.45	4.22	7.05	0.3	0.50
Glass-DX210	37.87	5.49	10.90	1.58	4.91	0.71	0.87	5.05	6.91	0.3	0.50
DX210-$BF_3$400	3.21	0.47	3.21	0.47	1.20	0.17	6.54	6.54	6.68	0.34	0

(a) HMS, high-modulus carbon fiber

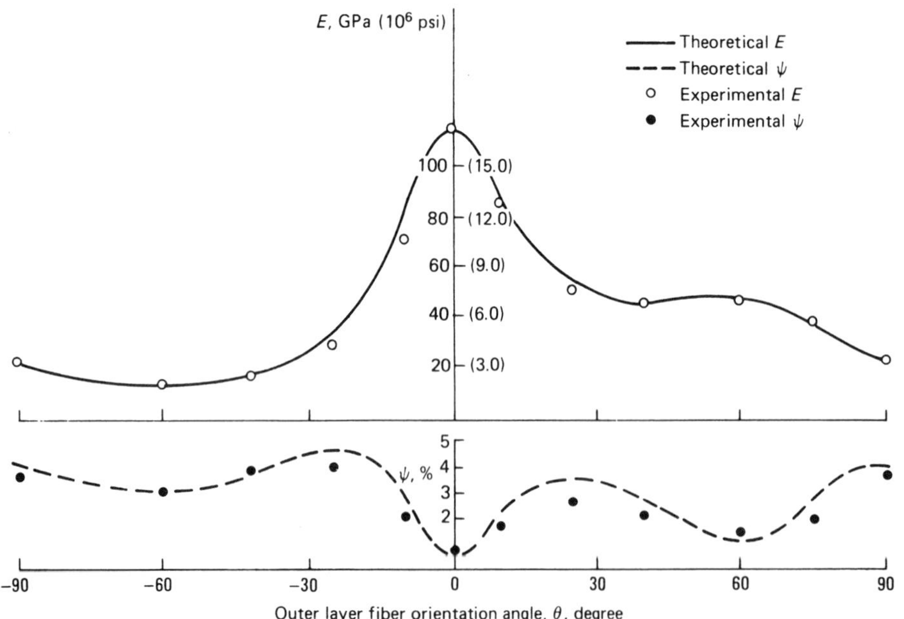

Fig. 12 Variation of flexural modulus (E) and damping (Ψ) with outer layer fiber orientation angle (θ) for $0°, -60°, 60°)_s$ made from high-modulus carbon fibers in DX210 epoxy resin

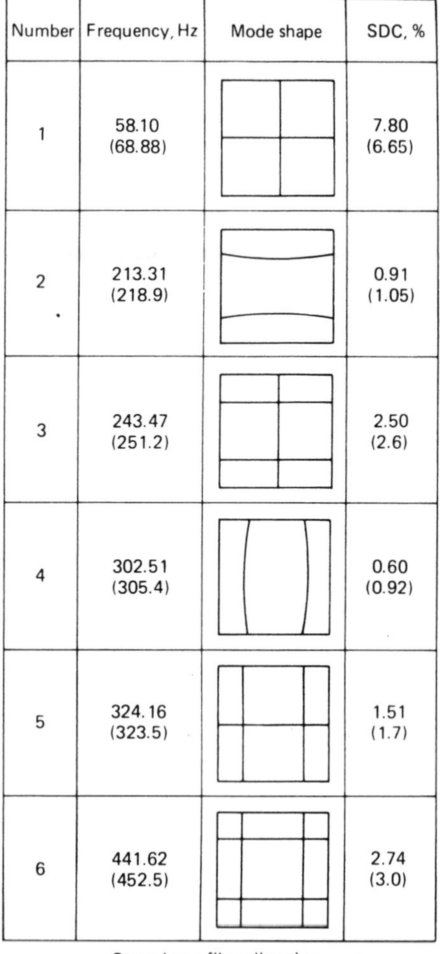

Fig. 13 Natural frequency and damping of various modes of an eight-layer $(0°, 90°, 0°, 90°)_s$ CFRP plate (plate 1). Experimental values in parentheses

the results for GFRP plates in free-free vibration. All show good agreement between prediction and measurement.

The effect of air damping and the additional energy dissipation associated with the supports affect the results of the very low damping modes, such as mode 4 of plate 1, mode 4 of plate 3, and so on. These are essentially beam modes in which the large majority of the strain energy is stored in tension/compression in the fibers and not in matrix tension or shear. However, the results for all the plates used are satisfactory, even when the specimens have imperfections, such as slight variations in thickness and the nominal angle of the fibers (±2° to (±3° error). It can be said that the more twisting there is, the higher the damping. For instance, for an eight-layer cross-ply (0°/90°) GFRP plate (Fig. 15), the two beam-type modes, that is, modes 2 and 3, appear to be similar, but the relationship of the nodal lines to the outer fiber direction means that the higher mode has much less damping than the lower one. The other modes of vibration of this plate all involve much more plate twisting, and hence matrix shear, than do modes 2 and 3, and so the damping is higher.

Design Considerations for Plates. It is important for designers to realize the significance of these results, which show that for all the plates, the damping values are different for each mode. For instance, for the all-0° square GFRP plate in Fig. 17, the damping of the first mode was over 14 times that of the sixth mode. Also, it should be noted that some modes may have much less damping than others, especially when most of the fibers are in one direction. If such a low-damping mode has its natural frequency close to or in the frequency range of any excitation, it may well lead to excessive motion and cause fatigue, noise radiation, component malfunction, and so on.

D.X. Lin, R.G. Ni, and R.D. Adams (Ref 14) showed how the prediction of natural frequencies and damping values could be simplified for geometrically similar structures by using a series of design charts. First, the damping is a function only of the mode shape. Thus, for a series of square plates with a given fiber orientation, the damping value of each mode is constant, irrespective of the dimensions of the plate. It should be noted that the damping of epoxy and similar high-performance resins is not frequency-dependent in the way that is normally associated with thermoplastics, except near the glass transition temperature, which would normally be outside the design range, even though aerospace structures have wide temperature range of operation. Furthermore the natural frequencies can all be scaled from a series of simple numbers, or read off a design chart. Figure 17 shows such a chart for an all-0° GFRP plate that has a volume fraction of 0.50. For a given mode, the natural frequency of the ith mode, f_i, is given by $f_i = k_i h/a^2$, where h is the plate thickness and a is its side length. Thus, it is possible, by using charts such as those in Fig. 17, to determine quickly and accurately the natural frequency and damping of any of the first six modes of a square plate with that particular fiber arrangement.

Because the volume fraction can also change, it is necessary to construct a further series of graphs to allow for this. Figure 18 shows the

Number	Frequency, Hz	Mode shape	SDC, %
1	165.17 (156.6)		1.44 (1.40)
2	279.14 (272.0)		0.93 (0.88)
3	387.8 (372.3)		0.63 (0.65)
4	432.57 (407.8)		1.23 (1.26)
5	511.43 (486.1)		0.98 (0.99)
6	800.37 (779)		0.92 —

Outer layer fiber direction ⟶

Fig. 14 Natural frequency and damping of various modes of a 12-layer (0°, –60°, 60°, 0°, –60°, 60°)$_s$ CFRP plate (plate 2). Experimental values in parentheses

Number	Frequency, Hz	Mode shape	SDC, %
1	66.42 (62.2)		7.16 (6.7)
2	131.62 (131.4)		2.47 (2.8)
3	164.46 (159.2)		1.62 (1.9)
4	189.79 (180.5)		4.87 (4.9)
5	208.87 (200.05)		3.73 (3.2)
6	347.16 (326.7)		5.09 (5.8)

Outer layer fiber direction ⟶

Fig. 15 Natural frequency and damping of various modes of an eight-layer (0°, 90°, 0°, 90°)$_s$ GFRP plate (plate 3). Experimental values in parentheses

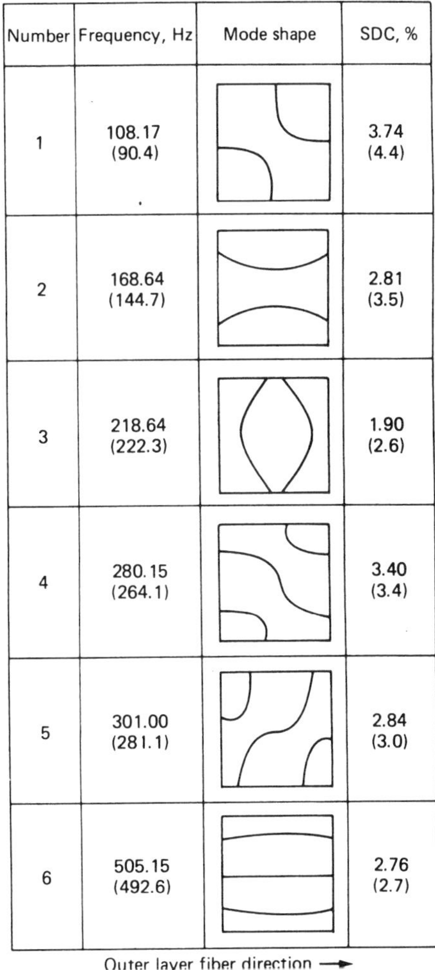

Number	Frequency, Hz	Mode shape	SDC, %
1	108.17 (90.4)		3.74 (4.4)
2	168.64 (144.7)		2.81 (3.5)
3	218.64 (222.3)		1.90 (2.6)
4	280.15 (264.1)		3.40 (3.4)
5	301.00 (281.1)		2.84 (3.0)
6	505.15 (492.6)		2.76 (2.7)

Outer layer fiber direction ⟶

Fig. 16 Natural frequency and damping of various modes of a 12-layer (0°, –60°, +60°, 0°, –60°, +60°)$_s$ GFRP plate (plate 4). Experimental values in parentheses

variation of natural frequency and damping of an all-0° GFRP plate with volume fraction. Again, the damping will not change with plate dimensions (h and a), although it does decrease as the volume fraction increases. Figure 18 is based on a plate for which $h/a^2 = 0.032\ m^{-1}$. Now, because:

$$f_i = k_i h/a^2$$

k_i must be some function of *inter alia*, the volume fraction. Thus:

$$\frac{f_i}{f_i'} = \frac{h}{h'}\left(\frac{a'}{a}\right)^2$$

and by cross-correlating from charts such as those given in Fig. 17 and 18, it is possible to predict the damping and frequency of a given mode as h, a, and V_f vary (Ref 14).

Woven Fibrous Composites

Woven fiber-reinforce plastics are becoming increasingly important because they have the following advantages over laminates made from individual layers of unidirectional material:

- Improved formability and drape
- Bidirectional reinforcement in a single layer
- Improved impact resistance
- Balanced properties in the fabric plane

The woven composite is formed by interlacing two sets of threads, the warp and the weft, in a wide variety of weaves and balances.

Figure 19 shows the damping results obtained by cutting a series of beans at various angles, θ, from a 16-ply plate of CFRP. The fibers were woven to a balanced five-harness satin weave pattern in which one weft thread was interwoven with every fifth warp thread. This weave is the most widely used in laminates, because it gives higher mechanical properties than do plain and twill weaves, due to reduced crimping. The damping increases from about 1% at θ = 0° and 90° to a maximum of about 6% at θ = 45°. R.G. Ni and R.D. Adams' prediction (Ref 11) for a 0°/90° cross-ply made from unidirectional laminae is also shown on Fig. 19, and is in reasonable agreement with the experimental data for the woven material. The damping of the woven material is modified because the twisting of the specimens is restrained internally by the perpendicular arrangement of the warp and weft threads.

While further work is necessary to characterize the various weaves, it appears that the results will, at first approximation, be similar to those for laminates made from unidirectional laminae with the same in-lane fiber orientations.

Sandwich Laminates

To maximize the stiffness of GFRP laminates, it is common to add thin skins of CFRP. R.G. Ni, D.X. Lin, and R.D. Adams (Ref 16) made mathematical predictions of the dynamic properties of such hybrid laminates. They obtained excellent agreement between their experimental results and their theoretical predictions for the damping and moduli of plates, and of beams cut from these plates. These authors also showed how to maximize both the stiffness of a laminate from the ratio of the amounts of glass and carbon, and their relative costs.

The theoretical analysis showed that the effect of the core material on the flexural modulus and damping of this type of hybrid is generally not great. This allows some freedom in choosing the orientation of the GFRP core, and even in the selection of core materials.

Effect of Temperature

Many composites are based on polymeric matrices, usually epoxy resins, for which there are temperature-dependent damping capacities and moduli. While the influence of frequency on damping and modulus is not as strong for epoxies as it is for the high-damping polymers, as used in constrained-layer and similar damping treatments, it is not negligible. Figure 20 shows the change of E_L, E_T, and G_{LT} of a unidirectional CFRP composite over the range of –50 to +200 °C (–60 to +390 °F). (The matrix material was DX209 epoxy resin cured for 2 h at 180 °C (355 °F) and postcured for 6 h at 150 °C (300 °F).) A logarithmic scale was used, and it can be seen that the 2 matrix-dependent moduli, E_t and G_{LT}, were significantly reduced at temperatures above 150 °C (300 °F). Indeed, the transverse specimen (90° orientation) could not be tested at temperatures above 150 °C (300 °F), as it sagged under its own weight. In contrast, the 0° modulus was essentially unaffected until the matrix became shear soft, at which point the deformation became more by shear than by bending and fiber deformation. Figure 21 shows damping on a logarithmic scale and the much higher damping levels that are available in shear and transverse loading than in longitudinal tension/compression. The Ψ_L damping is due not only to increased matrix damping, according to the rule of mixtures, but also to the enhanced shear deformation referred to previously. The damping

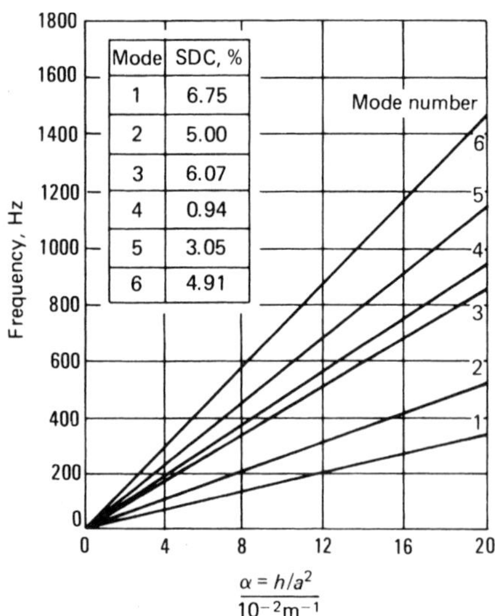

Fig. 17 Variation of natural frequencies and damping with the ratio of thickness to the area of a square plate (all 0°) GFRP. $V_f = 0.50$

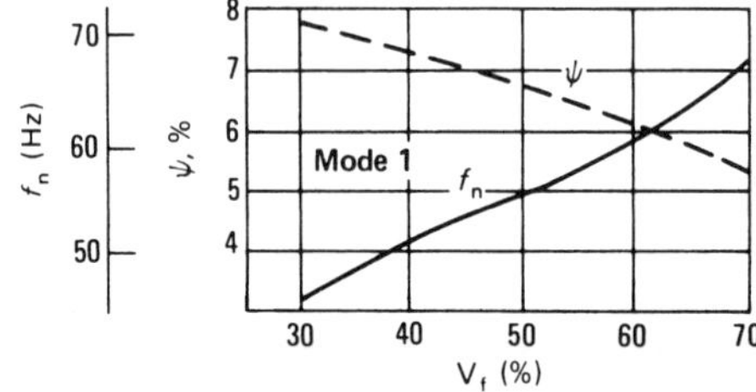

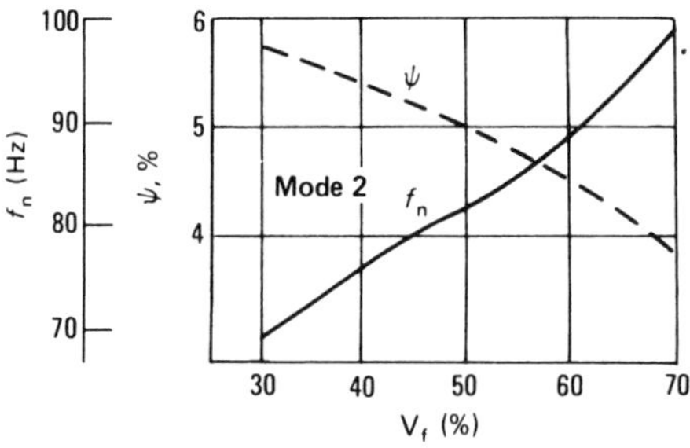

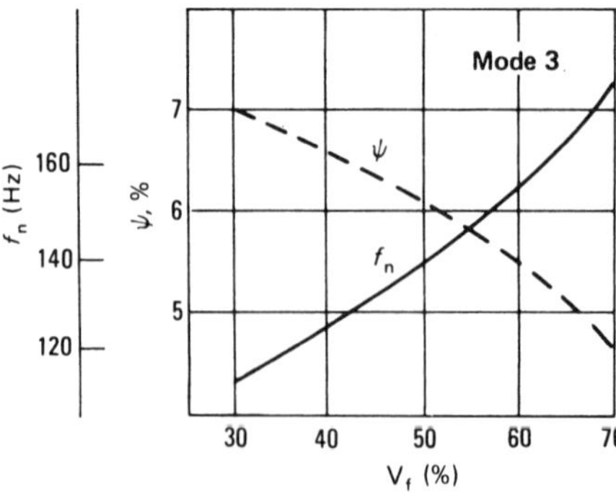

Fig. 18 Variation of natural frequencies (f_n) and damping (Ψ) of a GFRP (all 0°) plate with fiber volume fraction (V_f). $\alpha = h/a^2 = 0.32\ m^{-1}$

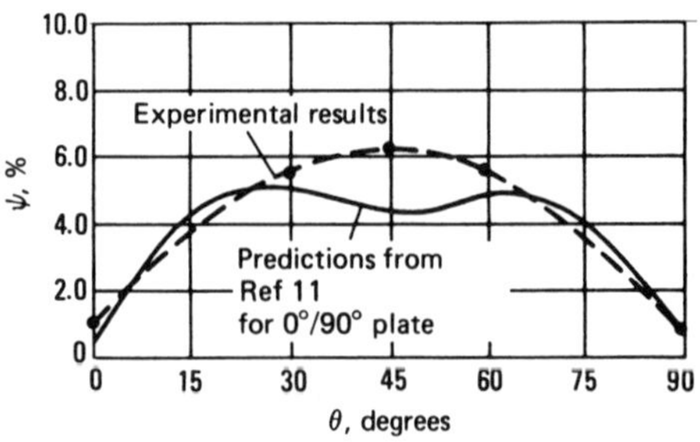

Fig. 19 Variation of specific damping capacity (Ψ) for a series of beams cut at various angles (θ) from a woven 16-ply CFRP plate

peak, at about 180 °C (360 °F), represents classical viscoelastic behavior. Testing beyond 200 °C (390 °F) was impossible because of charring.

At lower temperatures, the β relaxation phenomenon comes into effect. This is illustrated in Fig. 22 for a cryogenic grade, woven glass-fiber-reinforced epoxy material.

To achieve a wide range of resin properties, a standard resin was modified by the addition of a flexibilizer. By varying the proportions of resin to flexibilizer, precondensates with different glass transition temperatures were formed. Shell Epikote 828 (Shell Oil Co.) was used as the standard resin and flexibilized by the addition of Epikote 871 in the proportions 1:1 and 2:1 (828/871) by weight to give FO (pure 828), F50 (50% flexibilizer), and F33 (33% flexibilizer). The resin was made into prepreg with type II (high-tensile strength) carbon fiber and laminates pre-

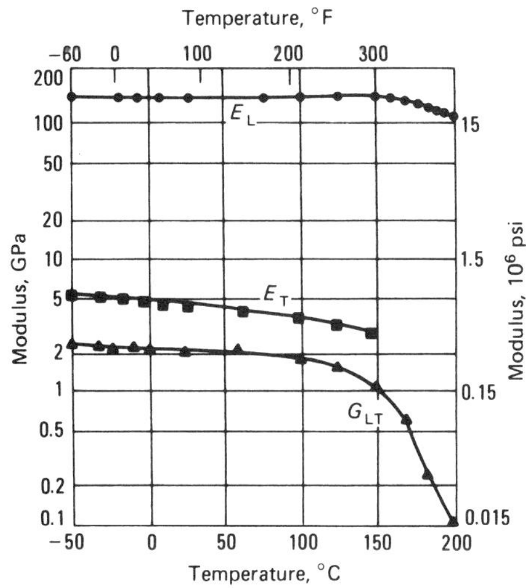

Fig. 20 Variation of longitudinal modulus (E_L), transverse modulus (E_T), and longitudinal shear modulus (G_{LT}) with temperature for high-modulus carbon fibers in DX209 epoxy resin. V_f = 0.5

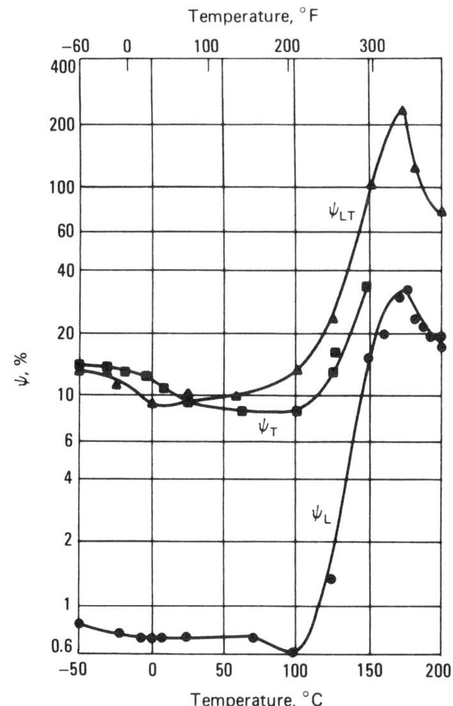

Fig. 21 Variation of longitudinal damping (Ψ_L), transverse damping (Ψ_{LT}) with temperature for high-modulus carbon fibers in DX209 epoxy resin. V_f = 0.5

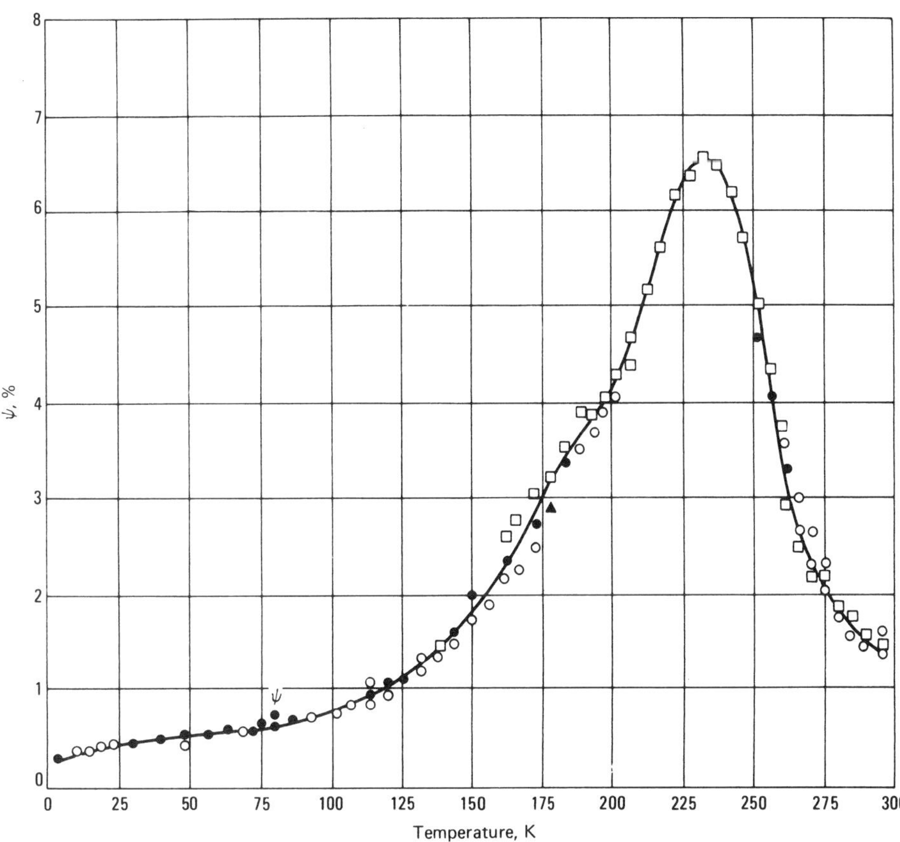

Fig. 22 Variation of specific damping capacity (Ψ) with temperature for a glass cloth-epoxy specimen

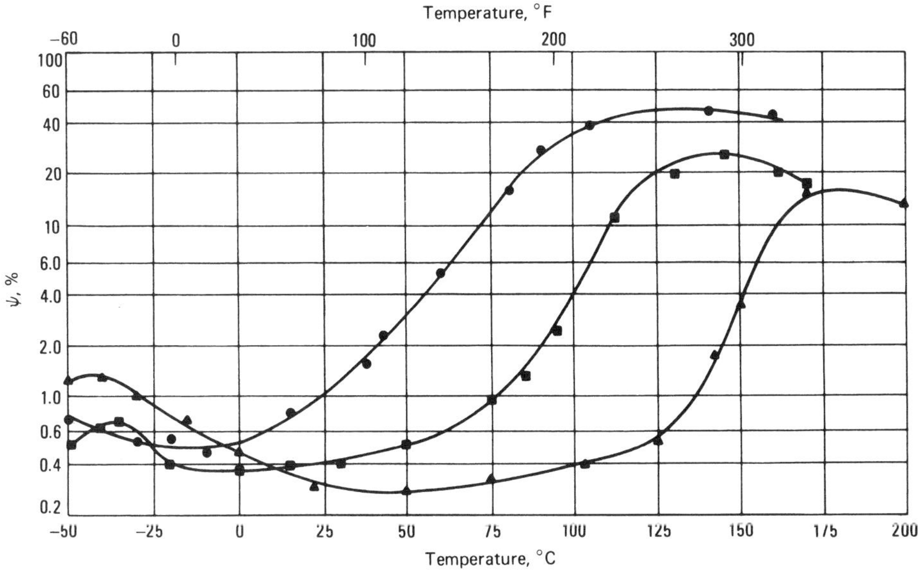

Fig. 23 Variation of specific damping capacity (Ψ) with temperature for 0° unidirectional composite made from Epikote flexibilized resin. V_f = 0.5

pared from it. Figure 23 shows that increasing the flexibilizer content increases the damping and decreases the glass transition temperature.

Figure 24 shows the combined effect of fiber orientation and temperature on the flexural damping of a series of beams cut at various angles from a unidirectional plate (type II carbon fibers in DX209 epoxy resin). The damping results of specimens with angles of 0° to 40° are presented in Fig. 24; specimens from 50° to 70° (not shown) showed very little difference in behavior. The frequency of vibration used in measuring the glass transition temperature varied from 324 Hz for the 0° specimen to 120 Hz for the 40° specimen. There was a reduction of the peak temperature of about 10 °C over the range of fiber angles of 0° to 20°.

The damping properties near the relaxation peaks for a range of frequencies are given for ±10° and ±20° specimens (Fig. 25). In both cases, there is a reduction of the damping peak with increase of frequency. A comparison of traces with approximately the same frequency at the peak (that is, 249 Hz, ±10° and 235 Hz, ±20°), showed that the damping was almost identical, at about 53% SDC, but that the peak temperature for the ±20° specimen was nearly 20 °C (36 °F) below that of the ±10° specimen. The contribution of shear damping for the ±20° specimen is much larger than is that for the ±10° specimen (Fig. 11), and the longitudinal tensile component is almost negligible. However, due to the fairly high flexural modulus of the ±10° specimen, $E\pm10$, and its relatively low torsion modulus, $G\pm10$, there will be shear deformation in flexure. The difference between the two types of shears is one of direction; the flexural shear is denoted by σ_{zx} where z is perpendicular to the plane of the laminate, and the shear that is due to the fiber angle is denoted by σ_{xy}. For 0° specimens, σ_{zx} and σ_{xy} lie in the plane of symmetry, and the effect will be identical, but for more complex laminates involving adjacent laminae at different angles, the result is not as obvious.

The effect of temperature on flexural modulus depends to a large extent on the lay-up; where the fiber angle is near 0°, there is only a small reduction at high temperatures, but at larger fiber angles (20 to 90°), the modulus can decrease by more than an order of magnitude.

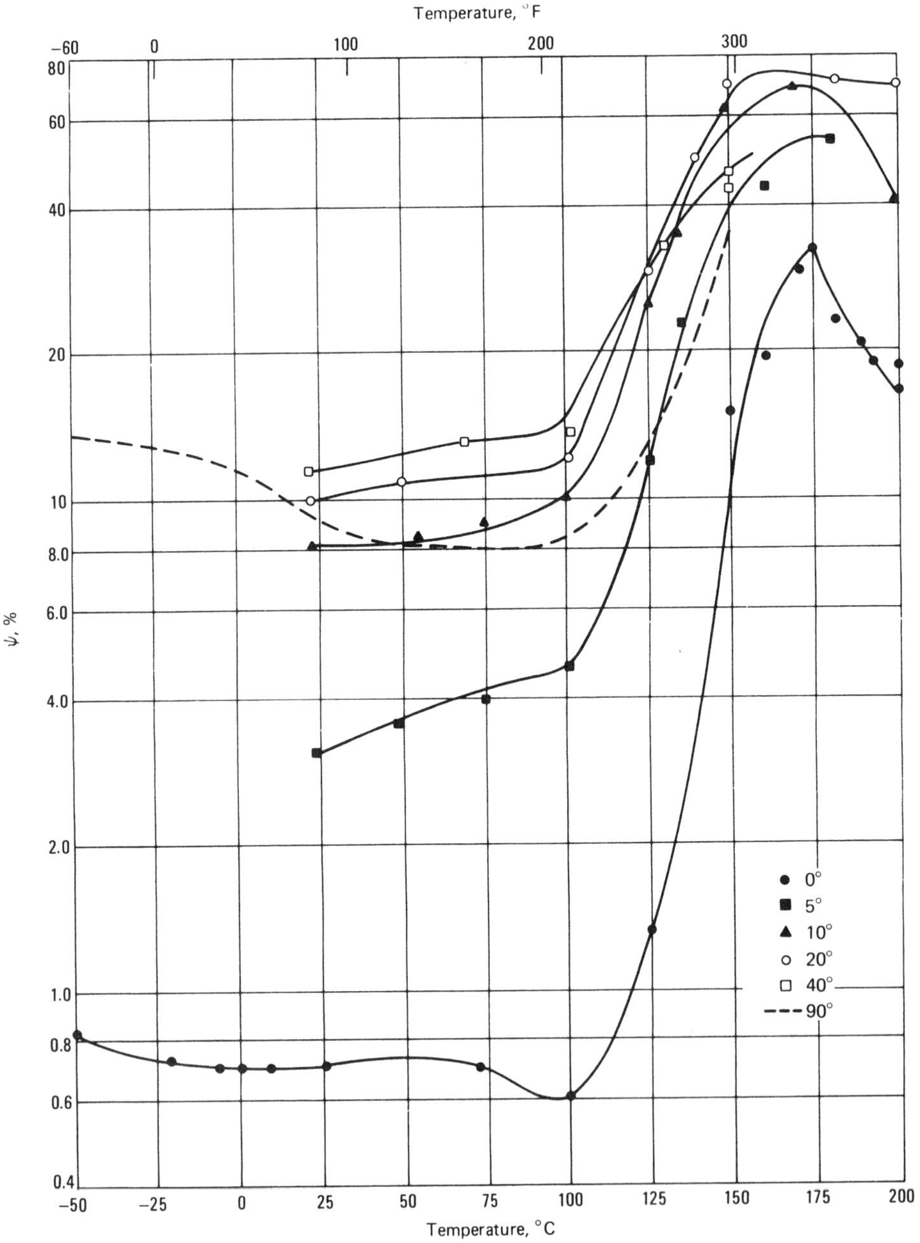

Fig. 24 The effect of fiber orientation on the variation of specific damping capacity (Ψ) with temperature for high-modulus carbon fibers in DX209 epoxy resin. $V_f = 0.5$

Relationship Between Damping and Strength

If improving damping properties of a laminate at no detriment to its mechanical properties is an objective, it is interesting to examine the differences between ±15° angle plies and 0°/90° cross plies. In flexure, the strengths and moduli are almost identical for the range of fibers, whereas the damping of the angle plies is double that of the cross plies. In torsion, the shear moduli of angle plies are largely dependent on the fiber modulus and are much larger than the cross-ply shear moduli, the values of which are nominally

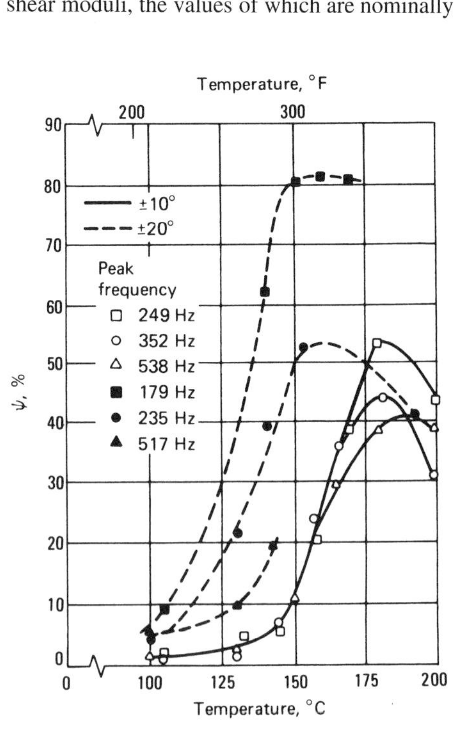

Fig. 25 Variation of specific damping capacity (Ψ) with temperature for ±10° and ±20° angle-plies made from high-modulus carbon fibers in DX209 epoxy resin. $V_f = 0.5$

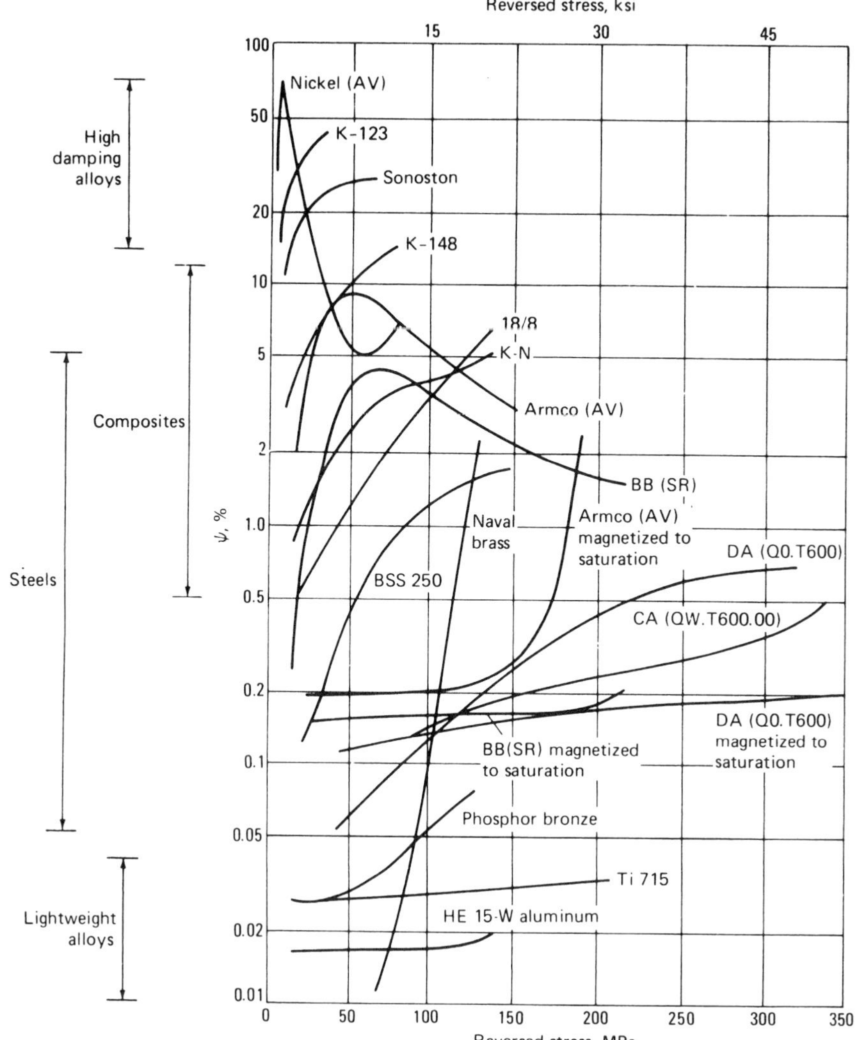

Fig. 26 Specific damping capacity (Ψ) versus stress for a range of ferrous and nonferrous metals. Nickel (AV), annealed in vacuum. K-123, K-148, K-N, grades of cast iron. 18/8, stainless steel. Armco (AV), low-carbon, iron, annealed in vacuum, BB(SR), 0.12% carbon steel, stress relieved. BSS 250, Naval brass, and phosphor bronze are copper-based alloys. CA, DA, high-carbon steels. HE 15-W, Duralumin aluminum alloy. Ti 715, titanium alloy

independent of fiber modulus. The damping of angle plies is, in this latter case, less than half that of the cross plies.

Thus, different lamination geometries and fiber moduli can be arranged to give some common properties between laminates while having very different properties in other modes. In design, this gives greater flexibility to cater for strength and stiffness in one direction, with optional properties in others, according to requirements, than can possibly be achieved with isotropic materials. The damping properties of laminates can now be added to these design parameters (Ref 17).

Composites Versus Metals

To put the damping of composites in context, a comparison should be made with the damping of metals. Figure 26 shows the variation of damping with cyclic stress amplitude for a range of common structural metals. The metallic specimens were tested in axial vibration (tension/compression) using the apparatus described by R.D. Adams and A.L Percival (Ref 18); more details of the results are given in Ref 19 and 20. Composites provide slightly higher damping than steels, but significantly less than conventional high-damping alloys. On the other hand, low-weight high-strength alloys such as aluminum and titanium give extremely low damping; values of less than 0.01% SDC have been reported (Ref 21).

ACKNOWLEDGMENTS

This article is adapted from R.D. Adams, Damping Properties Analysis of Composites, *Composites*, Vol 1, *Engineered Materials Handbook*, ASM International, 1987, p 206–217.

REFERENCES

1. S.A. Suarez, R.F. Gibson, C.T. Sun, and S.K. Chaturvedi, The Influence of Fiber Length and Fiber Orientation on Damping and Stiffness of Polymer Composite Materials, *Exp. Mech.*, Vol 26, 1986, p 175–184
2. R.D. Adams and D.G.C. Bacon, The Dynamic Properties of Unidirectional Fibre Reinforced Composites in Flexure and Torsion, *J. Compos. Mater.*, Vol 7, 1973, p 53–67
3. D.F. Adams and D.R. Doner, Longitudinal Shear Loading of a Unidirectional Composite, *J. Compos. Mater.*, Vol 1, 1967, p 4–17
4. Z. Hashin, Complex Moduli of Viscoelastic Composites, II, Fibre Reinforce Materials, *Int. J. Solids Struct.*, Vol 6, 1970, p 797–804
5. R.G. Ni and R.D. Adams, A Rational Method for Obtaining the Dynamic Mechanical Properties of Laminae for Predicting the Stiffness and Damping of Laminated Plates and Beams, *Composites*, Vol 15, 1984, p 193–199
6. R.D. Adams and D.F Short, The Effect of Fibre Diameter on the Dynamic Properties of Glass-Fibre-Reinforced Polyester Resin, *J. Phys. D. Appl. Phys.*, Vol 6, 1973, p 1032–1039
7. R.D. Adams, The Dynamic Longitudinal Shear Modulus and Damping of Carbon Fibres, *J. Phys. D., Appl. Phys.*, Vol 8, 1975, p 738–748
8. S.W. Tsai and H.T. Halpin, *Introduction to Composite Materials*, Technomic Publishing Co., Westport, CT, 1980
9. S. Chang and C.W. Bert, Analysis of Damping for Filamentary Composite Materials, *Composite Materials in Engineering Design*, B.R. Noton, Ed., American Society for Metals, 1973, p 51–62
10. R.D. Adams and D.G.C. Bacon, Effect of Fibre Orientation and Laminate Geometry on the Dynamic Properties of CFRP, *J. Compos. Mater.*, Vol 7, 1973, p 402–428
11. R.G. Ni and R.D. Adams, The Damping and Dynamic Moduli of Symmetric Laminated Composite Beams—Theoretical and Experimental Results, *J. Compos. Mater.*, Vol 18, 1984, p 104–121
12. M.M. Wallace and C.W. Bert, Transfer-Matrix Analysis of Dynamic Response of Composite-Material Structural Elements With Material Damping, *Shock & Vib. Bull.* 50, Part 3, Sept 1980, p 27–38
13. P. Cawley and R.D. Adams, The Predicted and Experimental Natural Modes of Free-Free CFRP Plates, *J. Compos. Mater.*, Vol 13, 1978, p 336–347
14. D.X. Lin, R.G. Ni, and R.D. Adams, Prediction and Measurement of the Vibrational

Damping Parameters of Carbon and Glass Fibre-Reinforced Plastics Plates, *J. Compos. Mater.*, Vol 18, 1984, p 132–152

15. D.X. Lin and R.D. Adams, Determination of the Damping Properties of Structures by Transient Testing Using Zoom-FFT., *J. Phys. E., Sci. Instrum.*, Vol 18, 1985, p 161–165
16. R.G. Ni, D.X. Lin, and R.D. Adams, The Dynamic Properties of Carbon-Glass Fibre Sandwich-Laminated Composites: Theoretical, Experimental and Economic Considerations, *Composites*, Vol 15, 1984, p 297–304
17. R.D. Adams and D.G.C. Bacon, The Effect of Fibre Modulus and Surface Treatment on the Modulus, Damping, and Strength of Carbon-Fibre-Reinforced Plastics, *J. Phys. D., Appl. Phys.*, Vol 7, 1974, p 7–23
18. R.D. Adams and A.L Percival, Measurement of the Strain-Dependent Damping of Metals in Axial Vibration, *J. Phys. D., Appl. Phys.*, Vol 2, 1969, p 1693–1704
19. R.D. Adams, The Damping Characteristics of Certain Steels, Cast Irons, and Other Metals, *J. Sound and Vibr.*, Vol 23, 1972, p 199–216
20. R.D. Adams, Damping of Ferromagnetic Materials at Direct Stress Levels Below the Fatigue Limit, *J. Phys. D., Appl. Phys.*, Vol 5, 1972, p 1877–1889
21. G.A. Cottell, K.M. Entwistle, and F.C. Thompson, The Measurement of the Damping Capacity of Metals in Torsional Vibration, *J. Inst. Metals*, Vol 74, 1948, p 373–424

Bolted and Bonded Joints

L.J. Hart-Smith, The Boeing Company

THE STRUCTURAL EFFICIENCY of a composite structure is established, with very few exceptions, by its joints, not by its basic structure. Joints can be manufacturing splices planned at predetermined locations in the structure or unplanned repairs that could be needed anywhere in the structure. Consequently, unless a specific application needs no provision for repairs or uses throw-away unrepairable components, the correct sequence for design is to first locate and size the joints, in fiber patterns optimized for that task, and then fill in the gaps (the basic structure) in between.

This sequence is a marked departure from normal practice for conventional ductile metal alloys and is necessitated by the relative brittleness of fiber-reinforced composites. Yielding of ductile metals usually reduces the stress concentrations around bolt holes so that there is only a loss of area, with no stress concentration at ultimate load on the remaining (net) section at the joints. With composites, however, there is no relief at all from the elastic stress concentration if the holes or cutouts are large enough. Even for small holes in composite structures, the stress-concentration relief is far from complete, although the local disbonding (between the fibers and resin matrix and local intraply and interply splitting close to the hole edge) does locally alleviate the most severe stress concentrations.

The reason for emphasizing the importance of joints in the design of composite structures is that the availability of large computer optimization programs and the highly deficient treatment of residual thermal stresses within the resin in most of the composite laminate theories have combined to create the illusion that optimized composite structures will necessarily be highly orthotropic and tailored precisely to match the load conditions and stiffness requirements. (There are no terms in most theories to allow for separate residual thermal stresses in the fibers or matrix of the monolayer, which serves as the building block for cross-plied laminate theories. The omission is due to the artificial homogenization of distinctly two-phase composite materials into mathematically simpler one-phase models. Fortunately, there is finally one mechanistic theory—see the article "Characterizing Strength for Structural Design" in this Volume and Ref 1 and 2—in which there is a proper distinction between the fiber and resin constituents in fiber-polymer composites. Separate characterization of each failure mechanism in each constituent has shown that only a few true materials properties are needed to explain what appear to be many different loading conditions at the laminate and lamina level. The progressively more widespread use of this approach will lead to far less reliance on empiricism and costly testing than has been necessary in the past.)

If composite structures were highly orthotropic and precisely tailored, the task of designing joints in composites would be much more difficult than it is now. The capability of bolted joints in such highly orthotropic materials is often unacceptably low. Hence, the laminate can never be loaded to the levels suggested by lamination theory for unnotched laminates.

Fortunately, or unfortunately, depending on one's point of view, the strength of composite structures with both loaded and unloaded holes depends only slightly on the fiber pattern (for nearly quasi-isotropic laminates); the stress-concentration factor increases almost as rapidly as the unnotched strength for slightly orthotropic patterns. Indeed, throughout the range of fiber patterns surrounding the quasi-isotropic lay-up, the bearing strengths and gross-section strengths are almost constant, which simplifies the design process considerably. A valid case can often be made for a small amount of orthotropy, within the shaded area in Fig. 1, particularly when there is a preferred load direction or stiffness require-

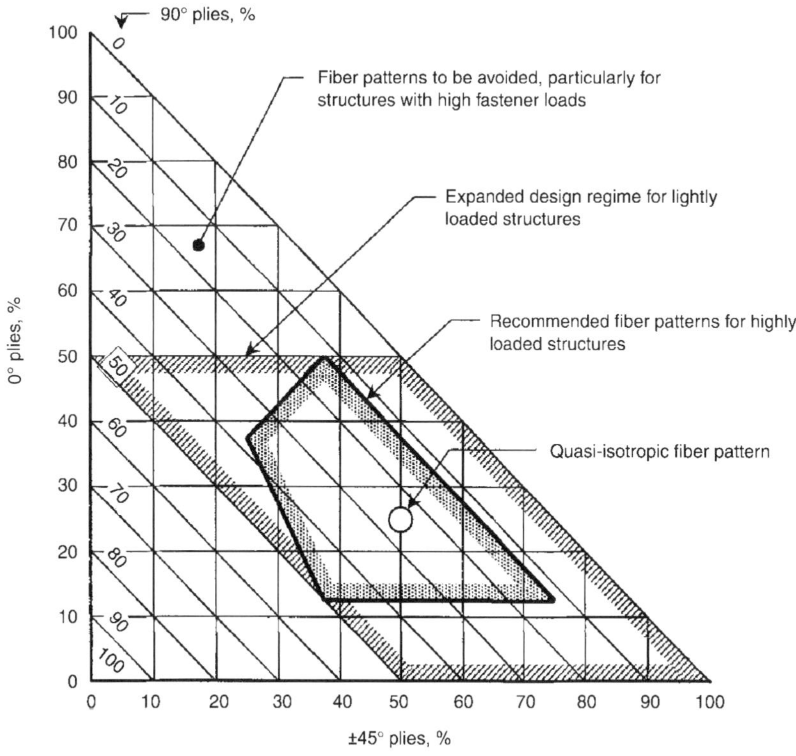

Fig. 1 Selection of lay-up pattern for fiber-reinforced composite laminates. All fibers in 0°, +45°, 90°, or −45° direction. Note: lightly loaded minimum gage structures tend to encompass a greater range of fiber patterns than indicated, because of the unavailability of thinner plies.

ment that must be met. The farther a laminate pattern is outside the shaded area, the more likely it is to fail prematurely by through-the-thickness cracks parallel to the maximum concentration of fibers.

Even for those few truly non-strength-critical uses of highly orthotropic fiber patterns, such as space structures with zero coefficient of thermal expansion and one-shot missiles, there must be a transition to nearly quasi-isotropic patterns around any bolt holes; the structural efficiency of bolted joints in highly orthotropic laminates is known to be inadequate. Therefore, the material presented here is applicable to all sensible composite structures, although it deliberately excludes mechanical joints in highly orthotropic materials. If joints were assessed in terms of an efficiency comparing the strength of the joint with the strength of the same unnotched laminate, far stronger composite structures would be designed than have been when this consideration has been overlooked. As is explained later, it is extremely difficult to attain a 50% joint efficiency (even with multirow bolted joints); even an efficiency of 40% in a single-row joint requires the use of the most appropriate pitch-to-diameter (w/d) ratio. Attention is confined to uniaxial membrane loading, because most of the relevant test data on bolted joints are similarly restricted, and because the analysis methods for off-axis loading and applied bending moments are still being developed.

The design of joints in nearly quasi-isotropic composites is straightforward, once the notion of joint efficiency as a function of geometry is accepted, although it is also necessary to allow for nonlinearities in the material behavior; linearly elastic analyses are far too conservative. The analysis of adhesively bonded joints using elastic-plastic adhesive models has advanced to the stage at which it can legitimately be called a science. The design of straightforward bonded joints has been reduced to following a few procedures and obeying a few simple design refinements to prevent premature failures due to induced peel loads. The design and analysis of the more complex stepped-lap bonded joints needed for much thicker and more highly loaded bonded structures is facilitated by the use of digital computer programs based on nonlinear continuum-mechanics solutions. Even the determination of the design load level for bonded joints is easy, regardless of the nominal applied loads. In no case should the strength of the joint be allowed to fall below that of the surrounding structure; otherwise, the bonded joint would have no damage tolerance and could act as a weak-link fuse. Fortunately, with the strong ductile adhesives typically used by the aerospace industry, the bond is inevitably stronger than the adherends for properly designed joints between thin members. Even for thicker structures, the bond can always be made stronger than the structure by using enough steps in the joint. It has been recognized that it is also necessary to prevent the accumulation of irreversible damage in the adhesive layer by using a sufficiently complex joint geometry to ensure that the application of design limit load does not exceed the linear elastic capability of the adhesive. Recent progress in the prediction of bonded joint strength and resistance to delamination in composite laminates includes the ability to include both shear and peel loads, as well as residual thermal stresses from curing at high temperatures, in the failure criteria (see Ref 2).

The design and analysis of bolted or riveted joints in fibrous composites, however, remains very much an art, because of the need to rely on empirical correction factors in some form or other. Mechanically fastened joints differ from bonded composite joints in one further aspect: the presence of holes ensures that the joint strength can never exceed the local laminate strength. Indeed, after years of research and development, it appears that only the most carefully designed bolted composite joints will be even half as strong as the basic laminate. The simpler bolted joint configurations will attain no more than a third of the laminate strength. However, because the adhesively bonded repair of thick composite laminates is often impossible or impractical (Ref 3), there is a real need for bolted composite structures quite apart from the greater ease of assembly at mechanically fastened manufacturing breaks between subassemblies. A further problem with the design of bolted composite structural joints is that fibrous composites are so brittle that there is virtually no capability for redistributing load, as is afforded by yielding of ductile metals. Consequently, it is very important to calculate accurately the load sharing between fasteners and to identify the most critically loaded one. There is a common misconception that one should always strive for the benign failures associated with bearing-critical bolted joints, because tension-through-the-holes failures are so abrupt. What is not widely appreciated is that the latter failure modes are also associated with far higher bolted composite joint strengths. Also, it is all but impossible to design a multirow bolted joint that *will* fail by bearing.

(The preference for bearing-critical joints also extends to mechanically fastened joints in metallic structures at some aircraft factories. While this might be attainable for virgin structures, the higher bearing stress needed to reduce the net-section stresses inevitably results in the earlier initiation of fatigue cracks at the fastener holes. In the presence of such cracks, late in the life of structures, failure by tension through the reduced net section will undercut any bearing failures, thwarting the original design approach. The point is that specific failure modes are associated with different joint strengths and lives, and that these associations need to be acknowledged when selecting joint geometries.)

Obviously, one can avoid the strength limitations of bolted or riveted composite joints by using such techniques as local pad-ups to thicken chordwise bolt seams on wing skins, for example, and glass softening strips in the skins over the spar caps. However, such an approach precludes the possibility of making repairs with mechanical fasteners throughout the remaining unprotected structure, unless one is prepared to accept a substantial reduction in strength.

This article starts with a discussion of adhesively bonded joints, covering the keys to durability, the elastic-plastic mathematical model for the adhesive in shear, the simple design rules for thin bonded structures, the computer programs for the more highly loaded stepped-lap joints, and the two-dimensional effects associated with load redistribution around flaws and with damage tolerance. Additional information is available in the article "Secondary Adhesive Bonding of Polymer-Matrix Composites" in this Volume.

Mechanically fastened joints are then discussed, starting with the elastic-isotropic geometric stress-concentration factors, the empirically established correlation factors to convert these elastic values to those observed in the composites at failure, the identification of optimal joint proportions for single-row joints, and the design and analysis of the stronger multirow joints, with particular regard to the bearing-bypass interaction. Additional information is available in the article "Mechanical Fastener Selection" in this Volume and in Ref 4 and 5.

Fundamentals of Shear Load Transfer through Adhesively Bonded Joints

Adhesively bonded joints can be strong in shear but are inevitably weak in peel, so the objective of good design practice is to arrange the joint to transfer the applied load in shear and to minimize any direct or induced peel stresses. The details of the design vary with the load intensity (and, hence, the thickness of the adherends), as shown in Fig. 2. The thinner members can be joined effectively by simple, uniformly thick overlaps, while thicker members require the more complex stepped-lap joints.

For each of the joints shown in Fig. 2, the potential shear strength of the bond—that is, the strength that the bond could have developed had the adherends not failed first—exceeds the direct strength of the adherends outside the joint, up to a determinable thickness. This characteristic is shown in Fig. 3, which also shows the loss of bond strength that is sometimes associated with flaws in or damage to the bond. Even with such degradation, the bond will be stronger than the members outside the joint, up to some lesser adherend thickness.

The key point of Fig. 3 is that for adherend thicknesses greater than that for which the bond and member strengths are equal, there can be absolutely no tolerance with respect to flaws, porosity, or damage. The slightest imperfection would lead to catastrophic unzipping of the entire bond area if sufficient load were applied. That is why it is so important that bonded joint strengths *must* exceed those of the adherends, even to the point of exceeding the strength by at least 50% to permit the occurrence of minor

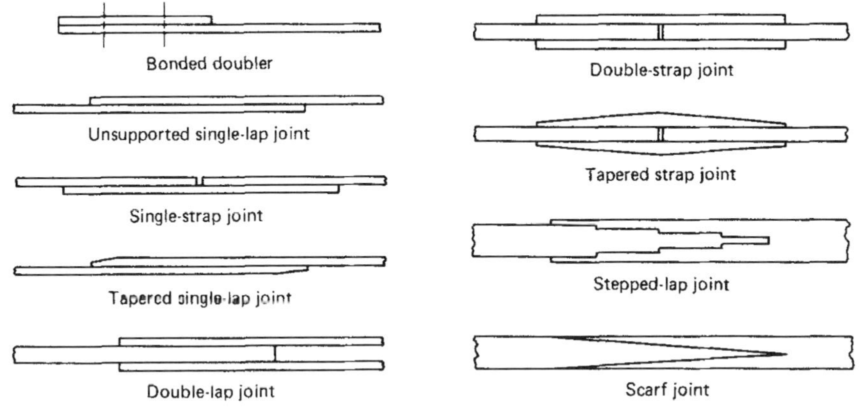

Fig. 2 Adhesively bonded joint types

manufacturing flaws or imperfections. Subject to that proviso, bonded joints between thin members have a remarkable insensitivity to very large local flaws, as explained in Ref 6. In this context, the term "thin" is adjusted to suit the complexity of the joint and refers to those sensible designs for which the nominally perfect bond is stronger than the members being joined. Such a design philosophy for bonded joints should always be followed, even when the nominal applied loads are less than the strength of the members. Otherwise, there will always be the possibility of a local flaw that is large enough to convert the nominally perfect bond into a weak-link fuse. A flaw in an underdesigned joint shares the characteristics of a through crack in a metal sheet, as shown in Fig. 4, except that it is much harder to find. Figure 4 refers equally to metal and composite structures, except that, for the latter, load redistribution around the bond flaw may also cause delaminations in the composite panel or possibly result in the unzipping of the bond.

Adhesive bonds must also be resistant to the environment in which they operate, which is typically thermal or chemical. This need has been demonstrated in the many in-service failures of secondary and, in at least two cases, primary bonded metal structures on U.S. aircraft made during the late 1960s and early 1970s. Those failures were not caused by poor design detailing; indeed, the most recent adhesives failures known to the author that were due to mechanical overloading of bonded aircraft structures occurred over half a century ago on glued wooden aircraft. There were also some structural failures on some wooden aircraft in the tropics during World War II, due to a poor choice of glue, which was very sensitive to moisture. However, those joints were properly proportioned, and even the glue worked adequately in Europe.

Bonded joint failures in metal structures have occurred when the absorption of moisture by some adhesives on the surface of the adherends hydrolyzed and subsequently corroded the oxide surface of clad aluminum alloys. This subject was explored in depth during the U.S. Air Force Primary Adhesively Bonded Structure Technology (PABST) program (Ref 7–9). It is now well known that aluminum alloys must be anodized, in phosphoric or chromic acid, to create a stable, durable oxide surface, and that the surface must be promptly coated with a corrosion-inhibiting primer, usually BR-127 or Redux liquid. Using clad 7075 aluminum alloys should be avoided. Similarly, titanium alloys and steels need appropriate surface preparations for reliable adhesive bonding, as do steels.

Somewhat surprisingly, the need for comparable attention to the preparation of fibrous composite surfaces for adhesive bonding has not received nearly as much publicity. The widespread use of inferior preparations, such as removing no more than a peel ply, or scuff sanding followed by solvent contamination, remains the norm. R.J. Schliekelmann, a pioneer of adhesive bonding of metal structures, has warned of the importance of this issue to composites (Ref 10). L.J. Hart-Smith et al. have strongly recommended light grit blasting as the best known treatment today (Ref 11). This view is shared by A.N. Pocius (Ref 12), who has also advocated mechanical abrasion with Scotch-Brite pads (3M Corporation). Promising work has also been done on composite surface preparation by so-called flash blasting, but no production applications are known yet.

Surprisingly, only the quality-control tests for adhesive bonding of *metallic* structures include both lap-shear tests to confirm the completeness of the cure process for the adhesive *and* wedge-crack (or other peel test) to confirm the *durability* of the joints, under a hostile (hot/wet) environment to accelerate the test. Specification for the manufacture of bonded *composite* structures includes only short-term strength tests and omits any requirements to confirm the durability of such bonds. The need for such additional tests is evident from service experience and is associated with two known phenomena. One is the transfer of release agents from peel plies (see Ref 13); the other is prebond moisture not removed by drying prior to bonding (see Ref 14 and 15). There is as great a need for a durability test as part of the quality-control program for bonded composite structures as there is for bonded metallic structures. Unless this is implemented, no inroads will ever be made on the enormous cost

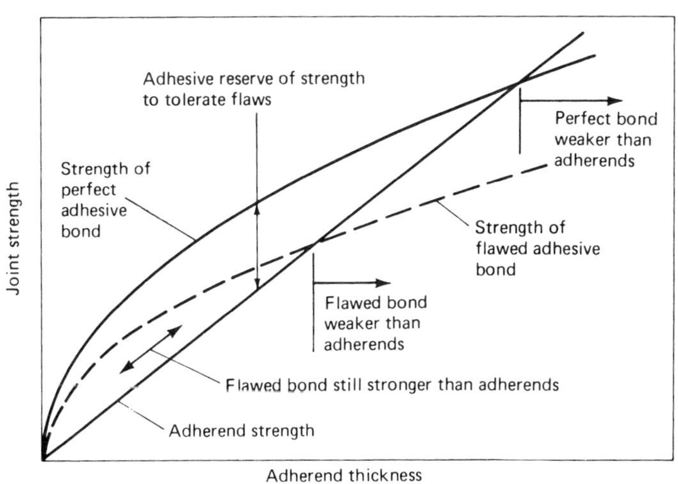

Fig. 3 Relative strength of adhesive and adherends, as affected by bond flaws. τ_p is the maximum shear stress, σ_∞ is the remote skin stress.

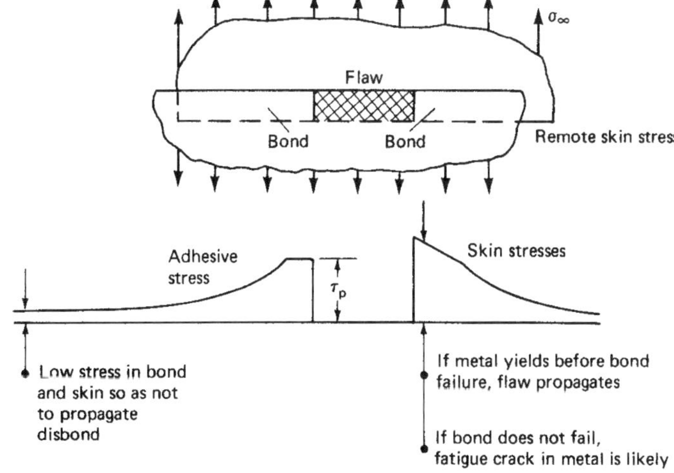

Fig. 4 Redistribution of load at flaws in bond

of inspections that can tell *nothing* about how well the adhesive is stuck (only whether or not a gap has opened up between the adherends). These inspections would be rendered unnecessary by assurance that potential interfacial failures between adhesive and adherends had been precluded by proper processing at the time of manufacture.

The subsequent discussion in this article assumes that the durability of the surfaces to be bonded has been ensured by appropriate preparation. Otherwise, just as for metal bonding, no reliable life can be established for adhesively bonded composite structures.

The subject of environmental durability of the adhesive layer itself, rather than of the interface, is much more straightforward and can benefit from the massive amount of testing already done for metal bonding. The adhesive resin can be regarded as a well-behaved engineering material up to some service temperature, which depends on the amount of plasticizing additives as well as on the base resin. That temperature, called the glass transition temperature, can be reduced slightly by the absorption of moisture. Increasing the glass transition temperature for bonding on supersonic aircraft, or near engines, has meant sacrificing most of the adhesive strength at lower temperatures by omitting the modification of the basic epoxy or phenolic resin by rubber, nylon, or vinyl additives. The analysis of adhesively bonded joints requires a nonlinear shear stress-strain curve for all adhesives, ductile or not, because even the brittle adhesives exhibit substantial nonlinear behavior at temperatures approaching their upper service limits. The strongest structural additives are suitable for most of the structure of subsonic aircraft, having an upper limit of about 70 °C (160 °F).

Even a small amount of moisture can be very harmful to bonded composites (Ref 16). Absorbed water in cured laminates must be removed by careful, gentle drying before any bonded repairs are performed. If such moisture is driven off too rapidly, it will delaminate the composite. Conversely, if it is not driven off completely, it will later react adversely with any uncured material (adhesive or resin) in the patch. Likewise, any moisture absorbed by the uncured resin (in a prepreg) or adhesive will prevent the proper curing of the material. Many uncured resins are hygroscopic. It is therefore very important that such materials be properly stored and, subsequently, thoroughly thawed out, so that there is no opportunity for them to absorb the condensate formed when they are removed from the freezer.

Today, rational engineering design of bonded structures is based on the measured adhesive stress-strain relation in shear for a thin layer of adhesive between thick aluminum adherends. Given these stress-strain data for a range of operating temperatures, it is now possible to calculate the actual adhesive stress distributions within the bonded joints, at least in the short term. More work will be needed to characterize the time-dependent changes in internal load distribution under sustained loads. However, the lack of such information does not prevent the satisfactory completion of most designs.

After the surface preparation issue has been resolved, the real key to the durability of adhesively bonded joints is that the minimum adhesive shear stress in a joint needs to be restricted to prevent failure of the joint by creep rupture, every bit as much as the maximum stress needs to be restricted to prevent static failure. This issue is of tremendous importance in interpreting data from test coupons. The prime objective of designing bonded structural joints should be to ensure that the bond will *never* fail, while the objective of designing test coupons is to ensure that the adhesive will *always* fail, at as uniform a stress state as can be established. Unfortunately, therefore, bonded test coupons are, in many ways, totally unrepresentative of the behavior of real structural joints. In particular, a highly nonuniform stress distribution in the adhesive is necessary if a structural joint is to attain an adequate life.

Nonuniformity of Load Transfer through Adhesive Bonds

The classical analysis by O. Volkersen (Ref 17) established in 1938 that the load transfer through adhesive bonds between uniformly thick adherends is not uniform, but peaks at each end of the overlap, as shown in Fig 5. This nonuniformity results from the compatibility of deformations associated with the variation of direct stress, within the adherends, from one end of the bonded overlap to the other.

A few years later, M. Goland and E. Reissner analyzed the distribution of the peel stresses induced in the adhesive layer by the eccentricity in load path associated with single-lap joints (Ref 18). Many investigators, including the author, have identified deficiencies in this work and derived "better" analyses. However, in a recent reassessment in which he corrected *both* the modeling errors by Goland and Reissner *and* the one he introduced in Ref 19 and 20 in correcting their mistake, L.J. Hart-Smith has shown in Ref 21 that their original analysis is numerically very close to perfection. Mention should also be made of the analyses published by N.A. de Bruyne (Ref 22) that have resulted from his work on Redux and its application in England during and after World War II.

L.J. Hart-Smith has built upon these pioneering investigations and added nonlinear adhesive behavior to the analysis and design of adhesively bonded joints in the form of an elastic-plastic adhesive model (Ref 23–25). Also, the A4E series of digital computer programs was developed for joints of various geometries, under contract to National Aeronautics and Space Administration (NASA) Langley and the laboratories at Wright-Patterson Air Force Base. The origins of these programs are given in Ref 26 and 27.

The knowledge imparted by the precise analyses on which Fig. 5 is based makes it possible to understand the differences between the behavior of adhesive bonds in test coupons and structurally configured joints (see Fig. 6). The key difference is that for the short-overlap test coupon, the minimum adhesive shear stress and strain are nearly as high as the maximum values, while for the long-overlap structural joint, the minimum adhesive shear stress and strain can be made as low as desired by using a sufficiently long overlap. Consequently, the short-overlap test coupon is extremely sensitive to failure by creep rupture (which accumulates under both steady and cyclic loads), because there is no mechanism for restoring the adhesive to its original state when the load is removed. While there

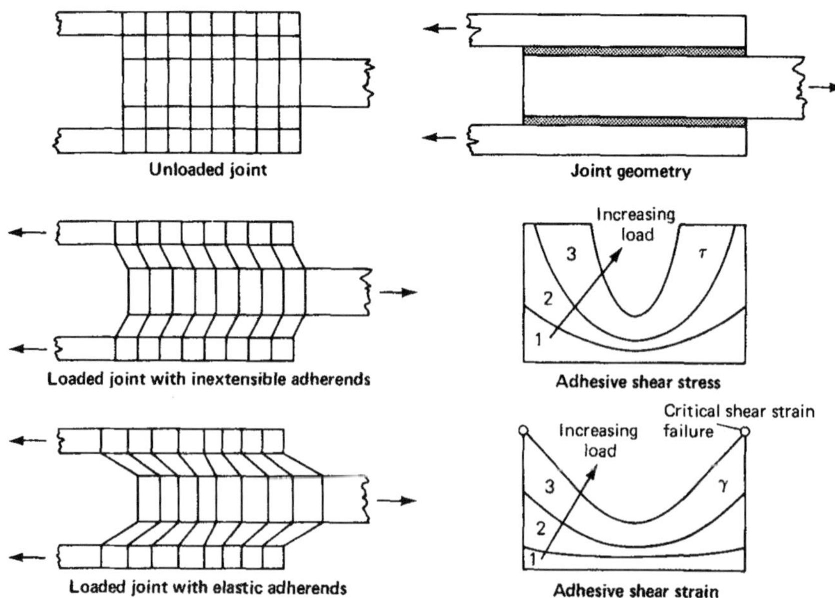

Fig. 5 Shearing of adhesive in balanced joints

is creep in the adhesive at the ends of the long overlap, between points F and G, where the stress (at J) is high, there can be none in the middle, between points D and E, if the stress (at A) is low enough. Consequently, the creep that does occur cannot accumulate, because the stiff adherends push the adhesive back to its original position whenever the joint is unloaded. This memory, or anchor, in part of the adhesive is the key to a durable bonded structure. Without it, there can be no successfully bonded structure. Such recovery during unloading does not imply that the adhesive suffers no damage at all when loaded slightly beyond the knee in the stress-strain curve.

The question of just how low a minimum stress should be has yet to be resolved scientifically. However, during the PABST program, the minimum was set at 10% of the maximum, and environmental testing on both coupons and complete structures showed no adverse effects, even though premature failures were commonplace with the standard half-inch-overlap test coupons. The influence of minimum stress on the design overlap, for standard double-lap or double-strap bonded joints, is shown in Fig. 7. The width of the elastic trough is adjusted so that the minimum stress is 10% of the maximum. This value is reached when the elastic trough has a total length of $6/\lambda$, where λ is the exponent of the elastic adhesive shear stress distribution. To that elastic overlap, which transfers a fraction $1/\lambda$ of the total applied load, a sufficient plastic zone must be added at each end to bring the total shear strength of the bond up to a level at least equal to the entire strength of the adherends, with the adhesive stressed to its maximum shear strength (for a particular environment). The maximum design overlap is normally associated with the highest service temperature for the bonded joint. (The formula established for the overlap during the PABST program was equal to the sum of the plastic zones sufficient to transfer the *total* load and the length $6/\lambda$ of the elastic trough. This gave no credit for the elastic load transfer. When this is included, the overlap can be reduced slightly to the sum of the lengths of the plastic zones, calculated the same way, and $5/\lambda$.)

It was found during the PABST program that, for the thicknesses of aluminum alloy suitable for bonding on subsonic transport aircraft, the overlap could be calculated at approximately 30 times the central adherend thickness in a double-lap joint. In addition, because the modulus of cross-plied carbon/epoxy laminates within the shaded area in Fig. 1 is on the same order of magnitude as for aluminum alloys, a similar overlap-to-thickness ratio would also be satisfactory for such laminates.

Actually, the static strength of bonded joints between uniform adherends is quite insensitive to the precise (long) overlap, as shown in Fig. 8. Any longer overlap beyond point "C" would be superfluous. This insensitivity of the joint strength to the total bonded area is important in recognizing the folly of designing joints with the old notion that the bond strength is equal to the product of the bond area and some fictitious uniform "allowable" shear strength.

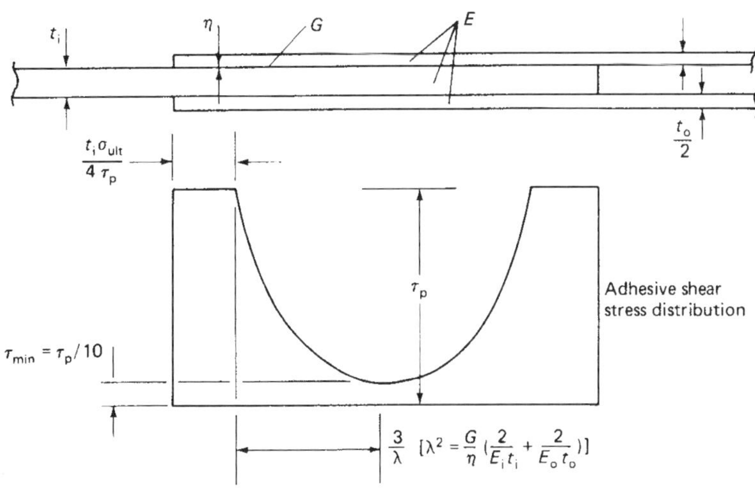

Fig. 7 Design of double-lap bonded joints. Plastic zones must be long enough for ultimate load. Elastic trough must be wide enough to prevent creep at middle. Adequate strength must be verified. G, shear modulus; E_i, elastic modulus of the center; E_o, elastic modulus of the outer pieces; η, adhesive thickness.

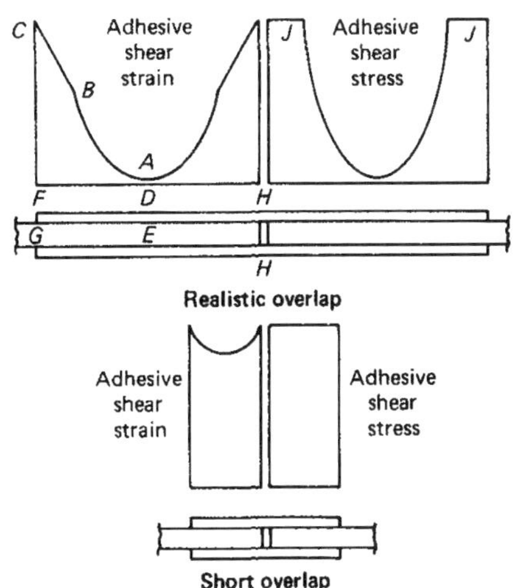

Fig. 6 Nonuniform stresses and strains in bonded joints. See text for discussion.

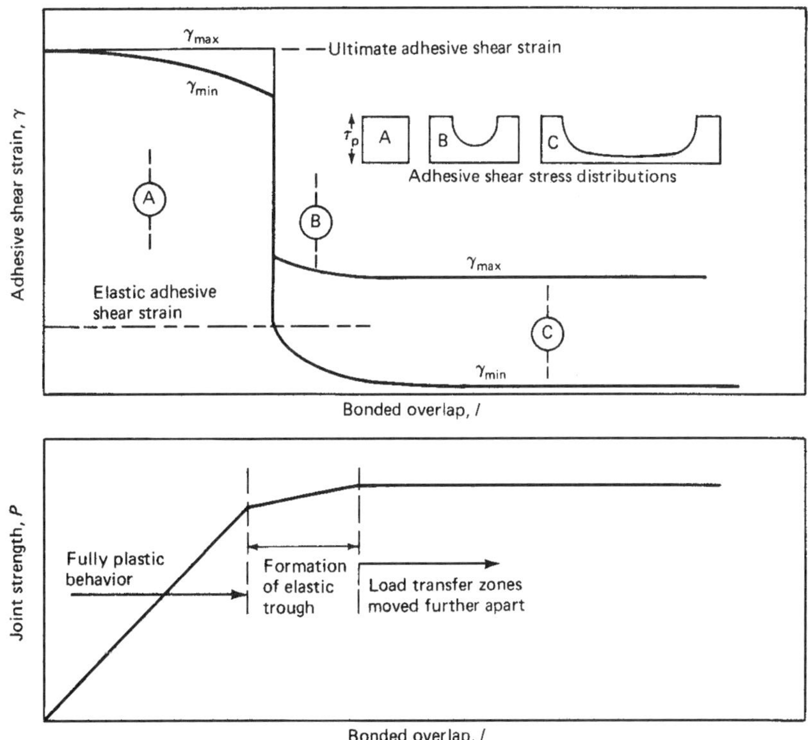

Fig. 8 Influence of overlap, l, on maximum and minimum adhesive shear strains in bonded joints

Another important point shown in Fig. 8 is that for all overlaps longer than the abrupt precipice in the upper diagram, the maximum strain in the adhesive is limited by the adherend strength to a value below that which would be needed to fail the adhesive. No such protection is afforded for short overlaps or thick adherends. This issue is explained more fully in Ref 28, where similar diagrams have been prepared for adherends of different thicknesses and adhesive properties appropriate for a range of thermal environments. It is shown there that if the adherends are too thick, the limit on the peak shear strain shown in Fig. 8 is removed. Therefore, a more complex stepped-lap joint is appropriate for adherends thicker than about 3.2 mm ($\frac{1}{8}$ in.). Also, it is found that the limiting strength of the joint is usually set by the lowest service temperature, while the design overlap is set by the highest service temperature, at which the adhesive is the softest.

Another consideration in the design of bonded joints concerns the need to restrict the maximum shear strain developed in the adhesive at the ends of the bonded overlap. Once the knee in the stress-strain curve has been exceeded, progressively more fractures (hackles) develop at 45° to the bond surfaces, as the result of the tensile stress associated with the shear deformations. It is therefore appropriate to ensure that the design limit load does not strain the adhesive beyond the knee in the stress-strain curve. Because the shear strength of the bonded joint is proportional to the square root of the adhesive strain energy in shear, a design ultimate load 50% higher than limit load would be associated with an ultimate shear strain almost twice that at the knee, as explained in Fig. 9. The remainder of the stress-strain curve for ductile adhesives would be reserved for damage tolerance and the redistribution of loads around local damage. For brittle adhesives, the limits on joint strength would be established by equating design ultimate load to the end of the stress-strain curve, which would not contain any distinct knee.

Having established the design overlap for simple bonded joints, the elimination of adverse peel stresses is addressed next. These peel stresses occur for single-lap and single-strap joints having a primary eccentricity in load path and for double-lap and double-strap joints, as shown in Fig. 10, even though there is no obvious eccentricity in the seemingly balanced joints. While some have argued that it is more appropriate to modify the adhesive failure criteria to account for an interaction between shear and peel stresses, the author contends that the presence of any significant peel stresses necessarily detracts from the shear strength of the joint. Therefore, to improve structural efficiency, those peel stresses should be removed from the structure by simple modifications in design detail rather than be included in a more complicated failure criterion. Such a philosophy also simplifies the analyses by separating the tasks of characterizing the adhesive stress components. Nevertheless, the importance of J.H. Gosse's new polymer failure criteria for quantifying the appreciable loss of shear strength inherent in designs in which adhesive layers *are* subject to intense peel stresses (explained in the article "Characterizing Strength for Structural Design" in this Volume) cannot be overstated.

The simple design modifications that reduce the peel stresses to insignificance are shown in Fig. 11. The idea is to make the tips of the adherends thin and flexible so that only negligible peel stresses can develop. Reference 29 discusses the effects of variations in bondline thickness, such as those shown in Fig. 11. The local thickening shown is beneficial, and, as could be expected, any pinch-off would be detrimental. Such local thickening of the adhesive layer must be used with caution with high-flow heat-cured adhesives, lest voids be created by capillary action. Additional adhesive or scrim fillers can be used, if necessary, to avoid any such problems.

The exact proportions in tapering the adherend or thickening the adhesive layer are not otherwise critical. If the overlap is long enough, it is impossible to overdo the peel-stress relief. This is demonstrated in Fig. 12, which shows that the joint strength remains constant with varying amounts of tapering, because the *other* end of the joint, where no peel stresses develop, is unchanged. The precise distribution of the shear stress transfer at the tapered end is modified, but the integral of those shear stresses is not. This insensitivity can also be deduced from

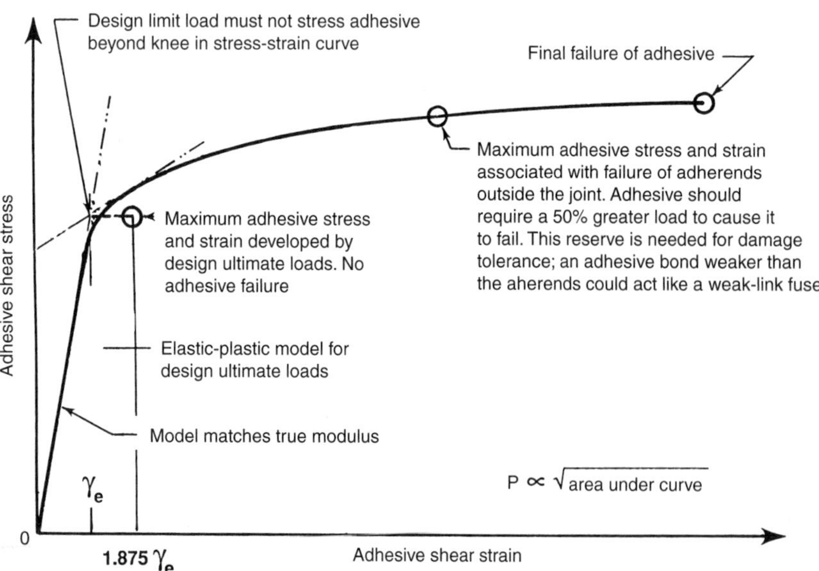

Fig. 9 Modeling of adhesives for design of shear joints. The design process must account for nonlinear adhesive behavior, but a precise stress-strain curve is not mandatory. An approximation, based on a similar adhesive, will usually suffice.

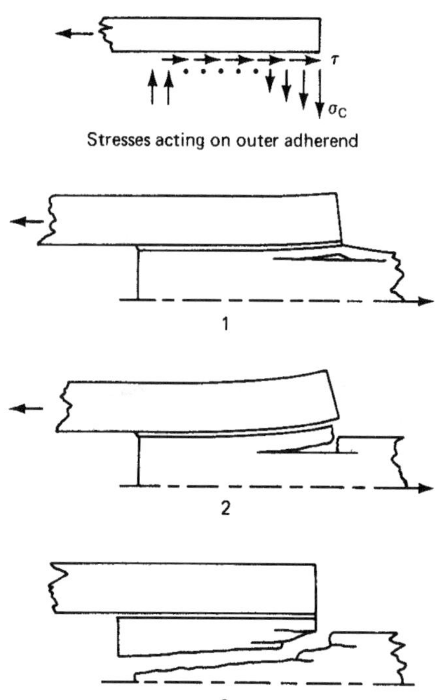

Fig. 10 Peel stress failure of thick composite joints, where 1, 2, and 3 indicate failure sequence

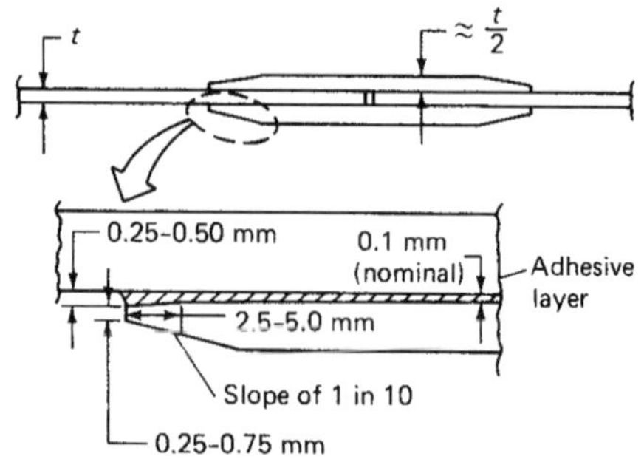

Fig. 11 Tapering of edges of splice plates to relieve adhesive peel stresses (slightly thicker tips permissible for aluminum)

the comparison of bonded joints and bonded doublers in Fig. 13. Compatibility of deformations for long overlaps requires that there be uniform strain at the middle of the joint, and that consequently, for stiffness-balanced joints as shown, half the load must be transferred at each end of the joint, even if the ends are not identical. For long-overlap bonded joints, it is fair to say that the adhesive at one end of the joint is unaware of the presence or absence of the other end of the joint. In other words, the adhesive stresses around the edges of bonded splices are the same as those around the periphery of wide-area doublers.

Elastic-Plastic Adhesive Shear Model

The linearly elastic analysis of bonded joints has been found to be far too conservative for the strong ductile adhesives used on subsonic transport aircraft. Of the possible nonlinear models that could have been proposed to characterize the actual adhesive behavior, only the simple elastic-plastic model has proved amenable to widespread application. This is because the mathematical simplicity permitted explicit closed-form solutions to be obtained for the simpler joints, and those results facilitated comprehensive parametric studies. In addition, those same closed-form solutions apply to each step of the more complex and stronger stepped-lap joints. The elastic-plastic model in Fig. 14 is shown in comparison with an actual stress-strain curve, which is now customarily measured on thick-adherend test specimens using a Krieger KGR-1 extensometer, shown in Fig. 15.

The mathematical model at ultimate load has the same peak shear stress and strain as the actual characteristic and the same strain energy (area under the curve). This was established as the appropriate model in Ref 31, in which the analysis for double-lap joints using the bilinear model shown in Fig. 14 reveals that the predicted joint strength would be the same for any two-straight-line adhesive model having the same strain energy. In other words, the only advantage of the bilinear model is that a single model would work for all load levels. The elastic-plastic model needs to be adjusted for less than ultimate loads, as shown in Fig. 14. Actually, it is usually sufficient to perform only two analyses: a linearly elastic one for limit load using the actual adhesive shear modulus, and an elastic-plastic model to predict the ultimate joint strength. The latter model is inappropriate for low load levels, because the initial shear modulus is too low then, and the elastic strain energy is too high. One must also pay attention to the effective limit imposed on *design* ultimate strength in Fig. 9.

It is important to understand that the simple elastic-plastic model in Fig. 14 is a mathematical *approximation*; it is far from the physical *reality* in which the softening is associated with the *linear elastic* bending of the short ligaments of adhesive tying the adherends together between adjacent hackles, as shown in Fig. 16. On unloading, while there is some hysteresis, there is almost complete recovery of the strain; it is far from the straight-line load reduction with a large permanent offset that is associated with the classical ductile yielding of metal alloys.

The hackles shown in Fig. 16 apply for monotonic loading. In the case of reversed loading, it is possible to try to develop such hackles at both ±45°, culminating in a saw-tooth fracture surface. It really is important to respect the limits spelled out in Fig. 9. In practice, this means a willingness to use stepped-lap bonded joints for thicker adherends. Doing so adds the further benefit of automatically reducing the adhesive peel stresses induced at the end(s) of the joint.

The adhesive stress-strain curves in shear vary with the operating environment, as shown in Fig. 17 for a typical ductile adhesive. While the individual properties, such as peak shear strength and strain-to-failure, vary greatly with the operating temperature, the areas under all three curves in Fig. 17 are quite similar. The ultimate strength of a long-overlap bonded joint between uniform adherends is shown by analysis to be defined by the strain energy of the adhesive layer

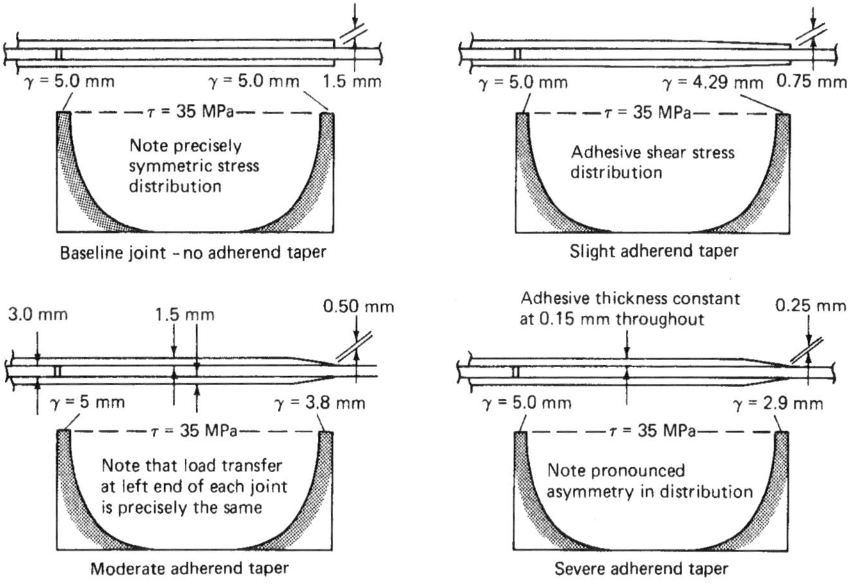

Fig. 12 Insensitivity of adhesively bonded joint strength to modifications at one end of joint only. Adhesive strain at right end of joint decreases with more taper.

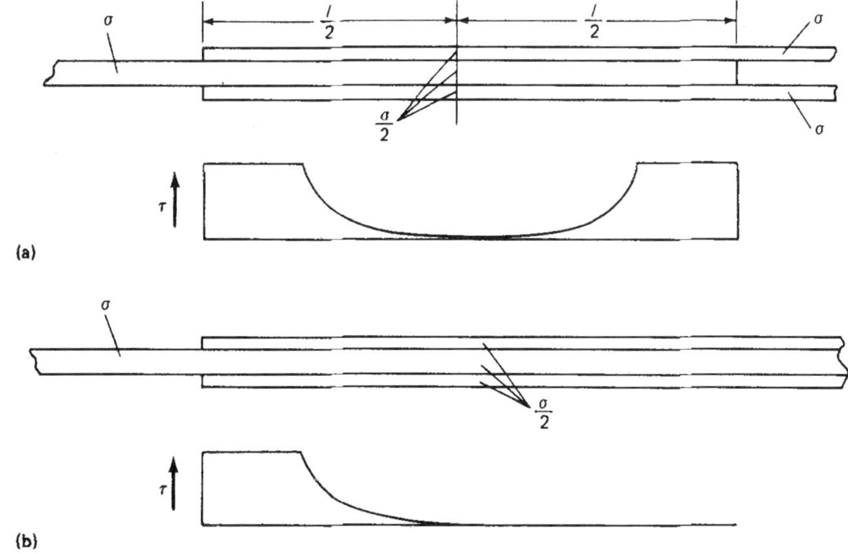

Fig. 13 Similarity of bonded stresses in joints and doublers. (a) Same adhesive stresses in each case. (b) Same maximum adhesive shear strain for same adherend and metal stresses

in shear, not by any individual properties, such as peak shear stress (Ref 31). The strain energy is proportional to the area under each of the curves in Fig. 17. Consequently, the strengths of realistically configured bonded joints are not very sensitive to the operating environment, provided that the temperature is kept below the glass transition temperature for each adhesive.

The difference between the behavior of ductile and brittle adhesives is characterized in Fig. 18. That difference is not as pronounced at the upper service temperatures, at which even the brittle adhesives are considerably ductile. It should also be noted that even at room temperature, the brittle adhesive characteristic is significantly nonlinear. The reasons that both ductile and brittle adhesives have been developed are that ductile adhesives are typically limited to service environments no greater than about 70 °C (160 °F), and that there are some applications (in proximity to engines or on supersonic aircraft) where brittle adhesive bonding is still viable, even if much of the strength has had to be sacrificed to attain much higher service temperatures.

Single-Lap Adhesively Bonded Joints

The eccentricity in load path inherent in unsupported single-lap joints decreases the joint strength below the level that could have been developed in the absence of the bending associated with that eccentricity. That loss of joint strength is quantified in Fig. 19, which shows, for example, that for the standard ASTM D 1002 lap-shear test coupon, for which the abscissa is about 2, the structural efficiency is limited to no more than one-third. (The structural efficiency is defined as the ratio of the direct membrane stress outside the joint to the sum of the stretching and bending stresses at the ends of the bonded overlap.) However, Fig. 19 also points the way to alleviating the problem, that is, by increasing the overlap from the 8 to 1 ratio used on the test coupon to about 80 to 1 for structural joints. The joint can never be as strong as the basic structure outside it. However, for long overlaps and thin adherends, the weakness is in the adherends rather than in the adhesive, and, in any case, the joint strength need only exceed the alternative, that is, riveting, which causes a significant loss of strength because of the holes.

A detailed analysis of single-lap bonded joints can be found in Ref 15. Naturally, if the joint is supported against out-of-plane rotations, the appropriate method of analysis would be to consider the actual joint as one side of a double-lap joint that was twice as thick. Normally, single-lap joints should not be considered for joints thicker than about 1.8 mm (0. 07 in.) of aluminum alloy or its equivalent. The same peel-stress relief techniques shown in Fig. 11 are equally applicable to single-lap and single-strap joints, except that protection is needed at both ends of the bonded overlap instead of only at one.

Stepped-Lap Adhesively Bonded Joints

Composite laminates that are too thick and hence too strong to be joined by simple uniform lap-splice bonded joints can be bonded together successfully by stepped-lap joints of the type shown in Fig. 20. (Glued scarf joints, which work well for wood at a slope of about 1 in 20 at most, are not as attractive for advanced composites, because the slope needs to be much shallower, at no more than about 1 in 50, resulting in scarf joints for thick laminates that are very large.)

Each step of the stepped-lap bonded joint is governed by the same differential equation that applies to double-lap joints. Consequently, there is a highly nonuniform shear stress distribution in the adhesive, with the load transfer concentrated at the ends of each step, as shown in Fig. 21.

The design and analysis of stepped-lap bonded joints have been made straightforward by the digital computer programs A4EG and A4EI, which are based on an elastic-plastic shear

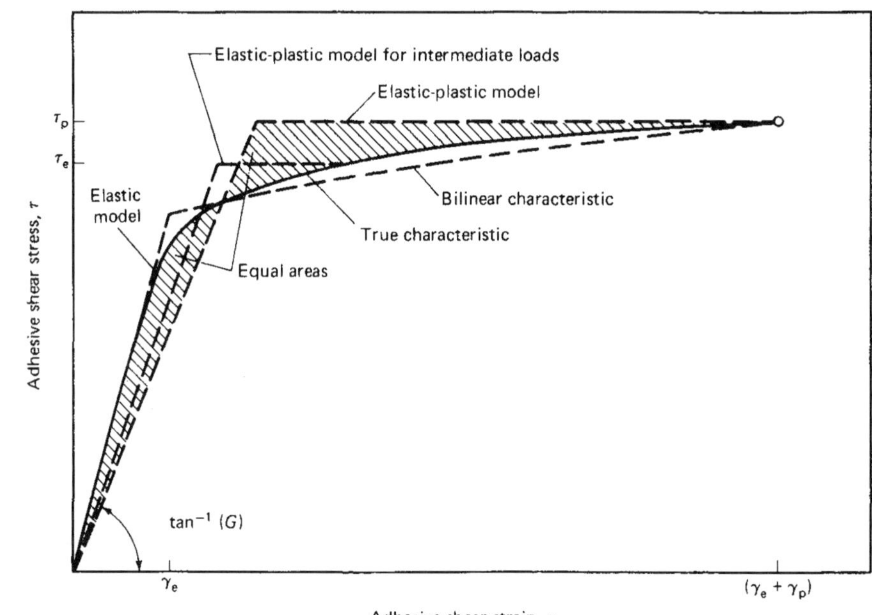

Fig. 14 Representations of adhesive nonlinear shear behavior

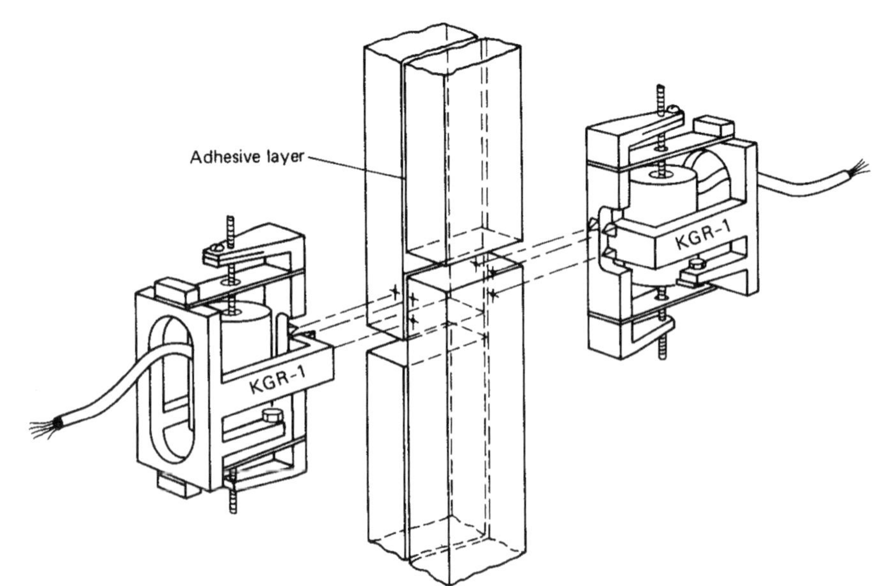

Fig. 15 KGR-1 extensometer and thick-adherend adhesive test specimen. Source: Ref 30

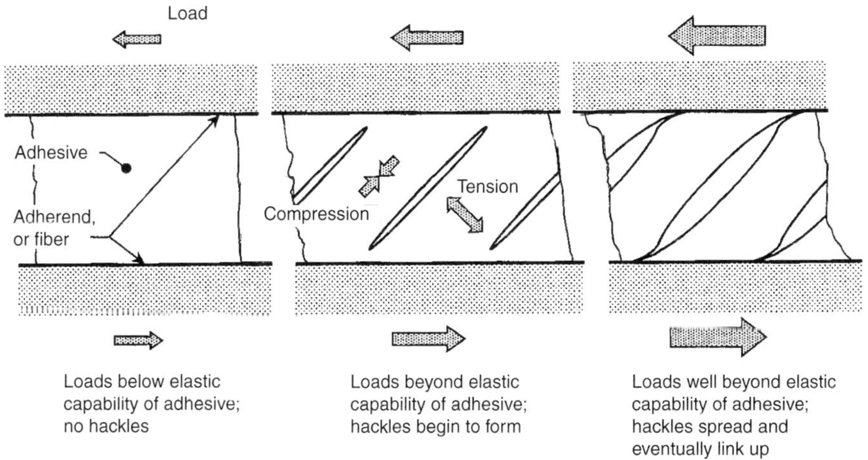

Fig. 16 Tensile hackle failures resulting from in-plane (or transverse) shear applied to constrained polymers in the form of thin films between fibers or adherends

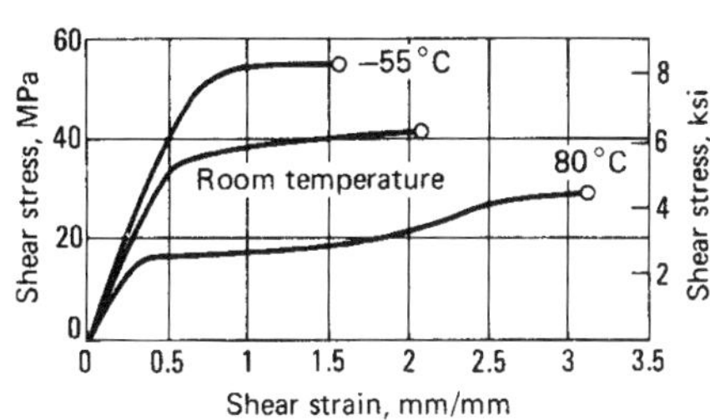

Fig. 17 Effect of temperature on adhesive stress-strain curves in shear. Nylon/epoxy adhesive (120 °C, or 250 °F, cure)

model (Ref 32, 33). The first program employs a uniform adhesive layer throughout the joint. The second program expanded on the first and incorporated variable adhesive properties, so that the effect of flaws and defects could be investigated (worked examples of joints analyzed by these programs are found in Ref 6, 26, 27, 29, and 34). It should be noted that the A4EG and A4EI programs do not merely predict the strength of joints of specified geometries, but also serve as valuable tools for improving the initial designs. Some rules of thumb for initial design are that the end steps must be neither too thick nor too long—0.76 mm (0.030 in.) thick titanium with a step length of 9.5 mm (0.375 in.) is typical, lest premature fatigue failures occur. Most of the other steps are usually 12.7 to 19.1 mm (0.50 to 0.75 in.) long, with step thicknesses no greater than 0.5 mm (0.02 in.) (and preferably much less) on each side of the joint, with one longer step near the middle of the overlap to provide creep resistance. The computer programs give enough detailed information about the internal stresses within the joint for the initial design to be improved upon by modifying design details. Any poorly proportioned step usually shows up rapidly. Once the proportions have been adjusted properly, the most powerful variable with which to increase the joint strength is the number of steps; merely increasing the bond area for the same number of steps is not effective. The strength continues to increase as the number of steps is increased to one per ply, and the number should always be sufficient to ensure that the bond strength (calculated by overriding the adherend strength limits while maintaining the same stiffnesses) exceeds the adherend strengths by at least 50%.

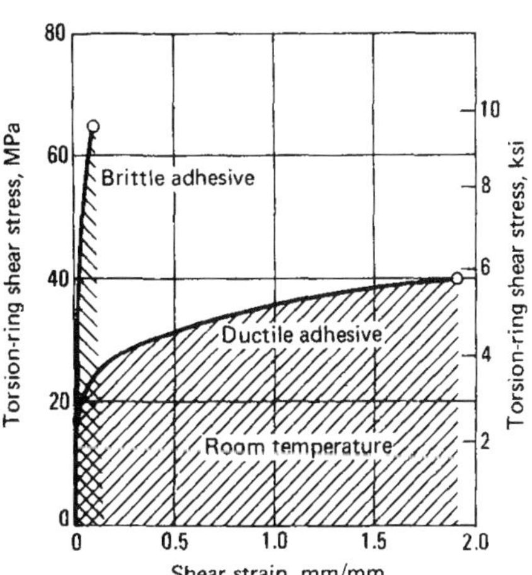

Fig. 18 Adhesive stress-strain curves in shear

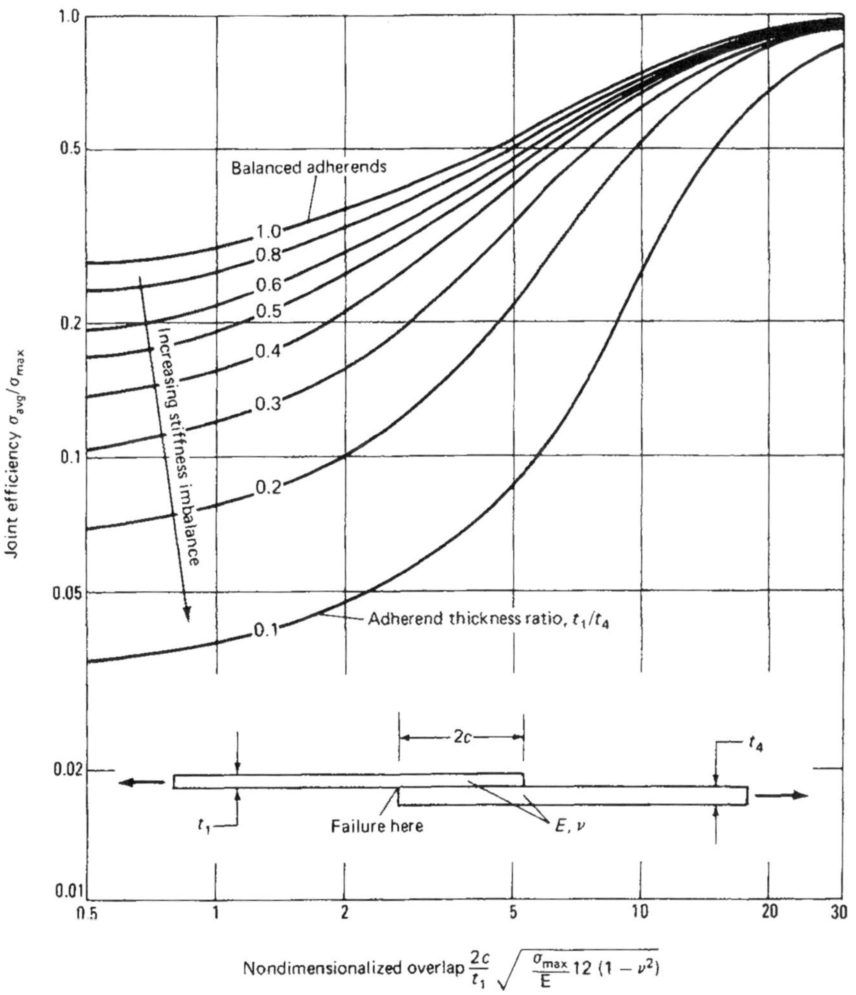

Fig. 19 Effect of adherend stiffness imbalance on adherend bending strength of single-lap bonded joints. Thinner adherend t_1 critical in combined bending and axial load at end of overlap

Load Redistributions with Flawed and Damaged Adhesively Bonded Joints

It is not sufficient to design bonded splices to a strength that is only adequate for the nominally applied loads, unless there is no need for damage tolerance. If a bonded splice is everywhere weaker than the local strength of the adherends just outside the joint, any load redistribution associated with local flaws in the bond or damage to it could cause the remaining bond to unzip catastrophically. This phenomenon is explained in Fig. 4; the uniform remote stress in the adherends must be kept lower for larger flaws or damage, lest the remaining bond become overloaded and fail just outside the ineffective bond area.

However, if the intact bond outside the weakened area was stronger than the adherends, no amount of load redistribution could ever fail the bond, as explained in Ref 6 and 26. Any subsequent failure would be transferred to the adherends, where it would become visible much sooner. The appropriate analysis for estimating the remaining life in the damaged bonded structure then pertains to the adherends and not to the adhesive. The same is true when structures so thick that they should not be bonded are bonded and then are protected by fail-safe mechanical fasteners. Any initial flaws or damage will unzip sufficiently to enable some of the fasteners to pick up the load through the defective area. From that point on, the basic load transfer is redistributed, as explained in Ref 26 and 33. The disbond will grow no further, and the subsequent life will be determined by the most severely loaded fastener through the area of defective bond.

A word of caution is in order about the current fashion of misapplying fracture mechanics theory (from cracked metal structures) to estimating the life of adhesively bonded structures. Such a malpractice is more likely to result in bonded structures inferior to those designed by classical nonlinear strength-of-materials approaches than it is to result in improvements. The key to designing bonded structures is that the nominally unflawed bond must never be weaker than the members being joined. If the bond is stronger, the adherends determine the structural life, whether there is a bond flaw or not. The notion that it is permissible to design weak-link fuse bonded joints and justify this practice by calculating a supposedly adequate finite fatigue life must be discouraged. The associated potential for instantaneous unzipping of the remaining bond area would place an intolerable burden on inspection. Finding cracks in metal structures has been difficult enough, and they are much easier to detect.

Further, the two situations (flawed bonds and cracked metal) are not at all comparable. The basis of the damage tolerance approach to cracked metal structures is that there will be a relatively long period of slow, stable crack growth before a critical crack length is reached. That usually allows sufficient opportunity to detect small cracks and repair them. In adhesive bonds, on the other hand, the measured disbond rates have either been so rapid that the bonds would need to be inspected several times on each flight to ensure that it was safe to continue, or so slow that no growth could be detected. There has been no in-between behavior that would lend itself to metallic damage tolerance techniques. This difference is explained in Fig. 22 (from Ref 35). Properly designed bonded joints, on the other hand, exhibit remarkable tolerance to quite large bond flaws. Fracture mechanics analyses can be valuable in this context when used to calculate thresholds below which initial damage will not propagate, rather than to calculate rates of damage growth.

Another beneficial use of fracture mechanics analysis of bonded and laminated composite structures is to identify design details and stacking sequences that should be avoided (see Ref 36). Special attention should be paid to the numerous publications on delaminations in composites by T.K. O'Brien at NASA Langley; one of these is included in Ref 36. The need for such an approach is accentuated by the current lack of capability in the standard composite laminate theories to account for residual thermal stresses in the resin, which is, after all, where the cracks and delaminations in fiber-reinforced composites occur. While a few of the published laminate theories (mechanistic rather than interactive) do an adequate job of predicting the fiber-dominated strengths of composite laminates under arbitrary in-plane loads, none of the published theories can do justice to resin-dominated strengths, and all are quite incapable of accounting for such things as stacking-sequence effects. Most laminate theories work only for uniaxial loading and are unacceptable for biaxial loads, although new

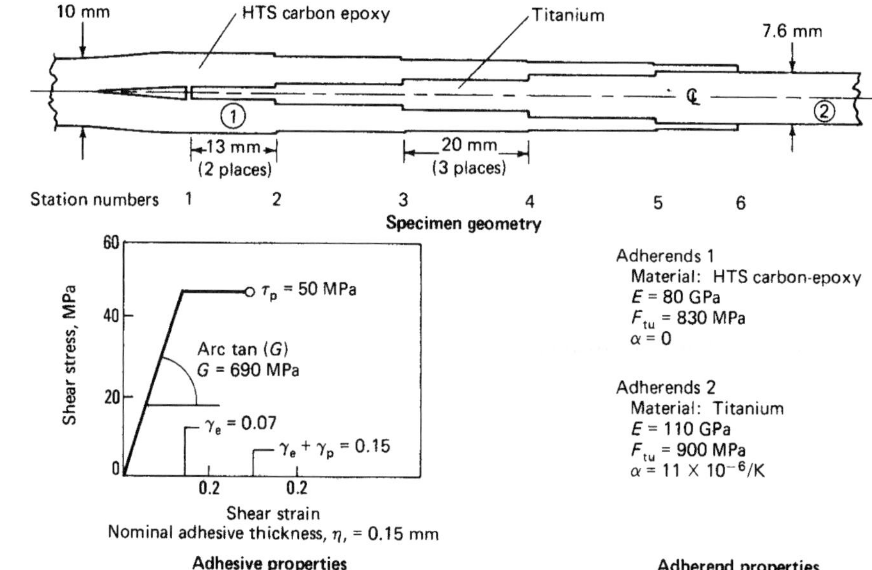

Fig. 20 Typical stepped-lap adhesively bonded joint

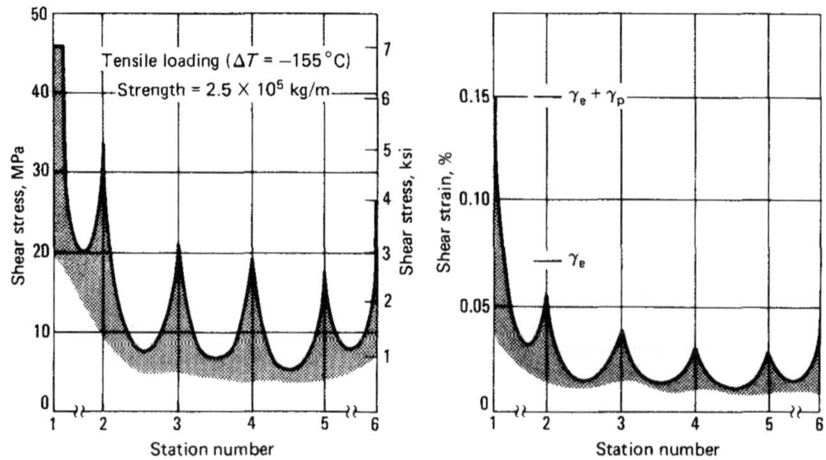

Fig. 21 Adhesive shear stresses and strains in unflawed bonded joint

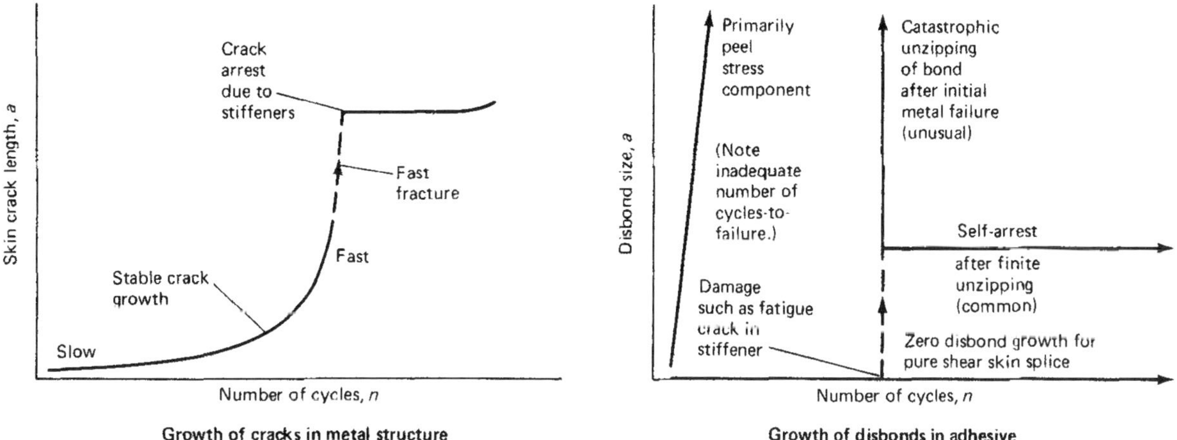

Fig. 22 Differences between growth of cracks in metal components and adhesive bonds. Source: Ref 35

and old cross-plied laminate theories that do work satisfactorily for biaxial in-plane loads are discussed in Ref 37 and 38. Such deficiencies in the laminate theories may be the reason that all bolted composite joint analyses have had to rely on substantial empirically determined correlation factors between theory and test.

Fundamentals of Shear Load Transfer through Mechanical Fasteners

Perhaps the most important thing to understand about mechanically fastened joints in fibrous composite structures is that the eventual failure of the composite occurs long after the laminate has stopped behaving like the one-phase homogeneous engineering material on which it is usually modeled. While the fibers and the resin matrix are both essentially linear until failure, the microcracks and delaminations around bolt holes in composite laminates cause substantial internal load redistributions that are not accounted for in conventional mathematical models of bolted or riveted composite joints. Thus, there appears to be substantial nonlinear behavior associated with the normal rivet or bolt sizes used in composite structures. However, while there are indeed softened zones at the microlevel, as shown in Fig. 23, this softening is unlike the yielding associated with ductile metal alloys in similar circumstances.

However, there are striking similarities in the behavior at the macrolevel. For example, the residual-stress zone around cold-worked holes in metal structures leads to very substantial increases in the fatigue life. Likewise, any increase in the albeit much smaller softened zone around fasteners in composites causes an increase in the static strength. Either the careful installation of interference-fit fasteners or the gentle fatiguing of bolted composite structures can increase the static tensile strength ever closer toward the unnotched net-section strength. The corresponding increase in compressive strength will not be as dramatic, because it is dominated more by bearing stresses than by net-section stresses. Indeed, with the more recent toughened resins that have been developed, a new failure mode has been detected—cracks right through the laminates that, if the nominal strain is high enough, grow under compressive cyclic loads in exactly the same manner as through cracks grow under tensile loads in metallic structures. The reason for this is that while the microdamage in the resin is benign under tensile loads, because it averages fiber strains in regions of high stress gradients, the same damage destabilizes axially compressed fibers. This phenomenon had never been noticed in the older, more brittle resins, because the entire laminate would fail before the necessary strains for this mode of failure could be developed.

There is a very strong similarity between the effects of design details on the fatigue strength of bolted or riveted metal structures and on the static strength of composite structures. Perhaps the strongest analogy is associated with the desirability of restricting the bearing stress. As shown in Fig. 24, at the elastic level the peak tension stress alongside the loaded bolt hole in an isotropic panel is on the same order of magnitude as the average bearing stress, P/dt. Keeping the bearing stress low is the key to structurally efficient bolted composite joints, particularly for multirow joints, as explained in the section "Multirow Bolted Composite Joints" in this article.

There are also some curious juxtapositions of behavior between metallic and composite components. For example, in metal aircraft structures, a severe application of load early in the life of the aircraft will retard the subsequent growth of cracks by creating a larger plastic zone at the crack tips or likely crack sites. Conversely, if all bolted composite aircraft were subjected to five lifetimes of fatigue testing before delivery, their ultimate strength would be increased significantly, perhaps by as much as a factor of 2.

Because of the distinctly two-phase material behavior of fibrous composites around both loaded and unloaded holes (Fig. 23), there will

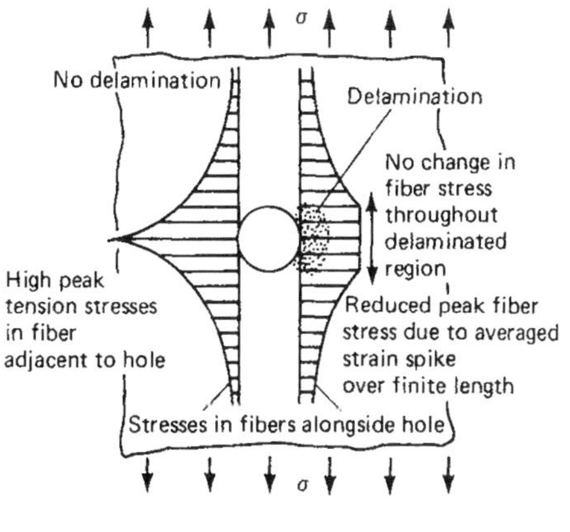

Fig. 23 Stress-concentration relief at small holes in fiber-reinforced composites

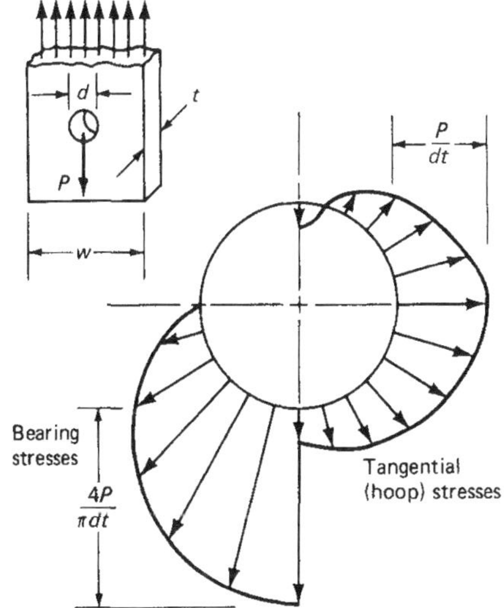

Fig. 24 Bearing and hoop stresses at bolt hole

be a continued need for a substantial empirically established correlation factor to reconcile test and theory for bolted composite joints. This can be done in a straightforward manner, as in the author's hypothesis (Ref 33, 39–41), in which the amount of stress-concentration relief is assumed to be proportional to the intensity of the original elastic stress concentration. That hypothesis leads to an easily calculated residual stress concentration for other geometries that have not been tested. With a correlation factor determined from single-hole test specimens as a starting point, this method has been shown to be effective in predicting the strength of highly loaded multirow bolted composite joints (Ref 42). In Ref 43, this method has been extended to in-plane shear loads on multirow joints. Reference 43 also contains some improved stress-concentration formulas for loaded and unloaded bolt holes that are simpler than those developed earlier, with no loss of accuracy. This method of analysis is presented here.

The literature on bolted composite joints contains another basic approach to this nonlinearity problem, usually referred to as the characteristic-length or characteristic-offset approach. The origins of this approach are the point-stress and average-stress failure criteria (Ref 44). With that method, the linearly elastic analysis is presumed to be valid outside some empirically determined softened zone adjacent to the hole. The basic drawback to that approach, which can, of course, always be shown to be capable of explaining any test results one at a time, is that the so-called characteristic dimension varies considerably with bearing stress, and that failure is being predicted at some place other than where it is known to occur. Nevertheless, both methods of analysis will continue to be used until it is possible to cover all joint geometries and bearing stress intensities with a single theory. At present, each approach covers some situations not covered by the other. Both have been used successfully in hardware applications, and both have led to increased understanding of stress concentrations around bolt holes in composite structures.

Single-Hole Bolted Composite Joints

The methods developed in Ref 39, 40, and 43 for the analysis and design of bolted or riveted composite joints call for a major empirical correlation factor. Once that is accepted, it makes sense to use analyses for elastic isotropic materials as reference points, because they are simple and widely available. Corrections for both the nonlinear behavior described in Fig. 23 and for orthotropy can be combined into a single factor, provided that the mode and location of failure do not change. Separate analyses are needed for bearing failures and for the tension-through-the-hole failure modes. The various modes of failure are illustrated in Fig. 25. Compression strengths tend to be higher and not as sensitive to stress concentrations, because some of the load can be transmitted through the fastener instead of the entire load going around it.

The other major failure mode, shear-out, does not occur within the shaded area of laminate patterns in Fig. 1. Outside that area, the wide-spread splitting accompanying shear-out and the low load level at which it occurs (see, for example, Ref 39 and 45) discourage the installation of fasteners in such highly orthotropic laminates. A weakness in shear-out cannot be corrected by adding more edge distance for the fasteners. Even an increase in thickness, without changing the troublesome fiber pattern, is not very effective. Any added thickness is better employed by changing to a more thoroughly interspersed, nearly quasi-isotropic pattern.

Reference 43 contains formulas for the elastic-isotropic stress concentration associated with a loaded bolt hole of diameter, d, in a finite strip of width, w. With respect to the average net-section tension stress, the peak stress-concentration factor on the net section immediately adjacent to the hole is:

$$K_{te} = \frac{w}{d} + \frac{d}{w} + 0.5\left(1 - \frac{d}{w}\right)\Theta \approx \frac{w}{d} + \frac{d}{w} \quad \text{(Eq 1)}$$

where

$$\Theta = \left(\frac{w}{e} - 1\right) \text{ for } e/w \leq 1,\ \Theta = 0 \text{ for } e/w \geq 1$$

provided that the edge distance, e, is adequate (that is, $e \geq w$). The cited reference contains modifications for short edge distances. R.B. Heywood gives the corresponding expression for the stress-concentration factor at an unloaded hole in the middle of a strip (Ref 46):

$$K_{te} = 2 + (1 - d/w)^3 \quad \text{(Eq 2)}$$

Reference 39 also contains formulas for stress conditions associated with holes in different geometries. A major benefit of having explicit expressions for these stress concentrations is that they facilitate parametric studies and identification of optimal joint geometries. The maximum strength of brittle, perfectly elastic strips loaded by a central bolt is 21% of the unnotched strength at an optimal w/d ratio of about 2.5. The bolts should be placed close together to minimize the peak hoop tension stress, which, as shown in Fig. 24, is on the same order as the average bearing stress.

Fortunately, at least for the small, typically 6.5 mm (0.25 in.) diameter, fasteners used in most aircraft structures, the pessimistic outlook for bolt holes in window glass materials does not occur in fiber-reinforced composites, because of the separate behavior of the two distinct constituents of such composites. There is then considerable relief of the stress-concentration factors, as shown in Fig. 26, which also includes the ef-

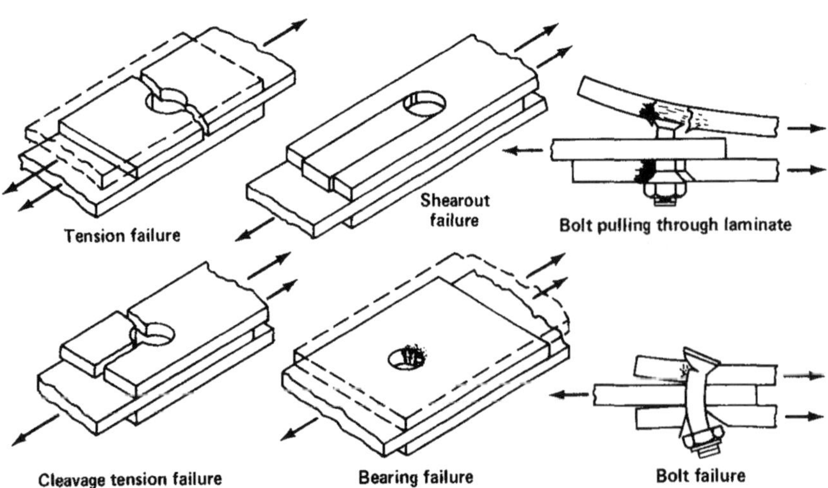

Fig. 25 Modes of failure for bolted joints in advanced composites

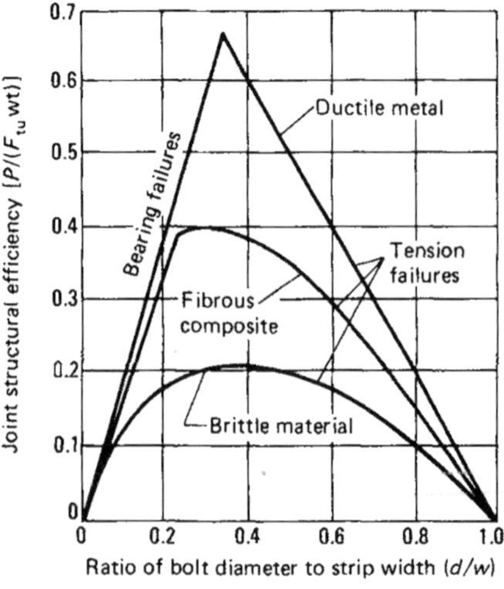

Fig. 26 Relationship between strengths of bolted joints in ductile metals, fiber-reinforced composites, and brittle materials

ficiency of bolted joints in highly ductile and perfectly brittle materials. It is evident that fibrous composite behavior cannot be predicted on the basis of a minor perturbation from either the elastic or plastic analyses shown. (It should also be noted that the strength increase shown in Fig. 26 for roughly 6.5 mm, or 0.25 in., diameter bolts in carbon/epoxy composites decreases asymptotically as the fastener diameter increases, and, for very large bolt holes or cutouts, the linearly elastic predictions would be expected to apply.)

The origin of this substantial stress-concentration relief for typical fastener sizes is explained in Fig. 27, in which the theoretical stress-concentration factors, K_{te}, are calculated according to Eq 1. The observed stress concentration at failure, K_{tc}, is calculated as:

$$K_{tc} = F_{tu}(w-d)/P \quad \text{(Eq 3)}$$

where P is the load at which the specimen failed, F_{tu} is the ultimate tensile strength, and the numerator is the unnotched net-section strength.

It was postulated in Ref 39, 40, and 43 that the amount of (nonlinear) relief would be proportional to the intensity of the original (elastic) stress concentration. Thus, the effective stress-concentration factor experienced by the composite laminate at loaded and unloaded bolt holes is taken to be:

$$K_{tc} = 1 + C(K_{te} - 1) \quad \text{(Eq 4)}$$

in which the correlation factor, C, varies with both the fiber pattern and the hole size. A value of 0 for C would indicate complete stress-concentration relief, as with ductile metals, while a value of 1 (for quasi-isotropic materials) would indicate no relief at all. As a useful *aide-memoire*, the value of the C factor has been found to be close to 0.25 for 0.25 in. bolts in three different carbon epoxy quasi-isotropic laminates, which fraction is the same as the percentage of 0° plies. Higher values have been deduced for orthotropic laminates. For 6.5 mm (0.25 in.) diameter fasteners in laminates within the shaded area in Fig. 1:

$$C \approx (\%\ 0^\circ \text{ plies})/100 \quad \text{(Eq 5)}$$

as shown in Fig. 28.

Absorbing the orthotropy factor into the single coefficient C can be justified only when the mode of failure does not change. Whether this effect of orthotropy were incorporated into an expanded abscissa or into a steepened slope of the line in Fig. 27, the result would be the same. This combination would be expected to become invalid for most of the fiber patterns outside the shaded area shown in Fig. 1, because of a predominance of shear-out failures.

For small d/w (or large w/d) ratios, the laminates will fail at a lower load in bearing under the bolt rather than by tension through the hole. Therefore, a lower-bound cutoff is needed to cover this failure mode. This is shown on the left of the middle curve in Fig. 26. Such bearing failures also occur for ductile metal alloys, as shown to the left of the top curve in Fig. 26.

The optimal w/d ratio, when allowance is made for the nonlinear behavior of the composite around the bolt holes, is approximately 3 to 1 for 6.5 mm (0.25 in.) diameter bolts, being slightly higher for smaller bolts and lower for larger ones. These optimal ratios pertain to single-row joints in which all of the load is transferred through a single row of fasteners; different values are given in the section "Multirow Bolted Composite Joints" in this article. Also, whereas the maximum strength for ductile metals occurs at the intersection of the bearing and tension strengths, the maximum efficiency for single-row bolted composite joints is developed by tensile failures of the net section, at a bearing stress that is typically only about three-fourths of the bearing stress the composite material could withstand at wider bolt spacings. The philosophy of simultaneous failures is definitely not applicable here.

The bearing strength of composite laminates is strongly influenced by the presence or absence of any through-the-thickness clamp-up, as shown in Fig. 29. There is a nearly 2 to 1 difference between the pin-loaded case, in which there is no clamp-up at all, and the finger-tight case, for which the bolt head and nut prevent any initially damaged composite material from unloading itself by deflecting sideways. Because all the material is confined under these circumstances, the joint continues to carry on to higher

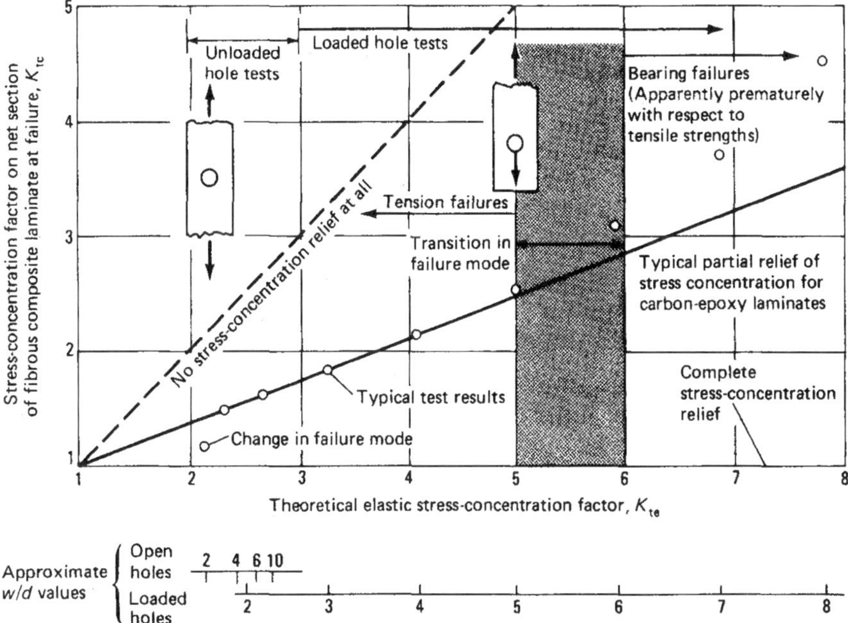

Fig. 27 Relation between stress-concentration factors observed at failure of fiber-reinforced composite laminates and predicted for perfectly elastic isotropic materials

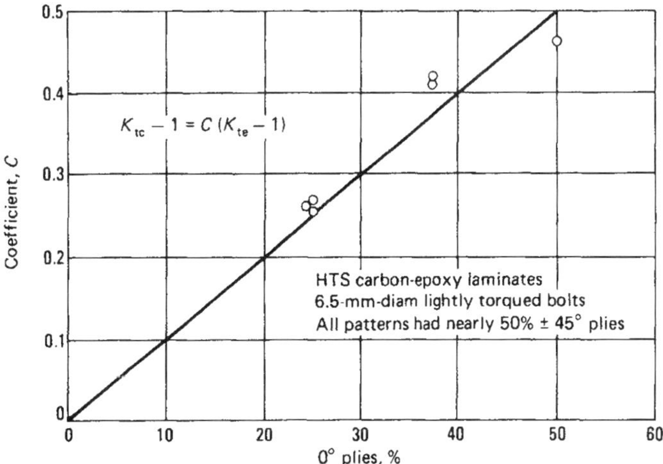

Fig. 28 Stress-concentration relief at bolt holes in composite laminates

loads, as shown. This improvement in strength is customarily accounted for in design. The even greater strengths achievable by torquing the bolts down tightly should not be relied upon for design purposes, because it would be very difficult to detect a single undertorqued fastener that would substantially reduce the static strength of the composite structure. In metal structures, on the other hand, the loss of such clamp-up would merely reduce the fatigue life, with no associated reduction in static strength. In any case, the improvement in bearing strength of composites due to additional bolt torque is often not realized, because tension-through-the-hole strength may govern the design, particularly for large fasteners.

Multirow Bolted Composite Joints

The limited structural efficiency of bolted composite laminates containing single-row splices is not sufficient for them to compete on a weight basis with well-designed aluminum alloy structures. This is indicated by Fig. 30, which points to the need for operating at higher strain levels. However, this need has sometimes been misinterpreted and has been responded to by changing to structurally inferior patterns to acquire the increase in strain, only to have that goal nullified by an associated reduction in modulus. Interestingly, diagrams similar to Fig. 30, but prepared for mildly orthotropic laminate patterns, have shown that the increase in strength associated with additional 0° plies (those in the primary direction of loading) are almost nullified by the associated reduction in strain-to-failure because of the higher stress-concentration factors, K. Likewise, the lower stress concentrations and higher strains-to-failure associated with softened laminates carry with them a balancing decrease in strength because of the lower modulus.

Tinkering with a good fiber pattern usually cannot substantially enhance the strength of fibrous composite laminates. A well-known exception is the use of local softening strips and pad-ups, which can virtually eliminate the effect of stress concentrations with respect to the basic laminate. However, such an approach leaves the structure outside those locally protected areas with little, if any, damage tolerance (because of the higher operating strain permitted by the softening strips and pad-ups) and severely limits the opportunity to perform repairs, so the situations in which such an approach is practical are limited.

An alternative technique for improving the structural efficiency of bolted or riveted composite structures is to improve the joints themselves, by using more than one row of fasteners in conjunction with tapered splice plates. The analyses in Ref 39, 40 and 43 pointed the way to almost accomplishing this in the 1980s, and considerable progress has since been made in the design and analysis of such joints. The validity of the methods has been confirmed by extensive testing of large, highly loaded bolted composite joints (Ref 42). The key to the analysis of multirow bolted composite joints is a formula for the bearing-bypass interaction. Such an interaction, for tensile loads, is shown in Fig. 31, where the terms "bearing load" and "bypass load" are defined. The bearing load is reacted at the particular bolt under consideration, while the bypass load, interrupted by the bolt hole, passes by and is reacted elsewhere. Figure 32 also covers compressive loading, for which the bearing-bypass interaction is more complicated.

When the bearing load is high enough, there is a bearing-stress cutoff for sufficiently wide fastener spacing, but for closer spacings, the failure will be in the net section whether the load is all taken out on that fastener (pure bearing) or all reacted at other fasteners in the joint (pure bypass). The extremities of the interactions could be established by test if a theory were not available. The real key to Fig. 31 is the linear interaction between bearing and bypass loads whenever the joint fails in tension through the hole; that is:

$$\sigma_{net}K_{tc} + \sigma_{brg}K_{tb} \le F_{tu} \text{ (and } \sigma_{brg} \le F_{brg}) \quad \text{(Eq 6)}$$

where K_{tb} is the bearing stress concentration factor and F_{brg} is the ultimate bearing strength.

The existence of this linear interaction has been known since about 1970 and confirmed by other analysis methods. Many curves similar to

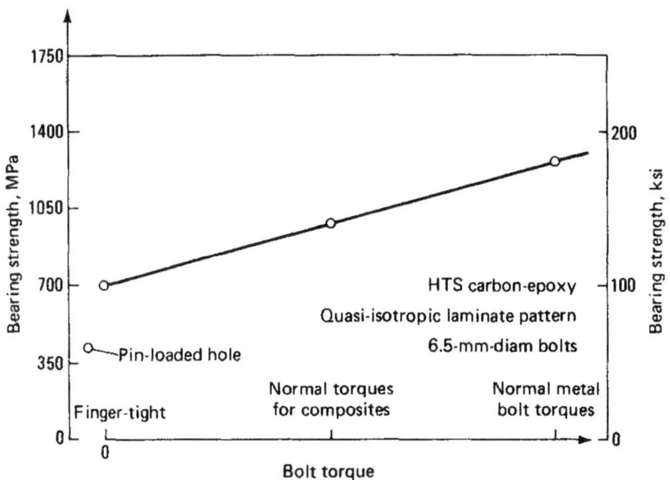

Fig. 29 Effect of bolt torque on bearing strength of fiber-reinforced composite laminates

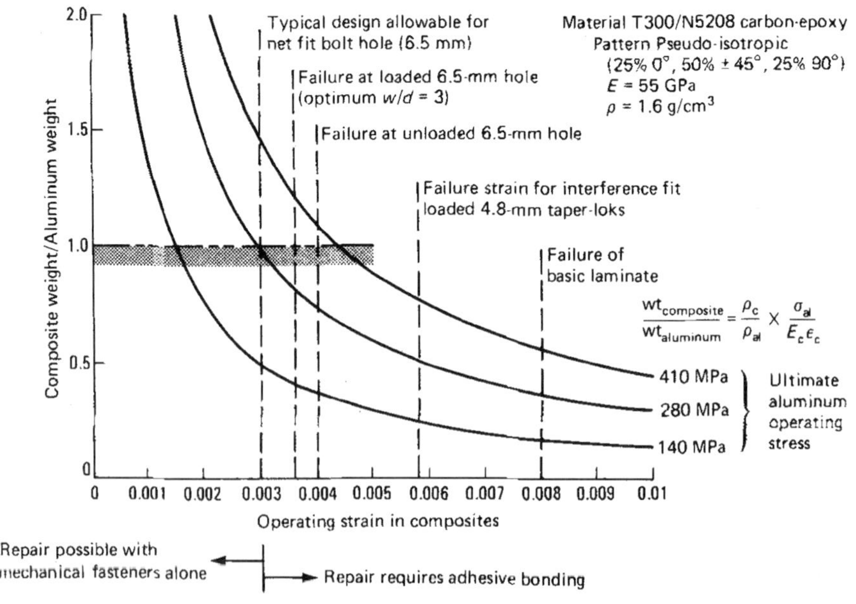

Fig. 30 Relative weights of aluminum and carbon/epoxy composite structures. Failure strains are less for loaded holes, for using statistical basis rather than average, and for larger holes. Reliance on benefit from interference-fit fasteners requires absolutely no net or loose-fit bolts. Otherwise, static strength will be reduced by a factor of 2. Multiple rows of bolts in uniformly thick members increase strength by only a few percent. Further strain limits for damage tolerance and impact resistance are not yet established.

Fig. 31 have been derived by the Bolted Joint Stress Field Model (BJSFM) computer program (such as Ref 47, 48) using the characteristic-offset analysis method, and the linearity has been confirmed by extensive testing reported in numerous documents. (The use of the BJSFM analysis method, with a fixed characteristic offset for all hole sizes, permits an assessment of the hole-size effect, which requires varying values of the coefficient C with the present method of analysis. The bearing-bypass interaction used with the BJSFM method is usually established for a fixed w/d ratio of 4 to 1, while the C-factor method can encompass such interactions that are permitted to vary with the w/d ratio, as demonstrated in Ref 43.)

Equations 1 to 5 permit the construction of joint efficiency charts of the type shown in Fig. 33, which covers all the intermediate cases for single-row joints between a pure bypass load along the upper envelope and a pure bearing load on the lowest curve. Figure 33 reveals that the only way to improve upon the efficiency of an optimized single-row joint is to move the fasteners in the most critical row further apart and simultaneously decrease the bearing stress on the same row of fasteners. The *last* row of a multirow joint in each member, where there is no bypass load left and a reduced total load, is best designed with the geometry for an optimized single-row joint.

These seemingly mutually contradictory requirements can be met only with the assistance of an accurate load-sharing program. Only one has been developed that covers nonlinear behavior in the fastener load-deflection characteristic. That is the A4EJ program derived in Ref 33 and described in Ref 26.

This nonlinear analysis code requires nonlinear characteristics for the fastener load-deflection curves. This may seem to limit the utility of the method. However, Fig. 34 shows that the method will work quite well with approximate models. Standard design practice limits the increase in hole diameter that can be tolerated to a standard offset of 2% of the fastener diameter. At that limit, there is little difference between the actual load carried (when known) and that carried by a model in which the secondary slope is set at one-fifth of the primary slope and the knee at a height of 85% of the maximum. It is important to differentiate between the maximum fastener load, established only with far greater damage to the hole, and the design ultimate load at the 2% of diameter offset. However, once that is done, even a total neglect of any nonlinear increment in the fastener would not cause a significant error. What the nonlinear analysis accomplishes is that the critical fastener loads are held constant, while additional load applied to the joint is able to increase (linearly) the lesser loads transferred through the more lightly loaded fasteners.

Comparative analyses of multirow bolted composite joints reported in Ref 42 have shown that if the basic structure is to be repairable, the optimal splices must contain uniformly thick skins with tapered splice plates, as shown in Fig. 35. Also, the diameter of the fasteners varies throughout the joint. The innermost bolts, adjacent to where the skins butt together, are largest, at about a w/d ratio of 3 to 1. There is no bypass load there in the skin, so that row is optimized as a single row joint. Obviously, that is the worst

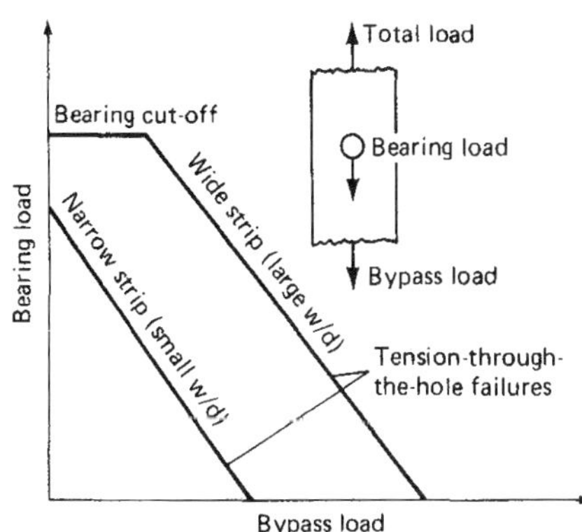

Fig. 31 Bearing-bypass load interaction for loaded bolts in advanced composites

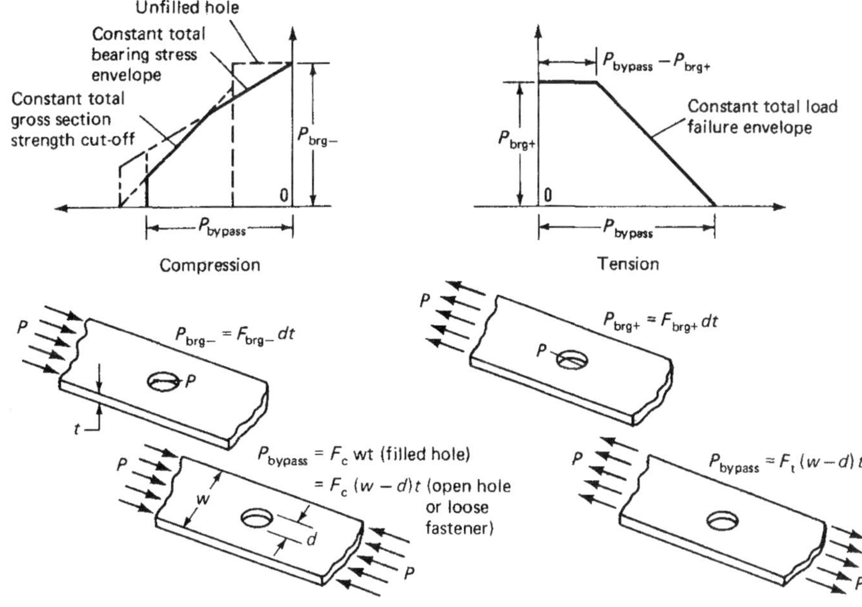

Fig. 32 Outer envelope of bearing-bypass load interactions. F symbols are all ultimate material strengths, dt is the bearing area.

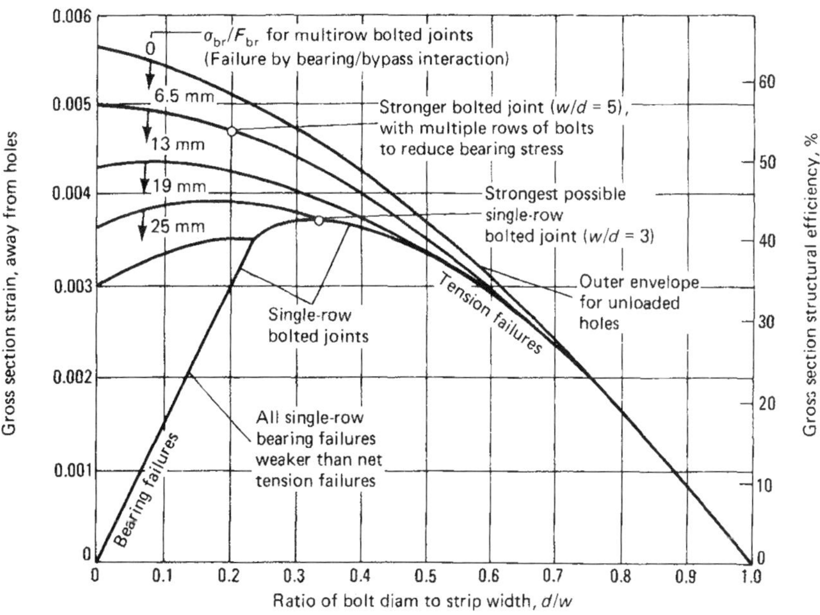

Fig. 33 Influence of bolted joint design on structural efficiency of carbon/epoxy composite structures

possible thing to do to the splice plates, because the maximum bearing and bypass loads coincide there. Consequently, the splice plates must be suitably reinforced. The weight penalty associated with an off-optimal splice plate is trivial in comparison with the substantial weight savings associated with maximizing the structural efficiency of the entire basic skin. This highlights a commonly used, but totally inappropriate, metric for joints whereby it is the weight of the splice that is minimized instead of the total weight of the structure.

The next two rows of fasteners are sized at a w/d ratio of 4 to 1, because there is some bypass load there, in all members. The critical fastener row is the outermost one, near a tip of the splice plate. The smallest, most flexible fasteners are used there ($w/d = 5$), and the tip thickness of the splice plate is limited to prevent those bolts from picking up too much load. It was found that the bearing stress in the skin on that critical row of fasteners could be kept under 25% of the ultimate bearing strength. The resulting high structural efficiency, at a gross-section strain of 0.005, is shown by Fig. 33 to be much higher than can be obtained with optimized single-row bolted composite joints. It is also much higher than can be achieved by nonoptimized multirow bolted composite joints. For example, adding a second row of fasteners in tandem, while retaining the optimal spacing for a single-row joint, would increase the joint strength by only about 10%, a rather small gain for having doubled the number, weight, and cost of the fasteners.

The strength increase is even greater with respect to off-optimal joints, with one or more rows of fasteners, proportioned in such a way as to enforce benign failures in bearing. While that is a noble goal, it must be recognized that there is an associated loss of about one-third of the ultimate strength to obtain that noncatastrophic indication of an overload.

Figure 36 shows how the strength of typical bolted composite structures varies with fiber pattern as well as with the efficiency of the joint design for mechanically fastened composite joints. It is apparent that the most efficient multirow joints are about 50% as strong as the unnotched parent laminate. Moreover, the joint strength is not very sensitive to the fiber pattern, even for a 6.5 mm (0.25 in.) diameter bolt, and becomes even less sensitive for much larger fasteners. The joint strength curves in Fig. 36 would tend to become much flatter and lower for larger bolt sizes for both joints, either with more than one row of fasteners or only one, if it were not that the critical fastener of a multirow joint has to be kept small to raise the structural efficiency by limiting the load it can accept.

Practical Considerations

To attain the high structural efficiency of bolted composite joints, each fastener must accept its correct share of the load. Because composites fail at a very low strain level, such proper load sharing is incompatible with loose-fit holes. On the other hand, the testing of interference-fit fasteners, which were either hammered in or twisted in, also left something to be desired. The obvious solution to this dilemma is the use of a loose sleeve that subsequently is expanded to fit properly when the fastener (bolt or rivet) is installed. Much valuable work on this subject has been performed by E.R. Speakman (Ref 49). A sleeved rivet is illustrated in Fig. 37.

A similar problem exists in composite laminates in regard to the use of countersunk fasteners, particularly single-shear fasteners. As indicated in Fig. 38, as the fastener rotates under low loads, the head moves out of contact with the laminate, and all of the load is reacted by bearing on the (parallel) shank. For this reason, the author advocates that, in the analysis of countersunk fasteners, the head be totally discounted. Such a procedure means restricting the depth of the countersink to no more than one-half the thickness of the outer member. Only after the shank area has failed in bearing does the head make contact with the laminate again.

Such a design procedure would imply a minimum skin thickness of twice the size of the countersunk head on the fastener, even though it has become common practice to countersink deeper, in some cases knife-edging the outer composite member. There is no universal analysis method to cover the design of such questionable joints, and there have been failures associated with such concepts, even though some tests show such a practice to be tolerable, while others have not. It is necessary to confirm the adequacy or inadequacy of such designs by specific testing. Alternatively, because this problem can arise only for relatively thin structures, adhesive bonding might well be considered instead.

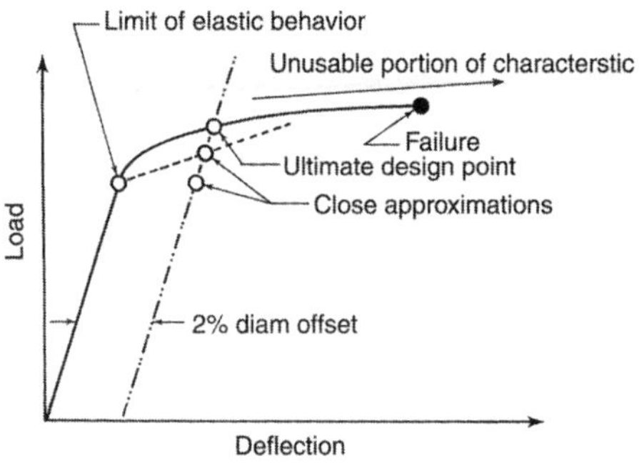

Fig. 34 Idealized fastener load-deflection characteristics

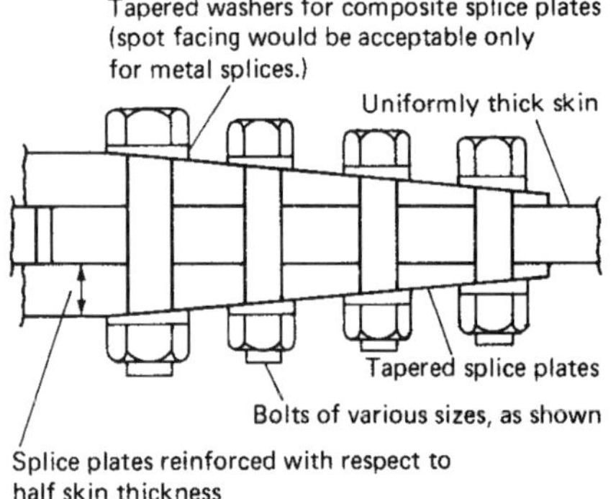

Fig. 35 Optimal proportions for multirow bolted composite joints

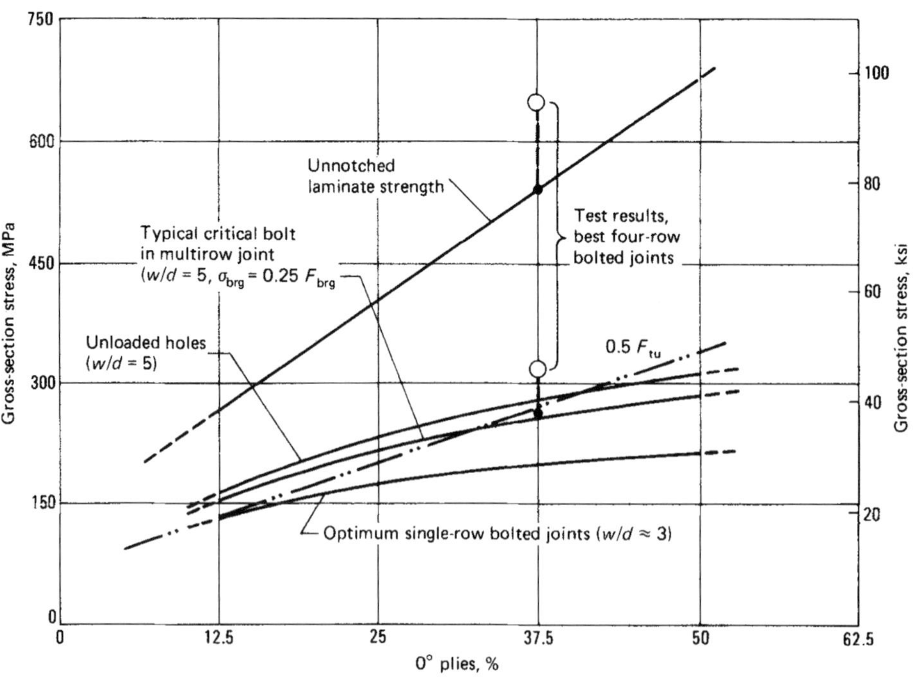

Fig. 36 Gross-section design stresses for bolted composite structures (carbon/epoxy laminates). Chart applicable for bolts up to 9.5 mm (37 in.) in diameter. Larger bolts are associated with progressively lower laminate stresses.

A related issue is the installation of fittings in composite control surfaces. Whenever such fittings occur behind cutouts in the leading edge of the surface, it is always permissible to use shallow protruding-head fasteners, as shown in Fig. 39. (The drag from the cutout masks that from the fastener heads.) Not only is there more effective bearing area on the shank than with countersunk fasteners, but the bolt-bearing allowable strength is also raised by about a factor of 2, because of the through-the-thickness clamp-up on the laminate. This substantial improvement on bearing strength is illustrated in Fig. 29.

A considerable simplification in the design process for mechanically fastened composite structures is afforded by the use of diagrams such as Fig. 40, which was prepared for older carbon fibers. Points A and B in the figure could probably be raised by a strain increment of 0.001 for the newer high-strain fibers. Such a simple chart, which can reasonably be applied when there are orthogonal load components also present, can safely cover all of the relatively lightly loaded fasteners, as at skin-to-spar and skin-to-rib seams on wings, leaving only the few major load-transfer splices requiring more detailed analysis of the kind discussed in the section "Multirow Bolted Composite Joints" in this article.

It is not possible to cover all that is known about joints in fibrous composite structures in a single article. Only some of the highlights have been addressed here, and the reader is referred to the references cited and the other copious literature on the subject for further information.

It has been explained here that adhesive bonding is more suitable than mechanical fastening for thin structures (both composite and metal), and that the strength of such joints can, and should, exceed the strength of the members being joined. The issue of the durability of bonded joints is just as important as the short-term static strength, and distinct, albeit simple, design features are needed to ensure that the adhesive bonds will not fail prematurely.

Either mechanical fastening or more complex, bonded stepped-lap joints are needed for thicker, more highly loaded structures; adhesive bonds would only act as weak-link fuses in thick structures. It is never acceptable to design an adhesively bonded joint that is weaker than the members being joined. On the other hand, bolted composite joints can never be as strong as the member being joined, either, unless one resorts to softening strips and local pad-ups, which leave the basic structure too highly stressed to be repaired. Indeed, designing to structural efficiencies of 50% is quite a challenge. Finally, it should be noted that the design of the joints should always precede the process of filling in the gaps (sizing the laminates), and that due consideration should always be given to designing structures that can be repaired.

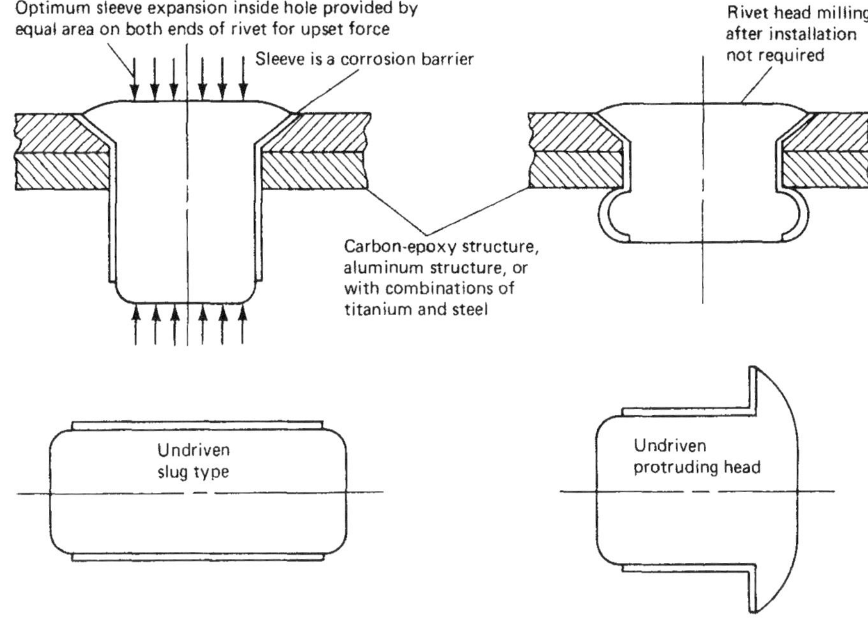

Fig. 37 Sleeved rivet

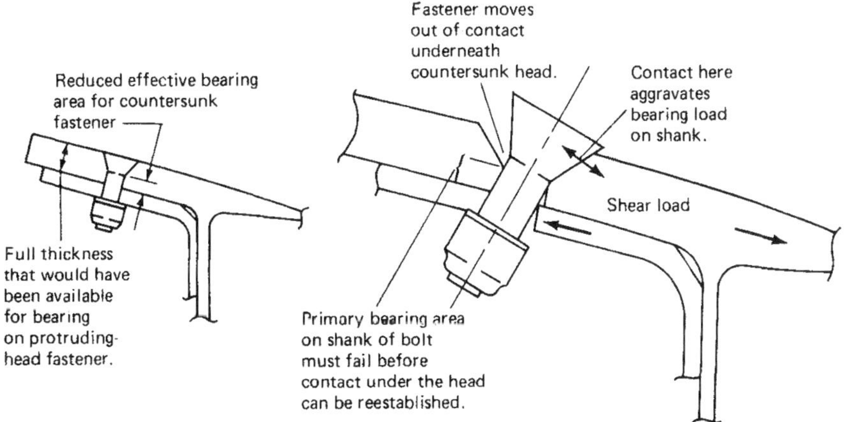

Fig. 38 Problems with using flush fasteners at fittings for composite structures

REFERENCES

1. L.J. Hart-Smith and J.H. Gosse, "Characterizing the Strength of Fiber-Polymer Com-

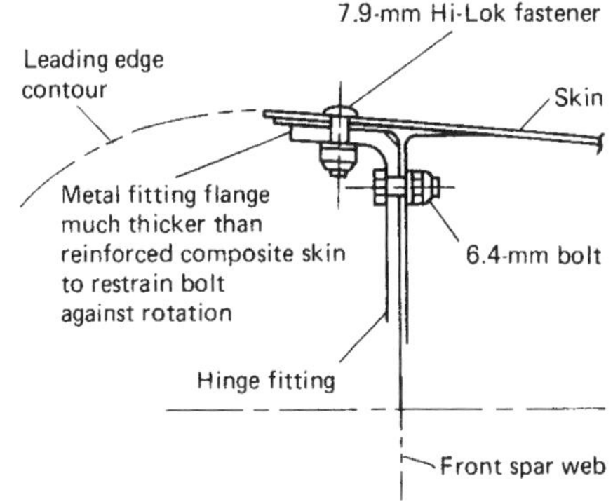

Fig. 39 Thickened hinge fitting flanges to minimize bolt bearing stresses. Hi-Lok (Hi-Shear Corp.)

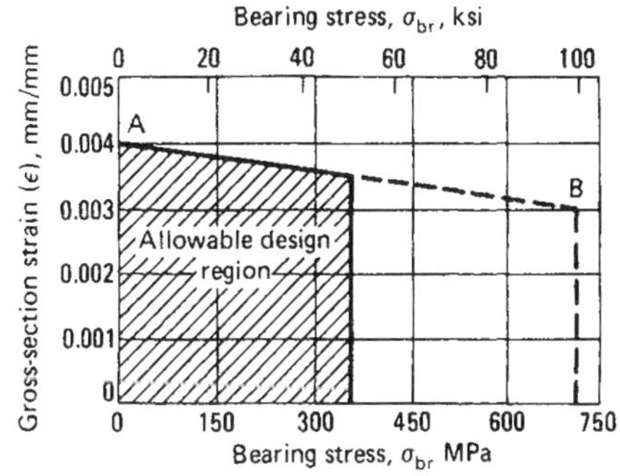

Fig. 40 Example of design guidelines for bolted carbon/epoxy structures

posites Using Mechanistic Failure Models," Boeing Paper MDC 00K0050, to be published in American Institute of Aeronautics and Astronautics, Textbook on composite materials, Murray Scott, Ed.

2. J. Gosse and S. Christensen, Strain Invariant Failure Criteria for Polymers in Composite Materials, AIAA-2001-1184, The Boeing Company, *Proc. 42nd American Institute of Aeronautics and Astronautics/American Society of Mechanical Engineers/American Society of Civil Engineers/American Helicopter Society/American Society for Composites Structures, Structural Dynamics, and Materials Conf.*, 16–19 April 2001 (Seattle, WA)
3. L.J. Hart-Smith, The Design of Repairable Composite Structures, *SAE Trans.* 851830, SAE Aerospace Technology Conf., Society of Automotive Engineers, 1985
4. E.W. Godwin and F.L. Matthews, A Review of the Strength of Joints in Fibre-Reinforced Plastics, Part 1: Mechanically Fastened Joints, *Composites,* Vol 11, 1980, p 155–160
5. F.L. Matthews, P.F. Kilty, and E.W. Godwin, A Review of the Strength of Joints in Fibre-Reinforced Plastics, Part 2: Adhesively Bonded Joints, *Composites,* Vol 13, 1982, p 29–37
6. L.J. Hart-Smith, Effects of Flaws and Porosity on Strength of Adhesive-Bonded Joints, *Proc. 29th SAMPE Annual Symposium and Technical Conf.,* Society for the Advancement of Material and Process Engineering, April 1984, p 840–852
7. E.W. Thrall, Jr., Failures in Adhesively Bonded Structures, *Bonded Joints and Preparation for Bonding,* AGARD-NATO Lecture Series 102, Advisory Group for Aerospace Research and Development, North Atlantic Treaty Organization, 1979, p 5-1 to 5-89
8. L.J. Hart-Smith, Adhesive Bonding of Aircraft Primary Structures, Douglas Paper 6979, *SAE Trans.* 801209, SAE Aerospace Congress and Exhibition, Society of Automotive Engineers, 1980
9. R.W. Shannon et al., "Primary Adhesively Bonded Structure Technology (PABST): General Material Property Data," United States Air Force, AFFDL-TR-77-107, Douglas Aircraft Company, Sept 1978, 2nd ed., 1982
10. R.J. Schliekelmann, Adhesive Bonding and Composites, *Progress in Science and Engineering of Composites,* Vol 1, T. Hayashi, K. Kawata, and S. Umekawa, Ed., *Fourth International Conf. Composite Materials,* (North Holland), 1983, p 63–78
11. L.J. Hart-Smith, R.W. Ochsner, and R.L. Radecky, Surface Preparation of Fibrous Composites for Adhesive Bonding or Painting, *Douglas Service Magazine,* first quarter, 1984, p 12–22
12. A.V. Pocius and R.P. Wenz, Mechanical Surface Preparation of Graphite-Epoxy Composite for Adhesive Bonding, *Proc. 30th National SAMPE Symposium,* Society for the Advancement of Material and Process Engineering, March 1985, p 1073–1087
13. L.J. Hart-Smith, G. Redmond, and M.J. Davis, "The Curse of the Nylon Peel Ply," McDonnell Douglas Paper MDC 95K0072, presented to 41st International SAMPE Symposium and Exhibition, 25–28 March 1996 (Anaheim), *Society for the Advancement of Material and Process Engineering; in Proc.*, p 303–317
14. L.J. Hart-Smith, "Effects of Pre-Bond Moisture on Interfacial Failures in Glued Composite Joints—and What to Do about It," presented to MIL-HDBK-17 Meeting, 30 March to 2 April 1998 (San Diego, CA); also to be presented to a future International Society for the Advancement of Material and Process Engineering Symposium and Exhibition
15. T. Kinloch, paper referenced in L.J. Hart-Smith paper for San Francisco Society for the Advancement of Material and Process Engineering
16. S.H. Myhre, J.D. Labor, and S.C. Aker, Moisture Problems in Advanced Composite Structural Repair, *Composites,* Vol 13, 1982, p 289–297
17. O. Volkersen, The Rivet-Force Distribution in Tension-Stressed Riveted Joints with Constant Sheet Thicknesses, *Luftfahrtforschung*, Vol 15, 1938, p 4–47
18. M. Goland and E. Reissner, The Stresses in Cemented Joints, *J. Appl. Mech., (Trans. ASME),* Vol 11, 1944, p A17–A27
19. L.J. Hart-Smith, "Adhesive-Bonded Single-Lap Joints," NASA CR-112236, Douglas Aircraft Company, Jan 1973
20. L.J. Hart-Smith, Stress Analysis: A Continuum Mechanics Approach, *Developments in Adhesives, 2,* A.J. Kinloch, Ed., Applied Science Publishers, 1981, p 143
21. L.J. Hart-Smith, "The Goland and Reissner Bonded Lap Joint Analysis Revisited Yet Again—but This Time Essentially Validated," Boeing Paper MDC 00K0036, to be published
22. N.A. de Bruyne, The Strength of Glued Joints, *Aircr. Eng.,* Vol 16, 1944, p 115–118, 140
23. L.J. Hart-Smith, "Analysis and Design of Advanced Composite Bonded Joints," NASA CR-2218, Douglas Aircraft Company, Jan 1973; reprinted, complete, Aug 1974
24. L.J. Hart-Smith, Design and Analysis of Adhesive-Bonded Joints, *Proc. First Air Force Conf. Fibrous Composites in Flight Vehicle Design,* AFFDL-TR-72-130, Air Force Flight Dynamics Laboratory, 1972, p 813–856
25. L.J. Hart-Smith, Advances in the Analysis and Design of Adhesive-Bonded Joints in Composite Aerospace Structures, *Proc. 19th National SAMPE Symposium and Exhibition,* Society for the Advancement of Material and Process Engineering, April 1974, p 722–737
26. L.J. Hart-Smith, Bonded-Bolted Composite Joints, *J. Aircr.,* Vol 22, 1985, p 993–1000
27. L.J. Hart-Smith, Adhesively Bonded Joints for Fibrous Composite Structures, *Joining Fibre-Reinforced Plastics,* F.L. Matthews, Ed., Elsevier, 1987, p 271–311
28. L.J. Hart-Smith, "Differences between Adhesive Behavior in Test Coupons and Structural Joints," paper presented at ASTM Adhesives Committee D-14 Meeting, March 1981 (Phoenix), American Society for Testing and Materials
29. L.J. Hart-Smith, "Adhesive Layer Thickness and Porosity Criteria for Bonded Joints," AFWAL-TR-82-4172, Douglas Aircraft Company, Dec 1982
30. R.B. Krieger, Jr., Analyzing Joint Stresses Using an Extensometer, *Adhes. Age,* Vol 28 (No. 11), Oct 1985, p 26–28
31. L.J. Hart-Smith, "Adhesive-Bonded Double-Lap Joints," NASA CR-112235, Douglas Aircraft Company, Jan 1973
32. L.J. Hart-Smith, "Adhesive-Bonded Scarf and Stepped-Lap Joints," NASA CR-112237, Douglas Aircraft Company, Jan 1973
33. L.J. Hart-Smith, "Design Methodology for Bonded-Bolted Composite Joints," AFWAL-TR-81-3154, Douglas Aircraft Company, Feb 1982
34. L.J. Hart-Smith, Further Developments in the Design and Analysis of Adhesive-Bonded Structural Joints, *Joining of Composite Materials,* STP 749, K.T. Kedward, Ed., American Society for Testing and Materials, 1981, p 3–31
35. L.J. Hart-Smith, Design and Analysis of Bonded Repairs for Metal Aircraft Structures, *Proc. International Workshop on Defense Applications of Advanced Repair Technology for Metal and Composite Structures,* Naval Research Laboratory, July 1981, p 251–260
36. W.S. Johnson, Ed., *Delamination and Debonding of Materials,* STP 876, American Society for Testing and Materials, 1985
37. L.J. Hart-Smith, Simplified Estimation of Stiffness and Biaxial Strengths for Design of Carbon-Epoxy Composite Structures, *Proc. Seventh Department of Defense/National Aeronautics and Space Administration Conf. on Fibrous Composites in Structural Design,* AFWAL-TR-85-3094, 1985, p V(a)-17 to V(a)-52
38. L.J. Hart-Smith, Simplified Estimation of Stiffness and Biaxial Strengths of Woven Carbon-Epoxy Composites, *Closed-Session Conf. Proc.,* 31st International SAMPE Symposium and Exhibition, Society for the Advancement of Material and Process Engineering, April 1986, p 83–102
39. L.J. Hart-Smith, Mechanically Fastened Joints for Advanced Composites—Phenom-

enological Considerations and Simple Analyses, *Fibrous Composites in Structural Design,* Fourth Conf. on Fibrous Composites in Structural Design, E.M. Lenoe, D.W. Oplinger, and J.J. Burke, Ed., Plenum Press, 1980, p 543–574

40. L.J. Hart-Smith, "Bolted Joints in Graphite-Epoxy Laminates," NASA CR-144899, Douglas Aircraft Company, Jan 1977
41. L.J. Hart-Smith, Design and Analysis of Bolted and Riveted Joints in Fibrous Composite Structures, *Joining Fibre-Reinforced Plastics,* F.L. Matthews, Ed., Elsevier, 1987, p 227–269
42. W.D. Nelson, B.L. Bunin, and L.J. Hart-Smith, Critical Joints in Large Composite Aircraft Structure, *Proc. Sixth Conf. Fibrous Composites in Structural Design,* AMMRC MS 83-2, Army Materials and Mechanics Research Center, 1983, p II-1 to II-38
43. L.J. Hart-Smith, "Analysis Methods for Bolted Composite Joints Subjected to In-Plane Shear Loads," McDonnell Douglas Paper MDC 96K0086, presented to AGARD 83rd Structures and Materials Panel, Bolted/Bonded Joints in Polymeric Composites, Specialists Meeting, 2–3 Sept 1996 (Florence, Italy), Advisory Group for Aerospace Research and Development; Bolted/Bonded Joints in Polymeric Composites, *AGARD Conf. Proc.,* AGARD CP-590, Jan 1997, p 8-1 to 8-11
44. J.M. Whitney and R.J. Nuismer, Stress Fracture Criteria for Laminated Composites Containing Stress Concentrations, *J. Compos. Mater.,* Vol 8, 1974, p 253–265
45. R.L. Ramkumar and E.W. Tossavainen, "Bolted Joints in Composite Structures: Design, Analysis and Verification; Task I Test Results—Single Fastener Joints," AFWAL-TR-84-3047, Northrop Aircraft Division, Aug 1984
46. R.B. Heywood, *Designing by Photoelasticity,* Chapman and Hall, 1952, p 268
47. S. P. Garbo and J. M. Ogonowski, "Effect of Variances and Manufacturing Tolerances on the Design Strength and Life of Mechanically Fastened Composite Joints," AFWAL-TR-81-3041, McDonnell Aircraft Company, April 1981
48. S.P. Garbo, "Effects of Bearing/Bypass Load Interaction on Laminate Strength," AFWAL-TR-81-3144, McDonnell Aircraft Company, Sept 1981
49. E.R. Speakman, Advanced Fastener Technology for Composite and Metallic Joints, *Fatigue in Mechanically Fastened Composite and Metallic Joints,* STP 927, J.M. Potter, Ed., American Society for Testing and Materials, 1986

Instability Considerations

Gerald Flanagan and Carol Meyers, Materials Sciences Corporation

THE ANALYSIS OF STABILITY for laminated composite plates owes much to theoretical developments for isotropic plates and shells. Indeed, much of the progress in understanding stability of composites has occurred by rederiving the isotropic results while taking into account all of the additional stiffness terms that can be present for a composite. While the additional terms greatly increase the length and complexity of the equations, the fundamental mechanics largely remain the same. Considerable basic information on the buckling of composite plates and shells may be found in Ref 1 to 6. In addition, an extensive review of literature can be found in Ref 7. This article focuses on the unique characteristics of composites and laminated plates. It also focuses on stability issues associated with practical, structural laminates. The study of instability can also include postbuckling behavior. However, in a brief article, postbuckling phenomena cannot be addressed.

Background

Instability in laminated flat plates or shells is a state of critical loading, such that a small perpendicular static load would result in a large transverse displacement. The laminate is said to buckle. In dynamic situations, loading on the laminate is such that the response to transverse vibratory input is much greater than if it were unloaded.

This article assumes a familiarity with lamination theory. For laminated plates, the most general relationship between in-plane force intensities (N_i), moment intensities (M_i), strains (ε_i), and curvatures (κ_i) is given by the expression:

$$\begin{Bmatrix} N_x \\ N_y \\ N_{xy} \\ M_x \\ M_y \\ M_{xy} \end{Bmatrix} = \begin{bmatrix} A_{11} & A_{12} & A_{16} & B_{11} & B_{12} & B_{16} \\ A_{12} & A_{22} & A_{26} & B_{12} & B_{22} & B_{26} \\ A_{16} & A_{26} & A_{66} & B_{16} & B_{26} & B_{66} \\ B_{11} & B_{12} & B_{16} & D_{11} & D_{12} & D_{16} \\ B_{12} & B_{22} & B_{26} & D_{12} & D_{22} & D_{26} \\ B_{16} & B_{26} & B_{66} & D_{16} & D_{26} & D_{66} \end{bmatrix} \begin{Bmatrix} \varepsilon_x \\ \varepsilon_y \\ \gamma_{xy} \\ \kappa_x \\ \kappa_y \\ \kappa_{xy} \end{Bmatrix} \quad \text{(Eq 1)}$$

where A_{ij}, B_{ij}, and D_{ij} are computed using standard lamination theory. The A_{ij} coefficients are the stretching stiffness terms, the B_{ij} terms represent stretching-bending coupling, and the D_{ij} terms represent bending stiffness. N_i has the units of force/per unit length, and M_i has the units of force times length per unit length. For a symmetric plate, the B_{ij} terms are zero. In this case, the in-plane forces and midplane strains decouple from the moments and curvatures.

Under thin-plate assumptions (Kirchhoff theory), the vertical equilibrium in the presence of in-plane loads is given by:

$$D_{11}\frac{\partial^4 w}{\partial x^4} + 4D_{16}\frac{\partial^4 w}{\partial x^3 \partial y} + 2(D_{12}+2D_{66})\frac{\partial^4 w}{\partial x^2 \partial y^2} + 4D_{26}\frac{\partial^4 w}{\partial x \partial y^3} + D_{22}\frac{\partial^4 w}{\partial y^4} = N_x\frac{\partial^2 w}{\partial x^2} + 2N_{xy}\frac{\partial^2 w}{\partial x \partial y} + N_y\frac{\partial^2 w}{\partial y^2} \quad \text{(Eq 2)}$$

where w is the out-of-plane deflection of the plate. Solutions of this equation form the basis of linear buckling theory for thin, symmetric, anisotropic plates.

Orthotropic Plates

In the full form of the plate equations, the terms D_{16} and D_{26} are bending-twisting coupling terms. If $D_{16} = D_{26} = 0$, then the plate is orthotropic in bending. Many composite laminates are not exactly orthotropic (see the subsequent anisotropic plate discussion). However, assuming orthotropic properties is often a reasonable assumption that leads to important simplifications to the governing equations. Simple-support (SS) boundary conditions will be satisfied by any term in the series:

$$w = C_{mn}\sin\left(\frac{m\pi x}{a}\right)\sin\left(\frac{n\pi y}{b}\right) \quad \text{(Eq 3)}$$

where a and b are the panel dimensions in the x and y directions, respectively, C_{mn} is a constant coefficient, and m and n are integers. For an orthotropic plate, and $N_{xy} = 0$, Eq 1 will be satisfied by any term of the series (Eq 2) if $N_x = N_{xcr}$, where:

$$N_{xcr} = -\frac{\pi^2\sqrt{D_{11}D_{22}}}{b^2}k \quad \text{(Eq 4)}$$

and k is a buckling coefficient for a compressive load. Here, the convention is adopted where a negative load is compressive. For the SS boundary condition, k is given by:

$$k = \frac{D_{11}m^4 + 2c^2(D_{12}+2D_{66})m^2n^2 + c^4D_{22}n^4}{\sqrt{D_{11}D_{22}}\,(c^2m^2 + c^4n^2R)} \quad \text{(Eq 5)}$$

where c is the aspect ratio, a/b, and R is the load ratio, N_y/N_x. The number of half-waves in the buckling mode shape are determined by the wave numbers m and n. One must find the values of m and n that yield the smallest value of k, and thus the smallest buckling load. If $R = 0$, then the minimum value of k_c occurs when $n = 1$. The value of m is a function of the plate aspect ratio and materials properties. This is illustrated in Fig. 1, in which the minimum buckling coefficient is plotted for the special case of $(D_{12} + 2D_{66})/D_{22} = 1$, and different values of D_{11}/D_{22}. For $D_{11}/D_{22} = 1$, the plate is isotropic.

For a given plate-aspect ratio, it is possible to plot the buckling coefficient as a function of the laminate stack. For a square plate ($a/b = 1$), the buckling coefficient as a function of the percentage of ±45° plies in a [±45/0/90] family laminate is shown in Fig. 2, where the 0° degree ply direction is parallel to the x-axis of the plate. In this plot, the buckling load is normalized by the layer fiber-direction modulus, (E_1). For a square panel, the optimal laminate for buckling uses all ±45° layers. The other counter-intuitive result is that the buckling load is independent of the relative percentage of 0° and 90° layers. The optimal laminate changes depend on the aspect ratio. Figure 3 shows a carpet plot of buckling coefficients for the same [±45/0/90] family of laminates, and $a/b = 0.25$. In this case, the optimal laminate contains all 0° plies. In the carpet plot format, the solid lines represent different percentage of 0° layers. The dashed line represents the limit of zero percentage of 90° layers.

The shear load case does not have a closed-form solution. Equation 3 still applies for SS boundary conditions, but Eq 2 is not satisfied by

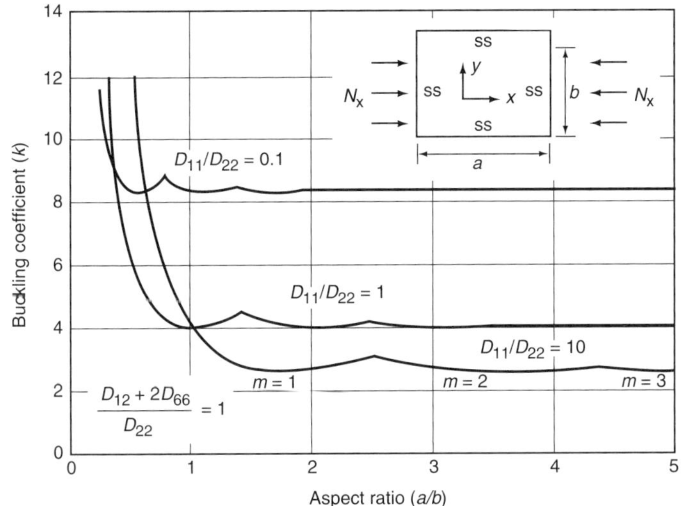

Fig. 1 Buckling coefficient for plate under uniaxial compression

a single term of the series. A typical approach is to use an energy method to obtain an approximate solution using a finite series. The buckling coefficient plot for shear load (N_{xy}) given in Fig. 4 was created using such an approach. Using this coefficient, the buckling load for shear is given by:

$$N_{xycr} = \frac{\pi^2 \sqrt[4]{D_{11} D_{22}^3}}{b^2} k_s \quad \text{(Eq 6)}$$

Materials properties for a typical intermediate modulus graphite/epoxy material ($E_1 = 21 \times 10^6$ psi, $E_2 = 1.6 \times 10^6$ psi, $G_{12} = 0.85 \times 10^6$ psi, $\nu_{12} = 0.35$) were used in the calculations for Fig. 4, and the curves are for specific stacking sequences. The plot assumes that the number of ply groups, n, is large, so that the laminate is effectively homogeneous through the thickness. For the shear case, there is a less distinct transition as the number of waves in the mode shape changes.

Approximate buckling coefficients for a variety of other boundary conditions and load cases can be found in the literature. One of the most complete collections available is contained in Ref 8.

Finite Stack Effects

Carpet plots can be generated assuming that the plate behaves as a homogeneous material. For example, one can compute the effective in-plane stiffness (the **A** matrix in Eq 1) using lamination theory. An approximation of the bending stiffness is:

$$D_{ij} = \frac{h^2}{12} A_{ij} \quad \text{(Eq 7)}$$

This equation assumes that the position of the ply in the stack is not important. In reality, the bending stiffness of a composite plate is a function of the stacking sequence. The importance of stacking sequence is particularly evident for thin laminates with a small number of layers. This effect is shown in Fig. 5 for a $[0/90]_{ns}$ laminate and a $[90/0]_{ns}$ laminate, where n is the number of times the basic ply pattern is repeated. In Fig. 5, the buckling load is normalized by the bending stiffness using a homogeneous assumption. As seen in the figure, for an infinite number of ply groups, the buckling coefficient for both patterns will approach 1. For a small number of ply groups, there can be a considerable error in the homogenous assumption.

Anisotropic Plates

Any composite laminate that uses angle plies ($\pm\theta$) in the stacking sequence will have some degree of anisotropy in the bending stiffness. This means that the D_{16}, D_{26} bending-twisting coupling terms will not be exactly 0, even if there are an equal number of plus θ and minus θ plies. The effect is demonstrated in Fig. 6. Here, the ratio of D_{16} to D_{11} is plotted as a function of the number of repeated ply groups in a $[\pm 45]_{ns}$ laminate. The relative magnitude of D_{16} rapidly decreases with the number of ply groups, but will never exactly reach 0. The presence of D_{16} and D_{26} generally decreases the buckling for an axially loaded plate, as shown in Fig. 7.

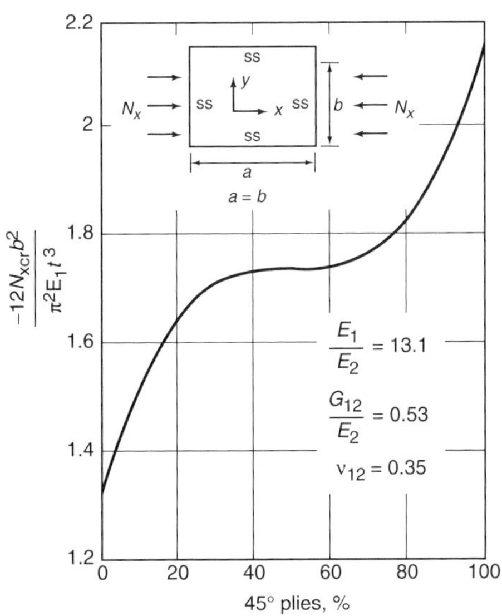

Fig. 2 Normalized buckling coefficient as function of percentage of ±45° plies. [±45/0/90] family laminate, square (a/b = 1). Uniaxial compressive load

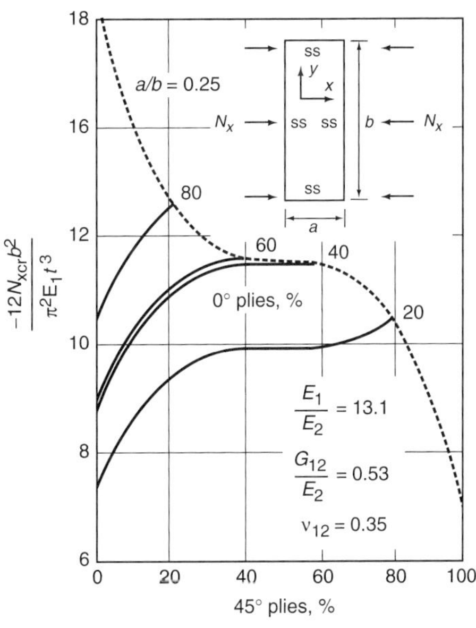

Fig. 3 Carpet plot of normalized buckling coefficient. [±45/0/90] family laminate with a/b = 0.25. Solid lines indicate different %0° plies. Dashed line is limit of 90° ply = 0%. (%90° = 100% –% 0°–%45°)

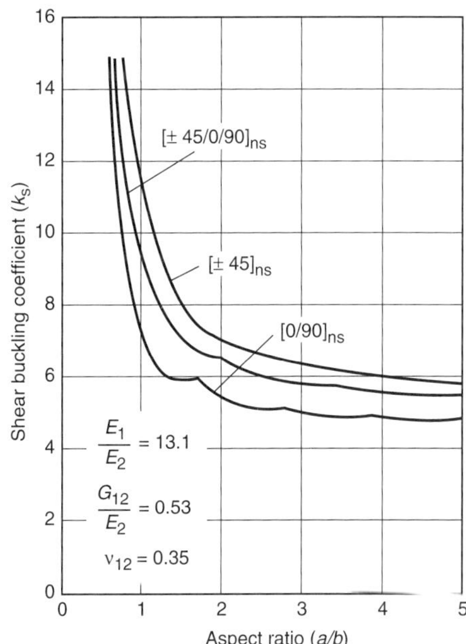

Fig. 4 Shear buckling coefficient for various graphite/epoxy laminates

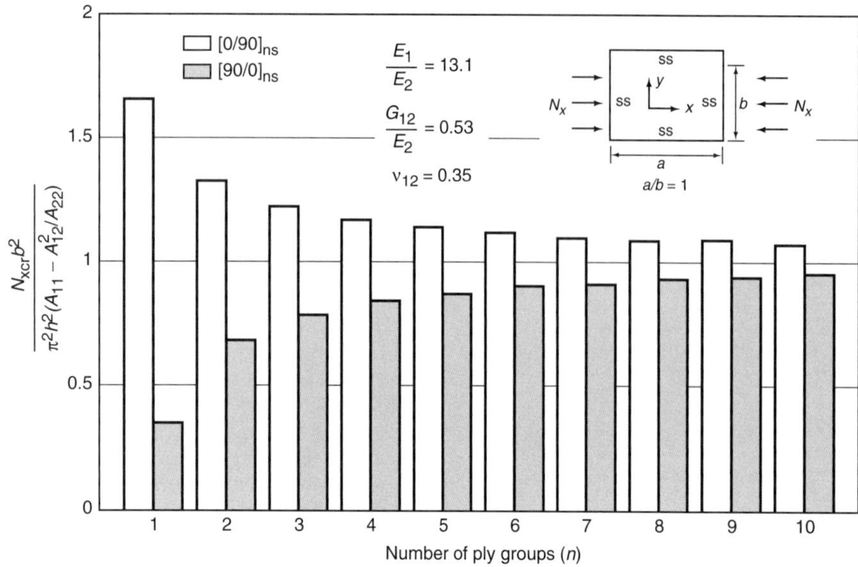

Fig. 5 Normalized buckling load for $[0/90]_{ns}$ and $[90/0]_{ns}$ laminates as a function of number of ply groups

Closed-form solutions can be obtained for the buckling of long (infinite) anisotropic plates. These solutions provide a lower bound for the

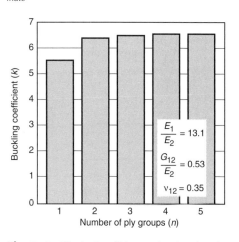

Fig. 6 Relative size of bending-twisting term as a function of number of ply groups for a $[\pm 45]_{ns}$ laminate

Fig. 7 Buckling load coefficient as a function of number of ply groups for a $[\pm 45]_{ns}$ laminate with $a/b = 1$

anisotropic effect. Parametric studies of the influence of D_{16} are given in Ref 9.

Another important difference between plates and shells with orthotropic or isotropic properties and those with anisotropic properties is the reflection symmetries of the mode shapes. While orthotropic plates exhibit reflection symmetry (or antisymmetry), allowing the use of quarter-plate models, anisotropic structures do not. Instead, anisotropic plates and shells exhibit inversion symmetry (or antisymmetry) with respect to the normal axis, resulting in a skewing of the mode shape, as shown in Fig. 8. This skewing of the mode shape results primarily from the presence of the twisting coupling terms, D_{16} and D_{26}, and is therefore a feature even in so-called quasi-isotropic laminates.

Under shear loading, an anisotropic plate will have different buckling loads for positive and negative shear.

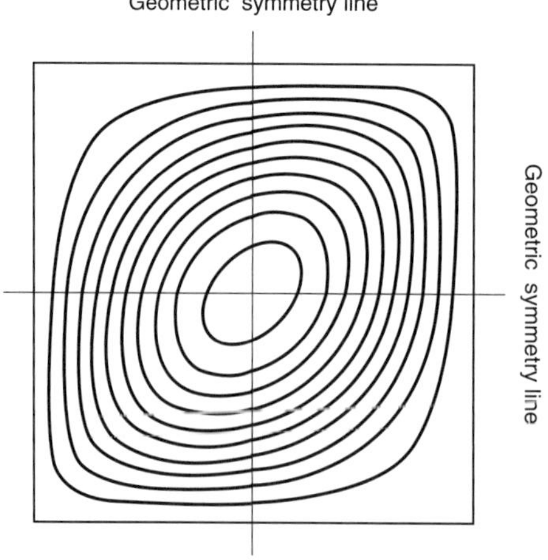

Fig. 8 Mode shape for $[\pm 45]_s$ laminate under axial load

Unsymmetric Plates

Most structural laminates are constructed using a stacking sequence that is symmetric about the geometric midplane of the plate. Using a symmetric laminate eliminates the bending-stretching coupling that can exist for a general laminate. The bending-stretching coupling is reflected by nonzero **B** matrix terms in lamination theory. The presence of a nonzero **B** matrix will usually reduce the theoretical buckling load of a plate. One should use caution with the concept of linear buckling for a nonsymmetric plate, because out-of-plane deflections will occur when in-plane loads below the buckling value are applied.

Nonsymmetry also adds an additional degree of complexity to the solution of the plate buckling equations. However, if the edge boundary conditions are such that there are no in-plane forces as a result of bending deflections, that is, the edges are free to translate in the plane of the plate, then one can use reduced bending properties in the equations for a symmetric plate. The reduced bending stiffness matrix, $\tilde{\mathbf{D}}$, is given by:

$$\tilde{\mathbf{D}} = \mathbf{D} - \mathbf{B}^{T}\mathbf{A}^{-1}\mathbf{B} \quad \text{(Eq 8)}$$

Transverse Shear Stiffness Effects

The interlaminar shear stiffness relative to the in-plane properties of a fiber reinforced composite is typically much smaller than for homogeneous materials. The reduced stiffness means that transverse shear effects are significant for much larger width-to-thickness ratios than for metal plates. Figure 9 shows the reduction in buckling coefficient as a function of b/t (width over thickness) for an axially loaded plate, and Fig. 10 shows a similar plot for a shear loaded

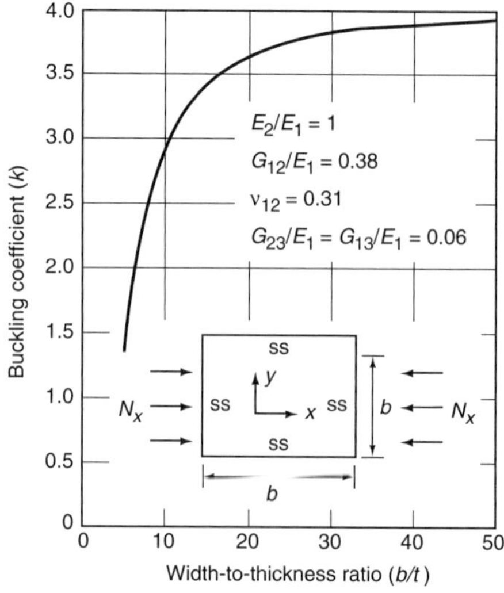

Fig. 9 Axial compression buckling coefficient as a function of width-to-thickness ratio (b/t) for a thick graphite/epoxy quasi-isotropic plate with $a/b = 1$

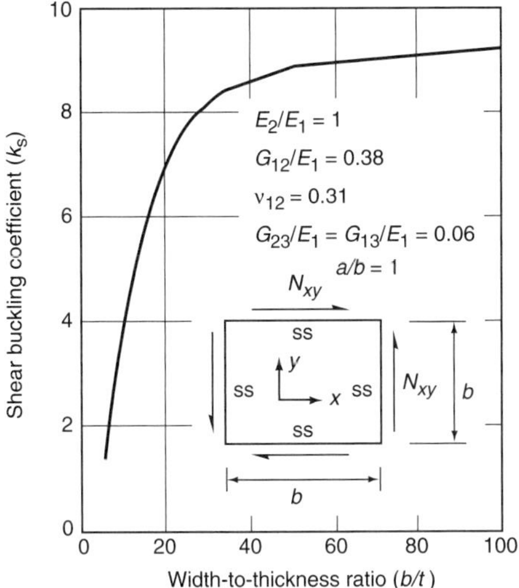

Fig. 10 Shear buckling coefficient as a function of width-to-thickness ratio (b/t) for a thick graphite/epoxy quasi-isotropic plate with $a/b = 1$

plate. The materials properties used for these plots are typical of graphite/epoxy quasi-isotropic laminates, where E_1, E_2, G_{12}, G_{13}, G_{23}, and ν_{12} are effective laminate properties. Because of this reduction in buckling load, it is important to use a finite element formulation that allows for shear deformation. These are sometimes referred to as thick-plate elements.

The most common thick-plate formulations allow for an additional rotation about the midplane of the plate in addition to the rotation related to the second derivative of w, as given by the Kirchhoff theory. Thus, there are additional degrees of freedom at a node in a finite element formulation.

The transverse shear stiffness of a laminated plate is also a function of stacking sequence. A commonly used method for determining the effective stiffness is given by Whitney (Ref 10). His approach involves determining the interlaminar shear stress distribution based in elasticity theory, and then finding the effective stiffness that yields the same strain energy for an assumed plate theory as for the exact stress distribution.

Edge boundary conditions require extra care when thick-plate formulations are used. For example, to specify a SS boundary condition along an edge parallel to the x-axis, one would normally only have to specify that w-displacement along the line is 0. In a thick plate, one can also specify whether rotation about the y-axis should be 0 or unconstrained along the same line.

Hygrothermal Buckling

Another consideration for composite structural stability is hygrothermal buckling. In this case, in-plane loads are induced at constrained edges by the expansion of the material due to thermal expansion and/or swelling of the matrix from moisture absorption. An interesting aspect of thermal buckling for graphite-fiber composites is that graphite fibers have a negative coefficient of thermal expansion, thus it is possible for plates with certain angle-ply lay-ups to buckle due to a decrease in temperature. Moisture absorption is a consideration for polymer-matrix composites, with the amount of swelling depending on the degree of molecular cross-linking in the polymer. The article "Hygrothermal Behavior" in this Volume expands on this topic.

Composite Sandwich Panels

Sandwich panels can be treated as conventional laminated plates where the core is a layer of the laminate with low stiffness properties. An extended discussion of sandwich panel instability is given in Ref 11. For a sandwich panel, it is even more important to account for the transverse shear effects using a thick-plate theory or a finite element with transverse shear flexibility. Sandwich panels also exhibit additional failure modes associated with instability of the facesheet due to insufficient elastic support from the core. One form of instability is buckling between the cell walls of a honeycomb core. Facesheet instability can also occur on foam cores. A simple, approximate equation for the mode was developed by Hoff and Mautner (Ref 12), given by:

$$\sigma_{crit} = c(E_f E_c G_{cz})^{1/3} \qquad \text{(Eq 9)}$$

where E_f is the facesheet in-plane modulus in the direction of the applied stress, E_c is the core through-thickness modulus, and G_{cz} is the core through-thickness shear modulus. The coefficient c is a constant and is usually assumed to be in the range of 0.5 to 0.65. More information on this topic can be found in the article "Analysis of Sandwich Structures" in this Volume.

Computer Codes

General-purpose finite element codes are typically used for the evaluation of stability for plates with more general shapes and boundary conditions. Modern finite element codes are usually acceptable for performing buckling calculations for composites if an appropriate thick-plate element is available. In addition to general-purpose codes, a number of specialized codes have been developed. The motivations for creating these codes are usually related to the ease of setting up problems, the solution speed, structural optimization, or more robust solutions for the post-buckling regime. Some of the more mature and easily obtainable codes are described.

There are several codes that start with the assumption that the structure is prismatic, that is, the geometry is uniform in one direction. This restriction allows one to assume that the deflections have a trigonometric dependence along the constant cross-section direction. The governing equations for the transverse direction then can be solved as ordinary differential equations. These equations can be solved by either exact or numerical methods.

A general-solution approach was first described by Wittrick and Williams (Ref 13). Their code, called VISPASA, was later incorporated into a stiffened panel optimization code called PASCO (Ref 14). The exact solution scheme allows for rapid solutions, which in turn makes the optimization process more practical. PASCO is particularly useful for stiffened composite panels in which both the laminate and geometry of the stiffener are design variables. The basic approach has been enhanced by later developments (Ref 15).

Another efficient panel optimization code is PANDA2 (Ref 16). PANDA uses a combination of closed-form equations and numerical approximations to check a number of potential failure modes.

Structural Analysis of General Shells (STAGS) (Ref 17) is frequently used when a postbuckling solution is needed. STAGS uses the finite element method, and therefore can be used for general shapes and boundary conditions. The strength in STAGS is in its robust nonlinear algorithms. There is a large body of literature that demonstrates STAGS for a variety of stiffened plate and shell problems.

Shell Panel Instability

Many of the general observations made about the effects of anisotropy and shear deformation on composite plate stability also hold for shells. Buckling characteristics of shell panels may be different from those of plates even in the case of isotropic materials, however, because of the coupling of in-plane and out-of-plane responses due to the shell curvature. This may be further complicated in the case of composites by the presence of anisotropy. The complexity of the shell theory used to address these issues depends on the thickness, coupling, and geometry for a given shell configuration. A detailed discussion of the issues is beyond what can be accomplished within a short article. References 5 and 18 through 21 contain more detailed discussions of this topic.

REFERENCES

1. S.G. Lekhnitskii, *Anisotropic Plates*, 2nd ed., S.W. Tsai and T. Cheron, Trans., Gordon and Breach Science Publishers, 1968
2. S.A. Ambartsumyan, *Theory of Anisotropic Plates,* Technomic, Lancaster, PA, 1970
3. J.M. Whitney, *Structural Analysis of Laminated Anisotropic Plates,* Technomic, Lancaster, PA, 1987
4. R.M. Jones, *Mechanics of Composite Materials,* 2nd ed., Taylor and Francis Group, New York, 1998
5. A.K. Noor, Mechanics of Anisotropic Plates

and Shells–A New Look at an Old Subject, *Comput. Struct.,* Vol 44 (No. 3), 1992, p 499–514

6. M.P. Nemeth, Importance of Anisotropy on Buckling of Compression-Loaded Symmetric Composite Plates, *AIAA J.*, Vol 24 (No. 11), Nov 1986, p 1831–1835
7. A.W. Leissa, "Buckling of Laminated Composite Plates and Shell Panels," AFWAL-TR-85-3069, Air Force Wright Aeronautical Laboratories, 1985
8. DOD/NASA Advanced Composites Design Guide, Prepared Under Contract F33615-78-C-3203 by Rockwell International Corp., Vol II: Analysis, July 1983
9. M.P. Nemeth, "Buckling Behavior of Long Symmetrically Laminated Plates Subjected to Shear and Linearly Varying Edge Loads," NASA TP 3659, July 1997
10. J.M. Whitney, Stress Analysis of Thick Laminated Composite and Sandwich Plates, *J. Compos. Mater.,* Vol 6, Oct 1972, p 426–434
11. J.R. Vinson, *The Behavior of Sandwich Structures of Isotropic and Composite Materials,* Technomic Pub., 1999
12. N.J. Hoff and S.E. Mautner, Buckling of Sandwich Type Panels, *J. Aeronaut. Sci.,* Vol 12 (No. 3), 1945, p 285–297
13. W.H. Wittrick and F.W. Williams, Buckling and Vibration of Anisotropic or Isotropic Plate Assemblies Under Combined Loadings, *Int. J. Mech. Sci.,* Vol 16, 1974, p 209–239
14. S. Stroud, W. Jefferson, and M.S. Anderson, "PASCO: Structural Panel Analysis and Sizing Code, Capability, and Analytical Foundations," NASA TM-80181, Nov 1981
15. M.S. Anderson and D. Kennedy, Inclusion of Transverse Shear Deformation in Exact Buckling and Vibration Analysis of Composite Plate Assemblies, *AIAA J.*, Vol 31 (No. 10), Oct 1993, p 1963–1965
16. D. Bushnell, Optimum Design of Composite Stiffened Panels Under Combined Loading, *Comput. Struct.,* Vol 55 (No. 5), 1995, p 819–856
17. B. Almroth, F. Brogan, and G. Stanley, "User's Manual for STAGS," NASA CR 165670, 1978
18. R. C. Tennyson, Buckling of Laminated Composite Cylinders: A Review, *Composites*, Vol 1, 1975, p 17–24
19. K.P. Soldatos, Nonlinear Analysis of Transverse Shear Deformable Laminated Composites Shells–Part I: Derivation of Governing Equations, *J. Pressure Vessel Technol.*, Vol 114 (No. 1), 1992, p 105–109
20. K.P. Soldatos, Nonlinear Analysis of Transverse Shear Deformable Laminated Composites Shells—Part II: Buckling of Axially Compressed Cross-Ply and Oval Cylinders, *J. Pressure Vessel Technol.,* Vol 114 (No. 1), 1992, p 110–114
21. I. Sheinman, D. Shaw, and G.J. Simitses, Nonlinear Analysis of Axially Loaded Laminated Cylindrical Shells, *Comput. Struct.,* Vol 16 (No. 1–4), 1983, p 131–137

Damage Tolerance

Mike R. Woodward and Rich Stover, Lockheed Martin Aeronautics Company

THE DAMAGE TOLERANCE DESIGN PHILOSOPHY has been required on all U.S. Air Force aircraft as a result of a catastrophic in-flight failure in the 1960s. This philosophy requires a fracture-mechanics-based analytical demonstration of the ability of the airframe to operate safely for a specified period of time with periodic inspections of the airframe. The initial design goal is to have an inspection interval equal to the desired life of the aircraft. However, if this is not achievable due to an increase in the severity of usage or analytical errors, the aircraft can be operated safely for an extended period of time with the imposition of periodic inspections. The frequency of these inspections is based on the analytically predicted life of critical airframe components.

This article addresses the issue of the implementation of composite damage tolerance requirements as it relates to military aircraft. The issue of damage tolerance is applicable to other aircraft and applications in other industries as well. A Federal Aviation Administration (FAA) proposed policy for the certification of materials for other planes, including acrobatic and commuter aircraft, recognizes that key properties of structural laminates must include impact-damage element strengths. The FAA recognizes that complementary test data and analysis are needed to account for the effects of damage as part of the material performance envelope for general aircraft (Ref 1).

This article includes a brief introduction of the concepts and definitions of damage tolerance and the closely related topic of durability. Also included is a discussion of the primary failure mode of interest, compression after impact (CAI). The methodology and issues associated with the development and analytical implementation of useful design allowables are also presented. Finally, since the damage tolerance criteria were developed for metallic structures, a discussion of certain shortcomings of current criteria, due to the unique growth and failure characteristics of composites, will be presented.

Definitions

Durability of a structure is its ability to maintain strength and stiffness throughout the service life of the structure (Ref 2). Durability also addresses such issues as corrosion resistance, fatigue, and thermal damage, which are discussed elsewhere in this Volume. The structure must have sufficient durability over its design life to meet its expected loads and environment without imposing an onerous maintenance or inspection burden upon the operator. The level of damage associated with the durability requirement is associated with typical impact events or manufacturing-induced flaws. Durability is primarily an economic issue and applies to all structures.

Damage tolerance is the ability of critical structures to withstand a level of service or manufacturing-induced damage or flaws while maintaining its function (Ref 2). However, the goal of this requirement is to allow operation of the aircraft over a specified period of time in order to assure continued safe operation. Safe operation must be possible until the defect is detected by routine scheduled maintenance or, if undetected, for the design life. The level of this damage tolerance and the initial flaw size for metals or required impact threat for composites is much greater than that required to meet durability requirements and represents worst-case type impact events or manufacturing-induced damage. Again, this requirement addresses a safety issue and applies only to *primary structures* necessary for safety of flight.

Durability and Damage Tolerance Criteria

Durability and damage tolerance are design philosophies in which the structure is designed to withstand a specified amount of damage or a specified damage threat. The amount of damage is a function of the structure of interest. While all procuring agencies impose damage tolerance criteria, the specifics of these criteria are tailored to the application. However, all criteria have the following in common.

Durability Impact Threat. This criterion requires that all composite structures have the capacity to withstand damage from a nuisance-type, low-velocity impact, typically 8 J (6 ft · lbf), without resulting in functional impairment. Functional impairment is defined as the presence of damage in a part that requires maintenance action. In addition, the diameter and shape of the impactor, typically 1.3 cm (0.5 in.) and hemispherical, are defined along with an impact velocity range, which assures that the impact is, indeed, low velocity. An example of the application of this criterion is the determination of the minimum thickness of a composite fuel boundary. This structure must be sized such that an 8 J (6 ft · lbf) impact does not result in a fuel leak.

Damage Tolerance Impact Threat. This criterion requires that critical, safety-of-flight structures are able to withstand damage from a worst-case, low-velocity impact without resulting in failure at a specified load level. The impact energy level is typically defined as one which results in barely visible damage up to an upper limit, typically 136 J (100 ft · lbf). Again, the diameter and shape of the impactor, typically 2.54 cm (1 in.) and hemispherical, are defined along with an impact velocity range, again assuring that the impact is, indeed, low velocity.

Other Damage Tolerance Damage Threats. Generally, other damage threats are defined. These include surface scratches of a certain length, depth, and orientation, and manufacturing defects, such as an inclusion in the laminate at the most critical location within the laminate. An inclusion could be a liner or paper backing that adheres to a prepreg. The relative criticality of the type of damage depends upon the type of structure, how it is loaded, and its location in the assembly.

Specific Criteria

Specific criteria from a current military aircraft program have been summarized as follows:

Damage tolerance criteria

- *Damage tolerance impact:* Interlaminar delamination damage resulting from a low-velocity impact is assumed to represent a worst-case threat for damage tolerance analysis and verification testing. This damage shall be assumed to be representative of that caused by a 2.5 cm (1 in.) diameter hemispherical impactor dropped normal to the surface from a height of 0.6–1.2 m (2–4 ft). The kinetic en-

ergy of the impact shall be the lower of a specified upper energy limit of 136 J (100 ft · lbf) or the energy required to produce damage clearly visible from a distance of 7.5 m (5 ft). This impact threat is applicable to all fracture critical structure. *Fracture critical structure* is defined as a structure whose failure would result in the loss of the aircraft or injury to ground personnel.
- *Damage tolerance scratch:* 100 mm (4.0 in.) long by 0.5 mm (0.02 in.) deep. This tolerance limit is also applicable to all fracture critical structures.
- *Damage tolerance single circular delamination:* 50 mm (2 in.) in diameter. This tolerance limit is also applicable to all fracture critical structures.
- *Residual strength requirement:* The structure must carry maximum spectrum load after two lifetimes of fatigue loading under the critical environmental conditions.
- *Statistical basis:* Typical

Durability criteria

- *Durability impact:* Low-velocity impact 1.3 cm (0.5 in.) diameter impactor; drop height 0.6–1.2 m (2–4 ft). The kinetic energy of the impact shall be 3.4–8.1 J (2.5–6 ft · lbf) depending on availability of access and function of structure. This requirement is applicable to all structures.
- *Residual strength requirement:* Must carry maximum spectrum load after two lifetimes of fatigue loading at the critical environment.
- *Functional impairment requirement:* Impact must not result in functional impairment, such as a fuel leak, interference, or requirement for repair.
- *Statistical basis:* Typical

Damage Tolerance Philosophy

The purpose of the damage tolerance design philosophy is to ensure that the aircraft can operate safely for a period of time with damage present within the airframe. Often, as the aircraft matures, internal loads are increased, or usage is determined to be more severe. In these cases, inspections may be imposed on the aircraft in order to assess the safety of continued operation of the aircraft. This usage tracking and management is a normal part of the flight test and the subsequent force management program. This philosophy is illustrated in Fig. 1 and 2 for a metallic structure and in Fig. 3 and 4 for a composite structure.

Metallic Structures. The damage tolerance design philosophy for metallic structures is characterized by the following:

- The flaws are assumed to be cracks inherent in the material or induced during the manufacturing process. They are assumed to be in the most critical location for a given structure. The initial size is determined by specification (based on historical data) or by inspection technique.
- Crack growth is stable and self-similar.
- The assumed initial flaw does not appreciably affect static strength.
- The goal is to preclude fleet maintenance activity by demonstrating by analysis that a crack growth life of two times the expected usage life (an inspection interval of one usage life) exists.

Figure 1 illustrates implementation of the damage tolerance process for metallic structure at the time of initial design. Crack length as a function of time is shown for an aircraft with an 8000 h design life (i.e., an 8000 h inspection interval; the inspection interval is one-half the analytical life). The initial flaw size is determined by specification and is a function of material and inspection technique.

Figure 2 demonstrates what happens when usage severity increases or when analytical errors are discovered after the aircraft are fielded. As shown, if loads increase, there is an increase in usage severity; if an analysis error occurred, the aircraft can be operated safely for a period of time by the imposition of an inspection. This initial inspection interval is one half of the analytically-predicted life using current spectra and loads. Subsequent inspection intervals are a function of the field inspection capability. Once the structure is inspected and found to be crack free, no further maintenance needs to be performed until the re-inspection interval occurs. This process can be repeated until the aircraft is

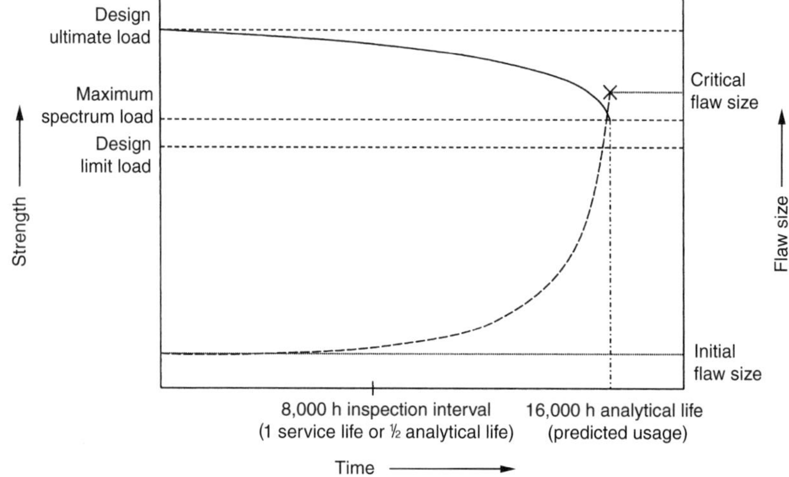

Fig. 1 Damage tolerance of a metallic structure based on initial design. Flaw size (broken line) and residual strength (solid line) are plotted versus time.

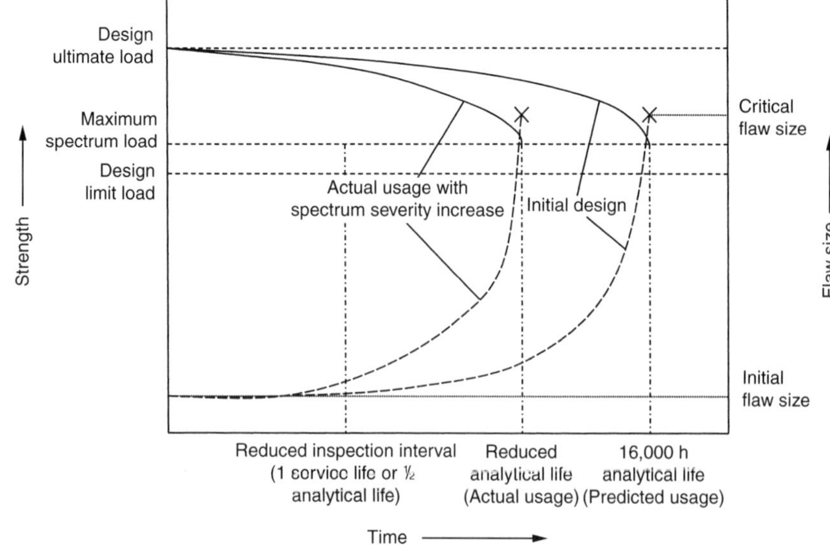

Fig. 2 Damage tolerance of a metallic structure based on actual usage. Flaw size (broken line) and residual strength (solid line) are plotted versus time. Analytical life is reduced due to increased loading, severity of usage, or the discovery of analytical errors in the original life prediction.

retired. Dealing with issues such as these is the function of the force management programs implemented for all aircraft that are designed using the damage tolerance philosophy.

Composite Structures. The damage tolerance design philosophy for composite structures is concerned with the following flaw types:

- *A large, undetected manufacturing defect:* This defect is assumed to be an inclusion within the laminate, resulting in a delamination.
- *A surface scratch:* The length and depth is specified. The location and orientation is assumed to be that which is most critical for a given structure.
- *Undetected impact damage:* The damage area is consistent with an impact of an energy that caused barely visible surface damage. This damage is assumed to be in the critical location. Since this is the critical flaw for most structures, the rest of this article will focus on issues associated with this flaw type.

In addition, the damage tolerance design philosophy for composite structures is characterized by the following:

- Flaw growth is unstable and is not self-similar.
- The initial flaw (impact damage) does appreciably affect the static strength.
- The goal is to preclude fleet maintenance activity by demonstrating, by analysis and testing, that the damage described does not constitute a safety risk over the expected usage life.

Figure 3 illustrates some of these points. The growth of impact damage is characterized by periods of little to no growth at the lower load levels, followed by relatively large growth increments associated with the highest load cycles in each block of cyclic loading. Failure under cyclic loading is often quasi-static and the scatter in life is large. One detrimental aspect of impact damage is the immediate loss in static strength once the impact occurs. This phenomenon, coupled with the residual strength requirement, and the uncertainty associated with its growth characteristics are where the current criteria fail. The response of impact-damaged structures to cyclic loading will be discussed later. In summary, compression after impact does not lend itself to analytical life predictions and associated inspection intervals.

Figure 4 demonstrates the effect of an increase in usage load level. Compression strength after impact is relatively insensitive to spectrum severity. As seen, this situation could lead to a possible static failure situation. Since there is not necessarily a reliable stable flaw growth period, imposition of an inspection interval will not alleviate this situation. This growth characteristic and other issues associated with impact damage prevent the management of the presence of flaws in composite structure from being treated in a manner equivalent to metallic structure.

Compression After Impact Failure Mode

Although, by specification, there are three types of damage tolerance flaws that are considered in the design of composite structure, the critical flaw is damage resulting from a low velocity impact.

Impact damage in a laminate is induced as a result of the contact force of the impactor and the deflection within the laminate. These contact forces result in localized crushing of the laminate resin and fiber (Fig. 5). The deflections, induced by the impact event, result in multiple delaminations resulting from interlaminar shear failures. The ply interfaces where these occur are a function of the stacking sequence of the laminate and tend to occur at interfaces at which there are large differences in the in-plane properties of the sublaminates. The size and location of the delaminations are a function of the material properties of the laminate, interlaminar shear strength, stiffness, mode II toughness, local panel stiffness, and impact energy. See the article "Fracture Mechanics of Composite Delamination" in this Volume for more information on the modes of delamination. The deflection of the

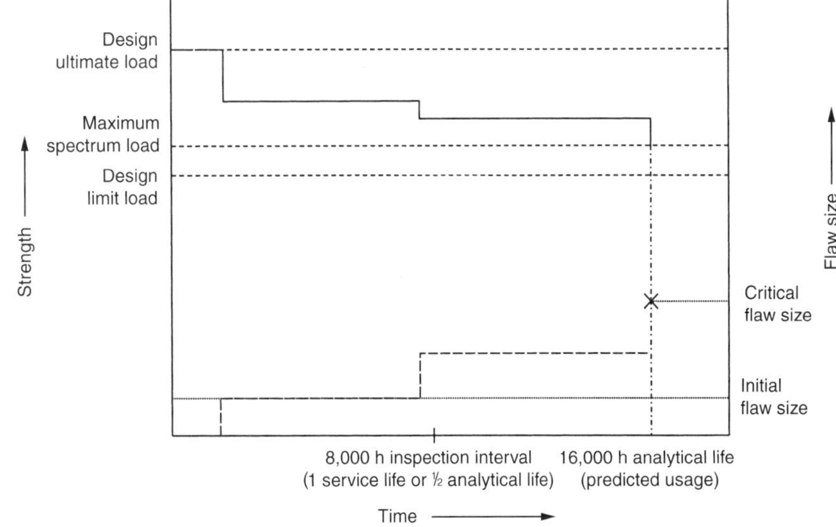

Fig. 3 Damage tolerance of a composite structure based on initial design. Flaw size (broken line) and residual strength (solid line) are plotted versus time. The step function nature of the curves represents large growths in the degradation associated with the highest load cycles in each block of cyclic loading. The design ultimate load is 150% of the design load limit.

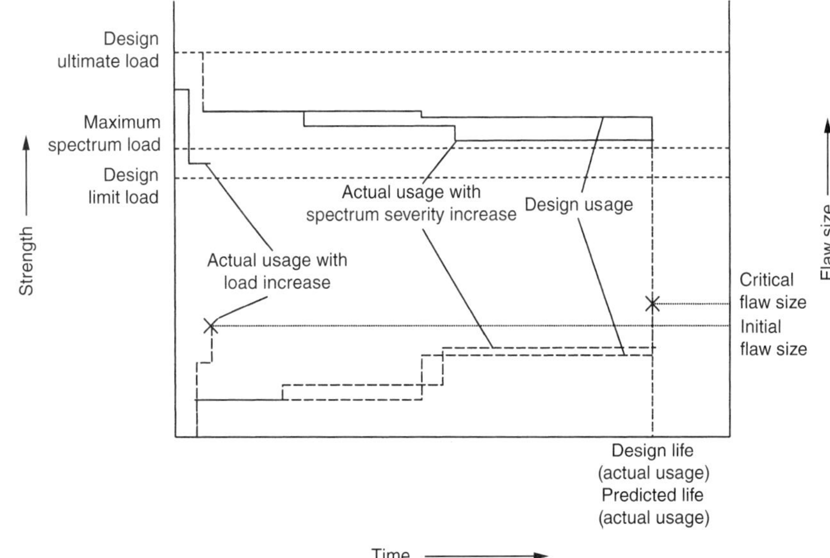

Fig. 4 Damage tolerance of a composite structure based on actual usage. Flaw size (broken line) and residual strength (solid line) are plotted versus time. Increased loading could lead to static failure. Increase in the spectrum severity does not affect the compression after impact failure mode.

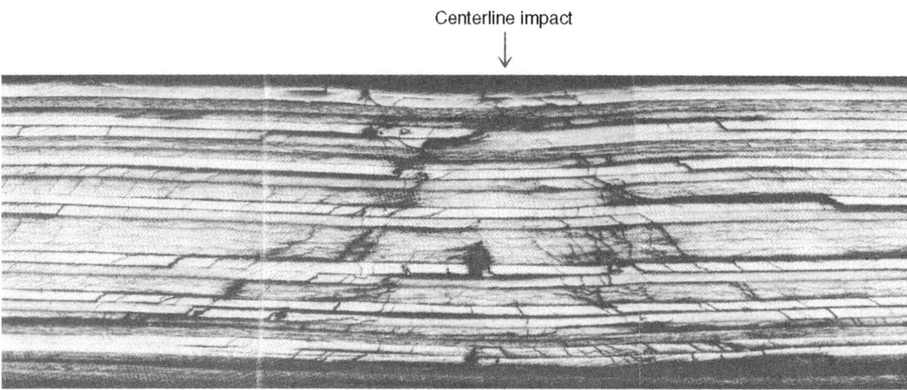

Fig. 5 Cross section of AS6/2220-3 graphite/epoxy laminate showing damage due to impact with energy of 40 J (30 ft · lbf). Diagonal shear cracks in matrix are seen and extensive delamination has occurred.

laminate may also result in the tensile failure of fibers. In most cases of low-velocity impact, the damage is confined to the matrix, and little fiber damage occurs. Therefore, the in-plane tension strength of the laminate may not be seriously degraded. However, even with impact levels that leave little indication of damage on the surface, the matrix damage may be significant, and, therefore, its ability to stabilize the fibers in compression may be seriously degraded. Because of this, tolerance to impact damage is often the critical design consideration and compression is the critical loading mode. Because this damage is insidious, the study of barely visible impact damage (BVID) is an important safety issue.

The critical failure mode for impact damage is CAI. It is a common misconception that this failure is a fiber failure, although there usually is fiber failure at final collapse. This failure has been shown, through testing, correlation, and observation of failures, to be able to be classified as an out-of-plane failure of the laminate due to buckling. In a postbuckled state, this compression results in out-of-plane loads around the perimeter of the delamination. These out-of-plane loads result in the sudden propagation of the delamination and subsequent collapse of the laminate. This CAI failure sequence is illustrated in Fig. 6.

It should be noted that, after initial buckling, it is possible to have additional sublaminates buckle. In addition, although Fig. 6 shows a relatively simple buckled mode shape, it is possible to have more complex buckling modes and contact between the top and bottom sublaminates. The complexity of the damage and failure mechanisms has increased the difficulty of the development and verification of adequate deterministic models of the compression after impact failure mode.

Impact Damage Growth Characteristics under Cyclic Loading. Composites respond differently to subcritical cyclic loads than metals. The fatigue curve for composites is relatively flat, compared to the curve for metals. For a constant-amplitude loading condition of $R = 10$ (that is, compression-compression) the 10^6 cycle endurance condition typically corresponds to a maximum cyclic stress (in compression) of 60 to 65% of the undamaged static ultimate (Fig. 7). The fatigue curve is much higher for spectrum-type loading, which is more representative of typical aircraft loading conditions. A typical transport loading sequence is also shown. The reason for the improvement in the spectrum load condition is that, for composites, only the high-level loads cause significant fatigue damage or damage growth. Consequently, typical aircraft loading is relatively benign compared to constant amplitude load cycling because of the few high-load or peak-load cycles encountered. This is in contrast to metals, for which the large number of low-stress cycles is the primary contributor to crack growth; the high-stress cycles may actually be beneficial. In metals, the higher compressive load levels may produce retardation of crack growth due to yielding at the crack tip. Because composites are only sensitive to the high-level loads, they have the advantage of being able to truncate spectrums drastically in simulating lifetimes of cyclic loading. Ironically, however, a large number of loading lifetimes may be required to obtain an *exceedance* confidence because of the characteristic flat cyclic loading curve of the material and the associated data scatter inherent in time-to-failure data. Exceedances are occurrences of loading in excess of the baseline loading used to determine the loading spectrum.

The CAI failure mode is essentially a mode I failure. (Fig. 2 in the article "Fracture Mechanics of Composite Delamination" in this Volume illustrates the three modes of delamination fracture.) Even toughened composites exhibit very high mode I crack growth exponents; this results in very little difference between the threshold strain energy release rate (G_{Ith}) and the critical

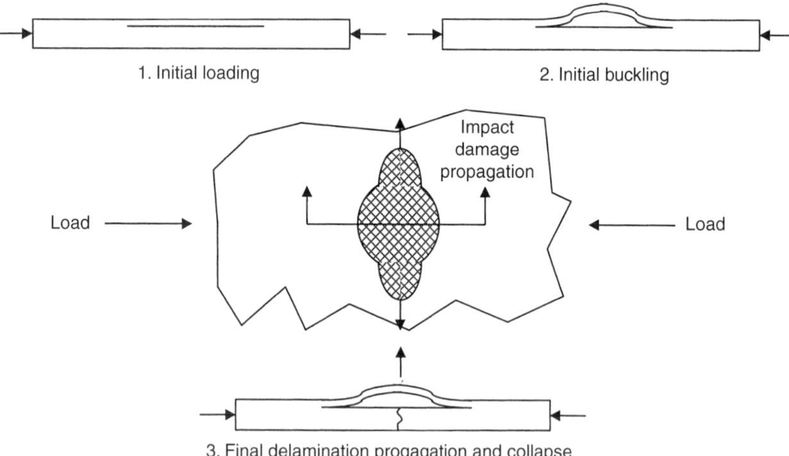

Fig. 6 The compression after impact (CAI) failure sequence. (1) At the beginning of the load cycle the damaged laminate remains stable. (2) The strain level becomes high enough to initiate buckling at one or more of the delamination interfaces, resulting in a thin, buckled sublaminate and a thicker, more stable sublaminate. (3) As the load increases, the thin sublaminate buckles and further out-of-plane loads result around the perimeter of the delamination. The postbuckling continues until the out-of-plane loads exceed the critical mode I strain energy release rate or the interlaminar tension allowable. The final failure occurs as the delamination propagates perpendicular to the principal strain direction and the laminate collapses.

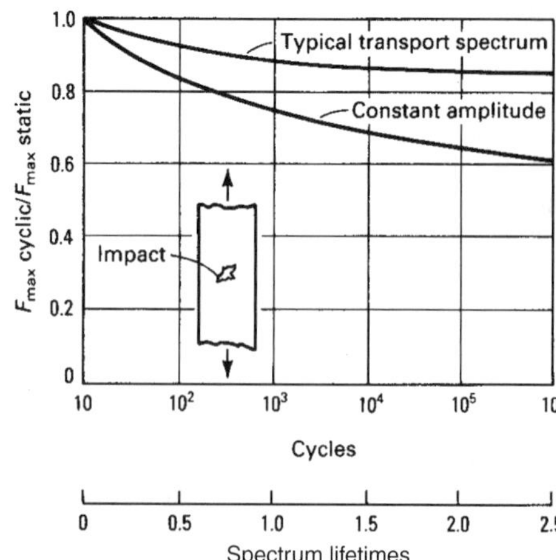

Fig. 7 Typical load cycle response for constant amplitude versus spectrum-loading fatigue testing. $R = 10.0$ (compression-compression).

strain energy release rate (G_{Ic}). This manifests itself in tests by the following:

- No flaw growth (except for rounding out of the delamination) at strain levels of 75 to 85% of the static failure strain.
- The CAI failure does not exhibit a slow stable period of flaw growth. The failure typically occurs by sudden extension of the delamination at the higher load levels, as demonstrated in Fig. 3 and 4. For a given configuration and strain level, failure sometimes occurs during the first application of the highest cycles; it may also occur later in the life in a seeming random manner. This results in large amount of scatter in life for a given maximum spectrum strain level. As stated previously, this characteristic prevents force management in a manner similar to metals.

Damage Tolerance Allowables Development

The general concept and development of design allowables is presented in the article "Design Allowables" in this Volume. The procedure for damage tolerance allowables development directly addresses the threats presented to the composite structure and the design criteria for the structure. Tool drops, rolling equipment strikes, and runway debris all act as possible threats to the integrity of a composite structural member. These threats fall into the category of low-velocity impacts (LVI). When they possess sufficient energy, they will develop into low-velocity impact damage (LVID). Since impacts are a way of life for any real-world large airplane, the following questions must be answered: "When does impact severity go from trivial to functional impairment?" and "Can defects causing structural impairment be detected during a non-mission-interrupting inspection?" For many other applications, impacts are likewise numerous. Tests must be developed that provide the analyst with design guidelines to assure safe, reliable structures.

As discussed previously, the two philosophies of damage tolerance and durability each result in unique levels of testing and differing guidelines. The damage tolerance tests incorporate the criteria of functional capability with damage level. Exactly how much damage is tolerable and how an inspection is performed to find such damage will drive the allowables tests. As mentioned previously, delamination damage can often be quite sizeable before it reaches the point of visibility, and the inspection of a large composite structural member such as a wing or vertical tail is complicated by the relative inaccessibility presented by the item. While it may be advisable to do an ultrasonic inspection when any known accidental LVI has occurred, it would be impractical and should not be necessary as a part of a routine preflight inspection. Most criteria employed today involve the concept of defining undesirable damage as that which is clearly visible by a trained observer at a set distance, for example 1.5 m (5 ft). This allows composite surfaces to be visually inspected in a time-efficient manner. Since damage areas can be sizeable without being clearly visible, the part must be designed to perform its function with the damage present. Usually, damage tolerance test impacts are performed with 12.7 mm (0.5 in.) diameter impactors, which tend to limit fiber breakage and maximize delamination damage. Other sizes may be used. To simulate large hail stone damage in composite sandwich airframe structures, a 63.4 mm (2.5 in.) impactor can be used (Ref 3).

Durability tests incorporate lower energy impacts and the concept of functional impairment. Besides strength, these test criteria include other impairments, such as moisture intrusion into honeycomb panels, or fuel leakage from a fuel tank. Usually, durability tests are performed with smaller impact heads, usually 12.7 mm (0.5 in.) diameter.

Defining the Range and Scope of Coupon Tests and Trial Impact Coupons. While the combinations of materials, laminate stacking sequences, and thickness are infinite, an allowables developer can perform only a limited number of expensive coupon tests in order to establish a reliable set of composite damage tolerance allowables. Varying parameters of thickness and stacking sequence are necessary, as is the establishment of maximum impact energy before damage is visible. If, for example, a criterion of visibility at 1.5 m (5 ft) is desired, a number of trial impact tests should be performed prior to any other mechanical testing. These trial impact tests will establish the impact energy level needed to be applied to mechanically tested coupons for BVID evaluation. A full range of laminate thickness and stacking sequences should be tested at various impact energies to correctly establish the relationship between panel attributes, impact energy, dent depth, and visibility. Visibility can be subjective, based on the viewing conditions and panel surface treatments. Often, a dent depth criteria can be established and matched to a visibility requirement. An upper limit on impact energy is usually established based on an analysis of threats found in the aircraft environment (Fig. 8).

There is usually a design range of laminate families available to the composite laminate designer. These range from hard laminates with a high percentage of 0° fibers, to laminates stiff in shear with a high percentage of cross-plies. Test programs should endeavor to sample a variety of laminates throughout the design space.

Impact Boundary Conditions. Care must be taken when applying boundary conditions to coupons being impacted. The effects of edge translational and rotational stiffness can drastically affect the resultant damage area and the residual strength. Standard test methods specify a specific size impact window, with the coupon being clamped at the periphery. The size of the window may depend on the level of impact energy and thickness of the panel being impacted. The ideal fixity is the actual adjacent structure, which may be difficult to reproduce. When defining tests are performed for damage resistance only (no moisture intrusion) thinner laminates can be tested. For damage tolerance, thicker laminates should be used.

Environmental and Cyclic Tests. Like most allowables development programs, a building block approach should be used. Once a set of criteria has been established, coupons are constructed and tested. These coupons should be conditioned to represent the extreme cases of exposure to environment effects: cold temperature dry (CTD), room temperature dry (RTD), elevated temperature dry (ETD), and elevated temperature wet (ETW). These are specified in the Advanced General Aviation Transport Experiments Consortium (AGATE) program (Ref 1). Next, cyclic fatigue effects should be established. When performing cyclic fatigue tests, test coupons normally are subjected to two lives of fatigue. Then, residual compression strength is determined at the end of the life with the coupon at elevated temperature and saturated moisture. Strain gages are applied to the compression panel in a judicious way (Fig. 9). Far field strains should be measured, as well as the strains over the delaminated portion of the coupon. Cyclic tests will usually be conducted at strain levels that result in postbuckling of the delaminated coupon. Strain gages monitor this activity. Rounding out the ragged damage area usually occurs during cycling. At some point, delamination growth becomes unrestrained and the panel fails. When enough tests are performed to quantify a fatigue reduction factor, the static failure loads are reduced by this factor to calculate allowables.

The Building Block Approach and Scale-Up Effects. In any good allowables program, a building block approach to allowables development may be used. The building block approach is explained in the article "Overview of Testing and Certification" in this Volume. At the beginning, trial impact tests assess the material damage areas. Next, compression-after-impact tests are performed to quantify basic coupon strength. Scale-up effects, such as the effects of adjacent

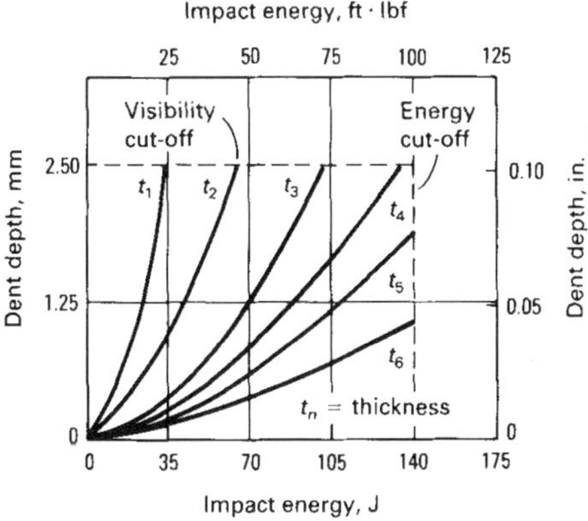

Fig. 8 Impact energy versus dent depth with energy and visibility cut-off limits. Source: Ref 4

fasteners, stitching, or other through-the-thickness binding methods, should be quantified with the use of multi-bay stiffened test panels. Normally, for airframe structures, a three-bay panel is tested with the damage applied at the center of the panel or over a stiffener. Often, application of impacts over stiffeners do not create large delaminations, because the substructure supports the impact forces. Off the supports, impact loads are carried by interlaminar stresses which may result in delaminations. Delamination growth at binding points may be restrained, but most often panel widths are greater than damage runout widths. Box beams are normally used to verify a design with combined shear-compression-pressure loads once a design concept has been chosen.

Designing a damage-tolerant composite structure that incorporates postbuckling during cyclic loading should be avoided. The bending moments and internal loads generated in a postbuckled structure make an accurate damage tolerance analysis extremely difficult.

Implementation of a Damage Tolerance Analysis Methodology

Compression after impact failure does not lend itself to prediction by a purely deterministic model. A semiempirical analysis methodology that has been successfully implemented is presented in the following paragraphs. This methodology combines a complex regression algorithm with a simplified analytical model of the failure.

Mechanics Based Model. Initial attempts at predicting CAI strength were accomplished purely analytically. The model (Ref 4) is a one-term Raleigh-Ritz approximation of a clamped elliptical plate under general biaxial loading in an infinite parent laminate. The model consists of an initial buckling solution and a postbuckled solution. The derivative of the total strain energy is taken with respect to delamination growth in the axial and transverse directions. A Newton-Raphson technique is then used to determine the strain level required to produce a strain energy release rate equal to the critical mode I strain energy release rate (G_{Ic}). This is the predicted static failure strain. This model was developed in a closed form in order to speed computation.

However, after an in-depth comparison with an extensive set of test data, it was determined that a purely analytical approach to the prediction of CAI strength was inadequate for the range of laminates being considered. Possible reasons for this include the following:

- *Delamination characteristics:* The impact damage was modeled as a geometrically exact single delamination. Examination of impact damage shows that the actual damage consists of multiple irregularly-shaped delaminations.
- *Shape function:* The assumed shape function was a one-term elliptical function. Although it was never confirmed experimentally, it is possible that this was inadequate in describing the postbuckled shape of the delamination.

As a result, it was determined that an empirical approach was needed.

The regression algorithm requires a set of CAI test data that adequately represents the range of laminate stacking sequences and thickness combinations that will be used for the design. The CAI strength of a given laminate is highly dependent on stacking sequence. Therefore, it is important that, during the design process, consistency must be maintained between the laminates used in the allowables development effort and those used in the actual design.

The regression variables include various laminate stiffness terms representing in-plane stiffness E_x E_y, bending stiffness G_{xy}, and the degree of stiffness stratification through the thickness of the laminate. The basic regression is of the form:

$$\sigma_c = a_0 \cdot a_1 \cdot a_2 \cdot a_3$$

where σ_c is the uniaxial CAI strength, a_0 is the open hole compression seed, a_1 is the CAI adjustment, a_2 is the impact energy term, and a_3 is the D matrix stratification term.

Further,

$$a_0 = (C_1 / a_{kt})(E_x{}^{C2} \cdot E_y{}^{C3} \cdot G_{xy}{}^{C4})$$

$$a_1 = (C5 \cdot E_x + C6 \cdot E_y + C7 \cdot G_{xy})(t^{C8})$$

$$a_2 = C9 \cdot E^{-C10t^{-C11}}$$

$$a_3 = (d_{11} / d_{11s}) \cdot (d_{33} / d_{33s})^{C13} \cdot (d_{22} / d_{22s})^{0.4675}$$

where $C1$–$C13$ are regression constants; E_x, E_y, G_{xy} are the effective axial, transverse, and shear moduli; t is thickness; E is impact energy; a_{kt} is the orthotropic stress concentration factor; d_{11}, d_{22}, and d_{33}, are laminate bending stiffness terms; d_{11s}, d_{22s}, and d_{33s} are smeared laminate bending stiffness terms.

Linear regression factors are applied to E_x, E_y, and G_{xy} moduli and to bending stiffness terms. Thickness and impact energy terms require exponents. As thickness is increased, failure stress is reduced. As impact energy is increased, failure stress is reduced.

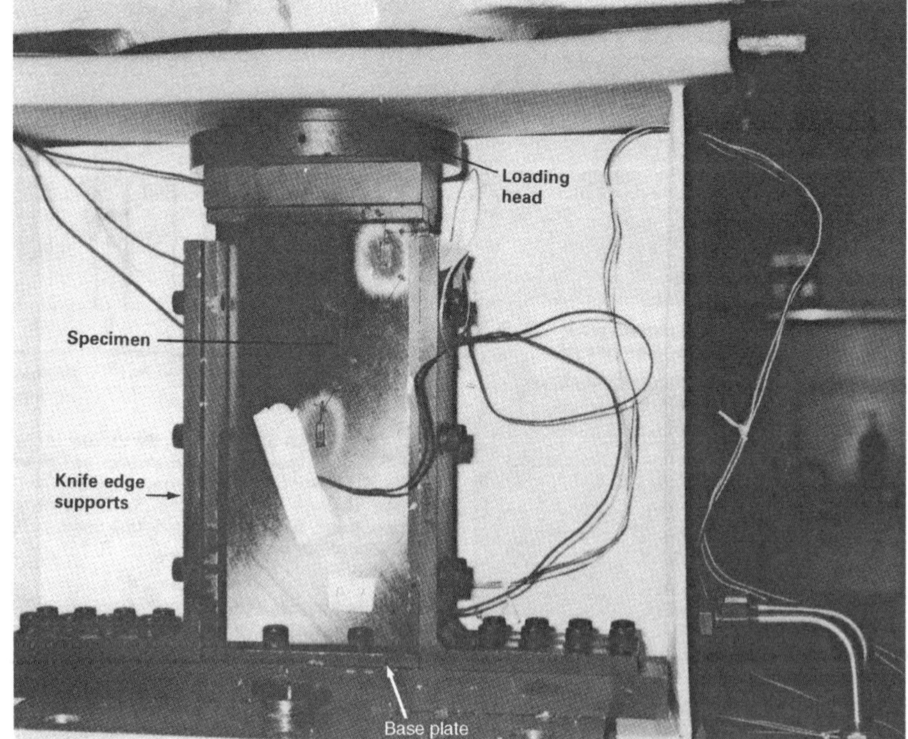

Fig. 9 Test set-up for compression testing of 125 × 250 mm (5 × 10 in.) laminate panels

Table 1 Assumed nondetectable flaw/damage

Type	Size
Scratches	A surface scratch that is 100 mm (4.0 in.) long and 0.50 mm (0.02 in.) deep
Delamination	An interply delamination that has an area equivalent to a 50 mm (2.0 in.) diameter circle with dimensions most critical to its location
Impact damage	Damage caused by the impact of a 25 mm (1.0 in.) diameter hemispherical impactor with 135 J (100 ft · lbf) of kinetic energy, or with that kinetic energy required to cause a dent 2.5 mm (0.10 in.) deep, whichever is least

Adapted from JSSG-2006 (Ref 5)

When dealing with a visibility or dent depth criteria, additional relationships are established which define the impact energy necessary to produce detectable damage for a given laminate type and thickness. The assumed conditions for nondetectable damage or flaws are given in Table 1. The combination of these two relationships will yield failure predictions.

Semi-Empirical Analysis Methodology. The final analysis methodology combines the analytical model and the regression algorithm. An initial uniaxial compression strain is calculated using the regression algorithm. This is then used to determine a calibrated critical strain energy release rate for the analytical model. This analysis is the run using the calibrated strain energy release rate, G_c, under the actual strain state (biaxial principal strains) to generate an initial static allowable. This allowable is then modified by an environmental and fatigue knockdown factor and a bending factor, resulting in the final CAI design allowable.

This process is automated to allow direct integration of loads and stacking sequences from a finite element model or it can be run on a case-by-case basis. Both the regression algorithm and the analytical model were developed with computational efficiency in mind.

REFERENCES

1. "Proposed Issuance of Policy Memorandum, Material Qualification and Equivalency for Polymer Matrix Composite Material Systems," DOT, FAA, 13 June 2000
2. *Composite Materials,* Vol 3, *Material Usage, Design, and Analysis*, MIL-HDBK-17-3E, U.S. Department of Defense, Jan 1997
3. "Review of Damage Tolerance for Composite Sandwich Airframe Structures," DOT/FAA/AR-99/49, Aug 1999
4. "General Specification for Aircraft Structures," MIL-A-872221, U.S. Air Force, Feb 1985
5. *Joint Service Specification Guide, Aircraft Structures*, JSSG-2006, Department of Defense, Oct 1998

SELECTED REFERENCES

- *Composite Materials,* Vol 3, *Material Usage, Design, and Analysis,* MIL-HDBK-17-3E, U.S. Department of Defense, Jan 1997
- D.Y. Konishi, "Delamination Growth in Composite Structures Under Inplane Compression Loading," AGARD-CP-355, 12–14 April 1983

Out-of-Plane Analysis

Jonathan Goering, Albany International Techniweave, Inc.

THE STRENGTH AND STIFFNESS of laminated composite materials is most often anisotropic. The methods of analyzing the directional dependence of the mechanical properties of composites, especially those perpendicular to the major plane of the laminate, are discussed in this article.

The Challenge

Laminated composite materials are often fabricated from stacks of plies (lamina) consisting of strong, stiff, reinforcing fibers, such as carbon, surrounded by a relatively weak, soft matrix, such as epoxy. The mechanical properties of these plies in the direction parallel to the reinforcement are controlled by the longitudinal properties of the fiber. The mechanical properties perpendicular to the fiber are controlled by the properties of the matrix. This results in unidirectionally reinforced plies that have substantially different properties in the directions parallel and perpendicular to the fiber (the longitudinal and transverse directions, respectively). The ratio of the longitudinal to transverse stiffness of an intermediate modulus carbon/epoxy ply, for example, can be on the order of 30 or 40 to 1. Differences in strength can be even more profound, and it is not uncommon to use plies with transverse strengths that are nearly two orders of magnitude less than the longitudinal strength.

Designers minimize the effects of these differences by employing stacking sequences that orient plies in several different directions in the plane of the laminate. In very simplistic terms, the directions of these plies will correspond to the directions of the primary loads, and the amount of reinforcing fiber in a given direction will be proportional to the magnitude of the load in that direction. While this technique can be used to optimize a laminate's ability to carry in-plane loads, it does very little to influence the strength or stiffness in the direction through the thickness of the laminate (the z-direction in Fig. 1).

In the through-thickness direction, a laminate can be characterized as a number of relatively weak, soft layers separated by layers of equally weak, soft matrix. This combination of weak layers coupled through weak layers leads to laminate out-of-plane strengths that are comparable to the transverse strength of a ply.

Relatively low laminate out-of-plane strengths can result in structures that fail in through-thickness modes, even though the primary loads are in-plane. In addition to direct out-of-plane loads, such as beams in three- or four-point bending and stiffener pulloff, the strength analyst must be cognizant of cases where primary loads in the plane of the laminate induce secondary loads that act in the through-thickness direction. Such cases include free-edge stresses in cross-plied laminates under axial loads, radial stresses in curved laminates subject to tangential loads and bending moments, and curling of axially loaded curved flanges.

Analytical models for calculating out-of-plane stresses due to direct and indirect loads have been developed for most cases of practical interest to structural engineers. The approaches used in these models have included simple mechanics of materials formulations, complex closed-form elasticity solutions, and computationally intensive numerical solutions. Each approach has its strengths and weaknesses, and the correct model for a given application depends on many factors. For example, a simple model based on beam theory may be adequate for predicting trends, while a more detailed finite element model may be required to accurately predict interlaminar stresses.

Regardless of the approach taken, the analyst must weigh the fidelity of the selected analytical model against the fidelity of the available materials properties data. Coupon tests that are used to measure out-of-plane strengths are generally

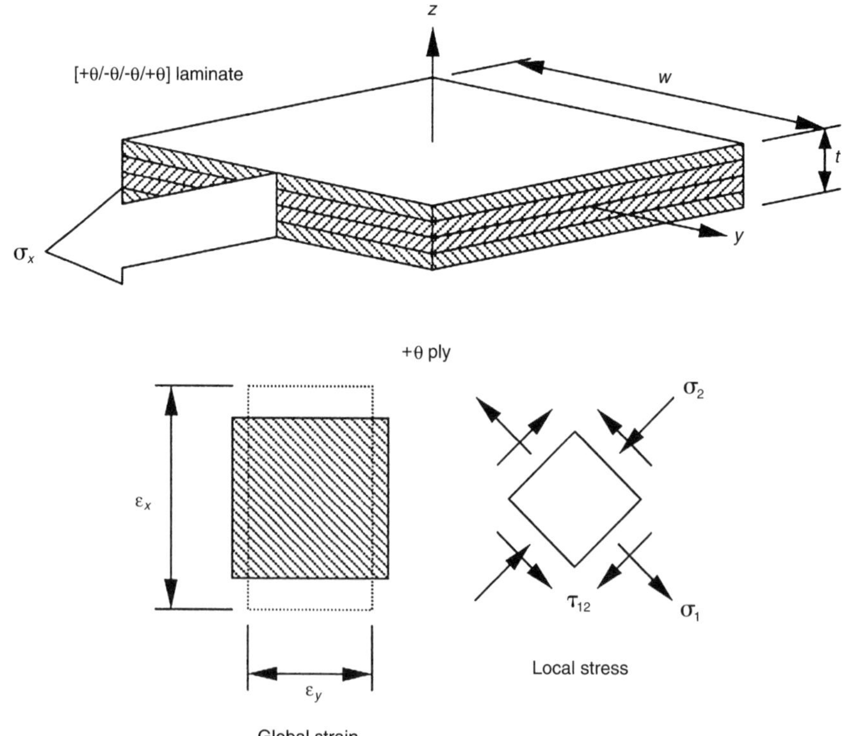

Fig. 1 Local shear stress in a symmetric laminate subject to a uniform axial stress in the x-direction (σ_x). The global strain is shown, but there is no in-plane shear strain (γ_{xy}). Local shear stress (τ_{xy}) is developed in each ply.

characterized by significant scatter, resulting in reduced "B-basis" statistical allowables. Out-of-plane tensile tests, in particular, are notoriously inaccurate and unreliable (see the article "Lamina and Laminate Mechanical Testing" in this Volume). It is therefore unreasonable to expect extremely accurate interlaminar strength predictions from any analytical model, regardless of its fidelity, if there is a high degree of uncertainty in the materials properties that are used. It is therefore recommended that a good degree of caution accompany any stress analysis intended to quantify out-of-plane failure modes.

Out-of-Plane Analysis Techniques

The following sections discuss some of the more common out-of-plane analysis techniques. These sections begin with some common indirect load cases, followed by direct out-of-plane load cases, and conclude with a brief discussion of composite materials that are reinforced in the z-direction (also known as three-dimensional, or 3-D composites). The intent of this article is to introduce some (but certainly not all) of the models available, to summarize the relevant concepts involved, and to discuss applicability. It is not intended to provide rigorous derivations of the theories behind the models considered. In most cases, references that include details of the derivation have been cited.

Free-edge stresses refer to interlaminar stress components that can develop at free edges of a laminate subject to in-plane loads. Classical laminated plate theory provides a good method for determining the states of stress and strain away from the edges of a laminate, but tends to break down near free edges. The basic problem is that the classical theory includes in-plane shear and extensional stresses that cannot exist on the free surfaces of edges parallel to the applied load. The classic example is a $[+\theta/-\theta]_s$ laminate subject to a uniform axial stress in the x-direction (σ_x). Since the laminate is balanced and symmetric, this strain will cause an extension in the x-direction (ε_x) and a contraction in the y-direction (ε_y), but there will be no in-plane shear strain (γ_{xy}) or bending (Fig. 1).

The problem becomes evident when a ply-by-ply analysis is performed to determine the local stress state for each ply. This process will predict a uniform shear stress (τ_{xy}) in each ply that exists even at the free edge. Since this condition is physically impossible, another stress component must develop to satisfy the imbalance in the moments due to the in-plane shear. For this particular case, a shear stress in the x-z-plane (τ_{xz}) develops in the vicinity of the free edge. The actual distributions of the shear stresses across the width of the laminate will be similar to those shown in Fig. 2.

A similar phenomenon occurs in cross-ply laminates (i.e. $[0/90]_s$). In this case, it is the mismatch in Poisson's ratios between plies, rather than shear coupling, that leads to transverse extensional stresses (σ_y) that cannot exist at the free edge. For this case, shear in the y-z-plane (τ_{yz}) and normal stresses (σ_z) develop to keep the moments in balance. Since laminates often possess a combination of shear coupling and mismatches in Poisson's ratios ($[0/90/\pm\theta]_s$ laminates, for example), the full compliment of interlaminar stresses can usually be expected. In all cases, these interlaminar stresses are restricted to a region that extends approximately a laminate thickness away from the free edge. Beyond that boundary, the classical laminated plate theory solution is valid.

A substantial number of researchers have investigated the free-edge stress problem, and a wide variety of models have been developed. This work was pioneered by Pipes and Pagano (Ref 1), who used finite difference solutions to calculate free-edge stress distributions. More recent models, such as that presented by Flanagan in Ref 2, use series solutions based on stress functions. Both approaches have benefits and drawbacks.

The finite difference (or finite element) approach can be applied to any geometry, but requires a new model for each new laminate. This drawback can easily be overcome by developing a preprocessor that automatically generates the finite difference grid or finite element mesh, and a postprocessor for interpreting the results. A more difficult problem is that this approach can require highly refined grids to characterize the very steep gradients of interlaminar stress distributions that may be singular. Convergence can therefore be very slow. The article "Numerical Analysis" follows in this Volume.

Solutions based on stress functions avoid this problem, but are more difficult to formulate. This approach generally requires the solution of an eigenproblem with several dozen degrees of freedom. Problems of this size present no real computational difficulties for even modest personal computers. When selecting a method of this type, care should be used to ensure that the model has not made restrictive assumptions regarding the distribution of various stress components.

A very simple alternative approach has also been developed for generating quick estimates of the interlaminar stresses. This approach is based on assuming simple shapes for the distributions of the interlaminar stress components and calculating the magnitudes required to keep all forces and moments in balance. This approach was suggested by Pagano in Ref 3, and the assumed shapes of the interlaminar stress distributions were guided by finite difference results. The assumed shape of the normal stress (σ_z) is shown in Fig. 3. The magnitudes of these distributions are chosen such that the resultant of σ_z is 0, and the moment due to σ_z balances the moment due to σ_y. This approach obviously provides a very rough approximation to the magnitude of the peak interlaminar stress, but it can be very useful for quickly determining trends when comparing various laminate families. This type of solution has been extended to other interlaminar stress components with different shapes assumed for their distribution. Reference 4 is a typical example.

Several authors have reviewed the existing body of work that has focused on modeling the free-edge stress problem. Details of the various approaches that have been taken to this modeling can be found in sources such as Ref 2 and 5. It should be noted that while free-edge failure is a real phenomenon, the free-edge stress analysis often becomes an academic exercise for real structures that are usually bonded or mechanically fastened to other structural members. This type of failure is, however, a practical concern in the test lab because it can preclude the desired failure modes for some types of coupon test (tensile tests of $\pm 45°$ laminates, for example).

Curved Laminates. Laminated composite structures often include corner details that can be treated as curved laminates. Web plies wrapping around a radius to form the flanges of a C-channel or I-beam are typical examples. When this type of structure is loaded, the applied loads can act to "open" or "close" the corner radii, depending on their direction (Fig. 4). This results in the development of interlaminar stresses in the radial direction, through the thickness of the composite. When the corner is being closed, the radial stress is compressive and typically not a concern, but when the corner is opened, the radial stress is tensile and can lead to delamination.

The development of this radial stress can be demonstrated by considering a two-ply curved laminate subject to a couple acting on either end (Fig. 5a). The free-body diagram of each ply re-

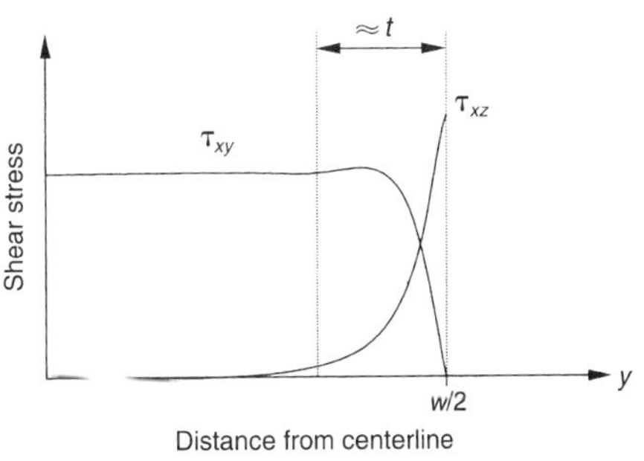

Fig. 2 Distribution of shear stresses across the width of a laminate. Free-edge stress distribution is limited to a region approximately one laminate thickness wide.

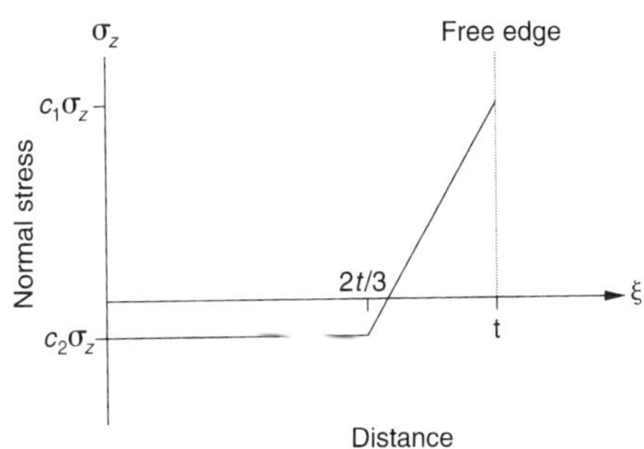

Fig. 3 Approximation of free-edge normal stresses

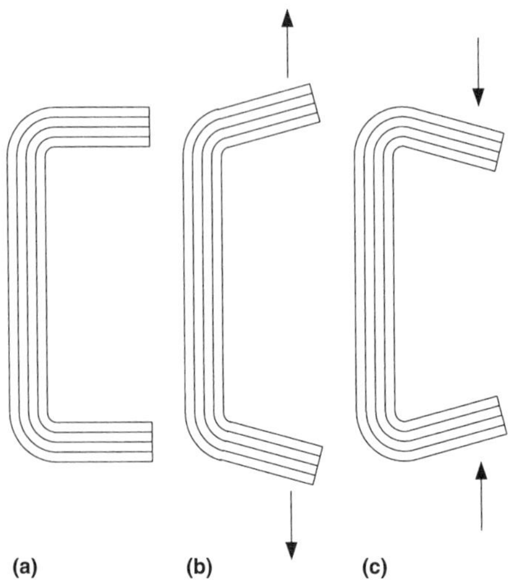

Fig. 4 A curved laminate "C" channel in various loading conditions. (a) Unloaded. (b) Radii open under tensile load. (c) Radii close under compressive load

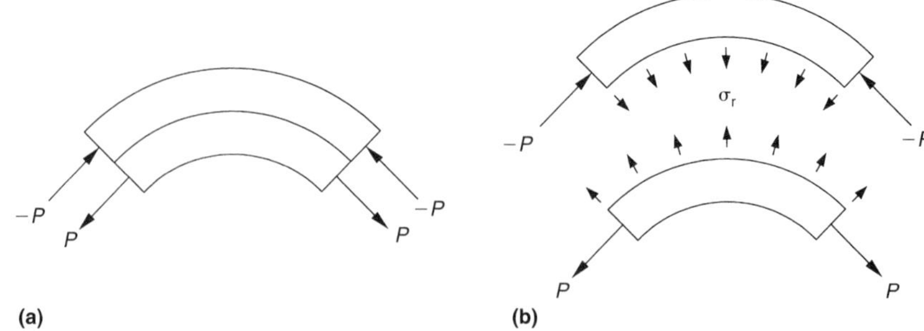

Fig. 5 Development of radial stresses in a curved laminate. (a) The force couples (−*P*, + *P*) act on the curved laminate. (b) The radial stresses (σ_r) must balance the vertical components of these loads.

veals the need for radial stresses to balance the vertical components of the tangential loads applied to the edges (Fig. 5b). For this simple case, the magnitude of the radial stress can be calculated by assuming some distribution (uniform, for example), integrating the vertical component of the radial stress over the surface of the interface, and setting the result equal to the vertical component of the applied load.

Real curved laminates in actual structures will more likely be loaded by some combination of end moments, in-plane loads, shear loads, and surface pressures (Fig. 6). Lekhnitskii presents an elasticity solution for a nonhomogeneous curved bar subject to an end moment or end load in Ref 6. Although this approach is formulated for a general nonhomogeneous material, specific solutions can only be found for materials that have certain restrictions on their anisotropic nature. The solution actually provided by Lehnitskii is only applicable to materials with properties that vary in proportion to their radial position.

A somewhat simpler, and arguably more useful, strength of materials solution for balanced symmetric curved laminates is developed in Ref 7. This solution is similar to classical laminated plate theory in that it assumes the tangential displacement varies linearly through the thickness. Since the laminate is curved, the tangential strain distribution is nonlinear. It is this nonlinear strain that makes the curved laminate analysis somewhat more complicated than the analysis of conventional flat laminates.

The magnitude of the tangential strain is determined by equating the applied tangential load to the resultant of the tangential stress, and the applied moment to the moment due to the tangential stress. In this process, the tangential stress in a ply is expressed as the product of the assumed tangential strain and the tangential stiffness of the ply. This formulation leads to quantities, analogous to the [*A*] and [*D*] matrices of classical laminated plate theory, which define the tangential strain distribution for a given tangential load and bending moment. The magnitude of the tangential stress in each ply can then be evaluated. Once the tangential stress distribution is known, the shear stress ($\tau_{r\theta}$) can be found by summing the moments about the center of curvature. The tangential and shear stress distributions are required to calculate the radial stress distribution, which is found by summing the radial forces.

This sounds like a complicated procedure, but in practice it is not that much more difficult than classical laminate plate theory. If done by hand, implementing this process would be a daunting task, but the method can be coded into a computer program with modest effort. Once done, the analysis of a curved laminate is no more difficult than a conventional flat laminate analysis.

Flange Curling. An out-of-plane phenomenon that is related to the analysis of curved laminates is the curling of curved flanges subject to tensile loads (Fig. 7). The loads applied to the web of the structure shown in Fig. 7 act to increase the radius of the web. When this happens, the flanges bend upward to try to remain at their initial radius. This bending of the flanges is referred to as flange curling. The curling of the flange tends to open the radius that is formed when web plies wrap around to form the flange. As described in the previous section, this induces radial stresses through the thickness of the laminate, which can lead to the delamination of the structure. A similar phenomenon occurs when the curved flange is put in compression, but this load causes the flanges to bend downward, which closes the web to flange radius, thereby inducing radial compression.

Simple models for this problem do not exist, and it is most easily handled using a numerical

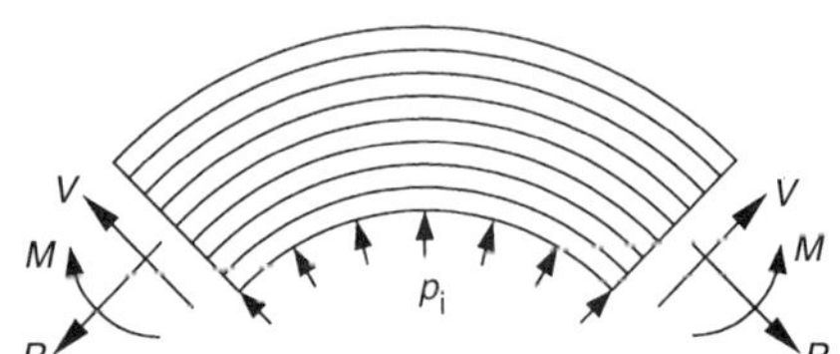

Fig. 6 Combined loads acting on a curved laminate. *P*, in-plane load; *V*, shear load; *M*, end moment; p_i, surface pressure

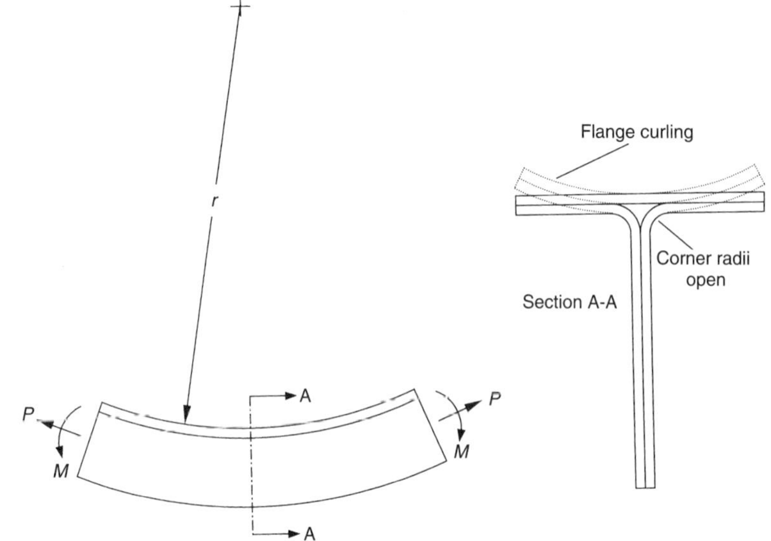

Fig. 7 Flange curling induced by loads on a curved substructure

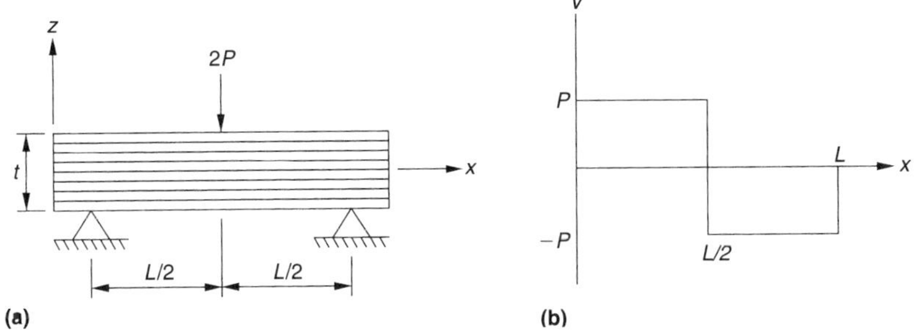

Fig. 8 Laminated beam in three-point bending. (a) Load diagram. (b) Shear diagram

technique such as the finite element method. A common approach uses the so-called global-local method. In this method, a relatively coarse global finite element model is generated and used to define the boundary conditions for more refined models of local details. For the flange curling problem, the global model can use laminated plate elements to define the shape that the corner radius takes on when it opens. This shape can then be used in a more refined analysis of the curved laminate that defines the corner.

Note that this problem only occurs in unsupported flanges. In practice, flanges are generally attached to some other structural component, such as a skin, that constrains curling. However, structural components such as frames or bulkheads are often tested in a free-standing condition. For these tests, it is important to perform a flange-curling analysis to ensure that the component will not fail prematurely in a mode that will not exist in the final structure.

Beams In Bending. One of the simplest examples of a structure subject to direct out-of-plane loading is a laminated beam in three-point bending. The shear diagram for this configuration, as shown in Fig. 8, identifies regions of constant shear between the point at which the load is applied and the supports. This leads to an average shear of *P*/*A*, where *A* is the cross sectional area of the beam. From beam theory, the distribution of this shear through the thickness is a simple parabola that satisfies the condition that the shear must be 0 on the traction-free surfaces. It can be shown that this distribution peaks in the center of the specimen at a value of 3/2 times the average shear.

This approach is fine for isotropic specimens, but researchers have shown that the parabolic distribution is not representative of the actual distribution in an orthotropic specimen. In Ref 8, Whitney presents a two-dimensional elasticity solution for the shear distributions in homogeneous orthotropic beams in three- or four-point bending in the form of an infinite series. Whitney shows convergence with 100 terms in the series, which presents little computational difficulty to a modern personal computer. The shear distribution predicted by this model shows that the peak shear is found near the applied load. The magnitude is greater than the peak calculated for a parabolic distribution, and its through-thickness location is shifted away from the centerline of the specimen, toward the side upon which the load is applied (Fig. 9).

The difference between the parabolic solution for an isotropic material and the more complex distribution for the orthotropic material accounts for the problems associated with using the three-point bending test as a method for determining interlaminar shear strength. The problem is that the parabolic distribution is assumed when backing the interlaminar strength out of the failure load. A better approach would be to perform an analysis that accounted for the beam being orthotropic, and using the resulting distribution to determine the peak stress at failure.

Methods for determining materials properties that rely on the use of an analysis tend to be frowned upon. There is a saying that no one believes analytical results except the person who performed the calculations, and everyone believes experimental results except the person who conducted the test. This could explain why hybrid experimental/analytical techniques tend to offend everyone's sensibilities. Such an approach could, however, lead to better quantitative results from a simple, inexpensive test that is generally considered only a qualitative test.

Stiffener Pulloff. A common direct out-of-plane load case is the transfer of a load from a composite skin into the supporting structure. A good example is the transfer of the pressure on the skin of an aircraft into the supporting ribs, frames, and spars (Fig. 10). The study of this load case is especially important for bonded or co-cured composite structures, because the loads must be carried across unreinforced (no *z*-direction fiber) interfaces. Being able to predict the peak value of the normal and shear stress distributions in the interface between the skin and substructure is essential.

One of the more simple models for this problem is based on treating the bonded or co-cured flange as a beam on an elastic foundation (Fig. 11). This problem has been studied extensively (Ref 9, for example), and solutions for many common load cases exist. Drawbacks to this type of solution are that bending in the skin is not accounted for, and the calculation of the foundation stiffness is very subjective. In addition, the beam on elastic foundation approach does not explicitly model the geometry of the so-called "noodle" or "nugget" of resin that exists in many skin-to-substructure joints (Fig. 12). The stress distribution in the interface can be

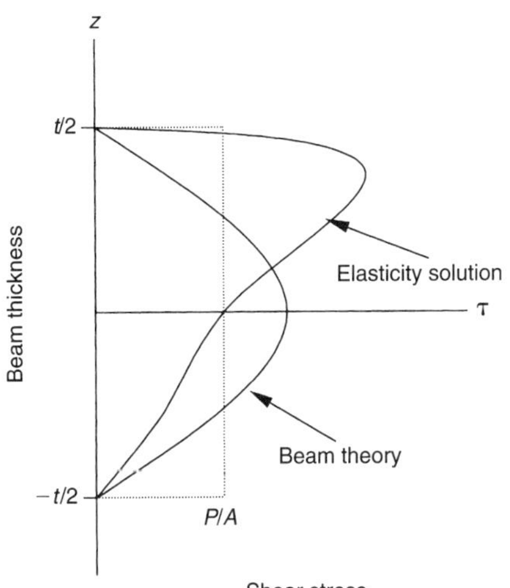

Fig. 9 Shear distribution through the thickness of an orthotropic beam

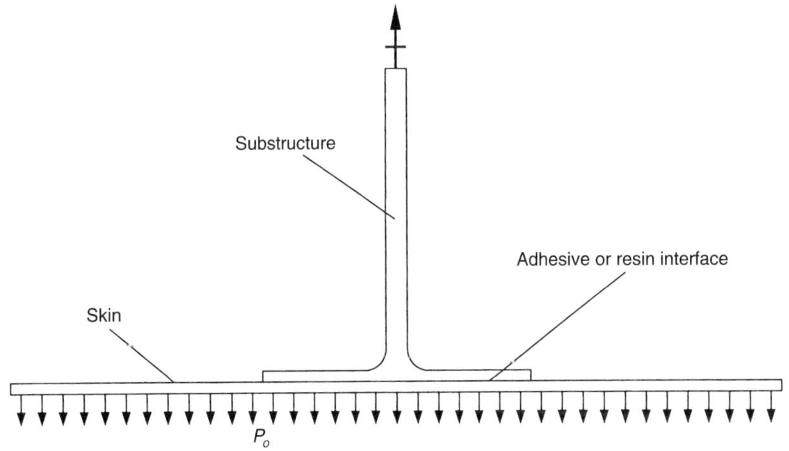

Fig. 10 Transfer of pressure loads on the skin through the substructure

sensitive to the geometry of this detail, and the peak stresses often occur in or near it. Because of these drawbacks, this formulation is not recommended for laminated composite materials.

The most direct approach to explicitly including the geometry of the interface in the pulloff analysis is to use the finite element method. The modeling effort can be simplified by using a two-dimensional model that represents a slice through the structure that is perpendicular to the substructure. It is common to assume that the model is in a state of plane strain. Using this approach, plies can be modeled individually using solid elements, or can be lumped together into plate elements. This technique, when combined with *p*-version finite elements, is particularly powerful and efficient. (In *p*-version finite element analysis, the polynomial degree of elements can be varied over a wide range. Thus, the error can be controlled not only by mesh refinement, but also by increasing the polynomial degree of all elements.)

A finite element approach that uses frame elements to model the skin and substructure, and membrane elements to model the interface is presented in Ref 7. The stress distributions predicted with this model were shown to correlate well with similar distributions predicted by very detailed models that used solid finite elements to explicitly model each ply. For either type of finite element model, the geometry is usually simple enough that a preprocessor for generating the finite element mesh can easily be developed.

The frame-and-membrane type model is obviously easier to generate, but the solid-element approach has the advantage of providing interlaminar stresses in the skin and substructure, along with the stresses in the interface. The substructure often includes curved laminates in areas where webs are folded to form flanges. Pull-off loads tend to open the radii of these details, and the solid element models will predict the resulting radial stresses in the same analysis that yields the interface stresses.

3-D Composites. As previously mentioned, the through-thickness axis typically represents the weakest direction of a conventional laminated composite. Various schemes have been devised for reinforcing this otherwise weak direction. These include 3-D weaving, stitching, and various proprietary techniques for inserting through-thickness reinforcement, such as "T"-forming and "Z"-pinning. See the article "Fabrics and Preforms" in this Volume for illustrations of 3-D composites. These 3-D composites, also known as n-directionally reinforced composites, can be analyzed using many of the tools used to analyze conventional two-dimensional composites, but the generation of effective properties for them is somewhat more complicated.

The typical approach to calculating effective properties for a 3-D composite is based on defining a representative volume element (RVE). The RVE is the smallest volume that fully characterizes the composite in terms of the total fiber content and the distribution and orientation of that fiber. The properties of the RVE are therefore representative of the bulk properties of the composite.

Most procedures for calculating the effective properties of the RVE are based on volume averaging properties of the constituents. For 3-D composites, it is advantageous to volume average the stiffness or compliance matrices, rather than individual engineering properties, because the matrices account for all of the coupling (i.e., shear-extensional, shear-shear, etc.) that may be present in the material. The expressions for the effective stiffness and compliance are given by the following equations, respectively:

$$[C]^* = \frac{1}{V}\sum_{i=1}^{n} V_i \cdot [C]_i \quad \text{(Eq 1)}$$

$$[S]^* = \frac{1}{V}\sum_{i=1}^{n} V_i \cdot [S]_i \quad \text{(Eq 2)}$$

In Eq 1 and 2, it is assumed that the composite is comprised of n-unidirectional fiber bundles. $[C]_i$ and $[S]_i$ are the stiffness and compliance matrices of the ith bundle transformed into global coordinates, V_i is the volume fraction of the ith bundle, and V is the total volume of the RVE. It can be shown that volume-averaging the stiffness matrices results in an upper bound on the effective properties, and volume-averaging the compliance leads to a lower bound. This process has been extended to other effective properties, such as coefficients of thermal expansion and conductivities (see Ref 10).

If the composite is orthogonal, the effective through-thickness properties can be extracted from individual terms in an orthotropic compliance or stiffness matrix. For example, the through-thickness modulus of elasticity can be calculated from the knowledge that the S_{33} term in the compliance matrix for an orthotropic material is given by $1/E_{33}$. These relationships do not hold for the more general anisotropic case, but the orthotropic assumptions can sometimes be used as a first-order approximation.

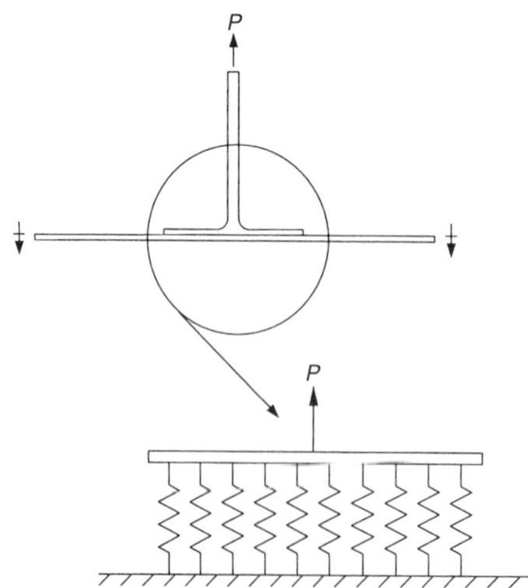

Fig. 11 Skin-to-structure interface modeled as a beam on an elastic foundation

It is important to bear in mind that the properties of the RVE only represent the composite if the fiber architecture does not change. For some 3-D composites, the fiber architecture is continuously variable. The architectures of integrally woven stiffeners or inserts are good examples. For these cases, there may be no single RVE that will provide the bulk properties of the composite. The typical approach used for these structures is to zone the component into a number of distinct regions and to define a unique RVE for each zone.

Conclusion

In spite of the problems associated with models for conducting out-of-plane analysis, composite structural development programs are usually successful. This success can be attributed to the efforts of competent structural engineers to minimize out-of-plane loading, their prior knowledge of design details, failure analysis of previous unsuccessful designs, and a reluctance to stray too far away from tried-and-true methods. Although the conservative approach adopted by many designers and analysts *has* been ridiculed by some, a certain amount of conservatism is warranted. Most out-of-plane analysis methods are still approximate at best, and determining allowable properties is difficult, which can lead to unreliable results.

It is therefore important to experimentally validate any analytical tool before using it in a design environment, to establish the limits of applicability of an analytical method, and to strictly stay within those limits. The importance of using analytical techniques that are consistent with the methods used to generate design allowable should also be reemphasized. It is very easy to be lulled into a false sense of security by analytical models that produce color contour plots of stress distributions and report peak values to four decimal places, and also very easy to forget that the input materials properties were only good to two significant digits.

On the bright side, out-of-plane analysis is an area that is still being actively researched. New, hopefully more accurate and reliable, modeling techniques are being developed. Accompanying this analytical work is an interest in developing

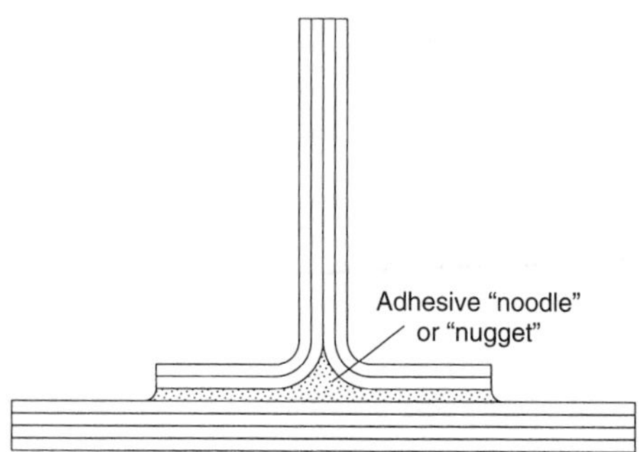

Fig. 12 Resin-rich region in a skin-to-structure interface

better test techniques. In the meantime, analysts should be cautioned to thoroughly understand the assumptions inherent in their models, and to verify the integrity of the experimental data they use.

REFERENCES

1. R.B. Pipes and N.J. Pagano, Interlaminar Stresses in Composite Laminates under Uniform Axial Extension, *J. Compos. Mater.*, Vol 4, Oct 1970, p 538–548
2. G. Flanagan, An Efficient Stress Function Approximation for the Free-Edge Stresses in Laminates, *Int. J. Solids Struct.*, Vol 31 (No. 7), April 1994, p 941–952
3. N.J. Pagano and R.B. Pipes, Some Observations on the Interlaminar Strength of Composite Laminates, *Int. J. Mech. Sci.*, Vol 15, 1973, p 697
4. P. Conti and A. De Paulis, A *Simple Model to Simulate the Interlaminar Stresses Generated near the Free Edge of a Composite Laminate,* STP 876, W.S. Johnson, Ed., American Society for Testing and Materials, Philadelphia, 1985, p 35–51
5. N.J. Salamon, An Assessment of the Interlaminar Stress Problem in Laminated Composites, *J. Compos. Mater. Sup.*, Vol 14, 1980, p 177–194
6. S.G. Lekhnitskii, *Theory of Elasticity of an Anisotropic Body*, Translated from the revised 1977 Russian edition, Mir Publishers, 1981, p 256–262
7. P.C. Paul, C.R. Saff, K.B. Sanger, M.A. Mahler, H.P. Kan, and R.B. Deo, "Out-of-Plane Analysis for Composite Structure Volume I," Report Number NAWCADWAR-94138-60 (Vol 1), Naval Air Warfare Center, Warminster, PA, 15 Sept 1994
8. J.M. Whitney, Elasticity Analysis of Orthotropic Beams under Concentrated Loads, *Compos. Sci. Technol.*, Vol 22, 1985
9. M. Hetényi, *Beams on Elastic Foundation*, University of Michigan Press, Ann Arbor, MI, 1946
10. Zvi Hashin, Analysis of Composite Materials—A Survey, *J. Appl. Mech.*, Vol 50, Sept 1983, p 481–505

Analysis of Sandwich Structures

Stephen Ward, SW Composites
Lawrence Gintert, Concurrent Technologies Corporation

A SANDWICH STRUCTURE is comprised of layered composite materials formed by bonding two or more thin facings or facesheets to a relatively thick core material. In this type of construction the facings resist nearly all of the in-plane loads and out-of-plane bending moments. The thin facings provide nearly all of the bending stiffness because they are generally of a much higher modulus material and are located at the greatest distance from the neutral axis of the component. The core material provides spacing and transmits shear between the facesheets so that they are effective in bending about a common neutral axis. The core also provides most of the through-thickness shear rigidity of the sandwich construction and stabilizes the facesheets so they can be loaded to stress levels higher than the limits imposed by general buckling of thin plates. Core materials are generally selected to be lightweight and to be compatible with the facesheet material and the face-to-core attachment methods used in fabrication. The face-to-core attachment method, such as an adhesive bond, braze, or weld, is generally based on structural and environmental requirements for the sandwich system. By proper choice of materials for facings and core, constructions with higher ratios of stiffness-to-weight and strength-to-weight can be achieved, in comparison to other types of construction. A sandwich structure is also very good in fatigue because the facings are continuously bonded to the core, resulting in minimal stress risers. In most cases, the main reason sandwich construction is used is to save weight, but it also may provide other benefits such as thermal and sound insulation, and reduced cost.

The following topics are discussed in this article:

- Sandwich panel failure modes
- Nomenclatures and definitions
- Strength checks
- Stiffness and internal loads
- Flat panels under pressure loading
- Curved sandwich panels
- Local strength analysis methods
- Flat panel stability

It is assumed that the reader is familiar with the general structural behavior of composite materials and is aware of the various combinations of materials that may be employed in the design of a composite component. Further information regarding the design and analysis of structural composites and sandwich composites may be found in MIL-HDBK-17, from which much of the information provided herein has been taken. Furthermore, at the time of this publication MIL-HDBK-17, Revision F, 2001, is in the process of incorporating a new section devoted to sandwich construction, combining sections of the canceled MIL-HDBK-23, which provided the basic principles from which sandwich analysis has evolved. These basic principles have been developed for polymer-matrix composites, but may be applied to metal-matrix composites and ceramic-matrix composites as well. Likewise many of the analytical procedures are specific to honeycomb core sandwich structures in which the facings are not truly continuously supported by the core. Each cell of the honeycomb leaves an unsupported portion of the facesheet and may constitute a critical parameter in the design of the sandwich structure, depending on the cell geometry and facesheet properties. Another source of analytical information is the series of Forest Products Laboratory Reports listed in Table 1.

While sandwich panels can be constructed in a variety of ways with a variety of materials, for the purposes of describing the structural analysis of sandwich panels, a honeycomb core panel with beveled core edges, as shown in Fig. 1, is used. The methods developed for the analysis of honeycomb sandwich panels of this type offer an example for describing the various failure modes of sandwich construction. The critical failure modes and properties for each of the panel constituents must be established in order to conduct the analyses as described herein. The panel constituents for this example include honeycomb core and orthotropic facesheets. The flat face is referred to as the tool side, and the opposite face is the bag side. The bag-side facesheet follows the contour of the core as it slopes down around the panel perimeter to meet the tool side. The sloping portion of the core is called the ramp region, and the solid laminate where the tool and bag faces come together is called the edgeband.

Sandwich Panel Failure Modes

Honeycomb panel failures can be divided into three categories: insufficient strength, local instability, and general instability.

Insufficient strength failure modes are described subsequently. See Fig. 2 for pictorial representations of these modes.

- *Facing failure* is simply characterized by cracked facesheets. This failure occurs when the facesheet strength is exceeded.
- *Transverse shear failure* can manifest itself as face-to-core debonding or as a shear failure in the core itself. This failure occurs when the core or the face-to-core adhesive has insufficient shear strength.
- *Flexural core crushing* is a concern when the facesheets tend to move toward each other under the influence of bending. This failure mode occurs when the core has insufficient compression strength.
- *Flatwise tension or compression* occurs in the ramp area where the bag-side facesheet changes direction. The flatwise, or interlaminar, stresses are induced at the ramp radii. A flatwise tension stress can cause face-to-core debonding, while a flatwise compression stress can cause core crushing.

Local instability includes the following two failure modes illustrated in Fig. 3:

- *Intracell buckling*, or face dimpling, is a local instability characterized by the buckling of a facesheet into or out of the confines of a single cell. This failure can occur when the facesheets are thin.
- *Face wrinkling* is a local instability characterized by the inward or outward buckling of the face, accompanied by core crushing, core tearing, or face-to-core debonding. This failure can occur when the core has a low density.

General instability failure modes are given subsequently and are shown in Fig. 4:

- *General buckling* of a sandwich panel resembles the classical buckling of plates or columns. The facesheets and core remain intact in this type of failure.

- *Shear crimping* is an instability that can occur if the wavelength of each buckle is of the same order as the cell size. The crimping phenomenon is characterized by a local core shear failure and the lateral dislocation of the facesheets. Since the wavelengths are so short, shear crimping appears to be a local instability failure, but it is really a form of general instability. This failure mode can occur when the core shear modulus is low.

Nomenclature and Definitions for Loads, Geometry, and Material Properties

The variables used throughout this section to represent the loads and characteristics applied to a flat sandwich panel are given in Table 2. Figure 5 gives a pictorial representation of the general load state for a flat sandwich panel. The geometry of the honeycomb sandwich is shown in Fig. 6.

Assumptions and Definitions. The analysis of honeycomb sandwich panels is made easier when a few assumptions are made. The following statements are considered true for every honeycomb sandwich analysis method, unless otherwise noted:

- The in-plane stiffness of the honeycomb core is negligible with respect to the facesheets: ($E_{x\text{core}} = E_{y\text{core}} = G_{xy\text{core}} = 0$).
- The centroid of the whole sandwich element is coincident with the centroid of the facesheets by themselves. This is implied by the previous assumption.
- The facesheets are thin, and the moments of inertia about their own centroids are negligible; that is, $t_{\text{t}}^3 = t_{\text{b}}^3 = 0$.
- The distance between the facesheet midplanes is considered to be equal to the distance between the face centroids.
- The point at which in-plane load is applied to the edgeband is considered to be halfway between the face centroids (midplanes).
- Normal (out-of-plane) shear forces are carried exclusively by the core and are distributed evenly through the core thickness.
- The honeycomb panels in this article are all rectangular, and the load coordinate system (x, y, z) is coincident with the core material system (L, W, T).
- The *midplane* of a sandwich element is located halfway between the face surfaces: $y_{\text{midplane}} = t/2$.
- The *centroid* of a sandwich element is located at the point where no bending strain occurs in a flat panel. When the facesheets have unequal thicknesses, the centroid does not coincide with the midplane:

$$y_{\text{centroid}} = \frac{\sum_{i=1}^{2} (t_i \cdot y_i)}{\sum_{i=1}^{2} (t_i)}$$

- The *neutral axis* of a sandwich element is similar to the centroid in that it is located at the point where zero strain is induced under the influence of bending loads. For a flat panel, the neutral axis coincides with the centroid, but, for a curved panel, the neutral axis does not coincide with the centroid.

Strength Checks

Edgeband and Ramp. Figure 7 shows the areas where a flat sandwich panel should be checked for adequate strength. Each fastener around the edgeband must be checked for adequate bearing/bypass strength.

In the area where the bag-side facesheet changes direction, the core is subject to flatwise tension and/or compression. In the case of flatwise tension, the face-to-core adhesive must provide an adequate bond, and in the case of flatwise compression, the core must have adequate crushing strength.

The shear force normal to the panel reaches a maximum at the fastener centerline. In the ramp region, the bag-side face and the honeycomb core both react to the shear load. The core is checked for adequate shear strength in the entire ramp region, but it is often critical at the top of the ramp when pressure is the only applied load. At this location, the core is assumed to carry 100% of the out-of-plane shear.

Analysis Overview of Panel Acreage. The following procedure is recommended for the stress analysis of sandwich panels in areas away from core ramps and edgebands. The center of the panel is exposed to a peak bending moment, and the facesheet strength, flexural core crushing, local instability, and general instability failure modes are often critical at this location.

1. Determine the sandwich panel and the stiffness properties of the individual faces as defined by their [A], [B], [D], [G] matrices. Use appropriate ply properties based on temperature and moisture environment. Determine allowable strengths for the facesheet, core, and adhesive materials.
2. Obtain internal loads acting on the sandwich panel, either through a finite element analysis

Table 1 Selected Forest Products Laboratory (FPL) reports related to sandwich structures

FPL report number	Title
1810	Wrinkling of the Facings of Sandwich Construction Subjected to Edgewise Compression
1810-A	Wrinkling of the Facings of Sandwich Construction Subjected to Edgewise Compression; Sandwich Constructions Having Honeycomb Cores
1815	Effect of Shear Strength on Maximum Loads of Sandwich Columns
1817	Short-Column Compressive Strength of Sandwich Constructions as Affected by the Size of the Cells of Honeycomb-Core Materials
1827	Edgewise Compressive Strength of Panels and Flatwise Flexural Strength of Strips of Sandwich Constructions
1828	The Bending of a Circular Sandwich Plate under Normal Load
1829	Flexure of Structural Sandwich Construction
1830	Buckling of Cylinders of Sandwich Construction in Axial Compression
1833	Critical Loads of a Rectangular, Flat Sandwich Panel Subjected to Two Direct Loads Combined with a Shear Load
1834	Behavior of a Rectangular Sandwich Panel under a Uniform Lateral Load and Compressive Edge Loads
1838	Stresses within a Rectangular, Flat Sandwich Panel Subjected to a Uniformly Distributed Normal Load and Edgewise, Direct, and Shear Loads
1840	Buckling of Sandwich Cylinders in Torsion
1844	Analysis of Long Cylinders of Sandwich Construction under Uniform External Lateral Pressure
1844-A	Analysis of Long Cylinders of Sandwich Construction under Uniform External Lateral Pressure; Facings of Moderate and Unequal Thicknesses
1845	Stresses Induced in a Sandwich Panel by Load Applied at an Insert
1845-A	Stresses Induced in a Sandwich Panel by Load Applied at an Insert
1845-B	Stresses Induced in a Sandwich Panel by Load Applied at an Insert
1846	Transfer of Longitudinal Load from One Facing of a Sandwich Panel to the Other by Means of Shear in the Core
1847	Deflection and Stresses in a Uniformly Loaded, Simply Supported, Rectangular Sandwich Plate
1847-A	Deflection and Stresses in a Uniformly Loaded, Simply Supported, Rectangular Sandwich Plate; Experimental Verification of Theory
1852	Elastic Stability of Cylindrical Sandwich Shells under Axial and Lateral Load
1854	Compressive Buckling Curves for Sandwich Panels with Isotropic Facings and Isotropic or Orthotropic Cores
1857	Elastic Buckling of a Simply Supported Rectangular Sandwich Panel Subjected to Combined Edgewise Bending and Compression
1857-A	Elastic Buckling of a Simply Supported Rectangular Sandwich Panel Subjected to Combined Edgewise Bending and Compression; Results for Panels with Facings of Either Equal or Unequal Thickness and with Orthotropic Cores
1859	Elastic Buckling of a Simply Supported Sandwich Panel Subjected to Combined Edgewise Bending, Compression, and Shear
1867	Compressive Buckling Curves for Simply Supported Sandwich Panels with Glass-Fabric-Laminate Facings and Honeycomb Cores
1868	Buckling of Simply Supported Rectangular Sandwich Panels Subjected to Edgewise Bending
1871	Torsion of Rectangular Sandwich Plate
1874	Torsion of Sandwich Panels of Trapezoidal, Triangular, and Rectangular Cross Sections
1876	Compressive Buckling Curves for Sandwich Cylinders Having Orthotropic Facings
2171	Wrinkling of Faces of Aluminum and Stainless Steel Sandwich Subjected to Edgewise Compression

USDA Forest Service, Forest Products Laboratory, Madison, WI, www.fpl.fs.fed.us

or with specialized closed-form solutions or computer programs.

3. Using the stiffness properties, determine the sandwich panel strains and curvatures. Determine the internal loads acting on each individual facesheet.
4. Determine the damage assumptions and associated strength requirements for durability and damage tolerance by referring to the appropriate design criteria.
5. Determine the margin of safety of each local failure mode:
   (a) Check both facesheets' in-plane failures resulting from tension, compression, and shear loads.
   (b) Check core transverse shear failure.
   (c) Check core crushing from local loads and flexure-induced crushing.
   (d) Check flatwise tension in core and adhesive.
   (e) Check face wrinkling on both faces.
   (f) Check face dimpling on both faces.
6. Determine, if necessary, the margin of safety for general instability:
   (a) Check general buckling.
   (b) Check shear crimping.

Stiffness and Internal Loads

Plate Stiffness Analysis. The first step in the analysis is to define the stiffness properties for the whole panel and for the individual faces. The best approach is to use a laminate analysis program to calculate the different stiffness matrices. Calculate first the [A], [B], and [D] matrices of the *whole panel*. Use the individual ply properties and assume that the core is a special type of ply with no in-plane stiffness, but with the correct transverse shear stiffness:

$$\begin{bmatrix} N \\ M \end{bmatrix} = \begin{bmatrix} A & B \\ B & D \end{bmatrix} \begin{bmatrix} \varepsilon \\ \kappa \end{bmatrix} \qquad \text{(Eq 1)}$$

Use a program that will also determine the transverse shear stiffness coefficients, A_{44}, A_{45}, and A_{55}, of the plate:

$$\begin{bmatrix} Q_x \\ Q_y \end{bmatrix} = \begin{bmatrix} A_{55} & A_{45} \\ A_{45} & A_{44} \end{bmatrix} \begin{bmatrix} \gamma_{xz} \\ \gamma_{yz} \end{bmatrix} = [\mathrm{G}] \begin{bmatrix} \gamma_{xz} \\ \gamma_{yz} \end{bmatrix} \qquad \text{(Eq 2)}$$

If such a program is not available, assume that the core alone provides the transverse shear stiffness. This is valid if the faces are thin compared to the core, say less than 5% of the core thickness. Calculate the coefficients as follows:

$$\begin{aligned} A_{55} &= cG_{xz\text{core}} \quad A_{45} = 0 \\ A_{44} &= cG_{yz\text{core}} \quad A_{54} = 0 \end{aligned} \qquad \text{(Eq 3)}$$

Using the same laminate analysis program or hand analysis formulae, determine the stiffness properties, that is, the [A], [B], and [D] matrices, of *each individual face*:

$$\begin{aligned} \begin{bmatrix} N \\ M \end{bmatrix}_1 &= \begin{bmatrix} A & B \\ B & D \end{bmatrix}_1 \begin{bmatrix} \varepsilon \\ \kappa \end{bmatrix}_1 \\ \begin{bmatrix} N \\ M \end{bmatrix}_2 &= \begin{bmatrix} A & B \\ B & D \end{bmatrix}_2 \begin{bmatrix} \varepsilon \\ \kappa \end{bmatrix}_2 \end{aligned} \qquad \text{(Eq 4)}$$

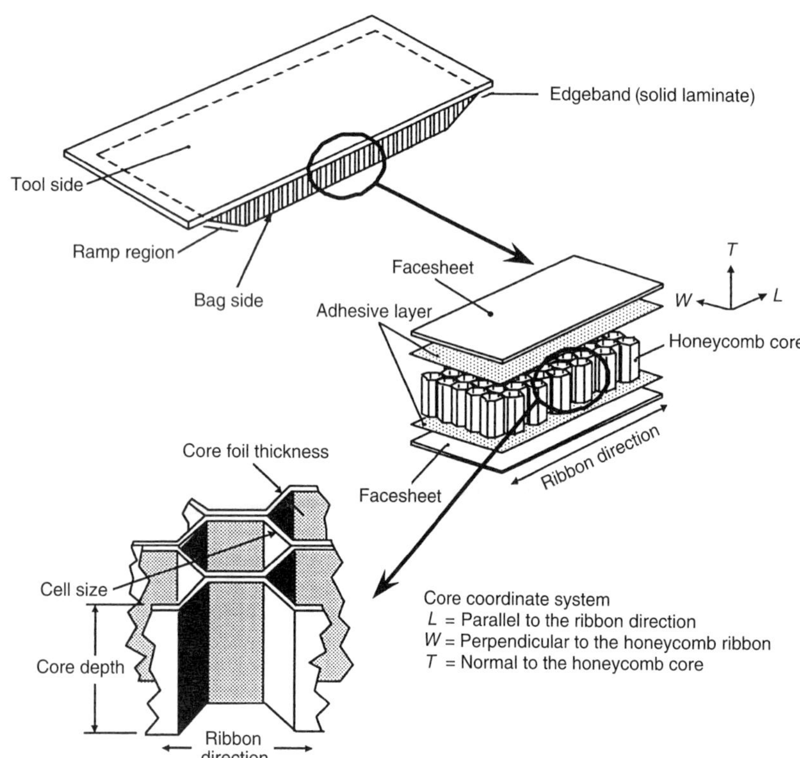

Fig. 1 Honeycomb sandwich construction

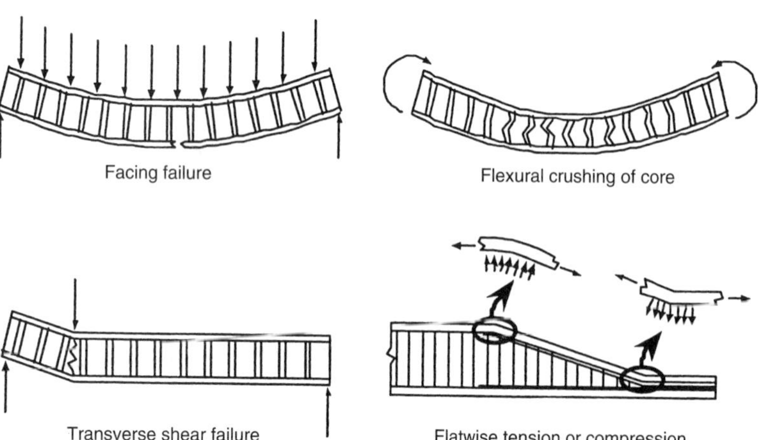

Fig. 2 Failures caused by insufficient strength

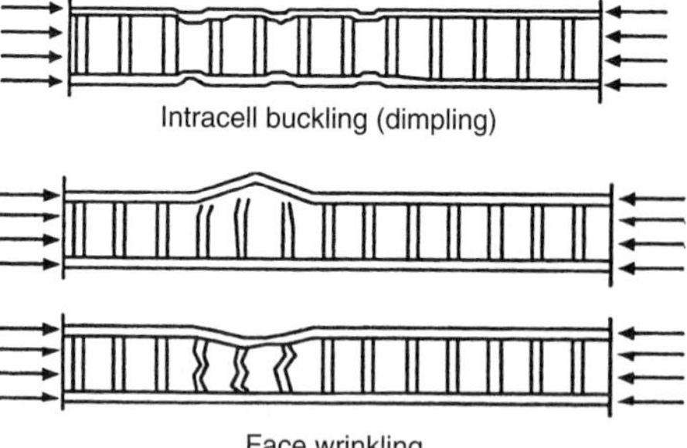

Fig. 3 Failures caused by local instability

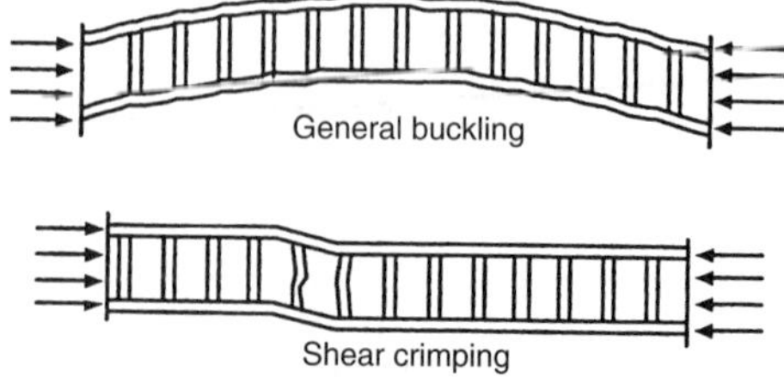

Fig. 4 Failures caused by general instability

Table 2 Nomenclature and definitions

Symbol	Definition	SI units	Customary units	Comment
c	Core depth at any point in the honeycomb panel	m	in.	For $x \leq L_{AB}$ $c = 0$ (no core) For $L_{AB} < x < L_{AC}$ $c = \frac{x - L_{AB}}{L_{AC} - L_{AB}} t_c$ For $x \geq L_{AC}$ $c = t_c$
C_{zx}, C_{zy}	Compliance factors for panel strips parallel to the x- and y-directions, respectively	1/MPa	in.^{3}/lb	...
d	Distance between the face midplanes at any point in the honeycomb panel	m	in.	$x \leq L_{AB}$ $d = t_e - \frac{t_t + t_b}{2}$ $L_{AB} < x < L_{AC}$ $d = (t_c - t_e + t_t + t_b) \frac{x - L_{AB}}{L_{AC} - L_{AB}} + \left(t_e - \frac{t_t + t_b}{2}\right)$ $x \geq L_{AC}$ $d = t_c + \frac{t_t + t_b}{2}$ $x \geq L_{AC}$ $d = t_c + \frac{t_t + t_b}{2}$
D_{zx}, D_{zy}	Flexural stiffnesses for panel strips parallel to the x- and y-directions, respectively	N/m	lb/in.	Per unit width
E_{cc}	Core compression modulus in the z-direction	MPa	psi	...
E_x, E_y, E_{xf}, E_{yf}	Facesheet elastic moduli parallel to the x- and y-directions, respectively	MPa	psi	"f" subscript indicates it is the modulus for the face being checked.
f_{xflat}, f_{yflat}	Flatwise tension or compression stresses at the ramp radii	MPa	psi	...
f_{xf}, f_{yf}	In-plane facesheet stress in x- and y-direction, respectively	MPa	psi	For face being checked
f_{xyf}	In-plane facesheet stress	MPa	psi	For face being checked
G_{xy}	Facesheet shear modulus in the xy plane	MPa	psi	...
G_{zx}, G_{zy}	Core shear moduli in the xz and yz planes, respectively	MPa	psi	...
H_{zx}, H_{zy}	Out-of-plane shear stiffnesses for panel strips parallel to the x- and y-directions, respectively	N/m	lb/in.	Per unit width
K_x, K_y	In-plane (axial) stiffnesses for panel strips parallel to the x- and y-directions, respectively	N/m	lb/in.	Per unit width
L_{AB}	Distance from the fastener centerline to the start of the ramp	m	in.	...
L_{AC}	Distance from the fastener centerline to the end of the ramp	m	in.	...
L_{AD}	Distance from the fastener centerline to the panel center	m	in.	...
L_x, L_y	Length of a rectangular panel in the x- and y-directions, respectively	m	in.	...
M_x, M_y	Edge bending moments per unit width	Nm/m	in. · lb/in.	M_x acts along the edge normal to the x-direction and induces compression in the tool side of the panel. M_y acts along the edge normal to the y-direction and induces compression in the tool side of the panel.
M'_x, M'_y	Bending moments caused by eccentric in-plane load	Nm/m	in. · lb/in.	Per unit width
M_x, M_y	Pressure-induced bending moments	Nm/m	in. · lb/in.	Per unit width
N_x, N_y, N_{xy}	In-plane panel forces per unit width	N/m	lb/in.	N_x acts along the edge normal to the x-direction and induces tension in the x-direction. N_y acts along the edge normal to the y-direction and induces tension in the y-direction. N_{xy} acts along all edges and induces tension in the +45° direction, where the x-direction is considered to be 0° and the y-direction is considered to be 90°.
N_{xt}, N_{yt}, N_{xyt}	In-plane loads for the tool-side facesheet	N/m	lb/in.	Per unit width
N_{xb}, N_{yb}, N_{xyb}	In-plane loads for the bag-side facesheet	N/m	lb/in.	Per unit width
P	Point load	N	lb	Concentrated load in classic beam formulas
p	Uniformly distributed load	N/m	lb/in.	Uniform distributed load in classic beam formulas
P_z	Uniform pressure	MPa	psi	P_z acts normal to the xy plane, in the downward direction ($-z$), and induces compression in the tool side of the panel.
P_{zx}, P_{zy}	Midspan pressures applied to the x-and y-beams, respectively	MPa	psi	$P_{zx} + P_{zy}$ P_z
R_{zx}, R_{zy}	Out-of-plane edge reactions	N/m	lb/in.	R_{zx} acts along the edge normal to the x-direction and is directed upward ($+z$). R_{zy} acts along the edge to the y-direction and is directed upward ($+z$).
s	Honeycomb cell size	m	in.	Measured side-to-side, see Fig. 1
t	Distance between the external face surfaces	m	in.	...
t_t, t_b, t_f	Facesheet thicknesses for the tool and bag sides, respectively, or the thickness of the face being checked	m	in.	t_1, t_2 are also used to indicate the face thicknesses in equations
t_e	Edgeband thickness	m	in.	...
t_c	Core depth outside the ramp region where the facesheets are parallel to each other	m	in.	...
V_{zx}, V_{zy}	Core shear loads for panel strips in the x- and y-directions, respectively	N/m	lb/in.	Per unit width
w	Deflection	m	in.	Deflection in beam formula
δ	Deflection	m	in.	Panel deflection
η_x, η_y	Rotational fixity factor for panel edges normal to the x- and y-directions, respectively	...	...	1.0 for fully fixed, 0.0 for simply supported
ν_{xy}, ν_{yx}	Facesheet Poisson's ratios	...	...	The term, ν_{xy}, is defined as the absolute ratio of strain in the y-direction to strain in the x-direction when load is applied uniaxially in the x-direction, $E_x \nu_{xy} = E_y \nu_{xy}$
ϕ	Ramp angle with respect to the tool-side face	Degree	Degree	
θ	Angle of bag-side facesheet at any point in the honeycomb panel	Degree	Degree	For x, L_{AB}, $\theta = 0$ $L_{AB} < x < L_{AC}$ $\theta = \phi/2$ at center of ramp radii $= \phi$ at flat portion of ramp $x \geq L_{AC}$ $\theta = 0$

Other symbols used in this section are common to plate analysis and matrix representations.

It is important to realize the difference between the face matrices (Eq 4) and the overall plate matrices (Eq 1), and to always use the appropriate matrices for each analysis. For instance, when checking global buckling, use the plate [D] matrix, but when checking face dimpling or wrinkling, use the facesheet [D] matrix. Some formulas, such as those for face wrinkling, call for the face extensional modulus E_x (Eq 6) or E_y, but since wrinkling involves face bending deformation, it is more accurate to use the flexural modulus (Eq 5) instead of (Eq 6):

$$E_{x\text{flex}} = \frac{12D_{11}}{t_1^3} \quad \text{(Eq 5)}$$

assuming that $B_{ij} = 0$ and $\kappa_y = 0$, $\kappa_{xy} = 0$.

$$E_{x\text{ext}} = \frac{A_{11}}{t_1} \quad \text{(Eq 6)}$$

assuming that $B_{ij} = 0$ and $\varepsilon_y = 0$, $\gamma_{xy} = 0$.

Equation 6 would be appropriate if the deformation involved only a face extensional deformation. Note also that these two definitions imply that the deformations (both curvatures and strains) are constrained in the transverse direction. Conversely, if the forces and moments are zero in the transverse direction, one should use

$$E_{x\text{flex}} = \frac{12}{t_1^3 D'_{11}} \quad \text{(Eq 7)}$$

for bending assuming that, $B_{ij} = 0$ and $M_y = 0$, $M_{xy} = 0$. For extension, one should use:

$$E_{x\text{ext}} = \frac{1}{t_1 A'_{11}} \quad \text{(Eq 8)}$$

assuming that $B_{ij} = 0$ and $N_y = 0$, $N_{xy} = 0$ and where:

$$\begin{bmatrix} A' & B' \\ B'^T & D' \end{bmatrix} = \begin{bmatrix} A & B \\ B & D \end{bmatrix}^{-1}$$

Thus, when using any equation which calls for a face stiffness modulus, use the definition of E_x, which corresponds to the mode of deformation.

Beam Stiffness Analysis. Many methods are available to calculate the deflections, bending moments, and shear force distribution in beams under various types of loading and boundary conditions. All these formulae require the use of the beam bending stiffness, D. First, calculate the overall plate bending stiffness matrix [**D**] as explained previously. Then, depending on the aspect ratio of the beam, which is the beam width (b) to thickness (d) ratio, use the following relations (where the "1" direction is along the beam length). For wide beams ($b/d > 6$): $D = D_{11}$ (assumes the transverse curvature, $\kappa_y = 0$). For narrow beams ($b/d < 6$): $D = 1/D'_{11}$ (assumes the transverse moment, $M_y = 0$). Note also that, in general, the transverse shear deformation of the core cannot be neglected.

For instance, the transverse deflection at the free end of a cantilevered beam subjected to a concentrated load, P, can be expressed as:

$$w_{\max} = \left(\frac{PL^3}{3Db} + \frac{PL}{A_{55}b} \right) \quad \text{(Eq 9)}$$

where the first term represents the deflection due to bending and the second term represents the additional deflection due to the transverse shear deformation.

Similarly, the maximum transverse deflection of a simply supported beam subjected to a uniform distributed load, p, can be expressed as:

$$w_{\max} = \left(\frac{5pL^4}{384Db} + \frac{pL^2}{8A_{55}b} \right) \quad \text{(Eq 10)}$$

The deflection of a general beam can be determined using the following differential equation:

$$\frac{d^2y}{d^2x} = \frac{M_x}{D} + \frac{1}{A_{55}} \left(\frac{dV_x}{dx} \right) \quad \text{(Eq 11)}$$

Once the maximum bending moment and shear resultant are obtained, determine the core stresses and facesheet line loads and strains, and then check all the potential failure modes shown in Fig. 2, 3, and 4.

Combined Transverse and In-Plane Loadings. If a plate or beam is subjected to both transverse loads (e.g., pressure) and in-plane compression or shear, additional deflections and stresses will be created beyond the simple superposition of the deflections and stresses created by each loading. If no computer program is available to handle this type of effect, use the following procedure:

1. Calculate the deflections and stresses created by the transverse loads.
2. Calculate the stresses due to the in-plane loads, P.

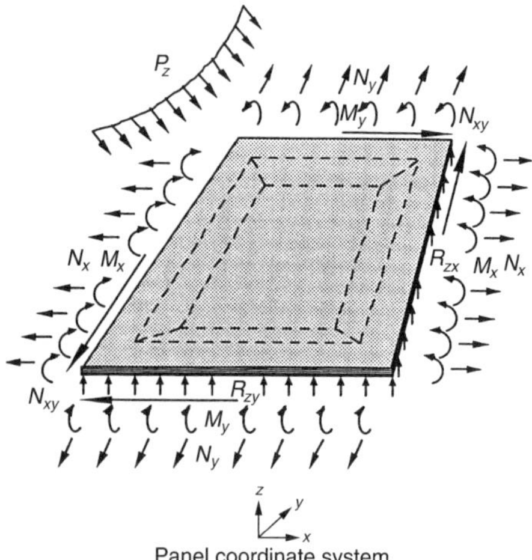

Fig. 5 Generalized load state for a flat sandwich panel. The loads are expressed in terms of the panel coordinate system, which may or may not be coincident with the core coordinate system shown in Fig. 1. Often the L-direction (parallel to the core ribbon) and the x-direction are identical and parallel to the short side of a rectangular panel.

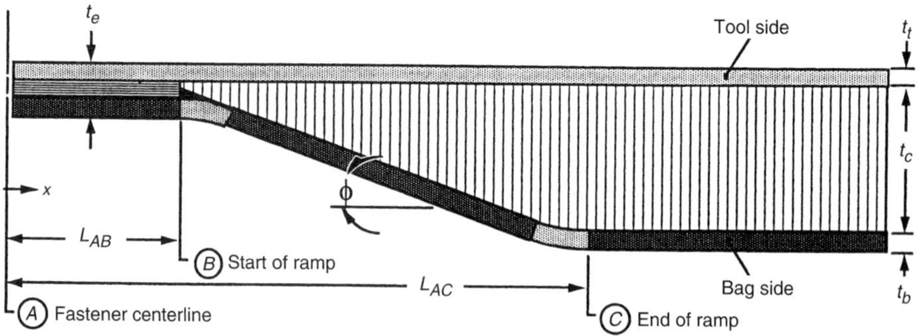

Fig. 6 Geometry of the honeycomb sandwich

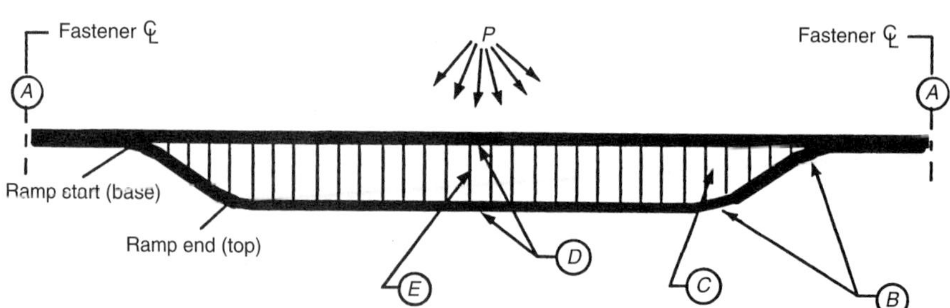

Fig. 7 Critical strength-check locations for a flat sandwich panel. A, bearing/bypass; B, flatwise tension and/or compression; C, core shear; D, face strength and instability; E, flexural core crushing

3. Calculate the critical (buckling) load under the in-plane loads, P_{cr}.
4. Multiply the stresses and deflections due to transverse loads by the ratio $R = 1/[1 - (P/P_{cr})]$ where (P/P_{cr}) is the buckling ratio.
5. Add together the stresses due to in-plane loads and the amplified stresses due to transverse loads.

Facesheet Internal Loads. Typically, the plate or beam stiffness properties will be input into a finite element (FE) model or into a specialized plate analysis program that will return the internal loads in the form of the plate force, moment, and transverse shear resultants. The sandwich plate strains and curvatures are calculated with the stress-strain relations shown previously or with the help of a laminate analysis program. The facesheet strains and loads can be calculated from:

$$\begin{bmatrix} \varepsilon_x \\ \varepsilon_y \\ \varepsilon_{xy} \end{bmatrix}_1 = \begin{bmatrix} \varepsilon_x \\ \varepsilon_y \\ \varepsilon_{xy} \end{bmatrix}_{\text{plate}} + \left(\frac{c+t_2}{2}\right) \begin{bmatrix} \kappa_x \\ \kappa_y \\ \kappa_{xy} \end{bmatrix}_{\text{plate}}$$

$$\begin{bmatrix} N_x \\ N_y \\ N_{xy} \end{bmatrix}_1 = [A]_1 \begin{bmatrix} \varepsilon_x \\ \varepsilon_y \\ \gamma_{xy} \end{bmatrix}_1 + [B]_1 \begin{bmatrix} \kappa_x \\ \kappa_y \\ \kappa_{xy} \end{bmatrix}_{\text{plate}} \quad \text{(Eq 12)}$$

Similar equations are used for the other face.

Flat Panel Internal Loads and Stresses—Pressure Loading

The analysis methods described in the following sections are formulated for flat rectangular honeycomb panels subject to in-plane loads (N_x, N_y, and N_{xy}) and uniform pressure (P_z). This section is intended to give an approximate solution for a pressure-loaded plate for instances where a more detailed analysis, such as a FE model, are not available or not required. The analysis steps are:

1. Idealize the panel as two wide beams perpendicular to each other and intersecting in the middle of the panel. Compute the flexural and shear stiffnesses for each of the beams.
2. Split the total pressure into two uniform parts. One part is carried exclusively by the x-beam, and the other part is carried exclusively by the y-beam. Compute the pressure split by equating the midspan deflections for each beam.
3. Impose an inverted triangular pressure distribution on each of the two beams. Each beam carries the full pressure magnitude at the supported ends, but, at the midpoint, they share the total pressure based on the split calculated in the previous step. Note that all internal loads are derived from the inverted triangular pressure distribution, and the uniform distributions in step 2 are only used to compute the pressure split between the two beams.
4. Compute the bending moment and vertical shear reactions at the beam ends. Use a factor to account for partial rotational fixity.
5. Develop a freebody diagram to derive in-plane facesheet loads and core shear loads at any point along the beams.

Flexural and Shear Stiffnesses. When uniform pressure is applied to a sandwich panel, it is useful to think of some of the pressure being carried by a panel strip from fastener line to fastener line in the x-direction and by another strip from fastener line to fastener line in the y-direction. In this way, the panel is idealized as two mutually perpendicular wide sandwich beams. See Fig. 8.

The flexural stiffness of a beam is a quantity that relates bending moment to curvature. So, for a beam parallel to the x-direction, the curvature at any point along the span, κ_x, is equal to the bending moment at that point divided by the flexural stiffness of the beam, D_{zx}.

For a narrow beam, D_{zx} is simply equal to E_xI_x. A wide beam, however, has greater flexural stiffness than a narrow beam, because the curvature in the plane normal to the applied moment is constrained to be negligible. Thus, for beam x, $\kappa_y = 0$, and for beam y, $\kappa_x = 0$.

The flexural stiffnesses, D_{zx} and D_{zy}, for the two mutually perpendicular panel strips are derived below. The subscripts, "t" and "b," refer to the tool-side and bag-side facesheets, respectively.

$$D_{zx} = \frac{d^2}{\left(\dfrac{1-\nu_{xy}\nu_{yx}}{E_x t}\right)_t + \left(\dfrac{1-\nu_{xy}\nu_{yx}}{E_x t}\right)_b}$$

$$D_{zy} = \frac{d^2}{\left(\dfrac{1-\nu_{xy}\nu_{yx}}{E_y t}\right)_t + \left(\dfrac{1-\nu_{xy}\nu_{yx}}{E_y t}\right)_b} \quad \text{(Eq 13)}$$

The shear stiffness of a beam is a quantity that relates shear force to slope. So, for a beam parallel to the x-direction, the slope at any point along the span is equal to the shear force at that point divided by the shear stiffness of the beam, H_{zx}.

The shear stiffnesses (H_{zx} and H_{zy}) for each of the two panel strips are derived below:

$$H_{zx} = cG_{zx}$$
$$H_{zy} = cG_{zy} \quad \text{(Eq 14)}$$

Midpanel Deflection and Pressure Split. As stated in the previous section, the total uniform panel pressure can be split between two mutually perpendicular beams in the x- and y-directions. The fraction of pressure carried by a beam is directly proportional to its stiffness, and the pressure split between the two beams can be determined by enforcing deflection compatibility at their midspans.

The deflection of a conventional panel subject to uniform pressure is usually a function of flexural stiffness only. However, since the low shear modulus of the core allows significant shear deformations, the deflection of a sandwich panel requires the consideration of *flexural stiffness and shear stiffness*. See Fig. 9.

It is useful to express the maximum midspan deflection of a beam in terms of a compliance factor. So, for a beam parallel to the x-direction, the midspan deflection, $\delta_{x\text{mid}}$, is equal to the amount of uniform pressure carried by the beam, P_{zx}, multiplied by the compliance factor of the beam, C_{zx}.

The out-of-plane compliance factors, C_{zx} and C_{zy}, for the two mutually perpendicular panel strips are derived below:

$$C_{zx} = \frac{(5-4\eta_x)L_x^4}{384D_{zx}} + \frac{L_x^2}{8H_{zx}}$$
$$C_{zy} = \frac{(5-4\eta_y)L_y^4}{384D_{zy}} + \frac{L_y^2}{8H_{zy}} \quad \text{(Eq 15)}$$

Note that the compliance factors are comprised of two terms. The first term represents the deflection due to flexure, and the second term represents the deflection due to shear.

Each of the beams carries the amount of uniform pressure required to equalize its midspan deflections. The pressure reacted by the x-beam, P_{zx}, plus the pressure reacted by the y-beam, P_{zy}, is equal to the total pressure, P_z. Deflection

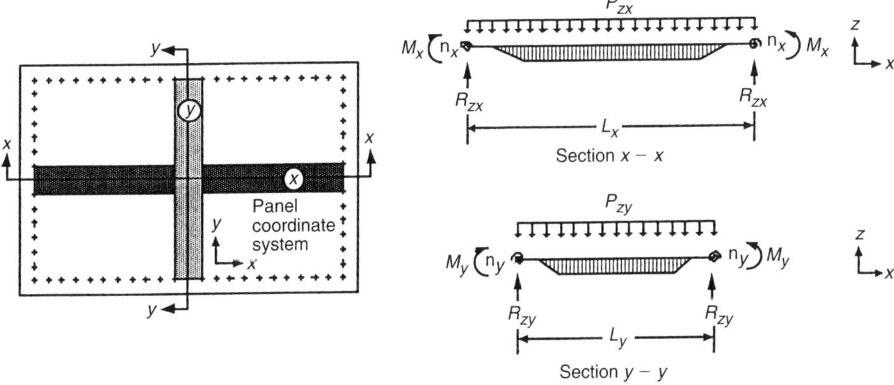

Fig. 8 A flat honeycomb panel is idealized by two mutually perpendicular wide sandwich beams

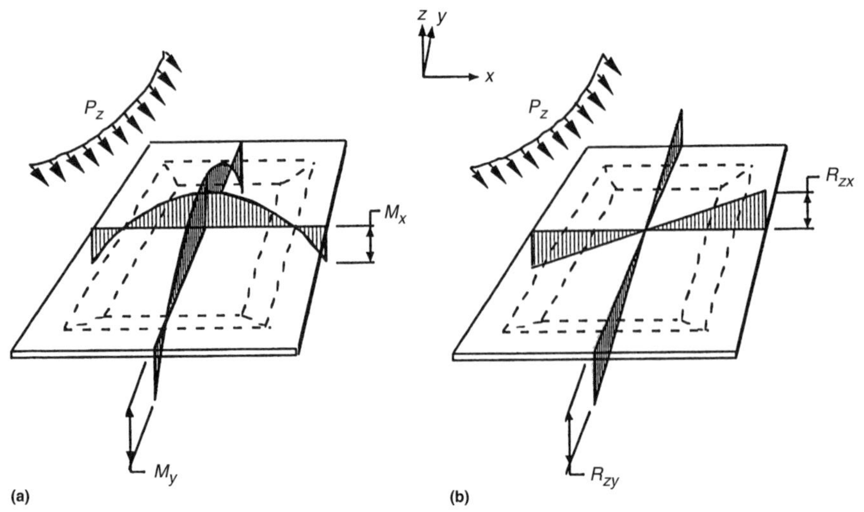

Fig. 9 Approximate midpanel moment (a) and shear (b) distributions for a flat panel exposed to uniform pressure (P_z)

compatibility:

$$\delta_{xmid} = C_{zx}P_{zx} = \delta_{ymid} = C_{zy}P_{zy}$$

Total pressure:

$$P_{zx} + P_{zy} = P_z$$

By combining the previous two equations, the pressure reacted by each beam can be derived:

$$P_{zx} = \frac{C_{zy}}{C_{zx} + C_{zy}} P_z$$
$$P_{zy} = \frac{C_{zx}}{C_{zx} + C_{zy}} P_z \qquad \text{(Eq 16)}$$

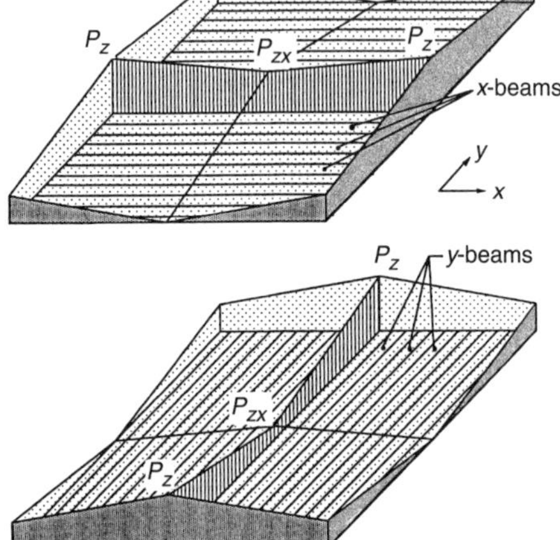

Fig. 10 The inverted triangular pressure distribution. The flat panel can be divided into any number of x-beams and y-beams, but the critical beams are the two that pass through the panel center. These midspan beams carry the full pressure magnitude at their ends, and they each react a percentage of the total pressure at their intersection point. The sum of the two inverted triangular pressure distributions equals the total uniformly applied pressure.

An approximate expression for the maximum deflection of a sandwich panel subject to uniform pressure is:

$$\delta_{max} = \left(\frac{C_{zx}C_{zy}}{C_{zx} + C_{zy}}\right) \cdot P_z \qquad \text{(Eq 17)}$$

Inverted Triangular Pressure Distribution. The pressure split derived in Eq 16 applies only at the intersection point of the two beams. Thus, the applied pressure at the midspan of the x-beam has a magnitude of P_{zx} and the applied pressure at the midspan of the y-beam has a magnitude of P_{zy}. It would not be appropriate, however, to say that the x-beam, for example, is subject to P_{zx} uniformly across its length. This is due to the fact that as the end of the x-beam is approached, it will tend to carry proportionately more pressure than the corresponding y-beam. In other words, when proceeding from the midspan to the end of the x-beam, the load path in the x-direction appears to get stiffer with respect to the y-direction.

Therefore, an inverted triangular pressure distribution is considered to be an appropriate model. The x-beam and the y-beam carry P_{zx} and P_{zy} at their respective midspans, and they carry the full pressure magnitude, P_z, at their ends. Between the midspan and the ends, the pressure distribution varies linearly. This is illustrated in Fig. 10.

The end reactions, both vertical shear and bending moment, are computed below for both the x-beam and the y-beam:

$$R_{zx} = (P_z + P_{zx})\frac{L_x}{4}$$
$$R_{zy} = (P_z + P_{zy})\frac{L_y}{4}$$
$$M_x = -\eta_x \frac{L_x^2}{96}(3P_z + 5P_{zx}) \qquad \text{(Eq 18)}$$
$$M_y = -\eta_y \frac{L_y^2}{96}(3P_z + 5P_{zy})$$

Note that the equations for the end moments, M_x and M_y, contain fixity factors for rotation, η_x and η_y. The fixity factors are equal to 1.0 for fixed ends, and they are equal to 0.0 for pinned ends. The fixity factors are equal to the actual end moments divided by the moment that would have been generated had the end been fully fixed.

A bending peak occurs at the midspan of the beam, as given by Eq 19. Also refer to Fig. 11 for a graphic representation of the pressure distribution and the resulting shear and moment distributions. Note that the midspan bending moments given below are distinguished by double tick marks. This means that the moments are a result of the applied pressure only, and the effect of the offset in-plane load, N_x, is not included. The moment contribution from the offset in-plane load is discussed in the following section.

$$M''_{xmid} = \frac{L_x^2}{96}[P_z(4 - 3\eta_x) + P_{zx}(8 - 5\eta_x)]$$
$$M''_{ymid} = \frac{L_y^2}{96}\left[P_z(4 - 3\eta_y) + P_{zy}(8 - 5\eta_y)\right] \qquad \text{(Eq 19)}$$

Internal Shear and Moment Distributions. Having established the pressure distribution and resulting end reactions, the internal shear and bending moment can be derived at any point

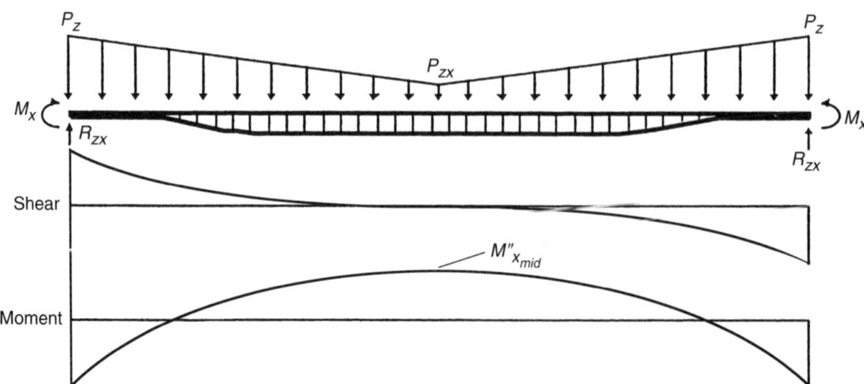

Fig. 11 Shear and moment diagrams for a panel strip. Notation is for the x-beam. The y-beam would be similar.

along either of the two mutually perpendicular beams. Before this is done, however, the effect of an applied in-plane load must be considered.

The in-plane load, N_x, is applied halfway between the face midplanes, and, because the halfway point shifts away from the tool side elsewhere in the sandwich beam, a bending moment is developed. The total moment at any point along the beam, therefore, is comprised of two components, namely, the component from the eccentric in-plane load, M'_x, and the component from the out-of-plane pressure load, M''_x. Both bending moment components, M'_x and M''_x, must be added together to arrive at the full bending magnitude.

The freebody diagram in Fig. 12 shows how to derive the moment due to an offset in-plane load. The in-plane load, N_x, induces no bending in the edgeband. From there, the bending moment varies linearly through the ramp region. The moment then becomes a constant value where the facesheets become parallel. The freebody diagram in Fig. 13 illustrates the bending moment due to applied pressure only. The freebody diagrams in Fig. 12 and 13 use notation for the x-beam parallel to the x-direction. The freebody diagrams for the y-beam are analogous.

The facesheets resist the entire bending and in-plane loads, while the core resists the vertical shear uniformly through its thickness. Figure 14 shows the general freebody diagram with the equations for the facesheet loads (N_{xt} and N_{xb}) and core shear (V_{zx}). In the ramp region, the bag-side facesheet changes direction, so the equations for facesheet loads and core shear are dependent on the angle of the bag-side face. The angle, θ, goes to zero at the top of the ramp where the faces become parallel.

At the ramp radius locations, flatwise stresses (f_{flat}) develop between the bag-side facesheet and the core. These stresses tend to either crush the core or pull the face away from the core, depending on their direction. The flatwise stress MPa (psi) is simply computed as the facesheet load N/m (lb/in.) divided by the ramp radius m (in.) for small angles. This calculation is illustrated in Fig. 14.

This analysis method can only approximate the internal load state for a honeycomb panel. The face-sheets are considered to be ineffective in reacting to vertical shear, and the core is considered to be ineffective in reacting to in-plane and bending loads. All bending moments are carried as a tension-compression couple in the facesheets, and the core shear is considered to be uniformly distributed through the core thickness. These and other simplifications are made to facilitate hand calculations. To obtain a more accurate picture of the internal load state, especially in the ramp region where some of the shear is reacted in the facesheets, a FE model may be required.

Core Shear Stress Distribution. The maximum vertical shear stress occurs at the panel edges. However, this does not necessarily mean that the core closest to the panel edge is exposed to the highest shear magnitude. This is because the bag-side facesheet can react to some of the vertical shear in the ramp area. The core shear needs to be evaluated at all points through the ramp area, to the point where the facesheets become parallel. Note that because the core thickness approaches zero at the base of the ramp, the core shear stress mathematically approaches infinity. To get a more accurate representation of

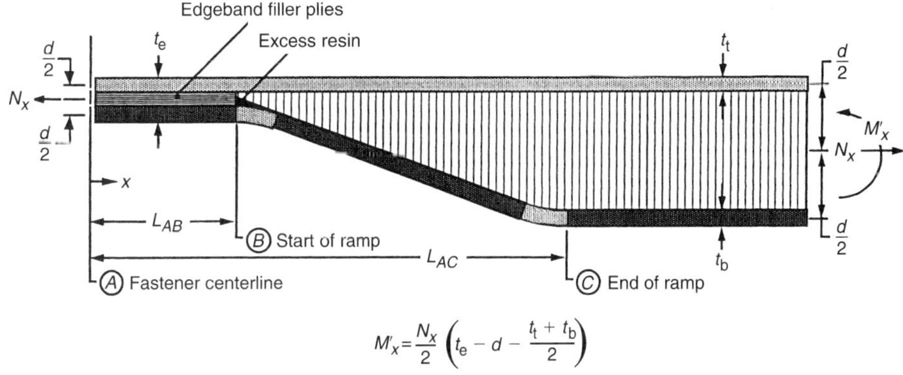

Fig. 12 Bending moments from in-plane load. The bending moment from offset in-plane load, N_x, is a function of the facesheet separation, d. The distance, d, varies linearly through the ramp region.

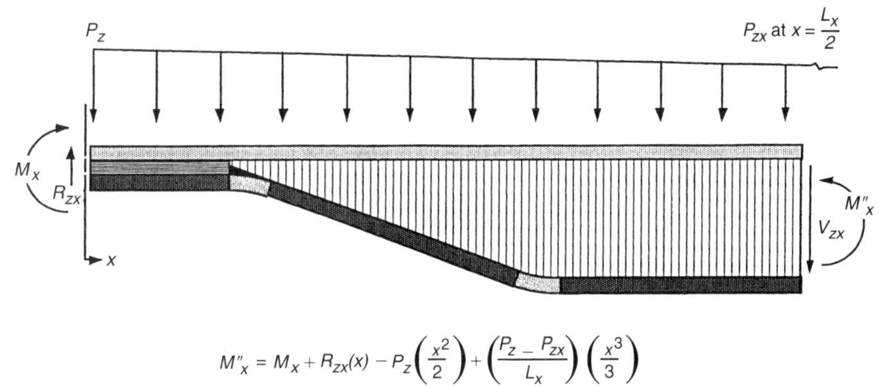

Fig. 13 Bending moments from pressure load

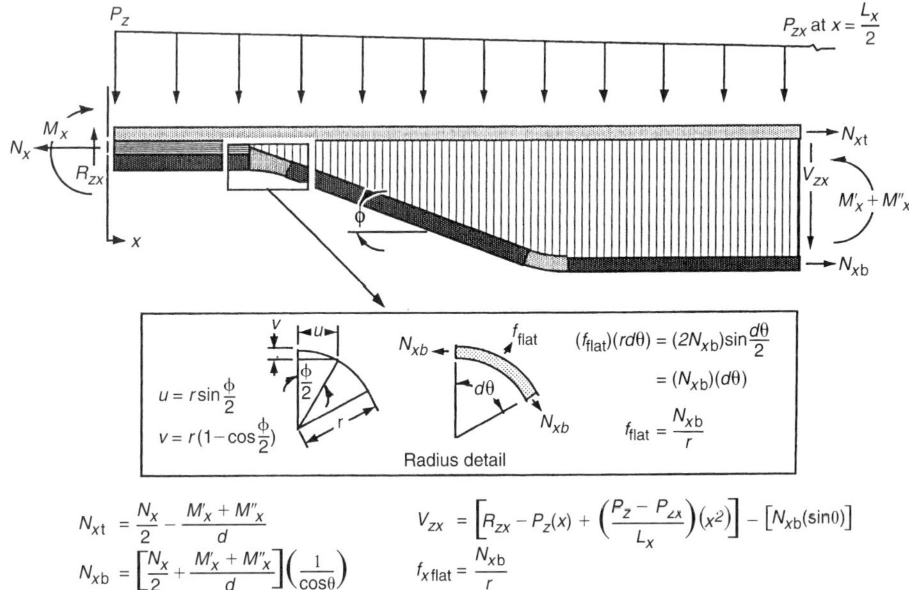

Fig. 14 Freebody for internal panel loads

the core shear stress distribution in the ramp area, a FE model may be required.

The face-to-core adhesive shear is considered to be equal to the shear in the core itself. However, the adhesive shear allowables are invariably higher than those for the honeycomb core, and a face-to-core shear failure is typically considered not to be a problem.

Facesheet Internal Loads and Stresses. The facesheet fiber strain (ε) is often critical at the center of a panel where the bending moment is high. The bending moment can also be large near the edges of a panel, so a moment diagram should be constructed for each of the two mutually perpendicular panel strips to make sure that the most critically loaded portion of the panel is analyzed. The following equations are based on an analysis at the middle of the honeycomb panel where the x-beam and the y-beam intersect each other. The bending moment is carried as a tension-compression couple in the facesheets. For each face, the in-plane loads are augmented or diminished by the bending loads, as shown by Eq 20. A positive moment puts tension in the bag-side face and compression in the tool-side face.

The applied shear load is split between the two facesheets in Eq 22, based on their relative in-plane shear stiffnesses. Note that the subscript, "t,"refers to the tool side, "b" refers to the bag side, and "f" refers to one face or the other.

$$N_{xf} = \frac{N_x}{2} \pm \frac{M'_x + M''_{xmid}}{d}$$
$$N_{yf} = \frac{N_y}{2} \pm \frac{M'_y + M''_{ymid}}{d} \qquad \text{(Eq 20)}$$
$$N_{xyf} = \frac{(N_{xy})t_f G_{xyf}}{t_t G_{xyt} + t_b G_{xyb}}$$

Add the terms for the bag-side face, and subtract the terms for the tool-side face. Nx_f, Ny_f, Nxy_f are the in-plane facesheet loads for the face being checked, N/m (lb/in.). M''_{xmid}, M''_{ymid} are the midspan bending moments from pressure load Nm/m (in. · lb/in.).

The x- and y-facesheet stresses are computed using the following equations, or a laminate analysis code:

$$f_{xf} = \frac{N_{xf}}{t_f}$$
$$f_{yf} = \frac{N_{yf}}{t_f} \qquad \text{(Eq 21)}$$

f_{xf}, f_{yf} are the in-plane facesheet stresses for the face being checked, MPa (psi). N_{xf}, N_{yf}, N_{xyf} are the in-plane facesheet loads for the face being checked, N/m (lb/in.).

The facesheet shear stress can be calculated with Eq 22. The sign of the shear stress does not matter in the margin calculation, so the absolute value is taken.

$$f_{xyf} = \left| N_{xy}\left(\frac{G_{xyf}}{G_{xyt}t_t + G_{xyb}t_b}\right)\right| \qquad \text{(Eq 22)}$$

f_{xyf} is in-plane facesheet shear stress for the face being checked, MPa (psi). N_{xy} is applied in-plane shear load at the panel edges, N/m (lb/in.).

Curved Sandwich Panel Internal Loads and Stresses

Up to this point, only flat honeycomb panels have been considered. This section includes an analysis to quantify the effect of significant panel curvature. It is convenient to idealize a panel as two mutually perpendicular strips. Each strip, then, is a sandwich beam and can be analyzed as such. Figure 15 shows the geometry for a curved sandwich beam. In addition to considering the effect of beam curvature, the effect of in-plane core stiffness is also included in the following analysis procedures.

General Equations and Analysis Method. The bending strain distribution for a straight beam is linear from one extreme fiber to the other, but a curved beam has a nonlinear bending strain distribution. For a curved beam, the strain (ε_θ) through the thickness is represented by a smooth curve passing through zero at the neutral axis. As with any composite, the stress distribution (σ_θ) is a step function that cannot be represented by a single equation. For this reason, the following general bending equation for composite curved beams is written for strain (ε_θ), not stress (σ_θ):

$$\varepsilon_\theta = K_r \cdot \frac{(M)(y)}{D_\theta} \qquad \text{(Eq 23)}$$

The K_r term is dependent on the fiber location in addition to the cross-sectional properties. K_r is greater than 1 for the fiber closest to the center of curvature, less than 1 for the fiber furthest from the center of curvature, and 0 at the neutral axis. As a beam looses its curvature and becomes more straight, the K_r term approaches 1.

$$K_r = \left(\frac{D_\theta}{K_\theta}\right)\left(\frac{1}{(R_c)(y)}\right)\left[1 + \frac{1}{Z_\theta}\left(\frac{y}{R_c + y}\right)\right] \qquad \text{(Eq 24)}$$

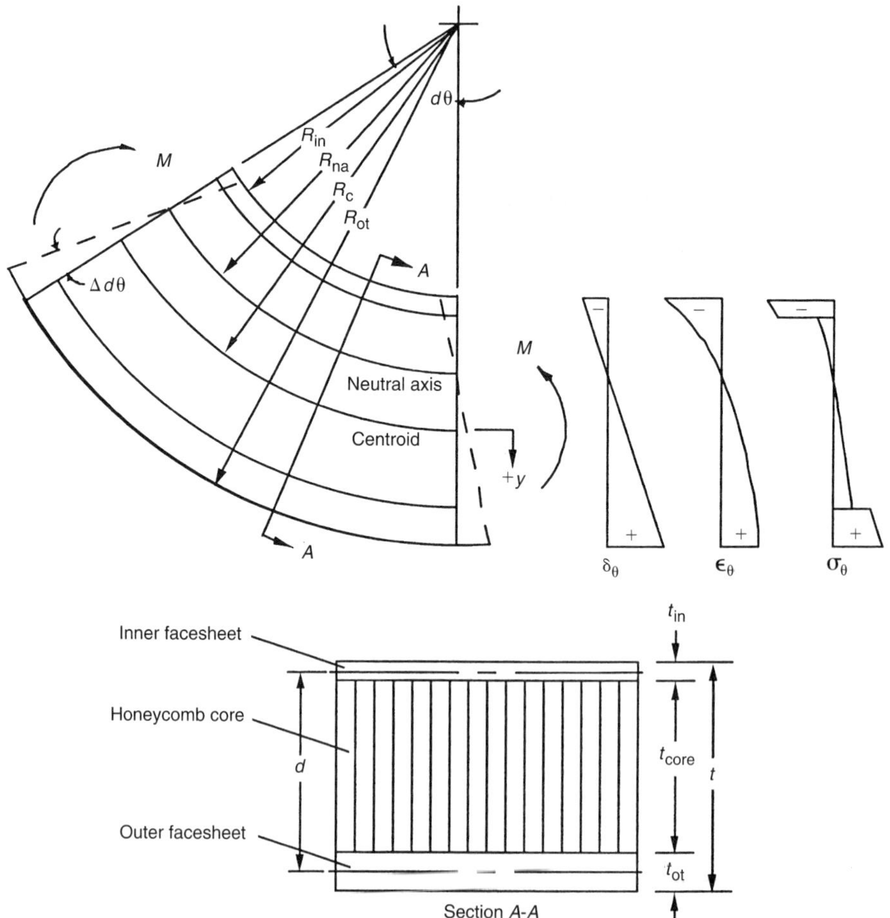

Fig. 15 A curved sandwich beam subjected to pure bending. A positive moment puts tension in the fiber furthest from the center of the curvature. Locations through the thickness of the beam are measured from the centroid, the positive direction being away from the center of the curvature. As the radius of a curved beam gets smaller, the neutral axis shifts from the centroid toward the center of curvature, and the bending strain distribution becomes increasingly nonlinear.

K_θ = Axial (circumferential) stiffness per unit width

$$\sum_{i=1}^{n}(A_i)(E_i)$$

with units of N/m (lb/in.).
D_θ = Bending stiffness per unit width

$$\sum_{i-1}^{n}(E_i)(I_i)$$

with units of Nm (lb · in.).
Z_θ = Dimensionless property

$$\sum_{i=1}^{n}-\frac{1}{t_i}\int_{t_i}\frac{y}{R_c+y}dt$$

M = Bending moment per unit width with units of Nm/m (in. · lb/in.).

A positive moment puts tension in the fiber furthest from the center of curvature. R_c = Radius of curvature to the sandwich centroid in m (in.). y = Distance from the sandwich centroid in m (in.). Measurements away from the center of curvature are positive. Measurements toward the center of curvature are negative.

The *axial, or circumferential, stiffness* of the curved sandwich beam is equal to the cross-sectional area times the modulus (AE) of the facesheets plus the AE of the honeycomb core. In this analysis, both faces are considered to have identical moduli, E_{face}. Note that the core modulus is very small compared to the facesheet modulus and is typically neglected. It is included in this and other calculations in order to quantify the effect of core stiffness.

$$K_\theta = E_{face}(t_{in}+t_{ot})+E_{core}t_{core} \quad \text{(Eq 25)}$$

E_{face} = Facesheet modulus in the circumferential direction, MPa (psi). E_{core} = Honeycomb core modulus in the circumferential direction, MPa (psi). E_{core} can be considered to be equal to $2 \cdot G_{core}$, where G_{core} is the shear modulus in the plane of the applied moment. t_{in}, t_{ot} = Inner and outer facesheet thicknesses, respectively, m (in.). t_{core} = Core thickness, m (in.).

The centroid dimension for a curved sandwich beam is computed in the same way as for a straight beam. However, unlike a straight beam, the centroid does not coincide with the neutral axis:

$$R_c = \frac{1}{K_\theta}\left[E_{face}(t_{in}+t_{ot})\left(R_{ot}-\frac{t_{ot}}{2}-\frac{(d)(t_{in})}{t_{in}+t_{ot}}\right) + E_{core}t_{core}\left(R_{ot}-t_{ot}-\frac{t_{core}}{2}\right)\right] \quad \text{(Eq 26)}$$

R_{in}, R_{ot} = Radii of curvature for the inner and outer facesheets, respectively, m (in.). d = Distance between facesheet midplanes, m (in.), $R_{ot} - R_{in} - (t_{in} + t_{ot}/2)$.

The flexural stiffness, or bending stiffness, D_θ, for a narrow sandwich beam is equal to the modulus times the moment of inertia (EI) for the facesheets plus the EI for the honeycomb core. A wide beam is stiffer in bending than a narrow beam, but the following equation does not take this augmented stiffness into account. The following equation for flexural stiffness is an approximation. The centroid and midplane of each facesheet are considered to be coincident. In addition, the centroid of the two combined faces is considered to be coincident with the centroid of the core, so their respective moments of inertia can be directly superimposed to obtain the moment of inertia for the entire sandwich element:

$$D_\theta = E_{face}\left(\frac{d^2 t_{in}t_{ot}}{t_{in}+t_{ot}}\right)+E_{core}\left(\frac{t_{core}^3}{12}\right) \quad \text{(Eq 27)}$$

The Z_θ term of Eq 24 is a property of the cross section somewhat similar to the moment of inertia. This dimensionless property is written for the sandwich section:

$$Z_\theta = -1+\frac{R_c}{K_\theta}\left[E_{face}\cdot \ln\left(\frac{R_{ot}}{R_{in}}\right)+(E_{core}-E_{face}) \times \ln\left(\frac{R_{ot}-t_{ot}}{R_{in}+t_{in}}\right)\right] \quad \text{(Eq 28)}$$

The facesheet stresses in the circumferential direction, σ_θ, are computed as follows:

$$\sigma_{\theta in} = K_{rin}E_{face}\left(\frac{(M)(c_{in})}{D_\theta}\right)$$

$$\sigma_{\theta ot} = K_{rot}E_{face}\left(\frac{(M)(c_{ot})}{D_\theta}\right)$$

$$K_{rin} = \left(\frac{D_\theta}{K_\theta}\right)\left(\frac{1}{(R_c)(c_{in})}\right)\left[1+\frac{1}{Z_\theta}\left(\frac{c_{in}}{R_c+c_{in}}\right)\right]$$

$$K_{rot} = \left(\frac{D_\theta}{K_\theta}\right)\left(\frac{1}{(R_c)(c_{ot})}\right)\left[1+\frac{1}{Z_\theta}\left(\frac{c_{ot}}{R_c+c_{ot}}\right)\right] \quad \text{(Eq 29)}$$

c_{in} = Distance from sandwich centroid to the midplane of the inner facesheet, m (in.) = $-[(R_c - R_{in} - (t_{in}/2)]$. c_{ot} = Distance from sandwich centroid to the midplane of the outer facesheet, m (in.) = $+[(R_{ot} - R_c\ (t_{ot}/2)]$.

The face-to-core bondline stresses in the radial or flatwise direction, σ_r, are computed below. The following equations consider $\sigma_{\theta in}$ and $\sigma_{\theta ot}$ to be uniformly distributed through the inner and outer facesheet thicknesses, respectively:

$$\sigma_{rin} = +\sigma_{\theta in}\frac{t_{in}}{R_{in}+t_{in}}$$

$$\sigma_{rot} = -\sigma_{\theta ot}\frac{t_{ot}}{R_{ot}-t_{ot}} \quad \text{(Eq 30)}$$

Local Strength Analysis Methods

The following subsections contain analysis methods for each of the various sandwich panel failure modes.

Facesheet Fiber Strain. Facesheet material allowables are often available in terms of strain values. Given facesheet internal loads calculated with either a closed form or finite element analysis of the panel, the loads in the facesheets can be converted to strains with Eq 31. The load-to-strain conversion and the strain rotation can also be accomplished by using a laminate analysis computer program:

$$\varepsilon_{xf} = N_{xf}\left(\frac{1}{tE_x}\right)_f - N_{yf}\left(\frac{\nu_{yx}}{tE_y}\right)_f$$

$$\varepsilon_{yf} = N_{yf}\left(\frac{1}{tE_y}\right)_f - N_{xf}\left(\frac{\nu_{xy}}{tE_x}\right)_f \quad \text{(Eq 31)}$$

$$\gamma_{xyf} = N_{xyf}\left(\frac{1}{tG_{xy}}\right)_f$$

ε_{xf}, ε_{yf}, γ_{xyf} = In-plane facesheet strains, 10^{-6} m/m (μin./in.). N_{xf}, N_{yf}, N_{xyf} = In-plane facesheet loads, N/m (lb/in.). E_x, E_y, G_{xy}, ν_{xy}, ν_{yx}, t = Material properties and thickness for the face being checked.

Each of the fiber orientations needs to be checked, and this may require rotating the x- and y-strains to other directions. The angle, α, is measured counterclockwise from the x-direction.

$$\varepsilon_{\alpha f} = \left(\frac{\varepsilon_{xf}+\varepsilon_{yf}}{2}\right)+\left(\frac{\varepsilon_{xf}-\varepsilon_{yf}}{2}\right)\cos(2\alpha) + \left(\frac{\gamma_{xyf}}{2}\right)\sin(2\alpha) \quad \text{(Eq 32)}$$

or

$$\varepsilon_{\alpha f} = \varepsilon_{xf}\cos^2\alpha+\varepsilon_{yf}\sin^2\alpha+\gamma_{xyf}\sin\alpha\cos\alpha$$

$\varepsilon_{\alpha f}$ = In-plane facesheet strain with respect to the fiber being checked, 10^{-6} m/m (10^{-6} in./in.). ε_{xf}, ε_{yf}, γ_{xyf} = In-plane facesheet strains, 10^{-6} m/m (10^{-6} in./in.). α = Angle of fiber being checked, in degrees.

Core Shear. For panels subjected to normal pressure loading, transverse shear loads, Q_x and Q_y, are carried by the core. Use a laminate analysis program that can determine the maximum transverse shear stresses, τ_{xz} and τ_{yz}, in the core caused by transverse shear forces, or use the simplified relations below. For panels with facesheet thickness less than 5% of the core thickness, assume that the core carries all the shear load:

$$\tau_{xz} = \frac{Q_x}{c} \quad \tau_{yz} = \frac{Q_y}{c} \quad \text{(Eq 33)}$$

If the facing thickness is greater than 5% of the core thickness, the faces will carry some of the shear and:

$$\tau_{xz} = \frac{Q_x}{c+\frac{t_1+t_2}{2}}$$

$$\tau_{yz} = \frac{Q_y}{c+\frac{t_1+t_2}{2}} \quad \text{(Eq 34)}$$

Calculate the core margin of safety (MS) based on the appropriate core shear allowables, F_{sl},F_{sw} (in ribbon longitudinal and ribbon transverse direction, respectively), or the face-to-core bond strength, with the following equation. Equation 35 assumes that the ribbon longitudinal direction is oriented along the x-axis:

$$MS = \frac{1}{\sqrt{\left(\frac{\tau_{xz}}{F_{sl}}\right)^2 + \left(\frac{\tau_{yz}}{F_{sw}}\right)^2}} - 1 = \frac{F_{sl}F_{sw}}{\sqrt{F_{sw}^2\tau_{xz}^2 + F_{sl}^2\tau_{yz}^2}} - 1 \quad \text{(Eq 35)}$$

Flatwise Tension and Compression. At the edges of a typical honeycomb sandwich panel, the bag-side facesheet ramps up over the core (Fig. 14). At the start and finish of the ramp, where the facesheet changes direction, interlaminar stresses (flatwise tension or compression) are induced at the face-to-core bondline. A flatwise tension stress can cause debonding between the face and the core, and a flatwise compression stress can induce core crushing. The flatwise stress should be computed at the center of each ramp radius. The following equations provide approximate magnitudes for the flatwise stresses. A *FE* model may be required to provide a more accurate assessment of the stress state in the ramp areas.

The subsequent equation is based on the assumption that the flatwise stress is uniformly distributed around the radius from the start of curvature to the end of curvature. Note that the computation requires the load in the bag-side facesheet, and this is dependent on, among other things, the distance between the faces and the angle of the bag side with respect to the tool side. The gap between the faces and the angle of the bag side are both variables in the ramp region, so the analyst needs to take care in obtaining the proper geometry.

The following equations use loads in the x-direction. The panel strip in the y-direction must also be checked, and similar equations can be written:

$$f_{x\text{flat}} = \pm\frac{N_{xb}}{R} \quad \text{(Eq 36)}$$

Use "+" for concave radii and "–" for convex radii. $f_{x\text{flat}}$ = Flatwise stress at radius, MPa (psi). N_{xb} = Load in the bag-side facesheet, N/m (lb/in.). R = Ramp radius, m (in.).

At the radius closest to the edgeband, the critical stress is considered to be interlaminar tension between the plies of the bag-side laminate. At the radius furthest from the edgeband, the failure modes are considered to be either separation of the bag-side face from the core due to flatwise tension or core crushing due to flatwise compression. Flatwise compression allowables are equivalent to the crushing strength of the core material, F_{cc}.

The flatwise tension and compression margin of safety is computed from the equation:

$$MS_{x\text{flat}} = \frac{F_{\text{flat}}}{f_{x\text{flat}}} - 1 \quad \text{(Eq 37)}$$

MS_{flat} = Flatwise stress margin of safety. F_{flat} = Flatwise stress allowable, MPa (psi). f_{flat} = Flatwise stress at radius, MPa (psi).

Flexural Core Crushing. As a sandwich panel bends, the core must restrain the facesheets from moving toward each other. In this way, a compressive or crushing force is induced in the core. This failure mode is checked at the location of the maximum bending moments. The core crushing stress is computed using:

$$f_{\text{crush}} = \frac{M_x^2}{d\,D_{zx}} + \frac{M_y^2}{d\,D_{zy}} + P \quad \text{(Eq 38)}$$

f_{crush} = Core compressive stress, MPa (psi). M_x,M_y = Bending moments from in-plane and pressure loads, Nm/m (in. · lb/in.). P = Normal pressure or locally applied load, MPa (psi)

The margin of safety is calculated using:

$$MS_{\text{crush}} = \frac{F_{cc}}{f_{\text{crush}}} - 1 \quad \text{(Eq 39)}$$

MS_{crush} = Core crushing margin of safety. f_{crush} = Core compressive stress, MPa (psi). F_{cc} = Core compressive strength, MPa (psi).

Intracell Buckling. *Intracell buckling*, or *face dimpling*, is a local instability failure where a facesheet buckles within the confines of a single cell. The honeycomb cell walls serve as nodal points while one or both of the faces buckle, inwardly or outwardly, within the unbonded region of the cell interior. Dimpling of the facings may not lead to failure, unless the amplitude of the dimples becomes large. This could cause the dimples or buckles to grow across core cell walls and result in wrinkling of the facings. Dimpling that does not cause total structural failure may be severe enough so that permanent dimples remain after removal of load.

Intracell buckling can be induced in facesheets subjected to in-plane compression or in-plane shear. The critical location normally occurs at the middle of the panel, where the bending moment is high. The following subsections contain simplified formula for intracell buckling analysis. Alternatively and for combined loading cases, a laminated plate buckling computer program can be used. The conservative approach is to assume a square simply supported plate with edge length equal to s, the core cell size, and use the stiffness properties for the individual facesheet being checked. Determine the loading acting on each individual face and apply these loads in the buckling analysis to determine the margins of safety. For curved panels, this approach remains valid, because the cell size is usually much smaller than the panel curvature.

The facing properties shall be values at the condition of use; that is, if the structure is at elevated temperature, then facing properties at that environment shall be used in design. The facing modulus of elasticity is the effective value at the facing stress. If this stress is beyond the proportional limit value, an appropriate tangent, reduced or modified compression modulus of elasticity, shall be used.

The following analysis methods assume that the panel faces are not subjected to normal pressure.

Compression Intracell Buckling. The *intracell buckling critical* stress is the same for both the x- and y-directions, and the expression is given:

$$F_{\text{Cdimple}} = \left(\frac{\pi^2}{12}\right)\left(\frac{E_x(1+\nu_{yx})+E_y(1+\nu_{xy})}{1-\nu_{xy}\nu_{yx}} + 4G_{xy}\right) \times \left(\frac{t_f}{s}\right)^2 \quad \text{(Eq 40)}$$

Equation 40 is valid for facesheets that are orthotropic. If the faces were quasi-isotropic (a homogeneous 25/50/25 lay-up), the previous expression reduces to:

$$F_{\text{Cdimple}} = \left(\frac{\pi^2}{3}\right)\left(\frac{E}{1-\nu^2}\right)\left(\frac{t_f}{s}\right)^2 \quad \text{(Eq 41)}$$

F_{Cdimple} = Compression intracell buckling critical stress, MPa (psi).

The margin of safety for compression intracell buckling is given below. Only compressive stresses produce buckling, and all tensile stresses should be ignored or set to zero in the following interaction equation:

$$MS_{\text{Cdimple}} = \frac{F_{\text{Cdimple}}}{f_{xf} + f_{yf}} - 1 \quad \text{(Eq 42)}$$

MS_{Cdimple} = Margin of safety for compression intracell buckling, MPa (psi). F_{Cdimple} = Intracell buckling critical stress, MPa (psi). f_{xf},f_{yf} = in-plane facesheet compression stresses for the face being checked, MPa (psi).

Shear Intracell Buckling. An empirical expression for the intracell buckling critical stress for shear is shown below.

$$F_{\text{Sdimple}} = (0.60)E_{xf}\left(\frac{t_f}{s}\right)^{1.5}$$

or

$$F_{\text{Sdimple}} = (0.60)E_{yf}\left(\frac{t_f}{s}\right)^{1.5} \quad \text{(Eq 43)}$$

F_{Sdimple} = Intracell buckling critical stress for shear, MPa (psi).

The intracell buckling margin of safety for shear is computed below. The allowable can be expressed in terms of the x- or the y-directions. Use the lowest of the two.

$$MS_{\text{Sdimple}} = \frac{F_{\text{Sdimple}}}{f_{xyf}} - 1 \quad \text{(Eq 44)}$$

$MS_{Sdimple}$ = Margin of safety for shear intracell buckling. $F_{Sdimple}$ = Intracell buckling critical stress for shear, MPa (psi)

Combined Compression and Shear Intracell Buckling. For facesheets with combined compression and shear loads, the following interaction equation may be used:

$$R_c = \frac{(f_{xf} + f_{yf})}{F_{Cdimple}}$$

$$R_s = \frac{f_{xyf}}{F_{Sdimple}} \qquad \text{(Eq 45)}$$

$$MS_{dimple} = \frac{2}{R_c + (R_c^2 + 4R_s^2)^{1/2}} - 1$$

Face Wrinkling. *Face wrinkling* occurs when the core material or the face-to-core bond does not adequately stabilize the facesheets. It is similar to the buckling of a facesheet into or away from the elastic foundation of the honeycomb core.

Face wrinkling can be induced in facesheets subjected to in-plane compression or in-plane shear, and the critical location normally occurs at the middle of the panel where the bending moment is greatest. Analysis of this localized buckling behavior is complicated by the unknown waviness of sandwich facings. Thus, the designer must, in effect, consider the buckling of a column (facing) that is supported on an elastic foundation (core), that is not initially straight. The initial curvature or deflection (waviness) is not easily defined or easily measured. Growth of initial waves causes stresses in the core and in the bond between the facings and core. Final failure may occur suddenly, and the facing may buckle inward or outward, depending on the flatwise compression strength of the core relative to the flatwise tensile strength of the bond between the facing and core. The analysis in this section should be used in conjunction with information on general buckling and instability. The final design should be checked to ascertain whether wrinkling of the sandwich facings might occur at the design load. Because of uncertainties in analysis and values of material properties, it is recommended that the final design be checked by tests of a few specimens.

As with other cases, the facing properties shall be values at the condition of use. If the structure is at elevated temperature, then facing properties at that environment shall be used in design. The facing modulus of elasticity is the effective value at the facing stress. If this stress is beyond the proportional limit value, an appropriate tangent, reduced or modified compression modulus of elasticity, shall be used.

Compression Face Wrinkling. The compression stress allowable for face wrinkling is given below for both the x- and y-directions. The following equations have been found to correlate well with test data from panels with relatively soft cores, such as Nomex (E.I. DuPont de Nemours & Co., Inc., Wilmington, DE). For very stiff metallic cores, these equations may produce unconservative results. In these cases, an analysis that includes facesheet waviness and core-to-facesheet bond strength may be required. These analyses can be found in MIL-HDBK-23. (This handbook is in the process of being converted and expanded by the MIL-HDBK-17 committee, and it will be released as a separate MIL-HDBK-17 volume in the future.)

In the x-direction, use the lower of:

$$F_{xfwrinkle} = -0.44(E_{xf}E_{cc}G_{xz})^{1/3}$$

$$F_{xfwrinkle} = -0.247(E_{xf}E_{cc}G_{xz})^{1/3} - 0.078\frac{G_{xz}^2}{G_L}\frac{t_c}{t_f} \qquad \text{(Eq 46)}$$

In the y-direction, use the lower of:

$$F_{yfwrinkle} = -0.44(E_{yf}E_{cc}G_{yz})^{1/3}$$

$$F_{yfwrinkle} = -0.247(E_{yf}E_{cc}G_{yz})^{1/3} - 0.078\frac{G_{yz}^2}{G_L}\frac{t_c}{t_f} \qquad \text{(Eq 47)}$$

$F_{xfwrinkle}$, $F_{yfwrinkle}$ = Face wrinkling allowables, MPa (psi). E_{xf}, E_{yf} = Elastic flexural moduli in the x- and y-directions for the face being checked, MPa (psi). E_{if} = $12D_{ii}/t^3$ (not necessarily equal to axial modulus, E_i = A_{ii}/t). For stresses above the material yield stress, use the reduced modulus for E_{if}. G_L = Core shear modulus in the ribbon direction, MPa (psi).

The MS for compression face wrinkling is computed subsequently. In flat panels, only compressive stresses produce buckling, and all tensile stresses should be ignored or set to zero in the following interaction equation. The following equation is used when f_{yf} is the maximum compressive stress. When f_{xf} is the maximum compressive stress, the y-term should be cubed instead of the x-term. If only one load is compressive, the cubed exponent is left off:

$$MS_{Cwrinkle} = \frac{1}{\left(\frac{f_{xf}}{F_{xfwrinkle}}\right)^3 + \left(\frac{f_{yf}}{F_{yfwrinkle}}\right)} - 1 \qquad \text{(Eq 48)}$$

$MS_{Cwrinkle}$ = Face wrinkling margin of safety. $F_{xfwrinkle}$,$F_{yfwrinkle}$ = Face wrinkling allowables, MPa (psi).

Shear Face Wrinkling. The shear wrinkling allowable can be expressed in terms of the x- or the y-directions. Use the lowest of the following four equations:

$$F_{Sfwrinkle} = \frac{0.44(E_{45f}E_{cc}G_{xz})^{1/3}}{\sqrt{3}}$$

$$F_{Sfwrinkle} = \frac{0.44(E_{45f}E_{cc}G_{yz})^{1/3}}{\sqrt{3}}$$

$$F_{Sfwrinkle} = \frac{0.247(E_{45f}E_{cc}G_{xz})^{1/3} + 0.078\frac{G_{xz}^2}{G_L}\frac{t_c}{t_f}}{\sqrt{3}}$$

$$F_{Sfwrinkle} = \frac{0.247(E_{45f}E_{cc}G_{yz})^{1/3} + 0.078\frac{G_{yz}^2}{G_L}\frac{t_c}{t_f}}{\sqrt{3}} \qquad \text{(Eq 49)}$$

$F_{Sfwrinkle}$ = Face wrinkling allowable for shear, MPa (psi). E_{45f} = Elastic flexural moduli in direction 45° to the x-direction for the face being checked, MPa (psi).

$$\frac{1}{E_{45f}} = \frac{1}{4E_{xf}} + \left(\frac{1}{4G_{xy}} - \frac{\nu_{xy}}{2E_{xf}}\right) + \frac{1}{4E_{yf}}$$

For stresses above the material yield stress, use the reduced modulus for E_{if}. G_L = Core shear modulus in the ribbon direction, MPa (psi).

The shear wrinkling margin of safety is computed with the following equation.

$$MS_{Sfwrinkle} = \frac{F_{Sfwrinkle}}{f_{xyf}} - 1 \qquad \text{(Eq 50)}$$

$MS_{Sfwrinkle}$ = Margin of safety for shear wrinkling. $F_{Sfwrinkle}$ = Wrinkling allowable for shear, MPa (psi).

Core Shear Crimping. *Core shear crimping* is a general instability failure that can occur when the core shear modulus is low. The compression and shear allowables for crimping are computed for the x-, y-, and xy-directions:

$$F_{xcrimp} = -(0.75)\left(\frac{d^2}{t_f t_c}\right)G_{xz}$$

$$F_{ycrimp} = -(0.75)\left(\frac{d^2}{t_f t_c}\right)G_{yz} \qquad \text{(Eq 51)}$$

$$F_{xycrimp} = -(0.75)\left(\frac{d^2}{t_f t_c}\right)\sqrt{G_{xz}G_{yz}}$$

F_{xcrimp}, F_{ycrimp}, $F_{xycrimp}$ = Crimping allowables, MPa (psi).

The shear crimping margins are computed subsequently. A suitable interaction equation for biaxial and/or shear loading is not known, so a margin of safety is computed for each direction individually. Only compressive stresses produce buckling, and all tensile stresses should be ignored.

$$MS_{xcrimp} = \frac{F_{xcrimp}}{f_{xf}} - 1$$

$$MS_{ycrimp} = \frac{F_{ycrimp}}{f_{yf}} - 1 \qquad \text{(Eq 52)}$$

$$MS_{xycrimp} = \frac{F_{xycrimp}}{f_{xyf}} - 1$$

MS_{xcrimp}, MS_{ycrimp}, $MS_{xycrimp}$ = Margins of safety for shear crimping. F_{xcrimp}, F_{ycrimp}, $F_{xycrimp}$ = Crimping allowables for shear, MPa (psi).

Flat Panel Stability Analysis Methods

The article "Instability Considerations" in this Volume offers a general treatment of composite panel buckling. General stability solutions are best obtained from a computer analysis, using either a closed-form buckling solution or a FE analysis. The analysis must include the influence of the core transverse shear flexibility. In most cases of sandwich panels with thin orthotropic facesheets, the panel stiffness matrix terms A_{16}, A_{26}, B_{ij}, D_{16}, and D_{26} are usually small or zero. Thus, the analysis method does not have to include the capability for including the effects of these terms. Most panel buckling codes, and all finite element codes, can analyze combinations of in-plane compression (axial or biaxial) and shear loads.

Some computerized buckling analysis tools will predict the shear crimping instability mode. This mode occurs when the core shear stiffness is low. This mode can be detected from the analysis output by either a large number of half-waves or a very short wavelength of the critical stability mode shape.

In most cases, linear eigenvalue buckling analyses will overstate the buckling load of panels and cylinders because panel imperfections and nonlinear responses are not included. Empirically derived correlation factors are often used to reduce the predicted buckling loads from an eigenvalue analysis to provide sufficient levels of conservatism. The NASA Langley Reseach Center has published an extensive number of documents on various advanced methods for predicting the stability of composite structures.

SELECTED REFERENCES

- "Aeroweb Honeycomb Sandwich Design," Instruction Sheet Number AGC.33e (Part 2), Ciba Composites, Anaheim, CA, Jan 1980
- H.G. Allen, *Analysis and Design of Structural Sandwich Panels,* Pergamon Press, 1969
- G. Bao, W. Jiang, and J.C. Roberts, Analytical and Finite Element Solutions for Bending and Buckling of Orthotropic Rectangular Plate, *Int. J. Solids Struct.,* Vol 34 (No. 14), Elsevier Science Ltd., 1997, p 1797–1822
- H. Becker, *Handbook of Structural Stability Part II—Buckling of Composite Elements,* National Advisory Committee for Aeronautics TN 3782, Aug 1957
- C.W. Bert, W.C. Crisman, and G.M. Nordby, Buckling of Cylindrical and Conical Sandwich Shells with Orthotropic Facings, *AIAA J.,* Vol 7 (No. 2), Feb 1969, p 250–25, *AIAA J.,* Vol 7 (No. 9), Sept 1969, p 1824
- M.P. Boyle, J.C. Roberts, P.D. Wienhold, G. Bao, and G.J. White, "Experimental, Numerical, and Analytical Results for Buckling and Post-Buckling of Orthotropic Rectangular Sandwich Panels," Symposium on Design and Manufacturing of Composite Structures, 5–10 Nov 2000 (Orlando, FL), ASMA International Mechanical Engineering Congress and Exhibition
- *Composite Materials Handbook,* MIL-HDBK-17, Materials Sciences Corp., University of Delaware, and U.S. Army Research Laboratory, April 2000
- O.B. Davenport and C.W. Bert, Buckling of Orthotropic, Curved Sandwich Panels In Shear and Axial Compression, *J. Aircr.,* Vol 10 (No. 10), Oct 1973, p 632–634
- O.B. Davenport and C.W. Bert, Buckling of Orthotropic, Curved Sandwich Panels Subjected to Edge Shear Loads, *J. Aircr.,* Vol 9 (No. 7), July 1972, p 477–480
- *Design Handbook for Honeycomb Sandwich Structures,* Hexcel, 1970
- G. Gerard, *Introduction to Structural Stability Theory,* 1962
- G. Gerard and H. Becker, *Handbook of Structural Stability Part I—Buckling of Flat Plate,*. National Advisory Committee for Aeronautics TN 3781, Aug 1957
- G. Gerard and H. Becker, *Handbook of Structural Stability Part III—Buckling of Curved Plates and Shells,* National Advisory Committee for Aeronautics TN 3783, Aug 1957
- N.J. Hoff and S.E. Mautner, The Buckling of Sandwich-Type Panels, *J. Aeronaut. Sci.,* July 1945, p 285–297
- J.M. Housner, and M. Stein, "Numerical Analysis and Parametric Studies of the Buckling of Composite Orthotropic Compression and Shear Panels," NASA TN D-7996, Oct 1975
- C. Kassapoglou, S.C. Fantle, and J.C. Chou, Wrinkling of Composite Sandwich Structures Under Compression, *J. Compos. Technol. Res.,* Vol 17 (No. 4), Oct 1995, p 308–316
- C. Libove and S.B. Batdorf, "A General Small-Deformation Theory for Flat Sandwich Plates," National Advisory Committee for Aeronautics Report 899, 1948
- C.H. Lu, Bending of Anisotropic Sandwich Beams with Variable Thickness, *J. Thermoplast. Compos.,* Vol 7, Oct 1994, p 364–374
- A.K. Noor, W.S. Burton, and C.W. Bert, Computational Models for Sandwich Panels and Shells, *Appl. Mech. Rev.,* Vol 49 (No. 3), March 1996, p 155–199
- N. Paydar and C. Libove, Stress Analysis of Sandwich Plates with Unidirectional Thickness Variation, *J. Appl. Mech.,* Vol 53, 1986, p 609–613
- N. Paydar and C. Libove, Bending of Sandwich Plates of Variable Thickness, *J. Appl. Mech.,* Vol 55, 1988, p 419–424
- F.J. Plantema, *Sandwich Construction,* John Wiley and Sons, 1966
- M. Stein and J. Meyers, "A Small Deflection Theory for Curved Sandwich Plates," National Advisory Committee for Aeronautics Report 1008, 1952
- M. Stein, and J. Meyers, "Compressive Buckling of Simply Supported Curved Plates and Cylinders of Sandwich Construction," National Advisory Committee for Aeronautics TN 2601, Jan 1952
- *Structural Sandwich Composites,* MIL-HDBK-23A, Dec 1968
- R.T. Sullins, G.W. Smith, and E.E. Spier, *Manual For Structural Stability Analysis of Sandwich Plates and Shells,* NASA CR-1457, Dec 1969
- J.R. Vinson, Optimum Design of Composite Honeycomb Sandwich Panels Subjected to Uniaxial Compression, *AIAA J.,* Vol 24 (No. 10), 1986
- J.R. Vinson and S. Shore, "Bibliography on Methods of Structural Optimization for Flat Sandwich Panels," Report NAEC-ASL-1082, U.S. Naval Air Engineering Center, April 1965
- J.R. Vinson and S. Shore, "Design Procedures for Structural Optimization of Flat Sandwich Panels," Report NAEC-ASL-1084, U.S. Naval Air Engineering Center, April 1965
- J.R. Vinson and S. Shore, "Methods of Structural Optimization for Flat Sandwich Panels," Report NAEC-ASL-1083, U.S. Naval Air Engineering Center, April 1965
- S.H. Ward and S.F. McCleskey, "Buckling of Laminated Shells Including Transverse Shear Effects," Paper AIAA-87-0728-CP, 28th AIAA SDM Conf., April 1987
- S. Yusuff, Theory of Wrinkling in Sandwich Construction, *J. R. Aeronaut. Soc.,* Vol 59, Jan 1955, p 30–36
- S. Yusuff, Face Wrinkling and Core Strength Requirements in Sandwich Construction, *J. R. Aeronaut. Soc.,* Vol 64, March 1960, p 164–167
- D. Zenkert, *An Introduction to Sandwich Construction,* EMas Publishing

Finite Element Analysis

Naveen Rastogi, Visteon Chassis Systems

MOST APPLICATIONS of advanced fiber-reinforced composite materials require detailed analysis and design at component, substructure, and system levels to evaluate the structural response under applied static, dynamic, fatigue, and impact loads. Accurate static load analysis and natural frequency extraction are often considered essential first steps in many design processes, before more complex analyses, such as transient, fatigue, dynamic durability, crash energy absorption, and shape and size optimization, are performed. This article provides an overview of finite-element-based analyses (FEA) of advanced composite structures highlighting the key aspects. Additional information on the general use of FEA is provided in the article "Finite Element Analysis" in *Materials Selection and Design,* Volume 20 of *ASM Handbook.*

The analysis and design of fibrous composite structures is hierarchical by nature. While the static stiffness and modal response can be computed from the macrolevel analyses, the computation of more complex structural characteristics, such as ultimate load-carrying capability under static and dynamic loads, static and dynamic fatigue life, and impact-crash energy absorption, require a very detailed knowledge of material behavior at the micro, or fiber-matrix, level. Thus, understanding the damage mechanisms at the micromechanical level is the key to successfully designing the fibrous composite structures. A reliable micromechanical analysis of properties of fibrous composite materials is the crucial first step in subsequent macromechanical analysis and design of structures manufactured from these materials. See the articles "Micromechanics" and "Macromechanics Analysis of Laminate Properties" in this Volume.

Because fibrous composite materials offer a wide range of fiber-matrix combinations in many forms, *analysis, rather than experimentation,* becomes a more practical procedure to obtain physical materials properties, such as elastic constants, coefficients of thermal and moisture expansion, viscoelastic properties, thermal conductivity, and static strengths. Thus, as Hashin (Ref 1) pointed out, the relevant methods for evaluating such properties are those of applied mechanics, rather than those of materials science.

The preceding statement is also true in performing the macrolevel analysis of structures manufactured from these highly tailorable fibrous composite materials. It is far more practical to analyze and optimize the design concepts for different materials combinations on a computer, rather than manufacturing and testing each concept. Use of appropriate, accurate, and efficient computer-aided engineering tools, rather than the costly and time-consuming physical testing, is the most cost-effective way to analyze, design, and optimize fibrous composite structures subjected to various types of applied load, such as static, dynamic, cyclic fatigue, and impact-crash. The National Aeronautics and Space Administration (NASA) and the defense, automotive, and civil infrastructure industries have been unrelenting in the development of advanced composite analysis and design tools, through individual efforts as well as through mutual cooperation and collaborations with universities.

Two classical examples from the mechanics of composite materials are solved in this article using FEA approach. These numerical examples illustrate the two unique aspects of the analysis of multilayered composite structures:

- The continuity of transverse stresses at the layer interfaces
- The free-edge, or boundary layer, effects

For an in-depth study, the reader is referred to various texts (e.g., Ref 2–17) covering a wide range of topics in the FEA of composite structures.

Overview of Finite Element Analysis

Finite element analysis has emerged as one of the most powerful tools to solve complex engineering problems and has become an integral part of every established computer-aided design, manufacturing, engineering, and optimization process. The acronyms CAD, CAM, CAE, and CAO have been "coined" to designate these processes, respectively. In their text, Bathe and Wilson (Ref 2) describe numerous ways to classify the finite element (FE) formulations, even when restricting oneself to the solution of structural mechanics problems based on variational principles. A FE formulation can be displacement-based, stress-based, mixed, or hybrid. The displacement-based FE formulation is the most widely used because of its simplicity, generality, and good numerical properties. Moreover, the convergence criteria for the displacement-based FE formulations are precisely established as compared to the other formulations. The concepts of FE method have been successfully used to develop a wide variety of beam, plate, shell, plane stress, plane strain, axisymmetric, and three-dimensional (3-D) solid elements.

In a FEA, the structure is represented as an assemblage of a finite number of elements. The principle of *virtual work* forms the basis of displacement-based FE formulations. The displacement field of each element is approximated in the form of a function whose unknown coefficients are treated as *generalized coordinates.* This type of FE formulation is often termed the *generalized coordinate finite element formulation.* However, in most standard commercial FE analyses, the generalized coordinates are further expressed in terms of the element *nodal displacements.* Depending upon the type of formulation used, either the generalized coordinates or the nodal displacements are unknowns in the analysis. First, the solution to these unknowns is obtained; subsequently, the displacements, stresses, and strains in the finite elements of the structure are computed.

Once the geometry definition (or the CAD data) of a component or substructure system is known, the following steps are required to perform FE-based structural analysis:

1. Select type of FEA: static, modal, dynamic, thermal, coupled-fluid structure, linear, or nonlinear.
2. Select type of FE: beam, plate, shell, plane strain/stress, axisymmetric or solid, and mesh (coarse or fine) discretization.
3. Define constitutive models: full 3-D orthotropic/anisotropic, two-dimensional (2-D) orthotropic/anisotropic, equivalent orthotropic, or laminate model.
4. Define static, dynamic, and/or cyclic applied loads of forces, moments, temperatures, accelerations, and so on.

5. Prescribe kinematical boundary conditions, the translational and rotational restraints.
6. Choose solution method (direct sparse, preconditioned conjugate gradient iterative, arctangent, etc.) and the solution control parameters.
7. Obtain the deformation patterns, strains, and stresses at various locations in the structure and evaluate the ultimate load-carrying capacity of the structure.

While all the above steps are common to the analysis of both the metallic as well as composite structures, steps 2, 3, and 7 make the FEA of composites different, tedious, and complex. Aspects of a detailed FEA that can seem overwhelming include:

- Input of fiber architecture definition
- Input of material data
- Extraction of stresses and strains in the material coordinate system
- Availability of many different criteria to determine the damage initiation and progression

The two key aspects of the FEA of composite structures are:

- Homogenization of materials properties to obtain the elemental constitutive law
- Post-processing of numerical results to recover strains and stresses in the principal material directions for subsequent failure prediction analysis

These are also the most important characteristics that distinguish the composite FEA from the metal FEA, and make the analysis of composites more complex and time-consuming. In the analysis of composite structures, the homogenization of materials properties occurs at two levels, one based on micromechanics and the other based on macromechanics. A structure created from different composite raw-material forms, such as unidirectional lamina, roving, braids, woven fabrics, sandwich, or chopped random mats (see the Section "Constituent Materials" in this Volume) may exhibit different macromechanical response. Thus, the computation of basic layer/lamina/ply-level elastic constants from its material constituents (fiber, matrix, and coatings) and the fiber architecture type (unidirectional roving, braids, braid angles, woven fabrics, fiber directions, and weave patterns) is an essential first step in any FEA of composite structures.

Homogenization

No real-life fibrous composite structure can be completely discretized at the microlevel, the level of its constituent fiber and matrix, in a single stress analysis. Even with the most sophisticated computers now available, it is not only computationally expensive, but also practically impossible to perform such a detailed microlevel discretization and analysis. Therefore, in practical applications of numerical analysis techniques such as FE methods, it becomes necessary to idealize and discretize a composite structure at the macrolevel. The important first step in this direction is to obtain the elastic constants of a ply/lamina/single layer by homogenizing materials properties at the microlevel. The reinforcement-fiber architecture types, such as unidirectional roving, woven fabrics, and braids, influence the homogenized properties at the microlevel. Fiber architecture plays a dominant role in determining the mechanical response of textile composite materials. Inhomogeneous local displacement fields develop within textile composite laminates, even under uniform extension, as a result of the interweaving and interlacing of the yarn bundles.

A convenient way to analyze a textile composite is to consider a unit cell, or *representative/repetitive volume element* (RVE), of the material. A unit cell is a unit of repeating fiber architecture that can be considered the building-block of the material. The size of the repeating unit cell is dependent on the tow size of the yarns, the angle at which they are intertwined or interwoven, and yarn spacing. Thus, for the textile composite material reinforcements, such as woven or braided composites, it is customary to obtain the 3-D on-axis material constants for a unit cell. (For more details on textile composite materials, see the article "Fabrics and Preforms" in this Volume.) Once the homogenized single-layer/lamina elastic constants are obtained, they are then used to derive the elemental constitutive laws at the macrolevel.

In a full *3-D analysis,* the fibrous composite structure is essentially discretized at the lamina level, rather than at the fiber-matrix level. Each ply is discretely modeled in space using 3-D solid elements. There are obvious variations to this approach, where all or some layers can be smeared into a single layer and modeled using effective 3-D anisotropic materials properties. As compared to the full microlevel analysis, a full 3-D analysis still does not greatly reduce the computational complexities, because the discretization of any real-life, multilayered composite structure at the ply (or single-layer/lamina) level is by no means an easy task.

While a full 3-D structural analysis may be possible in terms of computational power and resources, it is still prohibitively expensive and a waste of computational time and memory. It is prudent to analyze the real-life structures using 2-D shell or one-dimensional (1-D) beam-, bar-, or rod-type elements. One can always resort to a more detailed, global-local-type full 3-D analysis in highly stressed regions or regions of special interest, such as joints, ply drop-off, and areas where free-edge effects become prominent. In a typical 2-D analysis of multilayered composite structures, the layers are modeled as a smeared entity effective plate membrane, with bending and coupling stiffness constants derived from the classical laminated plate theory. In composite analysis, these stiffness constants are also known as the [**A**], [**B**], and [**D**] stiffness matrices relating plate-shell stress and moment resultants to the midsurface strains and curvatures.

One-dimensional beam elements are most often used in conjunction with 2-D plate-shell elements to model stiffeners and ribs attached to the skin in stiffened plates and shells. In civil engineering analysis applications, beam elements are independently used to model girders and frames. However, as compared to the metallic structures, the use of 1-D beam elements in the analysis of composite material structures is limited. In many structural analysis problems, 1-D beam elements fail to capture the anisotropy, the weakness in transverse shear direction, and the coupling effects associated with a typical composite material behavior. All these effects also complicate the mathematical theory involved in the derivation of composite beam section properties in stretching, bending, torsion, and warping. Thus, the use of beam elements in the analysis of composite structures should be evaluated on a case-by-case basis. One of the best uses of 1-D beam-element-based analysis is in the preliminary design of laminated composite beams and frames, where the analysis needs to be repeated a number of times in an optimization loop (Ref 18).

As in the case of metals, FEA of fibrous composite structure involves the use of various elements or combinations of elements:

- 3-D hexahedrons, bricks, tetrahedrons, and axisymmetric solids
- 2-D shells, plates, and plane stress-strain quadrilaterals
- 1-D beams, bars, rods, trusses, and springs

In case of composite FEA, it is of utmost importance to understand how the macrolevel homogenization is performed to obtain the material constitutive laws for the 3-, 2-, and 1-D finite elements. The types of assumptions and the mathematical theory used to derive the homogenized elemental material constitutive laws at different dimensional levels play an important role, because the subsequent recovery of strains and stresses after the analysis is very dependent on them. Furthermore, it is prudent to note that the mathematical problem of optimization of such a fibrous composite structure under applied loads is essentially an optimization of its constituent materials and the fiber architecture type through these homogenized material constitutive laws.

A general theoretical background for the displacement-based, linear elastic FEA of fibrous composite structures will be outlined, so that the elemental constitutive laws for 3-D solid, 2-D shell, and 1-D beam elements can be obtained through the homogenization process. An I-section beam structure, subjected to arbitrary static and kinematical boundary conditions, is considered as an example problem to demonstrate the relevance of obtaining material constitutive laws at various levels of FEA. This fibrous composite I-beam can be manufactured by pultrusion process using unidirectional roving, by laying up unidirectional fibers, by using fabric prepeg, or by using woven or braided perform consolidated in the resin transfer molding process. Irrespective of the type of constituents, the fiber architecture, or the manufacturing process, in order to proceed with the FEA of the I-beam under applied loads and constraints, it is essential to obtain an appropriate material constitutive law to generate the elemental and, subsequently, the global structural stiffness matrix. At each dimensional level, the fibrous composite constitutive laws are very different and more complex than the simple metallic isotropic constitutive laws.

3-D Solid Elements

Consider an I-section beam with its web and flanges discretized by solid brick elements for a full 3-D analysis (Fig. 1). The generalized strain vector for a typical 3-D solid element, in the elemental Cartesian coordinate system, is:

$$\vec{\boldsymbol{\varepsilon}} = [\varepsilon_{xx}, \varepsilon_{yy}, \varepsilon_{zz}, \gamma_{yz}, \gamma_{xz}, \gamma_{xy}]^T \quad \text{(Eq 1)}$$

Assuming small displacements and displacement gradients, the 3-D strain-displacement relations for the brick element are:

$$\varepsilon_{xx} = \frac{\partial U}{\partial x} \quad \varepsilon_{yy} = \frac{\partial V}{\partial y} \quad \varepsilon_{zz} = \frac{\partial W}{\partial z} \quad \gamma_{yz} = \frac{\partial V}{\partial z} + \frac{\partial W}{\partial y}$$
$$\gamma_{xz} = \frac{\partial U}{\partial z} + \frac{\partial W}{\partial x} \quad \gamma_{xy} = \frac{\partial U}{\partial y} + \frac{\partial V}{\partial x} \quad \text{(Eq 2)}$$

where $U = u(x,y,z)$, $V = v(x,y,z)$, and $W = w(x,y,z)$ are the element displacement fields in the three orthogonal coordinate directions.

Let the generalized stress vector for the brick element be:

$$\vec{\boldsymbol{\sigma}} = [\sigma_{xx}, \sigma_{yy}, \sigma_{zz}, \tau_{yz}, \tau_{xz}, \tau_{xy}]^T \quad \text{(Eq 3)}$$

Also, let ΔT and Δm represent the change in temperature and moisture content, respectively, of the element from some datum values. The hygrothermal effects may be important to consider in the analysis of composite structures, due to certain service conditions. (See the article "Hygrothermal Behavior" in this Volume.) The constitutive law for the brick element, including hygrothermal effects, is:

$$\vec{\boldsymbol{\sigma}} = [\mathbf{C}]\vec{\boldsymbol{\varepsilon}} - \{\mathbf{a}\}\Delta T - \{\mathbf{b}\}\Delta m \quad \text{(Eq 4)}$$

where C_{ij} denote the off-axis stiffness coefficients, a_i the off-axis thermal constants, and b_i the off-axis moisture or swelling constants. The coefficients C_{ij}, a_i, and b_i are given by (Ref 19):

$$\begin{aligned}[\mathbf{C}] &= [\mathbf{J}]^{-1}[\mathbf{S}']^{-1}[\mathbf{J}]^{-T}\\ \{\mathbf{a}\} &= [\mathbf{J}]^{-1}[\mathbf{S}']^{-1}\{\boldsymbol{\alpha}'\}\\ \{\mathbf{b}\} &= [\mathbf{J}]^{-1}[\mathbf{S}']^{-1}\{\boldsymbol{\beta}'\}\end{aligned} \quad \text{(Eq 5)}$$

In Eq 5, the on-axis compliance matrix $[\mathbf{S}']$ for orthotropic materials, in terms of engineering constants, is (Ref 3):

$$[\mathbf{S}'] = \begin{bmatrix} \frac{1}{E_1'} & -\frac{\nu_{12}'}{E_2'} & -\frac{\nu_{13}'}{E_3'} & 0 & 0 & 0 \\ -\frac{\nu_{21}'}{E_1'} & \frac{1}{E_2'} & -\frac{\nu_{23}'}{E_3'} & 0 & 0 & 0 \\ -\frac{\nu_{31}'}{E_1'} & -\frac{\nu_{32}'}{E_2'} & \frac{1}{E_3'} & 0 & 0 & 0 \\ 0 & 0 & 0 & \frac{1}{G_{23}'} & 0 & 0 \\ 0 & 0 & 0 & 0 & \frac{1}{G_{13}'} & 0 \\ 0 & 0 & 0 & 0 & 0 & \frac{1}{G_{12}'} \end{bmatrix} \quad \text{(Eq 6)}$$

Here, the major Poisson's ratio is denoted ν_{21}', and the minor Poisson's ratio is denoted ν_{12}'. The vectors representing the on-axis coefficients of thermal expansion and the on-axis coefficients of moisture expansion are:

$$\begin{aligned}\{\boldsymbol{\alpha}'\} &= [\alpha_1', \alpha_2', \alpha_3', 0, 0, 0]^T\\ \{\boldsymbol{\beta}'\} &= [\beta_1', \beta_2', \beta_3', 0, 0, 0]^T\end{aligned} \quad \text{(Eq 7)}$$

In Eq 5, $[\mathbf{J}]$ is the transformation matrix relating the off-axis material constants to the on-axis material constants, and is given by:

$$[\mathbf{J}] = \begin{bmatrix} m^2 & n^2 & 0 & 0 & 0 & 2mn \\ n^2 & m^2 & 0 & 0 & 0 & -2mn \\ 0 & 0 & 1 & 0 & 0 & 0 \\ 0 & 0 & 0 & m & -n & 0 \\ 0 & 0 & 0 & n & m & 0 \\ -mn & mn & 0 & 0 & 0 & m^2 - n^2 \end{bmatrix} \quad \text{(Eq 8)}$$

where $m = \cos\theta$ and $n = \sin\theta$, and θ is the lamina/ply/layer orientation with respect to the elemental x-axis. Figure 1 in the article "Macromechanics Analysis of Laminate Properties" in this Volume shows the orientation.

As mentioned previously, for many woven and/or braided fiber architecture types, it is often easier to obtain the on-axis stiffness coefficients, C_{ij}', directly as a result of the homogenization at microlevel using RVE concepts (Ref 20). However, the on-axis stiffness matrix $[\mathbf{C}']$ may no longer be orthotropic. Also, when smearing some or all the layers into a single layer, the effective 3-D materials properties may not be orthotropic, thereby resulting in an anisotropic on-axis stiffness matrix $[\mathbf{C}']$. In all these cases, the off-axis coefficients in the constitutive law, Eq 4, can be alternatively given as:

$$\begin{aligned}&[\mathbf{C}] = [\mathbf{J}]^{-1}[\mathbf{C}'][\mathbf{J}]^{-T} \quad \{\mathbf{a}\} = [\mathbf{J}]^{-1}[\mathbf{C}']\{\boldsymbol{\alpha}'\}\\ &\{\mathbf{b}\} = [\mathbf{J}]^{-1}[\mathbf{C}']\{\boldsymbol{\beta}'\}\end{aligned} \quad \text{(Eq 9)}$$

Once the elemental constitutive law given by Eq 4 is established, the statement of *internal virtual work* for the solid element, $\delta W^{\text{int}} = \iiint_V \delta\vec{\varepsilon}^T \vec{\boldsymbol{\sigma}} dV$, can be used to derive the elemental stiffness matrix in the usual manner (see Ref 2). Subsequently , the global stiffness matrix is assembled, and the numerical problem is solved to obtain the elemental and/or nodal displacements under applied static and/or kinematic boundary conditions The 3-D elemental strain-displacement relations in Eq 2 can then be used to obtain the strains. The 3-D element stresses are recovered using the constitutive law given by Eq 4. The element stress/strain vectors are further transformed into the material coordinate system using the transformation matrix, such as the one given by Eq 8. These stresses and strains can now be used in subsequent progressive damage and/or failure analysis.

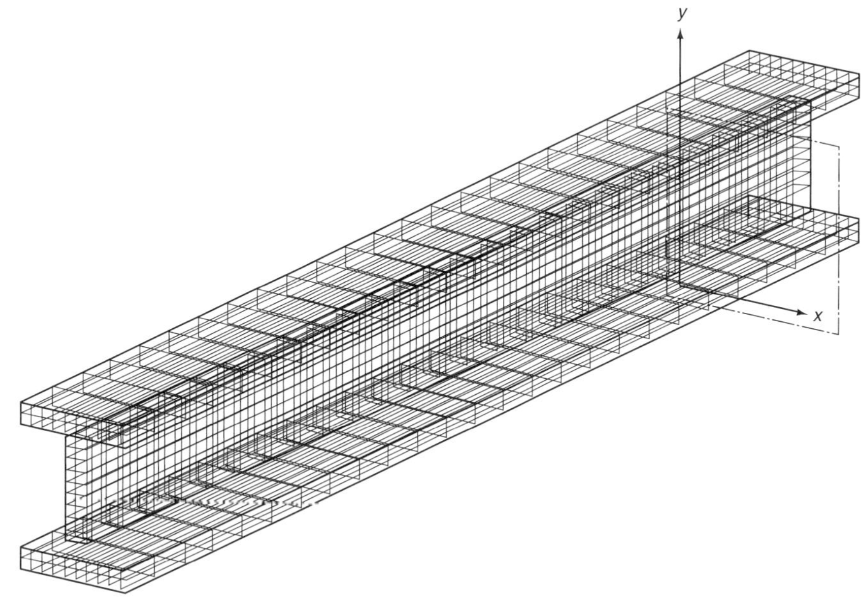

Fig. 1 An I-beam discretized with 3-D solid elements

Rastogi (Ref 21) developed variable-order 3-D solid elements using the formulations presented previously. Subsequently, a FORTRAN computer code called structural analysis using variable-order elements (SAVE) was written to perform 3-D analysis of laminated structures (Ref 22). Examples of some benchmark problems solved using the SAVE code and other commercially available FE codes are presented in the later part of this article.

2-D Cylindrical Shell Elements

Figure 2 represents the I-section beam whose web and flanges are discretized by 2-D shell elements. A shell is actually a 3-D body that is thin in one dimension. The concepts, which are generally applicable to the 3-D analysis, are also applicable to the shells. Thus, while working with shell theories, one tries to exploit the thinness of the shell and reduce the theories to a 2-D analysis. However, each shell analysis needs to be performed on a case-by-case basis. For an accurate analysis of thick composite shells, either a higher-order shell theory with shear deformation effects, a layer-wise theory (Ref 23), or a quasi-three-dimensional theory may be required. Consider that *G*/*E*, the ratio of shearing to extensional stiffness, is fixed for an isotropic material at 1/(2 + 2υ), or about 0.40 for most metals. By contrast, for a unidirectional lamina of high-modulus graphite-epoxy, the value of *G*/*E* can be as low as 0.01. Thus, it is apparent that the same loading will induce significantly more transverse shear deformation in composite structures than in their metal counterparts. Indeed, it is not difficult to find composite problems where transverse shear is the dominant response mode of the structure. It is important, therefore, to consider the transverse shear deformation effects in analyzing composite structures using 2-D shell/plate elements.

In order to derive the material constitutive law of a typical shell element, a consistent first-order transverse shear deformation shell theory, developed by Rastogi and Johnson (Ref 24), is used. Based on the assumption that the shell thickness, *t*, is relatively small and hence, does not change during loading, the displacement at any arbitrary material point in the shell element is approximated by:

$$U(x,\theta,z) = u(x,\theta) + z\phi_x(x,\theta)$$

$$V(x,\theta,z) = v(x,\theta) + z\phi_\theta(x,\theta)$$

$$W(x,\theta,z) = w(x,\theta) \quad \text{(Eq 10)}$$

where $u(x,\theta)$, $v(x,\theta)$, and $w(x,\theta)$ are the displacements of the points of the reference (or middle) surface, and $\phi_x(x,\theta)$ and $\phi_\theta(x,\theta)$ are the rotations of the normal to the reference surface, as shown in Fig. 3. The 3-D engineering strains are related to the displacements by:

$$e_{xx} = \frac{\partial U}{\partial x} \quad e_{\theta\theta} = \frac{1}{(R+z)}\left[\frac{\partial V}{\partial \theta} + W\right]$$

$$e_{x\theta} = \frac{\partial V}{\partial x} + \frac{1}{(R+z)}\frac{\partial U}{\partial \theta}$$

$$e_{zz} = \frac{\partial W}{\partial z} \quad e_{xz} = \frac{\partial W}{\partial x} + \frac{\partial U}{\partial z}$$

$$e_{\theta z} = \frac{\partial V}{\partial z} + \frac{1}{(R+z)}\left(\frac{\partial W}{\partial \theta} - V\right) \quad \text{(Eq 11)}$$

Substituting Eq 10 into Eq 11 and rearranging the terms results in the following expressions for the 3-D engineering strains:

$$e_{xx} = \varepsilon_{xx} + z\kappa_{xx} \quad e_{\theta\theta} = \frac{\varepsilon_{\theta\theta} + z\kappa_{\theta\theta}}{\left(1+\frac{z}{R}\right)} \quad e_{zz} = 0$$

$$e_{x\theta} = \frac{\gamma_{x\theta} + z\left(1+\frac{z}{2R}\right)\bar{\kappa}_{x\theta} + \frac{z^2}{2R}\tilde{\kappa}_{x\theta}}{\left(1+\frac{z}{R}\right)}$$

$$e_{xz} = \gamma_{xz} \quad e_{\theta z} = \frac{\gamma_{\theta z}}{\left(1+\frac{z}{R}\right)} \quad \text{(Eq 12)}$$

in which ε_{xx}, κ_{xx}, $\varepsilon_{\theta\theta}$, $\kappa_{\theta\theta}$, $\gamma_{x\theta}$, $\bar{\kappa}_{x\theta}$, $\tilde{\kappa}_{x\theta}$, γ_{xz}, and $\gamma_{\theta z}$ are the shell strains, independent of the *z*-coordinate. The transverse shear strains, e_{xz} and $e_{\theta z}$, given in Eq 12 were obtained through differentiation of Eq 10 with respect to *z*. However, Eq 10 is approximate in the *z*-coordinate, so differentiating with respect to *z* cannot capture the distribution of the transverse shear strains through the thickness of the shell. Since the material is assumed rigid in the *z*-direction (e_{zz} = 0), the distribution of the transverse shear strains, and consequently the distribution of the transverse shear stresses, does not influence the shell behavior. It is the integral of the transverse shear stresses through the thickness, or transverse shear resultants, that influences the shell behavior. Thus, the transverse shear strains in Eq 12 are the *average* values, evaluated at the reference surface (*z* = 0).

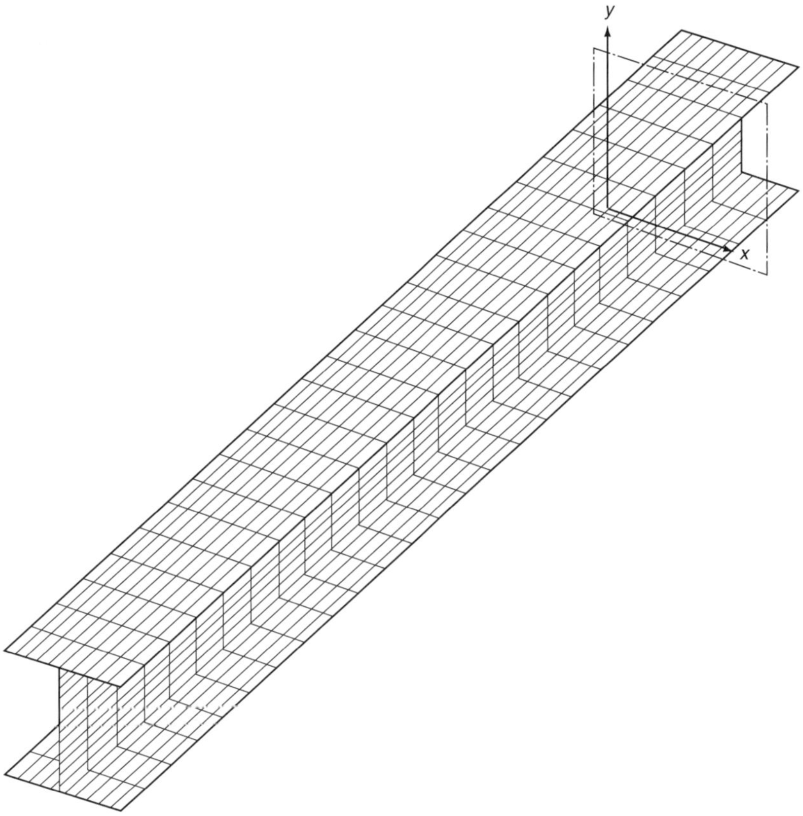

Fig. 2 An I-beam discretized with 2-D shell elements

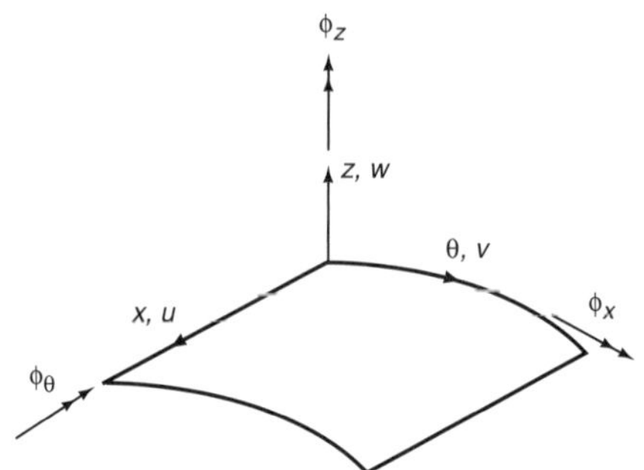

Fig. 3 Displacements and rotations for a shell element

Assuming small rotations, the 2-D, or shell strain measures, are defined as:

$$\varepsilon_{xx} = \frac{\partial u}{\partial x} \quad \varepsilon_{\theta\theta} = \frac{1}{R}\frac{\partial v}{\partial \theta} + \frac{w}{R} \quad \gamma_{x\theta} = \frac{\partial v}{\partial x} + \frac{1}{R}\frac{\partial u}{\partial \theta}$$
$$\kappa_{xx} = \frac{\partial \phi_x}{\partial x} \quad \kappa_{\theta\theta} = \frac{1}{R}\frac{\partial \phi_\theta}{\partial \theta} \quad \bar{\kappa}_{x\theta} = \frac{\partial \phi_\theta}{\partial x} + \frac{1}{R}\frac{\partial \phi_x}{\partial \theta} + \frac{1}{R}\frac{\partial v}{\partial x}$$
$$\tilde{\kappa}_{x\theta} = \frac{\partial \phi_\theta}{\partial x} - \frac{1}{R}\frac{\partial \phi_x}{\partial \theta} - \frac{1}{R}\frac{\partial v}{\partial x} \quad \gamma_{xz} = \phi_x + \frac{\partial w}{\partial x}$$
$$\gamma_{\theta z} = \phi_\theta + \frac{1}{R}\frac{\partial w}{\partial \theta} - \frac{v}{R} \qquad \text{(Eq 13)}$$

If the average transverse shear strains in Eq 12 are set to zero, the rotations about the normal are:

$$\phi_x = -\frac{\partial w}{\partial x} \quad \phi_\theta = \frac{v}{R} - \frac{1}{R}\frac{\partial w}{\partial \theta} \qquad \text{(Eq 14)}$$

so that

$$\kappa_{x\theta} = \bar{\kappa}_{x\theta} = -\frac{2}{R}\frac{\partial^2 w}{\partial x \partial \theta} + \frac{2}{R}\frac{\partial v}{\partial x} \quad \tilde{\kappa}_{x\theta} = 0 \qquad \text{(Eq 15)}$$

Hence, the thickness distribution of the in-plane shear strain reduces to:

$$e_{x\theta} = \frac{\gamma_{x\theta} + z\left(1 + \dfrac{z}{2R}\right)\kappa_{x\theta}}{\left(1 + \dfrac{z}{R}\right)} \qquad \text{(Eq 16)}$$

which results in a classical shell theory with no transverse shear deformation effects. It is evident from Eq 12 that three shell strain measures are needed to represent the distribution of in-plane shear strain through the thickness in the transverse shear deformation shell theory; whereas only two shell strain measures are required in classical shell theory to represent the shearing strain distribution through the thickness (refer to Eq 16).

In the 3-D shell theory, the *internal virtual work* for the shell is:

$$\delta W_{\text{int}}^{\text{shell}} = \iiint_V [\sigma_{xx}\delta e_{xx} + \sigma_{\theta\theta}\delta e_{\theta\theta} + \sigma_{zz}\delta e_{zz} + \sigma_{x\theta}\delta e_{x\theta} + \sigma_{xz}\delta e_{xz} + \sigma_{\theta z}\delta e_{\theta z}]dV \qquad \text{(Eq 17)}$$

where V denotes the volume of shell and $dV = [1 + (z/R)]dxRd\theta dz$. Substitute the variation of Eq 12 into Eq 17, and note that the virtual strains are explicit functions of z. Integrals of the stresses with respect to z give force and moment resultants conjugate to the shell strains. Hence, the volume integral in Eq 17 reduces to an area integral, and the internal virtual work for the shell element becomes:

$$\delta W_{\text{int}}^{\text{shell}} = \iint_S \delta\vec{\varepsilon}_{\text{shell}}^{\,T}\vec{\sigma}_{\text{shell}}dS \qquad \text{(Eq 18)}$$

where S denotes the area of the reference surface, with $dS = dxRd\theta$. The generalized 9 × 1 stress vector of the shell in Eq 18 is:

$$\vec{\sigma}_{\text{shell}} = [N_{xx}, N_{\theta\theta}, N_{\theta x}, M_{xx}, M_{\theta\theta}, \bar{M}_{x\theta}, \tilde{M}_{x\theta}, Q_x, Q_\theta]^T \qquad \text{(Eq 19)}$$

and the generalized strain vector for the shell is:

$$\vec{\varepsilon}_{\text{shell}} = [\varepsilon_{xx}, \varepsilon_{\theta\theta}, \gamma_{x\theta}, \kappa_{xx}, \kappa_{\theta\theta}, \bar{\kappa}_{x\theta}, \tilde{\kappa}_{x\theta}, \gamma_{xz}, \gamma_{\theta z}]^T \qquad \text{(Eq 20)}$$

The physical stress resultants and stress couples for the shell, some of which appear in Eq 19, are:

$$(N_{xx}, M_{xx}) = \int_h (1, z)\sigma_{xx}\left(1 + \frac{z}{R}\right)dz$$
$$(N_{\theta\theta}, M_{\theta\theta}) = \int_h (1, z)\sigma_{\theta\theta}dz$$
$$(N_{x\theta}, M_{x\theta}) = \int_h (1, z)\sigma_{x\theta}\left(1 + \frac{z}{R}\right)dz$$
$$(N_{\theta x}, M_{\theta x}) = \int_h (1, z)\sigma_{\theta x}dz$$
$$Q_x = \int_h \sigma_{xz}\left(1 + \frac{z}{R}\right)dz \quad Q_\theta = \int_h \sigma_{\theta z}dz \qquad \text{(Eq 21)}$$

In Eq 19, $\bar{M}_{x\theta}$ and $\tilde{M}_{x\theta}$ are the mathematical quantities conjugate to the modified twisting measures, $\bar{\kappa}_{x\theta}$ and $\tilde{\kappa}_{x\theta}$, respectively, and are defined in terms of the physical stress couples by:

$$\bar{M}_{x\theta} = \frac{1}{2}(M_{x\theta} + M_{\theta x}) \quad \tilde{M}_{x\theta} = \frac{1}{2}(M_{x\theta} - M_{\theta x}) \qquad \text{(Eq 22)}$$

The nine elements of the stress vector in Eq 19 and the relations of Eq 22 determine all the stress resultants and stress couples listed in Eq 21, except for in-plane shear resultant, $N_{x\theta}$. The shear stress resultant, $N_{x\theta}$, is determined from the moment equilibrium about the normal for an element of the shell. This so-called sixth equilibrium equation is:

$$N_{x\theta} = N_{\theta x} + \frac{M_{\theta x}}{R} \qquad \text{(Eq 23)}$$

Written in full, the *internal virtual work* for the shell element is:

$$\delta W_{\text{int}}^{\text{shell}} = \iint_S [N_{xx}\delta\varepsilon_{xx} + N_{\theta\theta}\delta\varepsilon_{\theta\theta} + N_{\theta x}\delta\gamma_{x\theta} + M_{xx}\delta\kappa_{xx} + M_{\theta\theta}\delta\kappa_{\theta\theta} + \bar{M}_{x\theta}\delta\bar{\kappa}_{x\theta} + \tilde{M}_{x\theta}\delta\tilde{\kappa}_{x\theta} + Q_x\delta\gamma_{xz} + Q_\theta\delta\gamma_{\theta z}]dS \qquad \text{(Eq 24)}$$

The material law for a lamina with one material axis in the normal direction is:

$$\begin{Bmatrix} \sigma_{xx} \\ \sigma_{\theta\theta} \\ \sigma_{x\theta} \end{Bmatrix} = \begin{bmatrix} C_{11} & C_{12} & C_{16} \\ C_{12} & C_{22} & C_{26} \\ C_{16} & C_{26} & C_{66} \end{bmatrix} \begin{Bmatrix} e_{xx} \\ e_{\theta\theta} \\ e_{x\theta} \end{Bmatrix} - \begin{Bmatrix} a_1 \\ a_2 \\ a_6 \end{Bmatrix} \Delta T(x, y, z) \qquad \text{(Eq 25)}$$

where the off-axis stiffness coefficients, C_{ij}, and the thermal constants, a_j, appearing in Eq 25 are given by Eq 5. Substitution of Eq 25 into Eq 21 in conjunction with Eq 22, and use of Eq 12 for the 3-D engineering strains, results in following *linear elastic constitutive law* for a laminated composite shell element:

$$\begin{Bmatrix} N_{xx} \\ N_{\theta\theta} \\ N_{\theta x} \\ M_{xx} \\ M_{\theta\theta} \\ \bar{M}_{x\theta} \\ \tilde{M}_{x\theta} \end{Bmatrix} = \begin{bmatrix} A_{11} & A_{12} & A_{16} & B_{11} & B_{12} & B_{16}^1 & B_{16}^2 \\ A_{12} & A_{22} & A_{26} & B_{12} & B_{22} & B_{26}^1 & B_{26}^2 \\ A_{16} & A_{26} & A_{66} & B_{61} & B_{62} & B_{66}^1 & B_{66}^2 \\ B_{11} & B_{12} & B_{61} & D_{11} & D_{12} & D_{16}^1 & D_{16}^2 \\ B_{12} & B_{22} & B_{62} & D_{12} & D_{22} & D_{26}^1 & D_{26}^2 \\ B_{16}^1 & B_{26}^1 & B_{66}^1 & D_{16}^1 & D_{26}^1 & D_{66}^{11} & D_{66}^{12} \\ B_{16}^2 & B_{26}^2 & B_{66}^2 & D_{16}^2 & D_{26}^2 & D_{66}^{12} & D_{66}^{22} \end{bmatrix} \times \begin{Bmatrix} \varepsilon_{xx} \\ \varepsilon_{\theta\theta} \\ \gamma_{x\theta} \\ \kappa_{xx} \\ \kappa_{\theta\theta} \\ \bar{\kappa}_{x\theta} \\ \tilde{\kappa}_{x\theta} \end{Bmatrix} - \begin{Bmatrix} N_{xx}^T \\ N_{\theta\theta}^T \\ N_{\theta x}^T \\ M_{xx}^T \\ M_{\theta\theta}^T \\ \bar{M}_{x\theta}^T \\ \tilde{M}_{x\theta}^T \end{Bmatrix} \qquad \text{(Eq 26)}$$

in which stiffnesses A_{ij}, B_{ij}, and C_{ij} are given in Table 1. Note that for the deep shells, large t/R ratios, the shell curvature can induce extension-bending and/or bending-twisting coupling even for balanced, symmetric laminated constructions, due to nonzero B_{ij} terms. Also, compare the expressions for A_{ij}, B_{ij}, and D_{ij} , as given in Table 1, with the simple membrane and bending stiffness expressions for metallic (isotropic material) shells. In Eq 26, the thermal stress resultants and stress couples, denoted by superscript T, are:

$$(N_{xx}^T, M_{xx}^T) = \int_h (1, z)a_1\Delta T(x, y, z)\left(1 + \frac{z}{R}\right)dz$$
$$(N_{\theta\theta}^T, M_{\theta\theta}^T) = \int_h (1, z)a_2\Delta T(x, y, z)dz$$
$$N_{\theta x}^T = \int_h a_6\Delta T(x, y, z)dz$$
$$\bar{M}_{x\theta}^T = \int_h z\left(1 + \frac{z}{2R}\right)a_6\Delta T(x, y, z)dz$$
$$\tilde{M}_{x\theta}^T = \int_h \frac{z^2}{2R}a_6\Delta T(x, y, z)dz \qquad \text{(Eq 27)}$$

The lamina material law relating transverse shear stresses and strains is:

$$\begin{Bmatrix} \sigma_{\theta z} \\ \sigma_{xz} \end{Bmatrix} = \begin{bmatrix} C_{44} & C_{45} \\ C_{45} & Q_{55} \end{bmatrix} \begin{Bmatrix} e_{\theta z} \\ e_{xz} \end{Bmatrix} \qquad \text{(Eq 28)}$$

where the transverse shear stiffnesses, C_{44}, C_{45}, and C_{55}, are given by Eq 5. Substitution of Eq 28 into the last two equalities of Eq 21, in conjunction with Eq 12 for the transverse shear strains, results in the following linear elastic constitutive law for a laminated composite shell element relating transverse shear resultants and strains:

$$\begin{Bmatrix} Q_\theta \\ Q_x \end{Bmatrix} = \begin{bmatrix} A_{44} & A_{45} \\ A_{45} & A_{55} \end{bmatrix} \begin{Bmatrix} \gamma_{\theta z} \\ \gamma_{xz} \end{Bmatrix} \qquad \text{(Eq 29)}$$

The transverse shear stiffnesses, A_{44}, A_{45}, and A_{55}, in Eq 29 are given in Table 1. Because Eq 12 represents average values of the transverse shear strains, the constitutive law relating transverse shear resultants and strains, Eq 29, can be viewed as a Hooke's law, based on the assumption of constant transverse shear strain distribution through the thickness. Alternatively, one can obtain the constitutive law relating transverse shear resultants and strains, based on the assumption of constant transverse shear stress distribution through the thickness. A detailed discussion on the subject is given in Chapter 2 of the text by Vasiliev (Ref 25). However, both methods result in a shear correction factor of one (as compared to 5/6 for isotropic materials).

For classical shell theory, the linear elastic constitutive law for a laminated composite shell element is reduced to:

$$\begin{Bmatrix} N_{xx} \\ N_{\theta\theta} \\ N_{\theta x} \\ M_{xx} \\ M_{\theta\theta} \\ \bar{M}_{x\theta} \end{Bmatrix} = \begin{bmatrix} A_{11} & A_{12} & A_{16} & B_{11} & B_{12} & B_{16} \\ A_{12} & A_{22} & A_{26} & B_{12} & B_{22} & B_{26} \\ A_{16} & A_{26} & A_{66} & B_{61} & B_{62} & B_{66} \\ B_{11} & B_{12} & B_{61} & D_{11} & D_{12} & D_{16} \\ B_{12} & B_{22} & B_{62} & D_{12} & D_{22} & D_{26} \\ B_{16} & B_{26} & B_{66} & D_{16} & D_{26} & D_{66} \end{bmatrix} \times \begin{Bmatrix} \varepsilon_{xx} \\ \varepsilon_{\theta\theta} \\ \gamma_{x\theta} \\ \kappa_{xx} \\ \kappa_{\theta\theta} \\ \bar{\kappa}_{x\theta} \end{Bmatrix} - \begin{Bmatrix} N^T_{xx} \\ N^T_{\theta\theta} \\ N^T_{\theta x} \\ M^T_{xx} \\ M^T_{\theta\theta} \\ \bar{M}^T_{x\theta} \end{Bmatrix} \quad \text{(Eq 30)}$$

in which stiffnesses A_{ij}, B_{ij}, and D_{ij} are the same as given in Table 1, and thermal stress resultants and stress couples are given by Eq 27.

The transverse shear deformation formulations given in the preceding paragraphs for the composite cylindrical shell element can be readily reduced for a laminated flat plate element by first replacing $R\theta$ with y and letting $1/R$ approach 0 in Eq 10 through 24. Note that the thickness distribution of the in-plane engineering shear strain for the plate element reduces to:

$$e_{x\theta} = \gamma_{x\theta} + z\bar{\kappa}_{x\theta} \quad \text{(Eq 31)}$$

Thus, in the transverse shear deformation shell theory, three shell strain measures are needed to represent the distribution of in-plane shear strain through the thickness (see Eq 12); whereas, only two strain measures are required in transverse shear deformation plate theory to represent the shearing strain distribution through the thickness (refer to Eq 31). Furthermore, because $\tilde{M}_{x\theta} = 0$, the linear elastic constitutive law for the laminated plate element will have the usual 6 × 6 stiffness matrix, instead of a 7 × 7 matrix, as given by Eq 26 for the shell element. The A_{ij}, B_{ij}, and D_{ij} expressions given in Table 1 will now have $1/R$ terms eliminated, reducing them to the simplified stiffness coefficients based on the classical laminated plate theory (Ref 4).

Once the elemental constitutive law is established for transverse shear deformable shell theory (Eq 26 and 29), or for classical shell theory (Eq 30), the statement of internal virtual work for the shell element (Eq 24) can be used to derive the shell element stiffness matrix in the usual manner. Subsequently, the global stiffness matrix for the structure is assembled, and the numerical problem is solved to obtain the shell element reference surface displacements and rotations as given by Eq 10. The element strain-displacement relations in Eq 11 can then be used to obtain the 3-D engineering strains. The stresses at any material point in the shell are then recovered, using the constitutive laws given by Eq 25 and 28. The stress/strain vectors may require further transformation in the material coordinate system for subsequent use in the progressive damage analysis and/or failure analysis. Johnson and Rastogi (Ref 26) successfully used the first-order shear deformable theory presented here to develop a shell superelement to analyze orthogonally stiffened composite cylindrical shells subjected to internal pressure loads.

1-D Beam Elements

Beams, such as hat, blade, angle, I-, C-, L-, J-, or F-sections, and circular or rectangular tubes, are commonly used in various industrial applications. Generally, beams are either used as stand-alone structures, or in combination with skins as stiffening elements. If either the wall thickness of the beam is small as compared to its cross-sectional dimensions, or the beam cross-sectional dimensions are sufficiently small compared to its length, a 2-D branched shell analysis may be performed to analyze the beams. A full 3-D analysis with solid elements is warranted for all other cases.

In cases where a 2-D branched shell analysis would suffice, the computational resources required for the analysis can still be very large, thereby making it cumbersome for a design optimization process. This is especially true when these beam sections are made of composite materials and attached to a sheet or skin as stiffening elements. For the purpose of preliminary design and optimization of structures, it may be prudent to model and analyze the beams as 1-D beam elements.

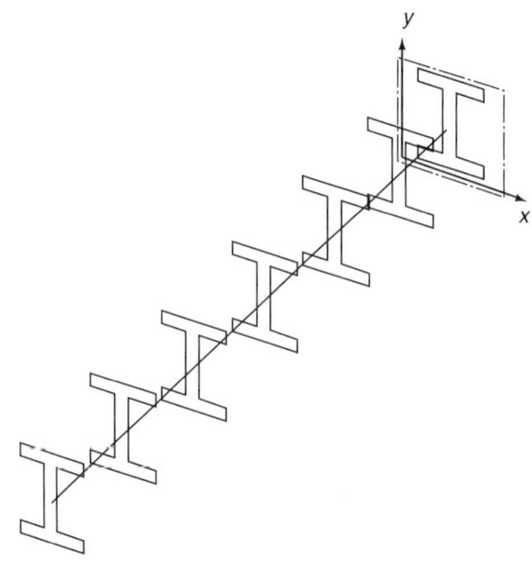

Fig. 4 An I-beam discretized with 1-D beam section elements

Consider the open-section I-beam discretized by 1-D beam section elements in Fig. 4. In order to obtain the constitutive law for composite beam elements, a thin-walled, open-section,

Table 1 Stiffness coefficients

$$\{A_{11}, B_{11}, D_{11}\} = \int_t C_{11}\{1, z, z^2\}(1 + \frac{z}{R})dz$$

$$\{A_{12}, B_{12}, D_{12}\} = \int_t C_{12}\{1, z, z^2\}dz$$

$$\{A_{22}, B_{22}, D_{22}\} = \int_t C_{22}\{1, z, z^2\}(1 + \frac{z}{R})^{-1}dz$$

$$\{A_{16}, B_{61}\} = \int_t C_{16}\{1, z\}dz$$

$$B_{16} = B^1_{16} = \int_t C_{16}z(1 + \frac{z}{R})dz$$

$$B^2_{16} = \int_t C_{16}\frac{z^2}{2R}dz$$

$$D_{16} = D^1_{16} = \int_t C_{16}z^2(1 + \frac{z}{R})dz$$

$$D^2_{16} = \int_t C_{16}\frac{z^3}{2R}dz$$

$$\{A_{26}, B_{62}\} = \int_t C_{26}\{1, z\}(1 + \frac{z}{R})^{-1}dz$$

$$B_{26} = B^1_{26} = \int_t C_{26}z(1 + \frac{z}{2R})(1 + \frac{z}{R})^{-1}dz$$

$$B^2_{26} = \int_t C_{26}\frac{z^2}{2R}(1 + \frac{z}{R})^{-1}dz$$

$$D_{26} = D^1_{26} = \int_t C_{26}z^2(1 + \frac{z}{2R})(1 + \frac{z}{R})^{-1}dz$$

$$D^2_{26} = \int_t C_{26}\frac{z^3}{2R}(1 + \frac{z}{R})^{-1}dz$$

$$A_{66} = \int_t C_{66}(1 + \frac{z}{R})^{-1}dz$$

$$B_{66} = B^1_{66} = \int_t C_{66}z(1 + \frac{z}{2R})(1 + \frac{z}{R})^{-1}dz$$

$$B^2_{66} = \int_t C_{66}\frac{z}{2R}(1 + \frac{z}{R})^{-1}dz$$

$$D_{66} = D^{11}_{66} = \int_t C_{66}z^2(1 + \frac{z}{2R})^2(1 + \frac{z}{R})^{-1}dz$$

$$D^{12}_{66} = \int_t C_{66}\frac{z^3}{2R}(1 + \frac{z}{2R})(1 + \frac{z}{R})^{-1}dz$$

$$D^{22}_{66} = \int_t C_{66}\frac{z^4}{4R^2}(1 + \frac{z}{R})^{-1}dz$$

$$A_{44} = \int_h C_{44}\left(1 + \frac{z}{R}\right)^{-1}dz$$

$$A_{45} = \int_h C_{45}dz$$

$$A_{55} = \int_h C_{55}\left(1 + \frac{z}{R}\right)dz$$

curved beam theory by Woodson, Johnson, and Haftka (Ref 27) is used. The development of a combined theory for torsion and flexure of thin-walled, open-section, curved beams is usually accredited to V.Z. Vlasov (Ref 28). Bauld and Tzeng (Ref 29) extended Vlasov's curved beam theory to straight beams having laminated composite material wall construction. Woodson, Johnson, and Haftka (Ref 27) contributed to further the work in this area by developing a Vlasov-type classical theory for laminated composite curved beams with thin-walled open sections. Later on, Johnson and Rastogi (Ref 26) added the effects of transverse shear deformation to this work. A brief description of this thin-walled, open-section, laminated curved beam theory will acclimatize the reader with the complexities of homogenization at the 1-D level required to obtain an accurate laminated beam constitutive law.

Let the coordinate system (x,θ,ζ) be located at the centroid of the curved beam, in accordance with the right-handed system shown in Fig. 5, in which ζ is the normal coordinate. Let the displacements of a material point on the beam reference axis in the x, θ, and ζ directions be denoted by $u(\theta)$, $v(\theta)$, and $w(\theta)$, respectively. Let the rotations about the x, θ, and ζ axes be denoted by $\phi_x(\theta)$, $\phi_\theta(\theta)$, and $\phi_z(\theta)$, respectively. The displacement of a generic material point in the beam is related to the displacement and rotations of the point on the reference surface by approximations:

$$\begin{aligned} U(x,\theta,\zeta) &= u(\theta) + \zeta\phi_\theta(\theta) \\ V(x,\theta,\zeta) &= v(\theta) + \zeta\phi_x(\theta) + x\phi_z(\theta) - \omega(x,\zeta)\tau(\theta) \\ W(x,\theta,\zeta) &= w(\theta) - x\phi_\theta(\theta) \end{aligned} \tag{Eq 32}$$

The cross section of the beam is in the $x\zeta$ plane normal to the θ axis, so that U and W are interpreted as in-plane displacement components. V is the out-of-plane component. It is assumed that the beam cross section is rigid in its own plane. In Eq 32, $\omega(x,\zeta)$ is the warping function of the beam cross section, and $\tau(\theta)$ is the twist rate. For laminated composite materials, $\omega(x,\zeta)$ not only depends upon the beam geometry, but also on the type, architecture, lay-up, and orientation of the composite material as well. The beam strains, curvatures, and twist rate are related to the displacements and rotations of the beam reference axis as:

$$\varepsilon_\theta = \frac{\dot{v}+w}{R_0} \quad \kappa_x = \frac{\dot{\phi}_x}{R_0} \quad \kappa_z = \frac{\dot{\phi}_z - \phi_\theta}{R_0} \quad \tau = \frac{\dot{\phi}_\theta + \phi_z}{R_0}$$
$$\gamma_z = \phi_x - \frac{(v-\dot{w})}{R_0} \quad \gamma_x = \phi_z + \frac{\dot{u}}{R_0} \tag{Eq 33}$$

where the overdot denotes an ordinary derivative with respect to θ. In Eq 33, ε_θ is the circumferential normal strain of the centroidal arc, κ_x is the in-plane bending rotation gradient, κ_z is the out-of-plane bending rotation gradient, γ_x is the transverse shear strain in the $x\theta$ plane, γ_z is the transverse shear strain in the $\theta\zeta$ plane, and R_0 is the radius of the beam reference arc. The *internal virtual work* is:

$$\delta W_{\text{int}}^{\text{beam}} = \int [N_\theta\delta\varepsilon_\theta + M_x\delta\kappa_x + M_z\delta\kappa_z + T_s\delta\tau + M_\omega\delta(\dot{\tau}/R_0) + V_x\delta\gamma_x + V_z\delta\gamma_z]R_0 d\theta \tag{Eq 34}$$

in which N_θ is the circumferential force, M_x is the in-plane bending moment, M_z is the out-of-plane bending moment, M_ω is the bimoment, T_s is the St. Venant's torque, V_x is the transverse shear force in the x-direction, and V_z is the transverse shear force in the ζ-direction. Due to the inherent assumption that the beam is a built-up shell structure, with shell branches representing various flanges and webs of the beam, the beam resultants in Eq 34 are fundamentally expressed as contour integrals of the shell resultants of each of its branch. The shell resultants for each branch are obtained in the usual way, by using an appropriate 2-D shell theory. For example, one can use the shell theory, such as the one presented earlier in this work, as the starting point to further develop the expressions for these beam resultants. Assuming that the transverse shear forces are decoupled from extension, bending, and torsional deformation, the Hooke's law for the composite material beam is:

$$\begin{Bmatrix} N_\theta \\ M_x \\ M_z \\ M_\omega \\ T_s \end{Bmatrix} = \begin{bmatrix} EA & ES_x & -ES_z & -ES_\omega & EH \\ ES_x & EI_{xx} & -EI_{zx} & -EI_{\omega x} & EH_c \\ -ES_z & -EI_{zx} & EI_{zz} & EI_{\omega z} & -EH_s \\ -ES_\omega & -EI_{\omega x} & EI_{\omega z} & EI_{\omega\omega} & -EH_q \\ EH & EH_c & -EH_s & -EH_q & GJ \end{bmatrix} \times \begin{Bmatrix} \varepsilon_\theta \\ \kappa_x \\ \kappa_z \\ \dot{\tau}/R_0 \\ \tau \end{Bmatrix} \tag{Eq 35}$$

and

$$\begin{Bmatrix} V_x \\ V_z \end{Bmatrix} = \begin{bmatrix} GA_{x\theta} & GA_{zx} \\ GA_{zx} & GA_{\theta z} \end{bmatrix} \begin{Bmatrix} \gamma_x \\ \gamma_z \end{Bmatrix} \tag{Eq 36}$$

The stiffness terms appearing in Eq 35 and 36 are commonly referred to as modulus-weighted section properties containing complex contour integrals and are given in Ref 26 and 27. However, a couple of brief comments are in order. First, the "*EH*" terms in Eq 35 are unique to the laminated thin-walled beams (Ref 29). Thus, the coupling between extension-bending and torsional deformation is unique to laminated composite beams. If the laminate construction for each branch, flanges and webs, of the beam is orthotropic, then "*EH*" terms are all equal to zero. Second, for the structural models in which the effect of warping of the beam cross section is excluded, the contribution of the bimoment, M_ω, to the virtual work of the beam in Eq 34 is neglected, and fourth row and column of the beam stiffness matrix, Eq 35, are ignored. Also, the warping function $\omega(x,\zeta)$ is taken as zero. In the limit as the radius of the beam reference arc, R_0, approaches infinity, the laminated, thin-walled curved beam theory presented here reduces for straight laminated beams. For further details on the laminated composite curved beam theory presented here, see Woodson's dissertation (Ref 18).

Reference 18 implemented the classical laminated, thin-walled curved beam theory via a displacement-based 1-D beam element having seven degrees of freedom (DOF) per node. The accuracy of the beam theory outlined here in isotropic and anisotropic beam analyses was demonstrated, and the practical usefulness of such an approach in preliminary design optimization process was established. Both Woodson (Ref 18) and Johnson and Rastogi (Ref 26) demonstrated the significance of modeling the restrained cross-sectional warping effects in accurately predicting the stresses in thin-walled open-section laminated beams. Warping is a distinctive feature of thin-walled open-section beams. Restraint of cross-sectional warping leads to additional longitudinal normal strains in beams subjected to torsion loads.

Once the elemental constitutive law (Eq 35 and 36) for transverse shear deformable curved beam theory is established, the statement of internal virtual work for the beam element (Eq 34) can be used to derive the beam element stiffness matrix in the usual manner. Subsequently, the global stiffness matrix for the complete structure is assembled, and the specified numerical problem is solved to obtain the beam element reference surface displacements and rotations given by Eq 32. The 3-D engineering strains can now be obtained by substituting the global beam displacements, Eq 32, into the 3-D elemental strain-displacement relations given by Eq 11. (Note that coordinate z is replaced by ζ, and R is replaced by R_0 in Eq 11.) The stresses at any material point in the beam webs and flanges, originally treated as the shell branches, are then computed using the lamina constitutive laws given for a shell element (Eq 25 and 28). Note that the stress/strain vectors may need to be further transformed into the material coordinate system for use in subsequent progressive damage and/or failure analysis.

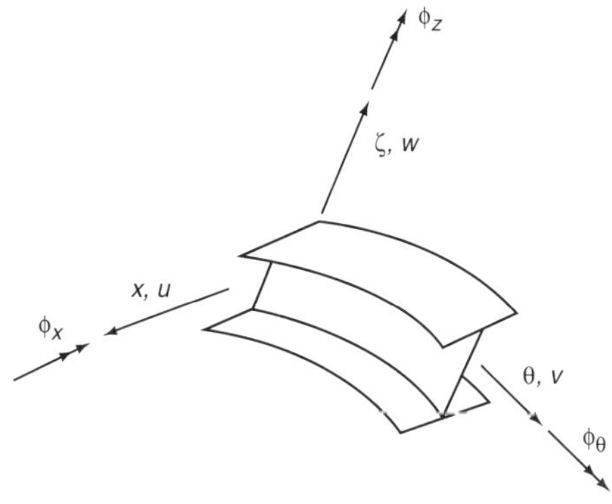

Fig. 5 Displacements and rotations for a curved beam element

Commercial Finite Element Analyses Codes

As has been stated, the two most fundamental and important aspects of FEA of composite structures are:

- *Homogenization* of material properties to obtain the elemental constitutive law at an appropriate level of analysis
- *Post-processing* of numerical results to recover strains and stresses in the principal material directions for subsequent failure prediction analysis

Note that an efficient postprocessing of numerical result is inherently tied with an accurate preprocessing of composite-material-related input information. Thus, a good commercial code for composite FEA is one that incorporates the homogenization process at appropriate level of analysis, as well as supports pre- and postprocessing of composite-material-related information in an efficient and user-friendly manner.

Table 2 lists some of the commercially available FE codes that can analyze composite structures under various loading conditions. All these codes fully support 3-D solid elements with complete anisotropic material constitutive law. They also support 2-D plate and shell elements, including transverse shear deformation effects with simplified laminated-plate-theory-based constitutive laws (Ref 4). However, this author is not familiar with any commercial FE code that supports the correct form of constitutive laws for 1-D, composite material beam elements.

The pre- and postprocessors of most of the commercial codes listed in Table 2 support the key aspects related to the analysis of fibrous composite materials. These include:

- Input of ply properties based on unidirectional as well as 2-D woven fiber architecture
- Ply lay-ups
- Vector orientations used to define ply orientation in space
- Computation of 3-D effective properties
- Computation of [**A**], [**B**], and [**D**] stiffness matrices for plate and shell elements
- Recovery of strains and stresses in various coordinate systems, such as global axis, local element axis, laminate axis, and lamina axis
- First ply failure based on either point stress/strain (maximum strain/stress) or quadratic failure (Tsai-Wu, Hill, Hashin) criterion

Some of the explicit analysis codes, such as LS-DYNA, MSC-DYTRAN, PAM-CRASH, and ABAQUS also provide progressive damage material models for ultimate failure load prediction. However, these computational progressive damage models have not been experimentally verified for a wide variety of structural applications. Based on the author's personal experience, ESI-SYSPLY is perhaps the most comprehensive and user-friendly pre- and postprocessor program currently available for composite FEA. However, in the current form, it does not have the interface with most widely used FEA solvers, such as NASTRAN and ABAQUS, thereby severely limiting its utility. Over the years pre- and postprocessing tools have been highly optimized for the FEA of metallic structures. These tools now need significant enhancement in their capabilities to accurately and efficiently analyze and design complex structures manufactured from advanced composite materials.

Numerical Examples

The continuity of transverse stresses at the layer interfaces and the free-edge effects are

Table 2 Commercially available finite element codes

Code	Company	Web address
Codes with built-in pre- and postprocessors for composites		
ABAQUS	Hibbitt, Karlsson & Sorensen, Inc., Pawtucket, RI	http://www.abaqus.com/products/
ALGOR	Algor, Inc., Pittsburgh, PA	http://algor.com/homepag2.htm
ANSYS	ANSYS, Inc., Canonsburg, PA	http://www.ansys.com/
CATIA/Elfini	IBM and Dessault Systemes, Newark, NJ	http://www.catia.ibm.com/prodinfo/cov.html
COSMOS	Structural Research & Analysis Corp., Los Angeles, CA	http://www.srac.com/products.html
EMRC-NISA II	Engineering Mechanics Research Corp., Troy, MI	http://www.emrc.com/webpages/composite/compov.html
ESI-SYSPLY	ESI Group, Paris, France	http://www.esi.fr/products/sysply/overview.html
ESRD-StressCheck	Engineering Software Research and Development, Inc., St. Louis, MO	http://www.esrd.com/CompositeAnalysis.htm
Pro/MECHANICA	PTC, Needham, MA	http://www.ptc.com/products/proe/sim/structural.htm
SDRC-IDEAS	Structural Dynamics Research Corp., Milford, OH	http://www.sdrc.com/nav/software-services/product-catalog/lamcomp.pdf
Codes using separate pre- and postprocessors		
LS-DYNA	Livermore Software Technology Corporation, Livermore, CA	http://www.lstc.com
MSC-NASTRAN/DYTRAN	MSC Software Corp., Costa Mesa, CA	http://www.mechsolutions.com/products/patran/lammod.html
VR&D-GENESIS	Vanderplaats Research & Development, Inc., Colorado Springs, CO	http://www.vrand.com/genesis_fact.htm
Pre- and postprocessors		
PATRAN	MSC Software Corp., Costa Mesa, CA	http://www.mechsolutions.com/products/patran/patran2000.htm
HyperMesh	Altair Engineering, Inc., Troy, MI	http://www.altair.com/

Table 3 Comparison between the results obtained for various a/h ratios for a $[0/90/0]_T$ simply supported laminate subjected to sinusoidal loading on the top surface

Quantity	$a/h = 2$	$a/h = 4$	$a/h = 10$	$a/h = 50$	$a/h = 100$	Source
$\bar{\sigma}_{xx}\left(\frac{a}{2},\frac{b}{2},\frac{h}{2}\right)$	1.436	0.801	0.590	0.541	0.539	(a)
	1.436	0.801	0.590	0.541	0.539	(b)
$\bar{\sigma}_{xx}\left(\frac{a}{2},\frac{b}{2},-\frac{h}{2}\right)$	−0.937	−0.754	−0.590	−0.541	−0.539	(a)
	−0.938	−0.755	−0.590	−0.541	−0.539	(b)
$\bar{\sigma}_{yy}\left(\frac{a}{2},\frac{b}{2},\frac{h}{6}\right)$	0.668	0.534	0.284	0.184	0.181	(a)
	0.669	0.534	0.285	0.185	0.181	(b)
$\bar{\sigma}_{yy}\left(\frac{a}{2},\frac{b}{2},-\frac{h}{6}\right)$	−0.742	−0.556	−0.288	−0.185	−0.181	(a)
	−0.742	−0.556	−0.288	−0.185	−0.181	(b)
$\bar{\tau}_{xy}\left(0,0,\frac{h}{2}\right)$	−0.0859	−0.0511	−0.0288	−0.0216	−0.0214	(a)
	−0.0859	−0.0511	−0.0289	−0.0216	−0.0213	(b)
$\bar{\tau}_{xy}\left(0,0,-\frac{h}{2}\right)$	0.0702	0.0505	0.0290	0.0216	0.0214	(a)
	0.0702	0.0505	0.0289	0.0216	0.0213	(b)
$\bar{\tau}_{xz}\left(0,\frac{b}{2},0\right)$	0.164	0.256	0.357	0.393	0.395	(a)
	0.164	0.256	0.357	0.393	0.395	(b)
$\bar{\tau}_{yz}\left(\frac{a}{2},0,0\right)$	0.2591	0.2172	0.1228	0.0842	0.0828	(a)
	0.2591	0.2172	0.1228	0.0842	0.0828	(b)

(a) From the SAVE analysis (Ref 21, 22). (b) By Pagano (Ref 30)

unique aspects in the analysis of multilayered composite structures. Finite element analysis of two classical examples from the mechanics of composite materials illustrates these aspects of multilayered composite structures. The first example is a problem of transverse bending of a simply supported $[0/90/0]_T$ laminated plate, the benchmark solution of which was obtained by Pagano (Ref 30). The second numerical example is of a $[0/90]_s$ laminated plate under uniform extension (Pagano, Ref 31, 32), illustrating the free-edge effects in multilayered composite structures.

Example 1: Transverse Bending of a Laminated Plate. A simply supported $[0/90/0]_T$ laminated plate is subjected to sinusoidal loading on the top surface. Laminated plates with two different aspect ratios are considered. For $a/h = 4$, the plate represents a thick multilayered structure. For $a/h = 50$, a thin-walled structure is represented. All layers are assumed to be of equal thickness. The material properties for the orthotropic lamina are (Ref 30): $E_1/E_2 = 25$, $E_2 = E_3$, $G_{12}/E_2 = G_{13}/E_3 = 0.5$, $G_{23}/E_2 = 0.2$, $\nu_{12} = \nu_{13} = \nu_{23} = 0.25$. The origin of the right-handed coordinate system is chosen at the corner of the middle surface of the plate, that is, $0 \leq x \leq a$, $0 \leq y \leq b$, and $-(h/2) \leq z \leq (h/2)$ (see Fig. 6).

This problem is analyzed by using the novel 3-D FEA tool SAVE, developed by the author (Ref 21, 22). For the laminated plate problem described previously, a quick comparison between 3-D elasticity solution of Pagano (Ref 30)

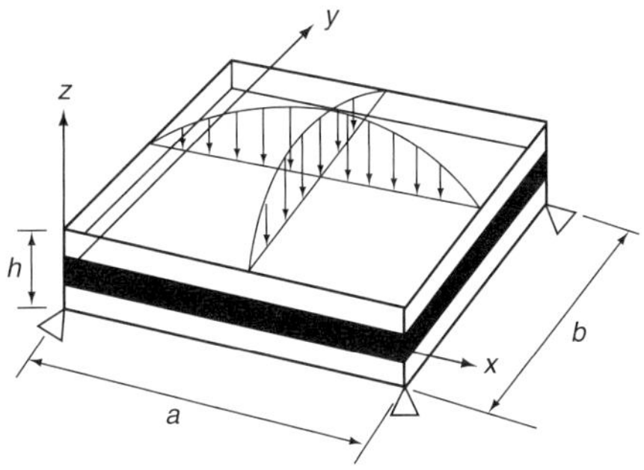

Fig. 6 A simply supported $[0/90/0]_T$ laminate subjected to sinusoidal loading on the top surface

Table 4 Comparison among the results obtained for $a/h = 4$ from various 3-D analyses for a $[0/90/0]_T$ simply supported laminate subjected to sinusoidal loading on the top surface

Quantity	SAVE, 1 × 1 × 1, $M = 6$, 1,805 DOF	ABAQUS, 20 × 20 × 4, C3D20, 61,200 DOF	ABAQUS, 12 × 12 × 2, C3D20, 11,664 DOF	NASTRAN, 12 × 12 × 2, CHEXA20, 11,664 DOF	I-DEAS, 12 × 12 × 2 (parabolic), 11,664 DOF	I-DEAS, 6 × 6 × 2 (parabolic), 2,916 DOF	I-DEAS, 12 × 12 × 2 (linear), 3,024 DOF	ABAQUS, 12 × 12 × 2, C3D8, 3,024 DOF
$\overline{\sigma_{zz}}(\frac{a}{2},\frac{b}{2},\frac{h}{2})$	1.0	1.005	1.02	1.02	1.02	1.025	0.950	0.826
$\overline{\sigma_{xx}}(\frac{a}{2},\frac{b}{2},\frac{h}{2})$	0.801	0.788	0.800	0.800	0.769	0.773	0.760	0.571
$\overline{\sigma_{xx}}(\frac{a}{2},\frac{b}{2},-\frac{h}{2})$	−0.754	−0.744	−0.750	−0.750	−0.725	−0.729	−0.716	−0.547
$\overline{\sigma_{yy}}(\frac{a}{2},\frac{b}{2},\frac{h}{6})$	0.534	0.528	0.532	0.532	0.516	0.521	0.514	0.483
$\overline{\sigma_{yy}}(\frac{a}{2},\frac{b}{2},-\frac{h}{6})$	−0.556	−0.550	−0.554	−0.554	−0.539	−0.543	−0.537	−0.514
$\overline{\tau_{xy}}(0,0,\frac{h}{2})$	−0.0511	−0.0508	−0.0509	−0.0498	−0.0500	−0.0504	−0.0492	−0.0519
$\overline{\tau_{xy}}(0,0,-\frac{h}{2})$	0.0505	0.0503	0.0503	0.0494	0.0496	0.0500	0.0487	0.0514
$\overline{\tau_{xz}}(0,\frac{b}{2},0)$	0.256	0.257	0.255	0.256	0.257	0.259	0.252	0.261
$\overline{\tau_{yz}}(\frac{a}{2},0,0)$	0.2172	0.2228	0.2400	0.2398	0.2408	0.2427	0.1743	0.1703

DOF, degrees of freedom; M, degree of polynomial

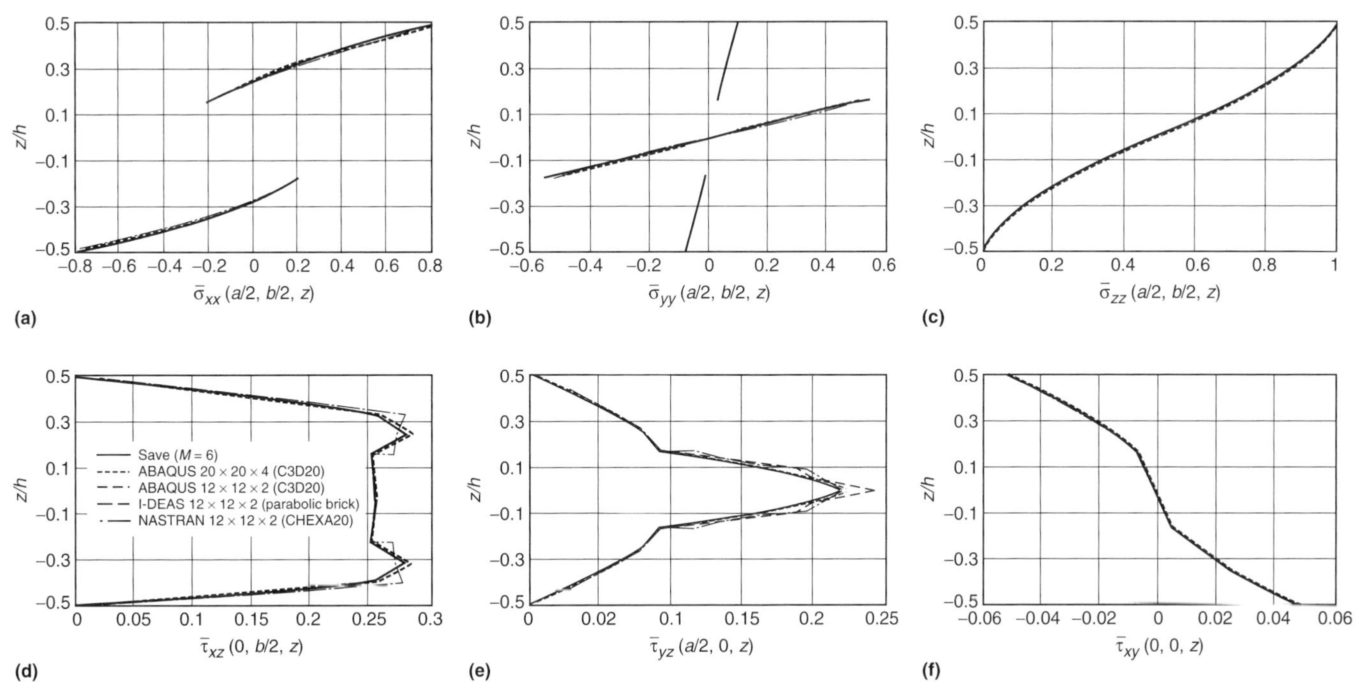

Fig. 7 Through-the-thickness distributions for $a/h = 4$. (a) σ_{xx}. (b) σ_{yy}. (c) σ_{zz}. (d) τ_{xz}. (e) τ_{yz}. (f) τ_{xy}. In the legend for these curves, M is the degree of the polynomial.

and the 3-D structural analysis code SAVE is presented in Table 3 for various a/h ratios. The normalized quantities used in Table 3 are described as: $\overline{\sigma_{xx}} = \sigma_{xx}/(q_0 s^2)$, $\overline{\sigma_{yy}} = \sigma_{yy}/(q_0 s^2)$, $\overline{\sigma_{zz}} = \sigma_{zz}/q_0$, $\overline{\tau_{xy}} = \tau_{xy}/(q_0 s^2)$, $\overline{\tau_{xz}} = \tau_{xz}/(q_0 s)$, $\overline{\tau_{yz}} = \tau_{yz}/(q_0 s)$, where $s = a/h$ and q_0 is the peak magnitude of the applied sinusoidal pressure load at the center of the laminated plate at the top surface. The results presented in Table 3 demonstrate the accuracy of SAVE analysis code in the 3-D analysis of multi-layered structures. Results from SAVE analysis can now be used as a basis to compare with the results obtained from commercial FEA codes.

Next, the example problem is analyzed using commercial FEA codes such as ABAQUS (Ref 33), NASTRAN (Ref 34), and I-DEAS (Ref 35). The solid elements—C3D8 and C3D20 in ABAQUS, and CHEXA and CHEXA20 in NASTRAN—and linear and parabolic brick in I-DEAS are used in the analyses. Results from the commercial FEA codes and the SAVE analysis are compared in Table 4 for $a/h = 4$. The mesh description shown in Table 4 represents the number of elements that are used to represent each composite layer in the three orthogonal coordinate directions. For example, a 12 × 12 × 2 finite element mesh represents 12 solid elements in x- and y-direction each, and 2 solid elements in the z-direction, in every single composite layer. As is shown in Table 4, the numerical values of the six stress components as obtained from the 3-D FEA using solid elements with quadratic shape functions (parabolic in I-DEAS, CHEXA20 in NASTRAN, and C3D20 in ABAQUS) are within 5% of the exact values. Only the transverse shear stress component, τ_{yz}, shows some significant difference (about 12 %) from the exact solution. However, as is shown in Table 4, the accuracy in the solution of this stress component is increased significantly by refining the FE mesh. In Table 4, compare the results obtained from I-DEAS and ABAQUS analyses with progressive mesh refinement (6 × 6 × 2, 12 × 12 × 2, and 20 × 20 × 4 meshes of parabolic solid elements). It is also worth noting that a sufficiently accurate solution to the problem being analyzed could be obtained by using parabolic brick elements in a coarse mesh (6 × 6 × 2 per layer) with 2916 DOF only. However, in spite of using a more refined mesh (12 × 12 × 2 per layer), solid elements with linear shape functions (linear brick in I-DEAS and C3D8 in ABAQUS) do not provide an accurate solution. For the numerical problem analyzed here, solid elements with linear shape functions, also known as constant strain elements, can be erroneous in the bending stress values by as much as 30%.

The through-the-thickness distributions of six stress components, as shown in Fig. 7, demonstrate many unique features of the 3-D stress state in multilayered laminated composite structures. Note the jump in the in-plane normal stress components σ_{xx} and σ_{yy} at the layer interfaces (see Fig. 7a and b). In multilayered laminated structures, in-plane stresses σ_{xx}, σ_{yy}, and τ_{xy} are discontinuous (hence, the in-plane strains ε_{xx}, ε_{yy}, and γ_{xy} are continuous) at the layer interfaces. On the other hand, the transverse stresses σ_{zz}, τ_{yz}, and τ_{xz} are continuous at the material interfaces, as shown in Fig. 7(c)–(e). However, the out-of-plane strains ε_{zz}, γ_{yz}, and γ_{xz} are now discontinuous (or jump) at these interfaces.

Continuity of the transverse normal and shear stresses at the layer interface, is a unique and important aspect in the analysis of multilayered laminated structures. Table 5 presents the actual numerical values of transverse stress components σ_{zz}, τ_{yz}, and τ_{xz} at the layer interfaces, thereby providing a deeper insight into the continuity of these interlaminar stresses. The notation "T" represents values computed at the interface approaching from the top; similarly, "B" represents values computed at the interface approaching from the bottom. While the SAVE analysis code is almost perfect in satisfying the continuity of interlaminar stresses at the interfaces, ABAQUS analysis with a very refined mesh (20 × 20 × 4 per layer with 61,200 DOF) is also reasonably good in achieving that goal. However, as the mesh size becomes coarser, the

Table 5 Interlaminar stresses as obtained at the ply interfaces from various 3-D analyses of a $[0/90/0]_T$ simply supported laminated plate ($a/h = 4$) subjected to sinusoidal loading on the top surface

Quantity		SAVE, 1 × 1 × 1 mesh ($M = 6$), 1,805 DOF	ABAQUS, 20 × 20 × 4, C3D20, 61,200 DOF	ABAQUS, 12 × 12 × 2, C3D20, 11,664 DOF	NASTRAN, 12 × 12 × 2, CHEXA20, 11,664 DOF	I-DEAS, 12 × 12 × 2 (parabolic), 11,664 DOF	I-DEAS, 6 × 6 × 2 (parabolic), 2,916 DOF	I-DEAS, 12 × 12 × 2 (linear), 3,024 DOF	ABAQUS, 12 × 12 × 2, C3D8, 3,024 DOF
$\overline{\sigma_{zz}}(\frac{a}{2},\frac{b}{2},-\frac{h}{6})$	T	0.269	0.267	0.258	0.258	0.264	0.266	0.382	0.389
	B	0.269	0.270	0.265	0.265	0.269	0.271	0.182	0.099
$\overline{\tau_{xz}}(0,\frac{b}{2},-\frac{h}{6})$	T	0.2575	0.2575	0.2575	0.2575	0.2575	0.2600	0.2533	0.2613
	B	0.2575	0.2625	0.2725	0.2725	0.2750	0.2770	0.2693	0.2730
$\overline{\tau_{yz}}(\frac{a}{2},0,-\frac{h}{6})$	T	0.0758	0.0828	0.1010	0.1005	0.1010	0.0967	0.1709	0.1643
	B	0.0758	0.0763	0.0778	0.0775	0.0780	0.0786	0.0645	0.0665
$\overline{\sigma_{zz}}(\frac{a}{2},\frac{b}{2},\frac{h}{6})$	T	0.718	0.719	0.719	0.719	0.722	0.728	0.808	0.881
	B	0.718	0.721	0.725	0.725	0.726	0.732	0.605	0.582
$\overline{\tau_{xz}}(0,\frac{b}{2},\frac{h}{6})$	T	0.2525	0.2575	0.2700	0.2700	0.2700	0.2733	0.2725	0.2680
	B	0.2525	0.2525	0.2525	0.2525	0.2525	0.2548	0.2508	0.2618
$\overline{\tau_{yz}}(\frac{a}{2},0,\frac{h}{6})$	T	0.0893	0.0898	0.0910	0.0910	0.0915	0.0922	0.0750	0.0738
	B	0.0893	0.0963	0.1145	0.1140	0.1145	0.1155	0.1778	0.1786

DOF, degrees of freedom; T, top; B, bottom; M, degree of polynomial

Table 6 Comparison among the results obtained for $a/h = 4$ from various 2-D analyses for a $[0/90/0]_T$ simply supported laminate subjected to sinusoidal loading on the top surface

Quantity	SAVE (3-D), 1 × 1 × 3 mesh ($M = 6$) 1,805 DOF	I-DEAS (2-D), 24 × 24 mesh (linear shell), 3,553 DOF	ABAQUS (2-D), 24 × 24 mesh, S4R, 3,553 DOF	MECHANICA, 2-D; $p = 6$	NASTRAN (2-D), 24 × 24 mesh, CQUAD4, 3,553 DOF
$\overline{\sigma_{xx}}(\frac{a}{2},\frac{b}{2},\frac{h}{2})$	0.801	0.397	0.397	0.398	0.396
$\overline{\sigma_{xx}}(\frac{a}{2},\frac{b}{2},-\frac{h}{2})$	–0.754	–0.397	–0.397	–0.398	–0.396
$\overline{\sigma_{yy}}(\frac{a}{2},\frac{b}{2},\frac{h}{6})$	0.534	0.592	0.592	0.592	0.592
$\overline{\sigma_{yy}}(\frac{a}{2},\frac{b}{2},-\frac{h}{6})$	–0.556	–0.592	–0.592	–0.592	–0.592
$\overline{\tau_{xy}}(0,0,\frac{h}{2})$	–0.0511	–0.0429	–0.0429	–0.0429	–0.0428
$\overline{\tau_{xy}}(0,0,-\frac{h}{2})$	0.0505	0.0429	0.0429	0.0429	0.0428
$\overline{\tau_{xz}}(0,\frac{b}{2},0)$	0.256	0.310	0.310	0.310	0.310
$\overline{\tau_{yz}}(\frac{a}{2},0,0)$	0.2172	0.2750	0.2750	0.0675	0.2750

DOF, degrees of freedom; M or p, degree of polynomial

commercial FE analyses results tend to become more distinct as well as less accurate at the interface (refer to Table 5). Once again, in all the commercial FE analyses, the transverse shear stress component, τ_{yz}, shows the most significant differences. As is shown in Table 5, the continuity of interlaminar stresses at the layer interfaces is the worst from the FEA with constant strain elements, thereby making them unsuitable for transverse bending analysis of multilayered composite structures.

In general, a 3-D analysis using discrete layer-by-layer representation of the laminate can be performed with reasonable accuracy, using solid elements with quadratic shape functions in any of the commercial FE codes evaluated here. However, due to limitations in the available computational resources, many times it may not be possible to discretize a complex, practical structure completely with 3-D solid elements. In addition, most of the real-life structures are thin-walled, so as to justify the use of 2-D shell elements in their analyses. However, the limitations, or bounds, of using 2-D shell elements to accurately analyze multi-layered composite structures needs to be well understood.

The thick laminated plate problem (a/h = 4) described previously is now analyzed using 2-D shell elements available in the commercial FE codes, namely, ABAQUS (S4R), NASTRAN (CQUAD4), I-DEAS (linear shell), and MECHANICA (p-type shell) (Ref 36). The type of shell element used in each analysis is mentioned in parentheses. The stress solutions obtained from various 2-D shell analyses are compared with the exact 3-D solution, as shown in Table 6. The 2-D shell analysis does not provide the transverse normal stress component, σ_{zz}. Note the very high numerical discrepancy among the stress values as obtained from exact 3-D solution and various 2-D analyses using shell elements. The largest discrepancy is in the magnitude of stress in the fiber direction in 0° layer, where the stress values from the 2-D analysis are almost 50% lower than the exact 3-D values. At the same time, the similarity among the 2-D analyses solutions is remarkable. Except for the values of transverse shear stress, τ_{yz}, as obtained from MECHANICA, the numerical results for the stresses obtained from the 2-D shell analyses are essentially the same. A systematic attempt was made to check the convergence of the 2-D solutions by increasing the order of shell elements

Table 7 Comparison among the results obtained for a/h = 50 from various 2-D analyses for a $[0/90/0]_T$ simply supported laminate subjected to sinusoidal loading on the top surface

Quantity	SAVE (3-D), 1 × 1 × 3 mesh, (M = 6) 1,805 DOF	I-DEAS (2-D), 24 × 24 mesh (linear shell), 3,553 DOF	ABAQUS (2-D), 24 × 24 mesh, S4R, 3,553 DOF	MECHANICA, 2-D; p = 6	NASTRAN, 24 × 24 mesh, CQUAD4, 3,553 DOF
$\bar{\sigma}_{xx}(\frac{a}{2},\frac{b}{2},\frac{h}{2})$	0.541	0.536	0.536	0.536	0.536
$\bar{\sigma}_{xx}(\frac{a}{2},\frac{b}{2},-\frac{h}{2})$	−0.541	−0.536	−0.536	−0.536	−0.536
$\bar{\sigma}_{yy}(\frac{a}{2},\frac{b}{2},\frac{h}{6})$	0.184	0.184	0.184	0.183	0.184
$\bar{\sigma}_{yy}(\frac{a}{2},\frac{b}{2},-\frac{h}{6})$	−0.185	−0.184	−0.184	−0.183	−0.184
$\bar{\tau}_{xy}(0,0,\frac{h}{2})$	−0.0216	−0.0215	−0.0215	−0.0215	−0.0215
$\bar{\tau}_{xy}(0,0,-\frac{h}{2})$	0.0216	0.0215	0.0215	0.0215	0.0215
$\bar{\tau}_{xz}(0,\frac{b}{2},0)$	0.393	0.394	0.392	0.388	0.392
$\bar{\tau}_{yz}(\frac{a}{2},0,0)$	0.0842	0.104	0.104	0.025	0.104

DOF, degrees of freedom; M or p, degree of polynomial

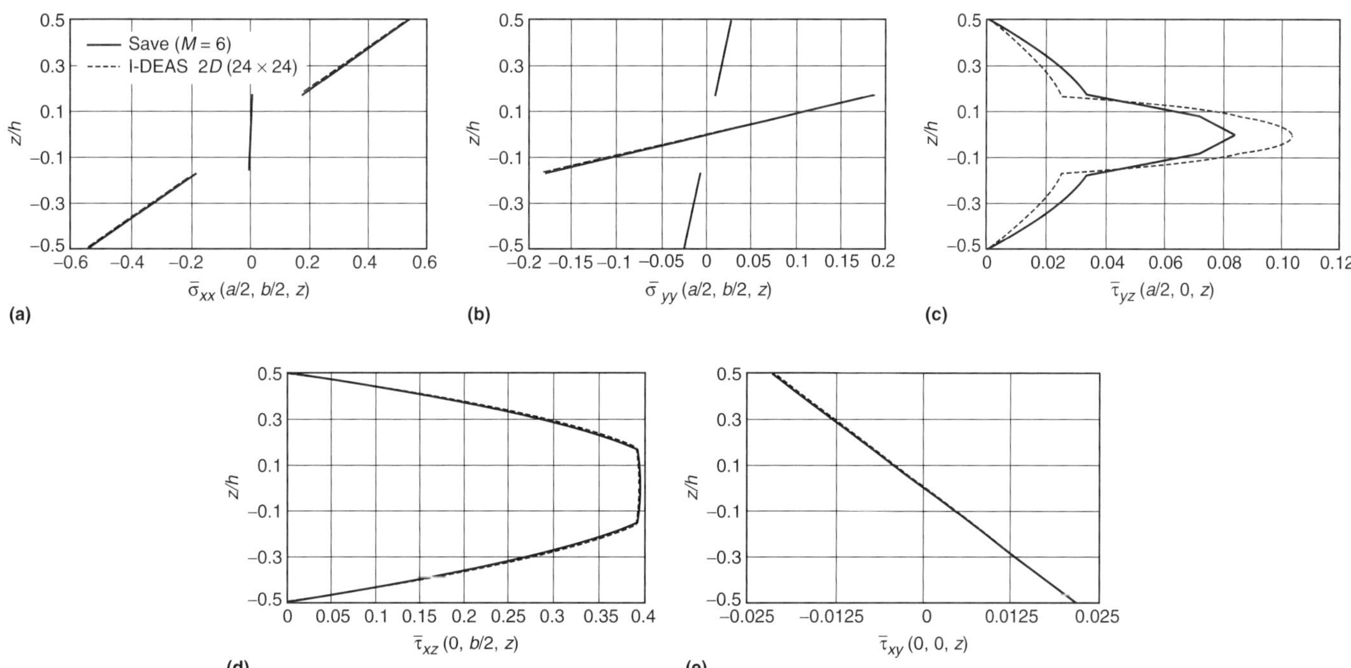

Fig. 8 Comparisons between 2-D and 3-D solutions for a/h = 50. (a) σ_{xx}. (b) σ_{yy}. (c) τ_{yz}. (d) τ_{xz}. (e) τ_{xy}. In the legend for these curves, M is the degree of the polynomial.

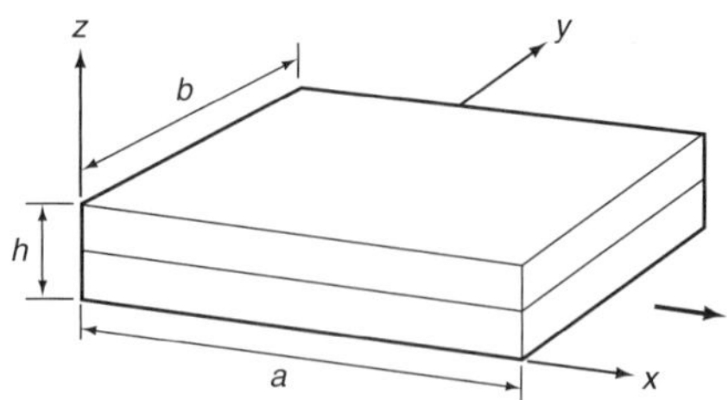

Fig. 9 A $[0/90]_S$ laminate subjected to uniform axial extension

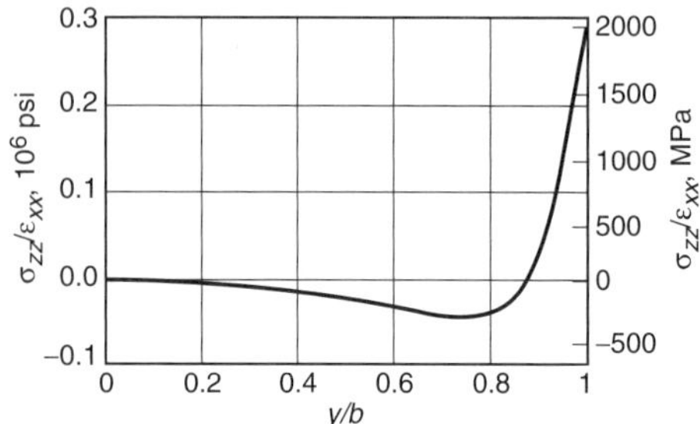

Fig. 10 Interlaminar normal stress, σ_{zz}, at the midsurface

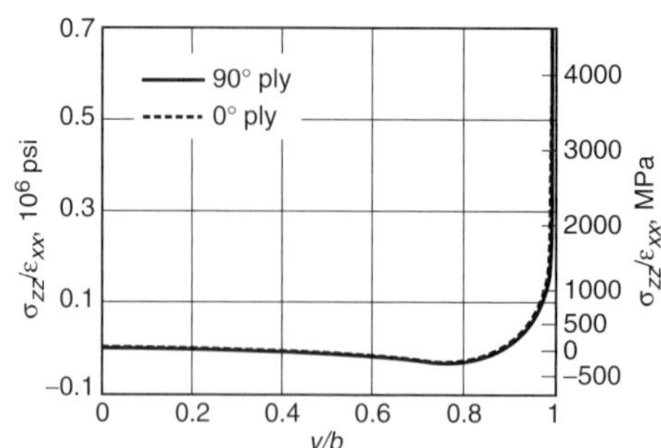

Fig. 11 Interlaminar normal stress, σ_{zz}, at the 0/90 interface

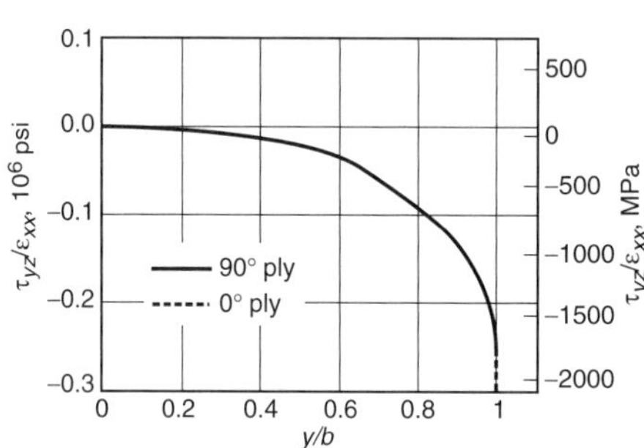

Fig. 12 Interlaminar shear stress, τ_{yz}, at the 0/90 interface

(e.g., S4R to S8R in ABAQUS, CQUAD4 to CQUAD8 in NASTRAN, and linear shell to parabolic shell in I-DEAS), as well as by refining the FE mesh in the model. No further improvement in the numerical solution of the problem was observed.

Further insight into this subject is gained by analyzing the laminated plate problem described previously with $a/h = 50$. The same 2-D shell elements and FE mesh are used during the analysis. Numerical results from a typical 2-D shell analysis using SDRC I-DEAS and the 3-D exact analysis SAVE are presented both in tabular form (Table 7) and as plots of stress distributions through the thickness of the laminate (Fig. 8). Except for the transverse shear stress component, τ_{yz}, numerical solutions obtained from the 2-D and 3-D analyses for this problem compare very well with each other. The numerical examples discussed here emphasize the need to understand the limits of 2-D shell elements in the analysis of anisotropic, multi-layered composite structures.

Example 2: Uniaxial Extension of a Laminated Plate. This example focuses on the free-edge effects in a $[0/90]_s$ laminated plate subjected to uniaxial extension (see Fig. 9). Pagano (Ref 31) presented the closed-form solution to this classical problem in 1974. Later on, Pagano and Soni (Ref 32) also solved this problem using a global-local variational model. Here, the results from the SAVE FE analysis program, performed using a 1 × 20 × 12 mesh of *variable-order* rectangular solid elements (Ref 21, 22), are presented.

Due to the symmetry of geometrical and materials properties and the applied loading, only one-eighth of the configuration of the $[0/90]_s$ laminated plate ($a = b = 4$ h; see Fig. 9) need be analyzed. The uniform extension of the laminated plate is achieved by applying a uniform axial displacement at the ends $x = a$. For the purpose of analyses, the following lamina elastic constants are taken (Ref 31):

$E_1 = 138$ GPa (20×10^6 psi)
$E_2 = E_3 = 14.5$ GPa (2.1×10^6 psi)
$G_{12} = G_{13} = G_{23} = 5.9$ GPa (0.85×10^6 psi)
$\nu_{12} = \nu_{13} = \nu_{23} = 0.21$

The distributions of interlaminar stresses as obtained from the analysis are plotted along the y-direction at $x/a = 0.5$. All the stress components are normalized by the applied axial strain. The distributions of the transverse normal stress, σ_{zz}, as obtained from the analysis at the midsurface of the $[0/90]_s$ laminate in the 90° layer, are shown in Fig. 10. The normalized peak value of 2.0 GPa (0.29×10^6 psi) for this stress component, which occurs at the free edge $y/b = 1$, compares very well with those obtained by Pagano (Ref 31) and Pagano and Soni (Ref 32). Next, the distributions of the normalized transverse normal stress component, σ_{zz}, as obtained from the analysis at the interface of the 0/90 layers, are shown in Fig. 11. Note that in Fig. 11 the numerical results from both 0° layer and 90° layer are plotted separately but appear superimposed. As is shown in Fig. 11, the continuity of the transverse normal stress component, σ_{zz}, is satisfied extremely well. Similar observations are made regarding the distributions of the transverse shear stress component, τ_{yz}, as shown in Fig. 12. Note the high gradients of interlaminar stresses that occur in the vicinity of the free-edge at $y/b = 1$ (see Fig. 11 and 12). These stresses are normally the primary cause of delamination failure in multilayered laminated structures.

REFERENCES

1. Z. Hashin, Analysis of Composite Materials—A Survey, *J. Appl. Mech.,* Vol 50, 1983, p 481–505
2. K.J. Bathe and E.L. Wilson, *Numerical Methods in Finite Element Analysis,* Prentice Hall, 1987
3. S.W. Tsai, *Introduction to Composite Materials,* Technomic, 1980
4. J.M. Whitney, *Structural Analysis of Laminated Anisotropic Plates,* Technomic, 1987
5. J.R. Vinson, *The Behavior of Sandwich Structures of Isotropic and Composite Materials,* Technomic, 1999
6. L.T. Tenek and J. Argyris, *Finite Element Analysis of Composite Structures,* Kluwer, 1998
7. J.N. Reddy and O.O. Ochoa, Finite Element Analysis of Composite Laminates, *Solid Mechanics and its Applications,* Vol 7, Kluwer, 1992
8. Z. Gurdal, R.T. Haftka, and P. Hajela, *Design and Optimization of Laminated Composite Materials,* Wiley, 1999
9. A.E. Bogdanovich and C.M. Pastore, *Mechanics of Textile and Laminated Composites,* Kluwer, 1996
10. A.G. Mamalis, D.E. Manolakos, G.A. Demosthenous, and M.B. Ioannidis, *Crashworthiness of Composite Thin-Walled Structural Components,* Technomic, 1998
11. S. Abrate, *Impact on Composite Structures,* Cambridge University Press, 1998
12. S.C. Tan, *Stress Concentrations in Laminated Composites,* Technomic, 1994
13. Y.-Y. Yu, *Vibrations of Elastic Plates: Linear and Nonlinear Dynamical Modeling of Laminated Composites and Piezoelectric Layers,* Springer, 1996
14. G. Cederbaum, I. Elishkoff, J. Aboudi, and L. Librescu, *Random Vibration and Reliability of Composite Structures,* Technomic, 1992
15. P. Zinoviev and Y. Ermakov, *Energy Dissipation in Composite Materials,* Technomic, 1994
16. R.F. Gibson, *Principles of Composite Material Mechanics,* McGraw Hill, 1994
17. N.K. Naik, *Woven Fabric Composites,* Technomic, 1993
18. M.B. Woodson, "Optimal Design of Composite Fuselage Frames for Crashworthiness," Ph.D. dissertation, Department of Aerospace and Ocean Engineering, Virginia Polytechnic Institute and State University, Blacksburg, Virginia, Dec 1994

19. E.R. Johnson and N. Rastogi, "Effective Hygrothermal Expansion Coefficients for Thick Multilayer Bodies," AIAA Paper 98-1814, Proc. of the 39th American Institute of Aeronautics and Astronautics/American Society of Mechanical Engineers/American Society of Civil Engineers/American Helicopter Society/American Society of Composites Structures, Structural Dynamics and Materials Conference, 20–23 April 1998 (Long Beach, CA)
20. R.A. Naik, "Analysis of Woven and Braided Fabric Reinforced Composites," NASA-CR-194930, June 1994
21. N. Rastogi, "Variable-Order Solid Elements for Three-Dimensional Linear Elastic Structural Analysis," AIAA Paper 99-1410, Proc. of the American Institute of Aeronautics and Astronautics/American Society of Mechanical Engineers/American Society of Civil Engineers/ American Helicopter Society/ American Society of Composites 40th Structures, Structural Dynamics and Materials Conference, 12–16 April 1999 (St. Louis, MO)
22. N. Rastogi, "Three-Dimensional Analysis of Composite Structures Using Variable-Order Solid Elements," AIAA Paper 99-1226, Proc. of the American Institute of Aeronautics and Astronautics/American Society of Mechanical Engineers/American Society of Civil Engineers/AHS/ASC 40th Structures, Structural Dynamics and Materials Conference, 12–16 April 1999 (St. Louis, MO)
23. J.N. Reddy and D.H. Robbins, Jr., Theories and Computational Models for Composite Laminates, *Appl. Mech. Rev.*, Vol 47 (No. 6), 1994, p 147–169
24. E.R. Johnson and N. Rastogi, "Interacting Loads in an Orthogonally Stiffened Composite Cylindrical Shell," *AIAA J.*, Vol 33 (No. 7), July 1995, p 1319–1326
25. V.V. Vasiliev, *Mechanics of Composite Structures,* Taylor & Francis, 1993
26. E.R Johnson and N. Rastogi, "Load Transfer in the Stiffener-to-Skin Joints of a Pressurized Fuselage," NASA-CR-198610, May 1995
27. M.B. Woodson, E.R. Johnson, and R.T. Haftka, "A Vlasov Theory for Laminated Circular Open Beams with Thin-Walled Open Sections," AIAA Paper 93-1619, Proc. of the American Institute of Aeronautics and Astronautics/American Society of Mechanical Engineers/American Society of Civil Engineers/ American Helicopter Society/American Society of Composites 34th Structures, Structural Dynamics and Materials Conference (LaJolla, CA), 1993
28. V.Z. Vlasov, *Thin-Walled Elastic Beams,* National Science Foundation, 1961
29. N.R. Bauld and L. Tzeng, A Vlasov Theory for Fiber-Reinforced Beams with Thin-Walled Open Cross-Sections, *Int. J. Solids Struct.,* Vol 20 (No. 3), 1984, p 277–297
30. N.J. Pagano, Exact Solutions for Bi-Directional Composites and Sandwich Plates, *J. Compos. Mater.*, Vol 4, 1970, p 20–34
31. N.J. Pagano, On the Calculation of Interlaminar Stresses in Composite Laminate, *J. Compos. Mater.*, Vol 8, 1974, p 65–77
32. N.J. Pagano and S.R Soni, "Models for Studying Free-Edge Effects," *Interlaminar Response of Composite Materials*, *Composite Materials* Series, Vol 5, N.J. Pagano, Ed., Elsevier Science Publishing Company, Inc., New York, NY, 1989, p 1–68
33. ABAQUS/standard version 5.8, Hibbitt, Karlsson and Sorensen, Inc., Pawtucket, RI
34. MSC/NASTRAN version 70.5, The MacNeal-Schwendler Corporation, Los Angeles, CA
35. I-DEAS master series 6, Structural Dynamics Research Corporation, Milford, OH
36. Pro/MECHANICA version 21, Parametric Technology Corporation, Waltham, MA

Computer Programs

Barry J. Berenberg, Caldera Composites

TRADITIONAL ENGINEERING MATERIALS are isotropic. Common engineering analyses can be performed with little more than a standard reference such as *Roark's Formulas for Stress and Strain* (Ref 1) and a scientific calculator. Laminated composites, on the other hand, are generally anisotropic. Performing a simple stiffness calculation, even for the case of an orthotropic laminate, is too complex for hand calculations.

Although somewhat lengthy, laminate calculations are relatively simple. They can be programmed into a spreadsheet with little difficulty. The challenge in this approach is verifying the calculations. The large number of variables involved, coupled with the anisotropic nature of composites, makes it difficult to prove the accuracy of the program for all types of laminates.

Fortunately, there are now a good number of high-quality commercial programs available for laminate calculations. Capabilities range from simple stiffness calculations and point-stress analysis to micromechanical modeling to shell buckling and other structural considerations. The problem now becomes one of finding a program that meets the user's needs.

Evaluation Criteria

Criteria for evaluating computer programs for composites structural analysis include database capabilities, types of engineering calculations supported, user, interface and operating systems, and technical support.

Databases

All composite programs, even the simplest ones for laminate stiffness calculations, deal with a large amount of data. Any program should therefore provide a means for storing and reusing this data. Database implementations can range from a simple text file that can be edited by hand to a fully relational database implemented in a commercial engine such as Microsoft Jet. Even when text files are used, the program can provide a graphical means of adding, editing, or deleting records.

The exact data to be stored depend on the calculations performed by the program, but usually include:

- Constituent material properties (engineering constants for reinforcements and matrices)
- Ply properties (engineering constants for individual lamina)
- Laminate definitions (lay-up sequences including material, orientation, and ply thickness)
- Results of calculations

If legacy databases exist, consideration must be given to importing old data into the new databases. Text files are the easiest to manipulate; commercial engines probably require a special utility, if conversion is even possible.

Engineering Calculations. For the purpose of selecting software, composite engineering calculations can be classified into three broad classes: micromechanics or material modeling, macromechanics or laminated plate theory, and structural analysis such as beam bending or joint failure. Some programs offer functions in only one of these classes, but it is becoming more common to offer all classes of calculations within a single package. If a needed function is not offered within the program, consideration must be given to how output from one program can be used as input to another program. For example, if a specialized program is used for buckling analysis, it must be able to read laminate properties (usually **ABD** matrices) from another program. Likewise, a laminate stiffness program might need to read ply properties generated by a micromechanics program.

Micromechanics programs take constituent material properties and generate ply properties. Calculations can be performed for different types of reinforcements (particulate, platelet, short fiber, long fiber, unidirectional, woven fabrics) and different types of matrices (polymeric, metallic, ceramic). For each material combination, there are several theories to choose from. Most general-purpose composite codes support only a subset of these materials and theories. To cover a more complete range of options, as well as user-defined theories, a specialized micromechanics program may be needed.

Macromechanics programs calculate laminate properties from ply or lamina properties using laminated plate theory. Inputs usually consist of engineering constants, obtained either from written sources—manufacturer's datasheets, open literature, *MIL-HDBK-17* (Ref 2)—or from micromechanics calculations. Outputs consist of, at a minimum, laminate engineering constants, including flexural constants. Most programs can also output constitutive equations such as the **ABD** and **Q** matrices.

Laminates are usually analyzed for both stiffness and strength, so these programs typically offer a point-stress capability. Loads are input as stress resultants or laminate strains; results are shown as ply stresses and strains in both ply and laminate coordinate systems. Failure criteria such as maximum stress or Tsai-Wu are used to calculate stress ratios or safety factors.

Temperature changes and moisture absorption can have a significant impact on composite behavior, so laminate programs should be able to handle environmental loads. Engineering constants should include laminate expansion coefficients, and stress/strain calculations should include temperature and moisture components.

Structural Analysis. Calculation of laminate properties and point-stress ratios is just the start of composite analysis. Once these preliminary screenings are complete, it is necessary to see how the laminate behaves under structural loads. Although finite-element analyses are often relied on for detailed design work, closed analytical solutions can be a powerful tool. Many types of structures can be analyzed this way, including beams, plates, shells, and pressure vessels. Solutions exist for stiffness, strength, stability, and dynamic conditions. Programs may also offer solutions for structural components, such as bolted or bonded joints, ply drop-offs, and stresses around cutouts.

Optimization. The goal of most design programs is to maximize strength or stiffness for a given set of loads while minimizing weight. This is an iterative process even for isotropic materials and is made more difficult by the large number of design variables available to the composites engineer. Some laminate and structural programs have tools to aid in the optimization process. In the simplest case, laminate properties and point-stress safety factors can be generated for a family of laminates. For example, a program might create a plot of modulus versus ply angle for the $[0/\pm\theta]_S$ family, where θ may vary from 0° to 90° in increments of 5°. In more complex cases, the program may be given a design goal and use an optimization algorithm to determine optimal materials, stacking sequence, and structural geometric parameters.

User Interface and Operating Systems

A good number of composite programs are now written for use under Microsoft Windows and sport a familiar graphical user interface (GUI). Graphic user interfaces are also common on programs written for UNIX systems, but some still use text-based interfaces. Macintosh programs are always GUI-based, but there are few composite programs written for that platform. It is important not to pick a program based solely on its interface: a slick cover may disguise a lack of capabilities.

Care must be taken to ensure programs are compatible with different versions of the operating system. UNIX programs should, of course, match the flavor of UNIX being run on the workstation. Most Windows 98 programs can run on Windows 95 systems, and vice-versa, but engineering programs especially often require Windows NT or 2000. Programs written for Windows 3.x may or may not run on Windows 9x or NT/2000 systems. Likewise, DOS-based programs may not run under any version of Windows, even a 9x version in DOS mode.

Support

Technical support should always be included with a software package, whether as part of the purchase price or for a maintenance fee. Support may be required not only for technical issues related to the calculations, but also for installation, system maintenance, and upgrades (software or hardware). If at all possible, arrange for a time-limited trial of the software before purchasing. Run some sample problems to test the features and make some support calls to determine the level of response that can be expected.

Few programs provide printed manuals anymore. On-line manuals should document all capabilities of the software, should be easy to navigate, and should have index and search functions. Theory manuals are not always included in the documentation, but are an important component. Some company standards require a specific theory to be used: in these cases there must be some way to determine what the software uses. Also, when comparing software results to the literature, discrepancies might be explained by differences in the theories used for the calculations. If theory manuals are not provided, this information should be available as part of the support agreement.

Reviews of Available Programs

Early programs for composite analysis tended to perform only one or a select few functions. Using ply properties from a micromechanics calculation in a laminate analysis, or laminate properties from a macromechanics calculation in a shell analysis, often required manually transferring the results from one program to another. Interfaces were text-based and linear: errors could not be corrected by backing up a step, and modifications to variables required an entirely new analysis. Storage of properties, if at all available, required the editing of a text file, often in a cryptic format.

Modern programs sport a graphical interface, built-in databases, and integrated modules for different types of analyses. Some programs even make it easy to add analysis modules, for those times when a specific type of calculation is not included in the program. Three of these comprehensive packages are reviewed in this section. Table 1 summarizes the capabilities of these programs.

CompositePro

CompositePro is one of the earliest comprehensive programs developed for the Windows operating system. First released in 1996, it is one of the few programs that will still run under any Windows version from 3.x to 2000.

The program has a multiple-document interface (MDI). The main window has a menu for accessing all of the analysis functions, a toolbar for quick access to the most common functions, and a window area for holding the individual analysis forms. There does not seem to be a built-in limit to the number of analysis forms that can be visible at once. Any single form can be printed as a graphical image, and a summary report can be generated for all analyses that have been run within a session.

The database uses a simple text format to store fiber, matrix, lamina, and core properties, as well as laminate sequences. One file stores properties for a single material, so a database of 50 materials requires 50 files. The files can be edited by hand, but it is easier to use the forms built into the program.

The only documentation for CompositePro is an on-line demo, which basically steps through the forms one at a time and explains how each works. The demo is similar to a help file, but it must be run sequentially, and there is no way to go directly to the guide for a specific form. Fortunately, the forms require little explanation, so the lack of printed or on-line help should not be missed. The theories used for the calculations are not specified, but the program author has been willing to provide this information via e-mail in the past.

Lamina and Laminate Analysis. Laminate properties can be generated using simple micromechanics calculations. Fiber and matrix materials are selected from the database, and lamina properties are calculated based on either volume or weight percent. The theory used is not specified. Resulting lamina properties can be saved in the lamina database for use in laminate calculations.

Lay-ups are entered in a tabular format, and special functions are available for creating symmetric laminates or rotating the entire laminate by some angle. These functions operate by simply copying plies, so it is not possible to undo a symmetry operation. Loads are entered as stresses, strains, or stress resultants (bending loads can only be entered as moment resultants, not as curvatures). The program also supports uniform temperature and moisture changes.

Output consists of constitutive matrices ($\bar{\mathbf{Q}}$, **ABD**, $\mathbf{ABD^{-1}}$) and engineering constants (both in plane and flexural, for two-dimensional thin laminates and three-dimensional thick laminates). Moduli and coefficients of thermal expansion in the principal directions can be shown in a bar graph. A complete set of stress analysis results are available, including: midplane laminate strains; stresses and strains in laminate and ply coordinates, at ply top, middle, and bottom surfaces; first-ply-failure (FPF) analysis; first-ply-failure survey; and progressive-ply-failure (PPF) analysis. All stresses and strains can be plotted.

The program provides three failure criteria: maximum stress, maximum strain, and quadratic or Tsai-Wu. The FPF analysis simply reports the first ply to fail under the applied load, including the failure mode (such as fiber tension or resin shear) and the factor of safety. The failure survey determines which ply will fail first under five basic loads (inplane tension and compression in the laminate X and Y directions, plus in-plane shear). Figure 1 shows the results of a failure survey on a simple laminate. Failure loads for each ply are listed in a table and plotted in a bar chart for comparison.

The PPF analysis is similar to a last-ply-failure (LPF) analysis, except that it reports the failure of each ply up to the last ply. The termination criterion can be either the first occurrence of fiber failure in a ply or failure of a specified number of plies in any mode. Degradation factors are specified individually for Young's modulus, E_{11} and E_{22}; shear modulus, G_{12}; and Poisson's ratio, ν_{12}. The report lists the plies in the order they fail and includes the reduced moduli, the safety factor, and the failure mode.

Structural Analysis. CompositePro provides functions for analyzing some simple types of structures: plates, sandwich plates, beams (with eight standard cross sections), shells, and pressure vessels.

All structural analyses begin with the definition of the geometry. For plates, this is length and width; for sandwiches, it also includes core thickness and material; for beams and shells, it is the dimensions of the cross section (radius, width, and height, as appropriate). Plate, facesheet, and wall thicknesses are all set by the laminate definition. Figure 2 shows an example of a hat-section definition. Dimensions are entered in a form, and section properties can be viewed in a separate window.

The structural results are somewhat limited, but cover the most common situations:

- *Plates:* Analyses include bending under a uniform pressure or concentrated load, buck-

Table 1 Capabilities of three programs for composites analysis

Program	Interface	Database	Micromechanics	Macromechanics	Structures	Design
CompositePro Version: 3.0 Beta OS: Windows 3.*x*, 9*x*, NT*x*, W2K Publisher: Peak Composite Innovations URL: http:// www.compositepro.com	MDI, printed report of all analyses (to printer only, no file option), English or SI units, on-line demo, no help files, no theory manuals	Simple text format. Store fiber (6), matrix (3), lamina (9), core (6) properties; laminate sequences. No references for included properties. Edit files or use program GUI.	Stiffness, thermal, strength, density. Theory not specified. Store results in database. Volume-fraction/weight-fraction converter; winding, fabric thickness (based on areal weight); roving converter; fabric properties (random, woven, stitched, based on weave style)	Stiffness, thermal properties; constitutive matrices; stresses, strains (top, middle, bottom); curvatures; FPF, LPF (max stress, max strain, quadratic); FPF failure mode survey; stress, strain, resultant, temperature, moisture loads	Plate (bending, stability, frequency); sandwich plate (bending, local and global stability); tubes/beams (bending, torsion, frequency; shell and Euler stability; thin- and thick-wall pressure vessels)	Thermal curvature; laminate surveys (tabular form of carpet plots); laminate parametric analysis (family studies)
Name: ESAComp Version: 1.5 OS: Windows 9X, NT4, W2K; UNIX Publisher: Helsinki University of Technology URL: http:// www.componeering.com	SDI (unlimited windows); screen, file, printed reports and plots; SI units; extensive help files (HTML format); full theory manual (PDF format and hard copy); Quick Start guide; built-in browser; API (documented on-line); fully customizable	Text format (not designed for simple editing). Adhesives; fibers; honeycomb and homogeneous cores; reinforced and homogeneous plies; matrix. Supports process specifications. Large database included	Unidirectional plies: thickness, engineering constants, thermal and moisture expansion from rule of mixtures. Save ply results into database	Ply: List and plot all constants and matrices. Laminates: All constants and matrices; FPF, LPF (8 failure criteria for composite plies; 4 each for homogeneous and core plies); sandwich wrinkling; laminate and layer stress and strain. FEA: Export laminate properties to ABAQUS, ANSYS, ASKA, I-DEAS, MSC/NASTRAN	Notched laminates; ply drop-offs; free-edge effects (built-in finite-element model)	Micromechanics: plot constants versus volume/weight fraction, fiber direction; multiple materials. Laminates: carpet plots; family studies; θ-laminates (variable angles); failure envelopes; strength and stiffness sensitivity studies (ply properties, orientation); multiobjective design (specify desired laminate properties, constraints, and objectives)
Name: V-Lab Version: 2.0 OS: Windows 9X, NT4, W2K Publisher: Applied Research Associates URL: http:// www.techpub.com	Outlook icon bar for selecting modules; tabbed dialogs within each module. Three-dimensional plots show failure envelopes. Extensive help files; minimal theory background. API, no documentation. Printed reports of individual analyses. SI or English units	MS Jet (access through program only). Fiber, matrix, lamina (8), and other materials (3); subcategories; temperature dependence; laminate sequences (4). Includes complete MIL-17 database	None, but database supports fiber and matrix properties	Lamina: constitutive matrices, stress/strain, failure (max stress, max strain, Tsai-Wu); no engineering constants. Laminate: constitutive matrices, stress/strain, moisture diffusion, free edge effects, plate with hole	Bonded joints (composite-composite, metal-composite).	Laminate carpet plots as part of lamina module.

ling under uniaxial or biaxial compression, and fundamental vibration frequency. Three types of boundary conditions are supported for each type of analysis. The bending analysis gives moments (*X, Y*, and *XY*) and maximum deflection at a user-specified point.

- *Sandwich plates:* Analyses include bending of a simply supported plate under uniform pressure and plate buckling under uniaxial compression. Both calculations include the local stability failure modes of face wrinkling and face dimpling. Maximum deflection only is given for the bending analysis.
- *Tubes and beams:* This section has the largest number of calculations. A full set of section properties can be displayed for the cross-section geometry. Beam calculations include bending, torsion, and vibration. Bending allows twelve boundary conditions and load-type combinations, with section *EI*, end-point reactions, rotations and moments, stresses (maximum and at a specified point), and maximum deflection included in the results. The torsion solution is for a free-clamped beam with an end torque and calculates beam properties (such as *GJ*), angle of twist, and shear stresses. Vibration allows eight boundary conditions (two with an end mass) and shows the frequencies of the first three modes. Stability analyses include shell buckling for cylindrical shells and column or Euler buckling for any cross section.
- *Pressure vessels:* Two modules provide solutions for thin-wall and thick-wall pressure vessels. The thin-wall module can analyze open or closed-end vessels with an internal pressure, axial load, and applied torque. The thick-wall module can analyze vessels under combined internal and external pressure, with an applied axial load and temperature change (no distinction is made between open and closed-end vessels). In both cases, ply stresses and strains are tabulated and plotted in the hoop, axial, shear (thin vessels only), and radial (thick vessels only) directions. The thin-wall module also calculates strength ratios and failure modes. The program gives no criteria for determining whether the vessel qualifies as thick or thin.

Several of the structural solutions use an *m, n* factor, such as plate bending (for iteration) or shell buckling (for buckle waves in the axial and circumferential direction). The user must specify maximum values for these factors. The results must be manually checked and, if the solution occurs at one or both of the maxima, the factors must be increased and the solution run again.

Utilities. CompositePro has several utility functions, most of which could be classified under micromechanics. The utilities include:

- *Converter* for volume fraction/weight-fraction conversions
- *Winding calculator:* Given a mandrel diameter and winding schedule, it calculates individual ply thicknesses. Results can be copied to the laminate definition form.

- *Fabric thickness:* Calculates layer thickness based on fiber volume, void volume, and areal weight
- *Roving converter:* Converts among various linear density units, such as cross-sectional area, yield, denier, and tex
- *Radius of curvature calculator:* Determines warping of a nonsymmetric laminate under a uniform temperature change
- *Fabric builder:* Calculates lamina properties for broadgoods (random continuous mat, woven fabric, stitched fabric) based on weave style (if appropriate), fiber volume, areal weight, fiber weight percent, and void volume percent. Resultant properties include lamina thickness, engineering constants, and strengths. The lamina properties can be saved in the database for use in laminate and structural analyses.

Design Utilities. Two design utilities were not yet available in the beta version supplied for this review: Laminate Surveys and Laminate Parametric Studies. The laminate survey form is basically a carpet plot in tabular form. Engineering properties and FPF strengths are calculated for $\theta_1/\theta_2/\theta_3$ laminates and tabulated at 10% ply-content increments (0%/0%/100%, 10%/0%/90%, 10%/10%/80%, etc.). The parametric study is similar to a carpet plot, but instead of adjusting ply content the ply angles are rotated. For example, applying a +5/0/+5 rotation to a 0/90/0 laminate would generate results for 0/90/0, 5/90/5, 10/90/10, . . ., 90/90/90 laminates.

ESAComp

Of the comprehensive programs reviewed here, ESAComp is the only one available on both Windows and UNIX systems. The standard UNIX distribution is for SGI platforms. Other UNIX platforms can be delivered on request, and a Linux version was in development at the time of this writing. ESAComp's focus is primarily on micromechanics and laminate analysis. Within those categories, it offers more features and analysis options than the other programs. An extensive set of design and optimization tools is provided. Version 2.0, scheduled for release in late 2000, will expand the design tools; add structural elements such as beams, plates, and shells; and include an improved interface for user extensions.

Because of its UNIX heritage, ESAComp uses a single-document interface (SDI) rather than a MDI. Most commands bring up a new window, which can be placed anywhere on the desktop. The program is fully documented on-line. Help files are in HTML format. They can be viewed in a standard browser or from within the program using the built-in, proprietary browser. A theory manual in portable document file (PDF) and printed format is also included. It details the theory used in all ESAComp analyses and even serves as a good stand-alone reference.

The interface is not as intuitive as other programs, making it difficult to use ESAComp without first reading the documentation. A Quick Start Guide (PDF and printed) is provided; working through it provides sufficient experience to run most analyses. The help documentation is comprehensive, but tends to describe the software more from a programmer's point of view than from a user's. This approach is probably necessary to show the full power of the program, but it does make the learning curve a bit steep.

Interface. ESAComp sessions work with a single case. Each case contains information about materials, plies, laminates, and loads. A case is set up by selecting one of those categories, defining the items for that category (selecting them from the database or entering new items into the database), and establishing the analysis options. Case setups are also saved in the database.

The main window also provides access to global program options. Options can be set for analysis, display, help, and units:

- *Analysis:* Failure criteria (eight for composite plies, four for isotropic plies, four for cores),

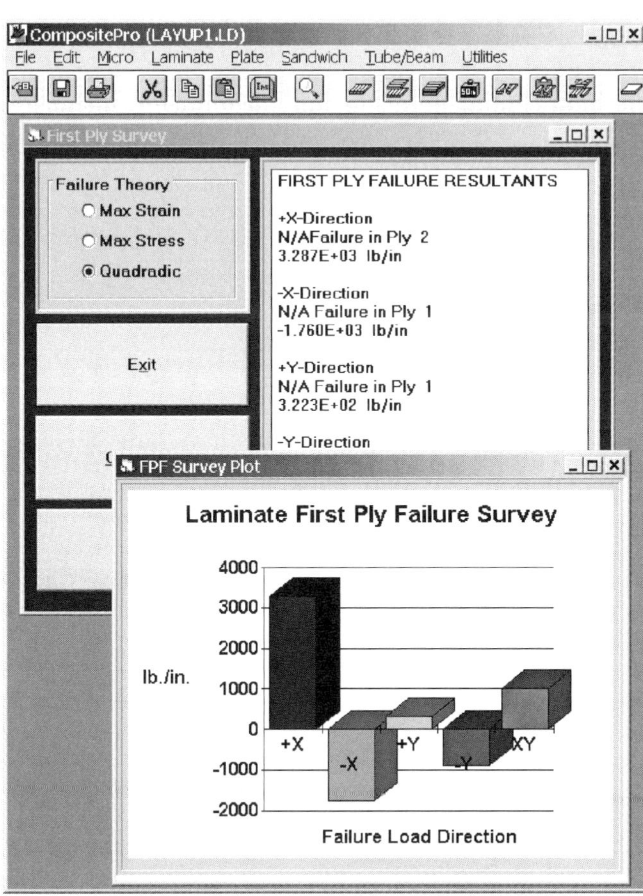

Fig. 1 Example of a laminate failure survey in the CompositePro software program

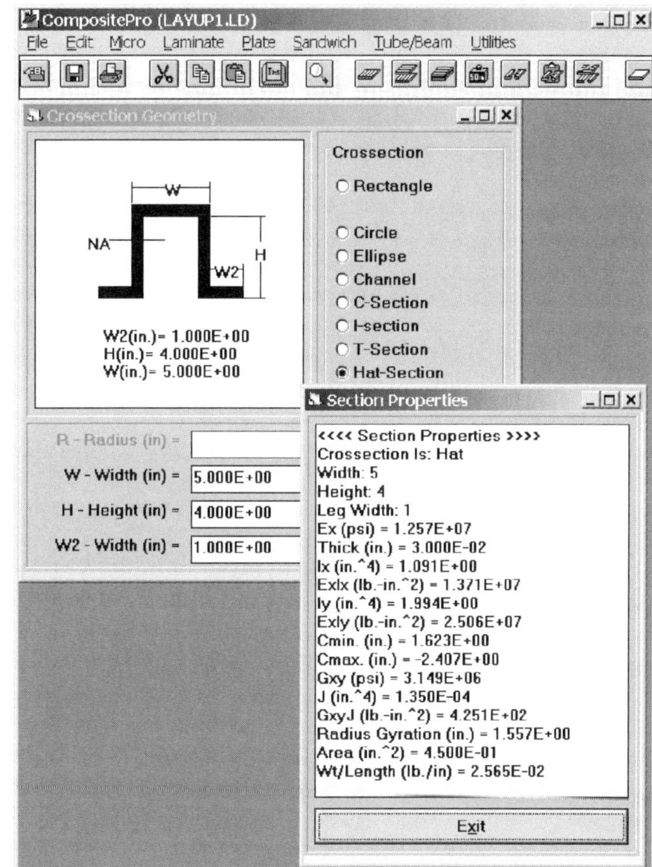

Fig. 2 Example of a beam definition in the CompositePro software program

factors of safety, sandwich wrinkling factor, stress/strain recovery plane

- *Display:* General; header; footer; line, bar, and layer charts (size, grid, scale); failure margins (expressed as margin or failure ratios)
- *Help:* Default to User Manual or Design Manual
- *Units:* Select default unit, format, and precision for all measurements (displacement, length, stress, coefficient of thermal expansion, pressure, etc.). Only SI units provided

Results of all analyses are displayed using the built-in HTML browser. The HTML pages are generated on the fly using a macro language. The global Display and Units options affect the results displays, and each results window has several options for altering the display. Users may also create their own macros for custom displays.

Database. ESAComp has been developed with the corporate user in mind, and nowhere is that more evident than in the database. Whether working with constituent materials, plies, laminates, or loads, three data levels are always available: User, Company, and ESAComp. The User level is for properties and analyses used by a single person, the Company level is for data shared by many, and the ESAComp level is for the extensive built-in collection of properties.

The database has also been developed with the manufacturer in mind. Each material is allowed six data categories, only one of which is mechanical data. The other categories are: Composition (physical properties), Operating Environment (temperature and pressure), Processing Data (cure cycle and applicable manufacturing processes), Product Data (manufacturer, type, specification, and price), and Comment. Keywords can be associated with each material, ply, or laminate; the list of built-in keywords includes categories, material types, and manufacturers. Items are referred to by an identification string, which can be built up from keywords. For example, a ply from one of the demonstrations is identified as "T300;Epoxy;UD-.200/210/60" with the keywords "Fiber;Carbon;Toray;Matrix; Epoxy;".

The ESAComp Data Bank is divided into seven categories: Adhesives, Fibers, Honeycomb Cores, Homogeneous Cores, Homogeneous Plies, Matrices, and Reinforced Plies. Each of those categories is further divided by material type. For example, fibers are categorized as Aramid, Carbon, or Glass. Material types are categorized by manufacturer, such as Akzo, DuPont, and Teijin for Aramid.

Constituent Materials. All analyses start by defining materials and loads. In the case of micromechanics, this means getting fiber and matrix properties from the database or defining new material properties.

The micromechanics analysis simply creates a ply property based on the selected fiber and matrix properties. Results include engineering constants, expansion constants, and strengths. If a mass per unit area of fibers is entered, the ply thickness will be calculated. The generated properties can automatically be entered into the database as a new ply material. Identification keywords are combined from the two materials, giving a default identifier; all processing and other information from the two materials is also included in the new ply definition.

The effects of volume or weight fractions and fiber directionality can be studied by specifying a range for one or both of these values. Any or all of the material constants can be plotted and tabulated against the selected variable. If both variables are chosen, the result is similar to a carpet plot with, for example, volume fraction on the X-axis and individual curves for the discrete angles.

Plies. The basic ply analysis simply calculates ply properties, engineering and expansion coefficients, stiffness and compliance matrices (two-dimensional and three-dimensional), invariants, and transformation matrices.

The basic analysis is made more powerful by specifying a ply angle. If a single value is specified, the results show the transformed properties. If a range of angles is specified, then all properties (including constitutive matrix components) can be plotted and tabulated against ply angle. In addition to the standard X-Y plots of property versus angle, ESAComp also offers a polar plot. The radial coordinate represents ply angle, and the circumferential coordinate represents the property. The X-component of the plot corresponds to the property in the 1-direction; the Y-component corresponds to the property in the 2-direction. For example, the polar modulus plot in Figure 3 shows E_1 on the horizontal axis and E_2 on the vertical axis.

Multiple materials can also be analyzed at once. Selecting more than one ply allows comparison bar charts and tables of properties to be generated. Comparison results can include all standard constants as well as specific moduli. An angle-range analysis can be combined with a multiple-material analysis to generate overlay

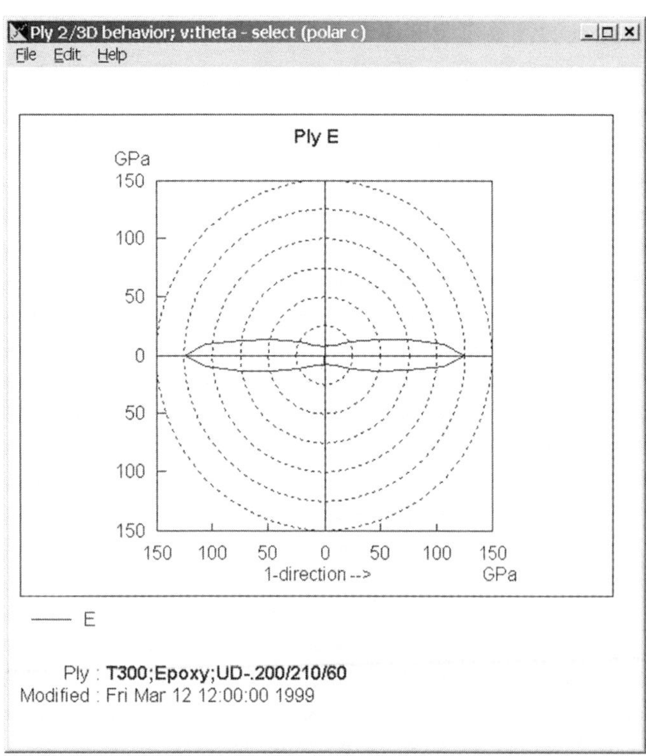

Fig. 3 Example of a polar modulus plot in the ESAComp software program

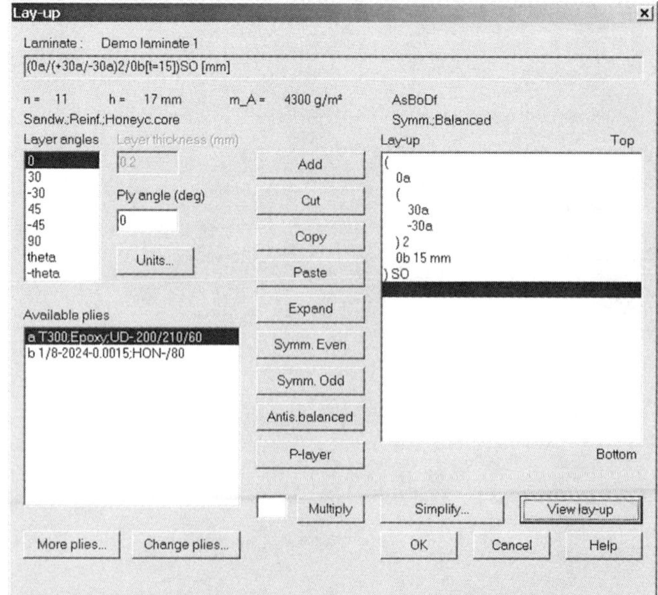

Fig. 4 Example of a laminate definition in the ESAComp software program

plots showing the variation of properties versus angle for all materials simultaneously.

Finally, the carpet plots can be generated for one material at a time. The laminate is of the format $[0/\pm\theta/90]_S$, where θ is specified by the user. Plot parameters (line spacing by percent for each angle) can be customized to generate dense or sparse plots. Any engineering, expansion, or strength constant can be plotted. For strength properties, any of the eight failure criteria may be used.

Laminates. As with other portions of the program, analysis of laminates starts by importing a laminate definition from the database or by defining a new laminate.

ESAComp has a rather unique but powerful method for defining laminates. The program uses standard laminate notation, with each ply entered as a single line in the laminate view. The line shows the material (designated by a letter) and the ply angle. Sublaminate delimiters and modifiers (such as "S" for symmetric) appear on their own lines. The laminate builder automatically recognizes special types of laminates, allowing the program to expand a lay-up, showing one ply per line. It can also contract a laminate, automatically inserting delimiters and modifiers as appropriate. Modifiers can be edited, so a symmetric laminate, for example, can be changed to an antisymmetric laminate with a single mouse click.

Figure 4 shows a sample laminate definition. It is a sandwich laminate with $[0/(\pm 30)_2]$ facesheets. The entire laminate is defined as Symmetric Odd (SO), which means that it is symmetric about the midplane of the core. The form shows the total number of plies (n), the total thickness (h), and the mass per unit area (m/A).

The basic laminate analysis is similar to the ply analysis, except that laminate properties are displayed. Multiple angles and multiple laminates can be analyzed at once. Results include the standard constants and matrices, plus normalized matrices, out-of-plane shear stiffnesses, layer (individual ply) properties, free-edge-effect estimates, and sandwich facesheet properties (if appropriate). Figure 5 shows a typical multiple analysis. In this case, two laminates are compared at four different angles. The longitudinal laminate modulus is plotted and tabulated for each laminate at each angle.

Strength analyses can be either FPF or degraded laminate failure (DLF), sometimes called last ply or ultimate failure. Strength results can be generated for a single laminate or for multiple laminates. Comparison results are plotted and tabulated for one property at a time. Failure envelope graphs show the failure region for a combination of any two load components and can be plotted for FPF, DLF, or both. The load types are the same as are available for load definitions (described later in this section). The plots can be generated for the entire laminate, for each layer, for a range of loads in one direction, or for multiple failure criteria.

If loads are defined, load-response results can be generated. Loads are stored in the database along with the case. They can be entered as forces and moments, normalized stresses, forces with zero curvature, or strains and curvatures. Loads can include external (physical) loads, temperature loads (constant through thickness or top and bottom surface temperatures), and moisture loads (constant or variable, as with temperatures). Tabulated and plotted load responses include layer stresses, layer strains, and margins of safety. Results can be generated for multiple laminates, multiple loads, and angle ranges.

Materials and laminates are never perfect, so ESAComp provides two types of sensitivity studies. The first shows the sensitivity of laminate properties to changes in ply properties. One ply property, such as E_1, is selected for the study and a $\pm$ tolerance is specified. Nominal, maximum, and minimum laminate properties (engineering constants, thermal and moisture constants, or strengths) are then tabulated and plotted. The second study shows the sensitivity to layer orientations. An orientation tolerance is entered for each ply (each can have a different tolerance); nominal, maximum, and minimum properties are then shown as for the ply properties study.

The laminate analysis includes three specialized solutions: notched laminate, layer drop-off, and free-edge stresses. The notched laminate solution can use either a defined load or a load ratio; notches can be circular or elliptical. The layer drop-off solver shows stresses where a ply is dropped from the middle of a laminate. Finally, the free-edge analysis is performed using a built-in finite-element solver and shows layer stresses at the free edge of a laminate.

Finally, laminate properties can be output to any one of five finite-element programs (ABAQUS, ANSYS, ASKA, I-DEAS, and MSC/NASTRAN). Output consists of a material definition in the appropriate input deck format. For example, the NASTRAN output is a PCOMP or PSHELL definition, and the I-DEAS output is a Universal File.

Design Features. ESAComp has several features to aid in the design and optimization of laminates. The easiest to use are the multiple-analysis options, described previously in the sections on materials, plies, and laminates.

Two special types of laminates can be defined: θ-laminates and p-laminates. Theta-laminates can have any number of plies specified as a variable angle, or "θ." In other words, θ-laminates define a family of laminates, such as $[0/\pm\theta/90]_S$. When running a basic laminate analysis, θ is automatically varied over a range, similar to a multiple-angle analysis.

For p-laminates, the total thickness of the laminate is assumed to stay constant, but the proportion of layers defined as p-layers is varied over a range. For example, if the nominal thickness of a $[0P/\pm 30]_T$ laminate is 0.015 in. (each ply with a thickness of 0.005 in.), a p-laminate study might set the 0° ply thickness to (0, 0.005, 0.010, 0.015). The corresponding thicknesses of the 30° layers would then be (0.0075, 0.005, 0.0025, 0). The basic laminate analysis then shows results over the range of p-values.

User Extensions. Although ESAComp does not emphasize program customization, interfaces are provided for extensive customization of the program. As described earlier, all results displays are created using a macro language. The macro files are in plain text format, allowing the macros for all built-in results to be used as examples (though they should not be modified). The macro language is capable of displaying any numerical result generated by ESAComp and of

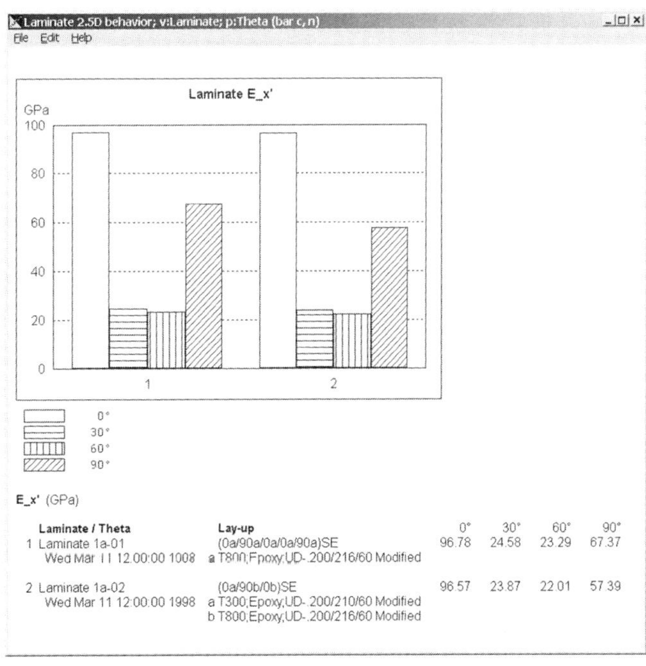

Fig. 5 Example of multi-laminate analysis in the ESAComp software program

creating line, bar, and polar plots of the results. Simple calculations can also be performed. Users can therefore customize the look of the results displays, combine results in ways not offered by the built-in macros, and even generate new results. The language is not fully documented, but the help file provides a fairly complex example of custom macro for combining the results from a basic laminate analysis and an FPF analysis.

For more complex analyses, user-defined procedures can be added. Procedures are written in the C Language Integrated Production System (CLIPS) designed at NASA/Johnson (National Aeronautics and Space Administration). Although few users are likely to be familiar with this language, the syntax seems rather simple. CLIPS documentation is available from a NASA Web site. The help file includes an example procedure that adds a failure criterion to the program. Although users could create other procedures by following this example, the lack of documentation specific to the ESAComp constructs would make this a difficult task. The next release is supposed to improve upon user extensions: if it does, this will become a much more useful feature.

V-Lab

A major shortcoming of most composite analysis programs is that they cannot perform all calculations. If the program does not support a type of analysis or specific theory, the only option is to use another program. With each program, though, comes the overhead of basic calculations such as laminate properties. If the analysis is highly specialized, it may not be available in a commercial package, forcing the user to write a customized program. To avoid the effort of developing an entire laminate program, it is common to export basic laminate properties (such as constitutive matrices) from a commercial package and import them into the user-written program.

V-Lab attempts to overcome this limitation by providing an interface for user-written calculations (called modules or Labs). The program ships with three Labs that provide standard functionality: ply or material analysis, laminate analysis, and bonded joint analysis. A Developer's Kit provides database documentation and an API, allowing the addition of user-created Labs. Unlike ESAComp, which mentions extensibility almost as an afterthought, V-Lab emphasizes user extensions as a selling point.

The program runs under Windows and has an Outlook-style MDI. The main program menu gives access to the Labs, program settings, and standard Windows functions. A simple toolbar provides open, save, print, and help functions, plus a switch between English and SI units. An Outlook-style icon bar on the left shows icons for each of the Labs. Each Lab has its own form; individual analyses are accessed through a tabbed interface on the Lab form. A report can be printed for each form showing any tabulated data and plots. Reports cover only the active tab and the active plot: several reports must be printed to cover all analyses in a Lab.

Full documentation is available in the on-line help files, with links to the appropriate sections from each form. The help files include theoretical overviews, but lack details of the specific implementations.

Databases are central to the functioning of V-Lab. The program supports multiple databases, but only a single database can be active or accessible at any one time. Each database stores both material properties and laminate definitions.

The view of a material within the database is called a data sheet. Although materials are classified by type (fiber, matrix, composite, coating, or isotropic), all data sheets hold the same set of properties. Each material can have multiple data sheets, representing properties at different temperature and moisture conditions, and the program can even create new data sheets by interpolating between existing environmental data sets.

V-Lab comes with two databases. The Sample database has a small number of materials and laminates, mainly for use in demonstrating V-Lab features. Of more use is the MIL-17 database. This database contains most (but not all) of the carbon composite properties from revision E of the handbook; it contains none of the glass, quartz, or other composite properties. Care must be taken when using the MIL-17 properties: the data sheets show normalized mean values, even when B-basis allowables are available. The MIL-17 file ships as a read-only database, but the data can be included in new databases by selecting an option in the New Session dialog.

Figure 6 shows a typical material datasheet from the MIL-17 database. The tabs across the bottom of the datasheet show that properties are defined at three or more temperature and moisture conditions. The MIL-17 properties have been imported into a new analysis, making them available for editing. Properties not already defined can be added to the datasheet, as shown in the Select Properties to Add window.

Material Lab. Although the V-Lab database defines categories for fibers and matrices, the program provides no micromechanics capabilities. The name of this Lab is a bit misleading: it is more for lamina analysis than for material analysis.

The Material Lab is used for creating or editing material data sheets, calculating constitutive properties (stiffness or compliance matrices), calculating strains from stresses or stresses from strains, performing a failure analysis (maximum stress, maximum strain, or Tsai-Wu), and generating carpet plots.

All analyses are performed on a single, unidirectional ply. The ply orientation can be rotated arbitrarily, but results cannot be plotted or tabulated versus ply angle. Carpet plots are generated for 0/90/±45 laminates only; properties that can be plotted are Young's modulus (E_{11} only), Poisson's ratio, shear modulus, thermal expansion coefficient, and open-hole tensile and compressive strength.

A major deficiency of many V-Lab analyses is a lack of numerical results. For example, the constitutive properties tab shows only stiffness and compliance matrices, not engineering constants. Also, the failure analysis tab provides only a qualitative result: the failure envelope is plotted in a graphics window, and the point-stress location is drawn in relation to that enve-

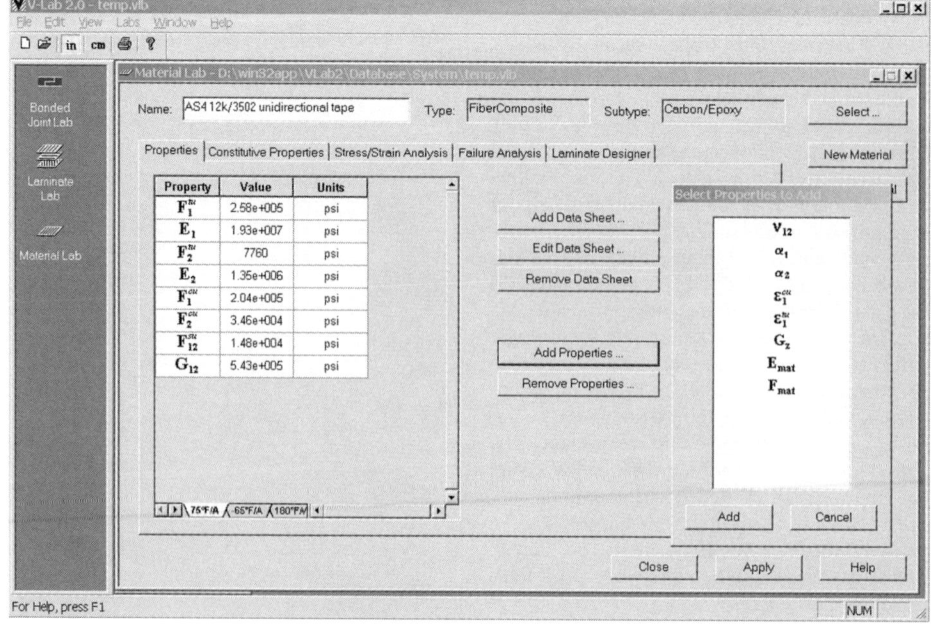

Fig. 6 Example of a material datasheet in the V-Lab software program

lope. If the point is green, the applied loads are below the failure loads. If the point is red, the applied loads are above the failure loads. No stress ratios, safety factors, or margins are shown, nor are they available in any reports or printouts.

The Laminate Lab is used to calculate laminate properties, perform point-stress analysis, run moisture-diffusion calculations, estimate free-edge effects, and determine strains in a plate with a hole.

Analysis starts with definition of the lay-up. Plies are entered in a grid, with buttons for adding and removing layers, and moving layers up and down in the sequence. Layers can only be added in the last row: there is no insert function. Laminate types include Symmetric, Antisymmetric, Symmetric/Midply, and Total. Stacking sequences can be stored in the database. Surprisingly, the database categorizes laminates differently than the definition form, allowing Any, Angle-Ply, Cross-Ply, and General.

Constitutive properties are given as **ABD** or $\mathbf{ABD}^{-1}$ matrices only: laminate engineering constants are available nowhere in the program. Furthermore, laminate thermal and moisture expansion properties are not shown at all, either as matrices or as engineering constants.

As in the Material Lab, stress, strain, and failure results are only shown graphically. Loads are input as stress and bending resultants or as laminate strains. Failure analysis results are shown using the same type of plot as in the Material Lab. As seen in Fig. 7, only one stress component can be viewed at a time. The thick horizontal line shows the location of the failure criterion calculation, plotted in the graph to the right. The box in the failure plot represents the failure envelope; the sphere represents the calculation point. In this particular case the ball is green, indicating no failure, even though it appears to be outside the envelope. The envelope plot indicates failure for these loads if the calculation line is moved up one more increment in the line chart. The lack of numerical results for laminate constitutive properties and stress/strain analyses, or even a quick "yes-no" flag for an entire laminate, severely limits the usefulness of V-Lab in engineering applications, where these numbers are usually required.

The moisture diffusion solution can be a useful tool for examining environmental effects. It depends on the laminate definition only for total thickness. Given an initial condition, a boundary condition (expressed as percent moisture concentration) and a laminate diffusivity, this module plots either a through-thickness moisture concentration profile or an average mass gain versus time curve.

The free-edge delamination module calculates the strain energy release rate (G value) for a crack extending from the free edge of a laminate. Inputs consist of a temperature change and an applied strain. Five different G values can be calculated (strain energy, virtual work, I, II, III). Results are shown in a bar graph, with one bar for each ply. Again, numerical results are not available, and no assistance is given in interpreting the results.

Finally, the Laminate Lab provides a module for calculating maximum strains in a plate with a hole. Input consists of the hole diameter, stress and bending resultants (which are independent of the stress/strain analysis), and optional bolt loads. The results are presented as maximum compressive and tensile strains and minimum margin of safety. Unlike the other analyses, this one gives a numerical result.

The Bonded Joint Lab shows the potential for the wide range of analyses that can potentially be performed with V-Lab. The Material and Laminate Labs provide the standard capabilities of a composites program; the Joint Lab is an added analysis type.

Using the Joint Lab can be a bit confusing and so is one case where it pays to first read the Help file. The analysis starts by defining joint materials. The module can examine composite-to-composite or composite-to-metal joints. For composite-to-composite joints, the parent material and the patch material must be the same (to simplify the terminology, all joints are treated as repairs). The laminate consists of 0°, 90°, and off-axis (user-defined angle) layers. All layers can be the same material, or each set of angles can be a different material. The laminate definitions are not linked at all to the Laminate Lab or the laminate database (but the database can store joint definitions).

The Lab supports only one joint geometry: a stepped double-lap joint, which is similar to a scarf joint. Steps are entered into a table. Each step definition consists of the number of 0°, 90°, and off-axis plies. The parent laminate and repair section can have a different number of layers of each angle in each step. Step lengths are defined in the parent laminate table.

Once the joint is fully defined, two analyses can be performed: joint strength analysis and applied loads analysis. The strength analysis view shows the allowables in each step plus the amount of the load carried by the repair. Results are given for axial loads and shear loads, with the joint loaded in either tension or compression. A factor of safety and a uniform temperature change can be specified. Three failure criteria are used to determine the strengths, as outlined in the Help file. The program will reset the step lengths during the strength analysis to meet minimum length requirements, but the criteria for setting minimum length are not given. With the allowables determined, the applied loads analysis calculates the margin of safety, critical step, and critical section (parent, adhesive, or patch) for a specified load expressed as axial and shear stress resultants.

Program Customization. One of the most appealing features of V-Lab is its expandability. The application programmer's interface (API) gives users access to the database, to the functions within existing Labs, and to V-Lab's user interface. If V-Lab does not provide a needed function or analysis type, users should be able to add their own routines without worrying about the standard overhead functions.

End users add functions through a Developer's Kit. The Kit includes definitions of the API functions and necessary header files for writing Labs. The calculation portion of user Labs can be contained in a dynamic link library (DLL). Any language that supports compilation to a DLL can be used, or existing DLLs from other programs or libraries can be reused. The actual interface to V-Lab must be handled through C++. This can make adding interfaces somewhat difficult because C++ is not an easy language to learn. The source file for a sample

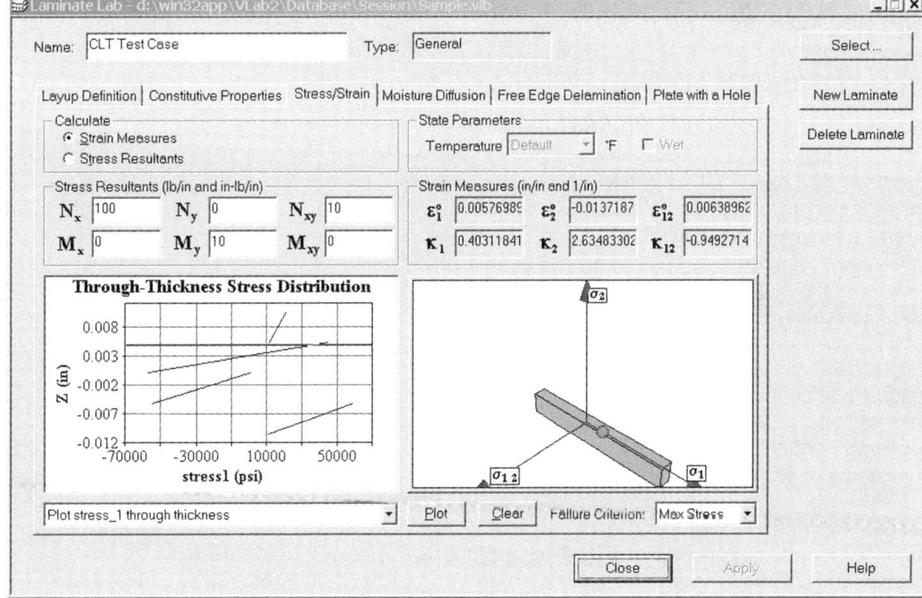

Fig. 7 Example of a stress analysis and failure plot in the V-Lab software program

Lab that simply displays the current units in a window takes up 7K or 235 lines of code.

Unfortunately, after more than one year since the release of V-Lab, the Developer's Kit has not yet been made available. No schedule has been set for its release, and no pricing has been set.

Other Programs

The programs reviewed above—CompositePro, ESAComp, and V-Lab—are only three of the many available. These three are the main comprehensive programs in use. Sometimes, though, a simpler program will do, or a specialized analysis must be performed. In that case, one of the programs listed in this section may provide an appropriate solution.

ASCA ASCA is a commercial Windows program published by AdTech System Research. Limited information about the program is available from http://www.adtechsystems.com/asca.html. The Web site also describes some additional programs available from AdTech.

ASCA has three modules: Composite Laminate Analysis (CLA), Free Edge Stress Analysis (FESA), and Transverse Crack Analysis (ALTRAC). The program includes a lamina material database system. The CLA module supports hygrothermoelastic point-stress analysis of laminates. Results can be viewed in tabular or graphical format.

CADEC is a program to accompany *Introduction to Composite Materials Design* (Ref 3). The license requires the user to own the textbook or to use it in a university course (either as an instructor or a student). The program runs on Windows systems. It may be downloaded from http://www.cemr.wvu.edu/~ejb/cadec.html.

Although organized around the book, the program can be used on its own. Calculations are divided into five chapters: micromechanics, ply mechanics, macromechanics, failure theory, and thin-walled beams. Each chapter has a contents page with links to individual calculation pages. In general, each calculation page carries out a single calculation. For example, the micromechanics chapter has 22 calculation pages, each covering a single material property. Alternate theories are covered on different pages: E_2 can be calculated using the rule of mixtures or Halpin-Tsai theory, but the results cannot be viewed simultaneously.

Because the program is meant to be a teaching tool, applicable formulas are shown on each page. In the case of E_2 mentioned above, the Halpin-Tsai formula is shown next to the calculations. Many pages also have graphs that are automatically generated. Most micromechanics pages, for example, plot the property versus fiber volume fraction.

Material properties and laminate definitions can be stored in files for later use. Properties generated from micromechanics analyses can be stored as ply materials. All ply and laminate constants, matrices, and results (stresses and strains) can be printed and plotted. The thin-walled beam chapter can handle arbitrarily shaped cross sections.

Help is available on a per-page basis—the entire help file cannot be browsed. The help tends to be terse, with many references to the textbook. In some cases, such as the thin-walled beam definition, reference to the text would be necessary in order to use the program.

CoDA is a commercial, modular program from the National Physical Laboratory (NPL) in Teddington, United Kingdom. Modules can be purchased and run separately or in any combination. CoDA runs under Windows 3.1 or higher. A multimedia demonstration file may be downloaded from http://www.anaglyph.co.uk/coda.htm.

The program consists of four modules: Material Synthesizer, Laminate, Panel, and Beam. The Material Synthesizer module performs full three-dimensional micromechanics calculations for unidirectional, random, continuous, and discontinuous fiber composites. Elastic, temperature, and moisture constants are calculated. Resulting ply properties can be used in the other modules.

The Laminate module is used to determine elastic, hygrothermal, and strength properties of laminated panels. The Panel module is used for the analysis of rectangular and circular panels under load. Panels are of arbitrary lay-up and may include rib stiffeners. The supported load types are point, line, and pressure. Results include stresses, deflections, and creep behavior. The Beam module is similar to the Panel module and supports several standard cross sections, load types, and boundary conditions.

COMPASS is a specialized program developed by The George Washington University and NASA Goddard. Executable binaries are freely available for HP, IBM, Sun, and SGI UNIX systems. The binaries and the User's Manual can be downloaded from http://mscweb.gsfc.nasa.gov/543web/compass/compass.html.

COMPASS performs a three-dimensional failure analysis of composite laminates. It uses a finite-element solution based on eight-node solid isoparametric elements. Layers may be composed of fiber reinforced composites or isotropic materials. Two solution approaches are available: (1) a nonlinear progressive failure analysis using the Von Mises criterion for isotropic plies and the Hashin criterion for composite plies and (2) delamination growth analysis using Griffith's criterion for the fracture mechanics approach.

ESDU International. Unlike the other products reviewed here, ESDU does not provide a single software package, but collections of engineering design data, methods, and software. The information is packaged in more than 1200 design guides that are grouped by Series. Most of the Series are related to mechanical and aerospace engineering. In addition to composites, other Series topics include dynamics, mechanisms, structures, and acoustics.

Each Series is further divided into Volumes, and Volumes are subdivided into Data Items. Each Data Item contains documentation in PDF format, FORTRAN source code for the calculations described in the document, a compiled DOS executable, and sample input and output files. The PDF documents provide the full theory for the Data Item, not just a description of the program. Thus, the Data Items also make a good basic reference.

The ESDU Web site at http://www.esdu.com provides a full listing of all Series, Volumes, and Data Items. Abstracts for each Data Item can be viewed at no charge; subscribers can download Data Items after logging in.

The Composites Series contains seven Volumes with 38 Data Items. Topics covered include basic laminate analysis, buckling of balanced and unbalanced plates, bonded joints, failure criteria, damping and acoustic loading, and natural vibration. Many special cases are covered, such as plates with holes, through-thickness shear stiffness, sandwich panels, edge delamination, and more.

The Laminator is a Windows shareware program for calculating laminate properties and performing point-stress analyses. It is available for download from http://tni.net/~mlindell/laminator.html.

The Laminator is a simple program, which makes it the right choice for a quick laminate analysis. Ply properties (engineering constants, thermal and moisture expansion coefficients, and strengths) are entered in a simple table. Up to ten properties may be stored in a file. The laminate is likewise entered in a table, with arbitrary materials, angles, and thicknesses for each ply. Loads include mechanical (forces and moments or strains and curvatures), temperature, and moisture components. Results are displayed in a plain text file and include all constants, matrices, stresses, strains, and load factors.

LAP is a commercial program from anaglyph Ltd., running on Windows 95 or higher. A program overview and a multimedia demo are available at http://www.anaglyph.co.uk/lap.htm.

LAP is used to perform point-stress analysis on laminates. It includes a database for storing ply properties and laminate definitions. Full hygrothermoelastic load conditions and results are supported, including residual curing strains. Two unique features of the program are calculation of the effects of deviation from nominal fiber volume and stiffness reduction factors based on layer failure. In the latter case, an iterative solution is used to give a nonlinear laminate stiffness response past the failure point. In addition to tabular and graphical output, interfaces are provided for export to text files, CoDA, and NASTRAN.

PROMAL. Like CADEC, PROMAL is a teaching program. It accompanies *Mechanics of Composite Materials* (Ref 4). PROMAL is distributed with the textbook, or course licenses are available directly from the author. Information about the book and the program can be found at http://www.eng.usf.edu/~kaw/promal/book.html.

PROMAL includes five separate programs, accessible from the master menu. The first program is a matrix calculator, mainly intended to aid in solving homework problems. The second is a database for holding lamina properties. Up to 100 materials are supported. Properties include engineering constants, lamina thickness, strengths, and thermal and moisture expansion coefficients. The third program is simply a utility for fixing database problems.

The fourth program performs micromechanical analyses. Elastic and hygrothermal properties are calculated; properties can be plotted against fiber volume fraction. The fifth and sixth programs perform macromechanical analyses of laminas and laminates, respectively. Results include all laminate constants, matrices, stresses, strains, and failure envelopes, in both tabular and graphical format.

SACL. The Stanford Structures and Composites Lab maintains a large collection of programs related to composites and structures. A full list of the programs, as well as contact information for the collections, is available from http://structure.stanford.edu/CodeDesc.html.

The general areas covered by the programs are Manufacturing, Impact, Joints, Delamination, Design, Smart Structures, and Environment. Most programs are distributed as FORTRAN 77 source code. A few are available in other languages or as Macintosh executables.

The Think Composites software package, developed by Dr. Stephen Tsai, includes the Mic-Mac spreadsheet, GenLam, and LamRank. Information about the package, plus a "lite" version of Mic-Mac, is available from http://www.thinkComp.com. That site also includes a downloadable version of *Theory of Composites Design* (Ref 5) in PDF format. Documentation for the Think Composites software is in the textbook.

Mic-Mac is a Microsoft Excel spreadsheet for performing point-stress laminate analysis. The spreadsheet is not protected, allowing it to be modified for additional calculations, but the lack of program documentation makes customization difficult. GenLam is a simple program for point-stress analysis, using simple text files as a database and for input. Finally, LamRank is a laminate-optimization program using the ranking method.

Internet Resources

Over the past few years, the Internet has become an invaluable source of both business and technical information. Its usefulness spans many industries, including composites. Within the composites industry, the Internet can be used for obtaining material data sheets, locating a manufacturer, and even researching and purchasing software.

On-line Programs

A few Web sites have started offering on-line programs. These are run directly from the remote site, usually as a Java applet. Although the current programs are of limited functionality, more capable programs should be expected in the future as the offerings of application service providers (ASPs) increases. Even now, major engineering tools such as Alibre Design (Ref 6) for three-dimensional computer-aided design (CAD) and e.VisualNastran 4D (Ref 7) for finite-element analysis are offered on-line on a subscription basis.

Classical Laminate Theory with Java (http://mlbf01.fbm.hs-bremen.de/java/applets/javalam.html). This is a little Java applet that calculates laminate stiffnesses, laminate strains, and ply stresses. Ply properties are calculated from a selection of five fibers and three matrices. Laminates can contain up to 20 plies. Loads are entered as stress and bending resultants, plus change in temperature. Results are printed in a tabular format. The program is very simple, with a promise of future extensions. A more powerful stand-alone version is available for download.

Think Composites (http://www.thinkComp.com). Dr. Stephen Tsai offers an on-line, interactive tutorial covering stress, strain, and ply properties transformations; failure criteria for plies and laminates; and laminated plate theory. There are 18 pages in all, each with a brief discussion of a single topic; some pages include a Java applet to demonstrate the principles. The Java applets run in the main browser window, so they cannot be viewed simultaneously with the text. The applets range from a Mohr's circle calculator to a laminate calculator showing constitutive matrices, engineering constants and failure envelopes (limited to the 11 materials from *Theory of Composites Design* and a four-θ laminate family). The site also offers *Theory of Composites Design* in PDF format, plus the lite version of the Mic-Mac spreadsheet. Free registration is required.

The University of Delaware's Center for Composite Materials (http://www.ccm.udel.edu/) offers eight on-line programs for analysis and learning. The programs are written in Java and are provided through an ASP server; the learning modules require Shockwave. The topics covered by the programs are composite properties analysis, preform properties analysis, cure-cycle design, mold-filling design, permeability analysis and laminate properties analysis. Each module has a descriptive overview, a theoretical overview with references and an applet. The modules load and run fairly quickly. Results are displayed in tabular or graphical format. A limited on-line database of material properties is available for each module, or users can enter their own properties. Inputs cannot be saved.

On-Line Resources

Software no longer has to be ordered through print catalogs; most publishers offer direct on-line sales. Some third-party sites offer downloads of engineering freeware, shareware, and demo programs; others provide summary or detailed reviews and categorized links to program home pages. A few on-line stores specialize in engineering and even composite programs. Some of the more useful sites are:

- About Composite Materials (http://composite.about.com/cs/software/): Comprehensive listing of composite and related engineering programs with links to publisher home pages and brief reviews. Offers detailed reviews of some programs.
- ASME Engineering Software Database (http://www.mecheng.asme.org): A large collection of engineering shareware and freeware. Browse by category or search by keyword.
- E-Composites.com (http://www.e-composites.com/software_store.htm): On-line composite software store divided into two categories: Analysis and Design, and Manufacturing.
- ER-Online (http://www.er-online.co.uk/software.htm) Brief reviews of engineering programs with links to publisher home pages.
- Lycos Directory, Software for Engineering (http://dir.lycos.com/Science/Technology/Software_for_Engineering/): Links to engineering software companies and download pages organized by category.
- NetComposites (http://www.netcomposites.com): On-line composite software and bookstore. Offers brief reviews of software and international ordering.
- Sector Systems Company (http://www.marblehead.com/business/034/mech.htm): CD-ROM of mechanical engineering shareware. On-line listing of programs only; no downloads.
- Simtel.net (http://www.simtel.net/simtel.net/win95/engin.html): Engineering section of this large, general archive.
- Softseek.com (http://www.softseek.com/Education_and_Science/Science_and_Engineering/): Engineering and science section of this large, general archive.

REFERENCES

1. W.C. Young and R.G. Budynas, *Roark's Formulas for Stress and Strain*, 7th ed., McGraw-Hill, 2001
2. *Composite Materials Handbook,* MIL-HDBK-17, U.S. Army Research Laboratory, Materials Sciences Corporation, and University of Delaware Center for Composite Materials, http://mil-17.udel.edu
3. E.J. Barbero, *Introduction to Composite Materials Design,* Taylor & Francis, 1999
4. A.K. Kaw, *Mechanics of Composite Materials,* CRC Press, 1997
5. S.W. Tsai, *Theory of Composites Design*, Think Composites, 1992
6. Alibre.com, Alibre Design, http://www.alibre.com
7. Engineering-e.com, e.visualNastran 4D, http://www.engineering-e.com/computing/

Testing and Analysis Correlation

Adam J. Sawicki, The Boeing Company

COMPOSITE STRUCTURAL STRENGTH is primarily driven by various forms of discontinuities. During design development, rigorous analyses are needed to predict load distribution and local stress concentrations. Many of the same structural details that cause fatigue concerns with metals require ultimate strength assessment for composites (e.g., cutouts and attachments). Finite element models with sufficient mesh refinement may be needed to predict composite stress concentrations, and reliable failure criteria must be in place for accurate sizing. Ideally, the latter should accurately predict the failure level and dominant failure mechanisms.

Many past composite design allowables approaches have used tension and compression data from uniaxially loaded small-notch coupons (e.g., open hole compression and filled hole tension) to write margins of safety for points in a structure. These approaches are only rigorously applicable to small notches in near-uniform stress fields. Alternative sizing methods, involving design values derived from analysis and test correlation, are likely needed for combined stress states and stress concentrations associated with local structural detail or significant damage. For example, test results have shown that the allowed local stresses near an access hole will likely exceed those for near-uniform stress fields. The associated concentrated stress fields for an access hole can result in localized damage formation and material softening without catastrophic failure.

Composite materials have complicated failure mechanisms; strain softening behavior is often involved in the local failure process. Accurate prediction of composite structural detail strength requires a detailed understanding of the significant failure mechanisms. For example, efforts to model composite interlaminar stresses, progressive damage growth, and other nonlinear effects require advanced modeling tools and accurate structural representation. It is typically not enough to develop good correlation for small coupons. Advanced analyses must be correlated with sub-component-level tests before they can be considered validated.

Detailed analyses and test correlations are typically required to support design development, structural sizing, and certification. The supporting test program should focus on design details, load cases, environmental conditions, damage types, and damage locations judged to be most critical or difficult to analyze. The test results should be used to scrutinize analytical predictions of deflections and strains up to and including the point of failure, as well as the actual failure sequence and mode. For most purposes, sufficient analytical validation is not achieved by merely obtaining test results that are greater than the required design load.

Critical local details (e.g., cutout, pad-up lay-ups, mechanical attachment areas, curved laminate radii, transversely loaded stiffener details, and post-buckled panels) should be evaluated at test scales large enough to address structural load paths and specific processes and material forms early in a program. The sizing analysis tools should be updated as required based on these test results. This approach should help support the design by eliminating "poor structural details" that could result in expensive, premature full-scale test failures.

The best available analyses should be performed to support definition of the test plan (e.g., loading sequence, gage placement, and instrumentation). Some differences between configured subcomponent test data and pretest predictions are likely. Possible sources of differences may occur near panel boundaries (load introduction points and edge effects), joints, damage, and other areas of load redistribution. It is important to understand these differences to:

- Ensure sufficient testing is performed to overcome analysis limitations
- Improve structural analysis schemes
- Develop scaling relationships with building block test results
- Ensure structural test parts have sufficient gage section
- Improve failure mode resolution and failure criteria accuracy

Final analysis schemes for configured composite structure should be aimed at predicting specific failure modes. For example, analytical methods should be able to distinguish between the following bolted-joint failure modes: net section, shear-out, end splitting, or pure bearing (compression). The methods development process is likely to involve several test and analysis iterations.

The "Building Block" Approach to Structural Qualification

In the design of aerospace composite structures, "building block" qualification programs are frequently conducted to verify the capability of the structure under design loads. This method utilizes a combination of tests and supporting analyses to minimize developmental risk, cost, and weight. A fundamental understanding of the purpose of the various levels of a building block program, along with the type and complexity of analyses used in interpreting test data at the various levels, is critical in achieving risk mitigation and cost minimization objectives.

Figure 1 presents a simplified overview of the building block method of structural qualification (Ref 1). The approach involves a testing sequence of progressively more complex structural coupons, elements, subcomponents, and so forth, throughout the design development process (Ref 2). Tests and supporting analyses of varying complexity are performed to fulfill four primary requirements:

- Generate strength and stiffness data to be used in structural analysis of the design
- Substantiate the load-carrying capability of the design
- Mitigate risk by testing specific design details prior to full-scale evaluation
- Verify accuracy of analysis predictions used in the design process

Tests and Analyses Vary with Building Block Level. The types of tests performed at each of the levels vary due to the different requirements and issues addressed at each level of the building block plan. At the material qualification level, tests are conducted to establish strength and stiffness data, verify environmental resistance, and generate specifications for procurement and quality control. Test specimens are primarily small coupons (notched and unnotched) with limited variation in lay-up (typically unidirectional, 0°; cross-ply, ±45°; and limited multidirectional lay-ups). Consequently, supporting analysis is generally limited to strength and stiffness calculation, along with general sizing analysis to promote the onset of a desired mode of failure.

At the other extreme of the building block plan, components and full scale articles are used to verify load distribution predictions (typically generated using a global finite element analysis), demonstrate load-carrying capability under a variety of design conditions, and assess failure modes for complex structures. Specimen boundary and load introduction conditions are more representative of the actual structure than in lower-level tests. The level of complexity permits incorporation of representative details (shear clips, cutouts, etc.) and thus allows examination of secondary loading effects. As verification of load path modeling is of primary importance, the effects of factors such as environment, damage, and defects are often not assessed at this level (Ref 1). It should be noted that tests performed at the structural element level and above produce data in support of a particular program or structure. Data produced in the material qualification and allowables phases are material related and are not, on their own, sufficient for structural qualification.

This article addresses issues concerning building block levels ranging from design-allowables coupons up through subcomponents, as these levels exhibit a wide variety of test-analysis correlation objectives. At these levels, enhanced analysis capability can be used most effectively in minimizing test complexity and cost while also reducing design weight and risk (Ref 3). Examples of tests for which good correlative capability has shown significant benefit are discussed. Additional information about the building-block approach is provided in the article "Overview of Testing and Certification" in this Volume.

Design Allowables Coupons

The primary purpose of tests conducted at the design allowables level is to generate strength data used for predicting the in-plane and out-of-plane strength capability of the structure. Consequently, analysis correlation work in this area centers on strength and failure-mode prediction. Examples of tests conducted at this level include notched (open and/or filled hole) tension and compression, inter/intralaminar shear and tension, and pin bearing. While many specimen details remain fairly generic, the lay-ups, stress concentrations, environmental effects, and failure modes tested are more representative of the actual structure than they are at the material qualification level.

Notched Laminate Strength Prediction Methods

The generation of notched strength allowables provides an excellent example of the benefits of good analytical correlation with test data. As these are generated as a generic design property, the data obtained must cover the envelope of permissible lay-ups utilized throughout the design. Unlike metals, little relief of the elastic stress concentration arising at an open or filled hole due to plastic deformation is observed in composites, resulting in a strong relationship between lay-up, failure mode, and associated strength (Ref 1, 2). An example of this is shown in Fig. 2, which exhibits the relationship between failure mode and the angle minus loaded (AML) plies laminate-configuration parameter (% ± 45° plies – % 0° plies) observed in open hole compression testing of several materials (Ref 4). Statistical testing across the complete laminate family to assess strength properties would be exorbitantly expensive. Therefore, an

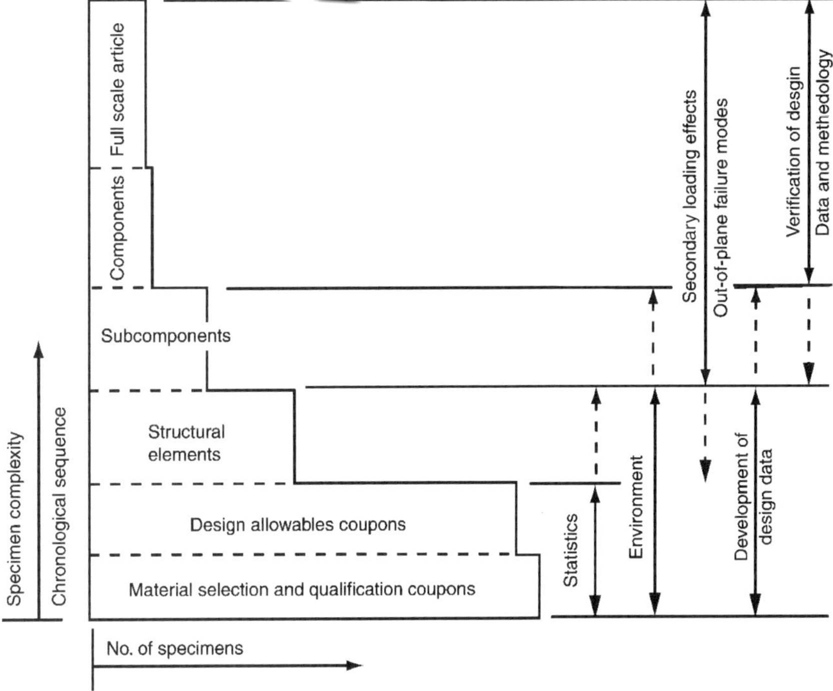

Fig. 1 Outline of the building-block methodology for qualification of composite structure. Source: Ref 1

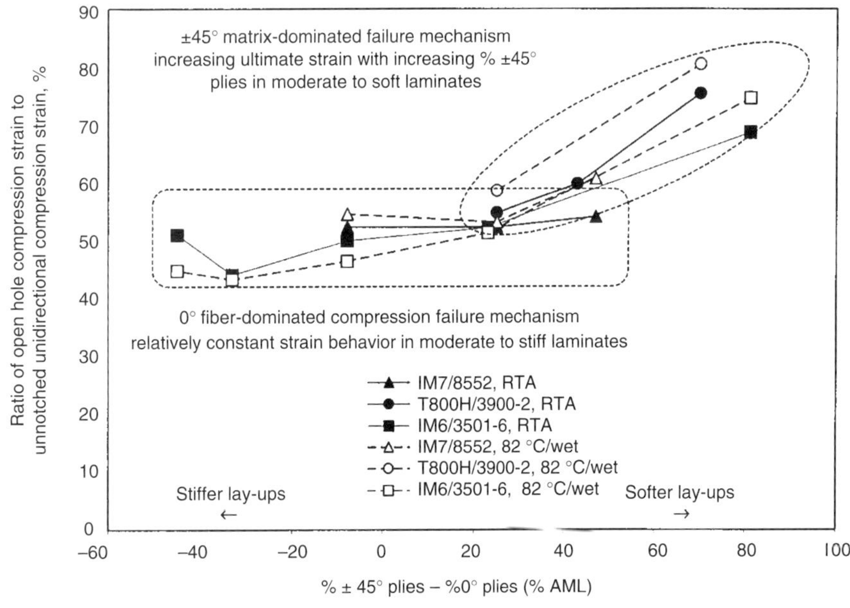

Fig. 2 Variation in failure modes for open hole compression specimens due to lay-up. RTA is Room Temperature ambient. Source: Ref 4

analytical method for relating strength to laminate-configuration is necessary to reduce the cost of generating these design data.

Stress and strain fields for notched anisotropic materials such as composite laminates can be determined using close-formed solutions such as those used by Lekhnitskii (Ref 5) or by finite element and finite difference techniques. Strength prediction is more complex due to the "hole-size effect," in which the ratio of notched to unnotched strength varies with hole diameter. This effect results from a number of factors, including greater localized stress gradients that promote stress-relieving subcritical damage formation near small holes, as well as the greater probability of defects and low strength material in the highly stressed region of a large hole (Ref 6).

Notched strength prediction has received much attention in the literature, and several predictive methods have been developed. Extensive reviews of models for predicting notched stress fields and strength for composites were documented in the mid-1980s by Crews (Ref 6), Curtis and Grant (Ref 7), and Awerbuch and Madhukar (Ref 8). Methods utilized up to that time included linear elastic fracture mechanics (Ref 9), two-parameter approaches including point and average stress criteria (Ref 10), and critical stress gradient (Ref 11). While successful in predicting the effect of hole size on strength for a given laminate configuration, such models are less effective in predicting the strength of lay-ups exhibiting significant stress-strain nonlinearity and subcritical damage formation.

Since the mid-1980s, additional notched strength predictive models utilizing progressive damage, finite element analysis (Ref 12, 13) and the spline variational technique (Ref 14) have been developed. These have utilized experimental data documenting subcritical damage formation to calibrate models for progressive damage formation and growth, as exemplified in Fig. 3 (Ref 13). Such models have been useful in predicting relationships between lay-up, failure mode, and far field failure strain semiempirically. Figure 4 shows an example of this provided by Bau (Ref 4), who used Chang's two-dimensional progressive damage methodology (Ref 12) to predict open hole compression failure of tape laminates.

Prediction of Strain Fields and Damage Formation

For notched laminates, test-analysis correlation is most frequently performed for prediction of strain fields and subcritical damage formation.

Strain Correlation. Localized strain data is most frequently obtained using strain gages; for notched coupons, axial strain gages are most commonly used. Gages are typically used in obtaining strain data local to the notch or hole at the location of peak axial stress concentration, in far-field locations, and in strain-gradient locations.

Gradients can also be assessed using photoelastic and shadow-moiré techniques, in which photoelastic sheets of material are bonded to the test specimen. As the specimen is strained, bands of differing color appear (as observed using an optical device). The bands correspond to the difference in principal strains within the specimen. An example of such an evaluation is Fig. 5, in which the shape and magnitude of photoelastic bands are compared to analysis predictions for the difference in principal strains in a uniaxially loaded coupon specimen containing a slit (Ref 15).

Test analysis correlation for local strains is influenced by several factors, among which are strain gradients, stress-strain nonlinearity, fastener-hole contact, and subcritical damage formation. Examples of how these factors influence test analysis correlation are provided by examining Fig. 6, which compares test data to finite-element-based predictions for strain at the edge of an open or filled hole under compressive loading (Ref 16). In strain fields with high gradients, correlation of predictions for specific strain levels with test data can be difficult due to the averaging effect of strain measurement under the area covered by the gage element. This accounts for the difference between measured and predicted strain seen in Fig. 6; despite the relatively small size of the gage element utilized in these experiments, there remains a finite distance from the hole over which strains are averaged in the gage measurement. Better correlation between predicted and measured strains can be achieved when the size of the elements used at the stress concentration approximates the size of the strain-gage element.

Nonlinearity in material stiffness properties results in the nonlinear strain measurement trend shown in Fig. 6 for both the open and filled hole cases. Such trends are not accounted for in analysis predictions when averaged stiffness properties are utilized; however, modern finite element codes can account for such nonlinear stiffness properties. The analyst must be aware of modeling assumptions regarding stiffness properties when assessing such nonlinearities.

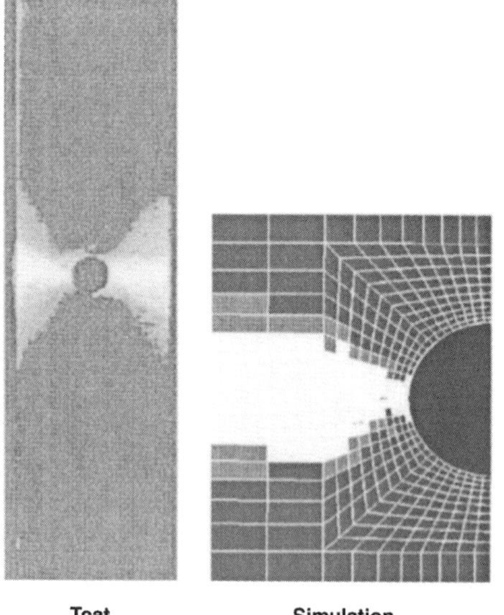

Fig. 3 Comparison of damage detected by X-radiograph with progressive damage finite element analysis prediction for open hole tension specimens. T800/3900-2 composite, $[(0°/\pm45°/90°)_2]_s$, 25 mm (1 in.) wide, 6 mm (0.25 in.) diam. Source: Ref 13

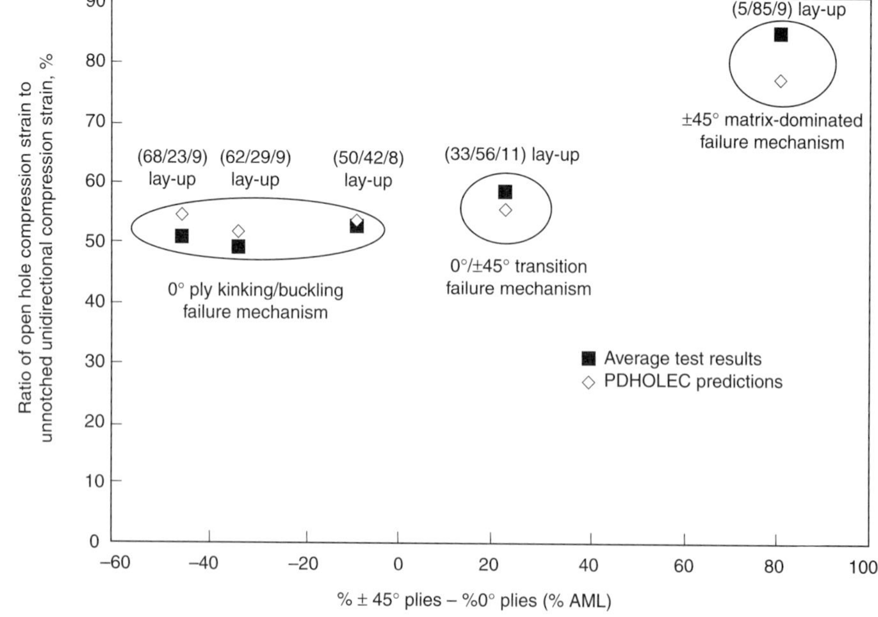

Fig. 4 Comparison of predicted and experimental strains and failure modes for IM6/3501-6 tape open hole compression specimens in 82 °C (180 °F)/wet conditions. Source: Ref 4

Fastener-hole contact is evidenced by the sudden change in load-strain slope exhibited by the filled hole specimens shown in Fig. 6. If a finite clearance is present in the specimen on manufacture, initially filled hole compression specimens will exhibit load strain behavior equivalent to that of open-hole compression specimens. When the laminate deforms such that the hole surface contacts the fastener, an alternative load path is formed (see Fig. 7). The onset of fastener-hole contact changes the strain and stress distribution about the hole, as shown in Fig. 8, as the peak stress concentration decreases and bearing stresses arise at the contact surfaces. This phenomenon occurred at different load levels for the Fig. 6 specimens due to differences in initial clearance. After fastener-hole contact was achieved, the rate of increase of strain with load decreased at the measured location, resulting in a steeper load-strain trend.

Subcritical, or noncatastrophic, damage formation is evidenced by sharp, sudden changes (most often decreases) in measured strain. In notched laminates, measurement of such subcritical failures is infrequently recorded by strain gages, because the relevant failure mechanisms (splits and delaminations) tend to change the measured strain gradients only slightly prior to final, catastrophic failure. This is especially true for notched compression failure, as the onset of subcritical damage tends to precipitate catastrophic failure. It should be noted that one set (curve 4) of filled-hole compression data in Fig. 6 did detect the onset of noncatastrophic damage, however.

Damage Correlation. Subcritical damage formation (fiber-matrix splits and delaminations) can be detected using destructive and nondestructive techniques. In both cases, tests are stopped at specified load levels such that the relative state and size of damage can be assessed incrementally. Destructive assessment is generally performed through sectioning of the laminate specimen at highly strained locations, followed by microscopic observation. Nondestructive assessment can be performed using x-radiographs (for splits and delaminations) and ultrasonic methods (most effective for delaminations). Nondestructive methods provide greater information on the overall state of damage than does destructive assessment but are less accurate in providing size and through-thickness location information than is destructive assessment. Such data are particularly useful in comparing progressive damage-analysis predictions using finite-element and cubic-spline techniques, as shown in Fig. 3.

Bolted Joints

Depending on the type of specimens, bolted joint tests can be conducted at either the design allowables level (for generation of design data) or the element level (for verification of joint sizing methodology). As with notched-strength coupons, analysis correlation work centers on strength and failure-mode prediction but also involves fastener-load distribution calculation. Specimen details are generally more representative of the actual structure than basic notched allowable coupons, as fastener type, clamp-up torque, and three-dimensional loading effects must be accounted for.

Bearing Strength Correlation

As with notched strength, bearing design data must cover the envelope of lay-ups used throughout the design. However, bearing deformation and damage are generally less sensitive to lay-up effects than is notched strength. Consequently, geometry-influenced failure modes

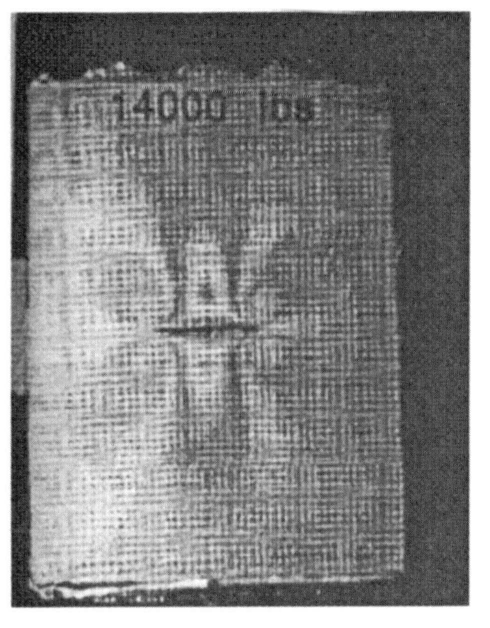

(a)

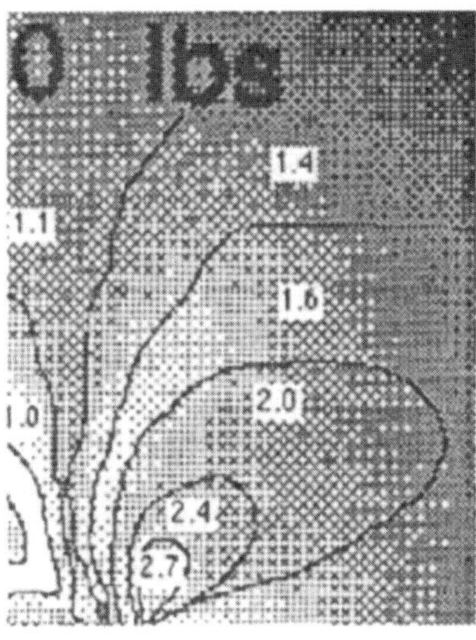

(b)

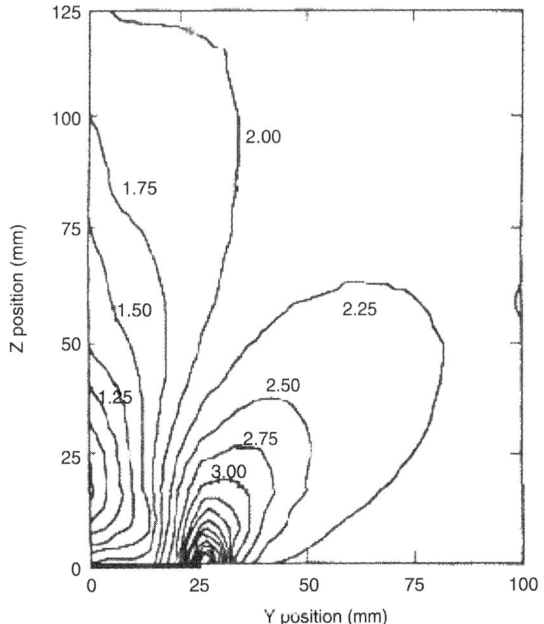

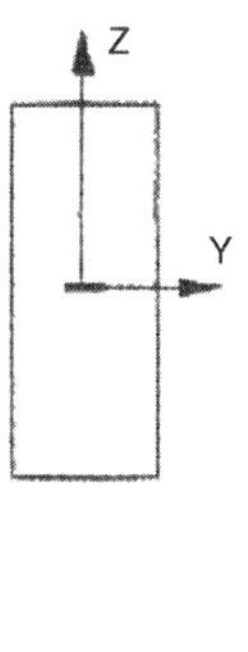

(c)

Fig. 5 Comparison of photoelastic fringe patterns with finite element analysis strain gradient predictions for a uniaxial coupon containing a slit. (a) Photograph of photoelastic test result. (b) Computer-enhanced image of test result. (c) Analysis prediction for photoelastic patterns. Source: Ref 15

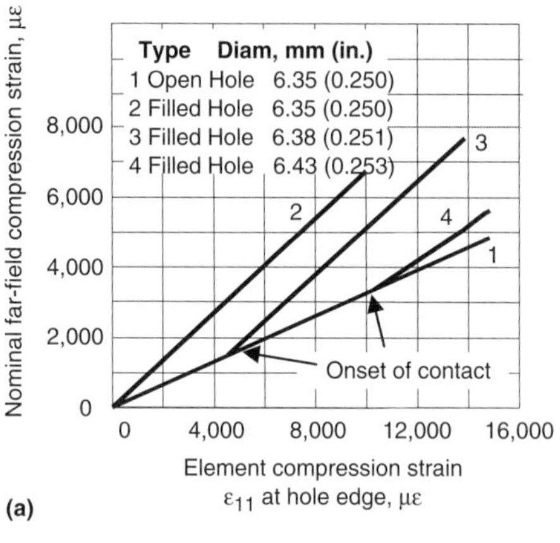

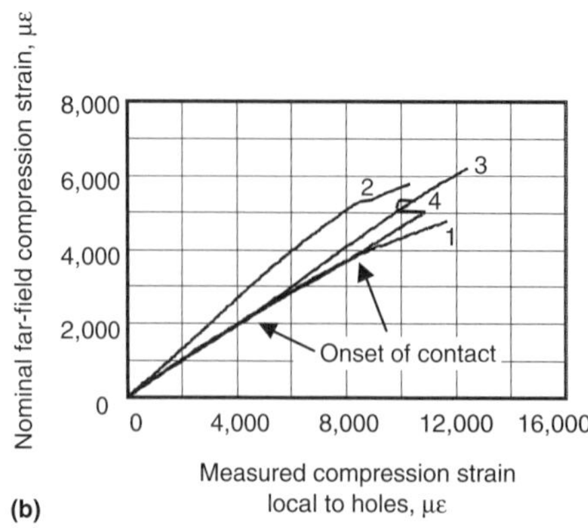

Fig. 6 Comparison of (a) predicted and (b) experimental load versus strain behavior for T800/3900-2 tape (angle minus loaded plies, AML, parameter = –8) open-hole and filled-hole compression specimens. Source: Ref 16

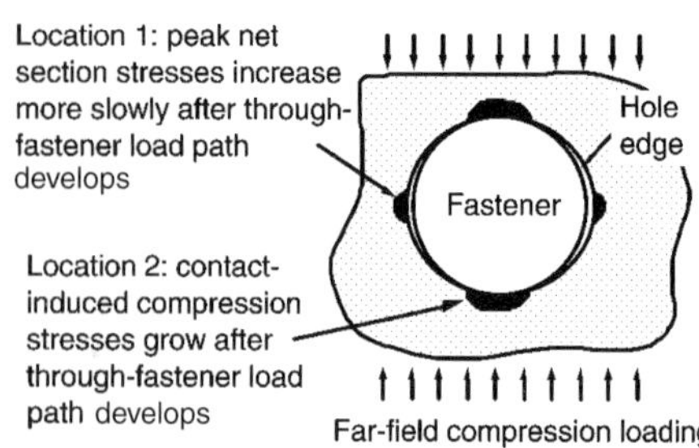

Fig. 7 Development of through-fastener load path at a filled hole under compression loading. Source: Ref 16

are more sensitive to the laminate configuration than is bearing damage (Ref 1). This is due to the significant amount of subcritical damage that forms as the fastener hole elongates. Final failure results from the onset of a geometry-influenced failure mode (shown in Fig. 1 of the article "Element and Subcomponent Testing" in this Volume), such as shear-out, cleavage, or net tension (Ref 17). Significant variations in bearing strength will tend to occur at extreme laminate configurations, due to the premature onset of a geometry-influenced mode of failure.

Bearing stress fields are not as easily determined as notched specimen stress fields. As discussed by Crews, this results from the need to model fastener-hole contact, friction, three-dimensional geometrical constraints, and through-thickness stress gradients (Ref 6). As with notched-strength prediction, bearing damage and strength prediction have been studied extensively. Early methods used several simplifying assumptions, such as a two-dimensional cosine distribution of bearing stress on the hole boundary (Ref 6); strength prediction methods included linear elastic fracture mechanics (Ref 18) and two-parameter approaches (Ref 19). Subsequently, progressive-damage finite-element analysis (Ref 13) and spline variational methods (Ref 20) have been developed.

Bearing strain field data can be obtained using strain gages, and correlation is influenced by factors such as strain gradients, stress-strain nonlinearity, fastener-hole contact, subcritical damage formation, and fastener deformation. However, subcritical damage formation (hole elongation) and fastener deformation are by far the greatest contributors to inelastic behavior, and correlation is most frequently performed using crosshead deflection or extensometer data. An example of this is provided in Fig. 9, which compares three-dimensional-finite element-based deformation predictions to load-deflection data (Ref 13). Subcritical damage formation is evidenced by gradual changes in the load-deflection curve slope. It should be noted that nonlinear load-deflection behavior of this type can also be caused by bending and plastic deformation of the fastener and that extraction of separate composite bearing and fastener load-deflection nonlinearities from such data is quite difficult.

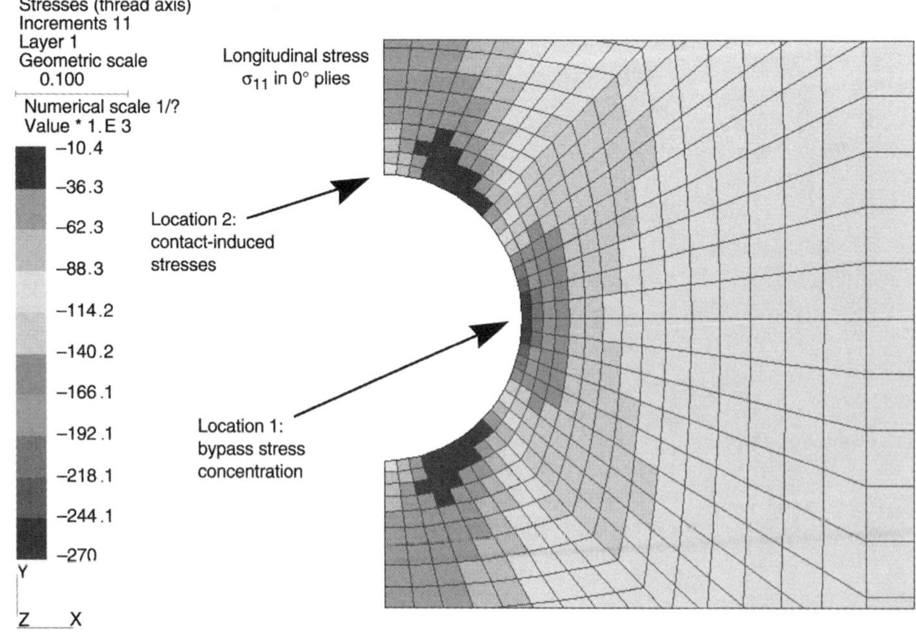

Fig. 8 Typical post-contact stress distribution in filled-hole compression specimen, demonstrating onset of contact-induced bearing stresses. Source: Ref 16

Bearing-Bypass Analysis

Multi-fastener joint specimens require a two-step analysis process. First, the load distribution between fasteners must be determined. Once this has been accomplished, the interaction of bypass and bearing stress fields, and its influence upon strength, can be determined.

Fastener Load Distribution. For composites, fastener load distributions are calculated using methods similar to those developed for metal

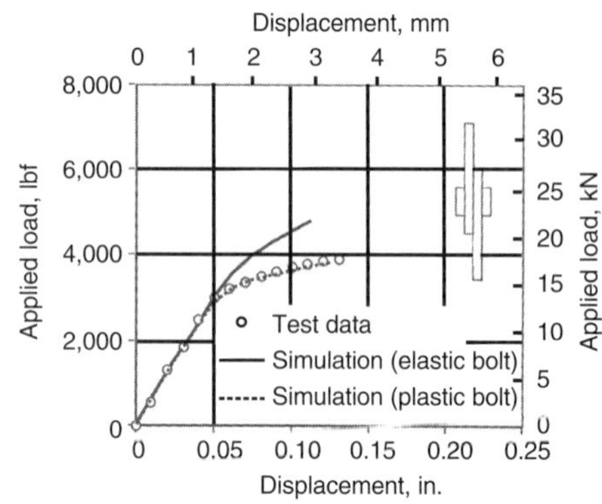

Fig. 9 Comparison of predicted and experimental load-displacement behavior for tension bearing specimen, single-lap joint. T800/3900-2 composite; $[(0°/\pm 45°/90°)_2]_s$; 50 mm (2 in.) wide, 6 mm (0.25 in.) diam; width-to-diameter ratio, 8; edge distance-to-diameter ratio, 6; clamp-up force, 3.6 kN (800 lbf). Source: Ref 13

joint structures, namely compatibility/equilibrium and finite-element-based solutions dependent upon adherend (plate) stiffness and fastener flexibility (Ref 21–22). Such models are developed through semiempirical calibration with test data to determine fastener flexibilities. Test analysis correlation is most frequently performed using axial strain gages located between fasteners. Due to the gradient nature of the strain field in these regions, calibration is often performed by testing the instrumented adherends with one or more of the joint fasteners removed, such that relationships between measured strain and load introduced through fasteners "ahead" of the gage can be obtained. Using the calibration data, the load distribution among joint fasteners can be monitored throughout the test (frequently, the load distribution changes as subcritical damage forms at the fastener holes).

Bearing-Bypass Strength. Stress distributions near a fastener hole can be approximated by the superposition of stresses for the unloaded hole (bypass) and loaded hole (bearing) cases. Once stresses have been calculated, they can be used with the various failure models for unloaded and loaded holes to calculate failure mode and strength (Ref 6), among these being those of Eisenmann (Ref 18), Garbo (Ref 19), Crews and Naik (Ref 23–24), and Hung and Chang (Ref 25). Predictions are usually presented in a graphical nature, providing an envelope of permissible bearing stresses and bypass strains (see Fig. 10). As would be expected, test-analysis correlation issues are a combination of those relevant for unloaded-hole (notched) coupons and bearing coupons. An additional source of variation in load-deflection nonlinearity is caused by load transfer; as shown in Fig. 11, the greater the amount of load transfer, the greater is the degree of load-deflection nonlinearity observed for the specimen due to greater subcritical bearing damage formation.

As with unloaded filled hole compression, fastener-hole clearance and contact can affect response, as evidenced by the test data shown in Fig. 12. As discussed by Crews and Naik (Ref 23) and Sawicki and Minguet (Ref 26), differences in clearance can affect both the failure mode and the strength of bearing-bypass specimens loaded in compression. The compression bearing-bypass "envelope" is characterized by a net-section compression-critical region (low bearing stresses) within which dual-sided fastener-hole contact occurs, and a bearing-critical region (high bearing stresses) within which dual-sided contact is lost (Ref 26). Proper measurement of hole and fastener diameters is necessary for accurate compression failure mode and strength prediction. It should be noted that this effect is of lesser importance for tension bearing-bypass failure.

Elements and Subcomponents

At the elements and subcomponents levels of testing, data representative of typical structural geometries are obtained (see the article "Element and Subcomponent Testing" in this Volume). Examples of the types of specimens tested are complex bolted and bonded joints, stiffened panels, beams, and sandwich panels. For elements, the data generated may be closely linked to an analysis methodology, enabling the development of design values. Frequently, the specimens are used to assess load and strain distributions near damage and defects (Ref 1). For subcomponent tests, verification of analysis and strength prediction is achieved, and critical design details (which cannot be addressed with confidence in a lower level test) are assessed (Ref 2). Statistical scatter and environmental effects may be derived from coupon and element-level test data.

Correlation Issues

Analysis correlation work for these types of specimens centers on strain distribution, strength prediction, and failure-mode prediction. Stress and strain distributions are commonly calculated using finite-element-based methods. However, the level of modeling detail is typically coarser than that in coupon-level tests. For example, rather than assessing the local strain level near a

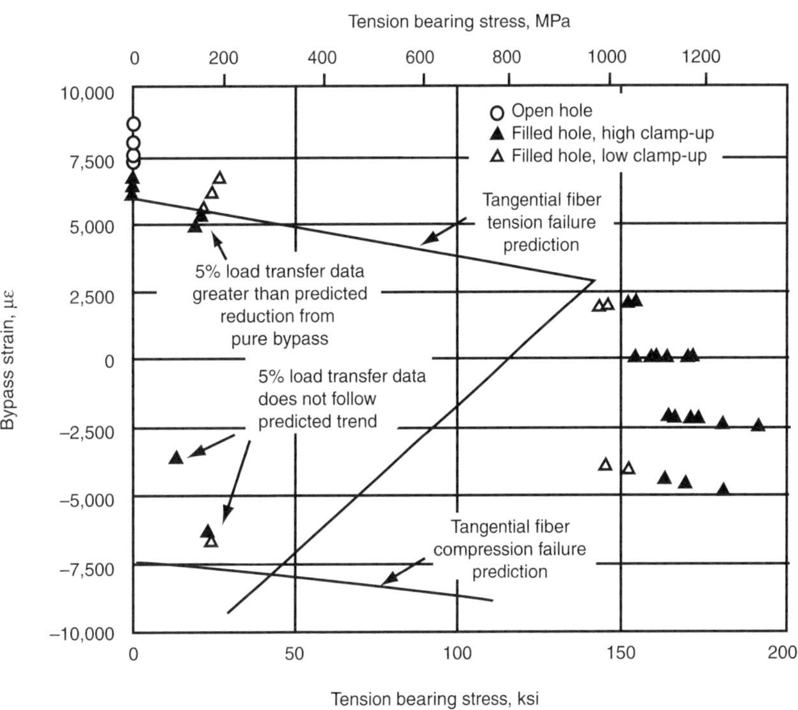

Fig. 10 Typical bearing-bypass interaction envelope and supporting test data for IM6/3501-6 tape laminates. Source: Ref 1

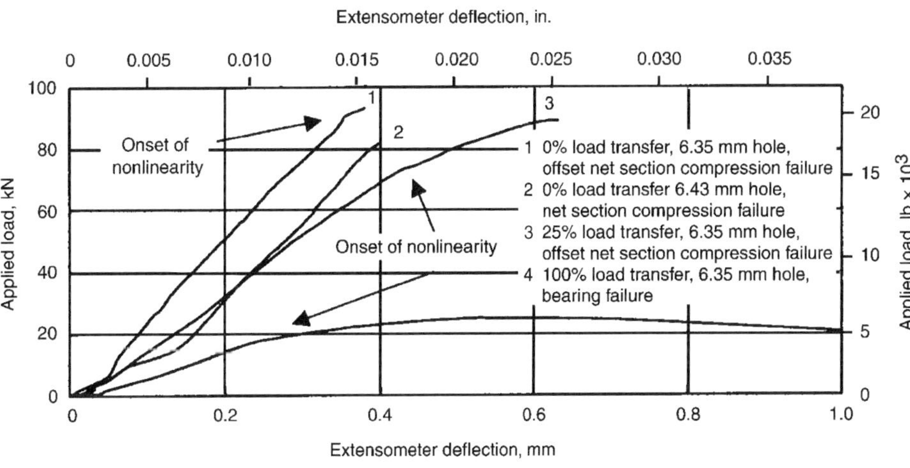

Fig. 11 Change in load-displacement nonlinearity for bolted joints with varying degrees of load transfer. Source: Ref 26

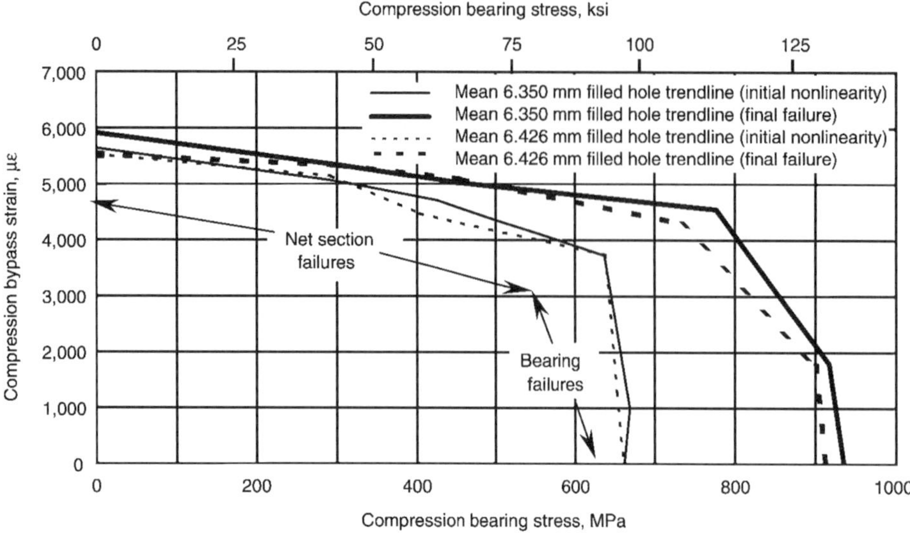

Fig. 12 Variation in compression bearing-bypass behavior due to differences in initial fastener-hole clearance. Source: Ref 26

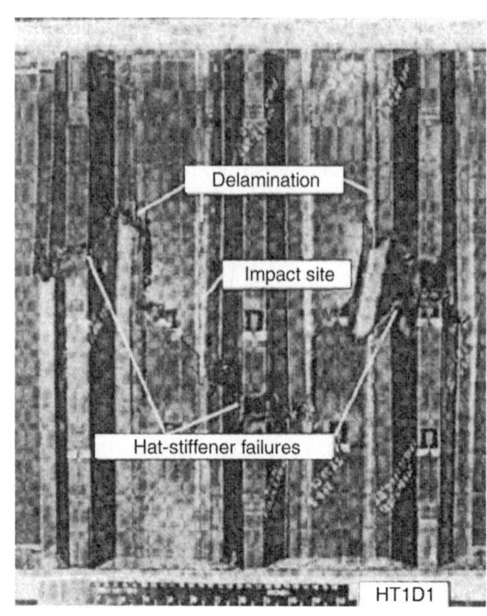

Fig. 13 Three-stringer element-level compression test specimen. Source: Ref 28

stress concentration at which failure will occur, comparisons will be made to notched far-field strain allowables obtained in the coupon-level tests. Similarly, failure mode prediction will be performed at a macro level (bearing or bypass failure) rather than at a coupon level (shear-out, fiber-dominated notched tension, etc.).

Strain and Damage Prediction. Localized strain data is most frequently obtained using strain gages; rosette strain gages are more frequently used than in simpler tests due to the need to quantify shear strains. Gages are typically used in obtaining basic section strain data, as well as in gradient locations and near stress concentrations and damage/defect locations. Gradients and damage growth can also be assessed using photoelastic coatings and shadow-moiré techniques.

Correlation issues for elements and subcomponents are similar to those for simpler specimens and include strain gradients, stress-strain nonlinearity, and subcritical damage formation/growth. It is at these levels, however, that nonlinearities related to stability are also assessed. For compression-loaded specimens (see Fig. 13), the onset of buckling frequently precipitates catastrophic failure, and strain correlation is centered on detecting and predicting the onset of buckling. Conversely, in stiffened shear panels (see Fig. 14), skins can effectively carry load through diagonal tension well past the onset of web buckling (Ref 27). For these specimens, strain correlation involves prediction of buckling as well as diagonal tension response. Stability-related strain nonlinearities are most frequently manifested through sudden changes in bending strain measurements.

Nonlinearities may also arise from the onset and growth of subcritical damage. Stiffened shear panels have exhibited good damage tolerance capability, operating well beyond the initiation of damage in webs and along stiffener bondlines. Strain gage data have been used effectively in monitoring the onset of damage growth; the stress levels at which growth begins are often used for damage-tolerant design purposes. Damage detection in these specimens primarily centers on nondestructive ultrasonic inspection while the test is being conducted, followed by destructive evaluation upon failure of the specimen.

Fig. 14 Three-stiffener element-level shear test specimen. Source: Ref 27

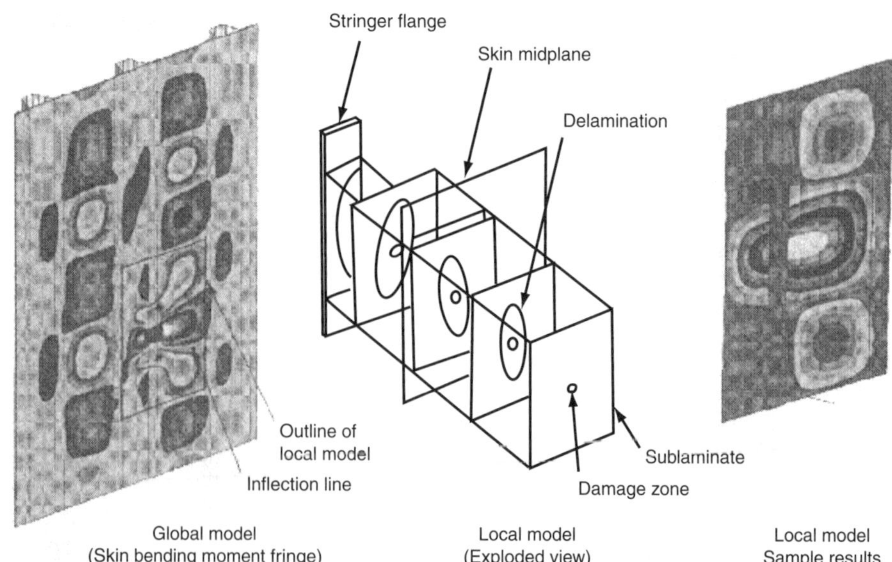

Fig. 15 Illustration of global-local modeling approach used for three-stringer compression test specimen. Source: Ref 28

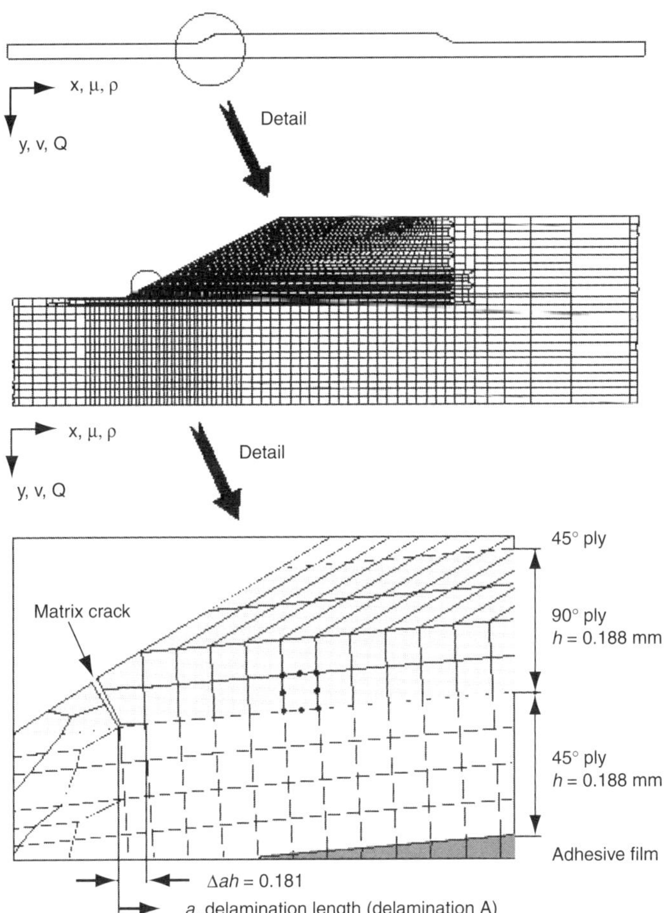

Fig. 16 Local finite-element model of a damaged bondline used in strain energy release rate calculation for bonded joints. Source: Ref 29

Failure Mode Prediction. Failure modes observed in these tests can differ from the critical failure mode as predicted by strength analysis using design allowables. This primarily results from differences in failure criteria, environment, and statistical sensitivity (Ref 1). With regard to failure criteria, some allowables are generated using conservative values for fastener torque, hole clearance, and so forth, which may not be present in a representative element or subcomponent test. For example, design strengths for net section tension and crippling are closely tied to catastrophic failure, whereas bearing and compression strengths are restricted to cutoff values, low clamp-up torque criticality, and so forth. Similarly, allowables developed for hot/wet or cold/dry criticality may not be critical in a room temperature test; subsequently, failure modes not as severely impacted by environmental effects may be found critical in a room temperature test.

Global-Local Modeling. Finite element methods have been highly effective in modeling element and subcomponent specimens containing defects, damage progression, and so forth, as they lend themselves to global-local modeling techniques. In such models, a coarse global mesh is used to account for the overall geometry, boundary conditions, loading conditions, and deformation (including post-buckled behavior) of the test specimen. Nodal deformations are monitored at the boundaries of a "patch," or group of elements locally surrounding the stress concentration. In the location of the patch, a fine local mesh is developed and modeled separately. In the local model, boundary conditions are forced to match the deformations calculated by the global model at the edge of the patch. Using the fine mesh, local stresses, strains, interlaminar strain energy release rates, damage progression, and so forth can be calculated. Stiffness changes calculated in the local model, due to damage onset and growth, are then "fed back" into the global model for use in the next iteration or load step. The global-local feedback process is then repeated until catastrophic failure is predicted.

Examples of global-local models are shown (Fig. 15 and 16). Figure 15 displays a global model containing a local patch for a stiffened compression panel, a local model of the skin containing delaminations, and local-model sample results (Ref 28). Figure 16 shows a local model for a bonded joint containing a matrix crack at the edge of the bondline. This model is used to correlate strain energy release rates to applied in-plane loads and moments for a given design detail. Data of this type are then used to predict the progression of bondline disbonds and delaminations in skin-stiffener panels (Ref 29).

Conclusions

The types of tests and analyses performed at the various building- block levels vary due to the different requirements and issues addressed at each level. Common techniques for stress, strain, strength, and failure-mode prediction can be used in the analysis of design-allowables coupons, elements, and subcomponents. Finite element techniques have proven especially useful in the modeling of contact, three-dimensional effects, postbuckling behavior, damage growth, and so forth. Model predictions are compared to data obtained from instrumentation (strain gages, photoelastic and shadow-moiré, etc.), nondestructive evaluation (ultrasonic, radiography), and destructive evaluation. As demonstrated in this article, recent finite element and cubic spline-based models have been used successfully in correlating predicted and actual damage progression in test specimens. However, more work in this area remains in transitioning these tools for use in general stress analysis.

ACKNOWLEDGMENTS

Much of the work discussed in this article would not have been possible without publication of notched strength, bolted joint, and element-level data and predictive correlation by personnel throughout the aerospace industry. Of particular note are those individuals from whose publications the author was able to obtain examples of test-analysis correlation, including P. Grant, H. Bau, J. Crews, F.-K. Chang, C. Rousseau, and P. Minguet.

REFERENCES

1. P. Grant and A. Sawicki, Relationship Between Failure Criteria, Allowables Development, and Qualification of Composite Structure, *Proc., American Helicopter Society National Technical Specialist Meeting on Rotorcraft Structures,* 30 Oct to 2 Nov 1995
2. D. Adams et al., Composites Qualification Criteria, *Proc., American Helicopter Society 51st Annual Forum,* Fort Worth, TX, 9–11 May 1995
3. A. Dobyns, B. Barr, and J. Adelmann, RAH-66 Comanche Building Block Structural Qualification Program, *Composite Structures: Theory and Practice,* STP 1383, ASTM, 2000, p 140–157
4. H. Bau, D. Hoyt, and C. Rousseau, Open Hole Compression Strength and Failure Characterization in Carbon/Epoxy Tape Laminates, *Composite Structures: Theory*

and Practice, STP 1383, ASTM, 2000, p 273–292
5. S. Lekhnitskii, *Theory of Elasticity of an Anisotropic Body,* Holden-Day, Ind. (San Francisco), 1963
6. J. Crews, A Survey of Strength Analysis Methods for Laminates with Holes, *J. Aeronaut. Soc. India,* Vol 36 (No. 4), 1984, p 287–303
7. A. Curtis and P. Grant, The Strength of Carbon Fibre Composite Plates with Loaded and Unloaded Holes, *Compos. Struct.,* Vol 2, 1984, p 201–221
8. J. Awerbuch and M. Madhukar, Notched Strength of Composite Laminates: Predictions and Experiments—a Review, *J. Reinf. Plast. Compos.,* Vol 4, 1985, p 3–159
9. M. Waddoups, J. Eisenmann, and B. Kaminski, Macroscopic Fracture Mechanics of Advanced Composite Materials, *J. Compos. Mater.,* Vol 5, 1971, p 446–454
10. J. Whitney and R. Nuismer, Stress Fracture Criteria for Laminated Composites Containing Stress Concentrations, *J. Compos. Mater.,* Vol 8, 1974, p 256–265
11. G. Caprino, J. Halpin, and L. Nicolais, Fracture Mechanics in Composite Materials, *Composites,* Vol 10, 1979, p 223–227
12. F.-K. Chang and L. Lessard, Damage Tolerance of Laminated Composites Containing an Open Hole and Subjected to Compressive Loadings: Part I—Analysis and Part II—Experiment, *J. Compos. Mater.,* Vol 25, 1990
13. X. Qing, H.-T. Sun, and F.-K. Chang, Damage Tolerance-Based Design of Bolted Composite Joints, *Composite Structures: Theory and Practice,* STP 1383, ASTM, 2000, p 140–157
14. E. Iarve, 3-D Stress Analysis in Laminated Composites with Fasteners Based on the B-spline Approximation, *Compos. Part A,* Vol 28A, 1997, p 559–571
15. A. Sawicki, "Damage Tolerance of Integrally Stiffened Composite Plates and Cylinders," master of science thesis, Department of Aeronautics and Astronautics, Massachusetts Institute of Technology, 1990
16. A. Sawicki and P. Minguet, Failure Mechanisms in Compression-Loaded Composite Laminates Containing Open and Filled Holes, *J. Reinf. Plast. Compos.,* Vol 18 (No. 18), 1999, p 1708–1728
17. MIL-HDBK-17-1E, *Polymer Matrix Composites,* Vol 1, *Guidelines for Characterization of Structural Materials,* Feb 1994
18. J. Eisenmann, "Bolted Joint Static Strength Model for Composite Materials, Third Conf. on Fibrous Composites in Flight Vehicle Design," NASA TM X-3377, April 1976
19. S. Garbo and J. Ogonowski, "Effect of Variances and Manufacturing Tolerances on the Design Strength and Life of Mechanically Fastened Composite Joints," Vol 1, *Methodology Development and Data Evaluation,* AFWAL-TR-81-3041, April 1981
20. E. Iarve and D. Mollenhauer, Three-Dimensional Stress Analysis and Failure Prediction in Filled Hole Laminates, *Composite Structures: Theory and Practice,* STP 1383, ASTM, 2000, p 231–242
21. Tate and Rosenfeld, "Preliminary Investigation of the Loads Carried by Individual Bolts in Bolted Joints," NACA-TN-1051, May 1946
22. H. Huth, Influence of Fastener Flexibility on the Prediction of Load Transfer and Fatigue Life for Multiple-Row Joints, STP 927, ASTM, 1986, p 221–250
23. J. Crews and R. Naik, Effects of Bolt-Hole Contact on Bearing-Bypass Damage-Onset Strength, *Proc. of the First NASA Advanced Composites Technology Conf.,* Nov 1990
24. R. Naik and J. Crews, Ply Level Failure Analysis of Graphite/Epoxy Laminates under Bearing-Bypass Loading, STP 1059, ASTM, 1990, p 191–211
25. C.-L. Hung and F.-K. Chang, Strength Envelope of Bolted Composite Joints under Bypass Loads, *J. Compos. Mater.,* Vol 30 (No. 13), 1996, p 1402–1435
26. A. Sawicki and P. Minguet, The Influence of Fastener Clearance Upon the Failure of Compression-Loaded Composite Bolted Joints, *Composite Structures: Theory and Practice,* STP 1383, ASTM, 2000, p 293–308
27. A. Sawicki, J. Sestrich, E. Schulze, and P. Minguet, Structural Response of Postbuckled Skin-Stiffener Panels Containing Unreinforced Penetration Holes, *Proc. 5th DoD Composite Repair Technology Workshop* (Coeur d'Alene, ID), Nov 2000
28. C. Rousseau, D. Baker, and D. Hethcock, Parametric Study of Three-Stringer Panel Compression-After-Impact Strength, *Composite Structures: Theory and Practice,* STP 1383, ASTM, 2000, p 72–104
29. R. Krueger, P. Minguet, and T. K. O'Brien, A Method for Calculating Strain Energy Release Rates in Preliminary Design of Composite Skin/Stringer Debonding Under Multiaxial Loading, *Composite Structures: Theory and Practice,* STP 1383, ASTM, 2000, p 105–128

Design Criteria

Greg Kress, Delta Air Lines

DESIGN CRITERIA are the decisive quantified goals that a product must attain. A product needs to achieve a certain level of safety, cost, and functionality. To achieve these design criteria, particular detailed considerations must be evaluated. Design considerations include what materials are used, the manufacturing processes, and the configuration that is selected. This article addresses criteria that are established in the engineering design phase of a composite structure. A broader overview of the entire design process is provided in *Materials Selection and Design*, Volume 20 of *ASM Handbook*.

Overview of Design Criteria for Composites

Design criteria are established in the initial phase of a design program, but may be changed throughout the development and production process. Products are manufactured and purchased to satisfy specific real or imagined needs. An airplane may be produced for high speed, large payload capacity, or flight endurance. An automobile is produced for ground transportation, but could be functionally classified as a sports car, luxury sedan, racing car, or cargo van. Similarly, rockets, boats, trains, sporting goods, medical devices, storage tanks, walking bridges, or highway overpasses are all produced for specific purposes. Composite materials have been used in every one of these industries, and in these applications, composites, as well as other materials, have met with successes and failures. To meet the intended function for a product, a designer needs to know clearly the expectations of the user, the expected life of the product, and the expected environment that the product will encounter. The way in which the designer applies the many design considerations will determine the margin of success that the application achieves.

Perhaps more than any other engineering material, composites, by their very nature, possess the flexibility to be tailored to achieve specific design requirements. However, there may be goals specified at the start of a design program that:

- Are more significant than others
- Are more achievable than others
- May only be accomplished at the expense of others

Design engineering is often the art of compromise.

Composites achieve their design flexibility from the large possible selection in material types, arrangements, and forms; the wide variety of processing methods available; and the many different variations available when choosing a structural configuration. Because composite design offers such a large selection, one can get lost in the details, and the result may be a final product that does not meet all of the original expectations. To ensure the correct design choices are made, it is best to take a methodical approach to evaluating the design requirements. To begin, for a particular application, the following design criteria might be determined to be the most relevant and should be listed in order of priority for the particular design:

- Cost
- Strength
- Stiffness
- Weight
- Size
- Repeatability and precision of parts
- Environmental constraints in processing, use, and disposal
- Aesthetics
- Manufacturability and production rates
- Assembly restrictions
- Life cycle durability and damage tolerance
- Maintainability and reparability
- Nonmechanical properties, such as flammability and electrical properties

From the prioritized design criteria, all of the engineering, material, process, and configuration options should be evaluated for their ability to fulfill the design requirements. One selection will not meet all of the prerequisites. However, based on the priority of the design criteria, the design team can more efficiently evaluate all of the options and more easily eliminate unacceptable alternatives.

Common composites material selection options are:

- *Fiber types:* Glass, carbon, aramid, boron, polyethylene, ceramic, tungsten
- *Fiber forms:* Unidirectional, woven fabric, random mat, chopped fiber, braided fabric
- *Polymer matrices:* Polyester, vinyl ester, epoxy, bismaleimide (BMI), polyimide, phenolic, cyanate ester. Polymers are classified as being thermoplastic or thermoset.
- *Other matrices*: Metal, ceramic, carbon, glass
- *Structural configurations:* Solid laminate, sandwich panels, stiffened panels
- *Core materials:* Honeycomb, foam, wood, syntactic

Processing options include:

- *Manufacturing methods:* Wet lay-up, prepreg lay-up, fiber placement, tape lay-up, pultrusion, resin transfer molding (RTM), vacuum-assisted resin transfer molding, filament winding, compression molding, injection molding, centrifugal casting
- *Processing equipment:* Vacuum bagging, molds, ovens, autoclaves, presses, mandrels, bladders

The application of composite materials in any industry has standard design criteria that will lead a designer toward choosing a particular design. Some criteria are mandated and are based on the collective experience within the industry. However, staying within the "standard industry guidelines" may produce results that are nearly identical to the competition. This may be the safe and possibly only path to follow, but will seldom result in industry advances or a competitive edge over any other available product. The negative aspect is that implementing a unique design comes with the risk that the design program will experience unplanned setbacks or potentially, a complete design failure. It is therefore necessary during product development that the design team fully research and understand the consequence of each design decision. The designer must evaluate the outcome that choosing one design option has on meeting its intended design criteria, as well as the effects that this option has on the other design criteria needed to make the product a success.

This article describes common design criteria and identifies the design considerations that have a significant effect on the end product. From the discussion, it should become obvious how seemingly independent design criteria and design considerations interact with one another. Used in conjunction with the detailed subjects covered elsewhere in this Volume, this article should help the designer make decisions in a design program that will enable it to achieve the maximum benefits of composite materials.

Cost

The cost versus benefit judgement is usually the prime factor in the choice of a design path. Factors contributing to the true cost are:

- Materials selection
- Component size
- Manufacturing methods
- Processing equipment

Cost alone may not be the primary design criteria driving new product development, but the respective costs associated with each consideration will affect the profitability of the project. A cost factor is associated with each step in the design process. Comparisons must take into account the number of parts being produced; their size; constituent materials; ancillary material costs, such as storage costs, energy costs related to curing temperature, and waste; and manufacturing techniques.

Materials Costs. Consider two composite structures, one made from glass fiber and polyester resin and another made from carbon fiber and epoxy. Fiberglass is the least expensive reinforcement, followed by aramid fiber, then carbon fiber, costing 5 to 10 times more. Similarly, polyester resins cost less than vinyl ester resins, and epoxy resins are the most expensive.

When considering the size of a fiber-resin part for a bicycle frame and a boat hull, a cost difference of converting from glass-polyester to carbon/epoxy would obviously result in a much larger dollar difference in the material cost of the boat. However, if the material costs of a bicycle selling for $200 were $5, an increase to $25.00 is a 500% increase in material costs and a 12.5% increase relative to the existing selling price. If a $200,000 yacht had a $5000 cost for the glass-polyester hull, the equivalent change would amount to a $25,000 cost. The $20 increase in the cost of the bicycle, which might be marked up considerably at the selling price, might be met with the same sales resistance as the $20,000 increase in the yacht, if there were no increase in the perceived value. For a racing bicycle, a 30% reduction in the weight of the frame may be perceived as a worthwhile design improvement. For a recreational bicycle or a yacht, the weight reduction may not be an acceptable benefit.

The value of a weight reduction will be evaluated based on the industry involved. A one pound weight reduction on a plane is evaluated in terms of the fuel savings over the life of the plane. A reduction of a pound in a rocket engine allows for one pound more payload and can be evaluated in those terms.

If mechanical performance is the design driver, characteristic property values are often normalized by density and cost to arrive at strength or stiffness per cost. This aids in the systematic evaluation of options. See the article "Cost Analysis" in this Volume.

Other design drivers, such as environment, manufacturability, or repairability, may require significant consideration over cost. The use of other fiber-matrix combinations made from boron, polyethylene, or quartz fiber with phenolic, BMI, polyimide, or cyanate ester resins, and metal-matrix, carbon-matrix, or ceramic-matrix materials should be considered.

Processing Costs. Although direct cost based on constituent materials may appear to be a large factor, other significant cost drivers are manufacturing considerations. Figures 1 and 2 show cost and cycle time comparisons for different manufacturing processes.

Wet lay-up, open molding is probably the least expensive process for a relatively small number of units. This is a common process for large-production marine manufacturing, where thick, heavy, woven fiberglass mat and random-oriented chopped fiber are hand or spray impregnated with polyester resin and cured at room temperature. Although conducive to large and inexpensive production, the optimization of fiber properties is not achieved, weight is often not minimized, and the level of precision is very operator-dependent.

Prepregs, fibers that are preimpregnated with mixed resin, optimize constituent properties by using a predetermined resin content and preferred fiber orientation. Prepregs are commonly used with both unidirectional and woven fabric forms. The resins contained in prepregs can often achieve higher service temperatures than their respective wet lay-up resins. However, they typically require frozen storage to prevent premature curing. Resin flow during cure is limited, so prepreg lay-ups will require vacuum bagging oven cures as a minimum and potentially press or autoclave pressure to achieve ply consolidation. Prepreg materials, frozen storage, short shelf lives, vacuum bagging, ovens, autoclaves, and presses all add significantly to the final cost. To relate this to the previous example, a prepreg fiberglass-polyester, vacuum-bagged, oven-cured composite can, in the end, become more expensive than a wet lay-up carbon/epoxy, open-molded, room-temperature-cured laminate.

Cost reduction measures have been developed through advances such as room-temperature-storage prepregs. A general aviation aircraft manufactured in Canada uses an impregnator. This equipment meters a specific quantity of resin onto the fibers as the fabric is pulled through it. This reduces the material cost of prepregs while still providing the desired precise resin content. Personnel are still needed to locate the material in the mold, ensure the reinforcement is completely saturated, and apply the vacuum bag.

Vacuum-assisted resin transfer molding involves liquid resin being drawn through prepositioned dry reinforcement under vacuum, using traditional single-tool surface molds. This manufacturing technology is designed to reduce the cost of hand lay-up, requiring less manpower, while providing a more predictable resin content and vacuum bag compaction. Vacuum-assisted

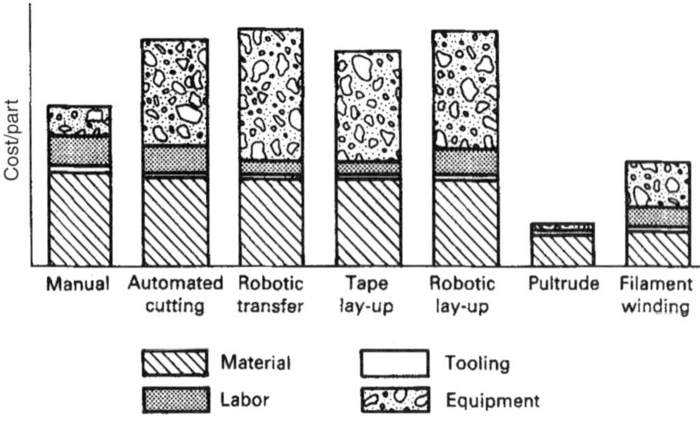

Fig. 1 Relative per unit cost for processing 0.4 m^2 (4 ft^2) 24-ply parts by different methods, based on 2000 units per year. Adapted from Ref 1

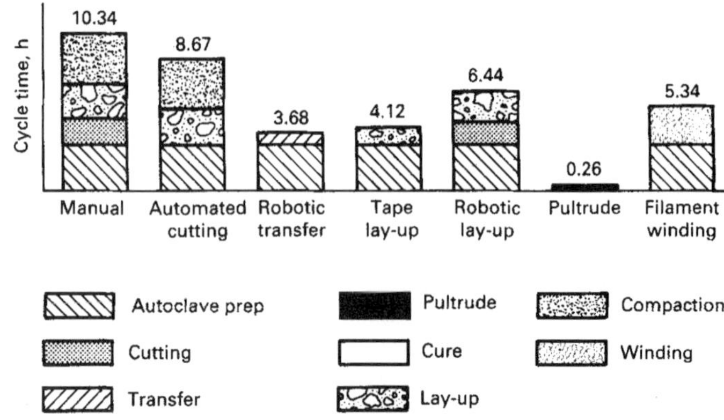

Fig. 2 Cycle time for a batch of 100, 0.4 m^2 (4 ft^2) 24-ply parts. Source: Ref 1

resin transfer molding has been used from low-cost manufacturing of small bicycle frame-sized components, to making objects as large as 20 m (65 ft) long train boxcar bodies and even larger boat hulls. Traditional RTM is a more costly process used to create composite parts to nearly net shape. Resin transfer molding is a closed-molded process where a dry fiber preform is placed in a two-sided (closed) mold, and heated resin is forced in under pressure. The mold part has a tooled surface on both sides, and hollow parts can be made with the use of mandrels and bladders. Resin transfer molding is ideal for small precision parts, where the size of the molds does not become cost-prohibitive.

Complex and accurate manufacturing often requires automation. This type of automation comes in the form of computer-controlled material cutters, ply-placement equipment, filament winding, pultrusion, tape wrapping, and fiber-placement machines. Although each has its own unique purpose, they all use large, computer-operated equipment that requires a significant capital investment. Even so, these advanced techniques have reached across the full spectrum of manufacturing, from filament winders for pipes, ducting, and storage tanks in industrial applications, to fiber-placement machines for advanced military aircraft.

Size

Size considerations impact both the manufacturing environment and the application of the composite in the final assembly. An advantage of composite structures is often the large size of the individual bonded assemblies. This extends from the ability of composite raw materials to be easily spliced with a simple overlap during lay-up. Complex contours that would typically require multiple metal parts can easily be molded into a single composite part. Additionally, one large mold can be less involved to construct than several smaller molds. Fabricating a single large component is less time-consuming, requires smaller inventory, and has fewer assembly joints than multiple smaller parts. No matter what the building material, joints are always a source of possible failure. Fewer joints result in material savings and weight savings, because the region around a joint requires material buildup to prevent the joint from failing first.

Excessively large size can become a detriment to a design. Large bonded panels can be cumbersome to handle and can get damaged easily while being moved during assembly. They can be cracked from bending, if not properly supported. Once in service, repairs to composite structures may require partial disassembly. The nature of composite construction makes panels stiff and resistant to bending. Whether adjacent panels are bonded together or mechanically fastened, these inherently stiff panels do not allow any deflection to provide access to within the structure. It is necessary to completely disassemble a panel at all of its joints to gain access within the structure. The larger a panel is, the more extensive the disassembly required to perform the repair. An example of this is a large commercial airline rudder. The composite assembly for the rudder is over 10 m (32 ft) in length (Fig. 3). Each side of the rudder is made from only two skin panels. The lower skin panel spans 5.87 m (19.25 ft) and requires removing mechanical fasteners 1.8 (6 ft) beyond the damage site to achieve enough bending in the panel to access the inside of the structure. It is wise to limit the size of components prone to wear or damage that will require replacement as a part of routine maintenance.

Large panel size stipulated as a design requirement can also lead to prohibitive manufacturing costs. Although lay-up tooling costs for prepreg and wet lay-up manufacturing may not give a compounded cost increase, the equipment costs for other fabrication methods may greatly increase. The complex equipment for filament winding, automated tape lay-up, RTM, and press, oven, and autoclave curing can become exponentially more expensive as individual components increase in size. Consideration must be given to residual stresses created in materials as they cool from elevated cure temperature. Larger parts are more prone to differential cooling.

The size of a final composite structure may be determined by some physical design requirement. For example, the number of joints, with their attendant costs and design challenges, may be reduced with larger components. Edges of laminates are subject to damage and stresses that cause delamination. Joints and edges can be reduced in number and located advantageously by adjusting the size of the components. The designer often has freedom to choose the size of the individual components. Instead of designing large composite panels just for the sake of being big, it is necessary to factor all of the design considerations to minimize the adverse effects.

Mechanical Properties

Stiffness, strength, and weight are functions of constituent materials, their relative quantities, and placement. The interactions between stiffness, strength, and weight design considerations can be misunderstood when applying composite materials to a new design. Noncomposite materials, such as metals, typically exhibit proportional properties. For example, the strength, stiffness, and weight of stainless steel are all greater than that of aluminum. The ratio of stiffness to density is approximately the same for steel and aluminum. However, the same is not true for composites. Of the primary reinforcement fibers, fiberglass, aramid, and carbon, each have stiffness, strength, and weight values that are not proportional. These considerations make composites material selection a more complex issue.

As weight is often the critical factor in evaluating the use of composites, the strength and stiffness are often listed as specific strength or specific modulus. The specific values are normalized by dividing the property value by the density. The specific values can also be normalized by dividing by the cost per mass or weight so a strength per cost comparison can be made.

It is easiest to categorize fiber selection by understanding several significant comparisons. These comparisons rank the fibers in a situation where all resins are equal, and stiffness and strength are evaluated based on weight, cost, and thickness. Laminate weight will obviously affect the final weight of the part, cost will relate the material investment, and thickness will compare the material characteristics per ply. Therefore, consider that currently:

- Fiberglass provides the greatest strength per dollar.
- Aramid provides the greatest strength per pound.
- Carbon provides the greatest stiffness per pound.
- Fiberglass and carbon provide comparable strength per ply thickness, both greater than aramid; however, fiberglass is considerably less stiff per ply than either carbon or aramid.

Weight is based primarily on the density of the fiber. Because nearly all resins fall within the same range, the fiber will determine the laminate weight where:

Constituent	Density	
	g/cm^3	lb/in.^{3}
Resin	1.15–1.35	0.0415–0.0488
Fiberglass	2.46–2.55	0.0900–0.0921
Aramid	1.44	0.0520
Carbon (graphite)	1.80	0.0650

Stiffness is presented with values that can be very deceiving when designing with composite materials. Once again, resin will not greatly impact laminate property differences during material selection, because resin has very low stiff-

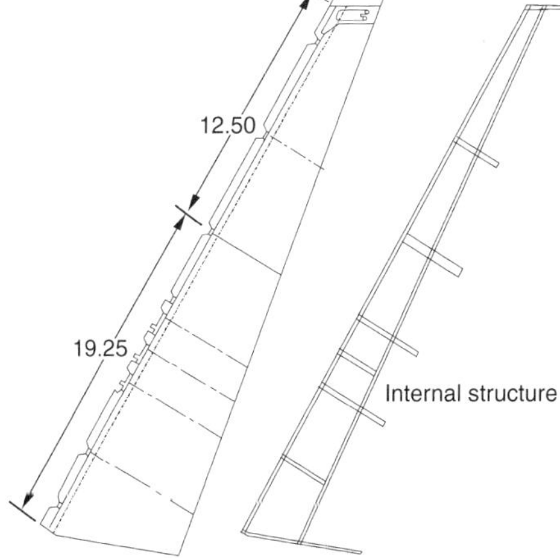

Fig. 3 Two large composite skin panels that make up the rudder of a large commercial aircraft. Dimensions are in feet.

ness. The fiber will be the primary factor in the laminate stiffness where:

Constituent	Modulus of elasticity GPa	10^6 psi
Resin	3.4	0.50
Fiberglass fiber	73.1–85.5	10.6–12.4
Aramid fiber	124–179	18–26
Carbon fiber	207–414	30–60
Graphite fiber	414–965	60–140

However, the previous numbers are for the fiber and the resin individually. When the fiber and resin are combined into either a unidirectional or woven fabric composite ply, the stiffness values will change drastically. Micromechanics will provide a calculated value, but material testing is typically required to evaluate the fiber-resin interface. Representative values for different ply materials are:

Ply material	Modulus of elasticity GPa	10^6 psi
Unidirectional fiberglass	34	5
Woven fiberglass	24	3.5
Unidirectional aramid	76	11
Woven aramid	38	5.6
Unidirectional carbon	124	18
Woven carbon	59	8.5

The previous differences represent the use of different fiber forms. This should be obvious, because unidirectional materials have fibers in only one direction (0°), and woven fabrics have fibers in two directions (0° and 90°). For symmetric weave fabrics, the stiffness may be identical in both the 0° and 90° directions. Unidirectional materials have considerable stiffness in the fiber (0°) direction and negligible stiffness transverse to the fiber (90°) direction. To determine the off-axis stiffness properties between the 0° and 90° directions, classical laminate plate theory uses equations representative of generalized Hooke's law and tensor transformation, in matrix form.

To achieve equal stiffness in all directions, as found in isotropic materials (metals), $[0°/90°/+45°/-45°]_s$ and $[0°/+60°/-60°]_s$ unidirectional laminates or $[(0° \text{ or } 90°)/\pm45°]_s$ woven fabric laminates are used. These laminates, called quasi-isotropic laminates, will have equal stiffness in all directions in the plane of the laminate, but not normal to the plane. Typical quasi-isotropic laminate stiffness values are:

Quasi-isotropic laminate	Modulus of elasticity GPa	10^6 psi
Fiberglass	19	2.8
Aramid	29	4.2
Carbon	41	6.0

Strength can be defined as the maximum stress value that the laminate can sustain. The strength that a structure must possess is based on the ultimate combination of loads that will be applied at the most severe environmental conditions for the structure. However, to ensure that the structure will not fail at this ultimate load condition, a *factor of safety* is applied. A typical factor of safety for metal aircraft structures is 1.5. This means that a structure designed to withstand a load of 6000 lbf will actually be designed to withstand 9000 lbf (6000 × 1.5 = 9000). For nonaerospace engineering applications where a weight penalty is not an issue, factors of safety of 6 to 10 may be applied. The factor of safety is often mandated by industry regulations.

A factor of safety is intended to account for engineering miscalculations, material and process flaws, or assembly defects. Early in aerospace applications of composite materials, a factor of safety of 2.0 was used. This meant that a composite structure was designed to be twice as strong as it really needed to be. This arose from the lack of precision in manufacturing techniques and the variability in material properties. As composite materials, processes, testing, and analytical techniques have improved, the factor of safety is often reduced to 1.5. A low factor of safety can be applied by purchasing composite materials to a stringent materials specification that ensures its properties and repeatability, and by employing well-defined and repeatable manufacturing techniques.

A *margin of safety* is another term associated with designing extra strength into a structure. For composite structures, once the factor of safety has been applied to the design load, and a laminate has been designed to withstand the loading condition, any additional load-carrying capability of the laminate is considered a margin of safety. An excessively high, positive margin of safety for composites can come from having a small selection of materials available where variations in ply and laminate thickness are limited.

A margin of safety is determined after the design of a laminate is completed and the laminate properties have been verified. The ability of a laminate to meet and exceed the required design strength or other criteria is identified by having a positive margin of safety. Verification of strength is often a controversial issue with composites. Stress is easy to calculate from basic mechanics as the load or force divided by the given area. The Système International d'Unités (SI) units of stress are N/m^2, called pascal, Pa, or in customary units, pound force per square inch, lb/in^2, or psi. For a given laminate comprised of known materials and orientations, the stress at failure strength, can be experimentally determined using standardized mechanical testing methods. The strengths are usually determined for a single load direction applied with the testing machine. Results will vary from test coupon to coupon, with different laminate configurations. See the Section "Testing and Certification" for a full treatment of data analysis and test methodology. It should be noted that multiaxial testing is done, but this testing capability is limited, and usually it is reserved for thick composites.

Detailed analysis can provide the solution to determining the strength at all locations throughout a composite structure. This analytical procedure can use one of several composite failure criteria. There are many failure criteria that exist, but none have proven to be applicable for all materials in all loading situations. The designer must consider situations of compressive loading and out-of-plane loading carefully.

Within a structurally acceptable range of resin content, the values for strength and stiffness will increase with lower resin content and higher fiber volume, because the fiber is the primary means for providing strength and stiffness in a composite. However, the normalized strength and stiffness multiplied by the ply or laminate thickness will indicate the actual strength and actual stiffness per ply in units of force per unit of width. Figure 4 and Table 1 use this concept. To avoid resin content effects in determining strength, it is easiest to look at composite failure based on elongation, or strain. Hooke's law illustrates that, to a certain limit, stress is directly proportional to strain. Because both stress and stiffness are in proportional units of force per unit area, the strain is independent of thickness, as shown in Fig. 4. Therefore, within the structurally acceptable range of resin content, the determining consideration for resin content should

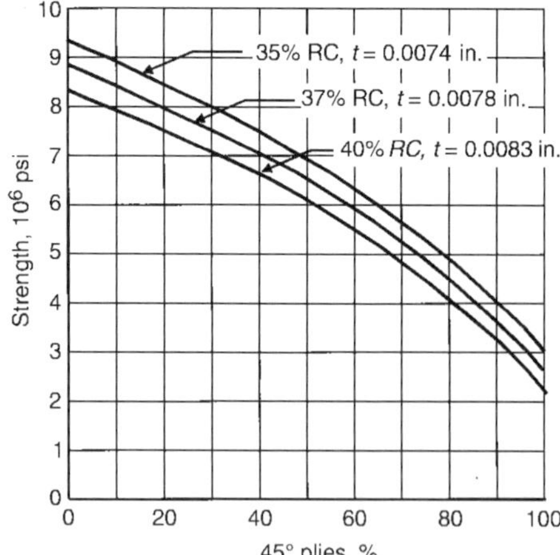

Fig. 4 Strength versus percent 45° plies for three lamina, with resin content (RC) and thickness (t) as indicated. Selected values are given in Table 1.

Table 1 Properties of lamina plotted in Fig. 4

Resin content, %	0° modulus, 10^6 psi	Ply thickness, in.	Actual modulus, 10^6 lbf/in.	Tensile strain in./in.	Strength per ply, lbf/in. of width
35	9.3	0.0074	0.06882	0.009	0.00062
37	8.8	0.0078	0.06864	0.009	0.00062
40	8.3	0.0083	0.06889	0.009	0.00062

not be the change in mechanical properties, but the weight considerations associated with higher resin content and the environmental considerations associated with lower resin content.

Example: Effect of Fiber Areal Weight on Material Usage and Other Design Considerations. Unidirectional carbon fiber used in aerospace structures is typically available in 95, 145, and 190 g/m^2 (0.31, 0.477, and 0.623 oz/ft^2) fiber areal weight (FAW). The FAW is the weight of dry reinforcement per unit area (width × length) of tape or fabric. Because a FAW of 95 g/m^2 (0.31 oz/ft^2) is half that of 190 g/m^2 (0.623 oz/ft^2), it also has half the thickness. Designing in three plies of 95 g/m^2 (0.31 oz/ft^2) unidirectional material will allow a more precise strength to be achieved compared to two plies of 190 g/m^2 (0.623 oz/ft^2) unidirectional tape if only 280 g/m^2 (0.91 oz/ft^2) of material is needed. If 145 g/m^2 (0.477 oz/ ft^2) material is available, only two plies would be required to supply the same amount of carbon fiber as three plies of 95 g/m^2 (0.31 oz/ft^2) material. Design considerations to be evaluated are the added cost and weight if unneeded material is used, the additional time in laminating more numerous plies, and the excess inventory that must be maintained if multiple variations of the same material type are used.

Repeatability and Precision

The level of repeatability and precision required in the final product must be considered in the initial design. On the production level, a tolerance for precision in size and shape will be set to assure proper fit of joined components. Manufacturing precision is achieved with proper materials selection, tooling, lamination sequence, processing control, and final trim.

Tooling considerations involve molds that retain accuracy after repeated cure cycles. Metal tooling has long been used for its ability to maintain a precise shape. Metal tooling is also the most expensive, because complex tool surfaces must be machined from the tooling metal. Metal tooling is often heavy, and the thick sections act as a heat sink, which can interfere with the proper curing of the composite materials. Metallic tooling methods involving deposited metals, such as electroformed nickel or cast aluminum, are able to produce thinner metal molds without large machining operations. Composite tooling is considerably easier to fabricate, using lay-up and fabrication techniques similar to manufacturing composite parts. Composite tooling typically cannot withstand the numerous repeated thermal cycling, nor are composite tools as resistant to damage as metal tools, but the reduced price will offset the lower life span. See the articles "Electroformed Nickel Tooling", "Elastomeric Tooling", "Design, Tooling, and Manufacturing Interaction", and "Composite Tooling" in this Volume.

Automation can increase manufacturing precision and increased productivity. Computer-operated cutting tables are used to quickly and accurately cut plies. These usually have software that nests plies along the length and width of the roll to reduce material waste. Computer-operated filament winding, tape wrapping, and tape-laying machines use numeric control to accurately laminate parts. Five-axis routers are used to quickly and accurately trim parts. Computerized equipment is available for all phases of fabrication, but at a significant cost that must be justified. Hand lamination is still a viable technique, but it is susceptible to operator variability. Increased accuracy can still be achieved. Using prepregs versus wet lay-up will ensure accurate resin content. Laser ply projection can be used to both accurately cut plies as well as accurately locate plies in a mold. Trim and drill fixtures can be incorporated to help guide the final trimming and drilling operation. The objective is to develop the optimal combination of automated technology and manual operations to produce the most cost-effective production.

Mechanical Properties. From a mechanical properties standpoint, precision is viewed as the ability to achieve a repeatable strength. The value used to statistically represent an achievable strength of a material is called an allowable. As identified in the previous discussion on strength, stiffness, and weight, composite design often uses strain or elongation to evaluate the strength. When determining at what point a ply will fail in elongation, numerous mechanical coupons are tested to achieve the design value. Calculating an average of all the test values yields a result where approximately half of the values have already failed. The average, or mean value, is typically not acceptable in determining the design allowable, because a 50% probability of failure is not acceptable; however, average values are used in test correlation to evaluate the accuracy of an analysis method.

The minimum specified mechanical property value is called the S-value.

Design allowables are chosen to select a value to ensure that failure will not occur. Statistics are applied to select an acceptable likelihood of failure. Typical statistical values are termed A-basis and B-basis. For A-basis, 99% of the test results should exceed the allowable value with a 95% assurance. For B-basis, 90% of the test results should exceed the allowable value 95% of the time. A-basis allowables are more conservative and used on single-load-path structures, where a failure of the part will result in failure of the structure. B-basis values are typically higher than A-basis values and are used where multiple load path exists, and failure of one part will not result in failure of the entire structure. Being based on statistics, the lower the spread between the minimum and maximum test values and the greater the number of values pooled in the statistical data, the higher the resulting allowable. Repeatability and precision are necessary to translate the test values into the final product. Detailed discussion on test methods and statistical reduction methods can be found in the article "Design Allowables" in this Volume, and in MIL-HDBK-17 (Ref 2).

Whether stress or strain is used to model the failure, only those values will be statistically reduced. Separate statistical allowables are usually determined for tension, compression, and shear. Axial stiffness (E_1), transverse stiffness (E_2), shear stiffness (G_{12}), and Poisson's ratio (ν_{21}) values will be determined from the test results. For many materials and applications, the stiffness and Poisson's ratio value will be an average between tension and compression tests. Only in cases where tension stiffness is significantly different from the compression stiffness will different values be used during the design analysis. Stiffness and Poisson's ratio are often only determined at room temperature. For a structure that experiences primarily room-temperature conditions, these elastic constants are acceptable. When the structure is subject to loads at sustained high or low temperatures, it is necessary to evaluate these elastic properties at these conditions.

Allowables must account for the environmental spectrum that the structure will be exposed to during its service life as well. Mechanical testing is performed with coupons conditioned at room temperature, the minimum and maximum temperature range, and with fluid contamination. Determining separate allowables for each environmental condition is recommended.

With the high costs and time-consuming nature of mechanical testing, determining a separate allowable with data pooled at each environmental condition has come under considerable scrutiny. The Advanced General Aviation Transportation Experiment (AGATE) program has implemented a methodology where normalized test data are pooled from all environmental conditions to determine allowables; this approach uses the statistical benefit of pooling large quantities of data (Ref 3). The AGATE methodology has made materials testing less of a burden for smaller companies.

Material allowables are typically generated for unidirectional material. The ultimate strength or ultimate strain has been shown to depend on the laminate stacking sequence. The 0° failure strain can be higher for laminates that have more ±45° plies. To account for this, some statistical models for determining allowables are based on percentages of 0°, 90°, and ±45° plies.

Damage Tolerance and Durability

Damage of a massive nature, as well as hidden damage and flaws, are considerations for the designer.

Massive Damage. If a structure is going to be operating in an environment where it may potentially become damaged, it is a concern that a catastrophic failure not occur before the damage is discovered and can be repaired. Significant damage that affects a large area may impact a primary load-carrying member of a structure and lead to immediate failure. To prevent this, a designer must employ multiple load paths so other structural members are present to carry the load.

Multiple-load-path structures require the use of B-basis material allowables. A single-load-path structure is one such that a single member failure would lead to a catastrophic failure of the structure. Single load path requires A-basis material allowables.

Minor Damage. Of equal concern to significant damage is small damage that can go unnoticed or is barely visible. This type of damage is often referred to as barely visible impact damage and is of great concern, because small damage can grow without being detected and eventually lead to a catastrophic failure. The study of damage growth is called fracture mechanics. Predicting damage growth with composites is very involved, because variability in fiber, fiber forms, ply orientation, matrix material, and laminate configuration will affect the results. Determining if the damage growth will lead to a catastrophic failure is the study of damage tolerance. Cyclic mechanical testing and analytical methods are used in damage tolerance calculations to help determine inspection intervals that would discover damage growth before failure occurs. Related to damage tolerance is damage resistance, which involves the materials selection and structural configuration categories of the design considerations. These considerations focus on designing a structure that is not prone to damage and likewise result in a structure that is more damage tolerant.

Damage growth in a composite typically occurs when delamination forms at the tip of a crack. The delamination grows with increasing severity of load cycles. The delamination can reduce the effective laminate modulus and cause a redistribution of stress that eventually leads to fiber breakage and finally, laminate failure. Damage tolerance can be improved by using toughened resin systems that resist crack propagation. The use of honeycomb core in frequent-impact areas needs to be closely evaluated. The choice of stiffened solid laminate substructures or sandwich panels will affect the damage resistance of a structure. Sandwich panels are significantly stiffer for the weight and amount of material used, but are more subject to impact damage normal to the plane of the panel. Increasing the compressive strength of the core provides greater impact resistance to the facesheets for low-energy impacts, but for high-energy impacts, the core properties have very little effect on penetration of the facesheet. The effects of impact damage on core panels can be seen in Fig. 5. See the article "Damage Tolerance" in this Volume.

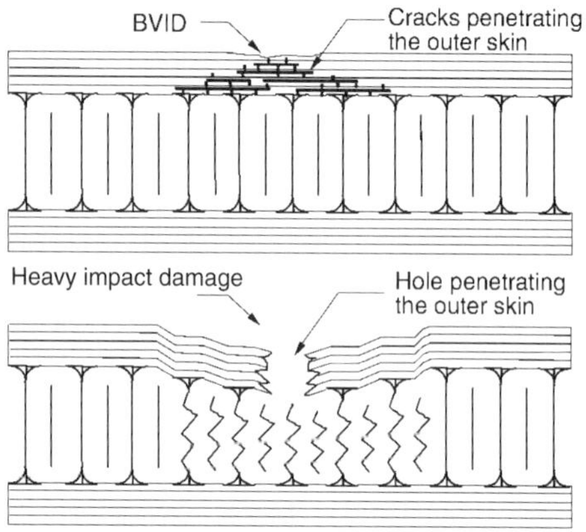

Fig. 5 Barely visible impact damage (BVID) and heavy impact damage on a sandwich structure with a honeycomb core

Environmental Constraints

Environmental factors, such as temperature, moisture, corrosive liquids, light, and other radiation, must be considered. If the environment of the final assembly is not known by the composite designer, the allowable service environment should be stipulated. Often, industries classify materials for use in specific environments.

The effect of environmental degradation on the mechanical integrity of a composite is significant. Moisture can also migrate through sandwich panel facesheets or enter as a result of impact damage and be absorbed in the honeycomb core, as shown in Fig. 6. Low-resin-content prepregs and sandwich panels with a low number of facesheet plies are easy candidates for moisture intrusion. Moisture can also seep through open-cell foam cores. Open-cell foams, as opposed to closed-cell foams, have an interconnected network of cells, similar to a sponge. Many foaming adhesives used to bond honeycomb core pieces together have an open-cell structure that allows water to migrate deep inside honeycomb core sandwich panels. The absorbed moisture can freeze, expand, and delaminate the skin from the core. The combination of low-resin-content aramid fiber sandwich laminates, using aramid paper core, assembled with open-cell foaming adhesives have been problematic.

Environmental considerations need to be addressed at all phases in the life cycle of a composite. In the production phase, uncured composites can be drastically affected by temperature, moisture, and contamination. B-staged prepregs and adhesives have limited storage times at frozen temperatures, typically 6 to 12 months at –18 to –12 °C (0 to 10 °F). At room temperature, the shelf life is reduced even more, typically 10 to 30 days. Prepregs are so sensitive to storage time at a given temperature that the time out of the freezer and at room temperature is usually tracked in hours. This is called the out time. Liquid resins and adhesives are also affected by temperature, by increasing or decreasing the working life of the material. Increasing the ambient temperature of a resin will decrease the pot life of the material. A standard rule, called the "10 degree rule," for resins states that increasing the temperature 6 °C (10 °F) from a specified temperature will reduce the working life of the resin by half.

Moisture affects uncured composite materials by being absorbed into the resin. Prepregs, while in frozen storage, are sealed in plastic bags to prevent frost from forming on the B-staged material. Because moisture condenses on objects removed from a frozen environment, prepregs are not removed from their plastic storage bags until after the material has warmed to the surrounding temperature. Out time is logged as the time from when the roll is removed from the freezer until it is resealed and placed back in the freezer.

Moisture, even humidity in the air, affects liquid resins by chemically altering the material. Absorbing moisture results in lowering the glass transition temperature, T_g. The T_g, which can be determined several ways, is an indication of the service temperature of a composite laminate. Moisture can also absorb into fibers and core and have an effect on elastic and strength properties. Aramid fibers and aramid paper core are known for absorbing moisture. This moisture must be removed prior to a high-temperature cure, to prevent delamination from moisture expansion. All aramid-based materials should be stored in a low-humidity environment. Fiberglass is also susceptible to moisture degradation. Common fiber finishes applied to fiberglass to promote resin adhesion are water soluble and can be removed if dry fiberglass material comes in contact with moisture.

Uncured composite materials are also very susceptible to environmental contamination. Oils, grease, or silicone-based products should not come in contact with dry material, prepregs, or core material. Compressed air and careless application of release agents are common sources of contamination. The need to limit heat, moisture, and contaminants have led to the use of "clean rooms" as the location where raw composites are processed. Clean rooms have strictly controlled temperature and humidity. The use of compressed air, release agents, and room pres-

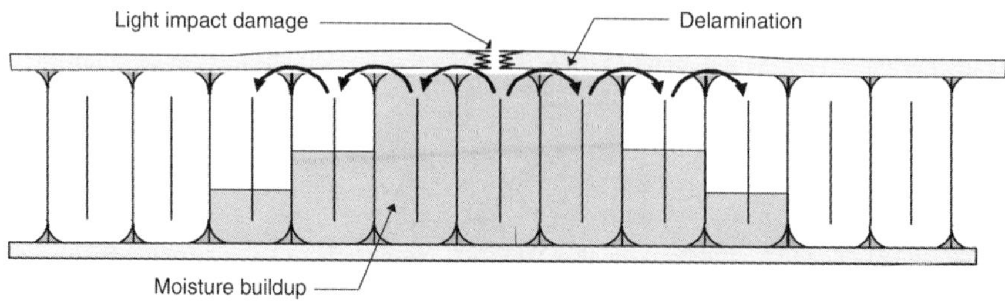

Fig. 6 Moisture propagation into a honeycomb core sandwich structure

sure are controlled to maintain the location free of contamination.

Cured composites are also susceptible to environmental degradation. In hot/wet conditions, the resin is typically attacked first; moisture absorbed into the cured resin lowers the T_g. At elevated temperatures when the T_g is reached, the resin softens to the point where load is not efficiently transferred through the laminate, and premature failure occurs.

Resins are the environmental "weak link" in a composite. Hydraulic fluid, brake fluid, paint strippers, and other corrosive chemicals soften and dissolve various resins. Small impacts, heat, and ultraviolet rays can erode away the resin on the surface of a laminate and leave the fiber reinforcement unsupported. Maintaining a proper surface finish, controlling service temperature, and keeping trimmed edges and fastener holes sealed mitigate the adverse effects of environmental degradation.

Conclusions

Composite materials offer a wide range of flexibility for the designer. Although so many possibilities give the designer many options, it needs to be remembered that some combinations will work better and cost less and will be easier to manufacture, easier to repair, stronger, stiffer, lighter, or more damage resistant. Having so many options also means that there is a greater opportunity to make the wrong decision. Because the widespread use of composites is still relatively new, there are many design considerations that have not been fully evaluated. Some applications evolved as replacements for parts made from metal or natural materials. The design was dictated by the characteristics of these materials. The possibilities of composites allow for imaginative designs. A designer can evaluate the past applications of composites and determine which combinations have produced better results. The designer should remain mindful of previous successes and failures, but also maintain a close watch on new developments and future trends. A designer must use sound engineering practices to ensure the integrity of a composite design. Applying these practices to modern composite technology will guarantee viability in the marketplace.

REFERENCES

1. S. Krolewski and T. Gutowski, Effect of the Automation of Advanced Composite Fabrication Processes on Part Cost, *Proc. 18th Society for the Advancement of Material and Process Engineering Technical Conf.,* Oct 1986, p 83–97
2. MIL-HDBK-17-1, *Guidance,* Vol 1, *Polymer Matrix Composites,* Department of Defense, Feb 1994
3. J. Tomblin et al., AGATE Material Qualification Methodology for Epoxy-Based Prepreg Composite Material Systems, Advanced General Aviation Transport Experiments, Feb 1999

SELECTED REFERENCES

- K. Potter, *An Introduction to Composite Products,* Chapman & Hall, London, U.K., 1997
- M. J. Owen, V. Middleton, and I.A. Jones, Ed., *Integrated Design and Manufacture Using Fibre-Reinforced Polymeric Composites,* Woodhead Publishing, Ltd., Cambridge, England, 2000
- *Delaware Composites Design Encyclopedia,* Vol 1–6, Technomic Publishing Company, Inc., Lancaster, PA, 1990
- R. M. Jones, *Mechanics of Composite Materials,* 2nd ed., Taylor & Francis, Philadelphia, PA, 1999

Design Allowables

Chris Boshers, Composite Materials Characterization, Inc.

DESIGN ALLOWABLES are statistically determined materials property values derived from test data. They are limits of stress, strain, or stiffness that are allowed for a specific material, configuration, application, and environmental condition. The selection of appropriate design allowables for structures composed of composite materials is essential for the safe and efficient use of these materials. To help ensure safety, the use of appropriate design allowables is required by regulatory agencies for aircraft structures, for example. An extensive discussion and guidelines for the development and use of design allowables is contained in MIL-HDBK-17 (Ref 1). While certain industries use different terms, and unfortunately, similar terms are assigned different meanings, the general concept of design allowables is applicable to other industries as well.

A design engineer or materials scientist is often faced with the difficult challenge of finding or generating these allowables. While more conventional structural materials, such as metals or plastics, have allowables, these materials are generally considered to be homogeneous, which limits the possible failure modes, and hence, the testing required to characterize the material. Composites are heterogeneous and show varying degrees of anisotropy, resulting in a larger variety of potential failure modes. Because composites are an engineered material, the designer often cannot simply look up composite design allowables in a handbook or generic database, but must rather make informed decisions as to the selection, computation, quality, and applicability of allowables. This article discusses:

- The need for design allowables
- The development of design allowables
- Important factors that affect the selection of allowables
- Lamina versus laminate allowables
- Extending laminate results
- Specific techniques used in the statistical development of allowable values

The selection of the appropriate degree of testing to achieve the proper balance of initial cost versus the degree of certainty required for design allowables is discussed briefly here and in more detail in the Section "Testing and Certification" in this Volume.

Need for Design Allowables

Design allowables are used to ensure the safe and successful operation of a part or structure. Design begins with a determination of the use of the structure. See the article "Design Criteria" in this Section. The anticipated static and dynamic loads as well as the environment are among the considerations. Conversely, failure is defined. This is not always obvious. Microscopic "failures" are a strain relief mechanism that may increase the toughness of a material. Structural analysis will determine the most likely failure modes. The mechanical failure of a structure or substructure is usually related to exceeding the strength or deformation capabilities. Whether strength or deflection controls the design, an allowable strength value is a specified stress or strain level that must not be exceeded. The design allowables are obviously a function of the constituent material, the amount, and the arrangement of that material.

Allowables are normally determined in a manner appropriate to the consequences of failure; the allowables for a component for which failure is cosmetic would be determined much differently than the allowables of a structure for which failure might lead to loss of life.

Design allowables are the statistically defined materials property allowable strengths, usually referring to stress or strain, that are determined by a well-documented test program. Design allowables must account for all materials property variability that can reasonably be expected in the manufacture and assembly of a composite component. They must also account for manufacturing process variations and acceptable anomalies and for structural analysis limitations. Often, design allowables are intimately tied to a particular analysis method and, in these cases, cannot be used with other analysis approaches.

The factor of safety (FOS) is the ratio of the allowable load that the structure can carry to the applied load on the structure. Regulatory agencies prescribe minimum FOS for specific structural applications. These regulatory minimum FOS are established to account for all the uncertainties in loading, geometry, workmanship, variations in use and environment, accuracy of the design mathematical models, and uncertainty in the knowledge of the materials property values.

Development of Design Allowables

Historically, calculation of composite material design allowables has been modeled after the techniques used for metals. In the aerospace industry and in other design venues, the use of *A*- and *B*-basis allowables, originally developed for use with metallics, is commonly accepted by most certifying authorities. Simply stated, the *A*-basis allowable of a given materials property is the value that 99% of the property value population is expected to exceed with 95% confidence. Similarly, the *B*-basis allowable is the value expected to be exceeded by 90% of the property value population, also with 95% confidence. For a given set of experimental data, the determination of *A*- or *B*-basis allowables is primarily affected by three parameters: the mean, the variability of the test data, and the number of tests. The specific distribution model for the variability of the data also has a large effect. For homogeneous materials, this approach works well. These allowables can be developed under a moderate degree of testing of relatively small samples, and allowables can be concisely summarized in a specification, database, or handbook. For composite materials, the situation is a great deal more complex.

Factors Affecting Design Allowables

Heterogeneity. Composite materials are, by definition, heterogeneous. This heterogeneity confers unique advantages to composites over homogenous materials, but complicates the development of design allowables. The number of potential failure modes of the material is increased due to the presence of multiple constituent materials. For example, in polymer-matrix composites (PMC), some failure modes are sensitive to matrix properties, some failure modes are dominated by reinforcing-fiber properties, and some failure modes are most strongly influenced by the properties of the fiber-matrix interface. The dependence of specific failure modes on polymer-matrix composites is shown in Table 1. It is vital to understand how failure modes are influenced by constituent properties so that tests can be properly configured to yield rational design allowables. It is also critical that multiple failure modes are not contained in a set of data used to calculate an allowable. Test results with different failure modes should be separated before allowables calculations are performed.

Anisotropy. As an engineered material, a composite can be designed to satisfy specific directionally based needs. The designer of a composite structure can modify the percentage of fibers aligned in a given direction to meet specific design requirements. This feature is one of the principal advantages of composite materials. This ability to customize the composite adds to the complexity of determining allowables. Composite structures can range in degree of anisotropy, from isotropic to fully anisotropic. Many laminated composites exhibit orthotropic behavior. Fibers are usually aligned within a two-dimensional plane, either uniaxially or cross-plied, thus imparting relatively high (but variable) stiffnesses and strength within this plane. Properties normal to this plane are dependent almost solely on the properties of the matrix and thus, are usually much lower.

Equipment and good design practice often limit the options of fiber lay-ups and stacking sequences. Fortunately, unsymmetric or unbalanced laminates are rarely found in actual components. The presence of extension-bending coupling or shear-extension coupling found in unsymmetric or unbalanced lay-ups can make the development of allowables significantly more difficult. Other design guidelines can further restrict the permissible design space, as is discussed later.

Stacking sequence effects are important, however, even in a symmetric, balanced laminate. For failure modes influenced by bending loads or for failure modes sensitive to free-edge stresses, the specific order of the plies has a significant effect and warrants consideration in the development of allowables.

Environmental Effects. The environment in which a composite material is used can have a significant effect on materials properties. Changes in temperature affect all materials, and constituent materials of composites can be influenced to differing degrees. This difference in thermal expansion will create residual stresses within the material. Other important environmental effects include moisture (especially for PMC), exposure to specific gases, liquids, or solids, or even exposure to ultraviolet light or high-energy particles. The article "Hygrothermal Behavior" in this Volume addresses thermal and moisture effects.

In determining allowables, one must obviously have knowledge of the projected environment. One will also need to know the degree of impact that a particular environment has on constituent materials. For example, moisture has very little influence on carbon fibers, but can significantly affect the properties of polymer-matrix materials. Such knowledge is vital to efficiently determine allowables over the entire range of expected design conditions. However, it is very important not to make unfounded assumptions about which environmental conditions are critical, especially with new materials systems. Sometimes, complex interactions between the fiber and matrix lead to unexpected environmental conditions becoming critical.

Consider the case of a carbon-fiber-reinforced PMC. For subsonic aircraft, a typical range-of-use temperature is –54 to 82 °C (–65 to 180 °F). A wide range of humidity conditions is to be expected, so the moisture content of a composite structure could range from fully saturated to completely dry. At lower temperatures, the matrix tends to become more brittle, and tensile properties can be reduced. The presence of moisture would serve to reduce brittleness, so one should expect that tensile properties would be more critical at lower temperatures under dry conditions. At the other extreme of temperature, the stiffness and strength properties of the fibers should remain largely unaffected, while matrix properties can degrade significantly, especially in the presence of high moisture content. One should therefore concentrate testing efforts on those failure modes that are influenced by the constituent most sensitive to environmental effects. For in-plane tensile properties, low-temperature, dry conditions are typically critical. For shear and compression failures, the critical environmental conditions are usually at elevated temperature and fully moisture-saturated conditions.

Lamina Versus Laminate Allowables

When developing a plan to determine composite material allowables, a decision must be made to develop allowables for lamina or laminate properties, or both. If allowables are developed for lamina properties only, the list of required properties is relatively brief, with only a few stiffness and strength terms required. Unfortunately, lamina properties by themselves are rarely sufficient for design of composite structure. Lamina data can be used to predict laminate behavior with certain analytical assumptions. The results can be used as a first step in the materials selection process, but this building-block testing approach may or may not result in what are considered "laminate allowables." The articles "Overview of Testing and Certification" and "Testing and Analysis Correlation" in this Volume address this testing approach.

Analytical limitations currently exist in predicting failure for important failure modes when moving from lamina properties to practical laminates. Important failure modes that dominate design, such as bolted joint design, compression after impact, and notched strength, embody complex geometries and stress states that are extremely difficult to predict on a general analytical basis. The practical approach in dealing with these failure modes is therefore to employ empirical or semiempirical prediction methodologies that use laminate design allowables that are "tuned" to a specific analytical approach. Accurate predictions can then be achieved over a prescribed design space for which properties and allowables have been determined.

Stiffness-based failure is one subset of failure predictions in which values derived analytically from lamina properties can be reliable. Failure modes, such as panel and local buckling or design requirements based on deflection or stiffness, can be adequately predicted based on lamina stiffness properties. Common practice is to establish stiffness properties on a lamina. Note that because excessive stiffness can alter load paths and result in unexpectedly high stresses, upper and lower bounds are often placed on lamina stiffness properties. Also, because of the potential for matrix nonlinearity, techniques to "linearize" certain nonlinear stiffnesses are often employed. For example, for PMC, the secant shear modulus of a lamina is often substituted for the initial shear modulus when assessing composite strength.

Table 1 Failure modes of composite materials

Property/failure mode	Dominant constituent	Stress-strain behavior	Factors affecting properties
Stiffness			
Elastic constants	Fiber	Linear (except shear)	Temperature
Buckling	Fiber	Linear	Fiber alignment
Crippling	Fiber	Linear	Element geometry
In-plane strength			
Tension	Fiber	Linear	Low temperatures
Compression	Matrix/interface	Some nonlinearity	Moisture/elevated temperature
Shear	Interface	Nonlinear	Moisture/elevated temperature
Pin bearing	Matrix/interface	Some nonlinearity	Element geometry
Bearing/bypass	Matrix/interface	Some nonlinearity	. . .
Out-of-plane strength			
Interlaminar shear	Matrix	Nonlinear	Elevated temperatures
Interlaminar tension	Matrix	Nonlinear	Moisture content
Free-edge failure	Matrix	Nonlinear	Chemical exposure
Durability/damage tolerance			
Notched tension and compression	Interface	Some nonlinearity	Elevated temperatures
Compression after impact	Matrix/interface	Nonlinear	Moisture content
Fatigue	Matrix (only for properties sensitive to fatigue)	. . .	Load history

Efforts are currently underway to develop general failure prediction methodologies based upon fundamental constituent materials properties and laminate geometry. Should these efforts result in accurate, robust failure predictions over a wide range of materials and failure modes, allowables development could be shifted to a lamina, unit cell, or constituent level, thereby reducing the effort in laminate allowables development (Ref 2).

Manufacturing Techniques and Constituent Forms. The use of certain manufacturing methods or constituent forms invalidates the concept of lamina or laminate. For example, the use of three-dimensional textile fiber forms in conjunction with injection molding processes produces a composite with no lamina or laminate in the conventional sense. Bulk molding compounds are another example of composites that are not laminates. The use of a unit cell concept in this context is more logical, and allowables generated for the unit cell might be an efficient approach.

Requirements for Laminate Allowables. As previously discussed, laminate allowables are employed due to the difficulty in predicting most strength-dependent failure modes using lamina properties. It is important to recognize that laminate allowables are usually developed for a specific analytical technique that has been proven to correlate to a particular failure mode. The test specimen geometry, the test procedure, experimental results, and the analytical methods used to predict failure are all interconnected, and the resulting allowables are appropriate only for use in that specified analytical method. An example of this analytical dependence is the prediction of bolted joint strength. Test data are collected on specific geometrical and loading conditions, then semiempirical analytical techniques are used to extend the test data to other geometries and loads. Several analytical techniques are in use today in the composite industry to predict bolted joint strength, with each technique requiring the collection of specific test data under specific experimental configurations (Ref 3). See the article "Bolted and Bonded Joints" in this Section for more information.

Extending Laminate Results

Extrapolation of design allowables, that is, the use of design allowables beyond the point for which supporting test data exist, can lead to very unconservative results. Because of unexpected changes in materials behavior and failure modes, extrapolation should *never* be used. Laminate allowables should be developed to the actual working loads. Certain failure modes exhibit dramatic changes beyond given points. Consider, for example, the case of the transverse tensile strength for a laminate as the percentage of 0° fibers increases. When the percentage of 0° plies increases to 100%, the transverse tension strength drops dramatically. Good design practice limits this sort of extreme example, but the dangers of extrapolation exist for most failure modes.

Interpolation between two or more values is acceptable as long as no significant nonlinearities or discontinuities are expected and the failure modes are the same. Certain failure modes can exhibit local minima or maxima, which could cause problems on interpolation. Obviously, caution must be employed, but one can usually deal with such behavior through increased testing, analytical treatment, and experience.

Design space includes a variety of variables, including lay-up, thickness, temperature, and other design or environmental effects. Laminate allowables must be developed across the *design space* for which one intends to use the selected material. Figure 1 illustrates the lay-up design space for a two-dimensional laminate composed solely of 0°, ±45°, and 90° oriented unidirectional tape plies. The design space meeting the guidelines is shaded. Possible laminates at which to evaluate design allowables are indicated. These identified laminates bound the laminate design space. Combined with other test data taken at the extremes of temperature, moisture content, and other environmental effects, one should be able to confidently use the resultant design allowables for all permissible structural configurations.

One can also quickly grasp the main problem associated with the use of laminate-based design allowables. A significantly greater degree of testing is needed to generate design allowables for laminates than for lamina allowables. The costs associated with a test program can be enormous, and if the budget will not support such a test program, there are two options: limiting the design space so that allowables are needed for fewer combinations of laminates and environmental condition, or using statistical techniques that reduce required testing. As an example of limiting the design space, the designer may specify that only quasi-isotropic laminates (25/50/25) will be used in a particular design, thus dramatically reducing the required scope of testing. Such a limitation can reduce the advantages composites have over other structural materials, however.

Hybrid methods can be a very cost-effective means of obtaining high-quality lamina or laminate allowables. As an example of a hybrid method, laminate mean values could be developed across the design space for all important failure modes, and using statistical data gathered through lamina testing, allowables could be determined. A lamina/laminate approach is under development and evaluation by a MIL-HDBK-17 committee at the time of this printing.

Carpet Plots. The ability to predict an infinite number of variations in laminates without sophisticated software could potentially constrain and confuse the design process. In the past, some companies had restricted themselves to the use of 0°, ±45°, and 90° lamina orientations. This is becoming less true, as a generalization, with the advance in composite technologies. Given specific angle orientations as a constraint and the assumption of a uniaxial load case, laminate data can be represented by *carpet plots*, which are maps of a laminate property versus the percentage of one of the lamina orientations. Figures 2, 3, and 4 show the axial stiffness, axial strength, and Poisson's ratio for a 0°, 45°, and 90° laminate family. The carpet plot is for a given design temperature and for a certain design strength criterion, such as *B*-basis for the ultimate properties. The carpet plots assume that the laminate is lin-

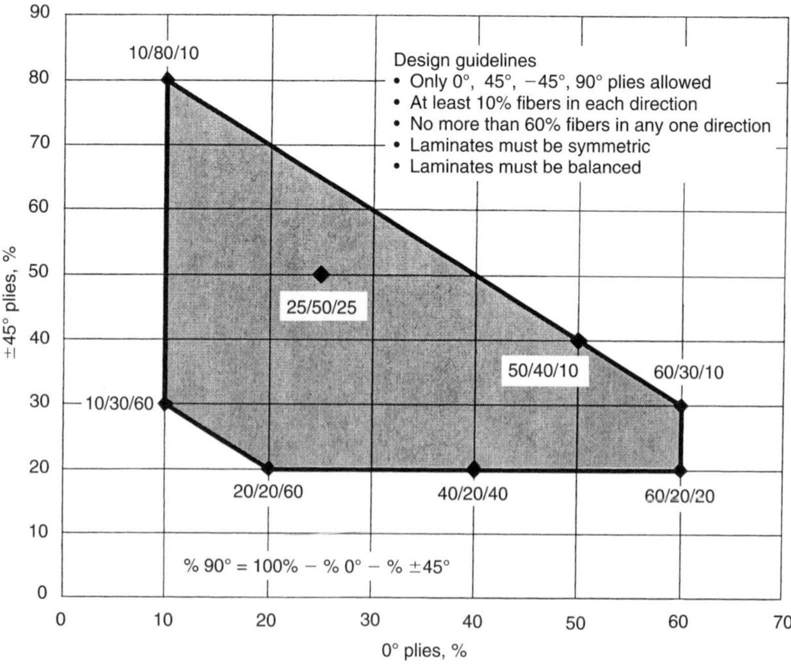

Fig. 1 Sample laminate design space

ear to failure (that is, no material nonlinearities, no ply cracks, and no extraneous failures such as free-edge stresses). For some materials, carpet plots of strength are inaccurate at the 0% 0° ply laminates.

Carpet plots are simple to use. One interested in a particular laminate property would first select the appropriate plot for the design application. Stiffness properties are given in Fig. 2. For a laminate composed of 40% 0° fibers, 50% ±45° fibers, and 10% 90° fibers, the stiffness is read at 26 GPa (3.8 × 10^6 psi). The procedure is to first find the percentage of ±45° plies, and then follow that value vertically until it intercepts the correct percentage of 0° or 90° plies, both at the same point. Then, the ordinate value for the laminate stiffness can be read.

Equivalence. Certification efforts that build on existing materials property information are also worthy of investigation. If one can demonstrate materials and process equivalence to a material in an existing materials property database, then potentially one can use the higher allowables determined for the combined data set. It has been recognized by agencies such as the Federal Aviation Administration (FAA) in the United States that a significant cost savings can be realized by industry and the FAA by sharing an approved central database and standardizing the engineering protocol to demonstrate materials equivalency (Ref 4).

The effect of the population size is illustrated in the example that follows in the next section. This approach offers dramatic cost and time savings. Details are found in the article "Test Program Planning" in this Volume.

Statistical Determination of Allowables

In this section, a brief overview of the procedure for computing *A*- or *B*-basis allowables is presented. A comprehensive treatment of the subject can be found in the MIL-HDBK-17-1E (Ref 1). Computer software and spreadsheets are also available from the MIL-HDBK-17 web site (www.mil17.org) to assist in establishing allowables. The flowchart from the Military Handbook that illustrates the *B*-basis procedure is reproduced in the article "Overview of Testing and Certification" in this Volume.

The actual computation of an allowable is conceptually quite simple. However, in practice, a high degree of experience and judgment related to testing, data analysis, and statistical calculations are required. The *A*- or *B*-basis values described earlier are functions of the following:

- Probability distribution
- Number of specimens tested
- Statistics describing the probability distribution

MIL-HDBK-17 contains a detailed description of the statistical procedures for determining allowables for composites. The simplest method for allowables calculation, using the normal distribution method, is described subsequently. Besides the normal distribution, the population may be better described by a Weibull or lognormal distribution, or if it fits none of these, a nonparametric calculation is used (Fig. 5). The *B*-basis value can be determined from the formulas given in MIL-HDBK-17 section 8.3 for each type of distribution.

Normal Method for Obtaining *B*-Basis Values. These examples consider the case of a set of data that are normally distributed, have no batch-to-batch variations, and have no outlier data points. If these assumptions are validated, the *B*-basis value is then calculated using the formula:

$$B = \bar{X} - k_B s$$

where $\bar{X}$ is the mean, s is the standard deviation, and k_B is the one-sided *B*-basis tolerance factor for a normal distribution, obtained from Table 8.5.10 of MIL-HDBK-17-1E.

Example: Effect of Number of Specimens Tested on *B*-Basis Values. Suppose that 12 specimens were tested. The data are a normal distribution with the mean and standard deviation computed as:

$$\bar{X} = 45.2 \quad s = 4.6$$

For the number of specimens tested (n = 12):

$$k_B = 2.211$$

and the *B*-basis value (B) can be computed as:

$$B = \bar{X} - k_B s$$

$$B = 45.2 - 2.211 \times 4.6$$

$$B = 35.0$$

As an illustration of the effect of a change in sample size, if the samples were doubled through more testing or finding valid database information, and the mean and standard deviation were still unchanged:

$$k_B = 1.854$$

and the *B*-basis value (B) can be computed as:

$$B = 45.2 - 1.854 \times 4.6$$

$$B = 36.7$$

This may not appear to be a great difference, but it does represent an almost 5% increase in the design allowable, with the same degree of confidence in the result.

If the population size were infinite, the largest B value would be attained by definition of the 90th percentile for a normal distribution:

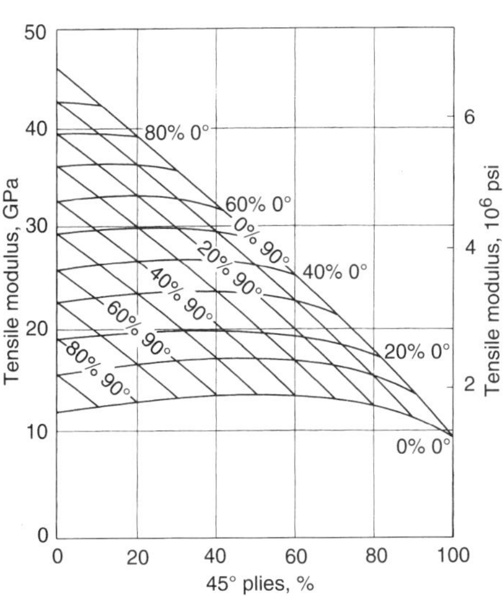

Fig. 2 Carpet plots illustrating tensile modulus of laminates

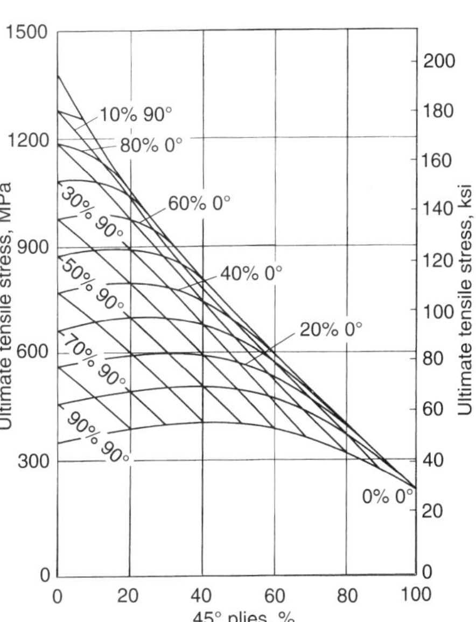

Fig. 3 Carpet plots illustrating tensile strength of laminates

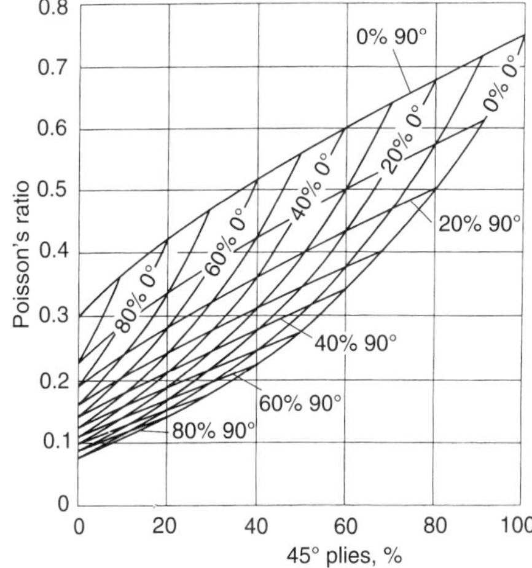

Fig. 4 Carpet plots illustrating Poisson ratio variation

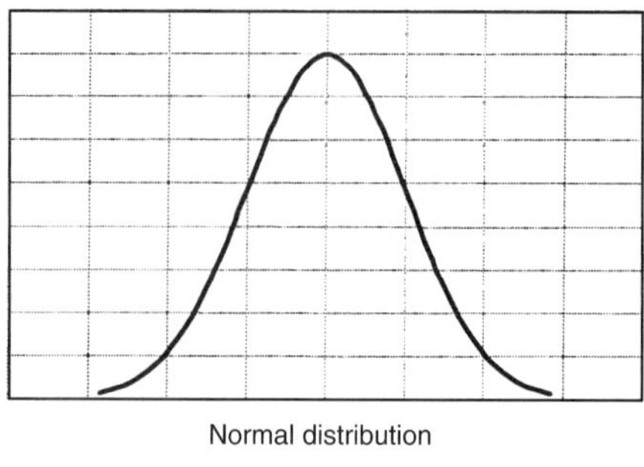

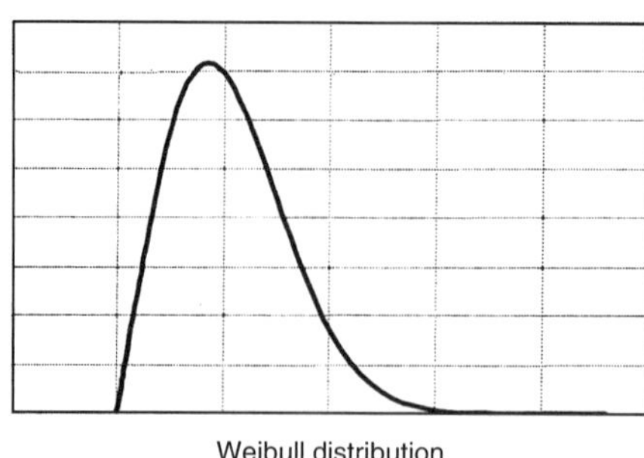

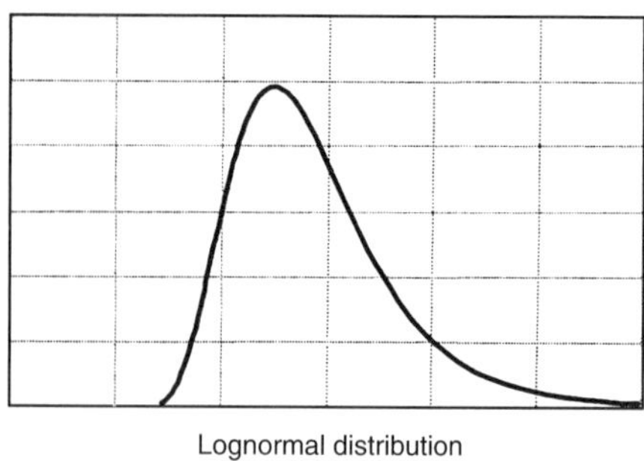

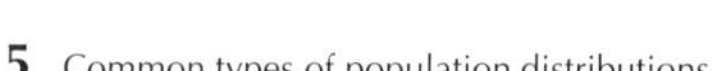

Fig. 5 Common types of population distributions

$$k_B = 1.282$$

and the B-basis value is:

$$B = 45.2 - 1.282 \times 4.6$$

$$B = 39.3$$

Each population distribution-type has a unique means of determining allowable values, but the basic procedures are similar.

Sample Size. The most common question when planning a test program to determine allowables is probably, "How many tests are enough?" As seen previously, the answer is significant. Unfortunately, the answer is not simple. The size of the test sample depends upon:

- Statistics used
- Expected variability exhibited by the material
- Anticipated use of the material
- Whether A- or B-basis allowables are required

An often-quoted number of individual tests at a given set of test and laminate conditions is 30 tests (six tests from each of five material batches) for the development of B-basis allowables for a particular property for a new material. For particular industries, standards or certifying organizations may have guidelines or mandates. Under the Advanced General Aviation Transport Experiments (AGATE) program, sponsored by the National Aeronautics and Space Administration (NASA) and the FAA, three batches of materials with 18 total specimens are recommended for B-basis allowables, and five batches with a total of 55 specimens are suggested for A-basis allowables (Ref 5).

If not bound by specific requirements, the answer to the question of sample size lies in the economics of the cost of the testing as compared to the cost of the reduced allowable values. As seen previously, reducing the sample size has a direct effect on allowables; for two samples with the identical mean and variability, the sample with fewer tests will have a lower allowable. If one has a rough expectation of the average and standard deviation, the impact of sample size can easily be evaluated, and sample size can be selected based on trade studies of testing costs versus the cost of lower allowables. The distribution of B-basis values as a function of sample size is shown in Fig. 6.

The use of regression, data pooling, or other statistical techniques can reduce sample size while not incurring the same negative impact on allowables normally incurred by performing fewer tests. These techniques can be more difficult to use, however, and may incur greater scrutiny from a certification authority such as the FAA.

Computational Procedures. While the example calculations for design allowables were simple, the steps leading up to that point are much more involved. These steps include:

- Determining whether the data is from a single batch or multiple batch, and whether there are statistically significant variations between batches
- Selection of the calculation based on whether data is structured or unstructured
- Detecting and evaluating outliers
- Selection of distribution type by analysis

Structured versus Unstructured Data Sets. The sources of variability in a composite material include the materials property variability of the constituent materials, batch-to-batch variability, panel-to-panel (or component-to-component) variability, or variability within a given panel or component. Since multiple test coupons could be composed from a single batch or machined from a given panel, if batch or panel variability is significant, the resulting data set is said to have structure. The presence of structure in a data set is undesirable—in effect, the size of the data set is reduced, thereby negatively affecting allowables.

The effect of structure within a data set can be dramatic. The best means of dealing with expected variability due to differences in material batches or panels is to include sufficient numbers of batches or panels, such that the variability of these effects can be assessed separately from the basic material variability. Five independent batches of material are commonly recommended for use in the development of allowables for a new material. Proper planning of the test program is also important. One can minimize the effects of panel variability by using test coupons taken from different panels for identical test conditions. Using larger numbers of smaller panels is also preferred over using fewer numbers of large panels.

Outliers in the Data Set. The data should be screened for possible *outliers*. These are data values that vary greatly from the rest of the population. Possible reasons for outliers are clerical or test procedural mistakes, mishandling of test samples, or simply poor-quality material. The outliers should be investigated to determine source of the discrepancy. If it is truly determined to be erroneous, it may be dropped for the data set. If no cause can be found for the discrepancy, the data must be kept as being a valid result. Statistical methods are available to define the deviation from the mean when compared to the standard deviation, which would categorize a data point as being an outlier.

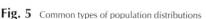

Selection of Proper Population-Distribution Type. Use of the population-distribution type, which best describes the specific failure mode results, is obviously very important in obtaining accurate design allowables. Proper selection is aided by statistical procedures that test whether the data fits a Weibull, normal, or lognormal distribution (Ref 4). The Weibull distribution is often considered to be the most appropriate for strength distributions of classical brittle materials and is appropriate for many composite failure modes. However, the normal distribution has been found to fit composite material data just as well as the Weibull distribution and is much easier to work with. Once the appropriate distribution is selected, one may compute an allowable value, using data set statistics and methods appropriate to the selected distribution.

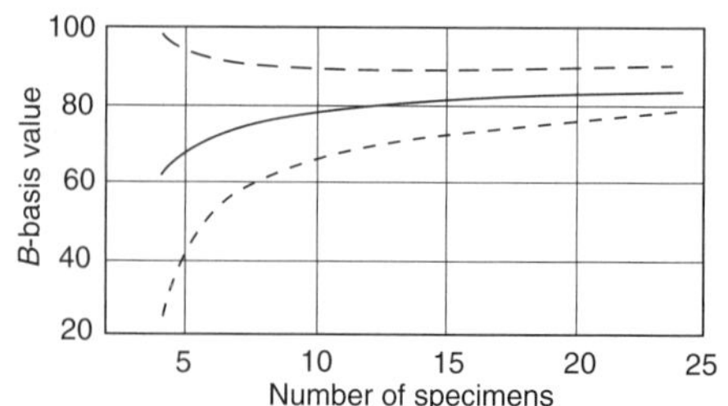

Fig. 6 Range of B-basis values as a function of the number of specimens. One sigma limits; mean = 100; standard deviation = 10. Source: Ref 1

Ensuring the Validity of Allowables

As the intent of determining design allowables is to promote reliability and safety of the structure, it is important to remember that a linkage must exist between the test population used to determine the results and the population of materials in the actual fabricated structures in service. The characteristics of composites that lead to the variability that challenges the determination of design allowables are still present, and these variables must be monitored in production and application. Obvious factors include:

- Changes in the constituent materials used in lamina
- Changes in suppliers
- Variations in manufacturing processes of making laminates and components
- Materials handling and storage that could degrade material

The responsible organization must have established and implemented procedures to ensure that the materials properties of the fabricated composite structures are the same as those of the materials used to develop allowables. This organizational effort is usually the responsibility of materials and process organizations as well as quality assurance experts. Details of this effort are beyond the scope of this article.

REFERENCES

1. *Composite Materials,* MIL-HDBK-17-1E, *Polymer Matrix Composites,* Vol 1, Guidelines for Characterization of Structural Materials, *Department of Defense Handbook,* Jan 1997
2. D.W. Sleight, N.F. Knight, Jr., and J.T. Wang, "Evaluation of a Progressive Failure Analysis Methodology for Laminated Composite Structures," AIAA Paper 97-1187, 38th AIAA/ASME/ASCE/AHS/ASC Structures, Structural Dynamics, and Materials Conference, 7–10 April 1997 (Kissimmee, FL)
3. *Composite Materials,* MIL-HDBK-17-3E, *Polymer Matrix Composites,* Vol 3, Material Usage, Design, and Analysis, *Department of Defense Handbook,* Jan 1997
4. "Material Qualification and Equivalency for Polymeric Matrix Composite Material Systems," proposed issuance of policy memorandum, Federal Aviation Administration, DOT, Federal Registery, Vol 65 (No. 114), 13 June 2000
5. J. Tomblin, Y. Ng, C. Yeow, and R. Suresh, "Material Qualification and Equivalency for Polymer Matrix Composite Material Systems," DOT/FAA/AR-00/47, April 2001

Computer-Aided Design and Manufacturing

Olivier Guillermin, VISTAGY, Inc.

CONTINUOUS FIBER COMPOSITE MATERIALS offer dramatic opportunities for producing lightweight laminates with tremendous performance capabilities. However, the high cost and complexity of designing and manufacturing composites have largely offset the benefits of using these materials. To unlock the full potential of lightweight laminates, new software applications have been developed that transform general computer-aided design (CAD) systems into a high-performance composite engineering environment for designing and manufacturing composite parts. These applications have evolved from software programs that originally attempted to model the draping of fabric onto complex curved surfaces.

Overview

History. As early as 1878, the mathematician Chebyshev made an attempt at modeling the fitting of a woven fabric onto a curved surface, assuming inextensible fibers and pivoting yarn crossover joints (Ref 1). Since then, the mapping of clothes to three-dimensional (3-D) surfaces has been the subject of constant research, especially in the textile industry, as exemplified in Mack and Taylor (Ref 2). More recently, the draping of fiber-reinforced composite sheets on curved tool surfaces has generated numerous research efforts. For example, important advances in analytical and numerical draping algorithms for compound curvature surfaces have been made by Robertson et al. (Ref 3, 4), Van der Weeen (Ref 5), Smiley and Pipes (Ref 6), Van West et al. (Ref 7), Heisey and Haller (Ref 8), Gutowski et al. (Ref 9), Tam (Ref 10), and Gelin et al. (Ref 11). In the last five years, the results of this research have been integrated in major CAD systems, which has led to the advent of commercial composite engineering software now used in production at large aerospace and automotive companies worldwide (Ref 12–15).

Challenges. Identifying shapes that can be easily draped, selecting lay-up processes that will minimize the amount of rework, and knowing how to design tooling ahead of time are all very valuable to the composite engineer. Being able to make decisions early on at the predesign stage, before the part is built, is even more valuable. Using composite engineering software in the design and manufacturing process of composite parts allows the engineer to design with composite features directly in the CAD system. Composite engineering software also provides a seamless link from the CAD model to structural and flow analysis and to the manufacturing applications, resulting in shorter overall design cycles.

Composite Features. State-of-the-art composite engineering software provides high-level composite features in the CAD system, allowing the engineer to efficiently manage the large amount of data generated during laminate design. The engineer works with familiar composite features, including zones, laminates, plies, cores, and ply orientation rosettes. The engineer can also manage the nongeometric attributes for these composite features, such as part number, materials specification, and ply or fiber orientation. Composite engineering software also maintains associativity between features. The part boundary, material, ply boundary, or the lay-up skin-related items, such as flat patterns, are easily updated when changes are made to the part. As the design progresses, the actual laminate can be analyzed and the number of plies, thickness, materials, and true fiber orientations can be verified.

Complete Part Definition. Accuracy of information throughout every stage of the design cycle is essential to the proper completion of a composite design. Composite engineering software maintains the complete definition of a composite part in the CAD model. For example, plies may have both a 3-D net and 3-D extended ply boundary with a corresponding flat pattern for each. In the event of a design alteration, accuracy is assured by verifying model consistency and alerting the user to elements that may require attention. The validity of the definition of each feature is also verified. For instance, it is ensured that ply boundaries are closed and on the tool surface.

Cost-Effective Changes. Composite engineering software makes it easy to discover potential design and manufacturing problems early in the development cycle. This allows changes to be made in the initial stages of design, instead of going undetected to the manufacturing floor where the costs incurred will be 10 to 1000 times greater.

Material Databases. Composite engineering software provides user-configurable material databases that include information such as material thickness, properties, producibility, and company specifications.

Computer-Aided Design, Manufacturing, and Engineering Functionality. Composite engineering software includes computer-aided design, computer-aided engineering, and computer-aided manufacturing modules. Design functionality may include core sample and ply stacking analysis, producibility and flat-pattern evaluations, laminate surface offset, and engineering documentation. Analysis functionality may include a structural analysis (finite-element analysis, or FEA) interface and a resin transfer molding (RTM) interface. In manufacturing, a flat-pattern export file generator for nesting systems and automated cutters, a fiber-placement interface, and a laser projection interface are examples of modules used to ensure a seamless link from design to the manufacturing floor. These functionality areas are discussed in more detail in the following sections.

Composite Draping Simulation

A draping simulation is used to generate fiber paths, identify areas of wrinkling and bridging, develop flat patterns, and allow the calculation of local ply orientations and the resulting laminate mechanical properties, such as stiffness, permeability, volume fraction, and thickness. The simulation is used as a design tool and manufacturing aid to guide the lay-up process, ensure repeatability, and minimize material waste. This section describes the kinematics of fabric deformation and explains the algorithms used in draping simulation.

Kinematics of Fabric Deformation. The ease of handling and drapability of continuous fiber fabrics lend themselves to the forming of deep-drawn and compound-curved shapes (Fig. 1 and 2). In woven fabrics, drapability is facilitated by the ability of the fabric to undergo large in-plane shear deformations, due to a trellising action of warp and weft yarns. In unidirectional fabrics, fibers slide relative to one another for in plane shear to occur, and it is generally assumed that the distance between the fibers remains constant, whereas the fibers of the woven fabrics come closer to each other under shear deformation. The draping process consists of forcing initially flat fabric to conform to a surface of any shape. Flat or developable surfaces can be draped with no fabric in-plane shear deformation, hence fiber paths are predictable without the aid of a material deformation model. On compound-curved surfaces, however, fiber paths depend on the fabric deformations and on the lay-up process. The ability to predict fiber paths using the appropriate material and process models has important practical applications:

- The true fiber orientations in the plies allow accurate calculation of laminate physical properties, such as stiffness, strength, and thermal expansion coefficients.
- Knowledge of fiber paths and shear deformations allows prediction of wrinkling and bridging in the fabric and indicates optimal locations for the cutting of relief darts.
- Exact fabric flat patterns can be developed from the draping simulation.
- The simulation can help define the best lay-up start point and keep track of this information to assure repeatability of ply lay-up and draping.
- A number of secondary physical properties can be determined from the draping simulation, including ply thickness, fiber volume fraction, outside mold definition, and mass properties.
- The simulation can be used as a design tool for optimizing a draping in terms of minimized total fabric shear deformation or specified fiber orientations at points on the surface, or for positioning unavoidable darts and splices at noncritical areas of the part.

Modeling Approaches. The existing models for draping simulation fall into one of the following two categories: mapping models and mechanical models. Mapping models assume a geometric mechanism to transform an initial unit square of fabric into the corresponding draped shape. Mechanical models use the equilibrium equations that balance the internal forces in the fabric with external applied loads. The mapping model algorithms rely on the CAD system for the necessary geometry data. They are not computationally intensive and can provide a quick answer. Design engineers mostly use this approach when choosing between several ply configurations. In contrast, mechanical models require the use of FEA. This approach is used by analysts and applied to the detailed study of composites forming and stamping. More information about FEA of composites can be found in the article "Finite-Element Analysis" in this Volume. Assumptions commonly made in the mapping approach include:

- The yarns are inextensible in the fiber direction.
- Tool-ply and ply-ply friction is neglected.
- Crossover points of warp and weft yarns act as pivoting joints for woven fabric, or the transverse spacing between fibers is constant for unidirectional materials.
- The composite ply maps perfectly onto the tool surface without out-of-plane wrinkles or discontinuities.
- The manufacturing process (hand lay-up, fiber placement, tape laying) defines how the composite sheet is "pinned" onto the tool surface.

For complete background information on the mathematical aspects of the mapping approach, including finite strain measures, 3-D geometric constraints, surface coordinates, and relevant concepts in differential geometry, the reader is referred to Ref 16.

Mapping Algorithms. Current mapping algorithms are usually a variation of the fishnet, mosaic, or least-squares algorithms (Ref 5–7).

In the fishnet algorithm, a net represents the fabric, with the knots simulating the warp and weft yarn crossovers. The net is draped onto the tool surface so that all the knots lie on the surface and the lines between the knots keep a constant length. The manufacturing process determines the order in which the net cells are applied onto the tool surface. Usually, the lay-up process will start from two perpendicular geodesic lines of predetermined knot locations or from one geodesic and a transverse progression rule. For a cell to be transformed from the initial flat shape to the applied final shape, three knots must already be pinned onto the tool surface, and the draping simulation engine then calculates the projection of the fourth knot (Fig. 3).

In the mosaic algorithm, the tool surface is modeled with facets, and geodesic lines cross the element edges at constant angle. This algorithm is a simpler version of the fishnet algorithm. Very fine meshes are necessary for a good result.

The least-squares algorithm is also a variant of the fishnet algorithm, in which the position of the fourth knot of a cell is obtained by minimization of the cell elastic strain energy. This approach presents some challenges related to the choice of an appropriate finite-element formulation and mesh size. The quality of a ply can be measured by the elastic shear deformation energy stored in the ply after draping. This is a function of the elastic shear modulus of the material and the shear deformation angles over the ply. The highest-quality draping of a surface may be considered that which has the least total shear strain energy, because it would be the easiest to drape, in terms of deformation effort, and would be the least likely to have wrinkling and bridging problems.

Composite Hierarchy

Laminate Definition. In the composite engineering environment, a laminate is a composite object that groups other composite objects together. The laminate can be viewed as an intuitive organization of components within the design that have unique attributes relative to the other laminates. A laminate is usually composed of a skin and a boundary associated to it. A lam-

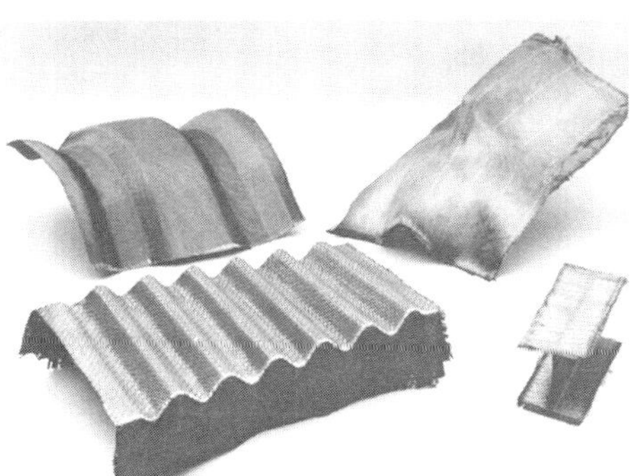

Fig. 1 Examples of woven fabric composite parts

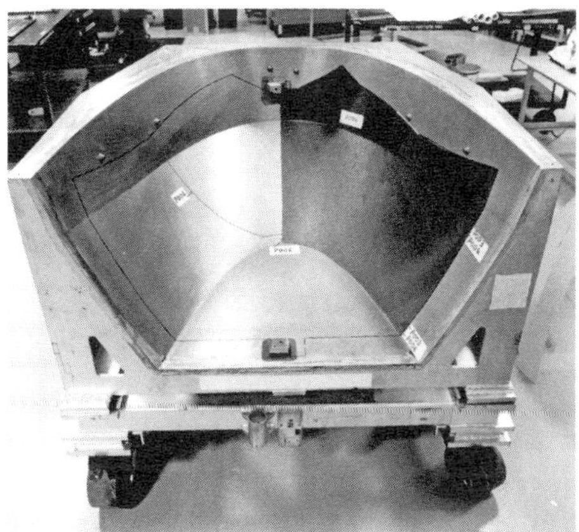

Fig. 2 Composite part showing compound curvature

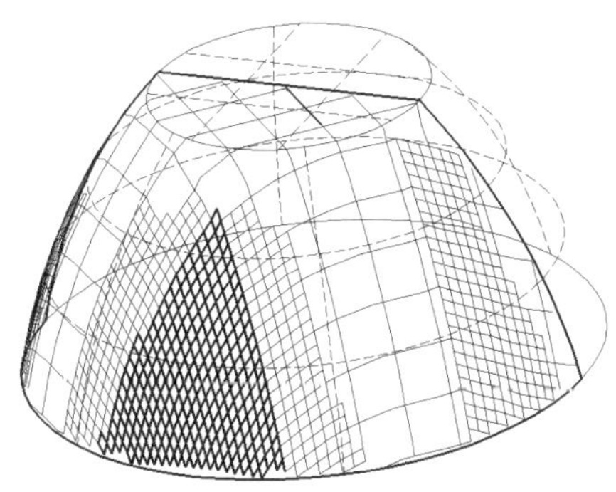

Fig. 3 Material scissoring shown by a draping simulation using the fishnet algorithm

inate can be defined as any organization of lower-level laminate components that aids in defining logical part assemblies. These lower-level components can be plies, cores, or additional groupings of other lower-level laminates.

One example of a laminate organization that is required for part-definition accuracy is the insertion of a core or insert object. Because inserts are usually very thick in nature, the inclusion of insert objects greatly affects the topology of the part for all plies/cores after its inclusion. Hence, a new laminate must be defined above the insert. All plies and inserts on this new laminate will be working off an accurate representation of the surface they are laid upon.

Ply Definition. A ply is the basic component of the composite hierarchy. A ply must be fabricated from a sheet of two-dimensional (2D) material. This cutout is known as a flat pattern (Fig. 4). The flat pattern is then laid up on a 3-D tool. There are several features in a 3-D ply that must be transferred accurately to the 2-D flat pattern. The composite engineering environment stores all the 2-D and 3-D information necessary to accurately define the ply. Typical ply information includes parent laminate name, lay-up sequence and step, material, fiber orientation rosette, stagger and drop-off indices, net or trimmed boundary, and holes or cutouts.

Core Sample and Ply Analysis

Core Sample. Composite design involves the bringing together of a large number of individual components (plies, cores) to satisfy various requirements (fiber orientations, thickness, stack-up, etc.) that change over the surface of the part. It is therefore necessary to be able to check the arrangement of critical areas of the part, to ensure that all design requirements are being met. A core sample is the term used to denote the design evaluation at given points of the laminate structure. A core sample "pierces" the structure at the given points and provides information about the laminate design at those points. Core sample results include information such as target and actual thickness and fiber orientations, orientation percentages, and ply counts (Fig. 5).

Ply Analysis. It is easy to calculate mass, area, and cost properties after the flat pattern of the ply has been generated. Parameters obtained from a ply analysis may include ply generation date, largest and average ply deformations, length of the flat-pattern outer periphery, flat-pattern total area, total material weight of the ply, total cost of the ply material, and ply center of gravity.

Producibility and Flat-Pattern Evaluations

Manufacturability Warnings. Producibility evaluations enable design engineers to balance part geometry, material, and process constraints by using draping simulation technology to predict how composite materials conform to complex surfaces (Fig. 6). By running producibility evaluations, engineers can visualize fiber orientations, predict manufacturing problems, and take corrective action during design. Producibility evaluations highlight areas where a ply will wrinkle during lay-up or exceed available material width. Material and process models are now available for many composites, including woven and unidirectional composites, dry and prepreg materials, and various processes such as hand lay-up, tape laying, fiber placement, or RTM. Input data typically consist of one or more surfaces representing the lay-up tool, 3-D ply boundary curves, materials specifications, and ply origin and orientations.

Darting and Splicing. There are two basic types of wrinkling that can occur during the lay-up process. The first type is called out-of-plane wrinkling, or puckering. This type of wrinkling is common in apparel. Out-of-plane wrinkling is caused by an excess of material in a given region of the surface. The second type of wrinkling is called in-plane bridging. In-plane bridging is caused by a lack of material in a given region. The material, not physically able to drape over the entire surface, spans or bridges regions of the surface. Splicing the ply into two or more pieces helps alleviate wrinkling. Splicing eliminates wrinkling by reducing the overall surface a single ply has to drape. Splicing must take into consideration the width of the material to minimize the number of splices (Fig. 7). Darting techniques attempt to eliminate wrinkling without dividing the ply into smaller pieces. Darting usually cuts the fibers that initiate the wrinkling and prevents them from propagating the wrinkling outward in the ply (Fig. 4). Darting techniques cannot be used in case of bridging, because they would generate an invalid flat pattern that overlaps onto itself.

Flat-Pattern Generation. A flat pattern is generated as follows: determine where each yarn intersects the ply boundary or internal cutout and map this information to a 2-D, orthogonal representation of the undraped fabric. As a result of the draping deformation, flat patterns for 0°/90° and ±45° on nonaxisymmetric compound-curvature parts will differ (Fig. 8). Flat-pattern generation also properly accounts for changes in surface area and density that occur when woven materials conform to compound-curvature shapes. The flat patterns are usually stored within the CAD model for output to ply nesting or cutting machines.

Laminate Surface Offset

As a result of the complex laminated structure of a composite part, the thickness of the final solid resulting from the lay-up varies throughout the part. Thus, even a part created on a very simple and smooth tool surface can produce a final volume with complex geometry, when all the details of laminate thickness changes, cores and inserts, ply boundaries, holes, drop-offs, and staggers are taken into account. It is very difficult to adequately model this solid in a CAD system, because it requires accurate knowledge of the distribution of thickness, as well as sophisticated

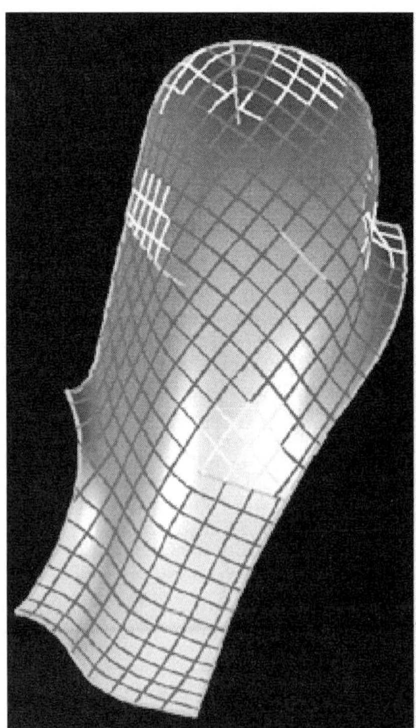

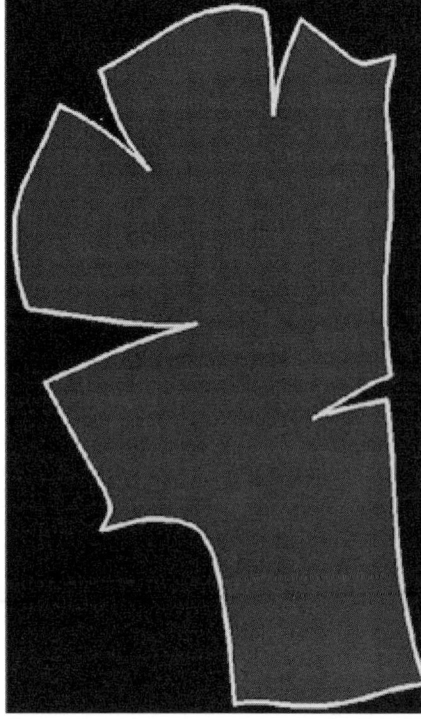

Fig. 4 Draping simulation and flat pattern for an aircraft wheel cover

surfacing capabilities. However, a model of the as-manufactured solid is very desirable, because it enables design of matched-mold tooling, machining of mating surfaces, and allows virtual assembly of parts to check for fit and serviceability.

Efforts to manually create the laminate offset surface in a CAD model are error-prone, and because of the difficulty of modeling the complex transitions between regions of different thickness, only an idealized representation of the laminate offset surface is generated with manual tools. At the same time, automatic modeling of all the ply drop-offs and core transitions results in extremely complex geometric models that strain the capabilities of modern CAD systems. Laminate offset surface capabilities address these issues through automatic optimization of the computed offset surface. Such a capability is built upon proven thickness calculation capabilities and advanced surfacing techniques to capture the thickness variations in the laminate without resorting to explicit surfaces for all ply transitions in the laminate. The laminate offset surface is developed from the original CAD surfaces that define the tool, and the drop-off regions are modeled through surface curvature rather than individual faces. This results in computationally efficient CAD models that have offset surface features that closely resemble the as-manufactured part, where transition regions are smoothly curved. The detail of the offset surface is thus ideally suited for all applications, including mating surfaces and mock-up.

Engineering Documentation

For composite parts, a difficult task facing the engineer is creating accurate design documentation. With composite design engineering software, once the information has been entered into a model, the engineer can use electronic documentation products to automatically generate engineering drawings, material tables, sequence charts, ply lay-up diagrams (Fig. 9), sequence charts (Fig.10), arrow text, laminate thickness and ply counts, and draped and schematic cross sections (Fig.11). Documentation is generated as CAD geometry that can then be plotted to hardcopy output. The format of the reports and drawings can be customized to follow drafting standards. The accuracy of the documentation is ensured, because it is generated directly from the data stored in the composite engineering environment. As the part definition is modified during the design process, the documentation elements can be quickly and easily updated to reflect these changes.

Flat-Pattern Export

Automatic Export. Flat-pattern export modules automatically generate a flat-pattern data file for export from the CAD workstation to the nest-

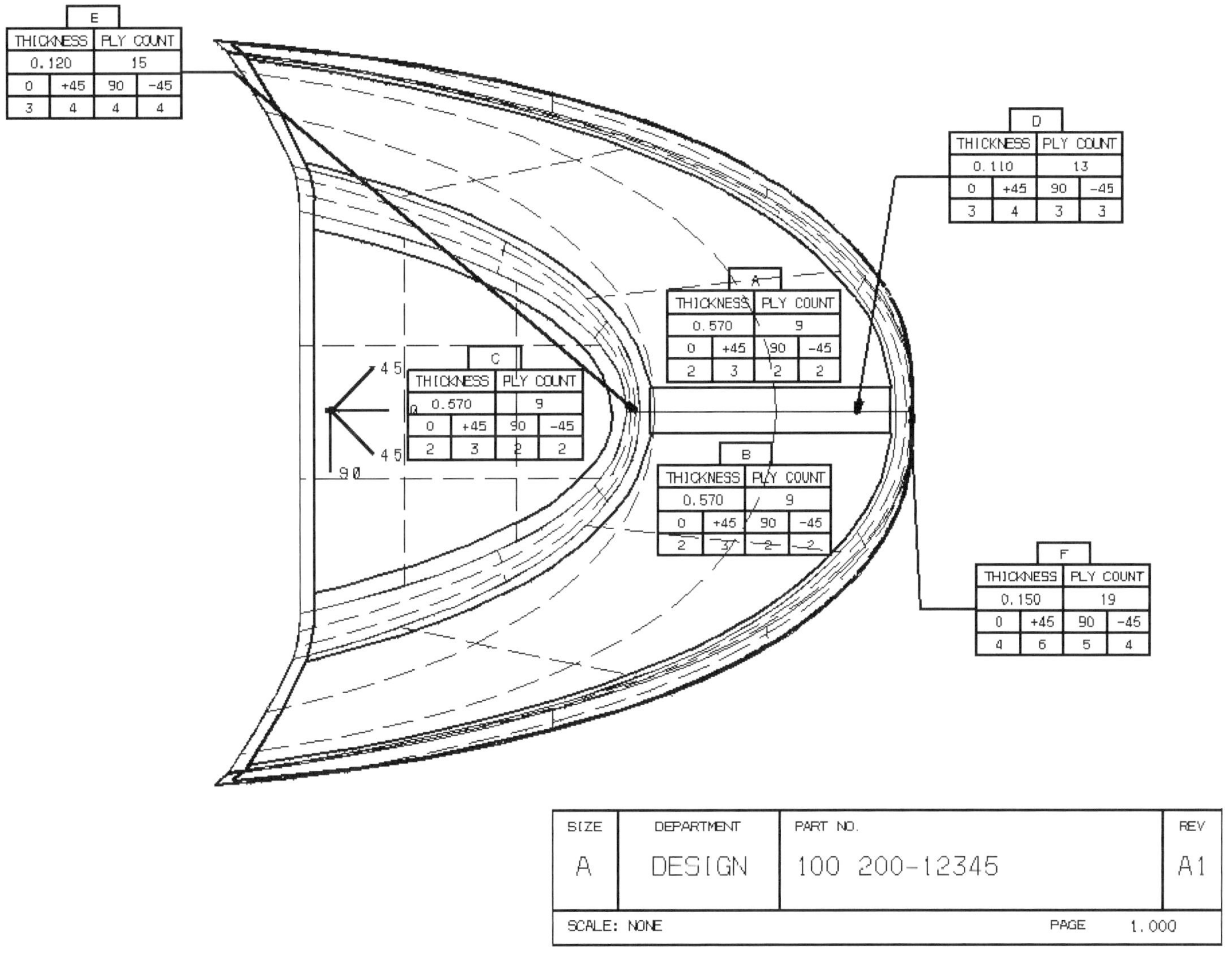

Fig. 5 Core sample results

ing software and cutting system. Working directly from the CAD system, flat-pattern export maintains file integrity and eliminates the need for manual manipulation of drawings and attributes in the transfer. Engineering changes are communicated quickly and correctly to the manufacturing floor through this automated process. Flat-pattern export automatically extracts flat patterns from the CAD model, eliminating the need for engineers to manually pick through data.

Flat-Pattern Optimization. Flat-pattern export may also enable users to fillet corners with a specified radius, in order to optimize manufacturing productivity. Corners that have been filleted decrease cutting time by eliminating stop-start sequences due to direction changes of the boundaries. Flat-pattern modules detect the sharpest corner of the flat pattern and start at that location. Subsequent corners with changes in direction that are larger than a user-specified angle are replaced by fillets, allowing the cutter to proceed at a smooth, consistent rate.

Structural Analysis Interface

A typical composite part is made of tens or hundreds of individual plies of various materials, each having a unique shape, orientation, and location. This complexity is compounded by the fact that in most cases, the final design of a part cannot be analyzed in its to-be-manufactured state. Analysis interfaces solve this dilemma by providing to the structural analyst a complete and detailed description of the final part design, enabling accurate verification of the performance of the part (Ref 17).

True Part Definition. The typical composite part design process starts with an analyst using FEA software to determine the requirements for the design, including laminate thickness, material, and so on, based on expected loads. Engineers can then use composite design engineering software to design the actual part in the CAD system. However, even with the best tools and most diligent efforts, the final design may differ significantly from the idealized part that was analyzed. Fibers in the resulting laminates may deviate significantly from the specified ply orientations, causing unknown variations in properties. The final design will also contain many details and modifications, including additional plies that were not considered in the original analysis. All of these issues can have a considerable effect on the performance of the final part. The analysis interface addresses this problem by enabling engineers to design a composite part in the CAD system, determine the state of the manufactured part using simulation technology, and then use the complete definition of a part in its to-be-manufactured form as input into the analysis software. The analyst can now rerun the analysis using the ply definitions and fiber orientations from the final part design, resulting in a more accurate assessment of the part. By linking the capabilities of the CAD system to the analysis software, the analysis interface allows designers to deliver the master model part definition that resides in the CAD system, complete

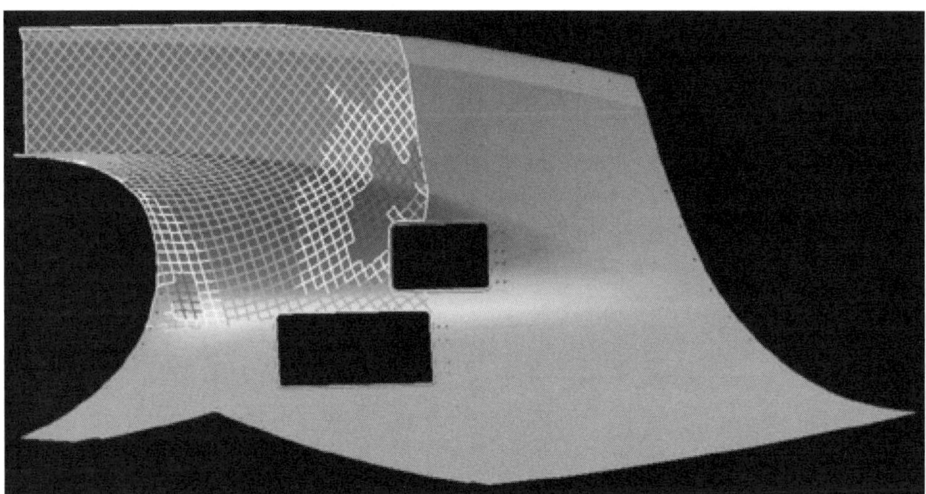

Fig. 6 Draping simulation to evaluate ply producibility for an aircraft cowling

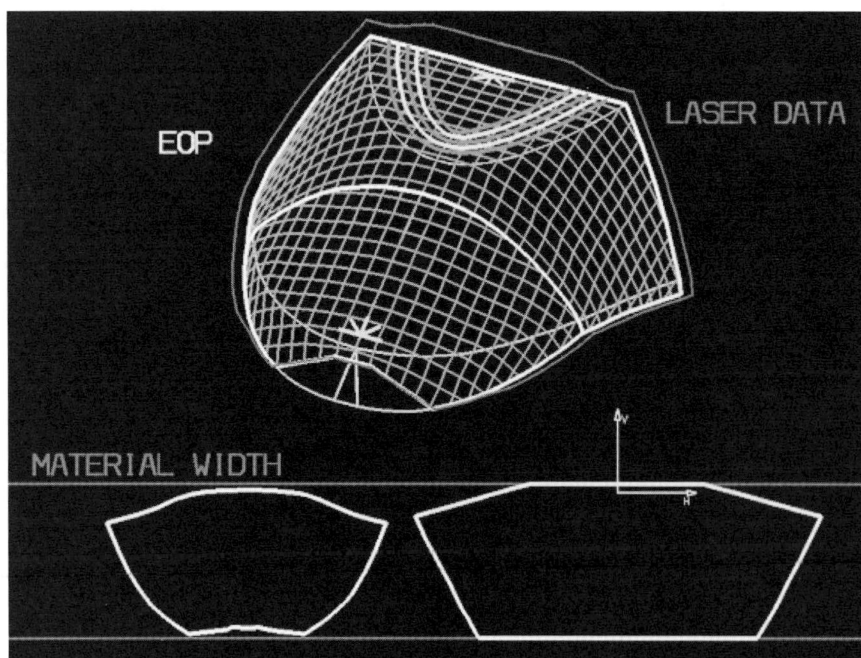

Fig. 7 Splicing of a full-body ply based on material width. EOP, edge of part

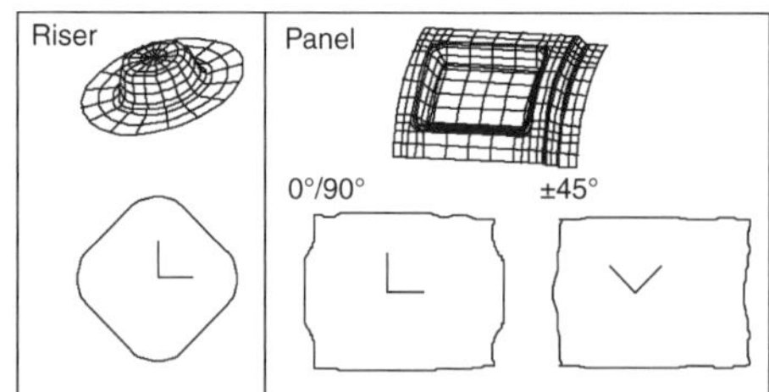

Fig. 8 Flat patterns as a function of fiber orientations

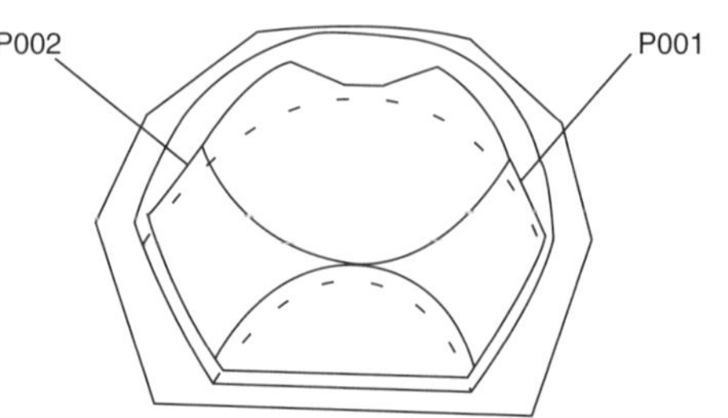

Fig. 9 Ply lay-up diagram

with fiber orientations and all other details, back to the analyst for verification that it meets all requirements.

Resin Transfer Molding Interface

RTM Process. Thermoset polymer composites can be produced by injection of reactive liquids into molds that contain dry reinforcement of continuous fibers. One process increasingly used for that purpose is RTM, in which the resin is injected at low pressure and sometimes under vacuum (Ref 18). Resin injection through a fibrous reinforcement is modeled as a flow through a porous medium and obeys Darcy's law, which states that the resin flow rate through a unit area of material is proportional to the pressure gradient in the mold (Ref 19). The coefficient of proportionality is the permeability of the porous medium (measured by appropriate experiments) divided by the viscosity of the resin (which varies in time with temperature and degree of cure). Permeability becomes lower when the fiber volume content of the composite increases, whereas viscosity decreases with temperature.

Figure 12 shows various aspects of the RTM simulation for a complex helicopter part, including the finite-element mesh and the successive resin front positions in time. The pressure field in the mold may also be displayed. A correct knowledge of mold filling allows adequate positioning of the injection ports and vents. There are three ways to facilitate the resin flow in the mold: decrease the fiber volume content (for example, by lifting slightly the mold cover during injection), increase the injection pressure, or heat the mold and/or the resin to reduce viscosity. Using the appropriate simulation software, these three parameters can be studied and tuned adequately. This is especially important in the case of large parts (of more than one square meter), complex parts with ribs, or parts with a high fiber volume content (between 50 and 60%). A RTM simulation software should contain the following four critical features (Ref 20):

- It must satisfy the exact conservation of resin mass during injection.
- It must be able to simulate race tracking, that is, the much faster resin flows that occur in specific areas of the mold, such as the edges.
- It must solve the heat transfer problem during resin injection (i.e., calculate the temperature field in the mold and in the part).
- Finally, it must simulate curing of the part.

Linking the RTM finite-element software to the composite engineering software through a RTM interface provides a more accurate description of the resin injection process by incorporating in the RTM model local variations due to the composite material draping process. Draping may generate local changes in ply thickness and directional variations in porosity and permeability due to material scissoring.

Fiber Placement and Tape-Laying Interfaces

Fiber-placement machines combine the advantages of filament winding, contour tape laying, and computer control to automate the production of complex composite parts that conventionally require extensive hand lay-up. Using fiber-placement machines can reduce costs, cycle times, structural weight, and handwork/rework when manufacturing composite parts, but creating data files to drive the machines is time-consuming and error-prone. With a fiber-placement interface, engineers can generate fiber-placement data files directly from the CAD model. The fiber-placement interface is a powerful functionality for designing parts manufactured by the fiber-placement process. The interface manages fiber-placement design and engineering entities, including slice axis, fiber axis, mandrel alignment points, and process regions.

Laser Projection Interface

Laser projection systems can reduce errors and shorten the lay-up time for composite parts by displaying ply outlines directly on the lay-up tool. These outlines aid in the location and orientation of plies during the lay-up process. With a laser projection interface, users can generate laser data files from within their CAD system directly from the 3-D model of the composite part. Laser projection interfaces use the CAD model of the composite part to generate the laser projection data and calibration files. Ply and sequence labels are also automatically included. However, as the lay-up of a composite part progresses, the accumulation of plies offsets the sur-

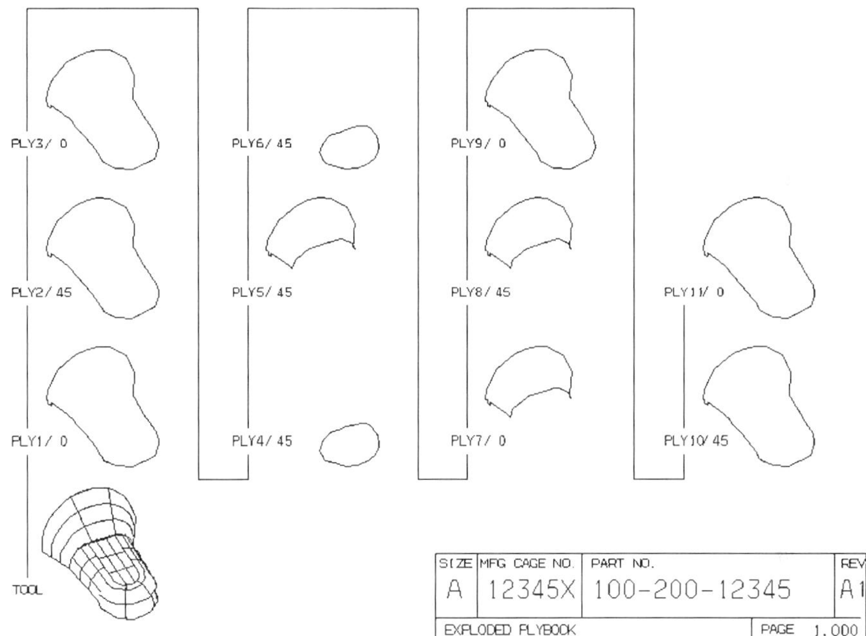

Fig. 10 Ply book showing lay-up sequences

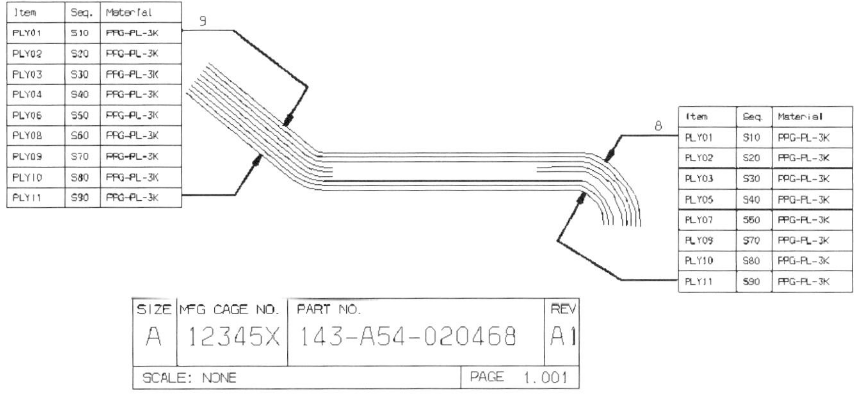

Item	Seq.	Material
PLY01	S10	PPG-PL-3K
PLY02	S20	PPG-PL-3K
PLY03	S30	PPG-PL-3K
PLY04	S40	PPG-PL-3K
PLY06	S50	PPG-PL-3K
PLY08	S60	PPG-PL-3K
PLY09	S70	PPG-PL-3K
PLY10	S80	PPG-PL-3K
PLY11	S90	PPG-PL-3K

Item	Seq.	Material
PLY01	S10	PPG-PL-3K
PLY02	S20	PPG-PL-3K
PLY03	S30	PPG-PL-3K
PLY05	S40	PPG-PL-3K
PLY07	S50	PPG-PL-3K
PLY09	S70	PPG-PL-3K
PLY10	S80	PPG-PL-3K
PLY11	S90	PPG-PL-3K

Fig. 11 Schematic cross section of composite part output from CAD system

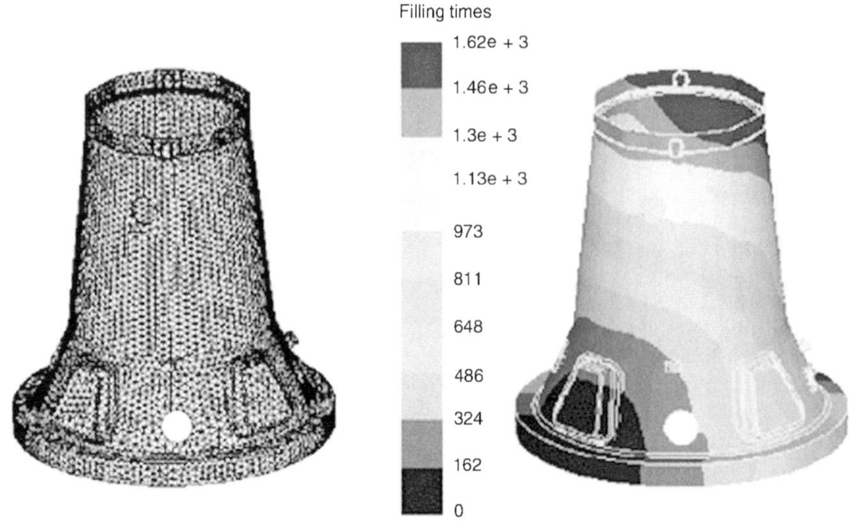

Fig. 12 Finite-element mesh (left) and resin flow-front simulation (right) for resin transfer molding injection

face on which the laser is projected. This results in considerable parallax error in the projected profile, especially in thick or highly contoured parts. Laser projection interfaces may automatically account for material thickness and offset due to ply buildup when generating the laser projection data. In addition, using the CAD model of the tool surface, the laser projection interface may provide additional data that will aid the programming of multihead systems for very large or highly contoured parts, where a single projection head may not meet the requirements.

REFERENCES

1. D.J. Struik, *Lectures on Classical Differential Geometry*, 2nd ed., Addison-Wesley, Reading, MA, 1961
2. C. Mack and H.M. Taylor, The Fitting of Woven Cloth to Surfaces, *J. Text. Inst.,* Vol 47, 1956, p 477–488
3. R.E. Robertson, E.S. Hsiue, E.N. Sickafus, and G.S.Y. Yeh, Fiber Rearrangements During the Molding of Continuous Fiber Composites, I: Flat Cloth to Hemisphere, *Polym. Compos.,* Vol 2 (No. 3), 1981, p 126–131
4. R.E. Robertson, E.S. Hsiue, and G.S.Y. Yeh, Fiber Rearrangements During the Molding of Continuous Fiber Composites, II: Flat Cloth to a Rounded Cone, *Polym. Compos.,* Vol 5, 1984, p 191–197
5. F. Van der Weeen, Algorithms for Draping Fabrics on Doubly-Curved Surfaces, *Int. J. Num. Meth. Eng.,* Vol 31, 1991, p 1415–1426
6. A.J. Smiley and R.B. Pipes, "Fibre Placement During the Forming of Continuous Fibre Reinforced Thermoplastics," Technical Paper EM87-129, The Society of Manufacturing Engineers, 1987
7. B.P. Van West, M. Keefe, and R.B. Pipes, The Draping of Bidirectional Fabrics Over Arbitrary Surfaces, *J. Text. Inst.*, Vol 81 (No. 4), 1990, p 448
8. F.L. Heisey and K.D. Haller, Fitting Woven Fabric to Surfaces in Three Dimensions, *J. Text. Inst.*, Vol 79, 1988, p 250–263
9. T.G. Gutowski, D. Hoult, G. Dillon, and J. Gonzalez-Zugasti, Differential Geometry and the Forming of Aligned Fibre Composites, *Compos. Manuf.*, Vol 2, 1991, p 147–152
10. A.S. Tam, "A Deformation Model for the Forming of Aligned Fiber Composites," Ph.D. thesis, Department of Mechanical Engineering, Massachusetts Institute of Technology, 1990
11. J.C. Gelin, A. Cherouat, P. Boisse, and H. Sabhi, FE Modeling of Glass Fiber Fabric Shaping Process, *Conf. Proc. Second Int. Symp. TEXCOMP2* (Leuven, Belgium), 1994
12. A.E. Trudeau and S.C. Luby, FiberSIM: Design for Manufacturing of Laminated Composite Parts at Sikorsky Aircraft, *Proc. American Helicopter Soc.*, Vol 2, 1995
13. B.P. Van West and S.C. Luby, Fabric Draping Simulation in Composites Manufacturing, Part 1: Description and Applications, *J. Adv. Mater.*, Vol 4, 1997, p 29–35
14. B.P. Van West and S.C. Luby, Fabric Draping Simulation in Composites Manufacturing, Part 2: Analytical Methods, *J. Adv. Mater.*, Vol 4, 1997, p 36–41
15. O. Guillermin, Closing the Loop Between Design, Analysis, and Manufacturing, *Proc. American Society for Composites 15th Technical Conf.*, Sept 2000, p 707–715
16. T.G. Gutowski, *Advanced Composites Manufacturing*, Wiley & Sons, 1997, p 297–372
17. J. Klintworth and O. Guillermin, Integrated Design, Analysis, and Manufacturing of Composite Structures, *Proc. 32nd International SAMPE Technical Conf.*, Society for the Advancement of Material and Process Engineering, Nov 2000
18. C.D. Rudd, A.C. Long, K.N. Kendall, and C.G.E. Mangin, *Liquid Moulding Technologies*, Woodhead Publishing Ltd., 1997, p 457
19. R. Gauvin and M. Chibani, The Modelling of Mold Filling in Resin Transfer Molding, *Int. Poly. Process.*, Vol 1 (No. 1), 1986, p 42–46
20. F. Trochu, R. Gauvin, and D.M. Gao, Numerical Analysis of the Resin Transfer Molding Process by the Finite Element Method, *Adv. in Polym. Technol.*, Vol 12 (No. 4), 1993, p 329–342

Design, Tooling, and Manufacturing Interaction

Anthony J. Vizzini, University of Maryland

THE USE OF COMPOSITE MATERIALS provides the designer with great flexibility with which to meet part performance requirements. Even after a composite material has been selected, the design must still address the microstructure of the component. The type of reinforcement—continuous fiber, short fiber, whiskers, chopped roving, woven or braided fabrics, and preforms—and its orientation greatly affect the performance of the component. Indeed, the ability to tailor a component increases its range of functionality as well as the complexity of the design. For example, the skin of an aircraft wing near its root may involve a hundred plies. Although the plies may all be the same material in the same format, it is the collective orientation of the plies that yields the desired extensional, flexural, and torsional stiffnesses. The design at the microscale is more important than simply the orientation of the reinforcement. Failure mechanisms such as delamination, fiber microbuckling, fiber kinking, and transverse cracking all occur on the microscale and are sensitive to manufacturing variations.

Just as the design must address the microstructure, the design must also address the macroscale. Composite materials can be formed into near-net shapes. Construction of components that often require many individual parts can be made in one step. Stiffeners can be staged, cocured, precured and integrated, or bonded. Sandwich construction with honeycomb or foam results in lightweight alternatives to discretely stiffened panels. As the part count is reduced, the complexity of the components is increased. The structural design may be as extensive as the aft fuselage of the V-22 Osprey (built by Boeing) or as simple as composite dimensional lumber made from recycled plastics.

Designing composites for structural performance initially involves meeting a set of desired performance specifications (typically weight in aerospace applications) at a minimum cost. When one introduces manufacturing costs as a constraint in addition to structural performance, the cost optimization process becomes more complicated. Designing composites for manufacturing is more involved than designing the part to be fabricated within specified dimensional tolerances. Indeed, the desired orientations of the reinforcement must be met with special attention paid to the presence and effects of anomalies or defects. Moreover, the prospect of large, integrated structures necessitates designing the manufacturing process concurrently with the component.

An indication of the difficulty in addressing this rather important issue is demonstrated by the material devoted in textbooks that specialize in composite structures. Since the 1975 release of *Mechanics of Composite Materials* by R.M. Jones, there have been many texts dealing with the mechanics of composite materials. A small number of these address manufacturing aspects along with the mechanics. Other texts are available with manufacturing or integrated design as their focal point. Those texts were surveyed to determine the amount of content devoted to manufacturing and are placed in chronological order in Fig. 1. Traditionally, those texts dealing with mechanics typically devote no more than 10% to manufacturing. Strong's text is the exception in that it updates much of his earlier text in manufacturing for a mechanics-based audience. In recent years, integrated manufacturing texts have been published, providing new sources. Thus, integrated manufacturing and structural design within academia is probably lagging behind structural design of composites by nearly twenty years.

Selection of Composites Manufacturing Processes

Often the design of a composite component is done in tandem with design of an equivalent metallic component to assess the cost/benefit of alternate materials. This can result in an unfair comparison as the designer employs such constraints as *black aluminum*, the use of quasi-iso-

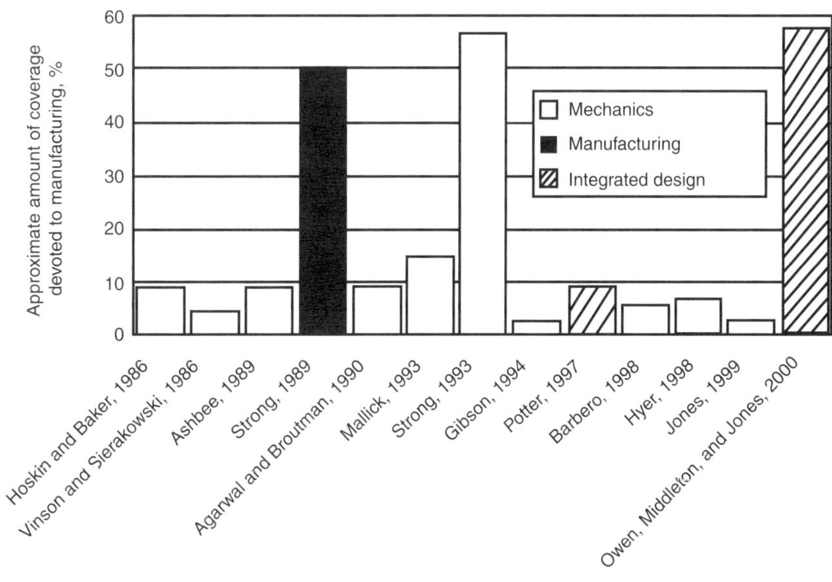

Fig. 1 Manufacturing coverage in composite texts

tropic layups to degrade the behavior of an orthotropic material to that of an isotropic material. Or the designer develops the manufacturing process concurrently with that for the metallic component. This design process does not take into account the tailorability of the composite material nor the potential advantages of the manufacturing process to increase performance, lower part count and weight, and decrease overall cost. The differences between composites and the materials they would potentially be replacing are significant enough to warrant independent development of the component and the manufacturing process.

Prior to the design of the composite component, many constraints may be imposed. Selection of the manufacturing process may be automatic based on available equipment and prior experience. The number of parts to be made may be known, thus limiting the time to manufacture and the expected costs per part. Overall dimensions (such as those for a boat hull) or dimensional constraints are specified. Surface finish and dimensional stability may be specified. The operating environment and general loadings should be known. Thus, many selections are made prior to the actual design of the component. The material system is most likely chosen based on the operating temperature, desired mechanical properties, material availability, and cost considerations. The manufacturing process will be selected based on surface finish, cycle time, and part cost. The selection of the material system often influences or limits the selection of the manufacturing process and vice versa.

The choice of material greatly influences the ability to design for manufacturing. The greatest latitude is afforded by polymeric resins. Structures that require ceramic, metallic, or carbon matrices will involve forming processes that introduce matrix into the reinforcement. In metal-matrix composites, for example, reinforcements increase strength, decrease the coefficient of thermal expansion, and improve the wear resistance at a cost of a reduction in ductility and in fracture toughness. Thus, the design of a component often will begin with the manufacturing process itself and will extend the available technology to incorporate the reinforcement. The goal is to improve the overall performance of the metal or ceramic rather than to create a material with different response than the base matrix. Thus, this article concentrates on design for manufacturing of polymeric composites.

Process Considerations

Independent of selections made prior to the design, many aspects of the manufacturing process are still unknown and are a function of the microscale and macroscale design of the component. The general composite manufacturing process can be subdivided into three separate stages. The first is preparation and involves handling the raw materials as well as mold fabrication and preparation. The second stage is the actual forming process. It is in this process that chemical reactions or phase changes occur or the constituents are consolidated into the desired component as outlined in the Section "Manufacturing Processes" in this Volume. Finally, additional fabrication may be required such as trimming, machining, bonding, finishing, or coating, as outlined in the Section "Post-Processing and Assembly" in this Volume.

Preparation

Two aspects of manufacturing that interact with the design are the handling qualities of the raw materials and characteristics of the mold. Prior to the manufacturing step, raw materials are acquired as individual constituents or in mixed form. As individual constituents they are either combined prior to the manufacturing process or combined as a result of the process. Materials premixed such as preimpregnated fabrics and tapes, sheet-molding compounds, and bulk-molding compounds may be assembled prior to the manufacturing process.

Handling Qualities. The ability of the preimpregnated ("prepreg") material to stick to itself and other materials is called *tack*. A tacky material will stay in place once it is situated on a mold or on top of another layer. Materials with little tack may require the use of a local heat source such as a heat gun to increase tack so that the materials can be held in place in the mold. Materials with too much tack increase the effort required by the operator to place the material in the correct position because errors in placement cannot be easily remedied. The degree of tack is influenced by ambient temperature, relative humidity, and the age and resin content of the material. Tack affects the design by limiting the size of the individual ply that can be handled and the ability to place it on the part. Although templates can be used for positioning individual plies, tacky materials must be placed accurately the first time, whereas low-tack materials may shift prior to consolidation, resulting in a disturbance in the location of a ply. The lay-up of dry fiber preforms for resin transfer molding often utilizes a "tackifier" compound in the form of a liquid or powder to add tack to otherwise tack-free materials.

The ability of the material (fabric, with or without resin) to conform to the shape of the mold is called *drape*. The greater the drape is, the more contour can be designed into the part. Therefore, drape limits the amount of compound curvature. This is separate from the concern of laying a planar material on a doubly curved mold or the reverse problem of representing in two dimensions a three-dimensional surface without distortions. Typically, thermoplastic materials have little drape, and, thus, are made to conform to the shape of the mold during the manufacturing process as is done in thermoforming. However, thermoplastic materials that have been cut into long, narrow strips and then loosely laid as a stretchable fabric do exhibit some degree of drape.

Because thermosets cure at any temperature, preimpregnated staged materials have a finite workable time out of storage, and wet lay-up resin systems, once mixed, have a finite pot life. Beyond these time limits, handling of the constituents becomes difficult and the mechanical properties of the resulting composite structure decrease. Thus, the time to complete the assembly must be addressed in the design of the component. If intricate ply lay-ups are required, then pre-kitting must be employed in forming the preform for wet systems or automation for cutting and material application for prepreg systems. The size of the structure may limit how much material can be applied without significant degradation of mechanical properties caused by exceeding out-time and shelf-life limits. However, there are manufacturing processes and materials well suited for long assembly times. Many of the closed-mold processes, vacuum-assisted resin-transfer molding (VARTM), or structural reaction injection molding (SRIM), when used with preforms, can result in reduced handling time of the resin. The dry reinforcement is placed in the desired orientation, and then the resin is introduced.

The ability of the resin to properly wet out the fibers, to consolidate individual layers, and to decrease void content is related to its viscosity. There is a trade-off between increased wet-out and handling characteristics. Low viscosity resins tend to pool in resin-rich areas for large parts or escape the part entirely, resulting in a lack of uniformity in, or very high, fiber volume. Resin systems must be tailored to provide low viscosity during winding processes or in flow periods of autoclave processes but must have sufficient viscosity to remain where placed within the structure during the process.

Tooling Considerations. The role of the tool or mold is to impart the shape to the composite part during the manufacturing process. Tool design is based on the requirements for the tool to maintain its shape during the manufacturing process and is a function of the processing temperature, applied loads, and curing time. In addition the number of replicates per tool affects its material of construction.

Here, consideration of the manufacturing process is very important. The geometry of the part is constrained by the ability to form the necessary tooling. Highly contoured surfaces will require a highly contoured tool. Making use of available geometries such as flats and tubes results in low-cost tooling. Complex tooling often requires manufacturing the desired master model shape using a rigid medium such as wood. The mold is then made using this machined master model shape or plug, often from composite materials.

One key aspect that must be incorporated into the mold design is compensation for the phenomenon referred to as *springback*. Springback is caused by segregation and shrinkage of the resin to one side in an area with a large change in radius. Because of differences in thermal expansion, residual stresses arise during the manufacturing process. When the part is removed from the tool, the part deforms to the state governed by the residual stress state. For example, springback results in a one or two degree change in an L-section and can be addressed by considering the residual stress state in the design of the tool.

Differences in the coefficients of thermal expansion (CTE) between the tool and the part are significant as indicated in Table 1. Most forming processes involved compliant material being placed on the tool at room temperature with a subsequent rise in temperature to cure or consolidate the material. From this *stress-free* point, the part and mold are cooled to room temperature and differential shrinkage occurs. This difference can be used as a means to release a part, such as with graphite/epoxy tubes on an aluminum or steel mandrel; however, the CTE of the tube in the hoop direction must be sufficiently smaller than that of the mandrel. In this way tubes with reinforcement in the hoop direction easily release from the mandrel, whereas highly longitudinally aligned tubes do not. To provide better dimensional stability, the CTE of the tool is matched to that of the structural component in many high-performance aerospace applications.

Forming Processes

Because the manufacturing process is to be designed concurrently with the component, design guidelines are flexible. Manufacturing of a designed component is often limited only by the creativity of the engineer and the budget of the project. Although currently not all conceivable parts can be made with composites, the constant stream of new products using composite materials attests to the ingenuity of manufacturing engineers.

In general, the manufacturing process can impose limitations on the microscale, such as the orientation of the reinforcement, and on the macroscale, such as the ability to form an integrated structure. Although an individual forming process has specific requirements on types of resins and reinforcements that can be used, the design considerations can be discussed among three areas. Laminated hand laid-up structures require extensive labor and tooling and thus are used only in those applications where the added performance can justify the relatively high costs. A second group of forming processes is that which makes use of dry reinforcements in a semicontinuous or continuous fashion such as filament winding, braiding, or pultrusion. The third group includes the closed-mold processes as discussed in the articles "Resin Transfer Molding and Structural Reaction Injection Molding," "Vacuum Infusion," and "Compression Molding" in this Volume.

Preimpregnated Tapes and Fabrics. Laminated preimpregnated materials often offer the greatest mechanical properties. High specific strength and stiffness are important in weight-constrained structures within the aerospace industry. Preimpregnation provides a consistent product with a uniform distribution of reinforcement and resin, with high fiber-volume fractions possible. Such laminated structures typically require a great amount of hand labor and autoclave processing. This results in a relatively high cost of manufacturing. Nevertheless, proper design of a composite component can decrease the overall manufacturing costs.

In laminated structures, the orientation of each ply is a design variable. This increases the complexity of the design process, and thus ply angles are often limited. Several common approaches include allowing only orientations that are multiples of 15° or, more stringently, laminates made up entirely of 0, +45, –45, and 90° plies. These design strategies limit the orientations that are involved if hand lay-up is to be used. However, limitation of angles may not be necessary. Templates can be used to cut material with the desired orientations and to place the plies on the tool. A trained worker can just as easily lay a 15° ply as a 17° ply. However, if the design requires many plies (shape and orientation), then additional care must be taken to sort the individual plies and to ensure that each ply is laid down in the correct sequence. It is also important that the sensitivity to a given angle is not greater than ±3°. Mylar templates or lasers often are used to indicate on the tool the location and orientation of each successive layer, thus eliminating much of the error in hand layup. However, variations between specified and as-manufactured orientation will always occur.

The cutting of plies can be automated to increase efficiency and quality. Techniques include water jets, lasers, reciprocating knife, and die cutting. Using these methods, intricate plies can be cut repeatedly with no limitation on orientation of the reinforcement. A water jet introduces moisture to the uncured composite, and extended exposure needs to be avoided. Laser cutting results in a heat-affected zone and may alter the local mechanical properties.

The contour of the tool is of great concern when using preimpregnated tapes and fabrics. Whenever there is a double radius of curvature, flat materials cannot be used without stretching or cutting and overlapping. The inverse problem is to take any shape with a compound curvature such as a hemisphere and flatten it without excessive straining of the surface (Fig. 2a). One can see that the initial planar material requires many discontinuities. Even if cutting is reduced to a minimum as in the cone in Fig. 2(b), the orientation about the structure cannot be prescribed. Thus, a requirement for all of the fibers in a layer of a cone to be in one direction and only have one joint per ply is impossible. The orientation of fibers in structures with realistic surface con-

Table 1 Coefficients of thermal expansion for mold materials

Material	Coefficient of thermal expansion	
	10^{-6}/K	10^{-6}/°F
Aluminum	22.5	12.5
Steel	12.1	6.7
Sand/polyvinyl alcohol	12.2	6.8
Sand/sodium silicate	11.5	6.4
Ceramic	12.1–12.6	6.7–7.0
Glass prepreg	11.7–13.1	6.5–7.3
Graphite prepreg	3.6	2.0
Invar	1.4–5.2	0.8–2.9
Monolithic graphite	0.2–1.8	0.1–1.0

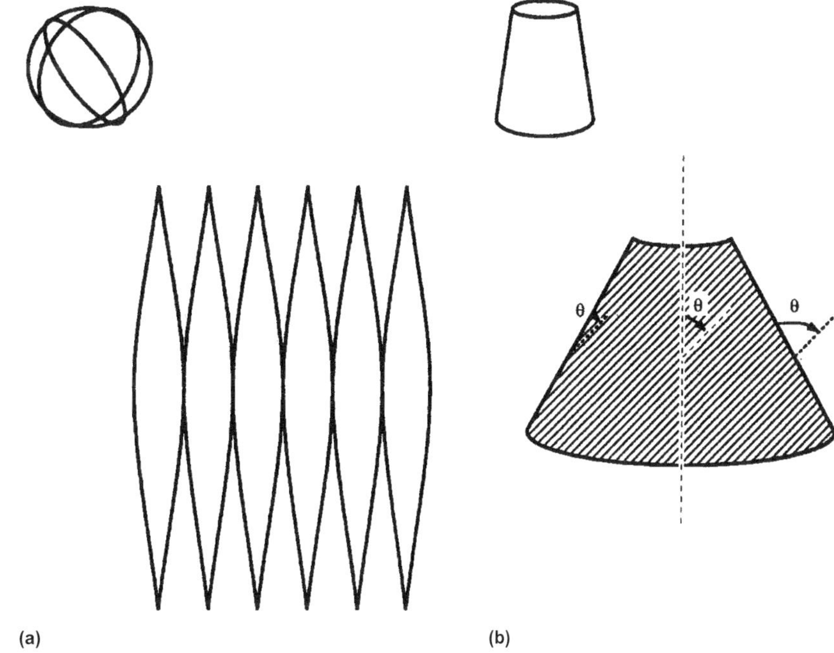

Fig. 2 Flattened contours. (a) Sphere. (b) Truncated cone

tours is a continuum problem that the designer must be aware of.

Many of the restrictions mentioned above can be overcome by using tow placement. Individual tows or strips of preimpregnated material can be laid down using a multiaxis, multi-degree-of-freedom robot arm. The material is tacked to the tool by applying pressure through the head of the tow placing arm. If this head is heated or an external heat source such as a laser is used, then thermoplastics can be used. Individual strips can be placed on the tool in the desired orientation. This process removes the variations inherent in hand processing, although it requires extensive programming and expensive fabrication equipment. Errors in orientations caused by the surface contour are limited by the width of the tow or strip being used.

Because most laminated structures are placed in a vacuum bag and cured with additional autoclave pressure, major concerns are maintaining the integrity of the bag during the forming process and proper transfer of the applied pressure to the part. In any concave portion of the part, the vacuum bag can form a bridge if it is locally of inadequate size. Thus, insufficient consolidation will occur in that section. One approach that reduces this effect is a reusable silicone rubber bag. The bag is originally formed on the tool. Even if the bag conforms as it should, a fillet should still be allowed in a corner; however, the fiber volume in the fillet will be lower than that in the surrounding material. For example, if an I-beam is constructed by laying up two separate C-channels, placing them together, and applying additional plies on the flanges, a small resin-rich pocket will form (Fig. 3a). To alleviate this resin-rich zone, additional material can be placed in that area to maintain the same fiber-volume fraction (Fig. 3b). In some cases, this remedy cannot be applied. Because plies have discrete thicknesses, the thickness of a part is changed using terminating plies, resulting in a resin-rich area that cannot be filled. A possible remedy is the use of a preform or bulk molding compound partially staged that can be cured with the overlaid flange plies.

Dry Fibers and Broad Goods. One major disadvantage of using preimpregnated tapes and fabrics is that they require batch processes that involve significant hand labor or, in the case of automated tape laying and fiber placement, significant programming and capital investment. Mixing the reinforcement with the resin system in situ during the fabrication process allows for three-dimensional reinforcements or continuous processing while increasing material utilization.

In wet filament winding, fibers are drawn through a resin bath and wound on a rotating mandrel. This is the primary manufacturing method for cylindrical or spherical pressure vessels, because continuous fibers can be easily placed in the hoop direction. Low-cost constant cross-section components can be made using a filament winder with two degrees of freedom, the rotation of the mandrel and the translation of the payout eye. Increasing the number of degrees of freedom in the process increases its complexity as well as the complexity of parts that can be created. Additional payout eyes increase the speed of the process as well as introduce the possibility of performing braiding in the process. Variations to the winding process can include varying cross-sectional geometries, post-winding forming that can alter a convex outer surface to an I-beam shape as in Fig. 4, and inclusion of fittings and bosses.

One concern in filament winding is the angle of the fibers. Hoop (circumferential) winding involves laying fibers at nearly 90° with respect to the longitudinal axis of the mandrel. This results in a cylinder with high hoop strength. Helical (off-axis) or polar (axial, near-longitudinal) windings provide reinforcement along the length of the structure. As these fibers are wound, they have a tendency to slip. One exception is the geodesic path, which is a straight line on the flattened equivalent surface. As the part is formed, its thickness will increase, thus changing the geometry of the process. Additional information on design considerations with this process is provided in the article "Filament Winding" in this Volume.

Pultrusion is used to produce indefinite-length constant cross-section components. Fibers, fabrics, and mats are pulled through a die with resin introduced at one end. The die is tapered to apply hydrostatic pressure to the resin, resulting in fiber wet-out. An exothermic reaction can occur or heat is added to result in curing of the component. Design limitations include the need for a large proportion of reinforcement in the longitudinal (axial) direction to enable the process to be run. Annular cross sections or holes increase the complexity and cost of the die; however, it is better to have them formed in the part rather than added by post-forming machining. (It should be noted, though, that holes can be formed only in the pull direction of hollow closed sections.)

Molding Processes. The last set of forming processes involves forming with a closed mold. Such processes include matched-die molding and resin-transfer molding. These processes frequently are used to fabricate parts in large quantities with short cycle times.

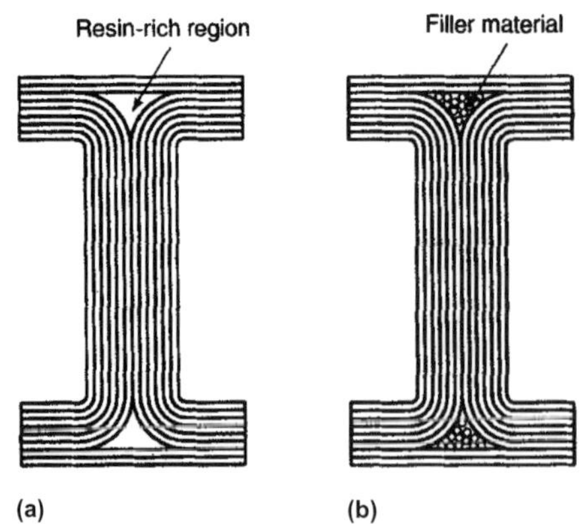

Fig. 3 Schematic drawing of a C-channel (a) with a resin-rich region and (b) with filler material to maintain fiber volume fraction

The constraints that are posed by the forming process are the methods by which the resin is introduced into the mold and how the chemical reaction is to occur. The flow characteristics are often non-Newtonian. Mold design is based on specialized design experience and may utilize sophisticated software to locate resin entry and exit ports and to account for flow patterns, velocity, shrinkage, and thermal expansion. Often the resin is curing as it is being introduced into the mold; thus its rheology is a nonlinear function of time. Clearly, there are limitations in the shape of the component. A high degree of compartmentalization of the mold increases the need for many entry ports.

The dry reinforcement is placed in the mold before the resin is introduced. Fabrics, mats, and preforms of various cross sections and geometries are possible by employing the expertise of textile engineers.

Post-Processing and Fabrication

Once the consolidation process is completed, the component usually requires additional fabrication steps to complete. The part is trimmed and holes are drilled. The surface may be prepped and painted. In addition, several parts may be bonded together to form a larger component, or secondary bonding is performed to yield a sandwich structure. The design of the component must also consider these steps and anticipate possible adverse effects.

Machining. The final shape and form of a metallic structure is realized in the machining process. Composite structures are formed prior to being machined. Machining is necessary to facilitate mechanical joints, cut small parts from stock items, and remove excess material. To avoid damage, composites should not be machined using metal techniques that use cutting, tearing, or shaving tools. Thus, if a cavity is required, it should be formed in the consolidation process and not by machining unless it is a thick-walled shape or has a "strong-back" composite or metal liner bonded in the cavity.

Cured composite materials can be cut using a number of techniques including mechanical

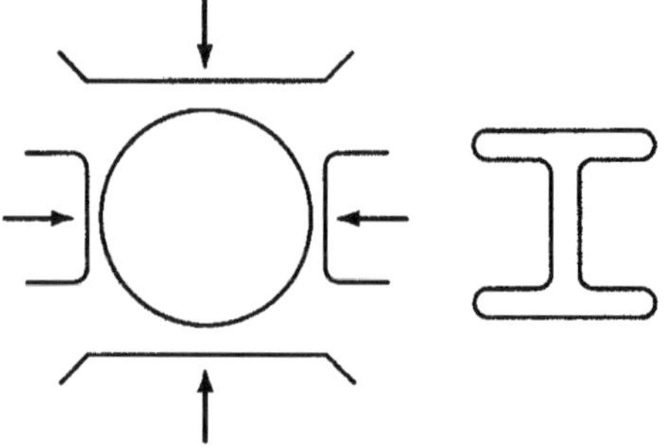

Fig. 4 Post-winding forming

methods and water jets. Mechanical methods require an increase in tool speed, a decrease in the feed rate, and a cooling lubricant. Often, carbide tip tooling is used; however, to prevent excessive damage or delamination to the composite structure, diamond-grit tooling should be used. Thus, the composite structure is machined using abrasives. Care must be taken to allow for particle removal and to prevent heating the part.

Water jets provide for a greater amount of complexity in cutting. Water jets can cut through a 25 mm (1 in.) thick structure at relatively fast feed rates (1.5 m/min, or 5 ft/min) and can be used for intricate details. The starting point of the water jet must be away from the part edge because of the possibility of delamination.

Because of the potential threat of damage during machining, designs should limit the amount of post-fabrication forming. Near-net-shape fabrication can result in a minimum amount of machining. Whereas holes can be drilled effectively, it is often better to incorporate a fixture into the component during its forming rather than to attach it through mechanical means later. However, difficulties arise when cocuring metal parts into composite parts due to the differences in CTEs.

Bonding. The ability to reduce the number of parts in an assembly is a clear advantage of using composite materials. Yet, if the manufacturing and design processes are developed independently of each other, this advantage will be severely diminished. An illustrative example of the choices available is a stiffened plate. In Fig. 5(a), the plate is made in three separate steps. The skin is fabricated, and the stiffener is fabricated. A secondary bond is performed. Although the stiffener fabrication may make use of a high-yield low-cost method such as pultrusion, performing the secondary bond reduces some of the cost benefit. One alternative is to cocure the stiffener with the skin. Film adhesive that has a similar cure cycle as the resin can be used to increase the integrity of the bond line. In Fig. 5(b), the stiffener may or may not be precured. A second variation has the stiffener now integrated with the skin. In Fig. 5(c), the macroscale of the design has increased, resulting in additional specifications on the microscale. Finally, the whole concept of skin with a blade stiffener can be abandoned, replaced by either a foam-filled hat section (Fig. 5d) or a sandwich construction.

Again, if one approaches a composite structure with the same limitations imposed by metal construction, the potential of the composite material is not achieved. For example, an aircraft fuselage is constructed using thin skin stiffened by longerons along its length and hoop stiffeners about its circumference. The intersections of these stiffeners are at right angles, out of fabrication necessity. This limitation is imposed primarily because the metal structure must be made in many pieces and assembled. The true design objective of flexural and torsional stiffness can be met more efficiently with a composite structure if the artificial constraint of right-angle stiffeners is removed and stiffness is achieved through other means (such as sandwich construction).

Sandwich structures provide high bending stiffness at low weight. Various core materials are used such as expanded polymer foam, balsa wood, aluminum or Nomex honeycomb, or syntactic closed-cell foams. The face sheets can be formed separately and bonded to the core, cocured with the core, or cured in separate steps layer by layer. Forming core to different contours requires additional fabrication. Foam and honeycomb cores can readily conform to flat and cylindrical sections, although anticlastic deformations may cause problems on relatively small radius-to-thickness ratios. Compound curvatures are more difficult to attempt. The core material determines the minimum radius of curvature. Lower density core materials tend to conform easily but may offer lower shear stiffness and strength. The use of in-place foaming, overexpanded honeycomb, or scored-foam boards allows complex curvature or shapes while maintaining structural integrity.

The manufacturing process will determine the consolidation pressures seen by the face sheets during their forming process. If cured separately, high pressures can be used. Secondary bonding then occurs at temperatures equal to or lower than the cure temperature of the face sheets and at significantly lower pressures so as not to compromise the core material. Curing face sheets on the core directly results in a slight dimpling and reduced mechanical properties if honeycomb cores are used. If a resin infusion method is being used, nonporous core material must be used.

When using sandwich structures, most applications require that the edges must be closed out to allow for joining and to prevent damage and water intrusion. Several techniques are used, and some require machining of the core. Solid cores such as foam and balsa wood can be readily cut or sanded into the desired shape. Honeycomb cores require special cutting tools. In some cases the machined-out core is then backfilled with a resin/filler edging compound and cured to create a closeout. In other cases a specially fabricated metal or composite edge member is cocured or postbonded in place.

Repair

An often-overlooked aspect of manufacturing with composites is repair. In addition to repair of damage inflicted in service, repair (or rework) is necessary if the component is damaged during manufacture or if a quality assurance check indicates that certain specifications are not met. The choice between repair or rejection depends on the ability to repair the structure effectively. This requires both access and proper procedures. Clearly, a proper design would anticipate likely damage events such as delicate areas being overstrained prior to final assembly or a tool drop on a composite surface. Poorly designed manufacturing processes yield a systematic flaw that may go undetected until the component is in the field.

General guidelines apply for composite repair as they do for repair of metallic structure. Convenient access should be provided. Thus, there is a trade-off between fully integrated structures and structures that are assembled with mechanical fasteners. Composite repair requires significant surface preparation. The damaged material is first removed, and the surrounding area is scarfed. A filler or a partially staged or cured bonded preform and a surface patch of several plies of fabric/resin prepreg is applied to return the strength and stiffness, to restore the contour of the surface, or to prevent water intrusion. Application is accomplished using a portable heating and vacuum bag unit. The core of sandwich structures is replaced if it is damaged. This necessitates an additional bonding cycle.

Conclusions

The scale of design of a composite structure is substantially broader than an equivalent metal

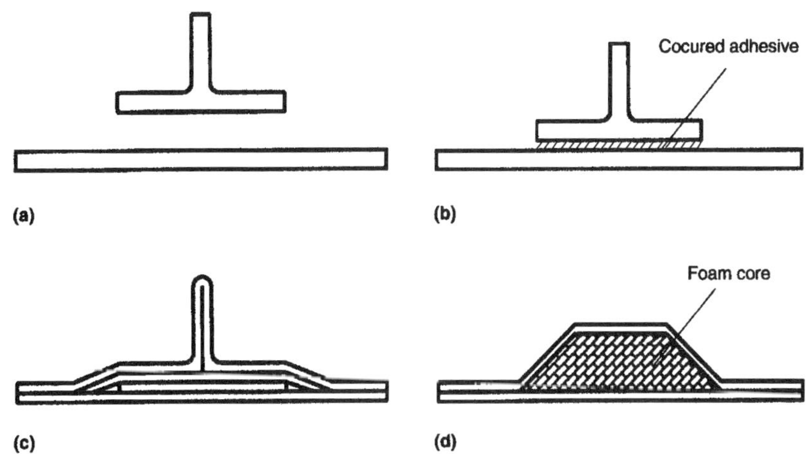

Fig. 5 Integration of stiffener and skin. (a) Mechanical/adhesive attachment. (b) Cocured. (c) Integrated lay-up. (d) Redesign

structure. This in turn increases the difficulty in the design process and is partly attributable to some of the advantages of composites, notably the ability to tailor the microstructure of the component and to integrate individual components into a single structure. This additional complexity is compounded by the relative scarcity of individuals who have knowledge of or experience with such materials. In addition the level of instruction at leading universities in manufacture of composite structures as compared to mechanics corresponds to the perception that research in manufacturing is less noble than research in mechanics. However, the recent emergence of texts specifically in integrated design may indicate a gradual reversal of this perception and an increase in awareness and research activity.

A vast pool of readily available experience aids the design of metallic structures. Clearly, the manufacturing practices of today involving milling machines, lathes, and drill presses have been honed in the preceding decades. Advanced composite materials are relatively new materials that pose new challenges to engineers. Moreover, it is unlikely that within an organization, the necessary expertise in materials, structures, and manufacturing will reside in a single individual. Even simple components may require a design team and consultants to cover adequately the many facets involved in the process.

A key point is the need to codesign the manufacturing process and tooling with the component. Failure to coordinate both activities results in higher costs and poorer performance. Indeed, manufacturing may offer alternatives to the design that an engineer biased by his or her experience with metals may not contemplate. The emergence of composite tooling for composite components clearly indicates the limited ability for conventional materials to be formed in other than conventional shapes.

One drawback of using composite materials is the apparent lack of guidelines to assist in the design for manufacturability. New applications result in new challenges with little or no previous experience on which to build. An exposition in composite materials (International Composites EXPO '97 in Nashville, TN) displayed many new products in major and emerging end-use markets. Examples included a front-end apron for passenger cars that replaces 44 steel parts at a 25% weight savings and a sheet molding compound, cross-vehicle beam that consolidates 20 steel and plastic pieces with a 10% weight savings. Such examples indicate the advantages of integrating large structures through the use of composites.

Almost all processes can be improved once implemented by controlling key parameters that affect the occurrence and development of defects. Temperatures and pressures can be monitored and controlled to reduce process variations, yet mechanical performance may not be as sensitive to the processing variables as it is to the process itself. Care must be taken not to simply incrementally progress along a given path for an old process, but also to explore alternative manufacturing methods. New raw materials, processing materials, and methods are continuously being developed. The increased role of textile science due to the emergence of braided preforms is an example of how advantages can be seen by those who are willing to exploit both old and new technology in different areas.

SELECTED REFERENCES

Books

- B.D. Agarwal and L.J. Broutman, *Analysis and Performance of Fiber Composites,* 2nd ed., John Wiley & Sons, Inc., 1990
- K. Ashbee, *Fundamental Principles of Fiber Reinforced Composites,* Technomic Publishing Company, Inc., 1989
- E.J. Barbero, *Introduction to Composite Materials Design,* Taylor & Francis, 1998
- *Delaware Composites Design Encyclopedia,* Vol 3, *Processing and Fabrication Technology*, Technomic Publishing Company, Inc., 1990
- R.F. Gibson, *Principles of Composite Material Mechanics,* McGraw-Hill, Inc., 1994
- T.G. Gutowski, Ed., *Advanced Composites Manufacturing*, John Wiley & Sons, 1997
- B.C. Hoskin and A.A. Baker, Ed., *Composite Materials for Aircraft Structures*, American Institute of Aeronautics and Astronautics, Inc., 1986
- D. Hull, *An Introduction to Composite Materials,* Cambridge University Press, 1981
- M.W. Hyer, *Stress Analysis of Fiber-Reinforced Composite Materials,* McGraw-Hill, Inc., 1998
- R.M. Jones, *Mechanics of Composite Materials,* 2nd ed., Taylor & Francis, 1999
- G. Lubin, Ed., *Handbook of Composites*, Van Nostrand Reinhold Company, Inc., 1982
- P.K. Mallick, *Fiber-Reinforced Composites,* 2nd ed., Marcel Dekker, Inc., 1993
- M.J. Owen, V. Middleton, and I.A. Jones, Ed., *Integrated Design and Manufacture Using Fibre-Reinforced Polymeric Composites,* Woodhead Publishing, Ltd., 2000
- K. Potter, *An Introduction to Composite Products,* Chapman & Hall, 1997
- M.M. Schwartz, *Composite Materials Handbook,* McGraw-Hill, Inc. 1984
- A.B. Strong, *Fundamentals of Composite Manufacturing: Materials, Methods, and Applications,* Society of Manufacturing Engineers, 1989
- A.B. Strong, *High Performance and Engineering Thermoplastic Composites,* Technomic Publishing Company, Inc., 1993
- J.R. Vinson and R.L Sierakowski, *The Behavior of Structures Composed of Composite Materials,* Martinus Nijhoff Publishers, 1986

Periodicals

- *Composites Technology,* Ray Publishing, Inc.
- *High-Performance Composites,* Ray Publishing, Inc.
- *Reinforced Plastics,* Elsevier Science Ltd.
- *SAMPE Journal,* Society for the Advancement of Material and Process Engineering

Cost Analysis

Stephen Mitchell, General Electric Aircraft Engines
Rebecca Ufkes, Ufkes Engineering

AFFORDABILITY is the key issue facing design engineers and manufacturers of composite components for current and next-generation aircraft, spacecraft, propulsion systems, and other advanced applications. To realize affordability goals, it is vital for engineering and manufacturing to accurately estimate manufacturing costs and risks at any stage of a program, but especially in the concept and preliminary design stage. Although the concept and preliminary design stages typically consume only 10% or less of program budget, over 80% of product cost is committed in these early stages.

In addition, lead times for design and fabrication of composite components often pace the development cycle. Consequently, a major priority is to reduce design cycle time and still produce the most efficient, lowest-risk component possible. Understanding the impact of critical cost elements on design features is a key step in reducing the overall cost of a component. It is critically important for the manufacturer to also quantify the cost elements of the manufactured part in order to reduce costs and simplify the manufacturing processes.

This article describes software tools available for modeling and analyzing costs associated with design and manufacturing options for advanced composites programs. An example is given of a composite exhaust nozzle shroud where the design and manufacture options were analyzed and adjusted, based on the use of cost analysis tools.

Composite Cost Tools

For decades, engineers have conducted their work without the benefit of fast cost feedback of their design concepts. However, over the past several years, a number of programs funded by the U.S. Air Force have resulted in the development of a variety of computer-based tools that allow for quick feedback of process cost. Two commercially available programs that have been used in recent Air Force-funded programs to develop composite process cost models are Cost Advantage by Cognition Corporation and SEER-DFM by Galorath Incorporated. Although a variety of software programs exist, most commercially available software can be categorized as either an open architecture, requiring user-provided rules and data, or a populated module with predefined equations based on industry standards.

In the Design and Manufacture of Low-Cost Composites for Engines (DMLCCE) Air Force program, General Electric Aircraft Engines (GEAE) used Cost Advantage as a framework to develop custom process cost models for filament winding and braiding of engine bypass ducts. In

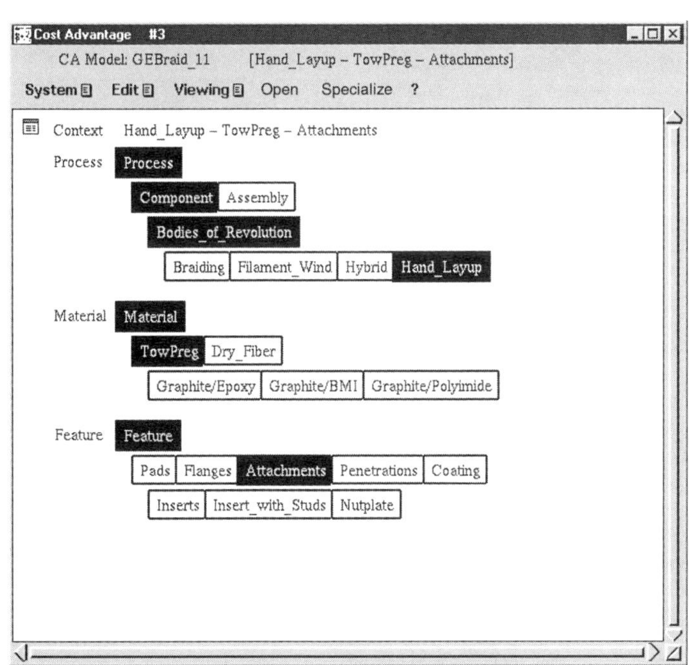

Fig. 1 Developed model hierarchy using Cost Advantage software

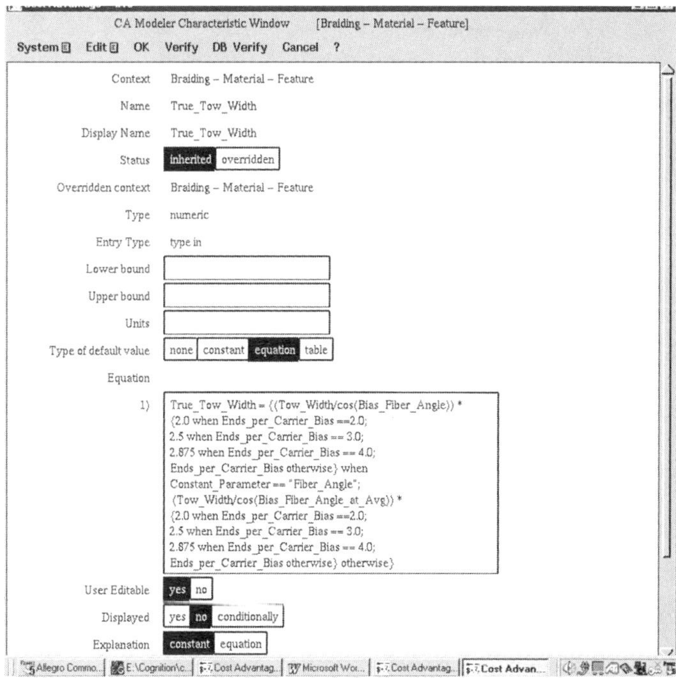

Fig. 2 Default model calculation for the braiding process, as created by a model builder

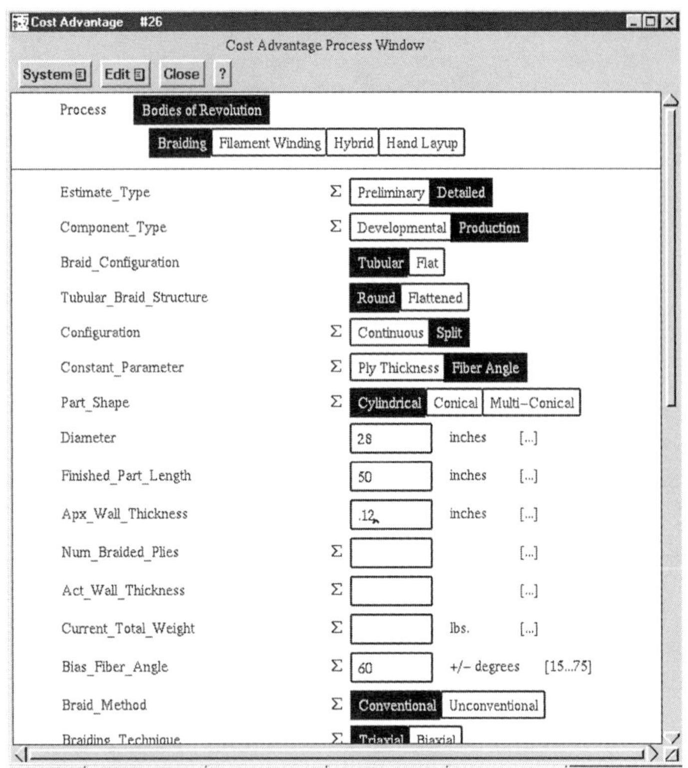

Fig. 3 Braid module process input window

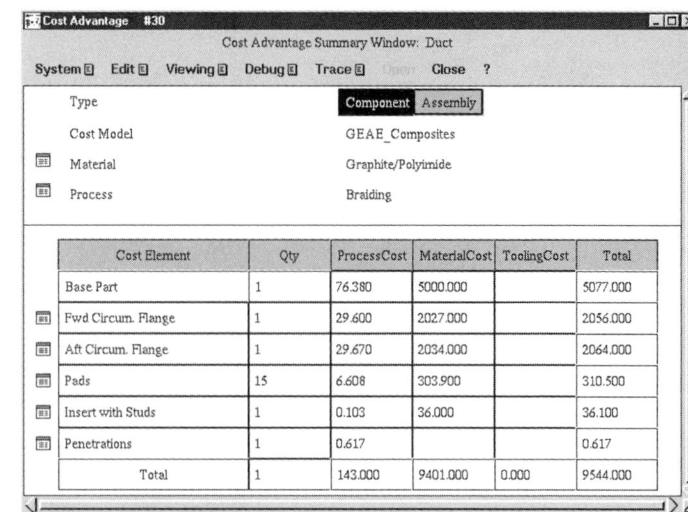

Cost Element	Qty	ProcessCost	MaterialCost	ToolingCost	Total
Base Part	1	76.380	5000.000		5077.000
Fwd Circum. Flange	1	29.600	2027.000		2056.000
Aft Circum. Flange	1	29.670	2034.000		2064.000
Pads	15	6.608	303.900		310.500
Insert with Studs	1	0.103	36.000		36.100
Penetrations	1	0.617			0.617
Total	1	143.000	9401.000	0.000	9544.000

Fig. 4 Output format from a Cost Advantage model

the DMLCCE program, GEAE directed the braiding and filament winding of a number of prototype composite ducts and captured the process steps and manufacturing data for each feature of the duct. These data were consolidated into algorithms, rules, and supporting data tables and programmed into Cost Advantage. The Cost Advantage software provides an architecture, or shell, to accept the rules, equations, and limits established by the engineer and manufacturer.

The flowchart of the desired model must be structured in the Cost Advantage software using the Process, Material, and Feature categories. The resulting flowchart for the General Electric Aircraft Engines DMLCCE composite model is shown in Fig. 1. Each node can have its own series of branches; however, it is impossible to show all branches, or paths, at one time in this view. Once there is an established flowchart, the model builder creates characteristics and corresponding relationships at various "contexts" within this framework. Figure 2 illustrates the interface for a model builder creating a characteristic for the braiding process. This example shows the interface for creating a default or programmed calculation. Note that this particular variable is not displayed to the user, but is derived using several existing user inputs. The true tow width of the braided tow is the value being calculated.

Once a model is completed and released by the "model builder," users can query the model. The resulting interface for the braid process as defined in the process windows can be seen in Fig. 3. The items noted with the sigma symbol (Σ) indicate that the variables are system defaults or system calculations.

Based on inputs and model calculations, rules and restrictions may be invoked to alert the user of a problem concerning the design and/or the manufacturing process. The alert may offer guidance to the user, for example: "Warning: A single end per carrier is not meeting your coverage requirements for this part. Please increase the Ends

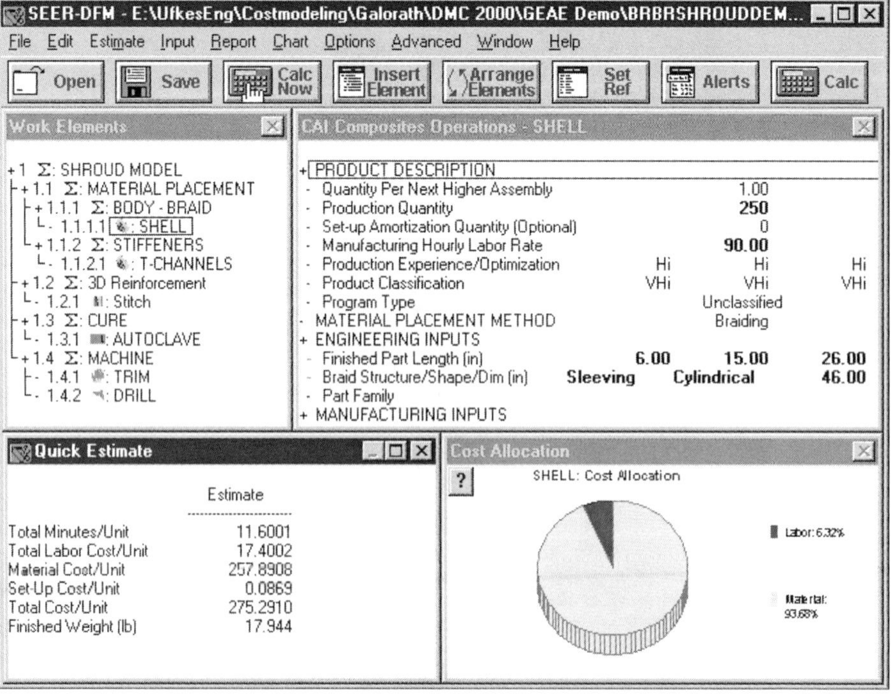

Fig. 5 Standard interface for SEER-DFM cost modeling software

per Carrier Bias variable or modify your coverage requirements."

Once the analysis is complete, the user is provided with a comprehensive summary. This summary identifies the total labor hours and material dollars as well as a cost breakdown per feature. This allows the user to quickly identify cost drivers. A summary window is shown in Fig. 4.

Under the U.S. Air Force-funded Composites Affordability Initiative (CAI), industry members from Boeing, GEAE, Lockheed Martin, and Northrop Grumman used SEER-DFM to develop comprehensive cost models for over 20 composite processes. Under this program, the CAI team members developed cost modules that plug into the existing SEER-DFM commercial software. This tool also guides the engineer through the composite process and, in many cases, identifies changes needed to avoid manufacturing problems or optimize manufacturing conditions. This software provides a variety of user-friendly features, such as a standard interface and detailed descriptions, graphics, pictures, and narrated videos. Figure 5 shows the standard interface for SEER-DFM.

The upper left corner allows the user to create a work breakdown structure for the part. Each work element, or process, has a specific parameter input window, as shown in the upper right corner. Outputs, reports, and charts are provided in the lower half of the screen.

The parameter window in Fig. 6 corresponds to the shell work element highlighted in Fig. 5. In this example, braiding is selected as the material placement method, and all of the required inputs for braiding are displayed.

Note that various inputs can be "bounded" by a range of values. This allows a user to perform a risk analysis on one or more variables, in the event that exact inputs are not known or defined at that time. Many of the values appearing in the window are system defaults derived from tables or equations; however, these values can be modified as needed.

Each variable in the parameter window will open into an input screen when selected. This screen will provide additional information to the user regarding the specific variable. Figure 7 shows graphical assistance to the user for the structure/shape/dimension variable shown in Fig. 6. In this case, the engineer has selected a "T"-channel as a stiffener by clicking the appropriate icon at the top of the screen.

Help modules are available throughout the model. The SEER-DFM software also has alerts built into the program that provide guidance to the user. A defined "Alert" button identifies all invoked alerts in red.

The output of the model can be displayed in report or graphic format. Output can be generated for either the top component level, the subassembly level, or the individual work element level. The software also includes a built-in "set reference" capability that allows the engineer to perform trade studies and sensitivity analyses relative to a baseline. An example of one of the detailed reports can be seen in Fig. 8.

Both Cost Advantage and SEER-DFM cost model software allow the engineer to evaluate different composite processes and can provide immediate cost feedback during all phases of design. The tools can also provide manufacturing and producibility guidance, assisting the engineer in designing affordable, low-risk designs. A key objective of implementing cost model software is to provide the engineer with electronic data concerning the manufacturing process and its critical elements so that smart, affordable decisions can be made early in the program in order to reduce downstream manufacturing costs.

Cost Savings

Cost modeling software makes it easier for engineers to perform cost estimates and choose among design alternatives, with the result being lower-risk, affordable components with reduced time-to-market. Figure 9 depicts the results of a trade study for an engine shroud where the advantages of braiding were compared against hand lay-up. The component is a continuous shell with integral internal "I-beam" stiffeners. The cost model allowed the engineer to examine the benefits of each process for both the shell and the stiffeners. Figure 10 shows the GE F110 composite exhaust nozzle shroud braided by A&P Technology using the lowest-cost process identified in the study.

In addition to component savings, a variety of significant program savings can also be realized through the use of cost models. The following lists some of the attributes found in various cost modeling software and the potential cost benefits:

Attribute	Cost benefit
Knowledge of critical process steps	Lower cost and faster development
Knowledge of alternative processes	Lowest-cost design
Design advice	Fast demonstration of performance
Manufacturing warnings and alerts	Reduced cost through reduced risk
Fast, user-friendly software	More studies per program dollar

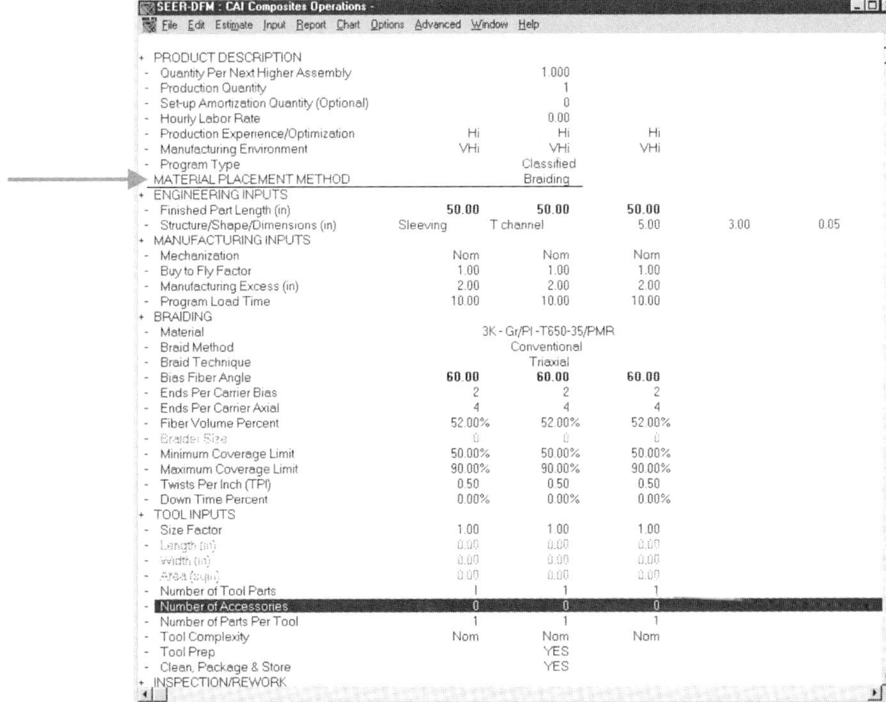

Fig. 6 Braiding parameter input window in SEER-DFM software

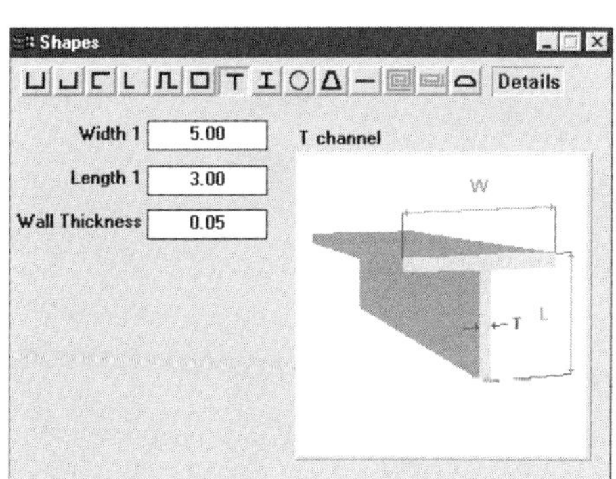

Fig. 7 Geometry input interface in SEER-DFM software

Industry has also documented a variety of savings within their respective companies. One key savings results when the engineer is provided electronic knowledge of alternative manufacturing processes and their critical elements. This up-front knowledge reduces program risk and downstream manufacturing costs. Another cost savings is the result of conducting cost studies faster than conventional methods. During the CAI validation phase, the CAI team documented several time savings that ranged from 88 to 95%. The trade study depicted in Fig. 9 was conducted using SEER-DFM in 10% of the time required for conventional consultation or quotation approaches.

Although the benefits are difficult to quantify, another cost savings is the ability to conduct more cost analysis trade studies within a fixed conventional schedule allocation. Some companies identified "10 times as many cost analysis trades" performed in the same time frame. Finally, the cost savings resulting from risk avoidance could provide significant benefits through fewer manufacturing iterations and faster development cycles.

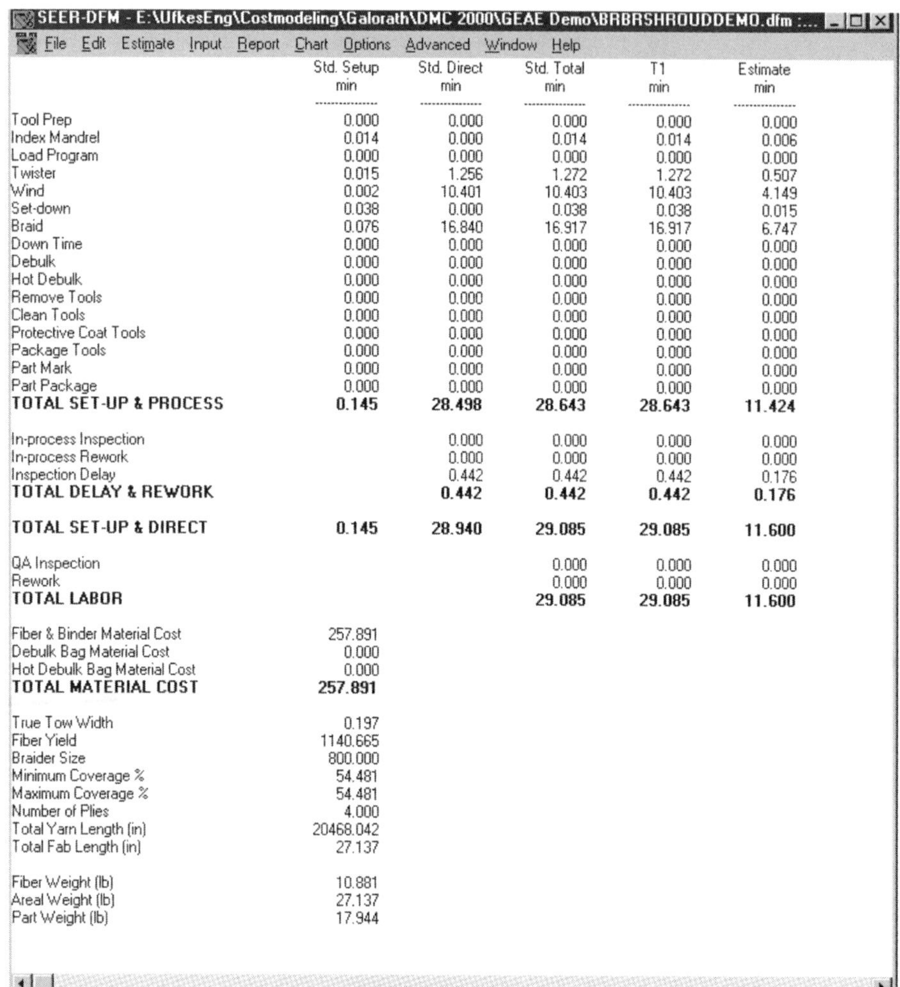

SEER-DFM - E:\UfkesEng\Costmodeling\Galorath\DMC 2000\GEAE Demo\BRBRSHROUDDEMO.dfm :...

File Edit Estimate Input Report Chart Options Advanced Window Help

	Std. Setup min	Std. Direct min	Std. Total min	T1 min	Estimate min
Tool Prep	0.000	0.000	0.000	0.000	0.000
Index Mandrel	0.014	0.000	0.014	0.014	0.006
Load Program	0.000	0.000	0.000	0.000	0.000
Twister	0.015	1.256	1.272	1.272	0.507
Wind	0.002	10.401	10.403	10.403	4.149
Set-down	0.038	0.000	0.038	0.038	0.015
Braid	0.076	16.840	16.917	16.917	6.747
Down Time	0.000	0.000	0.000	0.000	0.000
Debulk	0.000	0.000	0.000	0.000	0.000
Hot Debulk	0.000	0.000	0.000	0.000	0.000
Remove Tools	0.000	0.000	0.000	0.000	0.000
Clean Tools	0.000	0.000	0.000	0.000	0.000
Protective Coat Tools	0.000	0.000	0.000	0.000	0.000
Package Tools	0.000	0.000	0.000	0.000	0.000
Part Mark	0.000	0.000	0.000	0.000	0.000
Part Package	0.000	0.000	0.000	0.000	0.000
TOTAL SET-UP & PROCESS	**0.145**	**28.498**	**28.643**	**28.643**	**11.424**
In-process Inspection		0.000	0.000	0.000	0.000
In-process Rework		0.000	0.000	0.000	0.000
Inspection Delay		0.442	0.442	0.442	0.176
TOTAL DELAY & REWORK		**0.442**	**0.442**	**0.442**	**0.176**
TOTAL SET-UP & DIRECT	**0.145**	**28.940**	**29.085**	**29.085**	**11.600**
QA Inspection			0.000	0.000	0.000
Rework			0.000	0.000	0.000
TOTAL LABOR			**29.085**	**29.085**	**11.600**
Fiber & Binder Material Cost	257.891				
Debulk Bag Material Cost	0.000				
Hot Debulk Bag Material Cost	0.000				
TOTAL MATERIAL COST	**257.891**				
True Tow Width	0.197				
Fiber Yield	1140.665				
Braider Size	800.000				
Minimum Coverage %	54.481				
Maximum Coverage %	54.481				
Number of Plies	4.000				
Total Yarn Length (in)	20468.042				
Total Fab Length (in)	27.137				
Fiber Weight (lb)	10.881				
Areal Weight (lb)	27.137				
Part Weight (lb)	17.944				

Fig. 8 Detailed output report from SEER-DFM software

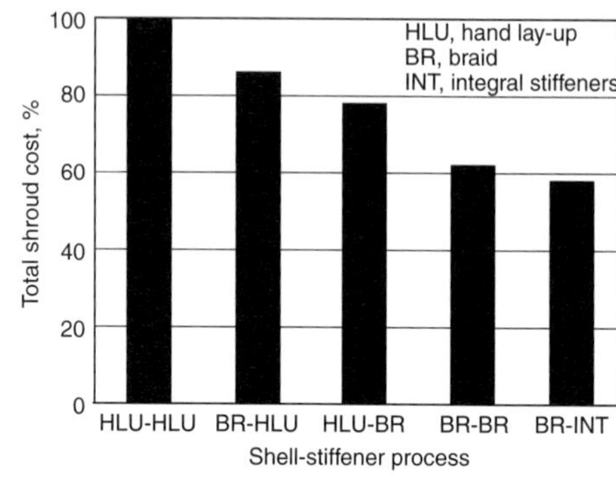

Fig. 9 Cost comparison (trade study) of different processes for manufacturing a composite shroud

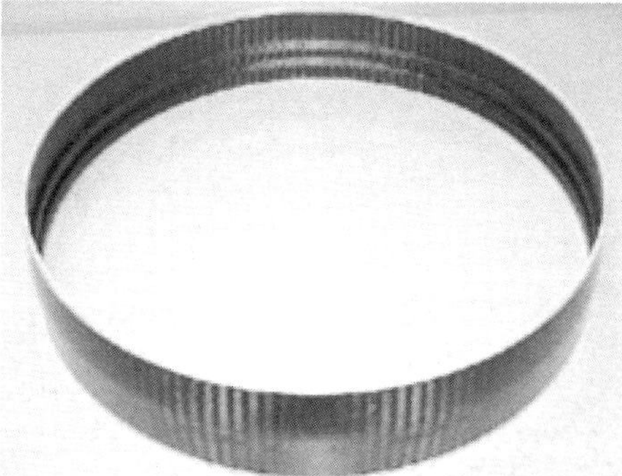

Fig. 10 Braided shroud with integral stiffeners. Approximately 1.2 m (4 ft) in diameter.

Rapid Prototyping

David L. Bourell and Joseph J. Beaman, Jr., The University of Texas at Austin
Donald Klosterman, University of Dayton
Ian Gibson, University of Hong Kong
Amit Bandyopadhyay, Washington State University

RAPID PROTOTYPING (RP)—also known as solid freeform fabrication, automated fabrication, layered manufacturing, and so forth—consists of a range of technologies that are capable of taking computer-aided design (CAD) models and converting them to a physical form or part. This process is automatic, generally independent of the model geometry, and does not require special tooling or fixtures. Complex, three-dimensional (3-D) contours are quantized in the form of stacks of two-dimensional, finite thickness layers or cross sections. If these layers are very thin, then the parts made will be sufficiently accurate to suit a range of applications. Nearly all RP parts can be characterized by a stair-step effect that approximates the original shape, which is most obvious on shallow slopes and curves. A most comprehensive classification of RP processes was proposed by J.P. Kruth (Ref 1), in which the focus is on the initial state of the raw materials used, namely solid, liquid, and powder-based manufacture. Other sources for more detailed information are included as Ref 2 to 6.

Review of Processes

Photopolymer Systems. Stereolithography (SLA) (Ref 7) is regarded as the first commercial RP process and uses liquid-based photopolymer resin as the raw material (Fig. 1). Polymerization occurs at a specific frequency of light, supplied by a laser source, which scans across the surface of the photopolymer. The laser intensity is matched to the absorption of the photopolymer so that solidification is limited to a short depth, representing the layer thickness. Parts are built on an elevator platform, which increments down from the surface as layers are added. Stereolithography was first commercialized by 3D Systems and is registered to their machines. There are, however, a number of variations from other companies that also use photopolymer resins. Parts made using SLA are surrounded by liquid resin during the build so there is a need to ensure that all layers, and parts of layers, are connected to each other and to the build platform at all times during the build process. Overhanging part features must therefore be connected using additional support structures, which are fabricated at the same time.

Powder Sintering. Selective laser sintering (SLS) uses powder as the raw material (Fig. 2). Parts are built on a platform, which indexes downward as more powder is added at the top. A laser melts or sinters the powder particles ac-

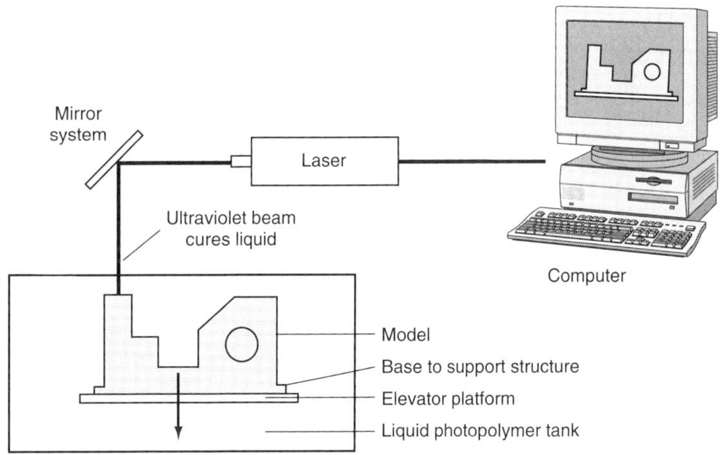

Fig. 1 Stereolithography (SLA) rapid prototyping system. Courtesy of Milwaukee School of Engineering

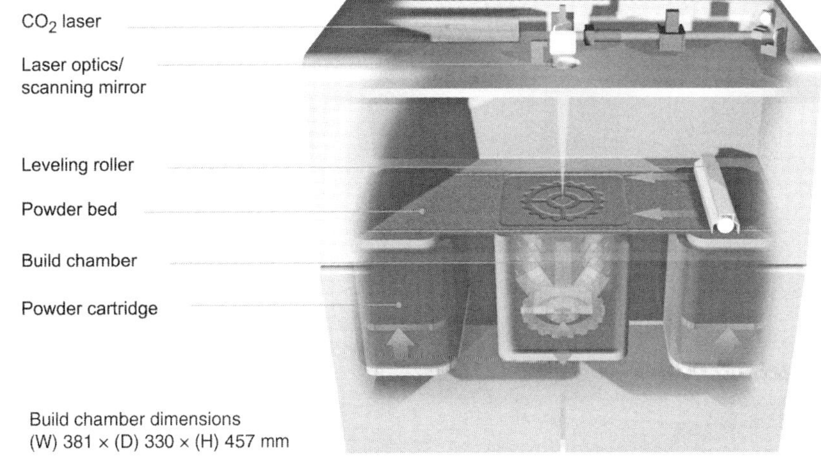

Fig. 2 Selective laser sintering (SLS) rapid prototyping system. Courtesy of DTM Corporation

cording to the cross section at a particular layer. Each layer cools rapidly, and laser penetration is such that it thermally bonds to the layer below. The powder material must therefore be thermoplastic in its behavior. The use of powders means that part surfaces have a granular texture, and there is also a tendency for parts to be porous. Loose powder surrounds the solid part, thus eliminating the need for specific support structures. Thermal processing also leads to very good part strength. Selective laser sintering is registered to machines manufactured by DTM Corporation (Ref 8), but similar machines are also made by EOS GmbH in Germany (Ref 9).

Hot Melt Extrusion. Fused deposition modeling (FDM) material comes in solid form as a filament. This is extruded through a heated nozzle, which deposits a thin "road" of material (Fig. 3). First, roads are extruded to form the outline of the part. These roads are then filled in to complete the layer. Since the material is optimally softened and not fully liquefied when it exits the nozzle, FDM generally uses amorphous polymers. Fused deposition modeling must also use support structures for overhanging features. Supports are extruded through a second nozzle and can therefore be held at a different temperature or made from a different material. This allows the supports to come away from the part easily. A recent development is the use of a soluble support material that can be removed with a minimum of mechanical damage to the part. Fused deposition modeling is currently commercialized by Stratasys Inc. (Ref 10).

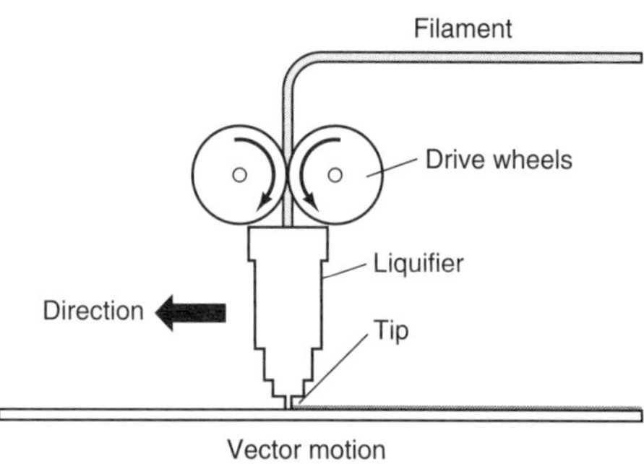

Fig. 3 The fused deposition modeling (FDM) hot melt extrusion process. Courtesy of Penn State University

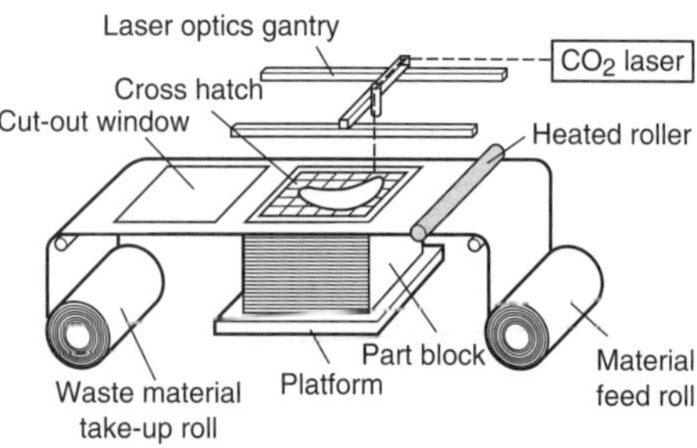

Fig. 4 Sheet lamination using the laminated object manufacturing (LOM) process.

Sheet Lamination. Laminated Object Manufacturing (LOM) (Ref 11) uses solid sheets of material, which are sequentially bonded together and cut to form the part (Fig. 4). The thickness of the sheet material, which is normally paper, represents the layer thickness. After each layer is bonded and cut, the part is separated from the feed material by cutting it around the outline. Further cuts or "cross hatches" are required to permit easy removal of the waste material after the entire part is complete. Thus, LOM parts are surrounded by solid material and do not require support structures during the building process. LOM was first commercialized by Helisys Inc., which used the approach described previously to cut and bond adhesive-backed paper that was delivered on a continuous roll. Another laminating machine, which uses single sheets of paper for each layer, photocopying technology to apply the adhesive, and a blade to cut the part outlines, is made by Kira in Japan (Ref 12).

Solid Ground Curing (SGC) (Ref 13), a process developed by Cubital in Israel, also fabricates parts from photopolymer resins but in a different way than stereolithography (Fig. 5). Resin is spread onto a platform, which is then exposed to ultraviolet light through a mask, which is printed from the layer data onto a glass plate. Uncured resin is vacuumed away, and the space is filled with molten wax. The wax solidifies and the whole layer is machined, level to the required layer thickness. Parts are therefore a combination of resin and wax and do not require supports. Wax is removed using a chemical bath or autoclave. Solid ground curing can be considered a hybrid system since it uses solid wax and liquid resin.

Three-Dimensional Printing (3DP). Developed and licensed by the Massachusetts Institute of Technology (Ref 14), 3DP can be found in a number of commercial forms. Powder is spread onto a build platform (Fig. 6). Liquid is then printed from an ink-jet print head. The liquid dries and binds the powder particles together to form the layer. 3DP is therefore another hybrid process using powders and liquid. Like SLS, the

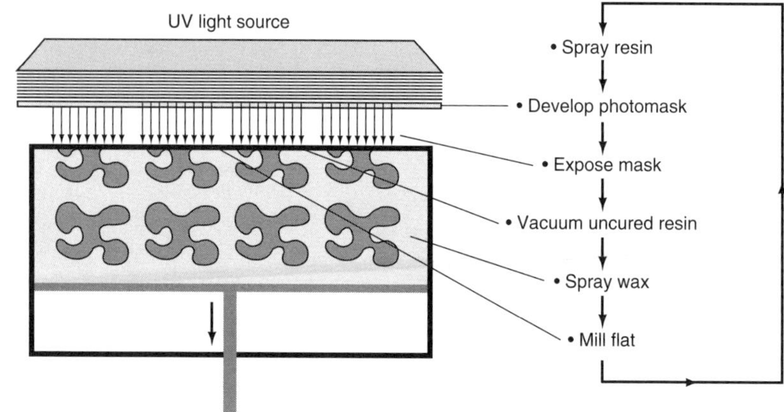

Fig. 5 The solid ground curing (SGC) process from Cubital. Courtesy of Penn State University

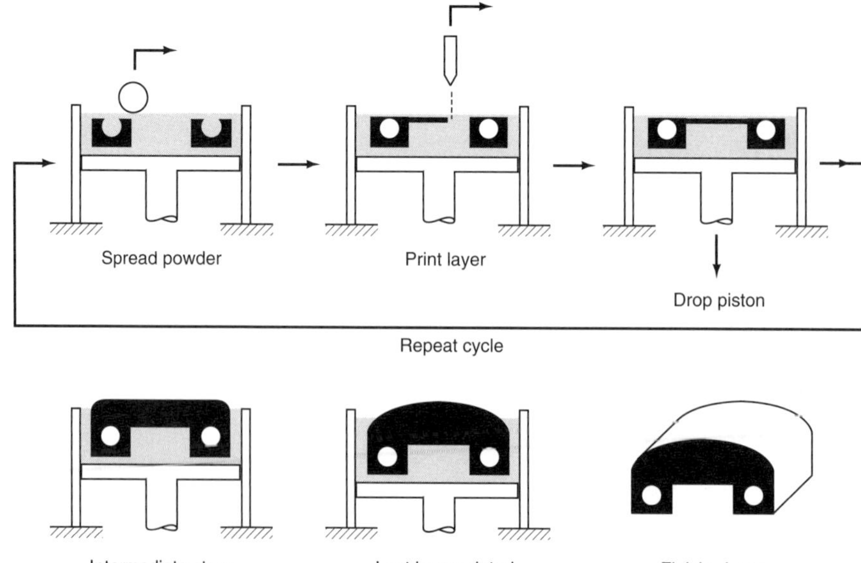

Fig. 6 The basic three-dimensional printing (3DP) process. Courtesy of MIT

use of different powders results in different applications. The most common machine is the Z402 from ZCorp, which uses multiple nozzle ink-jet print heads to print large areas in one pass, making it possible to create parts quickly. Like SLS, parts exhibit a granular texture and are porous. Three-dimensional printing parts generally require strengthening using a resin-based infiltrant.

Drop-on-drop systems, like 3DP, FDM, and others, use nozzles to create parts. The Sanders ModelMaker (Ref 15) (Fig. 7) and Thermojet (registered to 3D Systems) processes deposit material in a molten droplet form. This material then solidifies rapidly to allow further droplets to be applied. These processes generally use wax as the raw material. Sanders machines use two types of wax, one for support structures that can be removed from the part material at low temperature. Thermojet systems create supports from the same material, resulting in comparatively rough, down-facing surfaces.

Metal Systems. All of the above commercial systems concentrate on polymeric materials or materials with low melting points. A number of processes have been adapted so that they can process metals, but few of them have reached commercial status to date. It is not difficult to see how FDM, LOM, and SLS can be developed into metal systems. Direct sintering of metal powders is possible with the EOSint M machine, although the metals are, admittedly, relatively low melting point. The Laser Engineered Net Shape (LENS) directed material-deposition process commercialized by Optomec, Inc. (Ref 16) feeds metal powder into a head, which then melts and deposits in a similar manner to FDM. StratoConception (Ref 17) uses machining to create metal sheet laminates, which are bonded together like LOM. Obviously, high power, temperature, and atmosphere considerations make these direct methods difficult tasks to achieve.

Direct Fabrication of Composite Structures

Significant advances in the technology of rapid prototyping during the 1990s have produced a new capability for directly fabricating advanced material prototypes and end-use components. The list of advanced materials includes particulate and fiber-reinforced polymer, ceramic-matrix composites (CMCs), and metal-matrix composites (MMCs). Adapting the various RP processes for direct fabrication of ceramic materials has received the most effort because, compared to techniques for fabricating metals and polymers, traditional techniques for small-lot fabrication of complex-shaped ceramic components are difficult, time consuming, labor intensive, and expensive. Thus, RP technology was expected to yield the earliest and greatest payoff for direct fabrication of ceramic materials. Great strides, however, were also made with direct fabrication of polymer and metal components during this time period. Currently, a wide variety of RP processes exists for direct fabrication of particulate and fiber-reinforced composites.

Fiber-Reinforced Composites. Of all the RP techniques, LOM is the only one well-suited for direct manufacture of fiber-reinforced composites. Because LOM is essentially a sheet-processing method (Fig. 4), it is capable of handling common sheet preforms such as fabrics and prepregs that are traditionally used in composite fabrication.

Recent research efforts have established the viability of LOM for direct fabrication of continuous-fiber reinforced polymer-matrix composites (PMCs) and CMCs. With PMCs, a full discussion of the various issues involved is given elsewhere (Ref 18, 19). The general approach is to use the LOM machine to lay up and shape a green (partially cured and consolidated) composite, followed by additional off-line consolidation and cure using a heated vacuum bag or autoclave. Glass fiber/epoxy composites made with LOM using a commercially available prepreg, Scotch Ply (3M), exhibited approximately 85% of the strength (tension, compression, flexure, and interlaminar shear) of an autoclave cured panel. Figure 8 is a photograph of some PMC parts. The standard CO_2 laser of the LOM machine can be used without modification to cut glass fiber/epoxy prepregs. However, for higher performance fibers such as carbon or silicon carbide, an entirely different cutting mechanism is required. To this end, researchers have demonstrated high-quality cutting of continuous silicon-carbide (SiC) fibers via photoablation using a copper-vapor laser in a bench-top LOM process (Ref 20).

For CMCs, the LOM machine is used again only to lay up and shape a green composite. Ceramic-matrix composite prepregs must contain a polymer-ceramic precursor resin of sufficient tack, or a tackifier can be used in between prepreg layers. One study demonstrated the use of a novel preform comprised of a layer of SiC fiber/furfural unidirectional prepreg adhered to the top of a SiC ceramic tape (Ref 21). Regardless of the preform type, the green CMC must undergo significant postprocessing involving high-pressure consolidation, high-temperature resin-to-ceramic conversion, and possibly infiltration or reinfiltration with additional ceramic precursor resin or liquid metal.

Regardless of the material type, LOM and other RP processes are limited to building with flat, horizontal layers. While it is true that complex, curved geometries can be created with this process, they must be built up from thin, flat layers and then postmachined to get the final part. Thus, flat-layer RP processes are incapable of addressing the larger geometrical issues involved with fiber composite fabrication, namely fiber orientation and continuity. In response to this need, the first curved-layer RP process was developed. The new process, referred to as curved LOM, was motivated by the need for rapid fabrication of fiber-reinforced structures containing sloping, curved surfaces, especially thin curved-shell components. It is crucial to maintain fiber continuity along the curved surfaces of these components.

Details of the curved layer process are found elsewhere (Ref 22). It begins with production of a matched tool or mandrel for the intended part. This tool can be generated by any of several other RP processes, including the standard LOM process using LOM paper. The finished LOM mandrel is mounted to the flat building platform in the curved LOM machine. Size limitation is approximately 30 by 30 by 5.5 cm (12 by 12 by 3 in.). Sheets of the desired build material (e.g., composite prepreg) are loaded onto an external, rotatable feed table, picked up with a vacuum chuck, and shuttled to the mandrel. A flexible thermoforming mechanism laminates each new layer to the curved mandrel with steady, uniform vacuum pressure and heat. After the laminator retracts, a CO_2 laser cuts each layer, accounting for the sloped surface. The fiber orientation can be varied from layer to layer by programming the rotatable feed table. The process proceeds one layer at a time until the part is finished. If necessary, the laminator can be used to provide additional post cure to the final part. Subse-

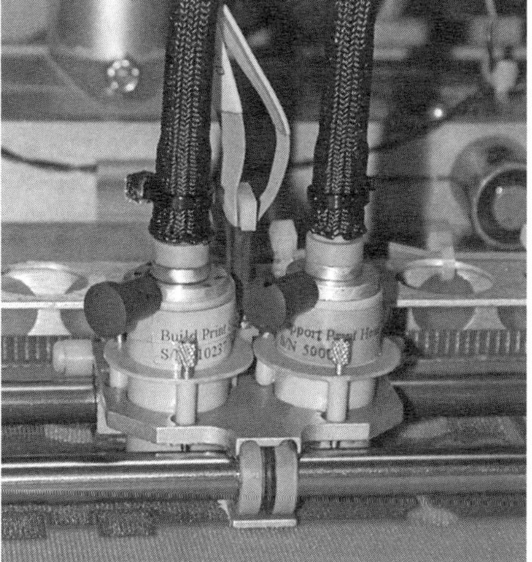

Fig. 7 Drop-on-drop system (Sanders ModelMaker) print jets, showing the two jetting heads above sample parts. Courtesy of Sanders Prototype International

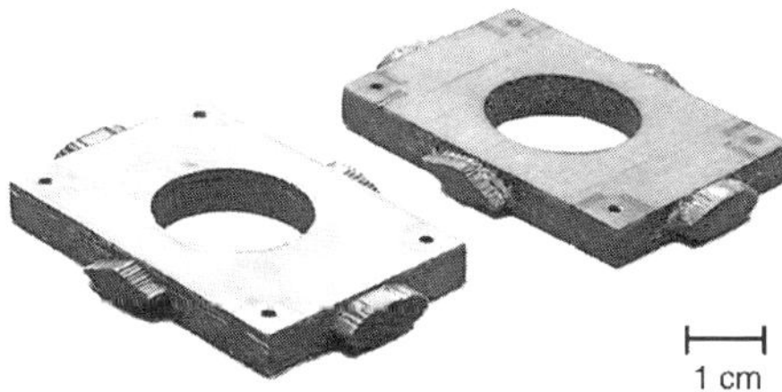

Fig. 8 Parts made with glass fiber/epoxy prepreg using laminated object manufacturing (LOM). The part on the right has been fully cured.

quently, the part is removed from the mandrel, and the excess material is manually stripped away (decubed). Suitable postprocesses are then performed to obtain a fully consolidated, cured, and/or densified PMC or CMC.

The viability of using curved LOM for production of PMC (Ref 23) and CMC (Ref 21, 22) structures has been established. Curved-layer CMC components are shown in Fig. 9. Widespread industrial use of LOM or curved LOM for direct fabrication of PMCs had not occurred by the year 2001, most likely because of size limitations and the availability of automated tape placement (ATP) machines (Ref 24) used in the aerospace industry (see the article "Automated Tape Laying" in this Volume). However, compared to ATP, the cost and ease of use of LOM machine is favorable for production of small (e.g., 60 by 30 by 15 cm, or 24 by 12 by 6 in.) articles. Thus, with regards to PMCs, LOM holds the most short-term potential for the consumer-goods industry. Ceramic and CMC articles are often not as large as PMC structures, and thus the potential benefits of LOM for these materials still remain for all applications.

Particulate-Reinforced Metal- and Ceramic-Matrix Composites. Processing of MMCs and CMCs presents unique opportunities for RP techniques due to the inherent nature of high-cost, low-volume production needs of value-added products. Net-shape fabrication of controlled microstructure parts has already been demonstrated, utilizing some of the commercial RP systems. Although extensive research and development work is still pending for tailoring these approaches to mature commercial techniques for industrial-scale production, some of the initial results show significant promise and are herein discussed.

Magnesium/Silicon Carbide Composites. Wohlert and Bourell (Ref 25) utilized the SLS process to fabricate particulate Mg/SiC metal-matrix composites (Fig. 10). In their approach, polymer-coated commercial SiC powders were used to produce porous SiC ceramic preforms. Preforms were binder removed and sintered, prior to metal infiltration. Porous SiC preforms were infiltrated with commercial die-casting AZ91D magnesium alloy under controlled nitrogen environment via pressureless metal infiltration. Composites with fine features having 40 to 50 vol% of SiC particles were successfully processed via this approach. The Mg/SiC composite microstructure showed little or no residual porosity for structures where the pore sizes were uniform and smaller in size. One of the problems in this two-stage approach is the selection of metal-ceramic combination. For the pressureless infiltration process to be successful, the surface tension of the liquid infiltrant must be lower than the surface energy of the solid matrix. Usually the surface energies of the ceramics tend to be quite low, causing difficulties in selecting the matrix metal for preforms of different ceramic compositions.

Metal-Ceramic Composites. Bandyopadhyay et al. (Ref 26, 27) reported the fabrication of interpenetrating phase metal-ceramic composites using FDM. Interpenetrating phase composites are those where both the metal and the ceramic phases are connected to itself in all three directions. In this approach, controlled porosity ceramic preforms were fabricated using the indirect FDM. Polymeric molds of desired parts were fabricated using ICW wax with different tool path variations. Molds were infiltrated with mullite ($Al_6Si_2O_{13}$) ceramic slurry or gel, and dried. The structures were then subjected to a binder removal and sintering cycle. The polymeric roads of the mold formed the pores in the controlled porosity mullite preform. By varying the tool path and the slice thickness of the mold, size, shape and distribution of the pores in the ceramic preform can be varied. Mullite preforms were then infiltrated using an Al metal via pressureless reactive metal infiltration to form mullite-Al or alumina-Al composites in which the metal phase filled the designed pores of the preforms. Uniform and functionally gradient composites with 20 to 50 volume percent metal contents were fabricated having various shapes and sizes. By varying the metal and the ceramic phases in the composites, the properties of the final part could be tailored for specific application.

Ceramic-Matrix Composites. Ceramics are hard and brittle, difficult to machine, and have low-volume production in numerous applications. During the mid- to late 1990s, extensive research was focused in the development of direct RP systems for ceramics and ceramic composites. The SLS is one of the commercially available processes where ceramic parts can be produced directly using polymer-coated ceramic powders. The parts require postprocessing, such as binder removal and sintering. In fused deposition of ceramics (FDC) (Ref 28), ceramic particle loaded thermoplastic filaments were used with commercial FDM systems to directly produce green ceramic components. In situ reinforced Si_3N_4, alumina, and lead zirconium titanate (PZT) are some of the ceramic materials that have been produced using this process. Postprocessing such as binder removal and sintering is necessary for the green FDC parts. Due to high volume fraction of thermoplastic binder content of the green part, parts greater than 15 mm (0.6 in.) thick are difficult to binder remove. The 3DP process was utilized to fabricate different structural, electronic, and bioceramic monoliths and composites. For small parts, most of these direct-deposition techniques are capable of achieving >98% theoretical density, but cracking and warpage during full densification of complex-shaped, large-size parts are still serious concerns. Attempts have also been made to directly produce functional ceramics and composites using other RP processes, and some of the efforts are still continuing for numerous applications.

Freeform Tooling for Composite Part Lay-Up

While some inroads have been made in the area of composite part production using freeform techniques, another strong area of application of these technologies is in production of tooling for composite part lay-up. This has been alluded to earlier in this article with the treatment of curved LOM. In the commercial sector, tools for injection and compression molding of composites represent a significant process expense, and limited success has been achieved in the application of toolless manufacturing processes to tool production. One example is SLS of epoxy-infiltrated

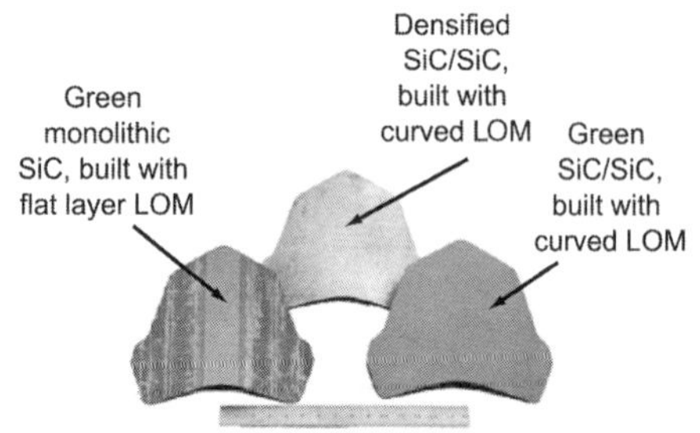

Fig. 9 Aircraft engine flame holders. The piece on the left illustrates the poor surface finish obtained with the flat-layer LOM process compared to the curved layer LOM process.

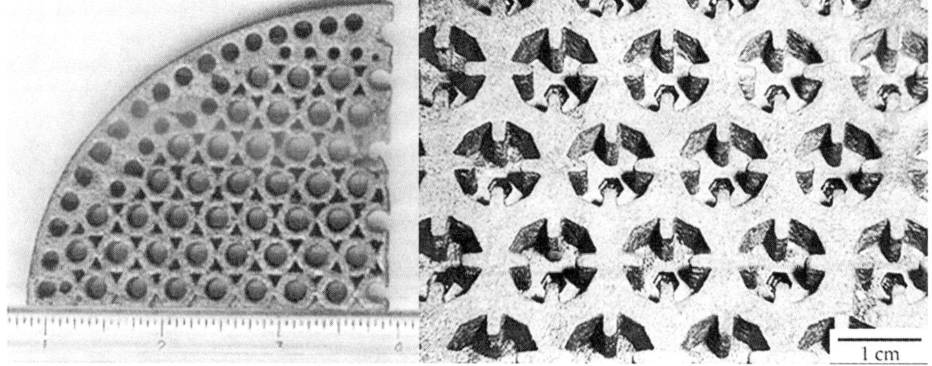

Fig. 10 Particulate composite parts produced by SLS processing of SiC preforms followed by liquid-metal infiltration of a magnesium alloy. Source: Ref 25

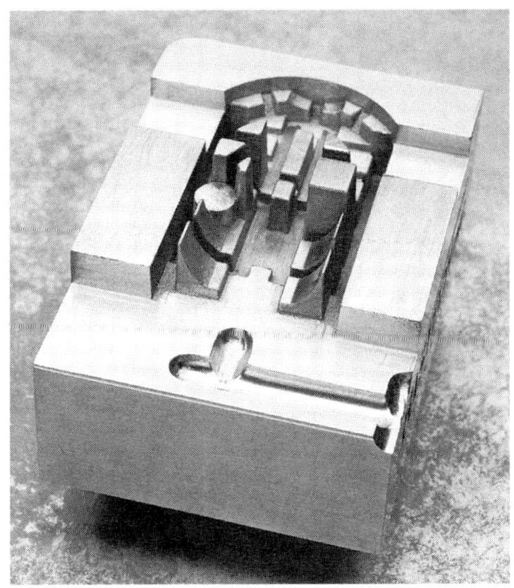

Fig. 11 Selective laser-sintered tool using stainless steel infiltrated with bronze. Courtesy of DTM Corporation

metal molds (Ref 29). Freeform fabrication may also be used to produce tools for a large number of "half-mold" processes including hydroforming, diaphragm forming, vacuum forming, resin-transfer molding, manual/mechanically-assisted lay-up and electroformed nickel tooling.

Virtually any freeform fabrication technique may be used to produce short-run tooling. Epoxy-backed SLA molds have been demonstrated for aerospace applications in a resin transfer molding (RTM) operation (Ref 30), and SLA parts have been used for a variety of soft tooling mold applications including RTM and vacuum forming (Ref 31, 32).

A limited number of commercial freeform-fabrication techniques are capable of producing metallic tools that can be operated for extended numbers of parts. These include selective laser sintering (DTM Corporation, EOS GmbH) and direct metal deposition (Optomec) (Ref 33). A sample tool is shown in Fig. 11. Here, Type 420 martensitic stainless steel powder is coated with a polymer binder and SLS processed. The part, composed of approximately 60% metal, is fired to burn off the binder and to infiltrate with a bronze alloy. The final part has tolerances as high as 0.51 mm (0.020 in.), so critical surfaces must be finished by some form of machining operation.

REFERENCES

1. J.P. Kruth, Material Increases Manufacturing by Rapid Prototyping Techniques, *Annals of the CIRP,* Vol 40 (No. 2), 1991, p 603–614
2. C.L. Thomas, Rapid Prototyping, *ASM Handbook,* Vol 20, *Materials Selection and Design,* ASM International, 1997, p 231–239
3. P.D. Hilton and P. Jacobs, *Rapid Tooling, Technologies and Industrial Applications,* Marcel Dekker, Inc., 2000
4. J.J. Beaman, J.W. Barlow, D.L. Bourell, R.H. Crawford, H.L. Marcus, and K.P. McAlea, *Solid Freeform Fabrication: A New Direction In Manufacturing,* Kluwer Academic Press, Boston, 1997
5. M. Burns, *Automated Fabrication—Improving Productivity in Manufacturing,* Prentice Hall, 1993
6. *Solid Freeform Fabrication Symposium Proc.* (Austin, TX), University of Texas, Aug 1990–2001
7. P.F. Jacobs, *Stereolithography and other RP&M Technologies,* Society of Manufacturing Engineers, 1996
8. DTM Corporation, www.dtm-corp.com, Internet research
9. Electro Optical Systems (EOS) GmbH, www.eos-gmbh.de, Internet research
10. Stratasys Inc., www.stratasys.com, Internet research
11. J. Park, M.J. Tari, and H.T. Hahn, Characterization of the Laminated Object Manufacturing (LOM) Process, *Rapid Prototyping Journal,* Vol 6 (No. 1), 2000, p 36–49
12. Kira Corporation, www.kiracorp.co.jp, Internet research
13. Cubital, www.cubital.com, Internet research
14. Three Dimensional Printing (3DP) Laboratory, Laboratory for Manufacturing and Productivity, Massachusetts Institute of Technology, anxiety-closet.mit.edu/afs/athena/org/t/tdp/www/index.html, Internet research
15. Solidscape, Inc., www.solid-scape.com, Internet research
16. Optomec Inc., www.optomec.com, Internet research
17. StratoConception, CIRTES (Centre d'Ingénierie de Recherche et de Transfert de l'Esstin à Saint-Dié-des-Vosges), www.cirtes.fr/strato/index.htm, Internet research
18. D. Klosterman, B. Priore, and R. Chartoff, Laminated Object Manufacturing of Polymer Matrix Composites, *Proc. Seventh International Conference on Rapid Prototyping,* April 1997 (San Francisco, CA), University of Dayton, p 283–292
19. B. Priore, "Fabrication of Polymer Composites Using Laminated Object Manufacturing," M.S. thesis, University of Dayton, Dec 1996
20. A. Lightman and G. Han, Laser Cutting of Ceramic Composite Layers, *Solid Freeform Fabrication Symposium,* Aug 1996 (Austin, TX), University of Texas, p 291–298
21. D. Klosterman, R. Chartoff, N. Osborne, G. Graves, A. Lightman, G. Han, A. Bezeredi, and S. Rodrigues, Direct Fabrication of Ceramics and Composites through Laminated Object Manufacturing (LOM), *Proc. 43rd International SAMPE Symposium & Exhibition,* 1–4 June 1998 (Anaheim, CA)
22. D. Klosterman, R. Chartoff, N. Osborne, G. Graves, A. Lightman, G. Han, A. Bezeredi, and S. Rodrigues, Development of a Curved Layer LOM Process for Monolithic Ceramics and Ceramic Matrix Composites, *Rapid Prototyping Journal,* Vol 5 (No. 2), 1999, p 61–71
23. D. Klosterman, A. Popp, R. Chartoff, M. Agarwala, I. Fiscus, E. Bryant, S. Cullen, and M. Yeazell, Direct Fabrication of Polymer Composite Structures with Curved LOM, *Proc. Solid Freeform Fabrication Symposium,* Aug 1999 (Austin, TX), University of Texas, p 401–409
24. W.P. Benjamin, The Fiber Placement Path Toward Affordability, *SAMPE J.,* Vol 34 (No. 3), May/June 1998
25. M. Wohlert and D.L. Bourell, Rapid Prototyping of Mg/SiC Composites by a Combined SLS and Pressureless Infiltration Process, *Proc. Solid Freeform Fabrication Symposium,* Aug 1996 (Austin, TX), University of Texas, p 79–88
26. A. Bandyopadhyay, Functionally Designed 3-3 Mullite-Aluminum Composites, *Advanced Engineering Materials,* Vol 1 (No. 3–4), 1999, p 199–201
27. R. Soundararajan, R. Atisivan, G. Kuhn, S. Bose, and A. Bandyopadhyay, Processing of Mullite-Al Composites, *J. Am. Ceram. Soc.,* Sept 2000
28. M.K. Agarwala, A. Bandyopadhyay, R. van Weeren, P. Whalen, A. Safari, and S.C. Danforth, Fused Deposition of Ceramics: Rapid Fabrication of Structural Ceramic Components, *Ceramic Bulletin,* Vol 11 (No. 60–65), 1996
29. J.J. Beaman, J.W. Barlow, D.L. Bourell, R.H. Crawford, H.L. Marcus, and K.P. McAlea, *Solid Freeform Fabrication: A New Direction in Manufacturing,* Kluwer Academic Press, Boston, 1997, p 143–151
30. S. Hayse, RTM Aerospace Components Developed Using Rapid Prototype Tooling, *Proc. 43rd International SAMPE Symposium,* 31 May–4 June 1998, p 1715–1723
31. M.R. Snyder, Rapid Toolers, Prototypers Aim to Eliminate Time-Consuming Steps, *Mod. Plast.,* April 2000, p 24–28
32. J. Male, H. Tsang and G. Bennett, A Time, Cost, and Accuracy Comparison of Soft Tooling for Investment Casting Produced Using Stereolithography Techniques, *Proc. Solid Freeform Fabrication Symposium,* Aug 1996 (Austin, TX), University of Texas, p 1–8
33. P. Dickens, *Rapid Prototyping and Tooling: Update on Rapid Manufacturing,* Vol 8 (No. 6), Time-Compression Technologies, 2000, p 56–58

Design Guidelines

John Bootle, Frank Burzesi, and Lynda Fiorini, XC Associates, Inc.

DESIGNERS have more freedom when using composite construction than they do when using other materials, because with composites they are free to select different fibers, flakes, or particles and to combine them with a choice of different resins, ceramics, or metals. The skin can be different than the core. The designers are free to determine the amount and distribution of the constituents. A composite laminate may be built to any thickness, and the fibers may be oriented to achieve the desired strength and stiffness. This article addresses the basic guidelines considered in designing a composite structure. More detailed information on many of the topics addressed in this article is available in other articles in this Volume.

In the materials selection part of the design process, a broad choice can be made between the use of composite construction, metals, unreinforced polymers, and natural materials. As a general guideline, if a part can easily be fabricated from traditional materials, such as aluminum, steel, wood, or plastic, this choice may represent the lowest-cost solution. Composite construction has many advantages, including weight reduction, high stiffness, and corrosion resistance in polymer-matrix composites (PMC), hardness and high service temperature in ceramic-matrix composites (CMC), and improved strength and stiffness in metal-matrix composites (MMC). It is also relatively easy to mold large, complex shapes, which often result in lower costs than metal fabrication. A comparison of typical materials properties is given in Table 1.

This is a general introduction to composites; it is intended to familiarize the reader with the general considerations necessary to design and construct a composite part. For convenience, many of the terms common to composites are defined in this article. A complete glossary is in the back of this Volume.

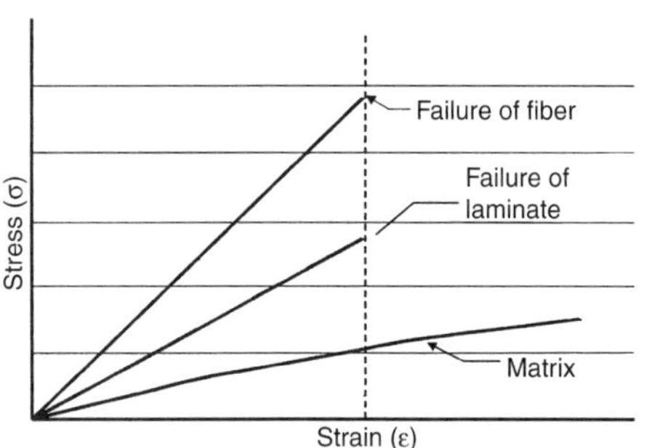

Fig. 1 Stress-strain relationship in a composite

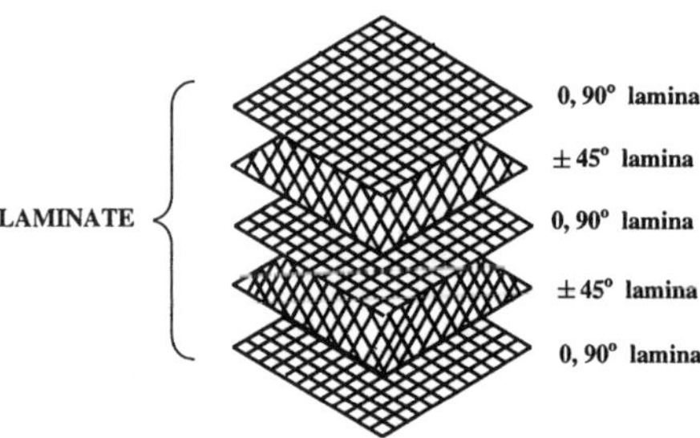

Fig. 2 Typical balanced-symmetric laminate

Definition of Composites

A composite material can be defined as a macroscopic combination of two or more distinct materials having a recognizable interface between them. However, because composites are usually used for their structural properties, the definition can be restricted to include only those materials that contain reinforcement (such as fibers or particles) supported by a binder (matrix) material.

Figure 1 shows a generalized diagram to illustrate the stress-strain relationship in a typical composite. Composite laminates can fail suddenly when the fibers break, unlike most metals, which have a plastic deformation region beyond the straight line "Hooke's law" relationship. Therefore, the strain limit of the fibers will determine the failure of the composite laminate.

Following are definitions of terms that apply to composites in general (additional definitions can be found in the "Glossary" in this Volume):

matrix. The essentially homogeneous resin, polymer, or other material in which the fiber system or other reinforcement of the composite is embedded. Both thermoplastic and thermoset resins may be used, as well as glass, ceramics, and metals.

reinforcement. The primary load-carrying or reinforcing element, usually fiber, embedded in the matrix. Chopped fibers, whiskers, particles, and flakes may also be used.

lamina. A single ply of a layered composite material

laminate. A product made by bonding two or more lamina to form a composite material. Figure 2 shows a typical balanced laminate of five lamina of plain weave cloth.

fiber orientation. The directional alignment of fibers in a composite. In composite construction, the designer has the freedom to align the fibers in any particular orientation to achieve specific laminate properties. The terms *isotropic*, *anisotropic*, and *quasi-isotropic* are used to describe the resulting laminate properties.

isotropic. A material having uniform properties in all directions, typically a metal

Table 1 Comparisons between typical properties of epoxy resin with various reinforcements and various metals

	Density		Ultimate unidirectional strength				Unidirectional tensile modulus	
			Tensile		Compressive			
Material	g/cm^3	lb/in.^{3}	MPa	ksi	MPa	ksi	GPa	10^6 psi
Carbon (AS4)	1.55	0.056	1482	215	1227	178	145	21.0
Carbon (HMS)	1.63	0.059	1276	185	1020	148	207	30.0
S-glass	1.99	0.072	1751	254	496	72	59	8.6
E-glass	1.99	0.072	1103	169	490	71	52	7.6
Aramid	1.38	0.050	1310	190	290	42	83	12.0
Aluminum (7075-T6)	2.79	0.101	570	83	570	83	69	10.0
Titanium (6Al-4V)	4.42	0.160	1100	160	1100	160	114	16.5
Steel (4130)	7.83	0.283	655	95	655	95	207	30.0

Composite properties are for general quasi-isotropic laminate and are dependent on fiber orientation.

anisotropic. A material having varying properties in different directions, typically a composite laminate. By orienting the fibers in a prescribed manner, the properties can be tailored to the exact loading and stiffness requirements of the design. Table 2 shows the directional properties of carbon fibers, which can be used to the designer's benefit to build an efficient structure.

quasi-isotropic. A material approximating an isotropic material, typically a composite laminate with the fibers oriented in the 0°, 90°, +45°, –45° to simulate isotropic properties.

Following are a list of common definitions relating to fibers and fabrics:

fiber. Basic unit of fibrous material
tow. An untwisted bundle of continuous fibers
roving. A number of tows collected into a parallel bundle with little or no twist
yarn. A number of twisted fibers assembled into a continuous length and suitable for weaving into a fabric
sizing. Finish applied to fibers that allows the resin matrix to adhere to the fibers
tape. Parallel tows of fibers held together in a prepreg or cross-stitching to form standard widths of unidirectional fibers
fabric. A textile structure produced by weaving tows of fibers. Figures 3, 4, and 5 show common fabric weaves.
warp. Longitudinal fibers of a fabric. The warp is the high-strength direction, due to the straightness of the fibers.
fill. Fibers running over and under the warp fibers at an angle of 90° to the warp direction. Also called woof and weft. The fill-direction is the lower-strength direction, due to the curvatures of the fibers.
nonwoven. A textile structure produced from a collection of tows in a random mat
prepreg. Typically fabric or tape that is preimpregnated with a resin and stored for use. The resin is partially cured to a "B" stage. This is an intermediate stage in the polymerization reaction of thermoset resins. A prepreg must be stored in a freezer and has a limited shelf life (usually six months).

The following terms apply to the resin used as a matrix as well as impregnating resins:

thermoset. A resin that is substantially fused and insoluble after being cured by either heat or chemical means
thermoplastic. A resin that can be softened by heating and hardened by cooling through a characteristic temperature range

Analysis of a Composite Laminate

There are a number of computer programs that may be used to analyze a composite laminate. These programs generally fall into two groups:

- *Group 1 codes:* These allow the user to specify the composite lay-up. The code will then predict the laminate properties. These properties may then be used in a typical finite-element analysis (FEA). This form of analysis is quick and is often used during the preliminary design of a composite structure. Because this form of analysis is dealing with the global laminate properties, it is not possible to predict the laminate failure conditions, such as interlaminar shear.
- *Group 2 codes:* These allow the designer to input the composite lay-up ply-by-ply directly into the FEA model of the complete structure. These codes have the advantages of making it possible to predict the detailed performance of each ply within the laminate and to calculate failure criteria, such as maximum strain, maximum stress, Hill-Tsai, and Tsai-Wu. The ply-by-ply approach leads to large models and is consequently used after the preliminary design has been established.

While these codes are available, it is always essential to have a good grasp of the basic equations governing the laminate performance, because this will aid the designer with a basic understanding essential to the design of an efficient structure. The basic laminate equations are presented in the following paragraphs.

Stress-strain relationships for metals and composites are defined below. For metals:

$$\sigma = E\varepsilon$$

where σ is stress, ε is strain, and E is Young's modulus. For composites:

$$\sigma_{ij} = Q_{ij}\varepsilon_{ij}$$

where Q_{ij} is the lamina stiffness.

The stiffness matrix for plane stress is called the reduced stiffness matrix, where, ij = 1, 2, and 6:

$$[Q] = \begin{bmatrix} Q_{11} & Q_{12} & Q_{16} \\ Q_{21} & Q_{22} & Q_{26} \\ Q_{16} & Q_{26} & Q_{66} \end{bmatrix} = \begin{bmatrix} \dfrac{E}{1-\nu} & \dfrac{\nu_{12}E_{22}}{1-\nu_{12}\nu_{21}} & 0 \\ \dfrac{\nu_{21}E_{11}}{1-\nu_{12}\nu_{21}} & \dfrac{E_{22}}{1-\nu_{12}\nu_{21}} & 0 \\ 0 & 0 & G_{12} \end{bmatrix}$$

where ν is Poisson's ratio, E is Young's modulus, G is shear modulus, and $Q_{16} = Q_{61} = Q_{26} = Q_{62} = 0$, for principal fiber directions.

Stress-Strain Load Relationships. The general stress-strain relationship is:

$$\sigma = E\varepsilon$$

For tension, compression, and shear:

$$\sigma = N/A \rightarrow E\varepsilon = N/A \rightarrow N = (EA)\ \varepsilon$$

where N is the stress resultant and A is the unit area. For bending:

$$\sigma = Mc/I \rightarrow E\varepsilon = Mc/I \rightarrow M \rightarrow (EI)\varepsilon/c$$

$$\rightarrow M = (EI)\ K$$

Fig. 3 Plain weave, yarn interlacing

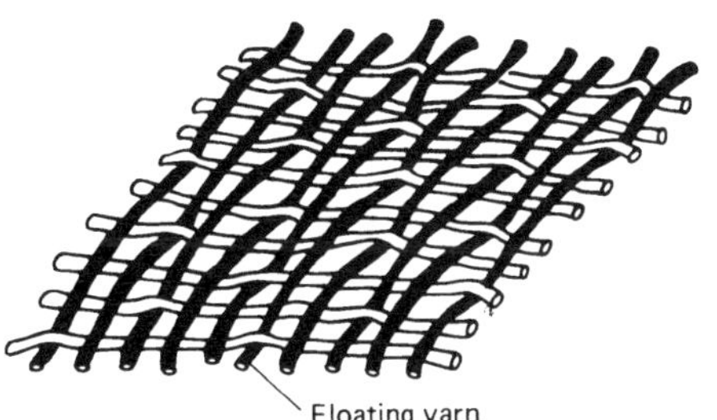

Fig. 4 Fiber-harness satin weave, interlacing

Table 2 Properties of carbon fiber

	Modulus		Ultimate unidirectional strength				Coefficient of thermal expansion	
			Tensile		Compressive			
Direction	GPa	10^6	MPa	ksi	MPa	ksi	10^{-6}/K	10^{-6}/°F
Axial	160	23.1	1724	250	1365	198	0	0
Transverse	11	1.6	41	6	228	33	22.5	12.5

For some carbon fibers, the axial coefficient of linear expansion is negative.

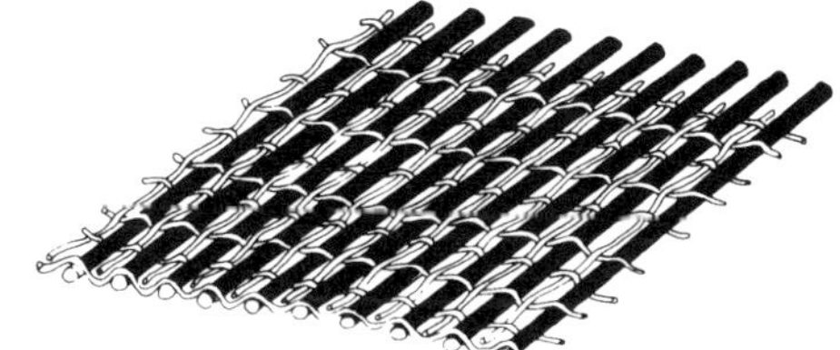

Fig. 5 Unidirectional weave

where M is the resultant moment, c is the distance from the neutral axis to the extreme fiber, I is the moment of inertia, and K is a curvature. The resultant stresses and moments are seen in Fig. 6.

General Load Displacement Case. These stress and resultant moments can be used, as is usual in plate theory, to develop a general load, strain, curvature relationship:

$$N = (EA)\varepsilon$$

$$M = (EI)\,K$$

In matrix form:

$$\begin{Bmatrix} N_x \\ N_y \\ N_{xy} \\ M_x \\ M_x \\ M_{xy} \end{Bmatrix} = \begin{bmatrix} A_{11} & A_{12} & A_{16} & \vdots & B_{11} & B_{12} & B_{16} \\ A_{21} & A_{22} & A_{26} & \vdots & B_{21} & B_{22} & B_{26} \\ A_{61} & A_{62} & A_{66} & \vdots & B_{61} & B_{62} & B_{66} \\ B_{11} & B_{12} & B_{16} & \vdots & D_{11} & D_{12} & D_{16} \\ B_{21} & B_{22} & B_{26} & \vdots & D_{21} & D_{22} & D_{26} \\ B_{61} & B_{62} & B_{66} & \vdots & D_{61} & D_{62} & D_{66} \end{bmatrix} \begin{Bmatrix} \varepsilon_x \\ \varepsilon_x \\ \varepsilon_{xy} \\ K_x \\ K_x \\ K_{xy} \end{Bmatrix}$$

where N terms are in-plane loads; M terms are moment loads; A, B, and D terms make up the laminate stiffness matrix; ε terms are the midplane strains; and K terms are curvatures.

The terms of the stiffness matrix are:

$$A_{ij} = \sum_{k=1}^{N} (\bar{Q}_{ij})(z_k - z_{(k-1)})$$

$$B_{ij} = \tfrac{1}{2}\sum_{k=1}^{N} (Q_{ij})(z_k^2 - z_{(k-1)}^2)$$

$$D_{ij} = \tfrac{1}{3}\sum_{k=1}^{N} (Q_{ij})(z_k^3 - z_{(k-1)}^3)$$

where $\bar{Q}_{ij} = Q_{ji}$ rotated into material coordinates from principal coordinate directions. The differences in z represent individual ply thicknesses, as seen in Fig. 7.

The equations may be simplified for a symmetrical and balanced lay-up:

$$\begin{Bmatrix} N_x \\ N_y \\ N_{xy} \\ M_x \\ M_x \\ M_{xy} \end{Bmatrix} = \begin{bmatrix} \begin{bmatrix} A_{11} & A_{12} & A_{16} & & & \\ A_{21} & A_{22} & A_{26} & & 0 & \\ A_{61} & A_{62} & A_{66} & & & \\ & & & D_{11} & D_{12} & D_{16} \\ & 0 & & D_{21} & D_{22} & D_{26} \\ & & & D_{61} & D_{62} & D_{66} \end{bmatrix} \end{bmatrix} \begin{Bmatrix} \varepsilon_x \\ \varepsilon_x \\ \varepsilon_{xy} \\ K_x \\ K_x \\ K_{xy} \end{Bmatrix}$$

where B terms = 0 for symmetrical laminate. The details of this characterization of a laminate composite using matrices is detailed in the article "Macromechanics Analysis of Laminate Properties" in this Volume.

Solution of General Load Case. The steps are:

1. Determine terms of modulus matrix, Q_{ij}, for *each* layer in lamina coordinates.
2. Transform Q_{ij} lamina into $\bar{Q}_{ij}$ laminate.
3. Calculate "EA" terms, A_{ij}, B_{ij}, D_{ij}, for laminate and set up stiffness matrix.
4. Set up load case, calculate strains and curvatures, then combine strains and curvatures to determine total strain of the laminate.
5. Transform laminate strains to lamina strains for *each* layer.
6. Calculate lamina stresses from lamina strains for *each* layer.
7. The use of computer codes greatly reduces the time required to solve these equations.

A two-stage approach for the analysis of composite structures is recommended:

- Use simple code to determine global laminate properties. These properties are then used for preliminary design and optimization.
- For design verification and structural analysis, the composite structure is modeled using a finite-element code in which each ply (lamina) will be modeled and the stresses and failure criteria determined.

Summary of Factors Affecting Composite Materials Properties and Allowables. Materials properties for composites are stated as design allowables that are statistically determined from test data. Factors affecting the materials property values for fiber-reinforced polymers include, but are not limited to:

- *Volume fraction (percent fiber to total volume):* Generally, the fiber volume will be in the range of 45 to 65%.
- *Temperature:* Generally, high cure temperatures are indicative of higher operating temperatures. The higher the cure temperature, the higher the cost of materials and processing. Therefore, it is important to understand the operational conditions and to specify the appropriate resin, to avoid adding unnecessary cost. Temperature differentials in processing and in service, combined with different coefficients of thermal expansion (CTE)

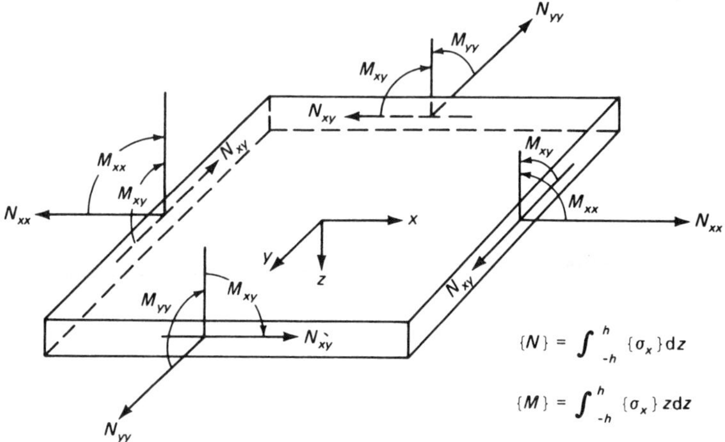

Fig. 6 Stress and moment resultants

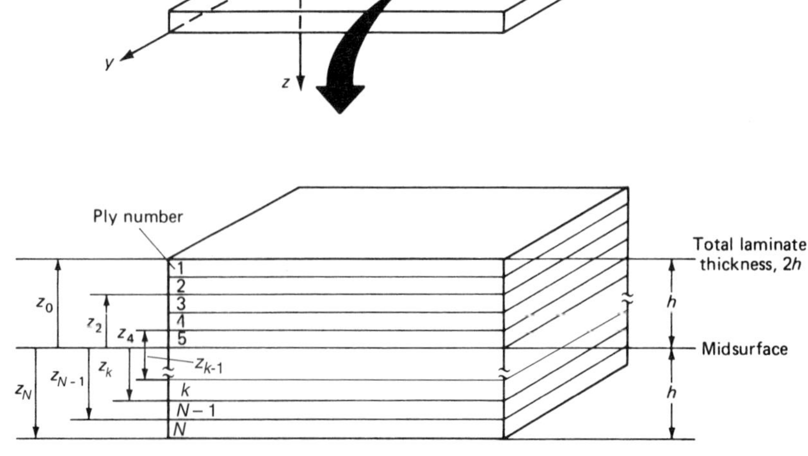

Fig. 7 Laminate construction with ply designations

of components, lead to internal thermal stresses.

- *Moisture absorption:* The matix, reinforcement, and their interface respond differently to moisture. This is called hygral behavior.
- *Orientation* of fibers in laminate
- *Test procedures*, number of tests, and analysis of data
- *Process control* relative to manufacture of composite laminate

Laminate Design. In order to minimize any residual thermal stresses caused during cure of the resin, it is always good practice to design a symmetrical, or balanced, laminate. Examples of balanced laminates are presented in Table 3. The first example uses unidirectional tape, and examples 2 and 3 are typical quasi-isotropic laminates fabricated from woven cloth.

Table 4 presents examples of the effects caused by nonsymmetrical laminates. These effects are most pronounced in laminates that are cured at high temperature in an autoclave or oven, due to the thermal stresses developed in the laminate as the laminate cools down from the cure temperature to room temperature. Laminates cured at room temperature using typical wet lay-up or vacuum-assisted resin transfer molding (VARTM) do not exhibit the same degree of distortion, due to the much smaller thermal stresses.

Mold Design

There are many types of molds that can be manufactured in order to produce a composite part. The type of tooling chosen will vary, based on several factors. These factors include:

- Molding process used. This includes autoclave, resin transfer molding (RTM), VARTM, and wet lay-up, which is defined subsequently.
- Temperature of cure
- Surface quality desired on finished part
- Budget
- Number of parts being produced from the tooling
- Size and complexity of the parts

Once these factors have been addressed, the type of tooling required can be determined.

Master Model. Depending on the complexity of the composite part and the type of tooling to be made, there are different routes to the production of the mold. The master model can be a physical representation of the actual composite part, computer-aided design (CAD) data, or drawing of the part. How a master model is defined is necessary in creating the tooling.

Metal Tooling. If the mold is to be made of a metal, the metal tool can be directly machined to the desired shape and size using CAD data or a drawing of the finished part. If the mold will be going through a cure cycle, the differences of the CTEs will have to be taken into account when selecting the material and defining the size of the mold.

Composite Tooling. When considering composite tooling, a physical mold master will need to be created to make the mold. The master can be made from the materials listed in Table 5, which includes the advantages and disadvantages of each.

Tool Care. No matter what type of tooling is used, the quality of the parts produced from the tooling will be a direct reflection of how the tool is treated in the working environment. Some common faults that will lead to degradation of the tool surface and reduced life of the tool are:

- Incorrect application of release agent
- Cutting on the tool surface
- Cleaning of the tool surface with inappropriate materials or equipment
- Impact damage to the tool surface

Matrix-Resin Selection

For resin-based composites, resin selection is an important step in designing the composite for use in a particular application. There are several general types of matrix-resin systems, and within each, there are countless variants that are commercially available. Selection of a basic resin group is based on general performance criteria of the application. It is important to note that a thorough investigation of a particular manufacturer's matrix-resin system must be undertaken prior to final selection and use.

The first step in the matrix-resin selection process is to determine the requirements of the final application. Requirements should be based on the envelope operation conditions of the application, including, but not limited to, the following:

- *Structural characteristics* of strength, stiffness, and toughness. While the reinforcement is the primary structural member, transverse properties, compression, and toughness requirements must be considered in resin selection.
- *Resistance* to corrosion, chemicals, moisture, and other environmental factors, such as ultraviolet radiation
- *Thermal characteristics,* including maximum and minimum temperatures, temperature differences, and thermal cycling
- *Fire, smoke, and toxicity*
- *Outgassing*

After the application requirements are defined, a number of fiber reinforcements and matrix-resin systems may satisfy them. A suitable matrix-resin system will have particular processing requirements and costs associated with it that may preclude its use on a particular application. Table 6 cross-references resin systems with performance and processing methods to aid the selection of resin systems.

Typical PMC Processes

Many different methods may be used to process composite components. A brief overview is presented in Table 7. The choice of processing method is determined by the materials and intended use of the composite part.

Wet lay-up is used in low-stress applications where performance and weight are not critical, but lowest cost is very important. Wet lay-up parts can be fabricated using continuous woven fiber and a roller to spread the resin and completely wet-out the fiber. The fiber reinforcement may also be applied to the mold using a chopper gun that sprays a mixture of resin and fiber di-

Table 3 Symmetrically balanced laminates

Example	Lamina	Written as
1	±45°, –45°, 0°, 0°, –45°, +45°	$(+45, -45, 0)_S$
2	±45°, 0°/90°, ±45°, 0°/90°, 0°/90°, ±45°, 0°/90°, ±45°	$(\pm 45, 0/90)_{2S}$
3	±45°, ±45°, 0°/90°, 0°/90°, ±45°, ±45°	$([\pm 45]_2, 0/90)_S$

Table 4 Examples of effects of nonsymmetry

Type	Example	Comments
Symmetrical, balanced	(+45, –45, 0, 0, –45, +45)	Flat, constant midplane stress
Nonsymmetrical, balanced	(90, +45, 0, 90, –45, 0)	Induces curvature
Symmetrical, nonbalanced	(–45, 0, 0, –45)	Induces twist
Nonsymmetrical, nonbalanced	(90, –45, 0, 90, –45, 0)	Induces twist and curvature

Table 5 Materials used as mold masters

Material	Advantages and disadvantages
Wood	Only usable at low temperature Easily worked Inexpensive materials Not very accurate or dimensionally stable Surface requires sealing to produce suitable mold surface
Urethane tooling block	More accurate Relatively cheap More stable than wood—still short term Will take in moisture over time Requires surface sealing Reaction problem to epoxy prepregs Capable of withstanding autoclave cures Requires machining
Epoxy tooling block	Price is variable depending on grade of block, but expensive compared to wood or urethane Surface coating not always necessary High-quality block extremely stable Capable of withstanding autoclave cures
Metal	Can be steel or aluminum, cast or fabricated, or a combination Excellent surface finish. Surface sealing is not required. Extremely heavy Large thermal mass to heat up and cool down Cost is relatively inexpensive Long-term stability is good if protected from corrosion Welded joints can leak

Table 6 Comparison of resin system performance and processing characteristics

Attribute	Polyester	Vinyl ester	Epoxy	Phenolic	Bismaleimide	Cyanate ester
Applications						
Typical applications	Marine, general	Marine, general	Aerospace, general	Fire, smoke, and toxicity applications	Aerospace, electrical	Aerospace
Performance						
Structural	Fair	Good	Better, tough	Good, brittle	Good, brittle	Good, brittle
Corrosion and chemical resistance	Poor	Excellent	Good	Excellent	Good	Excellent
Moisture absorption	Poor	Excellent	Good	Excellent	Excellent	Excellent
Glass transition temperature (T_g)(a), °C (°F)	70 (160)	70–163 (160–325) with postcure	95–175 (200–350) with postcure	70–120+ (160–250+) with postcure	150–220 (300–425) with postcure	175–230 (350–450) with postcure
Fire, smoke, and toxicity	...	Requires additives	Requires additives	Good	Good	Good
Processing(b)						
Hand lay-up	Yes(c)	Yes(d)	Yes	No	No	No
RTM	Yes(c)	Yes(d)	Yes(d)	No	No	No
VARTM	Yes(c)	Yes(d)	Yes(d)	No	No	No
Filament winding	Yes(c)	Yes(d)	Yes(d)	No	No	No
Sheet molding	No	No	Yes(d)	Yes	Yes	Yes
Press/autoclave molding	No	No	Yes(d)	Typical(e)	Typical(e)	Typical(e)
Cost						
Comparative cost(f)	1	2	3	4	5	5

(a) Actual T_g varies with each system and cure method. (b) "Yes" or "No" under "Processing" reflects typical uses. (c) Room-temperature cure. (d) Room-temperature and elevated-temperature cure. (e) Elevated-temperature cure. (f) Where "1" is low and "5" is high

rectly onto the mold. Because this process uses room-temperature cure resins, the mold tools may be manufactured from wood or glass fiber, with a gel coat to produce a high-quality finish.

The concerns for the tooling are not as great as for the other methods of manufacturing. The tool does not need to hold a vacuum, and there are no concerns of thermal mismatch. This leads to a relatively inexpensive tool.

Autoclave process is used to manufacture high-performance parts that are designed for the highest strength-to-weight ratios. It is necessary to use resins that require a high cure temperature; typically, the higher the operating temperature for the composite, the higher the cure temperature of a resin. Tooling is usually fabricated from metal or special tooling prepregs that can withstand the typical high-pressure, high-temperature cure cycles. Due to the high-temperature cure cycle, the tooling has to be designed so that it is dimensionally correct at the elevated-cure temperature rather than at room temperature. Special care must be taken to ensure that the part may be easily removed and will not become trapped as the tool cools.

When using an autoclave cure, the following factors must be considered:

- Thermal mismatch
- Thermal mass of the tool
- Number of parts being made from the tooling
- Budget
- Surface-quality requirements
- Tool must be able to maintain a vacuum

Resin transfer molding requires matched metal tooling. The cure can be done at room temperature. The resin may be heated to facilitate flow into the tool, so mismatched CTEs may be a concern.

Vacuum-Assisted Resin Transfer Molding. There are about 30 different variations of the process that have been developed to meet particular applications. In general, VARTM is used to fabricate very large components. Typically, the dry fibers and core material are laid into the mold, a vacuum bag is then used, and the air is sucked out. Once a good vacuum is achieved, resin is infused into the part. Balsa or foam cores are typically used; honeycomb core cannot be used. Because VARTM uses continuous fibers and is cured under typical vacuum pressure of 84 MPa (25 in. of mercury), the resulting laminate is very high quality, with properties similar to autoclave cure and with a lower void content. The process is limited by the resin selection to typically room-temperature resins with very low viscosity, to allow for infusion. New resins are presently being developed to achieve higher operating temperatures; the operating temperature of parts may be enhanced by postcuring the cured part in the oven. Because this process uses room-temperature cure resins, the mold tools may be manufactured from wood, or glass fiber with a gel coat may be used to produce a high-quality finish.

Besides surface-quality requirements for the finished parts, tooling design for VARTM must consider the number of parts being produced from the tooling, the cycle time, and the ability to maintain a sufficient vacuum throughout its life.

Table 7 Various manufacturing processes

Process	Comment	Typical applications
Hand lay-up	Low cost Lower strength components Large parts Relatively low-cost tooling	Large commercial parts, where cost is more important than high strength or low weight
Vacuum bag, oven cure	Similar to wet lay-up, but improved consolidation leading to higher strength	Large commercial parts, where cost is more important than high strength or low weight
Autoclave cure	High quality High strength Relatively high cost of tooling Size limited by autoclave	High-performance military and aerospace components and thermal cores
Resin transfer molding	High quality High strength Matched metal tooling Lower cost than autoclave	Military and aerospace applications Large-volume commercial parts Small enclosures and keyboards
Vacuum-assisted resin transfer molding	Room-temperature process Large parts High quality Low cost	Extensively used for Navy applications Large electronic equipment enclosures, operator consoles, etc.
Compression molding	High-cost tooling High quality Complex parts Low part cost	Electronic module covers and small electronic equipment enclosures
Bonded metal	Typically, aluminum honeycomb construction	Lightweight back planes and electrically conductive components Commercial applications

Electromagnetic Interference (EMI) Shielding and Electrostatic Discharge (ESD) Protection

Electromagnetic interference shielding and electrostatic discharge protection are required in numerous composite applications, such as computer cases to meet emission specifications, or aircraft wing structures to dissipate lightning strikes. Some common EMI shielding methods, with pros and cons, are listed in Table 8.

Many published articles claim that very high shielding levels are obtainable for panels by using these methods. In all EMI and ESD protection schemes, grounding of the composite panel to the main structure is the area requiring the most attention. The major issue for the embedded EMI protection systems is that the surfaces are often resin-rich. This forms a good electrical insulating barrier and prevents electrical contact to the main structure. The resulting gap will act like a slot antenna and radiate at specific frequencies. Therefore, particular attention must be given during the design and fabrication to ensure that any embedded metallic layer is extended beyond the laminate matrix to provide a good electric bond to the metal.

Metal Plating

Metal plating is often used to provide enhanced corrosion protection and EMI protection for composite laminates. There are three considerations:

- Ensure the part will fit into the plating bath; this may exclude large parts.
- Choice of resin system
- Release agent used

The basic plating system is comprised of up to 20 baths, each containing a different chemical. The general process is to clean, etch, activate the surface, electroless plate the base metal, then plate other metals once a conductive metal surface is established. Conventional electroplating can be used to build up thickness. Typically, the etching process attacks the surface and provides microscopic sites where the metal molecules can form a mechanical bond to the composite laminate. In some plastics, such as acrylonitrile-butadiene-styrene, this is easy, and excellent plating can be achieved. The reflectors for car headlights are a good example. Typical epoxy resins are a long polymer chain that is very resistant to chemical attack. It is therefore very difficult to etch the surface to provide the molecular sites for the metal to mechanically adhere to the laminate. The simplest test to verify adhesion is to apply masking tape to the plated surface. When the tape is removed, it should be free of metal particles. There are several proprietary systems that claim to work. The author has achieved success with the McDermot system. Plating is not a trivial matter, and it is recommended that the composite fabricator works with the plater and carries out a number of trials to ensure the plated surface will meet specification.

Fire Resistance

Where composite structures are used in aircraft interiors, maritime applications, and mass transit applications, some degree of fire protection is normally required:

- Typically, the aircraft industry uses a standard that requires a composite structure to self-extinguish within 60 seconds of the flame being removed.
- Marine and mass transit industries require that a composite will not significantly add to a fire and that it retains structural integrity for at least 15 minutes.

Generally, the use of composites for aircraft interior applications is well established with a clearly defined test requirement. With the recent growth in the use of composites in the marine and mass transit industry, standards and acceptable laminate systems are still being developed.

There are two main approaches to the design of a fire-resistant laminate: resin selection and surface treatments.

Resin Selection. Because the glass fiber or carbon-fiber reinforcement does not burn, the resin selection is the element that determines the fire characteristics of the laminate. Typical specifications for aircraft interiors are specified in Federal Aviation Regulation (FAR) 25 or 23. These require that after exposure to a flame, a composite panel will self-extinguish within 60 seconds of the flame removal. This requirement is typically satisfied with a phenolic resin or an epoxy resin that has a flame retardant added. These resins are relatively expensive and require 120 to 175 °C (250 to 350 °F) cure cycle temperatures. They are not particularly suitable for use in large mass transit or marine applications, due to cost and cure considerations.

Surface Treatments for Laminates. Composite laminates may be coated with intumescent paints or have intumescent layers embedded into the surface of the laminate. When exposed to intense heat or flame, these coatings bubble into a foam that protects the material underneath. The advantage of intumescent paints is that they can be easily applied to the surface of the laminate once it is cured. However, they have the potential disadvantage that they can be abraded from the surface due to normal wear and tear, and hence reduce the fire protection. Embedding an intumescent layer into the laminate has the advantage that it cannot be easily worn off by normal use. However, it has the disadvantage that the intumescent material will absorb resin, which will burn off of the surface before the intumescent material begins to work.

The use of intumescent materials embedded into the surface of a low-cost vinyl ester resin structure is relatively new, but has been approved for use by the U.S. Navy for some shipboard applications. Further development to enhance the performance is presently being carried out by the marine and mass transit industries.

The graph presented in Fig. 8 shows typical cone calorimeter tests for two laminates protected by an intumescent layer.

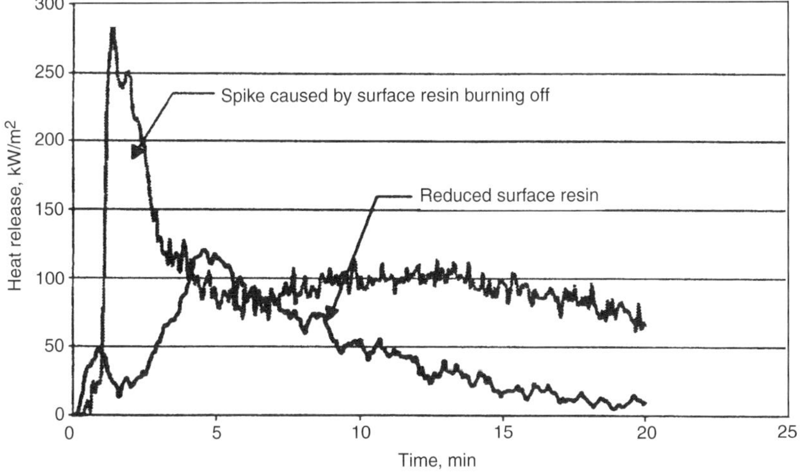

Fig. 8 Heat release averages from calorimeter tests for incident heat flux of 50 kW/m^2

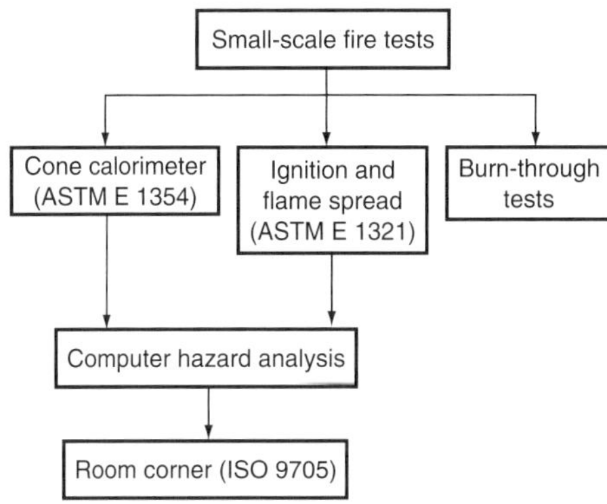

Fig. 9 Methodology for fire qualification

Performance Verification. For typical aircraft applications, there is a considerable database of experience, and it is often possible to verify performance of a laminate by carrying out coupon testing as defined in Boeing specification BSS 7230. For marine applications, some form of hazard analysis to verify that the composite structure will not add significantly to a fire is often required. The general methodology is described in Fig. 9. The small-scale testing could involve carrying out cone calorimeter testing in accordance with ASTM E 1354, for example. Typically, the cone calorimeter testing is carried out at incident heat fluxes of 25, 50, and 75 kW/m^2. The most important features for comparing the fire performance of laminates are the time to ignition and the heat released during the test. The results from the cone test are used as the input for a computer hazard analysis of the room where the composites are being used, to determine the effect of a fire on surrounding structures. If this analysis is inconclusive, then it will be necessary to carry out a full size test, typically an ISO 9705 corner test to determine the performance.

Table 9 lists a summary of some of the common fire-protection options and typical uses of each.

Thermal Conductivity

Pitch-based carbon fibers offer considerably higher thermal conductivity (K_L) than metals and have a much lower density. This comparison is shown in Table 10. The main use of these fibers is in space applications and thermal cores for electronic modules. The in-plane thermal conductivity for a ply of carbon fiber is determined by the rule of mixtures and is given by:

$$K_x = K_{FL} \cdot V_f \cdot \sin^2\alpha$$

$$K_y = K_{FL} \cdot V_f \cdot \cos^2\alpha$$

where V_f is fiber volume, K_{FL} is the longitudinal fiber thermal conductivity, and α is the angle of fibers in a particular ply.

The thermal conductivity through the thickness of the laminate K_z, is dominated by the resin and is typically in the region of 1.5 W/m · K (0.87 Btu/h · ft · °F). There are several equations to predict K_z, but presently they are approximations at best. It is recommended that the user

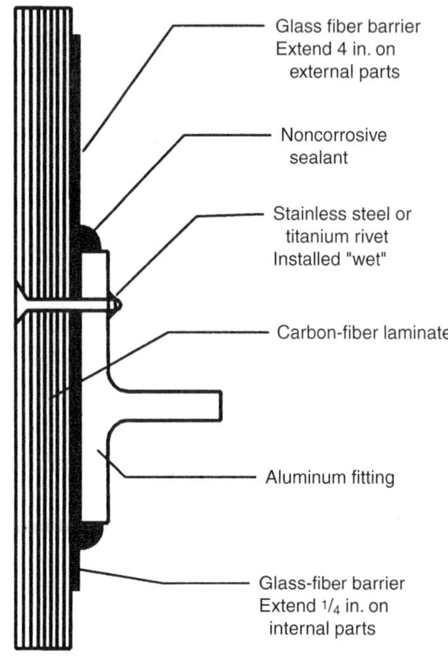

Fig. 10 Typical method of providing bimetallic corrosion protection

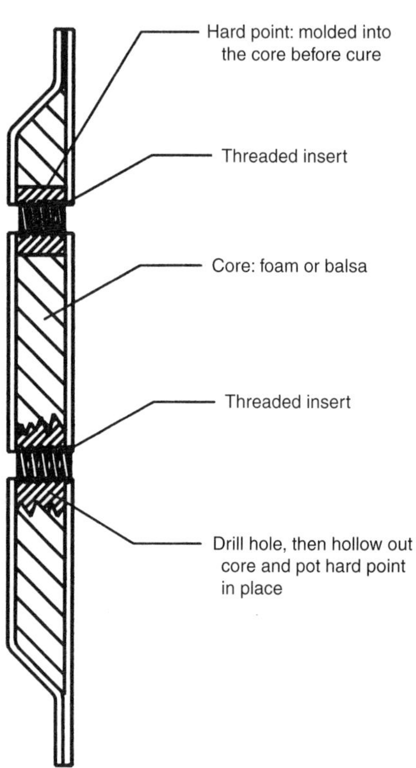

Fig. 11 One method of preparing laminate for threaded insert

Table 8 Common EMI shielding methods

Protection method	Comment
Carbon fibers	Carbon fibers are electrically conductive and, therefore, provide a low-level EMI shielding.
Nickel-plated carbon fibers	The electrical conductivity enhanced by nickel plating can provide higher levels of shielding, up to 70 dB. Good for ESD protection
Metal mesh	Metal meshes provide a high level of EMI shielding.
Electrically conductive paint flame spraying	This is an effective method, but has the disadvantage that it is a surface layer and needs to be protected from abrasion and corrosion.
Metal plating	See text

Table 9 Summary of fire-protection options

Resin	Comment	Use
Vinyl ester resins	Low cost Easy to process Low fire resistance	Use intumescent coating to meet typical commercial and maritime specifications
Epoxy resins	120 °C (250 °F) cure temperature	Can use fire inhibitors, but these produce fumes when burned. Meets FAR 25.853
Phenolic resins	175 °C (350 °F) cure temperature	Typically used for aircraft interiors

Table 10 Properties of various thermally conductive materials

		Fiber thermal conductivity (K_{FL})		Tensile modulus	
Fiber	Manufacturer	W/m · K	Btu/h · ft · °F	GPa	10^6 psi
K1100	Amoco	1060	613	965(a)	140(a)
P120	Amoco	640	370	830(a)	120(a)
K13C2U	Mitsubishi	620	360	900(a)	130(a)
P100	Amoco	520	300	724(a)	105(a)
XSH-70A	Nippon	250	140	738(a)	107(a)
Aluminum beryllium	...	210	120	190	28
Aluminum	...	187	108	70	10

(a) These are fiber values; the stiffness of a composite laminate will be less.

Table 11 Galvanic series

Anodic (most active)
Magnesium alloys
Galvanized steel
Aluminum
Mild steel
Cast iron
Lead
Tin
Brass
Nickel
Copper
Titanium
Nickel (passive)
Stainless steels (passive)
Silver
Gold
Carbon, graphite
Cathodic (least active)

base design calculations on previously measured data. K_z is dependent on the resin thermal conductivity and radial thermal conductivity of the fiber, K_{FR}. The problem is that K_{FR} varies, depending on the plane through the fiber. Therefore, a statistical term must be included for K_{FR}. The result is that, for practical purposes, it is better to work from measured data. Recent work has demonstrated that it is possible to increase K_z up to about 4 to 6 W/m · K (2.3 to 3.5 Btu/h · ft · °F) by adding boron nitride powder to the laminate.

Corrosion

Glass-fiber laminates exhibit excellent corrosion resistance and may be used with most common metals without using special precautions to prevent corrosion. When carbon-fiber laminates are used in conjunction with metal parts, special care must be taken to prevent bimetallic corrosion. Reference to the galvanic table, Table 11, shows that carbon fibers and aluminum are on opposite ends of the table, which indicates that particular precaution needs to be taken when aluminum fittings are to be used with a carbon-fiber structure. However, no special precautions need to be used when passivated stainless steel fittings are used.

Typical methods to provide bimetallic corrosion protection are shown Fig. 10. The glass fiber barrier extends at least 0.1 m (4 in.) beyond the aluminum fitting when the fitting is in an external location and exposed to water. This distance may be reduced to 0.063 m (0.25 in.) when used in a dry, internal location. The fasteners are dipped in epoxy resin and installed wet, so that the resin will cure to form a tight moisture barrier.

Aluminum mesh may be embedded into glass-fiber laminate to provide EMI shielding, but copper mesh or nickel-plated fibers should be used in carbon-fiber structures.

Fasteners

There are a large number of proprietary fasteners that have been designed to work with composite laminates. It is also possible to use traditional helical coil inserts, key inserts, and nut plates. If the position of the threaded inserts is known before fabrication, then hard points may be embedded into the laminate prior to cure. The hard point may be fabricated by simply filling the hole in the core with glass-fiber cloth during the lay-up in VARTM systems, or by embedding precured G10 or phenolic when using a prepreg system. This method is depicted in Fig. 11.

If the location of the fastener is not known prior to cure, a hole may be drilled through the laminate, and the core hollowed out and then filled with epoxy or other potting compound. Once this has cured, it is then possible to drill and insert the helical coil inserts or key insert.

Engineering Mechanics and Analysis of Metal-Matrix Composites

Bhaskar S. Majumdar, New Mexico Institute of Mining and Technology

METAL-MATRIX COMPOSITES (MMCs) differ from other composite systems primarily with respect to the inelastic deformation mechanisms of the matrix phase. Whereas the inelastic matrix strain in both ceramic-matrix composites (CMCs) and brittle polymer-matrix composites (PMCs) is dominated by the compliance from multiple matrix cracks, the matrix strain in MMCs arises from plasticity or viscoplasticity (or creep) of the ductile metal matrix. The difference between plasticity and viscoplasticity is that the former mechanism is essentially time-independent, whereas the latter is strongly time-dependent. Their relative magnitudes are governed by the temperature of loading, with viscoplasticity becoming significant at homologous temperatures (T/T_m, where T_m is the melting point), typically above 0.4. In titanium alloys, this temperature is slightly lower, approximately 0.35.

Important reasons for selecting MMCs over other composites in load-bearing applications are their high specific stiffness, strength, wear and environmental resistance, and toughness at temperatures between subzero and 650 °C (1200 °F). The higher temperature limit is based on currently available materials and may increase as new materials and processes become available. On the one hand, PMCs become inoperable above about 250 °C (480 °F), and on the other hand, CMCs have too low a strength without damage in this temperature domain. Thus, there is a range of temperatures where MMCs become strong candidates as the material of choice, and MMCs have indeed been considered enabling for a number of components and systems. The toughness advantage of MMCs derives from the ductility of the matrix. This advantage is reduced when the fiber volume fractions become high (>0.5) or the matrix becomes brittle, such as when the metal is an intermetallic with less than 3% elongation to failure. That is why the fiber volume fraction in most structural applications is typically less than 0.3, although there are a few exceptions. Specifically, higher volume fractions are used in wear, thermal, and electrical applications at the expense of toughness. It is important to bear these properties and the temperature range of application in mind while considering design with MMCs.

The difference between the thermal expansion coefficient of the metal-matrix and the ceramic-fiber or particulate reinforcement is typically large. (See tables in the article "Properties of Metal-Matrix Composites" in this Volume.) Hence, residual stresses from thermal mismatch have a significant effect on the overall deformation and damage response. Thermomechanical loading must be considered an integral aspect of any stress analyses with MMCs.

In addition to thermomechanical loading, it is also important to consider damage in the design of composites. This is because failure theories must realistically be based on the mechanisms of damage. In MMCs, there are essentially three types of damage. Two of the damage mechanisms are fiber-matrix debonding damage and fiber fracture, which are also present in other composite systems. The third form of damage is microvoid nucleation inside the matrix, followed by their growth and coalescence, leading to matrix rupture. The general sequence of damage is as follows:

- Damage initiated as interface crack or fiber crack
- Intense plasticity of the ductile metal matrix adjacent to damage site
- Microvoid nucleation in the matrix
- Microvoids grow and coalesce
- Matrix rupture and composite failure

The discontinuous MMCs are discussed later, but suffice to state that damage in many such composites involve either particle fracture or particle matrix separation followed by intense matrix plasticity and matrix rupture.

Inelastic analyses of MMCs have generally been restricted to interface and fiber damage and matrix plasticity and viscoplasticity. Matrix damage has generally not been considered, except in discontinuous systems whose ductility and toughness are significantly influenced by matrix-failure events. Even here, the analyses have been partial and will need to be expanded greatly to obtain an accurate predictive failure response of MMCs.

Micromechanics of Fiber-Reinforced MMCs

Micromechanics of composites are conducted at the fiber-matrix level to relate the lamina-level properties, such as stress-strain behavior and failure response, to the constituent properties of the reinforcement and matrix. The overall goal is to use the predictive methodology to develop tailored composites and also to make accurate predictions of their performance in service. Indeed, the current rapidly changing and cost-conscious technological environment has made such a predictive formalism essential. Note that this methodology is different from past approaches with PMCs, where the emphasis generally lay on lamina- and laminate-level testing and analyses. Here, a microscopic understanding of stress-strain evolution, damage nucleation, and growth at the fiber-matrix level is emphasized. Even in the case of PMCs, it is now widely recognized that design and development must be micromechanics-based, because testing at lamina and laminate level cannot keep pace with new materials development and the need to insert materials in untested stress-displacement-temperature domains.

The following results, based on the constitutive response of the reinforcement and the matrix, can be derived from micromechanics analyses:

- Overall stress-strain response of the composite under a wide range of load, temperature, time, and cycle conditions
- Stresses and strains at locations corresponding to potential sites of damage and failure

Micromechanics analysis is combined with experimental results at the single-fiber, or single-ply multiple-fiber level, to establish critical conditions for the initiation and propagation of failure. Some of these failure mechanisms are discussed briefly in the next section. However, it is relevant to point out here that damage initiation and failure are gradually being incorporated into micromechanical calculations, although there may be some debate as to whether such calculations fall within the realm of micromechanics or mesomechanics. The insertion of damage into micro- or mesoscale analyses has become possible, because of significant strides in computational power, novel multiscale algorithms, and new experimental insights on damage initiation and growth. Their description, however, is outside the scope of this article.

The following items are discussed subsequently, with reference to a unidirectional fiber-reinforced composite:

- Stiffness in the longitudinal and transverse directions
- Stress-strain response and stress distribution under linear elastic conditions
- Stress-strain response and stress distribution under elastic-plastic or elastic-viscoplastic conditions
- It should be pointed out, especially to those familiar with PMCs, that while MMCs are often fabricated from lamina, the processing is such that there is no discernable interface between the laminae. No concerns about interlaminar shear arise with MMCs, as is the case with PMCs.

Stiffness of MMCs

A rule of mixtures (ROM) formula, derived from a one-dimensional model, is generally adequate for determining the elastic modulus (E_c) of the composite in the fiber (longitudinal) direction:

$$E_c = V_f E_f + V_m E_m \qquad \text{(Eq 1)}$$

where V_f is the volume fraction of fibers, V_m is the volume fraction of the matrix ($V_m = 1 - V_f$), and E_f and E_m are the elastic modulus of the fiber and matrix, respectively. The corresponding Poisson's ratio can be determined using the concentric cylinder model (CCM) described later.

The analysis is slightly more complicated for the transverse modulus. In this case, one may consider various self-consistent models (Ref 1) using a composite cylinder assemblage. Alternately, one may use the NDSANDS computer program developed at the Air Force Research Laboratory (Ref 2, 3) and also based on the concentric cylinder analysis. As will be seen later, fiber-matrix debonding is often the critical damage mechanism for transverse loads.

Stress-Strain Response and Stress Distribution Under Linear Elastic Conditions

Longitudinal and Thermal Loading. It is assumed that a stress-free composite is subjected to a temperature change (ΔT), an applied stress (σ_c), or both. The mechanical loading is applied in the fiber direction, and the temperature is assumed to be uniform throughout. Also, while fibers are generally organized in a rectangular or hexagonal array inside the matrix, major simplification is obtained by considering a concentric cylinder assemblage. The resulting fiber-matrix CCM is illustrated in Fig. 1.

This is an axisymmetric problem, and the equilibrium equations in the r-, θ-, z-coordinate system reduce to:

$$\frac{d\sigma_r}{dr} + \frac{\sigma_r - \sigma_\theta}{r} = 0 \qquad \text{(Eq 2)}$$

The two independent displacements are u and w in the r- and z-directions, respectively. The strains are given by:

$$\varepsilon_r = \frac{du}{dr}, \quad \varepsilon_\theta = \frac{u}{r}, \quad \text{and} \quad \varepsilon_z = \frac{dw}{dz} \qquad \text{(Eq 3)}$$

Note that only ordinary derivatives are used, because u cannot be a function of z due to the infinitely long cylinders, and because w cannot be a function of r, otherwise isostrain conditions in the z-direction are violated. The displacement field given by Eq 3 can be used to write the compatibility condition for strains. The resultant compatibility condition is:

$$\frac{d\varepsilon_\theta}{dr} + \frac{\varepsilon_\theta - \varepsilon_r}{r} = 0 \qquad \text{(Eq 4)}$$

Equations 2 and 4 form the basis for elastic-plastic-viscoplastic analysis. Under linear elastic conditions, the equilibrium and compatibility requirements are identically satisfied if u has the form of Eq 5, where A and B are constants for each constituent:

$$u = \frac{A}{r} + Br \qquad \text{(Eq 5)}$$

Thus, A and B may be designated as A_f and B_f for the fiber and A_m and B_m for the matrix. Differentiation of Eq 5 according to Eq 3 provides the strains, and generalized Hooke's law is used to determine the stresses from the strains. When thermal strains are present, they must be subtracted from the total strains derived from Eq 5 and 3, in order to determine the stresses. The stress components then become:

$$\begin{aligned} \sigma_r &= \lambda(\varepsilon_r + \varepsilon_\theta + \varepsilon_z - 3\alpha\Delta T) + 2G(\varepsilon_r - a\Delta T) \\ \sigma_\theta &= \lambda(\varepsilon_r + \varepsilon_\theta + \varepsilon_z - 3\alpha\Delta T) + 2G(\varepsilon_\theta - a\Delta T) \\ \sigma_z &= \lambda(\varepsilon_r + \varepsilon_\theta + \varepsilon_z - 3\alpha\Delta T) + 2G(\varepsilon_z - a\Delta T) \end{aligned} \qquad \text{(Eq 6)}$$

where

$$\lambda = \frac{E\nu}{(1+\nu)(1-2\nu)} \quad \text{and} \quad G = \frac{E}{2(1+\nu)}$$

λ is a Lame's constant, and G is the shear modulus. The constants E, λ, G, ν, and α are specific to each material and are designated by subscripts "f" and "m" for the fiber and matrix, respectively. α refers to the thermal expansion, E is the Young's modulus, and ν is the Poisson's ratio of each constituent. The value of α will vary with temperature, so the value appropriate for the temperature range, ΔT, must be used. In Eq 6, the radial and circumferential strains are derived from Eq 5, and $\varepsilon_z = k$ is a constant for both the fiber and the matrix for maintaining isostrain conditions. The unknowns of the problem are the constants A_f, B_f, A_m, B_m, and k, requiring five independent boundary conditions. With the fiber radius, a, and matrix radius, b, as shown in Fig. 1, those boundary conditions are as follows:

- The displacement must be finite in the fiber at $r = 0$, hence $A_f = 0$.
- The radial displacements must be continuous across the interface, that is, $u_{\text{fiber}} = u_{\text{matrix}}$ at $r = a$.
- The radial stresses must be continuous across the interface, that is, $\sigma_r^{\text{fiber}} = \sigma_r^{\text{matrix}}$ at $r = a$.
- The radial stress must be zero at $r = b$; that is, $\sigma_r^{\text{matrix}} = 0$ at $r = b$.
- The sum of the axial stresses, normalized with respect to the respective areas, must be equal to the far-field applied stress in the fiber direction; that is, $V_f\sigma_z^{\text{fiber}} + V_m\sigma_z^{\text{matrix}} = \sigma_c$.

Once the constants are determined, they can be substituted into Eq 6 to obtain stresses at different locations. The strains can be used to determine the relevant material response, such as the effective elastic modulus and Poisson's ratio, under isothermal axisymmetric mechanical loading. Also, by holding $\sigma_c = 0$, the thermal expansion coefficient of the composite can be determined along both the axial and radial directions.

The set of equations for the remaining unknown constants, B_f, A_m, B_m, and k, can be represented through the following matrix equation:

$$\begin{vmatrix} a_{11} & a_{12} & a_{13} & a_{14} \\ a_{21} & a_{22} & a_{23} & a_{24} \\ a_{31} & a_{32} & a_{33} & a_{34} \\ a_{41} & a_{42} & a_{43} & a_{44} \end{vmatrix} \begin{vmatrix} B_f \\ A_m \\ B_m \\ k \end{vmatrix} = \begin{vmatrix} b_1 \\ b_2 \\ b_3 \\ b_4 \end{vmatrix} \qquad \text{(Eq 7)}$$

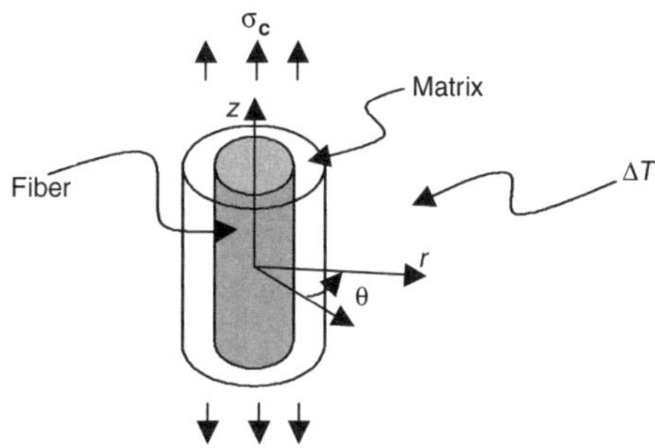

Fig. 1 The concentric cylinder model (CCM) for analyzing metal-matrix composites. The fiber radius is a, and the matrix radius is b, so the volume fraction of fibers is $V_f = a^2/b^2$. σ_c is the applied far-field stress.

where the constants a_{ij} and b_i are as follows:

$$a_{11} = a$$

$$a_{12} = -\frac{1}{a}$$

$$a_{13} = -a$$

$$a_{14} = 0$$

$$b_1 = 0$$

$$a_{21} = \frac{E_f}{(1+\nu_f)(1-2\nu_f)}$$

$$a_{22} = \frac{E_m}{(1+\nu_m)a^2}$$

$$a_{23} = -\frac{E_m}{(1+\nu_m)(1-2\nu_m)}$$

$$a_{24} = \frac{E_f\nu_f}{(1+\nu_f)(1-2\nu_f)} - \frac{E_m\nu_m}{(1+\nu_m)(1-2\nu_m)}$$

$$b_2 = \left[\frac{E_f\alpha_f}{(1-2\nu_f)} - \frac{E_m\alpha_m}{(1-2\nu_m)}\right]\Delta T$$

$$a_{31} = 0$$

$$a_{32} = \frac{E_m\nu_f}{(1+\nu_m)a^2}$$

$$a_{33} = \frac{E_m}{(1+\nu_m)(1-2\nu_m)}$$

$$a_{34} = \frac{E_m\nu_m}{(1+\nu_m)(1-2\nu_m)}$$

$$b_3 = \frac{E_m\alpha_m}{(1-2\nu_m)}\Delta T$$

$$a_{41} = \frac{2E_f\nu_f V_f}{(1+\nu_f)(1-2\nu_f)}$$

$$a_{42} = 0$$

$$a_{43} = \frac{2E_m\nu_m V_m}{(1+\nu_m)(1-2\nu_m)}$$

$$a_{44} = \frac{E_f(1-\nu_f)V_f}{(1+\nu_f)(1-2\nu_f)} + \frac{E_m(1-\nu_m)V_m}{(1+\nu_m)(1-2\nu_m)}$$

$$b_4 = \sigma_c + \left[\frac{E_f\alpha_f V_f}{(1-2\nu_f)} + \frac{E_m\alpha_m V_m}{(1-2\nu_m)}\Delta T\right] \quad \text{(Eq 8)}$$

Equation 7 can be solved, and the radial and circumferential stresses determined through Eq 6:

$$\sigma_r^{\text{fiber}} = \sigma_\theta^{\text{fiber}} = 2(\lambda_f + G_f)B_f + \lambda_f k - (3\lambda_f + 2G_f)\alpha_f\Delta T$$

$$\sigma_r^{\text{matrix}} = -2G_m A_m / r^2 + 2(\lambda_m + G_m)B_m + \lambda_m k - (3\lambda_m + 2G_m)\alpha_m\Delta T$$

$$\sigma_\theta^{\text{matrix}} = 2G_m A_m / r^2 + 2(\lambda_m + G_m)B_m + \lambda_m k - (3\lambda_m + 2G_m)\alpha_m\Delta T$$

$$\sigma_z^{\text{fiber}} = 2\lambda_f B_f + (\lambda_f + 2G_f)k - (3\lambda_f + 2G_f)\alpha_f\Delta T$$

$$\sigma_z^{\text{matrix}} = 2\lambda_m B_m + (\lambda_m + 2G_m)k - (3\lambda_m + 2G_m)\alpha_m\Delta T \quad \text{(Eq 9)}$$

Equation 9 provides accurate solution of the stress and strain fields, as well as the axial strain (k) and radial displacement (u at $r = b$) response of the composite, under any complex combination of thermal and mechanical load under linear elastic conditions. It is important to perform the calculations in Eq 7 with high precision, using double precision numbers so that rounding errors do not significantly affect the stresses and strains. Interface stresses are obtained by substituting $r = a$ in the final solution.

Under purely thermal loading, that is, $\sigma_c = 0$, and when $\nu_f = \nu_m = \nu$, a more concise solution is obtained (Ref 4) for the radial stress at the interface:

$$\sigma_r^{\text{interface}} = -\frac{(\alpha_f - \alpha_m)\Delta T E_m}{2\lambda_1}\left[\frac{V_m}{1-\nu_m}\right]$$

$$\text{where } \lambda_1 = \left(1 - \frac{1}{2}\left\{\frac{1-2\nu}{1-\nu}\right\}\left\{1 - \frac{E_c}{E_f}\right\}\right) \quad \text{(Eq 10)}$$

Here, E_c is the longitudinal modulus of the composite and can be computed using the ROM (Eq 1). Note that when ΔT is negative, such as when cooling from the processing temperature, and $\alpha_m > \alpha_f$, as is often the case, the interface stress is negative; that is, there is a compressive pressure or a clamping stress at the interface. The corresponding axial stresses in the matrix and fiber are:

$$\sigma_z^{\text{matrix}} = (\alpha_f - \alpha_m)\Delta T E_m \left[\frac{\lambda_2}{\lambda_1}\right]\left[\frac{E_f}{E_c}\right]\left[\frac{V_f}{1-\nu_m}\right]$$

$$\sigma_z^{\text{fiber}} = -\frac{V_m}{V_f}\sigma_z^{\text{matrix}}$$

$$\text{where } \lambda_2 = \frac{1}{2}\left[1 + \frac{E_c}{E_f}\right] \quad \text{(Eq 11)}$$

Note that the axial stresses remain independent of r in each of the constituents under elastic conditions. Also, the ratio of the radial stress at the interface to the axial stress in the fiber (both negative quantities) is simply $E_c/(E_f + E_c)$. This ratio is useful for experimentally estimating the radial residual compressive stress at the interface. Thus, the axial residual stress in fibers can be determined relatively easily by chemically dissolving a length of the matrix (Ref 5) and comparing the fiber length before and after removal of the matrix. The radial residual stress at the interface is then the axial residual stress multiplied by a factor derived from the CCM analysis. That factor is simply $E_c/(E_f + E_c)$, when the Poisson's ratios of the constituents are identical. Note that the radial residual stress at the interface is important for the transverse strength of unidirectional composite, as is discussed later. Because of complex viscoplastic deformation, it is often difficult to estimate residual stresses based on thermal processing history of the composite, and so direct measurements using etching, x-ray, or neutron diffraction procedures are necessary. If the bond strength is assumed to be zero, then the radial residual stress can also be estimated from the transverse tension test, from the knee in the stress-strain curve (Ref 6, 7).

Transverse Loading. The deformation is no longer axisymmetric under transverse loading. The finite-element method (FEM) is often employed on a unit cell representation of the structure, as illustrated in Fig. 2. Generalized plane strain is often used in the FEM calculations, and either a constant stress or a constant displacement boundary condition is specified on plane *BC*. The boundary condition on face *AB* is not well resolved. If the composite is thin, such that plane-stress conditions may be valid, then boundary *AB* is considered to be stress-free. Such analyses show that *AB* is curved and no longer parallel to *DC*. On the other hand, if the cell is embedded well inside a large composite, then face *AB* is considered to move parallel to *CD*, and this usually results in greater tensile stress being generated at the fiber-matrix interface. The type of boundary condition on *AB* has influence on the final local stress-strain fields and needs to be evaluated carefully.

The FEM procedure is particularly useful for any arbitrary direction of loading and is not restricted to a concentric cylinder geometry. Also, any elastic, plastic, or viscoplastic constitutive response can be built into the calculations. However, the procedure is computer time-sensitive compared with simpler calculations that can be done using calculators or simple computer programs. In particular, the FEM procedure can become fairly time-consuming and expensive if the longitudinal elastic-viscoplastic response has to be analyzed over tens or hundreds of thermomechanical cycles. Under those circumstances, models such as the CCM analysis or Eshelby's method of analysis for particulate composites remain particularly attractive. (The Eshelby method models metal inclusions or reinforcing particles with an ellipsoidal shape.)

A number of analytical techniques have also been developed to determine the stress-strain response and the local stresses under transverse loading. One such formulation is the NDSANDS program (Ref 2, 3). In Ref 8, a three-phase model was formulated for considering both thermal and transverse loading of the composite (Fig. 3). The

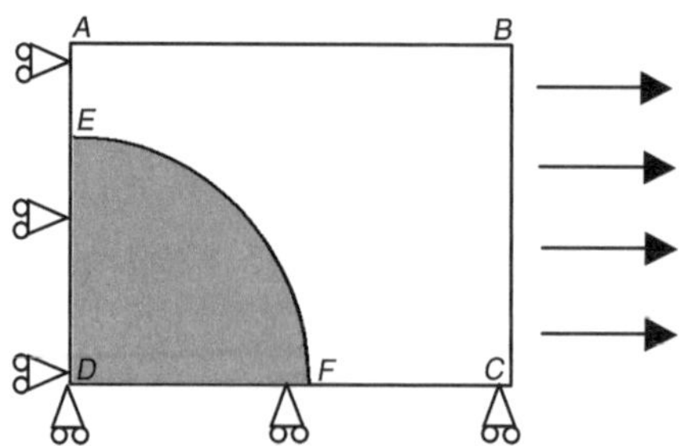

Fig. 2 Unit cell representation of the composite in finite-element calculations. The quarter-fiber is represented by the shaded area.

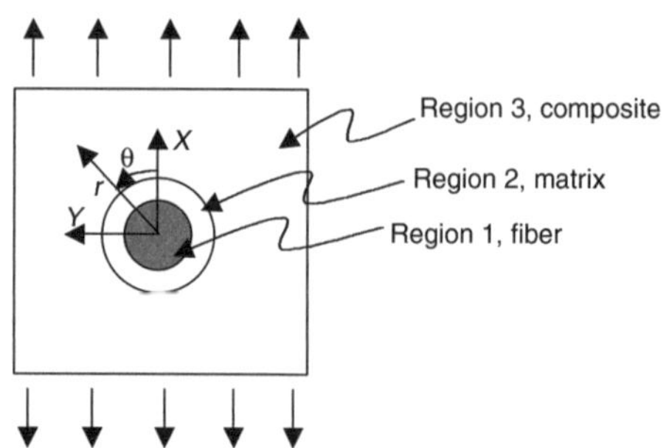

Fig. 3 Three-phase model for analyzing MMCs. Source: Ref 8

stress components in cylindrical coordinates are based on the plane-strain formulation in Ref 8 and 9, and are expressed as:

$$\sigma_{rr} = \left[\frac{A}{r^2} + 2B\right] + \left[-2D - 6\frac{F}{r^4} - 4\frac{G}{r^2}\right]\cos 2\theta$$

$$\sigma_{\theta\theta} = \left[-\frac{A}{r^2} + 2B\right] + \left[2D + 12Er^2 + 6\frac{F}{r^4}\right]\cos 2\theta$$

$$\tau_{r\theta} = \left[2D + 6Er^2 - 6\frac{F}{r^4} - 2\frac{G}{r^2}\right]\sin 2\theta \qquad \text{(Eq 12)}$$

Stress boundary conditions are used at each interface, and an initial guess is made for the region 3 composite properties. An iterative scheme is used to determine the constants in Eq 12, and reasonably good correlations were obtained with FEM solution for a MMC under thermal and transverse load.

When the fiber volume fraction is low or when a single-fiber composite is considered, one may consider a single fiber embedded in an infinite matrix. In this case, Eq 13 (Ref 9) may be used to determine the stresses in either the fiber or the matrix:

$$\frac{\sigma_{rr}^{\text{m}}}{\sigma_{a\theta}} = \frac{1}{2}\left[1 - \frac{\gamma R^2}{r^2} + \left(1 - \frac{2\beta R^2}{r^2} - \frac{3\delta R^4}{r^4}\right)\cos 2\theta\right]$$

$$\frac{\sigma_{\theta}^{\text{m}}}{\sigma_a} = \frac{1}{2}\left[1 + \frac{\gamma R^2}{r^2} - \left(1 - \frac{3\delta R^4}{r^4}\right)\cos 2\theta\right]$$

$$\frac{\tau_{r\theta}^{\text{m}}}{\sigma_a} = -\frac{1}{2}\left[1 + \frac{\beta R^2}{r^2} + \frac{3\delta R^4}{r^4}\right]\sin 2\theta$$

$$\frac{\sigma_{rr}^{\text{f}}}{\sigma_a} = \frac{1}{2}[\beta_o + \delta_o \cos 2\theta]$$

$$\frac{\sigma_{\theta\theta}^{\text{f}}}{\sigma_a} = \frac{1}{2}\left[\beta_o + \left(\frac{6\gamma_o r^2}{R^2} - \delta_o\right)\cos 2\theta\right]$$

$$\frac{\tau_{r\theta}^{\text{f}}}{\sigma_a} = \frac{1}{2}\left[\frac{3\gamma_o r^2}{R^2} - \delta_o\right]\sin 2\theta$$

where

$$\beta = -\frac{2(G_f - G_m)}{G_m + G_f\kappa_m}, \quad \gamma = \frac{G_m(\kappa_f - 1) - G_f(\kappa_m - 1)}{2G_f + G_m(\kappa_f - 1)},$$

$$\delta = \frac{G_f - G_m}{G_m + G_f\kappa_m}$$

$$\beta_o = \frac{G_f(\kappa_m + 1)}{2G_f + G_m(\kappa_f - 1)}, \quad \gamma_o = 0, \quad \delta_o = \frac{G_f(\kappa_m + 1)}{G_m + G_f\kappa_m}$$

$$\text{and } \kappa_m = 3 - 4\nu_m, \quad \kappa_f = 3 - 4\nu_f \qquad \text{(Eq 13)}$$

Here, σ_a is the far-field tensile stress perpendicular to the fiber, θ is zero along the direction of loading (Fig. 3), r is the radial distance from the center of the fiber, R is the radius of the fiber, the superscripts "f" and "m" refer to the fiber and matrix, respectively, G_f and G_m are their shear modulus, and ν_f and ν_m are the corresponding Poisson's ratios. The interface corresponds to the location $r = R$.

In MMCs, the fiber-matrix bond strength is generally kept *low,* because experiments show that the strength and toughness in the longitudinal direction is reduced substantially if the bond is strong. There are essentially two reasons for this behavior. First, a higher interface strength is usually accompanied with some chemical reaction at the interface, which in turn creates minute flaws in the strong fibers (typically > 2 GPa, or 290 ksi). This lowers the fiber strength, thus degrading the fiber-dominated longitudinal strength of the composite. Second, ceramic fibers have a statistical distribution of strengths. When the bond strength is low, premature failure of a weak fiber causes debonding along its sides, and the load in the broken fiber is efficiently distributed among many of its neighbors (global load sharing). In other words, stress concentration on the nearest neighbor is low, and thereby it is protected from immediate failure. On the other hand, when the bond strength is *high,* the load from the broken fiber is transferred mainly to the nearest fiber, causing it to break (local load sharing). This type of localized fracture sequence leads to premature failure of the composite, even though most of the fibers may be of significantly higher strength. There is, however, a penalty for this weak bond. Under transverse stress, a weak bond results in early fiber-matrix debonding. A typical stress-strain curve for a transversely loaded titanium-matrix composite is sketched in Fig. 4, where the knee in the stress-strain curve at B is associated with fiber-matrix debonding. Such a mechanism is confirmed by compliance measurements as well as by interpretation of changes in the Poisson's ratio (Ref 6, 7). The strain at B is usually low, about 0.3%, and the associated low strength poses a major limitation to the application of fiber-reinforced MMCs. Attempts are underway to improve this strength with minimal loss of longitudinal properties.

The residual radial stress at the interface has a strong influence on the stress corresponding to point B, because the local radial stress is simply the sum of the residual clamping stress and the local stress due to far-field transverse loading. Equations have been provided previously for calculating the residual stress as well as the stress due to a transverse applied load. There is also a need to model the postdebonded region, BC, when the material is primarily elastic. Reference 9 does provide equations for calculating displacements for a slipping fiber (similar to Eq 13 shown previously), and they may be used to calculate the postdebonded stress-strain behavior in region BC.

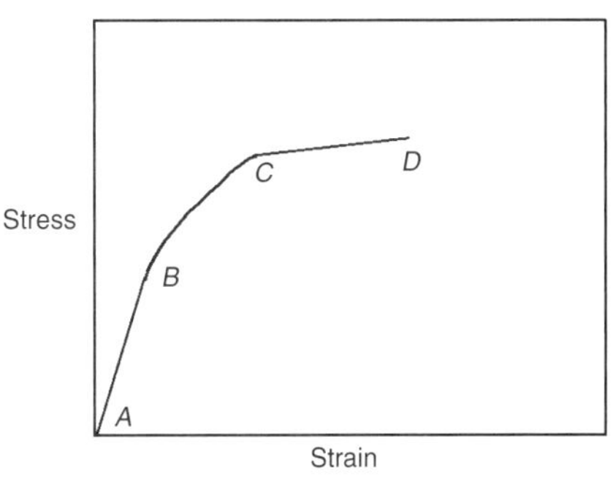

Fig. 4 A typical stress-strain curve under transverse loading when the interface bond strength is weak. Debonding initiates at a fairly low stress at *B*, and is accompanied with small-scale plasticity around the debonded fibers. Large-scale plasticity ensues at *C*, and failure occurs at *D*. Source: Ref 6, 7

Stress-Strain Response and Stress Distribution Under Elastic-Plastic and Elastic-Viscoplastic Conditions

Longitudinal and Thermal Loading. Axisymmetric conditions are maintained under longitudinal loading, and the CCM model is particularly advantageous. However, plasticity rules must be invoked. A method for incorporating plasticity and viscoplasticity into the CCM analysis is indicated in Ref 10 and 11. The calculations are based on the successive approximation approach of plasticity (Ref 12), as well as the elastic-plastic calculations performed earlier using a CCM model (Ref 13, 14). The matrix cylinder of Fig. 1 is divided into a series of thin concentric cylinders, and a finite-difference scheme is used to integrate Eq 2 and 4. Any arbitrary strain-hardening behavior can be modeled using the CCM formalism.

A simpler, but less accurate, method is to simply use a one-dimensional isostrain model. Essentially, the composite stress is expressed as:

$$\sigma_c = V_f\sigma_f + V_m\sigma_m \qquad \text{(Eq 14)}$$

where σ_f and σ_m are the stresses in the fiber and matrix, respectively. At any given strain, the stresses in the fiber and the matrix can be obtained from the respective stress-strain data, and the results summed according to Eq 14. This approach cannot account for the triaxial stress state around the fiber, but does provide a reasonably good estimate of the stress-strain plot.

A typical stress-strain plot for a longitudinally loaded composite is illustrated in Fig. 5. The onset of nonlinearity of the stress-strain curve is associated with yielding of the matrix, as confirmed by observation of slip bands and using transmission electron microscopy (Ref 6, 15). The yielding of the matrix is influenced by the residual axial stress in the matrix, which is usually tensile, and the yield strength of the matrix.

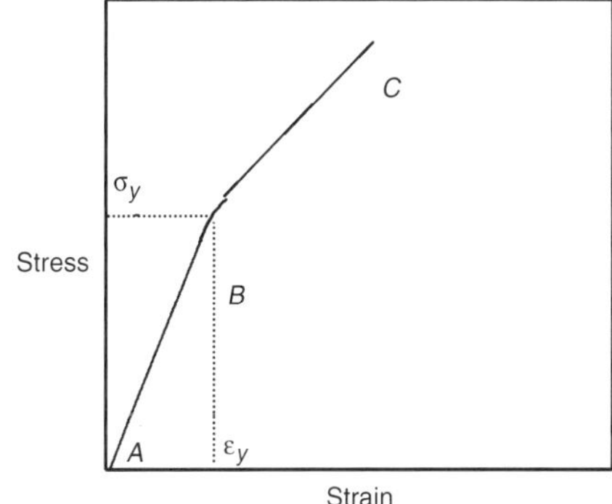

Fig. 5 Typical stress-strain curve for a longitudinally loaded MMC

If the stress-strain behavior of the fiber-free "neat" material is known, then the residual axial stress in the matrix can be estimated from the knee, as shown in Ref 6.

The postyield domain of the stress-strain plot is matrix-plasticity-dominated. However, toward the end of region *BC* in Fig. 5, fiber cracks start occurring, so that there is combination of plasticity and damage. Here, the statistical fiber-fracture model in Ref 16 and 17 can be used to incorporate the effects of fiber failure. Essentially, the fiber fracture model is used to determine an effective nonlinear stress response of the fiber (see subsequent equations), as indicated in Fig. 6. The effective stress-strain behavior of the damaged fibers can then be used either in the elastic-viscoplastic CCM model, as was done in Ref 18, or in a simple one-dimensional representation of the composite longitudinal response.

For time-dependent loading, viscoplastic or creep models have to be used. Among them, Bodner-Partom's viscoplastic model with directional hardening (Ref 19, 20) has been used extensively in the finite difference code for elastic-plastic analysis (FIDEP) computer code (Ref 10, 11) that is based on the CCM model. The model contains 12 unknown constants that are estimated from tension, fatigue, stress relaxation, and creep tests on the matrix-only "neat" material. Values for a number of titanium alloys are provided in Ref 11 and 21.

A number of other models have also been developed to determine the stress-strain response under viscoplastic deformation. These include the vanishing fiber diameter (VFD) model, (Ref 22–24), the method of cells (Ref 25), and the generalized method of cells (Ref 26). The computer code VISCOPLY has been developed based on the VFD model and using the viscoplastic model of Ref 27. Results from that code have been compared with experimental data on titanium matrix composites (Ref 28, 29). Comparisons of the different codes with Bodner-Partom's viscoelastic model were conducted in Ref 21 by considering both in-phase and out-of-phase thermomechanical fatigue loading. The models were compared with results from the FEM method.

Transverse Loading. The models referenced in the previous paragraph have been used to determine the stress-strain response under transverse loading. One problem in modeling is that at elevated temperatures, the residual clamping stress at the interface is reduced significantly. Combined with the fact that the transverse strength of the interface is maintained quite low to obtain damage tolerance in the fiber direction, interface debonding occurs quite early at elevated temperatures. However, because of the ductility of the matrix, debonding does not lead to failure. Consequently, plasticity and viscoplasticity with debonded fibers must be considered during transverse loading of a unidirectional composite.

As indicated earlier, the FEM method may be relied upon, provided the micromechanisms of deformation and damage (such as debonding) are adequately taken into account, and provided the inelastic deformation of the matrix is modeled accurately. However, FEM is not efficient for thermomechanical loading. In recent years, the method of cells has been extended to account for fiber-matrix debonding. Also, the VFD model has been modified to account for a debonded fiber. Details on these issues may be obtained from the references in the previous section.

Simplified equations of the stress-strain behavior under elastic-plastic conditions, based on FEM calculations, have been provided in Ref 30. A Ramberg-Osgood power law model is used to represent the matrix plastic behavior, and it is shown that the effective yield strength of a fully bonded composite is increased over that of the matrix material. Further details are presented in the section on discontinuous composites.

Multiaxial Loading. For loading other than in the 0° or 90° direction, one may refer to the work in Ref 31 and 32, where the plastically deformed composite is treated as an orthotropic elastic-plastic material. The flow rule here allows for volume change under plastic deformation, unlike the case of monolithic alloys. The approach has the advantage of collapsing data from different lamina on a single curve. However, the method is semiempirical and is not based on the constituent elastic-plastic deformation behavior of the matrix.

A more rigorous formulation based on a FEM technique was adopted in Ref 33 and 34. Standalone software, called IDAC, is available, such that any multiaxial stress state can be analyzed. Note that off-axis loading is simply a case of multiaxial loading of a unidirectional lamina. The input requirements for the program are the elastic, plastic, and viscoplastic parameters of the matrix and the tensile strength of the fiber-matrix interface. The latter is included because of the propensity for fiber-matrix debonding at low transverse stresses, which strongly influences the post-debond elastic-viscoplastic response of the composite.

Micromechanics of Discontinuously Reinforced MMCs

The stress-strain response of discontinuously reinforced composites (DRCs) is influenced by the morphology of particles, both in the elastic and elastic-plastic domain. Most of the applications of DRCs have been with discontinuously reinforced aluminum alloys (DRAs). The particle shapes of alumina or SiC reinforcements, employed most often in DRAs, are generally blocky and angular, rather than spherical or cylindrical. Whiskers are generally modeled as cylinders with a high aspect ratio, the ratio of height to diameter.

Elastic Deformation. Although the primary effects of particles are their modulus and volume fraction, their shape has influence on the modulus of the composite. The effects of particle shapes are discussed in Ref 35 and 36. Experimental data in Ref 36 to 39 show that the finite-element results of Ref 36 for a unit cylinder with an aspect ratio of unity provide best agreement with experimental data. The Hashin Shtrikman bounds for the elastic moduli (Ref 40) are too wide apart for making an adequate estimate. Rather, Mura's formulation (Ref 41), although developed for spherical particles, appears to match the unit cylinder FEM solution reasonably well up to a fiber volume fraction of 0.25. Beyond that volume fraction the deviation from the FEM result is large, and actual FEM results, such as those in Ref 36 should be used. Note also that the ROM (Eq 1) overestimates the modulus of DRCs and should not be used. The elastic moduli from Mura's analytical solution (Ref 41) are as follows:

$$G = G_m \left[1 + \frac{V_p(G_m - G_r)}{\left(G_m + 2(G_r - G_m)\dfrac{4-5\nu_m}{15(1-\nu_m)} \right)} \right]^{-1}$$

$$K = K_m \left[1 + \frac{V_p(K_m - K_r)}{\left(K_m + \dfrac{1}{3}(K_r - K_m)\dfrac{1+\nu_m}{1-\nu_m} \right)} \right]^{-1} \qquad \text{(Eq 15)}$$

and E and ν for the composite are obtained from:

$$E = \frac{9KG}{3K+G} \qquad \nu = \frac{3K-2G}{2(G+3K)}$$

Here, the subscripts "m" and "r" refer to the matrix and reinforcement, respectively, and G and K are the shear modulus and bulk modulus of the composite, respectively. V_p is the volume fraction of reinforcement.

In addition to the FEM approach, one may use Eshelby's technique to determine elastic modulus for various shapes and volume fractions of reinforcements. Such calculations are nicely illustrated in Ref 35, which provides a computer program at the end of the book. It is also relevant to mention that although particle distribution has negligible effect on elastic modulus at low volume fractions, the effect becomes larger at high volume fractions. The distribution effect is largely experienced through a change in the hydrostatic stress distribution in the matrix, and such a change is anticipated to be larger when

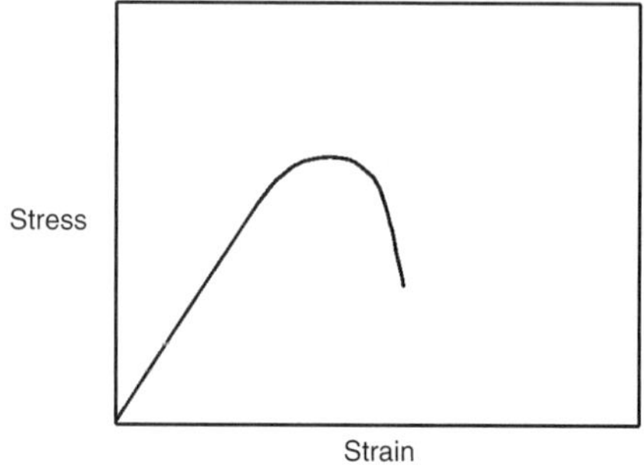

Fig. 6 Schematic of the effective stress-strain response for damaging brittle fibers, based on the statistical model of Ref 16, 17

the volume fraction of the matrix phase is smaller. However, experimental results are not available that can validate this distribution effect.

Elastic-Plastic Deformation. Analysis of elastic-plastic deformation with rigid, spherical particles has been considered in Ref 42 for an elastic-perfectly plastic (no strain hardening) matrix. The flow stress, σ_c, under dilute conditions ($V_p < 0.25$) may be expressed as:

$$\sigma_c = 1 + \beta V_p \quad \text{(Eq 16)}$$

where β was estimated to be approximately 0.375 for spherical particles.

In Ref 30, FEM analysis was conducted for different-shaped rigid particles. The σ_c for a perfectly plastic matrix reinforced with unit cylinders (loaded perpendicular to the axis of the cylinder) show β to be a function of V_p:

$$\beta = 9V_p - 0.16 \quad \text{(Eq 17)}$$

When matrix strain hardening is considered, the results in Ref 30 can be used. Essentially, the matrix is represented by the Ramberg-Osgood formulation:

$$\varepsilon = \frac{\sigma}{E_m} + \alpha\left(\frac{\sigma}{\sigma_o}\right)^n \quad \text{(Eq 18)}$$

where $\alpha = 3/7$, n is the inverse of the work-hardening exponent, N, of the matrix, E_m is the elastic modulus of the matrix, and σ_o is a normalizing parameter approximately equal to the yield strength of the matrix. The corresponding stress-strain response of the particulate-reinforced composite, based on FEM calculations (Ref 30), is estimated to be:

$$\varepsilon_c = \frac{\sigma_c}{E_c} + \alpha\left(\frac{\sigma_o^m}{E_m}\right)\left(\frac{\sigma_c}{\sigma_N}\right)^n \quad \text{(Eq 19)}$$

where the subscript "c" refers to the composite, "m" is the matrix, and σ_N is a reference stress, almost equal to the 0.2% yield stress of the composite. σ_N is a function of the volume fraction, work-hardening rate of the matrix, and the particle shape. It is expressed in Ref 37 as:

$$\frac{\sigma_N}{\sigma_o^m} = \xi\left[(1+\kappa N)(1+\beta V_p) - \kappa N\right] \quad \text{(Eq 20)}$$

where V_p is the volume fraction of particles, β can be obtained from Eq 17, and κ is a function of the shape and volume fraction of particles and is plotted in Ref 30. ξ is approximately 0.94 at small plastic strains (less than $3\varepsilon_o$, where ε_o is the yield strain of the matrix), but ξ becomes unity at large strains. Approximate values of κ are 3.1, 3.5, and 4.25 at V_p of 0.1, 0.15, and 0.2, respectively. All these quantities are valid only for unit cylinder particles, and they are considered here because this shape provides best correlation with the experimentally determined elastic modulus of DRAs. For particles of other shapes, one may refer to Ref 30. In summary, Eq 19 provides the entire stress-strain curve for the composite when the parameters E_m and n ($= 1/N$) in Eq 18 are known for the matrix. Results in Ref 37 and 38 for a silicon carbide particle, SiCp, reinforced 7093 aluminum alloy show that the previous estimation formulas provide reasonable correlation with the experimentally determined stress-strain response of the composite.

A few remarks are in order here. The formulas can only provide approximate values, and they were based on rigid particles with infinite elastic modulus. Experiments on composites with the same volume fraction of particles in the same matrix, but with different sizes of particles, show that the strength tends to increase with smaller particle size. This effect is not captured by FEM calculations, where the absolute size of particles do not influence the results. Possible effects of particle size include:

- The reduction of grain size of the matrix and, hence, an increased strength of the matrix
- The punching of dislocations from the particles and the associated strengthening, which would be more effective at small particle sizes
- The limitation of standard FEM solution when the size scales become small
- The matrix alloy may be affected by reaction with the particle.

These issues are not captured by current modeling practice, and hence the predictive equations provided previously should only be used for initial estimation.

The ductility of the composite is an important issue in DRCs, unlike fiber-reinforced systems, where debonding fibers can provide damage tolerance when loaded in the fiber direction. Ductility of DRCs can vary anywhere from 10 to 70% of the matrix, with ductility being affected significantly at volume fractions of 0.25 and higher. Recent discussions on these issues are available in Ref 35 and Ref 37 to 39. Important damage mechanisms include particle fracture and particle-matrix debonding (see the article "Fracture and Fatigue of DRA Composites" in *Fatigue and Fracture*, Volume 19 of *ASM Handbook*). Particle fracture is particularly dominant for high-strength matrices, such as peak or underaged 2*xxx* and 7*xxx* aluminum alloys, and is established by observing mirror halves of the fracture surface. Debonding is observed in lower-strength matrices, such as 6*xxx* aluminum alloys, although it is often difficult to establish whether failure occurred at the interface or whether it initiated in the matrix immediately adjacent to the interface. The latter mode mostly occurs when the bond is strong and the matrix is quite weak, such as aluminum alloys in the overaged condition.

Models of ductility have been proposed in Ref 37 and 39 to obtain initial estimates of ductility. The model in Ref 39 is based primarily on statistical particle fracture according to Weibull statistics and subsequent specimen instability according to the Considere criterion. (See the article "Uniaxial Compression Testing" in *Mechanical Testing and Evaluation*, Volume 8 of *ASM Handbook*, for an introduction to the Considere criterion.) The problem with this approach is that necking is essentially nonexistent in DRCs possessing any appreciable volume fraction of particles. Nevertheless, reasonable agreement was obtained with experiments conducted by the authors. The model in Ref 37 presupposes the existence of particle cracks, and failure is postulated based on rupture of the matrix between cracked particles. Once again, reasonably good agreement is obtained between the predictions of the model and experimental data on DRAs from a wide number of sources. However, the strain prior to particle fracture is neglected. Reference 39 also provides empirical equations for calculating the particle stress in a power-law hardening matrix at different values of imposed plastic strains. These formulas may be used to estimate the extent of damage as a function of applied strain. An alternate simplified methodology is suggested in Ref 37 for calculating particle stress and then determining particle strength based on the fraction of cracked particles. Such analyses suggest a Weibull modulus of approximately 5 and a Weibull strength of 2400 MPa (350 ksi) for 10 μm size SiC particles.

The previously mentioned elastic-plastic models assume a uniform distribution of particles. Although clustering may be considered small in well-processed powder-metallurgy-derived composites of volume fractions less than 0.2, nonuniformity and clustering is the rule rather than the exception. A Voronoi cell FEM approach has been developed in Ref 43 to assess elastic-plastic deformation of a multitude of unevenly distributed particles, rather than the uniform distribution assumed in unit cell FEM calculations. The analyses show that particle fractures occur early in regions of clusters, and this is accompanied with large plastic strains and hydrostatic stresses in damaged regions. These regions then become the locations for microvoid initiation, and because void growth is linearly proportional to the plastic strain and exponentially dependent on the level of hydrostatic tensile stress (Ref 44), the voids can rapidly grow to coalescence. A ductility model based on Voronoi cell computations remains to be established, but should provide a more accurate estimate of damage and failure for a nonuniform microstructure.

Local Failures of Fiber-Reinforced MMCs

Longitudinal Loading. Under monotonic tension loading, failure of the composite is determined by fiber fracture. Generally, fiber strengths follow weak-link Weibull statistics, where the probability of failure (P_f) of a fiber of length L is expressed as:

$$P_f = 1 - \exp\left[-\frac{L}{L_o}\left(\frac{\sigma}{\sigma_o}\right)^m\right] \quad \text{(Eq 21)}$$

where "m" is the Weibull modulus and σ_o is the Weibull (approximately average) strength for a fiber of length L_o.

For a ductile matrix, the matrix is always yielded, so that in a one-dimensional model, the composite ultimate strength, σ_c^U, is simply:

$$\sigma_c^{\,U} = V_f\sigma_f^{\,U} + (1 - V_f)\sigma_m^{\,flow} \qquad \text{(Eq 22)}$$

where σ_f^U is the effective strength of the fiber at instability of the composite, and σ_m^{flow} is the flow stress in the matrix at that value of composite strain, typically 0.8 to 1%. The value of σ_f^U depends on the mode of failure. If the interface is so weak that failure of a fiber at any location is equivalent to loss of load-carrying capability of the entire fiber, then σ_f^U may be equated to the dry bundle strength (σ_{dbf}) (Ref 45):

$$\sigma_{dbf} = \frac{\sigma_o}{\left(me\dfrac{L}{L_o}\right)^{1/m}} \qquad \text{(Eq 23)}$$

where e is the exponential term approximately equal to 2.718.

A more-realistic situation is the ability of the broken fiber to recarry the load after a sliding distance, δ, from the fiber break. In this case, one must consider the frictional sliding stress, τ, which can be independently determined from pushout or fragmentation tests. The associated effective fiber strength, according to Curtin's global load-sharing model (Ref 16, 17), is:

$$\sigma_{glf} = \sigma_{ch}\left[\frac{2}{m+2}\right]^{\frac{1}{m+1}}\left[\frac{m+1}{m+2}\right] \qquad \text{(Eq 24)}$$

where the characteristic fiber strength σ_{ch} is:

$$\sigma_{ch} = \left(\sigma_o^m \tau \frac{L_o}{r}\right)^{\frac{1}{m+1}} \qquad \text{(Eq 25)}$$

In Curtin's model (Ref 16, 17), the fragmenting fibers essentially follow the constitutive law:

$$\sigma_f = \varepsilon_f E_f\left[1 - \frac{1}{2}\left\{\frac{\varepsilon_f E_f}{\sigma_{ch}}\right\}^{m+1}\right] \qquad \text{(Eq 26)}$$

where the subscript "f" refers to the fragmenting fibers. At instability, this leads to an effective fiber strain (ε_f^U):

$$\varepsilon_f^{\,U} = \frac{\sigma_{ch}}{E_f}\left(\frac{2}{m+2}\right)^{\frac{1}{m+1}} \qquad \text{(Eq 27)}$$

The total strain in the composite at failure (ε_c^U) is then simply:

$$\varepsilon_c^{\,U} = \varepsilon_f^{\,U} - \varepsilon_f^{\,Res} \qquad \text{(Eq 28)}$$

where ε_f^{Res} is the residual strain in the fiber, being predominantly compressive and negative.

This model has been found to correlate quite well with the strength of a number of fiber-reinforced titanium alloys (Ref 17, 46, 47). However, local load-sharing has also been observed (Ref 48–50), where the density of fiber cracks was found to be far below those predicted by the global load-sharing model. Reference 50 provides a comparison of different models in the context of failure of an orthorhombic titanium alloy reinforced with SiC fibers. The local load-sharing situation is well captured by the second fiber fracture model of Zweben and Rosen (Ref 51), and the pertinent equations are also provided in Ref 50. The local load-sharing model gives effective fiber strengths that are slightly lower than the global load-sharing model. The lowest bound on the effective fiber strength is obtained from the dry bundle model. Although this may be overly conservative during room-temperature deformation, when there is significant clamping stress between the fibers and the matrix, the dry bundle model may provide a reasonable lower bound at high temperatures.

Transverse Loading. Under transverse loading, the onset of nonlinearity is determined by fiber-matrix separation, as discussed earlier. Debonding occurs when the local radial stress is greater than the bond strength of the interface. The local radial stress is simply the far-field stress ($\sigma^{far\text{-}field}$) multiplied by a stress-concentration factor (k) less the residual radial stress ($\sigma_r^{residual}$) at the interface. Stated mathematically:

$$\sigma_r^{\,local} = k\sigma^{far\text{-}field} - \sigma_r^{\,residual} \qquad \text{(Eq 29)}$$

Models for determining k and the thermal residual stress have been described earlier, with the single-fiber case being given by the analytical equations (Eq 22). Typical values of k are in the range 1.2 to 1.5.

The ultimate strength is governed by matrix rupture. If the fibers are not debonded, then the models described for discontinuous reinforced particles may be used without much loss of accuracy. Thus, Eq 16 with $\beta = 0.375$ may be used. When the fibers are debonded, then the strength of the composite is less than that of the matrix. In this case, one usually resorts to FEM analysis.

Macromechanics

Strength of Fiber-Reinforced Composites. The cases of tensile loading in the longitudinal and transverse directions have been described earlier. Figure 7 shows measured and predicted stress-strain plots for 0° SCS6/Ti-15-3 composites, where the sudden increase in the predicted strain response is interpreted as failure of the specimen (Ref 18). Modeling was conducted using the FIDEP code with both elastic-plastic and elastic-viscoplastic matrix using the Bodner-Partom model, which was modified to incorporate fiber fracture according to Eq 26. Figure 7 shows good agreement between the predicted stress-strain curves and strengths with experimental data. This type of correlation also was observed at elevated temperatures, when viscoplastic effects became important.

For off-axis or multiaxial loading, the IDAC (Ref 33) program may be used to compute the stress-strain response of the composite and the local stresses/strains in the constituents. The onset of failure can then be predicted based on the mechanisms, that is, fiber fracture, transverse failure, or shear failure, depending upon which mechanism can operate at the least value of the far-field load.

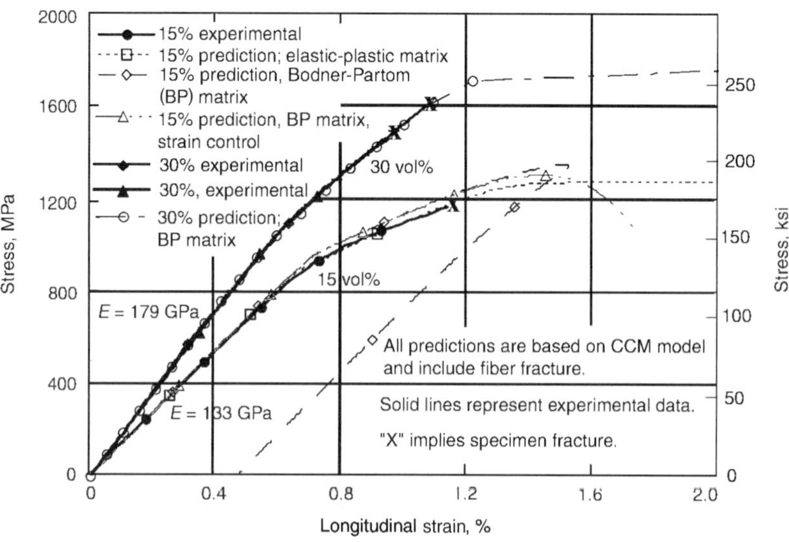

Fig. 7 Comparison of predicted and experimental stress-strain behavior of SCS6/Ti-15-3 composites at room temperature for 15% and 30% fiber volume fractions. Both elastic-plastic and elastic-viscoplastic analysis was conducted, and fiber fractures were incorporated into the model. The sudden increase in strain in the predicted curves signifies specimen failure. Source: Ref 18

Strength of Discontinuous Reinforced Composites. The stress-strain curve has been covered in an earlier section. The ultimate strength is dependent on the elongation to failure, which is generally much less than the matrix. Models of ductility have been presented earlier.

Fatigue of Fiber-Reinforced MMCs. The longitudinal fatigue life of fiber-reinforced MMCs can generally be grouped under three regimes, in a plot of stress or strain range versus the cycles to failure (N_f). They are illustrated in Fig. 8, which was first postulated for polymer-matrix composites (Ref 52). The regimes have also been confirmed in MMCs and exhibit distinct differences in failure mechanisms (Ref 53, 54).

Regime 1, with N_f typically between 1 and 1000 cycles, is dominated by fiber fractures without any matrix cracks. At elevated temperatures under isothermal fatigue conditions, fiber fractures appear to be precipitated by *progressive ratcheting* of the matrix under viscoplastic conditions. Essentially, matrix viscoplasticity results in the gradual transformation of the matrix strain range from tension-tension to fully reversed-loading tension-compression, where $R = -1$, although the composite may be subjected to only tension-tension loading at an R-ratio (minimum to maximum stress ratio on the composite) of 0.1, for example. The offloading of the matrix results in progressively increased loading being experienced by the fibers, as required by Eq 14, causing them to fail with an increased number of cycles. In this scenario, if the final fiber stress is insufficient to cause any significant breakage of fibers (well below the rounded region of Fig. 6), progressive fiber failure should be avoidable. Indeed, this maximum stress approximately delineates the boundary between regimes 1 and 2 under isothermal conditions.

The frequency of loading becomes an important factor in regime 1, because matrix creep can lower the maximum matrix stress attainable in both the tension and compression part of the cycle at low frequencies (<0.01 Hz). The result is an even greater load being carried by the fibers and a consequent poorer fatigue performance with lower frequency. The increased matrix creep and associated transfer of load to the fiber is manifested in the strain-ratcheting behavior of the composite, which shows increased ratcheting with reduced frequency at elevated temperatures. Thus, life prediction in regime 1 requires both a modeling of the composite response based on a good viscoplastic characterization of the matrix and adequate incorporation of fiber fracture using Weibull statistics. The CCM model for analysis has already been discussed, and reference has been made to the Bodner-Partom model for viscoplastic characterization of the matrix (Ref 10, 11, 21). The matrix responses have been integrated into the available FIDEP and IDAC codes.

Under in-phase thermomechanical fatigue (IP-TMF), the extent of matrix ratcheting and fiber damage is observed to be larger (Ref 18, 55, 56), and simultaneously the IP-TMF life is observed to be shorter than under isothermal conditions. One problem found with various investigations was that often the frequency of loading was smaller under IP-TMF than under isothermal conditions. In the extreme case, creep of the matrix may relax its value to zero at the end of the tension cycle. The result is that the entire applied load would then be carried only by the fibers, causing their stress to be significantly higher than under faster isothermal conditions. If all these factors are appropriately taken into account, then results under different test conditions (isothermal and IP-TMF) in regime 1 can be rationalized in terms of the maximum fiber stress (Ref 57). However, this does not clarify the entire picture, because the CCM model with Bodner-Partom constants accurately predicts the isothermal ratcheting response at the highest temperature, but significantly underpredicts the ratcheting response for IP-TMF at the same frequency (Ref 18). Thus, other factors may be present as well, and fiber damage due to molybdenum weaves was suggested for a SCS6/Ti-15-3 system (Ref 18, 55). However, this explanation may only be valid for panels with molybdenum weaves. Overall, a complete understanding of IP-TMF has yet to emerge, although current predictions are much closer to experiments.

At room temperature, when viscoplastic conditions are negligible, the previous explanation is inadequate to explain why fibers should fail after the first cycle. In Ref 53, an alternate mechanism was proposed for the initiation of fiber cracks. Microstructural observations suggested damage in the coating and in the reaction zone, leading to cracking of fibers.

Regime 2 is matrix-crack dominated, similar to monolithic alloys, but fiber stress also plays an important role. In this regime, the fatigue life can either be plotted as the stress range ($\Delta\sigma$) versus N_f, or as the strain range ($\Delta\varepsilon$) versus N_f. A plot of $\Delta\sigma$ versus N_f shows that fatigue life increases with fiber volume fraction and is mainly an effect associated with load transfer from the matrix to the higher-strength elastic fibers. Such a plot also shows that composites have fatigue performance superior to the matrix alloy. This behavior is also observed with discontinuous reinforcements. However, if the fatigue life is plotted as $\Delta\varepsilon$ versus N_f, as is most often done with monolithic alloys, then the MMC is generally found to have slightly poorer performance than the monolithic alloy. Fatigue tests with R-ratio of −1 show better performance than with an R-ratio of 0.1, at the same strain range (Ref 58). Microstructures show a greater density of matrix cracks, but the stress in the fibers are only half of what would occur under tension-tension loading. Because composite failure requires the breakage of fibers, life is improved under negative R-ratio compression conditioning. Models have been proposed to include both the composite strain range and the fiber stress for predicting fatigue life in regime 2 (Ref 53, 57–59).

In regime 2, matrix cracks can initiate anywhere between 10 and 30% of life, depending on the preparation of samples. In other words, the majority of life is spent in the fatigue crack growth (FCG) domain. A number of investigators have addressed FCG (Ref 60–63), and the common feature of their models is the reduction of the stress-intensity factor (shielding) at the matrix crack tip by the bridging fibers:

$$\Delta K_{local} = \Delta K_{applied} - \Delta K_{bridging} \quad \text{(Eq 30)}$$

The primary difference between the models is the way in which the shear lag analysis is conducted. Canonical equations are provided in Ref 64 to simplify calculations of fatigue crack growth. However, a factor that has not been considered in these models is the shielding of the crack due to higher-modulus fibers ahead of the crack tip. The effect of this shielding is analyzed in Ref 65, and it is observed that the interface tensile strength can have a substantial effect on the retardation of matrix crack growth in the low ΔK regime. The interface tensile strength then constitutes a microstructural variable, in addition to the friction shear stress parameter (τ), that could be used to control the crack growth kinetics.

Regime 3 represents the fatigue limit, which is the stress level below which the material can be cycled infinitely without damage. The matrix behavior is elastic in this region.

Fracture Toughness

Fiber-Reinforced Composites. In ductile matrix systems, a number of different behaviors have been observed, depending on the strength of the matrix, the fiber-matrix bond strength, and the volume fraction of fibers.

When the matrix strength is low, matrix-dominated shear deformation occurs prior to any fiber fracture. Indeed, in boron-fiber-reinforced aluminum composites, a shear deformation mode parallel to the fibers is observed (Ref 66–68). Here, an intense slip zone develops over a plastic zone of length L perpendicular to the crack plane. At a critical load, when L is on the order of 3 to 17 times the crack length, the damage zone stops propagating and is replaced by

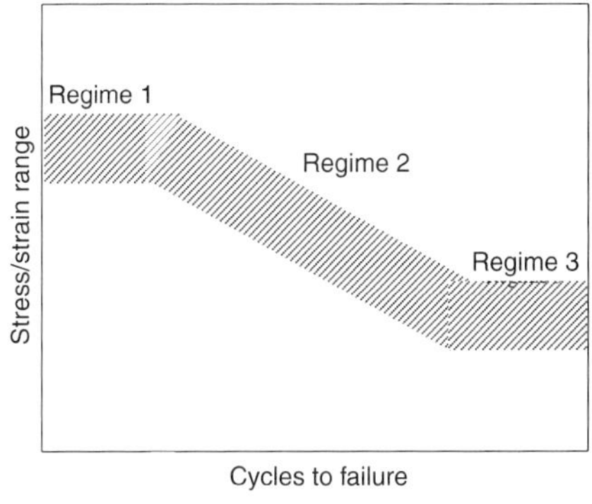

Fig. 8 Schematic showing the three regimes of fatigue of fiber-reinforced MMCs

failure of fibers at the crack tip. This in turn leads to catastrophic fracture of the composite along the original notch plane. Most notable is the fact that an H-shaped shear zone is created prior to crack extension, which is absent during propagation of the crack. The crack extension is not self-similar. A similar type of damage zone and crack extension has also been observed in glass-fiber-reinforced epoxy composites (Ref 69).

In the previous type of deformation mode, the effective toughening is extremely high, because the blunted, deflected crack tip attenuates the stress ahead of the crack tip over a distance of the order of the crack tip opening displacement. For crack lengths of a few millimeters or longer, toughness values of 100 MPa $\sqrt{m}$ (91 ksi $\sqrt{in.}$) have been realized for the boron aluminum system. The effect is reduced for a smaller crack length and approaches approximately 30 MPa $\sqrt{m}$ (27 ksi $\sqrt{in.}$) at a crack length less than 0.5 mm (0.02 in.). Thus, fracture toughness may not be the appropriate parameter for predicting failure in these systems, which do not obey self-similar crack growth. In Ref 66, an attempt was made to estimate the onset of fracture with H-shaped cracks, based on the attainment of a critical strain in the fiber direction a distance of over two fiber diameter ($2a$) ahead of the crack tip. It was found that the local strain in the representative volume element for specimens with different notch lengths all fell in the error band for the failure strain of unnotched composites. The following set of equations may be used to estimate the failure load, P_{ult}, for a center-cracked panel of width W and crack length $2a$ (Ref 70) and possessing an unnotched strength, $\sigma_{unnotched}$:

$$\frac{P_{ult}}{\left(1-\frac{2a}{W}\right)}+2\frac{\tau^*}{\pi(a_2-a_1)}\left[-a_1^2 Ln\left(\frac{1+\sqrt{1+a_2^2\beta^2}}{a_1\beta}\right) + a_2^2 Ln\left(\frac{1+\sqrt{1+a_2^2\beta^2}}{a_2\beta}\right)\right]=\sigma_{unnotched} \quad \text{(Eq 31)}$$

where

$$a_{1,2}^2=\frac{E_1}{2G_{12}}-\nu_{12}\pm\sqrt{\left(\frac{E_1}{2G_{12}}-\nu_{12}\right)^2-\frac{E_1}{E_2}} \quad \text{(Eq 32)}$$

and where + is for a_1^2 and – is for a_2^2, and

$$b\approx d\left(\frac{2\pi}{3\sqrt{3}\,c}\right)^{1/2} \qquad \beta=\frac{aP_{ult}}{b\tau^*}$$

Here, d is the fiber diameter, c is the volume fraction of fibers, τ^* is the in-plane shear strength of the unidirectional composite in the fiber direction, E_1 is the modulus in the fiber direction, E_2 in the transverse direction, G_{12} is the shear modulus, ν_{12} is the Poisson's ratio, and b is of the order of distance between two adjacent fibers.

When the matrix strength or the fiber volume fraction is high, the dominant damage mode is fiber fragmentation in the zone of intense matrix plastic deformation near the crack tip and ultimately, composite fracture. In order to predict the fracture toughness, some estimate of the flow stress and the critical displacement is needed. This was modeled in Ref 71 and 72 by considering that the periphery of fractured fiber tips acts as the nucleation center from which intense matrix plasticity develops. This is a form of macroscopic void growth, at a length scale that is significantly larger than the distance between intermetallic particles, which act as the void nucleation site for fracture of monolithic metallic alloys. The following estimated toughness (J_{Ic} is obtained (Ref 71):

$$J_{Ic}\approx\frac{1}{\sqrt{3}}(1-V_f)\sigma_Y L_D \quad \text{(Eq 33)}$$

where

$$L_D\approx\beta_n d\frac{(1-\sqrt{V_f})}{\sqrt{V_f}} \quad \text{(Eq 34)}$$

and β_n is approximately 2. Here d is the diameter of the fiber, V_f is the volume fraction of fibers, and σ_Y is the yield stress of the matrix.

Very few experiments have been conducted on the fracture toughness of titanium-matrix composites. In Ref 73, a toughness of approximately 71 kJ/m^2 (4900 ft · lbf/ft^2) was reported for a SiC-Ti alloy, which may be compared with a typical toughness of 40 kJ/m^2 (2700 ft · lbf/ft^2), based on K_{Ic} = 70 MPa $\sqrt{m}$ (64 ksi $\sqrt{in.}$) for monolithic Ti-6Al-4V alloy. Using Eq 33 with σ_Y = 1040 MPa (150 ksi), V_f = 0.32, and d = 100 μm, a toughness value of 63 kJ/m^2 (4.3 ft · lbf/ft^2) is estimated, which compares reasonably well with the experimental data.

It is useful to note that J_{Ic} predicted by Eq 33 and 34 is quite strongly dependent on the volume fraction of fibers. Thus, $(1-V_f)\cdot(1-\sqrt{V_f})/\sqrt{V_f}$ decreases from approximately 0.59 to 0.12 on increasing V_f from 0.3 to 0.6. High-volume-fraction alumina/aluminum composites are currently being developed for a variety of applications, such as high-tension electrical cables and piston rods. Because of the lower strength of the alloy and the high volume fraction of alumina fibers, toughness values significantly less than titanium-matrix composites are anticipated.

A final note is in order regarding the role of the fiber-matrix interface. Equation 33 shows that the toughness is an increasing function of L_D. Weak interfaces would permit greater fiber-matrix sliding, thereby increasing the fracture toughness. This effect was elegantly used in Ref 74 to toughen aluminum-based composites while maintaining acceptable transverse strengths. In SiC-reinforced titanium-matrix composites pullout lengths are typically less than one fiber diameter, even for weak carbon-based interfaces. This is largely because of the high radial compressive stress that is generated at the fiber-matrix interface at the tip of a cracked fiber. For strong interfaces, such as those formed without a carbon layer on the SiC monofilaments, the pullout length will be even shorter. However, the effect of a smaller L_D may be balanced by a higher flow stress associated with constrained yielding of the matrix in the fragmentation zone. Tensile tests on unnotched SiC-Ti-matrix composites with different interfaces indicate correlated fiber fractures, independent of the type of interface. Slip band observations and ultrasonic images of fiber breaks confirm that correlated fractures are a result of slip band interactions. A slip band impinging on a fiber localizes sufficient strain to fracture that fiber (Ref 49). Similar experiments have to be conducted with notched composites to provide an assessment of the role of interface strength on the toughness of composites with high matrix strength.

Discontinuously Reinforced Composites. Hahn and Rosenfield's ductile fracture model (Ref 75) is by far the most commonly used model for particulate MMCs. Assuming that crack growth will occur if the extent of heavily deformed zone ahead of crack tip becomes comparable to the width of the unbroken ligaments separating cracked particles, the fracture toughness can be expressed as:

$$K_{Ic}=\left[2\sigma_y E\left(\frac{\pi}{6}\right)^{1/3} d\right]^{1/2} V_p^{-1/6} \quad \text{(Eq 35)}$$

where K_{Ic} is the critical value of the stress-intensity factor, V_p is the volume fraction of particulates, d is the particle diameter, E is the composite modulus, and σ_y is the yield strength of the composite. A key validation point for the model was the $V_p^{-1/6}$ dependence observed in a number of monolithic aluminum alloys. A slight modification of the model was made in Ref 76 to account for the observed effect of specimen thickness on the fracture toughness of the material.

The main problem with Eq 35 is that it shows an increasing toughness with yield strength, σ_y, whereas the reverse is normally observed. A summary of toughness data with comparisons to models can be found in Ref 77. From a microstructural perspective, a higher strength is usually accompanied by concentrated and localized slip bands, which accelerates the initiation of microvoids in those bands. Mechanically, a higher strength is accompanied with a reduction in the work-hardening exponent, N. This effect was accounted for in the model of Garrett and Knott (Ref 78), which was essentially based on an earlier paper of Hahn and Rosenfield (Ref 79). The following equation was obtained in Ref 78:

$$K_{Ic}=N\sqrt{\frac{2EC\varepsilon_c^*\sigma_y}{(1-\nu^2)}} \quad \text{(Eq 36)}$$

Typical values of the parameters were C = 0.025 m and ε_c^* = 0.1.

This form does indeed show the correct inverse dependence of toughness on strength, because N generally decreases sharply with increasing strength. However, the problem with the analysis is that the results of Ref 80 illustrate that local strains along any orientation θ (measured with respect to crack plane) are extremely insensitive to the material parameters, rather than the strong *N* dependence that was assumed in Ref 78 and 79. A recent discussion on these models, in the context of the micromechanisms of fracture, is provided in Ref 37. This reference also presents an alternate model, based on localized slip, to explain the large decrease in toughness in the peak-aged condition of DRAs. Although reasonably good agreement was found with limited experimental data, further validation of the model is necessary.

Software

The following software programs are available for MMC analysis:

- NDSANDS, developed at Air Force Research Laboratory, Materials Directorate. Elastic analysis parallel and perpendicular to fiber axis, laminates
- FIDEP, developed at Air Force Research Laboratory, Materials Directorate. Elastic-plastic-viscoplastic concentric cylinder model
- VISCOPLY, developed at National Aeronautics and Space Administration (NASA) Langley Research Center. Elastic-viscoplastic model based on the vanishing fiber diameter analysis
- IDAC, developed at Research Applications Inc., San Diego, under Air Force contract. Elastic-plastic-viscoplastic analysis based on FEM procedure, with emphasis on multiaxial loading of laminas

REFERENCES

1. Z. Hashin and B.W. Rosen, The Elastic Moduli of Fiber Reinforced Materials, *J. Appl. Mech. (Trans ASME)*, Vol 31, 1964, p 223–232
2. N.J. Pagano and G.P. Tandon, Elastic Response of Multidirectional Coated-Fiber Composites, *Compos. Sci. Technol.*, Vol 31, 1988, p 273–293
3. G.P. Tandon, Use of Composite Cylinder Model as Representative Volume Element for Unidirectional Fiber Composites, *J. Compos. Mater.*, Vol 29 (No. 3), 1995, p 385–409
4. B. Budiansky, J.W. Hutchinson, and A.G. Evans, Matrix Fracture in Fiber-Reinforced Ceramics, *J. Mech. Phys. Solids*, Vol 34, 1986, p 167–189
5. S.M. Pickard, D.B. Miracle, B.S. Majumdar, K. Kendig, L. Rothenflue, and D. Coker, An Experimental Study of Residual Fiber Strains in Ti-15-3 Continuous Fiber Composites, *Acta Metall. Mater.*, Vol 43 (No. 8), 1995, p 3105–3112
6. B.S. Majumdar and G.M. Newaz, Inelastic Deformation of Metal Matrix Composites: Plasticity and Damage Mechanisms, *Philos. Mag.*, Vol 66 (No. 2), 1992, p 187–212
7. W.S. Johnson, S.J. Lubowinski, and A.L. Highsmith, Mechanical Characterization of Unnotched SCS6/Ti-15-3 MMC at Room Temperature, ASTM STP 1080, ASTM, 1990, p 193–218
8. A.L. Highsmith, D. Shee, and R.A. Naik, Local Stresses in Metal Matrix Composites Subjected to Thermal and Mechanical Loading, ASTM STP 1080, J.M. Kennedy, H.H. Moeller, and W.S. Johnson, Ed., ASTM, 1990, p 3–19
9. N.I. Muskhelisvili, *Some Basic Problems of the Mathematical Theory of Elasticity*, Noordhoff International, Leyden, The Netherlands, 1963
10. D. Coker, N.E. Ashbaugh, and T. Nicholas, Analysis of Thermo-Mechanical Cyclic Behavior of Unidirectional Metal Matrix Composites, ASTM STP 1186, H. Sehitoglu, Ed., 1993, p 50–69
11. D. Coker, N.E. Ashbaugh, and T. Nicholas, Analysis of the Thermo-Mechanical Behavior of [0] and [0/90] SCS-6/Timetal21S Composites, *ASME*, Vol 34 (No. H00866-1993), W.F. Jones, Ed., 1993, p 1–16
12. A. Mendelson, *Plasticity Theory and Application*, Macmillan, 1968
13. C.H. Hamilton, S.S. Hecker, and L.J. Ebert, Mechanical Behavior of Uniaxially Loaded Multilayered Cylindrical Composites, *J. Basic Eng.*, 1971, p 661–670
14. S.S. Hecker, C.H. Hamilton, and L.J. Ebert, Elasto-Plastic Analysis of Residual Stresses and Axial Loading in Composite Cylinders, *J. Mater.*, Vol 5, 1970, p 868–900
15. B.S. Majumdar, G.M. Newaz, and J.R. Ellis, Evolution of Damage and Plasticity in Metal Matrix Composites, *Metall. Trans. A*, Vol 24, 1993, p 1597–1610
16. W.A. Curtin, *J. Am. Ceram. Soc.*, Vol 74, 1991, p 2837
17. W.A. Curtin, Ultimate Strengths of Fibre-Reinforced Ceramics and Metals, *Composites*, Vol 24 (No. 2), 1993, p 98–102
18. B.S. Majumdar and G.M. Newaz, In-Phase TMF of a 0° SiC/Ti-15-3 System: Damage Mechanisms, and Modeling of the TMC Response, *Proc. 1995 HITEMP Conf.*, NASA CP 10178, Vol 2, National Aeronautics and Space Administration, 1995, p 21.1–21.13
19. S.R. Bodner and Y. Partom, Constitutive Equations of Elastic Viscoplastic Strain Hardening Materials, *J. Appl. Mech. (Trans. ASME)*, Vol 42, 1975, p 385–389
20. K.S. Chan and U.S. Lindholm, Inelastic Deformation Under Non-Isothermal Loading, *ASME J. Eng. Mater. Technol. (Trans ASME)*, Vol 112, 1990, p 15–25
21. D. Robertson and S. Mall, Micromechanical Analysis and Modeling, *Titanium Matrix Composites Mechanical Behavior*, S. Mall and T. Nicholas, Ed., Technomic Publishing Co., 1998, p 397–464
22. G.J. Dvorak and Y.A. Bahei-El-Din, Plasticity Analysis of Fibrous Composites, *J. Appl. Mech. (Trans. ASME)*, Vol 49, 1982, p 193–221
23. G.J. Dvorak and Y.A. Bahei-El-Din, Elastic-Plastic Behavior of Fibrous Composites, *J. Mech. Phys. Solids*, Vol 27, 1997, p 51–72
24. Y.A. Bahei-El-Din, R.S. Shah, and G.J. Dvorak, Numerical Analysis of Rate-Dependent Behavior of High Temperature Fibrous Composites, *Mechanics of Composites at Elevated Temperatures*, AMD Vol 118, American Society of Mechanical Engineers, 1991, p 67–78
25. J. Aboudi, A Continuum Theory for Fiber Reinforced Elastic-Viscoplastic Composites, *Int. J. Eng. Sci.*, Vol 20, 1982, p 605–621
26. S.A. Arnold, T.E. Wilt, A.F. Saleeb, and M.G. Castelli, An Investigation of Macro and Micromechanical Approaches for a Model MMC System, *Proc. 6th Annual HITEM Conf.*, NASA Conf. Publ. 19117, Vol II, National Aeronautics and Space Administration (NASA) Lewis, 1995, p 52.1–52.12
27. M.A. Eisenberg and C.F. Yen, A Theory of Multiaxial Anisotropic Viscoplasticity, *J. Appl. Mech. (Trans. ASME)*, Vol 48, 1991, p 276–284
28. M. Mirdamadi, W.S. Johnson, Y.A. Bahei-El-Din, and M.G. Castelli, Analysis of Thermomechanical Fatigue of Unidirectional TMCs, ASTM STP 1156, W.W. Stinchcomb and N.E. Ashbaugh, Ed., ASTM, 1993, p 591–607
29. W.S. Johnson and M. Mirdamadi, "Modeling and Life Prediction Methodology of TMCs Subjected to Mission Profiles," NASA TM 109148, National Aeronautics and Space Administration (NASA) Langley, 1994
30. G. Bao, J.W. Hutchinson, and R.M. McMeeking, Particle Reinforcement of Ductile Matrices Against Plastic Flow and Creep, *Acta Metall. Mater.*, Vol 39, 1991, p1871–1882
31. C.T. Sun, J.L. Chen, G.T. Shah, and W.E. Koop, Mechanical Characterization of SCS-6/Ti-6-4 Metal Matrix Composites, *J. Compos. Mater.*, Vol 29, 1990, p 1029–1059
32. C.T. Sun, Modeling Continuous Fiber Metal Matrix Composite as an Orthotropic Elastic-Plastic Material, ASTM STP 1032, W.S. Johnson, Ed., ASTM, 1989, p 148–160
33. J. Ahmad, S. Chandu, U. Santhosh, and G.M. Newaz, "Nonlinear Multiaxial Stress Analysis of Composites," Research Applications, Inc. final report to the Air Force Research Laboratory, Materials and Manufacturing Directorate, Contract F33615-96-C-5261, Wright-Patterson Air Force Base, OH, 1999
34. J. Ahmad, G.M. Newaz, and T. Nicholas, Analysis of Characterization Methods for Inelastic Composite Material Deformation Under Multiaxial Stresses, Multiaxial Fatigue and Deformation: Testing and Prediction, ASTM STP 1387, S. Kalluri and P.J. Bonacuse, Ed., ASTM, 2000, p 41–53
35. T.W. Clyne and P.J. Withers, *An Introduction to Metal Matrix Composites*, Cambridge University Press, Cambridge, 1993

36. Y.L. Shen, M. Finot, A. Needleman, and S. Suresh, Effective Elastic Response of Two-Phase Composites, *Acta Metall. Mater.*, Vol 42, 1994, p 77–97
37. B.S. Majumdar and A.B. Pandey, Deformation and Fracture of a Particle Reinforced Aluminum Alloy Composite, Part II: Modeling, *Metall. Trans A,* Vol 31, 2000, p 937–950
38. B.S. Majumdar and A.B. Pandey, Deformation and Fracture of a Particle Reinforced Aluminum Alloy Composite, Part I: Experiments, *Metall. Trans. A,* Vol 31, 2000, p 921–936
39. J. Llorca and C. Gonzalez, Microstructural Factors Controlling the Strength and Ductility of Particle Reinforced Metal-Matrix Composites, *J. Mech. Phys. Solids,* Vol 46, 1998, p 1–28
40. Z. Hashin and S. Shtrikman, *J. Mech. Phys. Solids,* Vol 11, 1963, p 127
41. T. Mura, *Micromechanics of Defects in Solids,* 2nd ed., Martinis Nijhoff, The Hague, 1987
42. J. Duva, A Self Consistent Analysis of the Stiffening Effect of Rigid Inclusions on a Power-Law Material, *J. Eng. Mater. Struct. (Trans. ASME),* Vol 106, 1984, p 317
43. S. Ghosh and S. Moorthy, Elastic-Plastic Analysis of Arbitrary Heterogeneous Materials with the Voronoi Cell Finite Element Method, *Comp. Methods Appl. Mech. Eng.,* Vol 121, 1995, p 373–409
44. J.R. Rice and D.M. Tracey, *J. Mech. Phys. Solids,* Vol 17, 1969, p 201–217
45. A. Kelly and N.H. Macmillan, *Strong Solids,* 3rd ed., Clarendon Press, Oxford, 1986
46. C.H. Weber, X. Chen, S.J. Connell, and F. Zok, On the Tensile Properties of a Fiber Reinforced Titanium Matrix Composite, Part I, Unnotched Behavior, *Acta Metall. Mater.,* Vol 42, 1994, p 3443–3450
47. C.H. Weber, Z.Z. Du, and F.W. Zok, High Temperature Deformation and Fracture of a Fiber Reinforced Titanium Matrix Composite, *Acta Metall. Mater.,* Vol 44, 1996, p 683–695
48. D.B. Gundel and F.E. Wawner, Experimental and Theoretical Assessment of the Longitudinal Tensile Strength of Unidirectional SiC-Fiber/Titanium-Matrix Composites, *Compos. Sci. Technol.,* Vol 57, 1997, p 471–481
49. B.S. Majumdar, T.E. Matikas, and D.B. Miracle, Experiments and Analysis of Single and Multiple Fiber Fragmentation in SiC/Ti-6Al-4V MMCs, *Compos. B: Eng.,* Vol 29, 1998, p 131–145
50. C.J. Boehlert, B.S. Majumdar, S. Krishnamurthy, and D.B. Miracle, Role of Matrix Microstructure on RT Tensile Properties and Fiber-Strength Utilization of an Orthorhombic Ti-Alloy Based Composite, *Metall. Trans. A,* Vol 28, 1997, p 309–323
51. C. Zweben and B.W. Rosen, A Statistical Theory of Material Strength with Application to Composite Materials, *J. Mech. Phys. Solids,* 1970, p 189–206
52. R. Talreja, *Fatigue of Composite Materials,* Technomic Publishing Company, 1987
53. B.S. Majumdar and G.M. Newaz, Constituent Damage Mechanisms in Metal Matrix Composites Under Fatigue Loading, and Their Effects on Fatigue Life, *Mater. Sci. Eng. A,* Vol 200, 1995, p 114–129
54. P.K. Brindley and P.A. Bartolotta, Failure Mechanisms During Isothermal Fatigue of SiC/Ti-24Al-11Nb Composites, *Mater. Sci. Eng. A,* Vol 200, 1995, p 55–67
55. B.S. Majumdar and G.M. Newaz, Damage Mechanisms Under In-Phase TMF in a SCS-6/Ti-15-3 MMC, *Proc. 1994 HITEMP Conf.,* NASA CP 10146, National Aeronautics Space Administration, 1994, p 41.1–41.13
56. T. Nicholas, An Approach to Fatigue Life Modeling in Titanium Matrix Composites, *Mater. Sci. Eng. A,* Vol 200, 1995, p 29–37
57. T. Nicholas, Fatigue and Thermomechanical Fatigue Life Prediction, *Titanium Matrix Composites Mechanical Behavior,* S. Mall and T. Nicholas, Ed., Technomic Publishing Co., 1998, p 209–272
58. B.A. Lerch and G. Halford, Effects of Control Mode and R-Ratio on the Fatigue Behavior of a Metal Matrix Composite, *Mater. Sci. Eng A,* Vol 200, 1995, p 47–54
59. B. Lerch and G. Halford, "Fatigue Mean Stress Modeling in a [0]32 Titanium Matrix Composite," Paper 21, HITEMP Review-1995, Vol II, NASA CP 10178, National Aeronautics and Space Administration, 1995, p 1–10
60. D.B. Marshall, B.N. Cox, and A.G. Evans, The Mechanics of Matrix Cracking in Brittle Matrix Fiber Composites, *Acta Metall. Mater.,* Vol 33, 1985, p 2013–2021
61. R.M. McMeeking and A.G. Evans, Matrix Fatigue Cracking in Fiber Composites, *Mech. Mater.,* Vol 9, 1990, p 217–227
62. L.N. McCartney, New Theoretical Model of Stress Transfer Between Fiber and Matrix in a Uniaxially Fiber Reinforced Composite, *Proc. R. Soc. (London) A,* Vol 425, 1989, p 215
63. J.M. Larsen, J.R. Jira, R. John, and N.E. Ashbaugh, Crack Bridging in Notch Fatigue of SCS-6/Timetal 21S Composite Laminates, ASTM STP 1253, W.S. Johnson, J.M. Larsen, and B.N. Cox, Ed., ASTM, 1995
64. B.N. Cox and C.S. Lo, Simple Approximations for Bridged Cracks in Fibrous Composites, *Acta Metal. Mater.,* Vol 40, 1992, p 1487–1496
65. S.G. Warrier and B.S. Majumdar, Elastic Shielding During Fatigue Crack Growth of Titanium Matrix Composites, *Metall. Trans. A,* Vol 30, 1999, p 277–286
66. G.J. Dvora, Y.A. Bahei-El-Din, and L.C. Bank, *Eng. Fract. Mech.,* Vol 34 (No. 1), 1989, p 87–104 and p 105–123
67. J. Awerbuch and G.T. Hahn, *J. Compos. Mater.,* Vol 13, 1979, p 82–107
68. E.D. Reedy, Analysis of Center-Notched Monolayers with Application to Boron/Aluminum Composites, *J. Mech. Phys. Solids,* Vol 28, 1980, p 265–286
69. J. Tirosh, *J. Appl. Mech. (Trans. ASME),* Vol 40, 1973, p 785–790
70. J.F. Zarzour and A.J. Paul, *J. Mater. Eng. Perform.,* Vol 1 (No. 5), 1992, p 659–668
71. J.B. Friler, A.S. Argon, and J.A. Cornie, *Mater. Sci. Eng.,* Vol A162, 1993, p 143–152
72. A.S. Argon, *Comprehensive Composite Materials,* A. Kelly and C. Zweben, Ed., Vol 1, Pergamon Press, Oxford, 2000
73. S.J. Connell, F.W. Zok, Z.Z. Du, and Z. Suo, *Acta Metall.,* Vol 42 (No. 10), 1994, p 3451–3461
74. A.S. Argon, M.L. Seleznev, C.F. Shih, and X.H. Liu, *Int. J. Fract.,* Vol 93, 1998, p 351–371
75. G.T. Hahn and A.R. Rosenfield, Metallurgical Factors Affecting Fracture Toughness of Aluminum Alloys, *Metall. Trans. A,* Vol 6, 1975, p 653–670
76. A.B. Pandey, B.S. Majumdar, and D.B. Miracle, Effects of Thickness and Precracking on the Fracture Toughness of Particle Reinforced Al-Alloy Composites, *Metall. Trans., A,* Vol 29, (No. 4), 1998, p 1237–1243
77. J.J. Lewandowski, Fracture and Fatigue of Particulate Composites, *Comprehensive Composite Materials,* A. Kelly and C. Zweben, Ed., Vol 3, *Metal Matrix Composites,* T.W. Clyne, Ed., Elsevier, 2000, p 151–187
78. G.G. Garrett and J.F. Knott, The Influence of Composition and Microstructural Variations on the Mechanism of Static Fracture in Aluminum Alloys, *Metall. Trans. A,* Vol 9, 1978, p 1187–1201
79. G.T. Hahn and A.R. Rosenfield, Sources of Fracture Toughness: The Relation Between K_{Ic} and the Ordinary Tensile Properties of Metals, *Applications Related Phenomena in Titanium Alloys,* ASTM STP 432, ASTM, 1968, p 5–32
80. R.M. McMeeking, Finite Deformation Analysis of Crack-Tip Opening in Elastic-Plastic Materials and Implications for Fracture, *J. Mech. Phys. Solids,* Vol 25, 1977, p 357–381

Fracture Analysis of Fiber-Reinforced Ceramic-Matrix Composites

F.W. Zok, University of California at Santa Barbara

ONE OF THE KEY ATTRIBUTES of continuous fiber-reinforced ceramic composites (CFCCs) is their ability to undergo inelastic straining upon mechanical loading (Ref 1). The mechanisms for these strains involve matrix cracking and debonding and sliding along the fiber–matrix interfaces. The inelastic strains impart a high toughness to CFCCs in essentially the same manner that dislocation plasticity imparts high toughness to metallic alloys. That is, the inelasticity reduces the local levels of stress around strain-concentrating features, such as cracks and notches, and hence increases the level of applied stress necessary to initiate fiber fracture at the crack tip. This phenomenon is referred to as *plastic shielding*. An additional attribute of CFCCs is the stochastic nature of fiber fracture within the composite. A consequence is that fiber failure occurs over a range of locations relative to the macroscopic crack plane. The subsequent *pullout* of broken fibers leads to additional shielding of the crack tip.

From a macroscopic viewpoint, the fracture properties of CFCCs differ from those of metals in three important respects, as listed in Table 1. These differences provide the impetus and the directions for modifying existing methodologies for damage-tolerant failure prediction (currently used for metallic components) such that they can be applied to CFCC components.

Some trends in the degree of damage tolerance, as manifested in the notch sensitivity of strength, are highlighted in Fig. 1, based on Ref 2–5. Results are presented for the net-section tensile strength, σ_N, of open-hole specimens for typical metals, CFCCs, and polymer-matrix composites (PMCs), all with the same normalized hole radius, a/w = 0.2. The metals listed exhibit no notch sensitivity for hole diameters approaching 10 mm (0.4 in.). This behavior is attributable to the extensive plasticity that occurs across the entire net section prior to fracture and the effects of this plasticity on reducing the stress concentration at the hole edge. At the other extreme, PMCs exhibit severe notch sensitivity. The strength diminishes rapidly with increasing hole diameter and eventually approaches the value predicted from the elastic stress concentration factor, k_σ. This notch sensitivity is largely a consequence of the absence of inelastic straining mechanisms in these composites. Continuous fiber-reinforced ceramic composites with high toughness exhibit intermediate behavior in the sense that their strength diminishes gradually with hole diameter and appears to saturate at a relatively high value, typically 70% of the unnotched strength.

The objective of this article is to review the mechanics of inelastic deformation and fracture of CFCCs, as needed for the development of damage-tolerant failure prediction methodologies for use in engineering design. An underlying theme pertains to the anisotropy in their mechanical properties and its effect on notch sensitivity of strength. The scope of the article is restricted to CFCCs with balanced 0°/90° fiber architectures, because of the emphasis on these architectures within the CFCC community.

Many of the concepts and models described here have been adapted from analogous problems in monolithic materials. Notable examples include: models of stress redistribution around strain concentrations due to inelastic straining; fracture resistance curves and the conditions associated with crack stability; cohesive or bridging zone concepts; and effects of material and structural size scales, leading to large scale bridging (LSB) or large scale yielding (LSY). Such connections are noted where appropriate.

The coverage in this article is organized as follows:

- A general framework for damage-tolerant design with structural materials is outlined. The

Table 1 Macroscopic differences in fracture properties of CFCCs and metals

Characteristic	CFCC	Metal	Consequence
Failure strains	The magnitude of the total straining capacity of CFCCs is limited to values of ≈1%.	In metallic alloys, failure strains in the range of 10–50% are common.	These differences have implications in the efficacy of plastic shielding in the two classes of materials.
Nonlinear behavior	Because the mechanism of inelasticity in CFCCs involves cracking, the process is driven largely by normal (tensile) stresses.	Plasticity in metals is driven by the deviatoric component (a) of the stress state and is essentially independent of the hydrostatic stress.	The constitutive laws for the mechanical response of metals and CFCCs in the nonlinear regime are fundamentally different from one another. A related feature is the mechanical anisotropy of CFCCs with most common (two dimensional) fiber architectures.
Fracture resistance	The increase in fracture resistance due to fiber pullout is typically much greater than the intrinsic composite toughness (in the absence of bridging). Additionally, the amount of crack growth needed to attain a steady-state resistance is typically of the same order as the dimensions of CFCC coupons or components of interest.	Fracture resistance is dictated largely by the behavior of an enclave of heavily deformed material at the crack tip. In most cases of practical interest, this enclave is very small in relation to other structural dimensions, and thus a *small-scale yielding* (SSY) treatment is adequate. The problem of *large-scale yielding* (LSY) arises in very tough metals, especially under plane-stress conditions.	A *large-scale bridging* (LSB) mechanics is needed to describe the structural response in CFCCs, including the conditions associated with crack stability.

(a) The stress component that is related to the difference in the stress and the mean stress. The hydrostatic stress is the mean stress. This terminology is used in modeling the observation that plastic deformation is a shear phenomena and not dependent on hydrostatic stress.

framework identifies two broad classes of phenomena that are obtained in such materials: *crack-tip inelasticity* prior to the onset of fracture initiation, and *crack bridging* during crack propagation.

- The common classes of fracture behavior of CFCCs are described. The classification system provides a rationale for selecting the pertinent features and mechanisms into the failure prediction methodology.
- The constitutive laws needed to describe crack-tip inelasticity are presented.
- The stress distribution section demonstrates the effects of inelasticity on crack-tip stress fields.
- Models for crack initiation are discussed.
- Crack propagation models are derived.
- Environmental degradation effects on damage tolerance are addressed.

General Framework for Fracture Analysis

It is instructive to begin by outlining a general framework for the description of fracture in structural materials in the presence of notches and cracks. There are two broad categories of phenomena (Fig. 2). The first involves *local inelastic straining* in the material surrounding the crack tip, which reduces the intensity of the stress singularity. Inelastic straining can occur by one of numerous mechanisms, including dislocation glide in metallic alloys, distributed microcracking in two-phase ceramics with large internal stresses, stress-induced phase transformations in stabilized zirconia alloys, and matrix cracking and interface sliding in CFCCs. The magnitude of the shielding effect can be computed using standard finite-element methods, provided suitable constitutive laws for the inelasticity are available.

The second category of phenomena pertains to the *fracture process zone* (FPZ). The FPZ represents the region directly ahead of the crack within which the strains become highly localized and lead to the initiation and propagation of a macroscopic crack. Generally, fracture initiation is stochastic when it involves fracture of brittle constituents. Indeed, stochastic behavior is obtained in CFCCs as well as in fiber-reinforced polymer-matrix composites. Following fracture initiation, the mechanical response of the material in the crack wake is characterized by a bridging traction law, as shown schematically in Fig. 2. Of the two steps in the fracture process, fracture initiation and crack propagation, the one requiring the higher stress dictates the notched strength.

This framework for fracture analysis has been used successfully in the context of numerous fracture mechanisms, including ductile rupture of metals, cleavage of inhomogeneous alloys, such as steels (Ref 6), and fracture along bimaterial interfaces (Ref 7). It is anticipated that the framework will be implemented by the CFCC design community once an understanding of the features specific to CFCCs reaches a suitably mature level. The remainder of this chapter focuses on the features needed for this implementation.

Classes of Material Behavior

Continuous fiber-reinforced ceramic composites exhibit one of three broad classes of deformation and fracture behaviors, designated class I, II, and III (Ref 8). The key features associated with each are shown schematically in Fig. 3. In CFCCs with 0°/90° fiber architectures, these behaviors are elicited by performing tension tests both with and without notches in two orientations: with the loading direction parallel to one of the two fiber axes, denoted the 0°/90° orientation; and with the loading direction oriented at ± 45° to the fiber axes.

Class I behavior is characterized by the propagation of a dominant matrix crack, accompanied by fiber pullout, but with otherwise negligible inelastic deformation. This behavior is obtained in materials with unusually high interfacial toughness and/or sliding resistance (as a consequence of oxidation of the fiber–matrix interfaces, for example) and yields relatively damage-intolerant behavior. Fiber pullout is manifested in the form of a *rising fracture resistance curve* (so-called *R*-curve). The fracture resistance starts at a value comparable to the fracture toughness of the matrix and increases with crack growth as the bridging zone develops. Once the broken fibers at the point furthest from the crack tip completely disengage from their respective matrix sockets, a steady-state fracture resistance is obtained. Because of the large length scales associated with the bridging, the extent of crack growth needed to attain steady state is rather large, typically approximately 10 to 100 mm (0.4 to 4 in.). An implication is that extremely large test specimens, on the order of 1 m (40 in.), are needed to obtain *small-scale bridging* (SSB) conditions and hence extract in a direct manner the intrinsic fracture resistance curve. In smaller test specimens and structures, the fracture resistance curve is influenced by structural dimensions. The connections between the macroscopic structural response and the fundamental parameters dictating the pullout process are made through a LSB mechanics (Ref 9). Some typical experimental results for the fracture resistance behavior of a class I material are shown in Fig. 4. For comparison, predictions based on both

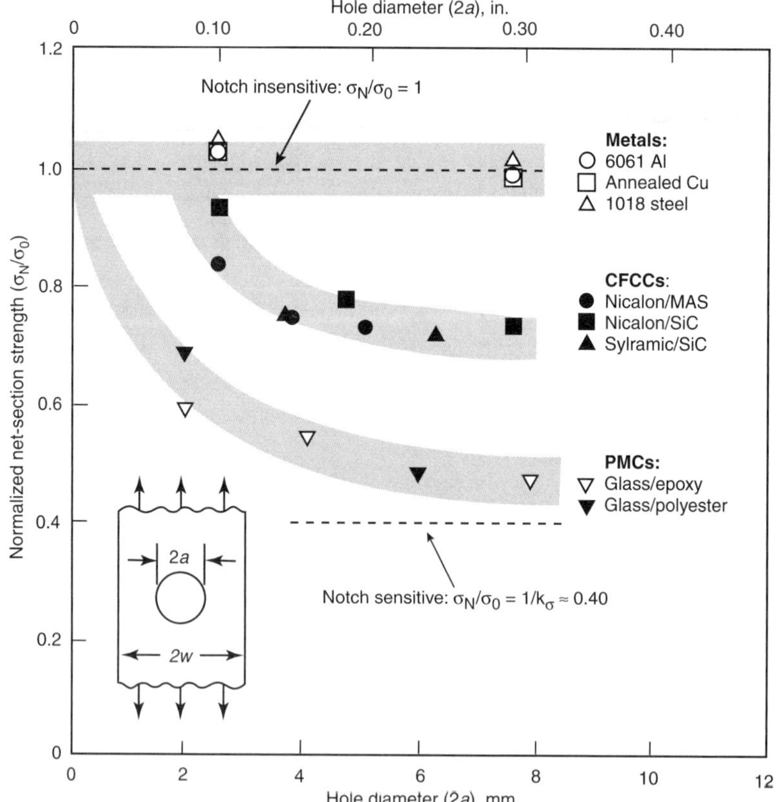

Fig. 1 Notch sensitivity. Effects of hole diameter on the tensile strength of metals, CFCCs (Ref 2, 3), and polymer-matrix composites (PMCs) (Ref 4, 5). The data are presented on the basis of the net-section strength, σ_N, normalized by the respective unnotched tensile strength, σ_0. The composites have two-dimensional (2D) fiber architectures (either laminated or woven), and the loads are applied parallel to one of the fiber axes. In all cases, the normalized hole diameter is a/w = 0.2. The lower limit on the notched strength is given by $1/k_\sigma$, where k_σ is the elastic stress concentration factor. Data on metals courtesy of J.C. McNulty, University of California, Santa Barbara

LSB and SSB models, described subsequently, are shown also.

Class II behavior is characterized by the formation of *multiple* matrix cracks in both 0°/90° and ±45° orientations, initially with negligible fiber fracture. The cracks are manifested macroscopically as inelastic strain. Some results for a Nicalon/SiC composite are shown in Fig. 5(a). The inelasticity serves to redistribute the stresses in notched specimens, such that the peak stress concentration is reduced from its initial (elastic) value. Once fiber fracture begins, the subsequent pullout leads to *R*-curve behavior in essentially the same manner as in class I materials; the main difference is that the extent of pullout in class II materials is greater than it is in class I materials, because the interfaces are weaker and hence the lengths over which debonding and sliding occur are greater. The combined effects of plastic shielding and fiber pullout lead to highly damage-tolerant and notch-insensitive fracture behavior. Large-scale bridging models can be used to simulate the fracture resistance behavior, although complications exist with regard to the coupled effects of the bridging and the inelastic straining.

Class III behavior materials exhibit essentially linear behavior up to fracture in the 0°/90° orientation, but significant inelasticity in the ±45° orientation. This behavior is obtained in CFCCs in which the matrix modulus is much lower than that of the fibers. In 0°/90° orientations, the contribution of the matrix to the initial elastic modulus of the composite is small, and hence any subsequent matrix damage has little effect on the composite response. In some cases, the low matrix modulus arises from the presence of a high level of matrix porosity, introduced intentionally to impart high damage tolerance in the absence of weak fiber coatings (Ref 12). In others, it is a consequence of the high density of matrix cracks and fine-scale porosity resulting from the constrained pyrolysis and densification of the matrix precursor material (Ref 13). In the ±45° orientation, the matrix modulus plays a more significant role in the initial elastic response, and hence the matrix damage that occurs as a consequence of loading is manifested in significant inelasticity. An example of this anisotropic behavior in a carbon-carbon (C-C) and an all-oxide CFCC are shown in Fig. 5(b) and (c). In notched geometries in the 0°/90° orientation, the inelasticity occurs in the form of long, slender shear bands aligned parallel to the loading direction. This deformation can reduce the stress concentration by a modest amount in some cases, although the efficacy of this deformation is considerably lower than that in class II materials, as demonstrated in the section "Stress Distributions in Notched Specimens" in this article. In other cases, the deformation has the effect of increasing the stress concentration (Ref 15). Fiber pullout and the associated *R*-curve are again obtained during fracture.

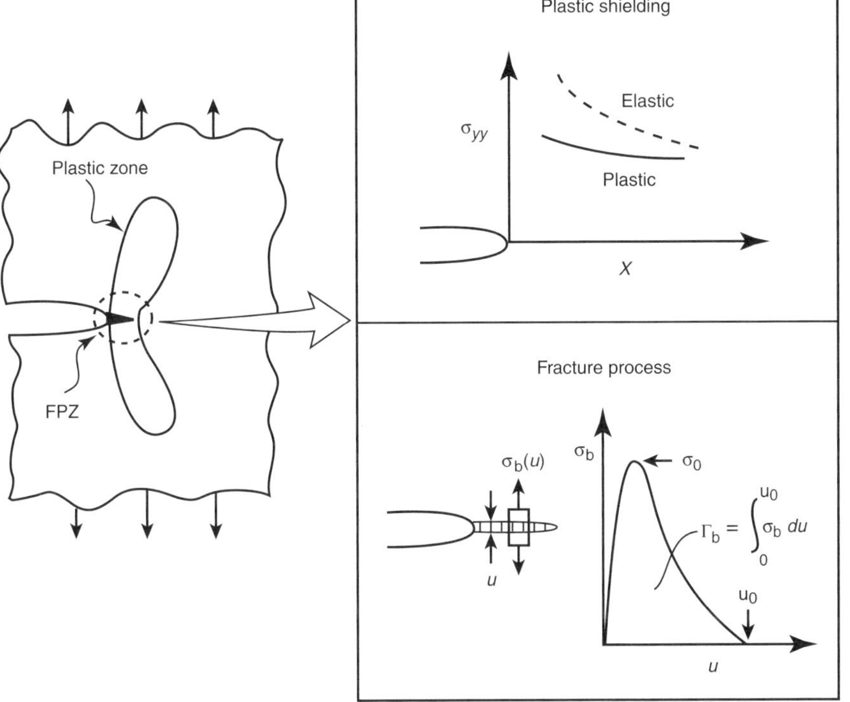

Fig. 2 The effects of inelasticity on the crack-tip stresses and the characterization of the fracture process zone (FPZ) through a bridging traction law. Here Γ_b is the steady-state toughness of the FPZ, independent of plastic shielding.

Class I
Matrix cracking and fiber pullout

Class II
Multiple matrix cracking

Class III
Shear damage by matrix cracking

Fig. 3 The three common classes of fracture behavior in CFCCs. Source: Adapted from Ref 8

Constitutive Laws for Inelastic Straining

The micromechanics of matrix cracking, interface debonding and sliding, and their roles in the macroscopic stress–strain response are very

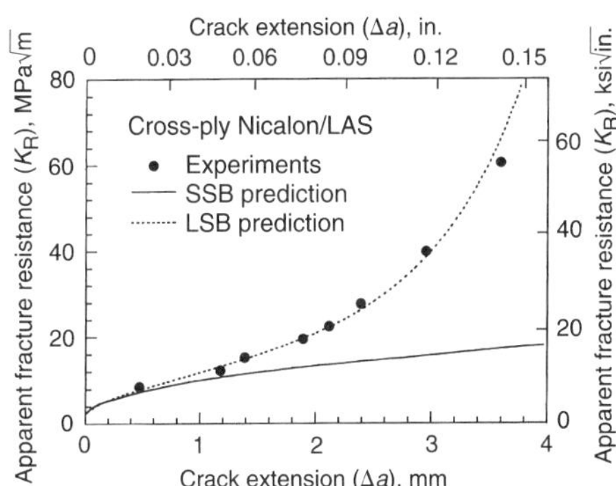

Fig. 4 Fracture resistance curve for a Nicalon/LAS (Li_2O-Al_2O_3-SiO_2) composite that had been subjected to an embrittling heat treatment in air of 16 h at 800 °C (1470 °F). Upon heat treatment, the carbon coating on the fibers is replaced with an oxide layer that inhibits interfacial debonding and sliding. The solid line shows a LSB prediction, based on a linear softening traction law (Eq 4) The bridging parameters are: τ = 270 MPa (39 ksi), E = 150 GPa (22 × 10^6 psi), ν = 0.25, h = 11 μm (4.33 × 10^{-6} in.), f_0 = 0.22, and R = 7 μm (2.75 × 10^{-6} in.); the initiation toughness is K_0 = 2 MPa $\sqrt{m}$ (1.8 ksi$\sqrt{in.}$). The dashed line shows the corresponding SSB prediction for the same bridging parameters. Source: Adapted from Ref 10

well understood. Indeed, there exists a vast scientific literature dealing with this class of problems (see, for example, Ref 16–18). Despite their large collective volume, most papers are restricted to unidirectionally-reinforced composites, subject to uniaxial loadings parallel to the fibers. Some have dealt with 2-D cross-ply and woven architectures, but again, subject to uniaxial loading along one of the fiber axes. Although these studies have yielded important insights into the mechanisms and mechanics of failure in CFCCs, they have not lead directly to the development of tools that are amenable for use in structural analysis, especially when off-axis and/or multitiaxial stresses are present.

With this recognition, two independent groups recently have developed engineering approaches to describe the inelasticity of CFCCs, specifically for use in structural analysis. The key papers were published almost simultaneously in 1997 (Ref 15, 19). Although the details of the two approaches differ considerably, both contain three key features:

- They faithfully (albeit approximately) represent the material behavior under *multiaxial* stress states.
- They can be implemented readily into finite-element codes that are used commonly in engineering design.
- They can be calibrated using a small number of standard mechanical tests.

Both approaches are based on a homogenized representation of the composite without an explicit dependence on the fiber architecture or the size scale of the microstructure, except insofar as these features influence the macroscopic properties obtained from the mechanical tests used for calibration and the macroscopic material symmetry. Preliminary assessments of their capabilities and use in engineering design have been encouraging. Selection of one over the other will be based ultimately on trade-offs between the level of complexity and the level of effort required for their calibration and implementation. The extent to which they explicitly incorporate the damage mechanisms and associated micromechanics also may have some bearing on the selection process, although the criticality of this feature in engineering design has yet to be established.

BHL Approach. The first approach, developed by Burr, Hild, and Leckie (Ref 19) and subsequently referred to as BHL, is couched in terms of continuum damage mechanics. To begin, the physical internal variables that characterize the damage state are identified. For 2-D laminates or weaves under biaxial stressing, ten internal variables are needed to fully characterize the extent of matrix cracking, interfacial sliding, and fiber damage in the two-ply types. State potentials are then derived in terms of the state variables. The derivations of these potentials are guided closely by micromechanical models of matrix cracking and interface sliding. The potentials are then used in a framework of irreversible thermodynamics to obtain the forces driving each of the damage mechanisms. The growth laws for each of the state variables are calibrated by performing uniaxial tension tests in both the 0°/90° and ±45° orientations along with periodic unloading-reloading excursions to measure hysteresis. The behavior of the composite in other loading directions or under multiaxial loading is obtained through an interpolation procedure. The behavior upon unloading also can be obtained. Once calibrated, the constitutive law can be implemented into a finite element code as a user material subroutine.

GH Approach. The second approach, developed by Genin and Hutchinson (Ref 15) and subsequently referred to as GH, is based on a purely phenomenological representation of the stress-strain response of a CFCC along the directions that coincide with the material symmetry: 0°/90° and ±45° for balanced 2-D laminates and weaves. It begins by partitioning the two in-plane strains for principal stressing in the 0°/90° orientation into two functions, with each function being dependent on only one of the two principal stresses. Similar partitioning is invoked for principal stressing in the ±45° orientation, yielding two additional strain functions. Because the principal axes are indeterminate for equi-biaxial loading, the strain functions obtained from principal stressing in the 0°/90° must match those obtained for principal stressing in the ±45° orientation. The latter requirement reduces the number of independent functions to three. The nonlinearity in these functions is couched in terms of 'stress deficits,' defined as the difference between the elastic stress that would exist at a prescribed strain and the one actually obtained. For other stress states, where the principal stress directions are at an arbitrary angle to the fiber axes, the stress deficits are obtained using an interpolation procedure. A summary of this procedure is given in the Appendix of this chapter. The constitutive law is calibrated through monotonic tension tests in the 0°/90° and ±45° orientations; no unload-reload excursions are required. The calibrated constitutive law is implemented into a finite-element code as a user material subroutine, similar to that of the BHL constitutive law. The GH law has the advantage of being somewhat easier to calibrate and implement; for balanced 2-D laminates, it requires only three independent strain functions, whereas the BHL law requires calibration of ten state functions.

Validation of the BHL and GH constitutive laws has been accomplished by performing tests other than those used for their calibrations and comparing the measured responses with the predicted ones. Two test types have been used. The first is the Iosipescu test, which is used to measure the response in pure shear parallel to the fibers. Comparisons between the BHL law and measurements made on a woven Nicalon/SiC composite are shown in Fig. 6. The agreement between theory and experiment is good (within about 5%). Similarly good agreement has been obtained between the predictions of the GH law and pure shear measurements made on a 0°/90° Nicalon/CAS ($CaO-Al_2O_3-SiO_2$) laminate (Ref 15). The second test geometry is an open-hole tensile specimen. Strains are measured at select points around the hole using small, 0.7 mm (0.025 in.), strain gages. Comparisons between these types of measurements on a 0°/90° Nica-

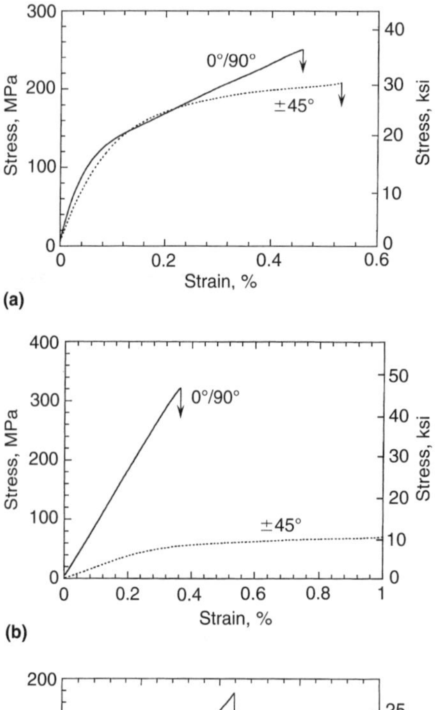

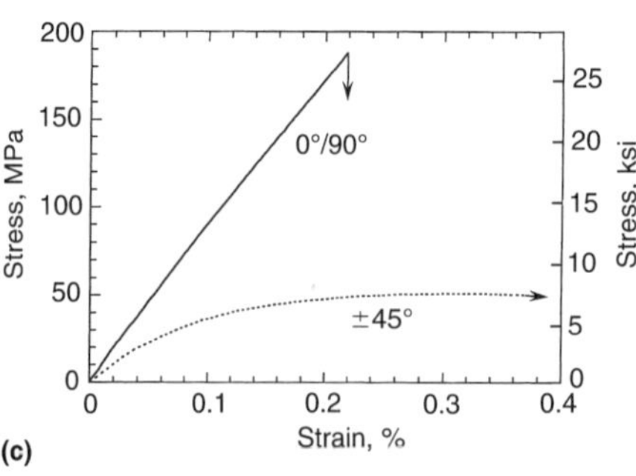

Fig. 5 Stress–strain behaviors of 2-D woven composites in 0°/90° and ±45° orientations (a) Nicalon/SiC (plain weave fabric). Source: Ref 11. (b) Carbon-carbon (plain weave). Source: Ref 13. (c) Al_2O_3/mullite (eight-harness satin weave). Source: Ref 14

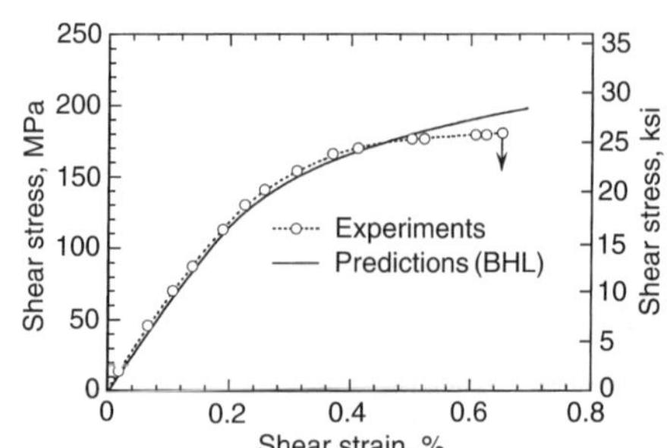

Fig. 6 Comparisons of measured and predicted shear responses of a Nicalon/SiC CFCC. The prediction is based on a finite-element calculation using the BHL constitutive law. Source: Adapted from Ref 19

lon/MAS ($MgO-Al_2O_3-SiO_2$) laminate and those predicted by the GH law are presented in Fig. 7. Again, the agreement is very good, thereby providing additional confidence in the predictive capability of the constitutive law. A related feature that emerges from the latter experiments is that the local strain at the hole edge (in the region of maximum stress concentration) can attain values that are considerably larger than the unnotched tensile failure strain. This difference highlights the importance of size scale and stress gradient effects in the onset of failure. This issue is addressed further in the section "Fracture Initiation" in this article.

Binary Model. One of the deficiencies of both the BHL and GH constitutive laws is the absence of an explicit dependence on the fiber architecture and the nonuniformity of the damage at the scale of the fibers and the fiber tows. This deficiency is expected to be important in cases where the stress gradients exist over distances that are comparable to or smaller than the length scales associated with the microstructure. An alternate modeling approach that provides a more rigorous numerical representation of the behavior of the fibers and/or the fiber tows and the intervening matrix is the so-called binary model (Ref 20, 21). The model can be implemented in two ways. In the first, one-dimensional spring elements are used to represent the individual fibers within a tow, and the surrounding matrix is represented by effective medium elements with the appropriate nonlinear behavior. In this implementation, the model is capable of simulating the interactions between fiber fracture events at the *microscale*, thereby providing a critical theoretical link between the properties of the individual fibers and the properties of the fiber *tows*. In the second implementation, spring elements are used to represent the fiber *tows* (rather than the individual fibers) and the surrounding matrix and transverse fiber tows by effective medium elements. In this implementation, the model represents the material behavior at the *mesoscale*, with information from the microscale computations integrated accordingly. The tow properties may encompass nonlinear deformation caused by fiber failure, matrix cracking, and interface sliding within the tow.

The binary model has numerous attractive features:

- It does not rely on periodicity in the fiber architecture.
- It can readily deal with large spatial variations in the stress.
- It can incorporate any arbitrary nonlinear response in the fibers and the matrix as well as statistical strength distributions.
- It can compute stress and strain distributions in the matrix and fiber elements.

It is ideal for capturing the interactions between stress concentration sites, fiber weave patterns, and multiaxial three-dimensional stress states. Generally, however, the model is more computationally intensive than the homogeneous model and does not lend itself to the simulation of full-scale subelements or components. Its role in structural analysis is expected to be limited to the representation and simulation of those material elements within a component that are most critically stressed and are likely to be the sites of component failure. In this context, the binary model would be combined with an appropriate homogenized constitutive law (such as the one of GH or BHL) to perform global/local analyses, closely analogous to those for textile polymer-matrix composites. (For global/local approaches to polymer composite structures, see, for example, papers by J.D. Whitcomb, A. Tabiei, and their coworkers). The implementation of this approach awaits further developments in the numerical codes and an assessment of the use of the codes in damage and failure prediction.

Stress Distributions in Notched Specimens

The homogeneous nonlinear constitutive laws can be used to calculate the spatial extent of inelastic straining around notches and holes and to assess the role of this inelasticity in mitigating stress concentrations. The results of some finite-element calculations of the crack-tip stresses and the inelastic zones under SSY conditions are plotted in Fig. 8 and 9. The examples are selected to be representative of the behaviors of class II and class III materials. All calculations are based on the GH model. For the purpose of these calculations, the in-plane properties of the class II material are assumed to be isotropic. The tensile stress–strain response is taken to bilinear, with the initial moduli $E_0 = E_{45}$. The change in slope occurs at a critical cracking stress, σ_c, and the tangent moduli beyond cracking are $E_0' = E_{45}' = 0.2E_0$. Similar properties are assumed for the class III material, with the exception that the response in the fiber direction is taken to be linear for all stress levels. Two pertinent features emerge:

- The shape of the inelastic zone for the class III material is distinctly elongated along the loading direction, because of the strong anisotropy of the inelasticity. The length of this zone is $\approx 0.1(K/\sigma_c)^2$. Furthermore, there is essentially no inelasticity directly ahead of the crack tip along the incipient fracture plane. By contrast, the inelastic zone in the class II material is essentially equiaxed and of a size $\approx 0.1(K/\sigma_c)^2$.
- The tensile stresses ahead of the crack in the class II material are reduced considerably to

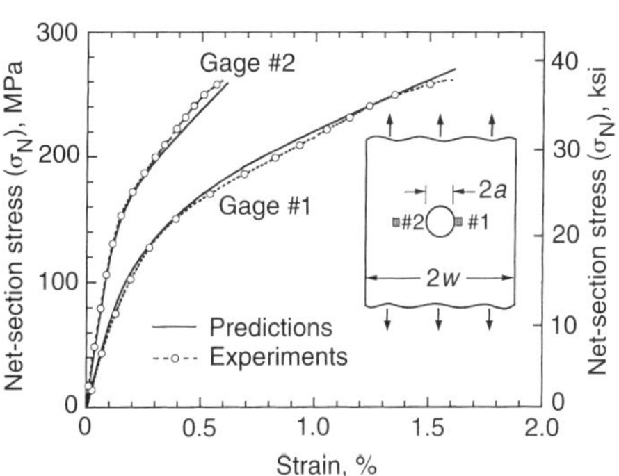

Fig. 7 Comparisons of measured and predicted strains at two locations in an open-hole tensile specimen of a $[0°/90°]_{3s}$ Nicalon/MAS CFCC. The predictions are based on finite-element calculations using the GH constitutive law. Source: Adapted from Ref 2

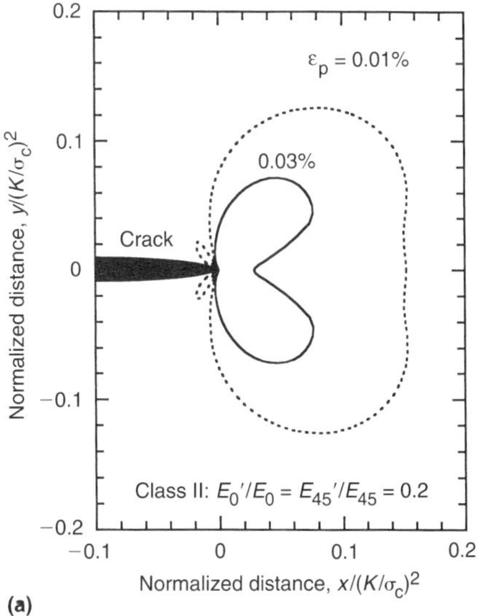

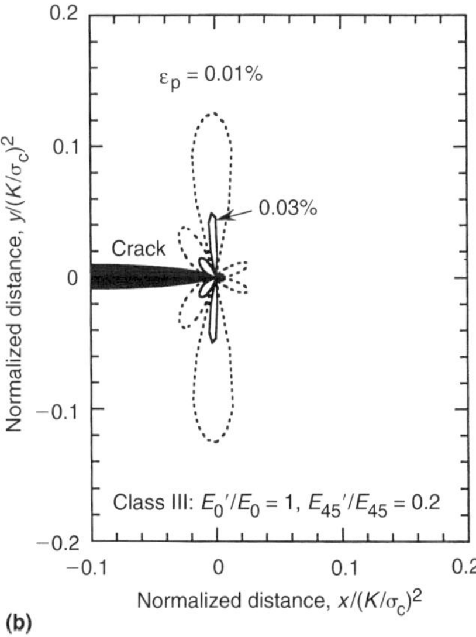

Fig. 8 Inelastic zones around a crack tip under SSY yielding conditions for (a) class II and (b) class III materials. The coordinates *x* and *y* are measured horizontally and vertically, respectively, from the crack tip, and the stresses are applied remotely along the *y*-direction. The effective plastic strain is denoted ε_p. The normalizing distance is $(K/\sigma_c)^2$, where *K* is the applied mode I stress-intensity factor and σ_c is the matrix cracking stress. Courtesy M.Y. He, University of California at Santa Barbara

about half of the elastic values, over distances that are comparable to the inelastic zone size. Only small reductions in stresses are obtained in the class III material, largely because of the absence of inelasticity ahead of the crack tip. Clearly, the efficacy of the inelasticity in stress redistribution is superior in class II materials.

The reduction in the peak stress concentration due to inelasticity in notched specimens can be determined in an approximate way using the method developed by Neuber (Ref 22). Neuber's rule states that the *stress* and *strain concentration factors*, k_σ and k_ε, following the onset of local nonlinear straining are related to the *elastic stress concentration factor*, k_e, through the relation $k_\sigma k_\varepsilon = k_e^2$. Neuber demonstrated this relation to be strictly valid for metals subject to antiplane shear loading (Ref 22). Subsequently, the law has been used extensively in predicting stress concentrations in metals for a variety of notch and loading configurations (Ref 23). A graphical representation of Neuber's rule is shown in Fig. 10. From an operational viewpoint, the law is implemented by finding the intersection point between the tensile stress-strain curve and a hyperbola described by $\sigma\ \varepsilon = k_e^2 \sigma_A \varepsilon_A$, where σ and ε are the local (maximum) stress and strain, and σ_A and ε_A are the corresponding applied values. The stress concentration factor, k_σ, is then the ratio of the stress at the intersection point to the applied stress. In applying Neuber's rule to CFCCs subject to remote loading in the 0°/90° orientation, the relevant stress-strain curve is taken to be the one measured in that same orientation.

Figure 11 shows the stress concentration factors obtained from finite-element calculations for a class II material and those from Neuber's rule for some typical notched geometries. The comparisons indicate that Neuber's rule provides an accurate description of k_σ over a wide range of applied stress and notch shape. The results can be used to estimate the notched strength by combining the stress concentration factor with the measured unnotched tensile strength, assuming the failure criterion to be deterministic. However, as demonstrated in the subsequent section, this approach yields overly conservative estimates of the notched strength and fails to predict size-scale effects. (Similarly conservative estimates are obtained when the stress concentration factors obtained through Neuber's rule are used to predict fatigue lives in notched metal components; empirical methods have been developed to account for these size-scale effects and have found use in fatigue lifing [Ref 23]). Nevertheless, when a conservative design is necessarily required, or as a first step in the design process, this approach is expected to provide some useful guidance.

Fracture Initiation

Fracture initiation occurs essentially when the peak tensile stress exceeds the fiber bundle strength and the inelastic strains become highly localized in the region of extensive fiber fracture. Experiments on several CFCCs indicate that the conditions for fracture initiation depend on the volume of highly stressed material. Direct evidence of these size effects has come from comparisons of the maximum strains that are attained in test specimens with varying stress gradients. For instance, in the $[0°/90°]_{3s}$ Nicalon/MAS composite, the unnotched tensile failure strain is 1.0%, the tensile failure strain in four-point flexure is ≈1.4%, and the failure strain at the edge of the hole in one a center-hole tensile specimen is ≈1.6% (Ref 2, 24). These measurements are consistent with the expectation that the failure strain increases with decreasing volume of material in the most heavily stressed region of a structure.

The volume-dependence of the fracture initiation condition has been modeled using two approaches. The first is based on the *point-stress failure* criterion. Here, fracture is postulated to initiate when a critical stress (taken to be the unnotched tensile strength) is attained over a characteristic length, *d*, ahead of the notch. This approach is analogous to that used to describe cleavage fracture in ferrous alloys containing carbide particles; in the latter case, the characteristic distance correlates with the particle spacing, and the critical stress is dictated by the particle strength (Ref 6). The procedures for its implementation and assessment include:

- Performing nonlinear finite-element calculations of the stresses around the notches
- Calculating the notched tensile strength using several assumed values of the characteristic distance, *d*
- Making comparisons between the predictions and the experimental data in order to infer the characteristic distance and to check on the consistency in the trends with various structural dimensions and geometric features

Figure 12 shows examples for the Nicalon/SiC system (Ref 2). The effects of hole diameter, 2*a*, at a constant value of *a/w* (Fig. 12a) and of specimen width at a constant value of hole diameter (Fig. 12b) are captured remarkably well using this approach, when the characteristic distance is selected to be *d* = 0.75 mm (0.030 in.) Furthermore, in situ observations indicate that strain localization does not occur prior to the ultimate strength, confirming that fracture coincides with the initiation event. Similarly good correlations have been obtained for other CFCCs, including Nicalon/MAS (Ref 2), Sylramic/SiC (Ref 3), and Al_2O_3/mullite (Ref 14). Interestingly, the inferred characteristic distances for these CFCCs lie in the rather narrow range of ≈0.50 to 0.75 mm (0.020 to 0.030 in.). This correlation suggests a commonalty in the size-dependence of fiber bundle failure and strain localization; however, quantitative connections between *d* and the size scales in fiber bundle failure have yet to be established. Nevertheless, the narrowness of the inferred range of *d* suggests that the approach is quite robust and probably applicable to other CFCCs of interest. From an engineering viewpoint, it has the further advantage of being relatively easy to implement and use.

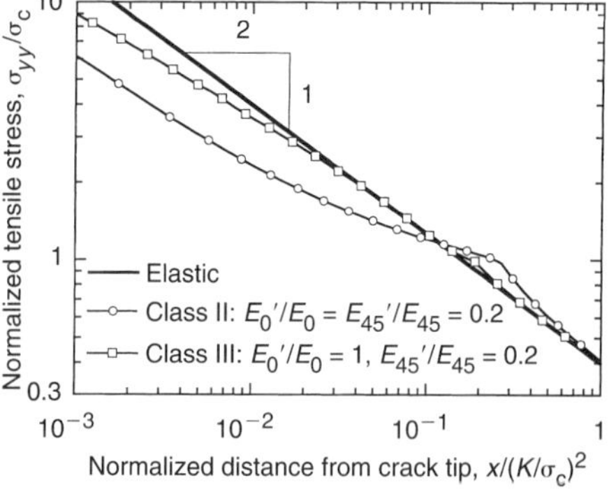

Fig. 9 Stress distribution along the incipient fracture plane, for class II and class III materials as well as in an elastic, isotropic material. The stresses are normalized by the matrix cracking stress, σ_c. The corresponding inelastic zones are plotted in Fig. 8. Courtesy M.Y. He, University of California at Santa Barbara

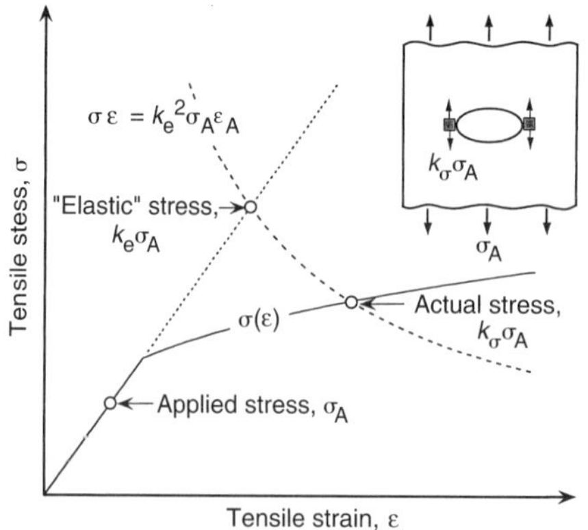

Fig. 10 The procedure used to implement the Neuber law in calculating the stress concentration factor in an elastic-plastic material

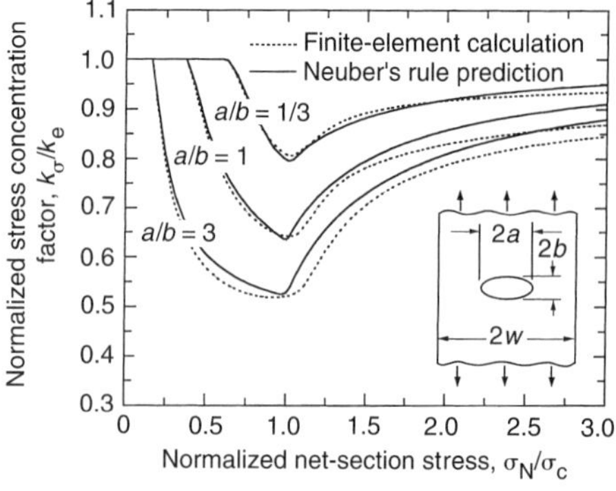

Fig. 11 Effects of inelasticity and notch shape on the stress concentration factors in a class II CFCC. The finite-element results are based on the GH constitutive law, assuming bilinear stress–strain behavior with the parameters shown in the inset of Fig. 8(a). Also shown for comparison are the predictions of the Neuber law. Courtesy X.-Y. Gong, University of California at Santa Barbara

Its main deficiency is in the lack of a sound physical basis.

To further illustrate the size effect, Fig. 12 also shows notched strength predictions stemming from a deterministic (size-independent) failure criterion (labeled $d = 0$). This prediction is based on the assumption that failure occurs when the maximum tensile stress (at the hole edge) reaches the unnotched tensile strength. These predictions strongly underestimate the measured notched strengths and fail to correctly predict the size-scale effects that are found experimentally.

An alternate approach to modeling fracture initiation is based on the premise that the composite strength is probabilistic and follows *weakest-link fracture statistics*. Figure 13 shows the results of a preliminary attempt to assess the probabilistic approach in failure prediction of a Nicalon/SiC CFCC. The predictions are based on finite-element calculations of the stresses in the notched specimens using the GH constitutive law and assuming that the composite strength distribution follows the Weibull function. The comparisons suggest that the composite Weibull modulus is $m = 15 \pm 5$, which is significantly higher than that of the fibers alone ($m \approx 3$–5). This approach is expected to be more robust than the point-stress failure criterion, because it has a stronger mechanistic basis, but is more cumbersome to implement. Furthermore, issues pertaining to the nature and the size of strength-limiting flaws in CFCCs and the broad applicability of weakest-link scaling approaches have yet to be addressed. For instance, the critical "flaw" that leads to fracture in CFCCs is not preexisting (as it is in monolithic ceramics), but rather "evolves" during the straining process and comprises clusters of numerous broken fibers. The size of these clusters dictates the minimum volume that can be used when applying weakest-link scaling laws at the macroscopic level (Ref 25). The binary model, which is described in the section "Constitutive Laws for Inelastic Straining" in this article, is expected to be well suited to addressing these issues.

Crack Propagation

The effects of fiber pullout on crack propagation can be modeled using well-established bridging or cohesive zone concepts. The general approach to this class of problem is to establish the integral equations that describe the crack-tip stress-intensity factor and the crack-opening displacement profile for the specimen geometry and loading configuration of interest, following standard procedures in the stress analysis of cracks. Solutions to these equations (normally obtained through numerical methods) yield results in the form of stress versus crack length. In this context, the key material properties are: the bridging law, which describes the relationship between the crack surface tractions, σ_b, and the crack-opening displacement, u; and the intrinsic crack-tip toughness, K_0.

Closely analogous problems associated with crack bridging in other materials systems have been studied extensively; the materials include ductile particle-reinforced ceramics, short fiber-reinforced cementitious materials, and monolithic ceramics, such as Al_2O_3 and Si_3N_4. (For details on the latter materials and a good treatment of the pertinent mechanics, see the book by B. Lawn, Ref 26, and the references therein.)

A useful pedagogical tool for representing the instability conditions for the propagation of a bridged crack is the tangent construction plot, shown in Fig. 14. (This construction has been used in the context of metals that exhibit R-curve behavior; see, for example, the books by D. Broek, Ref 27, and Kanninen and Popelar, Ref 28.) The plot contains two types of curves: the fracture resistance, K_R, plotted against the crack extension, Δa (beyond the initial notch length); and the stress-intensity factor, K_I, due to the applied load, plotted against the *total* crack length, $\Delta a + a_0$. In this context, the right side of the abscissa is interpreted as Δa and the left side as a_0. The fracture resistance curve initiates at the intrinsic fracture toughness, K_o, (at $\Delta a = 0$) and subsequently increases with crack extension as the bridging zone develops. Under SSB conditions, once the bridging elements furthest from the crack tip disengage, both the bridging zone length and the fracture resistance reach steady-state values, independent of additional crack growth. Using the J-integral, the steady-state resistance, K_{ss}, is given by:

$$\frac{K_{ss}}{K_0} = \sqrt{1 + \frac{\bar{E}\Gamma_b}{K_0^2}} \qquad \text{(Eq 1)}$$

where $\bar{E}$ is the plane-strain composite modulus and Γ_b is the bridging toughness:

$$\Gamma_b = \int_0^{u_0} \sigma_b(u)du \qquad \text{(Eq 2)}$$

The amount of crack extension, Δa_{ss}, needed to achieve the steady state under SSB conditions is dependent somewhat on the shape of the traction law, but scales with the quantity $u_0\bar{E}/\sigma_0$. For typical values of these parameters ($u_0 \approx 10$ to 100 μm, $\bar{E} \approx 100$ GPa, and $\sigma_0 \approx 100$ MPa), this bridging length is in the range of ≈10 to100 mm. The conditions for instability are:

$$K_I = K_R \text{ and } \frac{dK_I}{da}\ \frac{dK_R}{da} \qquad \text{(Eq 3)}$$

These conditions are satisfied when the curve K_I ($\Delta a + a_0$) is tangent to the curve K_R (Δa). The curves shown in Fig. 14 illustrate that when the initial flaw is small in relation to Δa_{ss}, the instability occurs when the crack has grown only a small amount. In this case, the bridging plays a negligible role in the strength. By contrast, when the flaws are comparable or larger than Δa_{ss}, the instability occurs when the crack has

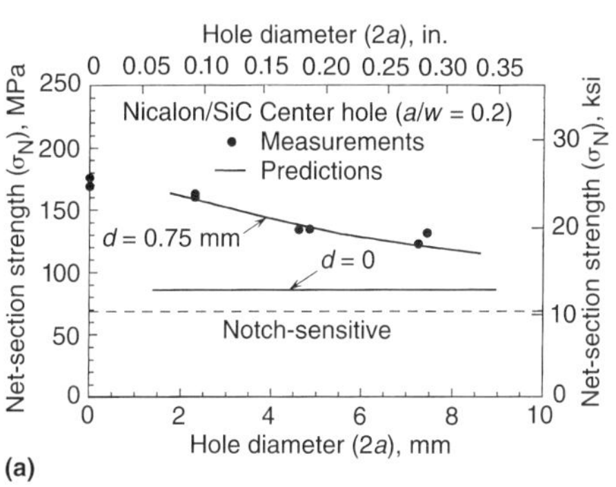

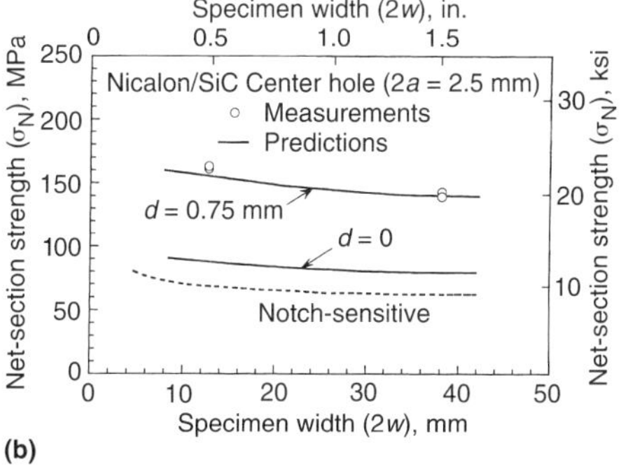

Fig. 12 Comparisons of measured strengths with predictions based on the point-stress failure criterion. The dashed lines show predictions based on the elastic stress concentration factor and the unnotched tensile strength. Hole is centered. d is the characteristic distance. (a) Hole-to-width ratio is constant. (b) Hole diameter is constant, $2a = 2.5$ mm (0.098 in.), as width varies. Source: Adapted from Ref 2

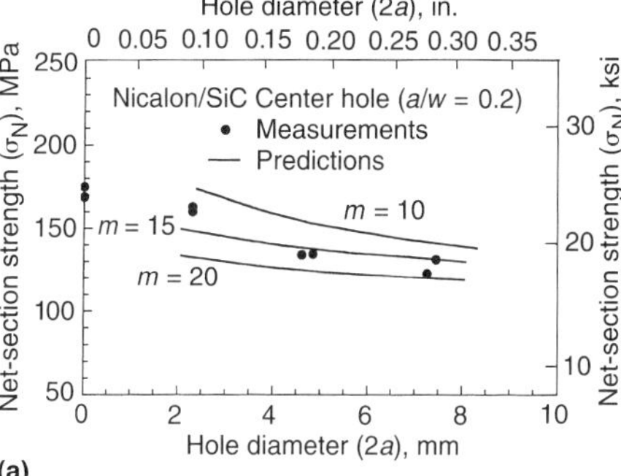

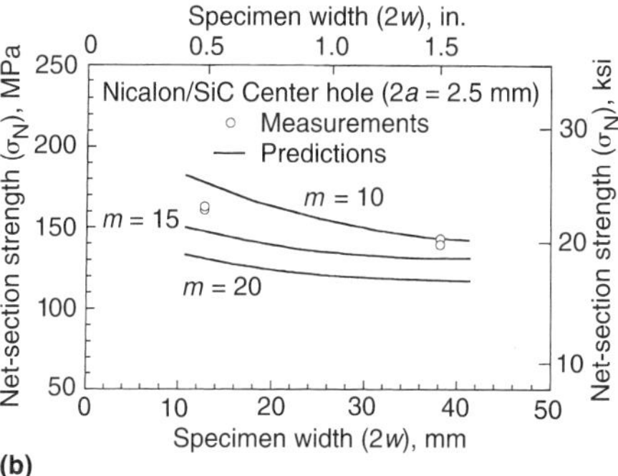

Fig. 13 Comparisons of measured strengths with predictions based on the probabilistic failure model. Hole is centered. (a) Hole-to-width ratio is constant. (b) Hole diameter is constant $2a = 2.5$ mm (0.98 in.), as width varies. Source: Adapted from Ref 2

extended by $\approx \Delta a_{ss}$. In this case, the steady-state toughness is almost fully used in the composite strength.

Rather comprehensive solutions exist for the crack propagation stress in uniaxial tension for a variety of traction law shapes, including rectilinear, linear hardening, linear softening, and parabolic (Ref 29–32). All are based on the assumption that the adjacent composite material remains *elastic*; the coupled effects of inelastic deformation and fiber pullout have yet to be explored. Representative results are plotted in Fig. 15 for center-cracked specimens of infinite width ($a/w \approx 0$) for the linear softening traction law (Ref 32). The latter traction law is selected here because it is consistent with the prediction from a shear lag analysis of a single bridging fiber. The result of this analysis is:

$$\sigma_b(u) = \frac{2\tau f_0 h}{R}\left[1 - \frac{u}{h}\right] = \sigma_0\left[1 - \frac{u}{h}\right] \quad \text{(Eq 4)}$$

where τ is the interfacial sliding stress, f_0 is the volume fraction of fibers that are aligned parallel to the loading direction, h is the fiber pullout length, and R is the fiber diameter. The results are presented in terms of the propagation stress, σ_p, normalized by the peak stress, σ_0, in the traction law and plotted against a nondimensional crack length, α, defined by (Ref 29, 32):

$$\alpha \equiv \frac{a_0\sigma_0}{u_0\bar{E}} \quad \text{(Eq 5)}$$

where $2a_0$ is the initial crack length and u_0 is the critical crack-opening displacement upon complete disengagement of the bridging elements (equivalent to h in the shear lag result in Eq 4). The normalizing crack length, $u_0\bar{E}/\sigma_0$, is the characteristic bridging-length scale that dictates Δa_{ss}. The effects of the intrinsic toughness are incorporated into a normalized toughness parameter, λ, defined by (Ref 32):

$$\lambda \equiv \frac{\Gamma_0}{\sigma_0 u_0} = \frac{K_0^2}{\sigma_0 u_0 \bar{E}} \quad \text{(Eq 6)}$$

where Γ_0 is the intrinsic fracture energy (related to the intrinsic fracture toughness, K_0, through the Irwin relation, $\Gamma_0 = K_0^2/\bar{E}$), and the normalizing fracture energy, $\sigma_0 u_0$, is proportional to the bridging toughness. The results show three main regimes of behavior, governed mainly by the value of α. When the initial crack length is very small ($\alpha \leq 0.01$), the propagation stress is dictated by the intrinsic toughness, K_0, in accordance with the Griffith relation (written in nondimensional form):

$$\frac{\sigma_p}{\sigma_0} = \left[\frac{\lambda}{\pi\alpha}\right]^{1/2} \quad \text{(Eq 7)}$$

The predictions of Eq 7 are plotted as a series of dashed lines on the left side of Fig. 15. In this regime, crack bridging has negligible effect on the crack stability, as illustrated by the tangent construction plot in Fig. 14. At the other extreme, where the initial crack length is very large ($\alpha > 1$), the propagation stress again follows the Griffith relation, except now the pertinent toughness is the steady-state composite toughness; this defines the SSB regime. In this regime, the relation between the strength and the initial crack length can be expressed as:

$$\frac{\sigma_p}{\sigma_0} = \left[\frac{\lambda + 1/2}{\pi\alpha}\right]^{1/2} \quad \text{(Eq 8)}$$

These predictions are shown by the dotted lines on the right side of Fig. 15. Between these extremes, the strength is predicted by a LSB model. The predictions of the LSB model converge with the nonbridging prediction and the SSB prediction when the initial flaw size approaches the respective limiting value, as required. Furthermore, because the flaws of interest are generally smaller than the characteristic bridging-length scale, $u_0\bar{E}/\sigma_0$, SSB conditions are rarely achieved, and hence the LSB model is needed to describe the notch sensitivity of the propagation stress.

The bridging law parameters can be determined in one of several ways. The first is based on micromechanical models, such as the shear lag model that leads to the result in Eq 4, coupled with independent measurement of the pertinent material parameters, including the sliding stress and the pullout length. The accuracy of the resulting bridging law depends on the accuracy of these measurements, recognizing that some are difficult to make in a manner that accurately reflects the fracture process. For instance, the sliding stress that is obtained by common measurement techniques, such as by fiber push-in (Ref 33) or push-through tests (Ref 34), is usually higher than the value that is representative of the pullout process. The discrepancy is the result of the difference in the sign of the Poisson strain; in some cases, it may also be associated with a dependence of the sliding stress on the extent of interface sliding (because of wear, for example, Ref 35). The accuracy of the bridging law depends also on the fidelity of the micromechanical model upon which the law is based. Notwithstanding these complications, micromechanical models are attractive and popular, because they form a critical link between the physics of the pullout process and the associated macroscopic mechanical response.

The second approach involves either direct or semidirect mechanical measurements. The most direct method is to perform a tensile test on a deeply notched specimen and measure the variation in the load with the crack-opening displacement in the regime beyond the load maximum (Ref 35, 36). Although direct, this type of test is prone to instabilities near the load maximum, a consequence of the elastic unloading of the material away from the crack plane when the load falls from its peak value. Indeed, in cases where the values of the bridging stresses and the pullout lengths are small, catastrophic fracture occurs *at* the load maximum, leading to complete separation of the two crack faces and the loss of all information about the bridging parameters. An example of a pullout test on a $[0°/90°]_{3s}$ Nicalon/MAS CFCC is shown in Fig. 16. Most

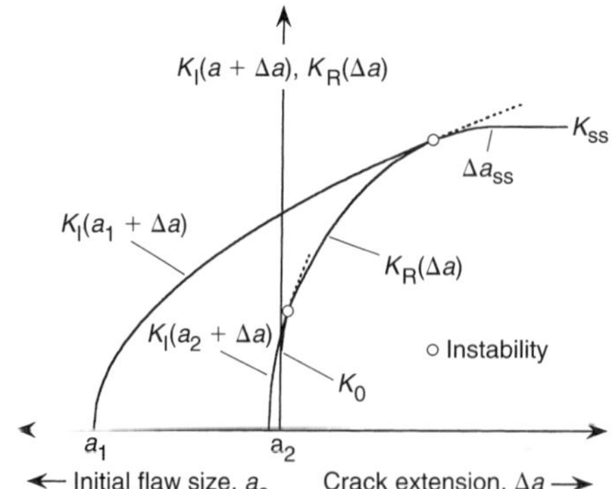

Fig. 14 Tangent construction plot used to represent the stability of bridged cracks. Fracture resistance (K_R) is plotted against crack extension (Δa). Stress-intensity factor, K_I, is plotted against total crack length.

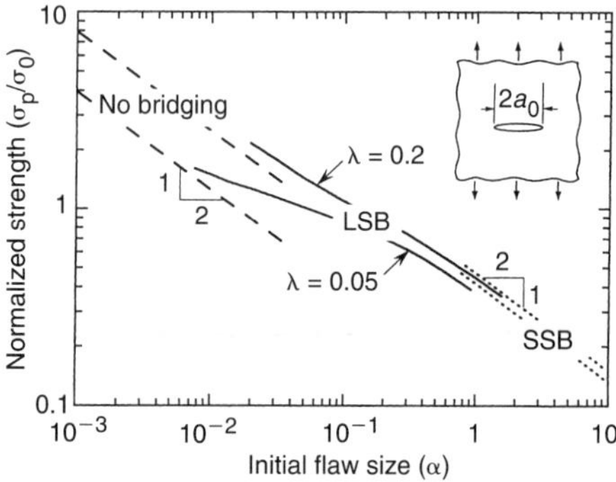

Fig. 15 Normalized strength vs. nondimensional crack length (α). Effects of flaw size (α) and the toughness (λ) on the crack propagation stress (σ_p) for $a/w << 1$. The bridging law is assumed to be linear softening, with a peak stress, σ_0. The dotted lines on the right are the SSB predictions and are applicable when $\alpha > 1$. The dashed lines on the left side represent the behavior in the absence of crack bridging and are applicable when $\alpha < 0.01$. Source: Adapted from Ref 32

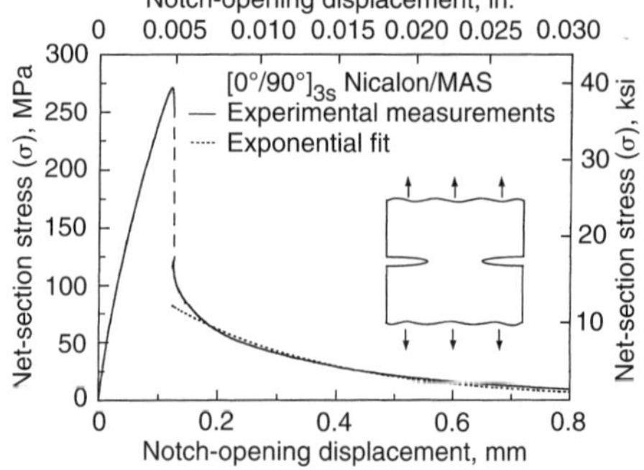

Fig. 16 Measurement of the pullout response of a $[0°/90°]_{3s}$ Nicalon/MAS CFCC and the fitting of the exponential function in the regime following complete fiber fracture (Eq 9). Source: Adapted from Ref 35

of the information about the bridging is extracted, with the exception of the portion immediately following the load maximum (shown by the dashed line). In this case, the bridging law in the pullout regime is well described by an exponential softening function, given by (Ref 35, 36):

$$\sigma_b = \sigma_* \exp(-u/u_*) \quad \text{(Eq 9)}$$

where σ_* is the peak pullout stress and u_* is a characteristic displacement. The inferred values of the bridging parameters are $\sigma_* \approx 100$ MPa and $u_* \approx 300$ μm. In addition to its use in fitting experimental data of this type, the use of the exponential function can be further justified on the basis of a micromechanical model of fiber *bundle* pullout through a shear lag analysis. The analysis is essentially identical to that used for pullout of a single fiber, but incorporates the distribution in pullout lengths. When this distribution is exponential, the analysis yields an exponential bridging law, essentially identical to Eq 9, with the characteristic displacement, u_*, being equivalent to the average pullout length, $\bar{h}$, and the bridging stress, σ_*, related to the other parameters by (Ref 35):

$$\sigma_* = \frac{2\tau f_0 \bar{h}}{R} \quad \text{(Eq 10)}$$

This direct approach is preferred for determining the bridging parameters.

In instances where the bridging parameters cannot be measured directly through notched tension tests, the parameters can be obtained through a semidirect method, using test geometries that promote stable crack growth and yield data that are amenable to analysis. One such method is based on edge-notched flexure tests. Measurements are made of the load–deflection response as well as the crack length. The bridging parameters are then inferred by fitting the data (in the form of an *R*-curve, for example) with the predictions of a bridging model, using an assumed form for the bridging law. One example is shown in Fig. 4 (Ref 10). In general, the uniqueness of such a fit may be questionable, because of the assumptions about the form of the traction law and the intrinsic toughness, and is therefore inferior to the more direct approach described previously. A related indirect method for deducing the traction law is through a combination of high-resolution crack-opening displacement measurements ahead of a notch and numerical simulations (Ref 37).

A variation on this semi-direct method involves measurement of either the load versus displacement response or the load versus *crack mouth-opening displacement* (CMOD) response of an edge-notched three-point flexure specimen once the matrix crack has propagated across the *entire* cross section (Ref 38). In this regime, the response is dictated entirely by fiber pullout, independent of the intrinsic toughness, K_0. This loading geometry can be analyzed fairly accurately using beam theory. For this purpose, the two halves of the broken composite are treated as rigid blocks; the bridged crack is assumed to be an infinitesimal plastic hinge, and the crack-opening profile is assumed to be linear across the cross section. If the traction law follows an exponential form (Eq 9), the predicted load-CMOD response in this regime is given by (Ref 38):

$$P = \frac{4B\sigma_* W^2 u_*^2}{S\delta^2} \times \left[1 - \left(1 + \frac{\delta(W-a_0)}{Wu_*}\right)\exp\left(-\frac{\delta(W-a_0)}{Wu_*}\right)\right] \quad \text{(Eq 11)}$$

where P is the applied load, B is the specimen thickness, W is the specimen width, a_0 is the notch depth, S is the loading span, and δ is the notch mouth-opening displacement. An analogous result can be derived for the load-displacement response. The fit of Eq 11 to the measured P-δ curve for a [0°/90°] Si_3N_4/BN composite is shown in Fig. 17.

The fracture stress is the larger of the critical stress needed for fracture initiation, σ_i, and that needed for propagation, σ_p. Comparisons of σ_i and σ_p for a $[0°/90°]_{3s}$ Nicalon/MAS CFCC are shown in Fig. 18. The traction law for this material is shown in Fig. 16, and the initiation condition is calculated using the point-stress failure criterion, as described previously. When the notches are short, the strength is dominated by the initiation event. A transition to propagation-controlled fracture occurs at a critical value of notch length, dependent on the value of the characteristic length in the point-stress criterion. Using a value, d = 0.5 mm (0.02 in.), that is consistent with the experimental data in the short notch regime, the transition is predicted to occur at $a \approx 80$ mm (3 in.). The transition shifts rapidly to larger values of crack length as the characteristic length increases. It also shifts in this direction when the notches are more blunt, for example, circular holes (Ref 2). These results suggest that fiber pullout (following fiber fracture) contributes negligibly to the notched strength of this particular CFCC, except in cases where the initial crack length is very large and probably outside the range that is relevant to most CFCC components. Given the rather large values of bridging stress and pullout lengths obtained in this composite, it is surmised that the pullout process is likely to be comparatively unimportant in the notched tensile strength of other class II CFCCs. However, it may play an important role in preventing catastrophic fracture under displacement-controlled modes of loading. Additional work is needed to confirm this hypothesis and to assess the importance of bridging in the fracture properties of other classes of CFCCs.

Environmental Degradation

One of the most significant problems hindering the widespread use of SiC-based CFCCs is their susceptibility to oxidation in the targeted service environments. A particularly insidious form of oxidation occurs internally within these CFCCs, without significant gain or loss of material. The process occurs by oxygen ingress through matrix cracks, followed by reaction of the oxygen with the fibers and the fiber coatings (Ref 3, 39–42). Commonly, the reactions result in the elimination of the fiber coatings (carbon or boron-nitrogen) and the formation of silicate glasses that bond the fibers to the matrix. Once bonding has occurred, the damage tolerance associated with sliding interfaces is lost. The problem is particularly severe at intermediate temperatures, 600 to 900 °C (1100 to 1650 °F) and is thus known as a "pesting" phenomenon. At lower temperatures, the reaction kinetics are too slow to have a substantial impact, and at higher temperatures, a protective oxide layer forms on the composite surface, which seals the surface and inhibits oxygen ingress. The embrittlement phenomenon can be overlooked during routine mechanical property characterization studies, which normally focus on ambient temperature and high-temperature properties, 1100 to 1300 °C (2000 to 2400 °F), with the tacit assumption

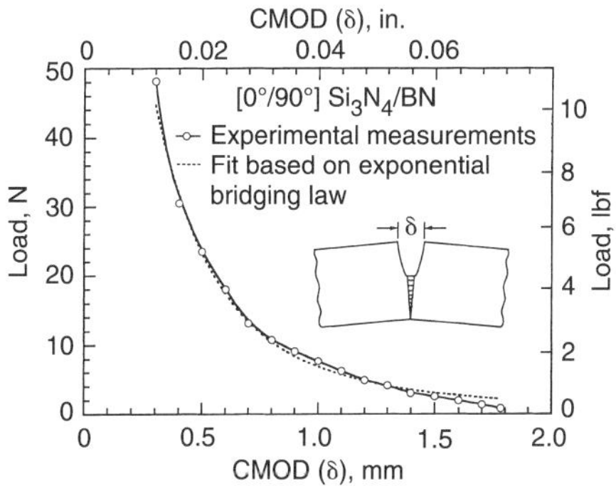

Fig. 17 Load vs. crack mouth-opening displacement (CMOD). Measurement of the traction law from the load-CMOD response following complete cracking in an edge-notched flexure specimen of a [0°/90°] Si_3N_4/BN composite. Source: Adapted from Ref 38

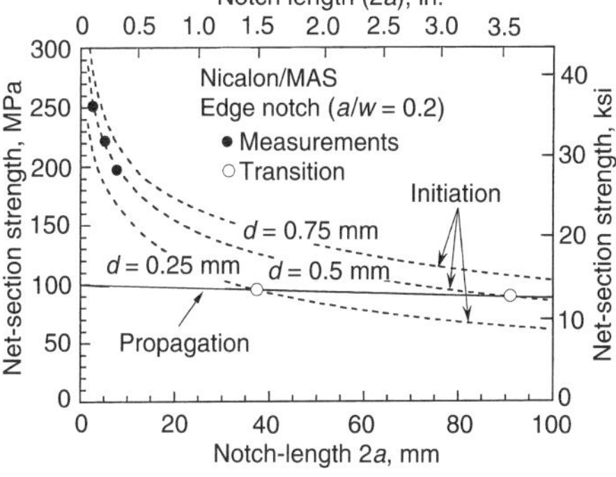

Fig. 18 Stresses required for fracture initiation and crack propagation in double-edge-notched tensile specimens of a Nicalon/MAS CFCC. The transition from initiation-controlled to propagation-controlled fracture occurs at the intersection points of the curves, indicated by the open symbols. Source: Adapted from Ref 2

that the properties vary monotonically with temperature. It can be identified experimentally by performing stress-rupture tests on tensile specimens subject to a temperature gradient along the specimen length that spans the embrittlement range, from less than 600 °C (1100 °F) to greater than 900 °C (1650 °F). The temperature at the location of failure corresponds with the most severe embrittlement at the prescribed stress level (Ref 39). Corroborating evidence of the embrittlement can be obtained from fracture surface examinations. Because oxygen ingress occurs along matrix cracks, the embrittlement problem is prevalent at stresses above the matrix-cracking limit and is exacerbated by conditions that accelerate the rate of oxygen ingress or compromise the integrity of the protective oxide layer. Such conditions are obtained during thermal and/or mechanical cycling.

The loss in damage tolerance associated with cyclic mechanical loading in notched specimens in the intermediate-temperature regime is demonstrated in Fig. 19. The material is comprised of Sylramic SiC fibers in a plain weave architecture and a SiC matrix. The unnotched *low cycle fatigue* (LCF) threshold at 815 °C (1500 °F) is dictated by the matrix-cracking stress, 150 to 160 MPa (22 to 23 ksi). Above the cracking stress, fracture occurs rapidly, typically in <100 hours. Moreover, the LCF curve for stresses slightly above the threshold is extremely shallow, indicating a very strong sensitivity of fracture time to applied stress. The matrix-cracking stress similarly dictates the LCF threshold for open-hole tensile specimens. That is, once the cracking stress is exceeded locally, even over a very small distance ahead of the hole, fracture ensues. Consequently, a reasonably accurate prediction of the threshold stress is obtained through the *elastic* stress concentration factor in combination with the matrix-cracking stress. This highly notch-sensitive behavior suggests the need for an extremely conservative design approach for CFCC structures containing holes when this embrittlement mechanism is operative. Furthermore, it precludes the exploitation of the inelastic straining mechanisms that operate in these materials and impart good damage tolerance in nonoxidizing environments.

The pathway for achieving significant improvements in the long-term durability of this class of composite remains ill-defined. One approach that has received renewed interest in recent years involves the use of environmental barrier coatings. The robustness of such coatings and their effectiveness in improving durability of the underlying CFCC structures remains to be demonstrated.

Conclusions

Many of the features needed for damage-tolerant design of CFCC components are available for use by the engineering community. The general framework is consistent with that used for other structural materials, most notably metals. The important features that have been developed specifically for CFCCs include: nonlinear constitutive laws for inelasticity at the macroscopic scale; rudimentary models of fracture initiation at a crack or notch tip, including the effects of size scales; and bridging models to describe the effects of fiber pullout on crack propagation. The models can be calibrated through the use of relatively straightforward test procedures. Ongoing activities in the development of numerical models to simulate the response of CFCCs at the microscopic and mesoscopic scales are expected to significantly enhance the predictive capability of the deformation and fracture models. The mechanics of other material phenomena, including oxidative embrittlement, creep, and fatigue, are expected also to emerge once CFCCs are used more extensively in thermostructural components.

Other characteristics of CFCCs are discussed in "Properties and Performance of Ceramic-Matrix and Carbon-Carbon Composites" in this Volume.

Appendix: The Genin-Hutchinson Constitutive Law

The Genin-Hutchinson constitutive law is valid for proportional in-plane loading of fiber composites with balanced fiber architectures. The following summary applies specifically to 2-D orthogonal architectures.

When the principal axes of loading (denoted I and II) are aligned with the two fiber axes, the principal strains, ε_I and ε_{II}, are assumed to be related to the principal stresses, σ_I and σ_{II}, through the functions, f_0 and f_{0T}, via:

$$\varepsilon_I = f_0(\sigma_I) + f_{0t}(\sigma_{II}) \quad \text{(Eq 12a)}$$

$$\varepsilon_{II} = f_0(\sigma_{II}) + f_{0T}(\sigma_I) \quad \text{(Eq 12b)}$$

The two functions represent the stress-strain measurements in a 0°/90° tension test, with f_0 obtained from the axial strains (parallel to the loading direction) and f_{0T} obtained from the transverse strains. Similarly, when the principal straining axes are at 45° to the two fiber directions, the principal strains and stresses are assumed to be related by:

$$\varepsilon_I = f_{45}(\sigma_I) + f_{45T}(\sigma_{II}) \quad \text{(Eq 13a)}$$

$$\varepsilon_{II} = f_{45}(\sigma_{II}) + f_{45T}(\sigma_I) \quad \text{(Eq 13b)}$$

where f_{45} and f_{45T} are obtained from a tension test performed in the $\pm 45°$ orientation. Consideration of the special case of equibiaxial tensile loading ($\sigma_I = \sigma_{II} = \sigma$) requires that the four functions be related through:

$$f_{45T}(\sigma) = f_0(\sigma) + f_{0T}(\sigma) - f_{45}(\sigma) \quad \text{(Eq 14)}$$

Hence, only three of the stress-strain curves are independent functions.

For the purpose of implementing the constitutive model into a finite-element program, Eq 12 and 13 are inverted such that:

$$\sigma_I = \Sigma_0(\varepsilon_I, \varepsilon_{II}) \quad \text{(Eq 15a)}$$

$$\sigma_{II} = \Sigma_0(\varepsilon_{II}, \varepsilon_I) \quad \text{(Eq 15b)}$$

for the 0°/90° orientation, and

$$\sigma_I = \Sigma_{45}(\varepsilon_I, \varepsilon_{II}) \quad \text{(Eq 16a)}$$

$$\sigma_{II} = \Sigma_{45}(\varepsilon_{II}, \varepsilon_I) \quad \text{(Eq 16b)}$$

for the $\pm$ 45° orientation. The reductions in the stresses due to matrix cracking (the so-called "stress deficits") are:

$$\Delta\sigma_I^0 = \frac{E_0}{(1-\nu_0^2)}(\varepsilon_I + \nu_0\varepsilon_{II}) - \Sigma_0(\varepsilon_I, \varepsilon_{II}) \quad \text{(Eq 17a)}$$

$$\Delta\sigma_{II}^0 = \frac{E_0}{(1-\nu_0^2)}(\varepsilon_{II} + \nu_0\varepsilon_I) - \Sigma_0(\varepsilon_{II}, \varepsilon_I) \quad \text{(Eq 17b)}$$

for the 0°/90° orientation, where E_0 and ν_0 are the Young's modulus and Poisson's ratio, respectively. Similarly, in the $\pm 45°$ orientation, the stress deficits are:

$$\Delta\sigma_I^{45} = \frac{E_{45}}{(1-\nu_{45}^2)}(\varepsilon_I + \nu_{45}\varepsilon_{II}) - \Sigma_{45}(\varepsilon_I, \varepsilon_{II}) \quad \text{(Eq 18a)}$$

$$\Delta\sigma_{II}^{45} = \frac{E_{45}}{(1-\nu_{45}^2)}(\varepsilon_{II} + \nu_{45}\varepsilon_I) - \Sigma_{45}(\varepsilon_{II}, \varepsilon_I) \quad \text{(Eq 18b)}$$

where E_{45} and ν_{45} are the corresponding Young's modulus and Poisson's ratio in the $\pm 45°$ orientation.

When the axes of the principal strains are oriented at an arbitrary angle, θ, to the fiber directions, the stress deficits along the principal strain axes are obtained through an interpolation be-

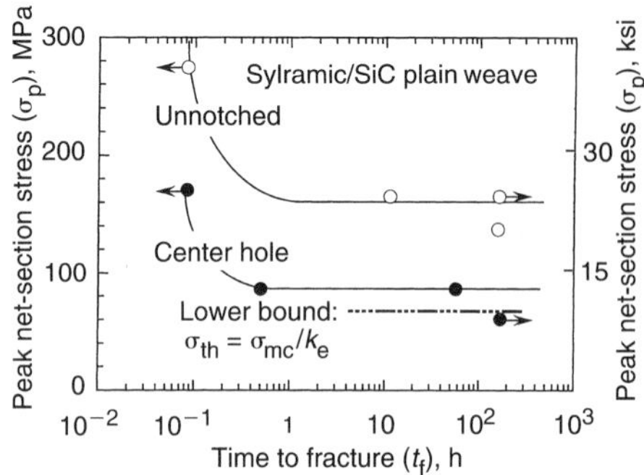

Fig. 19 Low cycle fatigue (LCF) behavior of a SiC-based CFCC at a temperature of 815 °C (1500 °F). Arrows pointing to the right indicate runout; arrows pointing to the left indicate test results obtained from uniaxial tension tests. The loading spectrum comprised relatively rapid loading and unloading (each taking about 1 min) and a hold time of 2 h at the peak stress. σ_{th} is the threshold stress in the open-hole specimen, and σ_{mc} is the matrix-cracking stress. Source: Adapted from Ref 3

tween the stress deficits in the 0°/90° and ±45° orientations in accordance with:

$$\Delta\sigma_I = \Delta\sigma_I^0 \cos^2 2\theta + \Delta\sigma_I^{45} \sin^2 2\theta \quad \text{(Eq 19a)}$$

$$\Delta\sigma_{II} = \Delta\sigma_{II}^0 \cos^2 2\theta + \Delta\sigma_{II}^{45} \sin^2 2\theta \quad \text{(Eq 19b)}$$

Upon transforming these stress deficits back to the fiber axes (denoted 1 and 2), the full in-plane stress-strain relations are obtained:

$$\sigma_1 = \frac{E_0}{1-\nu_0^2}(\varepsilon_1 + \nu_0\varepsilon_2) - \Delta\sigma_I \cos^2\theta - \Delta\sigma_{II}\sin^2\theta \quad \text{(Eq 20a)}$$

$$\sigma_2 = \frac{E_0}{1-\nu_0^2}(\varepsilon_2 + \nu_0\varepsilon_1) - \Delta\sigma_I \sin^2\theta - \Delta\sigma_{II}\cos^2\theta \quad \text{(Eq 20b)}$$

$$\tau_{12} = \frac{E_{45}}{2(1+\nu_{45})}\gamma_{12} - (\Delta\sigma_I - \Delta\sigma_{II})\sin\theta\cos\theta \quad \text{(Eq 20c)}$$

ACKNOWLEDGMENTS

The author gratefully acknowledges the Air Force Office of Scientific Research, under Contract F49620-99-1-0259 monitored by Thomas Hahn, for financial support of the activity on CFCCs at the University of California at Santa Barbara.

REFERENCES

1. A.G. Evans and F.W. Zok, The Physics and Mechanics of Fibre-Reinforced Brittle Matrix Composites, *J. Mater. Sci.,* Vol 29, 1994, p 3857–3896
2. J.C. McNulty, F.W. Zok, G.M. Genin, and A.G. Evans, Notch-Sensitivity of Fiber-Reinforced Ceramic Matrix Composites: Effects of Inelastic Straining and Volume-Dependent Strength, *J. Am. Ceram. Soc.,* Vol 82 (No. 5), 1999, p 1217–1228
3. J.C. McNulty, M.Y. He, and F.W. Zok, Notch Sensitivity of Fatigue Life in a Sylramic/SiC Composite at Elevated Temperature, *Compos. Sci. Technol.,* in press 2001
4. J.M. Whitney and R.J. Nuismer, Stress Fracture Criteria for Laminated Composites Containing Stress Concentrations, *J. Compos. Mater.,* Vol 8 (No. 3) 1974, p 253–265
5. J. Awerbuch and M.S. Madhukar, Notched Strength of Composite Laminates: Predictions and Experiments–A Review, *J. Reinf. Plast. Compos.,* Vol 4 (No. 1), 1985, p 3–159
6. R.O. Ritchie, R.F. Knott, and J.R. Rice, On the Relationship Between Critical Tensile Stress and Fracture Toughness in Mild Steel, *J. Mech. Phys. Solids,* Vol 21, 1973, p 395–410
7. J.W. Hutchinson and A.G. Evans, Mechanics of Materials: Top-Down Approaches to Fracture, *Acta Mater.,* Vol 48 (No. 1), 2000, p 125–135
8. F.E. Heredia, S.M. Spearing, T.J. Mackin, M.Y. He, A.G. Evans, P. Mosher, and P. Brønsted, Notch Effects in Carbon Matrix Composites, *J. Am. Ceram. Soc.,* Vol 77 (No. 11), 1994, p 2817–2827
9. F. Zok and C.L. Hom, Large Scale Bridging in Brittle Matrix Composites, *Acta Metall. Mater.,* Vol 38, 1990, p 1895–1904
10. F. Zok, O. Sbaizero, C.L. Hom, and A.G. Evans, The Mode I Fracture Resistance of a Laminated Fiber Reinforced Ceramic, *J. Am. Ceram. Soc.,* Vol 74, 1991, p 187–193
11. C. Cady, F.E. Heredia, and A.G Evans, In-Plane Mechanical Properties of Several Ceramic Matrix Composites, *J. Am. Ceram. Soc.,* Vol 78, 1995, p 2065–2078
12. C.G. Levi, J.Y. Yang, B.J. Dalgleish, F.W. Zok, and A.G. Evans, Processing and Performance of an All-Oxide Ceramic Composite, *J. Am. Ceram. Soc.,* Vol 81 (No. 8), 1998, p 2077–2086
13. K.R. Turner, J.S. Speck, and A.G. Evans, Mechanisms of Deformation and Failure in Carbon-Matrix Composites Subject to Tensile and Shear Loading, *J. Am. Ceram. Soc.,* Vol 78, 1995, p 1841–1848
14. J.A. Heathcote, X.-Y. Gong, J. Yang, U. Ramamurty, and F.W. Zok, In-Plane Mechanical Properties of an All-Oxide Ceramic Composite, *J. Am. Ceram. Soc.,* Vol 82 (No. 10), 1999, p 2721–2730
15. G.M. Genin and J.W. Hutchinson, Composite Laminates in Plane Stress: Constitutive Modeling and Stress Redistribution Due to Matrix Cracking, *J. Am. Ceram. Soc.,* Vol 80 (No. 5), 1997, p 1245–1255
16. D.B. Marshall, B.N. Cox, and A.G. Evans, The Mechanics of Matrix Cracking in Brittle Matrix Composites, *Acta Metall.,* Vol 33 (No. 11) 1985, p 2013–2021
17. J.W. Hutchinson and H.M. Jensen, Models of Fiber Debonding and Pullout in Brittle Matrix Composites, *Mech. Mater.,* Vol 9 (No. 2), 1990, p 139–163

18 A.G. Evans, J.M. Domergue, and E. Vagaggini, Methodology for Relating the Tensile Constitutive Behavior of Ceramic Composites to Constituent Properties, *J. Am. Ceram. Soc.,* Vol 77, 1994, p 1425–1435

19. A. Burr, F. Hild, and F.A. Leckie, Continuum Description of Damage in Ceramic-Matrix Composites, *Eur. J. Mech A-Solids,* Vol 16 (No. 1), 1997, p 53–78
20. M.A. McGlockton, B.N. Cox, and R.M. McMeeking, "A Binary Model of Textile Composites: High Failure Strain and Work of Fracture in 3D Weaves," to be published, 2001
21. M.A. McGlockton, R.M. McMeeking, and B.N. Cox, "A Model for the Axial Strength of Unidirectional Ceramic Matrix Fiber Composites," to be published, 2001
22. H. Neuber, Theory of Stress Concentration for Shear-Strained Prismatic Bodies with Arbitrary Non-Linear Stress-Strain Laws, *J. Appl. Mech., (Trans. ASME),* Vol E28, 1961, p 544
23. J.A. Bannantine, J.J. Comer, and J.L. Handrock, *Fundamentals of Metal Fatigue Analysis,* Prentice Hall, Englewood Cliffs, NJ, p 124–157
24. J.C. McNulty and F.W. Zok, Application of Weakest-Link Fracture Statistics to Fiber-Reinforced Ceramic Matrix Composites, *J. Am. Ceram. Soc.,* Vol 80 (No 6), 1997, p 1535–1543
25. M. Ibnabdeljalil and W.A. Curtin, Strength and Reliability of Fiber-Reinforced Composites: Localized Load-Sharing and Associated Size Effects, *Int. J. Solids Struct.,* Vol 34, 1997, p 2649–2668
26. B. Lawn, *Fracture of Brittle Solids,* 2nd ed., Cambridge University Press, Cambridge, 1993
27. D. Broek, *Elementary Engineering Fracture Mechanics,* 4th Ed., Martinus Nijhoff Publishers, Dordrecht, The Netherlands, 1986
28. M.F. Kanninen and C.H. Popelar, *Advanced Fracture Mechanics,* Oxford University Press, New York, 1985
29. Z. Suo, S. Ho, and X. Gong, Notch Ductile-to-Brittle Transition Due to Localized Inelastic Band, *J. Eng. Mater. Technol.,* Vol 115, 1993, p 319–326
30. B. Budiansky and Y.L. Cui, On the Tensile Strength of a Fiber-Reinforced Ceramic Composite Containing a Crack-Like Flaw, *J. Mech. Phys. Solids,* Vol 42 (No. 1), 1994, p 1–19
31. B.N. Cox and C.S. Lo, Simple Approximations for Bridged Cracks in Fibrous Composites, *Acta Metall. Mater.,* Vol 40 (No. 7), 1992, p 1487–1496
32. G. Bao and F. Zok, On the Strength of Ductile Particle Reinforced Brittle Matrix Composites, *Acta Metall. Mater.,* Vol 41 (No. 12), 1993, p 3515–3524
33. D.B. Marshall, An Indentation Method for Measuring Matrix-Fiber Frictional Stresses in Ceramic Composites, *J. Am. Ceram. Soc.,* Vol 67 (No. 12), 1984, p C259–C260
34. T.J. Mackin and F. Zok, Fiber Bundle Push-Out: A Technique for the Measurement of Interfacial Sliding Properties, *J. Am. Ceram. Soc.,* Vol 75, 1992, p 3169–3171
35. J.C. McNulty and F.W. Zok, Low Cycle Fatigue of Nicalon Fiber-Reinforced Ceramic Composites, *Compos. Sci. Technol.,* Vol 59, 1999, p 1597–1607
36. P. Brenet, F. Conchin, G. Fantozzi, P. Reynaud, and C. Tallaron, Direct Measurement of Crack Bridging Tractions: a New Approach to the Fracture of Ceramic Composites, *Compos. Sci. Technol.,* Vol 56, 1996, p 817–823
37. B.N. Cox and D.B. Marshall, The Determination of Crack Bridging Forces, *Int. J. Fract.,* Vol 49, 1991, p 159–176
38. J.C. McNulty, M.R. Begley, and F.W. Zok, In-Plane Fracture Resistance of a Cross-Ply Fibrous Monolith, *J. Am. Ceram. Soc.,* Vol 84, 2001, p 367–375
39. F.E. Heredia, J.C. McNulty, F.W. Zok, and A.G. Evans, Oxidation Embrittlement Probe for Ceramic-Matrix Composites, *J. Am. Ceram. Soc.,* Vol 78, 1995, p 2097–2100

40. T.E. Steyer, F.W. Zok, and D.P. Walls, Stress Rupture of an Enhanced Nicalon/SiC Composite at Intermediate Temperatures, *J. Am Ceram. Soc.,* Vol 81 (No. 8), 1998, p 2140–2146

41. G.N. Morscher, J. Hurst, and D. Brewer, Intermediate-Temperature Stress Rupture of a Woven Hi-Nicalon, BN-Interphase, SiC-Matrix Composite in Air, *J. Am. Ceram. Soc.*, Vol 83, 2000, p 1441–1449

42. R.H. Jones, C.H. Henager, C.A. Lewinsohn, and C.F. Windisch, Stress-Corrosion Cracking of Silicon Carbide Fiber/Silicon Carbide Composites, *J. Am. Ceram. Soc.*, Vol 83, 2000, p 1999–2005

Manufacturing Processes

Chairperson: B. Tomas Åström, IFP SICOMP AB, Sweden

Introduction to Manufacturing of Polymer-Matrix Composites

B. Tomas Åström, IFP SICOMP AB, Sweden

WHEN FABRICATING components and structures from traditional construction materials, manufacturing is usually a matter of machining, molding, or joining material that is already solid and in such forms as block, rod, plank, or sheet. With fiber-reinforced composites, the situation is different in that both the material and component are manufactured simultaneously. (There are some exceptions with both metals (e.g., casting, sintering, and extrusion) and composites (e.g., prepregs, molding compounds, and, in some cases, thermoplastic composites). Most often, the aim in composites manufacturing is to realize near-net-shape or, ideally, net-shape manufacturing, meaning that little or no post-manufacturing machining and trimming is needed, which improves both process economy and individual component properties.

When material and component are simultaneously manufactured, both designer and manufacturer should have a good understanding of how manufacturing conditions influence material properties, since there is often a notable processing–property dependency. In addition to working with an anisotropic material, the designer must also have a good understanding of the processing requirements of candidate raw materials and the specifics of potential manufacturing techniques to be able to estimate the final properties of the component. Obviously, a candidate manufacturing technique must be capable of producing a part with the required geometry, but it is also important to note that the technique selected influences surface finish, allowable reinforcement configurations, available resins and their properties as matrices, as well as a host of other properties, including cost. Table 1 illustrates some of the challenges facing the composite designer when selecting the raw materials and manufacturing technique for a particular design.

Metals are essentially isotropic and homogenous and have predictable properties; material selection and component design for metals normally precede manufacturing considerations. Using the same methodology with composites (which, unfortunately, is not uncommon), will often produce an unsatisfactory end product. This is one reason why composite parts are rarely successful as direct replacements for metal parts; to be successful, composite components must be designed with composites in mind from the onset of the design process. For this reason, the designer must have a good understanding of the candidate materials and must be well versed in the manufacturing techniques that may be employed. The basics of polymer chemistry and physics, as well as available material types and forms, are covered in the Section "Constituent Materials" in this Volume. The bulk of this Section aims to provide reasonably detailed insight into the commercially most relevant techniques to manufacture composites, as well as fabrication of molds for these techniques. The Section focuses on structurally capable (meaning continuous- or at least long fiber-reinforced) polymer composites. The intention of the articles is to explain the key features of each technique and provide the reader with sufficient insight to allow selection of a technically and economically feasible manufacturing technique for a composite design. With product development times constantly decreasing, the need for predictive capabilities and process robustness increases; the article "Process Modeling" provides an introduction to the topic.

Once the appropriate manufacturing technique and raw material type and form have been selected and a mold fabricated, success in composites manufacturing requires close control of temperature and pressure throughout the molding process and throughout the component. During molding, the key is to employ sufficient pressure to maintain the liquid reinforcement-matrix mass in the desired shape at a specified temperature until it becomes dimensionally stable. If the reinforcement needs to be impregnated as part of the process, a pressure gradient is required to force the matrix through the fiber bed. For thermoset matrices, the time interval from (preimpregnated) molding compound to demoldable part is on the order of a few minutes; however, when the raw material is prepreg or separate fibers and matrix, the time interval may be hours or even days. For thermoplastic matrices in the

Table 1 Manufacturing-related issues to consider in design

Requirements due to component performance specifications
Reinforcement
Type
Continuous or discontinuous
Random or oriented
Sizing, coupling agent, and surface treatment
Volume fraction
Weave style
Filament count
Yarn characteristics
Matrix
Thermoset or thermoplastic
Temperature tolerance
Environmental tolerance
Compatibility with reinforcement
Additives and fillers
Void fraction
Surface finish
Dimensional tolerance
Damage tolerance
Holes, undercuts, bosses, and ribs
Inserts, fasteners, and potting compounds
Repairability
Requirements on manufacturing technique imposed by raw material
Reinforcement
Continuous or discontinuous
Random or oriented
Volume fraction
Matrix
Viscosity
Temperature, pressure, and time requirements
Toxicity
Requirements on manufacturing technique imposed by geometry
Overall size
Thickness
Hollow or solid
Constant or varying cross-sectional shape
Single or compound curvature
Requirements on manufacturing technique imposed by economy
Production rate and total series length
Degree of automation
Post-molding machining, trimming, surface preparation, painting, and finishing
Cost of
Capital equipment
Mold
Raw material
Labor
Energy
Mold life

Source: Ref 1

form of preimpregnated reinforcement or molding compound, the time to demolding (excluding the preheating stage) may be less than a minute to a few minutes, since the part only needs to be cooled to achieve dimensional stability.

When trying to grasp the essentials of a composite manufacturing technique, consider the following questions:

- What is used as the mold to give the composite its shape?
- How is the raw material made to conform to the mold?
- How is the impregnation pressure gradient applied (if applicable)?
- How is the consolidation pressure applied?
- How is the temperature controlled?

The emphasis of this Section is on widely accepted and emerging techniques to manufacture polymer composites. However, any technique which maintains the liquid reinforcement-matrix mass in the desired shape, typically at elevated temperature, until it becomes a solid will produce a composite. Whether the composite properties are acceptable and whether the technique is cost-effective are entirely different issues. There is no reason why different manufacturing techniques cannot be combined to create a new technique, underscoring the fact that, with composites, the only limitation is the imagination. Not surprisingly, this imagination also applies to the terminology used in manufacturing, and there is rarely a universally accepted name or acronym for a given technique.

Outlook

When trying to envisage future developments in composites manufacturing, it is instructive to take a look at the previous edition of this Handbook (*Engineered Materials Handbook,* Volume 1, ASM International, 1987). While most techniques covered in the present edition also were described in the 1987 edition, some techniques now covered are new (vacuum infusion and several thermoplastic techniques), and a couple that previously were reported as representing recent developments are now well established (fiber placement and tape laying). This observation indicates that the field of composite manufacturing is developing, albeit not at breakneck speed. What may not be immediately obvious are more subtle developments, some of which are discussed here.

- Traditional open-mold techniques, such as wet hand lay-up and spray-up, are gradually being replaced with closed-mold techniques, such as resin transfer molding (RTM), structural reaction injection molding (SRIM), and vacuum infusion. The primary driver in this transition is reduction in volatile emissions to improve work environment and reduce factory emissions (or, alternatively, reduce air treatment costs); these techniques also provide improved and more consistent component properties and reduced matrix use.
- In manufacturing of competition yachts, the materials and manufacturing techniques used increasingly resemble those traditionally used in aerospace applications. More specifically, preimpregnated reinforcement is used, together with high-performance polymer foam and honeycomb cores, and the composite matrix is crosslinked under vacuum and at elevated temperature, sometimes even in an autoclave. In this case, the main driver is performance enhancements.
- In aerospace applications, hand lay-up of preimpregnated reinforcement is still the industry norm, but automated lay-up techniques and RTM are gaining ground in the drive to reduce cost and enhance repeatability.
- The trial-and-error approach has long been the way to optimize a technique, and to a significant extent, this is still the case. However, process modeling, which has been an active research field in academia for a couple of decades, is now maturing to the extent that it is gradually becoming commonplace in industry. The overall driver is cost reduction, which is made possible through automation and enhancements in cycle time, process robustness, and component properties.
- For expensive components with high requirements (e.g., aircraft components) it may be financially beneficial to embed, within the component, sensors that monitor factors like degree of mold filling or crosslinking; this allows processing conditions to be tailored in order to optimize properties. Such tailoring depends on real-time process modeling to interpret sensory output and determine the most appropriate course of action. Also, in this case, the driver is cost reduction through improvements in process robustness and component properties.

To some extent, all techniques to manufacture polymer composites are seeing gradual improvements to enhance their competitiveness. In addition to the improvements already mentioned, there are gains to be made in terms of more intricate geometries, more complex reinforcement orientations, reduced void content, improved surface finish, etc., all of which ultimately lead to cost reductions. Such gradual refinements may very well be more important to the overall competitiveness of composites than invention of entirely new techniques.

A comprehensive treatment of materials, manufacturing, and post-manufacturing issues relevant to polymer composites is provided in Ref 1.

REFERENCE

1. B. T. Åström, *Manufacturing of Polymer Composites*, Chapman & Hall, 1997

Process Modeling

Suresh G. Advani, University of Delaware
F. Murat Sozer, KOC University, Turkey

POLYMER COMPOSITES have been in use for a considerable part of the twentieth century. Their advantages over other materials for high-performance, lightweight applications have increased their use in many aerospace, automobile, infrastructure, sports, and marine applications. The path to design and manufacturing of composite structures was pursued in evolutionary as well as revolutionary ways. They ranged from using hand lay-up with labor- and cost-intensive autoclave processing to the use of automated processes such as injection molding and extrusion, which traditionally have been employed by the polymer processing industry (Ref 1–3).

In order for composites to be widely used, especially for consumer goods such as in the automotive and recreational industries, two major goals had to be achieved. First of all, the cost of raw materials had to be competitive. Secondly, manufacturing methods had to be developed to achieve high-volume production. The methods needed to be based on the fundamental understanding of the physics of the process, rather than on the accepted trial and error practice ingrained on the shop floor of manufacturing sites (Ref 1, 4). Since the 1980s, composites research has led to the development and improvement of manufacturing methods.

The objective of this article is to categorize various composite manufacturing processes based on similar transport processes and to briefly outline the modeling philosophy and approach that is useful in describing composite manufacturing processes.

Classification Based on Dominant Flow Process

Transport processes encompass the physics of mass, momentum, and energy transfer on all scales. Because the composites are heterogeneous materials, there are simultaneous transfers of heat, mass, and momentum at micro-, meso-, and macroscales. This often occurs with chemical reactions in a multiphase system with time-dependent material properties and boundary conditions.

Composites manufacturing processes can be grouped into three categories:

- Short-fiber suspension methods
- Squeeze flow methods
- Porous media methods

Figure 1 shows the types of flow expected in these processing methods.

Short-fiber suspension manufacturing methods consist of manufacturing processes that involve the transport of fibers and resin as a suspension into a mold or through a die to form the composite. In such processes, the fibers in the molten deforming resin can travel large distances and are usually free to rotate and undergo breakage. The microstructure of the final product is linked with the processing method and the flow of the suspension in the mold. Injection molding, compression molding, and extrusion processes fall under this category. The reinforcements are usually discontinuous glass, aramid, or carbon fibers, and the resin may be either thermoset or thermoplastic.

Squeeze flow manufacturing methods, or advanced thermoplastic composites manufacturing methods, usually involve continuous or long, aligned, discontinuous fibers either partially or fully preimpregnated with thermoplastic resin. In these processes, the fibers and the resin deform together, like a dough containing strands of continuous wires or wire screens under applied stress to form the composite shape. The presence of fibers creates anisotropic resistance to the applied load, and usually the viscosity can be over a million times that of water. This prevents large bulk movements of the composite. Thermoplastic sheet forming, thermoplastic pultrusion, and fiber tape-laying methods can be described by this physics (Ref 6, 7). The precursor materials can be in various forms. One such form is thermoplastic tapes impregnated with aligned and continuous or long discontinuous fibers (Ref 8–10). The other popular form is a preform weave of the polymer fibers commingled with glass or carbon fibers. Under applied heat and pressure, the polymer fibers melt and occupy the space between the reinforcing fibers (Ref 11). The polymer may also be in powder form attached to the fibers during the initial stages. Heat will melt and the pressure will help fuse and consolidate the fiber assembly (Ref 12–14). Thermoplastic

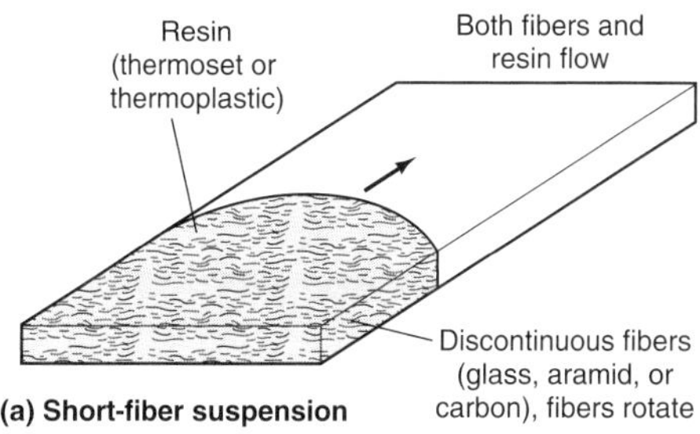

(a) Short-fiber suspension

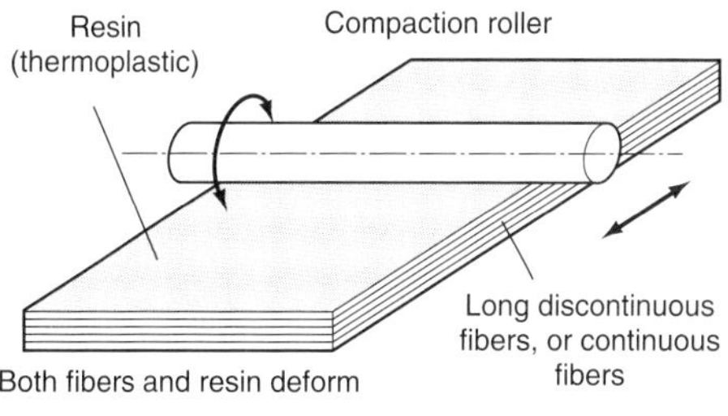

(b) Squeeze flow

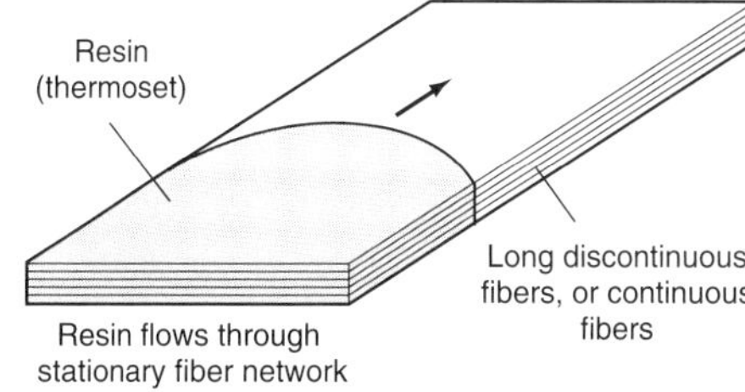

(c) Resin flow through porous media

Fig. 1 Schematic of types of flows expected in composites processing. (a) Short-fiber suspension manufacturing methods: flow of resin-fiber suspension in a mold or through a die. Examples are injection molding, compression molding, and extrusion. (b) Squeeze flow manufacturing methods (advanced thermoplastic composites manufacturing methods): compaction roller deforms both thermoplastic resin and preimpregnated fiber network. Examples are thermoplastic sheet forming, thermoplastic pultrusion, and tape laying. (c) Porous media manufacturing methods (advanced thermoset manufacturing methods): resin flows through stationary fiber network. Examples are liquid composite molding, thermoset pultrusion, filament winding, and autoclave.

resins cannot travel and infiltrate large distances due to their very high viscosity. Thus, the precursor material form has to accommodate a distributed resin percolation among the fiber architectural network.

Porous media manufacturing methods, or advanced thermoset composite manufacturing methods, involve usually continuous and nearly stationary fiber networks into which the resin will impregnate and displace the air, forming the composite in an open or a closed mold (Ref 1, 4, 15, 16). The resin in such processes is almost always a thermoset, due to its low viscosity. One does need to account for the complex chemical reactions that are prevalent in these methods. Liquid composite molding, thermoset pultrusion, filament winding, and autoclave processing are included in this category (Ref 7, 17–20). The materials can take various forms: partially impregnated prepregs, fibers with the liquid thermoset resin applied on the fly, or a stationary network of fibers impregnated with resin. The low viscosity of thermoset resin allows for this versatility. However, the disadvantage is introduction of complex chemical reaction and the gelling and curing phenomena.

Usefulness of Process Models

A model is an idealized mathematical representation of the physical process or the system. Manufacturing of composites has relied on intuition based on experience and trial and error methods when designing, developing, and producing new products. However, this approach has proven to be expensive in time and money when developing new prototype geometries. The risks involved have hindered the use of composite materials in many potential industrial applications. Use of process models can accelerate the path from conception to prototype development, thus making these materials and their processing operations cost-competitive with metals and other materials (Ref 5). The fundamentals in building process models for polymer-composite manufacturing methods, such as injection molding, pultrusion, and resin transfer molding are outlined in this section.

Composites processing models are built on the foundation of physical laws, appropriate assumptions, and boundary conditions based on an understanding of the physical phenomena and constitutive laws derived from experimental data. Once the model is well posed in mathematical equations, the behavior of the model in response to changes in the process and materials variables can be examined. This information can prove to be very useful in mold or die design, or in altering the manufacturing process to create a successful part. In order to investigate the behavior of a composite manufacturing process in a routine manner with minimum effort, the process model can be incorporated in a computer simulation. A computer simulation or a virtual processing scenario is a combination of:

- An idealized process model expressed in mathematical equations
- Numerical method to solve the equations
- Computer software to carry out the solution
- Software to display the results graphically, mimicking the physical behavior of the process

Such virtual composite processing scenarios can provide valuable and detailed information about the process and improve the understanding of the effects of process variables.

Example: Filling a Simple Mold. An L-shaped mold needs to be filled in minimum time without any "dry spots." There are three choices for injections, as shown in Fig. 2. Which one will provide the best results?

Different gate locations and conditions can be investigated to achieve the mold-filling goals. In the L-shaped mold shown in Fig. 2, three different gate locations under the same injection pressure are analyzed to find which location results in the minimum filling time, assuming that vent(s) will be placed at the last point(s) to be filled. In all three cases, the molds are filled through porous media under vacuum. The complete filling times are 51, 118, and 169 seconds in (a), (b), and (c), respectively. Actual trial and error tests would be expensive and take considerable design time. Incomplete filling can be avoided by choosing the gate location appropriately, and placing the vent(s) at the last points to be filled. One can conclude that 3, 1, and 2 vents are needed in (a), (b), and (c), respectively. During the design stage, engineers must analyze not only the injection time, but also the cost of gates, vents, and injection pressure. In each case, one gate and an injection pressure of 5×10^5 Pa (5 bar or 72.5 psi) were assumed. One can conclude that case (b) is a better choice than (c), because it takes less filling time and also requires fewer vents. By knowing the relative importance of filling time and vent cost, a design engineer could choose either (a) or (b).

Experimentation. Models are useful in understanding and codifying the manufacturing operation. Models provide detailed information about a process, such as flow front location, resin pressure, temperature, and flow rate. A model is like a scientific hypothesis that should be validated with experiments. If experiments conflict the hypothesis, the model continues to be revised until it agrees with the experiments. A scientist is more interested in understanding the physical world by using models, whereas a process engineer is usually interested in manipulating the model. A reliable mathematical model will reduce the scope of experiments by combining the effects of different variables and testing unproven design ideas. Finally, models can possibly provide more detailed information than an experiment. Models can provide information about variables that cannot be directly measured. Models do not replace experiments, but the combination of experiments, mathematical theory, physical laws, and models gives engineers and scientists insight to the process so it can be manipulated and tailored to meet their requirements (Ref 5).

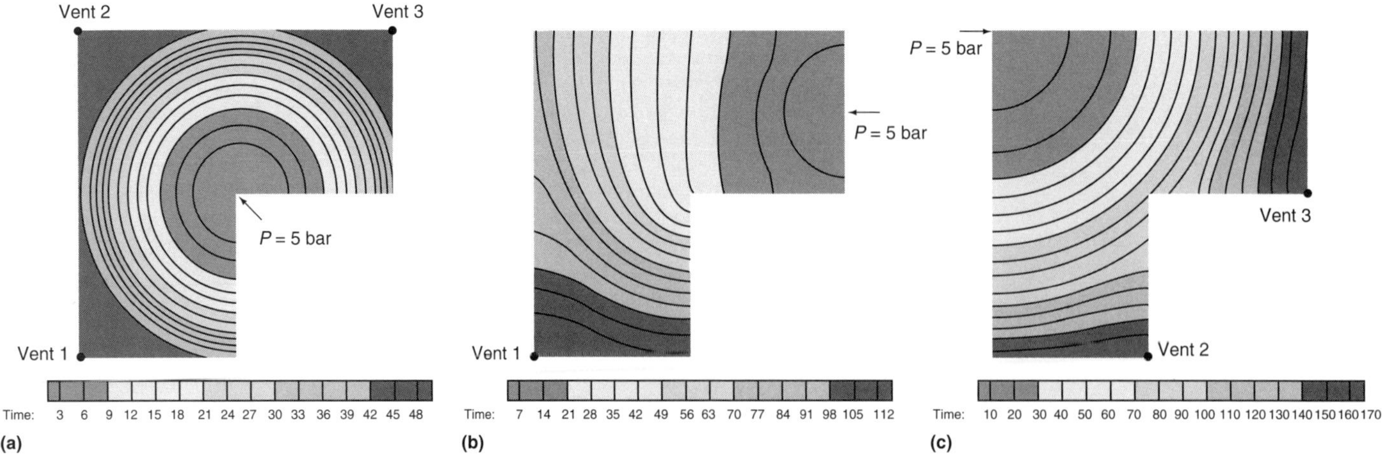

Fig. 2 Different scenarios in the mold-filling simulation code. Three different gate locations (arrows) are tried to find the minimum mold-filling time. The filling times are (a) 51 s, (b) 118 s, and (c) 169 s.

Resin transfer molding (RTM) provides an excellent example of the uses of process models (Ref 4, 15, 17, 18). In just the filling and curing of a RTM part, many physical phenomena transpire. A viscous polymer flows through a network of channels created between the fiber preforms to fill the mold cavity. Heat may enter the cavity by conduction from the mold walls. The resin molecules may start to react and form a cross-linked network, increasing the viscosity of the resin and also releasing heat, which needs to be dissipated. All these factors determine if the cavity will be completely filled, how long the part should be left in the mold, whether the part will wrap due to residual thermal stresses, and the final properties of the manufactured part.

As one cannot see inside a closed mold, it is difficult to know if the resin occupied all the empty spaces between the fibers, and if the part had cured sufficiently to retain its shape when it is demolded. A process model can let the engineer or the scientist "see" the filling pattern (as shown in Fig. 2) and the curing rate, thus quantifying the knowledge of the filling process. While learning more about the filling from the process model, an engineer does not need to run many experiments to find the best location for injection. The model can provide a few possible locations, which reduces the scope of experiments. Thus, a reliable model can reveal the performance and outcome of different mold designs, without the added expense and time of fabricating molds and testing every design.

Resin transfer molding simulations provide further benefits, such as characterization of preform and resin. From experiments, one can monitor the resin pressure, flow rate, and temperature by placing sensors at desired locations. A process model provides detailed information about the pressure field, flow-front shapes, temperature distribution, cure profiles, and velocity fields. These usually can be graphically displayed and easily interpreted to improve the understanding of the process and to identify the problem issues. However, computer simulations must be validated and verified if they are to represent the physical world. Also, one needs to conduct experiments to characterize permeability and cure kinetics that are used as inputs into the model. Thus, experiments are a necessary component in the construction of a process model.

Ingredients of a Process Model

A process model is constructed and verified from six main ingredients (Ref 1):

- Model or system boundary that identifies the system being studied
- Physical laws that ensure conservation of mass, momentum, and energy
- Constitutive laws to describe the materials and their phenomenological behavior. These are needed because we cannot completely describe, from first principles, some of the transport phenomena, such as the nonlinear material behavior of resin, the resin and fiber interactions, and resin cure kinetics at the macro scale.
- Boundary conditions to tailor the model to a specific composite manufacturing process
- Assumptions to simplify the process
- Experimental validation

These six ingredients are discussed in the following subsections.

Model or System Boundary

This is the region in which one should consider physical and constitutive laws. For example, if one wanted to model the material flow inside the screw of an extruder or injection molding machine, as shown in Fig. 3, one would identify the channel inside the screw as the system of interest. The external influences on the system, such as the rotation of the barrel and heat supply by the heaters, will be expressed as boundary conditions.

Physical Laws

Once the system is identified, one would express conservation of mass, momentum, and energy within the system boundaries (Ref 21, 22). The conservation equations are developed by choosing a small control volume within the system, such that the control volume is much smaller than the system being considered, but is much larger than the molecular volume so that the variables such as pressure, velocity, and temperature can be considered on a continuum scale.

The mass conservation equation is formulated by equating the difference between the rate at which the mass of the material is entering and leaving the system, to the rate at which the mass is increasing within the control volume:

$$\begin{pmatrix}\text{Rate of}\\ \text{mass increase}\end{pmatrix} = \begin{pmatrix}\text{Rate of}\\ \text{mass inflow}\end{pmatrix} - \begin{pmatrix}\text{Rate of}\\ \text{mass outflow}\end{pmatrix} - \begin{pmatrix}\text{Rate of mass lost}\\ \text{due to a sink}\end{pmatrix} \quad \text{(Eq 1)}$$

The momentum conservation is based on Newton's law that rate of change of momentum is equal to the forces acting on the control volume. The forces acting on the control volume are the shear stresses due to the viscous action of the deforming material, normal stresses due to the material deformation, the pressure within the material, and body forces due to any noncontact forces such as gravity or electromagnetism. This generates the equation of motion for the material in the system being considered. The equation of motion relates the velocity field of the material to the stresses and pressure acting on the system:

$$\rho \frac{DU}{Dt}(\text{Inertia force}) = -\nabla P(\text{Hydrodynamic force})$$

$$+\nabla \cdot \tau(\text{Force due to stresses}) + F_B(\text{Body force}) \quad \text{(Eq 2)}$$

where ρ is material density, U is the velocity vector, P is static pressure, τ is the viscous stress tensor, F_B is the body force vector, and t is time. However, one does need a relationship between stresses and the deformation of the fluid before one can solve for either pressure or velocities experienced by the fluid. The equations that describe this relationship are called constitutive equations.

For thermoset materials, where the viscosity is low, one can usually impregnate the resin within a stationary fiber preform bed and thus use the flow through porous media theory to describe the motion. Hence for such materials, the momentum conservation is not described by a physical law but by an empirical relationship between the velocity and the pressure gradient within the material.

Energy conservation allows one to determine the temperature field by considering the energy balance for a control volume within the

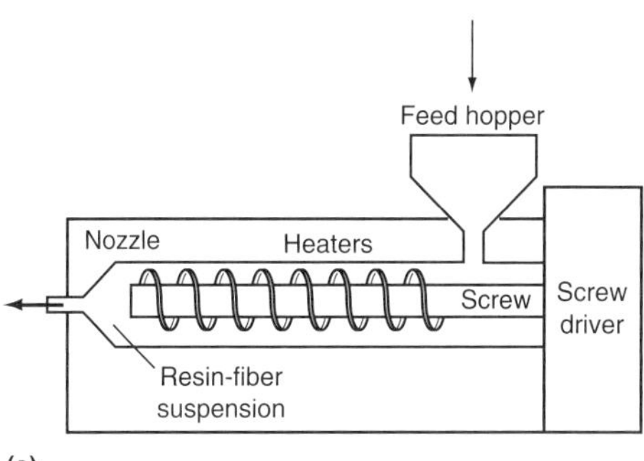

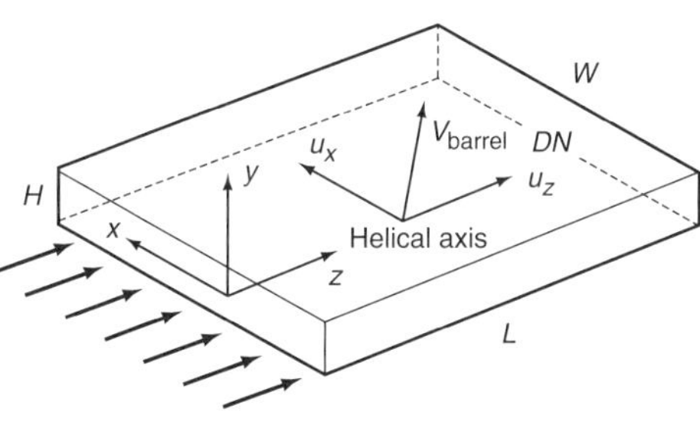

Fig. 3 Model of injection molding machine. (a) Flow of material inside the screw of an injection molding machine. (b) Model boundary and coordinate system. Instead of choosing a spiral coordinate system, which leads to complex mathematics, the screw is considered fixed, and the barrel is rotated in the opposite direction. The coordinate system is then fixed on the unwrapped channel of the screw. V_{barrel} is the velocity of the upper plate. u_x and u_z are components of this velocity in x and z directions respectively. $V_{barrel} = \pi DN$, where D is the diameter of the screw and N is the speed in revolutions per second.

system:

$$\begin{pmatrix}\text{Rate of increase}\\ \text{of internal and}\\ \text{kinetic energy}\end{pmatrix} = \begin{pmatrix}\text{Inflow flux}\\ \text{of internal and}\\ \text{kinetic energy}\end{pmatrix} + \begin{pmatrix}\text{Inflow flux}\\ \text{of heat}\end{pmatrix} + \begin{pmatrix}\text{Rate of energy}\\ \text{increase due to}\\ \text{total stress, } \sigma\end{pmatrix} + \begin{pmatrix}\text{Rate of energy}\\ \text{increase due to}\\ \text{body forces } \mathbf{F}_B\end{pmatrix} + \begin{pmatrix}\text{Rate of energy}\\ \text{generation due}\\ \text{to a source}\end{pmatrix} \quad \text{(Eq 3)}$$

where σ is the total stress tensor given by $\sigma_{ij} = \tau_{ij} - P\mathbf{I}_{ij}$. Here $\mathbf{I}_{ij} = 1$ when $i = j$ and $\mathbf{I}_{ij} = 0$ when $i \neq j$.

The energy produced within the system may be due to crystallization kinetics or to reaction kinetics. In the latter case, the energy generation term will be a function of the temperature, and the equation is nonlinear. For thermoplastics, due to their high viscosity, much of the heating of the material is caused by viscous dissipation. For example, in injection molding, although the heaters supply the heat to initially melt the polymer, a substantial amount of heat is generated as the material deforms through the narrow channels, generating heat due to viscous dissipation. Hence, this should be accounted for in the energy balance. Because composites consist of resin and fibers, laws of mixture are usually applied to calculate thermophysical properties, such as heat capacities and thermal conductivities.

Constitutive Laws

Constitutive equations are empirical relations between parameters of interest. They usually do not incorporate the physics, studied and analyzed at the micron and molecular level, into the equation at the macroscale (Ref 23).

These equations must be such that the relationships and the results do not change with the coordinate frame. Almost all constitutive equations require the researchers to characterize constants needed in the equation that are specific to the material and its state. For example, for a fluid subjected to a stress, if the stress is always directly proportional to the strain rate the fluid undergoes, the empirical constant of proportionality is called viscosity. This constitutive relation is known as Newtonian law, and the fluids that exhibit this behavior are called Newtonian fluids. Constitutive equations should also be stable in the processing regime to be consistent with the physics, as exhibited by the experiments.

Constitutive equations are necessary to describe the processing of composite materials due to their heterogeneous nature, the complex chemistry of the resin and its interaction with fibers and fillers, and simultaneous transport of mass and energy at the micro-, meso-, and macrolevels. Issues that are analyzed at the microscale, such as growth rate of a micron-size spherulite, can be represented at the macroscale level, for this case, in terms of crystallization kinetics, by use of appropriate constitutive equations. Constitutive equations describe the global picture of the process and the process parameters, which is of interest to the process engineer, instead of getting entangled in the details at the micron level (Ref 1). Constitutive equations invariably require the researchers to determine constants that are functions of the material and process conditions. Thus, independent characterization and cataloging of material constants for constitutive equations can become a daunting task, which slows down and undermines the modeling of such processes.

Some examples of constitutive equations in composites manufacturing processes are tabulated in Table 1.

The constitutive equations that are used to describe the material behavior along with the mass, momentum, and energy conservation equations form a system of eleven equations with eleven primary variables. These variables are pressure, three components of velocity, temperature, and six independent components of stresses. To solve this system of equations, one would need to prescribe boundary conditions.

Boundary Conditions

The external influences that affect the system or process are expressed by formulating boundary conditions for the variables. In general, there are two types of boundary conditions: kinematic, which deal with velocity, and dynamic, which deal with stress fields.

Considering the physical contact of the fluid at the boundary, boundary conditions can be further divided into five groups (Ref 28):

- Liquid-solid interface (contact at solid surface)
- Liquid-liquid interface
- Liquid-vapor interface
- Free surface
- Specified inlet and exit boundary conditions

Liquid-Solid Interface. At the liquid-solid interfaces, the relative velocity of a viscous fluid with respect to the solid boundary is assumed to be zero. That is, $\mathbf{U} = \mathbf{U}_{\text{Solid}}$. This is known as no-slip condition. Although this assumption is not always correct, that is, fluid may slip on the solid surface, the idea of no-slip approximation is supported by many experiments in the literature.

Some examples of fluid-flow problems with liquid-solid-interface-type boundary conditions are shown in Fig. 4. In all four cases, it was assumed that the fluid domains in z-direction (out of paper) are large so that there is no variation in z-direction. In Fig. 4 (a) and (b), a fluid is bounded by two parallel, infinitely long plates. The lower plate is stationary, but the upper one moves horizontally in x-direction. Due to the disturbance from the moving upper plate, there will be fluid flow. The upper plate is pulled with a constant speed, V, in Fig. 4(a). In Fig. 4(b), the pulling force is specified instead of the speed.

The no-slip condition can be directly applied in Fig. 4(a). If the plates are impermeable (nonporous), there is no fluid flow in the normal directions on the plates, which can be written as $\mathbf{U} \cdot \mathbf{n} = u_y = 0$ at $y = 0$ and $y = h$, where $\mathbf{U}$ is the fluid velocity vector, and $\mathbf{n}$ is the normal vector on the plate. The tangential velocity component, $u_x = V$ at $y = h$, and $u_x = 0$ at $y = 0$, considering the no-slip condition. These are kinematic boundary conditions because they only involve the velocity field.

The boundary condition on the upper plate of Fig. 4(b) is a dynamic condition. The pulling force applied on the plate is specified. The pulling force per unit area, F, can be calculated as $(\int \tau_{xy}|_{y=h} dxdz)/(\text{total plate area})$. In fact, this problem is a one-dimensional problem, because the velocity vector and stress tensor are functions of only y, not x. Hence, τ_{xy} is constant at $y = h$. The dynamic boundary condition is then $\tau_{xy} = F$.

Table 1 Examples of constitutive equations in some composites manufacturing processes: empirical relations between parameters of interest

The change in fiber orientation tensor, a_{ij}, due to flow (Ref 24):

$$\frac{Da_{ij}}{Dt} = -\frac{1}{2}(\omega_{ik}a_{kj} - a_{ik}\omega_{kj}) + \frac{1}{2}\lambda(\dot{\gamma}_{ik}a_{kj} + a_{ik}\dot{\gamma}_{kj} - 2\dot{\gamma}_{kl}a_{ijkl}) + 2C_I\dot{\gamma}(\delta_{ij} - 3a_{ij})$$

where $\omega_{kj} = (\partial u_j/\partial x_k) - (\partial u_k/\partial x_j)$ (the vorticity tensor)

$\dot{\gamma} = \sqrt{\frac{1}{2}\dot{\gamma}_{ij}\dot{\gamma}_{ji}}$ (magnitude of the rate of strain tensor)

C_I = interaction coefficient

λ = aspect ratio of the fiber

Approximation of a_{ijkl} in terms of a_{ij} (Ref 24):

$$a_{ijkl} = \frac{1-f}{35}(\delta_{ij}\delta_{kl} + \delta_{ik}\delta_{jl} + \delta_{il}\delta_{jk}) + \frac{1-f}{7}(a_{ij}\delta_{kl} + a_{ik}\delta_{jl} + a_{il}\delta_{jk} + a_{kl}\delta_{ij} + a_{jl}\delta_{ik} + a_{jk}\delta_{il})$$

here δ_{ij} is the Dirac delta function and f is the degree of alignment

Specific energy generated during cure of a resin system; $\dot{s}$, is

$\dot{s} = R_\alpha E_\alpha$

where E_α = the heat of reaction

$$R_\alpha = (A_1 e^{E_1/RT} + A_2 e^{E_2/RT}\alpha^m)(1-\alpha)^n$$

α = degree of cure

R = universal gas constant

m, n, A_1, A_2, E_1, and E_2 are empirical constants

Temperature-dependent resin viscosity (Arrhenius equation):

$$\mu = \mu_0 e^{-c(T-T_0)}$$

where T_0 is the reference temperature at which $\mu = \mu_0$.

Temperature and degree of cure-dependent resin viscosity (Ref 15, 25):

$$\mu = a_0 e^{-b_0\alpha_e(a+b\alpha)/RT}$$

where a, b, a_0, and b_0 are to be determined experimentally.

Permeability of a porous medium, K, by a capillary model (Ref 26, 27):

$$K = C\frac{\phi^3}{(1-\phi)^2} = \frac{1}{DS^2}\frac{\phi^3}{(1-\phi)^2}$$

where S = the specific wetted surface area

$\phi = 1 - V_f$ = the porosity of porous medium and V_f is the fiber volume fraction

$D = k_0(L_e/L)$ = the dimensionless shape factor (an experimental parameter)

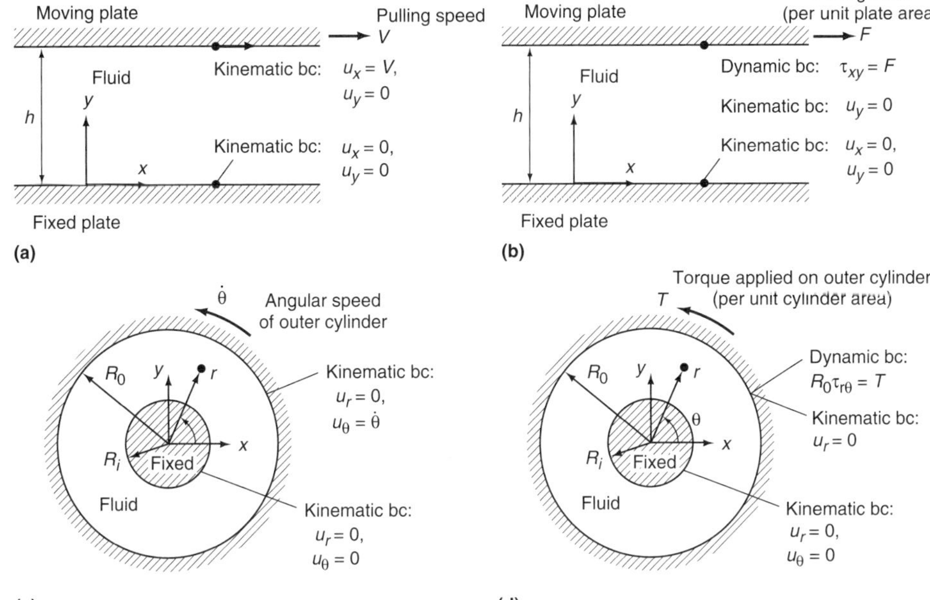

Fig. 4 Four example situations for different boundary conditions (bc). (a) Kinematic bc at the upper and lower boundaries of fluid flow within a rectangular channel. (b) The same as in (a), except that the pulling force, F, on the plate is specified instead of the speed. So, this bc on the upper boundary of (b) is dynamic. (c) Kinematic bc on the outer- and inner-cylinder boundaries of fluid flow within a concentric domain (R_o and R_i are the radii of the outer and inner cylinders, respectively, and u is the velocity). (d) The same as in (c), except that the torque, T, applied to the outer cylinder is specified instead of the angular speed. So, this bc on the outer boundary of (d) is dynamic.

In Fig. 4(c) and (d), the fluid domain is a concentric gap between a fixed inner cylinder and a rotating outer cylinder. Because the inner cylinder is fixed (it has a zero velocity vector), and the fluid will also have the same zero velocity vector on that cylinder, according to the no-slip condition. In Fig. 4(c), the angular velocity of the outer cylinder is specified as $\dot{\theta}$. The fluid will also have the same angular velocity, or equivalently the same tangential velocity component, $u_\theta = \dot{\theta} R_0$.

In Fig. 4(d), the external torque is applied to the outer cylinder. The torque per unit area, T, is calculated as $(\int r\tau_{r\theta}|_{r=R0}\, rd\theta)$/(total cylinder area) on the outer-cylinder surface where $r = R_0$. Here θ changes from 0 to 2π, and the total area is $2\pi R_0 L$, where L is the length of the cylinders in z-direction. This problem is only one-dimensional; the velocity and stress fields are functions of r only, hence $\tau_{r\theta}$ is constant at $r = R_0$. The corresponding dynamic boundary condition is then $R_0\tau_{r\theta} = T$.

Liquid-Liquid Interface. Consider the two immiscible fluids A and B within a rectangular channel, as shown in Fig. 5. The kinematic boundary conditions on the upper and lower plates are $u_{xB} = V$ at $y = h_A + h_B$, and $u_{xA} = 0$ at $y = 0$, respectively. Two more boundary conditions are needed at the liquid-liquid interface in order to uniquely solve this problem. For viscous fluids, the velocities are assumed to be continuous at their interface. $\mathbf{U}_A = \mathbf{U}_B$ in vectorial form, or $u_{xA} = u_{xB}$ and $u_{yA} = u_{yB}$ in scalar form at $y = h_A$. Considering the dynamic interactions of adjacent control volumes of fluids A and B, the viscous shear stress τ_{xy} must be continuous across the interface. Hence, $\tau_{xyA} = \tau_{xyB}$, which can also be written as $\mu_A\partial u_{xA}/\partial x = \mu_B\partial u_{xB}/\partial x$ at $y = h_A$ for Newtonian fluids.

The boundary conditions of mold filling during the resin transfer molding process are illustrated in Fig. 6. No leakage of resin along the wall is assumed, considering an impermeable mold wall. That corresponds to the normal component of velocity being zero:

$$\bar{u}_n = -\frac{1}{\mu}\left(K_{nn}\frac{\partial P}{\partial n} + K_{nt}\frac{\partial P}{\partial t}\right) = 0$$

where n and t denote the directions normal and tangent to the mold wall, respectively. However, the tangential velocity component is nonzero, allowing a slip on the wall. Pressure of resin is equal to the vent pressure, if it is directly connected to the vent. At the injection gate, either the pressure or the flow rate is specified.

Assumptions

In order to simplify the models, some assumptions are made. Certain assumptions can dramatically simplify a process model (Ref 1, 29). However, inappropriate simplifications can also lead to process behavior predictions that are not consistent with observations. Hence, it is important that the assumptions are well reasoned, based on experience, or validated with experiments. The common assumptions employed in one or more processes, depending on the phenomena of interest, are described in this section. These assumptions will not necessarily be employed for every process. For every phenomenon modeled, one should go through the exercise of justifying every assumption made to simplify the model.

Quasi-Steady State. Physically, a variable such as velocity, temperature, or pressure is in steady state. This means that from a stationary reference frame, the variable does not experience any change with time at that spatial location. Mathematically, steady state can be described by setting $\partial(\ )/\partial t = 0$. Quasi-steady-state assumption refers to approximating an unsteady or time-dependent flow with small inertial effects, as a

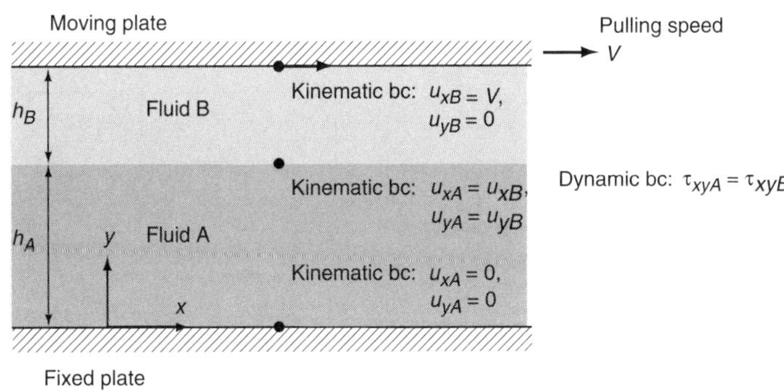

Fig. 5 Boundary condition (bc) at a liquid-liquid interface

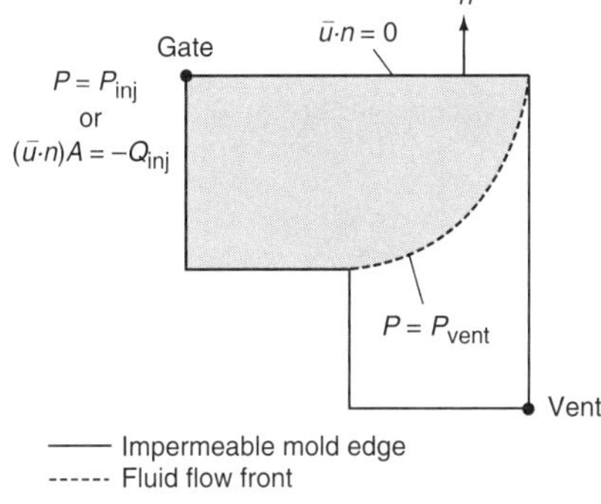

Fig. 6 Boundary conditions for a moving flow-front problem with Q_{inj} as the specified injection flow rate or P_{inj} as the specified injection pressure

succession of steady state flows. So, even if the problem contains time-dependent boundary conditions, one can solve it as a steady state problem at any instance of time, t. At that time, t, the boundary condition will be a constant value, so one can solve the steady state governing equation.

This is a reasonable approach if the momentum transfer from the boundary conditions is immediate and the material inertia plays an insignificant role. The kinetic viscosity v, usually governs the rate of momentum transfer. For polymers and polymer composites, this value is very high, as compared to water. The rate of momentum transfer can almost always be approximated as immediate at any instant in time. Another way to describe this is that when the viscosity is high and the process velocity is slow, the inertial effects will be insignificant.

Examples. A thermoplastic polymer is squeezed between two parallel disks with a constant force, F. It is desired to obtain the gap separation between the plates as a function of time. A quasi-steady-state assumption allows one to ignore the inertial terms in the momentum equation and solve the radial problem as a steady state problem at any time, t, for the instantaneous gap height. Other examples that use this assumption are the processes that simulate the mold-filling scenario. In these classes of problems, the solution domain in which one solves for the fluid pressure is bounded by the boundaries of the resin in the mold. The domain is bounded by the mold boundaries if the resin has reached the mold walls, and by the boundaries of the instantaneous resin front (also known as the flow front) if the resin has not reached the mold boundaries. After solving for the fluid pressure, one calculates the fluid velocities, advances the resin front based on the velocity field, and re-solves for the pressure for the new domain. This procedure is continued until the mold is filled. Thus the quasi-steady-state solution of the pressure is dependent only on the instantaneous material properties and the boundary conditions, which are functions of time.

Note that the justification of neglecting the transient terms in the equation of motion follows from the fact that the kinematic viscosity of polymers is high, and because the speeds are slow, the Reynolds number, which is the ratio of inertia forces to viscous forces, is low. However, the thermal diffusivity of polymers is low, so the heat transfer is much slower, and one cannot always ignore the transient terms in the energy equation. Prandtl number, which is the ratio of momentum transfer to energy transfer, is very high for polymers, on the order of 100 or more. Thus, for nonisothermal processes, one usually cannot ignore the transient term in the energy conservation equation.

Fully Developed Region and Entrance Effects. When a system variable does not change along a certain direction, one proclaims that the variable is fully developed with respect to that direction. For example, if the temperature profile does not change along the x-direction, one can physically assume that the temperature is fully developed along the x-direction. Mathematically, one can express this condition as $\partial T/\partial x = 0$.

The assumption "fully developed flow and insignificant entrance effects" is widely used while developing process models for polymer and polymer composites processing. This assumption is again related to the rate of momentum transfer. The higher the kinematic viscosity, the faster the momentum transfer will be, and the sooner the velocity profile will develop.

Consider flow in a tube from a reservoir or from a pressure pot, as shown in Fig. 7. The entrance region of length, δ, is the region in which the flow profile is rearranging from plug flow to a parabolic profile for a viscous Newtonian fluid. Usually, this region is proportional to the diameter, D, of the tube and the Reynolds number, $\text{Re} = UD\rho/\mu$, where U is velocity, ρ is density, and μ is viscosity:

$$\frac{\delta}{D} = 0.054\ \text{Re(approximately)} \quad \text{(Eq 4)}$$

If the Reynolds number is less than one, the entrance effects last for less than the tube diameter, and the assumption of fully developed flow will not influence the important physics or the solution.

Similarly, if one wanted to assume a fully developed temperature profile along the flow direction, the following criteria need to be met:

$$\frac{\delta_t}{D} \cong (0.03\ \text{to}\ 0.04)\ \text{Re Pr} \quad \text{(Eq 5)}$$

where δ_t is the length of the thermal developing region, and the Prandtl number is given by $\text{Pr} = c_p\mu/k$, where c_p is specific heat at constant pressure, μ is viscosity, and k is thermal conductivity. In composites processing, this assumption is easy to justify for long tubes or long characteristic flow directions, but not for short tubes, because the Pr number can be on the order of 1000 for most materials. Also, if the temperature boundary condition is changing with time, a fully developed temperature profile cannot be easily justifiable. The other important number is the Graetz number, which relates the thermal capacity of the fluid to convection heat transfer. When it is small, one can assume that both the velocity and temperature profiles are developed in the direction of flow.

Fully developed flow is a common assumption used in polymer and composites processing, as compared to the fully developed temperature profile due to low Reynolds number flows. One of the most common situations in which the fully developed flow is used is in conjunction with the lubrication approximation. This allows one to simplify the equations of motion considerably, and retain the important physics of the flow in the process model.

Lubrication Approximation. Osborne Reynolds (Ref 30) coined the term *lubrication approximation* when he was addressing hydrodynamic lubrication analysis. The key requirements to apply this theory are that the flow should be viscous (the Reynolds number should be small), and the flow should take place in narrow gaps. While processing composites, one usually is dealing with parts that are possibly meters in length and width, but only millimeters in thickness. Because they have low Reynolds number flows, lubrication analysis can be used to simplify the model.

Following is a review of how lubrication theory allows one to simplify the equations of motion for a Newtonian viscous material. The conditions that should be met before applying this analysis to a flow problem are:

- The material should be incompressible
- The flow should be isothermal
- The Reynolds number should be less than one (the inertial forces should be smaller than the viscous shear forces)
- The gap height should be very small compared to the in-plane dimensions
- If the gap height, h, is not a constant, it could vary very slowly with the in-plane dimensions. For in-plane dimensions x and y, dh/dx and $dh/dy << 1$.

An example is shown in Fig. 8. The parts manufactured by this process are about 2 to 3 mm

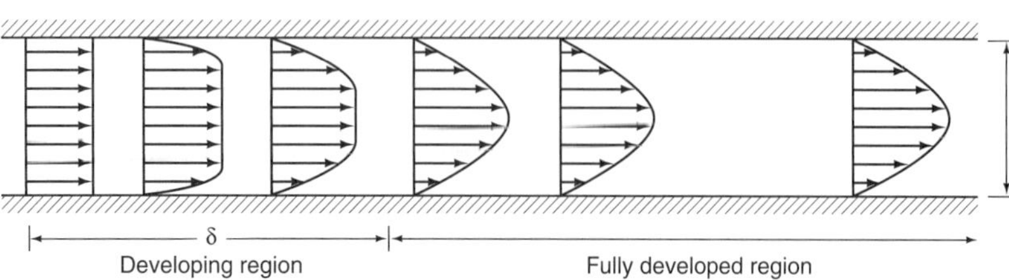

Fig. 7 Development of velocity profile

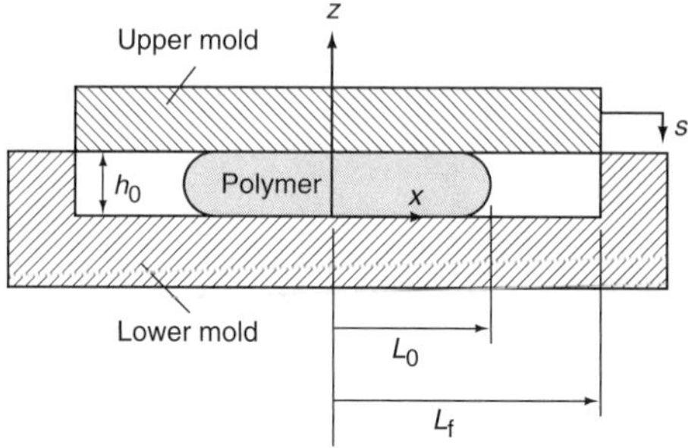

Fig. 8 Compression molding process can be modeled as a lubrication approximation, with $h << L$.

(0.08 to 0.12 in.) in thickness (h_0) and can be as long as 1 to 2 m (several feet). One also assumes that the material does not slip at the surface of the walls. These two assumptions make it possible to effectively treat compression molding as a lubrication problem.

Thin Shell Approximation. If the no-slip at the boundaries is not satisfied, it may be difficult to justify the lubrication approximation. When there is full-slip, it is possible to model the flow as plug flow through the cavity thickness. For example, when Darcy's law (Ref 31) for flow of thermoset resins through a network of fibers is considered, one assumes a full-slip boundary condition along the mold surfaces. In such cases, the flow in the thickness direction can be ignored if:

$$\left(\frac{h}{L}\right)^2 \frac{K_h}{K_L} << 1 \quad \text{(Eq 6)}$$

where h and L are the thickness and in-plane dimensions, and K_h and K_L are the permeabilities of fiber network in thickness and in-plane directions, respectively.

Experimental Validation

Almost all process models that are developed involve one or more assumptions, and many of them use constitutive or phenomenological equations to represent material behavior. Thus, it is important to check and see if the model predictions agree with experimental results.

If a simulation of a model has been developed, it can provide many details, such as the pressure and temperature distribution, and fiber orientation state at every location. An experiment can only measure finite quantities. Hence, the choice of which variables to measure, and where to measure them, becomes an important consideration.

There are many ways to validate a model. One may choose to monitor the history of just one of the governing variables in the experiment, or all of the field variables, and compare them directly with the predictions. For example, one may monitor the temperature of the resin at the midpoint of the mold as a function of time in injection molding process and compare it with the predictions from the nonisothermal simulations. Another approach may be to indirectly compare experimental findings with predictions. In curing a thermoset composite, one may monitor the final state of the cure after the composite is demolded by performing differential scanning calorimetry analysis on various samples cut from the fabricated composite (See the article "Thermal Analysis" in this Volume). The resulting cure distribution can be compared with the predictions of the model. A similar approach can be adopted for verification of the model for prediction of the crystallization state or fiber orientation state.

It is important to compare the proper variables when performing validation experiments. To validate the model for flow-induced fiber orientation, a simulation of injection mold filling is developed, assuming no variations in fiber concentration and fiber length distribution. A constitutive rheological model is used for stress-strain relationship, and fiber orientation is predicted. Next, the results are compared with the fiber orientation state measured from injection-molded samples. This is not a good validation of the flow-induced fiber orientation model, because in injection molding there are many other parameters that may have influenced the fiber orientation pattern. However, if one could create a suspension of fibers in simple shear flow, or other well-defined flows, and measure the orientation of the fibers in such flows, it would help validate the flow-induced fiber orientation model. Moreover, it would also elucidate the phenomena of fiber-fiber interactions, which could lead to refinement of the model (Ref 32).

Hence, the type of experiment is also an important factor in the validation studies of the formulated process model. Every process model usually consists of many phenomena and substeps, with assumptions at every sublevel. If possible, one should try to validate every submodel independent of the overall model. For example, in filament winding there are many submodels, such as thermochemical, fiber motion, stress, and void models. It will be useful to independently validate these models, rather than just comparing the final predicted mechanical properties with the measured properties. It is sometimes not feasible to validate every submodel, in which case one may want to consider indirect validation of some of the submodels.

It is crucial to validate the overall process model in addition to validating individual submodels, because this sheds light on the accuracy of the modeled interactions between the submodels. One may validate every submodel of the process model and assume that the process model is validated, but there may be assumptions about the interactions between the submodels that have not been verified. Thus, the validation of a process model is not complete until one also validates the final results with the predictions.

If the model predictions agree with the experiments, one has created a successful model that can be used for design, manufacturing, and control. One such example is shown in Fig. 9. The flow-front locations as predicted by the flow through porous media model for flow during resin transfer molding is on the right. A model experiment performed in a mold with transparent lid recorded the flow fronts seen on the left.

Reexamining the Parts of the Model

Reexamining Assumptions. In situations where the predictions and the experimental results do not agree, the modeler should revisit his assumptions and make sure the validation experiments honor those assumptions. The modeler should have verified the simulation or the model with closed form solutions or with mesh refinements. Next, the modeler should question the constitutive law that is being used to represent the phenomena. Sometimes, the modeler can learn enough from the experiments to modify the law. For example, if the model is using a power-law fluid to represent the material behavior, and the experiment involves very low shear rates, the experimental results and predictions will not match. One may need to refine the model to using a Carreau fluid. In the same way, the fiber-fiber interaction may have been represented with a constant parameter in the flow-induced fiber orientation model. However, the model experiments may show that the expected orientation behavior is slightly different than the predictions. This may induce the modeler to think that the interactions cannot be constant under all fiber orientation states. One would expect the fiber-fiber interactions to be higher when the orientation state is in complete disarray (random) as compared to when all the fibers are aligned. Thus, the modeler may use this insight to improve the fiber orientation model.

Revisiting Laws. Usually the models can be improved or refined by including more material parameters. For example, in the cases suggested previously that included a switch from power-law to Carreau fluid, three parameters are needed instead of two. Similarly, if the fiber interaction parameter is made dependent on orientation, an additional equation may be needed that will allow this relationship to be determined. At other times, one may need to completely reformulate the constitutive law to accommodate the new phenomena being observed. For example, a random fiber preform clearly obeys Darcy's law, because it has been validated many times. However, some of the stitched or tightly woven fabrics have two scales of pores: very small ones between fibers, and large ones between fiber tows, as shown in Fig. 10 (Ref 33).

When the fluid impregnates these preforms, the pores between the fiber tows are filled at a much earlier time than the smaller pores between the fibers. This would require reformulation of the model, because it has been discovered that the saturation of the porous media with dual-length scale is not instantaneous, as in random preforms (Fig. 10a).

Reexamining Boundary Conditions. Sometimes the culprit may be the incorrect application of the boundary conditions, or the boundary condition may be unknown. If a convective heat-transfer boundary condition exists on the outside of the mold, one would need to specify a convective heat-transfer coefficient that itself requires a constitutive law. One approach is to create validation experiments that do not use this boundary condition but use a specific temperature or heat flux.

Formulation of Models

Model formulations may vary, but they generally follow the plan outlined in Fig. 11 (Ref 5).

Problem Definition

The purpose of a model is to predict the behavior of a process for a range of inputs and conditions (Ref 34). Hence, one must define the physical process and its inputs. The physical process may not represent the complete composite manufacturing process, but may focus on a small aspect of the process during manufacturing. For example, in injection molding, mold filling is only one aspect of the manufacturing process. The model may treat the screw, the runner, and the spruce as only a source of fiber suspensions at a given flow rate. It is important to define the system that one is modeling and to draw a boundary around it. The other parts of the process, which can be modeled as other subsystems, can interact with the defined system by what they supply across the boundary (Ref 35).

The aim of the model should be defined, because it will influence what aspect of the model is emphasized. It is useful to identify the important responses of the process and what conditions and inputs should be represented. Depending upon the aim, different models for the same physical process can give different answers. For example, in processes such as RTM, some models merely relate the flow rate to the pressure. Others may provide detailed information about the flow-front locations in complex geometry. Still others may be limited to a few cavity shapes. Some models may even provide temperature histories and predict residual stresses. Models may only focus on the curing phase and ignore filling. Thus, there can be multiplicity of models for the same process. The model one chooses will depend on what issues are important and how much time and effort one can devote to finding the answers.

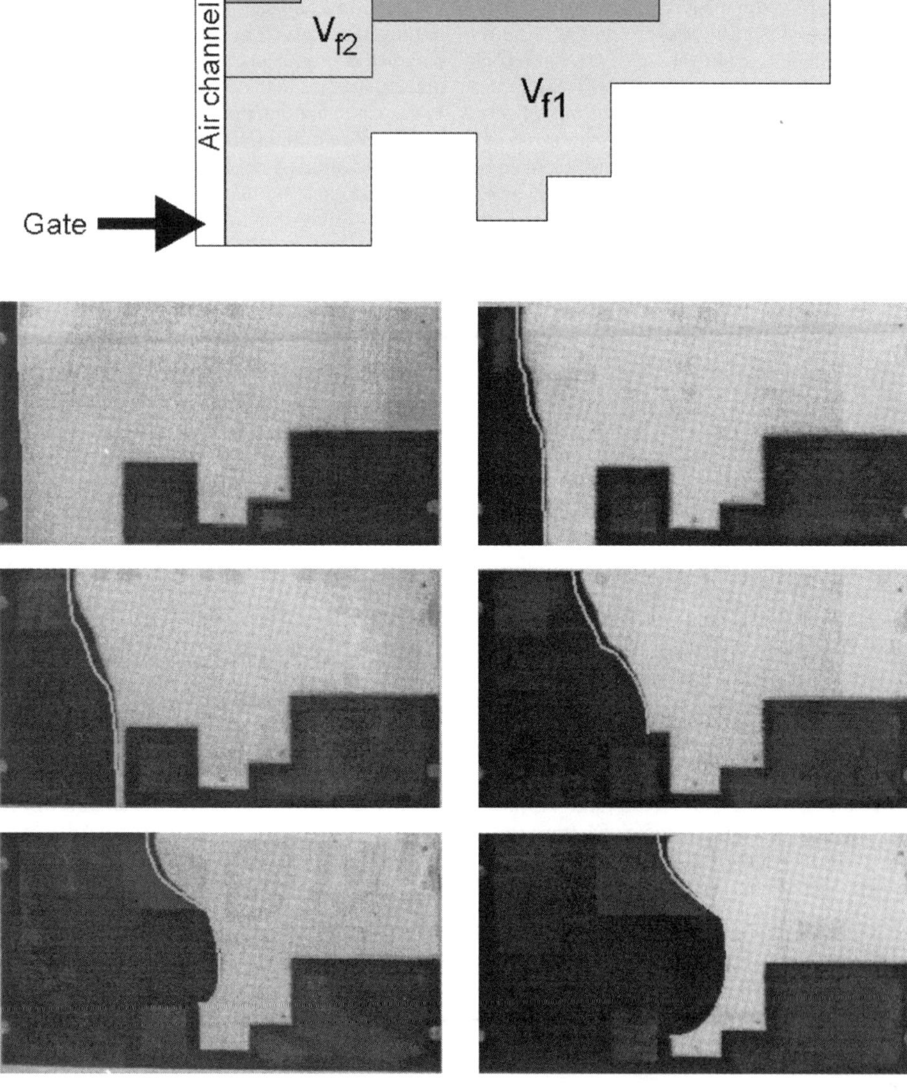

Fig. 9 Experimental validation of flow in an RTM. The mold configuration is shown at the top. The lower portion shows the numerically predicted flow fronts superimposed on the experimental images taken at 20 s increments. Source: Ref 33.

Building the Mathematical Model

Once the system is defined and the important quantities are identified, one can build the model from physical laws, empirical and phenomenological observations, and/or from analogies with other systems. A mathematical model, which represents the physical process, describes the system behavior by a set of mathematical equations, with the quantities of interest as primary or secondary variables. Interactions between the chosen system and the surroundings are included as boundary conditions of the model.

Most composites manufacturing process models combine the fundamental physical laws of mass, momentum, and energy conservation with empirical observations, such as viscosity or permeability laws. The models can become complicated if one tries to include every known effect. The skilled modeler will try to simplify the model by making assumptions that will retain the important effects, while making it easier to solve the mathematical equations. Simplifying the model will reduce the number of parameters required. The results may be more easily understood.

As an example, RTM flow is important only in the in-plane direction when filling thin cavities, so one can simplify the governing equations from three dimensions to two (Ref 4, 15). To solve the equations, one needs to provide the

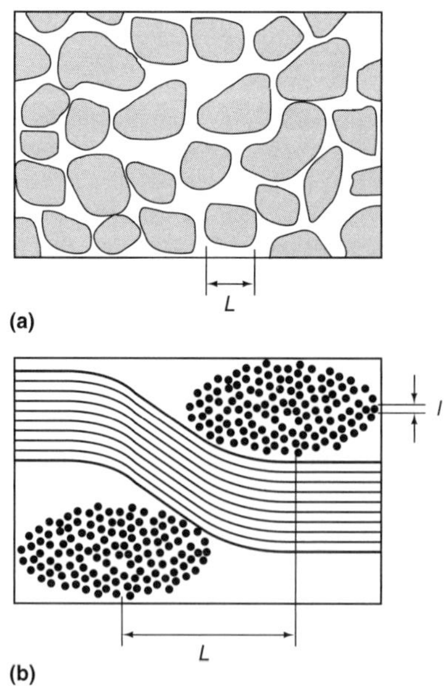

Fig. 10 Flow through porous media. (a) Schematic diagram of a simple porous medium exhibiting a single-length scale. (b) Schematic cross section of a woven fabric unit cell, demonstrating the dual-length scale porous medium

permeability tensor. For the two-dimensional case, one needs only two principal permeability values, rather than three. The case for using a viscosity model is similar. A Newtonian fluid needs only one material parameter. However, if one chooses to use the Carreau fluid model, four material parameters must be determined. In addition, the equations are nonlinear and more difficult to solve.

Solution of the Equations

The formulated mathematical model may be a simple, ordinary differential equation with one independent variable and one dependent variable, or it may be a system of complicated and coupled nonlinear, partial differential equations with two or more dependent variables that rely on more than one independent variable. The simple equations could be solved analytically if appropriate boundary or initial conditions are specified. For models with partial differential equations to be solved in complex geometry, one can select standard numerical methods, such as finite difference, boundary element, or finite element analysis (Ref 36–38). Special techniques may be required if the equations or boundary conditions are nonlinear, such as a moving boundary problem in the case of mold filling (Ref 39). The objective of the model also determines the method to be selected for solution, because the choice of numerical methods determines the time and cost of setting up and running a simulation. When implementing a numerical solution, it is important to consider pragmatic issues, such as reliability, portability, efficiency, and user interface of the computer software.

Model Assessment

Model assessment must consist of two parts: verification and validation.

Verification alludes to whether the selected method provides the correct solution to the formulated set of equations with the prescribed boundary conditions. One must always verify that the numerical technique does not have any programming errors or inconsistencies that can lead to inaccurate solution of the governing equations. If one has implemented a numerical solution, it can be compared to analytic or classical solutions for simplified geometry, or for steady state situations. If no analytic solution is available, one can refine the time step or the grid size over the domain and check for convergence of the solution. One can also perform global mass and energy balances over the domain to check if they are being conserved on a global scale.

Validation refers to how well the process model describes the physics of the selected phenomenon. Because assumptions were made, empirical relationships introduced, and boundary condition approximated, it is imperative to check that the important physics to be modeled are still retained in the model. Validation also allows one to check if any important phenomena have been missed in the process. At the same time, validation will uncover insignificant influences included in the process model that may not be necessary.

How does one validate a process model? The most common approach is with experiments. One can approach this at two levels.

First, to ensure the process model is capturing the correct physics, it is important to carry out a controlled laboratory experiment or a model experiment. If the goal is to validate the fiber orientation model due to flow in a Newtonian fluid, one could use a model fluid such as silicone oil and nylon fibers with tracer fibers to understand and record the orientation behavior. If the model results are compared directly with fiber orientation measurements taken from injection-molded plaques, other effects, such as viscoelasticity, fiber breakage, cooling of the polymer, and fiber clustering, may play a role in influencing fiber orientation in addition to the flow. Hence, it would be difficult to separate the influence due to flow on fiber orientation from these other effects that were not included in the process model.

Model experiments can many times reveal the underlying physics in a processing situation and block out the noise or deviations due to other effects. However, it is important to make sure that the noise is only noise and not an important effect in the process that the model is ignoring.

Although model experiments will provide useful information for validation of the "idealized model," one still needs to know how well the "idealized model" represents the reality of the factory floor. The second level of experiments should mimic the manufacturing situation. One could have used random preforms in model experiments to demonstrate how well Darcy's law captures the physics of the flow in closed molds in thermosets processing. However, if stitched or woven preforms are the reinforcement choice in manufacturing, it is important to validate that these materials also exhibit Darcy's law, and if not, how far do they deviate from it. Questions such as "Is it necessary to develop a new model for such materials?" or "Can one estimate the error introduced due to the dual-scale nature of the preform?" will arise and need to be addressed.

Revision of the Model

If the model agrees with the experimental results, one has a successful model that can make useful predictions. However, in most cases there will be disagreement between the model and the experiments. It is important to methodically explore the possible causes of the discrepancy. First, one must check that the solution method used is not flawed. This requires looking for errors in the implementation of the solution

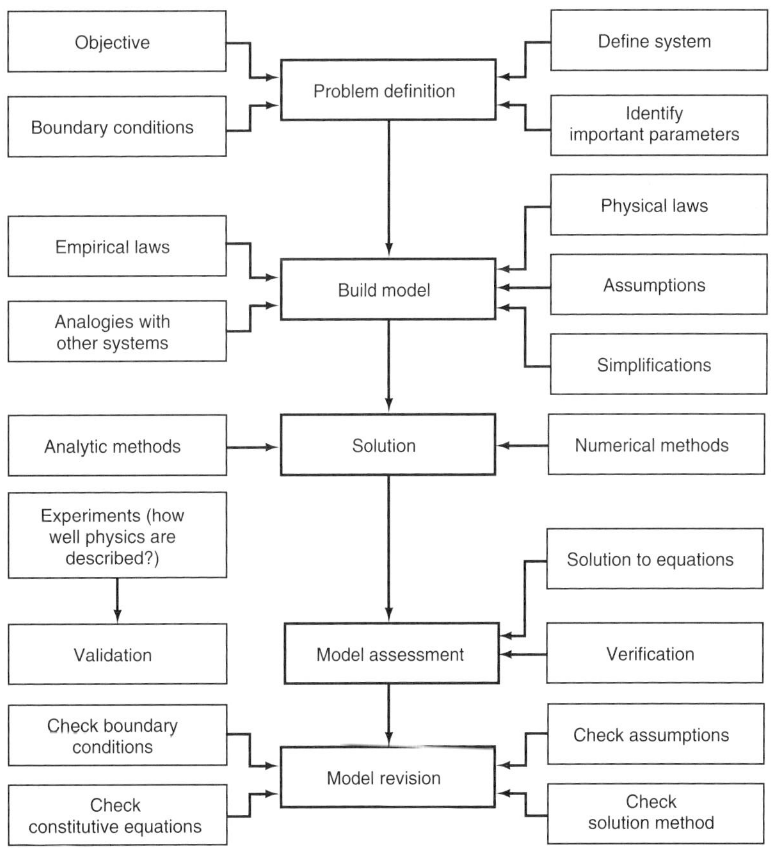

Fig. 11 Modeling flowchart

method for the governing equations. Next, one must check if there are deficiencies in the model. The model may have used an erroneous assumption, inappropriate empirical law, a false hypothesis, an oversimplification, or inaccurate boundary condition. For example, if it is assumed that the fiber-fiber interactions during the flow are not important, and the experimental results do not agree, then reexamining this assumption in the model might be necessary. Thus, it is important to separate the deficiencies in the model from those in the numerical methods, because both of these are packaged into a computer program, and it is very easy to regard them as one entity.

Another simple cause of disagreement could be inaccurate characterization of material parameters. For example, in RTM, the model may use a constant value for the permeability of the preform in the mold. However, in the experiment, the material may exhibit large variations. The result is that the experimental fill times or inlet pressures will be very different from the predicted ones. Thus, the process model may be correct, but incorrect specification of material parameters can cause disagreements. It is also useful to make certain that the physics embedded in the process model is the physics being described by the experiment.

There is a common saying that when a modeler is presenting results from a model, nobody believes them, except for the modeler. However, when an experimentalist presents the results, everyone believes them, except for the experimentalist. Thus, it is important to make sure that the experiment was conducted under the same conditions assumed in the model. It is important that the laboratory methods and practices assure accurate and consistent results: no inaccurate calibration of the measurement probes, leakage of the resin, fluctuations in the flow rate, or temperatures that would make the experimental boundary conditions different than the ones assumed in the model. These could be the root cause of disagreement.

Models routinely disagree with experiments, and revisions should be considered as a natural and necessary component of the modeling approach. The revisions can include additional physics in the model to explain the observations made in experiments. The refined model will thus more closely mirror the physical process.

REFERENCES

1. S.G. Advani and E.M. Sozer, *Process Modeling in Composites Manufacturing*, Marcel Dekker Publishers, New York, to be published 2002
2. S.G. Advani, Introduction, *Flow and Rheology in Polymeric Composites Manufacturing*, Suresh G. Advani, Ed., Elsevier Publishers, Amsterdam, 1994
3. T.G. Gutowski, A Brief Introduction to Composite Materials and Manufacturing Processes, *Advanced Composites Manufacturing*, T.G. Gutowski, Ed., John Wiley and Sons, New York, 1997
4. S.G. Advani and E.M. Sozer, Resin Impregnation in Liquid Molding Processes, *Comprehensive Composite Materials*, A. Kelly, Ed., Elsevier Science, 2000
5. C.L. Tucker III, Introduction, *Fundamentals of Computer Modeling for Polymer Processing*, C.L. Tucker III Ed., Hanser Publishers, Munich, Germany, 1989
6. C.M.O. Bradaigh, Sheet Forming of Composite Materials, *Flow and Rheology in Polymeric Composites Manufacturing*, Suresh G. Advani, Ed., Elsevier Publishers, Amsterdam, 1994
7. J.P. Fanucci, S. Nolet, and S. McCarthy, Pultrusion of Composites, *Advanced Composites Manufacturing*, T.G. Gutowski, Ed., John Wiley and Sons, New York, 1997
8. S. Shuler and S.G. Advani, Transverse Squeeze Flow of Concentrated Aligned Fibers in Viscous Fluids, *J. Non-Newton. Fluid Mech.*, Vol 65, 1996, p 47–74
9. T.S. Creasy, S.G. Advani, and R.K. Okine, Transient Rheological Behavior of a Long Discontinuous Fiber-Melt System, *J. of Rheology*, Vol 40, 1996, p 497–520
10. T.S. Creasy and S.G. Advani, A Model Long-Discontinuous Fiber Filled Thermoplastic Melt in Extensional Flow, *J. Non-Newton. Fluid Mech.*, Vol 73, 1997, p 261
11. W. Vanwest, R.B. Pipes, and S.G. Advani, Consolidation Mechanics in Co-Mingled Fabrics, *Polym. Compos.*, Vol 12, 1991, p 417–427
12. B.T. Åström, R.B. Pipes, and S.G. Advani, On Flow Through Aligned Fiber Beds and Its Application to Composites Processing, *J. Comp. Mat.*, Vol 26, 1992, p 1351–1373
13. J.D. Muzzy, Processing of Advanced Thermoplastic Composites, *Mfg. International '88*, ASME, Vol 4, 1988, p 27–39
14. J.D. Muzzy, X. Wu, and J.S. Colton, The Processing Science of Thermoplastic Composites, *Advanced Composites Manufacturing*, T.G. Gutowski, Ed., John Wiley and Sons, Inc., New York, 1997
15. S.G. Advani, M.V. Bruschke, and R. Parnas, Resin Transfer Molding, *Flow and Rheology in Polymeric Composites Manufacturing*, Suresh G. Advani, Ed., Elsevier Publishers, Amsterdam, 1994
16. C.L. Tucker III, Forming of Advanced Composites, *Advanced Composites Manufacturing*, T.G. Gutowski, Ed., John Wiley and Sons, New York, 1997
17. R.S. Parnas, *Liquid Composite Molding*, Hanser Publishers, Munich, Germany, 2000
18. L.J. Lee, Liquid Composite Molding, *Advanced Composites Manufacturing*, T.G. Gutowski, Ed., John Wiley and Sons, New York, 1997
19. A.C. Loos and J.T. Tzeng, Filament Winding, *Flow and Rheology in Polymeric Composites Manufacturing*, Suresh G. Advani, Ed., Elsevier Publishers, Amsterdam, 1994
20. G. Dillon, P. Mallon, and M. Monaghan, The Autoclave Processing of Composites, *Advanced Composites Manufacturing*, T.G. Gutowski, Ed., John Wiley and Sons, New York, 1997
21. R.B. Bird, R.C. Armstrong, and O. Hassager, *Dynamics of Polymeric Liquids*, John Wiley and Sons, New York, 1987
22. S. Middleman, *Fundamentals of Polymer Processing*, McGraw-Hill Book Company, New York, 1977
23. M.R. Kamal and M.E. Ryan, Models of Material Behavior, *Fundamentals of Computer Modeling for Polymer Processing*, C.L. Tucker III, Ed., Hanser Publishers, Munich, Germany, 1989
24. S.G. Advani and C.L. Tucker, A Numerical Simulation of Short Fiber Orientation in Compression Molding, *Polym. Compos.*, Vol 11, 1990, p 164–173
25. S.G. Advani and P. Simacek, Modeling and Simulation of Flow, Heat Transfer and Cure, *Resin Transfer Moulding for Aerospace Structures*, T. Kruckenberg and R. Paton, Ed., Kluwer Academic Publishers, Dordecht, The Netherlands, 1998
26. J. Kozeny, *Sitzungsberichte Wiener Akademie der Wissenshaft, Abt IIa*, Vol 136, 1927
27. P.C. Carman, Fluid Flow Through Granular Beds, *Institution of Chemical Engineers*, Vol 15, 1937
28. S. Middleman, *Fundamentals of Polymer Processing*, McGraw-Hill, 1977
29. C.-C. Lee and J.M. Castro, Model Simplification, Fundamentals of Computer Modeling for Polymer Processing, C.L. Tucker III, Ed., Hanser Publishers, Munich, Germany, 1989
30. O. Reynolds, On the Theory of Lubrication and Its Application to Mr. Beauchamps Tower's Experiments, *Philos. Trans. R. Soc.*, Vol 177, 1886, p 157–234
31. H. Darcy, *Les Fontaines Publiques de la Ville de Dijon*, Dalmont, Paris, 1856
32. C.L. Tucker III and S.G. Advani, Processing of Short-Fiber Systems, *Flow and Rheology in Polymeric Composites Manufacturing*, Suresh G. Advani, Ed., Elsevier Publishers, Amsterdam, 1994
33. S. Bickerton, "Modeling and Control of Flow during Impregnation of Heterogeneous Porous Media, with Application to Composite Mold Filling Processes," Ph.D. thesis, University of Delaware, 1998
34. M.M. Denn, *Process Modeling*, Longman, New York, 1986
35. Z. Tadmor and C.G. Gogos, *Principles of Polymer Processing*, John Wiley and Sons, Inc., New York
36. S.I. Guceri, Finite Difference Solution of Field Problems, *Fundamentals of Computer Modeling for Polymer Processing*, C.L. Tucker III, Ed., Hanser Publishers, Munich, Germany, 1989
37. M.R. Barone and T.A. Osswald, Boundary

Element Solution for Field Problems, *Fundamentals of Computer Modeling for Polymer Processing*, C.L. Tucker III, Ed., Hanser Publishers, Munich, Germany, 1989
38. J.F.T. Pittman, Finite Elements for Field Problems, *Fundamentals of Computer Modeling for Polymer Processing*, C.L. Tucker III, Ed., Hanser Publishers, Munich, Germany, 1989
39. H.P. Wang and H.S. Lee, Numerical Techniques for Free and Moving Boundary Problems, *Fundamentals of Computer Modeling for Polymer Processing*, C.L. Tucker III, Ed., Hanser Publishers, Munich, Germany, 1989

Composite Tooling

Louis C. Dorworth, Abaris Training Resources, Inc.

COMPOSITE TOOLING is the making of tools from composite materials. Since the early 1980s the "black art" of making high-performance advanced composite molds and fixtures has evolved from company proprietary methods to more conventional industry standards. The advent of low-temperature curing prepregs for high-temperature service has changed the course of the advanced composite tooling industry. The ability to lay-up and process a production prepreg tool laminate directly on a master model or plug has greatly improved the accuracy of these tools, and at the same time eliminated the cost of producing expensive intermediate tools.

While prepregs are preferred for high-performance tooling, "wet lay-up" materials and processes are still used for many other applications. Modern lay-up methods and vacuum bagging techniques can be employed with long pot-life resins to achieve acceptable tool laminates. Many of the wet lay-up methods and techniques parallel those used to fabricate prepreg tooling, which is the primary focus of this article.

Tool designers have also begun to adopt methods of component designers. The integration of stiffening flanges and other molded features in the design of composite tools has greatly contributed to increased dimensional stability as well as vacuum and pressure integrity of the composite tools. The goal is to minimize weight while maintaining stiffness of the tool laminate, thus reducing the size and mass of any supporting substructure. The resulting tools will have desirable thermal properties and will be efficient in production.

Many of the principles outlined in this article are currently recognized as standard shop practice for designing and fabricating quality composite tools in today's modern tooling shops.

Advantages of Composite Tools

The primary advantage of composite tooling is that it is lighter than metal tooling. This weight advantage makes for ease of handling, transportation, and storage of composite molds and fixtures. In many cases, light-duty carts and tugs can be employed instead of heavy-duty overhead cranes and forklifts. Most small-to-medium-size composite tools can be lifted onto tables, carts, and racks without additional handling equipment. The lower thermal mass contributes to more desirable heating and cooling rates than metals.

Composite tool laminates are generally manufactured to a relatively constant thickness. This provides for an ideal thermal gradient in the part. Compared to a machined metal tool that may have a varying cross-sectional thickness, the composite tool heats and cools more evenly and thus provides a more uniform temperature profile when processing a composite part.

Carbon-fiber-reinforced tool laminates have a very low coefficient of thermal expansion (CTE) and can be manufactured to more closely match the CTE of a carbon-fiber part. This is most important when molding complex shapes. Glass-fiber-reinforced tool laminates have a greater CTE than carbon fiber laminates and should only be considered for use in molding composite parts with very low process temperatures, or if the geometry allows for thermal differential. (See Table 1 for comparative material properties.)

The lower thermal mass of the composites translates into energy savings for all molds that are heated.

The facilities and equipment necessary for fabricating composite tools are virtually the same as that required for other composite manufacturing. This makes it possible for most composite component manufacturers to make their

Table 1 Thermal properties of selected tooling materials

		Specific heat		Thermal mass(a)		Thermal conductivity coefficient		Coefficient of thermal expansion	
Material	Specific gravity	J/kg · K	Btu/lb · °F	J/kg · K	Btu/lb · °F	W/m · K	Btu/h · ft · °F	10^{-6}/K	10^{-6}/°F
Metals									
Cast aluminum	2.70	962.8	0.23	2595.3	0.62	201.2	116.2	23.2	12.9
Steel	7.86	460.5	0.11	3600	0.86	51.9	30	12.1	6.7
304 stainless steel	8.02	502.3	0.12	4018.6	0.96	16.3	9.4	17.3	9.6
Nickel	8.90	418.6	0.10	3726	0.89	72.1	41.7	13.3	7.4
Invar 36	8.11	502.3	0.12	4060.4	0.97	10.47	6.1	1.4	0.8
Invar 42	8.13	502.3	0.12	4102.3	0.98	15.3	8.8	5.2	2.9
Plaster									
Gypsum-base	1.4–1.6	3516–4186	0.84–1.0	4939–6698	1.18–1.6	1.44	0.8	14.9	8.3
Composites									
Fiberglass/epoxy	1.8–2.0	1255.8	0.3	2260.4–2511.6	0.54–0.60	3.1–4.3	1.8–2.5	14.4–16.2	8.0–9.0
Carbon fiber/epoxy	1.5–1.6	1255.8	0.3	1883.7–2009.3	0.45–0.48	3.5–6.1	2.0–3.5	0–10.8	0–6.0
Graphite									
Monolithic	1.74–2.0	1130.22–1255.8	0.3–0.3	1967.42–2511.6	0.5–0.6	23.07–31.72	13.3–18.3	0.18–1.8	0.1–1.0

(a)Thermal mass is specific gravity times specific heat.

own tool laminates in-house. A substantial cost savings can be realized.

Another advantage of composite tooling is the relative ease of fabrication and duplication. Tool laminates can be laid-up on compound contours and complex shapes without much difficulty. Additionally, duplicate molds can be made off of the same model with precision and accuracy. This is a real benefit when multiple molds or fixtures are required for production. The turnaround time for a set of composite tools can be significantly less than for a set of machined metal tools of the same size and shape.

Disadvantages of Composite Tools

Composite tools have less durability and damage tolerance than metal tools. The biggest complaint throughout the advanced composite industry is that composite molds begin to lose their ability to maintain vacuum and/or pressure integrity. This problem can be attributed to several factors:

- The tool laminate is usually thermally cycled in production. This causes the resin to microcrack and eventually creates a path for vacuum or pressure leaks. This is primarily attributed to the difference in CTE between the resin matrix and the fiber reinforcement. Certain woven forms, such as large yarn or plain weave fabrics, are more prone to this problem because they have large, open areas at the intersecting yarns that are either void-filled or resin-rich. (See Fig. 1 and 2 for fabric void potential.)
- The use of knives or other sharp objects against the tool surface by the operator during the part lay-up can created fine scores in the resin layer at the surface of the mold, which contributes to the degradation of the laminate. This can be further aggravated when the part mechanically sticks to the scored surface upon demolding. Subsequently, the surface is fractured.
- Composite tooling can easily be damaged during transportation and should be handled using extreme care. Flexing the tool laminate or impacting the edges of the tool during transportation can propagate the internal microcrack path, leading to an increased leak rate.

Another disadvantage to composite tools is that they are not easily altered or adjusted. While it may be possible to weld or machine a joggle or other detail on a metal tool surface, this kind of alteration is more difficult with composites. Any machining of the molded tool surface is sure to lead to decreased vacuum or pressure integrity. Modifying the composite tool surface once it has initially been molded is not recommended.

Designing composite tools with turnbuckles and other adjustment devices has proven to be difficult. The composite tool laminate is not ductile like metal. When bending a composite laminate, there are fibers in tension at the outer layers and fibers in compression at the inner layers. These forces can lead to dimensional distortion, especially at elevated temperatures. (The shape that was achieved at room temperature is not necessarily maintained at higher temperatures.) In addition, the flexing of the matrix of the laminate while performing adjustments can cause cracking and contribute to the potential for vacuum or pressure leaks.

The quality of a composite tool is highly dependent on proper selection of materials and workmanship. Outside procurement of good quality composite tooling can be problematic due to the myriad of materials and processes available. One vendor's idea of a high-performance composite tool may differ greatly from that of another. A tool built using wet lay-up/vacuum bag techniques cannot compare to a tool made with prepregs in an autoclave process. It is wise to provide detailed tooling material and process specifications to all potential vendors, so that there are no questions as to what is expected in the tool construction.

Tool Design Overview

When designing composite tools, the first things to consider are the service requirements. Certain conditions such as the service temperature, vacuum/pressure requirements, production rate (number of parts or uses required), and engineering dimensional tolerances for the final part or assembly will govern the decision as to what materials and processes are used when building a tool laminate.

The actual tool laminate construction, including thickness, ply count, and orientation of fibers are determined by the size and shape of the tool as well as the static and dynamic loads that will be applied to the tool in service.

A shape that is inherently self-supporting, such as an aircraft radome (Fig. 3), can easily be designed with integrated stiffening features and less substructure. Shapes that are flat or slightly contoured usually require more detailed analysis of added stiffness and more substantial substructure to provide rigid support.

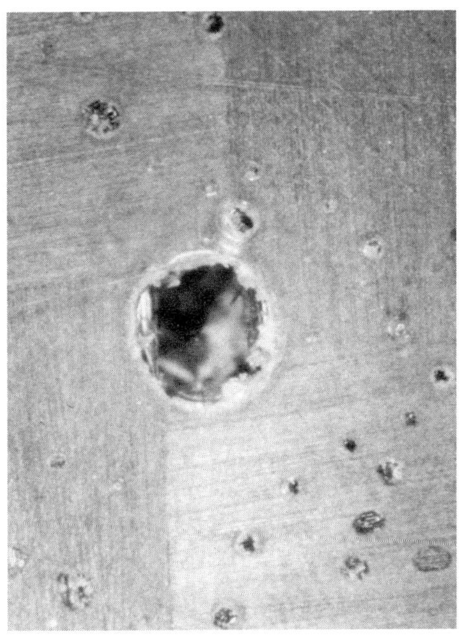
(a)

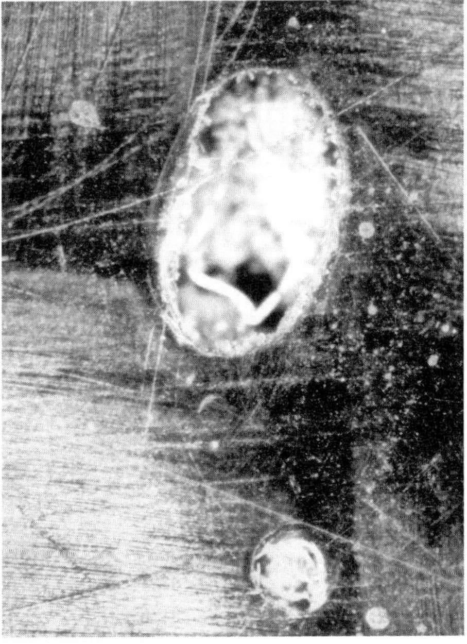
(b)

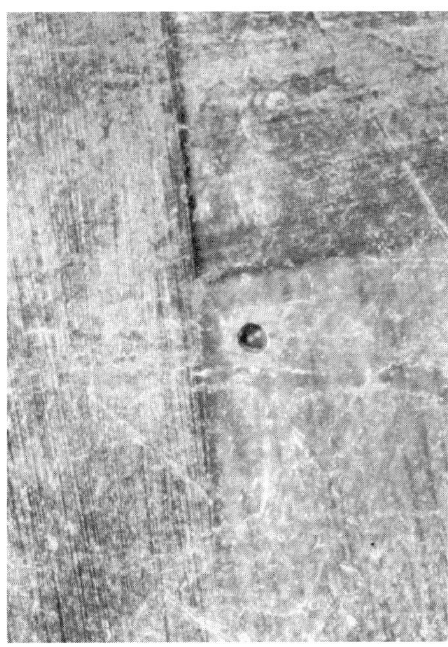
(c)

Fig. 1 Fabric influence on void potential. (a) 3K plain weave (b) 12K-2 × 2 basket weave (c) 6K-5HS satin carbon weave. 50×

Incorporating "bathtub" flanges that surround the tool laminate can be of great benefit to integrating stiffness into the design, especially for smaller molds and fixtures. Adding reverse flanges about the periphery so that the tool laminate does not directly sit on the edge will increase its durability (Fig. 4).

Simple add-on protective devices can preserve the integrity of a tool laminate. For example, the placement of an extruded rubber edge-guard material around the periphery of the tool laminate can protect the edge from minor impacts in production, such as contact with belt buckles.

Molded index fingers or locator buttons can be included in the design to provide accurate location for subsequent trimming, drilling, or assembly tools (Fig. 5). The use of standardized molded locators can improve vacuum and pressure integrity in high-performance tooling. Drilled locators and potted bushings or pins in these tools can lead to premature degradation of the tool laminate and often present maintenance problems in service.

Integrated bushings or pins can be molded in place, however these types of locators can also be problematic at elevated temperatures. If tooling holes and pin locations are necessary in the final part, drilling them from a secondary fixture may be more accurate. Care must be taken to account for thermal expansion when designing locator or index features so as to ensure proper part location in subsequent tools.

Provisions for wedging or otherwise extracting the part from the tool should also be considered at the design stage. Many composite tools and parts are designed with little or no thought about this issue and are subsequently damaged during the demolding process.

The final tool design may include a secondary structure, frame, or cart that may or may not be attached to the tool laminate. There are many concepts for design of substructure, from simple, light tubular or monocoque designs to heavier "eggcrate" structures. Additional features such as V-groove wheels for the autoclave rail track, or permanent vacuum bag/plumbing might be necessary to accommodate production-specific requirements.

Calculating differential linear thermal expansion is required for determining tooling hole and pin locations and for design of secondary structures when materials with differing CTE are used and the temperature will be cycled.

The coefficient of linear thermal expansion is symbolized α_l, and $\alpha_l = \Delta L/L$ per degree, where ΔL is a change in length. The change in length is therefore:

$$\Delta L = \alpha_l \cdot L \cdot \Delta T$$

where ΔT is the change in temperature.

The preferred units for α_l are 10^{-6}/K (SI) and 10^{-6}/°F (U.S. customary). Values can be converted using the factors shown below:

To convert	To	Multiply by
10^{-6}/K	10^{-6}/°C	1
10^{-6}/K	10^{-6}/°F	0.55556
10^{-6}/°F	10^{-6}/K	1.8

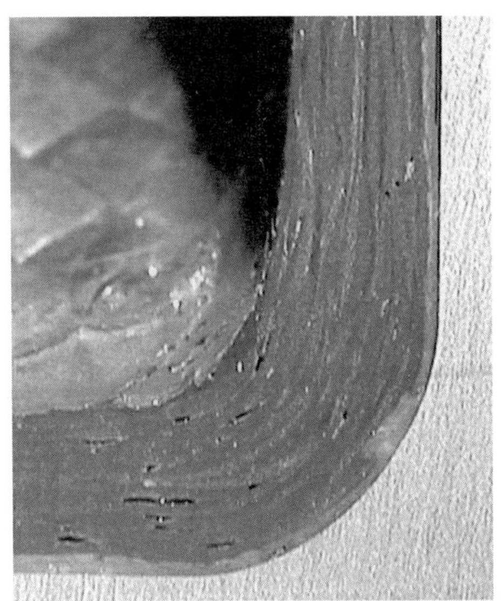

Fig. 2 Typical inner-laminar voids found in a laminate made with 3K plain weave carbon fabric. 200×

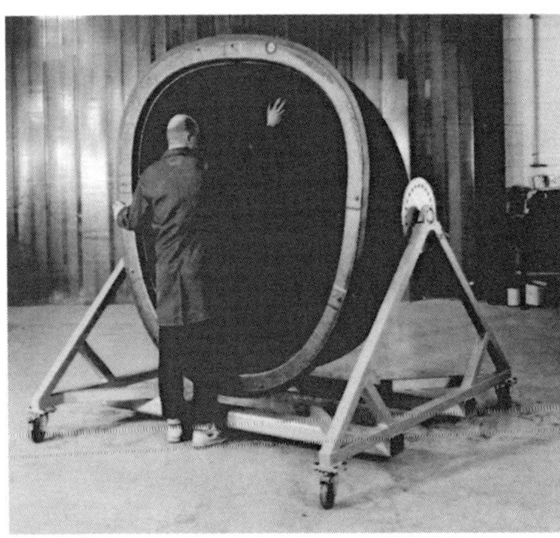

Fig. 3 Aircraft radome tooling. Courtesy of The Advanced Composites Group, Inc.

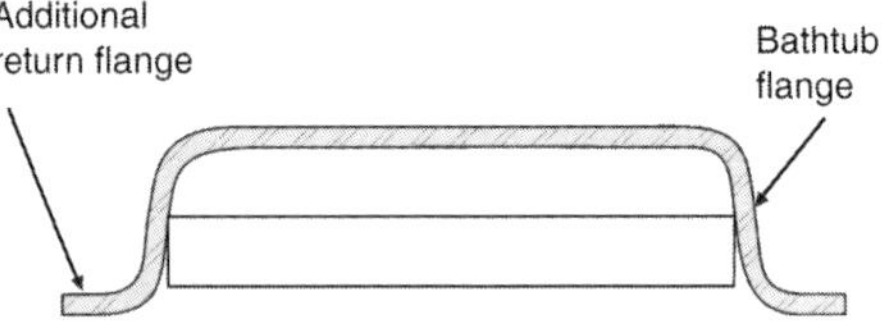

Fig. 4 Integral stiffening flanges

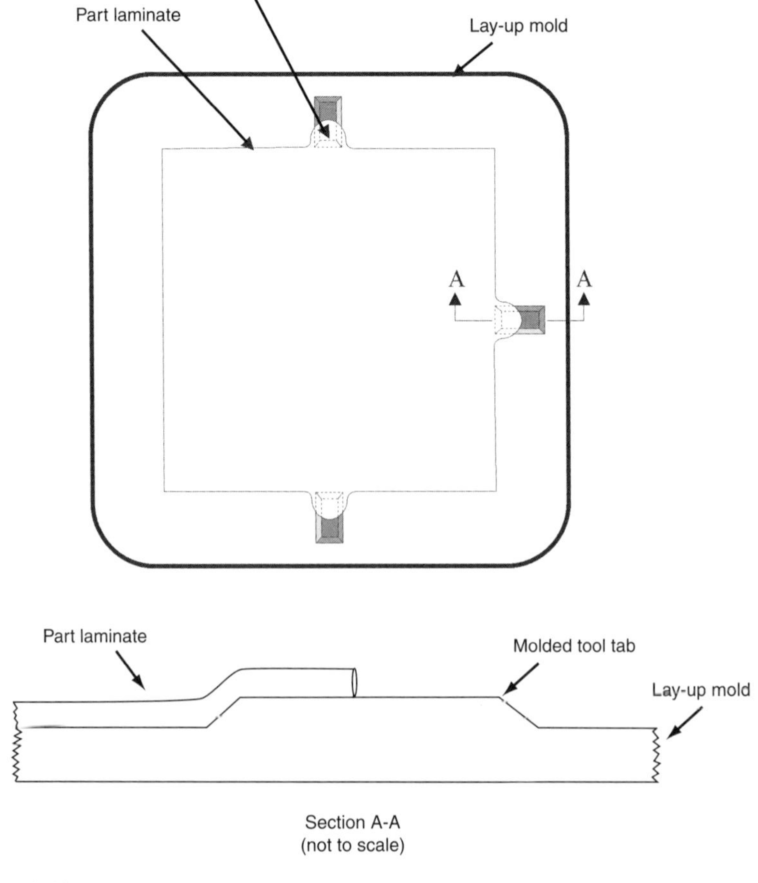

Fig. 5 Molded locator features

Example 1: Calculating the Differential Thermal Expansion for an Aluminum Substructure. An aluminum substructure of 122 cm (48 in.) is heated from an ambient temperature of 21 °C (70 °F) to the processing temperature of 177 °C (350 °F), so the change in temperature is 156 °C (280 °F). A typical CTE for this aluminum is 23.2×10^{-6}/K (12.9×10^{-6}/°F). Calculating the ΔL in SI units:

$$\Delta L = (23.2 \times 10^{-6}) \cdot 122 \cdot 156$$

$$\Delta L = 0.442 \text{ cm}$$

Calculating the ΔL in U.S. customary units:

$$\Delta L = (12.9 \times 10^{-6}) \cdot 48 \cdot 280$$

$$\Delta L = 0.173 \text{ in.}$$

Example 2: Calculating the Differential Thermal Expansion for a Carbon Fiber Reinforced Plastic (CFRP) Mold. A CFRP mold also 122 cm (48 in.) in length is subjected to the same thermal cycle as in Example 1. The CTE of the CFRP in the direction of interest is 3.6×10^{-6}/K (2.0×10^{-6}/°F). Calculating the ΔL in SI units:

$$\Delta L = (3.6 \times 10^{-6}) \cdot 122 \cdot 156$$

$$\Delta L = 0.069 \text{ cm}$$

Calculating the ΔL in U.S. customary units:

$$\Delta L = (2.0 \times 10^{-6}) \cdot 48 \cdot 280$$

$$\Delta L = 0.027 \text{ in.}$$

It should be noted that the CTE for composite tooling depends on the ply orientation.

Master Model or Pattern Design

The master model or pattern from which the tool laminate is to be made must provide for all the tool features, such as the molded flanges, locators, and indexes. It must also provide a suitable quality surface and be capable of withstanding the process conditions the tool laminate will require. The heat transfer capability and the service temperature of the model or pattern must be considered when processing at elevated temperatures. The model or pattern surface should not leak when subjected to vacuum or autoclave pressure or deform when heated. A pre-lay-up vacuum and/or pressure check is necessary prior to committing materials to the model surface.

Appropriate draft angles should be designed into the model or pattern to ensure ease of parting when the tool laminate is later removed. Prepositioned wedges or wax strips along the parting planes of the model or pattern may also be considered to minimize forces when demolding the tool laminate. This forethought can improve the final quality of the tool laminate.

Locations for removable fences or planks should be included on the model or pattern when multi-piece tools are to be built. Parting planes can include molded self-alignment features and be designed to minimize difficulties in tool fabrication and subsequent manufacturing.

Designing flat surfaces, flanges, or parting planes on or parallel to the primary *X*, *Y*, or *Z* axis planes can be useful for rigging or setup of the subsequent tooling that is made from the model or pattern. Various materials can be considered for construction of the master model. Cast polyurethane or epoxy tooling planks can be bonded together and numerical control machined to shape. Other materials, such as wood, metal, plaster, and foam, have also been used for this purpose. The choice of materials is often determined by the capabilities of the shop and their familiarity with the material.

The master model or pattern may require the application of a surface sealer, and assuredly, a mold release agent prior to molding. The materials selected for sealing and releasing the model or pattern should be tested and deemed compatible with the resin system to be used in the construction of the tool laminate.

Fiber and Fabric Selection

E-glass and high-strength carbon-fiber fabric reinforcements are typically used in the construction of rigid tool laminates. On the basis of cost per weight, E-glass is the less expensive of the two materials; however, E-glass is heavier (2.55 g/cm^3) than carbon (1.76 g/cm^3) and is less stiff. Laminates made with E-glass have a higher CTE and thermal mass than laminates made with carbon fiber (Table 2). Aramid fibers are usually not used for solid laminate tools. Aramid-fiber-reinforced elastomeric products are available for use in flexible and semirigid tool fabrication.

Long fiber fabric forms are preferred over short, random fiber (mat) materials for construction of high-performance tool laminates. Long fiber fabrics offer greater stiffness and strength. Unidirectional materials are generally not used in the construction of composite tool laminates. The incorporation of unidirectional layers in shear-web stiffeners or bathtub flanges may be useful, however.

The most popular fabric styles used in advanced composite tooling are twill, plain, and satin weaves. The plain and twill weave fabrics generally have a lower yarn count per inch than satin weaves. This makes the plain weave one of the least expensive fabric styles. The trade-off is that the plain weave is less drapable than the twills or the satin weaves, while providing less fiber load per ply. Another disadvantage of plain weave fabrics compared to the satin weaves is that they have a greater number of open areas at the intersecting yarns that are either void-filled or resin-rich (Fig. 1 and 2).

While helpful in quickly building thickness, the use of heavy double satin, 2 × 2 basket, modified plain, and leno weaves is discouraged for use in high-performance tool lay-ups because these materials tend to produce laminates with a very high resin and void content.

Resins

Epoxy resins are the most popular choice for high-performance tools, while polyester and vinyl ester systems are perhaps the most widely used resins for tooling outside of the aerospace industry. Other resins, such as bismaleimides (BMI) and polycyanates (cyanate esters), can also be used for constructing high-temperature (>200 °C or 392 °F) composite tool laminates.

Polyester resins have the lowest cost per kilogram of any of these systems, while the vinyl esters are a close second. The costs of epoxies vary depending on the formulation, but are considerably less expensive than the BMI or polycyanate systems.

Comparatively, epoxies offer medium-to-high-temperature capabilities, with generally greater strength and fiber adhesion properties than polyester or vinyl ester resins. While the temperature capabilities of epoxies are not as great as those of the BMI or polycyanate systems, they are adequate for use in many process applications (Table 2).

Surface Coat and Surface Ply

The use of surface coat resins are typical in wet lay-up construction but may or may not be required for prepreg tool laminates. Prepreg surface ply materials have been developed for use in non-autoclave and vacuum bag tool laminate construction by at least one prepreg manufacturer. The prepreg surface ply is preferred in lieu of a surface coat with that system because it provides more uniform resin content with a higher fiber volume at the tool surface. Surface coat resins are generally not required for autoclave-cured tool laminates.

If surface coat resins are to be used in the construction of high-performance laminates, then application of a thin, consistent layer is crucial. One to two layers, totaling up to 0.5 mm (0.02 in.) thick is recommended. Thicker applications can lead to cracking and crazing of the surface when exposed to elevated temperatures.

Table 2 Resin temperature comparison

	Cure temperature		Service temperature	
Resin	°C	°F	°C	°F
Polyester	RT–121	RT–250	60–140	140–285
Vinyl ester	RT	RT	49–149	120–300
Epoxy	RT–177	RT–350	65–191	150–375
Bismaleimide	177–288	350–550	204–316	400–600
Cyanate ester	121–177	250–350	93–288	200–550

RT, room temperature

To control the surface coat resin thickness, laminators estimate the area to be covered and calculate how much resin is necessary to cover the area at the prescribed thickness. Often, epoxy surface coats are applied by using hand squeegees and short bristle brushes to uniformly distribute the resin. Polyester surface coat resins are often sprayed on because they can be reduced to a spray-on consistency without affecting the surface quality.

As with any resin interface in the laminate, it is imperative that the surface coat resin be chemically active when the next layer is applied. Usually this means that the resin is allowed to partially gel and devolatilize prior to the application of the next layer. Timing the interface is critical to achieving a good bond.

Tool Laminate Construction Techniques

Precise lay-up of the composite tool laminate is the key to making a good production tool. A carefully laid-up laminate, employing much attention to detail, will result in a high-quality mold or fixture that resists leaks and will perform for many cycles.

As with other composite structures, it is recommended that a basic quasi-isotropic, balanced, and symmetrical laminate using 0°, 90°, +45°, and –45° angles of orientation be designated in most cases. For larger-sized tools, using either wet lay-up or prepreg processes, plies are generally cut into conveniently sized rectangles or "tiles" to make the lay-up more manageable. These tiles are cut with the warp yarns running in the long direction and then laid-up in such a manner that the warp yarns (or the length of the rectangle) match the orientation requirements for each layer.

It is accepted practice to overlap the finer (face) plies approximately 2 to 10 mm (0.08–0.4 in.) at all splice joints. The subsequent bulk plies are then butt spliced. Joint locations are then offset a minimum of 25 mm (1 in.) for each subsequent ply. Gaps between the butt joints can be filled with additional yarns if required to maximize fiber volume and to reduce the potential for voids or resin-rich pockets in the laminate.

Great care is taken to prevent bridging of the fibers in tight corners or joggles, both during lay-up and through subsequent processing. A good rule is to disallow continuous fibers through inside radii by splicing each layer at or near the corner. The use of separate 25 to 50 mm (1–2 in.) wide strips at these locations can aid in reducing bridging. The splice locations for these strips are typically alternated every ply so that no two adjacent plies are spliced in the same place.

Vacuum debulking is somewhat labor intensive but the benefits justify the labor involved in performing this operation. The use of a perforated release film, bleeder/breather materials, and a vacuum bag to debulk plies at selected intervals is one of the most valuable methods of reducing inner-laminar defects. Debulking every ply in the tool laminate stack allows the laminator to inspect every layer in-process. If there are any defects, such as small bridges in tight corners, gaps between butt-spliced pieces, or other abnormalities, these problems can be fixed prior to the application of additional layers.

It is important to be mindful of the working time or out time of the materials used in the construction of the tool laminate so that each layer or series of layers is applied within its recommended time. This will assure the best possible bond between each layer. For larger tools, if this is not possible, a portion of the laminate stack may be laid-up and partially processed prior to the completion of the lay-up. When this situation occurs, proper preparation of the previous surface is mandatory prior to proceeding. The use of a (non-release-treated) peel ply on the surface, then removed and followed by a careful scuff with a fine abrasive buffing pad is recommended to energize the backside surface prior to bonding. The surface should be cleaned and free of dust before additional layers are applied.

When using a wet lay-up process, an "interface coat" of laminating resin should be applied to the cleaned surface before proceeding. With prepreg materials, an interface coat is typically not necessary. (Consult the specific prepreg material manufacturer for recommendations.)

The final vacuum bag, bleeder, and breather stack should be designed to accommodate the materials and processing conditions to be used for curing the tool laminate. For example, a prepreg laminate with a net resin content that will be cured in the autoclave may require a "no-bleed" schedule that involves a release film layer sealed at all edges. It may also need to be covered with a thick, non-woven breather layer within the bag. A wet lay-up laminate with a high resin content, which is to be cured in an oven or under vacuum bag conditions at ambient temperatures, may require a porous peel ply, a bleeder layer, a separator film, and a breather layer within the vacuum bag.

Curing and Demolding

Depending on the resin system, curing may require allowing the laminate to sit at room temperature for a number of hours or days, or curing may occur in an oven or an autoclave at elevated temperatures. It is advisable to follow the resin manufacturer's instructions without deviation. Shortcutting the cure cycle can lead to a loss of structural and/or thermal properties in the tool laminate. Accelerating the cure with higher than recommended temperatures can also be detrimental. Generating an exothermic reaction in excess of the resin capabilities can lead to excessive shrinkage, reduced cross-linking, and/or microcracking within the laminate.

It is imperative that the initial cure be complete before the tool laminate is demolded. Often, low-temperature curing, high-temperature service resin systems require an initial cure cycle followed by an elevated temperature postcure cycle. The postcure is usually done after the substructure has been attached and the tool laminate is demolded from the model or pattern. This is called a "free-standing postcure." Because the resin system is weak and not entirely cross-linked prior to postcure, it can easily be damaged if flexed or impacted at this time. For this reason, extreme care should be taken to prevent excessive force on the tool laminate when demolding.

Cutting and Trimming

Any cutting or trimming of the tool laminate should be done only after it has been cured and/or postcured. For mold-quality tool laminates it is recommended that the lay-up be done in such a fashion that the postprocess trimming be limited to grinding or sanding off the sharp edges around the periphery. The vibration and heat generated during conventional machining operations can greatly affect the resin matrix at the edges of the tool laminate. This can lead to premature leaks in vacuum integral tool laminates.

If cutting or trimming is required, then the use of a high-speed circular saw or cutting wheel is preferred over a reciprocating saw. Carbide or diamond abrasive-coated steel blades work best for cutting carbon and glass-reinforced tool laminates. Waterjet cutting of the tool periphery might also be considered if available.

Substructure Design

Normally the direct substructure is built using the same or similar materials as that used in the construction of the tool laminate. Solid laminate panels or tubes are preferred over honeycomb-paneled substructures, because they are generally more durable.

If the tooling is to be used at elevated temperatures, then any potential differential thermal expansion between the tool laminate and the substructure should be examined. Dissimilar materials can be destructive at elevated temperatures if tied directly to the tool laminate. Some tool designers, however, have successfully used dissimilar materials such as steel framework, with advanced composite tool laminates by creating limited attachment points (Fig. 6).

The best substructure designs provide rigid support for the tool laminate with the minimal addition of weight and mass. The conventional eggcrate designs of yesterday have come under examination as being inefficient and costly. Tool designers today are getting away from the old "box-crate" designs and are instead using smaller-sized "box-trussing" techniques (Fig. 7) or modular, tubular structures.

Some of the most efficient designs tie the box-truss type components to the integrally molded bathtub flanges of the tool laminate. The cross supports in this design are attached with strips of resin-impregnated cloth to the inside surface

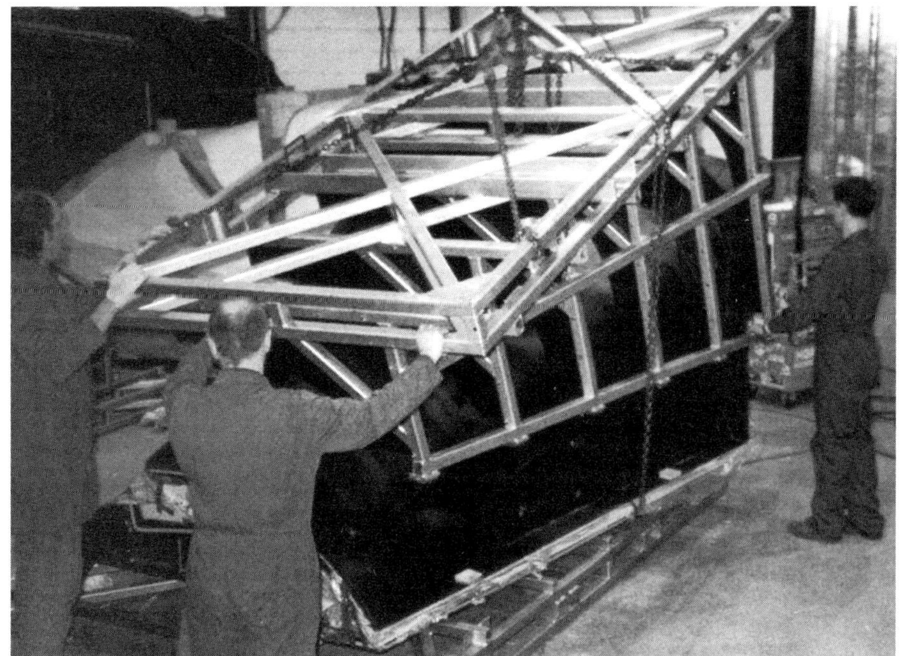

Fig. 6 Steel substructure attached to composite tool laminate. Courtesy of The Advanced Composites Group, Inc.

of the molded flanges at the base. These cross supports are typically only 25 to 50% of the height of the molded flange and may post up to the backside of the tool laminate as required to provide interim stanchions.

Another popular and effective substructure design includes the use of square or rectangular composite tubular components that are fastened and bonded together using factory-molded corners, tee fittings, and flat gusset plates. The modular design of these tubular structures makes construction fast and easy with minimal material waste. Like the box-truss-bathtub design, "spaceframe" tubular structures promote good airflow around the tool for elevated temperature processing in the oven or autoclave (Fig. 8).

The use of a rigid steel frame structure in conjunction with a minimized composite substructure, attached through "free-floating" attachments, can also be considered. This is probably the most economical way to facilitate large-scale tool designs (Fig. 9).

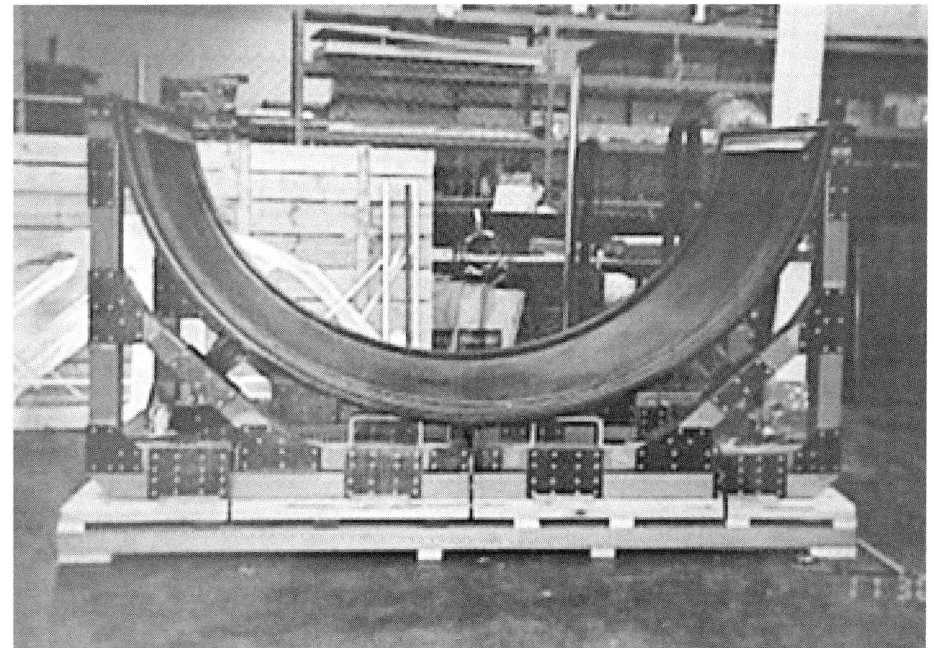

Fig. 8 Tubular spaceframe construction of substructure of cowl tool. Courtesy of Airtech International, Inc.

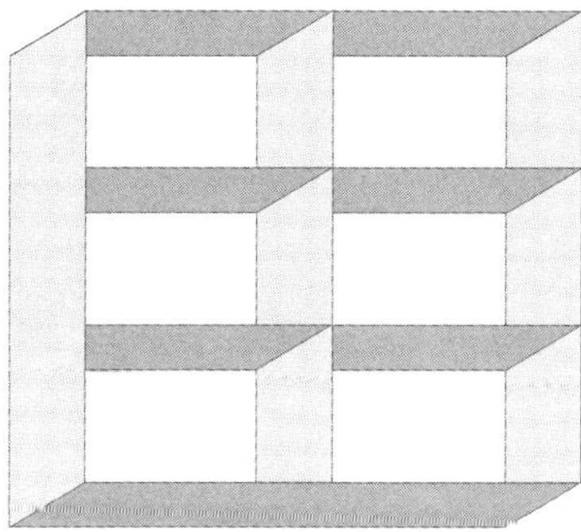

Box-crate design

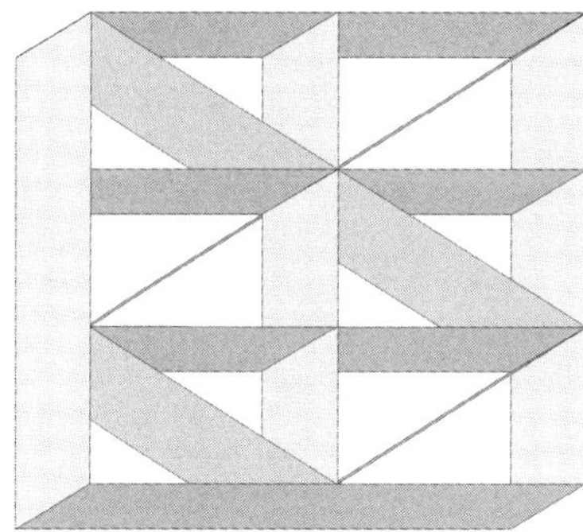

Truss-box design

Fig. 7 Conventional box-crate vs. truss-box design

Some manufacturers have created designs where the substructure is not tied into the tool laminate at all. This "cradle" approach usually requires a more substantial substructure because it does not fully use the load-carrying ability of the tool laminate itself.

There are many ideas on how to attach the substructure to the tool laminate. One concept involves attaching the structure to the tool laminate with a thin silicone bead and fillet. This idea allows for the difference in CTE (if applicable) to be taken up by the silicone rubber. With this method, it is important to have a uniform thickness (3–5 mm, or 0.12–0.20 in.) of rubber between the substructure and the backside of the tool laminate. Of course, the silicone rubber must meet the service temperature requirements.

Other designs use the wet-fabric-tie-in technique. Usually several strips of fabric are tied to the tool laminate at equally spaced increments, constituting an approximate 50% area of "tie-in." Standard practice is to leave a nominal 5 mm (0.20 in.) gap between any header stock and the backside of the tool laminate, so as to reduce direct force contact and to minimize the potential heat sink in the area of the attachment.

To minimize possible distortion or shrinkage, if the substructure is a composite, the subcomponents of the substructure should be postcured before assembly. This is especially important when cross supports are to be bonded between integrally molded flanges in a monocoque tool design. As a general rule, the substructure assembly itself is cured and/or postcured prior to attachment to the tool laminate.

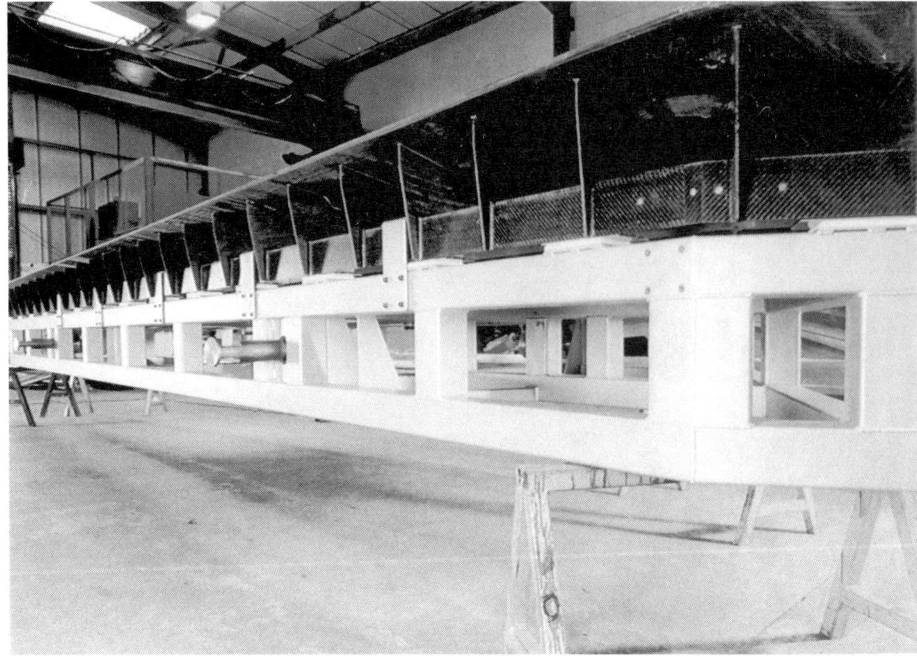

Fig. 9 Carbon-epoxy tool "free floating" on steel frame. Courtesy of The Advanced Composites Group, Inc.

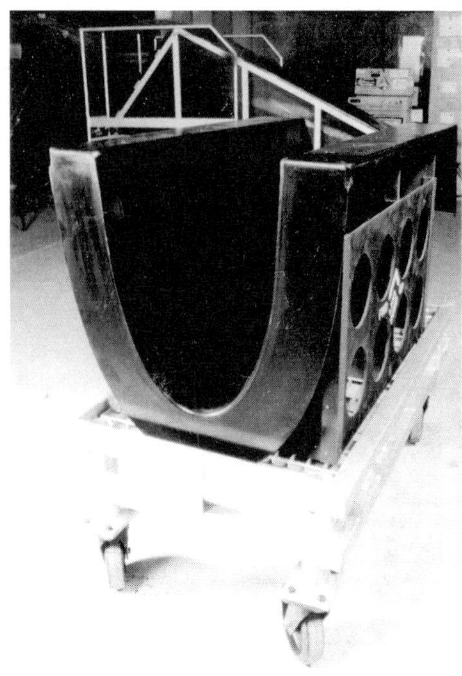

Fig. 10 Composite tool mounted on steel cart. Courtesy of The Advanced Composites Group, Inc.

Steel or aluminum carts can be used for transportation of composite tooling. The carts may or may not be designed with universal features to accommodate a range of tools/sizes (Fig. 10). For large tools, the carts can be designed with V-groove wheels to mount on a track in the oven or autoclave.

Future Outlook

The use of prepreg materials for tool construction will continue to grow. Materials manufacturers are continually improving existing products and creating new products for use in tooling. Development of resin systems that have extended work life and low-temperature cures will continue to dominate the tool fabrication industry because they will produce the most dimensionally stable tools.

There is much promise for low-expansion, high-temperature-capable resins, such as polycyanate formulas, to come to the forefront in the fabrication of high-performance tooling in the future. The strength, toughness, and low CTE of this type of resin system make it a viable choice for tool laminate construction. Such properties are ideal for use with carbon-fiber reinforcements beause the CTE are similar. The somewhat high cost of this resin system is a limitation, however the cost may be justified if the tool laminate has resistance to vacuum leaks provides for more parts in production.

The use of elastomers in conjunction with the construction of tool laminates for improved durability and leak prevention is a well-known concept that is still to come to fruition. Many companies have perfected the use of elastomeric membranes for use as leak barriers in high-performance tools, yet the application of this concept is still limited. The use of coprocessed elastomers in tool laminates that require hinge joints and/or other flexible features will also be more widespread. More development of these materials and processes will be seen in future tool laminate designs.

Manufacturers that have switched to metal alloys for production tooling will reconsider composites in the future. The lightweight advantage of composites combined with the lower costs and increased durability of the next-generation materials will encourage a swing in this direction.

SELECTED REFERENCES

- "Advanced Composite Tooling: Design & Fabrication" and "Composites: Technologies & Economics," 1999 Workbook, Abaris Training Resources, Inc.
- Fabric Handbook, Hexcel Fabrics, 1997
- Kevin S. Jackson, Low Temperature Curing Prepreg Systems for Composite Repair Tooling: A Method of Making Tools Directly From Parts, *ACG* Vol 166 (No. 2), The Advanced Composites Group,1994
- Materials & Products Catalog, Airtech International, May 2000
- John J. Morena, *Advanced Composite Mold Making,* Van Nostrand Reinhold Co., 1988
- Training Manual-LTM Mould Tool Manufacture, *ACG* Vol 124, (No. 1), The Advanced Composites Group, 1997
- "Zyvax Product Application Guide," (No. 1, Revision 1), Zyvax, Inc., 1999

Electroformed Nickel Tooling

Jim R. Logsdon, EMF Corporation

ELECTROFORMING is the production or reproduction of an article by electrodepositing a thickness of metal onto a form or shape called a mandrel and subsequently separating that deposit (or electroform) from the mandrel. Electroforming is a mature, well-recognized technology and is used in various applications including making printing plates for currency, rotary screens for printing textiles, intricate wave guides, high-precision solder masks, and molds of all sizes—from small, extremely complex molds for compact disk production to huge molds having surface areas greater than 18.6 m^2 (200 ft^2).

Electroformed molds offer a competitive alternative to aluminum, steel, and fiberglass/resin molds. Two factors considered in new mold procurement are the total cost (both initial cost and maintenance cost) and expected life of the mold. In the case of electroformed molds, it usually costs less and takes less time to produce a metal-faced mold by electroforming an approximately 5 mm (0.2 in.) thick metal shell, mounting the shell to a support structure, and adding heating/cooling lines, vacuum systems, and ejectors (if required) than machining a mold. It is possible using an electroformed mold to produce parts having a variety of contours at the pressures typically used in most molding processes.

Electroforming Process

While the initial process of electroforming is identical to electroplating, it is the preparation of the mandrel and the removal of the electroform that differentiates the two processes. The surface of the metal deposited against the mandrel will replicate the surface finish and contour of the mandrel exactly so that very fine details, textures, or other finishes on the mandrel surface will be reproduced in the electroform. For a variety of reasons, electroforming is commercially done with only a few of the metals that are used in electroplating. These metals are primarily nickel, copper, and to a lesser extent, gold or silver. Copper electroforms are primarily used in applications where high thermal and electrical conductivity is required, such as microwave guides or circuit boards. The higher strength, hardness, and versatility of nickel has made it the material of choice for electroforming large parts such as molds. The wide range of mechanical properties that can be incorporated in nickel electroforms is a function of the type of electrolyte and the knowledge and expertise of the electroformer. The electrolytes used for electroforming are basically the same as those used for electroplating and the properties of the deposit can be influenced by operating conditions and solution additives. For example, the current density (i.e., the total amperage placed on the mandrel divided by its surface area) employed during the deposition process can affect the appearance and mechanical properties of the deposit, as can electrolyte pH and temperature. The addition of organic sulfur containing "grain refiners" to the nickel bath increases the hardness of the deposit, but the incorporated sulfur limits the maximum usable temperature. However, the addition of cobalt to a nickel solution will improve the deposit hardness without any temperature limitations. Thus, the electroformer has a wide range of options to consider when making molds.

The values that are listed in Table 1 are specific for a sulfamate nickel plating solution that typically produces a deposit having the lowest stress levels of all of the nickel plating solutions. Typical values for both a normal and a "hard" sulfamate bath (i.e., one containing a grain refiner) are tabulated.

Once the range of nickel properties is deemed acceptable for a planned mold, then some additional factors need to be considered. These include the shape and size of the mold, the expected durability of the mold, the required delivery time, and the manufacture and cost of the necessary mandrel.

Shape of the Mold. There are some contour limitations when using electroforming for mold manufacturing. Usually the cavity or female mold half is the easier of the two halves to electroform since electrodeposition will take place on the outside surface of a male mandrel, whereas the female mandrel used for the core or male mold half requires deposition on the inside of the mandrel. Thus, the male molds are typically more difficult to produce due to current density distribution on the inside of the mandrel. An experienced electroformer will recognize difficult geometries and take the appropriate steps to ensure a good electroform. Figure 1 shows examples of the deposit thickness distributions that can occur on different mandrel geometries. The electroformer can use shielding on outside corners or projections and/or auxiliary anodes in recessed areas to improve thickness uniformity, and the use of these processing aids also reduces the time required to finish the electrodeposition phase of the mold manufacture. Experience shows that if a molder feels that the molded part can be removed from the mold without the use of movable cores or removable inserts, then the mold geometry probably would lend itself to the electroforming process.

Size of the Mold. The ability to produce large area molds by electroforming only requires an electroforming tank and solution that is large enough to submerse the mandrel for the amount of time required to deposit the desired thickness. Parts that have been produced by nickel electroforming have included lay-up molds in excess of 26 m^2 (280 ft^2) for aircraft part production and resin transfer molding (RTM) molds having a nickel area greater than 14 m^2 (150 ft^2) per mold half for making truck components. With nickel tanks as large as 11.3 by 4.3 by 4.3 m (37 by 14 by 14 ft) available in the United States, the electroforming capacity available for composite molds is almost unlimited.

Table 1 Typical properties of sulfamate nickel deposits at 25 °C (75 °F)

	Hardness,	Tensile strength		Elongation,	Internal stress		Purity,	Application temperature	
Deposit	HRC	MPa	ksi	%	MPa	ksi	%	°C	°F
Normal	16–23	414–758	60–110	10–20	14–42(a)	2–6(a)	99+	>980	>1800
Hard	30–50	862–1725	125–250	5–15	0–103(b)	0–15(b)	99+	>230(c)	>450(c)

(a) Tensile. (b) Compressive. (c) Depends on grain-refiner content

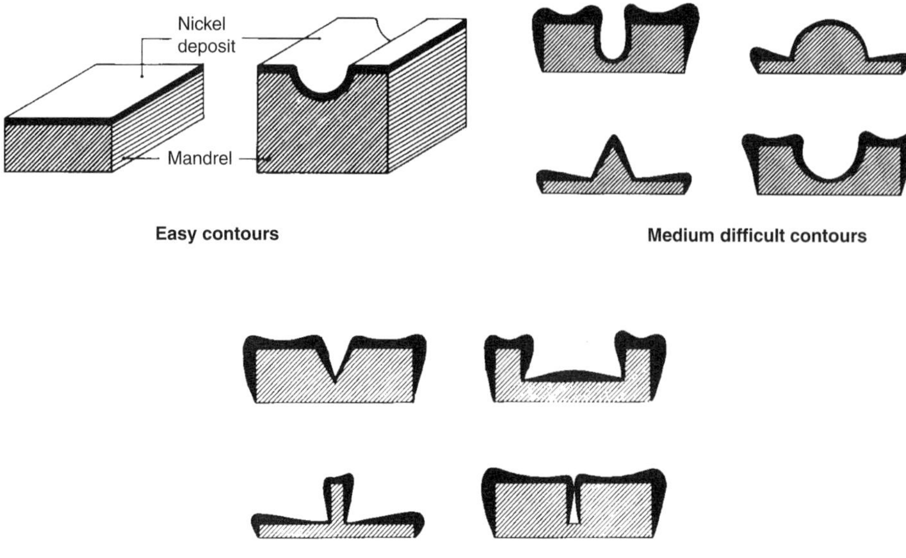

Fig. 1 Examples of deposit thickness distribution for various contours

Mold Fabrication Time. The time to complete a mold is a function of its size, shape, desired metal thickness, and type of mold. The metal thickness of an electroformed mold is a function of the average plating current during the deposition cycle and the total time of deposition. Typical thickness of nickel electroformed molds is approximately 5 mm (0.2 in.). For this thickness, an easy to medium-difficult geometry (see Fig. 1) may require 4 to 6 weeks for completion of the electroform. If the electroform is to be used for either autoclave tooling or an RTM preform mold as shown in Fig. 2 and 3, an additional 2 to 3 weeks may be required for final completion of the mold. If the electroform is to be the face sheet of a compression mold as shown in Fig. 4, then the addition of heating/cooling lines, ejectors, leader pins, and/or side locks can add an additional 4 to 8 weeks depending on the size of the nickel electroform. Electroforms having more difficult contours may require as long as 6 to 10 weeks to complete the deposition process depending on the exact contour.

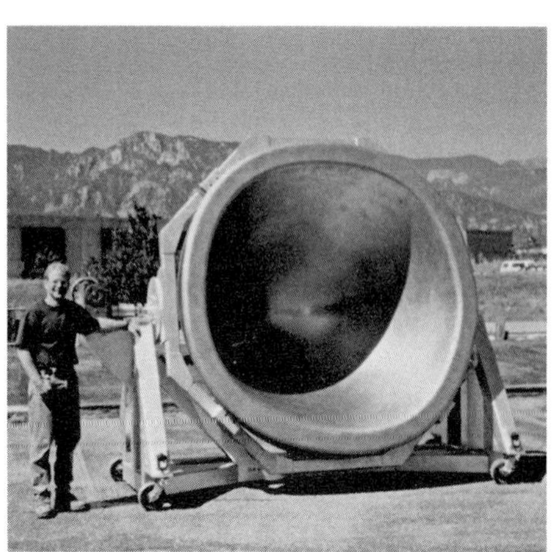

Fig. 2 Autoclave curing mold for aircraft radome

Durability of Nickel Molds. Nickel molds have demonstrated an increased damage tolerance compared to the softer aluminum or fiberglass/resin molds. Cleanup of a mold with a hand-held scraper to remove excess resin can gouge a soft face mold, but may only leave a rub mark on the nickel surface. It is possible to repair a damaged nickel surface by soldering or welding a damaged area and then repolishing to the original contour. Such repairs, however, may be visible on the surface of a high-gloss molded part, even though they are hardly noticeable on the nickel surface. Chrome plating of the nickel surface can further increase its surface hardness to the same value as a chrome-plated steel mold.

Mandrel Cost and Design Considerations

Mandrel fabrication guidelines can be supplied by most electroformers for customers furnishing the required mandrel. The manufacture of the mandrel and its surface is a critical stage in the production of electroformed molds. A poorly built, flimsy mandrel may distort during the electroforming process, resulting in contour variations in the electroform. Since the mandrel surface is exactly replicated by the electroform, surface blemishes such as pits and bumps will be reproduced in the surface of the electroform. This section briefly discusses mandrel fabrication by either the use of fiberglass/resins or by the machining of the mandrel directly from computer-aided design (CAD) data.

Fiberglass/Resin Mandrels. When a master model is available, the mandrel may be made by either making it directly off the model or by making a reverse or splash from the model and then making the mandrel from these expendable aids. In both cases, there may be some loss in contour tolerance due to the shrinkage of the resins used in the reverse and/or mandrel. If an existing mold needs to be replaced, it is sometimes possible to make the mandrel directly from that mold, depending on the surface quality of the mold. Again, some shrinkage of the resin may occur, resulting in the mandrel surface not exactly replicating the mold contour. The surface of the mandrel is usually manufactured with several layers of resin face coats backed with as much as 10 to 13 mm (0.4–0.5 in.) of fiberglass/resin. This face sheet must be supported in order to retain its contour, and this is done by a variety of methods. The two main ones use either laminates made of the same material as the face sheet that are attached to the back of the surface to give rigidity to the face sheet or steel or composite tubing or pipe attached to the back of the face. If a metal framework is used, it must be coated to prevent attack by the electroforming solution. All metal tubing must be sealed at the ends to prevent solution from entering and being trapped in the tube. This will eliminate carrying out the solution from the tank when the mandrel/nickel combination is removed from the tank and will also prevent contamination of the solution by the dissolved metal tubing.

The backup structure provides the electroformer with a means to suspend the mandrel in the electroforming tank, but it must also be capable of supporting the weight of the deposited nickel on the face of the mandrel. For a nickel thickness of 5 mm (0.2 in.), the weight of the nickel hanging on the mandrel will be approximately 44 kg/m^2 (9 lb/ft^2) of nickel area. Since the nickel shell is not removed from the mandrel until it is mounted in a mold chase or frame, the added weight from the mold components during buildup of the mold may add as much as 732 kg/m^2 (150 lb/ft^2) of additional weight on the mandrel.

The resins used in the construction of the mandrel must be stable in the nickel solution and fully cured before the mandrel is shipped to the electroformer. The expense of setting up and maintaining an electroforming tank to produce the low-stress deposits required for mold production is sizeable. The loss of production and expense of treating the solution in a large tank due to organic contamination from an uncured mandrel or use of an unproven resin could exceed $100,000. If the mandrel manufacturer is unsure of the materials being used, he or she should consult with the electroformer regarding the construction of the mandrel. A 30 by 30 cm (12 by 12 in.) sample can be easily placed in a small electroforming tank to check out the suitability of the proposed mandrel material.

The following guidelines, along with Fig. 1, can assist the mandrel manufacturer in producing a high-quality mandrel. Additional guidelines are provided in ASTM B 832 and the other sources cited in the list of Selected References at the end of this article.

- The quality of the face coat on the mandrel is important not only to ensure the correct contour, but also to produce a blemish-free nickel mold surface capable of producing the desired finish on the molded parts.
- External angles on the mandrel should be provided with as generous a radius as possible to avoid excessive buildup of nickel at these areas.
- Internal (concave) angles on the mandrel should be provided with a fillet radius at least equal to the thickness of the metal to be deposited. Where sharp internal angles are mandatory, the use of auxiliary anodes will be required and the electroforming time and the mold cost will increase.
- The mandrel should have additional area around the perimeter of the part to provide the desired mold run-out area and also to provide the electroformer with space to attach copper bus bar for electrical connection to the direct current (dc) rectifier.
- Silicone-based mold releases should be avoided in producing the mandrel. Such releases are difficult to remove completely from the mandrel and could result in separation of the nickel from the mandrel during the early electroforming stages. If separation occurs, the contour of the nickel in that area will be affected, which may necessitate the removal and disposal of the thin nickel deposit and starting the mandrel surface preparation anew.
- Types and locations of alignment pins and tooling balls for adjustment and location of the mold bases relative to the mold face and the other half of the mold should be coordinated with the electroformer to ensure the fabrication of acceptable molds.

Costs of fiberglass/resin mandrels typically are \$2690/m^2 (\$250/ft^2) or higher depending on the contour, size, and availability of a master model or splashes.

Machined Mandrels. At the time of publication, most companies have begun to use CAD in the design of their products. This widespread use of computers permits the transfer of data to vendors for the machining of master models or, in some cases, the direct machining of mandrels for the electroforming process.

The truck and automotive companies have preferred to generate a master model for their design personnel to approve, resulting in a fiberglass/resin mandrel being produced from that master with the possible loss of accuracy in the contour as described earlier. The aircraft companies, on the other hand, have begun to machine the electroforming mandrels directly from tooling boards or mass cast modeling pastes in order to improve the contour tolerances of the finished electroform. The ease of machining lightweight foam blocks appealed to the fabricators of mandrels, but the weight or density of these blocks presented a problem to the electroformer due to their buoyancy in the electroforming solution. This forced the electroformer to attach heavy weights to the mandrel to counteract the buoyancy. These weights hanging from the mandrel support sometimes resulted in the distortion of the mandrel surface. In addition, two other problems arose: (1) the porosity of the foam after machining sometimes resulted in porosity in the electroform, and (2) the necessity of gluing the foam blocks together sometimes resulted in either depressed or raised areas in the nickel surface due to a mismatch between the thermal expansions of the foam and the adhesive when the mandrel was immersed in the nickel solution. In recent years, several manufacturers have begun to produce tooling boards having densities exceeding that of the electroforming solution, thereby removing the buoyancy problems. The adhesives used to cement these blocks together have been developed to more closely match the thermal expansion of the foam, thereby greatly reducing the glue-line problems on the nickel surface.

Regardless of the density of the foam used, a property of these foam block materials that must be considered before machining is the high values of their coefficients of thermal expansion (CTEs). For example, a mandrel machined to net dimensions at room temperature 21 °C (70 °F) from a foam having a CTE of 42.5×10^{-6}/°C (23.6×10^{-6}/°F) that is immersed in the electroforming solution at 49 °C (120 °F) will yield a nickel electroform at room temperature with dimensions that are approximately 0.25 mm (0.010 in.) larger than desired for each 30.5 cm (12 in.) of length or width. If this mandrel had tooling pins located 152.4 cm (60 in.) apart, the separation of those pins would be incorrect on the nickel shell by approximately 1.3 mm (0.05 in.). Corrections to the mandrel dimensions to compensate for the large CTE of the mandrel material can be incorporated during machining and will help ensure that the resulting electroform has the correct contour. If necessary, tooling pins and/or other critical details can be installed in the finished electroform after it has been removed from the mandrel.

The cost of a machined mandrel can be \$5380/m^2(\$500/ft^2) or higher, depending on the tooling board or material that is to be machined, the labor costs for gluing and sealing the tooling boards, the hourly cost of the machine used, and the mandrel size and complexity.

Comparison of Nickel and Other Tooling Materials

A thorough discussion of electroformed nickel molds for composite production would be remiss

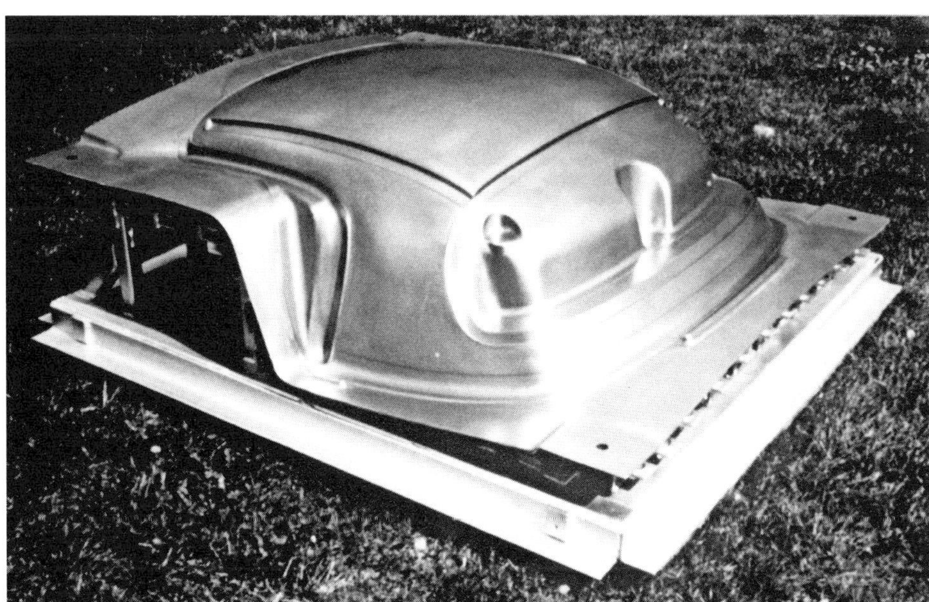

Fig. 3 Nickel shell male preform mold for composite auto roof

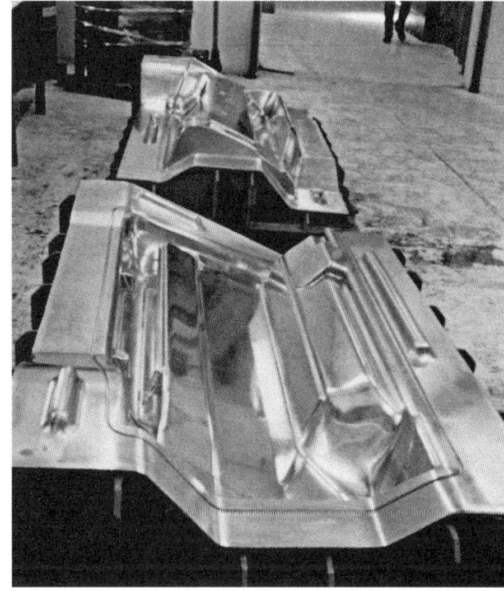

Fig. 4 Resin transfer molding molds for truck cab side fairings

Table 2 Coefficients of thermal expansion of selected tooling materials

Material	Coefficient of thermal expansion, 10^{-6}/K
Electroformed nickel	13.1
Steel	12–13
Invar-36	2.7
Aluminum	23.4
Fiberglass/epoxy (50–60 vol% fiberglass)	9–12.6

Table 3 Relative heat-up times for various materials

	Thickness		Weight		
Material	mm	in.	kg	lb	Relative heat-up time
Electroformed nickel	5	0.2	210	462	1
Steel	25	1	927	2040	4.9
Aluminum	25	1	330	726	3.4
Fiberglass/epoxy	25	1	202	444	1.6

without comparing nickel to competitive materials.

Coefficients of Thermal Expansion. A tabulation of the various CTEs of the materials discussed in this article is presented in Table 2 for the consideration of mold designers. The user of nickel molds can incorporate expansion or shrinkage factors into the molds through the mandrel construction in the same manner that steel, Invar, or aluminum molds are machined to incorporate these factors.

Thermal Cycles for Compression Molding. As faster cure times in the various compression molding processes are required by molders, the heat-up and cool down times of the molds used must be considered. The thermal cycling of nickel shell molds will be faster compared to machined steel and machined or cast aluminum molds due to the reduced mass of the nickel that must be heated or cooled. Cooling or heating lines located directly behind the thin nickel shell offer faster thermal responses than those molds having 1 or 2 in. of material between the lines and the face. Because the nickel shell can be thermally isolated to a great extent by using concrete or a resin behind the nickel, any heat generated during the cure cycle can be removed faster than if a large block of steel or aluminum had to be cooled. A rough calculation of the time required to heat various mold materials is based on the weight and heat capacity of each material. Table 3 shows the relative times that are required to raise the temperature of a 4.6 m^2 (50 ft^2) mold by 38 °C (100 °F) for a 5 mm (0.2 in.) thick nickel shell compared to three other mold materials. The amount of heat absorbed by each material was assumed to be the same, thereby permitting a comparison of the time required. Heat losses due to conduction, convection, or radiation into the support structure or backing materials were ignored for this calculation. Since the actual thickness of molds may vary depending on the material and the depth at which the cooling channels are drilled, Table 3 compares the thin nickel shell to a 25 mm (1 in.) thickness of the other materials.

Thus, a 100 mm (4 in.) thick aluminum mold could take almost 14 times longer to heat up than the thinner nickel shell. However, if the heating channels on the aluminum mold were very close to the mold face, then the mold-face temperature may reach the desired operating temperature while the rest of the aluminum mass is still warming up.

Thermal Cycles for Metal Autoclave Molds. The use of nickel, steel, or Invar molds in the autoclave curing of aircraft composite parts is appealing to the aircraft industry due to their unlimited lifetimes at cure temperatures of 150 °C (300 °F) and higher compared to resin molds. Invar-36 is a 64%Fe-36%Ni alloy that is widely used in the curing of graphite/epoxy parts since its CTE closely matches that of the graphite parts. Based on a comparison of 1999 prices, the cost of an Invar mold may be several times greater than a nickel or steel mold, but depending on the contour of the graphite part, that cost may be justified. A comparison of the costs and heat-up times of comparable steel, nickel, and Invar molds has to include the thickness of the face sheet, the weight of the support structure, and the contour of the mold. Table 4 compares the costs and relative heat-up times for the three metals for a mold having a wing leading edge contour. The cost for the nickel mold includes a machined master model, a fiberglass/epoxy mandrel and the finished nickel mold. The costs for the steel and Invar molds includes machining of the surface and the welding and related costs for the support structures. The heat-up times are again compared relative to the nickel mold. The area of this mold was 3.5 m^2 (38 ft^2), and the support structure for the metal face of the mold was assumed to be the same design for all three molds. The support structures on the nickel and steel molds were welded steel, while the support structure for the Invar mold was welded Invar as required. The total weight listed below includes the face sheet and the support structure. The cost for the Invar tool could not be obtained for this geometry, but two aircraft firms have stated that Invar molds are costing \$2000 to \$3500/ft^2 yielding a price for this comparison of about \$76,000 to \$130,000.

These relative heat-up times are strictly theoretical since actual autoclave data are not available. The numbers do show the improved cycle times that could be obtained in ideal conditions when using nickel molds. In reality, these heating times can be skewed if the air circulation in the autoclave favors a particular area or if the support structure design prevents good air circulation around the back side of the face sheet in the autoclave.

Table 4 Comparison of nickel, steel, and Invar autoclave molds

	Thickness		Total weight			
Face material	mm	in.	kg	lb	Total cost	Relative heat-up time
Nickel	6	0.24	1093	2410	\$39,400	1
Steel	9.5	0.38	1148	2530	\$77,440	1.06
Invar	12	0.5	1179	2600	(see text)	1.24

Future Developments

The electroforming process is well established for mold production and continual improvements are expected, especially in the area of new alloys having higher strengths and lower CTEs. For example, Invar has been successfully electroformed on a small scale, and with increased research it may be possible to produce electroformed Invar molds for graphite/epoxy part production. The addition of cobalt to the nickel bath will increase the hardness of the electroform and thus improve mold service lifetimes. Computer simulation of the electric fields around the mandrel will assist the electroformer in anode placement, which will improve the deposit distribution and result in faster deposition and lower electroforming times. While electroforming has not changed much in the last 50 years, new ideas and continual research into alloys and micromachine devices will make the future of electroforming very interesting.

SELECTED REFERENCES

- AESF Electroforming Symposium, March 1996, American Electroplaters and Surface Finishers Society
- G. Malone and M.F. Browning, Electroforming, *Surface Engineering*, Vol 5, *ASM Handbook*, ASM International, 1994, p 285–298
- R. Parkinson, *Electroforming—A Unique Metal Fabrication Process*, Nickel Development Institute, 1998
- W. Safranek, *The Properties of Electrodeposited Metals and Alloys*, 2nd ed., American Electroplaters and Surface Finishers Society, 1986
- A. Simonian, *Modern Electroforming*, Nickel Development Institute, 1990
- "Standard Guide for Electroforming with Nickel and Copper," B 832, *Annual Book of ASTM Standards*, Vol 02.05, ASTM
- S.A. Watson, *Applications of Electroforming*, Nickel Development Institute, 1990
- S. A. Watson, *Electroforming Today*, Nickel Development Institute, 1990

Elastomeric Tooling

R.C. Adams and Marvin Foston, Lockheed Martin Aeronautical Systems

ELASTOMERIC TOOLING uses rubber details to generate required molding pressure or to serve as a pressure intensifier during composite-part curing cycles. The rubber is made from castable room-temperature vulcanized (RTV) rubber compounds or calendered silicone rubber sheets (reinforced and unreinforced) in "B" stage form (fully compounded but uncured).

Composite materials are currently the materials of choice in the aircraft and many commercial industries. Composite parts have grown from simple-shaped parts to large, highly contoured co-cured structures. The fabrication of co-cured structures reduces or even eliminates fasteners, mate joints, part count, subassembly, and assembly operations.

Recently developed lean manufacturing approaches incorporate low-cost tooling methodologies in the Integrated Product Team component design. This includes a tooling policy that standardizes the hard-tool interface for all outer skins and substructure. The skins are hard tooled to inner mold line and substructure is hard tooled to outer mold line. This provides a controlled interface for assembly. This tooling approach with the increased usage of composites components has created new families of project tools, bag-side semirigid cauls.

These bag-side outer/inner mold-line cauls are required to improve surface quality, provide aerodynamic smoothness, and achieve more demanding part tolerances. The cauls reduce bagging time and eliminate bag wrinkles and the chance of a lay-up "bridge" that would result in bag failure, causing part rejection. To meet these requirements the bagside caul must be both rigid and flexible. Rigidity is required to achieve tolerance/configuration control, while flexibility ensures good compaction.

Bag-Side Elastomeric Cauls

Commercially available caul systems are provided in two forms:

- *Form 1:* calendered reinforced and unreinforced sheets of rubber
- *Form 2:* calendered unreinforced sheets of rubber in combination with graphite or fiberglass/epoxy prepreg, which is used to selectively reinforce the caul as required

Form 1 Caul. A form 1 caul system has several unique advantages for simple contoured parts. The materials are low in cost, easy to lay-up, and have a wide processing window of 110 to 175 °C (235–350 °F). The calendered sheets of rubber can be purchased fully compounded in

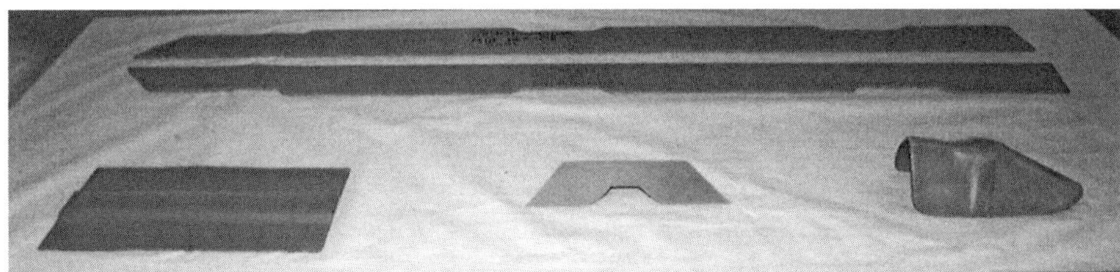

Fig. 1 Semirigid cauls built using form 1 caul system

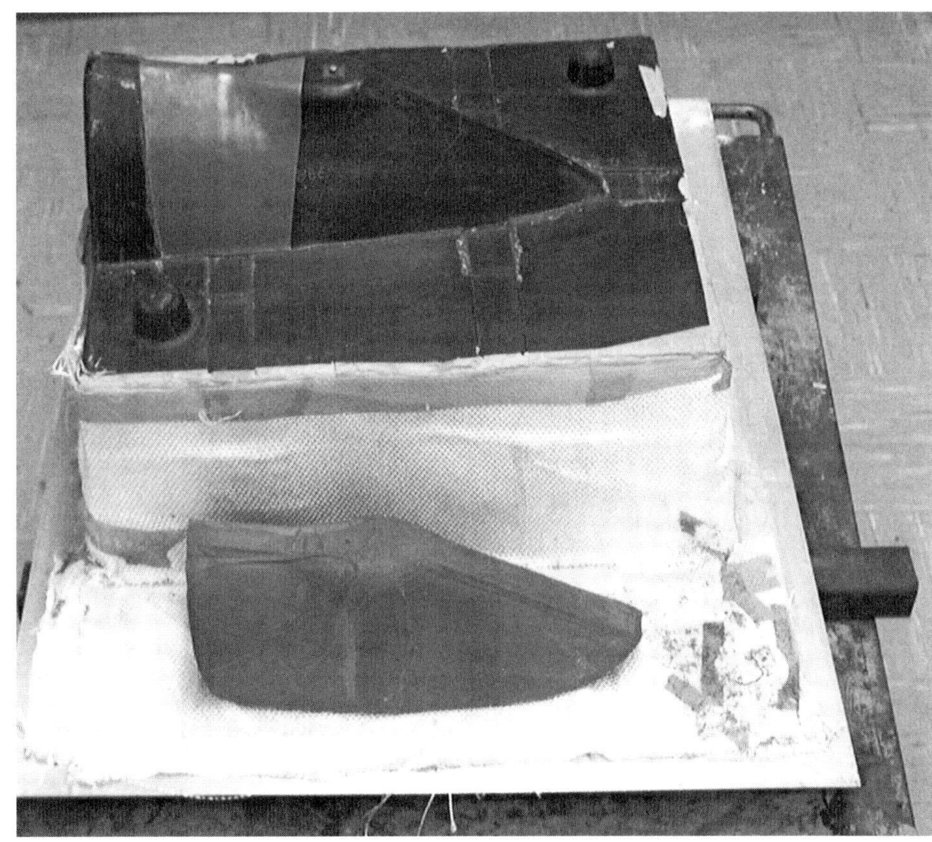

Fig. 2 Wax dummy part and curing tool

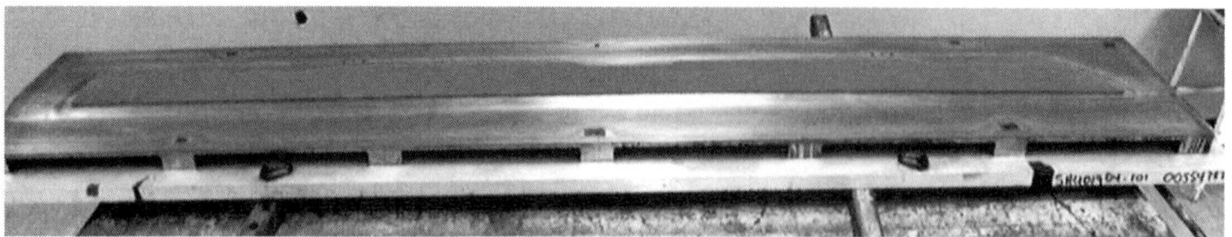

Fig. 3 Caul fabricated using part model initially built to make trim tools

"B" stage form with or without fiberglass reinforcement. Fiberglass reinforcement generally is not desired when high elongation is required. These materials are commonly used together.

Fabrication. Machined or plastic-faced plaster part models that represent the outer/inner mold line of the part should be used whenever possible to fabricate cauls, but cauls also can be fabricated on curing tools. The caul material can be cured at temperatures lower than 120 °C (250 °F). This advantage allows the use of sheet wax to produce an inexpensive "dummy" part that can be used to fabricate the caul. Figure 1 shows semirigid cauls built using the form 1 caul system. Figure 2 shows a curing tool that required a wax dummy part to fabricate the required reinforced caul, while the caul in Figure 3 was fabricated using a part model that was initially built to make trim tools. Both approaches eliminate the cost of building models specifically for use in caul fabrication. A review of the contour of the parts provides guidance as to which caul fabrication approach and caul system should be used.

To build cauls using the form 1 system, part model and curing tool surfaces are cleaned with alcohol to remove all dirt, grease, and oil. The curing tool is release coated and the part thickness laid-up with the required thickness of adhesive-backed wax sheet. Because adhesive is a silicone rubber contaminant, all butt joint seams between the wax sheets are filled with paste wax to isolate the adhesive. Adhesive contamination will prevent the rubber from curing in those areas. The surfaces of the part model and waxed curing tool are coated with a release agent, a commercial dishwashing detergent. A 5% detergent to 95% water mixture provides a good release for most rubber compounds.

Usually four plies are sufficient for this caul system, but the number of plies can vary. A combination of reinforced and unreinforced material is used to allow more expansion in tool radii. The basic lay-up is shown in Fig. 4. This orientation provides good surface smoothness and requires no special treatment for most ramps and drop-offs. Special treatment is required for most male and female radii areas, as shown in Fig. 5. This stacking arrangement creates a stretch joint to provide better radii compaction and caul elongation in two directions.

The calendered rubber sheet material is laid up in manageable pieces, taking care to apply the sheet to surfaces without wrinkles or trapped pockets of air. The first ply is debulked at room temperature under full vacuum, and lay-up completed as shown in Fig. 4 and 5. The curing cycle for cauls laid up on curing tool with waxed part model buildups is shown in Fig. 6. Cauls fabricated on part models that can withstand temperatures as high as 175 °C (350 °F) is shown in

Ply 4 Unreinforced silicone
Ply 3 Reinforced silicone
Ply 2 Reinforced silicone
Ply 1 Unreinforced silicone
Part model

Fig. 4 Typical caul lay-up system

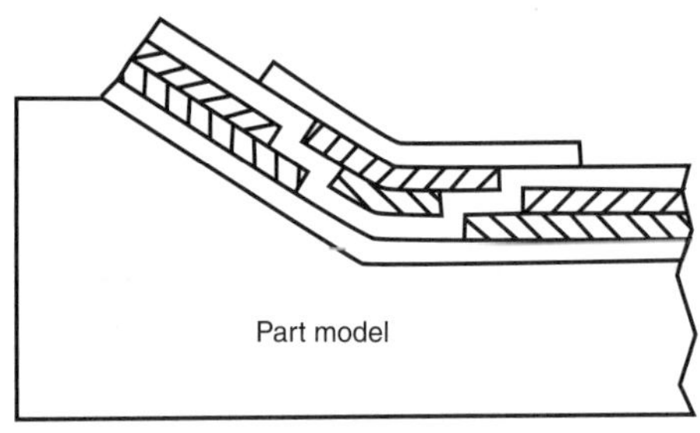

Fig. 5 Tooling radii stretch joint

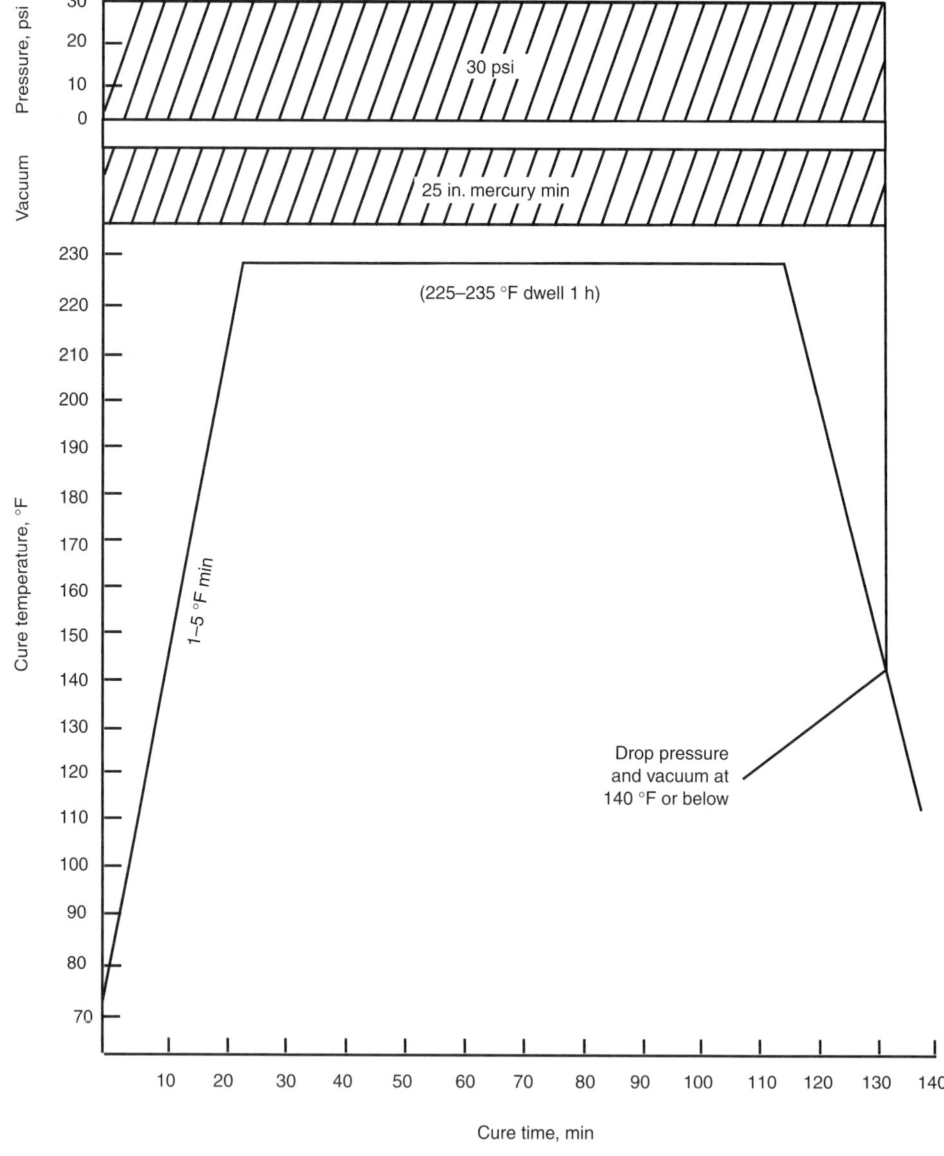

Fig. 6 Schematic of 110 °C (230 °F) cure cycle

Fig. 7. Cauls cured at low temperature are post-cured unrestrained in an oven for 1 h at 175 °C (350 °F).

Form 2 Caul. Some part configurations fabricated in the autoclave require a "matched-mold" type of caul to provide the bag- or caul-side part definition. Parts having one or more integral stiffeners or highly compound complex contour surfaces require cauls having tailored reinforcement in selected areas.

The caul system selected for matched-mold cases is a combination of pretreated calendered silicone and fiber/epoxy prepreg material that, when co-cured, provides a semirigid caul having predictable thermal expansion. The semirigid cauls built using this caul system are shown in Fig. 8. Figure 9 shows a stiffened graphite/epoxy panel with a ramped buildup around its periphery, which was successfully produced using a graphite/epoxy reinforced caul. This system was also used to fabricate the caul shown on the part model in Fig.10.

Fabrication. Building a caul with this system is similar to fabricating a simple contour caul. The exceptions are: The pretreated silicone requires a special release agent on the part models. A primer is needed on both sides of the graphite/epoxy reinforcements to achieve a good bond to the silicone rubber. A different caul ply stack-up and radii treatment (Fig. 11), and cure cycle (Fig. 7) are required.

These caul systems can be used during debulking cycles of resin transfer molding (RTM) preforms. The preforms are debulked to eliminate excess bulk so they can be easily loaded in the matched-mold RTM tool. Conventional vacuum bags pull preforms too tight around the corners of debulking mandrels, which, combined with the increased bag pressure, overcompacts the preform fibers in these areas. Reinforced cauls can be built by waxing up the required debulk thickness and building cauls to this offset. The cauls control the debulked preform thickness uniformly over the desired mandrel surface area, which eliminates resin-rich areas on the corners of RTM parts.

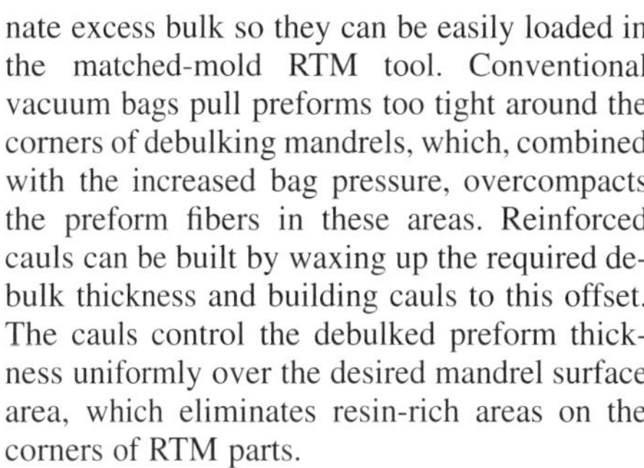

Thermal Expansion Molding Methods

Two basic methods use the principles of thermal expansion molding: the trapped, or fixed-volume rubber method, and the variable-volume rubber method.

The fixed-volume method exploits the large difference between the coefficient of thermal expansion (CTE) of the elastomer and the CTE of metals. The elastomer is confined within a closed metal tool cavity; when heated, it expands into the cavity, exerting the pressure required to compact a composite laminate. One of the chief benefits is that it allows the manufacturing engineer to apply adequate pressure with or without a vacuum bag or autoclave.

Elastomeric mandrel compounds have been formulated to meet a wide range of pressure requirements. Compounds are available that can generate controllable molding pressure ranging from less than 7 to greater than 13,800 kPa (less than 1 to greater than 2000 psi) at cure temperature.

The variable-volume method offers more flexibility than the fixed-volume method because a precisely calculated volume of rubber is not normally required. In most applications, the rubber is simply "set back" to allow for the bulk factor of the molding material during assembly of the tooling details. If excess pressure is generated during vacuum bag molding, it is vented against the vacuum bag. In press molding, the excess pressure causes the floating plate to retract the movable press platen.

In an airframe, thermal expansion molding is used primarily in boxlike structures such as rudders, vertical stabilizers, wing boxes, spoilers, and ailerons. Elastomeric tooling provides the means for fabricating integrally stiffened skins with a co-cured substructure in a single curing operation. Secondary bonding is thereby eliminated, substantially reducing direct manufacturing costs. The basic mechanism of thermal expansion molding is the transfer of uniform compaction pressure to an uncured composite laminate by an elastomeric tooling detail.

Molding Stages. During thermal expansion molding for a simplified, one dimensional case—using the fixed-volume rubber method—the rubber block freely expands across a gap and contacts the composite prepreg material, which

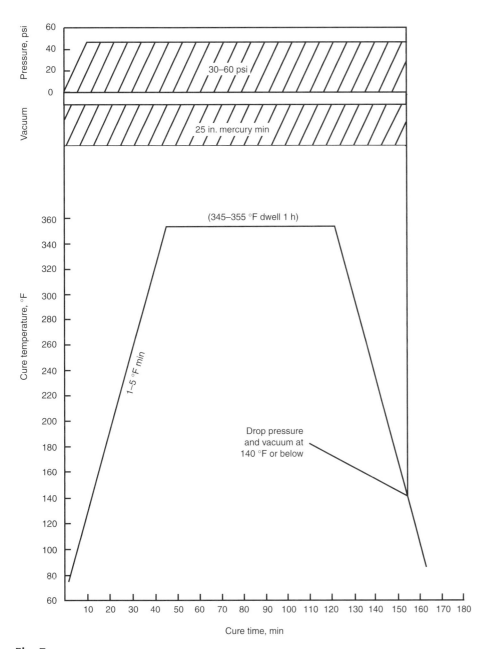

Fig. 7 Schematic of 175 °C (350 °F) cure cycle

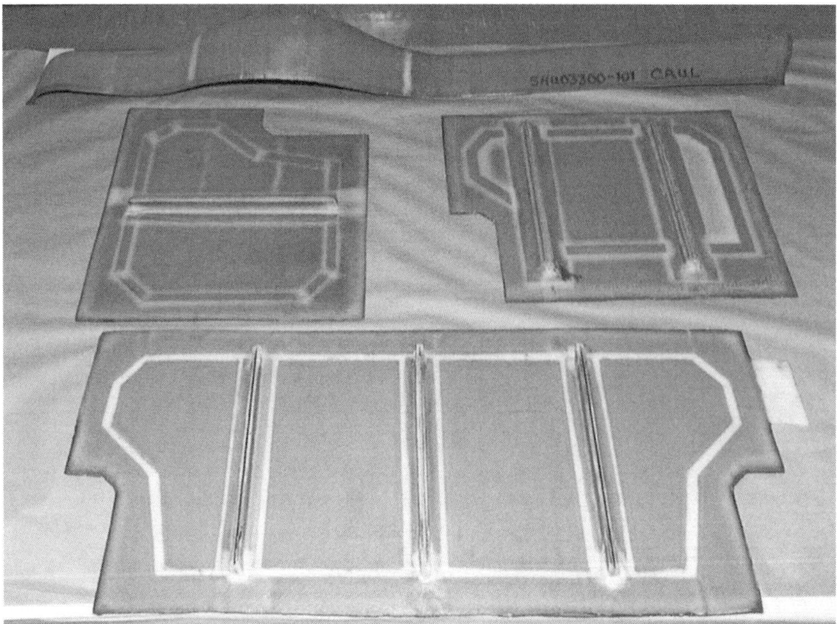

Fig. 8 Semirigid cauls built using form 2 caul system

is compacted under increasing pressure until the resin gels. At the gel point, the laminate has been compacted to its final molding thickness under pressure. The laminate is cured at the gel temperature for a time period determined from rheometric data. The cured laminate is then removed from the tooling and postcured unrestrained in an oven.

Postcuring following curing at the gel temperature eliminates the excessive pressure that would be generated if the temperature were raised to the final cure temperature, which could cause damage to parts.

Volumetric Analysis

The significant properties that are required to characterize elastomeric tooling material are CTE, bulk modulus, hardness, and dimensional stability under repeated cycles of pressure and temperature. The nature of the thermal expansion process with an elastomeric material can be obtained by putting pressure transducers on three faces of a rectangular mold to permit the monitoring of pressure exerted by a rectangular brick in three directions. Using data from the rectangular mold model, volumetric relationships can be derived that are valid for complex as well as for simple tooling configurations.

The controlling equations for pressure in the fixed-volume rubber method of thermal expansion molding can be reduced to a single equation when two characteristics of the elastomeric material being used are determined through accurate tests. These characteristics are the percentage of volume by which the elastomer shrinks between being poured and being cured, and the pressure generated per degree of increase in temperature of a confined elastomeric specimen. Once these properties are determined, the volume lost to shrinkage can be restored during use by adding a suitable ΔT to the nominal positive gradient. This differential is known as the shrinkage compensation factor, or Δt_s (delta temperature allowance for shrinkage).

Numerically, the Δt_s is obtained by dividing the percentage of shrinkage by the volumetric expansion factor of the rubber material:

$$\Delta t_s = \frac{(x)\%}{B_r} \qquad \text{(Eq 1)}$$

where x is rubber shrinkage and B_r is the volumetric expansion coefficient of rubber.

The pressure compensation factor, Δt_p, may also be offset by determining the amount of temperature increase required to provide the desired pressure:

$$\Delta t_p = \frac{P}{P/d} \qquad \text{(Eq 2)}$$

where P is the desired pressure and P/d is the pressure generated per degree increase in temperature.

The basic equation controlling the thermal expansion molding process is:

$$V_{r2} = V_{r1} + V_{r1} B_r \Delta T_e \qquad \text{(Eq 3)}$$

where V_{r2} is the volume of rubber at the cure temperature at which pressure is equal to 0, V_{r1}

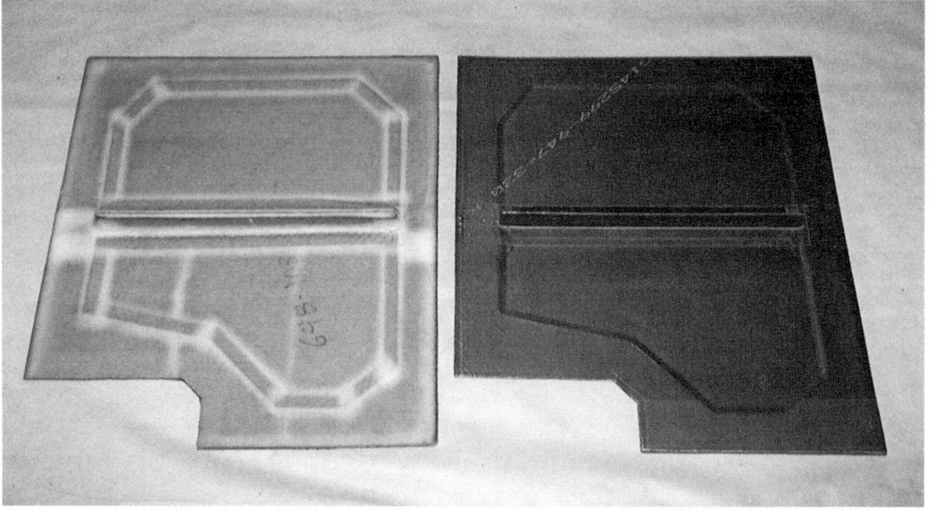

Fig. 9 Stiffened graphite/epoxy panel with ramped buildup around its periphery built using graphite/epoxy reinforced caul

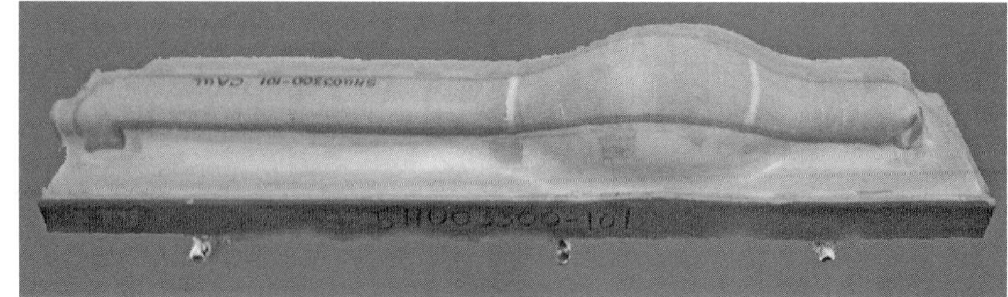

Fig. 10 Caul on part model built using graphite/epoxy reinforced caul

is the volume of rubber at room temperature (RT), and ΔT_e is the effective change in temperature, which is cure temperature ($-\Delta t_s - \Delta t_p$ – RT), where Δt_s and Δt_p refer to Eq 1 and 2. Note that Eq 3 is accurate to less than $\pm 1\%$ error.

The initial starting point in tool design for the thermal expansion molding process is at cure temperature. The geometry of the part at temperature is surrounded by the tool inner mold lines, and a cavity is then designed to hold the rubber detail.

The initial value for the volume of rubber at the cure temperature, V_{r2}, is obtained by subtracting the volume of the pan at temperature, V_{p2}, from the volume of the total tool cavity at temperature (V_{tc2}), with pressure equal to 0 psi:

$$V_{r2} = V_{tc2} - V_{p2}$$

where

$$V_{tc2} = V_{tc1} + V_{tc1} B_t \Delta T$$

$$V_{p2} = V_{p1} + V_{p1} B_p \Delta T$$

where B_t is the volumetric expansion coefficient of the metal details, B_p is the volumetric expansion coefficient of the material of the part, and

$$\Delta T = T_2 - T_1$$

where T_2 is the cure temperature (desired pressure application point) and T_1 is room temperature.

The clearance between the laid-up bulk thickness of the uncured part and the rubber at its room-temperature size should then be determined. This is to ensure that there is enough clearance for the tool assembly. If the clearance is inadequate, the depth of the tool cavity must be increased. This larger cavity, in turn, will call for a commensurately thicker rubber mandrel. Generally, the differences between the expansion factors of the hard tool material and the rubber is adequate for tool assembly.

After the proper tool cavity and rubber sizes are obtained, the rubber can be poured directly into the fabricated tool cavity. When this technique is used, the pan configuration and setback size are represented by wax. The volume of wax, V_w, required for setback is equal to the difference in rubber volumes:

$$V_{r2} - V_{r1} = V_w$$

The shrinkage can also be compensated for at any time after the rubber volume has been determined. One simply increases the physical dimensions by the percentage of shrinkage. Note that this volume of wax does not include the cured-part dimensions.

To ensure accurate geometry of the cured part, the tool designer must take into account the geometries of all three critical surfaces when the setback wax volume is distributed in the mold. The three geometries can be quite different when a strictly mathematical interpretation is taken. However, by using a two- or three-dimensional computer-aided design, maintaining the geometric configuration becomes straightforward.

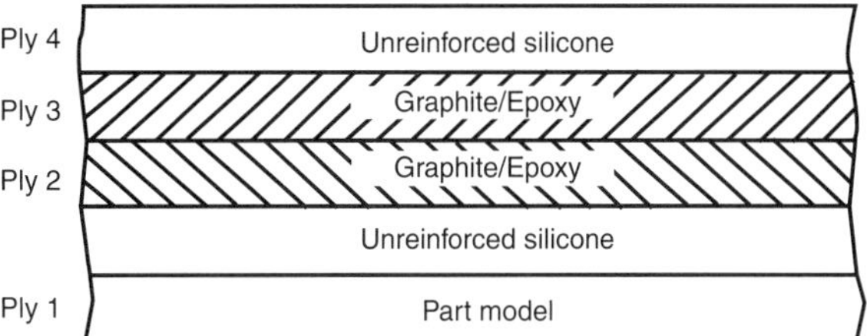

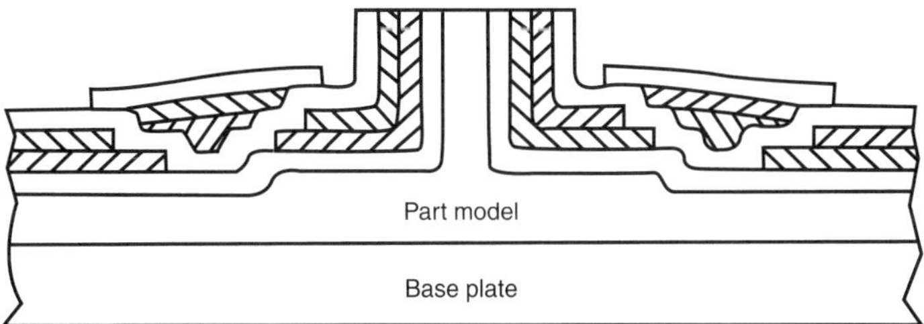

Fig. 11 Ply stack-up and lay-up system for dealing with joint radii

Open Molding: Hand Lay-Up and Spray-Up

Finn Roger Andresen, Reichhold AS, Norway

OPEN MOLDING, also known as contact molding, open laminating, and wet lay-up, is the method used longest in the polymer-matrix composites industry to make thermoset composite products, and it is still the selected production process for a wide range of composite products. It is a basic process that provides many of the advantages of composites processing, using relatively basic materials technology and processing methods.

The molding method involves placing reinforcements and liquid resin onto the surface of an open mold (which may or may not be precoated with gel coat), or onto other substrates, as, for example, when making a one-off sandwich construction, when making on-site repairs by applying a reinforcing vacuum-formed acrylic, corrosion-resistant lining on steel on-site repairs of tanks and pipes, and so on.

The hand lay-up version involves applying the reinforcements and resin by hand, while the spray-up version uses tailored spray equipment to deposit both reinforcements and resin on the mold or an alternative substrate.

Open molding is a process typically used for low- to medium-sized series (from a few to 200–300 parts/yr), offering a number of process and product advantages. Producing large, complicated shapes as well as smaller and simpler composite products is possible.

The hand lay-up process involves low investment costs and little prior working knowledge of the process, while spray-up involves some investment in tailored spray-up machines and spray guns. Well-trained operators and dedicated facilities are required to produce components and products having high quality.

Process Characteristics

Open molding offers a number of process and product advantages over other high-volume, complex application methods and is therefore used for a number of specialized products. Process advantages include:

- Freedom of design
- Easy to change design
- Low mold and/or tooling costs
- Low start-up costs
- Low to medium capital costs
- Regarded as a simple process
- Tailored properties possible
- High-strength large parts possible
- Large-sized parts possible
- On-site production (one-off) possible

Disadvantages associated with the open molding process include:

- Low to medium number of parts/year
- Long cycle times per molding
- Labor intensive
- Evaporation, exposure, and emission of volatile organic compounds (VOCs)
- Not the cleanest application process
- Only one surface has aesthetic appearance
- Operator-skill dependent
- Sharp corners and edges limited
- Long reworking time per molding
- Limited amount of filler to modify properties

Laminate properties depend on resin quality and reinforcement type, but a primary benefit of open molding is the ability to tailor the properties of thermoset composite products. However, this is dependent on both amount (fiber fraction) and type (direction) of reinforcements used, as shown in Fig. 1.

Note, that too high of a fiber fraction for a given reinforcement type can result in a laminate that is too dry, that is, there is not sufficient resin present to wet and/or impregnate all the fibers by the manual consolidation operation (homogenization process). Consequently, this will result in a drop of properties, as indicated in Fig. 1. The use of woven roving (WR) and multiaxial fabrics makes it possible to tailor the direction of the continuous fibers in these materials, enabling the fabricator to place the properties where and in which direction is desired.

Applications

Thermoset composite parts are used in applications requiring high strength-to-weight ratio, corrosion resistance, antimagnetic properties, thermal and electrical insulating properties, freedom of design, ease of transport and installation, and so forth.

Typical products manufactured using prefabricated molds and tools, include products that have small to large surface area and simple and complex shapes, and they are restricted in size only by practical handling of molds. Typical products include:

- Boat hulls and decks (Fig. 2)
- Tanks and vessels (Fig. 3)
- Components for the transport industry (auto and train parts)
- Industrial parts
- Building parts
- Electrical parts and covers

The so-called one-off moldings are nearly unlimited in size; applications and products include:

- Reinforcement of steel and concrete structures
- Corrosion-resistant liners
- Large vessels and boats, normally sandwich constructions (Fig. 4)
- Large surface area subsea covers, normally sandwich constructions (Fig. 5)
- Reinforcing vacuumed acrylic sanitary parts

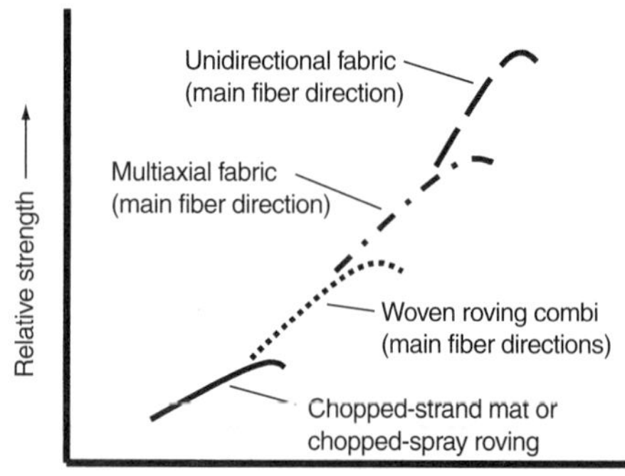

Fig. 1 Influence of reinforcement fraction and type on mechanical properties of open-molded fiber reinforced polymer-matrix composite laminate

Process Description

Open molding typically involves depositing the reinforcements and liquid resin onto a mold surface or depositing materials onto other substrates, which are then integrated into the final composite part. The laminating principles are similar. The mold surface quality is of utmost importance when surface aspect requirements are high because the composite part surface replicates mold surface quality.

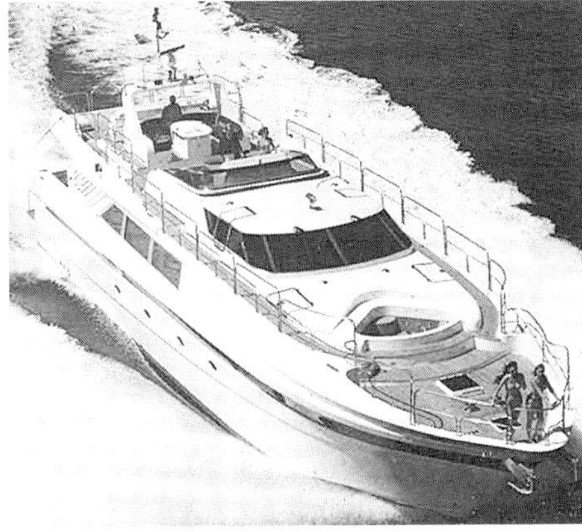

Fig. 2 Open-molded composite boat hull and deck for luxury cruiser. Courtesy of Gulf Craft-UAE

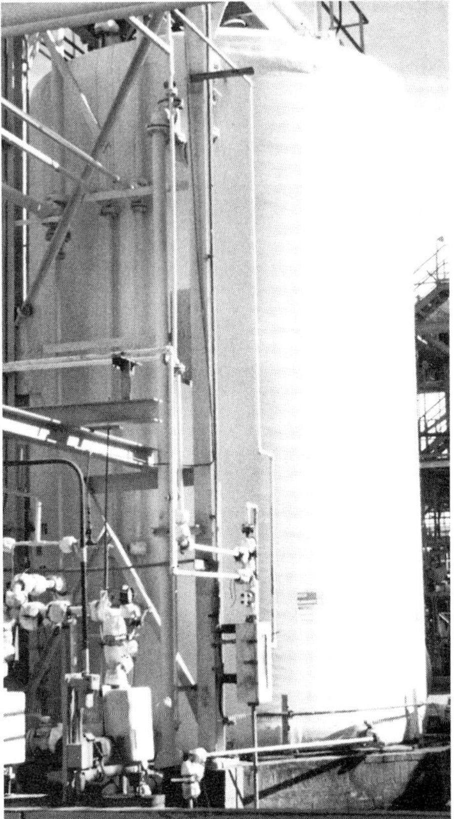

Fig. 3 Open-molded composite chemical storage tank. Courtesy of OxyChem

Molds and tools for the open-molding industry are often made of composite materials using a tailored mold and tool gel coat as the surface finish layer, which provides a durable, high-gloss surface. Cast molds, electroformed nickel-shell molds, and other metal molds are also used; these give a longer mold life in normal use.

The hand lay-up process is illustrated in Fig. 6. Before starting the actual laminating process, the mold surface has to be clean and prepared with a suitable mold-release agent, which must be properly cured before the catalyzed gel coat is applied. Gel coat is a tailored pigmented or nonpigmented resin that typically is applied as the first 400 to 700 m outer layer. It not applied as the first 400 to 700 μm outer layer. It not only provides the surface quality, but it also functions as a protective layer against weathering and other exposure, protecting the final underlying reinforced laminate from direct environmental attack and consequent possible unwanted degradation of laminate properties. The recommended type and amount of organic peroxide (typically 1.5–2 wt% of a good methyl ethyl ketone peroxide) must be added to the preaccelerated gel coat before use; however, it often is preaccelerated by the supplier.

In the case of pure hand lay-up, the gel coat is also applied by hand, using a suitable soft brush. Curing time is typically a few hours at ambient temperature, after which application of resin and reinforcements can start.

A suitable type and amount of a given curing system must be added to the resin before starting

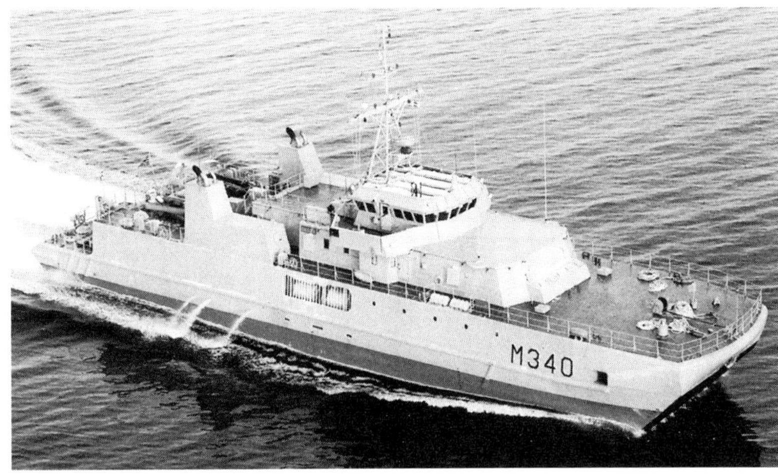

Fig. 4 Open molded composite (sandwich construction) Norwegian Navy mine hunter. Courtesy of Kvæner Mandal

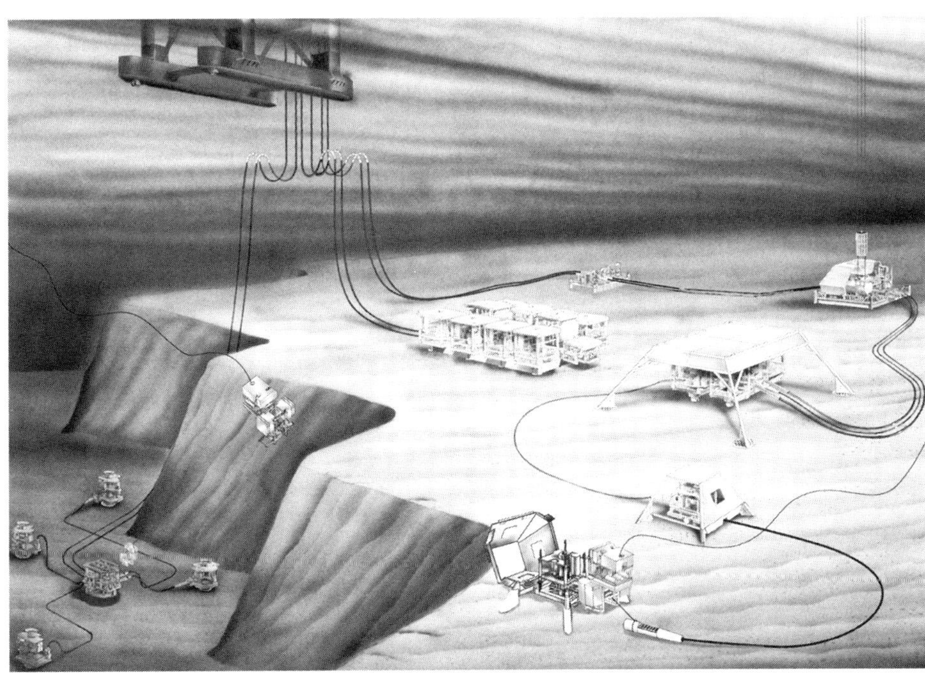

Fig. 5 Open-molded composite (sandwich construction) subsea covers. Courtesy of ABB Offshore System AS

the actual laminating operation. This depends on the type of resin used, so it is recommended that the supplier be consulted for specifics.

In fabricating composite laminates for use in marine applications where surface aspects and resistance to osmosis and blistering is important, a skin laminate is often applied behind the gel coat. This consists of 1 to 2 layers of a 20 to 30 Tex 450 g/m^2 chopped-strand mat (CSM) of the powder-bonded type, preferably impregnated with a low-styrene, high-quality resin (Fig. 7). Such a skin laminate has good hydrolytic stability, low shrinkage, good toughness, and good curing properties at ambient temperature. A grooved metal roller is used to consolidate the skin laminate, ensuring that all fiber filaments are wetted and all air entrapments are removed (Fig. 8).

After a curing 8 to 24 h at ambient temperature, the construction of the structural, or load-carrying, laminate can begin. Liquid resin, to which is added the recommended curing system, is applied onto the cured gel coat surface (or the cured skin laminate) using a suitable soft brush or synthetic hair roller. The resin system is applied manually from a container containing the catalyzed resin, or via a resin-dispenser roller system. The latter is a cleaner application method, but requires a resin-pumping and connected roller system. The first layer of dry reinforcement is placed into this liquid layer, and more liquid resin is applied, in a quantity sufficient to properly wet the reinforcement layer. Consolidation using the metal roller is again necessary, and this sequence is followed until the required laminate thickness/part construction is achieved.

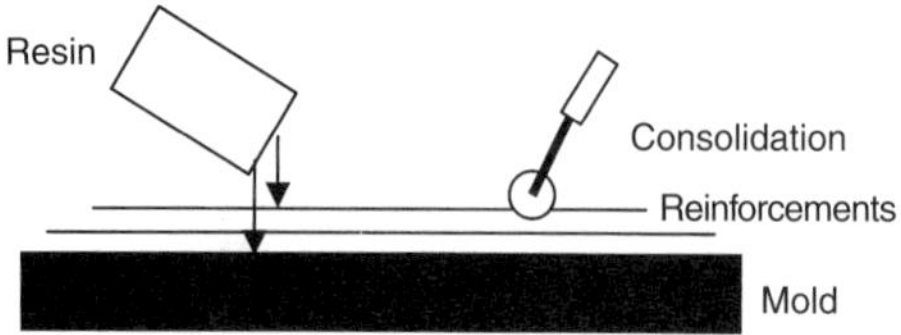

Fig. 6 Hand lay-up

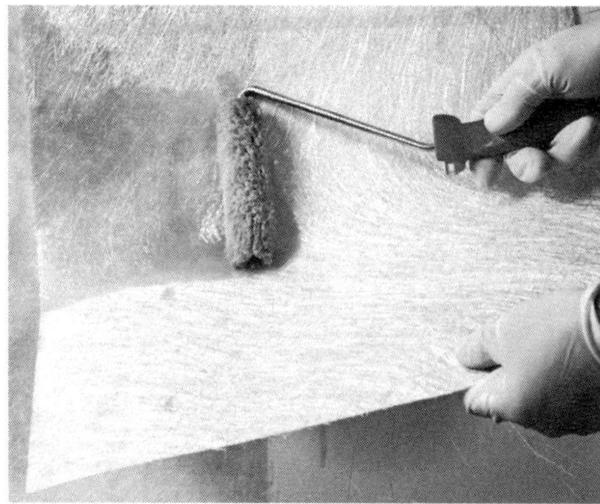

Fig. 7 Application of resin and chopped strand mat

The curing system added to the liquid resin will start the chemical cross-linking reaction. After a proper curing period, a top coat (also a pigmented or nonpigmented tailored resin) is applied, for both cosmetic purposes of the inner surface and the protection of the underlying laminate.

Hand lay-up allows a wide selection of reinforcement type. Generally, reinforcements are in the form of mats ranging from simple CSMs to the more complex and sophisticated WR and/or multiaxial fabrics also often combined with chopped fibers, the so-called combimats. The choice of reinforcement influences the final mechanical properties of the laminate.

In the spray-up version of the open-molding process, the liquid gel coat (when required) is applied in the correct wet-film thickness using tailored spray equipment (Fig. 9). After a proper curing period of the gel coat, liquid resin and chopped fibers are simultaneously deposited onto the gel coated surface from specialized spray equipment and spray guns (Fig. 10).

In fabricating laminates for use in marine applications, a 1 to 2 mm (0.04–0.08 in.) skin laminate can be applied using a silane-sized spray roving impregnated with a high-quality skin laminate resin system. After curing as with hand lay-up, building up the load carrying laminate can begin. The sprayed, catalyzed liquid resin will wet the reinforcement fibers, which are simultaneously chopped in the same spray gun. These chopped fibers replace the CSM typically used in hand lay-up. Additional reinforcements such as WR or multiaxial fabrics can be placed between the chopped-fiber spray-up layers, but these have to be wetted with liquid resin also, either by applying by hand or through the spray gun without chopped fibers. Between the individual layers of chopped fibers or WR/multiaxial fabric layer, the wet laminate is consolidated by rolling using a grooved metal roller. A typical chopped-fiber/resin laminate thickness between consolidations is 1.5 to 2 mm (0.06–0.08 in.) maximum. Spray-up, with or without hand-laid layers, is continued in this sequence until the total laminate thickness is applied. As for a hand-made laminate, the inner surface is often coated with a top coat after curing the main laminate.

Workmanship is important for hand lay-up and spray-up. Proper preparation of the mold surface using correct mold-release application and preparation plays a key role in demolding the product. It is essential that the gel coat layer is applied in the correct thickness and evenly distributed over the total area, to avoid unwanted surface irregularities and reduced long-term protection of the part. Gel coat quality should match the application (hand brush or spray) to avoid unwanted sagging and to get good air release and "hiding" power.

For hand (brushing) application, the total gel coat thickness typically is applied in two operations. The first application of ~400 μm (~16 mils) wet film is applied as evenly as possible. After a setting period, a second ~400 μm layer is applied in a crosswise direction to the first to obtain the most even total film thickness possible. Because brushing is time consuming and difficult, spraying is used more often. Recommended spray-gun tip size, is an opening of 455 to 660 μm (18–26 mils) with a 40° angle.

Good workmanship also is important in the application of the reinforcements and resin (load-bearing laminate construction) behind the gel coat. The reinforcement must be placed correctly and evenly so that tapered overlaps and laminate edges are created. This is especially important when using hand lay-up to achieve correct thickness changes. When impregnating the reinforcements, it is important that the resin is evenly distributed to obtain the same reinforcement fraction over the total surface area and to obtain the required thickness.

For each single or double layer of reinforcement mat, the wet laminate has to be consolidated using a grooved metal roller. This is necessary to obtain air release and to split the individual strands in the reinforcement. Good splitting is essential to achieve good mechanical

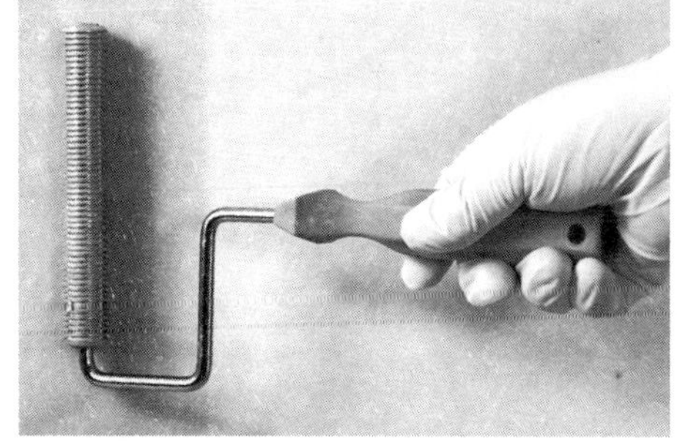

Fig. 8 Laminate consolidation using grooved metal roller

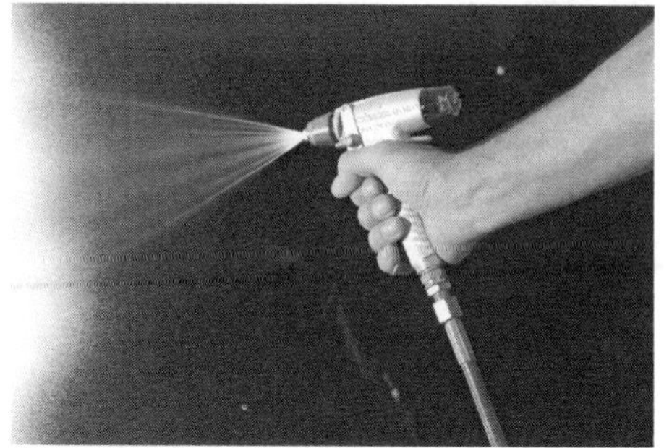

Fig. 9 Gel coat spray-up

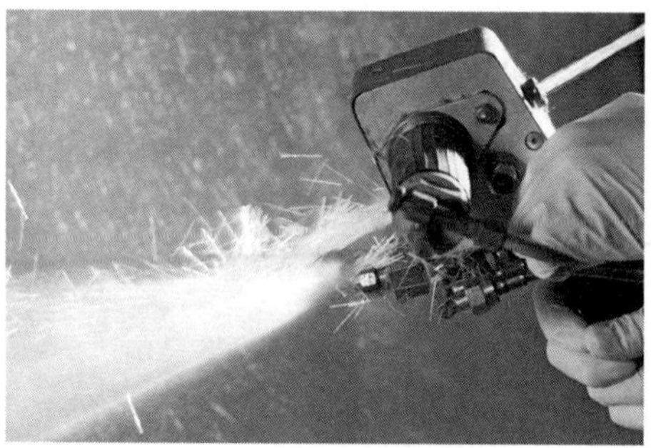

Fig. 10 Resin/glass spray-up gun

properties; the greater the fiber surface area available for the resin to impregnate and bond to, the better the properties will be.

Reinforcements in the form of mats make it difficult to handle corners and edges. Therefore, the design should have a sufficient radius in corners and over edges. Otherwise, the reinforcement mat tends to stretch in corners and buckle over edges, resulting in air pockets and/or resin-rich areas having low glass content. Corners and edges that are too sharp can also result in excessive rolling, causing thin laminates compared with the rest of the construction.

In the spray-up process, chopped-glass fiber and resin are deposited via a spray gun equipped on a custom pumping machine. It is important to follow the calibration and operation instructions set by the supplier. This is especially important for the resin spray patterns and the resin/glass ratio. The spray pattern will influence the uniformity of the wet laminate, and glass content (and corresponding mechanical properties) is controlled by adjustment of the chopper. Consolidation is also important here, and it is always recommended to consolidate with the grooved metal roller between each 1.5 to 2.0 mm (0.06–0.08 in.) wet laminate. This will secure proper air release and splitting of fiber strands. Achievable glass content using only chopped-fiber roving (normal for spray-up), is lower than for hand lay-up. However, it is possible to combine spray-up laminates with one or more layers of WR and/or multiaxial fabrics to achieve improved properties, either over the total area or in areas where the improved properties are required.

Regardless of the lay-up method used, the quality of the final part depends on the skills of the laminator, so trained workers will always be able to make better laminates and part-to-part consistency than untrained personnel.

Laminate quality is also affected by temperature, as viscosity and gel and cure properties are temperature dependent.

Resin viscosity guides the wet-out properties of a resin, and resin suppliers typically adjust the resins to optimal viscosity for the application process, generally for a temperature between 18 and 25 °C (65 and 77 °F). Too low of a temperature will result in higher viscosity, making it more difficult to consolidate and impregnate the laminate, and possibly causing unwanted air entrapment. Too high of a temperature causes viscosity to drop, which can cause sagging on more vertical areas. Low viscosity also tends to wet better, so the laminators automatically make less use of the metal roller, causing less fiber strand splitting and reduced mechanical properties.

Temperature also influences the gel and cure behavior of the resin. Low temperature inhibits gel and cure, which can affect part quality; the state of cure when the part is demolded and put into service is of utmost importance. High temperatures decrease gel time and increase reactivity; decreased gel time can cause the resin to solidify before proper part laminating is finalized, possibly resulting in a scrapped part. Increased reactivity (cure speed) can result in too high of a peak exotherm, which can cause discoloration, internal stress buildup, resin cracking and so forth. Therefore, control of material storage temperature and temperature of the work area is important.

Open molding using unsaturated polyester and epoxy vinyl ester laminating resins involves working in an environment containing styrene monomer, the reactive solvent in these resins. A certain amount of styrene will evaporate from the resin during processing. Because styrene is regarded and listed as a harmful constituent, precautions must be taken to protect workers from too-high styrene exposure. Maximum allowable styrene exposure levels are regulated nationally and vary from 20 to 100 parts per million (ppm). Using the so-called low-styrene emission (LSE) resins combined with adequate ventilation reduces styrene exposure and emission by at least 50% compared with a non-LSE laminating resin.

Optimal cross-linking (curing) reaction for open molding at room temperature might not be complete, so postcuring at elevated temperature is often recommended. Baking a part for a few hours at elevated temperature is often sufficient to achieve full cure; the temperature and baking time is dependent on resin quality. Table 1 lists necessary postcuring periods versus the heat-deflection temperature (HDT)—also known as the deflection temperature under load, or DTUL (as measured according to ISO 75, Method A)—of the resin system.

Materials

The predominant matrix-resin materials used for open molding as described here are unsaturated polyester resins and epoxy vinyl ester resins. Other matrix materials including phenolics and epoxies are also used in specialized applications. The resins are delivered and used in a liquid state, usually made thixotropic to prevent sag tendencies on more vertical areas. Glass fibers are the predominant reinforcement materials used, but more sophisticated reinforcements, such as aramid and carbon fibers, are often used in combination with glass fibers. Material selections are made based on both short- and long-term end-product requirements.

Unsaturated polyester resins and epoxy vinyl esters can be formulated to have a wide range of properties, depending on the raw material combination and polymerization process. Orthophthalic resins typically are selected for parts exposed to normal weather and water resistance (general-purpose laminating resins); these resins can also be formulated to have very good corrosion resistance in humid conditions (high-quality orthophthalic laminating resins).

Resin systems based on dicyclopentadiene (DCPD), alternatives to general-purpose orthophthalics, typically are used where improved part surface cosmetics are required. This is due to their improved ambient-temperature curing behavior and their ability to be formulated for reduced shrinkage. Isophthalic and terephthalic resins generally are selected for use in more aggressive exposures, as these in general have a better chemical resistance than the orthophthalics and DCPD-based systems. Epoxy vinyl esters are used in applications requiring high chemical resistance. Within these three categories, the mechanical and physical properties can be wide, especially with respect to rigidity and heat, corrosion, and fire resistance.

Reinforcements are available in a variety of qualities and fiber design. The simplest form of glass fiber reinforcements is CSM, typically used in the hand lay-up mode, and gun-roving and/or spray-up roving, typically used in the spray-up mode. The amount and type of reinforcement dictate mechanical properties of the laminate, but only to a certain extent, as the fiber fraction normally has to be kept below 40 wt%. More sophisticated fiber reinforcements, such as the WR, WR combi, multiaxial fabrics, and multiaxial fabrics combi, must be used for higher mechanical properties, which are dependent on the fiber fraction and direction. These are also delivered in the form of mats, so they have to be laid by hand regardless of application mode for the rest of the reinforcements.

Component Properties and Characteristics

Apart from being dependent on the component design, short- and long-term properties of a fiber reinforced composite laminate made using open molding may vary depending on material selection and workmanship. Material selection and workmanship and workshop conditions influence short-term properties. Long-term properties (i.e., how well the composite laminate can withstand different exposures and service loads during the expected lifetime) depend on the type and intensity of the exposure, as well as the ma-

Table 1 Recommended postcuring temperature and time based on resin heat deflection temperature (HDT)

Postcuring temperature		Postcuring time for indicated resin heat deflection temperature, h			
°C	°F	for HDT of 65 °C (149 °F)	for HDT of 85 °C (185 °F)	for HDT of 100 °C (212 °F)	for HDT of 130 °C (265 °F)
40	104	24	48	96	120
50	122	12	24	48	92
60	140	6	12	18	24
70	158	3	6	9	12
80	176	1.5	3	4	6

terial selection, workmanship, and state of cure when put into service. Typical short-term properties are:

- Mechanical properties
- Heat resistance
- Thermal conductivity
- Electrical properties
- Fire retardance
- Visual aspects

Typical long-term properties are:

- Weather resistance
- Water resistance
- Chemical resistance
- Heat aging
- Fatigue resistance
- Creep resistance

Mechanical Properties. The strength and stiffness of a composite laminate are dictated by the type, amount, and direction of the fiber reinforcement in the thermoset resin matrix. Glass fiber is the most widely used reinforcement for unsaturated polyesters and epoxy vinyl esters, but aramid and carbon fibers are used when increased mechanical properties are required. Glass fiber forms include CSM and spray roving, as well as WR, multiaxial fabrics/knitted fabrics, and unidirectional (UD) fabrics. Woven roving, multiaxial fabrics, and UD fabrics also are combined with chopped roving (combimats).

Woven roving, multiaxial fabrics and UD fabrics are normally used when increased mechanical properties are required, as glass content then is increased. Woven roving and multiaxial fabrics are used when increased properties in certain directions are necessary.

Woven roving aramid fibers are primarily used when lower laminate weight is required. Aramid improves mechanical properties, especially impact resistance, but at the expense of compression properties. Because aramid fibers are more expensive than glass fiber, they often are used together with glass fiber and are known as glass-aramid hybrids.

Carbon fiber is used as continuous roving or as certain fabrics and also often as a hybrid together with glass, due to its relatively high price. Carbon fiber increases mechanical properties; types having high modulus result in a laminate having low-impact properties and vice versa.

Table 2 lists representative properties for a standard laminate using a general-purpose orthophthalic laminating resin. Properties of laminates of different matrix resins reinforced with 30 wt% (17 vol%) CSM glass fiber are listed in Table 3. Table 4 lists properties of the same resins listed in Table 3, reinforced with WR combimat (800/100) of ~50 wt% (32 vol%) glass fiber. Expected achievable properties using a high-quality isophthalic/neopentyglycol (Iso/NPG) resin as the laminating resin are shown in Table 5. Carbon fiber is used in cases where requirements for high mechanical and stiffness properties are dominant, and expected laminate properties are shown in Table 6. The laminates are made using a rubber-modified vinyl ester, and carbon fiber multiaxial fabrics based on improved carbon fiber roving. Improved shear properties in vinyl ester laminates are also found (indicatively) if a smaller amount of chopped-glass fibers are used between the carbon fiber fabric layers.

Increased stiffness of a composite product can be optimized by intelligent design, by using stiffener ribs, making a sandwich construction, and/or making the laminate thicker. A significant weight saving compared with a similar steel construction can be realized (at least 50%) regardless of the type of polymer composite laminate construction.

Visual Aspects. Three main visual aspects are color, surface gloss, and surface print-through. Suitable pigment pastes are added if a colored laminate is required. As described earlier, the gel coat surface layer provides the surface visual aspects, and the quality of the mold surface and the gel coat quality will have great influence on visual quality. The part surface replicates the mold surface, so a high-quality, glossy mold surface is required. Gel coat formulation will have impact on the surface gloss, color appearance, and so forth.

Surface print-through is an important factor affecting the cosmetic nature of the surface. The fiber print-through appears on the surface (normally the gel coated surface) as print-through of the reinforcement fibers in the structural laminate. This typically is caused by resin shrinkage in the laminate after part demolding, so that any reduction of such shrinkage after demolding the part is essential. Sandwich constructions can also show print-through (a print-through of the core

Table 2 Representative open-molded laminate mechanical properties for general-purpose orthophthalic laminating resins

	Spray roving	Chopped strand mat	Chopped strand mat	Chopped strand mat	Chopped strand mat/woven roving	Test standard
Glass content, wt%	30–35	25–30	30–35	35–40	45–50	ISO 1172
Glass content, vol%	16–20	14–16	16–20	20–24	28–32	Calculated
Density, g/cm^3	1.45	1.40	1.45	1.50	1.68	ISO 1183
Tensile strength, MPa (ksi)	70 (10)	70 (10)	90 (13)	110 (16)	180 (26)	ISO 527
Tensile elongation, %	1.8	1.8	1.8	1.8	2.0	ISO 527
Tensile modulus, GPa (10^6 psi)	7.0 (1)	6.0 (0.9)	7.5 (1.1)	9.0 (1.3)	12.5 (1.8)	ISO 527
Flexural strength, MPa (ksi)	140 (20)	140 (20)	155 (22.5)	175 (25)	240 (35)	ISO 178
Flexural modulus, GPa (10^6 psi)	6.0 (0.9)	5.5 (0.8)	6.5 (0.95)	8.0 (1.2)	10.5 (1.5)	ISO 178
Impact, P 4 J(a), kJ/m^2	75	70	80	90	110	ISO 179
Compressive strength, MPa (ksi)	110 (16)	100 (14.5)	120 (17.4)	140 (20)	150 (22)	ISO 604
Compressive modulus, GPa (10^6 psi)	7.5 (1.1)	6.5 (0.95)	8.0 (1.2)	9.5 (1.4)	12.5 (1.8)	ISO 604

(a) P4J, 4J pendulum.

Table 3 Representative standard laminate mechanical properties for different resin qualities

	Tough ortho	Standard iso	Improved iso/NPG	Standard VE	Rubber modified VE	Test standard
Tensile strength, MPa (ksi)	95 (13.8)	95 (13.8)	100 (14.5)	100 (14.5)	95 (13.8)	ISO 527
Tensile elongation, %	2.0	2.0	2.1	2.1	2.1	ISO 527
Tensile modulus, GPa (10^6 psi)	7.0 (1)	7.0 (1)	6.3 (0.91)	6.3 (0.91)	6.1 (0.88)	ISO 527
Flexural strength, MPa (ksi)	160 (23.2)	160 (23.2)	160 (23.2)	160 (23.2)	155 (22.4)	ISO 178
Flexural modulus, GPa (10^6 psi)	6.0 (0.9)	6.0 (0.9)	5.9 (0.89)	5.9 (0.89)	5.8 (0.84)	ISO 178
Compressive strength, MPa (ksi)	115 (16.7)	115 (16.7)	135 (19.6)	140 (20.3)	140 (20.3)	ISO 604
Compressive modulus, GPa (10^6 psi)	6.8 (0.97)	6.8 (0.97)	6.0 (0.9)	6.0 (0.9)	6.0 (0.9)	ISO 604

Ortho, orthophthalic resin; iso, isophthalic resin; iso/NPG, isophthalic/neopentylglycol resin; VE, vinylester resin

Table 4 Representative laminate mechanical properties of a high-quality laminate using different resin systems

	Tough ortho	Standard iso	Improved iso/NPG	Standard VE	Rubber modified VE	Test standard
Tensile strength, MPa (ksi)	200 (29)	200 (29)	205 (29.7)	220 (31.9)	230 (33.3)	ISO 527
Tensile elongation, %	1.8	1.8	1.9	2.0	2.0	ISO 527
Tensile modulus, GPa (10^6 psi)	17.0 (2.5)	17.0 (2.5)	16.0 (2.3)	16.0 (2.3)	16.0 (2.3)	ISO 527
Flexural strength, MPa (ksi)	350 (50.7)	340 (49.3)	340 (49.3)	350 (50.7)	350 (50.7)	ISO 178
Flexural modulus, GPa (10^6 psi)	14.0 (2.0)	14.0 (2.0)	13.0 (1.9)	13.0 (1.9)	13.0 (1.9)	ISO 178
Compressive strength, MPa (ksi)	210 (30.4)	210 (30.4)	250 (36.2)	270 (39.1)	260 (37.7)	ISO 604
Compressive modulus, GPa (10^6 psi)	17.5 (2.5)	17.5 (2.5)	16.5 (2.4)	16.5 (2.4)	16.5 (2.4)	ISO 604

Ortho, orthophthalic resin; iso, isophthalic resin; iso/NPG, isophthalic/neopentylglycol resin; VE, vinylester resin

material on the surface) especially when square cut core material is used. The degree of print-through is dependent on:

- The gel coat quality (reactivity, HDT)
- Skin laminate: correct fiber type and fraction, resin quality (shrinkage and reactivity)
- Structural laminate: fiber fraction and resin reactivity
- Demolding: state of cure when demolding

The Long-Term Properties. The change in short-term properties with time and exposure is primarily dependent on the resin used in the laminate. However, parameters including fiber quality and fiber fraction, laminate construction, workmanship, and state of cure when put into service all can have important influence.

The weather resistance of a composite laminate is generally considered to be very good for a normal, good-quality laminate constructed and designed for outdoor exposure. A composite laminate will not corrode as will steel and aluminum, but the laminate surface will be subject to attack by rain, wind, and ultraviolet (UV) radiation, which can cause a change in color and surface gloss, and in some cases fiber blooming (one can see and feel fibers on the surface) for non-gel-coated parts.

Mechanical properties, of a good quality laminate with a proper surface protection are little influenced in the long term. Such laminates will retain >90% of their initial short-term values even after years of normal outdoor exposures, despite color and gloss changes. However, when a composite laminate gets or has a surface defect of some kind (which often is attributed to bad workmanship), the properties can be reduced more rapidly, as moisture and other "weather impurities" can penetrate into the laminate and thus cause breakdown in the structure.

To avoid this unwanted penetration, the structural parts of a laminate should always be protected, either by using a sufficiently pigmented gel coat layer or making a resin-rich surface by using one or two layers of a suitable surfacing veil. Making this resin-rich layer as free from voids (pinholes, craters, etc.) as possible is important to avoid possible sites for moisture penetration into the load-bearing structure of the laminate.

Two principle concerns with respect to water resistance are resistance to osmosis and blistering in parts such as boat hulls, swimming pools, bath tubs, and whirlpools, and so forth. Normal water resistance is discussed together with chemical resistance in general.

Blistering is generally caused by osmosis, and blister resistance is consequently determined by:

- Water quality: less osmosis in salt water than fresh water
- Gel coat quality: a high-quality, hydrolytic stable gel coat preferred
- Gel coat layer thickness: 500 μm (20 mils) min cured film preferred
- Gel coat layer porosity
- Gel coat layer state of cure
- Skin laminate quality behind the gel coat: fiber quality and resin quality, no air entrapments, and good state of cure. Postcuring at elevated temperature can be required.

Chemical resistance, including water resistance requires special attention, because the long-term behavior of a composite part exposed to aggressive conditions depends largely on resin system and reinforcement quality, laminate construction, curing/postcuring, workmanship, and so forth. Use of a general-purpose orthophthalic resin generally is not recommended in this case. Also the type and intensity (concentration and temperature) of the chemical exposure influences service life.

To achieve a good barrier between the structural laminate and the corrosive medium, it is always recommended to make a laminate having a chemical-resistant liner to protect the structural laminate from chemical exposures (Fig. 11). It is further recommended that the total laminate should be made with the same kind of resin used for the chemical-resistant liner. However, it is a well-accepted practice to build the structural laminate with a less chemical-resistant resin system to reduce total part price. For example, a suitable epoxy vinyl ester can be used for the liner, and the structural laminate made of a good isophthalic resin having good HDT.

To obtain the optimal chemical-resistance performance, a postcuring cycle at elevated temperature is recommended. A good postcuring cycle involves a 16 to 24 h cure at ambient temperature (>18 °C, or 65 °F) before postcuring at a higher temperature. Recommended postcuring temperature can be related to the chemistry of the resin and mostly related to the HDT of the resin (see Table 2).

Basic Design Guidelines

When designing a composite part, one should never try to make a part-to-part substitution of a metal part. For example, thermoset composite materials have lower stiffness (modulus) compared with metals, so a composite part has to be intelligently designed to overcome its lower stiffness. This can be accomplished by designing a part having ribs, a sandwich construction, and/or increasing section thickness where required.

Using the reinforcement possibilities intelligently will also contribute to overcoming the lower stiffness properties. That is, one can use directed reinforcements (unidirectional or multiaxial) placed strategically where the part is likely to encounter higher stresses.

In a sandwich construction, core materials are imbedded into the laminate where higher stiffness is required, while still keeping part weight low compared with a similar metal part.

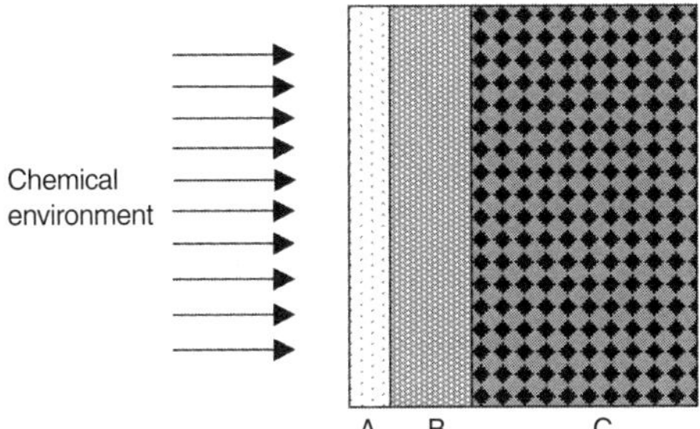

Fig. 11 Recommended chemical-resistant laminate construction. A, layer with surfacing veils impregnated with 90 to 95% resin; B, two-layer laminate having 450 g/m^2 powder-bonded mat, preferably with 20 Tex ECR fiber, or an equal thickness made of a silane-sized ECR spray roving (glass content should be 20–30%); A + B, chemical-resistant liner (preferably 2.5–3.5 mm, or 0.01–0.14 in. thick); C, structural laminate

Table 5 Representative laminate mechanical properties of high-quality laminates using an improved Iso/NPG resin

	Chopped strand mat	Woven roving combi	Biaxial 0/90	Biaxial unidirectional	Glass/aramid	Test standard
Fiber content, wt%	35	50	58	60	50	ISO 1172
Fiber content, vol%	20	32	41	42	31	Calculated
Density, g/cm^3	1.50	1.60	1.70	1.75	1.40	ISO 1183
Tensile strength, MPa (ksi)	125 (18.1)	205 (29.7)	350 (50.7)	600 (87.0)	225 (32.6)	ISO 527
Tensile elongation, %	1.9	1.9	2.5	2.4	2.0	ISO 527
Tensile modulus, GPa (10^6 psi)	8.0 (1.1)	16.0 (2.3)	20.0 (2.9)	28.0 (4.1)	17.0 (2.5)	ISO 527
Compressive strength, MPa (ksi)	150 (21.7)	250 (36.2)	280 (40.6)	540 (78.3)	210 (30.4)	ISO 604
Compressive modulus, GPa (10^6 psi)	7.5 (1.1)	16.5 (2.4)	20.5 (3.0)	29.0 (4.2)	14.0 (2.0)	ISO 604

Table 6 Representative laminate mechanical properties made with carbon fiber reinforced and rubber-modified vinyl ester resin laminate

	Unidirectional	Biaxial 0°/90°	Test standard
Fiber content, bulk wt%	50	45	ISO 1172
Fiber content, vol%	36	31	Calculated
Tensile strength, MPa (ksi)	1400 (203)	630 (91.3)	ISO 527
Tensile modulus, GPa (10^6psi)	80.0 (11.6)	40.0 (5.8)	ISO 527
Tensile elongation, %	1.9	1.7	ISO 527
Compressive strength, MPa (ksi)	700 (102)	400 (58)	ISO 604

Corners and edges of the laminate should always have a minimum radius of 6 mm (0.2 in.) for the lay-up to follow the surface and prevent the occurrence of resin-rich areas. Designs incorporating undercuts are difficult to mold, but not impossible if a multipart (split) mold is used. Draft angles should be a minimum of 2° to allow easy part demolding.

Proper placement of reinforcements is very important to preclude sharp changes in thickness where stress concentrations and consequent delamination and warping can occur. Such sharp changes are avoided by carefully tapering the lay-up plies. If the total laminate is made wet-in-wet, there is the possibility of part warpage.

Unsaturated polyester and epoxy vinyl ester have a certain shrinkage upon cure; therefore, a laminate tends to become marginally smaller than the mold it is built in. As an indication, the shrinkage of standard unsaturated polyester laminate is 1 mm/1000 mm (0.01 in./10 in.). This requires designing and building a mold to compensate for part shrinkage. Shrinkage is dependent on design, laminate thickness wet-in-wet, fiber fraction, and so forth.

Outlook

Use of fiber-reinforced thermoset composites as a competitive construction material is expected to grow. Open molding will likely continue to be an important fabrication method due to its competitiveness for short production cycles and large complex parts for a variety of end-product applications. However, this potential growth will be dependent on the evolution of better and easier-to-use application equipment and improved materials, both resin systems and reinforcements.

Open molding with styrenated resin systems causes evaporation, exposure, and emission of VOCs and hazardous air pollutants (HAPs). Therefore, it is important to reduce these hazards. This can be solved and/or improved by the use of both better application equipment and thermoset resin systems having low or no VOC/HAP, but still maintaining the good and easy application properties of the unsaturated polyesters and epoxy vinyl esters.

More effective spray-up equipment needs to be developed—easier-to-use spray guns and nonatomized applications—to reduce VOC/HAP emissions caused by the application equipment. Development of new resin systems must address low/no VOC/HAP requirements.

Further improvement in gel coat technology, that is, gel coats having improved water-weather and UV resistance, will enable the open-molding industry to make composite parts having improved long-term surface stability (color and gloss), which will be more competitive in applications requiring good, long-term surface-aspect stability (especially in the building industry),which is not achievable with existing technology.

ACKNOWLEDGMENT

The information in this article is to a large extent based on Reichold technology and experience with the open-molding method for manufacturing fiber reinforced polymer-matrix composite laminates.

SELECTED REFERENCES

- B.T. Åström, *Manufacturing of Polymer Composites*, Chapman & Hall, 1997
- N.L. Hancox and R.M. Mayer, *Design Data for Reinforced Plastics—A Guide for Engineers and Designers*, Chapman & Hall, 1994
- M. Holmes and D.J. Justin, *GRP in Structural Engineering*, Applied Science, 1983
- *Introduction to Composites*, The Composites Institute, 1995
- A.F. Johnson, *Engineered Design. Properties of GRP*, The British Plastics Federation, 1986
- G. Lubin, *Handbook of Composites*, Van Nostrand Reinhold, 1982
- S.T. Peters, *Handbook of Composites*, 2nd ed., Chapman & Hall, 1998

Custom Sailing Yacht Design and Manufacture

Richard Downs-Honey and Paul Hakes, High Modulus New Zealand Limited
Mark Battley, Industrial Research Limited, New Zealand

COMPOSITE MATERIALS are used in a wide range of marine vessel applications, from kayaks of a few meters in length up to military and commercial vessels of more than 70 m (230 ft). The reasons for the use of composites vary greatly, depending on the type of application. Composites dominate the market for mass-production small pleasure craft because of the flexibility and efficiency of manufacturing methods, good durability, and low maintenance requirements. For large luxury vessels, it is the ability to obtain a very high class finish, combined with low maintenance requirements and good performance from lighter weight structures, that drive the use of composites. In military applications, high specific strength, shock resistance, ability to incorporate stealth features, and low magnetic signature are key issues. For commercial craft, strength, stiffness, and durability provide composites with competitive advantages.

The most innovative use of marine composites is in the production of one-off custom sailing yachts, such as racing or luxury pleasure craft. For these vessels the high specific stiffness and strength, good toughness, high corrosion resistance, and excellent fatigue life of modern composites, combined with the development of very flexible manufacturing processes, have enabled composites to compete very successfully with aluminum. The availability of a wide range of specialized reinforcement and core materials and resin systems tailored to low-temperature manufacturing techniques have also been key factors in the growth of composites use in this field.

This article focuses on the design process, materials, and manufacturing techniques used for one-off and low-volume production sailing craft. These include racing yachts of typically 10 to 20 m (33 to 66 ft) length for short coastal events (Fig. 1), 20 to 25 m (66 to 82 ft) ocean racers (Fig. 2), 24 m (79 ft) America's Cup racing craft, multihull racers of 35 m (115 ft) or more (Fig. 3), and large (40+ m, or 130+ ft) luxury cruising craft.

Yacht Structure

A typical yacht structure can be considered to be comprised of three different types of components: the main hull/deck assembly (Fig. 4); the above-deck "rig" consisting of mast, boom, spinnaker pole, and sail furling systems; and the below-water appendages, the keel and rudder. Composites are used for all of these components; however the design requirements, structural solutions, and manufacturing methods are different for each.

The primary function of the hull and deck assembly is to provide a watertight buoyant structure that can maintain the correct hydrodynamic

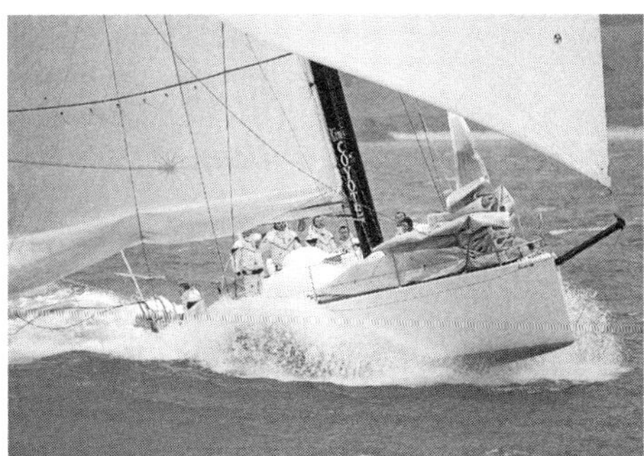

Fig. 1 Racing monohull (*Kiwi Coyote*) for coastal events. Courtesy of Ivor Wilkins

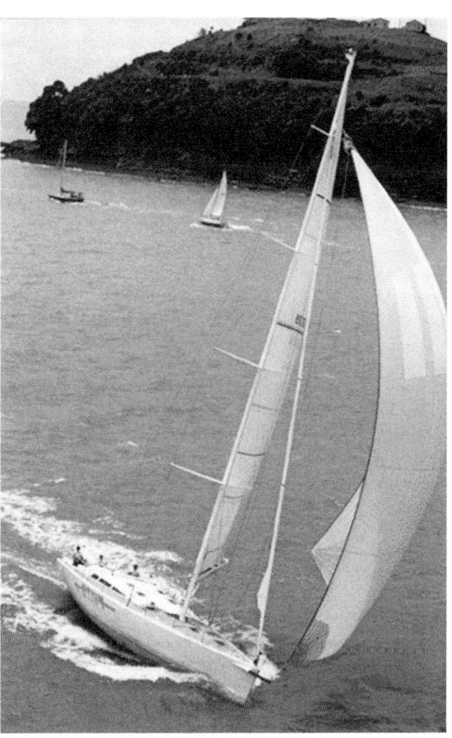

Fig. 2 Offshore performance cruising monohull (*Pinta*). Courtesy of Martin Yachts, New Zealand

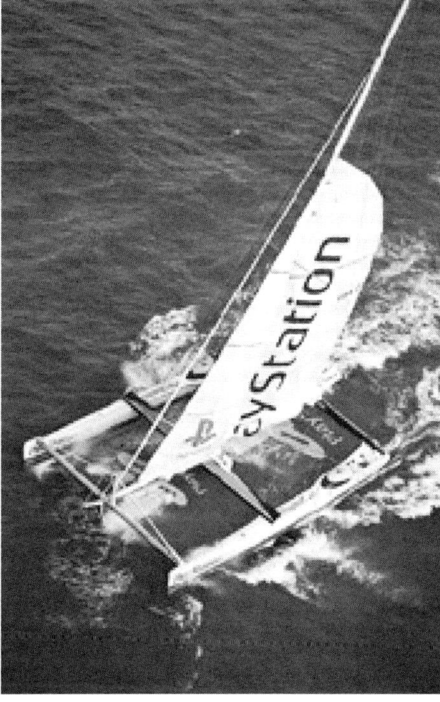

Fig. 3 Multihull racing yacht (*Playstation*) for around-the-world races. Courtesy of Steve Fossett Ocean Challenge

shape when subjected to applied loads from the water and from the rig and appendages.

The mast, in conjunction with its associated rigging, transfers the forces from the sails to the yacht hull, thereby propelling the vessel through the water. The pretension of the rigging results in extremely high compression loads in the mast tube and bending in the fore-aft direction, which is used to optimize the sail shape. In addition to distributed sail loads, the mast is also subjected to torsion from offset loads, such as the boom, and localized loads from the rigging.

Other tubular components include the boom, which is subjected to sail loads and concentrated loads from the mainsheet and vang, resulting in high compression and bending loads; the spinnaker pole, which is primarily subjected to compression; and the spreaders, which act to triangulate the rigging loads.

The purpose of the keel is to counteract the transverse aerodynamic force produced by the sails, thereby enabling the yacht to travel in a forward direction, and to provide stability by resisting the associated heeling moment. Shaped as a foil, the keel is subjected to hydrodynamic loads and also large bending loads, due to the mass of lead in the bulb. The rudder, which also provides lift to counteract the transverse aerodynamic forces and controls the steering of the yacht, is also subjected to large hydrodynamic loads, generating high bending loads at the top of the foil where it reduces in cross section to enter the yacht hull.

A yacht structure operates at the interface between water and air, making loads variable and very difficult to predict. Forces from wind and water can combine to produce dynamic loading on all of the structure at the same time. The loads are also significantly influenced by how the yacht is sailed, with human error being a significant factor in failures, particularly in the mast and rig.

The costs of manufacturing these types of vessels vary greatly depending on the intended use of the boat. As an example, Table 1 summarizes some indicative costs for typical high-performance 18 to 20 m (59 to 66 ft) monohull racing and performance cruising yachts. The racing yacht would have a very basic interior, with no joinery, mostly unpainted interior laminates, and only what is absolutely necessary to live on board. In the year 2000, the overall cost of such a boat was approximately $1.8 million, with a total of approximately 35,000 hours of labor involved in the design, construction, and fitting-out to the stage of launching the boat in the water. Labor constitutes approximately 40% of the total cost, the next largest component being materials for the hull, at approximately 34%. The cost of the cruising yacht would be approximately $2.0 million, with the interior being a much larger component of the total cost.

Design Guidelines

The structural design process for a sailing yacht endeavors to combine the geometry constraints, imposed by the hull shape and interior arrangement, with the material properties and construction processes to meet the applied loads with an acceptable safety margin. Considerable progress has been made in defining achievable materials properties, given the limitations of the building process. Similarly, there have been advances in design tools, such as finite-element analysis, enabling more refined analysis of complex geometries. However, the science is still severely constrained by the lack of in-depth understanding of the applied loads. The definition of the dynamic forces applied to a sailing yacht, particularly in extreme conditions, is complex. As a result, the design process is based on past experience, simplified load scenarios, gross assumptions, and acceptable safety margins.

Hull and deck shells are typically designed to resist a spectrum of static pressures. Decks are only occasionally subject to a head of water, typically in the order of 1 to 2 m (3 to 7 ft) at most. The hull bottom, especially forward, can be exposed to higher slamming loads when sailing in waves, and hence the design pressure might equate to a 5 to 8 m (16 to 26 ft) head. An arrangement of internal structural support (bulkheads, frames, and other local stiffeners) is developed with due consideration to the interior accommodation requirements. This is matched to a suitable plating specification (selection of core and skins dependent upon the unsupported panel span and design head), such that deflection criteria and safety margins are met. Overlaid on this is the localized treatment of high stresses generated by the mast and rigging attachments, deck hardware, keel and rudder, and the engine. This often involves additional patching and specific framing in order to spread the load into the surrounding structure. On larger (>20 m, or 66 ft) vessels, overall bending deflections under both rig and wave load scenarios may be calculated, because fore-and-aft rigidity is critical to sailing performance.

The definition of loads in the rig is a little easier than for the hull shell. Sail forces can be estimated, and from this, the rigging supporting the mast sized. Factors are then applied to account for inertial loads as the boat pitches in the fore-and-aft direction when sailing over waves. The major use of composites in rigs is in the mast tube itself, which can be treated as a supported column under compression. Given a slender section to minimize wind resistance, the design problem becomes one of buckling, often leading to the use of higher-modulus carbon reinforcements (Fig. 5). In addition to the specification of

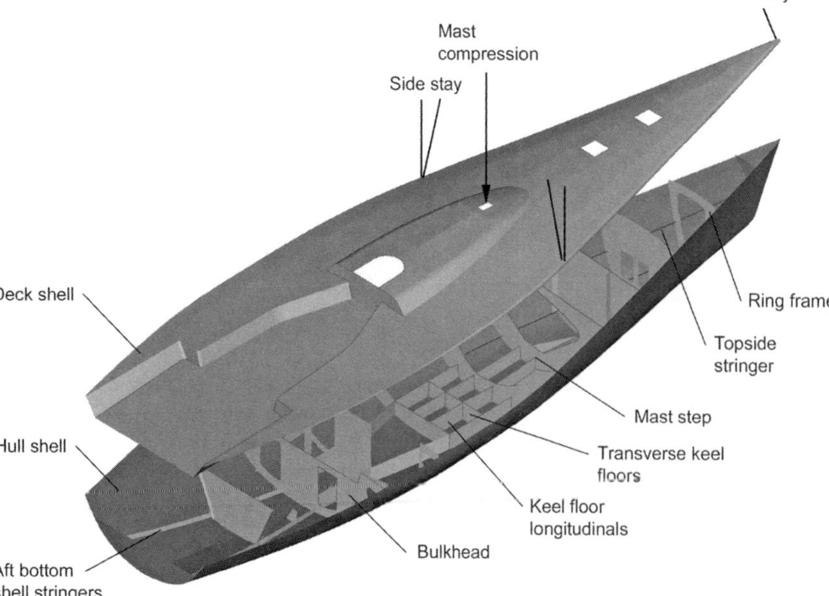

Fig. 4 Exploded view of typical yacht structure

Table 1 Cost comparison for typical 18–20 m (60–66 ft) racing and cruising yachts

Component	Racing, %	Cruising, %
Design	5	5
Tooling	4	5
Hull and deck structures	50	35
Equipment	10	20
Rig and sails	30	15
Interior	1	20
Total	**100**	**100**

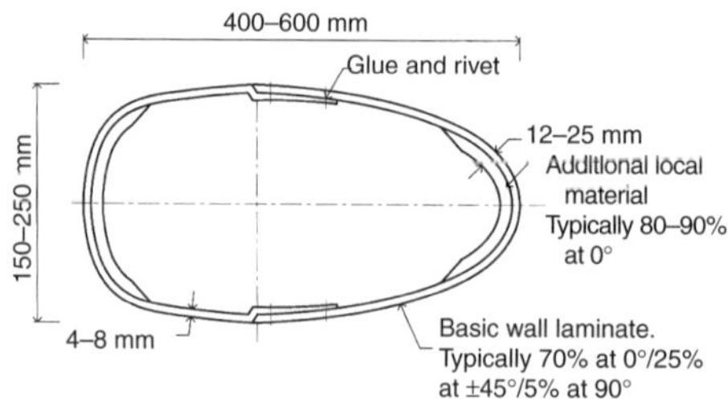

Fig. 5 Typical mast cross section

a section shape and laminate capable of sustaining the compressive forces, there are equally important secondary loadings to consider, such as at the interfaces with the supporting rigging. In a mast with a wall thickness of nominally 6 to 8 mm (0.24 to 0.31 in.), the reinforcement in the region of stay terminations can increase the thickness locally to 15 to 20 mm (0.59 to 0.79 in.).

Keels and rudders are similarly apparently straightforward. The maximum load that can be applied to a ballast keel can be estimated by a static analysis of a severe knockdown in which the vessel lies on its side. The hydrodynamic forces applied to the rudder can be calculated based on understanding of the section shape and expected speed. Often the angle of attack of the foil is limited by the ability of the steering system to apply sufficient torque, and this can result in a load lower than might be calculated from first principles. In order to produce efficient foil shapes for both the keel and rudder, there are restrictions on the section size, and hence the design becomes dimension-limited. In most cases, ultimate strength is the primary design constraint, but increasingly with deep slender foils, stiffness is also a concern, because excessive deflection can lead to loss of performance. As with the rigs, this drives the design toward the use of carbon-fiber reinforcements.

The design process is not entirely an "engineering" exercise. In addition to the loading scenarios and strength or stiffness criteria described previously, the specification has to take into consideration constraints imposed by the level of technology available to the builder, as well as the requirements of independent regulatory authorities and organizers of specific racing classes. These rules and regulations are usually a summary of the best available knowledge at the time and are intended to ensure safety and/ or control costs. However, they are sometimes unable to keep pace with developing technology, hence limiting opportunities for innovative structural solutions.

Yacht-building technology ranges from production female molded construction, based on materials and processes little changed since the 1980s (polyester resin, chopped strand mat and woven rovings, hand laminating), to elevated-temperature cure, vacuum consolidation, and unidirectional prepreg tapes with honeycomb cores. Most custom or one-off builders use epoxy-resin systems with some form of vacuum-assisted consolidation to reduce resin content. Sandwich construction is also widespread. Nevertheless, the design engineer needs to be aware of the fiber content the boat-building yard is capable of achieving with their processes. For a cross-ply, unidirectional glass laminate (either distinct plies or a multiaxial fabric), this could range from a low of 50 to 55% by weight through to better than 70%, depending on the resin rheology, form of the reinforcement, and consolidation process. The choice of core material can be influenced by the builder's ability to meet processing constraints. Elevated-temperature cure raises issues related to outgassing and stability of foam cores. Because most boats are manufactured in relatively uncontrolled working environments, humidity during the manufacturing process can be highly variable, leading to concerns over use of balsa or Nomex (DuPont) cores.

Material selection can also be influenced by the class rules for the particular yacht. Carbon-fiber reinforcements and honeycomb cores are not permitted in the Volvo 60 class for racing around the world (Ref 1). Consequently, the designs are based on aramid fibers, with some S-glass, and either foam or balsa cores. The intention, when the rule was written, was no doubt to limit cost. In the intervening period, carbon reinforcements have become more cost-competitive, yet the rules are slow to change, because this would penalize existing yachts. Even in the America's Cup (Ref 2), where cost is not a major constraint, the carbon used in the hull construction (Fig. 6) is limited to standard-modulus grades, although intermediate-modulus material is allowed in the rigs. Some rating rules try to assess the benefit that use of advanced construction materials can generate in terms of reduced weight and improved performance. While higher-performing materials are not excluded, their use is penalized in the handicap calculation. This can lead to use of lower technology than is optimal if the penalty is inconsistent with the actual performance advantages.

Given a portfolio of materials acceptable to the builder and allowable by the racing rules, the designer then addresses constraints that may be imposed by a scantling code, if applicable. For a period, racing yachts were covered by an American Bureau of Shipping (ABS) guide (Ref 3), and most events required plan approval prior to construction. This guide has been withdrawn, and ABS is no longer certifying racing yachts, although some event organizers and racing classes still require the yacht to be designed to meet these requirements. With modern sandwich design, the limiting factor tends to be the minimum outer skin thickness, a criterion based on durability and unrelated to frame spacing or shell properties. The design begins with the selection of an acceptable skin thickness, and from there develops core specification to suit the unsupported panel dimensions, or defines framing to suit the shell properties. Often the result is well in excess of the minimum requirements for local panel stiffness and strength, as laid down in the guide, and may appear "over-engineered" simply because the skin thickness constraint dominates.

Luxury performance craft not necessarily intended for racing may need to be built to comply with one of the international scantling rules (Ref 4–7). This can be a requirement of the owner for added surety in the design and build process and to reduce insurance premiums, or a statutory requirement if the vessel travels internationally. Most of these rules have been developed for a wide range of craft, and the intended construction method was conventional polyester chopped strand mat/woven roving (CSM/WR) female molding. Often the higher-fiber content, epoxy-based specifications devoid of any interlaminar chopped strand plies are more than adequate in terms of strength and stiffness, but fail to meet specific requirements aimed at a lower-technology process. An example would be the mandatory use of a chopped strand mat layer next to the core surface, desirable to improve adhesion in a production process, but unnecessary in a one-off process where the core is bonded using vacuum bag techniques and epoxy adhesives. While most scantling authorities allow some scope for variations, this is typically an expensive process, requiring significant analysis and testing to validate the proposed change.

Typical Design Solutions. Despite the constraints ranging from costs through scantling authority rules, there are still numerous possible solutions to the design of any vessel. Different emphasis on the trade-off between weight and cost, acceptable levels of toughness, and materials availability can result in widely varying specifications for what is essentially the same design. Individual designers also have preferences based on experience and can favor one ma-

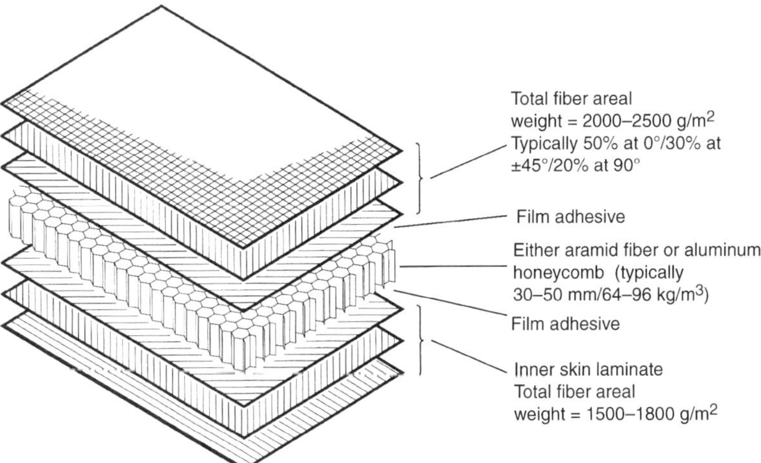

Fig. 6 Typical laminate for America's Cup hull skin

terial or style over another for no apparently rational reason. The following example is therefore not necessarily representative of the industry as a whole, nor ideal in all situations, however, it provides a general overview of a typical structure.

A 20 m (66 ft) performance cruising yacht, built with no regard to a specific racing rule, would most certainly be a sandwich construction, with a mixture of aramid, carbon, and E-glass reinforcements. The hull shell would be based on a core thickness of 30 to 40 mm (1.2–1.6 in.), depending upon the interior arrangement, with bulkheads and partitions providing support for the shell. Without secondary stiffeners, such as transverse frames or fore-and-aft stringers, a thicker core is likely. Core material is likely to be a rigid polyvinyl chloride (PVC) foam of 80 to 100 kg/m^3 (5.0–6.2 lb/ft^2) density, with either linear foam or higher-density end grain balsa used in the slamming areas toward the bow of the boat.

The outer skin would be in the order of 2.5 mm (0.010 in.) thick and consist of a combination of aramid and glass reinforcements, with individual plies in the 300 to 800 g/m^2 (1.0–2.6 oz/ft^2) areal weight range. The aramid is included for durability and to achieve a minimum skin thickness at low weight, and would constitute about 50 to 70% of the skin thickness. The fibers are likely to be aligned with the principle loads, with two-thirds running fore-and-aft and the balance athwartships. The glass fibers, possibly laid off-axis (±45), reduce cost and simplify the fairing process if used for the outermost ply, because sanding through the fairing compound into the aramid is not recommended. The inside skin is generally in the order of 70 to 80% of the thickness of the outer skin, due to reduced concern over impact. For this reason, carbon is likely to be specified, particularly in the bottom shell running fore-and-aft where it is most effective with regard to overall hull bending loads.

Allowing for additional reinforcement in the region of the keel, core bonding adhesive, and fairing compound, the average panel weight is in the order of 12 to 14 kg/m^2 (2.4–2.8 lb/ft^2), yielding a bare hull shell of less than 2 tonnes (2 metric tons, or 4400 lb).

The deck is of a lighter construction, with a core thickness in the 20 to 30 mm (0.8 to 1.2 in.) range, and varying depending upon the local support. If weight is of primary concern, 48 kg/m^3 (3.0 lb/ft^3) Nomex is favored over 80 kg/m^3 (5.0 lb/ft^3) foam, and there will be a higher percentage of carbon, with perhaps aramid used only in the high-traffic areas, such as the cockpit. With skin thickness of 1.8 mm (0.07 in.) outside and 1.1 mm (0.04 in.) inside, there is a requirement for considerable local reinforcement in the region of fittings, such as winches and sail tracks. Overall, an average panel weight of less than 10 kg/m^2 (2 lb/ft^2) can be expected, with a bare shell weight of around three-quarters of a tonne (1650 lb).

Internal structure consists of transverse bulkheads and longitudinal bottom girders, with local transverse floors in way of the keel and mast. The bulkheads and girders are sandwich, with a 15 to 25 mm (0.6 to 1.0 in.) core of either foam or possibly Nomex in some cases, with 1.5 to 1.8 mm (0.6 to 0.7 in.) E-glass skins (fibers typically at ±45) and local unidirectional carbon capping on exposed edges. Floors are typically 100 mm (4 in.) wide and 150 to 200 mm (6 to 8 in.) deep on centerline tapering outboard, of lower-density nonstructural foam, and covered with up to 5 to 8 mm (0.2 to 0.3 in.) of E-glass orientated at ±45 to carry shear loads in the webs. Bending properties are improved through capping of 7 to 10 mm (0.28 to 0.39 in.) of E-glass unidirectional, although in some cases a thinner carbon capping is justified on the basis of reduced weight.

The composites structure would weigh approximately 3.5 to 4.0 tonnes (3.9 to 4.4 tons), a small percentage of the overall weight of the vessel of typically 18 to 20 tonnes (20 to 22 tons), which can include as much as 6 to 10 tonnes (6.6 to 11.0 tons) of lead ballast at the bottom of the keel.

The carbon mast has a high percentage of 0° fibers, in the range of 65 to 70%, with a small percentage (5%) at 90° and the balance at ±45°. The tube itself is approximately 370 mm (14.6 in.) fore-and-aft by 195 mm (7.7 in.) transversely and has a basic wall thickness of 7 to 8 mm (0.28 to 0.31 in.) of carbon unidirectional prepreg, autoclave-cured at 3 bar (300 kPa) pressure to a volume fraction of 57 to 58%. This is designed as an Euler column subjected to a working load of approximately 500 kN (112 × 10^3 lbf), due to the forces exerted by the supporting stays. Transferring the high local loads from the stays, supporting spreaders, and other rigging into the tube demands quite detailed specific local reinforcing. Wall thickness in the region of openings and fittings could increase to 10 to 15 mm (0.4 to 0.6 in.), with the additional patching tending toward a quasi-isotropic laminate.

The rudder stock, or main spar, is a rectangular section to allow a relatively narrow (10 to 12% chord) foil shape (Fig. 7), with a buildup locally in the region of the bearing to approximately 300 mm (12 in.) diameter. The sides of the stock, where most of the transverse bending load is carried, are of the order of 25 to 30 mm (1.0 to 1.2 in.) thick at the intersection with the hull and are likely to have upwards of 60 to 75% of the fibers aligned with the stock, and the balance at ±45°. On the fore-and-aft faces, the 0° content is reduced, because these webs primarily carry shear. The laminate tapers considerably along the length, in line with the varying bending moment requirements. The stock is typically made over a non-structural, high-density foam former from standard-modulus carbon unidirectional, often in prepreg form and consolidated in an autoclave.

Material Types and Forms

The high-performance requirements of the modern sailing yacht are the primary drivers for lightweight construction, leading to a focus on high-fiber-content laminates based on advanced reinforcements. A range of techniques has been developed by custom yacht builders to achieve the relatively high fiber fractions required. Each of these processes creates its own constraints on the materials selection.

By far the simplest and most widespread is the "wet-preg" approach, which requires a long open-time resin system, can make use of a wide range of dry reinforcements (unidirectional tapes and broadgoods), and is compatible with most core materials. A prepreg construction is more restrictive in terms of material options. While broadgoods are available, they are more costly than collimated unidirectional tapes. There are few, truly low-temperature cure systems, and hence the selection of core materials is limited to those suitable for elevated cure.

Resin infusion has its own constraints. Open cellular cores are not readily adapted to this system, and depending upon the resin system used, some of the foam materials may also be excluded, due to interaction with styrene under vacuum. Reinforcements need to be designed to assist flow through the laminate during infusion, and consequently, tight, highly anisotropic unidirectional tapes are not favored.

Reinforcements. Despite the apparent drive toward high-performance fibers, the majority of hull and deck structures are built with a high proportion of E-glass. On a "cost per unit of weight saved" basis, it is rare that a project will warrant extensive use of carbon or aramid fibers, although there are many areas where selective placement is effective. Chopped strand mat and woven rovings have been almost universally replaced by multiaxial knitted reinforcements (0/90 biaxial, ±45 double bias, and triaxial), typically in the 600 to 1200 g/m^2 (2.0 to 4.0 oz/ft^2) range. Heavier quadraxials in excess of 2000 g/m^2 (6.6 oz/ft^2) are used in female molding; however, the side lap causes problems in one-off male molding. To minimize the side lap problem, some fabrics are supplied with tapered edges, where the warp fibers are removed along the side of the roll to reduce thickness buildup. Application of multiple plies of lighter unidirectional fabrics (250 to 400 g/m^2, or 0.8 to 1.3 oz/ft^2) is

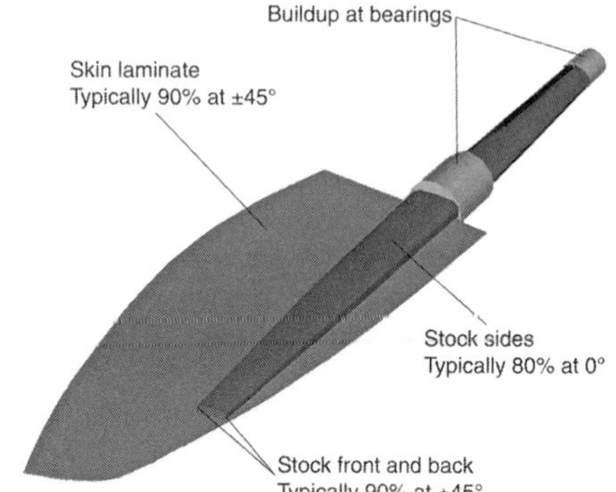

Fig. 7 Typical rudder stock and blade

still popular despite the increased labor, because adjacent layers can be butted to avoid sidelaps. While the design engineer might favor a particular form due to enhanced (potential) properties, it is often the builder's criteria with regard to handling, ease of wet-out, and the ability of the material to follow compound curves that dominate the selection decision.

Reinforcements of carbon and aramid are readily available in woven cloth (150 to 350 g/m^2, or 0.5 to 1.1 oz/ft^2) and unidirectional (200 to 500 g/m^2, or 0.7 to 1.6 oz/ft^2) forms, with limited multiaxial options, primarily double-bias ($\pm 45°$). The styles used are often those that have been originally developed for aerospace applications, which can be more costly than necessary due to the associated higher quality assurance requirements. A more limited but cost-effective range of marine-specific reinforcements is available, with specifications typically limited to the use of 200 and 300 g/m^2 (0.7 and 1.0 oz/ft^2) carbon or aramid unidirectionals, 200 g/m^2 (0.7 oz/ft^2) carbon cloth, and 175 and 300 g/m^2 (0.6 and 1.0 oz/ft^2) aramid cloth. There are a few glass/aramid hybrids, both cloth and unidirectional, also available in the 400 to 800 g/m^2 (1.3 to 2.6 oz/ft^2) range.

With dry reinforcements, the choice of carbon fiber is very limited, unless a significant volume justifies a custom production run. In general, the designs are based on high-strain, standard-modulus material, except for top-end, unlimited budget race boats. In prepreg construction, the options are much greater, and occasionally intermediate- or even high-modulus material is specified longitudinally in the hull and deck structure to improve rigidity, where the construction rule permits. The specific stiffness is particularly valued in the rigs, and here the use of higher-modulus fibers is quite common, especially in the larger (>40 m, or 130 ft) spars of superyachts (yachts 30 m, or 100 ft, or more in length).

Resins. The choice of resin system is very much based on practical considerations. Long working time, enabling the use of on-site impregnators and vacuum consolidation, compatibility with a wide range of cores, and low toxicity have driven the market toward epoxy systems, for both wet and prepreg applications. Some yards continue to use polyester resins; others have moved from polyester to the intermediate step of using vinyl-ester resins. Interestingly, the overall cost differential is negligible, despite the apparent two- to threefold cost increase associated with epoxy systems. As a proportion of the overall cost of materials, the resin is less than 25%. Cost increases from reduced resin use due to higher fiber content are offset by the elimination of the need for chopped strand mat (because of the better interlaminar properties of epoxy) and less waste due to more controlled processing techniques.

Cores. The most common core material used in one-off construction is closed foam, either rigid (cross-linked) PVC (Herex, Divinycell) or tougher, higher-elongation linear developments (Airex, Corecell). Typically, the minimum density used is 80 kg/m^3 (5 lb/ft^3), because thin skin laminates on lighter foams tend to bruise under local point loads. In the hull shell, it is not uncommon to see cores in the 100 to 130 kg/m^3 (6 to 8 lb/ft^3) range in the forward slamming areas. Selected-density end grain balsa has become an attractive option with prepreg construction, due to problems associated with outgassing and thermal stability of some foams. Honeycomb cores are also popular with prepreg construction. Nomex has been the most widely used, typically 48 to 64 kg/m^3 (3 to 4 lb/ft^3), both small-cell hexagonal and overexpanded. Recently, the higher specific performance of aluminum honeycomb has been attractive in the America's Cup and large offshore racing multihulls (such as the *Playstation*, Fig. 3), but there are concerns over the longevity of the core when combined with carbon skins due to electrolytic corrosion in a marine environment.

Technique Characteristics

The manufacturing techniques for the different components of a one-off or low-production yacht vary significantly to suit the requirements of each part of the structure. Manufacturing methods are generally highly labor-intensive, without extensive automation. Building conditions in most boatyards are much less well controlled than typical aerospace clean rooms. Approaches range from ambient or low-temperature cure wet lay-up, often using a "wet-out" machine, to autoclaved prepregs. The development of specialized materials, particularly lower-temperature cure resins with long out-life and low-temperature cure prepregs, has been a significant factor in the development of current manufacturing techniques. Autoclaves or vacuum bagging techniques are widely used to ensure good laminate consolidation and to minimize excess resin and hence, weight.

Hulls and decks are nearly always manufactured from either prepreg or wet preg materials. The latter is a development of traditional hand, wet lay-up techniques, but with a resin developed to have extended gelation time at room temperature. The reinforcements are passed through an on-site wet-out/impregnation machine, then taken directly from the machine and laid into the mold. This gives the builder the versatility of curing at low elevated temperatures (typically 50 °C, or 120 °F), the ability to control and vary resin content on-site, very good draping characteristics, and extended working time (typically 6 to 48 h).

The other major method widely used is based on low-temperature prepregs, which typically cure at 75 to 120 °C (170 to 250 °F). Prepreg-based processes (Fig. 8) provide the convenience of very clean working conditions and the luxury of long open times for the resin (typically 20 to 40 days), thus allowing smaller laminating teams. Fiber volume fractions and overall weight of the structure are also very well controlled, but are predetermined off-site when the prepreg is manufactured. This approach requires more care in tooling design and construction to ensure that the tooling will maintain adequate dimensional stability at the elevated curing temperatures. In addition to the higher cure temperatures, close management of the cure cycle is also required. Significant planning is required to order suitable materials ahead of time, particularly if particular volume fraction materials are required to meet racing-class rule constraints. Unlike wet lay-up materials, prepregs do not drape, therefore requiring careful cutting and placement to avoid overlaps. Debulking is also commonly required during the lamination process. These factors usu-

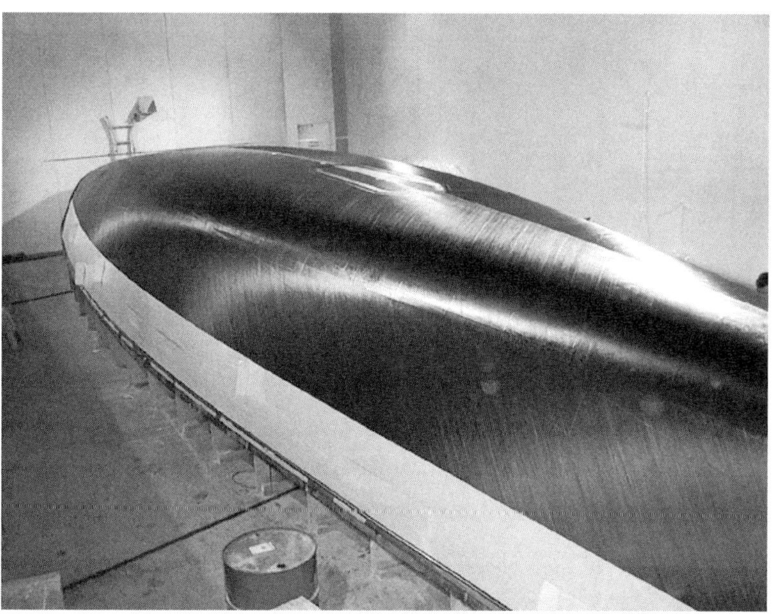

Fig. 8 Prepreg hull on male mold prior to consolidation

ally result in greater labor costs and higher use of materials, such as vacuum bagging consumables.

The requirements of tooling for the hull and decks of one-off or low-production vessels are very different from those for large-production components. Low cost is the primary constraint, long-term tooling durability is not a major issue, and the cycle time for laminating the component is not as critical as for high-production levels. The most cost-effective tooling for a hull or deck shell is often a mold constructed from particle board, timber stringers, plywood, and timber framing, using fabrication techniques reminiscent of traditional wooden boatbuilding. Male molds are commonly used for hulls, while female molds are generally used for decks. These types of molds are adequate for low-temperature cure; for higher-temperature prepregs, the selection of mold materials and fabrication techniques requires more care to ensure stability of the tooling at higher temperatures.

Spars are usually manufactured from prepreg materials and often autoclaved in custom-built, long autoclaves, typically at temperatures of 120 °C (250 °F) and pressures of 3 to 5 bar (300 to 500 kPa). The tooling requirements are quite different than for a hull or deck. If the structure is being autoclave-cured, the thermal stability of the tooling is critical, often leading to the use of carbon/epoxy for construction of the molds. Molds are often designed so that different-sized masts can be constructed from the same mold by using only part of the length or depth of the tool. The stock (shaft) of the rudder is also normally a single-skinned hollow section, so techniques similar to mast manufacture are often used. Other processes used for the rudder and minor components, such as spinnaker poles, booms, stanchions, tillers, steering wheels, winch driveshafts, and tubes for use internally, include resin infusion, closed mold with internal bladder, filament winding, and tube rolling. (Separate articles in this Section provide more information about these processes.)

Hulls and Decks. The following sections discuss tooling, laminating practice, curing, mold removal, and quality control for manufacturing hulls and decks using composites.

Tooling. The aim of the tooling for hull and decks is to build a low-cost, accurate tool that can withstand curing temperatures with little or no distortion and give a clean release to the molding. Tooling cost is very important, because it typically has to be amortized over very short production runs of one to twelve boats. The hull and deck can be built successfully in either a male or female mold; however, hull shells are commonly built on a male plug to achieve greater fairness of the hull shape and to minimize tooling costs. A well-faired male mold used with a well-prepared core can produce an immaculate paint job with an average of less than 0.5 mm (0.02 in.) of lightweight fairing compound, far lighter than most gel coats or similar products.

Male molds are generally constructed using techniques that have evolved from traditional wooden boatbuilding. Timber frames are constructed to define the section shape at regular intervals or stations. Each frame is often cut and shaped accurately as two half-frames alongside each other, which are then joined at the centerline of the boat to produce a totally symmetrical shape. Wooden bracing is then used to restrain the frames in their correct orientation and spacing. Accurate datum points are critical to enable the builder to constantly reference back to a known centerline, station, or waterline to ensure accuracy of the build. Not only does a one-off vessel need to be perfectly symmetrical for performance reasons, but many such vessels are subject to rating rules, such as the America's Cup, where the hull shape is measured to the millimeter.

A variety of wood-based materials are used for cladding of the mold. Sheet particleboard or plywood can be used for flat or single-curvature surfaces. Compound curves, such as on a female deck mold, will normally be either planked with two layers of diagonally orientated plywood, or strip-planked with cedar or similar straight-grained workable timber. In the case of molds that will be subjected to prepreg curing temperatures, it is imperative that cracks do not appear in the mold during the cure cycle, causing loss of vacuum integrity. For these molds, the sheet material will often be scarfed rather than joined with a butt join, and all timberwork (framing and cladding) will be sealed on both sides with a high-temperature resin. Once completely clad, the mold is sheathed with one to two layers of 200 to 300 g/m^2 (0.7 to 1.0 oz/ft^2) boat cloth (fine plain-weave E-glass cloth). The mold is then faired and painted prior to application of a release agent. Often a high-gloss surface is not required; as long as the surface is fair, even a non-gloss surface sanded with 120 grit can be perfectly adequate to get a release.

The male mold can be used to build the boat or as just the pattern to mold a female fiberglass or carbon-fiber tool. Female molds are used for some prepreg constructed hull and deck shells, where the increased cost is offset by advantages of weight savings, dimensional stability, and vacuum integrity during the high-temperature cure cycle. The release agent is applied to the mold surface just before the job commences, to reduce contamination risks.

Laminating of hull and decks is usually done manually by a team of laminators working from scaffolding above and alongside the mold (Fig. 9). Careful preparation and planning is the key to achieving a high-quality result, with each piece of reinforcement laid onto the mold in the correct orientation and position relative to adjoining layers. Wet lay-up materials have a limited working life, and prepregs need to be removed from refrigeration ahead of time in order to reach ambient temperature.

For both prepreg and wet preg laminates, the first layer is often a peel ply, either prepreg or dry fabric saturated with a controlled amount of resin through an on-site impregnator, commonly known as a wet-out machine (Fig. 10). These

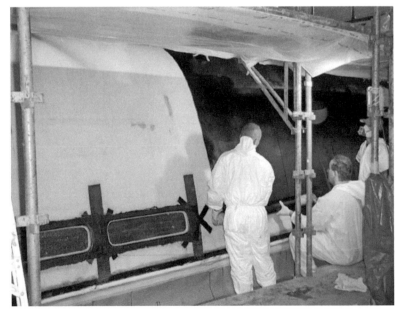

Fig. 9 Laminating a male molded hull

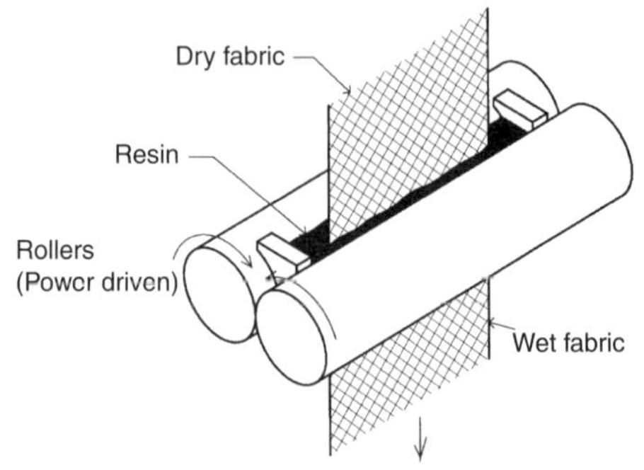

Fig. 10 Schematic of impregnator/wet-out machine

enable accurate control of fiber-resin ratios with wet resin systems. The dry fiber is saturated as it is pulled through the tight tolerance gap between two drive rollers, which contain a pool of catalyzed resin.

The rolls of reinforcement and resin are rolled out and initially compacted by hand, using small rollers and a rubber "squeegee" tool, then the edges trimmed. Width and length are constrained by handling considerations related to the weight of the impregnated roll. Rolls of up to 50 linear meters (165 ft) of unidirectional tape 200 to 300 g/m^2 (0.7 to 1.0 oz/ft^2) and 300 to 500 mm (12 to 20 in.) wide are typical. For wider broadgoods (1200 to 1500 mm, or 47 to 59 in., wide) and heavier weights (600 to 1200 g/m^2, or 2.0 to 4.0 oz/ft^2), lengths are restricted to approximately 10 linear meters (33 ft).

A hull shell will usually be laid up with full-length runs of unidirectional or cloth (0°, parallel with centerline or waterline), or off-axis transverse drops, with the only cutting and lapping necessary at the gunwale (sheer) and centerline. Decks often take much more careful detailing to cut, fit, and lap layers of reinforcement (often cloth rather than unidirectionals) into the corners of a mold.

Fitting sheets of core, whether structural foam or honeycomb, is a relatively straightforward process, typically performed by vacuuming the core down onto a predetermined amount of wet epoxy slurry or a prepreg glue film. A form of strapping or ties is often required for plain sheet foam or honeycomb that is bent around a male mold to hold it in place while the vacuum bag is sealed down and evacuated. Using female molds can provide an advantage, because the sheets will bend and can naturally lock themselves in place. Unlike typical production boat manufacturing, contoured, or scrimmed and cut, foam is rarely used for one-off vessels, because of reduced core mechanical properties and the addition of significant weight in the form of core adhesive. Once the core has been carefully faired with long sanding boards to remove any undulations, it is then rebated for any laps or thickness buildups for localized reinforcing in the next skin. Then the final laminate is applied and again, the entire assembly is bagged and cooked. The final cook may often be of longer duration to give all the laminates their full postcure, whereas on previous cures, it may have only been partial to preserve the mold.

Placing the vacuum bagging materials on a 80 to 250 m^2 (860 to 2690 ft^2) hull shell can take many hours. Layers of peel ply, release films, and breather/bleeder felts need to be carefully cut and fitted prior to the bagging material itself, which is usually a giant blown nylon or polythene vacuum bag.

Curing. The first stage of the curing cycle is to evacuate the air from the vacuum bag. This is, again, a combined effort from a team of workers to ensure that the bag is positioned correctly as it clamps down upon the laminate and vacuum stack. Without care at this stage, excessive wrinkling and small bridges or spans of vacuum bag across the internal radii of a deck mold can cause wrinkles and voids in the corners in the actual laminate.

An oven is erected around the mold, or the entire assembly moved into an existing oven. Ovens typically consist of thin alloy or plywood panels with a polystyrene core for insulation, or simply a polythene bag with fiberglass batts laid over for insulation. Heat is generated by gas furnaces, electricity, or steam. Requirements of a good oven are quick heating of the tool and air space and very even temperature dispersion. Quick ramp rates are essential for prepregs that may require ramp rates greater than 150 °C (270 °F) per hour. These can lead to high energy-input requirements and a number of fans and ducting when dealing with large structures, such as the hull shells.

Ovens will generally contain 12 or more movable thermocouples that can be attached to the vacuum bag or inserted into the laminate to check for even temperature distributions. Test "cooks" involving only the mold are often used to ensure that the oven will reach the desired temperature (typically 90 to 120 °C, or 195 to 250 °F) within the ramp rates required, and also that all parts of the mold heat evenly. This is particularly important for hull shells, where the centerline of an inverted hull shell may reach excessively high temperatures while 4 m (13 ft) lower in the oven the gunwale only reaches 70 °C (160 °F). Fans are used to circulate air into problem areas. If the tool entraps large pockets of cooler air, these can act as insulation, making it impossible to heat the surrounding air enough to achieve the desired ramp rate. Similarly, a thick tool with significant thermal mass can also cause heating problems.

Often, vacuum pressure monitoring equipment may be necessary to ensure that a bag does not leak during the cook. For a low temperature cook for wet preg boats (40 to 70 °C, or 105 to 160 °F), it is possible to enter the oven for brief periods to audibly check and make quick repairs to a bag; for the higher-temperature cooks, this is rarely an option, so everything must be correct and double-checked before the cook is started.

Removal from Mold and Fitting of Internal Structure. Prior to release from the tool, a thin layer of low-density, filled fairing compound is applied to the cured outer skin. Where weight is critical, care is taken to only fill the hollows, rather than cover the entire surface. The manual process of sanding, refilling, and resanding is time-consuming, hard labor, but necessary to achieve a smooth fair surface suitable for a high-gloss paint finish.

Throughout the process, consideration is given to releasing the item from the mold by ensuring that the molding has sufficient lifting points to raise it clear of the mold. This process can also be done by removing the mold from the molding using a crane with slings to lift and rotate both the mold and molding and then lifting the mold from the structure.

The molded shell structure (especially the hull) is relatively flexible without any internal framing, so it must then be braced, leveled, plumbed, and set up to the exact same beam widths as it was on the mold. Keel floors are then fitted and bonded in their correct positions. These can be manufactured in a variety of ways, from female molding keel floors and post-fitting, to hand laying them up in place over foam and timber formers. Timber may often be used in the region of the keel floors and mast step and then encapsulated in glass. In the case of the mast step, it will be used in an end grain orientation for its capacity to withstand the high compression loads. Bulkheads will often be manufactured on a flat table using the same processes as used on the main structures, that is, either prepreg or wet preg laminates vacuum consolidated and cooked on either side of a core. These will be accurately fitted and then secondary bonded in place. Secondary bonding will generally involve carbon or E-glass double-bias tapes hand-laminated in place.

Quality control is a crucial part of the laminating process. A mistake made in the laminating, or inadequate control of laminating processes and curing processes that lead to material not consolidating or curing correctly, can mean the scrapping of many costly materials, project time, and man hours. Scantling authorities often want to quantify the laminating premises and may also require the production of specimens before and during lamination for mechanical testing. When the laminating starts, the quality controls and procedures need to be well defined and understood by the laminating team. This includes prior testing of compatibility of release systems and resins. During the lamination, the humidity is monitored and controlled, if possible. All rolls of prepreg are recorded as used, so that traceability, weight, and waste control can be tracked.

Quality control plays a very important role in not only making sure that all material conforms as far as curing properly and meets established weight or quantity parameters, but also in ensuring that by having well-formatted plans and procedures accompanied with check lists, the laminating team can operate together efficiently. On completion of the laminate, this enables the builder to be sure that the team of workers placed all the required layers in the laminate, with the correct proportion of resin, in their correct positions and orientations.

Masts. Mast tools (Fig. 11) are typically constructed from a high degree of unidirectional fibers for length stability, and may often be constructed from four quadrants that bolt together to form the complete section, allowing flat sections to be added to the mold to increase the size of the section.

Conventional prepreg application processes need to be modified to cope with building a mast tube. Typically, the female tooling is in two parts, and a considerable number of layers need to be applied. In some areas, well over one hundred plies at varying angles are required to distribute local stress. Because of differential thermal properties of the tool (often low-cost glass composite) and the component and extreme dimensions (up to 50 m, or 165 ft, long), it is desirable to cure the laminate in one operation to avoid prerelease or demolding. This requires a long out-time prepreg, because the lay-up process can take a number of weeks, as well as careful intermediate debulk stages and critical control of the cure cycle to avoid potential excess exotherm of thick sections and to ensure adequate flow and consolidation.

While shorter off-axis plies can be precut, the longitudinal layers are taken directly from the roll in situ. Relatively low-tack prepregs are used, with local hot air flow required to aid drapability. Some hand consolidation with small rollers is necessary to avoid bridging across internal radii (Fig. 12). A stack of perforated release film and breathers intended for minimum bleed is applied, and a vacuum pulled. The complete tool is slid on rollers into the autoclave, typically 800 to 1000 mm (30 to 40 in.) in diameter, but up to 50 m (165 ft) long.

Cure is at 2 to 3 bar (200 to 300 kPa), and generally follows a slow, controlled ramp, with dwell periods to even out temperature. Maximum cure temperatures are in the order of 120 to 130 °C (250 to 265 °F). The two C-shaped sections are fitted internally with rigging, pulleys, and other components, such as instrumentation wiring, before being joined with adhesive in a single-lap detail on the mast sidewall. Rivets are used to provide clamping pressure for the wet, ambient-temperature cure adhesive.

Many other methods to produce mast tubes have been tested and, in some cases, developed to commercial level for specific size-range products. These include wet lay-up over tapered mandrels, bladder molding of prepregs for small internal sections, and filament winding or braiding for small components. However, for the larger vessels, the two-piece autoclaved approach has proven to be the most successful.

The rig consists of more than a bare tube. Intricate fittings, where rigging terminates and spreaders are used to support the mast column, create challenges for the use of composites. Geometry and high local loads lead to complex stresses, especially in areas subject to bearing loads and thick sections with tight radii of curvature. Construction techniques are very component-related and range from wet lay-up to prepreg autoclave cure and bladder molding.

Appendages. Manufacture of the rudder and the keel use almost all the skills the boatbuilder has to offer. Accurate sectional shape and profile are critical to the handling performance of the yacht. Great care has to be taken by the builder to achieve a shape that is symmetrical, dimensionally correct, and has a well-finished surface. A rudder blade or stock may be almost 4 m (13 ft) long for an America's Cup yacht, making it a challenging task to maintain its symmetry to the nearest millimeter during a 100 °C (210 °F) cure.

Keels come in many configurations, sometimes with a bulb at the base, or just as a straight fin. They can also be completely constructed from lead with an internal steel support frame, or only consist of lead in the lower half or bulb. In this case, the top part or all of the keel fin is typically constructed from either carbon fiber or high-tensile steel materials.

The requirement for accurate dimensional tolerances has lead to the widespread use of computer numerically controlled (CNC) machining for rudder and keel tooling. This is normally produced by machining a male pattern from laminated particle board or foam, with final surface preparation by the builder. Split female molds are then made from this pattern. In the case of a keel bulb and fin foundry, work is required, with tons of molten lead or steel being poured into concrete or sand molds, respectively, with all keel bolts and internal framework in place. The casting will require a great deal of surface finishing to achieve the desired end result; quite often the surface is initially cut back by CNC machining, followed by labor-intensive grinding, sanding, and painting.

Rudders are typically a complicated composite structure. The backbone or rudder stock (Fig. 13) is nearly always a rectangular carbon-fiber section that is built to the maximum dimensions that the diameter of the bearings and the thickness of the blade will allow. This shaft can be manufactured in much the same way as a spar: by laminating the carbon over a foam core. Other approaches include split female molding, using vacuum consolidation or inflatable bladders. Because the wall thickness is critical to both the shape and strength, accurate quality control is necessary to ensure that the correct fiber volumes are achieved. During the curing process, the stock or mold must be clamped into a jig that will stay straight. Localized buildups are then laminated in the region of the upper and lower bearings and machined in a lathe. The alignment of these bearings is crucial for correct operation of the rudder.

The blade is typically manufactured in either a female mold as two halves or hand shaped from a structural foam or Nomex honeycomb. When female molding, once the skins have been laminated, provision is made to accept the stock. The two halves are then glued and clamped about the stock, the remaining volume being filled with

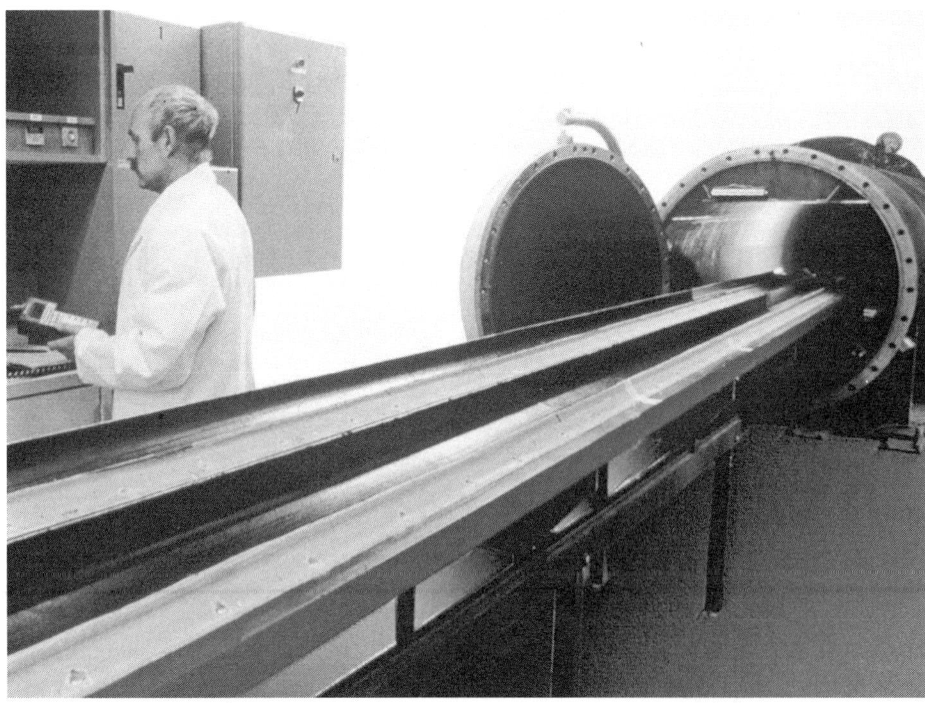

Fig. 11 Mast tooling. Courtesy of Marten Spars

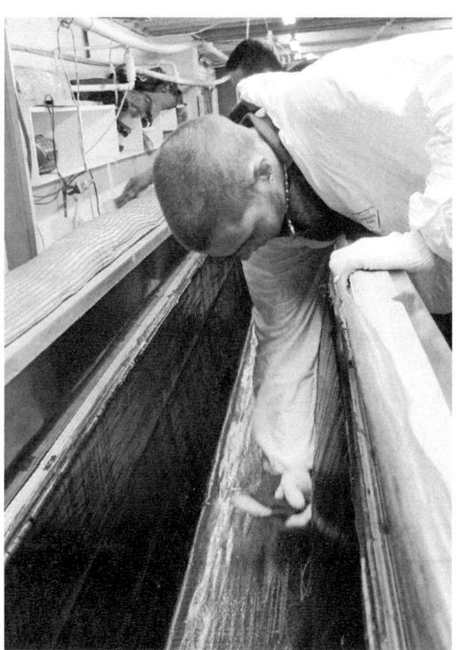

Fig. 12 Laminating a prepreg mast section. Courtesy of Southern Spars

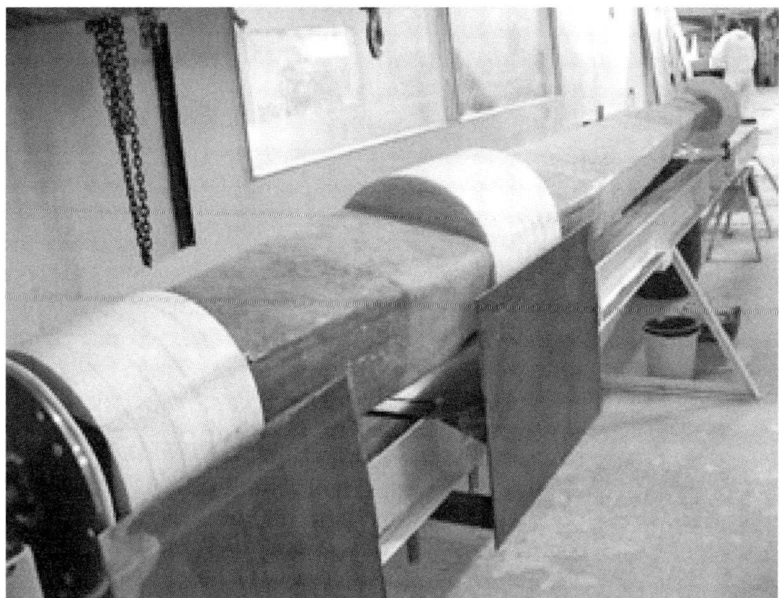

Fig. 13 Rudder stock. Courtesy of Yachting Developments

either structural foam or Nomex. In the case of shaped foam, two halves are typically used to help maintain symmetry about the centerline. The blank is bonded to the back of the stock, along with the nosepiece, and then the entire blade is laminated with a thin skin of carbon fiber. This is vacuum-consolidated and cured while clamped straight, to maintain an accurate shape. In both cases, the final manufacturing stages involve manual fairing and painting to achieve the correct shape with a high-quality surface finish. Accurate templates are used to check the sectional shape during the finishing processes.

Outlook

Custom, one-off construction will continue to be a part of the marine market. The opportunity to create a unique, tailored solution for the discerning client will always be attractive, particularly where cost is not necessarily the only criterion, be it a race boat with improved performance or a luxury cruising yacht designed to meet the specific requirements of the owner. In volume terms, one-off construction will always be small relative to the female molded production output, but will continue to be the incubator for development of new technologies. The trickle-down effect is well proven, with the mass market now accepting of sandwich construction and experimenting with resin infusion and wet-preg epoxy techniques.

In the near future, construction using prepreg systems is likely to increase as new lower-temperature cure cycles are developed to enable low-cost, stable, one-off tooling. Structural design tools will be refined, with more confidence in finite-element techniques as the definition of applied loads is improved. This may lead to more complex structural arrangements and details that are better suited to prepreg techniques, due to extended working time and the ability to apply selective unidirectional tapes in line with defined load paths. Environmental concerns over solvents and the health aspects of working with wet resins will also be a driver toward prepregs.

Despite reductions in the price of carbon as more high-volume, nonaerospace commercial applications become available, the likelihood is that the construction will still be dominated by E-glass. The full potential of this material is yet to be realized, and developments in forms that allow reduced resin content and higher properties along with improved design and building processes will see continued improvements in the performance of simple E-glass structures. Carbon and other advanced fibers will find greater acceptance in specific areas of the vessel, such as masts and appendages, where the higher cost can be justified due to significant weight savings.

REFERENCES

1. "The Volvo Ocean 60 Rule 2000," Volvo Event Management UK Ltd, 2000
2. "International America's Cup Class Rule 1995," Royal New Zealand Yacht Squadron and New York Yacht Club, 1995
3. "Guide for Building and Classing Offshore Racing Yachts," American Bureau of Shipping, 1994
4. "Rules for Classification of High Speed and Light Craft," Det Norske Veritas Classification AS, 1997
5. "Classification of Special Service Craft," Lloyds, 1996
6. "Rules for Classification and Construction, 1—Ship Technology, Part 3—Pleasure Craft," Lloyd Germanischer, 1996
7. "Boat and Ship Design and Construction," Australian Standard 4132.3 and 4132.1, 1993

Prepreg and Ply Cutting

Joe Lautner, Gerber Technology Inc.

MANUFACTURING PROCESSES for advanced composites share common attributes. Fibers and resins are engineered, and raw materials are cut, shaped, and cured to meet the performance requirements of the end products. As composite materials have evolved since the 1950s, so have the methods and practices used to manufacture and cut these materials. Automated cutting systems that can manage data efficiently and are compatible with computer-aided design (CAD) systems help to reduce labor requirements and work-in-progress (WIP) costs, reduce waste of costly materials, and increase the quality of composite parts.

This article briefly reviews the history of prepreg and ply cutting technologies as well as outlines the options available for creating the necessary data and for nesting, cutting, and kitting the plies. The article also discusses the ways these steps influence the workflow for various applications.

History of Composites Ply Cutting

Manufacturers first used fiberglass-reinforced plastics and epoxy resins during the 1950s to produce boat hulls and fishing poles. Makers of boats employed straight knives, scissors, or hand-held motorized rotary blades to cut dry, woven and nonwoven fiberglass (Fig. 1). Once cut, the fiberglass was then laid up by hand and "painted" with resin.

The 1970s gave birth to "advanced" composites, led by the development or refinement of materials such as carbon and aramid fibers and advanced matrix (resin) materials and spurred by the demand for lightweight, high-performance military aircraft. Manufacturers were required to cut these materials very accurately, according to the orientation of their innate fibers (Fig. 2). Once again, they turned to hand-held straightedge knives—using them to trace around aluminum templates placed on the composite material (Fig. 3). The process was slow, inaccurate, ergonomically incorrect, and inherently wasteful.

Not only was it necessary for hand cutters to cut each ply according to the specific orientation of the fiber, but to complicate the process even further, they were required to lay each ply in the correct order in the tool. Thus, hand cutters began to cut the materials in the order in which they would later be laminated (Fig. 4).

The first tools available to the industry that automated the nesting process were developed by Hughes Aircraft. ("Marking," "marker making," and "nesting" are terms used to refer to the process of efficiently marking ply shapes on material to maximize material use.)

During this time, automation providers introduced tools for fast and efficient nesting and cutting of apparel fabric, which, at that time, cost \$1 to \$3 per yard. How much could these tools save manufacturers in an industry where material costs were as high as \$300 per yard? The answer is hundreds of thousands of dollars.

The first automated nested and cutting systems for composites manufacture were sold to large aerospace companies at a cost per installation of approximately \$750,000; the costs were funded in part by government contracts. Shortly thereafter, manufacturers introduced ultrasonic cutting systems, which delivered cleaner cuts and higher tolerances at a cost of \$1 to \$2 million per installation.

Creating the Data

In a large composites manufacturing facility, cutting is merely one component in the overall process. Cutting personnel receive the material to cut and the data to define the cutting. After cutting, the pieces are usually labeled and removed. Efficiencies can be improved by improving the nesting, labeling, and unloading processes.

In order for composite parts to be manufactured successfully, they must mesh precisely when the final item is assembled. The composite part is usually designed using a CAD system. Computer-aided design data usually encompasses:

- A three-dimensional definition of the lay-up tool or a surface of the finished part

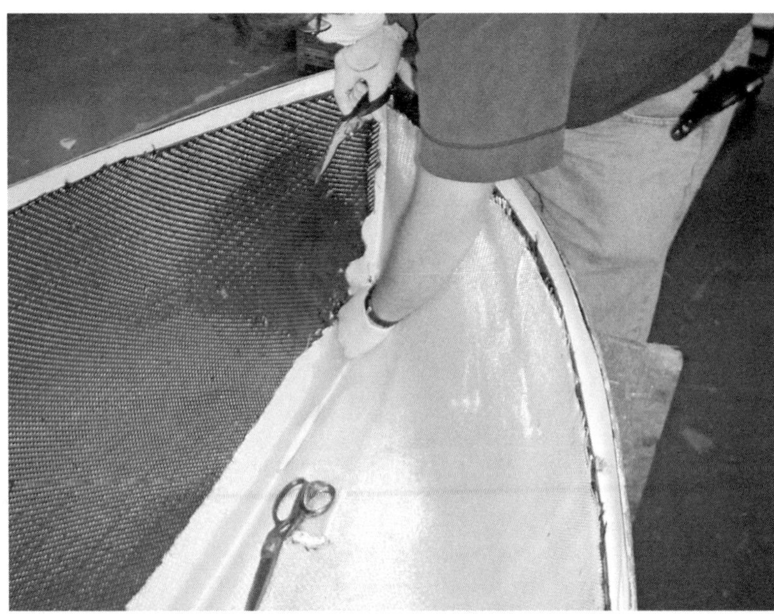

Fig. 1 Hand cutting of fabric

- A flat pattern for cutting that will result in the ply being the correct shape when laid on a curved tool (see Fig. 2 in the article "Manual Prepreg Lay-Up" in this Section)
- Rules or instructions indicating the precise location of each ply on the tool as the part is being assembled

If any of these three conditions is not precisely managed, finished parts will be flawed. Software packages, such as FiberSim (Vistagy Inc.), model the behavior of the material as it is draped on the tool. The bending and draping behavior is taken into account when the flat patterns are defined for cutting. Using such modeling approaches can result in plies that are matched to the lay-up sequence and meet tight tolerances (e.g., 0.40 mm, or 0.015 in.).

Nesting the Pieces

Material is one of the most costly components in composites manufacturing. Advanced composite material is expensive to produce. In addition, strict environmental regulations make the disposal of many epoxy resins as costly as the production of the actual material.

Advanced nesting of the entire table, rather than individual kits placed end to end, has yielded an 18% improvement in material use (Ref 1). Such improvements in use have significantly reduced the amount of raw material required and the amount of scrap material yielded (Fig. 4).

Overhead laser projectors can also improve material use by providing a preview of pieces to be cut. It is often helpful to view the cutting patterns while positioning material on the table, because, many times, a variance of only a few inches can mean the difference between complete and incomplete kits.

Kitting

Kitting is the process of assembling cut plies in the order in which they will be placed on tools to form laminates. When dealing with simple kits, operators can recognize and extract plies from the cutting table in the correct order. As kits become more complicated, operators must use maps to determine the order in which plies should be collected. Full table nesting presents one major problem—unloading cut parts becomes a very complicated and time-consuming task.

Technology has once again addressed this problem. Today, laser projectors guide operators in the proper order of removal of cut pieces. A single laser projector that meets U.S. Food and Drug Administration Center for Devices and Radiological Health (CDRH) class II laser safety regulations can cover an entire 15 m (48 ft) table. A hands-free remote control on the projector automatically advances the display to the next ply when the correct ply has been removed. This feature helps ensure that pieces are removed in the correct order for kitting (Ref 2).

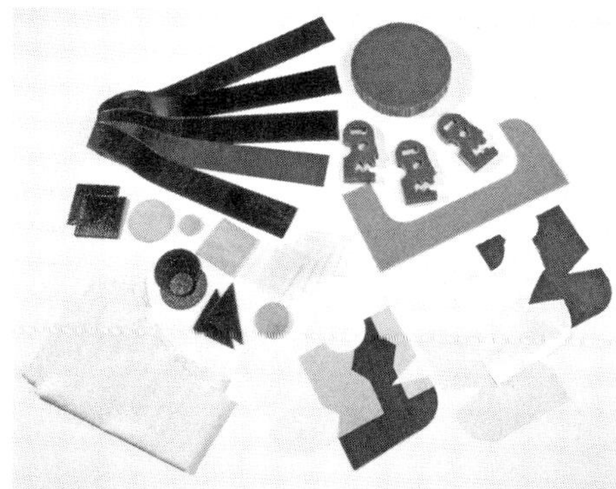

Fig. 2 Examples of cut shapes

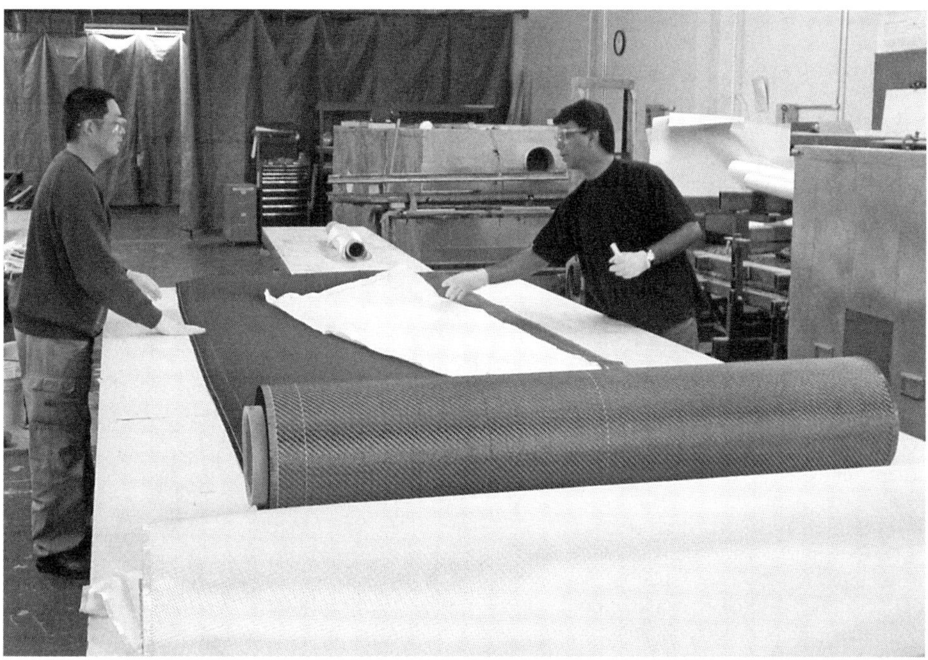

Fig. 3 Hand marking of plies

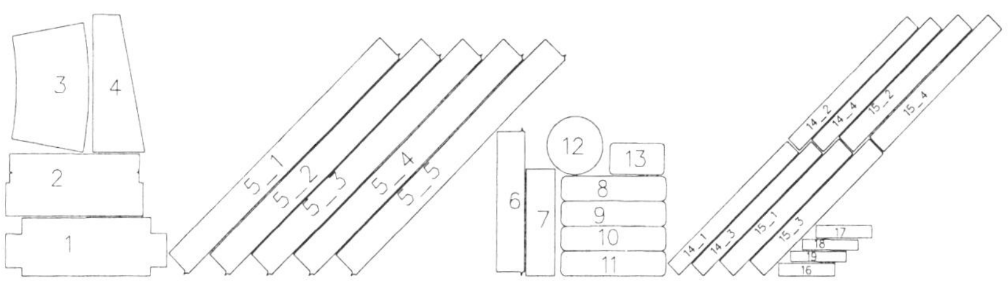

Nesting in kit order

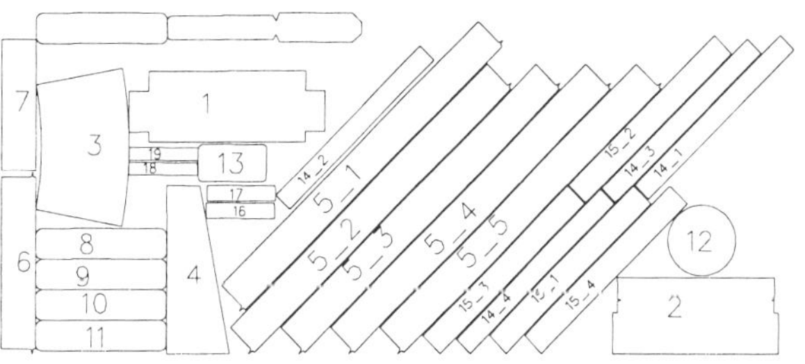

Nesting for material efficiency

Fig. 4 Nesting

Cutting

There are several options available to cut plies. When aerospace firms implemented automated cutting in the 1980s, reciprocating blade, multiply, "static" (meaning non-conveyorized cutting surfaces), and ultrasonic cutting systems were the only available technologies.

Manufacturers created work orders to meet their lengthy production schedules. For example, they typically cut and kit materials a month in advance to accommodate their production requirements. The steps in the process were:

1. Pull materials from the freezer.
2. Spread several layers of material on cutting surface.
3. Cut prenested plies in kit order.
4. Remove cut plies for off-line kitting and bagging.
5. Return kits to freezer.
6. Retrieve kits when ready to lay-up.

Because the technology was developed to cut many layers slowly, the equipment was only cost-effective when cutting multiple layers. However, this process increased WIP costs and included many "non-value-added" steps. It also did little to maximize material use. Parts from existing kits were often "borrowed" to complete orders, thereby leaving kits incomplete. Cut materials often went unused and were discarded when their shelf life was depleted.

This process violated many of today's current manufacturing concepts, such as just-in-time (JIT), cellular, and lean manufacturing principles. Existing automated companies were forced to change the way they cut and kit.

Simpler, less expensive, and faster single-ply static cutting systems were introduced in the 1990s. These new systems enabled manufacturers to cut material on demand, more accurately, with less waste, and with improved edge quality. This new cutting method streamlined the entire process. Table 1 compares the characteristics of different cutting methods.

Today, many composites fabricators can process work orders on a shift-by-shift basis, cutting what they need when they need it. This is what the process may look like today:

1. Generate daily work orders.
2. Pull material from the freezer, as needed.
3. Create efficient nests to meet daily work orders.
4. Cut material quickly.
5. Remove material from the table in the order it is to be kitted, and deliver it to the lay-up personnel.

This process satisfies most needs. However, there are some applications that require different approaches. For higher-volume applications, for example, interior floor and wall panels for major commercial airline companies, multiple-ply cutting is required to meet the high volumes.

In some cases, up to twenty layers of prepreg or woven carbon or up to 75 mm (3 in.) of honeycomb core are cut on a conveyorized reciprocating blade cutter and kitted off-line. The kits are then delivered directly to the crush core panel presses for fabrication in a JIT or lean manufacturing environment.

In other cases, cutting personnel may deliver parts to several lay-up areas. It may, therefore, be necessary to cut multiple plies of material, kit them off-line, and store them in freezers. In such cases, a conveyorized, or single-ply cutter, may be appropriate.

Fundamental differences exist between conveyorized and static cutting systems that should be considered when evaluating cutting systems.

Fundamentals of static single-ply cutting (Fig. 5) include:

- Allows manufacturers to label part numbers on each ply efficiently
- Material is either manually or automatically pulled onto the table.
- Pieces are picked off the table and assembled into kit order.
- Allows greater flexibility when changing materials often
- In most cases, is the best solution for JIT, lean, and cellular manufacturing
- Is a lower-cost technology
- Is available in a variety of lengths to satisfy requirements and floor constraints
- Delivers the best edge quality

Fundamentals of conveyorized single-ply cutting (Fig. 6) include:

- Allows manufacturers to label part numbers on each ply efficiently
- Reduces material handling, because material is automatically fed onto the table
- Material changes are more time-consuming than with static cutters.
- Parts are removed from the table in the order in which they were cut.
- If nesting plies for efficiency, a separate kitting station may be required. This means additional labor costs.
- Can accomplish higher production rates in higher-volume requirements with fewer product mixes
- If plies are nested in kit order, parts can be kitted as they are removed; however, material efficiencies will drop.
- Maximizes floor space
- Delivers best edge quality

Fundamentals of conveyorized multiple-ply cutting (Fig. 7) include:

- Piece identification requires an additional step.

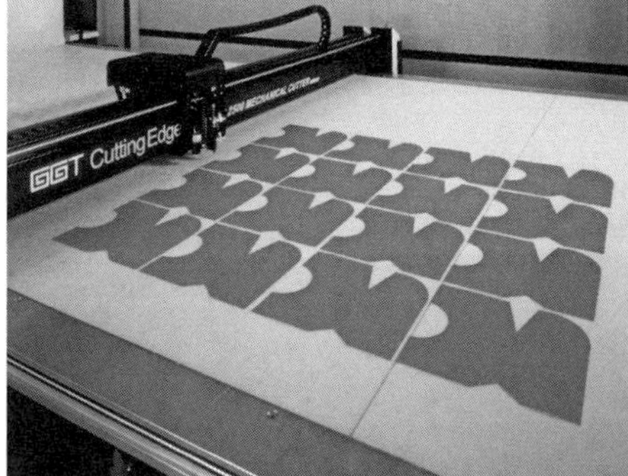

Fig. 5 Static single-ply cutting

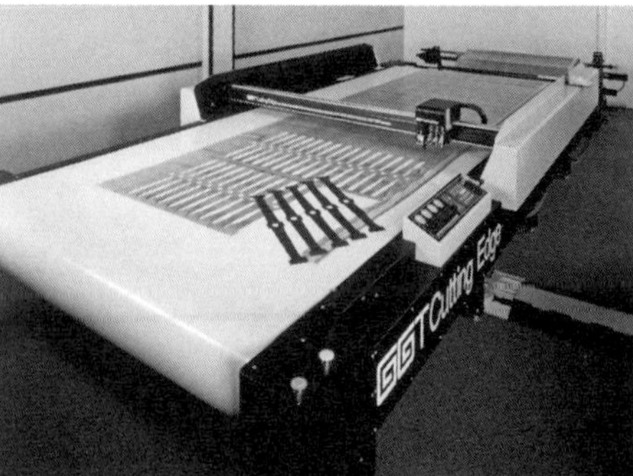

Fig. 6 Conveyorized single-ply cutting

Table 1 Characteristics of prepreg and ply cutting methods

Method	Capital cost	Advantages	Disadvantages	Data required
Hand cutting using templates	Low	Uncomplicated, low maintenance	Slow and inaccurate Ergonomically undesirable Requires the creation, maintenance, and storage of templates	Patterns reverse-engineered off of tooling
Automated reciprocating blade	Moderate to high	Multiple-ply cutting for higher volumes, dry aramids	Typically not suitable for lean, just-in-time (JIT), or cellular manufacturing Not suitable for low volumes Involves higher consumable costs and maintenance	Computer numerically controlled (CNC) data
Automated ultrasonic	Moderate to high	See above	Maintenance and consumables cost not justifiable for single ply cutting.	CNC data
Drag knife/ wheel cutter	Moderate	Best option for modern, lean, JIT, and cellular manufacturing	...	...
Dies	Moderate	Suitable for multiply cutting; accurate.	Lacks flexibility Requires the creation, maintenance, and storage of templates.	Typically CNC data

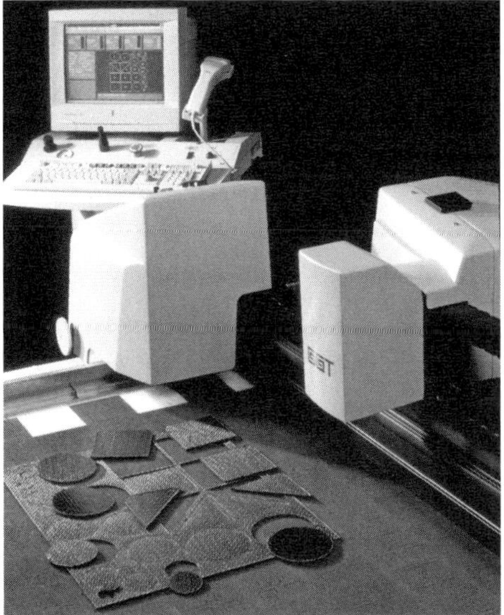

Fig. 7 Conveyorized multiple-ply cutting

- Off-line kitting is, for the most part, mandatory.
- Efficient only if cutting multiple plies
- Suited for high-volume cutting
- May require additional floor space to spread materials

Labeling

There are four primary ways to label cut plies when using an automated cutter (alphanumeric characters and bar coding are options):

- Inkjet part numbers directly on the plastic backing film
- Inkjet-printed, pressure-sensitive labels automatically applied to the cut plies
- Cutter-mounted pen
- Inkjet pressure-sensitive labels manually placed after cutting. (The laser projector system supports a wireless labeler worn on the belt of the cutter operator. When the correct piece is removed from the cutter, this device prints a label for the operator to adhere to the cut part.)

The labeling process typically uses existing label data and requires no new data generation. Labeling usually occurs on the cutter. Occasionally, if the cut pieces are smaller than the labels, an automatic labeler may cause small pieces to stick together. These challenges are easily addressed by an automation solution.

The laser projection system can also guide the sorting of partial kits by pointing to locations on sorting tables, located near the cutters, for partial kits unloaded from the cutter. This also speeds the cutter unloading process (Ref 1).

REFERENCES

1. A.E. Trudeau and S. Blake, *KitGuide: Putting Composite Plies In Lay-Up Order While Still on an N/C Cutter*, American Helicopter Society, 1998
2. S. Blake,"Laser Guidance for Hand Laid Composites: Past, Present, and Future," EM97-112, Composites '97, Society of Manufacturing Engineers, 1997

SELECTED REFERENCES

- B.A. Strong, *Fundamentals of Composite Manufacturing: Materials, Methods, and Applications*, Society of Manufacturing Engineers, 1989
- A.C. Marshall, *Composite Basics*, 4th ed., Marshall Consulting, 1994

Manual Prepreg Lay-Up

Andrew Mills, Composites Manufacturing Research Centre, Cranfield University, United Kingdom

WHEN THE FIRST PRODUCTION of carbon fiber occurred in the late 1960s, it was realized that very lightweight layers of nonwoven tape would be required to fabricate thin shell and blade components, the first targets for the new lightweight material. Without weaving, the fibers could not be handled once taken off a reel. Another limitation was that the long-established technology of wetting woven fabrics with liquid resins layer by layer was not feasible for thin-layer, lightweight structures, since at the optimal fiber proportion (60% by volume), distribution of the resin had to be accurately controlled. Another complication for the glass fabric, wet lay-up technology was its inability to provide laminated components with tightly packed, accurately aligned fibers. The "runniness" of liquid wet lay-up resins cannot hold fibers where placed by laminator tools.

To provide a stable material with combined resin in layers of typically 0.13 mm (0.005 in.) thickness, prepreg technology was developed by the 3M Company in the United States at the request of Rolls Royce Engines in the United Kingdom, which had started to produce carbon fiber in-house. Automation of fiber and resin combination provided material with near-straight fibers and consistent resin content in a form that had a tackiness suited to laying up multiple layers of material in complex-shape tools.

By 2000, a vast range of prepregs with different fiber types, fabrics, tape styles, resin types, and thicknesses became available, enabling the manufacture of most lightweight structures by hand lay-up. Prepreg hand lay-up has been an exceptionally successful technology.

The process requires very low investment but is a labor-cost-intensive approach. It is best suited to components with either annual production-materials consumption of less than approximately 1 tonne (2200 lb) or curvature that prevents any form of automated lay-up. It utilizes the extreme dexterity of human hands in positioning and conforming prepreg to double-curvature surfaces and tool details such as flanges, ribs, holes, and blades.

Prepreg lamination has become established as a respected craft of the modern age. Because of its versatility and reliability, almost all performance vehicles, racing cars, boats, planes, and spacecraft applications of composites depend on the prepreg hand lay-up process. Today, despite many research attempts, the hand lay-up of prepreg is the most cost-effective, highest quality approach to the manufacture of many large or small components.

Technique Characteristics and Applications

Prepreg Form. The two most common prepreg forms are unidirectional tape and woven fabric. Different lay-up techniques are required for each form.

For manufacturing-cost reasons, woven-fabric prepregs are used wherever possible despite the considerably lower laminate stiffness and strength achieved with these prepregs. The lower stiffness and strength result from crimp in the fiber tows as the weft yarns cross the warps. This bends the tows during fabric manufacture, and processing cannot recover their straightness. Also, at each yarn crossover, a fiber-free space is created that becomes filled with resin; hence the fiber volume fraction of woven laminates varies from 50% for heavy (24K and above) to 58% for near-unidirectional woven fabrics having 90 to 98% of fiber in the weft direction. For unidirectional prepreg with a multidirectional lay-up, the fiber volume fraction ranges from 58 to 63%. Consequently, woven prepreg laminates are both less stiff and strong and are heavier with the higher resin content than unidirectional tape laminates. Woven laminates also provide much greater damage tolerance than unidirectional laminates since the latter have low resistance to delamination crack growth during and after impact.

The lay-up attributes of woven prepregs are:

- Thicker (therefore fewer) layers and faster lay-up rate
- Much higher curvature conformability and hence lower susceptibility to wrinkling
- Greater material width of 1.25 or 1.7 m (4.1 or 5.6 ft) compared to 0.3 or 0.6 m (1 or 2 ft) for tape prepreg. (Tape prepreg is narrow since it has low conformability, and materials waste is high for wide tape.)
- Lay-up rates are therefore approximately 3 to 5 times higher than for unidirectional tape.
- No requirement to butt strip edges since fabrics are wider than the parts
- Less-precise ply orientation is required since the lay-up is less optimized; lay-up can therefore be faster.

Manufacturing disadvantages of woven prepregs are:

- Higher proportion of waste from the wider material
- Higher cost of low-thickness fabric prepreg since the weaving process preceding prepregging is an added cost. Thicker woven prepreg with a fiber areal weight (FAW) of 370 g/m^2 has become standard since the weaving cost is around half that of the conventional 285 g/m^2 fabric. These thick prepregs confer reduced stiffness to the resultant components.

As a result of the manufacturing-cost benefits of woven prepregs, they are used predominantly for hand lay-up, apart from very lightweight-niche applications. Unidirectional tape lay-up is better suited to automated tape layers that can rapidly cut and deposit material, provided the lay-up is flat enough (see the article "Automated Tape Laying" in this Volume). Recently, thicker unidirectional tape prepreg has been qualified for aircraft use so as to increase laminating rate of thick structures. However, the resulting restriction on thickness tailoring prevents the use of thick prepreg in many structures.

The other lay-up characteristics are resin tack and conformability of fabric style. These both determine the difficulty of manipulation of prepreg into tool recesses. For parts with shape complexity, a highly drapable, high-tack resin is preferred to produce a fully consolidated lay-up. For flat or single curvature parts, a less drapable fabric such as plain weave with a low tack (stiff) resin is better suited.

Placement Tolerance. Since hand lay-up is a craft skill using floppy materials, the placement tolerance cannot be specified very closely. The acceptable tolerance differs for woven and tape materials. For tapes, which are much stiffer and applied in strips of typically between 150 and 600 mm (6 and 24 in.), a positional tolerance of ± 1 mm (± 0.04 in.) and a straightness tolerance of $\pm 2°$ can be realistically achieved. For woven prepreg, tolerances of ± 2 mm (± 0.08 in.) for position and ±3° for straightness are realistically achievable.

Application Suitability. A great range of unidirectional and woven prepreg types have been developed to suit diverse applications. The original prepregs were developed for very highly optimized components in aerospace engines, and similar styles of very thin (0.125 mm, or 0.005 in., ply) prepregs are in use today in large volumes. The fighter aircraft and racing car markets use tape and woven prepregs made from very high-cost narrow tow fiber that provides laminate moduli up to 240 GPa (35 × 10^6 psi) for tape and up to 130 GPa (19 × 10^6 psi) for woven fabrics. Resins to suit these high-performance fibers have complex formulations tailored either for toughness or temperature resistance but have similar lay-up attributes to long established low-cost resins. These thin materials naturally have a low hand-deposition rate, but the labor cost represents a small proportion of the overall manufacturing cost. For low-volume production of thin structures, the manufacturing cost is dominated by mold tooling and assembly costs.

Over the past ten years there has been a rapid growth in the use of standard high-strength carbon tapes and fabrics. For performance cars, commercial aircraft, and sporting goods use, two standard prepregs have been established: thick unidirectional tape with a fiber weight of 270 g/m^2 and five-harness satin woven fabric with a fiber weight of 370 g/m^2. The use of prepreg thickness above these levels is not normally considered to be worthwhile, since the lay-up sequences needed to achieve balanced and therefore unwarped laminates result in a low level of thickness optimization.

Non-weight-critical applications such as wind turbines and lower cost sporting goods generally use glass fiber prepreg at as high a thickness as can be readily handled. For this reason thick unidirectional prepregs of up to 500 g/m^2 FAW and woven (and now multiaxial) fabric prepregs of up to 1000 g/m^2 FAW are being produced. The resin-content and void-level specifications are looser for such materials, which, combined with the high fiber weight, enable prepreg manufacture at up to 16 kg/min. The prepreg production cost is therefore very much lower than that for traditional thin prepregs.

Prepreg hand lay-up is well suited to all applications for structures where a stiffness of greater than around 15 GPa (2.2 × 10^6 psi) is required. Below this stiffness, components can be manufactured with far lower labor cost by low fiber volume fraction processes such as chopped fiber, spray up and wet lay-up with heavy (>1 mm, or 0.04 in., thick) fabrics.

The process is also uneconomic for simple-shape components of greater that several millimeters thick where more than one component per week is required. For components that have these factors, automated lay-up becomes attractive. However in lower economies, hand lay-up is still preferred for large, thick simple parts.

Technique Description

The process of lay-up definition through to bagging for resin-curing comprises the following five stages: lay-up definition, ply-kit cutting, lay-up, debulking, and preparation for curing.

Lay-Up Definition. The lay-up of a component is defined by the:

- Overall shape produced by the mold tool curvature
- Thickness in terms of the number of layers over the surface
- Ply outlines (drop offs) if the thickness is varying
- Orientation to suit the load paths

For most lightweight components, the lay-up instructions will be produced from a finite-element-analysis model of the component. The model will have the simulated design limit load introduced to the lay-up. The thickness and ply orientations are then modified until all regions of the component are shown to have less than maximum allowable strain in each ply. For structures with complex shape and/or loading, the specified lay-up is generally quasi-isotropic, meaning that there is an equivalent number of 0, 90, 45, and 135° plies. This is also preferred since it removes any complication of resin shrinkage symmetry. A so-called balanced lay-up will have a balanced or symmetric proportion of fibers at each angle about a midplane. This is critical for unidirectional tape materials but also important for satin and twill-weave fabrics; plain-weave fabrics are immune to lay-up imbalance but have lower drapability and stiffness than the former types.

The next step is to decide the size and shape of each prepreg piece. To minimize the number of pieces, software tools such as FiberSIM (VISTAGY Inc., Waltham, MA) were developed. These are used to assess the tool shape where prepreg pieces are to be positioned and, using data on the material drapability (ability to be sheared to conform to double curvature), indicate whether prepreg pieces are likely to wrinkle. After one or more iterations, a kit of pieces and their orientations are defined (Fig. 1 and 2).

Ply-Kit Cutting. The target for the cutting operation is to minimize waste as much as possible. Purchase cost and disposal cost is extremely high, even for low-glass prepregs. Offcuts can represent a hidden cost, which can result in the manufacturing process being unjustifiable.

Software applications such as FiberSIM have been developed to minimize cutting waste from the prepreg roll. The software is used to match the total kit of plies to the material-roll width and to define the cutter paths.

Users of large quantities of prepreg use an automated device that cuts the material and, in some models, stamps a bar code or number on it to identify the piece from CAD data. Ultrasonic machines (Fig. 3) using a vibrating knife are able to leave the lower surface backing film uncut, which reduces lay-up time during laminating. Manually, the pieces are stacked in order for lay-up. These kits may be sealed and stored in a freezer if a delay is incurred before use.

Lay-Up. The difficult part of the process is applying the reinforcement, any stiffening cores, and attachment inserts to the mold tool so as to confer the inherent stiffness or strength of the fibers to the molded component.

The kit of prepreg pieces is transferred to the mold tool by laminators, who use their fingers and spreading tools to force the tacky, stiff material into the corners of the tool and then smooth it over the flat or gently curving areas. For complex-shape parts such as racing car chassis, the backing film is peeled away progressively to prevent too much of the surface of the pieces from adhering too soon. Hot air blowers are sometimes used locally to soften the prepreg such that it can be conformed into tight recesses. Even with a fully precut kit, the laminator has to trim plies with a blade at the component edges since, for double curvature components, each layer of prepreg is unique in terms of how the plies shear (Fig. 4) (Ref 1). Sandwich structures, which include tapered edge rigid foam or honeycomb core pieces and any attachment inserts, can be placed directly into the lay-up, or placed into the lay-up with uncured film adhesive; in both instances the sandwich structures are cocured with both inner and outer skin. For accurate location of the core and attachment point inserts, the lay-up is cured three times; once for the outer (tool face) skin, once to bond the core and inserts with

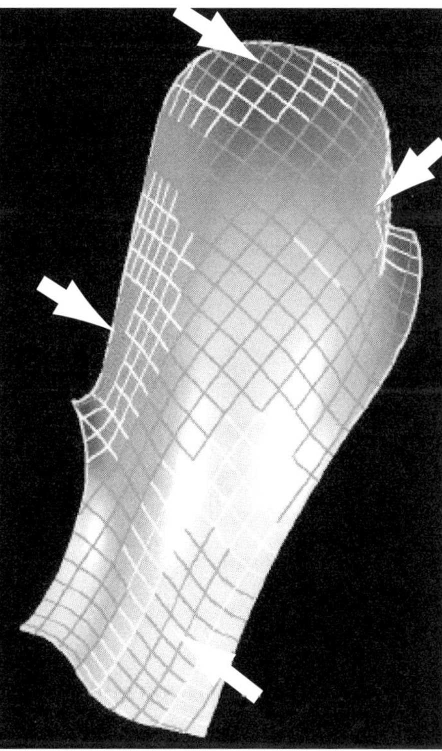

Fig. 1 FiberSIM model of woven-ply draping into fairing tool. Red zones (indicated by arrows) are areas of predicted fiber wrinkling. Courtesy of VISTAGY Inc.

film adhesives, and once for the inner (bag face) skin.

Listed are some essential stages or features of the lay-up process to achieve acceptable quality moldings:

- The mold tool must be suitably treated with a release agent to prevent bonding during cure. A solvent or (now increasingly for health and safety reasons) a water-based formulation is wiped onto the tool with a cloth. One coating is applied to each molding and three or more layers to a new or repaired tool.
- The prepreg must be neither too tacky to be "unrepositionable" (since complex-shape pieces need to be applied in stages) nor too dry such that it will not adhere to the tool or the lay-up. The tack level is dependent on the resin formulation itself, its out-life (the resin becomes harder with time at room temperature), and the lay-up room temperature.
- No bridging of prepreg can occur across tool corners such that during cure, the bagging materials fully compress the prepreg to the complete surface of the tool with no air pockets or resin filled corners.
- No air pockets can be trapped between layers since these may remain throughout the lay-up and cure resulting in cracking between layers.
- No wrinkling or folds can be introduced since the stiffness and strength of the component is dependent on the fibers being as straight as possible along the main load paths. Wrinkles will also act as stress concentrations and may cause failure below design-limit strain.
- Nothing can be allowed to contaminate the lay-up such as backing films, grease, insects, and litter. Any inclusion may prevent bonding, cause wrinkling, or produce gas during cure. It is exceptionally easy to leave pieces of thin polythene-backing film between layers. They are frequently brightly colored to help avoid this. Many inclusions are undetectable by nondestructive examination and may become partly bonded. Evidence of an inclusion can possibly only be detected through catastrophic disbonding in service. Such mistakes may be expensive, particularly with aircraft primary structure or space programs.

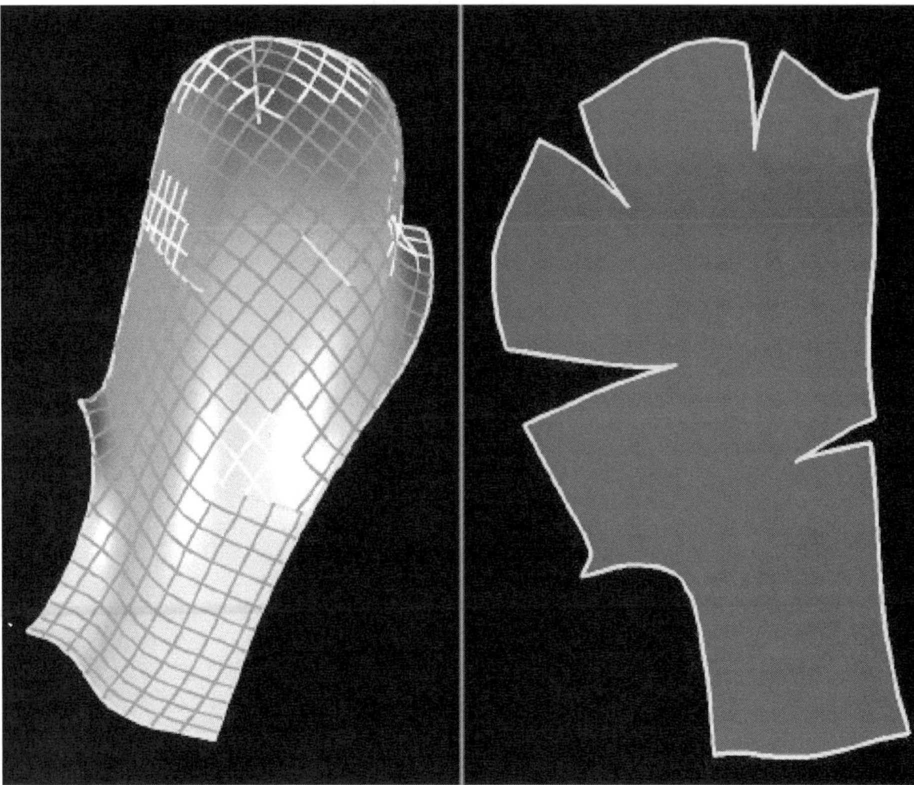

Fig. 2 FiberSIM model of woven ply draping into fairing tool after applied ply cuts. The shape on the right is the predicted flattened ply shape to be cut. Courtesy of VISTAGY Inc.

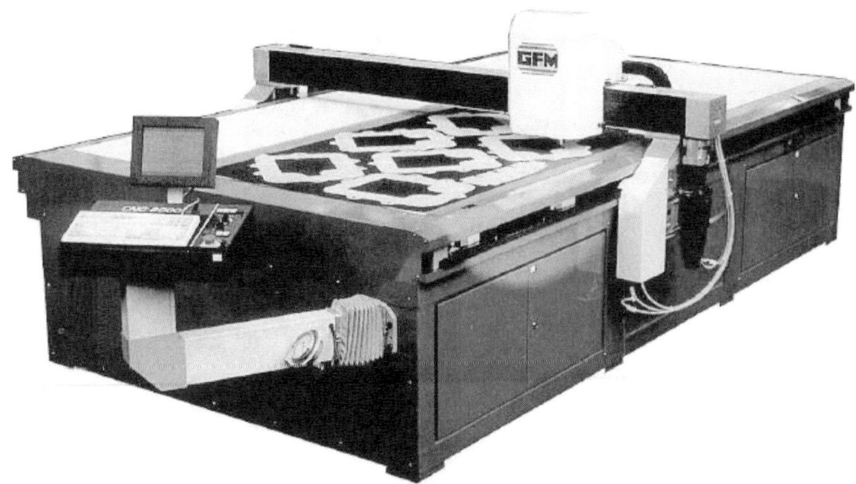

Fig. 3 Ultrasonic prepreg ply cutting machine. Courtesy of GFM (United Kingdom)

Ply Orientation and Position. In spite of the tacky nature of the prepreg and the complexity of many tool shapes, a laminator has to maintain the ply orientation and edge position. The criticality of this depends on the maximum working strain of the component, the area of structure, and the tooling approach used. Fortunately, there is usually an obvious inverse correlation between shape complexity and normal working strain. Highly loaded parts or areas of components are usually close to being flat and straight. The most complicated parts do not normally work at very high strain. The tooling approach is important because some critical components, such as wing skins, match ply edge positions (ply drops) to steps in tooling. This ensures that there is no resin-rich bead or possible void at ply edges. To allow the laminator to reach an acceptable deposition rate, two visual techniques are used to show where the prepreg piece edges should be positioned: foil templates and laser projection.

Before the introduction of laser projection, for components with critical lay-up, ply-drop positions, the laminator needed to apply a foil template over the tool and then over each applied layer and then mark the next ply-edge positions using a noncontaminating marker pen. The laminator starts lamination by laying each ply following the marked most critical edge and working outward to the component edge, trimming any excess.

Laser projection is a clever, yet essential and most effective innovation that greatly reduces lay-up time and improves quality. Instead of a laminator following a drawn outline, a laser and

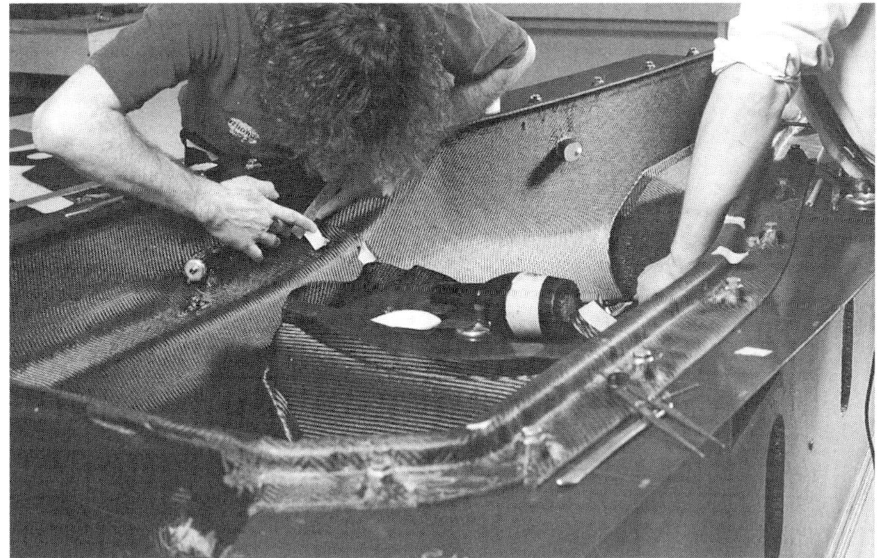

Fig. 4 Lola BMS-Ferrari Formula 1 car monocoque, manufactured by hand lay-up of woven carbon fiber prepreg. Courtesy of Nigel Macknight, Motorbooks International

mirror device causes very rapid precession of a laser point around the ply outline, which produces a static, bright red line. The line is produced by a suspended laser projector connected to a personal computer, which converts ply outline data with data on the tool curvature to provide the true ply edge (Fig. 5).

Debulking. An unfortunate result of the nature of high-quality prepreg is the inevitability of air entrapment between layers. Even after visible air pockets have been forced out, very thin pockets of air can remain. If these are not removed before the curing process, the resulting laminates can have entrapped air bubbles. If the concentration of bubbles or voids is high enough, the laminate is vulnerable to matrix cracking and delamination.

A process known as debulking is used to remove entrapped air. A reusable nylon, natural rubber, or silicone-rubber membrane is sealed around the tool periphery over the lay-up with a fabric breather cloth placed in between and a vacuum applied to the lay-up. The lay-up becomes compressed and, during a period of around 30 min, the layers are squeezed more tightly together and air removed. This process is carried out between every 0.5 and 2 mm (0.02 and 0.08 in.) of lay-up thickness. Although this step detracts from process efficiency, the laminator can use the interruption to organize documentation and materials.

The debulking process has a secondary benefit resulting from the additional compaction. After the debulking stage, the lay-up is consolidated to a thickness very close to that of the finished laminate. Consequently, when the fully laminated component is cured in an oven or autoclave, the outer plies should remain unwrinkled. Without debulking stages, the outer plies tend to wrinkle as the lay-up underneath compresses (Fig. 6).

Preparation for Curing. When the lay-up is complete and checked, it needs to be sealed such that it can be compressed and cured by the specified pressure and temperature cycle. This varies from vacuum only (oven) cure with 120 °C (250 °F) temperature applied for 1 or 2 h for non-weight-critical parts to autoclave cure with typically 5 bar (500 kPa) pressure with a carefully determined temperature-profile application lasting for 5 h or longer for critical parts such as airframe structure. Prepregs for vacuum (oven) cure have a slightly higher resin content than for high- (autoclave-) pressure cure; the laminate fiber volume fraction for woven-prepreg oven-cured laminates is approximately 54%.

For applications that can tolerate the high cost of the consumable materials, four layers of material are applied to the lay-up:

- *Peel ply (woven polyester fabric, sometimes with a corona-discharge electrical treatment to ease removal):* to provide a uniform surface that protects the surface during subsequent operations prior to bonding
- *Release film with small holes ("pin pricked" thin film):* to allow air and volatiles to escape

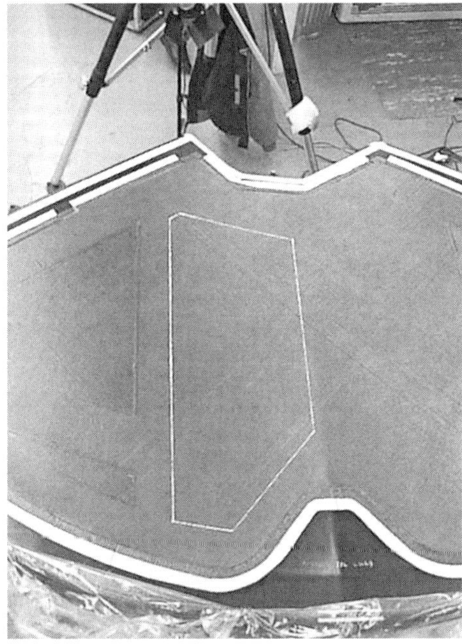

Fig. 5 Laser ply outline projection system in use on aircraft wing and fuselage fairing tool. Courtesy of Assembly Guidance Systems

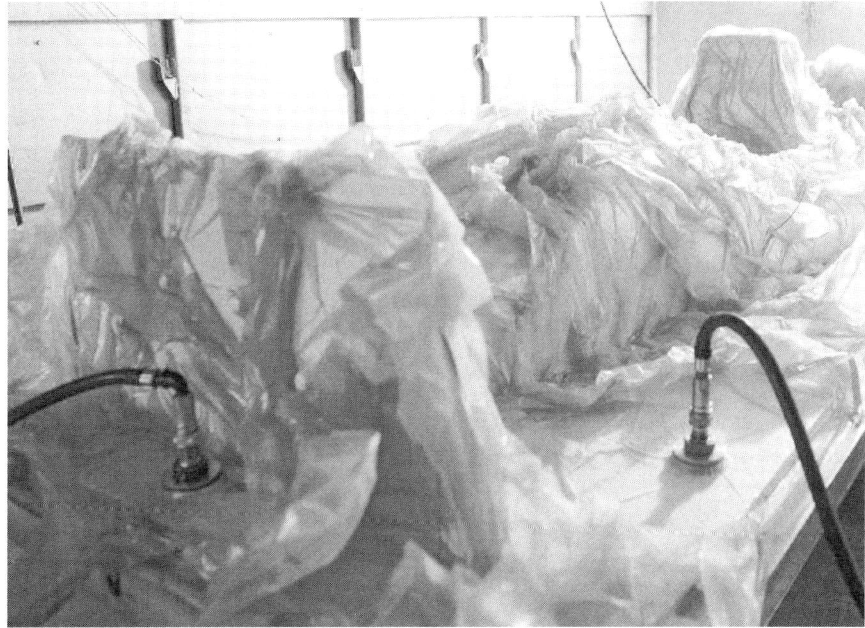

Fig. 6 Debulking of racing car monocoque lay-up. Courtesy of Nigel Macknight, Motorbooks International

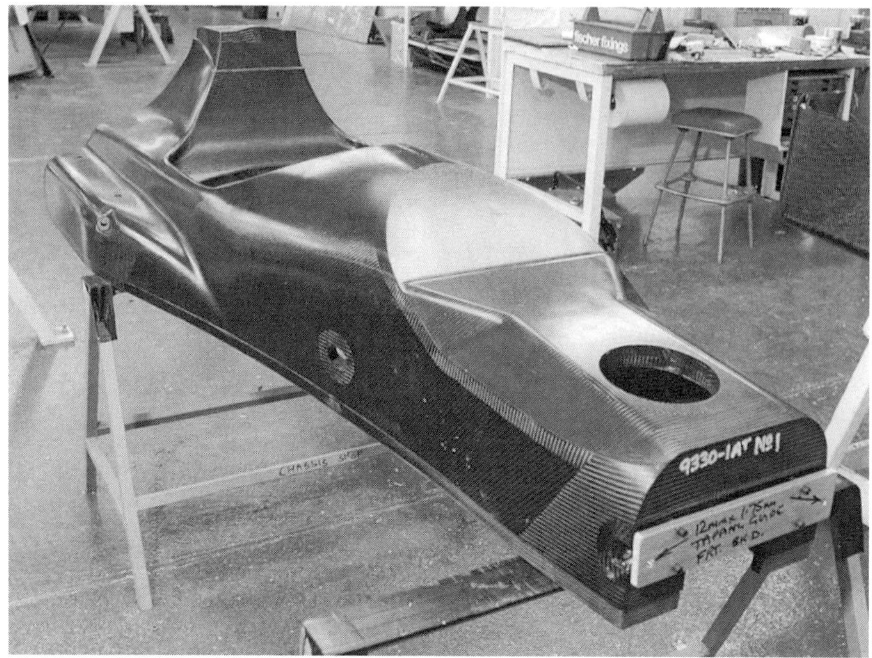

Fig. 7 Autoclave molded Lola Formula 1 car chassis upper half. Courtesy of Nigel Macknight, Motorbooks International

from the lay-up upper surface. Release films with perforations encourage resin removal (bleeding), whereas types without holes prevent bleeding.
- *Breather cloth (polyester fiber wadding):* to carry air and volatiles to be expelled through a vacuum pump
- *Vacuum bag (nylon film) with tacky rubber sealant gasket:* to seal the lay-up from the oven or autoclave hot air

This is a most difficult and costly process for both labor and materials. The total consumable cost varies from around $15/m^2 to $60/m^2, depending on the temperature and pressure applied. The vacuum-bag application is particularly difficult since for double curvature parts or those with raised details or tooling flanges, the bag needs to be folded with sealant tucks applied. Bag failures are common with less experienced operators. Consequently, where tooling budgets allow, custom silicone rubber bags are manufactured. These bags are made from 3 to 5 mm (0.12 to 0.20 in.) thick tough rubber that is bonded to a frame; the rubber can be stretched over the component surface by the applied vacuum. Their cost is in the order of $145/m^2 to $715/m^2 of tool surface, depending on the size and complexity. To reduce cure preparation time and the risk of puncture, very tough and "high elongation" consumable bagging films have recently been introduced.

Although preparation for cure appears to be a very complex and costly process, it improved with the introduction of nil-bleed prepregs in the 1980s. Prior to these, specific volumes of excess resin would be bled out of the lay-up into glass fabrics. These had to be applied in one or several layers between the peel-ply and release-film layers. Prepregs are now reliably produced with a highly controlled resin content of typically 34 $\pm$ 1% by weight. Figure 7 (Ref 2) shows a cured, demolded, and trimmed Formula 1 car chassis, upper half. Figure 8 shows the completed car of which all of the structure apart from the engine and gearbox is composite, predominantly manufactured using 120 °C (250 °F) curing epoxy-resin and woven intermediate-modulus (IM) fiber prepreg.

Component Properties

Over the history of composite structures, prepreg hand lay-up has been used to mold a great diversity of parts. Extremes of sewage tanks to satellite solar array supports and truck leaf springs to Formula 1 engine air inlet trumpets and fuel injector tubes are examples.

These diverse applications have had materials specifically tailored to provide extremes of performance. For instance aramid fibers in conjunction with resins with low-fiber adhesion can provide laminates that are impenetrable to low-velocity bullets. Space satellite structures are optimized for extreme low weight and just enough robustness to reliably survive launch vibrations; such structures can have laminate stiffnesses of up to 280 GPa (41 $\times$ 10^6 psi), more than double that of standard carbon fiber unidirectional laminates. One limitation with current polymer prepreg matrix resins is a maximum service temperature of around 270 °C (520 °F). Non-polymer-matrix materials are not amenable to prepreg hand lay-up since they are not tacky.

The prepreg hand lay-up process can use all types of reinforcement fiber in tape or fabric form. Fibers range in stiffness from E-glass, providing laminates with tensile moduli up to 42 GPa (6 $\times$ 10^6 psi), to ultrahigh-modulus pitch-based carbon, providing laminates with tensile moduli up to 490 GPa (71 $\times$ 10^6 psi) (Fig. 9). Any resin can be used that is capable of being formulated to provide a high viscosity such that the prepreg has tacky surfaces. The most common matrix resins are epoxies as a result of their strength, fiber adhesion strength, and slow curing, which provides a freezer out life (i.e., lay-up period) of up to many weeks. Their upper service-temperature-limit is around 150 °C (300 °F) in a hot, wet environment and hence for higher service temperatures, bismaleimide resins with a limit of around 200 °C (390 °F) and then polyimides with a limit of around 270 °C (520 °F) were developed (Ref 3) (see the articles "Bismaleimide Resins" and "Polyimide Resins" in this Volume). Figure 9 shows the range of laminate stiffnesses provided by a wide range of prepreg reinforcement types.

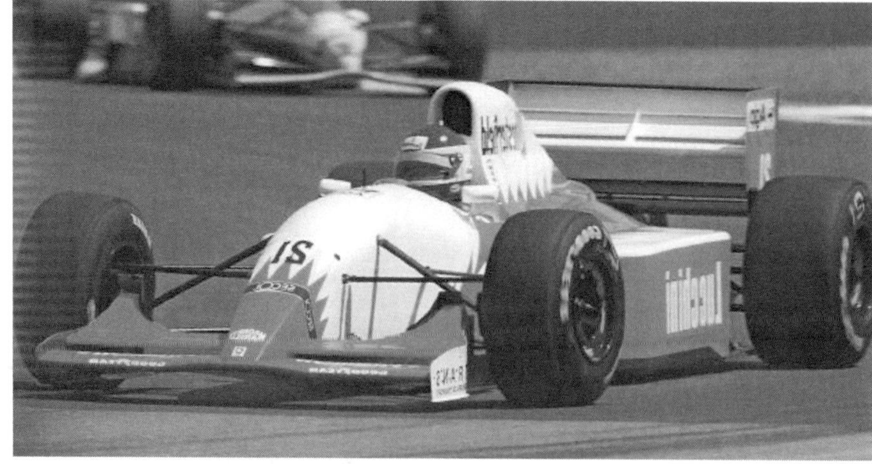

Fig. 8 Lola BMS Ferrari Formula 1 car. All structure, including wings, fairings, and monococque, is molded by hand lay-up of woven prepreg and autoclave cured. Courtesy of Nigel Macknight, Motorbooks International

Table 1 Prepreg types and lay-up characteristics

			Cure temperature		Typical thickness		Width		Maximum lay-up rate		Approximate cost		
Fiber type	Form(a)	Resin type	°C	°F	mm	in.	m	ft	kg/h	lb/h	$/kg	$/lb	Damage resistance
E-glass	UD	Epoxy	120	250	0.25	0.010	0.6	2.0	2	1	30	14	Medium
	Woven	Epoxy	120	250	0.37	0.015	1.7	5.6	10	5	25	11	Very high
	Woven	Phenolic	135	275	0.37	0.015	1.7	5.6	10	5	15	7	Medium
	Multiaxial	Epoxy	120	250	0.6	0.024	1.25	4.1	15	7	5	2	High
Aramid	Woven	Epoxy	120	250	...	...	1.7	5.6	...	...	...	...	Extremely high
Carbon	UD	Epoxy	120	250	0.25	0.010	0.6	2.0	2	1	40	18	Low
	UD	Epoxy	180	360	0.25	0.010	0.6	2.0	2	1	40	18	Very low
	Woven	Epoxy	120	250	0.37	0.015	1.7	5.6	6	3	50	23	Medium
	Multiaxial	Epoxy	120	250	0.6	0.024	1.25	4.1	9	4	35	16	Medium
Intermediate-modulus carbon	UD	Epoxy	180	360	0.13	0.005	0.3	1.0	1	0.5	70	32	Very low
	Woven	Epoxy	120	250	0.29	0.011	1.7	5.6	4	2	105	48	Medium
High-modulus carbon	UD	Epoxy	180	360	0.13	0.005	0.3	1.0	1	0.5	85	39	Extremely low
	Woven	Epoxy	120	250	0.29	0.011	1.7	5.6	4	2	135	61	Low

(a) UD, unidirectional tape with multi-angular lay-up. Multiaxial, fabric with 2 to 7 layers of tows at varying angles knitted into a drapable fabric (also called noncrimp fabric).

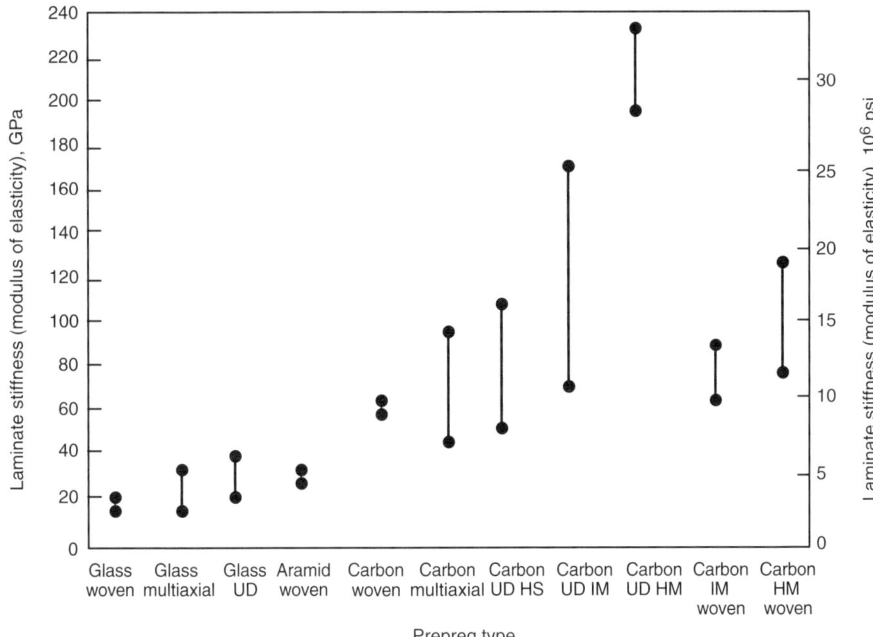

Fig. 9 Laminate stiffness provided by a range of prepreg reinforcement types. Range shows the effect of lay-up. UD, unidirectional; HS, high strength; IM, intermediate modulus; HM, high modulus

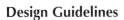

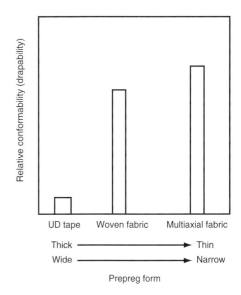

Fig. 10 Relationship between prepreg form and conformability to component curvature

Design Guidelines

Materials and process selection for lightweight composite materials is primarily driven by how much an industry will pay for weight reduction of components and how many parts will be made. For one-off structures and those with production levels of one or a few per month, the cost of the prepreg is usually greatly outweighed by the design, project engineering, and tooling cost.

Structures for which there is little incentive for weight reduction are rarely manufactured from prepreg, since wet lay techniques use much lower-cost composite materials.

Hand lay-up of prepregs is applied to a very wide field of industries and applications. At the industrial end with higher volume production in the order of five to ten parts per day, a thick prepreg, often using a multiaxial stitched (multilayer, multiangular, nonwoven) fabric with a lower-cost, faster-cure resin, will be used. The maximum service-strain levels will be low, and, hence, bubbles and the occasional wrinkle can be tolerated. This also allows the prepregs to be manufactured fast, having wider resin content tolerance bands. A good example of this is E-glass fiber/epoxy resin wind turbine blades. The thick (typically 600 g/m^2) stitched multiaxial fabric in a very tacky resin is able to conform to the blade curvature and to the root section where it joins the hub.

For low-volume, high-performance applications such as rocket launchers with skin features for attachment points, the lay-ups are complex and are provided by unidirectional-tape prepreg of very low thickness (typically 125 g/m^2 FAW). The fiber choice is high-modulus grade, and the resin is formulated to resist higher temperatures than epoxies can sustain. The bismaleimide carbon prepregs are up to 200 times the cost of the glass-epoxy wind-turbine materials.

Table 1 gives a comparison of prepreg types and their manufacturing attributes, costs, and laminate-damage resistance. Figure 10 indicates the level of curvature conformability that can be provided by prepreg reinforcement forms and its relationship with prepreg width and thickness.

Outlook

Despite many impressive research projects and facility investment in the United States and Europe, which have investigated and implemented production of molding processes considered to have the potential to offer cost reduction compared to prepreg hand lay-up, prepreg lay-up is not being replaced for low-volume applications except for low-surface-area parts with extreme lay-up complexity. Very successful examples where resin injection molding of dry preformed fabrics have been developed for propeller-blade molding by Dowty aerospace propellers in England; for sine wave spars and engine-intake ducts for fighter aircraft by Dow–UT (now GKN Westland Aerospace) in the United States and for regional aircraft control surfaces by Bombardier Shorts in Northern Ireland. These applications make use of the higher drapability of dry fabrics compared to prepreg and the use of matched metal tools to provide net-shape parts, which do not require shimming during assembly. The process-engineering simplicity of prepreg lay-up and cure using a vacuum bag and/or pressure is undeniably preferable to liquid molding processes. The downside of freezer storage and high prepreg cost if procuring small quantity continues to be overcome by the ability to make components simply and reliably.

For applications with low curvature, such as aircraft-wing and tailplane panels, prepreg tape laying by large machine tools will continue to replace hand lay-up. For applications with highly weight optimized, closed sections that can be rotated, such as small aircraft and helicopter fuselages, the fiber placement process as developed by Alliant Techsystems, Cincinnati Milacron, and Boeing will become further established (see the article "Fiber Placement" in this Volume).

There are two apparent trends for prepreg manufacture to further reduce the cost of hand lay-up:

- Scale up of production with low-cost carbon fiber to enter new markets such as low volume production cars, trains, larger wind-turbine blades, and infrastructure repair. Companies such as Zoltech and Hexcel are installing wider, faster prepreg lines.
- Introduction of thick multiaxial fabric prepregging is being made to capitalize on the stiffness of these laminates coupled with the very low manufacturing cost of the fabric.

REFERENCES

1. Nigel Macknight, *The Modern Formula 1 Race Car*, Motorbooks International, 1993, p 88–100
2. T.G. Gutowski, Ed., *Advanced Composites Manufacturing*, Wiley-Interscience, 1997, p 207–239
3. D.H. Middleton, Ed., *Composite Materials in Aircraft Structures*, Longman Scientific and Technical, 1990, p 17–38

Fiber Placement

Don O. Evans, Cincinnati Machine

FIBER PLACEMENT is a unique process combining the differential tow payout capability of filament winding and the compaction and cut-restart capabilities of automated tape laying. During the fiber placement process, individual prepreg fibers, called tows, are pulled off spools and fed through a fiber delivery system into a fiber placement head (Fig. 1). In the placement head they are collimated into a single fiber band and laminated onto a work surface, which can be mounted between a headstock and tailstock.

When starting a fiber band or course, the individual tows are fed through the head and compacted onto a surface. As the course is being laid down, the processing head can cut or restart any of the individual tows. This permits the width of the fiber band to be increased or decreased in increments equal to one tow width. Adjusting the width of the fiber band eliminates excessive gaps or overlaps between adjacent courses. At the end of the course, the remaining tows are cut to match the shape of the ply boundary. The head is then positioned to the beginning of the next course.

During the placement of a course, each tow is dispensed at its own speed, allowing each tow to independently conform to the surface of the part. Because of this, the fibers are not restricted to geodesic paths. They can be steered to meet specified design goals.

A rolling compaction device, combined with heat for tack enhancement, laminates the tows onto the lay-up surface. This action of pressing tows onto the work surface (or a previously laid ply) adheres the tows to the lay-up surface and removes trapped air, minimizing the need for vacuum debulking. It also allows the fiber to be laid onto concave surfaces.

Figure 2 is a diagram of a fiber placement system. This system has seven axes of motion and is computer numeric controlled. The machine consists of three position axes (carriage, tilt, crossfeed), three orientation axes (yaw, pitch, roll), and an axis to rotate the work mandrel. All of these axes are necessary to make sure the processing head is normal to the surface as the machine is laminating tows. The machine also has up to 32 programmable bidirectional electronic tensioners, which are mounted in an air-conditioned creel. These tensioners provide individual tow payout and maintain a precise tension. The fiber placement head is mounted on the end of the wrist. The head precisely dispenses, cuts, clamps, and restarts individual prepreg tows.

Applications

Fiber placement was developed during the mid-to-late 1980s. In 1990 the first production fiber placement machine was delivered to an aerospace company. The first company to implement fiber placement on a production aircraft was Boeing Helicopters. A U.S. government-funded program was conducted by Boeing and Hercules to develop the design and process for fiber placing the aft fuselage for the Bell/Boeing V-22 Osprey. This part was designed to take advantage of the unique capabilities of fiber placement. The first four prototype V-22 aft fuselages were made from nine hand-laid sections. Switching to single-fiber-placed monolithic structure

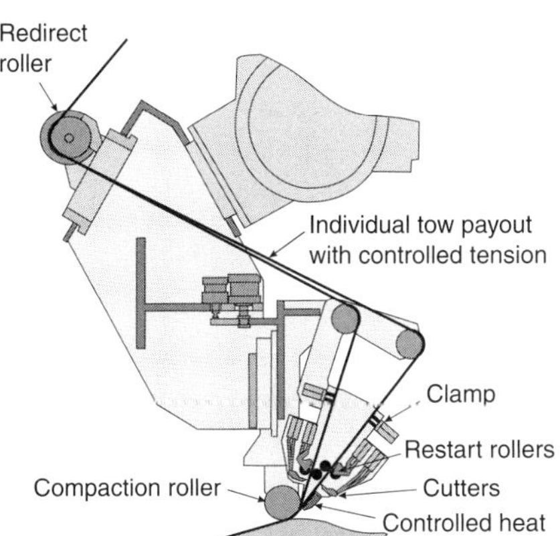

Fig. 1 Fiber placement head

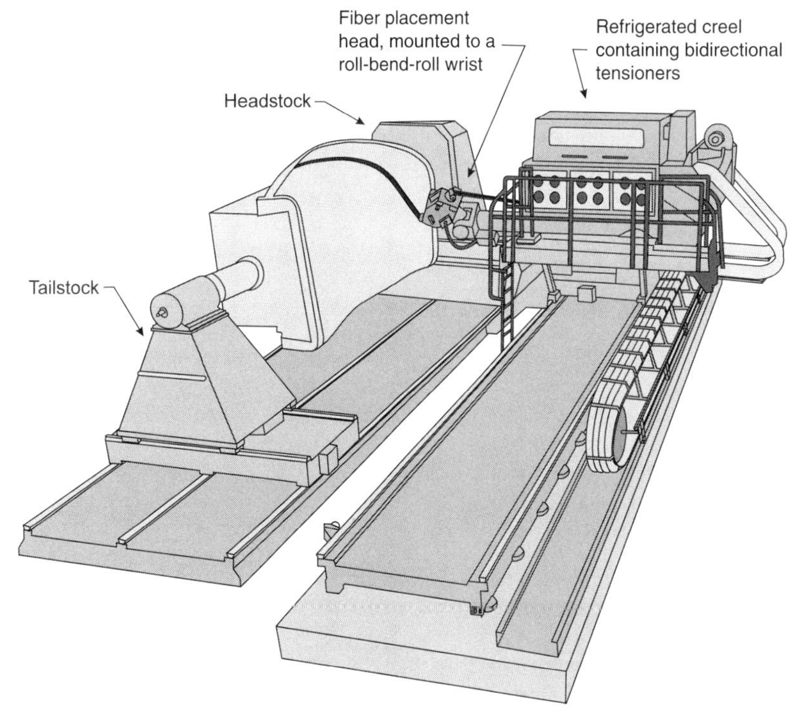

Fig. 2 Fiber placement system

cut the number of fasteners by 34%, and cut the trim and assembly labor by 53%. Through the combination of design optimization and fiber placement, Boeing also reduced the material scrap by 90%. Several other production V-22 parts are being fiber placed by the Bell/Boeing team. These components include the fuselage side skins, sponsons, drag angle, main landing gear doors, fuel boom, and the rotor blade grip (Ref 1).

Another military aircraft that is taking advantage of the unique capabilities of the fiber placements is the F/A-18 E/F Super Hornet. The U.S. Navy funded a program to further advance fiber placement by implementing it on a F/A-18 E/F fuselage skin (Fig. 3). The program implemented at Northrop Grumman realized a labor savings of 38% when compared to hand lay-up. Northrop Grumman is also using fiber placement for inlet duct skins, side skins, and covers for the F/A-18 E/F.

Fiber placement is also being used in commercial aircraft. Raytheon Aircraft in Wichita, Kansas, is using fiber placement to fabricate fuselage sections for the Premier I and Hawker Horizon business jets (Fig. 4). The fuselage is a honeycomb sandwich construction. Graphite facesheets inclose a Nomex (DuPont) honeycomb core for a total thickness of 20.6 mm (0.81 in.). This design creates a fuselage shell free of frames and stiffeners. The shells are also free of rivets and skin joints. Because the shells do not contain frames, there is more usable space for passengers or cargo.

By using the fiber placement process to fabricate the fuselages, Raytheon has realized weight savings, material savings, reduced part count, reduced tool count, reduced shop flow time, and increased part quality. The Premier I fuselage consists of only two cured parts. The forward shell extends from the radome bulkhead to the aft pressure bulkhead and is 8 m (26 ft) long. It includes the baggage area, cockpit, and cabin areas. The aft shell extends from the aft pressure bulkhead to the tailcone, and is about 5 m (16 ft) long. The Premier I shells weigh less than 273 kg (600 lb), whereas an equivalent metal aircraft would weigh at least 454 kg (1000 lb). This is a 40% weight savings. If the same two composite fuselage sections were made in a comparable metal design, they would contain more than 3000 pieces. It would be made up of stringers, stiffeners, bulkheads, clips, and external skins. This reduction in part count significantly reduces part fabrication time and the number of tools required to make and assemble the parts (Ref 2).

Material scrap for hand lay-up can be as high as 30 to 50%. Fiber placement has a typical material scrap of 2 to 7%. On a 273 kg (600 lb) fuselage, this material savings becomes very significant.

On the Premier I fuselage, quality assurance (QA) review found that the machine is very repeatable and maintains a tighter tolerance than the hand lay-up process. Because of this, QA personnel closely scrutinize the first production part to make sure that it meets all of the design requirements. If the part program builds a part that meets all of the design requirements, it is considered "bought off." As long as the part program is not changed, QA personnel needs to do only periodic inspections, instead of checking every ply as it is laid.

Materials

A fiber placement machine can dispense prepregged fibers that are commonly used by the aerospace industry, such as carbon, aramid, glass, and quartz. These fibers need to be fully impregnated with a resin and formed into tows or slit tape. The width of tow or slit tape used by fiber placement range from 3.2 to 4.6 mm (0.125 to 0.182 in.). A width of 3.2 mm (0.125 in.) is most common today. Tows are typically wound onto a 7.6 cm (3 in.) diameter by 28 cm (11 in.) long core in a helical pattern. A typical length for a 2.3 kg (5 lb) spool of prepregged IM7-12K tow, 3.2 mm (0.125 in.) wide, is 3350 m (11,000 ft).

Slit tape is fabricated by running a 7.6 cm (3 in.) wide tape through a slitter, creating smaller widths of slit tape. These narrow slit tapes are then wound onto a number of cores to form spools. When the slit tape is wound onto the core, a backing film, which is wider than the slit tape, must be added. If the backing film is not used, the slit tape cannot be removed from the spool, because of stringers that will occur during the despooling operation. A stringer occurs when the edge of the slit tape separates and stays on the spool while the rest of the slit tape is despooled. This will cause the slit tape to eventually break. During part fabrication, this backing film is removed before the fiber reaches the fiber placement head.

The tow width of the material is very important in controlling the gap between the prepregged tows. For example, if the fiber placement head is designed to lay down tows that are 3.2 ± 0.38 mm (0.125 ± 0.015 in.) wide, the tows will be compacted onto the surface in 3.2 mm (0.125 in.) spacings. If the tow is exactly 3.2 mm (0.125 in.) wide, there will be no gap between the tows. If the tows are 2.5 mm (0.100 in.) wide, there will be a 0.63 mm (0.025 in.) wide gap between the tows. If the tows are 3.8 mm (0.150 in.) wide, there will be a 0.63 mm (0.025 in.) overlap.

The ideal fiber placement material has no tack at 21 °C (70 °F) and high tack at 27 to 32 °C (80 to 90 °F). Low tack is needed when the material is being pulled off the spool and guided through a fiber delivery system and head, but high tack is needed when it is being compacted onto the surface.

Materials that have a low tack can be despooled with a fiber tension of 0.23 kg (0.5 lb) or less. These low tensions are achieved because the resin does not stick to the spool or the components of the fiber delivery system. This lower fiber tension is needed while fiber placing concave areas. A higher tension will cause the fiber to bridge over concave areas. Materials with low tack levels also have less tendency to deform or rope while being pulled through the fiber delivery system. They also transfer less resin to the components of the fiber delivery system and head. This reduces the number of times that these components need to be cleaned because of a resin buildup. Resin buildup in the head can cause it to malfunction.

Part Design Considerations

Fiber placement has the capability of reducing composite material and labor cost. To take advantage of these cost savings, the designer must take into consideration the unique capabilities and limitations of fiber placement. Some of the items that the designer must consider are ply shapes, tow steering, dropping and adding tows, and surface geometry. By optimizing ply shapes, the designer can eliminate the need to hand lay a piece of the ply that cannot be laid by the machine. The designer can also take advantage of the ability of fiber placement to steer tows so they can follow applied stresses, but the tows must not be steered less than 635 mm (25 in.) or they will buckle. The designer needs to take into consideration where the tows are added and

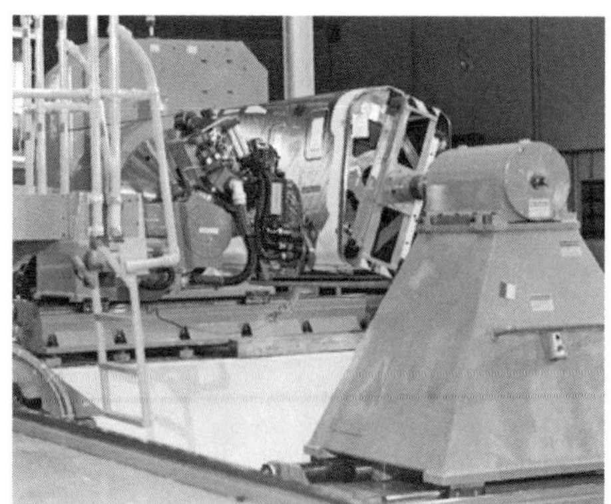

Fig. 3 Fiber placement of the Northrop Grumman F/A-18 E/F fuselage skin

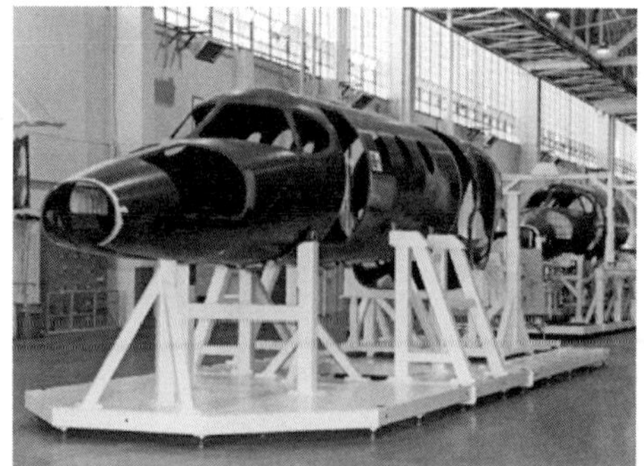

Fig. 4 Raytheon Premier I fuselage manufactured by fiber placement

dropped, making sure there are not too many gaps and overlaps in a small area. The surface geometry must be such that there are no head collisions and that the concave radii are not too small for the compaction roller to fit into.

When generating ply shapes, the designer must consider the shortest tow length the machine can lay down. This length is the distance from the start of the lay-down point to where the tow is cut in the head. This is called the minimum cut length. It varies from 63.5 to 152 mm (2.5 to 6 in.), depending on the head size and configuration. If the area that is to be filled with tows is less than the minimum course length, the machine cannot lay tow in these locations. These areas could be laid in by hand, or the ply shapes could be adjusted to overcome this limitation. Three techniques can be used to eliminate areas of missing tows (Ref 3):

- In the problem areas, the exterior ply boundaries can be extended past the required part shape, such as tabs on the corner of 45° plies. These extended areas are later removed.
- Curved interior plies can be reshaped to match the fiber angles.
- Some of the holes can be distributed to full-coverage plies having the same fiber angles.

Designers specify the fiber angles that are required to meet mechanical property requirements. Steering of the fibers is required to maintain these angles on a complex shaped tool. A typical fiber placement machine using 3.2 mm (0.125 in.) wide materials can steer a fiber band along a 63.5 cm (25 in.) radius without buckling the individual tows. The buckling occurs because the fibers on the outside steering radius are in tension and the fibers on the inside steering radius are in compression. When steering a radius smaller than 63.5 cm (25 in.), the tows will begin to buckle if laid on a flat or a convex surface, or 'Venetian blind' if laid on a concave surface. Venetian blinding occurs when the fibers on the inside steering radius of the individual tows are adhered to the surface and the fibers on the outside steering radius are in the air.

The designer needs to pay special attention to two surface geometry issues when designing a part that is to be manufactured by fiber placement. The first is concave surfaces, and the second is areas with small radii of curvature. When considering a part with a concave surface area, the designer must make sure the fiber placement head can fit into the concave area without hitting the surface of the part. There are some techniques that can be used to overcome some of these limitations. To help the head fit into a concave area, the off-line software has a feature known as collision avoidance. The part and head geometry are programmed into the software. The software constantly checks to see if the two are colliding. If they come close to colliding, the software will rock the head off the surface normal away from the collision. There are limits to how much the head can be rocked off the surface normal. If the head hits on both the front and back sides, the software cannot avoid the collision, and the area should be redesigned. Rocking the head to the front or back slightly affects the effective applied compaction force and the minimum cut length. Rocking the head sideways also affects the effective applied compaction force and requires extra compactor compliance.

Outlook

Because of the unique capabilities of fiber placement, many aerospace companies are using it to fabricate a variety of composite parts. In a relative short period of time, this approach has been developed into a widely accepted automated manufacturing process for affordable composite aerospace components. In the aerospace community, it is typically very difficult to obtain approval to change how a part is fabricated once the part has been qualified to be flight worthy. To change the part design or how it is fabricated requires the part to be requalified. This can be an expensive effort and makes it difficult to justify the change. The key to avoiding this requalification cost is to design the parts for fabrication by fiber placement from the beginning. As new aircraft and aerospace programs are introduced, fiber placement will be used to fabricate many more composite parts to gain the benefits of reduced cost, improved quality, and improved performance.

REFERENCES

1. C.G. Grant, Fiber Placement Process Utilization Within the Worldwide Aerospace Industry, *SAMPE J.*, July/Aug 2000, p 7–12
2. K.M. Retz, "Premier I: Success with Fiber Placement," SME Composites 1998 Manufacturing and Tooling Conf., 9–12 Feb 1998
3. D.O. Evans, "Design Considerations for Fiber Placement," 38th International SAMPE Symposium, 10–13 May 1993

Automated Tape Laying

Michael N. Grimshaw, Cincinnati Machine, A UNOVA Company

AUTOMATED TAPE LAYING is a mature process and is currently being used in both commercial and military aircraft applications. This article provides a brief history of the process and describes the use of commercially available flat and contour tape-laying equipment. The materials section describes feedstock materials suitable for automatic tape layer (ATL)-grade composite materials.

History

Advanced composites were introduced in unidirectional tape form in the early 1960s. Originally performed by hand, the lay-up process was labor intensive, and inconsistency with hand lay-up caused quality problems with the cured laminates. In the mid-1960s, there was a big push for automation by the aircraft industry. Early machines were home-built by aerospace companies and/or job shops under the direction of materials suppliers. Machine configurations ranged from hand-assisted tabletop prototypes to the first full computer numerically controlled (CNC) gantry-style tape layer, which was developed under U.S. Air Force contract by General Dynamics and the Conrac Corporation. This machine was used to make composite parts for the F-16 with 75 mm (3 in.) wide tape. During the late 1970s and early 1980s, machine tool builders produced the first commercially available flat and contour CNC tape-laying machines, which made aircraft parts for military programs such as the B-1 and B-2 (stealth) bombers (Fig. 1). Tape widths ranged from 75 to 150 mm (3–6 in.) on contoured surfaces and up to 300 mm (12 in.) on flat surfaces (Ref 1 and 2). In the late 1980s, the use of automated tape laying began to focus on commercial aircraft applications. Throughout the 1990s, the equipment, programming, lay-up techniques, and ATL-grade composite materials were further developed to make the tape-laying process more productive, reliable, and user friendly. As of 2001, there are approximately 40 to 45 commercially produced tape-laying machines in the field (Fig. 2).

Process Overview

Unidirectional graphite epoxy tape is supplied in roll form on backing paper and typically comes in 75, 150, and 300 mm (3, 6, and 12 in.) widths. Contour applications use 75 and 150 mm (3 and 6 in.) widths, while flat applications use 150 and 300 mm (6 and 12 in.) widths. The roll of material is loaded into the tape-laying head (Fig. 3). The tape head is mounted on a 4-axis gantry for flat applications or a 5-axis gantry for contour applications (Fig. 4). The gantry positions the tape head over and onto flat or contour tools for lay-up. A typical part consists of many plies of tape laid up at various ply angles. A "ply" consists of one layer of tape courses at a given angle (Fig. 5). Plies are laid or stacked on top of each other to create a laminate. For flat laminates (commonly called charges, blankets, or panels), once the lay-up process is completed, the laminates are typically removed from the lay-up bed and transferred to a CNC ply cutter where parts are cut out of the laminate. The cut pieces or part kits are stacked and hot drape-formed into structural parts, such as stringers, ribs, C-channels, I-beams, and so on, or stacked onto a contour skin tool to form a contour skin panel. The formed structural parts or skin panels are cured either as a separate structural part or skin panel, or assembled together and co-cured/co-bonded as a contoured skin panel with structural stiffeners (Fig. 6). Laminates that are laid as a contour part usually remain on the contour tool (Fig. 2). The contour tool and the laminate are transferred to the autoclave for curing or to an assembly area where they are mated with structural parts prior to curing.

Advantages. Tape layers compact plies of graphite/epoxy tape with exceptional consistency and greatly reduce fabrication costs com-

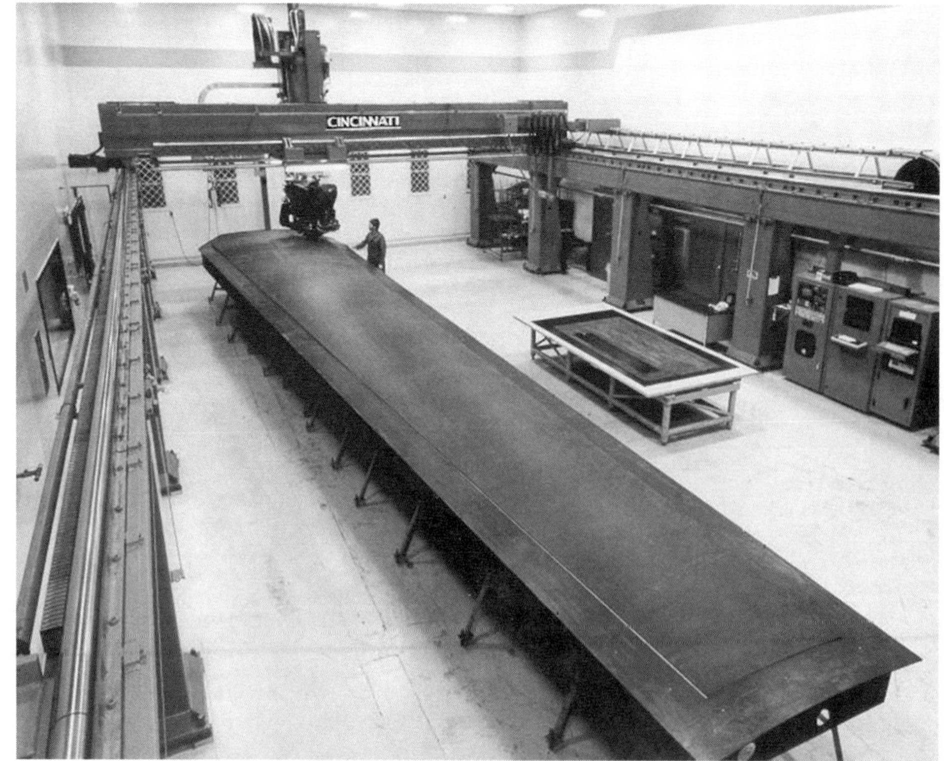

Fig. 1 Contour skin lay-up using a gantry-type automated tape layer

pared to hand lay-up. Users of tape-laying equipment have claimed reductions in personnel hours of up to 70 to 85% for flat charges versus hand lay-up, and lay-up rates as high as 1000 kg/week (2200 lb/week). See Fig. 7 for typical lay-up versus scrap rates for flat panels made from 150 and 300 mm (6 and 12 in.) tape widths. Lay-up rates for contour skin panels vary depending on contour complexity, accuracy required, part thickness, and width of tape used. Flat-to-medium contoured parts are well suited for tape laying. The bigger the part and plies, the more productive tape layers are.

Another advantage is that tape layers have $\pm 190°$ of head rotation; therefore, fiber angles are not limited—any ply angle can be laid up. Cut angles range from 0° to 85°. Tape slitting is used on nonfull width courses.

Disadvantages. Highly contoured parts are not suited for tape laying because the tape tends to buckle and bridge at plane transitions. Also, backing paper breakage can occur. Small plies also lower the productivity of the tape layer.

Applications

Examples of parts made from flat laminates are empennage structural parts (spars, ribs, stringers, C-channel, and I-beam stiffeners) on the Boeing 777, the Airbus A330/340 (shown in Fig. 6), and the Airbus A340-500/600. Examples of contour tape laid parts include horizontal/vertical stabilizer skins on the Boeing 777, the Airbus A330/340, and the Airbus A340-500/600 (Fig. 2 and 6); wing skins on F-22 fighters (Ref 3) (Fig. 8); V-22 *Osprey* tilt rotor wing skins; B-1 and B-2 bomber wing and stabilizer skins (Fig. 1); and Eurofighter upper and lower wing skins.

Description of Equipment

Tape Layer. The ten-axis gantry-type tape-laying machine shown in Fig. 4 is designed to lay composite tape materials on flat and contoured surfaces. All ten axis movements (five on the gantry and five on the tape head) are CNC to enable the tape to be laid on the contour of a mold surface automatically.

The high-rail gantry-type machine is constructed with x-axis ways in 3.7 m (12 ft) increments. This allows the use of multiple gantries on a common set of ways and permits lamination operations on different workpieces simultaneously. Another advantage of the gantry-type machine is the capability of loading and unloading workpieces on one end while continuing to laminate on the other end.

The x-axis gantry travels on two parallel sets of hardened-steel guide ways that are elevated and supported by two parallel sets of fixed uprights spaced in 3.7 m (12 ft) increments. The y-axis cross saddle and z-axis vertical slide assembly, which provide the transverse and vertical movement of the tape-laying head, are mounted to the gantry cross rail. The cross saddle travels on two parallel sets of guide ways mounted to the gantry cross rail. The z-axis vertical slide is located in the center of the cross saddle and travels perpendicularly to the cross saddle on a pair of ways mounted to the vertical slide. The c-axis supports and rotates the a-axis saddle and tape head and is assembled in the vertical slide. The a-axis saddle travels on radial ways mounted to a plate attached to the c-axis. Movement of the a-axis provides the tape-layer head tilt motion. The tape head is bolted to the a-axis saddle (Fig. 3).

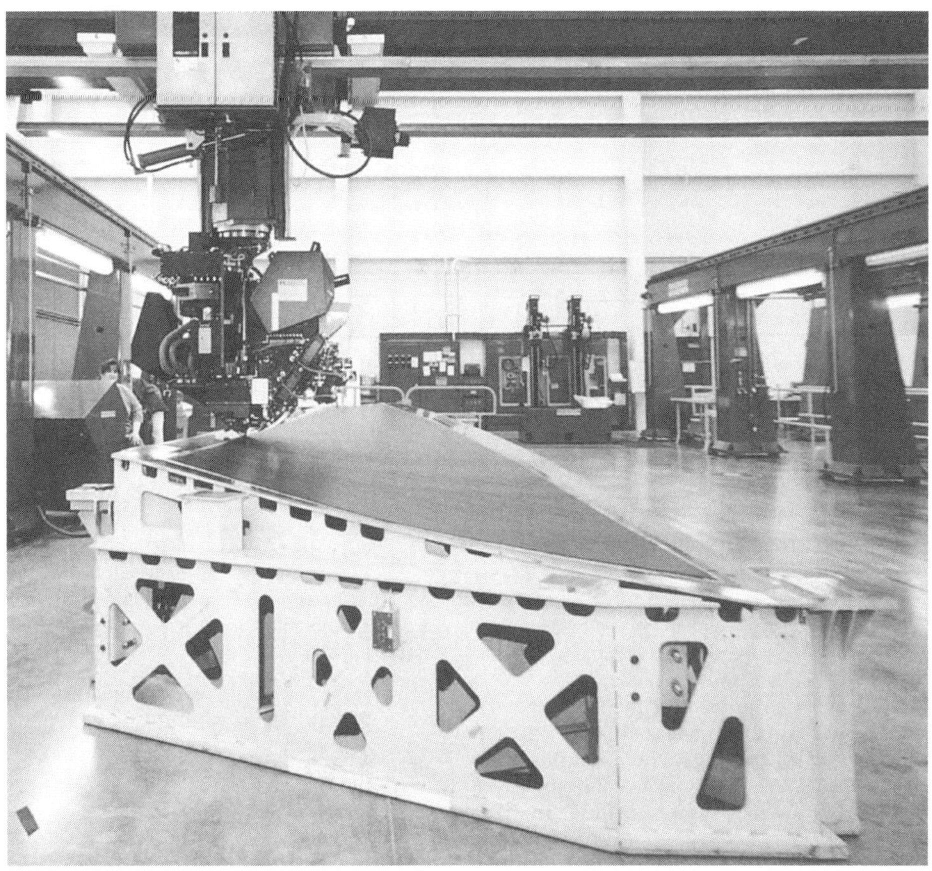

Fig. 2 Automated tape lay-up of a contour skin showing the integrated contour tooling

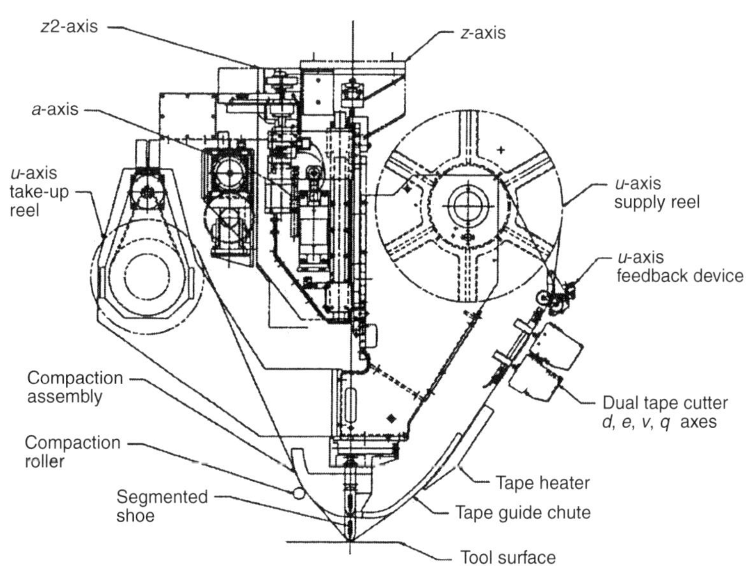

Fig. 3 Tape head for an automated tape layer

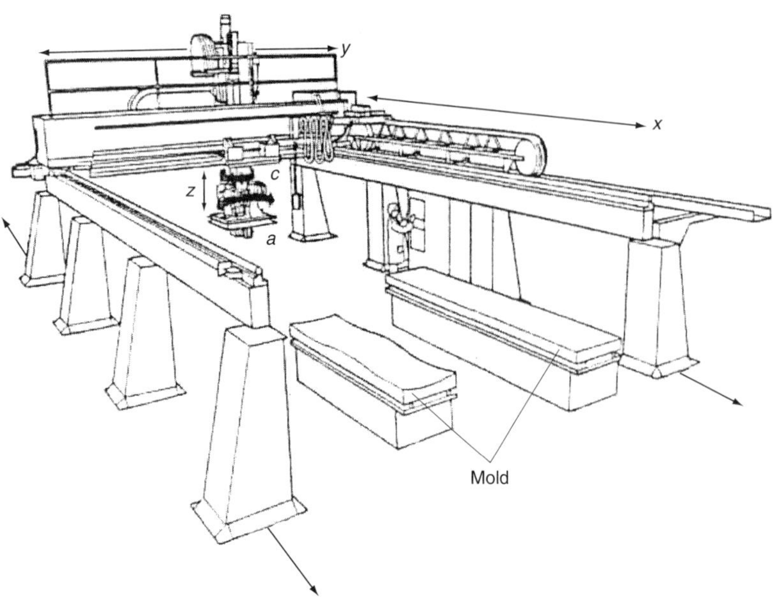

Fig. 4 Main machine axes of a gurney-type automated tape layer. The x-axis can be extended in 3.7 m (12 ft) increments.

Tape Head. A spool of tape is loaded on the supply reel located on the top front of the tape head (Fig. 3). Tape is fed past the tape position feedback device, over the upper tape guide chute, and past the cutters. It continues through the lower tape guides, under the segmented compaction shoe, and onto a backing paper take-up reel located on the rear of the tape head. The movement of composite tape through the tape head is called the *u*-axis. Both the supply reel and take-up reel motors control the tape.

The two linear cutter axes *v* and *q* are identical in construction and are mounted on the front of the head between the supply reel and the segmented compaction shoe. They slide in a direction perpendicular to the tape path. The two rotary cutter axes *d* and *e* orient the stylus cutters to the tape. These two axes are similar in construction. The *d*-axis is mounted on the *v*-axis and the *e*-axis is mounted on the *q*-axis. The *v*-*d*- and *q*-*e*-axes perform the motions to cut the desired angle on the tape. The *d*- and *e*-axes normally position simultaneously with *x*- and/or *y*-axis positioning for the next cut at start of course. Cutting is through the composite tape, but not through the backing paper.

The segmented compaction shoe is designed to lay composite tape over contoured surfaces such as pockets (Fig. 9), pad-ups, and overall skin contour while maintaining a fairly even compaction force distribution across the width of the shoe. A tail compaction roller accompanies the tape shoe. This roller is required when the end of the tape is cut diagonally into a long strip (tail) to suit the edge of the ply. A programmable tape-compaction system allows variable tape-compaction pressures to be applied during tape laying. Pressures are changed by the part program or by operator input.

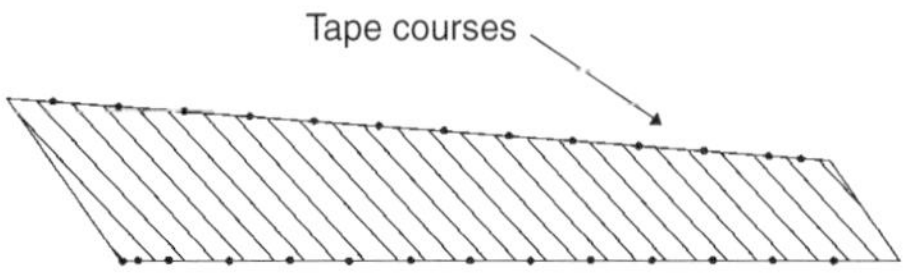

The tape head is equipped with an optical tape-flaw-detection system that signals the machine control to stop laying tape when a flaw marker on the tape has been detected. The tape head also contains a tape-heating system (Fig. 3). For bismaleimide and other dry resin systems that lack appropriate tack for tape-to-tape adhesion, the tape-heating system warms the prepreg to increase tack levels just ahead of the lay-down shoe/roller (Ref 4). Heated tape temperatures range from 26 to 43 °C (80–110 °F).

Control. The CNC is a multiblock buffered-contouring system, which is specifically designed for tape-laying applications. It contains no spindle or tooling functions that are associated with general purpose CNCs (since these are not needed by tape-laying machinery), but has additional functions and flexibility to accommodate different composite tape-laying heads. All operator controls, along with the monitor, are enclosed in a control console, which is located outside the work zone. In addition to the console, a hand-held pendant is provided allowing the operator to control various machine functions from within the working envelope.

Off-Line Programming System. The design and programming system (Fig. 10) aids the user in preparing input data for CNC composite tape-laying machines. Creating the part programs requires special programming techniques because the tape must follow the "natural path" determined by the contour of the tool. Also, individual courses of tape must be positioned to ensure the user's design criteria, including gap and fiber-orientation specifications, are achieved.

Tape courses

Fig. 5 One layer of angled courses for a vertical stabilizer ply

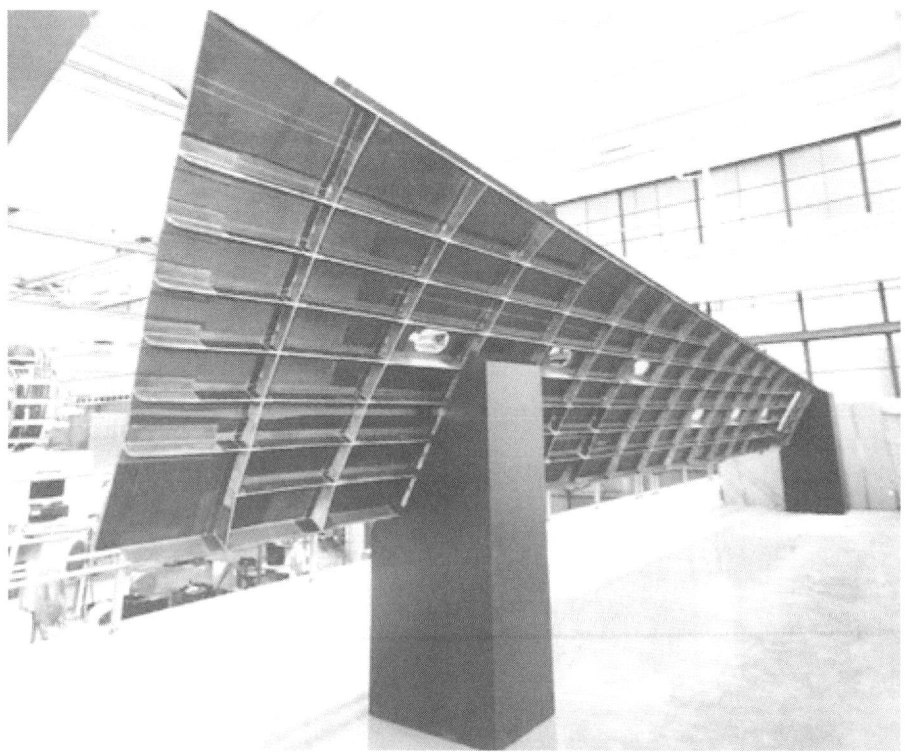

Fig. 6 Airbus A330/340 HTP contour lower skin with stringers, rib shear ties, and spar caps integrated

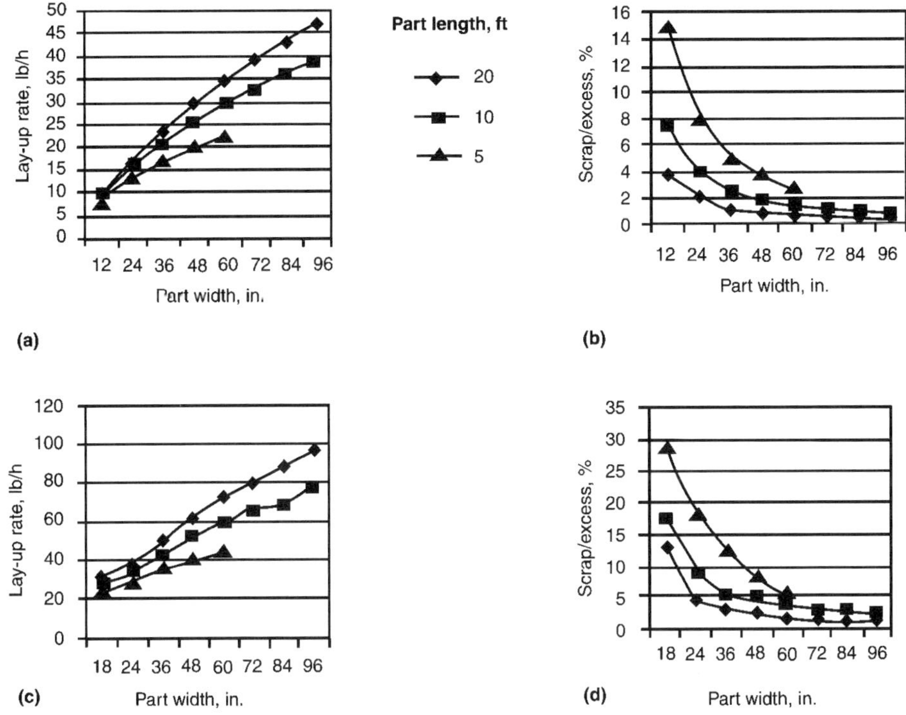

Fig. 7 Estimated flat lay-up and scrap rates for 150 and 300 mm (6 and 12 in.) tape widths. (a) Lay-up rate for 150 mm (6 in.) tape. (b) Scrap rate for 150 mm (6 in.) tape. (c) Lay-up rate for 300 mm (12 in.) tape. (d) Scrap rate for 300 mm (12 in.) tape

The user defines the surface of the tool, ply boundaries, design parameters, and machine processing parameters. Using these file inputs, a batch program creates an automatically programmed tool (APT) source code along with graphics data, log files, and a restart file. The results may be analyzed graphically. The APT source program may be processed by an APT compiler and postprocessor to create the numerically controlled part program for the tape layer.

Tape Laying Process Description

According to the part program, the proper codes and axis position commands are executed to place the tape head onto the mold surface. After touchdown, tape is laid on the mold surface in the manner desired through the use of CNC programmed movements of the machine *x*-, *y*-, *z*-,*c*-, *a*-, *d*-, *e*-, *q*-, *v*-, and *u*-axes.

As the tape is laid on the mold surface, the head is suspended above the tool, with the compaction force being applied by the compaction shoes/roller to the lay-up surface. This reduces tape wandering when traversing over breaks and through valleys (Fig. 8). Compaction force is programmable and is entered from the operator's console. The tape-compaction force across the full width for 150 mm (6 in.) wide tape ranges from 27 to 133 kgf (60–293 lbf), and the total-compaction force across the full width for 300 mm (12 in.) wide tape ranges from 27 to 273 kgf (60–601 lbf). These compaction ranges are used during normal tape lay-up mode.

Prior to the end of each tape course, the tape is cut to suit the angle at the edge of the ply. Cuts are made with either the tape head stopped for a zero-degree cut or with the tape head moving for an angled cut. This operation is performed by four programmed CNC drives (*q*-, *v*-, *d*-, and *e*-axes) that control movement of two cutters. The speed of each linear cutter axis is programmed to be in relationship to the tape speed to establish the angle of the cut. The other two drives provide for rotation of the two cutters about their shaft axis (*d* and *e*). This programmed cutter rotation assures the cutter always will be aligned along the direction of the cut. Cuts are made by cutting through the composite material but without cutting through the backing paper.

After the tape cut has been made, the last portion of the tape is laid either with the compaction roller (if on an angled cut) or with the segmented shoe (if on a zero-degree cut). The head then lifts from the mold surface and moves to the start of the next course of tape to be laid. Tape courses can be laid unidirectional or bidirectional. Typically, bidirectional is faster because it takes less time to rotate the tape head 180° and move to

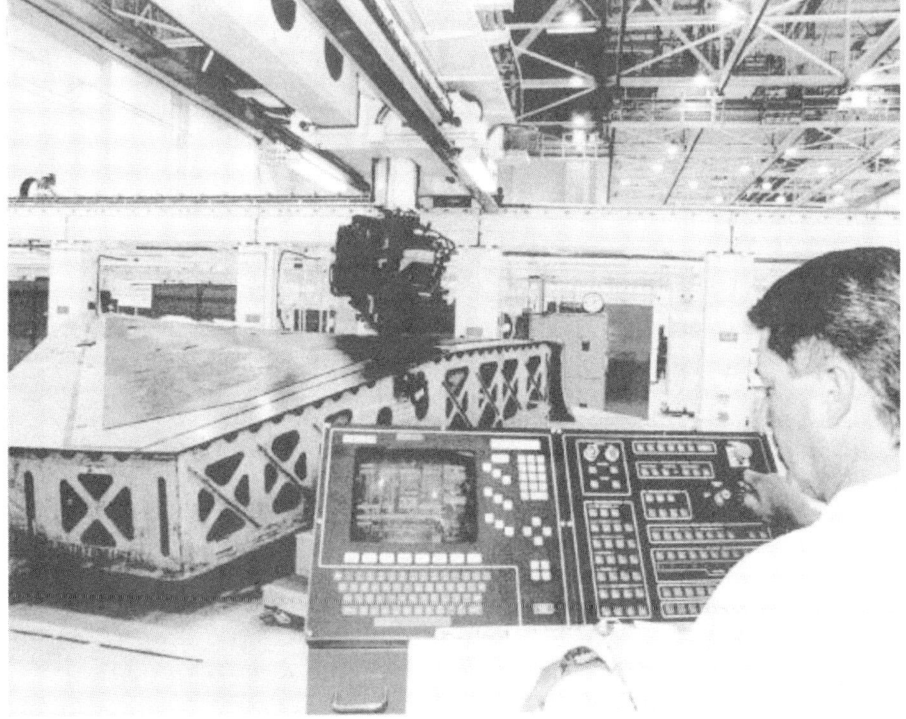

Fig. 8 Contour tape lay-up on an F-22 wing skin

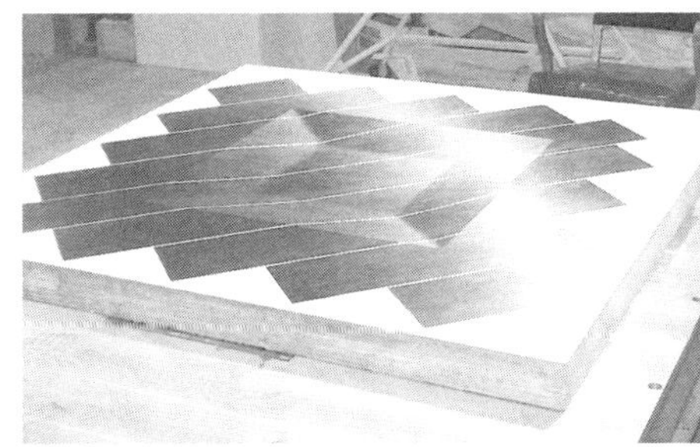

Fig. 9 Contour pocket test tool for automated tape lay-up

the next course than it takes to leave the tape head in the same orientation and move back to the start of the next course. For course lengths that are shorter than 1 m (40 in.), unidirectional and bidirectional lay-up take approximately the same amount of time moving between tape courses. This process repeats to create the finished ply. Plies are laid on top of each other to create the finished laminate.

Typical Material Types and Forms

In general, feedstock materials (tape) suitable for automated tape laying consist of unidirectional carbon fiber or glass impregnated with thermoset resin, supplied in roll form on a backing paper carrier material, on 255 mm (10 in.) inside-diameter cores, and with edges of impregnated fibers flush with backing paper.

Backing Paper and Resin Impregnation. Rolls of composite material for hand lay-up and automated tape lay-up have different requirements. The durability and release coatings of the backing paper carrier material are very important and make ATL-grade supply rolls successful for automated lay-up over material supply rolls for hand lay-up. For example, if the backing paper is not durable enough, problems with backing paper breakage will occur. When the backing paper breaks, the tape head will need to be rethreaded. Improper release coatings will affect how freely the tape will move through the tape head guide chutes and compaction devices. Also, improper release coatings will also affect how well the composite tape is maintained or stays on the backing paper in addition to how well the tape comes off the backing paper during compaction of the tape to the lay-up surface. If the impregnated composite tape separates from the backing paper prior to the cutting, guiding, and compaction devices, poor tape placement on the lay-up tool will occur. If the impregnated composite tape does not come off or separate from the backing paper during compaction, tape placement will also be affected.

Material tack is also a key factor for successful automated tape lay-up. The distribution of the resin through the fibers ("wet-through" or "wet-out") affects how well the tape will adhere to the lay-up tool and to itself when laminating subsequent plies. Prepreg with too little resin on the surface of the fibers will not adhere well to itself or to the lay-up surface and will require tape heating to increase material tack for lamination. Bismaleimides and other toughened epoxy resins also require tape heating to increase material tack for lamination because these resin systems tend to have very low tack. Good wet-out also aids in holding the fibers together during compaction. Prepreg with too much resin on the surface of the tape and too little resin in the center of the tape tends to pull apart or separate during compaction. For example, half of the composite tape may adhere to the lay-up surface while the other half stays on the backing paper. In other words, the tape tears apart.

Design Guidelines

Automated tape laying is among a variety of processing techniques that are used to fabricate composite parts. To best use the tape laying process, part geometry and the method that is used (flat or contour tape laying) must be considered. Depending on part complexity, size, and shape, tape-laid parts are usually flat-to-medium contour and fall into part categories mentioned earlier. Highly contoured aircraft parts such as fuselages, inlet ducts, nose cones, nozzles, sponsons, rotor blade grips, and so on are better suited for fiber placement than tape laying. When considering automated tape lay-up to manufacture a part, the following part features should closely match machine capabilities:

- Ply shapes/fiber angles should fall within the cutter angles available.
- Contour and mold clearance required must be relative to the tape head shape.
- Pad-ups/stiffeners or ramp angles must be accommodated, and the machine must be able to conform to the surface without tape buckling or bridging.
- Composite material formulation and form must be suitable for the part and the process.
- Process requirements such as tape heating need to be considered.
- The width of tape used should be selected to maximize lay-up rates while keeping scrap to a minimum when creating ply shapes.
- Adequate material choices must be available to meet the design requirements of the part.

In areas where the process required does not match the machine's capabilities, manual intervention will be necessary. To reduce manual intervention, it is best to consider the composite materials available, the equipment processing capabilities, and part flow through the plant at the start of a new program.

Consideration must also be given to the lay-up surface or tool. The choice of mold or table surface materials used for bismaleimide (BMI) tape lay-ups, which typically require tape heating, is important. For instance, on the tape-dispensing head itself, special materials are used to help maintain tape temperature once the tape is heated. These same considerations must also be applied to the mold surface. Materials that act as a heat sink must be avoided for BMI tape lay-up. Other typical lay-up surfaces include Invar (iron-nickel alloy) contour tools and aluminum flat tables with vacuum. Tape is laid up directly on the tool surface or on plastic films (Mylar, Tedlar, E.I. DuPont de Nemours and Co., Inc., Wilmington, DE; nylon; etc.) for flat lay-ups held in place with vacuum. Another film used for flat lay-ups is glass/polyphenylene ether (PPE) that is taped down to aluminum tables. The part is laid up and then removed from the glass/PPE film, which remains on the aluminum table.

Outlook

The tape-laying process has played an important role in advancing the use of composites for both commercial and military aircraft applications. Tape laying will continue to be a highly productive and cost-effective solution as more parts are converted from aluminum to composite and as new programs consider composites for added strength, light weight, and fabrication economy. Some examples of future applications could include composite wings for commercial aircraft, windmill blades, structural parts for civil

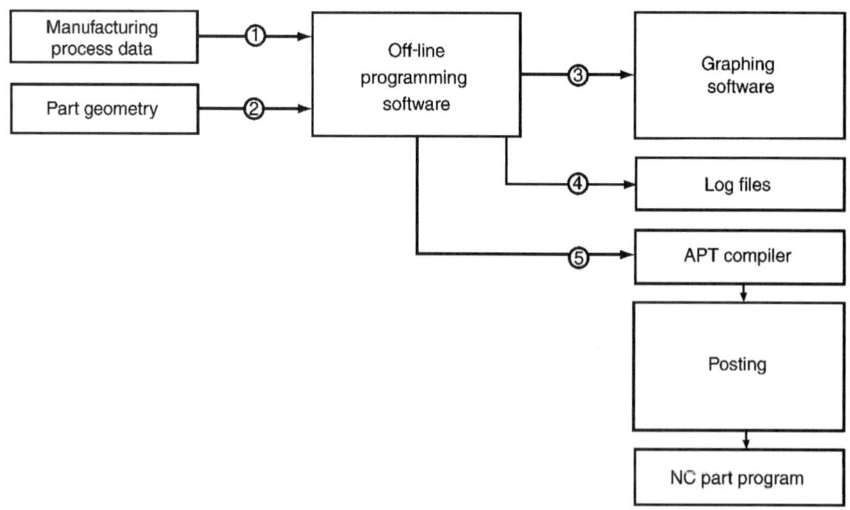

Fig. 10 Programming system block diagram for an automated tape layer. (1) Manufacturing process data include specifications such as tape width, tape thickness, fiber orientation, and gap tolerances. (2) Part geometry consists of numerical descriptions of the contoured surface and boundaries. (3) Graphics data, generated by the software, can be visually displayed with graphing software. (4) Log files are generated by the software and contain exception listings and the ply summary report. (5) APT source code is generated by the software for processing by an APT compiler. NC, numerical control

applications, and structural parts for the automotive and other transportation industries.

ACKNOWLEDGMENTS

The author would like to thank the following companies for reference photos: The Boeing Company, Construcciones Aeronauticas S.A., Aerostructures, and *High-Performance Composites* magazine.

REFERENCES

1. P.F. Pirrung, Flat Tape Laying, *Engineered Materials Handbook,* Vol 1, *Composites,* ASM International, 1987, p 624–630
2. L.A. Williams III, Contoured Tape Laying, *Engineered Materials Handbook,* Vol 1, *Composites,* ASM International, 1987, p 631–635
3. J. Heth, Inside Manufacturing: Automated Tape-Laying Excels for F-22's Wing Skin Panels, *High Perform. Compos.,* Vol 7 (No. 5), Sept/Oct 1999
4. M.N. Grimshaw, J. Beard, Jr., and M.D. Schulz, Automated Tape Layup of a BMI Vertical Stabilizer Skin, *Advanced Composites III: Expanding the Technology,* Proceedings of the Third Conference on Advanced Composites, ASM International and the Engineering Society of Detroit, 1987, p 173–182

Curing

CURING is the irreversible change in the physical properties of a thermosetting resin brought about by a chemical reaction, condensation, ring closure, or addition. Cure may be accomplished by the addition of curing or cross-linking agents, with or without the addition of heat and pressure.

Curing of resins can also be accomplished using ultraviolet radiation and electron beams, but these methods are used for very specific applications and are not commonly used for composite manufacturing.

Preparation for Curing

Processing materials must be added to a composite ply lay-up before autoclave curing. These materials control the resin content of the cured part and ensure proper application of autoclave pressure to the lay-up.

In selecting materials for use in preparing a laminate for curing, cure temperatures and pressures must be considered, as well as compatibility of the processing materials with the matrix system.

Material Types and Functions

The materials usually used in preparing a lay-up for autoclave curing are peel ply (optional), separator, bleeder, barrier, breather, dam (depending on laminate thickness and tooling), and vacuum bag. The materials shown in Fig. 1 and 2 represent complex lay-ups. A generality may be made concerning these materials: Each should be prevented from becoming a possible source of contamination to the composite laminate. Contamination can result in poor adhesion in subsequent bonding or painting operations; also, volatile contaminants can enter the laminate prior to gelation, resulting in porosity and consequent poor matrix-dominant properties. The materials must also be compatible with the maximum cure temperature and pressures required for the matrix system being cured. Each material is discussed subsequently. Maximum use temperatures can be determined by consultation with suppliers.

The peel ply, if used, is placed immediately on top of or under the composite laminate. It is removed just before bonding or painting operations so that a clean, bondable surface is available. It is usually a woven fabric and may be either nylon, polyester, or fiberglass. The fabric is treated with a release agent that must not transfer to the laminate; otherwise, subsequent bonding or painting operations may not be satisfactory. Nylon will not release from phenolics and is not satisfactory for high-temperature curing matrices, such as polyimides or bismaleimides, because its upper use temperature is about 177 °C (350 °F). Nylon can be used if the initial cure temperature is low and if it is removed before postcure. A peel ply can also be used between

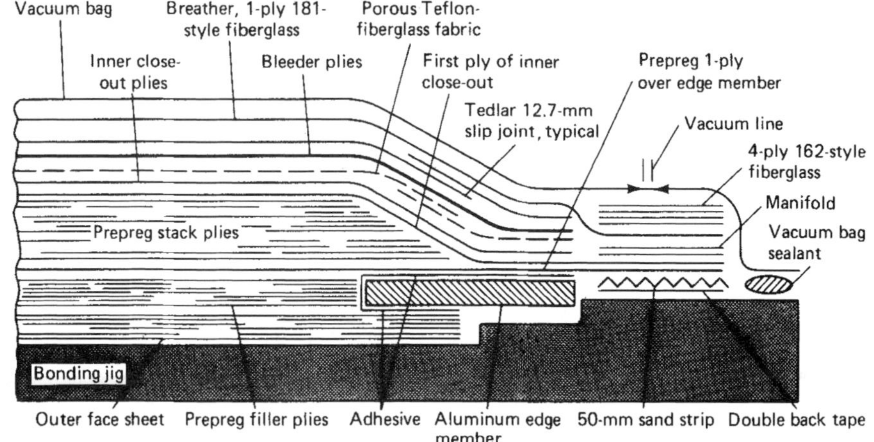

Fig. 1 Complex lay-up, including metal closeout

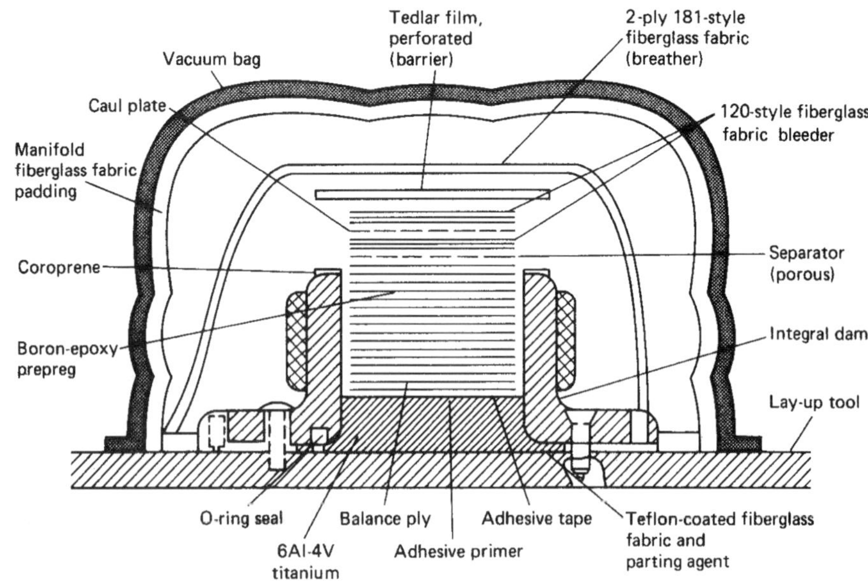

Fig. 2 Complex lay-up showing tool with integral dam. Shown before application of vacuum for clarity. After vacuum is applied, the vacuum bag and fiberglass padding conform to the shape of the tool/lay-up assembly. Note: Lay-up to be co-cured to titanium strap

the mold and a thick laminate to accept entrapped volatiles, thereby preventing porosity in the external composite plies.

A separator (release material) is placed on top of or under the laminate and peel ply (if peel ply is used). It allows volatiles and air to escape from the laminate and excess resin to be bled from the laminate into the bleeder plies during cure. It will also give the cured part a smooth surface, except for porous Teflon (E.I. DuPont de Nemours and Co., Inc.), which gives a slightly textured surface. After cure, the release material must be easily freed from the cured laminate without causing damage. Most separator materials are porous or perforated and contain fluorocarbon polymers. The size and spacing of perforations or the porosity of the material determines the amount of resin flow from the surface of the laminate, thereby lowering resin content (increasing the fiber volume) of the cured part. If no resin removal during cure is desired, totally unperforated separator film should be used. A prepreg with high flow will not be retarded by porous Teflon, which acts as a minibleeder ply and soaks up a small amount of resin.

Bleeder. The purpose of the bleeder material is to absorb excess resin from the lay-up during cure, thereby producing the desired fiber volume. Fiberglass fabric or other absorbent materials or fabrics are used for this purpose. The amount of bleeder used is a function of its absorbency, the fiber volume desired in the part, and the resin content of the prepreg material used in the lay-up. In advanced composites, essentially all excess resin is bled from the surface of the laminate, with edge bleeding being minimized by properly damming the lay-up edges. Personnel should establish tables giving plies of bleeder per ply of lay-up for each prepreg material. These tables are often set up for a particular bleeder material, and then equivalencies are given for other materials. For instance, 1 ply of 181-style fiberglass is considered equivalent to 2.5 plies of 120-style fiberglass fabric.

To determine the correct number of plies to use:

1. Determine resin content of prepreg from receiving inspection data or vendor certification data.
2. Obtain bleeder/prepreg ratio from the table for the given resin content.
3. Multiply number of plies in the lay-up by the bleeder/ply ratio.
4. Round off to the nearest low whole number; this is the number of plies of fiberglass fabric to be used as a bleeder.

For example, to determine the number of plies of 120-style fiberglass fabric required for a 24-ply laminate in which the graphite/epoxy has a resin content of 35.7%:

1. Round off 35.7% to 35%.
2. According to a user table, ratio of bleeder/ply of graphite/epoxy for 35% is 0.27.
3. $24 \times 0.27 = 6.48$
4. Round off to 6; this is the number of bleeder plies.

If the user is willing to tolerate a lower fiber volume with lower cured mechanical properties, bleeding may be eliminated. However, a significant weight increase may occur if the prepreg used in the no-bleed process contains more resin than remains in a cured part subjected to bleeding. An alternative is to obtain a prepreg with an existing fiber volume close to that of the desired final part. Either method eliminates the cost of the bleeder.

Barrier. A nonadhering material, called the barrier, or barrier film, is commonly placed between the bleeder plies and breather plies. In the case of epoxy resins, it is frequently an unperforated film, or barrier film so resin removal from the part can be controlled. For resins that produce volatile by-products during cure, a film with small perforations and large spacing is used to prevent the breather material from becoming clogged with resin and unable to perform its function. Often, a low-cost material such as Tedlar (DuPont) film is used instead of nonporous Teflon, because of the expense of the latter. Thermocouples are installed at the edge of the part between the barrier film and breather plies to monitor part temperature. They also provide the information needed to allow control of the heating medium operation in computer-controlled autoclaves.

The breather is a material placed on top of the barrier film to allow uniform application of vacuum pressure over the lay-up and removal of entrapped air or volatiles during cure. It may be drapable, loosely woven fabric, or felt. Care must be exercised in using coarse, open-weave fabrics, because if bridging of the vacuum bag occurs beyond the elongation properties of the bag material, bag failure will occur, which could result in loss of the part. Some lay-ups use an edge breather consisting of a single fiberglass tow laid along the edges of the composite and draped over the dams.

A dam is sometimes located peripherally to minimize edge bleeding. It may be an integral part of the tool or built in position using materials such as rubber neoprene cork pressure-sensitive tape, silicone rubber, or Teflon or metal bars. Dam height should be approximately the same as the lay-up thickness, including release and bleeder plies, to prevent rounding off of the part edge by the action of the vacuum bag.

The vacuum bag is used to contain any vacuum pressure applied to the lay-up before and during cure and to transmit external autoclave pressure to the part. It prevents any gaseous pressurizing medium used in the autoclave (air or inert gas) from permeating the part and causing porosity and poor or unacceptable part quality. Commonly, an expendable material such as nylon is used for this purpose. Because of the physical and chemical properties of the bag, nylon-6 cannot be used above 160 °C (325 °F), and nylon-6,6 cannot be used above 205 to 215 °C (400 to 420 °F). Neither of these materials is compatible with phenolic resins or certain other matrices. Kapton (DuPont) can be used with polyimides and other materials requiring high-temperature cures. For long runs and highly contoured parts, semipermanent bags may be used. Such bags are commonly made of molded-to-shape rubber. To provide a seal between bag and tool, the bag is commonly secured to the tool with a tape material (bag sealant) that adheres to both the tool and the bag.

The application of the vacuum bag is extremely critical. Bag perforation by the sharp edges of the tool and leakage due to improper sealing at the tool edges may result in a porous part. The complex contours of most aircraft parts often require folds in the bag to take up excess bag material. If these folds are not properly made, or if large wrinkles are left in the bag, undesirable wrinkles may develop in the cured part. Thus, this operation is probably the most critical single step to part quality and must be performed carefully by skilled mechanics.

Autoclave Cure Systems

An autoclave system allows a complex chemical reaction to occur inside a pressure vessel according to a specified time, temperature, and pressure profile in order to process a variety of materials. The evolution of materials and processes has taken autoclave operating conditions from 120 °C (250 °F) and 275 kPa (40 psi) to well over 760 °C (1400 °F) and 69,000 kPa (10,000 psi). The materials processed in autoclaves include metal bonding adhesives, reinforced epoxy laminates, thermoplastic laminates, and metal-ceramic-, and carbon-matrix materials. Although the autoclave system is tailored to specific process requirements, the basic design and subsystems described here are standard for most autoclaves.

The major elements of an autoclave system are a vessel to contain pressure, sources to heat the gas stream and circulate it uniformly within the vessel, a subsystem to pressurize the gas stream, a subsystem to apply vacuum to parts covered by a vacuum bag, a subsystem to control operating parameters, and a subsystem to load the molds into the autoclave.

Pressure Vessel

The pressure vessel shell provides the means to retain pressure inside the work space. The pressure vessel typically is fabricated from carbon steel and lined with galvanized or stainless steel. Plates up to 150 mm (6 in.) thick are rolled to shape and joined by arc welding. The dome-shaped heads or ends are fabricated from similar material and either press-formed or spun.

The most critical portion of the vessel is the closure, or breech lock. A silicone or fluorocarbon rubber material is normally used in this area to allow good sealing without requiring metal-to-metal contact at the door face. The door is usually hinged or carried to one side by a crane.

It is mandatory to design, fabricate, and test all pressure vessels to national and industry-recognized standards. These include material specifications and design stress levels allowable in the vessel.

The autoclave owner must have an approved organization modify or maintain the pressure vessel; any improperly made modification or repair may compromise the integrity of the vessel and subsequent safety. If properly maintained and inspected, the life of a pressure vessel should exceed 50 years.

Internal Structure. The vessel, upon completion and subsequent testing, is prepared for installation of the internal structure, which provides insulation, duct work, and support for all components to be mounted in the autoclave.

The insulation is used to reduce energy costs and keep the exterior at a safe temperature by preventing heat transfer to the vessel. It is typically a ceramic wool material, in sheet or blanket form, and should not be in direct contact with the autoclave atmosphere. The insulation is covered with sheet metal, normally 16- and 18-gage aluminized steel or stainless steel, which is attached in such a way as to allow thermal expansion and protect the insulation from the gas stream in the autoclave.

The duct provides a channel for the gas to be circulated in the autoclave. Provisions for tracks for carts to bring the molds into the autoclave are made.

Gas Stream Heating and Circulation Sources

Currently, several heating methods are available for autoclave systems. The most common method for large autoclaves is indirect gas firing, in which products of combustion from an external chamber are passed through an internal, stainless alloy coil. This system is reliable and can be controlled to allow thermal cycling. The gas-fired systems usually provide substantial operating savings over electrical systems, and are used in autoclaves with maximum operating temperatures of 450 to 540 °C (850 to 1000 °F).

Steam heating can be used for autoclaves operating in the 150 to 175 °C (300 to 350 °F) range. The superheated steam is passed through a coil in the autoclave to heat circulating gas.

Most small autoclaves (under 2 m, or 6 ft in diameter) are electrically heated. Electric heating elements are mounted in the circulating gas stream and configured not to radiate onto the workload in the autoclave. An advantage is the ease of temperature control.

Gas circulation within the autoclave is essential to provide mass flow for temperature uniformity and heat transfer to the part load. This is accomplished with a blower mounted in the rear of the autoclave. The gas is drawn into the blower through the cooling coil and heater, then returned down the length of the autoclave through the annular duct to the door, where it is then directed through the work space. In the modern autoclave system, the fan motor is mounted in a pressurized housing.

The air circulation should be from 1 to 3 m/s (250 to 500 ft/min) in the work space. Circulation any higher than 3 m/s (500 ft/min) may cause problems with the vacuum bags over the parts if they are not properly attached. Variable-speed fan systems are available for improved part heating performance.

Gas Stream Pressurizing Systems

Three pressurization gases are typically used for autoclaves: air, nitrogen, and carbon dioxide. Proportional inlet and vent valves allow autoclave pressures to be controlled and varied precisely. It is important that this very hot gas being introduced into the pressure vessel not impinge on the part load, because the gas stream could cause part damage due to thermal or mechanical shock.

Air is relatively inexpensive when supplied in the 690 to 1030 kPa (100 to 150 psi) range and is acceptable for most 120 °C (250 °F) cures. The main disadvantage of air is that it sustains combustion and thus, may be hazardous at temperatures above 150 °C (300 °F). Nitrogen is the gas most commonly used in autoclaves. The liquid nitrogen is stored in cryogenic form and then vaporized at approximately 1400 to 1550 kPa (200 to 225 psi). Higher-pressure tanks and systems are available. Nitrogen suppresses combustion and diffuses well into the air when the autoclave is opened. However, nitrogen costs can be significant if many autoclaves in a plant are using nitrogen and if the autoclaves are large and operating at high pressure. Carbon dioxide is the second most commonly used gas. It is stored as refrigerated liquid at approximately 2050 kPa (300 psi). Its primary disadvantages are high density, hazards to personnel, and physical flow-related problems. When using any nonlife-sustaining gas, care should be taken not to enter any vessel without ensuring that adequate oxygen is present.

Vacuum Systems

Most parts processed in autoclaves are covered with a vacuum bag, which is used primarily for compaction of laminates and to provide for removal of volatiles. The bag allows the part to be subjected to differential pressure in the autoclave without being directly exposed to the autoclave atmosphere. The vacuum bag is also used to apply varying levels of vacuum to the part.

New production methods have brought increasing complexity to autoclave vacuum systems. Originally, the vacuum systems consisted of a three-way valve that allowed application of vacuum to the part bag or venting of the bag to the atmosphere after pressure application. This proved to be adequate for simple laminates and metal bonding, but as the resin systems became more sensitive and quality control became more stringent, advanced vacuum systems were developed (Fig. 3).

The purpose of these systems is to provide fully computer-controlled manipulation and monitoring of part pressure, not just supply pressure. The ability to provide pressure on the part under the bag by means of vacuum has reduced void content by keeping the dissolved volatiles and water in solution in the resin system itself.

Loading Systems

Loading systems are probably the most perplexing aspect of production confronting the autoclave user. Because of the circular configuration of the vessel and the relatively small size of the components, carts must be designed to distribute parts horizontally and vertically in the autoclave. Other considerations are:

- The loaded parts should be accessible to enable repair of bag leaks.
- All vacuum source and vacuum sensor lines must be connected to the part when loaded on the cart, and vacuum must be maintained as the parts are introduced into the autoclave.
- The cart must be easily rolled or transported into the autoclave.

Designing a cart system to meet all the desired criteria is a challenge. The essential loading-system requirements must be determined, because including one feature will often preclude the inclusion of another. Typically, carts of various configurations are used, based on mold size and shape.

Modified Autoclaves for Specialized Applications

The development of thermoplastic-matrix composites has necessitated the design of specialized equipment for use within autoclaves to form thermoplastic materials. This need has been met with retrofittable processing fixtures that enable the processing of high-temperature materials in existing low-temperature autoclaves. Often, electrically heated molds are used. Autoclaves should be manufactured to incorporate design features that make transitions to new materials relatively simple.

The polyimides and related resin-matrix systems have created a new set of problems in the design of autoclave systems. Primarily, the vacuum control systems have had to be reengineered to accept the large amount of volatiles (resin solvent) released during cure. Also, additional computer interaction is required to process these materials properly.

Metal-matrix composites require systems operating from 480 to 700 °C (900 to 1300 °F) at 6900 to 69,000 kPa (1000 to 10,000 psi) to diffusion bond the matrix into a homogeneous mass. Because of the high-pressure requirement, autoclave systems for curing these composites are usually smaller than others.

Modified autoclaves are being used for processing carbon-carbon composites, both for impregnation and carbonization. These complex

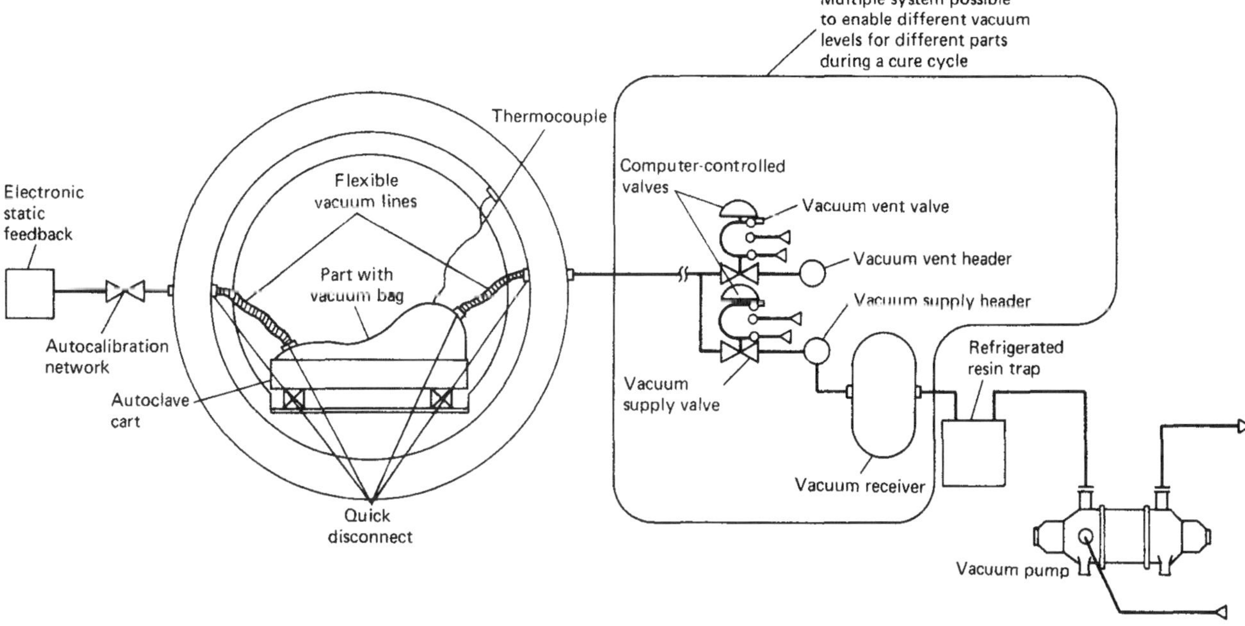

Fig. 3 Advanced vacuum system

autoclaves operate at temperatures up to 815 °C (1500 °F).

Phenolic parts have been processed as exit cones and throats for rocket motors in hydroclaves for many years. A hydroclave is similar to an autoclave, except that it is water flooded and pressurized. Hydroclaves are typically run at 6900 kPa (1000 psi) and 150 to 175 °C (300 to 350 °F).

The vacuum pressure chamber (Fig. 4) is a dedicated flexible process center designed for field repair and remanufacturing of composite parts. Future advances will necessitate more dedicated equipment that is directed to specific applications, yet is functionally similar to the autoclave.

Safety and Installation

It is usually standard to have redundant safety features on any autoclave because of the potential seriousness of any malfunction. Overpressure conditions are usually prevented by three different methods: a separate overpressure sensor and shutdown control, rupture disks designed to rupture at pressures above the operating pressure of the autoclave, and pop-off safety valves with the same function. A standard-production autoclave has all three. Vessels are usually proof tested to high margins of safety, but the danger posed by the possibility of a burst vessel cannot be overemphasized.

Overtemperature protection is not as critical an issue from an injury standpoint, but overtemperature conditions could damage the interior systems of the autoclave; therefore, overtemperature controls are usually provided. The vessel shell, because of the internal insulation, may not be rated to the maximum operating temperature of the autoclave. The external surface of the autoclave should not exceed 60 °C (140 °F), except at penetrations.

Control Systems

Recent developments in sensors and computer technology have greatly increased the ability to monitor and control cure cycles (see the article "Cure Monitoring and Control" in this Volume).

The cure cycle is controlled by feedback from thermocouples, transducers, and advanced dielectric and ultrasonic sensors. The software is growing in complexity, with features varying between suppliers of computer systems.

Autoclave curing of composites attempts to induce specific chemical reactions within polymers that result in predictable engineering properties. Accordingly, control of the curing process should be based on chemical engineering and fluid dynamic principles. This article describes a computerized approach to the simultaneous control of materials reaction behavior and consolidation dynamics, using an autoclave as the reaction vessel.

The primary objectives of computer control of the autoclave process are to improve cured-product quality and reduce fabrication costs by providing:

- Process optimization
- Reduced process inconsistencies and product rejections
- Accurate, real-time quality assurance with rapid error detection and correction
- Verification of process reaction behavior kinetics
- Nondestructive verification of cured properties
- Accurate, permanent process documentation
- Flexibility in adapting to new or modified processes

Aircraft structures are designed on the basis of allowables, which in turn are based on the testing of coupons cured by a specified procedure, which includes time, temperature, heat-up rate, pressure, and vacuum. In production, the parts are cured on tools that vary in geometry, materials, and mass and therefore can result in different thermal cycles. This variance can affect the quality and performance of the laminate. The product characteristics can differ from those in the engineering allowables database.

The computer is programmed to cure the parts according to an algorithm based on the specifications. If any parts cannot be cured properly because of the mass of the tool, the computer

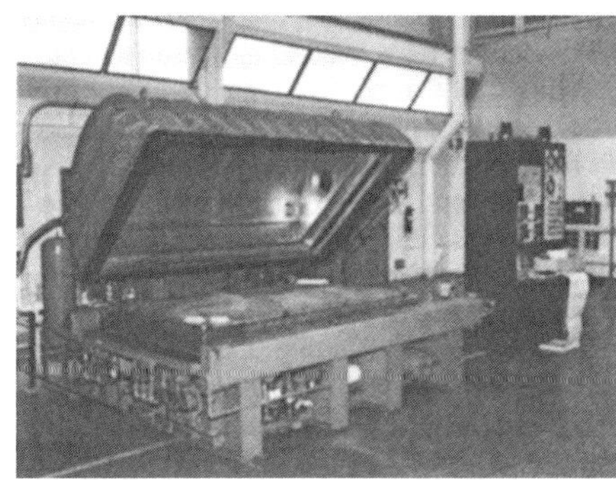

Fig. 4 Vacuum pressure chamber. Courtesy of Naval Air Rework Facility, San Diego

identifies them from its calculation and records the discrepancy in its memory. Thus, parts are cured properly and efficiently, and a proper quality control record is maintained.

Control Dynamics

Composite cure control begins with a basic understanding of the reaction process relationships. The primary regulating parameter for these reactions is temperature. More accurately, the thermal history of a material determines its kinetics, viscoelasticity, morphology, phase precipitation, cross-link density, glass transition properties, and polymer network structure. These are the factors that affect both the process behavior (flow consolidation consistency) and the structural-engineering properties evolved from the cured prepreg.

In addition, each material has different thermal reaction sensitivity characteristics, based on its composition, which define the most tolerant and effective thermal-cure profile. It is the total thermal-cure history that governs the consistency, uniformity, and quality of the chemical curing process, as illustrated in Fig. 5, which shows that a shift of 6 to 9 °C (10 to 15 °F) in temperature can affect the viscosity state a material exhibits during cure. This information, when combined with kinetic data, defines the thermal-control requirements of the process (heat rates, allowable thermal gradients across the entire load, and optimal pressurization time).

The chemistry data are also used to define heat transfer, fluid, and gas transport requirements for the specific part configuration being built. Resin viscosity and kinetics interact with gas diffusion processes and fluid hydrostatic pressure through the time-temperature cure cycle. The laminate quality depends on how well these interactions are controlled to favor void reduction rather than generation.

The autoclave vessel dynamics must also be recognized. The vessel represents a chamber in which air or inert gas is circulated. The vessel can heat or cool this air stream and increase the chamber pressure. Initially, the main reason for the use of autoclaves in composite manufacturing was to achieve uniform pressurization around complex shapes to consolidate the material. Although autoclaves accomplish their function well, autoclave air streams moving across part tooling surfaces create nonuniform air flow disturbance patterns inside the vessel. As a result, heat transfer dynamics to the part become variable and, when coupled with tooling mass variations, part thermal conformance to process requirements is not met. The challenge is to develop logic that recognizes the thermal-variation effects and can control interactively to maintain part conformance.

Temperature Control Logic. The approach to temperature control logic for chemically reactive material uses multiple thermocouple sensors to provide sufficient information for accurate computation of the critical characteristics of the load. The critical parameters that the system must compute are heat rate transfer and part temperature gradients. The heat rate transfer characteristics of the load determine the efficiency of the translation of the power level of the vessel into part temperatures. It is important to realize that this parameter is not constant during a run or repeatable between autoclave runs. It depends on tooling-mass differentials, autoclave loading geometry (air stream deflection and turbulence), vessel temperature, and vessel pressure. Variation in thermal transfer characteristics of the load results in temperature gradients in the parts and variant reaction behavior. The general chemical rule of thumb is that the reaction rates double for every 10 °C (18 °F). The computer calculates the maximum, average, and minimum load heat transfer characteristics dynamically during the process. This information is coupled with vessel temperatures that will optimize uniformity and process rates.

Part temperature gradients result from variable heat transfer characteristics and must be controlled to achieve uniform properties in the composite structure. The composite laminate undergoes the transitions from liquid to gel to glass (vitrification) as a function of the effect of temperature on kinetic behavior. Thus, allowing significant temperature gradients to exist at these transition functions can cause laminate cure stresses, nonuniform laminate consolidation, and trapped volatiles, all of which degrade performance properties.

The initial objectives are to collect sufficient information to characterize the thermal dynamics of the load in real-time and to control the temperature gradient distributions in the part (and, ultimately, the consistency of reaction cure behavior).

Pressure and Vacuum Control Logic. Vacuum, actually a subset of pressure, refers to the level of pressure in the part bag envelope. Pressure control follows a logic that is similar to that of temperature. This allows for diffusion control of volatiles, which can reduce the potential for laminate porosity. The process specification defines the vessel and bag pressurization requirements, based on cycle times and part temperature. The resultant control output signals are sent to the vessel and bag manifold regulating circuits, respectively.

Other real-time controls include monitoring resin viscosity, resin chemical characteristics, and ply thickness.

Other Process Cures

Room-temperature curing is the most advantageous in terms of energy savings and portability. Efforts continue to produce room-temperature cure resin systems with improved physical characteristics.

Oven curing is much like the autoclave method. Vacuum bagging is used for consolidation and the removal of trapped gasses. The pressure is limited to the difference to atmospheric pressure. Shrink-wrap tapes can be used to apply additional pressure to the composite. This is practical when the geometry is simple, such as a cylindrical composite sleeve being shrunk on a metal shaft.

Hot presses are used for bulk molding compounds and prepregs. The pressure, temperature, and cycle time are readily controlled. The metal tooling is heated internally. Good dimensional tolerances can be achieved.

Resin transfer molding may be used with room-temperature cure resins or may be cured at elevated temperatures.

Pultrusion uses a heated die to create shapes with constant cross sections. The geometry of the die and the pull rate determine the cure

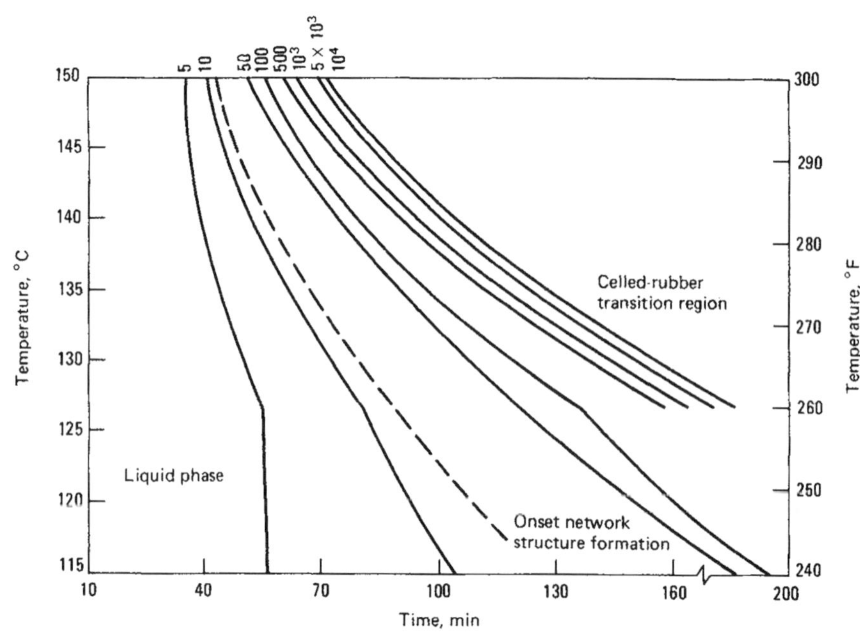

Fig. 5 Effect of temperature and time on material viscosity during cure

time. Cure time, temperature control, and material consistency is critical, because the material must be fully cured just as it exits the die.

Thermoplastic Composites

Thermoplastics are not cured, but they are heated to a sufficient temperature to be molded into the desired shape with vacuum and/or pressure. The processes of thermoforming reinforced thermoplastics does share some of the same challenges of temperature, pressure, vacuum control, and material consistency.

ACKNOWLEDGMENTS

This article was compiled, in part, from the following articles in *Composites,* Volume 1, *Engineered Materials Handbook,* ASM International, 1987:

- T.W. McGann and E.R. Crilly, *Preparation for Cure*, p 642–644
- T. Taricco, *Autoclave Cure Systems,* p 645–648
- R.J. Hinrichs, *Computerized Autoclave Cure Control,* p 649–653

Resin Transfer Molding and Structural Reaction Injection Molding

C.D. Rudd, University of Nottingham

RESIN TRANSFER MOLDING (RTM) and structural reaction injection molding (SRIM) belong to a family, sometimes denoted liquid composite molding. The common feature is the injection of a liquid polymer through a stationary fiber bed (Fig. 1). Impregnation relies on a pressure gradient, and the way that this is created, together with the nature of the tooling, defines the process. Several variants can be identified in addition to the two main processes given in the title. Many of these rely on subtly different applications of vacuum to drive the resin flow and are covered elsewhere in this Volume. This article reviews mainly those techniques that use hard tooling and positive (superatmospheric) pressures to produce structures.

Technique Characteristics

Main Features and Drivers. One of the principal advantages of liquid molding is the absence of a single, defined process. The tooling and process can be configured to suit the economics of the application. For one-off molding and large structures single-sided tooling with vacuum-driven impregnation is normal, while for high volumes reactive processing combined with matched steel molds and robotic assembly of fiber preforms provide the highest throughputs. This flexibility permits economic processing across a broad range of production volumes, although the principal range of interest is up to 35,000 and 100,000 units per year for RTM and SRIM, respectively.

Liquid molding competes with most of the open-mold and closed-mold alternatives. The significant advantages and disadvantages are listed in Table 1. The major shifts toward this family of process can be attributed to three important factors:

- New or threatened legislation concerning volatile organic compound (VOC) emissions. This is manifested largely in new applications for vacuum infusion for low-volume fabricators.
- Cost-reduction drives in the aerospace industry. Here the shift is away from high-cost prepregs toward lower-cost fabrics and epoxy resins using RTM, resin-film infusion (RFI), and vacuum infusion.
- Niche-market vehicles in the automotive industry. Low- and intermediate-volume vehicle bodies are uneconomic to manufacture in stamped metal. Below 35,000 units/yr attractive savings in investment costs are possible by using liquid molding instead of sheet molding compounds (SMCs).

Process Capabilities and Economics. Process throughput is largely a function of investment. Figure 2 shows a typical cycle breakdown for a large component. Aside from handling operations that benefit from investment in automation, the two main factors are injection and heating/curing times. Simple gravity or vacuum-driven injection systems may be useful for low-

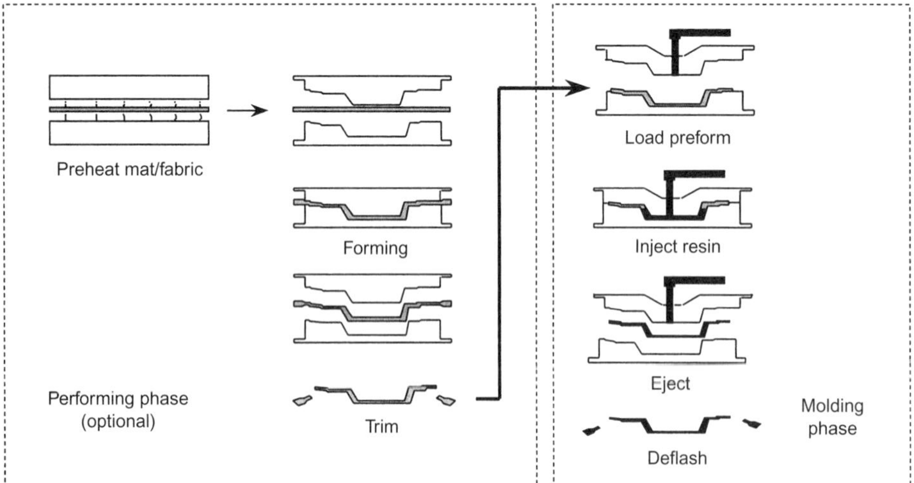

Fig. 1 Liquid molding process

Table 1 Advantages and disadvantages of liquid composite molding versus competitive processes

Advantages of liquid molding	Disadvantages of liquid molding
Versus open mold/wet laminating	
Reduction/elimination of VOC emissions	Higher investment costs–tooling and equipment
Improved uniformity, quality assurance	
Two cosmetic faces	
Reduced labor costs	
Versus prepreg processing/vacuum bag and autoclave	
Reduced materials costs	Higher tooling costs
Reduced labor costs	In-house resin formulation
Thick sections possible–easier debulking	Greater quality assurance responsibility (molder)
Direct control of thickness and fiber volume fraction	
Flexible use of reinforcement, resins	
Fewer shelf life issues	
Versus compression molding/SMC, BMC	
Reduced tooling costs	Longer cycle times
Fewer shelf life issues	In-house resin formulation
Use of structural performs	Greater quality assurance responsibility (molder)
	Greater floorspace requirement

volume or prototyping work, but most industrial operators rely on positive-pressure systems that operate between 2 and 10 bar. Typical filling rates are 1 to 3 L/min (0.26–0.79 gal/min), although exact values depend on the gating strategy, fiber fraction, and the nature of the injection system. SRIM metering systems may double these outputs. Heating and curing times vary with part thickness and resin formulation. Urethane-based SRIM resins may be sufficiently rigid for demolding within 40 s of mold fill, while thick sections or epoxy laminates may require several hours in the mold. Process times are generally competitive with SMC for small parts, where 3 min seems a reasonable target, while larger items (>1 m^2, or 10.8 ft^2) require 20 min or more.

Flexibility in the use of materials is one of the key attributes of liquid molding. Industrial applications involve a variety of reinforcement styles, although the main split is between the aerospace sector, using more or less exclusively fabrics, and the automotive industry, where random reinforcements are used for appearance and semistructural items. However, as vehicle manufacturers and their suppliers make further inroads toward fully structural composite bodies some convergence is likely. Whichever route is followed, a wide range of reinforcements styles can be incorporated, including the relatively narrow range of fabrics used in prepregging, as well as less conventional braids, three-dimensional weaves, for example. Fiber architecture imposes the main limit on achievable volume fraction of fiber (V_f); 65 vol% is feasible for flat panels (although 60% is a more realistic target), while for (continuous) random reinforcements 35 vol% represents a practical ceiling.

Cost reduction provides the rationale for the majority of new applications. Automotive manufacturers seek reductions in tooling costs, and this provides an operating window that competes with the lower band of SMC applications (typically up to 35,000 units). Conversely, aerospace operators look to offset the higher investment costs associated with RTM by lower-cost materials, since the manufacture of an intermediate prepreg is eliminated. One cost-saving feature that is common to both sectors is component integration, whereby several moldings or stampings can be combined with a substantial reduction in tooling investment. A simple example is the manufacture of a one-shot sandwich panel in RTM (Fig. 3) that replaces separately molded skins and a secondary bonding operation. Clearly, the same approach can be extended to much more complex structures as demonstrated by several studies from the automotive sector.

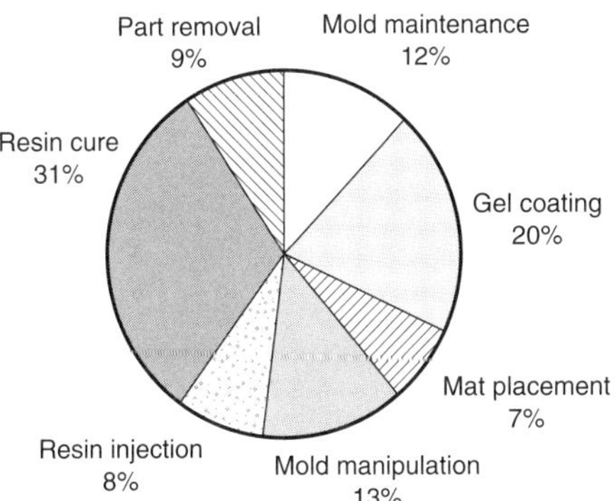

Fig. 2 RTM cycle time breakdown for typical industrial part

Applications

Automotive. Many of the prominent applications of liquid molding have been automotive. Lotus (U.K.) introduced vacuum-assisted resin injection (VARI) for the 1974 Elite, which continued for the 1990 Elan. The Dodge Viper (U.S.A.) is another example of a low-volume, high-performance vehicle with RTM body panels and SRIM bumper beams; similar is Aston Martin's DB7 (UK), with the hood, fenders, and deck-lid in RTM. The latter manufacturer extended its use of composites in the 2001 Vanquish with A pillars, front-crash structure, and transmission tunnel in RTM. Other low-volume applications of note include GM's Corvette (USA) and Alpha Romeo Spider (Italy) convertible hard tops, Ford Aeromax 120 (USA) and Mack (USA) truck hoods, Iveco (Europe) Eurocargo truck cab roofs, and BMW Z-1 (Germany) body panels.

In addition to mainstream passenger vehicle and truck parts, resin transfer molding has made successful inroads into low-volume niche vehicles for defense applications including the manufacture of all-terrain-vehicle bodies. Djurner and Palmqvist (Ref 1) describe one example of an all-terrain-vehicle body designed to withstand the high loads imposed during helicopter lift. Large panels were made using unsaturated polyester and acrylic resins with preformed continuous filament random mat (CFRM) reinforcement.

The Renault Espace (France) provides what is probably the most notable example at medium volumes. Matra produced the RTM body panels and closures for this vehicle, which were installed onto a galvanized steel space frame. The Espace became a victim of its own success when sales demand outpaced production capability, and body manufacture switched to SMC.

One of the first commercial applications for SRIM was a bumper beam for the 1989 Chevrolet Corvette. New application areas under investigation include underhood parts, for example, radiator supports, lamp housings, and oil pans. Other emerging application areas include structural cross-members, truck beds, and floor pans.

The most successful high-volume applications have been the manufacture of foam-cored spoilers by Sotira (France) using RTM and variants on that process for a variety of European vehicles. The process reached maturity for nonstructural parts with the introduction of RTM rear spoilers for the 1995 Ford Fiesta at projected annual volumes of up to 250,000 vehicles/yr. Front bumper beams for the General Motors' all-purpose vehicles (Lumina, Silhouette, and Trans Sport) have also been produced at annual volumes in excess of 115,000. Further potential high-volume applications include semistructural seating components such as the BMW (Germany) 300 series seat back.

Aerospace. Early examples of aerospace applications include the manufacture of radomes. These are generally produced in monolithic or syntactic cored laminates using a woven or knitted sock preform. A typical example is that of the (U.K.) Royal Air Force (RAF) Tornado fighter with an overall length of approximately 2 m and major diameter of 1.6 m. One of the best documented aerospace applications has been blading for aircraft and hovercraft propellers (Ref 2), using a complex preforming process that includes fabric, mat, foam injection, and braiding. Several successful airframe parts were produced for the (USA) F-22 and F117-A fighter aircraft. These replace, for example, hand-laminated sine-wave spars at a reported cost saving

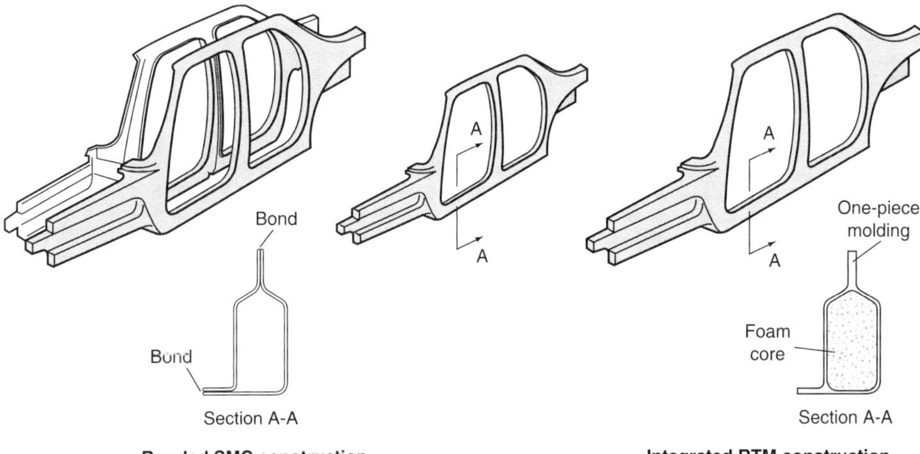

Fig. 3 Sandwich panel manufacture by liquid molding versus bonded SMC. Courtesy of Ford Motor Company

of more than $25,000 per aircraft. Other applications include engine inlet glands and fuselage frames, both of which are fracture critical, having equivalent or improved structural properties compared with prepregs and demonstrably lower void levels. Aeroengine applications have grown also. Boeing's blocker door replaced a 40-piece aluminum assembly with a six-piece carbon/epoxy fabrication manufactured in matched metal molds. Similarly, inlet and fan exit casings, thrust reversers, and cascades have also been produced by Dow-UT. Each of these parts is flight critical and has been certified by the Federal Aviation Administration (FAA), generally replacing titanium alternatives.

Technique Description

The basic approach consists of loading the mold cavity with the required level of reinforcement, closing to a predetermined cavity height, and injecting a liquid resin at positive pressure. The reinforcement (preform) may contain inserts of rigid foam or other materials, while the polymer phase is (usually) introduced as a thermosetting resin. As indicated earlier, there are many variants on this simple approach, which have been developed to speed production, to reduce tooling costs, or to improve properties. The more important variants are discussed briefly in the sections that follow.

Structural reaction injection molding (Fig. 4) relies on polyurethane chemistry. The high reactivity of the material, once mixed, demands rapid dispensing and close metering. The key to SRIM is the rapid delivery of low-viscosity reactants on a metered basis through (usually) an impingement mix head into a heated mold. Delivery is via a piston or lance system. The delivery rates are controlled to modify process times or polymer properties. The separate storage tanks are usually heated and agitated, while the reactants are recirculated to the mix head and back to the tanks periodically in order to maintain the entire system at uniform temperature. Many materials are moisture sensitive, which requires the reactants to be stored under a blanket of dry nitrogen. Although the reactants are stable in isolation, polymerization is extremely rapid once mixed. Thus it is necessary to clear the mixing device of any material following a molding shot. Self-cleaning impingement mix heads are now common.

Most commercial reactive processing facilities involve two streams. Occasionally a third stream will deliver pigments, and so forth. High flow rates mean that the dynamic response of the system needs to be very fast, and the delivery needs to be metered very carefully. For piston or lance-based pumps this is usually monitored using linear displacement transducers. Hydraulic actuation is used exclusively for the dispensing devices. Depending on the materials being processed, the reactant temperatures may be 30 to 200 °C (85–390 °F), although 50 to 90 °C (120–195 °F) is common for urethanes. The tanks and hardware are maintained at the necessary temperature by circulating hot oil or water, while the delivery lines are kept warm by circulating the reactants. For high-viscosity systems, trace heating is used on resin supply lines and fittings. A comprehensive review of RIM processing and processing equipment is provided by Macosko (Ref 3).

Vacuum-assisted resin injection has broad industrial applications. Lotus pioneered its use, although the original process is generally attributed to Hoechst. Vacuum-assisted resin injection molds are usually vented. A partial vacuum is applied to provide mold clamping, reinforcement compaction, and an increase in the forcing-pressure gradient. The reduced internal pressure minimizes mold deflections, which is particularly important when producing large-area moldings in low-cost, lightweight molds. Hayward and Harris (Ref 4) demonstrated a significant increase in laminate mechanical properties, attributed to reduced voidage resulting from the partial vacuum; removing air from within fiber bundles improved wet through and reduced voidage at a microscopic level.

Vacuum Infusion. A logical extension of VARI is to evacuate the mold cavity completely prior to impregnation. This technique has two main applications:

- The manufacture of aerospace composites with low void fractions
- Low-investment manufacture under flexible tooling

In the first case, the vacuum (1–5 mm Hg) is generally augmented by a positive resin supply pressure, while in the second case the resin supply is generally at atmospheric pressure. This process is popularly known as VARTM, RIFT, SCRIMP, and so forth and is covered in detail elsewhere in this Volume.

Vacuum-injection processes have been used for glider ailerons, railroad coachwork, and for a wide range of marine structures. The principle is that a sealed mold cavity, containing a preform, is created between the vacuum bag and a relatively stiff mold. This cavity is then evacuated, which compacts the reinforcement and removes the residual air. Resin is then introduced to the cavity (usually via a peripheral gallery) and impregnates the reinforcement as it advances toward the central suction point(s). Since the process is carried out at atmospheric pressure, the degree of rigidity required in the tooling is minimal. The mold is generally a gel-coated glass/epoxy laminate with a heating matrix embedded in an epoxy concrete backing. Since the available pressure difference is limited to around 1 bar, resin velocities are lower than those in conventional RTM. Although peripheral gating speeds up the filling phase, fill times can be prohibitive for large parts. Thus, flow-enhancing fabrics are used to increase effective preform permeability. While the creation of easy-flow channels within the preform is generally undesirable due to the difficulty of ensuring complete air removal, the presence of the vacuum means that the danger of air entrapment is greatly reduced. A useful review is given by Williams et al. (Ref 5).

Resin-Film Infusion (RFI). This process lies somewhere between traditional autoclave molding and vacuum infusion. A single molding tool is used in combination with a vacuum bag to drive the impregnation. The resin is introduced as a film or pelletized solid at the same time as the reinforcement. The raw materials are then enclosed as for conventional vacuum bagging, and

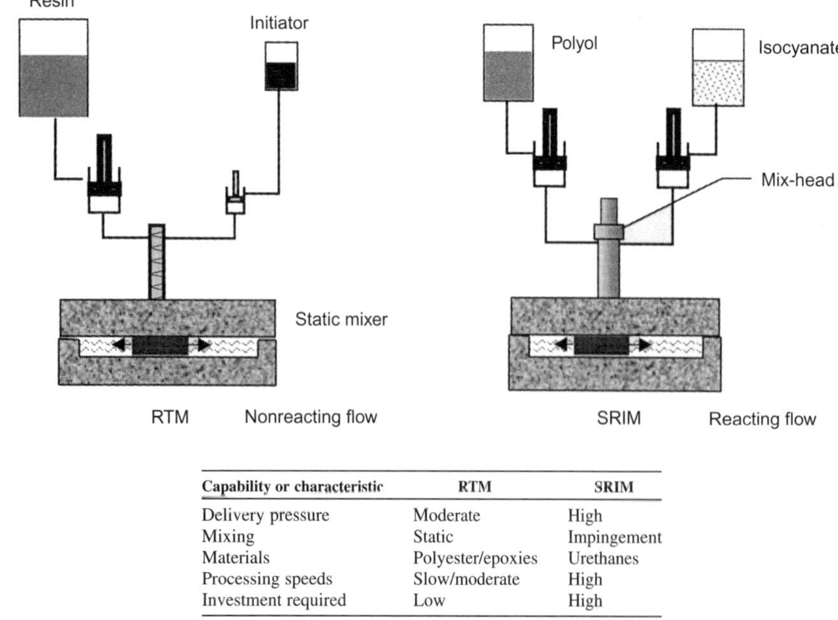

Capability or characteristic	RTM	SRIM
Delivery pressure	Moderate	High
Mixing	Static	Impingement
Materials	Polyester/epoxies	Urethanes
Processing speeds	Slow/moderate	High
Investment required	Low	High

Fig. 4 Comparison of RTM and SRIM processes

the resulting assembly is taken through a heat and pressure cycle to reduce the matrix viscosity sufficient for impregnation prior to gel and cure. Materials costs are lower than with prepreg, and through-thickness properties can be improved by stitching or three-dimensional fabrics. The main attraction of RFI is probably for parts of high surface area. Since the flow is through-thickness, the in-plane dimensions are relatively unimportant, whereas in conventional RTM they influence the filling time strongly.

Injection-compression molding involves loading the preform, partially closing the mold cavity (Fig. 5), and injecting a metered resin shot. The degree to which the mold halves are held apart during injection varies in practice, but is generally only a small fraction of the overall cavity height. A small increase in thickness results in a relatively large change in preform permeability; thus the resin can be injected relatively quickly. Since the resin charge is injected into an expanded cavity, it will only impregnate a portion of the final surface area of the part. The final compression stroke, which closes the cavity down to its final design thickness, provides the squeezing action necessary to cause the in-plane flow, which fills the cavity. A proprietary version of the process has been used with a high degree of success in the manufacture of automotive spoilers (Ref 6).

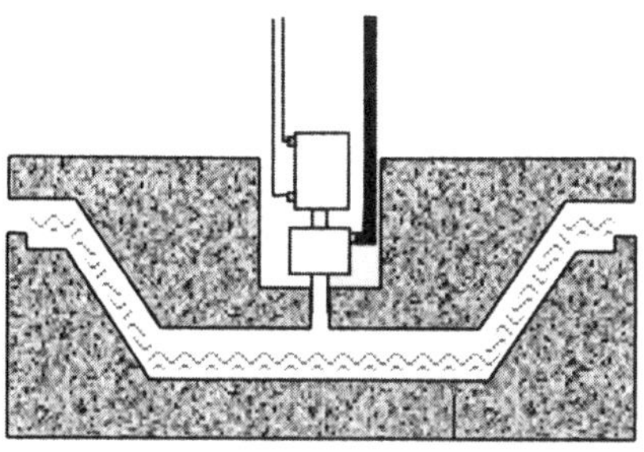

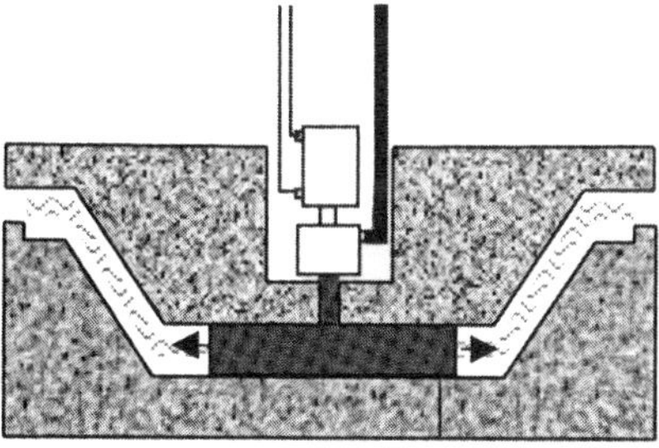

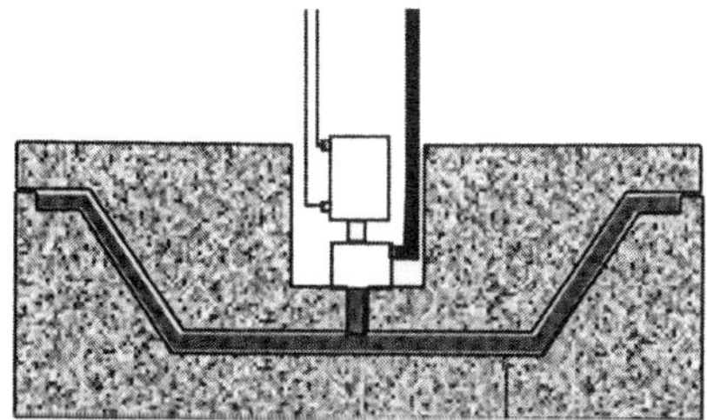

Fig. 5 Injection-compression molding. Initial stand-off enables rapid injection due to increased permeability. The final compression stroke provides rapid fill-out and void collapse.

Material Types and Forms

The materials used in liquid molding do not vary greatly from the conventional mats, fabrics, and resins used in wet laminating or press molding. Where significant differences occur, these generally involving adjustment of either the resin viscosity, gel time, or the reinforcement architecture to provide relatively easy flow during impregnation. This section provides a brief overview of the materials that are commonly used together with some of the processing characteristics that are important to processing speed and part quality.

Reinforcement Materials. Moldings can be made successfully using most conventional forms of mat and fabric reinforcements. The two important exceptions to this rule are chopped-strand mats, which are usually made with high-solubility binders and are therefore susceptible to fiber washing and dense preforms produced exclusively from monofilaments as these have very low permeabilities. Some fabrics are produced specifically for liquid molding. These are termed flow-enhancing fabrics and contain warp-bound tows that create local flow channels in an otherwise low-permeability region.

The major decision that impinges on structural design is the choice of preforming route. This influences the available fiber orientations and volume fractions. Low-volume parts or simple preforms are best assembled by hand in the mold using mats or fabrics. However, this is time consuming and introduces variability. Hand-placed reinforcements tend to be combined with a pinch-off, and this necessitates a postmold trimming operation. Alternatively, net-shape preforms can be produced conveniently by thermoforming the same materials using thermoplastic powder as a binder. Conventional systems use infrared ovens and low-cost stamping presses, which are often actuated pneumatically, since the pressures involved are limited to a few bar. The fiber volume fraction available with CFRM implies a maximum tensile modulus of approximately 10 GPa (1450 ksi) and tensile strength of up to 120 MPa (17 ksi). For higher performance, fabric reinforcements are used, and these include a wide range of woven products and the so-called zero crimp or engineered fabrics. Engineered fabrics offer greater flexibility depending on their method of construction and are produced as multilayer fabrics stitched together with nonstructural yarns. Standard configurations include quasi-unidirectional, 0°/90°, ±45°, and quasi-isotropic (0°/+45°/90°/–45° or –60°/+60°/120°). Custom arrangements can always be procured, although the setup costs tend to be prohibitive for short runs. The construction of both woven and engineered fabrics influences not only the mechanical performance of the part but the ease with which it can be formed into a complex shape (drapeability) and impregnated with liquid resin (permeability). Both of these issues are addressed in subsequent sections.

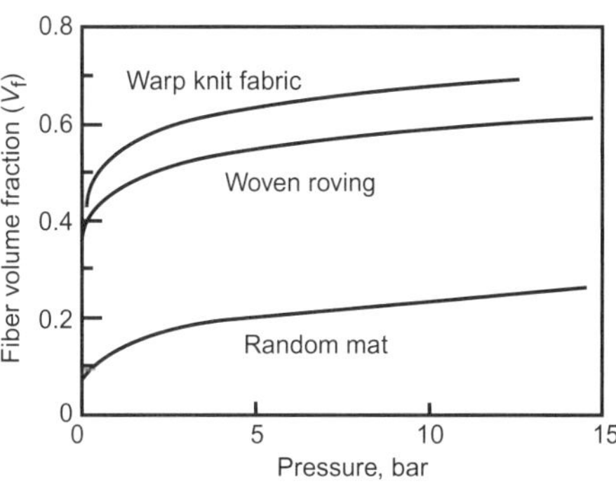

Fig. 6 Typical reinforcement compaction behavior at ambient temperature. Source: Ref 7

Large (e.g., marine) structures cannot be formed effectively to produce a handlable preform. These are often dealt with using combination mats or fabrics that are prestitched to reduce labor costs and assembly times. Typical examples include woven/chopped fiber assemblies and random mat skins fastened to a polyester felt to form a lightweight sandwich construction.

Unlike prepregs, liquid molding is relatively flexible in its use of different reinforcement styles. Thus, textile techniques such as braiding or three-dimensional weaving can be used to provide other fiber architectures. Braiding is useful for closed sections (especially tubular components) and provides either biaxial (±ϕ) reinforcement, which provides good torsional properties, or, when axial or bending loads dominate, 0° reinforcements can be inlaid using a triaxial braid. The principal advantage of three-dimensionally woven structures is for applications demanding high through-thickness or impact properties. Similar effects can be achieved by through-stitching with Kevlar. These techniques are likely to be of future interest for aerospace applications, where a degree of shaping potential, plus the facility to vary the balance of through-thickness and in-plane reinforcements, offers useful flexibility for structural design.

Reinforcement Processing Characteristics. The relationship between compaction pressure and fiber volume fraction is important since this dictates the mold-clamping force for a given laminate thickness (Fig. 6) (Ref 7). Compaction forces may be of the same order as the resin pressure. The transverse compliance is also a function of temperature and saturation arising from the heat-softening characteristics and lubrication effects, respectively. Compliance is relatively easy to measure directly using a mechanical testing machine or, in an industrial environment, a simple arrangement can be set up using a dial gage together with a series of weights.

Permeability is defined by Darcy's law and describes the ease with which the resin will impregnate the reinforcement. In general, permeability decreases exponentially with increasing fiber volume fraction and will also be higher for random reinforcements than aligned fiber materials (Fig. 7). This effect is tied to both the operating volume fraction and the reinforcement architecture. Reinforcement permeability is related strongly to wetted surface area and, as such, reduces dramatically as the fiber volume fraction is increased. The time necessary to impregnate a given geometry from a constant-pressure resin supply is generally proportional to the porosity (proportion of voidage) divided by the permeability. Conversely, when using a positive-displacement pump the pressure required to impregnate the same geometry will be proportional to the inverse of this relationship. Thus, the reinforcement design is linked closely to the characteristics of the processing equipment and the molding cycle time. Typical relationships between in-plane permeability and reinforcement volume fraction are illustrated in Fig. 7 (Ref 8).

Although quoted values of permeability provide a convenient basis for comparing reinforcements, it is worth remembering that this relies on a very approximate description of the impregnation process. The reinforcement structure is generally heterogeneous, which is to say that the pore space is not distributed evenly between the fibers. Large gaps may exist between adjacent yarns, while the spacing between filaments within these yarns is likely to be orders of magnitude lower. These variations may provoke "flow-fingering" during impregnation and subsequent entrapment of microvoids within the yarns. Such phenomena depend on the architecture of the reinforcement, the resin flow rate (or imposed pressure difference), and the viscosity and surface tension of the resin. Where microvoidage problems arise they can often be reduced (but not necessarily eliminated) by vacuum assistance and by reducing the flow rate to a value that approaches that of capillary action. However, the latter method may be impractically slow. Alternative strategies for void removal include purging with an excess of resin and "burping" or introducing several packing-venting cycles where the cavity pressure is alternatively raised and then vented following mold fill. Other potential sources of microvoids include the entrainment of air in liquid resin during mixing (which can be dealt with via a degassing phase) and the presence of volatiles within the mold cavity.

Where complex curvature exists in the part, it may be desirable to consider the formability of the reinforcement. Random reinforcements can tolerate uniaxial strains of around 30% before fiber straightening limits further stretching. Fabrics deform via a different mechanism due to the presence of the straight, inextensible tows. The dominant mechanism here is in-plane shear, and most materials exhibit nonlinear stress-strain behavior up to the so-called locking angle. Comparative measurements can be made using a simple parallelogram fixture. While the forces themselves are of relatively little interest, it may be useful to know the point at which locking occurs. This is usually taken as the point at which fabric wrinkling becomes evident and occurs at around 30°. The effective locking angle is a function of the fabric architecture (Fig. 8) (Ref 9) and, for zero crimp fabrics, is controlled by the presence of holding stitches.

Resin Systems. Most of the familiar resin types can be processed by liquid molding including polyesters, acrylics, phenolics, epoxies, and bismaleimides. The controlling factor here is viscosity and an upper limit of 0.8 Pa · s (similar to a heavy motor oil) provides a useful rule of thumb. Where the viscosity exceeds this value, it may be necessary to introduce either resin preheating or a low viscosity, reactive diluent. The latter are used widely for vacuum infusion due to the low-pressure gradients available in that process.

Unsaturated polyesters represent the largest tonnage and are used mainly in nonstructural parts. The low-viscosity requirement generally dictates a higher styrene content than normal laminating resins, although fillers and shrinkage control additives can be used in the usual way. Epoxies fall into three main categories: very-low-viscosity (0.3 Pa · s) formulations for vacuum infusion, which use reactive diluents to reduce fill times, medium-viscosity (0.5 Pa · s) formulations for RTM, and high-performance resins, which require substantial preheat temperatures to achieve the low viscosities necessary for injection. Epoxy formulations for SRIM have also been developed that combine low viscosity (using preheat) with a high reactivity hardener to give rapid fill and fast cure (<5 min), although significant applications have yet to emerge. Aerospace applications requiring higher-temperature performance usually use bismaleimides, and here again the high room-temperature viscosities usually require preheat temperatures in the region of 100 °C (210 °F) for injection.

Structural reaction injection molding relies almost exclusively on polyurethanes (although a number of other polymers can be processed in this way). These differ slightly from conventional RIM systems in that the gel time is extended to take account of the longer fill times that accompany the use of a preform. To provide a compromise between the rapid processing of polyurethanes and the ease of handling of polyesters, several hybrid resins have been developed for RTM. These use styrene monomer with an isocyanate component, together with conventional organic peroxide curing agents.

Although virtually all of the established processes use thermosets, there are several thermoplastics that can be processed via liquid molding. Since the major factor inhibiting impregnation with thermoplastic resins is their high viscosity, one potential solution is to impregnate using monomers and polymerize the thermoplastic in situ. The technology used here is that of RIM, for which–aside from urethanes–polyamide 6 is the best known application. Relatively few studies have been reported for fiber composites, and most of the development has focused on NYRIM, a variant patented by DSM. Related processing for polyamide 12 has been patented by EMS Chemie (Ref 10), which uses anionically polymerized laurolactam to produce either a fiber reinforced part directly or an intermediate, thermoformable prepreg. To overcome pot-life problems, a liquid-activator system was devel-

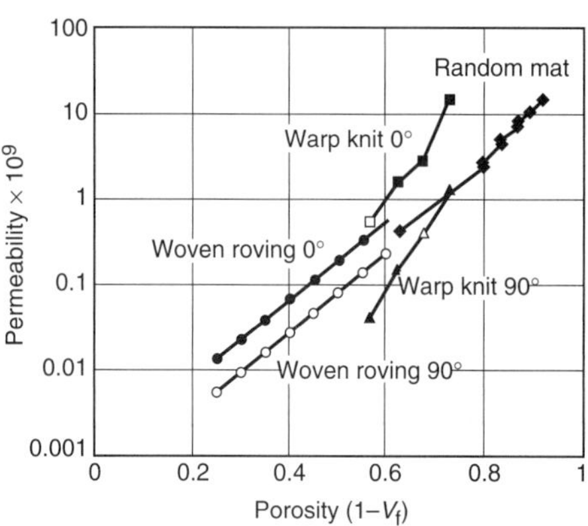

Fig. 7 Typical reinforcement in-plane permeability behavior. Source: Ref 8

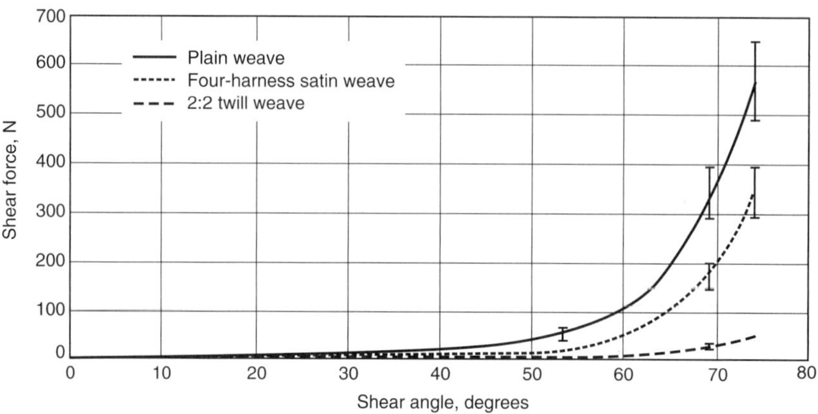

Fig. 8 Typical reinforcement in-plane shear behavior. 800 g/m^2 glass fiber fabrics. Source: Ref 9

oped containing both activator and catalyst. Both the liquid activator and the molten laurolactam can be stored indefinitely. A somewhat different approach is offered by "cyclics" technology (Ref 11). The concept here is to impregnate the reinforcements with a low-viscosity thermoplastic resin (prepolymer), which subsequently reacts in the presence of heat and a catalyst to increase its molecular weight via conversion of its short molecular chains to a linear structure in a ring-opening polymerization reaction. This technology has been demonstrated in the past for polybutylene terepthalate (PBT) and polycarbonates.

Curing. Unlike SMC compression molding, curing of liquid-molded parts takes place in a generally nonuniform pattern. This is due to the variations in thermal and chemical history of the resin from the injection gate to the vent. These differences are most noticeable in nonisothermal processes (i.e., when cold resin is injected into a heated mold). In most situations, the vent region will cure first and the (cooler) gate last. Drastic measures need to be adopted to correct or reverse this tendency. One possibility is to introduce variable initiator dosing (Ref 12), while another is to use a tapered resin preheating technique (Ref 13). For near-isothermal processes (or where the resin gel time is much longer than the fill time), the mold will generally reach an equilibrium temperature before curing commences, thus the cure progression will be more or less uniform. In-plane curing gradients do not appear to provoke any particular problems. Any arising variations in degree of cure can be dealt with by postcuring the part. Through-thickness problems can be more problematic. The main problem here is with relatively thick laminates that may be subject to overheating or interlaminar cracking during polymerization. The first problem may be addressed simply by adjusting the resin formulation (reducing the initiator concentration or adding inhibitors) to produce a less vigorous reaction. The second problem occurs mainly in curved shells (Ref 14) and is a function of resin shrinkage, fiber orientation, and thickness-to-diameter ratio. This can be resolved in many cases by adding flexibilizers, reducing the proportion of hoop reinforcement or redesign.

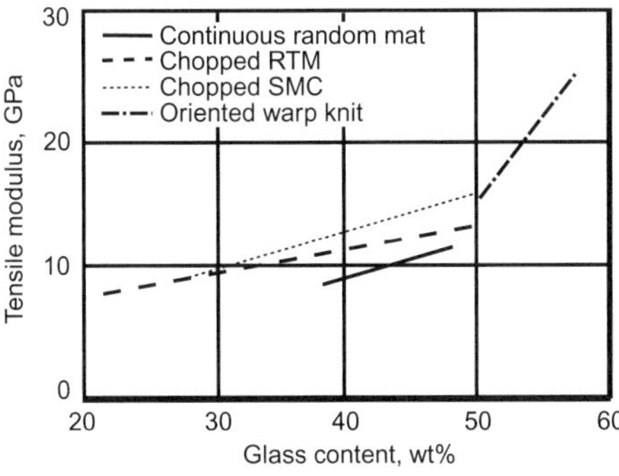

Fig. 9 Tensile modulus of various RTM material with E-glass reinforcement. Source: Ref 15

Representative Component Properties

In a well-organized process, the properties of RTM parts are determined in the usual way by the fiber reinforcement and the matrix resin (Fig. 9, 10) (Ref 15). The major factor, as in most processes, is the fiber volume fraction window at which a given reinforcement can be processed. A lower band is imposed here by the need to prevent fiber washing. This is achieved largely by imposing a compaction pressure in the mold. The process-specific factors that may also play a role include:

- Fiber volume fraction limitations imposed by the part geometry. These can be determined empirically or estimated with the aid of draping software.
- Fiber realignment arising from the preforming stage. Again, draping software may be useful here.
- Matrix modifications due to absorbed binders, for example. The solubility of any preform binders in the matrix resin may have a significant influence on the final toughness and glass transition temperature. Depending on the relative rates of filling and solution, this may produce a property gradient in the matrix.

Design Guidelines

Although processes vary widely, most rely on low-pressure impregnation. This makes the technology particularly attractive for large-area parts that would require expensive and heavy press tools for use with molding compounds. Other competing low-pressure, low-cost tooling routes include vacuum bag or autoclave molding. However, liquid molding offers two major advantages from a design perspective:

- Components can be made with two accurate, molded faces. Dimensional control is superior, which facilitates any subsequent assembly operations.
- Thick sections (or sandwich panels) are easier to produce since debulking is easier with dry fabrics than prepreg.

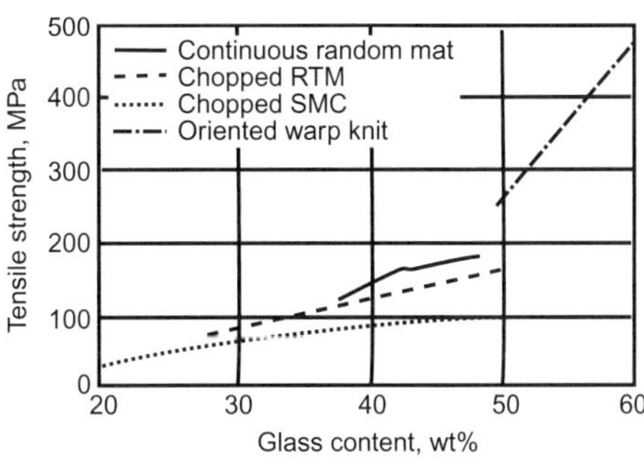

Fig. 10 Tensile strength of various RTM material with E-glass reinforcement. Source: Ref 15

Another advantage is the ability to produce relatively complex shapes. The dry mats or fabrics that are used can be formed or tailored fairly conveniently to complex curves and other forms. Geometric forms are generally limited by the same considerations regarding draft angles as conventional pressing operations, although it is possible to produce difficult shapes involving reentrants, for example, by special tooling techniques. These require the use of either flexible tooling based on elastomers, expendable cores such as low-melting-points alloys, water soluble plasters, or bladders. Some of these are subject to patent protection.

While the geometric form is generally unconstrained, it is usually sensible to maintain the thickness as uniform as possible. Change in thickness requires a step change in the number of layers of mat or fabric, and unless the superficial density is very low this may cause rippling in the laminate surface. The reinforcement preparation stage is also complicated, requiring multiple templates or robotic cutting. Step changes in thickness are especially undesirable due to the difficulty of ensuring that the reinforcement butts closely to the corner of the mold. Many attempts to ensure that the reinforcement is located with a high degree of accuracy are frustrated by reinforcement shifting during either mold closure or resin injection. Some of these problems can be overcome by adopting a separate preforming operation.

Sandwich Structures. Sandwich panels are generally easier to make by liquid molding than by using prepreg techniques. The reinforcement is assembled with any inserts or cores before impregnation in a single shot, with significant reductions in secondary foaming or bonding operations. Many of the successful RTM applications to date involve sandwich laminates, including automotive spoilers and propeller blades.

The decision to produce the structure as an integral molding or to manufacture the skins separately, followed by bonding or postfoaming, depends on the cost and difficulty of producing the foam core. The conventional way involves a separate molding (usually in polyurethane or polyetherimide foam) that is made to the dimensions of the component, minus an allowance for the skin thickness. The core is then enclosed by the reinforcement and impregnated. Failure to maintain the required fiber volume fraction is likely to result in core shifting (Fig. 11).

Foam cores play an important role in successful processing, and their quality should not be overlooked. Since they help to define the flow cavity, any inaccuracies may compromise molding quality. Undersize cores reduce the reinforcement volume fraction in the skins, causing resin richness and overweight parts. They also reduce the reinforcement compaction pressure. Since this is the only means of core location during resin injection, reduction in the holding force makes the core susceptible to movements under fluid pressure. Consequences include uneven skin thickness, dry patches, and overheating in

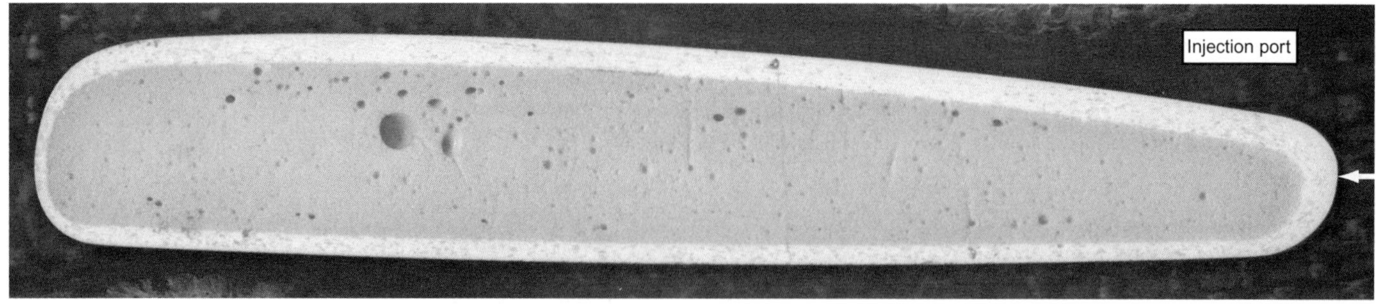

Fig. 11 Cross section through a foam-cored RTM component showing evidence of core shifting. Although specified with uniform skin thickness, the rigid polyurethane core has shifted under fluid pressure to produce approximately 2-to-1 right-to-left and upper-to-lower skin thickness ratios.

the thicker areas. Similarly, core-surface imperfections also result in resin-rich areas. These cause high local shrinkage or sink marks in the laminate surface.

The final design consideration concerns the skin-core adhesion. When the core is produced as a separate molding, its glossy skin does not support bonding. There may also be a significant carryover of release agent, which inhibits the development of a useful bond. Delamination may result during postcuring, painting, or in-service loading. Skin abrasion prior to RTM is normal using abrasive paper or by bead blasting. However, either route may reveal surface voids that must be filled prior to resin injection to avoid causing the sink marks described previously.

Hollow Laminates. Hollow structures offer a significant weight and cost saving compared with sandwich panels, but require more imagination to produce by RTM (Fig. 12) (Ref 16). A common technique here is to use an elastomeric bladder (which may be filled with particulates). The bladder is filled, loaded into the mold, and evacuated to rigidize the core. The preform skins are added, and the matrix resin is injected. Following resin cure, the core can be removed after releasing the vacuum. In a further variant, a positive pressure is applied to the bladder after the end of injection and prior to resin cure in order to consolidate the laminate. One potential advantage here is that the core may be formed with indentations in the surface that provide a runner system to aid resin distribution. These channels are destroyed when positive pressure is applied to the bladder, and the excess resin is bled out through the laminate. If particulates are used to stabilize the bladder, these can be extracted after venting. The bladder itself may be sacrificial or reusable.

Laminate/Preform Design. As with prepregs, the reinforcement dominates laminate stiffness and on-axis properties. When fabrics are used, it is simply necessary to generate design data at the relevant fiber volume fractions. Design calculations may then proceed in the usual way using laminate theory or finite element analysis. Complex shapes may dictate a need to take into account the effects of forming on the reinforcement architecture. This emerging discipline is discussed in detail elsewhere (Ref 17).

Inserts. One of the advantages of liquid molding includes the potential for incorporation of cores and inserts within a single-shot molding. In practice, the designer must decide whether inserts should be included at the preforming stage or fitted after molding. While the former may provide better mechanical integrity, it may be prohibitively expensive, in which case the molding may require subsequent drilling and bonding operations. When molded-in inserts are used, these may be located within the mold body, the preform or foam core. The situation is complicated by the need to ensure a reasonable level of fiber reinforcement around the insert when it is intended to transfer loads in and out of the structure. Bighead or other proprietary fasteners are commonly used in this respect. If inserts are to be used in this way, then the decision needs to be made at a relatively early stage to ensure they are accommodated in the design of the tooling.

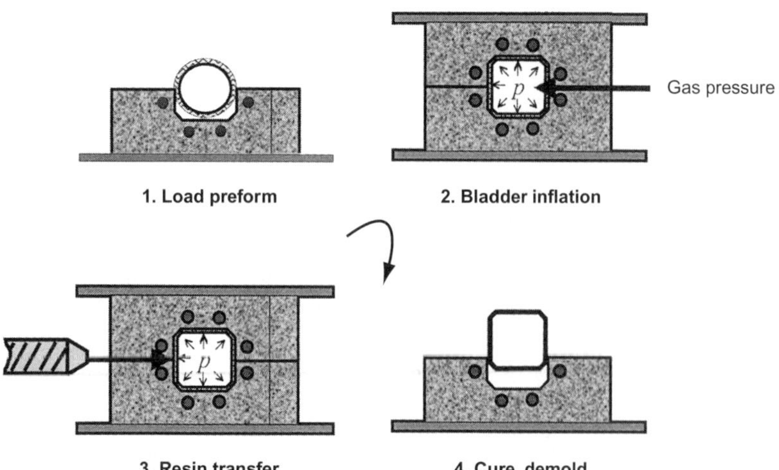

Fig. 12 Bladder inflation molding for hollow RTM structures. Source: Ref 16

Mold Design. The earliest decision that must be made concerns the mold material. This is governed almost entirely by the production volume. Serviceable prototypes for static testing can often be made using soft tooling (e.g., plaster, resin, resin/sand concrete, etc.). Here, the working life of the mold will only extend to a few parts, and the operating pressures and temperatures must be kept close to ambient. Low-volume manufacture (less than 1000 parts) relies heavily on glass reinforced plastic (GRP) tooling, which may be hand-laminated or vacuum-bagged glass fiber-epoxy. Secondary stiffening is usual via plywood or steel box-section, and this is laminated over the rear face of the tool.

Shell tooling (Fig. 13) is often used in medium-volume manufacturing (up to 40,000 parts), and this mimics GRP construction with the composite shell replaced by nickel or a nickel/copper laminate with a steel or aluminum stiffener. The nickel surface may be polished to a high degree and is considerably more durable than GRP. The shells themselves are manufactured traditionally by electroforming, although more recently chemical vapor deposition has gained in popularity.

Monolithic metal tools are the only realistic option for high-volume work (greater than 40,000 parts). Aluminum is commonly used at the lower end of this range, where its machinability and low density provide some economic benefits. However, the rapid wear that accompanies the use of glass fiber reinforcement and the difficulty of achieving the highest surface finishes make P20 tool steel the most popular material for high-volume automotive work.

The mold design loop needs to address the flow, thermal, and structural characteristics of the tool set. Failure to address each of these issues will result in lack of control over the part impregnation, curing, and dimensional control, respectively.

Flowpath Design. Gating and venting is an obvious area of concern with respect to part quality. The injection port(s) need to be sized and situated such that the cavity can be filled in an acceptable time and without any macroscopic air entrapment. Likewise, vents should be positioned adjacent to the last points to fill. This may be difficult to achieve when relying on intuition alone, but fortunately several commercial and semicommercial computer-based flow modeling packages (Ref 18, 19) are now available that predict flow front advancement (Fig. 14) and ease this aspect of the design process (Ref 20).

"Race-tracking" is a practical problem that most molders encounter at some stage. Here, the resin flows preferentially (usually at the periphery of the part) in the gap between the preform and the edge seal. This leads to short-circuiting between the gate and vent, and the resulting air entrapment is likely to scrap the part. The problem arises because of the large difference in permeabilities between the relatively dense preform and even small gaps (e.g., 1.0–2.0 mm, or 0.04–0.08 in.). It is worth recalling that a random preform has approximately the same flow resistance as a 0.2 mm (0.008 in.) channel. Clearly the solution lies in controlling both the dimensions of the preform and the cavity itself. In practical terms, this means close attention to preform fit using either steel-rule die cutting or an automated cutting table. At the same time, the mold body needs to be sufficiently rigid to restrain deflections due to either incoming fluid pressure or the reinforcement compression.

Heating. Electrical resistance heating, steam, hot water, or hot oil circulation are used commonly. Steam, water, and oil require a circulating path in the mold body. In the case of shell molds, pipes can be added to the rear face of the shell, while they can be cast-in-place for ceramic, Kirksite, or metal spray molds. Gun drilling is generally used to transport the fluid in monolithic molds. Fluid-circulating systems often incorporate a supplementary chiller. Electrical systems comprise resistance heating elements in the form of strips, cartridges, custom castings, fabrics, or embedded in rubber or mineral pads (in the case of polymer composite molds). Since poor thermal design can extend the overall cycle time, it is important that the heating system is matched to the temperature distribution that is required. For fluid systems this includes the location, depth, and size of the heating circuitry. It is also necessary to balance the flow rate through different areas of the heating circuit in order to achieve uniform heat transfer into the laminate. The siting and sizing of heating passages is usually done empirically. However, the use of relatively simple thermal analysis provides a much greater degree of confidence in heating circuit design.

Structural Design. Molds for RTM components typically have a large surface-area-to-volume ratio. Thus, the mold-bursting forces can be substantial. Even relatively low pressures (<5 bar) generate deflections that can seriously affect the component thickness and fiber fractions. The molds and their supporting structure must therefore be sufficiently stiff. Even when using precompacted reinforcements there can be significant loft remaining in the preform, and this has to be compressed in order to close the mold. The resulting compaction force maintains the preform integrity during impregnation, thus preventing fiber wash. Pressures in excess of 5 bar may be involved in order to achieve the desired fiber fraction.

Fluid pressures depend strongly on the materials and process. Structural reaction injection molding may involve cavity pressures at the injection point of up to 50 bar, while conventional RTM is generally a decade lower. Vacuum assistance will increase the driving pressure gradient for impregnation while using atmospheric pressure to resist mold separation. With high injection pressures monolithic metal molds are generally unavoidable and are usually press-mounted. Lightweight tooling options for high-quality components require careful design to ensure that mold deflections are within acceptable limits, and although hand calculations suffice for simple geometries, finite-element analysis is normally necessary for large and complex parts. Adequate joint support is also necessary to maintain seal integrity. This prevents resin overspill and loss in control over cavity pressure. Consideration should be given to the likely pressures during both impregnation and laminate curing, since the latter are often higher (Fig. 15).

With the exception of the vacuum infusion process, it is common to gate the mold in the center and vent in the corners or to gate and vent on opposite edges. The edge condition determines the control of the resin flow. Solutions range from pinching the reinforcement between the mold halves to create a restriction to a fully machined and telescoping flash-gap. Although the "pinch-off" is used widely, this is a low-volume manufacturing option and implies post-molding trimming stations. Investment in net edge tooling based on a carefully controlled flash gap or perimeter seal is preferable for most operations. However, this requires accurate reinforcement placement, which is unlikely to be achieved without investment in preforming equipment.

Outlook

Resin transfer molding was the subject of intense research and development during the 1990s (Ref 21). Early efforts were stimulated by the automotive industry via a series of high-pro-

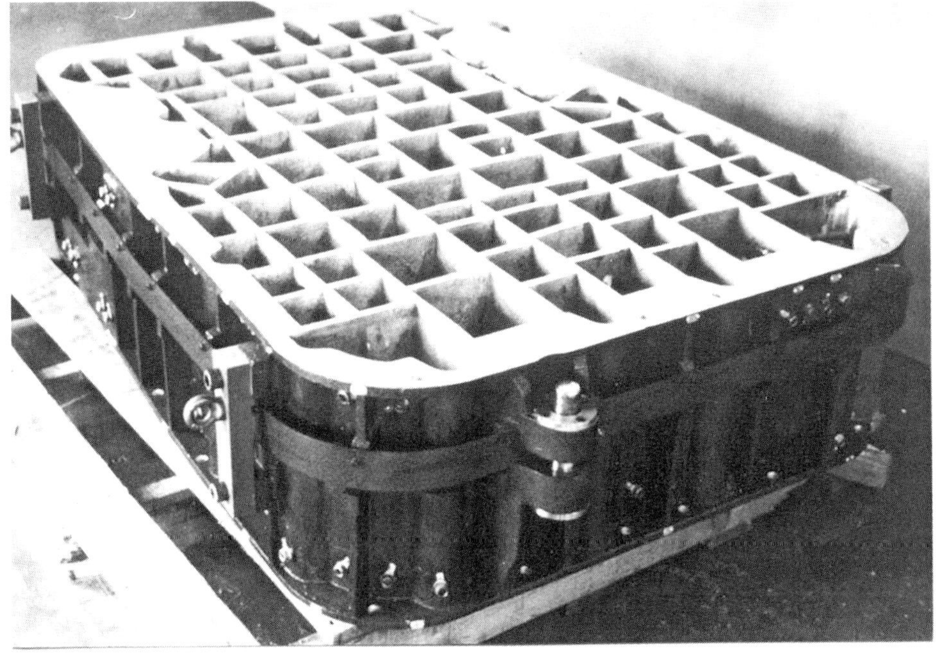

Fig. 13 Lightweight nickel shell mold with cast aluminum egg-crate stiffener. Courtesy of Ford Motor Company

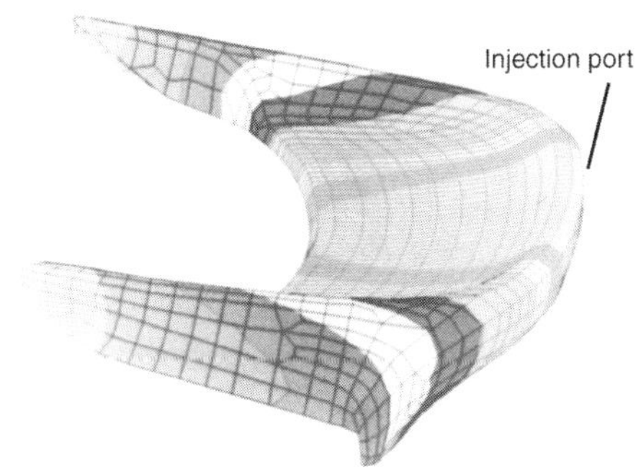

Fig. 14 Mold filling simulation showing fill time contours. Courtesy of Ford Motor Company

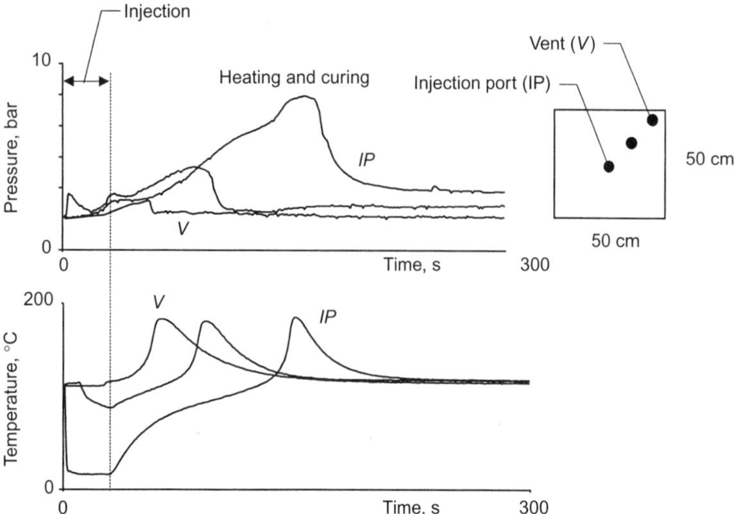

Fig. 15 Pressure and temperature cycles during nonisothermal RTM

file demonstrator studies. This has translated into significant new business for the supply base, although most RTM-intensive applications to date are confined to low production volumes. The 2000 European market for finished RTM parts was estimated at 30,000 tonnes (Ref 22). This is attributable in part to the supply infrastructure, since many of the existing molders are small, independent operators with limited capital budgets. Manufacture of cosmetic auto-body panels by RTM also runs into competition with alternative techniques as volumes increase beyond approximately 25,000 units/yr, where the lower materials costs associated with SMC and RRIM may become more attractive. Exceptions occur when the excellent potential of RTM for component integration can be exploited, exemplified by the high-volume manufacture of European automotive spoilers in the mid-1990s. The identification of markets where liquid molding offers a unique economic solution provides the most promising way forward. One such area undoubtedly includes vehicle structure. As pressures for emissions and mass reduction open up the market for lean-weight technologies, liquid molding offers the only feasible *low-cost* solution for building integrated body structures in composite.

The aerospace sector represents another important growth area for liquid molding. Much of the early interest was stimulated by the potential for cost reduction versus prepregs. As the technology developed it has become evident that opportunities extend beyond simple substitutions and that by using different textiles techniques new damage-tolerant structures can be developed that were previously restricted to metals. In this sense, RTM is likely to be used alongside existing prepreg processes. Resin-film infusion or vacuum-impregnation techniques will likely be used where prepreg is displaced for large structures and relatively simple shapes such as aerodynamic surfaces.

REFERENCES

1. K. Djurner and K. Palmqvist, Structural RTM for Automotive Parts, *Reinf. Plast.,* May 1993, p 24–27
2. R.F.J. McCarthy, G.H. Haines, and R.A. Newley, Polymer Composite Application to Aerospace Equipment, *Compos. Manuf.,* Vol 5 (No. 2), 1994, p 83–93
3. C.W. Macosko, *Fundamentals of Reaction Injection Molding,* Hanser Publishers, 1989
4. J.S. Hayward and B. Harris, The Effect of Vacuum Assistance in Resin Transfer Moulding, *Compos. Manuf.,* Vol 1 (No. 3), Sept 1990, p 161–166
5. C. Williams, J. Summerscales, and S. Grove, Resin Infusion under Flexible Tooling (RIFT); A Review, *Composites,* Part A, Vol 27a, 1996, p 517–524
6. G. Goulevant, D. Neveu, and B. Paumard, Patents WO92112846 (6.8.92), FR2672005 (31.7.92), AU9212773 (27.8.92), and PT100141 (29.4.94)
7. F. Robitaille and R. Gauvin, Compaction of Textile Reinforcements for Composites Manufacturing. I: Review of Experimental Results, *Polymer Compos.,* Vol 19 (No. 2), April 1998, p 198
8. Representative data from NIST Standard Reference Database 63 NIST Database on Reinforcement Permeability Values: Data on Composite Reinforcement Materials Used in Liquid Composite Molding. National Institute of Standards and Technology
9. B.J. Souter, Ph.D. thesis, University of Nottingham, U.K., 2000
10. R. Leimbacher and E. Schmid, "Thermoplastically Formable Composite Materials Based on Polyamide 12 Matrix," U.S. Patent 5837181, EMS-American Grilon Inc., Serial No. 858442, filed 19970519, issued 19981117
11. www.cyclics.com, Cyclics Corp., Rensselaer, NY
12. P.J. Blanchard and C.D. Rudd, Cycle Time Reductions in Resin Transfer Moulding Using Phased Catalyst Injection, *Compos. Sci. Technol.,* Vol 56, 1996, p 123–133
13. M.S. Johnson, C.D. Rudd, and D.J. Hill, Microwave Assisted Resin Transfer Moulding, *Composites,* Part A, Vol 29A, 1998, p 71–86
14. T.J. Corden, "Development of Design and Manufacturing Techniques for GRP Waste Water Treatment Equipment," Ph.D. thesis, University of Nottingham, U.K., 1996
15. C.F. Johnson, Resin Transfer Molding, *Composites,* Vol 1, *Engineered Materials Handbook,* ASM International, 1987, p 564–568
16. U. Lehmann and W. Michaeli, Automated Production of Hollow Composite Parts with Complex Geometry in RTM, *Proc. Int. Conf. Automated Composites (ICAC 97)* (Glasgow, U.K.), 4–5 Sept 1997, Institute of Materials, London, U.K., p 43–58
17. A.C. Long and C.D. Rudd, Fabric Drape Modelling and Preform Design, *Resin Transfer Moulding for Aerospace Structures,* T. Kruckenberg and R. Paton, Ed., Kluwer Academic Publishers, 1998
18. S.G. Advani and P. Simacek, *Resin Transfer Moulding for Aerospace Structures,* T. Kruckenberg and R. Paton, Ed., Kluwer Academic Publishers, 1998
19. A. Hammami, R. Gauvin, and F. Trochu, Modeling the Edge Effect in Liquid Composites Moulding, *Composites,* Part A, Vol 29 (No. 5–6), 1998, p 603–609
20. F. Trochu, P. Ferland, and R. Gauvin, Functional Requirements of a Simulation Software for Liquid Molding Processes, *Sci. Eng. Compos. Mater.,* Vol 6 (No. 4), 1997, p 209–218
21. M. Mehta, RTM and SRIM for Structural Composites: The Promise That Hasn't Been Realized, *Proc. ASM/ESD Advanced Composites Conference and Exposition* (Dearborn, MI), 6–9 Nov 1995, p 535–546
22. *Composites: A Profile of the Worldwide Reinforced Plastics Industry,* 3rd ed., Elsevier, Oxford, U.K., 2000

SELECTED REFERENCES

- B.T. Åström, *Manufacturing of Polymer Composites,* 1st ed., Chapman and Hall, London, 1997
- T. Kruckenberg and R. Paton, Ed., *Resin Transfer Moulding for Aerospace Structures,* Kluwer Academic Publishers, 1998
- C.W. Macosko, *Fundamentals of Reaction Injection Molding,* Hanser Publishers, 1989
- K. Potter, *Resin Transfer Moulding,* Chapman and Hall, London, 1997
- C.D. Rudd, A.C. Long, K.N. Kendall, and C.E. Mangin, *Liquid Moulding Technologies,* 1st ed., Woodhead Publishing, Cambridge, U.K., 1997, 457 pages

Vacuum Infusion

Arlen Hoebergen, Centre of Lightweight Structures TUD-TNO, The Netherlands
J. Anders Holmberg, SICOMP AB, Sweden

VACUUM INFUSION is a resin injection technique and is derived from resin transfer molding (RTM). A resin injection technique generally consists of the following production steps:

- Dry reinforcement is placed in a mold.
- The mold is closed.
- Resin flows through the mold and impregnates the reinforcement.
- The resin cures.
- The mold is opened and the product is demolded.

A general way of distinguishing between different resin injection techniques is how the pressure gradient is applied to force the resin to flow through the mold. In the case of vacuum infusion the pressure gradient is created by vacuum on the outlet port. The resin injection tank and inlet port are at ambient pressure, as opposed to resin injection techniques (such as RTM) where the resin injection tank is pressurized.

The use of vacuum as the driver behind resin flow has a large impact on the application of the technique and the actual process in the workshop. The major advantage of using vacuum is the absence of large forces on the mold. Standard RTM techniques require strong and stiff tooling. The larger the product, the more difficult and expensive this becomes. This is why the first success for vacuum infusion has been in large products that are made in small quantities. The major disadvantage of using vacuum is the sensitivity to leakage. A leak will result in air flowing into the mold. This often results in void-rich areas in the cured part. In RTM (with a pressurized resin tank and an outlet at ambient pressure), a leak in the mold would just result in resin spillage. Besides, air will flow into the mold much easier than resin will flow out of the mold (i.e., the viscosity of air is much smaller than the viscosity of the resin).

Although vacuum infusion is considered a recent development, the first production trials date back to the 1940s with a method called the Marco Process (Ref 1, 2). In the following years, a number of trials were carried out using vacuum as the driving force for resin injection. Developments increased in the 1970s and 1980s due mainly to the threat of environmental legislation. The main impetus for the development has always been the elimination of styrene emission. The technology was developed as an alternative to open-mold manufacturing processes like hand lay-up and spray-up. Vacuum infusion was considered as a low-cost alternative. Besides, with minor modifications the molds used for hand lay-up and spray-up could also be used for vacuum infusion. With new legislation coming into force, more and more companies switched to vacuum infusion in the 1990s. The legislation generally focused on the two elements of styrene emission. In many Western countries, the maximum allowable concentration of styrene at the workspot (mac value) has been reduced from about 100 to 20 or 25 ppm (Ref 3, 4). In addition, environmental emissions have been limited (exhaust) (Ref 5). For many companies with mainly open-mold manufacturing, this meant investing in ventilation equipment to keep the styrene level low and filters to remove styrene from the exhaust.

While the reduction of styrene emission is evident, the technology has a number of additional benefits. The quality consistency is an important benefit since it has allowed the technology to be used in the advanced composites industry as well. Currently, the aviation and even the aerospace industry are strongly interested in the application of this technology.

Although vacuum infusion has been in use since the 1960s, it is still a "new" technology and is not fully matured. The developments in this manufacturing technology have been enormous in the past 20 years, resulting in a large number of different injection processes described in the literature. The information about these developments often has focused to a great extent on their differences, and frequently new techniques were designated by new exotic abbreviations, such as vacuum-assisted resin injection (VARI) (Ref 6), bladder infusion process (BLIP), Seeman composite resin infusion molding process (SCRIMP) (Ref 7, 8), and others (Ref 9). However, the commonalties between these techniques must be acknowledged. Only then will it be possible to learn and understand the technology in full, and therefore to exploit modifications fully.

In this article, vacuum infusion as a process is detailed with respect to other manufacturing techniques for composite materials, including RTM. This includes mechanical properties, production volume and process economics, followed by a section showing different technological applications. Next, a comprehensive description of the technology is provided, starting with a theoretical section on the resin flow and how this can be enhanced, and continuing into a more practical description with concentration on how a part can be made. The practical focus is continued in a section that deals with equipment and materials requirements. Representative component properties and some brief design guidelines are presented. Finally, a brief outlook is made on new developments, markets, and applications of the technology.

Technique Characteristics

Vacuum Infusion Compared to Other Methods. From a technical point of view, vacuum infusion is a derivative of resin transfer molding. From a production and manufacturing point of view, RTM is considered as a competitor or an alternative to prepreg processing and compression molding using sheet molding compounds (SMCs); for example RTM can be considered viable when the production volume will not justify SMC press molding. Vacuum infusion, on the other hand, has been developed as an alternative to open-mold hand lay-up and spray-up techniques. However, developments in the technology have shown that vacuum infusion can also be an alternative to prepreg compression molding and prepreg vacuum bagging.

When choosing the most cost-efficient manufacturing technology for a certain part several criteria play a role. Important criteria are:

- The number of parts (production volume)
- The size and geometry of a part
- The required performance (i.e., stiffness and strength per unit weight)
- The required surface finish

In an ideal situation, the design, material, and manufacturing technique are selected and optimized to obtain the most advantageous performance-to-cost ratio for the part. In Fig. 1 several press molding, injection molding, and open-mold manufacturing techniques are shown schematically with respect to the possibilities of production volume and part performance. This figure shows that while vacuum infusion initially was developed to replace hand lay-up and spray-up in the area of small production volume of large parts with low performance, it is now clear that vacuum infusion actually is applicable in much wider areas:

- Up to an intermediate number of parts (i.e., 1000 a year)
- Small and large parts
- Low and high performance parts

Vacuum Infusion Versus RTM. Vacuum infusion is a derivative of RTM. From Fig. 1 it is clear that the areas of applicability of RTM and vacuum infusion overlap. In a way, the technologies also overlap as well. There is no clear boundary between RTM and vacuum infusion. The tooling and the method to apply the pressure gradient determine the technique, to a large extent. The tooling selection is obviously strongly related to the production volume and the product size (see Fig. 2), and the pressure gradient selection is subsequently related to the tooling. There is no confusion in the extreme conditions: RTM in a stiff mold with 500 kPa (5 bar) pressure on the resin inlet, vacuum infusion with a thin foil as one mold half, and only vacuum on the resin outlet. But what about a vacuum infusion process with one stiff mold half and a semirigid glass-fiber/polyester second mold half? To speed up the process, one can apply pressure on the inlet (e.g., +100 kPa, or +1 bar) during the initial stage of the injection. What kind of process is this? It is clear that it is not important how we name the technology, as long as the operator knows the process and the engineer understands the physics behind the process.

In a way resin injection techniques can suffer from the same problems plastics in general did in the 1950s. Because of bad design and bad applications, plastics were considered inferior by many. There are no bad resin injection techniques, only bad applications of them. The versatility of the technique must be understood; subsequently the part, the material, *and* the technique must be designed to get the optimal solution.

Possibilities and Limitations of Vacuum Infusion. The manufacturing method poses limitations on what can or cannot be achieved. Although it is said that virtually everything is possible with vacuum infusion, there are a few constraints.

Geometry. In principle, there are no geometrical limitations for vacuum infusion: three-dimensional curved, shelllike structures and closed hollow parts are all possible. The practicality and the accessibility to place the dry reinforcement in the mold system are the most important criteria to decide on the economical viability of the part. Details in the geometry can cause problems, such as:

- Sharp edges in the part can disturb the flow pattern of the resin (see the section "Technique Description" in this article).
- Thickness variations in the part can also cause disturbances in the flow pattern. However, the main problem lies with the resin system. A good cure of the thin part often results in a very large exothermal temperature rise in the thick part. The thickness of the laminate itself is not a problem, provided the resin has been selected carefully. Laminates of a few tenths of a millimeter as well as up to 100 mm (4 in.) have been manufactured with vacuum infusion.

Component Size. The manufacture of very large parts using vacuum infusion has been a matter of courage rather than technology development, due to the cost of scrap parts. When a part with a surface area of 100 m^2 (1075 ft^2) can be made, why not a part of 200 or 500 m^2 (2150 or 5380 ft^2)? Again, limitations are related to a practical problem: accessibility of the part (before and during the injection). In addition, the larger the part, the bigger the risk that something can go wrong. In general, to justify the greater risk, the manufacture in one-production shot must have clear advantages above the manufacture in two or more sections.

Parts Integration (Core Materials and Metal Inserts). Similar to other injection techniques, as well as to hand lay-up and prepregging, vacuum infusion can accommodate the application of various kinds of cores and inserts. However, honeycomb cores are usually not applied in vacuum infusion, although the honeycomb can be covered with some type of sealing foil to prevent resin from penetrating into the honeycomb. Cores must be made of closed-cell materials, but still can result in void-rich areas due to cell collapse. A small test on new material is always recommended.

Fiber Content. Two aspects determine the fiber content of the part: the fiber reinforcement used and the pressure applied. This is why parts with a broad range of fiber contents (15–65 vol%) can be made.

Surface Finish. The mold system used and the resin/reinforcement combination determine the surface finish of the part. In general, a good quality surface on one side of the part is very feasible.

Net Shape Molding and Tolerances. Net shape manufacture is rare with vacuum infusion. Usually, edges need to be trimmed. In addition, the foil side of the part can have sharp ridges of resin due to folds in the foil. In some cases these ridges need to be removed by sanding. Obviously, small tolerances can be best achieved with stiff tooling and, if required, special tooling is

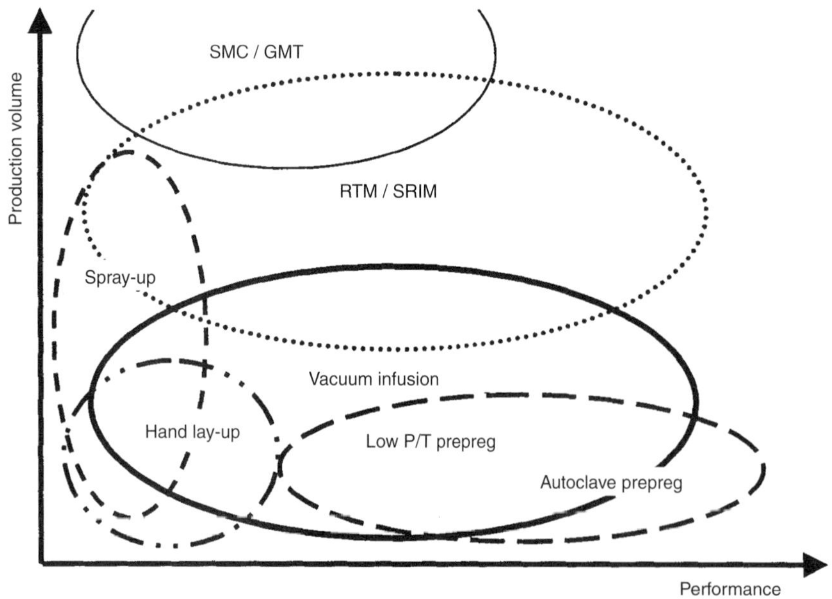

Fig. 1 Production volume and relative part performance that can be achieved with various production techniques. SMC, sheet molding compounds; GMT, glass mat thermoplastics; RTM, resin transfer molding; SRIM, structural reaction injection molding; P/T, pressure/temperature

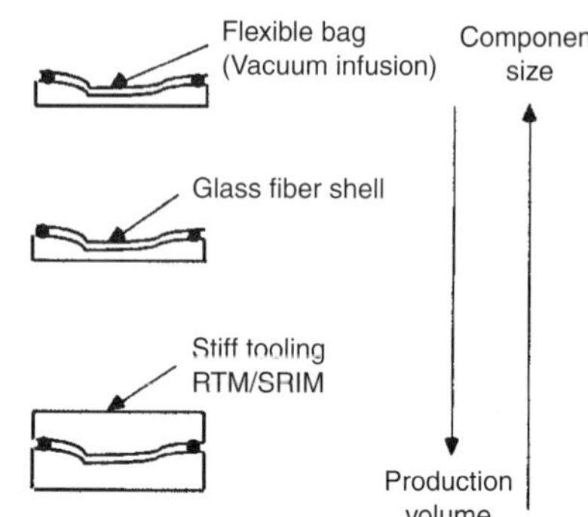

Fig. 2 Tooling selection related to production volume and component size

made to ensure small tolerances at specific spots in the part.

Economy. Table 1 gives a general overview of the different cost categories in the manufacturing process; of course, details will depend on specific product characteristics.

Workshop Requirements. For hand lay-up and spray-up, ventilation equipment is required. For prepregging, workshop conditioning (temperature and humidity) is usually required. When using vacuum infusion or RTM, workshop conditioning is not required, although some kind of temperature control is advised.

Equipment. For vacuum infusion, a small vacuum pump and an overflow vessel are sufficient. RTM requires injection equipment. Spray-up involves a spray gun, and hand lay-up can be done with a simple roller and brush. Low pressure/temperature (P/T) prepreg will require a vacuum pump as well, and it is usually combined with a simple oven. Autoclave prepreg obviously requires an autoclave.

Tooling. Tooling for vacuum infusion, hand lay-up, spray-up, and low P/T prepreg can be simple and relatively cheap. For autoclave prepreg, tooling usually gets a bit more expensive, and for RTM, tooling will be most expensive.

Ancillary Materials. Hand lay-up and spray-up do not really require ancillary materials, but vacuum infusion does involve a foil, sealant tape, tubes, and hoses. The same applies to the prepregging technologies where foils, peel ply, and bleeder materials are used.

Raw Materials. Vacuum infusion requires more-expensive reinforcement materials than spray-up, but is much cheaper than prepregging materials.

Labor depends very much on the part characteristics. Compared to hand lay-up, vacuum infusion can gain time in the placement of the dry reinforcement in the mold, but will lose time during the sealing of the foil on the mold and during the injection.

Advantages. Vacuum infusion has been developed as a low-cost technique that is able to compete in cost with spray-up and hand lay-up while having a number of advantages. The main advantage and impetus behind the development of the technology is the elimination of styrene emission, combined with the ability to work with a simple mold system (only one stiff mold, as with spray-up or hand lay-up). This results in an improved internal and external environment over open-molding techniques (Ref 10). Other advantages are:

- Improved laminate quality (better impregnation and higher fiber content)
- Improved consistency of the product properties (properties are less dependent on the craftsmanship of the employee). This can enable use of lower design safety factors, resulting in a more efficient design (Ref 11).
- Less material use (compared to hand lay-up and spray-up, less resin is used and there is less waste on the product edges, i.e., overspray).

Disadvantages. When a company decides to apply vacuum infusion, it must be recognized that the technique also poses requirements on the part design, processing conditions, and the training of employees. Good training of the employees is essential to prevent production failures. A main disadvantage of the technology is the absence of control tools that can be used to assist the workshop employees. For example, mistakes in laying down the dry reinforcement cannot be identified before the injection starts. Other disadvantages of the technology are:

- Sensitivity to leakage, which makes the process critical for mistakes
- A good surface finish can be difficult to achieve, especially when thin and thick laminates are combined. When the whole part is cured at once, a high exothermal temperature peak and large cure shrinkage may result, which increase the risk for print through.
- Waste. Many ancillary materials often are used only once (foil, sealant tape, tubes, hoses, valves) and discarded after demolding.

Applications

Early developments of vacuum infusion were mainly performed in the marine industry to reduce styrene emission from open-mold manufacturing. This is manifested by the fact that most successful applications demonstrated today are fiberglass-reinforced polyester boats and yachts. However, vacuum infusion is feasible for many more applications than just replacing hand lay-up and spray-up for marine applications. This has been demonstrated recently by new products manufactured with vacuum infusion. The new products range from fiberglass solar cell housings to carbon fiber stealth ships. Examples from different sectors are given in Table 2 (Ref 12–15).

In the following paragraphs, typical applications of vacuum infusion are presented with the purpose of showing the versatility of the process.

Sailing Yachts. The most well-known application for vacuum infusion is the manufacturing of hulls for sailing yachts. Both single shell and sandwich hulls have been manufactured. A representative example is the manufacturing of a 17 m (55 ft) sailing yacht at Conyplex, the Netherlands (Ref 12) (see Fig. 3). The hull consists of a gelcoat, unsaturated polyester resin, multiaxial glass fiber reinforcements, and a balsa core. To facilitate placement of the core in the female mold, contoured sheets of balsa are used. Slits in the balsa open up when the contoured sheets are bent. These slits play a role in shortening the fill time. Infusion of the resin is carried out in one step and with one resin injection tank, using a polyamide bag and a "fishbone" arrangement of resin distribution channels. In Fig. 4 the white glass reinforcement, not yet wetted with resin, can be clearly distinguished from the dark areas, already impregnated with resin, around the resin distribution channels. This type of infusion requires only one resin injection tank, which is easy to monitor. The outlet ports are located all around the flange of the hull.

At Conyplex, this resulted in a reduction of both labor cost and cycle time, besides the benefits generally linked to vacuum infusion, such as reduction of styrene emission and better quality. Other common applications of vacuum infusion for sailing yachts include decks and hatches. Popular resins other than polyesters are vinylester and epoxy.

Recreational boats are made in larger numbers than sailing yachts and are still mainly produced by spray-up or wet lay-up. However, stricter legislation on solvent emissions forces the producers to move toward closed-molding techniques. An example where the producer has shifted from spray-up to vacuum infusion for the manufacture of hulls for large recreational boats is Ryds in Sweden. To keep the process rational as they moved from spray-up to vacuum infusion, they used a thin glass fiber shell instead of a bag as the male mold. The female mold is similar to a spray-up mold that has a modified flange construction. The lay-up consists of a heavy combination fabric (a random mat material with

Table 2 Examples of applications and parts made with vacuum infusion

Sector	Applications
Marine	Hulls, decks, and hatches of yachts, hulls and decks of recreational boats
Transportation	Roof and floor of refrigerated container, automotive exterior body panels, train fronts
Aerospace	Rudder of small aircraft
Industrial	Fan blades, part for fish counting unit, toilet bowl, oil separator
Energy	Solar cell housings, wind turbine blades, electrical insulation materials
Infrastructure	Lighting columns, bridge deck
Military	Hull of composite armored vehicle, hull of stealth corvette

Table 1 Comparison of different cost categories for different manufacturing processes

	Vacuum infusion	RTM	Hand lay-up	Spray-up	Low P/T prepreg(a)	Autoclave prepreg
Workshop requirements	\$\$	\$\$	\$\$\$\$	\$\$\$\$	\$\$\$	\$\$\$
Equipment	\$\$	\$\$\$	\$	\$\$	\$\$\$	\$\$\$\$\$
Tooling	\$\$	\$\$\$\$	\$\$	\$\$	\$\$	\$\$\$
Ancillary materials	\$\$\$	\$\$	\$	\$	\$\$\$	\$\$\$
Raw materials	\$\$	\$\$	\$\$	\$	\$\$\$	\$\$\$\$
Labor	\$\$	\$	\$\$	\$	\$\$\$	\$\$\$

(a) P/T, pressure/temperature

a special internal feeder) supplemented by glass fiber weaves for additional strength and stiffness. The combination fabric has high permeability and is easy to manually place into the mold on top of a slightly tacky gelcoat layer. Rapid infusion and cure is facilitated by circumferential infusion of a low-viscosity polyester resin. The injection channel is visible on the untrimmed edge of the boat shown in Fig. 5. The cost estimates made after production of 150 boats showed that both material and labor costs are higher with vacuum infusion than spray-up (Ref 10). The reasons for this are cost and handling of the reinforcements. Noticeable savings when using vacuum infusion instead of spray-up can be found in areas of energy consumption for ventilation, maintenance, and spare parts for spray-equipment, maintenance and cleaning of work areas, clothing and personal protection equipment, and finally, a reduction of total waste and landfill costs. Other gains are an improved and more consistent laminate quality and a weight reduction.

Military Ships. A good example of cost-effective manufacture of high-performance composites with vacuum infusion is the hull panels for the Visby class corvette. The panels consist of carbon fiber/vinylester skins and polyvinyl chloride-based core. With ordinary wet lay-up, one side of the sandwich has to be laminated and cured first before the other side can be laminated. The rolling operation also requires a significant amount of labor for large surfaces. With vacuum infusion, on the other hand, the whole sandwich is impregnated with resin in one step and with reduced labor (see Fig. 6). In addition, the vacuum-infusion process for the hull panels results in a high fiber content and a consistent laminate quality. In a secondary operation, the hull panels are joined together to form larger parts (see Fig. 7). The principle of the manufacturing procedure is illustrated in Fig. 6. The bottom reinforcement, core material, and top reinforcement are placed on a large flat table. Resin inlets and a distribution channel are placed along one long side of the table (on the left in Fig. 6). For this application, slots machined in the core enhance the resin flow.

On the Visby corvette, the stern, hatches, and other parts are also made by vacuum infusion.

Armored Vehicles. Vacuum infusion has also attracted the attention of manufacturers of composite armored vehicles. Vosper Thornycroft, United Kingdom, has used vacuum infusion to manufacture a two-piece hull for a prototype Advanced Composite Armoured Vehicle Platform (Ref 15). The choice of vacuum infusion to inject epoxy resin into multiaxial E-glass was based on relative cost estimates and comparisons with wet lay-up, prepreg processing, and RTM for production numbers greater than 100. Benefits of vacuum infusion for this application include more consistent and higher quality than with wet lay-up, lower manufacturing costs than prepreg processing, and the option to use thicker fabrics than possible with wet lay-up.

Transportation. For a long time, small to medium quantities of body panels have been produced with different vacuum infusion techniques for cars, trucks, and buses. Low costs for tooling and part-specific equipment make these processes more economical than steel stamping for small series production. Usually the lay-up of body panels consists of a gelcoat layer followed

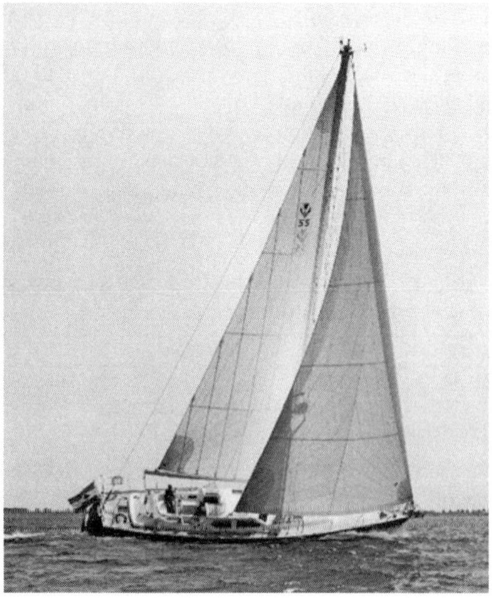

Fig. 3 Contest 55 sailing yacht with hull manufactured by vacuum infusion. Courtesy of Conyplex Shipyard, Medemblik, the Netherlands

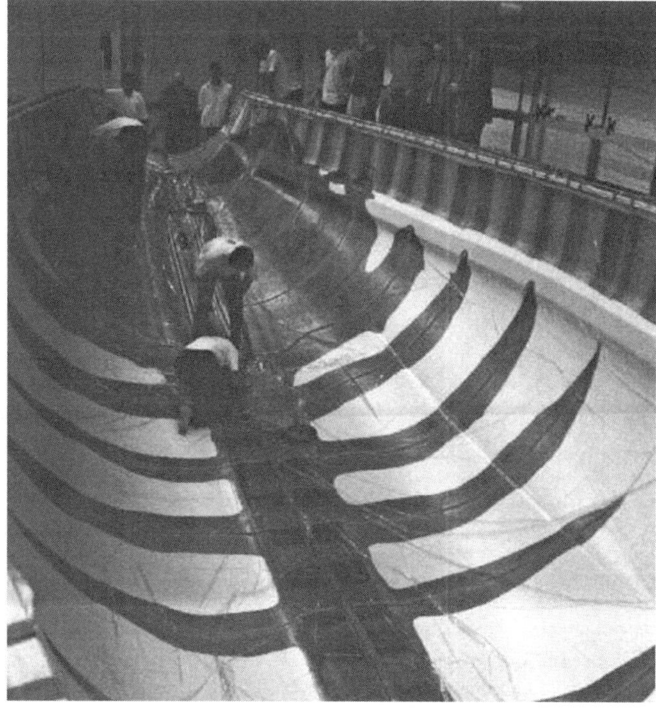

Fig. 4 Flow front progress during the infusion of a Contest 55 hull. Courtesy of Conyplex Shipyard, Medemblik, the Netherlands

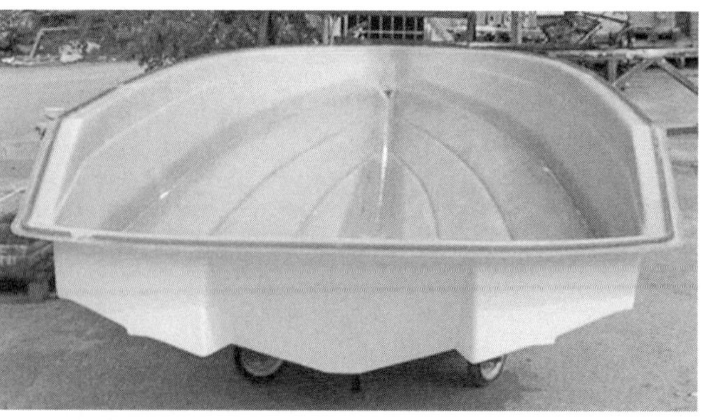

Fig. 5 Vacuum infused 5.1 m (17 ft) boat hull

by one or several layers of highly permeable reinforcement and cores. Gelcoat, dry reinforcement, and cores are applied manually into a female fiberglass mold. The second mold half is, in general, a flexible fiberglass shell. A small injection machine is commonly used to automate mixing of the resin components. The injection machine also shortens the cycle time due to pressurization of the inlet.

Body panels are also produced with hand lay-up and spray-up, but vacuum infusion has several advantages over these processes. The most important are cleaner production, more consistent quality, better laminate properties, and shorter cycle time for most applications.

Technique Description: Theory and Background

Flow of Resin. To use vacuum infusion technology, it is good to understand the basic physics behind the flow of a liquid through a porous medium. For a Newtonian liquid, the one-dimensional flow through a porous medium can be described by Darcy's law (Ref 16):

$$\frac{Q}{A} = \frac{K}{\mu}\frac{\Delta P}{\Delta x}$$

where

Q = volumetric flow rate (m^3/s)
A = cross section area (m^2)
K = permeability (m^2)
μ = viscosity of the liquid (Pa · s)
$\Delta P/\Delta x$ = pressure gradient (Pa/m)

What is the use of this law?

Before making a part using any resin injection technique, it is desirable to predict or assess the resin flow pattern. This is used in placement of the resin inlet and outlet ports. Other considerations are whether the part will be filled completely and how fast it will be filled. All of this is preferably known before the start of manufacture.

The fill time is important for both small and large parts. For small parts, the cycle time is critical to an economically viable production. Resin gel time can be critical in larger parts. Besides, the longer the injection lasts, the more things can go wrong. From Darcy's law we can easily conclude the following (assuming that other parameters remain constant):

- The bigger the pressure difference, the quicker the part is filled.
- The lower the resin viscosity, the quicker the part is filled.
- The higher the permeability, the quicker the part is filled.

What is obvious from Darcy's law is the influence of part geometry and injection strategy (location of inlet and outlet ports) through A and Δx on fill time. However, for specific geometries and injection strategies we must work out Darcy's law together with the equation of mass conservation to see this influence. Now, this all might seem very obvious, but, considering Darcy's law, where should the focus be in part manufacture?

In vacuum infusion, the maximum pressure difference is atmospheric pressure, about 100 kPa (1000 mbar). The absolute pressure of the vacuum in the mold during production can vary from about 2 to 40 kPa (20 to 400 mbar). The resulting pressure difference between inlet and outlet is then between 60 and 98 kPa (600 and 980 mbar). Consequently, the resulting influence on fill time cannot be more than a factor of two.

When a part is being made, most companies use a resin system that is developed for injection purposes. The resin viscosity usually varies from about 100 to 400 mPa · s (although resin systems with lower and higher viscosity are also used). Most of the time the resin has a viscosity of about 200 to 300 mPa · s. Consequently, the resulting influence on fill time is between a factor of two and four.

Although pressure difference and resin viscosity both influence the production, this influence is only minor when compared with the influence of the reinforcement permeability and injection strategies.

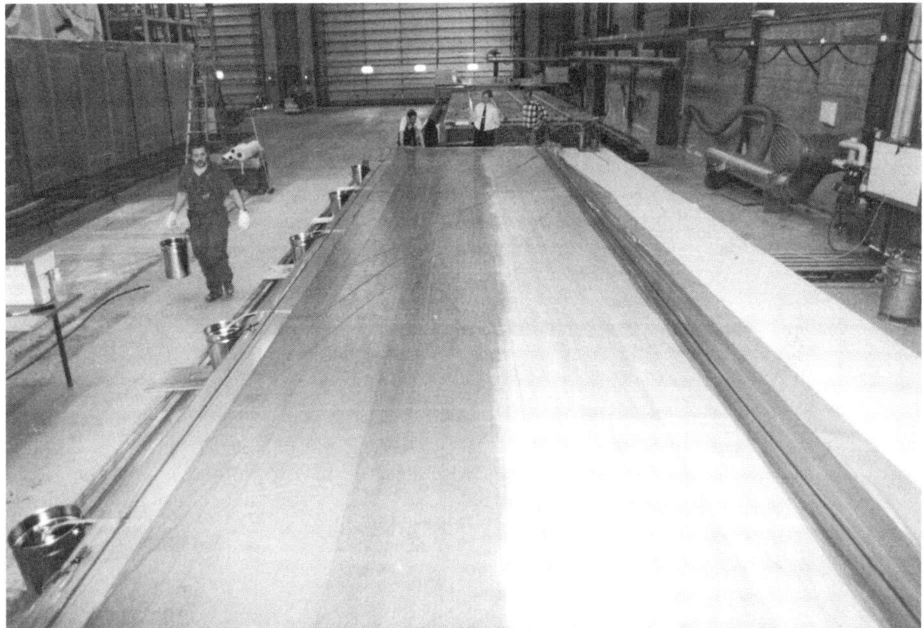

Fig. 6 Vacuum infusion of a 3.2 × 12 m (10.5 × 39 ft) glass fiber/vinyl ester sandwich illustrating the technique for creating a hull panel for the corvette shown in Fig. 7. Courtesy of Kockums Shipyard, Karlskrona, Sweden

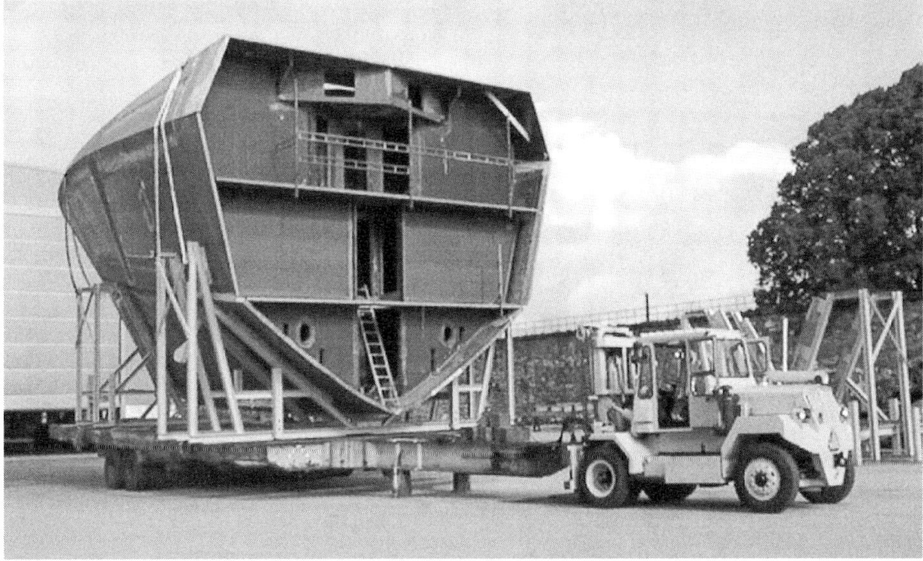

Fig. 7 Stern section of the Visby class corvette. Courtesy of Kockums Shipyard, Karlskrona, Sweden

Permeability is a geometrical property of the reinforcement and describes how easily the resin can flow through the material. It is often considered as a constant in Darcy's law. The permeability can be experimentally determined. However, since Darcy's law has been used for many industrial applications, much work has been done in predicting the permeability of a porous medium. The Carman-Kozeny model is most frequently used. This model relates the permeability to the porosity. In the case of fiber reinforcement, the permeability can be related to the fiber volume fraction (see also Fig. 8) with the following formula:

$$K = \frac{1}{C \cdot S^2} \cdot \frac{(1 - V_f)^3}{V_f^2}$$

where

K = permeability (m^2)
C = Kozeny constant
S = specific surface area (m^2/m^3)
V_f = fiber volume fraction

The Carman-Kozeny relation is an approximation, usually only valid for a limited range of fiber volume fractions. Therefore, this relationship can only be used accurately as an interpolation formula. The Kozeny constant still needs to be determined experimentally.

A major difference between matched-tooling RTM and vacuum infusion with a foil is the compression of the reinforcement. In RTM the reinforcement compression is dictated by the mold cavity, while in vacuum infusion the compression is related to the pressure (vacuum) in the mold cavity. The dry reinforcement in the mold is a resilient, compliant layer, which will be compressed upon evacuation of the mold. In general, random mat materials are more resilient, that is, compressed more at a given pressure than woven rovings or multiaxials. A typical compression graph of a random mat is shown in Fig. 9. Note that the compaction pressure available during processing is the ambient pressure (approximately 100 kPa, or 1000 mbar) minus the pressure within the vacuum bag. Although at a compaction pressure above 40 kPa (400 mbar) (absolute pressure within the vacuum bag below 60 kPa, or 600 mbar), the amount of compression seems not very significant, the influence on the fiber volume fraction and, consequently, the permeability is still of significance.

Reinforcement type and binder content influence the amount of compression. This is shown in Fig. 10. The type of random mat in this graph has a high binder content. This reinforcement is, consequently, relatively stiff and difficult to compress. The combination fabric (a random mat material with a special internal feeder) is easier to compress, and the woven roving can only be compressed initially. It must be realized, however, that wet and dry compression can differ significantly, for example, if the resin dissolves the binder. Theoretically, the compression of the reinforcement also causes the reinforcement to spring up a bit during the injection (as the flow front passes and the local pressure increases) (Ref 17, 18). This results in a decrease in fiber volume fraction and, consequently, an increase in permeability. Hence, in vacuum infusion, permeability is not a constant!

The Carman-Kozeny relationship shows that the variation in permeability for the same material, but at different fiber volume fractions, is very large. It is not unusual to obtain a factor of ten difference between different fiber contents. Between different materials, the differences can be even larger. This immediately shows the importance of the selection of the fiber reinforcement, since fill time is inversely proportional to the permeability.

The laminate in a part often consists of a few different layers of reinforcement. When porosity and permeability differences between the layers are not too large, the overall permeability can simply be calculated using a rule of mixtures (Ref 19). However, large differences between the layers result in a more complex situation with three-dimensional flow. A simple rule of mixtures, consequently, gives a too-optimistic value for the overall permeability. This is due to a three-dimensional flow that occurs when poorly permeable layers are impregnated by the resin flow from highly permeable layers. Knowing this effect, we can use highly permeable layers as resin feeder material. This can be applied either within the laminate using an internal flow layer (such as cores or a random glassmat) and thus creating a resin rich core, or outside the laminate with an external flow layer (using any feeder material). The external flow layer can be separated from the actual laminate using a peel ply and therefore, the flow layer can be removed from the laminate after cure.

Finally, it must be recognized that the reinforcements in the mold are not the only producers of resistance to the resin flow. Every tube, valve, and so on results in resistance to flow and can therefore also influence fill time. To compare these influences, it is possible to characterize all items in terms of permeability.

A tube can be characterized with permeability by using the relation:

$$K = 1/8\ r^2$$

where K is permeability (m^2) and r is inner radius tube (m). Clearly, when a tube is treated like a permeable medium it must be recognized that at constant pressure difference the fill time (for the tube) is also proportional to the squared length of the tube.

In conclusion, the permeability of the reinforcement being used has a large impact on the fill time of the part. Unfortunately, reinforcement suppliers do not give the permeability of their materials. In addition, measurement of the permeability is not straightforward and is influenced by the fiber volume fraction of the reinforcement (i.e., the amount of compression in vacuum infusion) (Ref 20, 21). However, an estimate of the reinforcement permeability can be made easily (see the discussion of reinforcements in the section "Equipment and Material Types and Forms" in this article). Approximate values of permeability of various materials are shown in Table 3.

Injection Strategy. How does the injection strategy, that is, the location of the resin inlet and outlet ports, influence the fill time of the part?

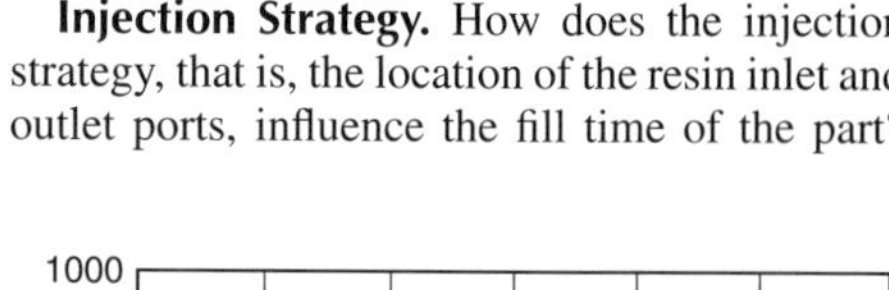

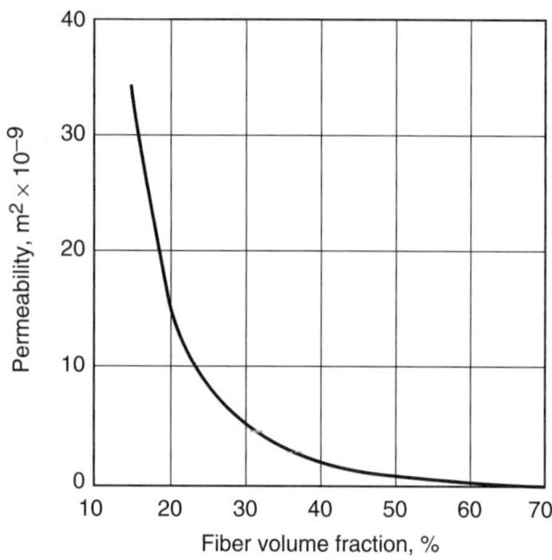

Fig. 8 Permeability as predicted by the Carman-Kozeny model

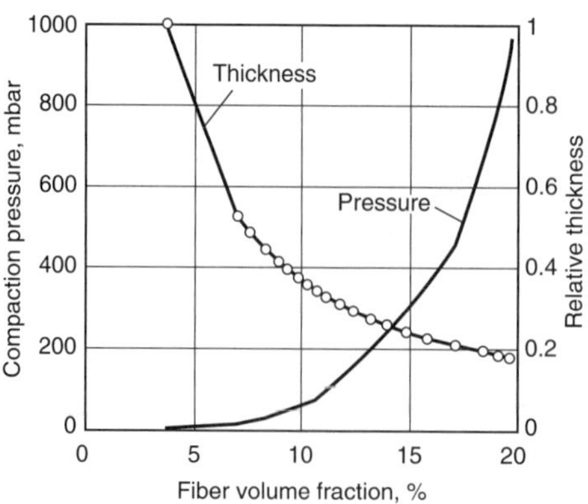

Fig. 9 Influence of compaction pressure on thickness and fiber volume fraction for a random mat reinforced composite

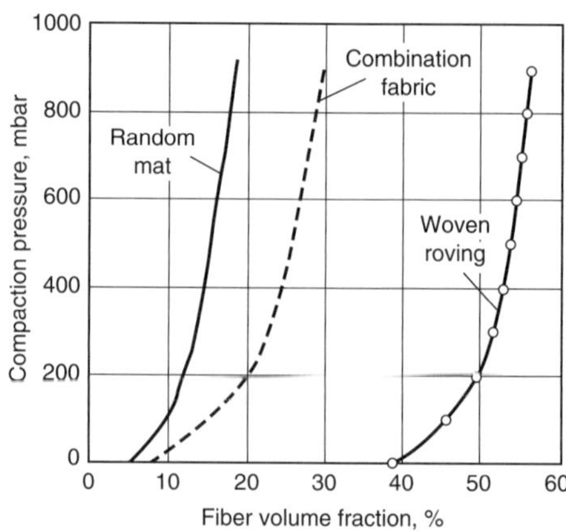

Fig. 10 Influence of compaction pressure on fiber volume fraction for three different reinforcements

There are three basic injection strategies to consider:

- Strip injection (edge injection of a rectangular plate) (Fig. 11a)
- Point injection of a circular plate (Fig. 11b)
- Circumferential injection of a circular plate (Fig. 11c)

Each injection strategy can be considered as a combination of these three.

For each of these injection strategies, we can work out Darcy's law in conjunction with mass conservation equations to get the flow front progression and fill time of the part. Consider the injection of flat plates with the following geometry and injection strategy:

- Strip injection of a rectangular plate, 1 m (3.3 ft) long
- Point injection of a circular plate, 2 m (6.6 ft) in diameter
- Circumferential injection of a circular plate, 2 m (6.6 ft) in diameter

The position of the resin flow front versus time for these three injection strategies is shown in Fig. 12. In this example, the vacuum in the mold cavity is set at 10 kPa (100 mbar).

The strip injection under this specific circumstance takes 1000 s. It can be seen that the flow front progress slows down in the course of the injection. This is due to the decrease in pressure gradient with flow front progression. The pressure difference between resin inlet and resin outlet, and the resulting pressure gradient with flow front progression is shown in Fig. 13. The point injection under these conditions takes over 4500 s. The flow front slows down much more than during the strip injection because the length of the flow front increases with flow front progress (the diameter of the flow front increases). The pressure gradient drops much quicker as compared with the strip injection of a rectangular plate (see Fig. 14). During circumferential injection the opposite takes place. The flow front actually speeds up at the end of the injection, and the part is filled in only 500 s. The pressure gradient is shown in Fig. 15.

The repercussions of the injection strategy on the fill time can be very significant. When we compare two injection strategies for a flat rectangular plate of 1 × 2 m (3.3 × 6.6 ft), edge injection from the short side will take about 25 times longer than a fishbone injection (as shown on the Contest hull in Fig. 3 and 4).

From these simple examples we can conclude that injection strategy parameters that influence fill time are:

- Injection distance
- Ratio of length of the injection channel and length of the flow front (The possible variation in this ratio during injection should also be considered.)

Dry Spot Formation. So far we have discussed the influence of resin, reinforcement per-

Table 3 Permeability of reinforcements, flow layers, and tubes

Material	Permeability, 10^{-9} m^2
Glass reinforcement	
Multiaxial	0.05–0.30
Woven roving	0.05–0.30
Random mat	1–4
Combination mat	4–8
Cores and flow layers	
Contoured balsa (25 mm, or 1 in.)	3
Flow layer grid	10
Flow layer braiding	50
Tubes	
Internal diameter 5 mm (0.2 in.)	800
Internal diameter 10 mm (0.4 in.)	3000
Internal diameter 25 mm (1 in.)	20,000

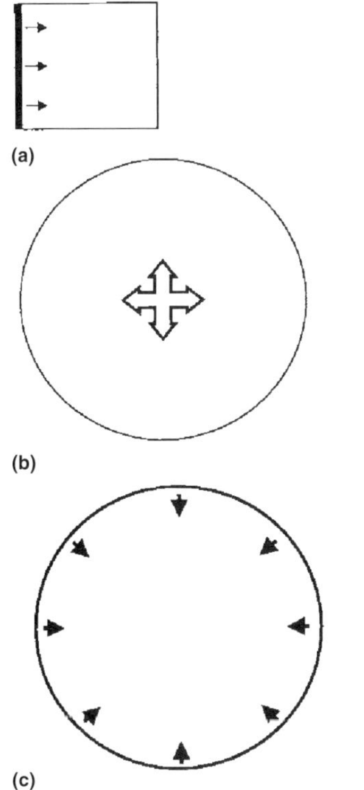

Fig. 11 The three basic injection strategies to consider. (a) Strip injection. (b) Point injection. (c) Circumferential injection

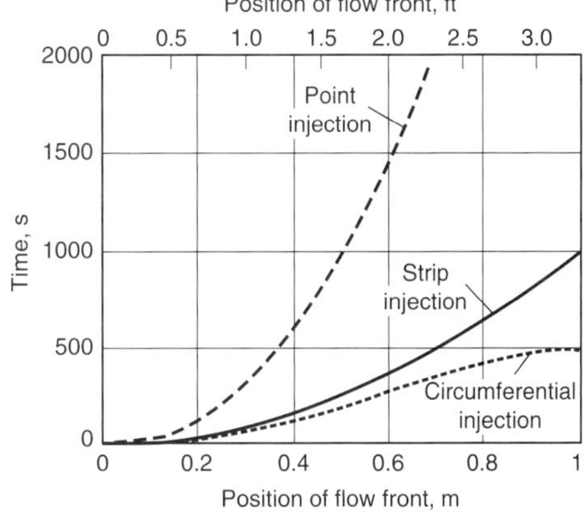

Fig. 12 Flow front progress, in time, for the three basic injection strategies

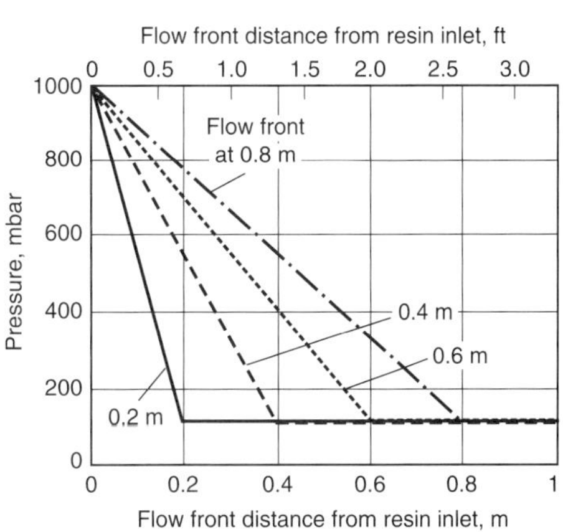

Fig. 13 Pressure gradient during strip injection of a rectangular plate at four flow front positions

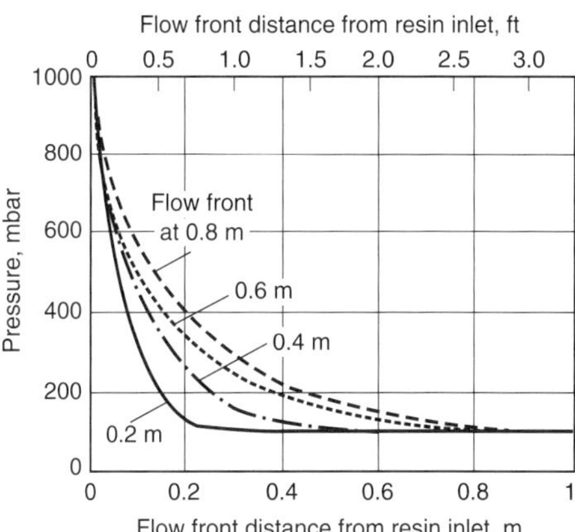

Fig. 14 Pressure gradient during point injection of a circular plate at four flow front positions

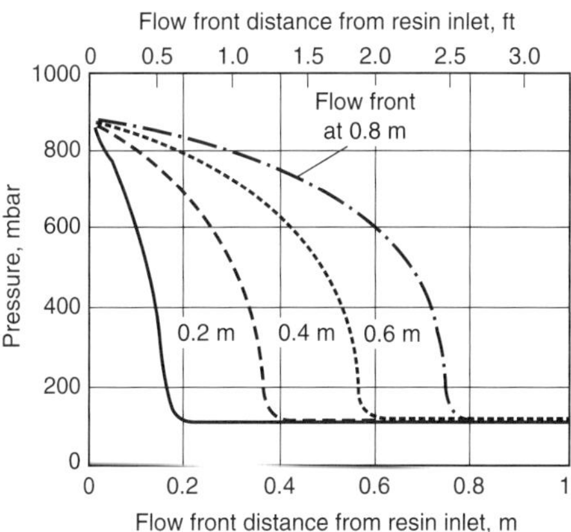

Fig. 15 Pressure gradient during circumferential injection of a circular plate at four flow front positions

meability, and injection strategy on the fill time of the part. However, a major issue concerning the injection strategy is to fill the part completely, without dry spots. Dry spots are formed when the resin flow front encloses part of the reinforcement that is not directly connected to an outlet. This results in entrapped air, which can result in either a none-impregnated spot or a void-rich area in the laminate. There are three major ways in which part of the laminate can become enclosed by resin:

- *Differences in injection distance:* In Fig. 16 a cover box is shown. When this part is injected from one side to the other there is a large difference in the distance that the resin needs to flow. Along the edge, the distance is much smaller than over the top of the box. Consequently, a dry spot will be formed.
- *Differences in reinforcement permeability:* In Fig. 17 a rectangular panel is shown. The central part consists of a poorly permeable fabric, while the rest consists of a highly permeable random mat. When this panel is injected from one side to the other, the resin will flow faster around the woven fabric than through the woven fabric, resulting in a dry spot.
- *Runner channels ("racetracking"):* In Fig. 18 a panel with ribs is shown. It can be difficult to drape the reinforcement around the ribs. This will result in a small gap (channel) between the edge of the rib and the reinforcement. This gap will have a high permeability, and resin will flow through this channel easily. Therefore, the area between the ribs can be enclosed.

The examples given previously are typical in plane problems. However, similar problems can occur through the thickness of the part. In Fig. 19 a cross section of a panel is shown. One side of the panel is quite thick, while the other side is thin. Because it is a large panel and the reinforcement has low permeability, a flow layer is placed on top of the laminate. When this panel is injected from the thick side to the thin side, the following can occur: the resin flows through the feeder material and starts impregnating the reinforcement. The through-thickness impregnation, however, is quite slow. Accordingly, the thin part is impregnated before the thick part, and a dry spot can be formed.

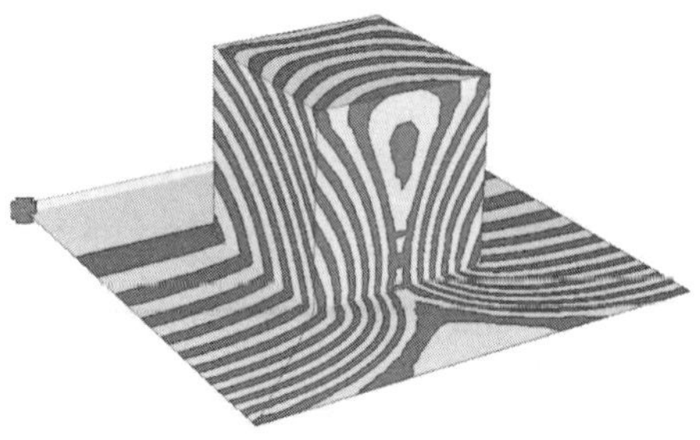

Fig. 16 Flow front simulation of the edge injection of a cover box

The mistakes in the examples mentioned previously are quite obvious. However, as the part complexity increases, similar problems can occur and they are not always as easily recognized. Fortunately, flow simulation software is available. Based on part geometry, permeability and injection strategy flow front progression in time is calculated. For complex geometries, this kind of software is very helpful to determine the appropriate injection strategy (Ref 12, 22–24).

Technique Description: How Parts Are Made

Vacuum infusion is a versatile technique. Before starting the production of a part, it first must be determined how the part will be made. It must be realized that vacuum infusion is just one option and that other techniques might be suitable as well. In the ideal situation, a comprehensive list of part requirements forms the basis for a concurrent development and selection of design, materials, and production technology. This ensures that the optimal solution can be obtained.

Injection Tests. When vacuum infusion has been selected for manufacturing the part, the following general testing sequence is advised:

- *Small scale injection tests (flat panels):* In order to judge both the reinforcement (handling, permeability) and the resin (handling, viscosity, impregnation of reinforcement, cure), simple injection tests can be carried out on small rectangular panels. This provides an initial screening of the materials (see also the section "Materials" in this article).
- *Full scale simplified injection tests:* Difficult sections in the part can be investigated with injection tests using relatively simple tooling on a 1 to 1 or 1 to 2 scale. For example, a change of thickness in the part can be investigated with an injection test on a flat panel. The same can be done with an insert or rib. A corner or an edge can be investigated using a simple bend aluminium plate as tooling.
- *Full scale section injection test:* Finally, a full scale section of the part can be made in the production mold. This final test ensures fine-tuning of the process and elimination of possible mistakes.

The injection tests are carried out concurrently with the development of the appropriate injection strategy. When the part is complex, a flow front simulation tool can also be helpful.

Mold Preparation. The mold must be cleaned properly. Damage to the mold must be repaired carefully so as to not affect the airtightness of the mold. Finally, a release agent must be applied. Careful cleaning and proper application of the release agent will greatly prolong the life span of the mold.

Application of Gelcoat and/or First Layer. Depending on the size and the requirements of the part, a gelcoat can be applied. The gelcoat should not be applied on the flange of the mold that is used for sealing. First, a hand lay-up layer can be applied on the gelcoat. This layer is applied either to get better durability properties (using a resin system other than the injection resin) or to protect the gelcoat layer during lay-up of the dry reinforcement and to assure good adhesion between the laminate and the gelcoat. Large parts often require several days or even weeks to

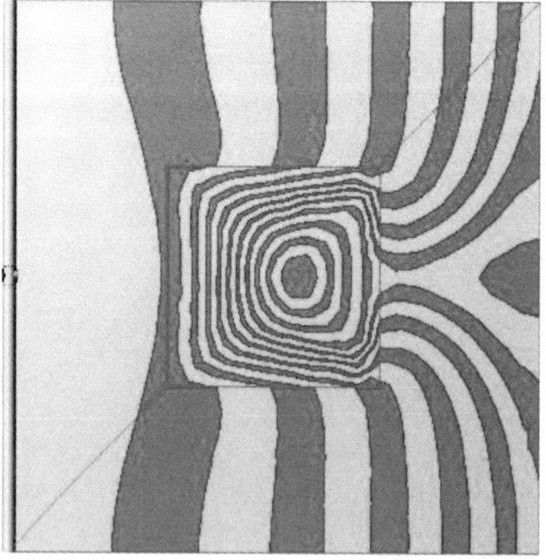

Fig. 17 Flow front simulation of a panel with a central part of a poorly permeable fabric

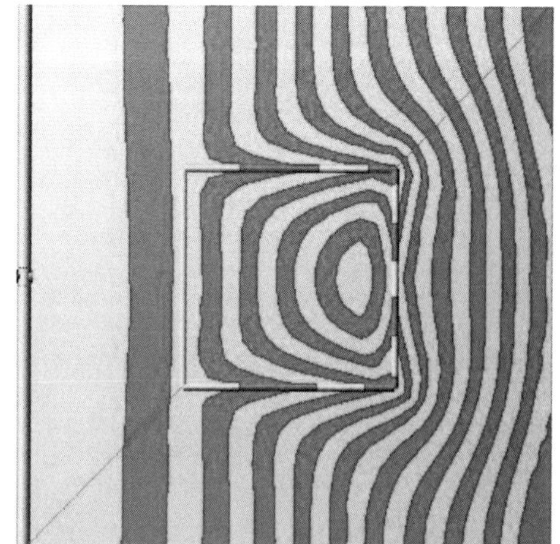

Fig. 18 Flow front simulation of a panel with ribs

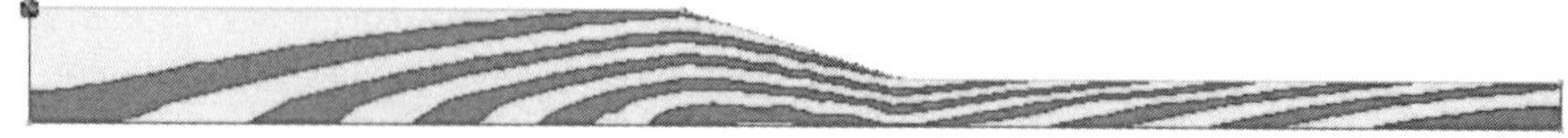

Fig. 19 Cross section of a panel with a thick and thin part and a flow layer on top of the laminate

put all the reinforcement in the mold. Without the hand lay-up layer, the gelcoat would be damaged and adhesion would be poor.

Placement of Dry Reinforcement and Cores in the Mold The dry reinforcement and cores (if used) are placed in the mold. For small parts, the reinforcement could be preformed to speed up the cycle time (as in RTM). For large parts, the reinforcement (sometimes precut) is placed in the mold and secured (if required). Securing the reinforcement and cores in the appropriate position can be difficult, especially with complex geometries and vertical surfaces. In order to secure the reinforcement, three methods can be used:

- Temporary clamps and fasteners (will be removed from the part before or after the infusion)
- Permanent mechanical fasteners, such as staples (will remain in the part)
- Adhesives, such as thermoplastic binders, hot-melts, or glue

A permanent securing method (mechanical fasteners or adhesives) can affect laminate properties (see also the section "Representative Component Properties" in this article).

Placement of Distribution Channels and/or Flow Layers. When a flow layer is used on top of the reinforcement, this layer is usually placed on the reinforcement with a peel ply in between. This enables the removal of the flow layer after infusion and cure of the resin. Based on the selected injection strategy, resin distribution channels (often plastic or steel helicoils) are placed on the reinforcement and/or flow layers. To ensure removal, the distribution channel is usually wrapped in a peel ply. This can also prevent the foil of the vacuum bag from being pressed between helicoils of the distribution channel and thus blocking the channel. However, it must be realized that the peel ply produces resistance to the resin flow. Multiple wrapping of the injection channel with a peel ply will result in a very slow injection. When an internal flow layer is used (reinforcement layer with high permeability), it is best to ensure that the resin distribution channel is in direct contact with this layer to ensure fast infusion.

Placement of Inlet. The resin inlet can be integrated into the mold and, in this case, the resin distribution channel must be properly connected to the resin inlet. In many cases the resin inlet is a plastic tube that is placed on the mold flange and sealed onto the mold with tacky tape. The tube must be properly connected to the distribution channels.

Placement of Outlet Ports on Top of the Reinforcement. The position of the outlet ports depends on the injection strategy. One can roughly distinguish two different ways:

- On the edge of the part
- Somewhere central on the part (not on the edge)

When the outlet ports are located on the edge of the part, the placement of an outlet port is very simple and easy. Often an "outlet channel" is placed around the part (sometimes only partially around the part). This channel can also be integrated in the mold. At the location where an outlet port is required, a simple connection is made between the reinforcement and the outlet channel. This connection can be made simply with some flow layer material.

If the outlet port is located somewhere on the part, it is slightly more difficult to properly realize an outlet port. Integration of the outlet in the mold is a foolproof solution. Obviously, if it is required to realize an outlet port through the vacuum bag, this can only be done after placement of the vacuum bag. Although there are special fittings available for this purpose, these outlets remain a possible location for leakage. Such a leakage might not destroy the part, but because it is located at the outlet it will be difficult to check the part for leakage prior to injection.

Closure of the Mold. Obviously, closing the mold also depends on the type of mold. When a flexible glass reinforced plastic shell is used, the seals are usually integrated in the mold. A slot in the mold with rubber or silicone o-rings is very effective. When a foil is used, the foil needs to be draped over the part and sealed onto the mold with tacky tape.

For any mold system it is possible to choose between a single or double seal. Because leakage is critical in vacuum infusion, a double seal is often the preferred solution. Flow layer material is placed in the cavity between the two seals and the cavity is evacuated, ensuring the absence of leakage (see Fig. 20).

Proper draping of the foil over the part is a critical step. Clearly, the foil needs to be big enough to follow the geometry and completely cover the part. This is especially critical when a foil is used that cannot be stretched (such as polyamide foils). When the part is complex, this usually results in folds in the foil. These folds will need to be properly sealed as well (see Fig. 21).

Application of Vacuum and Test for Leakage. When the mold is closed (foil is sealed onto the mold flange), the mold cavity can be evacuated. Clearly, the resin inlet hose must be closed. If a double seal is used, the cavity between the seals is evacuated first. The pressure (vacuum level) in this cavity and leakage must be checked. Although some companies rely solely on the pressure measured (if a certain pressure level is achieved, the seal is considered acceptable and there is not too much leakage), this is considered insufficient. To control the leak rate, the following method, applied by most companies, is considered simple and good: the hose to the pump is closed and the pressure decay is measured (after 1, 2, etc. minutes). This results in a leak rate of x mbar per minute, which is a good unit for deciding on acceptance of this leak rate. For the cavity between the seals, a leak rate of 100 or 200 Pa (1 or 2 mbar) per minute is often considered acceptable.

Then the mold cavity can be evacuated. When a fiberglass shell is used, this is a matter of starting the pump or opening a valve and waiting for the required injection pressure. When a foil is used, excess air has to be removed first. When the foil is just pressed onto the reinforcement, the valve to the pump is closed. The pressure in the mold cavity should be close to atmospheric pressure (approximately 99 kPa, or 990 mbar, absolute pressure). Now the position of the foil is checked. Along all edges, the foil and the glass reinforcement are manually pressed tightly into the edge. This can prevent unwanted racetracking channels. Finally the pressure is slowly decreased to reach the required injection pressure. Foil and reinforcement are pushed into the edges to prevent these from bridging over edges.

The leak rate is checked in the same manner described previously. A sonic leak detector is normally used to find the location of leaks. Leaks in the foil are closed with a little bit of tacky tape. A leak rate of about 500 Pa (5 mbar) per minute is usually considered acceptable for large parts, although a leak rate of 1000 Pa (10 mbar) and even up to 1500 Pa (15 mbar) per minute is sometimes accepted.

As mentioned previously, vacuum infusion is very sensitive to leakage. It can be disastrous for the part. Checking and searching for leaks can easily take a day for a large part (such as a 17 m, or 55 ft, hull).

Preparation of the Resin. The resin for the infusion must be in the workshop at least 24 hours before the infusion to allow the resin to reach the same temperature as the workshop. Only after the leak rate is considered acceptable can the resin components be mixed. Mixing needs to be done carefully to prevent dragging

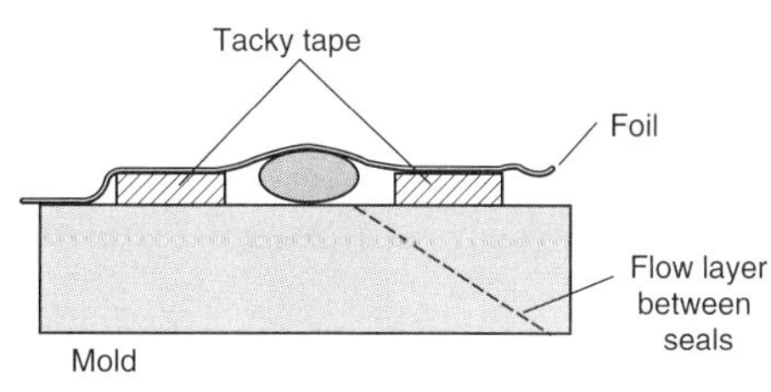

Fig. 20 Double sealing with a flow layer to evacuate the cavity between the seals

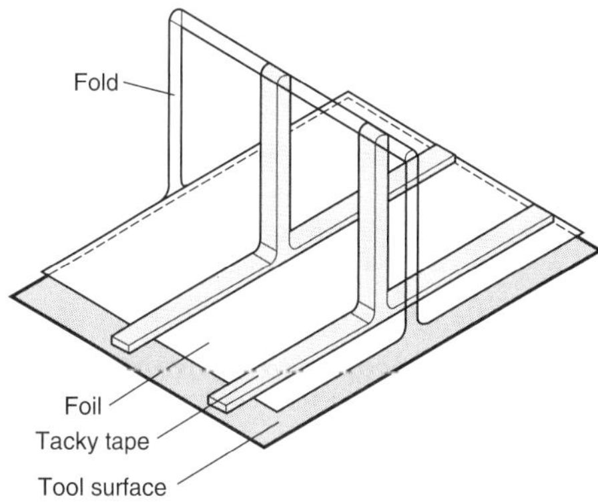

Fig. 21 Properly sealed folds in the foil

in excessive air (which can cause bubbles in the part). The resin can be degassed before and after mixing, depending on the purpose. Before mixing, the resin can be degassed thoroughly to remove dissolved air (Ref 25, 26). After mixing, degassing can be used to remove small bubbles that are dragged into the resin during mixing. Degassing can, however, affect resin cure. Checking the resin temperature, viscosity, and gel time is good practice to prevent mistakes, especially for large parts.

Infusion of the Resin. When the leak rate is acceptable, the injection pressure is set and checked, the resin is mixed and the temperature and viscosity of the resin is checked, then the infusion can start. In the simplest method, a hose is fixed in a bucket with resin. The hose is opened (valve, or removal of a clamp) and the resin flows into the mold.

Needless to say, the hose must remain in the resin during the whole infusion. The resin level in the bucket must be monitored. When the hose is pushed to the bottom of the bucket, the hose can be closed and the resin flow will slow down.

During the infusion, the process must be monitored. When a foil is used, the resin flow front can easily be seen. In large parts, operators can walk on the foil (no shoes!) to monitor the process. Bubbles in the resin indicate a leak in the foil. The bubbles can be visually traced back to the hole in the foil, and the hole can be sealed with tacky tape.

Racetracking channels can cause dry spots. These dry spots can be removed using an emergency outlet that ensures the dry spot is impregnated with resin (see also the section "Equipment and Material Types and Forms" in this article).

Finishing the Infusion. Even though the resin has filled the entire mold cavity, this does not mean that the infusion process is complete. Void content, thickness, thickness tolerances, and fiber content of the part are all affected by how the infusion is ended. The four main possibilities to finish the infusion are:

1. Close inlet
2. Close outlet
3. Close both inlet and outlet
4. Increase pressure at outlet and subsequently close inlet

To illustrate which option is good and which is not, we must look at the pressure in the mold cavity. Figure 22 shows the pressure in the mold cavity for a rectangular plate, just after the mold has been filled (the line labeled "mold filled"). At this moment, there is almost no compressive force on the reinforcement close to the inlet. This means that the laminate is thicker close to the inlet and contains excess resin, as compared to the vicinity of the outlet.

If the inlet is closed first, the pressure in the entire mold will decrease to reach the infusion pressure (the line labeled "Option 1"). Excess resin will flow toward the outlet and the thickness of the part will reduce, leading to a high and homogeneous fiber content. However, air bubbles present in the part will increase in size, and this will be most prominent in the part close to the inlet since the pressure drop close to the inlet is much larger than near the outlet. In addition, there is also the risk of degassing of the resin. This means that air, dissolved in the resin, will form bubbles since the amount of air that can be dissolved in resin is smaller at lower pressure. Clearly, this is not a desirable situation.

If the outlet is closed first, the pressure in the entire mold will increase to atmospheric pressure (the resulting pressure will depend on the relative position of the resin tank with respect to the mold; see the line labeled "Option 2"). Although this will cause bubbles to decrease in size, the thickness of the part will slowly increase due to the resilience of the reinforcement, resulting in a laminate with low fiber content. Gravity may also cause resin flow on vertical surfaces, leading to poor thickness tolerances. Again, this is not desirable.

Closing both inlet and outlet at the same time will result in pressure equilibrium somewhere in between the atmospheric pressure at the inlet and injection pressure at the outlet (the line labeled "Option 3"). This is a good way to end the infusion. However, in circumstances where a small leak persists, this method can result in a part with many voids and bubbles. In this case, Option 4 is more favorable. The pressure at the outlet is first increased (for example, from 10 to 40 kPa, or 100 to 400 mbar, absolute pressure). Then the inlet is closed. This will result in an equilibrium pressure, as shown with the line labeled "Option 4" in Fig. 22, and at a leak, a small pressure gradient will remain. In an optimized process, the inlet can be closed before the mold is entirely filled. If properly made, the excess resin present in the mold will flow toward the outlet during the pressure equalization and complete the infusion with a minimum of resin spillage through the outlet.

In conclusion, increase the pressure and close only the inlet. The outlet can be closed after gelation of the resin when flow no longer is possible. When the resin has cured, all ancillary materials (foil, hoses, etc.) can be removed and the part can be demolded.

Equipment and Material Types and Forms

Molds. One of the main benefits of vacuum infusion is that the process only requires one stiff mold half. The other half of the mold can be either a flexible bag or a thin shell. The stiff part of the mold can be manufactured by most of the materials and techniques developed for other composite fabrication processes, such as wet hand lay-up, spray-up, or RTM. There are, however, two requirements that must be considered during design and manufacture of the mold:

- The mold must be absolutely airtight. This requirement seems obvious, but it cannot be stressed enough since any leakage through the mold is likely to lead to severe manufacturing problems and waste of parts. If holes are drilled in a mold to realize a resin inlet or outlet, this may cause complex paths for leakage. The walls of such a hole should be sealed with resin; a seal at the outer edge of the hole may not be sufficient in this case.
- The mold must contain a flange to allow sealing of the bag or shell. The width of the flange depends on the details of the seal arrangement and the inlet/outlet design, but in general, 150 to 250 mm (6 to 10 in.) is sufficient.

The most cost-efficient mold type depends on the application. The most common type is composite tooling, and often wet lay-up molds can be converted to vacuum infusion molds by constructing a flange. Formed and welded sheet metal is often suitable for single curved shapes. Milled ureol blocks are feasible for complex shapes in a small series. In all these cases, it is important to make sure that all joints in the mold are airtight.

There are three main options for the flexible half of the mold:

- Disposable foil
- Reusable bag
- Thin glass reinforced shell

All three types are in common use today, and the selection depends on part geometry, resin system, and the number of parts to be produced. The disposable foils are usually made of polyamide (PA) or polyvinyl alcohol (PVA) and are of the same type as those used for prepreg consolidation. Re-usable bags are usually shaped or molded to the same geometry as the mold. The materials generally used are polyurethane and silicone. Like the stiff mold, reusable bags must be cleaned properly and may not be damaged. In addition, they can become charged with static electricity. A common problem for both disposable foils and reusable bags is the resistance to solvents in the resin system. Particularly, styrene is an aggressive solvent, and dissolution of the foil leads to either leakage or poor surface quality. Certain types of PA and PVA foils have proven to work well with styrene based resins.

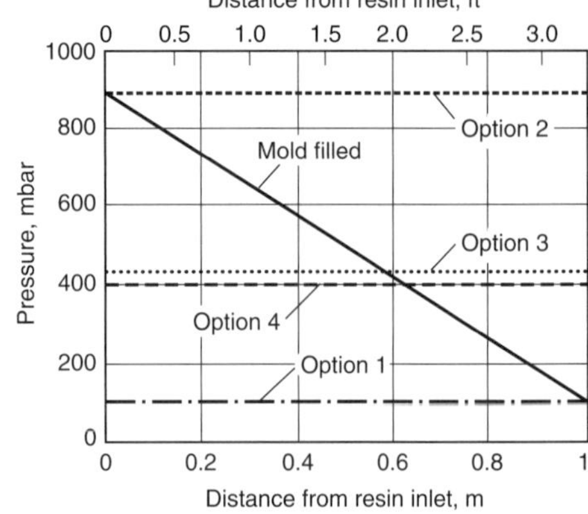

Fig. 22 Pressure in the mold cavity after filling the part and after ending the infusion. See text for discussion

Thin shells are usually made by applying tooling wax in the rigid mold half to build the part thickness. The tooling wax is then covered with a clear gelcoat followed by wet lay-up of glass reinforcement to a thickness of 1 to 5 mm (0.04 to 0.20 in.). The thickness of the shell should be such that it is rigid enough to handle, but still flexible enough to adjust for reinforcement overlaps and other irregularities in the mold and reinforcement. Finally, a layer of clear topcoat can be applied to ensure that the shell is airtight. The use of a clear gelcoat and topcoat is preferred since it allows observation of the mold-filling pattern during infusion.

Equipment. Vacuum infusion puts small requirements on investments in equipment. A basic setup is shown schematically in Fig. 23.

Vacuum Pump. The vacuum pump should be capable of an absolute pressure of less than 10 kPa (100 mbar) without large oscillations. The capacity is of little significance since a small vacuum pump has a capacity of 10 m^3/h (350 ft^3/h) or more. This is more than enough for most vacuum infusion applications. For large parts, however, a vacuum pump with a higher capacity will shorten the time required for evacuation of the mold cavity before infusion. A vacuum control valve should be connected to the pump to control the pressure in the mold cavity. This can, in the simplest case, be a valve to a leak. Finally, a relatively large vacuum accumulator can be an insurance against power breakdown. Without an accumulator, the part will most likely be scrapped if the vacuum pump shuts down during infusion.

Ancillary equipment for vacuum infusion is comprised of pressure transducers for process control, sonic leak detectors and other equipment for detection and location of leaks, mixing, degassing, and dispensing systems to reduce the amount of manual labor and open handling of the resins, and "emergency equipment."

The possibility to use emergency equipment, such as additional inlet and outlet ports to prevent failure of the infusion of a large, expensive part, is a big advantage to vacuum infusion as compared to other closed-molding processes. The equipment can be very simple, but still effective (see illustration of emergency outlet in Fig. 24). Consider the case of a large air inclusion that will result in a dry spot if no action is taken. If the needle of a simple syringe connected with a small hose to the vacuum pump is pushed through the foil at the centre of the dry spot, the remaining air can be evacuated. Tacky tape around the needle should be pushed against the foil to prevent leakage. In a similar way, incomplete mold filling caused by blocked injection channels or premature gelation can be remedied by applying one or several emergency inlets at the flow front. Although this is complicated, it has been used successfully.

Materials involved include resins, reinforcements, cores, inserts, and ancillary materials.

Resin types commonly used with vacuum infusion are unsaturated polyester and vinyl ester, but also some epoxy and phenolic resins have been demonstrated as feasible. The resin system selection is usually a trade-off between performance, cost, and processing characteristics. The main processing characteristics of resins for vacuum infusion are described by viscosity and reaction kinetics. For practical purposes, gel time and exothermal temperature peak usually indicate the reaction kinetics.

The mold fill time is proportional to the resin viscosity, and so a low viscosity is desirable. A viscosity range commonly considered suitable for vacuum infusion is 100 to 400 mPa · s, which is the same as the desirable viscosity range for RTM. Higher viscosity resins can be processed with vacuum infusion, but at the expense of a long fill time and possible poor impregnation of fiber bundles.

The gel time, after which no flow is possible, has to be long enough to provide sufficient time for starting the infusion, completing the mold filling, and, if necessary, extracting excess resin. The gel time should also include some safety margin to account for deviations from nominal temperature and other factors that affect the fill time and gel time. Usually the gel time is tailored to fit each specific application by changing the resin formulation. For free-radical polymerizing systems (such as the styrene-containing systems), small changes are easy to attain by varying the peroxide content. Common gel times range from 20 minutes to several hours, depending on the application.

Reinforcement. As for resin systems, the selection of reinforcements is a trade-off between performance, cost, and processing characteristics. Most reinforcements that can be used for hand lay-up or RTM can be used for vacuum infusion, even though special measures might be necessary for placement of dry reinforcements into the mold and for reaching reasonable fill times. This means that unidirectional fabric, multiaxial fabric, woven roving, and random mat are all feasible reinforcements for vacuum infusion.

The fiber type is normally not important for the process, and reinforcements based on glass, carbon, aramid, flax, sisal, and so on can all be used for vacuum infusion. For specific fiber types, the processing characteristics may be critical (i.e., moisture in natural fibers, difference in wet and dry permeability).

The processing characteristics of reinforcements are related to two steps in the production:

1. Placement of dry reinforcement in the mold
2. Infusion of the resin

To enhance placement of the dry reinforcement in the mold, two different properties can be identified: drapability and shape stability. Drapability describes the ability of reinforcements to con-

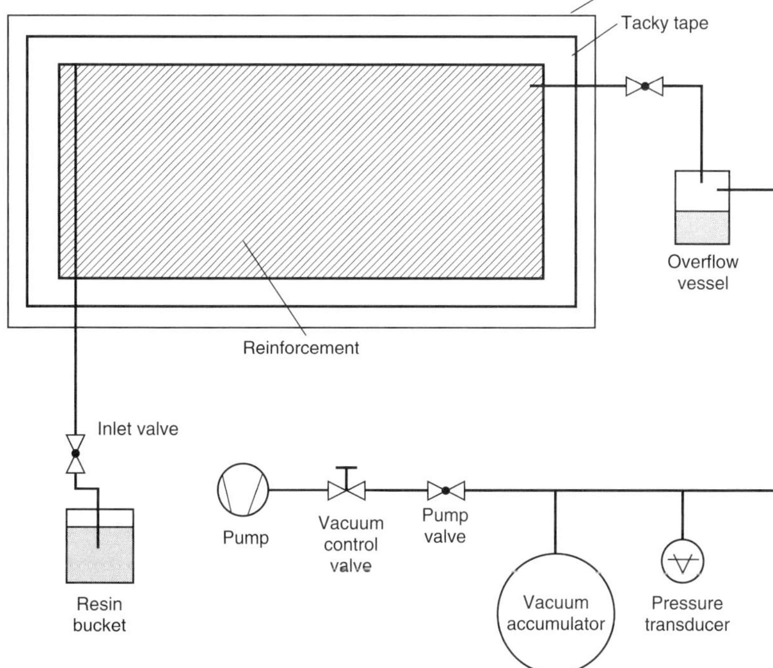

Fig. 23 Schematic of a basic vacuum infusion setup

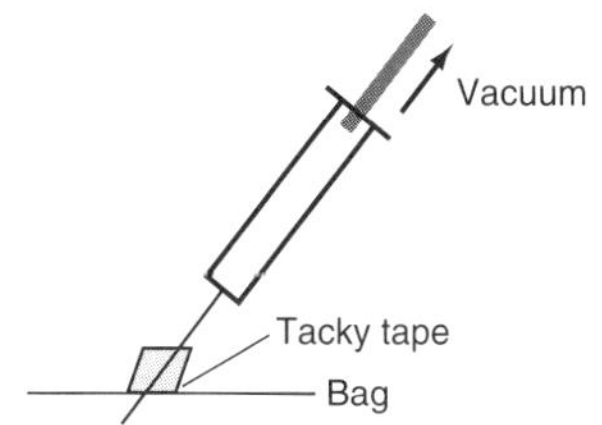

Fig. 24 A simple syringe with needle as emergency outlet

form to a double curved shape. Drapable reinforcements conform easily to a double-curved shape with little force and without wrinkles. On the other hand, poorly drapable reinforcements will require cutting and division into smaller pieces before they can be used to cover a complex surface. Draping will always affect fiber orientation (Ref 27, 28). For vacuum infusion, where the dry fabrics are usually placed in the mold manually through cut-and-paste forming, it is important that the reinforcement is easy to handle. In addition, it is important that the reinforcement stays in the correct shape and position after manual forming. We have chosen to denote this property as shape stability.

For the infusion of the resin, important properties are permeability and reinforcement compression behavior. The reinforcement is compressed due to the vacuum that is applied in the mold cavity, and because the tooling is flexible. The atmospheric pressure exerts the force on the reinforcement. This results in two effects. Due to the compression of the reinforcement in and on edges, the reinforcement can either bridge an edge or create wrinkles (see also the section "Application of Vacuum and Test for Leakage" in this article). In addition, it will affect the part thickness and fiber content and, consequently, the permeability of the reinforcement (see also the section "Permeability" in this article). Reinforcements with different architecture and binder content have significantly different compression behavior.

The permeability of reinforcement can vary significantly. Reinforcement suppliers do not (yet) provide data sheets with compression and permeability characteristics of their material. To obtain information about the permeability, flow experiments must be carried out. Several methods for this purpose are suggested in the literature (Ref 21, 29, 30). Two different methods can be distinguished: radial or parallel flow experiments. Both methods have their merits. Radial flow experiments give the whole permeability tensor in one experiment, while parallel flow experiments are less sensitive to errors and easier to interpret. With vacuum infusion it is easy to perform both types of measurements to obtain an estimate of the permeability (Ref 31). A convenient methodology to characterize permeability for a new reinforcement is:

- Carry out a point injection experiment (radial flow method). This will provide the principal directions of the permeability tensor (i.e., are there differences in permeability in different directions, and in which direction is the permeability highest or lowest).
- Carry out parallel flow experiments (strip injections) in the major and minor direction of the permeability tensor. This will provide estimates of the permeability in the principal directions.

These kinds of flow experiments can be easily carried out in a workshop to obtain rough estimates of permeability. When a reinforcement or reinforcement stack with known permeability is available, this can be done by comparative measurements. It is easy to carry out strip injections with a setup similar to the sketch in Fig. 25. The effective permeability of the lay-up in strip i is approximately:

$$K_i \approx \frac{t_{\text{ref}} K_{\text{ref}}}{t_i}$$

where K_i is permeability of strip i, K_{ref} is permeability of reference material, t_{ref} is fill time for the strip with reference material, and t_i is fill time for strip i. An important aspect in obtaining accurate results is to use the same size and length of injection hoses. The best result is obtained when the flow front progress in time is registered, and a plot of time versus the square of the flow front (t versus x^2) is made. The slope of the resulting line is a good indication for the permeability (which can be derived from Darcy's law; see the section "Flow of Resin" in this article).

There are a large number of reinforcements available on the market, and most of them can be used with vacuum infusion. The different reinforcement types do, however, exhibit significantly different processing properties with respect to vacuum infusion. The processing properties of the most common types are put in relation to each other in a qualitative manner in Table 4. Note that this table provides general information, and that for individual reinforcements, this can be different.

Cores. Some core materials selected to give the part strength and stiffness can be used to quickly distribute resin over the part surface. Contoured sheets of balsa or foam contain slits that enable the core to conform to double-curved shapes. The slits that open up when the core is bent are natural channels that can be used for rapid resin distribution. After complete mold filling and cure, the slits are filled with neat resin that joins the reinforcement cubes together but also adds significant weight to the product. If the slits are not wanted for resin distribution, they should be sealed with filler, as conventionally made for other composite manufacturing processes. A commercially available alternative to contoured cores are cores with machined grooves. Many small grooves will act as a flow layer, and a few large well-placed grooves can be used as resin distribution channels. Also, grooves in the core are a compromise that add weight to the product in order to gain processability.

For some applications, it is beneficial to use flow layer on only one side of the sandwich. In such cases, a perforated core should be used to allow resin to flow through to the other side of the sandwich.

Inserts. Metal or composite inserts can be conveniently used with vacuum infusion. As for other composite processes using molded-in inserts, it is important to choose materials and surface treatment such that the composite adheres well to the insert. Both the surrounding laminate and the insert have to be designed to avoid stress concentrations and thermal mismatch.

Ancillary Materials. A careful choice of ancillary materials for the vacuum infusion process can reduce costs and labor significantly. Pneumatic polyamide tubes, connections, and valves work well for many applications. They are easy to find, relatively low-cost, and rational to work with. All tubes, connections, and valves must, of course, be airtight and able to withstand vacuum pressure. Another important aspect is chemical resistance to the resin. The inlet valve must be possible to clean or cheap enough to dispose of after each injection. An effective and cheap inlet valve can be realized by using an inlet tube that can be folded and opened several times without breaking. Plastic or metal helicoil wires are ideal resin distribution channels.

For weight-critical applications, it may not be acceptable to use internal flow layers such as contoured core materials, continuous strand

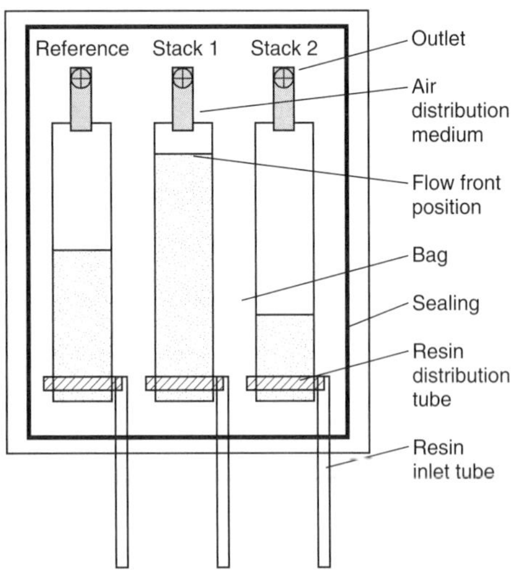

Fig. 25 Schematic of strip injection with multiple reinforcement stacks

Table 4 Processing properties of different reinforcement types

Reinforcement type	Drapability	Shape stability	Compaction(a)	Permeability
Continuous strand mat	Poor to good	Medium	Poor	High
Combination fabric	Very good	Very good	Poor	Very high
Woven roving (plain weave)	Poor	Medium	Good	Medium
Woven roving (satin weave)	Good	Medium	Very good	Low
Multiaial	Poor	Medium	Very good	Low

(a) The ability of the reinforcement to compact to a high fiber content under 1 bar pressure (vacuum)

mats, or combination fabrics. For such applications, an external flow layer is used with a peel ply between the flow layer and the structural reinforcement. The requirements of the flow layer are such that it should enhance the flow in a balanced manner without absorbing an excessive amount of resin. If the geometry is complex, the flow layer should also be highly drapable. Suitable external flow layers are therefore highly permeable thin textiles in the form of nonwovens, coarse weaves, or welded nets.

The glue for positioning dry reinforcement on vertical surfaces has to be compatible with the resin and possible to apply in small amounts where it is needed. The glue should also adhere quickly to the reinforcement to enable efficient lay-up.

Representative Component Properties

Mechanical Properties of Components. The mechanical properties of composite components are primarily depicted by the fiber reinforcement (orientation, fiber volume fraction) and, for a few properties, by the polymer matrix. In general, this implies that the mechanical properties of a component made with a specific manufacturing technology are related to the reinforcement that can be used and the fiber volume fraction that can be achieved. In Table 5 the range of fiber volume fractions for different glass reinforcement types and production techniques is given. Three different types of reinforcement are distinguished:

- Random mat: chopped-strand mat and continuous-strand mat, as well as spray-up roving
- Woven roving and woven fabric
- Unidirectional (UD) reinforcements: rovings and tapes, also including multiaxials; stitched UD layers in different orientations

In Table 6 the mechanical properties for three different glass reinforcement types are given in a common range of fiber volume fractions (V_f):

- Random mat (10 to 30% V_f)
- Woven roving (balanced 0/90, 30 to 50% V_f)
- UD (40 to 70% V_f)

Table 5 Common range of fiber volume fractions for different reinforcement types in various production techniques

Manufacturing technique	Fiber volume fractions (V_f), % Random mat Min	Random mat Max	Woven roving Min	Woven roving Max	Unidirectional and multiaxial Min	Unidirectional and multiaxial Max
Spray-up	10	20	...	...	...	...
Hand lay-up	10	20	25	40	40	50
Vacuum infusion	20	30	40	50	50	65
Resin transfer molding	20	30	40	50	50	65
Prepreg compression molding	...	...	40	55	50	70
Filament winding	...	...	...	...	50	70
Pultrusion	20	30	40	55	50	70

The values for mechanical properties given in Table 6 are averages based on literature data. Semi-empirical calculations result in slightly higher values for woven roving, UD (Ref 32), and random mat (Ref 33).

Influence of Production on Properties. The main influence of the production technique on the mechanical properties is related to the fiber volume fraction that can be achieved. Production techniques that result in similar fiber volume fraction will result in similar mechanical properties. However, matrix-dominated properties, such as interlaminar shear, can be influenced substantially by the production technique and by the way the technique is carried out in the workshop. Unfortunately, there are hardly any data available. In the subsequent paragraphs, the influences of two important vacuum infusion production parameters are discussed: the influence of processing conditions on cure and resin properties, and the influence of reinforcement adhesives on mechanical properties.

Influence of Processing Conditions on Cure and Resin Properties. The cure of the polymer matrix is influenced by the processing conditions. As with any manufacturing technique that uses thermoset resins, the temperature and relative humidity can affect the cure of the resin. However, there is also evidence that absorption of resin components and/or desorption of components on the reinforcement (e.g., sizing) or core material (e.g., absorption of water) influence the cure of the resin. In a workshop, this can usually be recognized as a difference between gel time in the mold and in the injection tank. The gel time in the mold can be shorter as well as longer!

The vacuum in the mold cavity results in another effect that is prominent with resins containing styrene. The free-radical polymerization reaction is inhibited by the presence of oxygen. However, with vacuum infusion there is hardly any oxygen present in the mold cavity. This can result in a higher degree of cure of the resin and, consequently, a slightly more brittle resin matrix. In addition, this can affect secondary bonding.

Influence of Reinforcement Adhesives on Properties. With the vacuum infusion process, dry reinforcements must be placed in the mold. When the part is complex or has vertical surfaces, it is not always easy to keep the reinforcement positioned until the mold is closed and vacuum is applied. One of the methods for keeping the reinforcement positioned is with the use of adhesives. Adhesives on the reinforcement need to be used with caution because little is known about the short or long term effect on laminate properties. However, there is evidence (Ref 12) that the use of adhesives adversely affects the interlaminar shear strength.

It is clear that this issue will require further research to prevent failure of parts due to unknown effects of processing conditions on mechanical properties.

Design Guidelines

Even though, with more or less effort, virtually any part can be made with vacuum infusion, it is important that development and selection of the materials, manufacturing technique, and design are carried out concurrently. When vacuum infusion is selected, the materials and design of the part must be tailored to the process. Design of a part or component is often made based on the functionality of the product, raw material price, and performance requirements such as weight, stiffness, or strength. All too often, production engineering aspects are only considered at the end of the development process, when the possibility to make design changes is limited. Considering the manufacturing process at an early stage makes it possible to drastically reduce future production costs. Important factors to consider during design and choice of materials are described below.

Type of Tooling. The number of parts to be made and the geometrical complexity decides if foil or glass fiber shell is the best tooling type. If a fiberglass shell is to be an option, there has to be sufficient draft angles all over the part (generally 1 to 3°). A fiberglass shell will cost more than foil for a single shot, but is reusable. The fiberglass shell also enables production of parts with two relatively good surfaces, requires less labor during mold closure, and is less prone to leakage than foils. Foils, on the other hand, give larger geometrical flexibility and the possibility to change the injection strategy without tool modifications.

Placement of Dry Reinforcement in the Tool. A drapable and formable fabric can be used in large sheets without extensive cutting and it conforms easily to complex shapes. This is in contrast to some of the high-performance fabrics that are difficult to drape and handle. Accepting more weight in the part may enable se-

Table 6 Mechanical properties for different reinforcement types and various fiber volume fractions

	Random mat			Woven roving (balanced)			Unidirectional			
Fiber volume fraction (V_f), %	10	20	30	30	40	50	40	50	60	70
E_1, GPa	4.8	8.4	12.0	13	18	24	31	37	43	49
E_2, GPa	4.8	8.4	12.0	13	18	24	9	10	12	13
G_{12}, GPa	2.5	2.5	2.5	3.3	3.3	3.3	3.4	4.2	4.9	5.6
ν_{12}, GPa	0.33	0.33	0.33	0.19	0.19	0.19	0.29	0.28	0.28	0.27

E_1, tensile modulus in the fiber direction; E_2, tensile modulus transverse to the fiber; G_{12}, shear modulus in the 1–2 plane; ν_{12}, Poisson's ratio in the 1–2 plane

lection of a reinforcement that results in a cheaper production.

Large radii and little double curvatures make preforming easier. Inner radii should be made larger than 12 mm (0.5 in.), if possible, and even larger for thick laminates.

Injection Strategy. What injection strategy should be chosen, and where should flow layers be placed? Can core materials be used for resin distribution? A slight modification of the design may not affect the performance of the product, but can result in a huge improvement in processability.

Another consideration is how the flow front pattern will develop and how inserts, potential channels at edges, reinforcement overlaps, and so on will affect it.

Cure. With vacuum infusion, the whole laminate is cured at once, in contrast to spray-up and wet lay-up techniques. Thick laminates with a low fiber content will therefore require special resin systems to avoid a detrimental temperature peak during cure. Variations in thickness in a part can cause problems as well. Either the thick part is exposed to a large exothermal temperature raise, or the thin parts show insufficient cure.

Parts Integration. Vacuum infusion is a process that enables a high degree of parts integration. Often the key to cost-effective production of products with vacuum infusion is parts integration, but there is a limit when further integration is no longer practical. Parts integration usually saves weight and reduces labor in secondary operations, but at the expense of more complex preforming or cutting and less robustness during infusion.

Outlook

Vacuum infusion is a technology still not fully matured. The research done since the 1980s has boosted the application of the technology. These applications, in turn, have revealed critical issues for the technology and have shown the need for further research and development. Two main areas for further research are:

- Material development
- Processing equipment and process control

Finally, the successful application of vacuum infusion and the material properties achieved (high fiber volume fraction and low void content) have triggered the attention of the aerospace industry.

New Applications. Vacuum infusion is expected to compete not only with autoclave prepregging but also with other traditional materials used in the aerospace industry. In recent years, developments have already focused on the application of vacuum infusion in this market segment. Until now, this has resulted mainly in small parts made for small aircraft, such as the manufacture of a rudder for the Euro Enaer Eaglet (see the section "Applications" in this article). Now that this has proven feasible, developments will focus on large parts for small aircraft, and it will not take long before an entire fuselage for a small aircraft can be made with vacuum infusion. Current developments also show that commercial application of small and large parts for large aircraft are within reach. These applications include spars, bulkheads, and control surfaces. This implies mainly carbon parts. Both relatively simple shapes (but rather thick parts—10 to 20 mm, or 0.4 to 0.8 in.) and complex shapes (such as a multirib design for a control surface with a top skin, bottom skin, and ribs) could be manufactured in one shot.

Besides these applications, the manufacture of high-temperature-resistant fairings for aerospace rockets also seems feasible. This would imply a vacuum infusion process carried out at elevated temperatures. Initial experiments carried out at the Centre of Lightweight Structures have shown the feasibility of such an infusion at temperatures as high as 150 °C (300 °F) with subsequent postcure at even higher temperatures. Obviously, the appropriate high-temperature-resistant ancillary materials have to be selected, and the process must be well controlled and monitored, but this is feasible.

Material Development. Both resin suppliers and reinforcement suppliers have been working on special systems for injection. For resin systems, this implies mainly a low viscosity system with well-controlled curing behavior. Resin development will and must continue to provide systems with both good mechanical properties and low viscosity in order to facilitate not only processing, but also low shrinkage for a good surface quality. In addition, these systems need to have well-controlled cure behavior to prevent a detrimental temperature peak in thick laminates and, at the same time, allow for a proper cure in thin laminates. This will facilitate the manufacture of highly integrated complex parts.

In addition to the development of better and easier-to-handle resin systems, the characterization of resins and their cured properties must be investigated. Influences of processing conditions on cure behavior and, consequently, on the cured resin properties must be determined to prevent part failure and a resulting lack of confidence in the material and the technology.

Reinforcement development has focused on both drapability/shape stability and permeability. At this moment, easy-to-apply reinforcements with a high permeability, to allow fast infusion of parts, are available. However, this is at the expense of low fiber volume fractions and a relatively high cost. Reinforcement suppliers should continue this development to realize highly permeable, high fiber volume fraction reinforcements.

Core materials currently under development show good permeability, combined with small resin uptake.

Processing Equipment and Process Control. Where can vacuum infusion equipment be obtained? Vacuum pumps, pressure transducers and overflow vessels can all be found, but unfortunately, there are few equipment suppliers capable of delivering a comprehensive vacuum infusion tool kit, including the required process control tools.

It is still difficult to monitor the process properly and to determine, before the infusion, if there are no mistakes in the part, such as unwanted racetracking channels, leaks, wrong filling pattern resulting in dry spots, or too-long fill time resulting in premature gelation of the resin.

However, based on current developments it is anticipated that this kind of equipment will be available within the next five years. This will further prevent production failures and the scrapping of parts. As a result, the confidence in the technology will grow, making it easier for companies to switch to vacuum infusion and resulting in more applications being realized with the technology.

REFERENCES

1. R.H. Sonneborn, A.G.H. Dietz, and A.S. Heyser, *Fiberglass Reinforced Plastics*, Reinhold Publishing Corporation, New York, 1954
2. I.E. Muskat, Method of Molding, U.S. Patent 2,495,640, 1945
3. The Occupational Safety and Health Administration in Sweden, *Occupational Exposure Limit Values*, AFS 1996:2, 1996
4. InfoMil Factsheet, "Styrene Emission in Polyester Processing," Factsheet LF10, Mar 1998
5. T. John, MACT, "Professional Boatbuilder," No. 60, Aug/Sept 1999
6. Group Lotus Cars Ltd., Vacuum Moulding Patent, G.B. Patent 1,432,333, March 1972
7. W.H. Seeman, Plastic Transfer Molding Techniques for the Production of Fiber Reinforced Plastic Structures, U.S. Patent 4,902,215, 1990
8. W.H. Seeman, Plastic Transfer Molding Apparatus for the Production of Fiber Reinforced Plastic Structures, U.S. Patent 5,052,906, 1991
9. Vacuum-Injection Process for Large GRP Mouldings, *Reinf. Plast.*, Vol 21 (No. 10), 1977, p 321–327
10. J. Pettersson, Implementing Vacuum-infusion Technique as Replacement for Spray-up in Boat Manufacturing, *Proc. 21st International SAMPE Europe Conference of the Society for the Advancement of Material and Process Engineering*, April 2000, p 405–412
11. J.L.Clarke, Ed., *Structural Design of Polymer Composites, EUROCOMP Design Code and Handbook*, E & FN Spon, 1996, p 38–41
12. A. Hoebergen, The Practical Application of the Vacuum Injection Technique in Boat Building, *Proc. 15th International Symposium on Yacht Design and Yacht Construction*, Oct 1998, p 1–19
13. A. Jacob, LM Glasfiber: Building on Blade Technology, *Reinf. Plast.*, Vol 44 (No. 2), 2000, p 26–30

14. M. Gan, A. Hoebergen, and N. Weatherby, Composite Lighting Columns, a Design that Saves Lives!, *Proc. 21st International SAMPE Europe Conference of the Society for the Advancement of Material and Process Engineering*, April 2000, p 477–486
15. M.A. French, Demonstrating the Potential Use of Composite Materials and New Modelling Techniques for Future AFVS, *Proc. 21st International SAMPE Europe Conference of the Society for the Advancement of Material and Process Engineering*, April 2000, p 3–14
16. R.A. Greenkorn, *Flow Phenomena in Porous Media—Fundamentals and Applications in Petroleum, Water and Food Production*, Dekker, 1983
17. A. Hammami and B.R. Gebart, Analysis of the Vacuum Infusion Moulding Process, *Polym. Compos.*, Vol 21 (No.1), 2000, p 28–40
18. A. Hammami and B.R. Gebart, A Model for the Vacuum Infusion Moulding Process, *Plast. Rubber Process. Appl.*, Vol 27 (No. 4), 1998, p 185–189
19. B.R. Gebart, P. Gudmundsson, L.A. Strömbeck, and C.Y. Lundmo, Analysis of the Permeability in RTM Reinforcements, *Proc. of the Eighth International Conference on Composite Materials*, July 1991, p 15-E
20. Z. Cai, Estimation of the Permeability of Fibrous Preforms for Resin Transfer Moulding Processes, *Compos. Manuf.*, Vol 3 (No. 4), 1992, p 251–257
21. A.S. Verheus and J.H.A. Peeters, The Role of Reinforcement Permeability in Resin Transfer Moulding, *Compos. Manuf.*, Vol 4 (No. 1), 1993, p 33–38
22. A. Hoebergen, E. van Herpt, and M. Labordus, The Manufacture of Large Parts Using the Vacuum Injection Technique, Practical Injection Strategies for Boat Building Used in the Manufacture of the Contest 55, *Proc. 20th International SAMPE Europe Conference of the Society for the Advancement of Material and Process Engineering*, April 1999, p 237–246
23. X. Sun, S. Li, and L.J. Lee, Mould Filling Analysis in Vacuum Assisted Resin Transfer Moulding. Part I: SCRIMP Based on a High-Permeable Medium, *Polym. Compos.*, Vol 19 (No. 6), p 807–817
24. J. Ni, S. Li, X. Sun, and L.J. Lee, Mould Filling Analysis in Vacuum Assisted Resin Transfer Moulding. Part I: SCRIMP Based on Grooves, *Polym. Compos.*, Vol 19 (No. 6), p 818–829
25. M. Labordus, M. Pieters, A. Hoebergen, and J. Soderlund, The Causes of Voids in Laminates Made with Vacuum Injection, *Proc. 20th International SAMPE Europe Conference of the Society for the Advancement of Material and Process Engineering*, April 1999, p 433–441
26. M. Labordus, A. Hoebergen, J. Soderlund, and T. Astrom, Avoiding Voids by Creating Bubbles, Degassing of Resin for the Vacuum Injection Process, *Proc. 21st International SAMPE Europe Conference of the Society for the Advancement of Material and Process Engineering*, April 2000, p 47–58
27. O.K. Bergsma, Computer Simulation of 3D Forming Processes of Fabric Reinforced Thermoplastics, *Proc. Ninth International Conference on Composite Materials*, July 1993, Vol IV, p 560–567
28. O.K. Bergsma, *Three Dimensional Simulation of Fabric Draping*, Delft University Press, 1996
29. T.S. Lundström, B.R. Gebart, and E. Sandlund, In-Plane Permeability on Fibre Reinforcements by the Multi-Cavity Parallel Flow Technique, *Polym. Compos.*, Vol 20 (No. 1), 1999, p 146
30. T.S. Lundström and R. Stenberg, In-Plane Permeability Measurements, A Nordic Round Robin Study, *Compos. Part A: Appl. Sci. Manuf.,* Vol 31 (No. 1), 1999, p 29–43
31. T.J. Corden and C.D. Rudd (1997), Permeability Measurements and Modelling Techniques for Vacuum Infusion, *Proc. Fifth International Conference on Automated Composites*, Sept 1997, p 231–242
32. R.M. Jones, *Mechanics of Composite Materials*, Taylor & Francis, 1999, p 151–157
33. C.S. Smith, *Design of Marine Structures in Composite Materials,* Elsevier, 1990, p 52–53

SELECTED REFERENCES

Flow phenomena in general

- R.A. Greenkorn, *Flow Phenomena in Porous Media Fundamentals and Applications in Petroleum, Water and Food Production,* Dekker, 1983

Processing of composites in general

- B.T. Åström, *Manufacturing of Polymer Composites*, Chapman & Hall, 1997
- R.S. Davé, A.C. Loos, Ed., *Processing of Composites*, Hanser, 1999
- "Tutorial on Polymer Composites Molding," Intelligent Systems Lab, Michigan State University, http://islnotes.cps.msu.edu/trp/

Liquid molding technologies and vacuum infusion

- B.R. Gebart and L.A. Strombeck, *Processing of Composites—Principles of Liquid Composite Moulding*, Hanser, 1999, p 358–387
- C.D. Rudd, A.C. Long, K.N. Kendall, and C.G.E. Mangin, *Liquid Moulding Technologies*, Woodhead Publishing Ltd., Cambridge, United Kingdom, 1997
- K. Potter, *Resin Transfer Moulding*, Chapman & Hall, London, United Kingdom, 1997

Overview articles

- A. Hoebergen, The Practical Application of the Vacuum Injection Technique in Boat Building, *Proc. 15th International Symposium on Yacht Design and Yacht Construction*, Oct 1998, p 1–19
- C. Williams, J. Summerscales, S. Grove, Resin Infusion under Flexible Tooling (RIFT): A Review, *Compos.,* Vol 27A, 1996, p 517–524

Compression Molding

Charles W. Peterson, Azdel bv, The Netherlands
G. Ehnert, R. Liebold, K. Hörsting, and R. Kühfusz, Menzolit-Fibron GmbH, Germany

COMPRESSION MOLDING is the single largest primary manufacturing process used for automotive composite applications today. The process is also used to manufacture parts and components for other industrial and consumer applications. This article describes the basic design, materials, processing equipment, and techniques used, together with some application examples and market volume information.

A typical manufacturing chain involves the conversion of composite constituent materials, often using a semifinished product (or preform), into an end-use application. Fully formed parts are molded in matched metal compression molds that give the final part shape; usually these undergo secondary operations such as deburring, hole punching, insert assembly, and, in some cases, painting, and adhesion priming or friction welding for tertiary assembly operations with other parts and components. This type of composite component manufacture is based on either thermoplastic or thermosetting matrix materials reinforced, in the overwhelming majority of instances, by glass fibers. Emerging new materials also use combinations with natural fibers and polymeric fibers.

The three main groups of materials that are compression molded are:

- Glass-fiber-mat-reinforced thermoplastics (GMT)
- Long-fiber-reinforced thermoplastics (LFT)
- Sheet molding compounds (SMC) (thermosets)

The processing and applications of each of these materials is discussed in some detail following a general overview of the compression molding process.

Process Description and Characteristics

Compression molding techniques use a flow-forming process where a measured amount by mass of formable composite molding material is placed into an open compression mold and formed into the final component shape under the action of a high-speed, high-pressure press. Figure 1 shows a schematic diagram of a press mold and also how the molding material spreads to fill the mold cavity during the forming cycle. Figure 2 shows schematically a typical fully automated compression molding production line.

Compression molding offers a number of attractive characteristics as a solution for particular applications. Important criteria that may influence the selection of a process are the number of parts produced, cost-effectiveness, and ability to produce physically complex parts.

Number of Parts Produced. The process hardware investments associated with compression molding become favorable from a minimum total production series of 100,000 parts per year, using single cavity tooling; for smaller series, other manufacturing technologies are often more cost-effective. In the automotive sector, annual volumes could reach a maximum of 1,000,000 parts per annum using several molding tools in parallel for one application.

Cost-Effectiveness. The cost effectiveness of a compression molded application depends on several factors, such as hardware amortization, raw material and energy costs, recycling of trimmed waste, series size, cost of automation versus manual labor, material and machine yields, packaging, secondary operations, and so on. Examples of the economies of scale for thermoplastic process can be found in Ref 1.

Part Complexity. Compression molding applications typically exploit the same design flexibility of molded plastics, such as injection molding. Most complex geometrical shapes can be realized, including:

- Large surface areas, for example, 0.1 to 4 m^2 (1 to 40 ft^2) or more, although typically less than 1 m^2 (10 ft^2)
- Wall sections as thin as 1.3 mm (0.05 in.) (ideally with some concavity for dimensional stability)
- Complex ribs (1 to 10 mm, or 0.04 to 0.4 in., in width) and corrugated structures (Fig. 3)
- Bosses, flanges, tabs, spigots, hollow sections, massive hinges, interlocking features, snap fittings, and undercuts (Fig. 3, 4) (Ref 2)
- Molded-in features, such as metallic threaded inserts, ferrules, film hinges, compatible elastomers for sealing lips, decorative fabrics, printed films, high-quality painted surfaces (e.g., in-molded coatings), and auxiliary high-

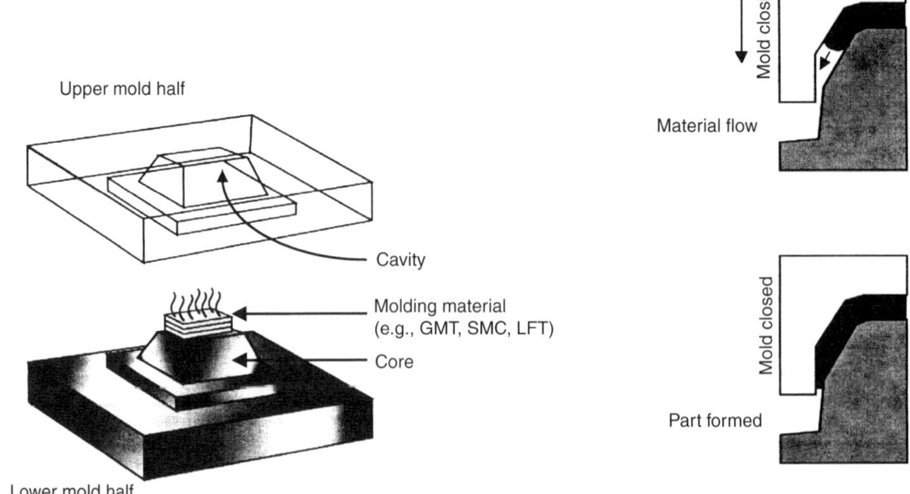

Fig. 1 Schematic diagram of mold cavity filling and part forming in compression molding

performance prepregs as local extra reinforcements (Ref 3)

- In-mold piercing of fixing holes and other openings
- Surface texturing, though the finest finishes are limited by glass fiber read-through
- Colored matrix materials in a broad range of colors for finished parts or base-coat colors for painted parts
- Welded assemblies to similar matrix materials (thermoplastics only), bonded structures, bolting, self-tapping screw bosses, snap fits, and riveting (Fig. 5)

Part Design and Process Engineering

Computer-Aided Part Design. A wide range of computer-aided design software packages is available that can be used to design and optimize composite structures. As for all fiber-reinforced composites, it is optimal to use a three-dimensional mechanical and physical property matrix to describe the material behavior. Optimal designs are found when the three-dimensional loading cases and where local material properties are known. For flow-molded parts, fiber reorientation and matrix segregation can be predicted with basic predictive software packages, in combination with flow-molding simulation software such as EXPRESS (M-Base, Aachen, Germany) (Ref 4) and CADpress (The Madison Group, Madison, WI) (Ref 5). As in most industries, a high degree of "evolution" exists whereby new applications copy and optimize features from predecessor and similar designs, thereby minimizing or eliminating complex computations. Materials suppliers and design agencies offer services and instruction ranging from simple approximations to full computational design facilities.

Process simulation is a modern and accurate technique for creating optimal designs and process productivity for large volume applications. Optimal designs are often the result of an iterative process involving a detailed, three-dimensional finite element model (FEM) that is first used for molding simulation and then for mechanical performance simulation. The model can be used to identify weak areas where failure is likely; the design of the part can then be strengthened in those regions and the model recalculated. The iteration process, assuming con-

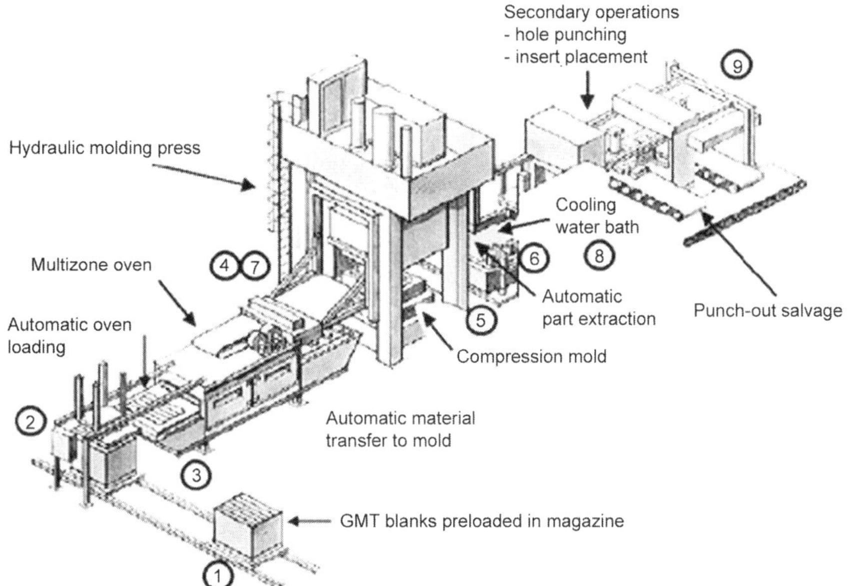

Fig. 2 Typical glass-mat thermoplastic (GMT) compression molding production line

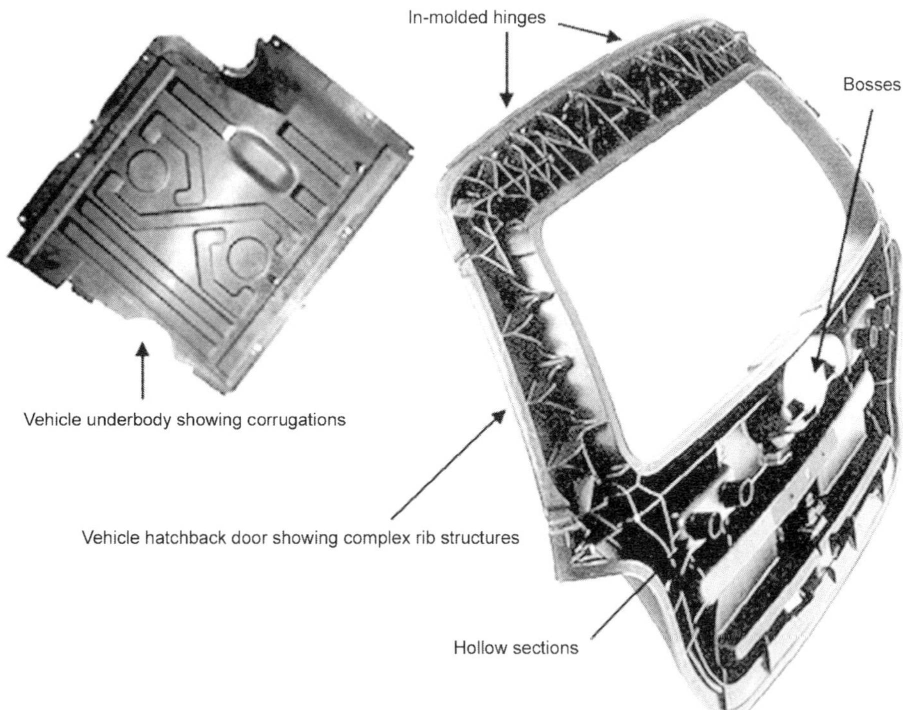

Fig. 3 Examples of corrugations and complex rib structures in compression molded parts

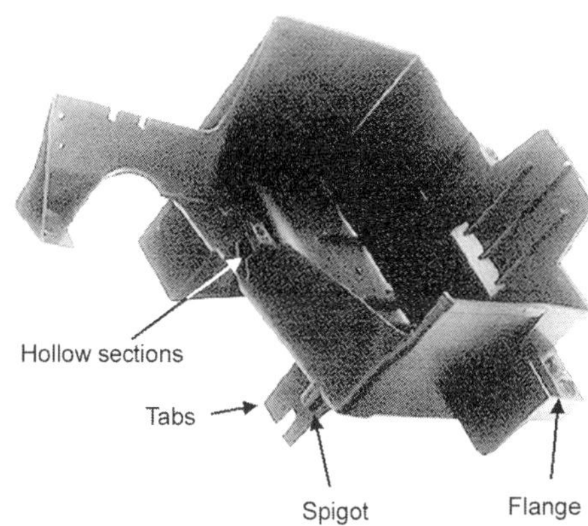

Fig. 4 Example of a compression molded part (a vehicle battery tray) incorporating special molded-in features

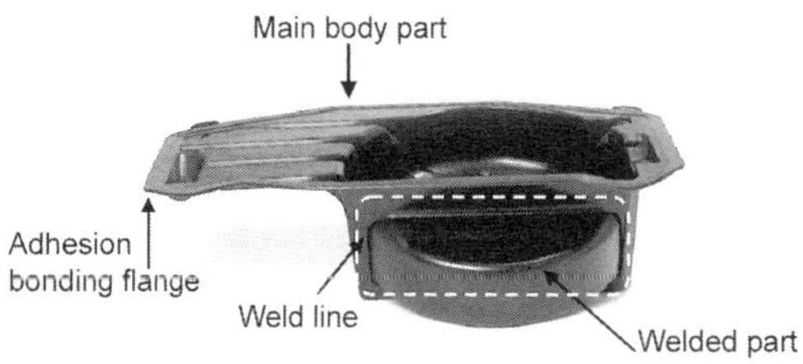

Fig. 5 Example of a GMT compression molded assembly (vehicle spare wheel well) incorporating welded parts

vergence, results in an optimal component. Processing design packages are able to predict fiber orientation, local cooling rates, and cavity pressures.

In compression molding, the properties of the final part depend significantly on the forming process itself. Important factors are flow patterns, fiber orientation, and effects such as freezing (thermoplastic material) or curing (thermoset material). These are not predictable for the engineer while designing the process and the mold; therefore, the use of modern simulation tools is very helpful and can eliminate the need for time-consuming trial-and-error methods.

One FEM-based software package that has been proven very useful is called EXPRESS, developed by the Institute for Plastics Processing (IKV) in cooperation with M-Base Engineering + Software. The program is embedded in the computer aided design and analysis environment and simulates the entire compression molding process; the software can be used to similate the curing effects of thermoset materials (sheet molding compounds/bulk molding compounds) as well as the freezing effects of thermoplastic materials (GMT/LFT). The process is made predictable, and the design of parts and molds made easier, faster, and more reliable. Geometric design and process conditions can be optimized before the mold is made.

EXPRESS enables the design engineer to study different variants and analyze the influences of input parameters at a very early stage of development. Therefore, errors in the process and failures of the final part can be predicted in the simulation, leading to shorter development time and minimized mold modifications. This enhances the quality of the final part and significantly reduces tooling and other costs.

One input parameter for the program is the part geometry. This is in the form of a 2.5D FEM mesh of the final product. Within this mesh, the positions of the molding material (known as blanks) are defined. Blanks can be multiple, overlapping, and can be applied with predefined fiber orientation. Also a very important issue for the simulation is the properties of the material. Rheological behavior, for example, is expressed by the Carreau-Model parameters as the fiber interaction coefficient determines how fibers interact with each other during flow. Data from the materials pressure-volume-temperature diagram is needed for the simulation of shrinkage and warp. Finally, processing conditions, such as mold and blank temperatures, have to be defined.

Using this input, EXPRESS calculates the position of flow fronts that can be analyzed to detect possible flow problems, such as uneven filling, weld lines, and air entrapments. When the flow simulation is done, a nonisothermal EXPRESS calculation generates the temperature distribution during the process. By considering the freezing effects when processing thermoplastic material, the program can also compute the resulting flow channel height throughout the mold, including the detection of early freezing problem areas. Another important result is the fiber orientation. This gives information about the non-isotropic character of the final part, because this is a very important item when processing long-fiber-reinforced plastics. Part warp is calculated from the predicted fiber orientation distribution and the cooling and curing (thermoset material) effects on shrinkage. This provides the engineer with useful information about the dimension stability of the final part. The program also calculates using anisotropic material properties, which can be imported to other computer-aided engineering processors for structural analysis of the part. Figure 6 shows a typical graphical output from EXPRESS.

Design for Manufacturing. Traditionally, the compression molding industry grew from a number of entrepreneurs in the 1960s and 1970s who first molded thermoset parts and later adapted their equipment for thermoplastics, which became commercially available in the 1980s. As the industry matured, companies and applications grew rapidly during the 1990s, and several major machinery manufacturers from the metal forming and plastic injection molding sectors installed the first complete turn-key production facilities. Smaller molders also grew their own infrastructure, building on in-house engineering expertise, and many novel process patents were applied for. Today, several major equipment suppliers have established the most flexible manufacturing systems adapted to the key compression molding processes. Figure 2 shows the main features of a typical compression molding production line.

Compression Molding of Glass Mat Thermoplastics

Process Description

GMT compression molding is a continuous line process for the manufacture of large-volume composite parts. The process is most economical when it is run continuously to make one type of part without need to change the process conditions or mold tool. The steps in the process are described subsequently and in Fig. 2.

Step 1: Loading the Blanks. GMT blanks, purchased from one of the leading materials suppliers, arrive at the molder and are repacked into custom mobile "magazines" in a configuration that orients the blanks in the appropriate pattern for being loaded into the GMT heating oven (Fig. 7).

Step 2: Delivery of Blanks to the Oven. The magazines are then rolled into place in front of the blank heating oven, guided by tracks, buffers, and end stops so as to position the blanks accurately underneath a two-dimensional pick-up-and-place robot system. At this point, the blanks are lifted by vacuum-assisted suction cups by the robot and placed down on an open steel wire mesh belt in the configuration appropriate to the charge pattern to be placed in the mold (Fig. 7).

Step 3: Heating ("Lofting") of the Blanks. The GMT blanks are transported on the wire mesh belt through a multizone heating oven. These ovens are typically long-wave infrared (IR) heating ovens. More recently, other methods of heating have become available, such as hot air impingement ovens, forced convection air ovens, ultraviolet flash ovens, contact ovens, and combination convection/IR ovens. Ovens are typically electrically powered; however, gas-flame heating is popular, especially in France. All have their relative merits; for example, hot air or convection ovens allow blanks of various thickness to be heated simultaneously at one temperature set point. This can be achieved with IR ovens, too, with locally adjusted oven segments for material of different thickness. Some ovens use internal pyrometers to feed back the temperature of the blank to the oven process controller, which adjusts the power distribution to optimize the heating conditions. The fundamentals of GMT heating are discussed in several technical papers (Ref 6).

A typical GMT oven cycle is shown in Fig. 8. In the first step, blanks are inserted cold and can be heated very aggressively until they absorb sufficient heat to approach the melting region of the thermoplastic matrix. Just before melting, the material should be moved to a cooler oven zone of lower radiation intensity, where the energy may stabilize through the material. During this

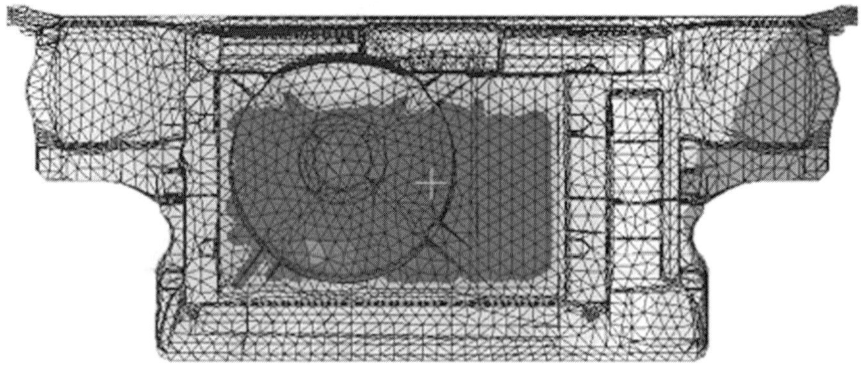

Fig. 6 Example of mold-filling simulation output from EXPRESS compression molding process simulation software

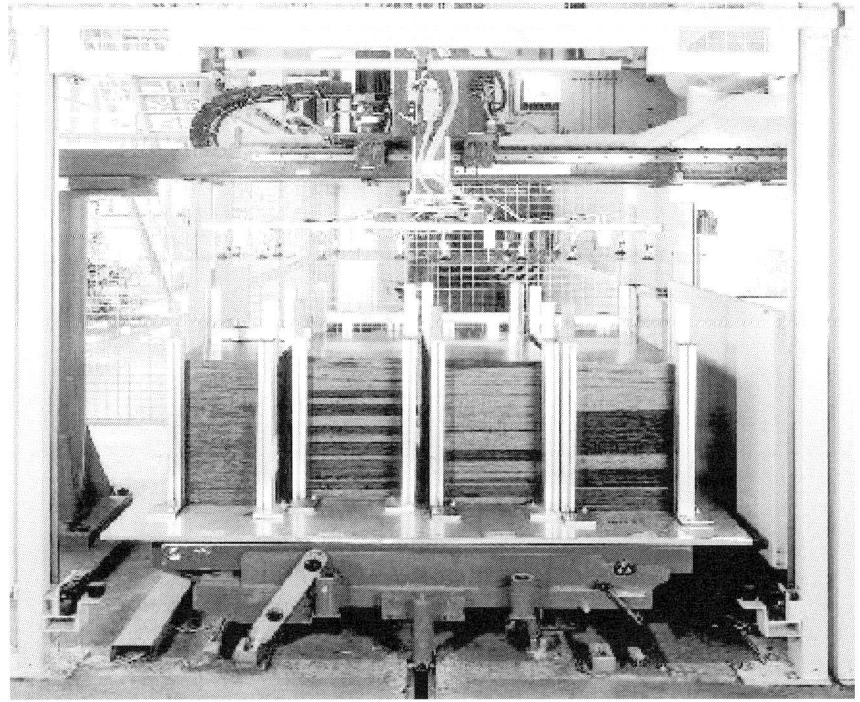

Fig. 7 GMT compression molding blanks under pick-up-and-place two-dimensional robot

phase, a lesser amount of heat is added, however sufficient to bring the material just above the melting point of the matrix. At the moment the matrix melts, the glass mat within the laminate begins to revert back to its original three-dimensional form in a process known as "lofting." Here the material thickness rises by a factor of two or three back to the original lofted height of the glass mats before lamination. In this state, the material now contains a lot of hot air, which is an insulating material and has poor heat conductivity. The material then moves on to the next oven zone and is further heated to the appropriate molding temperature about 40 °C (70 °F) above the melting point of the material.

Step 4: Transfer to the Mold. Once lofted and at the appropriate molding temperature, the material is transferred from the exit of the oven to the open mold cavity. This is typically automated, using needle grabber systems as shown in Fig. 9. Some novel patents exist in this area (Ref 7).

Step 5: Part Forming. As soon as the blanks are placed in the mold, the loading grabber is rapidly withdrawn, and the mold closes under the action of a high-speed hydraulic press. The press cycle begins with a high-velocity, controlled closing cycle. Once the closing velocity can no longer be maintained because the viscoelastic resistance caused by the flowing material is so great, the press is programmed to switch to force control, and the mold closes further at a slower speed until the cavity is filled and the part solidified and formed. The graph in Fig. 10 shows the variation in cooling time with part wall thickness. Press cycle design is the task of experts; however, it can be systematically developed with the aid of in-mold pressure sensors, which allow the programmer to link the viscoelastic behavior of the material in the mold to the hydraulic constraints of the press (Ref 8).

Step 6: Part Ejection. Once formed and solidified, the press opens and the part remains in one-half of the mold cavity, ready for ejection and transfer to secondary operations further downstream.

Due to their shape, some molded parts need to be forced to remain in one-half of the mold to enable a controlled removal. For such parts, small undercuts are strategically designed into the part to ensure that it remains on one-half of the mold tool. The part is then ejected from the cavity with classical ejector pins, sometimes in combination with air poppet valves. In this ejection mode, the part is also forced/lifted over the undercuts designed to hold the part in the cavity. For major undercut features, moving cores or slides need to be pulled out of their cavity or special feature before ejection can occur.

Step 7: Recharging. As soon as the part is ejected, the sliding cores are repositioned in the cavity, a new charge of material is laid into the mold as described in step 4, and the molding cycle is repeated.

Step 8: Immediate Postprocessing. Parts hot from the press can, if sufficiently dimensionally stable, be conveyed on to a deburring station. If controlled shrinkage is needed, parts can be fixed to a cooling jig, sometimes water-cooled in a bath, or sprayed with waterjets to remove the heat from the part and allow it to take on the desired final shape (Ref 9).

Step 9: Secondary Operations. Parts then continue on to other downstream operations, such as drilling, milling, water-jet cutting, and so on, where further complex and contour features are added. Waste collected from these sec-

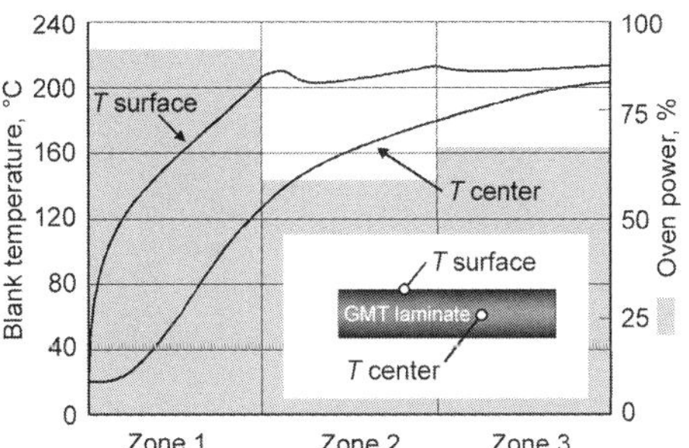

Fig. 8 Typical three-zone infrared oven cycle for heating of GMT blanks

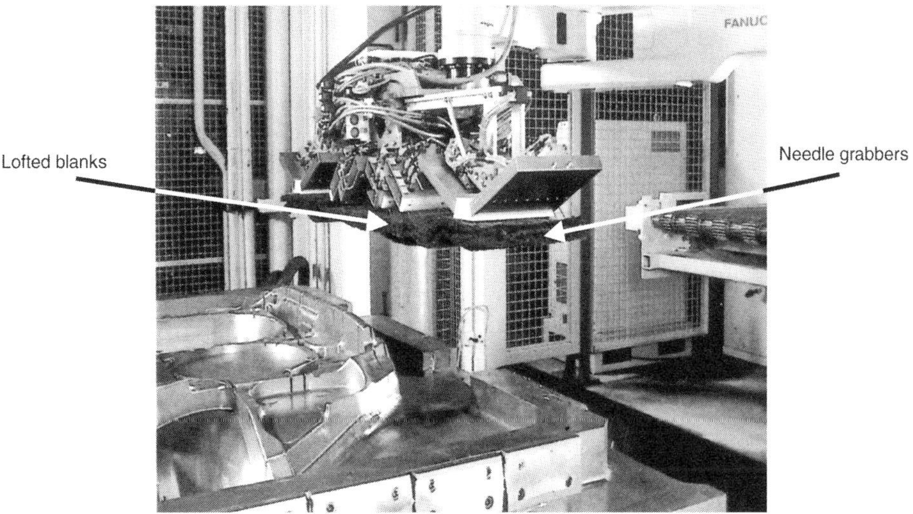

Fig. 9 Hot lofted GMT blanks being transferred from oven belt to the mold

ondary operations can be reprocessed either by the molder in an LFT or injection molding process, or returned to the material suppliers who add small amounts of such waste into their GMT laminates (Ref 10, 11).

Process Optimization. The steps mentioned previously constitute a typical GMT compression molding cycle. State-of-the-art molding equipment is available that can produce thin wall-section moldings in cycle times below 30 s, using double cooling circuits in the mold, which allows the fastest removal of heat during solidification.

Multiple cavity tooling is also used to enable optimal use of the commercially available presses. It can also be advantageous for moldings, which are consumed in pairs, for example, left and right parts, front and rear, or parts that connect to each other.

A technical troubleshooting guide (Ref 12) explains in detail how many of the items in steps 1 to 9 can be optimized, and Ref 13 focuses on dimensional stability.

Mold Tooling

Compression molds are mostly machined from steel. They are designed for a vertical closing action whereby the molding material flows to fill the cavity at the start of the molding cycle. A robust and multi-stage dynamic guide system is used in combination with a parallel controlled hydraulic press to ensure the mold closes bringing the material under the high pressures (5 to 30 MPa, or 1 to 4 ksi). Such high pressures are needed to move the reinforcement structure throughout the cavity and ensure a high degree of air expulsion and composite consolidation. The main features of a compression mold are shown in Fig. 11. Advanced processes, such as in-mold coating (Ref 14) and vacuum-assisted molding are practiced in a few cases where very high-quality surface finishes are required.

Secondary Operations

The most modern molds incorporate some trimming and hole-punching operations to take place in the mold cavity during molding (Ref 9). Once molded, parts typically undergo some or all of the following secondary operations often in the following order:

- Cooling in air or postcrystallization clamped to a cooling jig, sometimes under water or waterjet spray
- Deburring of flash from shear edges (e.g., manual knife tools, milling, routing, and flaming)
- Hole punching, drilling, contour milling, waterjet trimming, or laser trimming
- Plasma, corona, or fluoridation surface priming for adhesive bonding (Ref 15) and/or painting of parts
- Addition of subcomponents, for example, clip-on nuts, bolts/washers, crimp fixations, and so on
- Welding for thermoplastics to other compatible components, and bonding for thermosets to other materials

Tertiary Operations

Once the molded part has completed secondary operations, it can, in many cases be directly fitted or applied to its end-use application at the original equipment manufacturer (OEM). More often, a compression-molded part is part of a subassembly or multifunctional module. In such cases, the molder has additional manufacturing facilities on site to complete the operations. Alternatively the part is passed on to a tier 1 supplier who further integrates the part into a module assembly that is supplied to the OEM, who is often able to eliminate many detailed, complex process steps. Such operations include:

- Application of soft-touch foam layers, noise absorption layers (e.g., instrument panels and underbody shields)
- Bonding/welding to other components
- Fixation of subassemblies, for example, automobile front-end components (Ref 16)

GMT Market Information

A typical value chain for compression molded composites is shown in Fig. 12, which represents the tier supplier system typical to the automotive

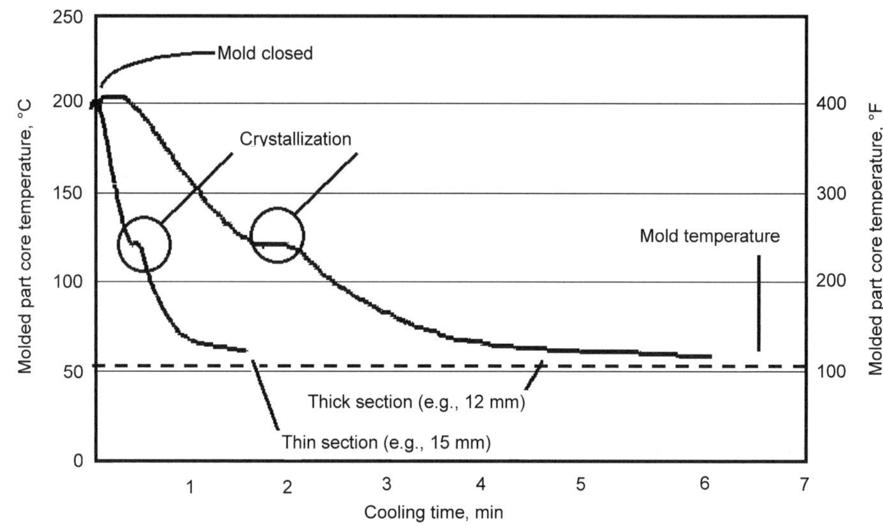

Fig. 10 Cooling curves for GMT moldings

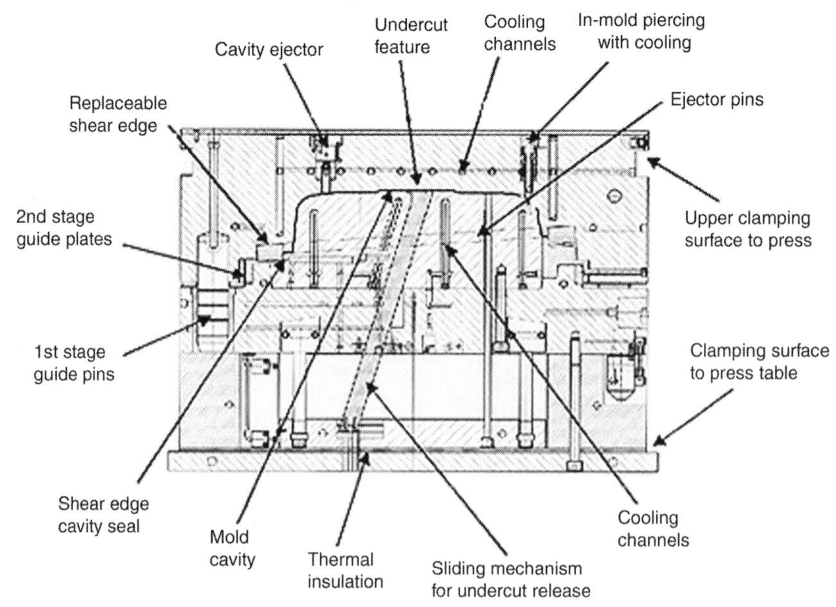

Fig. 11 Typical features of a compression mold (example shown is a mold design for forming a spare tire wheel well)

industry. Here a decentralized supply infrastructure exploits a wealth of global knowledge and competitive creativity, which can include design, predevelopment, and manufacture of parts and optimized processes, which make the most cost-effective composite solutions. Following governmental legislation in the 1990s, a functional infrastructure was created for recycling of process reject and end-of-life compression molded parts. Original equipment manufacturers, molders, and raw materials suppliers are motivated to reprocess waste arising from all steps of the compression molding process. Most applications contain some reprocessed production waste products, ranging from a few percent up to 50% recyclate (Ref 10).

The GMT market grew during the 1990s, with an average volume growth rate of 21% per year. In 2000, production volume was 39,000 tons in Europe and 12,000 tons in North America. The growth in the 1990s was driven by a variety of technical and economic factors. Automotive applications were expanded in a number of areas (Ref 17, 18), especially where compression molded parts were able to replace steel structures. The production volume growth rate was lower at the end of the 1990s, despite the wider use of GMT in a growing number of applications. This was attributed to molded parts becoming lighter and thinner due to the following factors:

- Improved blank weight and flow consistency, giving lower reject rate
- Improved mold filling, given by higher flow materials
- Improved predictive design capabilities, maximizing materials utilization
- Design "evolution," new applications exploiting advantages of predecessor designs
- Over-dimensioning of old designs being corrected, based on field performance data

GMT Material Advances

The rapid growth of the GMT industry has been firmly supported by materials development, which continues to move the frontiers of materials performance to new levels (Ref 1, 19, and 20). This allows parts to be designed and manufactured with improved economics and reduced system weight. These improved materials give direct savings on molded part costs due to advances in the following areas:

- *Development of materials with high flow capability:* The availability of very high flow materials allows parts to be designed with thinner walls and larger surface areas, thus reducing part weight and molding cycle times.
- *Development of improved glass mat technologies:* Glass mat reinforcements have developed to the point where they are very highly consistent in glass fiber distribution, blank weight distribution, local mechanical properties, and maximum load conditions.
- *Optimized matching of matrix and reinforcement:* The flow performance is a synergistic combination of fiber mobility and the viscoelastic characteristics of the thermoplastic matrix. Appropriate matching of the matrix and reinforcement allows predictable mechanical and physical properties, increased production part yields, design flexibility with detailed features, and wider process windows in secondary operations, such as adhesive bonding and hole punching.

Evolution of GMT Materials. The evolution of glass-fiber mat reinforcements can be illustrated by the development and use of four main types (Fig. 13):

- Needled continuous glass-fiber mat was a technology of the late 1980s and early 1990s. When judged by more recent standards, this material offers low consistency and low flow mobility. Applications were often robustly dimensioned and molded with long cycle times despite their good price-performance system costs. Such products remain popular because users have built up trust and experience with them. However, they are increasingly being superseded by more advanced technologies.
- Needled chopped glass-fiber mat (dry layed) was the most widely used glass mat technology in the 1990s. Through improved fiber dispersion techniques and double-sided needling methods, fiber mobility, blank weight consistency, and mechanical properties were significantly improved in both mean value and variation.
- Chopped fiber glass mat (wet layed) became much more widely used during the later 1990s, and further improvements were made to blank weight and fiber content consistency, as well as fiber mobility and mechanical property performance.
- Unidirectional/random hybrid glass mat (dry layed, needled) is a highly directionalized reinforcement structure made from a combination of unidirectional rovings and orthotropic fibers. Such composites have been successfully used in several generations of vehicle bumper beams, seat backs, and knee bolsters, where a highly directionalized reinforcement is desired in locations where high loads are carried in known directions.

Figure 14 shows x-ray photographs taken from rib fill testing of the first three types of glass mat reinforcement structures.

Parallel to these main generations of glass fiber mats are several significant hybrid reinforcements systems, such as:

- *Glass-fiber mineral-filled systems:* give a combination of high elasticity and toughness

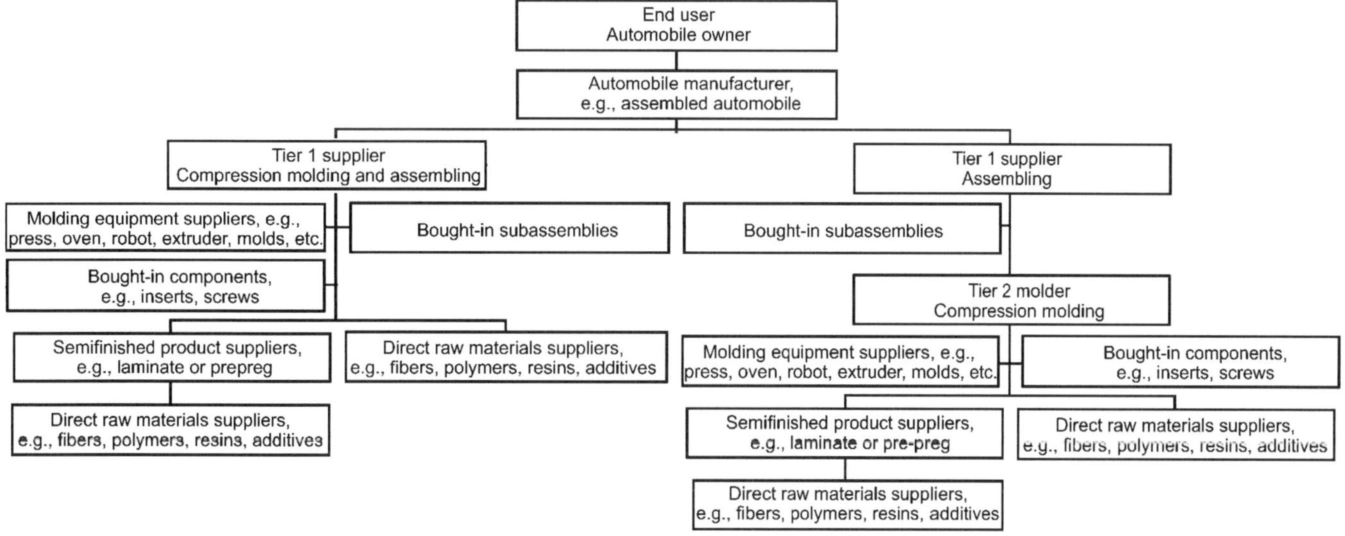

Fig. 12 Value chain for compression molding parts assembly

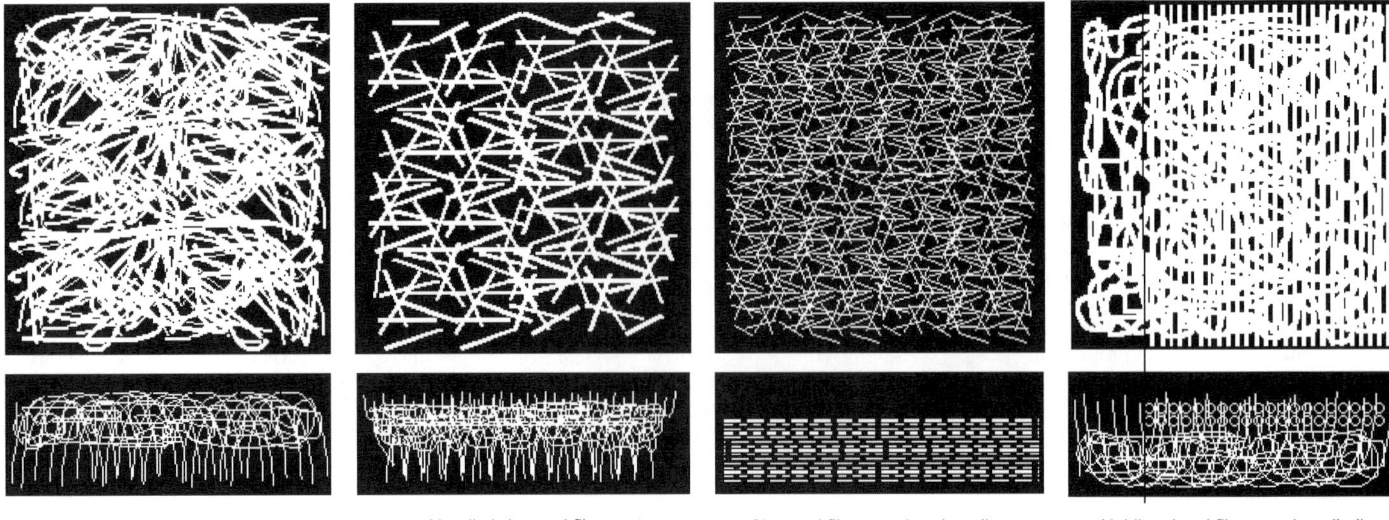

Fig. 13 GMT glass-fiber mat reinforcement types

in high-energy-absorbing bumper beams (Ref 21)

- *Very high flow laminates:* allow designs with minimum wall thickness and deep, thin rib structures while maintaining high property consistency in engine noise shields
- *Fabric-reinforced mat systems:* woven fabrics made of glass fiber or polymeric fiber laminated together with mobile mats, which allow locally extremely high loads to be absorbed and dissipated through a molded composite structure. These are used in off-road sports-utility vehicles (Ref 22) for underbody shields, bumper beams, and structural door modules.

GMT Recycling and Reprocessing

The GMT materials process is well suited to incorporate high usage of GMT recyclate. Materials maintain their consistency in molded parts, with all the advantages of a long-fiber-enforced composite allowing an attractive economic and environmental package ideal for the large volume turnovers of the automotive industry. Such materials have typically very high laminate consistency and extremely good flow performance. Matrix degradation is not a significant problem because materials are restabilized online during lamination.

Reference 10 reviews typical mechanical and performance properties of the previous groups, and Ref 11 and 23 give examples of practical processes used for reprocessing GMT.

Molder and postconsumer GMT recyclate is also reprocessed outside of the traditional compression molding industry, for example in LFT and injection molding processes. Figure 15 shows an example of a heavy-duty grating module system widely used in animal pen flooring. Based on polypropylene, this system gives excellent chemical resistance, long-term performance, and a rapid payback when compared to other competing thermoset molded or pultruded systems. Other examples include railway sleepers, and electrical insulators, and plastic lumber for "street furniture."

Compression Molding of Long-Fiber Thermoplastics

Around 1990, long-fiber-reinforced granulate (LFG) materials were introduced into the market (Ref 24). These granulate materials consist of glass-fiber bundles that are impregnated with thermoplastic material. The material is manufactured in a thermoplastic pultrusion process where the glass-fiber bundles are cut into lengths of 12.5, 25, and 50 mm (0.5, 1, and 2 in.). The material has to be melted again in an extruder before molding. The molten charge is then placed into the mold. This can also be regarded as a very costly process, especially when consid-

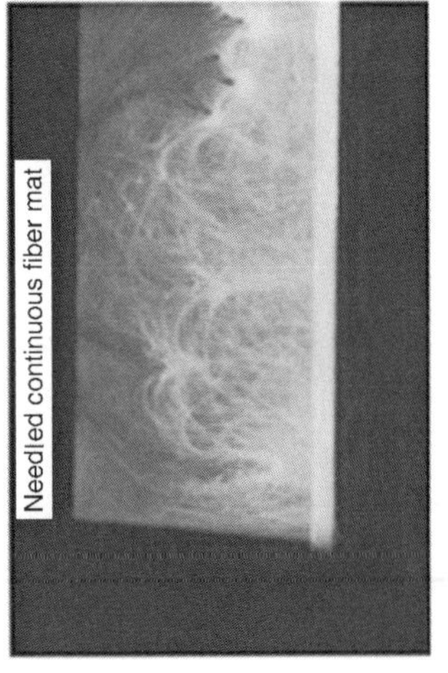

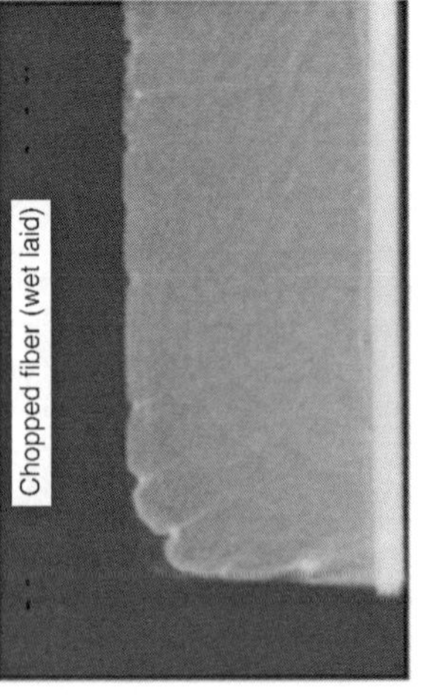

Fig. 14 Fiber mobility in deep ribs (3 × 38 mm, or 0.1 × 1.5 in.) for three different GMT reinforcement types

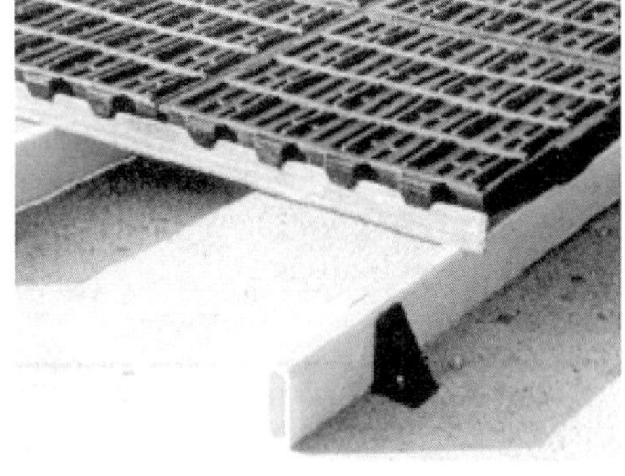

Fig. 15 Example of a for structural application using recycled GMT

ering the process parameter configuration (e.g., low rotational screw speed to maintain the fiber length of the granulate). For this reason, especially in the automotive industry, there was a demand for significant cost savings with similar or better material properties of the component. To reach this target, a direct process technology, avoiding the semifinished product manufacture and the double heating, was developed as a so-called long-fiber-reinforced thermoplastic (LFT) process. The direct LFT process contains continuous fibers (e.g., glass) and a thermoplastic matrix (e.g., polypropylene), which are fed into an extruder. The plasticated material is then extruded and cut. Afterwards, the plasticated material is directly placed into the compression mold and then formed into a component. In comparison to traditional processes (GMT, LFG, and SMC), the individual discontinuous production process steps are eliminated.

LFT Materials

For the direct LFT process, any kind of thermoplastic material can be used. The only requirement is that the compound tolerates a short time exposure to oxygen. For high-volume production, mainly polypropylene is used. The reason is that LFT penetrates the existing GMT market, which is based on polypropylene (PP). Other thermoplastic materials (e.g., polyamide, acrylonitrile-styrene-acrylate, and acrylonitrile-butadiene-styrene) can be used if required.

For the reinforcement, each type of glass roving (e.g., E-glass) with a compatible sizing suitable to the used thermoplastic matrix can be used. To get a good impregnation, a fiber of 1200 to 2400 tex usually is used for series production. Additional information can be found in the articles, "Glass Fibers" and "Thermoplastic Resins" in this Volume.

LFT Compression Molding Process

A customized extruder is used for virgin material. After plastication and homogenization of the thermoplastic pellets, the fibers are preimpregnated and cut into length in a proprietary process, followed by further homogenization at moderate back pressure (Fig. 16). Then the plasticated material charge is cut and transported to a handling device that feeds the molding press (Ref 25).

A continuous stream of compounded material leaves the extrusion line at a temperature of approximately 220 °C (430 °F) in the case of PP. The endless material output is cut to the correct length to deliver the molding input at desired charge weight. Equipment design and operating parameters are critical to maximize the molded component properties.

If recycled material is being used, scrap parts or cut-outs are first shredded to chips by using, for example, a single screw mill (Fig. 17). The maximum size of the chips (Fig. 18) depends on the size of the second extruder in the process chain. The recyclate then is plasticated in the second extruder and fed back into the virgin stream. This is a fully closed-loop recycling system.

LFT Applications

Typical applications can be found in the automotive industry for components such as front end support structures (e.g., Volkswagen Passat, Fig. 19a), floor panel covers (e.g., Skoda Fabia), trunk boxes, and battery covers. A nonautomotive application for LFT is a railroad car container.

Figure 19(b) illustrates the layout of a fully automated production line for the manufacture of the Volkswagen Passat B5 internal front end incorporating closed-loop recycling. Raw materials and recyclate are fed into separate extruders. Then, the plasticated material is placed into the compression mold. After molding, the untrimmed component is cooled before going on to secondary operations. After that, further holes and features are cut out in a four-step waterjet cutting process. The component is then washed and trimmed before transfer to the subcomponent assembly line. Several rivets are integrated into the component to ensure easy assembly (for example, of lamps, fan, and locking mechanism). As of 2000, the manufacturer was producing approximately 500,000 units per year. The molded component weight is nominally 4.2 kg (9.3lb); approximately 20% of the charge weight consists of cut-outs, which are recycled and reused.

Comparison of LFT with GMT and SMC

One of the main targets in the development of LMT compression molding was to achieve similar or better materials properties than those of GMT materials. One of the main criteria influencing the mechanical properties is the fiber length. The fiber length distribution in LFT is illustrated in Fig. 20, which indicates a peak fiber length of approximately 50 mm (2 in.). The LFT fiber-length distribution ensures optimal values for elastic modulus, tensile strength, and impact toughness (Ref 26). Traditionally, GMT is produced with a constant fiber length of 25 or 50 mm (1 or 2 in.) and often treated with a needle punching process. The mechanical properties of GMT, LFT, and SMC testpieces are compared in Table 1. The glass fiber volume fractions for the GMT and LFT testpieces are identical; the LFT material includes 30% recyclate. In comparison with GMT, LFT material features superior mod-

Table 1 Comparative properties of LFT, GMT, and SMC compression moldings

Property	LFT	GMT	SMC
Glass fiber content, wt%	40	40	30
Recyclate content, wt%	30	. . .	5
Tensile strength, MPa (ksi)	60 (8.7)	65 (9.4)	60 (8.7)
Tensile modulus, GPa (10^6 psi)	7.2 (1.0)	6.1 (0.9)	9.5 (1.4)
Flexural strength, MPa (ksi)	110 (16)	110 (16)	160 (23)
Flexural modulus, GPa (10^6 psi)	5.4 (0.8)	4.1 (0.6)	8.9 (1.3)
Impact strength, kJ/m^2	60	75	70
Density, g/cm^3	1.21	1.21	1.80

Note: All values measured on a testpiece taken from an automotive structural front end

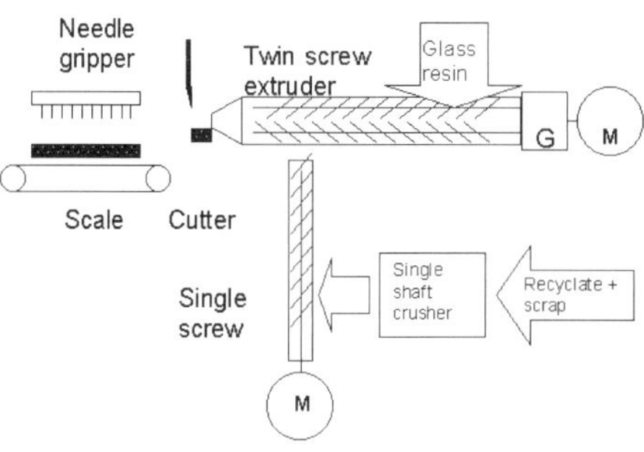

Fig. 17 LFT line including incorporation of recyclate

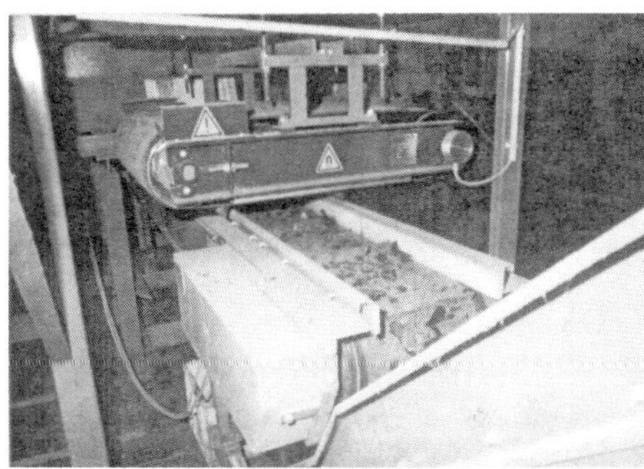

Fig. 18 Recyclate feedback in closed-loop LTF compression molding

Fig. 16 Direct LFT plastication process

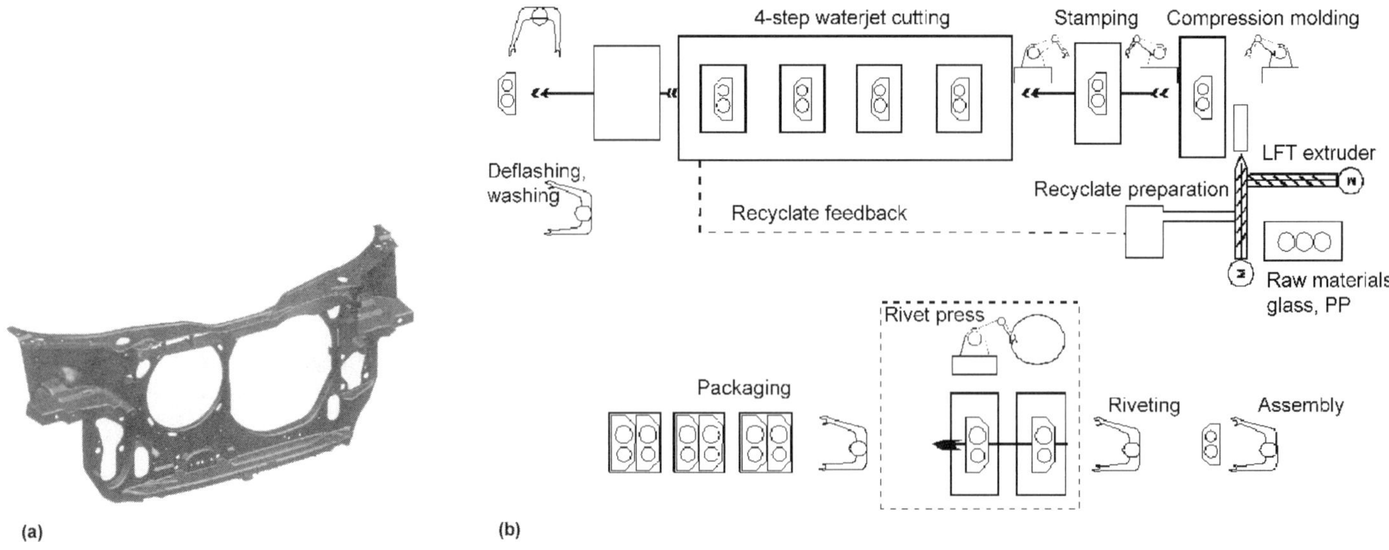

Fig. 19 Automobile front end technical support structure manufactured by LFT compression molding. (a) Volkswagen B5 Passat front end. (b) Production line

ulus of elasticity due to the more effective use of the longer fibers (>30 mm, or 1.2 in.). On the other hand, LFT materials exhibit poorer energy absorption/dissipation behavior than GMT materials.

The advantage of the LFT process and the LFT material can be summarized as follows: The process is much more cost-effective than GMT, not only due to the elimination of single process steps, but also because less manpower is needed for production. Also, cycle times have been reduced by 15% as a result of a better flowability of the plasticated material in comparison with the GMT. A further advantage of the LFT process is the component surface, where LFT avoids white spots of naked fibers occasionally found in GMT parts that result from poorly impregnated glass fibers, whereas the impregnation quality in the LFT process is superior.

GMT processing is also known for mold tool wear. The reason for this disadvantage is erosion caused by diesel effects, which occurs much less during LFT processing. Machinery stops also reduce the probability of undesirable materials degradation using the direct LFT extrusion process. A production line stop in GMT necessitates clearing the oven. This can also entail a high amount of material waste in the start-up procedure of the process. In extreme cases, waste has been reduced from about 6% with GMT to about 1% with LFT.

Some of the properties and characteristics of SMC, GMT, and LFT are compared in a spiderweb graph (Fig. 21). The economic efficiency can be calculated as a function of the component weight (Ref 1). Basis for the cost comparison of SMC, GMT and LFT is an annual production volume of 100,000 parts and a required molding pressure of 1,500 tons. All values illustrated in Fig. 22 are related to GMT, which was set to 100%. For lightweight parts (approximately 1 kg, or 2 lb), GMT shows cost advantages. LFT achieves break-even at a component weight of approximately 1.5 kg (3 lb), where LFT is favorable compared with GMT component costs.

Advances in LFT

The direct LFT technology was successfully introduced into the market by Menzolit-Fibron in 1997 with the Volkswagen Passat B5 front end. Today, there are many applications for the technology.

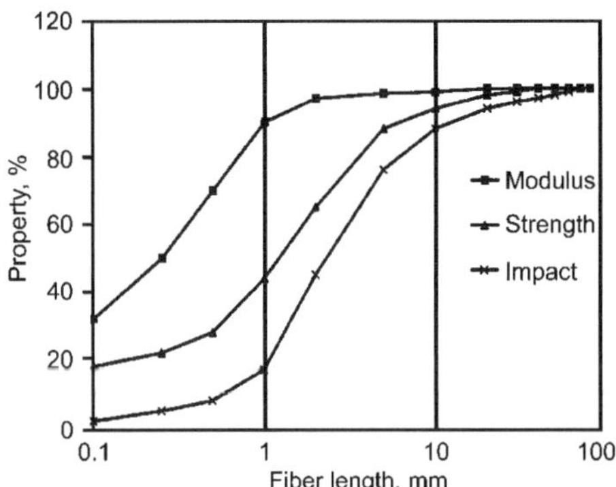

Fig. 20 Relationship between fiber length and properties for LFT materials

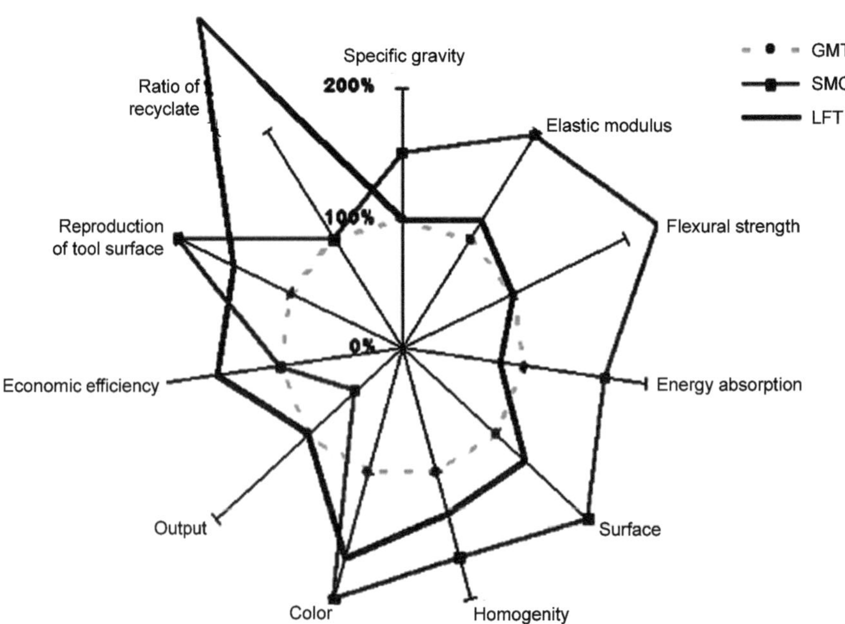

Fig. 21 Comparison of GMT, LFT, and SMC compression molding processes and materials properties

Currently, in the front end market, there is a tendency that requires metal inserts to fulfill the increased crash requirements. In this field, injection molded hybrid parts with metal inserts are also realizable (Ref 27), where LFT also fulfills these standards by using metal inserts.

Due to the high flexibility of the LFT process, it is very easy to investigate alternative fiber and matrix materials, for example, natural fiber reinforcements (e.g., flax, hemp, sisal) (Ref 28) required by the automotive industry. There is still a high potential for material and process improvements for new successful applications manufactured in the direct LFT process.

Compression Molding of Sheet Molding Compounds

The range of applications for SMCs comprises molded parts with a weight of a few grams up to several kilograms. The processing methods used, are injection molding or compression molding and depend on the size, complexity of shape design, strength requirements, or cost calculation of the molded part. The largest share of the material is processed in compression molding. Molded parts are used in many different sectors of the industry. The range of application stretches from molded electrical insulation parts to force-transmitting and force-absorbing molded parts to painted automobile body panels with a "Class A" surface finish. The excellent flow performance of SMC permits the integration of parts in the design of molded parts, which has a cost-saving effect in the production of molded parts.

The composition of the SMC material has a special status among plastics, because the share of organic components, such as resins and additives, may be reduced to a share of 25%, depending on the formulations used. The remaining shares are inorganic and consist of aggregates (fillers) and reinforcing glass fibers. A typical composition might consist of 25% unsaturated polyester (UP) resin, 25% glass fiber, and 50% filler. This resource-saving material composition of SMC is completely in line with modern ideas of what a material should be.

The following information shows how versatile the design possibility of reinforcing-fiber structures can be, and how materials characteristics can be influenced by them. The range of application variations used in SMC extend from random-fiber reinforcement (25 and 50 mm, or 1 and 2 in., fiber length) all the way to unidirectional glass-fiber reinforcement.

Additional information on SMCs is provided in the article "Molding Compounds" in this Volume.

Development of SMCs

In the 1950s, the possibility of thickening UP resins with alkaline earth oxides and hydroxides was discovered in the United States and the Federal Republic of Germany. This proved to be the foundation for the production of SMC. Initially, the material was manufactured by means of impregnating glass-fiber mats on simple two-roll systems. However, crack-free components with good surface finishes could only be manufactured later after the discovery of the vibration-reducing effect of polyethylene powder in the UP resin matrix. Applications in the electrical industry soon followed.

A new impregnation system with top-mounted wide cutters for glass-fiber rovings was developed in the United States, in order to avoid the use of expensive glass-fiber mats, to rationalize the manufacturing process, and to reduce the cost of the material. The American designation for sheet molding compound (SMC) was adopted as an international standard.

As early as the 1960s, cable distribution cabinets, strip lighting, and housings for electrical appliances were already being manufactured using SMC. Owing to the efficient molding technique, components able to carry higher loads soon followed, such as cylinder head covers or oil pan covers for diesel traction engines.

Studies of the effects of thermoplastics dissolved in styrene in UP resins led to the development of low-profile unsaturated polyester (LP-UP) resins in the 1970s. For the first time, this material was used successfully for the production of automobile body panels with an acceptable surface finish quality.

Various front ends of automobiles in the United States and the removable sunroof of the VW-Porsche 914 in Europe were the first serial production parts made from LP-SMC.

Due to the relatively high finishing costs after painting in cases of large-area SMC automobile body panels, the application of the material made slow progress in Europe. Only with the advent of the use of the IMC method in the early 1980s and the later introduction of the vacuum compression molding technique did more applications for passenger cars follow in Europe, such as, for example, the engine hood of the Citroen BX. However, a faster pace of development was set in the field of interior and exterior parts for commercial vehicles.

The high-strength SMC materials developed in the early 1980s which featured a combination of unidirectional glass-fiber strands, random fibers, and a fiber share of 60% by weight, resulted in the use of the material for the bumpers of several new automobile models.

Material Characteristics of SMCs

SMC consists of a resin matrix into which reinforcing fibers are embedded. The composition of the matrix is adapted to the required characteristic profile. The characteristics of the resin matrix that can be influenced include:

- Resistance to chemicals
- Resistance to weathering
- Surface structure
- Flexibility (module of elasticity)
- Dyeability
- Shrinkage
- Flame retardation
- Strength characteristics (pressure and impact resistance)
- Dynamic characteristics
- Surface hardness

The following characteristics can be influenced through reinforcing fibers (distribution and fiber structure):

- Strength and rigidity characteristics (depending on the fiber distribution and the predominant direction of the fibers)
- Shrinkage/warping (depending on the fiber distribution, the predominant direction of the fibers, or flow orientation)

The SMC material can be adapted to the specified requirement profile by changing its structure or its composition

SMC Matrix Resins

SMC is a variable system of components, which, depending on the intended purpose of use, may be composed according to their physical and mechanical characteristics and thus, is suitable for use in a wide range of applications. A wide selection of UP resins, additives, hardeners, fillers, and reinforcing fiber structures is available for the optimization of SMC formulations. A standard SMC paste formula is:

Component	Parts
Unsaturated polyester resin	100
Monostyrene	10
Hardener	1
Inhibitor	Depends on reactivity and flowability
Pigment	Depends on color desired
Fillers	80–210
Thermoplastic additive	10
Mold release agent	5
Thickener	1.5

Orthophthalic acid, isophthalic acid, terephthalic acid, and bisphenol-A resins are used as

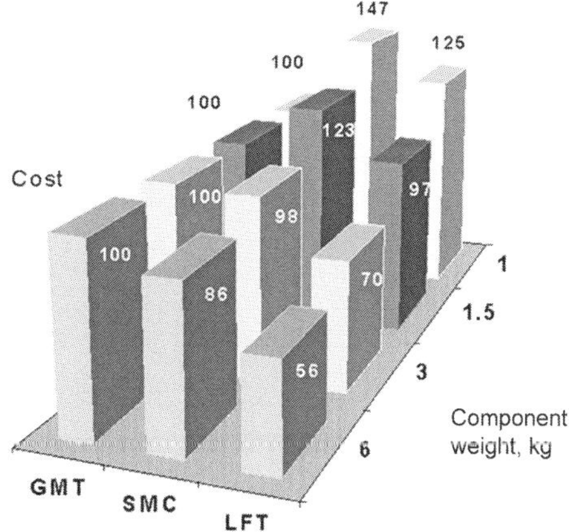

Fig. 22 Relative costs of GMT, LFT, and SMC compression molded parts

UP resins. Vinyl ester resins, which do not belong to the group of UP resins, have opened up another area of application for SMC, especially in the case of molded parts being subjected to dynamic or sudden impact loads.

With the development of the low-shrink (LS) and low-profile (LP) UP resins, it is now possible to manufacture molded parts with an excellent surface finish quality. Curing shrinkage has been reduced, and dimensional stability, dimensional accuracy, and surface finish quality have been improved significantly. Sensitivity to microcracking and sink marks above ribs or bosses has been reduced considerably.

Unsaturated polyester resins shrink during curing by about 6 to 9% by volume. Through the addition of 20 to 40% by weight of a high polymer dissolved in styrene, the curing speed during warm curing is reduced or eliminated completely. The chemical reaction usual for highly filled polymers for UP resins may be assumed as similar to unfilled systems. However, the kind of reaction as well as the start and duration of the reaction will be different.

Based on its curing shrinkage, SMC is classified in three groups (Table 2). Standard UP resins are always used in cases where mechanical or physical characteristics are given higher priority over surface finish quality. Dyeing is possible in a wide range of colors.

Low-shrink UP resins, like standard UP resins, can be dyed with pigments. However, the available range of colors is somewhat limited due to the two phases typical for this type of resin system. The shrinkage, which is reduced in comparison to standard resins, has a positive effect on the accuracy and warpage of the molded part as well as the quality of the surface finish.

Low-profile UP resins do not exhibit any shrinkage or even show an increase in volume. These resins cannot be dyed uniformly due to the whitening effect occurring during curing. This type of resin is often used in applications of molded parts that are later spray painted.

Monostyrene Additive. The addition of monostyrene to the formulation serves the purpose of reducing the viscosity of the resin paste in order to achieve good wetting of the glass strands and in order to add the styrene to the formulation, which escapes during manufacturing and processing.

Hardener. The hardener consists of an organic peroxide, which has a curing effect (polymerization) on the UP resin in the compression mold under supply of heat. In order to achieve optimal curing conditions for the molded part, several organic peroxides of different types may be combined.

Inhibitors. The addition of an inhibitor is intended to serve a two-fold purpose. On the one hand, it provides good shelf-life properties over a prolonged period of time for the resin matrix, and on the other hand, it can be used to vary the flow time of the SMC in the mold by modifying the concentration.

Fillers are used for the purpose of reducing thermal shrinkage, resulting in an improvement of the quality of the surface finish of the molded parts. Also, the transport of the reinforcing fibers during the flow process in the mold is improved, and the sensitivity of the matrix to cracking during the curing process is reduced. The most frequently used fillers for SMC formulations are calcium carbonate, aluminum trihydrate, and kaolin.

Calcium carbonates exhibit a low oil-absorption rate and thus may be added in a relatively large amounts to UP resins. They reduce thermal shrinkage and impart a smooth surface finish to the molded parts.

Aluminum trihydrate is a noncombustible, non-water soluble, and nontoxic white powder. When mixed with the UP resin, it adds flame-retardant characteristics to that material. The effectiveness of aluminum trihydrate is based on the disintegration into aluminum oxide and water:

$$Al_2O_3 3 \cdot 3H_2O \rightarrow Al_2O_3 + H_2O$$

The disintegration begins at 180 °C (350 °F) and ends at 600 °C (1100 °F). This is a strong endothermic process with 1970 kJ/kg (470 cal/g) aluminum trihydrate. The endothermic reaction cools the flame contact area and keeps it, with a sufficiently high share of aluminum trihydrate, below the disintegration temperature of the polymers. The water being released under the reaction reduces the combustion speed. Aluminum trihydrates as fillers have a flame-retardant effect, do not release any halogens when exposed to a flame, and exhibit a low level of flue gas density.

Kaolins are mainly used for molded parts in which high priority is given to chemical resistance.

Thermoplastic Additive. A finely ground polyethylene powder is added to standard SMC as a low shrink agent. Aside from improved flow characteristics of SMC, polyethylene reduces the shrinkage of the UP resins, which has a positive effect on the sensitivity to cracking and the quality of the surface finish of the molded parts.

Mold Release Agent. To guarantee trouble-free removal of the molded parts from the mold, parting compounds are added to the SMC paste. As a rule, these consist of zinc or calcium stearates. The function principle of stearates can be traced back to a change in the solubility between unhardened and hardened UP resins. During the curing process, the stearate at the surface of the UP resin becomes incompatible and causes the formation of a molecular zinc stearate layer between the molded part and the surface of the mold.

Thickeners. Thickening of UP resins is achieved with alkaline earth oxides or hydroxides (MgO, $Mg(OH)_2$, CaO, $Ca(OH)_2$) via the carboxyl groups of the UP resin (Ref 30). Thickening of UP resin with CaO is, in comparison to MgO, only possible with the addition of H_2O. Due to the sensitivity of the thickening behavior with CaO, the overall content of H_2O in the UP resin must be monitored and kept as constant as possible. In case of UP resins exhibiting poor thickening behavior, the addition of H_2O may also be required when MgO is used. The advantage of UP resin thickened with CaO lies in the lower absorption of H_2O when the molded parts are stored in water.

The so-called maturation time of SMC in order to increase viscosity can, depending on the formula and the storage temperature, be between one day and several weeks. Suitable compression molding viscosities depend on the application and are between 20 and 80 $\times$ 10^6 mPa · s. The thickening results in a nonsticking and relatively rigid semifinished SMC product, which is easy to handle and provides good resin paste and glass fiber transport during the flow process and avoids the concentration of resin.

Other Additives. More wear-resistant surface finishes can be achieved through the addition of solid microglass beads. The UP resin shrinks during curing, causing the glass beads to protrude above the surface. Owing to their hardness, the resistance to wear can be improved in this way.

For the purpose of reducing the density of SMC, a portion of the fillers may be replaced with hollow microglass beads. The addition of conductive carbon black (soot) improves the electrical conductivity.

Matrix Preparation. Mixing of the resin paste may take place according to different procedures:

- Batch-oriented mixing and continual addition of a thickening agent
- Continual mixing process for all components of the resin paste

SMC materials manufactured in Europe are mainly manufactured in batch-oriented mixing

Table 2 Classification of structural molding compounds according to their shrinkage behavior

SMC	Additive	Condition in the resin	Polymerization shrinkage, %
Standard SMC	Polyethylene powder	Two phases	0.15–0.3
Low-shrink SMC (LS-SMC)	Solution of polystyrene	Two phases	0.06–0.14
	Polycaprolactol in styrene monomer	Two phases	0.06–0.14
Low-profile SMC (LP-SMC)	Solution of polymethyl methacrylate (PMMA)	Two phases	≥0.04
	Polyvinyl acetate (PVAC)	Single phase	≥0.04
	Liquid rubber	Two phases	≥0.04
	Saturated polyester	Single phase	≥0.04
	Cellulose acetobutyrate in styrene monomer	Single phase	≥0.04

processes of the raw material components and subsequent continual addition of the thickening agent. This processing method has proven itself to be best suited in the manufacture of many different SMC formulas. Dissolvers and so-called turbulence mixers are used as mixing tools in the batch-oriented mixing process.

The resin compound is mixed in large containers, which are then transported to the SMC impregnation system. There, the resin paste is extracted by means of a pump, while the thickening agent is added continually. Mixing takes place either in a static mixer or in a dynamic mixing system.

The continual mixing method is used in production processes in which the entire demand of the production can be satisfied with one or only a few different SMC formulas.

SMC Material Manufacture

- The production of SMC comprises the following processing stages:
- Paste preparation
- Dosage of two- or three-component paste
- Creation of a reinforcing fiber structure and its impregnation and packaging
- Thickening of the paste

Paste Preparation. In a batch-oriented preparation of paste, the individual raw materials are stored in large containers, silos, or tanks, and the prescribed quantities are metered to the mixing devices by computer-controlled dosing stations. Low- or high-shear mixers, depending on the process, are used to mix the resin paste. In the case of high-shear mixers, high temperatures are generated in the shear area, which requires a fine balance of the hardener/inhibitor combination as well as the selection of hardener in order to prevent a premature hardener reaction during the mixing process. Low-shear mixers process the paste mixture much more gently, which is evident by considerably lower paste temperatures. In many cases, the low-shear mixer is equipped with an additional downstream homogenizer in order to dissolve any possibly existing agglomerations. If, in the case of resin pastes intended for dyeing, the dye paste is added during the preparation of the paste, it is possible to process the paste in a two-component paste dosage system in the SMC plant. It is common practice to work without any addition of dye paste when preparing the resin paste, in order to reduce the cleaning time of the containers and mixing aggregates and to omit the time-consuming weighing of the dye pastes.

Paste Dosage. From the paste preparation, the paste is transported in large containers to the paste dosing station, which is installed adjacent to the SMC plant. Aside from the commonly used two-component dosing stations, the use of three-component dosing stations has become more widespread.

The function of two-component dosing stations is to continually control the dosage of the resin paste and the thickening agent and, in the case of three-component systems, the dye paste as well. A sensor system monitors the accuracy of the dosage. The accuracy of the dosage is either controlled gravimetrically or according to the Coriolis principle. The individual flows from the dosing station are mixed either in a static mixing unit or in a dynamic mixer.

SMC Impregnation. The construction of the SMC plant consists of the flat-surface dosing of the resin paste by means of a squeegee, the cutter for the purpose of cutting and dosing in reinforcing fibers, and the impregnation unit (Fig. 23). Prior to entering the squeegee box, a thickener is added to the resin in a two-component pump system, and the two components are mixed with each other. One squeegee each is used to apply the resin paste to the surface of films, which enclose the chopped glass reinforcing fibers from above and below. The fiber rovings are metered according to the drawing speed of the cutter and cut to a length of 25 or 50 mm (1 or 2 in.). The two-dimensional, unoriented staple fiber structure is created in a free-fall from the cutter onto the film coated with resin paste.

The impregnating unit, consisting of twin belts and rollers, presses the resin paste applied to both films between the glass strands. At the end of the process, the impregnated SMC is wound up in coils or stored in containers in zigzag layers.

Cutting the Reinforcing Fibers. Cutting of the textile glass rovings takes place on a wide cutter. The essential components of the cutter are the feed roller, the rubber roller and the cutter roller. In this type of cutter (Fig. 24), the fiber is not really cut, but actually broken (Ref 31). The filament bundles are, depending on the roving quality, more or less connected to each other through the sizing material on the fibers. This cohesion between individual filaments of the fiber strands must be opened mechanically using a deflector device prior to the cutting procedure.

Technology of Modern SMC Facilities. System engineering of modern SMC manufacture has reached a high technical standard. The light construction of earlier systems has given way to more massive designs. This prevents elastic deformations in components of the systems, which may be caused by the forces occurring when the output capacity of the systems is increased. This has a positive effect on semifinished products made from SMC.

The quality of the SMC, is monitored by sensors that read, record, and further process the following parameters of a control circuit in the control unit of the SMC plant:

- Film tension
- Filling level at the squeegees
- Layer thickness of resin paste
- Distribution of reinforcing fibers
- SMC thickness
- Squeegee gap adjustment
- Winding tension of the SMC when winding into coils

The technology of the systems has been continually revised and improved in recent years (Ref 32). The following system components were the focal points in these endeavors:

- Impregnating section
- Automatic feed of winding cores
- Automatic packaging of SMC rolls
- Automatic transport of rolls to the maturation chamber

The impregnating units were extended, reinforced, and equipped with a high level of power reserves in order to improve the impregnating capabilities. Parallel guides guarantee an even thickness of the SMC.

Automatic feeding of winding cores and automatic packaging of the SMC rolls can also contribute to reducing the personnel requirements in production.

Immediately after packaging, the rolls are transported to the maturation chamber, which, for space-saving reasons, permits a continual vertical as well as horizontal throughput. The

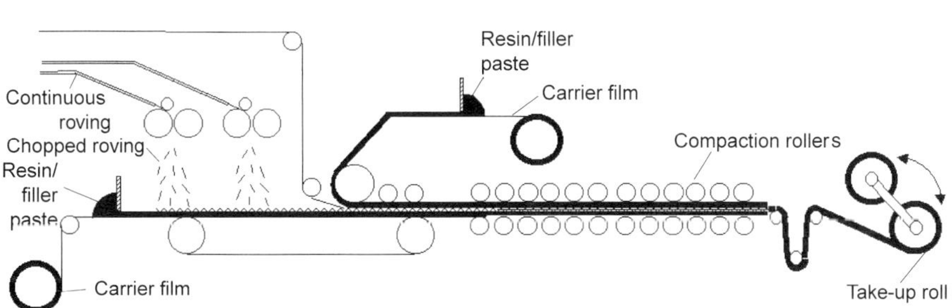

Fig. 23 Schematic diagram of the SMC impregnating system

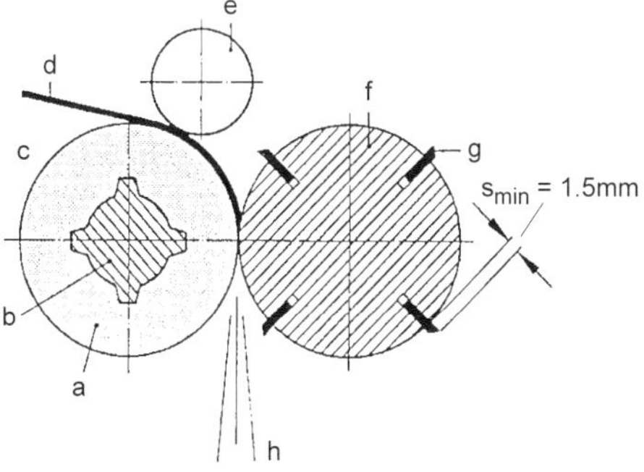

Fig. 24 Schematic diagram of cutting with feed rollers. (a) Rubber roller. (b) Hub. (c) Feed roller. (d) Fiber. (e) Tensioning roller. (f) Cutting roller. (g) Cutting edge. (h) Cut fibers

doctor blade control has been refined; however, the basic principle has not changed.

Maturation Process. Four of the rolls or pallets are placed on a pallet and then allowed to thicken for several hours in the maturation chamber. The matrix is thickened up to the point when the resin paste reaches the viscosity required for the flow process in the mold, the two films can be peeled off, and the SMC is ready for processing, free of sticking.

Fiber Reinforcement Structures

Impregnating systems with wide cutters for glass fiber roving are used for the manufacture of SMC. Randomly arranged glass strands 25 to 50 mm (1 to 2 in.) in length are used as reinforcement fibers. The initial products are textile glass rovings with 2400 or 4800 tex (weight in grams per 1000 meters). A roving consists of a grouping of several filament bundles with a fiber fineness (or strand titer) of 40 to 80 tex. The filament diameter is nominally 14 μm.

The structure of the SMC fiber is manufactured in the SMC plant and determines, aside from the fiber content, the mechanical characteristics. A distinction can be made between the following fiber structures:

- Randomly arranged chopped glass strands, mostly of a length of 25 to 50 mm (1 to 2 in.). For the purpose of influencing the flow characteristics in the mold as well as the surface finish quality, mixtures using fibers of both 25 and 50 mm (1 and 2 in.) can be used. The material designation for SMC with this fiber structure (Fig. 25a) is SMC-R (R = random).
- Randomly arranged chopped glass strands and continuous glass fiber strands with asymmetric fiber structure. The material designation for this structure (Fig. 25b) is SMC-C (C = continuous).

The SMC used in general applications is SMC-R. Of the three previously described fiber structures it is the one that allows the use of the simplest processing techniques due to its even flow characteristics. SMC-C is used for achieving a high level of mechanical properties. Due to the harder-to-control flow processes and material shrinkage, these materials are used predominantly for load-bearing components requiring higher levels of strength. These fiber structures are also known as multifiber structures.

SMC with Random Fiber Structure. The mechanical properties in SMC are predominantly determined by the structure of the reinforcing fibers. A two-dimensional, random fiber with largely even strength characteristics in x and y direction is most common. Changes toward one preferred direction, known as orientation, may occur during the flow process in the mold. In this respect, the design of the SMC blanks (dimensions, shape, number of layers) as well as the arrangement of the blank in the mold is of great significance. The aim is to retain the specified fiber structure in the SMC as much as possible throughout the flow process in the mold. Obstacles in the mold cavity (tapers, changes in cross section, ribs, spigots, dead ends, etc.) as well as the length of flow paths are taken into consideration when designing the SMC charge.

A reinforcing fiber content of up to 60% by weight can be achieved in the SMC while maintaining positive flow characteristics.

The mechanical properties of the molded parts change depending on the content of reinforcing fibers. However, the content of reinforcing fibers influences the compressive strength to a lesser degree than the tensile strength (Fig. 26). Should the glass fiber content exceed 65% by weight, the tensile strength values will surpass the compressive strength values. The bending strength, which is a mixed value from tensile and compressive strength, increases continually, but exhibits a flatter increase curve with a glass fiber content between 50 and 65 wt% due to the drop in compressive strength.

The resin matrix can influence the rigidity or the flexibility of an SMC material. The matrix controls the interaction between the reinforcing fibers and can be adjusted by changing the composition of the resin paste to make it more rigid or flexible. Therefore, the modulus of elasticity data shown in Fig. 27 are to be understood merely as examples for a special SMC material; the modulus can be adjusted to suit a special application by charging the matrix composition.

High-Performance Compound (HPC) with Unidirectional Reinforcement. A fiber structure with unidirectional glass-fiber strands is built up for molded parts with high requirements on strength and rigidity. The manufacture of such fiber structures is achieved through the introduction of glass-fiber roving strands in the direction of SMC production.

The amount of the unidirectional glass-fiber strands lying in the test direction determines the level of tensile and compressive strengths. In the case of tensile loads, the forces are transmitted directly to the reinforcing-fiber strands, so that the influences of the matrix are eliminated to a

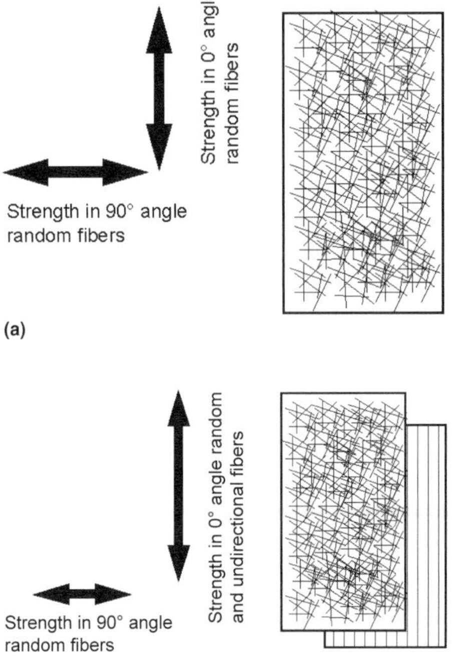

Fig. 25 Fiber patterns in SMC materials (fiber length 25 or 50 mm, or 1 or 2 in). (a) SMC with random reinforcing fibers (SMC-R). (b) SMC with random and unidirectional reinforcing fibers (SMC-C)

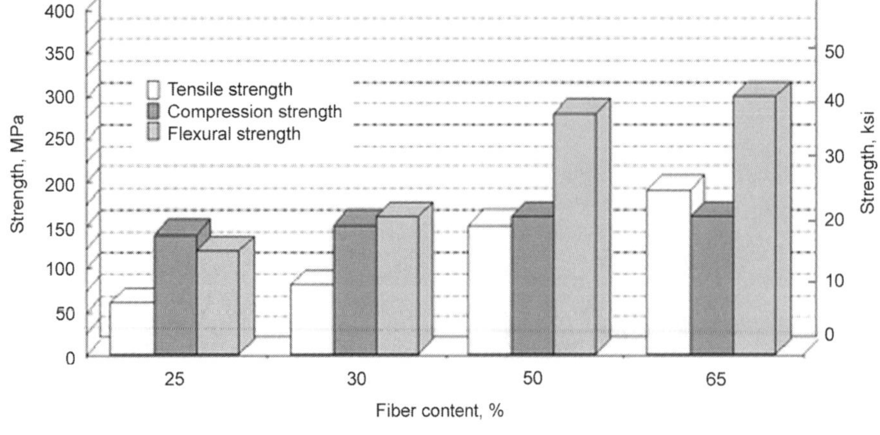

Fig. 26 Relationship between strength and reinforcing fiber content for SMC composites

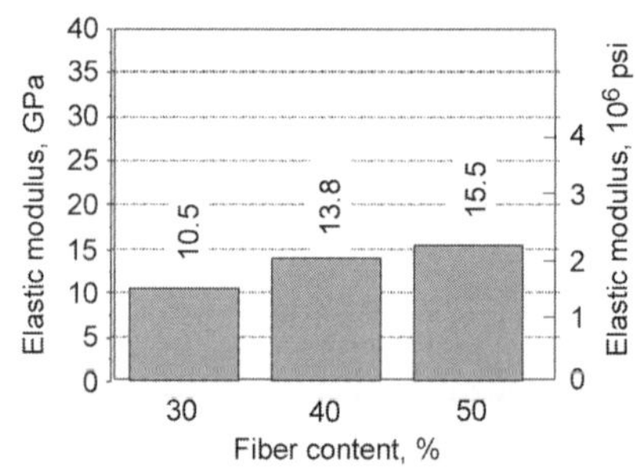

Fig. 27 Relationship between modulus of elasticity and reinforcing fiber content for SMCs with random fibers

large extent. In the case of compressive loads, the forces are acting vertically on the reinforcing fibers, which absorb part of the forces acting upon them. In this case, the matrix assumes a supporting function for the glass-fiber strands. This results in an increase of all values of strength characteristics.

An SMC material consisting solely of unidirectional glass-fiber strands only offers the strength of the matrix perpendicular to the fibers. In order to improve the transverse strength characteristics and to reduce inner stresses in the laminate, a random fiber structure is laid on top of the fiber strands (Fig. 25). This creates an asymmetrically reinforced-fiber structure (Fig. 28a), which can be partially compensated for by layering (Fig. 28b).

The flow characteristics of SMC are influenced by the introduced fiber structures. Generally speaking, the HPC flow processes require higher compressive forces than those required for SMC with random reinforcement. Also, consideration must be given to the fact that the higher the content of reinforcing fibers, the higher the compressive forces required for the flow process.

In a comparison of SMC material with 60% by weight, randomly arranged reinforcing glass fibers with an SMC material in which 40% by weight are unidirectional, the tensile strength of the latter is more than doubled at the same overall fiber content (Fig. 29). Depending on the required strength characteristics, the overall content of reinforcing glass fibers and the share of unidirectional reinforcing-fiber strands may be freely chosen according to the requirements of the application.

Similar to the tensile strength, the elastic modulus also increases with an increasing unidirectional glass-fiber content (Fig. 29).

This group of material is used under the designation HPC in the manufacture of automobile bumpers and as an additional material for bumpers of vans and trucks. This application has been established for many years and has proven itself in daily use.

SMC Materials Testing

Since the resin pastes for the continual production of SMC are manufactured in batches, the constant quality level of the batches of paste is of the utmost importance. For that reason, it is necessary to inspect each batch carefully before it is processed in the SMC plant.

The following inspections have been proven in practice:

- Viscosity, through the use of a Brookfield viscometer
- Color, according to DIN 5033
- Reactive behavior, according to DIN EN ISO 12114

The following parameters should be controlled during the production of SMC:

- Belt speed
- Cutter speed
- MgO dosage
- Height of squeegee gap
- Mass per unit area substance, according to DIN EN ISO 10352
- Glass content, according to DIN EN ISO 11667
- Fiber wetting, according to ISO/DIS 17771

The following inspections are required during thickening or maturation:

- Temperature in the maturation chamber
- Viscosity by means of paste samples
- Plasticity, according to DIN EN ISO 12115

Test samples can be made from process-ready SMC in accordance with ISO/CD 1268-8. From these test samples, depending on the requirements, the materials characteristics can be determined. The essential characteristics have been recorded in a universal materials database for fiber reinforced molding compounds known as the "FUNDUS" database. The test methods adopted for all of Europe by the European Alliance for SMC, most of which are derived from ISO or EN standards, comprise all essential characteristics in order to determine the properties of the material.

SMC Form of Supply and Storage Conditions

According to DIN 16913, the standard designation for SMC (resin mat) made from rovings is UP-GMSR, and for SMC made from glass fiber mats it is UP-GMSB. However, these designations have not yet gained general acceptance.

After the impregnating process, the SMC is rolled up into coils between layers of polyethylene film or stored in zigzag layers in containers to await further processing. During the storage time, the UP resin continues to thicken with the aid of the added alkaline earth oxides or hydroxides. Depending on the formulation structure, the SMC can be stored up to six months at room temperature.

SMC Compression Molding Processing Description

The largest quantity of SMC is processed according to the compression molding method. However, processing in injection molding methods with a special, easy-flowing SMC formula is gaining importance.

SMC is processed into molded parts in heated steel molds operated by hydraulic presses (Fig. 1). The pressures used in the molding process lie between 3 and 14 MPa (30 and 140 bar) and generally depend on the formula of the SMC and the shape of the molded part. SMC-quality grades with a high content of fillers of glass fibers require high molding pressures. Parts with high sidewalls, ribs, or spigots require higher pressure than flat molded parts.

The SMC is cut into blanks for the purpose of processing. The SMC blanks are smaller than the projected surface of the molded part. In most cases, the blank size is between 40 and 70% of the size of the molded part, depending on the degree of difficulty of filling out the mold. The blank will be placed in the mold in such a way that the flow paths to the edge of the molded part are equal in all directions, in order to prevent undesirable fiber orientations caused by change of the material flow directions. Through the calculation of the flow front and the resulting shape of the blank, it is possible to avoid weak areas caused by change of fiber orientation during the flow process in the mold.

The blanks are cut either mechanically on a cutter or manually at the press. After pulling off the separating film, several blanks are placed in layers until the input weight, corresponding to the weight of the molded part plus allowance for the flash to be trimmed off, has been reached.

The SMC blank is placed in the mold. Then, under pressure and temperature, the SMC is formed to the contours of the mold when the mold is closed. Mold temperatures of 135 to 160

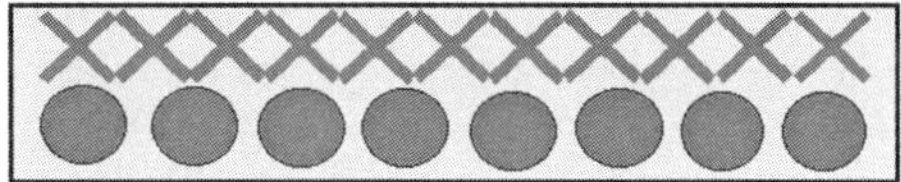

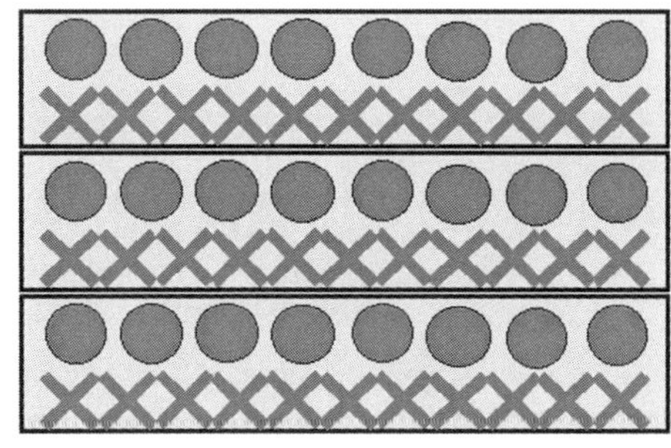

Fig. 28 High-performance SMCs with unidirectional reinforcements. (a) Asymmetric fiber structure. (b) Layering of the asymmetric structures prior to processing

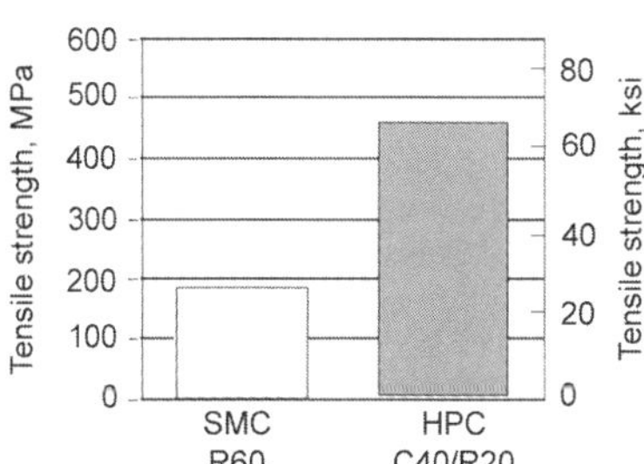

Fig. 29 Tensile strength comparison with SMC and HPC with identical content of reinforcing fibers (R, random; C, continuous)

°C (275 to 320 °F)—depending on the formula used—are common in this process.

The forming speed of the SMC inside the mold is selected to ensure that no damage of the glass fibers will occur. Once the cavity of the mold is filled, the full pressure is acting on the molded part. The press remains under pressure until the curing reaction is completed. The curing process can be traced through piezoelectric pressure sensors inside the mold, and the press can be opened automatically by a microprocessor control system at the end of the curing time.

Process Data Retrieval and Analysis. The technology of SMC processing is still characterized, to a large extent, by empirical studies. Analyses of defects are performed with the aid of molded parts in order to determine the cause of defects and to eliminate the cause through suitable measures by modifying the paste.

A new and decisive way for the future is to make the individual processes in the manufacture of molded parts more transparent through the observation of process signals and to use the information gathered in this way to derive a differentiated view of the technical procedures. An instrument developed for this purpose is the data retrieval system MEDAS (Ref 33), with appropriate amplification and sensors needed for the retrieval of process data.

The values to be monitored relate in particular to the function of the production plant, in which the dosage function and the forces required for this purpose are recorded. The dosage function consists of the closing motion of the press, its parallelism, as well as a possible elastic behavior of the equipment. In the further course of the molding process, it may be possible to solve shrinkage effects and other processing details.

From the retrieved data, it may be deduced whether the molding system, prior to the actual dosing procedure, may be allowed to perform its basic function undisturbed as set up, or whether new signal progressions may be observed by making changes to the process.

From the start of the molding process, the viscoelastic resistance of the material has an effect on the initiated forming process, allowing conclusions to be drawn with regard to the toughness as well as other characteristics of the molding material.

Similar information can be deduced from the observation of the cavity pressure of the mold. The closing force represents an indicative value for the overall resistance of the material, while locally measured mass pressures in the cavity may provide insights into the timing of filling as well as other local effects, which may also be taken into consideration as verification data for a simulation. By comparison of calculated local pressures and the displacement of the flow front, the plausibility of the simulation results may be verified with the aid of the measured data.

In addition, recording of interior mold pressures yields further information about the distribution of pressures during the liquid phase of the molding material as well as information on the temperature and local progress of reaction shrinkage.

Further essential information for the evaluations of the process procedures are the mold temperatures, which should be recorded and verified separately for each heating circuit. The entire sensory equipment to be used includes:

- Measuring of distances
- Measuring the force of the dosing unit
- Verification of parallelism
- Measuring the interior pressure of the mold
- Mold temperatures

In special cases, the mass temperature and the dielectric conductivity of the molding material may provide insight about the procedures in the interlacing reaction. With the use of special sensors for measuring heat flow, values such as thermal capacity or the reactive enthalpy of molding materials can be measured under controlled technical conditions.

The software permits retrieval and data storage of signals as well as the visualization of individual or several different curves on one screen. Comparison functions enable the comparison of a measurement with a good or poor processing result as well as the ability to diagnose possible causes.

An additional software add-on permits the statistical analysis as well as the quantitative determination of process signals. This includes, for instance, pressure and temperature, heights, pressure increase speeds, and many other characteristic signal progressions.

Tool Design

Molds are either made from steel or, in the case of preproduction, from aluminum. Flat guides have proven to be best suited as mold guides for larger molds. The guide surface should be about 6 to 15% of the projected surface of the molded part, depending on the degree of difficulty of the shape of the molded part. When the parting line of both halves of the mold is joined, 75% of the guide surfaces should be in contact.

The mold can be heated using electricity, oil, water, or steam. The most widespread heating methods are steam and oil, which provide a more even temperature distribution than an electric heating system.

The temperature differences between the male and the female should not exceed 5 to 10 °C (9 to 18 °F), depending on the SMC. The punch (male side) should have the lower temperature of the two in order to prevent any interference between the two halves of the mold.

For the purpose of easier ejection of the molded parts, the mold is equipped with ejectors, which are mechanically or hydraulically driven or designed as air ejectors. It is recommended, by means of selectively placed undercuts, to hold the molded part in one half of the mold and then lift the molded part from the mold with the aid of ejectors. This prevents damages to the molded parts caused by sticking in the mold.

Painting of SMC Molded Parts

Painting of molded parts of automotive body panels made from SMC is generally done using

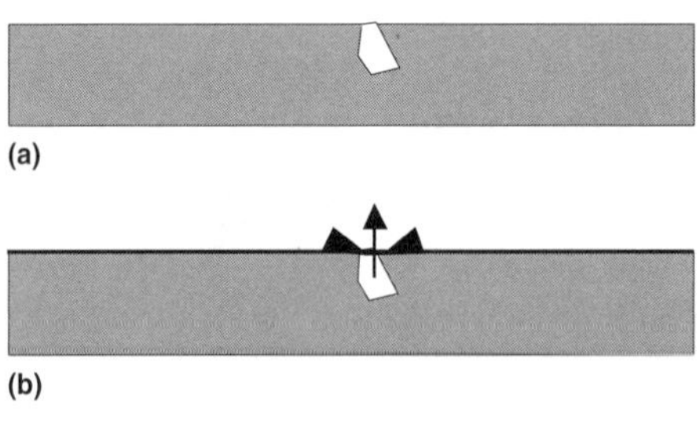

Fig. 30 Creation of paint defects due to inhomogeneities in the SMC surface finish. (a) Air inclusion in the surface of the molded part. (b) Expansion of air in the inclusion during drying forms a crater.

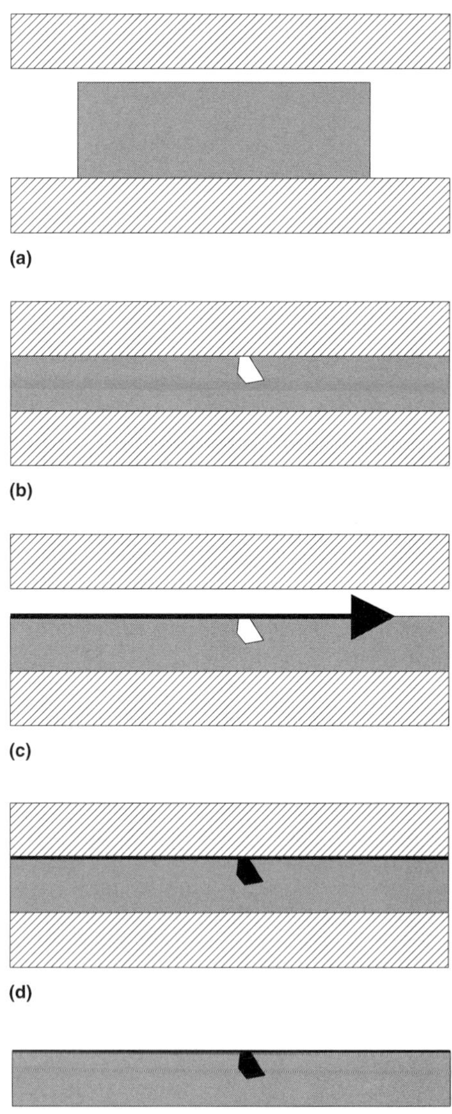

Fig. 31 Schematic diagram of the in-mold coating process. See text for description.

the same paints and at the same furnace temperatures as used for painting of sheet metal parts. In most cases, the molded parts are primer-coated by the manufacturer of the molded parts, and later a top coat is applied either off-line or on the production line of the automobile manufacturer. During the application of the primer, defects such as craters or pores in the primer coat can be caused by inclusions of air or styrene vapor, which must be removed by reworking the molded part. Air inclusions in the SMC molded part may occur for the following reasons:

- Molding-on stops the compression molding procedure.
- Styrene vapor bubbles may form, and existing air is not compressed.
- Air inclusions in the SMC
- Air inclusions caused by deep contours of the molded parts

Air inclusions in the surface of the molded part cannot be filled with a primer applied with a conventional spray-painting method (Fig. 30a). It may be possible to cover the defective area with paint in the spray-painting process, but, in the subsequent stage of drying in the drying furnace, a defect (crater) will appear due to the expansion of the air enclosed in the painted surface (Fig. 30b).

The in-mold coating (IMC) method is applied in order to reduce the occurrence of defects in the painted surface (Ref 32). The coating process is performed in a second pressure cycle on the still-hot SMC molded part in the following process steps:

- An SMC blank is inserted in the hot mold (Fig. 31a).
- The mold closes and forms the SMC molded part (Fig. 31b), which cures under pressure and temperature.
- After curing of the SMC, the IMC paint is injected. The mold opens slightly for this purpose (Fig. 31c).
- The mold recloses and distributes the paint on the surface of the molded part (Fig. 31d). The IMC paint cures under pressure and temperature.
- The mold opens and the coated molded part can be removed from the mold (Fig. 31e).

Air inclusions and cracks behave neutrally after filling with IMC paint in the drying furnace, and no longer lead to defective areas.

Applications of SMC Compression Molding

Electrical Industry. Cable and telephone branch boxes are among the oldest applications of SMC (Fig. 32). Aside from switch cabinets, millions of units of strip lighting (Fig. 33) which are used throughout every type of industry, have proven their value for more than 30 years in the electrical industry. These components have been proven for use in sanitary facilities and under wear and tear caused by aggressive media. The high technical standards can usually only be seen when looking at the interior of the components. The illustrated base plate (Fig. 34) serves as a footing for a curved lantern pole. All functional elements (stiffeners, mounting holes, sealing lips, and opening bolts) are integrated in the component. The SMC is dyed and designed for low shrinkage, so that they do not have a tendency to warp. The grained surface finish is long-term weather resistant, even without the protection of paint.

In the field of interior design and installations, various systems in different sizes are assembled to form complete units. The openings required for this purpose are preformed and can be cut out easily, if necessary (Fig. 35). It is important that the residual wall thickness is strong enough to guarantee the insulation, but also thin enough to permit easy cutting.

Satellite antenna manufactured by SMC compression molding gained access to sophisticated applications due to their excellent weather resistance and freedom of design, combined with outstanding dimensional stability. Their longitudinal expansion coefficient, which is close to that of steel, makes these antennas unaffected by extreme temperature fluctuations. However, a wire mesh must be embedded in the antenna dishes, because the SMC material alone does not reflect the radio waves.

Another advantage is the excellent flowability of the SMC materials, which not only allows the complete embedding of the wire mesh, but permits the inclusion of all attaching elements with reinforcing ribs at the rear.

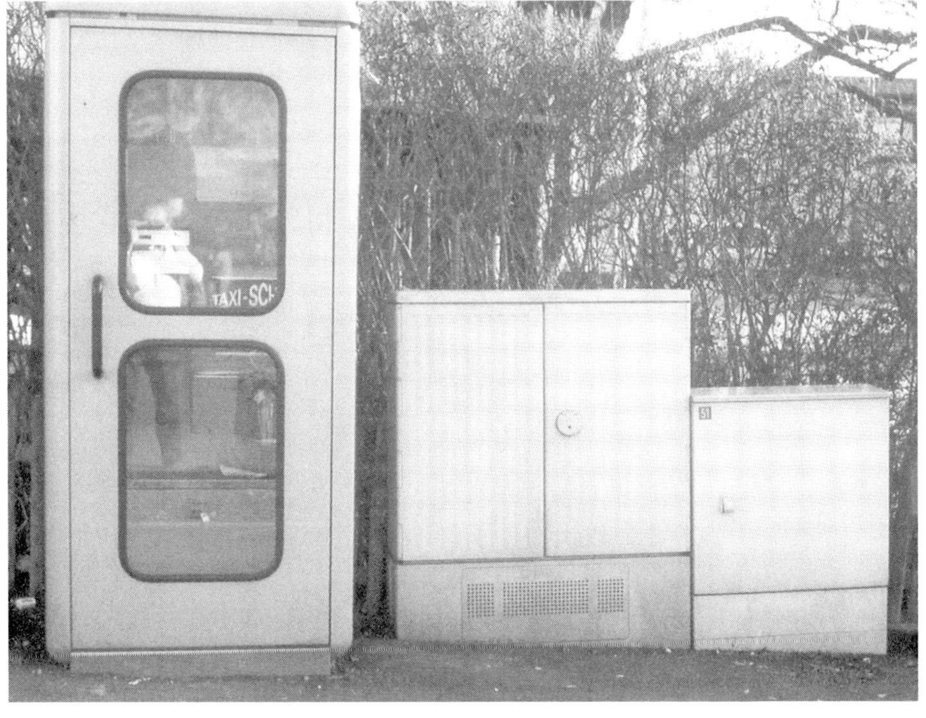

Fig. 32 Unpainted cable and telephone boxes manufactured by SMC compression molding. The boxes, exposed to the weather for 25 years, are shown next to an old painted telephone booth.

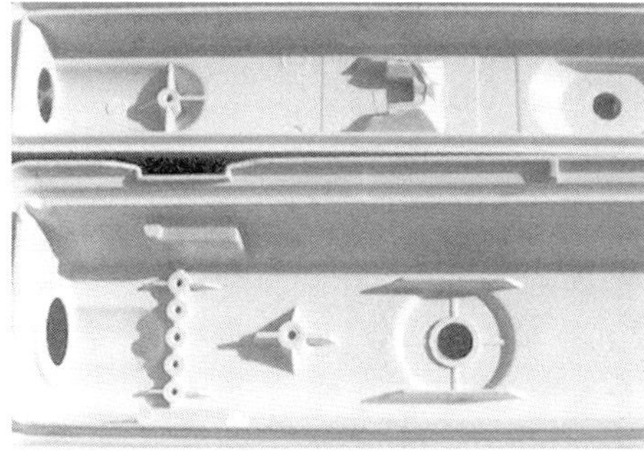

Fig. 33 Strip lighting units manufactured by SMC compression molding

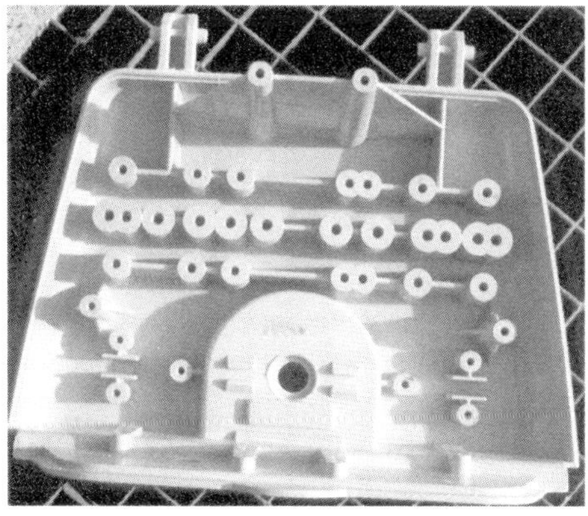

Fig. 34 Base plate for curved lantern pole. Manufactured by SMC compression molding

Automobile Industry. In the field of passenger cars, bumper supports made from high-strength SMC—so-called HPC or SMC–C—have proven their worth for many years (Fig. 36). With materials characteristics approaching those of high-end composites, high-strength SMC has secured a safe niche for itself for many years. The average vehicle owner will only become aware of the SMC supports when the vehicle is disassembled, because a closed fascia usually covers them (Ref 29).

The combustion behavior of SMC is of great importance for applications in the passenger compartment. In most cases, these parts are declared to be safety-related parts subject to mandatory documentation. This applies to, for example, hatchbacks, trunk lids, doors, and so on that are connected to the interior.

Parts manufactured SMC compression molding are able to meet the demands according to ISO 3795, DIN 75200, FMVSS 302, and many other vehicle-related standards without any special fire-protection measures.

For many years, structural supports made from SMC have been in use in the manufacture of passenger cars, lately also made from long-fiber-reinforced thermoplastic. As shown in Fig. 37, the components are delivered ready-for-assembly to the system supplier. The parts support the radiator, headlights, indicators, cables, and many other installed components.

For many years, spoilers have been a proven design in single-shell as well as double-shell design in passenger cars (Fig. 38). High Class A demands are made on the components, resulting in the frequent use of IMC as pressed-on primer.

Since the introduction of the Renault Espace, the first European minivan, its entire exterior body panels have been made from SMC (Fig. 39). The development of the Class A SMC can be traced through the history of this vehicle.

The particularly high demands of the German automobile industry can be met nowadays, proven by examples of trunk lids of Daimler-Chrysler cars made from SMC.

In the sector of commercial vehicles, the material has established itself due to its freedom from corrosion. The examples of the Mercedes-Benz Actros show that more than 30 SMC parts fulfill their intended functions (Fig. 40). The following components are made from SMC: bumpers, engine hood, doorsills, toolboxes and lids, fenders, top, and side covers. The side component shown in Fig. 40(b) in unfinished condition is equipped with the recesses for the headlights, flashers, fog lights, the ribbed stepping surface, all attaching elements, and the required stiffeners. High demands on strength and surface-finish quality are made on components such as side panels, toolbox lids, wheel arch, and other cover panels (Fig. 40c). Because all parts are painted together with the driver's cab, they must be supplied in a condition ready for topcoat painting. Reworking rates of topcoat painting are tolerated only up to 1%.

Other manufacturers use single-component bumpers, which are of very large dimensions due to the size of the vehicles. Battery covers of various designs and dimensions are used for various vehicle models (Fig. 41). The parts must be able to withstand persons standing on them and there-

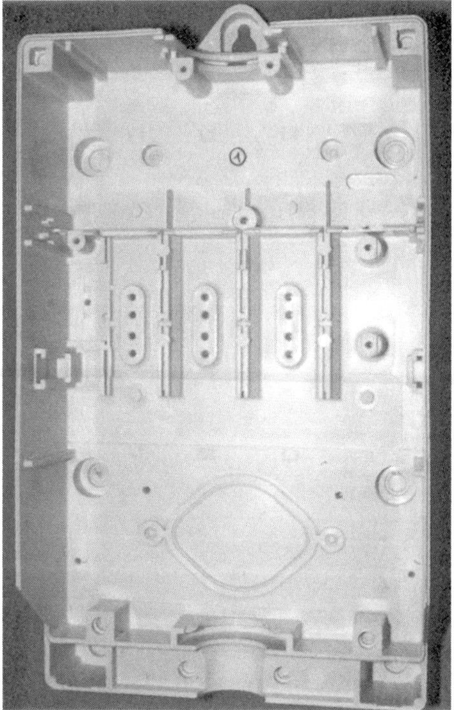

Fig. 35 Electrical switch cabinet for interior use. Manufactured by SMC compression molding

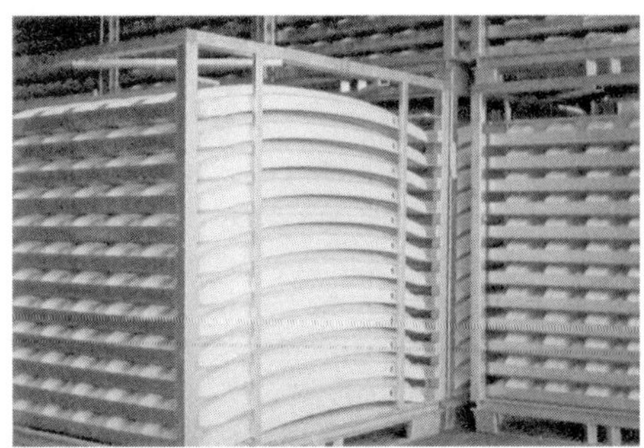

Fig. 36 Bumper support made from compression molded C-SMC

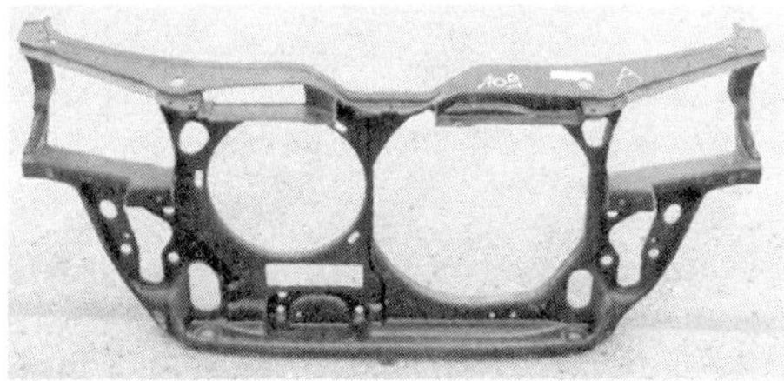

Fig. 37 Technical front end (structural support) for Ford Galaxy and Volkswagen Sharan manufactured by SMC compression molding

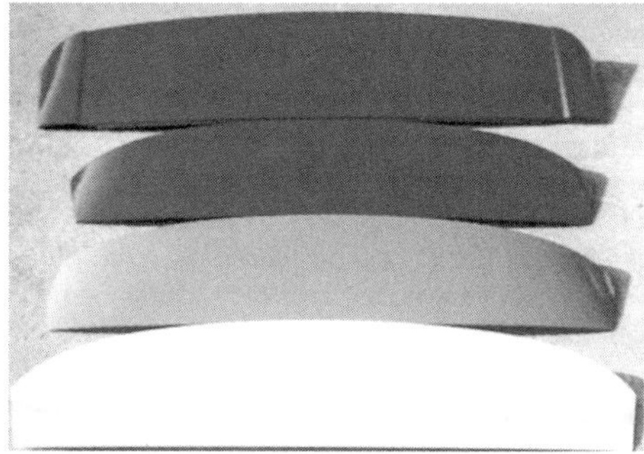

Fig. 38 Car spoilers manufactured by SMC compression molding and with the use of in-mold coating as primer for subsequent painting

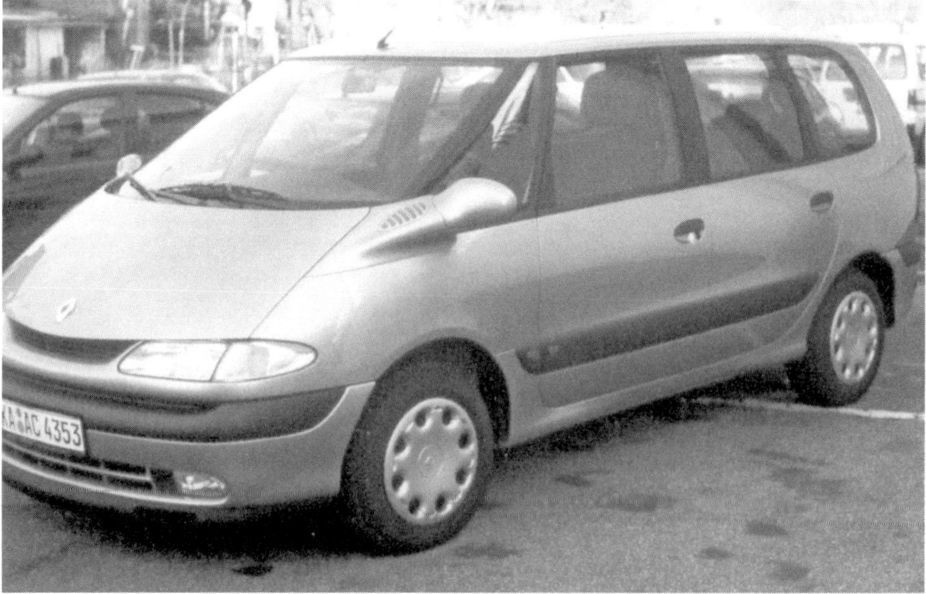

Fig. 39 Example of a minivan (Renault Espace) with exterior body panels made by SMC compressions molding

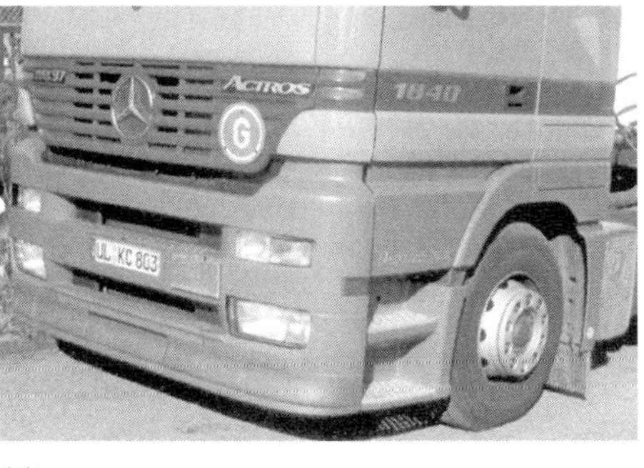

(a)

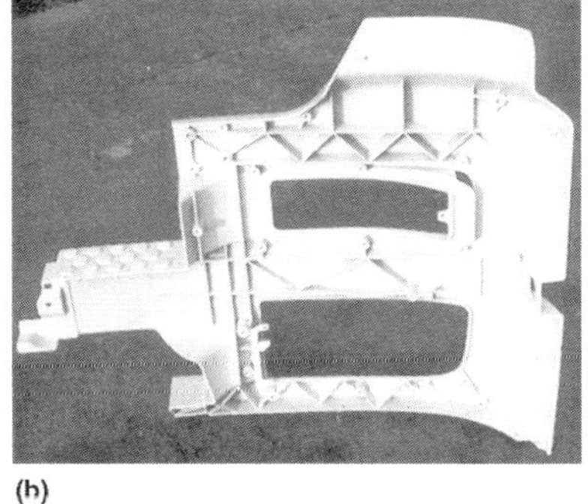

(b)

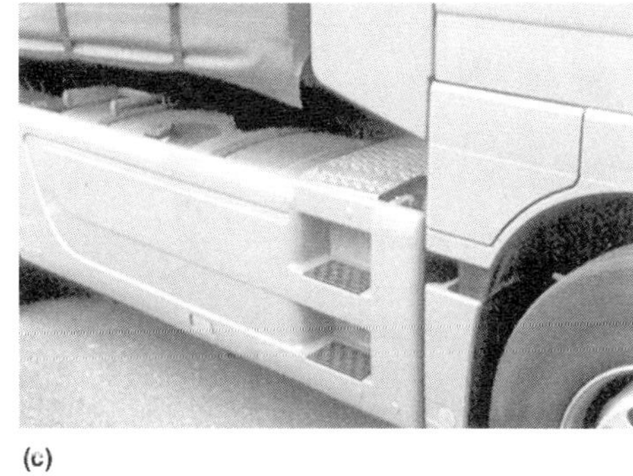

(c)

Fig. 40 Truck cab with multiple exterior components made from SMC (Mercedes-Benz Actros). (a) Front view. (b) Bumper side component. (c) Side panel with access ladder, toolbox lid wheel arch, and other parts

fore, they are designed with pyramid-shaped, raised patterns to improve grip.

Rail Vehicles. For many years, SMC components have made inroads, particularly as wall elements in the interior of many types of rail vehicles (Fig. 42). Most of the Interregio trains of the Deutsche Bahn (German Railway) are equipped with several different elements of self-extinguishing SMC material (Ref 32, 34).

Civil Engineering. Many application examples that are immediately connected to the building industry have already been mentioned in the electrical engineering applications. When it comes to particular resistance in moist conditions and exposure to aggressive media, cable trays and sewage pumps are made from SMC, for example.

Other Applications. SMC components are also used in the medical sector. They not only serve as cover panels for various devices, but they may also be used for parts subjected to considerable loads, such as the supporting part of a dentist's chair, shown from the rear in Fig. 43.

The pleasant surface finish of the patio table shown in Fig. 44 is achieved with the incorporation of recyclate particles.

Reduction of Emissions from Molded Parts

The problem of emissions in the interior of passenger cars has become a topic of decisive importance, particularly in the last ten years. With respect to this issue, components made from SMC have captured the focal point of interest. Figure 45 shows how styrene emission occurs during the compression molding cycle.

Because molding compounds are highly versatile materials with excellent materials properties, there has been a high degree of interest in finding ways to quantify and reduce emissions. Starting point initiatives were made by members of the automobile industry, who specified the first guidelines in defined test methods and limiting values (max 100 ppm).

Through the addition of suitable additives to the low-profile SMC formula, it was possible to lower toxic organic compound emissions from molded parts to the limiting value of max 100 ppm. The reduction is achieved during the curing process in the mold and requires no additional heat treatment. This method is pointing the way toward the use of molded parts without the necessity of a cost-intensive tempering process. Analyses of the emitted substances proved that no toxic substances were set free.

SMC Recycling and Reprocessing

The issue of recyclability of SMC has been addressed with particle recycling (Ref 32). The ERCOM recycling company has established particle recycling on an industrial scale. The objective was to build up a recycling concept interesting to the SMC industry, while creating material-specific advantages through the use of recycled materials. Avoiding disposal was the foremost consideration, but the declared objective was the exploitation of special characteristics of recycled materials. The aim was upcycling (creation of material with improved properties as compared with the original material); recycling (creation of material with equivalent properties) was accepted. Downcycling (creation of materials with reduced properties) was to be avoided.

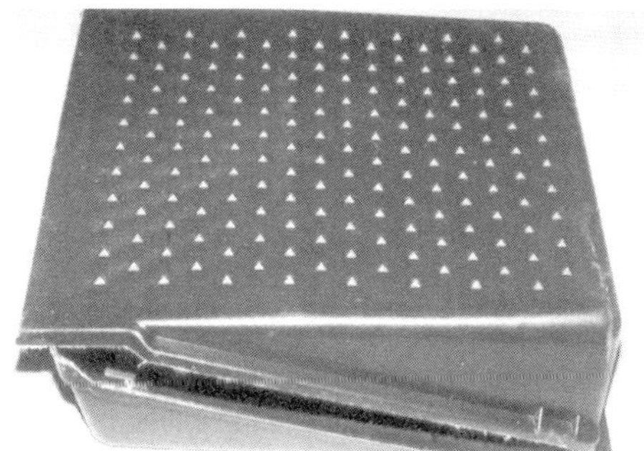

Fig. 41 Battery cover for commercial vehicles. Made from compression-molded SMC

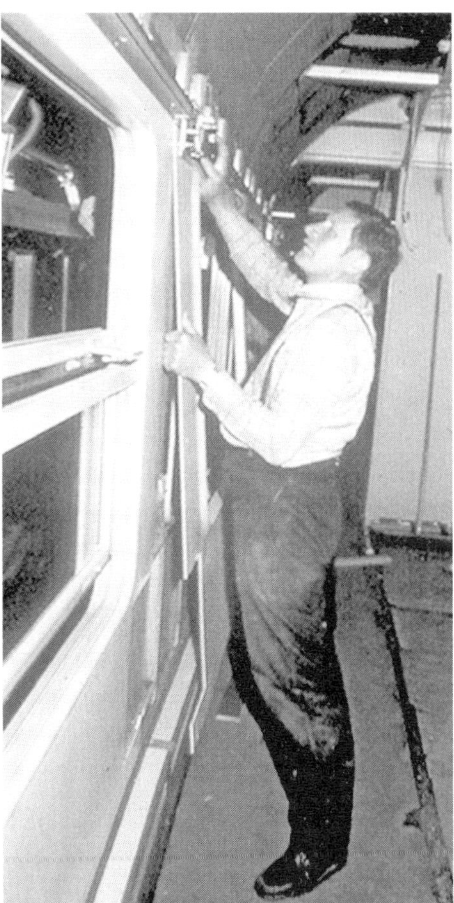

Fig. 42 . Assembly of SMC compression-molded interior wall elements in passenger rail cars

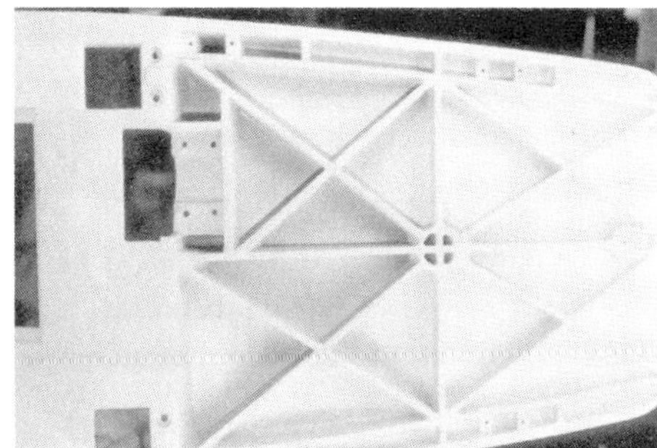

Fig. 43 Supporting part of a dentist's chair manufactured by SMC compression molding

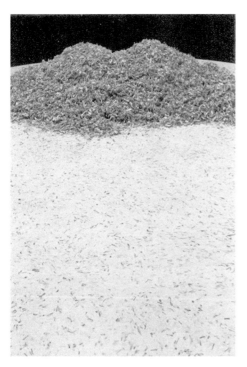

Fig. 44 SMC patio table containing recycling material (with loose recyclate shown on top of the table)

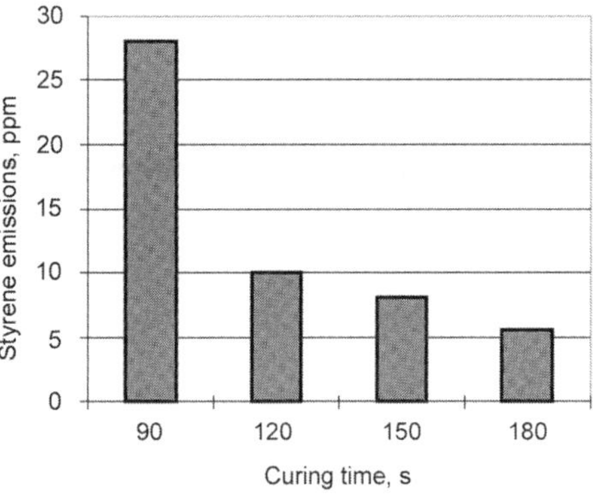

Fig. 45 Effect of curing time duration on styrene emissions from SMCs (mold temperature 160 °C, or 320 °F)

The advantages of recycled SMC are:

- Reduction of density
- Substitute for new glass-fiber material
- Decorative surface finishes
- Creation of structured surfaces

The costs of recycling were, in part, recovered through the selective use of recycled materials and improvement of properties. Recycling at zero cost is not possible. With the inclusion of certain characteristics, which are only available with recycled materials, recycling costs can be quite economical. In decorative applications, for example, the special structured surfaces of molded parts can only be achieved with the use of recycled materials (Fig. 44).

ACKNOWLEDGMENTS

The authors wish to thank the following people for providing input and information: U. Krause, Dieffenbacher Automation GmbH, Germany (molding plant equipment); P. Dankochick, Faroex Inc., USA (recycled GMT applications); G. Kaufmann, George Kaufmann AG, Switzerland (compression molds); E. Baur, M-Base Engineering + Software GmbH, Germany (EXPRESS compression molding software); R. Oosterhoff, PPG Industries Fiber Glass bv, The Netherlands; R. Mandos, Polynorm Plastics bv (compression molded GMT parts); O. Wallner, Schuller SMG GmbH, Germany (molding plant equipment); and G. Rothweiler, Schmidt und Heinzmann GmbH, Germany (SMC plant information).

REFERENCES

1. A. Oelgarth, H. Dittmar, W. Stockreiter, and H. Wald, GMT or LFT ?, *Kunstst. plast eur.*, April 1998, p 6–8
2. A. Tome, Direktverschraubungen in GMT (Screwing Directly into GMT), *Proc. Second International AVK-TV Conf.* 12–13 Oct 1999, B7–1
3. M. Novotny, Innovative GMT-System-Solutions for Automotive Applications, *Proc., PP '99 Polypropylene '99, Eighth Annual World Congress,* 14–16 Sept 1999, Maak
4. E. Baur, M. Ritter, and M. Michaeli, Prozesssimulation fuer das Fliessverfahren (Process Simulation of Flow Molding), *KU Kunstst.*, Vol 89, Aug 1999, p 70–74
5. T. Osswald, "Einsatz von CAE bei der Entwicklung von Pressbauteilen—Statusbericht fuer Europa und USA" ("Use of CAE in the Development of Compression Molded Parts—Status Report on Europe and USA"), Number 16, *Proc. 28th AVK Conf.*, 1–2 Oct 1997
6. M. Mahlke, Strategies and Plant Concepts for Pre-Heating GMT, *Proc. 22nd AVK Tagung,* May 1989, 13-1/7
7. Vorrichtung Zumgreiten von Flaechengebilden (Fixture to Grab Flat Articles), German Patent DE 43, 07, 142 C1
8. E. Semmler, A. Oelgarth, and W. Michaeli, GMT—Prozesse Modellieren (GMT—Process Modelling), *Plastverarbeiter*, Vol 47 (No. 8), 1996, p 24–25
9. G. Spur and St. Liebelt, Bearbeitung von GMT—ein Technologievergleich (Processing GMT—A Comparison of Technologies), *Kunstst.*, Vol 87, April 1997, p 442–450
10. C. Peterson and J. Jansz, GMT: Advances in Long Fibre PP Composites, *Polypropylene International Conf.*, 24–25 Oct 1994, p 27/1–27/14
11. V. Mattus, M. Neitzel, R. Dittmann, H. Hoberg, and H. Wallentowitz, Verwertung von GMT (Reprocessing of GMT), *Kunstst.*, Vol 88, Jan 1998, p 71–75
12. "Troubleshooting and Processing Guide for Azdel Molding," Azdel Inc., Shelby, NC, 1996
13. H. Giles, Reducing Shrinkage and Warpage in Glass-Mat Thermoplastic Composites, *Plast. Eng.*, Sept 1996, p 43–45
14. D. McBain, E. Strauss, and F. Wilczek, Advances in In-Mould Coatings, *Reinf. Plast.,* May 1997, p 34–39
15. T. Jud, H. Meinert, and R. Pettirsch-Tisler, Kunststoff-Ersatzradmulden (Plastic Spare Well Wells), *KU Kunstst.*, Vol 90, April 2000, p 108–112
16. S. Kupper and W. Selg, "GMT Front End for the VW Golf," *Proc. 21th AVK Conf,* Oct 1991
17. A Plastic Bumper Beam, Costing Less Than a Roll-Formed Steel Bumper Beam, *Plast. Bus. News,* Vol 22 (No. 42), 11 Nov 1998
18. B. Gilliard, W. Bassett, D. Featherman, E. Haque, C. Johnston, and T. Lewis, "I-Section Bumper Beam with Improved Impact Performance from New Mineral-Filled Glass Mat Thermoplastic (GMT) Composite, Paper Number 1999-01-1014, *Proc. Society Automotive Engineers,* 1999
19. H. Dittmar, J. Groen, F. Mooijman, and C. Peterson, Chopped Fibre Laminates—Latest GMT Developments, *Proc. Second International AVK-TV Conf.*, 12–13 Oct 1999, B4-1
20. M. Ericson, "Future Development Potentials for GMT's and LFT's," *Proc. Langfaserverstaerkte Thermoplaste im Automobil—Stand der Technik und Zukuenftige Perspektiven* (Proc. Long Fiber Reinforced Thermoplastics in Automobiles—State of the Art and Future Perspectives), 9–10 Nov 1999
21. E. Haque, "Development and Characterization of Thermoplastic SMC: Mineral-Filled GMT," Paper Number 20000-01-1076, *Proc. Society Automotive Engineers,* 2000
22. M. Seufert, U. Steuer, and D. Hebecker, Daempfungswannen aus GMT-PP (Resistant Underbody Pans Made from GMT-PP), *Kunstst.*, March 1998, p 325–329
23. V. Mattus, "Möglichkeiten und Grenzen der Verwertung langfaserverstaerkter Thermoplaste" ("Opportunities and Limits to the Reprocessing of Long Fiber Reinforced Thermoplastics"), *Proc. Langfaserverstaerkte Thermoplaste im Automobil-Stand der Technik und zukuenftige Perspektiven,* 9–10 Nov 1999
24. R. Kühfusz, *Langfaserverstärkte Thermoplaste* (Long Fiber Reinforced Thermoplastics), SKZ, Würzburg, Germany, Nov 1999
25. R. Brüssel, LFT—Direktverfahren von Menzolit-Fibron (LFT—Menzolit-Fibron Direct Process), *AVK-Tagung*, Baden-Baden, Germany, Sept 1998
26. P. Stachel, Long Fiber Reinforced Thermoplastics, 13th *Annual Advanced Composites Conf.*, Michigan, USA, Sept 1998
27. Front end in Hybridtechnik, *Kunststoffberater*, May 2000, p 6
28. R. Bräuning, Determination on Improvement of Mechanical Properties and Optim-

isation of Processing Conditions of Sisal Fiber Reinforced Polypropylene Compounds for Automotive Applications, diploma thesis, ICT, Pfinztal, Germany, April 2000
29. Fahrzeugteile vom Feld (Automotive Parts in the Field), "Hightech Report '99," Daimler-Chrysler, p 82
30. A.H. Horner and R.N. Brill, Some Factors Influencing Polyester Resin Behavior during the SMC Thickening Reaction, *Preprint 40th Annual Conf. SPI,* 1985, p 16-D
31. R. Kleinholz and R.M. Mai, *Kunstst.,* Vol 67, 1977
32. G. Ehnert, *Kunstst.,* Vol 71, 1983, p 455
33. H. Derek, printed information, SMC-Technologie, Stolberg, Germany
34. H. Wolf, G.P. Ehnertand, and K. Bieniek, New SMC-Generation for Molded Parts with Low C-Emission without Post Curing, *Preprint Internationale AVK-TV Tagung,*1998

Filament Winding

S.T. Peters, Process Research
J. Lowrie McLarty

FILAMENT WINDING is a process for fabricating a composite structure in which continuous reinforcements (filament, wire, yarn, tape, or other), either previously impregnated with a matrix material or impregnated during winding, are placed over a rotating form or mandrel in a prescribed way to meet certain stress conditions. When the required number of layers is applied, the wound form is cured and the mandrel can be removed or left as part of the structure.

High-speed, precise lay-down of continuous reinforcement in predescribed patterns is the basis of filament-winding. The filament-winding machine (Fig. 1) traverses the wind eye at speeds that are synchronized with the mandrel rotation, controlling the winding angle of the reinforcement and the fiber lay-down rate. The deposition can be controlled either by computer numerically controlled (CNC) machines or by simple mechanically controlled winders; the latter are less convenient, but require a lower capital investment. Figure 2 shows the basic six axes of the CNC machines. Figure 3 is a schematic of the optimized control systems for efficient wet filament-winding. Usually, the mechanical machines are limited to three axes or less, whereas the CNC machines can accommodate up to seven axes.

Thermoset resins, generally used as binders for reinforcements, can be applied to the dry roving at the time of winding, which is known as wet winding. They may also be applied prior to winding as a tow or tape prepreg and used promptly or refrigerated. Usually the cure of the filament-wound composite is conducted at elevated temperatures without vacuum bagging or autoclave compaction. Mandrel removal, trimming, and other finishing operations complete the process.

Aerospace and some other applications generally use untwisted fiber; in many commercial applications, twist is introduced by the composite manufacturer when the untensioned fiber is fed from a center pull container. The mandrel can be cylindrical, spherical, or any other shape as long as it does not have reentrant (concave) curvature—although several manufacturers have been able to incorporate complex reentrant curves in filament-wound structures (Fig. 4 and 5) (Ref 1). Large or thick-walled structures, particularly structures of revolution such as cylinders or pressure vessels, are most easily wound.

The reinforcement can be wrapped in adjacent bands or in repeating bands that are stepped the width of the band to eventually cover the mandrel surface. The technique, in process, looks somewhat like that shown in Fig. 6 and can be changed with both CNC and mechanical filament-winding machines to result in many different winding patterns (e.g., polar, helical, or hoop). The technique can vary winding tension, reinforcement material, wind angle, or resin content (if wet wound) in each layer until the desired thickness and resin content of composite is achieved with the required orientation. Multiple composite components can be fabricated simultaneously in the same equipment, with accurate fiber angles and good resin control. Figure 7 shows four square columns being fabricated. For small items, such as golf shafts, it is possible to wind up to 20 components simultaneously (Fig. 8).

The filament-winding industry, manufacturing processes, machines, and raw materials have undergone drastic changes during the time since the previous versions of this article (for the *Engineered Materials Handbook,* Volumes 1 and 2) were written. Many new manufacturers have emerged, primarily in the commercial and sporting goods sectors, and the emphasis has shifted from filament-winding of rocket motors to that of golf shafts, driveshafts, or drill risers. Some

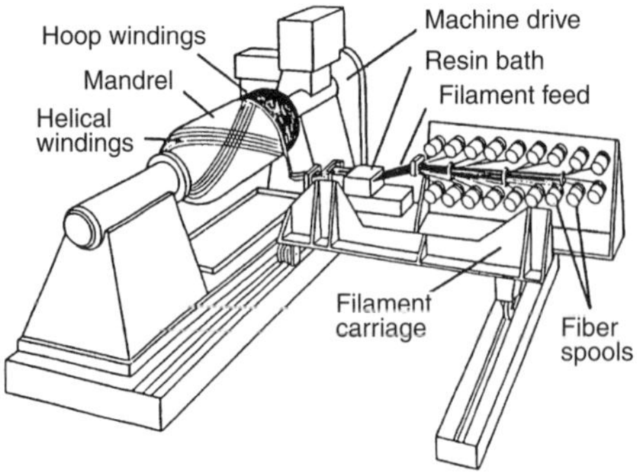

Hoop windings
Mandrel
Helical windings
Machine drive
Resin bath
Filament feed
Filament carriage
Fiber spools

Fig. 1 Typical filament-winding machine

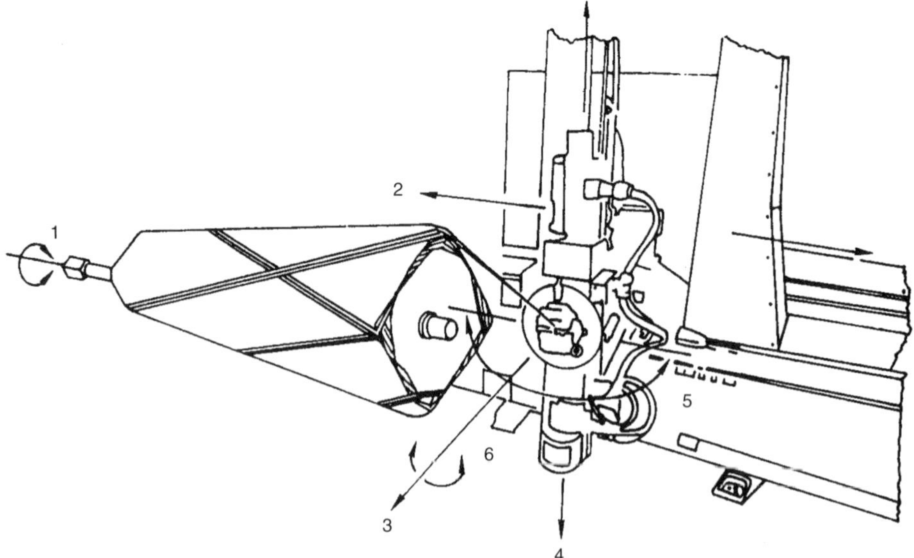

Fig. 2 Six axes of filament-winding machine motion. Courtesy of McClean Anderson, Inc.

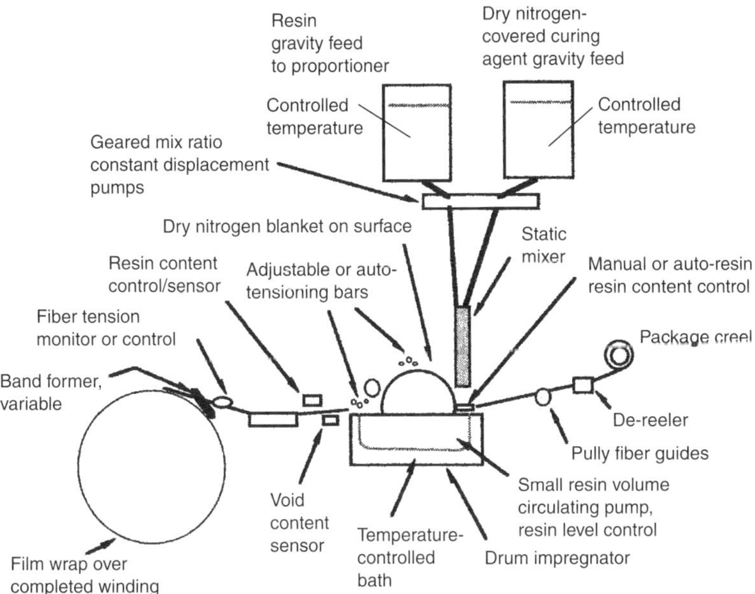

Fig. 3 Optimized controls for a wet-winding process

of the recent advancements in filament-winding include:

- The use of prepreg tows rather than impregnating the dry fibers. The change to prepreg has been driven by reductions in cost of the fibers (and the resultant prepreg), the need for minimal or no cleanup (long a problem for wet filament-winding), the reduced environmental impact, and faster wind speeds (no resin sling for hoops, no aeration of resin in impregnation bath).
- Increased strength and modulus of fibers, especially carbon-graphite fibers, versus those that were available in the 1980s
- Availability of fibers in larger tow sizes, making the process even more cost effective by increasing the speed of fiber deposition
- The evolution of new wet-winding resin systems and the increased availability of third party-formulated resins
- The evolution of cheaper towpregs, which has made their use cost-effective for many applications when compared to wet-winding resin systems
- The development of low-viscosity wet resin systems for resin transfer molding (RTM), and their subsequent adaptation for use in for filament-winding
- Improvements in filament-winding machines and controls. Seven axes of movement are commonly available, and most CNC machines feature easy-to-program software. The winding motions can now be programmed off-line much easier and faster, resulting in more cost-effective changeovers and layer modifications

Advantages and Disadvantages

Advantages. The most important advantage of filament-winding is its low cost, which is less than the prepreg cost for most composites. The reduced costs are possible in filament-winding because a relatively expensive fiber can be combined with an inexpensive resin to yield a relatively inexpensive composite. Also, cost reductions accrue because of the high speed of fiber lay-down.

Other advantages of filament-winding compared to other compacting and curing processes are:

- Highly repetitive and accurate fiber placement (from part to part and from layer to layer). The accuracy can be superior to that of fiber placement and automated tape-laying machines.
- The capacity to use continuous fibers over the whole component area (without joints) and to orient fibers easily in the load direction. This simplifies the fabrication of structures such as aircraft fuselages and reduces numbers of joints for increased reliability and lower costs.

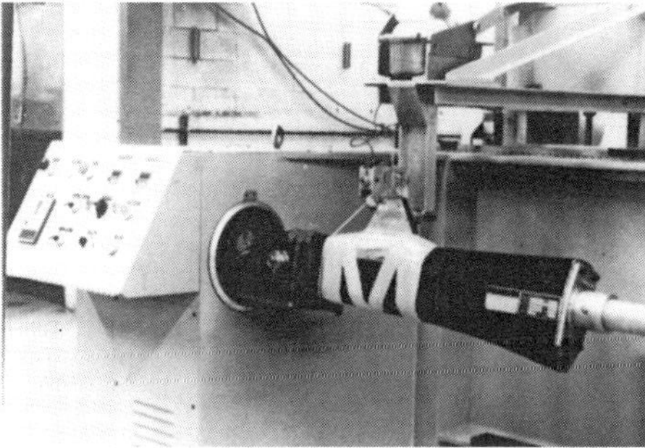

Fig. 4 Complex winding patterns for the V-22 grip assembly. Courtesy of McClean Anderson, Inc.

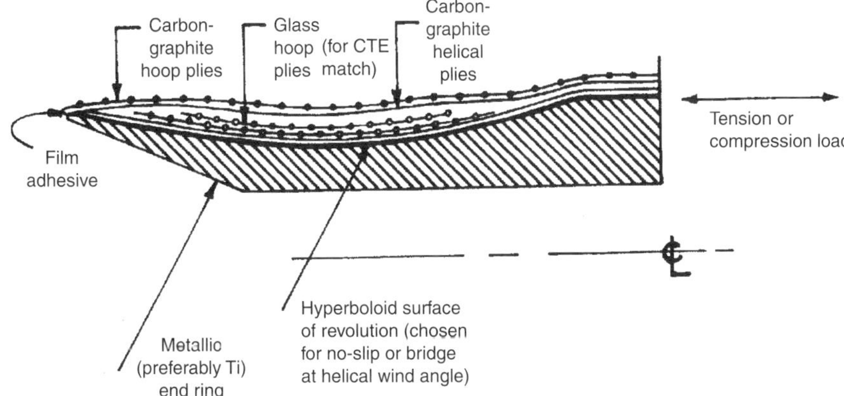

Fig. 5 In situ reentrant filament-wound joint

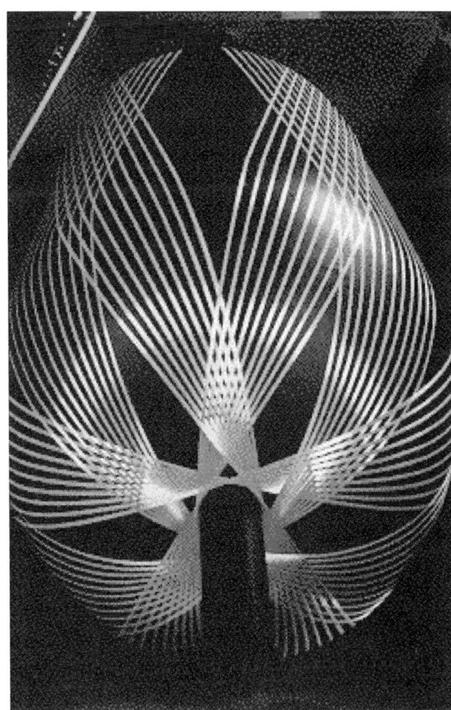

Fig. 6 End view of multipass, single-tow filament-winding. Courtesy of Entec Composite Machines, Division of Zoltek Inc.

- Elimination of the capital expense (and size restrictions) of an autoclave and the recurring expense for inert gas. Thick-walled structures can be built that are larger than any autoclave can accommodate.
- Ability to manufacture a composite with high fiber volume
- Mandrel costs can be lower than other tooling costs because there is usually only one tool, the male mandrel, that sets the inside diameter and the inner surface finish.
- Lower cost for large numbers of components because there can be less labor than many other processes. It is possible to filament wind multiple small components, such as up to 20 golf shafts at once (Fig. 8), leading to sharply reduced costs compared to flag rolling. Costs are eliminated for bagging and disassembly of the bagging materials, as well as the recurring costs of these materials.
- Costs are relatively low for material since fiber and resin can be used in their lowest cost form rather than as prepreg.

Disadvantages of filament-winding include:

- Need for mandrel, which can be complex or expensive
- Necessity for a component shape that permits mandrel removal. Long, tubular mandrels generally do not have a taper. Unless nonuniform shapes are capable of mechanical disassembly, mandrels must be made from a dissolvable or frangible material. Different mandrel materials, because of differing thermal expansion and differing composite materials and laminate lay-up percentages of hoops versus helical plies, will demonstrate varying amounts of difficulty in removal of the part from the mandrel.
- Difficulty in winding reverse curvature
- Inability to change fiber path easily (in one lamina)
- Poor external surface finish, which may hamper aerodynamics or aesthetics

It is important to note that most of the disadvantages are application-specific and, in many cases, have been circumvented by innovative design and equipment modifications.

Several factors offset the disadvantages associated with mandrels. Usually the mandrel is less expensive than the dies or molds for forming methods other than pultrusion or RTM.

Inexpensive mandrel materials, such as cardboard and wood, have been successfully used. Fabricators of large rocket motors have been using water-soluble sand mandrels or plaster mandrels that can be stripped, reduced in size, and passed out through relatively small ports.

Even though reverse curvature generally cannot be wound, three options are available for circumventing this restriction. The first involves winding the part, bridging the concave area, and then installing a reverse curvature caul plate and applying external pressure during cure. This technique may require dropping winding tension or cutting fibers in scrap areas. A variation of this is the use of a caul plate that is removed as the fiber band crosses the depression and is replaced immediately and held until the band passes the next circuit. This method maintains the placement and tension of the fibers and eliminates the need for cutting. A second approach is to wind the exact shape on a positive dummy mandrel insert, then remove the insert and place the fiber. The third option is to wind into a reduced section area by choosing the hyperboloidal curvature of the recess in conjunction with the selection of the helical fiber angle (Ref 1).

The fiber path cannot be changed easily, but it can be done by use of pins, sawtooths, or slip of the tow. Fiber placement is the only fabrication method capable of "steering" the fiber. Commercial pinrings are available (Fig. 9).

A better outside surface can be obtained by use of outer clamshell molds. (This was the technique used for the Beech Starship, shown in Fig. 10. A bladder on the male mandrel was used to expand the part into a female mold to attain an aerodynamic finish, Ref 2.) External hoop plies or thinner tows on the last ply can be used. Uncompacted helical plies tend to be more bumpy than hoops. Another option is to use shrink tape or porous tetrafluoroethylene-glass tape overwrap. Many aerospace fabricators have used these techniques. The result is a matte surface that tends to hide flaws or blemishes while imparting some smoothing.

Effects of Fiber Tension

In filament-winding, fibers are positioned under tension. This tension can be advantageous because fibers in tension can have twice the strength of those in compression. (Structural beams of carbon-graphite may have more fiber

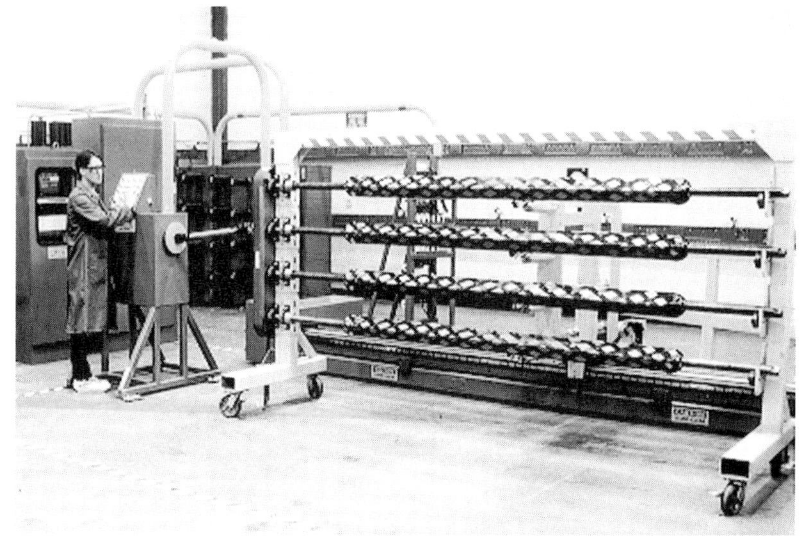

Fig. 7 Multiple component winding. Courtesy of CompositeTek, Inc.

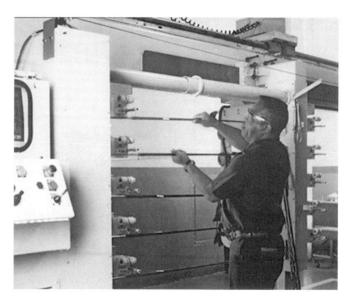

Fig. 8 CNC filament winding of multiple golf shafts. Courtesy of True Temper Sports Company

on the compression side to offset this fact. Fibers are added on the compression side by winding at zero degrees and retained by overwinds.) However, if the fibers in a laminate are not straight, the laminate will have reduced tensile and compressive strength values. Repetitive loads and other structural performance factors are also degraded by nonstraight fibers. That is, the straight fibers in a laminate will load and fail before the relaxed fibers are fully loaded. Fiber alignment is especially important for high-modulus fibers such as carbon-graphite because of their low strain-to-failure behavior. Correct use of fiber tension during winding is the only way to achieve straight fibers in a filament-wound structure.

Because the fibers are under tension, they can move or shift when there are cut ends in the part. It is possible to retain the wound wet fibers with tensioned circumferential fibers at each place that the fiber ends (such as a cut end or a ply drop-off). When the fibers are cut outboard of these positions, the fiber tension is reduced end-to-end of the structure, but the fibers remain straight and ready to equally assume the structural tension and compression.

It is sometimes advantageous to wind an outer hoop of dry glass at very low tension to absorb excess resin, or as material added for subsequent machining operations to avoid cutting structural fibers.

The effect of bands of fibers compressing the previously wound fibers, as the plies are placed upon one another, is to reduce the diameter of the uncured structure. The result of this reduced diameter is that the previously wound fibers are too long to remain straight and can be distorted, that is, crimped. Medium- and thick-wound walls must be wound with careful selection of tension to prevent crimping. Higher-tensioned fibers are placed on the inner plies. Since they are tight, they are resistant to further compaction. Succeeding plies have gradually reduced tension so as not to compress the inner plies.

The true fiber tension is that tension measured as the impregnated fiber exits the payout eye at the same speed in feet per minute used during winding the product. (This is called "dynamic" tension measurement.) Measuring the fiber tension at the creel is not accurate, even if all delivery contacts between creel and winding surface are via pulleys.

Materials

The filament-winding process allows choices in the selection of fibers, resins, and materials form (or delivery system)—that is, wet, prepreg tow, or prepreg tape.

Fibers

Fiberglass. The most widely used fiber for commercial filament-winding is fiberglass, which has been used in several grades in the United States for many years. Glass fibers used for filament-wound structures include types "E," "R," "S," and "C" (see the article "Glass Fibers" in this Volume). Fiberglass is used extensively where dimensional stability, corrosion resistance, and low-cost materials and processing are required.

Aramid fibers, specifically Kevlar 29, 49, and 149 (i.e., Du Pont de Nemours & Co., Inc., Wilmington, DE), exhibit exceptionally high strength-to-density and modulus-to-density ratios (known as specific strength and specific modulus). They also show great consistency with a low coefficient of strength variation, allowing high design allowables. Aramid composites have relatively poor shear and compression properties because of the fibrillar nature of the filaments, but find extensive use in pressure vessels and nonprimary loaded structures. Additional information is available in the article "Aramid Fibers" in this Volume.

Carbon/graphite fibers exhibit the largest range of available fiber mechanical properties. Constant improvements in fiber modulus, tensile strength, strain to failure, and surface finish have made handling for filament-winding easier. Although the modulus and tensile strength of graphite fibers have been dramatically improved over the past few years, increases in modulus have generally resulted in a decrease in tensile strength, and vice versa. The intermediate fibers have been the only exception. Increases in the amount of fiber graphitization result in increased modulus, which in turn results in increases in thermal and electrical conductivity. The cost of the fiber also increases, primarily because of lower demand for the high-modulus fibers and higher energy costs, and because large-scale production economies have not yet been imposed. All fibers, except ultrahigh-modulus pitch and extremely high-modulus pitch, have been successfully filament-wound. Additional information is available in the article "Carbon Fibers" in this Volume.

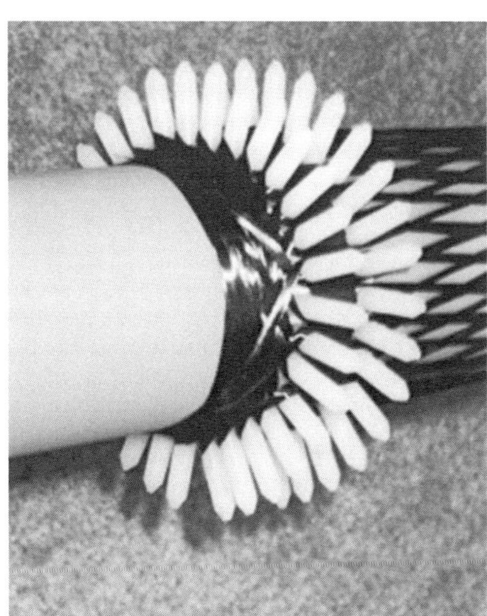

Fig. 9 Commercial preformed pinring. Courtesy of Advanced Composites, Inc.

Resins

The resin system in a filament-wound composite serves the same functions as it does in composite structures fabricated by other means, namely:

- Retaining the filaments in the proper position and orientation
- Transferring the load from filament to filament and ply to ply
- Protecting the filaments from abrasion (during winding and in the composite)
- Controlling electrical and chemical properties
- Providing the interlaminar shear strength

There are several handling criteria for a wet resin system that are unique to filament-winding:

- Viscosity should be 2 Pa · s (20 P) or lower
- Pot life should be as long as possible (preferably more than 6 h)
- Toxicity should be low

Important resin-matrix properties in the cured structure are adhesive strength, heat resistance, fatigue strength, chemical resistance, high strain to failure, and moisture resistance.

The introduction of aramid fiber in the early 1970s spurred new investigations into resin systems. Many resin systems that had worked well with glass were not appropriate for use with the new fibers. New types of resin systems were subsequently developed to address low-temperature cure, long pot life, high heat deflection, high elongation or strain to failure, and low toxicity. These five factors are somewhat exclusive, that is, a low-temperature cure does not usually result in high heat deflection properties, and high heat-deflection generally lowers strain capability.

Long pot life resin systems were developed to allow fabrication of large structures with an ex-

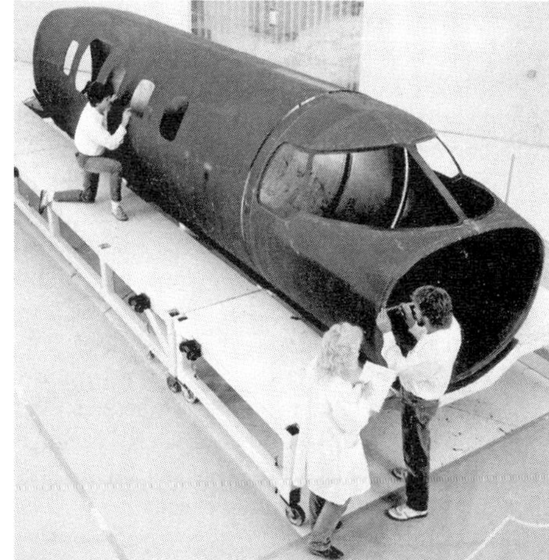

Fig. 10 Beech Starship filament-wound fuselage. Courtesy of Fibertek Division of Alcoa/TRE, Inc.

tended gel time and minimum exotherm. Generally, anhydride-cured systems have long pot lives, coupled with high-temperature cures and high heat-deflection temperatures. The high-temperature resin systems generally have higher cure temperatures and lower strain-to-failure capability.

Composite structure toughness is a concern for aircraft and all other long service life, impact-sensitive structures. Filament-wound aircraft structures, attractive because of the potential for large cost savings, must exhibit damage tolerance. Toughness can be incorporated into a composite structure by any of several methods:

- Introducing elastomer or thermoplastic particles
- Blending to result in an interpenetrating network
- Interleaving with thermoplastic film
- Decreasing cross-linking density
- Using special fiber orientations (including through-the-thickness reinforcement)
- Using a thermoplastic matrix

All toughened wet filament-winding resin systems depend on the addition of a prereacted epoxy resin and carboxy-terminated polybutadiene acrylonitrile rubber polymer to achieve toughness without shortening pot life. Generally, the addition of rubber also increases the viscosity of the resin system, which may be unacceptable from a processing standpoint. The toughened, long pot life and flexible formulations have lower heat-deflection temperatures (or glass transition temperatures) than do the high-temperature resin systems.

Another technique for increasing the fracture toughness of a filament-wound composite has been to use thermoplastic resins, because they offer outstanding interlaminar fracture toughness (G_{Ic}) and good compression strength after impact testing.

Delivery Systems

The three different impregnation methods commonly used are preimpregnated roving (prepreg), wet rerolled, and wet winding.

Prepregs. Preimpregnated rovings offer excellent quality control and reproducibility in resin content, uniformity, and band width control. These parameters can be determined well in advance of the filament-winding process; not on the factory floor where many of the quality control tests must be done for wet winding. Many high-performance resins that can only be impregnated using special processes, such as hot-melt, can be employed; however, the resin must be modified to reduce the adhesion between the resin-covered tow layers on the delivery package (usually tangential letoff rolls) because separator plies are not used for prepreg tows.

Most commercial prepregs may also use solvents or preservatives to extend storage life. These additives change the resin system from that which retains the same name but may be marketed for other applications that may enjoy broad qualification approval. Thus the filament-winding resin, because of the necessary minor modifications, may have to undergo detailed qualification testing. Some newer resin systems have been optimized for long out time, and some are marketed with essentially infinite storage time at room temperature, rather than in freezers.

Prepreg filament-winding resins are commonly thought to possess the following as advantages:

- Better resin-content control
- Encapsulation of carbon-graphite fibers (prevents small, airborne, graphite-fiber interference with electrical motors)
- Minimal fiber damage due to the protection offered by the resin and the use of roller redirects
- Better stability on a nongeodesic path
- More consistent composite properties

The commonly quoted disadvantages of prepreg tow are:

- Poor fiber availability. This is a result of adding another step to the manufacturing process.
- Requirement, generally, for refrigerated storage and control of out time
- Higher cost
- No room-temperature cures are possible.

Wet Rerolled. With wet-rerolled "prepreg," a controlled volume of resin is impregnated on fiber reinforcement and then respooled. Quality control can be performed away from the winding operation. Preservatives or solvents are not required, because the roving is either used immediately or stored in a freezer for future use. This can be a very cost-effective method for obtaining preimpregnated roving at the plant of the winder.

Wet Winding. The lowest-cost materials for composite processing are those that are brought together at the process by the composite manufacturer. Thus, if the design requirements allow wet filament-winding, it will always be less expensive than winding with prepreg, but the manufacturer must make some choices in terms of safety, cleanliness, and so on, before production. When a prepreg is used, there will be some limitations on the choice of fiber/resin; with wet impregnation the choices are unlimited.

Wet impregnation of fiber can be accomplished by either pulling the reinforcement through a resin bath or directly over a roller that contains a metered volume of resin controlled by a doctor blade. This low-cost system is widely used in commercial applications with polyester and epoxy resins. The resin content is affected by several parameters (most of which are interrelated): resin viscosity, the doctor blade setting, the interface pressure at the mandrel surface, winding tension, the number of layers, and the mandrel diameter.

Delivery systems for prepreg and wet-rerolled rovings are similar. Each includes a winding comb (or series of rollers) that is designed to collimate the several strands of roving into a single band width for delivery to the mandrel. Wet winding differs primarily in that the dry fiber roving passes from a creel (or tensioner) into a bath containing the winding resin and passes over a large drum that has a doctor blade that controls the thickness of the resin. Alternately, the roving passes through a series of rollers or rods that are submerged in the resin bath and are designed to flatten the roving strand and force resin into the fiber bundle. After leaving this type of bath, the band usually passes under a wiper or doctor blade to remove the excess resin. Next, the wet-out roving progresses to the winding eye, where it is deposited on the mandrel.

Often, the advantage of one delivery system over another is either lower cost or better resin content control. A major drawback of wet winding is that it is usually limited to horizontal winding operations.

Fiber Volume. Typical fiber volume fractions for several types of fibers in wet-wound composites are shown in Table 1. It can also be seen that the typical fiber volumes are similar to those for composites made by other methods, and that the fiber volume for helical and hoop fibers can be different. Fiber volume, for wet winding, can be changed by the composite manufacturer by resin content control and by more precise side-by-side fiber and fiber band lay-down than is possible with prepreg.

Void content for most wet-wound composites, unless special precautions are taken, are in the range of 3 to 6%. This has been of little concern to pressure vessel manufacturers who seek a composite that only experiences tension in the fibers at minimum weight, but it is of concern if the structure is to experience compression, bending, or shear.

Figures 11 and 12 and Table 2 provide some guidelines for choosing appropriate fibers, resins, and the form of starting materials.

Shapes

Filament-wound shapes generally include cylindrical, spherical, conical, or dome-end configurations. These bodies of revolution best exploit the advantages of high-speed winding. Any part with an axis of symmetry and without a concave surface can be filament-wound with state-of-the-art equipment. Cylindrical shapes with domes (or other provisions for turnaround) are ideal for winding. Additional information about typical shapes and components manufactured by filament-winding is provided in the section "Applications" in this article.

Table 1 Typical fiber volume fractions for helical winding and hoop winding

Fiber	Typical fiber volume fraction (V_f)	
	Helical winding	Hoop winding
Glass	0.55–0.60	0.65–0.70
Para aramid (Kevlar)	0.55–0.60	0.65–0.70
Carbon-graphite	0.50–0.55	0.60–0.65

Winding Patterns

The three basic filament-winding patterns are helical, polar (or planar), and hoop (see Fig. 13).

In helical winding, the mandrel rotates more or less continuously while the fiber feed carriage traverses back and forth at a speed regulated to generate the desired helical angle. The normal winding pattern provides a multicircuit helical. After the first circuit, the applied fibers may not be adjacent. If adjacent, it is called a one-circuit pattern. If three circuits are required to have the fiber band next to the starting fibers, it is a three circuit pattern. The helical pattern is characterized by fiber crossovers at certain points along the mandrel. The quantity of crossovers increases with the number of circuits per pattern. A layer is made up of a two-ply plus-and-minus angle-balanced laminate. The mandrel revolutions per circuit vary with the winding angle, band width, end dwell, and overall length of the vessel.

Winding of angle plies, if done with a helical program that does not completely cover the mandrel surface with each pass, results in a two-ply layer in which the two angles are interspersed. A polar-wind technique can apply laminate layers in a similar fashion, but the fiber is not deposited on a curved surface in the shortest length. This can cause increased tendency for fiber slippage and, possibly, reduced ultimate loads.

The advantage of helical winding is greater versatility. Almost any combination of diameter and length can be wound by trading-off wind angle and circuits to close the pattern. Minor adjustments can be made by changes in band width, wind angle, and dwell.

In polar winding, the fiber passes tangentially to the polar opening at one end of the chamber, reverses direction, and passes tangentially to the opposite side of the polar opening at the other end. A one-circuit pattern is inherent to polar winding. The windings are delivered by an arm while describing a great circle, and the laid-down pattern is planar. Because the mandrel is regulated to advance one band width for each rotation, succeeding band widths will lie adjacent to one another.

The main advantage of polar (or planar) winding is its simplicity. There is no carriage reversal, and an even winding speed can be maintained. However, because the fiber path is not a helix, it is not the shortest fiber distance between points. This can result in fiber slipping during wet winding and lower ultimate values in pressure vessels.

Hoop patterns are also known as girth, 90°, or circumferential (circ) winding. Strictly speaking, hoop winding is a high-angle helical winding that approaches an angle of 90°. Each full rotation of the mandrel advances the band delivery one full band width. The winding machine is much like a lathe in that the spindle speed is much more rapid than the carriage travel. Hoop windings are generally combined with longitudinal windings (helical or polar) to produce a balanced-stress structure. Hoop patterns are applied to the cylindrical section of a closed-end vessel, while helical and polar patterns reinforce both the cylinder and the domes.

Crossovers. One of the major differences between filament-wound composite laminates and those manufactured by other methods is the presence of crossovers. When a structure is helically wound with bands of fibers of a width such that in traversing from one end to the other the object is not covered completely, crossovers will result. Helical filament-winding patterns, rather than polar, are chosen for all structures where the length-to-diameter ratio equals or exceeds two, because polar-wind patterns can be expected to slip during fabrication and when cured and under load. The quantity of crossovers depends upon the width of the band and upon the number of circuits per pattern. The analysis for design of composites with crossovers is more involved than that for discrete layers.

When pressure vessels are loaded at very high rates (a matter of 10 to 20 microseconds from earth atmospheric to burst), they generally fail at the crossovers. There is some evidence that the cyclic fatigue resistance is reduced slightly when crossovers are used. Values when layers are five- to ten-thousandths of an inch thick are very close to those of structures having discrete layers.

In some evaluations, such as short beam shear tests, the crossovers appear to be of value in increasing the apparent shear stress to force the desired failure mode. In small rocket launch tubes, crossovers provide an additional benefit. If they are on the inner surface, they can prevent band or tows from unwinding or stripping from one end of the tube to the other. In parts that do not have crossovers, this is likely to happen, especially when individual fibers have not been completely attached to the resin matrix.

Also, a helical-wound tube without crossovers can fail under a tensile stress on the tube by transverse fiber pullout. Some have recommended an interior hoop layer to avoid this failure mode. Because the two helical layers that form each angle ply are interlaced at the crossovers, there is some degree of enhanced fracture toughness, at least between the angle plies.

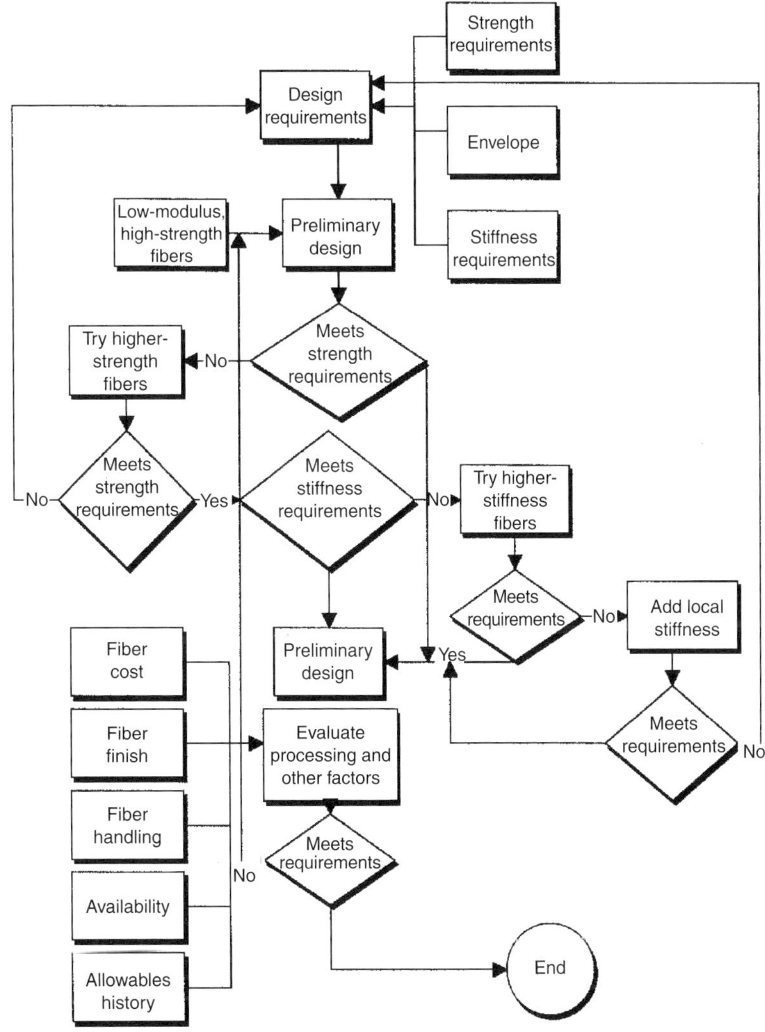

Fig. 11 Iterative process for selecting reinforcing fiber

Bands of tows can conform to extreme shapes without distortion or buckling or without having been strained (stretched). This is because each tow in a band can be any length relative to the others and can be free to slip, at least in wet-winding systems and in some prepreg when heated.

It is possible in filament-winding to have two bands, for example, that when they cross, the total thickness at the crossing may be less than the total thickness of the two bands, or less than the thickness of one band, due to the possibility of spreading. Of course, the band width at the nodes will be larger, related to the reduction in thickness. This technique can be used advantageously to build a practical structure such as an isogrid, without a complex grooved mandrel and without any additional fiber buildup at the nodes.

Tooling and Equipment

One of the big advantages of filament-winding over other composite manufacturing methods is the simplicity of tooling. The mandrel, which provides the part with accurate internal geometry, is generally the only major tool. Equipment and facilities required are usually simple and often consist of just a winding machine and curing oven.

Mandrel design can be as simple or as complex as the part requires. The factors that must be considered are production reusability, tolerances required, thermal expansion control, weight (equipment limitations), deflections (sagging), part removal from mandrel, and cost.

Low-cost mandrel materials such as cardboard or wood can often be used when winding routine parts. At the other end of the use spectrum, where critical parts require close tolerances, expensive steel mandrels designed for long-term use may be required. For high-temperature cure (315 °C, or 600 °F), graphite mandrels with low thermal expansion are advantageous. Gas-containment pressure vessels often require metal or plastic liners because composites are porous at high pressures; metal liners can also serve as mandrels.

Mandrel Types. Descriptions of the principal mandrel types used in the filament-winding industry are given below.

Water-soluble mandrels are primarily used in rocket motor cases and pressure vessels where mandrel removal through small openings is desired. The sand is cast into female molds that use preassembled components, such as insulation, wind axis, lightening tubes, and polar bosses. The sand is cured, and two mandrel ends are assembled and bonded. Two binder systems commonly used are polyvinyl alcohol and sodium silicate. The advantage of water-soluble sand mandrels is low cost for small production quantities and excellent dimensional reproducibility. The disadvantage is a high initial tooling cost.

Spider/plaster mandrels are often used to provide a high-tolerance mandrel surface in which a plaster sweep is used over removable or collapsible tooling. The plaster is cured, then overwrapped with a synthetic fluorine-containing resin tape or some other separator film. Following cure, tooling is removed, the plaster is chipped or washed out, and the release tape is removed, leaving the desired inside contour. Metal-supported plaster is generally used for relatively large parts (3 to 6 m, or 10 to 20 ft). For any larger size, the mandrel may be limited by torque or bearing strength of the wind-axis attachments.

Segmented-collapsible mandrels are specialized and expensive, but the advantages of their reusability and the continuous winding process renders expensive tooling worthwhile for high-production applications.

Cylindrical (tubular) steel mandrels are used to fabricate composites that are stripped (pushed or pulled) off the surface after curing. These tools must be of high quality for trouble-free usage. Chrome-plated, anodized, or hardened and polished surfaces assist in easy mandrel removal. A slight taper along the length of the mandrel also is beneficial. The tube mandrel may be as complex or as simple as economy dictates. Its size is limited only by the length of the winding machine bed.

Nonremovable liners in pressure vessels provide a lightweight pressure container that combines the high strength-to-density of composites with a thin, impermeable metal or plastic liner to contain high-pressure gas, such as helium, hydrogen, or oxygen (Fig. 14). Metal liners can be designed to carry either a large or small portion of the internal pressure, but in all cases the liner, which initially served as the winding mandrel, becomes a vital part of the pressure vessel.

Specialized mandrels include inflatable rubber (elastomeric) or plastic mandrels. These are limited by the explosive properties of the inflating medium. One approach is to fill the mandrel with a material such as sand and then draw a vacuum on it.

Winding Machines. In most winding machines, the mandrel is suspended horizontally between a head stock and a tail stock, much like a lathe (Fig. 1). The carriage travels lengthwise at speeds synchronized with the mandrel rotation to deliver the roving from a wind eye at various winding angles for the selected winding pattern. There is a great variety of winding equipment commercially available to wind helical, polar, or hoop patterns (refer to the Section "Winding Patterns" in this article). The bulk of production filament-winding is still performed using the mechanical gear-driven machines that evolved during the late 1950s. These machines will continue to be used because of their low cost. Polar winders with only two axes of rotation (mandrel and winding arm) still produce rocket motor

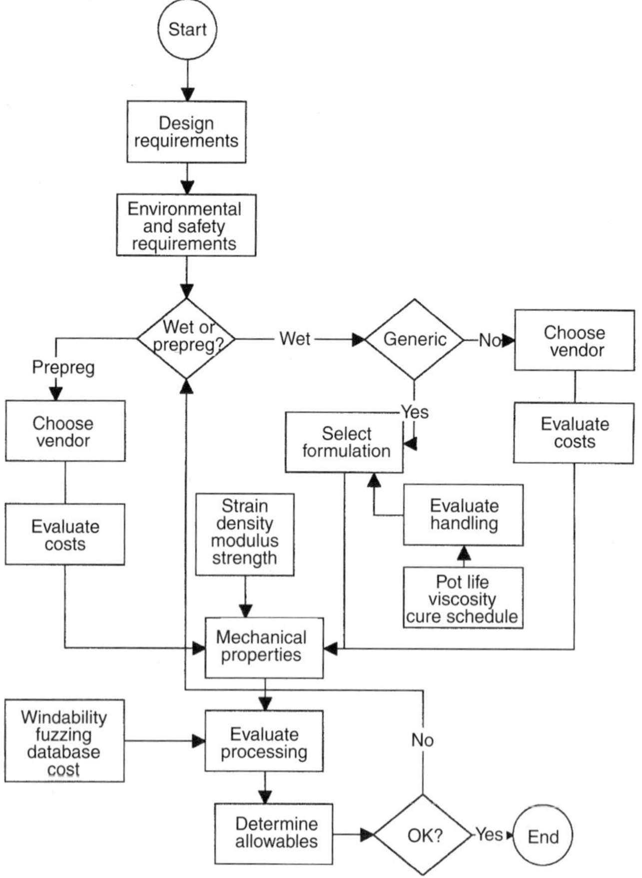

Fig. 12 Selection process for resin component

cases and spherical pressure vessels in great numbers.

Helical winders have progressed from two- to seven-axes machines (and some suppliers have promised eight-axes equipment). Helical winders may be either horizontal or vertical; the latter of which can be much simpler, because the load goes through the axis of rotation, minimizing mandrel deflections. Also, handling operations are simplified if the mandrel does not require horizontal-to-vertical rotation for installation of tooling or for B-staging (of rocket motor skirts).

Tensioners. Because most reinforcements are packaged on rolls, tension can be introduced at the roll. Magnetic or friction brakes, electronic rewind, and rotating scissor bars are the tension devices used. Because they rewind, the latter two allow the overtravel past the domes to be taken up, thus winding of low-angle patterns around end domes is possible.

The tensioners are often mounted on creels that are either remote to the winder or part of the carriage that actually travels with the delivery system. The tensioning devices should have as many of the following features as possible: variable but controlled tension levels, easily adjusted tensions, rewind capability to prevent fiber slacking, and uniform tension regardless of the size of the roll.

Ovens. The fabrication of the composite portion of the assembly is completed by the curing operation, although some resin systems are room-temperature cured and do not require an oven. Several equipment options for oven curing are available. The most commonly used are ovens (gas-fired, microwave, or electric) or autoclaves.

Most epoxy resin systems are cured in gas-fired ovens heated with either air or inert gas, without supplemental pressure. The use of vacuum bags and bleeder cloths has been implemented by some manufacturers, and the system is reported to produce void-free laminates with improved compaction. Autoclaves are commonly used with the more exotic resins, such as bismaleimides and polyimides. Bismaleimides require special considerations because of the high degree of compaction required to promote resin flow, while polyimides necessitate the removal of a high volume of volatile materials produced during cure. Generally, autoclaves are not

Table 2 Comparison of prepreg, wet winding, and wet-rerolled filament-winding materials systems

Parameter	Prepreg	Wet winding	Wet rerolled
Cleanliness	Best	Worst	Almost equal to prepreg. Mess is away from winder
Safety	Best; fibers and resin contained	Worst	Little better than wet. Impregnation can be done where it is convenient and safe.
Fiber availability	Poor; not all fibers available, some are special order	Best; any fiber that system can handle	Best; all fibers
Control of resin content	Best; constant speed and viscosity	Poor; speed of mandrel and resin viscosity varies	Better; process is away from winder and is faster; little viscosity change
Quality assurance	Highest; can be done in advance	Worst; imposes quality procedures onto factory floor and can lead to errors	Good; can be done ahead
Complex resin systems	Can use; hot melts are available	Very difficult; requires complex impregnators to remove solvents or liquefy hot melts	Difficult; still requires complex impregnators
Large data base systems	Yes	Commercial prepreg resin systems generally not available as liquids. Wet systems with large data bases are likely to be proprietary.	Same as wet winding
Graphite fibers encapsulated (to prevent electronic short circuits nearby)	Yes	No	They are not released at winder.
Storage	Must be refrigerated and storage records maintained	Easy mix at winder. Dry fibers have long shelf life.	Must be stored like prepreg, but for shorter time. Records must be kept
Pot life	Longest; can be adjusted	Short, not controllable	Same as wet
Cycle time	Adjustable; can be shortest	Limited control	Limited control
Fiber damage	Depends on impregnator; can be the least; fiber is handled twice	May require special equipment. Potentially the least, but seldom is	All handling of fiber is under control of the user.
Cost	Highest	Lowest	Above wet, but requires capital equipment for impregnation equipment
Large roving package	Depends on impregnator	Whatever is available dry from fiber sources	Same as wet
Room-temperature cure	Not possible	Possible	Possible
Simple resin formulation	Possible	Necessary	Necessary
Winding speed	Highest; resin throw and wetting are not factors	Lowest speed	Intermediate; resin can be staged to reduce resin throw
Stability on nongeodesic path	Highest possible	Lowest; wet resin may cause slippage	Intermediate; resin can be staged
Composite property variations	Least	Largest variations	Intermediate
Catenary	Not a problem	Dry fiber to impregnator may have catenary	Catenary would probably be found previously
Differential slip (e.g., to slip around or over pins)	Very difficult to have once the band is formed	Easy	Easy

Source: Adapted from Ref 6

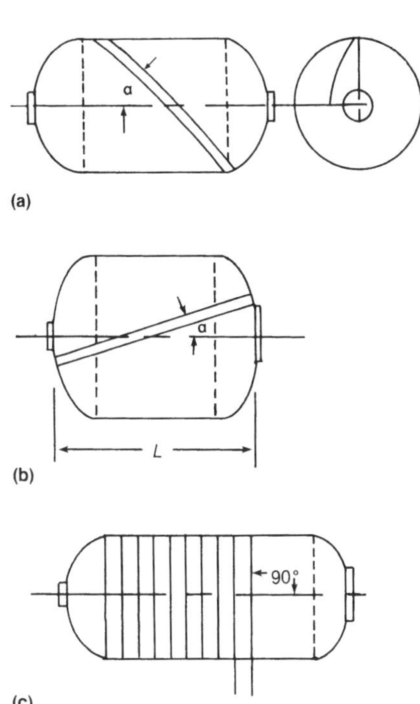

Fig. 13 Basic filament-winding modes. (a) Helical. (b) Polar. (c) Hoop. α, wind angle

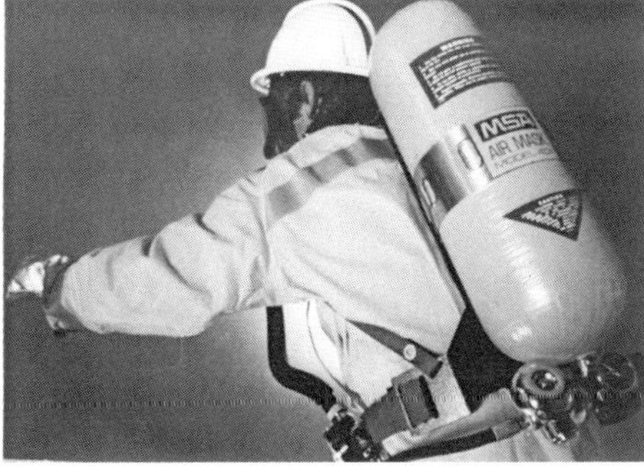

Fig. 14 Metal-lined filament-wound oxygen bottle. Courtesy of SCI, Astro Division of Harsco Corporation

used for pressure vessels such as pipes and tanks. If an autoclave is to be used for pressure vessels, care must be exercised to not bleed the resin too much. Excess bleed causes the filaments to relax and can even cause wrinkles, disturbing the load-carrying effectiveness of the filaments. Autoclaves are the state of the art for nonwound components, such as skins and panels for aircraft applications, for which the interface pressure between the continuous fibers and the thermally expanding mandrel may not otherwise develop during cure.

Microwave oven curing requires a high initial investment but provides life-cycle savings by dramatically reduced energy costs and significantly reduced cure times. However, special heating supplements, such as induction heaters, are often required at the composite-metal interfaces, and microwave cure works best with nonconductive fibers.

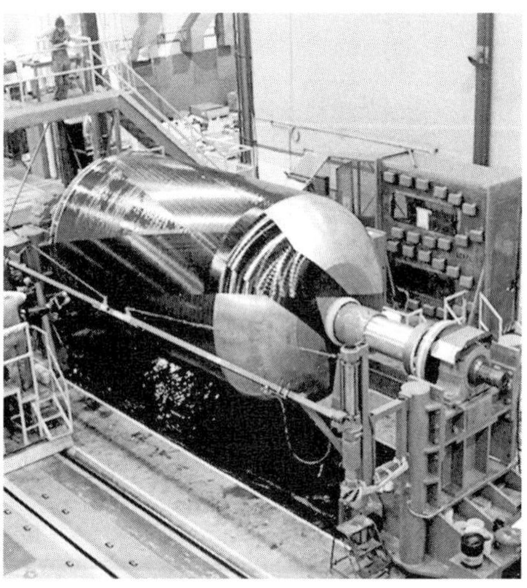

Fig. 15 Large winding for the Titan IV rocket motor. Courtesy of Alliant Techsystems, Inc.

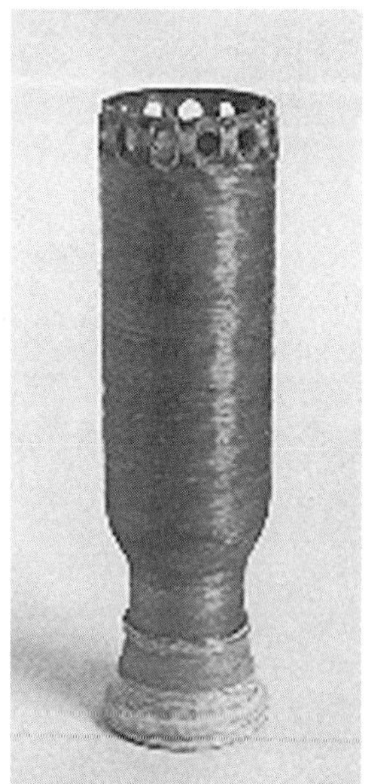

Fig. 16 Viper tactical rocket case with wound-in pin joint. Courtesy of Brunswick Defense Division (now Lincoln Composites)

Applications

Pressure vessels have been the most demanding and pervasive application for the technique. Filament-winding is the only fabrication technique for high-performance pressure vessels. The recent advances in increasing the strength of carbon-graphite and organic fibers have resulted in carbon-graphite fibers with a strength of almost 7000 MPa, or 1000 ksi (for example, Toray T-1000, [Toray Industries, Japan], 6370 MPa, or 924 ksi), and an organic fiber (PBO, manufactured under the trade name Zylon [Toyobo Co., Ltd., Japan]) has tensile strengths and moduli almost double those of p-aramid fibers. The performance factor of the fiber (fiber strength divided by density) using values quoted by the vendor shows the PBO fiber about 3% less efficient than T-1000 carbon-graphite fiber.

Rocket Motors. All new booster rocket motors manufactured in the United States are strong candidates for filament-winding. The Titan IV strap-on booster is now a filament–wound carbon-graphite-epoxy composite that has replaced the high-strength steel cases (Fig. 15). Strap-on boosters for Atlas and Delta rockets are also filament-wound. There are still no aircraft-launched tactical composite rocket motors in the United States in spite of their advantage of greater munitions insensitivity. Ground-launched tactical rocket motors have been in continuous production since the late 1970s when the Viper rocket motor concept was introduced. This was a glass-fiber reinforced structure with a 100% aft opening for introduction of a preformed propellant grain. The aft opening was closed with a closure that had removable pins inserted into the specially reinforced case end (Fig 16).

Natural Gas Vehicle (NGV) Tanks. A large market exists for composite-overwrapped NGV pressure vessels for mass and individual transportation. These vessels have used thick and thin steel and aluminum liners as well as thermoplastic liners. The fibers have been carbon-graphite and/or fiberglass with a variety of epoxy matrices (Fig. 17). The pressure vessels have performed well in service except for a very few problems. In 1985 there was an in-service failure of a hoop-wrapped high-pressure cylinder that necessitated recall and reinforcement of the dome-closure area. This was a metal failure. Only the cylindrical portion of this tank was filament-wound. Wound tanks use a process called autofrettage to expand the metal past yielding and place tension in the fibers. Without internal pressure, the steel is under compression and the fibers under tension. Under service pressure, the steel undergoes low tensile loading as the fibers sustain the high values.

Power Transmission Shafts and Rollers. The filament-wound power transmission shaft industry started because of corrosion problems with metallic shafts and poor durability in the corrosive atmosphere of water cooling towers. Also, composite shafts could be made longer, replacing two shafts with one composite shaft, eliminating the intermediate support and universal coupling with lower vibration concerns. Replacing of steel rollers (for slack take-up in paper mills and similar industries) resulted in higher throughput because of lower inertia in the roller (Fig. 18).

Sporting Goods. The effect on sporting goods of filament-wound composites has been immense. Virtually all tennis rackets are manu-

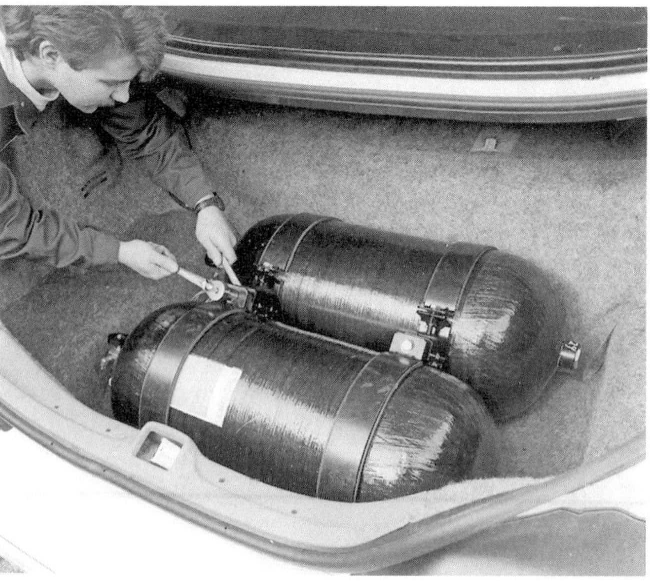

Fig. 17 Typical natural gas vehicle tanks. Courtesy of Lincoln Composites, Inc.

factured from composites. Many are made from a filament-wound preform (Fig. 19). The bulk of products are made from filament-wound broadgoods that are folded to result in a stacked prepreg with the desired fiber angles.

Boats. Most of the attempts to introduce filament-winding into the boating industry have been unsuccessful. Filament-winding was attempted as a technology by two contractors for large craft such as minesweepers, but failed because of fiber slip (Ref 3). However, the process has been successful for smaller craft.

A historical perspective on the applicability of filament-winding for diverse uses is illustrated by a small boat (Fig. 20) filament-wound in the 1950s. The boat has been in continuous use in rivers and lakes in the United States and Canada. It has never had to be repaired and has never leaked. The floor has recently increased its deflection. This may be due to the partial failure of the balsa bonded to the wound fibers or to the deterioration of the balsa. The many years of water transfer due to rain and time in water plus hull-bottom flexing are probably the significant factors.

The principal feature of this boat is the use of filament-wound material for molding complex shapes, that is, early preforms. The added feature was to combine this molding material with filament-winding to create an all filament-wound structure for any configuration.

The materials used were 250-yield glass rovings, epoxy resin, an epoxy curing agent, and three parts of green pigment. No other ultraviolet light protection was used. The war surplus end-core balsa varied between 140 and 220 g/cm^3 (5 and 8 lb/ft^3). No paint was used. Oarlock fittings and forward rope attachments were bronze.

The tooling consisted of hull-shaped boxes bolted together around a three inch steel tube. The boxes were small enough to be removed through the open section above the seats. Pockets were placed in the boxes as an internal detail for the seat supports. Materials needed for molding were filament-wound on a 0.9 m (3 ft) diameter mandrel. The mandrel surface had 1.6 mm (1/16 in.) deep circumferential grooves by using a plastic floor runner. This surface was for ease of materials removal without fiber displacement. Seat mandrels were of solid 25 mm (1 in.) balsa that were overwound at $\pm 65°$ and remained as part of the structure.

The winding pattern for the molding filament-wound material was $\pm 65°$ for two reasons. The fibers did not slip at end reversal. When used as a molding material, the $\pm 65°$ fiber orientation could be rotated to change the $\pm$ value. For example, the $\pm 65°$ would be $\pm 25°$ when rotated 90° and placed on the boat hull mandrel. During winding of the hull, fiber band placement was always on a nonslipping path. There were no circumferentials or longitudinals. The placement was based upon a design that should be flexible, that would have small changes in wind angle between the very few plies available, and would effectively distribute the load of the passenger and cargo within the hull and load on the outer hull due to beaching and to smooth rocks in shallow streams.

Representative Component Properties

Because most filament winders can use wet resin systems along with prepregs and preformulated wet resin systems, there is a need to verify the properties of the individual components of the composite as well as the fiber-resin combination and the cured component. Table 3 shows the test methods to verify the fiber-resin components.

Table 3 ASTM standards for fiber and matrix mechanical properties

ASTM No.	Title
Fibers	
D 3379	Test Method for Tensile Strength and Young's Modulus for High-Modulus Single-Filament Materials
D 2343	Test Method for Tensile Properties of Glass Fiber Strands, Yarns, and Rovings Used in Reinforced Plastics
D 4018	Test Method for Tensile Properties of Continuous Filament Carbon and Graphite Yarns, Strands, Rovings and Tows
D 885	Methods of Testing Tire Cords, Tire Cord Fabrics, and Industrial Filament Yarns Made from Man-Made Organic-Base Fibers
Matrix	
D 638	Test Method for Tensile Properties of Plastics
D 695	Test Method for Compressive Properties of Rigid Plastics
D 790	Test Methods for Flexural Properties of Unreinforced and Reinforced Plastics and Electrical Insulating Materials

Source: Ref 4

There are several reasons that filament-wound composites are not tested in the same manner as composites fabricated by other means. It is always preferable to test a laminate that has the same manufacturing method and lay-up as the component. This is relatively easy for common composites that generally have a flat surface that may replicate a surface of the component.

Filament-wound composites are generally surfaces of revolution, that is, curved, so that usually a portion of the composite will be impossible to test without bending. If the laminate could be wound onto a flat surface, if helical plies are used, the laminate can be expected to warp upon cure due to the lack of symmetry in a single-laminate wall. A further problem arises with flat filament-wound structures; the flat laminate is not adequately compacted across the flat surface, and the laminate center bulges during the winding. If it is desirable to wind a flat laminate that replicates the actual laminate, then that test part will have to be wound using a polar pattern for

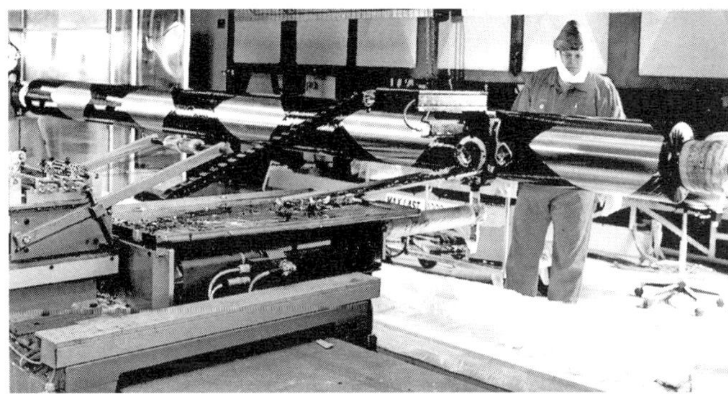

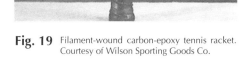

Fig. 18 Commercial roller filament-winding. Courtesy of Applied Composites AB, Celsius Group

Fig. 19 Filament-wound carbon-epoxy tennis racket. Courtesy of Wilson Sporting Goods Co.

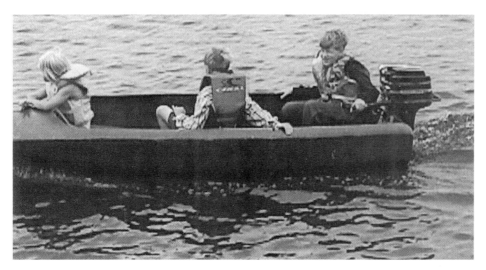

Fig. 20 Filament-wound car-top boat

the angle plies to avoid distortion of the laminate on cure and will probably have to be compacted by alternate means, depending on the thickness of the laminate. In either case, the manufacturing method is not representative of the actual part, and thus the properties are not representative.

To test a filament-wound structure, the general procedure has been to burst test a subscale bottle of the same laminate design and lay-up, because the bulk of filament-wound products have been pressure vessels. The raw materials can be tested as filaments, rings, and cylinders (Fig. 21). The filament or tow test results in somewhat higher values than those obtained by vessel testing. The ring-test specimen can also be cut up for short beam shear tests. These are for comparative shear values only and are not a true engineering shear. These shear values can be misleading with carbon/graphite fiber composites because of edge effects in a narrow ring and the nonuniformity of ply-to-ply strain. The ring tests are useful to develop ultimate tensile values, but not moduli. Three test methods have been adopted to evaluate unidirectional ply properties. These are transverse tension, compression, and in-plane shear. Table 4 shows these tests and a summary of the consensus standards for testing and evaluation of filament-wound components.

Design Guidelines (Ref 6)

The design process for any composite involves both laminate design and component design and must also include considerations of manufacturing process and eventual environmental exposure. These steps are all interdependent with composites, and the most efficient design must involve true concurrent engineering. These recommendations are directed towards the filament-winding design/manufacturing process. Other articles in this Volume address general design recommendations and those that relate to specific manufacturing methods.

Basic design guidelines include:

- Use the most appropriate fabrication method or methods for the part. Combine methods if necessary. Particularly for large structures, the relative cost of filament-winding is less than one-fourth that of hand lay-up and less than one-half that of tape laying.
- Choose the most appropriate starting material form. Use a wet resin, if appropriate and safe for the process, to further reduce the cost of manufacture.
- Consider fabrication requirements during preliminary design. Avoid designs that are technically elegant but cannot be built consistently or reliably.
- Design "net" parts. Reduce machining to a minimum. Try to incorporate composite-to-metal in situ joints in the winding process. *In situ* refers to a co-cured joint with possible failure-safe design. One joint technique (Ref 1) uses a reduced section to join a composite cylinder to an end fitting. The reduced section ensures that the joint is not totally dependent on the adhesive qualities of the bond and adds a measure of fail-safe performance because, without the adhesive, the components will remain joined. Whenever possible, co-cure adhesive-bonded assemblies and build in stiffeners.
- Take advantage of the flexibility of the filament-winding process. Ply thicknesses are not predetermined, as with unidirectional tape or woven fabric. They are a function, primarily, of the band width, the cross-sectional area of the filaments, the resin content, the filament count of the tow, and the number of tows. Some computer analysis programs, designed primarily for use with tape reinforcements, may only accommodate predetermined ply thicknesses in their included ply data tables. The user must know the techniques of circumventing these limitations or must use another analysis process.
- Select the simplest design to manufacture. If there is a hard choice between ease of analysis and ease of manufacture, choose the latter.
- Design for an entire composite structure rather than using composite as a substitute for a metal.
- Consider the possibilities of different fiber angles versus fabrication. If the design calls for very low angle helicals, but they would bridge or slip, consider absorbing a slight

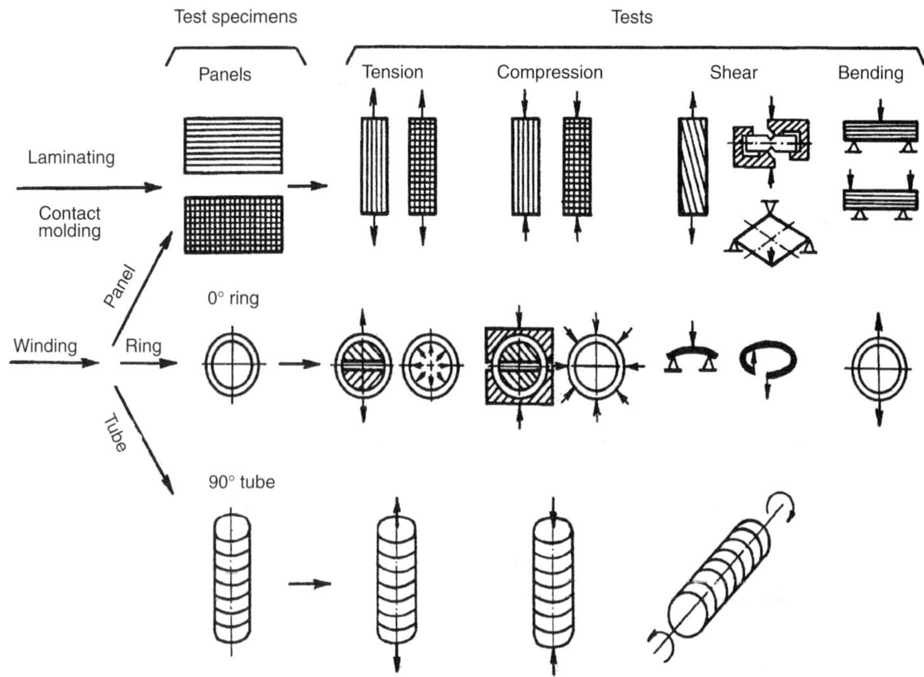

Fig. 21 Test specimens and test techniques for filament-wound composites. Source: Ref 5

weight penalty by designing with higher angle helicals to simplify fabrication.

Detailed design recommendations involve taking advantage of the orthotropic nature of the fiber composite ply:

- To carry in-plane tensile or compressive loads, align the fibers in the directions of these loads.
- For in-plane shear loads, align most fibers at ±45° to these shear loads.
- For combined normal and shear in-plane loading, provide multiple or intermediate ply angles for a combined load capability. Use resins that have the strain-to-failure values to match the fiber and fiber orientations and intra- and interlaminar forces. Intersperse the ply orientations. If a design requires a laminate with 16 plies at ±45°, 16 plies at 0°, and 16 plies at 90°, use the interspersed design $[90_2/\pm45_2/0_2]_{4S}$ rather than $[90_8/\pm45_8/0_8]_S$. Concentrating plies at nearly the same angle (0° and 90° in the previous example) provides the opportunity for large matrix cracks to form. These produce lower laminate allowables, probably because large cracks are more injurious to the fibers and more readily form delaminations than the finer cracks occurring in interspersed laminates. The preceding comments are true for most composite applications regardless of the fabrication method. Because of the (usually) axisymmetric nature of filament-winding, the resultant structure does not have to be symmetric with respect to the wall centerline unless more than one helical winding angle is used.
- Avoid extreme angle changes from ply to ply. It is recommended to step from 15° to 45° to 60° to 85° rather than directly from 15° to 85°.
- If a design requires all 0° plies, some 90° plies (and perhaps some off-angle plies) should be interspersed in the laminate to provide some biaxial strength and stability and to accommodate unplanned loads. This improves handling characteristics and serves to prevent large matrix cracks from forming. Use softening strips of lower-modulus fiber (such as cloth) at structure ends and in joints to reduce end stresses.
- Locally reinforce with fabric or mat in areas of concentrated loading. (This technique is used to locally reinforce pressure vessel domes.)
- Use fabric, particularly fiberglass or Kevlar, as a surface ply to restrict surface (handling) damage.
- Select the lay-up to avoid mismatch of properties of the laminate with those of the adjoining structures, or provide a shear/separator ply.
- Consider Poisson's ratio. If the transverse strain of a laminate greatly differs from that of adjoining structure, large interlaminar stresses are produced under load.
- Consider coefficient of thermal expansion. Temperature change can produce large interlaminar stresses if coefficient of thermal expansion of the laminate differs greatly from that of adjoining structure.
- The ply layer adjacent to most metal-to-composite bonded joints should not have fibers perpendicular to the direction of loading. Do not thicken the composite in the joint area. The essential stiffness (*EI*, where *E* is modulus of elasticity and *I* is moment of inertia) of all elements of the joint should not have abrupt changes. Glass fiber in carbon structures as well as various carbon fiber orientations can be used to achieve smooth transitions.
- Use multiple ply angles. Typical composite laminates are constructed from multiple unidirectional or fabric layers that are positioned at angular orientations in a specified stacking sequence. From many choices, experience suggests a rather narrow range of practical construction from which the final laminate configuration is usually selected. The multiple layers are usually oriented in at least two different angles, and possibly three or four (±θ°, 0°/±θ°, or 0°/±θ°/90° covers most applications, with θ between 30 and 60°). Unidirectional laminates are rarely used except when the basic composite material is only mildly orthotropic (e.g., certain metal-matrix applications), or when the load path is absolutely known or carefully oriented parallel to the reinforcement (e.g. stiffener caps, chain links and springs).

Table 4 ASTM standards for filament-wound composite mechanical properties

ASTM Designation	Title
Tensile properties	
D 5450	Transverse Tensile Properties of Hoop Wound Polymer Matrix Composite Cylinders
D 3039	Test Method for Tensile Properties of Fiber-Resin Composites
D 2585	Method for Preparation and Tension Testing of Filament-Wound Pressure Vessels (Discontinued 1996)
D 2290	Test Method for Apparent Tensile Strength of Ring or Tubular Plastics and Reinforced Plastics by Split Disk Method(a)
Compressive properties	
D 5449	Transverse Compressive Properties of Hoop-Wound Polymer Matrix Composite Cylinders
D 3410	Test Methods for Compressive Properties of Unidirectional or Crossply Fiber-Resin Composites
D 2586	Test Method for Hydrostatic Compressive Strength of Glass Reinforced Plastic Cylinders Transverse Compressive Properties of Hoop Wound Polymer Matrix Composite Cylinders (Discontinued 1996)
Shear properties	
D 5379	Shear Properties of Composite Materials by the V-Notched Beam Method
D 4255	Guide for Testing In-Plane Shear Properties of Composite Laminates(a)
D 2344	Test Method for Apparent Interlaminar Shear Strength of Parallel Fiber Composites by Short Beam Method

(a) Not in current ASTM catalog. Source: Ref 4

Fabrication Recommendations

This Section addresses the delivery and handling of the tow during filament-winding and was adapted from Ref 7. With only a small amount of attention and rudimentary engineering, carbon-graphite fiber tow can readily be spread evenly to its maximum width or any desired intermediate width. For a wet wound 12K tow, nominal width is about 3 mm (0.125 in.); for a 48 to 50K tow, it is 25 to 30 mm (1.00 to 1.25 in.). Good practice in fiber handling will result in wider band widths with resultant better control of layer thicknesses.

The tube package must be positioned horizontally, with the tube axis perpendicular to the direction of fiber feed. Fiber should never be pulled off the end because each revolution of feed introduces one twist. Twist is not acceptable for high-performance fibers because it decreases fiber volume and reduces some mechanical properties.

It is basically a matter of choice as to whether the fiber feed is taken from the top or bottom of the package unless a de-reeler is used to eliminate all tension. In that case it is better to have the fiber off the bottom to reduce the opportunity for material to slip off the package ends and become entangled on the support shaft. The dereeler uses slack for its operation and uses vertical side deflectors to eliminate end spill.

For guides, eyelets, and orifices that contact the tow:

- The bore diameter must not be less than 9 mm (0.375 in.).
- The entry and departure angles of the fiber through the guide should be minimized, never more than 20° from the normal. This prevents acute fiber abrasion.
- Ceramic guides are an excellent choice, but steel may be used (as in a "pigtail," for example) only if the guide is very well polished. Pigtail guides should not be of fine diameter and not used for carbon-graphite fiber. Pigtail guides allow the winder to move the fiber from one guide to the other without cutting fiber. Figure 22 shows some typical guides.
- Roller redirects, not guides or pigtails, should be used for prepreg. The best materials are Teflon (i.e., Du Pont de Nemours & Co., Inc., Wilmington, DE) or polyethylene (high-density polyethylene or ultrahigh molecular weight polyethylene). Radially grooved rollers of these materials have been found to be acceptable
- The first guide or pick-up point should be at least 400 mm (16 in.) from the package surface. If the guide is too close and a de-reeler is not used, the fiber scuffs laterally across the outer package surface, generally abrading and causing loose fiber. Additionally, if there are not vertical side restrictions, the first guide

should be on the horizontal centerline of the package to prevent fall-off of wraps at the edges and to minimize scuffing.

- Try to eliminate as many redirects (guides) as possible. The ideal fiber handling is zero touches between the creel to the wind eye, but this is generally impossible. The reason for reducing the number of redirects is that each redirect adds friction to the fiber with a multiplying effect. If fiber packages are tensioned, the control that should be exercised at the creel may not be possible.
- If the first guide from the package is shifted to either side of the centerline, the departure angle becomes more acute for material coming from the far end of the spool, which results in lateral slippage as it unwinds, scuffing the underlying fiber. This is especially prevalent with creel-tensioned fibers.
- Excessive tension, until the fibers have been wet with resin, should be avoided for a number of reasons. There is the possibility of increased self-abrasion over the roll surface and guides and possible breakage of the tow. The tow may imbed itself in underlying windings, producing a tangle that is unacceptable in a structure. Highest tension should be on the inner plies, with gradually decreased tension each ply until completion. This will prevent the outer plies from crimping the inner plies and making them ineffective in both tensile and compression loadings. The diameter or curvature of the product being wound and the winding angle determine the packing force normal to the surface; that is, use the lowest fiber tension that will assure straight fibers in the completed structure.
- If flat sheet is used as an orifice/guide plate, choices of materials should be limited to polytetrafluoroethylene (Teflon), high-density polyethylene, or nylon.
- The bore length of a guide is of little or no concern: It is the condition of the entry to the guide that determines success in handling.
- Carbon-graphite is a high modulus, and therefore a brittle and frangible material. There will always be some minor degree of fiber buildup at the guides and/or contact points. The essence of successful processing is what might be called "preventative housekeeping practices." In periods as short as 10 minutes elapsed processing time, any extraneous loose fiber buildup should be removed. If a small problem remains unattended, it will escalate very quickly into a serious problem, possibly resulting in tow breakage. Other fibers such as glass and aramid do not abrade or "fuzz up" as badly.
- Typically, loose fiber build-up problems are exacerbated with resin-wetted tow after it exits the resin bath, if tension is applied at the creel. Somewhat closer attention to "housekeeping" is demanded in this circumstance.
- Tube-packaged fiber is provided twist-free. However, "false twist" can occur. Typically, if the path length from the creel to the first process point is adequate (2.5 to 3 m, or 8 to 10 ft), especially with prepreg where false twist cannot be tolerated, the false twist will fall out.

Guidelines for spreading the fiber:

- Moving the fiber over a rolling surface does not increase spreading nearly as much as passing it over static surfaces. However, in either case, the surface should be polished to a surface roughness of 16 root mean square (rms) or better (comparable to drill rod stock, which may be used).
- The fiber bundle will assume a near-circular cross section 15 to 30 cm (6 to 12 in.) from band flattening. The distance shortens with tension. A wet fiber band should be deposited on the winding surface within a few inches of band forming.
- The lower the tension level on the tow, the wider the spread width will be. Ideally, only enough tension should be placed on the tow to prevent roving overruns when winding is stopped. For wet winding, a nonreversing mechanism on the impregnation roller or on the creel will prevent excessive spill problems with rewind tensioners when there are broken tows or lengthy reversals that drag the impregnated tow back over the roller.
- Diameters of static bars for band flattening should be no less than 12 mm (0.5 in.); 12 to 24 mm (0.5 to 1.0 in.) is a good working range. Usually, the larger the radius and the distance that the fiber passes over, the greater the spread of the fiber, although friction is increased.
- An "S" wrap, consisting of two static bars placed one over the other, is a very effective way to spread the fiber. The pair can be rotated as a unit to minimize or maximize the fiber contact or to provide tension in the fiber.
- The longer the fiber is in contact with the surface (residence time) on the static rods, the greater the spread width will be.
- Running speed has little or no effect on the spread width.
- The higher the back tension on the fiber, the more critical the sweep angle on unwinding becomes.
- If the package is mounted with a spring, washers, and nut arrangement (for tension control) on a shaft, the package should rotate in the direction that loosens the nut. (Otherwise, it will tighten the nut until the package is literally seized.)

Outlook

Technology. Filament-winding technology will shift to more dedicated equipment as the demand for more filament-wound products increases. Now, dedicated equipment is being used for filament-wound golf shafts, oil and water pipe, electrical fuses and interrupter tubes, commercial gas pressure vessels, chain links, transmission couplings, drive shafts and rotors, small spacers, and auto leaf springs.

Technology will be developed for maintaining the high structural strength values of the virgin fibers, such as carbon-graphite. For example, there will be increased use of de-reelers to eliminate tension at the creel, and tension will be applied only after fiber impregnation and will be controlled after band forming. New resin content sensors and controls will be developed.

The development will continue of apparatuses and processes to allow the dropping and starting of fibers in a wound structure (thereby allowing band widths and thicknesses to be changed).

Varying wall thickness and side-by-side fiber combinations can increase the number of products that can be economically wound, and will enable existing structures, such as bridge components, to use less material.

Prepreg tows and bands will become commercially available in thicknesses as small as 0.08 to 0.10 mm (0.003 to 0.004 in.). However, use of fibers this thin is not possible in wet winding. The very thin plies will increase the quantity of plies and strength of many structures. Many spacecraft structures use very thin plies for modulus-dominated quasi-isotropic structures.

Sensors and devices for controlling the resin content of wet-impregnated fibers will become more common. Use of these devices will reduce the resin waste and clean up now prevalent.

The use of wound material as a molding compound and as a primary bonded adjunct to filament-wound products is starting to be adopted for container corners and rotor bodies.

Applications. It is expected that filament-winding will be used increasingly to manufacture components in the following areas:

- *Transportation:* Railroad floor beams, door frames, pressure vessels, bus wheel wells (to prevent personnel injury from blown tires), over-the-road tankers for various liquids (in Europe and South America, not the United States), bridge beams, building columns

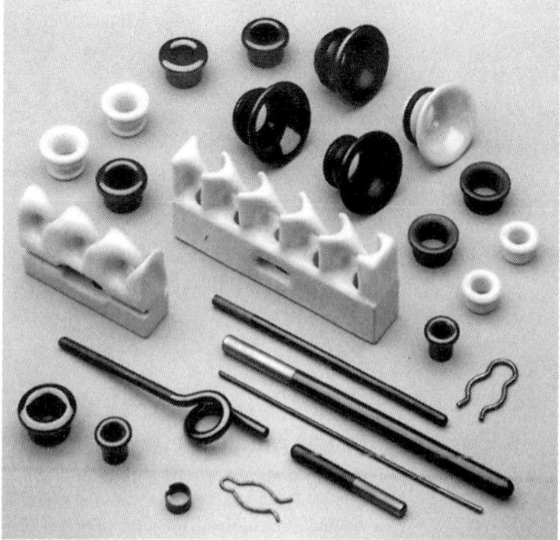

Fig. 22 Typical pigtail and ceramic guides. Courtesy of Texkimp, Ltd.

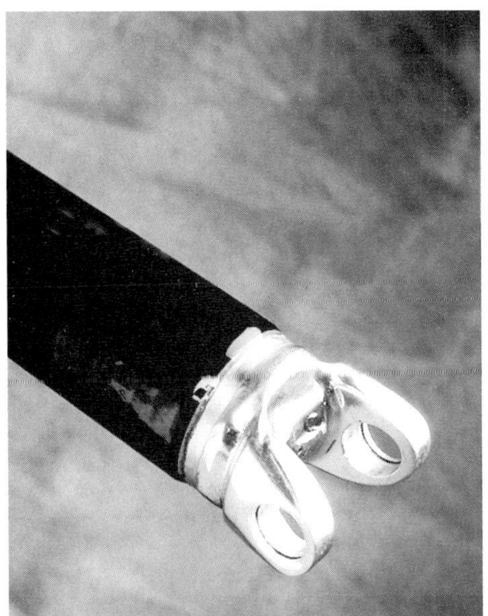

Fig. 23 Filament-wound composite driveshaft. Courtesy of ACPT

- *Springs.* In addition to leaf springs for autos and trucks, a spiral-wound spring is used for an aircraft door. Circular concave-wound disks are used in series as a shock absorber for glider landing gears.
- *Automobile Driveshafts:* When it was discovered that a composite driveshaft for an automotive application (the GMT-400 pickup truck) could be cost-competitive with its metallic counterpart, the effort was to find more applications on vehicles. Now many disparate vehicles, from garbage trucks to racecars, use filament-wound driveshafts (Fig. 23). In the future, these applications will transition more frequently to filament-winding, rather than other competing processes, because of the inherent cost-effectiveness of the process and because a more reliable joint technology exists for filament-wound shafts than for pultruded shafts.
- *NGV Tanks:* The trend has been to outfit more buses with the filament-wound tanks to comply with environmental restrictions. Automotive uses will increase greatly due to the recent qualification of type 2 cylinders (hoop-wrapped carbon-graphite fiber-epoxy over aluminum alloy 6061 high-pressure cylinders) for use in taxis and minivans. This is just the start of large-scale usage in automotive applications.
- *Automobile Flywheels:* As yet, the cost picture for employment of flywheels in automotive applications is not positive. More likely is the use of large composite flywheels for power plant storage of energy during off-peak hours. This concept is a great deal cheaper than building new power plants and would not encounter the environmental resistance that a new power plant would.

ACKNOWLEDGMENTS

Portions of this article have been adapted from two previous articles on filament-winding by W.D. Humphrey and S.T. Peters. The first appeared in *Composites,* Volume 1, *Engineered Materials Handbook*, ASM International, 1987, p 503–518. The second appeared in *Engineering Plastics,* Volume 2, *Engineered Materials Handbook,* ASM International, 1988, p 368–377.

REFERENCES

1. Peters et al. to Westinghouse, Method of Forming a Joint between a Tubular Composite and a Metal Ring, U.S. Patent 4,701,231
2. Larry J. Ashton, "Revisiting Cost Effective Filament-winding Technology," 44th International SAMPE Symposium (Long Beach, CA), May, 1999
3. Daniel N. Chappelar, Tak Aochi, and Robert J. Milligan, AD-A134577, Oct 1983
4. *Annual Book of ASTM Standards*, ASTM, West Conshohocken, PA
5. Yu. M. Tarnopol'skii and V.L. Kulakov in *Handbook of Composites*, 2nd ed., S.T. Peters, Ed., Chapman and Hall, London, 1998
6. S.T. Peters, W.D. Humphrey, and R.F. Foral, *Filament Winding, Composite Structure Fabrication,* SAMPE Publishers, Covina, CA, 1999
7. "Tips and Techniques for Handling Fortafil 50K Continuous Filament Carbon Fibers," Fortafil Fibers Inc., Salt Lake City, UT, 23 Feb 1996

SELECTED REFERENCES

- B.D. Agarwal and L.J. Broutman, *Analysis and Performance of Fiber Composites,* 2nd ed., Wiley Interscience, New York, 1990
- C. Harper, Ed., *Handbook of Plastics, Elastomers, and Composites,* 3rd ed., McGraw-Hill, New York, 1996
- P.K. Mallick, Ed., *Composites Engineering Handbook,* Marcel Dekker, New York, 1997
- S.T. Peters, Ed., *Handbook of Composites,* 2nd ed., Marcel Dekker, London, 1998
- S.T. Peters, W.D. Humphrey, and R.F. Foral, *Filament Winding: Composite Structure Fabrication,* 2nd ed., SAMPE, Covina, CA, 1999

Pultrusion

Joseph E. Sumerak, Creative Pultrusions Inc.
Jeffrey D. Martin, Martin Pultrusion Group

PULTRUSION is a cost-effective automated process for manufacturing continuous, constant cross-section composite profiles. Though developed in the early 1950s, pultrusion has gained a market and technical position of prominence in the 1980s and is now recognized as one of the most versatile of the composite production methods.

Pultrusion refers to both the final product and the process. Most simply, it refers to a method of manufacture wherein a collection of reinforcements saturated with reactive resin is pulled through a heated die that imparts the final geometry to the composite profile. In virtually every case, the continuous reinforcing fiber choices are integral to the processibility and the finished product properties. The resin matrix used is typically a liquid thermosetting resin, which reacts exothermically when heat is introduced to create a cross-linked polymer with exceptional engineering properties. The resulting thermoset composite profile cannot be reshaped or otherwise altered within its operating temperature range. In contrast, the extrusion of aluminum and thermoplastic materials generally involves unreinforced (homogeneous) materials that are heated and pushed through a die, then allowed to cool into the final solid shape. These materials may be reheated and reshaped numerous times with little loss of basic properties. Although a body of technology exists for thermoplastic pultrusion processing that enables post-pultrusion reshaping, it has not yet reached a position of commercial significance.

Despite the surge of commercial activity and study, there is still a significant amount of unpublished art in combining the continuous reinforcements and resins in a continuous operation that has kept the processor base small. During the 1980s, there was a dramatic increase in market acceptance, technology development, and pultrusion industry sophistication. In the 1990s, the number of technically competent personnel in pultrusion processing, materials supply, end use, and academia on a global basis has developed to the point where additional dramatic growth can occur. This coupled with increased awareness of the cost-competitive advantages of pultruded products and the availability of design standards and application specifications will enable pultruded composites to become a traditional material alongside steel, wood, and aluminum in the 21st century.

Technique Characteristics

Of the six basic elements in the pultrusion process, the three that precede the pultrusion machine are the reinforcement handling system (referred to as roving and mat creels), the resin impregnation station, and the material forming (or preforming) area. The pultrusion machine consists of component equipment that heats the input materials, cures the reactive resin, pulls the product through the die, and cuts the finished profile to a desired length.

The process begins when reinforcing fibers are pulled from a series of creels. The fibers are directed in a specific path through a resin bath, where they are impregnated with formulated resin. The resin-impregnated fibers are formed to the shape of the profile to be produced with excess resin being stripped from the fibers at this point. This consolidated material is then drawn into a heated steel die that has been precision-machined to the final shape of the part to be manufactured. The heated die initiates an exothermic reaction in the thermosetting resin matrix. The profile is continuously pulled and exits the mold as a hot, fully cured, constant cross-sectional area profile at a rate determined by the resin reactivity. Upon exiting the die, the profile cools in ambient or forced air, or is assisted by water spray, as it is continuously pulled by a mechanism that simultaneously clamps and pulls. The product emerges from the puller mechanism and is cut to the desired length by an automatic, flying cutoff saw. Either manual or automated part removal clears the product from the line for further value-added operations or for inspection and packaging. Very little additional cosmetic finishing is required for a properly processed pultruded profile.

Although pultrusion machines are available that can operate at rates that range from 25 mm/min to 5 m/min (1 in./min to 15 ft/min), typical production line speeds today are in the range of 0.6 to 1.5 m/min (2–5 ft/min). Higher effective output can readily be achieved by producing multiple streams (cavities) within one machine. Nearly 100% of the input raw materials exits the die as usable product. Pultrusion of high volume products can be executed with less than 2% raw material and finished product scrap.

Two general categories of pultruded products are: solid rod and bar stock produced from uniaxial reinforcements (0° orientation with respect to the machine direction), which deliver the highest axial tensile strength and stiffness, and structural profiles, which use a combination of uniaxial fibers and multidirectional fiber mats or fabrics to create a set of properties that meet the requirements of the application in the transverse (90°), off-axis (plus and minus angles other than 0 and 90°) and longitudinal (0°) directions.

More than 75% of all pultruded products are based on fiberglass reinforced polyester resin. When better corrosion resistance is required, vinyl ester resins are used and represent the next largest product segment. Both of these resin types are also available as flame-retardant versions. When a combination of superior mechanical and electrical properties is required, especially at elevated temperatures, epoxy resin is used. When applications require both high continuous-use temperature resistance and the highest mechanical properties, the use of epoxy resins reinforced with carbon or aramid fibers is the necessary option. Improved flame retardance, smoke suppression, and low toxicity can be achieved with selection of highly filled acrylic resin. The best overall flame, smoke, and toxicity performance coupled with high-temperature property retention is achieved with phenolic resin matrices. Toughness properties can be achieved with high elongation vinyl esters or thermoset polyurethane as well as with thermoplastic resins of various types. Each of the material selections has some processing expertise that must be well understood by the pultruder to make quality products.

Process Advantages

Pultruded composites exhibit all of the features found in products produced by other composite processes, such as high strength-to-weight ratio, corrosion resistance, electrical insulation, and dimensional stability. Additional advantages are derived from the process characteristics. One advantage is that the continuous nature of pultruded composites allows any transportable length to be produced. An example of such a product is the 1 to 3 mm (0.04–0.12 in.) diameter fiber-optic cable strength member rods that are pultruded in lengths of 2.2 km (1.4 miles) long and wound on a spool directly after the pultrusion gripper unit.

Another advantage is that complex, thin-wall shapes, such as those extruded in aluminum or polyvinyl chloride (PVC), are now possible because of recent process technology advances. Parts with multiple hollow sections can be produced using cantilevered steel mandrels and sophisticated forming guides. In addition to constant wall thickness profiles, which are always easier to pultrude, variable wall thickness in a constant cross section can be pultruded as well, providing a great deal of design flexibility. No other composite fabrication process can match the profile complexity possible with pultrusion.

Wire, wood, or foam inserts can be encapsulated on a continuous basis in pultruded products. In fact, any continuous feedstock may be encapsulated as long as sufficient bonding strength is present between the composite skin and the encapsulant in the application environment so as to prevent delamination.

A less obvious process advantage is the ability to use the widest variety of reinforcement types, forms, and styles with a broad selection of thermosetting resins and fillers. Virtually no other composite process offers as much materials versatility as pultrusion. Reinforcements can be placed precisely where they are needed for mechanical strength and consistency.

In addition, pultruded shapes can be made as large as required because equipment can be built in virtually any size. A corollary advantage of larger equipment is its ability to produce multiple cavities of the same or dissimilar profiles, which enables pultrusion to compete with traditional materials because of a relatively low resultant labor cost. Capital equipment costs of pultrusion and supporting equipment is low relative to aluminum or thermoplastic extrusion equipment. The cost of tooling for pultruded shapes is also low compared to other composite processes.

Applications

The versatility of the process has enabled pultrusions to penetrate such market areas as road and rail transportation, construction, infrastructure, marine, corrosion-resistant equipment, electrical/electronic, consumer, appliances/business equipment, aircraft, and specialty. With the newest forming technology, pultrusion can produce nearly any constant cross-sectional shape that can be extruded. Aluminum extrusions account for approximately 15% of all of the aluminum consumed, while pultrusions account for only 5% of all reinforced plastics produced; thus, pultrusion has much growth potential. However, pultrusions are rarely cost competitive based solely on shape replication since adjustments in strength factors usually require a wall thickness increase. There are several markets in which pultruded profiles have made a significant penetration that is not tied to just price competitiveness. Pultruded products are most successful when they provide corollary advantages that are not available with traditional competitive materials as previously described.

Two categories of pultruded shapes distinguish a processor's business focus. The first category, standard structural shapes, includes channels, tubes (round, square, and rectangular), I-beams, and wide-flange beams and solid bar stock that are produced for inventory in a variety of performance grades. Fabricators apply these standard shapes in designs for structures such as cooling towers, walkways, stairs and numerous other applications. A collection of standard structural shapes is shown in Fig. 1.

The second general category is custom profiles, where a pultruder assists the end user in designing a profile that suits a specific need and may be a consolidation of design functions replacing several parts or fabrication steps required with conventional materials. Custom shapes are generally not offered for sale to the general market because they are the proprietary property of the end user. A custom shape can also be a symmetrical geometry like a standard profile but may have special dimensions defined by the end user. Custom shapes are often nonsymmetrical and quite complex when the full potential for design consolidation is realized. Examples of custom pultruded profiles are shown in Fig. 2.

The highest-volume application of pultrusion at this time is the fabrication of nonconductive ladder rails for in-plant and communication and power utility use. The 1990s saw expansion of this product into the consumer market as well. Similarly, fiberglass tool handles, which were restricted to industrial use, now proliferate in retail outlets for garden and construction tools.

In highly corrosive environments, pultruded grating systems have become the standard because of their excellent mechanical properties and durability, replacing steel, aluminum, and even stainless steel systems. They are also used in elevated walkways and on steps where the supports are structural profiles, such as I-beams, channels, angles, and tubular shapes, that are often made to the same dimensions as steel or aluminum supports for ease of substitution of traditional materials. Cable trays of steel are being replaced by pultruded composite cable trays because of their superior corrosion resistance and better electrical insulation values. Corrosion-resistant fiberglass sucker rods have replaced steel in the extraction of oil.

Pultruded solid rectangular and square bars are being used in transformers, one of the oldest applications, to separate the windings and to permit air circulation. Utility market applications include guy strain insulators, standoff insulators, hot-line maintenance tools, and booms for electrical bucket trucks. Other electrical applications include high-voltage maintenance tool handles, bus bar insulator supports, fuse tubes, lighting poles, and cross-arms. Utility power poles up to 20 m (65 ft) in length are finding a competitive niche where traditional materials become cost prohibitive. High-voltage electrical power transmission towers as well as cellular communication towers are being introduced as low-maintenance designs for power companies. The digital communication revolution, which relies on high-speed fiber-optic cables for data transmission, also relies on pultruded cable tension members; the high tensile strength of these members ensures the strength of the cable and shields the fragile communication fibers from stress.

Dunnage bars that separate and isolate loads in trucks and railcars have been made from pultruded lineals for many years. The back doors that roll into the roof of the truck are also pultruded, as are the structural Z-sections between the inner and outer walls of a refrigerated truck trailer. Complete over-the-road trailers as well as rail cars have recently been produced using composite materials with a heavy content of pultruded profiles. One manufacturer has successfully tested a complete truck chassis as a pultruded beam fabrication with improved performance compared to steel.

Construction of residential and commercial buildings has successfully applied pultruded composite window and door framing, taking advantage of the superior thermal insulation, thermal expansion, and dimensional stability properties. Introduction of complete construction systems that include foam-filled or cellular paneling and functional connectors enable low-cost transport and assembly of structures for out-

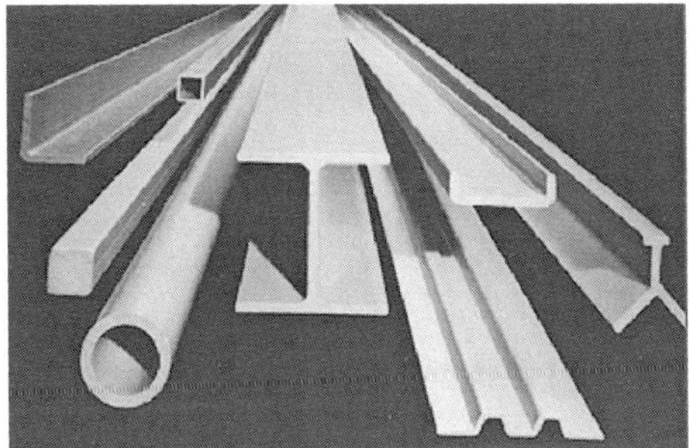

Fig. 1 Pultruded standard structural shapes. Courtesy of Creative Pultrusions, Inc.

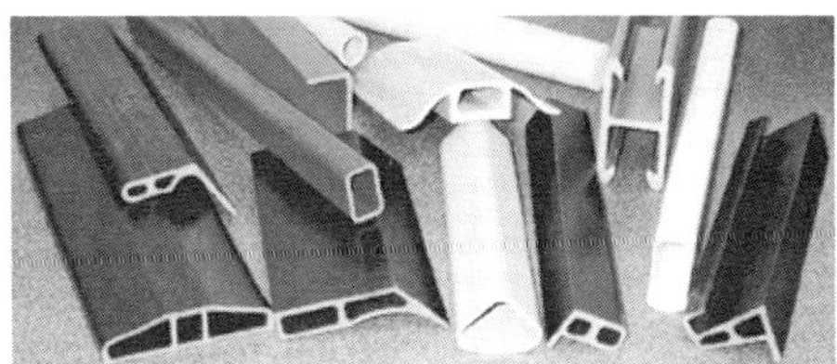

Fig. 2 Custom pultruded profiles. Courtesy of Creative Pultrusions, Inc.

buildings as well as low-cost emergency relief dwellings.

Flame-retardant pultruded composites have captured business in underground transit systems where low flame, smoke, and toxicity protect passengers in the event of fire. The Channel Tunnel, or Chunnel, project (connecting England and France under the English Channel) utilized a tremendous amount of pultruded product for electrical cable support systems and other structural applications. Offshore oil production platforms rely on flame-retardant phenolic pultruded gratings and structural shapes to provide corrosion resistance, structural function, and personnel protection.

In many buses, the luggage rack is pultruded. Hollow sections within the rack allow air to be passed for heating or cooling. Because of its continuous nature, the pultrusion process produces the rack in one piece to span the entire length of the bus. In another transit application, long lengths of electrically insulating coverboard are pultruded to cover the current-carrying third rail on rapid transit systems. Because of the design flexibility of composite profiles, the shape is designed to snap over the rail and yet support a load dropped from above or a railroad workman. On the highway, pultruded delineator posts that deflect without permanent deformation are now most often used instead of rigid rolled steel posts with plastic reflectors.

The recognition of the longevity potential of composites has opened vast new opportunities in the infrastructure market. Bridge decking to replace steel reinforced concrete is under intense study with many demonstration projects well into service-evaluation stages. Steel rebar is being challenged by composite rebar produced by hybrid pultrusion processes. Dowel bars that connect poured concrete slabs are also being tested as pultruded replacements for steel with much promise of greater durability. Highway guardrails are another very large potential where composites and specifically pultrusions are currently being evaluated. In all such applications, the higher initial cost of composites must be weighed against the life-cycle cost benefits afforded by the improved durability of the materials.

Key Technology Areas

There are three critical technology areas of equal importance: product composition, material forming, and control of process temperature.

Product Composition. Resin formulation and reinforcement selection determine composite properties that satisfy application needs. Reinforcements are selected to meet desired mechanical properties. The electrical insulation and the corrosion resistance of the composite are affected by the amount and type of reinforcement used. In many applications, compromise is required to meet all of the desired properties.

Pultrusion is a composite process that allows selective reinforcement of profile sections using different materials. This can be accomplished on a continuous basis with good consistency and repeatability. Base resin selection is important because the resin governs mechanical characteristics, operating temperature range, electrical insulation, corrosion resistance, and the flame and smoke properties of the profile. In addition, it governs process speed by its reactivity and can significantly control product aesthetics and tolerance capability. The resin matrix can be altered by chemical additives and fillers, which enhance its ability to handle higher temperatures; provide better electrical insulation, corrosion resistance, and dimensional stability; and lessen flame and smoke propagation. It is essential to the success of any pultruded profile that the polymer matrix be correctly engineered to meet the desired end-use properties and still provide those processing characteristics that are necessary to fulfill the economic goals of the application. This balance requires significant interaction between the end user and the pultruder.

Material Forming. The material-forming area usually comes after the reinforcements have been impregnated with resin. Reinforcements are precisely positioned using porcelain bushings, metal forms, or plastic guides that have been machined to allow axial and multidirectional reinforcements to pass from one to the next before entering the heated die. These guides, if properly designed, can ensure the consistent placement of the different reinforcement types. These forming guides can become very complex and interactive on large profiles and hollow sections. This necessitates engineering the reinforcements, their path, and their forming sequence. However, even with a fair understanding of materials, the techniques required to produce these forming systems can take years to develop. Even with experience, considerable on-line process engineering is required to fine-tune the material delivery and forming systems. This technology is fundamental to the consistency and optimization of mechanical properties and tolerances and is the most difficult aspect encountered by the beginning and novice pultruder.

Control of Process Temperature. With thermoset resins, it is important to control the rate and level at which heat is added to the matrix or removed from the profile. If too little heat is put into the die, the composite material will not reach its desired exotherm temperature, resulting in an incomplete cure and less than optimal properties in the finished profile. Too high a temperature can induce thermal stress cracking as the profile cools, resulting in a material that exhibits poor electrical insulation or corrosion-resistance properties.

The following discussion provides additional details of processing equipment and tooling, material composition, and process control essential for a basic understanding of the pultrusion process.

Process Equipment

The pultrusion process is depicted in Fig. 3. The basic elements of all pultrusion machines are very similar, but there are differences in the selection of heating components, power transmission, clamping devices, and cutoff saws. A full range of hardware as well as process control features are available from commercial machinery suppliers. These features designed from years of process insight help to bridge the gap between the art and experience of the established pultruders and the new companies entering the field. A pultruder must strive for a common denominator in establishing the processing system and its corresponding process control in a multimachine production facility.

Material In-Feed. Reinforcements are provided in packages designed for the best continuous runout of its material form. The continuous fiber creels are usually the first station on a process line. Continuous glass rovings are provided in center-pull packages that weigh 15 to 25 kg (33–55 lb) and are designed for a bookshelf-style creel. Creels of 100 or more packages are common and may be stationary or mobile. The glass roving is usually drawn from the package through a series of ceramic textile thread guides or drilled carding plates of steel or plastic. This allows them to be pulled to the front of the creel while maintaining alignment and minimizing fiber damage. Some creel designs allow multiple guide eyes (bushings) or guide bars to tailor the tension on each roving. The ease of servicing or replacing roving packages must be considered in selecting a creel design and package capacity since the process is never interrupted for material replacement.

While most center-pull rovings have a small twist useful for package formation, some fiberglass rovings are available as center-pull twistless; that is, the natural twist as a consequence of winding has been offset by a built-in reverse

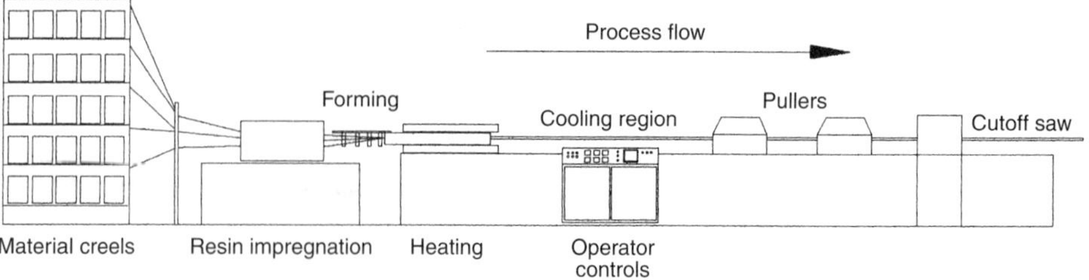

Fig. 3 Schematic of pultrusion process

twist. As an alternative, continuous fibers of glass, carbon, and organic polymers can also be supplied on packages with cardboard cores designed for outside payout to avoid twist. This style of package dictates the use of a multiple spindle creel design in which the packages are oriented horizontally. Ceramic bushings are again used to guide and protect fibers as they are delivered to the front of the creel. With this style creel, an additional consideration of package rotation and the resulting tension necessitates the use of a spindle bearing to provide uniform tension regardless of package size. Because packages in this configuration are usually smaller in diameter and weight, a greater number of packages may be found on such a creel design. It is not common to find both style creels used in the same facility due to the desire to standardize inventory and methods.

Directly after the roving creels is a creel designed to accommodate rolls of continuous strand mat, engineered fabric or surfacing veil. The roll materials are usually supplied in diameters between 305 and 610 mm (12 and 24 in.) with cores of 75 or 100 mm (3 or 4 in.) inside diameter. The creel must be able to accommodate both the size of the roll and the inside diameter of the core, along with appropriate spindle spacing and core bushings. The ability to lock the position of the roll in the desired lateral position will ensure consistent delivery of the material to the desired location in the profile. In many cases, it is also necessary to provide for the payout of web material in a vertical, rather than a horizontal, format. This requires independent roll stands with a vertical roll spindle and a roll support plate to support the material as the material pays off the roll.

As materials travel forward toward the impregnation area, it is necessary to control the alignment to prevent twisting, knotting, and damage to the reinforcements. This can be accomplished by using machined creel cards that have predefined specific locations for each material strand or ply. In some cases, these cards can be used for only one specific profile. An alternative approach uses a general-format creel card for roving and web locations that can be utilized and easily adapted for a variety of common profiles. While this is a less expensive approach, it requires more operator attention in order to confirm proper material input over the production period.

Resin Impregnation and Material Forming. The impregnation of reinforcements with liquid resin is basic to nearly every pultrusion process. The point at which resin is supplied and the manner in which it is delivered can take many different forms. A dip bath is most commonly used where fibers enter and exit a contained volume of resin with open top access only. With this design, fibers are passed over and under wet-out bars while immersed below the resin level, which causes the fiber bundles to spread and accept resin. This is suitable for products that are of an all-roving construction or for products that are easily formed from the resulting flat ply that exits the wet-out bath. In cases where it is impractical to dip materials into a bath, such as when vertical mats are required or hollow profiles are made, materials can pass directly into a "straight-through" resin bath. This design has entry-end and exit-end plates that have been machined for both passage and alignment of fibers as they pass through the resin. This alternative method provides the necessary impregnation without the need to move the reinforcements outside of their intended forming path. Since this type of bath has an open top as well as end plates that have a degree of resin leakage, a resin drip collection system and recirculation pump are necessary with this design. Due to recent attention to both industrial exposure limits to styrene for plant personnel as well as environmental volatile organic compound (VOC) emission regulations, emphasis has been placed on minimizing bath size, controlling airflow, and enclosing bath areas.

An alternative approach employing direct resin injection into the die is being used by many pultruders, but has substantial technical limitations regarding fiber permeability and maximum filler content as well as substantial hardware investment. This area of technology requires additional study before widespread use is possible.

Forming of reinforcing materials is usually accomplished directly after impregnation, although some initial steps can be carried out during the impregnation process as well. Forming guides are usually attached to the pultrusion die to ensure positive alignment of the formed materials with the die cavity. Forming is always accomplished progressively with consideration of continuous support for materials while maintaining operator accessibility for service. Sizing of the forming guide slots and holes and clearances between forming plates must be designed to prevent excess tension on the relatively weak and wet materials, but must allow for sufficient resin removal to prevent excessive hydraulic force at the die entrance.

In the case of tubular pultruded products, a mandrel support is necessary to extend the mandrel in a cantilevered fashion through the pultrusion die while securing it to resist the forward drag on the mandrel during processing. The mandrel support is typically attached to the die to achieve positive registration to the cavity and provide a platform for mounting forming guides. Materials must form sequentially around the mandrel in an alternating fashion to prevent weak areas due to ply overlap joints.

In the case of direct die injection, the reinforcements are formed dry and are fully compacted inside the die at the time of resin injection. Although this technique minimizes the problems associated with the wet bath systems, some limitations exist in the areas of wet-out, air entrapment, and maximum filler content. An alternative method pumps resin into a forming card prior to the die entrance and can be done at multiple forming stages to achieve better wet-out while minimizing exposed resin and the volume of resin committed to the process as compared to a bath system. A combination of techniques may be the answer for a specific profile, depending on its complexity, and each case requires special forming guide and impregnation consideration.

The materials commonly used for forming guides include fluoropolymers, ultrahigh molecular weight polyethylene, chrome-plated steel, and various sheet steel alloys. The pultrusion processor must employ a craftsman capable of converting sheet metal and plastic stock into forming guides with precise control to be most successful in processing complex shapes. Of all of the technologies employed by pultruders, the forming techniques and fabrication methods are perhaps the most proprietary and remain an unpublished art.

Die Heating. A number of different methods can be used to position and anchor the pultrusion die in the machine and to apply the heat necessary to initiate the reaction. The use of an open die bed with a yoke arrangement that allows the die to be fastened to the frame is the simplest arrangement. In all die-holding designs, the thrust that develops as material is pulled through the die must be transferred to the frame without allowing movement of the die or deflection of the frame. With this open-bed design, heating jackets that use hot oil or individual electrical resistance strip or plate heaters are positioned around the die at desired locations. Thermocouples are placed in the die to control the level of heat applied. Multiple individually controlled zones can be configured in this manner to achieve the greatest flexibility in heating design. This is the preferred method for complex nonsymmetrical profiles that have nonsymmetrical heating demands to achieve temperature uniformity around the cross section. This approach is well suited to single-cavity setups, but becomes more complex when the number of dies used simultaneously increases, since each die requires multiple heat sources and control thermocouple feedback provisions. To help alleviate this limitation, standardized wide heating jackets or wide heating plates can be designed to accommodate multiple dies.

Another popular die station design uses heated platens that have fixed zones of heating control with thermocouple feedback from within the platen rather than the die. The advantage of this method is that all dies can be heated uniformly with reduced-temperature cycling, because changes in temperature are detected early at the source of heat rather than at the load. In the same respect, however, a significant temperature drop will be common between the platen set point and the actual die temperature. Use of die monitor thermocouples identifies the differential and an appropriate controller set point can be established. When provided with the means to separate the platens automatically, the advantage of quick setup and replacement of dies can lead to increased productivity through reduced downtime with this heating design approach. A die mount height adjustment feature, found on many commercial open-bed and platen-based machines, allows the processor to exactly align the die centerline with the pulling mechanism to eliminate any product distortion associated with misalignment.

A source of cooling water or air is essential in the entry end of the die at start-up and during temporary shutdown periods to prevent premature gelation of the resin at the tapered or radiused die entrance. While the first section of the die is typically unheated to allow for some amount of natural cooling through convection, additional forced cooling is often applied by coring the die for fluid circulation, by using a detachable cooling jacket, or by utilizing the self-contained cooling zone within the heating platen. Such cooling is especially useful when high initial die temperatures are required, as with epoxy resins.

The most critical pultrusion process control parameter is the die-heating profile because it determines the rate of reaction, the position of reaction within the die, and the magnitude of the peak exotherm. Improperly cured materials will exhibit poor physical and mechanical properties, yet may appear visually identical to adequately cured products. Excess heat input may result in products with thermal cracks or crazes, which destroy the electrical, corrosion-resistance, and mechanical properties of the composite. Heat-sinking zones at the end of the die or auxiliary cooling may be necessary to remove exotherm heat prior to exit of the product from the die. The dynamics of the heat demands and reaction energy release have recently been modeled mathematically, empirically, and with the use of finite element analysis (FEA) methods, and graphical predictions of heat transfer balance can be used to guide the processor to optimal process conditions.

To increase process rates and to reduce temperature differentials between the die and the material that contribute to thermal cracking in large mass products, it is often desirable to preheat material before it enters the die. This may be accomplished by radio frequency, induction, or conventional conductive heating methods. Such heating devices are best applied as stand-alone devices that can be positioned before the die entrance when required.

The use of a process optimization instrument that allows tracking of external die temperature profiles and internal product temperatures as a function of die position during the curing process is highly desirable and a well-accepted test method. The data collected in a graphic format at a specific process speed represent a "snapshot" of steady-state process conditions that can be used for production troubleshooting, process engineering, and quality assurance documentation. There is a need for further process control developments of this nature that will provide improved process capability and production efficiency.

Clamping and Pulling Provisions. A physical separation of 3 m (10 ft) or more between the die exit and the pulling device is typically provided in order to allow the hot pultruded product to cool in the atmosphere or in a forced-water or air-cooling stream. This allows the product to develop adequate strength to resist the clamping forces required to grip the product and pull it through the die. The pulling mechanisms are varied in design among the hundreds of machines built by entrepreneurs or supplied by commercial machinery firms. Three general categories of pulling mechanisms that are used to distinguish pultrusion machines are the intermittent-pull single reciprocating clamp, continuous-pull dual reciprocating clamps, and continuous belt or cleated-chain puller.

The earliest pultrusion machines used a single clamp, which was hydraulically operated to grip the part between contoured pads. A carriage containing this clamping unit was then pulled by a continuous chain, which was driven by a variable-speed reversible drive train for a stroke of 3 to 4 m (10 to 13 ft). At the end of the stroke, the clamp released and the clamping carriage returned to its starting point. During this return interval, the product remained stationary until the clamping and pulling cycle could be reinitiated. Because of this pull-pause sequence, this style became known as an intermittent-pull machine. Variations of this design are still found in the industry, including multiple clamping heads for multiple-cavity production.

The continuous-pull reciprocating dual clamp machine has become the most popular style machine due to its versatility. Its alternating clamping, extension, and retraction cycles are synchronized between two pullers to provide a continuous pulling motion to the product. The value of using the intermittent-pull cycle with slow-cure materials or for purging die buildups is reflected in the fact that commercial reciprocating clamp machines also have selectable intermittent-pull sequences. Subtle variations exist in the use of different drive methods, such as direct-acting hydraulic cylinders, hydraulic motor driven chain drives or electrically powered recirculating mechanical ball screws. Methods of clamping can be hydraulic, pneumatic, or a mechanical wedge action. The basic prerequisite is that sufficient clamping pressure be available on the contoured puller block that is held within the clamping envelope. The longer the clamping unit, the lower the unit pressure on the pultrusion required to prevent slippage. Clamping units are available with lengths of 300 to 900 mm (12–36 in.). In addition, sufficient thrust must be provided to the clamping unit to overcome the pulling resistance and to maintain a uniform pulling speed. An advantage of the reciprocating clamp system is its need for only two matched puller pads to maintain a continuous pulling motion. These pads are easily changed and are generally fabricated of durable polyurethane for long life and mar resistance and are mounted on steel or aluminum bases.

Continuous-belt pullers have evolved from thermoplastic extrusion take-off pullers, but have been modified for higher pulling loads of pultrusion. These pullers are suitable for single-cavity or multiple-cavity production when all profiles are of the same physical size. Even with this restriction, uneven belt wear can result in slippage of adjacent cavities. As an advantage, the contact area of the belted puller is generally longer than that found with the reciprocating clamp pullers, which allows lower unit pressures on the pultrusion. A more flexible version of the continuous-belt machine is the cleated-chain (or caterpillar) puller, which has many individually contoured puller pads attached to chain ears along the chain length. This modification allows the production of complex shapes and multiple cavities by providing the necessary contoured pads. The number of individually contoured puller pads can vary widely, depending on the complexity of the part and the machine design. However, it is not uncommon to have several hundred contoured pads on a machine of this type, which makes the initial cost as well as the production setup time and cost substantial.

The space available within the gripper unit that determines the maximum possible size of profile is referred to as the machine envelope. Standard pultrusion equipment is available with production envelope sizes of 200 mm (8 in.) wide by 100 mm (4 in.) high to 1270 mm (50 in.) wide by 380 mm (15 in.) high. However, several machines have already been placed in production that can produce parts up to 2540 mm (100 in.) wide. More than 90% of all profiles can be produced on machines that have envelopes 760 mm (30 in.) wide and 305 mm (12 in.) high. Larger machines must have more power to pull the raw materials through the process. Power is especially important when the resin matrix begins its gel transition to final curing and the resultant part shrinkage occurs. The larger the surface area of the part and the lower the volumetric shrinkage, the more power is needed in the equipment. Standard pulling forces are in the range of 49 to 147 kN (5.5–17 tonf), but some machines are capable of up to 441 kN (50 tonf) of power.

One of the limitations to shape size within a given machine envelope is related to the forming area upstream of the die. When forming the raw materials for hollow shapes and especially for multicell hollow shapes, the size of the forming area is quite large. As wall thickness increases, this problem intensifies because there is more mat and roving material to deal with. The result is that the creel space width requirement at times may be far wider than the basic machine, limiting the machine product size capacity.

Cutoff Station. Every continuous pultrusion line requires a means of cutting product to length. Many systems employ radial arm or pivot saws on a table that moves downstream with the product flow and are activated manually when a length-limit switch activates a cutoff alarm. More sophisticated automatic cutoff saws are found on commercial machines, eliminating the need for operator attention. Both dry-cut and wet-cut saws are available, but regardless of design, a continuous-grit carbide or diamond-edged blade is used to cut pultruded products. Aramid-reinforced products present a special cutoff problem because of the toughness of the fiber. The use of conventional blades results in jagged edges and delamination. While water-jet cutting is satisfactory, a suitable cost-effective alternative is still being sought for these composites.

Process Tooling

Pultrusion tooling has two areas of consideration that are distinct, yet inseparable:

- The primary die, which is the precision-machined component that yields the final profile dimensions
- The devices required to align and form the input materials prior to entering the die as well as those required to clamp and draw the product through the die and to align the product during cutoff

All of the elements needed to produce a specific profile in addition to the primary die are referred to as secondary tooling items.

Primary Tooling. The pultrusion die is typically made from tool steel that can be purchased in an annealed condition or prehardened to 30 HRC. Pultrusion dies are usually multiple pieces that are machined and bolted together to form the desired profile cavity. Die pieces must be squared, rough machined, and then stress relieved to form the approximate cavity size. Each die component is then ground on a linear profile grinder to the finished dimension, with an as-ground finish of 0.50 to 0.65 μm. The die components are then aligned to form the finished cavity, and the pieces are doweled for positive parallel alignment within 0.025 mm (0.001 in.). Alternatively, an integral alignment groove can be provided along the length of the die near the parting line for a separate or integral key. The pieces are then drilled and tapped for bolts that are used to hold the die together against the internal pressure developed during processing.

After positive alignment and fastening, the exterior of the die is again ground flat. The die entrances are tapered or radiused to relieve pressures on the material as it enters the die and to decrease wear associated with fiber compaction at the entrance. The cavity surfaces are then polished to a 0.25 μm finish with buffing wheels and polishing compounds. The polished die is then plated with hard chrome to 0.025 to 0.038 mm (0.001–0.0015 in.) at 68 to 72 HRC hardness. Depending on profile complexity, additional grinding may be desirable after chrome plating on both the parting lines and the cavity.

An alternative to the softer steels described previously is the use of air- or oil-hardened steel, which can be heat treated to provide a 60 HRC hardness and does not require chromium plating if noncorrosive resin systems are processed. With resins of acidic pH, hard chrome may still be desirable on top of the hardened substrate to provide corrosion resistance, lubricity, and release characteristics. Also, with these steels, an allowance must be made for distortion upon heat treating prior to finish grinding. It is more difficult to modify a hardened tool after heat treating if additional tapped holes or grinding is required. The hardened tool is more prone to fracture at areas of stress or impact damage. The softer steel dies provide a tougher substrate resistant to brittle fracture and easily repaired. If chrome is the primary means of wear resistance, chrome-plated dies must be inspected frequently for complete surface coverage, because wear will proceed rapidly on the softer substrate steel once the chrome is removed.

It is difficult to predict die life, but a production quantity of 15,000 to 30,000 m (50,000–100,000 ft) is not uncommon for chrome-plated dies, which may be replated as necessary to extend their service lives. An equivalent or superior service life can be expected with hardened steel dies without chrome (if their design minimizes stress cracking and corrosion). Case hardening, ion implantation, and ceramic-base die alternatives have all been used with some success in an attempt to improve die life. Die lengths typically range from 610 to 1525 mm (24–60 in.), depending on the size, complexity, and tolerances required as well as the sensitivity to initial tooling cost, which increases rapidly for the longer die lengths.

Secondary Tooling. Forming technology is an art that develops over years of experience and is the most guarded area of processing technology. Improper execution will cause problems with chipping, cracking, poor reinforcement distribution, and frequent breakouts, all of which make continuous, economical processing very difficult. Properly executed, the constant, controlled delivery of material will in turn ensure reproducible quality and profitable production.

Various methods are used, such as step-sequence forms that are machined into steel or plastic plates that gradually collimate, align, and form the input materials. Continuous sheet metal forms can be used as an alternative or in conjunction with forming plates. Individual location guide eyelets and forming rods, tubes, or blades help to guide fiber to areas that are difficult to fill by other means. The guides that are used within the resin pan and on the creels are also considered part of secondary tooling if they are designed specifically for one profile. Although it is relatively easy to find a toolmaker who can manufacture a precision-machined pultrusion die, it is nearly impossible to find one with a pultrusion process insight that allows him to develop secondary tooling. Consequently, the design of secondary tooling is based on process experience with many forming system optimization trials, and fabrication is most often executed by the pultruder.

Clamping devices depend on the style of puller used. The continuous-belt cleat-style puller requires numerous custom urethane pads to conform to a complex profile. Reciprocating clamp-style pullers also require contoured puller blocks, but only for two clamping units. In either case, the design of clamping pads is such that adequate pressure can be applied to the product surface without cracking the profile. Consideration of shrinkage, angularity, and heat dissipation is often necessary in designing the clamping hardware.

Fixtures must also be provided at the cutoff saw to allow clamping before and after the blade to produce a quality cut. Insufficient guiding in this area can result in poor tolerances related to length and squareness as well as gouges caused by part movement relative to the blade.

Materials

One of the greatest advantages of the pultrusion process is that a wide range of materials can be used to provide a broad spectrum of composite properties. Given a specific profile geometry, the design engineer has a virtually unlimited supply of material options from which to construct a composite. The engineer must consider the intended function of the finished product, as well as the effects of temperature, atmosphere, environment, and time. Every selection, of course, carries an economic impact, and the optimal cost/performance options can be derived only with a proper understanding of the needs of the application and the available raw materials.

A composite is, by definition, a combination of reinforcement surrounded by a stress-transferring medium, or matrix, that allows the development of the full properties of the reinforcing fibers. The level of properties developed within a volume can be described approximately by the rule of mixtures, which, simply stated, predicts the resultant properties displayed in any direction to be proportional to the volume fraction of fibers aligned in that direction. Factors that influence composite property development include:

- The type of reinforcement fiber and its ultimate strength capability
- The form and style of reinforcement as it pertains to orientation of fibers
- The proportion of the selected reinforcement relative to the whole volume

In pultrusion, great versatility is possible with all three of these factors.

Reinforcement Types. The most widely used reinforcement has been and will continue to be glass fibers, because of ready availability and low cost. Electrical grade E-glass fibers are most commonly used, exhibiting a fiber tensile strength of approximately 3450 MPa (500 ksi) and a tensile modulus of 72 GPa (10.5×10^6 psi), but have relatively low elongation. Elongation of glass bundles ranges from 1.5 to 2%, while that of single strand is 3%. These properties of glass fiber result in composites with high strength and low elongation, with virtually no yield up to ultimate failure, which is by brittle fracture. A variety of fiber diameters and yields are available for specific applications. Recently, boron-free glass compositions have been developed for superior electrical and corrosion properties. A-glass compositions are also used, though primarily in continuous strand mat form. Higher tensile strengths can be achieved with S-glass fibers, which were developed for high-performance applications. These fibers exhibit a tensile strength of 4600 MPa (665 ksi) and a tensile modulus of 86 GPa (12.5 × 10^6 psi). Glass fiber surface sizing chemistry has been developed over many years to provide optimal wet-out and chemical bonding between the fibers and matrix resins, thus ensuring maximum strength development and retention.

Far greater stiffness can be achieved by using carbon fibers when their conductive nature would not be detrimental to the application. Carbon fibers are produced from a process of continuous graphitizing and stretching of a textile thread, such as polyacrylonitrile (PAN). The resultant fiber exhibits tensile strength from 2070 to 5500 MPa (300–800 ksi) and tensile modulus from 206 to 690 GPa (30–100 × 10^6 psi) with elongation of 0.5 to 1.5%. Normally, if high tensile strength is chosen, a lower tensile modulus must be accepted, and conversely. In addition to the mechanical properties cited, these fibers deliver unique properties, such as electrical conductivity, slightly negative thermal coefficient of expansion, high lubricity, and low specific gravity (1.8 versus 2.55 for E-glass). The price of carbon fibers is often the only limitation to their widespread use; however, recent advances in technology and production volume have dramatically reduced the price of commodity fibers (210 GPa modulus) to a reasonable level for many commercial applications. Carbon fibers do present some processing challenges as well, which limits the number of pultruders participating in this market segment.

High-modulus organic fibers, such as aramid fiber, are an attractive option for providing high tensile strength and modulus of 2750 MPa (400 ksi) and up to 131 GPa (19 × 10^6 psi), respectively, with elongation of up to 4%. The use of this fiber results in very tough composites that exhibit good flexural and impact strengths, which are well suited to ballistic applications and wherever energy absorption is necessary. The low specific gravity (1.45) of these fibers gives them one of the highest strength-to-weight ratios of any reinforcement available. Deficiencies in compressive strength and interlaminar shear strength are being addressed through improved surface chemistry and fiber treatment.

Other organic fibers have recently become available for use in pultrusion. Heat-stabilized and oriented polyester and nylon fibers with appropriate binders have been used as a replacement for glass in applications that would benefit from increased toughness and impact resistance, but where tensile and flexural strengths can be sacrificed. These fibers provide a low-modulus capability to composites, thus bridging the gap between thermoplastics and glass reinforced thermosets. With low specific gravity and only a moderate cost premium over glass, these fibers are well suited for certain commercial and industrial applications. A highly oriented polyethylene fiber geared toward higher specific strengths (high properties with low specific gravity) can also compete with the aramids in applications requiring stiffness, toughness, and light weight. All of the synthetic fibers have a lower use temperature capability than the inorganic fiber forms.

Reinforcement Styles. Once the fiber type has been selected, the next most important consideration is the ability to orient the fiber in the desired direction to utilize its properties most advantageously. A common denominator for all materials used in pultrusion is that they must be available in a continuous form to provide reasonably long payout lengths without defects, splices, or changes in cross-sectional volume.

The most common and lowest-cost form of continuous reinforcement is roving, which consists of continuous axial filaments in single and multiple-strand configurations. Glass rovings are designated by their yield, which is defined by the number of yards per pound of material or by the international designation, TEX, in grams per 1000 m. The two most commonly used yields are 4400 TEX (113 yd/lb) and 8800 TEX (56 yd/lb), the latter of which is the larger size tow of the two products. The rovings are typically supplied in 18 kg (40 lb) hollow cylindrical packages with a center payout that allows them to be stacked on a multiple-shelf (bookshelf) creel configuration. A similar package is available for the organic fibers previously described. Carbon fiber rovings, however, are provided in sizes designated by the number of filaments per tow, with the most common being 3K, 6K, and 12K, with K equal to 1000 filaments. The carbon tow areas are considerably smaller than the glass roving tow, and the package weights are 0.9 to 2.3 kg (2–5 lb), with an outside payout designed for a spindle-style creel system. This difference in material form, although of no consequence in the end product, does present some limitations to the processor with regard to creel style and capacity, splicing frequency, and product size limitations. Recently, larger tow options of 24K, 40K, 160K, and 320K, as well as assembled unidirectional webs held together with scrim or adhesive, reduce the creel limitations, allowing much larger parts to be manufactured.

The roving form allows maximum packing of fibers within a volume to yield the highest possible properties along the product axis, referred to as the longitudinal or machine direction. Maximum axial property development may be diminished by such factors as incomplete wet-out, improper fiber alignment, fiber damage due to creel or forming fixtures, and catenary (uneven fiber-to-fiber tension resulting in loops or nonparallel strands). Given near-perfect alignment, fiber fractions of 65 vol% are achieved (80 wt% for glass fibers). In such a product, there are no fibers oriented in the transverse direction (90° to the longitudinal axis), and the strengths exhibited by the composite in this direction reflect the strength of the matrix resin only.

To overcome this transverse strength deficiency, reinforcing fibers aligned in the transverse direction must be provided. Continuous-strand mat, which has fibers oriented randomly in all directions, is most commonly used to provide some level of transverse properties. These fibers are held together with a thermoset resin binder, which allows the mat to have sufficient tensile strength for processing.

Several mat styles can be used, but the most common is an E-glass mat that has fairly coarse fibers in an open or porous construction yet provides high overall structural efficiency. This mat is used on exterior surfaces and as a center ply to build a laminate with substantially improved transverse physical properties. The porous construction, however, results in a potential for composite surface porosity and provides a very noticeable fiber pattern on the finished product due to shrinkage of the large resin domains. When this is unacceptable, a fine-filament A-glass mat (or veil) is used as surfacing ply to bring more resin to the surface and to achieve a dense, aesthetic surface appearance. Recent strength improvements in fine-filament A-glass mats have allowed their use throughout the composite. Regardless of mat style, the processor depends on the mat manufacturer to provide control over fiber distribution, binder content and distribution, and defects that may have a serious impact on processing efficiency.

Random-fiber mats are generally used in weights of 150 to 600 g/m^2 (0.5 to 2.0 oz/ft^2). To accommodate the volume required by this lower bulk density type of reinforcement, it is necessary to remove fibers from the longitudinal direction. The resultant composite will have a slightly lower overall fiber content by volume because more resin is consumed to fill the open-structure mat described. As a result, the resultant increase in transverse and off-axis strengths is accompanied by a decrease in longitudinal properties. It is here that the engineer can exercise control over fiber proportions to achieve the properties necessary for the specific application. One restriction dictated by the nature of composites is the need to provide a symmetrical composite ply structure relative to the centerline of the thickness. This practice will prevent dimensional problems resulting from differential shrinkage of the plies of different reinforcement forms and styles.

Within the limits of design, glass mat and roving based pultrusions are the most common structural compositions, with typically 50 wt% fiber. By exercising control of the relative proportions, and the use of inorganic fillers, the overall fiber weight content can be varied between 40 and 80%. Mat construction is also available with carbon fibers having a fine-filament construction. Other mat-type products are produced by paper processing methods and can incorporate a variety of filament types for tailored properties.

Although the random-fiber orientation of a mat provides fiber orientation in all directions, a specific volume of fibers can be oriented transverse to the axis by means of biaxial fabric reinforcement. The traditional material used had been woven roving; however, problems associated with weave stability, wet-out, and ply edge fiber retention limited the effectiveness of this material in pultrusion. In addition, woven materials do not provide optimal properties due to fiber kink stresses during loading. The introduction of nonwoven biaxial fabrics employing fibers stitched or knitted together at the interstices has provided an effective solution to the problems mentioned above. The stitched fabrics can be supplied with any proportion of longitudinal-to-transverse orientation—even to the point of having a 100% transverse fiber continuous ply with only longitudinal stitch fibers. These materials are available from a large number of suppliers employing various techniques to ensure fiber directional stability, ply integrity, and thickness and weight control.

The biaxial fabrics are generally introduced as internal plies and used in conjunction with a mat as exterior plies. Although not impossible to apply, the use of these materials as exterior plies is somewhat limited because of the tendency for the transverse fibers to be distorted by friction at the die surface. This can be resolved to an extent by stitching a continuous strand mat to the biaxial fabric to create a stabilized three-ply fiber form referred to as a "complex" material. Multiaxis fabrics typically employing 0°, 90°, and ±45° orientations have also become available and provide additional direction strength as well as an improved level of fabric stability. Double-bias fabrics of ±45° without some amount of longitudinal fiber orientation for pulling strength and stability are impractical for pultrusion unless used strictly as an interior ply. Additional problems of splicing and fabric skewing make the use of these material forms more of a challenge to the pultruder.

In all of these multidirectional fabric styles, the supplier has the versatility of using every fiber type previously described (glass, carbon, or synthetic) in any or all of the directions possible or in an alternating fashion to provide hybrid composites with tailored properties. The challenge to the pultrusion design engineer becomes the identification of the most cost-effective style of reinforcement to use in an application not satisfied by the conventional mat/roving construction.

Because of the tendency toward ultraviolet degradation of the resin on surfaces of composites used outdoors, a condition known as fiber bloom will occur over time. This term refers to the exposure of fibers at the surface, which can be an irritant to human contact as well as an aesthetic detraction. To resolve this problem, surfacing fabrics of organic fiber composition, primarily polyester and nylon, are being used. The surfacing fabrics are available in a variety of weights and constructions and provide a corollary advantage of contributing to the impact strength and toughness of the composite. They also help the processor from the standpoint of providing a tough material to assist in carrying materials through the die while also protecting the die wall from the abrasive glass. The ability to provide a smooth resin-rich surface appearance without fiber patterns and the ability to be screen or roll printed with company logos, information, or wood grains make this surfacing material option an important element in many pultrusion composite designs.

Matrix Resins. Although the fiber type, form, and style determine the ultimate mechanical strength potential, the matrix resin determines the actual level of properties realized through effective coupling and stress transfer efficiency. There are composite properties, however, that are determined exclusively by the properties of the matrix resin. Among these are high-temperature performance, corrosion resistance, dielectric properties, flammability, and thermal conductivity. Selection of the resin, as well as formulation chemistry, becomes an important consideration that must be addressed very early in the design process.

Unsaturated polyester resins are most commonly used in pultrusion. Orthophthalic, isophthalic, and terephthalic acids or anhydrides, in combination with maleic anhydride and various glycols, are the basic backbone ingredients of polyester resins. The isophthalic polyester has dominated the supply by virtue of its well-rounded physical properties and economics. By adjusting the ratio of backbone chemical units, a variety of strength and elongation characteristics, as well as reactivity levels, can be achieved. A necessary characteristic of a pultrusion polyester is the ability to gel and cure rapidly to form the strong gel structure needed for adequate release at the die wall. Styrene monomer serves as a resin diluent and a reactive cross-linking agent necessary to form a thermoset polymer. Viscosities of 0.5 Pa · s (500 cP) are typical for highly diluted resins, or higher-viscosity, low-monomer versions can be blended at a later time with additional styrene to suit the processing need. The styrene level must be properly chosen to achieve good cross-link structure without leaving residual (unreacted) styrene in the finished composite. The final structure of the fully cured polyester resin is thermoset, resulting in the associated stability of the finished product to many adverse conditions.

Polyester resin properties differ based on their backbone compositions; the following generalizations can be made:

- Polyester resins exhibit good corrosion resistance to environments of aliphatic hydrocarbons, water, salts, and dilute acids and bases. They do not perform well when exposed to aromatic hydrocarbons and some concentrated acids. Corrosion-resistance guides provided by the resin supplier should be consulted for information on suitability to a specific chemical exposure.
- Because of the high unsaturation of the polyester chain and the resultant high cross-link density, polyesters exhibit volumetric shrinkage of up to 7%. This level can be reduced by using fillers and low-profile (thermoplastic) additives, which also help to control microcrack development and shrinkage-related sink marks.
- Polyester resins have glass transition temperatures ranging from 80 to 120 °C (175–250 °F). Exceeding this temperature threshold is accompanied by a rapid reduction in mechanical properties because of molecular chain movement. The actual continuous-use temperature must be defined in the context of the desired performance characteristics. Composites based on polyesters, for example, can be approved for continuous use at 150, 180, and even 200 °C (300, 355, and 390 °F) while retaining a high percentage of their electrical insulation properties, even though their ability to support mechanical stress decreases rapidly above the glass transition temperature. Chemical decomposition of polyesters will begin to occur at temperatures above 300 °C (570 °F).
- Polyester resins can be brittle or tough, depending on the backbone chemistry and the cross-link density. However, maximum elongation is in the 5% range; therefore, impact properties will depend greatly on fiber orientation, fiber type, and impact-modifying additives.
- Polyesters will support combustion without modification. Through the use of additives or molecular backbone bromination, the flammability and smoke-generation properties of polyesters can be greatly improved in order to satisfy many flammability codes.
- The electrical properties of polyesters make them suitable for use as primary insulators in many high-voltage applications. Secondary insulation applications abound for polyester-base composites. Retention of electrical properties at elevated temperatures has made polyester insulators the cost-effective material of choice in many applications.
- The weatherability of polyesters is fair to good, depending again on molecular backbone composition. Additional weatherability protection is usually sought through a variety of ultraviolet absorption additives, the use of polyester surface veils, and weather-resistant paints, such as polyurethane, applied in-line or as a secondary processing step.

Vinyl Ester Resins. When additional performance is required in the areas of corrosion resistance and elevated-temperature mechanical properties, vinyl esters are available as an alternative to polyesters. The chemical structure of vinyl ester resins is such that the reaction sites are at the end of each polymer chain rather than along the chain length, as with polyesters. This structure results in a thermoset resin that has a lower cross-link density and exhibits greater toughness properties, such as interlaminar shear and impact strength. In addition, there are fewer sites available for chemical decomposition along the vinyl ester molecule. The use of rigid molecular segments (like bisphenol A epoxy) along the polymer backbone results in the high-temperature capability of these materials.

In addition to being approximately 75 to 100% more expensive than polyesters, an added cost due to lower process speed is characteristic of vinyl esters used in pultrusion. This results from the slower reaction rate associated with its lower cross-link density. In every other respect, the processing of vinyl esters is very similar to that of polyester. Both resins require high-temperature initiation of catalysts to begin the reaction. The room-temperature pot life of these resins is usually 24 to 72 h.

Epoxy resins are used when physical properties of the highest level, as well as elevated-temperature property retention, are required, which is often the case in military and aerospace applications. Although they have increased continuous-use temperatures to about 150 °C (300 °F), composites made with epoxy resin are known for the poor toughness caused by their rigid structure. Much of this deficiency can be overcome with proper selection of reinforcements to provide impact strength. Epoxy resins do provide increased flexural strengths and interlaminar shear strengths greater than polyester and vinyl ester systems. In addition, their excellent electrical properties and corrosion-resistance also qualifies them for use in many commercial and industrial applications requiring superior performance.

Epoxy resins are expensive materials in a number of respects. The resins are three to six times more costly than polyesters and have a number of process-related costs not found with polyesters. Because they are cured by a stepwise reaction rather than an addition reaction, as with polyester resins, their reaction rate is very slow. The gelation of epoxy resins occurs at a later stage of reaction, and it is critical that the exotherm developed be contained within the die to avoid cracking. This dictates a slow process rate, which results in a higher labor and burden allocation to the product being produced. Unlike polyesters or vinyl esters, epoxy resin begins to react slowly as soon as it is mixed, resulting in a pot life measured in hours rather than days as viscosity begins to increase. The resin scrap rate is potentially higher if viscosity buildup affects wet-out to the extent that the bath must be recharged. The die temperature profiles used for epoxy are typically hotter than for polyesters in order to achieve reasonable pultrusion rates, and the resulting hot resin drip-off at the die entrance must often be discarded rather than recirculated to the resin bath to avoid bath gelation. Because of the tendency for the epoxy resin to bond strongly to the die wall, epoxy products often display surface defects, such as exposed fibers, chipping, or loss of dimension, all of which increase finished-product scrap rates. These additional material and processing costs place epoxy products in a class in which the end-use requirements must justify the high price and processing difficulty.

Much effort has been directed at developing more processible epoxy systems by using viscosity-modifying fillers, improved internal mold releases, and hybrid epoxy/vinyl ester structures. Some processors use slip sheets or release plies between the epoxy resin and the die wall to prevent bonding and to improve surface quality. Ultrasonic vibration of the die is one experimental method evaluated to reduce the adhesion tendency of epoxy resins. With improved methods, including selection of die materials and surface treatments, epoxy processing is now considered routine and cost competitive in high-performance applications.

Other resins in addition to the traditional three mentioned previously have achieved commercial significance. Resins based on methyl methacrylate and vinyl ester are quite attractive because they offer the advantages of higher physical properties, high filler loading due to very low viscosity, rapid processing speeds, smooth low-profile surfaces, and improved flame-retardant and weathering characteristics. Although the heat resin costs twice as much as polyesters, these resins have found use in applications that exploit their special properties. Most notably, methacrylate vinyl ester resins were used exclusively in the pultrusions produced for use in the Channel Tunnel project and other underground transit installations. The methacrylate resins are quite reactive and provide excellent processing speeds. Thus, the net cost premium is moderated, making these systems competitive with polyesters in many applications.

Phenolic resins have achieved a level of acceptance in applications where the highest level of flame, smoke, and toxicity performance are required. Another unique feature must be dealt with when processing these resin systems. Unlike any of the previous resins, which are 100% reactive with no reaction by-products, phenolic resins of the resole type are water and solvent diluted to provide workable viscosity and generate additional water as a reaction by-product during processing. As a result, phenolic products have a higher level of voids and a significantly lower mechanical property level than the previously mentioned resin systems. In addition, in order to achieve maximum strength potential, phenolic compatible roving and mat products must be used. Both acid-catalyzed and temperature-activated phenolics have now been processed successfully at rates that are comparable to vinyl ester resins. One of the very important considerations in processing these materials is the new demands on industrial hygiene and environmental emissions created by the presence of carrier solvent and phenol and formaldehyde components of the resin that are evolved during processing. As a result of all of these special needs, phenolic cannot be processed interchangeably by most pultruders and a fairly narrow supply base will exist for the near term.

Composite toughness has been a deficiency with the brittle matrices of polyester, vinyl ester acrylic, epoxy, and phenolic. While some high-elongation vinyl esters have been introduced, it is often with a sacrifice in reactivity, which affects process speed. Recent activity in two-component thermoset polyurethane pultrusion shows promise to increase elongation and toughness by a factor of two to five times that of polyester. Once again, the special equipment for meter-mix delivery of the reactive system along with special direct die injection hardware will limit this alternative to specialty processors or original equipment manufacturers (OEMs) with a specific product line that merits this investment.

A great deal of interest has developed in recent years in using thermoplastic resins as the matrix for pultruded profiles. The major driving force also comes from the desire for improved toughness as well as the additional benefit of postprocessing reformability. In addition, several of the engineering thermoplastic resins provide heat distortion properties that are superior to those of the epoxy systems currently used, making them very attractive for advanced composite applications. The technology for impregnating fibers with thermoplastic resins has been developed using a variety of methods, including hot-melt application, solvent solution impregnation, and fluidized bed particle application. Most of the success reported to date has been limited to the preparation of thin tapes or small-diameter rods, which are then used as molding materials in subsequent processing methods, such as compression molding. Limited success has been achieved with fairly simple shapes, but the surface quality and dimensional control is inferior to thermoset products at this time. Interest in this area is growing, however, and the advantages of these materials will undoubtedly result in the development of a viable pultrusion process. Recent new activity includes thermoplastic polyurethane as well as low-viscosity in situ polymerization of thermoplastic resins employing ring-opening chemistry. All thermoplastic approaches tout the substantially higher processing rates theoretically possible by eliminating the cure dependency of the thermoset polymerization reactions. In addition, pressures to provide recycling options by composite end users clearly favor thermoplastic systems.

Additives are used in all liquid resin systems to provide specific tailored performance. Although the thermoplastic processor often receives precompounded materials, the pultruder develops his own formulation and prepares it onsite for his own use. Resin suppliers have developed recommended formulations that are available to the general market, but the resin formulation is also a well-guarded secret of the pultruder and is often considered to be a competitive edge in cost or performance.

Fillers often constitute the greatest proportion of a formulation, second to the base resin. The most commonly used fillers are calcium carbonate, alumina silicate (clay), and alumina trihydrate. Calcium carbonate is primarily used as a volume extender to provide the lowest cost resin formulation in applications where performance is not critical. The clay fillers are used where improved corrosion-resistance and electrical properties are required. They also impart a superior surface finish to the pultruded product. Alumina trihydrate is a filler that is used for its ability to suppress flame and smoke generation and provide electrical-arc and track resistance. It is used in many applications to satisfy consumer

Table 1 General properties of fiberglass-reinforced pultruded products

Material	Specific gravity	Tensile strength, MPa	Tensile strength, ksi	Tensile modulus, GPa	Tensile modulus, 10^6 psi	Flexural strength, MPa	Flexural strength, ksi	Compressive strength, axial, MPa	Compressive strength, axial, ksi	Dielectric strength, parallel, kV/cm	Dielectric strength, parallel, kV/in.	Thermal conductivity, W/m · K	Thermal conductivity, Btu · in/h · ft^2·°F	Coefficient of thermal expansion, 10^{-6}/K	Water absorption, wt%
Solid rod and bar, 70% Wt_{fiber} all unidirectional fiber	2.00	690	100	41.4	6.0	690	100	410	60	23.6	60	0.30	2.0	3.0	0.25
Profiles, 50% Wt_{fiber} multidirectional reinforcement	1.80	242	35	17.2	2.5	242	35	138	20	7.87	20	0.576	4.0	4.4	0.6

Property(a): (a) The machine direction (lengthwise) properties given are typical of those attainable through the pultrusion process. Variations in glass content and orientation, as well as modifications to the resin system, can improve the properties. Composite systems can be developed to meet many custom physical, mechanical, chemical electrical, flame-resistant, and environmental properties. Source Ref 1

or governmental flammability codes for product safety. Other fillers, such as mica, talc, calcium sulfate, and various glass beads and bubbles are used by the pultruder for their specific property modification qualities, although they represent a small portion of total use.

Fillers can be incorporated into the resins in quantities up to 50% of the total resin formulation by weight (100 parts filler to 100 parts resin). The usual volume limitation is based on the development of processing viscosity, which also depends on the particle size and the characteristics of the resin. The low-viscosity acrylic resin, for example, can incorporate an additional 50 parts of filler beyond the polyester resin levels while maintaining processibility. Wetting agents have been developed that enable incorporation of a greater filler volume without increasing formula viscosity. These wetting agents and other surface modification agents can be added to the filler by the supplier or introduced as an additive by the pultruder. Air release agents are added to provide more efficient packing by reducing entrapped air in the liquid resin and void content in the finished product.

Another important category of materials in resin formulation are the initiators required to cure the thermosetting resins. The polyester, vinyl ester, and methacrylate systems are all cured by the elevated-temperature decomposition of organic peroxide catalysts. A variety of initiators that provide different levels of activation temperature are available. Pultrusion formulations typically employ a multiple-initiator system to provide rapid low-temperature initiation, followed by midrange acceleration and high-temperature reaction completion. This combination, which delivers the fastest processing speed, can also reduce resin pot life, especially in high ambient temperatures. The use of reaction inhibitors and the selection of catalyst type and quantity become important considerations in controlling resin scrap due to premature gelation of formulated resin. Catalysts for epoxy systems which are amine or anhydride cured, are usually supplied as a component that is matched in specific proportion to the epoxy resin system obtained from the supplier.

Mold releases are important in the development of adequate dynamic release of the curing material from the die wall to provide smooth surfaces and low processing friction. The mold release cannot leave a surface residual that interferes with bonding if subsequent painting or fabrication is necessary. These releases are added to the resin and are typically metallic stearates or organic phosphate esters suitable for high-temperature use.

Other special-purpose additives would include ultraviolet radiation inhibitor for improved weatherability, antimony oxide for flame retardance (used in combination with halogenated resins), pigments for coloration, and low-profile agents for surface smoothness and crack suppression characteristics. A variety of options are available in each of these material categories as well.

Properties of Pultruded Products

Mechanical Properties. The great amount of latitude that exists in selecting reinforcement type, form, style, and proportion allows a broad spectrum of mechanical properties. As noted, the directional strength in a pultruded composite can be greatly influenced by substituting longitudinal reinforcement for random mat or directional fabrics. A product with only longitudinal reinforcement will typically exhibit mechanical properties that are at least ten times greater than the same property measured transverse to the longitudinal fibers. In this type of composite, the properties of the fiber dominate the axial properties, but the properties of the resin dominate the transverse properties. As the volume fraction of fibers in the off-axis direction is increased, the longitudinal volume fraction, by necessity, must decrease; thus, the transverse properties are increased at the expense of longitudinal properties. This substitution method can be used to move the directionality of strength deliberately toward a one-to-one ratio, or even to the extent of achieving higher transverse properties when using some of the weft transverse orientation fabrics available. Accordingly, when evaluating pultruded product property data it is necessary to be aware that both lengthwise (LW or 0°) and cross-wise (CW or 90°) properties must be reported for an accurate representation of these nonisotropic materials. The magnitudes of typical properties for glass reinforced pultrusions from one supplier are given in Table 1 to illustrate the effect of orientation on property levels.

Table 2 indicates the effect on selected ultimate properties in the lengthening direction at an equal volume fraction of alternative continuous fibers. The specific contributions of fiber type become very apparent in the properties selected to illustrate this point. Because so many options exist, even among the unidirectional reinforcements, it is difficult to provide an all-inclusive list of properties. The designer must learn to exploit the specific fiber characteristics to achieve the desired performance properties, along with exercising the orientation options available from raw material suppliers. The end user must be aware that published values from any pultruder do not necessarily represent the limits of achievable properties.

The finished-product geometry often dictates the process to be used. A further comparison of selected pultrusion properties for different process methods is shown in Table 3.

Frequently, the decision to be made by an end user relates to the application of composite material as an alternative to such traditional materials as steel, aluminum, or wood. Selected relative properties of common alternative materials are listed in Table 4. Although Table 4 compares various materials in terms of absolute strength or stiffness, it is often desirable to determine the thickness of fiberglass reinforced plastic (FRP) necessary to achieve strength or rigidity equivalent to that of the traditional material. Such an analysis is shown in Table 5, using the data of

Table 2 Effect of fiber type on selected ultimate properties

Fiber type	Specific gravity	Tensile strength, MPa	Tensile strength, ksi	Tensile modulus, GPa	Tensile modulus, 10^6 psi	Compressive strength, MPa	Compressive strength, ksi	Thermal conductivity, W/m · K	Thermal conductivity, Btu · in./h · ft^2·°F
Fiberglass(a)	2.00	690	100	41	6.0	410	60	0.30	2.0
Carbon(b)	1.65	1000–1500	150–220	100–140	15–20	620–970	90–140	0.85–1.40	6–10
Aramid(c)	1.28	1400	200	80	12	280	40	0.15	1

Property, lengthwise. (a) E-glass unidirectional rovings. (b) Type AS carbon fibers (c) DuPont Kevlar 49 fibers. Based on 60% fiber volume. Source Ref 2

Table 3 Property comparison by process

		Property											
		Tensile strength		Tensile modulus		Flexural strength		Compressive strength		Impact strength		Thermal conductivity	
Processing method	Typical reinforcement composition	MPa	ksi	GPa	10^6 psi	MPa	ksi	MPa	ksi	J/m	ft · lbf/ft	W/m · K	Btu · in./h · ft^2·°F
Spray up(a)	30–50 wt% glass polyester resin ambient cure	60–120	9–18	6–12	0.8–1.8	110–190	16–28	100–170	15–25	210–640	48–144	0.17–0.23	1.2–1.6
Compression molding(a)	15–30 wt% glass-polyester SMC hot press	55–140	8–20	11–17	1.6–2.5	120–210	18–30	100–210	15–30	430–1150	96–264	0.19–0.25	1.3–1.7
	25–50 wt% glass mat-polyester wet layup, hot press	170–210	25–30	6.2–14	0.9–2.0	70–280	10–40	100–210	15–30	530–1050	120–240	0.19–0.26	1.3–1.8
Filament winding(a)	30–80 wt% glass roving-epoxy resin, variable angle	276–550	40–80	21–41	3.0–6.0	276 –550	40–80	310–480	45–70	2150–3200	480–720	0.27–0.33	1.9–2.3
Pultrusion rod and bar(b)	60–80 wt% glass roving only	414–690	60–100	31–41	4.5–6.0	345–552	50–80	276–414	40–60	2150–2687	480–600	0.27–0.33	1.9–2.3
Pultrusion profiles(b)	40–55 wt% glass roving/continuous strand mat	83–207	12–30	6.9–17	1.0–2.5	103–242	15–35	104–207	15–30	537–1075	120–240	0.28–0.57	2.0–4.0
	50–65 wt% glass roving/continuous strand mat/fabric	207–310	30–45	27–31	3.9–4.5	138–345	20–50	97–380	14–55	1020–2310	228–516	0.28–0.57	2.0–4.0

Note: Range of property values reflect transverse and machine direction anisotropy as well as reinforcement ranges possible. (a) Source Ref 3 (b) Source Ref 1

Table 4 and contributions of section geometry to strength and stiffness ultimate values. When the application does not require property equivalency, the product thickness can be reduced accordingly to yield savings in material and processing costs. A similar analysis can be conducted for the alternative fiber types to determine equivalent thickness factors for the high-strength high-modulus materials. The relative costs per unit volume can then be readily determined.

Physical Properties. The thermal conductivity of pultruded composites reflects both matrix and fiber characteristics. Generally, the fiberglass reinforced composites are excellent insulators for thermal and electrical environments. This is also true of the organic fiber composites, regardless of the matrix employed. The use of conductive carbon fibers, however, results in composites that exhibit greater thermal and electrical conductivity. This reduces their potential as insulators but creates new opportunities because of their static and heat dissipation characteristics.

Although fiberglass reinforced composites display a modest positive coefficient of thermal expansion, both aramid and carbon reinforced composites display a slightly negative coefficient of thermal expansion. This characteristic can be used to advantage in aerospace structures and in producing very tight tolerance parts. The thermal expansion characteristics can result in molded-in stresses in multidirectional reinforcement systems when dissimilar fiber types (hybrids) are used in the profile. Upon exiting the die, residual stress is relieved in the form of dimensional distortion that can be either cross sectional (angularity or flatness) or axial (warp, twist, or bow). Carbon reinforced composites are also noted for their lubricity and wear resistance, which makes them suitable for use as bearing materials. Their capacity for heat dissipation is advantageous in this application.

Specific gravity is a key consideration when strength-to-weight ratios are important, as in aircraft and aerospace applications. The specific strength of carbon and aramid reinforced composites excel because of their low specific gravity and high strength and stiffness characteristics. High-modulus polyethylene fibers also have very low specific gravity and high strength and stiffness properties at room temperature and have the potential to provide the highest specific strength available at lowest cost.

The impact resistance of organic fiber reinforced composites is quite high, making them suitable for energy-absorption applications, such as ballistic shielding. The impact resistance of carbon fibers is generally low, and advanced composites that use carbon rely on the tough resin matrix for impact properties. Fiberglass reinforced composites are also relatively poor in impact performance compared to the organic fibers, but are superior to carbon reinforced composites. The fatigue resistance of graphite reinforced composites is superior to that of the fiberglass reinforced composites, particularly when used with epoxy resins.

Chemical and corrosion-resistance characteristics of pultruded composites are predominantly attributed to the resin matrix. In considering a particular resin system for an intended environment, the degree of exposure, the concentration of the corrosive element, and the temperature of the environment must be known. Resin companies servicing the corrosion markets generally publish a list of chemical environments tested at various concentrations and temperatures, as well as recommendations for the use of their resins. The areas of suitability for polyester, vinyl ester, and epoxy resins are described in the section "Matrix Resins" in this article.

Chemical and corrosion attack can occur at the product surface or at the end of the profile. The presence of a resin-rich barrier layer on the surface can provide a greater degree of corrosion-resistance. Although this is readily achievable in the wet lay-up or filament-winding process, the nature of the pultrusion process requires a high fiber volume and significant internal pressure to fill the die volume and to minimize porosity. To achieve a resin-rich surface, a synthetic veil or mat that is typically of polyester fiber is used on the surface of the product when pultruded. The layer can range from 0.15 to 1.0 mm (0.005–0.040 in.) thick, depending on the barrier thickness required. In pultrusion, therefore, a resin-rich layer does not mean a fiber-free layer, it means that the fibers in the surface layer are organic fibers rather than inorganic reinforcing fibers.

The end cut of the profile is particularly vulnerable to corrosion because fibers are exposed

Table 4 Material property comparison of FRP versus alternative materials

	Property					
	Tensile strength		Tensile modulus		Flexural strength	
Material	MPa	ksi	GPa	10^6 psi	MPa	ksi
Wood						
Maple	100	15	12.4	1.80	55	8
Pine	60	9	12.1	1.75	35	5
Thermoplastics						
Unreinforced (typical)	55	8	3.4	0.5	55	8
Reinforced (typical)	100	15	6.9	1.0	140	20
FRP pultrusions						
50% wt mat and roving	242	35	17.2	2.5	242	35
70% wt unidirectional roving	690	100	41.4	6.0	690	100
Metals						
Aluminum	280	40	70	10	280	40
Steel	690	100	210	30	690	100

Source: Ref 4

to the corrosive agent. Any matrix crazing or resin-fiber debonding in this area will promote wicking of the chemical along the fiber surface. Therefore, it is a common practice to dip or brush coat the end cuts of pultruded profiles (as well as any fabricated holes along the product length) with resin to seal them from corrosive attack. If this is not done, the corrosion resistance of the fiber itself becomes an important consideration because the resin does not effectively protect the fiber from attack along the fiber/resin interface in damaged or machined areas.

As previously stated, of the glass fibers available, C-glass is by far the best in all-around chemical resistance, while ECR glass (modified E-glass) is excellent in most acids. Standard E-glass is relatively inferior in concentrated acidic and alkaline environments, and A-glass is poor in water resistance. Standard E-glass is the most popular and is available in pultrusion rovings and mats, while A-glass and C-glass veil is generally utilized for surface coverage. Aramid fibers are resistant to fuels, solvents, and lubricants and are superior to glass fibers in many strong acids and bases. Carbon fibers are resistant to alkaline and salt solutions, but are subject to attack by strong oxidizing agents and halogenated chemicals, particularly at elevated temperatures. It is important, therefore, to consider the chemical resistance aspects of both the reinforcement and the matrix when considering the application of any composite material in corrosive environments.

Design Guidelines

The design of any pultruded profile requires a thorough understanding of the material and processing contributions that affect the product design. Although many material options exist for use in pultrusion, some limit the configuration of the resulting profile. The primary characteristics of a pultruded product and process are listed in Table 6.

Table 7 shows many of the geometry guidelines for designing pultruded products. The pultrusion process can produce virtually any shape that can be extruded. The part must be consistent in cross section over its length. Tapered shapes cannot be produced. Some moderately curved shapes have been developed, but generally, the equipment required for this activity differs from a standard pultrusion machine and commercial success has been limited. Any length can be produced that can be transported.

There is theoretically no limit to the size of profile that can be pultruded; however, raw material (mat and fabric) width availability and maximum die sizes present practical limits as does the in-feed capacity of the process line. As mentioned, continuous-strand mat is available only to 3050 mm (120 in.) in width. Conversely, parts having total product perimeter dimensions less than 25 to 32 mm (1–1.25 in.) are difficult to manufacture with mat reinforcement. Cutting a continuous-strand mat less than 100 mm (4 in.) wide eliminates the continuous nature of the strands in the product and reduces the critical processing tensile strength. Woven tapes and cloth can be employed at the lower limits of size as a replacement for mat. Axially reinforced products (all roving) can be produced as small as 0.76 mm (0.030 in.) in diameter.

Because thermoset resin composites are exothermic in nature and dependent on conductive heat transfer for reaction initiation, it is more difficult to produce thick-wall products economically. When mat and roving are used in shapes, wall thickness is limited to approximately 25 mm (1 in.). With radio frequency preheating, all-roving reinforced solid rods up to 75 mm (3 in.) diameter have been successfully pultruded. If not properly processed, however, these thicker profiles are prone to crack or delaminate because of lack of control of exothermic temperatures and shrinkage.

The pultrusion process does not impose any limits on the cross-sectional draft angles designed into a part. A common condition referred to as toe-in is often seen when die angles are not properly compensated for by considering material shrinkage, especially at corners and at thickness transitions. Undercuts can be incorporated into the design of a part by using multipiece steel dies as long as the die can readily be disassembled for service in case a part should freeze (lock up) in the die cavity.

Longitudinal ribs and corrugations are possible, but care should be taken in any composite part to provide sufficient radius where one wall or rib section makes a transition to another. This permits a transfer of load without a concentrated stress in a sharp corner. Another reason for using a radius is related to pultrusion process considerations. Generally, with pultrusion dies that are chrome plated for wear resistance, it is difficult to obtain chrome that will plate in sharp corners or shallow ribs. Additionally, any sharp corner or parting line will wear significantly when fiberglass materials pass over them. It is good practice to radius mat-reinforced profiles by a minimum of 1.5 mm (0.06 in.) and roving reinforced shapes by a minimum of 0.76 mm (0.03 in.).

Isolated bosses cannot be produced unless they are longitudinal in nature, in which case they would be more properly described as a rib. Localized features, such as through-holes, cannot be molded in. Longitudinal inserts (or encapsulants), such as antenna wire, plywood, or polyurethane foam, can be accommodated with appropriate in-feed equipment.

It is desirable to maintain a uniform wall thickness when designing a profile. However, variations in thickness within a part are possible and common as long as proper forming control is executed that avoids mat folding and structural defects at the thickness transition. The pultruder must produce the profile at the speed required to cure the thickest section. With good communication and planning, the end user and pultruder can arrive at a part design that will meet the functional and performance requirements of the end user and also give the pultruder the best opportunity to design an efficient and highly productive pultrusion process.

Once a pultruded profile is produced, it can be fabricated in the same manner as aluminum or steel. However, because of the abrasive nature of

Table 5 Equivalent thickness factor of FRP fabricated by pultrusion relative to traditional structural materials

		Steel			Aluminum			Wood		
Pultrusion composition	Specific gravity	Tensile strength	Tensile modulus	Flexural strength	Tensile strength	Tensile modulus	Flexural strength	Tensile strength	Tensile modulus	Flexural strength
Profiles, 50% wt_{fiber} multidirectional reinforcement	1.80	2.5	2.15	1.82	1.0	1.49	1.16	0.25	0.79	0.45
Solid rod and bar, 70% wt_{fiber} all unidirectional fiber	2.00	1.0	1.71	1.12	0.4	1.19	0.71	0.10	0.63	0.27

Source: Ref 4

Table 6 Pultrusion product characteristics

Size	Equipment pulling envelope and forming guide width influence size on specific machinery
Shape	Constant cross-section, straight profiles; hybrid processes allow some curvature and local variable cross-section features
Length	Only limited by transportation limits. Flexible product can be coiled in very long lengths, e.g., 1 kilometer 2 mm diam fiber-optic strength member rods
Reinforcements	Fiberglass, carbon, aramid, thermoplastic polyester, polyethylene, and nylon, natural fibers—jute, flax, sisal
Reinforcement content, wt%	All roving from 40–80% by weight, mat and roving from 35–65% by weight, roving/mat/fabric to 70% by weight
Resin systems	Polyester, vinyl ester, epoxy acrylic, phenolic, polyurethane, and thermoplastic matrices
Mechanical properties	Anisotropic for all unidirectional, near-isotropic with multiaxial reinforcements including engineered fabrics
Labor content	Low to medium depending on the number of streams and machines tended by one operator. Also product size and speed dependent
Production rates	Typically 0.5–1.5 m/min (1.5– 5 ft/min), depends on thickness and resin type
Tooling costs	Low to medium depending on part complexity and forming guide complexity
Equipment costs	Medium to high depending on product size. Typically less than extrusion or injection equipment. Also depends on control sophistication

fiberglass, continuous-rim diamond tools are recommended. Wet cutting with diamond tools reduces heat buildup and degradation of the composite material. When composites incorporating aramid fibers are fabricated, water-jet cutting is highly recommended and is the preferred technique to provide clean edge cuts. Joining techniques include mechanical fastening and adhesive bonding. When using adhesive bonding, care must be taken to sand or otherwise prepare the surface before applying the adhesive. The guidelines provided by the adhesive manufacturer should be followed with regard to clamping time and the temperature of the adhesive under clamp pressure. Adhesive bonding, when properly done, is as reliable as mechanical fastening.

Painting of a finished profile is often necessary when outdoor use is considered. In such cases, both on-line and off-line methods are used. Both cases require environmental control from the standpoint of cleanliness to avoid paint defects and to handle fumes from paint systems. Technology has been developed for water-based paints as well as 100% solids powder coating systems for use with pultrusions that minimize these issues. Paint adhesion is enhanced through formulation of both the paint and the substrate pultrusion resin system.

Future Outlook

The 1990s saw remarkable growth in capability as the knowledge base of pultrusion has expanded. A flood of published investigations of process and materials topics in the 1990s has finally provided a sound literature base for most topics of interest to current and prospective pultruders. Continued commercial and academic contributions to the literature base is expected to bring pultrusion process science to a level on par with other well-established plastics processing methods.

Processors will continue to utilize engineered materials to achieve optimized properties with the intention of minimizing composite product weight and cost, which will be key to penetrating markets held by conventional materials. The palette of new resin and fiber forms has expanded dramatically and tailored properties can be achieved cost effectively by matching application needs to material capabilities.

Computer-aided design tools for both profile design and laminate property analysis have been a key development and are now commonly used by pultrusion process engineers. The integration of FEA methods with solid modeling software now enables design optimization of finished composite products and structures rather than simply the basic profiles.

Pultrusion machinery has evolved in terms of control capability and envelope such that the most complex of shapes of very large size can now be addressed. The capability to monitor the process and product quality at a new level has recently emerged, and further advances are expected until a truly closed-loop-process quality-control capability is achieved. A recognition of the value of vertical integration to provide end users with a finished or near-finished product as opposed to a raw pultruded profile will continue to present new opportunities for pultruders to capture margin and secure a proprietary position. Both on-line and off-line fabrication as well as painting and assembly will be employed to achieve these goals.

Hybrid processes will continue to evolve, blurring the lines between conventional pultrusion and compression molding, injection, filament winding, and other useful thermoset and thermoplastic production processes. Products with three-dimensional features are now enabled with process-parameter manipulation and clever die and machine design approaches. In short, the future of pultrusion is very promising as one of

Table 7 Pultrusion design guidelines

Feature	Pultrusion
Minimum inside radius	0.79 mm roving shapes, 1.6 mm mat shapes
Molded-in holes	No
Trimmed-in mold	Yes
Core pull and slides	Yes
Undercuts	Yes
Minimum recommended draft	No limitation
Minimum practical thickness	Roving, 1.0 mm. Mat, 1.5 mm
Maximum practical thickness	Roving, 75 mm. Mat, 25 mm
Normal thickness variation	As required
Maximum thickness buildup	As required
Corrugated sections	Yes, longitudinal
Metal inserts	No
Bosses	No
Ribs	Yes, longitudinal
Molded-in labels	Yes, but not recessed
Raised numbers	No
Finished surfaces (reproduces mold surface)	Two
Hollow sections	Yes, longitudinal
Wire inserts	Yes, longitudinal
Embossed surface	No

Source: Ref 5

the most cost-effective continuous production methods available to produce composite solutions to design problems.

REFERENCES

1. The Pultex Pultrusion Design Manual, Creative Pultrusions, 1999
2. Compiled data, Handbook of Fillers and Reinforcements for Plastics, Van Nostrand Reinhold, 1978
3. Commercial data sheets. Owens Corning Fiberglass, with permission
4. The Pultrusion Process Seminar Notebook, Martin Pultrusion Group, 1999
5. "Standard Specification for Dimensional Tolerance of Thermosetting Glass-Reinforced Plastic Pultruded Shapes," D 3917, Annual Book of ASTM Standards, American Society for Testing and Materials

SELECTED REFERENCES

- R.A. Anderson and R. Riddell, Effects of Pigments on Pultrusion Physical Properties and Performance, *Proc. Society of the Plastics Industry Reinforced Plastics/Composites Institute 38th Meeting,* Feb 1983 (Houston, TX), Society of the Plastics Industry, Inc.
- G.L. Batch and C.W. Macosko, Integrated Cure Characterization and Analysis for Pultrusion Processors, *Proc. 43rd Annual Society of the Plastics Industry Conference,* Feb 1988 (Cincinnati, OH), Society of the Plastics Industry, Inc.
- J.J. Beckman, R.N. Lehaman, et al., A Method of Producing Ladder Rail Using High Pressure Injection Die Impregnation, *Proc. 50th Annual Society of the Plastics Industry Conference,* Feb 1995 (Cincinnati, OH), Society of the Plastics Industry Inc.
- R. Birsa and P. Taft, A New Materials Approach for Providing Transverse Strength in Pultruded Shapes, *Proc. 39th Annual Society of the Plastics Industry Conference,* Jan 1984 (Houston, TX), Society of the Plastics Industry Inc.
- H.J. Buck, L.T. Blankenship, and C.Y. Lo, An Optimal Curing Approach for Pultruded Vinyl Ester Parts, *Proc. 44th Annual Society of Plastics Industry Conference,* Feb 1989 (Dallas, TX), Society of Plastics Industry Inc.
- N.H. Douglas and S.P. Walsh, Cure Systems for Highly Filled Pultrusions, *Proc. 49th Annual Society of Plastics Industry Conference,* Feb 1994 (Cincinnati, OH), Society of Plastics Industry Inc.
- K.J. Elias and D.K. Watkins, EPA Requirements for Hazardous Waste and Emission Controls in a Pultrusion Facility, *Proc. 42nd Annual Society of Plastics Industry Conference,* Feb 1987 (Cincinnati, OH), Society of the Plastics Industry Inc.
- H. Engelen and S. Li, Experimental Comparison of Resin Injection Methods for Pultrusion, *Proc. 54th Society of the Plastics Industry, International Composites Exhibitors Conference,* May 1999 (Cincinnati, OH), Society of the Plastics Industry Inc.
- European Pultrusion Technology Association (EPTA), Sleuithek 6, 3831 PB Leusden, The Netherlands
- D.J. Evans, Designing with Pultrusions from the Idea to the Application, *Proc. Society of Plastics Industry Reinforced Plastics/Composites Institute 38th Meeting,* Feb 1983 (Houston, TX), Society of the Plastics Industry Inc.
- G.W. Ewald, Curved Pulforming—A New Manufacturing Process for Composite Automotive Springs, *Proc. Society of Plastics Industry Reinforced Plastics/Composites Institute Meeting,* Feb 1981 (Washington, D.C.), Society of the Plastics Industry Inc.
- W.B. Goldsworthy and D.W. Johnson, Cutting Through the Glass Ceiling: A Report on the Development of an Innovative In-Line Machining Center to Economically Fabricate Pultrusions for Civil Engineering Applications, *Proc. 53rd Annual Society of Plastics Industry Conference,* Feb 1998 (Cincinnati, OH), Society of Plastics Industry Inc.
- R.D. Howard and S.J. Holland, Methacrylate Resins in Pultrusion: Factors Affecting Pulling Force, *Proc. 43rd Annual Society of Plastics Industry Conference,* Feb 1988 (Cincinnati, OH), Society of Plastics Industry Inc.
- G.A. Hunter, Pultruding Epoxy Resin, *Proc. 43rd Annual Society of Plastics Industry Conference,* Feb 1988 (Cincinnati, OH), Society of Plastics Industry Inc.
- B.H. Jones, Pultruding Filamentary Composites—An Experimental and Analytical Determination of Process Parameters, *Proc. 29th Society of Plastics Industry Reinforced Plastics/Composites Institute Meeting,* Feb 1974 (Washington, D.C.), Society of the Plastics Industry Inc.
- R.R. Joshi, L. Varas, et al., Polyurethanes in Pultrusion: Styrene Free Alternative Systems, *Proc. 54th Society of the Plastics Industry, International Composites Exhibitors Conference,* May 1999 (Cincinnati, OH), Society of the Plastics Industry Inc.
- E. Lackey ad J.G. Vaughan, Effects of Fillers on Pultrusion Processing and Pultruded Properties, *Proc. 54th Society of the Plastics Industry, International Composites Exhibitors Conference,* May 1999 (Cincinnati, OH), Society of the Plastics Industry Inc.
- R. Lopez-Anido and D.L. Troutman, Fabrication and Installation of Modular FRP Composite Bridge Deck, *Proc. 53rd Annual Society of Plastics Industry Conference,* Feb 1998 (Cincinnati, OH), Society of the Plastics Industry Inc.
- A.K. Maji, L. Sanchez, and R. Acree, Processing Variables and Their Effect on Pultruded Composites, *J. Adv. Mater.,* Vol. 31 (No. 4), Oct 1999
- J.D. Martin, Pultruded Window Lineals—Persistence Pays Off, *Proc. European Pultrusion Technology Association World Conference,* Oct 1996 (London, U.K.)
- J.D. Martin, Pultrusion Processing Technologies—Endless Surprises, *Proc. European Pultrusion Technology Association World Conference,* Oct 1996 (London, U.K.)
- J.D. Martin, Select the Right Pultrusion Machine, *Compos. Fabr.,* March 2000
- J.D. Martin and J.E. Sumerak, A Review of the Markets for Pultruded Applications and Factors Affecting Its Growth, *Proc. Society of Plastics Industry Reinforced Plastics/Composites Institute 38th Meeting,* Feb 1983 (Houston, TX), Society of the Plastics Industry Inc.
- J.D. Martin and J.E. Sumerak, Pultruded Composites—The Case against Aluminum Extrusions, *Proc. 39th Annual Society of Plastics Industry Conference,* Jan 1984 (Houston, TX), Society of the Plastics Industry Inc.
- T.S. McQuarrie and J.H. Hickman, The Pultruders Guide to Resin Selection, *Proc. 42nd Annual Society of Plastics Industry Conference,* Feb 1987 (Cincinnati, OH), Society of the Plastics Industry Inc.
- R. Meyer, *Handbook of Pultrusion Technology,* Chapman and Hall, 1985
- K.M. Miller, Pultrusion Provides Solutions to World's Decaying Infrastructure, *Proc. European Pultrusion Technology Association World Conference,* Oct 1996 (London, U.K.)
- A.S. Mossallam, Connection and Reinforcement Design Details for Pultruded Fiber Reinforced Plastic Composite Structures, *Proc. 49th Annual Society of Plastics Industry Conference,* Feb 1994 (Cincinnati, OH), Society of the Plastics Industry Inc.
- Pultrusion Industry Council (PIC), Composite Fabricators Association, 1655 North Fort Meyer Drive, Suite 510, Arlington VA 22209
- G.S. Rogowski and M.A. Tallent, Design Flexibility in Pultruded Parts Through Utilization of Thermoplastic Fibers, *Proc. 44th Annual Society of Plastics Industry Conference,* Feb 1989 (Dallas, TX), Society of the Plastics Industry Inc.
- D. Shaw-Stewart, Production of Pultruded Tubing by the Pultrusion Process, *Proc. 35th Society of Plastics Industry Reinforced Plastics/Composites Institute Meeting,* Feb 1980 (New Orleans, LA), Society of the Plastics Industry Inc.
- T. Starr, Ed., *Pultrusion for Engineers,* Woodhead Publishing Ltd., Cambridge, England, 2000
- B. Sturman–Mole and J.D. Martin, Integral Core Filled Pultrusion Processing Technology Offers Costs Competitive with Wood and PVC While Improving Numerous Mechanical Properties, *Proc. of 53rd Annual Society of Plastics Industry Conference,* Feb 1998 (Cincinnati, OH), Society of the Plastics Industry Inc.
- J.E. Sumerak, Understanding Pultrusion Process Variables for the First Time, *Proc. 42nd*

Annual Society of Plastics Industry Conference, Feb 1987 (Cincinnati, OH), Society of the Plastics Industry Inc.

- J.E. Sumerak, Pultrusion Die Design Optimization Opportunities Using Thermal Finite Element Analysis Techniques, *Proc. 49th Annual Society of Plastics Industry Conference,* Feb 1994 (Cincinnati, OH), Society of the Plastics Industry Inc.
- J.E. Sumerak, Pultrusion Process Optimization Using On-Line and Off-Line Techniques, *Compos. Manuf.,* Vol 13 (No. 2), 1997
- J.E. Sumerak and P.H. Hartman, Selective Interval Pulshaping—Introducing Variable Cross-Section Geometry Features to Thermosetting Pultruded Products, *Proc. 45th International Society of the Advancement of Material and Process Engineering Symposium,* May 2000 (Long Beach, CA), Society for the Advancement of Material and Process Engineering
- J.E. Sumerak, Y.R. Chachad, and J.D. Martin, Unlock Pultrusion Speed Potential with Thermally Optimized Pultrusion Dies, *Proc. 51st Annual Society of Plastics Industry Conference,* Feb 1996 (Cincinnati, OH), Society of the Plastics Industry Inc.
- J.E. Sumerak and J.D. Martin, Applying Internal Temperature Measurement Data to Pultrusion Process Control, *Proc. 41st Annual Society of Plastics Industry Conference,* Jan 1986 (Atlanta, GA), Society of the Plastics Industry Inc.
- J.E. Sumerak and J.D. Martin, The Pulse of Pultrusion—Pull Force Trending for Quality and Productivity Management, *Proc. 46th Annual Society of Plastics Industry Conference,* Feb 1991 (Cincinnati, OH), Society of the Plastics Industry Inc.
- J.E. Sumerak and K. Taymourian, Pultrusion Quality Control—A Comprehensive Approach, *Proc. 44th Annual Society of Plastics Industry Conference,* Feb 1989 (Dallas, TX), Society of the Plastics Industry Inc.
- R.I. Werner, Fiberglass Ladders and Pultrusion: A Challenge to a Young Industry, *Proc. 33rd Society of Plastics Industry Reinforced Plastics/Composites Institute Meeting,* Feb 1978 (Washington, D.C.), Society of the Plastics Industry Inc.
- R.I. Werner, Improvements in Means of Evaluating Weathering Characteristics of Pultrusions, *Proc. 35th Society of Plastics Industry Reinforced Plastics/Composites Institute Meeting,* Feb 1980 (New Orleans, LA), Society of the Plastics Industry Inc.
- R.I. Werner, Properties of Pultruded Sections of Interest to Designers, *Proc. 34th Society of Plastics Industry Reinforced Plastics/Composites Institute Meeting,* Jan 1979 (New Orleans, LA), Society of the Plastics Industry Inc.

Tube Rolling

Robert J. Basso, Century Design, Inc.
Paul A. Roy, Vantage Associates, Inc.

TUBE ROLLING is the most widely used method of producing composite tubular parts that require high strength-to-weight properties as well as high production capabilities. The tube rolling process utilizes prepreg materials having accurate resin content, which are produced on very precise prepreg and filming machines. The combination of accurate resin content and good fiber areal weight in prepreg materials offers designers a method to produce structurally sound tubular parts at a very rapid rate using relatively unskilled factory labor.

Tube rolling has many advantages over other methods of producing composite tubes. High production rates of 5 to 10 s per part are common—some manufacturers of golf shafts produce quantities up to 30,000 shafts per day using semiautomated rolling tables. Part-to-part consistency is high, and excellent surface finish is obtained, using a light sanding/polishing operation after curing. In addition, the process uses inexpensive durable mandrels. Part shapes can be cylindrical, conical, circular, oval, or any combination of these shapes. Fiber orientation can range from 0 to 90°. Disadvantages include size limitation and higher material costs. Part sizes range from 0.76 to 609 mm (0.030 to 24 in.) diameter and 7.3 m (24 ft) maximum length. Material costs for rolling prepreg tubes are greater than those for wet-wound and pultruded parts due the requirement for the prepreg stage. However, higher production rates and lower labor costs can offset the difference in material costs in many instances.

Typical products produced using tube rolling include the following:

- Golf shafts
- Arrows
- Ski poles
- Tennis racquets
- Antennas
- Aerospace components
- Fishing rods
- Bicycle components
- Telescopes
- Launcher tubes
- Masts

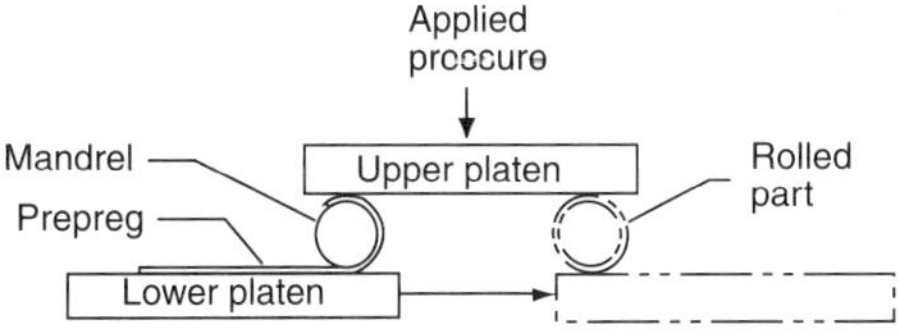

Fig. 1 Table rolling

Process Description

The first step in the tube-rolling process is to prepare a mandrel with a release agent and/or a tacking agent. Cut-to-size prepreg patterns are attached to the mandrel by hand pressure or warm tacking iron. Mandrel and pattern are placed on a rolling table surface and subsequently rolled into a compacted and densified laminate. Compaction and densification of the material during the wrapping process is accomplished using contact pressure between the mandrel, the prepreg, and the rolling table surfaces as shown in Fig. 1. Rolled parts are spirally wrapped with shrink tape under controlled tension to further debulk the laminate, and parts are cured in a curing oven. After curing, the mandrel is extracted and shrink tape removed. Parts are cut to length, and the exterior of the part is sanded, ground, and/or painted.

Process Equipment and Techniques

The same process and equipment are used to produce parts that are table rolled. Diameter and length of parts being produced dictate the size of the equipment required.

Mandrels. A variety of materials have been used for tube rolling mandrels. To produce small-to-intermediate-diameter tubing in volume, steel is commonly used because of its strength and stiffness. Steel mandrels are usually hardened and polished or chromed for ease of removal. Because the thermal expansion of steel is relatively low, heavy-duty mandrel pullers are required to remove the tube from the mandrel after cure.

Aluminum, which also has been used as a mandrel, is desirable for larger tubing because of its lower weight. Moreover, for a graphite tube that is greater than 50 mm (2 in.) in diameter, no puller is required because the differential expansion is sufficient to allow part removal after it has cooled. For fiberglass and aramid tubing, however, a mandrel puller is still required. In most instances, mandrel pulling is best attempted when the part is still hot, because cold parts are usually more difficult to pull.

Metal mandrels are used when external pressure is applied during cure. For thick-walled tubing where external pressure causes fiber wrinkling or where tube-geometry changes require internal pressure during cure, alternative mandrel materials are available. Female molds are usually used when internal pressure is required during cure.

Both Teflon and solid silicone rubber have been used as materials for mandrels undergoing internal pressure molding. The high thermal expansion coefficient of these materials can be used to exert exceptionally high pressures when the materials are properly confined. The amount of pressure applied is dependent on the cure temperature, mandrel volume, and restrictions imposed.

If more precise pressure control is required, a thin silicone rubber sleeve or a similar bladder material is placed over the mandrel, and the part is rolled over the sleeve. The sleeve can then be removed from the mandrel, with the uncured tube in place. The tube and rubber liner are then placed in a closed mold and the bladder is inflated during the cure. This method is particularly useful for fabricating irregularly shaped tubes. For round tubes, the mandrel can be left in place, and air can be applied through a port in the mandrel.

Sheeting. All rolling operations must start with sheet goods that are subsequently cut into patterns. Sheet cutting can be as simple as using a straight edge and a razor knife. For narrow sheets up to 460 mm (18 in.) wide, standard paper cutters fitted with hardened steel blades for longer life have been used. Outfitted with a creel for material feed, paper cutters can be a very efficient method of cutting large quantities rapidly. A method for cutting angle sheets (Fig. 2) has been used for many years to cut huge quantities of angle sheets.

In the area of automated equipment, high-speed sheet cutters are available. The typical fully automatic prepreg sheeter (Fig. 3), which digitally controls length of cut, can cut patterns at any angle automatically.

Pattern cutting, like sheet cutting, can be done manually or with automated equipment. Razor knives and templates, though primitive, are still used to cut small quantities of material. The trick is to stack multiple sheets of material and cut several patterns at one time. Stacks of up to 20 sheets of graphite-epoxy tape can be cut this way. When complex or extremely long patterns are required or when higher-speed cutting is necessary, the options range from steel-rule dies and roller presses (Fig. 4) to computer-controlled knives and water-jet cutters.

Tube Rolling. Tube rolling can be accomplished by hand or with rolling equipment. Rolling tables such as that shown in Fig. 5 are widely used to make tubular products such as golf shafts, fishing rods, and other tubes up to 9 m (30 ft) in length. The mandrel, with pattern tacked in place, is placed on the lower platen of the table. With the push of a button, the pneumatically controlled top platen drops to contact the mandrel, after which the movable lower platen slides back to totally envelop the pattern. The top platen is articulated to accommodate rolling either cylindrical or tapered tubes.

Shrink Tape Debulking and Cure. Heat shrinkable tapes such as cellophane, polypropylene, or nylon are used to incrementally debulk composite tubing after rolling. They are also used to apply the pressure during cure of noncritical parts such as golf shafts and fishing rods. The amount of actual pressure applied during cure depends on the type of tape used, its thickness, the number of layers applied, and the tension at which the tape is applied.

Typical shrink tapes of nylon, cellophane, polypropylene, and Tedlar (polyvinyl fluoride film, DuPont, Wilmington, DE) are readily available in appropriate widths and thickness. Polypropylene is limited to curing temperatures up to 145 °C (290 °F). Degradation of properties occurs above this temperature. Automatic shrink tape wrapping machines provide consistent tape-tension control as well as uniform spacing (pitch) of tape wraps.

One tape wrapping machine that is used extensively in the production of golf shafts, fishing rods, and other tubular parts is shown in Fig. 6. It can accommodate parts from 1 to 150 mm (0.04 to 6 in.) diameter and has adjustable pitch (overlap) from 0.75 to 25 mm (0.03 to 1.0 in.).

Finishing. Tubular products lend themselves to high-speed finishing methods. After cure, some amount of sanding or grinding is usually required. Sanding produces a good quality surface for cosmetic purposes, whereas centerless grinding is used when precise diameter control is required. Centerless sanders are widely used for high production rate items such as golf shafts and fishing rods. The machine shown in Fig. 7 is designed to provide uniform material removal for both straight and tapered parts at rates of up to 0.30 m/s (1 ft/s). Material removal is controlled by pressure application and feed rate. Sanding is performed with water as a coolant to improve the final finish quality and to eliminate fiber "dust."

Material Forms

Preimpregnated (prepreg) materials are most suitable for tube rolling when their form is either a fabric or unidirectional tape. Typically, fabrics are used when a 0/90° fiber orientation is required. Tubes made with this fiber orientation have good longitudinal and circumferential properties but poor torsional properties. Variants in longitudinal and circumferential mechanical properties depend on the fabric style selected. For example, the standard 181 style glass fabric will produce a tube with nearly equal properties in the two directions, whereas a 1543 weave style will produce a tube with a property imbalance of 8 to 1. Therefore, caution should be exercised when rolling fabrics to ensure that the warp and fill yarns are always wrapped in the proper orientation with respect to the tube axis.

Unidirectional tapes are used for tubes that require a higher degree of refinement in structural properties. It is possible to achieve any

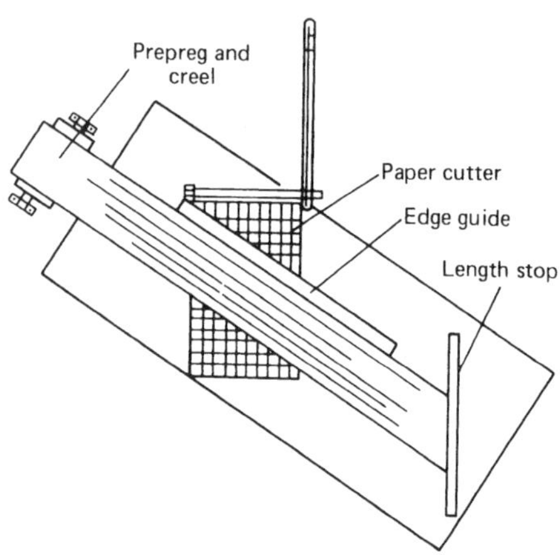

Fig. 2 Paper cutting for angle sheet cutting

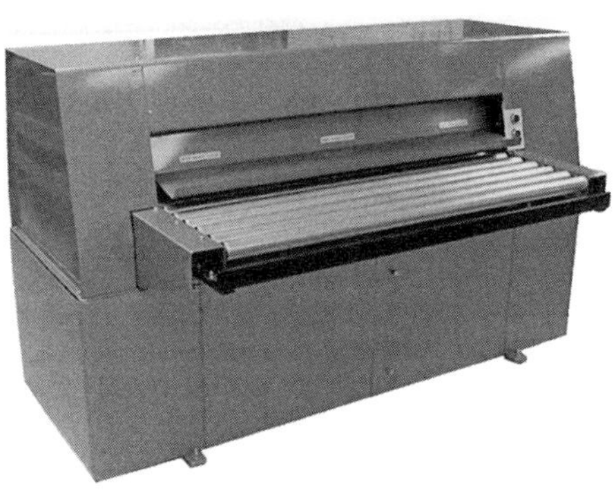
Fig. 4 Roller press with steel-rule dies. Courtesy of Century Design

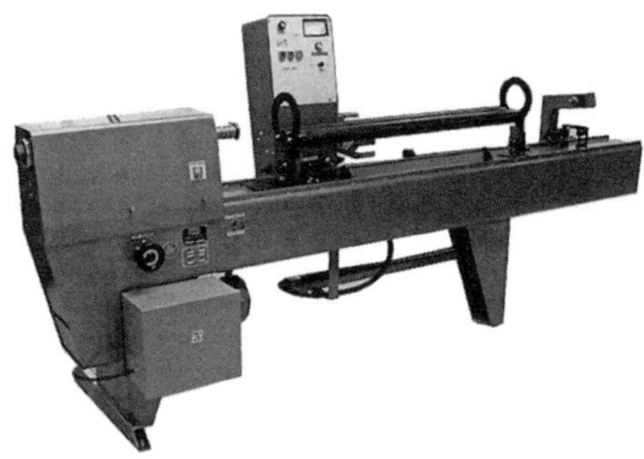
Fig. 6 Automatic shrink tape wrapping machine. Courtesy of Century Design

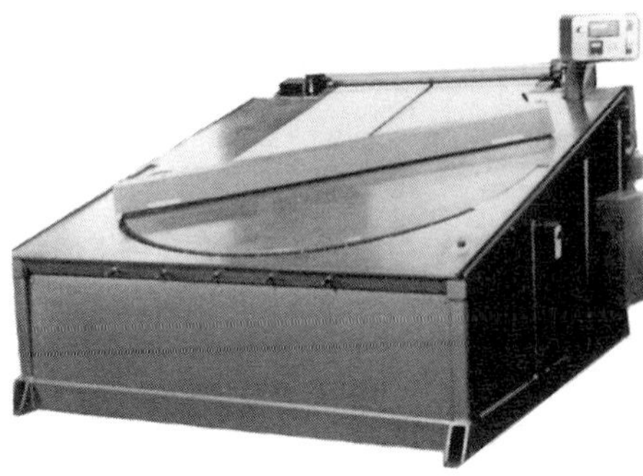
Fig. 3 Automatic angle-cutting prepreg sheeter. Courtesy of Century Design

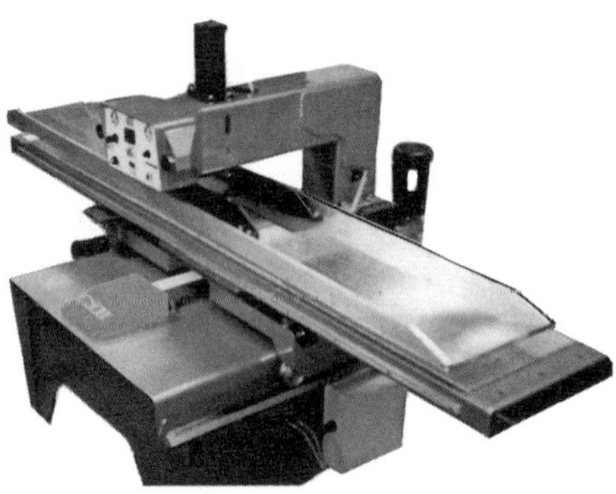
Fig. 5 Tube rolling table. Courtesy of Century Design

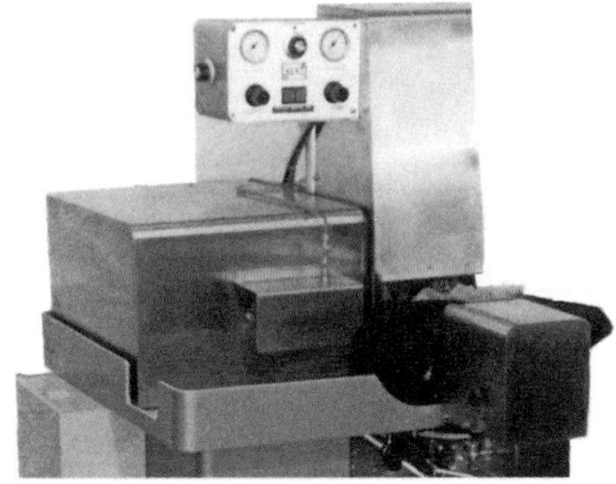
Fig. 7 Centerless sander. Courtesy of Century Design

combination of axial, hoop, and torsional mechanical properties with unidirectional tapes by using a predetermined combination of wraps. Unidirectional tape also provides better fiber translation than do fabrics and yields a more weight-efficient tube.

Both material forms require cutting of patterns in preparation for rolling. Prepreg pattern design is determined by the product being fabricated, the material form employed, and the equipment being used for fabrication. Generally, tubes made from prepreg fabrics are convolute wrapped, whereas tubes based on unidirectional prepreg tapes can be either convolute or spiral wrapped.

Wrapping Techniques

Convolute wrapping of cylindrical (constant-diameter) tubes is by far the fastest and simplest method of rolling. A rectangular sheet of material with a length equal to the desired number of circumferential wraps is continuously wrapped around the mandrel. For thin-walled shapes, a tube can be wrapped in one operation. When making thick-walled tubing or when using materials with a high bulk factor, it is desirable to wrap the tube in multiple wrap increments, debulking in between wraps by applying and removing shrink tape on automated tape wrapping machines with consistent tape-tension control.

Fabrics, as noted earlier, offer a simple and extremely rapid method of rolling tubes that have a 0/90° fiber orientation. Patterns are sized to the tube length, and an integral number of circumferential wraps are placed on the rolling surface. The prepreg pattern is heat-tacked to the mandrel on a work table commonly referred to as a "tacking table." The pattern/mandrel combination is transferred to a rolling table, and the prepreg pattern is tightly rolled with controlled pressure.

Unidirectional prepreg tape is the preferred material when a combination of longitudinal and helical wraps is desired. Longitudinal wraps are easily accomplished by cutting sheets to the desired tube length and splicing them together to form a single, wide sheet for the desired number of wraps. Splicing can be done by butting the plies. Figure 8 illustrates the procedure for rolling longitudinal (0°) plies. The release paper is removed, the mandrel is tacked in place, and the pattern is simply rolled up. It is generally preferable to lay the pattern on the table with the release paper side up, because it usually has more tack, which makes it easier to start the mandrel.

Preparing the pattern is slightly more difficult if circumferential (90°) patterns are required. Typically, because tube length is greater than the width of standard materials, patterns must be spliced together. Although overlap splices are normally out of the question, thin glass tape may be acceptable, or the patterns can be butted and "tacked" together with a warm iron.

A workable solution is to combine the hoop patterns with other patterns to form an integral unit that facilitates alignment and release paper removal. For example, if the tube design dictates a 0/90° construction, the two patterns can be combined as depicted in Fig. 9. The best way to accomplish this is to lay one pattern face down on top of the next pattern. The overlap zone should be firmly pressed together, using heat if necessary, to form a good bond. For volume production these patterns can be stacked for later use, at which time the release paper can be removed. Because the overlap is accomplished with the second pattern on top of the first, rolling is easier. If the overlap were on the underside, it could peel as it winds around the mandrel. The amount of overlap to use is at the designer's discretion. If the tube design indicates a precise ply-stacking sequence allowing no commingling of plies, the most exacting designer would not want to allow any overlaps in which case spiral wrapping should be considered. In convolute wrapping, at least one circumferential wrap overlap should be used.

With thin prepregs, a full overlap (double ply) could be used, although it is usually easier to start wrapping with a one-ply thickness before moving into the two-ply-thick material. Good design practice dictates that the overlap be made in equal circumferential wrap increments. If overlapping is used, the pattern size should be adjusted to accommodate the change in thickness.

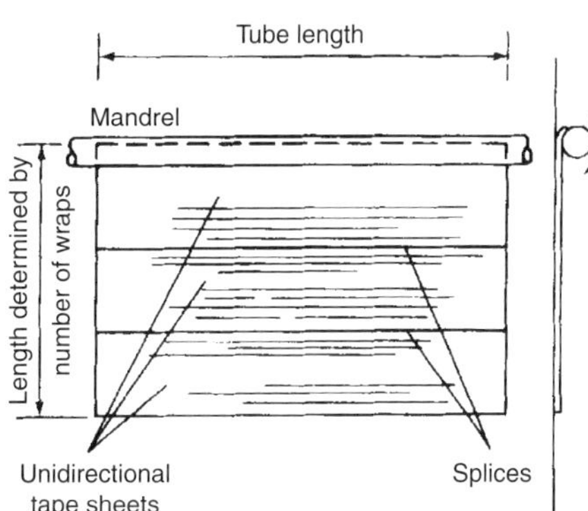

Fig. 8 Unidirectional tape, longitudinal ply rolling

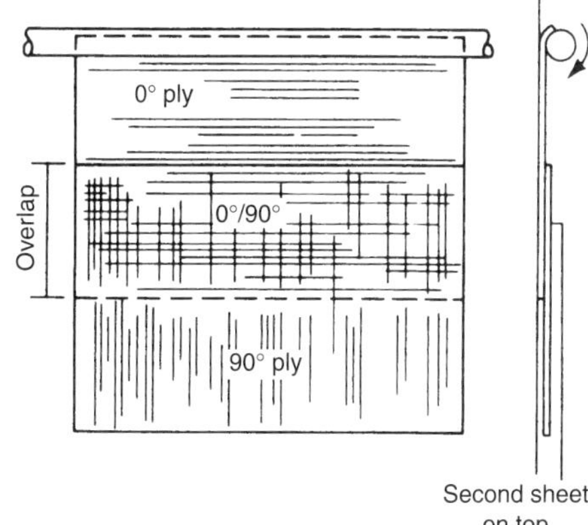

Fig. 9 Unidirectional tape, 0/90° rolling

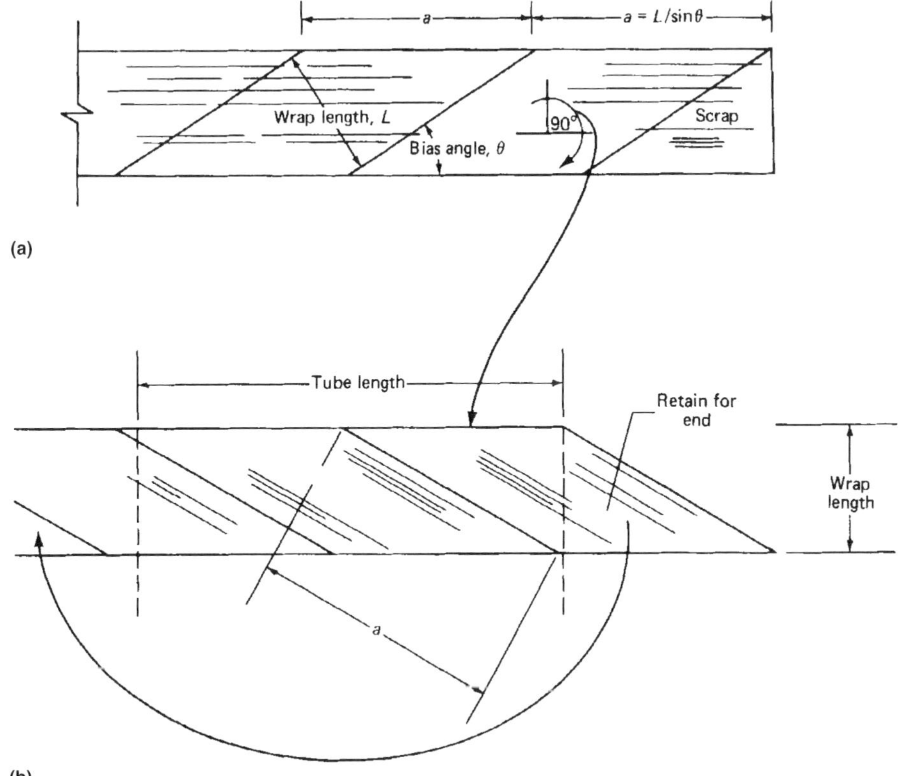

Fig. 10 Generating bias tape from unidirectional tape. (a) Unidirectional tape, bias cuts. (b) Bias tape lay-up

For angle patterns, the unidirectional tape must be converted into a bias tape (Fig. 10). Unidirectional tape is cut at the desired bias angle, with the length of each sheet being determined by the number of wraps desired. The bias sheets are then rotated 90° and spliced together to create a continuous bias tape that can then be cut into the desired patterns. Taping together the sides with the release paper is preferable. By exercising care in the cutting operation, precise angle control can be maintained.

Once the patterns are cut, it is usually best to overlap the opposing angle patterns before rolling. This facilitates release paper removal and helps maintain pattern integrity. The amount of overlap is a matter of choice, but integral multiples of the circumference (clocking) are desirable. Although overlapping is considered undesirable by some because of the commingling of plies, it is usually superior to rolling individual plies. Overlapping helps to align the plies, remove release paper, and hold the pieces together during handling and rolling. These benefits should outweigh any detrimental effects of ply commingling.

Convolute wrapping of tapered tubes is similar to rolling constant-diameter tubes, except that tapered patterns are used and provisions must be made to allow the mandrel to roll along a curvilinear path during rolling, as shown in Fig. 11. Commercially available rolling tables compensate for this lateral shift.

If precise fiber alignment is required, multiple convolute wrapping can present a problem. This is best illustrated by considering a multiple wrap using unidirectional tape. Figure 12(a) presents the usual approach of cutting a symmetrical pattern from the tape without regard to scrap. A close examination of the pattern shows that not all fibers are continuous, which could be a problem, although overlapping during wrapping can provide good fiber translation.

Starting the mandrel so that it is parallel to the fibers and then rolling it straight, on the mandrel, turns out to be difficult, as illustrated in Fig. 12(b). Because the mandrel is tapered, it must roll along an arc, which causes the fibers to be off-axis. Also, an uneven buildup on the mandrel would make it difficult to roll or to obtain good compaction. Starting the mandrel parallel to an edge, as shown in Fig. 12(c), improves the quality of rolling but does not alter the fiber misalignment problem. Moreover, starting the rolling with short discontinuous fibers is sometimes difficult. Figure 12(d) presents an alternative for one who accepts the fact that one must live with some fiber misalignment when convolute-wrapping taper tubes. In Fig. 12(d), the pattern is cut with one side parallel to the fiber direction. With the continuous fibers along the starting edge, the rolling process is easier to start, as shown in Fig. 12(e).

Figure 12(f) presents the preferred no-scrap method for cutting multiple tapered patterns. A sheet is sized for an even number of patterns, and a simple flip-flop cutting procedure will quickly and easily produce a large number of patterns.

Patterns that are cut as in Fig. 12(a) tend to compensate with a ± angle variation in increments of three layers, whereas wrapping with plies that are cut as in 12(d) and 12(f) tends to result in the accumulation of wrap in one angular orientation. This unbalanced angular wrap could cause problems with part stiffness and/or straightness if the angular deviation becomes too great. A greater than 5° angle change should be avoided. One solution is to wrap with single-layer patterns. This slow process is easily accomplished with longitudinal wraps but is much more difficult with high-angle wraps. A more desirable approach is to use spiral wrapping.

Path of mandrel

(a)

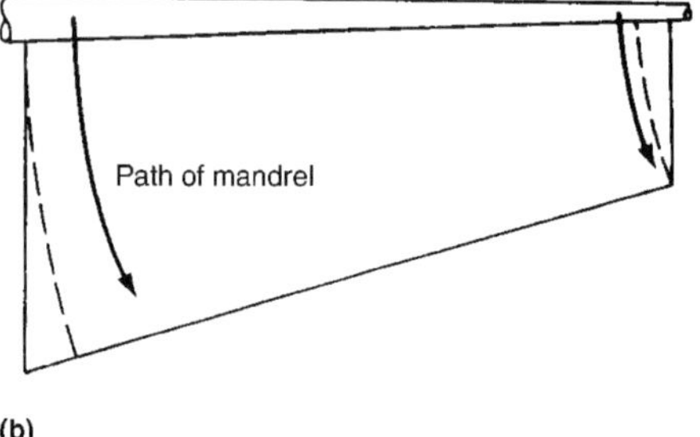

Fig. 11 Cylindrical versus tapered tube rolling. (a) Cylindrical mandrel. (b) Tapered mandrel

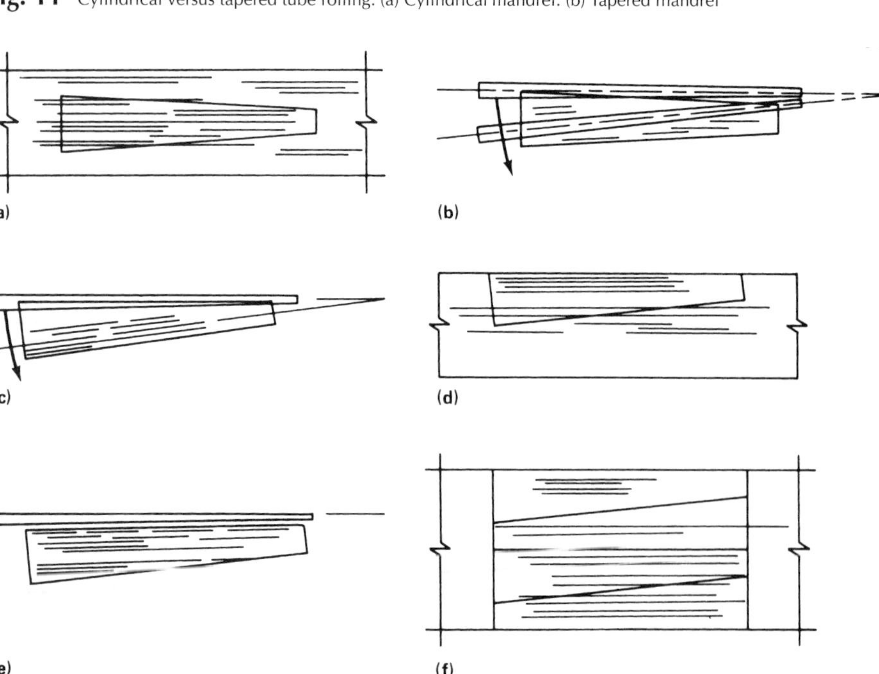

Fig. 12 Tapered tube pattern cutting and rolling. See text for discussion.

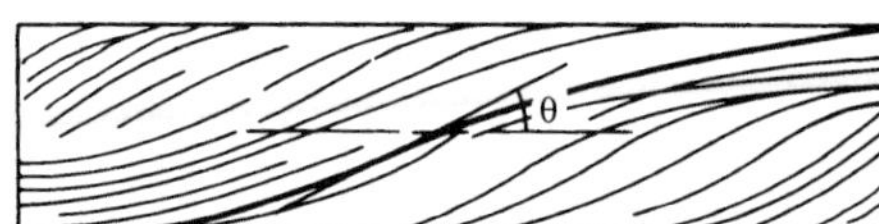

Fig. 13 Large-diameter shallow-angle wrap

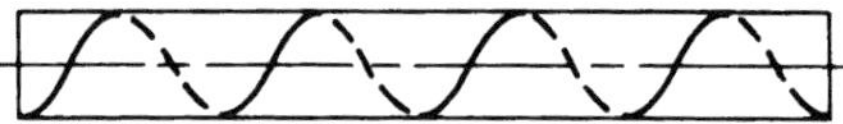

Fig. 14 Small-diameter high-angle wrap

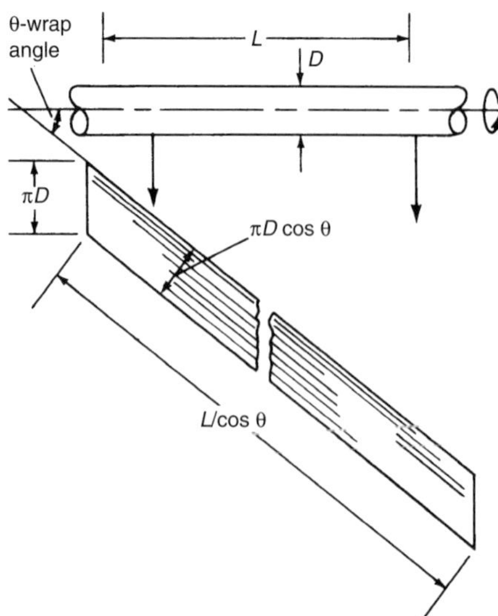

Fig. 15 Spiral wrap pattern, cylindrical tube

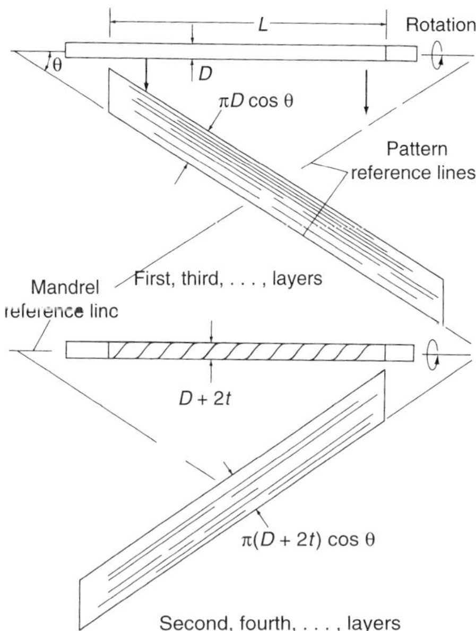

Fig. 16 Multiple spiral wraps

Spiral wrapping is an alternate method for making tubular shapes from composite materials. Hand or table rolling using spiral wrapping is slower than convolute wrapping because only one ply at a time is rolled. With automated wrapping equipment, however, spiral wrapping can be very competitive with convolute wrapping.

Spiral wrapping should be considered for thin-walled tubes to avoid overlaps or gaps in plies that could cause variations in circumferential stiffness (spine) or whenever precise dimensional control is required.

Single-ply angle-wrap applications also favor spiral wrapping because the fibers can be wrapped continuously from end to end with no overlaps or butts. Using ultrahigh-modulus fibers could also dictate the need for a spiral wrap design.

In the strictest sense, spiral wrapping can be used with fabrics, unidirectional materials, or even paper. In fact, most cardboard cores are spiral wrapped. The following discussion is restricted to structural tubing in which fiber continuity from end to end is required. Therefore, only unidirectional tape will be considered.

Spiral Wrapping of Cylindrical Tubes. The significance of spiral wrapping to structural tubing is in the application of angle plies. Longitudinal plies in spiral or convolute wrapping are equivalent with angle plies, however, spiral wrapping enables the designer to use the full capability of the composite by having continuous helical fibers with no overlaps or gaps. Spiral wrapping involves the use of long strips of material of a width determined by the tube diameter and the wrap angle. For short tubes or shallow angles, the wrap may not make one complete circumferential circuit around the mandrel, as shown in Fig. 13, whereas for long tubes or high angles, several spiral circuits around the mandrel will be needed, as illustrated in Fig. 14.

Figure 15 shows the pattern configuration and rolling procedure for spiral wrapping an angle pattern on a cylindrical mandrel. The pattern shown is a parallelogram with continuous fibers, and its width is a function of the mandrel diameter and the wrap angle. The pattern length is determined by the tube length and the fiber wrap angle. A few simple calculations show that as the wrap angle increases, the pattern width decreases and the pattern length increases. For very steep angles, long, thin patterns are needed.

The difficulty encountered in spiral wrapping multiple angle-plied tubes is that the width of each successive ply must be slightly larger to account for the diameter change introduced by the preceding layer, if a gap-free lay-up is to be achieved. Additionally, the mandrel should always be rolled in one direction, as in convolute wrapping. Reversing the rolling direction may loosen the ply previously wrapped, resulting in a poorly wrapped tube. With respect to spiral wrapping, this means that each successive ply should be started from opposite ends of the mandrel, as shown in Fig. 16. The first layer starts at the left end of the mandrel, with the pattern trailing off to the right. The second, opposing angle layer is rolled from the opposite end of the mandrel, maintaining consistency in the number of mandrel rotations. Also shown are reference lines, which are usually inscribed on the rolling table to facilitate mandrel and pattern alignment. Correct sized patterns and proper alignment should produce gap-free wraps around the mandrel.

Spiral wrapping of tapered tubes is similar to wrapping cylindrical tubes, with the exception that the patterns must be tapered to conform to the change in diameters of the tapered mandrel. Tapered patterns are generally cut on commercial roller presses that utilize simple steel-rule dies. Pattern lengths up to 12 m (40 ft) can be cut by this method.

For tubes with large diameter or steep tapers, spiral wrapping becomes less desirable because of the pattern shapes required. Not only are the patterns tapered, but because of the taper, the edges are curved (Fig. 17) and the advantage of end-to-end fiber continuity is lost.

To facilitate wrapping, it is usually desirable to start at the small end and work up the taper. This can be accomplished by starting the first ply on the under surface of the mandrel and the second layer on the top and by alternating for each successive layer (Fig. 18). In this way, the mandrel rotation direction is better maintained and compaction is achieved.

Outlook

Prepreg materials development is a continuous endeavor and the benefits of improved prepreg properties translate into newer and novel applications. Thermoplastic prepregs are working their way into advanced versions of parts that formerly comprised thermoset prepregs. The processing machinery is also changing to accommodate the higher temperatures required for thermoplastic prepregs. Production processes are being fully automated to reduce labor costs and to maintain part-to-part consistency.

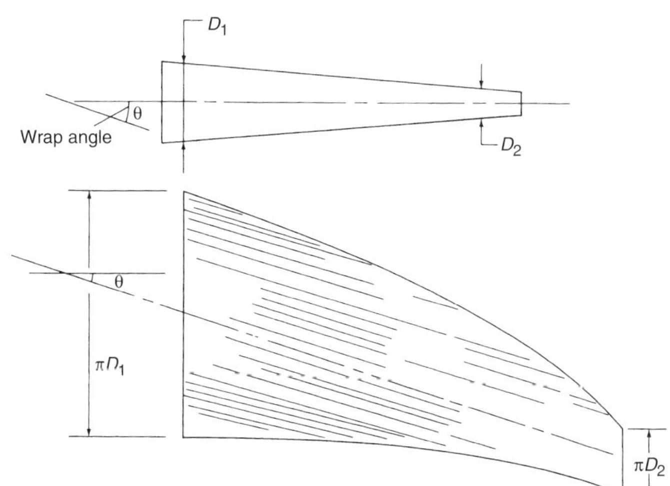

Fig. 17 Curved and tapered patterns for spiral wrapping large-diameter or steeply tapered tubes

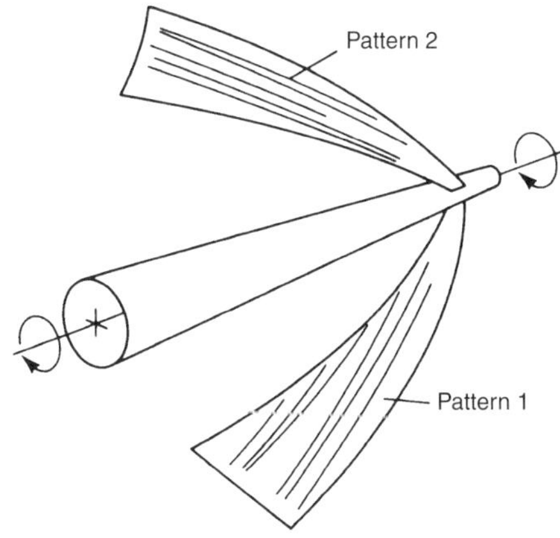

Fig. 18 Spiral wrapping of tapered mandrel

Thermoplastic Composites Manufacturing

B. Tomas Åström, IFP SICOMP AB, Sweden

THE GREATER PART of the "Manufacturing Processes" Section in this Volume is devoted to widely accepted and commercially important manufacturing techniques for polymer composites, and it so happens that with one notable exception (compression molding), these techniques almost entirely rely on the matrix being a thermoset polymer. The main reason for the lack of widespread acceptance of thermoplastic matrices is that they tend to be more difficult to process into a composite than thermosets. However, this fact does not mean that there are no techniques to manufacture composites with thermoplastic matrices. In fact, a number of techniques have been developed and are in limited use, and intense research and development efforts are underway to develop both new techniques and more easily processable thermoplastics. This article provides an overview of the more common techniques to manufacture structural thermoplastic composites. The term "structural" is used to refer to the ability to support substantial mechanical loads, meaning that structural composites are reinforced with continuous or at least relatively long fibers, thus deliberately excluding, for example, injection molding.

Characteristics of Thermoplastic Composites

What sets the materials discussed in this article apart from materials discussed in all but one of the other articles of the "Manufacturing Processes" Section in this Volume is that the matrix is a thermoplastic rather than a thermoset. It is relevant, thus, to first consider what influence the matrix type has on composite properties, processability, and cost.

There are small differences in the engineering properties of neat (unreinforced) thermosets and thermoplastics, although thermosets tend to be somewhat stiffer and more tolerant of elevated temperatures, courtesy of their (covalent) intermolecular crosslinks. Thermoplastics, on the other hand, have considerably higher strain-to-failure values, meaning that they are usually more damage tolerant. These differences between matrix types largely transfer into similar differences in the reinforced polymers. However, in-plane mechanical properties of composites are generally strongly fiber-dominated, meaning that any difference in the mechanical properties of the matrix tends to be obscured. In contrast, for out-of-plane properties and temperature-tolerance characteristics, which are usually matrix-dominated, such a difference may well be apparent.

Among the many issues that influence processability are matrix viscosity, processing requirements (e.g., in terms of temperature, pressure, and time), and worker health concerns. Low viscosity facilitates reinforcement impregnation, where each reinforcing fiber ideally should be surrounded by matrix without any voids. Fully polymerized thermoplastics have very high molecular weights, meaning that their melt viscosities are at least two orders of magnitude higher than melt viscosities for thermosets, which makes impregnation significantly more difficult. While some thermosets may be crosslinked at ambient temperature, other thermosets and all thermoplastics require a high processing temperature that must be precisely controlled to achieve consistent and expected properties. The higher viscosity of thermoplastics means that higher pressures tend to be required to achieve the same degree of material flow as with thermosets, but in many cases this difference is not dramatic. Whereas thermoplastics only need to be melted, shaped, and then cooled to achieve dimensional stability in a matter of seconds at the one extreme, thermosets may take several days to fully crosslink at the other extreme. In reality, the difference is considerably smaller, but it is generally true that thermoplastic composites may be manufactured more rapidly than thermoset ones. The very nature of thermosets makes them unpleasant to work with since chemical reactions involving volatile and potentially toxic substances are involved. In contrast, the molecular structure of fully polymerized thermoplastics makes them chemically inert if processed correctly, meaning that no hazardous substances need to be considered. Table 1 summarizes manufacturing-related properties and processing requirements for some representative matrices.

The costs of neat thermosets and thermoplastics are comparable, unless tolerance to high temperature is an issue. Then, thermosets are advantageous. Also when the starting point for a given manufacturing technique is some semifinished material form where part or all of the reinforcement impregnation has already been accomplished, thermoset-based materials are generally less costly (courtesy of their lower vis-

Table 1 Typical manufacturing-related properties and requirements for selected thermoplastic and thermoset matrices

Matrix type	Viscosity(a) Pa · s	Viscosity(a) cP	Temperature(b) °C	Temperature(b) °F	Pressure(b) MPa	Pressure(b) psi	Time(c)	Health concerns(a)
Thermoplastics								
PP	100	100,000	180–230	360–450	1	100	Minutes	None
PEEK	500	500,000	360–400	680–750	1	100	Minutes	None
Thermosets								
UP	0.1–1	100–1,000	20	70	0.1	10	Minutes–hours	Inhalation, contact
EP	0.1–1	100–1,000	20–80	70–180	0.1	10	Hours	Contact
	Up to 100(d)	Up to 175(d)	Up to 0.6(d)					

PP, polypropylene; PEEK, polyetheretherketone; UP, unsaturated polyester; EP, epoxy. (a) Matrix material prior to and during processing. (b) Requirements during consolidation (not conditions during, for example, preheating, flow, or cooling). (c) Relates to the entire processing cycle. (d) Refers to partly cross-linked matrix in semifinished raw material form. Source: Ref 1

cosity, which simplifies impregnation). However, under the right circumstances, the final component cost may end up lower for a thermoplastic composite due to faster, simpler, and, thus, cheaper manufacturing.

While thermosets clearly dominate in structural composite applications, the interest in thermoplastics is driven by several potential advantages, as summarized in Table 2. When considering this table it is important to keep in mind that no such sweeping comparison can ever be absolutely fair. For example, a high-performance thermoplastic matrix will contribute to better composite properties than a standard-performance thermoset (except in terms of cost).

Material Forms

The two main constituents in a polymer composite are the matrix and the reinforcement. The general types, forms, and representative properties are treated in the Section "Constituent Materials" in this Volume. However, for the purpose of this article, a brief recapitulation of material forms and representative composite properties is appropriate. Broadly speaking, possible raw material forms for use in composites manufacturing are the following:

- Reinforcement and matrix separately (for in-process impregnation)
- Molding compound (randomly oriented, continuous or discontinuous reinforcement at a volume fraction typically in the range 0.1 to 0.3, reinforcement partly or completely impregnated)
- Prepreg (short for preimpregnated reinforcement; oriented and usually continuous reinforcement at a volume fraction up to 0.6, reinforcement partly or completely impregnated)

In manufacturing of thermoset composites, separate reinforcement and matrix forms and molding compounds are the most common, whereas prepregs are the norm in high-performance applications. In contrast, in manufacturing of thermoplastic composites, use of reinforcement and matrix separately was more or less unheard of, due to impregnation difficulties, and molding compounds or prepregs were essentially always required. However, it is possible to impregnate the reinforcement as part of manufacturing starting out with a liquid monomer, which has low molecular weight and, thus, also viscosity. Following impregnation, the monomer is polymerized (but *not* crosslinked) to achieve high molecular weight (and thus structurally useful properties). This concept is not new, but it has essentially never made it out of the laboratory to see any significant commercial success until recently, due to unforgiving processing requirements that now appear to have been relaxed. Such in situ polymerizable thermoplastics may be used in many conventional thermoset manufacturing techniques, thus opening up a whole range of new opportunities for thermoplastic composites. However, with in situ polymerizable thermoplastics, the previously discussed good work environment facilitated by an inert matrix can no longer be taken for granted.

Fully polymerized thermoplastics are solids at ambient temperature and may be obtained in the form of pellet, powder, film, or fiber. Monomers intended for in situ polymerization are typically also solids at room temperature and, thus, need to be melted prior to mixing with the catalyst and initiator required to achieve polymerization. Courtesy of its low molecular weight, the melt temperature of a monomer is notably lower than that of the fully polymerized (high-molecular–weight) thermoplastic.

In both thermoplastic molding compounds and prepregs, the reinforcement may either be completely impregnated with the fully polymerized matrix (through melt or solvent impregnation) or just intimately physically mixed (through powder impregnation or commingling of reinforcing fibers with matrix fibers). In the latter case, melt impregnation must be accomplished at a later stage, either in an intermediate consolidation step or as part of final component molding. Fully impregnated thermoplastic prepregs are generally supplied as wide sheet or narrow tape on rolls. In most cases, the reinforcement is unidirectional (in the longitudinal direction), but woven and braided material forms are also available. Powder-impregnated and commingled prepregs are supplied as yarns, often woven or braided into a fabric, although fabrics may also be powder impregnated. Melt-impregnated molding compounds are supplied as rigid sheet, often cut to specification. In contrast, powder-impregnated molding compounds are flexible and usually delivered on rolls. Material forms that are already fully impregnated are bound to yield more complete consolidation and lower void content in the composite, but powder-impregnated and commingled prepregs have advantages in lower cost and better drapeability and in that they are easily woven and braided into fabrics.

Tables 3 and 4 provide indicative tensile properties of thermoplastic composites manufactured from different raw material types and forms with some thermoset composites included for references. Note that the tensile properties given are strongly fiber dominated.

Table 2 Qualitative comparison between thermoset and thermoplastic matrix composites

Property	Composite(a)	
	Thermoset	Thermoplastic
Cost	+	
Temperature tolerance	+	
Thermal expansion	+	
Volumetric shrinkage	+	
Stiffness	+	
Strength	+	
Toughness		+
Fatigue life	+	
Creep	+	
Chemical resistance		+
Available material data	+	
Raw material storage time (shelf life)		+
Simplicity of chemistry		+
Viscosity	+	
Processing temperature	+	
Processing pressure	+	
Processing time		+
Processing environment		+
Mold requirements	+	
Reformability		+
Recyclability		+

(a) "+" denotes a comparative advantage. Source: Ref 1

Technique Descriptions

Composite manufacturing requires precise control of temperature and pressure throughout the manufacturing cycle and throughout the material. The basic requirement on any manufacturing technique is to apply sufficient pressure to maintain the liquid reinforcement-matrix mass in the desired shape at a specified temperature for the time required for it to achieve dimensional stability. If the reinforcement is also to be impregnated as part of the process, a pressure gra-

Table 3 Representative tensile properties of glass-reinforced composites

Reinforcement form	Matrix type	Matrix/raw material form	Fiber volume fraction	Modulus		Strength		Failure strain, %
				GPa	10^6 psi	MPa	ksi	
Thermoplastic composites								
Mat(a)	PP	Melt-impregnated molding compound (GMT)	0.20	3.5	0.51	55	8.0	1.8
			0.30	4.5	0.65	70	10	1.8
			0.40	6.0	0.87	90	13	1.7
UD	PP	Melt-impregnated prepreg	0.35	28	4.1	620	90	2.1
UD	PP	Commingled yarn	0.35	28	4.1	700	100	. . .
			0.52	38	5.5	800	120	. . .
Fabric(b)	PP	Commingled yarn	0.35	15	2.2	350	51	. . .
Fabric	PA 12	Partly melt-impregnated fabric	0.52	26	3.8	350	51	1.6
Thermoset composites								
Mat	UP	Liquid (impregnated in process)	0.2	8.8	1.3	130	19	1.5
Fabric	UP	Liquid (impregnated in process)	0.35	16	2.3	240	35	1.5

PP, polypropylene; PA, polyamide; UD, unidirectional reinforcement; UP, unsaturated polyester. (a) Nominally in-plane isotropic reinforcement with randomly oriented fibers. (b) Balanced, woven fabric. Source: Ref 2-8

dient is first required to drive the matrix through the reinforcement. Manufacturing of thermoplastic composites involves the following steps:

1. Heat the matrix until it is liquid (or, alternatively, heat the monomer until it is liquid and mix it with catalyst and initiator)
2. Apply pressure gradient to impregnate the reinforcement (unless molding compounds or prepregs are used)
3. Apply pressure to make the impregnated reinforcement conform to the mold
4. Allow time for polymerization (if applicable)
5. Cool the material until the matrix solidifies and the component is dimensionally stable
6. Remove the component from the mold

With the exception of compression molding, which essentially always employs molding compounds, the following treatment concentrates on use of prepregs (containing fully polymerized thermoplastics) as raw material since prepregs have been and still are the starting point in most cases. With prepregs, composite manufacturing may be batchwise or more or less continuous. In batch techniques, the route from prepreg to final component may be divided into three basic steps: layup, consolidation, and molding. In the first step the number of prepreg plies required to form the desired postconsolidation thickness are laid up. The second step is to consolidate the plies into a monolithic laminate, and the third step is to form the sheet into the final geometry. In some cases two or even all three of these steps may be combined into one operation, but more commonly the steps are distinct and separate. In the continuous techniques, prepreg layup usually becomes an integral part of the consolidation step and sometimes also the molding step, which are accomplished on line through localized application of heat and pressure. This has given rise to the term on-line consolidation.

The mechanism responsible for bonding between thermoplastics is called autohesion and may yield virgin strength across a material interface in a fraction of a second, provided the surfaces are at sufficiently high temperature to allow significant molecular mobility and instantaneously are brought into intimate contact. While virgin strength may be achieved very rapidly in laboratory composite consolidation experiments, it is rarely possible to realize equally short consolidation times in real manufacturing situations. In most cases it is not autohesion that limits processing rate; it is the time required to heat and cool the material, since it has very low thermal conductivity.

While this article concentrates on relatively well-known manufacturing techniques, there are few limitations to what means may be employed to manufacture a composite. Thus, any process in which the liquid reinforcement-matrix mass is subjected to sufficient temperature and pressure is likely to result in a composite; whether the resulting composite properties fulfill requirements and the technique is economically feasible are entirely different issues. In attempting to understand the essential technical aspects of a composite manufacturing technique, considering answers to the following questions should prove helpful:

- What is used as a mold to give the composite its shape?
- How is the raw material made to conform to the mold?
- How is the impregnation pressure gradient created (if applicable)?
- How is the consolidation pressure applied?
- How is temperature controlled?

It deserves notice that most of the techniques discussed later in this article are known by more than one name, and the designations used herein are not necessarily the most common ones.

Prepreg Lay-Up. The most straightforward way of laying up prepreg plies to gradually build up a composite is to cut the prepreg by hand and, likewise, to lay up the plies by hand. However, in many cases automated equipment is used to cut the prepreg to size (see the article "Prepreg and Ply Cutting" in this Section). Layup of thermoplastic prepreg is similar to the thermoset counterpart (see the article "Thermoplastic Composites Manufacturing" in this Section), but a major difference is the complete lack of tack (stickiness) in thermoplastic prepregs, which may be artificially achieved through localized melting of adjacent plies using, for example, a soldering iron or a hot air gun. For melt-impregnated and solvent-impregnated prepregs the drape (formability) is also poor, and to permit conformation to the mold during layup, drape may also be artificially achieved through localized heating. Fabrics made from powder-impregnated and commingled material forms, in contrast, possess drape, but tack must still be artificially created. Following layup, the prepreg stack is consolidated and molded employing techniques described below.

Hand layup is naturally very time-consuming, but is nevertheless quite common due to the research and development status of many manufacturing operations. However, there are also automated means to layup thermoplastic prepreg tapes. Equipment conceptually similar to that used for automated layup of thermoset prepreg tapes (see the article "Automated Tape Laying" in this Section) may also be used to layup thermoplastic prepregs directly onto the mold. In this case the mating surfaces are first heated and then joined under pressure; see Fig. 1. If both the previously laid ply and the incoming tape have completely melted surfaces when they are joined, a separate consolidation step may not be needed, and the component thus is ready for removal from the mold as soon as layup is completed (meaning that layup, consolidation, and molding are simultaneously accomplished). However, due to the localized and highly nonuniform heating, it is most difficult to avoid residual stresses and component warpage, and it may therefore be more appropriate to only aim for partial (and thus more rapid) consolidation to ensure that the prepregs stay in place and then complete consolidation and molding in separate steps (as outlined in the following).

Table 4 Representative tensile properties of carbon-reinforced composites (fiber type varies between materials)

Reinforcement form	Matrix type	Matrix/raw material form	Fiber volume fraction	Modulus, GPa	Modulus, 10^6 psi	Strength, MPa	Strength, ksi	Failure strain, %
Thermoplastic composites								
Fabric	PA 12	In situ polymerizable liquid (impregnated in process)	0.54	63	9.1	790	110	1.3
Fabric	PA 12	Commingled yarn	0.56	65	9.4	830	120	1.3
UD	PEEK	Melt-impregnated prepreg	0.61	140	20	2100	300	. . .
Thermoset composites								
UD	EP	Solvent-impregnated prepreg	0.6	160	23	2700	390	. . .

PA, polyamide; PEEK, polyetheretherketone; UD, unidirectional reinforcement. EP, epoxy. Source: Ref 9–12

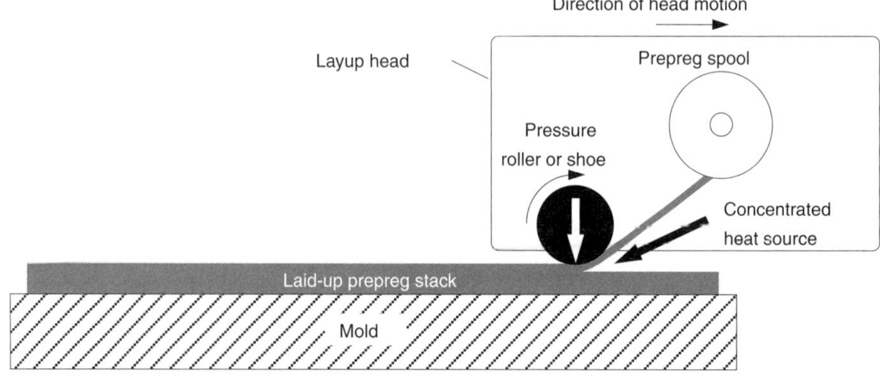

Fig. 1 Schematic of automated thermoplastic prepreg layup (resulting in partial or complete consolidation)

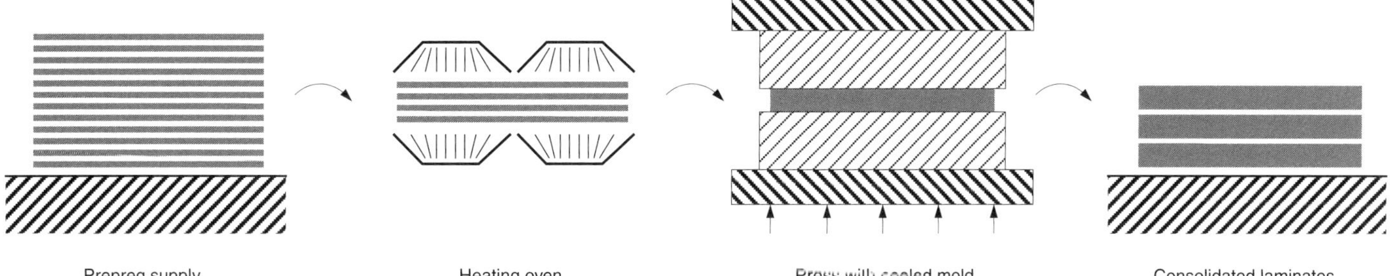

Fig. 2 Schematic of thermoplastic matched-die consolidation in press

Prepreg Consolidation. While a range of techniques is technically feasible to consolidate a stack of laid-up thermoplastic prepregs into a flat laminate (Ref 13), only a few are likely to be economically feasible for longer series: matched-die consolidation, double-belt-press consolidation, and calendering.

In matched-die consolidation, one or more hydraulic presses are used to consolidate the prepreg stack in a flat mold. One version of this technique employs an oven to heat the prepregs to melt the matrix, whereupon the prepreg stack is quickly transferred to a press with a cooled mold (Fig. 2). The press then very rapidly closes to apply sufficient consolidation pressure during cooling. This consolidation technique is best suited for fully melt-impregnated prepregs, and cycle times of less than a minute may be achieved assuming the matrix is completely melted when exiting the oven. In intermittent matched-die consolidation the incoming prepregs are heated in an oven to melt the matrix, whereupon the molten material is indexed into a press with a cooled mold, which closes to consolidate the prepreg stack (Fig. 3). The press then opens, the material is indexed again, and the process is repeated to gradually produce a continuous component.

A double-belt press offers one of the most efficient means of continuously consolidating prepregs into flat laminates (Fig. 4). The prepregs enter the press and are heated under pressure until the matrix melts, whereupon the laminate is cooled under pressure so as to exit the press fully consolidated. In this case, prepreg layup and consolidation are essentially performed simultaneously since the incoming prepregs are uncoiled from rolls of material through the forward motion of the belts of the press. In the related technique of calendering, the prepregs are heated in an oven to melt the matrix before they are consolidated in the nips between pairs of cooled calendering rolls (similar to rollforming as described subsequently, but with constant-diameter rolls).

These techniques to consolidate prepregs into flat laminates should be seen as a way to produce semifinished raw material for other techniques, including autoclave molding, diaphragm forming, compression molding, and rollforming, which are addressed separately subsequently. At least the latter three of these tend to yield better composite properties if the raw material is already fully consolidated rather than consisting of a stack of unconsolidated prepregs.

Autoclave Molding. In autoclave molding, prepregs are laid up onto a contoured mold, meaning that already during lay-up, the component more or less receives its final shape. This layup may either be performed manually or with some form of automated tape-laying equipment. The laid-up prepreg stack is then vacuum bagged in essentially the same way as thermoset prepregs, except that processing temperatures are so high that conventional bagging materials cannot be used. The prepreg stack is compacted and consolidated in an autoclave in a time frame of a few hours; consolidation and molding consequently occur simultaneously.

Since much of the early interest in thermoplastic composites had its origin in the military aerospace industry, autoclave consolidation has been used extensively. Although a technically feasible way to manufacture a range of aircraft components, the technique is not in widespread commercial use since it appears to offer no processing advantage over the thermoset relation. The only reason to select this route would be to exploit the inherent properties of the thermoplastic matrix, such as excellent damage tolerance.

Diaphragm forming may be seen as a derivative of autoclave molding. The main characteristic of the technique is that deeply drawn and geometrically complex components may be molded; examples include various aircraft components. The raw material is first placed between two flexible diaphragms. The diaphragms, but not the raw material, are then clamped around the entire perimeter, using a clamping frame, and the air is evacuated between the diaphragms.

In one version of the technique, the diaphragm-material stack is placed in an oven and heated to melt the matrix. The stack is then rapidly placed onto a one-sided female mold, and vacuum is drawn in the enclosed space between the lower diaphragm and the mold and/or pres-

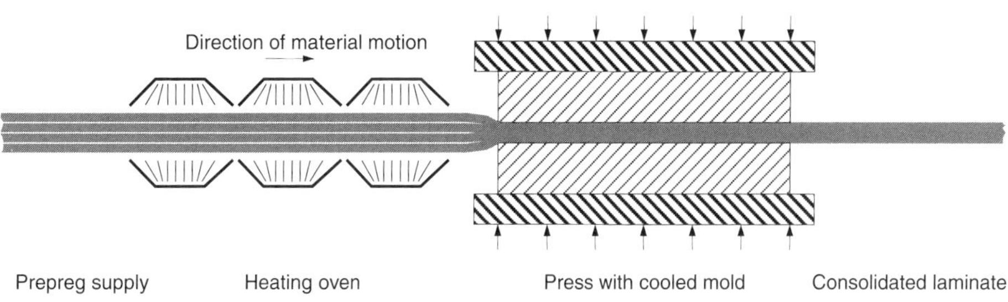

Fig. 3 Schematic of thermoplastic intermittent matched-die consolidation

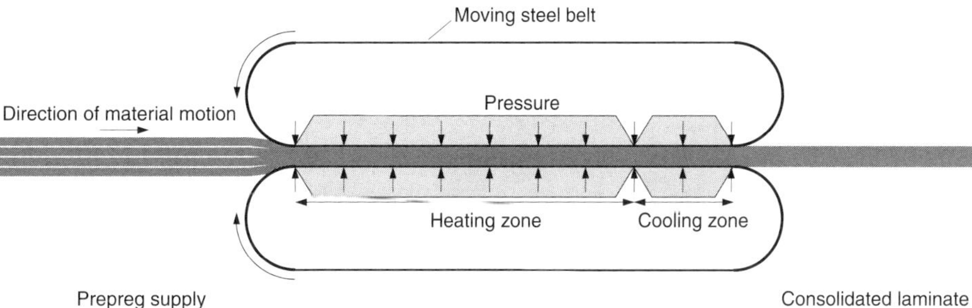

Fig. 4 Schematic of double-belt–press consolidation

sure applied above the upper diaphragm to force the material to conform to the mold (Fig. 5). Since the mold is likely unheated, the component solidifies quickly after coming into contact with the mold. With this technique, forming times are measured in seconds and cycle times in minutes (excluding preheating).

In another version, the diaphragm-material stack is fixed to the top of the thin-walled female mold and the entire assembly is then placed in an autoclave. Following evacuation of the air between the diaphragms, the internal autoclave atmosphere is heated to melt the matrix, whereupon vacuum below the lower diaphragm and pressure above the upper diaphragm make the material conform to the mold (Fig. 6). When forming is completed, the autoclave temperature is reduced to solidify the component. With this technique, forming takes only a few minutes, but the full cycle time is an hour or more. This version of diaphragm forming permits molding of more complex geometries than the previously described one since forming times are much longer.

Most types of prepregs have been used in diaphragm forming, but it appears as if investigations using melt-impregnated prepregs and fabrics woven from commingled and powder-impregnated yarns have been particularly successful. Diaphragms may be superplastic aluminum, sheet rubber, or polymer films. Rubber diaphragms have an advantage in that they may be reused, whereas aluminum and polymer films are permanently deformed.

Compression molding of thermoplastic composites is covered in more detail in the article "Compression Molding" in this Section, but for completeness, a discussion is also included in this article. Techniques to compression mold thermoplastic composites may be differentiated by whether they involve a significant amount of material flow to fill the mold or whether the material predominantly is deformed to conform to the mold. Randomly reinforced molding compounds, often called glass-mat–reinforced thermoplastics (GMT), permit flow since no straight, continuous fibers prevent it. In contrast, prepregs reinforced with continuous and aligned fibers cannot flow in the fiber direction without fracturing fibers, which is usually unacceptable.

The raw material is heated in an oven to melt the matrix and then stacked to form a charge that is rapidly placed in the cooled mold. Alternatively, long-fiber–reinforced thermoplastic (LFT) pellets may be fed into an extruder, which produces a charge that is quickly transferred to the mold. The press then quickly closes

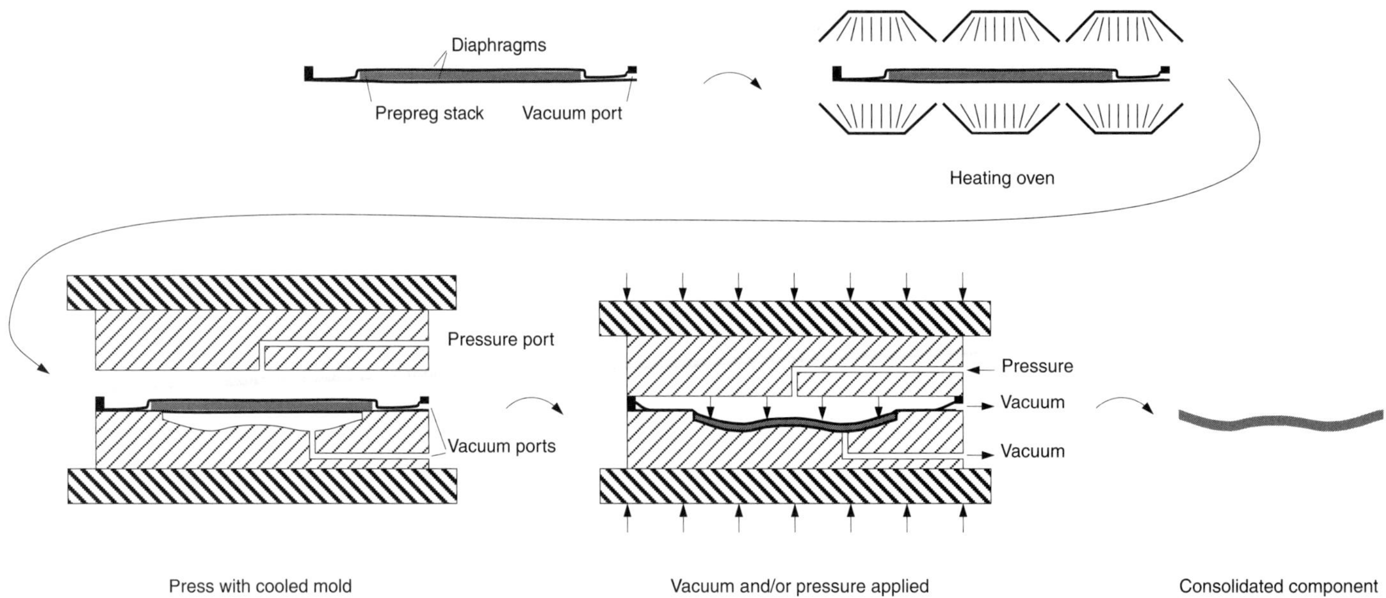

Fig. 5 Schematic of thermoplastic diaphragm forming in press

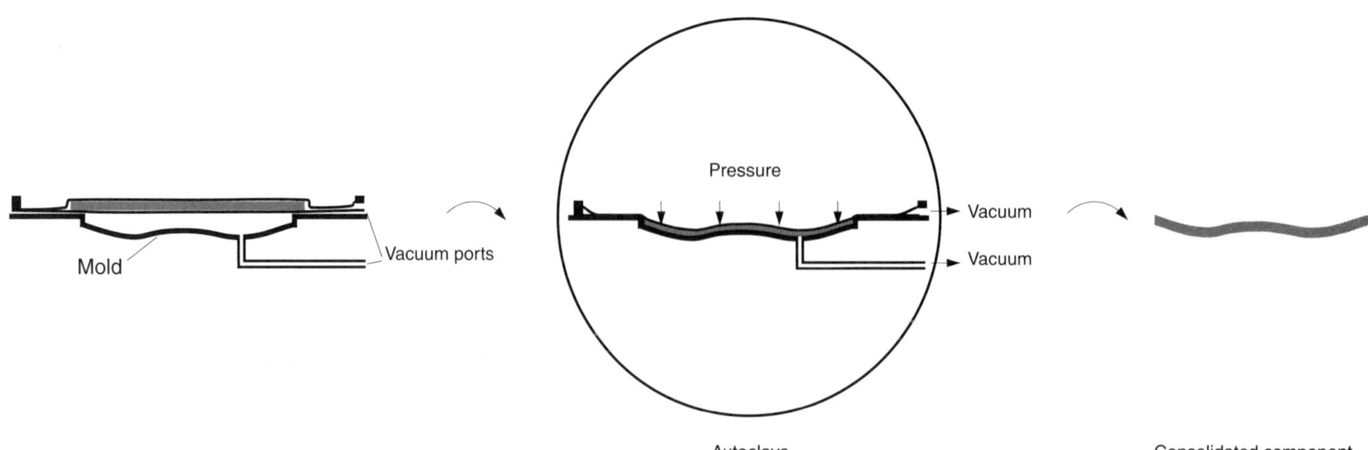

Fig. 6 Schematic of thermoplastic diaphragm forming in autoclave

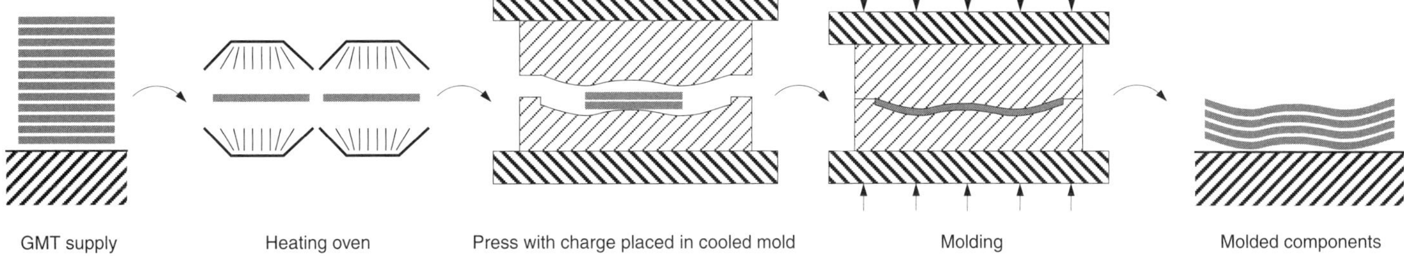

Fig. 7 Schematic of thermoplastic compression molding with molding compound. GMT, glass-mat reinforced thermoplastics

to mold the component before it solidifies and is ejected (Fig. 7). With GMT, the charge only covers about half the mold surface, meaning that material flow is notable. Since flow is significant, so is reinforcement orientation, and properties therefore may vary significantly within a component. In contrast, with continuously fiber-reinforced raw material, the charge must have at least the same in-plane dimensions as the component, and it is difficult to manufacture components with complex or deeply drawn geometries, which is relatively straightforward with GMT. Much work is ongoing to combine the good structural properties of prepregs with the straightforward manufacturing of GMT through a combination of the two material forms (but generally with the same matrix and fiber types in both materials). This may, for example, be realized by placing prepreg plies between sheets of GMT, where the latter flow to generate a complex component geometry. Work is also underway to develop compression molding techniques to manufacture all-thermoplastic sandwich components in which the foam, tube, or honeycomb core is based on the same polymer as that in the faces.

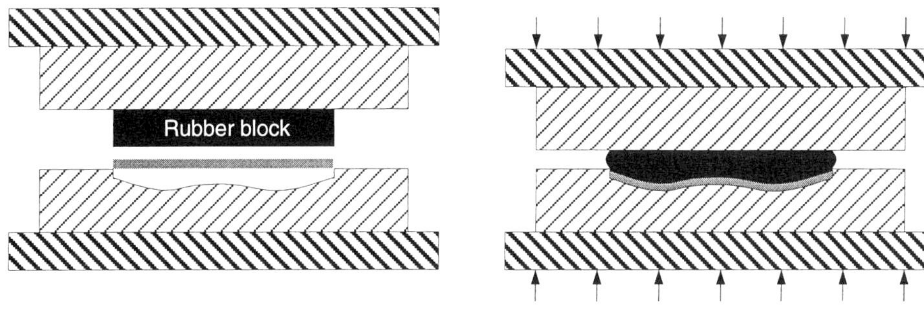

Fig. 8 Schematic of rubber-block molding

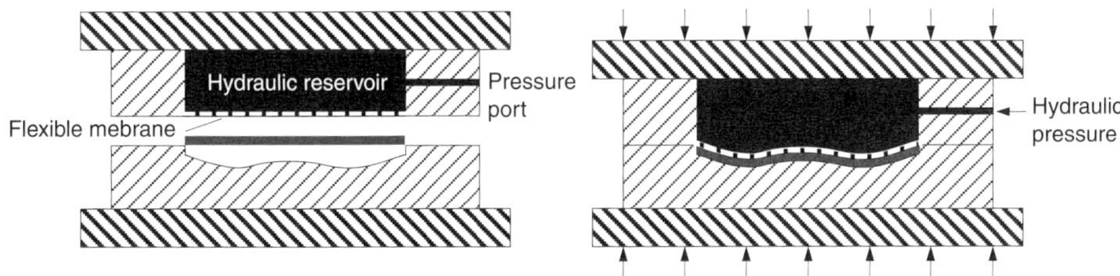

Fig. 9 Schematic of hydroforming

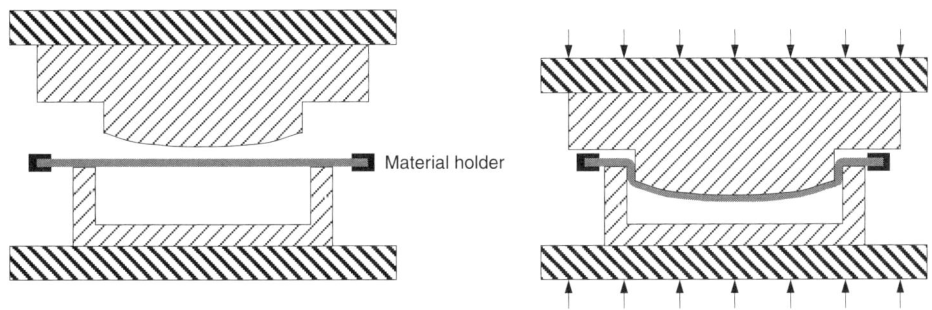

Fig. 10 Schematic of deep drawing

Compression molding of GMT is currently the only commercially widespread technique to manufacture thermoplastic composites with any appreciable fiber length. The technique is mainly used in the automobile industry, where the similarities with sheet metal stamping and thermoset compression molding have facilitated widespread acceptance.

Several modifications to conventional compression molding have been developed to permit molding of prepregs. Figure 8 illustrates rubber-block molding and Fig. 9 hydroforming, both of which reduce the risk of wrinkles in the component and employ cheaper molds. In hydroforming, a pressurized liquid is contained behind a flexible membrane that is capable of conforming to the shape of the lower mold half. Pressures may be significantly higher in hydroforming than in rubber-block molding.

In deep drawing the material to be formed is mounted in a frame that keeps it under tension until forming is completed. As the molten material leaves the preheater it is placed over a female "mold" essentially consisting of a frame the shape of the projected final product (Fig. 10). A male mold then rapidly punches the molten material through the frame and, since the male mold is cooled, the material quickly solidifies.

Melt-impregnated GMT is the most commonly used material form, but powder-impregnated GMT is also available. While it is the norm that GMT sheets are bought from a dedicated raw material supplier, in-house manufacture of thermoplastic molding compounds is becoming increasingly common. In molding of continuously reinforced composites, results are likely improved if preconsolidated composite panels are used rather than stacks of individual prepregs, since the time allowed for consolidation in most compression molding cases is very brief.

Roll Forming. In roll forming, several consecutive pairs of contoured, matching rolls, normally four or more, gradually deform the melted raw material to the desired shape (Fig. 11). The rolls, which are driven, are normally unheated, and they consequently cool the component. Roll forming is potentially capable of manufacturing any constant cross-section geometry, and components may be curved if desired. Nevertheless,

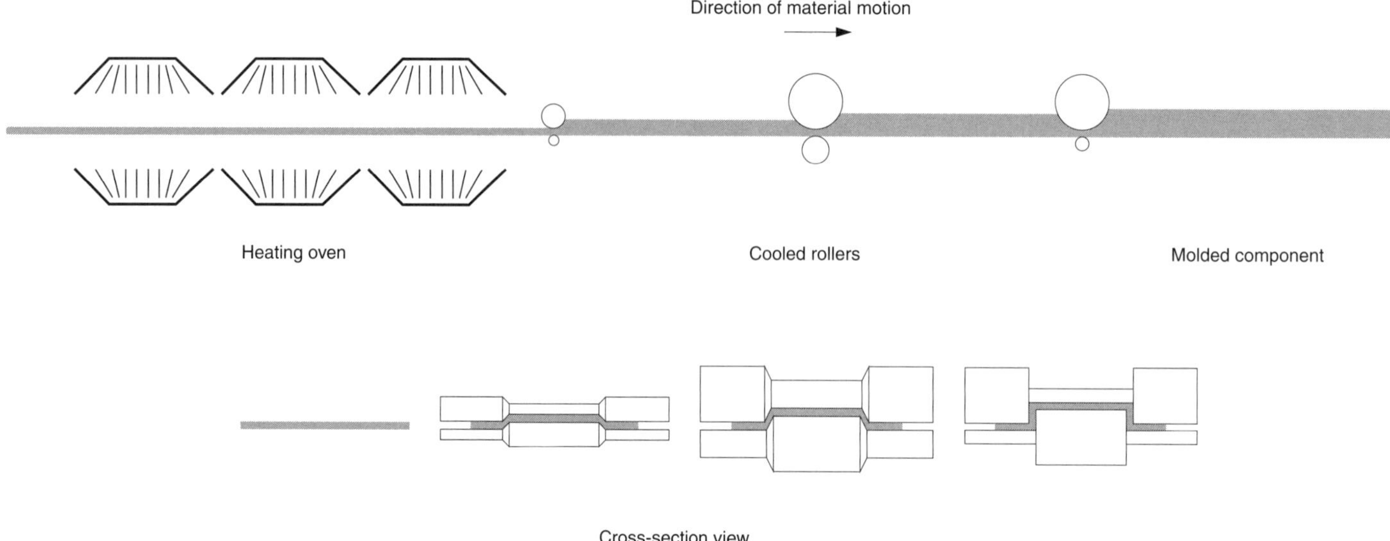

Fig. 11 Schematic of roll forming

so far thermoplastic composite roll forming has only been used to manufacture simple cross-sections, such as hat and Z-shapes. Most work to date has utilized preconsolidated panels as raw material, despite there being little reason why consolidation of prepregs should not be continuously carried out (e.g., with calendering rolls) in line with the actual roll-forming operation. Compared to most of the other manufacturing techniques described herein, little work on roll forming appears to be ongoing despite the technical feasibility of the technique having been proven.

Bladder molding is used to manufacture hollow products by means of an internal, pressurized bladder compacting the raw material against an external mold (Fig. 12). The raw material, usually in the form of a hollow braid made from commingled yarns, is draped over the bladder and is placed in the mold, which is closed. The bladder is then pressurized and the mold heated to melt the matrix fibers. When the matrix is melted and the reinforcement fully impregnated, the mold is cooled while maintaining bladder pressure. The mold temperature only needs to be reduced to where the composite is dimensionally stable, meaning that subsequent heating cycles need not commence from ambient conditions, thus reducing cycle time and energy requirements.

The liquid molding processes that may yield structurally capable thermoset composites, that is, resin transfer molding (RTM), vacuum infusion, and structural reaction injection molding (SRIM), all require that the matrix has very low viscosity to permit impregnation of the reinforcement present in the mold. Since fully polymerized thermoplastics have very high melt viscosities, direct adaptation of the conventional thermoset liquid molding techniques is not possible. (In injection molding, the short fibers are already intimately mixed with the fully polymerized thermoplastic, and this mixture is injected into the empty mold.) However, with in situ polymerizable thermoplastics, liquid molding may be realized since polymerization can be put off until the reinforcement is completely impregnated; Fig. 13 schematically illustrates such a process.

Filament Winding. Most thermoplastic filament-winding facilities have the elements of Fig. 14 in common. The prepreg tape is preheated on its way to the rotating mandrel. At the contact point the previously wound layer is heated and the incoming prepreg often given a further thermal boost. To ensure good consolidation, both surfaces must have melted surfaces when brought in contact. Heating sources that have been successfully used include hot-gas guns, infrared heaters, lasers, and open flames. To compensate for the low thermal conductivity of thermoplastics, the preheating oven may need to be quite long, and the mandrel may also be heated.

As long as only convex surfaces are wound, it may be sufficient to use back tension on the prepreg as the sole means of compaction. However, since the prepreg tape may be on-line consolidated in a fraction of a second, flat and concave surfaces may be wound without sacrificing consolidation quality or experiencing tape bridging, provided that an external pressure source, such as a pressure roller or sliding shoe, is used. Apart from permitting concave winding, on-line consolidation also virtually eliminates the need to follow the geodesic path to avoid slippage, thus allowing much greater freedom in geometries and reinforcement orientations than thermoset filament winding. Moreover, on-line consolidation may result in considerably lower thermally induced residual stresses than if the entire component concurrently went through the thermal cycle from processing temperature to ambient conditions. It is thus at least theoretically possible to build up any wall thickness without much worry of thermally induced residual stresses.

Since the matrix is melted for such a short time, it is natural that fully melt-impregnated prepregs result in better component properties than when commingled or powder-impregnated yarns are used, although all material forms have been used with success. Hoop winding speeds in excess of 1 m/s (3 ft/s) have been realized with laser and open flame heating using melt-impreg-

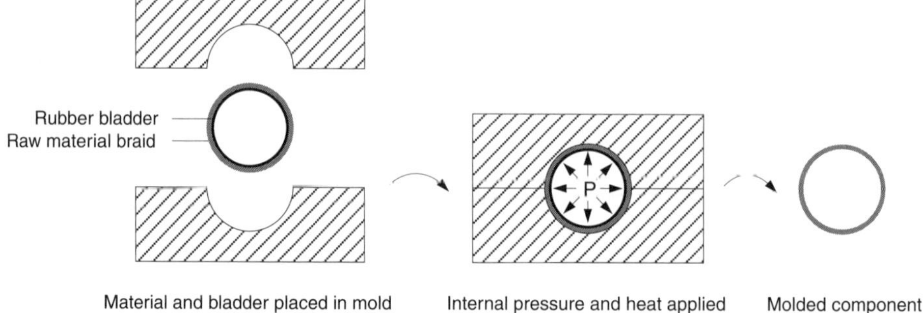

Fig. 12 Schematic of bladder molding

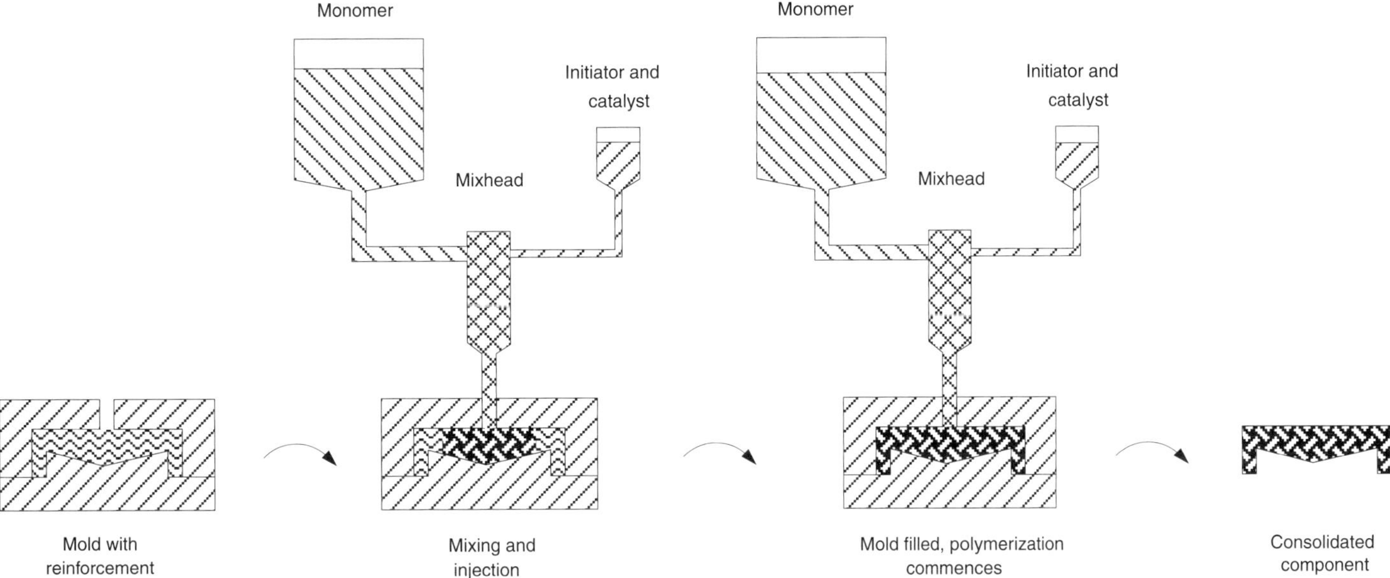

Fig. 13 Schematic of thermoplastic liquid molding. Source: Ref 10

nated prepregs, but lower speeds are the norm. Attempts at on-line impregnation with polymer powder and liquid impregnation with in situ polymerizable thermoplastics have also been carried out but have not been widely accepted.

Pultrusion. A basic thermoplastic pultrusion facility is schematically illustrated in Fig. 15. The raw material in prepreg form is pulled into a preheater and then enters a heated die, which has a taper where the material is gradually shaped to the final cross-section geometry before it is consolidated in a cooled die. Although one-piece dies have been tried, it is more common that at least two separate dies are used to allow higher temperature gradients. Consolidation is a gradual process that starts in the taper of the heated die and continues until the cooled die solidifies the matrix. The consolidation time is therefore a function of die lengths, die temperatures, and pulling speed. While speeds near 100 mm/s (4 in./s) have been reported for pultrusion of simple components using melt-impregnated prepregs, speeds an order of magnitude lower are more common. Ultrasonically vibrating dies are said to allow higher pulling speeds when melt-impregnated prepregs are used.

All prepreg forms have been tried, but there is little doubt that melt-impregnated prepregs result in the best component properties and the highest pulling speeds as long as the reinforcement is essentially longitudinal. To include nonlongitudinal reinforcement, it may be necessary to employ woven and braided material forms, and these are more readily available based on powder-impregnated and commingled yarns.

In order to improve process economy, the reinforcement should of course ideally be impregnated as part of the process in analogy with the thermoset technique. While various methods have been tried, use of in situ polymerizable thermoplastics in injection pultrusion is a technically proven solution that is being commercialized (Fig. 16).

Postforming. Localized postforming offers a simple yet effective means of making limited changes to already consolidated thermoplastic composites. For example, sheet and bar stock may be folded, flattened, and so forth through localized heating and subsequent forming. Despite the fact that if continuous reinforcement fibers are involved they are likely to buckle or fracture, line heating and subsequent folding of sheets and even sandwich panels has proven commercially viable in certain applications.

Outlook

While techniques to manufacture thermoset composites to a significant degree must be considered mature, most techniques to manufacture thermoplastic composites are significantly less developed, and the scope for technique improvements and innovation of completely new techniques is vast. The techniques described above have all been technically proven, but in most cases (with the exception of compression molding of GMT and the odd prepreg-based technique), they have failed to be economically competitive, which is generally due to the prohibitively high cost of thermoplastic prepregs. From this perspective, the introduction of relatively easily processable in situ polymerizable thermoplastics offers a very attractive opportu-

Preheater
Optional pressure roller
Prepreg spool
Concentrated heat source
Mandrel

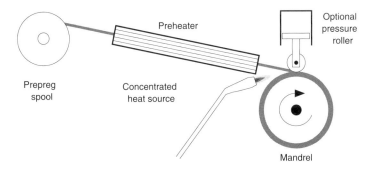

Fig. 14 Schematic of thermoplastic filament winding

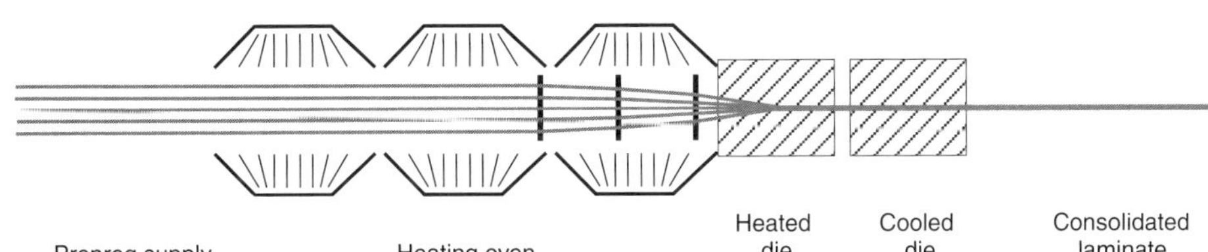

Fig. 15 Schematic of thermoplastic pultrusion

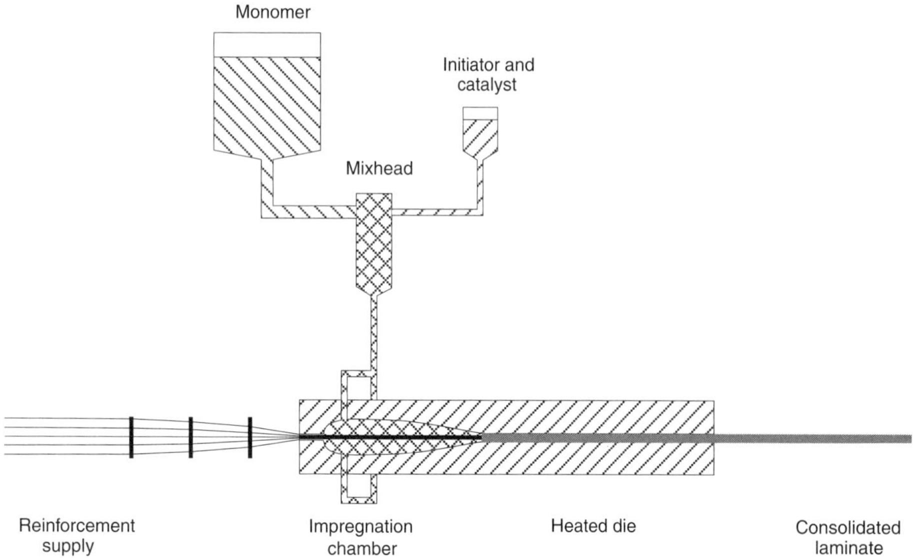

Fig. 16 Schematic of thermoplastic injection pultrusion. Source: Ref 10

nity, which is likely to bring on a transformation of the industry. While there will continue to be niche markets for composites manufactured from materials containing fully polymerized thermoplastics, in situ polymerized thermoplastics have a chance to capture volume markets since price and cycle times are competitive with the thermoset alternatives.

REFERENCES

1. B.T. Åström, *Manufacturing of Polymer Composites*, Chapman & Hall, 1997
2. N.L. Hancox and R.M. Mayer, *Design Data for Reinforced Plastics—A Guideline for Engineers and Designers*, Chapman & Hall, 1994
3. GMT Breaks Through in Automotive Structural Parts, *Reinf. Plast.*, April 1992
4. L.A. Berglund and M.L. Ericson, Glass Mat Reinforced Polypropylene, *Polypropylene: Structure, Blends and Composites, Vol 3, Composites*, J. Karger-Kocsis, Ed., Chapman & Hall, 1995, 202–227
5. "Plytron GN 638 T, Unidirectional Glass-Fibre/Polypropylene Composite," Borealis, Stathelle, Norway, 1995
6. "Commingled Glass/Polypropylene Roving," Vetrotex, Chambery, France, 1998
7. "Commingled Fabrics Glass/PP (Polypropylene)," Vetrotex, Chambery, France, 1998
8. "Product Information Vestopreg," Hüls AG, Marl, Germany, 1994
9. "Fibredux 6376," Ciba-Geigy Plastics, Cambridge, United Kingdom, 1991
10. "Advanced Composites with In Situ Polymerised PA 12," Ems-Chemie, Domat/Ems, Switzerland, 1998
11. "EMS Hybrid Yarns," Ems-Chemie, Domat/Ems, Switzerland, 1998
12. F.N. Cogswell, *Thermoplastic Aromatic Polymer Composites*, Butterworth-Heinemann, 1992
13. B.T. Åström, Thermoplastic Composite Sheet Forming: Materials and Manufacturing Techniques, *Composite Sheet Forming*, D. Bhattacharyya, Ed., Elsevier, 1997, p 27–73

SELECTED REFERENCES

Thermoplastic composite sheet forming

- D. Bhattacharyya, Ed., *Composite Sheet Forming*, Elsevier, 1997

In situ polymerization of thermoplastic polymers

- R.S. Davé, K. Udipi, and R.L. Kruse, Chemistry, Kinetics, and Rheology of Thermoplastic Resins Made by Ring Opening Polymerization, *Processing of Composites*, R.S. Davé and A.C. Loos, Ed., Hanser, 2000, p 3–31

Processing of Metal-Matrix Composites*

METAL-MATRIX COMPOSITES (MMCs) are a class of materials with a wide variety of structural, wear, and thermal management applications. Metal-matrix composites are capable of providing higher-temperature operating limits than their base metal counterparts, and they can be tailored to give improved strength, stiffness, thermal conductivity, abrasion resistance, creep resistance, or dimensional stability. Unlike polymer-matrix composites, they are nonflammable, do not outgas in a vacuum, and suffer minimal attack by organic fluids such as fuels and solvents.

In an MMC, the matrix phase is a monolithic alloy (usually a low-density nonferrous alloy), and the reinforcement consists of high-performance carbon, metallic, or ceramic additions. Reinforced intermetallic compounds, such as the aluminides of titanium, nickel, and iron, are also under development. Reinforcements, characterized as either continuous or discontinuous, may constitute from 10 to 70 vol% of the composite. Continuous fiber or filament (f) reinforcements include graphite, silicon carbide (SiC), boron, aluminum oxide (Al_2O_3), and refractory metals. Discontinuous reinforcements consist mainly of SiC in whisker (w) form, particulate (p) types of SiC, Al_2O_3, and titanium diboride (TiB_2), and short or chopped fibers (c) of Al_2O_3 or graphite.

This article discusses primary processing methods used to manufacture MMCs. A general introduction to MMCs is provided in the article "Introduction to Composites" in this Volume. Additional information on reinforcements and matrix alloys is provided in the Section "Constituent Materials." Extrusion, considerations are discussed in the article "Extrusion of Particle-Reinforced Aluminum Composites." Extensive property data are provided in the article "Properties of Metal-Matrix Composites." Other coverage of MMCs in this Volume can be found by referring to the table of contents and index.

Processing of Discontinuously Reinforced Aluminum

Most of the commercial work on MMCs has focused on aluminum as the matrix metal. The combination of light weight, environmental resistance, and useful mechanical properties has made aluminum alloys very popular; these properties also make aluminum well suited for use as a matrix metal. The melting point of aluminum is high enough to satisfy many application requirements, yet low enough to render composite processing reasonably convenient. Also, aluminum can accommodate a variety of reinforcing agents. Although much of the early work on aluminum MMCs concentrated on continuous fiber types, most of the present work is focused on discontinuously reinforced (particle or whisker) aluminum MMCs because of their greater ease of manufacture, lower production costs, and relatively isotropic properties. As shown in Fig. 1, however, higher performance composites are produced by more expensive, continuous fiber reinforcements. At the opposite end of the cost/performance spectrum are the particle-reinforced molten (or cast) metal composites. In between lie medium-priced composites, including those produced by preform infiltration and powder metallurgy (P/M) techniques.

The most commonly used reinforcement materials in discontinuously reinforced aluminum composites are SiC and Al_2O_3, although silicon nitride (Si_3N_4), TiB_2, and graphite have also been used in some specialized applications. For example, aluminum-graphite alloys have been developed for tribological applications because of their excellent antifriction properties, wear resistance, and antiseizure characteristics. Table 1 lists properties of materials used to reinforce aluminum alloys.

Processing methods for discontinuous aluminum MMCs include various casting processes, liquid metal infiltration, spray deposition, and P/M. Each of these processes is briefly reviewed in the following sections.

Casting

Virtually every casting method that can be used with unreinforced aluminum has been used with aluminum MMCs. These include the sand, gravity die (permanent mold), investment, squeeze, and lost foam casting processes as well as high-pressure die casting, which is emphasized subsequently. However, experience has shown that several modifications must be made to the normal melting and casting practice in order to produce high-quality castings from a com-

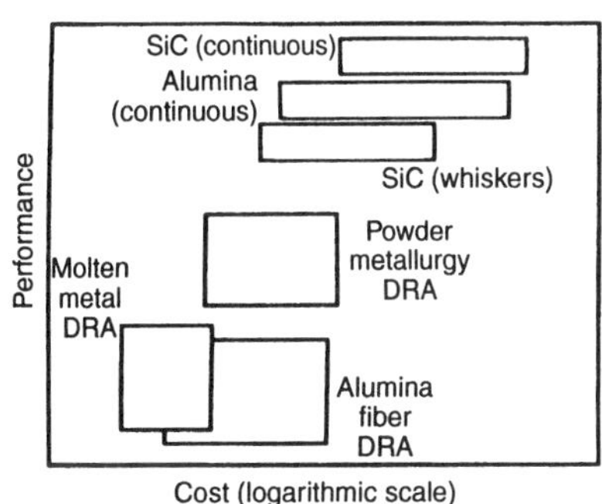

Fig. 1 The material cost versus performance of various aluminum-matrix composites. DRA, discontinuously reinforced aluminum

Table 1 Typical properties of particulate (p), whisker (w), and chopped fiber (c) reinforcements

	Reinforcement						
Property	SiC_p	Al_2O_{3p}	TiB_{2p}	Si_3N_{4p}	Al_2O_{3c}(a)	SiC_w(b)	Si_3N_{4w}
Density, g/cm^3	3.21	3.97	4.5	3.18	3.3	3.19	3.18
Diameter, μm	...	...	...	...	3–4	0.1–1.0	...
Coefficient of thermal expansion, $10^{-6} \cdot K^{-1}$	4.3–5.6	7.2–8.6	8.1	3.0	9	4.8	3.8
Tensile strength, MPa (ksi)	100–800(c) (14.5–116)(c)	70–1000(c) (10–145)(c)	700–100(c) (101.5–145)(c)	250–100(c) (36–145)(c)	>2000 (>290)	3,000–14,000 (435–2030)	13,800 (2,001)
Young's modulus, GPa (10^6 psi)	200–480 (29–70)	380 (55)	514–574 (75–83)	304 (44)	300 (43.5)	400–700 (58–101.5)	379 (55)
Elongation,%	...	...	...	...	0.67	1.23	...

(a) Saffil (ICI Americas, Inc.) (96% Al_2O_3-4%SiO_2). (b) >98% SiC. (c) Transverse rupture strength of bulk

*Portions of this article are adapted from M.M. Schwartz, *Composite Materials,* Volume II, *Processing, Fabrication, and Applications,* Prentice Hall PTR, ©1997. Used by permission of Pearson Education, Inc., Upper Saddle River, NJ. For additional credits, see "Acknowledgments" at the end of the article.

posite. Some of the differences in composite foundry practice are (Ref 1):

- Melting under an inert cover gas is at the discretion of the caster. Conventional degassing techniques, such as plunging tablets or gas injection, can cause nucleation of gas bubbles on the SiC particles and subsequent dewetting of the ceramic. Salt fluxing removes the SiC. On the other hand, a rotary injection system is available that can successfully flux and degas the melt. It uses an argon-SF_6 gas mixture. Additionally, simply bubbling argon through the melt using a diffuser tube can be used to remove hydrogen that has been absorbed by the melt.
- Close control of melt temperature is needed to avoid overheating and subsequent formation of aluminum carbide.
- The melt must be gently stirred during casting to maintain a uniform dispersion of SiC particles. The ceramic particles do not melt and dissolve in the matrix alloy, and because they are denser than the host alloy, there is a tendency for the particulate to sink to the bottom of the furnace or crucible.
- Turbulence during casting must be minimized to avoid entrapping gas.

By heeding these general guidelines, MMC ingots can be successfully remelted and cast using the current casting methods mentioned previously. Additional information on casting of aluminum MMCs can be found in Ref 2 to 11.

Melting. Aluminum MMCs are melted in a manner very similar to that used for unreinforced aluminum alloys. Conventional induction, electric-resistance, and gas- and oil-fired crucible furnaces are suitable. If a protective gas is used, the crucible should be charged with the gas prior to adding dry, preheated ingots. The ingots are dried at a temperature above 200 °C (390 °F) to drive off unwanted moisture, which could contaminate the melt. All furnace tools, such as skimmers, ladles, and thermocouples, also must be coated and thoroughly dried and preheated before use.

Melt-temperature control is standard, and, in general, pouring temperatures are similar to those used for unreinforced alloys. However, care must be taken to avoid overheating, which can cause the formation of aluminum carbide via the reaction $4Al + 3SiC \rightarrow Al_4C_3 + 3Si$. This reaction occurs very slowly at temperatures to about 750 °C (1380 °F), but accelerates with increasing temperatures from 780 to 800 °C (1435 to 1470 °F) for matrices containing a nominal 9% Si. The Al_4C_3 precipitates as crystals that adversely affect melt fluidity, weaken the cast material, and decrease the corrosion resistance of the casting.

Stirring. Because the SiC particles are completely wetted by liquid aluminum, they will not coalesce into a hard mass but will instead concentrate on the bottom of the furnace if the melt is not stirred. The density of most aluminum alloys is approximately 2.7 g/cm^3, while the density of SiC is ~3.2 g/cm^3. Therefore, the use of a stirrer that disperses the particles throughout the melt is recommended. (Any steel utensils immersed in the melt must be coated to prevent iron contamination and dried and preheated to avoid hydrogen generation.)

The stirring action must be slow to prevent the formation of a vortex at the surface of the melt, and care must be taken not to break the surface, which could contaminate the bath with dross. A scooping action, whereby the lower portion of the melt is gently but firmly made to rise, is the best method of hand stirring. Use of a slowly rotating, propeller-like mechanical stirrer is preferred by some foundries. In fact, results of laboratory studies indicate that the mechanical properties of the casting are maximized by continuous stirring versus intermittent (hand) stirring. When induction melting, the natural eddy-current stirring action of the furnace usually is sufficient to disperse the particles, although supplementary hand stirring (with the power off) is recommended to ensure that no particles have congregated in potential "dead" zones.

After stirring, the settling rate of the SiC particles is quite slow, due partially to thermal currents in the melt and to the "hindered settling" phenomenon. After 10 to 15 min, however, approximately the top 30 mm (1.2 in.) of the unstirred bath becomes devoid of SiC particles, although the distribution remains uniform throughout the balance of the melt. Consequently, it is important to stir the metal immediately before pouring, regardless of whether it was stirred during the melting and holding stages.

Fluxing and Degassing. A patented method of fluxing and degassing composite melts has been developed that uses a rotating impeller-like device to both stir the bath and inject a blend of argon and SF_6 gases. It also can be used to keep the SiC particles in suspension. The system employs a six-blade graphite impeller, which is connected to a threaded graphite drive shaft. A 610 mm (24 in.) diameter crucible requires the use of a 205 mm (8 in.) diameter impeller. Ten minutes of operation at a speed of 200 rpm usually is sufficient to shear the argon-SF_6 bubbles into an effective size. The thick, foamy dross that results is removed after the cycle is completed. Additional information on rotary fluxing and degassing can be found in the article "Nonferrous Molten Metal Processes" in *Casting,* Volume 15 of *ASM Handbook.* The melt can also be degassed by simply bubbling argon through the melt via a diffuser tube designed to provide a distribution of small bubbles. The melt should be stirred while bubbling the argon through the melt. A degassing time of 20 min at an argon flow rate of approximately 0.30 m^3/h (10 ft^3/h) can effectively reduce the hydrogen content of the melt to less than 0.10 mL/100 g for a 225 kg (500 lb) batch of molten composite. Some degree of melt cleansing or oxide removal is observed due to the attachment of oxides to the rising argon bubbles. The thick, frothy dross generated by bubbling argon through the melt should be continuously skimmed from the melt surface during the degassing period. Subsequent to degassing, the melt should be allowed to "rest" for 30 to 45 min without stirring to allow any remaining bubbles to float to the melt surface.

Pouring. It is neither practical nor necessary to maintain either an inert gas cover or stirring action while the liquid metal is transferred from furnace to pouring station. The recommended sequence of operations is to stir the bath thoroughly, skim off dross in the furnace, and then transfer the liquid to the pouring ladle (or remove the crucible). If the metal transfer involves pouring from, for example, a tilting furnace into a ladle, it is important to minimize turbulence in the metal stream to avoid entrapping gas. Tilting furnaces, however, generally are not recommended for use with composite melts. Pouring practice is the same as for unreinforced aluminum.

Gating Systems. The basic rules of running and feeding also apply to castable MMCs, including the use of filters that pass the SiC particles but trap oxides. However, the viscous melt behaves as though partially solidified, and the ceramic particles impede the free flow of gases. The composite is far less forgiving of turbulence than conventional aluminum. Thus, a poorly designed gating system can cause the formation and entrapment of gas bubbles in the liquid that remain in the solidified casting. Optimal running and feeding systems for castable MMCs are being developed, although many sound castings have been produced using existing schemes. More detailed information on gating systems for cast aluminum MMCs can be found in Ref 2, 5, and 12.

High-Pressure Die Casting

One casting process that aluminum MMCs have proved to be especially adaptable to is high-pressure die casting (Ref 8). The extremely rapid solidification rates achieved in die casting produce a very fine dendritic structure that is nearly pore-free and yields excellent mechanical properties.

Die Design. Aluminum MMCs have been high-pressure die cast without any changes to the die cast machines or dies (Ref 13). The dimensional shrinkage factor for these composite materials is in the range of 0.6%, which is similar to that of unreinforced aluminum alloys. In some cases, there is no need for alterations to the gating and venting of the dies that are currently used for conventional aluminum alloys. These composite materials can also be run with or without vacuum.

Flow Characteristics. Aluminum MMCs may be up to 50 times more viscous than their matrix alloy due to the fact that they are semisolid materials (molten metal/solid particle mixtures). The thixotropic behavior of these aluminum semisolid composites can best be used in high-pressure die casting. This is due to the fact that shear rates that are applied to the semisolid melt in order to inject it into the die cavity improve its fluidity. This combined with the fact that semi-solid materials are more viscous than their aluminum-matrix alloy means that they enter the die cavity with much less turbulence and less entrapped air.

To best use the thixotropic behavior of aluminum MMCs, a minimum gate velocity of 30 m/s (100 ft/s) is recommended. With this velocity, the composite material enters the die in an almost laminar flow, which has produced castings that are of a higher quality (less porous) than castings from unreinforced aluminum alloys poured under the same conditions.

Die Wear. A concern of the high-pressure die casters of aluminum composites is the effect of SiC particles on die life. The presence of hard (2400 HK) SiC particles in the melt raises questions about die wear and the effect on die casting equipment. However, analysis of studies done on aluminum composites show that each of the SiC particles are completely wetted by the molten aluminum. As the molten metal is shot into the die, only the aluminum, not the SiC, comes into contact with the die and/or die cast equipment. Therefore, aluminum MMCs should not lead to premature wear of the die or die casting equipment, because only molten aluminum is coming into contact with the die. As a result, conventional die steels, such as H13 hot work tool steel, are recommended for aluminum MMC die-casting dies.

Die Hold Time. High-pressure die casters have observed that productivity can be increased due to shorter cycle times. The shorter cycle times may be attributable to the unique properties of these materials. There are several factors that contribute to these shorter cycle times.

Because up to 20% of the melt is solid ceramic, less heat of fusion must be removed during solidification, and the thermal conductivity is greater due to the addition of the SiC particles. Therefore, with less heat being removed more quickly, the casting will solidify faster, resulting in shorter cycle times.

Aluminum composites can be poured at low temperatures (as low as 650 to 675 °C, or 1200 to 1250 °F), which is much lower than the normal pouring temperature of 705 to 730 °C (1300 to 1350 °F) for high-silicon (16 to 18 wt% Si) A390 alloy. These lower temperatures result in less thermal shock to the die and decreased die casting cycle times. A cycle time reduction of up to 20% has been observed. These factors can also result in increased die life due to less thermal stress on the die.

Compocasting

When a liquid metal is vigorously stirred during solidification, it forms a slurry of fine, spheroidal solids floating in the liquid. Stirring at high speeds creates a high shear rate, which tends to reduce the viscosity of the slurry even at solid fractions as high as 50 to 60% volume. The process of casting such a slurry is called *rheocasting*. The slurry can also be mixed with particulates, whiskers, or short fibers before casting. This modified form of rheocasting to produce near-net shape MMC parts is called *compocasting* (Ref 14–21).

The melt reinforcement slurry can be cast by gravity casting, die casting, centrifugal casting, or squeeze casting. The reinforcements have a tendency to either float to the top or segregate near the bottom of the melt, because their densities differ from that of the melt. Therefore, a careful choice of casting technique as well as of mold configuration is of great importance in obtaining uniform distribution of reinforcements in a compocast MMC (Ref 22, 23).

Compocasting allows a uniform distribution of reinforcement in the matrix as well as a good wet-out between the reinforcement and the matrix. Continuous stirring of the slurry creates intimate contact between them. Good bonding is achieved by reducing the slurry viscosity as well as by increasing the mixing time. The slurry viscosity is reduced by increasing the shear rate as well as by increasing the slurry temperature. Increasing the mixing time provides a longer interaction between the reinforcement and the matrix.

Compocasting is one of the most economical methods of fabricating a composite with discontinuous fibers. It can be performed at temperatures lower than those conventionally employed in foundry practice during pouring, resulting in reduced thermochemical degradation of the reinforced surface.

Pressure Infiltration Casting*

Pressure infiltration casting (PIC) is an MMC fabrication technique that involves infiltrating an evacuated particulate or fiber preform with molten metal subjected to an isostatically applied gas pressure (Ref 24–28). As in more traditional casting processes, PIC produces components to near-net shape. This is an important attribute for producing MMC components, because it reduces the amount of machining needed for these often difficult-to-machine materials. One of the most common composite materials fabricated using the PIC process is discontinuously reinforced aluminum (DRA) (Ref 24–26).

The greatest number of components fabricated via PIC are DRA electronic packages used to house and mount integrated circuits and multichip modules (Ref 29–31). The benefits of DRA to this application include a controlled coefficient of thermal expansion (CTE), which closely matches that of directly mounted integrated circuits, and a high thermal conductivity, which aids removal of the heat generated by these components. Components have also been prototyped for a number of applications in the automotive (e.g., brake rotors, connecting rods), aerospace (e.g., hydraulic manifolds, control links), gas turbine engines (e.g., stator vanes), and space propulsion (e.g., pump housings, flanges) industries.

*Written for this edition by Joseph M. Kunze, Triton Systems, Inc.

Process Description. Although there are several variations to the PIC process (Ref 26) for fabrication of near-net shape DRA components, all involve the infiltration of molten aluminum into a free-standing, evacuated preform by an external isostatically applied inert gas. The PIC process begins by inserting a reinforcement preform into a mold, which is placed inside a metal canister (Fig. 2). The metal canister is used to maintain vacuum inside of the mold and preform during the pressurization stage of the process. For the top-fill version of the process (Ref 24, 26), the canister typically extends above the mold to contain the molten aluminum charge. The entry port to the mold is sealed with molten aluminum through the use of a filter with sufficient surface tension to maintain the molten aluminum head.

An early experimental variation of the process is known as bottom fill (Ref 26, 27). In this variation, the mold assembly is sealed within the metal canister, and a tube extends down to a separate crucible containing the aluminum charge. The entry to the mold is sealed when the aluminum melts, and the end of the tube is submerged in the aluminum.

In both variations, the mold and the preform within it are evacuated. The most common method of evacuating the mold and preform is to place the entire mold assembly in a vacuum/pressure vessel and evacuate both the mold and vacuum/pressure chamber. The aluminum charge is then melted under vacuum, thus sealing the entry port to the evacuated mold.

In a variation of the top-fill approach, the aluminum is melted in a separate crucible and poured into the metal canister and onto the filter outside of the vacuum/pressure vessel (Ref 32). A tube leading through the filter and into the mold is then used to evacuate the mold and preform. After sufficient vacuum is attained, the tube is crimped and sealed. The entire assembly of both the mold and molten aluminum is placed inside a pressure vessel.

Regardless of the setup used, the mold and preform are heated to a predetermined temperature, so that the molten aluminum does not solidify upon contact and choke off infiltration (Ref 25). After the mold is preheated and the

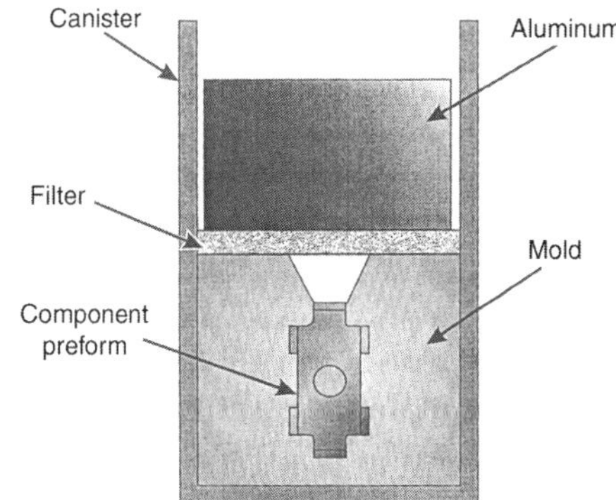

Fig. 2 Schematic of assembly for top-fill pressure infiltration casting

aluminum melt has reached the desired superheat temperature, inert gas pressure in the range of 2 to 10 MPa (300 to 1500 psig) is applied. The pressure difference between the gas outside of the mold and vacuum within the mold overcomes the surface tension forces of the reinforcement and drives the aluminum into the preform (Ref 33–35). As liquid aluminum infiltrates into the preform, the pressure acting on the mold quickly approaches the isostatic state. Hence, the mold only supports the pressure difference for a very short period of time so that large, expensive, and cumbersome molds are not needed (Ref 24, 26). To aid filling-shrinkage porosity, the mold is cooled directionally, and pressure is maintained until the entire casting is solidified.

DRA Materials Produced by PIC. The PIC process can produce DRA parts with a wide range of reinforcement types and volume fractions using both conventional casting and wrought aluminum alloys as the matrix (Ref 24, 26).

Matrix Alloys. Most traditional casting alloys increase their fluidity through the addition of elements such as silicon. Because PIC is a pressure casting process, it does not need to rely on the inherent fluidity of the molten aluminum in order to fully fill the mold and preform. This allows the use of off-the-shelf commercial alloys, which helps lower the cost of DRA parts due to the widespread availability of the alloys. Additionally, using commercial alloys enables the performance gain of the DRA to be easily ascertained. Discontinuously reinforced aluminum components have been successfully fabricated using familiar aluminum alloys, such as 2024, 6061, and A356, as the matrix (Ref 26, 33).

Reinforcements. Discontinuously reinforced aluminum fabricated using a preform provides a uniform reinforcement distribution with no segregation of the reinforcement during solidification. In PIC, the preform acts as a nucleation site for solidification and inhibits large grain growth during solidification and cool down, resulting in a very fine cast microstructure between the reinforcement particles (Ref 25, 36, 37). Additionally, because the preform is evacuated and the mold is directionally cooled, properly designed and processed components can be produced without porosity.

Preforms have been fabricated and pressure infiltration cast in a range of reinforcement levels varying from 30% to greater than 70%. Current technology does not provide for lower reinforcement volume fractions, because the preform must have sufficient reinforcement content to produce a stable geometry. A number of particulate reinforcements have been used to make preforms for the PIC process (Ref 24, 26, 33, 35). The most common reinforcements used are SiC and Al_2O_3 particulates. With a density only slightly lower than that of aluminum, boron carbide (B_4C) has also been investigated as a reinforcement—the close match in density means that settling of the reinforcement is avoided. However, at this time, boron carbide is not widely used in PIC, primarily due to its cost.

The Future of Pressure Infiltration Cast DRA. The ability to produce quality DRA components with the desired properties using PIC has been well documented (Ref 26, 29–33). The performance gains enabled by this class of material have been demonstrated by the number of prototypes that have been manufactured and successfully tested. As with most new materials and processes, the primary barrier to increasing the number of pressure infiltration cast DRA components in use tends to be the initial high insertion cost. Currently, cost issues are being addressed through the application of new technologies, such as rapid prototyping/manufacturing methods and computer modeling and simulation software. These technologies have the potential to reduce the cost and time associated with the manufacture of pressure infiltration cast DRA components. For example, new rapid prototyping and manufacturing processes are being applied to the manufacture of particulate preforms directly from a three-dimensional computer-aided design solid model and do not require any tooling. Computer modeling and simulation software enables the design and selection of initial processing parameters and thereby reduces the expensive trial-and-error approach to determining the optimal manufacturing process. In conclusion, as costs are reduced and the economics of various systems demand higher performance (e.g., greater service life, lighter weight, etc.), the number of pressure infiltration cast DRA components will increase accordingly.

Liquid Metal Infiltration

The pressureless metal infiltration (Primex, Advanced Materials Lanxide) process is based on materials and process controls that allow a metal to infiltrate substantially nonreactive reinforcements without the application of pressure or vacuum. Reinforcement level can be controlled by the starting density of the material being infiltrated. As long as interconnected porosity and appropriate infiltration conditions exist, the liquid metal will spontaneously infiltrate into the preform.

Key process ingredients for the manufacture of reinforced aluminum composites include the aluminum alloy, a nitrogen atmosphere, and magnesium present in the system. During heating to infiltration temperature (~750 °C, or 1380 °F), the magnesium reacts with the nitrogen atmosphere to form magnesium nitride (Mg_3N_2). The Mg_3N_2 is the infiltration enhancer that allows the aluminum alloy to infiltrate the reinforcing phase without the necessity of applied pressure or vacuum. During infiltration, the Mg_3N_2 is reduced by the aluminum to form a small amount of aluminum nitride (AlN). The AlN is found as small precipitates and as a thin film on the surface of the reinforcing phase. Magnesium is released into the alloy by this reaction.

The pressureless infiltration process can produce a wide array of engineered composites by tailoring of alloy chemistry and particle type, shape, size, and loading. Particulate loading in cast composites can be as high as 75 vol%, given the right combination of particle shape and size. Figure 3 shows a typical microstructure.

The most widely used cast composite produced by liquid metal infiltration is an Al-10Si-1Mg alloy reinforced with 30 vol% SiC. The 1% Mg present in this alloy is obtained during infiltration by the reduction of the Mg_3N_2. This composite system is being used for all casting processes except die casting. The composite most used for die casting is based on this system, with the addition of 1% Fe. Alloy modifications can be made to the alloy prior to infiltration or in the crucible prior to casting. The only universal alloy restriction for this composite system is the presence of magnesium to allow the formation of the Mg_3N_2. For the SiC-containing systems, silicon must also be present in sufficient quantity to suppress the formation of Al_4C_3. Composites consisting of Al_2O_3-reinforced aluminum that exhibit low excessive wear rates are also produced.

An important application area for pressureless molten metal infiltration is Al-SiC_p packages, substrates, and support structures for electronic components. Typical requirements include a controlled CTE to reduce mechanical stresses imposed on the electronic device during attachment and operation, high thermal conductivity for heat dissipation, high stiffness to minimize distortion, and low density for minimum weight. Compared with conventional aluminum alloys, composites having high loadings of SiC particles feature greatly reduced CTEs and significantly higher elastic moduli, with little or no penalty in thermal conductivity or density.

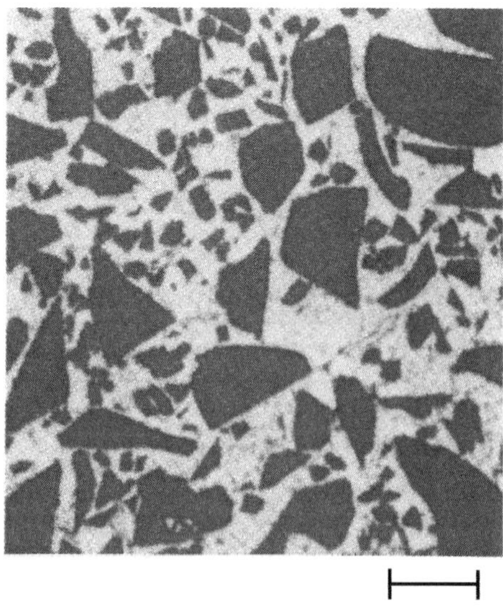

Fig. 3 Discontinuous Al-SiC MMC (60 vol% SiC) produced by the liquid metal infiltration process

Spray Deposition

Spray deposition involves atomizing a melt and, rather than allowing the droplets to solidify totally as for metal powder manufacture, collecting the semisolid droplets on a substrate. The process is a hybrid rapid solidification process, because the metal experiences a rapid transition through the liquidus to the solidus, followed by slow cooling from the solidus to room temperature. This results in a refined grain and precipitation structure with no significant increase in solute solubility.

The production of MMC ingot by spray deposition can be accomplished by introducing particulate into the standard spray deposition metal spray, leading to codeposition with the atomized metal onto the substrate. Careful control of the atomizing and particulate feeding conditions is required to ensure that a uniform distribution of particulate is produced within a typically 95 to 98% dense aluminum matrix.

A number of aluminum alloys containing SiC particulate have been produced by spray deposition. These include aluminum-silicon casting alloys and the 2xxx, 6xxx, 7xxx, and 8xxx (aluminum-lithium) series wrought alloys. Significant increases in specific modulus have been realized with SiC-reinforced 8090 alloy. Products that have been produced by spray deposition include solid and hollow extrusions, forgings, sheet, and remelted pressure die castings.

Spray deposition was developed commercially in the late 1970s and throughout the 1980s by Osprey, Ltd. (Neath, United Kingdom) as a method of building up bulk material by atomizing a molten stream of metal with jets of cold gas. Most such processes are covered by their patents or licenses and are now generally referred to as Osprey processes (Ref 38–40). The potential for adapting the procedure to particulate MMC production by injection of ceramic powder into the spray was recognized at an early stage and has been developed by a number of primary metal producers (Ref 41, 42).

A feature of much MMC material produced by the Osprey route is a tendency toward inhomogeneous distribution of the ceramic particles. It is common to observe ceramic-rich layers approximately normal to the overall growth direction. Among the other notable microstructural features of Osprey MMC material are a strong interfacial bond, little or no interfacial reaction layer, and a very low oxide content. Porosity in the as-sprayed state is typically about 5%, but this is normally eliminated by secondary processing. A number of commercial alloys have been explored for use in Osprey route MMCs (Ref 43–45).

Spray forming in the Osprey mode involves the sequential stages of atomization and droplet consolidation to produce near-net shape preforms in a single processing step. The as-sprayed material has a density greater than 98% of the theoretical density and exhibits a uniform distribution of fine equiaxed grains and no prior particle boundaries or discernible macroscopic segregation. Mechanical properties are normally isotropic and meet or exceed those of counterpart ingot-processed alloys. A major attraction of the process is its high rate of metal deposition, typically in the range 0.2 to 2.0 kg/s (0.4 to 4.4 lb/s).

Commercial viability mandates close tolerances in shape and dimensions, as well as consistency in microstructure and product yield. This requires an understanding of and control over the effects of several independent process parameters, namely: melt superheat, metal flow rate, gas pressure, spray motion (spray scanning frequency and angle), spray height (distance between the gas nozzles and the substrate), and substrate motion (substrate rotation speed, withdrawal rate, and tilt angle).

Powder Metallurgy Methods

Powder metallurgy processing of aluminum MMCs (Ref 46, 47) involves both SiC particulates and whiskers, although Al_2O_3 particles and Si_3N_4 whiskers have also been employed. Processing involves (1) blending of the gas-atomized matrix alloy and reinforcement in powder form; (2) compacting (cold pressing) the homogeneous blend to roughly 80% density; (3) degassing the preform (which has an open interconnected pore structure) to remove volatile contaminants (lubricants and mixing and blending additives), water vapor, and gases; and (4) consolidation by vacuum hot pressing or hot isostatic pressing. The hot pressed cylindrical billets can be subsequently extruded, rolled, or forged.

Whisker-reinforced aluminum MMCs may experience some whisker alignment during extrusion or rolling (Fig. 4). Control of whisker alignment enables production of aluminum MMC product forms with directional properties needed for some high-performance applications. Cross rolling of sheet establishes a more planar whisker alignment, producing a two-dimensional isotropy. The mechanical properties of whisker-reinforced aluminum MMCs are superior to particle-reinforced composites at any common volume fraction (Fig. 5).

Powder metallurgy methods involving cold pressing and sintering, or hot pressing, to produce MMCs are shown in Fig. 6 and 7 (Ref 48–50). The matrix and the reinforcement powders are blended to produce a homogeneous distribution. The blending stage is followed by cold pressing to produce what is called a *green body,* which is about 80% dense and can be easily handled. The cold pressed green body is canned in a sealed container and degassed to remove any absorbed moisture from the particle surfaces. The final step is hot pressing, uniaxial or isostatic, to produce a fully dense composite. The hot pressing temperature can be either below or above that of the matrix alloy solidus.

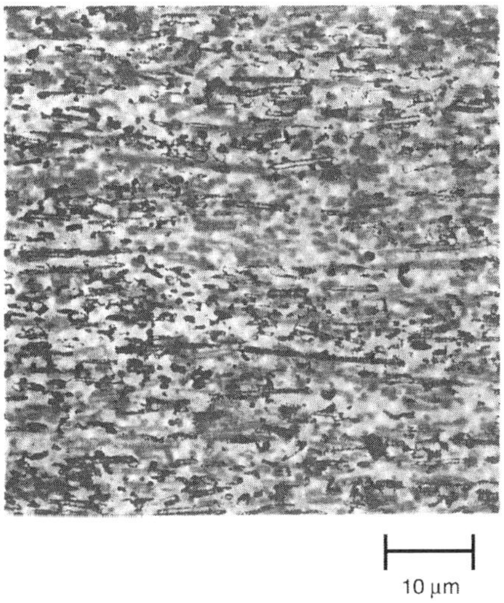

Fig. 4 SiC whisker-reinforced (20 vol% SiC) aluminum alloy sheet with the whiskers aligned in the direction of rolling

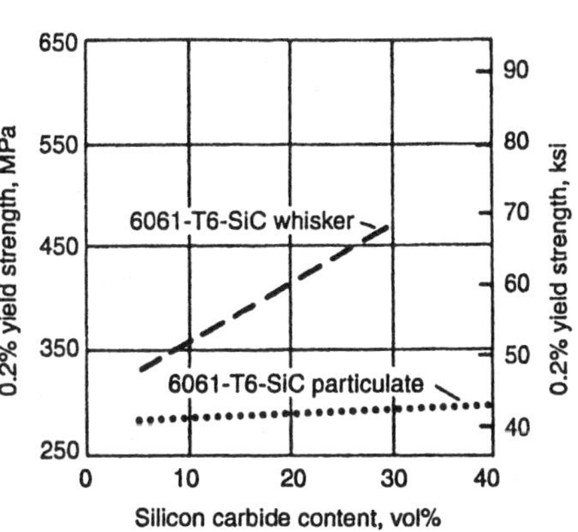

Fig. 5 Yield strength comparison between whisker- and particulate-reinforced aluminum MMCs

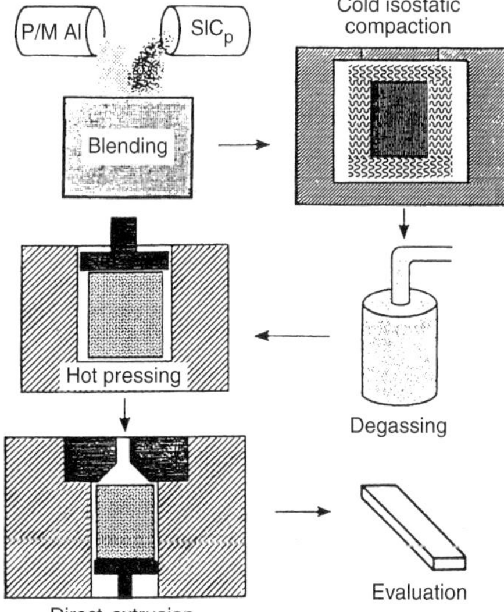

Fig. 6 Schematic interpretation of the processing route for P/M Al-SiC$_p$ composites. Source: Ref 48

The P/M hot pressing technique generally produces properties superior to those obtained by casting and by liquid metal infiltration (squeeze casting) techniques. Because no melting and casting are involved, the powder process for MMCs is more economical than many other fabrication techniques and offers several advantages, including the following:

- A lower temperature can be used during preparation of a P/M-based composite compared to preparation of a fusion metallurgy-based composite. This results in less interaction between the matrix and the reinforcement, consequently minimizing undesirable interfacial reactions, which leads to improved mechanical properties.
- The preparation of particulate- or whisker-reinforced composites is, generally speaking, easier using the P/M blending technique than it is using the casting technique.

This method is popular because it is reliable compared with alternative methods, but it also has some disadvantages. The blending step is a time-consuming, expensive, potentially dangerous operation. In addition, it is difficult to achieve an even distribution of particulate throughout the product, and the use of powders requires a high level of cleanliness, otherwise inclusions will be incorporated into the product with a deleterious effect on fracture toughness and fatigue life.

Processing of Continuous Fiber-Reinforced Aluminum

As shown in Fig. 1, aluminum MMCs reinforced with continuous fibers provide the highest performance/strength. Because of their high cost, however, most applications have been limited to the aerospace industry.

Aluminum-boron is a technologically mature continuous fiber MMC (Fig. 8). Applications for this composite include tubular truss members in the midfuselage structure of the space shuttle orbiter and cold plates in electronic microchip carrier multilayer boards. Fabrication processes for aluminum-boron composites are based on hot press diffusion bonding of alternating layers of aluminum foil and boron fiber mats (foil-fiber-foil processing) or plasma spraying methods.

Continuous SiC fibers are often used as replacements for boron fibers, because they have similar properties (e.g., a tensile modulus of 400 GPa, or 60×10^6 psi) and offer a cost advantage. One such SiC fiber is the SCS series, which can be manufactured with any of several surface chemistries to enhance bonding with a particular matrix, such as aluminum or titanium.

Hot molding is a low-pressure, hot pressing process designed to fabricate Al-SiC parts at significantly lower cost than is possible with a diffusion-bonding/solid-state process. Because the SCS-2 fibers can withstand molten aluminum for long periods, the molding temperature can be raised into the liquid-plus-solid region of the alloy to ensure aluminum flow and consolidation at low pressure, thereby eliminating the need for high-pressure die molding equipment.

The hot molding process is analogous to the autoclave molding of graphite/epoxy, in which components are molded in an open-faced tool. The mold in this case is a self-heating, slip cast ceramic tool that contains the profile of the finished part. A plasma-sprayed aluminum preform is laid into the mold, heated to near molten aluminum temperature, and pressure-consolidated in an autoclave by a metallic vacuum bag.

Aluminum-SiC MMCs exhibit increased strength and stiffness as compared with unreinforced aluminum, with no weight penalty. In contrast to the base metal, the composite retains its room-temperature tensile strength at temperatures up to 260 °C (500 °F).

Aluminum-graphite MMC development was initially prompted by the commercial appearance of strong and stiff carbon fibers in the 1960s. Carbon fibers offer a range of properties, including an elastic modulus up to 966 GPa (140×10^6 psi) and a negative CTE down to -1.62×10^{-6}/°C (-0.9×10^{-6}/°F). However, carbon and aluminum in combination are difficult materials to process into a composite. A deleterious reaction between carbon and aluminum, poor wetting of carbon by molten aluminum, and oxidation of the carbon are significant technical barriers to the production of these composites. Two processes are currently used for making commercial aluminum MMCs: liquid metal infiltration of the matrix on spread tows and hot press bonding of spread tows sandwiched between sheets of aluminum. With both precursor wires and metal-coated fibers, secondary processing, such as diffusion bonding or pultrusion, is needed to make structural elements. Squeeze casting also is feasible for the fabrication of this composite. Precision aerospace structures with strict tolerances on dimensional stability need stiff, lightweight materials that exhibit low thermal distortion. Aluminum-graphite MMCs have the potential to meet these requirements. Unidirectional P100 Gr/6061 aluminum pultruded tube exhibits an elastic modulus in the fiber direction significantly greater than that of steel, and it has a density approximately one-third that of steel.

Aluminum-Al_2O_3 MMCs can be fabricated by a number of methods, but liquid or semi-solid-state processing techniques are commonly used. A fiber-reinforced aluminum MMC is now used in pushrods for high-performance racing engines. The 3M Company produces the material by infiltrating Nextel 610 (3M Corporation) alumina fibers with an aluminum matrix (fiber volume fraction is 60%). Hollow pushrods of several diameters are made, where the fibers are axially aligned along the pushrod length. Hardened steel end caps are bonded to the ends of the MMC tubes. Additional information is available in the article "Automotive Applications of Metal-Matrix Composites" in this Volume.

Diffusion Bonding and Filament Winding. Fabrication of complex-shaped components is commonly achieved by diffusion bonding of monolayer composite tapes. The tapes may be prepared by a number of methods, but the most commonly used is filament winding, where the matrix is incorporated in a sandwich construction by laying up thin metal sheets between filament rows or by the arc spraying technique developed by the National Aeronautics and Space Administration (NASA) Lewis (now NASA Glenn) Research Center. In the latter process, molten matrix alloy droplets are sprayed onto a cylindrical drum wrapped with fibers. The operation is carried out in a controlled atmosphere chamber to avoid problems of oxidation and corrosion. The drum is rotated and passed in front of an arc spray head to produce a controlled porosity monotape. When lamination of the fibers between matrix alloy sheets is adopted to produce the monotape, a binder is used to hold the

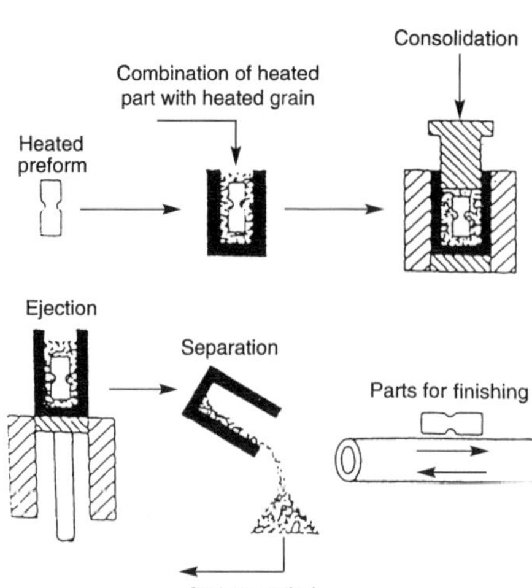

Fig. 7 Schematic illustration of the Ceracon technique for fabricating P/M MMCs. Source: Ref 49, 50

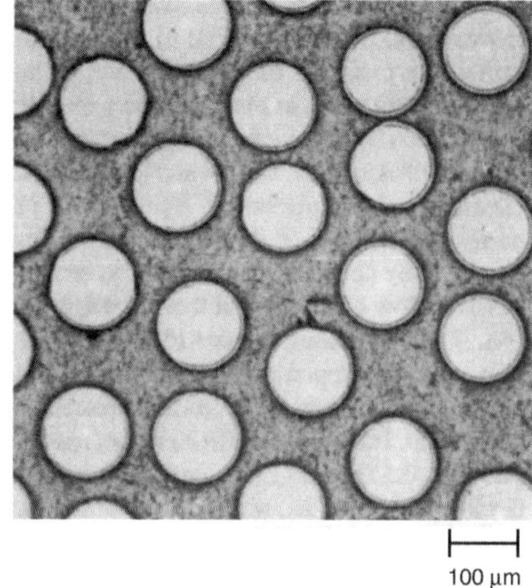

Fig. 8 Cross section of a continuous fiber-reinforced aluminum-boron composite. Shown here are 142 μm diam boron filaments coated with B_4C in a 6061 aluminum alloy matrix.

fibers in place prior to consolidation. This technique can also be combined with consolidation by hot isostatic pressing (HIP). Filament winding and monotape lay-up into multiple layers permit close control over the position and orientation of the fibers in the final composite.

A combination of the arc spray technique and diffusion bonding using SCS-6 SiC monofilament fibers was used to produce composites for various prototype applications in the aerospace and defense sectors of the market. In one example, a rocket motor shell was produced by filament winding of SCS-6 fibers and plasma spraying with an aluminum alloy. The rocket motor was reported to have been successfully fired and to have withstood the extreme temperatures, pressures, and vibrations associated with missile firing. In addition, the assembled motor, using the MMC shell, weighed about 10% less than a conventional steel motor.

Processing of Discontinuously Reinforced Titanium

Since the late 1980s, the unique benefits of the solid-phase processing of P/M titanium alloys have been used in the development of discontinuously reinforced titanium-matrix composites. For example, titanium carbide and titanium diboride powders have been added to both commercially pure titanium and the common titanium alloys using the blended elemental (BE) technique (Ref 51–55). The BE technique is a pressing and sintering P/M technique. It involves cold pressing or cold isostatic pressing a blend of fine elemental titanium and master alloy powders that have been sintered. Ceramic particles are included in the blend to produce particulate-reinforced metal-matrix composites (PR-MMCs); the reinforcements provide improved wear resistance, elastic modulus, creep, fatigue, and corrosion properties with less than a 3% change in alloy density. Elongation and, to a lesser extent, fracture toughness decrease in the trade-off. The following examples typify several titanium PR-MMCs, both in current production and under development; however, it should be noted that most of these examples are research projects and have not achieved commercial use.

Among the first titanium-base PR-MMC materials introduced to the commercial market was CermeTi-C (Dynamet Technology Inc.). These composites are created by the BE technique with the addition of titanium carbide (TiC) to prominent titanium alloys, such as Ti-6Al-4V and Ti-6Al-6V-2Sn. The titanium alloy matrix is formed during sintering by diffusion-driven solid-state alloying, typically at temperatures less than 250 °C (450 °F) above the β transus, or 1230 °C (2245 °F) for Ti-6Al-4V. As opposed to melt processing, the thermal decomposition of the TiC reinforcing particulate (melting point 3065 °C, or 5550 °F) can be limited to a practical extent during the sintering cycle. The resultant PR-MMC displays improved strength and elastic modulus, reflecting the load-sharing contribution of the tightly-bonded TiC particulate (density of 4.48 g/cm^3, elastic modulus of 145 GPa, or 21 $\times$ 10^6 psi, and hardness of 44 HRC) (Ref 56).

From 5 to 20 wt% TiC is added to commonly used titanium alloys. As an alternative to HIP or in addition to HIP operation, hot working (including forging, rolling, and extrusion) further increases the density and mechanical properties of the titanium alloy PR-MMC. The mechanically homogenized particulate distribution and the refined acicular α-β microstructure are retained by air cooling from the forging or extrusion temperature with a commensurate increase in tensile strength and ductility.

The addition of TiB_2 particulate by the BE technique is also done (Ref 57, 58). During normal sintering at 1200 °C (2190 °F), the TiB_2 particulate, in contact with the elemental titanium powder, reacts extensively or completely to form TiB. On cooling, the resultant TiB phase platelets extend beyond the boundaries of the prior titanium particles and bridge multiple α-β colonies.

At the Toyota Central Research and Development Laboratories, Inc., Saito et al. have continued efforts to reduce the cost of BE TiB_2-based PR-MMCs of titanium alloys (Ref 59–65). When 5 wt% TiB_2 is added to BE-derived, metastable β matrix, composed of Ti-4.3Fe-7.0Mo-1.4Al-1.4V, a derivative of Timetal LCB (TIMET, Denver, CO), the resultant 10% TiB_2 reinforcement forms a stable, crystallographically-oriented, coherent interface boundary, increasing the strength, stiffness, hardness, fatigue properties, and heat resistance of the matrix. Deformation flow stress of this material at 700 °C (1290 °F) approximates that of medium carbon steel, aiding producibility. This material is used for automotive engine valves and is the most commercially significant application of titanium PR-MMCs. Additional information is provided in the article "Automotive Applications of Metal-Matrix Composites" in this Volume.

Processing of Continuous Fiber-Reinforced Titanium*

Continuous fiber-reinforced titanium-matrix composites (CF-TMCs) offer the potential for strong, stiff, lightweight materials for usage temperatures as high as 800 to 1000 °C (1500 to 1800 °F). The principal applications for this class of materials would be for hot structure, such as hypersonic airframe structures, and for replacing superalloys in some portions of aerospace engines. The use of CF-TMCs has been somewhat restricted by both the high cost of the materials and the fabrication and assembly procedures.

Foil-Fiber-Foil Process

One method that has been used to fabricate CF-TMCs is the "foil-fiber-foil" method, depicted in Fig. 9. In this method, the silicon-carbide fiber mat (Fig. 10) is held together with a cross weave of molybdenum, titanium, or titanium-niobium wire or ribbon. The fabric is a uniweave system in which the relatively large-diameter SiC monofilaments are straight and parallel and held together by a cross weave of metallic ribbon. The Ti-15V-3Cr-3Sn-3Al foil is normally cold rolled down to a thickness of 0.11 mm (0.0045 in.). The plies are cut, laid up on a consolidation tool, and consolidated by either vacuum hot pressing or HIP.

*The sections "Foil-Fiber-Foil Process" and "Green Tape Process" were written for this edition by Flake C. Campbell, The Boeing Company, St. Louis. The section "Metal Wire Process" was written for this edition by Daniel B. Miracle, Air Force Research Laboratory.

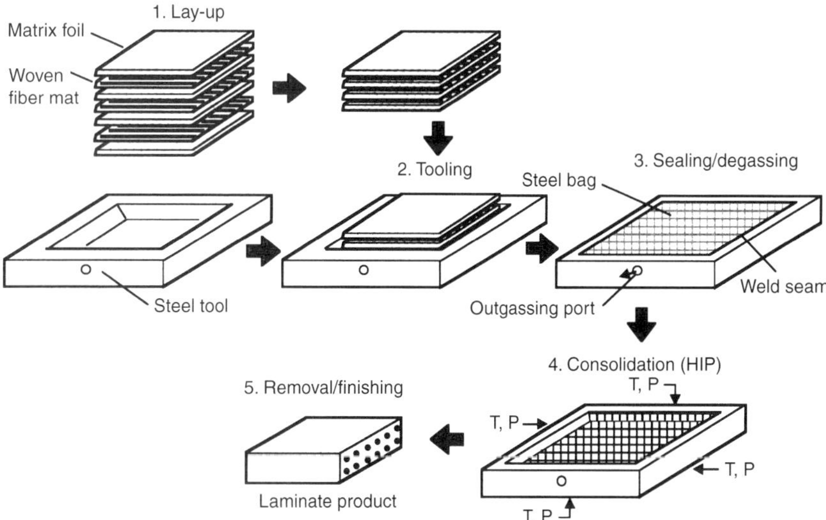

Fig. 9 Foil-fiber-foil method for titanium-matrix composite fabrication. HIP, hot isostatic pressing; P, pressure; T, temperature

Consolidation Procedures. The two primary consolidation procedures are vacuum hot pressing and HIP. High-temperature/short-time roll bonding was used some years ago, but only to a very limited extent. Typical fiber contents for CF-TMC laminates range from 35 to 40 vol%.

Vacuum Hot Pressing. In the vacuum hot pressing technique, the lay-up is sealed in a stainless steel envelope and placed in a vacuum hot press. After evacuation, a small positive pressure is applied via the press platens. This pressure acts to hold the filaments in place during the initial 450 to 550 °C (800 to 1000 °F) soak used to decompose the binder and remove it under the action of a dynamic vacuum. The temperature is then gradually increased to a level where the titanium flows around the fibers under an increased pressure and the foil interfaces are diffusion bonded together. Each fabricator uses a specific set of consolidation parameters, although a typical range is 900 to 950 °C (1650 to 1750 °F) at 41 to 69 MPa (6 to 10 ksi) pressure for 60 to 90 min.

Hot isostatic pressing has largely replaced vacuum hot pressing as the consolidation technique of choice. The primary advantages of HIP consolidation are that the gas pressure is applied isostatically, alleviating the concern about uneven platen pressure; and the HIP process is much more amenable to making complex structural shapes. Typically, the part to be hot isostatically pressed is canned (or a steel bag is welded to a tool), evacuated, and then placed in the HIP chamber. For titanium, typical HIP parameters are 850 to 950 °C (1600 to 1700 °F) at 103 MPa (15 ksi) gas pressure for 2 to 4 h. Since HIP processing is a fairly expensive batch processing procedure, it is normal practice to load a number of parts into the HIP chamber for a single run.

Green Tape Process

Another method for making CF-TMCs involves placing a layer of titanium foil on a mandrel and filament winding the silicon-carbide fiber over the foil in a collimated manner, as to produce a unidirectional single ply. An organic fugitive binder, such as an acrylic adhesive, is used to maintain the fiber spacing and alignment once the preform is cut from the mandrel. In this method (Fig. 11), often called the "green tape" method, the fibers are normally wound onto a foil-covered rotating drum, oversprayed with resin, and the layer cut from the drum to provide a flat sheet of monotape. The organic binder is "burned off" prior to the HIP cycle or during the early portions of the vacuum hot pressing cycle.

Plasma spraying replaces the resin binder with a plasma-sprayed matrix. Plasma spraying removes the potential of an organic residue causing contamination problems during the consolidation cycle and speeds the process by not having to outgas an organic binder. One potential disadvantage of plasma spraying is that titanium, being an extremely reactive metal, can pick up oxygen from the atmosphere, potentially leading to embrittlement problems. This method has been primarily evaluated for titanium-aluminide-matrix composites, due to the difficulty of rolling these materials into thin foil.

Metal Wire Process

A CF-TMC manufactured by a novel metal wire process has been developed to replace stainless steel in a piston actuator rod in Pratt and Whitney F119 engine for the F-22 aircraft. A Ti-6Al-2Sn-4Zr-2Mo (Ti-6242) alloy is hot drawn in a conventional wire drawing process to a diameter of 178 μm (0.007 in.). The Trimarc-1 SiC monofilament reinforcement is 129 μm (5.07×10^{-3} in.) in diameter and is produced by a chemical vapor deposition process on a tungsten wire core. An outer carbon-base coating protects the fiber from chemical interaction with the matrix during consolidation and service. The Ti-6242 metal wire is combined with 34 vol% of the SiC monofilament by wrapping on a rotating drum. The wires are held together with an organic binder and are then cut and removed from the drum to make a preform "cloth." This cloth is wrapped around a solid titanium mandrel, so that the SiC and Ti-6242 wires are parallel to the long axis of the mandrel. A short Ti-6242 cylinder, with an outer diameter of 10 cm (4 in.) and 5 cm (2 in.) high, is placed around one end of the cloth-wrapped mandrel, from which the piston head will be formed. After HIP consolidation, the piston head is machined from the stocky cylinder at one end of the piston, and a threaded connection is machined from the titanium mandrel at the other end. The remainder of the mandrel is removed by gun drilling. The final component is 30.5 cm (12 in.) long, and the shaft is 3.79 cm (1.49 in.) in diameter (see Fig. 6a in the article "Aeronautical Applications of Metal-Matrix Composites" in this Volume). The use of a titanium-matrix composite in the actuator piston is a landmark application and represents the first production aerospace application of TMCs.

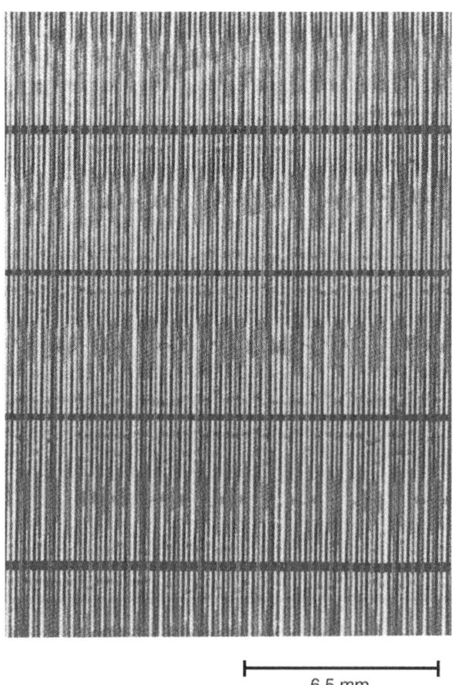

Fig. 10 SiC uniweave fabric showing cross weave

Based on the experience gained from the success of the TMC actuator piston rod, TMCs have been certified as nozzle links on the General Electric F110 engine, which is used for F-16 aircraft. The original link was produced from a square tube of Inconel 718, which was formed from sheet and welded along it length. The manufacturing process for the TMC nozzle links begins by winding Trimarc-2 SiC monofilament, which is similar to Trimarc-1 but is produced on a carbon core, on a drum as for the piston rod. Rather than using metal wire, Ti-6242 powder is sprayed with an organic binder over the wound SiC fibers to produce a preform cloth. This cloth is then cut and removed from the drum, as before, and wrapped around a mandrel. Ti-6242 fittings are added at each end for a clevis attachment and a threaded end, and the entire assembly is consolidated via HIP. After machining the clevis and the threaded end, the mandrel is removed. (A finished part is shown as Fig. 6b in the article "Aeronautical Applications of Metal-Matrix Composites" in this Volume.)

Processing of Other Metal-Matrix Composites

In addition to aluminum and titanium, several other metals and alloys have been investigated as matrix alloys for MMCs. This section describes work done to develop magnesium, copper, and superalloy MMCs. These MMCs have found only limited commercial application to date.

Magnesium-Matrix Composites

Magnesium-matrix composites are being developed to exploit essentially the same properties as those provided by aluminum MMCs: high stiffness, light weight, and low CTE. In practice,

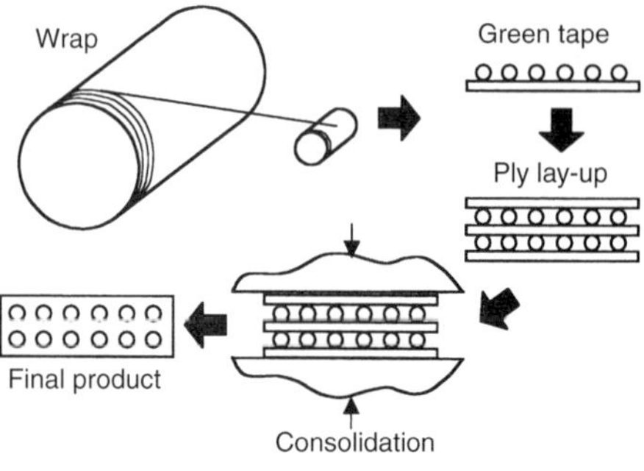

Fig. 11 Green tape method for titanium-matrix composite fabrication

the choice between aluminum and magnesium as a matrix is usually made on the basis of weight versus corrosion resistance. Magnesium is approximately two-thirds as dense as aluminum, but it is more active in a corrosive environment. Magnesium has a lower thermal conductivity, which is sometimes a factor in its selection. Magnesium MMCs include continuous fiber graphite/magnesium for space structures, short staple fiber Al_2O_3/Mg for automotive engine components, and discontinuous SiC or B_4C/Mg for engine components and low-expansion electronic packaging materials. Matrix alloys include AZ31, AZ91, ZE41, QE22, and EZ33. Processing methods parallel those used for the aluminum MMC counterparts.

Copper-Matrix Composites

Copper-matrix composites have been produced with continuous tungsten, silicon carbide, and graphite-fiber reinforcements. Of the three composites, continuous graphite/copper MMCs have been studied the most.

Interest in continuous graphite/copper MMCs gained impetus from the development of advanced graphite fibers. Copper has good thermal conductivity, but it is heavy and has poor elevated-temperature mechanical properties. Pitch-based graphite fibers have been developed that have room-temperature axial thermal conductivity properties better than those of copper. The addition of these fibers to copper reduces density, increases stiffness, raises the service temperature, and provides a mechanism for tailoring the CTE. One approach to the fabrication of graphite/copper MMCs uses a plating process to envelop each graphite fiber with a pure copper coating, yielding MMC fibers flexible enough to be woven into fabric. The copper-coated fibers must be hot pressed to produce a consolidated component. Graphite/copper MMCs have the potential to be used for thermal management of electronic components, satellite radiator panels, and advanced airplane structures.

Superalloy-Matrix Composites

In spite of their poor oxidation resistance and high density, refractory metal (tungsten, molybdenum, and niobium) wires have received a great deal of attention as fiber-reinforcement materials for use in high-temperature superalloy MMCs. Although the theoretical specific strength potential of refractory alloy fiber-reinforced composites is less than that of ceramic fiber-reinforced composites, the more ductile metal-fiber systems are more tolerant of fiber-matrix reactions and thermal expansion mismatches. When refractory metal fibers are used to reinforce a ductile and oxidation-resistant matrix, they are protected from oxidation, and the specific strength of the composite is much higher than that of superalloys at elevated temperatures.

Fabrication of superalloy MMCs is accomplished via solid-phase, liquid-phase, or deposition processing. The methods include investment casting, the use of matrix metals in thin sheet form, the use of matrix metals in powder sheet form made by rolling powders with an organic binder, P/M techniques, slip casting of metal alloy powders, and arc spraying.

ACKNOWLEDGMENTS

In addition to the sources cited as footnotes, selections from the following served as the basis for portions of this article:

- S. Abkowitz, Particulate Reinforced Titanium, *Powder Metal Technologies and Applications,* Vol 7, *ASM Handbook,* ASM International, 1998, p 882–883
- Metal-Matrix Composites, *Metals Handbook Desk Edition,* 2nd ed., J.R. Davis, Ed., ASM International, 1998, p 674–680
- Selection of Material for Forming Metal-Matrix Composites, *ASM Specialty Handbook: Tool Materials,* J.R. Davis, Ed., ASM International, 1995, p 268–273
- P. Rohatgi, Cast Metal-Matrix Composites, *Casting,* Vol 15, *ASM Handbook,* ASM International, 1988, p 840–854

REFERENCES

1. D.O. Kennedy, SiC Particles Beef Up Investment-Cast Aluminum, *Adv. Mater. Process.*, June 1991, p 42-46
2. D. Doutre, P. Enright, and P. Wales, The Interrupted Pour Gating System for the Casting of Metal Matrix Composites, *Proc. 26th Int. Symposium on Automotive Technology and Automation* (Aachen, Germany), 1993, p 539–544
3. P. Enright, D. Doutre, and P. Wales, Rapid Induction Melting of Discrete Volumes of MMC—An Economic Alternative to Bulk Metal Handling, *Proc. 26th Int. Symposium on Automotive Technology and Automation* (Aachen, Germany), 1993, p 545–551
4. D. Doutre, Foundry Experience in Casting Aluminum Metal Matrix Composites, *AFS Trans.*, Vol 101, 1993, p 1070–1076
5. B. Cox et al., Advances in the Commercialization of the Shape Casting of Aluminum Composites, *Proc. Second International Conf. on Cast Metal Matrix Composites* (Des Plaines, IL), D.M. Stefanescu and S. Sen, Ed., American Foundrymen's Society, 1994, p 88–99
6. D. Weiss and D. Rose, Experimental Design of Interrupted Flow Gating for Cast Metal Matrix Composites, *Proc. Second International Conf. on Cast Metal Matrix Composites* (Des Plaines, IL), D.M. Stefanescu and S. Sen, Ed., American Foundrymen's Society, 1994, p 194–203
7. W. Savage, Process, Technology, Plant and Equipment Requirements for the Large Scale Production of Aluminum Based Particulate Reinforced MMC's, *Proc. Second International Conf. on Cast Metal Matrix Composites* (Des Plaines, IL), D.M. Stefanescu and S. Sen, Ed., American Foundrymen's Society, 1994, p 100–109
8. B.M. Cox, Processing of High Pressure Die Castable Aluminum Matrix Composites, *Transactions 16th International Die Casting Congress and Exposition* (River Grove, IL), North American Die Casting Association, 1991, p 363–369
9. D.E. Hammond, Metal Matrix Composite High Pressure Die Castings As-Cast and Heat Treated, *Trans. 16th International Die Casting Congress and Exposition* (River Grove, IL), North American Die Casting Association, 1991, p 49–54
10. B.M. Cox, High Pressure Die Casting of Aluminum Metal Composites, *Diecast. Manag.*, Vol 11 (No. 5), 1993, p 23
11. D.J. Lloyd, Particulate Reinforced Composites Produced by Molten Metal Mixing, *High Performance Composites for the 1990s*, S.K. Das, Ed., TMS-AIME, 1990, p 33–45
12. "Gating Manual," Duralcan USA, San Diego, CA, 1991
13. N.R. Wymer, Die Casting Duralcan Aluminum Composites, *Diecast. Eng.*, May/June 1990
14. T.W. Clyne and P.J. Withers, *An Introduction to Metal Matrix Composites,* Cambridge University Press, Cambridge, 1993
15. S. Abis, *Compos. Sci. Technol.*, Vol 35 (No. 1), 1989
16. D.B. Spencer, R. Mehrabian, and M.C. Flemings, *Metall. Trans.*, Vol 3, 1972, p 1925
17. R. Mehrabian and M.C. Flemings, *AFS Trans.*, Vol 80, 1972, p 173
18. E.F. Fascetta, R.G. Riek, R. Mehrabian, et al., *AFS Trans.*, Vol 81, 1973, p 81
19. R. Mehrabian, R.G. Riek, and M.C. Flemings, *Metall. Trans.,* Vol 5, 1975, p 1899
20. Z. Zhu, A Literature Survey of Fabrication Methods of Cast Reinforced Metal Composites, *ASM Int. Meet. Cast Reinf. Met. Compos.*, S.G. Fishman and A.K. Dringra, Ed., Sept 1988 (Chicago, IL), 1988, p 93–99
21. B.N. Keshavaram, P.K. Rohatgi, R. Asthana, et al., Solidification of Al-Glass Particulate Composites, *Solidification of Metal Matrix Composites,* P. Rohatgi, Ed., Minerals, Metals and Materials Society, Indianapolis, IN, 1990, p 151–170
22. P. Rohatgi, Cast Aluminum-Matrix Composites for Automotive Applications, *J. Met.*, Vol 43 (No. 10), 1991
23. P.K. Balasubrainanian, P.S. Rao, B.C. Pai, et al., Synthesis of Cast Al-Zn-Mg-TiO_2 Particle Composites Using Liquid Metallurgy (LM) and Rheocasting (RC), *Solidification of Metal Matrix Composites,* P. Rohatgi, Ed., Minerals, Metals and Materials Society, Indianapolis, IN, 1990, p 181–190
24. J.T. Blucher, Discussion of a Liquid Metal Pressure Infiltration Process to Produce Metal Matrix Composites, *J. Mater. Pro-*

cess. Technol., Vol 30 (No. 2), 1992, p 381–390
25. A. Mortensen, V.J. Michaud, and M.C. Flemings, Pressure-Infiltration Processing of Reinforced Aluminum, *JOM*, Vol 45 (No. 1), 1993, p 36–43
26. A.J. Cook and P.S. Werner, Pressure Infiltration Casting of Metal Matrix Composites, *Mater. Sci. Eng. A*, Vol A144, 1991, p 189–206
27. A. Mortensen, L.J. Masur, J.A. Cornie, and M.C. Flemings, Infiltration of Fibrous Preforms by a Pure Metal: Part I. Theory, *Metall. Trans. A*, Vol 20, 1989, p 2535–2547
28. L.J. Masur, A. Mortensen, J.A. Cornie, and M.C. Flemings, Infiltration of Fibrous Preforms by a Pure Metal: Part II. Experiment, *Metall. Trans. A*, Vol 20, 1989, p 2549–2557
29. J.J. Stanco and A.J. Paul, Flexible Manufacturing System for Casting MMC Avionics Parts, *AFS Trans.*, Vol 93, 1995, p 829–836
30. C. Zweben, Metal-Matrix Composites for Electronic Packaging, *JOM*, Vol 44 (No. 7), 1992, p 15–23
31. M.K. Premkumar, W.H. Hunt, Jr., and R.R Sawtell, Aluminum Composite Materials for Multichip Modules, *JOM*, Vol 44 (No. 7), 1992, p 24–28
32. N. Salmon and J. Cornie, Advanced Pressure Infiltration Casting of Automotive Components, *Proc. 29th International Symposium on Automotive Technology and Automation*, Vol 1, 1996, p 199–206
33. J. Narciso, C. Garcia-Cordovilla, and E. Louis, Pressure Infiltraion of Packed Ceramic Particulates by Liquid Metals, *Acta Mater.*, Vol 47 (No. 18), 1999, p 4461–4479
34. E. Candan, H.V. Atkinson, and H. Jones, Effect of Alloying Additions on Threshold Pressure for Infiltration and Porosity of Aluminum-Based Melt Infiltrated Silicon Carbide Powder Compacts, *Key Eng. Mater.*, Vol 127–131 (Part 1), 1997, p 463–470
35. S.Y. Oh, J.A. Cornie, and K.C. Russell, Particulate Wetting and Metal: Ceramic Interface Phenomena, *Ceram. Eng. Sci. Proc.*, Vol 8 (No. 7–8), 1987, p 912–936
36. V.J. Michaud and A. Mortensen, Infiltration of Fiber Preforms by a Binary Alloy, Part II: Further Theory and Experiment, *Metall. Trans. A*, Vol 23A, 1992, p 2263–2280
37. A. Mortensen, J.A. Cornie, and M.C. Flemings, Columnar Dendritic Solidification in a Metal-Matrix Composite, *Metall. Trans. A*, Vol 19A, 1988, p 709–721
38. R.W. Evans, A.G. Leatham, and R.G. Brooks, The Osprey Preform Process, *Powder Metall.*, Vol 28, 1985, p 13–19
39. A.G. Leatham, A. Ogilvey, P.F. Chesney, et al., Osprey Process-Production Flexibility in Materials Manufacture, *Met. Mater.*, Vol 5 (No. 140), 1989, p 3
40. P.F. Chesney, A.G. Leatham, R. Pratt, et al., The Osprey Process—A Versatile Manufacturing Technology for the Production of Solid and Hollow Rounds and Clad (Compound) Billets, *Proc. First European Conf. Adv. Mater. Process.*, H.E. Exner and V. Schumacher, Ed., (Aachen, Germany), DGM, 1989, p 247–254
41. T.C. Willis, Spray Deposition Process for Metal Matrix Composite Manufacture, *Met. Mater.*, Vol 4, 1988, p 485–488
42. W. Kahl and J. Leupp, Spray Deposition of High Performance Al Alloys Via the Osprey Process, *Proc. First European Conf. Adv. Mater. Process.*, H.E. Exner and V. Schumacher, Ed., (Aachen, Germany), DGM, 1989, p 261–266
43. J. White and T.C. Willis, The Production of Metal Matrix Composites by Spray Deposition, *Mater. Des.*, Vol 10, 1989, p 121–127
44. J. White, N.A. Darby, I.R. Hughes, et al., Metal Matrix Composites Produced by Spray Deposition, *Adv. Mater. Technol. Int.*, Vol 58, 1990, p 9–42
45. A.G. Leatham and A. Lawley, The Osprey Process: Principles and Applications, *Int. J. Powder Metall.*, Vol 29 (No. 4), 1993, p 321–329
46. D. Huda, M.A. El Baradie, and M.S.J. Hashmi, Metal-Matrix Composites: Manufacturing Aspects, Part 1, *J. Mater. Process. Technol.*, Vol 37 (No. 1–4), 1993, p 513–528
47. A. Ghosh, In *Fundamentals of Metal-Matrix Composites*, S. Suresh, A Mortensen, and A. Needleman, Ed., Butterworth-Heinemann, Newton, MA, 1993, p 23–41
48. C.W. Brown, Particulate Metal Matrix Composite Properties, *Proc. P/M Aerosp. Def. Technol. Conf. Exhibit.*, F.H. Froes, Ed., 1990, p 203–205
49. B.L. Ferguson and O.D. Smith, Ceracon Process, *Powder Metallurgy*, Vol 7, *Metals Handbook*, 9th ed., ASM International, 1984, p 537
50. B.L. Ferguson, A. Kuhn, O.D. Smith, et al., *Int. J. Powder Metall. Powder Technol.*, Vol 24, 1984, p 31
51. S. Abkowitz and P. Weihrauch, Trimming the Cost of MMC, *Adv. Mater. Proc.*, Vol 136 (No. 1), July 1989, p 31–34
52. S. Abkowitz, H.L. Heussi, and H.P. Ludwig, Titanium Carbide/Titanium Alloy Composite and Process for Powder Metal Cladding, U.S. Patent 4,731,115, 15 March 1988
53. S. Abkowitz, P.F. Weihrauch, and S.M. Abkowitz, Particulate-Reinforced Titanium Alloy Composites Economically Formed by Combined Cold and Hot Isostatic Pressing, *Ind. Heat.*, Vol LX (No. 9), Sept 1993, p 32–37
54. S.M. Abkowitz, P. Weihrauch, S. Abkowitz, and H. Heussi, The Commercial Application of Low-Cost Titanium Composites, *JOM*, Vol 47 (No. 8), Aug 1995, p 40–41
55. S.M. Abkowitz et al., P/M Titanium Matrix Composties: From War Games to Fun and Games, *Eighth World Conf. on Titanium*, 23–26 Oct 1995, (Birmingham, England)
56. R. Boyer, G. Welsch, and E.W. Collings, Ed., *Materials Properties Handbook: Titanium Alloys*, ASM International, 1994, p 1141
57. S. Abkowitz, H.L. Heussi, H.P. Ludwig, D.M. Rowell, and S.A. Kraus, Titanium Diboride/Titanium Alloy Metal Matrix Microcomposite Materials and Process for Powder Metal Cladding, U.S. Patent 4,906,430, 6 March 1990
58. S. Abkowitz, H.L. Heussi, H.P. Ludwig, D.M. Rowell, and S.A. Kraus, Titanium Diboride/Titanium Alloy Metal Matrix Microcomposite Materials and Process for Powder Metal Cladding, U.S. Patent 4,968, 348, 6 Nov 1990
59. T. Saito, T. Furata, T. Yamaguchi, and K. Ogino, *Proc. 1993 Powder Metallurgy World Congress—PM '93,* Y. Bando and K. Kosuge, Ed., JPMA-JSPM, Vol 1, 1993, p 642
60. T. Saito, T. Furata, and T. Yamaguchi, *Development of Low Cost Titanium Matrix Composite Metallurgy and Technology of Practical Titanium Alloys,* S. Fujishiro, D. Eylon, and T. Kishi, Ed., TMS, 1994
61. T. Saito, A Cost-Effective P/M Titanium Matrix Composite for Automobile Use, Adv. Perf. Mater., Vol 2 (No. 2), 1995, p 121–144
62. T. Saito, T. Furuta, and T. Yamaguchi, Fatigue Properties of TiB Particle Reinforced P/M Titanium Matrix Composite, *Recent Advances in Titanium Metal Matrix Composites*, F.H. Froes and J. Storer, Ed., TMS, 1995, p 133
63. T. Furata and T. Saito, Fatigue Properties of TiB Particle Reinforced P/M Titanium Matrix Composite, *Proc. of Fourth Conf. on P/M Aerospace, Defense, and Demanding Applications*, F.H. Froes, Ed., Metal Powder Industries Federation, 1995, p 173–180
64. T. Saito, H. Takamiya, and T. Furuta, Thermomechanical Properties of P/M β Titanium Metal Matrix Composite, *Mater. Sci. Eng. A*, Vol 243 (No. 2), 1998, p 273–278
65. F.H. Froes and R.H. Jones, *Light Met. Age*, Vol 57 (No. 1, 2), 1999, p 117–121

Processing of Ceramic-Matrix Composites

K.K. Chawla, University of Alabama at Birmingham
N. Chawla, Arizona State University

CERAMIC-MATRIX COMPOSITES (CMCs) have ability to withstand high temperatures and have superior damage tolerance over monolithic ceramics (Ref 1, 2). A significant hurdle in realizing the full potential of CMCs, however, has been in the area of processing and manufacturability. Ceramic-matrix composites can be processed either by conventional powder processing techniques, used to process polycrystalline ceramics, or by newer techniques developed specifically for CMCs. Several of the most important or promising techniques are summarized in Table 1. In this article, the term "ceramic" encompasses crystalline ceramics, glass-ceramics, and amorphous materials, such as silica-based glasses. Some of the important processing techniques for CMCs are described, and the advantages and disadvantages of each technique are highlighted to provide a comprehensive understanding of the achievements and challenges that remain in this area.

Cold Pressing and Sintering

Cold pressing of a matrix powder and fiber mixture followed by sintering is a natural extension from conventional processing of ceramics. Shrinkage is a common problem associated with sintering of most ceramics. This problem is exacerbated when a glass-or ceramic-matrix is combined with a reinforcement material. Thus, after sintering the matrix generally shrinks considerably, and the resulting composite exhibits a significant amount of cracking. One of the reasons for high shrinkage after sintering is that fibers and whiskers—that is, reinforcements with high aspect ratio (length/diameter)—can form a network that may inhibit the sintering process. Depending on the difference in thermal expansion coefficients of the reinforcement and matrix, a hydrostatic tensile stress can develop in the matrix on cooling, which will counter the driving force (surface energy minimization) for sintering (Ref 3, 4). Thus the densification rate of the matrix will, in general, be retarded in the presence of reinforcement (Ref 5–9).

Hot Pressing

Hot pressing is frequently used in a combination of steps or in a single step in the consolidation stage of CMCs. Hot pressing is an attractive technique because the simultaneous application of pressure and high temperature can significantly accelerate the rate of densification, resulting in a pore-free and fine-grained compact. An example of a common hot-pressed composite is silicon carbide (SiC) whisker-reinforced Al_2O_3, used in cutting tool applications.

A common variant of conventional hot pressing is the slurry infiltration process. It is perhaps the most important technique used to produce continuous fiber reinforced glass and glass-ceramic composites (Ref 10–14). The slurry infiltration process involves two main stages: (1) incorporation of the reinforcing phase into a "slurry" of the unconsolidated matrix and (2) matrix consolidation by hot pressing.

Figure 1 shows a schematic of the slurry infiltration process. The first stage involves some degree of fiber alignment, in addition to incorporation of the reinforcing phase in the matrix slurry. The slurry typically consists of the matrix powder, a carrier liquid (water or alcohol), and an organic binder. The organic binder is burned out prior to consolidation. Wetting agents may be added to ease the infiltration of the fiber tow or preform. The fiber tow or fiber preform is impregnated with the matrix slurry by passing it through a slurry tank. The impregnated fiber tow or preform sheets are similar to the prepregs used in fabrication of polymer-matrix composites (PMCs) (Ref 2). The impregnated tow or prepreg is wound on a drum and dried. This is followed by cutting and stacking of the prepregs and consolidation by hot pressing. The process has the advantage that, just as in PMCs, the prepregs can be arranged in a variety of stacking sequences, for example, unidirectional, cross-plied (0°/90°/0°/90°, etc.), or angle-plied ($+\theta/-\theta/+\theta/-\theta$, etc.). Figure 2(a) shows an optical micrograph of a transverse section of a unidirectional alumina-fiber/glass-matrix composite (some residual porosity can be seen in this micrograph), while Fig. 2(b) shows the pressure and temperature schedule used during hot pressing of this composite.

As mentioned above, the slurry infiltration process is well suited for glass- or glass-ceramic-matrix composites, mainly because the processing temperatures for these materials are lower than those used for crystalline-matrix materials. The hot-pressing process does have the limitation of not being able to produce complex shapes. Application of a very high pressure during hot pressing can also easily damage the fibers and decrease the strength of the composite. The fibers may also be damaged by mechanical contact with refractory particles of a crystalline ceramic or from reaction with the matrix at very high processing temperatures. The matrix should have as little porosity as possible in the final product, as porosity in a structural ceramic material is highly undesirable. To this end, it is important to completely remove the fugitive binder and use a matrix powder particle smaller than the fiber diameter. The hot-pressing operational parameters are also important. Precise control

Table 1 Summary of CMC fabrication processes and examples of typical composite systems fabricated by these processes

Process	Examples
Slurry infiltration (ply stacking and hot pressing)	SiC/glass ceramic, carbon/glass-ceramic, C/glass, mullite/glass
Powder processing and hot pressing	SiC/Al_2O_3, Al_2O_3/Al_2O_3
Gas-liquid metal reaction (Lanxide)	SiC/Al_2O_3, SiC/SiC
Sol-gel (infiltration and sintering/hot pressing)	C/glass, mullite/mullite
Chemical vapor infiltration (infiltration of a woven preform)	SiC/SiC, C/SiC
Polymer conversion (infiltration and pyrolysis)	C/C, C/SiC, SiC/Si-C-N

within a narrow working temperature range, minimization of the processing time, and utilization of a pressure low enough to avoid fiber damage are important factors in this final consolidation part of the process. Fiber damage and any fiber/matrix interfacial reaction, along with its detrimental effect on the bond strength, are unavoidable attributes of the hot pressing operation.

In summary, the slurry infiltration process generally results in a composite with fairly uniform fiber distribution, low porosity, and relatively high strength. The main disadvantage of this process is that one is restricted to relatively low-melting or low-softening point matrix materials.

Whisker reinforced CMCs are generally made by mixing the whiskers with a ceramic powder slurry, dried, and hot pressed. Sometimes hot isostatic pressing (HIP) rather than uniaxial hot pressing is used. Whisker agglomeration in a green body is a major problem; mechanical stirring and adjustment of pH level of the suspension (matrix powder/whiskers in water) can help minimize this. Addition of whiskers to a slurry can result in very high viscosity. Also, whiskers with large aspect ratios (>50) tend to form bundles and clumps (Ref 15). Obtaining well-separated and deagglomerated whiskers is of great importance for reasonably high-density composites. Use of organic dispersants (Ref 16) and techniques such as agitation mixing assisted by an ultrasonic probe and deflocculation by a proper pH control (Ref 17) can be usefully employed.

Most whisker-reinforced composites are made at temperatures in the 1500 to 1900 °C (2730–3450 °F) range and pressures in the 20 to 40 MPa (3–6 ksi) range (Ref 18, 19). Figure 3 shows a scanning electron micrograph of a hybrid composite, consisting of SiC fibers (Nicalon) and whiskers in a glass-ceramic-matrix (Ref 20).

Reaction-Bonding Processes

Reaction-bonding processes similar to the ones used for monolithic ceramics can also be used to make ceramic-matrix composites. These have been used mostly with silicon carbide or silicon nitride matrices. The other advantages are:

- Little or no matrix shrinkage occurs during densification.
- Large volume fractions of whiskers or fiber can be used.
- Multidirectional, continuous fiber preforms can also be used.
- The reaction-bonding temperatures for most systems are generally lower than the sintering temperatures, so that fiber degradation can be avoided.

One great disadvantage of this process is that high porosity is hard to avoid.

A hybrid process involving a combination of hot pressing with the reaction-bonding technique can also be used (Ref 21, 22). Figure 4 shows the flow diagram for this process (Ref 22), while Fig. 5 shows a micrograph of a composite (SCS-6 fiber/ Si_3N_4) made by this process (Ref 23). Silicon cloth is prepared by attrition milling a mixture of silicon powder, a polymer binder, and an organic solvent to obtain a "dough" of proper consistency. This dough is then rolled to make a silicon cloth of desired thickness. Fiber mats are made by filament winding of silicon carbide with a fugitive binder. The fiber mats and silicon cloth are stacked in an alternate sequence, debinderized, and hot pressed in a molybdenum die and in a nitrogen or vacuum environment. The temperature and pressure are adjusted to produce a handleable preform. At this stage, the silicon matrix is converted to silicon nitride by transferring the composite to a nitriding furnace between 1100 and 1400 °C (2010 and 2550 °F). Typically, the silicon nitride matrix has about 30% porosity, which is not unexpected in reaction-bonded silicon nitride. Note also the matrix-density variations around fibers in Fig. 5.

Infiltration

Infiltration of a preform made of a reinforcement can be done with a matrix material in solid (particulate), liquid, or gaseous form. Liquid Infiltration is very similar to liquid polymer or liquid metal infiltration (Fig. 6). Proper control of

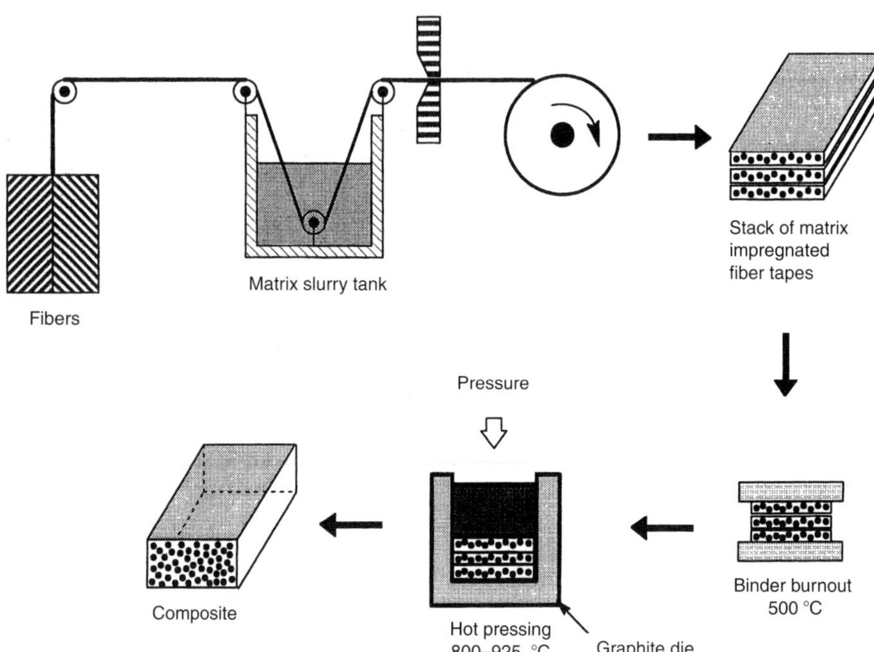

Fig. 1 Schematic of the slurry infiltration process followed by hot pressing

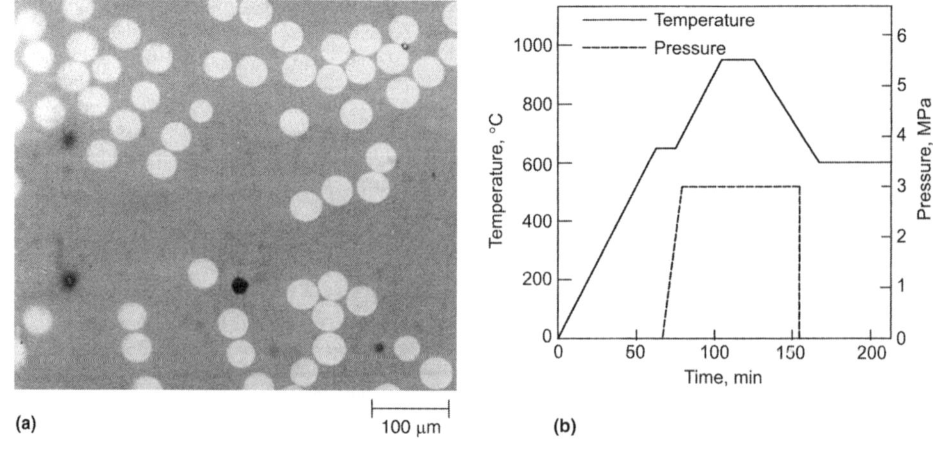

Fig. 2 Unidirectional alumina-fiber/glass-matrix composite formed by slurry infiltration followed by hot pressing. (a) Light micrograph of transverse section (some porosity can be seen in this micrograph). (b) Pressure and temperature schedule used during hot pressing of this composite

the fluidity of liquid matrix is, of course, the key to this technique. It yields a high-density matrix, that is, no pores in the matrix. Almost any reinforcement geometry can be used to produce a virtually flaw-free composite. The temperatures involved, however, are much higher than those encountered in polymer or metal processing. Processing at such high temperatures can lead to deleterious chemical reactions between the reinforcement and the matrix. Thermal expansion mismatch between the reinforcement and the matrix, the rather large temperature interval between the processing temperature and room temperature, and the low strain to failure of ceramics can add up to a formidable set of problems in producing a crackfree CMC. Viscosities of ceramic melts are generally very high, which makes the infiltration of preforms rather difficult. Wettability of the reinforcement by the molten ceramic is another item to be considered. Hillig (Ref 24) has discussed the melt infiltration processing of ceramic-matrix composites in regard to chemical reactivity, melt viscosity, and wetting of the reinforcement by the melt. A preform made of reinforcement in any form (for example, fiber, whisker, or particle) having a network of pores can be infiltrated by a ceramic melt by using capillary pressure. Application of pressure or processing in vacuum can aid in the infiltration process.

Assuming that the preform consists of a bundle of regularly spaced, parallel channels, one can use Poissuelle's equation to obtain the infiltration height, h:

$$h = \sqrt{\frac{\gamma r t \cos\theta}{2\eta}}$$

where r is the radius of the cylindrical channel, t is the time, γ is the surface energy of the infiltrant, θ is the contact angle, and η is the viscosity. Note that the penetration height is proportional to the square root of time and inversely proportional to the viscosity of the melt. Penetration will be easier if the contact angle is low (i.e., better wettability), and the surface energy (γ) and the pore radius (r) are large. However, if the radius of the channel is made too large, the capillarity effect will be lost.

The advantages and disadvantages of different melt infiltration techniques can be summarized:

Advantages

- The matrix is formed in a single processing step.
- A homogeneous matrix can be obtained.

Disadvantages

- High melting points of ceramics mean a greater likelihood of reaction between the melt and the reinforcement.
- Ceramics have higher melt viscosities than metals; therefore, infiltration of preforms is relatively difficult.
- Matrix cracking is likely because of the differential shrinkage between the matrix and the reinforcement on solidification. This can be minimized by choosing components with nearly equal coefficients of thermal expansion.

Directed Oxidation (Lanxide) Process

A version of liquid infiltration is the directed oxidation process, or Lanxide process (Lanxide is a trademark of Advanced Materials Lanxide LLC, Newark, DE) (Ref 25). A schematic of the directed metal oxidation process called DIMOX is shown in Fig. 7. The first step in this process is to make a preform. In the case of a fibrous composite, filament winding or a fabric lay-up may be used to make a preform. A barrier to stop growth of the matrix material is placed on the preform surfaces. In this method, a molten metal is subjected to directed oxidation, that is, the desired reaction product forms on the surface of the molten metal and grows outward. The metal is supplied continuously at the reaction front by a wicking action through channels in the oxidation product. For example, molten aluminum in air will get oxidized to aluminum oxide. If one wants to form aluminum nitride, then molten aluminum is reacted with nitrogen.
The reaction can be represented as:

$$Al + air \rightarrow Al_2O_3$$

$$Al + N_2 \rightarrow AlN$$

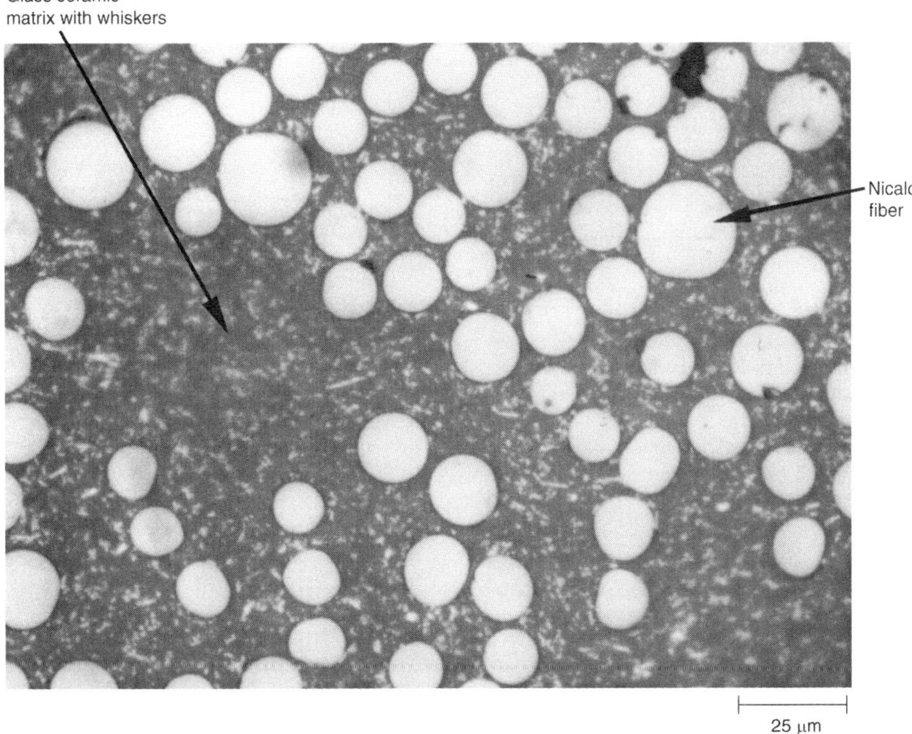

Fig. 3 Scanning electron micrograph of a hybrid composite, consisting of SiC fibers (Nicalon) and whiskers in a glass-ceramic-matrix. Source: Ref 20

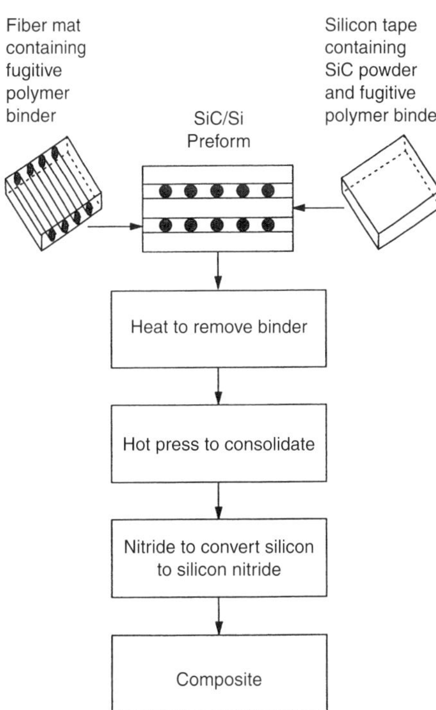

Fig. 4 Flow diagram of the reaction bonding process for processing SCS-6 fiber/Si_3N_4 composites (after Ref 22)

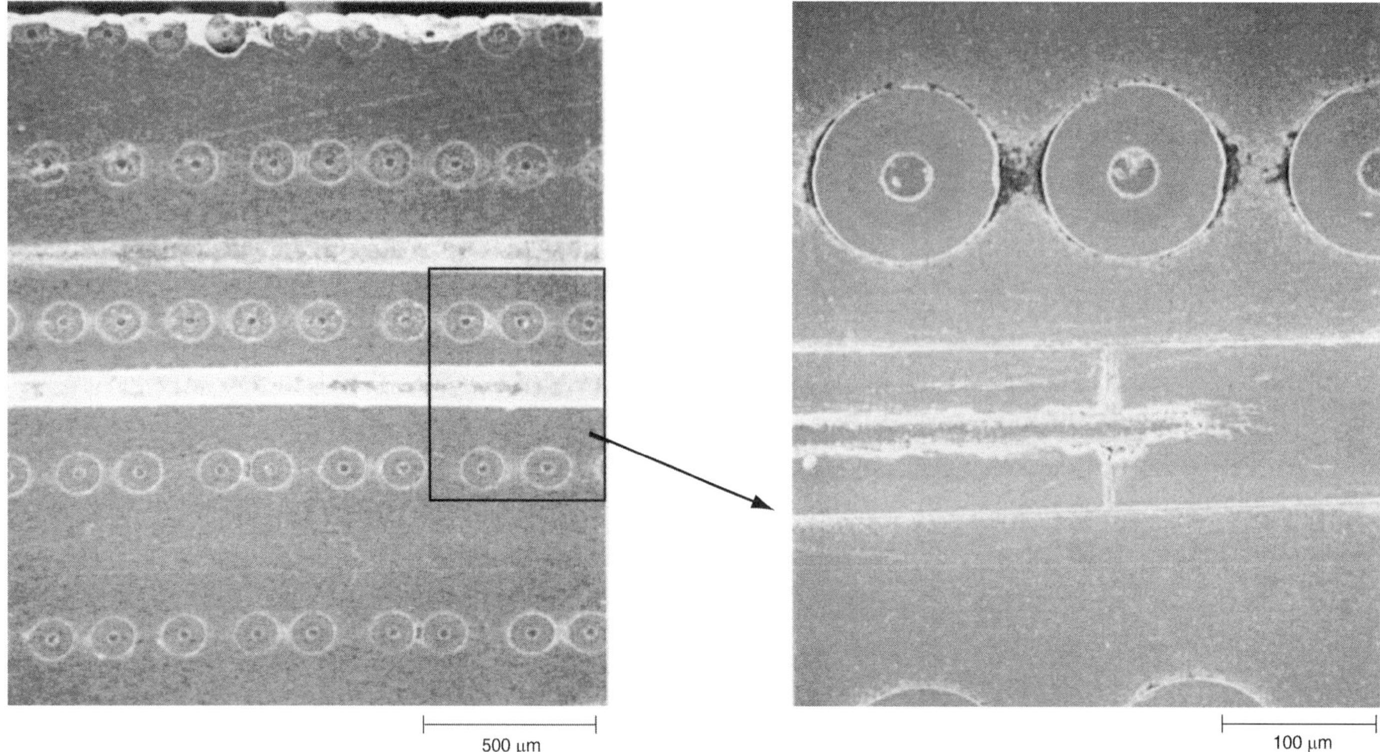

Fig. 5 Microstructure of reaction-bonded SCS-6 fiber/Si_3N_4 composite showing uniform fiber distribution and small amounts of residual porosity around the periphery of the large-diameter fibers

The end product in this process is a three-dimensional, interconnected network of a ceramic composite plus about 5 to 30% of unreacted metal. When filler particles are placed next to the molten metal surface, the ceramic network forms around these particles. As mentioned previously, a fabric made of a continuous fiber can also be used. The fabric is coated with a proprietary coating to protect the fiber from highly reducing aluminum and to provide a weak interface, which is desirable for enhanced toughness. Some aluminum (6–7 wt%) remains at the end of the process. This must be removed if the composite is to be used at temperatures above the melting point of aluminum (660 °C, or 1220 °F). On the other hand, the presence of a residual metal can be exploited to provide some fracture toughness in these composites.

Proper control of the reaction kinetics is of great importance in this process. The process is potentially a low-cost process because near-net shapes are possible. Also, good mechanical properties (strength, toughness, etc.) have been reported (Ref 25). The main disadvantages of this process are:

- It is difficult to control the chemistry and produce an all-ceramic matrix by this method. There is always some residual metal that is not easy to remove completely.
- It is difficult to envision the use of such techniques for large, complex parts, such as those required, for aerospace applications.

In Situ Chemical Reaction Techniques

In situ chemical reaction techniques to produce CMCs are extensions of those used to produce monolithic ceramic bodies. The most important methods are chemical vapor infiltration (CVI) and different types of reaction-bonding techniques.

Chemical Vapor Infiltration (CVI). When chemical vapor deposition (CVD) is used for infiltration of rather large amounts of matrix material in fibrous preforms, it is called chemical vapor infiltration (CVI). Common ceramic-matrix materials used are SiC, Si_3N_4, and HfC. The CVI method has been successfully employed by several researchers to impregnate fibrous preforms (Ref 26–30). The preforms can consist of yarns, woven fabrics, or three-dimensional shapes. Figure 8 shows a filament-wound Nicalon tube and a braided Nextel tube before CVI and after CVI.

Chemical vapor infiltration has been used extensively for processing near net shape CFCMCs and CMCs. The first attempts at using CVI as a processing technique were in densifying porous graphite bodies with carbon (Ref 31). In fact, about half of the commercially available carbon-carbon composites today are made by CVI (Ref 32). Chemical vapor infiltration can be thought of as a bulk form of CVD, which is widely used in depositing thin coatings. The process involves deposition of the solid matrix over an open-volume, porous fibrous preform by the reaction and decomposition of gases. An example of a CVI reaction is the deposition of titanium diboride,

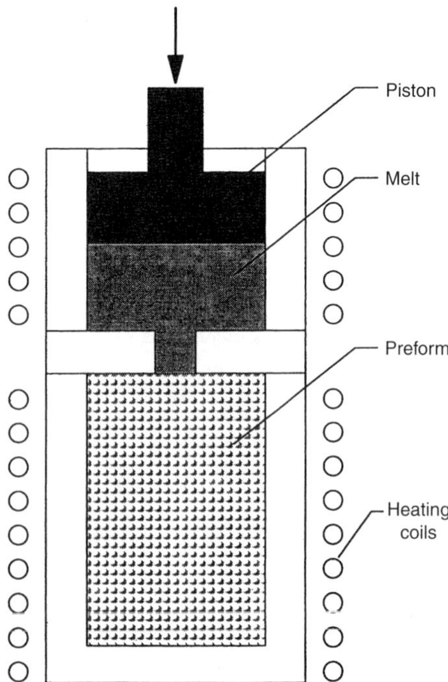

Fig. 6 Schematic of liquid infiltration processing. The technique is very similar to liquid polymer or liquid metal infiltration

which has a melting temperature of 3225 °C (5835 °F) but can be deposited at 900 °C (1650 °F) via CVI:

$$TiCl_4 + 2\,BCl_3 + 5\,H_2 \rightarrow TiB_2 + 10\,HCl$$

The resulting HCl by-product is very common in CVI-type reactions. The solid materials are deposited from gaseous reactants onto a heated substrate. A typical CVD or CVI process would require a reactor with the following parts:

- A vapor feed system
- A CVD reactor in which the substrate is heated and gaseous reactants are fed
- An effluent system where exhaust gases are handled

Figure 9 shows such a reactor in its simplest form. One can synthesize a variety of ceramic-matrices such as oxides, glasses, ceramics, and intermetallics by CVD. Table 2 shows several examples of ceramic composites fabricated by CVI (Ref 32). There are two main variations of CVI. Isothermal chemical vapor infiltration (ICVI) relies on diffusion for deposition (Ref 33, 34). The preform is maintained at a uniform temperature while the reactant gases are allowed to flow through the furnace and deposit the solid species. To obtain a uniform matrix around the fibers, deposition is conducted at low pressures and reactant concentrations. When the CVI process is carried out isothermally, however, surface pores tend to close first, restricting the gas flow to the interior of the preform. This phenomenon, sometimes referred to as canning, necessitates multiple cycles of impregnation, surface machining, and reinfiltration to obtain an adequate density. One can avoid some of these problems by using a forced gas flow and a temperature gradient approach to chemical vapor infiltration (Ref 35–37). Forced chemical vapor infiltration (FCVI) uses a combination of thermal gradients and forced reactant flow to overcome the problems of slow diffusion and permeability obtained in ICVI. This can eliminate, to some extent, the need for multiple cycles. Thus, FCVI processes typically yield much shorter infiltration times, while still obtaining uniform densification of the matrix and low residual porosity. As a comparison, a 3 mm (0.12 in.) part infiltrated by ICVI could take several weeks, while the same part infiltrated by FCVI would only take several hours. As is true with all CVI processes, with increasing densification a point of diminishing returns occurs, such that after a certain time the incremental increase in density is not proportional to the time required for deposition.

In FCVI, a graphite holder in contact with a water-cooled metallic gas distributor holds the fibrous preform. The bottom and side surfaces thus stay cool, while the top of the fibrous preform is exposed to the hot zone, creating a steep thermal gradient. The reactant gaseous mixture passes unreacted through the fibrous preform because of the low temperature. When these gases reach the hot zone, they decompose and deposit on and between the fibers to form the matrix. As the matrix material gets deposited in the hot portion of the preform, the preform density increases, and the hot zone moves progressively from the top of the preform toward the bottom.

When the composite is formed completely at the top and is no longer permeable, the gases flow radially through the preform, exiting from the vented retaining ring. To control deposition, the rate of deposition must be maximized while minimizing density gradients. Deposition reaction rate and mass transport are competing factors, so very rapid deposition results in the exterior of the preform being well infiltrated, while severe density gradients and a large amount of porosity are present within the preform. Very slow deposition rates, on the other hand, require long times and are not economically feasible. A balance between the two factors is required for optimal infiltration.

Consider the process of decomposition of a chemical compound in the vapor form to yield SiC ceramic-matrix on and in between the fibers in a preform. For example, methyltrichlorosilane (CH_3SiCl_3), the starting material to obtain SiC, is decomposed between 1200 and 1400 K:

$$CH_3Cl_3Si \rightarrow SiC(s) + 3HCl(g)$$

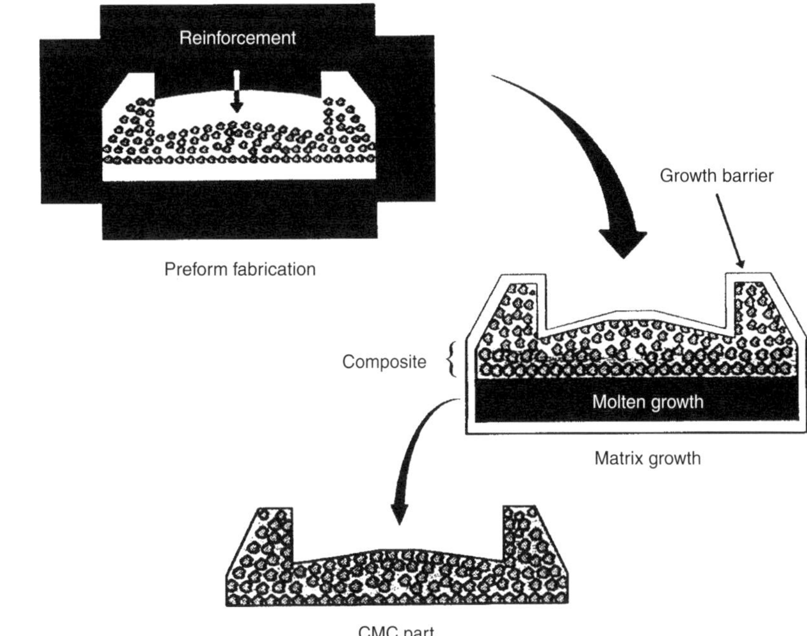

Fig. 7 Schematic of the directed metal oxidation (DIMOX) process. Courtesy of Lanxide Corporation

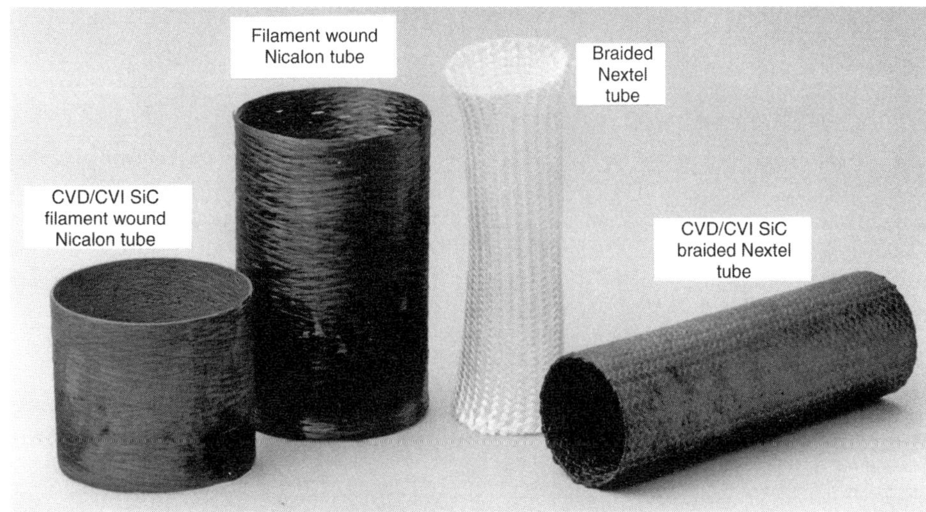

Fig. 8 Filament-wound Nicalon tube and a braided Nextel tube before and after being processed by chemical vapor infiltration. Courtesy of Thermo Electron Corporation

The vapors of SiC deposit as solid phases on and between the fibers in a freestanding preform to form the matrix. The CVI process is very slow because it involves diffusion of the reactant species to the fibrous substrate, followed by outflow of the gaseous reactant products. The CVI process of making a ceramic-matrix is, indeed, a kind of low-stress and low-temperature CVD process and thus avoids some of the problems associated with high-temperature ceramic processing. Using CVI, when processing CFCMCs one can deposit the interfacial coating on the fibers as well as the matrix in situ. For example, for Nicalon/SiC composites with a carbon interface, the carbon layer is deposited first, and then the SiC matrix is infiltrated without changing the preform conditions. The fibrous preforms are stacked layer by layer between perforated plates, through which the gases pass during infiltration. The carbon coating is typically deposited by means of a hydrocarbon gas at around 1000 °C (1830 °F) and reduced pressure to protect the fibers.

The graphitic coating on the fibers has a characteristic aligned structure of the basal planes. These basal planes are parallel to the fiber direction, but perpendicular to the incoming crack front, so deflection of cracks at the weakly bonded basal planes takes place instead of fracturing the fibers. The softer *c*-axis of the graphite is also aligned in the perpendicular direction to accommodate the thermal residual stresses that arise from processing. The matrix consists of a nucleation zone in a small region at the coating/matrix interface. After this, long columnar grains perpendicular to the surface of the fiber are seen. The preferred orientation is such that the (111) planes are aligned parallel to the fibers. The grains are composed predominantly of β-SiC with a cubic structure with small disordered regions of α-SiC. For CVI composites reinforced with woven fiber fabrics, the nature of the porosity is trimodal. Macroporosity is found between fiber bundles and between layers of fabric, with pore sizes less than 100 μm. Microporosity occurs between fibers in the fiber bundle, and the pore size is usually on the order of 10 μm. Lowden et al. (Ref 32), found that 70% of the pore volume was in the form of microporosity within the fiber bundle, 25% between the cloth layers, and 5% as holes between layers of the fabric.

This variant of CVI that combines forced gas flow and temperature gradient avoids some of the problems mentioned earlier. Under these modified conditions, 70 to 90% dense SiC and Si_3N_4 matrices can be impregnated in SiC and Si_3N_4 fibrous preforms in less than a day. Under conditions of plain CVI, it would take several weeks to achieve such densities; that is, one can reduce the processing time from several days to less than 24 h. One can also avoid using binders in this process with their attendant problems of incomplete removal. The use of a graphite holder simplifies the fabrication of the preform, and the application of a moderate pressure to the preform can result in a higher-than-normal fiber volume fraction in the final product. The final obtainable density in a ceramic body is limited by the fact that closed porosity starts at about 93 to 94% of theoretical density. It is difficult to impregnate past this point.

Advantages of a CVI technique or any variant thereof include:

- Good mechanical properties at high temperatures
- Large, complex shapes can be produced in a near-net shape
- Considerable flexibility in the fibers and matrices that can be used (oxide and nonoxide)
- It is a pressureless process, and relatively low temperatures are used, for example, compared to the temperatures involved in hot pressing.

Among the disadvantages, one should mention that the process is slow and expensive.

Reactive Consolidation or Liquid Phase Sintering. The term reaction bonding is used rather loosely in literature. Some researchers use it to encompass all processes not involving hot pressing. In this article the term is restricted to processes involving chemical reaction(s) between components to produce the desired end product. Reactive consolidation or liquid phase sintering are the other more descriptive terms of such processes. Some commercial success has been obtained in making silicon carbide based composites by reaction bonding. Siliconized silicon carbide is the name given to a composite of SiC grains in a silicon matrix. Commercially, such composites are available under different designations (e.g., K-T, Refel, and NC-435) from different producers.

Polymers are used to bond the preforms containing carbon in the form of carbon and silicon

Table 2 Typical chemical reactions for a variety of matrix materials made by CVI

Matrix	Fiber/reinforcement	Typical reactions
SiC	Nicalon, Nextel, carbon, Al_2O_3, SiC	$CH_3SiCl_3 \xrightarrow{\text{in } H_2} SiC + 2HCl$
TiC	Carbon	$TiCl_4 + CH_4 \xrightarrow{\text{in } H_2} TiC + 4HCl$
B_4C	Carbon	$4BCl_4 + CH_4 \xrightarrow{\text{in } H_2} B_4C + 12HCl$
ZrC (HfC)	Carbon	$ZrCl_4 + CH_4 \xrightarrow{\text{in } H_2} ZrC + 4HCl$
Cr_3C_2	Al_2O_3	$CrCl_x + CH_4 \xrightarrow{\text{in } H_2} Cr_3C_2 + HCl$
TaC	Carbon	$TaCl_5 + CH_4 \xrightarrow{\text{in } H_2} TaC + HCl$
Si_3N_4	Carbon, Nicalon, Nextel	$3SiCl_4 + 4NH_3 \xrightarrow{\text{in } H_2} Si_3N_4 + 12HCl$
BN	BN, SiO_2, Nextel, carbon	$BX_3 + NH_3 \xrightarrow{\text{in } H_2} BN + 3HX$ ($X = Cl,F$)
TiB_2	Carbon, Nicalon, Al_2O_3	$TiCl_4 + 2BCl_3 \xrightarrow{\text{in } H_2} TiB_2 + 10HCl$
ZrO_2	Al_2O_3, mullite, carbon	$ZrCl_4 + 2CO + 2H_2 \longrightarrow ZrCl_4 + 2H_2O + 2CO \longrightarrow ZrO_2 + 2CO + 4HCl$
Al_2O_3	Nextel, Al_2O_3, carbon	$2AlCl_3 + 3CO_2 + 3H_2 \longrightarrow 2AlCl_3 + 3H_2O + 3CO \longrightarrow Al_2O_3 + 3CO + 6HCl$

Source: After Ref 31

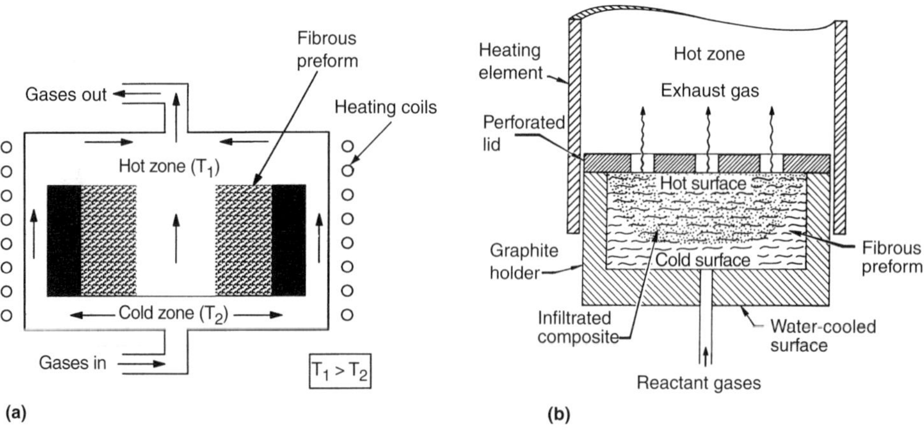

Fig. 9 Schematics of chemical vapor infiltration processes. (a) Isothermal chemical vapor infiltration. (b) Forced chemical vapor infiltration

carbide, followed by pyrolysis of the polymer to give more carbon (Ref 38, 39). The Refel material, developed in the United Kingdom (Ref 38), is formulated to give a minimum of free silicon, which in practice is limited to about 10 vol%. The infiltration is done under reduced pressure at temperatures up to 1700 °C (3090 °F) and for several hours. Hillig et al. (Ref 40) used a low modulus carbon fiber instead of carbon powder in the preform. Molten silicon reacts with carbon fibers to form SiC. The original geometry of the carbon fibers is retained. A big advantage of SiC/Si composite is that the constituents are in chemical equilibrium, and they have closely matched thermal expansion coefficients. Carbon fiber in the form of cloth, tow, felt, or matte is used as a precursor. A preform is made of carbon fiber and infiltrated with liquid silicon. Silicon reacts with carbon fibers to form SiC fibers in a silicon matrix. Typical composition of the resultant composite is Si (30–50%) + SiC fiber. Silicon matrix limits the use temperature to about 1400 °C (2550 °F).

In another version of this process, a liquid phase forms as a result of an exothermic reaction between elemental powders. A good example is that from the field of intermetallics, for example, nickel aluminides. The following steps are involved:

1. Mix nickel and aluminum in stoichiometric proportions.
2. Cold isostatic press to 70% theoretical density to obtain a green body.
3. Vacuum encapsulate the green body in a 304 stainless steel can.
4. Subject the canned material to reactive HIP.

Sol-Gel Techniques

Sol-gel techniques, which have been used for making conventional ceramic materials, can also be used to make ceramic-matrix materials in the interstices of a fibrous preform. A solution containing metal compounds—for example, a metal alkoxide, acetate, or halide—is reacted to form a sol. The sol is converted to a gel, which in turn is subjected to controlled heating to produce the desired end product: a glass, a glass-ceramic, or a ceramic. Characteristically, the gel-to-ceramic conversion temperature is much lower than that required in a conventional melting or sintering process. A schematic of a typical sol-gel process for processing CMCs is given in Fig. 10. It is easy to see that many of the polymer handling and processing techniques can be used for sol-gel as well. Impregnation of fibrous preforms in vacuum and filament winding are two important techniques. In filament winding, fiber tows or rovings are passed through a tank containing the sol, and the impregnated tow is wound on a mandrel to a desired shape and thickness. The sol is converted to gel, and the structure is removed from the mandrel. A final heat treatment then converts the gel to a ceramic- or glass matrix.

Some of the advantages of sol-gel techniques for making composites are the same as those for monolithic ceramics, namely, lower processing temperatures, greater compositional homogeneity in single phase matrices, potential for producing unique multiphase matrix materials, and so forth. Specifically, in regard to composite material fabrication, the sol-gel technique allows processing via liquids of low viscosity such as the ones derived from alkoxides. Covalent ceramics, for example, can be produced by pyrolysis of polymeric precursors at temperatures as low as 1400 °C (2005 °F) and with yields greater than those in CVD processes. Among the disadvantages of sol-gel are high shrinkage and low yield compared to slurry techniques. The fiber network provides a very high surface area to the matrix gel. Consequently, the shrinkage during the drying step frequently results in a large density of cracks in the matrix. Generally, repeated impregnations are required to produce a substantially dense matrix.

The sol-gel technique can also be used to prepare prepregs by slurry infiltration. The sol in the slurry acts as a binder and coats fibers and glass particles. The binder burnout step is thus eliminated because the binder, being of the same composition as the matrix, becomes part of the glass matrix.

Polymer Infiltration and Pyrolysis

Polymeric precursors can also be used to form a ceramic-matrix in a composite. Because of the generally high cost of processing CMCs, polymer infiltration and pyrolysis (PIP) is an attractive processing route because of its relatively low cost while maintaining small amounts of residual porosity and minimal degradation of the fibers (Ref 41–43). Moreover, this approach allows near-net-shape molding and fabrication technology that is able to produce nearly fully dense composites (Ref 44, 45). In PIP, the fibers are infiltrated with an organic polymer, which is heated to fairly high temperatures and pyrolyzed to form a ceramic-matrix. Due to the relatively low yield of polymer to ceramic, multiple infiltrations are used to densify the composite.

Polymeric precursors for ceramic-matrices allow one to use conventional polymer composite fabrication technology that is readily available and to take advantage of processes used to make polymer-matrix composites (Ref 42, 43). These include complex shape forming and fabrication. Furthermore, by processing and pyrolyzing at lower temperatures (compared to sintering and hot pressing, for example) one can avoid fiber degradation and the formation of unwanted reaction products at the fiber/matrix interface. French (Ref 42) lists some desirable characteristics in a preceramic polymer:

- High ceramic yield from polymer precursor
- Precursor that yields a ceramic with low free-carbon content (which will oxidize at high temperatures)
- Controllable molecular weight, which allows for solvent solubility and control over viscosity for fabrication purposes

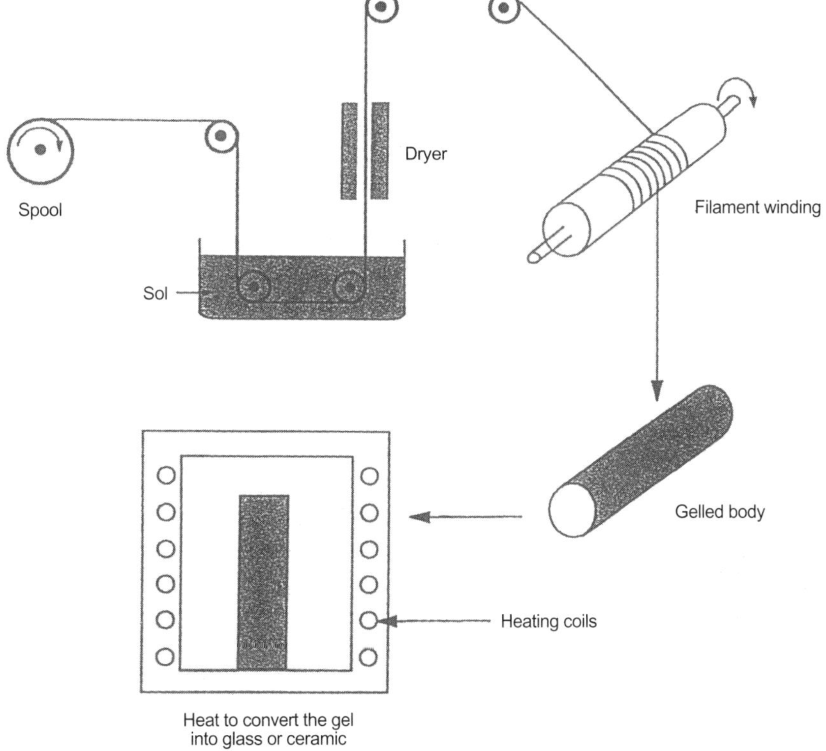

Fig. 10 Schematic of sol-gel process

- Low-temperature cross-linking of the polymer that allows resin to harden and maintain its dimensions during the pyrolysis process
- Low cost and toxicity

Most preceramic polymer precursors are formed from chloro-organosilicon compounds to form poly(silanes), poly(carbosilanes), poly(silazanes), poly(borosilanes), poly(silsesquioxanes), and poly(carbosiloxanes) (Ref 41). The synthesis reaction involves the dechlorination of the chlorinated silane monomers. Since a lot of the chlorosilane monomers are formed as by-products in the silicone industry, they are inexpensive and readily available. The monomers can be further controlled by an appropriate amount of branching, which controls important properties such as the viscosity of the precursor as well as the amount of ceramic yield.

All silicon-based polymer precursors lead to an amorphous ceramic-matrix, where silicon atoms are tetrahedrally arranged with nonsilicon atoms. This arrangement is similar to that found in amorphous silica (Ref 42). High-temperature treatments typically lead to crystallization and slight densification of the matrix, which results in shrinkage. At high temperatures, the amorphous ceramic begins to form small domains of crystalline phase, which are more thermodynamically stable (Ref 46). Silicon-carbide matrices derived from polycarbosilane begin to crystallize at 1100 to1200 °C (2010–2190 °F) while Si-C-O (polysiloxanes) and Si-N-C (polysilazanes) remain amorphous to 1300 to 1400 °C (23670–2550 °F).

Typically, the molecular weight range of the polymer is tailored, followed by shaping of the product (Ref 41). The polymer is then cross-linked and finally pyrolyzed in an inert or reactive atmosphere (e.g., NH_3) at temperatures between 1000 to1400 °C (1830 and 2550 °F). The pyrolysis step can be further subdivided into three steps. In the first step, between 550 and 880 °C (1020 and 1620 °F), an amorphous compound of the type $Si(C_aO_bN_cB_d)$ is formed. The second step involves nucleation of crystalline precipitates such as SiC, Si_3N_4, and SiO_2 at temperatures between 1200 and 1600 °C (2190 and 2910 °F). Grain coarsening may also result from consumption of any residual amorphous phase and reduction of the amount of oxygen due to vaporization of SiO and CO. Porosity is typically of the order of 5 to 20 vol% with pore sizes of the order of 1 to 50 nm. It should be noted that the average pore size and volume fraction of pores decrease with increasing pyrolysis temperature, since the amount of densification (and shrinkage) becomes irreversible at temperatures above the maximum pyrolysis temperature.

The main disadvantage of PIP is the low yield that accompanies the polymer-to-ceramic transformation and the resulting shrinkage, which typically causes cracking in the matrix during fabrication (Ref 41–45, 47, 48). Due to shrinkage and weight loss during pyrolysis, residual porosity after a single impregnation is of the order of 20 to 30%. To reduce the amount of residual porosity, multiple impregnations are needed. Reimpregnation is typically conducted with a very-low-viscosity prepolymer, so that the slurry may wet and infiltrate the small micropores that exist in the preform. Usually, reimpregnation is done by immersing the part in the liquid polymer in a vacuum bag, while higher-viscosity polymers require pressure impregnation. Typically, the amount of porosity will reduce from 35% to less than 10% after about five impregnations.

Significant gas evolution also occurs during pyrolysis (Ref 42). Thus, it is advisable to allow these volatile gases to slowly diffuse out of the matrix, especially for thicker parts. Typically, pyrolysis cycles ramp to 800 to 1400 °C (1470–2550 °F) over periods of 1 to 2 days to avoid delamination. Recall that pyrolysis must be done at a temperature below the crystallization temperature of the matrix (or large volume changes will occur) and below the degradation temperature of the reinforcing fibers. The pyrolysis atmosphere is most commonly argon or nitrogen, although in ammonia a pure amorphous silicon nitride with low amounts of free carbon can be obtained (Ref 49). Such an atmosphere may also lead to the formation of nitrides from the reaction of filler particles (Ref 50). With the formation of the ceramic, the gaseous by-product reaction can be written as (Ref 41):

$$P(\mathrm{s,l}) \xrightarrow{\Delta} C(\mathrm{s}) + G(\mathrm{g})$$

where P is the polymer, C is the ceramic, and G is the gaseous by-product. With the loss of the volatile gaseous products, the ceramic yield, α, is just the ratio of ceramic formed and the initial amount of polymer:

$$\alpha = \frac{m(C)}{m(P)} = 1 - \frac{m(G)}{m(P)}$$

where m represents the mass of a component (ceramic, polymer, or gas). The density ratio of the ceramic product, $\rho(C)$, to that of the polymer precursor, $\rho(P)$, is given by:

$$\beta = \frac{\rho(P)}{\rho(C)}$$

Two extreme cases of polymer-ceramic conversion can be considered. If the volume is not constrained, then diffusional flow will cause the pores to be filled, but a high amount of shrinkage will take place. The maximum volume change that occurs during conversion can be written as:

$$\psi = \alpha\beta - 1$$

If the volume is constrained (i.e., $\psi = 0$) then shrinkage does not occur, but a large amount of residual porosity is present. The maximum amount of porosity can be written as:

$$\pi = 1 - \alpha\beta$$

It has been reported that for filler-free pyrolysis of poly(silazane) to form bulk Si_3N_4, either a large amount of porosity (>8%) or a large amount of shrinkage (20%) took place (Ref 51). Fitzer and Gadow (Ref 28) used repeated infiltration and in situ thermal decomposition of porous reaction-bonded ceramics, such as silicon carbide and silicon nitrate with silazanes and polycarbosilanes, to process Si_3N_4/SiC composites. A typical sequence of steps taken in processing the composites is as follows:

1. Porous SiC or Si_3N_4 fibrous preform with some binder phase is prepared.
2. Fibrous preform is evacuated in an autoclave.
3. Samples are infiltrated with molten precursors—silazanes or polycarbosilanes—at high temperature (780 K), and the argon or nitrogen pressure is slowly increased from 2 to 40 MPa (0.3–5.8 ksi). The high temperature results in a transformation of the oligomer silane to polycarbosilane and simultaneous polymerization at high pressures.
4. Infiltrated samples are cooled and treated with solvents.
5. Samples are placed in an autoclave, and the organosilicon polymer matrix is thermally decomposed in an inert atmosphere at a high pressure and at temperature in the 800 to 1300 K range.
6. Steps 2 through 5 are repeated to obtain an adequate density. To produce an optimal matrix crystal structure, the material is annealed in the 1300 to 1800 K range.

Polymer-derived ceramic-matrix composites, similar to carbon/carbon composites, typically have a cracked matrix from processing as well as a number of small voids or pores. The large amount of shrinkage and cracking in the matrix can be contained, to some extent, by the additions of particulate fillers to the matrix, which, when added to the polymer reduce shrinkage and stiffen the matrix material in the composite (Ref 41). Figure 11 shows a schematic of filler-free versus active filler pyrolysis. Figure 12 shows the microstructure of a PIP CMC, indicating some residual porosity and a clear "filler network" in the matrix of the composite (Ref 52). Particulate or whisker ceramics used as fillers in the polymeric matrix can serve a variety of purposes (Ref 42):

- Reduce and disrupt the formation of matrix cracks that form during shrinkage of the polymer
- Enhance ceramic yield by forming reaction products during pyrolysis
- Strengthen and toughen the weak amorphous matrix and increase the interlaminar shear strength of the composite

The filler must be submicrometer in size in order to penetrate the tow bundle, and the coefficient of thermal expansion of the filler must match that of the polymeric matrix. It should be noted that the filler must not be used in very high fractions, and the slurry should not be forced into the reinforcing fibers since abrasion of the fiber fabric may take place. This is especially true with hard, angular fillers or ceramic whiskers. Typically, the volume fraction of filler is 15 to 25% of the matrix volume fraction. High filler loading may result in an increase in interply spacing and lower volume fraction of fibers.

When an "active" filler phase is added to the polymer, it reacts with solid or gaseous decomposition products to form new carbide phases (Ref 41):

$$P(\mathrm{s,l}) + T(\mathrm{s}) \xrightarrow{\Delta} C(\mathrm{s}) + M(\mathrm{s}) + G(\mathrm{g})$$

where T is the active filler, and M is the carbide phase formed. The other symbols have the same meaning as described in the previous expression. The maximum volume change of a precursor containing an active filler, ψ^*, can be expressed as (Ref 41):

$$\psi^* = \left(1 - \frac{V_T}{V_T^*}\right)(\alpha\beta - 1) + V_T\,(\alpha^{TM}\beta^{TM} - 1)$$

where V_T^* is the critical volume fraction of filler that determines maximum particle packing density of the reacted filler phase in the pyrolyzed product, α^{TM} and β^{TM} describe mass change of the filler phase and density ratio. For α^{TM} and $\beta^{TM} > 1$, volume expansion of the filler phase may compensate for polymer shrinkage during pyrolysis.

If one assumes isotropic dimensional changes, the linear shrinkage ε is related to the volume shrinkage ψ by (Ref 41):

$$\varepsilon = (\psi + 1)^{1/3} - 1$$

Thus, by controlling the amount of filler, the degree of shrinkage can be controlled.

Fiber architecture may have an impact in regard to PIP. One of the key factors is wetting of the fiber bundles. During pyrolysis, the precursor shrinks around the fibers, so cracks are introduced. For example, two-dimensional woven fabrics seem to have less propensity in developing interlaminar cracks than do cross-ply or unidirectional architectures. Satin weaves are preferred versus plain weaves because more uniform cracking is achieved and large cracks between weave crossover points are avoided (Ref 53). Due to the looser nature of the satin weave (it is more drapable), better wetting and densification may take place, although the loose nature of the weave also makes it more difficult to handle.

Self-Propagating High-Temperature Synthesis

Self-propagating high-temperature synthesis (SHS) can be used to produce a variety of refractory materials. The main disadvantage is that SHS products are very porous because of the fairly large porosity present in the original mix of reactants and because of the large volume change that results when the reactants transform to the products. Any adsorbed gases at the elevated temperatures used during this process can also add to the porosity of the final product. Synthesis concomitant with densification can improve the situation to some extent. This involves application of high pressure during the combustion or immediately after the completion of the combustion reaction when the product temperature is still quite high. Hot pressing, rolling, and shock waves are some of the techniques used to apply the necessary pressure.

The SHS technique involves synthesis of compounds without an external source of energy. One exploits exothermic reactions to synthesize ceramic compounds, which are difficult to fabricate by conventional techniques. For example, one can mix titanium powder and carbon black, cold press the mixture, and ignite the compact at the top in a cold-walled vessel. A combustion

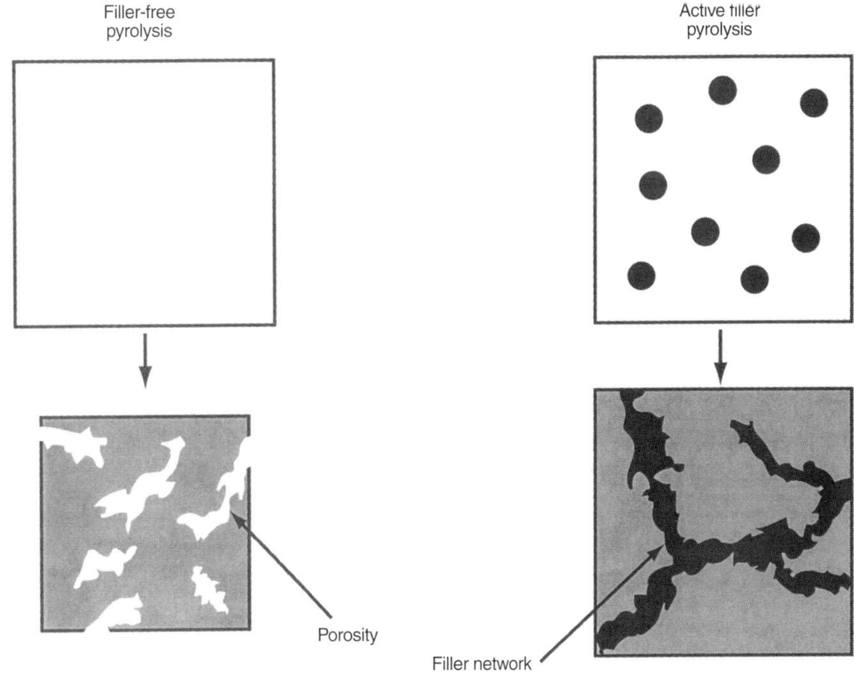

Fig. 11 Schematic of filler-free versus active filler pyrolysis. Source: Ref 52

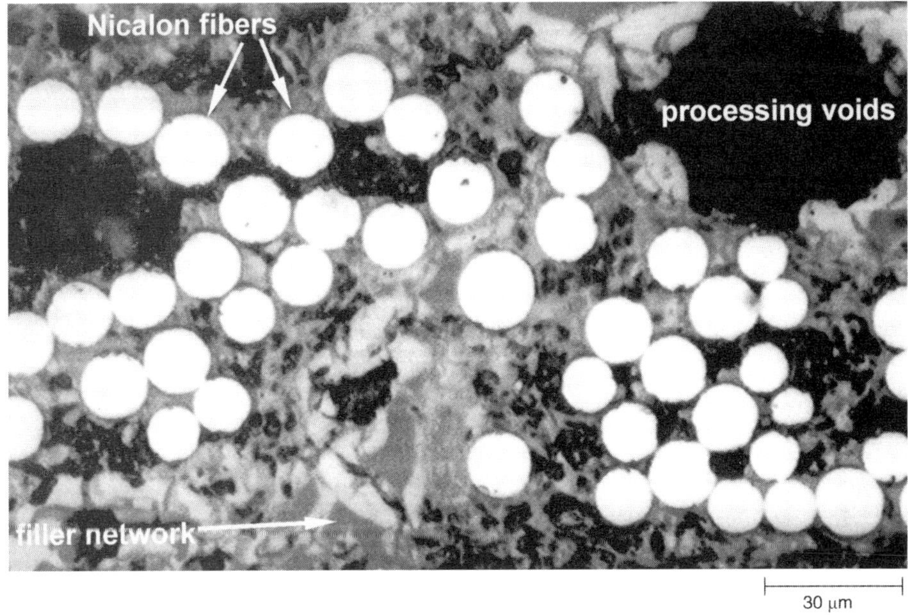

Fig. 12 Microstructure of a woven Nicalon/Si-C-O-N matrix composite with a SiC filler. Small amounts of residual porosity and a clear filler-free network can be seen in the matrix of the composite.

wave will pass through the compact, giving titanium carbide.

Among the salient features of SHS are:

- High combustion temperature (up to 4000 °C, or 7230 °F)
- Simple, low-cost equipment
- Good control of chemical composition
- Ability to obtain different shapes and forms

Many ceramics such as borides, carbides, nitrides, silicides, and sialons as well as composites such as SiC_w + Al_2O_3 have been synthesized by means of SHS. The SHS process gives a weakly bonded compact. Therefore, the process is generally followed by breaking the compact, milling, and consolidation by some technique such as HIP. Explosive or dynamic compaction can result in a relatively dense product. A good example of an SHS process to make composites is the proprietary process of Martin Marietta Corporation (Baltimore, MD), called the XD Process, wherein exothermic reactions are used to produce multiphase alloy powders. These are hot pressed at 1450 °C (2640 °F) to full density. Reinforcement in the form of particles, whiskers, and platelets can be added to the master alloy to make a composite. A good example is that of TiB_2 particles, about 1 μm diameter, distributed in intermetallic matrixes such as TiAl, TiAl + Ti_3Al, NiAl, and so forth.

Electrophoretic Deposition

The phenomenon of electrophoresis has been known since the beginning of the 19th century, but its applications in processing of ceramics and ceramic composites is relatively recent. Electrophoretic deposition (EPD) should not be confused with electroplating. In electroplating, ions are the moving species and they undergo ion reduction on deposition. In EPD, on the other hand, solid particles migrate with no charge reduction on deposition. Also, the deposition rate in EPD is ~1 mm/min while in electroplating it is ~0.1 μm/min. Electrophoretic deposition is a relatively simple and inexpensive technique, which can be profitably exploited for infiltration of tightly woven fiber preforms (Ref 54). Electrophoretic deposition makes use of nanoscale ceramic particles in a stable nonagglomerated form (such as in a sol or colloidal suspension) and exploits their net surface electrostatic charge characteristics while in suspension. On application of an electric field the particles will migrate toward and deposit on an electrode. If the deposition electrode is replaced by a conducting fibrous preform, the suspended particles will be attracted into and deposited within it, providing an appropriate means of effectively infiltrating densely packed fibrous bundles. A schematic diagram of the basic EPD cell is shown in Fig. 13. The movement of ceramic sol particles in an aqueous suspension within an electric field is governed by the field strength, and the pH, ionic strength, and viscosity of the solution (Ref 54). The electrophoretic mobility of charged particles in a suspension is given by the Smoluchowski equation (Ref 55):

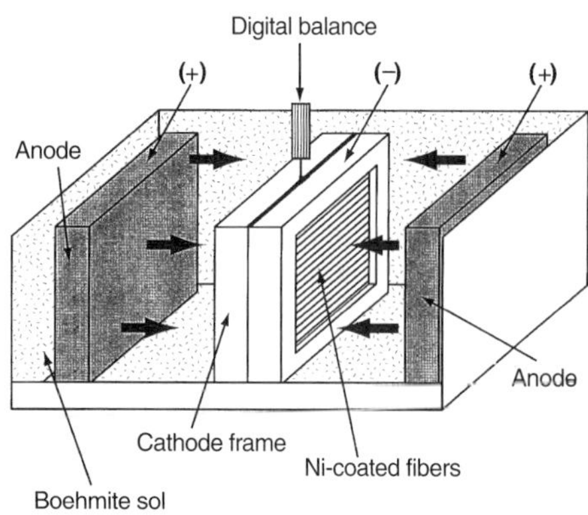

Fig. 13 Schematic of a basic electrophoretic deposition (EPD) cell (after Ref 56)

$$\text{Electrophoretic mobility} = \frac{U}{E} = \frac{\varepsilon\zeta}{4\pi\eta}$$

where U is the velocity, E is the field strength, ε is the dielectric constant, ζ is the zeta potential, and η is the viscosity. The zeta potential is a parameter for characterizing a suspension. It can be determined by measuring particle velocity in an electric field. According to the Smoluchowski equation, a suitable suspension for EPD should have a high particle surface charge, a high dielectric constant of the liquid phase, and a low viscosity. In addition, a low conductivity of the suspending medium to minimize solvent transport would be desirable (Ref 56).

REFERENCES

1. K.K. Chawla, *Ceramic Matrix Composites,* Chapman & Hall, London, 1993, p 4–10, 176, 314
2. K.K. Chawla, *Composite Materials,* 2nd ed., Springer-Verlag, 1997
3. R. Raj and R.K Bordia, *Acta Metall.,* Vol 32, 1989, p 1003
4. B. Kellett and F.F. Lange, *J. Am. Ceram. Soc.,* Vol 67, 1989, p 369
5. R.K. Bordia and R. Raj, *J. Am. Ceram. Soc.,* Vol 71, 1988, p 302
6. L.C. De Jonghe, M.N. Rahaman, and C.H. Hseuh, *Acta Metall.,* Vol 39, 1986, p 1467
7. M.D. Sacks, H.W. Lee, and O.E. Rojas, *J. Am. Ceram. Soc.,* Vol 70, 1987, p C-348
8. M.N. Rahaman and L.C. De Jonghe, *J. Am. Ceram. Soc.,* Vol 70, 1987, p C-348
9. K.M. Prewo, in *Tailoring Multiphase and Composite Ceramics,* Vol 20, Materials Science Research, Plenum Press, 1986, p 529
10. D.C. Phillips, in *Fabrication of Composites,* North-Holland, Amsterdam, 1983, p 373
11. J.A. Cornie, Y.-M. Chiang, D.R. Uhlmann, A. Mortensen, and J.M. Collins, *Am. Ceram. Soc. Bull.,* Vol 65, 1986, p 293
12. K.M. Prewo and J.J. Brennan, *J. Mater. Sci.,* Vol 15, 1980, p 463
13. J.J. Brennan and K.M. Prewo, *J. Mater. Sci.,* Vol 17, 1982, p 2371
14. R.A.J. Sambell, D.C. Phillips, and D.H. Bowen, in *Carbon Fibres: Their Place in Modern Technology*, The Plastics Institute, London, 1974, p 16/9
15. H.Y. Liu, N. Claussen, M.J. Hoffmann, and G. Petzow, *J. Eur. Ceram. Soc.,* Vol 7, 1991, p 41
16. S.J. Barclay, J.R. Fox, and H.K. Bowen, *J. Mater Sci.*, Vol 22, 1987, p 4403
17. M. Yang and R. Stevens, *J. Mater. Sci.*, Vol 25, 1990, p 4658
18. J. Homeny, W.L. Vaughn, and M.K. Ferber, *Am. Ceram. Soc. Bull.*, Vol 67, 1987, p 333
19. P.D. Shalek, J.J. Petrovic, G.F. Hurley, and F.D. Gac, *Am. Ceram. Soc. Bull.,* Vol 65, 1986, p 351
20. N. Chawla, K.K. Chawla, M. Koopman, B. Patel, C.C. Coffin, and J.I. Eldridge, *Compos. Sci. Technol.,* 2001, in press
21. R.T. Bhatt, NASA TN-88814, National Aeronautics and Space Administration, 1986
22. R.T. Bhatt, *J. Mater. Sci.*, Vol 25, 1990, p 3401
23. N. Chawla, *Metall. Trans. A,* Vol 28A, 1997, p 2423
24. W.B. Hillig, *J. Am. Ceram. Soc.,* Vol 71, 1988, p C-96
25. A.W. Urquhart, *Mater. Sci. Eng.,* Vol A144, 1991, p 75
26. E. Fitzer and D. Hegen, *Angew. Chem.*, Vol 91, 1979, p 316
27. E. Fitzer and J. Schlichting, *Z. Werkstofftech.*, Vol 11, 1980, p 330
28. E. Fitzer and R. Gadow, *Am. Ceram. Soc. Bull.*, Vol 65, 1986, p 326
29. D.P. Stinton, A.J. Caputo, R.A. Lowden, and T.M. Besmann, *Ceram. Eng. Sci. Proc.*, Vol 7, 1986, p 983
30. C.V. Burkland, W.E. Bustamante, R. Klacka, and J.-M. Yang, in *Whisker- and Fiber-Toughened Ceramics,* ASM International, 1988, p 225
31. R.L. Bickerdike, A.R.G. Brown, G. Hughes, and H. Ranson, *Proc. Fifth Conference on Carbon*, S. Mrosowski, M.C. Studebaker, and P.L. Walker, Ed., Pergamon Press, 1962, p 575
32. R.A. Lowden, D.P. Stinton, and T.M. Besmann, in *Handbook of Continuous Fiber Ceramic Matrix Composites*, American Ceramic Society, Inc., 1993, p 205
33. R. Naslain, *Euro-CVD-Four,* The Centre, Eindhoven, 1983, p 293
34. R. Naslain, *Ceramic Matrix Composites,* R. Warren, Ed., Chapman and Hall, London, 1992, p 199
35. D.P. Stinton, A.J. Caputo, and R.A. Lowden, *Am. Ceram. Soc. Bull.*, Vol 65, 1986, p 347
36. A.J. Caputo, D.P. Stinton, and R.A. Lowden, *Am. Ceram. Soc. Bull.*, Vol 66, 1987, p 368

37. T.M. Besmann, B.W. Sheldon, R.A. Lowden, and D.P. Stinton, *Science,* Vol 253, 1991, p 1104
38. C.W. Forrest, P. Kennedy, and J.V. Shennan, *Special Ceramics,* Vol 5, British Ceramic Research Association, Stoke-on-Trent, U.K., 1972, p 99
39. P.A. Willermet, R.A. Pett, and T.J. Whalen, *Am. Ceram. Soc. Bull.*, Vol 57, 1978, p 744
40. W.B. Hillig, R.L. Mehan, C.R. Morelock, et al., *Am. Ceram. Soc. Bull.,* Vol 54, 1975, p 1054
41. P. Greil, *J. Am. Ceram. Soc.*, Vol 78, 1995, p 835
42. J.E. French, in *Handbook of Continuous Fiber Ceramic Composites,* American Ceramic Society, 1996, p 269
43. F.I. Hurwitz, J.Z. Gyekenyesi, and P.J. Conroy, *Ceram. Eng. Sci. Proc.*, Vol 10, 1989, p 750
44. K. Sato, H. Morozumi, A. Tezuka, O. Funayama, and T. Isoda, *High Temperature Ceramic-Matrix Composites* II, A.G. Evans and F.W. Zok, Ed., American Ceramic Society, 1995, p 199
45. M.F. Gonon, G. Fantozzi, M. Murat, and J.P. Disson, *J. Eur. Ceram. Soc.,* Vol 15, 1995, p 185
46. J. Lipowitz, J.A. Rabe, L.K. Frevel, and R.L. Miller, *J. Mater. Sci.,* Vol 25, 1990, p 2118
47. R. Lundberg, R. Pompe, and R. Carlsson, *Comp. Sci. Tech.*, Vol 37, 1990, p 165
48. F. Sirieix, P. Goursat, A. Lecomte, and A. Dauger, *Comp. Sci. Technol.*, Vol 37, 1990, p 7
49. G.T. Burns and G. Chandra, *J. Am. Ceram. Soc.,* Vol 72, 1989, p 334
50. T. Erny, M. Seibold, O. Jarchow, and P. Greil, *J. Am. Ceram. Soc.*, Vol 76, 1993, p 207
51. R. Riedel, G. Passing, H. Schonfelder, and R.J. Brook, *Nature*, Vol 355, 1992, p 355
52. N. Chawla, Y.K. Tur, J.W. Holmes, J.R. Barber, and A. Szweda, *J. Am. Ceram. Soc.,* Vol 81, 1998, p 1221
53. F.J. Hurwitz, NASA Tech. Memo 105754, National Aeronautics and Space Administration, Oct 1992
54. T.J. Illston, C.B. Ponton, P.M. Marquis, and E.G. Butler, *Third Euroceramics,* Vol 1, P. Duran and J.F. Fernandez, Ed., Faenza Editirice Iberica, Madrid, 1993, p 419–424
55. D.R. Brown and F.W. Salt, *J. Appl. Chem.*, Vol 15, 1965, p 40
56. C. Kaya, A.R. Boccaccini, and K.K. Chawla, *J. Am. Ceram. Soc.,* Vol 20, 2000, p 1189

Processing of Carbon-Carbon Composites

CARBON-CARBON COMPOSITES (CCCs), high-density carbon fibers in a carbon matrix, began replacing fine-grained graphite as nose tips in rockets in the mid-1960s. They were subsequently introduced for applications that require their high specific strength and stiffness, in combination with their thermoshock resistance, chemical resistance, and fracture toughness, especially at high temperatures.

This article describes the manufacture, post-processing, fabrication, and properties of CCCs. Detailed information about CCC constituent materials is provided in the articles "Carbon Fibers" and "Carbon Matrices" in this Volume. Information about applications is provided in the article "Applications of Carbon-Carbon Composites" in this Volume.

Preform Fabrication

All types of carbon fibers can be used as reinforcements in many different architectures: random fibers; two-directional fabrics in stacked, stitched, or pierced configurations; three-directional geometries (cartesian or cylindrical coordinates) to increase the off-axis strength; or three-directional and multidirectional (4 to 11) weaves to minimize the empty spaces between the rod junctions. Unidirectional orientation has no importance for technical applications, but many basic investigations have been carried out using unidirectional composites as models (Ref 1–6).

Both three-directional and multidirectional composites are generally too expensive for industrial applications. Two-directional and multiaxial fibers usually suffice. Manufacturing techniques are listed in Table 1 with respect to the processibility of different geometries. In some cases, combinations of the main processing techniques are reasonable for manufacturing complex structures.

Multidirectional Woven Preforms

The main advantage of multidirectional CCCs is the freedom to orient selected fiber types and amounts to accommodate the design loads of the final structural component. Multidirectional fabrication technology provides the means to produce tailored composites.

The simplest type of multidirectional preform is based on a three-directional orthogonal construction, which is normally used to weave rectangular, block-type preforms. As shown in Fig. 1, this preform type consists of multiple yarn bundles located on cartesian coordinates. Each of the yarn bundles is straight in order to achieve the maximum structural capability of the fiber.

Table 1 Processing techniques for different geometries

Geometry	Axial pressing, 2-D	Vacuum-sack, 2-D	Autoclave, 2-D	Winding, 2-D	Weaving, 2.5/3-D
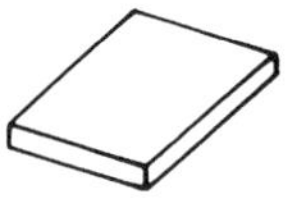	Easy	Easy	Easy	Possible	Possible
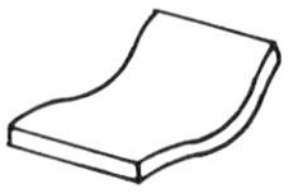	Easy	Easy	Easy	Not possible	Possible
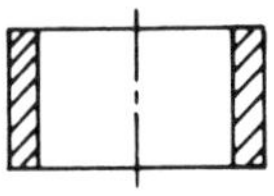	Not possible	Possible	Possible	Easy	Possible
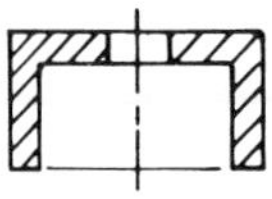	Not possible	Possible	Possible	Easy	Possible
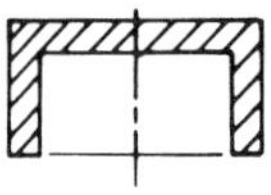	Not possible	Possible	Easy	Not possible	Possible
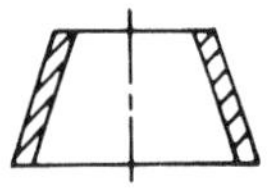	Not possible	Possible	Possible	Easy	Possible
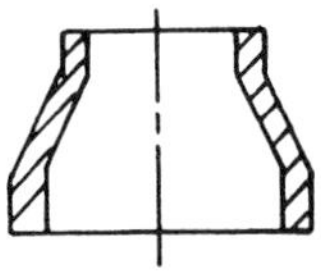	Not possible	Possible	Possible	Easy	Possible
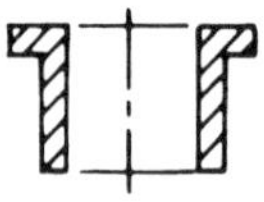	Not possible	Possible	Easy	Not possible	Possible
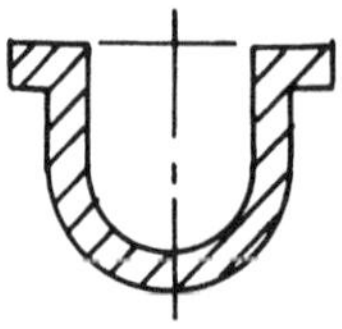	Not possible	Possible	Easy	Not possible	Possible
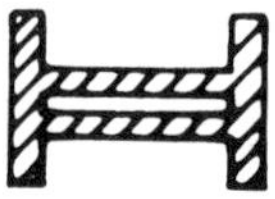	Not possible	Not possible	Possible	Not possible	Possible

Preforms are described by yarn type, number of yarns per site, spacing between adjacent sites, volume fraction of yarn in each direction, and preform density.

Several modifications of the basic three-directional orthogonal construction are available in order to achieve more isotropic preforms. This is accomplished by introducing yarns in additional directions. For example, a five-directional construction can be achieved by adding two reinforcement directions that are ±45° with respect to the yarns within the *X*-*Y* plane of the preform. Another option is to introduce diagonal yarns across the corners and/or across the faces of a rectangular three-directional preform to achieve a nonplanar multidirectional construction (Ref 7).

The type of multidirectional preform construction typically used for cylinders and other shapes of revolution (shown in Fig. 2) is a three-directional construction with yarns oriented on polar coordinates in the radial, axial, and circumferential directions. As with orthogonal block preforms, yarn type, spacing, and volume fraction can be varied in all three directions.

Fiber Selection. Fibers are normally available as yarns or tows containing 1000 to 12,000 filaments per strand. Fibers selected must be compatible with the weaving and densification process and must provide the physical and structural properties required in the composite.

The highest-modulus fibers have been subjected to the highest heat treatment temperature during manufacture. The properties of these high-modulus fibers are less affected by temperature exposure during carbon-carbon processing than high-strength intermediate-modulus fibers that have not been previously exposed to graphitizing temperatures.

In most cases, fiber properties are degraded by various handling and processing steps that occur during CCC fabrication. Small amounts of polymeric coatings or finishes are used to reduce handling damage and to improve fiber-matrix compatibility.

Manufacturing. The original multidirectional preforms used precise tooling to locate yarns, but the weaving operations were performed manually. Weaving operations have now been automated, but many details regarding equipment and procedures are proprietary.

Most multidirectional preforms used for CCCs are represented by the orthogonal or polar constructions shown in Fig. 1 and 2, respectively, or by some modification of these constructions. The techniques used to manufacture these preforms include weaving dry yarns (Ref 8), piercing fabrics (Ref 9, 10), assembling resin-rigidized yarns (Ref 11), and filament winding (modified) (Ref 12).

Block Preforms. One method of weaving three-directional orthogonal block preforms involves setting up a precisely spaced rectangular array of thin-walled metal tubes or solid rods representing the location of each *Z* direction reinforcing yarn (Ref 8, 13). Alternate *X* and *Y* layers of yarn are built up between the rows of metal tubes, as illustrated in Fig. 3. After the height of the preform has been established by *X*-*Y* layers, each *Z* direction tube (or rod) is replaced by yarn to establish the *Z* direction of the preform.

A modified three-directional orthogonal block construction is produced by using a two-directional woven fabric instead of *X*-*Y* yarn layers. These preforms are fabricated by piercing multiple layers of fabric over a precisely spaced rectangular array of metal rods. These metal rods, which represent the *Z* direction of the preform, are replaced with carbon yarns or precured (rigidized) yarn-resin rods as the final step of the process (Ref 10).

Shapes of Revolution. Fully automated computer-controlled equipment for fabricating three-directional cylindrical, conical, and contoured preforms has been developed both in the United States and in France. One version of this type of equipment is three-axis computer numerically controlled to define the preform configuration accurately and to place reinforcing fibers in the radial, axial, and circumferential directions (Ref 14). The outside surface defines the inside surface of the preform. Such machines can make preforms up to 2000 mm (84 in.) in diameter.

Automated equipment has also been developed to fabricate cylindrical preforms completely from dry yarns (Ref 13, 15). To weave preforms, this type of loom locates yarns in the circumferential and radial directions within an array of axial metal rods, which are then replaced by dry yarns.

Densification Processing

Generally, the best CCCs result from a densification process that fills the open volume of the preform with a dense, well-bonded carbon-graphite matrix. The actual densification process

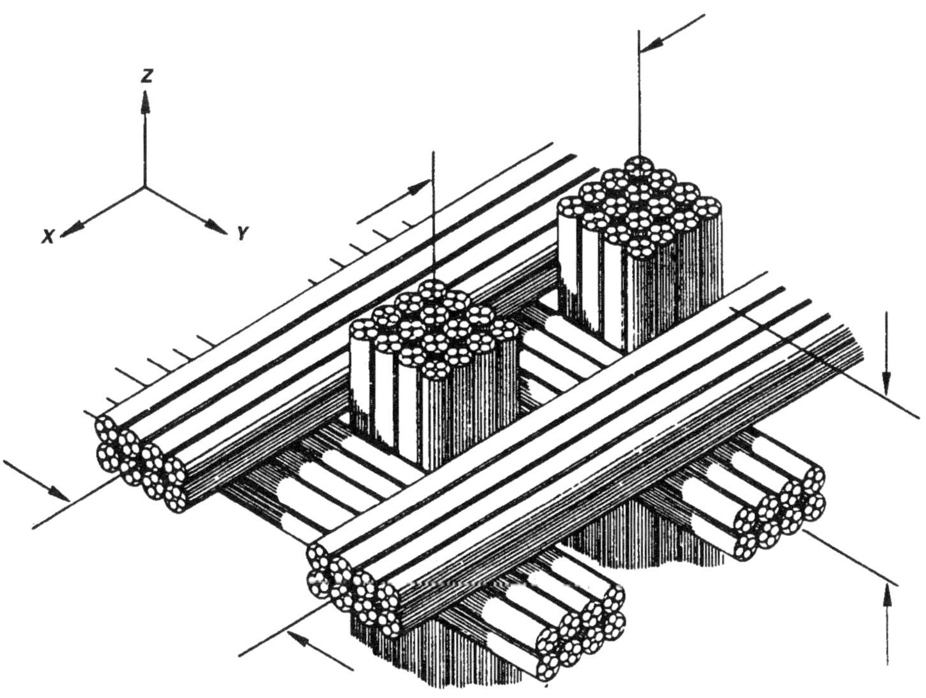

Fig. 1 Three-directional orthogonal preform construction. Source: Ref 7

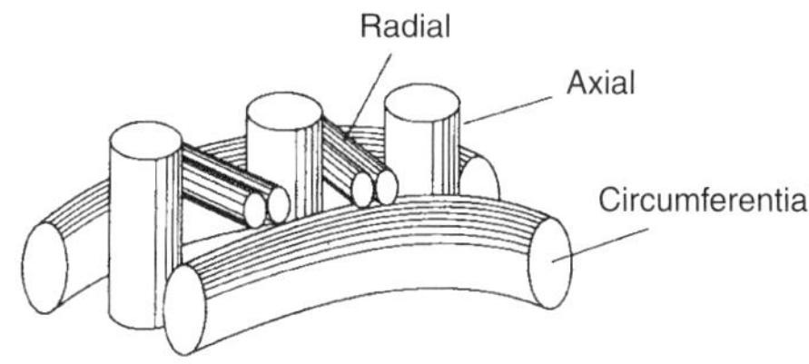

Fig. 2 Three-directional cylindrical preform construction. Source: Ref 7

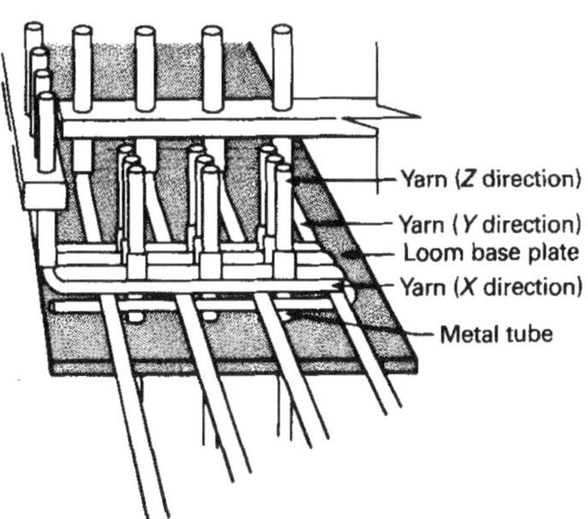

Fig. 3 Three-directional orthogonal weaving. Source: Ref 8

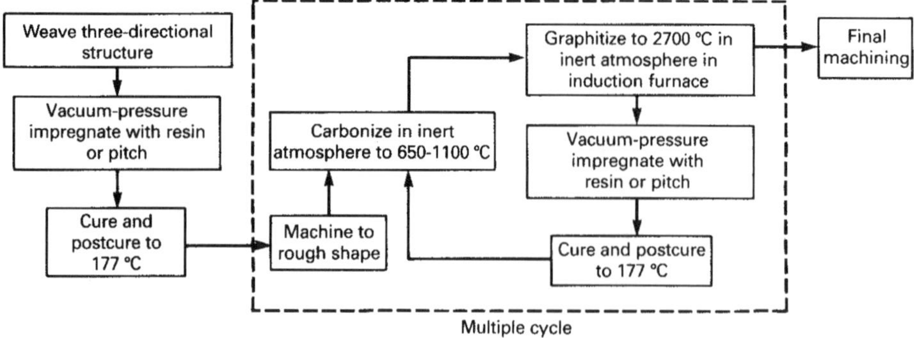

Fig. 4 Typical carbon-carbon densification process. Source: Ref 16

is dictated by the characteristics of the preform (Fig. 4). Four of the most important factors are carbon fiber type, fiber volume, preform thickness, and void size distribution within the preform.

Matrix Precursor Impregnants. The two general categories of matrix precursors used for carbon-carbon densification are thermosetting resins, such as phenolics and furfurals, and pitches based on coal tar and petroleum. The thermosetting resins polymerize to form cross-linked, infusible solids. As a result of pyrolysis, these resins form amorphous (glassy) carbon. The carbon yield at 800 °C (1470 °F) is about 50 to 60 wt%.

The coal tar and petroleum pitches are mixtures of polynuclear aromatic hydrocarbons. From their softening point up to about 400 °C (750 °F), the liquefied pitches undergo various changes, including volatilization of low-molecular-weight fractions, polymerization, cleavage, and rearrangements of the molecular structure. At temperatures above 400 °C (750 °F), mesophase spheres are formed in the isotropic liquid pitch. These mesophase spheres deform, coalesce, and solidify to form regions of extended order. The lamellar arrangement of the molecular structure in these regions favors the formation of a graphitic structure on further heating to above 2000 °C (3630 °F).

Coke yield from coal tar and petroleum pitches is about 50 wt% after pyrolysis at atmospheric pressure. However, pyrolysis of coal tar pitch at 600 °C (1110 °F) under 6.9 MPa (1 ksi) of pressure gives a coke yield of 90% (Ref 17). An increase in pyrolysis pressure does not increase coke yield over the 90% level.

Liquid Impregnation. The general processing technique using organic liquid impregnants as carbon matrix precursors involves multiple cycles of preform impregnation and heat treatment to produce a densified composite. Impregnant viscosity and coke yield, density, microstructure, and degree of graphitization must be considered (Ref 18). All of these factors are influenced by the time-temperature-pressure relationships encountered during processing.

The process can be modified by performing the carbonization step under pressures ranging from 6.8 to 103 MPa (1 to 15 ksi). This modified process has been designated as the pressure-impregnation-carbonization (PIC) process. Modified hot isostatic pressing equipment is used to impregnate and densify the composite effectively during the melting and coking stages of the carbonization process (Ref 19, 20). Isostatic pressure forces pitch into the small pores that are not filled during initial vacuum impregnation. As the pitch begins to pyrolyze, high isostatic pressure maintains the more volatile fractions of the pitch in a condensed phase. This reduces the amount of liquid forced out of the composite by pitch pyrolysis products.

The curves in Fig. 5 illustrate the advantage of PIC versus atmospheric-pressure carbonization to achieve high-density, multidirectional CCCs.

Chemical vapor infiltration (CVI) (Ref 21) of carbon uses gaseous hydrocarbons such as methane, propane/propylene, and benzene to deposit a carbon matrix internally in a carbon fiber preform. The process can be performed using three different methods. In the most commonly used technique (Fig. 6a), natural gas or other carbonaceous gases are flowed past and through a carbon fiber preform located in a low-pressure isothermal furnace. Uniform deposition throughout the preform can be achieved by operating at a temperature sufficiently low to permit rapid gaseous diffusion, compared to deposition of carbon. However, the deposition time is usually very long. Mass transfer through the fiber preform can be improved by inducing a pressure gradient through it (Fig. 6b). The deposition rate can be much higher. Enhanced deposition rates can be achieved also by using a temperature gradient deposition process (Fig. 6c).

A major problem with CVI is to achieve the uniform deposition of the carbon matrix throughout a thick preform. Mass transfer from the bulk gas must be sufficiently high in the fiber preform to keep a relatively constant concentration of carbon-containing molecules throughout. Hence, the rate at which carbon is deposited must be slow compared to the mass transfer of carbon into and throughout the preform.

Mass transfer of carbon-containing molecules into the preform is usually by diffusion, which slowly increases with temperature. The deposi-

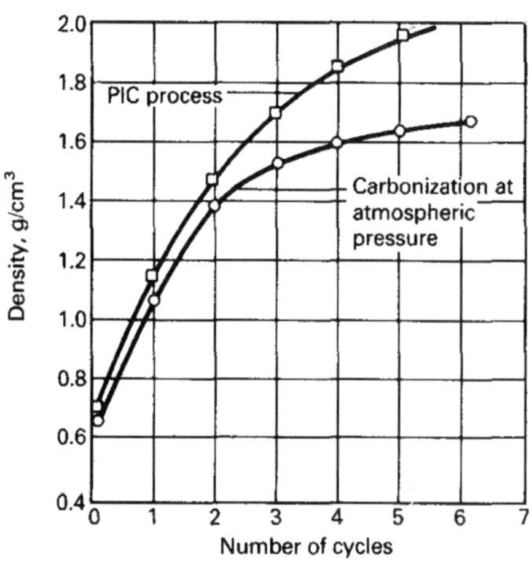

Fig. 5 Comparison of the pressure-impregnation-carbonization (PIC) process with carbonization at atmospheric pressure. Source: Ref 7

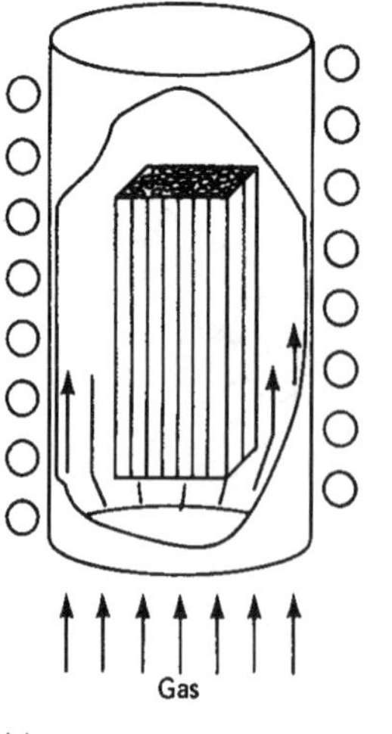

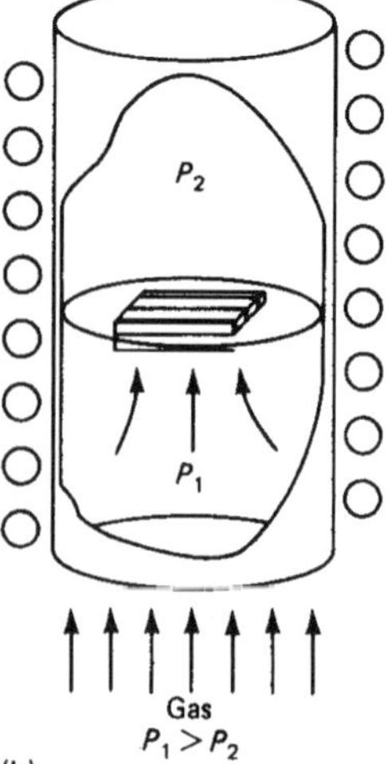

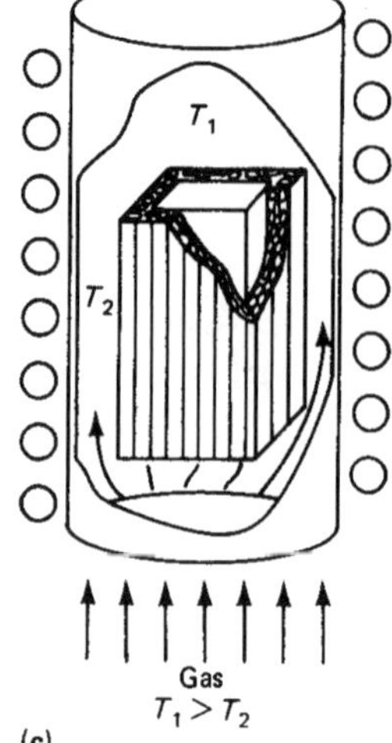

Fig. 6 Chemical vapor infiltration process

tion of carbon is complex, but the overall process has a high temperature coefficient. Hence, the relative rates of the two processes can be varied by adjusting the temperature. A temperature of 1000 to 1100 °C (1830 to 2010 °F) is commonly used, along with a pressure of 500 to 3000 Pa (5 to 30 mbar), to achieve a relatively uniform deposition of carbon throughout a part 10 mm (0.40 in.) thick.

More rapid mass transfer can be achieved by placing a pressure drop across the fiber preform (Fig. 6b). However, the deposition rate decreases as the pressure decreases, which produces nonuniform deposition through the preform. A pressure gradient process can be used at the end of a conventional cycle when mass transfer through tiny pores is extremely slow.

An alternative is to use a temperature gradient, such that carbon is deposited at a moving boundary that sweeps through the thickness (Fig. 6c). The deposition time can be significantly decreased, because mass transfer of the deposition gases is mostly through parts of the preform that have not yet been deposited upon. Unfortunately, the technique produces a variation in microstructure because deposition occurs at different temperatures.

A problem with all present CVI processes is closed pore formation caused by the sealing off of bottleneck pores, and, more insidiously, delaminated regions. However, high-temperature heat treatment may be employed to induce microcracks in the matrix to be filled in the subsequent CVI process. Using liquid impregnation to produce relatively uniform open pores, followed by CVI, is another attractive alternative.

Protective Coatings

Coating technology for carbon-carbon has been driven primarily by the aerospace and defense industries, in applications where the composite is exposed to high-temperature oxidizing environments. Advanced applications include hot-section components for limited-life missile engines, exhaust components for fighter aircraft, hypersonic vehicle fuselage and wing components, and structures for space defense satellites (Ref 22). The most notable application of coated carbon-carbon is for the nose cap and wing leading edges of the Shuttle Orbiter vehicle (Ref 23–25). Several dozen successful missions have been flown, demonstrating the flight worthiness of coated carbon-carbon in reentry applications. References 26 to 37 provide information about the historical development of methods for protecting carbon bodies.

Fundamentals of Protecting Carbon-Carbon

Carbon-Carbon Constituents and Microstructure. Applications requiring coatings typically use carbon fibers in laminated woven cloth or three-dimensional woven reinforcements. The fibers used are derived from rayon, polyacrylonitrile (PAN), or petroleum pitch and have a wide range of properties. For example, the elastic modulus along the fiber axis ranges from approximately 41.4 GPa (6×10^6 psi) for rayon fibers to 414 GPa (60×10^6 psi) for heat-stabilized PAN to 690 GPa (100×10^6 psi) for pitch fibers. The axial fiber expansion coefficients become lower as the fiber modulus increases.

The characteristics of the matrix vary, depending on the method of densification. Generally, the matrix microstructure spans a range from being glasslike, with small, randomly oriented crystallites of turbostratic carbon, to having strongly oriented and highly graphitized large crystallites. Weak interfaces usually exist between the fibers and matrix, because strong covalent atomic bonding prevents the carbon constituents from sintering, even at very high temperatures. Because the mechanical properties of the matrix are substantially inferior to those of the fibers, the fibers generally control the mechanical performance and expansion characteristics of the composites. A rayon-fabric-reinforced laminated construction typically exhibits the following in-plane properties: a tensile strength of 51.7 MPa (7.5 ksi), a tensile elastic modulus of 13.8 GPa (2×10^6 psi), and a coefficient of thermal expansion (CTE) of 2.4×10^{-6} °C^{-1} (1.3×10^{-6} °F^{-1}). Laminated constructions that have high-performance fibers exhibit the following typical in-plane properties: a tensile strength of 276 MPa (40 ksi), a tensile elastic modulus of 90 GPa (13×10^6 psi), and a CTE of 1.4×10^{-6} °C^{-1} (0.8×10^{-6} °F^{-1}).

Matrix Inhibition. Carbon begins to oxidize at measurable rates at approximately 371 °C (700 °F). Carbon-carbon composites exhibit high internal surface areas due to the porous nature of the structure (typical levels of interconnected porosity are 10 to 15%). Adding inhibitor phases to the matrix has become an important facet of an overall oxidation protection system, because inhibitors allow some control of oxidation that can occur through defects in coatings. Inhibitors can also prevent catastrophic oxidation failure due to coating spallation at high temperatures.

Additions of boron, boron compounds, and phosphorus compounds have been effective in protecting carbon bodies (Ref 38–43) by true chemical inhibition and by formation of internal and external glass layers that act as diffusion barriers. The practice of making boron additions to carbon-carbon for improved oxidation resistance was first disclosed in a 1978 patent (Ref 44). Since that time, many improvements and variations on this theme have been reported (Ref 45–54).

Internal chemical modifications can be made either by mixing the carbonaceous and nonoxide inhibitor powders and consolidating the constituents to form the carbon body, or by impregnating the porous body with liquids that contain the inhibitors, usually in oxide form. Boron and many nonoxide boron compounds are quite refractory, so the powder mixing and carbon processing route has often been used (Ref 41–43). In composite fabrication, submicron refractory compound additives are normally carried within impregnating resins and are dispersed through the fiber tows as well as between the fabric plies.

Coating Selection Principles. The most critical component of any coating architecture is the primary oxygen barrier. The oxygen barrier prevents oxygen ingress to the underlying composite by providing a physical permeation barrier and, in some cases, by gettering oxygen in the process. The critical parameters that guide the selection of the oxygen barrier are its oxidation characteristics, CTE, and inherent oxygen permeability. A material that forms an adherent, low-permeability oxide scale is preferred as an oxygen barrier because it oxidizes slowly and has the potential to self-heal. An Arrhenius plot of rate constants for oxidation of refractory materials typically considered for coating applications (Ref 55, 56) is presented in Fig. 7. Scale growth as a function of time can be estimated from Fig. 7 using the relationship $x^2 = Kt$, where x is the scale thickness, K is the parabolic rate constant, and t is time in hours. The silicon-based ceramics exhibit substantially lower oxide growth kinetics than the aluminum-, hafnium-, or zirconium-based ceramics. Time and temperature of service dictate material selection and coating thickness. However, from the standpoint of forming thin protective scales in thermal cycles with peak temperatures in the range of 1400 to 1700 °C (2550 to 3090 °F), only Si_3N_4 and SiC exhibit sufficiently low-rate constants for oxide growth over extended time periods.

Figure 8 compares the thermal expansion behavior of refractory coating candidates with that measured for high-performance, fabric-reinforced carbon-carbon (Ref 55–57). The expan-

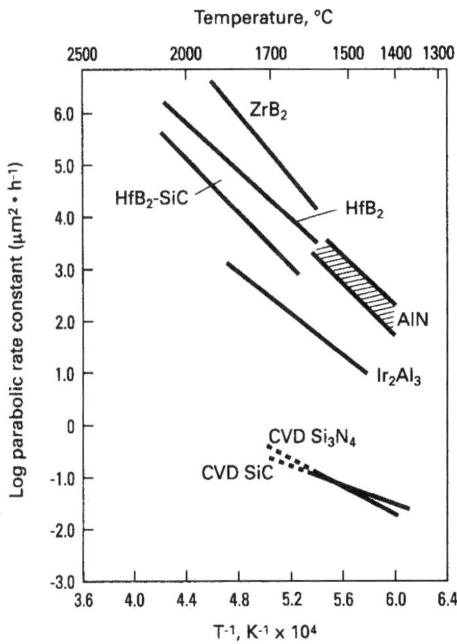

Fig. 7 Oxidation kinetics of refractory materials. CVD, chemical vapor deposition

sion of carbon-carbon in the in-plane directions is substantially lower than that for any of the refractory ceramics. This expansion difference, coupled with the high modulus of the refractory materials, results in significant thermal mismatch stresses when they are employed as coatings.

The properties of refractory materials that have been used in deposition studies are summarized in Table 2. Figure 9 presents the thermal stresses calculated as a function of temperature when these coatings were deposited onto high-performance, two-dimensional carbon-carbon laminates. For the refractory ceramics, Si_3N_4 provides the lowest thermal mismatch stresses of any of the ceramic coating candidates, but these stresses are still high enough to cause cracking. Therefore, it is usually found that deposited ceramic coatings exhibit microcracking and that the crack pattern depends on the coating thickness and deposition temperature. Iridium metal deposited by electron beam physical vapor deposition techniques can have low thermal mismatch stresses upon cooling. However, such a coating must then be able to withstand extremely high compressive stresses upon heating. In previously reported work (Ref 56), it has been shown that iridium-based coatings deposited by this technique onto high-performance carbon-carbon fail by compressive spalling at elevated temperatures.

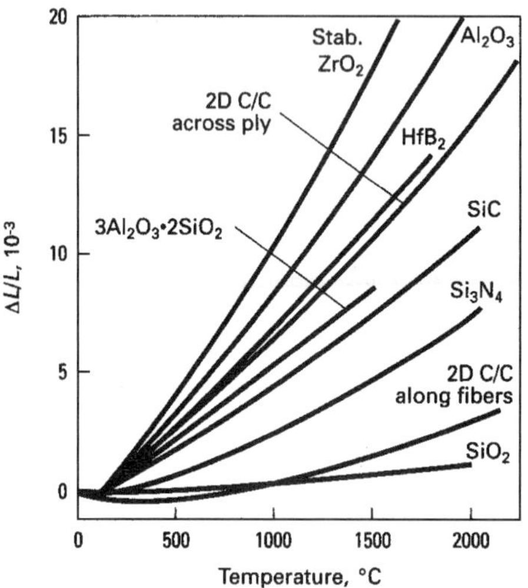

Fig. 8 Thermal expansion characteristics of ceramics and carbon-carbon laminates. 2D, two-directional; C/C, carbon-carbon laminae; *L*, specimen length

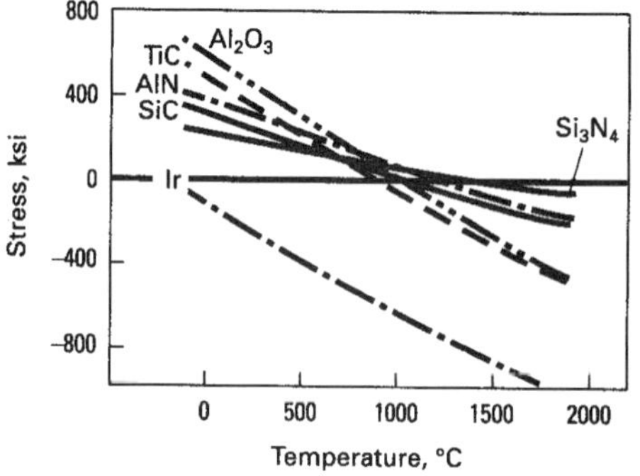

Fig. 9 Calculated thermal stresses for thin coatings on high-performance carbon-carbon laminates. Ratio of substrate thickness to coating thickness = 20.

Preferred Coating Approaches

Coating approaches are dictated by application requirements and fundamental behavior. Generally speaking, SiC- and Si_3N_4-based coatings have found broad use at temperatures below 1700 °C (3090 °F) because of minimum thermal mismatch stresses and low oxide-scale growth kinetics. In the higher temperature range, 1700 to 2200 °C (3090 to 3990 °F), refractory carbides and borides have been used for short time periods. Coating deposition techniques that have been used include pack cementation, CVD, and slurry processes. Coating architectures are normally built using combinations of these techniques. In the following sections, typical coating architectures are discussed in accordance with the process used to deposit the primary oxygen barrier.

Pack Cementation. The coating system used on the Shuttle Orbiter vehicle is the preeminent example of the use of a pack process to create an oxidation protection system for carbon-carbon (Ref 25). In this process, the carbon-carbon part is packed in a retort with a dry pack mixture of alumina, silicon, and SiC. The retort is placed in a furnace, and under argon atmosphere a stepped time-temperature cycle is used to activate conversion of the carbon-carbon surface to SiC. Peak process temperature is approximately 1760 °C (3200 °F). This creates a porous SiC surface nominally 1.0 to 1.5 mm in thickness. Multiple impregnation and curing with an acid-activated tetraethoxysilicate liquid produces SiO_2 coating of the porous surfaces. A surface sealant consisting of a mixture of a commercial alkali silicate bonding liquid filled with SiC powder is then applied.

This system was designed to provide protection during multiple reentry cycles where surface temperatures of 1540 °C (2800 °F) are anticipated. The success of the shuttle missions and further testing (Ref 23–25) have proven this to be an effective approach for low-performance rayon-based composites. Attempts to use similar coatings modified with boron (Ref 58, 59) for other aerospace applications requiring high-performance carbon-carbon have met with only limited success.

Chemical Vapor Deposition. Attempts to expand carbon-carbon use to turbine engine hot-section and exhaust components fostered the need for protective coatings that could be applied as thin layers over the structural components without compromising mechanical performance. The coating architectures developed have been dependent on the application lifetime as well as on dynamic or static structural requirements. The CVD coatings are normally applied in multiple cycles to ensure even deposition rates over curved surfaces. A substrate pretreatment is normally used to enhance adherence. Silicon nitride overlay coatings have been shown to be effective for limited-life (<20 h) cycles where heating above the deposition temperature occurs rapidly and peak temperatures reach 1760 °C (3200 °F) (Ref 55, 56, 60). For these coatings a thin reaction layer of SiC (formed in a pack process, of the order of 5 μm) has been used as a reaction barrier and to enhance adherence. The Si_3N_4 has been applied in thicknesses ranging from 125 to 250 μm (0.005 to 0.010 in.) in a multiple-step process.

Other applications require that carbon-carbon withstand hundreds of hours of exposure to peak temperatures in the range of 1400 to 1500 °C (2550 to 2730 °F) and undergo thermal cycling to temperatures in the range of 600 to 1200 °C (1110 to 2190 °F). In these extended-life applications, a boron-rich inner layer is used to provide a glassy phase to seal microcracks in the outer coatings. Elemental boron, B_4C, and combinations of boron compounds mixed with SiC or silicon are inner layer approaches. These layers are deposited in thicknesses normally in the range of 25 to 50 μm (0.001 to 0.002 in.) using CVD, conversion of the carbon surface, and slurry coating (Ref 61–63). Depositing SiC or Si_3N_4 by CVD is the preferred method to provide hard, erosion-resistant surfaces that cover the boronated inner layers and inhibit vaporization of borate glass sealants (Ref 64, 65). Overlay thicknesses in the range of 200 to 300 μm (0.008 to 0.012 in.) are normally deposited in a multiple-step process. A typical coating architecture on an inhibited composite is shown schematically in Fig. 10.

Silicate glazes are frequently applied to fill the microcrack network existing in SiC and Si_3N_4

Table 2 Properties of refractory materials deposited on carbon-carbon composites

		Deposition temperature		Bulk properties				
				Modulus			CTE (20–1900 °C)	
Material	Deposition process	°C	°F	GPa	10^6 psi	Poisson's ratio	10^{-6}/°C	10^{-6}/°F
SiC	CVD	1050	1920	448	65	0.19	5.2	9.4
TiC	CVD	1000	1830	448	65	0.19	9.5	17.1
Al_2O_3	CVD	1050	1920	400	58	0.28	10.3	18.5
AlN	CVD	1250	2280	345	50	0.3	6.1	11.0
Si_3N_4	CVD	1420	2590	317	46	0.3	3.6	6.5
Ir	Sputtering	250	480	524	76	0.3	7.9	14.2
HfO_2	EBPVD	1000	1830	138	20	0.25	10.6	19.1

CTE, coefficient of thermal expansion; CVD, chemical vapor deposition; EBPVD, electron-beam physical vapor deposition coatings. Although the glaze is applied externally and is susceptible to vaporization and physical removal, it has been shown to improve cyclic oxidation lifetimes. Glaze overcoats are normally applied as aqueous sols incorporating boron and silicon that can be painted, sprayed, or dip coated. Typical processing involves air drying and firing above 1038 °C (1900 °F) in an argon atmosphere (Ref 64). The glaze can be periodically replenished.

Slurry coatings are produced by dispersing appropriate ceramic or metal powders in a liquid vehicle to make the slurry, applying the slurry as a paint to the component surface, evaporating or gelling the liquid to harden the coating, and then heating to a high temperature to stabilize and densify the coating. Slurries are applied by brushing, spraying, or dipping. The liquid can be water or volatile organics with organic binders in solution, inorganic or organic sols or solutions that form oxides, or thermosetting preceramic polymers or polymer solutions (Ref 66, 67).

Hardening produces a coating composed of powder particles, bound together and bonded to the substrate by the solid that is precipitated or condensed from the liquid. Heating to a high temperature decomposes the binder phase to form carbon or a ceramic. The shrinkage associated with binder decomposition and incomplete solid-state sintering of the powder particles produces a cracked, porous, and often weakly bonded coating unless a flowable and wetting liquid is formed by one of the constituents. This can be a glass, molten metal, or ceramic melt.

Coatings meant to provide oxidation protection for graphite and CCC articles at temperatures below 1000 °C (1830 °F) often contain large amounts of boron in the form of elemental boron, B_4C, BN, metal borides, or B_2O_3 (Ref 68, 69). Employing B_2O_3 glass provides a wetting liquid at low temperatures on initial heating, and the nonoxides rapidly oxidize in use to produce the same result. Coatings composed mostly of refractory oxide particles bound together with small amounts of borate glass have shown utility at temperatures in the range of 1200 to 1500 °C (2190 to 2730 °F) in configurations where evaporation of the B_2O_3 is inhibited (Ref 47). When such coatings are made, the boron can be present in the powder constituents, the liquid vehicle, or both. Water or alcohol solutions of boric acid and liquid boron alkoxides are often used (Ref 47, 53). Solutions of preceramic boron polymers are also a possibility (Ref 70, 71).

Slurry coatings meant for higher temperatures, in which borates are replaced by glassy alkali silicates or aluminum phosphate, are prominent (Ref 37, 58). The use of siloxane fluids as preceramic polymers has also been disclosed (Ref 72). Converting the carbon surface to SiC is often recommended as a pretreatment to ensure the adherence of glassy borate, silicate, and phosphate coatings (Ref 37, 58).

The bonding and densification of slurry coatings with molten metal and melted ceramic phases have been used to produce protective layers with intermediate to very high temperature capabilities. Dense, very adherent coatings capable of extreme-temperature service can be made from paints containing fine refractory boride particles (Ref 30). The coatings are fully stabilized by heating the borides in contact with the carbon surface to temperatures over 2000 °C (3630 °F) in an inert environment to form a boride-carbon eutectic liquid. Coatings made by melting certain combinations of metal powders and reacting these with the carbon surface to form refractory carbides (Ref 73) are protective to 1800 °C (3270 °F). Work of this type (Ref 74), using a mixture of silicon, hafnium, and chromium powders reacted with the carbon surface at 1450 °C (2640 °F), has produced carbide coatings that provide excellent oxidation protection for short times at 1200 °C (2192 °F).

Other Methods. Coatings have been applied using other techniques, including sputtering and plasma spraying. Plasma spraying has been used successfully to coat CCCs with HfC, with the goal of improving surface hardness and erosion or corrosion resistance (Ref 75). Mechanical properties of the composites are retained after a thermal treatment under vacuum of 2h at 1000 °C (1830 °F).

Practical Limitations of Coatings

As mentioned above, CCCs can be used as structural materials to at least 2200 °C (4000 °F). At the time of this writing, viable coating concepts to match this capability have not been consistently demonstrated, especially for times greater than a few hours. Silicon carbide and Si_3N_4 are limited thermodynamically to temperatures of approximately 1800 to 1815 °C (3270 to 3300 °F). At higher temperatures, the SiO_2 layers that form and protect these materials are disrupted by CO and N_2 interfacial pressures that become greater than 10^{-1} MPa (1 atm), causing the coatings to erode by uncontrolled oxidation (Ref 56, 57). Use of more refractory materials such as HfC or HfB_2 is limited by the very rapid oxidation rates pointed out in Fig. 7. Rapid conversion of these films to high-expansion oxides leads to severe spallation in thermal cycles. Thus, above approximately 1760 °C (3200 °F), coating lifetimes are currently limited to a few hours.

For the range of applications where coating architectures incorporating borate sealant glasses are used, coating use temperatures are limited to approximately 1500 to 1550 °C (2730 to 2820 °F). When B_2O_3 contacts carbon at atmospheric pressure, the CO reaction product pressure exceeds 10^{-1} MPa (1 atm) at approximately 1575 °C (2870 °F). Borate glasses also cause dissolution of the protective SiO_2 scale forming on SiC or Si_3N_4, leading to more rapid corrosion because of the high oxygen permeability of the mixed glass. Experience in test cycles with peak temperatures about 1400 °C (2550 °F) has shown that accelerated dissolution of coatings along microcrack boundaries eventually causes gross oxidation of boron-based inner layers, leading to massive dissolution of the silicon-based overlays.

Moisture sensitivity of borate glasses (Ref 76) can be a major limitation. Hydrolysis at low temperatures in moist air converts adherent B_2O_3 containing layers into loosely bonded boric acid particulate. Under long-term exposure, sealant glasses forming beneath the hard overlays undergo moisture attack that leads to spallation. Subsequent heating cycles that rapidly release moisture can cause catastrophic failure. Finally, high-temperature exposure to moist environments makes borate glass susceptible to vaporization by the formation of HBO_2 (Ref 53).

Joining

Various aerospace systems, currently in the development stage, make use of structures and components that are fabricated from CCCs and monolithic graphite materials. These proposed systems use carbon-based materials for ground- and space-based interceptor propulsion components, satellite structural components, space truss structures, and hypersonic vehicle propulsion and skin assemblies. In all cases, advanced joining methods need to be developed in order to fully exploit the capabilities of the CCCs and graphite materials and to obtain the performance characteristics desired. During the last half decade, technological advancements in CCCs and their product forms have made the issue of component assembly and joining methods ever more important.

Depending on the specific application, joints accomplished by brazing methods can have a number of advantages over mechanically fastened joints, including:

- The size and weight of brazed assemblies can be significantly less.
- Brazing permits the use of designs involving small, compact, multipart components.
- The use of high-temperature braze materials allows components with brazed joints to function at higher operating temperatures.

Components assembled by brazing methods have been designed primarily for various rocket

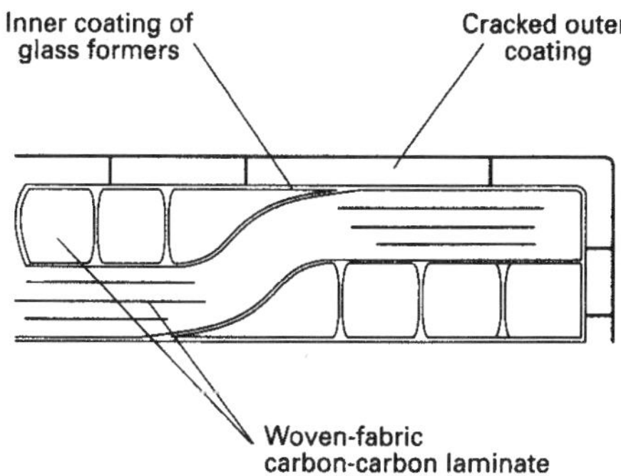

Fig. 10 Schematic of coating architecture used to protect carbon-carbon for extended-life applications

propulsion applications, including hot gas valve component joints and injector/thrust-chamber joints. Joining schemes for assembly of CCC parts for the national aerospace plane have also been developed, as have joining schemes to allow use of CCC and graphite armor tiles in the large vacuum vessel/plasma chamber for the Doublet 3 fusion research device (Ref 77).

These applications represent a wide range of operating temperatures, so a number of different braze materials and techniques have been developed in order to achieve system design requirements and enhance the capabilities of the joined components. Some of the materials investigated for brazing CCC and graphite include silver-based filler metals, gold-based filler metals, zirconium metal, hafnium metal, and hafnium diboride/hafnium carbide powder mixtures. Other researchers have investigated brazing and diffusion bonding of CCC using titanium metal, silver-based filler metals, copper-based filler metals, various silicides ($MoSi_2$, BSi_2, and $TiSi_2$), and various proprietary materials (Ref 78–81).

For moderate-temperature applications, both silver- and gold-based braze filler metals have been used to join CCC panels to other CCC panels and to join graphite materials to refractory metals. Typical brazing temperatures have ranged from roughly 800 to 1250 °C (1470 to 2280 °F) for such applications. For high-temperature applications, zirconium braze materials have been used successfully with both CCC and graphite materials; typically, braze temperatures of approximately 1850 °C (3360 °F) have been employed. Finally, for very high-temperature applications, joints have been fabricated using both hafnium metal and HfB_2 powder braze materials to join both CCC and graphite materials; brazing temperatures of approximately 2200 to 2550 °C (3990 to 4620 °F) have been used. These braze material/operating temperature combinations are summarized in Table 3.

Metals suitable for joining CCCs by graphite formation are those that react with carbon to form a carbide that decomposes upon heating to higher temperatures, leaving a metal-free carbon-carbon joint (Ref 82). However, metals with high vapor pressures, which readily oxidize at very low partial pressures of oxygen, and/or which form carbides that dissociate at very high temperatures (>2000 °C, or 3630 °F), seem to be unsuitable as interlayers for joining by this method.

One study (Ref 83) used brazing and solid-state diffusion bonding of three-dimensional CCC with silicon, Si_3N_4, SiB_4, boron, and $TiSi_2$ joining materials. The primary criteria for selecting these systems were:

- These materials and their carbides possess desirable high-temperature mechanical properties and thermal stability at temperature ranges greater than 1038 °C (1900 °F) and less than 1928 °C (3502 °F).
- Elements with low atomic numbers are involved in these systems.
- Joining by solid-state diffusion bonding and carbide formation was expected to be possible.
- Joining temperatures below 2205 °C (4000 °F) were expected.

The first three materials (silicon, Si_3N_4, and SiB_4) produced no bonding or very weak bonds. Thus, it was determined that only the latter two systems (boron and $TiSi_2$) were suitable for producing joints of sufficient shear strength ($\gamma >$ 3.4 MPa, or 0.5 ksi). Due to the difficulty of melting the boron interlayers, only solid-state diffusion bonding with boron was studied.

The optimum conditions for joining were determined to be 1995 °C (3625 °F), 15 min, and 7.2 MPa (1 ksi). The shear strengths of the joints made under optimum conditions increased with the testing temperature from an average value of 5.8 MPa (0.8 ksi) at room temperature to 18.1 MPa (2.6 ksi) at 1660 °C (3020 °F). $TiSi_2$ exhibited excellent wettability and penetrability during the brazing operations. The optimum temperature for brazing was 1490 °C (2715 °F). The maximum shear strength of an optimum joint was 406 MPa (59 ksi) at 1165 °C (2130 °F). The strength decreased at lower test temperatures, and at ambient temperature the average joint shear strength was 15.4 MPa (2.2 ksi) (Ref 83).

Another study investigated the solid-state diffusion bonding of CCCs by using boride and carbide interlayers (Ref 84). The maximum joint strength was achieved for CCCs bonded at 2000 °C (3630 °F) with a 2:1:1 mole ratio of titanium, silicon, and B_4C powders. These powders reacted in situ to produce interlayers of TiB_2 + SiC + B_4C. The joint shear strength increased with temperature, from 8.99 MPa (1.3 ksi) at room temperature to an average value of 14.51 MPa (2.1 ksi) at 2000 °C (3630 °F).

Properties of Carbon-Carbon Composites

Carbon-carbon composites have many of the desirable high-temperature properties of conventional carbons and graphites, including high strength, high modulus, and low creep. In addition, the high thermal conductivity and low CTE, coupled with high strength, produce a material with low sensitivity to thermal shock. Also characteristic of CCCs are a high fracture toughness and a pseudoplasticity, the latter of which bears a resemblance to fiber-reinforced polymers. These attributes make CCCs uniquely useful at temperatures as high as 2800 °C (5070 °F). The major problems have been high-temperature oxidation and off-fiber-axis properties.

Unidirectional CCCs can approach the same strengths and moduli as those achieved with resin matrix composites. Moreover, because their properties are maintained to 2000 °C (3650 °F), they represent the premier material for inert atmosphere or short-time high-temperature applications. Table 4 shows typical mechanical properties of unidirectional CCCs.

Decisive influences on the mechanical, thermal, and electrical properties of CCCs come from the fiber type, fiber volume fraction, fiber architecture, precursor, and processing cycle (Tables 5–7). With an increasing number of redensification cycles, porosity decreases and density, strength, and stiffness increase (Fig. 11). The final heat treatment temperature influences fracture behavior and physical properties such as the CTE, resistivity, and conductivity (Table 7).

All properties of CCCs are anisotropic. This originates from the carbon fibers, which are extremely anisotropic because of their graphite

Table 3 Carbon-carbon and graphite joining

Primary substrates joined	Operating temperature	Braze material	Temperature for initiation of melting, °C	Temperature for initiation of melting, °F
Graphite to refractory metal	Moderate	Silver, copper, titanium alloy	780	1435
Graphite to refractory metal	Moderate	Gold, palladium alloy	1190	2175
C-C to C-C, and graphite to graphite	High	Zirconium	1823	3315
C-C to C-C, and graphite to graphite	Very high	Hafnium	2180	3955
C-C to C-C, and graphite to graphite	Very high	HfB_2, with and without HfC	2260	4100

C-C, carbon-carbon. Source: Ref 77

Table 4 Mechanical properties of unidirectional carbon-carbon composites (~55 vol%)

	Parallel		Perpendicular	
	HTU	HMS	HTU	HMS
Modulus, GPa (10^6 psi)				
Tension	125 (20)	220 (30)	...	...
Compression	10 (1.5)	250 (35)	7.5 (1.1)	...
Strength, MPa (ksi)				
Tension	600 (90)	575 (85)	4 (0.60)	5 (0.75)
Compression	285 (40)	380 (55)	25 (4)	50 (7.5)
Bend	1250–1600 (180–230)	825–1000 (120–145)	20 (3)	30 (4.5)
Shear	20 (3)	28 (4)	...	...
Fracture toughness, kJ/m² (ft · lbf/ft²)	70 (4800)	20 (1370)	0.4 (30)	0.8 (55)

HTU, high tensile untreated surface; HMS, high modulus surface treated

Table 5 Mechanical properties of two-directional carbon-carbon composites at various final heat treatment temperatures

Fiber orientation	HTT °C	HTT °F	Density, g/cm³	Flexural strength MPa	Flexural strength ksi	Modulus GPa	Modulus 10^6 psi	ILSS MPa	ILSS ksi	Strain to failure, %
±15° tow	1200	2190	1.55	520	75.4	90	13.0	18	2.6	0.4
±15° tow	2200	3990	1.60	470	68.2	130	18.9	12	1.7	0.3
Cloth, 8 H/S	1200	2190	1.50	250	36.3	75	10.8	16	2.3	0.4
Cloth, 8 H/S	2200	3990	1.60	230	33.4	80	11.6	12	1.7	0.3
Cloth, 8 H/S	2500	4530	1.65	210	30.4	85	12.3	10	1.5	0.3

HTT, heat treatment temperature; ILSS, interlaminar shear strength; H/S, harness/satin

crystal lattice. Along the fiber axis, stiffness, strength, and electrical and thermal conductivity are excellent. Across the axis, these properties are poor. In the case of two-directional reinforcement, the ratio of anisotropy amounts to between 5/1 and 10/1.

The flexural strength of industrially manufactured CCCs with different fiber architectures varies between 100 and 600 MPa (15 and 90 ksi) (parallel to the laminates/fibers). A characteristic feature of carbon-carbon materials is that the ratio of flexural/tensile strength is 1/1.4. Wound tubes with fiber angles of ±15° and ±45° (normal to the axis) exhibit tensile strength values of 540 MPa (80 ksi) and 430 MPa (60 ksi), respectively. The strength values of three-directional reinforced weave structures range from 150 to 300 MPa (22 to 44 ksi). The strengths of felt and randomly oriented short fiber reinforcements are between 50 and 100 MPa (7.5 and 15 ksi).

Fatigue behavior is very attractive. Under alternating flexural loads, 70 to 80% of the ultimate flexural strength is still available (Ref 86, 87). Moduli values range from 40 to 150 GPa (6 to 22 × 10^6 psi) for two-directional and three-directional weaves, respectively. Besides the fiber type and orientation, the type of matrix precursor and the final heat treatment temperature decisively influence the modulus value. If the graphite layers of the matrix are oriented parallel to the fiber axis, then they can contribute to the composite modulus nearly in the same order of magnitude as the fibers.

A high-temperature strength capability is attractive for many structural applications. Although other high-temperature materials significantly lose strength at temperatures greater than 1300 °C (2370 °F), carbons and graphites keep their mechanical properties up to 2000 °C (3630 °F) (Ref 88). Ongoing tests clearly show increasing values up to the testing temperature of 1600 °C (2910 °F) in an order of magnitude of 40 to 50% (Ref 89), as shown in Fig. 12. The interlaminar shear strength increases about 70% (from room temperature to 1800 °C, or 3270 °F), and the modulus increases approximately 10%.

The physical and thermophysical properties of CCCs are also of great interest for specific applications. In one direction, along the fibers or laminates, the material acts as a heat conductor, but in the other direction (across) it acts as an insulator. The processing history of the composites is important to the final property values. Graphitization treatment increases conductivity and decreases resistivity (Table 7). This is still more pronounced if graphitizing matrices, such as pitch-based carbon or pyrolitic graphite, are used. In three-directional and multiaxial structures, the properties are balanced to a more isotropic behavior. However, the ratio of isotropy is

Table 6 Electrical resistivity and thermal conductivity parallel and perpendicular to the laminates of two-directional carbon-carbon composites

HTT °C	HTT °F	Electrical resistivity, μΩ · m Parallel	Electrical resistivity, μΩ · m Perpendicular	Thermal conductivity, W/m · K Parallel	Thermal conductivity, W/m · K Perpendicular
200	390	33–37	98–114	36–43	4–7
800	1470	8–12	68–81	127–134	39–46

HTT, heat treatment temperature

Table 7 Typical properties of three-directional orthogonal carbon-carbon composites

Property	Direction Z	Direction X-Y
Density, g/cm³	1.9	1.9
Tensile strength, MPa (ksi)		
at RT	310 (45)	103 (15)
at 1900 °K (2950 °F)	400 (58)	124 (18)
Tensile modulus, GPa (10^6 psi)		
at RT	152 (22)	62 (90)
at 1900 °K (2950 °F)	159 (23)	83 (120)
Compressive strength, MPa (ksi)		
at RT	159 (23)	117 (17)
at 1900 °K (2950 °F)	196 (28)	166 (24)
Compressive modulus, GPa (10^6 psi)		
at RT	131 (19)	69 (10)
at 1900 °K (2950 °F)	110 (16)	62 (90)
Thermal conductivity, W/m · K (Btu/ft · h · °F)		
at RT	246 (142)	149 (12)
at 1900 °K (2950 °F)	60 (5)	44 (4)
Coefficient of thermal expansion, 10^{-6}/°F (10^{-6}/K)		
at RT	0 (0)	0 (0)
at 1900 °K (2950 °F)	3 (5)	4 (7)
at 3000 °K (4950 °F)	8 (14)	11 (20)

RT, room temperature. Source: Ref 85

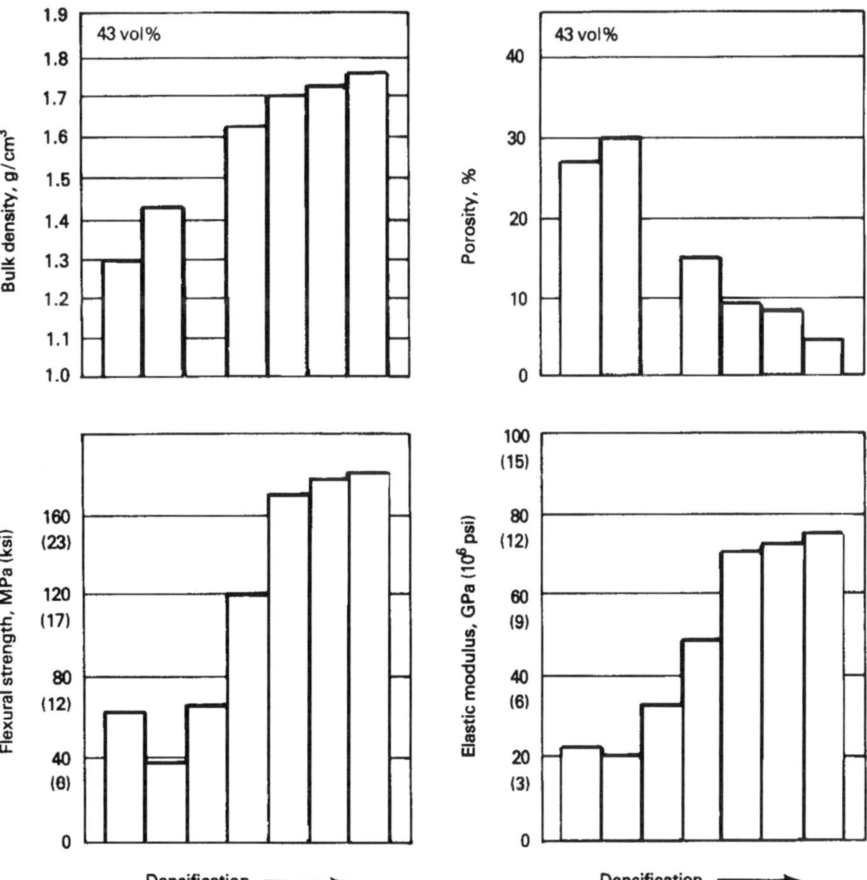

Fig. 11 Change of properties with number of redensifications (two-directional weave, 8 harness/satin)

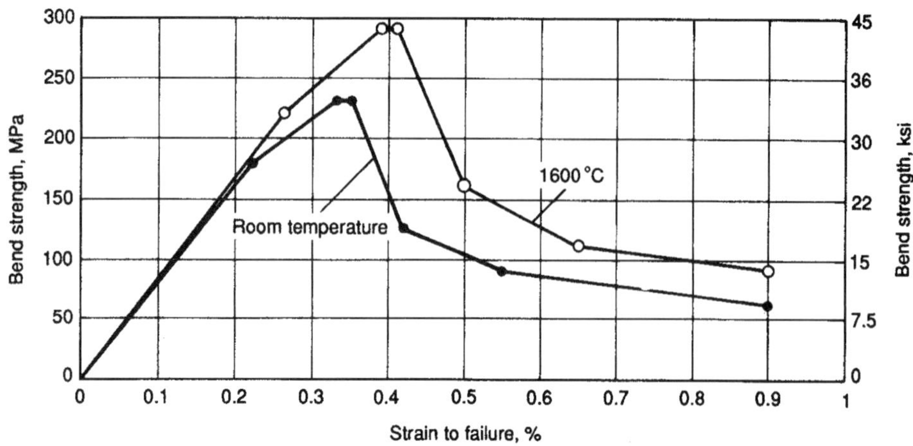

Fig. 12 Comparison of bend strength at room temperature and 1600 °C (2910 °F) (two-directional weave, 8 harness/satin in inert atmosphere)

dependent on the balance of fiber volume fraction in the *x*, *y*, and *z* directions. At high temperatures, electrical resistivity decreases and the composites show negative thermal conductivity behavior. Thermal conductivity also drops with higher temperatures.

Thermal expansion parallel to the laminates of two-directional CCCs is negative up to 800 °C (1470 °F). Across the laminates, a positive CTE is present. In general, however, the CTE data are low and can be tailored by the fiber architectures to a balanced expansion of nearly zero in the plane (Fig. 13).

Fracture Behavior. High fracture toughness values and pseudoplastic fracture behavior are most attractive for numerous applications. Both brittle, catastrophic failure by overstressing and critical stress concentrations at notches can be excluded. This high damage tolerance can be demonstrated by nailing a composite. No catastrophic, brittle failure occurs as one might expect for ceramic materials. Only the area around the nail shaft is delaminated. Bend tests on three-directional composites have shown enormous strains, up to 5% (Ref 90). The reasons originate from the complex minimechanical and micromechanical behavior of the several interfaces that are present in a CCC: fiber-fiber, fiber-matrix, and matrix-matrix interfaces (Ref 91). The crystalline structure of the matrix itself also influences toughness (Ref 92, 93). The micromechanics are not yet fully understood, but weak interfacial bondings seem to be a precondition for producing tough CCCs (Ref 1, 94). Bonds between fiber and matrix that are too good induce excessive damage and promote fast crack propagation through the fibers. The composite fails in a brittle mode, and no strengthening effect is achieved. The mechanism of load transfer is not well understood, either, but if the interfacial forces are low, no brittle fracture occurs. Because the shear and transverse strengths are very low, one could assume that the loads are transferred across the interfaces primarily by friction. In addition, mechanical interlocking of cracked matrix parts and particles can occur.

One can also assume that microcracking is still in service when loads are applied on the composite. However, the debonded and weak interfaces avoid the crack propagation through the fibers. The energy dissipation is additionally promoted by poorly bonded matrix-matrix interfaces, which act as a type of "duplex mechanism" (Ref 95) and increase the fracture toughness.

The influence of the graphitic matrix structure on toughness values was demonstrated in model experiments (Ref 96). Three-directional billets were graphitized to different extents to produce matrix structures that ranged from slightly to highly graphitic. In Fig. 14, the ability of the matrix to absorb energy is expressed as relative toughness. The maximum is reached at 2400 °C (4350 °F). The explanation for this is given by different lamellar structures of the pitch-based matrix. Less ordered microstructures allow crack propagation over long distances along the filaments, and energy dissipation is low with consequent low toughness. At 2400 °C (4350 °F), an intermediate stage exists where the microstructure is sufficiently ordered to accommodate some slip from shear forces, but is disordered

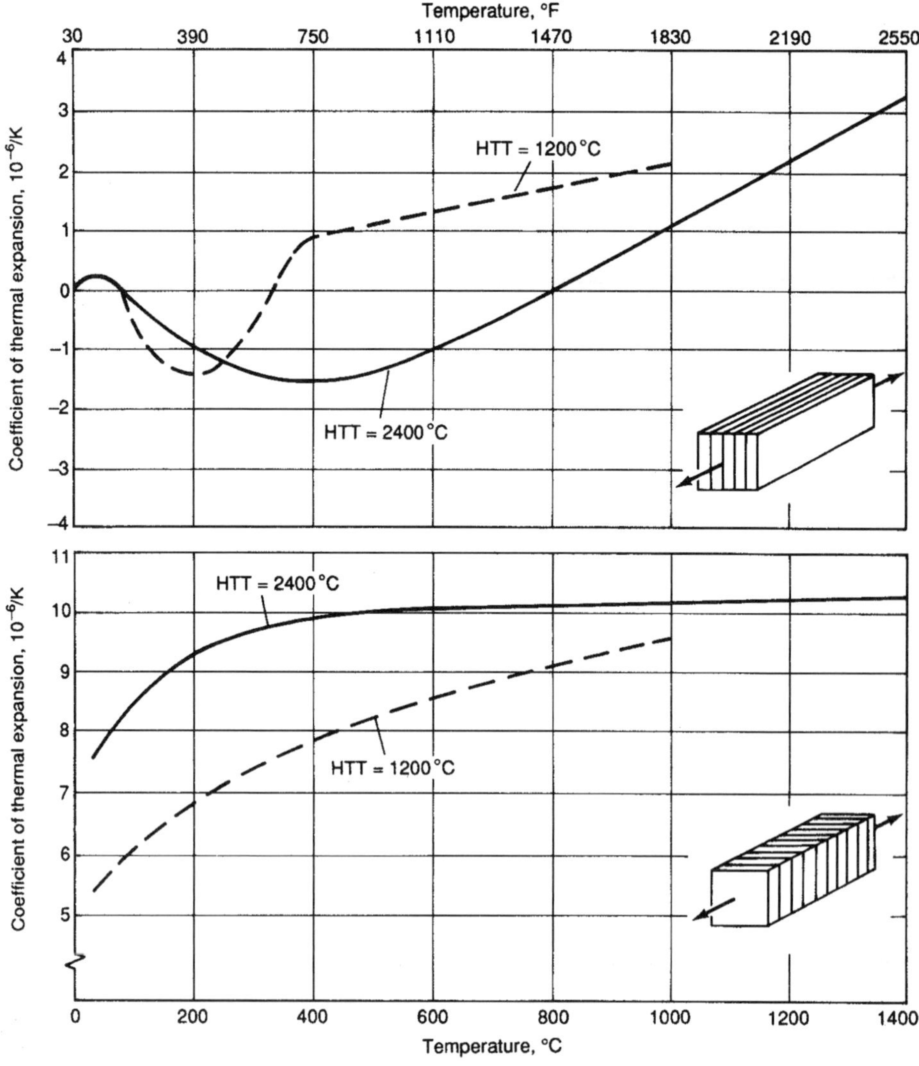

Fig. 13 Coefficient of thermal expansion, parallel and perpendicular to laminates of two-directional weave carbon-carbon composite with final heat treatment temperature (HTT) of 1200 and 2400 °C (2190 and 4350 °F)

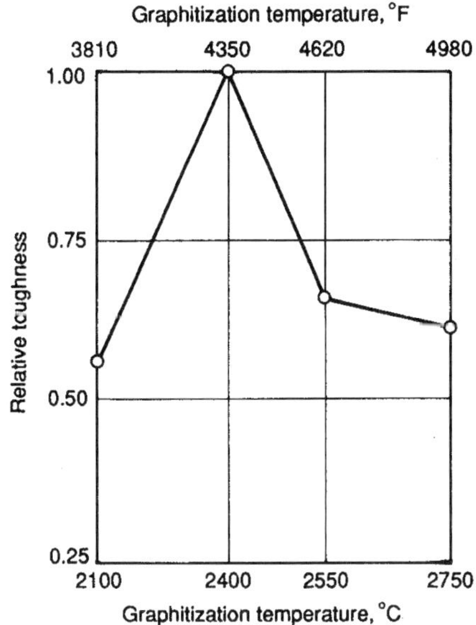

Fig. 14 Relative toughness as function of graphitization temperature (pitch-based matrix, three-directional, carbon-carbon). Source: Ref 97

enough to prevent long-range slip. Energy absorption and, therefore, toughness are high. A good graphitic order of the matrix decreases against toughness, because there is more extensive microcracking in the matrix and the chance for multiple fracturing is the greatest.

Oxidation of CCCs can begin at temperatures as low as 400 °C (750 °F). The rate of oxidation depends on the perfection of the carbon structure and its purity. Highly disordered carbons, such as carbonized resins given low-temperature heat treatments, oxidize at appreciable rates at 400 °C (750 °F). Highly graphitic structures, such as pitch-based carbon fibers, can be heated as high as 650 °C (1200 °F) before extensive oxidation occurs. At these low temperatures, carbons are very susceptible to catalytic oxidation by alkali metals, such as sodium, and multivalent metals, such as iron and vanadium, at extremely low concentrations. Therefore, the oxidation rate often is determined by the initial purity of the CCC or by in-service contamination. Borates and particularly phosphates have been found to inhibit oxidation up to about 600 °C (1110 °F) (Ref 98). Oxidation at higher temperatures becomes more rapid, and by 1300 °C (2370 °F), it is completely limited by mass transport of oxygen to the surface and transport of carbon monoxide and dioxide away from the surface.

Carbon-carbon composites can be attacked by strongly oxidizing acids, but they are inert to most other acids and to all alkalis, salts, and organic solvents.

ACKNOWLEDGMENTS

The information in this article is largely taken from the following articles in *Composites*, Volume 1, *Engineered Materials Handbook*, ASM International, 1987:

- H.D. Batha and C.R. Rowe, Structurally Reinforced Carbon-Carbon Composites, p 922–924
- R.J. Diefendorf, Continuous Carbon Fiber Reinforced Carbon Matrix Composites, p 911–914
- L.E. McAllister, Multidirectionally Reinforced Carbon/Graphite Matrix Composites, p 915–919

In addition, information was taken from:

- M.M. Schwartz, Joining MMCs, CMCs, CCCs, and Specialty Composites, *Joining of Composite-Matrix Materials*, ASM International, 1994, p 111–113
- J.R. Strife and J.E. Sheehan, Protective Coatings for Carbon-Carbon Composites, *Surface Engineering*, Vol 5, *ASM Handbook*, ASM International, 1994, p 887–891
- G. Ziegler and W. Hüttner, Engineering Properties of Carbon-Carbon and Ceramic-Matrix Composites, *Ceramics and Glasses*, Vol 4, *Engineered Materials Handbook*, ASM International, 1991, p 835–844

REFERENCES

1. W. Huettner, Ph.D. thesis, University of Karlsruhe, 1980
2. H. Brueckmann, Ph.D. thesis, University of Karlsruhe, 1979
3. E. Fitzer and M. Heym, *Z. Werkstofftech.*, Vol 8, 1976, p 269–279
4. C.R. Thomas and E.J. Walker, *High Temp.-High Press.*, Vol 10, 1978, p 79
5. E. Fitzer and W. Huettner, *Sprechsaal,* Vol 6, 1980, p 451
6. E. Fitzer and W. Huettner, Structure and Strength of C/C-Composites, *J. Phys. G, Appl. Phys.*, Vol 14, 1981, p 47–71
7. W.L. Lachman, J.A. Crawford, and L.E. McAllister, Multidirectionally Reinforced Carbon-Carbon Composites, *Proceedings of the International Conference on Composite Materials,* B. Noton, R. Signorelli, K. Street, and L. Phillips, Ed., Metallurgical Society of the American Institute of Mining, Metallurgical, and Petroleum Engineers, 1978, p 1302–1319
8. R.S. Barton, A Three Dimensionally Reinforced Material, *SPE J.*, Vol 4, May 1968, p 31–36
9. L.E. McAllister and A.R. Taverna, A Study of Composition-Construction Variations in 3-D Carbon-Carbon Composites, *Proceedings of the International Conference on Composites Materials,* Vol I, E. Scala, E. Anderson, I. Toth, and B. Noton, Ed., Metallurgical Society of the American Institute of Mining, Metallurgical, and Petroleum Engineers, 1976, p 307–315
10. L.E. McAllister and A.R. Taverna, Development and Evaluation of Mod-3 Carbon-Carbon Composites, *Proceedings of the 17th National SAMPE Symposium,* Society for the Advancement of Material and Process Engineering, 1972, p III-A-3
11. P. Lamicq, "Recent Improvements in 4-D Carbon-Carbon Materials," Paper 77-882, presented at the AIAA/SAE 13th Propulsion Conference, Orlando, 1977
12. C.K. Mullen and P.J. Roy, Fabrication and Properties Description of AVCO 3-D Carbon-Carbon Cylinder Materials, *Proceedings of the 17th National SAMPE Symposium,* Society for the Advancement of Material and Process Engineering, 1972, p III-A-2
13. P.S. Bruno, D.O. Keith, and A.A. Vicario, Jr., Automatically Woven Three-Directional Composite Structures, *Proceedings of the 31st International SAMPE Symposium,* Society for the Advancement of Material and Process Engineering, 1986, p 103–116
14. H.D. Batha, Fiber Materials Inc., private communication, May 1986
15. Y. Grenie and G. Cahuzac, Automatic Weaving of 3-D Contoured Preforms, *Proceedings of the 12th National SAMPE Symposium,* Society for the Advancement of Material and Process Engineering, 1980
16. L.E. McAllister and A.R. Taverna, "The Development of High Strength Three Dimensionally Reinforced Graphite Composites," paper presented at the 73rd Annual Meeting, American Ceramic Society, Chicago, 1971
17. L.E. McAllister and R.L. Burns, Pressure Carbonization of Pitch and Resin Matrix Precursors for Use in Carbon-Carbon Processing, *16th Biennial Conference on Carbon, Extended Abstracts,* American Carbon Society, 1983, p 478–479
18. L.E. McAllister and W.L. Lachman, Multidirectional Carbon-Carbon Composites, *Fabrication of Composites,* Vol 4, A. Kelly and S.T. Mileiko, Ed., North-Holland, 1983, p 109–175
19. R.L. Burns and J.L. Cook, Pressure Carbonization of Petroleum Pitches, *Petroleum Derived Carbons,* M.L. Deviney and T.M. O'Grady, Ed., Symposium Series 21, American Chemical Society, 1974, p 139
20. W. Chard, M. Conaway, and D. Neisz, Advanced High Pressure Graphite Processing Technology, *Petroleum Derived Carbons,* M.L. Deviney and T.M. O'Grady, Ed., Symposium Series 21, American Chemical Society, 1974, p 155
21. W.V. Kotlensky, Deposition of Pyrolytic Carbons in Porous Solids, *Chemistry and Physics of Carbon,* Vol 9, P.L. Walker, Jr. and P.A. Thrower, Ed., Marcel Dekker, 1973, p 173
22. L. Rubin, in *Carbon-Carbon Materials and Composites,* J.D. Buckley and D.D. Edie, Ed., Noyes, 1993, p 267
23. H.G. Maahs, C.W. Ohlhorst, D.M. Barrett, P.O. Ransone, and J.W. Sawyer, in *Materials Stability and Environmental Degradation,* MRS Symp. Proc., Vol 125, A. Barkatt, E.D. Verink, and L.R. Smith, Ed., Materials Research Society, 1988, p 15

24. R.C. Dickinson, in *Materials Stability and Environmental Degradation,* MRS Symp. Proc., Vol 125, A. Barkatt, E.D. Verink, and L.R. Smith, Ed., Materials Research Society, 1988, p 3
25. D.M. Curry, E.H. Yuen, D.C. Chao, and C.N. Webster, in *Damage and Oxidation Protection in High Temperature Composites,* Vol 1, G.K. Haritos and O.O. Ochoa, Ed., ASME, 1991, p 47
26. H.V. Johnson, Oxidation Resisting Carbon Article, U.S. Patent 1,948,382, 20 Feb 1934
27. K.J. Zeitsch, in *Modern Ceramics,* J.E. Hove and W.C. Riley, Ed., John Wiley, 1967, p 314
28. S.A. Bortz, in *Ceramics in Severe Environments,* W.W. Kriegel and H. Palmour, Ed., Plenum, 1971, p 49
29. E.M. Goldstein, E.W. Carter, and S. Klutz, in *Carbon,* Vol 4, 1966, p 273
30. J. Chown, R.F. Deacon, N. Singer, and A.E.S. White, in *Special Ceramics,* P. Popper, Ed., Academic Press, 1963, p 81
31. J.M. Criscione, R.A. Mercuri, E.P. Schram, A.W. Smith, and H.F. Volk, "High Temperature Protective Coatings for Graphite," ML-TDR-64-173, Part II, Materials Laboratory, Wright-Patterson Air Force Base, Oct 1974
32. *High Temperature Oxidation Resistant Coatings,* National Academy of Sciences and Engineering, 1970, p 112
33. K. Mumtaz, J. Echigoya, T. Hirai, and Y. Shindo, Iridium Coatings on Carbon-Carbon Composites Produced by Two Different Sputtering Methods: A Comparative Study, *J. Mat. Sci. Lett.,* Vol 12 (No. 18), 1993, p 1411–1412
34. D.C. Rogers, D.M. Shuford, and J.I. Mueller, in *Proceedings of the Seventh National SAMPE Technical Conference,* Society of Aerospace Material and Process Engineers, 1975, p 319
35. D.C. Rogers, R.O. Scott, and D.M. Shuford, in *Proceedings of the Eighth National SAMPE Technical Conference,* Society of Aerospace Material and Process Engineers, 1976, p 308
36. Surface Seal for Carbon Parts, *NASA Technical Briefs,* Vol 6 (No. 2), MSC-18898, 1981
37. D.M. Shuford, Enhancement Coating and Process for Carbonaceous Substrates, U.S. Patent 4,471,023, 11 Sept 1984
38. M.J. Lakewood and S.A. Taylor, Oxidation-Resistant Graphite Article and Method, U.S. Patent 3,065,088, 20 Nov 1962
39. E.M. Goldstein, E.W. Carter, and S. Klutz, in *Carbon,* Vol 4, 1966, p 273
40. W.E. Parker and J.F. Rakszawski, Oxidation Resistant Carbonaceous Bodies and Method for Making, U.S. Patent 3,261,697, 19 July 1966
41. R.E. Woodley, in *Carbon,* Vol 6, 1968, p 617
42. H.H. Strater, Oxidation Resistant Carbon, U.S. Patent 3,510,347, 5 May 1970
43. K.J. Zeitsch, in *Modern Ceramics,* J.E. Hove and W.C. Riley, Ed., John Wiley, 1967, p 314
44. L.C. Ehrenreich, Reinforced Carbon and Graphite Articles, U.S. Patent 4,119,189, 10 Oct 1978
45. T. Vasilos, Self-Healing Oxidation-Resistant Carbon Structure, U.S. Patent 4,599,256, 8 July 1986
46. P.E. Gray, Oxidation Inhibited Carbon-Carbon Composites, U.S. Patent 4,795,677, 3 Jan 1989
47. D.W. McKee, in *Carbon,* Vol 25, 1987, p 551
48. J.F. Rakszawski and W.E. Parker, in *Carbon,* Vol 2, 1964, p 53
49. D.W. McKee, C.L. Spiro, and E.J. Lamby, in *Carbon,* Vol 22, 1984, p 507
50. R.C. Shaffer, Coating for Fibrous Carbon Materials in Boron Containing Composites, U.S. Patent 4,164,601, 14 Aug 1979
51. R.C. Shaffer and W.L. Tarasen, Carbon Fabrics Sequentially Resin Coated with (1) A Metal-Containing Composition and (2) A Boron-Containing Composition Are Laminated and Carbonized, U.S. Patent 4,321,298, 23 March 1982
52. I. Jawed and D.C. Nagle, Oxidation Protection in Carbon-Carbon Composites, *Mat. Res. Bull.,* Vol 21, 1986, p 1391
53. D.W. McKee, in *Carbon,* Vol 24, 1986, p 737
54. J.E. Sheehan and H.D. Bartha, "C-C Composite Matrix Inhibition," paper presented at the 16th National Technical Conference, Society of Aerospace Material and Process Engineers, Oct 1984
55. J.R. Strife, in *Damage and Oxidation Protection in High Temperature Composites,* G.K. Haritos and O.O. Ochoa, Ed., American Society of Mechanical Engineers, 1991, p 121
56. J.R. Strife, in *Proceedings of the Sixth Annual Conference on Materials Technology,* M. Genisio, Ed., Southern Illinois University at Carbondale, 1990, p 166
57. J.R. Strife and J.E. Sheehan, in *Ceramic Bulletin,* Vol 67 (No. 2), 1988, p 369
58. D.M. Shuford, Composition and Method for Forming a Protective Coating on Carbon-Carbon Substrates, U.S. Patent 4,465,777, 14 Aug 1984
59. T.E. Schmid, "Oxidation Resistant Carbon/Carbon Composites for Turbine Engine Aft Sections," AFWAL-TR-82-4159, Materials Laboratory, Wright-Patterson Air Force Base, Oct 1982
60. J.R. Strife, "Development of High Temperature Oxidation Protection for Carbon-Carbon Composites," NADC Report 91013-60, Naval Air Development Center, Warminster, PA, 1990
61. D.M. Shuford, Composition and Method for Forming a Protective Coating on Carbon-Carbon Substrates, U.S. Patent 4,465,888, 14 Aug 1984
62. R.A. Holzl, Self Protecting Carbon Bodies and Method for Making Same, U.S. Patent 4,515,860, 7 May 1985
63. D.A. Eitman, Refractory Composite Articles, U.S. Patent 4,735,850, 5 April 1988
64. H. Dietrich, in *Mater. Eng.,* Aug 1991, p 34
65. J.E. Sheehan, in *Carbon-Carbon Materials and Composites,* J.D. Buckley and D.D. Edie, Ed., Noyes, 1993, p 2
66. C.W. Turner, Sol-Gel Process–Principles and Applications, *Ceram. Bull.,* Vol 70, 1991, p 1487
67. R.W. Rice, in *Ceram. Bull.,* Vol 62, 1983, p 889
68. N.A. Hooton and N.E. Jannasch, Coating for Protecting a Carbon Substrate in a Moist Oxidation Environment, U.S. Patent 3,914,508, 21 Oct 1975
69. G.R. Marin, Oxidation Resistant Carbonaceous Bodies and Method Producing Same, U.S. Patent 3,936,574, 3 Feb 1976
70. W.S. Coblenz, G.H. Wiseman, P.B. Davis, and R.W. Rice, Emergent Process Methods for High-Technology Ceramics, *Mater. Sci. Res.,* Vol 17, 1984
71. L.G. Sneddon, K. Su, P.J. Fazen, A.T. Lynch, E.E. Remsen, and J.S. Beck, in *Inorganic and Organometallic Oligomers and Polymers,* Kluwer Academic Publishers, 1991
72. M.S. Misra, Coating for Graphite Electrodes, U.S. Patent 4,418,097, 29 Nov 1983
73. A.J. Valtschev and T. Nikolova, Protecting Carbon Materials from Oxidation, U.S. Patent 3,348,929, 24 Oct 1967
74. H.S. Hu, A. Joshi, and J.S. Lee, *J. Vac. Sci.,* Vol A9, 1991, p 1535
75. M. Boncoen, G. Schnedecker, and J. Lukwicz, HfC Plasma Coating of C/C Composites, *Cer. Eng. Sci. Proc.,* Vol 13 (No. 7–8), 1992, p 348–355
76. P.B. Adams and D.L. Evans, in *Mater. Sci. Res.,* Vol 12, 1978, p 525
77. P.G. Valentine and P.W. Trester, Development of Brazed Joints in Carbon-Carbon, Graphite, and Refractory Metal Components for Rocket Propulsion and Spacecraft Applications, *Proc. 15th Conference on Metal Matrix, Carbon, and Ceramic Matrix Composites,* NASA CP-3133, Part I, J.D. Buckley, Ed., 1990, p 39–55
78. "Joining of Carbon-Carbon and Ceramic Matrix Composites," NSWC Presentation from the Interagency Planning Group Meeting, E. Becker, Ed., IDA Memorandum Report M-312, T.F. Kearns, Ed., April 1987
79. "Joining of Carbon-Carbon and Ceramic Matrix Composites," Materials Innovation Labs Presentation from the Interagency Planning Group Meeting, S. Yalof, Ed., IDA Memorandum Report M-312, T.F. Kearns, Ed., April 1987
80. P. Dadras, Joining of Carbon-Carbon Composites by Using $MoSi_2$ and Titanium Interlayers, *Proc. 14th Conf. on Metal Matrix, Carbon, and Ceramic Matrix Composites,*

NASA CP 3097, Part 2, J.D. Buckley, Ed., 1990

81. P.G. Valentine and P.W. Trester, Reaction Sintering: A Method for Achieving Adherent High-Temperature Coatings on Carbon-Carbon Composites, *Proc. 15th Conf. on Metal Matrix, Carbon, and Ceramic Matrix Composites,* NASA CP-3133, Part II, J.D. Buckley, Ed., 1991, p 811–820
82. P. Dadras and G. Mehrotra, Joining of Carbon-Carbon Composites by Graphite Formation, *J. Am. Ceram. Soc.,* Vol 77 (No. 6), 1994, p 1419–1424
83. P. Dadras and T. Ngai, Joining of C-C Composites by Boron and Titanium Disilicide, *Proc. 15th Conf. on Metal Matrix, Carbon, and Ceramic Matrix Composites,* NASA CP-3133, Part I, J.D. Buckley, Ed., 1991, p 25–38
84. P. Dadras and G. Mehrotra, Solid-State Diffusion Bonding of Carbon-Carbon Composites with Borides and Carbides, *J. Am. Ceram. Soc.,* Vol 76 (No. 5), 1993, p 1274–1280
85. A. Levine, "High Pressure Densified Carbon-Carbon Composites, Part II: Testing," Paper FC-21 presented at the 12th Biennial Conference on Carbon, Pittsburgh, 1975
86. Schunk Kohlenstofftechnik GmbH, Giessen, Germany, product information
87. U. Soltesz, private communication, 1988
88. J.R. Strife and J.E. Sheehan, *Am. Ceram. Soc. Bull.,* Vol 67 (No. 2), 1988, p 369–374
89. R. Meistring, private communication, 1989
90. L.E. McAllister and W.C. Lachmann, *Handbook of Composites,* Vol 4, A. Kelly and S.T. Mileiko, Ed., North Holland, p 139
91. J. Jortner, *Carbon,* Vol 24 (No. 5), 1986, p 603–613
92. J.E. Zimmer et al., *Molecular Crystals, Liquid Crystals,* Vol 38, 1977, p 188
93. J.E. Zimmer et al., *Advances in Liquid Crystals,* Vol 5, H. Brown, Ed., 1983, p 157
94. E. Fitzer, K.-H. Geigl, and W. Huettner, *Carbon,* Vol 18 (No. 6), 1980, p 383
95. J.G. Morley et al., *J. Mater. Sci.,* Vol 9, 1974, p 1171
96. R. Meyer et al., *Proceedings of the International Symposium on Science and Applications of Carbon Fibers,* Toyohashi University, Japan, 1984
97. G.H. Campell, M. Rühle, B.J. Dalgleish, and A.G. Evans, Whisker Toughening: A Comparison between Aluminium Oxide and Silicon Nitride Toughened with Silicon Carbide, *J. Am. Ceram. Soc.,* Vol 73 (No. 3), 1990, p 521–530
98. A. Gkogkidis, Ph.D. thesis, University of Karlsruhe, 1986

Post-Processing and Assembly

Chairperson: Flake C. Campbell, The Boeing Company

Introduction to Post-Processing and Assembly

Flake C. Campbell, The Boeing Company

ONE OF THE PRIMARY ADVANTAGES of composite designs is that they can achieve part-count reductions of up to 60% compared to equivalent metallic designs. However, even with these significant reductions, almost all composite structures require some type of post-processing and/or assembly operations. Since both of these operations add to the total cost of the final product in many instances, it is advantageous to minimize these operations if possible. In addition, many of the post-processing and assembly operations, such as trimming, drilling, and fastening, are more expensive for composites than metals. Trimming requires greater care because dull tools or incorrect feeds can cause heat damage or delaminations. Drilling is complicated by the abrasive nature of carbon fibers that can result in accelerated tool wear and splintering of the surface plies. During assembly, composites will tend to delaminate if excessive force is used to pull out gaps often encountered during assembly.

Polymer-Matrix Composites

This Section starts with the overview article "Machining, Trimming, and Routing of Polymer-Matrix Composites." This article is first because these are typical operations performed after composite curing but prior to other major post-processing or assembly operations. Machining of polymer-matrix composites (PMCs) can be accomplished using either traditional solid tools or with newer technologies, such as abrasive waterjet trimming. Even if traditional methods are used, special tools and parameters are required due to the abrasive nature of carbon fibers and the danger of overheating or delaminating the workpiece. Therefore, the tool materials, geometries, feeds, speeds, and rigidity requirements are generally more stringent and less forgiving than normally encountered in metallic structure.

The next two articles, "Secondary Adhesive Bonding of Polymer-Matrix Composites" and "Processing and Joining of Thermoplastic Composites," cover major assembly operations. Secondary adhesive bonding can be used either as a structural fabrication process (e.g., for honeycomb structure) or as an assembly method for attachment to other structure. The two critical variables in secondary adhesive bonding are adhesive selection and surface preparation. Adhesive selection is driven by a rather extensive list of variables, such as static and dynamic strength, modulus, temperature capability, and operating environment (e.g., humidity and moisture). Surface preparation is absolutely critical to obtaining a high-strength durable bond. This includes not only the composite parts to be bonded, but also any core materials or metallic details as well.

Thermoplastic composite materials offer potential post-processing advantages compared to thermoset composites. As a natural result of their structure, thermoplastic composites can be reformed into structural shapes after their initial consolidation. In addition, novel joining technologies such as induction welding are available for assembly operations. "Processing and Joining of Thermoplastic Composites" covers the different types of thermoplastic composites, processing methods, thermoforming methods, and joining technologies.

Although secondary adhesive bonding and thermoplastic composite joining processes offer significant cost advantages compared to mechanical assembly, mechanical fastening is and will remain an important assembly method for composite structures. First, in many instances, mechanical fasteners are the only feasible method for assembling composite parts to other major pieces of structure, and second, mechanical fasteners are often the only reliable method for highly loaded primary structure with complex load paths. Two articles cover this important assembly method for polymer-matrix composites—"Hole Drilling in Polymer Matrix Composites" and "Mechanical Fastener Selection." The article on hole drilling discusses shimming, drilling techniques (manual, power feed, and automated), reaming and countersinking operations, and hole-quality considerations. The article on mechanical fastener selection and installation covers fastener types and considerations, different types of fits, and special fasteners, such as blind fasteners, screws and nutplates, and temporary fasteners. It also covers a number of fastener installation methods and typical equipment.

The last article on post-processing and assembly of polymer-matrix composites, "Environmental Protection and Sealing," covers this important area with discussion of galvanic corrosion, thermal expansion considerations, different sealing methods, and painting. Although this article is the last article in this Section on polymer-matrix composites, environmental considerations and protection systems should be considered early in the design process to ensure success.

Metal-Matrix and Ceramic-Matrix Composites

The final two articles in this Section address post-processing and assembly of metal-matrix composites and ceramic-matrix composites. The article "Extrusion of Particle-Reinforced Aluminum Composites" addresses special considerations involved in extrusion operations for MMCs. The article "Post-Processing and Assembly of Ceramic-Matrix Composites" addresses finishing, coating, joining and other assembly methods, and nondestructive evaluation.

Machining, Trimming, and Routing of Polymer-Matrix Composites

Lawrence F. Kuberski, Fischer U.S.A.

POLYMER-MATRIX STRUCTURES are commonly fabricated to near-net shape. Therefore, by far the highest percentage of machining operations are trimming or roughing operations to remove the undesirable edge material from the cured part. Actual machining operations such as milling are used much less frequently, occasionally to mill seal grooves in parts or machine parts for improved fit during assembly.

Thermoset and thermoplastic composite parts are similar in machining characteristics but do exhibit some differences. Both materials contain high-strength fibers in a resin matrix. Both materials require the use of carbide tools, as a minimum, due to the extremely abrasive nature of the carbon reinforcing fibers. Tool wear during machining of thermoplastic composites is actually more severe than when machining thermoset composites. However, the most obvious difference between the two materials is the chip form. Thermoplastics form a folded ribbon type of chip compared to the dust particulate produced by machining of thermoset composites. Both material classes are similar in that they are susceptible to surface and/or exit delaminations, especially when the cutting tool becomes dull.

Machining Operations

A significant amount of work has been conducted to understand the complete machining process; that is, drilling, reaming, routing, trimming, and machining (end milling, slot milling, and facing) of carbon fiber-reinforced epoxy, or carbon/epoxy, thermoset composite materials. Some general guidelines for machining of carbon/epoxy composites are the following:

- Carbon/epoxy is abrasive by nature. Therefore, precautions should be taken to ensure that the carbon/epoxy particulate does not propagate into the precision machine/ground ways of the machine tool. The carbon/epoxy particulates can cause not only premature tool wear but machine wear as well.
- Carbon/epoxy dust can cause electrical components to short out or malfunction. All electronic components should be tightly sealed and have filter systems installed to prevent problems. Since thermoplastic composites generally form chips rather than particulates, electrical problems have not been experienced with these materials.

The aforementioned machining processes can be completed dry (with vacuum) or wet. When machining dry, a vacuum system must be used to collect the dust particulates to prevent them from becoming airborne. The vacuum system normally used is an ultrahigh-efficiency cartridge-type dust collection system providing capacity of 8.5 m^3/min (300 ft^3/min, or CFM, at an external static pressure of 7.5 kPa at 20 °C (30 in. H_2O at 70 °F) with an overall efficiency of 99% down to a 0.5 μm particle size. Even with this high efficiency system, it is imperative to remain vigilant of heat buildup or baking of the carbon epoxy particulate to the cutting tool. This problem can cause catastrophic part failure due to degradation and delaminations.

Enhanced tool life results when these operations are accomplished wet. Typical coolants are tap water or Bio-Cool 500 (Westmont Products, Dallas, TX) mixed at a 20-to-1 ratio, applied as flood. Another very important point for consideration is how the coolant will be recirculated during the machining processes. If the machine is not going to be dedicated to carbon/epoxy machining, then every consideration should be given to an auxiliary tank. This will prevent contamination of the coolant tank of the machine, an important point because dust particulates and not a chip form are generated during machining. The particulates form a sludge clogging filters and impeding coolant flow.

If the machine is not dedicated and an auxiliary tank will be used, the tank should be designed to provide a sludge and filtration system that will ensure adequate particulate-free coolant to be delivered to the cutting tool. This type of system will prevent contamination of the primary coolant delivery system of the machine and will also prevent severe corrosion to internal components.

Cutting Tools For Machining

Solid carbide cutting tools can be used; however, their life is very limited due to the abrasive nature of carbon/epoxy. Slot milling with solid carbide tools is not a cost effective process. During full slot milling of cuts with surface speeds in the range of 30.5 to 46 m/min (100 to 150 surface feet per minute, or sfm), overall tool life was typically less than 914 mm (36 in.) before delaminations occurred on the part surface. In addition, no conventional coatings, such as titanium nitride (TiN), titanium carbon nitride (TiCN) or titanium aluminum nitride (TiAlN) have proved advantageous for machining carbon/epoxy.

Diamond plated cutting tools offer little advantage over carbide tools when machining carbon/epoxy. This can be best explained with a little understanding of the plating process. The plating process lays down a single layer of bonding material, usually tin. This layer almost encapsulates the diamond particles leaving approximately 10 to 20% of the diamonds exposed. The problem with this type of tool occurs when the tool begins to generate heat during the cutting process. Once the tin bonding layer becomes hot, the diamonds lose adhesion, and, consequently, the tool is left with no cutting edges.

Brazed diamond cutting tools do have a significant advantage over carbide and plated diamond tools. The diamond braze process is also a layer process; however, nickel is used rather than tin and the application temperature is much higher because of the nickel. In addition, bonding of the nickel to the diamond is quite good, requiring only 10 to 30% of the diamond particles to be encapsulated, leaving 70% or more of the diamond exposed for cutting purposes. These tools can be fabricated into a wide variety of shapes and diameters. In selected applications, tools of diameters 50.8 mm (2 in.) and greater can be operated above 1,070 m/min (3,500 sfm) and at 5,080 to 10,160 mm/min (200–400 in. per min, or ipm) feedrate or more. A diamond brazed cutting tool with slots to break up the constant contact of the tool to the part surface is shown

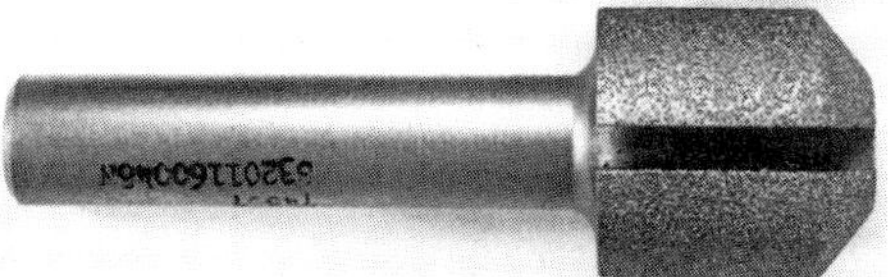

Fig. 1 Typical diamond brazed cutting tool

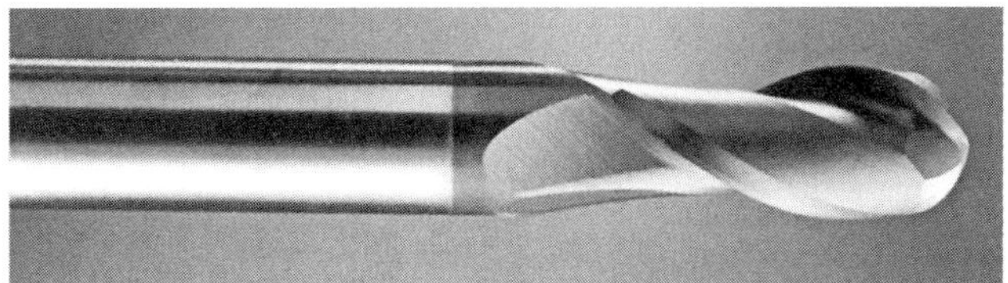

Fig. 2 Solid carbide end mill with thin film diamond coating

in Fig. 1. These slots can also carry coolant to help keep the tool cool, reducing carbon/epoxy buildup on the surface and subsequent delaminations or catastrophic failure.

Diamond Coated Carbide Tools. The latest thin film diamond coatings have shown good potential for machining carbon/epoxy. However, it is important to point out that the life of these coated tools does not approach the life of solid polycrystalline diamond (PCD) tools. They can be used successfully in the range of 612 m/min (2,000 sfm) with 0.025 to 0.051 mm per tooth (0.001–0.002 in. per tooth, or ipt) feedrate and are substantially less expensive than polycrystalline diamond tools. In addition, they can be used in dry-machining operations, but a high capacity vacuum system is required to keep the carbon/epoxy particulates from becoming airborne. A mist type coolant will prolong the life of these tools if the coolant can be tolerated on the part piece. A typical solid carbide end mill with a thin film diamond coating is shown in Fig. 2.

Polycrystalline cutting tools have a solid polycrystalline wafer brazed onto a high-speed steel (HSS) or carbide body. These tools present an interesting alternative to conventional cutting materials, such as carbides and brazed or plated tools, combining a very hard and wear resistant solid-diamond cutting edge. In many cases, their higher cost can be justified. Under certain conditions it is not unusual to experience 30 to 50 times longer tool life of solid carbide tooling. The main drawback to PCD tools is that the diamond is fragile and prone to chipping and breakage. They cannot be handled the way HSS, carbide, plated, or brazed tools are handled. Due to the fragile nature of these tools, extremely rigid setups, such as automated machine tools, are required.

Polycrystalline diamond tools can be operated at the higher surface speeds similar to brazed diamond tooling. However, polycrystalline tools have flutes rather than multiple cutting edges. Therefore, the surface finish obtained will be somewhat dependent on the feed rate or advance per revolution. Surface finishes of 40 R_a or better have been achieved.

Peripheral Milling

The cutting tool materials used for slot machining are also applicable to peripheral milling. Because the tool is not in constant contact with the workpiece, it is possible to achieve higher surface speeds during peripheral milling. However, increasing the surface speed also increases the incidence and severity of possible surface delaminations. Tool wear in all of these operations will cause delaminations and costly rework. Therefore, a thorough knowledge of the process and predictable tool life is extremely important to the end user. Ideally the surface produced by milling, routing, drilling, or countersink should be free of delaminations, as shown in Fig. 3. This carbon/epoxy sample had three machining operations performed– drilling, countersinking and milling of the top surface.

Face Milling

As with peripheral milling, face milling can be accomplished with the same type of cutting tools. However, as described in the section on brazed diamond cutting tools, these tools can be produced in a wide variety of shapes and sizes and can be easily custom fitted to milling operations. However, PCD tools are not as readily shaped and are significantly more expensive. An example of the machining parameters for facing operations is shown in Table 1. However, the tool should be balanced when operating at high sfm because balance can become an issue. Vibrations, which are either self-excited (tool problem) or forced resonant vibration (part vibration), can damage the spindle and the workpiece. So, as in any other high-speed machining operation, these types of vibrations must be recognized and properly dealt with to prolong both spindle and tool life.

In summary, there are several important points to remember when machining carbon/epoxy composites.

- To prolong tool life, prevent heat damage, and contain the carbon/epoxy particulate, the machining operations must be accomplished wet. Always use sharp tools.
- It is extremely important for programmers and operators to be familiar with the geometry of plated or brazed diamond tool shapes. Never exceed the length of the cutting edge.
- If intricate part shapes are involved, use of carbide tooling may be necessary. Tool life

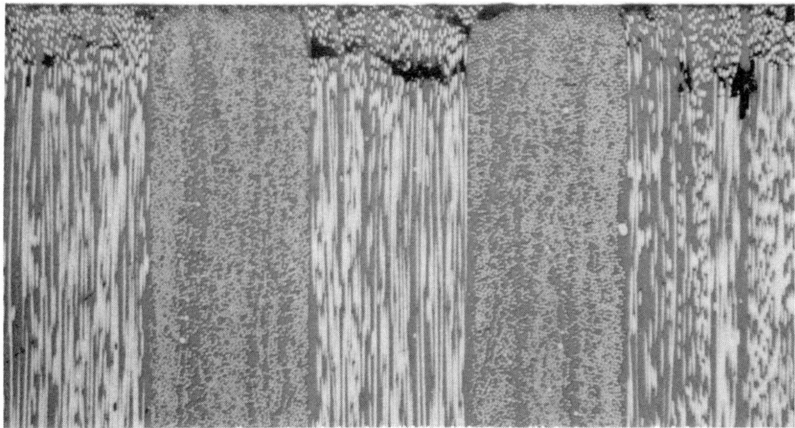

Fig. 3 Typical machined surface of carbon/epoxy composite

Table 1 Typical face-milling parameters for carbon fiber-reinforced epoxy composites

Tool diam		Speed(a)		Axial depth of cut		Radial depth of cut		Feed rate	
mm	in.	m/min	sfm	mm	in.	mm	in.	mm/min	in./min
63.5	2.5	320	1048	3.8	0.015	63.5	2.5	1524	60
		478	1572	2.54	0.100	63.5	2.5	1016	40
		638	2100	1.52	0.060	63.5	2.5	762	30
		638	2100	0.76	0.030	63.5	2.5	1016	40
101.5	4.0	510	1677	1.27	0.050	63.5	2.5	762	30

Note: Water used as flood coolant. (a) Tools can be operated at higher surface-feet-per-minute values when lighter cuts are taken.

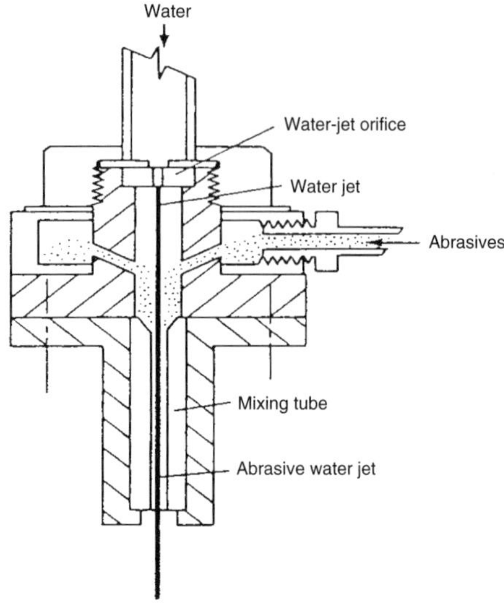

Fig. 4 Typical abrasive waterjet head configuration

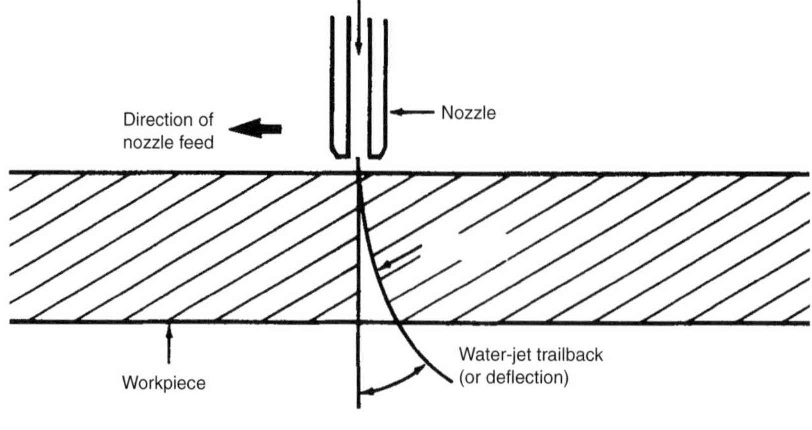

Fig. 5 Waterjet cutting

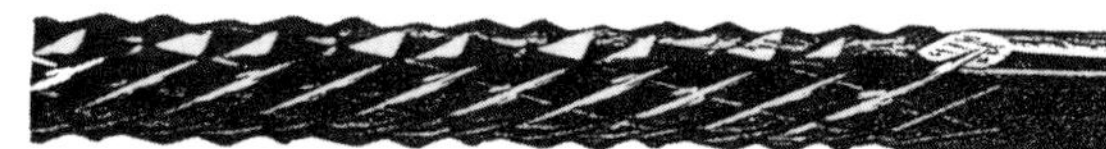

Fig. 6 Typical router bit

with carbide tooling is short. Therefore, the operator/programmer must be prepared to change tools frequently to prevent delaminations and subsequent rework.

- Brazed diamond tools can be fabricated in a wide variety of shapes and sizes but require adequate lead-time for procurement.
- Brazed diamond tooling can be cleaned with a soft wire brush or wheel to extend tool life.
- If PCD tools are used, the operators must be properly trained regarding handling of these costly tools. Rigid setups are also needed with polycrystalline diamond tools to preclude edge chipping or breakage.

Table 2 Partial list of materials cut with abrasive waterjet

Metals
718 Inconel
625 Inconel
6AL-4V titanium alloy (3.2 mm, or 0.125 in., thick)
Commercially pure titanium
Hastelloy
321 CRES (75 mm, or 3 in., thick)
15-7 PH CRES
301 half hard CRES
301 full hard CRES
Chromoloy
ESCO 49M-high nickel/high chrome alloy (170 mm, or 6.75 in., thick)
Mild steels
Glass (25 mm, or 1 in., thick)
Aluminum (140 mm, or 5.5 in., thick)
Peel shim stock
304L CRES (13 mm, or 0.5 in., thick)
Composites
Metal matrix
Graphite
Aramid
Glass
Laminated glass
Ceramics

Trimming

Abrasive waterjet is the preferred method for trimming carbon/epoxy composites. Cut quality and trim accuracy is best controlled using this method. A typical head configuration is shown in Fig. 4. These systems typically have 345 MPa (50 ksi) pressure capability at the pump. The orifice is made of sapphire that has a 1 mm (0.04 in.) diameter hole through which the high-pressure fluid flows. The 1 mm diameter hole typically diminishes pressure to 303 to 310 MPa (44–45 ksi) at the nozzle tip. The fluid is filtered to 0.05 μm and is pumped in relatively low volumes, typically 0.96 to 1.98 L/min (1–2 gal/min). The system uses an abrasive material, such as a No. 80 garnet grit that is introduced into the waterjet after the primary jet is formed. Some typical examples of abrasive waterjet trimming parameters on carbon/epoxy materials are given in the following table:

Material thickness		Feed rate		
mm	in.	mm/min	in./min	Surface finish (R_a)
≤12.7	0.5	381	15	50–70
25.4	1.0	254	10	50–70
25.4–50.8	1–2	127–152	5–6	50–70

Waterjet cutting produces less cutting force than most of the mechanical machining methods and generally requires only clamping to secure the part, virtually eliminating the need for intricate fixturing methods. In addition, the waterjet produces no heat affected zone and can dwell in one spot for some time without widening the cut width. However, the process is quite noisy (requiring ear protection), requires good filtration equipment for the water, must be carefully monitored for jet wear (the most common jet material is sapphire), and has a tendency to produce trailback, especially in thicker materials, as shown in Fig. 5. This trailback or deflection results in an angled cut on the edge of the workpiece but can usually be decreased to acceptable levels with a slower feed rate. As shown in the table above, the feed rates are significantly slower as the material thickness increases. This is to ensure that as little deviation as possible occurs from the top to the bottom of the part, as the waterjet has a tendency to spread as it penetrates thicker material. Also, as the feed rate increases, the waterjet can lag behind in thicker cuts. Several other difficult-to-machine material types are easily cut or trimmed by abrasive waterjet. A partial list is shown in Table 2.

Routing operations are conducted both by machine and by hand. When conducted by machine, routing by using PCD tools is possible. However, when the operation is conducted by hand, too many variables enter into the process to use PCD tools. Therefore, either a brazed diamond tool or a carbide router bit with diamond-shaped facets (Fig. 6) is often used.

Routers are frequently operated at speeds up to 30,000 rpm. In hand operations, the feed rate is adjusted by the individual operating the hand router. With sharp tool bits, this feed rate can be as much as 305m/min (1,000 ft/min). Using the same type tool in a robot or machine tool operation, the feed rate can be 610 m/min (2,000 ft/min) or more in trimming operations. In full slot cuts, the feed rate will drop approximately 50%. This is necessary to flush the particulate away from the tool. Unlike diamond brazed tools, which can be cleaned with a wire brush, or the PCD tools, which can be resharpened, these types of tools must be considered disposable. As with the other tool bits used for machining carbon/epoxy, the main criterion for tool life is evidence of any delaminations.

SELECTED REFERENCES

- T.O. Blankenship and L. Kuberski, "Routing and Near-Net Trimming of Carbon/Epoxy Composite Materials," Advanced Manufacturing Fabrication Facility R & D Report, McDonnell Douglas Aerospace, 1983
- S. Higgins and L. Kuberski, "Thermoplastic Milling Evaluation," Advanced Manufacturing Fabrication Facility R & D Report, McDonnell Douglas Aerospace, 1988
- J. Korican, *Water-Jet and Abrasive Water-Jet Cutting,* Sundstrand Corp., 1988
- L. Kuberski, "General Guidelines for Machining Carbon/Epoxy Composite Materials," Advanced Manufacturing Technology, Machinability and Cutter Development Group Bulletin, 1991
- L. Kuberski and W. Luebbert, "Machining Carbon/Epoxy Composite Materials," Advanced Manufacturing Fabrication Facility R & D Report, McDonnell Douglas Aerospace, 1982
- L. Kuberski and W. Luebbert, "Machining Seal Grooves and Trimming Composite Skins," Advanced Manufacturing Fabrication Facility R & D Report, McDonnell Douglas Aerospace, 1989
- L. Kuberski and K. Waymack, "Parameters For Water-Jet Machining of Carbon/Epoxy Composites," Advanced Manufacturing Technology, Machinability and Cutter Development Group Bulletin, 1991
- A. B. Strong, *Fundamentals of Composites Manufacturing: Materials, Methods, and Applications,* Society of Manufacturing Engineers, 1989

Secondary Adhesive Bonding of Polymer-Matrix Composites

Flake C. Campbell, The Boeing Company—St. Louis

ADHESIVE BONDING frequently is used to assemble composite components into larger structures. In addition, finished components that are damaged during assembly or service are often repaired with adhesive-bonding techniques.

Adhesive bonding is used only if subsequent disassembly of the subcomponents is unlikely. Bonded joints may be preferred if thin composite sections are to be joined when bearing stresses in bolted joints would be unacceptably high, or when the weight penalty for mechanical fasteners is too high. In general, thin structures with well-defined load paths are good candidates for adhesive bonding, while thicker structures with complex load paths are better candidates for mechanical fastening.

Adhesive Joint Design

In a structural adhesive joint, the load in one component must be transferred through the adhesive layer to another component. The efficiency with which this can be done depends on the joint design, the adhesive characteristics, and the adhesive/substrate interface. In order to transfer loads through the adhesive, the substrates (or adherends) are overlapped to place the adhesive in shear. Figure 1 shows some typical joint designs for adhesively bonded joints of composite-to-metal substrates.

Figure 2 shows a typical stress distribution for a double lap shear joint. Note that the adhesive is required to withstand relatively high local loads near changes in the joint section (i.e., at the ends). Therefore, adhesives designed to carry high loads need to be strong and tough, especially if there is any bending in the joint that would induce peel loads. Adhesives are frequently rubber modified; this practice sacrifices modulus in order to improve fracture toughness and fatigue life. However, in well-designed, toughened adhesives (e.g., second-phase toughening), only moderate reductions of the continuous-phase modulus occurs.

The criteria for selecting an adhesive must be considered in view of the joint design. The joint design must ensure that the adhesive is loaded in shear as far as possible. Tension, cleavage, and peel loading (Fig. 3) should be avoided when using adhesives.

Selection Criteria

The first criterion for selecting an adhesive is the capability to withstand the required stresses in the full range of environmental conditions to which the component may be exposed. The class of adhesive may be dictated by the loading conditions. For example, if high peel loads are unavoidable, a highly flexible adhesive would probably be more suitable than a rigid epoxy.

In-service environmental conditions should also be considered as a selection criterion because, for example, flexible polyurethane adhesives are more sensitive to moisture degradation than the equivalent polychloroprene (neoprene) rubber formulations.

Long-term stress conditions can also affect adhesive selection. Thermoplastic adhesives and highly flexibilized epoxy systems may be susceptible to creep under sustained load. On the other hand, rigid, glassy adhesives may have limited resistance to cyclic load conditions.

The practicality of the application process must also be considered, specifically, the method of surface preparation; the restriction on handling prepared surfaces before bonding; the method of mixing (if necessary) and applying the adhesive to the joint; the procedure for melting or curing the adhesive; the tooling necessary for support of the joint during bonding; and the methods for cleaning the joint after bonding, if necessary, and cleaning application equipment.

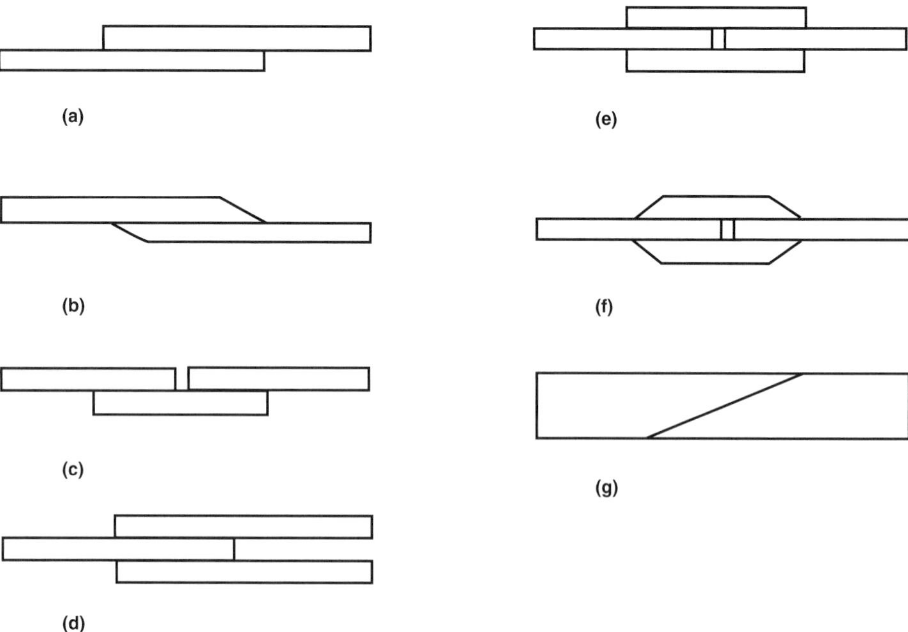

Fig. 1 Typical secondary adhesively bonded joint configurations. (a) Single lap joint. (b) Tapered single lap joint. (c) Single strap joint. (d) Double lap joint. (e) Double strap joint. (f) Tapered double strap joint. (g) Scarf joint

Adhesive characteristics are listed in Tables 1 and 2. Adhesive selection and use criteria are summarized as follows:

- The adhesive must be compatible with the adherends and able to retain its required strength when exposed to in-service stresses and environmental factors.
- The joint should be designed to ensure a failure in one of the adherends rather than a failure within the adhesive bondline.
- Thermal expansion of dissimilar materials must be considered. Due to the large thermal expansion difference between graphite composite and aluminum, adhesively bonded joints between these two materials have been known to fail during cool-down from elevated-temperature cures as a result of the thermal stresses induced by their differential expansion coefficients.
- Proper joint design should be used, avoiding tension, peel, or cleavage loading whenever possible.
- If peel forces cannot be avoided, a lower modulus (nonbrittle) adhesive having a high peel strength should be used.
- Tapered ends should be used on lap joints to feather out the edge-of-joint stresses. Refer to Fig. 1(b) and (f) for examples.
- Selection tests for structural adhesives should include durability testing for heat, humidity (and/or fluids), and stress, simultaneously.
- Surface preparation should be conducted carefully, avoiding contamination of the bondline with moisture, oil, and so on.
- When received, the adhesive should be tested for compliance with the purchase specification. This may include both physical and chemical tests, such as infrared, moisture content, resin content, base resin, secondary resins, curing agent, and accelerator.
- The adhesive should be stored at the recommended temperature.
- Cold adhesive should always be warmed to room temperature in a sealed container.
- Liquid mixes should be degassed, if possible, to remove entrained air.
- Adhesives that evolve volatiles during cure should be avoided.
- The humidity in the lay-up area should be below 40% relative humidity for most formulations. Lay-up room humidity is adsorbed by the adhesive and is released later during heat cure as steam, yielding porous bondlines and interfering with the cure chemistry.
- The recommended pressure and the proper alignment fixtures should be used. The bonding pressure should be great enough to ensure that the adherends are in intimate contact with each other.
- The use of a vacuum as the method of applying pressure should be avoided whenever possible, since an active vacuum on the adhesive during cure can lead to porosity or voids in the cured bondline.
- Heat curing is almost always preferred, because it yields bonds that have greater strength, heat, and humidity resistance.
- When curing for a second time, such as during repairs, the temperature should be at least 28 °C (50 °F) below the earlier cure temperature. If this is not possible, then a proper and accurate bond form must be used to maintain all parts in proper alignment and under pressure during the second cure cycle.
- Traveler coupons should always be made for testing. These are test coupons that duplicate the adherends to be bonded in material and joint design. The coupon surfaces are prepared by the same method and at the same time as the basic bond. Coupons are also bonded together at the same time with the same adhesive (mix lot, and so on) of the basic joint and subjected to the same curing process simultaneously with the basic bond.

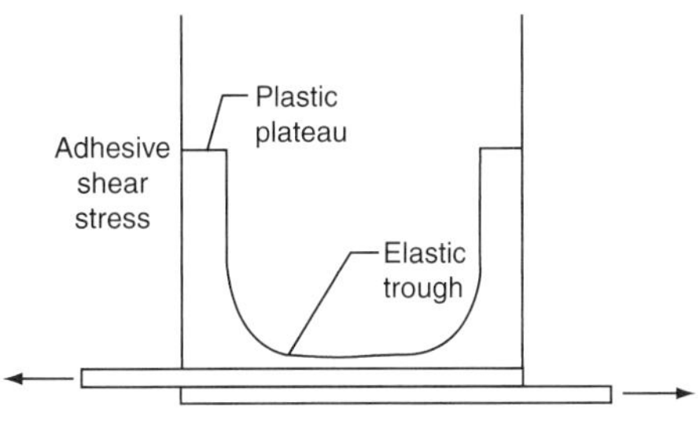

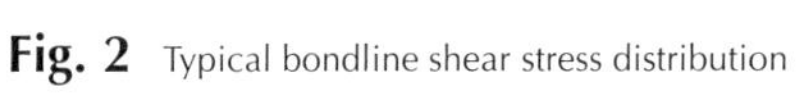

Fig. 2 Typical bondline shear stress distribution

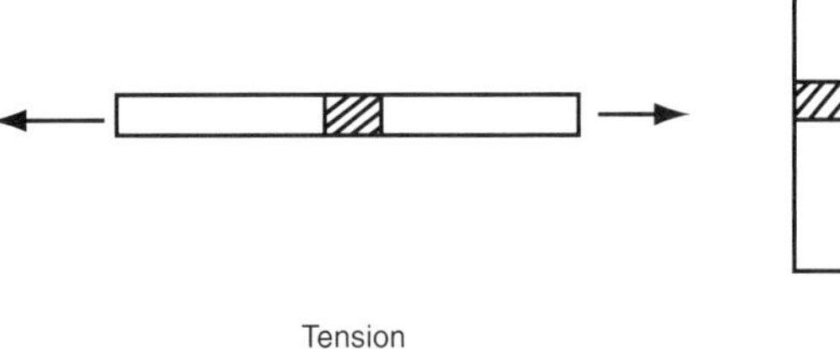

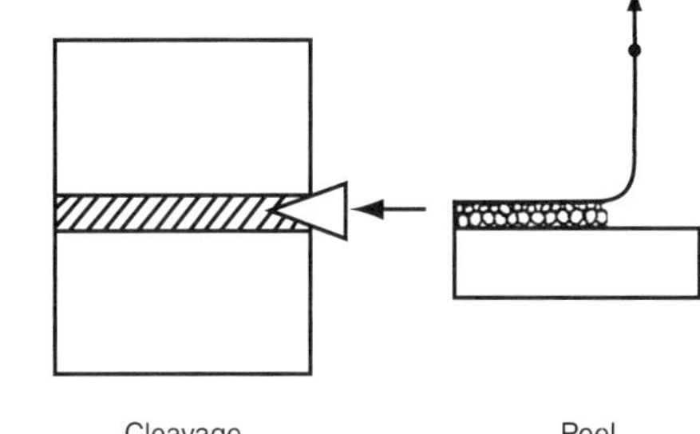

Fig. 3 Load paths to avoid in adhesive use

Table 1 Typical characteristics of adhesive types

Type	Form	Cure temperature, °C (°F)	Maximum use temperature, °C (°F)	Advantages	Disadvantages
Epoxy	Two-part paste	Room or accelerated at 93–178 (200–350)	Generally below 82 (180)	Ease of storage at room temperature; ease of mixing and use; long shelf life; gap filling when filled	Not generally as strong or environmentally resistant as typical heat-cured epoxies
	One-part film	121 (250) 149 (300) 178 (350)	To 82 (180) 149–177 (300–350)	Covers large areas; bondline thickness control; wide variety of formulas; higher-temperature curing materials; better environmental properties	Store at 18 °C (0 °F); short shelf life; high-temperature cure; brittle and low peel strength
Acrylic	Two-part liquid or pastes	Room to 100 (212)	105 (221)	Fast setting; easy to mix and use; good moisture resistance; tolerant of surface contamination	Strong, objectionable odor; limited pot life
Polyurethane	One or two parts	Room or heat cure	. . .	Good peel; good for cryogenic use	Moisture sensitive before and after cure
Silicone	One- and two-part pastes	Room to 260 (500)	To 260 (500)	High peel and impact resistance; easy to use; good heat and moisture resistance	High cost; low strength
Hot melt	One-part	Melt at 190–232 (375–450)	49–171 (120–340)	Rapid application; fast setting; low cost; indefinite shelf life; nontoxic; no mixing	Poor heat resistance; special equipment required; poor creep resistance; low strength; high melt temperature
Bismaleimide (BMI)	One-part paste or film	>178 (350) and 246 (475) postcure	177–232 (350–450)	Structural bonds with bismaleimide composites; higher temperature than epoxies; no volatiles; good shelf life	Brittle and low peel
Polyimide	Thermoplastic liquids; one- and two-part pastes	260 (500) and postcure	204–260 (400–500)	High-temperature resistance; structural strength	High cost; low peel strength; high cure and postcure temperatures; volatiles for some forms
Phenolic-based	One-part films	163–177 (325–350)	To 177 (350)	High-temperature use	Low peel strength

Table 2 Use-temperature guide to structural adhesives

Peel: L, low; M, medium; H, high. Lap shear: P, poor; Mod, moderate; G, good; V, very good; E, excellent. Peel is indicated first, followed by lap shear: peel/lap shear.

	Use temperature, °C (°F)								
Adhesive	−253 (−423)	−196 (−320)	−73 (−100)	−54 (−65)	Room	82 (180)	149 (300)	216 (420)	260 (500)
Epoxy-nitrile modified	L/V	L/V	L/E	L/E	H/E	M/V	L/Mod	. . .	. . .
Epoxy-nylon	L/E	L/E	L/E	L/E	H/V	L/G	L/Mod	. . .	. . .
Epoxy-phenolic	. . .	. . .	L/V	L/V	L/V	L/V	L/G	G	G
Vinyl-phenolic	. . .	. . .	. . .	L/V	M/E	H/E	L/Mod	. . .	. . .
Nitrile-phenolic	Mod	E	E	L/E	H/V	M/G	L/Mod	. . .	. . .
Bismaleimides	. . .	. . .	. . .	Mod	L/G	L/G	L/G	L/V	. . .
Polyimides	. . .	. . .	. . .	L/V	L/G	L/G	L/G	L/G	L/G
Polyurethanes	H/V	H/V	H/V	H/G	H/G	H/Mod	H/P	. . .	. . .
Acrylics	. . .	. . .	. . .	L/P	H/E	M/G	L/P	. . .	. . .

Ideally, traveler coupons are cut from the basic part, on which extensions have been provided.

- The exposed edge of the bond joint should be protected with an appropriate sealer, such as an elastomeric sealant or paint. Honeycomb assemblies should be hermetically sealed.

Highly Loaded Joint Considerations

For highly loaded structural applications, it is fundamental to compare the strength and durability properties of those adhesives that are candidates for selection. It is necessary to know the allowable stresses for the adhesive and to be able to calculate the design stresses on the adhesive in service. Unfortunately, the traditional lap shear test shown in Fig. 4 does not produce the true ultimate stress. Also, this test produces no data for adhesive shear modulus, which is required for a stress analysis of a bonded joint.

The lap shear strength is reported as the failure stress in the adhesive, which is found by dividing the failing load by the bond area. Since the stress distribution in the adhesive is not uniform over the bond area (it peaks at the edges of the joint as shown in Fig. 2), the reported shear stress is lower than the true ultimate strength of the adhesive.

However, lap shear data do have value from a comparative standpoint. One can determine if a certain adhesive has superior strength compared to another even though the actual design strength is not obtained. Also, lap shear values are useful for quality control, such as receiving inspection or as a proof of correct manufacturing processes (i.e., traveler coupons).

The development of the thick adherend test specimen and the KGR-l extensometer allows accurate shear stress and shear strain data to be obtained in the laboratory. Figure 5 and Ref 1 describe the procedures. This test produces a complete, accurate curve of adhesive shear stress versus shear strain for any environment reproducible in the laboratory up to 260 °C (500 °F).

Because the metal is so thick and the metallic adherend strains are therefore small, the thick adherend specimen produces an essentially uniform shear stress over the test area, allowing an accurate experimental determination of the adhesive shear stress-strain response.

The adhesive shear stress distribution for a typical bonded joint (Ref 2) is shown in Fig. 6. The joint shown has been simplified by using a single metal alloy, a single thickness, and a single value of G, the adhesive shear modulus. Note that changes in the adhesive shear modulus or bondline thickness will change the peak (critical) shear stress, with no change in load on the structure. This is unique and fundamental to the adhesive-selection process. It enables the designer to select the best adhesive for any environment. When the shear stress-strain curve ceases to be linear—that is, where the shear modulus is no longer constant—much can still be learned. Figure 7 shows a typical shear stress versus shear strain curve with explanations of several characteristics as they predict adhesive performance, while Fig. 8 shows the effects of temperature on the stress and strain properties of a typical structural adhesive.

Bonding to composites rather than to metals introduces significant differences in criteria for adhesive selection for two reasons: (1) compos-

Fig. 4 Single lap shear specimen. P, load

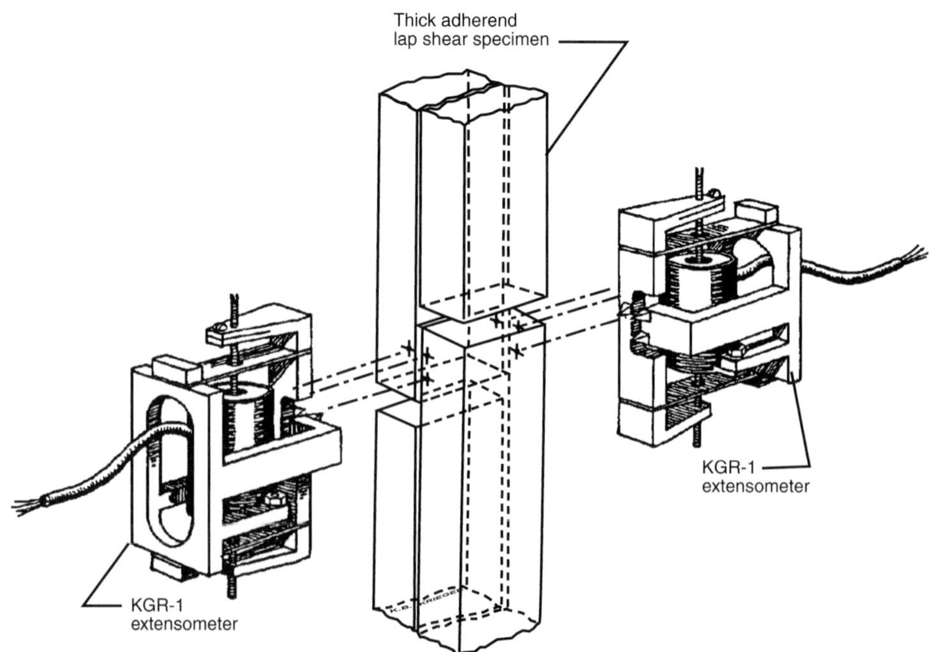

Fig. 5 KGR-1 extensometer with thick adherend specimen. Source: Ref 1

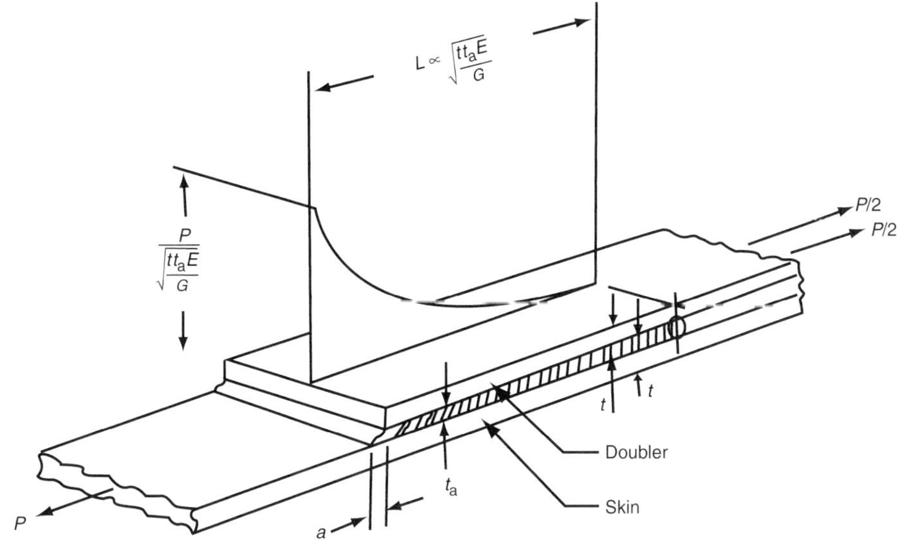

Fig. 6 Adhesive shear stress distribution for skin-doubler specimen. *E*, tensile modulus of adherends; *G*, shear modulus of adhesive. Source: Ref 2

ites exhibit a large drop in interlaminar shear stiffness compared to metals and (2) composites have a much lower shear strength than metals. This occurs because the interlaminar shear stiffness and strength depend on the matrix properties and not the higher properties of the fibers. The exaggerated deformations in a composite laminate bonded to a metal sheet and placed under tension are shown in Fig. 9. The adhesive passes the load from the metal into the composite until, at distance *L*, the strain in each material is equal. In the composite, the matrix resin acts as an adhesive to pass load from one fiber ply to the next. Because the matrix shear stiffness is low, the composite plies deform unequally in tension as shown. Failure tends to initiate in the composite ply next to the adhesive near the beginning of the joint or in the adhesive in the same neighborhood. The highest failure loads are achieved by an adhesive with a low shear modulus and high strain to failure, as shown in Fig. 6. This results because *L* will be the largest and the maximum shear stress will be lowest. It should also be noted that there is a limit to the thickness of the composite that can be loaded by a single bondline; however, multiple steps in the composite thickness giving multiple bondlines may be necessary for thick material.

Basic design practice for adhesive-bonded composite joints should include ensuring that the surface fibers in a joint are parallel to the direction of load to minimize interlaminar shear, or failure of the bonded substrate layer. In designs in which joint areas have been machined to a step-lap configuration, for example, it is possible to have a joint interface composed of fibers at an orientation other than the optimal 0° orientation to the load direction. This tends to induce substrate failure more readily than would otherwise occur.

To determine fatigue and creep performance (including under hostile environment) there are many tests, which like lap shear, do not present accurate shear failure stresses. For these conditions, one can again turn to shear stress versus shear strain data for allowable stresses, as described in Fig. 7 and 8. These allowable stresses can be compared to calculated stresses on the structure using the approach shown in Fig. 7.

The adhesive stress-strain curves can also be used on a comparative basis, that is, to determine whether adhesive A is better or worse than adhesive B. Here Fig. 7 can be used together with shear stress versus shear strain. Comparing *LL* stress values for fatigue performance is not a complete method, since shear modulus (*G*) can be different for the adhesive being compared. It is more accurate to compare *LL* stress (τ_{LL}) adjusted by the square root of *G*, for the two adhesives.

Much has been written about joint design. Experience and predominant applications point to using the adhesive in shear as the most effective method. Figure 10 shows a variety of designs. Figures 10(a) to (d) joints are all loaded in shear, while Fig. 10(e) is loaded in tension and Fig. 10(f) is loaded in peel. Note that Fig. 10(e) and (f) exhibit large tensile stress peaks in the adhesive. These peaks can be much higher than those in shear loading and are far less forgiving. Also, these peaks are very sensitive to small eccentricities. These problems make tension and

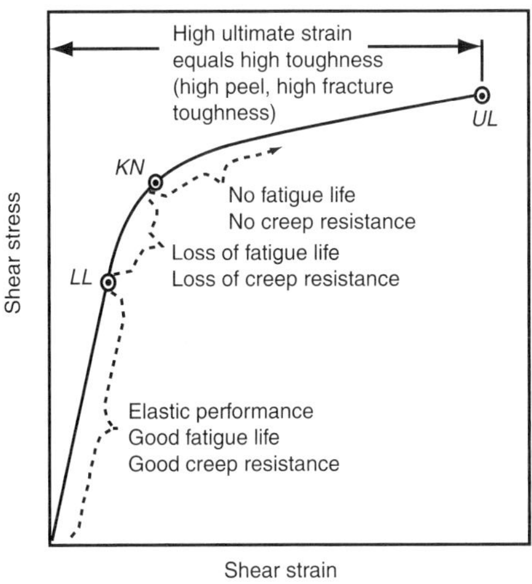

Fig. 7 Some general properties of adhesives relative to shear stress and strain. *LL*, end of straight line region; *KN*, maximum rate loss of stiffness; *UL*, ultimate strength

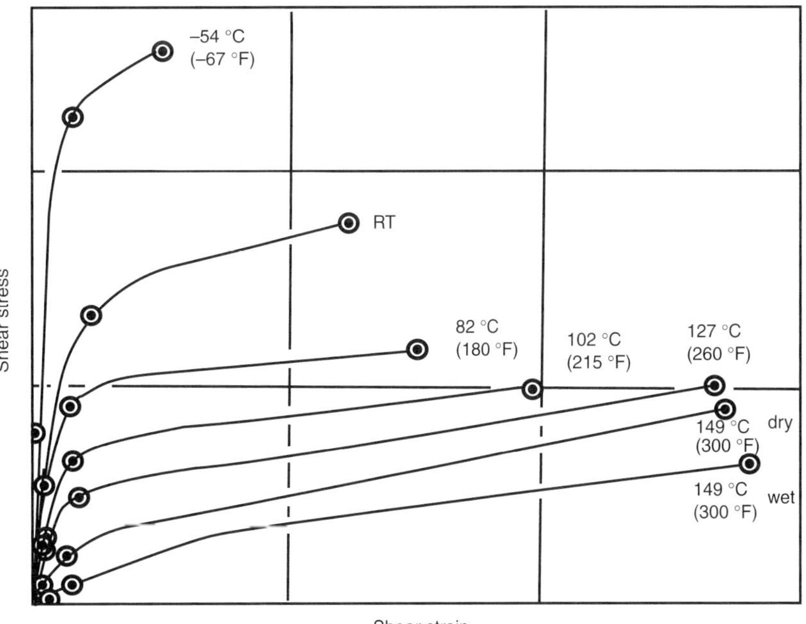

Fig. 8 Shear stress and strain at various temperatures for a typical structural adhesive. RT, room temperature

peel, at best, very questionable load paths. Figure 10(d) shows a scarf joint often used for damage repair. It is impressive in that there are no shear peaks in the adhesive stress distribution (i.e., a constant shear stress).

Durability can be evaluated in the adhesive-selection process by using the adhesive shear stress versus shear strain curves as obtained by the KGR-1 extensometer. As stated earlier, environments are easily obtained in the laboratory, which include temperatures from below –57 to 260 °C (–70 to 500 °F) and after any fluid saturation assumed to be experienced by the aircraft. Similar to the curves shown in Fig. 8, the shear stress-strain curves for these environments all have the same fundamental shapes and can be evaluated as to adhesive capability in the same way as described for ambient conditions. As shown in the Fig. 8 curve for the test conducted at 149 °C (300 °F) after humidity exposure (wet), hostile environments degrade the structural performance of most adhesives. This again emphasizes the point that it is important to conduct test programs for adhesives using the actual anticipated service environment.

It should be emphasized that bonding to cured composites presents a serious complexity for accurate stress analysis, because the composite has disproportionately low interlaminar shear stiffness and shear strength when compared with isotropic metals. This may well call for tests to verify the analysis for any critically bonded structure. For a more thorough discussion of adhesive-bonded joint design, refer to the article "Bolted and Bonded Joints" in this Volume.

Epoxy Adhesives

Epoxy-based adhesives are the most commonly used materials for bonding or repair of composite structures. The existence of a large variety of materials—to fit nearly any handling, curing, or performance requirement—results in an extensive list from which to choose. Epoxy adhesives impart high-strength bonds and long-term durability over a wide range of temperatures and environments. The ease of formulation modification makes it fairly easy for the formulator to employ various materials to control specific performance properties, such as density, toughness, flow, mix ratio, pot life/shelf life, shop handling characteristics, cure time/temperature, and service temperature.

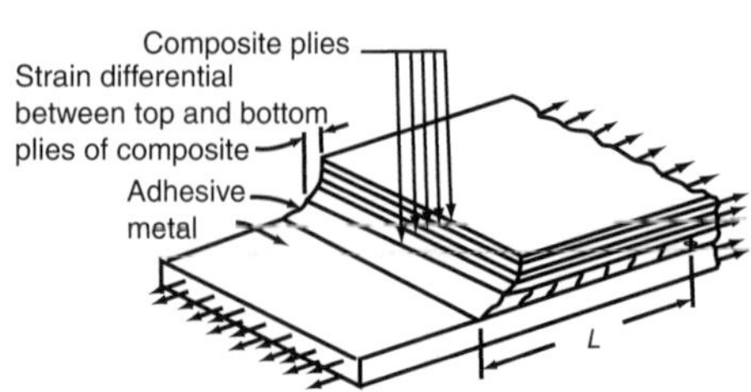

Fig. 9 Exaggerated deformation of composite plies and adhesive when bonded to metal

Advantages of epoxy adhesives are excellent adhesion, high strength and modulus, low or no volatiles during cure, low shrinkage, and good chemical resistance. Disadvantages include cost, brittleness unless modified, moisture absorption that adversely affects properties, and rather long cure times.

A wide range of one- and two-part systems

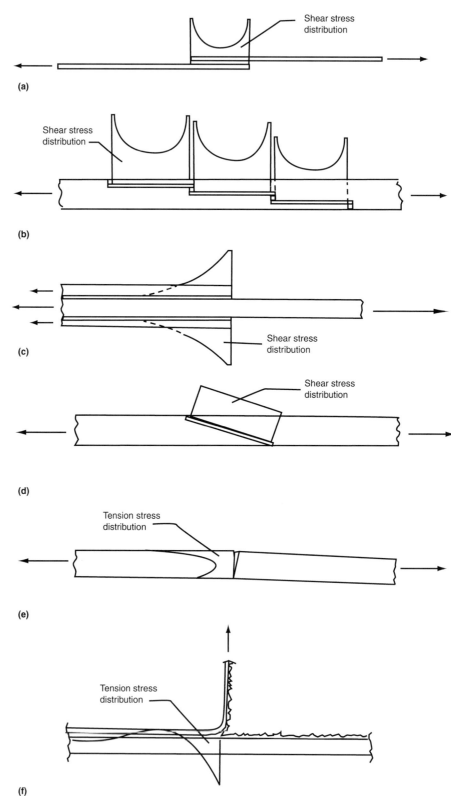

Fig. 10 Various bonded joint configurations. (a), (b), and (c) Shear. (d) Scarf. (e) Tension. (f) Peel

are available. Some systems cure at room temperature, while others require elevated temperatures.

Chemistry. Epoxy resins used as adhesives are generally supplied as liquids or low-melting-temperature solids. They commonly contain bifunctional epoxy groups, although higher functionalities are available. They can be cured by a variety of curing procedures, including admixture with the stoichiometric proportion of polyfunctional primary amine or acid anhydride. The amine or anhydride groups react with the epoxy groups by a simple addition reaction to give a densely cross-linked structure. Some epoxy compositions can be cured through a homopolymerization reaction initiated by strong organic bases (or rarely, acids). These compositions are less sensitive to the mix ratio, but are seldom encountered as two-part systems. The rate of the reaction may be adjusted by adding accelerators in the initial formulation or by increasing the temperature. To improve structural properties, particularly at elevated temperatures, it is common to cure temperatures close to (or preferably over) the maximum-use temperature for the structure.

Epoxy resin systems are usually modified by a wide range of additives that control particular properties. These additives include accelerators, viscosity modifiers and other flow-control additives, fillers and pigments, flexibilizers, and toughening agents. The versatility of these materials has led to the development of a wide range of epoxy adhesives for specific applications.

Epoxy-based adhesives are available in two basic cure chemistries: room temperature and elevated temperature. Within each cure type, there is a wide range of formulated resins to cover specific application and performance requirements.

One-Part Elevated-Temperature Curing Epoxy Liquid and Paste Adhesives. These materials typically require an elevated-temperature cure of 120 to 177 °C (250–350 °F). The primary chemistry of one-part systems usually consists of a mixture of bifunctional and multifunctional resins with noncatalyzed or imidizole catalyzed dicyanimide. As such, the normal room-temperature shelf life ranges from 15 to 30 days for catalyzed materials and up to six months for noncatalyzed systems. Service temperatures for these materials are generally close to their respective curing temperatures; however, the actual service temperature should always be determined by testing at the expected service conditions.

Typical packaging for the one-part adhesives includes pint, quart, gallon, and five-gallon containers. In addition, for ease of application, most are supplied in cylindrical polyethylene sealant gun cartridges that, depending on their size, can contain up to 500+ g of material. Since the chemistry and performance of some one-part paste adhesives are similar to that of film adhesives, these materials are often referred to as "film adhesive in a tube."

Two-Part Room-Temperature Curing Epoxy Liquid and Paste Adhesives. These systems are most commonly used when a room-temperature cure is desired. They are available as clear liquids or as filled pastes with a consistency ranging from low-viscosity liquids to heavy-duty putties. Typical cure times are 5 to 7 days; however, in most cases 70 to 75% of the ultimate cure can be achieved within 24 h, and, if needed, the pressure can usually be released at that point. Under normal bondline thickness conditions (0.125–0.250 mm, or 0.005–0.010 in.), cure can be accelerated with heat without fear of exotherm. A typical cure would be 1 h at 82 °C (180 °F). For higher-temperature applications, there are also two-part adhesives that require a high-temperature cure of at least 82 °C (180 °F).

Two-part systems require mixing a part A (the resin and filler portion) with a part B (the curing agent portion) in a predetermined stoichiometric ratio. Two-part epoxy adhesives usually require mixing in precise proportions to avoid a significant loss of cured properties and environmental stability. The amount of material to be mixed should be limited to the amount needed to accomplish the task. The larger the mass, the shorter the pot, or working, life of the material. The pot life is defined as the period between the time of mixing the resin and curing agent and the time at which the viscosity has increased to the point when the adhesive can no longer be successfully applied as an adhesive. To avoid potential exotherm conditions after application, excess mixed material should be removed from the container and spread out in a thin film. This prevents the risk of mass-related heat buildup and the possibility of a fire or the release of toxic fumes.

Many of the bifunctional and multifunctional resin types formulated into one-part systems are also employed in part A of the two-part systems. However, the ability to cure, or cross link, at room temperature is due to different curing agent (part B) chemistries. These are generally mixtures, to various degrees, of modified and unmodified aliphatic amines, polyamides, and modified cycloaliphatic amines. Curing of higher-temperature service two-part systems, which require an elevated-temperature cure, is usually accomplished singularly or with mixtures of aromatic and unmodified cycloaliphatic amines. A number of these materials are primary skin sensitizers, and some caution is necessary to avoid direct contact.

Some of the more reactive aliphatic amines will react with ambient water and carbon dioxide, and, if left exposed too long in the mixed condition prior to part mating, a carbonate layer may form on the adhesive surface. If this occurs, it will inhibit good substrate-to-adhesive contact and will significantly decrease mechanical properties. The opportunity for carbonate formation can be limited by avoiding high-humidity bonding conditions and mating the parts as soon as possible after adhesive application. In cases where carbonate formation cannot be avoided, covering the exposed area with polyethylene film until mating the parts will help minimize carbonate formation. Troweling the surface prior to mating can also be an effective method of disrupting any carbonate formation.

In addition to the packaging methods described for the one-part materials, meter mix equipment is available for continuous application where applicable, usually involving large areas. Mixing of the two parts can be accomplished by pumping material through either a hydraulic mixer or a static mixer. For smaller applications, dual cartridge kits, in which both part A and B are manually pushed through a static mixer, are also available for most two-part systems. Two-part adhesives can usually be stored at room temperature; however, part A may contain resins that can self-polymerize and require cold storage.

Due to their versatility, two-part resin systems are frequently used to repair damaged composite assemblies. Low-viscosity versions can be used to impregnate dry graphite cloth for repair patches or to inject into cracked bondlines or delaminations. Thicker pastes are used to bond repairs where more flow control is required. For example, if the material has too low a viscosity and is cured under high pressure, the potential for bondline starvation exists due to excessive flow and squeeze out. Viscosity control of two-part adhesives is usually done with metallic and/or nonmetallic fillers. Fumed silica is frequently added to provide slump and flow control. For more information on composite repair, see the Section "Product Reliability, Maintainability, and Repair" in this Volume.

Many adhesives are of the same resin and curing chemistry family; however, different versions are manufactured (nonfilled, metallic or nonmetallic filled, thixotroped, low density, and toughened) for specific performance requirements. For example, a nonmetallic-filled adhesive may be preferred over a metallic-filled adhesive if there is concern for possible galvanic corrosion in the joint. In thin composite structures where bending or flexing is a concern, a toughened adhesive may be warranted.

In addition to composite bonding and repair applications, two-part epoxy paste adhesives are also used for liquid shim applications during mechanical assembly operations. The ability to tailor flow, cure time, and compressive strength have made these materials ideal for use in areas of poor fit-up.

Epoxy Film Adhesives. Structural adhesives for aerospace applications are generally supplied as thin films supported on a release paper and stored under refrigerated conditions (–18 °C, or 0 °F). Film adhesives are available using high-temperature aromatic amine or catalytic curing agents with a wide range of flexibilizing and toughening agents. Rubber-toughened epoxy film adhesives are widely used in the aircraft industry. The upper temperature limit of 121 to 177 °C (250–350 °F) is usually dictated by the degree of toughening required and by the overall choice of resins and curing agents. In general, toughening of a resin results in a lower usable service temperature. Film materials are frequently supported by fibers that serve to improve handling of the films prior to cure, control adhesive flow during bonding, and assist in bondline thickness control. Fibers can be incorporated as short-fiber mats with random orientation or as woven cloth. Commonly encountered fibers are polyesters, polyamides (nylon), and glass. Adhesives containing woven cloth may have slightly degraded environmental properties because of wicking of water by the fiber. Random mat scrim cloth is not as efficient for controlling film thickness as woven cloth, because the unrestricted fibers move during bonding, although spun-bonded nonwoven scrims do not move and are therefore widely used.

Surface Preparation

Surface preparation of a material prior to bonding is the keystone upon which the adhesive bond is formed. Extensive field service experience with structural adhesive bonds has repeatedly demonstrated that adhesive durability and longevity depend on the stability and bondability of the adherent surface. Combinations of heat, moisture, and stress have been shown to be particularly effective in discriminating among the various surface preparations used in the prebond conditioning or treatment of both metallic and composite surfaces.

Although it should be understood that the satisfactory performance of the bonded joint is the primary objective, technology has made it possible to characterize in detail the chemical and physical properties of surface oxide layers on metals. Instrumental techniques—such as scanning electron microscopy and transmission electron microscopy—and surface analysis techniques—such as Auger and ion microprobe analysis—can be used to gain an intimate knowledge of the influence of surface preparation variables on the oxide that is produced. Therefore, with the availability of these powerful analytical tools, a significantly increased understanding of the required chemical and physical characteristics of a metal prebond surface can be expected.

In the past, surface treatment evaluation techniques were limited to the stressed exposure of lap shear specimens or, perhaps, hot/wet peel testing. These tests, however, did not readily discriminate among surface treatments of varying durability. A test for the discrimination of surface preparations finally became available with the development of the wedge-opening (double-cantilever beam).

In general, high-performance structural adhesive bonding requires that great care be exercised throughout the bonding process to ensure the quality of the bonded product. Chemical composition control of the polymeric adhesives; strict control of surface preparation materials and process parameters; and control of the adhesive lay-up, part fit-up, tooling, and the curing process are all required to produce, for example, airworthy structural assemblies. Of course, this is in contrast to the mechanical joining of components, which requires a lower level of cleanliness control to obtain satisfactory performance. Given this situation and the inherent advantages of adhesive bonding compared to mechanical attachment, surface preparations are required that provide optimal adhesion and maximum environmental resistance, at least for critical aerospace applications.

Great care is needed to obtain the best product possible using state-of-the-art technology to produce adhesive-bonded flight hardware, both primary and secondary structure. This usually requires the development of and strict adherence to detailed and comprehensive materials and process specifications, as well as end-item nondestructive inspection.

Composite Surface Preparation. The first consideration that occurs in preparing a composite part for secondary adhesive bonding is moisture absorption of the laminate itself. Absorbed laminate moisture can diffuse to the surface of the laminate during elevated-temperature cure cycles, resulting in weak bonds or porosity or voids in the adhesive bondline and, in extreme cases where fast heat-up rates are used, actual delaminations within the composite laminate plies. If honeycomb is used in the structure, moisture can turn to steam resulting in node bond failures or blown core. Relatively thin composite laminates (3.17 mm, or 0.125 in., or less in thickness) may by effectively dried in an air-circulating oven at 121 °C (250 °F) for 4 h minimum. Drying cycles for thicker laminates should be developed empirically using the actual adherend thicknesses. After drying, the surface should be prepared for bonding and then the actual bonding operation conducted as soon as possible. It should be noted that prebond thermal cycles, such as verifilm cycles to check for part fit-up prior to actual bonding, can serve as effective drying cycles. In addition, storage of dried details in a temperature- and humidity-controlled lay-up room can extend the time between drying and curing.

Numerous surface-preparation techniques are currently used prior to the adhesive bonding of composites. The success of any technique depends on establishing comprehensive material, process, and quality-control specifications and adhering to them strictly. One method that has gained wide acceptance is the use of a peel ply. In this technique, a closely woven nylon or polyester cloth is used as the outer layer of the composite during lay-up; this ply is torn or peeled away just before bonding or painting. The theory is that the tearing or peeling process fractures the resin-matrix coating and exposes a clean, virgin, roughened surface for the bonding process. The surface roughness attained can, to some extent, be determined by the weave characteristics of the peel ply. Some manufacturers advocate that this is sufficient, while others maintain that an additional hand sanding or light grit blasting is required to prepare the surface adequately. Abrasion increases the surface energy of the surfaces to be bonded and removes any residual contamination, while surface roughening increases the bond area and mechanical interlocking. The abrading operation should be conducted with care, however, to avoid exposing or rupturing the reinforcing fibers of the surface.

The use of peel plies on composite surfaces to be structurally bonded certainly deserves careful consideration. Factors that need to be considered include: the chemical makeup of the peel ply (e.g., nylon versus polyester) as well as its compatibility with the composite-matrix resin, the surface treatment used on the peel ply (e.g., silicone coatings that make the peel ply easier to remove also leave residues that inhibit structural bonding), and the final surface preparation (e.g., hand sanding versus light grit blasting) employed. The reader is referred to Ref 3 and 4 for a more in-depth analysis of the potential pitfalls of using peel plies on surfaces to be bonded. The authors of Ref 3 and 4 maintain that the only truly effective method of surface preparation is a light grit blast after peel ply removal. Nevertheless, peel plies are very effective at preventing gross surface contamination that could occur between laminate fabrication and secondary bonding.

A typical cleaning sequence would be to remove the peel ply and then lightly abrade the surface with a dry grit blast at approximately 138 kPa (20 psi). After grit blasting, any remaining residue on the surface may be removed by dry vacuuming or wiping with a clean, dry cheesecloth. Although hand sanding with 120 to 240 grit silicon carbide paper can be substituted for grit blasting, hand sanding is not as effective as grit blasting in reaching all of the impressions left by the weave of the peel ply on the composite surface. In addition, the potential for removing too much resin and exposing the carbon fibers is actually higher for hand sanding than it is for grit blasting.

If it is not possible to use a peel ply on a surface requiring adhesive bonding, the surface may be precleaned (prior to surface abrasion) with a solvent such as methyl ethyl ketone (MEK) to remove any gross organic contaminants. In cases where a peel ply is not used, some type of light abrasion is required to break the glazed finish on the matrix resin surface. The use of solvents to remove residue after hand sanding or grit blasting is discouraged due to the potential of recontaminating the surface.

Another method can be used to avoid abrasion damage to fibers. When the graphite composite is first laid up, a ply of adhesive is placed on the surface where the secondary bond is to take place. This adhesive is then cured together with the laminate. To prepare for the secondary bond, the surface of this adhesive ply is abraded with minimal chance of fiber damage; however, this sacrificial adhesive ply adds weight to the structure.

Surface-conditioning techniques can be automated for use in high-production situations. All surface treatments should have the following principles in common. The surface should be thoroughly cleaned prior to abrasion to avoid smearing contamination into the surface. The glaze on the matrix surface should be roughened without damaging the reinforcing fibers or forming subsurface cracks in the resin matrix. Any residue should be removed from the abraded surface. The prepared surface should be bonded as soon as possible.

Metal Surface Preparation. The following surface preparations are used for various metals to be bonded to the cured composite. Although seemingly adequate bond strength can often be obtained with rather simple surface treatments (e.g., surface abrasion or sanding of aluminum adherends), long-term durable bonds under actual service environments can suffer significantly if the metal adherend has not been processed using the proper chemical surface preparation.

Several methods are used with titanium. Any method developed for titanium should undergo a thorough test program prior to production implementation and then must be monitored closely during production usage. A typical process used in the aerospace industry involves:

1. Solvent wiping to remove all grease and oils
2. Liquid honing at 275 to 345 kPa (40–50 psi) pressure
3. Alkaline cleaning in an air agitated solution maintained at 93 to 100 °C (200–212 °F) for 20 to 30 min
4. Thoroughly rinsing in tap water for 3 to 4 min
5. Etching for 15 to 20 min in a nitric-hydrofluoric acid solution maintained at a temperature below 38 °C (100 °F)
6. Thoroughly rinsing in tap water for 3 to 4 min followed by rinsing in deionized water for 2 to 4 min
7. Inspecting for a water-break-free surface
8. Oven drying at 38 to 77 °C (100–170 °F) for 30 min minimum
9. Adhesive bonding or applying primer within 8 h of cleaning

The combination of liquid honing, alkaline cleaning, and acid etching results in a complex chemically activated surface topography containing a large amount of surface area for the adhesive to penetrate and adhere. The adhesive bond strength is a result of both mechanical interlocking and chemical bonding.

Another method used to prepare the surface of titanium for bonding, called dry chromic acid anodizing, involves:

1. Degreasing using solvent-wipe (acetone or MEK may be used) if the metal surface is contaminated with oil or grease
2. Soaking/cleaning metal parts in alkaline cleaner bath until a water-break-free surface is obtained (10–15 min)
3. Rinsing with hot water (>43 °C, or 110 °F) for 5 min.
4. Etching in a nitric-hydrofluoric acid bath for 1.5 min
5. Rinsing with cold water for at least 5 min
6. Anodizing in a chromic acid bath for 20 min at 5 V potential, with a current density of 13.45A/m^2 (1.25 amp/ft^2)
7. Rinsing with cold water for at least 5 min.
8. Drying using hot air (66 °C, or 150 °F)

Several different methods are also used to prepare aluminum alloys for adhesive bonding. Forest Products Laboratory (FPL) etching is a chromic sulfuric acid etch, and its procedure is found in ASTM D 2651. It is perhaps the earliest method developed for preparing aluminum for bonding. Chromic acid anodizing is a later method and is perhaps more widely used than the FPL etch. Different manufacturers use minor variations of this method, usually in the sealing steps after anodizing. Phosphoric acid anodize (PAA) is the most recent of the well-established procedures and has an excellent service record for environmental durability. It also has the advantage of being very forgiving of minor variations in procedure. A detailed procedure of this surface preparation can be found in ASTM D 3933.

Because metallic cleaning is such a critical step, dedicated processing lines are normally constructed, and chemical controls, as well as periodic lap shear cleaning control specimens, are employed to ensure in-process control. Automated overhead conveyances are used to transport the parts from tank to tank under computer-controlled cycles to ensure the proper processing time in each tank.

Due to the rapid formation of surface oxides on both titanium and aluminum, the surfaces should be bonded within 8 h of cleaning or primed with a thin protective coat of epoxy primer. For parts that will undergo a severe service environment, priming is always recommended because today's primers contain corrosion-inhibiting compounds that enhance long-term durability. Once the primer has been cured, the parts may be stored in an environmentally controlled clean room for quite long periods of time (e.g., up to 50 days or longer would not be unusual). All cleaned and primed parts should be carefully protected during handling or storage to prevent surface contamination. Normally, clean white cotton gloves are used during handling, and wax-free Kraft paper may be used for wrapping and longer storage.

Sandwich Structures

Sandwich construction has been used extensively in the aerospace industry because it is an extremely lightweight structure that exhibits high stiffness and strength-to-weight ratios. A typical sandwich structure consists of two thin, high-strength facings bonded to a thick, lightweight core. Each component by itself is relatively weak and flexible, but when combined into a sandwich panel they produce a structure that is stiff, strong, and lightweight. A honeycomb sandwich panel, formed by adhesively bonding thin skins to honeycomb core, is shown in Fig. 11.

The basic concept of a sandwich panel is that the facings carry the bending loads and the honeycomb core carries the shear loads. In most cases, the facing stresses are uniformly distributed. Facing materials that are normally used are aluminum, fiberglass, graphite, and aramid. Typical aerospace structure has relatively thin facing sheets (0.25–3.17 mm, or 0.010–0.125 in.) with core densities in the range of 61 to 128 kg/m^3 (3.8–8.0 lb/ft^3).

Supported film adhesives are normally used to bond composite structural honeycomb assemblies. The primary considerations for selecting an adhesive system are strength requirements, service temperature range, and ability to form a fillet at the cell wall ends. Sandwich panels are typically used for their structural, electrical, and energy absorption characteristics, or a combination thereof.

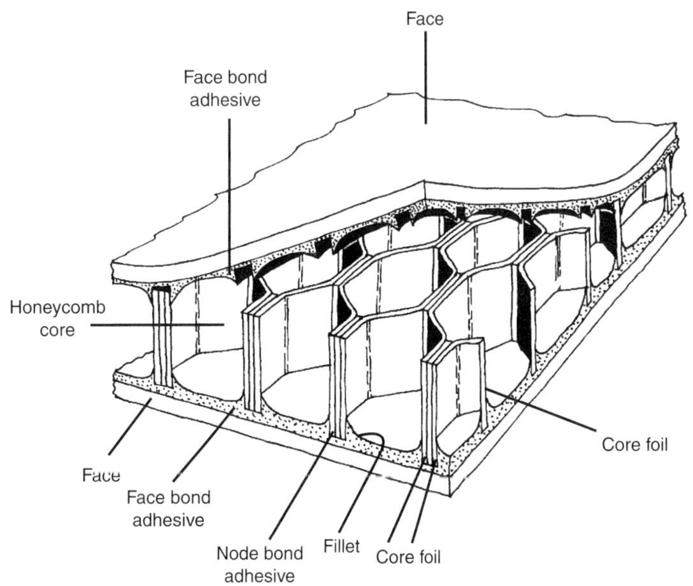

Fig. 11 Components of a honeycomb panel

Honeycomb Core

Most honeycomb used today is adhesively bonded aluminum hexagonal-cell honeycomb core that is subsequently bonded to facings to form a sandwich panel. The most common nonmetallic core materials are Nomex or Korex (aramid), fiberglass, or graphite. Nonmetallic core is normally dipped in liquid phenolic, polyester, or polyimide resin to achieve the final density, although other resin systems can be used. There are three basic cell configurations: hexagonal, overexpanded, and flexible. For a more in-depth discussion of honeycomb core and its properties, refer to the article "Lightweight Structural Cores" in this Volume.

Aluminum honeycomb assemblies have experienced serious in-service durability problems, the most severe being moisture migrating inside the assemblies and causing corrosion of the aluminum core cells. Honeycomb suppliers have responded by producing corrosion-inhibiting coatings that have improved durability. A typical corrosion-inhibiting arrangement is shown in Fig. 12. The core foil is first anodized with phosphoric acid and then coated with a corrosion-inhibiting primer. However, corrosion can still be a serious issue with aluminum honeycomb assemblies, and proper sealing methods are imperative. It should also be noted that the freeze/thaw cycles encountered during a typical aircraft flight can cause skin-to-core delaminations if liquid water is present in the honeycomb cells.

Honeycomb Processing

Honeycomb processing before adhesive bonding includes: perimeter trimming, mechanical forming, heat forming, core splicing, contouring, and cleaning.

Trimming. The four primary tools used to cut honeycomb to plan dimensions are serrated knife, razor blade knife, band saw, and a die. The serrated and razor edge knives and die cutter are used on light-density cores; white heavy-density cores and complex-shaped cores are usually cut with a band saw.

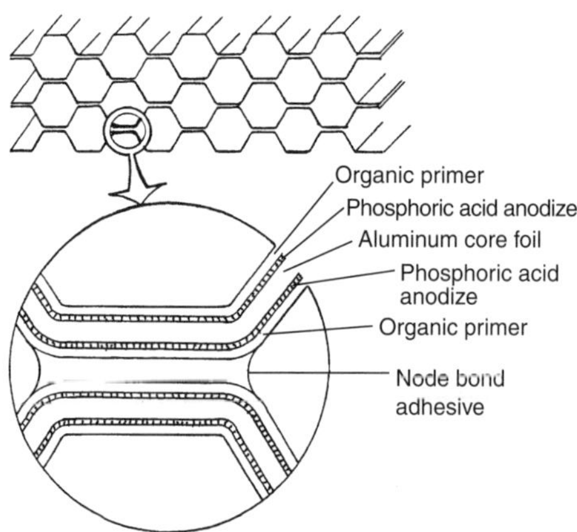

Fig. 12 Corrosion-resistant honeycomb core

Forming. Metallic, hexagonal honeycomb can be roll- or brake-formed into curved pans. The brake-forming method will crush the cell walls and densify the inner radius. Overexpanded honeycomb can be formed to a cylindrical shape on assembly. Flexcore usually can be shaped to compound curvatures on assembly.

Nonmetallic honeycomb can be heat formed to obtain curved parts. Usually the core slice is placed in an oven at high temperature for a short period of time. The heat softens the resin and allows the cell walls to deform more easily. Upon removal from the oven, the core is quickly placed on a shaped tool and held there until it cools.

Splicing. When large pieces of core are required, or when complex shapes dictate, smaller pieces can be spliced together to form the finished part. This is usually accomplished with a foaming adhesive, as shown in Fig. 13. Core splice adhesives normally contain blowing agents that produce gases (e.g., nitrogen) during heat-up to provide the expansion necessary to fill the gaps between the core sections. Different core types, cell sizes, or densities can be easily interconnected in this manner.

Machining. In many sandwich panel applications, such as air foils, honeycomb must have its thickness machined to some contour (Fig. 14). This is normally accomplished using valve-stem-type cutters on expanded core. Occasionally, the solid honeycomb block is machined using milling cutters. Typical machines used for contour machining (carving) are gantry, apex, three-dimensional tracer, or numerically controlled (NC) five-axis. With five-axis NC machining, the cutting head is controlled by computer programs, and almost any surface that can be described by x, y, and z coordinates can be produced. These machines can carve honeycomb at speeds of up to 1.27 m/s (50 in./s) with extreme accuracy. A standard contour tolerance of an NC machine is ± 0.13 mm (± 0.005 in.).

Cleaning and Drying. It is preferable to keep honeycomb core clean during all manufacturing operations prior to adhesive bonding; however, aluminum honeycomb core can be effectively cleaned by solvent vapor degreasing. Nonmetallic core, such as Nomex or Korex (aramid), fiberglass, and graphite core, readily absorbs moisture from the atmosphere. Similar to composite skins, nonmetallic core sections should be thoroughly dried prior to adhesive bonding. A further complication is that since the cell walls are relatively thin and contain a lot of surface area, they can reabsorb moisture rather rapidly after drying.

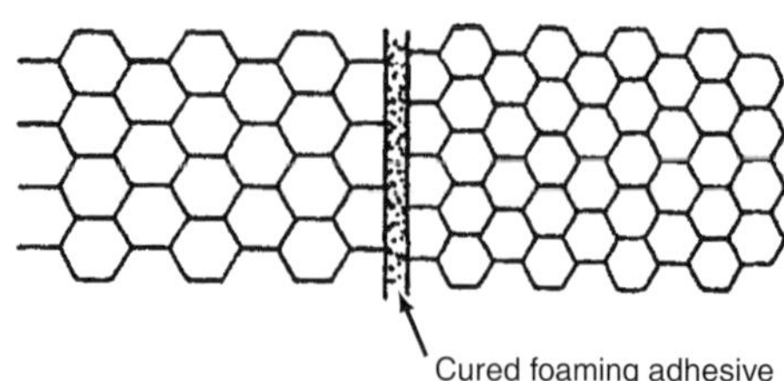

Fig. 13 Core splicing

Syntactic Core

Syntactic core is sometimes used as an alternate to honeycomb core. Syntactic core consists of a matrix (e.g., epoxy) that is filled with hollow spheres (e.g., glass or ceramic microballons). Syntactic cores are generally much higher in density than honeycomb, with densities in the range of 482 to 1284 kg/m^3 (30–80 lb/ft^3). They are used to make sandwich panels over a wide thickness range, including much thinner than is practical for honeycomb. They can also be used as fillers in honeycomb to increase local compression strength and as edge stiffening prior to machining core. When cured against precured composite details, syntactics do not need an adhesive. However, if the syntactic core is already cured and requires adhesive bonding, it should be scuff sanded and then cured with a layer of adhesive.

Foam Core

A third type of core material frequently used in adhesively bonded structure is foam core. The material is usually supplied in block form that is easily cut or machined to shape. Sections may be bonded together using either two-part paste adhesives or adhesive films. Both open- and closed-cell materials are available; however, closed-cell materials are normally used for bonded structure. Sections can also be heat formed to contour using procedures similar to those for nonmetallic honeycomb core. Core densities normally range from about 48 to 642 kg/m^3 (3–40 lb/ft^3). A wide range of materials is available made from resins such as polymethylacrylimide, polyvinyl chloride, polyurethane, and polyisocyanurate. Depending on their chemistry, these core materials can be used in the temperature range of 66 to 204 °C (150–400 °F).

Adhesive-Bonding Process

The basic steps in the adhesive-bonding process are:

1. Collection of all the parts in the bonded assembly, which are then stored as kits

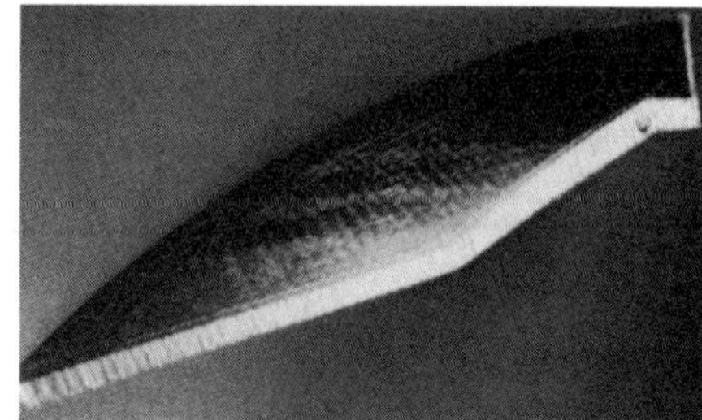

Fig. 14 Machined honeycomb parts

2. Verification of the fit-to-bondline tolerances
3. Cleaning of the parts to promote good adhesion
4. Application of the adhesive
5. Mating of the parts and adhesive to form the assembly
6. Application of a force to produce a good fit
7. Application of force concurrent with application of heat to the adhesive to promote a chemical reaction, if needed
8. Inspection of the bonded assembly

Prekitting of Adherends. Many adhesives have a limited working life at room temperature, and adherends, especially metals, are contaminated by exposure to the environment. Thus, it is normal practice to kit the adherends so that application of the adhesive and buildup of the bonded assemblies can proceed without interruption. The kitting sequence is determined by the product and production rate.

Bondline Thickness Control. Controlling the thickness of the adhesive bondline is a critical factor in bond strength. This control can be obtained by matching the quantity of available adhesive to the size of the gap between the mating surfaces under actual bonding conditions (heat and pressure). Higher applied loads during bonding tend to reduce bondline thickness. A slight overfill is usually desired to ensure that the gap is totally filled. Conversely, if all the adhesive is squeezed out of a local area due to a high spot in one of the adherends, a disbond can result.

Fortunately, most bonds do not require optimal strength and can tolerate some local disbonds. For these bonds, an attempt should be made to produce faying parts to a tolerance of 0.8 mm (0.03 in.), and enough adhesive should be applied to fill the gap. The use of excess adhesive adds weight and unnecessary material cost: it also increases cleanup costs. However, these negative factors must be tolerated in order to avoid disbonds during service.

Some of the most critical structural bond applications are found in highly loaded aircraft structures. For these applications, the adhesive used is in the form of a calendered film with a thin fabric layer. The fabric maintains the bondline thickness by preventing contact between the adherends. In addition, the carrier acts as a corrosion barrier between graphite skins and aluminum honeycomb core. Voids are not usually permitted. In the most common case, the bondline can vary from 50 to 230 μm (2–9 mils). Extra adhesive can be used to handle up to 510 μm (20 mils) gaps. Larger gaps must be accommodated by reworking the metal parts; tolerances are achieved by reworking of the various details so that they fit as required.

Prefit Evaluation. A prefit-checking fixture is often used in high-precision bonding. This fixture simulates the bond by locating the various parts in the exact relationship to one another as they will appear in the actual bonded assembly (see Fig. 15). For high-value assemblies, a verifilm operation is frequently conducted. The bondline thickness is simulated by placing a vinyl plastic film or the actual adhesive encased in plastic film in the bondlines. The assembly is then subjected to the heat and pressure normally used to chemically react the epoxy adhesive to form the bond. The parts are disassembled, and the vinyl film or cured adhesive is then visually or dimensionally evaluated to see what corrections are required. These corrections can include sanding the parts to provide more clearance, reforming metal parts to close the gaps, or applying additional adhesive (within permissible limits) to particular locations in the bond.

Verification of bondline thickness may not be required for all applications. However, the technique can be used to validate the fit of the mating parts prior to the start of production or to determine why large voids are produced in repetitive parts. When using paste adhesives, the adhesive thickness can be simulated by encasing the adhesive in plastic film (as mentioned previously) or aluminum foil. Once the fit of mating parts has been evaluated, the necessary corrections can be made. For cases in which the component parts can be dimensionally corrected, it is much more efficient to make the correction than risk having to scrap the parts or having them fail in service.

Adhesive Application

The application of adhesives and the accuracy of the application have a major impact on cost and quality. Enough adhesive must be applied to form an acceptable joint, but any excess represents wasted material. The labor and equipment costs should also be kept to a minimum. The method of application is a function of the physical form of the adhesive. The choice of method is also influenced by the volume and sophistication of the work.

The most commonly used adhesives are supplied as liquids, pastes, or prefabricated films. The liquid and paste systems may be supplied as one- or two-part systems. The two-part systems must be mixed before use and thus require scales and a mixer. The amount of material to be mixed should be limited to the amount needed to accomplish the task. The larger the mass, the shorter the pot or working life of the mixed adhesive. To prevent potential exotherm conditions after application, excess mixed material should be removed from the container and spread out in a thin film. This will prevent the risk of mass-related heat buildup and the possibility of a fire or the release of toxic fumes.

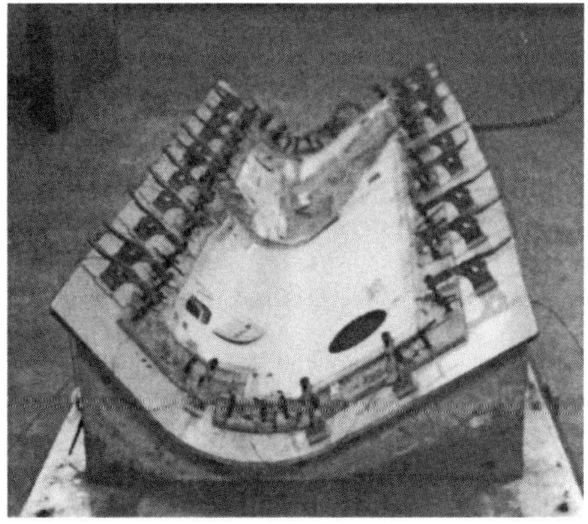

Fig. 15 Prefit fixture used for a complex-contour aircraft door

The storage facility plays a vital role in a production bonding operation. Many one-part adhesives and film adhesives must be stored at temperatures below ambient. Adhesives containing organic solvents must be segregated to reduce the risk of fire, and others containing polymers and solvents must be shaken periodically to prevent settling or gelation.

One factor that must be considered in adhesive application is the time interval available between adhesive preparation and final assembly of the adherend. This factor, which is referred to as pot, open, out-time, or working life, must be matched to the production rate. Obviously, materials that are ready to bond quickly are needed for high-rate applications, such as those found in the automotive and appliance industries. It should be noted that many two-part systems that cure by chemical reaction often have a limited working life before they become too viscous to apply.

Application of liquid adhesives can be accomplished using brushes, rollers, manual sprays, or robotically controlled sprays. A robot (Fig. 16) can apply tightly controlled quantities of adhesive to specific areas. Solvated two-part systems are sprayed using equipment with two pumps; preset quantities of each component are pumped through the spray head where they are blended into a single stream. Of course, many plants use several different application systems simultaneously for their various job shop requirements.

Application of paste adhesives can be accomplished by brush, by spreading with a grooved tool, or by extrusion from cartridges or sealed containers using compressed air. For the latter, the combination of the orifice diameter and the applied pressure controls the size of the bead applied to the work. Robots can move the application head in a constant path at a repetitive surface speed to enhance the accuracy of bead placement and size. The use of robots to apply paste adhesive is analogous to their use to locate

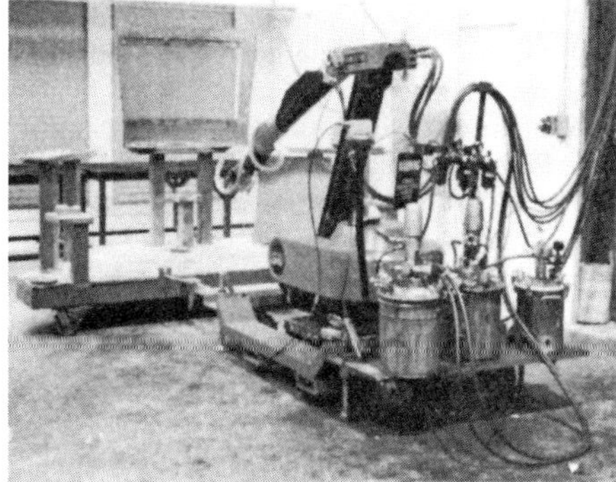

Fig. 16 Robot used for spraying adhesive

spot welds. In the automotive industry, several vans with plastic skins bonded to a steel structural frame are assembled using paste adhesives applied by robots.

Film adhesives are costly and thus are used mainly in aircraft applications. They consist of an epoxy, bismaleimide, or polyimide resin film and a fabric carrier. The fabric guarantees a bondline because it prevents contact of the adherends. These adhesives are manually cut to size, usually with knives, and placed in the bondlines.

Tooling

Adherends must be in the specified relationship to one another during bond formation. Slippage of one of the constituents of the bonded assembly will result in a need for costly reworking, or the entire assembly might be scrapped. When a paste or liquid adhesive is used, it is usually helpful to have a load applied to the joint to deform the adhesive to fill the bondline. In applications such as aircraft parts, higher pressures are used to force the adherends to fit to within small tolerances. The adhesives used in high-pressure bonding typically do not have a high flow; they contain a thin scrim fabric to ensure that a bondline is maintained. Fixtures can be used to maintain part alignment, or fixtureless concepts can be used in which some other method provides the required alignment.

Fixtures. Bonding fixtures can represent a large investment in tooling and have a significant impact on cost. Every time they are used, they must be loaded with parts, unloaded, cleaned, and maintained. Fixtures can be used for both high- and low-rate production. A bonding fixture contains several basic elements:

- A tooling surface matching the contour of the bonded panel (face sheet)
- A series of jig points, side rails, and pressure blocks as needed
- A support structure to prevent warpage of the face sheet for contoured tools
- A dolly or removable wheels to permit moving the fixture if needed

Press-Bonding Fixtures. Many flat panels are bonded in press-bonding fixtures. The face sheet of the fixture is flat, and the alignment rails are usually thinner than the thickness of the structural panel. For very thin panels, the rails may be higher than the panel to ensure that alignment is maintained. In this type of fixture, a pressure plate is used to take up the space between the panel and the top of the rails. The pressure plate fits within the alignment rails (see Fig. 17). Often, press-bonding tools are made to standard thickness so that several tools can be placed in the press cavity at the same time.

Pressure Bag Fixtures. Parts with significant contour must be bonded using a pressure bag process, because the thickness of the tooling needed for the parallel flat surfaces of press-bonding fixtures is excessive for these parts. Also, the extra thickness causes problems with thermal uniformity, tool cost, and handling.

In the pressure bag process, a plastic-film bag, usually a modified nylon for temperatures up to 190 °C (375 °F), is attached to the face sheet of the tool and sealed in place. The air under the bag is evacuated by a vacuum pump to produce a pressure of 96 kPa (14 psi). The heat required to chemically react the adhesive is provided by an oven. If higher pressure is needed, the tool is placed in a heated pressure vessel called an autoclave. The additional pressure required to obtain a good bond is obtained by pressurized air or an inert gas. As the pressure is applied, the vacuum under the bag is vented to prevent damage to the honeycomb assembly from entrapped vacuum.

Additional vacuum ports must be provided to evacuate the vacuum bag. Typically, two holes are drilled in the face sheet and tapped with pipe thread. A pipe sealed with Teflon tape is mounted in each hole. Quick-disconnect fittings and hoses are used to connect the tool to the vacuum systems in the oven or autoclave. One port is used to apply vacuum, and the second is connected to a recorder that monitors the pressure under the bag.

The rails are pinned to the face sheet so that they stay in place despite the side loads produced by the applied pressure. If the rails were to move, damage to the panel would result.

Panels with straight edges can be bonded using only the edge rails. However, many panels have one skin that projects beyond the core and second skin. Usually, the central core is enclosed by Z-shape members that are bonded to both the larger external skin and the smaller internal skin. The bonding fixture for these panels is configured to place the larger skin next to the face sheet of the tool. The rails surround the larger skin. The space between the rail and the vertical edge of the Z-shape member is filled with removable pressure blocks. Wedges are placed between the side rails and pressure blocks to force the blocks inward to ensure good contact with the Z-shape member. Blocks are also required when a space is needed between the skins for attachment of a fitting (see Fig. 18).

Pressure bag fixtures (Fig. 19) are more complex than press-bonding fixtures. These fixtures are fitted with a base to support the tooling surface in the proper contour. The base must contain provisions for moving the tools, such as removable wheels or hoist points for lifting the tool on the dolly or platens for positioning the tool in the autoclave (Fig. 20) or an oven. Flat tables are often used because they can accept tools of any configuration, provided there are several flat areas in the tool base. To prevent warpage, the base must be configured to maximize airflow under the face sheet.

Fixture Design. Several secondary rules apply to the design of a successful bonding fixture:

- The tooling surface must be precisely machined to the desired contour so that the skin fits well into the cavity produced by the face sheet and the rails.
- The face sheet must be free of nicks and gouges that could damage the skin.
- The side rails must be easily detachable from the face sheet; this can be accomplished by using pins or screws to attach the rails.
- The bonding fixture should be coated with Teflon to prevent adhesion before the tool is used for the first time.
- Mold release or fluorocarbon film must be applied before each use to prevent sticking of the blocks to the adhesive squeeze-out.

Including tapped, threaded holes in the bonding blocks to permit the use of a "T" wrench will simplify block removal. Also, jig points, locating blocks, or precisely located alignment pins must be provided for each major solid detail located within the honeycomb. These devices ensure that the parts are always in the same location

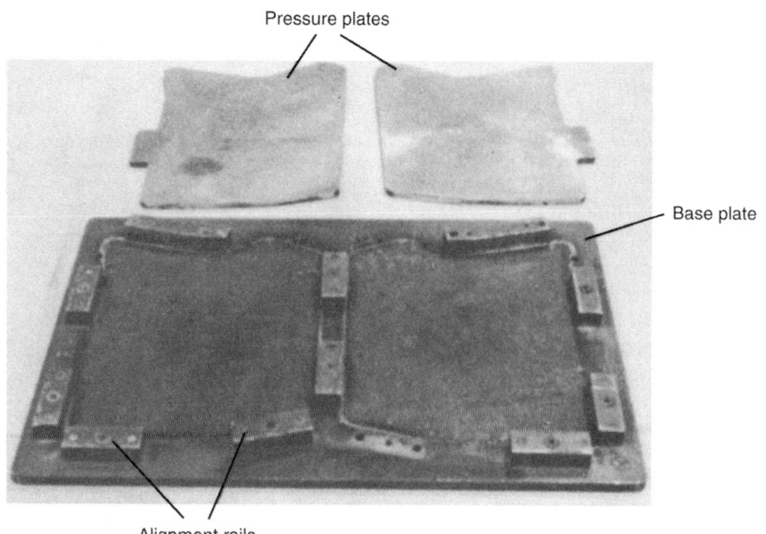

Fig. 17 Press-bonding fixture

so that the prefit operation performed before the panel is disassembled for cleaning will be valid for the panel when it is reassembled with adhesive after cleaning.

The coefficient of thermal expansion of the face sheet of the fixture and that of the panel skins should match so that the relative position of the tooling and skins is maintained during elevated-temperature curing of the adhesive. This is especially important for a sandwich structure. Both bonds of such a structure should be formed by chemical reaction within a narrow temperature range. As soon as one skin is bonded to the core, the relative positions of these bond constituents are locked in. As the assembly is heated further, the skins and core continue to expand thermally until the second skin is bonded. Because the second skin has expanded more than the first skin prior to bond formation, the panel has thermally induced warpage when cooled to ambient.

The solution to this problem is to use a fixture of minimum mass and provide a uniform flow of heated air above and below the tool surface. Typically, aluminum panels are bonded in aluminum fixtures and composite panels are bonded on composite, steel, or Invar fixtures. Composite tools for composite parts have the closest match in thermal expansion; however, composite tools are not as durable as metal tools for large production runs. Therefore, Invar or steel fixtures can be used to replace composite fixtures because the coefficients of thermal expansion of the two materials are closely matched; electroformed nickel tools are the next best choice.

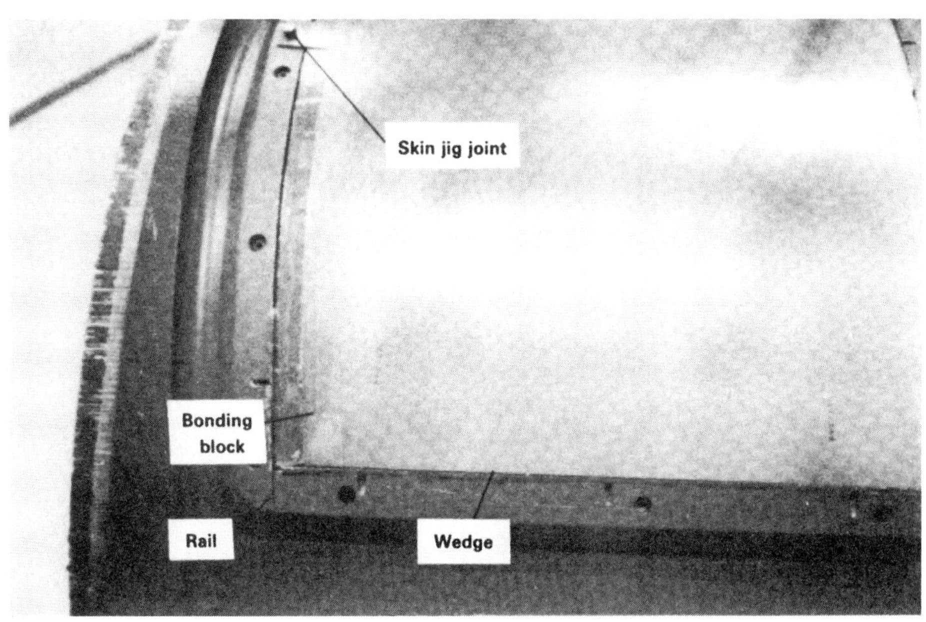

Fig. 18 Detail of a pressure bag bonding fixture

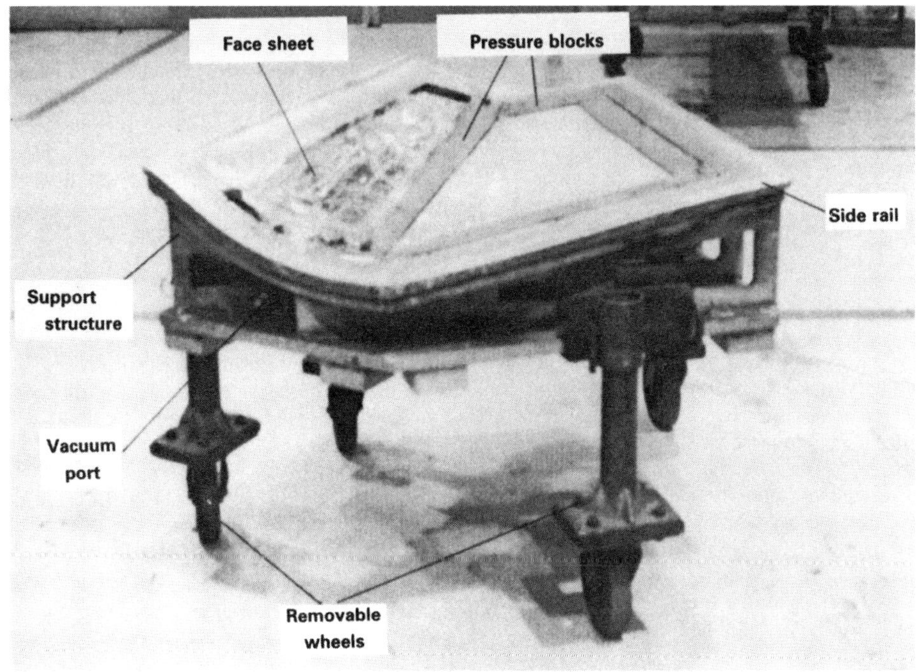

Fig. 19 Autoclave bonding fixture

Because the fixtures for large panels are heavy, handling equipment is required in a production bonding area. Cranes or forklifts are needed, and the tools must be fitted with the proper hoist points. Because the tools must be moved from the clean room (where the adhesive is applied to the individual parts) to the curing equipment, dollies or removable wheels must be provided. Some fabricators use permanently attached steel wheels to move the tools. If large platens are used, steel tracks in the floor and steel wheels on the platen are needed to move the plate in and out of the curing equipment.

Fixtureless Bonding. Alternatives to the use of fixtures are desirable for both high- and low-rate production. One method involves using the fully assembled part as the fixture, as in the case of some metallic automotive panels. Once the adhesive is applied to the edge of the internal skin and the external skin is folded over, the skins are locked into position and cannot move relative to each other. Another example is the various forms of insert bonding used to assemble electronic connectors and circuit boards.

Another fixtureless method for maintaining alignment of the adherends during bonding involves drilling precision alignment holes in the workpiece, applying the adhesive, and installing temporary fasteners. The fasteners are coated with mold release to prevent them from bonding to the assembly. The fasteners also apply force to the joint to produce adhesive flow. However, excessive clamp-up force with temporary fasteners can result in resin-starved bondlines in the vicinity of the fastener. A similar concept is used to mate the decks and hulls of small fiberglass boats. After bonding, the alignment holes are often enlarged to receive structural fasteners.

Pressure Applicators. A common approach for applying bonding pressure involves using clamping devices, such as C-clamps or woodworker's clamps, to hold the adherends in place. A fiberglass panel bonded with C-clamps is shown in Fig. 21.

Spring-loaded clamps that are similar to old-fashioned laundry clamps are also used for certain bonding applications because they can be installed and removed rapidly. One patented type of clamp has one movable surface and one fixed surface; the adjustable clamps are permanently attached to a base, and the movable jaws open and close as required. In high-rate production, pneumatically actuated clamps are used to accelerate the loading of parts or the removal of the assembly from the fixture.

Mechanical screw jacks can also be used to apply load and align adherends. For example,

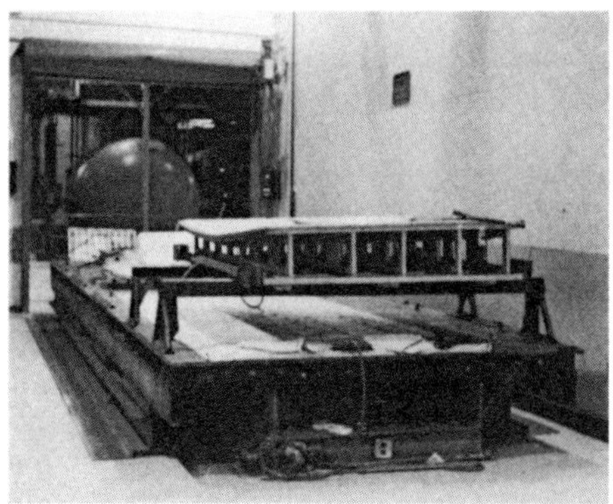

Fig. 20 Flat and contoured bonding fixtures mounted on a platen

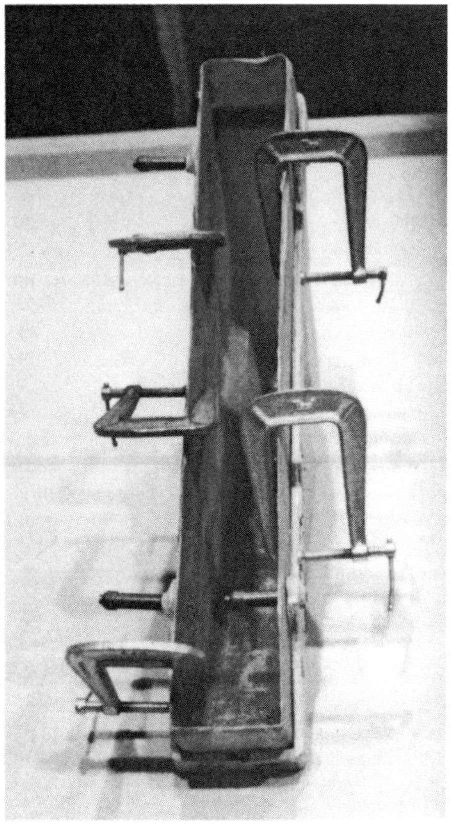

Fig. 21 Fiberglass assembly bonded using clamps and temporary fasteners

blocks of honeycomb material are often spliced in the vertical direction with a foaming adhesive that expands to fill the space between mating blocks. The operation is done in a fixture that defines the horizontal surface of the assembly. Pressure plates, strong backs, and screw jacks are used to push the core blocks toward the horizontal surface as the adhesive is cured in an oven (see Fig. 22).

Curing Equipment. Various types of curing equipment are used for adhesives requiring heat for polymerization. Conventional ovens and full or partial vacuum are used for lightweight assemblies with thin skins. A variation of this concept is used in the automotive industry: heated tunnels concurrently cure adhesives and exterior paint in automobile bodies. Multicavity platen presses (Fig. 23) are used to bond flat panels under heat and pressure. In the aircraft industry, most panels have a complex geometry and are bonded by the pressure bag technique. The bond may occur in an oven or an autoclave.

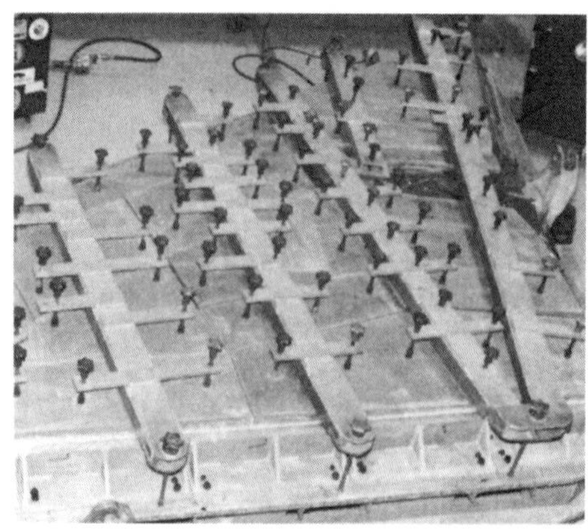

Fig. 22 Honeycomb splicing fixture using screw jacks to apply load

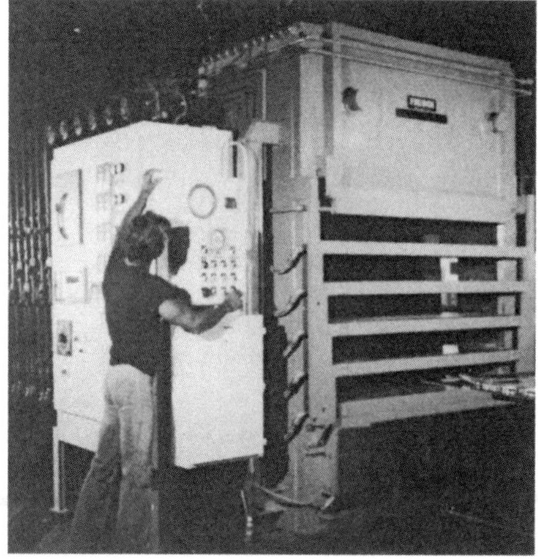

Fig. 23 Flat-panel bonding press. Courtesy of M.C. Gill Corporation

Inspection

Adhesively bonded joints and assemblies are normally nondestructively inspected after all bonding operations are completed. Radiographic and ultrasonic inspection methods are typically used to look for defects in both the bondlines and the honeycomb core portions of the assemblies. For a description of these test methods, as well as others, refer to the Section "Quality Assurance" in this Volume. In addition to these methods, it is quite common practice to leak check honeycomb-bonded assemblies by immersing the assembly for a short time in a tank of hot water (e.g., 66 °C, or 150 °F). The hot water heats the residual air inside the honeycomb core, and any leaks can be detected by air bubbles escaping from the assembly.

ACKNOWLEDGMENTS

A major portion of this article is derived from *Composites,* Vol 1 of the *Engineered Materials Handbook,* specifically "Adhesives Selection" by John Williams, Naval Air Development Center, and Weldon Scardino, Air Force Wright Aeronautical Laboratories; "Adhesive Bonding Surface Preparation" by Theodore J. Reinhart, Air Force Wright Aeronautical Laboratories; and "Honeycomb Structure" by John Corden, Hexel Corporation, Structural Products Division, and from *Adhesives and Sealants,* Vol 3 of the *Engineered Materials Handbook,* specifically "Adhesive Bonding Preparation, Application, and Tooling" by Hans J. Borstell and Valerie Wheeler, Grumman Aircraft. Sid Quick of Dexter Adhesives & Coating Systems supplied a significant amount of material on epoxy adhesives. Finally, Raymond B. Krieger Jr. of Cytec Fiberite Inc. contributed the section "Highly Loaded Joint Considerations" and material on surface preparation.

REFERENCES

1. KGR-1 Extensometer Operating Manual, Cytec Fiberite Inc., Havre de Grace, Maryland, 1978
2. R.B. Krieger, Evaluating Structural Adhesives under Sustained Load in Hostile Environment, *SAMPE Conference,* Oct 1973, Society of Material and Process Engineers
3. L.J. Hart-Smith, D. Brown, and S. Wong, Surface Preparations for Ensuring that the Glue Will Stick in Bonded Composite Structures, *10th DOD/NASA/FAA Conference on Fibrous Composites in Structural Design,* 1–4 Nov 1993 (Hilton Head Island, SC)
4. L.J. Hart-Smith, G. Redmond, and M.J. Davis, The Curse of the Nylon Peel Ply, *41st SAMPE International Symposium and Exhibition,* 25–28 March 1996 (Anaheim, CA), Society of Material and Process Engineers

SELECTED REFERENCES

- A.J. Kinlock, *Adhesion and Adhesives: Science and Technology,* Chapman & Hall, 1987
- A.V. Pocius, *Adhesion and Adhesives Technology,* Hansen Gardner, 1996
- *Adhesives and Sealants,* Vol 3, *Engineered Materials Handbook,* ASM International, 1990
- D.J. Damico, T.L. Wilkinson, and S.L. Niks, "Composites Bonding," STP 1227, ASTM, 1994
- L.-H. Lee, *Fundamentals of Adhesion,* Plenum, 1991
- E.M. Petrie, *Handbook of Adhesives and Sealants,* McGraw Hill, 1999
- B. Hussey and J. Wilson, *Structural Adhesives Directory and Databook,* Chapman & Hall, 1996

Processing and Joining of Thermoplastic Composites

Douglas A. McCarville and Henry A. Schaefer, Boeing Military Aircraft & Missile Systems

THE SPORTING GOODS, medical, automotive, chemical, and aerospace industries have applications that require materials with good combinations of impact resistance, fracture toughness, and elevated temperature endurance. Advanced thermoplastic composites (ATPCs)—meltable engineering resin/fiber mixes typically containing approximately 60 vol% continuous carbon, glass, quartz, and so on—possess these properties, and because of their melt-fusible nature, lend themselves to low-cost rapid thermoforming and joining methods.

Economic Considerations

In an effort to meet requirements on future aircraft such as the F-22 Raptor, X-33 Reusable Launch Vehicle, V-22 Osprey, and Joint Strike Fighter, the aerospace industry has been the primary driver for advanced high strength composite product forms (Ref 1, 2). Emphasis on weight minimization as a means of enhancing aircraft performance and reducing life cycle cost has pushed the use of composites in lieu of heavier, but in general, lower manufacturing cost, metals. Automated processes such as pultrusion, fiber placement, filament winding, and contoured tape laying have systematically reduced the cost of fabricating parts using traditional thermoset (TS)—materials that undergo chemical reaction during cure—resin systems. There remain, however, pocket applications that require better target properties (i.e., use temperatures greater than 105 °C, or 220 °F, enhanced environmental resistance or improved damage tolerance) than TS materials can deliver. In response, various combinations of high-performance thermoplastic (TP) matrix resins (Table 1) and continuous fiber reinforcements (Table 2) have been offered to the industry.

Advanced TP resins have relatively high molecular weights and, hence, melt viscosities (10^3 to 10^6 Pa · s), and are typically more challenging to prepreg than TSs (Ref 4). This means that, in small lots, TP raw materials are typically 2 to 5 times more expensive than mass produced TSs and 10 to 50 times more expensive than metals. In large production lots (i.e., thousands of kg/year), this cost difference between TPs and TSs can be negated, but to date, ATPC use remains low (a few percent of the U.S. advanced composite market) and said economies of scale remain unrealized.

Further impeding the penetration of TPs into the aerospace market are costs associated with

Table 1 Candidate matrix resins for thermoplastic advanced composites

Polymer	Glass transition temperature °C	Glass transition temperature °F	Melt temperature °C	Melt temperature °F
Semicrystalline				
Polyetheretherketone	143	290	343	650
Polyphenylene sulfide	88	190	290	555
Poly aromatic ketone	205	400	358	675
Polyetheretherketone	143	290	334	635
Liquid crystal				
Polyester	...	...	415	780
Amorphous thermoplastic				
Polysulfone	190	375	...	...
Polyether sulfone	225	437	...	...
Polyetherminide	215	420	...	...
Polycarbonate	140–150	285–300	...	...
Poly aromatic sulfide	204	400	...	...
Pseudothermoplastics				
Polyimide	255	490	...	...
Polyamideimide	275	525	...	...

Source: Ref 3

Table 2 Thermoplastic resin/fiber mix options

Product form	Description
Postimpregnated(a)	
Film stacked	Alternating sheets of fiber and resin film stacked and melt fused together
Co-woven	Narrow slit film woven with fibers
Co-mingled	Fine resin filaments interwoven with fibers
Powder coated	Resin powder attached to fiber tows
Dry preimpregnated(b)	
Tape	Boardy unidirectional fiber form typically 15 or 30 cm (6 or 12 in.) wide
Slit tape	Tape that is slit to width
Slit woven	Slit tape woven into rattanlike broadgood rolls to improve drapability
Wet preimpregnated(c)	
Tape	Tacky unidirection fiber
Slit tape	Tape that is slit to width
Tow	Yarnlike fiber bundles
Fabric	Woven tow

(a) Fiber and resin placed in physical contact then fused together during processing. (b) Fibers completely preimpregnated with resin, melt fusible. (c) Pseudothermoplastics with tack and drape, chemistry advances during processing.

creating allowable databases. Before a manufacturer can certify a new material for flight hardware, millions of dollars must be spent on element tests covering all conceivable operating environments (i.e., moisture soak, hot/wet temperature, fuel/solvent resistance, fatigue, etc.). This data must not only be based on the specific resin/fiber mix undertaken but must also be generated using any equipment developed or specifically modified to take advantage of the rate-independent processing parameters associated with melt-fusible TPs.

To avoid the cost of developing unique manufacturing equipment and methods specifically for converting dry TP material forms, many companies have chosen to direct their efforts toward assimilating pseudothermoplastics (PUTPs), such as Avimid K (E.I. DuPont de Nemours & Co. Inc., Wilmington, DE), Torlon (Amoco Performance Products Inc., Chicago, IL), or LARC-TPI (NASA Langley Research Center thermoplastic imide), into existing processes. These materials are prepreged as wet tacky broadgoods with the look and drapability of traditional TSs. Therefore, in theory, a fiber placement machine that is used one day to lay down epoxies could, with modifications to head pressure, backing removal, and heat application, be used later to place PUTPs. In practice, however, PUTPs are more sensitive than TSs to process variability and require much longer high-temperature cures; typically 10 to 24 h at 340 to 430 °C (645–805 °F), versus 4 to 8 h at 120 or 180 °C (250–355 °F). High raw material costs, tight process control requirements, the release of volatiles, extended cure cycles, and expensive shop expendables (autoclave bagging, breather, release, sealant, etc.), in general make PUTP parts cost two to four times that of equivalent TS or metal parts. In certain weight or performance critical applications (i.e., fighter wings, launch vehicle tanks, etc.), this cost difference is acceptable, but in others it has driven manufacturers to research potentially lower-cost dry TP processing options.

True (or dry) thermoplastics (TTPs), in which there are no chemical changes during processing, can be rapidly heated, remelted, shaped, consolidated, and cooled. These relatively rate-insensitive process parameters lend themselves to innovative lay-up, forming, and joining techniques that in certain applications slash process times from hours to minutes. Several industry and government-directed prototype efforts (Fig. 1) have been conducted that demonstrate the potential economic benefits of ATPC materials and methods, but full-up production of primary aircraft components has been hindered by the lack of long term, high-volume production contracts.

Material Options

Since ATPCs possess high melt viscosity resins and high volume fractions of continuous inelastic fibers, traditional thermoforming methods that rely on material flow during softening, such as injection molding, blow molding, compression molding, resin transfer molding, vacuum forming, and so on, cannot be used. Rather, these advanced material forms must either be placed directly to final shape or stacked in such a manner that individual plies can slip to shape during thermal forming. Further complicating manufacture is the fact that most TP parts are designed for weight-critical applications by tailoring thickness throughout to match loading requirements. Unlike metals, where material is machined or chemically milled away after processing to achieve a desired thickness, advanced composites require individual oriented plies to be cut to shape and sequentially stacked in precise locations (Fig. 2).

Pseudothermoplastics, or pseudo TPs, in which there are molecular-weight-increasing chemical reactions and volatile release during final processing, are preimpregnated in wet/tacky tape or fabric form similar to traditional TS materials. PUTPs are usually laid to shape by hand or with automated equipment (i.e., contoured tape lay-up machines or fiber placement machines). Individual full plies and partial padup plies (typically 0.14–0.30 mm, or 0.005–0.01 in., thick each) are sequentially placed on a shaped tool and vacuum compacted every 1 to 3 plies to reduce bulking. Once a layup is complete, it is vacuum bagged using high-temperature film and fiberglass breather to assist in the removal of solvents and volatiles (water, ethanol, etc.). PUTPs require slow controlled heat-up rates (0.5–1.6 °C/min to ~370 °C, or 1–3 °F/min to ~700 °F), extended holds (2 to 8 h), and precise pressure application (initial slight vacuum changing to ~1400 kPa, or ~200 psi, during hold) to achieve desired target properties. If a matched closed tool is used to make a tight tolerance part such as a rib or spar, special provisions must be made for volatile removal to ensure porosity-free laminates (Ref 5). Due to the extended nature of these cures and the fact that PUTPs possess melt viscosities an order or two magnitude greater than dry melt fusible TPs, these materials do not lend themselves to rapid processing methods such as pultrusion, press, rolling, or diaphragm forming. Figure 3 illustrates typical manufacturing flows for PUTP processing.

Postimpregnated thermoplastics (PITPs), in which the fiber and resin are placed in close physical contact then fused together during processing, are usually dry drapable fabric forms, similar to a burlap bag. Examples include commingled fabrics where both the reinforcement and resin are in fiber form, and powdered resin fabrics where resin powder is electrostatically deposited on the reinforcing fibers. PITPs lend themselves to layup directly on shaped consolidation tools. To achieve consistent fiber wetout, hence optimal structural properties, PITPs require longer fusion times and higher consolidation pressures than preimpregnated dry TPs. PITPs are compliant but cannot be vacuum com-

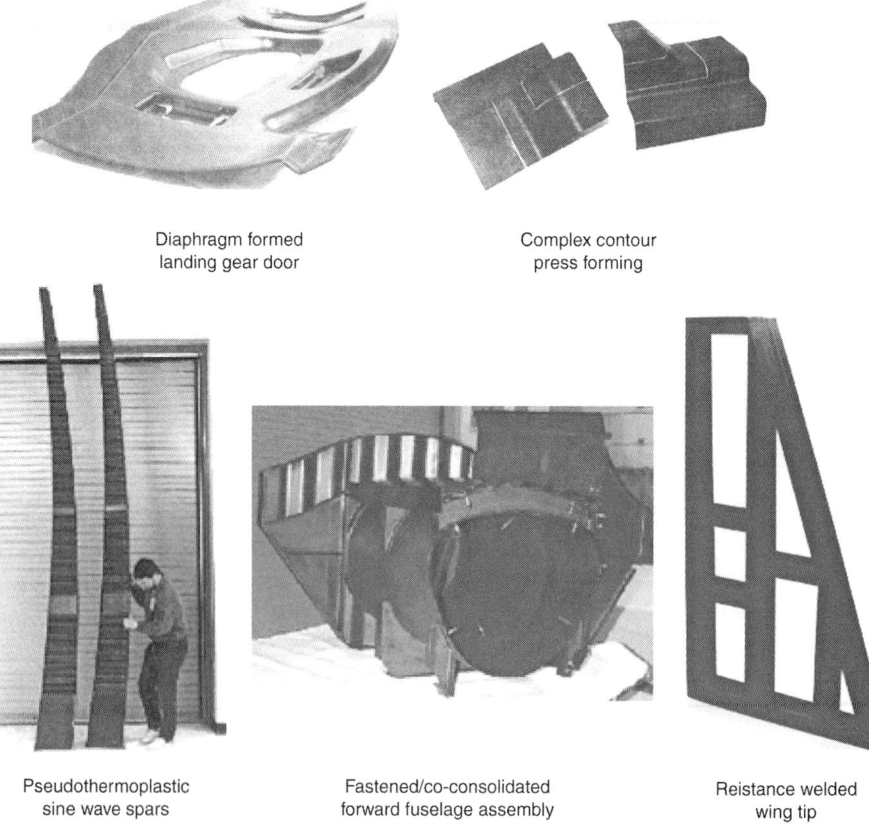

Fig. 1 Advanced thermoplastic aerospace components

pacted like wet composites. Therefore, precise ply cutout, kitting, and locating is somewhat labor intensive, and ramped plies have a tendency to shift during high-pressure thermal cycling. The PITP product form is most useful for making contoured constant thickness parts where slight variations in fiber/resin volume mix are acceptable. In these cases, short thermal cycles can be achieved and processing options include high temperature/pressure autoclaving (in the 370 °C, or 700 °F, 1400 kPa, or 200 psi, range), extended hold pressing, or diaphragm consolidation. Another PITP product form that circumvents lay-up difficulties is woven, or braided, tow shapes (Tee, J, C, etc.), which can be consolidated in heated, matched metal molds (Ref 6).

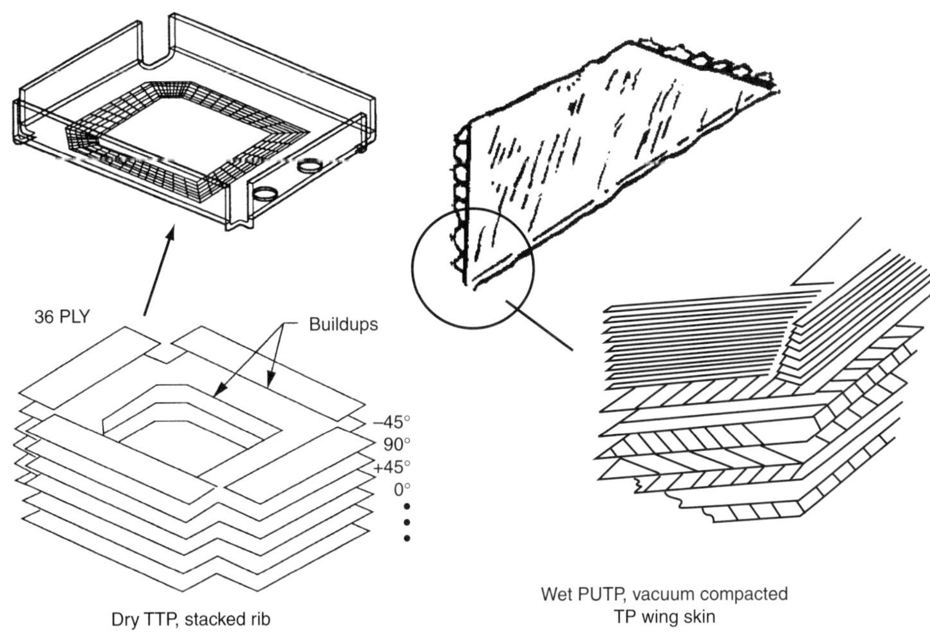

Fig. 2 Ply Stacking/orientating. TTP, true thermoplastic; PUTP, pseudothermoplastic; TP, thermoplastic

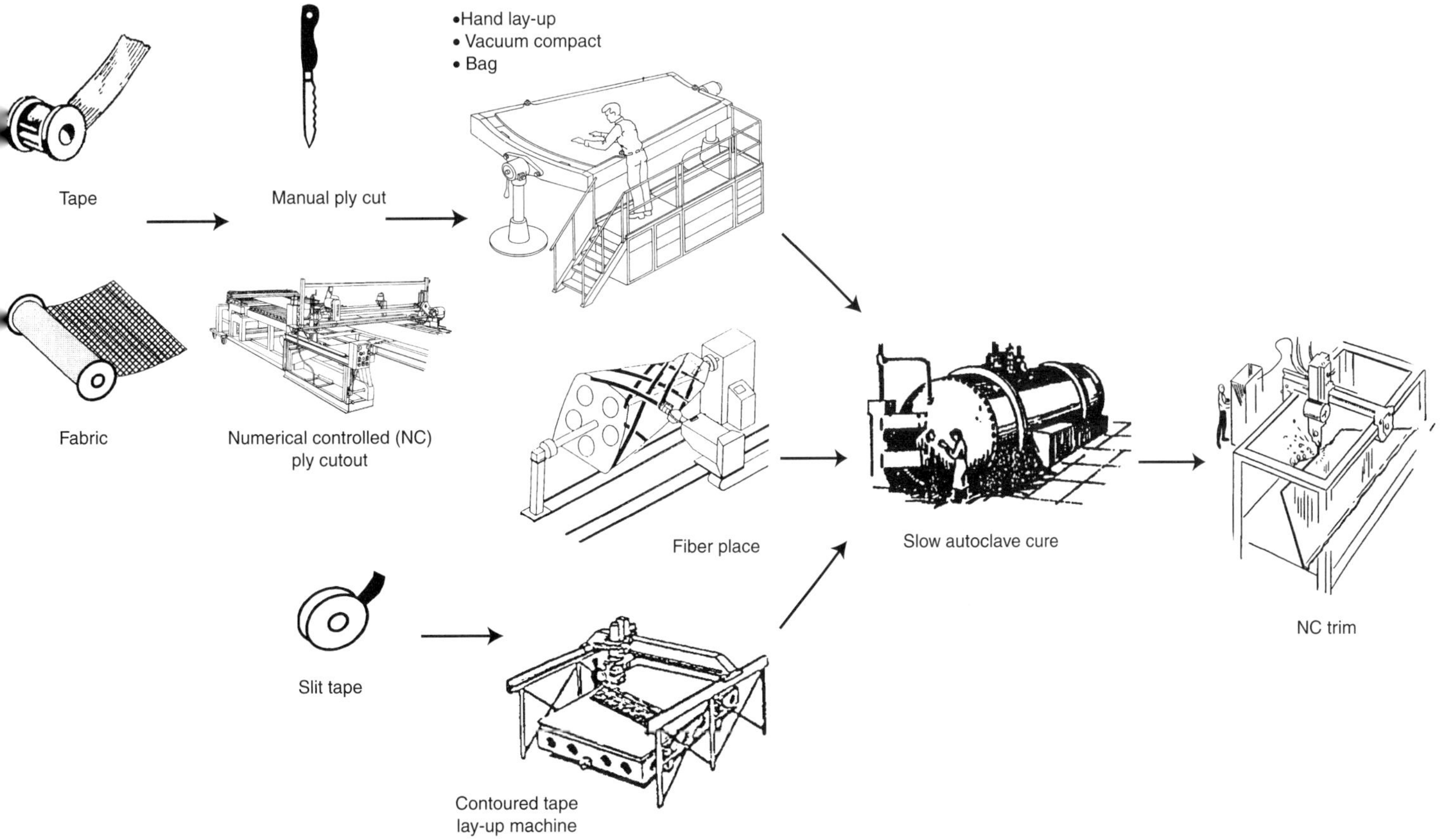

True (or dry) thermoplastics (TTPs), in which the continuous fiber reinforcement is completely wetted with a linear chain polymer resin that does not require further chemical reaction during processing, are preimpregnated as 150 or 300 mm (~6 or 12 in.) wide boardy tape rolls. This tape can be slit, slit woven, or seamed together to create product forms that lend themselves to rapid automated processing methods. Unlike TSs and PUTPs, dry thermoplastic raw material forms have indefinite shelf life at room temperature and do not require refrigeration. Further, processing parameters (heatup rate, hold during high-pressure thermal forming, and cool-down rate during consolidation) are mostly rate insensitive and rapid forming cycle times as low as 10 min are achievable. An exception is when slow cool-down rates are required to control crystallinity in a semicrystalline resin such as PEEK (polyetheretherketone) and transcrystallinity, which enhances resin adhesion to reinforcing fibers. Heating to above melt tempera-

Fig. 3 Pseudothermoplastic processing

ture can be accomplished by traditional methods such as two-sided infrared, convection, conducting platens, and so on. Shaping can be accomplished using a wide variety of modified TS or metal-forming methods such as hand layup, autoclaving, pultrusion, laminating, press forming, diaphragm forming, roll forming, and hydroforming. Laying up TTPs on compound curved tools is more difficult than with TSs because of the "boardy" nature of TTP prepregs and lack of tack. Secondary thermoforming equipment can be used to convert flat material layups to shaped parts via the following mechanisms:

- Moving the inelastic reinforcing fibers to shape without wrinkling or excessive waviness (the main forming mechanisms include interply slip, which occurs above the resin melt temperature, and intraply slip where fibers slide relative to one another)
- Applying adequate consolidation pressure (typically 700 to 7000 kPa, or 100 to 1015 psi)
- Cooling the material at a slow enough rate to avoid part warpage and also a rate that supports construction of the desired morphology in semicrystalline materials such as PEEK (polyetheretherketone) and PPS (polyphenylene sulfide).

Processing Methods

Pseudothermoplastics require extended cure cycles that allow time for matrix resin advancement and volatile removal. Therefore, PUTPs almost always are processed in an autoclave where the heat can be precisely controlled and byproducts can be removed with a vacuum system.

Postimpregnated thermoplastics usually are stacked constant thickness (possibly to shape) and consolidated in a manner so that the resin has sufficient time above melt temperature to fully wet the fibers (i.e., extended-hold autoclave, press, or diaphragm).

The objective when processing TTPs is to use the materials melt fusible characteristics to automate ply handling and forming. Tight tolerance ply locating is required for weight-critical aerospace designs, and parts usually are created by sequential placement of oriented (within ± 5° of desired) full plies intermixed with structure-enhancing pad-up plies. For example, a 2.54 mm (0.1 in.) thick laminate with stiffening might consist of a series of full tape plies at +45°, 90°, –45°, 0°, +45°, –45°, –45°, +45°, +45°, 0°, 90°, –45°, +45°, and 0° mixed with 3.8, 3.9, 4.0, and 4.1 cm (~1.5 in.) wide pad-up plies. Table 3 lists equipment prevalent in the industry for accomplishing such tasks as:

- Modifying incoming dry TP tape rolls to more useable product forms
- Placing or forming plies to shape
- Providing final consolidation heat and pressure

Weaving. Because of the high viscosity, high-temperature conditions required to melt impregnate true thermoplastics, it is difficult to prepreg TTP fabric forms directly. An alternative to using PUTP or PITP fabrics is to create a dry TP fabric by first slitting unidirectional prepeg tape then weaving it into wider roll stock. In this manner, 30 cm (12 in.) wide tape rolls can be converted into a semidrapable 300 cm (120 in.) wide mat amenable to automated ply cutout methods using dies, ultrasonic knives, water jets, and so on.

Seaming. Weaving reduces the load-carrying capability of unidirectional tape. An alternative width-increasing method is to butt weld or seam multiple tape rolls side by side. This can be done by hand with hot irons (400 to 600 °C, or 750 to 1110 °F) during prototyping efforts and in production with automated seaming equipment. There are 0° seamers that pull, guide, and seam up to five tape rolls at a time at rates as high as 20 m/min (65 ft/min) rolls 300 cm (118 in.) wide made in this fashion can then be cut into 0° or 90° plies using automated cutting equipment. Since 45° oriented plies are typically combined with 0° and 90° plies to create a layup, seamers have been made that repeatedly pull out a length of tape, butt seam it to a 45° oriented roll start, cut the new seamed section, and advance the section onto a roll. Throughput on these 45° seamers is slower, and the controls required to align, seam, and advance the tape are more complex than those of a 0° seamer. Therefore, in most cases, other than extremely high-volume efforts, it is cheaper to take 0° roll material and cut it to ±45° orientation during kitting.

Autoclaving. Other than considerations for higher temperatures (340–430 °C, or 645–805 °F) and pressures (700–2100 kPa, or 100–305 psi), laid-to-shape TPs can be consolidated in an autoclave using thermoset cure methods. The autoclave serves as a heated pressure vessel where vacuum, heatup, cooldown, and pressure application can be controlled to within precise limits. These high temperatures and pressure runs require the use of costly shop expendables (bagging, breather, release, and bag sealant), and the risk of a bag failure is greater than that of 180 °C (355 °F) cure TSs.

Preconsolidation. Within broad limits (each material has a specified process window developed by the supplier), most TPs can be heated and cooled repeatedly without affecting final component morphology. Thermoforming equipment (roll, press, and diaphragm formers) rely on ply and fiber slippage as the mechanisms for converting flat ply stacks into formed components. In most cases, this stack can be either loose (with spot seams to hold sequential plies relative to one another), fully preconsolidated (already melt fused into a solid stack), or some combination of a preconsolidated base with loose stack padups. Using preconsolidated planks eliminates manual ply-by-ply stackup and can dramatically cut costs during high-volume production. Preconsolidation can be accomplished using a laminator, press, autoclave, or a roll consolidator. The roll consolidator is an efficient way to make constant thickness sheet stock. In this apparatus, TP tape is pulled directly off preseamed, to width and orientation, rolls, heated in an infrared, conductive, or convective oven, and consolidated and cooled under a series of pinch rolls. The material often is contained within rigid metal plates as it passes under the rolls to ensure consistent pressure application and to avoid fiber distortion. In most cases, since the material will be subsequently thermoformed, only partial compaction is required, and rates of

Table 3 Thermoplastic processing equipment

Process	Description
Raw material modification	
Weaving	Tape is slit to 0.3 to 0.6 cm (0.1–0.2 in.) wide then woven to create a semidrapable form.
Hand seaming/tacking	Tape is butted together and seam welded to wider widths with a handheld iron. Also, ply stacks can be tack melted together.
Automated seaming	Equipment takes multiple 30 cm (12 in.), 0° tape rolls and butt seams them to wide (i.e., 300 cm, or 118 in.) 0° or 45° roll stock.
Sheet consolidating	Wide roll 0° and 45° roll stocks are stacked together and melt fused into sheet stock.
Autoclave	Material is laid to shape, vacuum bagged; autoclave heats TP to melt, applies pressure, and cools to consolidate.
Continuous processes	
Pultrusion	Slit tape stacks are pulled through a heated pressure die to generate continuous cross section Ts, Js, etc.
Roll forming	Similar to pultruding, but uses rollers to shape, consolidate, and cool the material
Fiber laminating (FL)	0.5 cm (0.2 in.) wide slit tape rolls are placed and melt fused to prior layers on a contoured mold tool (may autoclave after to get full compaction).
Contoured tape laminating	Similar to FL, but uses wider slit tape (7 cm, or 2.75 in.), better for large gentle contour parts such as wing skins
Thermoforming	
Press	Sheet or tack seamed stacks are heated in an oven, shuttled into a matched die, then formed/cooled under pressure.
Hydro	Similar to press, but hydrostatic fluid replaces one die half
Diaphragm	Sheet or tack seamed stacks are placed between extendable plates or bagging, heated in a one-sided die, and pressure blown to shape.
Induction	Similar to diaphragm, but an electromagnet field is used to heat the extendable plates, not the tool, thereby reducing cycle time

TP, thermoplastic. Source: Ref 7–9

1.5 to 3 m/min (5 to 10 ft/min) are achievable (rates are limited by how fast the composite can be heated and cooled).

Roll Consolidation. Unlike TSs and PUTPs, which can be compacted to within 5 to 15 % of their final cured thickness, dry, boardy thermoplastics cannot be vacuum compacted to remove bulk. Typically, spot seamed and stacked TPs exhibit bulk factors 2 to 4 times final consolidated part thickness. Therefore, hand laying up thick, highly padded parts, such as a wing skins or large cylinders, is impractical. One option for placing such components is to use modified thermoset fiber placement equipment. Fiber placement combines the differential tow payout of filament winding and the compaction and cut-restart capabilities of automatic tape laying (Ref 10). As shown in Fig. 4, TTP lamination (melt fusion on the fly) can be accomplished by feeding slit tape or tow from creel rolls onto a lay-up mandrel, heating the tape to above melt temperature, and cooling and consolidating the new layer to the previously placed stack with a pressure roller. This process sometimes is called in-situ consolidation and uses hot gas or a sweeping laser beam as the heat source. On flat parts, high fiber placement rates (several cm/s) and low void content (less than 1%) can be achieved. On highly contoured parts or parts with extensive ply drops, however, it is best to count on the laminator to only partially compact the stack (to within a 5% void content) and to subsequently achieve full consolidation by running the part through a high pressure/temperature autoclave cycle.

Roll Forming/Pultruding. Constant cross-section TP components (Tees, Js, Cs, Zs, or hats) can be made by pultruding or roll forming. A roll former operates in the same manner as the roll consolidator described previously. But, instead of using wide roll stock and flat rollers, it uses slit tape or narrow sheet stock and shaped roller dies. Typically, it is desired to fully consolidate during roll forming, so higher pressures and slower feed rates are used versus roll consolidation.

A pultruder uses a gradually changing cross section heated die through which tape stacks can be pulled, heated, formed to shape, and cooled. The die must contain a zone that allows the material to be heated to above melt temperature prior to forming and a subsequent zone that cools the laminate to shape under pressure. Because TP prepreg fibers are incompressible and there is minimal flow with high molecular weight TP resins, the die must have built-in gap width compliance in order to maintain compaction pressures of 700 kPa (100 psi) or greater. The roll and pultrusion processes can produce laminate at rates from 0.2 to 0.6 m/min (0.7 to 2 ft/min), which generally is slower than TS pultrusion. This factor combined with the fact that most aircraft components are weight optimized (composed of thickness variations) and contain compound contours has limited the infiltration of TP pultrusion and roll forming as a means of fabricating production hardware (Ref 11).

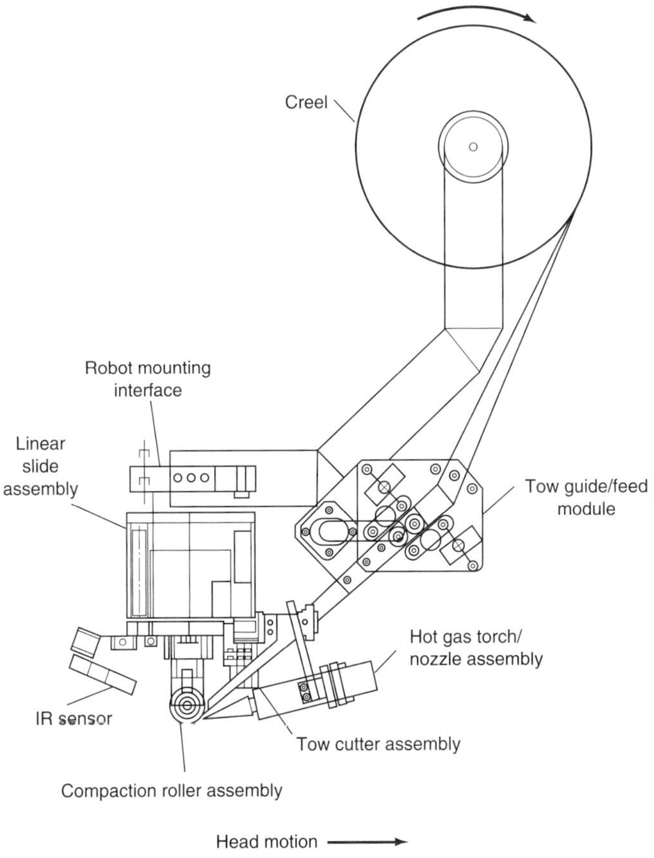

Thermoforming. In TP thermoforming processes (press, diaphragm, hydro, and induction), loose stack plies or preconsolidated sheet stock are formed and consolidated to shape in a single step. With TTPs, process heatup and cooldown rates have minimal effect on final part morphology; therefore, cycle times are far shorter than those used when autoclaving (Fig. 5). But in full-up production, thermoforming throughputs can be duplicated with an autoclave by loading several rate tools into a single run. Hence, rapid cycle times are not the primary driver for using thermoforming processes. Rather, the time saved by placing material flat versus laying it to shape is the main economic contributor (Fig. 6).

Press. During the press forming process (Fig. 7), flat stacked TP prepreg is heated to above melt temperature (340 to 430 °C, or 645 to 805 °F) in an oven, rapidly (within 1 to 10 s) shuttled to a forming die, pressed to shape, and consolidated and cooled under pressure (700 to 7000 kPa, or 100 to 1000 psi). In production, press forming dies usually are matched male-female sets constructed of steel or aluminum. But, during prototyping, rubber, wood, phenolics, and so on can be used. The die set can be maintained at room temperature throughout the forming/consolidation cycle. But, the use of a hot die (between 120 and 200 °C, or 250 to 390 °F) allows control of the cooldown rate (avoiding part warpage and controlling morphology in semicrystalline TPs such as PEEK and PPS) and extends the forming window, promoting better ply slip. The main disadvantage with this method is that the press only applies pressure in one direction, and hence, it is difficult to make complex shaped (i.e., beads, closed corners, etc.) parts or parts with legs that approach vertical. Since the temperature of the die set need not be cycled with each part, rapid forming times of between 10 min and 2 h are achievable with press forming (Ref 12).

Hydroforming. Hydroforming is similar to press forming, except that one die side is replaced with a flexible fluid diaphragm. Similar to the press, this allows for heating the prepreg in a separate oven, shuttling it into the forming zone, and forming and consolidating in a die. Unlike the press, consistent hydrostatic pressures can be applied to all part surfaces, and complex shapes and vertical flanges are obtainable. The primary drawback with this apparatus is that it is costly to scale up high-pressure hydraulics and associated containment mechanisms.

Diaphragm forming can be used to create shapes (beads, compound contour, etc.) that would be labor intensive to layup or are beyond the formability limits of press forming. The process starts by placing loose stack plies or preconsolidated sheet stock between two aluminum sheets that can plastically deform or between two plastic films that can elongate at high temperature. This stackup is placed in a diaphragm for-

Fig. 4 Thermoplastic laminating. IR, infrared. Source: Ref 10

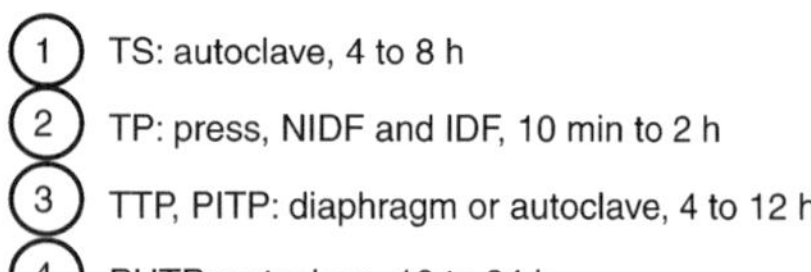

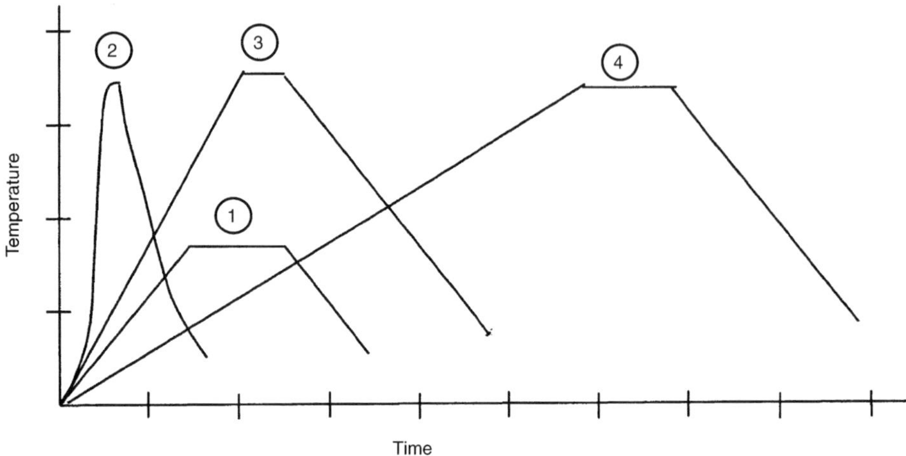

Fig. 5 Thermoplastic cycle times. TS, thermoset; TP, thermoplastic; NIDF, nonisothermal diaphragm forming; IDF, induction diaphragm forming; TTP, true thermoplastic, PITP, postimpregnated thermoplastic; PUTP, pseudothermoplastic

mer that consists of a one-sided metal die, a pneumatic pressure source, a means of evacuating the air from within the stackup, heating and cooling elements, and a clamping arrangement (Fig. 8). The stackup is heated and formed in place, and for sake of economy, an autoclave or press usually is used to apply heat and/or clamping pressure (Ref 13). Much like superplastic forming of aluminum sheet, diaphragm forming works by heating the material to above softening temperature while holding it under tension, then slowly applying pressure to one side to force it to take the shape of the forming mold. In TP diaphragm forming, the inelastic continuous reinforcement fibers prevent material stretching, but at forming temperature the stack becomes soft and pliable and can, for many geometries, be slipped into shape without wrinkling or splitting. In certain severe contours (beads, closed corners, etc.), this controlled reorganization will result in variations in laminate thickness. But unlike the press, pressure application is fluid and all laminate surfaces receive equivalent compaction force. The formation of wrinkles and split-

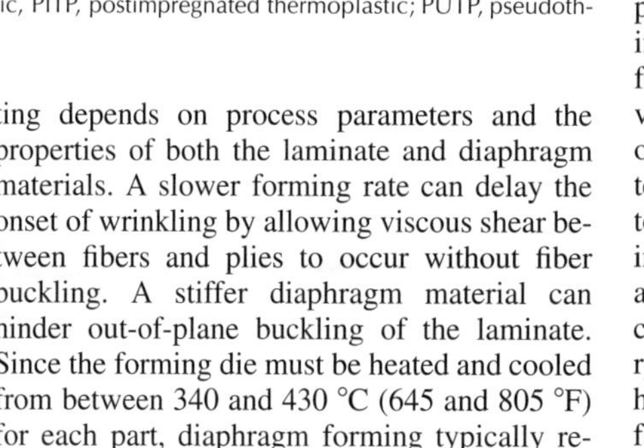
ting depends on process parameters and the properties of both the laminate and diaphragm materials. A slower forming rate can delay the onset of wrinkling by allowing viscous shear between fibers and plies to occur without fiber buckling. A stiffer diaphragm material can hinder out-of-plane buckling of the laminate. Since the forming die must be heated and cooled from between 340 and 430 °C (645 and 805 °F) for each part, diaphragm forming typically requires 4 to 8 h.

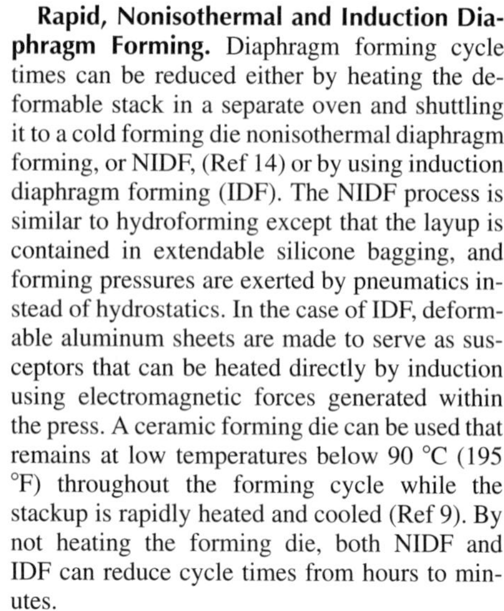
Rapid, Nonisothermal and Induction Diaphragm Forming. Diaphragm forming cycle times can be reduced either by heating the deformable stack in a separate oven and shuttling it to a cold forming die nonisothermal diaphragm forming, or NIDF, (Ref 14) or by using induction diaphragm forming (IDF). The NIDF process is similar to hydroforming except that the layup is contained in extendable silicone bagging, and forming pressures are exerted by pneumatics instead of hydrostatics. In the case of IDF, deformable aluminum sheets are made to serve as susceptors that can be heated directly by induction using electromagnetic forces generated within the press. A ceramic forming die can be used that remains at low temperatures below 90 °C (195 °F) throughout the forming cycle while the stackup is rapidly heated and cooled (Ref 9). By not heating the forming die, both NIDF and IDF can reduce cycle times from hours to minutes.

Joining

Although advanced composite process developments have made it possible to create one-piece, co-cured/co-consolidated structures with integral features not attainable or economically feasible with metals, secondary joining of individual components is still the prevalent means of creating complex assemblies. Mechanical fastening is a well understood and predictable way to join, but it involves undesirable drilling, and in some cases, countersinking operations, which are costly, cut continuous fibers, create stress concentrations, and degrade in-plane load-carrying capabilities. Consequently, manufacturers have pursued methods that replace traditional fastening techniques with noninvasive bonding and welding processes.

Fig. 6 Wing rib production cost comparison

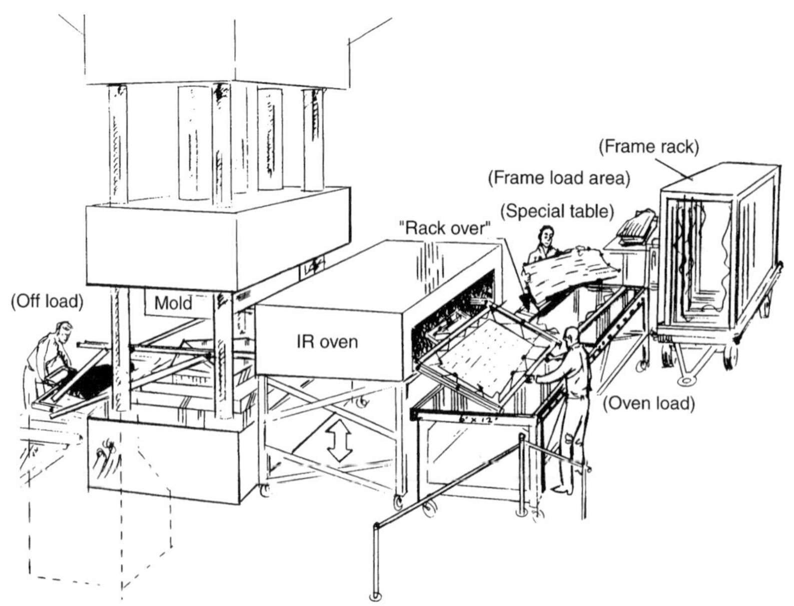

Fig. 7 Thermoplastic press forming

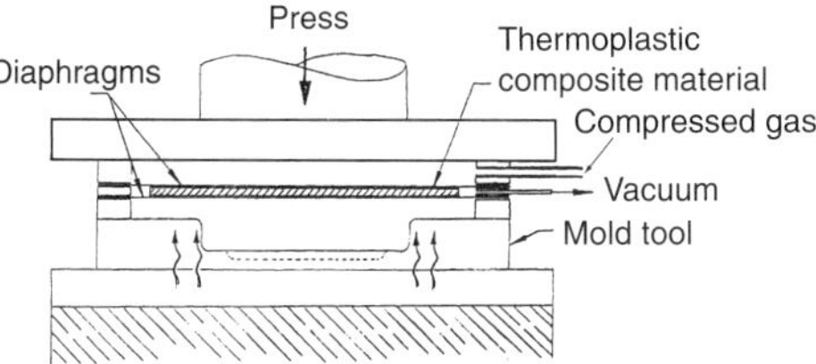

Fig. 8 Thermoplastic diaphragm forming

Within the aerospace industry, secondary bonding with 120 or 180 °C (250 or 355 °F) structural adhesives is the most used nonmechanical method for joining TS components. Well-characterized adhesives and surface treatments (to remove contaminants, increase contact area, and improve wetout) are used routinely to join large, highly loaded assemblies. Attempts to transition these methods to ATPCs, however, have been only marginally successful. Primarily, this is because thermoplastic substrate resins are relatively inert and do not lend themselves to the type of chemical attack required to facilitate a cohesive bond. Further, bonding adhesives in general have glass transition temperatures, fracture toughness, and environmental-resistive capabilities inferior to those of the TP components being assembled.

An attractive alternative for joining preconsolidated TP components is to melt fuse them together. Subsequently, manufacturers have pursued dual polymer bonding and co-consolidation methods, which seek to meld resin-rich TP surfaces together under heat and pressure. Surface treatment needs are limited to removing mold release contaminants and increasing bondline surface areas (i.e., by peel ply or mechanical abrading followed by a solvent wipe). This type of joining can be accomplished using various techniques, the more popular being autoclave, press, diaphragm, ultrasonic welding, resistance welding, and induction welding. Several manufacturers rely on these processes to join commodity grade thermoplastics, where consolidation pressures and temperatures are low compared with those of ATPCs. Widespread integration of these processes by the aerospace industry has been limited by a lack of production volumes and perceived risk levels associated with creating flawless, inspectable, durable bondlines.

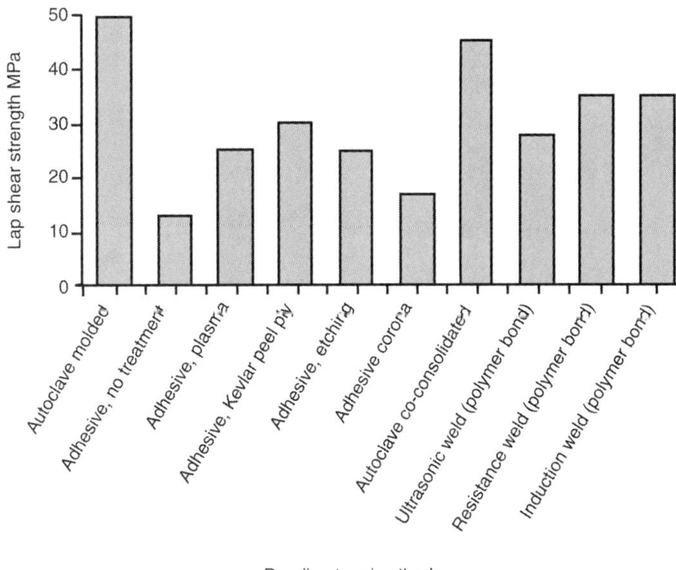

Fig. 9 Comparison of lap shear strength for various bond types/methods. Source: Ref 21, 23–29

Joint Types

Fastened. Since failure mechanisms are well understood and predictable, manufacturing methods are similar to those used on TS materials, and repair procedures exist, mechanical fastening is the most popular way to join TP aerospace components. Still, fastening is inherently costly. In general, drilled fastener holes are tightly spaced (approximately one every 3.8 cm, or 1.5 in.), require close diameter hole tolerances (±0.025–0.075 mm, or ±0.001–0.003 in., accomplished by step drilling and reaming), and necessitate two-sided installation and inspection access.

Since most aerospace grade ATPCs use abrasive continuous graphite fibers, short-duration expensive tungsten carbide or diamond grit drill bits are required to create precision fastener holes. Quality problems commonly associated with drilling TPs include surface delaminations, internal delaminations, fiber breakout, and degradation of the resin around the hole due to excessive heating. In response, several techniques and specialty bits have been developed to prevent such defects and to address specific applications such as drilling composite-metal stackups (Ref 15).

Equally important is fastener life cycle endurance. Traditional aluminum and steel fasteners do not work well in combination with graphite reinforcing fibers due to galvanic corrosion concerns. This problem necessitates the use of titanium, Inconel or austenitic alloys with graphite-compatible electromotive properties (Ref 16). During fastener installation, shank-to-hole interference fit must be maintained, and clamp-up loads must not exceed the compression strength of the composite materials being joined. Further, due to the sensitivity of graphite fiber to bearing loads, optimized countersinking configurations differ from those used on metal components (Ref 17).

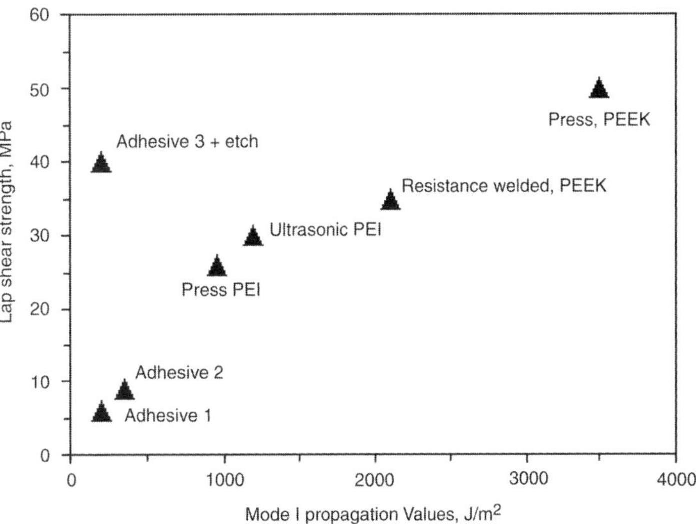

Fig. 10 Comparison of fracture toughness to lap shear strength for various bond types/methods. PEEK, polyetheretherketone; PEI, polyetherimide. Adhesive 1, Ciba Geigy AV138M, 100 °C (210 °F) cure; adhesive 2, Ciba Geigy AY103, 100 °C (210 °F) cure; adhesive 3, Ciba Geigy AV118, 180 °C (355 °F) cure. Source: Ref 25

Table 4 Comparison of selected thermoplastic-joining methods

Joining method	Advantages	Disadvantages
Press	Good for small, flat lap joints	Only applies pressure in one direction. Requires heating of tool and entire part. Hard to scale up
Diaphragm	Can apply fluid pressure. Can adapt to complex structures	Requires heating of tool and entire part. Requires dedicated tool
Autoclave	Even pressure throughout article Can adapt to complex structures	Requires heating of tool and entire part. Long heatup and cool down
Ultrasonic welding	Localized heating. Can use room temperature fixturing. Fast bond times (<10 s)	Hard to scale up. Not practical on complex geometries
Resistance welding	Localized heating. Can use room temp. fixturing. Good for 2–30 cm (0.75–12 in.) lap joints	Foreign object in bondline. Inconsistent heating as length increases
Induction welding	Localized heating. Can use room temperature fixturing. Potential to make running long welds	Foreign object in bondline

Adhesive Bonded. Adhesive bonding offers inherent advantages over mechanical fastening since load-carrying fibers are not cut and smooth aerodynamic surfaces can be maintained. Consequently, manufacturers have used bonding extensively when assembling TS aerospace hardware. By far the most popular product form is thin film epoxy resin systems carried on scrim fiberglass reinforcement. The bonding scenario consists of preparing and cleaning the bond surfaces, applying adhesive film, bringing the surfaces together and curing the adhesive under heat and pressure (normally 120 or 180 °C and 315 to 595 kPa, or 250 or 355 °F and 45 to 85 psi). Properly bonded articles can have joint strengths as good or better than fastened assemblies, and long term hot/wet capabilities at a temperature of approximately 105 °C (220 °F) are achievable. Bondlines can be inspected using traditional nondestructive techniques, but underlying cohesive quality cannot be determined without the use of destructive testing. Therefore, manufacturers must rely on extensive allowable databases and rigid process controls to ensure part-to-part integrity.

A good structural bond starts with clean, suitable bond surfaces. To create a bond surface, the substrates must be roughened to increase bond area. This can be accomplished by mechanical abrading, but more commonly, a finely woven peel ply is consolidated with the part, which, when removed, provides a uniformly textured, contaminant-free bond surface. If abrading (by grit blasting, sanding, etc.) is used, the bond surfaces must be wiped clean with a solvent to remove contaminants (Ref 18). Another essential to creating a good bondline is to maintain compaction pressure between the bonding surfaces during the bond cure cycle. On small, simply shaped parts, mechanical clamping can be used, but with large complex parts autoclave fixturing may be required. Even under autoclave pressure tight radii, joggled areas, and so on are difficult to confine. Small misalignments can result in gaps in the bond surfaces, creating poor bonds and, in turn, premature structural failure.

Standard surface preparation methods normally are not enough to promote wet out and chemical bonding when using ATPC resin systems. Rather, to achieve a structural bond, the chemical makeup of the TP part surface must be altered. Various methods have been used to accomplish this task, including flame treatment, corona discharge, plasma activation, and chemical etching (Ref 19). These methods have shown promise in producing bonded elements with room temperature bond strengths equivalent to those of bonded TS composites (Ref 20–23), especially when combined with standard abrading practices (Ref 24). Because of additional surface treatment costs, inconsistent or unpredictable bond quality, and the reduction in environmental and fracture toughness properties associated with lower temperature capable TS adhesives, secondary bonding of ATCPs has yet to meet with wide scale production acceptance.

Dual Polymer Bonded. Dual polymer bonding provides a high use temperature alternative to adhesive bonding. In this case, a resin film with a melt temperature, or in the case of amorphous polymers, a glass transition temperature (T_g), less than that of the TP parts to be joined is placed at the bond interface instead of a TS adhesive film. Optimally, to circumvent surface preparation problems and to obtain maximum adhesion between the resin film and base laminate, this bonding polymer is adhered to the bond interface of each part during an initial preconsolidation cycle. Typically, the bond surfaces are placed in intimate contact, fixtured or bagged and heated to above the melt temperature of the bonding resin, but below that of the individual components while compaction pressure (typically 700 to 1400 kPa, or 100 to 200 psi) is maintained. The resin-rich mating surfaces are fused together creating a structural assembly. The major drawbacks to this joining method are that the properties of the assembly are reduced to those of the polymer used for bonding and that the entire assembly must be fixtured/heated within a narrow process window to achieve good structural results. If the parts get too hot, the preconsolidated laminates may deform or delaminate, and if they are not hot enough, they will not stick together.

Co-consolidated. Co-consolidation involves the melt fusion of individual TP articles into a one-piece assembly. In this case, the TP matrix resin provides the bond mechanism. Usually, to enhance flow and fitup, a layer of resin film is placed at the mating surfaces prior to consolidation. This process creates assemblies that have properties consistent to the base components, but like dual polymer bonding requires careful fixturing and heatup while maintaining consistent pressure.

Welded. TP welding is the joining of two or more parts wherein only the areas being fused together are heated. The weld mechanism can be either dual polymer bonding or co-consolidation,

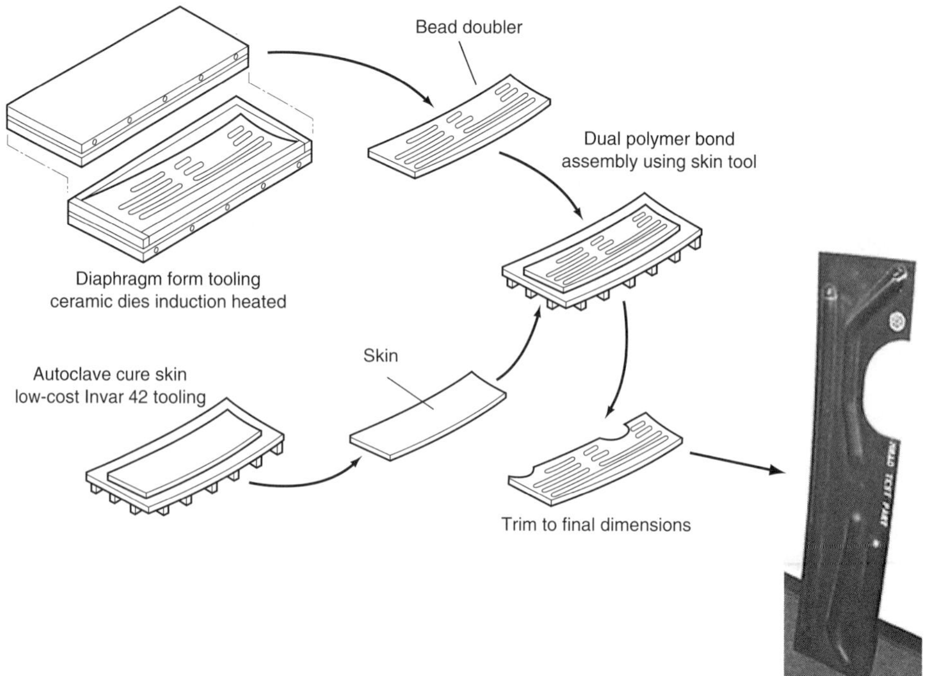

Fig. 11 Dual polymer bonded V-22 Osprey door

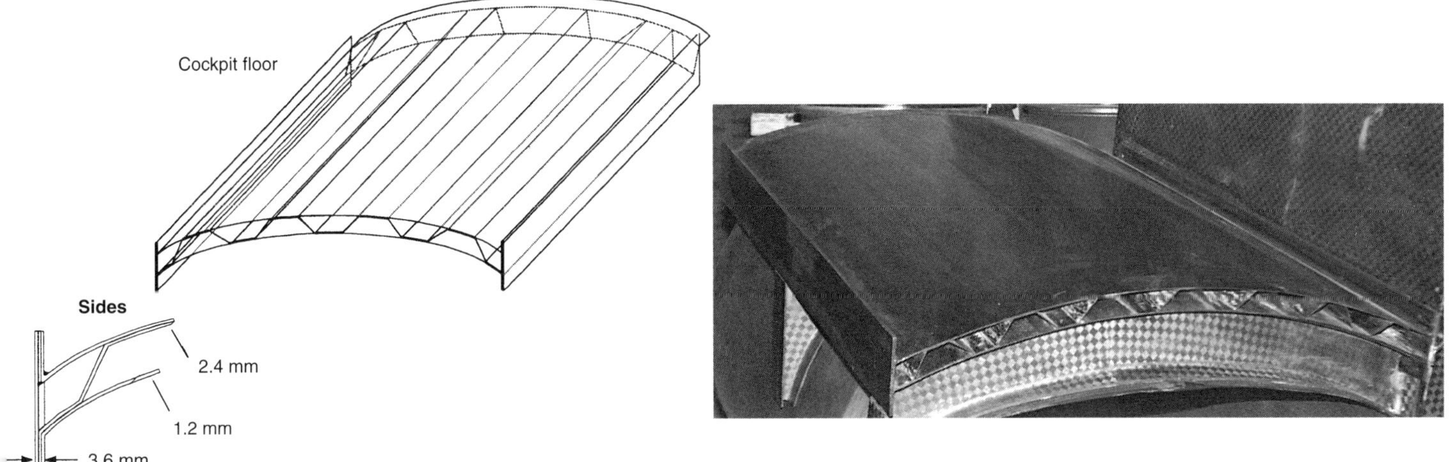

Fig. 12 Co-consolidated cockpit floor

and process methods include ultrasonic (heating by rapid vibration), resistance (heating with electric current), or induction (heating with magnetic field). Welding can be used to join preconsolidated parts ranging from, hat stiffeners, I-beams, and so on to large panels such as wing skins. This method has an advantage over pressing, diaphragming, and autoclaving because the bulk of the surface area of the parts need not be heated, and lay-up mandrels and fixture tooling materials are not limited to those compatible with the TPs at elevated temperatures. Figure 9 compares lap shear strengths reported for various bond types and methods, and Fig. 10 relates fracture toughness to lap shear strength. Table 4 summarizes the thermoplastic-joining techniques, indicating the relative advantages and disadvantages.

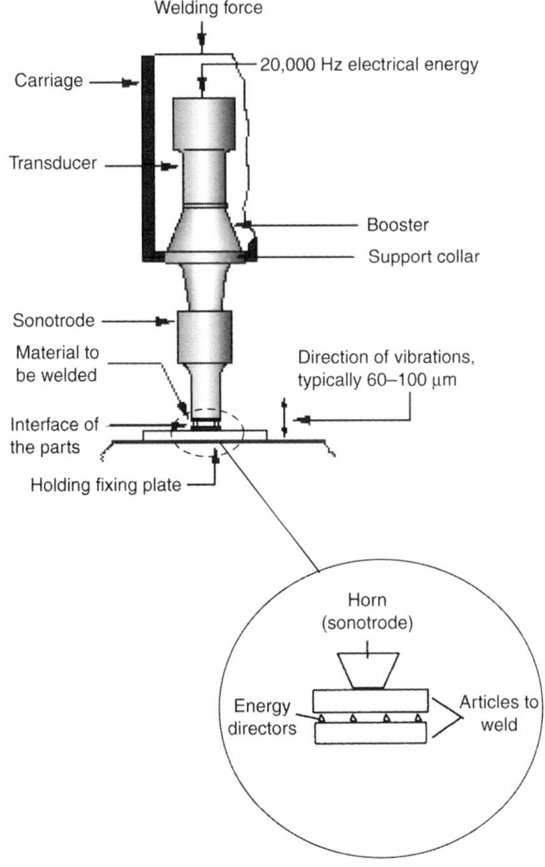

Fig. 13 Schematic for ultrasonic welder and multiunit weld machine. Source: Ref 30, 31

Joining Methods

Press, Diaphragm, and Autoclave. To facilitate a dual-polymer or co-consolidation TP bond, parts must be placed in intimate contact, heated to above melt temperature, and fused together under consolidation pressure (typically 700 to 1400 kPa, or 100 to 200 psi). Often the most difficult part of this process is to position and maintain the parts relative to one another while still allowing some degree of movement during the compaction/joining cycle. Simple lap shear specimens require this pressure and movement in only one direction and can be joined in a press using heated platens with stepped plates.

Complex contoured parts require fluid pressure application and are better joined in a diaphragm or autoclave. In these instances, locating dies can be used to hold the parts relative to one another and the entire assembly can be confined within a bag or bladder. For example, the V-22 Osprey aircraft landing gear door shown in Fig. 11 illustrates how a diaphragm former can be used to consolidate a base laminate, form a bead stiffened panel, and then join the two into an assembly via the dual polymer bonding process.

An autoclave is a large hollow pressure vessel that can in theory accommodate an infinite variety of dual polymer or co-consolidation assembly configurations. In practice, the constraining factor becomes the thermal expansion of the materials being bonded compared with that of the tooling being used to fixture the parts. Dual polymer bonding requires heatup from room temperature to approximately 230 °C (445 °F), and co-consolidation cycles go as high as 430 °C (805 °F). Over these temperature ranges aluminum and tool steels have incompatible coefficients of thermal expansion compared with those of the TP composites being joined. These temperatures limit tool choices to materials such as Invar 42 (an iron-nickel alloy), ceramic and monolithic graphite, which have coefficients of thermal expansion in the 4 to 5 μm/m/°C (2.2 to 2.8 × 10^{-6}in./in./°F) range over the range of the bonding cycle. Figure 12 displays an experimental cockpit floor co-consolidated in an autoclave.

Ultrasonic Welding. In ultrasonic welding vibration energy (typically 20–40 kHz) is used to heat the TP bondline. Figure 13 shows a schematic of an ultrasonic welder. During the welding process, the ultrasonic machine converts electric power to mechanical vibration through a horn (or sonotrode), which is placed in physical contact with the back face of one of the TP components being joined. Vibration focused through the horn causes this component to rapidly move relative to another fixed component and the resultant friction generates heat at the joint interface. The objective is to focus the heat at the bondline and keep the remainder of the part interior and the heat-affected zone, or HAZ (the area next to the bond) from deconsolidating. Since this method only heats the parts in the area being bonded, pressure only needs to be maintained directly under the horn and any associated HAZs. Pressure between 500 and 1400 kPa (70 and 200 psi) must be maintained until the part has cooled to below the T_g of the matrix resin.

Ultrasonic welding (especially in spot applications) of unreinforced TPs is used widely in the automotive and medical industries, and total weld times of less than 10 s are achievable (Ref 32). With ATPC materials a resin rich layer usually is added to enhance the polymer film-to-laminate bond, decrease melt viscosity, and lower melt-temperature requirements at the bond interface. In addition, researchers have developed molded-in energy directors that make heat up more efficient (Ref 33). The weld time to get a sufficient bond is a function of pressure, vibration amplitude of the horn, and thickness of the material. Care must be taken not to have too great of a weld time since this could cause the interior of the laminate to heat to above melt temperature and excessive squeeze-out could result. Although ultrasonic is perhaps the fastest TP welding technique, lap shear strengths (25–30 MPa, or 3625–4350 psi for PEEK components) are typically lower than for other methods, and it is difficult, if not impossible, to scale the process to complex and/or large geometries (Ref 25).

Resistance Welding. Figure 14 shows a schematic for the TP resistance welding process, in which electrical current is passed through conductive fibers or strands to create heat at the bond interface. This heating element (or susceptor) usually is made from metal (typically copper) or, preferably, graphite fibers identical to those used to reinforce the ATPC. The purpose of the susceptor is to focus heat locally at the bond interface, thereby minimizing laminate interior and adjacent bond area heating. As with ultrasonic welding, pressure must be maintained on the HAZ during part heat up and cooldown to avoid deconsolidation.

Weld times vary depending on the power supply and characteristics of the susceptor being used. But, total cycle times in the 30 s to 5 min range are achievable. Like most TP joining processes, resistance-welded parts usually have a resin-rich area at the bond interface. The process has been shown to be very efficient on small 2 to 30 cm (0.75–12 in.) flat joints and lap shear strengths for dual polymer resistance bonded articles can range from 30 to 35 MPa (4350–5075 psi), while strengths for co-consolidated resistance-welded articles are typically between 35 and 40 MPa (5075 and 5800 psi) (Ref 25, 26). As part length and curvature increases, differential edge and nonlinear heat-up effects often encroach. This phenomenon is less of a factor when dual polymer bonding, given the temperature required to fuse the bonding resin is lower than the T_g of the matrix resin. Scaling-up resistance welding to large aerospace structures is further complicated by the fact that consolidation pressures (700–1400 kPa, or 100–200 psi) must be maintained over the entire bond surface during heat up (Ref 34, 35). As shown in Fig. 15, however, wing tip substructure rib to spar joints lend themselves to resistance welding as long as joint length is relatively short and access for a pressure tool can be accommodated.

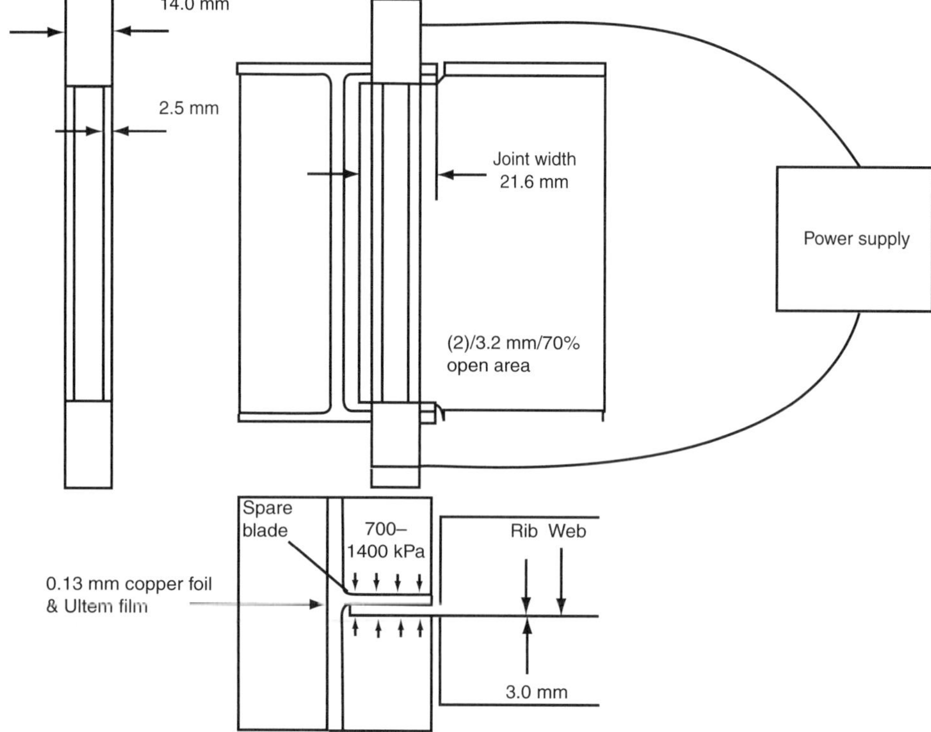

Fig. 14 Schematic for resistance weld of rib to spar

Induction Welding. Figure 16 shows the schematics of a moving head of an induction welder. During induction welding, the bond interface is heated by utilizing an electromagnetic field in conjunction with a susceptor embedded at the surface of one of the bond articles. Heating occurs, either by eddy current (EC) dissipation in an electrically conductive susceptor or by hysteresis losses in a magnetic susceptor, giving rise to particle interaction frictional heat. Since heating takes place only in the vicinity of the magnetic field, the HAZ and associated bond pressure can be focused exclusively on the area being joined. Early fabrication trials used thin magnetic/conductive metal susceptors (i.e., iron or nickel base) that provided rapid heatup, but graphite fibers (Ref 27, 28) and copper mesh also have been used to avoid corrosion concerns. In either case, a foreign material is being added to the bondline, and some degradation in structural properties compared with a co-consolidated joint is inevitable.

Typically, heat-up times (5 to 30 min) for induction welding are longer than either ultrasonic or resistance. Cycle times are dependent on the melt temperature one is trying to achieve, pressure applied (material contact as melt progresses improves conduction), input power, and susceptor type. As with all localized welding techniques, pressure on the part must be maintained above consolidation levels (350–1400 kPa, or 50–200 psi) to achieve good bond quality. Lap shear strengths between 30 and 35 MPa (4350 and 5075 psi) have been reported by a variety of research programs (Ref 25).

Induction welding has been widely pursued by the aerospace industry since it has potential for being adapted to long line weld applications, such as wing to spar or stiffener joints. Figure 17 displays a schematic of an induction welder used to bond sine wave spars to a fighter wing skin. Figure 18 shows an induction-welded article, consisting of a K3B skin and stringer. Like most TP process techniques, however, implementation of induction welding has been hindered by the lack of allowable databases, per-

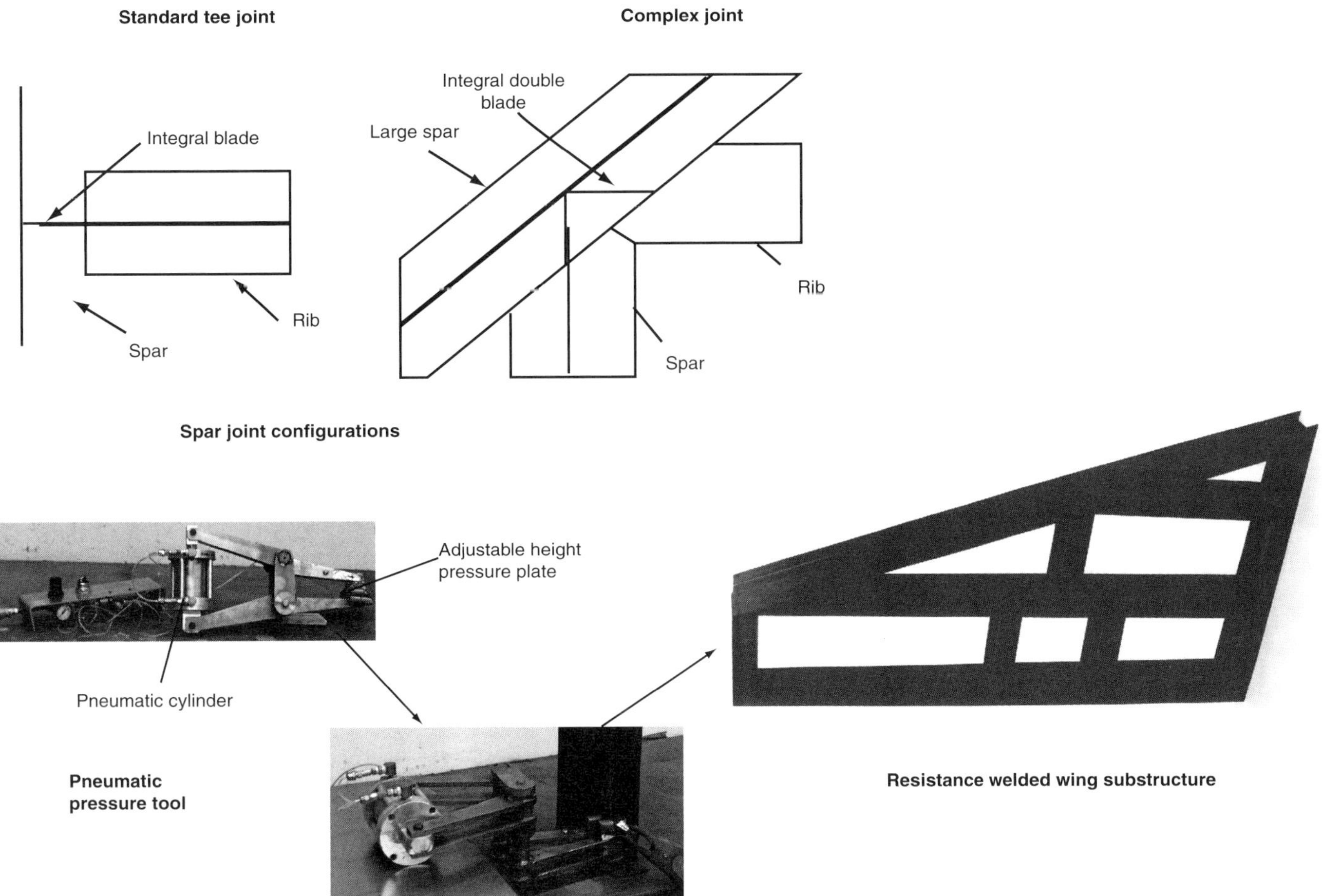

Fig. 15 Resistance welding wing substructure using copper foil and amorphous thermoplastic (Ultem, GE Company, Pittsfield, MA) resin

ceived life-cycle risks, and the lack of large-volume production contracts.

REFERENCES

1. Y.C. Chang, C.L. Ong, and M.F. Sheu, The Development of the Thermoplastic Composite Nose Landing Gear Door of a Fighter Aircraft, *42nd International SAMPE Symposium,* May 1997, p 1520–1530
2. A.J. Barnes, J. Harper-Tervet, S. Reeve, J. Schwarz, R. Stratton, F. Tervet, and T.B. Tolle, Superplastic Diaphragm Forming of Thermoplastic Complex Shaped Composites as a Cost Effective Manufacturing Process, *29th International SAMPE Technical Conference,* Oct 1997, p 383–394
3. M.T. Harvy, Thermoplastic Matrix Processing, Vol 1, *Engineered Materials Handbook, Composites,* ASM International, 1986, p 544–553
4. R.B. Gosnell, Thermoplastic Resins, Vol 1, *Engineered Materials Handbook, Composites,* ASM International, 1986, p 97–104
5. D.A. McCarville, I. Medoff, and J.L. Sweetin, Breathable Tooling for Forming Parts from Volatile-Emitting Composite Materials, U.S. Patent 5,709,893, Jan 1998
6. R.K. Okine, Processing of Thermoplastic Matrix Composites, Vol 11, *Composites Engineering Handbook, Materials Engineering,* Marcell Dekker, Inc., 1997, p 579–629
7. D.A. McCarville and J.A. New, Apparatus and Method for Joining a Plurality of Thermoplastic Tape, U.S. Patent 4,931,126, June 1990
8. D.A. McCarville and D.C. Rocheleau, Apparatus for Forming Laminate into a Predetermined Configuration, U.S. Patent 4,913,910, April 1990
9. M.R. Matsen, D.A. McCarville, and M.M. Stephan, Fastenerless Bonded Wingbox, U.S. Patent 5,847,375, Dec 1998
10. W.R Cox, R.W. Grenoble, N.J. Jonhnston, J.M. Marchello, and T.W. Towell, Thermoplastic Fiber Placement Machine for Materials and Processing Evaluations, *41st International SAMPE Symposium,* March 1996, p 1701–1711
11. M. Hou, Y. Mai, and L. Ye, Advances in Processing of Continuous Fibre Reinforced Composites with Thermoplastic Matrix, *Plastics, Rubber and Composites Processing and Applications 23,* McCrum, 1995, p 279–293
12. B.E. McKillop, Thermoforming of Thermoplastic Composites, *23rd International SAMPE Technical Conference,* Oct 1991, p 1006–1020
13. A.R. Offringa, Thermoplastic Composites—Rapid Processing Applications, *4th International Conference on Automated Composites,* Sept 1995, p 329–336
14. W. Michaeli and C. Pohl, Automated Diaphragm-Forming-Line for the Processing of Thermoplastic Composites with Reduced Cycle Time, *43rd International SAMPE Symposium,* May 1998, p 1979–1991
15. J.L. Phillips and R.T. Parker, Fastener Hole Considerations, Vol 1, *Engineered Materials Handbook, Composites*, ASM International, 1986, p 712–715
16. J.D. Pratt, Blind Fastening, Vol 1, *Engineered Materials Handbook, Composites,* ASM International, 1986, p 709–711
17. R.T. Parker, Mechanical Fastener Selection, Vol 1, *Engineered Materials Handbook, Composites,* ASM International, 1986, p 706–708
18. T. J. Reinhart, Adhesive Bonding Surface Preparation, Vol 1, *Engineered Materials Handbook, Composites,* ASM International, 1986, p 681–682

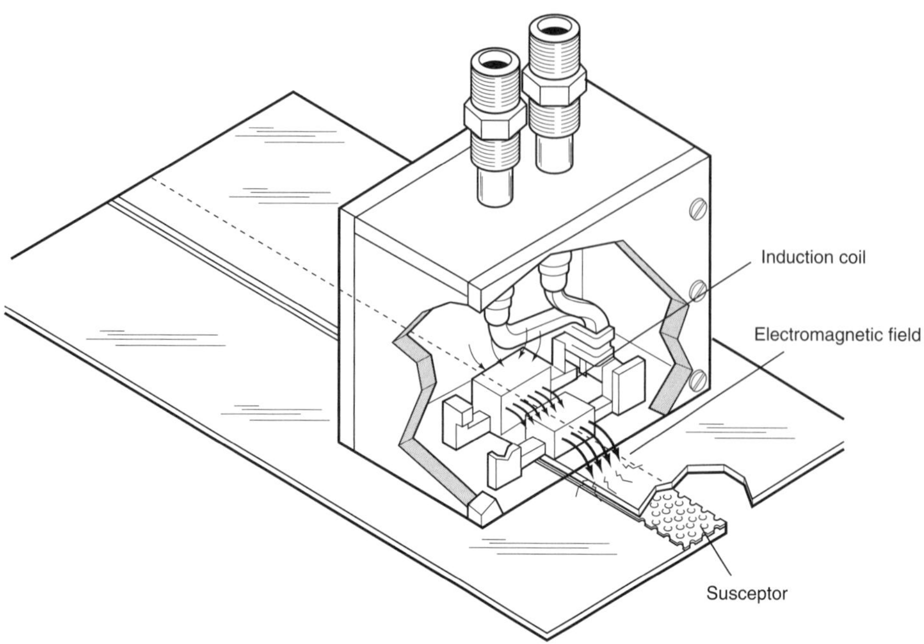

Fig. 16 Induction welder schematic

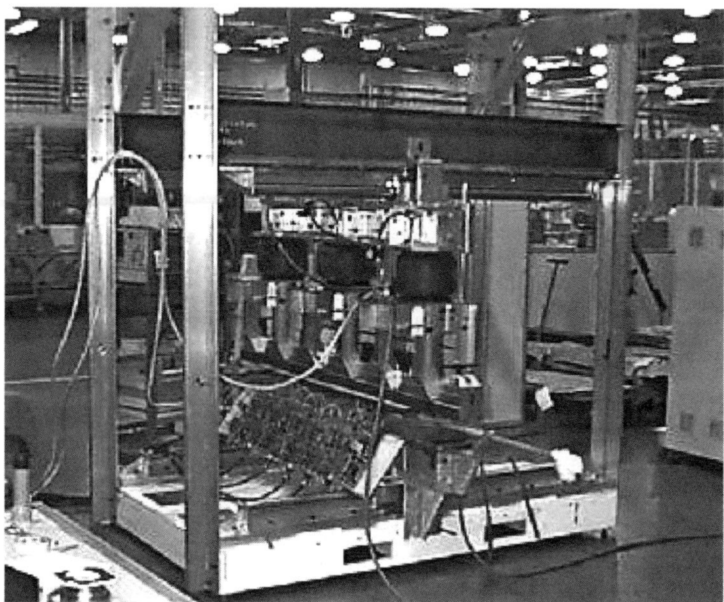

Fig. 17 Induction weld machine

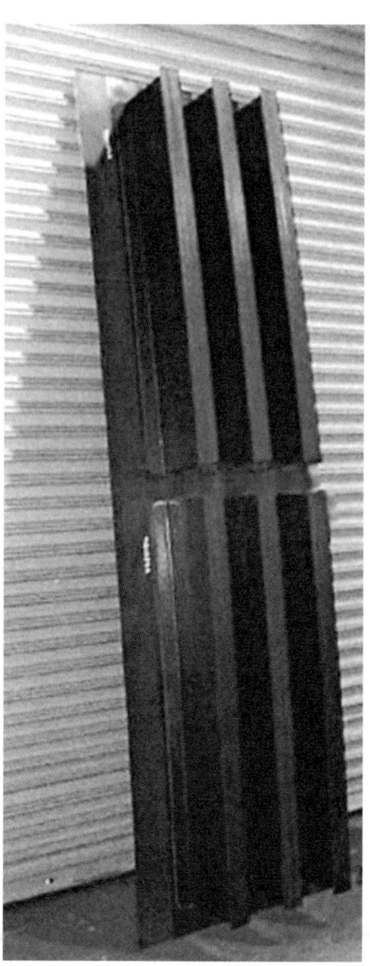

Fig. 18 Induction welded K3B skin/stringer using Avimid K3A at the bond interface

19. A.H. Landrock, Surface Preparation of Adherents—Chapter 4, *Adhesives Technology Handbook*, Noyes Publications, 1985, p 84–106
20. A.J. Kinloch, G.K.A. Kodokian, and J.F. Watts, Relationships Between the Surface Free Energies and Surface Chemical Compositions of Thermoplastic Fibre Composites and Adhesive Joint Strengths, *Journal of Materials Science Letters 10*, July 1991, p 815–818
21. S.Y. Wu, Adhesive Bonding of Thermoplastic Composites 2. Surface Treatment Study, *35th International SAMPE Symposium*, April 1990, p 846–858
22. B.R.K. Blackman, A.J. Kinloch, and J.F. Watts, The Plasma Treatment of Thermoplastic Fibre Composites for Adhesive Bonding, Vol 25, *Composites, Number 5*, May 1994, p 332–341
23. J.W. Powers and W.J. Trzaskos, Recent Developments in Adhesives for Bonding Advanced Thermoplastic Composites, *34th International SAMPE Symposium*, May 1989, p 1987–1998
24. B.R. Bonazza, Adhesive Bonding of Improved Polyphenylene Sulfide Thermoplastic Composites, *35th International SAMPE Symposium*, April 1990, p 859–870
25. P. Davies and W.J. Cantwell, Bonding and Repair of Thermoplastic Composites—Chapter 11, *Advanced Thermoplastic Composites- Characterization Processing*, Hanser, 1993, p 337–366
26. R.C. Don, Fusion Bonding of Thermoplastic Composites by Resistance Heating, *Center for Composite Materials Technical Report 90-13*, University of Delaware, 1990, p 1–56
27. J. Border, Induction Heated Joining of Thermoplastic Composites Without Metal S*usceptors, 34th International SAMPE Symposium,* May 1989, p 2569–2578
28. W.A. Lees, A Review-The Design and Assembly of Bonded Composites—Chapter 36, *Composite Structures*, Elsevier Applied Science, 1991, p 471–506
29. M.M. Schwartz, Joining of Polymer Matrix Composites and Resin Matrix Composite—Chapter 2, *Joining of Composite Matrix Materials*, ASM International, 1994, p 35–87
30. The Welding Institute, Ultrasonic Welding

Techniques, *The Welding Institute*, July 1997
31. Applied Technology Group, Ultrasonic Systems, *Product Literature from Branson Ultrasonic Corporation*, Dec 1998
32. A. Benatar, Ultrasonic Welding of Advanced Thermoplastic Composites, *Ph.D. Thesis*, Massachusetts Institute of Technology, 1987, p 1–315
33. E.C. Eveno, Investigation of Resistance and Ultrasonic Welding of Graphite Reinforced Polyetheretherketone Composites, *Masters Thesis*, University of Delaware, 1988, p 1–200
34. S.H. McKnight, S.T. Holmes and J.W. Gillespie, Jr., Scaling Issues in Resistance Welded Thermoplastic Composite Joints, *Center for Composite Materials Technical Report 97-08*, University of Delaware, 1997, p 1–47
35. S.H. McKnight, S.T. Holmes, and J.W. Gillespie, Jr., Large Scale Bonding of PAS/PS Thermoplastic Composite Structural Component Using Resistance Heating, *Center for Composite Materials Technical Report 93-03*, University of Delaware, 1993, p 1–23

Hole Drilling in Polymer-Matrix Composites

Michael J. Paleen and Jeffrey J. Kilwin, The Boeing Company, St. Louis

GOOD HOLE-DRILLING PROCESSES are key to joining composite parts with other composite parts or with metal parts. Poor hole quality can affect the strength and durability of structures. To consistently obtain good hole quality, it is important to identify four factors before selecting the optimal techniques, tools, and drill parameters. First, identify the material types in the assembly stack-up. For composite structures, the material type and fiber type must be known in addition to fiber orientation. For example, the hole preparation techniques and tools will differ between a carbon/epoxy composite part and an aramid fiber (Kevlar)/epoxy composite part. Also there may be different techniques and tools for unidirectional (tape) products and woven (cloth) products. When unidirectional carbon/epoxy materials are used on the part surface, the fibers are prone to splintering and fiber breakout from the hole-drilling process, especially if the surface is resin starved. This splintering or fiber breakout is much less of a problem with woven materials. Unidirectional fiber materials do offer some benefits over woven materials in their ability to be oriented in the direction of the structural load, which can keep weight to a minimum. Also unidirectional fiber materials typically have less waste than woven products, unidirectional products lend themselves to automated lay-up in tape-laying machines, and unidirectional products may provide a smoother aerodynamic external surface than woven products. It is not uncommon to mix composite types and fiber materials to better utilize the advantages of the materials. For example, composite structures can be a combination of unidirectional inner plies to keep weight to a minimum and woven surface plies for reduced impact damage or hole preparation damage, and the woven material adjacent to mating metal structure could be fiberglass to be more compatible with aluminum.

Any metallic structures in a joint must also be known. Often, the metallic structure serves as a backup for drilling and will help reduce or eliminate fiber breakout problems. Required hole size, hole tolerance, and the available equipment also influence hole-drilling process selection.

Part Fit-Up

Gaps detected between parts of an assembly must be evaluated to determine if they are acceptable "as is" or if they need to be shimmed. Gaps between mating parts may entrap drill chips and debris and also can allow fiber breakout and/or delaminations in the composite structure; this is discussed further in the Section "Hole Quality" in this article.

Shimming is the process of filling the gap between mating parts using either solid shims, liquid shim (moldable plastic), or a combination of both. Typically, engineering should evaluate an assembly to determine if some minor gaps can be tolerated and when shimming will be required. With this determined, additional guidelines may be established to identify when assembly personnel may automatically fabricate and install shims and when engineering is required to evaluate a gap. For example, in some aircraft assemblies, gaps up to 0.13 mm (0.005 in.) may be left unshimmed, gaps from 0.15 to 0.76 mm (0.006–0.030 in.) may be liquid (moldable plastic) shimmed, or a combination of a flat solid shim plus liquid shim may be used to accommodate tapered gaps. Gaps exceeding 0.76 mm (0.030 in.) require engineering evaluation. When determining if gaps are present, specific load application requirements must be specified in order to uniformly preload the parts to an acceptable level and not damage the parts. The amount of preload should be specified by engineering and may be limited to "thumb and forefinger" pressure, or the tightening of temporary fasteners or clamps to specified torque levels. Any gaps remaining after application of controlled preload are evaluated for shimming.

Solid shims can be fabricated from either solid metal, prelaminated metallic sheets, or from prefabricated laminated composite material. Assembly personnel must be given guidelines as to which materials will be acceptable. When specifying solid or laminated metallic materials, material compatibility must be considered to eliminate "built-in" corrosion problems. For example, aluminum shims should not be used if they will be in contact with carbon/epoxy composite structure. Since assembly personnel will be required to adjust the shim thickness if the gap is tapered, choose shim materials that can be easily shaped or cut in the production environment.

Liquid shim materials are often more advantageous than attempting to fabricate a complex tapered shim from solid materials. Assembly personnel fill gaps with the liquid shim, clamp the parts together under proper preload, and remove excess shim material squeezed from the joint. Since liquid shim materials are usually filled two-part epoxies, the elapsed time for the shimming operation may be as long as 8 to 24 h due to the cure time before additional assembly operations can continue.

When using solid or liquid shims, the shim material should be bonded to one surface of the mating parts. The key to good adhesion is surface preparation. Carefully follow the manufacturer's surface preparation procedures. Once shimming operations are completed, hole generation can begin.

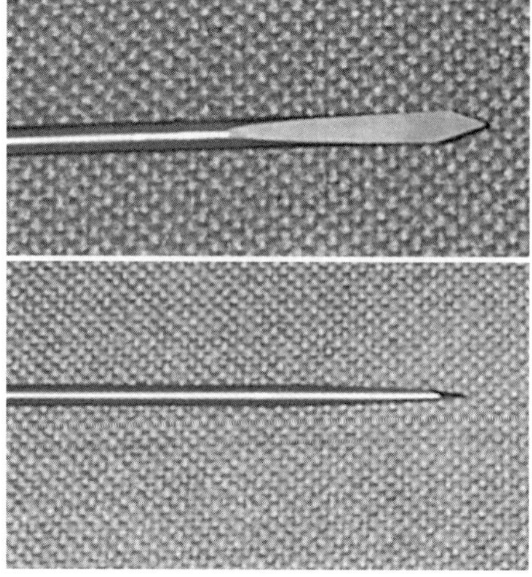

Fig. 1 A flat flute drill for drilling carbon/epoxy composites

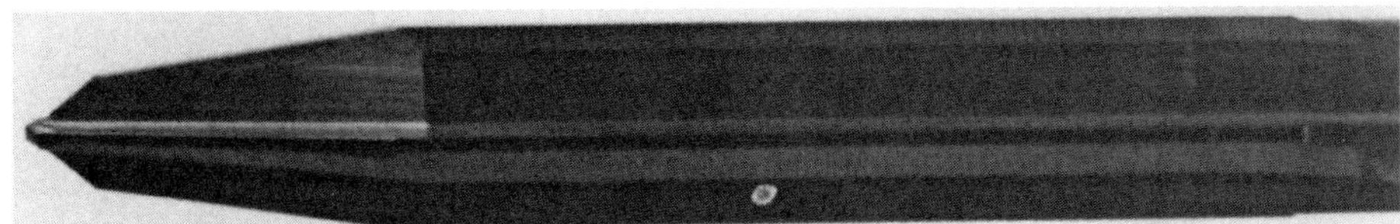

Fig. 2 Four-flute drilling/reaming cutter for carbon/epoxy composites

Drilling Considerations

Hole generation is very dependent on the materials in the joint and their stack-up. If the joint is all carbon/epoxy composite, special flat flute drills or similar four-flute drills have successfully produced quality holes in equipment operating from 2000 to 20,000+ rpm. Figure 1 shows a flat flute drill commonly used by hand-drilling techniques in 2000 to 3000 rpm drill motors. A four-flute drill used for hand drilling at 18,000 to 20,000 rpm usually with hard tooling is shown in Fig. 2. One key to successful hole drilling is feed control. If the cutters are hand fed through the materials with no controls, composite materials are susceptible to breakout damage and delaminations. Two methods to reduce this damage are: use of a hydraulic dash pot or control feed equipment (Fig. 3), which restricts the surging of the drill as it exits the composite material, and use of woven materials or barrier plies. One or two layers of woven material, which is less susceptible to breakout, can be designed into the part at its outer plies. If a composite part is in contact with a metallic part such as carbon/epoxy mated to aluminum, the woven ply on the composite part that mates the aluminum part can be a fiberglass ply, which provides corrosion protection in addition to reducing fiber breakout. For cases where no metallic structure provides backup support, it may be necessary to use a metallic plate or sheet as backup to avoid breakout. Figures 4 and 5 show the effect of proper utilization of a metallic backup plate in reducing exit-hole breakout.

Back counterboring is a condition that can occur when carbon/epoxy parts mate metal substructure parts. The back edge of the hole in the carbon/epoxy part can be eroded or radiused by metal chips being pulled through the composite. The condition is more prevalent when there are gaps between the parts or when the metal debris is stringy rather than small chips. Back counterboring can be minimized or eliminated by changing feeds and speeds, cutter geometry, better part clamp-up, adding a final ream pass, using a peck drill operation, or combinations of these.

If a composite part is sandwiched between two metallic parts, minimal drilling difficulties should occur. When drilling combinations of composite parts with metal parts, the metal parts may govern the drilling speed. For example, even though titanium is compatible with carbon/epoxy material from a corrosion perspective, slower drilling speeds (about 0.12 m/s, or 25 sfm) are required in order to ensure no metallurgical damage occurs to the titanium.

Carbon/epoxy is very abrasive to cutters, so carbide tools are a must for any significant drill life. Small diameter high-speed steel (HSS) drills, such as No. 40 drills used to manually drill pilot holes, are typically used because carbide drills are relatively brittle and are easily broken. The relatively low cost of these small HSS drills offsets the limited life expectancy. High-speed

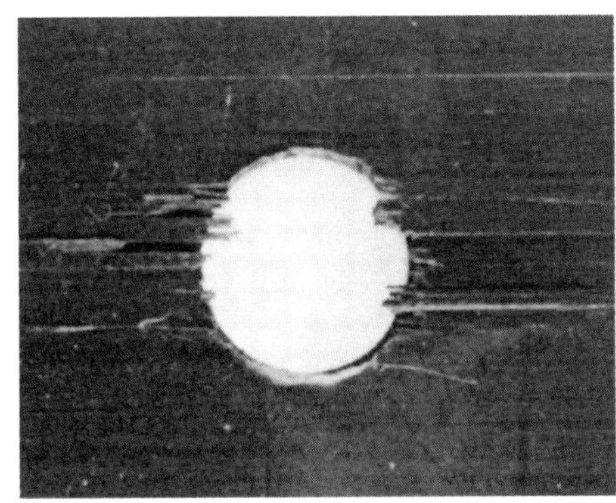

Fig. 4 Typical hole exit splintering damage from drilling without a backup

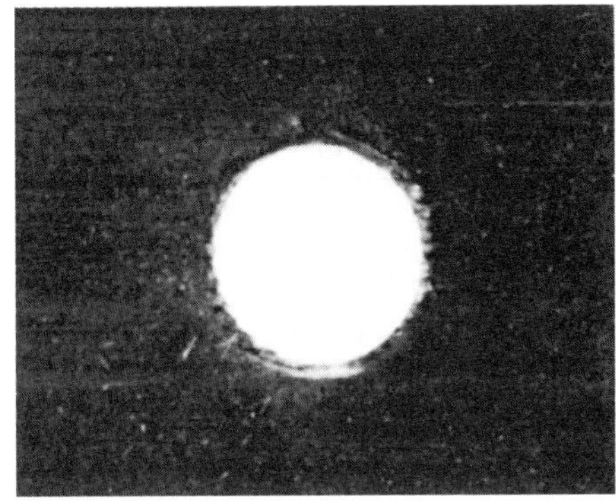

Fig. 5 Clean hole exit condition when using a backup

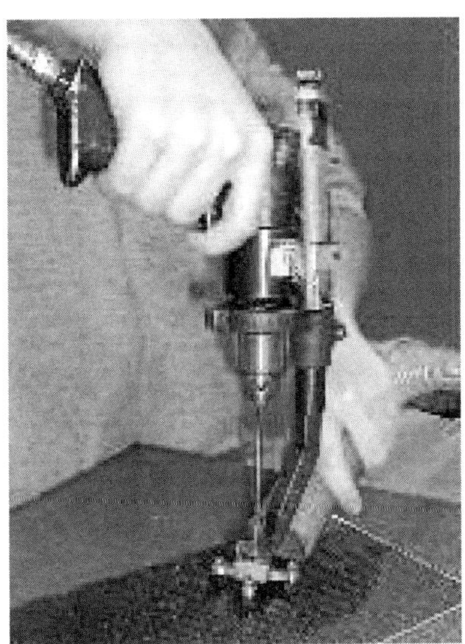

Fig. 3 Hand-feed drill motor with hydraulic dash pot for feed control

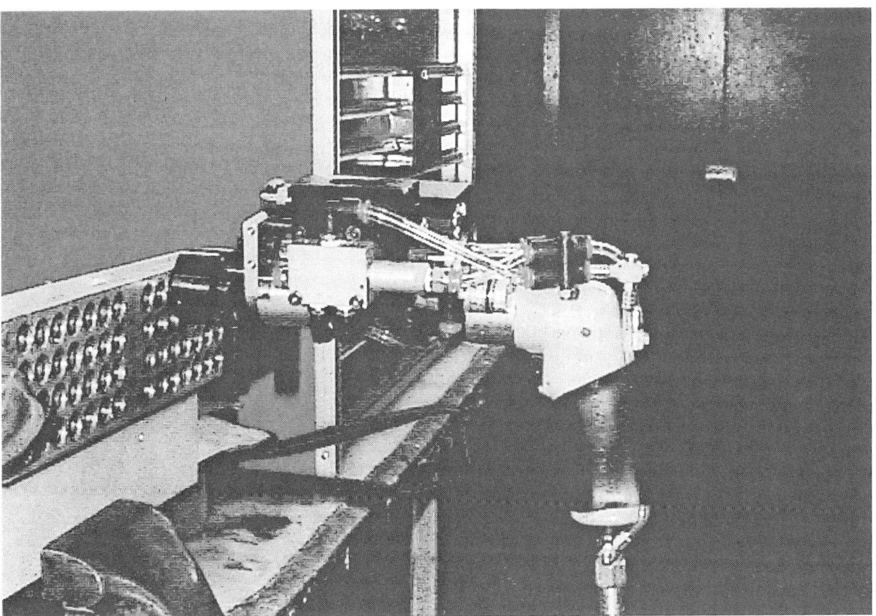

Fig. 6 Power feed tool with hard tooling plates

steel drills may last for only one hole. The most common problem with carbide cutters used in hand-drill operations is handling damage (chipped edges) to cutters. A sharp drill with a slow constant feed can produce a 0.1 mm (0.004 in.) tolerance hole through carbon/epoxy plus thin aluminum, especially if a drill guide is used. With hard tooling, tighter tolerances can be maintained. When the structure under the carbon/epoxy is titanium, drills can pull titanium chips through the carbon/epoxy and enlarge the hole. In this case, a final ream operation may be required to hold tight-hole tolerances.

Aramid fiber (Kevlar)/epoxy composites are difficult to drill unless special cutters are used because the fibers tend to fray or shred unless they are cut clean while embedded in the epoxy. Thus, drills with special "clothes pin" points and "fish tail" points have been developed that slice the fibers prior to pulling them out of the drilled hole. If the Kevlar/epoxy part is sandwiched between two metal parts, standard twist drills can be used.

Use of power-feed drill motors with hard tooling (Fig. 6) is very beneficial for drilling holes in composite or composite/metal joints because the uniform feed rate can prolong the drill life and control fiber breakout as the drill exits the composite. Again, speeds of 2000 to 3000 rpm with a 0.05 to 0.1 mm/rev (0.002–0.004 in./rev) feed rate have been very successful. Slower or faster speeds and feed rates may prove better for some applications.

Peck drilling is a method that uses hard tooling and a power-feed drill motor with lock-in type nose bushings. Peck drilling is a repetitive process of the drill advancing to ever-increasing depths and then withdrawing from the hole to clear the debris and dissipate heat. This "woodpecking" action continues until the hole is complete (Fig. 7). For deep holes, the drill can be rapid advanced almost to the surface to be cut, then slows to the preset drilling feed rate to complete another peck cycle. The rapid advance reduces the drilling time, and stopping the rapid advance short prevents damage to the drill, which extends drill life. Peck drilling can be advantageous for drilling through material stack-ups as thick as 38 mm (1.5 in.).

Automated drilling/fastener installation equipment has been successfully used with composite structures due to its controlled clamp-up, speeds, feed rates, drill/countersink combination cutters, repeatable fastener insertions, and collar swaging/tightening that are designed into the equipment. Automated equipment using numerical control (NC) programs can use hole-drilling techniques and benefits of hard tooling type operations without the hard tooling costs. The equipment can be combined with vision systems that can scan and "memorize" substructure locations prior to laying skins in position for drill-out. Another type of vision system can be used to locate key index or clamp holes tying a skin to substructure with the vision system "correcting" the programmed hole pattern to the actual key index/clamp hole positions. Many automated systems offer controlled clamp-up capabilities to minimize or eliminate gaps between parts. Most automated systems are extremely rigid, allowing drilling through thick stack-ups while using comparatively brittle cutters. Just as carbide cutters offer cutter life benefits over HSS cutters, polycrystalline diamond (PCD) cutters offer improved cutter life over carbide drills. Due to their brittle nature, PCD cutters require a rigid setup such as that offered by automated equipment to take advantage of their longer tool life.

Automated equipment can be programmed for fixed speeds and feed rates, for peck drilling, or for combinations of both. With correct selection of drills, feeds, and speeds, holes with a 0.076 mm (0.003 in.) tolerance can be produced in carbon/epoxy over aluminum structures using automated equipment. The drill/countersink combination cutters are especially beneficial as they ensure good alignment between the hole and countersink. These cutters have not been very successful in hand-drilling operations as hole size tolerance can be lost when the countersink portion of the cutter begins cutting. Automated equipment can be used just to prepare the holes, such as the Boeing F/A-18 C/D Wing Automated Drilling System (ADS) (Fig. 8), or the equipment can prepare the holes and install the fasteners, such as the Boeing F/A-18 E/F Wing Automated Drilling System (ADS) (Fig. 9).

Cutting fluids are not normally used or recommended for drilling thin (less than 6.3 mm, or 0.25 in. thick) carbon/epoxy structure. The

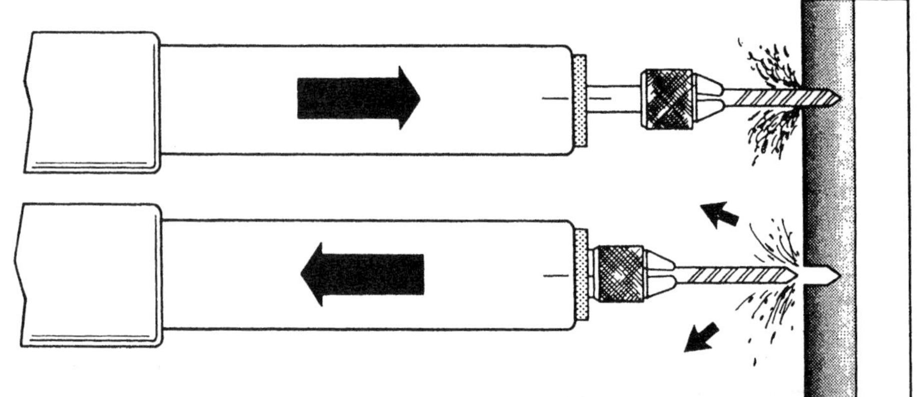

Fig. 7 Peck drilling in which drill advances into material, retracts, cools, and cleans chips before repeating the process

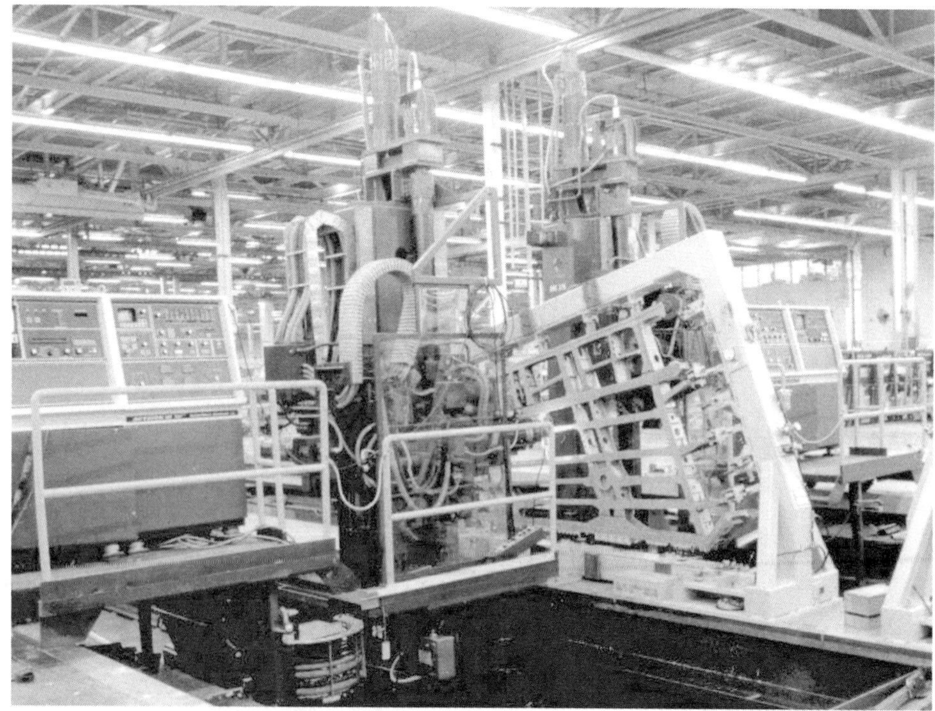

Fig. 8 Automated system for drilling fastener holes in wings

"dust" resulting from the drill process is broken fibers still encapsulated in resin so that they do not float freely in air. Industry practice has been to use a vacuum fixture or hose at the point of drilling and to use a vacuum to clean the structures after drilling. If cutting fluids are used, flood application is preferred to a light spray mist to avoid the dust from collecting or building up on the cutting tool, as this may result in an oversized hole.

Reaming

When acceptable hole tolerances cannot be maintained from a hole-drilling process, a reaming operation is needed. As with drilling, carbide cutters are needed for holes through carbon/epoxy composite structure. In addition, the exit end of the hole needs good support to prevent splintering and delaminations when the reamer removes more than about 0.13 mm (0.005 in.) on the diameter. The support can be the substructure or a board held firmly against the back surface. Typical reaming speeds are done at about one-half of the drilling speed. When the reamer removes about 0.13 mm (0.005 in.) or less on the diameter and surge control is used, the hole can be reamed without backup with little or no splintering or fiber breakout, especially if the composite parts have woven materials as outer layers or if there are bonded-on shims.

Countersinking

Countersinking a composite structure is required when flush head fasteners are to be installed in the assembly. For metallic structures, a 100° included angle shear or tension head fastener has been the typical approach. In composite structures, two types of fasteners are commonly used: a 100° included angle tension head fastener or a 130° included angle head fastener. The advantage of the 130° head is that the fastener head can have about the same diameter as a tension head 100° fastener with the head depth of a shear-type head 100° fastener. For seating flush fasteners in composite parts, it is recommended that the countersink cutters be designed to produce a controlled radius between the hole and the countersink to accommodate the head-to-shank fillet radius on the fasteners. In addition, a chamfer operation or a washer may be required to provide proper clearance for protruding head fastener head-to-shank radii. Whichever head style is used, a matching countersink/chamfer must be prepared in the composite structure.

There are three recommended choices of cutting tools for producing a countersink in carbon/epoxy structure: standard carbide insert cutters, solid carbide cutters, or PCD insert cutters. For carbon/epoxy structure, the countersink cutters usually have straight flutes similar to those used on metals. For aramid fiber/epoxy composites, testing has shown that a countersink that incorporates S-shaped positive rake cutting flutes produces a fuzz-free countersink edge. If straight-fluted countersink cutters are used, a special thick tape can be applied to the surface to allow for a clean cutting of the Kevlar fibers, but this is not as effective as the S-shaped fluted cutters, as shown in Fig. 10. Use of piloted countersink cutters is recommended because it ensures better concentricity between the hole and the countersink with less chance of gaps under the fasteners due to misalignment or delaminations of the part. A combination drill/countersink cutter ensures a good fit; however, thus far these cutters have been successful only in automated equipment scenarios. Typical countersinking operations are done at about 500 to 1000 rpm (depending on countersink diameter—larger countersinks are done slower) with vacuum attachments to catch debris.

Depth control for countersinking can be obtained by inserting the countersink cutter in a microstop cage (Fig. 11) and adjusting accordingly. Proper countersink size can be measured using commercially available countersink diameter/depth gages, but only with a gage designed for the correct countersink included angle. A countersink gage designed for 100° included angle countersinks cannot be used on 130° included angle countersinks as incorrect readings will occur. Another inspection technique is to verify the countersink size with the same type of fastener specified for the hole fully clamped in the part and check the flushness. When a piloted countersink cutter is used, the pilot must be periodically checked for wear, as wear can cause reduction of concentricity between the hole and countersink. This is especially true for countersink cutters with only one cutting edge.

For piloted countersink cutters, position the pilot in the hole and bring the cutter to full rpm before beginning to feed the cutter into the hole and preparing the countersink. If the cutter is in contact with the composite before triggering the drill motor, splintering may result.

Hole Quality

The quality of the drilled hole is critical; therefore, each hole should be visually inspected to ensure correct hole size and location and proper normality, as well as the absence of unacceptable splintering or fiber breakout, fiber pullout, delaminations, back counterboring, evidence of heat damage, and microcracking.

Delamination, separation of bonded composite plies, may occur at the drill entrance due to

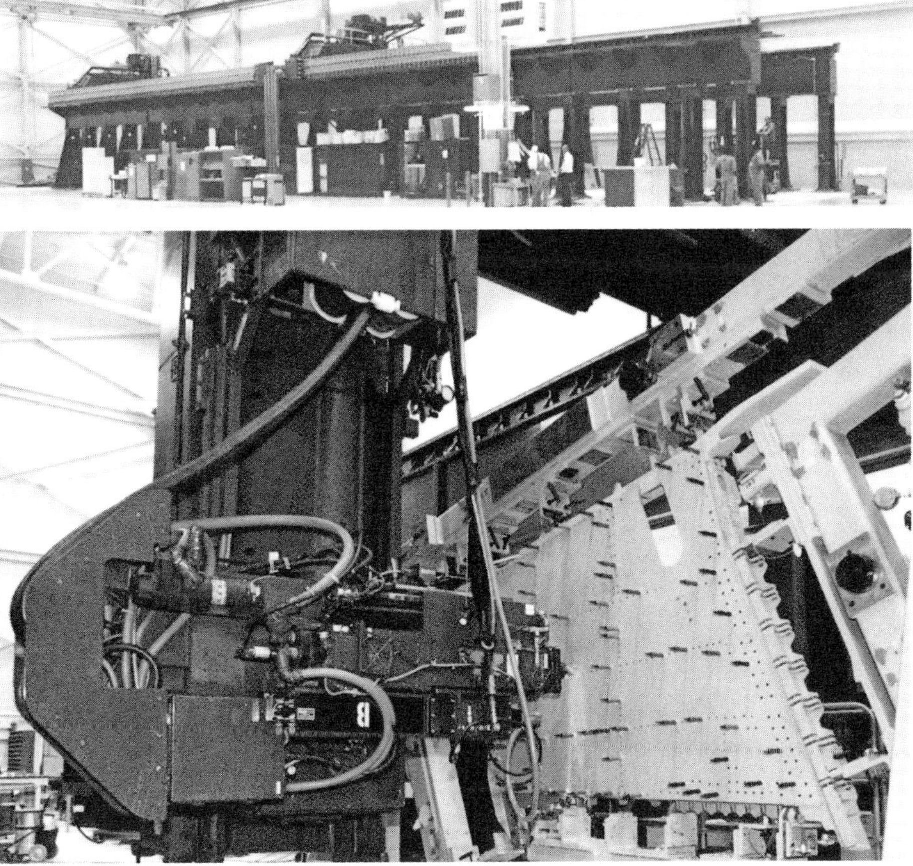

Fig. 9 Automated system for drilling holes and installing fasteners in wings

too fast of a feed rate for the speed, or at the drill exit due to too much feed force on unsupported materials. Splintering or fiber breakout conditions, fibers that break free from the surrounding resin matrix, may occur at the drill entrance or exit, especially in unidirectional material (Fig. 4). Fiber/resin pullout is a tear or breaking out of fibers and/or resin within a hole or machined edge. Microcracking is the creation of small cracks in the resin surrounding the fibers. Visual discoloration or partial melting of material surrounding a hole (usually worst on the drill exit side) is an indication of heat damage.

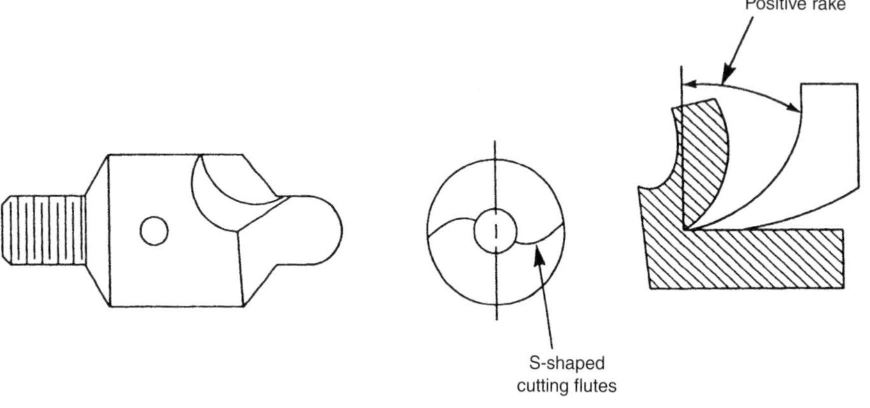

Fig. 10 Optimal countersink cutter for aramid fiber-reinforced composites

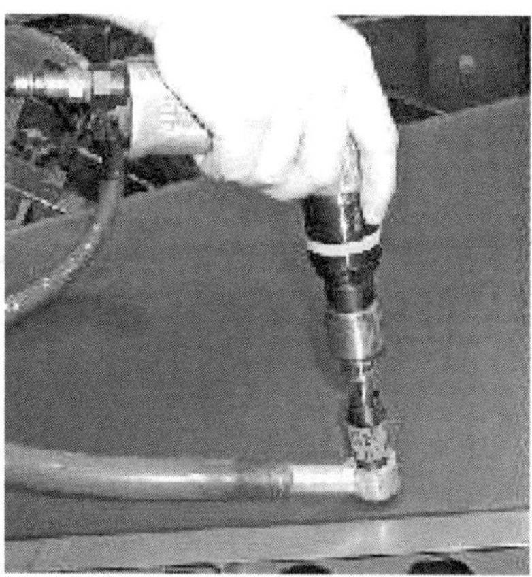

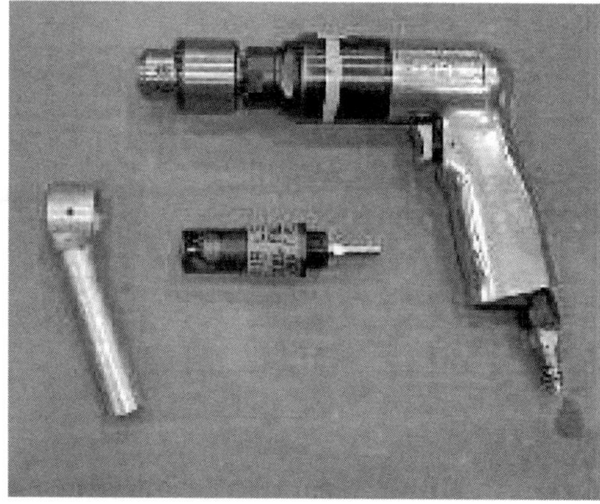

Fig. 11 Microstop cage for adjustable, controlled-depth countersinking

The required hole quality for the product must be defined to ensure the product will meet structural requirements and desired cosmetic requirements. Following is a general rule for acceptance of anomalies.

Defects smaller than a defined size (for example, 0.76 mm, or 0.03 in.) are acceptable "as-is." Defects a little larger but within a specified range (for example, 0.76–2.54 mm, or 0.03–0.10 in.) are rejectable but are automatically repaired, while those greater than the rejectable limit (for example, 2.54 mm, or 0.10 in.) are submitted to Engineering for determination if a repair (such as oversize fastener or filling of the defect) is an option or if part scrapage is required. The size limits may be dependent on location, structural loads, and cosmetics. If repairs are required for structural or cosmetic reasons, care must be taken to make good quality repairs. If repair materials are not carefully applied, the repaired part may be weaker than the damaged part. An example of such a condition is if the repair causes a buildup on one side of a fastener and thus a bad fit. The bad fit can produce bending loads in the fastener and highly concentrated bearing loads in the composite.

In addition to visual checks, the normal inspection methods and techniques for meeting dimensional requirements of the hole and countersink should be used.

SELECTED REFERENCES

- J.A. Boldt and J.P. Chanani, Solid-Tool Machining and Drilling, *Composites*, Vol 1, *Engineered Materials Handbook,* ASM International, 1987, p 667–672
- J.J. Kilwin, "Machining and Drilling Composites," Process Specifications (PS) 14111, Boeing—St. Louis, 1999
- J.L Phillips and R.T. Parker, Fastener Hole Considerations, *Composites*, Vol 1, *Engineered Materials Handbook*, ASM International, 1987, p 712–715

Mechanical Fastener Selection

Robert T. Parker, Boeing Commercial Airplane Company

FASTENER REQUIREMENTS for joining fiber reinforced composite structures differ from those for joining metallic structures. Fastener selection considerations for joining composites include corrosion compatibility, fastener materials, strength, stiffness, head configurations, importance of clamp-up, hole fit, and lightning protection.

When fiber reinforced composite materials began to be used in aerospace and aircraft structures, the inadequacy of conventional fasteners became apparent. Alloy steel was not compatible, cadmium plating quickly corroded away, reduced shear head fasteners pulled through during installation, and rivets crushed the composite or expanded in the hole and caused delamination of the laminated plies. A new set of requirements had to be established to determine which characteristics were optimal and which were detrimental. This article focuses mainly on carbon fiber composites; however, many of the principles discussed apply to aramid and glass fiber composites also. Corrosion compatibility would be less of a problem with noncarbon fibers, but then lightning-strike behavior may be more of a concern.

Additional information about general fastener selection criteria can be found in the article "Mechanical Testing of Threaded Fasteners and Bolted Joints" in *Mechanical Testing and Evaluation*, Volume 8 of *ASM Handbook*.

Corrosion Compatibility

Neither fiberglass nor aramid fiber reinforced composites cause corrosion problems when used with most fastener materials. Composites reinforced with carbon fibers, however, are quite cathodic when used with materials such as aluminum or cadmium, the latter of which is a common plating used on fasteners for corrosion protection.

Titanium and its alloys appear to be the fastener materials most compatible with carbon fibers. Fortunately, titanium alloys have the most desirable strength/weight ratio. Austenitic stainless steels, superalloys such as A286, multiphase alloys such as MP35N or MP159, and nickel alloys such as alloy 718 also appear to be very compatible with carbon fiber composites. Pitting corrosion has been seen in A286 under certain conditions. Copper-bearing alloys such as copper-nickel or Monel have a tendency to generate heavy corrosion products, although damage or loss of strength appears to be minimal.

Fastener Materials and Strength Considerations

Titanium alloy Ti-6Al-4V is the most common alloy for fasteners used with carbon fiber reinforced composite structures. Ultimate tensile and shear strengths for Ti-6Al-4V are 1100 and 660 MPa (160 and 95 ksi), respectively. Ti-3Al-2.5V and commercially pure titanium are used for some components of fastening systems. When higher strength is required, materials such as A286 or alloy 718 that have been strengthened by cold working can be used. Cold worked A286 fasteners can be obtained with an ultimate tensile strength of 1400 MPa (200 ksi) and an ultimate shear strength of 760 (110 ksi). The respective values for alloy 718 (cold worked) are 1515 and 860 MPa (220 and 125 ksi). Multiphase alloys

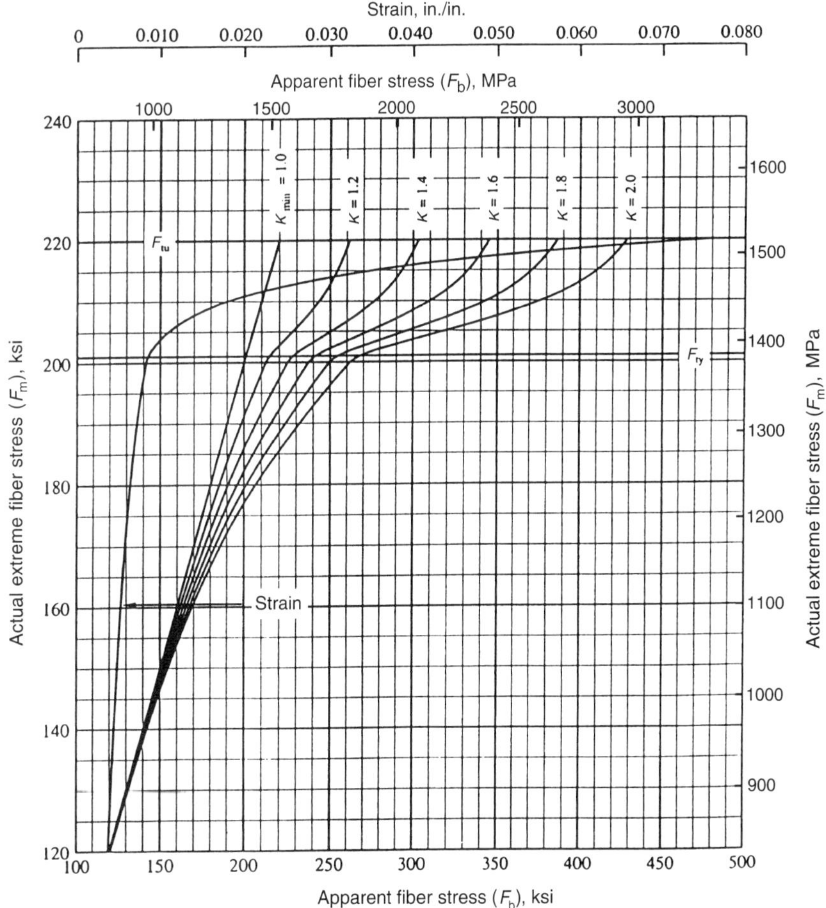

Fig. 1 Example of plastic bending curves for nickel alloy 718. F_{tu}, ultimate tensile strength; F_{ty}, yield strength.

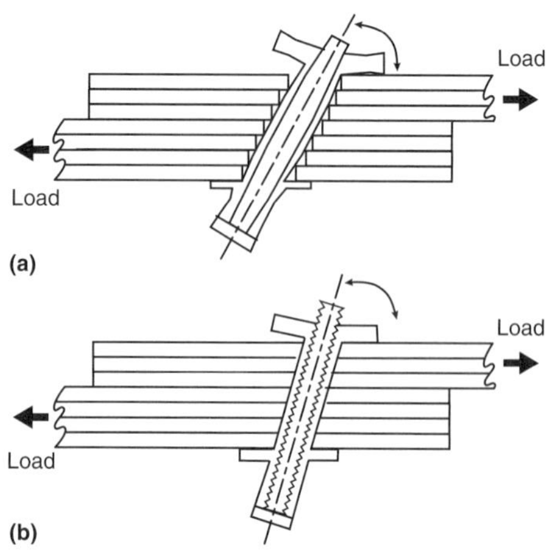

Fig. 2 Blind fastener bolt bending and deflection. (a) Smooth bore allows little resistance to bolt bending in multiple piece fasteners such as blind fasteners. The multiple pieces act as axial laminates and slide over each other. (b) The effect of the threads on the corebolt "lock" the corebolt to the other components and improve stiffness of the joint. However, the notches (threads) can be detrimental in fatigue if the loads are high enough to cause significant deflections.

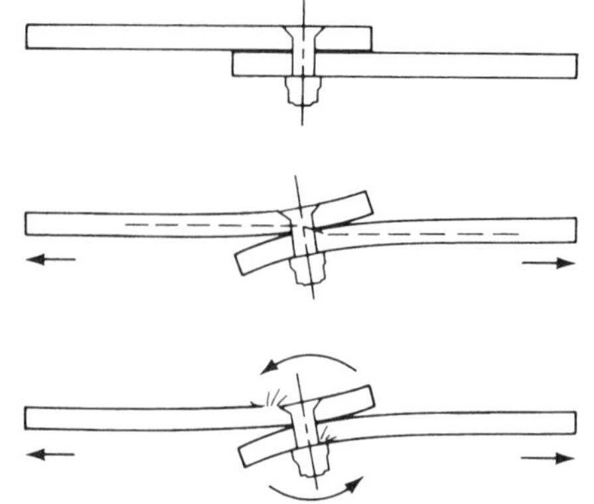

Fig. 3 Single fastener lap shear specimen in uniaxial tension

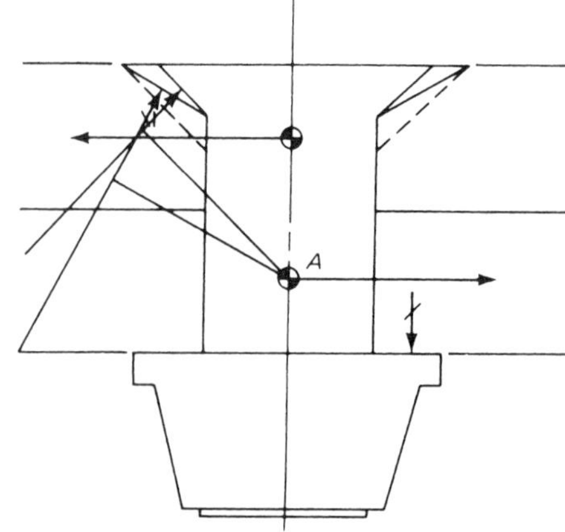

Fig. 4 Reaction loads of a flush head fastener in uniaxial tension

can be obtained with a tensile strength up to 1800 MPa (260 ksi). In the past, multiphase alloys were only used as blind fastener stems or corebolts where ultra-high strength was required for the fastener to function. Today, multiphase bolts are being considered to replace alloy 718 where loads are increasing due to growth of some aircraft models. However, in composite structure, it takes a very thick structure to warrant the high shear strength (F_{su} = 910 to 1000 MPa, or 132 to 145 ksi) of multiphase alloys.

Bolt Bending

Bolt bending is a much more serious issue in composite structure than in metal structure. Due to the increased interlaminar shear between the composite plies (similar to playing cards in a deck sliding past each other during bending), bending of the bolt occurs more easily. High-modulus and high-tensile-strength fastener material is desired where bending may occur. Stress-strain curve shape factor also plays a role. An example of a plastic bending curve is shown in Fig. 1 for alloy 718 cold reduced to tensile strength of 1515 MPa (220 ksi). Susceptibility of bolt bending in composite structure introduces higher reaction loads on the fastener head; this requires more careful consideration of head configuration.

Bending must also be considered in multiple-component fasteners such as blind fasteners. A threaded core bolt resists bending much better than a smooth bore pull-type blind fastener (Fig. 2); however, where fatigue loads may be present, the notches from the threads may influence the joint life. The threaded core bolt is usually capable of higher clamping forces (good for fatigue), but if eccentricity in the joint exists, the bending of the threads may still be undesirable. The designer must consider all of these variables, and then testing is required to evaluate the performance of the selected fasteners versus the design requirements.

Head Configuration Selection

Many fastener head styles exist in industry today: 100° reduced shear, 100° tension, AN 509, low-profile protruding, 12-point fatigue rated, and so forth. Because of their viscoelastic matrix resin properties, carbon fiber reinforced composites are more sensitive to high bearing loads than are metals. This means fastener heads (as well as nuts and collars) should be designed with as much bearing surface area as practicable.

The 130° reduced-height shear head originated during development of a suitable blind fastener specifically designed for composite structures and introduced to the industry in 1980 (Ref 1). By examining a single-fastener lap shear joint specimen loaded in uniaxial tension (Fig. 3), it can be seen that as the load is transferred through the fastener, an eccentricity begins to develop, and fastener tipping, or "cocking," occurs. This specimen was used to optimize flush head configurations and measure the contribution of the fastener to the stability of the specimen by delaying cocking and eventual pull-through. Figure 4 shows the reaction loads on the head. Assuming that the specimen loads act through the centroids of the fastener, and taking moments about *A*, it can be shown that very little change is noted by changing the angle of the head; the big difference is in the area of bearing that supports the reaction load. From this analysis, the 130° flush

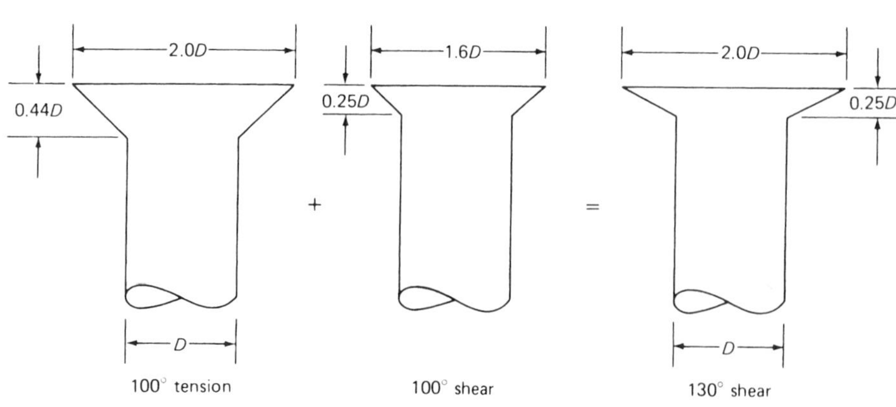

Fig. 5 Development of 130° head for shear

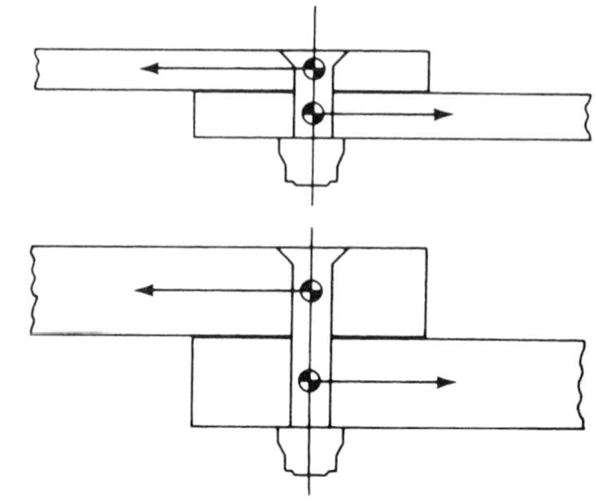

Fig. 6 Load distribution in fasteners joining thin and thick laminates

head was developed. The maximum area for a reduced-height shear head was obtained by using the tension head outer diameter; this resulted in 130°, as shown in Fig. 5. As the distance between the centroids becomes greater, however, the reaction loads go up in value, as demonstrated in Fig. 6. Therefore, the 130° is limited to thin laminates as shown in Fig. 7 where a standard shear head would cause a knife-edge condition, and the 100° reduced-height shear head would pull through more easily. As the laminate gets thicker by design, the standard shear head can be considered (up to 70% of the laminate thickness). It is best to use the tension head where possible (laminate thickness permitting) since that head will do best in bolt bending or pull-through. The smaller heads (lower head height) should only be used to accommodate thin laminates and prevent a knife-edge condition.

Several protruding head configurations are available, but are not as sensitive as flush heads in joint performance. Cole (Ref 2) used different testing and analyses, including fatigue, and arrived at essentially the same conclusions.

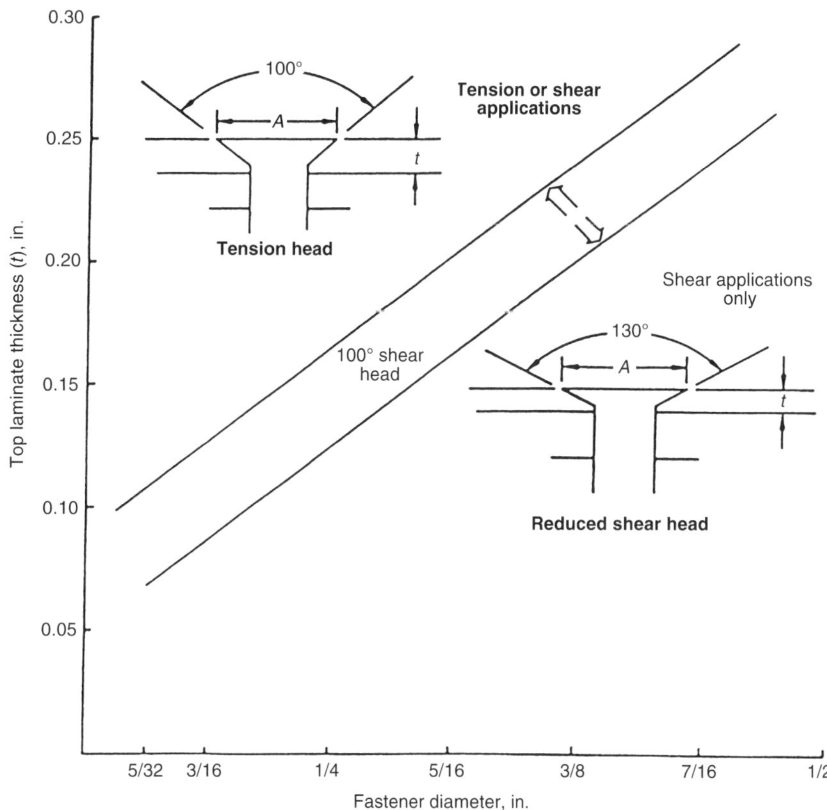

Fig. 7 Flush head applications for composite structures. The fastener head height should not exceed 70% of t, where t is the top sheet thickness. Head diameter, A, is the same for 100° tension and 130° reduced shear fasteners. Head diameter is 0.88 to 0.93A for 100° shear head fasteners.

Clamp-Up

When clearance fit holes are used, high clamp-up appears to be beneficial for joint strength and fatigue life. The clamping forces, however, must be spread out over a sufficient area so that the compressive strength of the resin system is not exceeded and the composite crushed. The role played by high clamp-up produces friction load transfer and delays cocking of the fastener in a loaded joint, which in turn may reduce ratcheting during cyclic loading. An improvement in fatigue performance has been shown from high clamp-up. Pratt (Ref 3) also found that high fastener preload, as well as large head bearing areas, were key factors influencing high lap shear joint strengths in composite structures. Phillips (Ref 4) found that load transfer fatigue testing with carbon fiber composites shows that gross load and stress concentration factors (K_t) at holes are not as critical. What is critical is bearing stress, because most failures are bearing-type failures caused by the fastener cocking under load and producing a high localized bearing stress. High clamp-up also delays slippage of the composite plies, which contributes to the high concentration of bearing stresses, as illustrated in Fig. 8. On the downside, continuous high clamp-up cannot be assumed or guaranteed over long periods of time. The time-dependent nature of composites can result in significant clamp-up relaxation during typical service lifetimes. Often, design data must be generated to account for this, by testing joints with fasteners installed at typically 50% of normal installation torque (Ref 5).

Chamfering of Holes

Whether or not chamfering should be required for composite structures to accommodate the head-to-shank fillet radius of protruding head fasteners has been debated. This author has seen data that show no obvious detrimental effects and an actual slight increase in lap joint strength with a measurable higher yield by not chamfering. In theory, the deformation of the material under the fillet radius of the fastener compresses the composite down into the hole-clearance, making a tighter fit and reducing fastener cocking. A comparison is shown in Fig. 9. Another theory is that the compression and bending of the fibers at the entrance of the hole "softens" the composite, reducing the theoretical stress concentration factor (K_t) and letting the composite behave in a less brittle manner. Part of the debate is "damage is damage," and water or other contaminants can migrate in. On the other hand, chamfering causes a loss of bearing area.

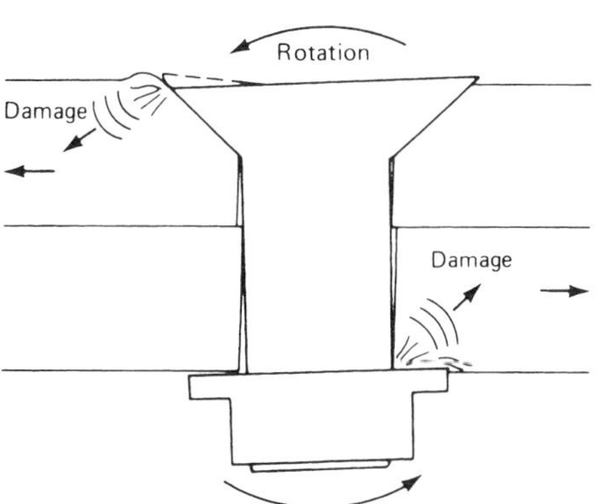

Fig. 8 Slippage of composite plies under load

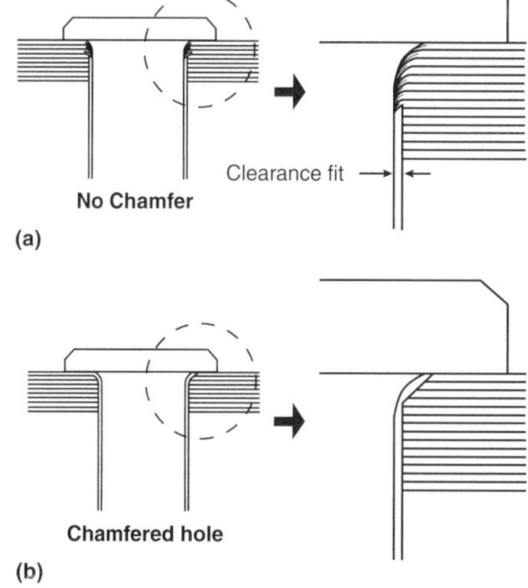

Fig. 9 Effect of chamfering holes. (a) Without chamfer, the composite material is compressed (displaced by fastener radius) and forced into hole clearance giving the effect of a net fit at the top of the hole. (b) Loss of composite material (chamfer) reduces bearing area and allows fastener to slip back and forth in clearance hole.

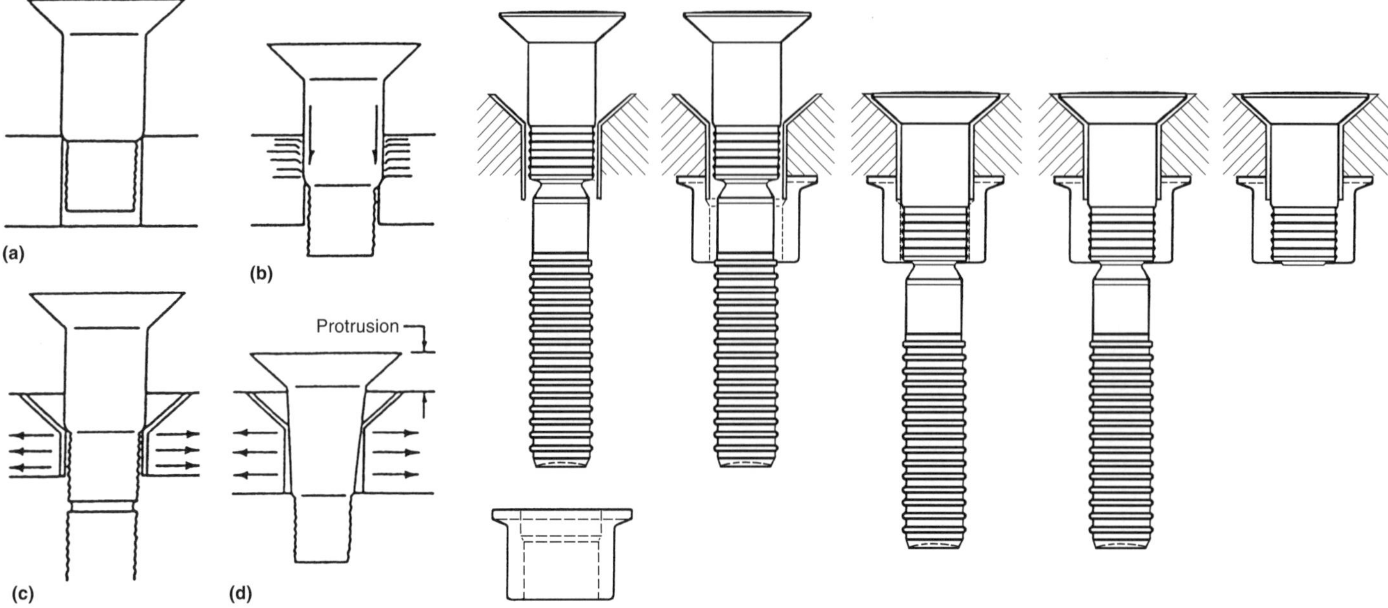

Fig. 10 Interference fit. See text for discussion.

Fig. 11 Sleeve-type Lockbolt installation sequence

Nonchamfering should be limited to shear-type protruding head fasteners. Tension and fatigue rated protruding head type fasteners, with a large head-to-shank radius, still require a chamfered washer under the head.

Interference Fit Fasteners

Another method of delaying cocking of the fastener under joint loading is to support the fastener for its full length. A net fit would be ideal, although impractical. Fastener manufacturers, working together with airframe companies, have developed methods of accomplishing an interference fit without detriment to joint performance. However, its advantages must be evaluated with regard to added cost and weight. In aluminum structures, bolts are frequently installed in "transition" fits, where, because of tolerance overlap, the bolt may be larger than the hole some percentage of the time. The bolts are pressed in or driven in with a rivet gun, with interference fits up to 0.0760 mm (0.003 in.). Not only does this interference fit in aluminum structures lock up the structure, but the hoop tensile stresses generated reduce the amplitude of the cyclic stresses next to the hole and improve the fatigue life of the joint.

With composite structures, however, driving the same bolt into interference causes high shearing forces on the reinforcing fibers and bends them down, breaking the matrix resin, as illustrated in Fig. 10(a) and (b). Work by Shoe (Ref 6) showed damage at as little as 0.01780 mm (0.0007 in.) of interference by this method. Because composite fibers will accommodate much more compression, a controlled expansion of a sleeve that remains statically in contact with the fibers (as shown in Fig. 10c and d) can produce interference up to 0.1525 mm (0.006 in.). This method was tested on major prototype hardware with excellent results. Unlike aluminum structures, however, composite structures gain no benefit from the greater interference. All that is desired is a "net" fit. The interference is used to absorb the tolerances on the hole and the fastener. Therefore, the interference limit need only be the total accumulation of tolerances to always ensure, at least a net fit, as a minimum.

The major advantages of the net/interference fit are lower joint deflection, equal fastener load sharing, reduction of relative fastener flexibility that causes localized high bearing stresses, and reduction or delay of hole growth/degradation (which can become excessive). An additional advantage is lightning-strike protection, which is a design consideration that is covered in the next section of this article. This author believes that major composite structures, such as a wing or large stabilizer, should have a certain percentage of sleeve-type interference fit fasteners to lock up the structure. Fasteners with all clearance holes can ratchet to one side when the structure is loaded, causing severe permanent deformations. Sleeve-type fasteners (interference fit) could be strategically located to aid in electrical continuity or lightning-strike protection.

Several sleeve-type fasteners are available that are either intended for composite structure or adaptable with hole-size adjustment. Figure 11 shows a Lockbolt (Huck International, Inc.) fastener incorporating a sleeve. The pintail is much

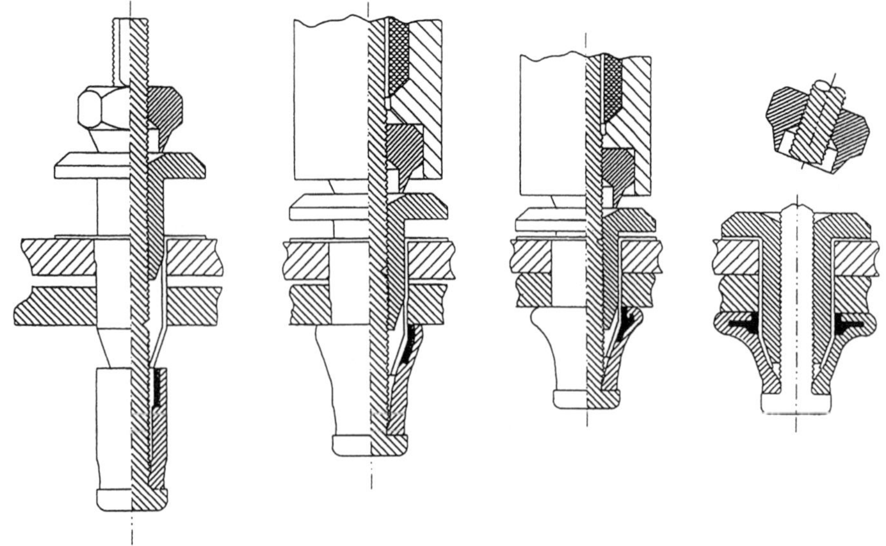

Fig. 12 Radial-Lok sleeve-type blind fastener installation sequence

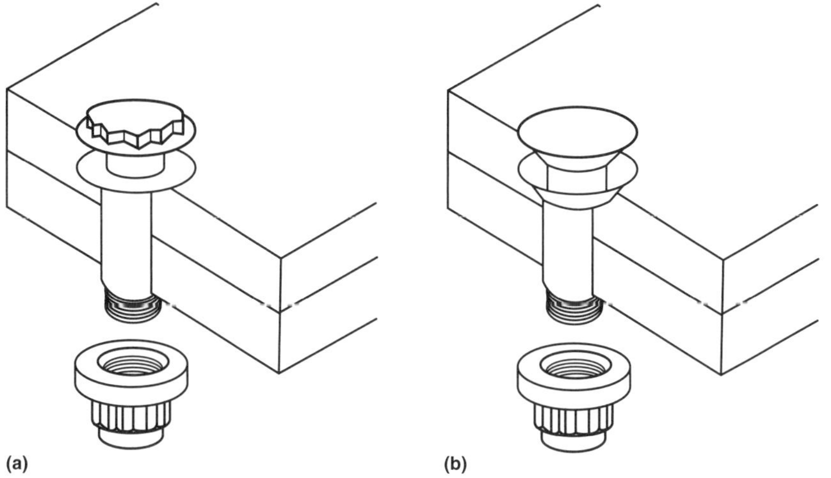

Fig. 13 Typical head styles of the SLEEVbolt fastener. (a) 12-point protruding head. (b) Flush head

longer (function of grip length) since the whole grip protrudes out of the sleeve before installation. The assembly drops into the hole; as the Lockbolt is pulled into the sleeve, the sleeve expands radially a controlled amount to generate the interference. This same principle is incorporated into a threaded-corebolt blind fastener, the Radial-Lok (Monogram Aerospace Fasteners Inc.). With this fastener, the formation of the backside components pull the fastener body into the sleeve, expanding the sleeve and generating interference. Figure 12 shows the installation sequence. Another permanent fastener that has been used in interference in composite structure is the SLEEVbolt (Paul R. Briles Corp.). This fastener consists of a tapered shank bolt in an internally tapered sleeve that is cylindrical on the outside. The 48-to-1 internal taper keeps the bolt travel short during installation. Sufficient exposed threads are engaged with a nut, and the bolt is essentially "jacked" into place. Figure 13 shows two head styles available. Although this bolt was designed for metal structure, it can easily be adapted to composite structure by enlarging the hole and reducing the resultant interference by about 50%. Radial expansion in composites should not exceed about 0.15 mm (0.006 in.) on the diameter.

When interference fit fasteners are required in mixed stack-up structure (composite laminate and metal sheet or plate), the structure is usually disassembled and the holes enlarged in the composite to prevent interference in that portion of the stack-up. Interference fit sleeves can solve this problem. The higher cost of the fastener can be offset by preventing disassembly, enlarging holes, and reassembly. However, caution needs to be exercised in eccentrically loaded joints of mixed stack-ups (thick composite skin with thick metal fitting) when using sleeved fasteners. Due to the low interlaminar shear modulus of laminate composite and the fixity of the metal fitting under cyclic eccentric loading, a concentration of bending occurs at the interface. Under cyclic loading, localized strain hardening of the sleeve at the joint interface occurs, eventually leading to cracking of the sleeve at the interface (Fig. 14).

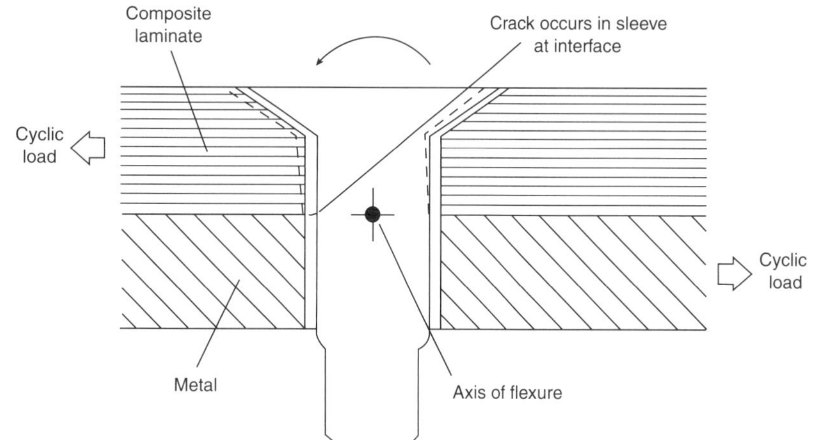

Fig. 14 Strain hardening of sleeved fastener in stack-up of mixed modulus materials, resulting in cracking under cyclic loading

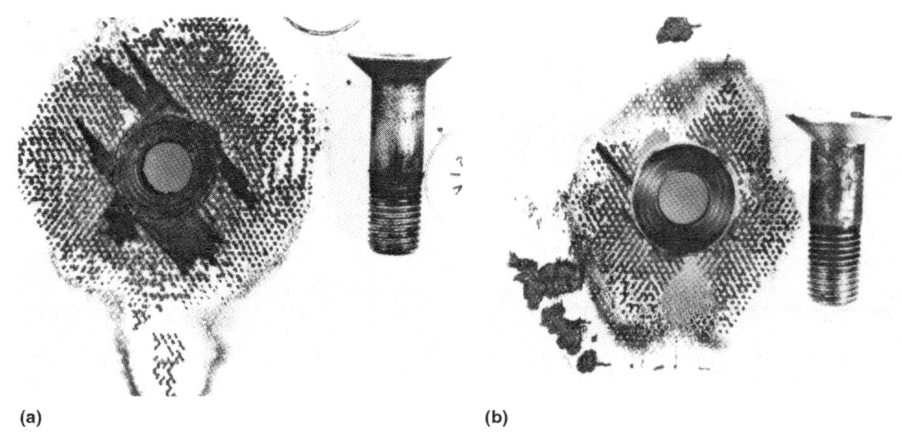

Fig. 15 Effect of corrosion-protection coatings on the lightning-strike resistance of fasteners for composites. (a) Fastener with corrosion protection finish, struck by 100,000 A. Heavy damage to composite. (b) Bare fastener struck by 100,000 A. No damage to composite

Lightning-Strike Protection

An aluminum airplane is quite conductive and is able to dissipate the high currents resulting from a lightning strike. A carbon fiber reinforced composite airplane would act like an anisotropic conductor, that is, not as conductive in all directions. Also, carbon fibers are 1000 times more resistive than aluminum to current flow, and epoxy resin is 1 million times more resistive (i.e., perpendicular to the skin). If the lightning strike attaches to a fastener, the current must be dissipated through the fibers perpendicular to the hole. If the fastener is not in intimate contact with the sides of the hole (clearance fit), the instantaneous heat energy ionizes the air in the gap and creates an arc plasma that blows out, severely damaging the structure. Intimate contact of a bare fastener (and/or sleeve) is the best combination found to date for electrical current dissipation. "Hiding" the fastener from the lightning may also be a solution. A swept-stroke lightning strike (defined as a zone 2 strike) attaching to a fastener head can produce currents

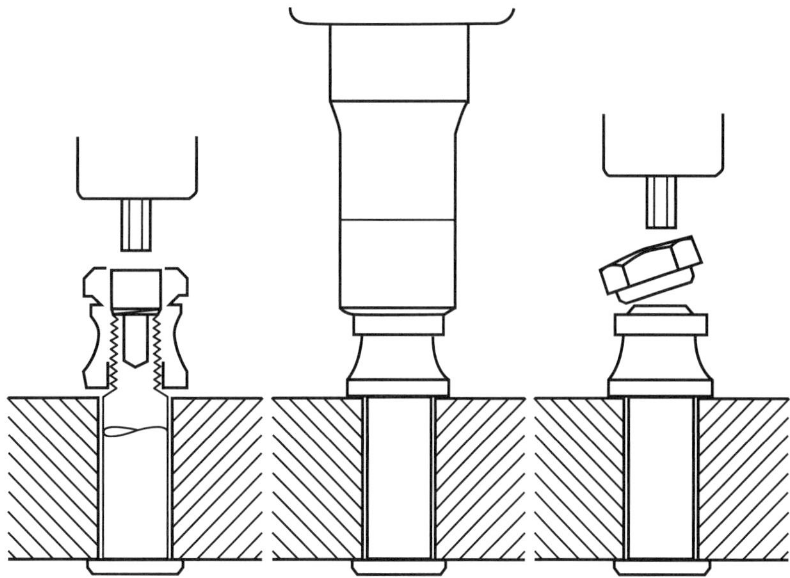

Fig. 16 Typical installation sequence for Hi-Lok fasteners

as high as 100,000 A. This current is conducted for a very short period of time (approximately 0.05 seconds maximum dwell time), but then it must be dissipated in that short time to minimize damage. Brick (Ref 7) has developed a fastener area-current relationship to predict whether a fastener has a large enough countersink and diameter to dissipate lightning-strike currents without arc plasma blowby. Although Ref 7 was directed more toward fuel environment, the method can also be used to minimize damage to the composite from lightning strike. Investigators Brick and Gosinsky (Ref 8) have determined that large countersinks (tension heads) with high clamping forces or an interference fit are important factors in the choice of fasteners in a potential lightning-strike area.

Fasteners with corrosion-protection coatings, such as NAS 4006 aluminum-phenolic coating or equivalent, are not recommended in potential lightning-strike areas. Figure 15(a) shows a fastener with a corrosion-protection finish that has been artificially struck with approximately 100,000 A of current. Because the protective finish was an insulator, the current avoided the fastener and attempted to dissipate into the top fibers of the composite with a high-concentration gradient. The composite was heavily damaged several plies deep. In Fig. 15(b), a bare fastener that was struck with identical current intensity shows more damage to the fastener, but almost no damage to the composite plies. It is much easier to replace the fastener than to repair the composite. The grid pattern shown in Fig. 15(a) and (b) is a copper mesh overlay used to help dissipate the current on the surface. A bare finish is preferred on the fastener for maximum conductivity; however, depending on the fastener material, a phosphate fluoride or a passivated finish appears to be acceptable and is usually required for paint adhesion or electrical ground return.

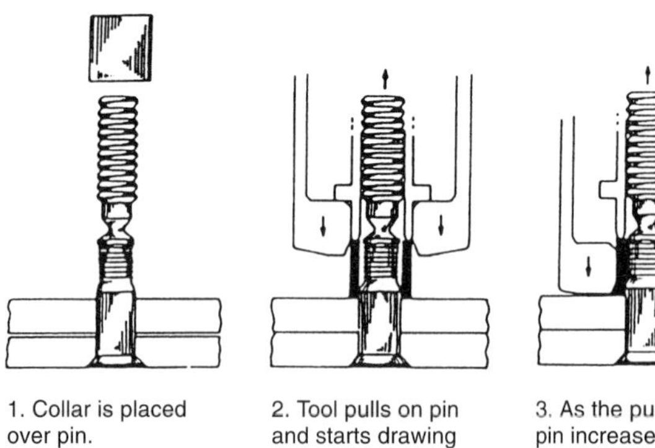

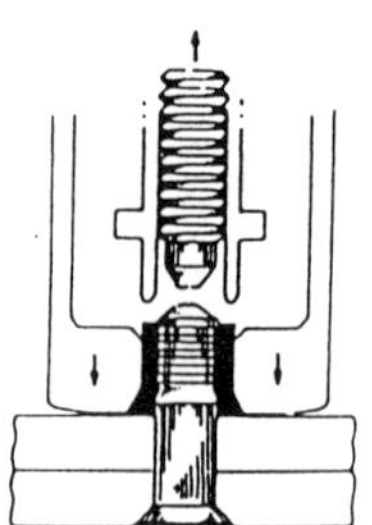

1. Collar is placed over pin.
2. Tool pulls on pin and starts drawing sheets together.
3. As the pull on the pin increases, tool anvil swages collar into locking grooves and a permanent lock is formed.
4. Tool continues to pull until pin breaks at the breakneck groove and is ejected. Tool anvil disengages from swaged collar.

Fig. 17 Typical installation sequence for pull-type Lockbolt fasteners

Hi-Lok and Lockbolt Fasteners

Most composite structures for the aircraft industry are fastened with Hi-Loks (Hi-Shear Corp.) or Lockbolts (Huck International, Inc.), for permanent installations. The Hi-Lok is a threaded fastener that incorporates a hex key in the threaded end to react the torque applied to the collar during installation. The collar includes a frangible portion that separates at a predetermined torque value. Figure 16 shows a typical installation sequence. The Lockbolt incorporates a collar that is swaged into annular grooves. It comes in two types: pull-type and stump-type. The pull-type (Fig. 17) is the most common, where a frangible pintail is used to react the axial load during the swaging of the collar. When the swaging load reaches a predetermined limit, the pintail breaks away at the breakneck groove. The installation of the Hi-Lok and the pull-type Lockbolt can be performed by one mechanic from one side of the structure.

The stump-type Lockbolt, on the other hand, requires support on the head side of the fastener to react the swage operation. This method is usually reserved for automated assembly of detail structure where access is not a problem.

The specific differences in these fasteners for composite structure in contrast to metal structure are small. For the Hi-Lok, material compatibility is the only issue; aluminum collars are not recommended. Standard collars of A286, 303 stainless steel, and, with special lubricants and or finishes, titanium alloy are normally used. The Lockbolt requires a hat-shaped collar that incorporates a flange to spread the high bearing loads during installation. The Lockbolt pin designed for use in composite structure has six annular grooves as opposed to five for metal structure.

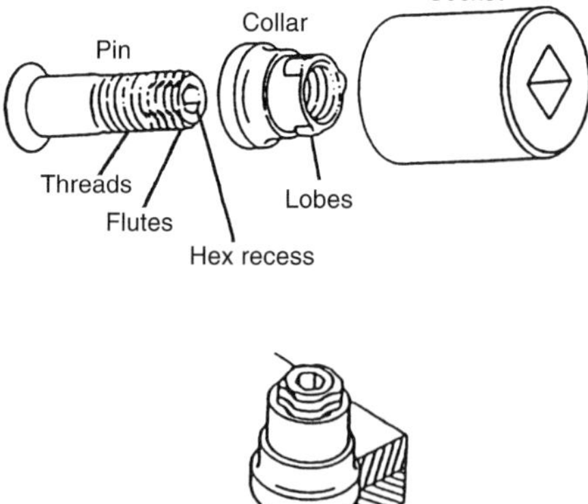

Fig. 18 Eddie Bolt installation process. As the collar is tightened against the structure and the correct preload is approached, the collar lobes begin to deform and roll into the flutes on the pin. Mechanical lock is achieved by filling at least one flute. A washer is required between the collar and the composite surface to prevent damage.

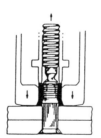

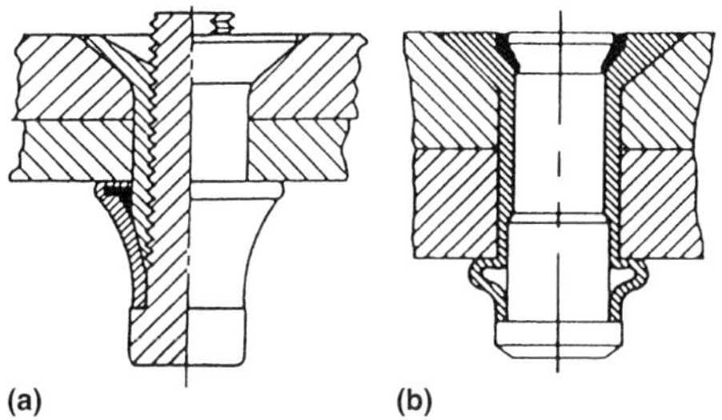

Fig. 19 Blind fasteners for joining composite structures. (a) Threaded-corebolt type. (b) Pull type

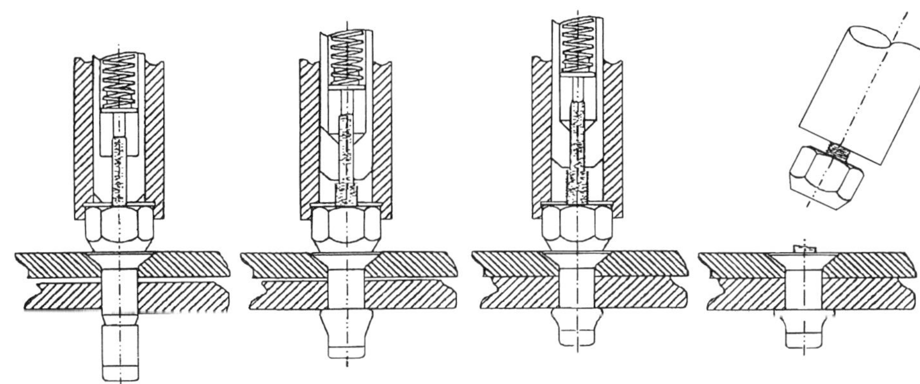

Fig. 20 Installation sequence for a threaded corebolt-type blind fastener

Eddie-Bolt Fasteners

Although Eddie-Bolt fasteners (Fairchild Corp., Dulles, VA) are similar to Hi-Loks, they are a natural choice for carbon fiber composite structures. The Eddie-Bolt pin is designed with flutes in the threaded portion, which allows a positive lock to be made during installation using a specially designed mating nut or collar. The mating nut has three lobes that serve as driving ribs. During installation, at a predetermined preload, the lobes compress the nut material into the flutes of the pin and form the locking feature. Figure 18 shows the installation process. The natural advantage for composite structure is that titanium alloy nuts can be used for compatibility and weight saving without the fear of galling. The nuts spin on freely, and the locking feature is established at the end of the installation cycle. Other threaded-fastener systems usually have a crimp in the nut or collar that elastically deforms to create friction and act as a locking feature. The friction can be a problem with titanium rubbing against titanium, as this material is very sensitive to galling without special finishes or lubricants. Then again, the lubricant defeats the purpose of the friction lock.

Blind Fasteners in Composite Structures

As composites were introduced into structural components, fewer fasteners were required. Stiffeners and doublers were co-cured with the skins, eliminating many fasteners. Panels became larger pieces; many times, this size increase caused accessibility problems. Blind fasteners or screws and nutplates must be used in areas with backside inaccessibility.

There are some advantages in using blind fasteners over nutplates:

- Faster installation
- Only one hole per fastener
- Tighter class of hole fit
- Usually lighter
- More easily replaced for defective installation

Several versions of blind fasteners have been developed for joining composite structures. The Composi-Lok (MAG Aerospace Industries, Inc., New York, NY) (Fig. 19a), is an example of a threaded corebolt type; the Ti-Matic (Huck International, Inc.) (Fig. 19b), is an example of a pull-type blind fastener.

The threaded-corebolt-type blind fastener has the highest clamping forces (advantage for joint fatigue strength) due to the mechanical advantage of the threads and very little relaxation at the end of the installation cycle. The corebolt threads "lock" the corebolt axially, improving the bolt-bending characteristics. Bolt bending is a common problem in composite structure due to the low interlaminar shear modulus of laminated composites. The high clamping forces are distributed over the large footprint on the backside. This particular blind fastener was designed specifically for use in composite structure; how-

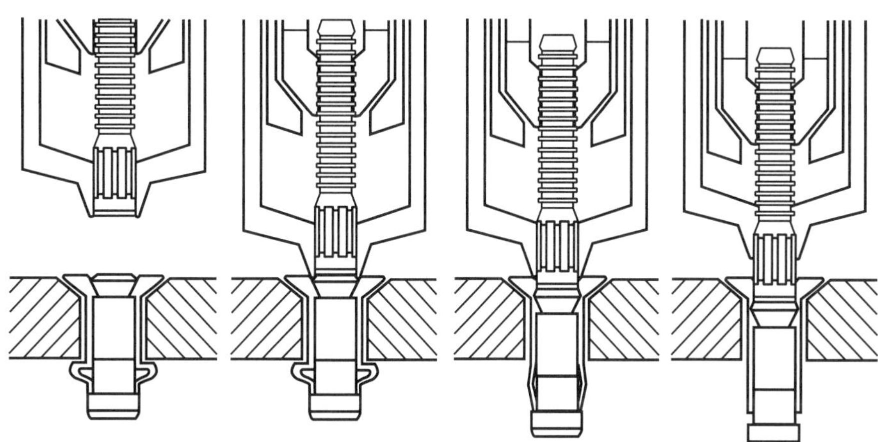

Fig. 21 Installation sequence for a pull-type blind fastener.

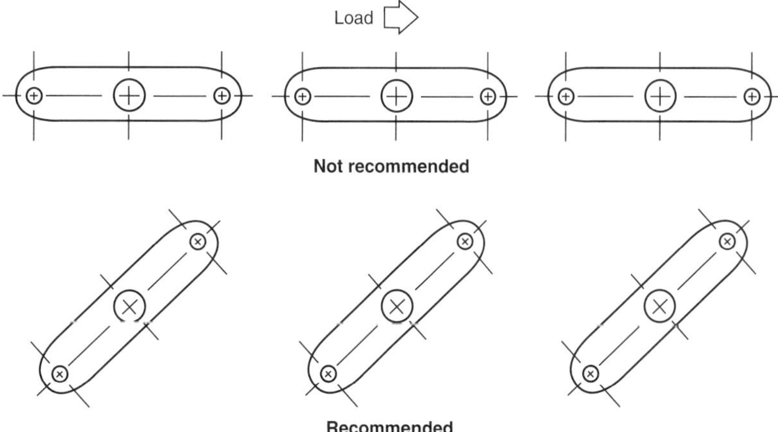

Fig. 22 Eliminating the effects of "tearing along the dotted line" with nutplates

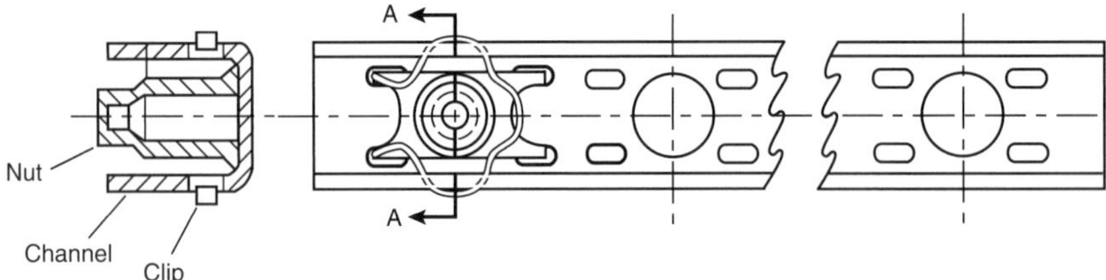

Fig. 23 Gang channel nuts

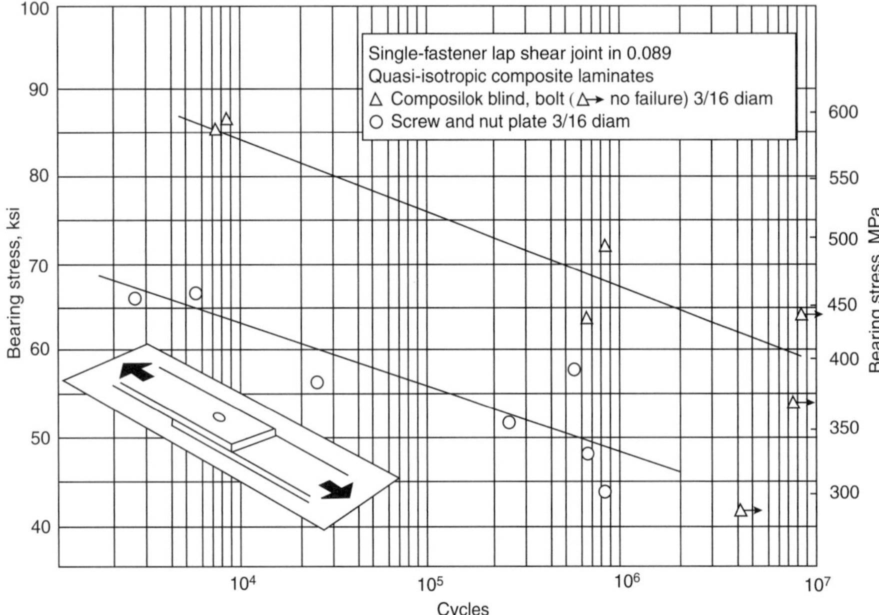

Fig. 24 *S-N* curve comparing blind fasteners with screws and nutplates in composite laminate

ever, it could be used in metal structure as well. Figure 20 shows the installation sequence. A sleeve is "jacked" (by the threaded corebolt) down over the tapered end of the fastener body and collapsed against the blind side of the structure. A small nonmetallic insert (not shown) keeps the sleeve deformation in the proper direction. Locking is provided by indents in the fastener body producing elastic deformation that increases friction and prevents the corebolt from loosening, much like a standard self-locking nut. The disposable drive-nut provides ease of installation and common tooling for both flush head and protruding-head configurations.

The pull-type blind fastener depends on a straight pull to provide the axial force necessary to collapse the sleeve or thin-walled portion of the fastener body. As the core pin is pulled upward, a groove, strategically placed, becomes positioned just in time for a locking ring to be forced into the groove. The locking ring provides retention of the core pin. Figure 21 shows the installation sequence. At completion of the installation, the excess core pin breaks away in tension and is discarded. The clamping forces are less than for the threaded-corebolt type, and the footprint is much smaller. However, the pull-type blind fastener installs more quickly, is usually lighter, and is less expensive. Joint fatigue testing has shown that the pull-type blind fastener does not perform nearly as well as the threaded-corebolt type, probably due to less clamp-up, smaller footprint, and greater susceptibility to bolt bending. Structural performance requirements should govern the choice of blind fastener type. It has been the philosophy of the design community that blind fasteners used in primary structure in aircraft be inspected on the backside (with a borescope) for proper formation.

Screws and Nutplates in Composite Structures

If removal of a closeout panel is anticipated in the life of the structure, screws and nutplates are recommended in place of blind fasteners. Nutplates used in composite structures usually require three holes, two for attachment of the nutplate and one for the removable screw. Other methods of attachment used in metal structures (Davis Press Nut, Rivnut, etc.) have not been successful in composites. A major disadvantage with nutplate attachment is the alignment of holes. "Hole out," net area stress, and "tear along the dotted line" are problems of concern for the designer. For close fastener spacing, rotating the nutplate attachment can reduce the "dotted line" effect, as shown in Fig. 22. Rotation of the nutplate, however, requires more edge margin, but then that in itself reduces the net area stress. Another method of minimizing the number of attachment holes is to use gang channel nuts, shown in Fig. 23. Gang channel made of composite material has been used in military airplanes where the nut element is replaceable. The channel is attached to the structure at much longer increments than if individual nutplates are used. The screw and nutplate assembly does not compare favorably with blind fasteners for structural performance in composite structure. Reference 9 was a study that compared static and joint fatigue performance for screws and nutplates with threaded-corebolt-type blind fasteners. Static joint tension ultimate strength for screws and nutplates was about 85% of the blind fastener capability; however, yield strength suffered the most with approximately 67%. The lower yield is due to the increased joint deflection and compliance of the fastening system. For the same reasons, joint fatigue strength is also much lower as shown in Fig. 24. For these reasons, screws and nutplates are not normally used or recommended for high-load transfer joints.

REFERENCES

1. "Qualification Test Results of Big Foot Blind Fasteners for Boeing Aircraft Co.," Report 518, Monogram Aerospace Fasteners, Division of Monogram Industries, Oct 1980
2. B. Cole, "Special Fastener Development for Composite Structures Program," paper presented at the National Aerospace Standards Committee Standardization Meeting, May 1982
3. J.D. Pratt, "Blind Fastening of Advanced Composites," paper presented at CogSME, Fastening Advanced Composites Conference (Renton, WA), Oct 1986
4. J. Phillips, "Fastening Composite Structures with HUCK Fasteners," Technical Paper, Huck Manufacturing Co., 1984
5. P. Grant, N. Nguyen, and A. Sawicki, "Bearing, Fatigue, and Hole Elongation in Composite Bolted Joints," 49th Annual Forum, American Helicopter Society, May 1993
6. D.M. Shoe, Internal report, Boeing Commercial Airplane Co., 1981
7. R.O. Brick, "Multipath Lightning Protection for Composite Structure Integral Fuel Tank Design," paper presented at the Tenth International Aerospace and Ground Conference on Lightning and Static Electricity (Paris, France), 1985
8. R.O. Brick and J.R. Gozinsky, Internal report, Boeing Commercial Airplane Co., 1986
9. "Results of Static Joint Lap Shear and Lap Shear Fatigue Tests Performed on Composi-Lok II and Nutplates and Screws," Test Report No. 562, Monogram Aerospace Fasteners, 1987

Environmental Protection and Sealing

Leslie A. Hoeckelman, The Boeing Company, St. Louis

ENVIRONMENTAL EFFECTS of ground and flight environments, including temperature extremes, damage by chemical fluids, moisture, and so forth, that affect the durability of polymer-matrix composites are an ongoing concern of aircraft manufacturers and operators. Carbon fiber reinforced polymer-matrix composites (or simply, graphite composites) present a special problem for assemblies that are bolted and bonded to metal structures because graphite, together with metals and alloys is in the electromotive series of alloys commonly used in aircraft structures (Table 1). A galvanic cell thus can form in the presence of moisture or other electrolytes between a carbon fiber reinforced composite and any of these metals that it contacts. Graphite, which is at the cathodic end of the series and which functions as a noble metal, is impervious to corrosion itself, but will accelerate corrosion in the adjacent less-noble metal.

Table 1 provides a guide for material selection based on the criterion of potential for galvanic corrosion. For example, there is considerably more difference in the galvanic potential between carbon fiber reinforced composite (CFRC) and aluminum than between CFRC and titanium or stainless steels. Likewise, there is considerably more difference in galvanic potential between CFRC and nonstainless steels than between CFRC and stainless steels. In addition, clad alloys and certain aluminum alloys have more galvanic potential than others.

Joining a CFRC to aluminum presents a potentially serious corrosion problem. The assembly of CFRC to aluminum is not prohibited, but it does require some special considerations and procedures.

Corrosion Control

Control of galvanic corrosion in aircraft structures usually involves either corrosion prevention or retardation of the corrosion rate. Prevention methods include barriers, material changes, and isolation (elimination of the moisture). Retardation methods include leaching of anticorrosion materials and consumable materials.

Barriers are the predominant method for corrosion prevention, applied either during fabrication or assembly. Fabrication-applied preventatives include materials such as fiberglass ply being co-cured onto the CFRC part surface. Another fabrication barrier would be a primer coat of paint or other organic coating applied to the part after machining and before assembly. This prevents the two materials from coming into contact. The primer or organic coating could also be in the retardation category, since anticorrosion compounds could be added to their chemistry. Assembly-applied preventatives include sealants and gaskets. A wet curing sealant, called a fay seal, is applied between the parts making up the assembly. A wet curing sealant, called a butt joint seal, is applied between the ends of two parts. A wet curing sealant can also be applied around the fastener shank and/or fastener head; this is called a wet installation. In some cases, an O-ring rubber seal can be placed on the fastener shank to form the seal. Seals around removable doors can use a form-in-place seal (FIP) or a formed gasket installed.

Materials Changes. Corrosion prevention via material selection includes using a more cathodic material in place of the aluminum with the carbon fiber reinforced composite. However, when using CFRC, aluminum, titanium, or stainless steel in aircraft structures, thermal expansion within the joint must also be considered along with the galvanic potential difference of the above materials. A comparison of thermal expansion coefficients is given in Table 2. The combination of CFRC and aluminum would result in the greatest thermal expansion mismatch, which would increase loads on the fasteners, adhesives, or sealants as the joint is subjected to in-service temperature variations. A thermal expansion mismatch also results in bonded joints when the bonding or co-curing is accomplished at elevated temperatures. In fact, adhesive bonds between CFRC and aluminum have been known to fail when exposed to subzero temperatures (e.g., –54 °C, or –65 °F), due to the large thermally induced stress gradient. The design of a CFRC-metal joint thus involves finding a balance between low cost, lightweight, availability, ease of fabrication, material mechanical property match, galvanic potential match, and thermal match. A good alternative consideration would be a CFRC-CFRC joint. However, the CFRC-CFRC joint still presents a galvanic corrosion problem with the metallic fastener, since they will be in contact with the carbon fiber ends.

Isolation (elimination) of the moisture or electrolyte is the final method of corrosion pre-

Table 1 Electromotive series of aircraft alloys, in descending order of tendency to corrode

Electrolyte is seawater.

Anodic (most active)
Magnesium alloys
Zinc
Alclad 7000 series aluminum alloys
5000 series aluminum alloys
7000 series aluminum alloys
Pure aluminum and alclad 2000 series alloys
Cadmium
2000 series aluminum alloys
Steel and iron
Lead
Chromium
Brass and bronze alloys
Copper
Stainless and heat-resistant steels
Titanium
Silver
Nickel and nickel alloys
Gold
Carbon fiber reinforced polymer composites
Cathodic (least active)

Source: Ref 1

Table 2 Thermal coefficient of expansion for composite and metallic materials

	Coefficent of thermal expansion, 10^{-6}/K	
Material	Longitudinal	Transverse
Carbon-fiber-epoxy (0°)	0.43	29.2
Carbon-fiber-epoxy (0°/ ±45°/90°)	3.4	3.4
Carbon-fiber-epoxy fabric (24 × 23 – 8HS)	2.7	4.0
E-glass epoxy (0°)	8.6	. . .
E-glass-epoxy (181-style weave)	9.9	12.1
Aramid-epoxy (0°)	–5.4	. . .
Aramid-epoxy (181-style weave)	–1.8	–1.8
Aluminum alloys	23.4	
Steel	10.8	
Titanium	10.1	
Stainless steel	18	

Values for composite laminates may be taken as typical; however, actual values for specific materials, especially in the graphite-epoxy system, can vary widely from these values. Source: Ref 1

vention. This essentially is the "keep it out and keep it in" philosophy. Fay surface, fillet, and butt joint seals satisfy this requirement. These sealing methods are discussed in the section "Sealing" in this article.

Retardation of the corrosion rate includes leaching of anticorrosion materials or a coating of a consumable/sacrificial material. The leaching compound may be found in the primer on fabricated parts or in the sealant that is applied during the assembly of the parts. Generally, the leachant has been a compound of cadmium or chromium. Due to environmental concerns, the current requirement is for an anticorrosion compound without cadmium or chromium. The material manufacturers are working to make this formulation. A sacrificial material is generally a very thin layer of a material (e.g., pure aluminum) applied to a part via ion vapor deposition during the fabrication process.

Design Considerations

Sealant joint design and installation workmanship usually are not the first consideration when structures requiring joints are designed. Therefore, sealants in joints often fail, resulting in a significant cost to replace or, in some cases, a complete joint redesign. Since most joint designs are unique to the rest of the structure design, some general guidelines are useful.

Shear, tension, and compression stresses are typically encountered in the sealant joint. Thermal expansion or contraction, structure movement, and environmental forces are the source of these stresses, which can deform the sealant and cause strain. Sealants must be able to accommodate a certain amount of movement; this property of a sealant is called percent elongation. Figure 1 shows a simple butt joint and the extension/compression experienced by the sealant. Figure 2 shows a simple fay surface joint and the lateral movement experienced by the sealant in the joint.

Good joint design is dependent on the mechanical and chemical resistance properties of the sealant material, the characteristics of the materials forming the joint (substrates), and on the joint configuration. Assuming that the general sealant properties such as chemical resistance and temperature capability are suitable for the joint application, there are certain other sealant and substrate material characteristics that must be considered by the designer, including sealant adhesion capability to the substrate, cohesive strength of the sealant material, percent elongation, and cohesive capability of the substrate.

Adhesion of the sealant to the substrate is an inherent property of the sealant/substrate interface and may be enhanced by the use of a primer (generally called an adhesion promoter). The cohesion (resistance to tearing) is an internal physical property of the sealant material. This will determine the minimum cross-sectional area of the joint. Percent elongation and elastic recovery is the ability of the cured sealant material to stretch. Cohesive strength of the substrate is usually associated with composite materials. A substrate that does not have sufficient strength to support the stresses that develop at the sealant/substrate interface will fail internally.

There are several important design considerations for the joint itself (Ref 2):

- Sufficient sealant/substrate interface to provide adequate adhesion
- Sufficient cross-sectional area to avoid cohesive failures
- Maximum surface area to volume ratio to reduce strain
- Accessibility for seal installation
- Accommodations for sealant cure requirements

Because sealant may fail either cohesively or adhesively, both properties are important and must be balanced to the joint requirements.

Sealing

Common methods used to seal aircraft structures are: fay surface, fillet, butt joint, and form-in-place (FIP) seals (Fig. 3). While there are various tools and equipment available, various dimensions to be held, various materials to use, and an adhesion promoter and a detackifier to use before and after application, there is one requirement that cannot be stressed enough: the sealing surfaces must be clean. The water break free test is the most common method to verify that a surface is clean. However, it should be noted that a water break free test cannot be used in many production operations. Many procedures have been developed to obtain a water break free surface. The area to be sealed, primed, or coated must be free from all grease, oil, dirt, and other foreign materials that can hinder the adhesion of the applied material.

Cleaning of the structure can take the form of a water and detergent scrub, followed by a solvent material wipe and then the "two-wiper cleaning" process. This last step removes the foreign materials (contaminant) that might be left behind if the cleaner was left to evaporate. In this cleaning process, one wiper is dampened with the solvent and the other is dry. The dampened one is applied to the part first, and, before

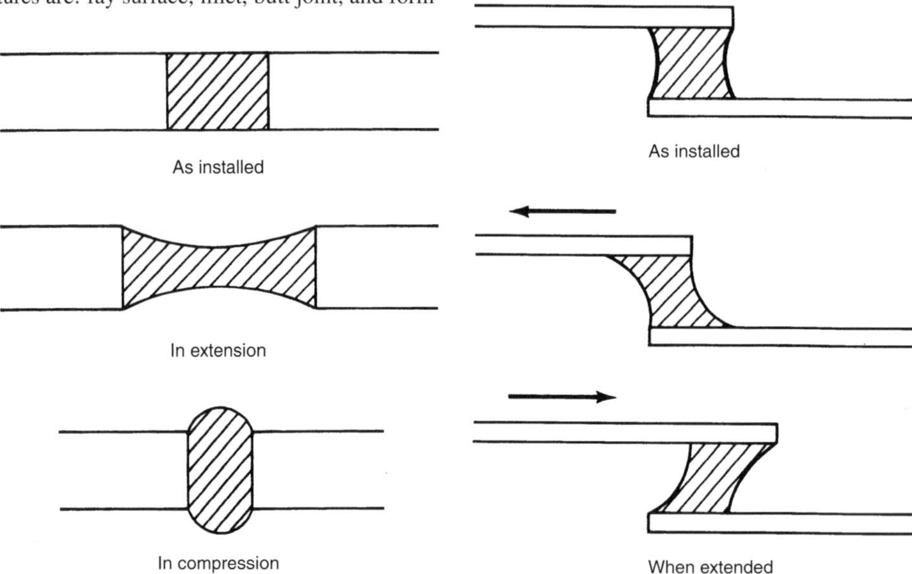

Fig. 1 Simple butt joint. Source: Ref 2

Fig. 2 Simple lap joint. Source: Ref 2

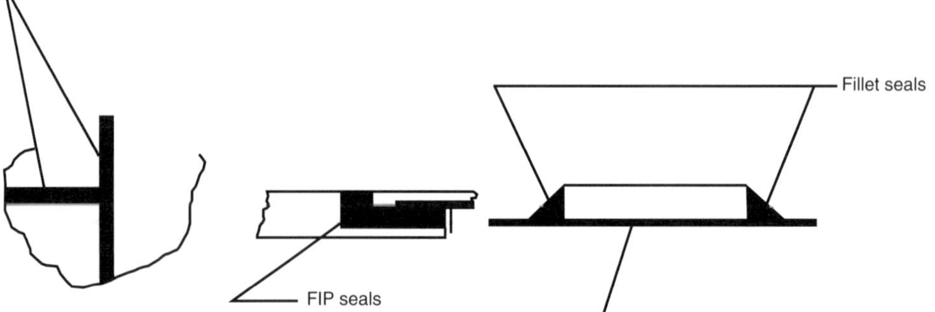

Fig. 3 Seal types

the solvent can evaporate, the second dry wiper is used to dry the part. Repeated turning of the wiper presents a new surface to the part. In some instances, the surface is lightly abraded and re-cleaned prior to sealing. In some cases, the water and detergent scrub are skipped as part of the cleaning process.

Sealant materials are categorized into several groups: base material types, temperature ranges, fuel wetted surfaces, and noncorrosion ability. The most common base material is polysulfide. The polysulfides typically use an accelerator material to cure the base rubber. This material is available within a normal temperature range of –55 to 120 °C (–65 to 250 °F) with short time exposure to 180 °C (360 °F). These sealants are available in a wide variety of types, including those specifically formulated for fay surface sealing and wet fastener installation. Other types are specifically formulated for fillet seals, butt joint seals, fuel tank sealing, and low density, low adhesion for removable panels. Formulations are also available for other special conditions. Within each of these categories, there are short and long application times (pot life) fast cure, minimum/low viscosity applications (spray or brush), and extrusion gun or spatula grades. It should be noted that the polysulfide sealants vary somewhat in their maximum service temperature and their continuous versus peak temperatures. Material suppliers and company/military/commercial specifications should be consulted for specific selections. The second-most-used material is the silicone category. These materials typically are used for the next higher temperature regime, in the range of –60 to 260 °C (–80 to 500 °F). The silicones use two different cure mechanisms, either catalytic or moisture (from humidity).

Fay surface sealing is a process that seals two surfaces that come into contact with each other in a fastened joint (Fig. 4). The fay seal is mandatory for adequate corrosion protection. Wet sealant fastener installation is also mandatory. The two surfaces are cleaned, and an application of an adhesion promoter may be applied to the two surfaces. Sealant material is next applied in a manner to coat one of the entire mating surfaces, monitored by material squeeze-out on the edges of the party boundary. Lower-viscosity materials are used for fay sealing thin sheets. When thick parts are assembled, a higher-viscosity material is used. Longer assembly time materials are required for large assemblies, such as large skins over spars, ribs, stringers, and longerons. Figure 5 shows examples of application tools for fay sealing. The roller often is used to obtain a uniform preassembly sealant thickness. The comb nozzle is used for small and/or narrow parts that need to be fay sealed. The notched comb also is used to apply a uniform preassembly sealant thickness.

Fillet sealing is a process that seals the edge of two surfaces that come into contact with each other in a fastened joint (Fig. 6). The fillet seal is used to prevent fuel, water, or air from getting out of where it should be or getting in where it should not be. The fillet seal constitutes the primary seal (backed up by the fay seal) in many joint designs. Fillet seals are usually located inside of the aircraft mold line. Wet sealant fastener installation is also mandatory. The two surfaces are cleaned, and an application of an adhesion promoter may be applied to the two surfaces. Sealant material is next applied in a manner to cover the interface of the one part to the other (Fig. 6). This is monitored by checking the dimensions "a," "b," "c," "d," or "e" as appropriate and shown in Fig. 6. A high-viscosity material is used for fillet seals, so that the fillet shape will be retained with the thixotropic properties of the material. Short assembly times are desired for the fillet application. A detackifier may be used over the sealant material to allow work to resume over the fillet, before the fillet seal is cured enough to be tack free. The detackifier minimizes the potential for drilling chips to stick to the sealant material. Special filleting tools are used to obtain the correct size and shape of the fillet bead.

Brush sealing is used to overcoat the collar, buck rivet tail, or other nut element of the installed fastener (Fig. 7). This process uses a lower-viscosity material and short assembly times. Detackifier may be used over the brushable sealant. This process is used in pressure areas, such as the cockpit, crew station, or cabin areas. Spray sealing is beginning to replace brush sealing for large areas. The spray is produced using a 14 MPa (2000 psig) pump and an airless spray head. The orifice and the spray cap determine the fan size and shape. The spray uses a low-viscosity, brushable grade, polysulfide material and further thins it with a solvent to obtain a specific Zahn cup time. Two to four applications are required with a solvent flash off time between applications. The same cleaning process is used for spray sealing. A nonwater-based adhesion promoter is spray applied prior to the actual spray seal process. The spray is applied approximately halfway up a spar web and 50 to 100 mm (2–4 in.) out onto the inner mold line of the skin.

Butt joint sealing and FIP seals are the last sealing processes during assembly. The butt joint

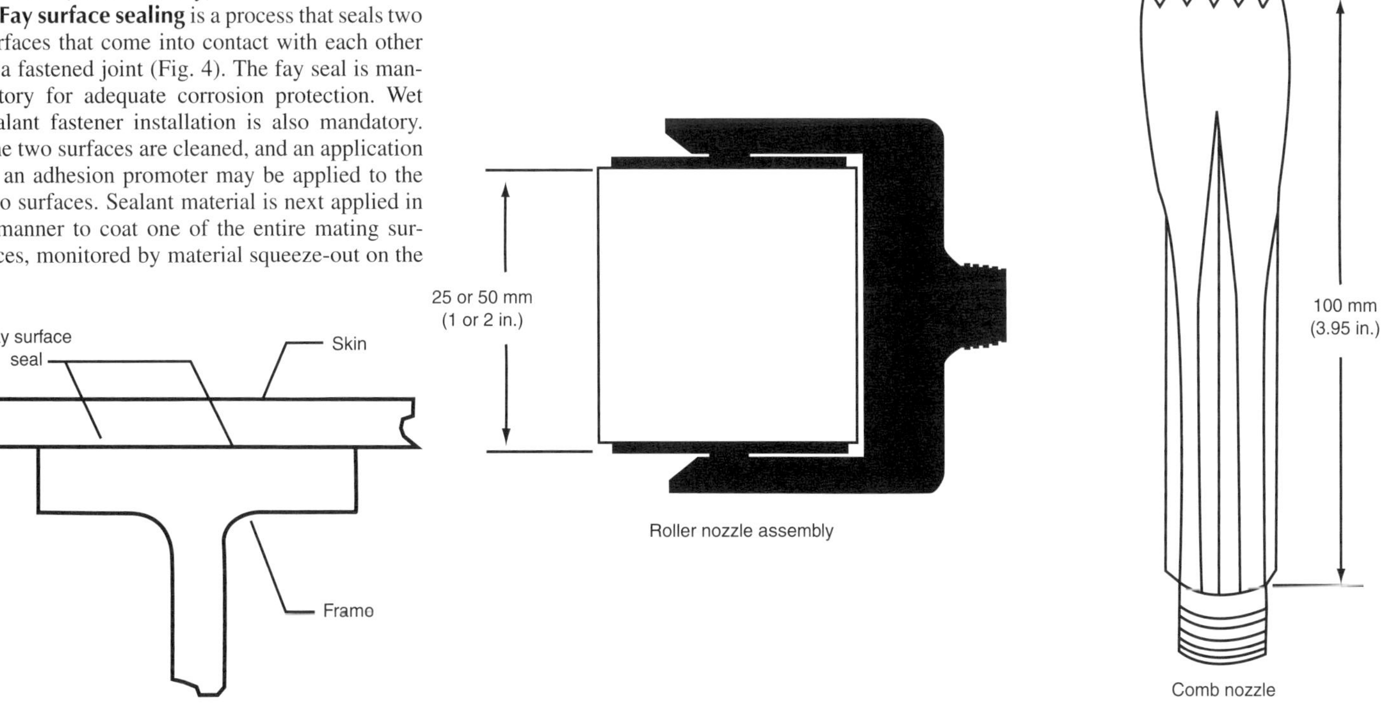

Fig. 4 Fay-surface seal

Fig. 5 Fay-seal nozzles

seal is applied between the edges of two parts (Fig. 8). This fills in the gaps between them. Nozzles are used to apply the sealant in the gap between the two skins. The FIP seal is used to seal access bay doors and removable doors and panels (Fig. 9). The door sill is cleaned like the other sealing processes. Spacers are attached to the sill to provide a specific seal thickness when completed. The location can be around the fastener using a donut-shaped spacer, or it can be located away from the fastener using the hole of the donut or some other shape (Fig. 9). When the second location is used, the volume where the spacer was removed is then filled in with the sealant used for the seal. The width of the FIP seal is dictated by the general design requirements for the assembly, but is usually approximately 13 mm (0.5 in.). After all of the spacers are located, the sill then has an adhesion promoter applied, and it is allowed to dry. Any puddling of the adhesion promoter must be soaked up with a wiper. During this time, the door has mold release applied to the edge and the sealant contact surface and then allowed to dry. Two or three coats of mold release may be required, depending on the specific mold release used. The door and the skin area around the door has masking tape applied to facilitate cleanup. Sealant is applied to the doorsill and the door installed with a specific sequence of fasteners. When the sealant is cured, the door is removed with the aid of a plastic wedge. Care is required to prevent damage to the seal. After the door is removed, the excess cured sealant and the mold release is cleaned up, and a powder parting agent is applied to prevent the door from resticking to the sealant.

Many fuel tanks use a noncuring sealant injected into a seal groove. This is considered to be a repairable fuel-boundary seal. It can be a polysulfide or a fluorosilicone material, called the groove or channel sealant. The channel sealant can have beads or chopped rubber, as a filler, mixed into the paste sealant. The filler material will migrate in the sealant when a flow of fuel begins to swell the paste. The filler material then moves to where the flow is exiting. The filler material forms a "log jam" at this point, and the sealant flows around them, resealing the groove. This material is injected into a channel that goes around the periphery of the tank. The material is injected in such a manner as to apply pressure to the sealant in the channel groove. Injection of this material is done at elevated pressures of 14 to 28 MPa (2000–4000 psig) at the nozzle tip. The tip pressure is dependent on the material thickness of the skin and frame, thicker parts have higher allowed tip pressure. This sealing method is generally used in conjunction with fay and fillet seal described above. A typical wing tank without a bladder would use fay seal be-

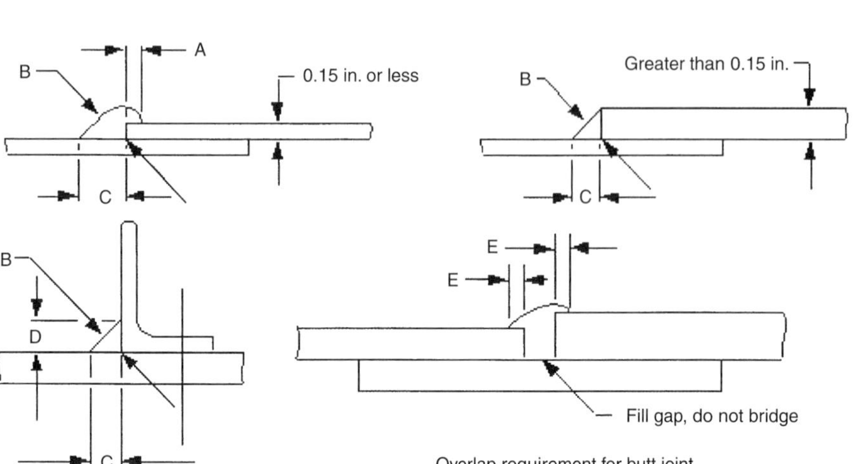

Material type	A and B, in.	C, D, and E, in.
Metals	0.10–0.15	0.15–0.25
Carbon fiber reinforced epoxy composite joined to dissimilar metals (such as aluminum)	0.15–0.25	0.2–0.3

Note: When upper material is greater than 0.15 in., then A = 0.

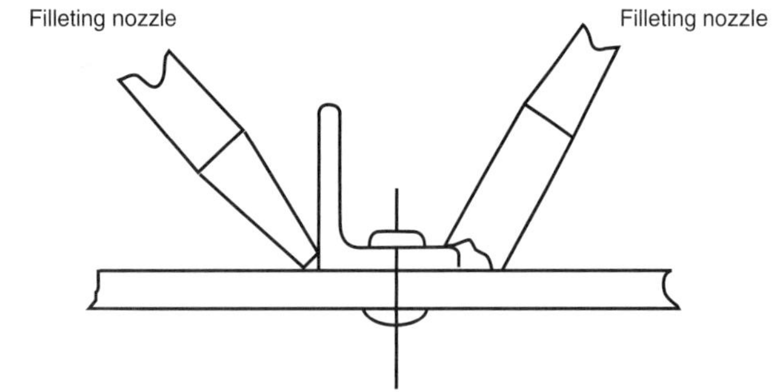

Fig. 6 Filleting criteria

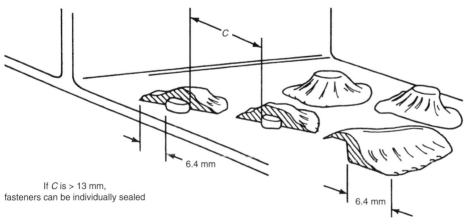

Fig. 7 Sealant overcoat of fasteners. Source: Ref 3

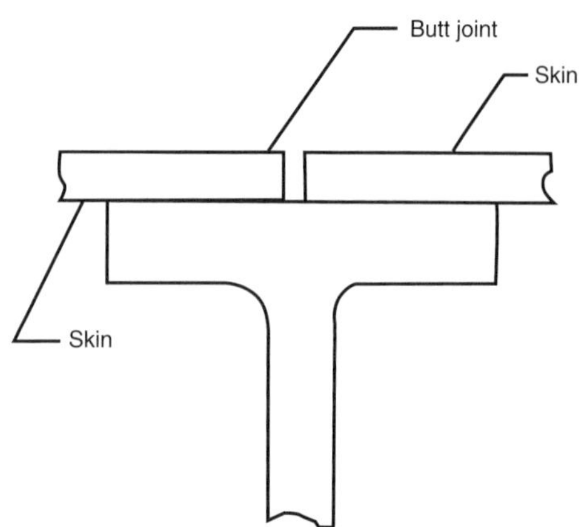

Fig. 8 Butt-joint seal

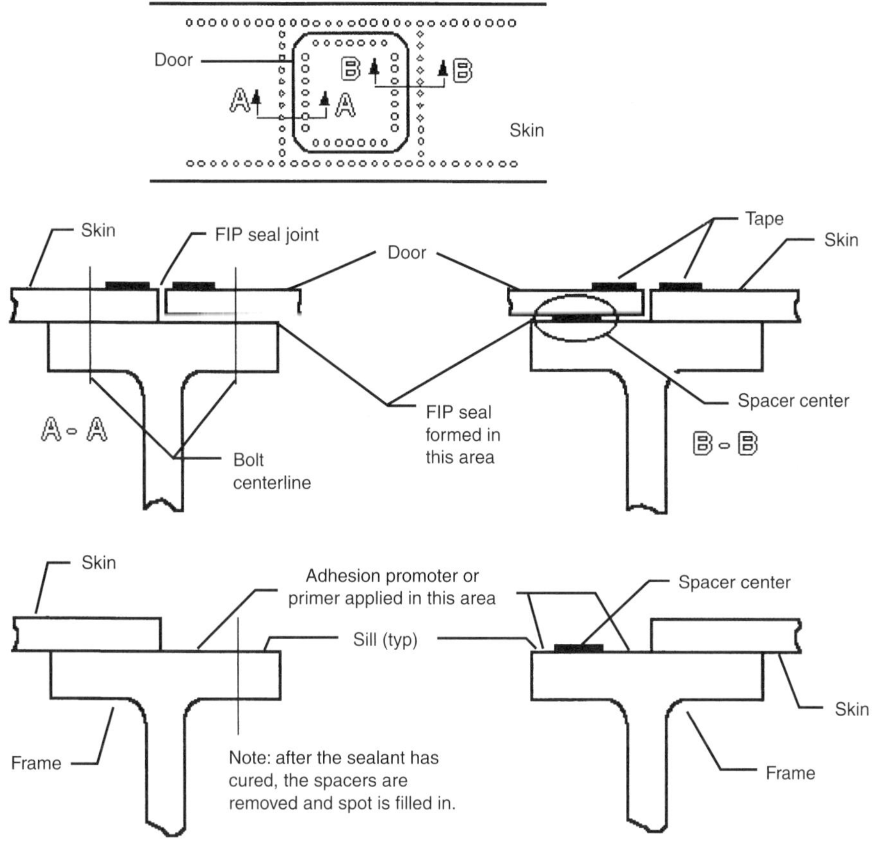

Fig. 9 Form-in-place (FIP) seals

tween the skin and the spar caps, then a fillet seal at the edge of the spar cap of the wet side of the wing skin. This would be followed by either a brush overcoat of the fasteners with sealant or spray sealing over the fasteners, up the spar web, and out over some of the inner mold line of the skin. After the polysulfide has all cured, then the channel seal material would be pumped into the channel

Channel seals require a channel groove machined or formed into the spar cap (Fig. 10). The width, depth, and location are determined based on the structural loading, volume contained in the channel groove, and the general design requirements. If the groove follows the fastener pattern, then the width will be greater than if the groove is on one side or the other of the fastener pattern. Groove depth must be minimized because the groove is counted as a gap in the fastener design. However, the groove needs to be deep enough to contain a sufficient volume of sealant material to maintain a good seal. Injection of sealant into the groove also must be considered because sealant materials are very viscous and require a significant amount of pressure to move them through the groove, typically 14 to 28 MPa (2000–4000 psig) nozzle tip pressure. Injection points need to be designed at approximately every 100 to 150 mm (4–6 in.). The injection can take place through the fastener, through a fastener hole with an injection tool (Fig. 11), or through a hole in the skin that gets plugged.

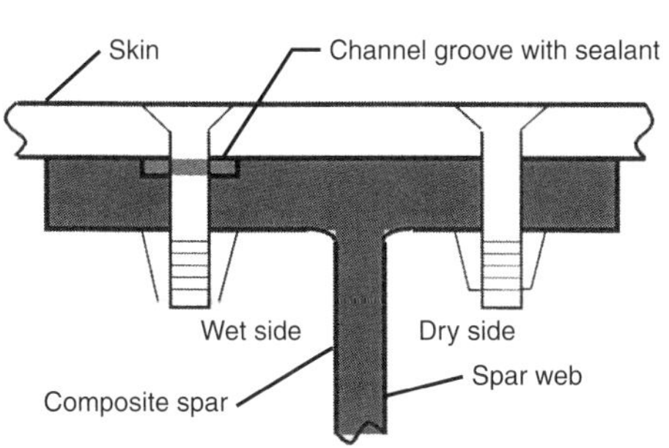

Fig. 10 Channel seals

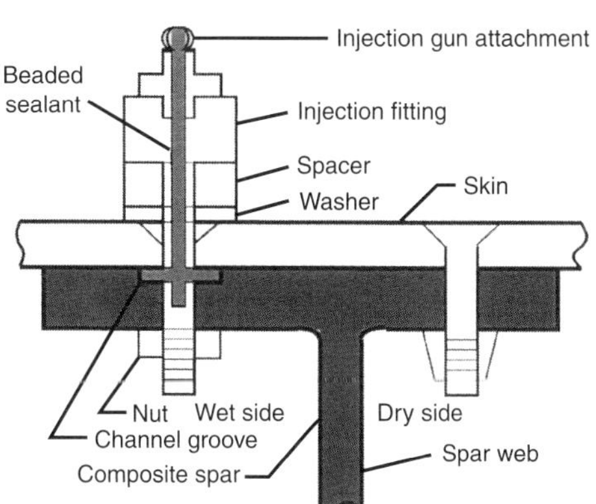

Fig. 11 Channel seal injection

Sealant application equipment includes pneumatic application guns with different sealant extrusion nozzles and with various size sealant cartridges ranging from 0.03 to 0.6 L (1–20 fl oz), pneumatic channel sealant injection equipment with a pressure regulator and gage for reduced tip pressures (used for sealing short lengths of channel groove and for field repairs), and airless spray sealing equipment. Sealant filleting and scraping is done using various hand tools.

Primer and Topcoat Systems

The primer and topcoat function as a system; therefore, the topcoat must be chemically and physically compatible with the primer system. The ability of the system to meet the user performance requirements is determined by how well the surface is prepared prior to coating.

Surface Preparation. Carbon fiber reinforced composite surfaces are prepared by scuff sanding or grit blasting to obtain visual dense scratches and loss of gloss. Priming or painting is conducted as soon as possible after surface preparation, and painting must take place within 36 h. If the part will not be painted within 12 h, it should be wrapped in clean roll paper prior to painting. Abrasive cleaning (grit blasting) is the preferred method of preparing unpainted CFRC surfaces (it is required for the mold-line surface) followed by dry wiping. Parts containing close tolerance holes are grit blasted and primered prior to drilling holes in the detail skin. Carbon fiber reinforced composite parts that are not grit blasted such as parts with complex geometry and/or locations inaccessible to grit blasting, reworked areas, and parts with thin, unsupported cross sections, are processed by removing any peel ply if present on the surface, dry wiping the composite surface, scuff sanding with 150 or 180 grit sandpaper by hand or with a pneumatic sander, and removing all sanding dust from the surface by dry wiping. Care must be taken not to sand into a free edge because it may cause edge delamination.

The entire primed or painted exterior composite surface is sanded using 180 grit or finer sandpaper to remove all surface gloss and contamination using an air-driven sander attached to an air-driven high-efficiency particulate air (HEPA) vacuum. Hand sanding is permissible for areas of less than 0.4 m^2 (4 ft^2) where mechanical sanding is not feasible.

Aircraft exterior mold-line surfaces are cleaned with detergent using the following process:

1. Wet down the aircraft, spray detergent on the surfaces, and scrub previously sanded areas with nylon abrasive pads. The detergent is allowed to set approximately 2 to 3 min on the aircraft, but not allowed to dry.
2. Rinse the aircraft with hot water 50 to 60 °C (120–140 °F) until the runoff water is free of detergent residue and evidence of the detergent (bubbling) on the aircraft is gone.

Table 3 Recommended primer and topcoat thicknesses

Application	Thickness			
	min		max	
	mm	mil	mm	mil
Interior (primer only), 2 coats	0.02	0.8	0.03	1.4
Exterior (primer), 1 coat	0.01	0.4	0.025	1.0
Exterior (topcoat), 2 coats	0.03	1.4	0.05	2.0
Exterior nonmold-line—primer and topcoat	0.04	1.8	0.08	3.0
Exterior mold line—primer topcoat, primed skins	0.04	1.8	0.10	4.0
Mold line leading edges—primer and topcoat	0.12(a)	4.6(a)	0.18(a)	7.0(a)

(a) Greater thickness is achieved by spraying on additional topcoat for abrasion resistance.

3. Wipe the exterior mold line using clean wipers (it is not necessary to wipe dry). The wiper is visually examined for contamination, if the aircraft surface still appears dirty. After the second cleaning, areas still dirty are allowed to dry and are locally hand cleaned.

Following detergent cleaning, the aircraft exterior mold-line surfaces are steam cleaned using a minimum steam pressure of 1379 kPa (200 psig), and the surfaces are raised using ambient-temperature clean tap water. Proper steam cleaning of intersecting surfaces and door fastener areas is particularly important. Surfaces should not be touched or contacted in any way after steam cleaning without personnel wearing proper protective clothing/coverings, such as gloves, overalls, boots, and protective caps. The aircraft is allowed to dry for a minimum of 4 h before painting, and surfaces to be painted are inspected for water and aircraft fluid drips and surface contamination immediately before painting.

Application of Primer. For all CFRC Parts requiring primer, one smooth, wet, continuous coat of the applicable catalyzed primer is applied to achieve 0.02 to 0.035 mm (0.8–1.4 mils) dry film thickness, a wet film thickness of approximately 0.09 to 0.13 mm (3.5–5 mils) will achieve the desired dry film thickness. The primer is allowed to dry a minimum of 5 min before applying additional primer to meet thickness requirements. Parts are cured 6 h prior to further processing. If more than 24 h elapse between primer applications, the surface must be hand solvent cleaned and scuff sanded prior to applying any additional primer coat(s).

Primer drying time depends on the atmospheric temperature and humidity conditions. Curing of a waterborne primer requires that the water evaporate first, which is achieved in the quickest way by air movement over the part. Elevated-temperature drying cycles may be used instead of air drying. Baking a part before the water evaporates will cause small blisters. Follow the material manufacturer's recommendation for elevated-temperature cure (Cure temperatures must not exceed 121 °C, or 250 °F, for composite parts). To ensure that drying is satisfactory:

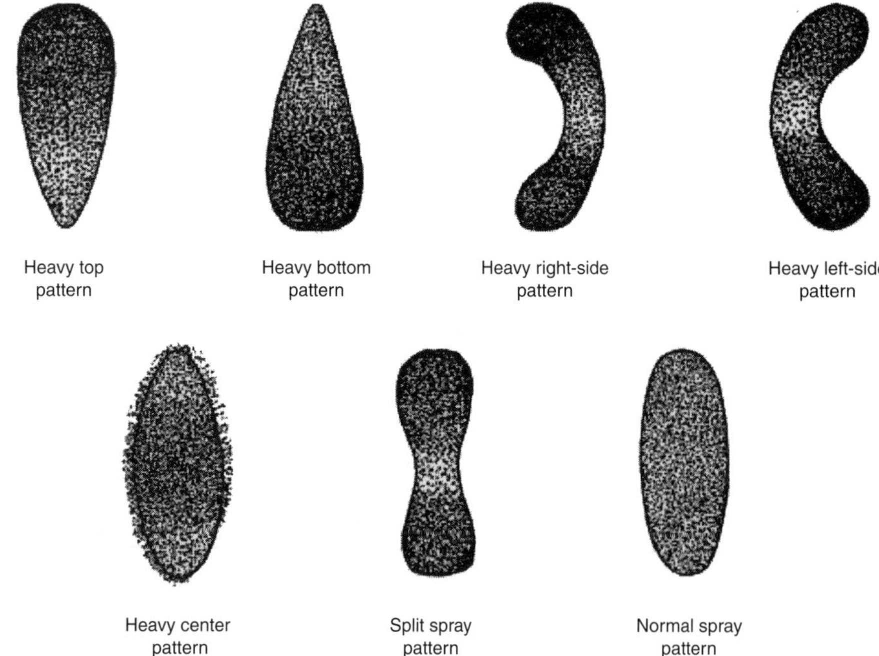

Fig. 12 Spray-painting patterns

- Primer film may not show any sign of solvent pop or blistering due to insufficient flash-off time.
- Primer film must resist marring by no. 250 tape and to pass a dry tape test upon cooling to room temperature.

Application of Topcoat. Parts should be at room temperature before topcoat applications. Surface roughness or overspray is removed by sanding with nylon abrasive pads or 320 grit or finer sandpaper after the primer has dried sufficiently to allow sanding. Areas containing excessively heavy roughness, runs, or sags are sanded using 240 grit sandpaper, and sanding dust is removed from seams by blowing with air and from skin surfaces by wiping with wipers dampened with TT-N-95 aliphatic naphtha. If the time interval between primer and topcoat application exceeds 24 h, areas must be sanded using 320 grit or finer sand paper, cleaned, and have a primer applied and allowed to dry a minimum of 1 h before applying the topcoat.

The topcoat should be allowed to dry for a minimum of 8 h at 24 °C (75 °F) minimum and less than 90% relative humidity before the aircraft is removed from the paint booth. Allow 16 h minimum dry time if the aircraft will be exposed to moisture after moving from the paint booth. If outdoor temperatures average less than 18 °C (65 °F), the aircraft is dried for a minimum of 48 h in a heated indoor area before storing outdoors. Time limits apply from the last paint application on the aircraft, excluding touch-up.

Primer and Topcoat Testing. Primed aircraft mold-line surfaces are wet-tape tested per ASTM D 3359, "Standard Test Methods for Measuring Adhesion by Tape Test," prior to final painting. Test locations are specified by engineering. The primer on the part should be air cured for a minimum of 12 days prior to testing.

ASTM D 3359 dry tape tests also are performed to determine the adhesion of the aircraft exterior finish. A minimum of 48 h air cure is required prior to testing.

Gloss measurements, taken only on the aircraft mold line, are made on flat surfaces only; measurements are not required on composite surfaces. The gloss readings at any location measured with a 60° gloss meter should be (a) gloss colors, 90 minimum; (b) semigloss colors, 15 minimum 50 maximum; (c) lusterless colors, 7 maximum; (d) lusterless black, 3 maximum.

The dry film thickness of the coating must fall within the minimum/maximum dimensions shown in Table 3. The coatings may be applied in any number of coats, provided the thickness and other requirements are met.

The maximum exterior mold-line dry film thickness should be determined by averaging individual measurements evenly distributed over the entire aircraft mold line as required by engineering. Individual maximum thickness values greater than those listed in Table 3 provided the average is within the range shown. Measurement locations should be representative of the general overall mold line. Thickness measurements are

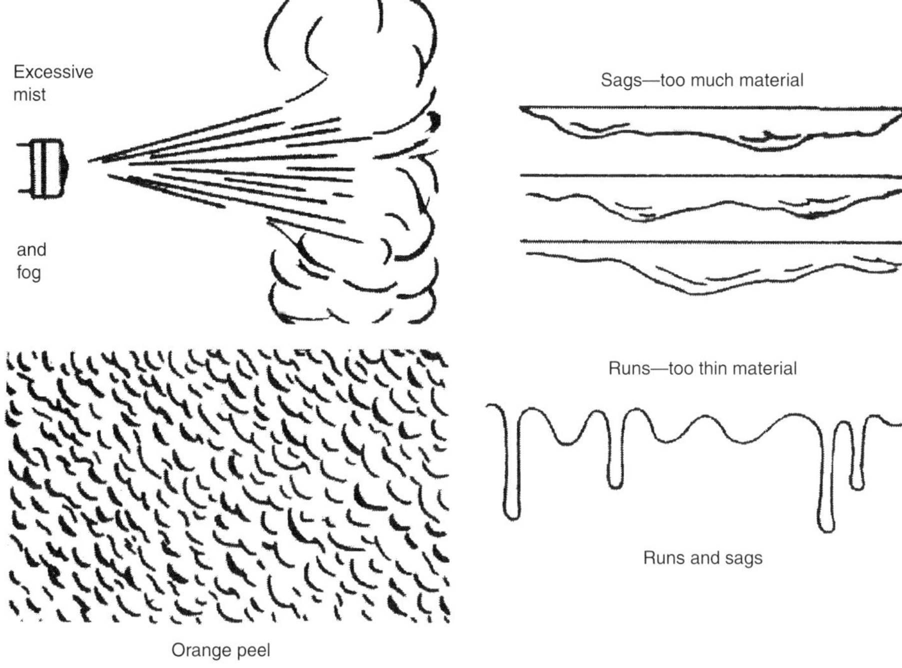

Fig. 13 Typical paint application defects

not taken on surfaces sprayed from multiple directions, demarcation line areas (color overlap areas), surfaces topcoated prior to final paint, and leading edges.

Defects in cured primer that are cause for rejection include non-continuous film and blistering, and lifting. The substrate can be visible through the primer, provided the minimum film thickness requirements are met.

Defects in cured topcoat that are cause for rejection include noncontinuous film; blistering, lifting, and fisheyes; runs and sags; streaks; blushing; film contamination; and gross orange peel.

Primer and Paint Application Equipment. Spray application of primers and topcoats is performed using only high-volume, low-pressure (HVLP) spray gun pressure or siphon feed, or electrostatic spray guns. Interior, hard-to-reach, and limited access spaces are excluded from the HVLP mandatory requirement.

Spraying at a distance of less than 150 mm (6 in.) between spray nozzle and part will cause poor atomization, a distance of more than 250 mm (10 in.) can cause dry spray, or orange peel with gloss topcoats. Figures 12 and 13 show spray painting patterns and common surface finish defects.

Maintaining records of the paint and solvents used on the mold line of each aircraft for final painting and paint detail parts by paint booth is recommended. This excludes paints used for markings, insignias, and touch-up. The record should include:

- Aircraft model and unit number
- Date of painting
- Date and time of mixing (for each paint)
- Paint specification
- Vendor name
- Vendor product number, batch number, date of manufacture for each component (i.e., base, curing, solution, thinner)
- Quantity of each component mixed
- Date and time of application of each paint
- Temperature and humidity conditions
- Date and time of aircraft removal from paint shop

Viscosity measurements should be taken only on materials mixed in quantities larger than 3.78 L (1 gal) for use in final painting of mold-line surfaces. Viscosity checks in paint shops are approximate measurements; standard ASTM procedures are not required. All records should be kept on file in accordance with environmental, contractual, and quality assurance requirements or as appropriate.

Chemical safety information on sealants, primers, and topcoats can be found in Material Safety Data Sheets (MSDS), which are required by OSHA Regulation 29 CFR 1910.1200 HAZARD COMMUNICATION to be furnished by the material supplier.

Classes of materials and chemicals that may be toxic, flammable, or otherwise harmful and therefore require appropriate personal protective equipment and safe work procedures include adhesion promoters, paint removers and strippers, polyurethane paint and coating systems, cleaners, solvents, acids, oxidizers, and alkalines.

REFERENCES

1. *Design Handbook,* Lockheed-California Co., Nov 1983
2. J.E. Thompson, Design Considerations Unique to Sealing, *Adhesives and Sealants,* Vol 3, *ASM Handbook,* ASM International, 1990, p 545–550
3. K. Adams, Application for Sealants, *Adhesives and Sealants,* Vol 3, *ASM Handbook,* ASM International, 1990, p 604–612

Extrusion of Particle-Reinforced Aluminum Composites

William C. Harrigan, Jr., MMC Engineering, Inc.

THE EXTRUSION of particle- and whisker-reinforced aluminum composites is similar to the extrusion of the matrix alloy. The presence of the reinforcements increases the shear strength at the extrusion temperature and increases the pressure requirements for the extrusion. The high pressures required for the extrusions and the high shear strength of the composites lead to higher heat generation during the extrusion. Alloys such as 7075 that are susceptible to "hot short" tearing have the same tendencies when used as matrix alloys for composites. Precise billet preheat temperature control and low speed control of the extrusion are necessary to avoid overheating of the composite during the extrusion. Presses designed for "hard-alloy" extrusions are needed for the composites.

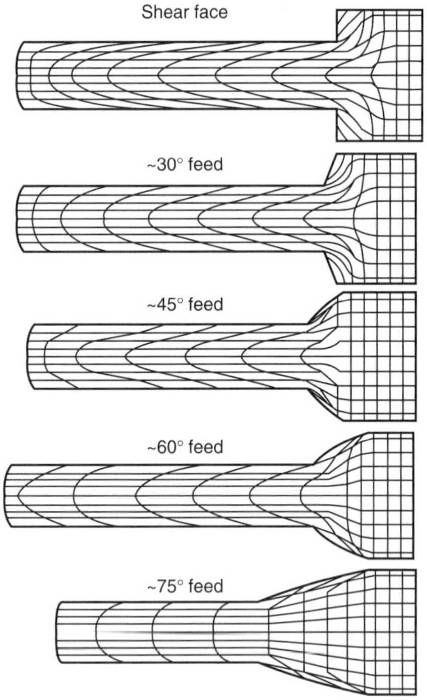

Fig. 1 Cross section of billets with embedded mesh extruded through dies with feed angles between 0° and 75° showing flow characteristics of the various die shapes

Dies and Shapes

Extrusions have been made with shear-face dies, conical-feed dies, and with bridge dies. Cross sections of billets with embedded mesh extruded through dies with feed angles between 0 and 75° are shown in Fig. 1.

The material flow pattern for each of these dies demonstrates the complex flow for the 0°, shear-face die to the uniform flow through the 75° die. The 75°-type die is often referred to as a streamline die. The uniform flow through the streamline dies minimizes damage to reinforcements in whisker-reinforced composites and aligns the whiskers in the extrusion direction. These dies have been used to maximize the mechanical properties of whisker-reinforced aluminum composites in the extrusion direction; however, the mechanical properties in the transverse directions are reduced by the alignment. A further consequence of the streamline die is the greater amount of "butt" loss in the long entrance to the final shape. This material-loss cost must be weighed against the property improvement in any application.

Hollow shapes have been made with forward extrusion with a die and mandrel and with "bridge" dies as well as backward extrusion. An example of a die and mandrel setup is shown in Fig. 2. The hole for the mandrel to pass through may be created by drilling billets or by piercing the billet in the extrusion press. This type of die produces seamless tube. The concentricity of the outer and inner diameters is a problem with this type of extrusion, and precise wall tolerances require drawing the tube after extrusion. An example of a "bridge" or "port hole" die setup is shown in Fig. 3. This type of die produces "seamed" tube that has good wall-thickness tolerance and thin-wall products. Examples of products made with bridge dies are thin-wall tubes for bicycle frame manufacture and a triple-hollow airfoil extrusion used for the exit guide vanes for the 4*xxx* engines produced by Pratt & Whitney Corporation for the Boeing 777 aircraft.

Parts have been made with multiple holes per die. A small angle extruded for electronics racks is shown in Fig. 4. A six-hole die was used to produce this part from a 150 mm (6 in.) diameter billet. The multihole extrusion was used in order to keep the area ratio between the product and the container to between 30 to 1 and 45 to 1. This range of extrusion ratios has been found to result in good control of the extrusion process

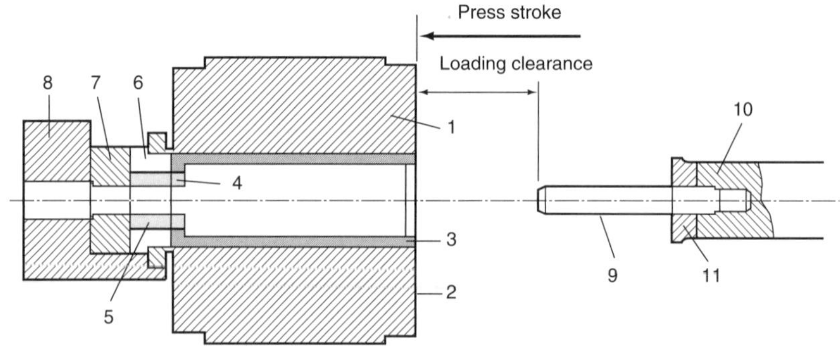

Fig. 2 Schematic of a die and mandrel extrusion setup for producing a single tubular product. Press and die components shown are 1 and 2, container; 3, liner; 4, extrusion die; 5, die backer; 6, die holder; 7, bolster; 8, press body; 9, mandrel; 10, extrusion stem; 11, seal block.

and produces a product that has well-defined mechanical properties. Extrusions have been made with extrusion ratios between 5 to 1 and 150 to 1 with satisfactory results. This product was solution treated in 12 m (40 ft) lengths, stretch straightened, and aged before being delivered. The amount of stretch is dependent upon the reinforcement level. The angles contained 25 vol% silicon carbide particles and remained in straightness tolerance after 1.5% stretch. Lower reinforcement levels require larger stretch amounts to bring the extrusions into tolerance.

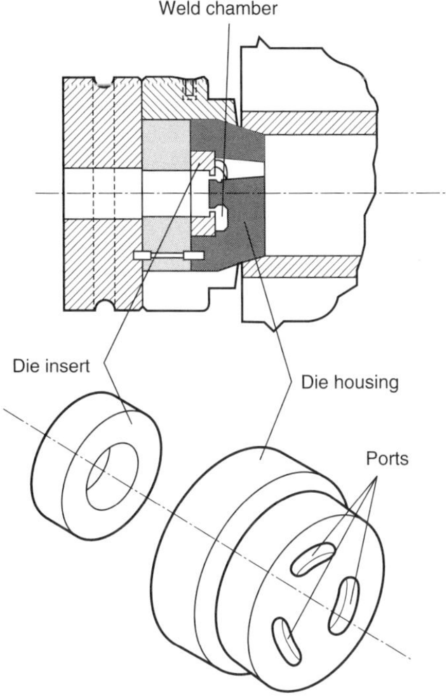

Fig. 3 Schematic diagram of a bridge or port die for extrusion of a shape containing a hollow

Effects of Reinforcements

The ceramic particles in the composite interact with the dies in two ways. The most immediate interaction is the wearing of the dies by the hard ceramics. The second interaction is the removal of the oxides from the die surface, which allows the clean iron to react with the aluminum matrix. The resulting brittle iron aluminide is very brittle and causes tears in the surface of the extrusions; such tearing includes hot shortness at high temperatures as well as ductility-related tearing at lower temperatures and speeds (Ref 1). The use of surface lubricants and conical dies minimizes the surface reaction, but results in nonsmooth surfaces caused by trapped excess lube. A second way of protecting the dies from the composite is the application of a ceramic coating on the die surface. The first successful coating system was a combination titanium carbide/titanium nitride deposited on the dies by a chemical vapor deposition (CVD) process. The dies need to be heat treated after the coating is applied to them. This coating produces parts with good surface quality while the coating remains intact. The ceramic particles in the composite wear the coating off quite rapidly. Approximately 76 m (250 ft) of 25 vol% composite can be extruded through a coated die before the coating is worn off. Another way to deal with the wear of the composite is the use of insert dies. A steel die body is made to hold a wear-resistant insert that has the desired shape cut in it. Such an insert is shown in Fig. 3. The insert is sacrificial and is replaced when the composite wears the opening beyond the part tolerance. Several materials were evaluated for wear during the extrusion of Duralcan 6061/Al_2O_3/20p composites. This study (Ref 2) demonstrated that cermet and ceramic inserts resist wear by the composite better than CVD or nitrided steel inserts.

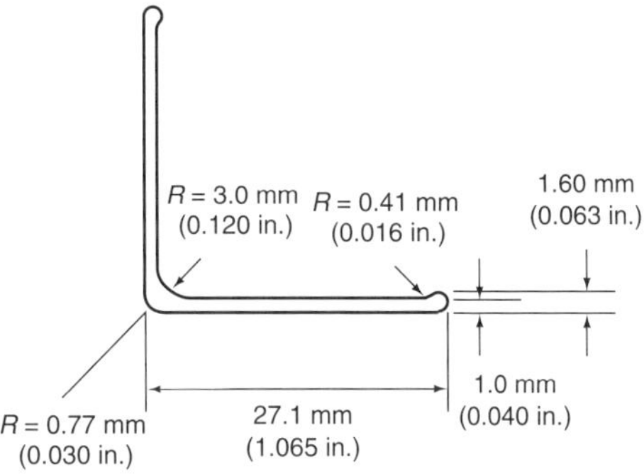

Fig. 4 Drawing of extruded angle for electronic rack. *R*, radius

REFERENCES

1. P.K. Saha, *Aluminum Extrusion Technology*, ASM International, 2000, p 204–208
2. P.W. Jeffrey and S. Holcomb, Extrusion of Particulate-Reinforced Aluminum Matrix Composites, *Conf. Proc. Fabrication of Particulates Reinforced Metal Composites*, ASM International, 1990, p 181–186

Post-Processing and Assembly of Ceramic-Matrix Composites

David Lewis III, Naval Research Laboratory
M. Singh, QSS Group, Inc., NASA Glenn Research Center

POST-PROCESSING of ceramic-matrix composites (CMCs) can be as critical to the successful and cost-effective use of these materials as the processing involved in producing the materials themselves. In only rare cases can these materials be produced in the finished form in which they are used. In nearly all cases, some form of post-processing is required. Post-processing, as defined here, includes those various processes that might be required to produce finished components from the CMC materials, such as:

- Machining or finishing operations
- Coating of the CMCs for thermal, chemical, or other reasons
- Joining of CMCs into CMC assemblies, or joining of CMC components to other components
- Assembly operations involving CMC components and other materials
- Nondestructive evaluation of CMCs, CMC components, or assemblies incorporating CMCs

This is illustrated schematically in Fig. 1. The path followed depends on whether the initial CMC processing is used to produce stock for fabricating components or to produce the components or assembly directly. Note that in the case of direct fabrication of assemblies, there can be significant inclusion of joining technology in the initial processing stage. Joining could include a variety of techniques, such as adhesive bonding, brazing or welding, and assembly with mechanical fasteners.

This article discusses the specific needs for science and technology in these areas, and the current state-of-the-art relative to the goal of employing CMCs in a variety of applications. One comment is appropriate: there is a large body of work relative to post-processing of CMCs and related materials (carbon-carbon [C-C] composites) that is very difficult to access because of classification, export control laws, and research and development that is deemed to be proprietary. There is, for example, extensive work on machining, joining, and coating of C-C composites for various military applications, which could be accessed by those with the appropriate clearances and need to know. The National Aeronautic and Space Administration (NASA) programs on the high-speed civil transport program and its successor on hypersonic vehicles have provided extensive development in the areas noted previously, but much of it is proprietary to the companies involved in the programs. Similarly, there are U.S. Air Force programs for high-temperature CMCs for engines and hypersonic structures and U.S. Navy programs on use of CMCs in various naval applications, such as engine components, that contain much relevant, but rather inaccessible information. The primary obstacle with much of this information is its restricted dissemination under U.S. export control laws.

Machining and Finishing of CMCs

Science and Technology Needs. While there are some processes capable of producing CMC components to near-net shape, such as the Lanxide direct metal oxidation process (High Performance Materials Group, MSE Inc., Newark, DE) (Ref 1), various solid freeform techniques (Ref 2, 3), and other techniques, such as injection molding (Ref 4), gel casting (Ref 5), and matrix infiltration into fiber preforms (Ref 6, 7), none of these has the capability of producing components to the tolerances and surface finishes typically required, for example, dimensional tolerances of 2 to 200 μm and surface finishes better than 25 μm root mean square (rms). The Lanxide process is the closest to net shape, producing a product very close in dimensions and shape to a starting aluminum-ceramic fiber preform, but is restricted in the choice of constituents for the composite. The techniques involving matrix or matrix-precursor infiltration into a fiber preform are limited in precision by two factors: the precision in forming of the fiber preform and the stability and dimensional tolerance retention of the preform during the matrix incorporation and consolidation step. The other techniques cited all involve substantial shrinkage on removal of organic binders and liquids and during sintering to final density. The linear shrinkage involved is typically on the order of 20 to 30% and depends on local density and geometry, thus limiting the precision achieved in the final component. As a result of the problems with various types of CMC processing, post-processing machining will generally be required to achieve the necessary dimensional tolerances, which, of course, depend on the particular application and requirements. Machining may also be necessary to achieve the surface finish required by a particular application; again, this is very sensitive to the particulars of the application. Finally, post-processing machining may be required to achieve contours or geometries not amenable to the particular CMC processing used or more readily done via post-processing.

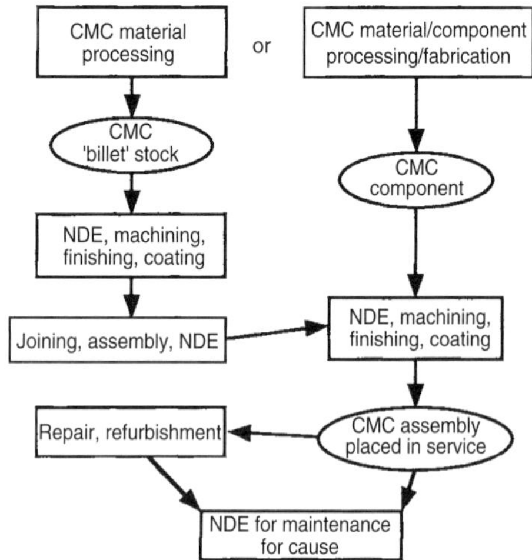

Fig. 1 Flow chart for postprocessing of CMCs, with two possible variants related to use of either "billet" stock followed by conventional processing—machining, joining, etc.—or near-net shape processing with joining during processing. Note occurrence of nondestructive evaluation (NDE) in several different areas of postprocessing.

Available Machining Technology. Unfortunately, in recent years there has been very little in the published literature on this subject, despite a large number of publications of processing and measurements of various properties of CMCs. There is one recent and comprehensive review article (Ref 8) on this topic, and one can find some information in the proceedings of the National Institute of Standards and Technology-sponsored meetings on ceramic machining (Ref 9). The conclusion that presumably can be drawn from this is that conventional ceramic machining procedures, or modifications of such procedures, can readily be used for machining and finishing of CMCs. This has been the authors' experience in approximately 20 years of work on these materials. With the use of appropriate tools, primarily diamond, these materials can be machined nearly as easily as conventional ceramic materials. In some ways, these materials (CMCs) are easier to machine, because they are typically designed for damage tolerance and thus are less susceptible to machining damage, permitting faster machining in many cases. On the other hand, with some types of CMCs, such as unidirectional fiber materials with the fibers weakly bonded to the matrix to achieve high toughness, there is a tendency for fiber pullout when the direction of the cutting media is parallel to the length of the fibers. Very rough machining can produce extensive fiber-matrix debonding and thus damage the CMC.

Some work published on laser machining (Ref 10–16) has been successfully applied to other materials in the past. This certainly shows promise for cutting and drilling CMCs with little damage to the materials, but requires modification to existing laser machining systems to achieve the high fluence necessary to ablate or vaporize refractory ceramic materials. Other techniques that have been explored for machining CMCs include ultrasonic cutting and waterjet cutting (Ref 17), both of which have advantages and disadvantages for particular uses. In addition, electrical discharge machining (Ref 18) can be used effectively for composites with sufficiently high electrical conductivity. All of these techniques can be competitive with conventional diamond machining for CMCs, and in many cases, they may be substantially cheaper, because of the high cost of consumables in diamond tooling for CMCs.

It is very likely that with those commercial operations actually using CMC components in systems, standard machining techniques have been developed. However, it may be necessary to wait for a larger and more mature CMC industry before such techniques are not deemed to be valuable proprietary information, and these techniques are set down in handbooks of standard machining practice or disclosed by manufacturers of CMC "billet stock" goods. One additional complication, which is also present in the polymer-matrix composite industry, is the wide variation in the nature of CMCs. These can be made from a wide range of fiber types, fiber architectures, and a wide range of matrices, the effect being that the machining parameters for various CMCs could also vary widely. A commercial entity using CMCs would likely have focused on a single material or related class of materials, where both the processing parameters and those for post-processing could be developed. This information may or may not be applicable to other types of CMCs.

The possibility exists of finishing some of these materials in the green state, where lower-cost tooling (carbide, high-speed steel) can be used, and any damage from the machining or finishing operation can be healed during the sintering or subsequent heat treatment. This may preclude the need for more extensive machining or finishing operations on the final product (Ref 19).

Coating and Surface Treatments for CMCs

Science and Technology Needs. While CMCs have been extensively promoted as the solution to high-temperature materials problems, existing CMCs may, in fact, also need protection themselves to survive particularly aggressive environments, or for other reasons. Most current CMCs are not stable for long periods in environments that attack the fiber-matrix interphase material. For example, the boron nitride (BN) and BN/SiC coatings developed by the authors and coworkers are subject to oxidative degradation, converting the boron nitride interphase from a debond coating into one that bonds the fiber strongly to the matrix, eliminating one of the primary toughening mechanisms in CMCs. In other cases, use of thermal barrier coatings may be necessary, either to protect the CMC itself from extremely high-temperature environments, or, in the case of a high-conductivity CMC, to protect an underlying metal or polymeric structure. There could be other reasons for the use of coatings on CMC components as well, with very different motivations, such as the use of conversion coatings to change the emissivity of the material and control the wavelength of the radiation emitted by the material when hot. This could be of importance for CMCs used as radiators in cooling systems or in heating systems, for example, in radiant burner tubes. There are a number of critical considerations that must be addressed to achieve a successful coating system for a CMC. These include chemical and thermal compatibility of the coating with the CMC, in addition to the coating meeting the requirements for its intended use, for example, effectively blocking oxygen transport in an antioxidation coating. One of the critical needs with coatings that has been addressed is that of the thermal mismatch stresses between a CMC substrate and coating, which can be modeled effectively using finite element methods and closed form techniques (Ref 20). These permit coating selection and design to minimize the stresses, which can greatly limit the service life of a coated CMC component.

Available Coating and Surface Treatments. There are a multiplicity of ways to produce coatings for CMCs, ranging from very low-cost techniques such as fired-on painted, dipped, or sprayed coatings (Ref 21); through techniques such as flame or plasma spraying (Ref 22); to the more exotic techniques such as physical vapor deposition, chemical vapor deposition, and so on. The particular appropriate technique is controlled by two factors—the cost tolerance of the application, and the ability to put down the required coating materials in the desired form. There are also several limitations with regard to some coating techniques, such as difficulty in coating complex shapes, and with the effects of the coating environment (e.g., high temperature and aggressive environment in a chemical vapor deposition reactor, and high temperatures associated with plasma spray). As a last resort, where coatings are impractical or impossible, the CMC itself may be modified to meet the particular requirements, although at some sacrifice in other properties, for example, incorporating oxidation barriers into the CMC itself, rather than relying on coatings (Ref 23).

Joining of CMCs

Science and Technology Needs. Joining is a critical need when either the requisite shapes cannot be produced directly from CMCs, or when the components or assemblies are larger than can be fabricated with the CMC process technology. Effective use of joining typically requires that:

- The joint and joining process does not degrade the properties of the CMC component.
- The joint must be as strong and as durable as the CMC components.
- The joint does not introduce any deleterious residual, thermal, or mechanical stresses.
- Some quality assurance method is available to ensure the quality of the joint after fabrication, and possibly during service.

Joining may also be required to transmit various types of loads, necessitating different kinds of joint designs and joint technologies, for example, shear stresses in large-area lap joints or tensile stresses in butt joints or tee joints. See Fig. 2 for schematic representations of various joint configurations. In the large-area lap joint, shear loads can be accomplished with a relatively low-strength joint, considering the relatively low shear strengths of most CMCs. It is much more difficult with a simple butt joint or tee joint, where the joint material must be as strong in tension as the CMC, which can have very respectable tensile strengths.

Available Joining Technologies. Joining, as noted previously, can encompass a variety of techniques, as required by application needs or by material and processing constraints. This can include adhesive bonding, which might be appropriate for locations seeing only moderate temperatures, but is unlikely to be used for

CMCs, which are typically selected for use at high temperatures. For higher-temperature applications, bonding via glass ceramics and preceramic polymers (Ref 24–29) or reaction bonding (Ref 30–36) is feasible and has been widely studied for both CMCs and C-C composites. Some forms of such bonding can be accomplished during the initial fabrication step, as in the use of melt infiltration to join fiber preforms into a complex assembly during the matrix infiltration step. Several examples of this are shown in Fig. 3 for the joining process developed at NASA Lewis Research Center (now NASA Glenn Research Center) (Ref 36) and Fig. 4 for CMC heat exchanger components (Ref 35). Joining of CMC components can also be achieved through mechanical fasteners, where a variety of high-temperature fastening systems has been developed for this purpose. There are extensive research and many publications and reports in this area, both in the open literature and in the restricted literature (Ref 29, 37–44). One interesting development has been the use of microwave energy for CMC joining, which has some great advantages over conventional heating in being able to locally heat joints without subjecting the entire assembly to high temperatures (Ref 45). At this point in time, for some classes of CMCs, joining appears to be a relatively mature area, with much technology available from which to choose. Readers should also consult the article on joining in the previous edition of this Volume (Ref 46), which covers much of the earlier work in this area, and the review articles listed in the references (Ref 47–49).

Assembly of CMCs

Science and Technology Needs. As noted previously, when CMC components required for applications are either too large to be fabricated in one piece with existing process technology, or the shapes are too complex to be fabricated, or it is required to assemble CMC components and other parts into a large and complex assembly, techniques for doing so will be required, including tooling, fixtures, alignment methods, and joining and fastening techniques. Some of these are probably transferable from metal and polymer-matrix composite technology, but the CMCs may introduce some special problems. These relate to the higher hardness of these materials, which may cause abrasive wear on fixturing and tooling; their higher stiffness and lower strain capability, which reduces the ability to force-fit parts; and their thermal expansion behavior, which differs from that of metallic and polymeric materials, requiring consideration of thermal expansion differences if substantial temperature differences are encountered in the assembly process, as in a brazed assembly.

Available Assembly Technologies. As noted previously, there is very little information published, either in the open or restricted literature, on this topic, though the nature of some programs would suggest that the problems associated with assembly of CMC components into large structures have been solved, to a large degree. For example, Fig. 5 shows two large disk brake assemblies, one using CMC bolts to join CMC disks, the other using bolts and ribs for the same purpose—to provide internal cooling passages in a CMC brake disk. These two components were produced by assembly and joining of a fairly large number of CMC subcomponents—disks, bolts, and ribs (Ref 35). The U.S. Navy currently uses CMCs in various forms in several aircraft and aircraft engines; these materials are presumably used in hot sections on the various stealth aircraft. Ceramic-matrix composite assemblies are being tested in helicopter engine applications, and CMCs are being actively considered for a number of uses in fusion power systems. In all of these cases, it is likely that the final component must be assembled from a number of smaller subunits, with provision for attachment to adjacent metallic or polymeric structures. Three examples found include two aerospace applications (Ref 50, 51) in the restricted literature, and one related to fusion power (Ref 52). Hopefully, in the future we will see more information published regarding this area of the technology required to use CMCs.

Nondestructive Evaluation

Science and Technology Needs. Nondestructive evaluation (NDE), in its general sense, appears several times in Fig. 1 and is a key need for use of CMCs, especially in critical applications where material or component failure would pose unacceptable risks. Nondestructive evaluation may be desirable in judging the quality of CMC material or components initially produced, and would normally be used as a process control device, if feasible and affordable. In addition, effective NDE techniques are desirable after machining, joining, coating, and assembly operations, again to ensure the quality of the postpro-

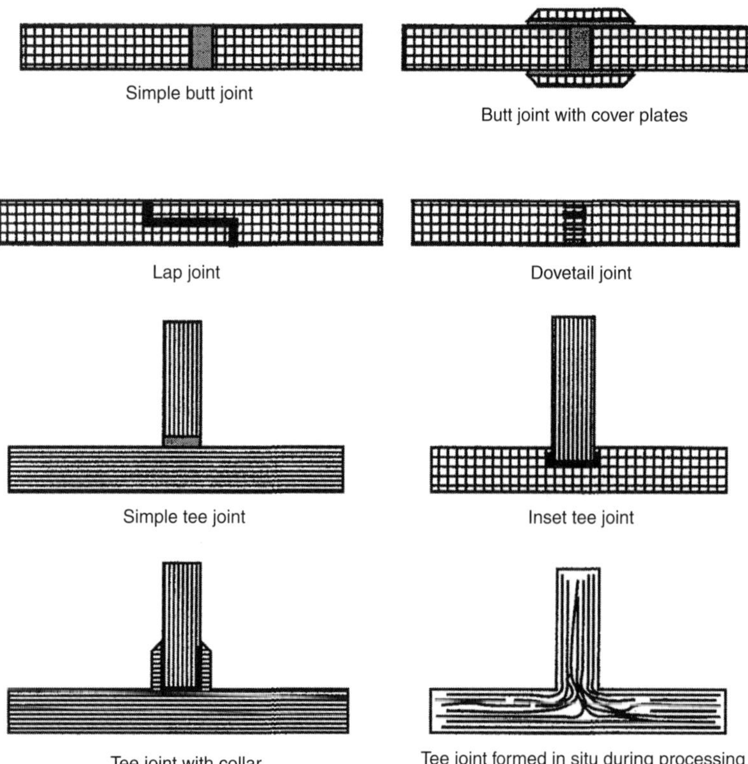

Fig. 2 Schematics of various types of joint designs for CMCs used to carry either tensile or shear loads. Different joint designs involve greatly varying amounts of cost and effort in joint fabrication and have greatly varying joint properties; some joints can be formed during processes such as reaction forming, rather than in postprocessing.

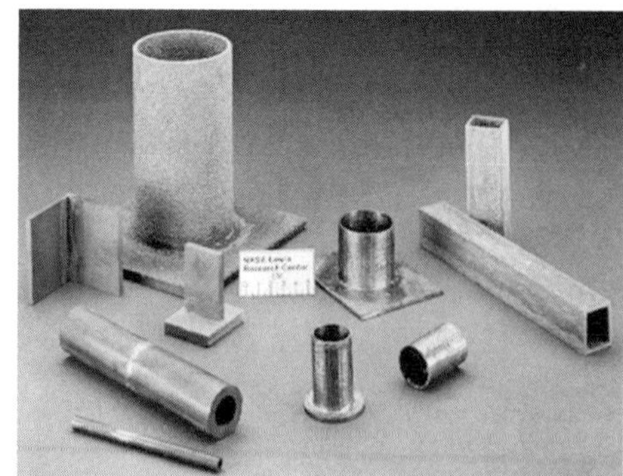

Fig. 3 Illustrations of various SiC and SiC composites joined using melt infiltration, a reaction-forming process to make various components. Courtesy of M. Singh, NASA Glenn Research Center

cessing steps. Finally, when the CMC component or assembly is placed in service, it may be necessary or preferable to have an NDE technique capable of determining whether, during service, property degradation or some form of damage has occurred that would require replacing or repairing the CMC material. In many applications, where repair or replacement costs are high and the costs of failure in service are similarly high, it is advantageous to have a technique that indicates when a component is about to fail. The component can then be replaced just in time (that is, not too late and not prematurely). In the same vein, if a CMC component is repaired in service, it would be desirable to have an NDE technique capable of judging the success of the repair.

Available NDE Technologies. In this area, there is a very large body of work performed and published, but no definitive results regarding the most appropriate NDE techniques for various types of CMCs. There is extensive work published on ultrasonic NDE (Ref 53–62) but no satisfactory way of doing this on large CMC articles. Ceramic-matrix composites are typically very lossy at the acoustic frequencies required to detect critical flaws, for example, 100 kHz to 100 MHz, and it is difficult to couple enough energy into materials to get effective NDE, especially for large components. With the additional complication of complex shapes and rough surfaces, the real need is for a noncontact method for ultrasonic NDE, with sufficient energy input and sensitivity to be effective. However, this does not yet exist (Ref 60). A variation on the ultrasonic method is the use of mechanical resonance measurements, that is, measurement of the complex mechanical impedance of a component (resonant frequencies and width of resonance peaks) (Ref 55–57, 61–67). This measurement can be sensitive to certain types of defects and in-service damage, and in some cases can be used as an effective process control system and for characterization of in-service damage and degradation. The typical changes seen are shifts in the resonance peaks, broadening of the peaks with defects and damages, and appearance of new peaks with significant defects or damage.

Another NDE technique, which has advantages in being noncontact and capable of large-area coverage but suffers in resolution, is thermal imaging—effectively, a measure of local thermal diffusivity in a material. This has been demonstrated to be useful for detection of certain types of defects in CMCs, where the defects are of sufficiently large size and differ substantially in thermal diffusivity from the base material (Ref 58, 61, 62, 67–69). Yet another technique, which has been explored by a number of investigators, is that of microradiography and computed x-ray tomography. These can certainly be effective for detection of relatively small defects, where there is sufficient atomic number contrast, but they suffer from problems with the scale of components that can be characterized (Ref 58, 59, 61, 62, 70–72). With conventional x-ray energies, the penetration depth is limited to a few centimeters for most CMC materials, greatly limiting the scale of products that can be characterized in this manner. The solution to this problem, increasing the x-ray energy via synchrotron sources, and so on, is hardly practical for industrial situations. Some other techniques have been explored as well for NDE of CMCs, including neutron diffraction for measurement of residual stresses and in neutron radiography (Ref 59, 73), the classic method of dye penetrants (Ref 71), and optical techniques employing laser scattering (Ref 59, 62), but with little promise of wide applicability at this point. There are several review articles and comparisons of different techniques available on this subject (Ref 58, 59, 61, 62, 74). Another good source of information on NDE, at present, is the NDE Working Group at NASA Glenn Research Center (Ref 75), which has had a great deal of experience applying NDE techniques to the CMCs involved in the NASA and Air Force programs on the high-speed civil transport and hypersonic vehicle programs.

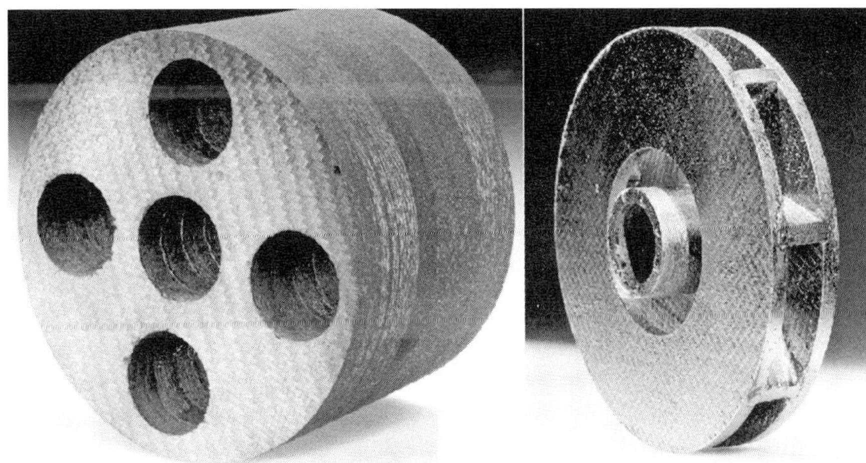

Fig. 4 Heat exchanger subassembly (left) and prototype radial outflow pump wheel (right) made by joining CMC components. Heat exchanger subassembly formed from eight individual CMC disks; pump wheel fabricated from CMC disks, plates, and tubes. Courtesy of W. Krenkel, German Aerospace Research Center

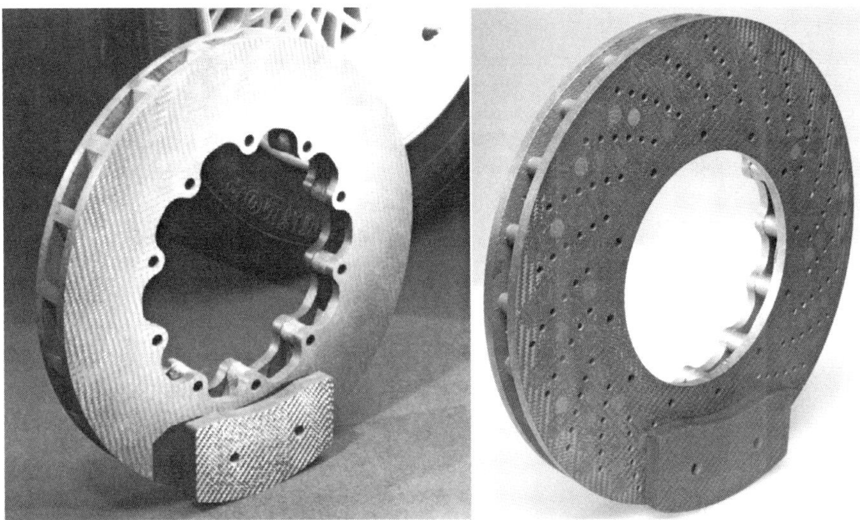

Fig. 5 Prototype C/SiC CMC disk brake assembly fabricated from CMC disks, bolts (right), and ribs (left). CMC brakes are now in use on two German production automobiles and provide greatly improved braking performance over metal disks. Courtesy of W. Krenkel, German Aerospace Research Center

REFERENCES

1. G.H. Schiroky, D.V. Miller, M.K. Aghajanian, and A.S. Fareed, Fabrication of CMC's and MMC's Using Novel Process, *Key Eng. Mater.*, Vol 127–131, 1997, p 141–152
2. C. Gasdaska, V. Jamalabad, M. Ortiz, B. Mitlin, and D. Twait, Solid Freeform Fabrication of Advanced Ceramics, *Ceram. Eng. Sci. Proc.*, Vol 21 (No. 4), 2000, p 135–142
3. D.L. Bourell, J.L. Beaman, R.H. Crawford, H.L. Marcus, and J.W. Barlow, Ed., *Solid Freeform Fabrication Symposium*, Univ. of

Texas at Austin, 1999 (also see volumes from preceding and succeeding years from same meeting)

4. R. Fischer, R. Gadow, and G.W. Schäfer, Manufacturing of Aluminum Nitride Heat Exchangers by Ceramic Injection Molding, *Ceram. Eng. Sci. Proc.,* Vol 20 (No. 4), 1999, p 595–602
5. J.J. Nick, D. Newson, R. Masseth, S. Monette, and O.O. Omatete, Gelcasting Automation for High Volume Production of Silicon Nitride Turbine Wheels, *Ceram. Eng. Sci. Proc.,* Vol 20 (No. 3), 1999, p 225–232
6. F.I. Hurwitz, J. Riehl, J. Madsen, T.R. McCue, and D.L. Boyd, Characterization of In Situ BN Interface Formed by Nitridation of Nextel 312, *Ceram. Eng. Sci. Proc.,* Vol 20 (No. 4), 1999, p 3–10
7. M. Kotani, A. Kohyama, K. Okamura, and T. Inoue, Fabrication of High Performance SiC/SiC Composite by Polymer Impregnation and Pyrolysis Method, *Ceram. Eng. Sci. Proc.,* Vol 20 (No. 4), 1999, p 309–316
8. R. Komanduri, Machining of Fiber-Reinforced Composites, *Mach. Sci. Technol.*, Vol 1 (No. 1), 1997, p 113-152 (comprehensive review article)
9. S. Jahanmir, Ed., Machining of Advanced Materials, *Proc. International Conf. on Machining of Advanced Materials* (Gaithersburg, MD), National Institute of Standards and Technology (NIST), 1993; also Ceramic Machining Consortium, NIST, www.ceramics.nist.gov
10. P. Tuersley, A.P. Hoult, and I.R. Pashby, The Process of a Magnesium-Aluminosilicate Matrix, SiC Fibre Glass-Ceramic Matrix Composite Using a Pulsed Nd-YAG Laser, Part I: Optimization of Pulse Parameter, *J. Mater. Sci.*, Vol 31 (No. 15), 1996, p 4111–4119
11. P. Tuersley, A.P. Hoult, and I.R. Pashby, The Processing of SiC/SiC Ceramic Matrix Composites Using a Pulsed Nd-YAG Laser, Part I: Optimisation of Pulse Parameters, *J. Mater. Sci.*, Vol 33 (No. 4), 1998, p 955–961
12. P. Tuersley, A.P. Hoult, and I.R. Pashby, Nd-YAG Laser Machining of SiC Fibre Borosilicate Glass Composites, Part II: The Effect of Process Variables, *J. Mater. Sci.*, Vol 33 (No. 4), 1998, p 963–967
13. P. Tuersley, A.P. Hoult, and I.R. Pashby, Nd-YAG Laser Machining of SiC Fibre Borosilicate Glass Composites, Part I: Optimisation of Laser Pulse Parameters, *Composites Part A: Appl. Sci. Manuf.*, Vol 29 (No. 8), 1998, p 947–954
14. P. Tuersley, A.P. Hoult, and I.R. Pashby, Nd-YAG Laser Machining of SiC Fibre Borosilicate Glass Composites, Part II: The Effect of Process Variables, *Composites Part A: Appl. Sci. Manuf.*, Vol 29 (No. 8), 1998, p 955–964
15. X. Chen, W.T. Lotshaw, A.L. Ortiz, P.R. Staver, C.E. Erikson, M.H. McLaughlin, and T.J. Rockstroh, Laser Drilling of Advanced Materials, *J. Laser Appl.,* Vol 8 (No. 5), 1996, p 233–239
16. J.W. Carroll, J.A. Todd, W.A. Ellingson, and B.J. Polzin, Laser Machining of Ceramic Matrix Composites, *Ceram. Eng. Sci. Proc.*, Vol 21 (No. 3), 2000, p 323–330
17. Waterjet Technology, Inc., www.waterjet-tech.com
18. C.C. Liu, Wire Electrical Discharge Machining and Mechanical Properties of Gas Pressure Sintered $MoSi_2/Si_3N_4$ Composites, *J. Ceram. Soc. Jpn.*, Vol 108 (No. 5), 2000, p 469–472
19. T.E. Easler, A. Szweda, and V.A. Black, Green Machining of Sylramic Ceramic Matrix Composites, Advances in Ceramic-Matrix Composites V, *Ceram. Trans.,* Vol 103, 2000, p 593–602
20. M.-J. Pindera, J. Aboudi, and S.M. Arnold, Thermomechanical Analysis of Functionally Graded Thermal Barrier Coatings with Different Microstructural Scales, *J. Am. Ceram. Soc.*, Vol 81 (No. 6), 1998, p 1525–1536
21. M. Ferraris, M. Salvo, C. Isola, M.A. Montorsi, and A. Kohyama, Glass-Ceramic Coating and Joining of SiC/SiC for Fusion Applications, *J. Nucl. Mater.*, Vol 263 (Part B), 1998, p 1546–1550
22. W.Y. Lee, K.M. Cooley, C.C. Berndt, D.L. Joslin, and D.P. Stinton, High-Temperature Chemical Stability of Plasma-Sprayed $Ca_{0.5}Sr_{0.5}Zr_4P_6O_{24}$ Coatings on Nicalon/SiC Ceramic Matrix Composite and Ni-Based Superalloy Substrates, *J. Am. Ceram. Soc.*, Vol 79 (No. 10), 1996, p 2759–2762
23. F. Lamouroux, S. Bertrand, R. Pailler, R. Naslain, and M. Cataldi, Oxidation-Resistant Carbon-Fiber-Reinforced Ceramic-Matrix Composites, *Compos. Sci. Technol.*, Vol 59 (No. 7), 1999, p 1073–1085
24. P. Colombo, B. Riccardi, A. Donato, and G. Scarinci, Joining of SiC/SiC_f Ceramic Matrix Composites for Fusion Reactor Blanket Applications, *J. Nucl. Mater.,* Vol 278 (No. 2-3), 2000, p 127–135
25. M. Ferraris, M. Salvo, C. Isola, M.A. Montorsi, and A. Kohyama, Glass-Ceramic Joining and Coating of SiC/SiC for Fusion Applications, *J. Nucl. Mater.,* Vol 263 (Part B), 1998, p 1546-1550
26. L.A. Xue, Electrically Insulating Joining of Carbon-Carbon Composites for High Temperature Applications, *Ceram. Eng. Sci. Proc.,* Vol 18 (No. 3), 1997, p 167–175
27. W.J. Sherwood, C.K. Whitmarsh, J.M. Jacobs, and L.V. Interrante, Joining Ceramic Composites Using Active Metals/HPCS Preceramic Polymer Slurries, *Ceram. Eng. Sci. Proc.,* Vol 18 (No. 3), 1997, p 177–184
28. S. Fareed and C.C. Cropper, Joining Techniques for Fiber-Reinforced Ceramic Matrix Composites, *Ceram. Eng. Sci. Proc.,* Vol 20 (No. 4), 1999, p 61–70
29. I.E. Anderson, S. Ijadi-Maghsoodi, O. Unal, T. Barton, W.E. Bustamente, B.C. Mutsuddy, and A. Szwerda, Low Temperature Joining of SiC Ceramics and CFCC Materials, *Proc. 20th Annual Conf. on Ceramic, Metal and Carbon Composites, Materials and Structures,* Naval Surface Warfare Center, Carderock Division, 1996, p 703–729
30. W. Krenkel and M.R. Nedele, Novel Concept of a High Temperature Heat Exchanger, *Ind. Ceram.* (Italy), Vol 19 (No. 2), 1999, p 109–111
31. P. Dadras, T.T. Ngai, and G. M. Mehrota, Joining of Carbon-Carbon Composites Using Boron and Titanium Disilicide Interlayers, *J. Am. Ceram. Soc.,* Vol 80 (No. 1), 1997, p 125–132
32. M. Singh, S.C. Farmer, and J.D. Kiser, Joining of Silicon Carbide-Based Ceramics by Reaction Forming Approach, *Ceram. Eng. Sci. Proc.,* Vol 18 (No. 3), 1997, p 161–166
33. C.A. Lewinsohn, R.H. Jones, M. Singh, T. Shibayama, T. Hinoki, M. Ando, and A. Kohyama, Methods for Joining Silicon Carbide Composites for High-Temperature Structural Applications, *Ceram. Eng. Sci. Proc.,* Vol 20 (No. 3), 1999, p 119–123
34. M. Singh and E. Lara-Curzio, Design, Fabrication and Testing of Ceramic Joints for High Temperature SiC/SiC Composites, *J. Eng. Gas Turbines Power (Trans. ASME),* Vol 123, 2001, p 288–292
35. W. Krenkel and T. Henke, Modular Design of CMC Structures by Reaction Bonding of SiC, *Proc. Joining of Adv. and Specialty Mater. II,* ASM International, 2000, p 3–9
36. M. Singh, Joint Design and Testing Issues in Reactively Joined SiC-Based Ceramics and Composites, *Adv. Brazing and Soldering Technology,* (IBSC-2000), American Welding Society and ASM International, 2000, p 322–329
37. T.F. Kearns, Ed., "Joining of Carbon-Carbon and Ceramic Matrix Composites," Institute for Defense Analyses Memorandum Report M-312, Institute for Defense Analyses, Alexandria, VA, 1987
38. A. Nagar and C. Foreman, Thermomechanical Fatigue and Strength of CMC Structural Joints, *Proc. 21st Annual Conf. on Ceramic, Metal and Carbon Composites, Materials and Structures,* Naval Surface Warfare Center, Carderock Division, 1997, p 337–347
39. L.H. Chiu and D. Nagle, Reaction Bonding of Advanced Materials, *Proc. 21st Annual Conf. on Ceramic, Metal and Carbon Composites, Materials and Structures,* Naval Surface Warfare Center, Carderock Division, 1997, p 349–358
40. S.I. Maghsoodi, I.E. Anderson, O. Unal, M. Nosrati, and T.J. Barton, Processing and Properties of Low Temperature Joints Between SiC/SiC Composites, *Proc. 21st Annual Conf. on Ceramic, Metal and Carbon Composites, Materials and Structures*, Naval Surface Warfare Center, Carderock Division, 1997, p 361–373
41. M.K. Brun, W.A. Morrison, and G.S. Corman, Joining of Toughened Silcomp Composites, *Proc. 21st Annual Conf. on Ce-*

ramic, Metal and Carbon Composites, Materials and Structures, Naval Surface Warfare Center, Carderock Division, 1997, p 383–390
42. B.H. Rabin and J.K. Weddell, Joining of CVI SiC/SiC CMC's Using Reaction Bonding, *Proc. 20th Annual Conf. on Ceramic, Metal and Carbon Composites, Materials and Structures,* Naval Surface Warfare Center, Carderock Division, 1996, p 579–599
43. C.H. Henager and R. Jones, Joining of SiC Ceramics Using Displacement Reactions, *Proc. 20th Annual Conf. on Ceramic, Metal and Carbon Composites, Materials and Structures,* Naval Surface Warfare Center, Carderock Division, 1996, p 647–661
44. R.J. Miller, J.C. Moree, D.C. Jarmon, M.E. Palusis, and R.E. Warburton, Development and Validation of Attachment Concepts for High Temperature Composites, *Proc. 21st Annual Conf. on Ceramic, Metal and Carbon Composites, Materials and Structures,* Naval Surface Warfare Center, Carderock Division, 1997, p 311–321
45. S. Aravindan and R. Krishnamurthy, Joining of Ceramic Composites by Microwave Heating, *Mater. Lett.,* Vol 38 (No. 4), 1999, p 245–249
46. A.G. Razzell, Joining and Machining of Ceramic Matrix Composites, *Composites,* Vol 1, *Engineered Materials Handbook,* ASM International, 1987, p 1–9
47. *Review of Ceramic Joining Technology,* Advanced Materials and Processes Technology Information and Analysis Center (AMPTIAC), Rome, NY, 1995
48. J.M. Howe, Bonding, Structure and Properties of Metal/Ceramic Interfaces, Part 1: Chemical Bonding, Chemical Reaction and Interfacial Structure, *Int. Mater. Rev.,* Vol 38 (No. 5), 1993, p 233–270
49. M.K. Brun, Formation of Tough Composite Joints, *J. Am. Ceram. Soc.,* Vol 81 (No. 12), 1998, p 3307–3312
50. C.H. Henager, B.C. Mutsuddy, and A. Szweda, Shear Testing of Joined Ceramic Composites, *Proc. 20th Annual Conf. on Ceramic, Metal and Carbon Composites, Materials and Structures,* Naval Surface Warfare Center, Carderock Division, 1996, p 601–616
51. C.R. Foreman, D.M. Box, and G.R. Corcoran, Development and Flight Testing of a Ceramic Matrix Composite Heat Shield for the AV-8B Harrier, *Proc. 20th Annual Conf. on Ceramic, Metal, and Carbon Composites, Materials and Structures,* Naval Surface Warfare Center, Carderock Division, 1996, p 817–842
52. K. Matsumoto, N. Fujioka, T. Hayakawa, N. Kawamura, and K. Sato, The Development of a Combustion Chamber Liner Utilizing a Long-Fiber Reinforced Composite Material Made Using the Polysilazane Impregnation Method and the Chemical Vapor Deposition Method, *High Temp. Ceram. Matrix Compos. III,* Vol 164 (No. 1), 1999, p 49–52
53. B.R. Tittmann, M.C. Bhardwaj, L. Vandervalk, and I. Neeson, Non-Contact Ultrasonic NDE of Carbon-Carbon Composite, *Ceram. Eng. Sci. Proc.,* Vol 20 (No. 3), p 325–332
54. K.H. Im, H. Jeong, and I.Y. Yang, A Study of the Ultrasonic Nondestructive Evaluation of Carbon/Carbon Composite Disks, *Korean Society of Mechanical Engineers Int. J,* Vol 14 (No. 3), 2000, p 320–330
55. W.A. Ellingson, E.R. Koehl, J.G. Sun, C. Deemer, H. Lee, and T. Spohnholtz, Development of Nondestructive Evaluation for Hot Gas Filters, *Mater. High Temp.,* Vol 16 (No. 4), 1999, p 213–218
56. V. Helanti, P. Pastila, A.P. Nikkila, and T. Mantyla, NDE Methods to Evaluate Ceramic Hot Gas Filters, *Ind. Ceram. (Italy),* Vol 20 (No. 1), 2000, p 33–35
57. Y.C. Chu, A. Lavrentyev, S.I. Rokhlin, G.Y. Baaklini, and R.T. Bhatt, Ultrasonic Evaluation of Time/Temperature Effect of Oxidation Damage in Ceramic Matrix Composites, *Rev. Prog. Quant. Nondestruct. Eval.,* Vol 13 B, 1994, p 1221–1228
58. J.G. Sun, D.R. Petrak, T.A.K. Pillai, C. Deemer, and W.A. Ellingson, Nondestructive Evaluation and Characterization of Damage and Repair of Continuous Fiber Ceramic Composite Panels, *Ceram. Eng. Sci. Proc.,* Vol 19 (No. 3), 1998, p 615–622
59. D. Allen, M. Mets, D. Lorey, J. Griffin, and D. Carlson, Nondestructive Evaluation Techniques for Ceramic Matrix Composites, *Ceram. Eng. Sci. Proc.,* Vol 19 (No. 3), 1998, p 631–638
60. M.C. Bhardway, I. Neeson, M.E. Langron, and L. Vandervalk, Contact-Free Ultrasound: The Final Frontier in Non-Destructive Materials Evaluation, *Ceram. Eng. Sci. Proc.,* Vol 21 (No. 3), 2000, p 163–172
61. R.M. Aoki, G. Busse, K. Eberle, C. Hansel, P. Schanz, and D. Wu, NDI Evaluation of Local Oxidised C/C-SiC Specimens, *Insight,* Vol 40 (No. 10), 1998, p 706–711
62. W.A. Ellingson, J.S. Steckenrider, and J.B. Stuckey, Preliminary Results of Applying Several NDE Methods to Ceramic Joints, *Proc. 20th Annual Conf. on Ceramic, Metal and Carbon Composites, Materials and Structures,* Naval Surface Warfare Center, Carderock Division, 1996, p 683–702
63. V. Kostopoulos, Y.Z. Pappas, and Y.P. Markopoulos, Fatigue Damage Accumulation in 3-Dimensional SiC/SiC Composites, *J. Eur. Ceram. Soc.,* Vol 19 (No. 2), 1999, p 207–215
64. R. El Bouazzaoui, S. Baste, and G. Camus, Development of Damage in a 2D Woven C/SiC Composite under Mechanical Loading, Part 2: Ultrasonic Characterization, *Compos. Sci. Technol.,* Vol 56 (No. 12), 1996, p 1373–1382
65. Y.M. Liu, Y. He, F.M. Chu, T.E. Mitchell, and H.N.G. Wadley, Elastic Properties of Laminated Calcium Aluminosilicate/Silicon Carbide Composites Determined by Resonant Ultrasound Spectroscopy, *J. Am. Ceram. Soc.,* Vol 80 (No. 1), 1997, p 142–148
66. C. Aristégui and S. Baste, Load Induced Change in the Elastic Symmetry of a Ceramic Matrix Composite Under Off-Axis Tensile Loading, *Rev. Prog. Quant. Nondestruct. Eval.,* Vol 17 B, 1998, p 1131–1138
67. Y.-L. Wang, J.E. Webb, and R.N. Singh, Evaluation of Thermal Shock Damage in 2-D Woven Nicalon-Al2O3 Composite by NDE Techniques, *Ceram. Eng. Sci. Proc.,* Vol 19 (No. 3), 1998, p 607–614
68. C. Deemer, J.G. Sun, W.A. Ellingson, and S. Short, Front-Flash Thermal Imaging Characterization of Continuous Fiber Composites, *Ceram. Eng. Sci. Proc.,* Vol 20 (No. 3), 1999, p 317–324
69. J.G. Sun, C. Deemer, and W.A. Ellingson, Thermal Imaging Measurement of Lateral Thermal Diffusivity in Continuous Fiber Ceramic Composites, *Ceram. Eng. Sci. Proc.,* Vol 21 (No. 3), 2000, p 179–185
70. Z. Guo, Q. Ye, J. Tian, and C. Zhang, High-Resolution CT Tests Ceramic Parts, *B. Am. Ceram. Soc.,* Vol 79 (No. 1), 2000, p 59–61
71. E.R. Generazio, Nondestructive Evaluation of Ceramic and Metal Matrix Composites for NASA's Materials Programs, *Advanced Ceramic Matrix Composites,* Technomic Publishing Co. Inc., Lancaster, PA, 1996, p 169–204
72. NDE of Tapes and Composites, *Bull. Am. Ceram. Soc.,* Vol 78 (No. 1), 1999, p 20
73. E. Martinelli, R.A.L. Drew, E.A. Fancello, R. Rogge, and J.H. Root, Neutron Diffraction and Finite-Element Analysis of Thermal Residual Stresses on Diffusion-Bonded Silicon Carbide-Molybdenum Joint, *J. Am. Ceram. Soc.,* Vol 82 (No. 7), 1999, p 1787–1792
74. M.H. Van de Voorde, Non-Destructive Evaluation (NDE) of Carbon-Carbon (C-C) and Ceramic Composite Materials, *Br. Ceram. Trans.,* Vol 97 (No. 6), 1998, p 287–292
75. NASA NDE Working Group, NASA-Glenn Research Center, Cleveland, OH

Quality Assurance

Chairperson: G. Aaron Henson III, Design Alternatives, Inc.

Introduction to Quality Assurance

Grover Aaron Henson III, Design Alternatives Inc.

THE COMPOSITES INDUSTRY is vast and far-reaching. Technology integration around the globe has enabled materials and manufacturing companies to intermingle ideas in design and development, manufacturing, and, of course, quality. The leading question is always, what is quality? Quality is *flawlessness.*

To achieve flawlessness, a quality system must be in place. This system is initially developed with four critical steps: integration of quality processes and procedures at the design phase, imposed traceability, documented continuous improvement, and *customer satisfaction.*

Quality assurance for composites is progressively changing. Many analysis tools and manufacturing methods continue to be developed to improve the quality of composite products. This Section of the Handbook discusses various quality processes and techniques that readers can implement with some assurance that they are not alone. It also examines various aspects of the quality life cycle, starting with characterization of the fiber and resins through understanding what was manufactured via nondestructive evaluation.

In-Process Monitoring

The quality of composite laminates has traditionally been determined in the cured state, which does not allow for process correction of a nonconforming condition. The quality of the composite material was based on validating the physical and mechanical properties of that structure after cure. A greater focus now is being placed on understanding the critical resin impregnation process during the fabrication stage. This effort supports the concept of "predicting" quality at the earliest point in the process. Much of the quality analysis performed in year 2000 begins its evaluation at the dry fiber level and continues through to a cured state. The reader is presented the importance of progressing from post-manufacturing inspection/verification (noncorrectable) to in-process inspection/verification (correctable-predictor) methods. This philosophy is critical to process improvement, cost reduction, and schedule enhancement goals.

Validation of composite products to a level of flawlessness begins with the design identification and selection of the correct resin and fiber. The entire manufacturing process must be considered during this selection process, to minimize quality cost and schedule impacts.

Resin studies define the constitution and chemical makeup, which categorizes resins into various families. These families dictate the processing environment requirements, manufacturing properties, and structural application of each resin. This information provides the designer with reliable choices in processing, cost, and life cycle performance.

The fiber selection process takes into consideration design strength and modulus requirements. Typical fiber configurations include continuous and discontinuous, woven, unidirectional tape, and three-dimensional braided preforms. Fiber materials include graphite, glass, aramid, and others. The fiber configuration and material are major components when analyzing the mechanics of fiber-reinforced composites.

Structural integrity requires the correct resin, fiber, orientation, and cure. Material orientation is a critical factor when using composite material for load-bearing structure. The ability to "tailor" material orientation allows the designer to create structure that is lighter weight than traditional aluminum structure. Therefore, verification of lay-up orientation process is key to the structural integrity. Ply orientation is verified and controlled with laser alignment equipment that guarantees accuracy and repeatability. Use of laser noninvasive verification processes greatly improves process efficiency and quality at the lay-up touch labor level.

The next generation of composite products will embrace more noninvasive methods of in-process validation and verification of material properties. The ideal of reducing and eliminating post-process end-item inspection and verification should be the goal of all existing and potential composite manufacturers. Quality assurance is the facilitator of product conformity to all other support organizations. Quality must be an integral member of the design effort to ensure quality is designed in with minimal impact and maximum benefit to the product.

Quality Assurance Factors

All engineering support groups must understand what constitutes a quality product for all other support groups. Therefore, a typical composite laminate lay-up process would include review and confirmation of the following items:

- Incoming raw material(s) conformity
- Released engineering requirements (includes process specifications and acceptance criteria)
- Approved tooling
- Approved planning documents
- Trained process operators and inspectors to enable self-inspection of ply orientation and configuration location
- In-process controls of critical processes and parameters, such as material out time and cure parameters (time, temperature, and pressure)
- Statistical process control (SPC) data collection of key process variables to ensure process capability and performance
- Nondestructive evaluation
- Verification of dimensional and configuration conformity

Each of these aspects is critical to the quality of a laminate.

Tooling and Assembly Considerations

Until recently, fabrication procedures for composite laminates were almost exclusively focused on autoclave processing. With the increased focus on next-generation composite processing affordability, out-of-autoclave curing has become a common goal. Processes such as vacuum-assisted resin transfer molding, resin transfer molding, electron beam curing, room-temperature curing, oven curing, and resin-fiber infusion are being adopted to meet the new affordability objectives.

The tooling concepts for out-of-autoclave processing are much more affordable and faster to fabricate. New materials include foam, lightweight wood, pressure-formed thin steel and aluminum, and thin composite materials. This type of tooling approach allows for rapid change capability in development programs and lower cost at the production levels. Longevity and accuracy are among the benefits of these new tooling concepts.

Traditional composite cure tooling is fabricated from steel, aluminum, or high-temperature composite materials. These types of materials are required to withstand the temperature and pressure of typical thermoplastic cure process. Their cost is high, and they require significant lead time to manufacture. Change is not a viable option with conventional autoclave-type tooling.

Year 2000 three-dimensional engineering offers reduced tooling cost by using computer-generated models to dictate radii, control surface geometry, and streamline complex surface contouring. This technology is integrated with numerical-controlled equipment to make tools much faster than conventional methods, as well as real-time inspection capability.

Process operators are becoming the "process owners," because they provide source-controlled quality based on real-time SPC data. Data are collected real time as the process runs, and the operator is notified to make authorized adjustments to the process to maintain conforming product. All of these features are effective in reducing the time required to manufacture new tooling and in eliminating end-item inspection.

As various industries explore the fabrication techniques of larger unitized structures for aircraft, ships, and other transportation vehicles, monitoring and controlling the composite laminate is essential. Less and less is the quality (flawlessness) of a laminate totally in the hands of the materials manufacturers, because resin infusion is becoming real time during the final fabrication stage. Several methods have been developed for real-time monitoring and controlling of liquid molding processes. The objective is to have real-time knowledge of resin location during processing. Combining resin monitoring with flow modeling greatly reduces or eliminates end-item inspection.

As these industries evolve to use larger structures, in-process inspection of bonding quality of joints begins to play a vital role in the unitization of structures. The quality arena is again challenged with the verification of joint quality, the understanding of contaminates, and the levels of acceptability. Methods to detect and verify them are being studied and expanded.

Adhesive bonding is a very complex arena; it has proven to be extremely difficult to gain acceptance in many of the high-tech markets. Many aspects of the bonding process come into play when analyzing structures for bonding compatibility, including bonding surface tension, surface preparation, roughness, contaminate levels, moisture content, and surface conditioning. In high-tech markets, all aspects have to be monitored and controlled to verify quality and to maintain and expand the use of composites for critical applications. For less-demanding applications, these aspects must be monitored to improve scrap rates and reduce returns.

Quality Assurance for Commercial Applications

Composite materials are becoming increasingly common in commercial products, such as bicycles, baseball bats, golf clubs, tennis rackets, automotive parts, and high-performance water and land race vehicles. The commercial industry uses approximately 65% of the graphite fibers produced, with aerospace companies and airframe manufacturers using the remaining 35%.

Commercial market requirements on quality are normally less demanding than for aircraft and transportation businesses. Nevertheless, control of the processes is still very important in reducing scrap-related costs. Industries that use advanced materials systems to build products for aircraft and other transportation markets are driven by structural integrity requirements. These industries recognize the need for structural validation and the necessity of continuous advancements in nondestructive analysis. There have been great strides in understanding and characterization of flaws, increasing our ability to identify and locate delaminations, voids, matrix cracking, and porosity in composite structures.

Nondestructive Testing and Data Fusion

In year 2000, nondestructive inspection/test methods such as pulse-echo and through-transmission ultrasonics are the technologies of choice in determining composite quality. Continuous improvement research has developed additional inspection methods, such as leaky Lamb wave, polar backscattering, nonlinear acoustics, ultrasonic, radiography, computed tomography, and infrared thermography, to name a few. The continued development of these technologies could effectively make huge improvements in some markets.

Data fusion systems are designed to provide nondestructive analysis data from fabrication and assembly processes for each individual composite part. The importance of these systems cannot be underestimated; collecting this manufacturing data provides not only a historical record (traceability) for fabrication and assembly, but, when properly mined, can also provide an essential source of information for engineering process analysis. Material review boards can use this technology to provide a data-supported disposition for "reworked" or "accept-as-is" nonconforming conditions.

Data integration systems will someday provide a single source of process information that can be used to determine product quality acceptance. The vision is that this technology will allow for in-process product acceptance without operator intervention. Statistical process control tools will play a vital role in the implementation of this technology. The "key" controllable process parameters can be monitored to provide the opportunity to disposition potential nonconforming conditions at the "correctable" level in the process. This concept is the "adhesive" that will bind all process quality elements to one source.

Conclusions

The articles in this Section have been written with the objective of sharing years of experience and technical knowledge. Many of the writers are renowned in their industries for being innovative and creative. Much of the technology is proven as of year 2000; however, some of the next-generation methods described are in their experimental state. The reader is encouraged to satisfy curiosity raised by this Volume by consulting the references cited in the individual articles that follow. The reader should endeavor to understand the level of maturity of the processes described and judge their merit for the application being considered. The future of composites quality will be guided by those who share and embrace the concepts described in this Handbook.

Resin Properties Analysis

John D. Russell, Air Force Research Laboratory

MOST RESINS USED IN COMPOSITE MATERIALS are blends or systems of ingredients, each of which is added to give some desired benefit for processing or for properties of the cured composites. Tests are performed on the resin in all stages of composite fabrication, including individual component materials, mixtures of ingredients that later become part of the final blend, the blend in its final composition, b-staged resin on impregnated fabric, and cured resin in a composite laminate.

Polymers with chemically different functions are used to categorize resin families. Early industrial polymers were resole type phenolics and polyesters based on styrene condensation. Epoxy and bismaleimide-based polymers are the most common resins used today in the aerospace industry. Other systems including polyimides, cyanate esters, polysulfides, and vinyls are used for specialized applications. This article focuses on epoxy because this resin category has widespread use and because it is tested using quality control measures typical of most resin systems.

Component Material Tests

Since each component of a resin system contributes to the final properties of the composite, it is essential to identify the individual component properties, define acceptable measurement ranges, and use appropriate test methods to determine these properties. A typical resin system will consist of one or more epoxy resins, a curing agent (such as an amine or anhydride), and a catalyst to control the rate of reaction. In addition, fillers or additional modifiers may be used to alter specific properties. Typically, the resin manufacturer will perform testing on the individual components of a polymer blend.

Resins

Resins may be tested to determine chemical content, moisture content, thermal behavior, chemical functionality, and other characteristics.

Epoxy per Equivalent Weight (EEW). Epoxy resins are chemically reacted to determine the epoxide content per unit weight of resin by wet chemical titration. Epoxide content is a measure of potential crosslink density.

Hydrolyzable Chloride. Epoxy resins are frequently made from chlorinated compounds. Any residual hydrolyzable chloride compound can poorly affect the reactivity and therefore the cured resin properties. The chloride content is measured by titration of a soluble sample.

Moisture. Since epoxies are hygroscopic and since absorbed moisture affects reactivity, moisture content is measured by drying or by titration using a Karl Fisher apparatus.

Melting Point. The melting point temperature of the resin influences how it is processed, and it should be measured using a calorimetric or dilatometric technique.

Softening Point and Viscosity. Because the viscosity of the resin affects system processibility and can be a measure of average molecular weight, the point at which the resin softens should be measured using a technique such as a cone and plate viscometer, a Brookfield viscometer, or a dilatometer.

Infrared (IR) Spectroscopy. This test is a rapid method for identifying chemical functionality, which is useful in differentiating epoxies with similar EEWs. A thin film of resin is placed on a crystal, and IR light is passed through the crystal and film at varying frequencies. Functional groups absorb at certain defined frequencies. The test is usually qualitative, but because absorption is proportional to quantity and intensity, quantitative results are also possible. This technique can also identify impurities or advancement of the polymerization reaction that may affect overall reactivity or final resin properties.

High-Performance Liquid Chromatography (HPLC). This test is performed by dissolving the resin in a solvent and depositing it into a packed column. The resin is then eluted selectively using a polar-nonpolar solvent mixture. This selective elution occurs as the equipment changes the ratio of solvents in a closely programmed system, providing a highly reproducible chromatogram. The detector is usually either an ultraviolet or refractive index technique. Separation is also possible by diverting selected fractions during elution. Like IR, this technique can identify impurities or advancement of the polymerization reaction that may affect overall reactivity or final resin properties.

Gel Permeation Chromatography (GPC). This test is similar to the HPLC test except that it displays separation by molecular weight groups rather than functional groups.

Other Techniques. Gas chromatography, mass spectrometry, and nuclear magnetic resonance (NMR) can be used in organic synthesis and to identify unknown organic mixtures but are not routinely used for quality control.

Curing Agents

Curing agents can be liquids or powders. An amine equivalent test should be performed in which liquid or solid amine curing agents are dissolved in a liquid media and titrated to determine the number of reactive hydrogens per unit weight. Techniques are available to determine primary, secondary, or tertiary amines. Reactivity decreases as the available hydrogen atoms move from primary to secondary. Only ammonia has an available third hydrogen. However, amines form what is known as quaternary salts with an anion, which can change the behavior of the material. Other analytical and chemical tests, such as IR, ultraviolet analysis, GPC, and melting point determinations may be used to determine the quality of the curing agents.

Catalysts

Many catalysts of epoxy reactions are molecular complexes with a Lewis acid, which is usually BF_3 and a tertiary amine. The complex is a quarternary salt, with the BF_3 acting as the anion and the amine acting as the cation. Tests include atomic absorption to quantitatively determine boron concentration; moisture to assess water content, which tends to degrade the complex; and IR, to identify the amine form.

Fillers and Modifiers

Fillers are often used in the form of ground or pulverized inorganic materials to improve dispersion and reactivity or provide increased surface area for flow control. Screens of increasing size are stacked to separate the particles by size. Finer particles can be evaluated by particle analysis, whereby the sample is dropped in a liquid and the rate and quantities of falling particles are measured optically. Very fine particles can also be analyzed in a column of controlled dry gas, using a sensitive balance to plot weight gain versus time.

Typical modifiers include:

- Flow control agents, such as finely divided silicon dioxide, clays, and high molecular weight polymers
- Tack enhancers, such as low molecular weight resin or polysulfide, a naturally tacky resin
- Adhesive ingredients, such as soluble rubbers, polysulfides, and dienes
- Flame retardants, such as halogenated resins with cobalts, phosphates, and other inorganic materials
- Color agents, such as pigments and dyes
- Toughening agents such as thermoplastic particles

Mixed Resin System Tests

After the components are mixed, tests are performed to document the presence of each ingredient and to ensure that the proper chemical reaction state has been obtained. These resins can be used to make preimpregnated reinforcing fibers (prepreg) or to infiltrate a fiber preform via resin transfer molding, vacuum assisted resin transfer molding, or resin film infusion. Testing on the resin blends are performed by either the resin manufacturer or the end user.

Gel Time and Viscosity. Gel is defined as the point when a three dimensional polymer network is formed. At this point, the viscosity of the polymer is essentially infinite, meaning the resin will neither flow nor wet out the dry or precured surfaces. Various techniques are available, including a Brookfield viscometer with thermocel, a cone and plate viscometer, and a rheometer type viscometer using oscillating parallel plates. Knowledge of gel time and viscosity is useful for predicting resin shop life and for determining resin cure characteristics.

Moisture tests are performed on neat resin using a titration method known as Karl Fisher. A moisture meter with P_2O_5 is also available to measure moisture.

HPLC and IR. Both chromatographs and spectrograms are used to "fingerprint" the resin blend. These techniques are also used to identify impurities or polymerization reaction advancement that may affect overall reactivity or final resin properties.

Solids and Volatile Content. When the resin is in a solution impregnation, the solids level is measured by evaporation of the solvents in an explosion-proof oven.

GPC. A chromatograph is used to define and fingerprint the molecular weight distribution of the resin. Reaction advancement can also be determined by this method.

Prepreg Tests

Resins that have been impregnated onto fibers are placed there via a solvent bath or by melt infusion. In either case, the resin can be heated, resulting in advancing the polymerization reaction to some degree. The resulting resin is referred to as *b-staged* resin. Both the manufacturer and the user typically run these tests to ensure that the prepreg contains the proper amount of acceptable component materials to meet user specifications.

Gel Time and Viscosity. Knowledge of gel time and viscosity is useful for predicting resin shop life and for determining resin cure characteristics. It is also useful for looking at an increase in molecular weight caused by resin advancement during the prepreg process.

IR Spectroscopy. This test is repeated on the resin after impregnation to ensure that no major change has occurred. Although the test is usually qualitative, techniques can be developed to obtain quantitative results.

HPLC. This test provides a signature of the components, separated by chemical functionality. Both quantitative and qualitative results can be obtained.

Atomic Absorption. When inorganic ingredients are used, they can be measured at low levels by atomic absorption.

Resin content. The amount of active resin, including the volatiles, is determined using acid digestion or by burning the resin off of the fibers. This test is used to determine if there is enough resin available to form suitable composite components. The quantity of active resin is expressed as a percentage of the total weight.

Volatile Content. For epoxies, the volatile level is usually less than 1% and results from residual solvents in any upstream process as well as absorbed water. Some resins, such as phenolics and polyimides, contain substantial volatiles in the form of water and alcohol reaction by-product or high boiling point solvents such as n-methyl pyrrolidone. Generally, a sample of prepreg is heated for a specified period of time at or near the temperature where volatile by-products are evolved. The weight before heating is compared to the weight after heating. Volatile content is expressed as a percentage of the original weight.

Fiber Areal Weight. This parameter is the weight of dry reinforcing fiber in the prepreg per unit area. The fiber weight, in conjunction with the resin solids content, allows the manufacturer and user to predict the theoretical ply thickness and the resultant fabricated part thickness. This property is obtained from the same sample as the resin content.

Resin Flow. Samples of plied product are exposed to pressure and heat (sometimes with bleeder) to measure the resin lost because of the flow of the resin at a specified temperature and pressure condition.

Tack. This test evaluates a subjective sticky characteristic of the prepreg. The most widely used test requires that a ply of prepreg be "tacked" to a tool and that subsequent plies be tacked to the first ply. The normal requirement is that the second ply shall be capable of being removed and repositioned if necessary. Tack is affected by many factors, including type of resin, resin content, and degree of resin advancement; temperature, and humidity (most epoxies are hygroscopic, and absorbed moisture increases tack). Therefore it is important to specify the conditions and methods of evaluation. Tack causes more problems for both the manufacturer and user than any other prepreg characteristic.

Drape. Like tack, drape is subjective. It is also greatly influenced by tack. Drape is the ability of a prepreg to be formed around defined radii and stay tacked to the tool for specified periods of time.

Room Temperature Out Time. This parameter is the period of time at ambient temperature for which a prepreg can maintain enough tack and drape to be used to make components in the production environment. This is important for building large parts by laying up prepreg. This could take several days depending on the part, and the resin must not have advanced beyond a usable level.

GPC. This technique is used for resin control after prolonged out time or storage to determine whether the resin has advanced beyond a usable level.

Table 1 Typical resin and prepreg property tests

Property	Test
Tensile strength, modulus, and strain	ASTM D 651 for resin ASTM D 3039 for composite
Poisson's ratio	ASTM E 132
Compressive strength, modulus, and strain	ASTM D 3410
In-plane shear strength, modulus, and strain	ASTM D 3518
Flexural strength and modulus	ASTM D 790
Impact toughness	ASTM D 3398
Fatigue	ASTM D 256 or user defined test
Density	ASTM D 1895
Thermal properties, including glass transition temperature, coefficient of thermal expansion, and weight loss at temperature	User defined
Chemical exposure to acetone, chlorinated solvents, oils, hydraulic fluids, jet fuel, body fluids, alcohol	User defined
Moisture effects	User defined
Flammability	User defined

Cured Resin and Prepreg Mechanical Properties

Mechanical properties that are typically measured during the development and use of an epoxy resin system are shown with the appropriate test methods in Table 1. Because these properties form the basis of subsequent composite properties, the tests are often performed on composite samples as well as neat resin samples. These properties are also frequently measured after exposure to moisture saturation, to chemical exposure, to thermal exposures, and to impacts at a known energy level.

Many test procedures are defined by ASTM methods. Any prior conditioning parameters are typically defined by the ultimate end use to which the composite will be subjected in actual service and are specified by the user.

Tooling and Assembly Quality Control

TOOLING AND ASSEMBLY METHODOLOGIES for advanced composites have steadily improved as a result of advancements in materials, through the use of computer-aided design/computer-aided manufacturing (CADCAM) technology, and through application of sophisticated design for manufacturing and assembly concepts. This article reviews techniques and technologies that are used to control the quality of tooling and assembly methods for composite components.

Tooling Quality Control

Jeff L. Ware, Lockheed Martin Aeronautics Company—Fort Worth

Fabrication methodologies for advanced composite tooling have benefited from advances in tooling materials and through the use of CADCAM technology. The thermomechanical properties of tooling materials have evolved such that they more closely match those of the production part to be fabricated. In addition to improvements in materials properties, today's tooling materials offer lower fabrication and materials costs. The advancements in CADCAM models have also provided opportunities for improved fabrication and inspection methods.

The use of CADCAM (also known as three-dimensional, or 3-D, engineering) technologies have helped to eliminate many of the conventional tooling methodologies once widely practiced up until about 1990. Conventional tooling methods of hand fairing plaster or plastic faces over aluminum lofting templates for fabrication of master models and then producing secondary control tools from reverse splashes are being replaced with electronic master models that exist in a computer-generated engineering tooling model. The 3-D engineering models provide all the control surfaces and coordination points to fabricate tooling associated with the engineering part. The 3-D engineering part model provides the tooling fabricator with the ability to design, plan, and program the data as needed. Often these data are fed into recognition databases that support numerically controlled fabrication and inspection work centers, including multiaxis machining and cutting centers, and high-precision measurement systems.

The advancements in electronic modeling, and the use of 3-D engineering models have shifted the conventional inspection methods from the inspector to the machinist or toolmaker. The inspector's role in relation to dimensional criteria has been greatly reduced, and in many instances, placed with the operator. The requirements for quality control are still as prevalent today as they were in the past, but the emphasis on quality control for the tool has shifted from a check of the end product quality to one of in-process monitoring. The use of sophisticated software and optimization programs along with modern fabrication and inspection systems means that the owner of a particular task (for example, designer, numerical control programmer, machine operator, or toolmaker) can readily inspect his or her own work by comparing the actual measured data to an engineering model. Toolmakers can fabricate and assemble details, perform and record in-process inspections of their own work, and provide inspection reports showing the actual tolerance conditions for acceptance by the inspector or auditor.

The tooling inspector's role is changing from one involving conventional hands-on dimensional and process inspection to that of an auditor. These new responsibilities include verifying engineering data for compliance through electronic configuration management systems, performing visual inspection according to pre-established inspections criteria, performing random in-process inspections, verifying traceability of materials certifications, and assuring that the quality records for the tool meet the company and customer requirements. Due to the complexity of some inspection systems, a company may elect to have a quality inspector or auditor perform the inspection while operating equipment such as coordinate measuring machines and laser imaging systems. The following sections in this article cover typical quality control points that an inspector or auditor would review during the fabrication of a tool used for curing advanced composites.

Documentation

The tooling inspector's or auditor's role in assuring quality control documentation of the tool fabrication process is mostly confined to the tool planning sheet or tool shop order. The planning sheet or shop order may be documented on a paper system or may reside on an electronic retention system. In the case of large or complex tools, a tooling logbook is used in conjunction with the tool planning sheet or shop order. The tooling logbook contains the complete work history of the tool, including changes that occurred after the tool was fabricated and any periodic inspections. It should remain with the tool or should be filed in the tooling shop office. The logbook is a good resource when trying to determine what has happened during the life of a particular tool. A third form of quality control documentation is a separate inspection buy-off sheet, which is used when a detailed planning sheet or shop order is not provided to build the tool. In the fabrication of a composite tool, whether graphite-epoxy prepreg or a wet lay-up is used, certain checkpoints can be universally used as inspection verification points through the fabrication of the master model, the pattern taken from it, and the composite tool made from the pattern.

Hand-Faired Master Models

When building a master model from plaster or hand-faired epoxy, the primary areas of concern to the inspector or auditor should include the following:

- *Base plate:* The base plate should be flat and without twist; this should be verifiable using a coordinate measuring machine (CMM) or manual measurement method.
- *Templates:* Each should be within tolerance on its contour.
- *Reference system:* If scribed on the base plate, it should be correct and within tolerance. If an optical reference system is used, it must be verified, and the date of optical equipment calibration must be checked.
- *Rigging:* The rigging should be checked to verify that the rigged templates are located properly and are vertical (not bowed or twisted).
- *Faired surface:* The surface should be free of flat spots, dips, and irregularities.
- *Scribe lines:* Trim and reference lines should be verified and checked for sharpness.
- *Final contour check:* It can be verified in its entirety through the use of a CMM.

- *Master documentation and identification:* These are the final items to be checked.

Machined Master Models

The inspection process is streamlined considerably when inspecting master models that have been machined on a computer numerically controlled lathe or mill. The inspector or auditor basically checks to confirm that no gross programming errors (such as the slip of a decimal point) have been made, and determines whether any items should be added to the tool after machining, such as scribe lines and identification. On smaller and simple machined master models, hand-held precision instruments, such as dial calipers and height gages, can be used to check dimensions. Templates are used to show any discrepancies in contours. A CMM, if available, can be used to check contours, hole locations, and scribe lines.

On large or complex machined master models, the contours can be checked with templates or with a CMM. To verify the proper location of tooling holes, scribe lines, and reference point templates, a CMM or optical measuring equipment can be used.

Second-Generation Patterns

When a pattern is to be taken from the master model, the inspection is similar to that for a plaster splash, plastic-faced plaster, or epoxy laminate. This is true for inspection both before and during fabrication of the pattern.

Before releasing the master model in order to make the pattern, the inspector or auditor may verify that:

- The surface of the master model is in an acceptable condition. It should be free of chips, cracks, or other surface blemishes that will affect the surface of the pattern.
- The required reference lines are clean and complete.
- The master reflects the latest engineering changes verifiable through the company or customer's configuration control management system. If the master model does not incorporate the latest engineering changes, it may be futile to fabricate any tooling from it.

The inspector or auditor may also verify that the toolmaker has the correct location on the master model taped off for his pattern and that it is large enough to make a tool, as determined by the tool-planning sheet. During pattern fabrication, the inspector or auditor should be concerned with each of the areas described subsequently.

Release. The master model should be released properly because it is critical that its surface be preserved for future tooling. A poorly released tool will usually result in destroying the master model tool face and destroying the transfer tool.

Fabrication. If a company or the customer has a formal fabrication procedure and requires that all patterns be fabricated according to the procedure, then the services of the inspection department are to ensure that the quality requirements of the company or customer are met.

Preremoval Inspection. Before the pattern is removed from the master model, an inspector/auditor should verify that the pattern has received the proper cure time and is tight to the surface of the master model. This indicates that no warping or twisting of the pattern occurred during cure. If it is difficult to see the edge where the surface of the master model and the pattern meet, the inspector can use a 0.05 mm (0.002 in.) feeler gage to determine if the pattern has lifted off the master.

Cleanup and Scribe Lines. After the pattern has been pulled from the master model, its surface should be cleaned of any release residue, and the scribe lines, which are now high male lines, will have to be reversed back into the surface of the pattern. This reversing procedure is critical and should be monitored to verify that the scribe lines are within the tolerance of the original lines. This can be accomplished by leaving 6.4 mm (0.25 in.) long male witness lines every 75 to 100 mm (3 to 4 in.). After verification, these lines are then reversed.

Composite Tooling

Graphite/epoxy or high-temperature glass cure tools generally fall into two categories:

- Wet lay-up tooling
- Tooling consisting of prepreg face sheets with a composite laminate eggcrate or tubular back-up structure

The inspection criteria are generally the same for both except that wet lay-up tooling requires a gel coat. The inspector or auditor may inspect the gel coat for thickness and proper gel time prior to the application of the first ply of fabric by the toolmaker.

The inspector or auditor must check or verify the following items:

- Quality of the control tool through the use of a CMM or by some other method before lay-up begins
- Control surface finish
- Scribe line depth and uniformity
- Bushing installation
- Identification of tools, thermocouple connectors, vacuum connectors, tooling and control bushing holes
- Vacuum integrity while under vacuum, service temperature, and autoclave pressure
- Compliance of the tool to the design and/or to fabrication specification manual
- Materials certifications
- Materials out-time logs
- Documentation regarding waterjet or laser cutting of support structure
- Surface control data forms high-precision measurement equipment
- Fabrication planning for compliance of each operation and completeness in the tool build process

Metallic Tooling

Metallic tooling made from Invar (a low-expansion iron-nickel alloy), steel, aluminum, and electroplated materials are becoming more popular for production composite cure tools. Metallic tools generally cost more than a composite wet or prepreg lay-up tool, but offer some advantages by eliminating the need for control/transfer tools, by extending service life, and by providing higher durability characteristics.

The inspector or auditor is responsible for checking or verifying the following items for metallic tooling:

- Surface finish through the use of visual or manual means
- Scribe line depth and uniformity
- Bushing installation
- Tool identification and identification of thermocouple connectors, vacuum connectors, and tooling and control bushing holes
- Vacuum integrity of the tool while under vacuum; service temperature and autoclave pressure
- Materials certifications
- Weld and weld heat treatment quality assurance through the use of penetrant, magnetic particle, ultrasonic, or visual inspections according to the relevant specification manuals or tool design requirements
- Surface control data from high-precision measuring systems
- Fabrication planning for compliance of each operation and completeness in the tool build process
- Compliance of the tool to design or fabrication specification manual requirements

There are other types of composite tools, such as bond, drill, trim, and assembly fixtures. Inspection of these types of tools will vary from type to type. The general responsibility of the toolmaker and of the inspector or auditor to build in quality will remain the same, regardless of the type of tools and the materials used. Technology advancement will continue in the development of software and support systems to assure compliance to design standards and to facilitate the involvement of all development and fabrication personnel in the quality process.

Composites Assembly Quality Control

Robert Moore and Dennis Bowles,
Northrop Grumman Corporation

Composite assembly methods often rely on the use of metallic fasteners for joining composite details and assemblies. Fastener installation usually requires hole drilling and countersinking of the composite material, which necessitate attention to quality issues such as delamination around holes and hole surface quality. The continued use of complex and costly "old school" assembly tooling and fixturing technology further complicates quality assurance of assembly operations. However, the on-going implementation of "up stream" assembly process enhancements has provided significant benefits in the areas of design and detail fabrication. Process improvements include, but are not limited to, the use of co-cured laminates, co-bonding of details, and the development of liquid molding processes. These improvements benefit assembly processes by enabling the incorporation of part details into larger subassemblies, thus reducing "down stream" assembly requirements. The best way to ensure the quality of assembly operations is to reduce or eliminate the need for mechanical assembly wherever possible.

Ideally, composite details and subassemblies would be designed and fabricated so that they can be assembled as snap-together modules. Thermoset composite materials that are not manufactured using resin transfer molding methods cannot normally meet the accurate, repeatable, and reproducible dimensional requirements for snap-together modules. However, composite parts can be designed and fabricated using localized "high-tolerance" tooling that will support self-locating assembly. This approach is affordable and allows the use of determinant assembly concepts (defined subsequently) without the aid of complex tooling and fixturing.

Methods for Simplifying and Improving Assembly Operations

Design for manufacture and assembly (DFMA) methods can be used to advance the minimal assembly concept and otherwise improve assembly operations. The DFMA process brings together design and manufacture personnel at the critical initial concept level of a new program or project. The early interaction between the groups ensures a concurrent and collaborative development effort that takes into account the manufacturing and assembly issues at the design concept level. This approach replaces the traditional manufacturing industry practice of "throwing it over the wall," which often results in the inclusion of nonproducible details in part designs and production nonconformities. The end result is high tooling costs, long process flow times, and significant design rework. DFMA tools are used to evaluate the product process from initial design through completed assembly. The DFMA process helps identify manufacturing and assembly quality issues and provides up-front engineering to avoid nonconforming process conditions. Process unity ensures products are designed with the correct form, fit, and function from the basic design to final product assembly. This process identifies and eliminates hidden costs and labor to benefit both the composite producer and customer.

Additional information about DFMA concepts and tools is provided in *Materials Selection and Design,* Volume 20 of *ASM Handbook.*

Determinant assembly (DA) involves the use of engineering-controlled, one-position molded-in or machined-in features on each individual composite detail. The one-position feature controls the fit and location of independent composite items to one another. The use of DA ensures that correct, quick, and accurate assembly of composite details and subassemblies is accomplished without the need for complex tooling or fixtures. Other DA process features include items such as engineering-controlled self-locating joints and numerically controlled (NC) machine-drilled holes and locating features. (It should be noted that when NC holes are used in the DA process, only a very limited number of holes are drilled in the details prior to assembly. These holes are used as an aid to provide accurate and repeated assembly capability. The holes may or may not receive fasteners as part of the assembly process, depending on other DA locating features.)

The DFMA and DA process concepts described previously support one of the major goals of the composites industry—toolless assembly. Assembly tooling will never be completely eliminated, but it can be minimized significantly by the use of DFMA and DA processes.

Flexible tooling is another concept that helps reduce the high tooling cost associated with composite assembly efforts. This tooling methodology is developed in concert with the engineering design phase to ensure the support of multiple configurations of the same part as well as parts in other component families. This concept must be an integrated approach, and it relies on high levels of "touch experience" and on the use of simulation software to identify quality concerns at the detail, subassembly, and assembly phases. Up-front dedication is mandatory from design, tooling, quality engineering, manufacturing engineering, and manufacturing groups for this process to be successful. Early identification of assembly quality issues results in reduced tooling cost and assembly time.

Assembly Process Monitoring

The process concepts and tools described previously also involve the application of functional real-time, operator-level, and decision-capable statistical process control tools. These tools must be employed to verify and maintain in-process control. Process monitoring must be nonintrusive at the operator level. Variable data collection of process parameters must occur at a point in the process where correction can be made. This is critical to minimize the creation of noncorrectable nonconformance conditions that require engineering disposition, possible repair, and schedule adjustment.

Quality concerns must be addressed, as the composite assemblies become larger. Verification requirements must be based on in-process performance, not after-the-fact detection of nonconformities, which may be uncorrectable. Nonconformance detection may result in significant repair cost and schedule delays or even total loss. Nonintrusive types of process control must be used to minimize the risk of process failure. Every effort should be made to use the process tools mentioned in this Volume to ensure all assembly and detail processes are conforming to engineering/customer requirements. These requirements must be evaluated at the design level and tailored by engineering to promote successful in-process verification and eliminate end-item evaluation/inspection requirements at the detail and assembly level. Additional information is provided in the article "Nondestructive Testing" in this Volume.

Outlook for Composites Assembly

Existing composite assembly methods are adequate for the types of structures currently being manufactured. However, new designs are implementing fewer details, larger sub-assemblies, and more self-locating final assemblies. Bonding of these assemblies will require application of more innovative design, manufacturing, process control, and assembly concepts. Manufacturing processes must develop to the point that if products are manufactured within statistically accepted process parameters, no final verification is required. The goal of eliminating the end-item verification step will require the application of advanced but easy-to-apply engineering and quality tools. Those who embrace the challenge of determinant assembly methods and design for manufacture and assembly concepts will benefit in the area of composite assembly.

ACKNOWLEDGMENTS

Portions of this article were adapted from material written by Steven F. Hanson, Composite Tooling International, Inc., for the previous edition of this Volume. Jeff L. Ware wishes to thank Greg Dean, Doug Bruner, and Andy Smith from Lockheed Martin Aeronautics Company—Fort Worth for their contributions to this article.

Reinforcing Material Lay-Up Quality Control

Barry P. Van West, The Boeing Company, Seattle

IN-PROCESS INSPECTION during composite material lay-up is essential if the structural, dimensional, and environmental performance designed into a part is to be consistently achieved. The inspection techniques are usually based on governmental standards, company processing specifications, quality assurance requirements, and what are generally known as good shop practices. Although inspection techniques vary from one company or facility to another depending on prescribed contractual requirements, available equipment, level of personnel training, and documentation systems used, they all fulfill the following criteria. The materials to be used in part fabrication must conform to drawing and material specifications, must have been stored and handled properly, and must be within specified shelf life and processing out-time limitations. Processing aids used in the shop must comply with accepted material standards, and lay-up procedures must be controlled to ensure proper material handling and consistent dimensional accuracy of the completed laminate. The processing environment must conform to requirements for cleanliness, temperature, and humidity; also, equipment must be qualified and within specified calibration limits. To ensure the above requirements are met, the processor must develop a set of standards that control facilities and equipment operation, procedures, and training for the sequence of tasks associated with the lay-up process. Figure 1 is an abbreviated flow chart of tasks associated with the lay-up process covered by this section. Cure process quality control following lay-up is covered in the article "Cure Monitoring and Control" in this Volume. Figure 2 is a cause-and-effect diagram for defects in composite lay-ups that are described in this article.

Facilities and Equipment

The facilities in which composite parts are laid up must meet requirements for cleanliness, temperature, and humidity. The requirements depend on the sensitivity to the environment of the materials being laid up, their limits on out-time and temperature, their tack, drapability, and tendency to absorb moisture. Dust particles must be limited because they become nucleating sites for void formation caused by moisture and entrained air. Aerosols and other contaminating materials must be avoided as they may act as releasing interfaces between plies, reducing the interlaminar strength of the finished part.

Controlled-Contamination Areas. Lay-ups must be performed in enclosed areas. All incoming air is filtered, and positive air pressure in the controlled-contamination area is required with respect to adjoining areas of lesser cleanliness. Compressed gas introduced into the area must be free of oil, condensed moisture, and particulate matter. Doors that open directly outside the building are used only in emergency situations. The airborne particulate count must meet preset requirements and be monitored at set intervals. Temperature and relative humidity are monitored continuously. Typical temperature and humidity requirements are shown in Fig. 3. Contamination-controlled environments are classified according to the allowable airborne particulate count. The number used for identification of each class in FED-STD-209 (Ref 2) corresponds to the maximum number of particles 0.5 μm or larger, permitted in 0.03 m^3 (1 ft^3) of air. A typical lay-up-controlled area classification is 400,000, with requirements shown in Table 1. The international standard is ISO 14644 (Ref 3).

Floors in the area are sealed or covered with nonflaking, easily cleaned material, such as plastic, paint, or vinyl tile. Walls and ceilings are covered with a high gloss or semigloss enamel. Autoclaves, ovens, and vacuum system equipment are generally not in the controlled area, but if so the outlets from this equipment are vented to the outside. Outlets are positioned or covered so that outside condensate cannot enter the outlet and are positioned away from air-conditioning intakes. Waste containers are emptied outside the controlled-contamination area, or liners are closed and removed from the container within the area. Cleaning schedules must be maintained within the controlled-contamination area. Cleaning methods are limited to water cleaning using mops, cloths, or rags, vacuuming with exhaust air vented outside the area or filtered to the same quality as the incoming air, chemical mopping using mops commercially treated with either propylene glycol, polyethylene glycol, or slightly tacky epoxy resin, and cleaning with water-based commercial glass cleaner. Protective clothing is worn over personal clothing when uncured parts are exposed to direct contact. If the protective clothing is removed from the controlled-contamination area, it is either cleaned or discarded. Requirements should be established concerning cleaning, frequency of changing, and storage of protective clothing. Protective gloves are worn when handling prepregs, adhesives, or precured details that will be bonded.

The following materials or procedures are generally prohibited in the controlled-contamination area: materials, tools, parts, or equipment

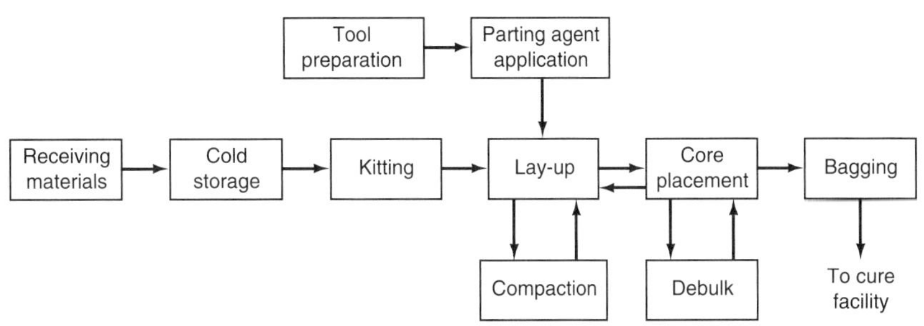

Fig. 1 Sequence of tasks associated with lay-up process

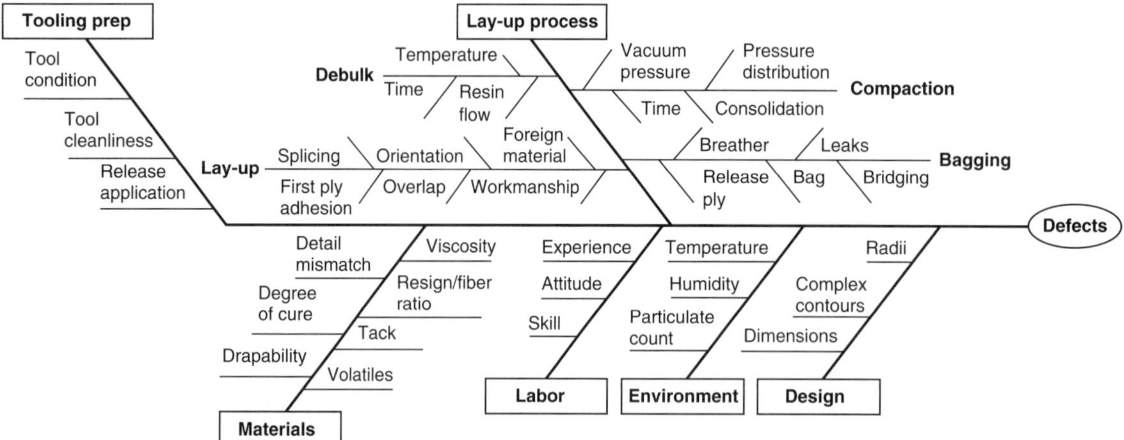

Fig. 2 Cause-and-effect diagram for defects in composite lay-ups. Source: Ref 1

that have visible contaminants such as dirt, grease, or oil on their exterior surfaces; processes or operations that produce uncontrolled spray, dust, fumes, or particulate matter (i.e., grinding, machining, sanding or milling); uncured parting agents (liquid mold releases); hand-cream dispensers; unapproved aerosol dispensers; waxes; compounds containing uncured silicone or any material detrimental to adhesion; unapproved cleaning solutions or methods; operations that generate hydrocarbons; some personal hygiene items (especially hair gel products); smoking, eating, chewing tobacco, or consuming beverages; and the operation of internal combustion engines. Similar requirements are enforced in core machining areas.

Procedures that are allowed in the controlled-contamination area include solvent cleaning of cured composite surfaces and peel ply removal from cured parts at a distance from any uncovered prepreg or uncured film adhesive, removal of particles by vacuuming or solvent wiping, hand-sanding to prepare cured bond faying surfaces for bonding if done away from any uncovered prepreg or uncured film adhesive and the sanding particles are vacuumed, inkjet marking, the application of tackifier solution to tool surfaces with minimum overspray, spraying water-based commercial glass cleaner for cleaning away from uncovered prepreg, uncured film adhesive or contact-use material, and drinking from permanently installed drinking fountains. Portable vacuum systems must be approved and have special filters if outlets are within the controlled area.

During controlled-contamination-area shutdowns, uncured parts, prepreg, and film adhesive materials are placed in a sealed bag and stored in the freezer or in the controlled-contamination area if their temperature is monitored continuously and exposure units continue to accrue during shutdown periods.

Process and Equipment Qualification. The following steps in the qualification process are recommended. All equipment used to perform critical operations on deliverable materials should be qualified. Each processing facility desiring to manufacture parts should be qualified. Each family of parts to be manufactured at a facility should undergo preproduction verification.

A part/tool thermal profile should be performed after the processor's autoclave has been qualified, except for parts built on thin (less than 25 mm, or 1 in.) aluminum flat plates. The thermal profiling requires sufficient thermocouples to identify the leading and lagging temperature locations in the part during heating and cooling. This ensures that the heat-up rate, cure temperature, cure time, and cool-down rate of all areas of the part can be maintained within specification requirements in all future identical parts by referring to just leading and lagging thermocouples for process control. A permanent lagging

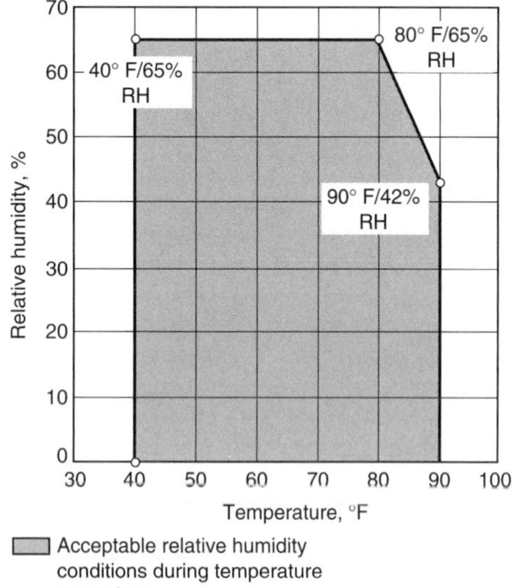

Fig. 3 Controlled-contamination-area temperature and relative humidity requirements

Table 1 Facility requirements and controlled area conditions

Controlled environment class	400,000 classification
Mass airborne particle count (≥0.5 μm)	400,000 per 0.03 m^3 (per ft^3)
Temperature	22 ± 3 °C (72 ± 5 °F)
Humidity	30–60% RH
Air pressure differential	Positive pressure with respect to adjacent areas of lesser cleanliness
Change rooms	Not required
Unidirectional air flow	Not required
Operation of internal combustion engines	Prohibited
Use of motors and equipment that spray or throw lubricants	Prohibited
Generation of nonvolatile residue	Controlled
Compressed gas use	Controlled
Cardboard	Limited
Exposed wooden surfaces	Allowed if no visible damage and coated with smooth nonflaking finish
Pencils and erasers	Not allowed
Carbon paper, paper pads	Allowed
Nonwork-related materials	Not allowed
Working in area	Trained
Cosmetics, perfume, cologne, aftershave, etc.	Most allowed, but may not be applied in the area. Certain items, such as hair gels, not allowed
Cleanroom clothing and shopcoats	May be required
Eating, drinking, and smoking	Not allowed
Dust, dirt, and debris	
Active work station	Visibly clean from 0.6–0.9 m (2–3 ft)
All other stations	Visibly clean from 1.8–2.4 m (6–8 ft)

thermocouple can be attached to the underside of the tool after thermal profile testing with multiple thermocouples ensures that this location represents the slowest heating area of the part. Insulation around the thermocouple can be used to increase lag time. The leading thermocouple can be placed in the excess at the edge of the laminate after the thermal profile testing with multiple thermocouples around the periphery of the part identifies the leading location.

All tools should receive leak checks after applying breather, vacuum bag sealing tape, and bagging materials to the tool in the same configuration that will be used in production. Each part should have an approved manufacturing plan, and a first-part qualification should be performed including a part inspection. Documentation from the first-part qualification should include a record of dimensional and nondestructive inspections, special engineering drawing allowances or exceptions, and cure records for vacuum, temperature, autoclave pressure, and pressure under the bag. The manufacturing plan includes definition of all operations related to part fabrication, including thermal processing, forming and inspection, and operations that ensure the correct orientation of prepreg fibers and core ribbon direction. Where automated processing uses computer controls, the processor must ensure software verification and security.

Equipment requiring qualification includes autoclaves, automated tape-laying machines, automated prepreg-cutting machines, drape-forming machines, inkjet-marking machines, and projection ply-locating machines. Qualification of an autoclave should include the determination of an upper limit on thermal mass that can be contained within the autoclave and still meet thermal rate requirements. Ovens, heat guns, and tacking irons need not be qualified, but must be calibrated and certified for temperature uniformity and control. Heat guns and tacking irons are certified not to exceed a maximum operating temperature that may be different for prepregs and adhesives. Heat blankets, used for repair and rework, must be calibrated and certified.

Material Control

One of the most significant areas in which quality-control personnel can be effective in preventing production problems is in material control. Controls must be in place to ensure arriving materials are to specification, to provide material traceability, to ensure conformance to shelf-life and out-time limits, and to ensure that handling procedures comply with specified practices. A quality-control manual must contain details on how to enforce these controls and verifications.

The purpose of receiving inspection is to ensure that each lot of material falls within key chemical, processing, and end-product parameters. For prepregs these include component percentages (such as resin, fiber, and catalyst), contents of impurities, volatiles and voids, resin flow parameters, and gel time. The temperature at which the material was shipped must be confirmed. For core materials, receiving inspection would include density measurements. Materials requiring end-product property testing must be laid up into panels and mechanically tested. Typical tests include compression, tension, and short-beam shear strengths.

Unused rolls, precut kits, partially laid-up parts, or partially used rolls of prepreg or adhesive materials are stored in sealed moistureproof bags or containers. Identification labels accompanying the material should contain the following information: supplier name, material specification number, material type, class, grade or style, batch number, lot number, date of kit preparation, and date of material manufacture. For precut kits, a means of providing traceability of the above information to each kit is necessary. Uncured lay-ups are bagged when transported outside of the controlled-contamination area.

A record must be kept of accumulated times in and out of refrigeration. When removed from refrigeration for use, the material must remain sealed until it reaches near-ambient temperatures such that no condensation forms on the outside of the film wrapper when wiped dry. Both handling life and mechanical life accumulate from the date and time the material is removed from the freezer. Handling life accumulates until the material is formed to final contour. If forming operations such as hot-drape forming are required, the handling life requirements continue until those forming processes are completed. Mechanical life accumulates until the autoclave cure is initiated. Typically, air-temperature excursions above the required freezer storage temperature are allowed as long as the excursion does not exceed specified temperature and time limits. Exposure units do not have to be added to accumulated life for temperature excursions within these limits. Figure 4 shows the relationship among storage, handling, and mechanical lives of a prepreg. The refrigeration temperature is usually −18 °C (0 °F) or lower.

Honeycomb core is packaged and stored in a manner that does not cause damage or contamination from water, grease, oil, dirt, or other foreign material detrimental to bonding. It must be identified using materials that will not contaminate subsequent core bonding.

Lay-Up

The lay-up process involves the handling of materials, the use of processing aids and equipment, the prevention of contamination, the use of procedures to control sequences and tolerances, and the upkeep of records. A set of operating regulations should be developed by the processor, describing the lay-up process and process-control methods, controlled-contamination area requirements, in-process inspection methods, and a training program. All personnel, including supervision and maintenance personnel who are working in the controlled-contamination area must receive training on the area requirements and on the special requirements for handling processing aid-materials.

Processing aids that come into contact with or are in the vicinity of the materials being laid up must not contaminate them. Processing aids are categorized as contact-use materials approved for use in direct contact with the part lay-up, and noncontact-use materials approved for use as aids to processing but not in contact with the lay-up. Contact-use materials include parting films, mold release materials, protective gloves, marking pens and pencils, rigid and flexible sweeps, peel ply, protective clothing, aprons and shoe-covers, ink-jet marking inks, and backing plates. Some tapes may be approved for contact use. Noncontact-use materials include vacuum bags, solvents, breathers, sealing compounds, pressure-sensitive tapes, identification marking labels, photogrammetry targets, alkaline cleaners, and absorbent wipers. Noncontact materials may contact the part outside of the net trim line. Table 2 lists commonly used materials. Special care should be taken when using processing-aid materials to ensure they are not inadvertently incorporated into the lay-up. It is important to make sure all film materials (backing paper, peel ply, nylon bagging films, etc.) are removed. Some of these materials are not detectable during end-item nondestructive inspection. The main issues that reduce detectability are: thin materials are less detectable than thicker materials, materials that absorb prepreg resin or bond well to resin are less detectable than those that do not, and all foreign materials are more difficult to detect when porosity (even at acceptable levels) is present in the cured laminate.

In-Process Control. Prepregs, adhesives, partially laid-up materials, and uncured parts removed from refrigeration are kept in sealed, moistureproof containers until they have thawed and warmed to room temperature. Protective gloves, clothing, and footwear (when required) are worn by material handlers. Prior to part fabrication, tool surfaces that come into contact with prepreg, resin, or adhesive during cure are either covered with nonperforated parting film or prepared with a release agent. Each section of unrolled material must be visually inspected prior to incorporation into a part. Material suppliers commonly attach markers identifying discrepant areas within an individual roll of mate-

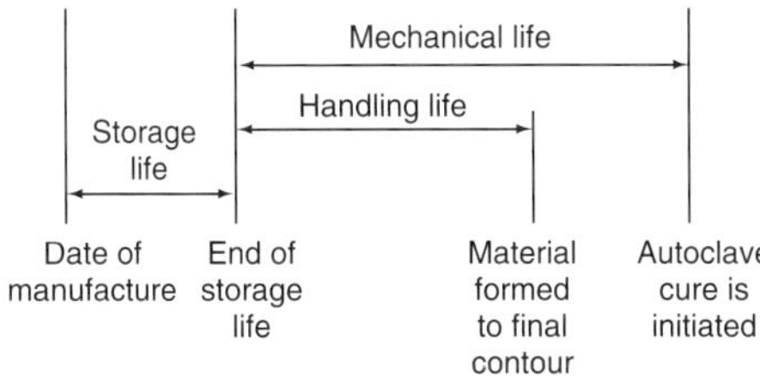

Fig. 4 Relationship of storage, mechanical, and handling lives of a prepreg. Prepreg and adhesives may be returned to storage one or more times provided their handling lives have not been exceeded.

rial. Fiber breakage and resin-poor areas are among the most common defects encountered.

Prepreg materials may be warmed to facilitate manufacturing operations. In addition to the handling and mechanical life allowances, prepreg materials may be exposed to an external heat source within temperature and time limitations. The time accumulated from each exposure is defined as the time from initial application of heat to the time the prepreg material has cooled to the temperatures allowed for normal handling. The use of automated tape-laying heated guide chutes or heat guns and tacking irons for heating prepregs is exempt from the cumulative time limit requirement, and exposures resulting from this use need not be monitored. Film adhesive materials should not be exposed to temperatures in excess of approved temperatures prior to cure except when heating the adhesive using heat guns and tacking irons certified for use on adhesives. The heat guns and tacking irons are kept in motion in small circles over the area to be tacked, at least 76 mm (3 in.) away from the adhesive surface. Prepreg plies may be removed for repositioning by using portable filtered cold-air blowers, compressed cold-air guns, or other cold sources but without lowering the temperature of prepreg material to a point where visible condensation forms on the part.

When trimming and laying up new plies, precautions must be taken not to cut previously applied materials. For example, protective metal strips can be placed under material being cut with a blade, or the ply can be marked, partially lifted, and cut with scissors. Compaction is recommended after lay-up of several plies and for the ply preceding core lay-up. Compaction is suggested for each ply in a tape laminate part that has been laid up by hand. For sandwich parts, once core is in place, it is recommended to limit subsequent use of compaction vacuum to a maximum of 33.8 kPa (10 in. Hg), primarily to prevent core movement. Debulking may be performed in an autoclave under vacuum, pressure, and heat. For typical sandwich parts, pressure is limited to 310 kPa (45 psig). The debulk temperature should not exceed 65 °C (150 °F) for 30 min, but may be less if resin properties require it.

The following information is recorded for each part: composite prepreg and adhesive specification numbers; material manufacturer's batch number, roll number, date of manufacture, and total accumulated exposure units of handling; mechanical and storage life; autoclave load or run number; part number; tool identification number; traceability to the cure cycle information; and discrepancy corrections accomplished. Similar traceability must be established for core material.

Peel ply is usually required on surfaces that will be adhesively bonded and on surfaces that are cured against breather and bagging materials. Peel ply is optional on surfaces cured against tooling substrates that will impart an untextured, smooth finish (e.g., metal, composite, or elastomeric surfaces). Cured laminates that have a textured surface (which comes from being cured against breather mats) are difficult to adequately prepare for bonding by sanding because the sandpaper tends to just hit the peaks.

Cleaning of honeycomb core may be accomplished by dust collection during machining, removal of dust and machine debris by vacuum cleaning and blowing with dry filtered air (electrostatic attraction of dust during machining and cleaning operation must be eliminated), or honeycomb core washing or vapor degreasing using solvents to remove oils or other visible contaminants.

Quality control of the lay-up process must verify that tool surfaces have been prepared, that materials are per specification and within time-history limits, that parts are fabricated in accordance with approved procedures, in particular that no foreign material contamination exists in the lay-up, that information is maintained for each part, that discrepancies that are accepted or reworked meet requirements, that rework is performed in accordance with the approved methods, that bagging is done correctly, and that thermocouples are placed at the correct locations.

Draping. Tools frequently have an orientation rosette marked on them at which point ply lay-up is initiated at the orientation specified on the drawing. On compound curved tools the fiber orientation will vary away from the initiation point, as shown in Fig. 5. This variation is the result of the kinematics of the draping process and cannot be avoided without inducing wrinkling or bridging. Wrinkling and bridging may occur anyway if the contour is severe enough, and darting and splicing are necessary to force the ply to conform to the tool surface. Darting and splicing are also used to limit the deviation in orientation of the fibers, in effect creating gores. The locations of darts and splices are critical to the strength of the part and must be approved by stress analysis. Software is available that simulates the draping process and defines the lay-up initiation point and orientation, predicts where wrinkling and bridging will occur, and shows how the introduction of darts and splices alleviates wrinkling and bridging problems (Ref 4, 5).

Voids form by mechanical entrapment of gases or by nucleation. Gases can be trapped by the resin-mixing operation, as a result of ply bridging and wrinkling, near wandering tows, fuzz balls, and broken fibers, and at ply drop-offs, overlaps, and splices. Nucleation occurs

Table 2 Processing aid materials for prepreg lay-up

Contact-use materials

Peel ply:
- Nylon and polyester fabric, fiberglass with release coating

Parting films:
- Fluorinated ethylene propylene (FEP), polytetrafluoroethylene (PTFE), or tetrafluoroethylene (TFE), polyvinyl fluoride (PVF), polyethylene, polymethylpentene, Teflon-coated glass fabric

Gloves:
- Latex rubber, polyethylene, cotton.

Rigid sweeps:
- Polyethylene, polyacetal, polyurethane, nylon

Flexible sweeps:
- Tedlar and polyethylene film, supercalendared silicon-coated paper

Protective clothing:
- Nylon net caps, reusable low-lint shopcoats, pants, boots, sleeves, coveralls, disposable polypropylene and olefin

Noncontact use materials

Vacuum bags:
- Nylon, polyethylene, latex rubber, silicon rubber, neoprene

Solvents:
- Methyl ethyl ketone (MEK), acetone, toluene

Breathers:
- Fiberglass fabric, polyester mat and fabric mesh, embossed blankets, Dacron, porous TFE-coated fiberglass, paper

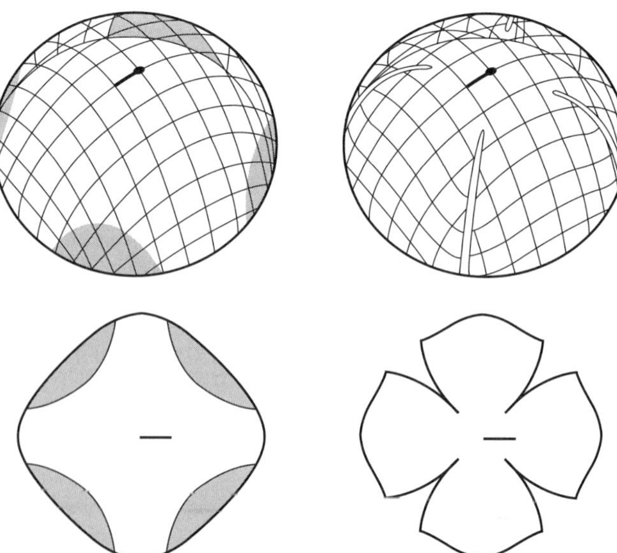

Fig. 5 Variation of fiber orientation with location on a compound-curved surface. Orientation will change if darts are cut and spliced to create gores. Flat patterns will also change. (Courtesy of Composite Design Technologies, Inc., Waltham, Mass.)

within the resin or at resin/fiber/particle interfaces. Water vapor, air, volatiles, and foreign particles can provide void nucleation sites in prepregs. Vacuum pressure sealed in honeycomb core can lower the hydrostatic resin pressure locally, allowing volatiles to emerge from solution. Lay-up and bagging procedures must ensure these imperfections are minimized. First-ply adhesion to the tool surface is especially important in female radii locations. Periodic compaction will consolidate plies and remove air if done correctly. Care must be taken not to trap air in the compaction process.

Vacuum Bagging. Wrinkles in the vacuum bag film frequently transfer to the part surface. Inadvertent wrinkles in the bag film should be avoided. When pleats are used to help the bag conform to part contour, they should be positioned to minimize effects in the part surface or provided with extra padding to prevent transferring to the part surface. Sharp contours must be padded to minimize the risk of bag failure. Breather materials must allow vapors to flow freely through the resin to escape as vented gas. An unrestricted vacuum path must be allowed to all areas of the part. The part should be left connected to an active vacuum source after completion of the bagging procedure. Leaving parts disconnected from vacuum for extended periods of time may result in ply wrinkles, voids, and other defects. Before starting the cure cycle, each vacuum bag is checked for leaks while connected to the autoclave system. A minimum vacuum of 74 kPa (22 in. Hg) is applied, and then vacuum sources are shut off. The vacuum gage reading should not drop more than 17 kPa (5 in. Hg) in 5 min.

Thermocouples are positioned in the lay-up for connection to the autoclave junction box. At least one thermocouple in the part must be identified as the lagging or slowest thermocouple during heating and cooling, and at least one must be identified as the leading or fastest thermocouple during heating and cooling. The thermocouples are electrically checked, and identification and locations are recorded. The combined accuracy of the thermocouple junction box and recorder should be ±3 °C (+6 °F) or better from 38 to 185 °C (100–365 °F).

Tolerances. The fiber orientation and location of each ply must be verified during lay-up. Precision templates can be constructed to aid in the alignment and positioning of plies. The templates for flat parts are commonly made of Mylar, rubberized fabric, or other flexible but inextensible material, and molded fiberglass is used for contoured parts. Eyebrow cutouts in the templates mark the edges of core and plies, and indexing holes fit over pins in the tool to establish orientation. Figure 6 shows examples of flexible and rigid templates. There are two scenarios for the use of these templates, one involving rough-cut plies and one involving plies cut on a ply-cutting machine. If a ply is rough cut and laid up with excess at the edges, the template is placed on the ply and the cutouts are used to hand mark the edge of ply on the ply itself, followed by cutting it to shape in place. The ply must have been marked with an orientation line that is lined up with marks on the tool edge or a rosette. If the ply is precision cut to net shape using flat pattern software, it can be laid up on the previous ply or tool surface, which has the outline and orientation of the ply hand marked on it using the template. In lieu of using templates, plies can also be inkjet marked by the cutting machine with the outline and orientation of the following ply. Optical lay-up templates using scanning laser lines projected from overhead are increasingly being used to project orientation and positioning information as a lay-up aid and for inspection. Tolerances depend on the specific program requirements. Typical values are shown in Table 3. Full plies are generally oversize to allow for trimming of the cured part. All splice joints should be offset from any other splice joint among any six consecutive plies through the thickness of the lay-up. Wrinkles are generally not permitted in fabric plies, which must be smoothed out. Tape splices should have no cut fibers; that is, the splices should be parallel to the fiber direction. Splices may cross within a lay-up except as specified by the drawings. There should be no overlaps in areas that will become faying surfaces, as shown in Fig. 7.

Discrepancies in prepreg material during lay-up include cuts, wrinkles, and fabric distortion. Typically, cuts should not exceed 2.5 mm (0.10 in.) in length in any 0.9 m (3 ft) of material and may be patched with an overlay of material 13 to 25 mm (0.5–1 in.) around the cut. Wrinkles may be up to 305 mm (12 in.) in length, but must be removed by smoothing with no fiber damage. Yarn deviation in fabrics should be less than 6 mm (0.25 in.) from nominal path, but may be more if the length of deviation is greater than 10 times the deviation.

Discrepancies in honeycomb core include cell tear-out (Fig. 8), frayed or burred areas, edge waviness, node bond separation, and core surface depressions. Typical discrepancy acceptance criteria are shown in Table 4. Discrepancies may be reworked by filling damaged areas or sweeping the surface with potting compound or by splicing in new core.

Statistical quality control may be used to apply statistical methods to determine the acceptance of ply lay-up operations with a minimum of inspection effort. Key characteristics and process parameters must be determined on which to base a quality appraisal. Key process parameters (KPP) include those parameters in each stage of the manufacturing process that have the greatest influence on the key characteristics and the performance of the final product. A nominal target value and control limits for each KPP must be established as well as the inspection method and monitoring frequency. The frequency of monitoring is a variable that depends on the acceptance rate of previously inspected work. In a simple example, if a specified number of consecutive plies are found to be within location and orientation tolerances, then only one of every m plies needs to be inspected. If a specified number of those are acceptable, then only one of every

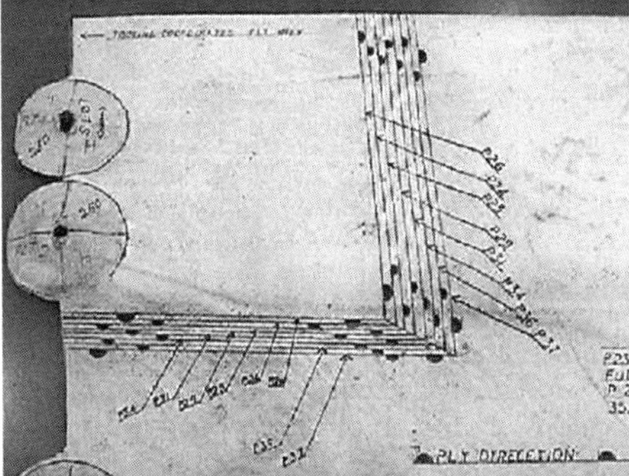

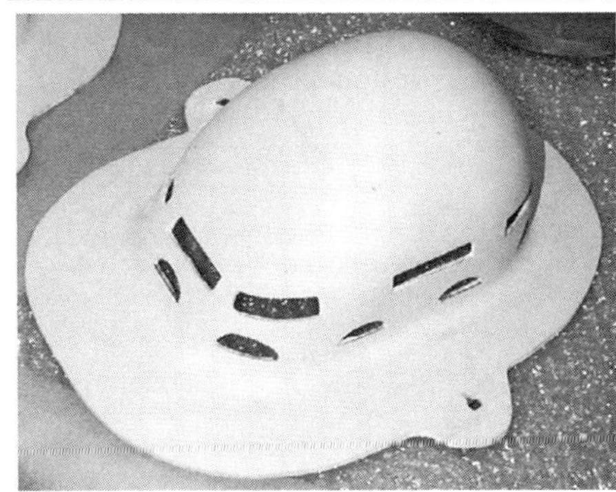

Fig. 6 Flexible and rigid ply locating templates with indexing cutouts denoting edges of plies and honeycomb core. Templates are used as lay-up guides and inspection tools.

Table 3 Typical tolerances for lay-up

	Tolerance
Orientation	
Fabric	±5°
Tape	±3°
Core (ribbon direction)	±5°
Position	
Full plies	Oversize
Partial plies and doublers	±0.25 mm (±0.010 in.)
Splicing	
Fabric	
Butt	No overlap, to 2.5 mm (0.10 in.) gap
Overlap	13–25 mm (0.5–1.0 in.)
Offset	25 mm (1.0 in.) min
Tape (no cut fibers)	
Butt	No overlap, to 2.5 mm (0.10 in.) gap
Overlap	None
Offset	13 mm (0.50 in.) min
Film adhesive	
Butt	No gap
Overlap	0–25 mm (0–1.0 in.)
Core	
Thickness	
Up to 50 mm (2 in.)	±0.15 mm (±0.006 in.)
50–100 mm (2–4 in.)	±0.25 mm (±0.010 in.)
Over 100 mm (4 in.)	±1.6 mm (±0.063 in.)
Position	±0.25 mm (±0.010 in.)
Chamfer angle	±3°

Note: Actual tolerances depend on specific program requirements.

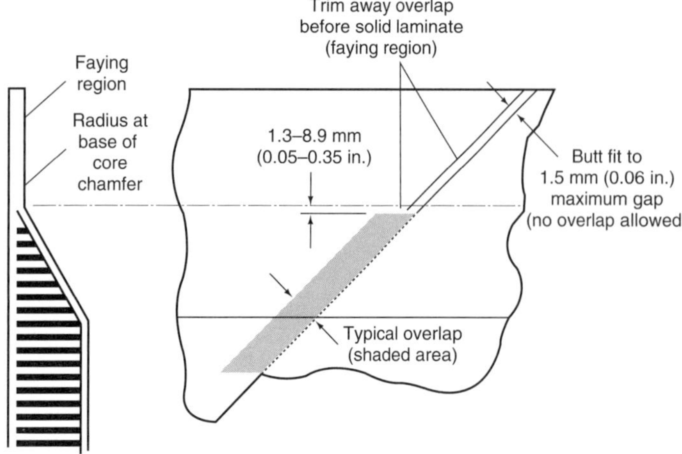

Fig. 7 Overlapping splices cut back to form butt splices in the faying region, maintaining a smooth faying surface

n plies needs to be inspected (with $n > m$), and so on. If discrepancies are found, the inspection rate reverts to previous levels of frequency.

A program of manufacturing self-examination may be instituted whereby the personnel doing lay-up tasks are specially trained to perform quality examinations of their own work according to specific procedures. This does not eliminate the need for auditing inspections, but reduces the workload on inspectors who would otherwise be required to inspect every ply for a number of tolerance parameters. This program is coupled with statistical quality control to determine the inspection rate.

Automated Tape Laying and Fiber Placement

Automated tape laying and fiber placement are prepreg lay-up processes that automatically control fiber orientation, ply position, and shape. With automated tape laying, a wide band of tape is drawn from a spool and laid down under pressure by a heated head, whereas with fiber placement individual prepreg tows of material are drawn from spools within a controlled-temperature chamber and collated into a single band of material at the head of the machine. Gentle contours can be laid up by tape-laying machines with deviations from a flat plane of more than 20°. Complex contours can be laid up and individual tows of material terminated and added due to the steering and cutting capability of fiber-placement machines. The processes still require hand lay-up of peel ply, fabric plies, small doublers, and isolation fiberglass for which ply sequence and orientation must be verified and lack of moisture and defects confirmed. The locations for these plies may be marked using an optical lay-up template or the machine-mounted laser.

In the fiber-placement process, gaps larger than a specified width and length are filled by manual insertion of tow to fill the gap, by removal and reapplication of the defective tow, or by manual adjustment of adjacent tows. Gaps resulting from tow convergence must be limited in width. Spliced ends are overlapped at least 25 mm (1 in.). Tow splices must be offset from other splices along the length of a tow and laterally from other splice locations. Each ply of the lay-up is visually examined for defects such as missing tows, wrinkled tows, fuzz balls, contamination/inclusions, or other defects. Nonconforming areas have the individual tows replaced by hand or the machine or the entire course replaced by the machine. Wrinkled tows and puckers are limited in width perpendicular to the fiber direction and in area. Folded and twisted tows are acceptable if the ply meets gap requirements. Bridged tows in the fiber direction are acceptable up to a maximum specified length.

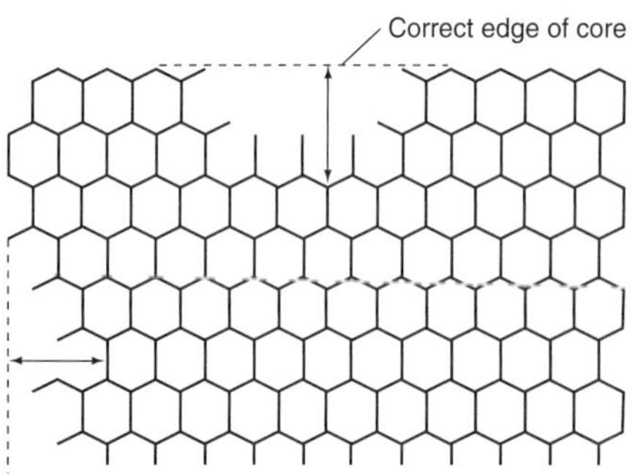

Fig. 8 Cell tear-out in honeycomb core

Table 4 Typical honeycomb core discrepancy limits

Discrepancy	Acceptable limits
Multiple discrepancies	No two within 152 mm (6 in.) and a maximum of 10% core area
Cell tear-out	161 mm^2 (0.25 in^2) max area or 13 mm (0.5 in.) max width from edge
Frayed or burred areas	No fiber fuzz after sanding
Edge waviness	Within 1.3 mm (0.05 in.) of nominal core edge
Node bond separation	Number of nodes: <10% partial and <1% total separation
Surface depressions	0.5 mm (0.02 in.) deep, 13 mm (0.5 in.) long

Actual limits depend on specific program requirements.

Numerically Aided Lay-Up

Modern lay-up processes are progressing toward automation that utilizes computers to facilitate each step of the process. This reduces error due to human intervention, reduces cycle times, increases the consistency of the finished parts, and reduces material waste and part rejections. The part is designed using a CAD system that defines part geometry, ply shapes, orientations, and sequences. For parts other than those made on automated tape laying or fiber-placement machines, such as parts made of fabric with a high degree of contour, an orientation rosette, and its location on the tool is defined. The design dataset is fed to a flat pattern simulator, which does a kinematic analysis of the plies being draped on the tool and computes the flat pattern shape for each ply. These data are fed to a nesting program that determines the least wasteful arrangement of plies within the bounds of the broadgoods from which the plies are cut. The nesting program provides instructions to a cutting machine to cut the nested plies. Each ply is marked with a part or ply number and reference points or lines to aid in initiating the draping process. Although not commonly utilized at present, pick-and-place machines can pick up individual plies and store them in specific locations for later retrieval. More likely, the plies will be kitted and stored by hand. At the time of part lay-up, an overhead laser projection system scans lines onto the tool and ply surfaces, defining the ply boundaries, orientations, and starting points, and compensating for any complex contour in the lay-up geometry and for the change in surface elevation due to ply and core thickness. The ply is laid up by hand with the aid of sweeps, using the laser projections as guides. Variations can occur in the way a ply is laid up due to the actions of the operator doing the lay-up. Variations in the sequence in which areas of the ply are swept onto the surface or the amount of stretching force applied to a fabric can cause variations in the resulting fiber paths. To minimize this variation, the sequence and technique of lay-up should be defined with marked or projected lines and the operators trained accordingly. In lieu of hand lay-up, pick-and-place machines could be used to select and position plies on the tool, using a vision system that can identify ply boundaries or reference points on the ply to control and verify position and orientation. Diaphragm-forming cells are used to form the ply or plies to the tool surface, although this process is currently limited to simple or gentle contours. Such a fully automated system would reduce quality-control requirements to first-part qualification, limited process monitoring, and final inspection.

The use of automated tape-laying or fiber-placement machines further automates the process by continuing the numerical process through the final lay-up and eliminates the need for flat patterns, nesting, precutting, marking, kitting, laser projection, and pick-and-place operations. Quality inspection requirements are reduced accordingly. However, automated tape laying and fiber-placement processes are restricted by part contour limitations.

ACKNOWLEDGMENTS

The author wishes to thank Donald A. Anderson and Kevin D. Summerfield of the Boeing Company for their assistance in producing this article and Lawrence A. Lang for excerpts taken from the previous edition of this article. Figures and tables are courtesy of the Boeing Company unless otherwise noted.

REFERENCES

1. J. Ou, Quality in Composite Sandwich Fabrication, Masters Thesis, Dept. Of Chemical Engineering, Massachusetts Institute of Technology, May 1994
2. "Airborne Particulate Cleanliness Classes in Cleanrooms and Clean Zones", FED-STD-209E, *Department of Defense,* 1992
3. "Cleanrooms and Associated Controlled Environments," ISO 14644, International Organization for Standardization, 1999
4. FiberSIM software, Composite Design Technologies, Inc., Waltham, MA
5. PAM-FORM software, ESI North America, Troy, MI

SELECTED REFERENCES

- "Calibration Systems," ASQ M1, American Society for Quality, 1996
- "Control Chart Method of Controlling Quality During Production," ASQ B3, American Society for Quality, 1996
- "Guide to Inspection Planning," ASQ E2, American Society for Quality
- "Introduction to Attribute Sampling," ASQ S2, American Society for Quality
- H.-J. Mittag and H. Rinne, *Statistical Methods of Quality Assurance*, Chapman & Hall, 1993
- "Model for Quality Assurance in Design, Development, Production, Installation and Servicing," SAE AS 9100, Society of Automotive Engineers
- D.C. Montgomery, *Introduction to Statistical Quality Control,* John Wiley & Sons, 1991
- *Polymer Matrix Composites Volume III. Materials Usage, Design, and Analysis,* MIL-HDBK-17\3E, Department of Defense, 1997
- "Product Cleanliness Levels and Contamination Control," MIL-STD-1246C, Department of Defense, 1994
- "Quality Assurance for Measuring Equipment," ISO 10012, International Organization for Standardization
- "Quality Control System Requirements," FED-STD-368A, Department of Defense, 1979
- "Quality Management and Quality Assurance Standards," ISO 9000, International Organization for Standardization.
- "Quality Management—Guidelines," ISO 10005/6/7, International Organization for Standardization.
- "Quality Systems—Models and Guidelines," ISO 9001/2/3/4, International Organization for Standardization, 1994
- "Safe Handling of Advanced Composite Materials," Suppliers of Advanced Composite Materials (SACMA), 1996
- "Sampling Procedures," FED-STD-358, Department of Defense, 1975
- "Specification of General Requirements for a Quality Program," ANSI/ASQ C1, American Society for Quality, 1996

Cure Monitoring and Control

Dirk Heider, Roderick Don, and E.T. Thostensen, University of Delaware
Kirk Tackitt, U.S. Army Research Laboratory
John H. Belk, The Boeing Company
Thomas Munns, ARINC

ACHIEVING PERFECT PARTS every time is an elusive goal. Industry has responded by choosing its battles carefully, gradually increasing its abilities by creating new materials and processes aimed at improved production of parts of increasing complexity and difficulty. Now that many variations on these few processing approaches have been mastered, it may be time to go to the next level. Composites manufacturers are now quite good at making a few kinds of parts with few defects at acceptable cost. If composites manufacturing is to be extended to more types of parts and into more markets, the technical capabilities of manufacturers will need to be expanded dramatically.

One way to enable this expansion is to further monitor the process as it unfolds, making in-process decisions as opposed to making only post-manufacturing inspection-based decisions. This will enable manufacture of more difficult parts by tuning the process for a particular part with a particular material on a particular day.

Generally, this takes the form of modeling the process, modeling the part, modeling the chemistry and kinetics, and attempting to combine all this information into something that can be used on the shop floor. This article deals with the current attempts of industry to create sensing approaches for this vision and includes those currently in use and some of the sensing approaches that are being investigated but have a reasonable chance at adoption. The reader should note that all of these sensing approaches share one key ingredient: all are based on the philosophy that sensors are valuable only if there is something to control.

Due to its current use and rising importance, dielectric sensing is covered in detail. Also, microwave curing is covered in somewhat more detail than the reader might expect. This is in part due to its potential near-term importance, but it also serves as a general conceptual model for electron-beam curing and ultraviolet curing, which are therefore not covered in any substantial detail as a result.

Process Control

Process control requires a sufficient knowledge of the entire manufacturing process to make the correct choices at the correct times. Recipe-based control requires sufficient knowledge of previous parts to extrapolate a plan that will, for the most part, result in a good part. Recipe-based control has worked very well for a long time and will continue to play a valuable role, especially in batch-based processes. On-line real-time process control will simply add new capabilities, allowing more part types, additional materials, and the ability to correct for variations in real time.

How will this process control work? It consists of modeling, sensing, and then control. Good models must be available for the parts, materials, tooling, and processes before one can hope to generate a recipe or build a control system. Fortunately, composites manufacturers know how to make good models of all these and simply need to tie them together and learn how to make and carry out good decisions.

Sensing is most useful when placed in the overall context of the manufacturing process, including part design, tool design (including locations of inlets, outlets, thermocouples, resin runners, etc.), cure cycle design (accounting for both the part and any tooling), and the infusion plan (including control of the process). Many of these interrelated elements must feed the infusion and cure process to be controlled. Sensing should not be intrusive to the part and should not affect part dimensions or properties. In addition, sensing must not significantly increase the difficulty of part manufacture or the overall part cost, after the decrease in scrap or increase in quality is factored in.

Numerous customized aids have been produced to facilitate efficient production of these designs and plans, including the Automated Tooling Manufacture for Composite Structure (ATMCS) design package (Prescient Technologies, Inc., Boston, MA). Another such aid is autoclave batch filling software in the form of COBRA (Lockheed Martin Corp.) and cure codes in the form of both COMPRO (University of British Columbia) and Computer Aided Curing of Composites (CACC) (McDonnell Aircraft Company) (Ref 1), all developed primarily for autoclave processes. These are of course in addition to the more common computer-aided design programs and various finite element packages that start the design process. As the composites industry migrates toward larger, more complex integrated structures, there will be a more pronounced need for process control because the industry simply cannot afford to throw away even one large part.

There are a host of properties that can be measured for use in real-time control, including tool or part temperature (Ref 2), pressure, vacuum level, resin viscosity, flow rate, resin position, degree of gelation, degree of cure, moisture content, and residual stress and strain. For each of these there are multiple sensors that might be considered in a control scenario, depending on the specifics of the manufacturing process and the level of confidence required.

For liquid molded parts, including those made via resin transfer molding (RTM), SCRIMP (TPI Technology Inc., Warren, RI), or vacuum-assisted RTM (VARTM), resin flow paints much of the picture. Current sensor-based process control procedures use dielectric sensing (Ref 3, 4), which would readily transfer to liquid molding applications.

Resin Cure Sensing

Several methods exist to begin the process of curing a composite resin system. Of course the most common is application of heat. However, several alternatives are finding niches or showing promise including ultraviolet (UV), electron beam (EB) (Ref 5), and microwave curing. Microwave curing is rising in importance and is used here to illustrate non-direct-heat approaches. Electron beam curing is discussed in the section "Dosimetry-Based Resin Cure Sensors" in this article to illustrate how non-direct-heating approaches can be addressed in cure-sensing schemes.

Microwave Curing of Thick-Section Composites

Microwave heating has been shown to minimize difficulties during thick-section composite cure through in situ volumetric deposition of energy (Ref 6). Thermal gradients during the ramp segment can be minimized and, because microwave heating is instantaneous, heat generation due to microwaves can be precisely controlled. Therefore, temperature excursions in the cure cycle can be minimized, and undesirable spatial solidification can be eliminated. Current research results indicate that microwave heating can substantially reduce the cycle time required to obtain an *inside-out* cure. Microwave cure cycle times are approximately one-third of the required cycle time for autoclave curing.

Research on curing of thick-section composites focuses on numerical process modeling and experimental investigations of microwave and conventional, autoclave curing. The process models combine aspects of transient heat transfer, microwave/materials interactions, and chemical reaction kinetics to model cure behavior in microwave and conventional processing (Ref 7). Models for the interaction of microwaves with laminated composites were developed to account for the influence of fiber orientation on the internal electric field within the composite. Numerical and experimental work focused on a model system of a cross-ply glass/epoxy laminate. Experimental investigations were conducted to develop a cure kinetics model (using epoxy resin EPON 862/curing agent W) for input into the numerical simulation and for validation of the numerical simulations through manufacturing experiments in a conventional autoclave and a state-of-the-art microwave furnace.

To compare the thermal and cure behavior of thick composite laminates during conventional and microwave curing, numerical simulations were performed for 25 mm (1 in.) thick cross-ply glass/epoxy laminates subjected to the same cure cycle (5 °C/min, or 9 °F/min to 165 °C, or 330 °F, for 2 h). Figure 1(a) shows numerical results for conventional curing. As expected, a significant thermal lag between the center and surface of the laminate exists. From the transient cure behavior, it is clear that the thermal gradients result in differential curing where the surface cures faster than the center. There is also a significant exothermic overshoot due to heat liberated from the chemical reaction. These thermal gradients combine to create the undesirable *outside-in* cure. Figure 1(b) shows numerical results for the same laminate subjected to microwave heating. Volumetric heating due to microwaves results in elimination of the thermal lag. Because the laminate is exposed to free convection in the unheated microwave cavity, the surface of the laminate is cooler and these thermal gradients promote the desired *inside-out* cure. In addition, the ability to control instantaneous microwave heat generation eliminates the temperature overshoot in the cure cycle. Thus, direct, volumetric heating due to microwaves significantly improves control over spatial solidification temperature excursions in the laminate.

Figures 1 (c) and (d) show cross-sectional micrographs of autoclave- and microwave-processed laminates, respectively. The importance of controlled spatial solidification is clear. The *outside-in* solidification of the thick laminate results in significant matrix cracking. Stresses in the thickness direction result from the shrinkage associated with curing a thermoset. When surfaces of the laminate cure first, the shrinkage of resin in the center of the laminate is constrained and results in tensile stresses in the thickness direction. In microwave cured laminates, where the center cures first, there is no buildup of tensile stresses due to resin shrinkage because the surfaces have not solidified. This explains why the microwave-processed laminate is crack-free.

Resin Cure Sensors

For resin cure monitoring, a robust, embeddable, or standoff sensor is desired that is capable of interrogating for degree of cure with a resolution sufficient to discriminate between, for example, 90 and 95% degree of cure for military structures. Robust egress and relatively inexpensive readout of the signal appropriate for the production environment should also be available. Several methods that have been demonstrated in the past for resin cure monitoring are given in Table 1 and should be considered.

The manufacturing process greatly affects the choice of sensing approach. The only approaches available commercially as part of commercially available control systems are thermocouple and dielectric. Dosimetry and nuclear magnetic resonance approaches have specific process alignments that may bring them to fruition in the near future.

Dielectric Cure Sensors. Dielectric measurements have been used for many years to characterize the electrical properties of materials and to study chemical reactions (Ref 8–10). Since they are the only readily available method for monitoring the cure process at this fidelity, this method is discussed here in detail. Readers must decide whether their needs warrant developing one of the other approaches listed previously or whether dielectric sensors will suffice. For organic polymer systems, dielectric measurements have been shown to strongly correlate with various quantities such as molecular mobility, dynamic moduli, extent of crystallization, viscosity, the buildup of glass-transition temperature (T_g), and the extent of cure. These correlations have resulted in increased interest in applying dielectric methods for process monitoring and control during the cure of composite materials.

Dielectrometry is commonly performed using either matched parallel plate or comb electrodes that may be embedded in the bulk material or located on the sample surfaces. An alternative probe technology is the microdielectrometer, which consists of an interdigitated electrode deposited on a semiconductor substrate. To determine the dielectric constant, a time-varying voltage is applied and the output voltage or current waveform is measured. The excitation voltage is usually a sinusoid in the frequency range from 10^{-4} to 10^{7} Hz. In general, the material will cause an attenuation of the output signal with an ac-

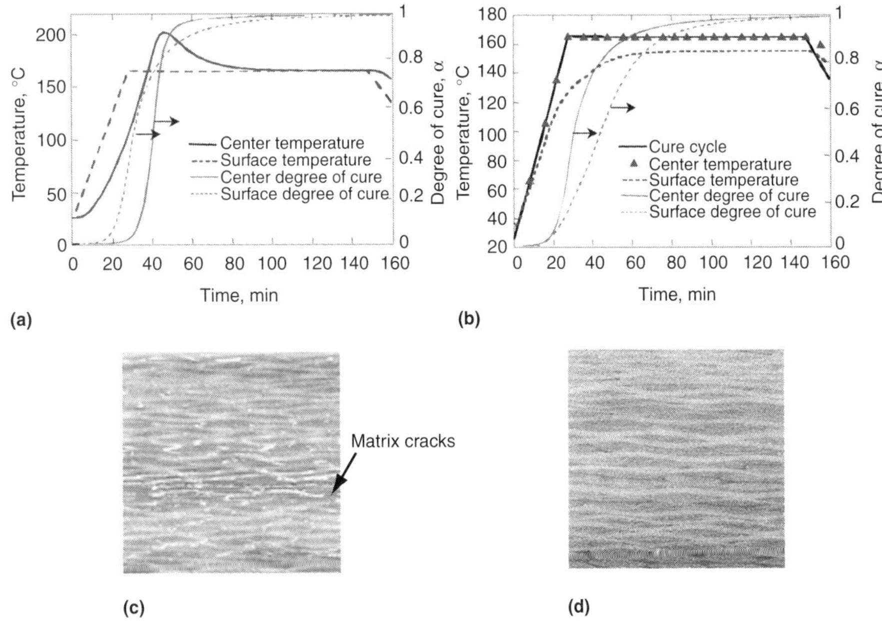

Fig. 1 Numerical results for (a) conventional and (b) microwave processing of a 25 mm (1 in.) thick glass/epoxy laminate and cross-sectional micrographs of (c) conventional and (d) microwave-processed laminates. Significant matrix cracking is seen in the autoclave-processed laminate, resulting from outside-in solidification stresses.

companying phase shift. The severity of these effects is determined by the sample conductance and capacitance, from which the complex dielectric constant may be determined via a model that incorporates the electrode geometry and an appropriate equivalent circuit representing the material under test. For polymers, the equivalent circuit is typically a collection of capacitive and resistive elements connected in parallel and/or in series. A basic example of this type of representation is given in Fig. 2. In this circuit, circuit C_1-C_2-R models the dipolar relaxations, and the addition of R_{ion} in parallel models ionic conductivity.

Dielectric Constant. The complex relative dielectric constant, ε*, is a measure of how much electromagnetic energy can be stored within a material and how much energy is absorbed or lost. The term "relative" in this instance comes from the fact that ε* is referenced to the permittivity of free space, so that $\varepsilon^* = \varepsilon/\varepsilon_0$, where $\varepsilon_0 = 8.85 \times 10^{-14}$. Farads/cm. Equation 1 defines ε* and shows the real and complex components, which are the dielectric permittivity, ε′, and the dielectric loss, ε″, respectively.

$$\varepsilon^* = \varepsilon' - i\varepsilon'' \quad \text{(Eq 1)}$$

For polymers, ε′ represents the polarizability of dipoles plus additional capacitance due to ionic charge accumulation and ε″ represents the losses associated with both dipole orientation and ionic conduction. Expressing this fact mathematically gives:

$$\varepsilon^* = (\varepsilon'_i + \varepsilon'_d) - i(\varepsilon''_i + \varepsilon''_d) \quad \text{(Eq 2)}$$

where ε'_i and ε'_d are the respective ionic and dipolar contributions to ε′, and ε''_i and ε''_d are the respective ionic and dipolar contribution to ε″.

Dipole Polarization. When a time varying voltage is applied to a sample, dipoles that are attached to polymer-backbone molecules will rotate to align themselves with the field. The time required for dipoles to align fully with the field is a characteristic of the dipole mobility and is referred to as the relaxation time, τ. The relaxation time is influenced by the following factors: temperature, viscosity, dipole size, dipole distribution, and the mobility of the segment to which the dipole is attached. In general, as temperature and segment mobility increase, τ decreases, and when dipole size or viscosity increase, τ increases. In reacting systems, for example, epoxy-amine, τ typically starts out low but then begins to increase as the reaction continues due to the motion-hindering mechanisms.

If a reacting system without any conducting ions were to be monitored versus time with a single frequency, the permittivity would be seen to remain initially at a constant level while the loss would be low. Early in the reaction, dipoles have sufficient mobility to quickly orient themselves to the applied field so full polarization can be achieved. Little energy is lost through alignment. As the reaction progresses, the permittivity would decrease, and the loss factor would increase to a maximum before falling again. This behavior is related to the increase in τ that results from the increased restriction of the dipole mobility due to the developing network. The point of maximum loss in this situation corresponds to the point where the period of the excitation voltage equals τ. Debye was the first to develop an analytical expression to describe hindered dipole motion in systems that possess a single relaxation time. Incorporating ionic conduction effects on the dielectric constant with the Debye model gives the following:

$$\varepsilon'_i = \frac{A}{\omega^{n=1}}\left(\frac{\sigma}{\varepsilon_0}\right)^2 \quad \text{(Eq 3)}$$

$$\varepsilon'_d = \varepsilon_u + \frac{\varepsilon_r - \varepsilon_u}{1 + (\omega\tau)^2} \quad \text{(Eq 4)}$$

$$\varepsilon''_i = \frac{\sigma}{\omega\varepsilon_0} - \frac{B}{\omega^{n=1}}\left(\frac{\sigma}{\varepsilon_0}\right)^2 \quad \text{(Eq 5)}$$

$$\varepsilon''_d = \frac{\omega\tau(\varepsilon_r - \varepsilon_u)}{1 + (\omega\tau)^2} \quad \text{(Eq 6)}$$

$$\varepsilon'' = \frac{\sigma}{\omega\varepsilon_0} + \frac{\omega\tau(\varepsilon_r - \varepsilon_u)}{1 + (\omega\tau)^2} \quad \text{(Eq 7)}$$

$$\sigma = \sum_i z_i q n_i \mu_i \quad \text{(Eq 8)}$$

where A and B are constants dependent on the electrode/material interface and electrode polarization, ω is the excitation frequency in rad/s, σ is the ionic conduction in $(\Omega/\text{cm})^{-1}$, z_i is the valence of the *i*th ionic species, q is the electron charge, n_i is the concentration of the *i*th species, μ_i is the ionic mobility, ε_r is the relaxed dielectric constant (defined as the value ε* reaches when the maximum possible dipole polarization has been achieved for the given conditions), and ε_u is the unrelaxed dielectric constant (defined as

Table 1 Recently investigated cure monitoring technologies

Resin cure monitoring method	Investigators	Comments
Thermocouples	Stanford University and most others	If you know the temperature history, you can predict degree of cure.
Dielectric	Micromet Instruments; Beijing University of Aeronautics and Astronautics (China); NASA-Langley; College of William and Mary; Lockheed	The standard method at this time. See text for more.
Ultrasonic	Micromet; Rockwell (laser based)	No part contact required; stitches can return anomalous signals.
Frequency dependent electromagnetic sensing (FDEMS)	NASA-Langley; Virginia Polytechnic Institute and State University; College of William and Mary; U.S. Air Force Materials Directorate; Hughes	Similar to dielectric
Fluorescence	National Institute of Standards and Technology (NIST); Johns Hopkins University; McDonnell Douglas (now Boeing); Duke Engineering Group; Northwestern University	This gets to the heart of the chemistry but sometimes requires dopants to get sufficient fluorescence of the host resin.
Acoustic waveguides (AWG)	Westinghouse Science and Technology	This is an offshoot in many respects of ultrasonic methods. "Leaky" AWGs interrogate part.
Fiberoptic index of refraction	Brunel University, Northrop Grumman, NIST	. . .
Fiberoptic strain sensors	Naval Research Labs; McDonnell Douglas (now Boeing); Lockheed Martin	Uses various relatively expensive fiberoptic sensors to measure strain at points.
Fourier transform infrared (FTIR) spectroscopy	NIST; Foster-Miller, Brunel University	This also gets to the heart of the chemistry but uses expensive fiber that you cannot reuse because it is embedded. Lower cost fibers are becoming available.
Near infrared (NIR) spectroscopy	Northwestern University, Brunel University	This builds on FTIR approach but works with telecom fiber. Uses neural networks to interpret data.
Direct current conductometry	University of Delaware; University of Dayton; General Electric; ASC Process Systems; Hughes Aerospace; U.S. Air Force Materials Directorate; U.S. Army Research Laboratories	Often requires ionic doping to decrease resistivity. Can be combined with SMARTweave resin flow monitoring.
Dosimetry	Adherent	For EB processing, film coatings or coated optical fiber versions indicate exposure levels by color changes in the film layer. See text for more.
Nuclear magnetic resonance (NMR)	Boeing	Rising in importance for fiber placement

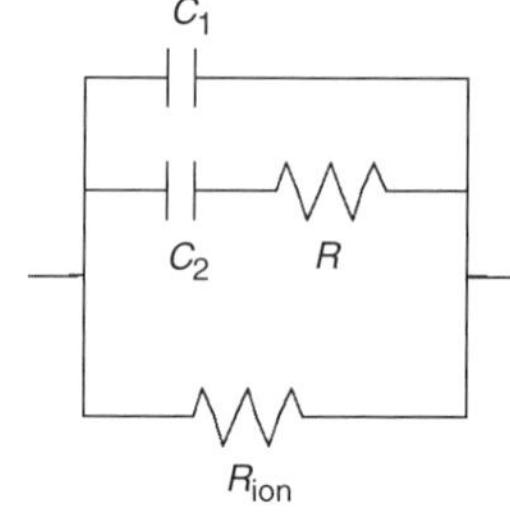

Fig. 2 Schematic of an equivalent circuit for a conducting polymer resin

the value of ε^* at infinite frequency, i.e., the base value of ε^* without dipole or charge migration included).

While Debye's model is sufficient for systems with one relaxation time, for example, a monodisperse, single-component monomer solution, real polymers typically exhibit a distribution of relaxation times. Therefore, the strict Debye equations no longer apply. For systems with a distribution of relaxation times, the Havrlik-Nagami (HN) equation is often used:

$$\varepsilon^* = \varepsilon_u + \frac{\varepsilon_r - \varepsilon_u}{\left[1+(i\omega\tau)^{1-\alpha}\right]^{\beta}} \quad \text{(Eq 9)}$$

where α is a parameter describing the width of the relaxation, and β is a parameter that describes the asymmetry of the relaxation. These shape parameters can be calculated by fitting Eq 3 to experimental data.

Ionic Conduction. Many of the resin systems used for composite materials, for example, epoxy-amine, contain impurity ions or are easily ionizable. The ions present in the resin will move under the influence of the applied electric field and absorb energy. As Eq 3 shows, the absorbed energy contributes to the dielectric loss. For highly conductive resins, the contribution of σ to ε'' can completely mask the losses due to dipole orientation. For these systems, the dielectric loss is given by Eq 10.

$$\varepsilon'' = \frac{\sigma}{\omega\varepsilon_0} \quad \text{(Eq 10)}$$

If ionic concentration does not change during cure, then the resin conductivity is a direct measure of the ionic mobility. The dependence of σ on ion mobility provides a powerful tool for monitoring the extent of cure, as the movement of ions through the polymer network will decrease as the network densifies. Prior to gelation, ionic mobility is high, and the conductivity is, in general, inversely proportional to the viscosity. At the gelation point, the macromolecule forms, viscosity becomes essentially infinite, and ionic mobility is drastically reduced. However, after gelation, ionic conduction does not become constant, as would be expected if viscosity were the sole determining factor. Instead, σ remains finite with a gradual decrease. This behavior corresponds to the further densification of the network that occurs as vitrification is approached. The existence of a measurable conductivity suggests that the local motion of polymer chain segments on the order of the ion size is sufficient to allow for conduction. Ionic conductivity is the most widely used parameter for cure monitoring because it is sensitive to the polymer viscosity, the concentration and type of molecular species present, and the microstructure of the polymer over a wide range of the cure. Measurement of ionic conductivity is typically accomplished through measuring the dielectric loss. Figure 3 shows a schematic of a typical plot of dielectric loss versus frequency, and Fig. 4 shows the typical behavior versus curing time.

Electrode Polarization. The analysis of dielectric data for cure monitoring can be difficult to interpret due to a phenomenon known as electrode polarization. This effect, which manifests itself under direct current conductivity measurements or low-frequency dielectrometry, is the result of the accumulation of ionic charge at the electrodes. Due to the blocking nature of the electrode/polymer interface, the accumulated ions cannot discharge, thereby creating a charged boundary layer that adds to the specimen capacitance. This increased capacitance adds to the permittivity and lowers the apparent loss. The electrode polarization effect can be modeled by adding two capacitances in series with circuit C_1-C_2-R from Fig. 2, as shown in Fig. 5, where these two capacitances are combined into a single capacitor of thickness $2t_b$. Assuming that the permittivity of the blocking layer is the same as the material, the blocking capacitance, C_b, is given by:

$$C_b = \frac{\varepsilon_0 \varepsilon' A}{2t_b} \quad \text{(Eq 11)}$$

where A is the area in cm^2, and t_b is the thickness of the polarized layer in cm.

Electrode polarization may become significant when the admittance of the equivalent circuit, $1/R$, becomes greater than ωC_b. If this situation is avoided, then the sample behaves as a simple dielectric. However, if this situation occurs, for example, for highly conductive resins, then charging of the electrodes through R masks other circuit responses. When $1/R$ becomes large, electrode polarization becomes significant when the following inequalities are satisfied:

$$\cot(\phi) > 1 \quad \text{(Eq 12)}$$

and

$$\cot(\phi) > \frac{L}{2t_b} - 1 \quad \text{(Eq 13)}$$

where L is the specimen length in cm. Experimentally, electrode polarization effects can be seen through the linearization of the plot of frequency versus loss factor, illustrated schematically in Fig. 6.

In composite materials, the presence of fillers such as fiber reinforcement may act as additional blocking interfaces that become polarized. These interfaces exhibit Debye-like phenomena known as the Maxwell-Waner (MW) relaxation. Heterogeneous systems that produce MW relaxations can be modeled as multiple-layered heterogeneous capacitors.

The Cole-Cole Plot. A convenient tool for displaying dielectric data is the Argand, or Cole-Cole, plot. This diagram is constructed by plotting ε'' versus ε' for various frequencies. For a resin with no ionic conductivity and a single relaxation time (Debye behavior), the Cole-Cole

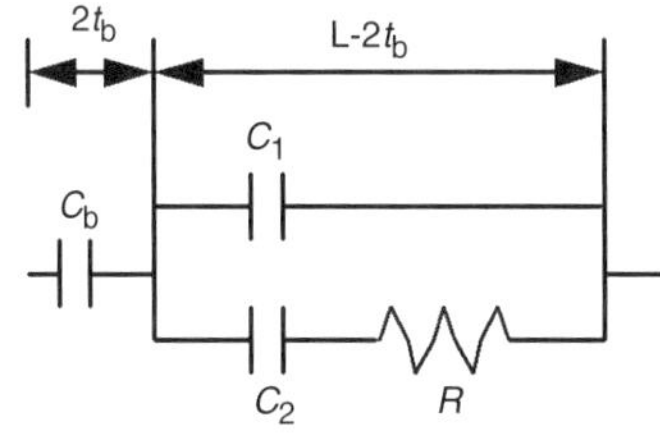

Fig. 5 Schematic of an equivalent circuit for a polymer sample of length L, with blocking layers

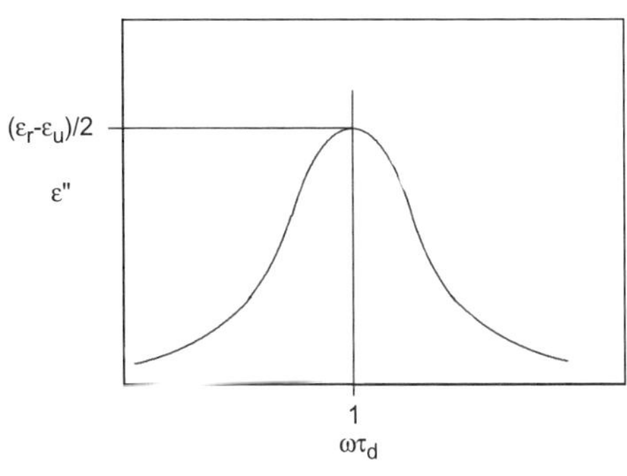

Fig. 3 Dielectric loss versus frequency for a typical epoxy resin

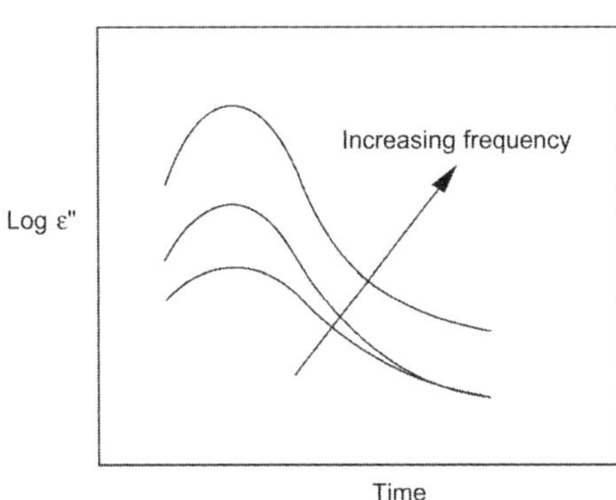

Fig. 4 Dielectric loss versus cure time for typical epoxy resins

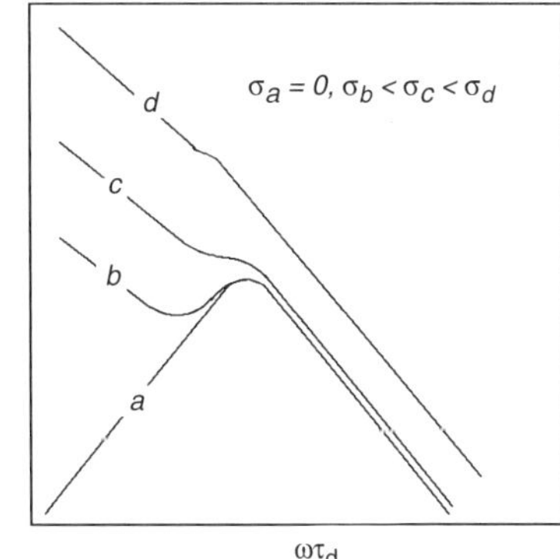

Fig. 6 The effect of ionic conductivity on the dielectric loss versus frequency

plot is a semicircle with its center on the axis and intercepts at ε_u and ε_r as Fig. 7 illustrates. A distribution in the relaxation times would transform the plot from a semicircle to a more complex trace that can be described via the HN equation (Eq 9). From a Cole-Cole plot, the effects of multiple relaxation times, conductivity, and electrode polarization can be quickly and easily determined.

Ionic conduction and the presence of blocking layers will alter the Cole-Cole plot. High levels of ionic conduction will result in an almost linear plot (Fig. 8). The effect of electron polarization is opposite to the effect of ionic conductivity. The presence of blocking layers causes the Cole-Cole plot to become semicircular, mimicking a single Debye relaxation. Figure 9 shows the effect of boundary layer thickness on the Cole-Cole plot.

Fiberoptics-Based Resin Cure Sensors. Fiberoptics may offer an inexpensive, robust method of monitoring resin-cure sensing. Various optical fiber approaches have been investigated, including monitoring the chemical changes within the resin via fluorescence, infrared spectroscopy, near-infrared spectroscopy, evanescent wave transmission (Ref 11), and tracking strain and temperature. All have been achieved at a level appropriate for laboratory use but none have really gained widespread acceptance.

The most simple of this class of sensors uses inexpensive optical fiber to monitor the changes that occur during cure in the index of refraction of the resin. Optical fiber with removable cladding (the part of the fiber that surrounds the light-carrying core of the fiber) has its cladding replaced in sensing locations with a high-refractive-index material, higher in index than the resin it is to be embedded within. This provides a large change across the entire cure but as the cure approaches completion, its index changes very little. For aerospace parts, this approach does not offer the resolution needed in the range desired but it may offer a low cost method for other industries.

The setup for achieving this comprises a laser, a power source for the laser, an optical detector, and some means of performing data collection and analysis. This approach has been done by several researchers in the past and recent availability of optical fibers with removable cladding may renew excitement over this approach.

Ultrasonics-Based Resin Cure Sensing. Ultrasonic techniques can be applied to monitoring the changes in mechanical response that result from the cure of thermosetting polymer matrix resins. Most of the techniques have focused on monitoring changes in viscosity in epoxy resins and composites undergoing thermal cure.

Fundamentally, ultrasonic cure monitoring methods involve introducing a pulsed ultrasonic signal to a curing system and measuring transit time for the signal to reach a receiving transducer. A signal velocity (and attenuation) is calculated from the transit time, amplitude, and distance. Changes in the ultrasonic signal velocity are analytically related to the density, thickness, and stiffness at the interface between the matrix and the transducer or waveguide.

Figure 10 shows a typical signal velocity trace for a carbon/epoxy composite under representative processing conditions (Ref 12). These basic relationships have been observed for a number of ultrasonic techniques with different coupling geometry (Ref 13, 14). An initial decrease in signal velocity is attributable to the decrease in viscosity of the matrix resin resulting from initial heating. This transition ends when the signal velocity reaches a minimum, corresponding with minimum viscosity. Then, the signal velocity increases as the effects of the cure reaction dominate the process (i.e., gelation and increasing cross-link density). Finally, the response levels off as cross-link density reaches a steady state.

Fiber ultrasonics is a technique that uses embedded filaments as sensing elements to characterize interfacial properties. The technique is based on guided-wave ultrasonics that were developed almost 60 years ago, when ultrasonic waves were used to propagate along transmission lines (Ref 15). When a high-frequency ultrasonic pulse (typically 0.5 MHz to 10 MHz) impinges on a rod, the ultrasound travels along the rod as a guided wave at specific velocities characteristic of the material properties of the rod. Analogously, if an ultrasonic pulse is applied to an unconstrained small-diameter fiber and the frequency of the ultrasound used for interrogation is chosen such that the corresponding wavelength is much smaller than the diameter of the fiber, the ultrasound will propagate along the length of the fiber as a guided wave. The properties of the ultrasonic wave propagation are characteristic of the fiber material properties (Ref 16, 17).

In cases where the fiber is constrained along its axial radial boundaries, the guided ultrasound leaks from the fiber to the surrounding media, thereby altering the observed ultrasonic response. The rate and nature of the ultrasonic leakage is a function of the density, thickness, and stiffness of the fiber-matrix interface region (Ref 18, 19). Therefore, analysis of the waveguide propagation provides a direct measure of the fiber-matrix interfacial characteristics.

The primary advantage of this method is that it offers a direct measure of stress-wave transfer within the material, which could enable both in-process material characterization and in-service condition analysis. In addition, a reinforcing fiber can be directly used as the primary sensor in the structure. Although there has been specialized application of guided-wave ultrasonic cure monitoring (Ref 20), fiber ultrasonic techniques that employ reinforcing fibers as the waveguides are still in development.

In conclusion, ultrasonic cure monitoring technologies allow the state of cure to be monitored without intrusive sensors. Commercial systems are available (Ref 12), even though most

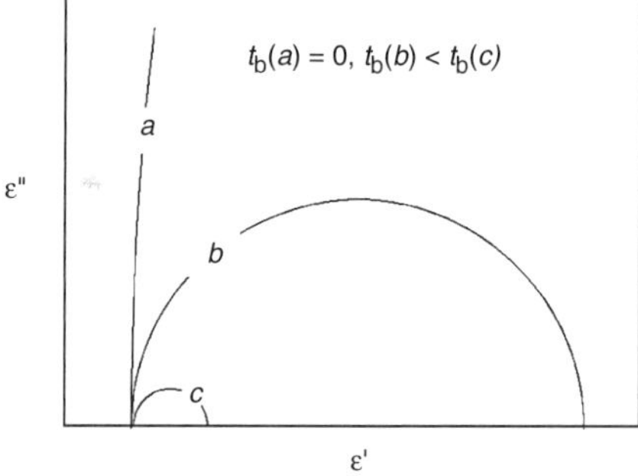

Fig. 9 The effect of boundary layer thickness on the Cole-Cole plot

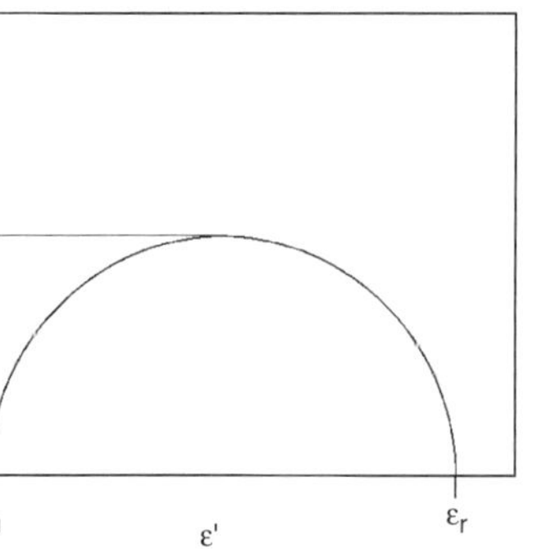

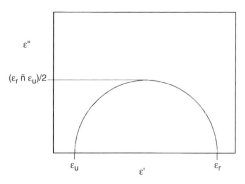

Fig. 7 A Cole-Cole plot

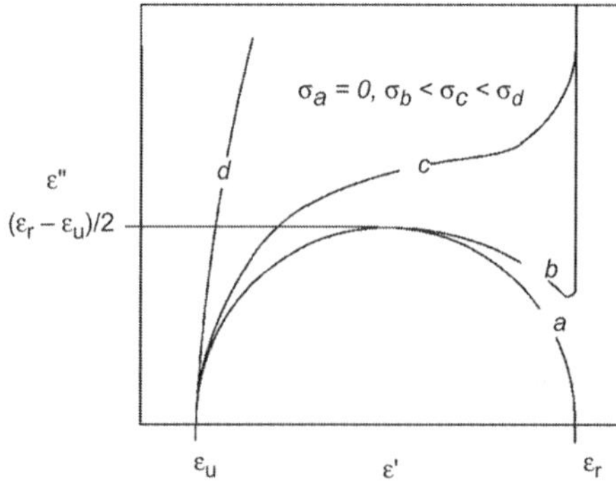

Fig. 8 Cole-Cole plot showing the effects of ionic conductivity

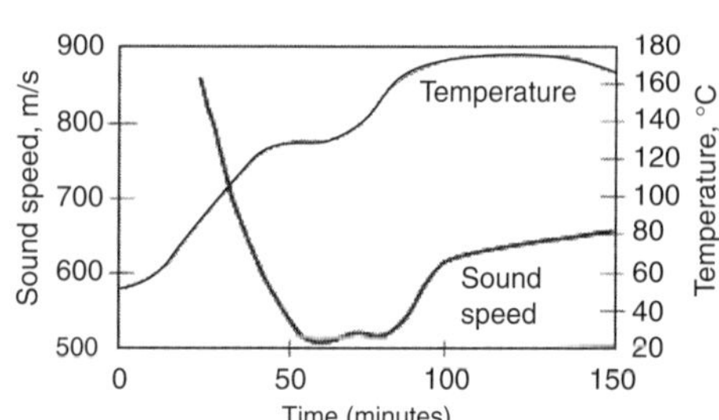

Fig. 10 Changes in ultrasonic signal velocity during processing of a compression molded carbon/epoxy prepreg laminate. Source: Ref 12

applications have been in research and process-development environments. Ultrasonic cure monitoring is being evaluated for production implementation for a range of composite processes.

Dosimetry-Based Resin Cure Sensors. Electron-beam curing of carbon fiber composite materials promises to be very economical while providing significant manufacturing options that are not possible with the conventional autoclave cure process. Advantages of EB curing include dimensional stability of cured parts, potential for secondary bonding after partial cure, speed of cure operation, lower cost, compatibility with complex assemblies, and low-cost tooling. If this technology makes it to maturity, conventional cure sensing approaches will not suffice because EB cure processes must be monitored for accumulated dose values to determine if adequate levels of radiation have penetrated the laminate being cured. This is a significant departure from current practice in autoclave and liquid molding processes.

This monitoring is currently performed as a post-process verification using film as the verification medium. This does not allow for the collection of in-process control data nor in-process adjustment of the process to ensure conforming results. The film is developed and the density compared to a known reference standard to determine the amount of accumulated radiation that has passed through the laminate. If the value is below or above the specification level, a nonconformance is generated and engineering must disposition the part. The cost of this nonconformance is determined by the type. Overcured laminates normally do not require any additional curing. Undercure nonconformances normally require additional post curing at a nominal temperature. The undercure and overcure are an inherent risk of using the film method of monitoring degree of cure in EB laminates.

Fiber optic dosimetry holds the potential to be used to predict cure-acceptance parameters, in-process and real-time. This capability would provide manufacturing the visibility of the cure process to partial cure laminates to specific glass-transition temperature (T_g) values. This partial cure capability should be predictable, repeatable, and reliable for production level EB curing operations. Current fiber optic dosimeters (Ref 21) have a limited life based on current technology development, but their cost appears to be dropping rapidly based on the sharing of development costs with the medical industry.

Reducing the need for post-EB cure physical verification such as T_g could also be accomplished by developing a statistical database that correlates the accumulated cure dose to the appropriate thermal T_g value. Once the correlation is established, the risk of a cure nonconformance could be eliminated except for catastrophic process failures such as equipment failures or blatant operator error. This concept becomes increasingly important as the unionization of composite parts into large structures continues and manufacturing nonconformance risks increase. Using the accumulated dose as a method of determining the degree of cure also improves the manufacturing process flow by eliminating the hold time for testing. Support labor cost will also drop due to a lack of post-process verification requirements.

Resin Cure Control

For autoclave, RTM, SCRIMP, VARTM, and other heat-activated cure processes, control is exercised over the temperature or pressure or both. None of these should require extreme measures to increase the overall degree of cure unless the cure is sufficiently nonuniform that a global cure cannot be performed. For other processes where energy is supplied via UV, microwave, or EB energy, additional exposure would be used to increase the degree of cure in localized areas.

Flow Sensing

As resin infiltrates the fibers in any of the infusion processes, it must follow a path that completely fills the part. This is more difficult than it appears due to variations in the permeability of the materials along its path. The most obvious problems are encountered when resin finds an easy path along the edge of the cloth in what is termed racetracking. The resin front path can be modeled, mapped, and, to some degree, controlled.

Flow Modeling

Resin-flow front mapping is useful for locating and identifying problems, but its full value cannot be achieved until the identified problem is fixed and the reasons for the sensed abnormalities are understood and accounted for in future components. Resin-flow modeling must be used in coordination with design and modeling to minimize the occurrences of flow-related problems and to optimize inlet and outlet locations as well as runner size and location. The University of Dayton Research Laboratory, the U.S. Army Research Laboratory, Stanford University, the University of Connecticut, and the University of Delaware all were active in flow modeling at the time of publication.

Flow Mapping

Process control will require improved resin-flow-front sensing methodologies tuned to the needs of high-quality composites. These flow mapping technologies must of course be mated with models and controls systems in the rest of the process to achieve the best part quality and cost. But the first step in achieving flow control is being able to track resin flow. Most of this work has concentrated on SMARTweave (developed by the Army Research Laboratory and licensed to Holometrix Micromet, Bedford, MA) but there has been some work in fiberoptic and infrared flow mapping that may well become important in the near future. SMARTweave and methods of a similar electrical nature have been found to work quite well in nonconductive materials, and some work has been done to extend this approach to carbon-fiber-based composites. Infrared flow monitoring has been demonstrated on heated tables but lags significantly in utility in the other bagged processes like VARTM and SCRIMP. Optical flow-front monitoring has also been demonstrated with various schemes to fill air gaps in the fiber with resin, but none have made it anywhere near production. At this time, the only method that has shown significant development and promise is SMARTweave.

SMARTweave for resin-flow front mapping was developed to monitor resin-flow-front progression and provide data for control of resin flow in large RTM fiberglass parts. The SMARTweave resin-flow-front monitoring process is well developed and commercially available for most current composites manufacturing processes. It consists of a grid of conductors, half of which are located between two plies in one orientation. The other half are located between two other plies and oriented orthogonally. The resistance between two conductors gives an indication of resin presence or absence at the point at which the conductors are closest. For carbon fiber composites, the fibers themselves are conductive, and so care must be taken to insulate the SMARTweave grid from the surrounding reinforcement. The U.S. Army Research Laboratory and the University of Delaware Center for Composite Materials have demonstrated that this can be accomplished by using a sensor grid composed of overbraided copper wires. Research has also shown that the SMARTweave technique can be accomplished using carbon tows as sensor elements to reduce the impact of the sensing grid on material performance. However, the use of carbon tows does not reduce the number of electrodes that must egress from a mold or vacuum bag.

While generally not a concern for processes that are not sensitive to minor pressure loss, resin loss, or air infiltration and embedded wiring, the point of egress of each sensing and excitation wire are potential resin or air-leak paths for VARTM and other highly vacuum-sensitive processes. Therefore, care must be taken to mitigate this risk. A potential solution has been found by reducing the number of wires needed to perform the multiplexing of the sensor grid to a three-wire set coupled to a signal-processing circuit board. These modifications to the process allow SMARTweave to be implemented on aerospace-quality structures as long as the wiring dimensions do not result in unacceptable strength degradation.

To further the acceptance of SMARTweave for monitoring the manufacture of strength critical components, further studies are needed to demonstrate that this method can be implemented without deleterious effects on structural performance. However, this technology has demonstrated sufficient reliability and performance that

Micromet Inc. (Bedford, MA) currently offers commercially available SMARTweave resin-front tracking systems based on the systems originally conceived by the U.S. Army Research Laboratory (Ref 22) and further developed by the University of Delaware Center for Composite Materials (Ref 23).

Resin Flow Control

There are currently no methods to modify the resin-flow front beyond altering the application of resin pressure at various inlets or the incoming resin temperature. For many cases, adjusting resin pot temperature or pressures works well, and controlling inlets and temperature is mostly straightforward. However, localized disturbances in the flow field cannot currently be addressed except by introducing more resin or cycling the resin to remove any pockets that are created. This is a known and identified gap in available technology.

Practical Issues in Sensing Resin Cure and Flow

Tool-Mounted Sensors. Most resin-cure-sensing efforts have either placed a sensor under the bagging material in autoclave processing or passed a sensor through the tool in RTM processing. Either of these tends to result in a mark of some sort in the surface of the part. Tool-mounted sensors tend to have less trouble with the wires or fibers moving or breaking. Tool-mounted sensors also tend to meet some resistance due to increased tool costs or fear that cleaning the tool surface will damage the sensor. Both of these objections have indeed been overcome in some instances (Ref 24), so tool mounting is still considered a viable option for production composite part manufacture.

Ingress/Egress. Sensors must have power to work. Usually they use electrical power; sometimes they use optical energy instead. In either case, any sensor that is in contact with the resin system must have available electrical or optical energy that will typically pass through the tooling or bagging used to contain and shape the part. This presents a major obstacle, especially when this is not considered until late in process design.

Resin under pressure tends to find a way out of the bag or tooling at these ingress points unless care is taken to seal the resin in over the entire temperature and pressure range. This thins the part or allows gasses to enter or collect. The designer must also consider that the fibers and resin will move during processing, sometimes shearing off the lead in wire or fiber so carefully designed into the tool. Both optical and electrical sensors have been used successfully in situ, but the designer must account for this as early as possible in the design of the tooling and, preferably, the part.

ACKNOWLEDGMENTS

The authors gratefully acknowledge the assistance of Shawn Walsh of the U.S. Army Research Laboratories and Renee Kent of ARINC for their help in the preparation of this article.

REFERENCES

1. M. Thomas et al., "Computer Aided Curing of Composites," McDonnell Aircraft Company Final Report, WRDC-TR-89-4084, 1989
2. P.R. Ciriscioli and G.S. Springer, *Smart Autoclave Cure of Composites,* Technomic Publishing Co., 1990
3. F. Stephan, A. Fit, and X. Duteurtre, In-Process Control of Epoxy Composite by Microdielectrometric Analysis, *Polym. Eng. Sci.,* Vol 37 (No. 2), 1997, p 436–449
4. J.M. Griffith and T. Hackett, F/A-18 C/D and E/F Implementation of Dielectric Sensor Adhesive Staging, *Proc. 45th International SAMPE Symposium,* Society for the Advancement of Material and Process Engineering, 21–25 May 2000, p 1267–1281
5. F. Abrams and T.B. Tolle, An Analysis of E-Beam Potential in Aerospace Composite Manufacturing, *Proc. 42nd International SAMPE Symposium,* Society for the Advancement of Material and Process Engineering, 1997, p 526–536
6. W.I. Lee, and G.S. Springer, Microwave Curing of Composites, *J. Compos. Mater.,* Vol 18, 1984, p 387–409
7. E.T. Thostenson and T.-W. Chou, Microwave Processing: Fundamentals and Applications, *Compos. Part A,* Vol 30 (No. 9), 1999, p 1055–1071
8. D. Kranbuehl, S. Delos, E. Yi, J. Mayer, and T. Jarvie, Dynamic Dielectric Analysis: Nondestructive Material Evaluation and Cure Monitoring, *Polym. Eng. Sci.,* Vol 26 (No. 5), 1986, p 338–345
9. D. Hunston, "Assessment of the State-of-the-Art for Process Monitoring Sensors for Polymer Composites," NISTIR 4514, U.S. Department of Commerce, National Institute of Standards and Technology, Materials Science and Engineering Laboratory, Polymers Division, 1991
10. P.R. Ciriscioli and G.S. Springer, Dielectric Cure Monitoring—A Critical Review, *SAMPE J.,* Vol 25 (No. 3), May/June 1989, p 35–42
11. M.A. Druy et al., "Fourier Transform Infrared (FTIR) Fiber Optic Monitoring of Composites during Cure in an Autoclave," *Adv. Compos.,* Sept 1989
12. D.S. Shepard and K.R. Smith, A Complete Ultrasonic Measurement System for In-Process Cure Monitoring and Control of Composites, *Conf. Proc. NDE Applied to Process Control of Composite Fabrication,* Nondestructive Testing Information Analysis Center, 1–2 Oct 1996
13. E.C. Johnson, J.D. Pollchik, and S.L. Zacharius, "An Ultrasonic Testing Technique for Monitoring the Cure and Mechanical Properties of Polymeric Materials," Report TR-93(3935)-12, The Aerospace Corporation, El Segundo, CA, 1993
14. R.M. Kent, Fiber Ultrasonics for Health Monitoring of Composites, *Proc. 19th Digital Avionics Systems Conf.,* IEEE, in press
15. D. Bancroft, The Velocity of Longitudinal Waves in Cylindrical Bars, *Phys. Rev.,* Vol 59, 1941
16. R.M. Kent and M.J. Ruddell, The In-Situ Sensor-Guided Process Characterization of Advanced Composite Materials, *JOM,* Vol 48 (No. 9), 1996
17. R.M. Kent and R.E. Dutton, Utilizing an In Situ Sensor to Monitor the Densification of a Borosilicate Glass Matrix Composite, *Proc. SPIE,* Vol 2948, The Society of Photo-Optical Instrumentation Engineers (SPIE), Vol 2948, 1996
18. E. Drescher-Krasicka, J.A. Simmons, and H.N.G. Wadley, Fast Leaky Modes on Cylindrical Metal-Ceramic Interfaces, *Review of Progress in Quantitative Nondestructive Evaluation,* D.O. Thompson and D.E. Chimenti, Ed., Vol 9A, Plenum Press, 1990, p 173–180
19. E. Drescher-Krasicka, J.A. Simmons, and H.N.G. Wadley, Leaky Symmetric Modes in Infinitely Clad Rods, *J. Acoust. Soc. America,* Vol 92 (1992), p 1061–1090
20. Y. Li and S. Menon, Ultrasonic Sensing of Composite Materials during the Heat-Cure Cycle, *Sensors Magazine,* Feb 1998
21. A.E. Hoytm et al., Scintillator Based Fiber Optic Dosimeters for Electron Beam Processing, *Proc. 45th International SAMPE Symposium,* Society for the Advancement of Material and Process Engineering, 2000, p 526–536 and p 1855–1862
22. S. Walsh and M. Charmchi, Free-Surface Flow Observations in the Resin Transfer Molding (RTM) Process, *Heat and Mass Transfer in Materials Processing and Engineering,* D. Zumbrunnen et al., Ed., American Society of Mechanical Engineers,-ASME HTD Vol 261, 1993, p 147–156
23. D. Heider, C. Hofmann, and J. Gillespie, "Automation and Control of Large-Scale Composite Parts by VARTM Processing," *Proc. 45th International SAMPE Symposium,* Society for the Advancement of Material and Process Engineering, 21–25 May 2000, p 1567–1575
24. B.P. Rice, "Composite Cure Monitoring with a Tool-Mounted UV-VIS-NIR Fiber Optic Sensor," *Proc. 39th International SAMPE Symposium,* Society for the Advancement of Material and Process Engineering, 1994

Nondestructive Testing

ASM International Committee on Nondestructive Testing of Composites*

COMPOSITE MATERIALS, because of their nonhomogeneous, anisotropic characteristics, pose significant challenges for defect detection and materials property characterization. Throughout their life cycle, composites are susceptible to the formation of many possible defects, primarily due to their multiple-step production process, nonhomogeneous nature, and brittle matrix. These defects include delaminations, matrix cracking, fiber fracture, fiber pull-out, and impact damage. Table 1 shows some of the defects that may appear in composite laminates and their effect on the structural performance. While the emphasis of most practical nondestructive evaluation (NDE) is on detection of delaminations, porosity, and impact damage, Table 1 shows that other defects can also have critical effect on the host structures.

This article introduces the principal methodologies and some advanced technologies that are currently being applied for NDE of composite materials. The primary discussion and examples are for fiber-reinforced polymer-matrix composites. Many of the techniques have general applicability to other types of composites, such as metal-matrix composites and ceramic-matrix composites. However, there may be specific application differences and limitations that are not addressed.

Ultrasonics

The most common method of NDE for composite materials is ultrasonic inspection. The measurement of ultrasonic parameters can provide a wealth of information on the quality of composites. Ultrasonics can generally detect delaminations, inclusions, matrix macrocracks, and voids in composites structures. The ultrasonic method itself uses longitudinal, shear, Lamb, Rayleigh, or guided waves for various measurements on composite materials. Wave parameters, including acoustic attenuation and speed, can be used to determine materials properties and characteristics, such as void fraction, stiffness, and, if the density is known, moduli. The reader is referred to other texts and articles to obtain detailed information on the fundamental aspects of ultrasonics as well as advanced methodologies for measurements using ultrasound (Ref 1–5).

The acoustic impedance of the media and frequency of the vibrations determine the ultrasound propagation through materials and the behavior at interfaces. The acoustic impedance (Z) of a material is defined as:

$$Z = \rho c \quad \text{(Eq 1)}$$

where ρ is the material density, and c is the acoustic velocity in the material. The frequency and wavelength are related by the equation:

$$f\lambda = c \quad \text{(Eq 2)}$$

where f is frequency, and λ is wavelength. At interfaces, the sound energy transmitted or reflected depends on the acoustic impedance of each media. The transmission (T) and reflection (R) of sound energy from media 1 to media 2 for a normal incidence sound beam is given by:

$$T = 4Z_2Z_1/(Z_2+Z_1)^2 \quad \text{(Eq 3)}$$

and

$$R = [(Z_2-Z_1)/(Z_2+Z_1)]^2 \quad \text{(Eq 4)}$$

respectively, where Z_1 and Z_2 are the acoustic impedances of media 1 and media 2. Table 2 provides some typical acoustic characteristics of materials, and Table 3 gives the relative wavelength as a function of the frequency. For example, at the interface between water and a graphite/epoxy interface, the transmission and reflection of sound energy will be 152% and 52%, respectively. The sound energy in the composite material will be greater than in the water. At an interface between graphite/epoxy and air, the transmission is 0.017%, and the reflection is 100%. It is this change in the acoustic impedance that allows ultrasound to be used to detect defects in materials. Delaminations and cracks represent air interfaces that transmit very little sound and provide a large reflection. Inclusions must have a sufficient difference in acoustic impedance from the composite material in order to be detected.

In solid homogeneous material, both longitudinal (compression) and transverse (shear) waves can be created and monitored independently. In composite materials, however, the separation of longitudinal and transverse waves is much more difficult. Composites are anisotropic media. The plane waves moving through the anisotropic media are often only quasi-longitudinal or quasi-transverse (containing both longitudinal and shear characteristics), because of the wave interactions at the many matrix and the reinforcing material interfaces. In fiber-reinforced composites, the ultrasonic waves can travel along fibers, and therefore, the technique can be highly sensitive to the fiber orientation in the structure. This feature can be used as a means of charac-

Table 1 Effect of defects in fiber-reinforced composite materials

Defect	Potential effect on structural performance
Delamination	Catastrophic failure due to loss of interlaminar shear strength. Typical acceptance criteria require the detection of delaminations with a linear dimension larger than 6.4 mm (0.25 in.).
Impact damage	Loss of compressive strength under static load
Ply gap	Strength degradation depends on stacking order and location. For $[0, 45, 90, -45]_{2S}$ laminate, strength is reduced 9% due to gap(s) in 0° ply and 17% due to gap(s) in 90° ply.
Ply waviness	For 0° ply waviness in $[0, 45, 90, -45]_{2S}$ laminate, static strength reduction is 10% for slight waviness and 25% for extreme waviness. Fatigue life is reduced at least by a factor of 10.
Porosity	Degrades matrix-dominated properties. 1% porosity reduces strength by 5% and fatigue life by 50%.
Surface notches	Static strength reduction of up to 50%. Strength reduction is small for notch sizes that are expected in service.
Thermal over-exposure	Embrittlement and reduction of toughness up to complete loss of structural integrity

**Chairpersons*: R.H. Bossi, The Boeing Company and D.E. Bowles, Northrop Grumman Corporation. *Contributors*: Y. Bar-Cohen, Jet Propulsion Laboratory; T.E. Drake, Lockheed Martin Aerospace; D. Emahiser, GKN Aerospace; R.W. Engelbart, The Boeing Company; G.E. Georgeson, The Boeing Company; E.G. Henneke II, Virginia Polytechnic Institute and State University; R.D. Lawson, The Boeing Company; S.-S. Lih, Jet Propulsion Laboratory; P.W. Lorraine, GE Corporate Research & Development; A.K. Mal, University of California at Los Angeles; S.M. Shepard, Thermal Wave Imaging, Inc.; and J. Tucker, Southern Research Institute.

terization of the structure (Ref 6). However, for the general inspection of fiber-reinforced composites, the most common inspection is with ultrasonic waves perpendicular to the fiber tape or fabric planes.

As the ultrasonic beam passes through a material, it will be attenuated due to scattering, absorption, and beam spreading. The anisotropic properties of composites can make them strong scatters of ultrasound, depending on the wavelength. As shown in Table 3, for ultrasonic frequencies between 1 and 10 MHz, the wavelength will be between 0.3 and 0.03 mm (0.01 and 0.001 in.). Features in the composite larger than one-tenth the wavelength will contribute to scatter. Features smaller than this will not be detectable. Absorption occurs due to the conversion of the sound energy into heat. Beam spreading is due to the geometric principles of the ultrasonic beam size, frequency, angle, and distance. Considering the attenuation due to scatter and absorption, the sound pressure of a plane wave in the far field can be represented by:

$$p = p_0 e^{-\alpha d} \quad \text{(Eq 5)}$$

where p is the end pressure, p_0 is the initial pressure, α is the attenuation coefficient, and d is the distance traveled. The attenuation coefficient in dB/m is obtained from Eq 5, such that:

$$\alpha d = 20 \log (p_0/p) \quad \text{(Eq 6)}$$

where 20 log (p_0/p) is the ratio in decibels of the initial-to-final pressure. The use of the logarithmic dB parameter is customary for attenuation or gain in ultrasonic inspection, because it allows significant ranges to be measured. A change of 6 dB represents a factor of 2 between the initial pressure and the end pressure; a change of 20 dB is a factor of 10, and a change of 80 dB is a factor of 10,000. Figure 1 shows an example plot of the attenuation of a fiber-reinforced graphite/epoxy material as a function of thickness measured at 5 MHz. Actual attenuation coefficients will vary as a function of the fiber, matrix, and lay-up. The acoustic attenuation for the example shown is on the order of 1300 dB/m (33 dB/in.).

The most common inspections of composite structures are through-transmission (TT) ultrasonics and pulse-echo (PE) ultrasonics. The TT method uses two transducers, one on each side of the part, to measure the acoustic attenuation through the structure. One transducer is the transmitter and is electronically pulsed to produce an ultrasonic signal, and the other transducer is the receiver, typically aligned opposite to the pulser. The coupling media of the ultrasound to the composite is usually water. This may be performed by immersing the sample in a water tank or by using water-squirter systems. For TT examinations, the pulser often employs a tone burst (several cycles of the waveform), so that significant ultrasonic power is available. Through transmission is the most common ultrasonic examination method for fiber-reinforced composites. Trough transmission is relatively simple to implement, much more forgiving than automated PE on alignment of the transducers to the part under test, typically has a wide dynamic range (>120 dB on some systems), and easily detects problems in multilayered structures. By comparing TT signal loss in adjacent good areas, porosity, unbonds, wrinkles, delaminations, and most inclusions can be detected. In the case of porosity, the signal loss can be correlated to standards. For example, porosity in the 1 to 2% range corresponds to a change of 4 to 8 dB in signal level for approximately 6 mm (0.25 in.) of graphite/epoxy material at 2.25 MHz. Through transmission methods cannot determine the depth or layer of detected defects. This must be accomplished using pulse-echo ultrasonic methods. However, data from TT methods are normally presented in the C-scan mode, which presents an image of the part with gray scale or color values relating to the attenuation experienced. This is perhaps the easiest ultrasonic presentation to interpret.

Pulse-echo ultrasonic methods typically use a single transducer as both the pulser and receiver of the ultrasound signal. The ultrasound is commonly coupled into the part using a couplant, such as water, glycerin, and other materials. Typical noncontact systems used to couple PE transducers to the parts are hand-held devices, immersion tanks, water-bubbler systems, or water-squirter systems. Any of these systems can be automated.

The advantages and limitations of the coupling methods for automated water-coupled systems are summarized in Table 4.

For PE inspection, the sound is reflected from the front and back surfaces of the composite material as well as from internal defects. Usually, a narrow electronic spike pulse is used in PE inspections to generate a short burst of ultrasound, so that a time-based waveform display (A-scan) can show the difference in the interfaces. While this presentation is not as intuitive as the C-scan, it has the advantage that defect depths can be determined and also, for a trained inspector, provides some information about the nature of the defect. Figure 2 shows a PE ultrasonic waveform at 5 MHz of composite structure. The first pulse is the front surface echo of the part (the interface between the coupling media and the part). The second pulse is the back surface echo of the part. Any reflective defects will show up as echoes between the front and back surfaces. The height of the echo correlates to the size, depth, surface geometry, and impedance mismatch of the defect to the composite. Delaminations (air interfaces) will essentially block all sound from going any further into the composite. Therefore, PE is usually limited to detection of the first occurring defect. By knowing the wave speed in the composite part, or through the use of reference standards, thickness or defect depth can be measured. Carbon/epoxy composite materials have a characteristic wave speed of around 3.2 mm/μs (0.125 in./μs). This can vary by as much as 5% in parts of the same material, so care must be used when using PE ultrasound for absolute thickness measurements. Automated PE inspection usually generates plan-view images of the time of flight from front surface to the next significant reflector (back wall or defect). Different colors or gray scales indicate part thickness or depth. Amplitude images can also be generated by gating on the back wall, a reflector plate, or gating after the front reflection. Parts with varying thickness have to use the latter method. Care must be taken in evaluating PE amplitude images, because defect reflections or multiples of the defect can occur within the gate. Porosity

Table 2 Acoustic characteristics of selected materials

Material	Longitudinal velocity, 10^5 cm/s	Acoustic impedance (Z), g/cm^2 · s	Density, g/cm^3
Air	0.3	40	0.0012
Water	1.5	1.5×10^5	1.00
Epoxy resin	3.0	3.9×10^5	1.30
Graphite/epoxy	3.0(a)	4.7×10^5	1.55
Aluminum	6.3	1.7×10^6	2.71
Titanium	6.1	2.7×10^6	4.60

(a) Sound beam normal to fiber orientations

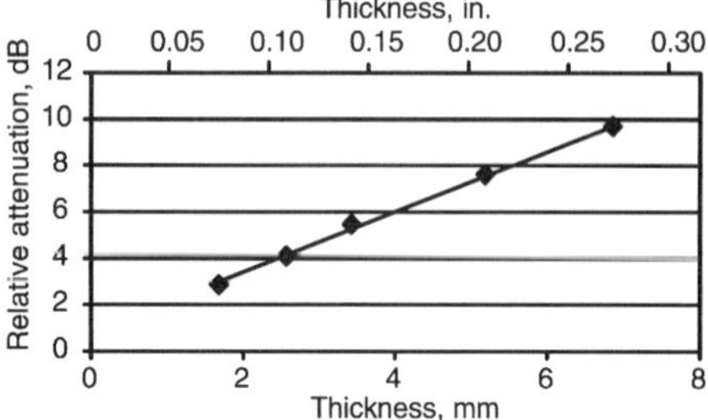

Fig. 1 Acoustic attenuation at 5 MHz for a graphite/epoxy composite as a function of material thickness

Table 3 Acoustic wavelengths in materials

	Air		Water		Epoxy resin		Graphite/epoxy		Aluminum		Titanium	
Frequency	mm	in.	mm	in.	mm	in.	mm	in.	mm	in.	mm	in.
50 kHz	0.66	0.026	2.96	0.12	6	0.24	6	0.24	12.6	0.50	12.2	0.48
100 kHz	0.33	0.013	1.48	0.06	3	0.12	3	0.12	6.3	0.25	6.1	0.24
500 kHz	0.066	0.0026	0.296	0.012	0.6	0.024	0.6	0.024	1.26	0.050	1.22	0.048
1 MHz	0.033	0.0013	0.148	0.006	0.3	0.012	0.3	0.012	0.63	0.025	0.61	0.024
5 MHz	0.0066	0.00026	0.0296	0.0012	0.06	0.0024	0.06	0.0024	0.126	0.0050	0.122	0.0048
10 MHz	0.0033	0.00013	0.0148	0.0006	0.03	0.0012	0.03	0.0012	0.063	0.0025	0.061	0.0024

detection with PE amplitude is usually more sensitive than TT, due to the back-wall reflection having gone through the part twice. Also, the dynamic range (~35 dB) in PE mode is usually limited, due to sound continuing to reverberate in the good layers of the composite. For these reasons, porosity over 1 to 2% usually cannot be quantified in PE mode.

Pulse-echo ultrasound is very sensitive to angle of the transducer to the part under test. The rule of thumb is that the transducer should be within 2° of normal to the composite. Maintaining 0.5° alignment provides better data quality (less variation) and is highly recommended. In comparison, TT data can be evaluated with up to about 10° of part misalignment. Automated systems for PE scanning thus usually require more axes of motion and more complex motion software or require contact with the part surface, with the transducer mounted in a free-gimbaled bubbler (which limits inspection near the edges). Pulse-echo is mainly used in the industry when access is limited to one side or when film-type foreign material inclusions are possible. These foreign materials have acoustic impedance very close to the composite and thus do not cause much difference in TT attenuation (less than 0.5 dB). However, these materials will generate significant reflections (20 to 30% of front wall) in PE mode. For automated PE inspection of thick composite parts (>13 mm, or 0.5 in., thick), time-corrected gain (often called distance amplitude correction) is required to keep PE defect sensitivity constant throughout the composite thickness. The electronic gain applied to the raw ultrasonic signal is increased as a function of time to compensate for the natural attenuation of the composite. Thus, defects near the back wall of the composite are brought up to the same amplitude as a near-surface defect. Newer-generation systems allow the operator to tailor this curve to the specific composite and lay-up in use.

In the aerospace industry and other industries as well, automated ultrasonic inspection is the principle inspection method for testing and accepting fiber-reinforced composites. Automated scanners are employed that acquire TT, PE, or combined ultrasonic measurements over an entire structure at high speed.

Automated ultrasonic scanning systems take many forms and sizes. They range from small tabletop immersion tanks to large overhead gantry systems. Figure 3 shows a small, flat panel scanner where the parts under test are suspended on a cable bed. The cables are smaller in diameter than the defect class size required. This is a TT-only water-squirter system and uses two channels of TT data to decrease inspection time. For more complicated composite structures, ultrasonic systems have been developed to track part contour. Figure 4 is a large overhead gantry system, with nine axes of motion to follow part curvature in two directions. The part contour is programmed, taught, or brought in via computer-aided design surface data. The mechanism moves the system over the part surface, following and keeping the squirters normal to the part contour. The system indexes at the end of each scan pass. For laminate composites, data is typically acquired at 1 mm (0.04 in.) spacing in the scanning direction and 2 mm (0.08 in.) spacing in the index direction. The transducers are pulsed at each 1 mm (0.04 in.) interval, and the ultrasonic signals are received, converted to digital data, and stored in a computer file. Imaging soft-

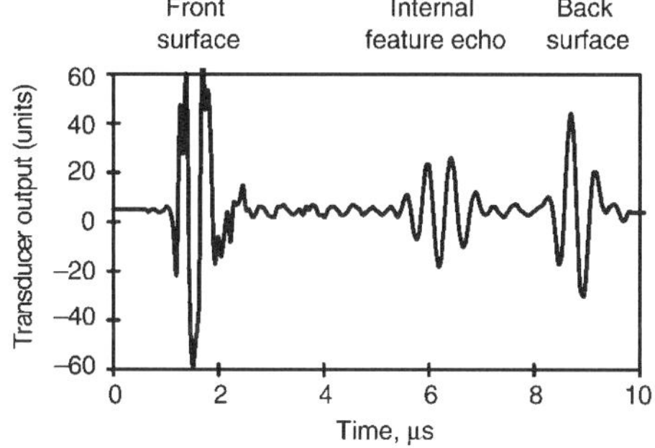

Fig. 2 Example ultrasonic waveform in a composite sample

Table 4 Advantages and limitations of automated system water-coupling methods

Method	Advantages	Limitations
Immersion systems	• Excellent signal quality, no moving water, very clean and stable • Good spatial resolution at a prescribed focal zone of the transducer • Large stand-off distances are possible • Can be used in TT and/or PE mode • Best resolution available using focused transducers	• Buoyancy and loading stresses on the part must be considered. • Part size, plus tooling and viewing the test under water, are issues. • Tank depth • Scanning speed
Water-squirter systems	• No immersion required (buoyancy not a problem) • Large stand-off distances (e.g., 200 mm, or 8 in.) are possible. • Resolution/power transfer of TT sound can be tailored for the application. • Fastest scanning • Can be used in TT and/or PE mode	• Manipulator systems can be complex to maintain surface alignment. • Water squirters must be properly designed and matched to the transducer application. • Scan quality can suffer due to water splash and air in squirter system. • Cannot effectively use focused transducers
Bubbler/dribbler systems	• Excellent signal quality • Low implementation cost	• Edge/cutout inspection limitations, due to the contacting nature of the bubbler scans, cannot cover the full part surface. • Speed limitations. Bubblers have been used at up to 50 cm/s (20 in./s) surface speed. Squirters are used up to 100 cm/s (40 in./s). • Cannot effectively use focused transducers • Can only be used in PE mode • Not effective for parts with complex shapes • Limited penetration capability

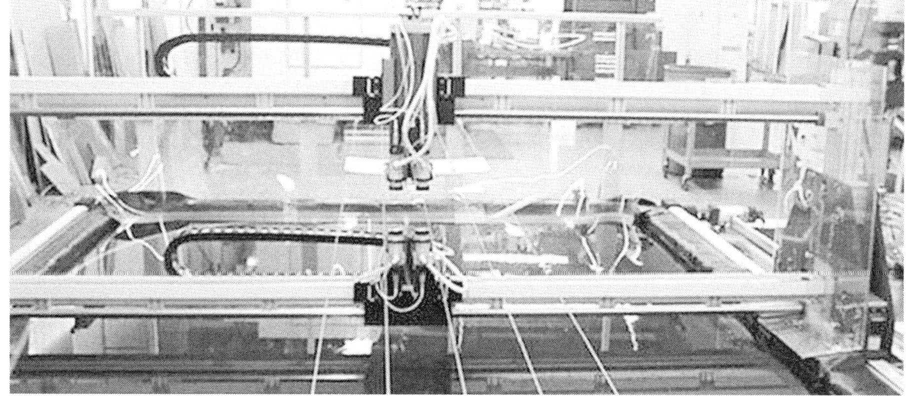

Fig. 3 Automated ultrasonic two-channel flat panel through-transmission system

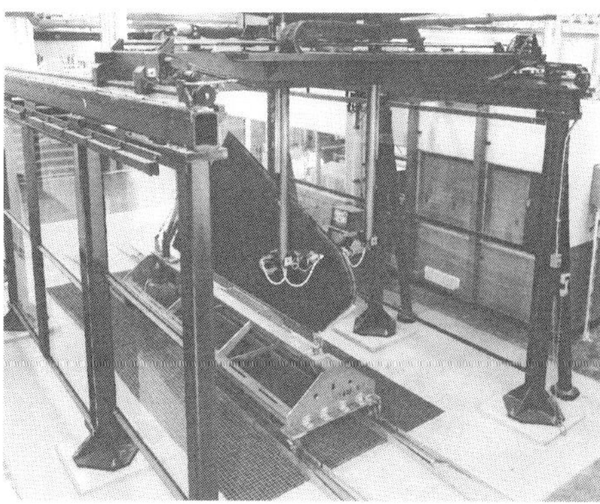

Fig. 4 Overhead gantry automated ultrasonic scanning system

ware is provided to view the data on a computer screen in shades of gray or color.

Most large gantry systems have maximum scan speeds of 76 cm/s (30 in./s) for flat parts. Part contour can slow motion down to the 38 cm/s (15 in./s) range. This provides for overall scan speeds in the 2.3 to 4.6 m^2/h (25 to 50 ft^2/h) range. On relatively flat parts, a second set of squirters (and the associated electronics) can be added to double this rate to 9.3 m^2/h (100 ft^2/h). These rates are calculated at 2 mm (0.08 in.) per index. When comparing methods, the data resolution must be considered for proper comparisons. Current-generation scanners and the associated acquisition electronics can scan at up to 100 cm/s (40 in./s) while maintaining 1 mm (0.04 in.) data spacing in the scan direction.

For round or nearly round composite parts, the most cost-effective ultrasonic scanning method is obtained by placing the part on a rotating turntable fixture under a gantry system. If the system is properly designed, the turntable should be able to rotate continuously to maintain 100 cm/s (40 in./s) movement of the squirters over the part. Turntables, combined with dual nozzles, can therefore provide 190 ft^2/h of scan speed at 1 by 2 mm (0.04 by 0.08 in.) data spacing. Figure 5 shows a turntable scanner system.

The latest generation of automated ultrasonic scanners has gone to independent machines on each side of the part to be tested. Advantages to these types of scanners are independent surface following from each side, much improved "reach-in" capability, overall stiffness, and reduced ceiling height. An example is shown in Fig. 6.

An important feature when choosing an ultrasonic scanning system is the ability of the system to provide 1 to 1 flaw sizing on complex curved structures. Figure 7 shows a TT image of the internal structure for the composite C-17 landing gear pod fairing shown in Fig. 6. The data have been acquired such that the two-dimensional image accurately represents the three-dimensional surface of the part, similar to map layouts. The lighter areas are laminate-only areas (less attenuation); the darker areas are fiber-honeycomb buildup areas. With the TT dynamic range of this system, both types of areas can be inspected with a 5 MHz transducer frequency. Honeycomb areas are typically scanned at 1 or 2.25 MHz. Multilayer (septumized) honeycomb or foam-filled structures are scanned at 250 kHz, 500 kHz, or 1 MHz. Because resolution suffers at lower frequencies, parts are generally scanned with the highest frequency that can provide penetration through the part. Laminate-only parts are generally scanned at 5 MHz for both TT and PE. In thin PE applications, 10 and 15 MHz are sometimes used.

The terms A-scan, B-scan, and C-scan are used throughout the nondestructive testing (NDT) industry to describe the types of data images being acquired. Figure 7 is considered a C-scan image, which is a plan view of the part. The colors or gray scales of a C-scan image can represent TT amplitude, PE depth, PE amplitude, and numerous other data types. An A-scan image is a single ultrasonic waveform display, as shown in Fig. 2, where the horizontal scale represents time, and the vertical scale represents amplitude. A B-scan image is a plot of distance along the surface of the part on the horizontal axis, with time plotted vertically and amplitude data represented in gray-scale shades or colors.

A- and B-scans are generally not acquired for production inspections of composite structures. The magnitude of data storage requirements for acquiring the full waveform data required for A- and B-scans has limited production applications—1 to 3 C-scan parameters per pixel (image files in the megabytes) versus 512 to 2048 waveform samples per pixel (image files in the gigabytes). Very critical composite and bonding applications, such as high-bypass fan blades and shuttle solid rocket motors, are where waveform acquisition is currently used in production. As computing and disk capacities increase, more systems will provide waveform capability at production inspection speeds. The advantage of waveform acquisition is verification and quantification of defects without separate inspection processes (such as hand A-scan).

Figure 8 shows A-, B-, and C-scan image examples. The C-scan image is the background image. This particular C-scan is PE amplitude data from the interface between a laminate and honeycomb substructure. The line over the defect in the upper right of the C-scan image shows the location of the B-scan image, which is shown in the left inset. The top sets of lines in the B-scan image are the front surface-part reflection. Below that are echoes from the internal composite structure. The defect shows up as a much stronger echo than the surrounding good area. The right inset is an A-scan trace over one point of the defect. The front and defect echoes are readily seen. Flaw detection is much easier using C-scan imaging, because the gray or color image provides a view of the defect and surrounding good areas for easy comparison.

Air-Coupled Ultrasonics

In many instances, it is beneficial to inspect some types of composite materials without contacting the surface with water or other coupling liquid used in the standard ultrasonic inspection system approach. One method to accomplish this is with air-coupled ultrasonic testing (UT). The technique can be used very effectively on composite materials, such as laminates, honeycombs, and foams. Air-coupled ultrasound inspection has been performed using frequencies from 50 kHz to 5 MHz (Ref 7–10). While the attenuation of ultrasound by air is an issue at high frequencies (at 1 MHz it is over 100 dB/m), it is the large acoustic impedance difference at the air-solid interfaces that has the greatest influence on the signal amplitude at the receiving transducer. As noted earlier, the transmission of ultrasound from graphite/epoxy composite to air is only 0.017%; whereas the transmission of ultrasound from graphite/epoxy composite to water is on the order of 93%. This nearly 4 orders of magnitude

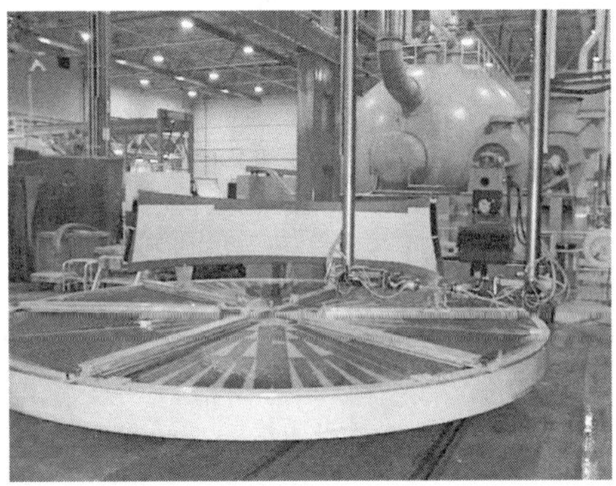

Fig. 5 Automated ultrasonic inspection system with a turntable

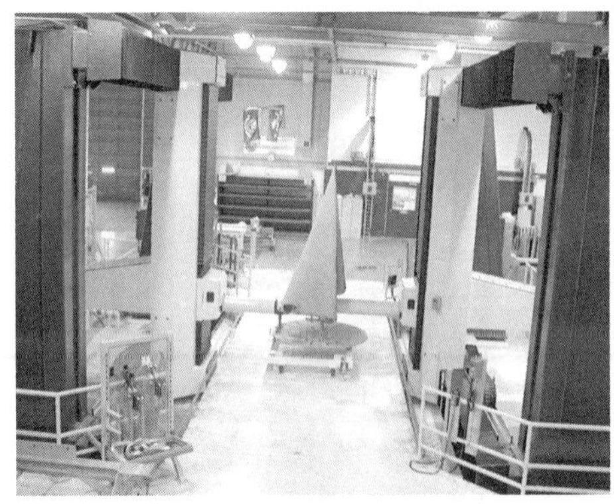

Fig. 6 Independent side automated ultrasonic scanning system

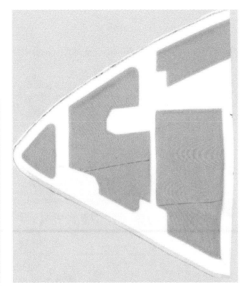

Fig. 7 C-17 pod fairing through-transmission ultrasonic data image

difference in transmission characteristics requires some significant differences in air-coupled UT systems from conventional equipment.

Materials with lower acoustic impedance (generally lower-density materials) are well suited for air-coupled UT inspection. Thick or multilayered sandwich panels with foam or honeycomb core construction are good examples. It is not unusual to find air-coupled UT effective through structures such as these that are 150 to 200 mm (6 to 8 in.) thick or more, using frequencies of a few hundred kilohertz. For solid laminate material and higher-frequency inspection, it is necessary for the ultrasonic transducers and electronics to have very high sensitivity.

Air-coupled UT can be performed with piezoelectric transducers or with microelectromechanical (MEM) transducers (Ref 10–13). The MEM transducers typically exhibit a significantly lower acoustic impedance than piezoelectric transducers and so provide a better acoustic match to air (Ref 12). However, MEM transducers are relatively new and have not yet been implemented in commercial instruments. The use of impedance matching layers for piezoelectric transducers has been demonstrated to transmit ultrasound through air with only 30 dB signal loss, compared to conventional contact transmission (Ref 9). The development of the efficient acoustic matching layers, high-intensity tone burst generators, and low-noise electronics allows the high interface losses in the air-coupled approach to be overcome with adequate sensitivity for air-coupled piezoelectric transducer application (Ref 14).

The use of high-power tone-burst operation and the reflection of most of the energy at the first interface back to the transducer suggest that air-coupled UT implementation should use the TT ultrasound or pitch-catch operational modes. Figure 9 shows the configurations commonly employed. The transducer is usually positioned close to the part (within an inch at frequencies above 400 Hz and within several inches for lower frequencies), with the beam focused in the part. Figure 9(a) shows the TT method. Figure 10 shows a comparison of a 400 kHz air-coupled inspection and a 5 MHz water-coupled TT inspection of a composite bonded assembly containing an internal void region. The air-coupled sensitivity to features in this application is very good. Figure 9(b) demonstrates a transducer setup using an angled beam. The angle beam can create shear waves in the part. The TT method, with the angle beam in particular, is an excellent technique on a number of materials inspections, such as honeycomb core structures where low frequency inspection (below 1 MHz) is necessary for penetration. However, for optimal signal levels, care should be taken on the selection of the angle to the surface. Because of the path of the shear waves in the part, an offset between the axes of the transducers is often necessary. The size of this offset will depend upon the type and structure of the composite and its thickness. Figure 9(c) shows one possible pitch-catch arrangement. A barrier is needed between the transducers to prevent direct communication of the transmitted acoustic wave through air. In fact, a common problem with air-coupled ultrasound is the need to protect against signals leaking around the edges of objects, limiting the quality of the inspection at those edges. Low-density foam can be taped along the edge to significantly reduce this edge effect. Figure 9(d) shows both a single-sided guided-wave technique and alternate two-sided configuration, with the second transducer on the opposite side. The single-sided pitch-catch technique is best for inspecting skins and skin-to-core bonds in sandwich panels, while the two-sided pitch-catch technique works best for thin laminates. To produce plate waves, the transducers are set at a low angle to the part and relatively far apart (150 mm, or 6 in., or more). Most air-coupled inspections can be performed using hand-held yoke systems or with the transducers mounted on robotic scanners.

Laser Ultrasound

Laser UT is a method for evaluating materials properties based on the analysis of ultrasound

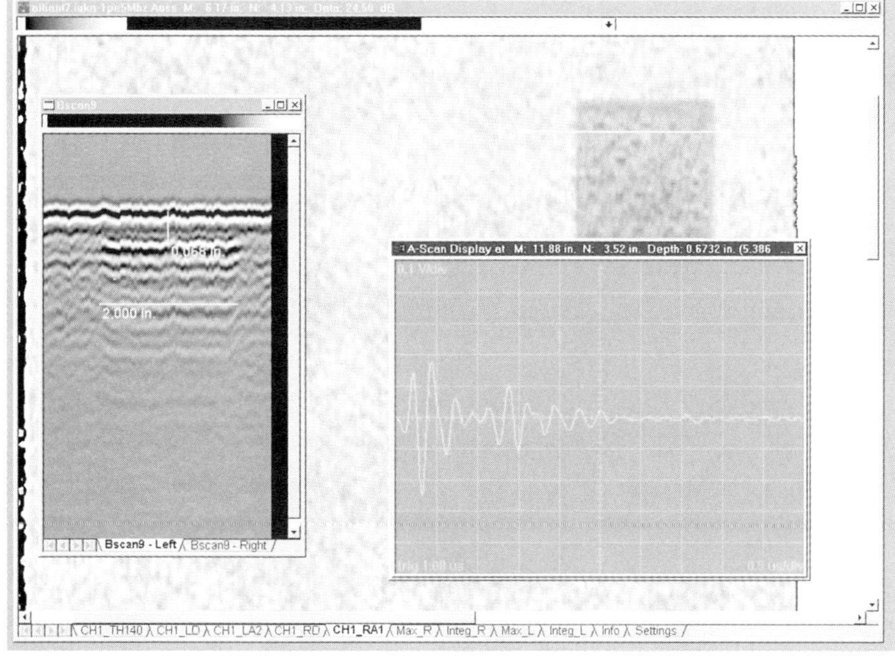

Fig. 8 A-, B-, and C-scan ultrasonic images

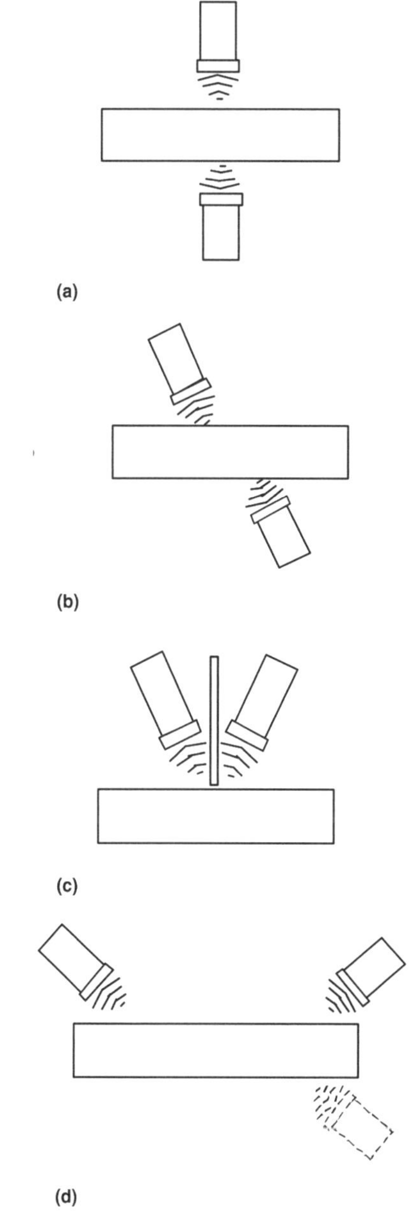

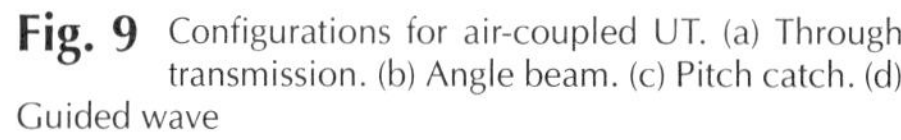

Fig. 9 Configurations for air-coupled UT. (a) Through transmission. (b) Angle beam. (c) Pitch catch. (d) Guided wave

that is generated and detected using lasers (Ref 15, 16). Although this field is very broad in terms of various implementation techniques and materials applications, this review is restricted to methods that are similar to conventional PE water-coupled UT systems and specifically applied to organic-matrix composite materials. Laser UT provides the same type of measurement information obtained with conventional ultrasonic systems, such as the presence of internal defects, bond integrity, part thickness, and other basic materials properties. The motivation for replacing conventional water-coupled piezoelectric transducers with laser-based systems varies with material types and the specific NDE requirements. In the aerospace industry, speed and flexibility are the primary benefits for testing composite materials with laser systems, while the noncontact remote-sensing feature is most important for process-control applications in the steel industry. For many composite materials and configurations, laser UT can be faster than other ultrasonic approaches and should be considered as an alternative to conventional water-coupled UT.

A brief introduction to the fundamentals is presented in this section, with a more detailed discussion to follow. Basically, laser ultrasonic systems use two lasers: one laser is used to generate ultrasound in the part by a mechanism called thermoelastic expansion, and a second laser is used to detect these vibrations as they return to the top surface (Ref 17–19). A diagram of a typical configuration is shown in Fig. 11. In the thermoelastic generation process, the absorbed laser energy is converted into heat in the top 10 to 100 μm (0.0004 to 0.004 in.) of the surface. The resulting temperature rise creates a local expansion of the material. If the heating laser pulse duration is short (10 to 100 ns), then the expansion will be in the frequency of ultrasound (1 to 10 MHz). The important feature is that the ultrasound will propagate perpendicular to the surface, independent of the laser angle of incidence. This allows generation of ultrasound in complex-shaped parts at angles as high as ±45° off-axis, compared to conventional water-coupled transducers that must remain within a few degrees of normal.

The detection laser is coaxial with the generation laser and illuminates the same point where the ultrasound is produced. Unlike the generation laser that is ideally absorbed by the composite, this laser is scattered off of the composite surface. The collected scattered light is analyzed by an interferometer to extract the ultrasonic signals that are "imprinted" on the laser as phase and frequency modulations caused by the moving surface. The ultrasonic signals extracted are basically the same as those obtained with conventional systems and can be analyzed using similar methods. Finally, the two laser beams are indexed over the composite surface with an optical scanner to produce standard C-scan images.

Laser Generation. The detailed mechanism of ultrasound generation by a laser pulse is relatively straightforward to illustrate (Ref 20). The key variables that determine performance are the laser pulse temporal duration, optical wavelength, energy, and the properties of the composite structure being tested. Figure 12 shows how absorbed laser light causes a temperature rise and therefore, a localized expansion of the composite material. If the pulse is temporally short, then the thermal expansion will generate ultrasonic waves, as shown in Fig. 13. The signal-to-noise ratio (SNR) of the resulting data improves linearly with the amplitude of the ultrasound; thus it is important to consider how to optimize generation methods.

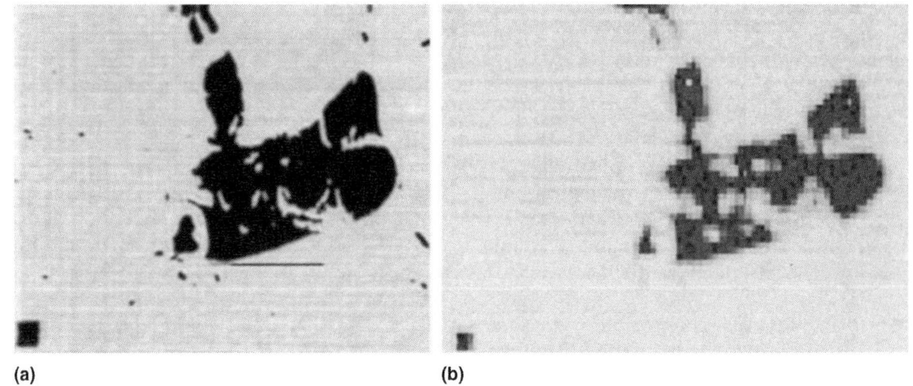

Fig. 10 Example scans of a graphite/epoxy paste-bonded laminate panel (approximately 200 × 175 mm, or 8 × 7 in.). (a) 400 kHz air-coupled. (b) 5 MHz water-coupled

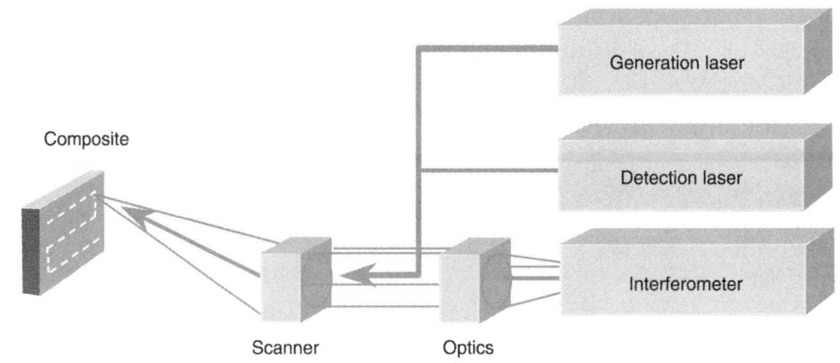

Fig. 11 A laser ultrasound system is composed of a generation laser, detection laser, interferometer, optical scanner, and computer controller.

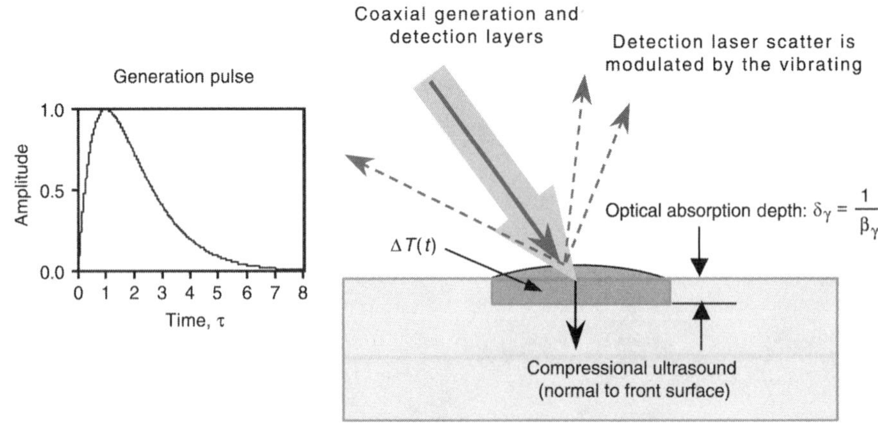

Fig. 12 Ultrasound generation by laser pulse. Ultrasound is generated in an organic composite by the absorption of energy from a pulsed laser, and the resulting surface vibrations can be monitored with a detection laser and sensitive interferometer. The resulting signals are equivalent to conventional pulse-echo ultrasonic signals. τ, rise time; β_λ, wave-length-dependent optical absorption coefficient.

Ultrasound is generated in the small volume of material where the laser energy is absorbed. The objective is to generate as much ultrasound as possible without exceeding temperatures that could damage or alter the appearance of the material. In a composite, there are potentially two different absorption mechanisms, corresponding to laser absorption within the polymer volume and absorption by the fibers. For a simple model that leads to most of the important considerations, consider two layers consisting of a resin layer over a fiber-resin layer. Laser light will penetrate into the resin and be absorbed at some rate, thereby creating a local temperature rise. If the resin is thin or particularly transparent to the laser wavelength, then any residual energy will be absorbed at the opaque resin-fiber interface. In the case where the light is primarily absorbed below the resin layer at the fiber interface this produces what is termed as a buried source. As a simplification of this general mechanism, buried sources will not be considered, but it is assumed that the light is exponentially absorbed in the resin layer only. Thermal conductivity can carry heat away, but is not significant over ultrasonic time scales less than 100 μs and may be ignored. Given these assumptions, the temperature profile can be modeled as:

$$T(x,t) = \frac{\beta_\lambda I_0}{\rho C_p} e^{-\beta x} \int_0^t f(t',\tau)dt' \quad \text{(Eq 7)}$$

where β_λ is the wavelength dependent optical absorption coefficient (m^{-1}), I_0 is the absorbed energy density of the laser (J/m^2), ρ is the material density, C_p is the specific heat, and $f(t'\tau)$ is the normalized laser pulse temporal profile with a characteristic rise time of τ. Some time after the laser pulse has deposited all of its energy, the peak surface temperature is reached. As a numerical example, the temperature rise would be about 80 °C (145 °F) for a typical epoxy resin with an absorption depth of 50 μm (0.002 in.) subjected to a 100 mJ laser pulse deposited over a 5 mm (0.2 in.) spot. For a volume absorber, the peak temperature, and therefore the maximum allowed energy density, is primarily influenced by β_λ and is independent of the temporal properties of the laser. The maximum allowed laser irradiation scales with energy density and not with peak laser power, which is an important point, because very short-pulsed lasers can be used without the risk of inducing surface damage for volume absorbers.

In addition to calculating the temperature rise of the surface modeled by Eq 7, a model is needed to predict how much ultrasound is actually generated in the material. The front surface displacement, u, is simply estimated as the product of the peak temperature rise, the coefficient of thermal expansion, α, and the optical penetration depth:

$$u_{\max} = \alpha I_0 / \rho C_p \quad \text{(Eq 8)}$$

As a numerical example, assume that 15% of a 100 mJ CO_2 pulse is in the first 100 ns, a 5 mm spot size, $\alpha = 5.5 \times 10^{-5}$/K, $\rho = 1250$ kg/m^3, and $C_p = 1050$ J/kg · K; this produces a front surface displacement of about 32 nm. Equation 8 does not contain the optical absorption coefficient, which might lead one to interpret this as meaning that β_λ does not influence the amount of ultrasound produced, except by limiting how much energy can be absorbed without excessive heating. Also, the role of the temporal profile of the generation laser does not alter the maximum temperature or displacement—so how important is the shape of the laser pulse? To address these issues, the complete wave equation must be modeled along with the laser-induced temperature rise; this shows that the amplitude of ultrasound that propagates through the material is dependent on β_λ, the velocity of sound, v, and the characteristic rise time, τ, of the laser pulse. For the case of an absorbing layer of sufficient thickness, a general rule can be expressed so that, if satisfied, the strength of ultrasound produced will be a maximum for a particular material and laser combination:

$$\beta_\lambda \cdot v \cdot \tau \leq 1 \quad \text{(Eq 9)}$$

Large acoustic amplitudes require a short-pulse laser tuned for the absorption in the resin layer. The frequency content of the ultrasonic pulse will obviously not exceed that of the generation pulse, so a sufficiently fast pulse must be used to generate the frequencies of interest. A general rule would be to use a pulse such that $\tau \leq (4f_{\max})^{-1}$. The ideal source laser would include the freedom to dynamically adjust the temporal and optical character of the pulse based on part material needs, which may be determined by thickness, defect nature, and the optical/mechanical properties of the part surface. A composite designer or manufacturer can improve laser UT results by assuring that the surface peel ply or resin depth is on the order of 100 μm or more. Figure 14 compares the relative amplitude of ul-

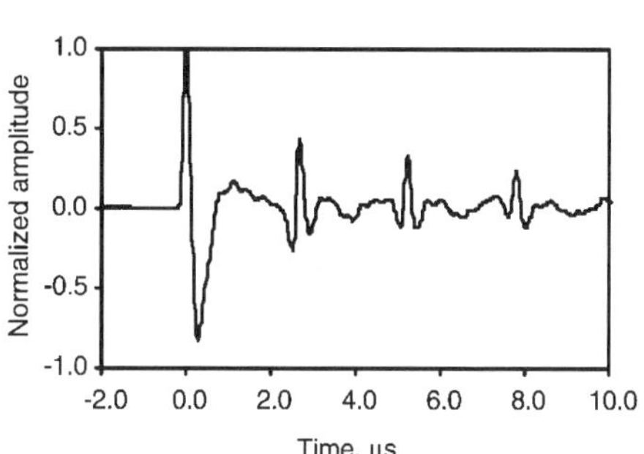

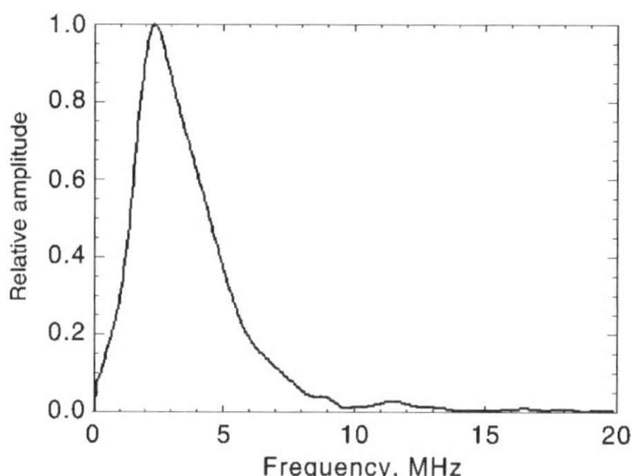

Fig. 13 Laser ultrasonic signal from a 3 mm (0.12 in.) thick graphite/epoxy composite showing the front surface signal and a series of back surface echos. The frequency spectrum of a typical back surface signal shows a center frequency near 2.5 MHz, with most of the energy well below 10 MHz.

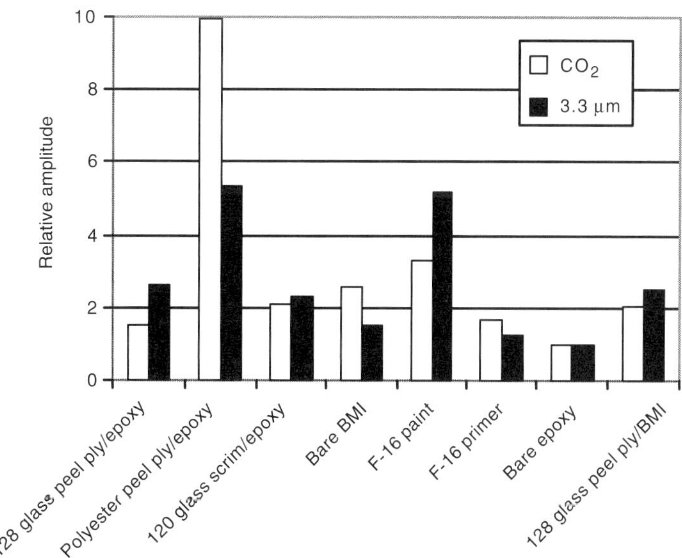

Fig. 14 Relative amplitude of ultrasound generated in a graphite/epoxy composite for various surface conditions. The data is normalized to the bare epoxy signal for both laser wavelengths (i.e., the CO_2 and 3.3 μm data cannot be directly compared). This shows there is considerable variance in signal strength for different surface conditions. BMI, bismaleimide

trasound generated for different surface conditions. As can be seen, different peel ply layers and paints can significantly alter the amplitude of the signals.

The short-pulse transversely excited atmosphere (TEA) carbon dioxide laser has made possible the inspection of many composite components (Ref 17, 18), because large longitudinal ultrasound pulses can be created without damage. However, carbon dioxide lasers do pose several problems, including the handling of gases consumed by the laser, the large size and cost of higher repetition rate units, and the problem that 10.6 μm radiation from the TEA carbon dioxide laser cannot be easily handled by fiber optics due to unacceptable attenuation. In addition, although the TEA carbon dioxide laser has been a popular choice, the optical wavelength and temporal pulse shape are not necessarily optimal (Ref 21). The temporal pulse width from an improved TEA carbon dioxide laser yields a useful energy for ultrasound generation in the first 100 ns that varies between 6 and 15% of the total energy.

Recent research has identified the use of mid-infrared lasers in the 3 to 4 μm (120 to 160 μin.) band, where the penetration depth corresponds to a volume absorption (Ref 22). A 3 μm (120 μin.) absorption arises from the OH molecular vibrational mode, which, while present in all composites, can vary widely by manufacturing and ambient atmospheric conditions. Instead, the 3.5 μm (140 μin.) CH vibrational mode is universal to polymer composites and does not suffer the same variations as the OH mode. Also, new fiber optic materials have been demonstrated with excellent propagation properties in the 3 to 4 μm (120 to 160 μin.) band, enabling the use of fiber delivery for remote access applications.

There are many lasers available that will provide surface absorption on the fibers, including the 1.06 μm (41.7 μin.) neodymium:yttrium-aluminum-garnet (Nd:YAG) laser and its doubled 0.532 μm (20.9 μin.) harmonic. While effective generators of ultrasound, these lasers have lower-energy damage thresholds for composites and are considered risky.

Laser Detection. An ultrasonic wave originating within the part that reaches the surface causes a small displacement—typically on the order of Angstroms (10^{-10} m) at frequencies of several MHz. Amazingly, these small displacements are detected routinely with piezoelectric transducers and can be detected with optical interferometers. In order to measure such small displacements, the quality of the detection laser and the interferometer are both critically important. The general detection scheme is to direct a bright laser at the part, collect the scattered light, and use a interferometer to analyze laser photons to measure the small phase or frequency shifts caused by the vibrating surface. One of the first considerations is how bright the detection laser needs to be to detect the laser-generated ultrasound. To estimate this, one must consider the fundamental limits of laser detection of a vibrating surface. First, the photons obey Poisson statistics—the number, N, arriving in an interval has an uncertainty or shot noise of roughly $N^{1/2}$—while the signal is proportional to N, yielding a fundamental SNR proportional to $N^{1/2}$. In addition to shot noise, amplitude and phase noise are present on the detection laser, with a linear dependence on N. These last two sources of noise can be reduced by appropriate selection of an interferometer or careful specification of the detection laser. In practice, the part surface is not mirror smooth, and the interferometer must deal with optical speckle—the random variations in phase of the arriving light across the detection aperture, due to small variations in the optical path length. A general expression for the SNR of shot noise limited detection of ultrasound is given as:

$$\mathrm{SNR} = 4\pi u(f)S(f)\sqrt{\frac{P_{\mathrm{det}}QE}{2\lambda hcBW}} \quad \text{(Eq 10)}$$

where $u(f)$ is the frequency-dependent surface displacement, λ is the detection laser wavelength, $S(f)$ is the response function of the interferometer (a Michelson interferometer has a $S(f)$ of 1.0), P_{det} is the laser power collected from the composite and delivered to the detector, QE is the detector quantum efficiency, h is Plank's constant, c is the speed of light, and BW is the detection bandwidth. Equation 10 shows the linear relationship of SNR with surface displacement, which was previously shown to be linear with the absorbed energy density of the generation laser. Assuming that an optimal generation laser is used, then only the response sensitivity of the interferometer, the detection laser wavelength, and the amount of detection laser power collected remain as important design variables. Note that the QE only varies over a small range for properly chosen detectors (40 to 90%), and the BW must be on the order of 10 MHz. Equation 10 can be inverted to solve for the minimum detectable displacement, which will give a good estimate of the sensitivity and dynamic range limit. As a conservative approximation, the root mean square (RMS) signal-to-noise ratio can be changed to a peak-to-peak value, where the noise is about 6.6 times the RMS value. Most UT systems operate on peak thresholds, so this is a valid approximation. Using a Nd:YAG 1.064 μm laser, 5 mW of detected power at a 50% QE, a 10 MHz BW, and a 50% interferometer sensitivity gives $u_{\min} \approx 40$ pm. If the induced ultrasound is on the order of 40 nm, then the amplitude dynamic range is 60 dB. This number is below many conventional UT systems, but is adequate for most aerospace composite testing requirements.

Next consider the amount of light collected from a diffuse target with a detection laser of power P_0, using a lens aperture of Φ_{lens} located a distance D_{target} away:

$$P_{\mathrm{det}} = \frac{P_0}{4}\left(\frac{\Phi_{\mathrm{lens}}}{D_{\mathrm{target}}}\right)^2 \eta_{\mathrm{loss}}(1-A)\cos\theta \quad \text{(Eq 11)}$$

where η_{loss} accounts for general system losses, A is the diffuse target absorption, and θ is the incident angle. Although this ideal diffuse model is an approximation to what is typically a much more complex reality, it does show that one would desire a powerful detection laser, a large collection aperture, and to operate close to the composite surface. For most detection systems, optical powers delivered to the interferometer in excess of a few mW are limited by laser noise, and additional power will not improve SNR. The required detection laser intensity can be estimated based on the particular application configuration. For example, collecting 5 mW of laser power using a 50 mm (2 in.) aperture positioned 2 m (6.6. ft) from an absorbing (90%) diffuse target tilted at 45° would require a peak power of over 900 W at the target, for a typical collection loss of 50%. Continuous-wave lasers of this power are impractical and would damage the surface, due to excessive heating. Therefore, long-pulsed (≈100 μs) detection lasers are used to produce high peak-power intensities during the short time interval of the ultrasonic event, while the average power remains at a safe level. The duty cycle for a 100 μs pulse at 400 Hz would make a 1 kW peak laser only 40 W in average power. Although the small aperture and large working distance of this example severely reduces the collected light level, these parameters establish an optical system with a large depth of field, allowing the system to scan complex parts without active focus control. Real composite surfaces do not behave as diffuse targets, but instead are mixtures of diffuse and specular (mirrorlike) properties. Specular surfaces can be several times brighter than a perfect diffuse reflector on-axis and then quickly drop off by a factor of 100 in intensity in just a few degrees off-axis. This extreme dynamic range requires both a large peak power detection laser and an active intensity control system to reduce brightness when operating on-axis with specular surfaces.

Multiple types of interferometers are possible, but two designs are of practical interest for remote scanning of rough parts. The confocal Fabry-Perot is the most important type of interferometer today, with excellent sensitivity, where $S(f) \geq 0.5$ from 1 to 10 MHz, and it has the ability to handle rough surfaces (Ref 23). The Fabry-Perot is a homodyne interferometer, consisting of two mirrors that form a resonant cavity that analyzes the phase and frequency of the returned light. A typical implementation is two spherical mirrors with a reflectivity of 95% spaced 1 m (3.3 ft) apart. This interferometer can be configured to reject common-mode amplitude noise produced by a less-than-perfect detection laser. The output of the interferometer is composed of light that has reflected back and forth 10 to 100 times within the cavity—achieving full sensitivity requires a single longitudinal mode detection laser with a sufficiently long coherence length. Either the Fabry-Perot cavity length or the laser must be adjusted dynamically to track the Fabry-Perot resonant pass band with the laser line frequency.

A new interferometer employing a photorefractive demodulator is emerging and may be important in the future (Ref 24). The photorefractive interferometer employs a nonlinear crystal to "correct" the speckled wavefront. The best designs today are within a factor of 4 of an ideal Michelson interferometer. The major benefits are the compact size (fitting within a 13 to 46 cm, or 5 to 18 in., rack mount package), robustness to vibrations, and potential tolerance of lower-quality lasers. The disadvantages are a loss of two times in sensitivity against the Fabry-Perot, and a requirement that the lateral velocity of the laser spot over the inspected part not exceed a value determined by the properties of the nonlinear crystal. The photorefractive interferometer performance will improve with additional developments, which may make it a preferred solution in the future. Additional interferometer types, such as the Michelson and Sagnac, exist but are limited to niche applications, such as laboratory measurements of materials properties, optical near-contact probes, and embedded as fiber optic sensors within structures.

LaserUT System. Any technology that is perceived as "new" must balance expectations with realistic performance. Although research and development have steadily progressed in this field since the invention of the laser in the early 1960s, there have been few practical implementations of this technology. One example of laser ultrasonics meeting expectations is the LaserUT system (Lockheed Martin), shown testing a complex composite duct in Fig. 15 (Ref 25). This system has been in full-time production use for testing composite inlet structures for the F-22 fighter since June 2000.

Lockheed Martin has developed two LaserUT systems, referred to as Alpha and Beta, for testing advanced aerospace composite structures. Both systems are similar in design, except that the work envelope of the Alpha gantry robot is much larger than that of the Beta robot. A short-pulsed TEA carbon dioxide laser generates ultrasound, and a long-pulsed, diode-pumped Nd:YAG laser with a dual differential confocal Fabry-Perot interferometer is used for detection. These lasers are optically combined to produce a coaxial beam that is about 5 mm (0.2 in.) in diameter at the composite surface. Inspection depth of field is fairly large and allows the part standoff distance to vary between 1.5 and 2.5 m (4.9 to 8.2 ft) from the optical scanner. Beam indexing (optical scanning) is done with a two-mirror galvanometer scanner that has a 50 mm (2 in.) clear aperture. A five-axis gantry robot moves the inspection head to the best position for scanning each region of a part. Scan coverage can be as large as 2 × 2 m (6.6 × 6.6 ft) for a single inspection view. Parts with significant contour are typically sectioned into a series of smaller scans, such that each subsection remains within the constraints of the system. Scanning constraints can be material-dependent, based on generation efficiency and optical scattering properties, but typical values are ±45° angle of incidence and a nominal working distance of 1.8 m (5.9 ft) from the surface.

All ultrasonic waveforms are digitally captured, processed, and permanently stored as the inspection point is indexed over the composite surface. Figure 16 shows the graphical display from the system for a composite part with a series of inclusion defects. The current LaserUT system operates at a maximum inspection rate of 400 points per second and is limited by the pulse rates of the lasers. As faster lasers become available, the scan rate will improve accordingly. Inspection coverage rate is obviously related to the index step size required for the material under test, which is usually influenced by the size of defect that must be found. A conservative rule is to index at a resolution three times higher than the reject flaw size dimension. For example, an index size of 2.0 mm (0.080 in.) is typically used for a 6.3 mm (0.25 in.) flaw reject criteria. A 400 Hz scan rate at 2.0 mm (0.080 in.) steps gives a maximum area coverage of 6 m^2/h (64 ft^2/h). This system typically inspects complex composite parts ten times faster than the previous conventional water-coupled PE or TT methods, because part teaching and setup procedures are much less critical, and the inspection results are more consistent from part to part.

If the need is to test large, flat composite panels, then conventional systems will operate as fast or faster and provide equivalent results. Conversely, if a component with even, gentle contour requires ultrasonic testing, then a laser system may be the most cost-effective method. Recall that the composite part must have at least a small layer of an organic material at the surface for efficient laser generation of ultrasound. If the surface is machined or totally resin-starved, then a laser system may have only limited success, unless some form of a surface treatment is applied. LaserUT will work better with some materials than others, based on the material type and the design of the system, and in all cases the candidate material should be evaluated to establish compatibility, both in terms of desired SNR performance and to verify that the surface is not damaged or visibly altered by the laser interactions.

Ultrasonic Spectroscopy

The primary use of ultrasonic spectroscopy is to evaluate the effect of changing wavelength on material interaction. Wavelengths that are large (low frequency) relative to a defect tend to be unaffected by it. However, wavelengths that are

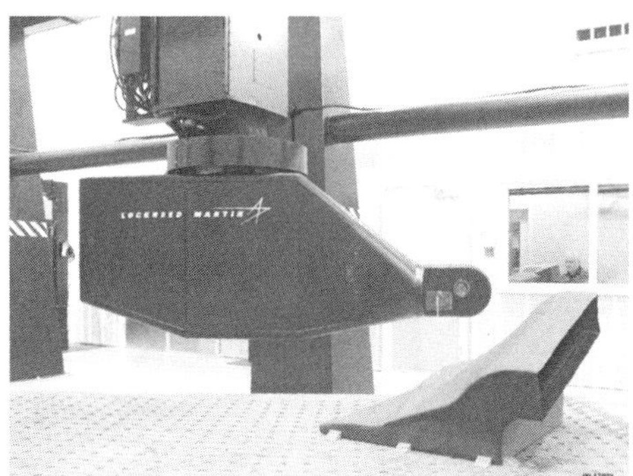

Fig. 15 Lockheed Martin Laser UT system testing a complex composite duct. This system routinely inspects parts ten times faster than conventional water-coupled UT systems and does not require expensive tooling to hold the part under test. The inspection head would be positioned above the part, approximately 2m (6 ft) away during a scan.

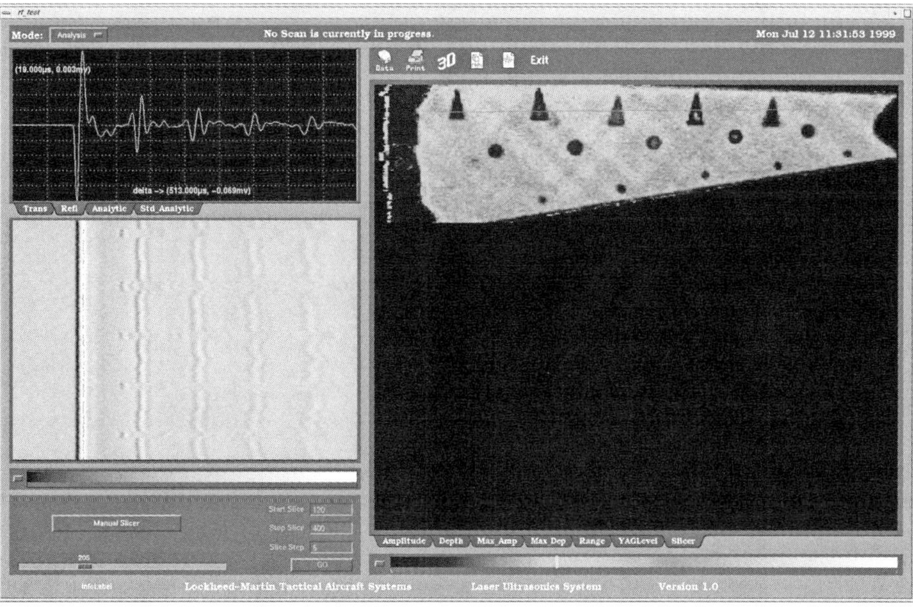

Fig. 16 LaserUT A-scan, B-scan, and C-scan images of a graphite/epoxy composite test part with inclusion materials. Each of the inclusions is clearly visible in the B-scan image.

comparatively small (high frequency) tend to interact. The degree of attenuation or scatter is a function of the wavelength-to-defect size. In the simplest case of internal porosity of uniform size, the porosity will act as a filter that will pass wavelengths below a certain frequency, partially attenuate wavelengths over a frequency range, and completely block all wavelengths over a given frequency.

Traditional ultrasonic spectroscopy methods have used broadband ultrasonics to permit taking data over a range of frequencies in a single test (Ref 26). This allows determination of the interaction of various frequencies with the tested materials. Typical broadband ultrasonic methods use a short, narrow pulse as the input signal. This provides a limited range of frequencies to be transmitted through the materials being tested. The short length of the pulse limits the total energy. The low energy results in an output signal with low SNR. More-recent work has resulted in a method of ultrasonic spectroscopy that uses a swept-frequency input signal (Ref 27). The signal can cover a wide, user-definable range of frequencies without compromising energy. The higher energy results in an output signal with a robust SNR in the frequency domain. This method provides a SNR over ten times greater than the traditional pulse method. Also, the spectrum can be designed to provide a uniform input over the range of frequencies. With multiple layers of varying material, how the ultrasonic waves respond (transmit or reflect) at the interfaces will depend on the relative acoustic impedances of the materials. This can provide the ability to inspect multiple layers and evaluate the nature of the interface.

Another aspect of ultrasonic spectroscopy is the phenomenon of resonance. Resonance is the result of constructive and destructive interference of standing waves in an ultrasonic medium that can be locally modeled as a plate. Positive interference happens when an integral number of half-wavelengths occur in the medium, which will happen periodically throughout a typical spectrum. Destructive interference occurs at odd quarter-wavelengths. Where this interference occurs in the frequency spectrum is a function of the thickness and velocity of the inspected part. For a given velocity, the spacing between resonance peaks (harmonics) is inversely proportional to thickness. If material velocity is known, material thickness can be determined from resonance spacing, and vice versa.

Starting with the fundamental equation for relating velocity (v) to frequency (f) and wavelength (λ):

$$v = f\lambda \qquad \text{(Eq 12)}$$

Knowing that the fundamental resonance occurs when there is half of a wavelength in a plate, then twice the plate thickness can be substituted for wavelength in the equation. Further, because higher-order resonance peaks (harmonics) are spaced at integer multiples of the fundamental frequency, then the spacing of any two successive peaks can be substituted for frequency. Thus:

$$v = f2d \qquad \text{(Eq 13)}$$

where v is the longitudinal velocity of the plate, f is the fundamental frequency or the spacing of any two successive resonance peaks, and d is the plate thickness. The significance of this relationship is that a very precise thickness measurement can be made using ultrasonic spectroscopy simultaneously with the spectral evaluation.

The magnitude (peak height-to-width ratio) of the resonance in a spectrum is a function of acoustic impedance mismatch on each layer of the part being inspected. The greater the mismatch, the more energy reflects back into the part and the more pronounced the resonance peaks (higher impedance mismatch means sharper peaks). When multiple plates are stacked and inspected using ultrasonic spectroscopy, each plate in the stack will resonate according to its thickness and velocity. The intensity of the resonance for each plate will be determined by the impedance mismatch at the boundaries and by the effects of internal damping of that plate.

Ultrasonic spectroscopy can use the resonance behavior of each material in the frequency domain. It has proven to be a very effective inspection technique for debonds and kissing debonds in multiple-layer composites. Also, the resonance behavior provides an easier and more-accurate interpretation capability for thickness or velocity measurements in single or multiple-layer structures. This is shown in the case of a 19 mm (0.75 in.) composite liner bonded to a graphite/epoxy 3.8 mm (0.15 in.) outer layer, as illustrated in Fig. 17 and 18. One of the samples is well bonded, and the second has a kissing debond. In the well-bonded sample, the resonant behavior in the spectrum is dominated entirely by the silica phenolic inner layer (80 kHz spacing). The full spectrum penetrates the bond, resonates the inner layer, and penetrates the bond again. In the debonded sample, the spectra graph shows the resonant behavior of the outer layer only. The full spectrum of energy is not penetrating the bond to resonate the inner layer (Fig. 18).

Ultrasonic spectroscopy has the capability to define attenuation as a function of frequency, allowing the user to establish signatures for various materials. The signal of each new sample can be compared to these signatures and evaluated for atypical responses caused by microstructure changes, porosity, microcracking, cracks, delaminations, fiber volume fraction, velocity (elastic modulus), and so on. Figures 19 and 20 show composite samples containing different levels of microcracking. The frequency cutoff varies with severity of microcracking, and surface roughness value increases. The micrograph is shown with the corresponding signal.

Lamb Waves

Lamb waves, also known as plate waves, are wave modes that propagate through layered me-

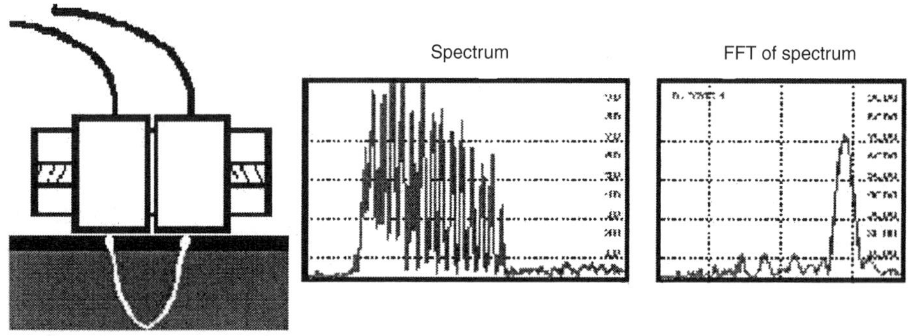

Fig. 17 Ultrasonic spectroscopy response of well-bonded multilayer composite. FFT, fast Fourier transform

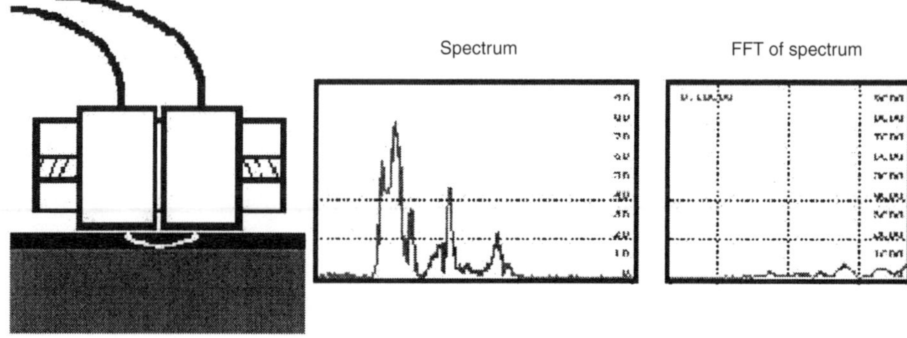

Fig. 18 Ultrasonic spectroscopy response of debonded composite. FFT, fast Fourier transform

Spectrum

1.885MHz cutoff

Nm

90 80 70 60 50 40 30 20 10 0

0.000 0.500 1.000 1.500 2.000 2.500

Frequency, MHz

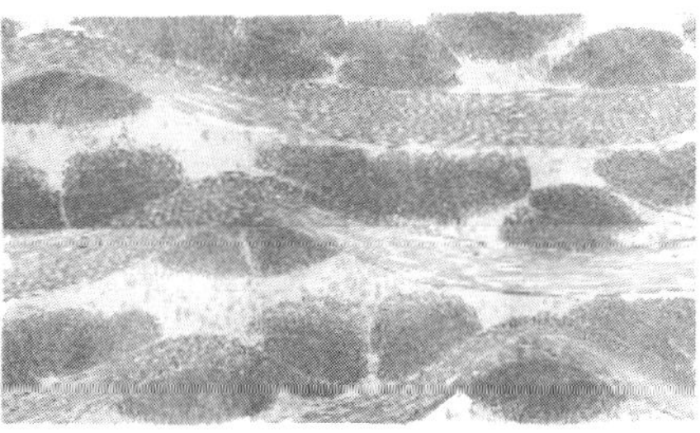

Fig. 19 Transmission of higher frequencies in a composite with no microcracking

dia with thickness that is only a few wavelengths. Lamb waves consist of a complex vibration that occurs throughout the thickness of the material. The propagation characteristics of Lamb waves depend on the density, elastic properties and structure of the material, as well as the thickness of the testpiece and the frequency. Their behavior in general resembles that observed in the transmission of electromagnetic waves through waveguides. There are two basic forms of Lamb waves: symmetric and antisymmetric. The form is determined by whether the particle motion is symmetric or antisymmetric with respect to the neutral axis of the testpiece. Theoretically, there are an infinite number of specific velocities at which Lamb waves can travel in a given material. Within a given plate, the specific velocities for Lamb waves are a complex function of the plate thickness and frequency. In symmetric (dilatational) Lamb waves, there is a compressional (longitudinal) particle displacement along the neutral axis of the plate and an elliptical particle displacement on each surface (see Fig. 21a). In asymmetric (bending) Lamb waves, there is a shear neutral axis of the plate and an elliptical particle displacement on each surface (Fig. 21b). The ratio of the major to minor axes of the ellipse is a function of the material in which the wave is being propagated.

Lamb waves can be induced by contact transducers and received after traveling through the material over a known distance. In such a case, only the first one or two symmetric and antisymmetric modes may be induced. The signal can provide useful information about the integrity of the material over the traveled distance and may prove superior to simple PE or TT because it allows faster scanning of the test part. Using a pair of transducers that transmit and receive normal to the test article surface allows inducing various Lamb wave modes and can provide qualitative information. This method is widely known as the acousto-ultrasonics (see the section "Acousto-Ultrasonics" in this article). Alternatively, one can use immersion coupling and induce Lamb waves to obtain quantitative data about the part; the related NDE technique is known as the leaky Lamb wave (LLW) method.

The LLW phenomenon is induced when a pitch-catch ultrasonic setup insonifies a platelike solid immersed in fluid (Ref 28). The phenomenon is associated with the resonant excitation of plate waves that leak energy into the coupling fluid and interfere with the specular reflection of the incident waves. The destructive interference between the leaky waves and the specularly reflected waves modifies the reflected spectrum, introducing a series of minima in the spectra of the reflected waves. The LLW experiment for composite laminate specimens involves measurement of the reflected field and extraction of the minima in the reflected spectra at various angles of incidence and orientations (polar angles) with respect to the laminate. The data is presented in the form of dispersion curves showing the phase velocity (calculated from Snell's law and the angle of incidence) of the LLWs as a function of frequency. The sensitivity of the dispersion curves to variations in the properties of the composite material, namely its anisotropy, layers thickness, stiffness constants, and the presence of defects, has made this phenomenon an attractive NDE method.

Bar-Cohen and Chimenti (Ref 29) investigated the characteristics of the LLW phenomenon and its application to NDE, focusing on the experimental documentation of observed modes and the effects of various types of defects on the measurements. Their study was followed by numerous theoretical and experimental investigations of the phenomenon (e.g., Ref 30–36). A method was also developed to invert the elastic properties of composite laminates from the LLW dispersion data (Ref 32, 37, 38), and the study was expanded to the NDE of bonded joints (Ref 39).

The experimental acquisition of dispersion curves for composite materials requires accurate control of the angle of incidence/reception and the polar angle with the fibers. The data acquisition involves the use of sequentially transmitted tone bursts, each of a specific frequency, spanning a selected frequency range. The reflected signals are acquired as a function of the polar and incidence angles and saved in a file for

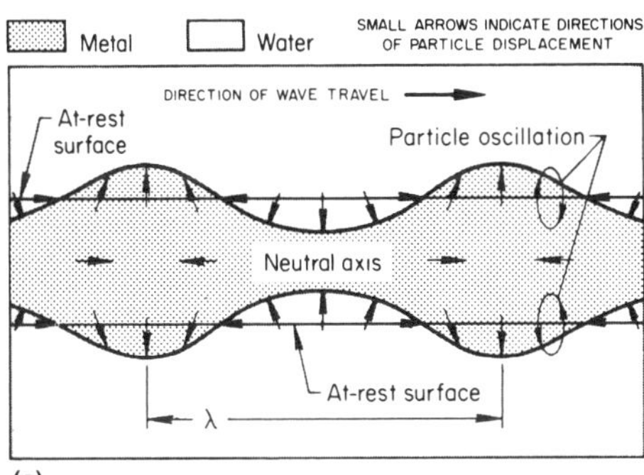

(a)

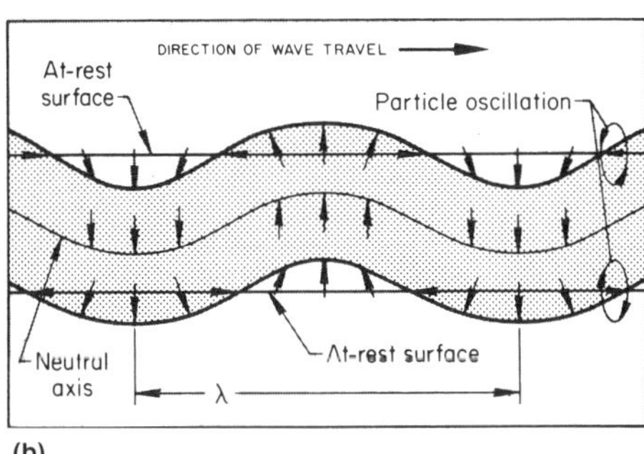

(b)

Fig. 21 Schematic diagram showing the two Lamb wave basic modes. (a) Symmetric. (b) Asymmetric

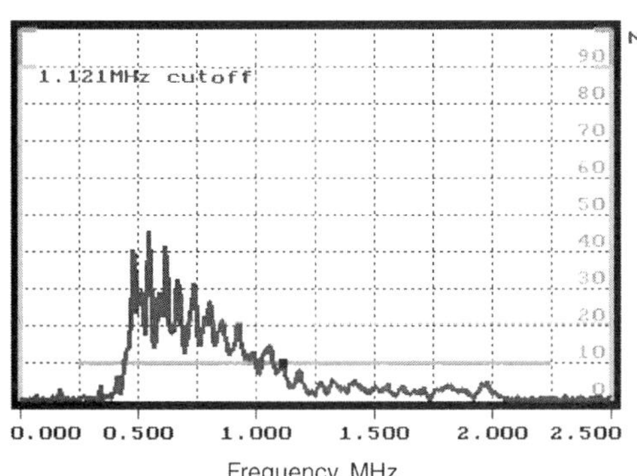

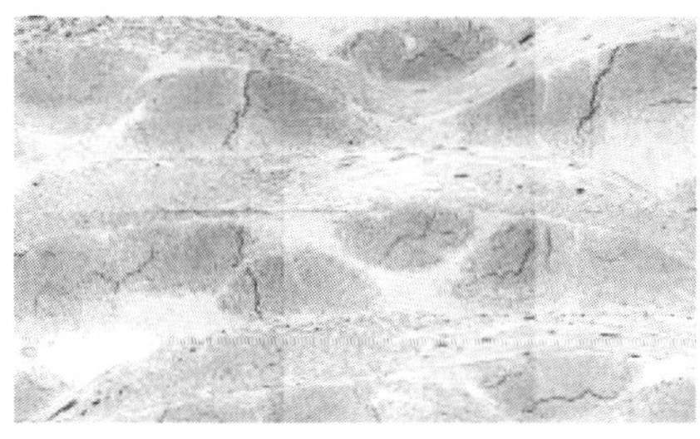

Fig. 20 Effect of pervasive microcracking on frequency response

analysis and comparison with theoretical predictions. The minima in the acquired reflection spectra represent the LLW modes and are used to determine the dispersion curves (phase velocity as a function of frequency). The incident angle is changed incrementally within the selected range, and the reflection spectra are acquired. For graphite/epoxy laminates, the modes are identified for each angle of incidence in the range of 12 to 50°, allowing the use of free-plate theoretical calculations. At each given incidence angle, the minima are identified, added to the accumulating dispersion curves, and plotted simultaneously on the computer display.

The capability to invert the elastic properties using LLW data is limited to the matrix-dominated stiffness constants (Ref 39). This limitation can be partially overcome if the incidence angles of 10° or smaller can be used in the experiments, but this is difficult, if not impossible, to achieve in practice with a single scanner. An alternative methodology based on pulsed ultrasonics was developed by Bar-Cohen, Mal, and Lih (Ref 28). Using pulses in pitch-catch and PE experimental setups, it was shown that all five elastic constants of a unidirectional laminate could be determined with a fairly high degree of accuracy.

The behavior of ultrasonic waves propagating through fiber-reinforced composites is determined by the material stiffness and dissipative characteristics. Theoretical modeling of this behavior requires several simplifying assumptions regarding the properties of the material. First, the unidirectional bulk material is treated as homogeneous, because the fiber diameter (e.g., graphite 5 to 10 μm and glass 10 to 15 μm) is significantly smaller than the wavelength. (For frequencies up to 20 MHz, the wavelength is larger than 100 μm.) Each layer of a composite laminate is assumed to be transversely isotropic, bonded to its neighboring layers with a thin layer of an isotropic resin at their interfaces. The mechanical behavior of the material of each lamina is described by an ensemble average of the displacements, the stresses, and the strains over a representative volume element (Ref 40). The average strains are related to the average stresses through the effective elastic moduli.

Calculation of the effective elastic constants of composite materials has been the topic of many studies. Extensive discussions of the bounds for the effective elastic moduli of fiber-reinforced composites can be found in (Ref 40) and other associated literature cited therein. For low frequencies and low fiber concentration, the theoretical prediction of the effective elastic constants is in good agreement with experimental results. On the other hand, for high frequencies the theoretical estimates are not satisfactory, because the effect of wave scattering by the fibers becomes significant. For fiber-reinforced composite materials, dissipation of the waves is caused by the viscoelastic nature of the resin and by multiple scattering from the fibers as well as other inhomogeneities. Both dissipation effects can be modeled by assuming that the stiffness constants, c_{ij}, are complex and frequency-dependent(Ref 41). Because the effects of dissipation on the velocity of the waves are usually quite small, the material is often assumed to be perfectly elastic in the application of the LLW technique.

An experimental system is shown schematically in Fig. 22. The height, rotation angle, and the angle of incidence of the transducer are computer controlled. The control of the angle of incidence allows simultaneous changes in the transmitter and receiver angles while maintaining a pivot point on the part surface and assuring accurate measurement of the reflected ultrasonic signals. The signals are transmitted by a function generator that frequency-modulates the required spectral range. This generator also provides a reference frequency marker for the calibration of data acquisition when converting the signal from time to frequency domain. A digital scope is used to acquire the reflection spectra after being amplified and rectified by an electronic hardware. The signals that are induced by the transmitter are received, processed, and analyzed by a personal computer after being digitized. As discussed earlier, the reflected spectra for each of the desired angles of incidence is displayed on the monitor, and the location of the minima (LLW modes) are marked by the computer on the reflection spectrum. These minima are accumulated on the dispersion curve, which is shown in the lower part of the display in Fig. 23. The use of the frequency-modulation approach introduces a significant increase in the speed of acquiring the dispersion curves. In this approach, 20 different angles of incidence can be acquired in about 45 s in contrast to over 15 min using the former approach. Once the dispersion data is ready, the inversion option of the software is activated, and the elastic stiffness constants are determined, as shown in Fig. 23.

Various defects can be detected and characterized based on the quantitative data that is available from the dispersion curves. In Fig. 24(a) the response from a defect-free graphite/epoxy laminate tested at the 0° polar angle is shown. In Fig. 24(b), the response from an area with a layer of simulated porosity (microballoons) is presented. As expected, at low frequencies the porosity has a relatively small effect, and the dispersion curve appears similar for the two cases. On the other hand, as the frequency increases, the porosity layer emulates a delamination and modifies the dispersion curves to appear as those for a laminate with half the thickness of the undamaged laminate.

To further enhance the accuracy of the dispersion data, a method has been developed to acquire and to display them as an image. Examples of such dispersion curves are shown in Fig. 25(a) and (b) for a 3.125 mm (0.12 in.) thick unidirectional laminate tested at 0 and 45° polar angles, respectively. This method has been found to allow viewing modes with amplitude levels that

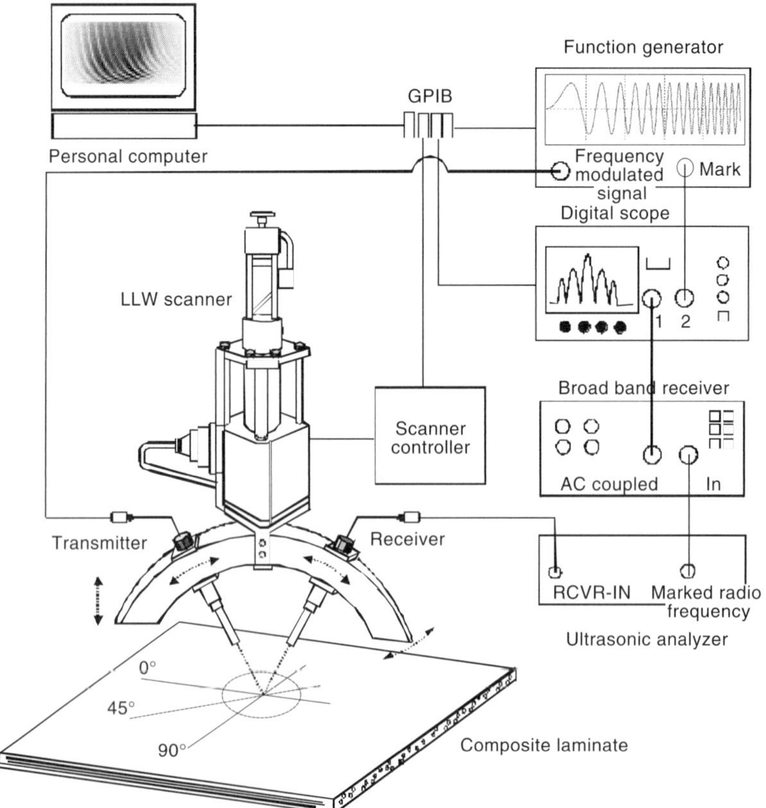

Fig. 22 A schematic view of the rapid LLW test system

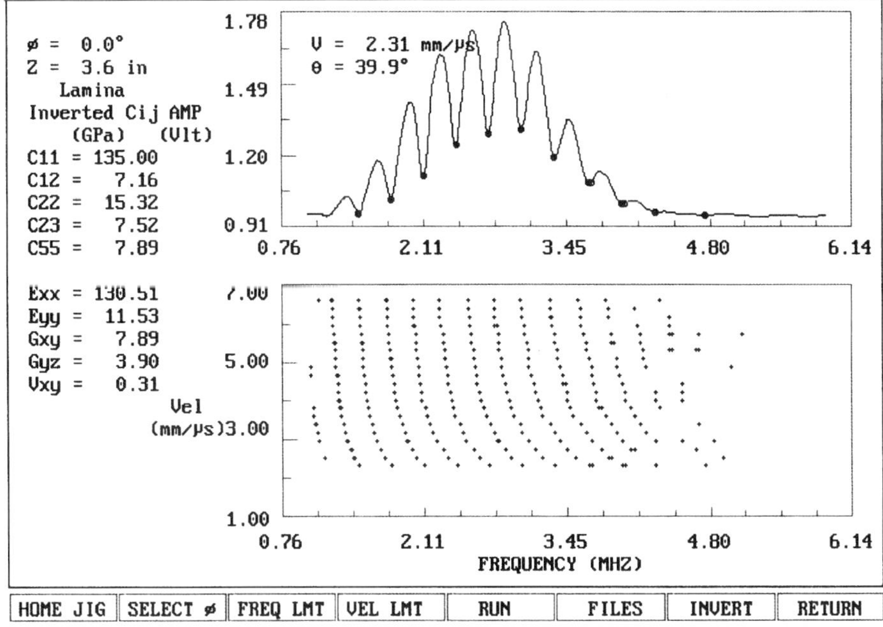

Fig. 23 Computer display after the data acquisition and inversion completion. The elastic stiffness constants are inverted from the dispersion curve and are presented on the left of the screen

are significantly smaller than what has been observed before. The white curved lines show the modes of the dispersion curve. In the case of propagation at 45° to the fibers (Fig. 25b), it can be seen that the modes that would otherwise be considered noise are clearly identified using this approach.

The LLW method has been studied by numerous investigators since 1990, and this has resulted in a good quantitative understanding of the behavior of the waves in composite materials. However, this knowledge base has yet to be translated into the development of practical NDE methods for production or field applications.

Nonlinear Ultrasonics

Standard ultrasonic inspection is based on linear acoustics. Under this condition, the acoustic waves transmit across an interface with equal intensity during the compression and tension mechanical motions at the interface. However, when the interface is imperfect, the transmission in the tension mode may not be fully supported, perhaps by the opening of microimperfections that change the surface area in contact at the interface. This change in characteristics of the interfaces in a structure between compression and tension results in harmonic signals that are characteristic of the nonlinear acoustic transmission of material (Ref 42). This nonlinear elastic behavior of interfaces provides a method for materials characterization, and in particular, the evaluation of bonded interfaces (Ref 43–45).

There are several ways to perform nonlinear ultrasonic inspection. One basic method uses two beams of ultrasonic energy at different tone burst frequencies. When the two acoustic signals interact, harmonics will be created. The presence of a signal at sum and difference of the two input frequencies is an indicator of nonlinear characteristics. Figure 26 shows this measurement configuration. The signal can be used for the detection of nonlinear features in material samples. Another approach is to use a high-amplitude tone burst as a probing signal frequency and a second signal created by vibration of the test article, also at high-amplitude, to stress an interface of interest. When the two signals interact, sidebands are generated. The sidebands to the probing frequency are at plus and minus the vibration frequency value. A Fourier transform display of the detected signal will show the sideband effects when nonlinear processes are present in the test objects. Figure 27 shows this configuration. Cracks, delaminations, and poorly bonded interfaces should serve as sources for the nonlinear effect and be detected.

Acousto-Ultrasonics

Acousto-ultrasonics, a technique originally developed by A. Vary and coworkers, is basically a pitch-catch method that uses two transducers, one to generate a wave and one to receive it after it has progressed along the material (Ref 46–48). It differs from the normal pitch-catch ultrasonic technique in that the two transducers are not placed in sight of one another to receive body waves. Rather, the two transducers are

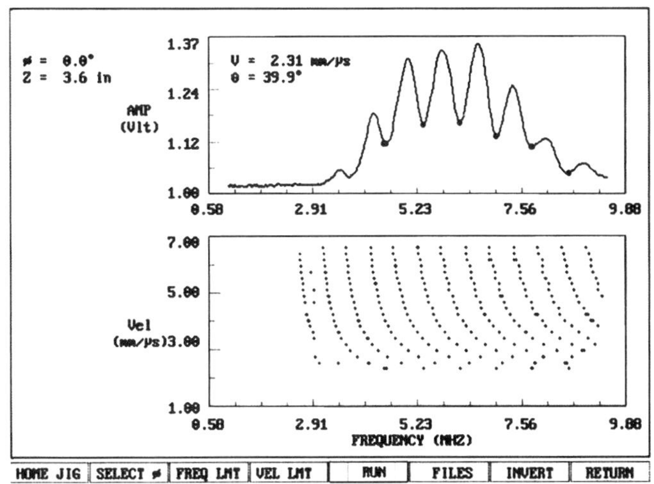

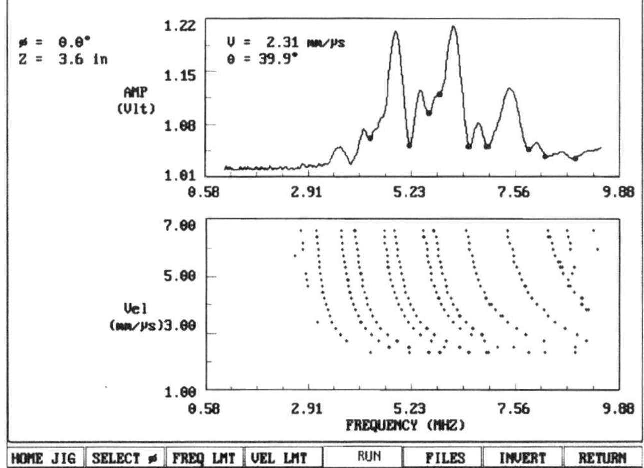

Fig. 24 Leaky Lamb wave characterization. (a) The reflection at 39.5° incidence angle and the dispersion curve for a graphite/epoxy $[0]_{24}$ laminate with no defects. (b) The response at a defect area where simulated porosity was introduced in the middle layer using microballoons

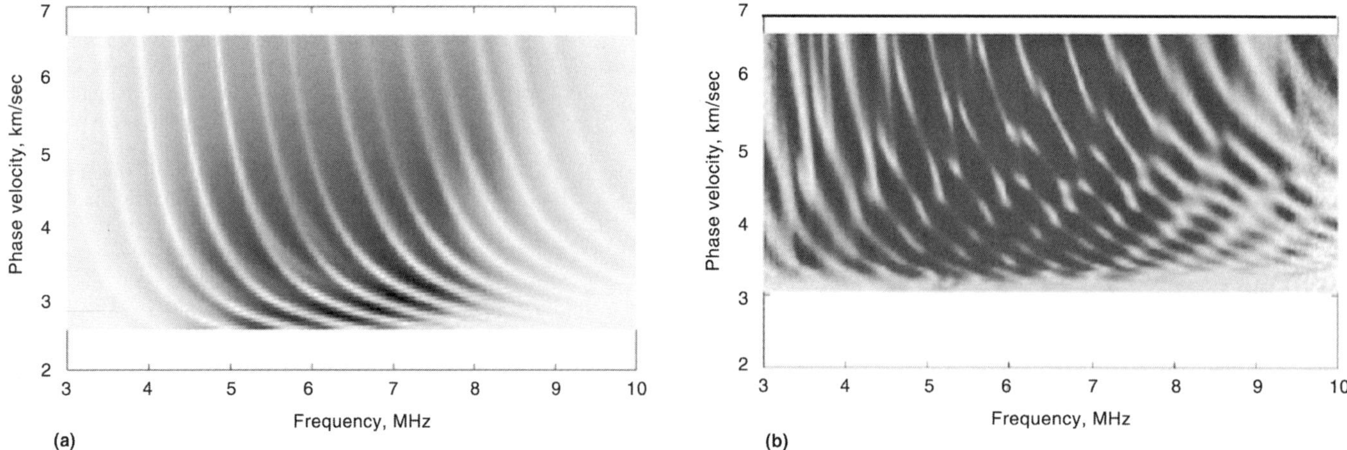

Fig. 25 Leaky Lamb wave dispersion curves for a unidirectional graphite/epoxy composite. (a) Curve showing wave propagation along the fibers generated by an imaging method. (b) Curve showing wave propagation at 90° to the fibers

placed on the same side of a plate, shown in Fig. 28, and the receiver responds to plate (Lamb) waves that are generated by the transmitter. The transmitter simultaneously generates body waves that are either partially converted into plate waves or reflected back and forth between the front and back faces of the plate under the transmitting transducer until all of their energy is thermally dissipated. The signal received by the second transducer has been found to correlate well with the location of the final catastrophic failure site and with stiffness changes during fatigue (Ref 49, 50). Various signal analysis procedures can be used to obtain more reproducible results from the technique (Ref 51).

Acousto-ultrasonic measurements are made by stimulating stress waves in the material and measuring a stress wave factor (SWF) (Ref 52). The SWF can be measured in several ways, such as the ring-down count, peak voltage, or energy. This is similar to acoustic emission testing. Lower values of SWF indicate higher material attenuation, related to microcracks, porosity, cure state, bond quality, morphology, and microstructure. Figure 29 presents typical results comparing changes in the RMS of the energy of an acousto-ultrasonic signal with stiffness during a fatigue test of a graphite/epoxy specimen. The acousto-ultrasonic technique may find application as a sensitive indicator of degradation of composites due to damage, fatigue, or other forms of material attack. However, this knowledge base has yet to be translated into the development of practical NDE methods for production or field applications.

Radiography

Radiography is a well-established production process with many variables in image formation and interpretation (Ref 53). The equipment performance, personnel qualifications and certification, test criteria, and test procedure scope must be identified and documented, if reliable and repeatable test results are to be achieved. Well-defined test criteria and high-quality reference images are needed to separate unacceptable material from acceptable materials with confidence. Radiography can be used with composite materials. It provides a permanent record of the test specimen in the image, reveals fabrication, assembly, and structural defects, and often suggests a corrective action in the process used. Digital data files can be easily communicated and shared. Digital data can be rescaled to accurately reconstruct engineering values of material density and size.

Radiographic testing involves exposing a media to x-ray radiation that has penetrated the specimen of interest, developing an image from the media, and interpreting the image developed.

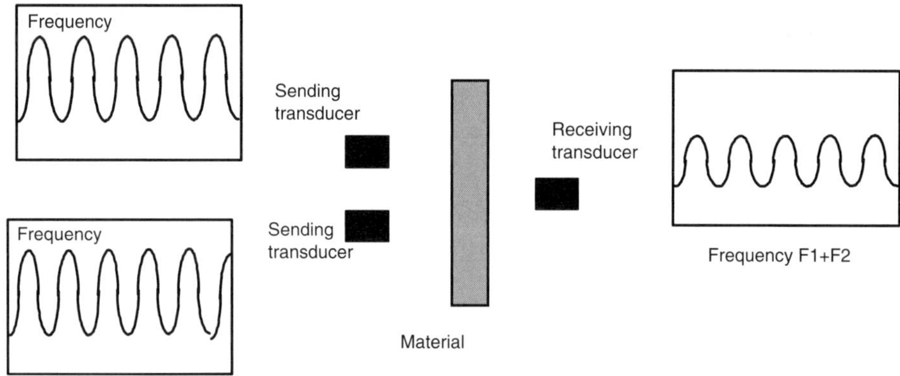

Fig. 26 Diagram for nonlinear ultrasonic measurement using two input beams

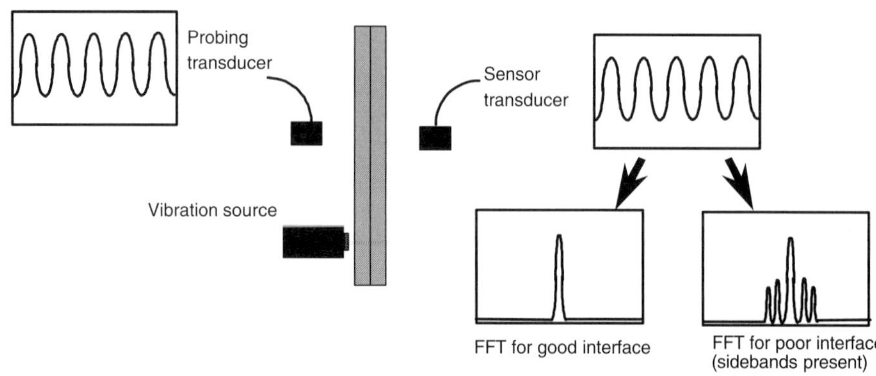

Fig. 27 Diagram for nonlinear ultrasonic measurement using a vibration source. FFT, fast Fourier transform

The general equation for the absorption of x-rays through material is:

$$I = I_0 e^{-\mu(E)x} \quad \text{(Eq 14)}$$

where I is the transmitted intensity, I_0 is the initial intensity, μ is the linear attenuation coefficient as a function of energy (E), and x is the material thickness. The variation in the transmitted radiation field (detected as image features) is the result of variable attenuation, due to changes in the material makeup or construction of the composite structure. Sensitivity to these feature changes are improved with lower x-ray energy and larger feature size. Higher x-ray energy is required to penetrate thicker or denser structures.

Radiographic testing can be applied to assure the maximum reliability of fiber-reinforced composite products and bonded assemblies, both with and without honeycomb. It is complementary to ultrasonic inspection, in that these methods can detect different types of defects, and data from one method can often be used to help interpret results from the other. Existing processes involve tube-type constant potential or rectified radiation sources for production radiography, and many systems are capable of operating at low energy ($<$ 50 kV). Radiographs are normally produced on a high contrast, small-grain-size medium capable of meeting the flaw detection requirements of the applicable product inspection and acceptance specification. Film radiography typically uses the human eye for a detector. Films are interpreted by passing sufficient quantities of light through the film during observation. If the radiograph has sufficient contrast and spatial resolution, it will be possible to detect small variations within the specimen. Contrast variations of 2% and spatial details of 0.50 to 1.25 mm (0.020 to 0.050 in.) are easily detected in most composite materials.

Radiographic contrast is actually a combination of subject contrast and film contrast. Subject contrast is directly affected by the energy of the ionizing radiation used, the density and thickness of the specimen, and the atomic number of the specimen material(s). Always apply the lowest practical energy level to maximize radiographic contrast. Film contrast is a function of the behavior of the film when it is exposed to varying quantities of radiation. Film contrast values are expressed as a relationship between film exposure and the resulting film density. Film radiography normally requires a darkroom to prepare film cassettes for exposure and to stage film in an automatic processor for development. There are many variables to control in this process; for example, exposure to light will compromise the quality of the radiographs, as will unsuitable film-processing chemistry.

Nonfilm methods, such as computed radiography (CR) and digital radiography (DR), can be employed as an alternative to x-ray film (Ref 54–56). The CR systems employ a plate coated with phosphor, which consists of barium fluorohalide containing a minute quantity of bivalent europium ions. The phosphor exhibits a phenomenon called photostimulable luminescence. Once the imaging medium is exposed to radiation, it is processed by scanning the image medium by laser in an image plate reader. The photostimulated luminescent light thus emitted is converted to a digital number representing the intensity. Once the stored photon energy has been extracted, the image plate is erased and ready for reuse. Digital radiography systems include charge-coupled device (CCD) arrays, amorphous silicon, and amorphous selenium. The CCD and amorphous silicon systems use an x-ray-to-light conversion layer (phosphor) and then a silicon imaging detector array. Amorphous selenium array detectors have a direct x-ray-to-light conversion process (Ref 57). The quality of these systems is dependent, among other things, on the combination of the x-ray sensing layer performance, the array pixel size, and, the readout system capability. The digital data from both CR and DR systems can be input to image processors for enhancement, archived, and/or converted to a hard copy image.

The use of an image quality indicator or reference standard is normally required for each inspection. Required image quality levels should be documented in a written inspection procedure, and image quality verification shall demonstrate a radiographic process capable of producing results with the level of quality necessary for detection of anomalies within the test material. Image quality indicators can contain naturally occurring or artificially produced flaws and/or holes or wires. The image quality indicators, which are sensitive to both contrast and definition factors, should be placed on the test specimen in the area of interest for each radiograph.

Radiographic testing of composites involves two primary processes: static, or stationary, radiography and in-motion radiography. Static radiography involves placing imaging medium under a test specimen and exposing the medium

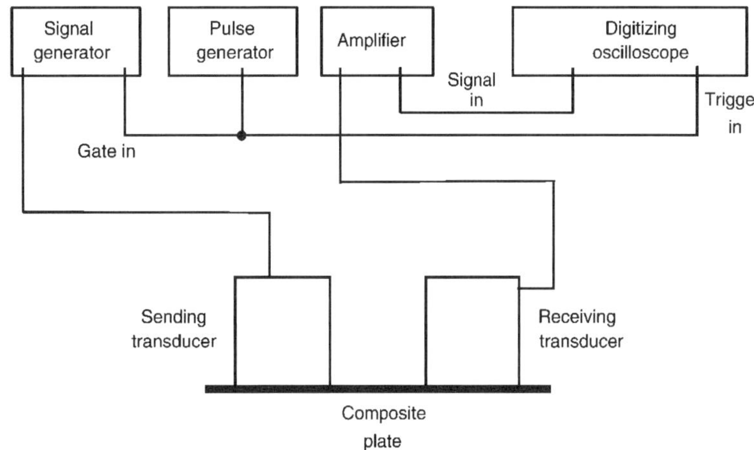

Fig. 28 Acoustic-ultrasonic experimental configuration

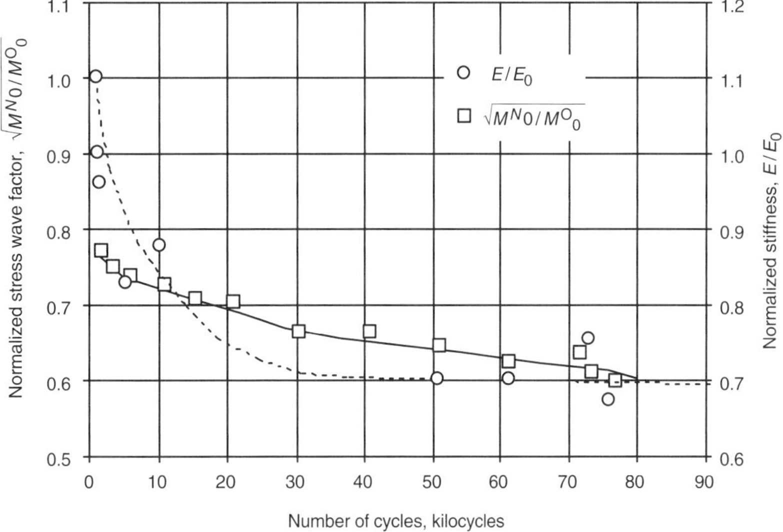

Fig. 29 Change of acousto-ultrasonic stress wave parameter during fatigue test of a graphite/epoxy specimen

without any specimen or source movement. Figure 30 shows a view of a radiation cell for composites material inspection. Radiation beam orientation and the number of exposures for any part or material are governed by the test object geometry and the size and location of the various types of anomalies to be detected. For most structures, the beam of radiation should be perpendicular to the inspection surface in the area of interest. A static exposure depicting minute voids averaging 0.635 (0.025 in.) in diameter in a composite structure is shown in Fig. 31.

In-motion radiography employs a robotic or electrically driven tube head support system to provide vertical motion as well as longitudinal and transverse motion of the x-ray tube. Typically, in-motion equipment is computer controlled, which provides a programmable means of varying the x-ray parameters in addition to velocity of the tube head motion. The motion system shall provide a smooth contiguous transition at all speeds, and the radiation energy system shall provide a degree of stability that will not cause radiation intensity banding within the radiograph. Figure 32 shows an example of an in-motion radiography facility.

For bonded honeycomb assemblies, the assembly should be oriented with the honeycomb cells (depth) parallel to the central ray of the x-ray beam. The long axis of the slit in the collimator should be aligned perpendicular to the direction of motion and the longitudinal axis of the x-ray tube. When radiographing metallic or composite close-out or web structures for adhesive or core tie-in, the x-ray beam shall be oriented parallel to the close-out or web structure. The long axis of the slit in the collimator shall be aligned perpendicular to the direction of motion and the longitudinal axis of the x-ray tube. Measuring the imaged web or close-out thickness on the radiograph and comparing it to the nominal web thickness, per the part drawing, shall verify critical beam alignment. Typically, if the imaged structure is 0.75mm (0.030 in.) over the blueprint nominal thickness, beam realignment should be preformed. Off-angle shots can obscure defects, such as lack of tie-in, voids, short core, and so on, due to geometric image enlargement on the medium. This being the case, accurate defect measurements cannot be performed. When parts are radiographed to detect cracks, only the area of the part within a cone of radiation with a maximum plane angle of 10° should be considered valid for interpretation. An in-motion exposure optimally aligned on a bonded honeycomb assembly depicting three areas of adhesive tie-in defects is shown in Fig. 33.

Geometric unsharpness is the foundation for establishing the quality needed to read and interpret radiographic images. Geometric unsharpness, as applied to in-motion and static radiography, is a derived numerical value from a specifically defined equation. In stationary radiography, the geometric unsharpness shall satisfy the following:

$$U_g = Ft/d \quad \text{(Eq 15)}$$

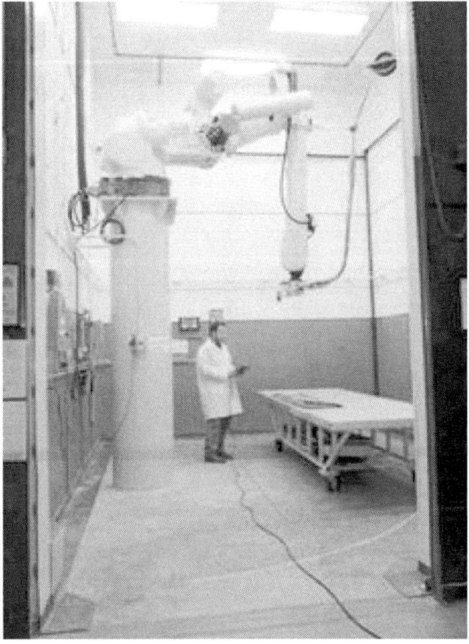

Fig. 30 Radiation cell for composites material inspection

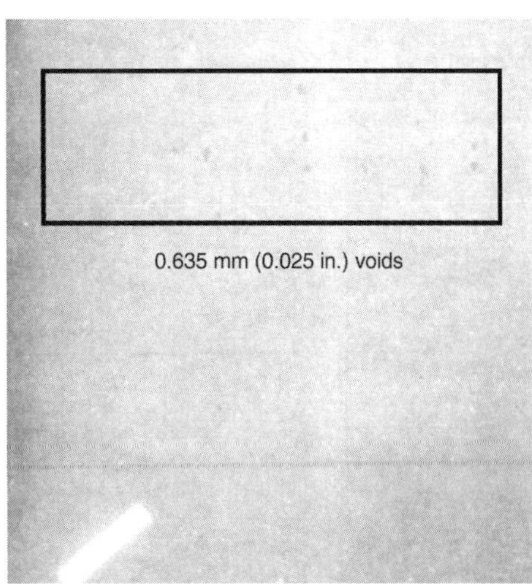

Fig. 31 Example of a radiograph of composite material containing voids

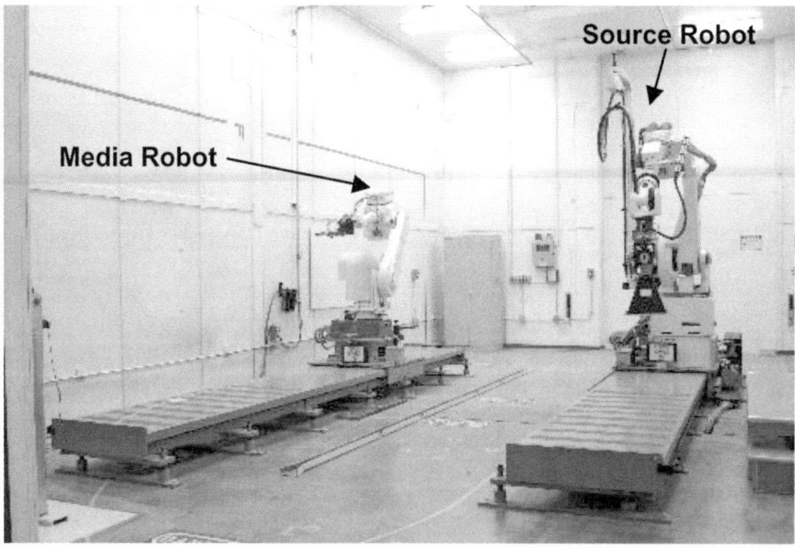

(a)

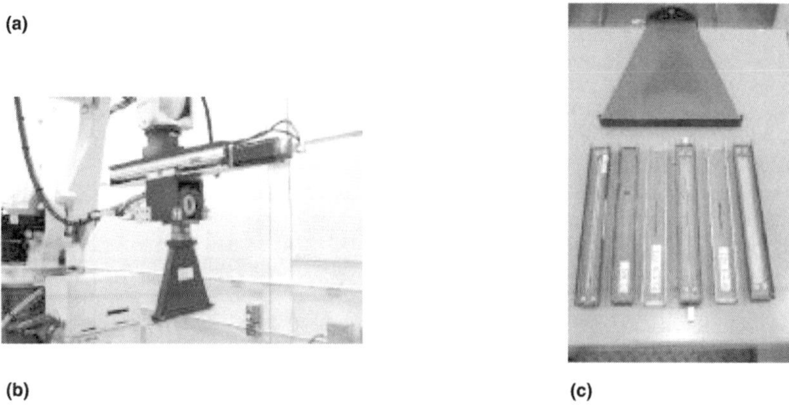

(b) (c)

Fig. 32 Example of an in-motion radiography facility showing (a) the facility, (b) a close-up of the source robot, and (c) the collimator and slits

where U_g is the geometric unsharpness, F is the maximum dimension of radiation source size, t is the thickness of the part (assuming that the film is against the part, otherwise it is the sum of the thickness of the part and the distance between the film and the part), and d is the distance from the source to the source side of the object.

For in-motion radiography, the unsharpness must meet the Eq 15 requirement, but an additional unsharpness criterion in the direction of motion must be satisfied. Geometric unsharpness for the in-motion method in the direction of motion is calculated as follows:

$$U_m = [T(F + S)]/C \quad \text{(Eq 16)}$$

where C is the minimum focal spot to collimator slit distance (collimator length), T is the distance between the imaging medium and the surface to the part farthest from the imaging medium to be interpreted, F is the effective focal spot size, and S is the collimating opening slit width in the direction of travel. The slit width is the opening at the distal end of the radiation collimator responsible for the focusing of the image.

Radiation energy levels should be selected in accordance with the standard x-ray potential curve based on equivalent material thickness. Figure 34 shows energy selection curves for x-ray inspection as a function of material and thickness. When radiographing a test specimen containing multiple materials, determine the predominate material and calculate the radiographic equivalence factor of the secondary materials to the predominate material equivalent thickness. Now the x-ray potential curve can be used for a single equivalent material thickness.

Computed Tomography

X-ray computed tomography (CT) can play an important role in the evaluation of composite materials and structures. Thick graphite- or plastic-fiber composites, multilayer bonded structure, honeycomb, and ceramic and metallic composites can exhibit difficult-to-interpret indications from standard NDE methods. Computed tomography can be used to detect and measure features, such as delaminations, porosity/voiding, resin-rich/resin-poor, bondline fill, cracking, dimensions, and so on, providing useful information during the composite structure development or the evaluation of nonconforming articles.

X-ray CT was invented in the 1960s and developed for medical applications in the 1970s and 1980s (Ref 58–63). Industrial application of CT has followed the medical developments, perfecting the technology for the evaluation of objects as small as an optical fiber to objects as large as an intercontinental ballistic missile. Medical CT systems are designed for high throughput and low dosages specifically for humans and human-sized objects. These systems can be applied to industrial objects, such as composite structure, that have low atomic number and are less than one-half meter (20 in.) in diameter (Ref 64). In the late 1970s and 1980s, industrial CT systems were specifically developed and applied to a variety of hardware items (Ref 65–67). Both medical and industrial CT systems are applicable to composites object inspection, depending on the object size, constituents, and features of interest (Ref 68–71).

While conventional radiography, as shown in Fig. 35(a), creates a shadowgraph containing superposition of information, x-ray CT uses measurements of x-ray transmission from many angles around a component to compute the attenuation coefficient of small volume elements. This data, as shown in Fig. 35(b), is pre-

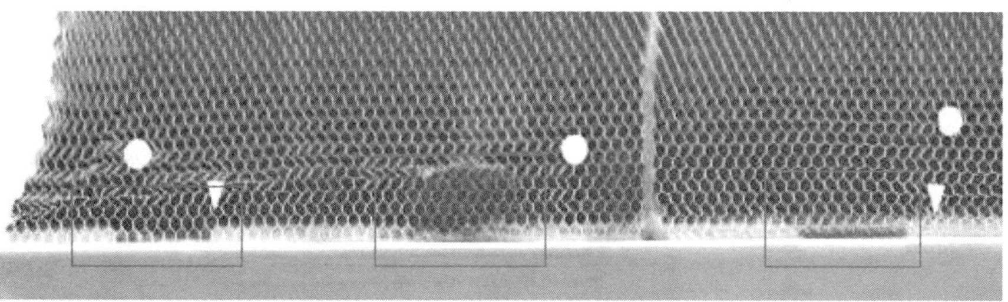

Fig. 33 Example of an in-motion radiograph depicting three areas of adhesive tie-in defects

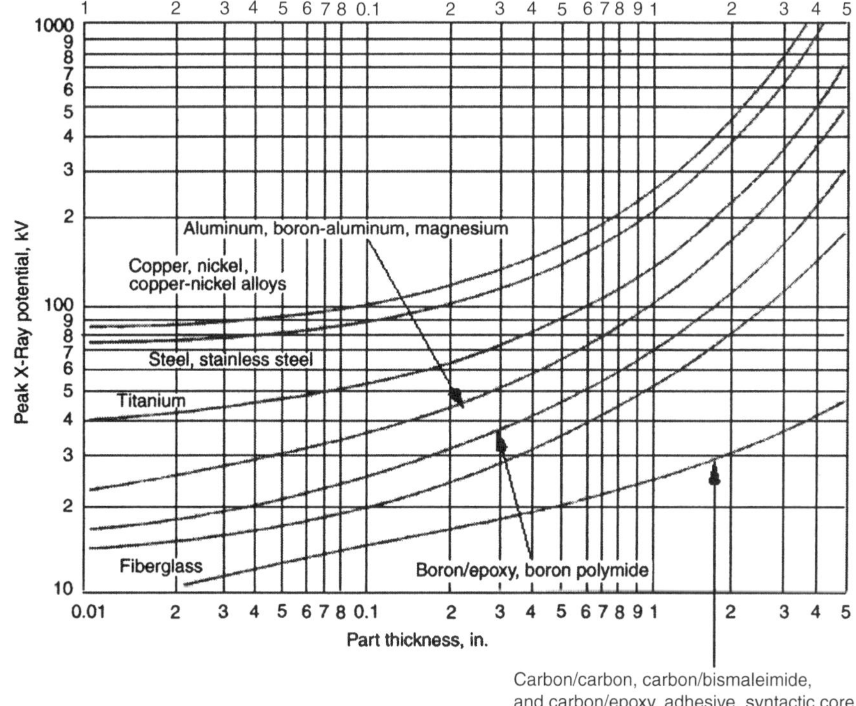

Fig. 34 Chart for the selection of x-ray energy as a function of material and thickness

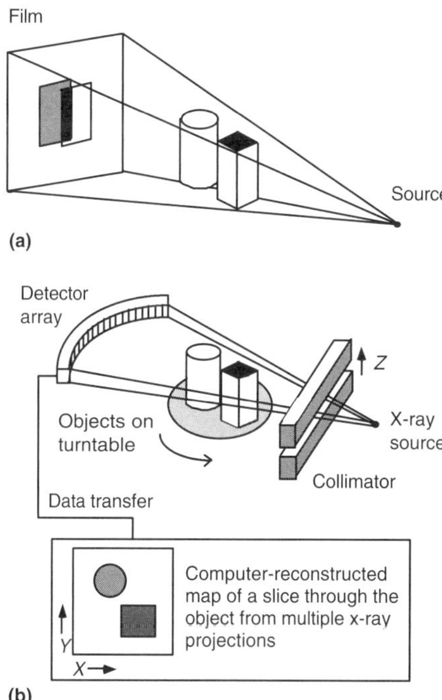

Fig. 35 Comparison of radiography and computed tomography (a) Conventional projection radiography. (b) CT using slit collimation

sented as a cross-sectional image map of the object. The clear images of interior planes of an object are achieved without the confusion of superposition of features. Computed tomography results are easy to interpret for feature detection and placement. Computed tomography can provide quantitative information about the density/constituents and dimensions of the features imaged. Figure 36 demonstrates the application of CT to a composite tail cone. The image on the left is a radiograph. The CT slice on the right, taken near the top of the cone, shows the internal configuration, dimensions, and material variation without the confusion of superposition of information in the radiograph. Multiple CT slices at sequential locations along the vertical axis are required to image the entire cone with CT.

X-ray CT can be considered the high-end application of radiation measurements, because the data obtained are quantitative measures (directly related to the x-ray linear attenuation coefficient) for each volume element throughout an object. The sensitivity can be high, because each reconstructed volume element is composed of back-projected rays from many orientations about the object. Equation 17 shows an estimate of the SNR in a voxel element (a unit of graphic information that defines a point in a three-dimensional space) as a function of various CT system characteristics for a reconstruction of cylindrical object (Ref 70):

$$SNR = 0.665\,\mu d^{3/2}[(vnt/\Delta p)e^{-2\mu R}]^{1/2} \qquad \text{(Eq 17)}$$

where μ is the linear attenuation coefficient, d is the x-ray beam width, v is the number of views, n is the photon intensity rate at the detector, t is the integration time of the detectors, Δp is the ray spacing, and R is the radius of the object. Equation 17 shows that the SNR improves with larger beam width, number of views, x-ray beam intensity, and integration time. The SNR will also be improved by decreasing the ray spacing and object diameter. These CT system characteristics reflect the trade-offs in optimizing a CT system. Fast scan times, fine resolution, high contrast sensitivity, and large object size are mutually exclusive, requiring compromise in system design.

Because of the high signal-to-noise in any voxel, CT can detect features below the resolution limit of the image (voxel size). For features that are larger than a single voxel, the contrast sensitivity improves by the square root of the number of pixels making up the feature. For a feature smaller than a pixel, the apparent density is averaged over the image voxel, and therefore, the signal for that image voxel is reduced. This is called a partial volume effect. Although the signal is reduced by the partial volume effect, the feature may still be detected. This is a significant point about the application of CT, because very often relatively large image voxels (compared to very fine defects) may be used, but small features are still detected, although they are not necessarily resolved. The contrast sensitivity typically provided by CT is in the range of 0.1 to 1%.

Computed tomography requires more sophisticated equipment for data acquisition and reconstruction than conventional radiography. The total time required to inspect an object volumetrically is relatively long, making CT a significantly more expensive inspection. Computed tomography has several variations from its basic concept of Fig. 35. The most useful forms for composite structure are second-generation and third-generation CT. The second-generation, rotate/translate scheme is commonly used for industrial objects, because objects larger than the x-ray beam fan angle can be accommodated. The third-generation, or rotate-only, scanning approach is used on small industrial objects, because it is faster than second-generation. Both the second- and third-generation methods use a one-dimensional detector array and only image one slice location through the part in a single CT scan. That slice inspection volume is the size of the fan beam height collimation. Another method, "volume CT" or "cone beam CT," uses a two-dimensional area detector and an uncollimated cone of radiation, such that the entire object may be inspected in one scan. This technique sacrifices some detail in the image quality for a higher throughput when the entire object must be inspected with CT and has limitations on the applicable part size (Ref 72, 73). It also generally works well only for relatively small objects. Limited-angle, tangential, and annular reconstruction CT are also methods that can be beneficial to large composite structure. Limited-angle CT does not require that the CT data be taken from all angles completely about the part. This can be particularly advantageous for large planar composite structure (Ref 74). Tangential and annular reconstruction offer advantages for large cylindrical structures where information is only needed along annular rings, particularly near the outside of the structure (Ref 75, 76).

Computed tomography data allows accurate evaluation of dimensions and locations in three-dimensional object space or material density (as related to x-ray linear attenuation coefficient) to be performed in any orientation throughout the volume of an object that has been scanned with the CT system. Tables 5 and 6 list the benefits and limitations of CT for composite materials and structures that result from the capability and

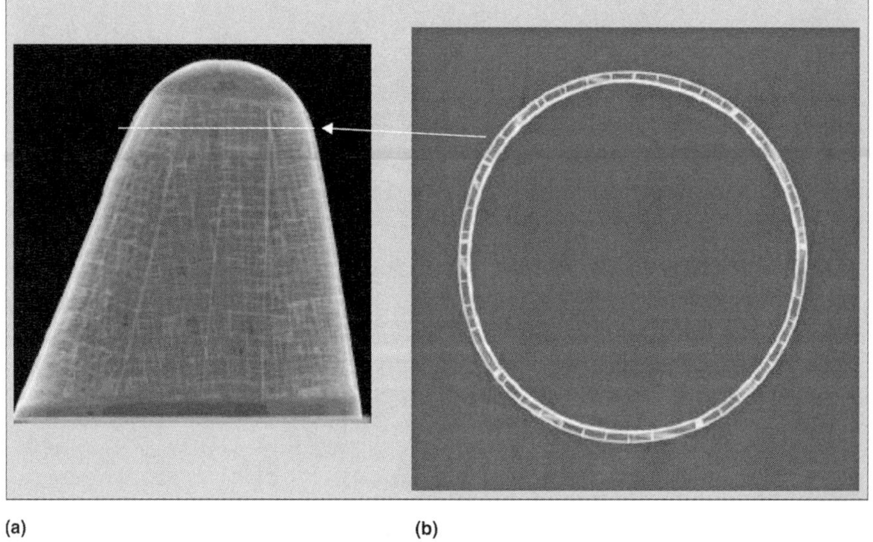

Fig. 36 Example of a composite tail cone approximately 800 mm (31.5 in.) tall and 50 mm (2 in.) in diameter at the midplane. (a) Radiograph of the sample. (b) CT slice near the top

Table 5 Capabilities of computed tomography for NDE of composites

Evaluation parameter	CT capability
Material consolidation uniformity (mixture distribution), voiding, porosity, dry ply, resin/fiber distribution, flow characteristics	Quantitative measurement of density and variation over a three-dimensional volume
Foreign material	Detection, location, and quantification
Bonds (inaccessible to other NDE methods)	Location, extent, variations (limited to bond separation)
Internal structures/reinforcements	Detection and measurement of placement, interface quality, shape, and condition
Damage and testing (impacts, environment, loading, etc.)	Volumetric feature detection measurement
Coatings	Thickness, variation, interface quality
Anisotropic fiber structure	Fiber direction, tow alignment, wrinkles, waviness
Dimensional measurements	Noncontact, internal, external measurement
Repairs (honeycomb)	Adhesive location and amount

complexity of the CT measurements (Ref 77). Figure 37 demonstrates the sensitivity of CT to features in composite structure. The CT image of the composite "J"-stiffener shows how the variations in the consolidation and the ply layups can be evaluated, particularly at T-junctions.

Thermography

Infrared thermography offers an ideal, cost-effective NDE solution for a wide range of in-service and manufacturing composites applications (Ref 78–82). It is fast, noncontact, can be single-sided, and offers wide area coverage of flat or curved parts. It is used for composite NDE applications, including detection of delaminations, impact damage, water entrapment, inclusions, density variations, and evaluation of adhesive bonds. Thermographic NDE systems range from a simple heat gun-infrared (IR) camera combination to fully automated inspections systems capable of thickness or defect measurement and advanced materials characterization.

In thermographic NDE (TNDE), a surface of the component under test is actively heated, and the subsequent surface temperature response of the part to the stimulation is monitored with an IR camera. Although there are many possible configurations for TNDE (e.g. TT, cooling stimulation, and step or modulated heating, to name a few), the same basic principles apply. The physical process can be reduced to three steps in which energy is converted to various forms:

- The surface of the component is uniformly heated. Typically this is accomplished using light, although forced air, steam, hot water, electrical current, electromagnetic induction, and acoustic energy have been demonstrated for particular applications.
- As thermal energy from the heated front surface diffuses toward the cooler interior and back surface of the component, the front surface temperature of the component falls. However, areas of the front surface that are located above subsurface defects (discontinuities in the material density, thermal conductivity, or heat capacity) will cool at a different rate than defect-free areas. Figure 38 graphically depicts this scenario for regions with and without subsurface defects.
- An image of the surface temperature of the heated component is monitored using an IR camera, which collects IR radiation from the surface of the sample. Defect areas will exhibit anomalous cooling behavior, which will appear in the infrared IR of the surface.

It is important to understand the energy conversion processes described previously, because ineffective conversion in any of these steps will adversely affect the result. For example, a component with an optically reflective surface will not absorb light efficiently, and may have to be treated with a removable paint or heated using a nonoptical source. A material that is a poor thermal conductor will respond to the heat stimulus very slowly, while the image of a sample with poor IR emissivity will be relatively weak.

Although it is possible to find large or shallow subsurface defects using a heat gun and an IR camera, pulsed IR thermography is the most widely used approach for industrial applications, because it offers the best combination of speed, sensitivity, repeatability, depth and spatial resolution, and quantification. In pulsed thermography, the surface is typically heated using flashlamps that provide a spatially uniform light pulse with a duration of a few milliseconds. A continuous image data sequence is acquired from the IR camera, beginning just before flash heating occurs and continuing until the sample reaches a steady-state temperature. (The duration depends on the thermal properties of the sample.) In most cases, digital data from the camera is acquired and stored on a personal computer for subsequent processing and analysis. Commercial pulsed thermography software analyzes each pixel individually to identify defects and measure physical properties. Figure 39 shows an example of a pulsed thermograph image of a honeycomb composite compared to x-ray and ultrasonic images.

Unlike imaging systems where resolution and sensitivity can be defined in absolute terms based on detector characteristics, characterization of resolution capabilities of TNDE requires consideration of sample material and defect depth, diameter, and composition, as well as the IR camera. Although a particular IR camera may be capable of extremely high spatial resolution of the sample surface, the true critical defect size is limited by the aspect ratio (minimum width-to-depth ratio) of the defect. The minimum detectable defect size is proportional to the aspect ratio. Although it is possible to image weaker defect responses using various signal processing methods, defects with aspect ratio greater than 2 are readily detectable with modern TNDE systems.

In many respects, composites are ideal materials for TNDE. Their optical reflectivity, IR emissivity, and thermal diffusivity generally fall within a range that allows evaluation without surface preparation or high-speed IR cameras. (This is often not the case for metals, where these

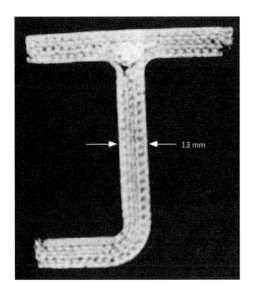

Fig. 37 Computed tomography image of a graphite/epoxy woven "J"-stiffener, showing ply condition and consolidation

Table 6 Limitations of computed tomography for NDE of composites

Attribute	Technical limitations
Volumetric measurement	Disbond must have separation
Detail sensitivity	
Resolution	Large structures: typically 0.5 mm (0.02 in.) features are resolved, smaller high-contrast features can be detected Small structures: (<250 mm, or 10 in.) typically resolves 1 to 2 parts in 500
Density measurement	Multiple materials must differ in x-ray linear attenuation coefficients (density and atomic number) for detection (0.01% to 0.1% for large, > 1 mm, areas)
Artifacts	Large aspect ratios cause streak artifacts (>15:1 is difficult). Detail sensitivity in low-density material near high-density features is compromised.
Part handling	
Penetration	X-ray transmission is limited by size, density, and atomic number of the part and by the available x-ray energy.
Size/shape	Access to 360° around the part

(a)

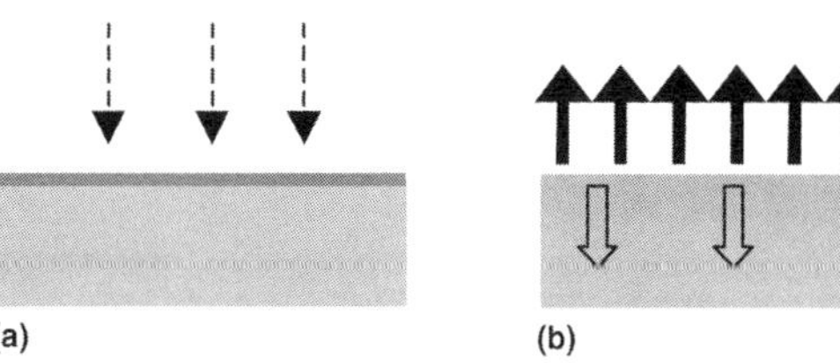
(b)

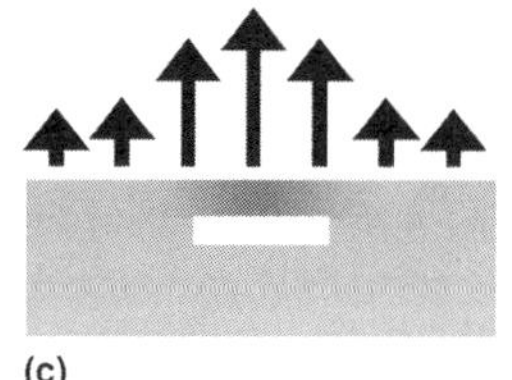
(c)

Fig. 38 Energy conversion in pulsed thermography. (a) A brief light pulse uniformly heats the sample surface. (b) Infrared radiation is emitted uniformly from the surface as thermal energy from the surface diffuses toward the interior of the sample. (c) Increased infrared radiation at the surface above a buried defect is due to interruption of the flow of heat into the sample by the defect

measures are routinely applied.) Common composites applications for TNDE include detection of voids, delaminations, inclusions, density variations, impact damage, bonding irregularities, and trapped moisture. Since IR radiation is emitted most strongly in the direction perpendicular to the surface, pulsed thermography is well suited to large planar structures or curved components with large radii of curvature. It can be applied to lay-ups or randomly oriented fiber materials. Defect contrast varies in proportion to the contrast between the thermal diffusivity of the defect and surrounding material. As a result, applications where the defect presents a composite-to-air, -vacuum, -metal or -water interface offer better performance than situations where materials such as a material inclusion are to be detected. For most composite applications, pulsed thermography systems are capable of evaluating an area of 0.1 m^2 (1 ft^2) in 5 to 20 seconds, depending on the thickness and thermal diffusivity of the material. (Low diffusivity materials require longer inspection times.) As thicker samples are inspected, it may be necessary to provide more input energy. In general, samples thicker than approximately 13 mm (0.5 in.) are not considered practical for thermographic inspection.

Low-Frequency Vibration Methods

Techniques that use frequencies lower than ultrasonic methods can be used to inspect composite structures (Ref 83). The adhesive bond between the skin and core of a composite sandwich structure can be inspected with one of a variety of low-frequency vibration techniques. In certain instances, solid laminate structure can also be inspected for impact damage or internal delaminations. The advantage of these vibration-based techniques over the higher-frequency methods is that a couplant between the probe and the test-piece is not required. They also generally require access to only one side of the structure and can be used when the material is too attenuative for PE or TT ultrasonic testing. Some of the most common vibration techniques are discussed subsequently.

The tap test uses the human ear as a sensor (which can pick up vibration in the 15 Hz to 20 kHz range), and is perhaps the oldest of all low-frequency vibration inspection methods. This method uses a coin or small hammer to "tap" the surface of a laminate or bonded composite while listening to the sound it makes (Ref 83). This method works because of the difference in the sound produced when a "good" versus "bad" region is tapped. A "good" region tends to "ring," while a "bad" region will sound "dead." The sound difference is due to the difference in the nature of the tap impact response. Damage, such as a disbond, results in a local decrease in the mechanical impedance of the structure, which changes the force-time curve caused by the tap near the flaw. The tap test is, in essence, related to the local stiffness. Tap testing is routinely used to detect disbonds, delaminations, and water in honeycomb core cells (Ref 84). However, it cannot detect small voids or disbonds smaller than about 13 mm (0.5 in.), and its sensitivity decreases with thickness to a depth of about 6 mm (0.25 in.) under a stiff material, after which it is totally unreliable. Tap testing is also very susceptible to changes within the structure of the part under test. Ply-thickness changes, core details, core fillers, bonded substructure, and edges are some of the features that can cause false calls. Knowledge of the design of the internal structure is essential to determining if tap testing will be effective and for effectively interpreting the inspection.

In recent years, instruments such as the Mitsui Woodpecker and the WichiTech RD^3 (digital) Tap Hammer have been developed to improve upon traditional tap inspection by providing quantitative data that are independent of inspector experience and ear sensitivity. These instruments make use of the amplitude, duration, or frequency response of the impact curve, because all are affected by the local stiffness. One or more of these features can be flagged as indicators of defects or damage.

Mechanical Impedance Analysis. Another method that senses the changes in the local stiffness due to flaws is called mechanical impedance analysis (MIA), which has been shown to be very effective at finding delaminations in composites (Ref 85). With MIA, a transducer contains a piezo-electric element subjected to an alternating current. The element causes the probe to physically vibrate at a low—and often audible—frequency. When the probe is placed on a structure, it vibrates the local area in a characteristic fashion, depending on the local mechanical impedance. The presence of a disbond below the probe will change the impedance of the structure, which will be measured by a second piezo-electric element in the probe. A popular instrument incorporating the MIA technique is the Staveley BondMaster (Staveley Instruments).

Velocimetric Methods. A family of test instruments exists that takes advantage of the flexure wave generated when an oscillating force is applied to a platelike structure. The speed of propagation and amplitude of these waves will depend upon the thickness and materials properties of the structure. Changes in the speed and amplitude can be monitored over a short distance by the use of low-frequency transducers. A typical probe will have a sending and receiving transducer set at a fixed distance (approximately 13 to 19 mm, or 0.5 to 0.75 in.) apart. Several examples of velocimetric instruments are the Zetec Sondicator (Zetec Inc.) and the Staveley BondMaster, when operated in its pitch-catch mode.

Higher-Frequency Bond Testers. A variety of bond testers operate in the range of 100 kHz to about 1 MHz. These operating frequencies are below typical ultrasonics, but above the low-frequency methods. They have a vibrating transducer that operates at one frequency or over a small range of frequencies near the natural resonance of the part. When the transducer is touching the part, its vibration characteristics are determined by the local impedance of the part. Local flaws or changes in the structure will change the resonance of the transducer. The Fokker Bond Testers, which have been used for bond inspection for many years, operate on these principles (Ref 86). They work by forcing the bonded structure to resonate. Disbonds within a joint or delaminations in a laminate will cause a shift in the resonant frequency and/or amplitude, which can then be detected and displayed.

The Bondascope is another well-known bond tester. Manufactured by NDT Instruments, it measures the amplitude and phase of the local mechanical impedance and displays the result on an oscilloscope (Ref 87).

Acoustic Emission

Acoustic emission is the transient release of elastic waves when materials undergo deformation. In composite materials, the sources of these emissions include matrix cracking, delamination, and fiber breakage. Acoustic emission can be a very sensitive measure, responding to microstructural variations, and has received significant attention as a technique for monitoring damage development in composites (Ref 88, 89). Acoustic emission is most often applied during structural testing, but can be used in process control and in-service monitoring.

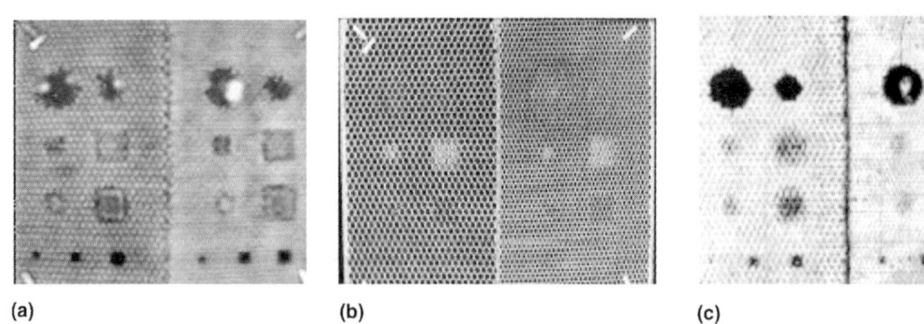

Fig. 39 Comparison of pulsed thermography. (a) X-ray. (b) Through-transmission ultrasound. (c) Images of a carbon/epoxy 5-ply laminate with aluminum core. Intentional defects include (top to bottom) synthetic fluorine-containing resin inserts in the laminate, synthetic fluorine-containing resin inserts at the skin-core interface, and potted core and simulated disbonds in the laminate

The stress waves, created by the acoustic emission of a sample under a load, travel along a sample and can be detected by piezo-electric crystals placed on the sample. The signals must be of short duration and sufficient energy. Acoustic emission from fiber breakage in composites is actually quite loud and is often heard audibly. Research indicates that there are three distinct energy-level groupings that indicate the different amounts of energy emitted from fiber breakage, matrix cracking, and delamination (Ref 90). By using multiple sensors and time-based triangulation methods, the location of the emission in the sample can be determined. An important phenomenon in acoustic emission in the Kaiser effect. When a sample is loaded, it will generate acoustic emission signals as internal breakage occurs. If the loading is stopped and released, the acoustic emission signal will go to zero. As the sample is reloaded, acoustic emission signals will not occur until the level of load exceeds the previous highest loading level.

As the signals are detected from acoustic emission tests, the amplitude data may be recorded as counts above a threshold energy, level in the detector. Measurements of interest include the count rate, the total counts, the total energy, and the ring-down of the counts from a loading step. The data are most often plotted against the load level on the test sample. Acoustic emission has been shown to be useful to predict failure loads for composite pressure vessels (Ref 91).

Eddy Current

Although eddy current testing (ET) is a common means of flaw inspection in metals, it can also be used in composites to find flaws or damage (Ref 92–94), as long as the composite contains electrically conductive materials, such as graphite fibers. Eddy current testing can also be used to determine the thickness of nonconductive coatings and the local conductivity of conductive coatings, both of which are often applied to composites.

The physics of ET are based upon well-known electromagnetic theory, as defined by Maxwell's equations (Ref 95). A wire containing a time-varying electrical current (i.e., alternating or pulsed current) produces a corresponding magnetic field variation that will induce electrical currents in any conductive material in close proximity to it. These currents, called "eddy" currents, are sensitive to the local electrical conductivity of the material in which they are generated. Perturbation of these eddy current paths due to flaws can be detected by an impedance change in the coil (the exciting coil, or a separate nearby pick-up coil) and measured by standard electrical bridge circuit in line with the coil.

The ET skin-depth equation describes the depth of penetration of eddy currents in an isotropic material:

$$\delta = 1/(\pi f \mu \sigma)^{1/2} \qquad \text{(Eq 18)}$$

where δ is skin-depth, f is frequency of inducing current in the ET probe, μ is magnetic permeability, and σ is electrical conductivity of the material being measured.

This equation shows that lower frequencies penetrate further. However, lower frequencies lose sensitivity to flaws, because the signal is essentially being averaged over a larger volume. It also shows that eddy currents will penetrate composites well, because polymer composites are much lower in conductivity than metals.

However, this equation is an approximation, because composites are not isotropically conductive. The fibers (rather than the matrix) are generally the conductors within composites. Often these fibers are continuous with the composite layers (plies) as the elements of unidirectional tape laid up in various orientations or as bundles of fibers woven together into a fabric form. In either case, the fibers are generally parallel to the surface of the structure to be inspected. Therefore, the composite will have a relatively high conductivity in the planes parallel to the surface, and low conductivity normal to the plies. This produces a tight, deep region of eddy current penetration in composites, which can sometimes be advantageous. However, it also means that the eddy currents will tend to run parallel to the plies (and surface) regardless of the ET coil orientation. This means that ET will be relatively insensitive to planar flaws, because the eddy current paths are altered little. Eddy current testing does not work well for identifying small delaminations or common composite foreign objects (such as composite bagging materials, tape, or misplaced adhesive), unless they produce significant local alteration of the ply orientations. It is also insensitive to porosity and matrix cracking, because both occur in the (ordinarily) nonconductive matrix. However, ET is very effective in finding cracks produced by fiber breakage and ply wrinkles (Ref 96) in composites. It has been shown to be particularly effective at detecting composite damage caused by low-energy impacts (Ref 97). Because cracks and wrinkles can be very difficult to find using other common nondestructive inspection methods, such as ultrasonic or radiographic techniques, ET of composites enjoys a small, but growing composites inspection market.

Eddy current systems are portable, easy to operate, and relatively inexpensive. Most provide an alternating, continuous current to the excitation coil, but some produce a pulsed signal that can produce greater penetration (which is not generally needed in most composite structures). The probe that is used to interrogate the part can contain the excitation coil that also senses the impedance changes. A separate pick-up coil is also common and can be located within the probe head, adjacent to the first probe, or on the opposite surface. Coils come in various shapes and size, and are manufactured to function at various frequencies. Generally, composite flaw inspection is done at frequencies between 100 kHz and about 30 MHz. The lower frequencies work best for carbon-carbon composites, which are highly conductive (but still orders of magnitude less conductive than metals), while the less-conductive graphite/epoxy composites are generally best suited to the mid-to-high end of the range. The electrical impedance changes sensed by the coil and accompanying bridge circuit are generally displayed on an oscilloscope as amplitude and phase or electrical resistance and reactance components. If the probe is attached to an x-y bridge, maps of the inspected area can be developed, which facilitate interpretation (Ref 98). Experimentation with the probes, drive frequencies, and standards with known flaws is necessary to determine the effects on the received signal.

Like other inspection methodologies, flaw identification must be based on calibration standards, and care must be taken to eliminate or account for other sources of signal change. Eddy currents are sensitive to nonrelevant parameters, such as minor dimensional changes, surface roughness, lift-off (probe-to-part distance), and proximity to real part features (edges, flanges, fastener holes, etc.). Signal changes due to flaws can often be separated from those produced by these features using phase or frequency adjustments provided by the ET hardware.

A special application for ET in composites is the measurement of conductive coatings thickness or conductivity. If the thickness can be determined using another method (such as pulse-echo UT), the conductivity can be measured. If the conductivity is constant within the coating, the thickness can be measured with a calibration block. Eddy current testing coating inspection requires sufficient conductivity difference between the coating and composite substrate. When a laminate is covered with a conductive coating, the composite itself will have to be evaluated with another method.

Optical Holography and Shearography

Optical holography is a technique that uses coherent light to generate interference patterns of the surface that change under small amounts of stress (Ref 99). By using a laser light, dual-exposure holograms are acquired before and after stressing the part. The interference patterns recorded can measure very small surface displacements, due to internal flaws. The stress is applied through heating, acoustic vibration, or service-type loads. With composites, this method is used to detect disbonds and delaminations. Its disadvantages are that it is less sensitive than ultrasonics, and the holographic apparatus must be isolated from vibration.

Laser shearography is a more recent variation of optical holography that monitors differential motion (Ref 100). As with optical holography, the part must be placed under stress. The constructive and destructive optical interference of the incident laser forms a speckle pattern on the stressed surface. The image is viewed by a video camera through an optical shearing device. When two sets of sheared images are compared electronically, surface changes are detected based upon the change in the speckle patterns. The output takes the form of an image-processed video display of the contour of the derivative of the displacement—a fringe pattern. This technique can be used to locate and size defects, such as disbonds or delaminations. Shearography is much less sensitive to vibrations than optical holography, making it much more portable and useful for field applications. Shearography can be used in the field with a vacuum chamber that has an open end, which seals to the skin of the structure under inspection. As a vacuum is pulled in the chamber, a measurable strain is produced that can be imaged.

Because they are mechanical-strain based, these methods work best with thinner composites, where internal flaws are close enough to the surface to be detected. Detectability and resolution decrease with defect depth, and a critical aspect ratio (flaw size-to-flaw depth) determines detectability. They are also blind to defects open to the surface when the surrounding-vacuum stressing method is used, and they have trouble finding bonded foreign material and contaminated bonds, because insufficient surface displacement occurs. On the other hand, these methods can be used to evaluate very large areas very quickly and are much faster than other inspection methods. In addition, they can be used to detect defects in large honeycomb structures that ultrasonic methods are incapable of penetrating. Shearography is regularly used to find impact damage in sandwich structures (Ref 101) and delaminations between plies in laminated composites (Ref 102).

Data Fusion

Data fusion can be applied to composite materials to improve data reduction and analysis for NDE. (Ref 103–109). The term "data fusion" in the NDE context refers to the process of integrating data from diverse process measurements and nondestructive observations of an object into a consistent description of the condition of the object (Ref 104). The objective of data-fusion methods is to coregister, colocate, and combine multiple data sets into useful forms. Combining carefully selected "modes" or alternative views of process and NDE data leads to reduced ambiguity by overcoming limitations of some inspection methods through the visualization of complementary information. Combining data from different process steps and NDE tests requires systematic engineering methodologies that are often outside the norms of conventional (i.e., single-mode) data analysis. In particular, precise cross-registration techniques and techniques for normalizing, cross-calibrating, and resampling are necessary. Of these, systematic registration of data with respect to the evaluated part is the fundamental requirement.

Data-fusion processing draws on technology in signal processing often used in target recognition or other processes. Statistical and probabilistic algorithms are used to reduce multimodal data for prediction of the material condition. Bayesian methods and Dempster-Shafer evidence theory are examples of methods that are being used for data fusion (Ref 105, 106). Figure 40 shows the levels of data fusion. Once registration of data is obtained, various mathematical algorithms can be applied to the data.

Managing the data from diverse measurements that may use differing frames of reference can be a formidable problem. An approach for the data handling that has been very successful replaces the familiar "image" data model with an "object" or finite-element data model (Ref 105). In the object model, not only the value of data is described, but also its geometry. Essentially, the data acquired from process monitoring or NDE operations are expressed in a part-fixed coordinate system, using techniques commonly used in finite-element analysis. Features of interest can be calculated by appropriate combinations of inputs from the various sources, which are transformable in a common coordinate system. The results can be mapped back onto any of the original test system representations or presented in standard computer graphics, visualization, or database representations.

Figure 41 demonstrates the registration of NDE data on a solid rocket motor nozzle. This figure shows that the visualization of ultrasonic, computed tomography, and eddy current test data can be presented together in part-fixed coordinates. The rocket nozzle exit cone shape is shown as a surface with features from each methodology displayed over the critical (i.e., highly stressed) forward region of the nozzle exit cone. The quantitative parameters evaluated here are eddy current impedance, minimum CT density through the wall, CT density averaged through the wall, and ultrasonic amplitude.

The importance of the multimodal data in the evaluation of a carbon-carbon composite rocket nozzle is shown in Fig. 42. Each inspection modality (e.g., CT or UT) can indicate the presence of an anomaly without necessarily distinguishing the material defect. For example, CT images of a dry ply and a delamination on two different parts are essentially indistinguishable. Con-

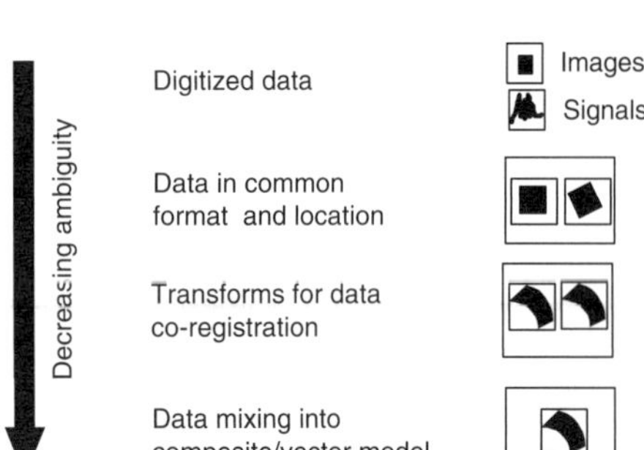

Fig. 40 Levels of data fusion

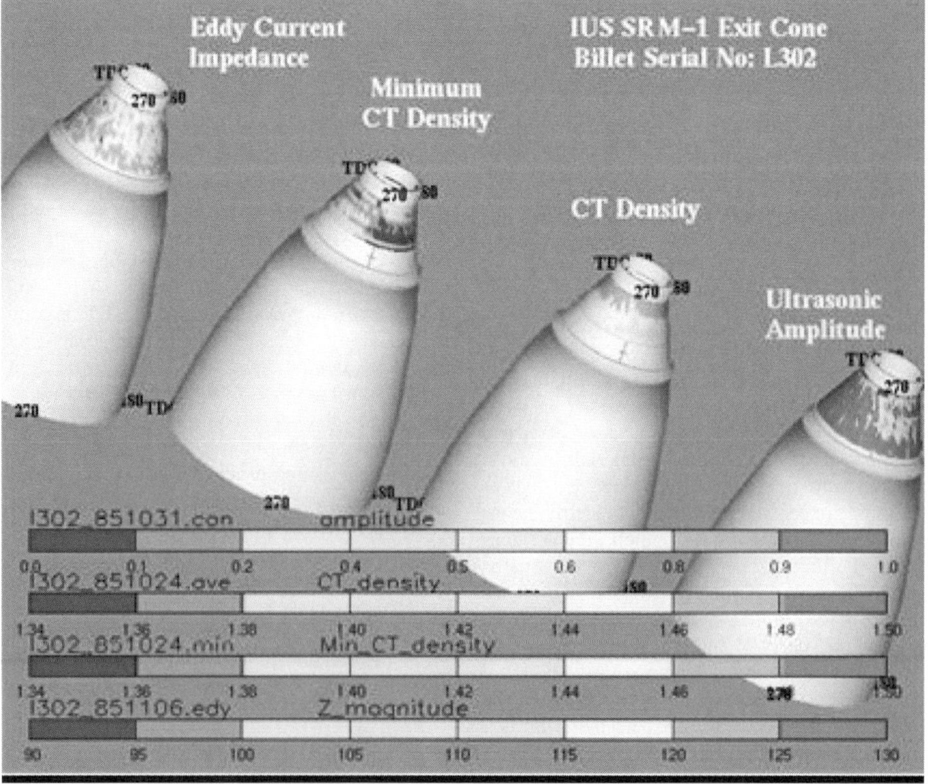

Fig. 41 Nondestructive evaluation multimode data fusion for a carbon-carbon rocket nozzle exit cone

versely, different NDE modalities may respond to an anomaly in differing degrees. Low-density CT indications can be due to wrinkling, dry-ply conditions, or delaminations. The dry ply condition can have sufficient across-ply tensile and interlaminar shear strengths to support the mission loading. A delamination, however, could result in mission failure if misdiagnosed as a dry ply. Only by considering complementary features of the ultrasonic data and the CT data can the two conditions be distinguished. In Fig. 41, the eddy current scan allows a correct interpretation of an otherwise benign low-density indication in the CT scan as a wrinkle whose presence would almost certainly lead to flight failure.

Another example of data fusion for a complex process is the integration of process monitor data and NDE measurements for thermoplastic induction welding. Time, temperature, and pressure are the critical parameters that must be sufficient for welding but not overprocessed enough to cause voiding. During welding, thermocouples are used to monitor the time and temperature at specific locations in the weld zone and may be adjusted by the induction coil controls. The time at temperature for the weld interfaces has been determined to be the most important measurement for the process control. The pressure to the tooling is a fixed value assigned for specific welding conditions. The temperature data is obtained from thermocouples placed at various locations along the weld. The equivalent time (in minutes) to a process target temperature is calculated for each thermocouple and is plotted as a function of position along the weld.

Ultrasonic inspection of the weldline is performed using PE ultrasonics with a full waveform digitizing scanning system. This full waveform data is processed to compare signal strengths from the weldline and the back of the spar cap to similar data taken from the skin surface. Figure 43 is an illustration of combining test data from both the final ultrasonic inspection and the processing time at temperature, as described subsequently. This data-fusion workstation display shows the geometric configuration of a welded skin to a T-spar. The geometry data includes chalkmarks for position information. The data-fusion workstation display in this case shows a three-dimensional view of the weld. The time at temperature data are shown at the top of the Fig. 43 image display by colored squares at the position of thermocouples in the test object. The depth locations in the object are very close, but can be shown by manipulation of the image display and also by the use of increasing square size with depth. The ultrasonic models shown in the lower portion of Fig. 43 are processed image data that are overlaid onto the geometry model of the weld. The bottom model is the ratio of the weldline echo to the front-face surface echo. Low intensity (dark) level is the most desirable. The middle model is a "weld factor" calculation, which is a point-by-point calculation of the ratio of the difference of the back of the spar cap signal and the weldline signal to the sum of the back of the spar cap signal and the weldline signal. This value is positive for a good weld and negative for a poor weld, although, because there is no back of the spar cap signal over the web of the T-spar, the weld factor along this longitudinal region is not a valid representation. This weld factor model is processed data, which essentially fuses ultrasonic amplitude data information from different depths in the part.

The data-fusion approach can be used to provide visualization of multimode NDE data and process information. The fundamental requirement for NDE data fusion is the coregistration of data obtained from various techniques or at different times and locations in part-fixed coordinates. This allows mapping the data to a geometry model of the part and allowing that data to be reviewed in a single workspace. Mathematical processes can then be performed to combine data types for evaluation purposes, such as estimation of feature size and criticality.

Standards

The internal structural quality of every composite detail, subassembly, and assembly must meet baseline quality criteria that design engineering establishes to ensure that the fabricated composite configuration meets the performance requirements. Internal quality that does not meet design performance requirements may result in failures at various stages of manufacture and life cycle. Nondestructive evaluation, inspection, and testing are used to determine the internal quality of composite configurations. Ultrasonic and radiographic methods are most commonly used to make this determination in composite materials. Technicians are certified to the specific customer requirements and most likely to the requirements of the American Society for Nondestructive Testing level II certification. The technician, using validated reference standards that contain known representative induced anomalies, calibrates equipment. Calibration ensures that the equipment is capable of detecting unacceptable conditions defined by the customer requirements. The technician then reviews and evaluates the results provided by the nondestructive method used to inspect/test the composite configuration and assesses the internal quality of the composite configuration. Ultrasonic and radiographic reference standards are critical quality tools of the composite manufacturing process. Without these tools the inspector would be unable to accurately evaluate the internal quality

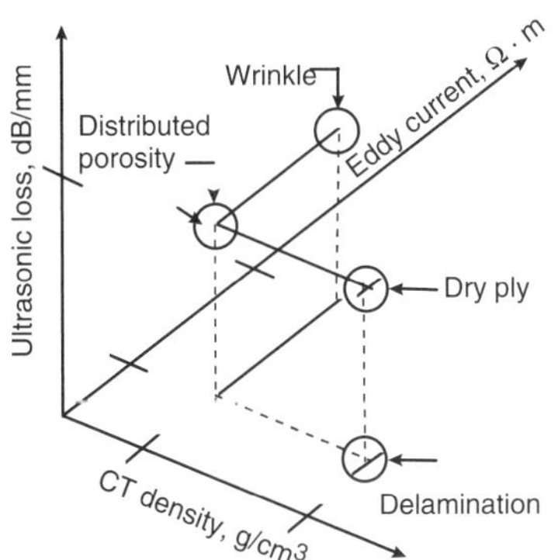

Fig. 42 Nondestructive evaluation parameter representations of anomalies

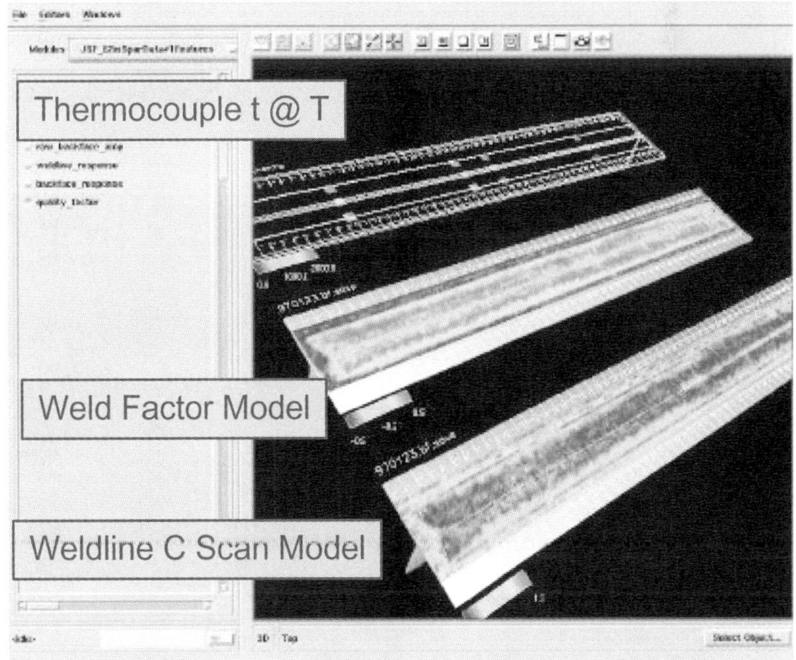

Fig. 43 Induction welding data fusion models of process data and NDE measurements

of the part. Composite configuration and engineering acceptance requirements are used to develop reference standards.

Reference standards can be fabricated in the environmental-controlled areas where normal composite lamination and bonding processes are performed. However, specific methods of inducing or creating known anomalies may require special areas to perform the required operation. Examples would be grinding of metallic and nonmetallic materials, milling of notches, or spraying of specific release agents. No special equipment is normally required to support the fabrication of composite ultrasonic or radiographic reference standards.

Ultrasonic Standards. The basic purpose of the ultrasonic reference standard is to provide the nondestructive inspection/test technician the capability to calibrate ultrasonic detection equipment to known anomalies. Once the selected system has been calibrated, the composite component can be evaluated to determine the internal quality. This determination is made by comparing the values obtained from the component being evaluated with those obtained from the "validated" reference standard. Customer requirements provide the amount of deviation allowed from the reference standard to the actual part values. The reference standard provides the operator with the capability to characterize the detected anomaly by the location, depth, size, and type. This information is then used to evaluate the component for acceptance and rejection.

Ultrasonic reference standards must be designed with as much versatility as possible. The reason is that composite configurations sometimes vary during the manufacturing process. If this occurs, the material thickness may change, bond lines become thicker or thinner, or the void content (porosity) may increase. Therefore, when designing an ultrasonic reference standard, one must ensure that the critical verification points are included in the basic design. Once standards are fabricated, they can sometimes be modified to represent missed or new conditions. Reference standard design, manufacture, and verification information should be accurately documented using written and graphic medium.

Typical methods of fabrication for cured composite laminate reference standards include, but are not limited to, milling flat-bottom holes or notches from the opposite side of the laminate and side-drilled holes into the side of a cure laminate. A typical laminate reference standard configuration containing typical induced defects is shown in Fig. 44. Precure methods of inducing laminate-type defects present a risk factor and should be created by personnel with extensive fabrication experience to ensure success. Duplicate standards are recommended when building precured laminate or adhesive bondline-type standards so that one can be destructively evaluated after verification to ensure that the defect is as intended. The process of inducing material to create between-ply laminate or bondline anomalies requires placing a "foreign" material between two plies or at adhesive bondline. The following materials have been used effectively for this purpose: synthetic fluorine-containing resin-coated fiberglass (0.075 mm, or 0.003 in.), synthetic fluorine-containing resin film, metallic shim stock (copper or stainless steel, 0.25 mm, or 0.010 in.), or precured, single-ply, extremely high-fiber content composite material. When using inserts, the adjacent ply should be cut out to minimize the bump due to inclusion of the induced defect. Metal shim stock works well, if the shim surface is prepared with a release agent.

The design of the reference standard must consider the ultrasonic evaluation method. The primary methods used in industry are PE and TT. Pulse-echo standards are used to perform defect characterizations, such as depth, size, and defect type (i.e., delamination, porosity, unbonds, etc.). Through-transmission standards are not normally designed to determine location. They are designed to identify areas that are later reevaluated using contact PE methods to characterize the defect in accordance with accept/reject criterion. Pulse-echo standards can be fabricated using several of the defect-induction methods mentioned previously. Care needs to be taken when developing PE induced defects. The induced defect must be representative of the defect induced during the manufacturing process. If induced defects are not representative of manufacturing defects, the chance of defects being accepted or good parts being rejected increases. Design and fabrication processes need to take into consideration the need to remove metallic and nonmetallic inserts used to create voids. This choice is normally made by the NDT engineer who has the ultimate responsibility of determining the reference standard design to meet evaluation requirements. Nondestructive testing standard design should be a part of the initial design phase process to ensure inspectability during fabrication and at completion of the product.

Validation of reference standards is a choice normally made by the customer and contractor. The standards should be scanned and the results documented. Signal response and location of each induced and noninduced anomaly must be documented for production inspection/test use of the standard. Confirmation of defect size and location by other methods, such as radiography, should also be considered. Customer specifications or government specifications provide the minimum requirements for signal response. Photographs are an excellent mode of documentation for both initial and destructive evaluations.

Radiographic reference standards are used to evaluate the internal quality of composite components that contain typical anomalies (porosity, cracks, adhesive voids, etc.) and "other" materials, such as honeycomb, metallic components, foam details, foreign material, and water inclusion. Typically, standards are not developed for foreign material, such as Exacto blades, washers, nuts, bolts, and other common items in the fabrication area that are readily recognizable when mistakenly included in a part. Radiographic reference standards are typically designed for various levels of porosity, cracks, nonmetallic inclusions, and honeycomb core defects (crushed, condensed, blown, cut, etc.). The radiographic standard is not used to calibrate the

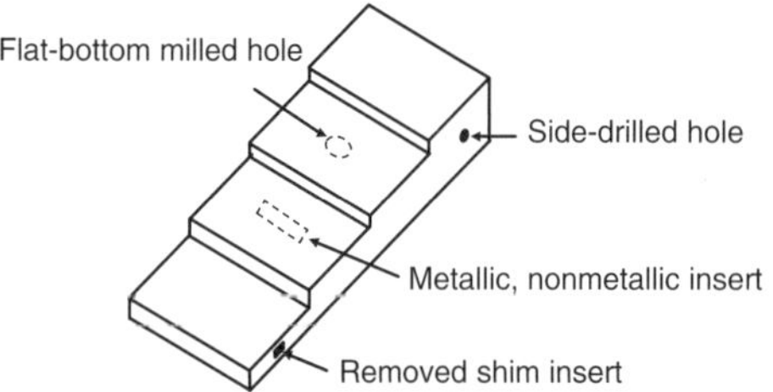

Fig. 44 Typical laminate reference standard configuration containing typical induced defects. Standard configuration should represent the configuration being evaluated and induced defects positioned in accordance with the NDT engineer's direction

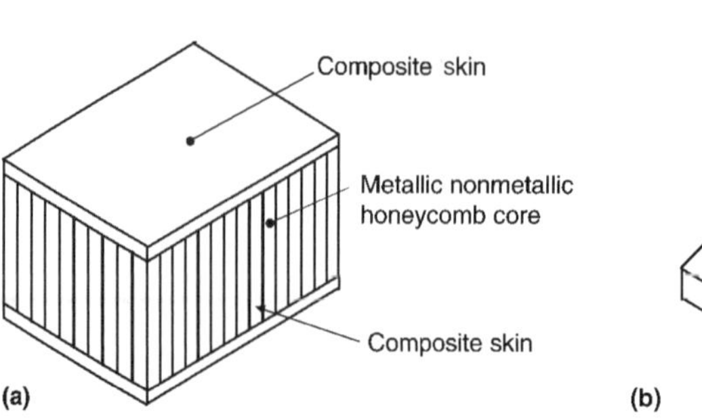

Composite laminate

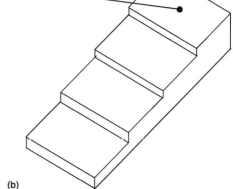

(b)

Fig. 45 Typical radiographic reference standard configurations. (a) Laminate skin honeycomb core sandwich configuration. This configuration also may be used in ultrasonic evaluation. (b) Laminate stepped wedge configuration

x-ray system. These reference standards are used as a post-process comparison to evaluate radiographic images from the composite component and to determine the internal quality. These standards provide the evaluator with a traceable record by which quality decisions can be made and supported. Reference standards are required to provide a uniform evaluation guideline from technician to technician.

Normally, radiographic reference standards are provided by specific sources and customers. Composite laminates typically exhibit porous conditions that are evaluated by comparison-type radiographs. The production radiograph is compared to the reference radiograph to determine the internal quality of the laminate and to determine acceptance. Radiographic standards are also used to evaluate the internal quality of adhesive (film and paste) bondlines for voids, porosity, and inclusions. Foreign material standards containing materials common to the composites fabrication process are normally developed by the manufacturer.

Porosity reference standards are difficult to fabricate repetitively. The major problem is controlling the amount of porosity. These standards can be used for radiographic as well as ultrasonic evaluation.

Composite radiographic reference standards are used to evaluate the internal quality of laminates, encapsulated metallic and nonmetallic details (honeycomb core, phenolic core, machine details, and others), adhesive bondlines, and cocured composite details. Typical honeycomb core defects include condensed core, blown core, node separation, cut core, and crushed core. Other defects characterized by radiographic reference standards include various types of foreign material, bond-line porosity, and laminate porosity. These defects are positioned in accordance with the NDT engineer's direction. Figure 45 shows typical radiographic reference standard configurations.

Nondestructive testing reference standards are fabricated in many configurations to support the verification needs of the customer. The aforementioned examples provide a basic look at those configurations. The NDT and design engineers must coordinate as early as possible in the design phase to ensure that the design is inspectable using identified NDE methods. The documentation of reference standards is critical to the inspection process. Begin this process during the design phase and continue updating as the standard is periodically reevaluated. All NDT standards should be reevaluated periodically to ensure that they continue to provide the correlation established when the standard was approved for use. Standards that do not maintain this correlation must be documented and the area(s) of failure controlled to prevent use. This information should be part of the quality plan.

REFERENCES

1. J. Krautkramer and H. Krautkramer, *Ultrasonic Testing of Materials*, 4th ed., Sringer-Verlog, New York, 1990
2. Y. Bar-Cohen and A.K. Mal, Ultrasonic Inspection, *Nondestructive Evaluation and Quality Control*, Vol 17, *ASM Handbook,* ASM International, 1989
3. Ultrasonic Testing, *Nondestructive Testing Handbook,* 2nd ed., American Society for Nondestructive Testing, 1991
4. E.K. Henneke II, Ultrasonic Nondestructive Evaluation of Advanced Composites, *Non-Destructive Testing of Fibre-Reinforced Plastic Composites*, Vol 2, John Summerscales, Ed., Elsevier Applied Science, New York, 1990, p 55–159
5. J.L. Rose, *Ultrasonic Waves in Solid Media*, Cambridge University Press, Cambridge U.K., 1999
6. Y. Bar-Cohen, NDE of Fiber-Reinforced Composite Material—A Review, *Mater. Eval.*, Vol 44, March 1986, p 446–454
7. J. Strycek and H. Loertscher, "Ultrasonic Air-Coupled Inspection of Advanced Material," 44th International SAMPE Symposium, May 1999 (Long Beach, CA)
8. M. Castaings, P. Cawley, R. Farlow and G. Hayward, Single Sided Inspection of Composite Materials Using Air Coupled Ultrasound, *J. Nondestr. Eval.,* Vol 17 (No. 1), 1998
9. M.C. Bhardwaj, "High Transduction Piezo-electric Transducers and Introduction of Non-Contact Analysis," *Encyclopedia of Smart Materials*, J.A. Harvey, Ed., John Wiley and Sons, NY, due in Oct 2000
10. W.A. Grandia and C.M. Fortunko, "NDE Applications of Air-Coupled Ultrasonic Transducers," 1995 Institute of Electrical and Electronics Engineers Ultrasonics Symposium, Nov 1995 (Seattle, WA)
11. D. Schindel, D. Hutchins, L. Zou, and M. Sayer, The Design and Characterization of Micromachined Air-Coupled Transducers, *Institute of Electrical and Electronics Engineers Trans. Ultrasonics, Ferroelectrics, and Frequency Control*, Vol 42 (No. 1), Jan 1995, p 42–50
12. I. Ladabaum, X.C. Jin, and B.T. Khuri-Yakub, Miniature Drumheads: Microfabricated Ultrasonic Transducers, *Ultrasonics*, Vol 36, 1998, p 25–29
13. B. Khuri-Yakub, Air Coupled Transducers, *Ultrasonic Testing*, Vol 7, *Nondestructive Testing Handbook,* 2nd ed., A.S. Birks and R.E Green, Jr., Ed., American Society for Nondestructive Testing, 1991, p 320–325
14. A.J. Rogovsky, Development and Application of Ultrasonic Dry-Contact and Air-Contact C-Scan Systems for Nondestructive Evaluation of Aerospace Composites, *Mater. Eval.*, Vol 49 (No. 12), Dec 1991, p 1491 1497
15. C.B. Scruby and L.E. Drain, *Laser-Ultrasonics: Techniques and Applications,* Adam Hilger, Bristol, 1990
16. J.-P. Monchalin, *Review of Progress in Quantitative Nondestructive Evaluation,* Vol 12, D.O. Thompson and D.E. Chimenti, Ed., Plenum, New York, 1993, p 495
17. T.E. Drake, Jr., K.R. Yawn, S.Y. Chuang, M.A. Osterkamp, P. Acres, M. Thomas, D. Kaiser, C. Marquardt, B. Filkins, P. Lorraine, K. Martin, and J. Miller, in *Review of Progress in Quantitative Nondestructive Evaluation,* Vol 17, D.O. Thompson and D.E. Chimenti, Ed., Plenum, New York, 1998, p 587
18. J.-P. Monchalin, C. Néron, J.F. Bussière, P. Bouchard, C. Padioleau, R. Héon, M. Choquet, J.-D. Aussel, C. Carnois, P. Roy, G. Durou, and J. Nilson, in *Phys. Can.*, Vol 51, 1995, p 122
19. A.D.W. McKie and R.C. Addison, Jr., *Ultrasonics*, Vol 32, p 507
20. M. Dubois, F. Enguehard, and L. Bertrand, *Phys. Rev. E.*, Vol 50, 1994, p 1548–1541
21. M. Dubois., P. Lorraine, R. Filkins, T.E. Drake, Jr., and K.R. Yawn, in *Review of Progress in Quantitative Nondestructive Evaluation,* Vol 19, D.O. Thompson and D.E. Chimenti, Ed., Plenum, 2000
22. P. Lorraine, M. Dubois, A. Bauco, R. Filkins, T.E. Drake, Jr., and K.R. Yawn, in *Review of Progress in Quantitative Nondestructive Evaluation,* Vol 19, D.O. Thompson and D.E. Chimenti, Ed., Plenum, 2000
23. J.-P. Monchalin, *Institute of Electrical and Electronics Engineers Trans. Ultrason., Ferroelectrics, Freq. Contr.,* UFFC-33, 1986, p 485
24. A. Blouin, P. Delaye, D. Drolet, L.-A. de Montmorillon, J.-C. Launay, G. Roosen, and J.-P. Monchalin, *Nondestructive Characterization of Material VIII*, R.O. Green, Jr., Ed., Plenum Press, New York, 1998, p 13
25. K.R. Yawn, T.E. Drake, Jr., M.A. Osterkamp, S.Y. Chuang, P. Acres, M. Thomas, D. Kaiser, C. Marquardt, B. Filkins, P. Lorraine, K. Martin, and J. Miller, in *Review of Progress in Quantitative Nondestructive Evaluation,* Vol 18, D.O. Thompson and D.E. Chimenti, Ed., Plenum, New York, 1999, p 387
26. D. Fitting and L. Adler, *Ultrasonic Spectral Analysis for Nondestructive Characterization*, Plenum, 1981
27. J. Koenig, J. Tucker, and K. King, "Application of Ultrasonic Spectroscopy to Rocket Motor Composites," JANAF Conf., Oct 1999
28. Y. Bar-Cohen, A. Mal, and S.-S. Lih, NDE of Composite Materials Using Ultrasonic Oblique Insonification, *Mater. Eval.*, Vol 51 (No. 11), 1993, p 1285–1295
29. Y. Bar-Cohen and D.E. Chimenti, Leaky Lamb Waves in Fiber-Reinforced Composite Plates, Vol 3B, *Review of Progress in Quantitative Nondestructive Evaluation*, D.O. Thompson and D.E. Chimenti, Eds., Plenum Press, New York and London, 1984, p 1043–1049

30. P.B. Nagy, W.R. Rose, and L. Adler, A Single Transducer Broadband Technique for Leaky Lamb Wave Detection, *Review of Progress in Quantitative Nondestructive Evaluation*, Vol 6A, 1987, p 483–490
31. A.H. Nayfeh and D.E. Chimenti, Propagation of Guided-Waves in Fluid-Coupled Plates of Fiber-Reinforced Composite, *J. Acoust. Soc. Am.*, Vol 83 (No. 5), May 1988, p 1736–1747
32. A.K. Mal and Y. Bar-Cohen, Ultrasonic Characterization of Composite Laminates, *Proc. Joint American Society of Mechanical Engineers and SE Meeting*, AMD-Vol 90, A.K. Mal and T.C.T. Ting, Eds., American Society of Mechanical Engineers, 1988, p 1–16
33. S.I. Rohklin and W. Wang, Critical Angle Measurement of Elastic Constants in Composite Materials, *J. Acoust. Soc. Am.*, Vol 85, (No. 5), 1989, p 1876–1882
34. V. Dayal, and V.K. Kinra, Leaky Lamb Waves in an Anisotropic Plate. I: An Exact Solution and Experiments," *J. Acoust. Soc. Am.,* Vol 85 (No. 6), 1989, p 2268–2276
35. K. Balasubramanian and J. Rose, Physically Based Dispersion Curve Feature Analysis in the NDE of Composite Materials, *Res. Nondestruct. Eval.*, Vol 3 (No. 1), 1991, p 41–67
36. D.P. Jansen and D.A. Hutchins, Lamb Wave Immersion Topography, *Ultrasonics*, Vol 30, 1992, p 245–254
37. A.K. Mal, Wave Propagation in Layered Composite Laminates under Periodic Surface Loads, *Wave Motion*, Vol 10, 1988, p 257–166
38. J.-H. Shih, A.K. Mal, and M. Vemuri, Plate Wave Characterization of Stiffness Degradation in Composites During Fatigue, *Res. Nondestruct. Eval.*, Vol 10, 1998, p 147–162
39. Y. Bar-Cohen et al. Ultrasonic Testing Applications in Advanced Materials & Processes, *Ultrasonic Testing*, Vol 17, *Nondestructive Testing Handbook*, A. Birks and B. Green, Jr., Ed., American Society for Nondestructive Testing, 1991, p 514–548
40. R.M. Christensen, *Mechanics of Composite Materials*, Wiley, New York 1981
41. A.K. Mal, Y. Bar-Cohen, and S.-S. Lih, Wave Attenuation in Fiber-Reinforced Composites, *Proc. M3D*, V.K. Kinra, Ed., ASTM STP 1169, 1992, p 245–261
42. D.C. Hurley, W.T. Yost, E.S. Boltz, and C.M. Fortunko, A Comparison of Three Techniques to Determine the Nonlinear Ultrasonic Parameter β, Vol 16, *Review of Progress in Quantitative Nondestructive Evaluation*, D.O. Thompson and D.E. Chimenti, Ed., Plenum Press, New York, 1997, p 1383–1390
43. S.U. Fassbender and W. Arnold, Measurement of Adhesion Strength of Bonds Using Nonlinear Acoustics, Vol 15, *Review of Progress in Quantitative Nondestructive Evaluation*, D.O. Thompson and D.E. Chimenti, Ed., Plenum Press, New York, 1996, p 1321–1328
44. T.P. Berndt and R.E. Green, Jr., Feasibility Study of a Nonlinear Ultrasonic Technique to Evaluate Adhesive Bonds, *Nondestructive Characterization of Materials VII*, R.E. Green, Jr., Ed., Plenum Press, New York, 1998, p 125–131
45. M.A. Sutin and D.M. Donskoy, Nonlinear Vibro-Acoustic Nondestructive Testing Technique, *Nondestructive Characterization of Materials VII*, R.E. Green, Jr., Ed., Plenum Press, New York, 1998, p 133–138
46. A. Vary and K.J. Bowles, "Ultrasonic Evaluation of the Strength of Unidirectional Graphite-Polyimide Composites," NASA TM-X-73646, National Aeronautics and Space Administration, 1977
47. A. Vary and K.J. Bowles, "Use of an Ultrasonic-Acoustic Technique for Nondestructive Evaluation of Fiber Composite Strength," NASA TM-73813, National Aeronautics and Space Administration, 1978
48. A. Vary and R.F. Clark, "Correlation of Fiber Composite Tensile Strength with the Ultrasonic Stress Wave Factor," NASA TM-X-78846, National Aeronautics and Space Administration, 1977
49. E.G. Henneke, J.C. Duke, W.W. Stinchcomb, A. Govada, and A. Lemascon, "A Study of the Stress Wave Factor Technique for the Characterization of Composite Materials," Contractor Report 3670, National Aeronautics and Space Administration, Feb 1983
50. A.K. Govada, J.C. Duke, E.G. Henneke, and W.W. Stinchcomb, "A Study of the Stress Wave Factor Technique for the Characterization of Composite Materials," Contractor Report 174870, National Aeronautics and Space Administration, Feb 1985
51. R. Talreja, A. Govada, and E.G. Henneke, Quantitative Assessment of Damage Growth in Graphite Epoxy Laminates by Acousto-Ultrasonic Measurements, Vol 3B, *Review of Progress in Quantitative Nondestructive Evaluation*, D.O. Thompson and D.E. Chimenti, Ed., Plenum Press, 1984, p 1099–1106
52. A. Vary, The Acousto-Ultrasonic Approach, *Acousto Ultrasonic Theory and Application*, John Duke, Ed., Plenum Press, NY, 1988
53. *Radiography and Radiation Testing*, *Nondestructive Testing Handbook,* 2nd ed., American Society for Nondestructive Testing, 1985
54. D. Wysnewski and R. Wysnewski, Computed Radiography, *NDE of Aging Aircraft, Airports, Aerospace Hardware and Materials*, SPIE Vol 2455, T. Cordell and R. Rempt, Ed., 1995, p 125–132
55. E. Anderson, M. Hartney, and R. Weisfield, Amorphous Silicon Imaging System for Improved X-Ray Image Capture in Nondestructive Evaluation, *Process Control and Sensors for Manufacturing*, SPIE Vol 3399, R. Bossi and D. Pepper, Ed., 1998, p 180–187
56. D. Gilbolom, R. Colbeth, M. Batts, and B. Meyer, Real-Time X-Ray Imaging with Flat Panels, *Process Control and Sensors for Manufacturing*, SPIE Vol 3399, R. Bossi and D. Pepper, Ed., 1998, p 213–223
57. P. Soltani, D. Wysnewski, and K. Schwartz, "Amorphous Selenium Direct Radiography for Industrial Imaging," American Society for Nondestructive Testing Fall Conf., 11–15 Oct 1999 (Phoenix, AZ)
58. A.M. Cormack, Representations of a Function by Its Line Integrals, with Some Radiological Applications," *J. Appl. Phys.*, Vol 34 (No. 9), Sept 1963, p 2722–2727
59. A.M. Cormack, Representations of a Function by Its Line Integrals, with Some Radiological Applications, II," *J. Appl. Phys.*, Vol 35 (No. 10), Oct 1964, p 2908–2913
60. G.N. Hounsfield, Computerized Transverse Axial Scanning (Tomography), Part I: Description of System, *Br. J. Rad.*, Vol 46, 1973, p 1016–1022
61. T.H. Newton and D.G. Potts, Ed., *Radiology of the Skull and Brain.* Vol 5, *Technical Aspects of Computed Tomography,* C.V. Mosby, St. Louis, MO, 1981
62. A. Macovski, *Medical Imaging*, Prentice-Hall Inc., 1983
63. A.C. Kak and M. Slaney, *Principles of Computerized Tomographic Imaging*, Institute of Electrical and Electronics Engineers Press, New York, 1987
64. K.D. Friddell, A.R. Lowrey, and B.M. Lemprier, Application of Medical Computed Tomography (CT) Scanners to Advanced Aerospace Composites, Vol 4, *Review of Progress in Quantitative Nondestructive Evaluation*, D.O. Thompson and D.E. Chimenti, Ed., Plenum Press, New York, 1985
65. P. Burstein, R. Mastronardi, and T. Kirshner, Computerized Tomography Inspection of Trident Rocket Motors: A Capability Demonstration, *Mater. Eval.*, Nov 1982, p 40
66. R.A. Armistead, CT: Quantitative 3D Inspection, *Adv. Mater. Process.*, March 1988, p 42–48
67. M.J. Dennis, Industrial Computed Tomography, *Nondestructive Evaluation and Quality Control*, Vol 17, *ASM Handbook,* ASM International, 1989
68. "Standard Guide for Computed Tomography (CT) Imaging," E 1570, *Annual Book of ASTM Standards,* ASTM, 1993
69. D. Copley, J. Eberhard, and G. Mohr, Computed Tomography Part 1: Introduction and Industrial Applications, *J. Mater.*, Jan 1994, p 14–26
70. R.H. Bossi, K.D. Friddell, and A.R. Lowrey, Computed Tomography, *Non-Des-*

ructive Testing of Fibre-Reinforced Plastics Composites, J. Summerscales, Ed., Elsevier Science Publishers, London, 1990

71. R. Bossi, K.K. Cooprider, and G.E. Georgeson, "X-Ray Computed Tomography of Composites," WRDC-TR-90-4014, *Wright Research Development Center*, July 1990
72. L.A. Feldkamp, P.J. Kubinski, and G. Jesion, Application of Magnification to 3D X-Ray Computed Tomography, *Review of Progress in Quantitative Nondestructive Evaluation*, IS-4923, D.O. Thompson and D.E. Chimenti, Ed., Williamsburg, VA, June 1987
73. B.D. Smith, "Cone-Beam Tomography: Recent Advances and a Tutorial Review," *Opt. Eng*., Vol 29 (No. 5), May 1990
74. J.E. Boyd, Limited-Angle Computed Tomography for Sandwich Structures using Data Fusion," *J. Nondestr. Eval.*, Vol 14 (No. 2), p 61–76
75. Perceptics Corporation, "High-Resolution Three-Dimensional Computed Tomography," U.S. Air Force, Wright Laboratory Final Report, WLTR-96-4117, Oct 1996
76. N. Gupta and V. Alreja, "Tangential Scanner for Waste Drum Inspection," American Society for Nondestructive Testing Industrial Computed Tomography Topical Conf., 13–15 May 1996 (Huntville, AL)
77. R.H. Bossi and G.E. Georgeson, Composite Structure Development Decisions Using X-Ray CT Measurements, *Mater. Eval.*, 1995
78. X.P.V. Maldague, *Nondestructive Evaluation of Materials by Infrared Thermography*, Springer-Verlag, 1993
79. V.P. Vavilov, Infrared Techniques for Materials Analysis and Nondestructive Testing, *Infrared Methodology and Technology*, Monograph Series International Advances in NDT, X. Maldague, Ed., Gordon and Breach, U.S., 1994, p 230–309
80. S.M. Shepard and T. Ahmed, Characterization of Active Thermographic System Performance, *Proc. SPIE Thermosense XXI*, Vol 3700, April 1999, p 388–392
81. S.M. Shepard, B Rubadeux, and T. Ahmed, Automated Thermographic Defect Recognition and Measurement, *Nondestructive Characterization of Materials IX, American Institute of Physics Conf. Proc. 497*, R.E. Green, Ed., 1999, p 373–378
82. Y.A. Plotnikov and W.P. Winfree, Visualization of Subsurface Defects in Composites Using a Focal Plane Infrared Camera, *Proc. SPIE Thermosense XXI*, Vol 3700, April 1999, p 26–31
83. P. Cawley, Low Frequency NDT Techniques for the Detection of Disbonds and Delamination, *Br. J. Non-Destr. Test*., Vol 32 (No. 9), Sept 1990, p 455–461
84. A.L. Seidl, Inspection of Composite Structures Part 1, *SAMPE J*., Vol 30 (No. 4), July/Aug 1994, p 38–44
85. P. Cawley, The Sensitivity of the Mechanical Impedance Method on Non-Destructive Testing, *NDT Int.*, Vol 20 (No. 4), Aug 1987, p 209–215
86. R.J. Schliekelmann, Non-Destructive Testing of Bonded Joints; Recent Developments in Testing Systems, *Nondestruct. Test*., Vol 8, 1975, p 100–110
87. C.C.H. Guyor, P. Cawley, and R.D. Adams, The Non-Destructive Testing of Adhesively Bonded Structure: a Review," *J. Adhes*., Vol 20, 1986, p 129–159
88. *Acoustic Emission Testing*, *Nondestructive Testing Handbook,* 2nd ed., American Society for Nondestructive Testing, 1987
89. M.A. Hamstad, A Review: Acoustic Emission, a Tool for Composite Materials Studies, *Exp. Mech.*, Vol 26 (No. 1), March 1986, p 7–13
90. J. Awerbuch, M.R. Gorman, and M. Madhudar, Monitoring Acoustic Emission During Quasi-Static Loading-Unloading Cycles of Filament-Wound Graphite-Epoxy Laminate Coupons, *Mater. Eval.*, Vol 43 (No. 6), 1985, p 754–764
91. E. Hill and T. Lewis, Acoustic Emission Monitoring of a Filament Wound Composite Rocket Motor Case during Hydroproof, *Mater. Eval.,* Vol 43 (No. 7), June 1985, p 859
92. G.L. Workman and C.C. Bryson, "Eddy Current Inspection of Graphite Fiber Components," NASA Technical Memorandum, NASA TM-103514, Oct 1990
93. S.N. Vernon and P.M Gammell, Eddy Current Inspection of Broken Fiber Flaws in Non-Metallic Fiber Composites, Vol 4B, *Review of Progress in Quantitative Nondestructive Evaluation*, Plenum Press, 1985, p 1229–1237
94. X.E. Gros, "Eddy Current Inspection of Composite Materials," NDT Summary Report from Eurocopter Collaboration, 1994
95. J.D. Jackson, *Classical Electrodynamics*, John Wiley and Sons, New York, 1962
96. G.E. Georgeson, B.M. Lempriere, E. Normand, and S.A. Galt, "Eddy Current Techniques," Inders Phase IV Final Report, D180-32000-1, Contract NAS9-16960, Dec 1989
97. X.E. Gros, Review of NDT Techniques for Detection of Low Energy Impacts in Carbon Reinforcements, *SAMPE J*., Vol 31 (No.2), March/April 1995
98. D.W. Lowden, X.E. Gros, and P. Strachan, Visualising Defect Geometry in Composite Materials, *Proc. Internat. Symp. Advanced Materials for Lightweight Structures*, European Space Research and Technology Centre (ESTEC) (Noordwijk, The Netherlands), 1994
99. P. Cielo, Optical Techniques for Nondestructive Testing: A Critical Review, *Int. Adv. Nondestr. Test*., Vol 12, 1986, p 231–350
100. J.W. Newman, "Inspection of Aircraft Structure with Advanced Shearography," presented at the American Society of Nondestructive Testing Fall Conf., Oct 1990
101. C. Bohn, Shearographic Nondestructive Inspection on the B-2 Program, *Nondestructive Evaluation of Aging Aircraft, Airports, Aerospace Hardware, and Materials, Proc. SPIE,* Vol 2455, 1995, p 218–225
102. H.M. Shang, S.L. Toh, F.S. Chau, V.P.W. Shim, and C.J. Tay, Location and Sizing Disbonds in Glassfibre-Reinforced Plastic Plates Using Shearography, *J. Eng. Mater. Technol*., Vol 113, Jan 1991, p 99–103
103. X.E. Gros, *NDT Data Fusion*, John Wiley, New York, 1997
104. R. Bossi and J. Nelson, Data Fusion for Process Monitoring and NDE," *Nondestructive Evaluation for Process Control in Manufacturing*, Proc. SPIE 2948, R. Bossi and T. Moran, Ed., 1996, p 62–71
105. X.E. Gros, J. Bousigue, and K. Takahashi, NDT Data Fusion at the Pixel Level, *Nondestruct. Test. Eval. Int*., Vol 32 (No. 5), July 1999, p 283–292
106. A. Dromingny-Badin, S. Rossatu, and Y.M. Zhu, Radioscopic and Ultrasonic Data Fusion via the Evidence Theory, *Trait. Signal*, Vol 14 (No. 5), 1997, p 499–510
107. J. Nelson, D. Cruikshank, and S. Galt, A Flexible Methodology for Analysis of Multiple Modality NDE Data, Vol 8A, *Review of Progress in Quantitative Nondestructive Evaluation*, 1989, p 819–826
108. R. Bossi and J. Nelson, NDE Data Fusion, *43rd International SAMPE Symposium and Exhibition,* H.S. Kliger, B.M. Rasmussen, L.A. Pilato, and T.B. Tolle, Ed., Society for the Advancement of Material and Process Engineering, Vol 1, 1998, p 489–497
109. G.E. Georgeson, B.M. Lempriere, and J.E. Shrader, "Integrated Nondestructive Evaluation Data Reduction System (INDERS)," JANAF, Silver Springs, MD, Oct 1989

Quality Assurance of Metal-Matrix Composites

William C. Harrigan, Jr., MMC Engineering, Inc.

QUALITY ASSURANCE of metal-matrix composites (MMCs) is similar to that of polymer-matrix composites (PMCs) in that the matrix and reinforcements need to be inspected and characterized prior to the manufacture of the composite, and the completed composite must also be inspected and characterized (see preceding articles in this Section for detailed information on quality assurance methods used for PMCs). Also, many of the techniques (and the exisiting infrastructure) used to assure the quality of monolithic-matrix alloys (e.g., aluminum alloys) can be used for particle-reinforced MMCs. This article describes characterization techniques, mechanical tests, and nondestructive evaluation methods commonly used for MMCs.

Characterization Techniques

For particle-reinforced aluminum composites, the reinforcements are characterized for chemical composition and particle size distribution. The matrix alloys are analyzed to ensure they are appropriate for the alloy and incoming form. Casting alloys are analyzed as ingots by spectrochemical techniques (Ref 1). Powder metallurgy alloys are characterized for particle size distribution and chemically analyzed by spectrographic methods for the melt or by inductively coupled plasma (ICP) methods (Ref 2) for the powder.

Composites manufactured from these components must also be chemically analyzed by appropriate methods. Composites containing silicon carbide cannot be analyzed by spectrographic methods due to the silicon signal coming from the reinforcement. The most reliable method is the ICP method. Since the ICP method involves dissolving the sample, a volume fraction analysis can be conducted on the same sample (Ref 3). The chemistry of the alloys and the microstructure of the resulting part control, to a large extent, the mechanical and physical properties of these alloys. The addition of the fine ceramic particles to the matrix alloy results in the maintenance of a fine microstructure. The ceramic particles act as grain nucleation sites for castings and as grain boundary pins in wrought alloys.

Ceramic particle reinforcements are single-crystal or polycrystalline particles that have well-defined physical and mechanical properties. The performance of the particles in the matrix is dictated by the particle shape and size distribution. Several methods are used for measuring the size distributions for particles in the 1 to 100 μm size range. Several of the common methods for particle size analysis are listed in Table 1 (Ref 4).

One method uses a laser to pass a light beam through a suspension of particles. Dispersing the particles in a liquid, such as water, produces a suspension. The analysis is conducted by passing the light beam through the suspension. An alternate method is to disperse the particles in air and pass the suspension through the laser beam. The diffraction pattern that is produced by the interaction of the laser beam with the suspension is analyzed to determine the size distribution of the particles in the suspension. This analysis method produces a measure of the actual size of the particles. Other methods, such as the Coulter counter, using electrical resistivity, present data for a calculated diameter for a spherical particle with the same volume that was detected by the instrument. For spherical or near-spherical particles, these two analysis methods result in similar particle size distributions. However, for irregular particles, these two methods differ in the size that they present. For an irregular particle with dimensions 2.5 by 1 by 2 μm, the laser scattering device will report a particle size of 2.5 μm while an electrical resistivity device will report a particle size of 2.12 μm. A plot of the spherical equivalent diameter for particles with fixed dimensional relationships of 2.5 to 2 to 1 is shown in Fig. 1. In applications where an absolute maximum size, such as 30 μm, is needed, a laser measurement will result in a particle size of 30 μm while a spherical equivalent device will measure only 25.5 μm. For some applications, these differences are very important, and one must understand the values presented by a given analysis technique.

Commercially available silicon carbide, alumina, and boron carbide powders are measured by techniques defined in the British Abrasive Federation standard FEPA 42-GB-1984 (Ref 5). Typical particle size distributions for silicon carbide powders classified as F400, F600, and F800 are shown in Fig. 2. These powders will be blended with aluminum alloy powders to create a metal-matrix composite. The size of the ceramic reinforcement must be compatible with that of the matrix in order for mixing to occur. The particle size distribution for a commercially available 6061 aluminum powder is also shown in Fig. 2. These powders have compatible size distributions and are typically used for production of aluminum-matrix composites. Submicron-sized ceramic particles have presented problems in blending with commercial matrix powders.

The appropriate size of ceramic particles for composites made by molten processing is influenced by several factors. Silicon carbide can react with molten aluminum to form aluminum

Table 1 Typical methods of particle size and size distribution measurement

Measuring principle	Method	Approximate useful size range, μm
Mechanical or ultrasonic agitation	Sieving	5–125 mm
Microscopy	Optical	0.5–100
	Electron	0.001–50
Electrical resistivity	Coulter counter	0.5–800
	Electrozone	0.1–2000
Sedimentation	Sedigraph	0.1–100
	Roller air analyzer	5–40
	Micromerograph	2–300
Light scattering	Microtrac	2–100
Light obscuration	HIAC particle counter (Pacific Scientific Instruments)	1–9000
Permeability	Fisher subsieve sizer	0.2–50
Surface area	Gas adsorption (BET)	0.01–20

BET, Brunauer-Emmett-Teller. Source: Ref 4

carbide and free silicon. Aluminum carbide is a very brittle phase that renders the composite unusable. In order to reduce the chances for the formation of this undesirable phase, particles with a minimum surface area are desirable. This leads to the use of larger particles. The strain-to-failure and strength of the composite has been found to be a function of the particle size. Each reinforcement has a critical particle size above which the probability of having a critical flaw increases markedly. For commercial silicon carbide and alumina particles, this size is approximately 20 μm. Composites made with reinforcements above the critical size tend to have low strain-to-failure and low strength. This limits the maximum size for the manufacture of structural aluminum-matrix composites. For cast composites it is important to know the relationships between strength, strain-at-failure, and reactivity as a function of particle size. It is also important to monitor the microstructure of these composites during processing in order to avoid or control reactions. The metallographic practices for these composites require standard practice (Ref 6), with care taken to polish the mount in a manner appropriate for a soft metal with hard particles in it.

Additional information about particle characterization techniques can be found in *Powder Metal Technologies and Applications,* Volume 7 of *ASM Handbook.* More information about characterization techniques, in general, for a broad range of materials is available in *Materials Characterization,* Volume 10 of *ASM Handbook.*

Mechanical Testing

Mechanical testing of wrought or cast composites can be done using appropriate metallic material test procedures. A list of relevant tests and associated standards is given in Table 2. Tensile testing is done with reduced-section specimens as defined in ASTM B 557 (Ref 8). The machining of samples should be done with diamond tools. The use of carbide or coated steel tools has been unsuccessful since these tools are dulled by the ceramic particles in the composite. Dull or worn tools result in torn surfaces or surfaces with highly disturbed metal. These surfaces result in widely variable mechanical properties. The same comments are appropriate for fatigue samples. A good example of consistent fatigue test results is the $R = -1$ tests (where R is the ratio of minimum stress to maximum stress) done on a 6090/SiC/25p composite by DWA Aluminum Composites Inc. in an Air Force Title III test program. Samples for this study were not hourglass shape, but had a con-

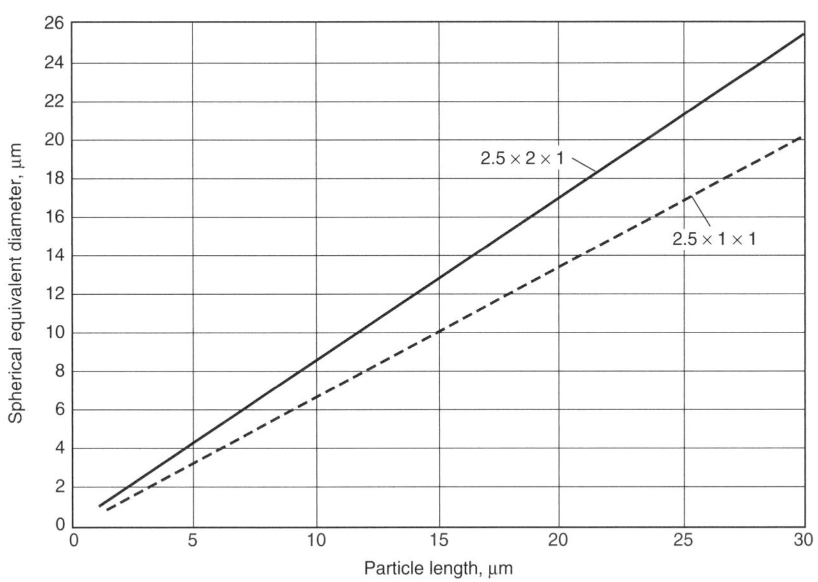

Fig. 1 Plot of spherical equivalent diameter as a function of maximum particle dimension for an irregular particle with relative dimensions of 2.5 to 2 to 1

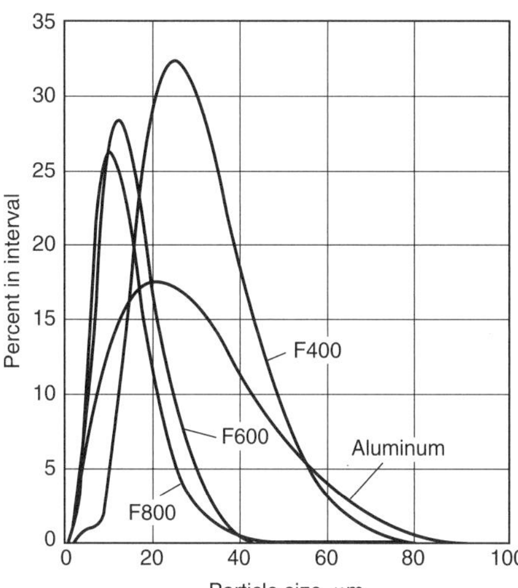

Fig. 2 Particle size distribution for F400-, F600-, and F800-grit silicon carbide particles and commercial 6061 aluminum powder

Table 2 Mechanical test specifications for aluminum-matrix composites

Property	Specification	Sample	Special considerations
Tensile strength	ASTM E 8 (Ref 7), ASTM B 557 (Ref 8)	Reduced section, round or rectangle	Similar to aluminum
Elastic modulus	ASTM E 111 (Ref 9)	Reduced section, round or rectangle	Similar to aluminum
	Ultrasonic velocity	Round or rectangular section	Similar to aluminum
Compression strength	ASTM E 9 (Ref 10)	Rectangle or cylindrical, constant section	Similar to aluminum
Fracture toughness	ASTM E 399 (Ref 11)	Compact tension	Precrack difficult due to non-straight crack front
	ASTM E 1304 (Ref 12)	Subsize samples	Valid due to low ratio of plane-strain fracture toughness to yield strength
Fatigue	ASTM E 466 (Ref 13)	Hourglass, reduced section	Polish test section with scratches in test direction
Shear	ASTM B 769 (Ref 14)	Rectangular sheet samples	Similar to aluminum
Pin bearing	ASTM E 238 (Ref 15)	Sheet with high-quality drilled holes	Hole quality must meet specification, pin strength must be high enough for composite

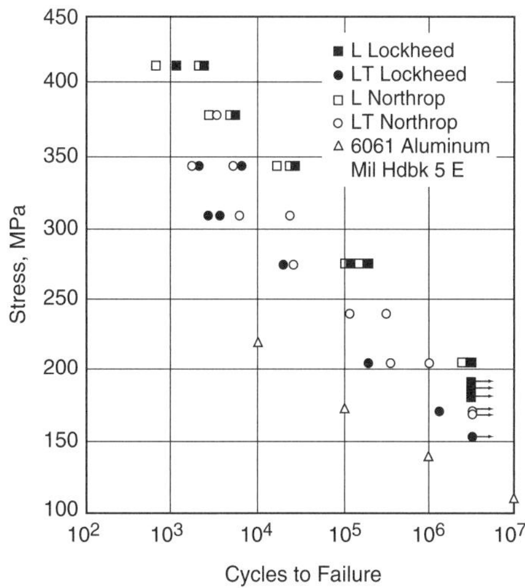

Fig. 3 Fully reversed ($R = -1$) fatigue test data for 6090/SiC/25p-T6P composite

stant gage section diameter of 5.1 mm (0.20 in.) diameter and were 25 mm (1 in.) long. The samples were accurately machined with diamond tools and tested at two laboratories, Northrop Aviation and Lockheed Aeronautical Systems. The data from this study are presented in Fig. 3. The uniformity of these data from two laboratories demonstrates the value of careful machining to ensure reproducible data.

The elastic modulus is an important attribute of these composites. The measurement of the modulus can be achieved by methods described in ASTM E 111 (Ref 9). Ultrasonic velocity measurements and resonant frequency measurements have also been used to determine the elastic modulus. By using appropriate ultrasonic transducers, the longitudinal and shear sound velocities can be measured. The Young's modulus and shear modulus can be calculated from the relationship:

$$E = 4\rho V_S^2 \left[\frac{3/4 - (V_S / V_L)^2}{1 - (V_S / V_L)^2} \right]$$

$$\gamma = \rho V_S^2$$

where E is Young's modulus, γ is shear modulus, V_L is longitudinal sound velocity, V_S is shear wave sound velocity, and ρ is density.

More detailed information about mechanical testing methods and data analysis is available in *Mechanical Testing and Evaluation,* Volume 8 of *ASM Handbook.*

Nondestructive Evaluation

Nondestructive assessment methods that have been successfully applied to particulate-reinforced aluminum composites are listed in Table 3. Ultrasonic techniques have been very successful in assessing the blending quality present in these composites. A paper by Shannon et al. (Ref 22) describes the ultrasonic inspection of large (349 mm, or 13.7 in. diam) billets containing 25 vol% silicon carbide in a 6000 series aluminum alloy. A through-diameter edge scan is shown in Fig. 4, and a through-thickness axial scan is shown in Fig. 5. The billet volume containing several of the indications found in this inspection were removed from the billet for microstructural examination. A small indication located at point "G" in Fig. 5 was one of the cut sections. A low-magnification optical micrograph from this area, Fig. 6, shows a localized high volume fraction of silicon carbide. A higher-magnification scanning electron micrograph, Fig. 7, demonstrates that this region contains silicon carbide particles with little or no matrix aluminum. The size of this matrix-starved region is on the order of 30 μm. This demonstrates that the ultrasonic test method is capable of detecting very small regions of poor blending.

Other test techniques that are appropriate for aluminum alloys have also been shown to be appropriate for particulate-reinforced aluminum composites. These methods and the appropriate test standards are listed in Table 3. Eddy currents measure electrical conductivity and can be calibrated to assess matrix alloy as well as volume fraction of the reinforcement. Holography techniques that employ stressing the component and

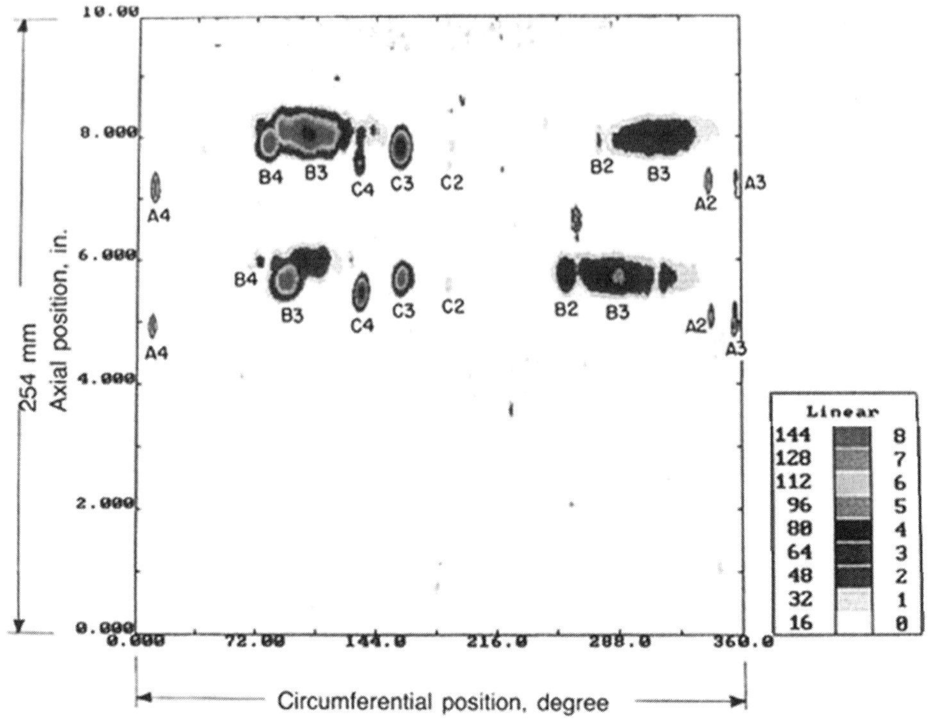

Fig. 4 Circumferential ultrasonic C-scan using 5 MHz transducer from the circumference of a 6090/SiC/25p billet

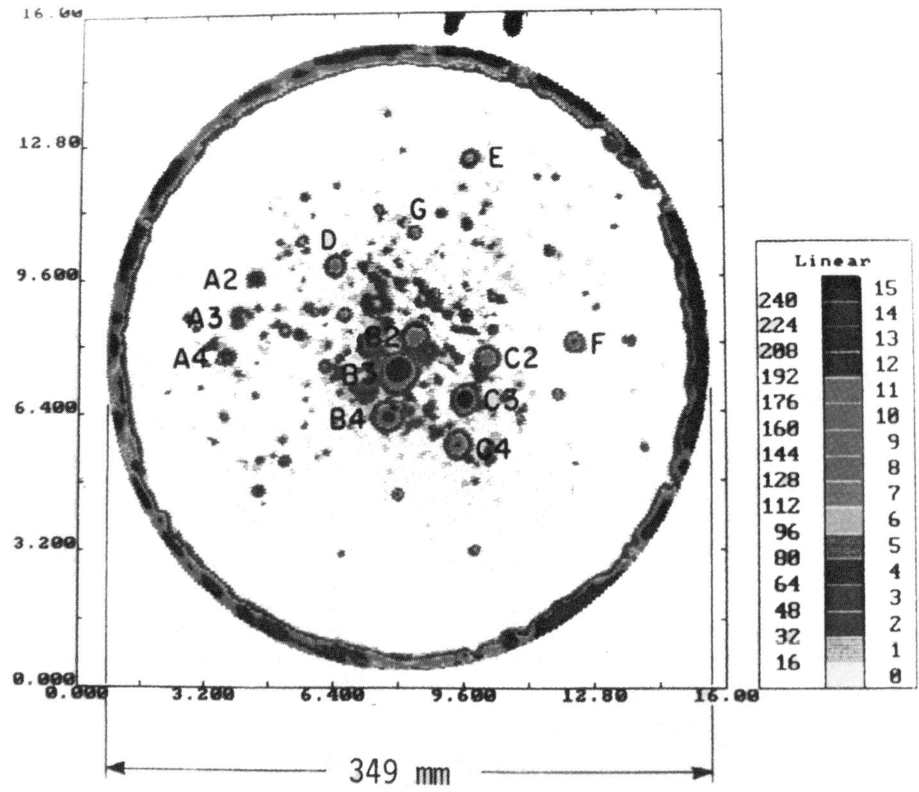

Fig. 5 Axial ultrasonic C-scan using 5 MHz transducer from the top of a 6090/SiC/25p billet

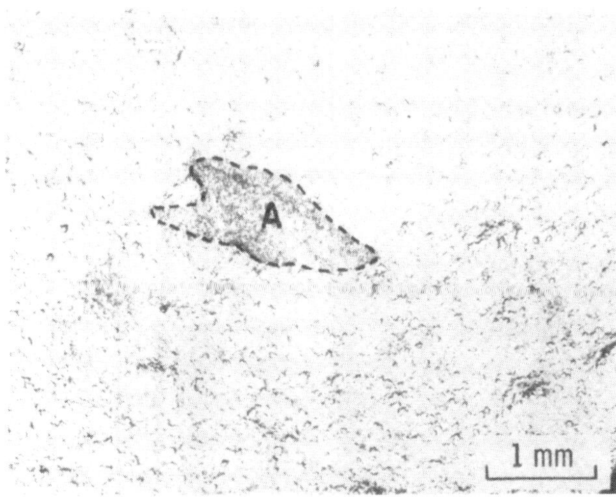

Fig. 6 Optical micrograph of a section cut from the 6090/SiC/25p billet at location G in Fig. 5

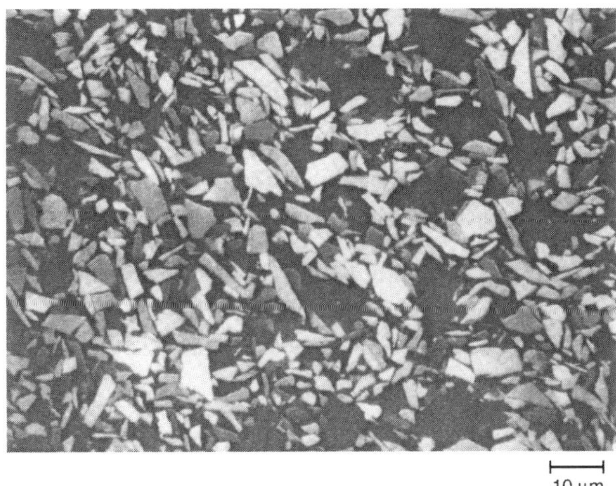

Fig. 7 Scanning electron micrograph of section "A" of Fig. 6 showing a small area of matrix-free silicon carbide particles

Table 3 Quality assurance techniques for aluminum-matrix composites

Type	Test methods	Comments
Ultrasonic	C-scan and velocity, ASTM E 1001 (Ref 16), ASTM E 127 (Ref 17)	Similar to aluminum; C-scan very sensitive to mixing
Eddy current	ASTM E 215 (Ref 18)	Similar to aluminum; sensitive to matrix alloy and volume percent
Optical methods	Holography	Appears to be effective for some shapes
Electrical conductivity	...	Similar to aluminum
Hardness	ASTM E 18 (Ref 19)	Similar to aluminum
X-ray	ASTM E 1030 (Ref 20)	Similar to aluminum
Liquid penetrant	ASTM E 165 (Ref 21)	Similar to aluminum

Source: Ref 22

calibrating a response appear to be useful in some shapes made with composites. The change in electrical conductivity during the age process of the matrix alloy can be used to track the age condition of these composites. Similarly, the change in hardness with heat treatment can be useful in assessing the heat treatment of these composites. X-ray inspection of these composites will yield results similar to that found in the unreinforced aluminum-matrix alloy. The x-ray cross section of silicon carbide is similar to aluminum and no contrast will be expected for localized areas of high volume fraction. The x-ray cross section for boron carbide may be sufficient for detection of mixing anomalies, however, appropriate standards must be provided for correct interpretation. Liquid penetrant inspection has been successfully applied to these composites. The addition of the ceramics to the aluminum matrix does not alter the performance of standard penetrants.

Information about nondestructive testing of PMCs is provided in the article "Nondestructive Testing" in this Volume. Additional information about nondestructive testing is available in *Nondestructive Evaluation and Quality Control,* Volume 17 of *ASM Handbook.*

REFERENCES

1. "Standard Test Method for Optical Emission Spectrometric Analysis of Aluminum and Aluminum Alloys by the Point-to-Plane Technique," E 227, *Annual Book of ASTM Standards,* ASTM
2. "Standard Test Methods for Chemical Analysis of Aluminum and Aluminum-Base Alloys," E 34, *Annual Book of ASTM Standards,* ASTM
3. "Standard Test Method for Fiber Content by Digestion of Reinforced Metal Matrix Composites," D 3553, *Annual Book of ASTM Standards,* ASTM
4. R.G. Iacocca, Particle Size and Size Distribution, *Powder Metal Technologies and Applications,* Vol 7, *ASM Handbook,* ASM International, 1998, p 234
5. "Standard for Bonded Abrasive Grains of Fused Alumina and Silicon Carbide," FEPA 42-GB-1984, The British Abrasive Federation, P. O. Box 58, Trafford Road, Trafford Park, Manchester M17 1JD, Great Britain
6. "Standard Practice for Preparation of Metallographic Specimens," E 3, *Annual Book of ASTM Standards,* ASTM
7. "Standard Test Methods for Tension Testing of Metallic Materials," E 8 (E 8M Metric), *Annual Book of ASTM Standards,* ASTM
8. "Standard Test Methods of Tension Testing Wrought and Cast Aluminum- and Magnesium-Alloy Products," B 557, *Annual Book of ASTM Standards,* ASTM
9. "Standard Test Method for Young's Modulus, Tangent Modulus, and Chord Modulus," E 111, *Annual Book of ASTM Standards,* ASTM
10. "Standard Test Method for Compression Testing of Metallic Materials at Room Temperature," E 9, *Annual Book of ASTM Standards,* ASTM
11. "Standard Test Method for Plane-Strain Fracture Toughness of Metallic Materials," E 399, *Annual Book of ASTM Standards,* ASTM
12. "Standard Test Method for Plane-Strain (Chevron-Notch) Fracture Toughness of Metallic Materials," E 1304, *Annual Book of ASTM Standards,* ASTM
13. "Standard Practice for Conducting Force Controlled Constant Amplitude Axial Fatigue Tests of Metallic Materials," E 466, *Annual Book of ASTM Standards,* ASTM
14. "Standard Test Method for Shear Testing of Aluminum Alloys," B 769, *Annual Book of ASTM Standards,* ASTM
15. "Standard Test Method for Pin-Type Bearing Test of Metallic Materials," E 238, *Annual Book of ASTM Standards,* ASTM
16. "Standard Practice for Detection and Evaluation of Discontinuities by the Immersed Pulse-Echo Ultrasonic Method Using Longitudinal Waves," E 1001, *Annual Book of ASTM Standards,* ASTM
17. "Standard Practice for Fabricating and Checking Aluminum Alloy Ultrasonic Stan-

dard Reference Blocks," E 127, *Annual Book of ASTM Standards*, ASTM
18. "Standard Practice for Standardizing Equipment for Electromagnetic Examination of Seamless Aluminum-Alloy Tube," E 215, *Annual Book of ASTM Standards*, ASTM
19. "Standard Test Methods for Rockwell Hardness and Rockwell Superficial Hardness of Metallic Materials," E 18, *Annual Book of ASTM Standards*, ASTM
20. "Standard Test Method for Radiographic Examination of Metallic Castings," E 1030, *Annual Book of ASTM Standards*, ASTM
21. "Standard Test Method for Liquid Penetrant Examination," E 165, *Annual Book of ASTM Standards*, ASTM
22. R.E. Shannon, P.K. Liaw, and W.C. Harrigan, Jr., Nondestructive Evaluation for Large-Scale Metal-Matrix Composite Billet Processing, *Met. Trans. A*, 23, 1541, May 1992

Introduction to Testing and Certification

Richard E. Fields, Lockheed Martin Missiles and Fire Control

ENGINEERS commonly want to predict the *future* performance of a material (or structure) using a property determined by measuring the test response of a current *or* past sample of the material (or structure), but it can be difficult to understand how to obtain reliable test data. The definitive resource for testing and certification of advanced composites is the multivolume U.S. Department of Defense (DoD) *Composite Materials Handbook,* Military Handbook 17 (MIL-HDBK-17). The Handbook is constantly being updated. Print copies of released versions are available through the DoD Single Stock Point (Philadelphia, PA) or from Technomic Publishing Company (Lancaster, PA). Released and working versions are publicly available on the Internet at http://www.mil17.org.

MIL-HDBK-17 was initiated in the 1950s to provide design data for plastics and glass-reinforced plastics. In 1988 the scope was updated to focus only on polymeric composites, and then in the mid-1990s was extended to metal matrix and ceramic matrix composites. MIL-HDBK-17 is now a multivolume set that describes in rigorous detail the aerospace industry consensus approaches for the testing and use of composite material data in structural applications. While MIL-HDBK-17 continues to be reviewed and distributed by the U.S. DoD, support has recently increased to include civil authorities such as the U.S. Federal Aviation Administration, other regions of the world such as Europe, Canada, South America, and Japan, and even nonaerospace industries and applications.

While MIL-HDBK-17 was developed with a focus on aerospace primary structure, its philosophies can be adapted to less critical aerospace structures as well as nonaerospace applications in other industries such as marine, ground transportation, and civil infrastructure.

The mammoth size of MIL-HDBK-17 illustrates the complexity of the subject. Further, the size and complexity are barriers to many that would benefit from MIL-HDBK-17. Despite ongoing efforts to improve the readability of MIL-HDBK-17, a competent engineer can still have trouble understanding enough content to follow its intent.

Section on Testing and Certification

In this Section, the content of the testing and certification philosophies of MIL-HDBK-17 Volume 1 are distilled down to the most important concepts, written by a number of the contributors to MIL-HDBK-17. In a condensed and hopefully more readable format this Section covers the basics of what to test, how to test, and how many to test to obtain specific properties of common advanced composite materials. MIL-HDBK-17 prefers the full-consensus standard test methods developed by ASTM Committee D-30 on Composite Materials, and so the discussions on test methods focus on ASTM standards, where they are available.

This Section begins by reviewing some important general concepts, then addresses more specific concerns and provides coverage of testing concepts for each major topical area. The Section includes the following articles:

Article	Topics addressed
Overview of Testing and Certification	The significance of certification The MIL-HDBK-17 "building-block" approach to testing Test result correlation, basic statistics, property normalization, and basic design allowables
Test Program Planning	Potential testing problem areas Test method selection Common and developing testing standards Test matrix planning and population sampling Factors that affect test results and design values Factors that affect schedule and cost of testing programs
Constituent Materials Testing	Standard test methods and testing issues for common properties of composite prepreg, fibers, and matrices
Lamina and Laminate Nonmechanical Testing	Standard test methods and testing issues for physical, thermal, and moisture properties of advanced composites
Lamina and Laminate Mechanical Testing	Standard test methods and testing issues for strength and modulus testing of lamina/laminate forms, including tests for tension, compression, shear, fracture, and fatigue
Element and Subcomponent Testing	Why element and subcomponent tests are performed Standard test methods and testing issues
Full-Scale Structural Testing	Why full-scale tests are performed Test methods and testing issues Results correlation

For additional details and more direct guidance on the application of these concepts in practice, the reader can refer to the relevant sections of MIL-HDBK-17.

Testing and Certification

Chairperson: Richard E. Fields, Lockheed Martin Missiles and Fire Control

Overview of Testing and Certification

Richard E. Fields, Lockheed Martin Missiles and Fire Control

COMPOSITES are complex engineered materials that often behave differently than common isotropic materials. As a result, the testing of composites remains something of an art rather than a science. Before testing a composite material, or before ordering or supervising such testing, the responsible party should first review the following considerations, each of which is covered in more detail in the following sections of this article:

- The differences between testing of composites and testing of isotropic materials
- The role of certification agencies and the importance of their early involvement
- The building-block approach to composites testing
- Determining the purpose of testing
- The need to normalize results, where feasible
- The use and application of basic statistics
- Other factors that influence design allowables

Related subjects are discussed in the next article in this Section, "Test Program Planning," which is followed by additional articles on specific types of tests.

Differences Between Testing of Composites and Testing of Isotropic Materials

The physics of composites testing may appear to be similar to the physics of testing isotropic materials, but the differences are significant (Ref 1). Laboratories that are expert and experienced at testing other materials are *not* automatically qualified to achieve good results when testing composites. Why is the testing of advanced composites so different, and often so difficult? The reasons include the following.

Material Anisotropy. The properties of a test sample made of composite materials are often significantly different in different directions; consequently, special testing methods may be required. For example, uniaxial mechanical tests never produce a pure uniaxial stress state throughout an entire test specimen; three-dimensional stresses always exist at discontinuities and loading points. The combination of multiaxial stresses and low strengths in directions other than the test direction can result in premature or erratic failure, which lowers the mean and increases scatter in the data. Careful attention to both test specimen design and testing practices are often required to overcome this problem. While the example mentioned previously is a mechanical test, similar difficulties can be experienced when testing other properties, such as in thermal or electrical testing.

Complicated and Nonintuitive Failure Modes. A correctly executed test for a strength- or fracture-based property should produce an expected failure mode, but multiple failure modes are possible in some tests, and some failure modes are not unique to correctly executed tests. Some failure modes can be so explosive (such as uniaxial tension strength) that they disguise potential testing or specimen preparation problems and provide few clues to test acceptability. Other failure modes (compression) are often ambiguous, with physical appearance of the failure being similar for both correctly and incorrectly run tests.

Unintentional Inhomogeneity. Many (though not all) isotropic materials are created as bulk material and then later formed into the end product. However, most composites are consolidated into the final materials form at the same time that the end product is produced. This can introduce additional process variation into the basic material. For example, local fiber volume changes are common, especially at part edges and in radii. Fiber orientation changes are another example of unintentional inhomogeneity—for example, the nominal 90° angle between warp and fill yarns of an orthogonal fabric can change drastically as the fabric is spread over a complex contoured surface.

Environmental Sensitivity of a Constituent. Many of the constituents of composite materials are sensitive to environmental conditions that do not affect many competing materials, such as metals. This is especially true of moisture in the case of polymer-matrix composites and organic-fiber composites, such as those that use aramid fiber.

Developing Nature of Composites Testing. While there have been a number of testing advancements and considerable progress toward consensus standards, the field of composites testing and certification is still maturing. Test methods are being developed that are less sensitive to some of the issues presented here, but more development is required to perfect the existing test methods. New materials systems, analysis methods, and structural applications continue to require new developments in test methods, test configurations, testing matrices, and data reduction approaches. If the reader is new to composites testing, he or she should seek help from or the advice of someone who has previous experience in composites testing.

Involvement of Certification Agencies

If a property is used to verify system capabilities, *especially* when human safety is involved, testing usually becomes an integral part of a process that is commonly called certification. The engineering of certain critical structures typically follows a specific approval process under the authority of an organization other than the designer. The approving organization can be the end user (especially in the case of a military application, where the process might be called *qualification*) or a government regulatory agency, in the case of publicly regulated structures. (An example of very stringent requirements for certification is seen in the U. S. Federal Aviation Administration requirements for design or modification of passenger-carrying aircraft.) Since both *certification* and *qualification* are also used with other specific meanings, MIL-HDBK-17 (Ref 2) has recently begun using the term "structural substantiation" to mean the generic process of validating the integrity of a structure, regardless of the agency in charge.

Certification requirements exist in many other industries, although often under a different name and certainly with different rules. In the United States, railroad equipment must meet Federal Railway Administration requirements, automotive equipment must meet Department of Transportation/National Highway Transportation Safety Administration requirements, pressure vessels must meet the codes of the American Society of Mechanical Engineers, civil engineering structures must meet their respective codes, and so on. However, in industries where design with composites is not yet common, composites applications are not always specifically addressed in certification requirements.

When a structure is developed that requires certification, the preapproval of the certification agency should be sought for the design database (or the plan for creating it, if design data does not exist) and the analysis and testing process. Even so, before committing to a specific process, the entire process should be understood. For example, there are parts of the MIL-HDBK-17 statistical flowchart that remain, at this writing, at least partially open-ended. This means that if the test results fail certain statistical tests and if it was agreed upon to literally follow MIL-HDBK-17 statistics to the letter, substantially more testing than was originally planned may ultimately be required in order to satisfy the flowchart. This can be disastrous to both cost and schedule, so it is advisable to both clearly understand the full process as well as to fully define—perhaps with sampling limits or alternative statistical methods—how to deal with statistical decision points.

Understanding the Building-Block Approach

The same factors that often make composites difficult to test, combined with the lack of validated and widely applicable standard analytical methods, result in distrust of structural substantiation by analysis alone. A specific combination of analysis and testing is most often used, with test results providing input to the analyses as well as confirming the analyses. This is called the *building-block approach* to design development testing, so named because it starts with large numbers of simple, focused tests and, in each succeeding level, builds on the level below with fewer, but more-complicated tests. The building-block approach is discussed in detail in Chapter 2 of MIL-HDBK-17 Volume 1.

The pyramid of Fig. 1 illustrates the building-block concept. At the lowest levels, the basic materials properties are determined using large quantities of test specimens, and multibatch population scatter is estimated. At each succeeding level, progressively more-complicated structures are built and tested, and the failure mode and load are predicted by analysis based on the lower-level data. When more data are obtained, the structural analysis models are refined as needed to agree with the test results. As the test structures become more complex, the number of replicates (repeated specimens of the same type and environment) and the number of environments are reduced. The culmination of the building-block pyramid is often a single confirming test of a full-scale component or a full-scale structural assembly.

Upper-level (especially full-scale) tests are not always performed at the worst-case design environment. Data from the lower levels of the building-block approach can be used to establish environmental compensation values to be applied to the loads of higher-level room-temperature tests. Similarly, other lower-level building-block tests determine truncation approaches for fatigue spectra and compensation for fatigue scatter at the full-scale level. The building-block approach can be summarized in the following steps:

- Procure and process materials to a specification that includes controls on constituent, prepreg, and lamina/laminate physical properties.
- Determine multibatch materials properties at the lamina and/or laminate level, and calculate the statistical basis values and preliminary design allowables.
- Based on the design/analysis of the structure, select critical areas and design features for subsequent test verification.
- For each design feature, determine the load/environment combination that is expected to produce a given failure mode with the lowest margin. Special attention should be given to matrix-sensitive failure modes (such as compression, out-of-plane shear, and bond lines) and potential "hot spots" caused by out-of-plane loads or stiffness-tailored designs.
- Design and test a series of test specimens, each of which simulates a single selected failure mode and load/environment condition. Compare test results to previous analytical predictions and adjust analysis models or design properties as necessary.
- Conduct increasingly more-complicated tests that evaluate more-complicated loading situations with the possibility of failure from several potential failure modes. Compare to analytical predictions and adjust analysis models as necessary.
- Conduct, as required, full-scale component (or assembly) static and fatigue testing for final validation of internal loads and structural integrity. Compare to analysis.

Building-Block Levels

Early in the test-planning process, decisions must be made about which building-block levels to test and the relative importance of each level in comparison to the other levels. Factors in these decisions include: manufacturing process, structural application, corporate/organizational practices, and/or the procurement or certification agency. While testing a single level of the building-block may suffice in rare instances (e.g., some noncritical, filament-wound applications subjected only to tensile loading), most applications will require at least two building-block levels, and it is very common to use three or more levels.

Coupon Tests. This class of testing can be further subdivided into the levels of constituent, lamina, and laminate testing.

Constituent testing evaluates the individual properties of fibers, fiber forms, matrix materi-

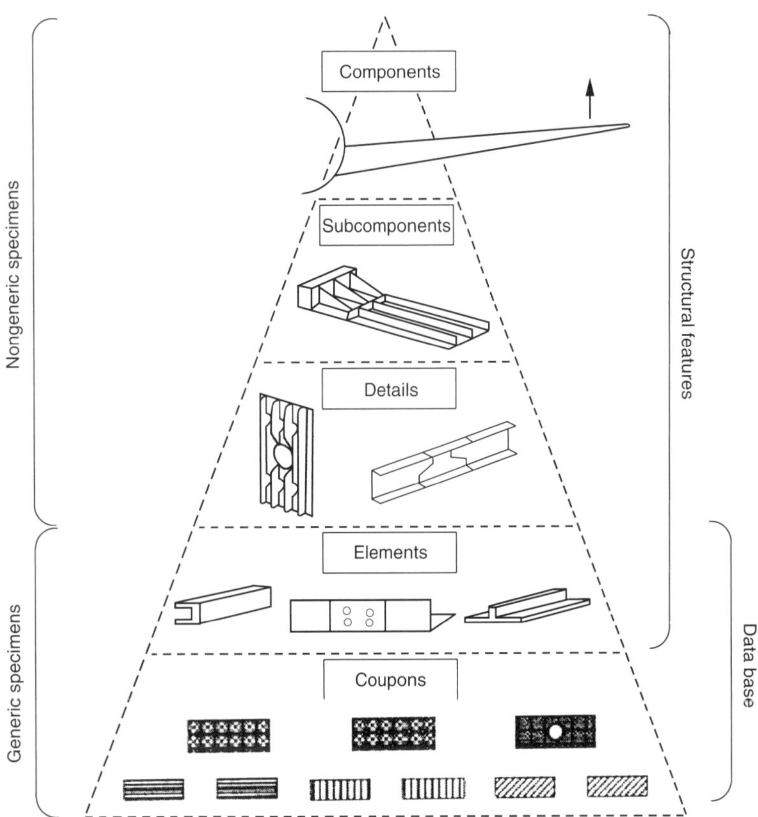

Fig. 1 The building-block pyramid for testing of composites

als, and fiber-matrix preforms. Key properties of both matrix and reinforcement include density, tensile strength, and tensile modulus. Most constituent tests are conducted using ASTM standardized test methods.

Lamina testing determines the properties of the fiber and matrix together in the composite materials form. Prepreg properties are included in this level, although they are sometimes included in the constituent level or even broken out into a separate level. Key properties include fiber areal weight, matrix content, void content, cured ply thickness, lamina tensile strengths and moduli, lamina compression strengths and moduli, and lamina shear strengths and moduli. Interlaminar fracture toughness is often tested at this level, but may also be tested at the laminate level. Depending on the design/analysis philosophy, the lamina level may be the primary source of structural design data, or the data may mostly be used for analysis confirmation and correlation and specification support. Most lamina tests are conducted using ASTM standardized test methods.

Laminate testing characterizes the response of the composite material in a given laminate orientation design. It is sometimes combined with lamina testing due to test method similarities. Key properties include laminate tensile strengths and moduli, laminate compression strengths and moduli, laminate shear strengths and moduli, interlaminar fracture toughness, and fatigue resistance. Depending on the design/analysis philosophy, this level may focus on confirming the ability of analysis methods to predict response from the lamina properties, or it may be the primary source of the design data. Most laminate tests are conducted using ASTM standardized test methods.

Structural Feature Tests. This class of testing can be further subdivided into the levels of structural element, detail, subcomponent, and component/full-scale testing.

Structural Element Testing. This level evaluates the abilities of the material to tolerate common laminate discontinuities and of analysis tools to predict the response(s). Key properties include open- and filled-hole tensile strength, open- and filled-hole compression strength, compression-after-impact strength, and joint-bearing and bearing-bypass strengths. Some of these properties may have full statistical test samples at all major environments; other properties may use truncated samples and/or environments. ASTM has standardized the simplest of these tests (with others being considered for standardization at the time of this writing), while some of the more-complicated tests may be application specific.

Detail Level Testing. More-complicated generic discontinuities are evaluated in special *structural detail* specimens that are designed to mimic many of the behaviors of complicated structural configurations that produce three-dimensional stress states. None of these tests are standardized as of 2001, but within an industry or within the engineering organization of a particular manufacturer, some quasi-standard test configurations may be common.

Subcomponent Level Testing. At the next level, the emphasis begins to shift from focusing on single failure modes to evaluation of the general structural response. A subcomponent test article may be an actual production hardware piece, or it may be a special design piece that includes a number of generic features of the typical subcomponents of concern. These test configurations are strictly application dependent.

Component/Full-Scale Level Testing. The highest level looks at the behavior and failure mode of increasingly more-complex structural assemblies. It typically uses the data from the lower levels of the building-block pyramid to simplify testing loads and/or environments. The details of these tests are application specific and are not specifically covered by MIL-HDBK-17.

Determining the Purposes of Testing

In addition to grouping material property tests by building-block level, collections of material property test data can be grouped by purpose into the five categories of screening, qualification, acceptance, equivalence, and structural substantiation. MIL-HDBK-17 calls these "data application categories."

Screening Data. The purpose of screening testing is initial evaluation of new material systems under worst-case environmental and loading test conditions. The MIL-HDBK-17 Volume 1, Chapter 2 screening test matrix results in small-sample mean values for various strengths, moduli, and physical properties and includes key properties at both lamina and laminate levels. It is designed to both eliminate deficient material systems from the material selection process and to reveal promising new material systems before planning subsequent, more in-depth evaluations.

Material Qualification Data. This collection of tests defines the requirements necessary for a material to meet a procurement specification. Ideally, material qualification testing is a subset of, or directly related to, the design allowables testing performed to satisfy structural substantiation requirements. The objective is quantitative statistics for key material properties. The resulting statistics are used in establishing material acceptance, equivalence, quality control, and design basis values. At the time of this writing, MIL-HDBK-17 does not yet fully define this testing, however, there are recommended guidelines that should be considered and requirements on those portions of the data that will be used for design allowables.

Acceptance Data. These tests are normally a subset of material qualification. They serve to verify material consistency by periodic sampling of material product and evaluation of key material properties. Test results from small sample sizes are statistically compared with control values established from prior testing to determine whether or not the material production process has changed significantly.

Equivalence Data. This testing category assesses the equivalence of an alternate material to a previously characterized material, usually for the purpose of using an existing design property database. In general, the alternate material is substantially the same as the known material, but may have minor process changes to the raw material or minor changes in the final end-object process due to processing at a different site by different equipment and operators. Key properties are tested in quantities large enough to provide an engineering conclusion, but small enough for significant cost savings (if equivalence is shown) as compared to generating an entirely new, self-sufficient database.

Structural Substantiation Data. These are all data used in the engineering assessment of the ability of a given structure to meet the requirements of a specific application. The development of design allowables, ideally derived or related to statistical data obtained during a material qualification task, is a subset of this category.

Data Normalization

Most composite material properties are dependent on the relative proportion of reinforcement and matrix that make up the composite material. If the specimens in a test sample have somewhat different proportions of the composite constituents, statistical conclusions about test results for some properties may not be entirely valid. *Normalization* is a post-test data adjustment process that seeks to eliminate unrealistic artificial variation in certain measured properties caused by local changes in constituent content. The details of the process of adjusting fiber-dominated results to a reference fiber volume (or, via a related procedure, a reference ply thickness) are summarized here and described in more detail in MIL-HDBK-17 Volume 1, Chapter 2.

In an oriented-fiber composite, a portion of the variation of a property value is simply due to locally changing fiber volume rather than variation in fiber, matrix, or fiber-matrix interface properties. For many processes, the fiber content is relatively fixed and the variation in fiber volume is due to locally greater or lesser amounts of matrix. Fiber volume can change enough to affect test results—even for the same nominal material—certainly between batches, commonly between panels of the same batch, and even between specimens within the same panel.

For many composites properties measured in the direction parallel to reinforcing fiber ("fiber-dominated properties"), the relation between property and fiber volume is essentially linear. This makes possible a procedure for adjusting raw test values so that the normalized values appear to have resulted from specimens at the same fiber volume content (or, via a related procedure, at the same ply thickness). The following sections discuss the theory, methodology, and practical application of this type of normalization. (The properties of other types of composites, such as randomly oriented, discontinuously reinforced composites, are also dependent on constituent content, but their property-constituent relationships are more complicated, and normalization procedures for these have not been widely adopted as of 2001.)

Normalization Theory. Composites properties that are dominated by the properties of the reinforcing fiber are dependent on the volumetric proportion (expressed either as a fraction or as a percentage) of fiber in the laminate. In the common "rule of mixtures" model, 0° tensile strength of a unidirectional laminate, for example, is assumed equal to the matrix tensile strength at 0% fiber volume and equal to the fiber tow tensile strength at 100% fiber volume:

$$F = V_f F_f + (1 - V_f) F_m \qquad \text{(Eq 1)}$$

where F is strength of the composite, F_f is strength of the fiber tow, F_m is strength of the matrix, and V_f is the fiber volume fraction.

The fiber volume fraction fiber is the same as the area fraction of fiber in the specimen cross section. Neglecting the effects of matrix starvation at high-fiber contents, the relationship between fiber volume and laminate ultimate tensile strength is therefore assumed to be linear for all proportions of fiber and matrix between 0 and 100% in this model. Given that the typical fiber properties are more than an order of magnitude higher than the matrix properties (less true for MMCs and CMCs), a common assumption is that the matrix properties are negligible compared to the fiber properties. With this assumption, the model relationship simplifies further to:

$$F = V_f F_f \qquad \text{(Eq 2)}$$

The model for elastic modulus follows the same behavior.

To apply this to laminate normalization, consider two laminates made from the same amount of the same fiber, but with slightly different fiber volumes (due to a slight difference in matrix content, which is manifested by a slight difference in thickness). Therefore $F_1 \neq F_2$, and a relationship exists that can adjust fiber-dominated properties between two different fiber volumes:

$$F_f = \frac{F_1}{V_{f1}} = \frac{F_2}{V_{f2}} \qquad \text{(Eq 3)}$$

Normalization Methodologies. Given the basic simplified theory above, a number of variants can be developed for practical application.

Direct Approach. One obvious method of application is to determine, post-test, the actual fiber volume of each test specimen by an appropriate test method and to adjust the raw data values by the ratio of the common fiber volume fraction to the measured values, as shown:

$$F_n = F \times \frac{V_{fn}}{V_f} \qquad \text{(Eq 4)}$$

where F_n is strength of composite, normalized; F is strength of composite, actual/measured; V_{fn} is fiber volume fraction, normalization value; and V_f is fiber volume fraction, actual.

This direct approach has a significant limitation. For large sample sizes, it is very expensive and generally impractical to accurately and directly measure fiber volume for each individual test specimen. Normally, only representative pieces from each test panel are used to estimate the typical panel fiber volume, and the within-panel matrix content (and fiber volume) variation is not directly assessed.

Cured Ply Thickness (CPT) Approach. Another method of data normalization employs the relationship between fiber volume and laminate CPT and requires some further derivation. Composites are commonly composed of three constituents: fiber, matrix, and (usually unintentionally) void. For such a composite with a given void and fiber content, laminate fiber volume is entirely dependent upon matrix content. This means that panel thickness (and hence CPT) is also dependent only upon matrix content. From this it can be shown that, for constant fiber areal weight, CPT is solely dependent upon fiber volume fraction. This dependency permits normalization of each individual test specimen by its ply thickness (total thickness divided by number of plies).

To create a useful working equation, start by defining the theoretical equivalent thickness of fiber that would result if the fiber could be shaped into a solid sheet of uniform thickness with no matrix or voids:

$$h_f = \frac{\text{FAW}}{\rho_f} \qquad \text{(Eq 5)}$$

where (when using consistent units) h_f is the equivalent thickness of solid fiber material in one ply, FAW is the fiber areal weight of one ply, and ρ_f is the density of fiber.

The fiber volume fraction for the ply (and the laminate, because it is assumed here that all plies are the same type) is this theoretical fiber thickness divided by the overall ply thickness (and this relationship applies to both the actual laminate and the normalizing laminate):

$$V_f = \frac{h_f}{\text{CPT}} \qquad \text{(Eq 6a)}$$

and

$$V_{fn} = \frac{h_{fn}}{\text{CPT}_n} \qquad \text{(Eq 6b)}$$

Substituting Eq 5 for h_f, yields:

$$V_f = \frac{\text{FAW}}{\text{CPT} \times \rho_f} \qquad \text{(Eq 7a)}$$

and

$$V_{fn} = \frac{\text{FAW}_n}{\text{CPT}_n \times \rho_f} \qquad \text{(Eq 7b)}$$

And then inserting these into the direct approach, Eq 4, results in a useful normalization equation in terms of FAW and CPT:

$$F_n = F \times \frac{\text{FAW}_n}{\text{FAW}} \times \frac{\text{CPT}}{\text{CPT}_n} \qquad \text{(Eq 8)}$$

To express Eq 8 in terms of normalized fiber volume rather than CPT, substituting Eq 7(b) back into Eq 8 (or, alternately, not inserting it in the first place) results in:

$$F_n = F \times \frac{\text{FAW}_n}{\text{FAW}} \times \frac{\text{CPT}}{\text{FAW}_n} \times V_{fn} \times \rho_f \qquad \text{(Eq 9)}$$

or

$$F_n = F \times \frac{\text{CPT} \times \rho_f}{\text{FAW}} \times V_{fn} \qquad \text{(Eq 10)}$$

One common view is that FAW variation should not be included in statistical variation, because FAW variation is commonly limited in the materials specification by physical tolerances. This view holds that if FAW variation is to be included in the data results, then it is best done as a uniform adjustment after data analysis, rather than additional variation. However, others may require that FAW variation be included in the data scatter, with the view that this variation is "real" and therefore should be considered in the data. (The author will not attempt to harmonize these two different views.) To include FAW variation in the data scatter, eliminate the first ratio of Eq 8 from the normalization, resulting in the simplest form of CPT normalization:

$$F_n = F \times \frac{\text{CPT}}{\text{CPT}_n} \qquad \text{(Eq 11)}$$

Compare Eq 11 to Eq 4 and note that CPT and fiber volume are inversely related, as confirmed by Eq 7(a) and (b).

Other normalization forms based on these same physics can be derived for special purposes.

Practical Application Notes. The FAW is assumed to be the actual fiber areal weight for each individual specimen, but, like fiber volume, this measurement is not made on a specimen basis. However, since FAW does not usually vary greatly within a batch of material, the batch average (or roll average, if available) FAW is generally sufficient for normalization. In the case of laminates made by resin transfer molding or other nonprepreg processes, lot or roll average areal weights for the fabric or preform would be used.

The derivations mentioned previously assume a consistent set of units. In actual practice, FAW is commonly reported in grams per square meter (g/m^2) and fiber density in grams per cubic centimeters (g/cm^3) or megagrams per cubic meter (Mg/m^3), while ply thickness is commonly reported in millimeters or inches. To use common, but inconsistent units, the appropriate conversion factors must be added to the equations.

As stated earlier, void content affects fiber volume. If porosity is "added" to a laminate without changing the absolute amounts of fiber or matrix, the thickness will increase and the fiber volume will decrease. However, for a given FAW, the change in fiber volume will be the same regardless of the source of a thickness change (matrix content change or void content change). Thus, when normalizing with these equations, there is no need to make any adjustment for void volume. (This assumes, of course, that the void content is not so large or localized that basic load-carrying capability is reduced.)

Common practice is to normalize fiber-dominated lamina and laminate strengths (both unnotched and notched) and moduli for laminates fabricated from tapes, fabrics, and rovings. Although fiber volume does affect, to a lesser extent, various matrix-dominated properties (in-plane and interlaminar shear, for example), as of 2001 there is no widely accepted normalization model for these effects, and such properties are not normalized by MIL-HDBK-17. In MIL-HDBK-17, normalized values for all mechanical strength and stiffness properties are presented except: 90° (transverse) tension and compression properties of unidirectional laminates, interlaminar tension and shear properties, in-plane shear properties, short beam strength, bearing and bearing-bypass properties, strain energy release rate, and Poisson's ratio.

Laminates fabricated from rovings and similar forms using a winding process present a unique situation relative to normalization. Such constructions do not have plies in the usual sense: the wound "ply" thickness depends upon tow band width, wind spacing, and tow spread during winding. Since nominal ply thickness and FAW are not directly applicable, normalization by ply thickness and FAW is not possible. Test data for these materials must be normalized using the direct approach based on the panel average fiber volume.

When fiber-dominated properties are normalized, data scatter should decrease compared to the un-normalized values, because variability due to fiber volume fraction differences is being reduced. Thus, coefficients of variation should be lower after normalization. However, this is not always observed, and there are a number of reasons why the reduction in scatter expected from normalization is not invariably realized:

- If measured CPT is close to the normalizing thickness and FAW is close to nominal, correction factors will be small and may be nearly the same magnitude as errors in measuring these quantities.
- Compression strength generally increases as fiber volume increases (over a practical range of fiber volume), but compression failure does not result in a "strength" in the same sense as tensile strength—compression failure is a form of buckling. The linear normalization model is sometimes inconsistent for compression strength, though it tracks well with compression modulus.
- Poor testing practices or badly prepared test specimens will cause premature failures. Inconsistent failures will result in erratic normalization results. (But such testing problems should be corrected anyway.)
- If the coefficient of variation is already small (less than 3%, for example), further reduction in variation as a result of normalization should not be expected, because this level of variability is about the minimum usually observed for most composites properties.

Lack of change in data scatter after normalization is usually not a cause for concern. However, if data scatter increases significantly after normalization, the reason should be investigated, because a testing problem may be the cause.

Statistical Data Reduction

Virtually all engineers have had at least some exposure to basic statistics, so this article does not concentrate on the science (any decent statistics textbook will take care of those details) but on specific engineering application of statistics to composite materials (and structure) properties. This article goes into depth on this topic, because understanding the basics of what will be done with the data is critical to understanding issues in planning and execution of testing.

A series of property tests of a given type, evaluated on what is nominally the same material, will normally yield slightly different results from each test. This isn't a surprise, because materials properties are expected to have some inherent variation that is manifested by a range of test results. The greater the number of tests, the greater the confidence that the test data reasonably represents the larger population of all possible outcomes.

One test result gives a minimum indication. Two or three test results confirm (hopefully) that the first test result was not an anomaly and begin to qualitatively indicate the variation in the data. However, it takes a far larger amount of data to give any reasonably accurate quantitative estimate of the variation. Exactly how much data are required is an engineering trade-off between the number of assumptions, the level of confidence required for a given need, and the cost associated with obtaining large amounts of data. Some issues of sampling versus statistics are briefly discussed subsequently and in more detail in MIL-HDBK-17.

One would like statistical data reduction to be straightforward and easy, but in actual practice, of course, this is often not the case. Some of the more significant problems include:

- Variation in data can come from a number of other sources (Ref 2). This added variation in the data distorts our view of the property. The actual property may best fit one statistical distribution, but with added external variation, the test data may best fit a different (incorrect) distribution. It is hard to tell from the data itself if this is a problem; one must look at the physical test evidence and monitor the testing closely to discern indications of problems that create external variation. In some cases this requires extensive training, experience, and direct observation of the testing in question.
- The test sample may not reflect the broader current/future population that is being characterized. This may be due to a defect in sampling; for example, material may have been sampled that has a different distribution from the nominal material, or it may be due to future changes in the properties of the broader material resulting from some change or loss of control in the process that creates the material. The MIL-HDBK-17 attempts to address the first issue by requiring multibatch sampling. The second issue is one of materials specification control; while the details of it are beyond the scope of this article, the message is that the specification must properly control the material via key characteristics of the process, materials result, or both.

Given a set of results from valid testing, one can make some statistical assumptions, apply some basic (or advanced) math, and arrive at common quantities that describe the properties of the test data variation, such as (for the normal distribution) the *sample mean*, $\bar{x}$, and *sample standard deviation, s*. These are called point estimates of the exact, but unknown, values of mean and standard deviation of the total population. Other important statistics are the *basis values*, which are interval estimates of a given percentile of the total population. The first two terms are well defined in any basic statistics book, but basis value requires further explanation, given subsequently.

Basis Value. A basis value is an estimate of a given percentile value of a materials property. There are two commonly used basis values, *A*-basis and *B*-basis, illustrated in the example shown in Fig. 2. Figure 2 shows a normal (Gaussian) probability density curve, which is familiar as the "bell-shaped" curve. (Other probability curves, such as the Weibull distribution, can and are used to improve fit to test data, but this article focuses on the common normal distribution for these examples.) The normal probability density curve is an exponential function:

$$f(x) = \frac{1}{\sigma\sqrt{2\pi}} e^{-\frac{1}{2}\left(\frac{x-\mu}{\sigma}\right)^2}$$

The example shows a normal probability density curve for a sample of unspecified test data with sample mean, $\bar{x}$, of 100, and sample standard deviation, *s*, of 8 (coefficient of variation of 8%). The sample mean of this distribution is the *x*-axis value at the center of the distribution. Dashed vertical lines drawn on either side of the mean show ± 1 sample standard deviation. The area under the curve between any two *x*-axis values is the probability that a test result will fall between those two values.

Despite agreement on the general definitions, *as of 2001, there is not universal agreement* on the specific details of the sampling methods or data reduction procedures for calculating basis values. A number of different sampling and statistical data reduction methods are in use by different organizations. In particular, the approach selected for composites by the MIL-HDBK-17 (Ref 2) committee is distinctly different from that selected for metals by the MIL-HDBK-5 (Ref 3) committee.

10th/1st Percentile Values. Those points where 90 and 99%, respectively, of the total population have a greater value than the percentile value are defined as 10th/1st percentile values. Looking at the example, if the sample accurately reflected the total population, the dark vertical dashed line at the *x*-axis value of 89.74 shows the 10th percentile value, and the similar line at a value of 81.39 shows the 1st percentile value. The areas under the curve to the right of each line equal 0.90 and 0.99, respectively. Correspondingly, 10 and 1%, respectively, of the total population have lower values, and the areas under the curve to the left of each line equal 0.10 and 0.01, respectively. With a 10th percentile value, it is expected that 10% of the total population will be below it. Likewise, with a 1st percentile value, it is expected that 1% of the population will be below it.

***B*-Basis Value.** This is a type of 10th percentile value, but it is not *the* 10th percentile value. The *B*-basis is a conservative estimate of the 10th percentile value, given that it cannot be trusted that the limited test data are completely representative of the broader population. The B-basis value in the example, for a small sample size of 18, is 84.2 and considerably lower than the theoretical 10th percentile value of 89.74.

The 10th percentile value for the sample equals the *B*-basis value only when the sample exactly mirrors the broad population; but this would be a poor assumption, especially with a small number of replicates. With limited data, one can't be sure of the true 10th percentile value, so a conservative estimate of the 10th percentile value is used instead.

The *B*-basis value is a *lower bound estimate* of the 10th percentile value, and thus the *B-basis value is almost always lower than the actual 10th percentile value*. Common aerospace design practice for *B*-basis is a 95% confidence estimate of the 10th percentile, which means 95 times out of 100 the *B*-basis will be at or below the true 10th percentile. Put another way, in only 5 times out of 100 will the *B*-basis estimate be above the true 10th percentile.

B-basis strengths are commonly used in design allowables for structures where it is tolerable that 10% of the material might have lower strengths. These structures might include those with any one of, or combination of, the following: conservative design factors, high margins, structural redundancy, and noncritical structure.

***A*-Basis Value.** Similarly to the *B*-basis value, the *A*-basis value is a type of 1st percentile value, but it is not *the* 1st percentile value. The *A*-basis value is a conservative estimate of the 1st percentile value, given that it cannot be trusted that limited test data completely represent the broader population, and is commonly given as a 95% confidence estimate. The *A*-basis value in the example, for a small sample size of 18, is 73.0 and considerably lower than the theoretical 10th percentile value of 81.39.

A-basis strengths are commonly used when deriving design allowables for critical structures, such as aerospace primary or flight-critical nonredundant structure, where there must be little chance of the materials strength being lower than the basis value. The possibility that 1% of the material might have a lower value is tolerable, given other conservatisms in engineering calculations.

***S*-Basis Value.** In addition to the previous two basis values, there is a third "basis" value that, as of 2001, isn't guaranteed to be a statistical value at all. The *S-basis* value is a specification minimum value that, in general, has no statistical basis. Note that recent changes to MIL-HDBK-5 are attempting to apply some rigor to this definition by steering users toward a small sample, normal distribution, 99-percentile estimate, which is normally lower than an *A*-basis from the larger sample that MIL-HDBK-5 requires. However, this is not yet an industry-wide practice, has not yet been adopted by MIL-HDBK-17 for composites, and historical *S*-basis values in existing specifications may have been determined by a different method.

Effect of Sample Size on Basis Values. As has been repeated several times, the more test data one has, the greater the confidence that the test data reflect the total population. The result of this greater confidence is that the basis value comes closer to the percentile value for the population, meaning that the basis value increases. A larger basis value is desirable in strength-critical designs, but there is a trade-off between the costs of the additional testing needed to increase the sample size and the increase in usable design strength. Figure 3 illustrates how the *B*-basis value increases as a function of sample size for three different coefficients of variation (CV). Very small samples (<10) take a huge "hit" in basis value, compared to the sample mean, with basis values for 9% CV at less than one-half of

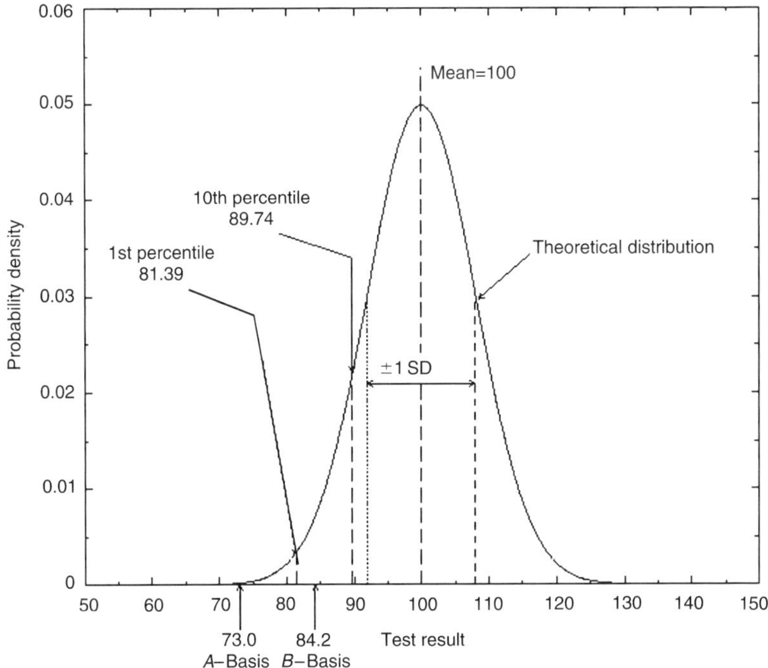

Fig. 2 Example of test results showing basis values for the normal distribution. Normal distribution (n) = 18; mean = 100; standard deviation (SD) = 8

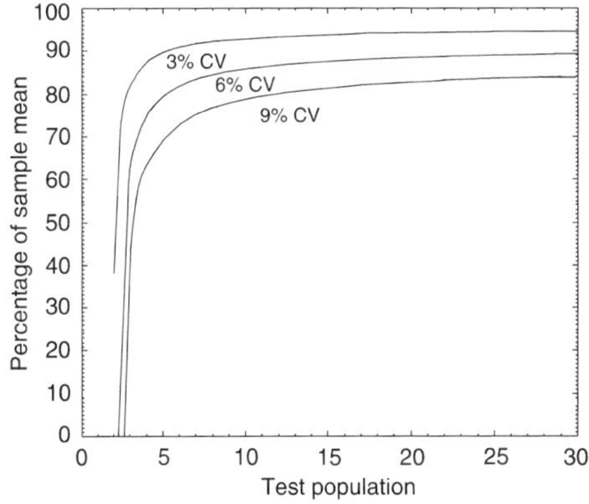

Fig. 3 Example showing how sample size influences *B*-basis values for the normal distribution. CV, coefficient of variation

the mean for a sample size of 3. (Meaningful assessment of test scatter doesn't exist at this sample size.) However, at sample sizes of 18 or more, basis values level off and there is little increase in the basis value for larger sample sizes (although the sample may better reflect the total population).

While testing matrices and related topics on statistics are discussed further in the next major Section, additional details on sampling requirements and calculation methods for *A*-basis and *B*-basis values for composites can be found in Volume 1 of MIL-HDBK-17, Chapter 8 on statistical methods.

ACKNOWLEDGMENTS

The author would like to acknowledge the contributions to this chapter from *The Composite Materials Handbook* Committee; ASTM Committee D-30 on Composite Materials; his employer, Lockheed Martin Missiles and Fire Control–Orlando, which supported his efforts in writing this article and organizing and editing this Section; and particularly, Mr. John Adelmann of Sikorsky Aircraft, his former co-chair in the MIL-HDBK-17 PMC Testing Working Group and source of much of the subsection on normalization.

REFERENCES

1. R.E. Fields, Improving Test Methods for Composites, *ASTM Standardization News,* Oct 1993, p 38–43
2. *Composite Materials Handbook,* MIL-HDBK-17, Vol 1, *Polymer Matrix Composites: Guidelines for Characterization of Structural Materials,* http://www.mil17.org/, a U.S. DOD Military Standardization Handbook
3. MIL-HDBK-5, *Metallic Materials and Elements for Aerospace Structures,* a U.S. DOD Military Standardization Handbook

Test Program Planning

Carl Rousseau, Bell Helicopter

ALL SIGNIFICANT TESTING PROGRAMS should begin with preparation of a detailed test plan document. A test plan specifies material properties to be evaluated, selects test methods, eliminates options offered by standard test methods by selecting specific specimen and test configurations, and defines success criteria. It is prepared by the contractor, approved by the certifying agency, and is the focal point for understanding between the contractor and certifying agency. A clearly written, well-prepared test plan is also a primary management tool used to define the scope of the work, degree of success, and progress toward completion.

Regulatory requirements/guidance and past experience provide starting points for test plan preparation. At minimum, data are required to provide quality control of the material being procured. These data serve as a statistical basis for procurement specification minima and/or acceptance testing conformity. Subsequent levels of the building block process (see Fig. 1 in the article "Overview of Testing and Certification" in this Section) are required for design allowable data, programmatic risk reduction, and analytical model validation. Specific requirements for these intermediate-to-high level building blocks vary widely with application and industry, but once the need for a specific level of testing is identified, a test matrix for those tests must be developed and included in the test plan. Typical types of composite test matrices are shown in Table 1.

This article discusses a number of testing objectives that affect the execution of testing programs. Topics covered include development of test matrices, testing standards, specimen preparation, environmental conditioning, instrumentation and data acquisition, failure modes, and data interpretation and recording.

Development of Test Matrices

The test plan primarily consists of the required test matrices. A separate matrix of tests is usually required for each material or structural form at each level of the building block process. This section focuses on general issues that must be considered in developing these test matrices. Subsequent sections cover the specifics of standard test methods, specimen preparation, and so on.

Property Needs. First, identify the material or structural properties requiring measurement. Complete characterization of all possible material properties at a given level or scale is rarely necessary. However, good engineering judgement should be used to balance the critical/minimum design needs with potential unforeseen downstream data needs. For example, the need for a full set of elastic properties may not be obvious in the test planning stage but may become necessary as detailed analytical models are developed in the later stages of design.

Environmental Conditions. Determine the environmental conditions under which the required material properties need to be developed. Room temperature and ambient moisture conditions are almost always required. Other temperature, moisture, and/or atmospheric conditions may be required in order to provide critical design properties or isolate key aspects of material behavior. Environmental conditioning approaches and requirements are discussed in more detail in a subsequent section.

Test Methods. The type of test method must be indicated for each property in the test matrix. A detailed description of how to execute each method should be provided elsewhere in the test plan document. Test method requirements are discussed in more detail in subsequent paragraphs.

Statistics. Perhaps the most contentious and difficult-to-understand aspect of test matrix development is defining the number of test specimens per condition (and per batch of material, if multibatch data are being developed) in order to assure an appropriate level of statistical significance. Much of the detailed test planning guidance found in MIL-HDBK-17, Volume 1 focuses on guidelines for establishing basis values for strength and strain-to-failure properties (see the article "Overview of Testing and Certification" in this Volume for a definition of basis values). Sampling schemes for this and other types of data usage, such as material screening, equivalency testing, and so on are detailed in MIL-HDBK-17, Volume 1. A specific statistical methodology for calculating basis values from test results, illustrated in Fig. 1, is recommended for general use in reducing data and is required for evaluation of data published in MIL-HDBK-17, Volume 2.

Depending on both the application and the procuring or certifying agency, modifications to the baseline MIL-HDBK-17 approach may be justified when developing new material data. In such cases, the handbook guidelines remain useful for support and reference. Alternate sampling and statistical approaches to development of basis values may be justified in certain instances, though they are less commonly used. These alternate approaches directly affect test matrix development and generally require a relatively sophisticated knowledge of both statistics and the material behavior of the specific material system. When using such alternate approaches, advance approval of the procurement or certification agency is strongly recommended.

Regardless of the sampling scheme, for small sample populations, the result of any basis value calculation is strongly dependent on the sample size. Smaller sample populations are obviously less costly to test, but there is a price of a different kind to pay since, as the population size decreases, so does the calculated basis value. Figure 2 shows, for example, the effect of sample size on the calculated B-basis value for samples of various sizes drawn from a given infinite population that is normally distributed. In the limit, for very large sample sizes the B-basis (ten percentile) value for this example would be 87.2. The dotted line in the figure is the mean of all possible B-basis values for each sample size; this line can also be interpreted as the estimated B-

Table 1 Typical types of composite test matrices

Constituent physical properties
Constituent mechanical properties
Prepreg physical properties
Lamina physical properties
Lamina mechanical properties
Unnotched laminate mechanical properties
Notched laminate strengths
Bearing/bypass joint strengths
Fastener pull-through strengths
Generic subelement testing
Design-specific subelement testing
Component testing
Full-scale static test article
Full-scale fatigue test article

basis value as a function of population size for a fixed sample coefficient of variation (CV) of 10%. The dashed lines represent the one-sigma limits for any given sample size (a two-sigma limit would approximately bound the 95% confidence interval). Not only does the estimated B-basis value increase with larger sample sizes, but, as the one-sigma limits illustrate, the expected variation in the estimated B-basis value significantly decreases. The lower one-sigma limit is farther from the mean B-basis value than the upper one-sigma limit, illustrating a skew in the calculated B-basis value that is particularly strong for small sample sizes. As a result of this skew, for small populations the calculated B-basis value is substantially more likely to be overly conservative than under conservative, increasing the significant penalty in B-basis value paid by use of small populations. While similar examples for nonnormal distributions would have different quantitative results, the trends with sample size can be expected to be similar.

Table 2 is an example of a typical test matrix.

Testing Standards

In addition to the test matrices, a detailed test plan will also include guidance on what standard test methods to use and specifics on how to use them (e.g., specifying which of the various options in the method to use in practice). The test plan also provides reference to appropriate documentation for nonstandard test methods.

At the coupon testing level, the results are either an intrinsic material property (like material compression modulus or tensile strength) or a generic structural response (like quasi-isotropic laminate open hole tension strength) from a small and relatively simple specimen. This result is often used as input to a simulation of the response of a larger and more complicated specific structure. At and above the subelement test level in the building block process, the testing is usually design-specific, thus no standard test methods are available. In most cases, structural test descriptions are either included in the test plan document or prepared separately and referenced by the test plan.

Coupon test methods, historically developed for metals or plastics, in most cases cannot be directly applied to advanced composite materials. While the basic physics of test methods for composites may be similar to their unreinforced counterparts, the heterogeneity, orthotropy, moisture sensitivity, and low ductility of typical composites often lead to significant differences in testing requirements, particularly with the mechanical tests.
The significant differences include the following:

- The strong influence of constituent content on material response, creating a need to measure the material response of every coupon
- A need to evaluate properties in multiple directions
- A need to condition specimens to quantify and control moisture absorption and desorption
- Increased importance of specimen alignment and load introduction method

Other distinguishing characteristics of many composite materials also contribute to testing differences. These characteristics include the following:

- Compression strength that is often lower than tensile strength (though specific material systems like boron/epoxy may behave counter to this)
- Operating temperatures that are closer to material property transition temperatures (compared to metals)
- Shear stress response that is uncoupled from normal stress response
- Heightened sensitivity to specimen preparation practices

A good overview of the mechanics of testing laminated Composites is given in Ref 1.

One measure of a test method is the theoretical ability of a perfect test to produce a desired result, such as a uniform uniaxial stress state throughout the conduct of the test. However, the

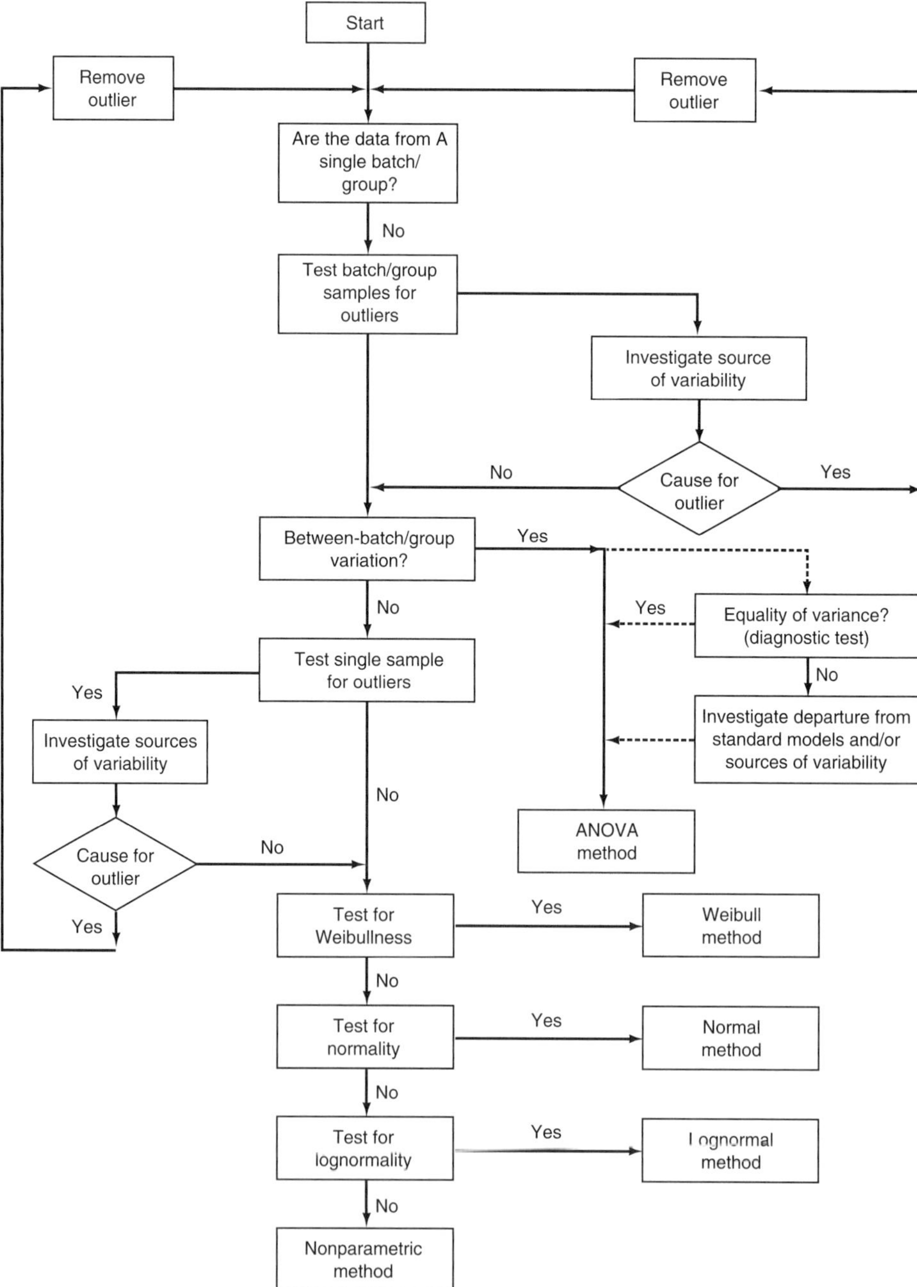

Fig. 1 Statistical methodology for calculating basis values from test results. ANOVA, analysis of variance. Source: MIL-HDBK-17

above factors tend to increase the sensitivity of composites to a wider variety of testing parameters than is seen with conventional materials. Therefore, test method robustness, or relative insensitivity to minor variations in specimen and test procedure, is just as important as theoretical perfection. Robustness, or lack thereof, is assessed by interlaboratory testing and is measured by *precision* (variation in the sample population) and *bias* (variation of the sample mean from the true average). The term *accuracy* is often used as a generic combination of aspects of both precision and bias. The terms *precision* and *bias*, being more specific, are preferred for use where appropriate. The precision and bias of test methods are evaluated by comparison testing, often called "round-robin" testing, both within laboratory and between laboratories. The obvious ideal is high precision (low variation) and low bias (sample mean close to true average) for test results both within laboratory and between laboratories. Such a test method would repeatedly produce reproducible results without regard to material, operator, or test laboratory. However, quantification of bias requires a material standard for each test, none of which is currently available for composites. As a result, bias of composite test methods can currently only be qualitatively assessed.

The effect on precision and bias of variation in test specimen size and geometry is somewhat separate from the precision and bias of a test method (for a given specimen) but more relevant to subelement and component-level testing. For heterogeneous materials, physically larger specimens can be expected to contain within the coupon a more representative sample of the material microstructure. While this effect is desirable, a larger specimen is more apt to contain a greater number of microstructural or macrostructural defects than a smaller specimen and, thus, can be expected to produce somewhat lower strengths (though possibly with lower variation, as well). Variations in specimen geometry can also create differing results. Size and geometry effects can produce statistical differences in results independent of the degree of perfection of the remaining aspects of a test method or its conduct; such effects should be expected. Therefore, even though the specimen response may not (and probably will not) be identical to that of the structure, the ideal test method will incorporate a specimen geometry that can be consistently correlated with structural response.

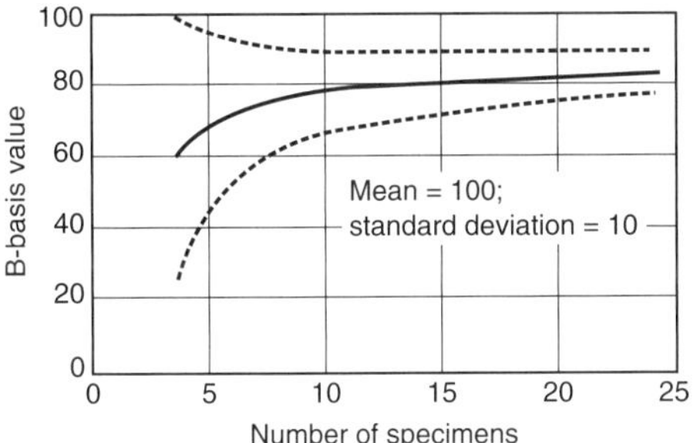

Fig. 2 Normal B-basis values with one-sigma limits. SD, standard deviation. Source: MIL-HDBK-17

As the criticality of various test parameters is still being researched and understood (even for relatively common tests) and as "standard laboratory practices," on close examination, are actually found to vary from laboratory to laboratory, it is critical to control or document as many of these practices and parameters as possible. ASTM Committee D-30, responsible for standardization of advanced composite material test methods, tries to consider all of these factors when improving existing standard test methods and developing new ones (Ref 2). Due to both their completeness and their status as full-consensus standards, ASTM D-30 test methods are emphasized in this Volume, where applicable.

Failure to minimize test method sensitivities, whatever their cause, can cause the statistical methods used to develop the necessary design basis values to break down, as all variation in data is implicitly assumed by the statistical methods to be due to material or process variation. Any additional variation due to specimen preparation or testing procedure is added to the material/process variation, which can result in extraordinarily conservative basis-value results.

Test methods, with emphasis on ASTM standards for advanced composites, are discussed in subsequent articles in this Section. The advantages and disadvantages of the various test methods for composites are discussed, including, for completeness, nonstandard but often referenced methods that have appeared in the literature. Test methods for which MIL-HDBK-17 currently accepts data are summarized in Table 3.

Specimen Preparation

After the test matrices and test methods have been developed/identified, the next step in test planning is to ensure representative and repeatable specimen preparation. As discussed elsewhere in this Volume, composite materials and structures are the products of complex multistep manufacturing processes. Thus, there are many sources for property variation simply in the preparation of test specimens. This variation must be identified and controlled to the greatest extent possible. Variations inherent in the normal product manufacturing process should be faithfully reproduced in the various levels of certification testing. Variations unique to test specimen fabrication and testing should be minimized or eliminated. To this end, ASTM Committee D-30 produced and maintains ASTM D 5687, "Standard Guide to the Preparation of Flat Composite

Table 2 Typical composite material test matrix

Mechanical property	Suggested test procedure(a)	Test condition and number of tests per batch(b)			No. of tests
		Min temp dry	RT dry	Max temp wet	
0° tension	ASTM D 3039	6	6	6	90
90° tension	ASTM D 5450	6	6	6	90
0° compression	ASTM D 3410 (Method B)	6	6	6	90
90° compression	ASTM D 5449	6	6	6	90
In-plane shear	ASTM D 5448	6	6	6	90
Interlaminar shear	ASTM D 5379	6	6	6	90
Total					**540**

min, minimum; max, maximum. (a) Refer to the article "Lamina and Laminate Mechanical Testing" in this Volume and MIL-HDBK-17, Volume 1, Section 6.7, Mechanical Property Tests, for more information on these ASTM test methods. (b) Tests shall be performed on each of the five batches. Minimum and maximum temperature tests shall be performed within ±2.8 °C (±5 °F) of the nominal test temperature. Nominal test temperatures will be as agreed to by contractor and certifying agency. Dry specimens are "as-fabricated" specimens that have been maintained at ambient conditions in an environmentally-controlled test laboratory. Wet specimens are environmentally-conditioned by exposing them in a humidity chamber until they attain an equilibrium moisture content agreed to by the contractor and certifying agency, and then packaging them in a heat-sealed aluminized polyethylene bag until required for test. Tests shall be performed in a manner which maintains the moisture content in specimens at the levels agreed to by the contractor and certifying agency. Source: MIL-HDBK-17

Table 3 Standard test methods from which MIL-HDBK-17 currently accepts data

Test category, lamina/laminate mechanical tests	Source of test method(a)	
	ASTM	SACMA
0° Warp tension	D 3039	RM 4, RM 9
90°/Fill tension	D 3039, D 5450	RM 4, RM 9
0°/Warp compression	D 3410, D 5467, D 6641	RM 1, RM 6
90°/Fill compression	D 3410, D 5449, D 6641	RM 1, RM 6
In-plane shear (b)	D 3518, D 5448, D 5379	RM 7
Interlaminar shear	D 5379	...
Short beam strength	D 2344	RM 8
Flexure	(c)	(c)
Open-hole compression	D 6484	RM 3
Open-hole tension	D 5766	RM 5
Single-shear bearing	D 5961	...
Double-shear bearing	D 5961	...
Compression after impact	(Draft)	RM 2
Mode I fracture toughness	D 5528	...
Mode II fracture toughness	(Draft)	...
Tension/tension fatigue	D 3479	...
Tension/compression fatigue	...	...

(a) SACMA (Suppliers of Advanced Composite Materials Association) test methods, in many cases, are subsets or supersets of the referenced ASTM test methods and, in other cases, have either a different scope or use a different testing methodology. For cases where a SACMA test method exists and either there is no ASTM test method covering the same property or the existing ASTM test method uses a different methodology, ASTM is considering adopting a form of the SACMA test method. For properties where there is more than one test method listed for either ASTM or SACMA, the different test methods either apply to different material forms or use different testing methodologies. SACMA is no longer active, and its test methods are not being maintained. (b) ASTM D 4255 will also be accepted for in-plane shear modulus of flat panels. (c) See MIL-HDBK-17, Volume 1, Section 6.7.7

Panels with Guidelines for Specimen Preparation" (Ref 3). While this standard is specific to organic matrix composites, much of its guidance is also applicable to laminated continuous fiber-metal and ceramic-matrix composites.

ASTM D 5687 describes the general process flow for preparation of flat composite panels and provides specific recommended techniques that are generally suitable to laminated fibrous organic polymer-matrix composites for each of the process steps in test specimen fabrication. The specific techniques included in this guide are the minimum recommended for common composite material systems as represented in the scope of this guide. For a given application, other techniques may need to be added or substituted for those described by this guide.

Specimen preparation is modeled in the 8-step process presented in Fig. 3. Laminate consolidation techniques are assumed to be by press or autoclave. It is assumed that the materials are properly handled by the test facility to meet the requirements specified by the material supplier(s) or specification, or both. Proper test specimen identification includes designation of process equipment, process steps, and any irregularities identified during processing.

The techniques described in ASTM D 5687 are recommended to facilitate the consistent production of satisfactory test specimens by minimizing uncontrolled processing variance during specimen fabrication. Steps 3 through 8 of the process may not be required for particular specimen or test types. If the specimen or test does not require a given step in the process of specimen fabrication, that particular step may be skipped. A test specimen represents a simplification of the structural part. The value of a test specimen lies in the ability of several sites to be able to test the specimen using standard techniques. Test data may not show properties identical to those obtained in a large structure, but a correlation can be made between test results and part performance. This may be due, in part, to the difficulty of creating a processing environment for test specimens that identically duplicates that of larger scale processes.

Specimen preparation practices should reflect those used on an applicable part, to the greatest extent practical. However, due to scaling effects, processing requirements for test laminates may not exactly duplicate the processes used in larger scale components. The user should attempt to understand and control those critical process parameters that may produce a difference in material response between the test coupon and the structure. It is important to also note that laminate quality is directly related to the prevention of contamination during lay-up and processing.

Regarding the eight steps shown in Fig. 3, the ASTM D 5687 procedure section provides guidance on the following:

- *Laminate lay-up:* Clean room requirements, dimensional considerations, lay-up materials and tooling, ply cutting and stacking (e.g., assuring proper ply orientations and staggering butt-spliced plies), and bagging considerations. In particular, standard nomenclature, notations, and coordinate systems are specified (consistent with those shown elsewhere in this Volume).
- *Laminate consolidation:* Recommended practices for temperature, pressure, and vacuum
- *Initial cutting of laminates/specimens:* Guidance on cutting and machining equipment.
- *Bonding of tabs:* If required, test specimen tabs strongly influence the success or failure of a particular test. This is because tabs are generally used to introduce load into very notch-sensitive orthotropic materials. Thus, failure to properly tab specimens generally results in tab-section rather than gage-section-failures. ASTM D 5687 provides detailed guidance on tab design, application, and machining.
- *Specimen machining/final cutting:* Further machining guidance focused on tolerance and quality control issues
- *Applying coatings/treatments:* Coatings are sometimes required prior to environmental conditioning. ASTM D 5687 simply states that coating manufacturer recommendations be followed.
- *Specimen conditioning:* ASTM D 5687 guidance simply consists of references to other documents. This subject is addressed in more detail elsewhere in this section.
- *Strain gaging:* ASTM D 5687 guidance points to other references, and this issue is also addressed elsewhere in this section.

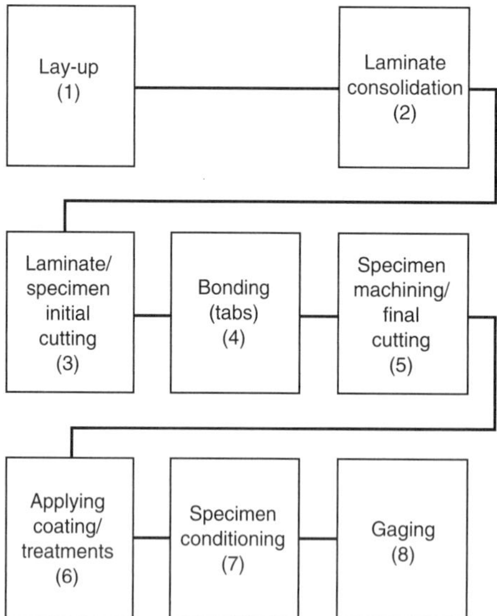

Fig. 3 Eight-step test specimen preparation model. Material identification is mandatory. Continuous traceability of specimens is required throughout the process. Process checks may be done at the end of each step to verify that the step was performed to give a laminate or specimen or satisfactory quality. Steps 4 and 5 may be interchanged. For aramid fibers, step 5 routinely precedes step 4. Steps 6, 7, and 8 may be interchanged. Source: ASTM D 5687

- *Process checks:* Finally, ASTM D 5687 also provides quality control guidance as described subsequently.

Each facility may develop a set of nondestructive examination (NDE) or other processing checks to assure that each step of the specimen preparation process has been performed satisfactorily. If the specimen fabrication process is shown to be sufficiently controlled to eliminate deviations from acceptable specimens, then control of the process indicates control of the specimen. In these cases, inspection is only an occasional verification of the process. In cases where the process has not shown that acceptable specimens are made by following process steps, inspection protocol, which defines inspections to be performed, should be initiated and every specimen evaluated until there is confidence that the process shall make adequate specimens. Process capabilities should be periodically checked if there is any doubt that specimens will meet the requirement. Nondestructive and destructive process checks are described in ASTM D 5687.

The contact surface of the material and the measuring device will determine the measured dimensions. Bridging of surface discontinuities and accounting for dimples (less than 0.8 mm, or 0.03 in.) can substantially affect the data produced. Figure 4 demonstrates this effect. Use of nonstandard devices on the same tests within a facility can create typical test data variations (not material variations) of 5 to 15%, due solely to measurement inconsistencies. Calibration of the measurement devices should, therefore, be traceable.

The precision of the dimensional examination of the specimen required depends on the specific type of measurement device. In performing dimensional examinations, the accuracy of the overall test should be considered. A propagation of error analysis for the test may demonstrate the level of accuracy required in the dimensional tolerances of a specific test.

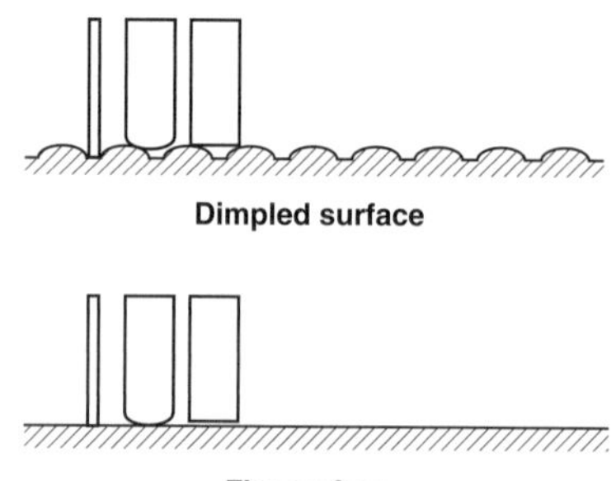

Fig. 4 Measuring of laminate surfaces. Each example shows the use of two different sizes and two different types of measuring probes. For a dimpled surface, if when too narrow a probe is used, minimum thickness rather than average thickness will be measured; if when too wide a probe is used, maximum thickness rather than average thickness will be measured. For a flat surface, probe width has minimal effect. Source: ASTM D 5687

Environmental Conditioning

Another step in test planning is specifying the details required to environmentally condition the test specimens. This testing should include all relevant environmental effects on material and structural behavior and may be necessary to establish the material operational limit (MOL). Properties of polymer-matrix composites are influenced markedly by temperature and moisture. Generally, matrix-dominated mechanical property values decrease with increases in moisture content and increases in temperature above room temperature. For properties that are highly dominated by reinforcement (fiber) properties (unidirectional tension, for example), this reduction may be reversed, absent, or minimal over reasonable temperature ranges. For properties influenced by the organic matrix (shear and compression, for example), the degradation of properties can be significant. Furthermore, the degradation is not linear. At a given moisture content, it becomes more severe with increasing temperature until a temperature is reached where dramatic property reductions begin to occur and beyond which these reductions may become irreversible. It is desirable to specify this onset of dramatic reduction as a characteristic temperature, which is also defined as the MOL or the maximum operating temperature. The purpose of establishing the MOL is to assure that materials are not operated in service under conditions where a slight increase in temperature might cause a significant loss in strength or stiffness and to absolutely avoid irreversible property changes. Similar operational limitations, due to temperature and oxidation rather than moisture, are also observed in ceramic-matrix composites.

There are not yet any fixed criteria for establishment of a MOL. One method (Ref 4–6) utilizes the glass-transition temperature (T_g) as determined from dynamic mechanical analysis (DMA) or similar data, reduced by some temperature margin ΔT. For epoxy-matrix composites, 28 °C (50 °F) is commonly used for the value of the temperature margin, but it can be argued that smaller margins may be acceptable for particular applications when supported by other data. While T_g is a useful tool, it should not be the sole basis for establishing MOL. Glass transition frequently occurs over a range of temperatures, and it is well known that measurement of T_g is test method dependent. Other data that are useful in establishing MOL include field experience (for established materials) and mechanical testing conducted over a temperature range that includes the $\pm\Delta T$ range around the measured T_g.

Evaluating the behavior of a matrix-dependent mechanical property in the appropriate wet condition as a function of temperature is considered a reliable method for verifying a MOL that has tentatively been determined from T_g data. Various investigators have used short beam strength, in-plane shear strength, in-plane shear modulus, and quasi-isotropic open hole compression strength for this purpose, with the latter two being most successful as MOL indicators. Four or five temperatures are typically chosen to provide trend lines for the selected property. Figure 5 shows three possible scenarios where mechanical testing is used to verify the MOL determined from T_g data. In the first instance, mechanical data corroborate the chosen T_g. In the second case, mechanical data suggest that the MOL predicted by T_g is conservative. In the third example, mechanical data do not support the MOL determined from T_g data and indicate that a lower MOL should be chosen. One approach to determining the MOL from mechanical property data is to use the temperature at which the property versus temperature plot deviates from linearity by a given percentage. An example of this can be found in Ref 7. However, a specific criterion for determining MOL that includes results from both T_g and mechanical testing has not been standardized and is still being discussed. Nevertheless, the MOL value predicted from T_g measurements that are verified or modified by mechanical property data provide a practical approach for defining the MOL of a material.

In addition to establishing the MOL, environmental testing must also be planned to quantify all critical physical and mechanical property changes that are the result of environmental effects. These effects can be broadly categorized as temperature, moisture (water), and fluid (other than water). The following three sections address test planning details for each category.

Temperature. Test planning for environmental conditions should include testing at room temperature, the maximum and minimum service temperatures, and intermediate and/or elevated (beyond service use) temperatures, as well. Guidance is usually available from the certifying agency regarding what temperatures are required. All critical physical and mechanical properties should be measured at the first three noted temperatures, at least. As noted in the MOL discussion, the combined effects of elevated temperature and moisture often dictate the critical design conditions for composites; thus, testing is often conducted under hot-wet conditions. Elevated temperature testing at dry conditions is sometimes performed in order to get an early indication of hot-wet performance, since moisture conditioning of test specimens may take a month or more. For example, 120 °C (250 °F)/dry and 80 °C (180 °F)/wet conditions yield similar laminate strength results for certain 175 °C (350 °F) curing carbon/epoxy prepregs. Minimum service temperature for many air vehicles is specified as –55 °C (–65 °F), thus, the majority of cold-temperature data resulting from atmospheric air vehicle programs are derived at this temperature. Since moisture effects at cold temperatures are less critical, these specimens usually are not moisture conditioned.

Moisture. Absorbed moisture itself can be considered a separate environmental condition that must be addressed in test planning. Most polymeric materials, whether in the form of a composite matrix or a polymeric fiber, are capable of absorbing relatively small but potentially significant amounts of moisture from the surrounding environment. The physical mechanism for moisture gain, assuming there are no cracks or other wicking paths, is generally assumed to be mass diffusion following Fick's law, the moisture analog to thermal diffusion. While material surfaces in direct contact with the environment absorb or desorb moisture almost immediately, moisture flow into or out of the interior occurs relatively slowly. The moisture diffusion rate is many orders of magnitude slower than heat flow in thermal diffusion. Nevertheless, after a few weeks or months of exposure to a humid environment, a significant amount of water will eventually be absorbed by the material. This absorbed water may produce dimensional changes (swelling), lower the glass transition temperature of a polymer, and reduce the matrix and matrix/fiber interface-dependent mechanical properties of the composite. This effectively lowers the maximum use temperature of the material.

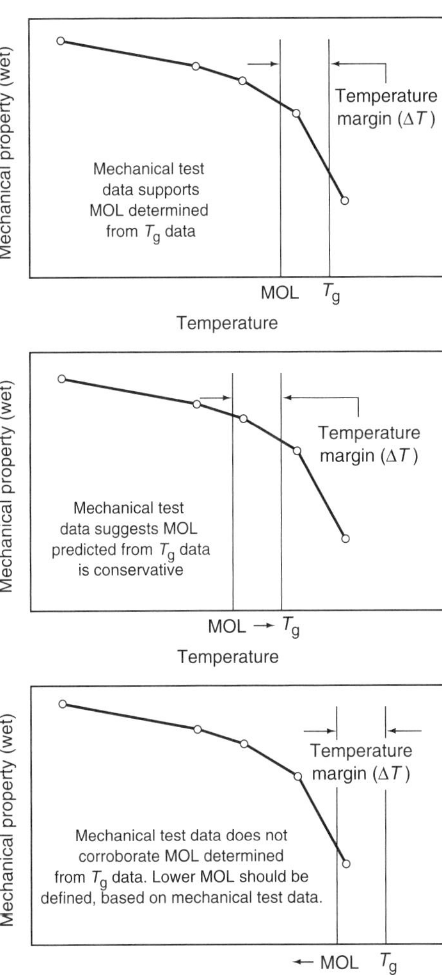

Fig. 5 Use of mechanical and glass-transition temperature (T_g) data to determine material operational limit (MOL). Source: MIL-HDBK-17

Since the amount of moisture absorbed by a material depends upon the thickness and time of exposure, fixed-time conditioning methods should not be followed for small, flat test coupons on which most moisture-conditioned testing is done. (However, fixed-time conditioning may be appropriate for thick components.) Instead, a conditioning procedure such as ASTM D 5229/D 5229M (Ref 8) should be followed because it accounts for the diffusion process and terminates with the moisture content nearly uniform through the thickness. Moisture equilibrium content is weakly related to temperature and is usually assumed to be a function only of relative humidity. The largest value of moisture equilibrium content for a given material under humid conditions occurs at 100% relative humidity; this is also often called the *saturation content.*

Another point to be emphasized is that moisture absorption properties under atmospheric humidity conditions are generally not equivalent to exposure to either liquid immersion or pressurized steam. These latter environments alter the material diffusion characteristics, producing a higher moisture equilibrium content, and should not be used unless they simulate the application environment in question.

To evaluate worst-case effects of moisture content on material properties, tests are performed with specimens preconditioned to the design service (end-of-life) moisture content, which is assumed equivalent to equilibrium at the design service relative humidity. The preferred conditioning methodology uses ASTM D 5229/D 5229M. Unless specified by the procuring or certifying agency, the design service moisture content is determined in one of several ways. It can be derived from semiempirical calculations that consider secondary effects on a particular type of structure, or it can be more conservatively established by simpler assumptions.

An example of the first case (semiempirical calculations) is documented in Ref 6, where worldwide climatic data and United States Air Force (USAF) aircraft-basing data were combined to define runway storage environmental spectra for each of the three classes of USAF air vehicles—fighters, bombers, and cargo/tankers. The study applied a ranking procedure to select baseline and worst-case locations with respect to the absorption of moisture by typical carbon/epoxy composite structures. Such data can be used to establish design service moisture content for a particular application; a typical specific design service relative humidity (RH) might be 81% RH for a tropically-based supersonic aircraft.

Another, more conservative, approach is to use the average relative humidity for a selected diurnal cycle taken from a reference such as MIL-STD-210 (Ref 9), the United States military guide to worldwide environmental exposure conditions. This usually leads to a higher design service relative humidity (88% RH is typical), since dry-out due to solar radiation, flight excursions (supersonic excursions, in particular), and seasonal climatic changes are not considered.

Given these and other historical considerations, the MIL-HDBK-17 Coordination Group has agreed that a reasonable upper-bound value for aircraft design service relative humidity is 85% and that this value may be used when a specific determination of design service moisture content has not been established for a specific aircraft application. Use of a design service moisture content of 85% RH will obviate extrapolation of data when test coupons are conditioned to equilibrium at this moisture level. Accepted design service moisture levels for other applications have not yet been established.

Fluids. Finally, it is important to characterize the physical and/or mechanical property degradation effects of fluids (or other forms of chemicals) commonly found in contact with the composite structure. The evaluation should account for different exposure levels of aircraft structure to fluids.

Two fluid exposure classifications are suggested, with example fluids cited for each group (Table 4). Group I fluids have the potential to pool or be in contact with the material for an extended period of time. Group II fluids include those that are applied and wiped off, those that evaporate or those that do not contact the material for an extended period of time. Exposure by immersion prior to testing or before evaluating weight loss is also recommended: a different exposure level should be used for each group:

- *Group I:* Immerse material in fluid until it reaches equilibrium weight gain (saturation). The MIL-S-8802 Sump Water corrosion test is an exception.
- *Group II:* Immerse material in fluid for 15 days to determine worst case effects.

Follow up with tests that simulate a more realistic exposure including accidental extended exposure. Both mechanical and physical testing should be done.

Mechanical testing should include open hole compression tests on quasi-isotropic lay-up specimens and $\pm 45°$ tension specimens. The open hole compression test has a meaningful relationship to design values and is sensitive to matrix degradation. The use of a $\pm 45°$ tension test is commonplace in industry for comparison of matrix properties. It is a sensitive test that will identify potentially harsh fluids. It provides an indication of whether sufficient shear stiffness has been retained to ensure acceptable matrix-fiber property transfer. While a material stiffness loss criterion is material and application specific, a 20–40% loss in shear modulus is generally considered significant and should be further investigated. A minimum of five specimens should be tested after exposure at room temperature and at the maximum use temperature. The results should be compared with unexposed controls. A more economical alternative to open hole compression and $\pm 45°$ tension testing is interlaminar or short beam shear tests. The specimens for these tests are easily fabricated, machined, conditioned, and tested. Although not as generally related to design properties, short beam strength tests are sensitive to matrix degradation and can be valuable indicators for material evaluation. As with the $\pm 45°$ tension tests, results after exposure should be compared to unexposed controls at room and elevated temperature to obtain fluid exposure effects.

Physical testing should include weighing to measure weight change, taking photomicrographs to examine for microcracks, and, where practical, using scanning electron microscopy to examine for surface crazing. Relative to the former, it should be noted that, because a saturation condition has apparently been reached, it does not automatically follow that further degradation of properties has ceased. Especially where new matrix systems are involved, tests with long-term exposure to critical fluids should be conducted. Due to the long exposure times involved, these tests should be started early in the evaluation process.

If water or moisture is proven to be the most property-degrading fluid, then fluid exposure tests involving other than moisture conditioning are not included in subsequent design testing; this has been the acceptable standard in the past. In effect, if the properties of the material after fluid exposure are better than after moisture exposure, then subsequent testing accounts for moisture only. If a fluid other than water is more critical, then subsequent testing must include evaluation with that fluid. In the case of Group II wipe on/wipe off fluids, the procedure is somewhat different, since water is not a good comparison. Consequently, comparison to a matrix

Table 4 Fluid exposure classifications

Fluid	Specification
Group I fluids	
JP-4 jet fuel	MIL-PRF-5624
JP-5 jet fuel	MIL-PRF-5624
JP-8 jet fuel	MIL-DTL-83133
Hydraulic fluid	MIL-H-5606 MIL-H-83282
Polyalphaolefin (PAO) cooling fluid	MIL-C-87252
Engine lubricating oil	MIL-PRF-7808 MIL-PRF-23699
Ethylene glycol/urea deicer (Class I)	SAE AMS 1435 (superseding SAE AMS 1432 and MIL-D-83411)
Sump water	SAE AMS S-8802 (superseding MIL-S-8802)
Methylene chloride	ASTM D 4701 (superseding MIL-D-6998)
SO_2/salt spray	. . .
Group II fluids	
Alkaline cleaner (Types 1 and 2)	MIL-C-87937 (superseding MIL-C-87936)
Methyl ethyl ketone (MEK) washing liquid	ASTM D 740 (superseding TT-M-261)
Dry cleaning solvent (Type 2)	MIL-PRF-680 (superseding P-D-680)
Hydrocarbon washing liquid	ASTM D 471 (superseding TT-S-735)
Polypropylene glycol deicer (Type 1)	MIL-A-8243
Isopropyl alcohol deicing agent	TT-I-735

that has an acceptable service history is recommended.

Instrumentation and Data Acquisition

A final step in test planning is specifying the necessary instrumentation and data acquisition. Instrumentation such as multi-element strain gages, can significantly increase the cost of any test; plan on 1-to-1.5 ratio for installation personnel hours per gage element, including the associated wiring. Thus, the test planner needs to have a clear understanding of the purpose (or multi-faceted purposes) of each test being specified, in order to efficiently plan the instrumentation needs. Similarly, the test planner also needs an a-priori understanding of the intended use of the resulting test data, in order to specify an appropriate form and format for the test data acquisition. This point is important, since a great deal of manpower can be expended (i.e., wasted) in simply handling and reformatting the large volume of certification test data to get it in a usable form for the necessary post-test engineering analysis. This manpower requirement can be greatly reduced if the experimental data is acquired, processed, and stored in a useful format to begin with. The two following sections give additional details regarding these topics.

Instrumentation. The purposes for doing the different types of certification testing vary widely, but the most common measurement categories are physical property, strength, and strain/displacement field correlation (with analytical/numerical models). Most physical property testing (density, coefficient of thermal expansion, T_g, elastic properties, etc.) is done via standardized coupon testing and the test standards provide detailed guidance regarding instrumentation. Strength testing always requires load monitoring and sometimes requires strain/displacement measurement, as well, in order to isolate multiple damage modes and/or reduce data. However, the large test matrices required to get high statistical confidence in basic lamina- or laminate-level strength properties offer a good opportunity to minimize strain-gage instrumentation, since strength-only measurements are often all that is needed. Strain/displacement field correlation is often, but not always, done on large, complex element and component tests. Careful up-front coordination with the stress analyst (and the certifying agency) is required for this aspect of test planning in order to capture critical forces, moments, surface strains, out-of-plane displacements, and structural stiffnesses in the test article without using an excessive amount of unnecessary instrumentation. Good generic guidance on experimental mechanics of composites is given in Ref 1.

Data acquisition techniques can range from manually reading instruments and recording the results in a lab notebook to use of specialized million dollar digital signal processing/computing/storage devices. The techniques chosen for use should simply be the ones most appropriate for the intended use of the data. The lab notebook approach is often suitable when a few raw data points will be used directly by the analyst. Simple non-strain-gaged subelement strength tests often fall into this category. On the other hand, a digital system that can automatically postprocess and store a large volume and/or high rate of data is essential for both complex full-scale test articles and large (more than 10,000 specimens) statistical design data coupon-testing programs. In both of these cases, it is important to efficiently and automatically transform the tremendous amount of raw data into useful engineering information, as well as archive the raw data for future unanticipated needs. Careful up-front planning of this task is essential, since it strongly influences the cost and schedule of what is often a program-pacing effort (i.e., structural allowables development).

Failure Modes

An important consideration in interpreting and reporting all composite material and structural test results is the isolation of one or more dominant failure modes. Standardized coupon test methods generally yield only one dominant failure mode; many test methods provide specific guidance in identifying failure modes and, thus, verifying the validity of a particular data point. In structural element and component testing, multiple failure modes are acceptable and often the norm. One of the most common uses of element and component test data is validation of analytically predicted failure mode (and load), or, conversely, the issue of identifying/isolating failure modes other than those predicted by analytical methods. Thus, correctly identifying and isolating the failure mode or modes is of prime importance and must be carefully documented in post-test data reports. Further details of failure mode identification are provided in subsequent articles in this Section. A useful global reference for structural failure is the USAF Composite Failure Analysis Handbook (Ref 10, 11), which contains fractographic data from failed test specimens, as well as case histories of failed composite structures.

Data Interpretation and Recording

Finally, the overall issues of data interpretation, recording, and reporting require consideration. Assuming that specimen preparation, environmental conditioning, testing, and laboratory reporting of relevant issues such as failure modes are properly completed, post-test data analyses are typically performed in order to interpret the data in a manner useful to the design engineer and/or certifying agency. This data analysis necessarily includes appropriate recording and reporting. Few standards for composite material data recording exist, other than ASTM E 1309 (Ref 12) and E 1434 (Ref 13) for coupon-level electronic database architecture. Good engineering practice should be used in determining the details of structural test data recording. Reporting should be documented in a manner that complements the test planning document(s) and meets all customer and/or certifying agency requirements. The following sections detail technical issues of post-test data analysis that require careful consideration and appropriate documentation.

Issues of Data Equivalence. Evaluation for data pooling (i.e., whether data from two possibly different subpopulations are enough alike to be combined) and material equivalence (i.e., whether a material with common characteristics to another is sufficiently alike to use its data for design) are similar issues of data equivalence. Both require statistical procedures to assess the similarities and differences between two subpopulations of data. These, and other related issues, are covered in more detail in MIL-HDBK-17, Volume 1.

Assessment of data equivalence begins by examining key properties for various within-batch and between-batch statistics. The ability to pool different subpopulations of test data is highly desirable, if for no other reason than to obtain larger populations that are more representative of the universe. Equally desirable is the ability to show one material without basis values equivalent to another that already has established basis values. Requirements for the use of pooled data or equivalent materials are normally established for each application during discussions with the certifying agency.

Before determining statistical degree of equivalence, basic engineering considerations should be satisfied; the two materials should be of the same chemical, microstructural, and material form families. To some extent, the criteria for this may be application-dependent. For example, property data from two composite systems with the same matrix and similar fibers may not warrant pooling if the fiber/matrix interface is distinctly different, even if the fibers have similar modulus and tensile strength. Data equivalence is typically evaluated for datasets that differ due only to relatively minor changes in precursor manufacturing or material processing. These changes include the following:

- Minor changes in constituents or constituent manufacturing processes
- Identical materials processed by different component manufacturers
- Identical materials processed at different locations of the same manufacturer
- Slight changes in processing parameters
- Some combination of the changes listed previously

Statistical data equivalence methods currently assume that between- and within-laboratory test method variation is negligible. When this assumption is violated, this test-method-induced artificial variation severely weakens the ability of the statistical methods to meaningfully compare two different datasets.

Hot Wet Testing—Reporting Moisture Content at Failure. Specimen static strength, tested hot/wet, is usually preconditioned to equilibrium moisture content. Typically, the test results report this equilibrium moisture content rather than the actual content at failure. One consideration during testing should be to minimize dry-out during the process and, thus, the potentially severe through-thickness moisture distribution at failure. This consideration must be traded off against others, such as heat-soaking the specimen long enough prior to testing to ensure a uniform thermal profile through the thickness. There are several ways to minimize the moisture dry out during hot/wet testing. These include testing in a humidity cabinet, using high-rate heating (via quartz lamps, for instance) to minimize total environmental chamber out-time, and/or using relatively thicker test specimens. Although these procedures are not practical to perform on every test specimen, it is important that for each series of hot/wet tests, some indication of moisture content at failure be obtained. This data may be obtained via (a) witness or traveler coupons that follow a test specimen through a representative testing process, (b) use of modeling to predict dry-out, given specimen time-temperature history from environmental chamber to failure, or (c) post-test moisture content measurement on an undamaged portion of an actual test specimen. This moisture content at failure should always be reported in conjunction with each series of hot/wet tests.

Strain Gage Calibration for Structural Test Articles. Another post-test data interpretation issue, which is specific to complex structural test articles, is strain gage calibration with associated internal loads models. While properly installed and instrumented strain gages give relatively accurate direct indications of point surface strains, this information is of limited use on complex multiaxially loaded static and fatigue test articles. Rather, relevant information from these test articles must generally be in a form compatible with the associated internal loads models, verification of which is often a primary objective of the structural testing. Thus, surface strain data must be converted into pointwise forces, moments, and displacements, since these are the fundamental results of typical plane-stress two-dimensional finite element models. In order to perform these calibrations, both local and overall elastic response of the structure is required. Detailed pointwise laminate analysis of the structure, as well as global finite element results, are required to obtain this calibration input. In order to accurately match structural test data, these analyses must often be run with separate tensile or compressive ply moduli, rather than the average values used in the internal loads and stress analysis activities performed for overall certification. Once the calibration factors are obtained to transform raw strain gage data into the required forces, moments, and displacements, they may be automatically applied, via computerized post-processing, to the raw stain data files from a large number of applied load cases and load levels.

REFERENCES

1. J.M. Whitney, I. M. Daniel, and R.B. Pipes, *Experimental Mechanics of Fiber Reinforced Composite Materials,* The Society for Experimental Mechanics Monograph No. 4, revised ed., Brookfield Center, CT, 1984
2. R.E. Fields, Improving Test Methods for Composites, *ASTM Standardization News,* Oct 1993, p 38–43
3. "Preparation of Flat Composite Panels with Guidelines for Specimen Preparation," D 5687/D 5687M, *Annual Book of ASTM Standards,* ASTM
4. I.G. Hedrick, and J.B. Whiteside, "Effects of Environment on Advanced Composite Structures," AIAA Conference on Aircraft Composites: Emerging Methodology for Structural Assurance, (San Diego, CA), American Institute of Aeronautics and Astronautics, 1977
5. P.J. Schneider, *Conduction Heat Transfer,* Addison-Wesley, 1955
6. J.B. Whiteside et al., "Environmental Sensitivity of Advanced Composites," Environmental Definition, Vol I, AFWAL-TR-80-3076
7. R.S. Whitehead and R.W. Kinslow, "Composite Wing/Fuselage Program," Test Results and Qualification Recommendations, Vol IV, AFWAL-TR-88-3098
8. "Moisture Absorption Properties and Equilibrium Conditioning of Polymer Matrix Composite Materials," D 5229/D 5229M, *Annual Book of ASTM Standards,* ASTM
9. MIL-STD-210C, "Climatic Information to Determine Design and Test Requirements for Military Systems and Equipment"
10. "Composite Failure Analysis Handbook," USAF Report No. WL-TR-91-4032, final report, contract F33615-85-C-5010
11. G. Walker, "Composite Failure Analysis Handbook Update No. 1," USAF Report No. WL-TR-93-4004, final report, contract F33615-86-C-5071, April 1995
12. "Standard Guide for Identification of Composite Materials in Computerized Material Property Databases," E 1309, *Annual Book of ASTM Standards,* ASTM
13. "Standard Guide for Development of Standard Data Records for Computerization of Mechanical Test Data for High-Modulus Fiber-Reinforced Composite Materials," E 1434, *Annual Book of ASTM Standards,* ASTM

Constituent Materials Testing

Shari Bugaj, FiberCote Industries, Inc.

A COMPOSITE is composed of some form of reinforcement combined with a matrix material, and the performance of the composite depends to a large part on the properties of these constituent materials. This article describes the most significant chemical, physical, and mechanical tests used to characterize the properties of constituent materials; the focus is on constituents for resin-matrix composites reinforced with continuous fibers or fabrics, but many of the techniques apply to constituents of other types of composites as well. Additional information on fibers, fabrics, matrix resins, and prepregs is available in the Section "Constituent Materials" in this Volume.

Tests for Reinforcement Fibers and Fabrics

Reinforcing fibers can be tested in the form of single filaments, tows, unidirectional tape, or fabric. While typical reinforcements are made up of bundles of filaments, it is possible to isolate single filaments to determine their properties. Academically this is interesting, but such testing has not allowed prediction of composite performance. Testing the single tow or bundle allows an evaluation of the reinforcing fiber in its simplest form and is valuable in across-the-band variability studies. Because many fibers are woven into fabrics for use in composites, physical tests may be used to characterize the fabrics, but it is recommended that mechanical tests also be performed on laminates of impregnated material. Unidirectional tapes are a convenient form for testing mechanical properties of fibers. Columnated tows of fiber are impregnated with an appropriate resin, and the resultant tape is cured with heat and pressure to form a laminate, which is subsequently machined into test specimens.

Chemical Tests

Surface characteristics and polymer analysis can be accomplished with x-ray photoelectron spectroscopy (XPS), generally regarded as an important technique. Also known as electron spectroscopy for chemical analysis, this key technique provides a total elemental analysis, with the exception of hydrogen and helium, of the top 10 to 200 Å (depending on the sample and instrumental conditions) of any solid surface that is vacuum stable or can be made vacuum stable by cooling. It also provides chemical bond information. Of all the presently available instrumental techniques for surface analysis, XPS is generally regarded as being the most quantitative, the most readily interpretable, and the most informative with regard to chemical information. It is relatively simple and straightforward. It can be used to determine surface sensitive (10 to 200 Å) characteristics and elemental sensitivity (parts per 1000) for all elements, except hydrogen and helium. Although the method requires relatively sophisticated and expensive instrumentation, many universities, industrial research and development groups, and commercial service laboratories provide access to their instruments on a collaborative or fee-for-service basis.

The information content in a typical XPS spectrum is enormous. There are various hierarchies of spectral interpretation: simple elemental analysis, detailed considerations of chemical shifts and chemical bonding nature in the surface region, and loss or relaxation structures that provide further information on the chemical nature of the surface. Many potential artifacts, often related to the preparation of samples, are also made available in an XPS experiment. The interpretation becomes progressively more difficult as one considers more-complex surfaces, such as those of multicomponent and multiphase materials. Some disadvantages of XPS include the need for a large analysis area of several mm^2 (although an instrument being developed will have an analysis area of about a 150 μm, or 5900 μin., diameter), a high vacuum requirement (10^{-6} to 10^{-9} Pa, or 10^{-8} to 10^{-11} torr), lengthy test time ($\frac{1}{2}$ to 8 h per sample), and low resolution (~0.1 to 1.0 eV). Charging and energy referencing can also be a problem. It may be necessary to consult the literature and examine a large number of spectra to obtain practical experience with spectral interpretation and analysis for a wide range of sample types. Other instrumental surface analysis techniques that are available and widely used include Auger electron spectroscopy (AES) and secondary ion mass spectroscopy. The Auger technique is actually much older in practical application than XPS. Because AES uses an electron beam, it is generally highly damaging to organic polymer surfaces, but, as a form of electron spectroscopy, it is complementary to XPS. Secondary ion mass spectroscopy has been applied to polymer surfaces, but is not yet used routinely nor is it as easily interpreted as XPS. Secondary ion mass spectroscopy is undergoing extensive development and may prove to be useful for routine polymer surface analysis. Table 1 compares the features of numerous techniques.

The carbon assay is done according to ASTM C 571 (Ref 1, discontinued in 1995) or ASTM C 831 (Ref 2) and basically involves combustion of the product to form carbon dioxide and an absorption train to collect and compute the original carbon content.

Sizing/Finish Content. High-strength fibers may have sizing applied to their surfaces to improve bonding, handling, or resin-fiber interface characteristics. Determining sizing content is very direct: the fibers are weighed, the sizing removed, and the fibers are weighed again. Typical methods include extraction with an appropriate

Table 1 Comparison of instrumental techniques for surface analysis of fibers

Technique	Quantitative analysis	Structure	Electronic levels	Vibrational levels	Depth profiling	Spatial resolution	Adsorption energy	In situ fingerprint
Auger electron spectroscopy	+	+	+		+	+		
Low-energy electron diffraction		+						
X-ray photoelectron spectroscopy	+	+	+					
Electron energy loss spectroscopy		+		+	+			
Secondary ion mass spectroscopy	+				+	+		
Scanning electron microscopy						+		
Thermal desorption mass spectroscopy	+						+	
Fourier transform infrared spectroscopy		+		+				+

solvent to achieve total solvation of the size, but with no attack on the fiber, and pyrolysis at a temperature that will burn off the sizing but not affect the fiber. It should be noted that both methods are overly idealistic from a practical viewpoint. Extraction frequently does not solvate all of the sizing, while pyrolysis frequently results in fiber weight loss.

For glass or quartz fibers, a size is typically applied in the fiber manufacturing stage to aid in processing the fibers into the final fabric form. The sizing may then be removed and a coupling agent added to aid resin-fiber bonding. This final application is typically referred to as a "finish" for these fiber types.

Physical Tests

Seven physical characteristics of reinforcements and the tests that measure them are described subsequently.

Density is best measured by means of ASTM D 792 (Ref 3) using displacement, ASTM D 3800 (Ref 4) using Archimedes principle, or ASTM D 1505 (Ref 5) using a density gradient column. These are all well-established methods that can be used with confidence.

Weight Per Length (Yield). A simple test is accomplished by weighing a known length of fiber. It is typically reported in g/μm (lb/μin.).

Filament diameter can be measured in two ways, direct and calculated, both of which are limited to round cross sections. The direct method is to view the fiber under a microscope or by microprojection in accordance with ASTM D 578 (Ref 6). Alternatively, the average filament diameter can be calculated from the following equation:

$$D = (4WPL)^{1/2}/(\pi \cdot \rho_f \cdot k)$$

where D is the filament diameter, WPL is the weight per length, ρ_f is fiber density, and k is the number of filaments per tow. Other methods of measurement include cross-sectional microscopy and image analysis with a vibroscope. Irregular cross sections are microphotographed and measured planimetrically.

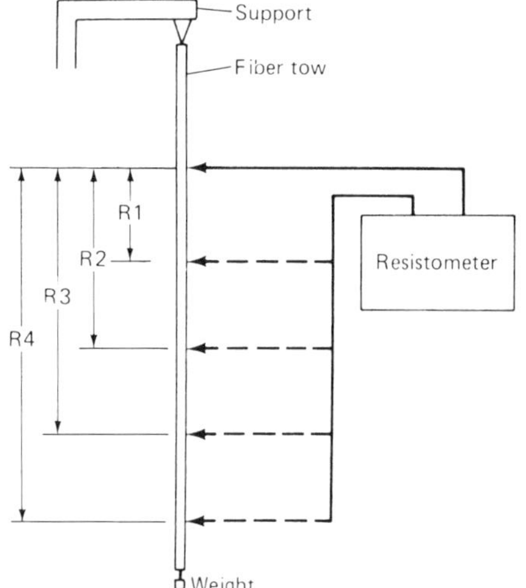

Fig. 1 Typical test setup for measuring electrical conductivity of fibers

Electrical conductivity can be measured by means of a simple resistance probe. A test setup similar to Fig. 1 may be used. The weight is hung to preclude wrinkling of the fiber. The resistance is measured at 25, 50, 75, and 100 mm (1, 2, 3, and 4 in.) intervals. Resistance versus distance plotted and the slope of line indicate the resistivity of the fiber. Because the resistivity is also a function of the cross-sectional area, the necessary filament data, that is, the number of filaments per tow and the filament diameter, should also be reported.

Thermal Expansion. Many thermal expansion procedures exist, but none give consistent, reproducible data when measuring fibers.

The number of twists per unit length of a carbon-fiber tow is determined by a twist test. The sequence is:

- Any frayed surface fiber is removed from the carbon fiber to be tested.
- Spool to be sampled is placed on spool holder.
- Fiber is unspooled, while being kept from twisting, and locked in the fixed clamp at the end of the cutting board.
- The free clamp is attached at the 1220 mm (48 in.) cutting edge, but sample is not cut from spool.
- A fine, pointed, polished stylus is inserted into the center of the sample at the opposite 1220 mm (48 in.) cutting edge, where the free clamp is located.
- The stylus is drawn down the sample, splitting the tow to the free clamp (making sure the movable clamp does not rotate).
- The stylus is backed off approximately 25 mm (1 in.) from the free clamp, and the number of fiber rotations to the free clamp is observed. The twist per mm (in.) (tpmm, or tpi) equals the number of rotations of fiber/1220 mm (48 in.).
- Results are reported to two significant digits. Example: 1.5 rotations/1220 mm (48 in.) = 0.0012 tpmm (0.031 tpi)

Fabric Weave. When fibers are woven into fabrics, the physical properties listed subsequently are measured.

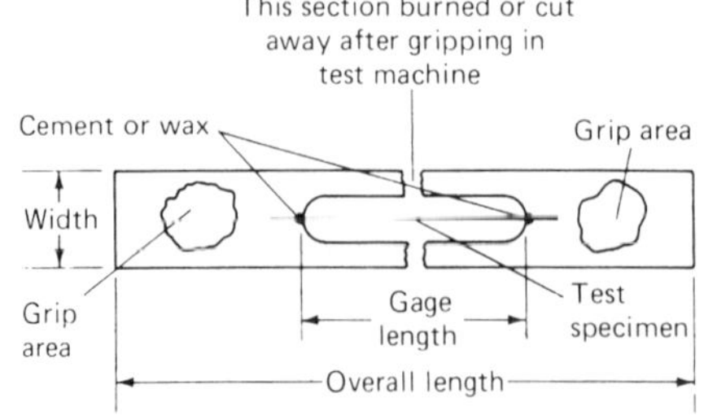

Fig. 2 Schematic showing typical specimen-mounting method for determining single-filament tensile strength

Yarn count is defined as the number of tows/mm (tows/in.) in both the warp and fill directions. This is done by simply measuring the dimensions of an undistorted fabric and removing and counting each thread. Data should be reported as the number of warp threads/mm (warp threads/in.) and number of fill threads/mm (fill threads/in.).

Fabric areal weight is measured by weighing a piece of undistorted fabric and measuring its surface area. The data is reported as g/m^2 (oz/yd^2).

Tensile strength of dry fabric may be measured using ASTM D 579 (Ref 7); however, it would be better to measure the tensile strength of an impregnated laminate, because the translation of dry fabric properties to composite properties is poorly understood.

Mechanical Tests

It is important to note that mechanical properties of fibers are very test-dependent. For example, Table 2 shows the difference in tensile strength of a typical fiber tested as a filament, tow, and laminate, all reduced to 100% fiber volume. These data emphasize the importance of identifying the test method when reporting test data.

Single-filament tensile strength can be determined using ASTM D 3379 (Ref 8), which can be summarized as a random selection of single filaments made from the material to be tested. Filaments are centerline-mounted on special slotted tabs (Fig. 2). The tabs are gripped so that the test specimen is aligned axially in the jaws of a constant-speed movable-crosshead test machine. The filaments are then stressed to failure at a constant strain rate. For this test method, filament cross-sectional areas are determined by planimeter measurements of a representative number of filament cross sections as displayed on highly magnified photomicrographs. Alternative methods of area determination include the use of optical gages, an image-splitting microscope, or the linear weight-density method.

Tensile strength and Young's modulus of elasticity are calculated from the load/elongation records and the cross-sectional area measurements. Note that a system compliance adjustment may be necessary for single-filament tensile modulus.

Tow Tensile Testing. Using ASTM D 4018 (Ref 9) or an equivalent is recommended. This is summarized as finding the tensile properties of continuous filament carbon and graphite yarns, strands, rovings, and tows by the tensile

Table 2 Effect of test method on fiber properties

	Nominal tensile strength					
	AS4		IM6		IM7	
Test	MPa	ksi	MPa	ksi	MPa	ksi
Filament	4100	595	4950	715	5400	780
Tow	4000	580	5050	730	5450	790
Laminate	3850	555	4300	625	4600	665

loading to failure of the resin-impregnated fiber forms. This technique loses accuracy as the filament count increases. Strain and Young's modulus are measured by extensometer.

The purpose of using impregnating resin is to provide the fiber forms, when cured, with enough mechanical strength to produce a rigid test specimen capable of sustaining uniform loading of the individual filaments in the specimen.

To minimize the effect of the impregnating resin on the tensile properties of the fiber forms, the resin should be compatible with the fiber, the resin content in the cured specimen should be limited to the minimum amount required to produce a useful test specimen, the individual filaments of the fiber forms should be well collimated, and the strain capability of the resin should be significantly greater than the strain capability of the filaments.

ASTM D 4018 method I test specimens require a special cast-resin end tab and grip design to prevent grip slippage under high loads. Alternative methods of specimen mounting to end tabs are acceptable, provided that test specimens maintain axial alignment on the test machine centerline and that they do not slip in the grips at high loads. ASTM D 4018 method II test specimens require no special gripping mechanisms. Standard rubber-faced jaws should be adequate.

Laminate Properties. The most generally representative procedure for measuring composite properties is to combine the fiber and resin and to test the composite as a cured laminate, because this is the form in which the materials are used. It is important to understand that laminate properties are a function of fiber, resin, and interface properties. Table 3 shows the dependence of mechanical properties on the resins used. Another factor to consider is the fiber volume fraction of the laminate. A fiber volume of 55 to 65% has been found to allow consistent measurement of properties. Because tensile properties are fiber-dominated, it is recommended that tensile strength and modulus be normalized to a constant fiber volume. A normalized fiber volume of 100% is common. This is done simply by using the following equation:

$$\text{Property (100\%)} = (\text{property} \times 100)/(\text{fiber volume, \%})$$

Laminate tensile testing should be conducted in accordance with ASTM D 3039 (Ref 10) or ASTM D 638 (Ref 11) for quartz or glass. Major concerns when conducting this test are:

- *Verification of collimation of fibers*: The specimens should be cut 0° ± ¼° from the fiber direction
- *Machining quality*: Specimens should be cut with a diamond blade circular saw, 180 grit minimum, using a water coolant. Specimens should be inspected to verify that no specimen damage was caused by machining.
- *Surface quality*: The panel should have a resin-rich surface to preclude fiber splitting. This can best be done by using an appropriate peel ply. Burlington peel ply 51789, style 52006, has been found to yield excellent results.

The apparent interlaminar shear test (previously referred to as a "short beam shear" test) is of little value to a designer, because apparent interlaminar shear strength is not necessarily representative for a pure shear test. However, this test is an inexpensive, easily done measurement of the quality of the laminate and fiber interface. It should not be used to compare fiber-resin systems. For example, a true shear test run on the systems shown in Table 3 would show 2220-3 resin-AS4 fiber to have higher shear strength than 3501-6 or 3502 resin. The test, however, is sensitive to changes within a product; because it has been shown to be a very valuable quality control test to identify changes in fiber-resin interfacial quality, it may be used to monitor product changes.

The short beam shear strength should be determined in accordance with ASTM D 2344 (Ref 12). This is a simple three-point bending test with a span-to-depth ratio of 4 to 1 and a nominal thickness of 2.03 mm (0.08 in.).

See the article "Lamina and Laminate Mechanical Testing" in this Volume for additional information on generating laminate mechanical property data.

Tests for Matrix Resins and Prepregs

This section defines some of the basic materials used for thermoset and thermoplastic resin matrices and their most significant chemical and physical tests. The individual characteristics are identified along with the test methods normally used for their determination. Many of the recommended tests are directed at the chemical properties of the resin. A complete evaluation of physical properties must also be performed to ensure that controls are adequate. Properties can be varied rather widely by the selection of the matrix resins, curing agents, and modifiers. Therefore, it is important to understand what these properties are and what effect they have on the resin matrix, impregnated fiber, and processing of the product. All tests described in this article are relative to uncured components and uncured and cured matrix systems. More detailed information about these resins is available in the Section "Constituent Materials" in this Volume.

Thermosets

The term *matrix* refers only to the nonfiber component of a composite. The key function of the matrix is to aid in the handling and processing of the fibers while translating the properties of the fibrous component in the composite. The matrix must also perform in a desired temperature envelope specified by the end-use application. The thermoset resins most widely used for composite matrices are epoxies, bismaleimides, phenolics, polyesters, vinyl esters, and polyimides. The properties of the uncured resins that are of most interest are the equivalent weight and viscosity, or rheological, values. When the equivalent weight is known, it is possible to calculate the optimal amount of curing agent required for the resin. The viscosity of the resin is a convenient index for its handling and flow characteristics during cure. Other properties of more limited interest include softening point, melting point, molecular weight, molecular weight distribution, specific gravity, refractive index, and chlorine content.

Of the thermoset systems being considered, only polyesters, vinyl esters, and epoxies require the addition of other ingredients to facilitate polymerization. There are other ingredients in some systems, particularly epoxies and bismaleimides, that serve as modifiers and, as such, may or may not enter into the chemical reactions during curing.

Epoxies are among the most widely used resins, because of their overall balance of properties. Their mechanical properties are superior to those of polyesters and phenolics, and they offer improvements in environmental/moisture resistance, fatigue resistance, and interlaminar shear strength. They also provide a combination of cross-link density and elongation that yields a balance of suitable properties over a broad temperature range. Because of this versatility, epoxies are finding increased use as matrix materials.

There are a large number of epoxy resins commercially available. The diglycidyl ether of bisphenol A (DGEBA), epoxy novolac, and tetraglycidyl-4,4′ diamino diphenyl methane (TGDDM) are the most commonly used epoxy resins for matrix formulation. Key property tests are listed in Table 4.

The bismaleimide (BMI) resins available commercially are limited. These resins have backbones similar to those of epoxies, but contain different functional end groups. The most basic and widely used resin is the bismaleimide of methylene dianiline (bis F). Bismaleimide resins cure by means of addition polymerization with little or no evolution of volatiles. They are prime candidates for matrix resins because of their high-temperature resistance, environmental stability under hot/wet conditions, superior smoke/toxicity properties, and epoxy-like processing. They tend to be more brittle than epoxies, but can be formulated to achieve various combinations of cross-link density and elonga-

Table 3 Effect of resin on laminate properties

Material		Tensile strength		Tensile modulus		Short beam shear	
Fiber	Resin	MPa	ksi	GPa	10^6 psi	MPa	ksi
AS4	2220-3	3650	527	221	32.1	106	15.4
AS4	3501-6	3450	500	225	32.7	124	18.0
AS4	3502	3000	435	223	32.4	134	19.4
AS4	4502	3000	432	220	31.9	102	14.8

Note: Tensile data normalized to 100% fiber volume

tion that provide matrix resins with balanced properties.

Bismaleimides are being used in applications that require temperature performance between that of state-of-the-art epoxies and polyimides. Key property tests are listed in Table 4.

Phenolic resins are available commercially in a wide variety of types. The two main types are a single-stage resole and a two-stage novolac. The resole phenolic is the most widely used, because of its handling characteristics in the impregnated form. It cures by means of a condensation-type reaction in which water is formed as a by-product. The resultant matrix is highly cross linked, but can be formulated with a wide variety of materials. The volatile by-products limit the use of resole phenolic for some composite applications. Phenolics have high heat and chemical resistance, good dielectric properties, dimensional and thermal stability, and surface hardness. They yield low smoke and toxicity properties after combustion, which is important for many applications. Key property tests are listed in Table 4.

Polyesters. Of the wide variety of polyester resins commercially available, those most commonly used are alkyd and unsaturated polyesters. These resins can be combined with monomers, such as styrene, to form a cross-linked matrix. Both alkyd and unsaturated polyester matrices can be used for diverse composite applications. Alkyd polyesters have good arc-track resistance and show outstanding retention of dielectric strength up to 175 °C (350 °F). Their highly cross-linked resin structure gives good dimensional stability at elevated temperatures. However, the percentage strength retention at elevated temperature is not as great as for some of the other matrix resins. In general, polyesters yield moderate composite properties and have poor chemical and hydrolytic resistance compared to other materials. Higher levels of matrix shrinkage during cure are also a detriment for some applications. Because polyesters can be cured quickly by means of a free-radical process and generally are less costly, there is incentive for using them in composites when their mechanical properties suit the application. Key property tests are listed in Table 4.

Polyimides. There are a limited number of polyimide resins available for use as composite matrices. These systems cure by means of a condensation reaction with evolution of a high level of volatiles. The two types of polyimide resins most widely used are PMR-15 and the family of pyromellitic dianhydride/oxydianiline polymers. These materials possess exceptionally high thermooxidative stability. However, the higher the oxidative stability, the more difficult they are to process. Polyimides are being used in composites applications that require temperature performance at temperatures (110 to 190 °C, or 230 to 375 °F) above the capabilities of BMIs. Their use is limited, because of the high volatile levels given off during cure. These volatiles pose severe processing problems for applications requiring large, thick composite parts. Nevertheless, the commercial success of polyimides in a variety of high-technology applications can be attributed to resin matrices with a good balance of thermooxidative stability, high glass transition temperature, and processing parameters. Key property tests are listed in Table 4.

Cyanate Esters. Another thermoset resin that is currently finding increasing potential as a matrix material is the cyanate ester. These resins perform in the same temperature range as epoxy resins, but offer a different balance of properties. Cyanate esters provide different formulation opportunities, because of their unique cure chemistry. They also are capable of co-curing with certain other thermosets, thus increasing formulation latitude.

Other Thermoset Resins. A wide variety of other matrix materials is also commercially available to provide specific end-use properties. For example, polybutadiene has excellent low-loss electrical properties with very flexible processing.

Formulations

Matrices or neat resin systems are mostly blended with ingredients that are added to impart a desired property to the prepreg and/or cured composite. Proper formulation of resin compounds requires knowledge of the molecular structure of the resins as well as their chemical/physical properties and curing reactions. The structure of the resin determines its physical and chemical properties. The number and location of the reactive sites determine the functionality and the cross-linking density. These properties establish the rigidity, thermal stability, solvent resistance, and other properties of the cured system. Resin structure also determines the viscosity of the resin, an important factor for processing. Resins are only building blocks in the development of a matrix formulation. A formulation may ultimately involve several resins combined with curing agents, catalysts, and modifiers such as fillers, flow control agents, or flexibilizers. Each component contributes to the final properties of the prepreg and cured composite and represents a major variable. Once the performance requirements of an application are known, an appropriate neat resin matrix can be formulated.

It is essential to identify key properties and define an acceptable range for each one before assigning a suitable test to measure those properties. Tests are typically performed on the individual components as well as on the uncured final formulation in order to better understand and characterize the resin system. Various chemical and physical tests are run on all types of resin matrices to ensure overall consistency and correct ingredient amounts, functional groups, molecular weight distribution, kinetics, and advancement levels.

To exemplify a neat resin matrix formulation, a typical epoxy matrix would contain epoxy A, epoxy B, a catalyst, and a curing agent. For example, most applications requiring a service temperature up to 120 °C (250 °F) would combine DGEBA (epoxy A) and/or DGEBA with epoxidized phenol novolac resins (epoxy B) with a dicyandiamide curing agent and tertiary amine salt catalyst.

An example of a current state-of-the-art epoxy-matrix system suited to a service temperature up to 177 °C (350 °F) would have TGDDM as epoxy A, diaminodiphenylsulfone as the curing agent, and a salt of BF_3 as the catalyst. Elastomer modifiers or flexible resins would be added as needed to improve toughness. For both of these examples, high-performance liquid chromatography (HPLC), differential scanning calorimetry (DSC), infrared spectroscopy, and rheometric dynamic scanning (RDS) viscosity tests are run to characterize the resin and ensure the quality of the molecular weight distribution,

Table 4 Properties and tests for thermoset resins and modifiers

Ingredient	Property	Test method
Epoxy resins		
Epoxy resins	Epoxide content	Titration
	Viscosity/ softening point	Viscometer/Duran or rheometer
	Residual chlorides	Titration
	Moisture content	Titration/Karl Fisher
	Molecular weight distribution	GPC
	Characterization	HPLC/infrared spectrosopy
Hardener (amine)	Amine content	Titration
	Purity	Melting point refractive index, HPLC
Catalyst	Purity	Melting point
	Cation	Atomic absorption
Modifier (inorganic)	Particle size	Sedigraph/particle sizer
	Moisture	Moisture analyzer/Karl Fisher
Modifier (organic)	Viscosity	Rheometer
	Reactivity	Titration
Bismaleimide resins		
Bismaleimide resin	Viscosity	Rheometer
	Composition	HPLC/infrared spectroscopy
Modifier (organic)	Viscosity	Rheometer
	Molecular weight	GPC
Phenolic resins		
Phenolic resin	Phenol	Titration
	Molecular weight	GPC
	Characterization	HPLC/infrared spectroscopy
	Solids	Evaporation
Modifier (organic)	Viscosity	Rheometer
	Molecular weight	GPC
Polyester resins		
Polyester	Reactivity	Titration of peroxide
	Molecular weight	GPC
	Purity	HPLC
		H_2O determination
Polyimide resins		
Polyimide resin	Ingredient ratio	HPLC/infrared titration
	Purity	HPLC
	Functional groups	Titration

GPC, gel permeation chromatography; HPLC, high-performance liquid chromatography

cure kinetics, functional groups, and rheological behavior for each batch of material. The chemical properties normally reported for these neat resin systems are those given in Tables 4 and 5. Chemical and physical property testing is performed on uncured neat resin systems prior to impregnation and on impregnated systems after cure. During system development, some properties are also measured on cured neat resin.

A typical BMI could contain a bis F, divinyl benzene (DVB), and thermoplastic resin. This example is a formulated matrix for applications requiring service temperatures up to 230 °C (445 °F). The bis F resin provides high-temperature properties, the thermoplastic resin modifies the rheology, and the DVB provides both matrix toughness (elongation) and tack. Applicable property tests are listed in Table 5.

A typical phenolic matrix would combine resole phenolic, ethyl alcohol, polyamide resin, and a catalyst. Resole phenolics, available in an alcohol solution, can be used directly as a matrix material with an inorganic acid catalyst. Nylon 6,6 polyamide resin can be added to improve matrix toughness and flow characteristics. Applicable property tests are listed in Table 5.

A typical polyester matrix would have an unsaturated polyester resin, styrene monomer, hydroquinone, and a promoter. A large variety of thermoset polyesters are commercially available that already contain styrene monomer. Inhibitors (such as hydroquinone) and promoters are added for gel- and cure-time control. Additional resins, such as isocyanates, can be added to improve toughness. Applicable property tests are listed in Table 5.

As discussed previously, only a limited number of polyimide resins are available for use as a matrix for composites. The complex processing technology required narrows the number of resins that would be useful for a matrix resin. One of the most commonly used resins is PMR-15. Applicable property tests are listed in Table 5. The presence of MDA (methylene dianiline), a suspected carcinogen, in PMR-15 has severely limited the number of end-use applications of PMR-15 in recent years. Some polyimide resins that do not contain MDA have been developed (see the article "Polyimide Resins" in this Volume).

Prepreg Forms

All five of the major families of matrix resins can be used to impregnate various fiber forms. The resin is then no longer in a low-viscosity stage, but has been advanced to a B-stage level of cure for better handling characteristics. The type of prepreg form is highly dependent on the end-use requirement. Four of the main forms of composite materials are unidirectional fiber tapes, woven fabrics, roving, and chopped mat. Fiber reinforcement may be in the form of strands that are composed of a number of very fine filaments. Strands can be gathered into continuous roving, chopped to provide mats, or twisted into yarns and woven into cloth. Fiber type can be glass, carbon, quartz, or aramid. Resin content in all forms must be tested, because it is one of the critical parameters for composite performance. The resin content is dependent on the laminating pressure and is of major importance, because, in conjunction with the fi-

Table 5 Properties and tests for uncured and cured thermoset-matrix resins and prepregs

Material	Property	Test method
Epoxy resins		
Uncured resin	Composition	HPLC
		Infrared spectroscopy
		GPC
	Processibility	RDS viscosity
		Gel time
		Volatile content
		Moisture content
	Reactivity	DSC ARC
Cured neat resin	Completeness of cure	Glass transition
		DSC
	Solvent/H_2O resistance	Glass transition, wet
		Moisture weight gain
		Solvent weight gain
		Interlaminar fracture toughness (G_{Ic})
	Resin toughness	Residual compression strength after impact
Uncured impregnated system	Characterization	HPLC
		Infrared spectroscopy
		DSC
	Processibility	Flow
		Gel
		RDS viscosity
		Volatiles
		Moisture
		Tack/drape
		Resin content
		Fiber weight
Cured impregnated system	Completeness of cure	DSC
		Glass transition
	Thermal properties	TGA
		Flammability
		Heat distribution temperature
	Electrical properties	Dielectric
Bismaleimide resins		
Uncured resin	Composition	HPLC
		Infrared spectroscopy
		GPC
		DSC
	Processibility	RDS viscosity
		Gel time
		Volatile content
Cured neat resin	Completeness of cure	Glass transition
	H_2O/solvent resistance	Glass transition, wet
		Moisture weight gain
		Solvent weight gain
	Resin toughness	Interlaminar fracture toughness
Uncured impregnated system	Characterization	HPLC
		Infrared spectroscopy
		DSC
	Processibility	Resin content
		Fiber content
		Flow
		Gel
		RDS viscosity
		Volatiles
		Tack/drape
Cured impregnated system	Completeness of cure	Glass transition
		DSC
	Moisture resistance	Weight gain
	Thermal properties	Thermal conductivity
	Laminate properties	Ply thickness
		Fiber volume
Phenolic resins		
Uncured resin	Composition	HPLC
		Infrared spectroscopy
		GPC
	Processibility	Solids
		Gel
		Volatile content
	Chemical activity	DSC

(continued)

HPLC, high-performance liquid chromatography; GPC, gel permeation chromatography; RDS, rheometric dynamic scanning; DSC, differential scanning calorimetry; ARC, accelerated rate calorimeter; TGA, thermogravimetric analysis

ber, it determines the strength of the ultimate laminate. Likewise, fiber areal weight is monitored, because the amount of fiber present in a composite laminate affects the ultimate strength. Property tests for the four prepreg forms are discussed subsequently.

Composites may also be processed by other techniques, such as wet lay-up or resin transfer molding, where the composite is made by combining the dry reinforcement directly with the liquid resin and curing—eliminating the preimpregnation step. These techniques offer particular advantages in appropriate situations and also allow a greater variety of reinforcement forms to be used, such as net-shape three-dimensional braids. For these process techniques, the resin and reinforcement are characterized separately, using the following guidelines as appropriate. The final composite properties are then determined as appropriate, often via element or subelement testing.

Unidirectional Tapes. Numerous fiber strands (tows) are creeled and spread while being combined with the resin matrix to produce a unidirectional tape prepreg. Once a tape is produced, the physical tests of resin content, fiber areal weight, volatile content, gel time, and flow can be run to characterize the system and ensure consistency. Chemical tests performed include HPLC, DSC, and infrared spectroscopy, as shown in Table 5. Unidirectional tapes are more commonly fabricated via a hot-melt method, although some solvent production lines are currently in use.

Woven fabrics provide more-uniform but lower composite strength properties than do tapes, but are nonetheless used extensively, because of the ease of fabrication and strength in both directions. Fabrics are produced in a broad range of styles, widths, and lengths. Woven fabrics can be impregnated either by means of a hot-melt or solution method, with the solvent being subsequently removed. The physical and chemical tests used to characterize woven fabrics are the same as those used for tapes.

Continuous strand rovings lend themselves to automated fabrication techniques by means of winding. Rovings may be impregnated in a solvent process and then wound on a core after the removal of solvent. Wet winding of low-viscosity blends of completely reactive components (containing no nonreactive solvents) is also widely done. Prepreg rovings typically provide better resin content control than that provided by wet winding. Physical tests include resin content, volatiles, band width, gel time, and yield (m/kg). Chemical tests are the same as those used for tapes and fabrics.

Chopped mat is a form that produces lower-cost structures with uniform strength characteristics. Composite strength properties are generally lower than those of woven fabrics. Physical tests should include resin content, areal weight (g/m^2), volatiles, gel time, and flow. Chemical tests should be run according to the applicable resin family (Table 5).

Table 5 (continued)

Material	Property	Test method
Phenolic resins		
Cured neat resin	Completeness of cure	Glass transition Solvent extraction
Uncured impregnated system	Characterization	HPLC Infrared spectroscopy DSC
	Processibility	Resin content Volatile content Flow Gel Tack/drape Fiber weight
Cured impregnated system	Completeness of cure	DSC
	Thermal properties	TGA Flammability
	Electrical properties	Dielectric
Polyester resins		
Uncured resin	Composition	Infrared spectroscopy HPLC
	Processibility	RDS viscosity Gel Volatile content
Cured neat resin	Completeness of cure	DSC
Uncured impregnated system	Characterization	HPLC
	Processibility	Resin content Flow Gel Tack/drape Fiber weight
Cured impregnated system	Completeness of cure	DSC
	Laminate properties	Ply thickness Fiber volume Hardness
Polyimide resins		
Uncured resin	Composition	HPLC Infrared spectroscopy GPC
	Processibility	RDS viscosity Gel time Volatile content
Cured neat resin	Completeness of cure	Glass transition DSC
	H_2O/solvent resistance	Glass transition, wet Solvent weight gain
Uncured impregnated system	Characterization	HPLC Infrared spectroscopy DSC
	Processibility	Resin content Fiber weight Flow Gel RDS viscosity Volatiles Tack/drape
Cured impregnated system	Completeness of cure	Glass transition DSC
	Moisture resistance	Weight gain
	Thermal properties	TGA Thermal conductivity
	Laminate properties	Ply thickness Fiber volume

HPLC, high-performance liquid chromatography; GPC, gel permeation chromatography; RDS, rheometric dynamic scanning; DSC, differential scanning calorimetry; ARC, accelerated rate calorimeter; TGA, thermogravimetric analysis

Thermoplastics

In conventional applications of thermoplastics, data from the physical and chemical property tests listed subsequently are usually offered by the resin supplier to inform the user of the behavior of the material:

- Tensile strength, yield, and break
- Elongation, yield, and break
- Tensile modulus
- Linear thermal expansion
- Electrical properties, including dielectric strength, dielectric constant, volume resistivity, dissipation factor
- Flexural strength, yield, and break
- Compressive strength
- Izod impact, notched

- Hardness (Rockwell)
- Water absorption, 24 h
- Thermal conductivity
- Continuous service temperature
- Processing temperature or melting point
- Heat-deflection temperature
- Solvent and chemical resistance
- Environmental resistance

Each thermoplastic polymer application has a need for some data from this list of tests. The processing method or the end use usually requires specific information about the chemical and physical nature of the material.

Impact Strength. Some of these tests assume special importance and even criticality for fiber-reinforced thermoplastics. For instance, the consideration of impact strength is significant in advanced composite applications. In fact, the behavior of thermoplastics in terms of their stress-strain relationship is the underlying reason for their consideration in impact-resistant and damage-tolerant applications. Looking at the stress-strain behavior of neat conventional thermosets, such as diaminodiphenysulfone-cured epoxies, one sees low strain and a steep curve all the way to failure. In the case of thermoplastics, strain is usually greater, but a unique behavior is observed before failure.

This phenomenon is the special involvement and the changes in molecular orientation that are known as yield. At the yield point, the average axis of molecular orientation begins to conform increasingly with the direction of the stress. Other terminology, such as draw, is sometimes used. There is usually a break in the stress-strain curve as it begins to flatten out, and more strain is observed with a given increased stress. The result is that the macromolecules begin to align and cooperate in their resistance to the applied stress. Frequently, there is a final increase in the slope of the curve (*strain hardening*) just before ultimate failure (Fig. 3). The extent to which this orientation takes place varies from one linear thermoplastic to the next, but the effect is quite significant in the behavior of such materials in these fiber-reinforced systems. Even the smallest amount of the orientation effect imparts greatly improved impact resistance and damage tolerance. In thermoplastics, there is much more area under the stress-strain curve; this area is a direct function of the work-to-failure.

Conventional thermosets do not behave this way and can be thought of as rigid networks that have a more glassy failure mode with much less area under the stress-strain curve. Thermoplastic resins being considered today as matrices for composites have relatively high values for their modulus or low strain-stress ratios. The molecular orientation effects are small but nevertheless quite important in their effect on toughness. Values for Young's modulus approaching 3450 MPa (500 ksi) have been reported. Such numbers are comparable to those of the thermosets. When these new, stiffer, and tougher resins began to appear, the need developed for more discriminating testing to evaluate the toughness and damage tolerance of composites fabricated with them.

Toughness and Damage Tolerance. Both National Aeronautics and Space Administration (NASA) and industry representatives have selected and standardized a set of five common tests for characterizing the toughness of fiber-resin composites. As the development of new, tougher thermoplastic-matrix resins is reduced to specific applications, these identified tests will become the standards for characterizing the new thermoplastic-based composites.

For interlaminar fracture toughness (G_{Ic}), the edge delamination and double cantilevered beam tests have been defined as appropriate. For damage tolerance, open-hole compression, open-hole tension, and compression after impact have been defined.

It should be noted that each test has its own set of problems. For example, failures in the double-cantilever beam test seldom occur solely in mode I (peel). In the past, different laboratories have used composite specimens with different resin content and fiber types, as well as different specimen dimensions and impact stress levels. In spite of these problems, test refinements have been made and reliable test data have begun to emerge. See Table 6 for G_{Ic} values.

Creep and Environmental Resistance. Special supplemental tests will be needed to assess thermoplastic resins as advanced composite matrices and to provide design assurances in the areas of temperature versus creep and environmental-stress cracking. Because the uncross-linked nature of thermoplastics means a departure from the familiar behavior of thermosets, tests will be needed to provide assurance of service life and reliability. For example, the differences in the failure behavior of many thermoplastics in the stressed and unstressed condition are dramatic, especially when the environmental effects of agents such as solvents and surface-active organics are present.

Creep in thermoplastics will have to be appropriately addressed if these resins are to become reliable matrices for advanced composites. The rigid, random network of the thermosetting resin is, by nature, a significantly different system than the collection of amassed, large, linear molecules in a thermoplastic. Test procedures and a test data bank will be required.

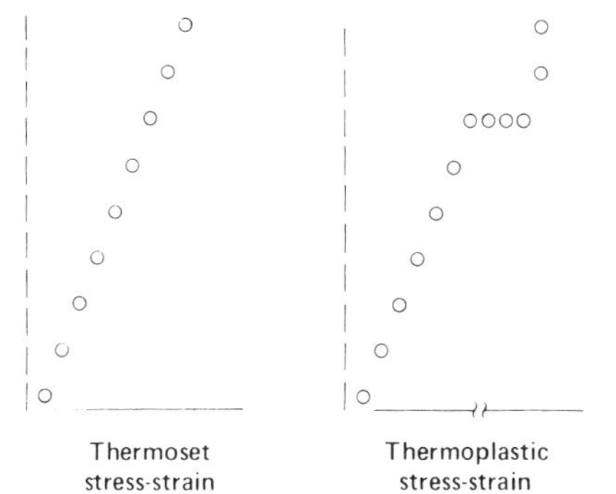

Fig. 3 Thermoset versus thermoplastic stress-strain behavior

Creep occurs in thermoplastics, because, unlike thermoset molecules, the molecules of thermoplastics are not bonded together by primary (covalent) bonds. Thus, thermoplastic molecules can make, break, and remake associations with their molecular neighbors. Such behavior allows subtle changes in form and shape. Corresponding reversible changes in thermosets are not possible, because the primary covalent chemical bond is the mainstay for retention of form and shape; once the limit of load-carrying ability is reached, bonds break and the thermoset fails catastrophically. Break and remake of bonds is not possible. The integrity of thermoplastic molecules can be attributed to simple mechanical entanglement, but a great deal of this integrity is due to reversible associations of ordered molecules by van der Waals forces, dipole-dipole interactions, and crystalline lattice energy. Some of the new thermoplastics rely on a high crystalline content for stiffness and creep resistance. The polyphenylene sulfides, for example, exhibit some of the best of both worlds and seem to be tough and damage tolerant.

One of the most difficult test configurations that could be used to define thermoplastic-matrix creep behavior would be a static load on a ±45° tensile coupon. This test would place a sustained load on the thermoplastic polymer, which would require the association forces within and between the polymer molecules to have enough strength and integrity to resist slow deformation and maintain the spatial configuration in this scissoring plane. This situation, difficult enough for the thermoplastic polymer, would be made even more severe by the imposition of an elevated temperature. Unfortunately, this most-difficult scenario for a test coupon can be a real-life load situation for an advanced composite structural component. Similarly, a beam in a static flexing load represents another very difficult real-life configuration in which retention of shape and form would be of critical importance. The influence of the composite designer can be significant in terms of selecting fiber configurations in the composite lay-up that would permit the fiber to handle this stress and let the thermoplastic resin synergistically contribute its best innate features.

Solvent and Chemical Resistance. Because the associative forces of thermoplastics are, by nature, completely different from the strong covalent chemical bond acting as the principal associative force in thermosets, the weaker forces of the thermoplastics can be much more suscep-

Table 6 Interlaminar fracture toughness (G_{Ic}) values of thermoplastic resins

Material	J/m²	ft · lbf/ft²
Polyphenylene sulfide	720	50
Polyetherimide	950	65
Polyamideimide	1050	70
Polysulfone	1175	80
Polyether etherketone	1600	110

tible to disruption by solvents. For example, any solvation around a polar site would alter molecular spacing and upset van der Waals association. Similarly, the strongest of these forces, the crystalline lattice energy, would also be disrupted if a solvent were present with enough solvating ability to come into the interstices in the crystalline structure of the ordered polymer. Thermosets are not immune to such disruption of molecular associative forces, however. It is well documented that the intrusion of water will reduce the glass transition temperature of a typical epoxy system. In fact, water is an agent that also must be considered in thermoplastic matrices.

Resistance to hydraulic fluids, lubricants, fuel, and solvents, especially when under stress, is an important requirement of composites used on aircraft. Many amorphous thermoplastics, such as polyetherimide and polysulfone, are prone to attack by hydraulic fluid and paint strippers, such as methylene chloride. When the crystallinity of a polymer is increased, its resistance to solvents improves. Consequently, polymers such as polyphenylene sulfide and polyether etherketone show better solvent resistance than other, less-crystalline polymers. The long-term suitability of such crystalline polymers in contact with solvents is yet to be determined.

Tests to evaluate solvent resistance have usually been before-and-after assessments of a given mechanical property after immersing the thermoplastic resin in the solvent or agent. A quick, reliable test consists of determining the weight picked up after a period of immersion. Also, dimensional changes can be measured after exposure, especially on neat resins. As described previously, solvent intrusion into polymer matrices disrupts the associative forces and consequently, swells the polymer. This can be detected by a simple measurement of sample dimensions and a calculation of volume change. This will provide an indication of the extent to which the composite may be affected by the solvent; however, mechanical testing is required to determine the true impact on performance. Screening may be done by apparent interlaminar shear testing in accordance with ASTM D 2344 in order to determine the worst-case solvent, which is most commonly water for thermosets. If required, a one-batch mechanical test matrix is then run after exposure to determine the potential knockdown during service. Some thermoplastic resin suppliers provide some information on water, with data on weight increase after a 24 h immersion in water. A more severe test is the 24 h water boil; however, there is some disagreement as to whether the water-boil test is representative of real-life aging.

The intrusion of solvent or any other agent, including water, may also interfere with the associative or adhesive forces at the interface between the resin and the fiber. This is true for both thermosets and thermoplastics. Such interference may be more severe for thermoplastics, because there is typically less functionality to assist in forming special adhesion sites on the fiber. With thermoplastics, the surface-surface strength is more a problem of physical interactions and classical adhesion. Testing interlaminar shear or transverse mechanical properties can assess the detrimental effects of such solvent or water intrusion.

Thermal Expansion. In another volume-change phenomenon, thermosets undergo a significant amount of volume shrinkage when the polymer is formed from its monomeric precursors. This change can be in the range of 3 to 5% of the volume of epoxies. In some addition-type unsaturated polymers, such as BMIs, it can be even higher and can become a source of difficulty by initiating microcracks. This behavior represents a potential advantage for thermoplastics in that such shrinkage is a possible source of microcracking in composite fabrication, especially in fabric or cross-plied laminates. Because the polymerization of thermoplastics is already over at the processing stage, the shrinkage caused by packing improvements on a molecular scale is minimal. The shrinkage that remains is due to contraction upon cooling, which is reported in the supplier's standard data as mold shrinkage or as a coefficient of linear thermal expansion.

Viscosity measurements on thermoplastic candidates for composite matrices are all taken at elevated temperature and, consequently, are not routinely provided by the resin suppliers. The melt values reported in Table 7 give some information as to how the resin will flow under laminating conditions, but the real nature of flow is important in good composite fabrication. If the flow is merely a sintering, there will be a discontinuity between plies, and voids will most likely be present. In processing composites, a good rule of thumb is that some degree of edge flow or bleed will be visible. If this is not the case, voids are likely to be present, because of air entrapment. Some fabricators use unrealistic pressures to prepare study samples; resins that require such treatment will not be suitable for producing good-quality composite structures. Brute force and the preparation of 75 × 75 mm (3 × 3 in.) test laminates are not suitable approaches for evaluating a resin for use in composite fabrication. In addition to the requirement for flow, there is a need for a workable viscosity for good tow wet-out during the initial prepreg process. The viscosity test values shown in Table 7 will change, usually downward, if thermal mistreatment of the polymer occurs during the prepreg or lamination processes or during rework of the finished composite.

When melting a thermoplastic resin in the prepreg process or, more importantly, in the final fabrication step, all crystalline order is erased (except in unique liquid crystalline polymers). Subsequently, during cooldown, the polymer reestablishes crystalline lattice order. The degree to which this order is reinstated is a function of the viscosity and mobility of the cooling system. If the cooling is fast, there is little time for the molecules to find their appropriate positions in the growing lattice structure. Many of the molecules will lose their mobility as the temperature is decreased and, being unable to move into the proper position to form the crystalline state, will be stranded in an amorphous condition. Conversely, if the cooling rate is slow, most of the molecules, or segments of molecules, will maintain freedom long enough to find their appropriate position in the crystalline state.

Characterization Methods. Some common characterization tests used for oligomers and polymers are not appropriate for the class of thermoplastics being considered for high-performance composite matrices, because the test methods require that the material be in solution. If the thermoplastic composite is to have solvent resistance, it cannot be soluble in any solvent. This is the case for inherent viscosity, for example, because this measurement is made in solution. Similarly, HPLC cannot be used as a characterization method. In composite applications that do not require a high degree of solvent resistance, the methods described might be used. With thermosets, HPLC has been used as a fingerprint characterization and quality-control tool. This analytical technique could be used for soluble thermoplastics.

Other methods, such as infrared spectroscopy, are more suitable for routine characterization or fingerprinting of thermoplastics. Before the advent of Fourier transform infrared (FTIR), infrared spectroscopy was difficult to use as a quantitative tool for measuring subtle changes in structure and concentration. Now that FTIR has been supplemented with im-

Table 7 Melt values of viscosity for selected thermoplastic resins

Material, temperature	Viscosity Pa · s	Viscosity P
Polyamideimide at 350 °C (662 °F)	10^6	10^7
Polysulfone at 300 °C (570 °F)	10^4	10^5
Polyetherimide at 305 °C (580 °F)	10^5	10^6
Polyphenylene sulfide at 313 °C (595 °F)	10^4	10^5
Polyether etherketone at 400 °C (750 °F)	10^3	10^4

Table 8 Useful property data for a typical carbon-resin composite

Property	Typical value
Fiber density, g/cm^3	1.80
Tow yield, m/kg (yd/lb)	1100 (565)
Cured resin density, g/cm^3	1.2
Prepreg density, g/cm^3	1.5
Prepreg thickness/ply, mm (in.)	0.15 (0.0067)
Resin film thickness, mm (in.)	0.085 (0.0034)
Resin film areal wt, kg/m^2 (oz/yd^2)	0.099 (2.946)
Fiber areal wt, kg/m^2 (oz/yd^2)	0.149 (4.420)
Prepreg resin content, %	40
Tow count, tows/mm (tows/in.)	0.17 (4.3)
Fiber volume fraction, %	49
Prepreg yield, m^{2}kg (ft^{2}lb)	4.00 (19.55)
Flow, %	5
Cured ply thickness, mm (in.)	0.15 (0.0061)
Fiber vol% (cured), %	53

Table 9 Typical acceptance and revalidation tests required for suppliers and users

Property	Testing required: Production acceptance (supplier)(a)	Production acceptance (user)(a)	Revalidation (user)(a)	Specimens required per sample
Prepreg properties				
Visual and dimensional	X	X	...	...
Volatile content	X	X	...	3
Moisture content	X	X	X	3
Gel time	X	X	X	3
Resin flow	X	X	X	2
Tack	X	X	X	1
Resin content	X	X	...	3
Fiber areal weight	X	X	...	3
Infrared analysis	X	...	...	1
Liquid chromatograph	X	X	X	2
Differential scanning calorimetry	X	X	X	2
Lamina properties				
Density	X	...	...	3
Fiber volume	X	...	...	3
Resin volume	X	...	...	3
Void content	X	...	...	3
Per ply thickness	X	X	X	1
Glass transition temperature	X	X	X	3
Short beam shear or ±45° tension	X(b)	X(b)	X(b)	6
90°/0° compression strength	X(c)	X(c)	X(b)	6
90°/0° tension strength and modulus	X(b)	X(b)	X(b)	6

(a) Supplier is defined as the prepreg supplier. User is defined as the composite part fabricatior. Production acceptance tests are defined as tests to be performed by the supplier or user for initial acceptance. Revalidation tests are tests performed by the user at the end of guaranteed storage life or room-temperature out-time to provide for additional use of the material after expiration of the normal storage or out-time life. (b) Tests shall be conducted at room temperature/dry. (c) Tests shall be conducted at room temperature/dry and maximum temperature/dry (see MIL-HDBK-17 Volume I, Section 2.2.2).

proved surface reflectance methods, this technique has become very viable for characterizing and studying thermoplastic resins and is informative for finished thermoplastic composites.

Perhaps the most important characterization methods for both thermoplastic and thermoset composites and composite precursors are gravimetry and mensuration. The values obtained are the criteria most critical to the outcome of successful composite components. Table 8 gives the type of data that are of vital significance to the prepregger, designer, and fabricator.

The basic mechanical performance and/or quality of polymer, fiber, prepreg, or composite is primarily determined by mechanical testing of a test coupon to attain the truest assessment of the performance of the material. The coupon test method is thoroughly described in the article "Lamina and Laminate Mechanical Testing" in this Section of the Volume.

Quality Conformance Testing. The previous discussion did not distinguish between characterization, qualification, and quality conformance testing. Quality conformance tests are needed to assure the continued integrity of a previously characterized material system. The tests performed must be able to characterize each batch/lot of material, so that a proper assessment of critical properties of a material system can be made. These critical properties provide information on the integrity of a material system with regard to material properties, fabrication capability, and use. Additionally, the test matrix must be designed to economically and quickly evaluate a material system.

Quality control in a production environment involves inspection and testing of composites in all stages of prepreg manufacture and part fabrication. Tests must be performed by the material supplier on the fiber and resin as separate materials, as well as on the composite prepreg material. The user of the prepreg must perform receiving inspection and revalidation tests, in-process control tests, and nondestructive inspection tests on finished parts. The sampling frequency and specific tests performed for a given resin system may well depend on a statistical analysis of the history of the material. Table 9 provides the typical test scenario required.

ACKNOWLEDGMENTS

This article was updated from G.E. Hansen, Tests for Reinforcement Fibers, p 285–288, and L.C. Hopper and G.L. Sauer, Properties Tests for Matrix Resins, p 289–294, *Engineered Materials Handbook,* Volume 1, *Composites,* ASM International, 1987.

REFERENCES

1. "Standard Methods for Chemical Analysis of Carbon and Carbon-Ceramic Refractories," C 571, American Society for Testing and Materials (note: standard discontinued in 1995)
2. "Standard Test Methods for Residual Carbon, Apparent-Residual Carbon, and Apparent Carbon Yield in Coked Carbon-Containing Brick and Shapes," C 831, *Annual Book of ASTM Standards*, American Society for Testing and Materials
3. "Standard Test Methods for Density and Specific Gravity (Relative Density) of Plastics by Displacement," D 792, *Annual Book of ASTM Standards*, American Society for Testing and Materials
4. "Standard Test Method for Density of High-Modulus Fibers," D 3800, *Annual Book of ASTM Standards*, American Society for Testing and Materials
5. "Standard Test Method for Density of Plastics by the Density-Gradient Technique," D 1505, *Annual Book of ASTM Standards*, American Society for Testing and Materials
6. "Standard Specification for Glass Fiber Strands," D 578, *Annual Book of ASTM Standards*, American Society for Testing and Materials
7. "Standard Specification for Greige Woven Glass Fabrics," D 579, *Annual Book of ASTM Standards*, American Society for Testing and Materials
8. "Standard Test Method for Tensile Strength and Young's Modulus for High-Modulus Single-Filament Materials," D 3379, *Annual Book of ASTM Standards*, American Society for Testing and Materials
9. "Standard Test Methods for Properties of Continuous Filament Carbon and Graphite Fiber Tows," D 4018, *Annual Book of ASTM Standards*, American Society for Testing and Materials
10. "Standard Test Method for Tensile Properties of Polymer Matrix Composite Materials," D 3039, *Annual Book of ASTM Standards*, American Society for Testing and Materials
11. "Standard Test Method for Tensile Properties of Plastics," D 638, *Annual Book of ASTM Standards*, American Society for Testing and Materials
12. "Standard Test Method for Short-Beam Strength of Polymer Matrix Composite Materials and Their Laminates," D 2344, *Annual Book of ASTM Standards*, American Society for Testing and Materials

SELECTED REFERENCES

- W. Brostow, Ed., *Performance of Plastics,* Hanser-Gardner, 2001
- S.B. Driscoll, Physical, Chemical, and Thermal Analysis of Thermoplastic Resins, *Engineering Plastics,* Vol 2, *Engineered Materials Handbook,* ASM International, 1988, p 533–543
- Evaluation of Reinforcement Fibers, *Guidelines for Characterization of Structural Materials,* Vol 1, *Composite Materials Handbook,* MIL-HDBK-17, Materials Sciences

Corporation, University of Delaware, Army Research Laboratory, www.mil17.org/

- D.K. Hadad and C.A. May, Physical, Chemical, and Thermal Analysis of Thermoset Resins, *Engineering Plastics,* Vol 2, *Engineered Materials Handbook,* ASM International, 1988, p 517–532
- H. Ishida, Ed., *Characterization of Composite Materials,* Butterworth-Heinemann, 1994
- *Materials Characterization*, Vol 10, *ASM Handbook*, ASM International, 1986
- Matrix Characterization, *Guidelines for Characterization of Structural Materials,* Vol 1, *Composite Materials Handbook,* MIL-HDBK-17, Materials Sciences Corporation, University of Delaware, Army Research Laboratory, www.mil17.org/
- Mechanical Testing of Polymers and Ceramics, *Mechanical Testing and Evaluation,* Vol 8, *ASM Handbook,* ASM International, 2000, p 26–48
- M.M. Millard, Fibers and Polymers, *Industrial Applications of Surface Analyses,* Vol 199, *American Chemical Society Symposium Series*, L.A. Casper and C.J. Powell, Ed., American Chemical Society, 1982, p 143–202
- T.A. Osswald and G. Menges, *Materials Science of Polymers for Engineers,* Hanser-Gardner, 1996
- C.D. Wagner, W.M. Riggs, L.E. Davis, J.F. Moulder, and G.E. Muilenberg, *Handbook of X-Ray Photoelectron Spectroscopy,* Perkin-Elmer Corporation, 1979

Lamina and Laminate Nonmechanical Testing

John Moylan, Delsen Testing Laboratories

CHARACTERIZATION of nonmechanical properties is performed in the testing and certification of composite materials for two primary purposes:

- To provide the designer with information of a nonmechanical nature that may be important in the final application. Among these are physical attributes such as thickness and density, thermal properties such as thermal conductivity and diffusivity, electrical properties, and flammability properties.
- To provide quality control characteristics of laminates for certification of materials and for quality assurance and control of final parts

In this article, properties with general interest that are commonly investigated will be discussed:

- Per ply thickness
- Constituent content
- Density
- Coefficient of thermal expansion (CTE) and coefficient of moisture expansion (CME)
- Glass transition temperature (T_g)
- Thermal conductivity, diffusivity, and specific heat

Unlike fabrication of parts using metallic materials, fabrication using composites generally involves a final cure of the material. Because this final cure step is often performed by the fabricator, and because the composites materials properties depend on this step, rigorous process quality control is required for critical parts. The physical attributes and constituent measurements described in this article can be used as quality verification tools.

Also in contrast to metallic alloys, the characterization of the composite material is dependent upon the size level at which the material is tested. As explained earlier in this Volume in the article "Overview of Testing and Certification," testing can be carried out at the constituent, lamina, laminate, and larger levels. Usually, economy is achieved by testing at the lowest level for which results can be analyzed and applied to the finished part.

MIL-HDBK-17, *Polymer Matrix Composites*, Volume 1, *Guidelines* considers all of the previously mentioned nonmechanical properties to be lamina physical properties. Certainly care must be taken in applying properties such as CTE derived at a lamina level to a full-sized component. Variations in the makeup and cure of a large part, intended and unintended isotropy, and residual stresses could affect the CTE of the final part.

It is recognized that there are composites for which the lamina and laminate distinction is not applicable. Small, representative samples of composite materials, such as bulk molded compounds or ceramics reinforced with discontinuous fibers, can be used for materials characterization.

Per Ply Thickness

The thickness of a composite part is an important property from the standpoint of weight and dimensional compliance and fit in applications that interface other parts, such as hardware. Additionally, thickness per ply is useful as a measure of resin content achieved during cure or consolidation. Part thickness is governed by the number of plies in the lay-up, the amount of matrix resin present (resin content), the amount of reinforcing fiber (fiber volume), and the amount of porosity (void volume). In the case of resin transfer molding, the tool dimensions dictate thickness (by controlling resin content). If it is assumed that the amounts of resin, fiber, and porosity do not vary from one ply to another within the structure, then the thickness per ply times the number of plies is representative of the part thickness. In practice, the proportions of resin, fiber, and porosity may vary somewhat from ply to ply. The magnitude of this variation is largely a function of processing parameters. Generally there is a nominal target thickness per ply that is achieved under normal processing. If more resin is bled off, the final thickness will be lower, the resin content lower, and the fiber content higher.

Measurement of per ply thickness is useful as an indication of resin content and a quality control check on the fabrication process. Thickness measurements are required for mechanical properties testing to determine the cross-sectional area of material under test. Methodology for this measurement is given in Suppliers of Advanced Composite Materials Association (SACMA) SRM 10R-94. This group is no longer active, but the standards are still in use.

In measuring thickness per ply, consistent use of the same type of measuring device is required. A double ball micrometer with 6 mm (0.25 in.) diameter balls is called out in the SACMA standard and is commonly used. Note that a flat anvil micrometer will generally give thicker readings, especially on fabrics, due to the weave causing local regions of the part to be thicker. Other surface texture properties may also give rise to local variations in thickness measurements. The micrometer should have a deep throat, allowing measurement of the center of larger panels. In making the measurement, care should be taken to keep the panel perpendicular to the micrometer. This becomes a greater issue with larger panels. Other methods for measuring thickness include ultrasonic and noncontacting optical methods.

Constituent Content

Polymer-matrix composites may contain two or more of the following: a polymer or resin matrix; fibers of polymer, carbon, glass, or other inorganics; and inorganic fillers. Most commonly, the composite consists of one type of fiber and one type of resin. Determination of resin content, along with void content, is useful in characterizing cure and in evaluation of mechanical test results. Reliable test methods exist for determining constituent content in simple composite systems with one fiber and one resin.

ASTM D 2584. For resin matrix/glass composites, ASTM D 2584, "Test Method for Ignition Loss of Cured Reinforced Resins," is commonly used. In this method, a composite specimen is predried and weighed. The specimen is then placed in a tared crucible and inserted in a muffle furnace to burn off all organic material. Following ignition in the furnace, the crucible is cooled in a dessicator and reweighed. The remaining material will include glass reinforcement along with inorganic fillers.

In some cases, the procedure may be modified to differentiate between the inorganic fillers and the glass fibers. The inorganic fillers may be dissolved in acid and the remaining material filtered. This approach may be successful in identifying calcium carbonate fillers, for example. This type of protocol depends on the chemical composition of the fillers and needs to be developed for each system.

ASTM D 3171. Resin-matrix composites may be analyzed using ASTM D 3171, "Fiber Content of Resin Matrix Composite by Matrix Digestion." The method employs standard digestion techniques to digest or remove the resin matrix without dissolving the fiber. Method A, a hot nitric acid digestion, and method B, a sulfuric acid/hydrogen peroxide digestion, are commonly used on carbon-fiber composites. Method C is a sodium hydroxide digestion that is designed for aramid-fiber composites. Other variations of the acid digestion procedure use microwave energy and pressure to speed the digestion process. In any of these methods, it is prudent to evaluate a fiber blank when testing a new or different material. Use of the blank will determine the extent that the fiber is attacked during the digestion process.

Hybrid Composites. More complex composites can be difficult to analyze, depending on the specific makeup of the hybrid. Combinations of the methods discussed previously may be useful to determine constituent content. For instance, for a glass-carbon hybrid, one might first perform an acid digestion to determine total fiber content and then burn off the carbon fibers in a muffle furnace to determine glass content.

Microscopic Evaluation. Another method for characterizing constituent content is through "metallographic" cross-sectioning followed by microscopic evaluation. This evaluation may be enhanced by the use of computer-based image analysis techniques. A small section of the composite is cut and then processed through a series of grinding and polishing steps to ensure an optical finish. When performed correctly, there should be no smear or rounding of the various materials, and the entire surface should be in the same plane. Once polished, the fibers, resin, and voids are visually apparent. Sometimes tougheners in two-phase resin systems may be apparent. One can also verify lay-up and ply count. Computerized image analysis may be used to scan the image and sum the areas of each constituent. The advantages of these methods include the ability to verify ply count and lay-up and to discern through-the-thickness variations in resin and void distribution. These methods eliminate the need for hazardous chemicals and thus eliminate the hazardous waste generated by methods such as the acid digestion method. The disadvantage of the method is that the analysis is limited to the single plane of cross-sectioning. The computer-based image analysis tools can require a significant investment in software and hardware. The imaging methods are not standardized, but there are currently efforts in ASTM D-30 and MIL-HDBK-17 to formalize and standardize these methods.

Measuring Voids. Void volume of composites may be calculated if the composite density, cured resin density, fiber density, and resin and fiber content by weight are known. The cured resin and fiber density must be known with precision, $\pm$ 0.001 g/cm^3. These properties are usually available from the materials supplier and should be obtained for the specific lot of material being evaluated. The calculation for void volume is found in ASTM D 2734, "Void Volume of Reinforced Plastics." Void volume can also be measured directly when using an image analysis approach.

Density

ASTM D 792. The density of cured composites is usually measured by a water displacement technique. This technique is found in ASTM D 792, "Specific Gravity and Density of Plastics by Displacement." The test method uses Archimedes' principle to determine the volume of the material. The mass is determined through direct weighing, and density is calculated from mass divided by the volume. The density of metal-matrix composites and ceramic-matrix composites can also be determined with this method. This method works well on materials with relatively smooth surfaces. Air bubbles can bias the measurement, particularly if they accumulate in surface imperfections or voids.

ASTM D 1505. Other techniques for measuring density include a gradient column technique, where specimens are suspended in a column with layers of materials of known densities. The density is determined from the level the specimen is supported in the column. The density within the column is verified by standard density floats. The method is described in ASTM D 1505, "Density of Plastics by the Density-Gradient Technique." This method is very accurate when performed correctly, but requires skill and practice to obtain optimal results. It is less commonly performed in actual practice.

Helium pycnometry has also been reported as a method for determining composite density. The accuracy of the technique is dependent on the ratio of the volume of sample to the volume of the chamber. This method may not be as accurate as the liquid displacement technique when the liquid displacement test is performed by an experienced operator. The required equipment is relatively expensive and not commonly found in composites laboratories, but may be justified when large quantities of specimens are to be tested without the need of extreme accuracy.

Coefficient of Thermal Expansion and Coefficient of Moisture Expansion

The dimensional stability of composite parts is primarily a function of the CTE and the CME. The CTE is the slope of the expansion versus temperature curve and is usually expressed in Système International d'Unités (SI) units of 10^{-6}/K or 10^{-6}/°C, or customary units of 10^{-6}/°F. It is assumed to be linear over the reported range. The CME is the slope of the expansion versus moisture content curve and is usually expressed in units 10^{-6}/% moisture.

Like other composite properties, CTE is highly isotropic in composite materials. Generally, coefficients of linear thermal expansion are measured in the in-plane (x and y) and out-of-plane (z) directions. The out-of-plane CTE is generally much larger than the in-plane CTE. Within the xy plane, the CTE can be expected to vary with the fiber lay-up. Three methods are commonly used to measure CTE in composites: dilatometry, strain gage measurements, and optical measurements.

Dilatometry and its related technique, thermomechanical analysis (TMA), are described in ASTM D 696 and E 831, respectively. In dilatometry, a small composite specimen is placed in a quartz tube with a quartz rod resting on its surface. As the sample is heated, the relative displacement of the tube to the rod is measured. The dilatometer uses a generally larger sample and was originally designed to measure displacement using dial indicators. A linear variable differential transformer can also be used by this method to measure the displacements. Accuracy is attainable down to several parts per million per degree Celsius. Precision between laboratories using the ASTM D 696 method is 1.5 to 2%. The TMA is an automated instrumental approach to the CTE measurement. Either instrument is calibrated with known standards, such as copper. More accurate measurements are needed in some applications (such as spacecraft). In such cases, optical measurements are performed. MIL-HDBK-17 accepts the D 696 method for in-plane CTE and the E 831 method for out-of-plane measurements.

Strain gages may also be used to determine CTE. This technique is generally slow and expensive for making materials property measurements. It is useful for measuring local CTEs on structures. The unknown specimen and a known material, usually quartz, are tested. The strain gages should be as nearly identical as possible. Both the reference material and the unknown specimen are placed together in an oven or temperature chamber. Care must be taken that the temperature is stable and that both the reference and the unknown sample are at precisely the same temperature. The CTE may then be determined from relative change in strain gage output between the two materials. The process is repeated at several temperatures over the range of interest.

Optical measurement techniques fall into two categories, interferometers and optical levers. Both of these techniques lend themselves to very accurate low-level CTE measurements. With care, accuracies to 0.01×10^{-6}/°C have been reported. Interferometer use is covered by ASTM E 289. The method uses interference patterns that relate directly to the wavelength of light used to measure very small changes in dimensions.

The other optical approach is to use an optical lever. The unknown material is placed together with a known material, such as quartz. The specimen is arranged so that the relative movement of the unknown specimen with respect to the known specimen deflects a laser beam, and this deflection is measured. It should be noted that significant edge effects may be present for composites, particularly at very low CTEs, so specimens representative of the actual size in use are sometimes required.

Moisture Expansion. No ASTM standard for CME currently exists. Investigators commonly test two identical specimens together at the same time, measuring dimensional change in one and specimen and weight change (moisture content) in the other. Effects of moisture gradients through the specimens must be considered. It must also be noted that CME may vary with temperature, so CME measurements at more than one temperature may be required. Besides causing swelling, absorbed moisture in a composite can change the T_g of the polymer and affect the mechanical properties. The means of measuring the rate of absorption (moisture diffusivity) and the total moisture content (moisture equilibrium) are discussed in ASTM D 5229/D 5229M, "Test Method for Moisture Absorption Properties and Equilibrium Conditioning of Polymer Matrix Composite Materials." These topics are addressed in the article "Hygrothermal Behavior" in this Volume.

Glass Transition Temperature

The glass transition of a polymer-matrix composite is a temperature-induced change in the matrix material from the glassy to the rubbery state during heating, or from a rubber to a glass during cooling. A change in matrix stiffness of two to three orders of magnitude can occur during the glass transition, due to the reduction of long-range molecular mobility of the polymer chains. The temperature range over which the glass transition occurs is a function of the molecular architecture and the cross-link density of the polymer chains. The observed glass transition is dependent on the basic test method, on details such as the heating or cooling rate, and on the test frequency, if a dynamic mechanical technique is employed. In addition to the change in stiffness, the glass transition is marked by a change in the heat capacity and a change in the CTE of the material.

The glass transition is frequently characterized by a T_g, but because the transition often occurs over a broad temperature range, the use of a single temperature to characterize it may give rise to some confusion. The experimental technique used to obtain the T_g must be described in detail for the measurement to be meaningful. The method by which T_g is calculated from the data must also be clearly stated. Reported T_g may reflect onset of the glass transition or midpoint temperature, depending on the data reduction method.

The T_g is also affected by environmental conditions, such as absorbed moisture. Upon exposure to high-humidity environments, polymer matrices will absorb environmental moisture and be plasticized by it. This will lower the T_g. Measurement of the T_g in a composite material plasticized by absorbed moisture poses some difficult experimental challenges. Heating the test specimen, as required for the measurement, will drive off at least some of the absorbed moisture, thereby affecting the measured properties.

Due to the decrease in matrix stiffness that occurs at the glass transition and the low strength of these polymer matrices in the rubbery state, the matrix can no longer function as effectively to transfer load to the fibers or suppress fiber buckling above the glass transition. The glass transition temperature is, therefore, frequently used to define the upper-use temperature of a reinforced composite structural material.

A safety margin of 28 °C (50 °F) between the T_g and the material operational limit (MOL) is a commonly used criterion in industry and is a guideline given in MIL-HDBK-17 for epoxy matrices. This should only be used as an initial estimation for a MOL, however. Testing of critical properties at the MOL temperature and long-term aging followed by additional testing are certainly appropriate. Creep behavior, in particular, will be substantially different above and below the T_g.

Several different methods are commonly used to characterize the glass transition in fiber-reinforced materials.

Differential Scanning Calorimetry (DSC). Because the heat capacity of a composite material changes at the glass transition, DSC may be used to determine T_g. The glass transition is detected as a shift in the heat flow versus temperature curve (Fig. 1). Many calorimeters are supplied with software that may be used to calculate T_g. In some resin systems, this change in heat flow at T_g is pronounced; on others it can be difficult to observe. In composite specimens, the resin content in the specimen is small, and the more highly cross-linked the resin, the smaller the change in heat capacity. It is, therefore, sometimes difficult to detect T_g.

Thermomechanical analysis techniques, such as expansion, flexure, or penetration, may also be used to determine T_g. In expansion TMA, the coefficient of linear thermal expansion is measured in the *z*-axis (through the thickness) as a function of temperature. As noted previously, heat capacity undergoes a change during the glass transition. In flexural TMA, a rectangular specimen is loaded in bending, and the dimensional change is measured as a function of temperature. The results of this determination will depend highly on the applied load and specimen geometry, so large laboratory-to-laboratory variation can be expected, unless a very specific protocol is followed. In penetration mode TMA, a sharp probe, similar to that used in a hardness test, is applied to the specimen under constituent load, and the specimen is heated. Near the T_g, the probe will begin to penetrate the surface of the sample, causing an inflection on the TMA curve. Like flexure TMA, the results depend highly on the applied load and specimen geometry.

Dynamic Mechanical Analysis (DMA). Several types of DMA have been used with composites, including torsion pendulum analysis, other resonant techniques, and forced oscillation measurements in tension, torsion, and shear. These forced measurements are made using a number of DMA instruments manufactured by DuPont, Perkin Elmer, Polymer Laboratory, Rheometrics, TA Instruments, and others. All these DMA techniques produce curves of dynamic storage, loss modulus, and loss tangent as a function of temperature. They reflect the amount of energy dissipated during each cycle of loading and go through a peak value during the glass transition.

The glass transition temperature may be determined from DMA data in several different ways, and this may be a source of differences in the reported values for T_g. The T_g may be determined as the temperature at the onset or the midpoint of the transition based on :

- Storage modulus curve
- Maximum in tan delta
- Maximum in loss modulus

The method used for calculating will produce markedly different values for the same set of DMA data, up to 28 °C (50 °F) difference. The temperature scanning rate and frequency employed will also affect the results.

The lowest DMA value, usually the onset of the observed T_g in the storage modulus curve, will often be the closest estimate of the tempera-

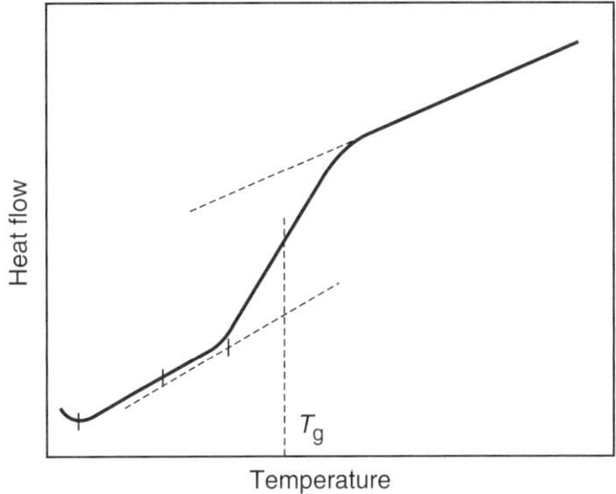

Fig. 1 Heat flow vs. temperature. Glass transition temperature, T_g, is determined by differential scanning calorimetry. Glass transition is marked by a change in heat capacity. Glass transition temperature is characterized as being the midpoint of the transition range. Source: MIL-HDBK-17, Volume 1

ture where a dramatic fall-off in mechanical properties is observed.

Direct Methods. The T_g is also sometimes measured by performing a series of mechanical tests at temperatures near the expected T_g. Matrix-dominated properties, such as ±45 in-plane shear modulus or flexural modulus, are often used. The results are then plotted at 5 °C (10 °F) intervals. The T_g will be apparent as a rapid fall-off of these properties.

Thermal Conductivity, Diffusivity, and Specific Heat

Thermal conductivity, diffusivity, and specific heat are important for predicting heat flow and are used in the design of electronic heat sinks, satellite structural buses, and other applications where prediction of temperature or heat flow is important. Direct thermal conductivity measurement methods are generally made under steady-state conditions. Transient methods actually are determinations of the thermal diffusivity, from which the thermal conductivity may be derived. These are described later in this article. To perform this derivation, specific heat and density must also be known. Specific heat is generally determined by DSC.

Thermal Conductivity

In the steady-state methods, the material is allowed to reach steady-state equilibrium. The test specimen is held in a system with a constant thermal gradient. The temperatures on either side of the specimen are constant, as is the energy to maintain the gradient. On reaching this steady state, the thermal conductivity, λ (W/m · K, or Btu/h · ft · °F), of a specimen in the thickness direction is determined from the Fourier relation:

$$\lambda = Q/(A\ \Delta T/L)$$

where Q is heat-flow rate in the metered section (W, or Btu/h), A is the metered section area (m^2, or ft^2) normal to the heat flow, ΔT is the temperature difference (K, or °F) across the specimen, and L is specimen thickness (m, or ft).

Several ASTM test methods are available for steady-state thermal transmission characterizations. The methods are summarized subsequently.

ASTM C 177, known as the guarded hot-plate method, is an absolute determination method covering the measurement of heat flux and associated test conditions for flat-slab specimens. The specimen surfaces are in contact with solid, parallel boundaries held at constant temperatures. This test method is good for low-thermal-conductivity materials and is applicable to a wide variety of specimens and a wide range of environmental conditions. It is most accurate for materials with low conductivity, λ less than 0.5 W/m · K (0.3 Btu/h · ft · °F). Figure 2 shows the main components of the idealized system: two isothermal cold surface units and a guarded hot plate. The guarded hot plate is composed of the metered area centerpiece and a concentric guard ring. Some apparatuses have a coplanar secondary guard. Sandwiched between these three units is the material to be measured. The measurement, in this case, produces a result that is an average of the two pieces, and therefore, it is important that the two pieces be as identical as possible. A single-sided mode of operation can be used in which the specimen consists of one piece placed on one side of the hot-surface assembly.

The arrangement of Fig. 2 demands that precautions be exercised concerning heat-flux losses and proper use of the thermal guard ring. Care is necessary for the accurate measurement of temperature differences and the temperature sensor separation. The guarded hot plate provides the power in watts for the measurement and defines the actual test volume, that is, that portion of the specimen that is actually being measured. The function of the primary guard ring is to reduce lateral heat flow within the apparatus.

Steps must be taken to ensure that the heat flows uniformly into the specimen and that there are good thermal contacts at all interfaces. Air gaps must be avoided.

ASTM E 1225, or guarded longitudinal heat-flow technique, is a comparative test method. Hence, reference materials or transfer standards with known thermal conductivities must be used. This test method is for materials with effective conductivities, λ, from approximately 0.2 to 200 W/m · K (0.1 to 115 Btu/h · ft · °F) over the approximate temperature range of 90 to 1300 K (–300 to 1099 °F). It can be used outside these ranges with decreased accuracy.

The general features of the technique are shown in Fig. 3. A test specimen is inserted under load between two similar specimens of a material of known thermal properties, the meter bars. A temperature gradient is established in the test stack by maintaining the top at an elevated temperature (z_1) and seating the bottom on a heat sink at temperature (z_6). Heat losses are minimized by use of a longitudinal guard having approximately the same temperature gradient. At steady-state equilibrium, the thermal conductivity is derived in terms of the measured temperature gradients in the respective specimens and the thermal conductivity of the reference materials.

The thermal conductance, the ratio of thermal conductivity to length, of the reference material should match the thermal conductance of the specimen as closely as possible to ensure similarity in temperature gradients and better accuracy. When the meter bars and the specimen are right circular cylinders of equal diameter, the technique is described as the cut-bar method. When the cross-sectional dimensions are larger than the thickness, it is described as the flat-slab comparative method. Essentially any shape can

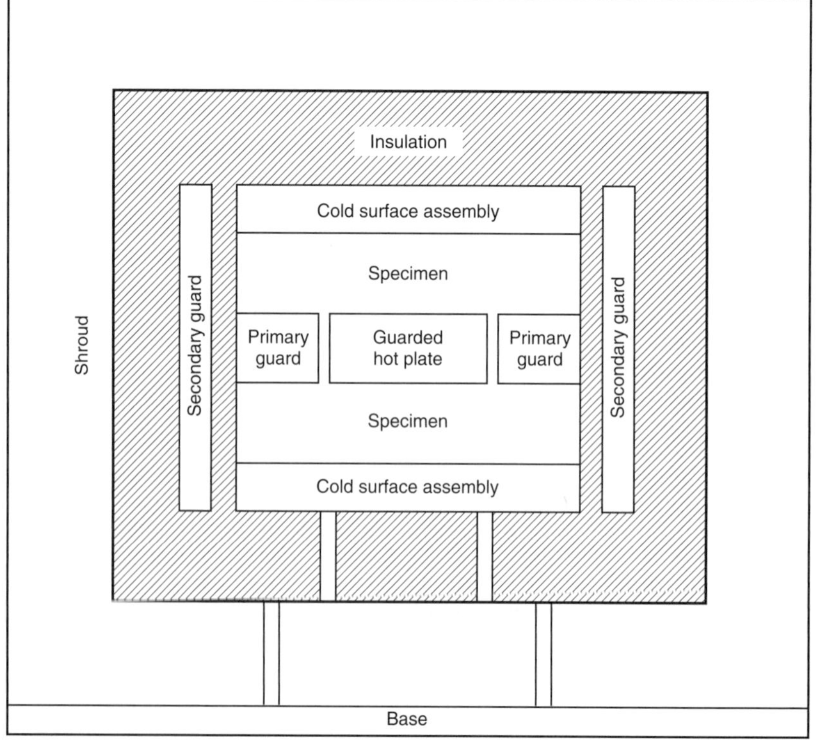

Fig. 2 General arrangement of specimens within a controlled environmental chamber for thermal conductivity measurements using the ASTM C 177 method. This is known as the guarded hot-plate method.

be used, as long as the meter bars and specimen have the same conduction areas.

This test method requires uniform heat transfer at the meter bar to specimen interfaces, which is normally attained by use of an applied axial load in conjunction with a conducting medium at the interfaces. The stack is surrounded by an insulator and enclosed in a guard shell. At steady state, the temperature gradients along the sections are calculated from measured temperatures along the two meter bars and the specimen. This result is a highly idealized situation, because it assumes no heat exchange between the column and insulation and uniform heat transfer at each meter bar/specimen interface. The errors caused by these assumptions are discussed in the ASTM standard.

ASTM C 518 describes the measurement of the steady-state thermal transmission through flat-slab specimens using a heat-flow meter apparatus. This is a comparative, or secondary, method of measurement, because specimens of known thermal transmission properties are required to calibrate the apparatus. The test applies to low-conductivity materials. To meet the requirements of this test, the thermal resistance of the test specimen shall be greater than 0.10 m^2 K/W (0.57 °F · ft^2 · h/Btu) in the direction of the heat flow, and edge heat losses shall be controlled using edge insulation and/or a guard heater.

The important features of the heat-flow meter apparatus are two isothermal plate assemblies, one or more heat-flux transducers, and equipment to measure temperature and the output of the heat-flux transducers. Either one or two specimens are used. Three common experimental configurations are depicted in Fig. 4. Equipment to control the environmental conditions is employed when needed.

A heat-flux transducer is a device that produces a voltage output, which is a function of the heat flux passing through it. The various types of heat-flux transducers are described in ASTM C 1046. The gradient type, commonly used in ASTM C 518, consists of a core across which the voltage is measured, normally with a thermopile. Appropriate calibration of the heat-flux transducers with calibration standards and accurate measurement of the plate temperatures and plate separation are required. These procedures are detailed in ASTM C 518.

The experimental procedure is to establish a steady-state, unidirectional heat flow through the test specimen(s) held between the isothermal parallel plates, one hot plate and the other a cold plate. The heat-flow rate, Q, is obtained from the measured voltage output over the heat-flux transducer. The thermal conductivity is calculated knowing Q; the separation between the hot and cold plates, L; the cross-sectional area, A; and the temperature difference across the specimen, ΔT.

The ASTM C 518 method has been used at ambient conditions of 10 to 40 °C (50 to 104 °F), with specimen thickness up to approximately 25 cm (10 in.), and with plate temperatures from –195 to 540 °C (–320 to 1000 °F) at 2.5 cm (1 in.) thickness.

ASTM E 1530 is similar in concept to ASTM C 518, but is modified to accommodate smaller test specimens having a higher thermal conductance. This method is relevant for specimens having a thickness less than 1.2 cm (0.5 in.), with a thermal conductivity in the range of 0.1 to 5 W/m · K (0.05 to 3 Btu/h · ft · °F).

Specific Heat

The heat capacity is the change in the internal energy of a material per degree temperature change per unit mass of material. The specific heat capacity is the ratio of the heat capacity to that of water. In practice, the specific heat capacity at constant pressure, C_p, is the measured quantity, with values reported in

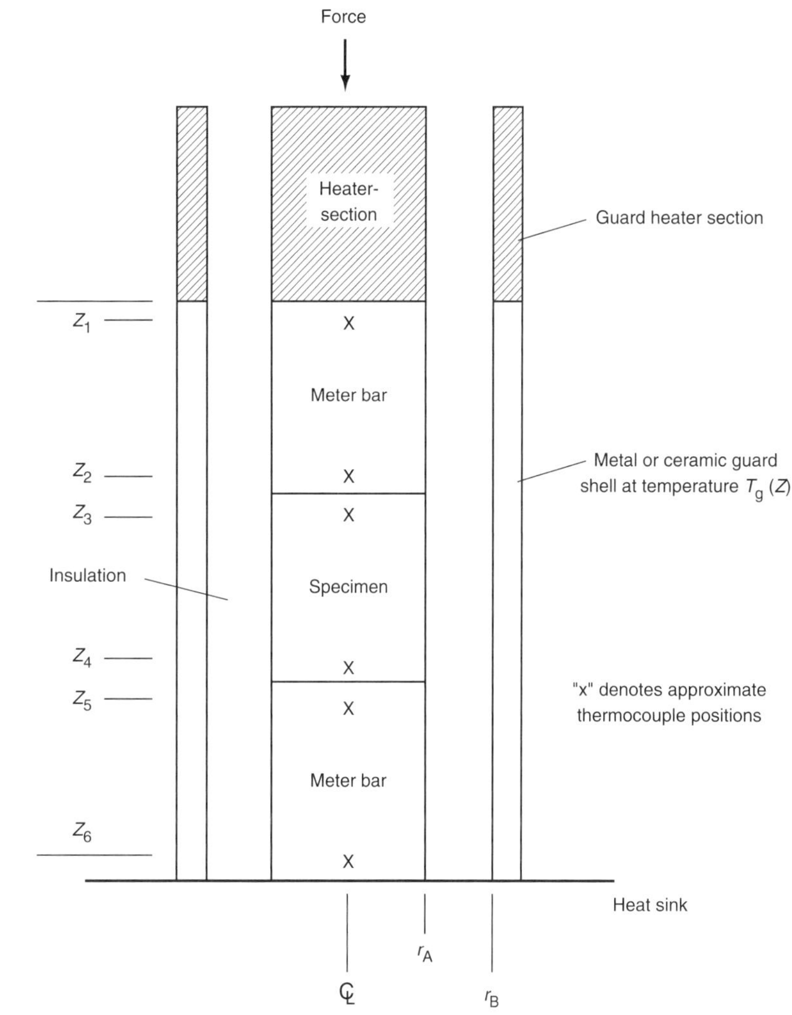

Fig. 3 General arrangement of test specimen and known specimens, the meter bars, in the guarded longitudinal heat flow technique for determining thermal conductivity by the ASTM E 1225 method. z_1 to z_6 are temperatures. For the method known as cut-bar, the specimens are right cylinders with radius r_A

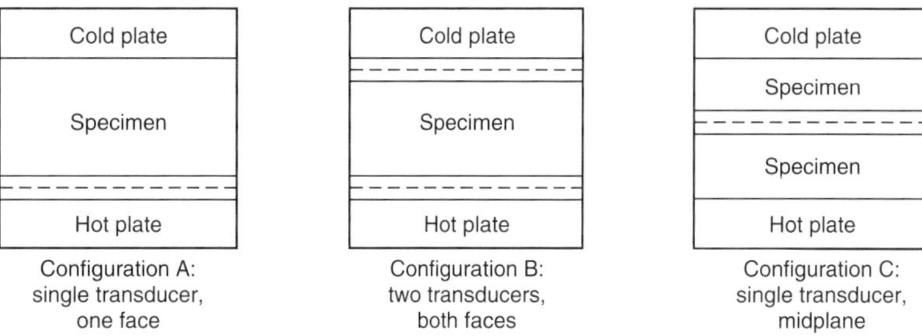

Fig. 4 Typical arrangements for measuring heat flow with heat-flux transducers under the ASTM C 518 method

J/kg · K in SI units, or Btu/lb · °F in customary units.

ASTM E 1269 is the standard test method for measuring the specific heat of polymer-matrix composites. It is based on DSC. This test is generally applicable to thermally stable solids and has a normal operating range from –100 to 600 °C (–150 to 1100 °F). The temperature range may be limited or extended, depending upon the instrumentation and specimen holders used.

A brief summary of the DSC test method is as follows:

1. Empty aluminum pans are placed in the specimen and reference holders. An inert gas atmosphere, such as nitrogen or argon, is typically used as the blanketing atmosphere.
2. An isothermal baseline is recorded at the lower temperature, and the temperature is then increased by adding heat, Q(W), in a programmed manner over the range of interest.
3. An isothermal baseline of the difference in energy required to heat the pans is recorded at the higher temperature, as indicated in the lower part of Fig. 5.
4. The procedure is then repeated with a known mass of specimen, M, in the specimen pan, and a trace of energy absorbed against time is again recorded.

The data so produced at this point are theoretically sufficient to calculate the specific heat of the specimen, but in practice, a calibration procedure with a standard material is important. Sapphire standards are commonly used.

A quantitative measurement of energy imparted to a test specimen as a function of temperature must be obtained to determine specific heat. Thus, the instrument used for these measurements must be calibrated in both the heat-flow and temperature modes.

Temperature Mode. Because specific heat is not a quickly changing function of temperature, the temperature mode of the instrument is ordinarily calibrated and checked only occasionally. Temperature calibration is achieved by observing the melting transition of reference materials. This calibration should be performed over the temperature range to be covered in the specific heat measurement of the unknown specimen. Materials commonly used as DSC temperature calibration standards include tin and indium, but other pure metals may be used.

Heat Flow Mode. Calibration in this mode is achieved through the use of a standard material whose specific heat is well established. The calibration procedure is known as the ratio method. The recommended standard material is synthetic sapphire (α-aluminum oxide).

Notable features of the DSC method are comparatively short test times and milligram specimen sizes. Because such small quantities of specimen material are used, it is essential that specimens be homogeneous and representative. The latter condition may be difficult to achieve if specimens are removed from a polymer-matrix composite panel of large size, due to manufacturing variability from one area of the panel to another. The problem may be addressed by measuring a number of specimens taken from different panel locations and averaging the results.

Thermal Diffusivity

Thermal diffusivity is a thermal response property of a material derived from transient heat-flow conditions. If the density and specific heat are known, the thermal diffusivity, α, may be used to calculate the thermal conductivity of a material from the relationship:

$$\lambda = C_p \alpha \rho$$

where λ is thermal conductivity in W/m · K (Btu/h · ft · °F), ρ is density in kg/m^3 (lb/ft^3), C_p is specific heat in J/kg · K (Btu/lb · °F), and α is thermal diffusivity in m^2/s (ft^2/s).

Two standard test methods are used. ASTM E 1461 is a more-detailed form that has applicability to much wider ranges of materials, applications, and temperatures, with improved accuracy of measurement. ASTM C 714 method applies only to carbon and graphite.

ASTM E 1461, the flash method, exists for the determination of thermal diffusivity of homogeneous, opaque, solid materials. With special precautions, the method can also be used on some transparent and composite materials. Thermal diffusivity values ranging from 0.1 to 1000 $\times$ 10^{-6} m^2/s (1 to 10,000 $\times$ 10^{-6} ft^2/s) have been measured by this technique, and measurements can be made from about 100 to 2500 K (–280 to 4000 °F). Normally this is done in a vacuum or inert gas environment. The flash method is the most common method reported in the literature for measurement of thermal diffusivity of polymer-matrix composites.

This test method is considered an absolute method of measurement, because no heat-flux reference standards are required. The essential features of the apparatus used in the flash method are the flash source, sample holder and environmental control chamber, temperature response detector, and data collection and analysis system. The flash source may be a laser, a flash lamp, or an electron beam. The usual specimen is a thin, circular disc with a front surface area less than that of the flash beam. The initial temperature of the specimen is controlled by a furnace or cryostat. The detector can be a calibrated thermocouple attached to the rear face of the specimen, an infrared sensor, or an optical pyrometer focused on the rear face and filter which is protected from the flash beam.

To conduct the flash test, the source is pulsed on the front surface of the specimen, and energy is absorbed by the specimen. The resulting rear face temperature rise is recorded. The measured temperature rise curve, Fig. 6, is examined to determine the baseline temperature, the maximum temperature rise, ΔT_{max}, and the time of initiation of the thermal pulse.

Thermal diffusivity values are calculated from the specimen thickness, L, and the time required for the rear face temperature to reach a certain percentage of its maximum value.

Round-robin test arrangements have shown that a measurement precision of ±5% can be attained for the thermal diffusivity of a variety of materials. Major sources of experimental uncertainty exist:

- *The determination of thickness (L).* This uncertainty is significant, because test specimens are relatively thin, and diffusivity varies with the square of the thickness.
- *The response time of the detector and its associated amplifiers,* which must be no more than 0.1 of the half-time value, $T_{1/2}$. In general, optical instruments have an acceptable response time. Thermocouples tend to be slower and should be carefully checked for response time against a calibrated source or chopped beam.
- *Nonuniform heating of the laser pulse,* which research shows can be a major source of error (>5%). Heat loss correction is required for the data analysis, especially at high temperatures. For temperatures below 400 °C (750 °F), there is a significant nonlinear effect of

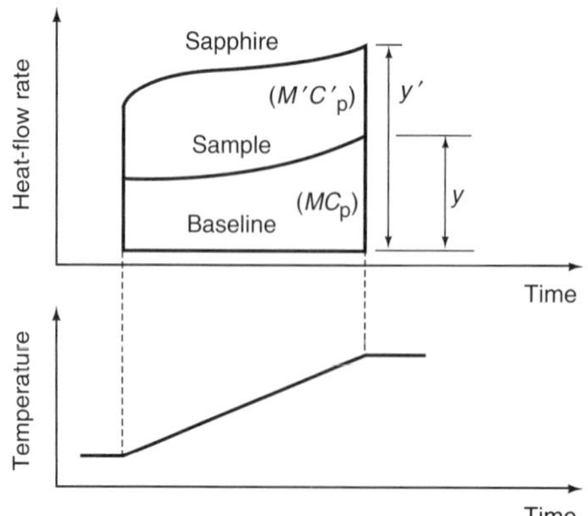

Fig. 5 Determination of specific heat by the ratio method (ASTM E 1269)

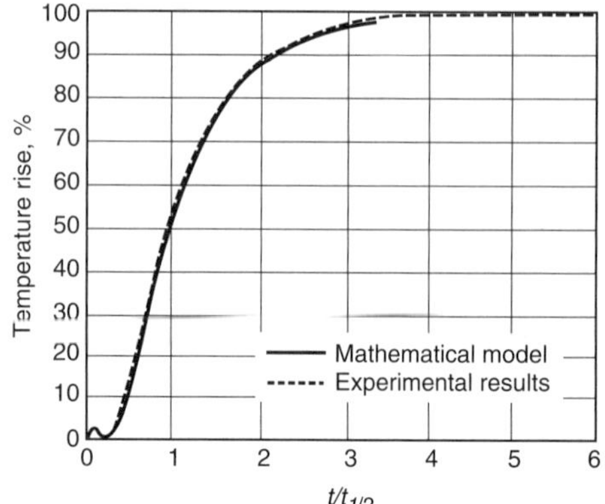

Fig. 6 Time-temperature curve from flash method for determining thermal diffusivity

the infrared detector on the measurements, which requires special corrections.

Advantages of the flash method are the simple specimen geometry, small specimen size, rapidity of measurement, and the ease of using a single apparatus to handle materials having a wide range of thermal diffusivity values. Furthermore, the short measurement time reduces chances of contamination and change of specimen properties due to exposure to high temperatures. The flash method has been extended to two-dimensional heat flow, so that large samples can be measured and the diffusivity in both the axial and radial directions can be measured.

Problems that can arise when applying the flash diffusivity method are partial transparency to the light beam exhibited by a specimen material, and different magnitudes of heat transmission manifested by the components of a multiphase specimen material, such as the reinforcement fiber and matrix of a composite.

The first situation is commonly dealt with by coating the front surface of the specimen with a thin layer of a light-absorbing material, such as graphite. If the second situation exists, the thermal pulse tends to move preferentially through the component phase having the higher thermal diffusivity, with the result that the temperature profile may be nonplanar at the specimen rear surface and depart noticeably from the theoretical model. This effect is sometimes observed, in practice, for composites having a large fraction of high-thermal-conductivity fibers oriented along the heat-flow direction. In this event, the flash method is not applicable.

ASTM C 714. This test method covers the determination of the thermal diffusivity of carbons and graphite to an accuracy of ±5% at temperatures up to 500 °C (900 °F). It requires a circular disk specimen of the order of 1.0 cm (0.4 in.) diameter and 0.5 cm (0.2 in.) thick. The method has the sensitivity to use small samples to analyze very low sulfur contents in graphite and, therefore, is relevant to nuclear reactors where sulfur, even in low concentrations, is a concern.

The method is summarized as follows. A high-intensity, short-duration thermal pulse from a flash lamp is absorbed on the front surface of a specimen, and the rear surface temperature change as a function of time is recorded. Thermal diffusivity is calculated from the specimen thickness and the time required for the temperature of the back surface to rise to one-half of its maximum value. The theoretical considerations and experimental caveats of ASTM E 1461 apply directly to ASTM C 714 and should be consulted.

ACKNOWLEDGMENTS

The material in this article has been adapted from MIL-HDBK-17. The author would like to acknowledge Don Adams, John Adelmann, Al Bertram, and other members of the committee who wrote the underlying MIL-HDBK-17 sections.

SELECTED REFERENCES

- D.S. Cairns and D.F. Adams, "Moisture and Thermal Expansion of Composite Materials," Report UWME-DR-101-104-1, Composite Material Research Group, University of Wyoming, Nov 1981
- "Density of Plastics by the Density-Gradient Technique," ASTM D 1505, *Annual Book of ASTM Standards,* ASTM
- "Determining Specific Heat Capacity by Differential Scanning Calorimetry," ASTM E 1269, *Annual Book of ASTM Standards,* ASTM
- "Fiber Content of Resin Matrix Composite by Matrix Digestion," ASTM D 3171, ASTM
- J.L. McNaughton and C.T. Mortimer, Differential Scanning Calorimetry, Perkin Elmer Order Number L-604, reprinted from *Physical Chemistry Series 2,* Vol 10, IRS, 1975, p 12, with permission from Butterworths, London
- MIL-HDBK-17, Department of Defense
- "Practice for In Situ Measurement of Heat Flux and Temperature of Building Envelope Components," ASTM C 1046, *Annual Book of ASTM Standards,* ASTM
- "Practice for Using the Guarded-Hot-Plate Apparatus in the One-Sided Mode to Measure Steady-State Heat Flux and Thermal Transmission Properties," ASTM C 1044, *Annual Book of ASTM Standards,* ASTM
- SACMA SRM 10R-94, Suppliers of Advanced Composite Materials Assoc.
- "Specific Gravity and Density of Plastics by Displacement," ASTM D 792, ASTM
- "Standard Test Method for Evaluating the Resistance to Thermal Transmission of Thin Specimens of Materials by the Guarded Heat Flow Meter Technique," ASTM E 1530, *Annual Book of ASTM Standards,* ASTM
- "Steady-State Heat Flux Measurements and Thermal Transmission Properties by Means of the Guarded-Hot-Plate Apparatus," ASTM C 177, *Annual Book of ASTM Standards,* ASTM
- "Steady-State Thermal Transmission Properties by Means of the Heat Flow Meter Apparatus," ASTM C 518, *Annual Book of ASTM Standards,* ASTM
- "Test Method for Ignition Loss of Cured Reinforced Resins," ASTM D 2584, *Annual Book of ASTM Standards,* ASTM
- "Test Method for Linear Thermal Expansion of Plastics Between –30 and 30 °C," ASTM D 696, *Annual Book of ASTM Standards,* ASTM
- "Test Method for Linear Thermal Expansion of Solid Materials by Thermomechanical Analysis," ASTM E 831, *Annual Book of ASTM Standards,* ASTM
- "Thermal Conductivity of Solids by Means of the Guarded-Comparative-Longitudinal Heat Flow Technique," ASTM E 1225, *Annual Book of ASTM Standards,* ASTM
- "Thermal Diffusivity of Carbon and Graphite by a Thermal Pulse Method," ASTM C 714, *Annual Book of ASTM Standards,* ASTM
- "Thermal Diffusivity of Solids by the Flash Method," ASTM E 1461, *Annual Book of ASTM Standards,* ASTM
- "Void Volume of Reinforced Plastics," ASTM D 2734, *Annual Book of ASTM Standards,* ASTM

Lamina and Laminate Mechanical Testing

Rod Wishart, Integrated Technologies, Inc. (Intec)

THE USE OF COMPOSITE MATERIALS continues to increase as new performance, reliability, and durability requirements drive structural designs to higher levels of efficiency. Because composite materials inherently require a large number of design variables, the use of analytic models to validate designs is of particular importance. Unfortunately, these analytic models are not yet capable of using lamina (single ply) properties to predict full-scale structural behavior. It is therefore typically necessary to validate all stages of design, from elements to full-scale structure, with both lamina and laminate (two or more plies bonded together) test data.

This article provides very general mechanical testing guidelines for the characterization of lamina and laminate properties. Because of the variety of composite materials currently in use, the test methods discussed in the article may not be appropriate for all material types. Where possible, the limitations of the existing test methods are discussed, but it should be noted that most of the methods discussed here are intended for use on polymer-matrix composites. A more thorough treatment of this topic can be found in Ref 1.

In order to develop and follow a test plan that will produce valuable data, much thought must be given to issues beyond the test methods themselves. The goal of the test program must be to produce data that will represent the structure ultimately being built throughout its performance envelope. To that end, issues such as specimen preparation, environmental conditioning, and instrumentation must all be considered. Brief discussion of some of these items is included in portions of this article, but far more complete treatments can be found in the article "Overview of Testing and Certification" in this Volume and Ref 1.

This article contains lamina and laminate testing guidance for the following general test types:

- Tensile property test methods
- Compressive property test methods
- Shear property test methods
- Flexure property test methods
- Fracture toughness test methods
- Fatigue property test methods

Numerous test methods of varying degrees of standardization are in use in the composite materials industry. This article describes only a select few that have gained industry-wide acceptance; the standards discussed in this article are listed in Table 1. In general, these methods are ASTM or other industry standards that should be consulted directly in order to judge their appropriateness for a given materials evaluation. Though methods created by the Suppliers of Advanced Composite Materials Association (SACMA) are briefly mentioned, this organization is no longer functioning, and their specifications are not maintained.

Failure Mode Analysis

When selecting and using a particular mechanical strength test method, the importance of obtaining the proper failure mode cannot be overemphasized. While universal definitions of "proper" and "valid" have not been established for most types of tests, careful evaluation of failure modes is critical to all test data analysis. Failure modes must be reported and identified in a consistent manner to enable comparisons of data. Data should be discarded when analysis indi-

Table 1 Selected standards for lamina and laminate mechanical testing

Designation	Title
ASTM standards(a)	
C 393	Standard Test Method for Flexural Properties of Sandwich Constructions
D 638	Standard Test Method for Tensile Properties of Plastics
D 695	Standard Test Method for Compressive Properties of Rigid Plastics
D 790	Standard Test Methods for Flexural Properties of Unreinforced and Reinforced Plastics and Electrical Insulating Materials
D 2344	Standard Test Method for Apparent Interlaminar Shear Strength of Parallel Fiber Composites by Short-Beam Method
D 3039/D 3039M	Standard Test Method for Tensile Properties of Polymer-Matrix Composites
D 3410	Standard Test Method for Compressive Properties of Polymer-Matrix Composite Materials with Unsupported Gage Section by Shear Loading
D 3479	Standard Test Method for Tension-Tension Fatigue of Polymer-Matrix Composite Materials
D 3518/D 3518M	Standard Practice for In-Plane Shear Response of Polymer-Matrix Composite Materials by Tensile Test of a $\pm 45°$ Laminate
D 3846	Test Method for In-Plane Shear Strength of Reinforced Plastics
D 4255	Standard Guide for Testing In-Plane Shear Properties of Composite Laminates.
D 5379	Standard Test Method for Shear Properties of Composite Materials by the V-Notched Beam Method
D 5467	Standard Test Method for Compressive Properties of Unidirectional Polymer-Matrix Composite Materials Using a Sandwich Beam
D 5528	Standard Test Methods for Mode I Interlaminar Fracture Toughness of Unidirectional Fiber-Reinforced Polymer-Matrix Composites
D 6415	Standard Test Method for Measuring the Curved Beam Strength of a Fiber-Reinforced Polymer-Matrix Composite
ISO standard(b)	
527	Plastics—Determination of Tensile Properties
SACMA standards(c)	
SRM 1	Compressive Properties of Oriented Fiber-Resin Composites
SRM 4	Tensile Properties of Oriented Fiber-Resin Composites
SRM 6	Compressive Properties of Oriented Cross-Plied Fiber-Resin Composites
SRM 7	In-Plane Shear Stress-Strain Properties of Oriented Fiber-Resin Composites
SRM 8R-94	Apparent Interlaminar Shear Strength of Oriented Fiber-Resin Composites by the Short-Beam Method
SRM 9	Tensile Properties of Oriented Cross-Plied Fiber-Resin Composites

(a) Published in the *Annual Book of ASTM Standards*, American Society for Testing and Materials, West Conshohocken, PA. (b) Published by the International Organization for Standardization, Geneva, Switzerland. Available in the United States from the American National Standards Institute (ANSI), New York, NY. (c) Published by the Suppliers of Advanced Composite Materials Association (SACMA), Arlington, VA. These standards are no longer maintained.

cates an unacceptable mode. The reader is advised to be conscientious regarding the documentation of failure modes, and to refer to examples provided within specific test methods where such examples exist.

Careful consideration must be given to the applicability of a given test standard to the material being evaluated. *When a test method consistently results in invalid failure modes for a given material, the testing should be repeated using a different method that is better suited to the material in question.*

Tensile Property Test Methods

The basic physics of most tensile test methods are very similar: a prismatic coupon with a straight-sided gage section is gripped at the ends and loaded in uniaxial tension. The principal differences between these tensile test coupons are the coupon cross section and the load-introduction method. The cross section of the coupon may be rectangular, round, or tubular; it may be straight-sided for the entire length (a "straight-sided" coupon) or width- or diameter-tapered from the ends into the gage section (often called "dogbone" or "bow-tie" specimens). Straight-sided coupons may use tabbed load application points. This section briefly discusses the most common tensile test methods that have been standardized for fiber-reinforced composite materials. Reference 1 includes a more detailed discussion and briefly reviews several nonstandard methods as well.

By changing the coupon configuration, many of the tensile test methods are able to evaluate different material configurations, including unidirectional laminates, woven materials, and general laminates. However, some coupon/material configuration combinations are less sensitive to specimen preparation and testing variations than others. Perhaps the most dramatic example of this is the unidirectional coupon. Fiber versus load axis misalignment in a 0° unidirectional coupon, which can occur due to either specimen preparation or testing problems or both, can reduce strength as much as 30% due to an initial 1° misalignment. Furthermore, bonded end tabs intended to *minimize* load-introduction problems in high-strength unidirectional materials can actually *cause* premature coupon failure (even in nonunidirectional coupons) if not applied and used properly. Because of these and similar issues, tensile testing is subject to a great deal of "art" in order to obtain legitimate data. Alternatives to problematic tests, such as the unidirectional tensile test, are often available, and careful attention must be paid to the test specification for recommendations. Reference 1 is also an excellent resource for test optimization suggestions.

In-Plane Tension Test Methods

Straight-sided coupon tension tests include:

- ASTM D 3039/D 3039M, "Standard Test Method for Tensile Properties of Polymer-Matrix Composites"
- ISO 527, "Plastics—Determination of Tensile Properties"
- SACMA SRM 4, "Tensile Properties of Oriented Fiber-Resin Composites"
- SACMA SRM 9, "Tensile Properties of Oriented Cross-Plied Fiber-Resin Composites"

ASTM D 3039/D 3039M, originally released in 1971 and updated several times since then, is the original standard test method for straight-sided rectangular coupons. It is still the most commonly used in-plane tension method. ISO 527 parts 4 and 5 and the two SACMA tensile test methods, SRM 4 and SRM 9, are substantially based on ASTM D 3039 and as a result, are quite similar. Care should be taken, however, not to substitute one method for another, because subtle differences between them do exist. In general, the ASTM standard offers better control of testing details that may cause variability, as discussed subsequently. For this reason, it is the preferred method.

In each of the previous test methods, a tensile stress is applied to the specimen through a mechanical shear interface at the ends of the coupon, normally by either wedge or hydraulic grips. The material response is measured in the gage section of the coupon by either strain gages or extensometers, subsequently determining the elastic material properties.

If used, end tabs are intended to distribute the load from the grips into the specimen with a minimum of stress concentration. A schematic example of an appropriate failure mode of a multidirectional laminate using a tabbed tension coupon is shown in Fig. 1. Because the straight-sided specimen provides no geometric stress-concentrated region, such as would be found in a specimen with a reduced-width gage section, failure often occurs at or near the ends of the tabs or grips. While this failure mode is not necessarily invalid, care must be taken when evaluating the data to guard against unrealistically low strengths resulting from poorly performing tabs or overly aggressive gripping.

Design of end tabs remains somewhat of an art, and an improperly designed tab interface will produce low coupon strengths. For this reason, a standard tab design has not been mandated by ASTM, although unbeveled 90° tabs are preferred. Recent comparisons confirm that the success of a tab design is more dependent on the use of a sufficiently ductile adhesive than on the tab angle. An unbeveled tab applied with a ductile adhesive will outperform a tapered tab that has been applied with an insufficiently ductile adhesive. Therefore, adhesive selection is most critical to bonded tab use. Furthermore, the use of a softer tab material is usually preferred when testing high-modulus materials (such as fiberglass tabs on a graphite-reinforced specimen).

The simplest way to avoid bonded tab problems is to not use them. Many laminates (mostly nonunidirectional) can be successfully tested without tabs, or with friction rather than bonded tabs. Flame-sprayed unserrated grips have also been successfully used in tensile testing without tabs.

Other important factors that affect tension testing results include control of specimen preparation, specimen design tolerances, control of conditioning and moisture content variability, control of test machine-induced misalignment and bending, consistent measurement of thickness, appropriate selection of transducers and calibration of instrumentation, documentation and description of failure modes, definition of elastic property calculation details, and data reporting guidelines. These factors are described in detail by ASTM D 3039/D 3039M.

Limitations of the straight-sided coupon tensile methods are described subsequently.

Bonded Tabs. The stress field near the termination of a bonded tab is significantly three-dimensional, and critical stresses tend to peak at this location. Much research has been done on minimizing peak stresses, but it is impossible to make general recommendations that are appropriate for all materials and configurations. Furthermore, improperly designed tabs can significantly degrade results. As a result, tabless or tabbed configurations that use unbonded tabs are becoming more popular, when the resulting failure mode is appropriate.

Specimen Design. There are, particularly within ASTM D 3039, a large number of coupon design options included in the standard, which are needed to cover the wide range of materials systems and lay-up configurations within the scope of the test method. Great care should be taken to ensure that an appropriate geometry is chosen for the material being tested.

Specimen Preparation. Specimen preparation plays a crucial role in test results. While this is true for most composite mechanical tests, it is particularly important for unidirectional tests, and unidirectional tension tests are no exception. Fiber alignment, control of coupon taper, and specimen machining (while maintaining alignment) are the most critical steps of specimen preparation. For very low strain-to-failure materials systems or test configurations, like the 90° unidirectional test, flatness is also particularly important. Edge machining techniques (avoiding machining-induced damage) and edge surface

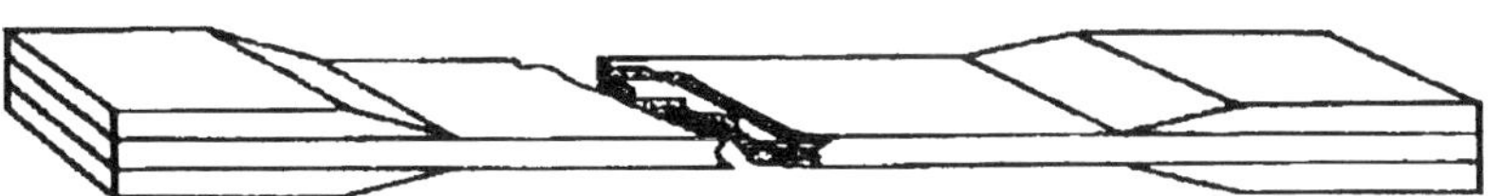

Fig. 1 Typical tension failure of multidirectional laminate using a tabbed coupon

finishes are also particularly critical to strength results from the 90° unidirectional test.

Unidirectional Testing. All the elements that make tensile testing subject to error are exacerbated in the unidirectional case, particularly in the 0° direction. This has led to the increased use of a much less sensitive $[90/0]_{ns}$-type laminate coupon (also known as the "crossply" coupon) from which unidirectional properties can be easily derived (Ref 2). Properly tested crossply coupons often produce results equivalent to the best attainable unidirectional data. While unidirectional testing is still performed, and in certain cases may be preferred or required, a straight-sided, tabless, $[90/0]_{ns}$-type coupon is now generally believed to be the lowest cost, most reliable configuration for lamina tensile testing of unidirectional materials. This straight-sided tabless configuration also works equally well for nonunidirectional material forms and for other general laminates. Another advantage is that, unlike with 0° unidirectional specimens, $[90/0]_{ns}$-type coupon failures do not usually mask indicators of improper testing/specimen preparation practices.

Width tapered coupon tension tests are standardized in ASTM D 638, "Standard Test Method for Tensile Properties of Plastics." The test, developed for and limited to use with plastics, uses a flat, width-tapered tensile coupon with a straight-sided gage section. Several geometries are allowed, depending on the material being tested. Figure 2 shows a schematic of one general configuration. Despite its heritage, this coupon has also been evaluated and applied to composite materials. The coupon taper is accomplished by a large cylindrical radius between the wide gripping area at each end and the narrower gage section, resulting in a shape that justifies the nickname of the "dogbone" coupon. The taper makes the specimen particularly unsuited for testing of 0° unidirectional materials, because only about half of the gripped fibers are continuous throughout the gage section. This usually results in failure by splitting at the radius, due to inability of the matrix to shear the load from terminated fibers into the gage section.

While the ASTM D 638 coupon configuration has been successfully used for fabric-reinforced composites and with general nonunidirectional laminates, some materials systems remain sensitive to the stress concentration at the radius. For its intended use with plastics, the coupon is molded to shape. Likewise, discontinuous fiber composites can be molded to the required geometry. To ensure valid results, care must be taken that the molding flow does not create preferentially oriented fibers. For laminated materials the coupon must be machined, ground, or routed to shape. The coupon also has the drawback of having a relatively small gage volume and is poorly suited for characterization of coarse weaves with repeating units larger than the gage width of 6.4 to 13 mm (0.25 to 0.50 in.). The standardized procedure, due to the intended scope, does not adequately cover the testing parameters required for advanced composites.

Limitations of the ASTM D 638 method are described in the following paragraphs.

Standardization. While the ASTM D 638 test is standardized, it was not developed for advanced composites and is primarily applicable to relatively low-modulus, unreinforced materials, or low-reinforcement volume materials incorporating randomly oriented fibers.

Specimen Preparation. Special care is required to machine the taper into a laminated coupon.

Stress State. The radius transition region can dominate the failure mode and result in reduced strength results. The width-tapered coupon is not suitable for unidirectional laminates, and is limited to fabrics or nonunidirectional laminates when gage section failures can be attained.

Limited Gage Section Volume. The limited gage width makes it unsuitable for coarse fabrics.

The sandwich beam test is standardized as ASTM C 393, "Standard Test Method for Flexural Properties of Flat Sandwich Constructions." While primarily intended as a flexural test for sandwich core shear evaluation, the scope also allows use for determination of facing tensile strength. While this use is not well documented within the test method, it has been used for tensile testing of composite materials, particularly for 90° properties of unidirectional materials, or for fiber-dominated testing in extreme nonambient environments. This test specimen is claimed by some to be less susceptible to handling and specimen preparation damage than D 3039-type 90° specimens, resulting in higher strengths and less test-induced variation.

In order to assure failure in the tensile facesheet, the compression facesheet is often manufactured from the same material, but at twice the thickness as the tensile facesheet.

Limitations of the ASTM C 393 method are described subsequently.

Cost. Specimen fabrication is relatively expensive.

Stress State. The effect on the stress state of the sandwich core has not been studied in tension and could be a concern.

Standardization. While this test technically is standardized, its practical application and limitations are not well studied or documented.

Environmental Conditioning. Conditioning is problematic because of the difficulty of assuring tensile facesheet moisture equilibrium due to the moisture protection offered by the compression facesheet and the core. The extended conditioning times required also often cause adhesive breakdown prior to testing.

Out-of-Plane Tension Test Methods

ASTM D 6415, "Standard Test Method for Measuring the Curved Beam Strength of a Fiber-Reinforced Polymer-Matrix Composite," is currently the only published standard for out-of-plane tensile testing specifically relating to composites, though modifications to ASTM C 297, C 633 and D 2095 are also often employed. These methods are not discussed here, and the reader is referred to Ref 1 and the test standards for more information.

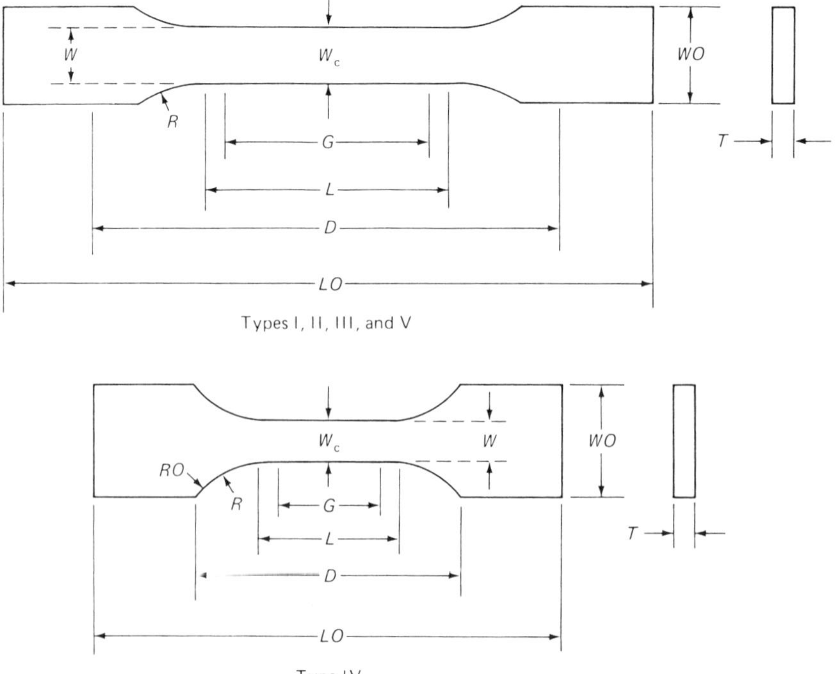

Fig. 2 Schematic of typical ASTM D 638 test specimen geometry. *W*, width; W_c, width at center; *WO*, width overall; *T*, thickness; *R*, radius at fillet; *RO*, outer radius; *G*, gage length; *L*, length; *LO*, length overall; *D*, distance between grips

Compressive Property Test Methods

The compression response of composite materials has been the subject of research efforts and test programs since the early 1960s. Even with this long-term study, there exist numerous methods to test composites in compression and no consensus on a single most-recommended test method to use. Compression tests are conducted on composite materials, using appropriate instrumentation, to determine compressive modulus, Poisson's ratio, ultimate compressive strength or strain-at-failure. These properties are determined through the use of test fixturing that is typically designed to be as simple to use and fabricate as possible, to minimize stress concentrations, to minimize specimen volume, and to introduce a uniform state of uniaxial stress in the specimen test section.

Compression testing is inherently influenced by test fixturing. Sufficient restraint must be provided by fixturing to inhibit undesirable failure modes, such as end brooming and column buckling. However, if excessive restraint is used, the resulting failure strengths may be artificially high. For this reason, consensus on the preferred test method has not been reached, and there are significant differences of opinion on the "proper" way to perform compression testing for a given material form. Selection of a compressive test method depends on the material being tested, the test environment, and the goals of the testing program. The quality of the test results can often be judged by the coefficients of variation in strength and modulus and the failure modes of the test specimens.

The measured compression strength for a single material system has been shown to differ when determined by different test methods. Variation in results can usually be attributed to one of the following parameters: fabrication practices, control of fiber alignment, improper coupon machining and specimen preparation, improper placement of coupons in test fixtures or fixtures in testing machines, and improper use of test fixtures.

The numerous in-plane compression test methods available can be broadly classified into three groups: (1) those that introduce load into the specimen test section through shear; (2) those that introduce load into the specimen test section through end-loading; and (3) those that introduce load into the specimen test section through a combination of end-loading and shear.

In-plane compression test methods can be further classified as having a supported or unsupported test section. An unsupported test section is defined as one inherently free from global buckling, with the faces of the specimen in the test section remaining unrestrained throughout the test. A supported test section is one with support on the specimen faces in the test section provided by the test fixture or ancillary equipment. All of the test methods discussed in this section require specimens with unsupported test sections, with the exception of ASTM D 5467, the sandwich beam method. A more complete discussion of compression test methodology and a description of test methods not covered here can be found in Ref 3–7.

In-Plane Compressive Test Methods

In-plane compressive test methods are standardized as:

- ASTM D 5467, "Standard Test Method for Compressive Properties of Unidirectional Polymer Matrix Composite Materials Using a Sandwich Beam"
- ASTM D 3410, "Standard Test Method For Compressive Properties of Polymer-Matrix Composite Materials with Unsupported Gage Section by Shear Loading"
- ASTM C 393, "Standard Test Method For Flexural Properties of Sandwich Constructions"
- ASTM D 695, "Standard Test Method for Compressive Properties of Rigid Plastics"
- SACMA SRM 1, "Compressive Properties of Oriented Fiber-Resin Composites"
- SACMA SRM 6, "Compressive Properties of Oriented Cross-Plied Fiber-Resin Composites"

The in-plane compression test methods described in this section can be used to generate the ultimate compression strength, strain-at-failure, longitudinal modulus, and Poisson's ratio of [0], [90], and orthotropic coupons, over a typical thickness range of approximately 1 to 6 mm (0.040 to 0.200 in.) With the exception of ASTM D 5467 (sandwich beam method), all of the test methods discussed subsequently will also accommodate $[0/90]_{ns}$-style laminates. Testing of these laminates and performing subsequent data reduction has become a popular means for eliminating specimen and fixture-related sensitivities associated with unidirectional specimens. A discussion on the use of [0/90] laminates for determining lamina properties and associated data-reduction methods can be found in Ref 2 and within SACMA method SRM 6. (Note again that SACMA methods are no longer maintained and should be used with care.) Test methods for specimen thicknesses greater than those covered by the test methods discussed here exist, but have not been standardized, and additional information on test methods for laminates thicker than 10 mm (0.400 in.) can be found in MIL-HDBK-17 (Ref 8).

Limitations of in-plane compression testing are described subsequently.

Test Method Sensitivity. It has been shown that different test methods do not measure the same compression strength for a single material system. Such differences can be attributed to the effects of specimen alignment, specimen geometry, and fixtures. For example, the variation in test results between the two procedures in ASTM D 3410 and the one procedure in ASTM D 5467 can be found in Ref 9.

Material and Specimen Preparation. Compression modulus and especially compression strength are sensitive to poor material fabrication practices, damage induced by improper coupon machining, and poor fiber alignment. Great care should be taken to minimize all these sources of error.

ASTM D 3410/D 3410M, "Compressive Properties of Polymer-Matrix Composite Materials with Unsupported Gage Section by Shear Loading." Two compression procedures are published by ASTM in test method D 3410 and have historically been called the Celanese (D 3410 procedure A) and the Illinois Institute of Technology Research Institute (IITRI) (D 3410 procedure B). The Celanese and IITRI procedures, as with many other published procedures, originally carried the names of the organizations under which the procedure was developed. The Celanese and IITRI procedures address the use of tabbed or untabbed rectangular coupons and the transfer of load into the specimen through shear via wedge-type grips.

General limitations of the ASTM D 3410 method are described herein.

Material Form. The test is limited to continuous-fiber or discontinuous-fiber reinforced composites for which the test direction is parallel to one of the principal material directions.

Test Fixture Characteristics. Although both procedures A and B transmit load to the specimen via tapered wedge grips, the wedges in procedure A are conical and the wedges in procedure B are rectangular. The conical wedges from procedure A are known to be prone to cone-to-cone seating problems (Ref 9). The rectangular wedge grip design used in procedure B was employed to eliminate this wedge-seating problem. In addition to these differences, the fixture used for procedure A is much smaller in size and weight than the fixture used for procedure B. (However, significantly smaller modified fixtures for procedure B have been developed and used with good success. The Wyoming Modified IITRI compression test fixture weighs roughly 25% of the ASTM D 3410 procedure B fixture but is essentially identical in function. It is limited to specimens of 13 mm (0.5 in.) or less in width and a thickness range of approximately ±2.5 mm (±0.10 in.) (per wedge set.) Fixture modifications to the Procedure A geometry are also available that alleviate the cone-to-cone seating problems with the specification-defined fixture (Ref 7, 10, 11).

A fixture characteristic that can have a significant effect on test results is the surface finish of the mating surfaces of the wedge grip assembly. Because these surfaces undergo sliding contact, they must be polished, lubricated, and free of nicks and other surface damage.

Strain Measuring Devices. While extensometers are not ruled out, practical considerations make the use of strain gages essentially required. Back-to-back gages are required for procedures A and B, although the standard relaxes this requirement for large numbers of test specimens.

ASTM D 3410, procedure A requires a test fixture that consists of a pair of matched conical wedge grips that are seated in a cylindrical housing (Fig. 3). The test specimen used in this fixture is a tabbed coupon of rectangular cross section. The specimen dimensions are nominally 140 mm (5.5 in.) long and 6 mm (0.25 in.) wide. The total thickness of specimen plus tabs is variable, but is toleranced to only ±0.05 mm (±0.002 in.) for a given wedge geometry. After placing the specimen in the test fixture, a compressive load is applied to the ends of the fixture in a standard testing machine. The load applied to the fixture is transferred from the wedge grips to the specimen tabs and then to the specimen through shear. The complex stress state in the tabbed region of the specimen changes to uniaxial compression in the specimen test section. Compression strength is determined from load at failure, while modulus and strain-at-failure are determined when strain gages are employed.

Limitations of ASTM D 3410, Procedure A. In general, this test method is highly susceptible to testing irregularities because of the problems discussed subsequently. Because of this, and because the addition to the standard of the more forgiving procedure B, procedure A has become a rarely used method.

Specimen Dimensions. Due to the conical geometry of the wedge grips in this test method, a given set of wedges will accommodate only a single specimen thickness. The total specimen thickness tolerance for a given wedge set is only ±0.05 (±0.002 in). This limitation and restrictive tolerance requires surface grinding of specimens to final thickness, as well as maintaining enough wedge sets to accommodate multiple specimen thicknesses.

Fixture Seating. The fixture design for the test method makes it susceptible to cone-to-cone seating problems on the conical wedge grips, as mentioned previously.

Material Form. The fixed gage length and width of this specimen make it inappropriate for fabric-based materials with unit cell sizes larger than the smaller specimen dimension.

Tabbing and Tolerances. The data resulting from this test method have been shown to be sensitive to the flatness and parallelism of the tabs, so care must be taken to ensure that the specimen tolerance requirements are met. This usually requires precision grinding of the tab surfaces after bonding them to the specimen. The fixture for this procedure requires tight manufacturing, assembly, and installation tolerances.

ASTM D 3410, Procedure B. The fixture design, specimen configuration, and loading principal for this test procedure are based on the same concepts as procedure A described previously. The fixture for this test method was designed primarily to eliminate the seating problems associated with the conical wedge grips in procedure A (Ref 9). In place of conical wedge grips, the fixture for this test method consists of a pair of matching rectangular wedge grips seated in a rectangular housing (Fig. 4). The fixture for this method is much larger and heavier than for procedure A. The test specimen used is typically tabbed, with a rectangular cross section having recommended dimensions of 140 to 155 mm (5.5 to 6.0 in.) long, 10 to 25 mm (0.50 to 1.0 in.) wide, and with a 10 to 25 mm (0.5 to 1.0 in.) gage length. Specimens tested with this procedure have a minimum required thickness, specified as a function of gage length, material modulus, and expected material strength, with an absolute minimum thickness of 1 mm (0.040 in.). As with the procedure A, the load that is applied to the fixture is transferred from the wedge grips to the specimen tabs through shear, and from the tabs to the test specimen through shear. The complex stress state in the tabbed region of the specimen changes to uniaxial compression in the specimen test section. Compression strength is determined from load at failure, while modulus and strain-at-failure are determined when strain gages or extensometers are employed.

Limitations of ASTM D 3410, Procedure B. The data resulting from this test method have been shown to be sensitive to the flatness and parallelism of the tabs, so care should be taken to ensure that the specimen tolerance requirements are met. This often requires precision grinding of the tab surfaces after bonding them to the specimen. The fixture for this procedure requires tight manufacturing, assembly, and installation tolerances.

ASTM D 5467, "Compressive Properties of Unidirectional Polymer Matrix Composites Using a Sandwich Beam." This method uses a honeycomb-core sandwich beam that is loaded in four-point bending, placing the upper facesheet in compression (Fig. 5). The upper sheet is loaded in compression and is usually a six-ply unidirectional laminate. The lower facesheet is typically the same material, but twice as thick in order to drive failure into the compressive facesheet. The two facesheets are separated by and bonded to a deep honeycomb core (usually aluminum). Failure of the compressive facesheet enables measurement of compression strength, compression modulus, and strain-at-failure if strain gages or extensometers are employed.

Limitations of the ASTM D 5467 method are described subsequently.

Material Form. This test procedure is limited to unidirectional material only.

Specimen Complexity. The specimen is much larger, and specimen preparation is more complex and expensive than for the two procedures in ASTM D 3410.

Compression Strength. Compression strength for unidirectional materials are typically higher (10 to 15%) than for the two procedures in ASTM D 3410. This is believed to be attributable to the one-sided support provided by the core material in the test specimen.

Poisson's Ratio. The validity of Poisson's ratio from this method has been questioned, due to anticlastic bending.

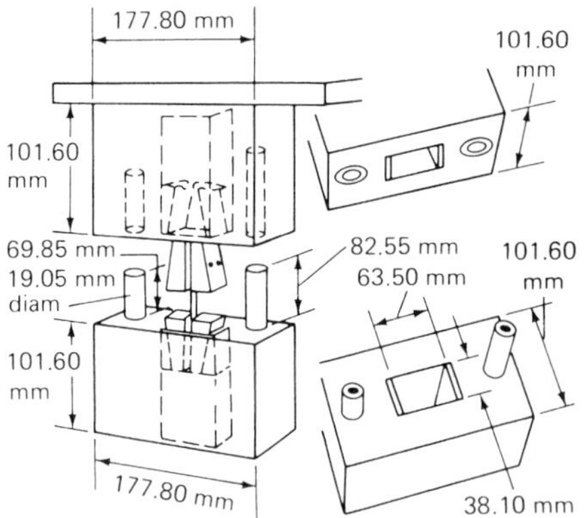

Fig. 4 Schematic of compression test fixture with pyramidal wedges (ASTM D 3410, method B)

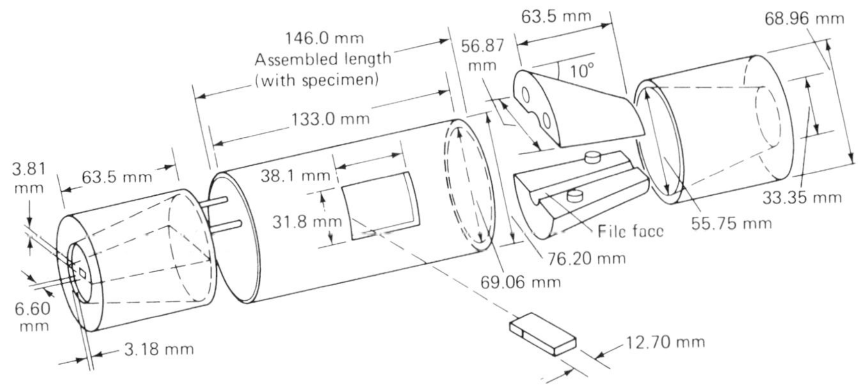

Fig. 3 Exploded view of compression test fixture (ASTM D 3410, method A)

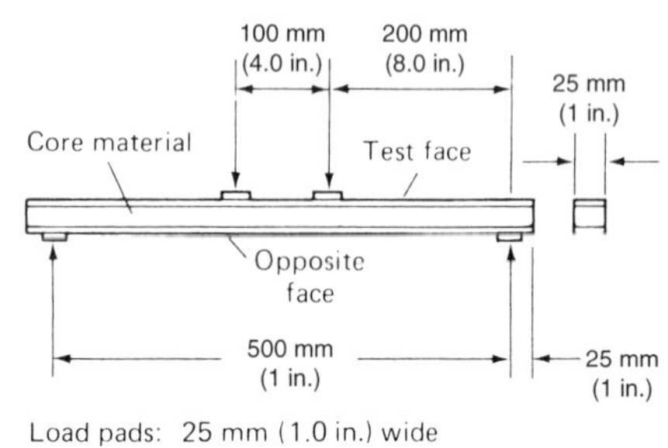

Fig. 5 Schematic of typical longitudinal sandwich beam compression specimen (ASTM D 5467)

ASTM C 393, "Flexural Properties of Flat Sandwich Constructions." ASTM C 393 is one of a series designed to test sandwich constructions, and covers the determination of the properties of flat, sandwich constructions subjected to flatwise flexure in the same manner as ASTM D 5467. ASTM C 393 expands on the properties measured by ASTM D 5467, and provides methodology to determine the flexural and shear stiffness of the entire sandwich, the shear modulus and shear strength of the core, or the compressive or tensile strength of the facesheets.

There are no limitations on the core or skin materials for this test method. The specimen is rectangular in cross section, and the core, facesheet, and span geometries are designed to achieve the desired failure mode according to the material property being measured. While not widely used for the determination of composite materials properties, this test method does allow for the design of a test specimen not covered by ASTM D 5467. Caution should be exercised in using this test for composite materials properties, because the equations for determining the material properties may not be applicable for some specimen geometries or core-facesheet combinations.

The use of this test method to determine the tensile properties of [90°] laminates is covered in MIL-HDBK-17 (Ref 12).

Limitations of the ASTM C 393 method are described in the following paragraphs.

Material Form. This test method is not limited in the material form of the core material or facesheet material. Equations for determining the material properties may not be applicable for some specimen geometries or core-facesheet combinations.

Specimen Geometry. This test method is limited to rectangular sandwich constructions, and the core, facesheet, and span geometries are allowed to vary in order to achieve the desired failure mode according to the material property being measured.

ASTM D 695, "Standard Test Method for Compressive Properties of Rigid Plastics." This method was developed by ASTM Committee D-20 for compression testing of unreinforced and reinforced rigid plastics. Two types of specimens can be used for this method. The first is typically used for unreinforced plastics and is in the form of a right cylinder or prism whose length is twice its principal diameter or width. Preferred specimen sizes are 12.7 by 12.7 by 25.4 mm (0.50 by 0.50 by 1.0 in.) for a prism and 12.7 mm diam by 25.4 mm (0.50 in. diam by 1.0 in.) for a cylinder. Smaller diameter rods or tubes may also be tested, provided they are of sufficient length to allow a specimen slenderness ratio of 11:1 to 16:1. The specimen is tested by placing it between the hardened-steel faces of a compression tool and loading it to failure.

The second test specimen in the standard is documented as intended for "reinforced plastics, including high-strength composites and highly orthotropic laminates" less than 6.4 mm (0.125 in.) thick. It uses a flat, untabbed specimen with a reduced width test section, as shown in Fig. 6. Two I-shaped support plates with longitudinal grooves are clamped to the faces of the specimen and are slightly shorter than the specimen. (See Fig. 7, which illustrates the same fixture, but a different specimen geometry.) After positioning the specimen between the support plates, a compressive load is applied to the end of the specimen until failure to determine ultimate compression strength. An extensometer may also be mounted to the specimen edge to determine compression modulus.

The dogbone specimen geometry has been evaluated with mixed results for its use with fiber-reinforced composites (Ref 9). Results indicate that while the shaped specimen works for some forms of fiber-reinforced composites, it is not appropriate for use with other relatively high modulus materials. In an attempt to modify this portion of the test method for use with high-modulus composites, a straight-sided, tabbed coupon has been developed to measure strength, and a similar specimen without tabs has been developed to measure modulus. In addition, an L-shaped base to support the fixture-specimen assembly has also been added to the test method. This method is often referred to as the "modified" ASTM D 695 method and is well represented by the SACMA SRM 1 method discussed subsequently.

Limitations of the ASTM D 695 Method. The published scope of this document states it is limited to unreinforced and reinforced rigid plastics, including high-modulus composites. Round-robin testing conducted by Committee D-30 found this method unacceptable for the measurement of strength of high-modulus composites (Ref 9).

SACMA SRM 1, "Compressive Properties of Oriented Fiber-Resin Composites." A variation on the ASTM D 695 test method for continuous high-modulus fiber composites has been developed and documented by SACMA as SRM 1. While essentially retaining the simple fixturing of the ASTM D 695 method, the variation uses straight-sided tabbed specimens for compression strength and an untabbed specimen for the measurement of modulus. An L-shaped base supports the fixture-specimen assembly. Both specimens are 80 mm (3.18 in.) long, 6.4 mm (0.5 in.) wide, and 1 to 3 mm (0.040 to 0.120 in.) thick. A schematic of the strength specimen installed in the fixture is shown as Fig. 7. The unsupported test section in this method is the shortest test section of any test method of this class and measures only 4.8 mm (0.188 in.) long. This may contribute to the higher values of compression strength typically measured with this method than from ASTM D 3410 procedures A and B.

Limitations of the SACMA SRM 1 method are described subsequently.

General. SACMA is no longer in existence, and its methods are not currently maintained. Therefore, referencing this specification should be done with care. Separate strength and modulus specimens are required for this test method. The short gage length and narrow width of the strength specimen result in a small test section volume.

Material Form. The material form is limited to polymer-matrix composites reinforced with oriented, continuous, high-modulus (>21 GPa, or 3 × 10^6 psi), fibers, and made primarily of

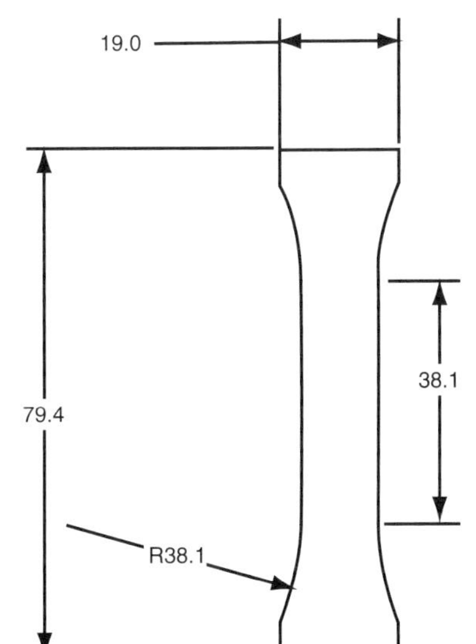

Fig. 6 ASTM D 695 specimen for thin materials. Dimensions in millimeters

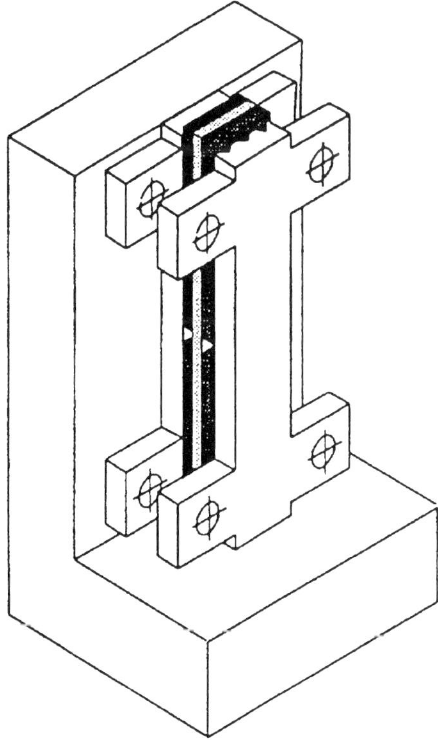

Fig. 7 Schematic of SACMA SRM 1 test fixture and strength specimen

prepreg or similar product forms. This test method is applicable to fabric-based materials only when the unit cell size of the coupon weave/braid is smaller than the 4.8 mm (0.188 in.) gage length of the coupon.

Compression Strength. Measured compression strengths from this test method are typically higher than for the methods in ASTM D 3410. This is believed to be due to the short and narrow gage length of this test specimen, and to the effect this geometry has in suppressing failure mechanisms that are present in longer, unsupported gage lengths such as in ASTM D 3410 procedures A and B.

This test method has been successfully used for strength measurement of unidirectional carbon-reinforced composites. However, one must be very careful to follow proper specimen preparation procedures, tabbing procedures, fixture/specimen alignment practices, and fixture loading practices, many of which have not been standardized or documented in SACMA SRM 1R-94 and are factors that will affect the results from this test method.

Strain-at-failure is not available because the gage region of the strength specimen is not large enough for a strain gage, and the modulus specimen geometry is not suitable for loading to failure. Consequently, stress-strain response, including monitoring of coupon bending strains as commonly done to assess proper gage section loading, cannot be observed over most of the actual curve.

SACMA SRM 6, "Compressive Properties of Oriented Cross-Plied Fiber-Resin Composites." This test method is identical to SACMA SRM 1R, with the exception that it is limited in material form to cross-plied laminates. This limitation is applied because the method is intended for the determination of unidirectional compression strength by applying a back-out factor to the strength determined from the cross-plied laminate. A method for backing out unidirectional properties is included in the standard and in MIL-HDBK-17 (Ref 2), although the two methods are slightly different, with the SACMA method using a greater degree of approximation.

Limitations of the SACMA SRM 6 method are the same as those listed previously for SACMA SRM 1. In addition, the use of the back-out factor in this test method assumes a linear elastic response of the material to which it is being applied. Also, the test is limited to cross-plied versions of the materials previously referenced in SACMA SRM 1.

Through-Thickness Compressive Tests

Because through-thickness compression data is rarely required, there are no standardized or widely accepted test methods to determine compression strength, modulus, or Poisson's ratio of composite laminates in this direction. These data have been reported to a limited extent in the literature, (Ref 13, 14), and in general, simple rectilinear specimens cut from thick-section laminates have been used to obtain these properties.

Shear Property Test Methods

Shear testing of composite materials has proven to be one of the most difficult areas of mechanical property testing in which to define a rigorously correct test, especially in the out-of-plane direction. A number of test methods have been devised, only some of which are described herein. Many of these methods were originally developed for materials other than continuous fiber-reinforced composites, such as metal, plastic, wood, or adhesive. Several of the methods are not yet fully standardized for composite materials, and none of the methods is without deficiency or limitation, though some are clearly more desirable than others.

While there is general agreement regarding the accuracy of shear modulus measurements (for properly conducted tests), determination of shear strength is far more problematic. The presence of edge effects, material coupling effects, nonlinear behavior of the matrix or the fiber-matrix interface, imperfect stress distributions, or the presence of normal stresses make shear strength determination from existing shear test methods highly questionable. Due to this uncertainty, shear strength data to be used for structural applications must be reviewed on a case-by-case basis.

A growing body of experience with composite shear testing, both published and unpublished, has led to a greater understanding of the strengths and weaknesses of each test method. The following conclusions have been offered by ASTM Committee D-30 (Ref 15). These philosophies are being included in existing and future ASTM standard shear test methods:

- There are no known standard (or nonstandard) test methods that are capable of producing a perfectly pure shear stress condition to failure for every materials system, although some test methods can come acceptably close on specific materials systems, as judged by the end user for a given engineering purpose.
- The strengths resulting from test methods that do not consistently produce a reasonable approximation of pure shear, or that do not fail via a shear failure mode, should not be termed "shear strength."
- Because ultimate strength values from existing shear tests are no longer believed able to provide an adequate criterion for comparison of materials systems, the addition of an offset strength is now recommended (0.2% offset, unless otherwise specified).

With the highly nonlinear stress-strain behavior of many filamentary composites, and especially with high-elongation materials systems, it is common to terminate a shear test prior to actual coupon failure. ASTM D-30 currently recommends ending shear tests at 5% shear strain if failure has not previously occurred. The rationale for this includes the following general statements, which are covered in more detail in MIL-HDBK-17 (Ref 16):

- *Practical use in structural laminates:* Shear strains in fiber-reinforced structures of 5% is a practical upper bound, even with the most ductile fibers available.
- *Limitations of common shear test methods:* Realignment, or scissoring, of fibers during both the $\pm 45°$ tensile shear and the V-notched beam shear tests (ASTM D 3518 and D 5379, respectively) makes data questionable past 5% shear strain.
- *Strain gage instrumentation limitations:* Strain gages are typically limited to about 6% shear strain, making this a practical limit for shear strain measurement.
- *Laminate restrictions:* While several of the shear test methods discussed herein are capable of determining a substantial portion of a laminate stress-strain curve and, with it, a shear modulus, there is no standard test method that has been shown to adequately determine the ultimate shear strength of a multidirectional laminate.

In-Plane Shear Tests

In-plane shear tests are standardized as:

- ASTM D 3518/D 3518M, "Standard Practice for In-Plane Shear Response of Polymer-Matrix Composite Materials by Tensile Test of a $\pm 45°$ Laminate"
- SACMA SRM 7, "In-Plane Shear Stress-Strain Properties of Oriented Fiber-Resin Composites"
- ASTM D 5379, "Standard Test Method for Shear Properties of Composite Materials by the V-Notched Beam Method"
- ASTM D 4255, "Standard Guide for Testing In-Plane Shear Properties of Composite Laminates"

ASTM D 3518/D 3518M, "Standard Practice for In-Plane Shear Response of Polymer-Matrix Composite Materials by Tensile Test of a $\pm 45°$ Laminate." This test uses a modified ASTM D 3039 tensile test coupon with a lay-up of $[\pm 45]_{ns}$ to measure in-plane shear properties. The in-plane shear stress in this coupon can be shown to be a simple function of the average applied tensile stress, allowing for straightforward calculation of the shear response of the material. This test method uses a simple test coupon, requires no fixturing, and measurement of strain can be performed using either extensometers or strain gages.

The 1994 release of the standard now contains many features missing in previous versions and should therefore be preferred over any older version. The SACMA version is a restricted subset of the ASTM standard. This fact, together with the unmaintained nature of SACMA specifications, should discourage the use of the SACMA SRM 7 method.

Limitations of the ASTM D 3518 method are described in the following paragraphs.

Material and Laminate Form. The material and laminate form is limited to fully balanced and symmetric ±45° materials. As discussed previously, the stacking sequence, ply count, and ply thickness have a direct effect on coupon strength, making it important to follow the recommendations of the specification.

Inhomogeneous Materials. The material is assumed homogeneous with respect to the size of the test section. Material forms with features that are relatively coarse with respect to the test section width, such as woven or braided textiles with a coarse repeating pattern, require a larger specimen width than is currently standardized.

Impurity of Stress State. The material in the gage section is not in a state of pure in-plane shear, because an in-plane normal stress component is present throughout the gage section, and a complex stress field exists near the free edges. Although the coupon is believed to provide reliable initial material response and can establish shear stress-strain response well into the nonlinear region, the calculated shear stress at failure does not represent the material strength. This is why the ASTM standard terminates the test at 5% shear strain.

Effects of Large Deformation. The extreme fiber scissoring that can occur in this specimen in ductile coupons changes the fiber orientation progressively with increasing strain, conflicting with the fiber orientation assumptions used in the calculation of results. This is a second reason why the test is terminated at 5% shear strain.

ASTM D 5379/D 5379-93, "Test Method for Shear Properties of Composite Materials by the V-Notched Beam Method." The V-notched beam shear test is often called the Iosipescu shear test, after one of its originators (Ref 17–19). The original concept was developed for metals testing in the late 1950s and early 1960s (Ref 20–22) and was refined and modified for fiber-reinforced composites during the early 1980s, which ultimately led to the release of the current ASTM standard (Ref 23–26).

In this method (Fig. 8), a material coupon in the form of a rectangular flat strip with symmetrical, centrally located V-notches is loaded in a mechanical testing machine by the fixture shown in Fig. 8(a). Either in-plane or out-of-plane shear properties may be evaluated, depending upon the orientation of the material coordinate system relative to the loading axis. When testing specimens of relatively thin cross section (generally less than 2.5 mm, or 0.10 in., thick), tabs are recommended. Tabs are bonded to either end of the specimen, away from the test area, to provide increased stability in the load introduction regions.

The specimen is inserted into the fixture with the notch located along the line-of-action of loading. The upper head of the fixture is attached to and driven downward by the cross head of the testing machine. The resulting relative displacement between the two fixture halves introduces the load into the specimen and develops a shear plane between the notches. By placing two strain gage elements, oriented at ±45° to the loading axis and centered between the notches, the shear response of the material can be measured. Further details about the mechanics of the specimen can be found in MIL-HDBK-17 (Ref 27).

Limitations of the ASTM D 5379 method are described subsequently.

Inhomogeneous Materials. The material is assumed homogeneous with respect to the size of the test section. Materials that have relatively coarse features with respect to the test section dimensions, such as fabrics using large filament count tows (12K or more) or certain braided structures, should not be tested with this method.

Uniformity of Strain Field. The calculations assume a uniform shear strain state between the notches. The actual degree of uniformity varies with the level of material orthotropy and the direction of loading. A new strain gage grid configuration has recently been developed especially for use with this test method. The active grid on this gage extends from notch-to-notch and provides an improved estimation of the average strain response. Especially when using conventional strain gages, the most accurate measurements of in-plane shear modulus for unidirectional materials have been shown to result from the $[0/90]_{ns}$ specimen.

Load Eccentricity. Twisting of the specimen during loading can occur, affecting strength results and especially elastic modulus measurement. It is recommended that at least one specimen of each sample be tested with back-to-back rosettes to evaluate the degree of twist. The use of tabs can often alleviate twisting problems associated with thin specimens.

Determination of Failure. Failure is not always obvious in certain materials or configurations. The test specification gives guidance in this area.

Instrumentation. Strain gages are required.

ASTM D 4255-83, "Guide for Testing for In-Plane Shear Properties of Composite Laminates." This test standard is one of the more expensive and complex shear methods currently standardized. It has also historically been subject to relatively high scatter, especially between laboratories. ASTM Committee D-30 is currently considering a revision that is intended to remove the most significant sources of that scatter.

The standard contains two methods: a two-rail method and a three-rail method shown schematically in Fig. 9 using specimens measuring 76 × 152 mm (3.0 × 6.0 in.) and 137 × 152 mm (5.375 × 6.0 in.), respectively. Each specimen type is loaded in bearing using steel fixturing and fasteners 12.7 mm (0.5 in.) in diameter. The two-rail configuration pulls each longitudinal edge of the specimen in opposite directions, creating a shear plane along the longitudinal centerline of the specimen. The three-rail configuration loads the outer two longitudinal edges of the specimen and the centerline of the specimen in opposite

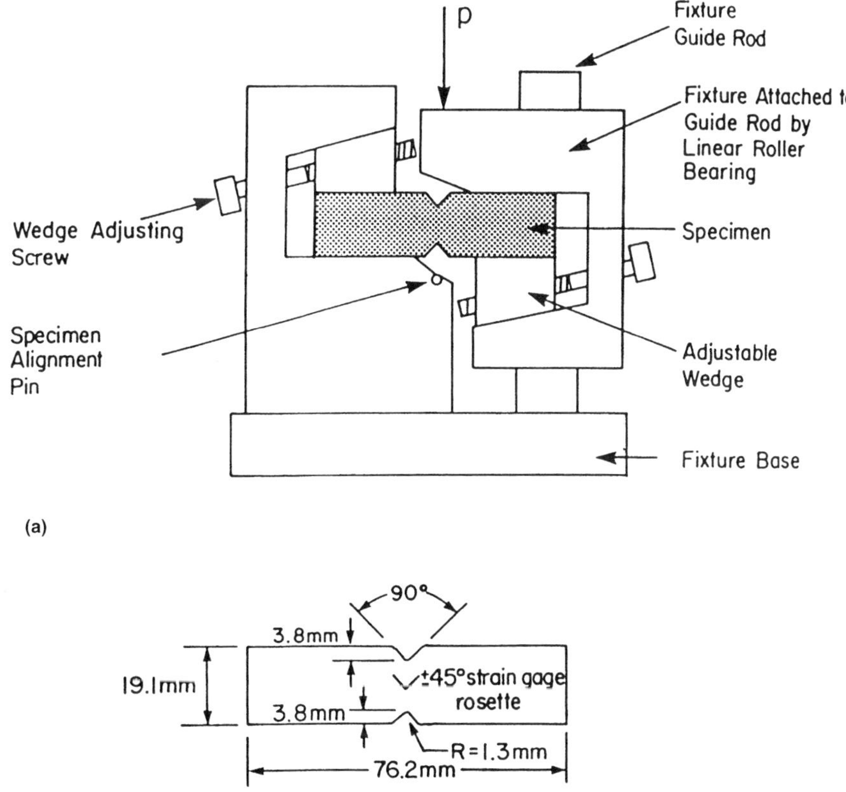

Fig. 8 Iosipescu V-notched beam shear test (ASTM D 5379). (a) Testing configuration. (b) Specimen

directions, creating two shear planes. In both cases, strain gages are typically used to measure applied shear strain.

Because the shear stress state is not uniform through the coupon, and because failures are often noted to begin outside the center of gage section (such as at the restrained corners of the plate), this test as currently standardized does not always produce reliable shear strength data (Ref 28). The three-rail test has a purer state of stress (Ref 29), although it requires a larger specimen size of approximately 150 × 150 mm (6 × 6 in.).

Limitations of the ASTM D 4255-83 method are described subsequently.

Specimen Size. Both versions require larger specimens than other shear tests.

Instrumentation. Strain gages are required.

Stress State. The stress state is known to be nonuniform, and the failure mode is typically influenced by nonshear failures starting outside of the gage section.

Data Scatter. High data scatter from round-robin tests casts doubt upon the reliability of the current version.

Out-of-Plane Shear Tests

Out-of-plane shear tests are standardized as:

- ASTM D 2344-84, "Standard Test Method for Apparent Interlaminar Shear Strength of Parallel Fiber Composites by Short-Beam Method"
- SACMA SRM 8R-94, "Apparent Interlaminar Shear Strength of Oriented Fiber-Resin Composites by the Short-Beam Method"
- ASTM D 5379, "Standard Test Method for Shear Properties of Composite Materials by the V-Notched Beam Method"

ASTM D 2344, "Standard Test Method for Apparent Interlaminar Shear Strength of Parallel-Fiber Composites by Short-Beam Method." ASTM Test D 2344, commonly known as the short-beam shear (SBS) test, attempts to quantify the interlaminar (out-of-plane) shear strength of parallel-fiber-reinforced composites. The specimen for this test is a short, relatively deep beam cut from a flat laminate. The specimen is mounted as a simply supported beam and loaded at the midpoint of the span of the specimen. The intent is to minimize bending stresses while maximizing out-of-plane shear stresses by using a short, deep "beam." However, the contact stresses induced at the load points greatly interfere with the strain distribution, both through the depth of the beam and axially along the length of the beam. The resulting failure is rarely, if ever, a true pure shear failure, but instead results from the complex stress state present in the specimen (Ref 30).

Despite its significant limitations, this test has commonly been used to develop design allowables for structural design criteria. This practice is not recommended. The ASTM D 5379 V-notch shear method discussed previously is the much-preferred choice. The short-beam shear test should only be used for qualitative testing, such as materials process development and control. As a quality control test, testing of laminate configurations other than unidirectional is common and acceptable, although they are currently nonstandard. A revision to the ASTM method is currently underway to allow the standard SBS testing of balanced and symmetric laminates.

A related (but unmaintained and less-preferable) method is SACMA SRM 8R-94.

Limitations of the ASTM D 2344 method are described in the following paragraphs.

Stress State. The stress state is known to be significantly disruptive and three-dimensional. The resultant strengths are a poor estimation of the out-of-plane shear strength.

Failure Mode. The failure mode is often multimode.

No Modulus/Material Response. Instrumentation of this specimen is not practical; therefore modulus and stress-strain data cannot be obtained.

ASTM D 5379, "Standard Test Method for Shear Properties of Composite Materials by the V-Notched Beam Method" (as applied for out-of-plane shear testing). This test method and the specimen geometry are described for the section "In-Plane Shear Tests" in this article. When testing for out-of-plane shear properties, the orientation of the fibers in the laminate is changed so as to cause a shearing action in the desired transverse plane. This test method is the only acceptable out-of-plane shear test available. The out-of-plane testing of laminates with fibers off-axis to the test direction, such as three-dimensional textiles, is subject to the same restrictions and limitations that are discussed in the section on in-plane testing.

ASTM D 3846-79, "Test Method for In-Plane Shear Strength of Reinforced Plastics." ASTM test method D 3846, despite the title, is *not* normally used as an in-plane shear strength test, but is in fact an out-of-plane shear strength test and as such is covered in this section.

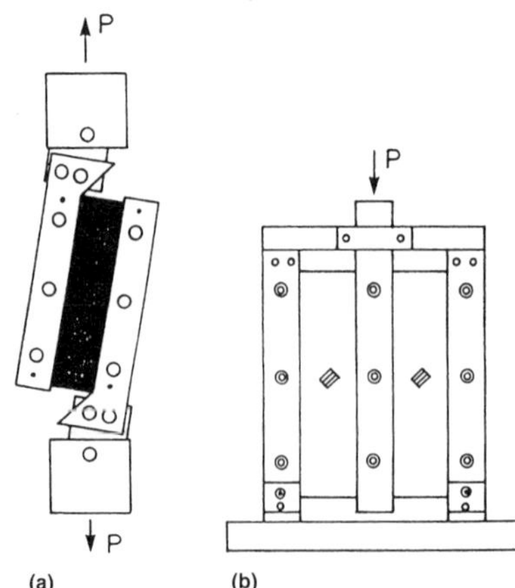

Fig. 9 Rail shear test (ASTM D 4255). (a) Two-rail configuration. (b) Three-rail configuration

This test is primarily intended for use on randomly dispersed fiber-reinforced thermosetting sheet plastics as a substitute to the short-beam shear test method ASTM D 2344 described previously. The test consists of a doubly notched specimen loaded in compression in a supporting jig as shown in Fig. 10. (The fixture is the same as is used in the ASTM D 695 compression test.) Failure occurs in out-of-plane shear in the plane of the specimen between the two notches. While this specimen can be (and has been) used for testing continuous-fiber laminated-reinforced plastics, it is not recommended for use on advanced composite laminates. The notches, which are machined into the specimen to force failure of the laminate in shear, have been shown to negatively influence the stress distribution in the coupon (Ref 31). As a result, a nonuniform, multiaxial stress state exists in the gage section, making a true strength calculation suspect at best.

Limitations of the ASTM D 3846 method are described herein.

Stress State. A highly three-dimensional, nonuniform stress state in the gage section causes strength values from this test to be unusually poor estimations of the true out-of-plane shear strength.

No Modulus/Material Response. Instrumentation of this specimen is not practical; therefore modulus and stress-strain data cannot be obtained.

Flexure Property Test Methods

There is considerable debate concerning the validity of flexural testing of fiber-reinforced composite materials. Measured flexural proper-

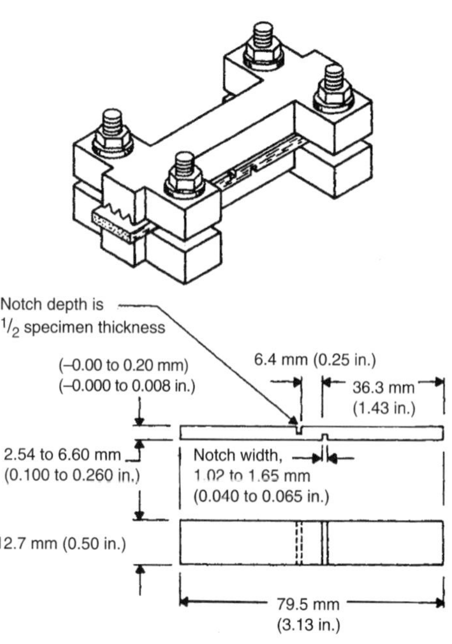

Fig. 10 Schematic of ASTM D 3846 test specimen and fixture

ties are often highly dependent on stacking sequence, as is illustrated by the fact that for highly orthotropic laminates, the maximum stress of a flexure specimen may not occur in the outermost fibers. In these cases, assumptions based on homogeneous beam theory that enable simple data analysis do not hold, and more detailed analysis based on laminated beam theory must be applied. Other aspects of flexure testing that may have significant influence on the accuracy of the properties measured include interactions with the loading surface geometry, end forces developed by large support span-to-specimen depth ratios, and shear deflections that result from low span-to-depth ratios. Because of the complexity of some of these effects, it is difficult to make broad recommendations that apply to the majority of candidate materials. It is for these reasons that laminate flexure testing should be used primarily for quality assurance and materials specification purposes.

ASTM D 790, "Standard Test Methods for Flexural Properties of Unreinforced and Reinforced Plastics and Electrical Insulating Materials." This specification was originally written for plastics, but has since been modified and approved for composites. It includes provisions for measuring maximum fiber stress, flexural strength, and flexural modulus. The basic test method consists of simply supporting a straight-sided, rectangular cross-section specimen on two supports symmetrically placed about the transverse centerline and loading in flexure with a third point placed on the transverse centerline. The specification includes two procedures that differ only by the applied strain rate. Procedure A is used primarily for measurement of flexural modulus and uses an outer fiber strain rate of 0.01 mm/mm/minute. Procedure B is restricted to measurement of flexural strength only and uses a strain rate ten times greater than procedure A (0.20 mm/mm/minute).

The span-to-depth ratio recommended by the specification depends upon the material stiffness and depth. Typical ratios are from 16:1 to 40:1, although some highly anisotropic composites require ratios of up to 60 to 1 in order to more accurately measure flexural modulus.

While many of the properties measured by this standard are subject to inaccuracies due to the complex stress states induced, particularly for highly anisotropic materials, the test method is useful for comparison purposes, provided all tests are performed using the same specimen geometry, span, and loading point arrangement. The reader is encouraged to read the specification carefully for guidance in performing this test and to critically review the data obtained.

Limitations of the ASTM D 790 method are described subsequently.

Highly Orthotropic Material Stress Distribution. The test method may not induce the maximum stress in the outer fibers of highly orthotropic laminates, making the calculations for maximum fiber stress inaccurate.

Maximum Fiber Strain Limitation. The method is only valid for materials that fail below 5% fiber strain.

Absolute Properties Are Often Not Measured. Due to the complex stress state that is often induced in this test, it should generally be used only as a quality assurance test rather than a source of absolute properties.

Fracture Toughness Test Methods

Fracture in structural solids is usually initiated by some crack or notch-like flaw, which induces high stresses in its immediate vicinity. The development of fracture mechanics has gained wide acceptance in metals, but because of the anisotropy of composite materials and the vast range of material behaviors represented in composites, their fracture behavior is still relatively poorly understood. A reasonable introduction to the basics of fracture mechanics can be found in MIL-HDBK-17 (Ref 32).

Fracture testing can be categorized into three types, based upon the manner in which crack tip stresses are developed. These three "modes" are defined by the relative displacement of the upper and lower crack surfaces with respect to each other. These modes are shown in Fig. 11. The primary property measured in fracture testing is the strain energy release rate, which is defined as the reduction in strain energy (or increase in potential energy) due to an infinitesimal self-similar extension of a crack. Catastrophic propagation of the crack will occur when this rate reaches a critical value, often referred to as the material toughness. Various test methods have been devised to measure the toughness of a given material in each of the three loading modes. However, though considerable work has been done in this area, as well as attempts to create methods for developing *R*-curves for modeling stable delamination growth as a result of both increasing static load and cyclic loading, only one test method (for mode I behavior) has been standardized. The following section describes only the standardized method for mode I testing, and the reader is referred to Ref 32 for information regarding several nonstandard methods.

Mode I test methods are standardized as ASTM D 5528, "Standard Test Methods for Mode I Interlaminar Fracture Toughness of Unidirectional Fiber-Reinforced Polymer-Matrix Composites." The test, commonly referred to as a double-cantilever beam test, is shown schematically in Fig. 12. The specimen measures 125 mm (5 in.) long, 20 to 25 mm (0.8 to 1 in.) wide, and 3 to 5 mm (0.12 to 0.20 in.) thick and uses a nonbondable film insert placed at the specimen midplane during panel manufacture to create an initial crack length of approximately 63 mm (2.5 in.). The applied load, *P*, to the two arms, the corresponding displacement, δ, and typical load-displacement traces obtained are shown in Fig. 12(c). The numbers on these traces indicate results for various delamination lengths and are obtained as the delamination progresses. Various procedures for data reduction, other details, and restriction on specimen dimensions to avoid geo-

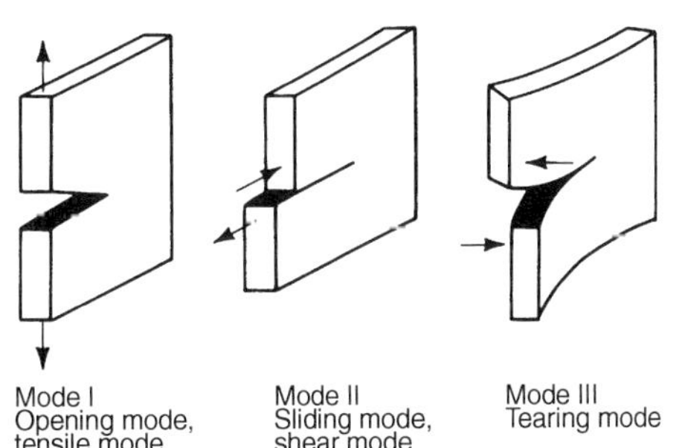

Fig. 11 Basic modes of crack extension

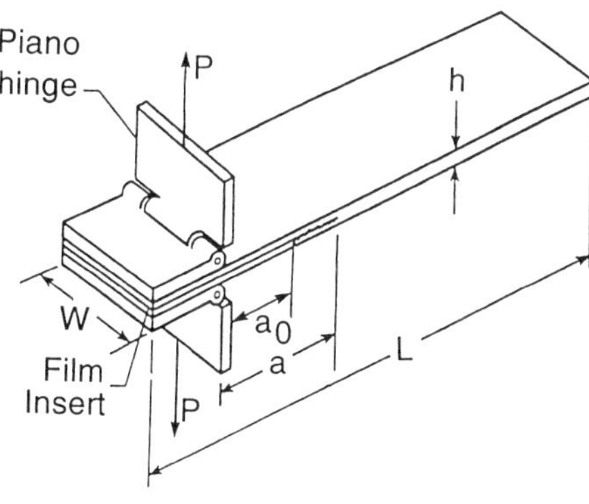

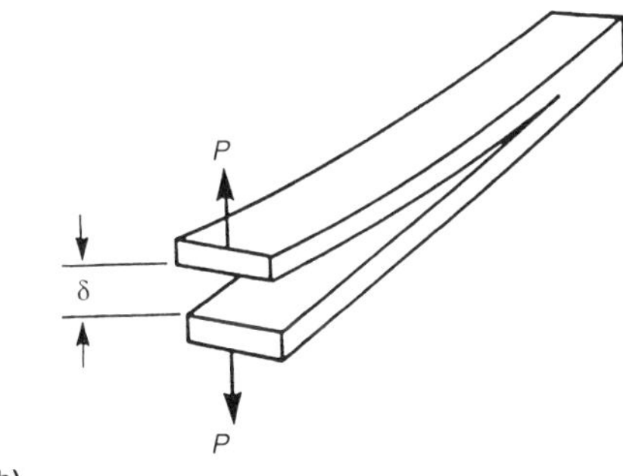

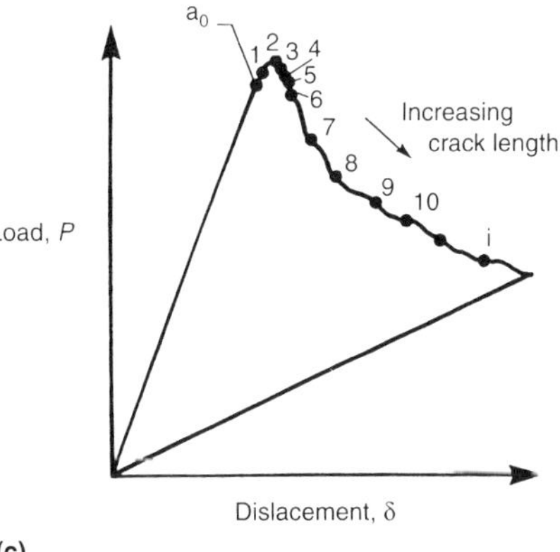

Fig. 12 Double-cantilever beam test (ASTM D 5528). (a) Specimen geometry. (b) Definition of crack-opening displacement. (c) Load-displacement trace during crack growth. a_0, initial crack growth

metric nonlinearities are documented in the standard.

Toughness values may vary depending on the tendency of the delamination to grow out-of-plane. For this reason, testing of nonunidirectional laminates is prohibited. However, some unidirectional laminates may allow considerable fiber bridging across the delamination plane. These bridging fibers may increase the measured toughness for all data past the initial crack, and the toughness value for initiation should therefore be identified separately from those at later stages of delamination growth.

In materials not strongly influenced by fiber bridging, a competing mechanism may dominate. When the delamination starts to grow from the insert, the initial toughness may be higher than that measured for subsequent growth. Data analysis in these cases requires that the initial toughness be disregarded as artificially high and that subsequent data be used instead.

Limitations of the ASTM D 5528 mode I method are described subsequently.

Material. Testing should be limited to unidirectional materials or at least laminates in which the delamination grows between two unidirectional plies aligned with the crack growth direction.

Failure Mode. Fiber bridging and artificially high initial toughness values (depending on the material being tested) require close attention to failure modes for proper interpretation of the data. Furthermore, propagation of the delamination front that "wanders" off the specimen midplane may result in high scatter.

Crack Growth Monitoring. Monitoring of the crack tip for growth is often difficult and requires great care. Observance of both sides of the specimen is important, because delamination fronts can grow asymmetrically. Application of a thin white film on each side of the specimen is often helpful, but great care should be taken to minimize the thickness of this film and to create as uniform a film surface as possible.

Fatigue Property Test Methods

Static lamina test data is often used to predict the properties of application-specific laminate materials by the use of lamination theory. However, there are not yet well-established methods for doing the same for fatigue properties. For this reason, fatigue design properties for a given structural application usually must be generated using laminates representative of that structure. Furthermore, expansion of coupon data using element and structural component specimens in a "building-block" approach is often required. Because of the design-specific nature of most fatigue testing, there are very few standardized test methods for fatigue characterization of composite materials. The methods that do exist are tension-tension methods that do not consider compression loading. This is primarily due to the fact that most fatigue driven structures are tension-critical, and that the buckling-sensitive nature of compression fatigue testing makes most tests specific to an application and inappropriate for standardization.

Fatigue testing is usually performed using a constant-amplitude oscillatory stress or strain applied about some mean load. Other fatigue tests called "spectrum" or "block-spectrum" tests are not constant amplitude and are designed to reflect the full spectrum of loads that a structure might experience during a representative service cycle. (For example, the service cycle of an aircraft structure typically extends from take-off to landing.) Because of the application-specific nature of spectrum testing, it is not discussed here.

Coupon-level fatigue testing is most often used to establish the characteristic curve of a laminate, relating the maximum applied oscillatory stress (S) or strain (ε) to the number of cycles to failure (N). These curves are called "stress-life" (S-N) or "strain-life" (ε-N) curves, respectively. The applied stress or strain is usually expressed as a percentage of the static material strength or failure strain.

In defining a fatigue test series, several variables must be considered, and all must be defined with regard to the intended use of the structure being evaluated. They include the following:

- *Upper cycle count limit, or "runout:"* Because it is possible to set the maximum oscillatory load low enough to cycle a specimen essentially forever without failing, a runout should be defined as a stop point to prevent the unnecessary time and expense of running a specimen longer than is appropriate for the application. At runout the residual strength of the specimen may be measured statically to determine property degradation compared to uncycled baseline specimens.
- *R-ratio:* This is the ratio of the minimum to the maximum applied stress or strain. For example, a tension-tension fatigue test with oscillatory stresses of 10 to 100 kN (2,250 to 22,500 lbf) has an R-ratio of 0.1. A reverse-loaded (tension-compression) test with oscillatory stresses of 50 kN to –50 kN (11,240 to –11,240 lbf) has an R-ratio of –1.0. Therefore, tension-tension tests have positive R-ratios between zero and 1, while compression-compression test R-ratios are positive and greater than 1.
- *Frequency:* Although most materials are generally insensitive to frequency, it is good practice to generate a given S-N curve using the same frequency for each specimen. Of particular concern is ensuring that the frequency used is not so fast that unacceptable heating of the specimen occurs. Each laminate has its own characteristics regarding frequency dependent heating. A general guideline is to limit frequency induced heating to 10 °C (20 °F) above ambient.
- *Waveform:* Most fatigue tests apply load using a sinusoidal waveform.

ASTM D 3479 "Standard Test Method for Tension-Tension Fatigue of Polymer-Matrix Composite Materials." The ASTM D 3479 test method uses the specimen geometry defined by ASTM D 3039 and provides for development of S-N curves as well as the characterization of damage growth, such as microcracking, delamination, or fiber damage due to fatigue cycling. Because of the gradual damage growth usually typical of fatigue testing, it is especially important to minimize the critical issues affecting test results for straight-sided tension testing, including tabbing, specimen machining, and grip alignment. (See the section "In-Plane Tension Test Methods" in this article.)

ACKNOWLEDGMENTS

Much of this section was borrowed from work others have done in support of MIL-HDBK-17. Of particular help were the MIL-HDBK-17 sections on tension and shear, written by Richard Fields; the compression section, originally written by Gene Camponeschi and recently revised by Donald Adams; and the fracture toughness section, written by S.N. Chatterjee.

REFERENCES

1. *Composite Materials,* Vol 1, Chapter 6, MIL-HDBK-17-1E, Department of Defense Handbook
2. Use of Crossply Laminate Testing to Derive Lamina Strengths in the Fiber Direction, *Composite Materials,* Vol 1, Chapter 6, MIL-HDBK-17-1E, Department of Defense Handbook
3. E.T. Camponeschi, Jr., Compression of Composite Materials: A Review, *Fatigue and Fracture of Composite Materials (Third Conference),* ASTM STP 1110, T.K. O'Brien, Ed., ASTM, 1991, p 550–580
4. G.A. Schoeppner and R.L. Sierakowski, A Review of Compression Test Methods for Organic Matrix Composites, *J. Compos. Technol. Res.,* Vol 12 (No. 1), 1990, p 3–12
5. M.G. Abdallah, State of the Art Advanced Composite Materials: Compression Test Methods, *Proc. JANNAF, CMCS, SM & BS Meeting,* 1984 (CA Institute of Technology, Pasadena, CA)
6. J.M. Whitney, I.M. Daniel, and R.B. Pipes, Experimental Mechanics of Fiber Reinforced Composite Materials, *SEM Monograph,* Vol 4, 1982
7. J.S. Berg and D.F. Adams, "An Evaluation of Composite Material Compression Test Methods," Report UW-CMRG R-88-106, University of Wyoming Composite Materials Research Group, June 1988
8. *Composite Materials,* Vol 3, Chapter 7, MIL-HDBK-17-3E, Department of Defense Handbook
9. K.E. Hofer and P.N. Rao, A New Static Compression Fixture for Advanced Composite Materials, *J. Test. Eval.,* Vol 5 (No. 4), 1977

10. D.F. Adams and E.M. Odom, Influence of Test Fixture Configuration on the Measured Compressive Strength of a composite Material, *J. Compos. Technol. and Res.,* Vol 13 (No. 1), Spring 1991, p 36–40
11. "Compression Test of Fiber Reinforced Aerospace Plastics: Testing of Unidirectional Laminates and Woven-Fabric Laminates, DIN 65 380, Deutsches Institut fur Normung, Koln, Germany, 1991
12. *Composite Materials,* Vol 1, Chapter 6, Section 6.7.4.2.5, MIL-HDBK-17-1E, Department of Defense Handbook
13. M. Knight, Three-Dimensional Elastic Moduli of Graphite/Epoxy Composites, *J. Compos. Mater.,* Vol 16, 1982, p 153–159
14. V. Peros, "Thick-Walled Composite Material Pressure Hulls: Three-Dimensional Laminate Analysis Considerations," master's thesis, University of Delaware, Newark, Dec 1987
15. ASTM Committee D-30 meeting, section D30.04.03 minutes for fall 1991 and spring 1993
16. *Composite Materials,* Vol 1, Chapter 6, Section 6.7.6.1, MIL-HDBK-17-1E, Department of Defense Handbook
17. M. Arcan and N. Goldenberg, "On a Basic Criterion for Selecting a Shear Testing Standard for Plastic Materials," ISO/TC 61-WG 2 S.P. 171, Burgenstock, Switzerland, 1957 (in French)
18. N. Goldenberg, M. Arcan, and E. Nicolau, On the Most Suitable Specimen Shape for Testing Shear Strength of Plastics, *Proc. International Symposium on Plastics Testing and Standardization,* ASTM STP 247, American Society for Testing and Materials, 1959, p 115–121
19. M. Arcan, Z. Hashin, and A. Voloshin, A Method to Produce Uniform Plane-Stress States with Applications to Fiber-Reinforced Materials, *Exp. Mech.,* Vol 18 (No. 4), April 1978, p 141–146
20. D.F. Sims, In-Plane Shear Stress-Strain Response of Unidirectional Composite Material, *J. Compos. Mater.,* Vol 7, Jan 1973, p 124
21. N. Iosipescu, "Photoelastic Investigations on an Accurate Procedure for the Pure Shear Testing of Materials," *Rev. Mec. Appl.,* Vol 8 (No. 1), 1963
22. N. Iosipescu, New Accurate Procedure for Single Shear Testing of Metals, *J. Mater.,* Vol 2 (No. 3), Sept 1967, p 537–566
23. D.E. Walrath and D.F. Adams, The Iosipescu Shear Test as Applied to Composite Materials, *Exp. Mech.,* Vol 23 (No. 1), March 1983, p 105–110
24. D.E. Walrath and D.F. Adams, "Analysis of the Stress State in an Iosipescu Test Specimen," Department Report UWME-DR-301-102-1, University of Wyoming, June 1983
25. D.E. Walrath and D.F. Adams, "Verification and Application of the Iosipescu Shear Test Method," Department Report UWME-DR-401-103-1, University of Wyoming, June 1984
26. D.F. Adams and D.E. Walrath, Further Development of the Iosipescu Test Method, *Exp. Mech.,* Vol 27 (No. 2), June 1987, p 113–119
27. *Composite Materials,* Vol 1, Chapter 6, Section 6.7.6.2.1, MIL-HDBK-17-1E, Department of Defense Handbook
28. R. Garcia, T.A. Weisshaar, and R.R. McWithey, An Experimental and Analytical Investigation of the Rail Shear-Test Method as Applied to Composite Materials, *Exp. Mech.,* Aug 1980
29. Y.M. Tarnopol'skii and T. Kincis, *Static Test Methods for Composites,* Van Nostrand Reinhold Company, New York, 1985
30. C.A. Berg, J. Tirosh, and M. Israeli, Analysis of Short Beam Bending of Fiber Reinforced Composites, *Composite Materials: Testing and Design, Second Conf.,* ASTM STP 497, American Society for Testing and Materials, 1972, p 206
31. C.T. Herakovich, H.W. Bergner, and D.E. Bowles, A Comparative Study of Composite Shear Specimens Using the Finite-Element Method, *Test Methods and Design Allowables for Fibrous Composites,* ASTM STP 734, American Society for Testing and Materials, 1981, p 129–151
32. *Composite Materials,* Vol 1, Chapter 6, Section 6.7.8, MIL-HDBK-17-1E, Department of Defense Handbook

SELECTED REFERENCES

- L.A. Carlsson and R.B. Pipes, *Experimental Characterization of Advanced Composite Materials,* 2nd ed., Technomic, 1997
- I.M. Daniel and O. Ishai, *Engineering Mechanics of Composite Materials,* Oxford University Press, 1994
- C.H. Jenkins, Ed., *Manual on Mechanical Testing of Composites,* 2nd ed., Fairmont Press, 1998
- Lamina and Laminate Characterization, Chapter 6, *Composite Materials Handbook,* Vol 1E, MIL-HDBK-17, Materials Sciences Corporation, University of Delaware, and U.S. Army Research Laboratory, www.mil17.org/
- D.W. Wilson and L.A. Carlsson, Mechanical Property Measurement, Chapter 7, *Composites Engineering Handbook,* P.K. Mallick, Ed., Marcel Dekker, New York, 1997
- D.W. Wilson and L.A. Carlsson, Mechanical Testing of Fiber-Reinforced Composites, *Mechanical Testing and Evaluation,* Vol 8, *ASM Handbook,* ASM International, 2000, p 905–932

Element and Subcomponent Testing

Lawrence A. Gintert, Concurrent Technologies Corporation

STRUCTURAL TEST SPECIMENS designed to characterize composite material behavior for failure modes not addressed in flat coupon specimens are known as *elements* (for smaller, more standard specimen configurations) and *subcomponents* (for nonstandard and typically larger specimens). The materials data presented in the previous Section can be used to design tests for structural elements and subcomponents tailored to represent the actual structural components being studied experimentally. These tests are used for allowable verification and for fulfillment of structural-integrity requirements specific to the materials and geometry of the component under consideration. These tests are necessary because the behavior of composites is not adequately characterized using two-dimensional coupon testing as in homogeneous or isotropic materials, especially in areas of structural joints and complex geometry.

It is assumed that the reader is familiar with the general structural behavior of composite materials and has been introduced to the "building-block" approach to composite materials certification discussed in the previous articles in this Section (see, in particular, the article "Overview of Testing and Certification"). This discussion focuses on experimental characterization of composite structures at the element and subcomponent level of complexity of the building-block approach described in *Composite Materials,* MIL-HDBK-17. The elements discussed characterize laminates, bolted and bonded joints, and damage tolerance behavior that is needed for design of composite structures, while subcomponents characterize structural behavior unique to specific design features of the full-scale structure. General discussion on analysis and design of bolted and bonded joints can be found in MIL-HDBK-17, Volume 3, Section 5, while damage tolerance is covered in Volume 3, Section 6.2.4. A complete description of the building-block methodology is provided in MIL-HDBK-17, Volume 1.

This article begins with an overview of why structural element and subcomponent testing are conducted, including a discussion on the different types of failure modes in composites. An overview of the testing methodology, fixturing, instrumentation, and data reporting is provided, followed by a description of various standard elements used to characterize composite materials for the various failure modes. Simple structural-element testing under in-plane unidirectional, multidirectional, and combined loading as well as out-of-plane loading are discussed. Simple bolted joints and bonded joints are discussed as well as data correlation with analytical predictions. Some of the standard testing methods are briefly discussed, and a list of ASTM testing standards applicable at the element level of testing for both polymer-matrix composites and metal-matrix composites is also included. Examples of subcomponent test specimens are also provided. The article ends with a brief discussion on durability and damage tolerance testing. Testing used to characterize damage applies to typical composite structures, assuming common design practices are employed such that damage incurred is typical of relatively balanced laminates of reasonable quality and integrity. This testing, known as compression after impact (CAI) testing, is used widely in the aerospace industry to gage damage tolerance potential of composite materials. It is discussed as being applicable to solid laminates as well as sandwich construction laminates.

The methodology provided herein is generally applicable to composites designed with standard composite practice employed, such as material buildup for mechanical fastening, adequate fastener edge distance, and fastener pitch. Refer to MIL-HDBK-17 for a more thorough discussion regarding composite design practice and certification guidelines.

Test Methodology and Considerations

The purpose of element and subcomponent testing is to characterize failure modes not addressed in lower-level testing. These failure modes are typically those that are influenced by stresses applied in the weakest direction of the composite materials being used, normally through the thickness for layered composites.

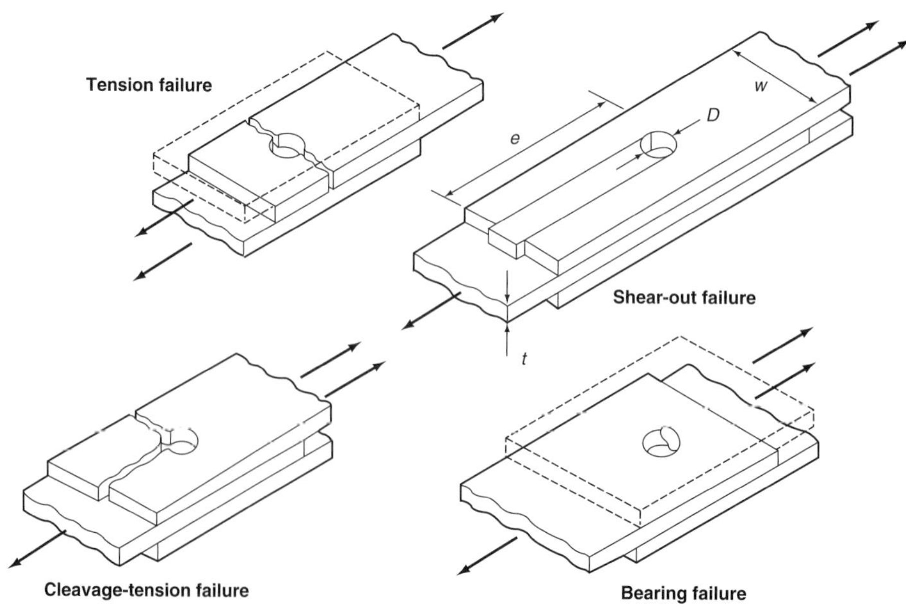

Fig. 1 Typical failure modes for bolted joints in advanced composites

The results of this testing are correlated with analysis to verify strength methodology as it applies to failure modes and magnitudes. Subcomponent tests usually represent a full-sized or scale-model segment of the real structure being evaluated.

Testing and analysis of composite joints and other elements are essential for establishing the structural integrity of composite structures and ensuring their reliability. Due to the inherent weakness of composite materials in the through-thickness direction, any joint in a composite structure is a potential failure site. Without proper design a joint can act as a damage initiation point, which can lead to a loss in structural strength and eventual failure of the component. Two types of joints in common use are mechanically fastened joints and adhesively bonded joints. The guidelines discussed subsequently from MIL-HDBK-17 define test types, laminates, environments, and replication that are needed for sound joint design.

For mechanically bolted joints, tests are recommended that characterize the joint for various failure modes: bearing, notched tension/compression, bearing/by-pass, shear-out, and fastener pull-through. Test matrices are provided in MIL-HDBK-17. A straightforward test method to determine material bearing strength is provided. The bearing strength measured by this test is the upper bound value that can be achieved in a realistic structural joint. The test is useful for qualification purposes or for material-to-material comparisons. A detailed analysis of the stress distribution around a fastener hole is available in MIL-HDBK-17, Volume 3, Section 5.3. Discussion on both theoretical and empirical approaches to the stress analysis of bolted joints in composite materials can be found in Ref 1.

For bonded joints, two types of tests are described. The first type determines adhesive properties that are needed in design. These tests provide adhesive stiffness and strength properties needed for analysis and design methods of MIL-HDBK-17, Volume 3, Section 5.2. The second type is used to verify specific designs. Examples of such tests are shown.

Failure Modes. An important consideration in element and subcomponent testing and analysis is the selection of the type of test method, with due attention to the failure mode that is likely to result with a specific design in a particular composite system. The various failure modes for bolted joints described subsequently provide an example of how this needs to be considered.

The occurrence of a particular failure mode is dependent primarily on joint geometry and laminate configuration or lay-up. Composite bolted joints may fail in various modes, as shown in Fig. 1. The likelihood of a particular failure mode is influenced by bolt diameter (D), laminate width (w), edge distance (e), and thickness (t). The type of fastener used can also influence the occurrence of a particular failure mode. Net section tension-compression failures occur when the bolt diameter is a sufficiently large fraction of the strip width. This fraction is about one-quarter or more for near-isotropic lay-ups in graphite/epoxy systems. It is characterized by failure of the plies in the primary load direction. Cleavage failures occur because of the proximity of the end of the specimen. This type of failure often initiates at the end of the specimen rather than adjacent to the fastener. In some instances, the bolt head may be pulled out through the laminate after the bolt is bent and deformed. This mode is frequently associated with countersunk fasteners and is highly dependent on the particular fastener used. Finally, it is important to note that for any given geometry, the failure mode may vary as a function of lay-up and stacking sequence or laminate configuration.

In order to design against the different failure modes and the interactions between them, the capability of the composite material has to be determined by tests. These are described in MIL-HDBK-17 to provide guidance as to amount of testing that would be typical, but not necessarily the minimum. These properties may be different for each distinct laminate, fastener type, and environmental condition. The properties also change depending on ply orientations (or typically the percentage of 0°, 90°, or ±45° direction plies) in the laminate. The number of laminates to be tested is governed by analysis capability and degree of confidence in extrapolation from test results.

The shear-out mode of failure is usually avoided in design by providing sufficient edge distance between the holes and at the free edge, and by using a balanced laminate configuration. Shear-out critical joints sometimes cannot be avoided, especially in rework situations. In those situations, a test program must be undertaken to

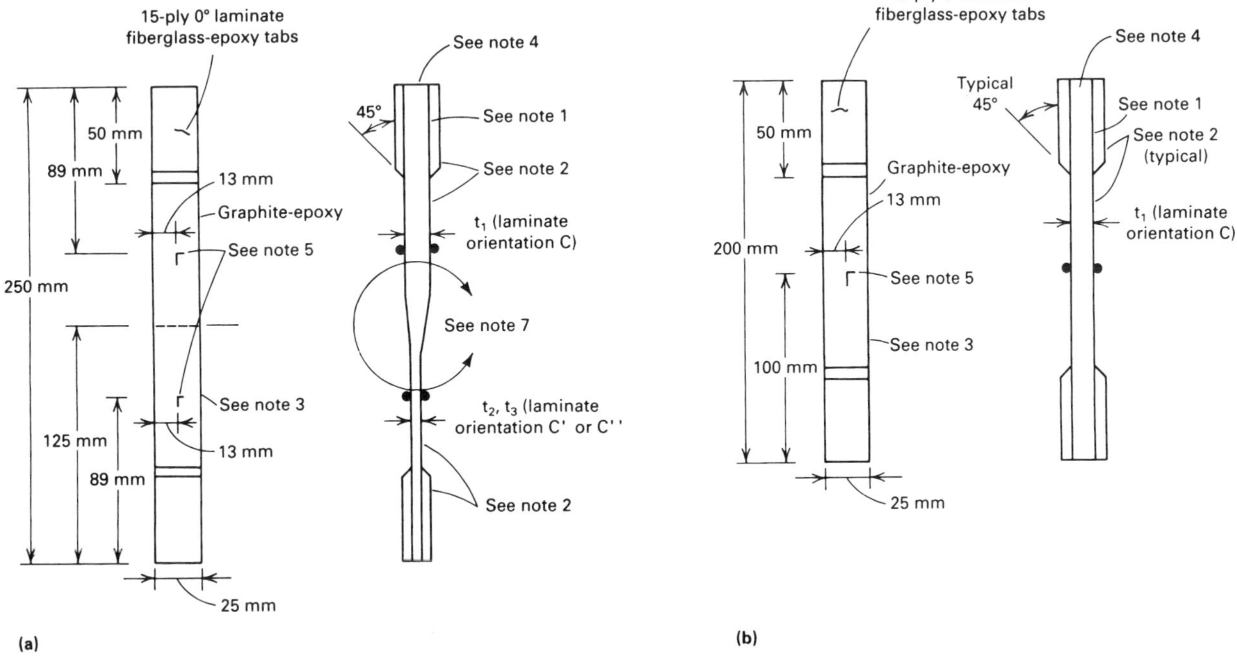

Fig. 2 Longitudinal or transverse tensile static and fatigue specimens. (a) Ply drop-off specimen. (b) Plain specimen. (1) Bond glass-epoxy tabs with an epoxy film adhesive. (2) Specimen thickness shall not vary more than ±0.13 mm (0.005 in.) from nominal. (3) Specimen longitudinal edges shall be parallel to 0.13 mm (0.005 in.). (4) Top end and bottom end surfaces shall be flat and parallel to 0.25 mm (0.010 in.). (5) Strain gages shall be micromeasurements EA 03-250BF-350 or equivalent, located as shown. (6) Testing shall be in accordance with ASTM D 3039 (Ref 2). (7) Location of ply drop-off

establish the materials properties for this failure mode. (See MIL-HDBK-17, Section 7.2.8 for further discussion.)

Net tension-compression and shear-out strengths are a strong function of laminate configuration, joint geometry, and hole size, but are only marginally dependent on fastener type, joint configuration, or environment. On the other hand, bearing and fastener pull-through strengths are greatly influenced by the type of fastener used and its characteristics, such as clamp effects, bolt stiffness, head and tail areas, countersinking, and so on. The laminate lay-up and stacking sequence do not affect bearing or pull-through strengths significantly unless extreme lay-ups are used, the extreme being defined as a laminate having highly concentrated plies or plies in only two directions.

Fixturing. Load introduction and support structures (i.e., fixturing) must be carefully designed to simulate those of the real structure, yet must not fail before the element or subcomponent does. Jigs and fixtures for subelements are usually custom-designed, while many standard fixtures for elements are governed somewhat by the standards for those test configurations. The test fixture should fully support the specimen against buckling in compression between tabs and might need to provide floating support features in order to avoid interference or unwanted load paths. Loading should represent design static or durability (fatigue) load cases based on the internal loading calculated for the particular structural segment, and therefore, the fixturing or load introduction apparatus would need to easily withstand this loading. Boundary conditions should also be representative of those provided by the surrounding structure, mandating a consideration of relative stiffness for the fixturing. Data to be recorded should be understood and planned for during fixture design so that instrumentation can be located in an effective manner that is easily accessed for inspection and troubleshooting. Anticipated strains and deflections at critical points in the structure should be considered as well.

Instrumentation. Instrumentation may be as simple as that shown in Fig. 2 for tensile elements, but will usually include a number of back-to-back biaxial strain gages used to measure the material and element behavior under more complex loading conditions. It may also include extensometers and deflection gages, especially if the test objectives include measurement of deformation or buckling of critical elements.

Instrumentation is usually greater for static than for fatigue testing, and to some extent, the static test results will influence the location and type of instrumentation to be used in the fatigue testing. Certainly the highest stress (strain) and deflection areas observed in the static test need to be monitored at least periodically, if not continuously, in fatigue testing. For surviving subcomponents, added instrumentation may be desirable for static residual-strength testing so that an accurate comparison can be made with the original static strength. Special instrumentation may be required for subcomponents that exhibit elastic buckling before reaching design ultimate load. Back-to-back biaxial gages or three-gage rosettes are preferred for nonbuckling compression testing, but are a necessity for compression buckling testing. A divergence of the strain readings of the back-to-back compression gages of more than ±10% from the mean strain usually indicates buckling.

Loading and recording equipment should be of a type that allows continuous reading, such that constant monotonically increasing loading rates, or deflection or strain rates, at critical points can be maintained to failure. Preliminary instrumentation static checkout runs should not exceed 20% of predicted design ultimate failure load. For fatigue loading of subcomponents, the temperature increases of the structure at high-strain areas should be monitored; if increases exceed 3 °C (5 °F), either the temperature or the fatigue-loading rate should be reduced.

For a monotonically increasing load, strain, or deflection-controlled static test, the important properties to measure at critical points are load-strain and load-deflection behavior to failure. Also, the failure mode, location, and type should be recorded photographically.

Data Analysis and Reporting. Materials property data should be collected, reduced, and analyzed, as well as simple element mechanical-behavior data. Load versus strain and load versus deflection data from static tests should be tabulated and continuous plots of their behavior curves recorded to failure. This data may represent not only materials properties, but also im-

Table 1 ASTM standards applicable to element-level testing of composites

Standard designation(a)	Title of standard	Property
C 297	Flatwise Tensile Strength of Sandwich Constructions	Flatwise tension
C 363	Delamination Strength of Honeycomb Core Materials	Peel
C 364	Edgewise Compressive Strength of Flat Sandwich Constructions	Edgewise compression
C 365	Flatwise Compressive Properties of Sandwich Cores	Flatwise compression
C 393	Flexural Properties of Sandwich Constructions	Flexure
C 394	Shear Fatigue of Sandwich Core Materials	Shear fatigue
C 480	Flexure-Creep of Sandwich Constructions	Flexual creep
D 3039/D 3039M	Tensile Properties of Polymer Matrix Composite Materials	In-plane tension
D 3410/D 3410M	Compressive Properties of Polymer Matrix Composite Materials with Unsupported Gage Section by Shear Loading	In-plane compression
D 3479/D 3479M	Tension-Tension Fatigue of Polymer Matrix Composite Materials	Tension-tension fatigue
D 4255	Testing Inplane Shear Properties of Composite Laminates	In-plane shear
D 5379/D 5379M	Shear Properties of Composite Materials by the V-Notched Beam Method	Shear
D 5448/D 5448M	Inplane Shear Properties of Hoop Wound Polymer Matrix Composite Cylinders	In-plane shear
D 5449/D 5449M	Transverse Compressive Properties of Hoop Wound Polymer Matrix Composite Cylinders	Transverse compression
D 5450/D 5450M	Transverse Tensile Properties of Hoop Wound Polymer Matrix Composite Cylinders	Transverse tension
D 5467	Compressive Properties of Unidirectional Polymer Matrix Composites Using a Sandwich Beam	In-plane compression
D 5766/D 5766M	Open Hole Tensile Strength of Polymer Matrix Composite Laminates	Open-hole tensile strength
D 5961/D 5961M	Bearing Response of Polymer Matrix Composite Laminates	Bearing
D 6115	Mode I Fatigue Delamination Growth Onset of Unidirectional Fiber-Reinforced Polymer-Matrix Composites	Mode 1 fatigue fracture
D 6264	Measuring the Damage Resistance of a Fiber-Reinforced Polymer Matrix Composite to a Concentrated Quasi-Static Indentation Force	Damage resistance
D 6415	Measuring the Curved Beam Strength of a Fiber-Reinforced Polymer Matrix Composite	Flatwise tension
D 6416	Two-Dimensional Flexural Properties of Simply Supported Sandwich Composite Plates Subjected to a Distributed Load	Plate flexure
D 6484	Open-Hole Compression Strength of Polymer Matrix Composites	Open-hole compression strength
Z 5370Z	Compression After Impact Strength of Fiber-Resin Composites	Compression after impact
Z 7225Z	Mixed Mode I-Mode II Interlaminar Fracture Toughness of Unidirectional Fiber Reinforced Polymer Matrix Composites	Mixed-mode fracture
Z 7254Z	Out-of-Plane Tension Test for Fiber-Reinforced Polymer-Matrix Composites	Flatwise tension
Z 8025Z	Determining the Compressive Properties of Polymer Matrix Composite Materials Using the Combined Loading Compression (CLC) Test Fixture	In-plane compression
Z 8517Z	Filled-Hole Tensile and Compressive Testing of Polymer Matrix Composite Laminates	Filled-hole tensile and compression strength
Z 8320Z	Determination of the Mode II Interlaminar Fracture Toughness of Unidirectional Fiber Reinforced Polymer Matrix Composites Using the Four Point Bend End Notched Flexure (4ENF) Specimen	Mode 2 fracture
Z 8297Z	In-Plane Shear Strength of Sandwich Panels	In-plane shear
Z 8300Z	Static Energy Absorption Properties of Honeycomb	Damage resistance

(a) The "Z" designation denotes standards that have been balloted but not yet approved at the time of this writing.

portant element behavior under loading, such as linearity range, deformation at elastic limit, and load versus deformation behavior beyond the elastic range to failure. Failure modes and their classification and relation to materials behavior become even more important than in coupons because they more closely resemble selected discrete areas of failure in the subcomponent test. Failure modes should be analyzed visually and microscopically, and selected critical failure surface areas should be studied with cross-sectional photomicrographs to determine the character, cause, and progression of the fracture at the microstructure level that leads to the macrostructural failure causing the subcomponent structural failure. Such study of the microstructure can provide information on materials, processing, or design defects that might cause premature failure. Accurate analytical prediction of failure load and mechanical behavior of structural elements is also more important than at the coupon level, because the element behavior may represent a discrete part of the subcomponent and lead to the development of analytical methodology for the subcomponent. Laminate lay-ups that have too many plies of the same orientation laid up together can also cause premature failure under certain loading conditions, such as hot/wet compression, which can be identified along with the microfailure mode.

Key points on the load-strain or load-deflection curves should be tabulated. These might be the end of linearity, any points of sudden load, strain, or deflection changes, and the initial straight-line slope, which gives the elastic-range structural stiffness. Recorded experimental data will need to be reported in detail, along with explanations of what data were obtained and how, when, and where. In addition, the data should be compared with analytical predictions of stresses, strains, and deflections at various points along the load path, and the predicted and actual failure load and mode should be compared. Once the body of the report is complete, conclusions can be drawn and the meaning and importance of the test results detailed. These will include such things as whether the structure performed in the manner for which it was designed, along with discussion of the meaning of any discrepancies in behavior. The concluding remarks should also state whether the testing met its scope of work and whether the test results satisfied the test plan objectives.

Standard Elements

Standard elements are those that characterize the general behavior of materials systems under in-plane loading, normal and bending loading, and at joints. Data from these standard element tests are useful to the designer for applications using the materials system in areas where this type of loading is expected, such that structural sizing may be established using the data and analytical techniques correlated with the testing results. This approach enables the design to proceed with structural substantiation by analysis correlated with these results, provided that the same critical parameters, such as material orientations, ply sequencing, edge distances, processing parameters, and general sound design practice are employed. Out-of-plane loading conditions and areas of nonstandard geometry must be considered separately, using subcomponent or full-scale testing. Environmental effects are typically addressed as part of the standard element testing because it is more economical to do at this level, but is only useful for addressing the failure modes characterized by those test methods.

Various test methods for solid laminates, sandwich laminates, and joints are discussed subsequently. Table 1 provides a list of ASTM testing standards applicable to composites at the element level of the building-block approach.

In-Plane Loaded Elements

In many respects, simple element testing under uniaxial tension and compression loading resembles coupon testing. However, the specimens are usually larger and occasionally contain discontinuities such as holes, notches (slots), ply drop-offs or joggles. These elements typically

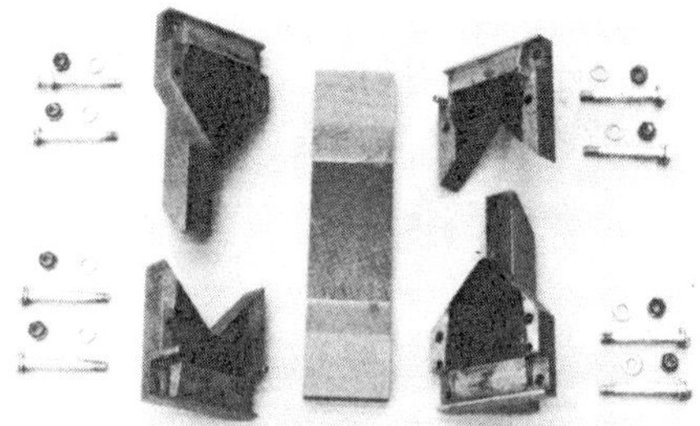

Fig. 4 Support fixture for compression static and fatigue testing

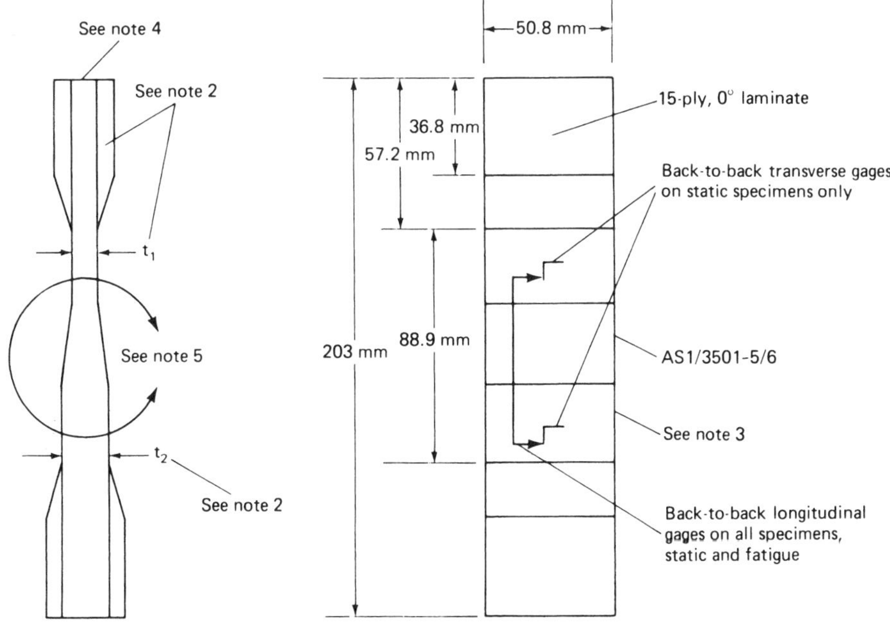

Fig. 3 Static and fatigue ply drop-off test specimen. (1) Bond fiberglass-epoxy tabs with epoxy film adhesive. (2) Specimen thickness shall not vary more than ±0.13 mm (0.005 in.). (3) Specimen longitudinal edges shall be parallel to 0.13 mm (0.005 in.). (4) Top end and bottom end surfaces shall be flat and parallel to 0.025 mm (0.001 in.). (5) Location of ply drop-off

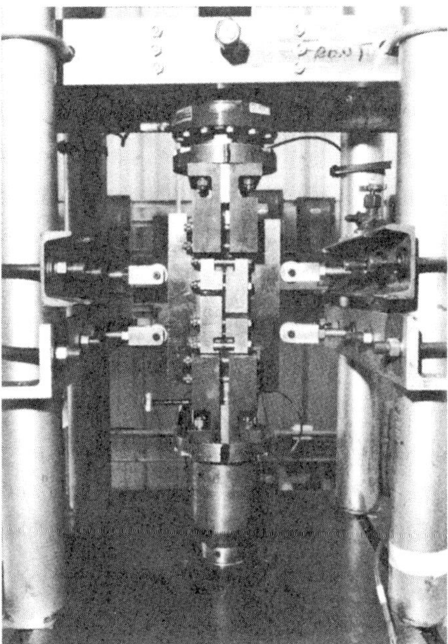

Fig. 5 Machine set-up for compression static and fatigue testing

have more instrumentation than do simple coupons, and more effort is required to provide adequate design of the load introduction and test fixtures, because few standard methods are available at the element level. In this case, adequate design means that the load introduction and test fixture configuration will allow the specimen to be loaded to the required stress (or strain) level at failure. Such design will also allow an acceptable failure mode to occur; that is, one that is expected in the full-sized structure (component and subcomponent).

Different types of elements are discussed subsequently. Note that for each type of element and subcomponent, adequate material must be incorporated into the grips or load introduction tabs in order to develop the loading such that the appropriate failure mode is experienced at specimen failure. For more information regarding the design of tabs and grips see MIL-HDBK-17, Volume 1, Section 7.

Tension-Loaded Elements. Although much information on tension-loaded coupons is given in ASTM D 3039 (Ref 2) that may be useful in design and testing of tension elements, additional work on load-introduction tabs, consideration of discontinuities, and added instrumentation are usually necessary. In the laminate evaluation longitudinal-tension specimens with and without a thickness discontinuity illustrated in Fig. 2, the discontinuity is a ply drop-off, but it could have been a center hole or a combination of both.

Effects of such discontinuities are covered in Ref 3 and 4. Small reductions in static compression strength and no reduction in fatigue strength are observed in these ply drop-off tests.

Compression-Loaded Elements. A typical compression-loaded element with ply drop-off defects is shown in Fig. 3. The clamped platen-supported fixture for these specimens is shown in Fig. 4. Load introduction is by bearing on the ends of the specimen, which is machined flat and parallel to within 0.025 mm (0.001 in.). The test set-up, which can be used in compression loading for both the static and fatigue test conditions, is shown in Fig. 5.

Because load introduction in these compression specimens is primarily by end bearing on the specimen and the tab, the bonded-area quality is not as critical as before. However, grinding the ends flat and parallel to ≤0.025 mm (≤0.001 in.) is critical, and both ends of every specimen should be inspected on a surface plate after machining. Those that do not meet this requirement should be rejected and reground, because nonuniform bearing can cause premature failure of the end-pad bonds.

Combined Load Elements. Combined in-plane loaded composite materials test elements and methodology can be as simple as the rail-shear test detailed in ASTM D 4255 (Ref 5) for obtaining shear stress-strain curves to failure of simple, unnotched, unidirectional, or multidirectional laminates. A picture frame test set-up shown in Fig. 6 is used for testing notched and unnotched multidirectional laminates in shear. With proper instrumentation (strain gages or deflectometers), this gives a shear stress-strain curve to failure. More complex testing includes biaxially loaded notched or unnotched multidirectional laminates. Such tests are usually combinations of compression and compression or tension and compression loading, each at 90° to the other.

Normal and Bending Loaded Elements

At the element level, these tests include bending of beams, transverse shear, transverse tension (or peel), and transverse compression (core compression in sandwich laminates). These beams may be solid laminates, stiffened sections (blade, hat, I), or sandwich beams with composite faces. Beam technology, in general, is well documented. Simple sandwich beams are discussed in Ref 6 and 7.

Testing composite and sandwich beam elements differs from testing isotropic material (metal) beam elements in that shear stresses (or strains) and deformations must be taken into consideration when designing, testing, and analyzing them. In addition, load and support-point softness should be considered in load introduction, as should the requirement for load pads to prevent local crushing, especially in sandwich beams with honeycomb or foam cores that are relatively weak in flatwise compression strength.

Long Beam Flexure. A four-point loaded simple sandwich beam element is shown in Fig. 7, with the applicable equations for calculating maximum face stress, core shear stress/bondline shear stress, and core shear modulus. Such elements may be tested according to ASTM C 393 and are used to measure core or face properties or to perform quality assurance testing, and are tested as structural elements representing larger beam-bending sandwich structures. For relatively long spans, the testing is sometimes referred to as "long beam flexural" testing. The same testing method, however, may be used to characterize transverse shear properties by shortening the span such that a panel shear failure

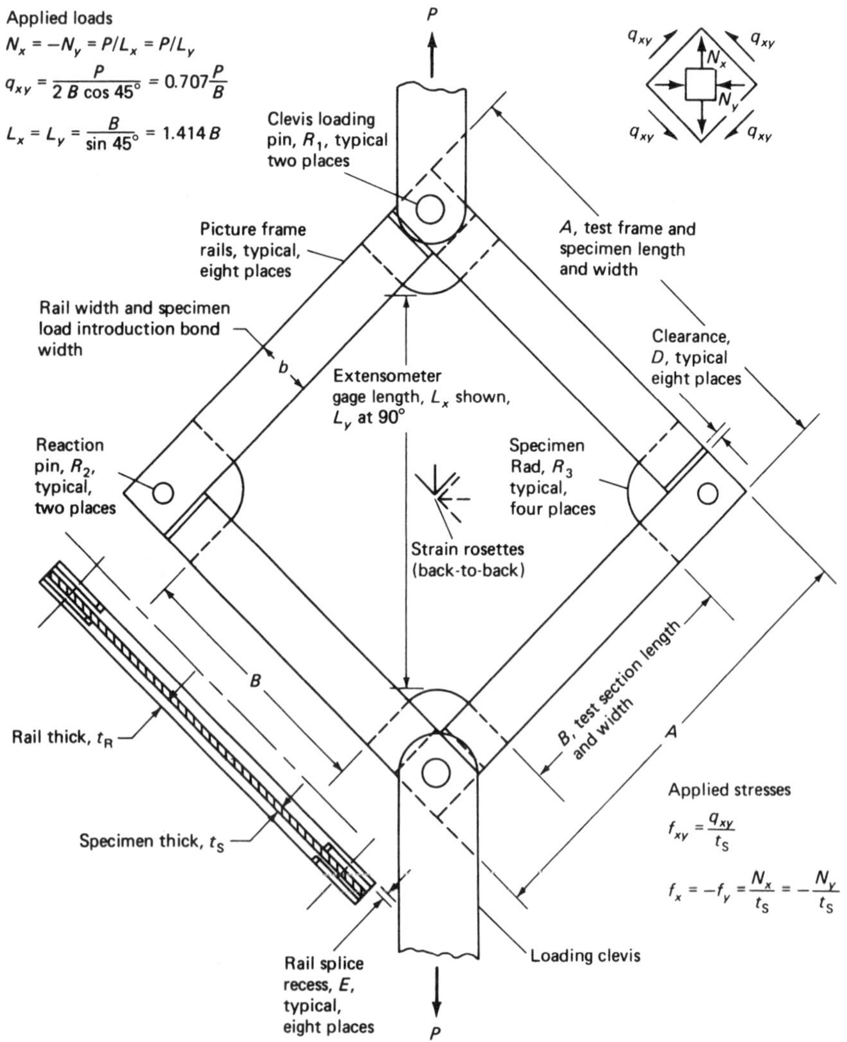

Fig. 6 Picture frame test set-up and specimen

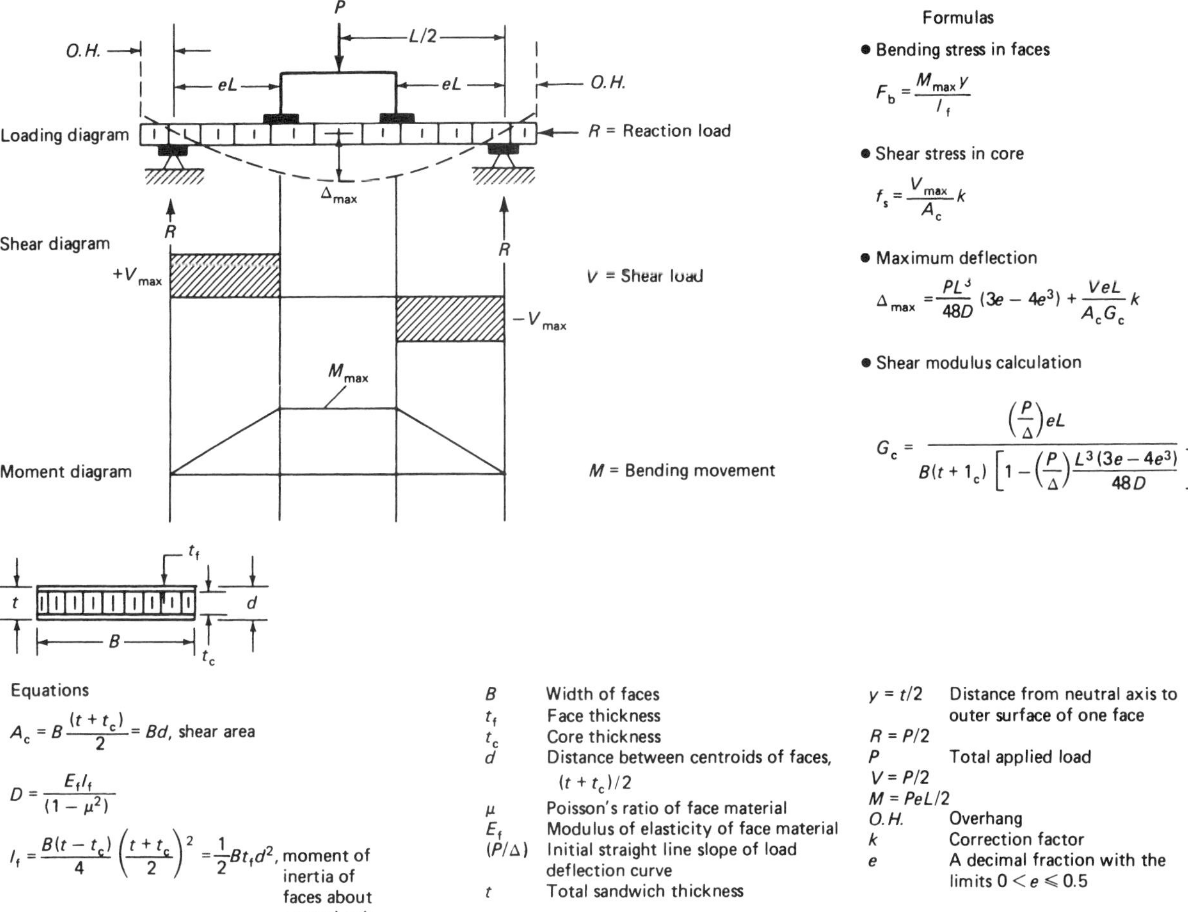

Fig. 7 Sandwich beam four-point load test

mode is experienced as discussed subsequently. Generally, the sandwich flatwise tension strength and the flatwise compression strength and modulus are required for complete analysis, in addition to similar sandwich core shear and facesheet properties. This is because of the need for face-wrinkling analysis plus intercellular-buckling analysis of honeycomb core sandwich specimens on the compression face (Ref 6). In addition, the core flatwise compression strength is used to calculate the load/support pad area necessary for use in testing the beam. Once the properties of all the sandwich constituents are known, the maximum load at failure can be calculated, and then the load pad size can be calculated.

Panel Shear. The same four-point loading setup is shown in Fig. 8, using a shorter span ratio such that a transverse shear failure occurs. This testing (also according to ASTM C 393) is used to characterize core shear properties for sandwich laminates and may require testing with the core material in specific orientations if the materials properties vary relative to the orientation, as with honeycomb core, for example.

Transverse Tension. The transverse tension strength of composites is one of the most important properties to characterize for sound design, because it is inherently the weakest direction for the material. While there are numerous approaches to characterize these properties, an example of one approach to this type of testing is provided in Fig. 9, showing a set-up for climbing drum peel testing in accordance with ASTM D 1781. This test literally peels one of the facesheets away from the core to establish the bond strength between the constituent materials. Other methods include flatwise tension of rectangular specimens and angle specimens with a precise bend radius, which is tested such that the radius is subjected to interlaminar tension stresses by pulling the legs of the specimen apart so that the radius tries to open.

Transverse Compression. The transverse compression test is generally conducted in accordance with ASTM C 365 in order to determine the core compression strength of a core material used in sandwich laminates. This strength

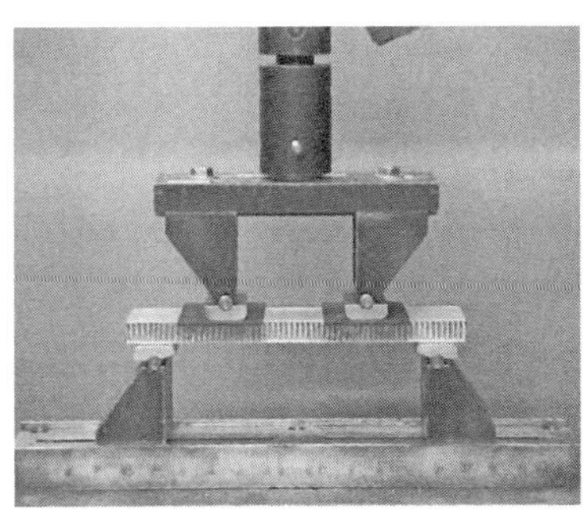

Fig. 8 Sandwich panel shear test set-up

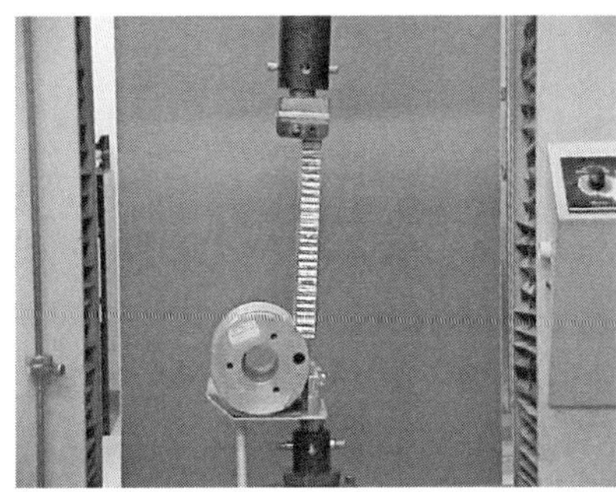

Fig. 9 Climbing drum peel testing for sandwich composites

may then be used in design to determine the required footprint to support a direct bearing load on a sandwich panel. It may also be used to establish allowable bending loads for a curved sandwich shell where kick loads tend to crush the core.

Joint Elements

The joint elements discussed in this section include mechanically fastened (or bolted) and bonded joint configurations used in the tests described in Ref 8 and 9. The various failure modes for bolted joints discussed earlier in this section will not be repeated here, but the testing used to characterize these failure modes is briefly covered. The bolted-joint discussion includes an example of analytical correlation of predicted strength values generated using an aerospace-approved method of analysis for bolted joints in composites. It should be noted that for composites, a joint that is both bonded and bolted would generally perform structurally superior to one that is either bonded or bolted. The bolt helps prevent a peel-type failure of the bond, and the bond reduces the tendency of the bolted joint to shear out. Testing of a bonded-bolted joint may be considered as a nonstandard joint and thereby tested as a subcomponent.

Material Bearing Strength. A simplified test introduces the bearing load in a double-shear configuration. In actual applications, load transfer in a single-shear configuration is more commonplace, resulting in larger stress concentrations in the thickness direction and lowering the realizable bearing strength. These single-shear tests are discussed later in this section. In other words, the bearing strength values measured in the double-shear test cannot be applied to single-shear joints. The double-shear arrangement is shown in Fig. 10.

Only a tensile loading condition is proposed for evaluating bearing failures. Under compression, the larger edge distance ($e >> 3D$) should only minimally influence the bearing stress at failure, unless a shear-out mode of failure is possible (e.g., a laminate with a large percent of 0° plies).

Both final bearing failure and bearing deformation are needed for materials characterization purposes. Therefore, it is recommended that the bearing stress variation as a function of hole deformation be documented, and that bearing stress values corresponding to the proportional limit, yield bearing (see MIL-HDBK-17, Volume 1, Section 7.2.1), and ultimate failure are recorded.

In summary, bearing strength, as measured by the double-shear test, is considered a materials property for relative evaluation and design. In realistic structural joints, factors like geometry, fastener type, and load eccentricity will significantly influence the realizable fraction of the bearing strength measured in the proposed test. Bearing strength tests more appropriate in design of joints are discussed later in this section as well as in MIL-HDBK-17, Volume 1, Section 7.2.5.

Single-Shear Bearing Strength of Joints. This section describes single-shear test specimens required to obtain bearing strength of single-lap joints. The resulting test data can be applicable either for the selection and screening of fasteners, the design of bolted joints, or both. If the actual joint configuration is double-shear, the test specimen and procedure described previously would be more appropriate.

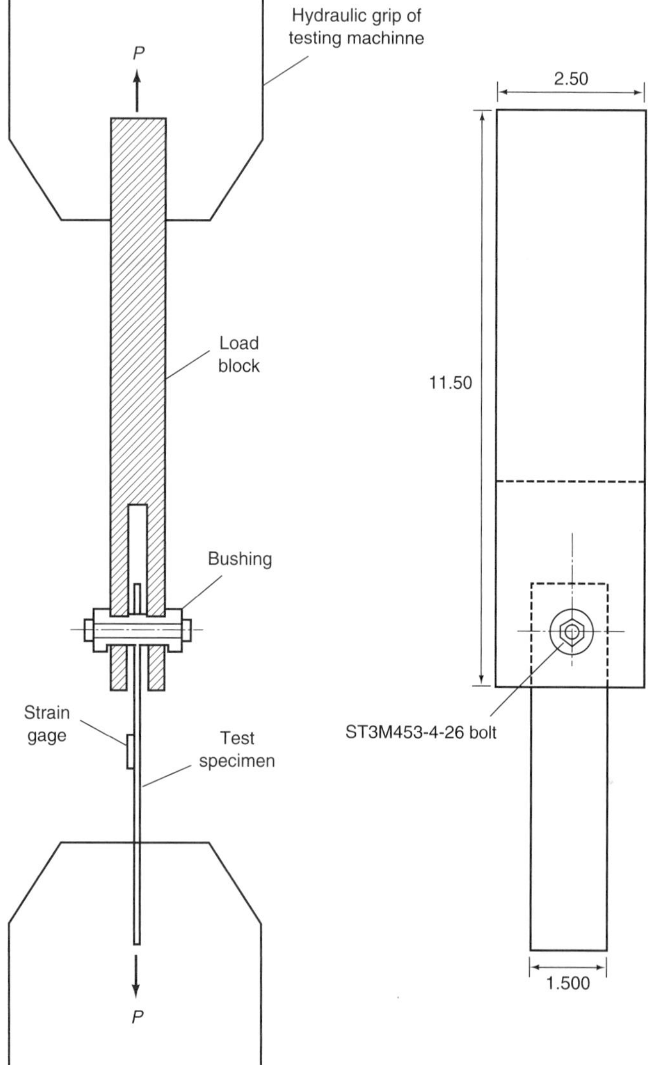

Fig. 10 Material bearing strength testing. Dimensions in inches

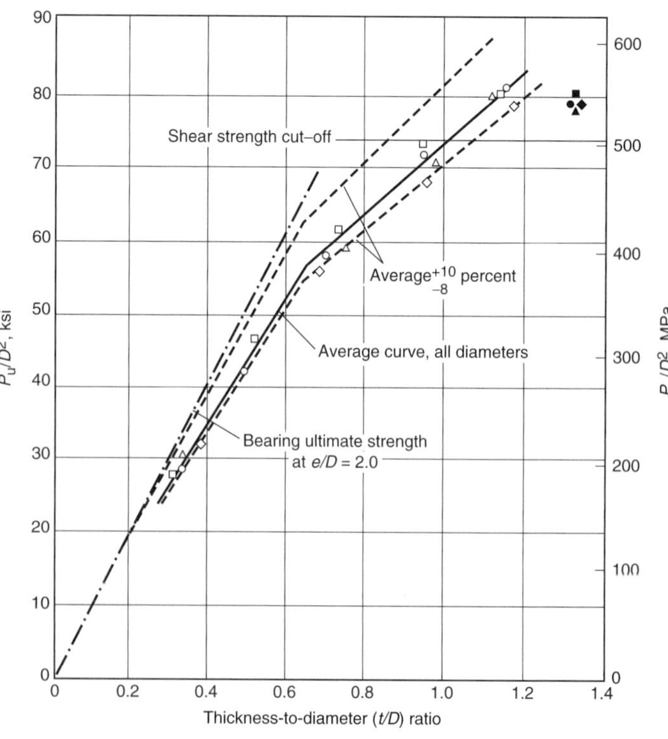

Fig. 11 Average ultimate-load analysis. P_u, ultimate load; D, diameter; t, thickness; e, edge distance

Bearing strength is a function of joint geometry and stiffness of the members and the fastener. It should be noted that for a 0/±45/90 family of laminates with 20 to 40% of 0° plies and 40 to 60% of ±45° plies, the bearing strength is essentially constant. In addition, fastener characteristics such as clamp-up force and head and tail configuration have a significant effect. However, for a specific laminate family, a specific fastener, and equal-thickness laminajoining members, the parameter with the greatest influence is *t/D*. This was recognized by the aircraft designers, and all the bearing data for metals is presented in MIL-HDBK-5 (Ref 10) in terms of the *t/D* parameter, Fig. 11. The slope of this nondimensional curve is the bearing strength, which decreases with increased *t/D* until, for sufficiently thick laminates, shear failure occurs in the bolt. The data generated using the recommended test specimens, procedures, and test matrices will produce equivalent data for composite joints.

In the design process, there may be instances where the joint configuration may not correspond to the test configurations recommended here, that is, unequal-joining members, gaps, solid shims, or fuel sealing provisions. These effects on bearing strengths should be evaluated by modifying the specimen geometry as needed. The test procedures presented here are still applicable.

Recommended composite-to-composite and composite-to-metal bearing specimen geometry are shown in Fig. 12 and 13. Both are single-lap geometry. Although it is generally more difficult to test than the double-lap configuration, the single-lap test configuration is more representative of most critical aircraft bolted-joint applications. The single-lap induces both bending and shear loads on the fastener, while the double-lap induces mostly shear loads.

The joint configurations shown in Fig. 12 and 13 may be used to generate both design and fastener screening data. In some cases, the fastener supplier and/or the requester may want to evaluate fastener behavior in a single-fastener configuration. The recommended single-fastener joint configuration is shown in Fig. 14. This is the same specimen specified in MIL-STD-1312-X (Ref 11).

It should be recognized that this joint configuration might be subject to high bending due to the load eccentricity transmitted through the bolt. Increasing the stiffness of the two laps, through increased thickness or material stiffness, can reduce the bending. It should also be noted that the single-fastener joint is generally not representative of multifastener joint applications (e.g., joint rotation, deflection). Therefore, it should be used mostly for fastener screening purposes.

When tested, the specimen geometry shown in Fig. 12 and 13 are intended to result in composite bearing failures (as opposed to tension or cleavage failures). Fastener pull-throughs and fastener failures, though not acceptable as a measure of composite bearing strength, do provide a measure of joint strength for a particular fastener type.

The metal tongue and doubler dimensions (Fig. 12 and 13) are specified to align the load path along the interface between the two laps. The doublers and the tongue shall be bonded to the composite bearing specimens prior to loading, or prior to specimen conditioning for environmental hot/wet tests. Fiberglass-epoxy can be substituted for metal doublers.

Pull-Through Strength. The test specimen configuration to determine pull-through strength is shown in Fig. 15, 16, and 17. It may be used for composite joints fastened by bolt/nuts, pin/collars, or comparable fastening devices. Pull-through is defined as the load level at which the composite specimen being tested can no longer support an increase in load. The test procedures are provided in MIL-HDBK-17, Volume 1, Section 7.2.9.

Bolted-Joint Element and Analysis Correlation. The bolted-joint structural element shown in Fig. 18 represents a static and fatigue specimen that was used to evaluate joints for aircraft wing structures. The joint was designed to fail at 1.58 MN/m (9000 lbf/in.). The grip tabs on the graphite-epoxy composite end represent an effective bonded area of 3.03 × 10^3 mm^2 (4.70 $in.^2$). At 15 MPa (2 ksi), the bonded area allowable used above the joint will be safe for at least 1.65 MN/m (9400 lbf/in.). The steel ends were tied directly with screws to the load plate on the test machine.

Failure of the specimen was designed to be gross thin-section tension (away from the joint), thick-section bolt bearing, or both. Stress in the thin, unnotched, gross composite area (outside the joint buildup) is 418 MPa (60.6 ksi) at design failure, whereas the unnotched stress allowable is 1048 MPa (152 ksi).

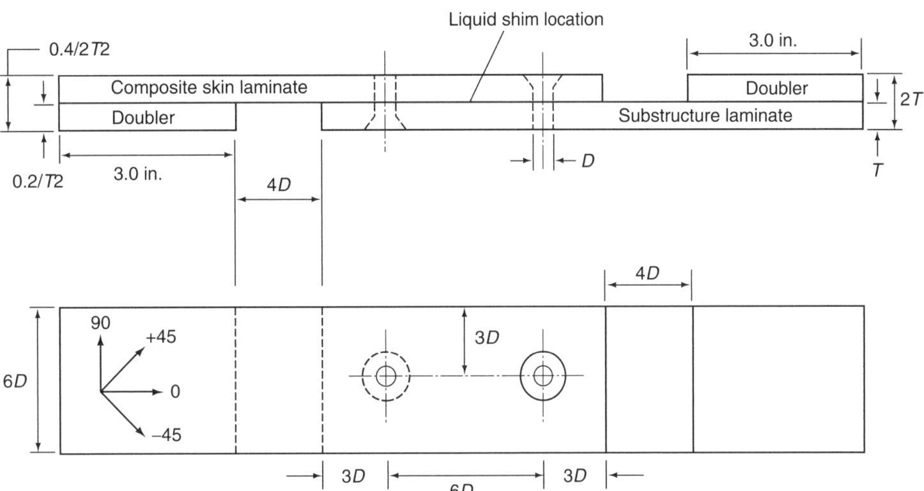

Fig. 12 Composite-to-composite joint configuration

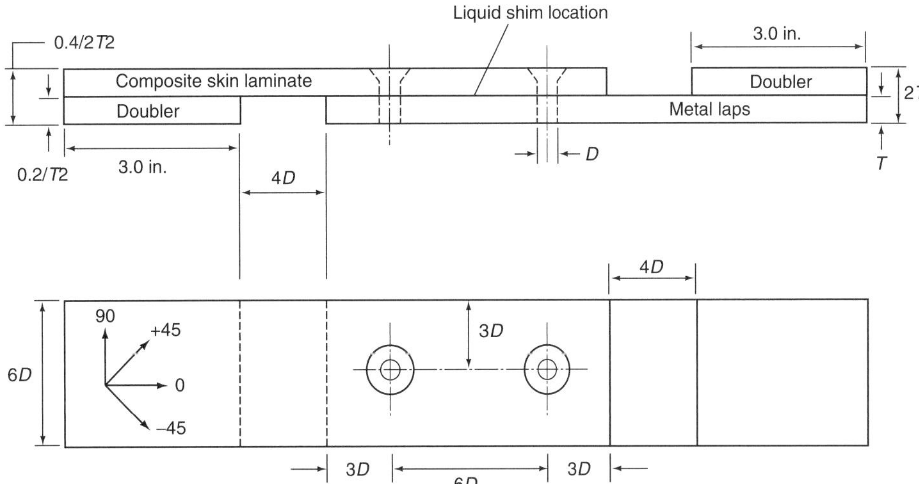

Fig. 13 Composite-to-metal joint configuration

Using properties given in Ref 12, the bolted joint of Fig. 18 was analyzed with a bolted-joint stress field model (BJSFM) computer program at a net area through the first hole (from the taper) in a load-net area analysis summarized in Fig. 19. The tension test data are slightly above the analytical bearing-failure values predicted by BJSFM. When the net tension analysis is compared with the test failure, a stress-concentration factor of approximately 2 is observed for this joint. Although the most obvious specimen failure was net tension through the first bolt hole, subsequent inspection of the failed specimens showed the onset of bearing failure that correlates to a reasonable degree with the BJSFM-predicted bearing (yield) failure. A finite element analysis of this joint, assuming that half the load is taken by each of the two fasteners, accurately predicted the failure load and mode as net tension through the first hole from the thickness taper. Therefore, both modes of failure, net tension through the first hole from the taper and bolt bearing at the same location, are applicable.

Bonded Joints. In principle, bonded joints are structurally more efficient than those that are mechanically fastened. Bonded joints eliminate hole drilling for fastener installation, resulting in a structure without notches that cause stress concentrations. Composite structures can have bonded joints fabricated by three different processes: secondary bonding, co-bonding, and co-curing. Secondary bonding uses a layer of adhesive to bond two precured composite parts (see the article "Secondary Adhesive Bonding of Polymer-Matrix Composites" in this Volume). Thus, this type is most similar to metal bonded joints in structural behavior and fabrication method. Co-curing is a process wherein two parts are simultaneously cured. The interface between the two parts may or may not have an adhesive layer. In the co-bonding process, one of the detail parts is precured, with the mating part being cured simultaneously with the adhesive. Surface preparation is a critical step in any bonded joints and must be clearly defined before any bonding is performed. This is particularly important in secondary and co-bonding processes. More detail on bonded joint fabrication is given in MIL-HDBK-17, Volume 3, Section 2.9.

The type of bonded joints addressed in this section are secondarily bonded and co-bonded. For these types of joints, knowledge of mechanical properties, particularly stiffness of the adhesive, is a design imperative. Well-designed adhesive joints in aircraft structures are not critical in the adhesive layer, but in the adherends, whether they be metal or composites, but this does not obviate the need to know the strength capability of the adhesive in shear and tension. The composite adherends are, in most cases, well-constructed laminates with sufficient number of plies in the principal load directions, ensuring that the failure mode is fiber-dominated. The adhesives are formulated to be much more ductile than the resins used as matrices in composites, because they are not required to provide support to fibers, particularly under compression

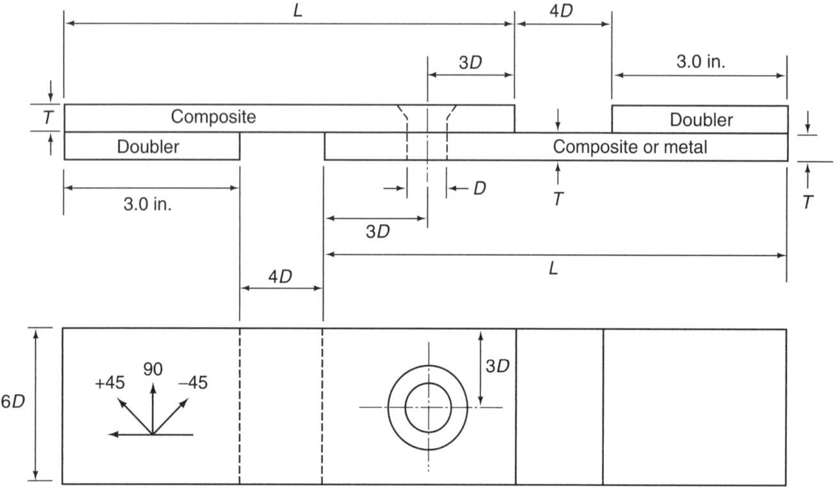

Fig. 14 Single-fastener lap joint

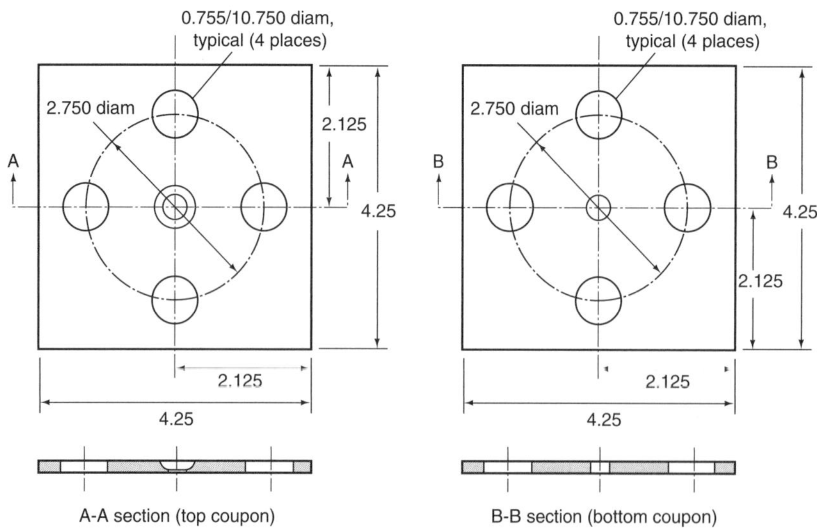

Fig. 15 Fastener pull-through screening test plate configurations. Dimensions in inches

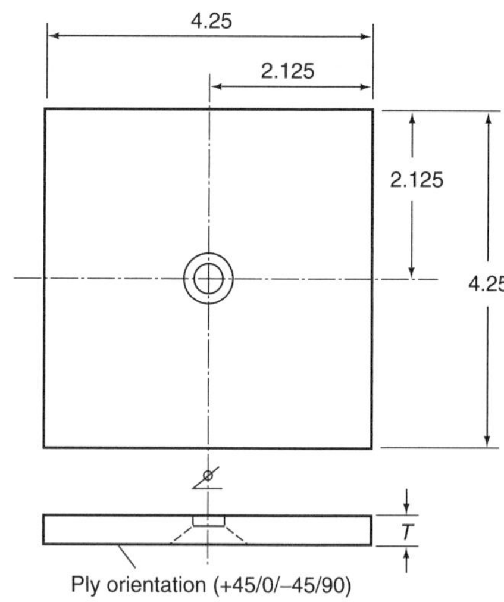

Shank diameter		Suggested minimum specimen thickness (*T*) for tensile testing(a) 100° tension head		130° shear head		Clearance hole	
mm	in.	mm	in.	mm	in.	mm	in.
4.0	5/32	2.44	0.096	1.40	0.055	33.3	1.31
4.8	3/16	2.82	0.111	1.55	0.061	38.1	1.50
6.4	1/4	3.81	0.150	2.03	0.080	50.8	2.00
7.9	5/16	4.83	0.190	2.69	0.106	63.5	2.50
9.5	3/8	5.82	0.229	3.23	0.127	76.2	3.00

(a) Thickness dimensions represent standard design criteria that allow the countersink to penetrate a maximum depth equal to 70% of the sheet thickness.

Fig. 16 Fastener pull-through design test plate configuration. Dimensions in inches

loading, thus steering the joint failure to the adherends. The fibers also constrain the resin so that the behavior of the matrix is also more brittle than the resin by itself. This may shift the composite bonded-joint failure to a transverse, through-the-thickness, tension failure of the composite laminate.

Two distinct types of tests are needed to characterize the behavior of a bonded joint and obtain sufficient mechanical data to perform structural analysis: shear properties and tensile properties. It is assumed that the mechanical properties of the composite adherends are known. For simplicity and standardization goals, the tests to determine adhesive properties make use of metal adherends. The results of these tests provide properties of adhesive for design and analysis, comparative data, and surface preparation effectiveness, but in no way represent the strength of a composite structural bonded joint. This is obtained by testing specimen configurations with composite and/or honeycomb adherends, which are more application-representative.

Adhesive Characterization. Adhesive strength and stiffness data is required if successful bonded joints are to be designed. Because the behavior of the adhesive is elastic-plastic, it is not sufficient to characterize the adhesive by ultimate strength and initial tangent modulus. The data that are needed include stress-strain curves in shear and tension at the service temperature and humidity environments. The test methods currently favored by the industry to obtain these data are the thick adherend test pioneered by Krieger (Ref 13 and 14) for the shear properties, and the tensile strength by means of bar and rod specimen described by ASTM D 2095 (Ref 15). None of the tests are completely satisfactory, for various reasons. These test methods are more thoroughly discussed in MIL-HDBK-17, Volume 3, Section 7.3.

Moisture-conditioning of adhesive specimens to equilibrium (uniform moisture content of the entire bondline) before wet testing requires prohibitive duration times—several years. This is because of low values of moisture diffusivity of common adhesives and the use of test specimens with moisture-impervious metal adherends, for which water can only enter the adhesive through exposed bondline edges. Fortunately, adhesive failures usually initiate at bond edges, due either to shear stress peaking or to peel (tensile) stresses. Thus, as long as a reasonable depth of adhesive near the edges has approached the desired equilibrium moisture level, test results will be representative of a fully equilibrated bondline. The common practice of exposing test specimens to the required relative humidity at reasonably high temperatures (71 to 82 °C, or 160 to 180 °F, for epoxies) for 1000 hours (42 days) achieves this goal. An alternative method to determine the effect of absorbed moisture on adhesives is to perform tension and compression testing on cast adhesive neat-resin specimens. Because, in this case, the entire specimen is exposed, the times to reach equilibrium are significantly less.

Characterization of adhesive shear properties by the thick adherend test method is accomplished using the KGR-1 extensometer, which is attached to a specimen of geometry shown in Fig. 20. Because of the KGR-1 design and use of aluminum adherends, the test method is limited to150 °C (300 °F).

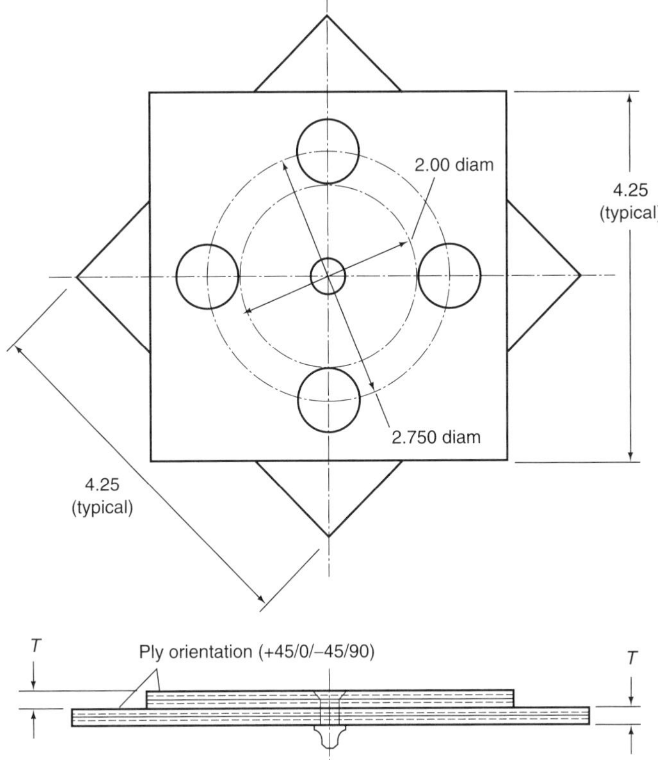

Fig. 17 Fastener pull-through screening test plates in assembled configuration. Dimensions in inches

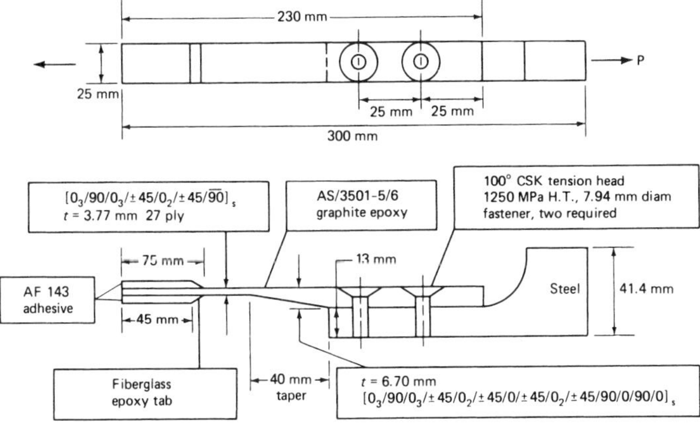

Fig. 18 Bolted-joint test specimen

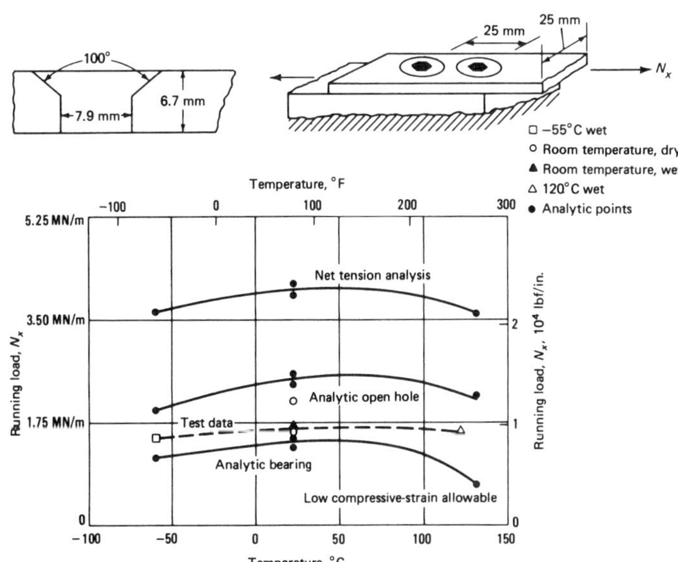

Fig. 19 Correlation of bolt-bearing data and analytical models

An alternate method to obtain shear strength and stiffness is by use of a tubular specimen loaded in torsion. The basis of the test is a narrow, annular ring of adhesive subjected to uniform shear loads around the circumference. Because the thickness of the tube is small compared to its radius, the shear stress across it is considered constant. Although the test provides pure shear distribution, the test apparatus is complex and specialized testing know-how is required, which have led to disuse of this test method. A test method using the tubular specimen is ASTM E 229 (Ref 16). It uses narrow but large-diameter adherend tubes and measures angle of twist by an Amsler mirror extensometer. Details of the test are described in the standard.

Tensile strength of the adhesive can be obtained by the ASTM D 2095 method, Fig. 21 (Ref 15). Either bar or rod specimen can be used in this test method. The design of the specimens and specimen preparation is described in ASTM D 2094 (Ref 17). The tensile strengths obtained by this test method should be used with caution, because the test specimen is susceptible to peel-initiated failure at the specimen edges. The adhesive failure strength can be used in an approximate peel analysis, as proposed in Ref 18. Because good bonded-joint design practice minimizes peel stresses, the exact knowledge of tensile strength capability is not that critical. An independent measurement of the Young's modulus of the adhesive is needed, because the adhesive often does not obey laws of isotropic material and thus cannot be derived from shear modulus measurement.

Tests for adhesive properties should be performed at room temperature, ambient conditions, and at low- and high-use temperature extremes, as discussed in MIL-HDBK-17, Volume 1, Section 2.2.8. The replication should be a minimum of five at each test condition.

Bonded-Joint Elements. Tests of bonded-joint configurations representative of actual joints must be tested to validate the structural integrity of the joint. Because these specimens quickly become point-design oriented, it is difficult to standardize. Thus the discussion will be limited to the simplest specimens that contain the important parameters of the bonded composite joint. A more complete discussion may be found in MIL-HDBK-17, Volume 3, Section 7.

Single-overlap specimens are similar to those described in the previous section. However, because single-overlap specimens induce additional peel stresses due to bending, the length of the joint must be longer to minimize that effect. This effectively eliminates usefulness of single-step specimens to determine strength property of realistic joints. Single-step single-overlap joints, however, are used for comparison between different adhesives and for quality control. The simplest, 25 mm (1 in.) wide, multistep or scarfed specimen has been developed to assure integrity of bonded repairs using "wet" lay-up for composite panels. This specimen, shown in Fig. 22, is referenced in a preliminary European Aircraft Industry Standard prEN 6066 (Ref 19). This standard also defines types of failures that are possible with such a specimen (Fig. 23).

Two-step and scarfed verification specimens are shown in Fig. 24 and 25 for the same spar-to-skin joint shown in Fig. 26. Such a specimen should be developed to validate any major joint design.

Double-overlap specimens range between single-step type to ones containing many steps, and are usually loaded in tension. The complexity is dependent on what type of data is to be obtained or the structural application. An example of a specimen derived from ASTM D 3528 (Ref 20) is shown in Fig. 27. This test specimen is useful

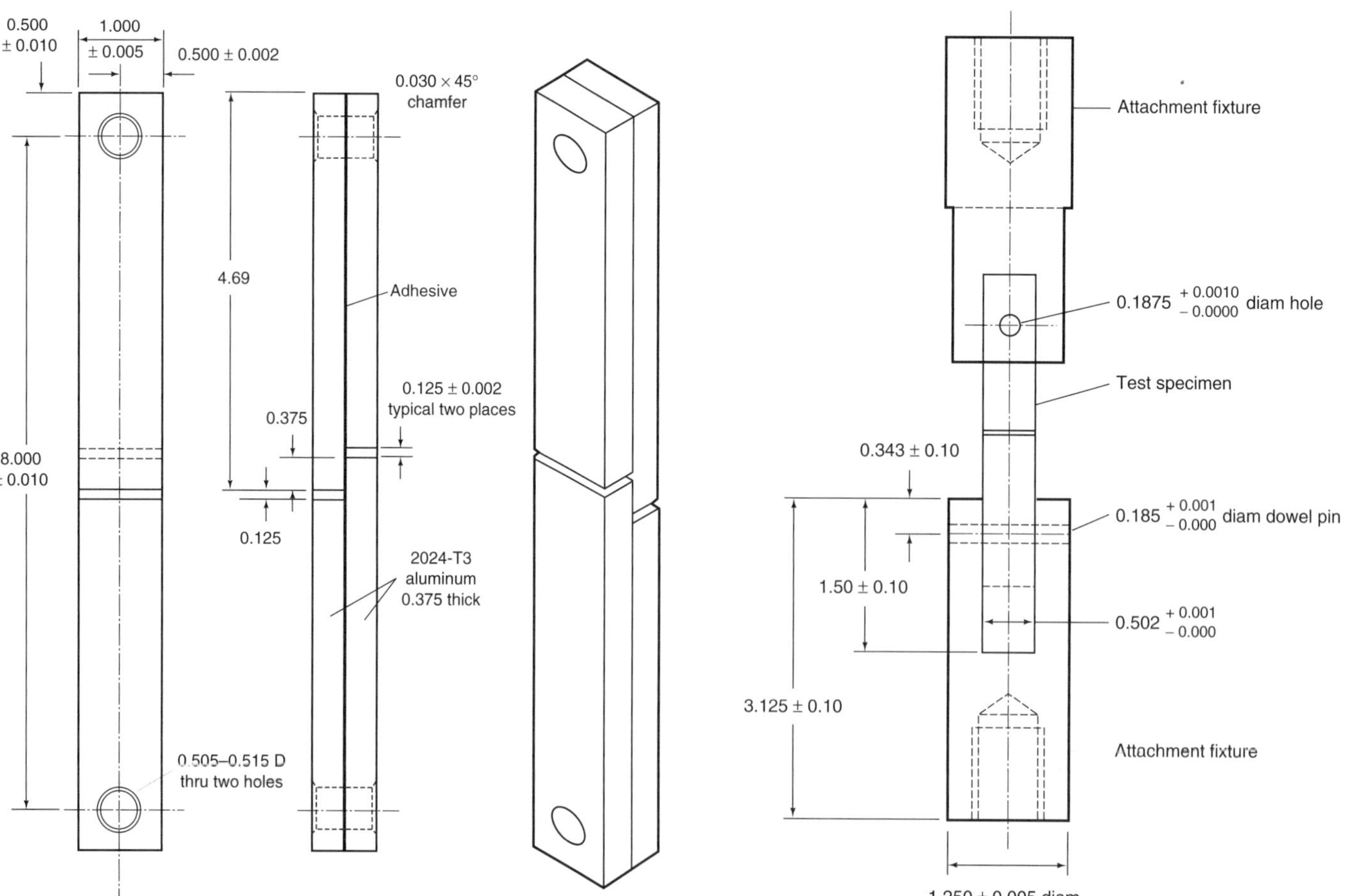

Fig. 20 Thick adherend specimen for characterizing the shear properties of adhesives. Dimensions in inches

Fig. 21 Test specimens and attachment fixtures for characterizing adhesive tensile strength

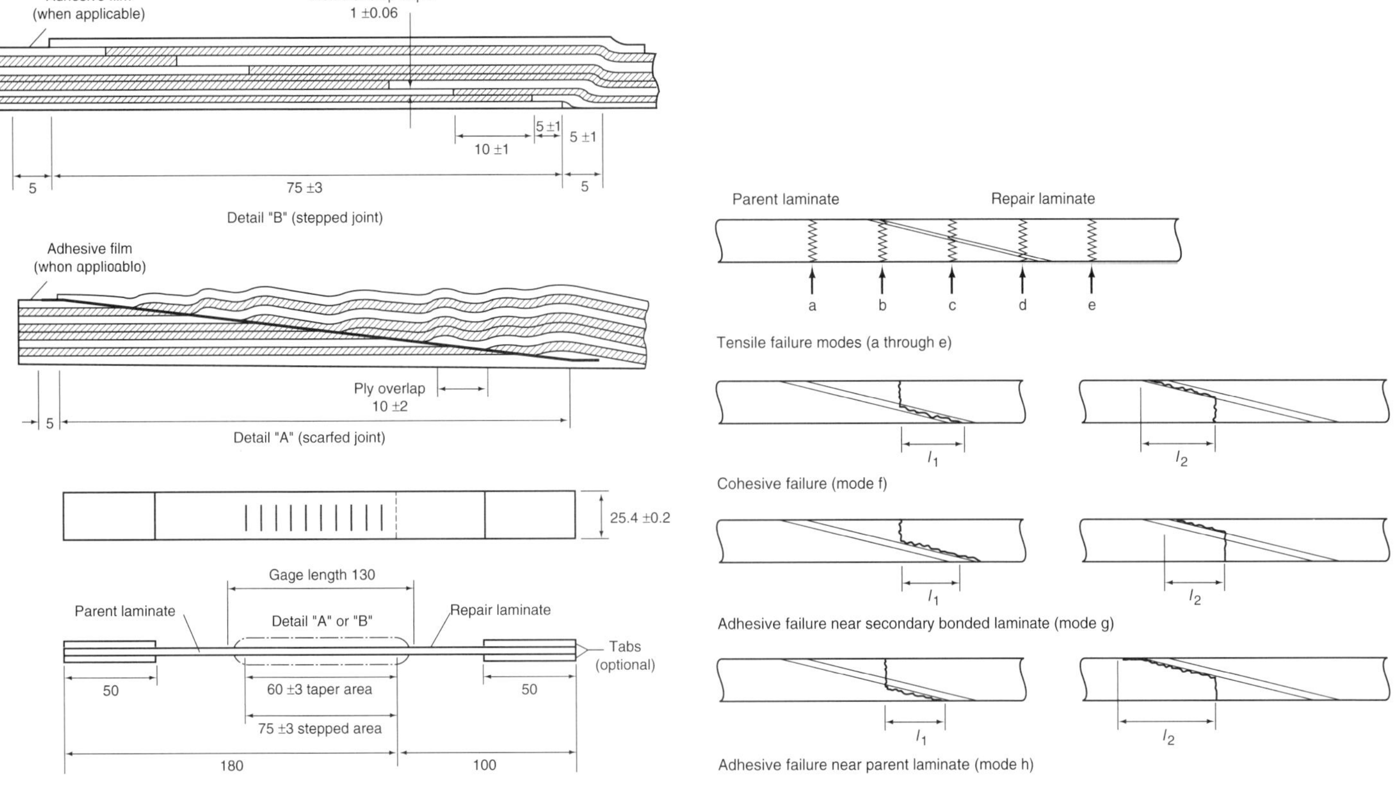

Fig. 22 Scarfed and stepped joint specimens. Dimensions in millimeters

Fig. 23 Failure modes and dimensions for joint specimens shown in Fig. 22

for determining adhesive shear strength, because the double-shear configuration reduces peel stresses. This configuration is not usually used in design, because the load transfer capability can be increased significantly by tapering the outside adherends. For higher load transfer, double-lap joints will contain many steps. To validate this type of joint, specimens shown in Fig. 28 have been used. These types of specimens are quite expensive to fabricate and hence, are not replicated in large numbers. Because these specimens are to represent a particular design, care must be taken that the specimen is manufactured using the same processes as the actual joint. Another example of a joint-verification specimen is shown in Fig. 26 and 29. It represents a chordwise connection between a composite skin and a titanium spar, and is a double-lap two-step joint. The multistep joint specimen could be converted to scarf joint specimen if that was the actual design.

Nonstandard Elements and Subcomponents

Examples of nonstandard elements and subcomponents are discussed subsequently. Each nonstandard element or subcomponent should be designed to represent an area of the structure having relatively complex load paths or failure modes, which are not easily characterized by simpler standard elements. The test specimen needs to be fabricated using materials and processes that are representative, if not identical, to those of the full-scale structure. As in element testing, adequate design consideration must be given to fixturing and load-introduction techniques, such that the proper failure mode is experienced during testing. For more specific information regarding fixturing, see MIL-HDBK-17, Volume 1, Section 7.

Skin-to-Stiffener Bond Tests. To assess the strength of skin-to-stiffener bonded joints in situations where out-of-plane loads are being developed, that is, fuel pressure and postbuckling, fairly simple tests are being used in the industry. Although these tests cannot completely represent the behavior of the actual structure, they provide design data and early assessment of the adequacy of selected materials and geometry before commitment to large component validation tests. The maximum benefits from these tests are obtained when the specimens represent as closely as possible the geometry and fabrication processes of the simulated component. The schematics of two such tests are presented here. The "T" pull-off test shown in Fig. 30 is similar to the test de-

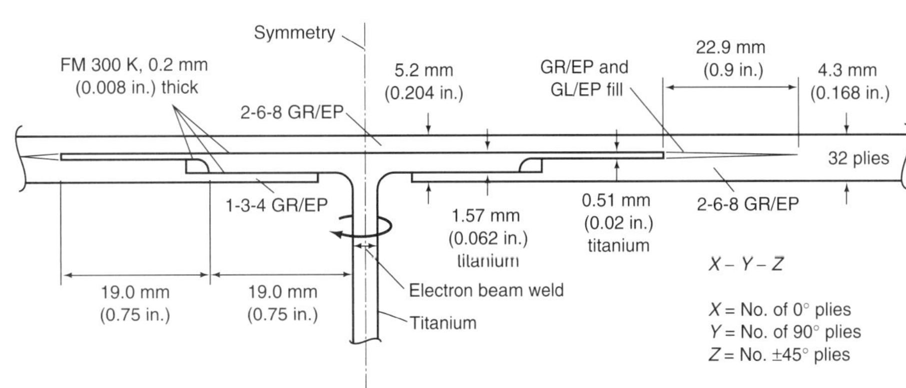

Fig. 24 One-sided specimen for a spar-to-skin joint. GR/EP, graphite/epoxy; GL/EP, glass/epoxy

scribed in ASTM C 297, except that only one block is needed. Because the bending of the skin and stiffener flanges are suppressed by the rigid loading block, the disbond failure will generally occur in the heel of the stiffener and not at the flange ends. This is a serious deficiency of the specimen if, in component tests, the failure is at flange ends. The location of the failure is strongly dependent on the ratio of stiffener/skin stiffness; the lower the ratio, the more useful is the test.

Using rollers to resist the pull-off load instead of the rigid block, shown in Fig. 31, can be a better method if the skin is more flexible. There is the problem how far apart to place the rollers to match the skin displacement. The specimen in Fig. 31 can be used to apply a moment to the bonded joint. This is represented by P_1 loads and R_1 reactions in Fig. 31. Postbuckling of shear panels introduces significant twisting moments in the interface, and the capability of the joint against them must be determined as part of the structural analysis.

Blade-Stiffened Subcomponent. A typical in-plane tension-loaded or compression-loaded blade-stiffened composite subcomponent structure is shown in Fig. 32. This subcomponent and test set-up may be used for both static and fatigue testing, although the load-introduction equipment and the instrumentation may differ for the two testing modes. Servo-hydraulic load-introduction equipment with load, strain, or deflection feedback and control may be used for either type of testing, but the power requirements and the test equipment cost may be relatively high. Electromechanical test equipment for deflection or strain-controlled fatigue testing requires less power and a lower financial investment. For either static or fatigue testing, computerized electronic monitoring/controlling is always the best method.

Load-introduction attachments to subcomponent ends and side supports are designed to simulate those used in the full-size structure, which may take tension, compression, or both types of loading. The blade-stiffened subcomponent shown in Fig. 32 is typical, but the structural configuration might also be a plain, solid laminate, a sandwich panel with composite facesheets, a double-skin corrugation, or other configuration. Environmental (temperature and humidity) conditioning may be done before installation in the test fixture or in the environmental chamber used in the testing. Such a chamber requires additional expense and design effort.

Durability and Damage-Tolerance Testing

Damage characterization is a key parameter in the use of composite materials. Damage such as internal delaminations may not even be visually apparent, and therefore must be considered in the design of a component, assuming that the damage exists and is undetected. Generally, a strain threshold at which damage does not propagate is established for a materials system based upon testing. Approaches for consideration of damage in design and certification are found in MIL-HDBK-17, Volume 3, Section 5.0.

Damage characterization can be divided into two groups: the resistance of a material to damage from impact (damage resistance), and the ability of a material or structure to perform safely after damage (damage tolerance). Damage may occur during the manufacturing process, while in use, or during maintenance operations. This damage can be the result of manufacturing defects or foreign body impacts. Impact and indentation tests that are commonly performed to evaluate the damage resistance and tolerance of candidate composite materials are discussed subsequently, as well as damage tolerance testing.

Impact Resistance. Damage resistance of a material is generally considered to be the material's resistance to impact damage. Impacts may

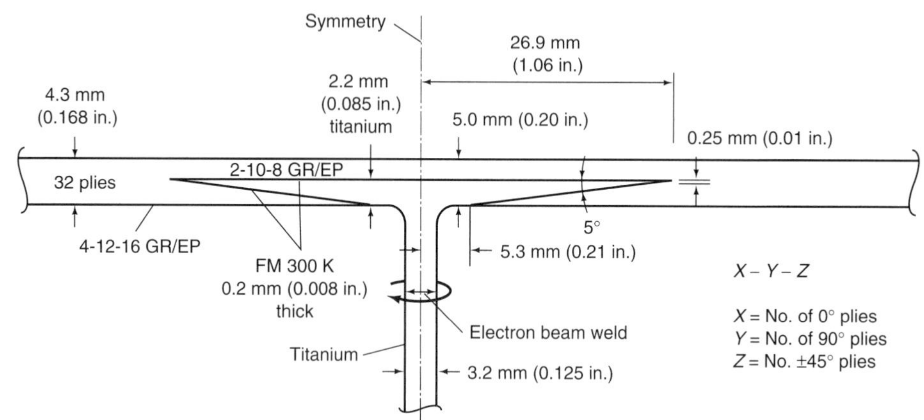

Fig. 25 Scarfed joint specimen for a spar-to-skin joint. GR/EP, graphite/epoxy

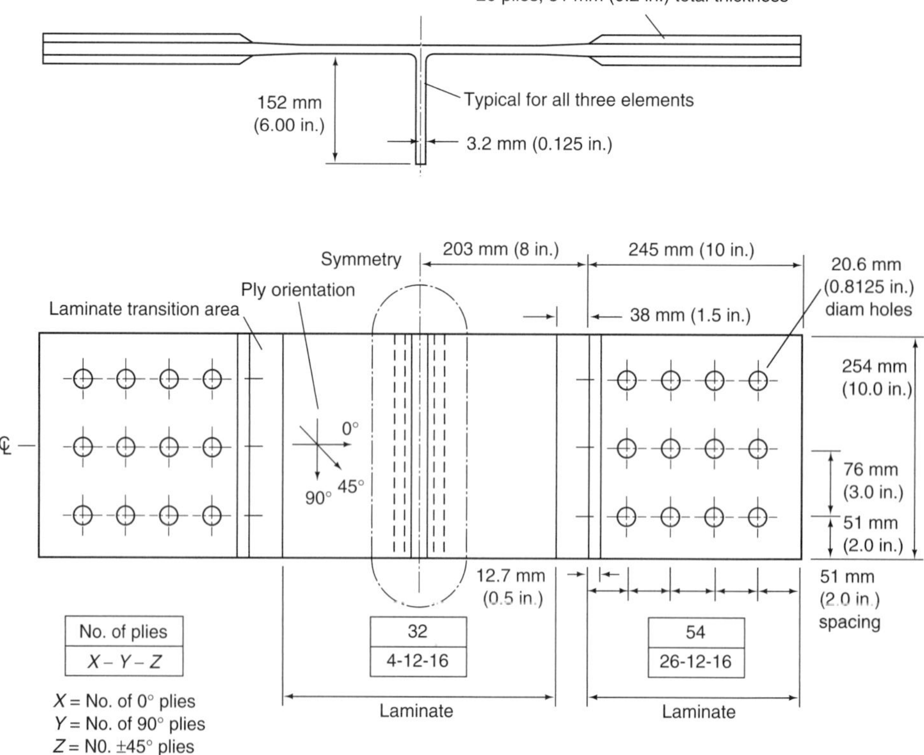

Fig. 26 Double-lap, two-step joint specimen configuration

arise from dropped tools, foreign objects such as rocks on runways, from hail and ice, and from ballistics. Impact testing at differing energy levels is commonly used to screen materials for damage resistance, damage tolerance, and as a part of larger element and subcomponent testing.

A common method for investigating impact resistance is the falling weight test. This type of impact is included as a portion of the compression after impact (CAI) testing discussed in MIL-HDBK-17. Generally, a flat panel is impacted normal to its surface. Commonly, a 13 to 25 mm (0.5 to 1 in.) diameter hemispherical tup (or striker) is used. Quasi-isotropic laminates approximately 5 to 10 mm (0.2 to 0.4 in.) thick are often used to screen materials for aircraft structural applications.

Energy levels for the falling dart test are generally given in foot-pounds or foot-pounds per inch of thickness. With variations of velocity, the damage may vary even with constant energy. This phenomenon is related to the type of damage, the rate it propagates in the specimen, and the deformation of the specimen during impact.

The falling weight used for CAI testing is generally dropped from a few feet, with a mass of 4.5 to 9 kg (10 to 20 lb), and is considered a low-velocity impact. Low-velocity tests such as a falling dart do not adequately simulate ballistic damage. Occasionally, investigators may accelerate the drop with elastic cords to gain a somewhat higher velocity. If very low velocity impacts are to be studied, a long fulcrum pendulum may be used to impact the specimen with a much higher mass.

Following the impact, an assessment of the damage is performed. Criteria for damage assessment may include measurement of the visually apparent damage area, measurement of dent depth, and non-destructive testing evalua-

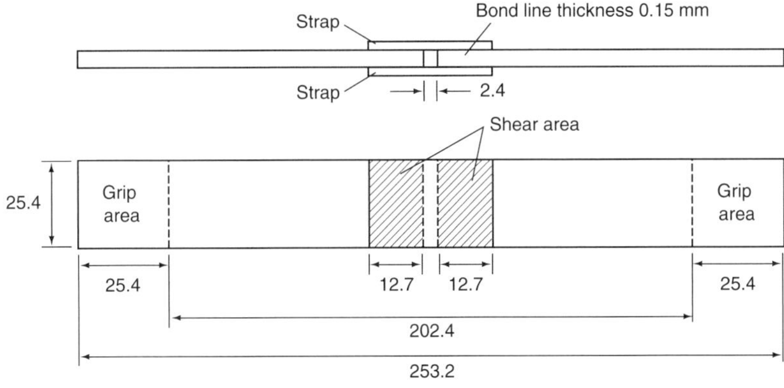

Fig. 27 Geometry of double-lap test specimens. The adherend is $[0]_{16}$ or $[0/90/-45/+45]_{2S}$ carbon/epoxy. The strap is $[0]_8$ or $[0/90/-45/+45]_S$ carbon/epoxy. Dimensions in millimeters

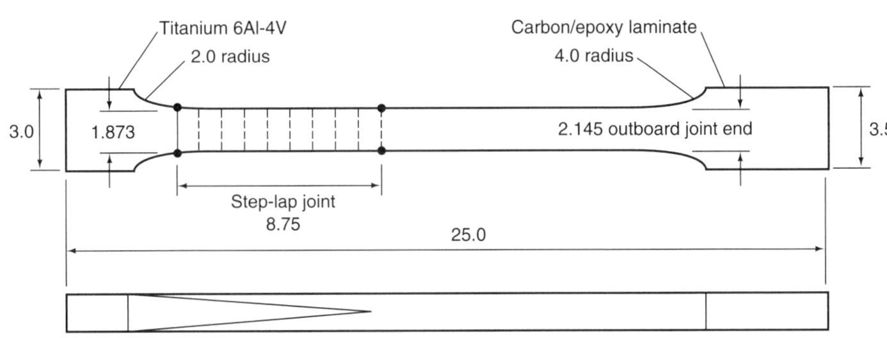

Fig. 28 Step-lap joint specimen example. Dimensions in inches

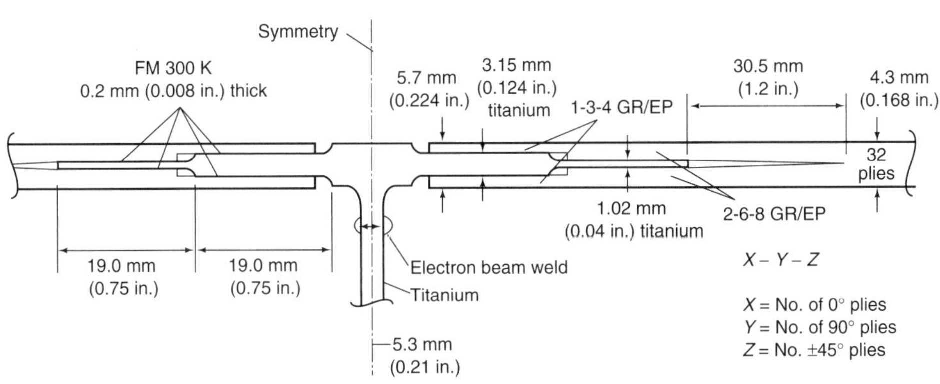

Fig. 29 Detail of the two-side stepped joint specimen

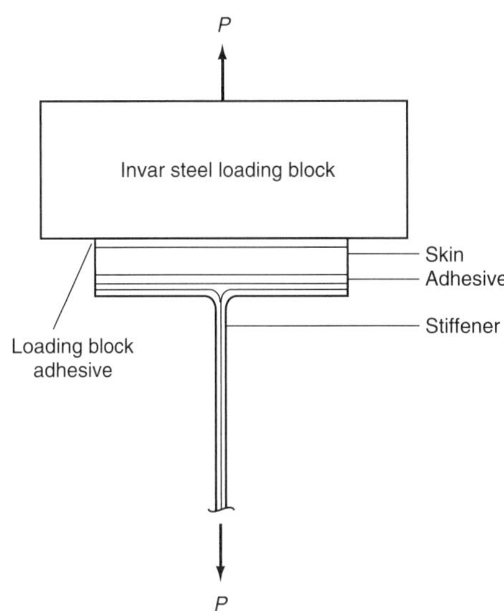

Fig. 30 "T" pull-off specimen for assessing the strength of skin-to-stiffener bonded joints

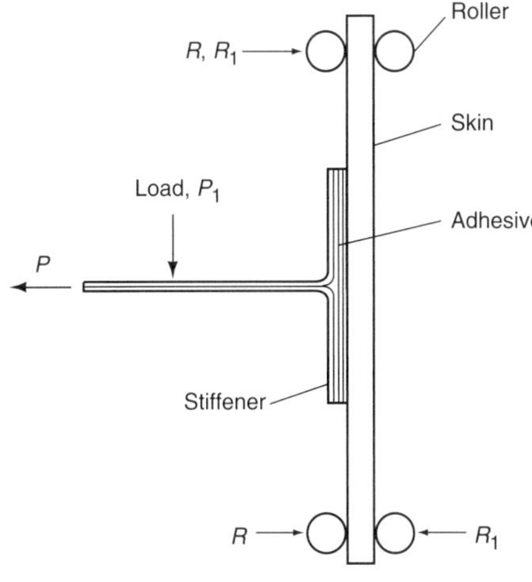

Fig. 31 "T" twist-off specimen for assessing the strength of skin-to-stiffener bonded joints

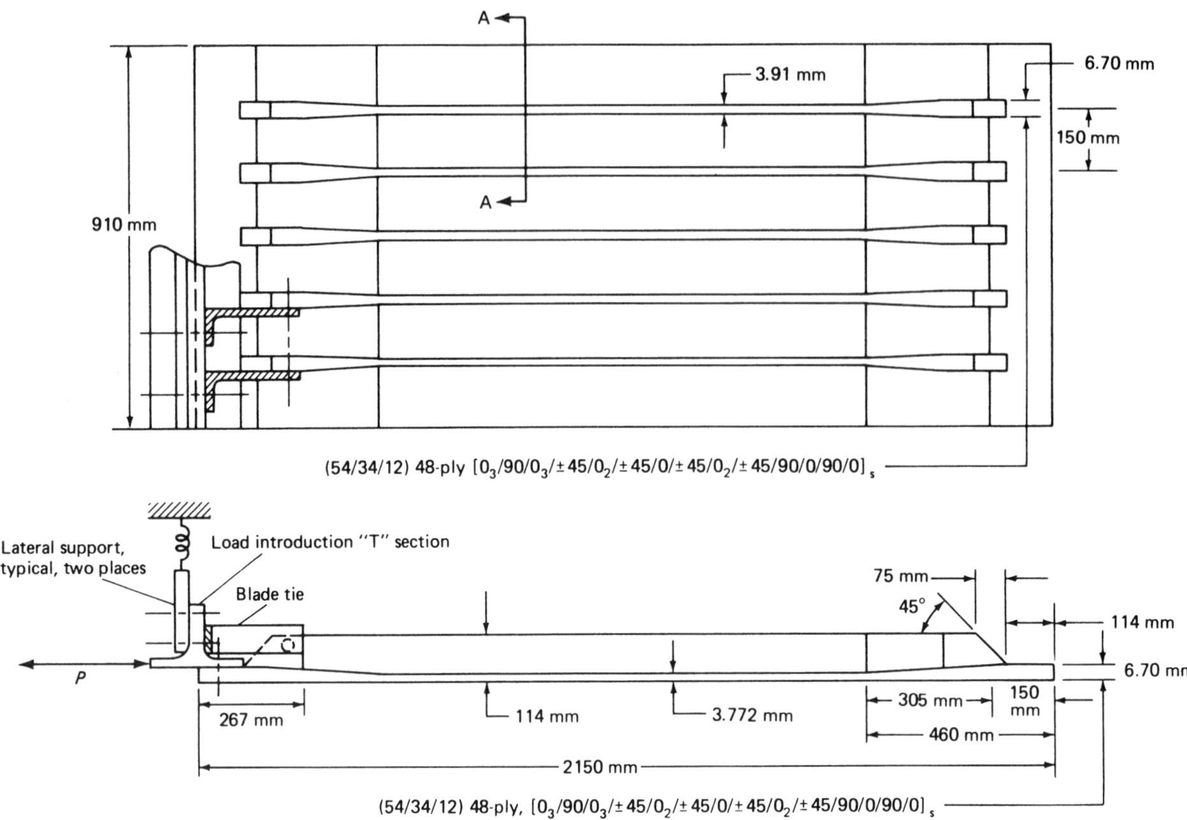

Fig. 32 Blade-stiffened subcomponent

tion for the internal damage area. Following this assessment, additional mechanical tests such as CAI or fatigue may be performed.

Other Damage Resistance/Tolerance Tests. Other impact tests are often included at higher levels of the building-block approach. These may include ballistic impact, ice/hail simulation, bird strike simulation, and other program-specific tests. These are often accomplished through the use of an air gun that fires a projectile at the test specimen. Details of these tests have not been standardized and are not discussed in detail here.

Quasi-static indentation tests may be performed by supporting a flat panel in a frame and indenting the center of the panel with a tip attached to a universal-testing machine. Load and deflection are measured during the test.

Specialized tests are also performed to evaluate a material's performance and durability in specific applications. These include roller cart and spiked-heel resistance tests for flooring.

ACKNOWLEDGMENTS

A significant portion of the material presented in this article has been adapted from the original article written by G.C. Grimes, K.W. Ranger, and M.D. Brunner that appeared in *Composites,* Volume 1, *Engineered Materials Handbook,* ASM International, 1987, p 313–345. Likewise, a great deal of material has been adapted from MIL-HDBK-17, Section 7, which features contributions from a number of composites industry experts.

REFERENCES

1. "DOD/NASA Advanced Composites Design Guide," Vol 1-A, Air Force Wright Aeronautical Laboratories, Dayton, OH, 1983
2. "Standard Test Method for Tensile Properties of Fiber-Resin Composites," D 3039, *Annual Book of ASTM Standards,* American Society for Testing and Materials
3. G.C. Grimes, D.F. Adams, and E.G. Dusablon, "The Effects of Discontinuities on Compression Fatigue Properties of Advanced Composites," CN. N0001979-C-0275 and 0276, Final Technical Report NOR 80-158, Northrup Aircraft Division, Oct 1980
4. G.C. Grimes and E.G. Dusablon, Study of the Static and Fatigue Compression Properties of Graphite/Epoxy Composites With Discontinuities Under Severe Environmental Exposures, *Composites Materials: Testing and Design,* STP 787, I.M. Daniel, Ed., American Society for Testing and Materials, 1982
5. "Standard Guide for Testing Inplane Shear Properties of Composite Laminates," D 4255, *Annual Book of ASTM Standards,* American Society for Testing and Materials
6. Structural Sandwich Composites, *Military Handbook* 23A, Department of Defense, Dec 1968
7. G.C. Grimes, Honeycomb Structures, *Handbook of Adhesive Bonding,* C.V. Cagle et al., Ed., McGraw-Hill, 1973
8. L.L. Jeans, G.C. Grimes, and H.P. Kan, Fatigue Sensitivity of Composite Structure for Fighter Aircraft, *Proc. AIAA/ASME/ASCE/AH 22nd Structures, Structural Dynamics, and Materials Conference,* 1981; also, *J. Aircr.,* 1982
9. R.L. Ramkamar, G.C. Grimes, D.F. Adams, and E.G. Dusablon, "Effects of Materials and Process Defects on the Compression Properties of Advanced Composites," Technical Report NOR 82-103, Northrop Aircraft Division, May 1982
10. Metallic Materials and Elements for Aerospace Structures, MIL-HDBK-5E, *Military Standardization Handbook,* 1 June 1987
11. "Fastener Test Methods," MIL-STD-1312
12. G.C. Grimes, K.W. Ranger, and M.D. Brunner, Element and Subcomponent Tests, *Composites,* Vol 1, *Engineered Materials Handbook,* ASM International, 1987, p 313–345
13. Raymond B. Krieger, Jr., "Stress Analysis of Metal-to-Metal Bonds in Hostile Envi-

ronments," *Proc. 22nd National SAMPE Symposium,* San Diego, CA, 26–28 April 1977

14. Raymond B. Krieger, Jr., "Stress Analysis Concepts for Adhesive Bonding of Aircraft Primary Structure," *Adhesively Bonded Joints: Testing, Analysis and Design,* ASTM STP 981, W.S. Johnson, Ed., American Society for Testing and Materials, Philadelphia, 1988, p 264–275
15. "Test Method for Tensile Strength of Adhesives by Means of Bar and Rod Specimens," D 2095, *Annual Book of ASTM Standards,* Vol 15.06, American Society for Testing and Materials, West Conshohocken, PA
16. "Shear Strength and Shear Modulus of Structural Adhesives," E 229, *Annual Book of ASTM Standards,* Vol 15.06, American Society for Testing and Materials, West Conshohocken, PA
17. "Preparation of Bar and Rod Specimens for Adhesive Testing," D 2094, *Annual Book of ASTM Standards,* Vol 15.06, American Society for Testing and Materials, West Conshohocken, PA
18. L.J. Hart-Smith, "Adhesive Bonded Single Lap Joints," NASA CR-11236, Jan 1973
19. "Determination of Tensile Strength of Tapered and Stepped Joints," European Aircraft Industry Standard prEN 6066 (preliminary)
20. "Strength Properties of Double Lap Shear Adhesive Joints by Tension Loading," D 3528-92, *Annual Book of ASTM Standards,* Vol 15.06, American Society for Testing and Materials, West Conshohocken, PA

Full-Scale Structural Testing

John E. McCarty, Composite Structures Consulting

STRUCTURAL DESIGN requires a continual assessment of structural functions to determine whether or not their requirements have been satisfied. First to be assessed are the initial functional requirements of the concept or configuration. The design is reassessed throughout the design process, as material selection, structural element identification, structural arrangement, manufacturing and quality-assurance methods, and in-service maintenance are defined and their effects on performance are quantified. The successful incorporation of each design element is determined by the in-service performance of the structure.

Because development and production involve a substantial financial commitment, the expected in-service performance must be assessed before the structure enters its service environment. Therefore, tests are performed throughout the developmental cycle to establish a database for the design and to evaluate the potential in-service performance of the selected elements. Full-scale testing of the completed structure (Fig. 1), or testing of large segments as a single unit (Fig. 2), is the major test in an extensive series. At their current stage of development, composite structures are very dependent on all levels of test in the validation process. This article describes the role of the full-scale testing in assessing composite structural systems of aircraft and qualifying them for in-service use.

The designer's first step in selecting an approach is to understand the need that the design is to fulfill. To define this specific need and ensure that the end product satisfies it, the designer must have a set of design requirements. The requirements usually do not define the structure itself, but rather its performance. Performance requirements are divided into two categories: those related to structural function (for example, the structural wing box, which transmits lift forces to the body for payload support) and those imposed to ensure safety and durability of the structural component. This article focuses on the second set of requirements. The full-scale test is one of the primary means of demonstrating how successfully a structure meets these structural performance requirements and is extremely important because it tests all combined relationships of the critical elements of the structure in the most realistic manner.

In airframe production, the full-scale structural test is most often performed on one of the first three or four airframes manufactured. This places the full-scale test either well into the production commitment or critical to initiation of the production commitment. Timing of this test in the overall schedule if an unexpected failure were to occur has the potential to impact both the cost of the airframe and the delivery schedule to the customer. If major redesign and/or tooling changes were required, costs would increase and the delivery schedule would slip, which could involve financial penalties and customer dissatisfaction.

The full-scale test enables the internal load distribution and the stress-strain level of each structural element to be imposed correctly. As it is the best representation of the true structural performance of the system, it must be a significant part of the certification or qualification process. It is imperative, therefore, that the purpose of each test element in the process be defined.

There are two basic approaches to full-scale testing for certification: the structure is certified by analysis and supported by test evidence, or the structure is certified by a successful full-scale test validation of the structure and the analysis. Regardless of which approach is taken, full-scale testing is usually required to satisfy the requirements of the agency conferring qualification or certification. Depending on the approach, there may be some difference in the test steps or their sequence and in the data required from the full-scale test.

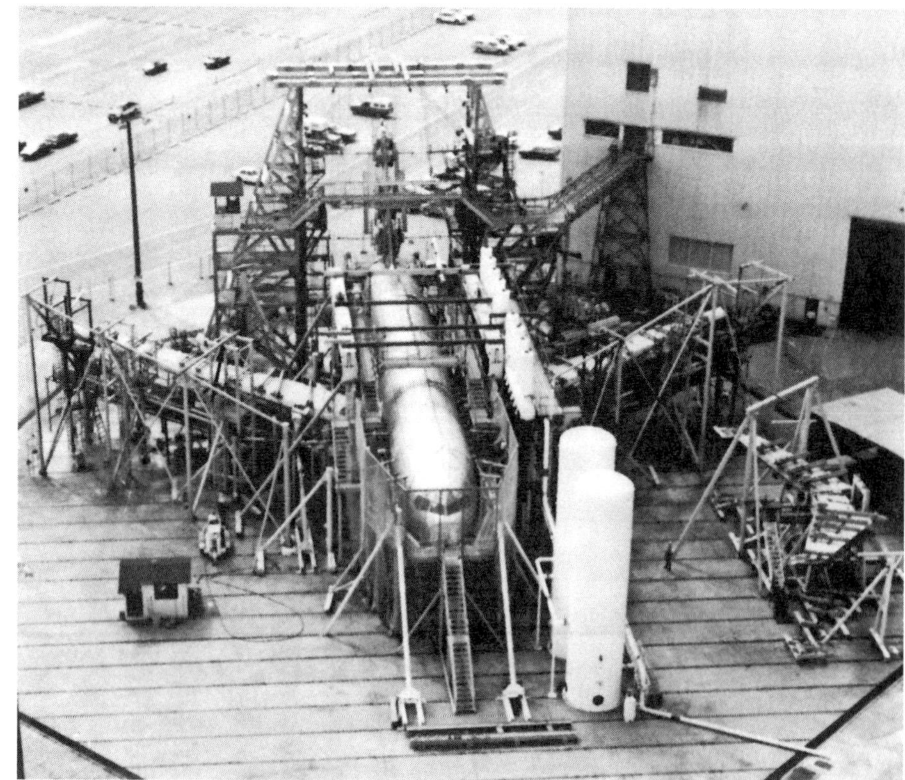

Fig. 1 Commercial aircraft full-scale fatigue test

Typical full-scale tests are static, durability (fatigue), and damage tolerance, the last of which may not require a full-scale test. These full-scale tests are designed to address the following questions about the structure:

- Is the analysis of the internal load distribution correct?
- Have there been any errors or omissions in design, manufacture, or quality-assurance measures?
- Are there any unexpected deflections that impose functional constraints?
- Have composite structures that are sensitive to out-of-plane or through-thickness loads been correctly or adequately covered by analysis or lower-level testing?
- Are there any deflections that significantly alter the load path and increase the stress-strain level of a structural element (that is, are there large displacement effects)?
- Has the assessment of durability been correctly made for composites, metals, and the combined structure, particularly in the interface areas?
- Has the damage tolerance of the structure been correctly evaluated by testing and analysis? For composite structures in particular, have the nonvisual flaw or damage effects on the structures been adequately assessed?

The use of full-scale tests must recognize the unique characteristics of composite structures and their response to the expected in-service conditions as simulated by these tests. Each test type described in the following sections is oriented to aircraft testing requirements, with emphasis on the special considerations needed for testing composite structures. The aircraft structure was selected as the basis for discussion because it is the most generic type of vehicle structure that uses composites.

Static Test

The full-scale static test is the most important test in qualifying composite structures because of their brittle nature, sensitivity to stress concentrations, and insensitivity to fatigue cycling. The parameters to consider when developing the basic requirements for the static test are the type of test article, the type and number of load conditions, the usage environment to be simulated, the load level, and the type and quantity of data to be obtained. The ability of the test data to meet certification requirements must be inherent in each of these static test requirements.

The full-scale test article, whether it is a major component or an entire airframe, is considered representative of the production structure. This implies both that it has been fabricated according to production drawings using specification-controlled materials on production tooling and following fabrication and assembly specifications and that it has been inspected according to production quality-control requirements. This inspection level represents the detection, acceptance, or rejection of manufacturing anomalies as required by the specifications and directed by the material review board.

To ensure that test data are a useful part of the certification database, additional special inspections are performed that further establish the test data validity. For composites, ultrasonic and x-ray inspection procedures are required to detect processing flaws such as porosity and delamination. This same level of additional inspection is performed after each critical test sequence.

Material Considerations. The type of test article used depends on its material composition, function, size, structural configuration, and the degree to which it represents the entire airframe or its full-sized major components.

The material composition of the test article can affect the test procedures and the load level. Carbon/epoxy is the composite material that is currently most commonly used. Properties unique to carbon/epoxy materials, as compared to metals, are displayed in Table 1. Carbon/epoxy materials are known to be generally linear to failure in their response to monotonic loading. This brittle nature of composites must be considered in selecting testing levels for test setup and checkout, strain surveys, limit load conditions, and the sequence of ultimate load conditions.

Moisture and Temperature Effects. Composites are also sensitive to temperature and can absorb moisture from in-service environmental

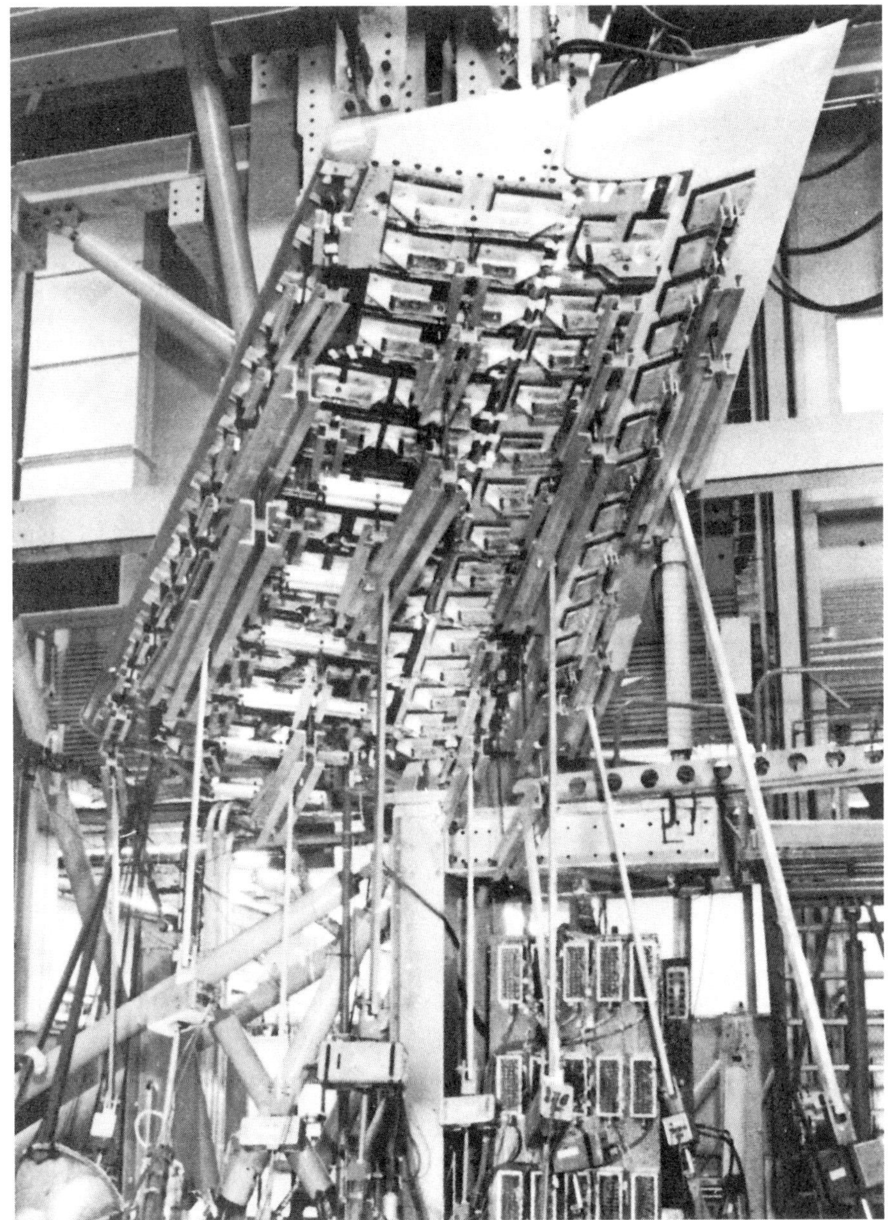

Fig. 2 Aircraft composite horizontal stabilizer full-scale test

exposure. As a full-scale test of even a small aircraft in a fully simulated environment would be very expensive and time consuming, alternative ways to determine environmental effects must be found. Although testing at room temperature and in ambient moisture is the most economical way to test a large structural system, it does not account sufficiently for environmental effects. The elements of the hot/wet (temperature and absorbed moisture) environmental test involve the same environmental considerations for both subsonic and supersonic flight environments. For flight and ground environments, only the temperature levels, time at temperature, and absorbed moisture content of the composite material will vary in magnitude.

The temperature profile of the structure as a function of heat input and its material and structural response must be accounted for by means of the analyses and tests required for certification. Changes in stress-strain caused by moisture absorption also must be accounted for by the same generic analysis and test sequences. The induced stresses and strains are caused by two levels of structural response. The first level is due to the physical compliance of the laminate, which is usually accounted for by ply-level properties and analysis at the laminate level or by laminate-level properties that include the effect of both moisture and temperature. The inclusion of this effect in the analysis of the structure can be accounted for by increased design stress-strain and by reduced allowables. The second level is introduced at the structural element or component level. It is induced by nonlinear temperature or moisture profiles imposed on the structure, the nonuniform coefficient of expansion of the composite elements due to different ply orientations, and the inherent structural redundancy of a complex airframe structure.

Because satisfying both moisture and temperature requirements is difficult at the full-scale level, most composite structures have required a "building-block" testing approach (Fig. 3), in which environmental effects are addressed at the analysis, coupon, structural element, subcomponent, component, and full-scale levels. The sums of these levels of analyses and tests must be consolidated in such a way as to validate the consideration of environmental effects on the composite structure. The methods that have satisfied this requirement at the full-scale level are to:

- Select the maximum environmental factor (that is, allowable reduction factor) used to correct the room-temperature allowables for the effect of environment and factor up the critical load conditions by the reciprocal of this factor
- Select the environmental factor used with the minimum margin of safety in the structure for each load condition being tested
- Select the environmental factor from the elements of the structure that are loaded in such a way that the type of loading and/or the structural load paths are the most sensitive to either the magnitude or the rate of change in capability with change in the environment
- Select the environmental factor from the elements of the structure that are loaded in such a way that the type of loading or the structural load paths are through the area of the structure where the effects of environment are the most severe or are the most poorly defined in the allowables used to establish that margin of safety
- Test to the ultimate load for each condition considered critical, use the strain-gage results to extrapolate the strains that would be added by the environmental effects, and require that these extrapolated strains still show a positive margin of safety

All these methods are suitable for an all-composite structure. In structures containing metal structural elements, these methods would impose the penalty of either overdesigning the metal structure or necessitating two test articles: one with an augmented metal structure for the environmentally factored composite test and one with no factors on the metal being tested to the ultimate load level to validate the metal elements. The only method that avoids these penalties is the last one given in the list. The selection of the environmental factors by any of the listed scenarios is dependent on analysis. The effect on failure mode and location should be considered in the selection of test environmental factors.

Structure Size. There are two considerations in choosing the size of the test structure: the cost of testing to get the environmental information on "allowables" to the statistical level usually considered acceptable and the cost of testing a full-scale small component in a simulated environment. If the component is small enough that a full-scale environmental test would be less costly than developing a large database that includes all relevant environmental allowables, combined with analysis to certify the structure, then testing in the environment is justified. Other considerations, such as type of structure (primary or secondary), type and complexity of loading, and structural configuration also play a role in the environmental conditioning required.

Critical Test Condition Selection. The steps in full-scale composite structure test procedure follow the same generic path as in a metal structure test procedure. These steps start with a review of the analysis of the structure. The selection of the most critical load conditions for the structure is based on this analysis.

The critical conditions selected are usually not based solely on the minimum safety margins, although this is the main consideration. Additional considerations may include:

- Stability-critical structures that have low but not minimum margins of safety
- Combined loading conditions that are difficult to analyze

Table 1 Behavior of carbon-epoxy versus metals under various conditions

Condition	Carbon-epoxy behavior relative to metals
Stress-strain relationship	More linear strain to failure
Static notch sensitivity	Greater sensitivity
Fatigue notch sensitivity	Less sensitivity
Transverse properties	Weaker
Mechanical properties variability	Higher
Sensitivity to aircraft hygrothermal environment	Greater
Damage growth mechanism	In-plane delamination instead of through-thickness cracks

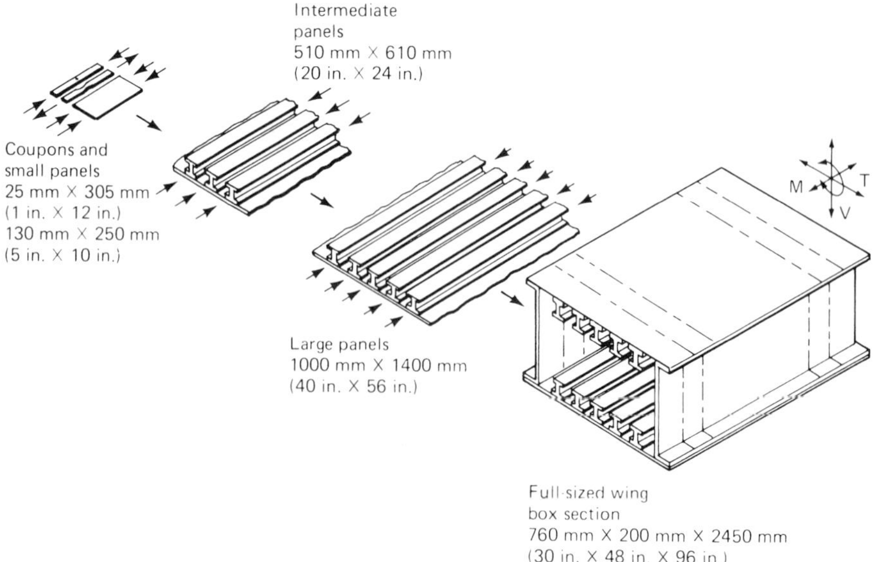

Fig. 3 Building-block testing approach

- Major structural joints or intersections that are difficult to analyze
- Areas where the building-block approach to certification must be demonstrated, such as when there is concern for a failure mode change between testing in the simulated environment and testing in an ambient condition
- Areas where the environmental factors methods described previously must be demonstrated

Load Application Alternatives. Once the critical conditions have been selected, the means of load application must be established to facilitate the most cost-effective method of simulating the real flight and ground loads application. The details of the methods of loading a composite structure need careful consideration because most composites have weak through-thickness strength and sensitivity to stress concentrations. Selection of a load application method must take into account composite structure sensitivity, the engineer's desire for the truest simulation of the load distribution, and the cost of the test setup. Loading methods include: formers that contact the structure on the exterior where the surface is supported by substructure, direct fastening to the substructure by penetrating the surface panels, and bonding or mechanically fastening to the surface panels.

Formers (Fig. 4) usually concentrate the loading more and do not give as good a representation of the distributed air load as the other methods. This method usually has a less complex loading setup and is therefore often the least costly.

Direct attachment to the substructure is usually similar in loading simulation and cost to the former method. However, for both composite and metal structures, care must be taken in the method of attachment to the substructure. If the attachment can be made at the same fastener locations that are used for attaching the surface panels and substructure elements together, the procedure is relatively easy. However, if special access holes are needed, this method is less acceptable for both metals and composites. The effects of holes are particularly bad for composites because of their stress concentration sensitivity.

Direct surface attachment (Fig. 5) usually offers a better chance of uniform load representation. This closer representation of the real vehicle structural load usually involves a more complex test setup. The application of the load directly to a composite surface must be done more carefully than to a metal surface because of stress concentration sensitivity and through-thickness weakness.

Loading setup is now controlled mostly by computers, which control not only the loading applied by each hydraulic jack but also the rate of loading. They also check the displacement of the jack or the load cell to prevent overload of the specimen. Computer control of load application has allowed more complex test setups and load application in a truly representative manner.

Instrumentation Requirements. Once the load application method and test setup have been selected, the instrumentation required to collect data (for submittal as part of the qualification base for the structure) must be defined. The data display must:

- Ensure correct application and introduction of the load
- Allow monitoring of the testing in real time and protect the test article from being incorrectly loaded
- Validate that the loads applied produce not only the correct loading, but also the correct deflected shape
- Validate that the correct interaction of the applied load is being made in the correct ratio and magnitude for combined load conditions
- Provide a means to automatically terminate loading when loading errors are detected, including a human reaction to the error and avoiding loss of the test article
- Validate that the internal strain distribution is as predicted by analysis

The types of instrumentation that are often applied in full-scale testing are strain gages; deflection measurement indicators; stress coats; photo stress, moiré fringe, and acoustic emission detectors; and accelerometers. All data are electronically recorded, and computers can be used to enhance the data at critical locations.

Test Procedure Considerations. Establishing test procedures and test sequencing requires that all test participants have defined responsibilities both in planning the test and during the test itself. As specific assignments will vary from company to company, they will not be detailed here except to state that they generally include test planning, test fixture design and setup, test functional checkout, and test conducting and monitoring for continuance/discontinuance during a particular test loading. Deciding who will make the critical decision to stop loading or to proceed is the key to providing maximum protection of the test article during critical portions of the test.

Selecting and establishing the test sequence is generic to most large-scale tests and is particularly important to composite structures. The test sequence usually starts with a checkout of the test setup, which involves functional testing of loading jacks, instrumentation, data recording, and real-time critical data displays. A simple loading case at low load levels is applied to ensure that loads are being introduced as expected. The unique features of each test may require more functional monitoring, data recording, and tracking procedures.

Following checkout of the test setup, a strain and deflection survey is usually run to determine whether the strain distributions and deflections are as predicted. This survey checks the analysis

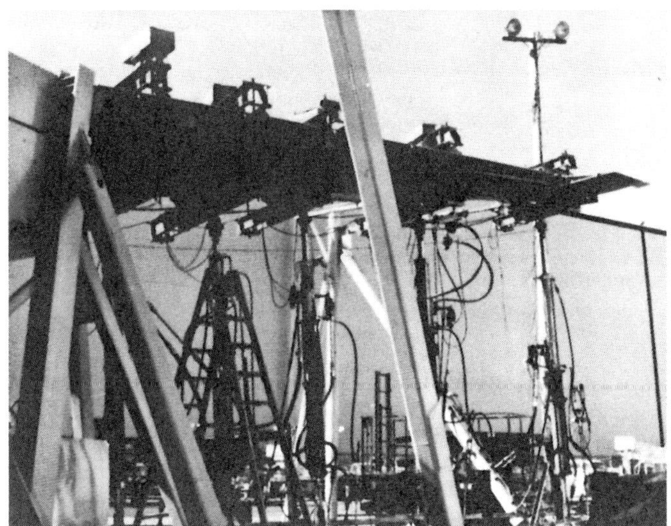

Fig. 4 Use of formers for loading aircraft horizontal stabilizer

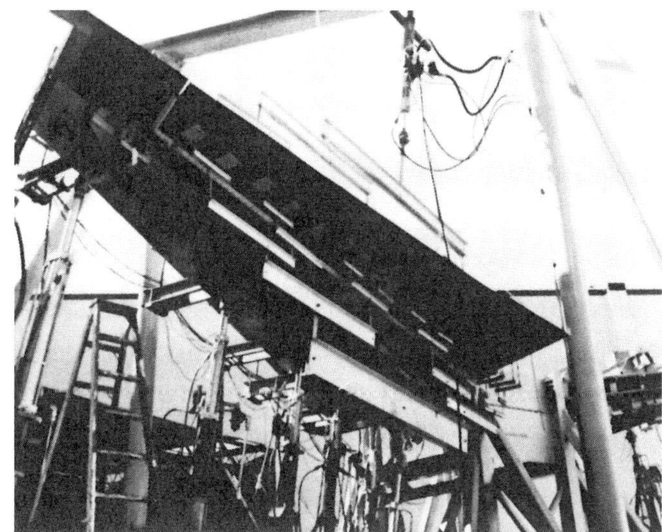

Fig. 5 Use of skin pads for loading aircraft elevator

of the structure and the test setup again and is usually done at a loading level that will not affect the certification test results. For composite structures, the testing load level is usually in the range of 30 to 50% of the design ultimate load level. The load conditions applied are simple singular (not combined spectrum, or cyclic) types used to determine whether the strains for these simple cases agree with the analysis. Then, low load levels of the selected critical certification loads are applied.

These results can then be extrapolated to the design ultimate load levels to determine whether the structure can sustain ultimate load as predicted. If these extrapolations continue to show positive margins of safety comparable to the analysis, testing can proceed. If the extrapolations show negative margins of safety or deviations from the expected load distribution, then testing is delayed until these problems are resolved. A serious problem arises when the deviations are small but critical and there is some risk of failure before reaching the required design load level. A review should be conducted before proceeding.

With the stress and/or strain at the proper level and the test anomalies resolved, testing can proceed through the design certification critical load tests. These tests run in sequence, with the conditions for which there is the highest confidence of success usually being run first and those with the highest risk of premature failure being run last. The first loading cases are often the most simple, which minimizes the loading complexity before running critical combined loading cases.

Ultimate Load Requirements. It is necessary at this point to discuss the type of load levels required by the qualifying or certifying agencies to meet their validation requirements. The static test load level requirement for U.S. Federal Aviation Administration (FAA) certification is based on experience the manufacturer and the FAA have had with a particular type of structure. To meet FAA requirements, conventional metal structures are usually tested only to the limit load. This may also be true for composite structures if the manufacturer has had experience with similar composite structures; otherwise, testing to the ultimate load level is required. Various U.S. Department of Defense (DoD) agencies require the ultimate load level for the static test in order to qualify most structures.

After completing the required testing, whether to limit or ultimate load, the manufacturer often picks the most critical condition and tests the article to destruction. This destruction test further validates not only the ability of the analysis to predict the load distribution but also the strength of the structure. If the destruction test failure load exceeds the required ultimate load, vehicle performance growth is warranted.

Test Results Correlation. The final step in the static test sequence is a review of the data obtained from the test and evaluation of its correlation with the stress analysis. The structure is also carefully inspected using nondestructive techniques to determine whether damage that has occurred cannot be readily detected visually. This is of particular importance to composite structures because many of their failure modes and sequences are interlaminar and thus may not be visible.

Durability (Fatigue) Test

The effects of cyclic loading on current carbon-epoxy composites have generally been shown to be noncritical, due to the static load sensitivity of composite structures to stress concentration. In addition, the load level threshold at which composites become sensitive to cyclic loading is a very high percentage of their static failure load. Because this threshold is so high and most vehicles do not experience repeated loads that approach their ultimate loads, composite structures are not fatigue critical. Even if they were to experience loads near this threshold, or slightly above, there are so few of these high cycles in the spectrum life of the vehicle that no significant fatigue damage would occur that would affect structural capability. No industry acceptable-damage rule has been developed for fatigue of composite structures because of this noncritical factor of fatigue loading and the complexity of the fatigue mechanism for composite materials.

Some of the new "tougher" matrix resin systems being used in composites may have characteristics that make them more fatigue-sensitive than the current epoxy systems. If this is true, the importance of the full-scale fatigue test for composite structures will grow significantly, along with the need to develop an acceptable-damage rule.

Spectrum Loading Considerations. To date, cyclic testing of composite structures has been conducted to evaluate a metal structure used with a composite structure. Lacking an accepted damage rule, validation of the durability of composite structures has generally used spectrum loading that represents a compromise between the spectra most critical for composites and metals. This compromise, necessitated by the difference in response of composite and metal structures to the magnitude of repeated loads in the applied spectrum, is particularly valid at the full-scale test level. Composites are cyclic-sensitive to loads high in the spectrum, which produce the most fatigue damage and shortest test life. Both the high and low loads in the spectrum can damage a metal structure. However, the high-spectrum loads that damage composites produce a generally unconservative test life (longer than the in-service life) for metal components of the structure.

In general, full-scale cyclic testing has been limited to two to four lifetimes of spectrum loading, including a spectrum load enhancement factor. The flat stress versus cycles curve for composite materials would require, from a statistically significant point of view, consideration of the large scatter in repeated load life in order to technically validate the fatigue performance of composite structures. This may be accomplished through a life and/or load factor.

Most of the test setup and performance considerations for the full-scale static composite structures test discussed in the previous section apply to the fatigue test. Only those requirements unique to the fatigue test are discussed in the following two sections.

Testing and Inspection Requirements. Selecting the loads to be applied represents a compromise for both the composite and metal structural elements. It is very easy to apply a random sequence of spectrum loads using computers to control the loading jacks. Most full-scale fatigue tests, if not all, are spectrum loaded. The methods of loading, attachment of load fixtures, instrumentation, data recording, and checkout of the test setup are all similar to those used in static tests. The fatigue test has the additional feature of inspection intervals throughout the test life. These inspections are conducted to determine whether any damage is progressing because of cyclic loading, to obtain fatigue performance of the structural details, and to catch a critical damage growth that could cause loss of the test article during load cycling.

Stiffness change of a composite structure has been found to be an indicator of fatigue damage. Therefore, stiffness checks should be conducted at various times throughout the test, in a manner similar to the imposed inspection sequence. Because a significant stiffness change in a full-scale test article is very difficult to detect, nondestructive (primarily ultrasonic and x-ray) inspection methods are commonly used to detect damage and monitor its growth throughout the fatigue test.

Accounting for Environmental Effects. After selecting the spectrum loading for a composite structure, a decision must be made as to a way to apply environmental effects during the fatigue test, or account for them in the test results. The cost of either conditioning or applying a real environment to a full-scale test article generally is prohibitive. Enhanced or factored spectrum loads are the easiest means of accounting for environmental effects. Although mechanically loading the full-scale structure in a manner that truly represents the effects of environmentally induced strains is very difficult, if not impossible, the factored spectrum load approach is currently the only real option. Modifying the test results by analysis will not be feasible until an acceptable-damage rule for composite structure fatigue is developed. With the full-scale fatigue test, as with the static test, a post-test inspection of the test article is very important to ensure that no fatigue damage has occurred.

Damage Tolerance Test

The damage tolerance test, like the static test, is a qualification requirement of both the FAA and the DoD. In the past, fatigue testing was not required by the FAA for structures designed as fail safe and/or damage tolerant, but was required for all so-called safe-life structures. Now, fatigue testing is required by the FAA if there is the possibility of widespread fatigue damage in service. To date, most composite structures have shown good fatigue resistance behavior, so there is little likelihood of widespread fatigue damage in service. However, because there is no large in-service database for composites in primary structural applications in commercial aircraft, the FAA most likely will require fatigue testing until such a database is available. As composites have been used in the primary structures of commercial aircraft since the late 1980s, the service data are becoming available. With industry review, the database will continue to improve. Also, because most of the current composite structures include metal components, the interaction of the metal and composite structural elements needs to have a good fatigue database from testing and in-service monitoring. Although the load level required by the FAA and the DoD varies, both specify residual strength requirements that vary with the flaw damage assumption, ability to inspect damage, type of in-service inspection used, and type of aircraft. The loading requirement must be carefully reviewed to establish the damage tolerance test residual strength requirements.

Testing composite structures for damage tolerance is particularly important, because it addresses the concerns associated with both the static and fatigue tests. As with the static test, the brittle nature and notch sensitivity of composites is a concern in the damage tolerance test. As in the fatigue test, the critical flaw or damage may be associated with either its initial state or its growth after cyclic loading. Because the full-scale damage tolerance test has many other similarities with the static and fatigue tests, information on instrumentation, load application, loading control, data display and recording, test setup and checkout, and test assignment responsibilities are not repeated; only concerns unique to the damage tolerance test are discussed.

The types of flaws or damage that are critical to current composite structures are penetrations, delaminations, and low-velocity impact damage. The following discussion is limited to impact damage, since it is currently the most critical type of damage for composite structures and its concerns are representative.

Cycling and Inspection Requirements. The damaged full-scale structure should be subjected to cyclic loading that substantiates a statistically significant life. Because structural response to impact damage is unique to composites, the imposed spectrum can be tailored to the needs of the composite structure only. Full-scale flaw or damage cyclic testing of a metal structure is not regularly done; therefore, the spectrum imposed for the damage tolerance test of composite structures can be tailored to a composite-sensitive spectrum. The repeated inspections required for the fatigue test are also required for this test.

The phasing of loads may be significant to crack growth in areas such as fastener holes. The phasing should be considered and, when justified, included in full-scale testing.

Accounting for environmental effects of temperature and absorbed moisture is a necessary part of the damage tolerance test. For the residual strength part of the test, the approaches noted for the static test can be applied here as well. The damage effect is usually so dominant that temperature and moisture do not have a strong effect on residual strength. However, the question of environmental effect during the cyclic test portion of the damage tolerance test is not easily addressed. Load enhancement of the spectrum, as suggested for the fatigue test, is currently the only option.

For verification of other damage tolerance, such as lightning strike protection, full-scale testing of certain components may be required.

Residual Strength Test. Once the lifetime spectrum loading requirements have been completed, the required residual strength loads are applied. As in the static test, there will be more than one type of loading required, and a critical loading selection must be made. If the structure successfully passes these residual strength tests, one option is to load it to failure to further integrate its damage tolerance capability. As for the other full-scale tests, a detailed inspection is made before the destruction test. The resulting test data are reviewed and correlated with the analysis as part of the certification of the structure for damage tolerance requirements.

SELECTED REFERENCES

- "Aircraft Structures," JSSG-2006, Department of Defense, Oct 1998
- "Composite Aircraft Structure Advisory Circular," AC-107A, Federal Aviation Administration, U.S. Department of Transportation, April 1984
- R.W. Johnson, J.E. McCarty, and D.R. Wilson, "Damage Tolerance Testing for the Boeing 737 Graphite-Epoxy Horizontal Stabilizer," paper presented at The Fifth Conference on Fibrous Composites in Structural Design (New Orleans, LA), Department of Defense/National Aeronautics and Space Administration, Jan 1981
- R.W. Johnson, J.E. McCarty, and D.R. Wilson, "737 Graphite-Epoxy Horizontal Stabilizer Certification," Paper 82-0745, presented at the 23rd Structures, Structural Dynamics and Materials Conference (New Orleans, LA), AIAA/ASME/ASCE/AHS, May 1982
- J.E. McCarty and D.R. Wilson, "Advanced Composite Stabilizer for Boeing 737 Aircraft," paper presented at The Sixth Conference on Fibrous Composites in Structural Design, Department of Defense/National Aeronautics and Space Administration, Jan 1983

Properties and Performance

Chairperson: Jeffrey Schaff, United Technologies Research Center

Properties and Performance of Polymer-Matrix Composites

THE DESIGN AND ANALYSIS of composite components and assemblies require a detailed knowledge of materials properties, which, in turn, depend on the manufacturing, machining, and assembly methods used. This article selects, from the many available composite fiber-resin combinations manufactured by conventional processing methods, a few that are representative of the common, high-volume types as well as a few of the more specialized types. These materials are identified and briefly described, and their properties are presented in graphic and tabular form. This collection of data is not intended to be comprehensive, but instead is meant to provide a general overview of the performance capabilities of selected polymer-matrix composite materials.

Materials and Properties Description

Composite components are in the form of fibers, resins, and fiber-resin combinations, as shown in Fig. 1. The fiber starts with single filaments grouped by 1000 to 12,000 into a fiber bundle, which can be chopped into short (3.2 to 50 mm, or $\frac{1}{8}$ to 2 in.) fibers, woven into fabric, or further combined into a fiber tow containing as many as 40,000 to 300,000 filaments. Fabrics and tows can be further processed into chopped 12.7 × 12.7 mm ($\frac{1}{2} \times \frac{1}{2}$ in.) fabric squares, or 6.4 to 12. 7 ($\frac{1}{4}$ to $\frac{1}{2}$ in.) chopped fiber tows, respectively.

Figure 2 illustrates four common types of fabric weave. In the plain weave, yarns are interlaced in an alternating fashion over and under every other yarn to provide maximum fabric stability and firmness and minimum yarn slippage. The thinnest and lightest-weight fabrics are also achieved by use of the plain weave. Fabrics as fine as 25.4 μm (1 mil) are being produced for the electrical industry for mica backing. The plain weave is the primary weave used in the coating industry.

The leno weave maintains uniformity of threads and minimizes distortion of threads where a relatively low number of threads is required. Grinding wheel reinforcements, lightweight membranes, and laminating fabrics used the leno weave to good advantage.

The eight-harness satin weave, a very pliable weave that conforms readily to intricately contoured planes, can also be woven with more threads per inch to achieve a high density. Satin weaves are used to best advantage in the reinforced plastic field, especially for prepregs for aircraft and missiles. Satin weave fabrics require more threads per inch to retain stability and are generally produced in the medium and heavy weight range (200 to 610 g/m^2, or 6 to 18 oz/yd^2).

In the crowfoot satin weave, one warp yarn weaves over three and under one fill yarn. It is used primarily in unidirectional fabrics for fishing rod reinforcement. Crowfoot weave fabrics also conform easily to contoured surfaces.

Resin forms are categorized as liquid, powder, or solid pellets. They can be combined with fiber or have fillers, such as carbon, graphite, calcium carbonate, clay, hydrated alumina or silica powder, added to them.

The fiber-resin forms in a majority of structural component applications are either filament-wound fiber bundles or tows, unidirectional fiber tape laydown (tape wrapped), woven fabric, chopped fiber molding compound, or lay-up fabrics that are all either combined with a staged (partially cured) liquid resin or impregnated with a wet resin during the fabrication process.

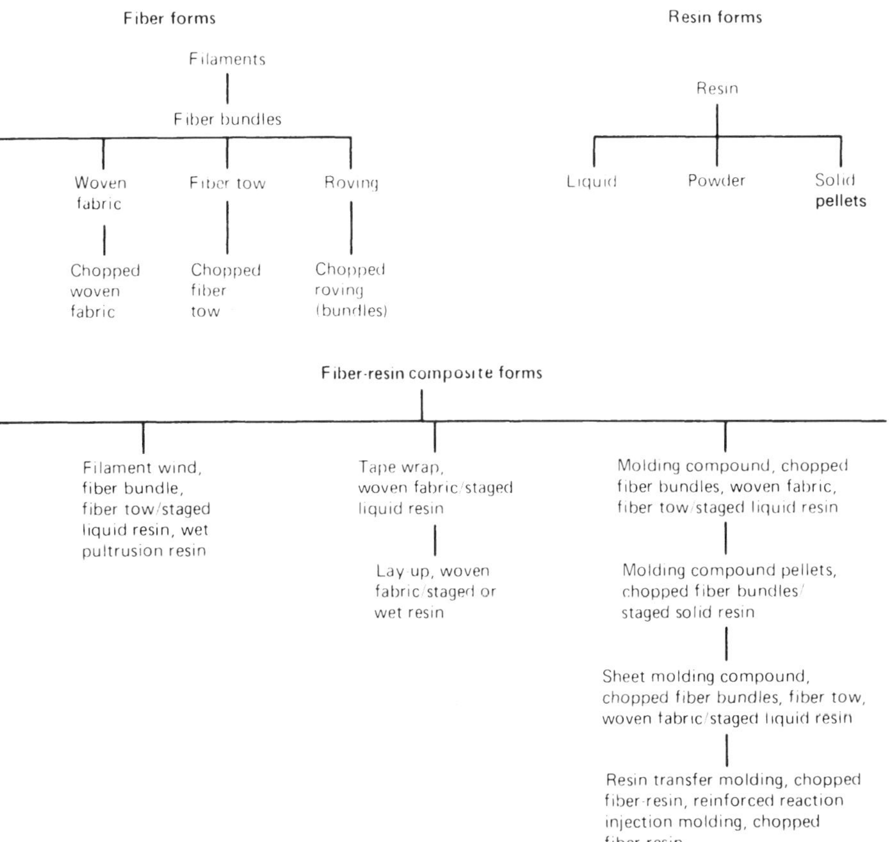

Fig. 1 Composite forms

The physical, mechanical, thermal, and electrical properties and in-service conditions of the forms that are presented in this article have been obtained from a survey of technical literature and publications and corporate product engineering data sheets and reports. Where a mulitude of data points exist for a given material property, multiple curves are drawn and the user can interpret the information based on the references.

Table 1 lists key physical, mechanical, thermal, and electrical properties and in-service conditions of concern for resin-matrix composites, many of which are covered in the following sections in this article.

The following general statements on material properties versus temperature represent guidelines for composite material use:

- Mechanical properties of fibers, resins, and fiber-resin composites decrease with temperature.
- Most mechanical properties of fiber-resin composites are higher than those for resin properties, but lower than those for fiber properties.
- Most thermal properties from room temperature to 260 °C (500 °F) increase with temperature.
- Carbon and graphite fibers increase the thermal and electrical conductivity of a fiber-resin composite material system.
- Properties may be different in all three planes, depending on fiber configuration.
- Factors that affect mechanical properties are resin-to-fiber ratio, resin and fiber types, resin-fiber interface, type of composite processing (filament winding, tape wrapping, or molding), and type of composite cure (autoclave, hydroclave, vacuum bag molding, extrusion, or compression or injection molding).

In addition, these observations on material properties in respect to form of reinforcement should be considered:

- Maximum properties in load direction 1 are achieved by unidirectional lamination of continuous fiber reinforcement (Fig. 3).
- In a unidirectional laminate, mechanical properties in load directions 2 and 3 are much lower than in load direction 1 and are highly dependent on the matrix resin.
- Bidirectional reinforcement can be achieved by cross-plying unidirectional tapes or broad goods, and by using woven fabric reinforcement.
- Strength can be tailored to end-use requirements by directional placement of individual plies of reinforcement, such as 0°/90°/60°/60°/90°/0° or 0°/45°/45°/0°.
- Mechanical properties of discontinuous-fiber-reinforced composites (chopped-fiber or chopped-fabric molding compounds) are usually substantially lower than those of continuous-filament-reinforced composites.
- Properties of composites made from molding compounds are generally omnidirectional in the plane of the part, unless flow in molding causes directional orientation of the reinforcing fibers.

Some data references for resin-fiber composites may not give fiber percentage by volume or weight, fiber length or diameter, resin type, supplier, or cure cycle. Despite the fact that complete data on these general properties are unavailable, the information given is intended to inform the engineer of the effects of fiber reinforcement. For individual applications of a fiber-resin composite, specific property data must be generated for design analysis, as well as to assist in manufacturing processes. More data references are available from raw material suppliers, the research and development laboratories of the user corporation, contract laboratories that ser-

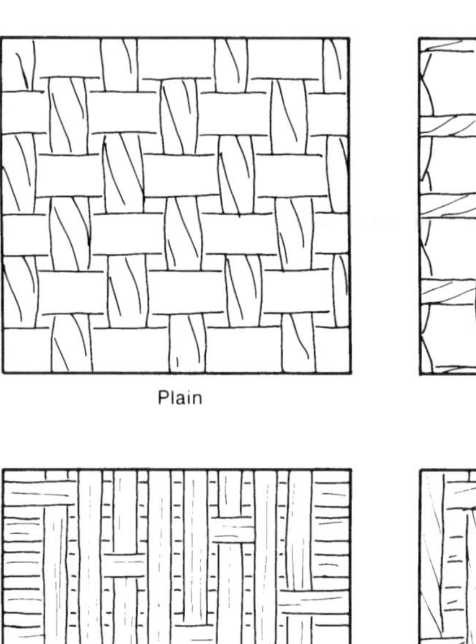

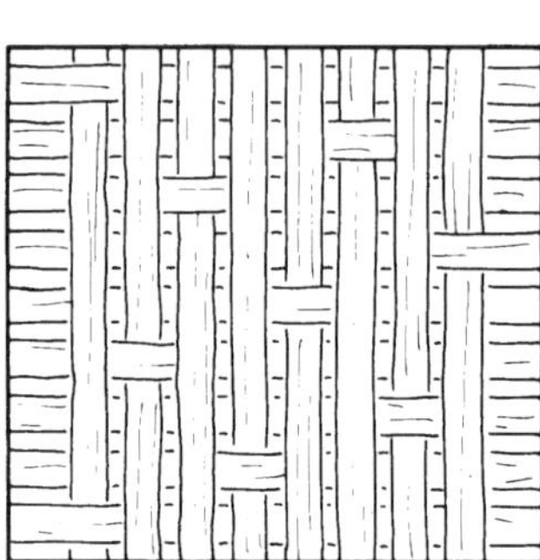

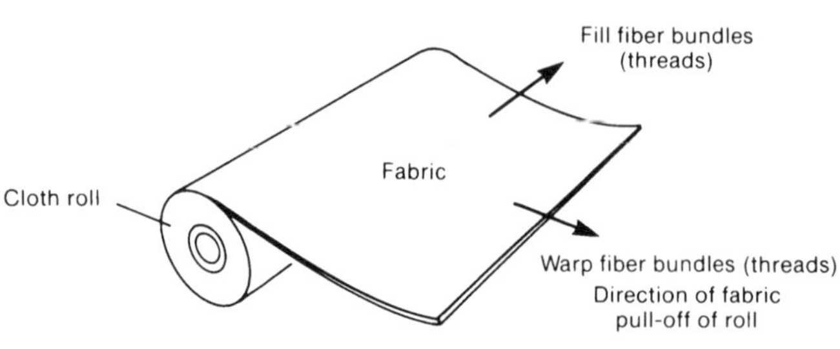

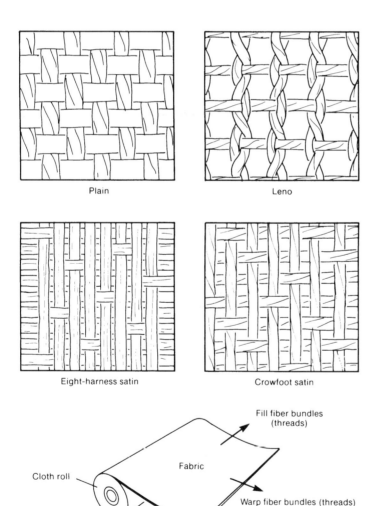

Fig. 2 Typical fabric weaves. Source: J.P. Stevens & Company, Inc.

Table 1 Important fiber-resin composite properties

Physical
Specific gravity
Density
Mechanical
Tensile strength
Tensile modulus
Poisson's ratio
Compressive strength
Compressive modulus
Shear strength
Shear modulus
Thermal
Coefficient of thermal expansion
Thermal conductivity
Specific heat
Elecrical
Dielectric constant
Dielectric strength
Dissipation factor
Volume resistivity
In-service conditions
Service temperature
Thermogravimetric analysis (stability temperature)
Temperature allowed on all standard loads
Flammability resistance
EMI/RFI protection

EMI/RFI, electromagnetic interference/radio-frequency interference

vice government and industry needs, and unclassified or nonproprietary documents. Basic material property data on a specific design application can be obtained by making a request to these information sources or by obtaining the necessary classification clearance, although designers will have to "flesh out" the data by property testing in their own test laboratories.

This article also contains descriptions and data that characterize each generic material according to its composition and method of manufacture. Because the composition and manufacture of virtually all materials are subject to change by their manufacturers, a composite may bear the same name for several years, but its mechanical and thermal properties may be modified appreciably.

Data sets for a particular material property may contain a single allowable curve. The curve and its extrapolation are based on knowledge of the material combined with engineering judgment. For this article, no attempt was made to derive an analytical function through the data set.

To assess properties, these factors need to be considered:

- Major axis of directionality
- Type of fabrication for component
- Fiber or fabric type, length, and fiber percentage by weight or volume
- Fiber finish and strength; fabric weave pattern
- Number of filaments and twist in fiber bundle
- Resin type and manufacturer
- Resin-to-fiber ratio, percent of filler, percent of volatile content, and percent of resin flow
- Test panel preparation and cure
- Test specimen preparation, test method, and number of tests
- Test specimen design, test fixture, and load ratio
- Test specimen condition, dry or wet

Axes Definitions, Symbols, and Special Property Calculations

Because composite materials can have different properties in each of the three directions, definitions of test axes are very important. Each test axis is defined as 1, 2, or 3 for unidirectional fiber, fabric, and fiber or cut-fabric molding compounds, as shown in Fig. 3. Directions 1 and 2 are usually either the direction of the fiber reinforcement or the direction transverse to the fiber, while direction 3 is perpendicular to the fiber or fabric layers, or across ply. Composite material shapes also have directional properties as illustrated in Fig. 3(d), with direction 1 being axial or longitudinal, direction 2 being hoop or circumferential, and direction 3 being radial or transverse. Figure 3(b), for example, indicates that ultimate tensile strength, with ply, could be expressed as σ_{tu1}, σ_{tu2}, σ_{tu12}.

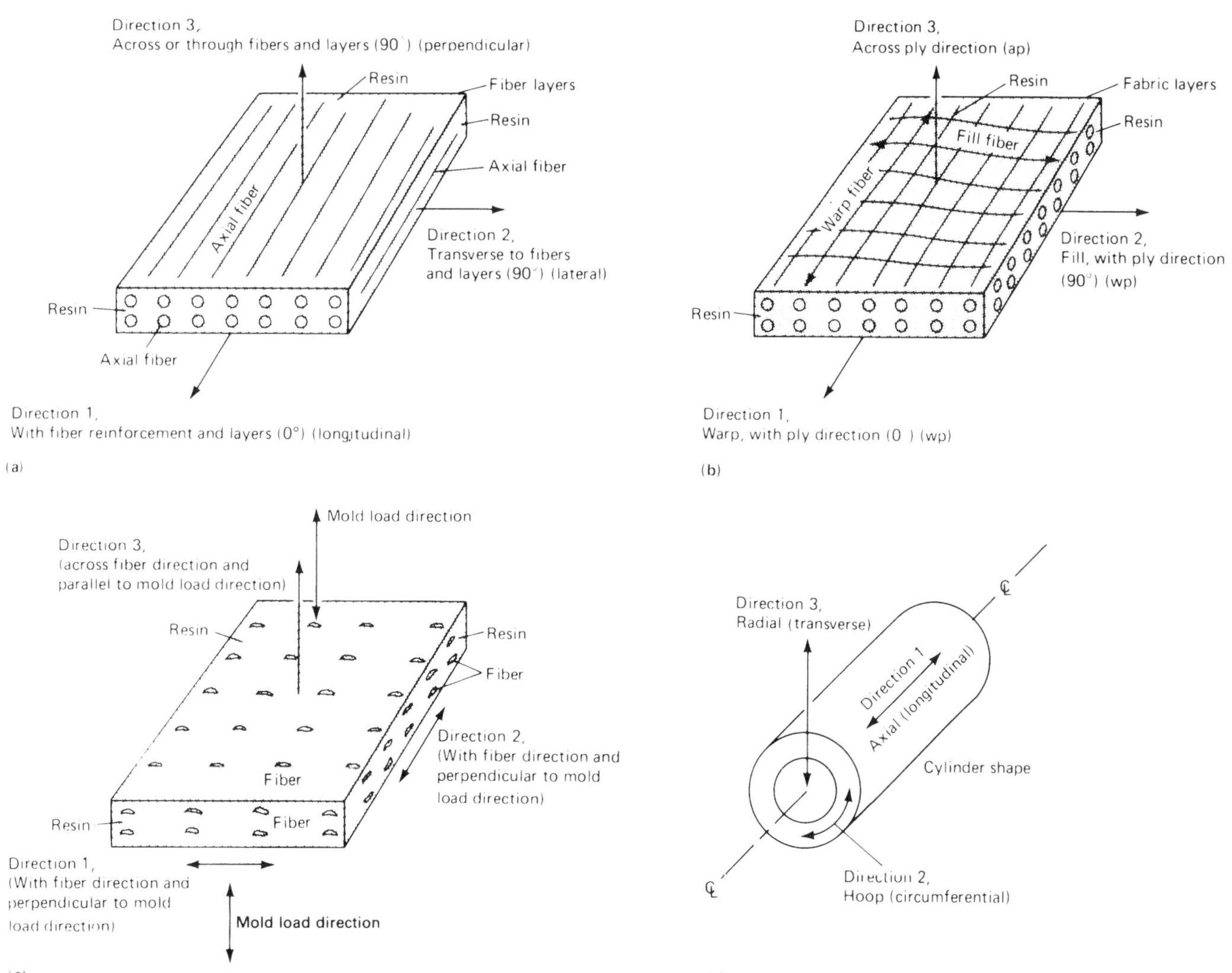

Fig. 3 Definitions of test axes for various composite types. (a) Unidirectional continuous fiber-resin composites (filament wind, tape lay-down, pultrusion). (b) Fabric-resin composites (tape wrap, lay-up). (c) Chopped fiber or fabric-resin molding compounds. (d) Shape components

For Poisson's ratio, ν, numeric subscripts are used:

$$\nu_{12} = \frac{\text{Strain in direction 2}}{\text{Strain in direction 1}}$$

where direction 1 is tension loaded and direction 2 is perpendicular to load application. Poisson's ratio, by convention, is expressed as a positive number even though the strain is actually a negative value, because most material shrink in the lateral direction when stretched in the longitudinal direction.

The coefficient of thermal expansion, α, is defined in Fig. 4 as the slope of the secant line from a reference temperature (20 °C or 70 °F, no expansion) to the expansion or contraction at the temperature of interest.

Definitions of the electrical properties used as standards for comparison of resins, fibers, and resin-fiber composites are:

- *Dielectric:* An insulating medium between two conductors to store and release energy
- *Dielectric constant:* Pure number indicating capability to store energy per unit volume
- *Dielectric strength:* The voltage that an insulating material of a given thickness can withstand before breakdown occurs
- *Volume (electrical) resistivity:* The electrical resistance between opposite faces of a unit cube of material
- *Dissipation factor (power factor) or loss tangent:* Multiplier used with apparent power to determine how much of the supplied power is available for use, that is, a measure of power loss in the material
- *Electromagnetic interference/radio-frequency interference (EMI/RFI) protection:* Provided by a material that will conduct an electrical signal away from the component that needs shielding or dissipate a localized electrical strike over a large surface area

The introduction of carbon fibers to all resin composite material will ensure a better EMI/RFI protective characteristic.

The definition of flammability characteristics of plastic materials is given by Underwriters' Laboratory (UL) rating tests for flammability of plastic materials. A typical test specimen for all ratings is 125 mm (5 in.) long by 12.7 mm (½ in.) wide by 12.7 mm (½ in.) thick. A Bunsen burner is applied at one end of a specimen that is held at the opposite horizontal or vertical end. Table 2 identifies the specifications for flammability ratings. Generally, a UL 94 V-0 rating is satisfactory, while 94 HB, 94 V-1, and 94 V-2 are less satisfactory. A 94 V-5 is the highest rating.

Overview of Constituent Materials

For a standard composite panel or structural shape, the ratio of matrix material to the fiber reinforcement ranges approximately from 1:2 to 2:1. The fiber is the main tailoring element for the design properties, while fiber orientation and fillers can provide secondary fine tuning for the product application.

The resin matrix provides stable dimensional control to the fiber laminate, a small participating component for properties, and a shear resistance between reinforcing fibers. A coupling agent enhances resin matrix-to-fiber bonding, while the filler can fine tune such properties as density, cost/pound, processing viscosity, strength, and flame-retardant characteristics.

Reinforcing-fiber characteristics such as density; fiber diameter, strength, and modulus; fiber filament bundle size; and woven-fiber fabric type or chopped-fiber form are initially optimized approximately by the "rule of mixtures" to help meet the composite properties needed for the design application engineering criteria for product operation and performance.

In addition, the selection of the ratio of matrix to reinforcement constituents is influenced by the loading patterns to the product, environmental operating conditions, the standard manufacturing-processing methods, reinforcement forms, costs, and completion time for the particular company and industry.

Currently, twelve or more fiber-reinforcement systems are available for resin-matrix composite fabrication into industrial, commercial, and aerospace products. Figure 5 shows a comparison of the properties of four of the most widely used fiber types: glass, aramid, carbon, and graphite. Density ranges from 1.44 to 2.48 g/cm³, strength from a minimum of 2200 MPa (320 ksi) to a maximum of 4585 MPa (665 ksi), modulus from 85 to 345 GPa (12 to 50 × 10^6 psi), and service-temperature capability in inert atmospheres from 500 to 3040 °C (930 to 5500 °F).

More detailed property data for fibers are provided in the article "Introduction to Reinforcing Fibers" and in the articles on specific fiber types in the Section "Constituent Materials" in this Volume.

Resin systems include at least 36 types or hybrid combinations, divided into thermoplastics (heat affected) or thermoset (heat permanently cured) divisions. The baseline room-temperature properties and service temperatures of three thermoplastic and three thermosetting resins in Fig. 6 show the ranges of density from 1.14 to 1.43 g/cm³, tensile strength from 53 to 112 MPa (7.7 to 16.2 ksi), tensile modulus from 875 to 4135 MPa (127 to 600 ksi), and service temperature from 130 to 370 °C (266 to 700 °F).

Table 2 Burn test criteria for Underwriters' Laboratory flammability ratings

Rating test	Specimen	Burn criteria(a)
94HB	Horizontal	<38 mm (1.5 in)/min burn for 3–13 mm (0.120–0.500 in. thickness
		<75 mm (3.0 in.)/min burn for <3 mm (0.120 in.) thickness
		No burn >100 mm (4.0 in.) specimen length
94 V-0	Veritcal	<10 s burn after each of two FA
		<50 s burn for 10 FA
		No total burn of specimen
		No dripping burn of cotton 305 mm (12 in.) below specimen
94 V-1	Vertical	<30 s after second FA
		<30 s burn after each of two FA
		<25 s burn for 10 FA
		No total burn of specimen
		No dripping burn of cotton 305 mm (12 in.) below specimen
84 V-2	Vertical	<60 s glow after second FA
		<30 s burn after each of two FA
		<290 s burn for 10 FA
		No total burn of specimen
		Brief dripping burn of cotton 305 mm (12 in.) below specimen
95 V-5	Vertical	<60 s glow after second FA
		<60 s burn after fifth FA
		No drip specimens

(a) FA flame applications, 10 s

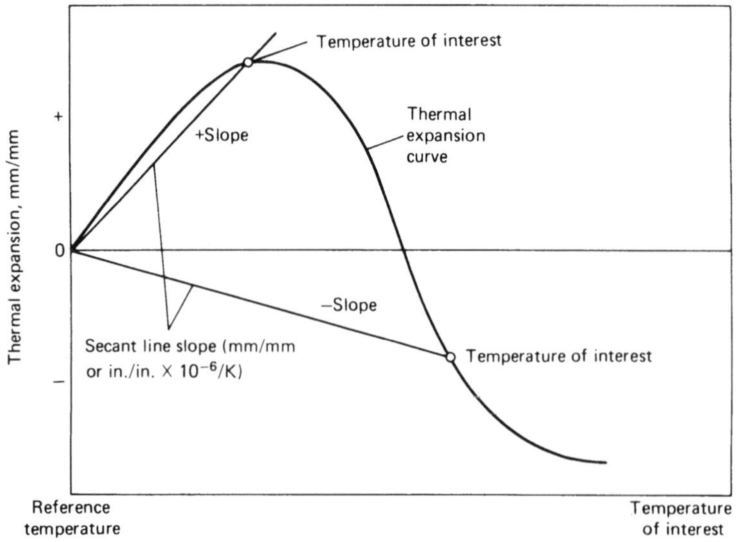

Fig. 4 Coefficient of thermal expansion is calculated as the slope of the secant line between the reference temperature (room temperature) and the temperature of interest. 10^{-6}/K × 5/9 = μin./in. × °F

Most matrix materials commonly used are preformulated at the supplier for the preimpregnated fiber, resin, curing agent, and coupling system. However, the manufacturer will often add small amounts of a filler to aid in the processing; change surface texture, color, and thermal and electrical conductivity; provide moisture resistance; and serve as an antioxidant. Modifications to the composition, however, must be tested for compatibility and successful cure processing to achieve properties tailored to meet specific product performance and service operation requirements.

Additional data on neat and reinforced resins are provided in the following sections in this article and in the Section "Constituent Materials" in this Volume.

Thermoplastic-Matrix Composites

Thermoplastic Polyester Resins and Fiber-Resin Composites (Ref 1–11). Three polyester resin systems—aromatic copolymers, polybutylene terephthalate (PBT), and polyethylene terephthalate (PET)—are used to describe the family of properties of thermoplastic polyester resins (Table 3, Fig. 7 to 14). Short-length glass and carbon-fiber reinforcements of up to 55% of the fiber-resin composite are used to improve or alter the properties in molding compounds. The UL service temperature of the unfilled resins ranges from 120 to 240 °C (253 to 474 °F). Applications are electrical/electronic components, chemical processing and oil field equipment, aerospace and transportation vehicles, appliance and consumer products, furniture, and bottles for toiletries and food products. More information on these resin systems is available in the articles "Thermoplastic Resins" and "Thermoplastic Composites Manufacturing" in this Volume.

Thermoplastic Polyamide Resins and Fiber-Resin Composites (Ref 12, 13). Some variations of polyamide (nylon) resin include alloys of polyolefin and other copolymers to tailor properties for specific uses. The melt point varies with the different product families but is between 212 to 270 °C (414 to 518 °F). Polyamide resins are discussed further in the article "Thermoplastic Resins" in this Volume. Short-length carbon and glass-fiber reinforcements of up to 43% of the fiber-resin composite are used to alter or improve the properties in molding compounds. The range of properties listed in Table 4 and shown in Fig. 15 to 24 include unreinforced and reinforced polyamide resin systems.

It should be noted that because all nylons pick up moisture, final design properties and dimensions will change depending on the relative humidity.

Thermoplastic Polysulfone Resins and Fiber-Resin Composites (Ref 8, 14, 15). Polysulfone resin exhibits the highest service temperature (150 to 205 °C, or 300 to 400 °F) of any melt-processable thermoplastic. The resin is strong, noted for high heat deflection temperatures, and stable in the presence of moisture. Care must be taken not to expose material to excessive ultraviolet rays or organic solvents. Polysulfone resins are discussed further in the article "Thermoplastic Resins" in this Volume. Glass-fiber reinforcements of up to 40% of the fiber-resin composite are used to alter properties. Property values listed in Table 5 and shown in Fig. 25 to 34 include resin with and without reinforcement. Applications include medical instrumentation, food processing equipment, chemical processing equipment, camera and watch cases, automotive and aerospace components, and water purification devices.

Thermoset-Matrix Composites

Thermoset Polyester Resins and Fiber-Resin Composites (Ref 1, 8, 16–23). Thermoset polyesters are low-temperature resins generally produced from the reaction of an organic alcohol (glycol) with both a saturated (isophthalic) and an unsaturated (maleic or fumaric) organic acid. The polyester is then dissolved in a liquid reactive monomer such as styrene, and the solutions are sold as polyester resins. Some polyesters are supplied as pellets or granular solids, and some are premixed with glass fiber for bulk molding compounds (BMCs) or sheet molding compounds (SMCs). Polyester resins with fiber reinforcements can be formulated to provide different mechanical, thermal, electrical, and flammability properties.

Because of their low cost, ease of processing, and good performance characteristics, unsaturated polyesters are the most extensively used type of thermoset resin. See Table 6 and Fig. 35 to 46 for properties. Unsaturated polyesters are generally combined with chopped, continuous, or woven glass fibers, as well as fillers and additives, to alter the properties to fit the application.

Thermoset polyesters are widely used in transportation, construction, electrical, and consumer products. In addition, the versatility of polyesters allows them to be used in a broad variety of processes. Through appropriate selection of the cross-linking initiator, these resins can be cured at any temperature from ambient to 175 °C (350 °F). Resin and glass fibers are combined at the "mold" in hand lay-up, spray-up, filament winding, pultrusion, and resin transfer molding. Both BMCs and SMCs, as well as other molding compounds, are used as input materials for compression, injection, and transfer molding processes. Because the fibers are not "preplaced" in the later molding operations, fiber orientation caused by molding compound flow can produce variable anisotropy in the finished parts. Molding compounds are available from many manufacturers.

Thermoset Phenolic Resins and Fiber-Resin Composites (Ref 1, 18, 24–42). Pheno-

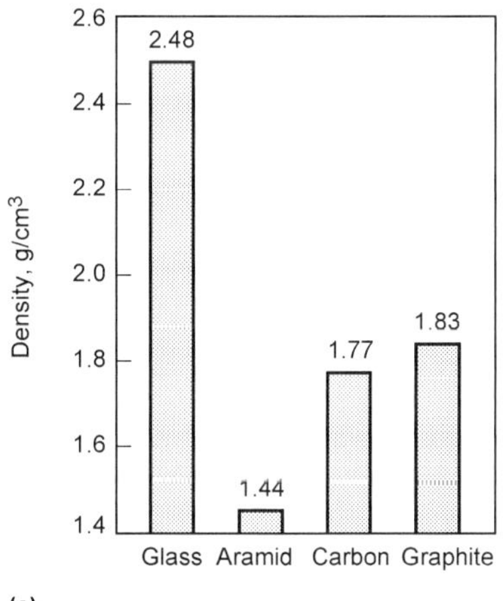

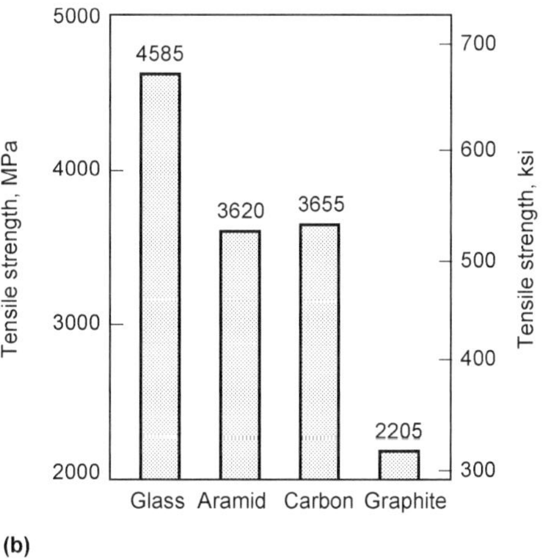

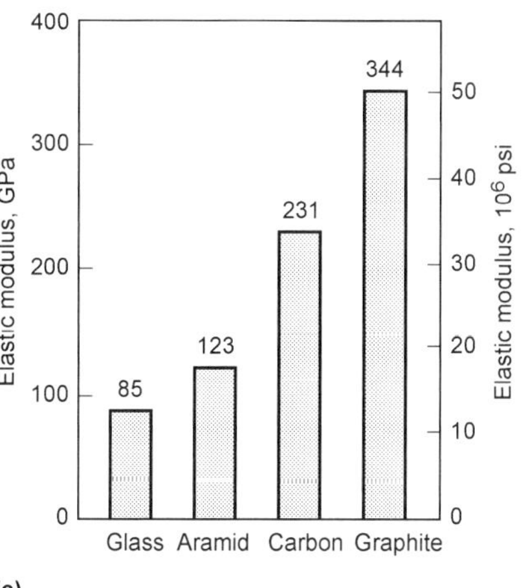

Fig. 5 Mechanical properties of selected reinforcement fibers. Inorganic fibers: glass (maximum temperature 970 °C, or 1780 °F) and aramid (maximum temperature 500 °C, or 930 °F). Organic fibers: carbon (maximum temperature 2500 °C, or 4500 °F) and graphite (maximum temperature 3000 °C, or 5500 °F). (a) Density. (b) Tensile strength. (c) Elastic modulus

lic resin systems are medium-temperature thermoset resins formulated from the reaction between phenol and formaldehyde. The two main resin types are resoles and novolacs. Two-stage phenolic resins (novolacs) are used for general-purpose molding compounds, while hybrids of the novolacs are used as impregnating resins with glass, carbon, and graphite cloth for tape wrapping or hand lay-up of aerospace components, rocket nozzle ablative, and insulation liners. Chopped-fiber molding compounds are used mostly in the automotive, appliance, and electrical component markets. General characteristics of these materials that make them suited for the previously mentioned applications are high service temperatures, good electrical properties, excellent moldability and dimensional stability, and good moisture resistance.

The following sections of this article describe three types of tapes for tape wrapping and lay-ups: glass fabric-phenolic tape, carbon fabric-phenolic tape, and graphite fabric-phenolic tape.

Table 7 and Fig. 47 to 64 give specific mechanical, thermal and electrical properties for each type of phenolic resin thermoset. Physical properties are identified in the table, but some test data and references are described in the following sections.

Glass-fabric-reinforced phenolic resin is used for lay-ups, tape wrapping, and molding compounds in the chopped cloth (12.7 mm × 12.7 mm, or ½ in. × ½ in.) version.

Carbon-fabric-reinforced phenolic resin reinforcement materials include the base fiber, which is a special variation of high-tenacity rayon tire cord reinforcement, pitch fibers, and polyacrylonitrile fibers. The base fiber is woven into plain leno, and satin weaves and subsequently carbonized at below 1650 °C (3000 °F). Polyacrylonitrile fibers are processed in much the same way as rayon, but in the base process the pitch fibers are carbon, which need no further carbonization after cloth weaving. The material is supplied either as a broad goods roll that is 965 to 1200 mm (38 to 48 in.) wide and approximately 20 to 45 kg (50 to 100 lb) per roll, or as a slit tape roll width. The raw material is used for hand lay-ups, tape wrapping, and molding compounds in the chopped cloth (12.7 mm × 12.7 mm, or ½ in. × ½ in.) version.

The tensile, compressive, and shear (strength and modulus) mechanical properties decrease in value with an increase in temperature.

The conductivity and specific heat thermal properties increase with a temperature increase. The coefficient of thermal expansion (CTE) with the ply has the same characteristics versus temperature, except for a decrease around 540 °C (1000 °F) due to the phenolic weight loss and conversion to a carbon char. The CTE across the ply, directly related to the phenolic resin, increases to 400 °C (750 °F), decreases to 815 ° (1500 °F), then increases again to 1926 °C (3500 °F).

No electrical properties are currently available, because carbon fabric phenolic is too highly conductive for most electrical industry applications.

Graphite-fabric-reinforced phenolic resin is manufactured in a manner similar to that for the carbon fabric-phenolic resin, except that the rayon-based fabric is graphitized at over 2205 °C (4000 °F). Graphitization at a higher temperature stabilizes the fabric from further thermal shrinkage at application temperatures (about 3315 °C, or 6000 °F) in aerospace components and rocket nozzles, increases thermal conductivity, and lowers the strength levels.

Mechanical, thermal, and electrical properties of graphite-fabric-reinforced phenolic resin are much the same as for the carbon-fabric-reinforced type.

Additional information is provided in the article "Phenolic Resins" in this Volume.

Thermoset Epoxy Resins and Fiber-Resin Composites (Ref 1, 8, 43–65). Epoxies are high-strength, medium-temperature resin systems that can be formulated into compounds, such as diglycidyl ether of bisphenol A (DGEBA); multifunctional epoxies, such as phenolic novolac; and aliphatic epoxies, such as cycloaliphatic. Temperatures up to 230 to 260 °C (450 to 500 °F) can be used for the latter two types of resin systems for short periods of time. At 540 °C (1000 °F), the hydrogen and oxygen have been driven off, leaving a weak carbonaceous char. Reinforced epoxy structures provide high strength-to-weight ratios and good thermal and electrical properties. Filament winding and machine or hand lay-up processes are used for advanced aircraft fuselages, wing and control surface panels, rocket motor cases, rocket nozzle structural shells, and commercial pressure vessels, tanks, and pipe. Glass fiber-fabric, carbon, graphite, quartz, and aramid fibers are used in molding compounds, hand lay-ups, and fiber-fabric prepreg composites for different applications to match pressure, temperature, service life, weight, and cost requirements (Ref 1, 8, 43).

This section focuses on seven fabric forms:

- Epoxy resin with and without E-glass fiber reinforcement
- Glass-fabric-reinforced epoxy resin
- S-glass-fiber-reinforced epoxy resin
- Quartz-fabric-reinforced epoxy resin
- Kevlar-49-fiber-reinforced epoxy resin
- Carbon-fiber-reinforced (T300) epoxy resin
- Graphite-fiber-reinforced (HM) epoxy resin

Table 8 shows specific characteristics of several of these materials, including specific gravity, useful temperatures, and reinforcement percentage. The remaining mechanical, thermal, and electrical properties are shown in Fig. 65 to 97.

Epoxy Resin with and without Reinforcement Fibers, and Molding Compounds. Epoxy resin characterization includes DGEBA, phenolic novolac, and aliphatic epoxies without fibers or fillers, as well as other resin systems with glass-fiber reinforcement or asbestos fibers and aluminum filler.

Glass-fabric-reinforced epoxy resin, used as a lay-up, provides a structural material with a large variety of epoxies and at least two glass fibers (E and S). Characterization includes mechanical, thermal, and electrical properties.

S-glass-fiber-reinforced epoxy resin is used as a filament-winding prepreg to manufacture pressure vessels, tanks, tubes, and cones. Characterization includes mechanical, thermal, and limited electrical properties.

Kevlar-49-fiber- and fabric-reinforced epoxy resin is used as a lay-up fabric for boats, aircraft surface panels, and electrical circuit boards. The fiber prepreg is also used in filament winding pressure vessels, tanks, tubes, and cone shapes.

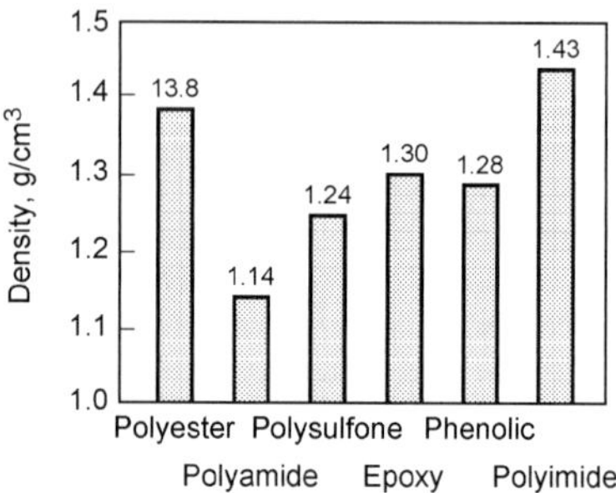

(a)

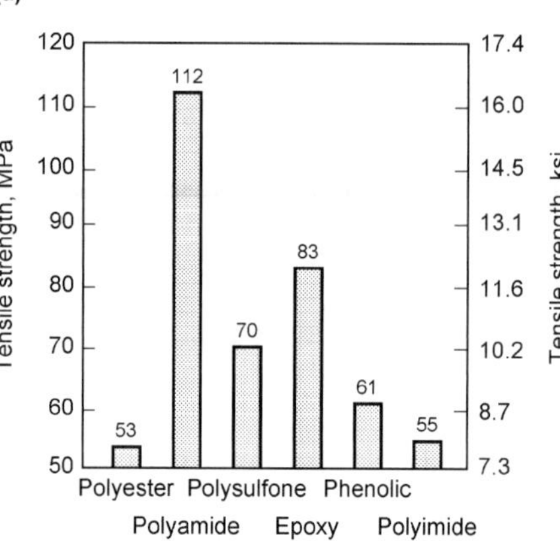

(b)

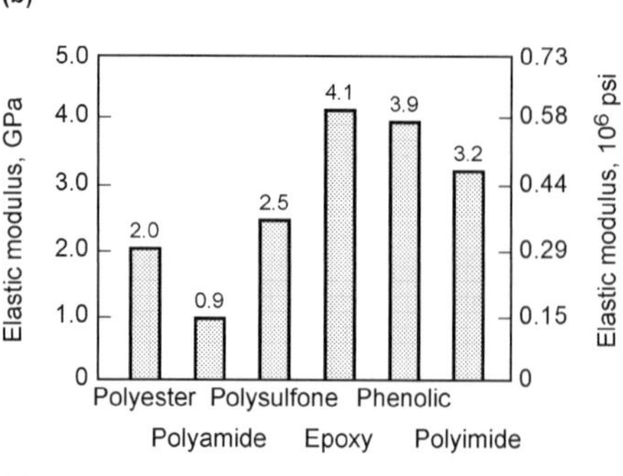

(c)

Fig. 6 Mechanical properties of selected matrix resins. Thermoplastics: polyester (unfilled; maximum temperature 140 °C, or 284 °F), polyamide (nylon 6/6, unfilled; maximum temperature 130 °C, or 266 °F), and polysulfane (standard; maximum temperature 160 °C, or 320 °F). Thermosets: epoxy (unfilled; maximum temperature 260 °C, or 500 °F), phenolic (unfilled; maximum temperature 230 °C, or 450 °F), and polyimide (unfilled; maximum temperature 370 °C, or 700 °F). (a) Density. (b) Tensile strength. (c) Elastic modulus

Carbon-fiber- and fabric-reinforced epoxy resin is reinforced with carbon fibers to form unidirectional prepreg tapes suitable for filament winding of components such as pressure vessels, tanks, and pipes, as well as shapes of revolution. It is also used for aircraft external structural panels and space structures.

Graphite-fiber-reinforced epoxy resin is reinforced with graphite fibers and supplied as unidirectional fiber prepreg tapes suitable for filament winding of components or as fabric prepreg rolls suitable for hand lay-ups.

Quartz-fabric-reinforced epoxy resin is reinforced with woven quartz (S/557 unidirectional fabric and S/581 eight-harness satin weave fabric).

Additional information is provided in the article "Epoxy Resins" in this Volume.

Thermoset Polyimide Resins and Fiber-Resin Composites (Ref 1, 8, 18, 66–72). Polyimide thermoset resins reinforced with fillers and short fibers are used as molding compound. In addition, continuous fibers or fabric that is preimpregnated with resin polymer is used for lay-ups, filament winding, and tape wrapping. Resin polymer is popular for its high-temperature characteristics (315 °C, or 600 °F), for long durations, and 480 °C, or 900 °F, for short durations), low-temperature properties at –195 °C (–320 °F) for long durations, and low creep and deflection under load at temperature. In addition, its electrical properties are excellent. Properties information is provided in Table 9 and in Fig. 98 to 104. Major applications are in the aerospace and electrical industries.

Additional information is provided in the articles "Polyimide Resins" and "High-Temperature Applications" in this Volume.

Thermoset Bismaleimide Resins and Fiber-Resin Composites (Ref 73–76). The bismaleimide thermoset resins, which may be cured at the lower epoxy cure temperature (175 °C, or 350 °F) and pressure (690 kPa, or 100 psi), do not have gaseous byproducts and thus provide void-free parts. They also offer a new polymer system to combine with various fiber types for improved composite designs. Table 10 and Fig. 105 to 108 show properties data. Applications include aerospace wing skin ribs, helicopter firewalls, and printed wiring boards.

Additional information is provided in the article "Bismaleimide Resins" in this Volume.

ACKNOWLEDGMENTS

The information in this article is largely taken from the Section "Forms and Properties of Composite Materials" in *Composites*, Volume 1, *Engineered Materials Handbook*, ASM International, 1987, p 353–415. The Section Chair was R.C. Laramee; contributors were R.G. Adams, R. Bacon, D. Beckley, P. Blanchard, R. Boudreau, D.L. Denton, L.E. DeShields, W.B. Hall, G.E. Hansen, K. Jacobs, J.R. Koenig, P.R. Langston, M.J. Michno, E.P. Rossa, M.E. Sauers, J.E. Theberge, and S. Witschen. The section "Overview of Constituent Materials" is adapted from R. Laramee, "Effects of Composition, Processing, and Structure on Properties of Composites," *Materials Selection and Design*, Volume 20, *ASM Handbook*, p 457–469.

REFERENCES

1. *Modern Plastics Encyclopedia*, Vol 62 (No. 10A), McGraw-Hill, 1985–1986
2. "Xydar—High Performance Engineering Resins, SRT-500, FC-Series," Dartco Manufacturing Inc.
3. E. Galli, New Thermoplastics Perform at Very High Temperatures, *Plast. Des. Forum*, March-April 1985
4. "Valox Engineering Thermoplastic Properties Guide," Plastics Group, Composite Polymers Products Department, General Electric Company
5. "Designing with Plastics," *Design Handbook*, DuPont Engineering Plastics Module IV Rynite, Polymer Products Department, E.I. DuPont de Nemours & Company, Inc.
6. Generic Thermoplastic Polyesters, 1986 Materials Reference Issue, *Mach. Des.*, 17 April 1986
7. "Carbon Fiber Reinforced Thermoplastic Composites," Engineering Plastics, LNP Corporation
8. Material Selector 1985, *Mater. Eng.*, Dec 1984
9. *The International Plastics Selector, Extruding and Molding Guides, Dest Top Data Bank*, Cordura, 1977
10. "Zytel Nylon Resins," General Guide to Products and Properties, DuPont Engineering Plastics, Polymer Products Department, E.I. DuPont de Nemours & Company, Inc.
11. "Carbon Fiber Reinforced Thermoplastic Composites," Engineering Plastics, LNP Corporation
12. "Nylon," *Modern Plastics Encyclopedia*, Vol 62 (No. 10A), McGraw-Hill, 1985–1986
13. H.R. Clausen, *Encyclopedia/Handbook of Materials, Parts and Finishes*, Technical Publishing, 1976
14. "Thermocomp—GF Series," LNP Corporation
15. "Udel-Polysulfone," Engineering Polymers Product Data, Union Carbide Corporation
16. "Industrial Glass Fabrics," Glass Fabrics Division, J.P. Stevens & Company, Inc.
17. D.L. Denton, "Mechanical Properties of an SMC-R 50 Composite," Owens-Corning Fiberglas Corporation, 1979
18. 1986 Materials Reference Issue, *Mach. Des.*, April 1986
19. "Plenco Molding Compounds," Plastics Engineering Company
20. "Fiberite Reinforced Molding Materials," Fiberite Corporation
21. "Plastics for Aerospace Vehicles," *Military Handbook 17A*, Department of Defense, Jan 1971
22. R.R. Barnet, "Evaluation of Glass Fabric Reinforced Plastic Laminates," Navord Report 2669, U.S. Naval Ordnance Laboratory, Jan 1953
23. S.S. Wang, D.P. Goetz, and H.T. Corten, *J. Compos. Mater.*, Vol 18 (No. 2), 1984
24. Resinox SC1008 Phenolic Product Data Sheets, Plastics Division, Monsanto Chemical Company
25. "Reinforced Molding Compounds," Fiberite Corporation
26. *1970 Guide to Plastics, Modern Plastics Encyclopedia*
27. G. Lubin, Ed., *Handbook of Fiberglass and Advanced Plastics Composites*, Van Nostrand Reinhold, 1969
28. K. Boller, "Tensile and Compressive Strength of Reinforced Plastic Laminates after Rapid Heating," Wright Air Development Division Report WADD-TR-60-804, Aug 1960
29. F.R. O'Brien and S. Oglesby, Jr., "Investigation of Thermal Properties of Plastic Laminates," Wright Air Development Center Report WADD-TR-54-306, 1955
30. *Military Handbook 17, Plastics for Flight Vehicles*, Department of Defense, June 1955
31. K. Boller, "Strength Properties of Reinforced Plastic Laminates at Elevated Temperatures," Wright Air Development Center Report WADD-TR-59-569, July 1959
32. "Mechanical Properties of MXB-6001 Phenolic Resin Impregnated Glass Cloth," Fiberite Corporation, May 1965
33. "Mechanical Properties of FM-5042 Glass Fabric Reinforced Prepreg Employing a MIL-R-92299 Resin," U.S. Polymeric Chemical Inc., June 1964
34. R.R. Barnet, "Evaluation of Glass Fabric Reinforced Plastic Laminates," Navord Report 2669, U.S. Naval Ordnance Laboratory, Jan 1953
35. L. Holliday, Ed., *Composite Materials*, Elsevier, 1966
36. Research and Development Laboratory Report LWR 278149, Morton Thiokol, Inc., Aug 1977
37. "Elevated Temperature Properties of Carbonaceous and Silica Fabric Reinforced Phenolic Composites," Table III, AGC MF-054, Aerojet General Company, 1964
38. "Various Mechanical and Thermal Properties of Carb-I-Tex and Carbon Phenolic," SoRI, for Lockheed Propulsion Laboratories, 1971
39. "Mechanical Properties Test Data Package," FM5064, FM5055, FM5014, U.S. Polymeric
40. "Subscale Ring Shearout Load Data," Report TWR-9071, Morton Thiokol, Inc., 1975
41. "Subscale Ring Shearout Test," Report TWR-20393, Morton Thiokol, Inc., 1977
42. Data Sheet, MXG175, MX4926, Fiberite Corporation

43. Epon 934 Product Data Sheet, Shell Chemical Company
44. Molding Compound Product Data Sheets, Fiberite Corporation
45. Epoxylite 5403 Product Data Sheets, Epoxylite Corporation
46. E-710 Data Sheet, U.S. Polymeric, 1965
47. "Thermal Conductivity for Nine Glass and Asbestos Reinforced Plastics," Research Paper FPL-36, U.S. Forest Service, Aug 1965
48. ANC-17, Plastics for Aircraft, June 1955
49. Short Beam Shear, Thiokol Laboratory Report, Morton Thiokol, Inc., Jan 1979
50. Short Beam Shear, Lockheed Laboratory Report, Lockheed Corporation, March 1979
51. M.L. White, "Design and Fabrication of an Improved Performance, Low Cost, Composite Main Rotor Blade for the Cobra Helicopter," Kaman Aerospace Corporation, 1977
52. W.T. Freeman and G.C. Kuebeler, Mechanical and Physical Properties of Advanced Composites, *Composite Materials: Testing and Design (Third Conference),* STP 546, American Society for Testing and Materials, 1974, p 435–456
53. L. Holliday, Ed., *Composite Materials,* Materials Science Series, Elsevier
54. "Data manual for Kevlar 49 Aramid," Textile Fibers Department, E.I. DuPont de Nemours & Company, Inc., 1974, 1986
55. "AS4/3502 Graphite Prepreg Tape and Fabric Module," Hercules, Inc.
56. Yeow et al., "On Time-Temperature Behaviour of Carbon-Epoxy," Fifth ASTM Conference Composite Materials, American Society for Testing and Materials
57. "Advanced Composite Development Studies of Graphite Epoxy," Lockheed Missiles and Space Company, Inc.
58. J.C. Ekvall and C.F. Griffin, Design Allowables for T300/5208 Graphite Epoxy Composite Materials, *J. Aircr.*, Vol 19 (No. 8), Aug 1982
59. D.N. Yates, R.D. Torczyner, and D.R. Sidewell, "Design and Development of Woven Structures Products for Aerospace Structures," paper presented at American Institute of Aeronautics and Astronautics/American Society of Mechanical Engineers/Society of Automotive Engineers 16th Structures, Structural Dynamics, and Materials Conference, Denver, May 1975
60. AS/3002, in *Advanced Composites Design Guide,* Vol IV, 3rd ed., 1973
61. W.T. Freeman and G.C. Kuebeler, Mechanical and Physical Properties of Advanced Composites, *Composite Materials: Testing and Design (Third Conference),* STP 546, American Society for Testing and Materials, 1974
62. "Magnamite Graphite Fibers," Hercules, Inc.
63. HM-HMS Graphite Epoxy Product Data Sheets, Hercules, Inc.
64. D.M. Mazenko and R.J. Milligan, "Epoxy For Structural Composites," SAMPE Technical Conference, Society for the Advancement of Material and Process Engineering, Oct 1980
65. Astro Quartz II Data Product Sheets, J.P. Stevens & Company, Inc.
66. "Thermid Polyimide Resin Product Sheets," National Starch and Chemical Corporation
67. "Vespel, Avimid Product Sheets," E.I. DuPont de Nemours & Company, Inc.
68. "Polyimide Molding Compounds," Fiberite Corporation
69. "Kinel Polyimide Molding Compounds," Rhone-Poulenc Inc.
70. Astroquartz Polyimide, *Military Handbook 17A,* Part 1, Sept 1973
71. R.V. Wolff and S.F. Monroe, Vacuum Cured Polyimide Laminate Properties, *SAMPE J.,* Aug-Sept 1969
72. W.T. Freeman and M.D. Campbell, Thermal Expansion Characteristics of Graphite Reinforced Composite Materials, *Composite Materials: Testing and Design (Second Conference),* STP 497, American Society for Testing and Materials, 1972
73. "'Compimide,' A Family of Bismaleimide Resins," The Boots Company
74. M.S. Hsu, T.S. Chen, J.A. Parker, and A.H. Heimbuch, NASA New Bismaleimide Matrix Resins for Graphite Fiber Composites, *SAMPE J.,* July-Aug 1985
75. M. Chaudhari, T. Galvin, and J. King, "Characterization of Bismaleimide System XU-292," Ciba-Geigy; also, Matrimid 5292 System, *SAMPE J.,* July-Aug 1985
76. "V-378A Addition Cured Bismaleimide Matrix Resin," and XV-388 Addition Cured Modified Bismaleimide Matrix Resin," Hitco

Table 3 Physical properties and service characteristics of thermoplastic polyester resins and resin-matrix composites

	Aromatic copolyester		PBT		PET	
Properties	Resin	40% glass fiber composite	Resin	15–40% glass fiber composite	Resin	30–45% glass fiber composite
Heat deflection temperature at 1820 kPa (264 psi), °C (°F)	355 (671)	. . .	55 (130)	205 (400)	. . .	225 (435)
UL in-service temperature rating, °C (°F)	240 (464)	. . .	120 (248)	140 (284)	140 (284)	150–180 (302–356)
Processing melt temperature, °C (°F)	400–450 (750–840)	. . .	270 (520)	. . .	290 (550)	. . .
Specific gravity	1.35	1.70	1.31	1.53	. . .	1.56–1.69
Density, g/cm³ (lb/in.³)	1.35 (0.049)	1.70 (0.061)	1.31 (0.047)	1.53 (0.055)	. . .	1.56–1.69 (0.056–0.061)
UL flammability rating	94 V 0	94 V-0	94 HV/94 V-0	94 HB/94 V-0	94 HB/94 V-0	94 HB/94 V-0

PBT, polybutylene terephthalate; PET, polyethylene terephthalate; UL, Underwriters' Laboratory

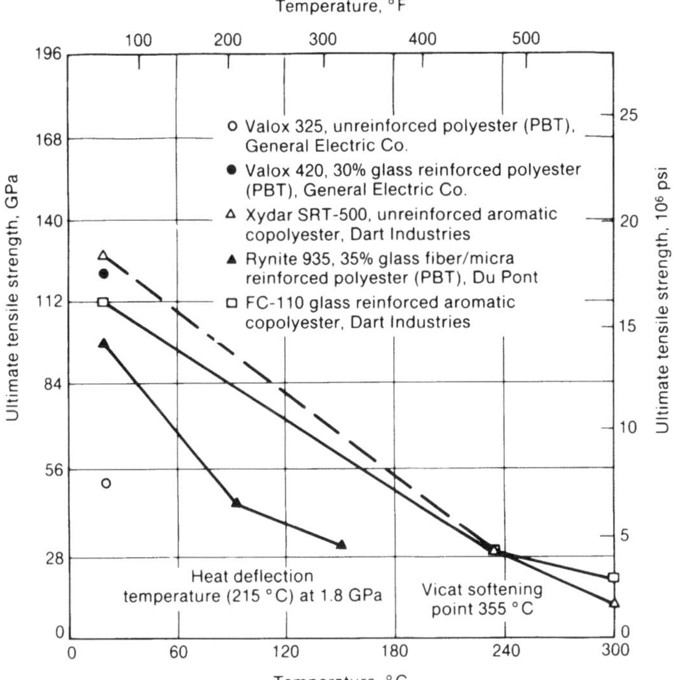

Fig. 7 Ultimate tensile strength versus temperature for thermoplastic polyester resin and resin-matrix composites

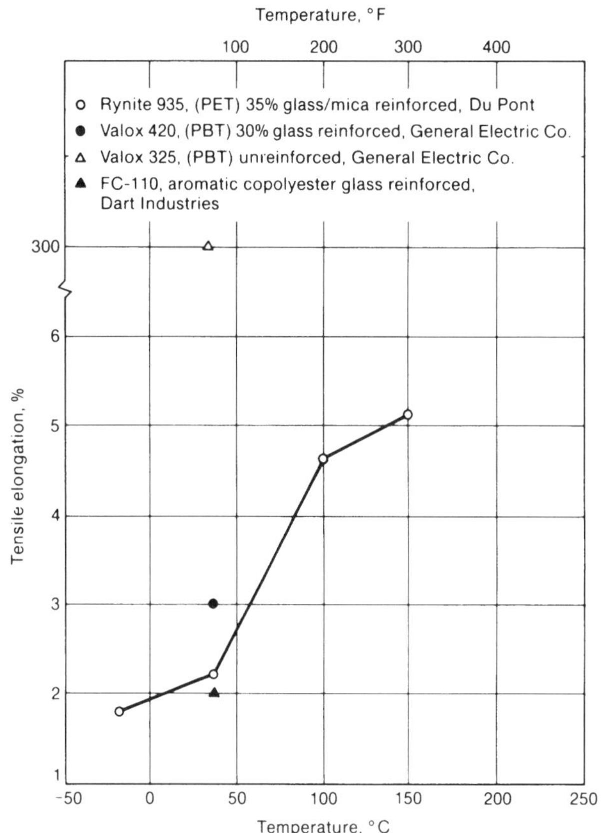

Fig. 8 Tensile elongation versus temperature for thermoplastic polyester resin and resin-matrix composites

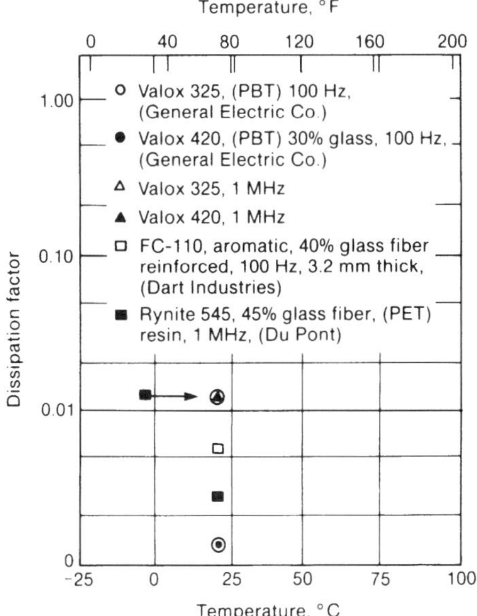

Fig. 9 Dissipation factor versus temperature for thermoplastic polyester resin and resin-matrix composites

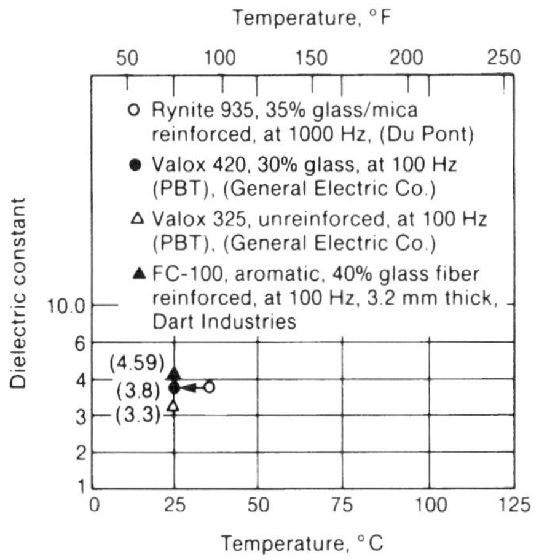

Fig. 10 Dielectric constant versus temperature for thermoplastic polyester resin and resin-matrix composites

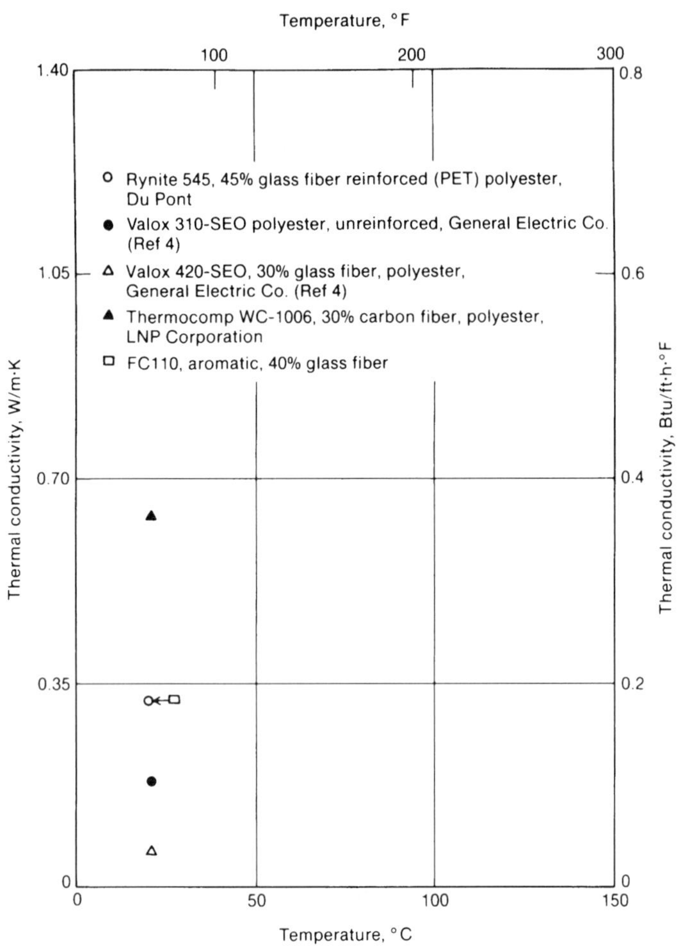

Fig. 11 Thermal conductivity versus temperature for thermoplastic polyester resin and resin-matrix composites

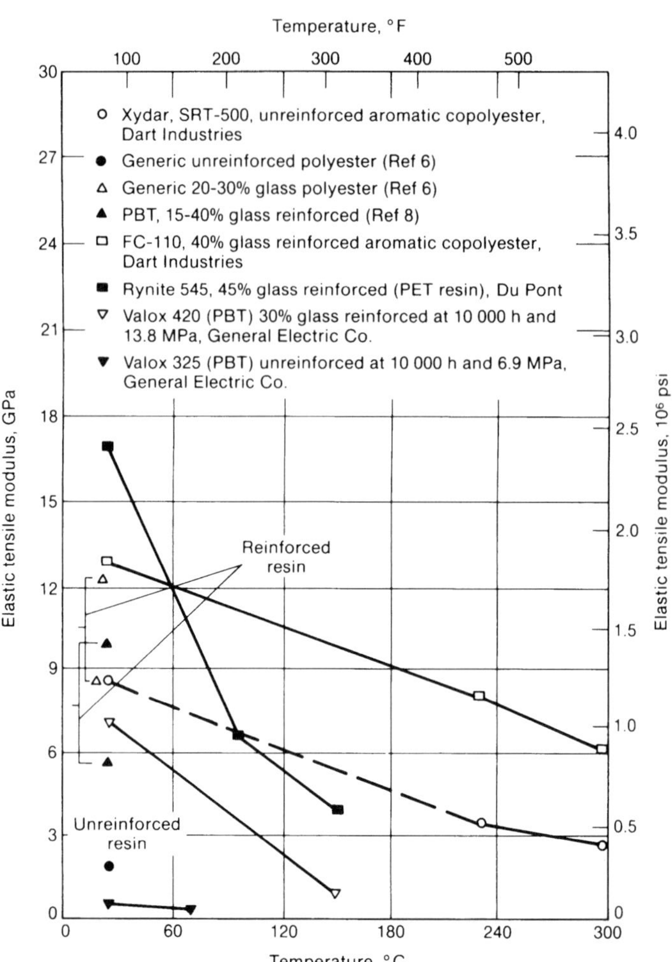

Fig. 12 Elastic tensile modulus versus temperature for thermoplastic polyester resin and resin-matrix composites

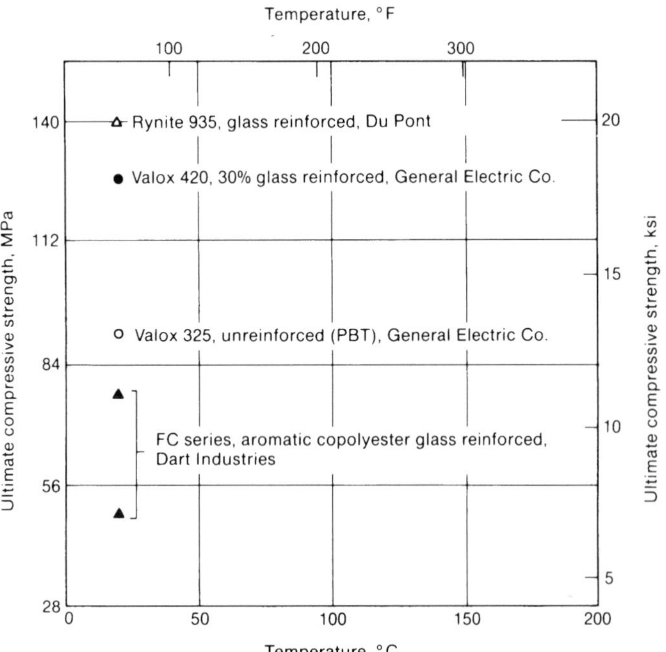

Fig. 13 Ultimate compressive strength versus temperature for thermoplastic polyester resin and resin-matrix composites

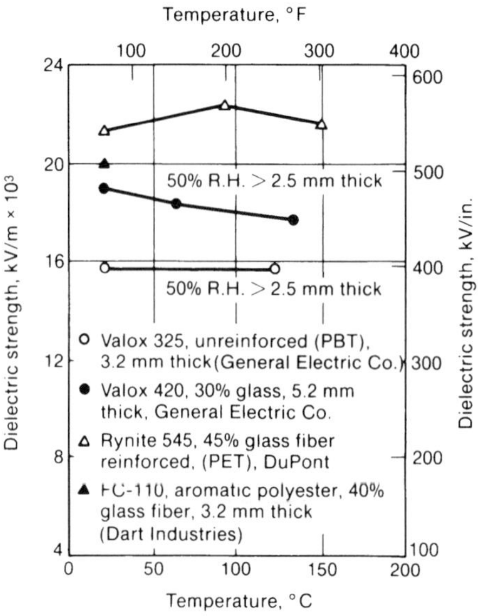

Fig. 14 Dielectric strength versus temperature for thermoplastic polyester and resin and resin-matrix composites. RH, relative humidity

Table 4 Physical properties and service characteristics of thermoplastic polyamide nylon 6/6 resin and fiber-resin composites

	Nylon 6/6		
Properties	Resin	30% carbon fiber composite	43% glass fiber composite
Specific gravity	1.14	1.28	1.51
Density, g/cm³ (lb/in.³)	1.14 (0.041)	1.28 (0.046)	1.51 (0.055)
UL in-service temperature rating, °C (°F)	130 max (266 max)	...	...
Heat deflection temperature at 1820 kPa (264 psi), °C (°F)	90 (194)	...	...
UL flammability rating	94 V-2	...	...

UL, Underwriters' Laboratory

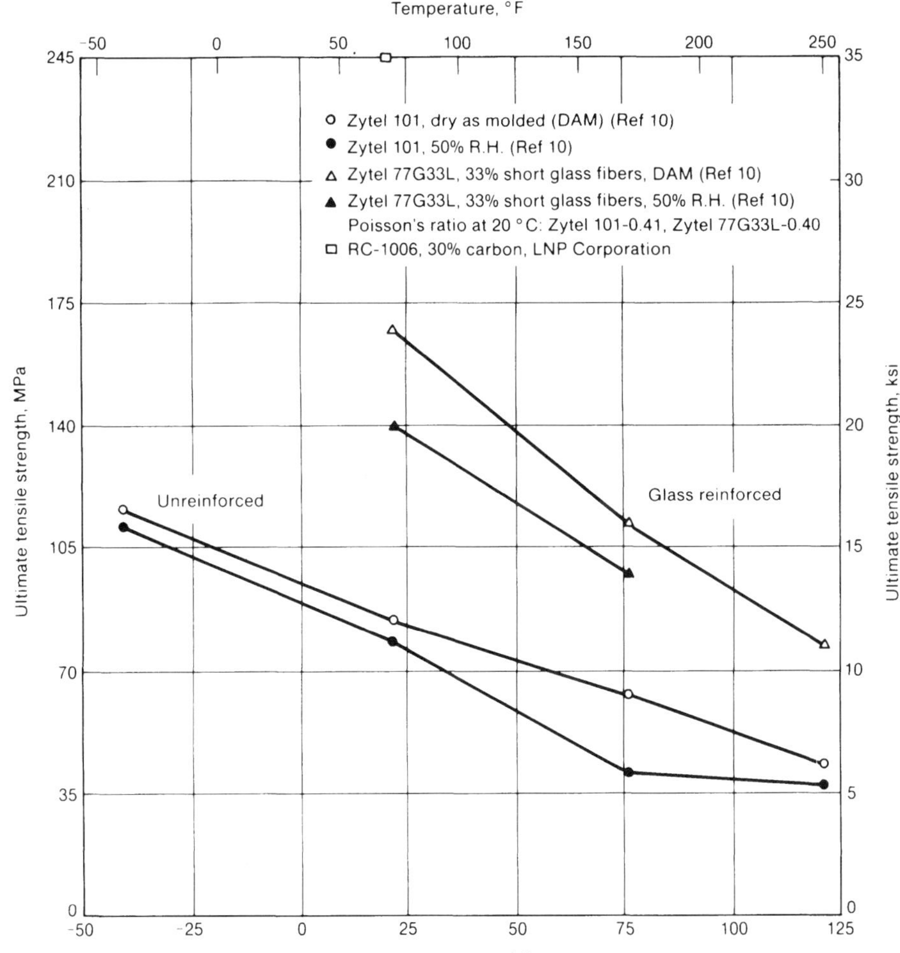

Fig. 15 Ultimate strength versus temperature for polyamide (nylon) resin and resin-matrix composites

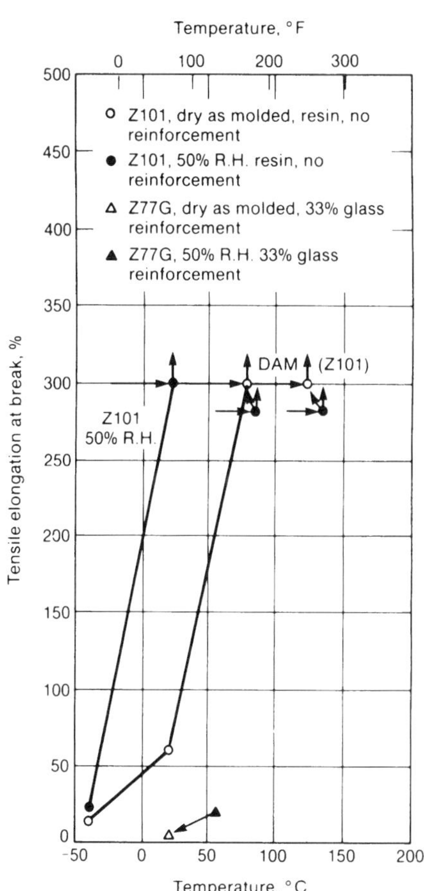

Fig. 16 Tensile elongation at break versus temperature for polyamide (nylon) resin and resin-matrix composites. DAM, dry as molded

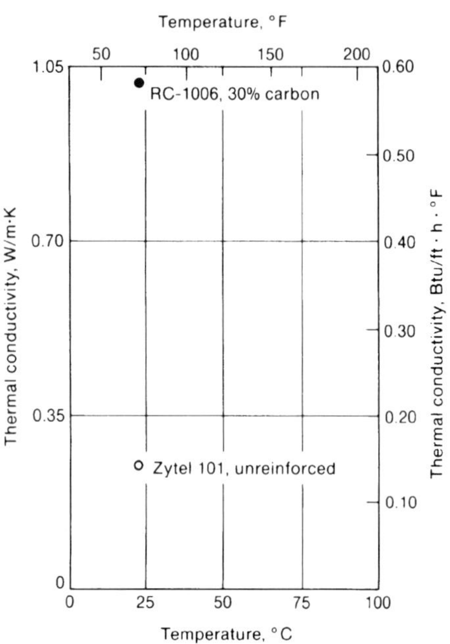

Fig. 17 Thermal conductivity versus temperature for polyamide (nylon) resin and resin-matrix composite

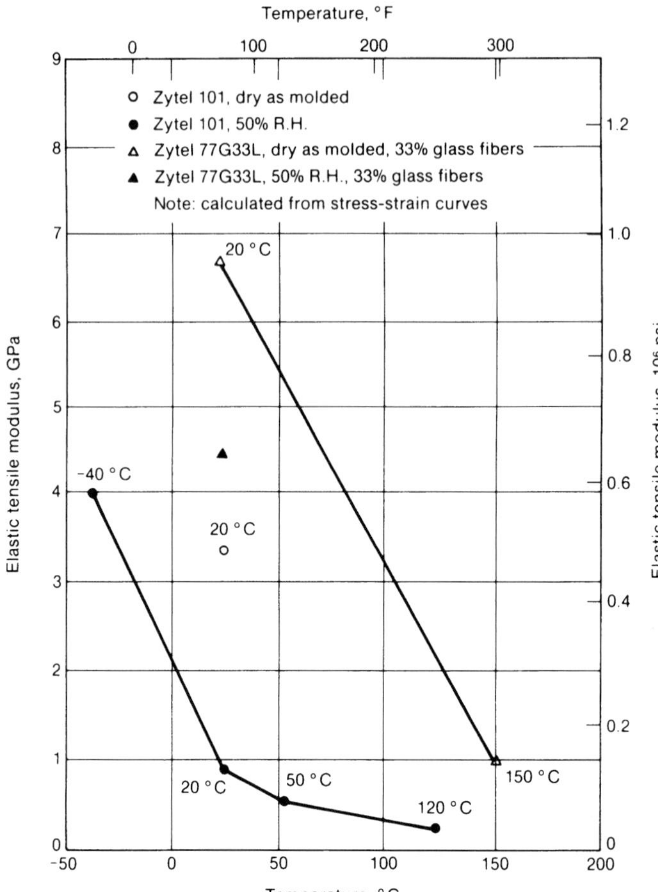

Fig. 18 Elastic tensile modulus versus temperature for polyamide (nylon) resin and resin-matrix composites

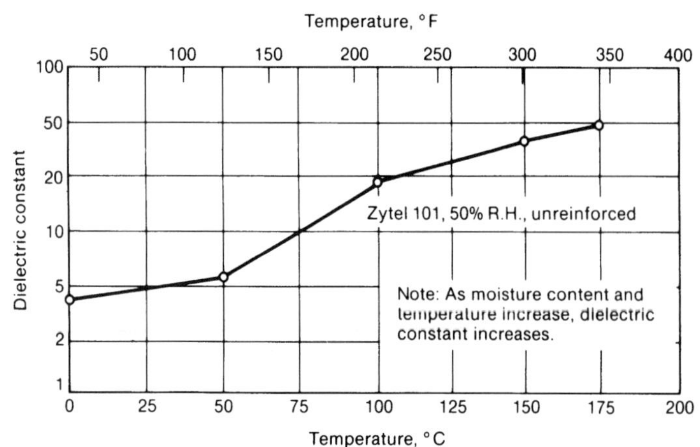

Fig. 19 Dielectric constant (100 Hz) versus temperature for unreinforced polyamide (nylon) resin

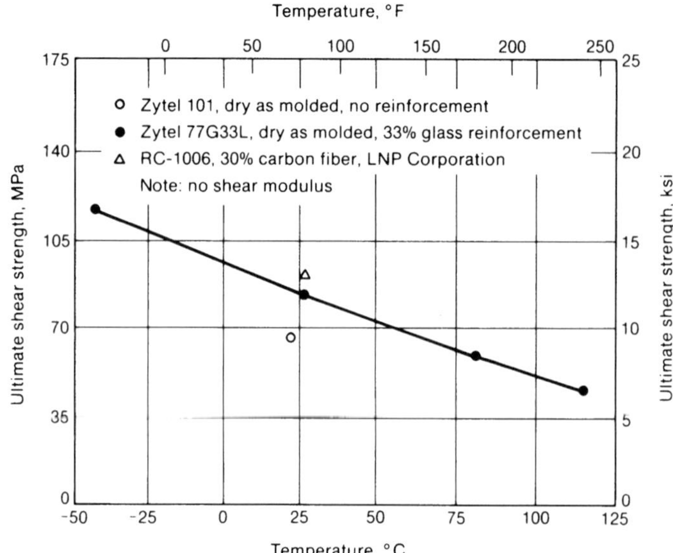

Fig. 20 Ultimate shear strength versus temperature for polyamide (nylon) resin and resin-matrix composites

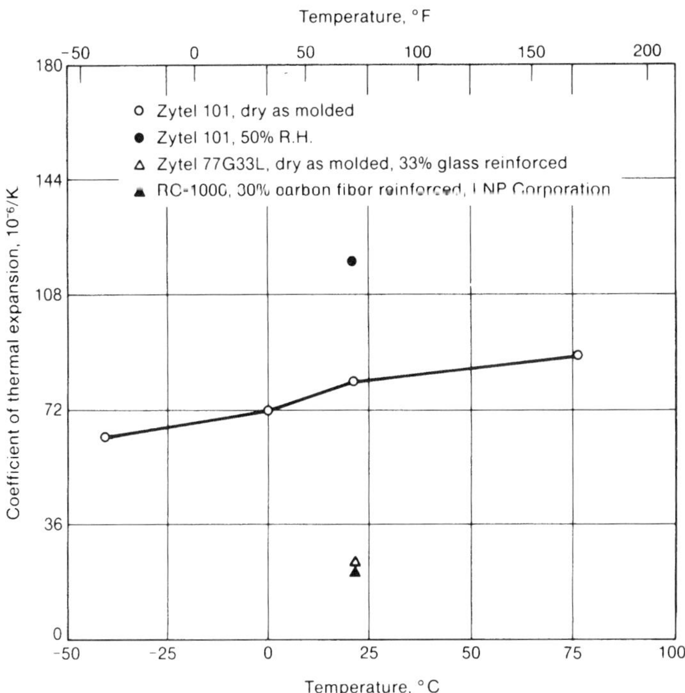

Fig. 21 Coefficient of thermal expansion versus temperature for polyamide (nylon) resin and resin-matrix composites. $10^{-6}/K \times \frac{5}{9} = \mu in./in. \times °F$

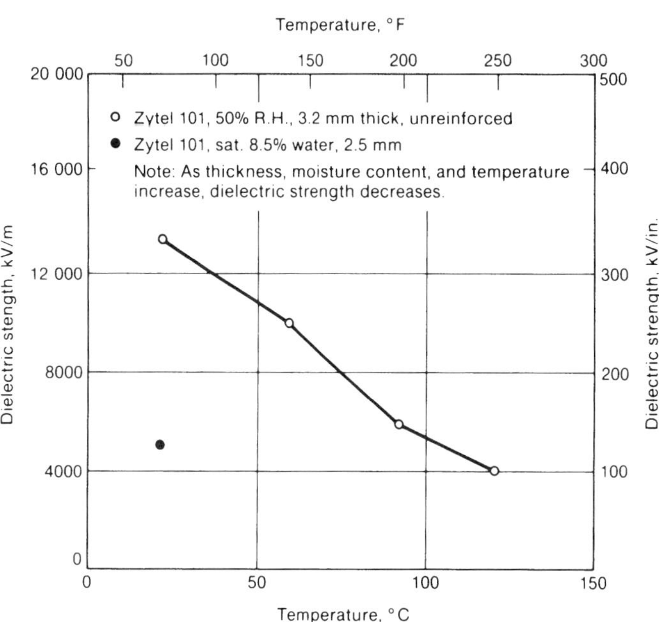

Fig. 22 Dielectric strength versus temperature for unreinforced polyamide (nylon) resin

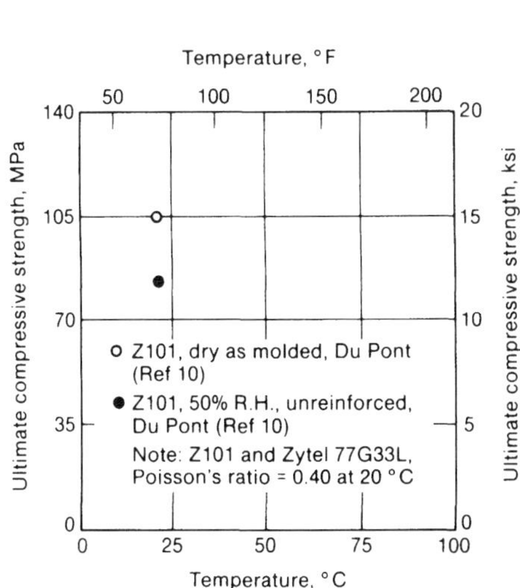

Fig. 23 Ultimate compressive strength versus temperature for polyamide (nylon) resin and resin-matrix composite

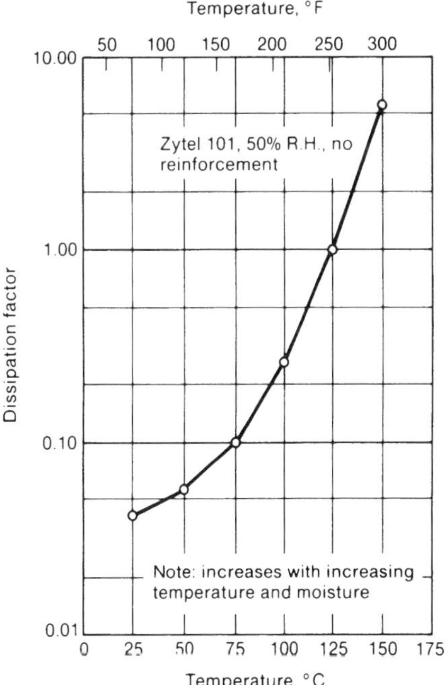

Fig. 24 Dissipation factor (100 Hz) versus temperature for unreinforced polyamide (nylon) resin

Table 5 Physical properties and service characteristics of polysulfone resin and fiber-resin composites

Properties	Neat resin	30% glass fiber composite	30% carbon fiber composite
Specific gravity	1.24	1.45	1.37
Density, g/cm^3 (lb/in.^{3})	1.24 (0.045)	1.45 (0.052)	1.37 (0.049)
UL in-service temperature rating, °C (°F)	160 (320)	...	...
Heat deflection temperature at 1820 kPa (264 psi), °C (°F)	175 (345)	185 (365)	185 (365)
In-service temperature °C (°F)	150–205 (300–400)	...	...
UL flammability rating	94 V-0	94 V-0	94 V-0

UL, Underwriters' Laboratory

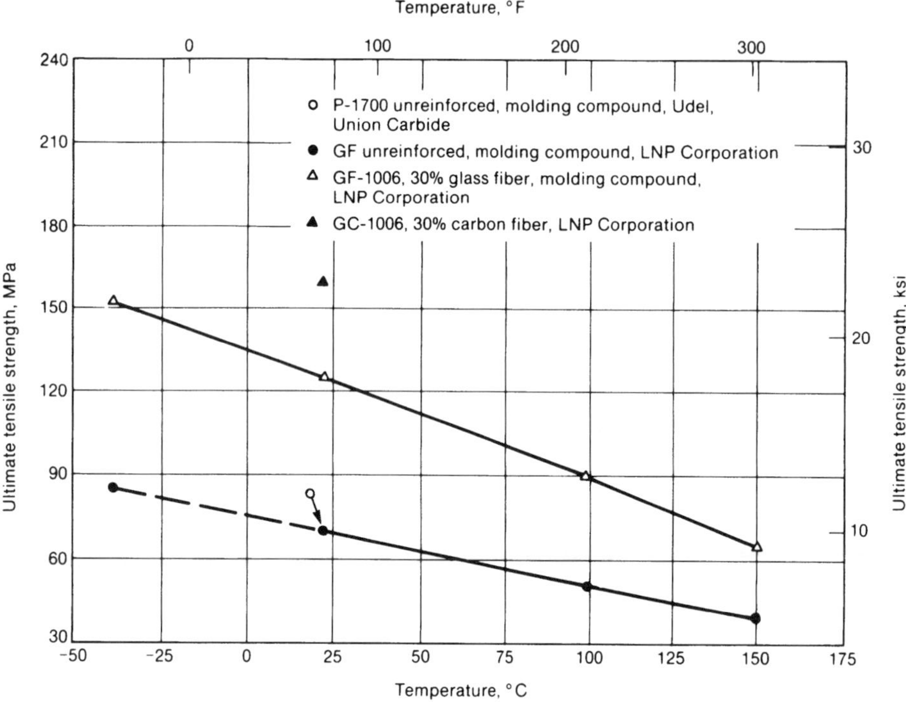

Fig. 25 Ultimate tensile strength versus temperature for polysulfone resin and resin-matrix composites

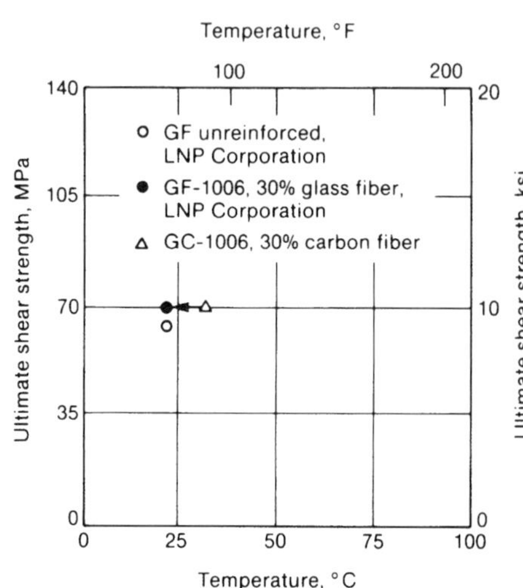

Fig. 26 Ultimate shear strength versus temperature for polysulfone resin and resin-matrix composites

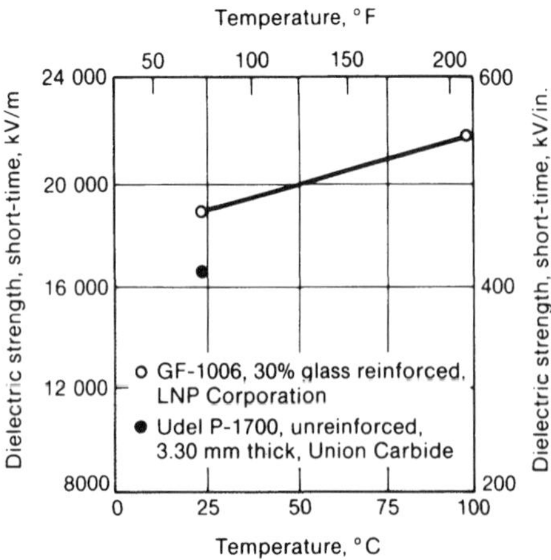

Fig. 27 Dielectric strength versus temperature for polysulfone resin and resin-matrix composite

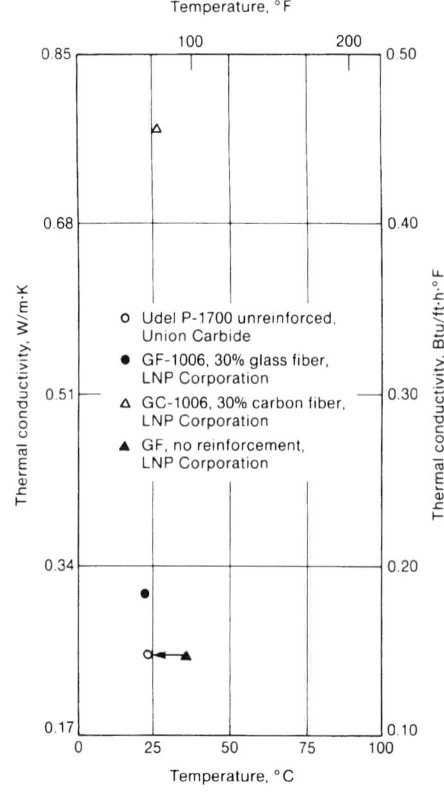

Fig. 28 Thermal conductivity versus temperature for polysulfone resins and resin-matrix composites

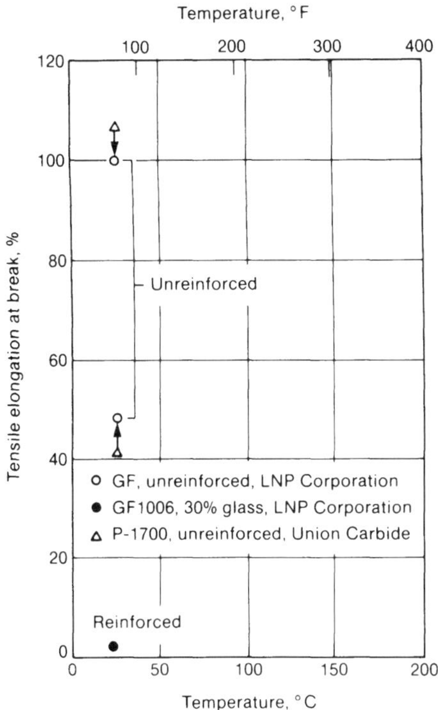

Fig. 29 Tensile elongation at break versus temperature for polysulfone resins and a resin-matrix composite

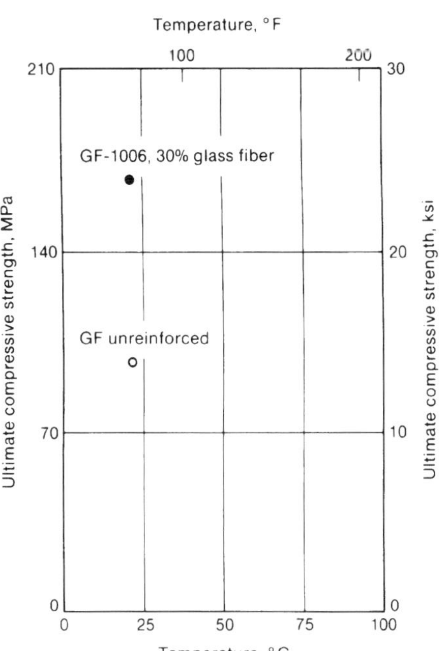

Fig. 30 Ultimate compressive strength versus temperature for polysulfone resin and resin-matrix composite

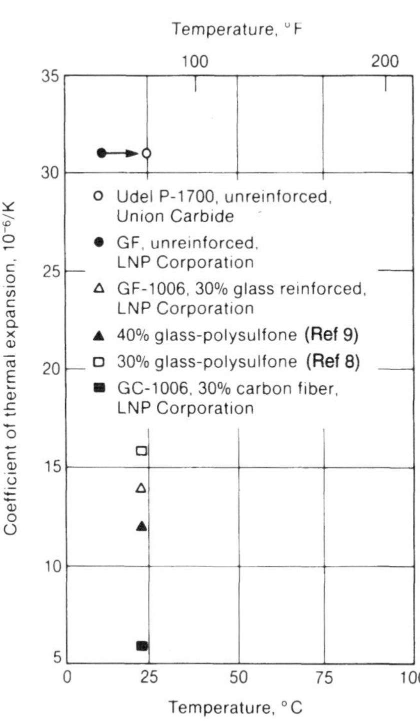

Fig. 31 Coefficient of thermal expansion versus temperature for polysulfone resins and resin-matrix composites. 10^{-6}/K × $\frac{5}{9}$ = μin./in. × °F

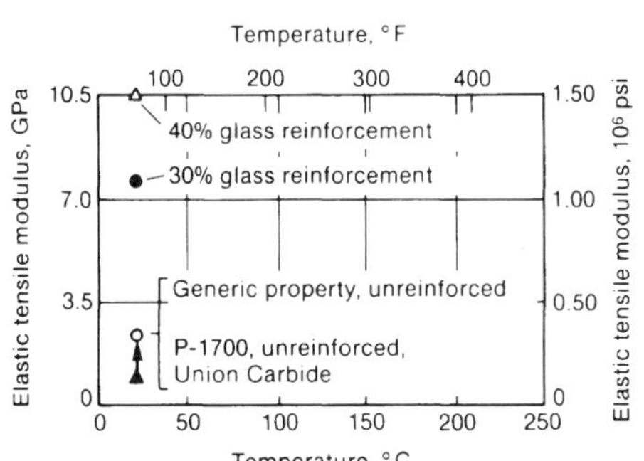

Fig. 32 Tensile elastic modulus versus temperature for polysulfone resin and resin-matrix composites. Source: Ref 8

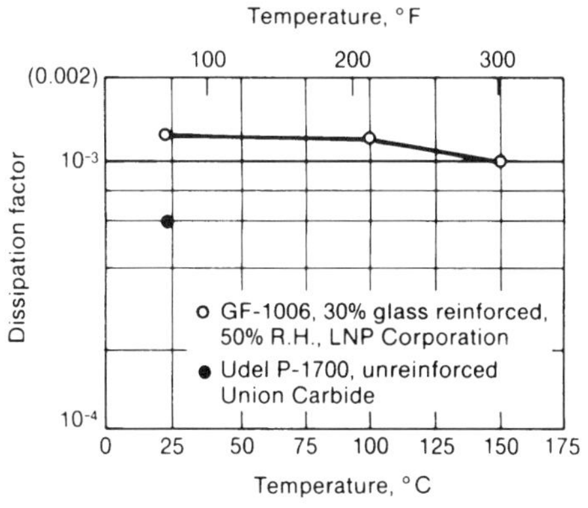

Fig. 33 Dissipation factor (60 Hz) versus temperature for polysulfone resin and resin-matrix composite

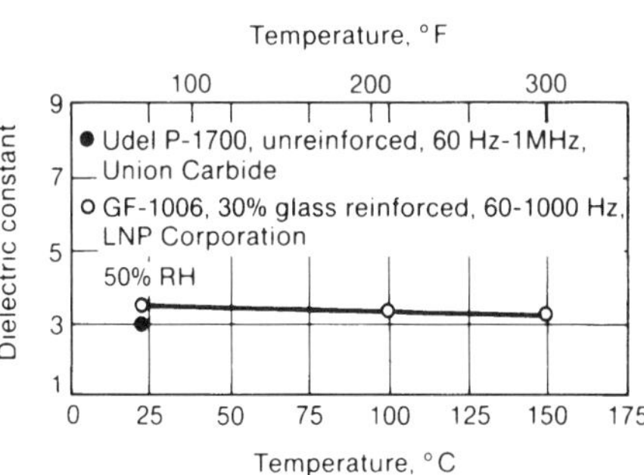

Fig. 34 Dielectric constant versus temperature for polysulfone resin and resin-matrix composite

Table 6 Physical properties and service characteristics of low-temperature polyester thermoset resin and resin-matrix composites

Properties	Neat resin	10–40 wt% glass fiber composite
Specific gravity	1.2–1.4	1.6–1.9
Density, g/cm^3 (lb/in.^{3})	1.2–1.4 (0.043–0.051)	1.6–1.9 (0.058–0.069)
In-service temperature, °C (°F)	120–150 (250–300)	120–205 (250–400)
Heat deflection temperature at 1820 kPa (264 psi), °C (°F)	50–205 (120–400)	190–205 (375–400)
UL in-service temperature rating, °C (°F)	180 (356)	...
UL flammability rating	...	...

UL, Underwriters' Laboratory

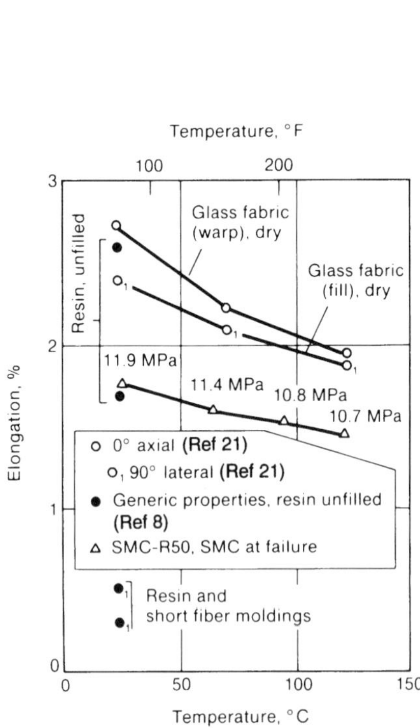

Fig. 35 Percent elongation versus temperature for thermoset polyester resin and resin-matrix composites

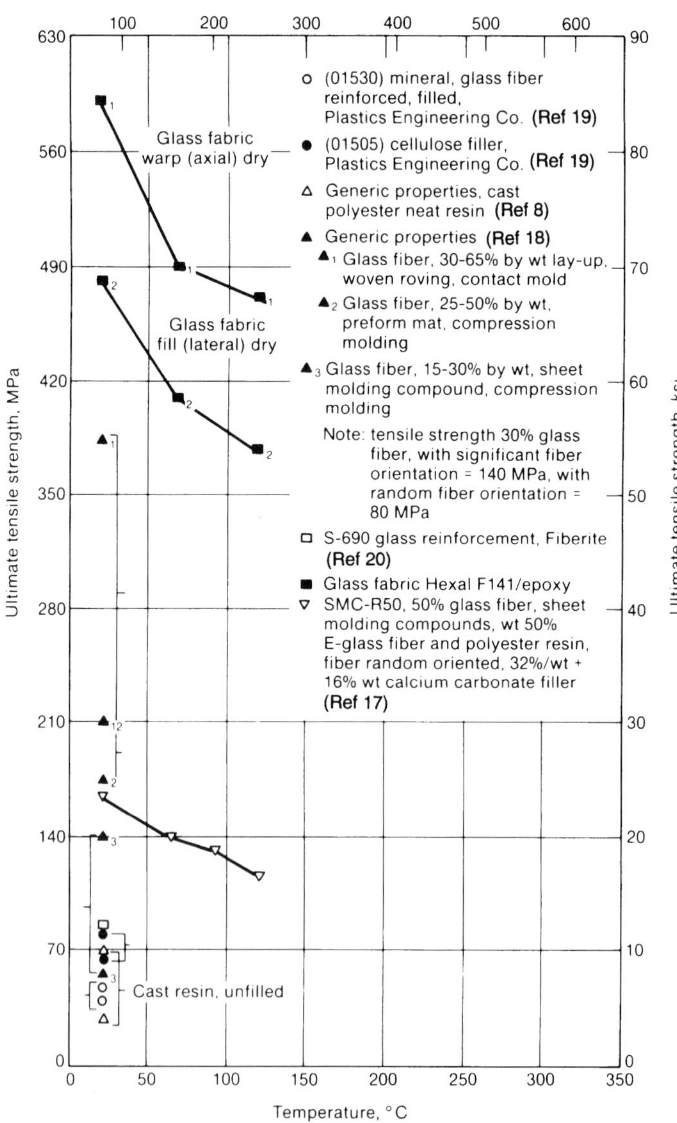

Fig. 36 Ultimate tensile strength versus temperature for thermoset polyester resin and resin-matrix composites. Ranges are due to property differences among compression, transfer, and injection molding processes.

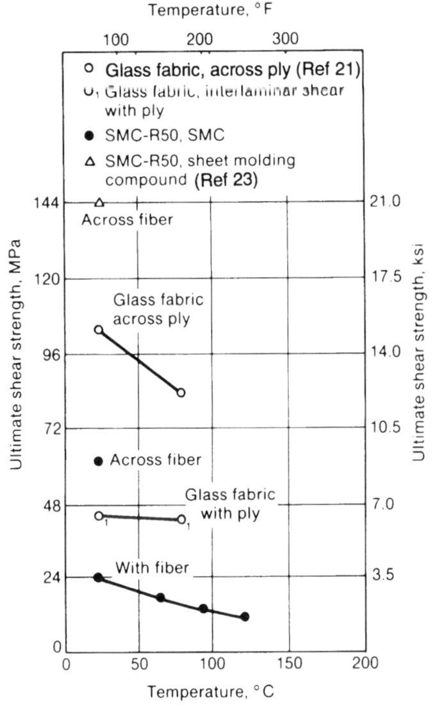

Fig. 37 Ultimate shear strength versus temperature for thermoset polyester-matrix composites

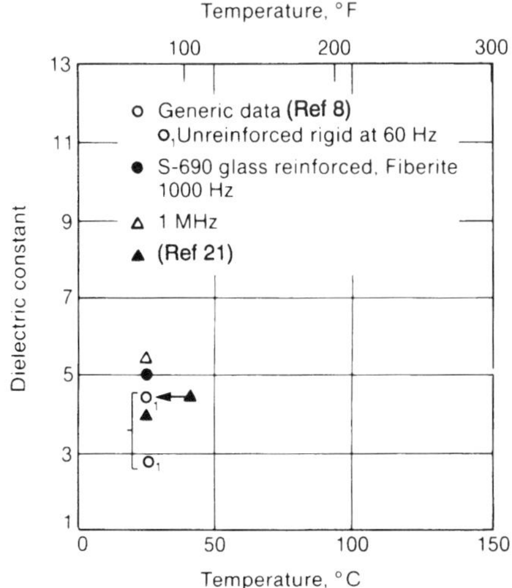

Fig. 38 Dielectric constant versus temperature for thermoset polyester resin and resin-matrix composites

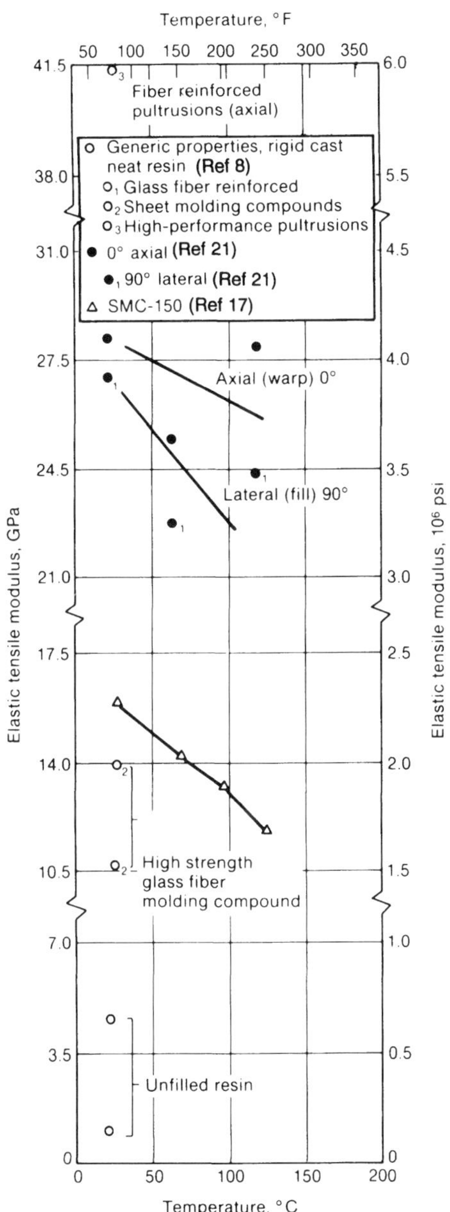

Fig. 39 Elastic tensile modulus versus temperature for thermoset polyester resin and resin-matrix composites

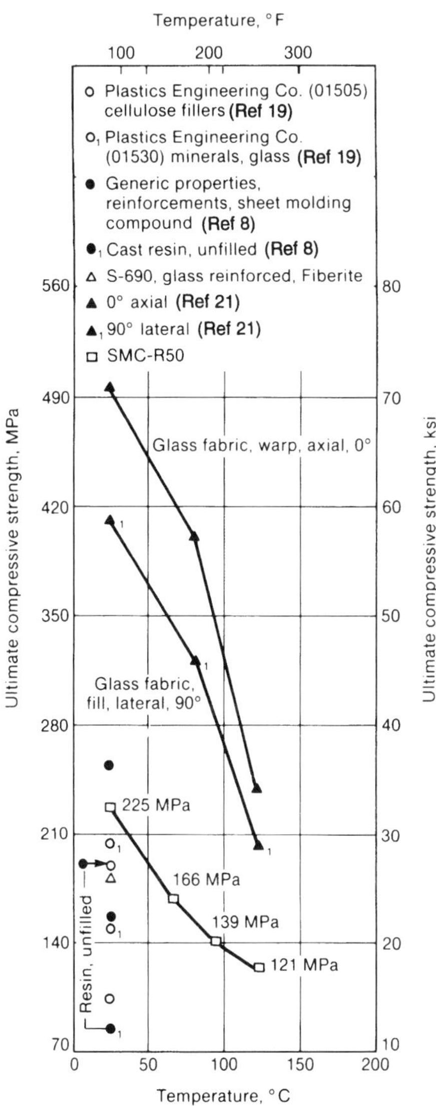

Fig. 40 Ultimate compressive strength versus temperature for thermoset polyester resin and resin-matrix composites

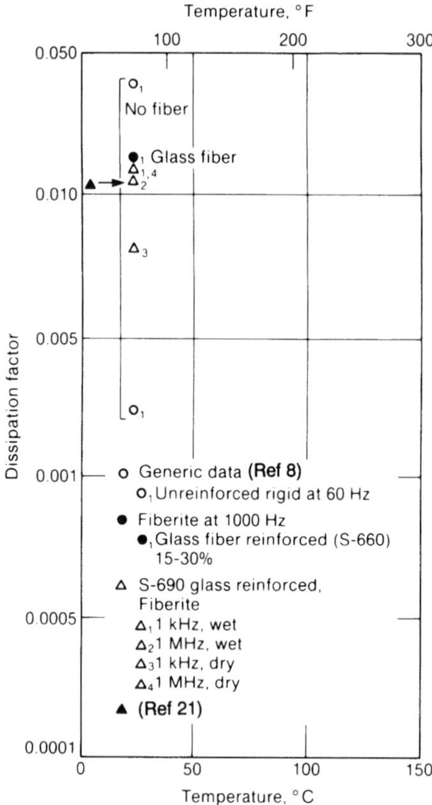

Fig. 41 Dissipation factor versus temperature for thermoset polyester resin and resin-matrix composites

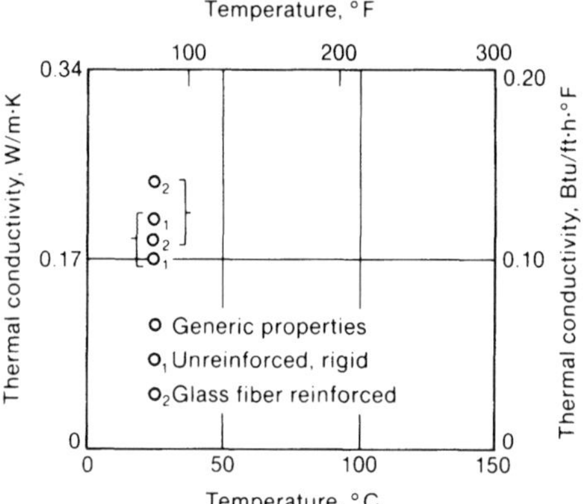

Fig. 42 Thermal conductivity versus temperature for thermoset polyester resin and resin-matrix composites. Source: Ref 8

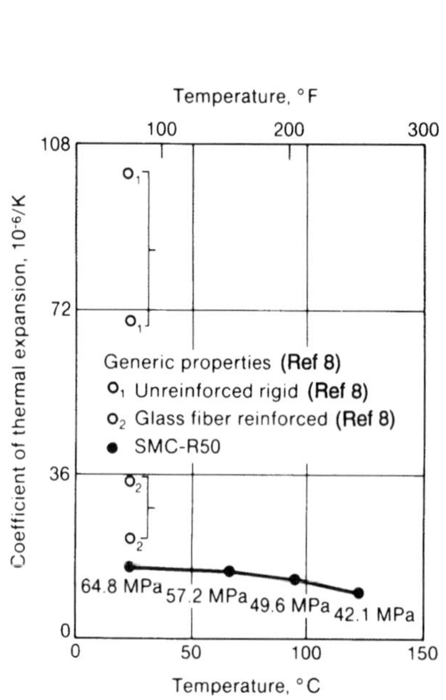

Fig. 43 Coefficient of thermal expansion versus temperature for thermoset polyester resin and resin-matrix composites. $10^{-6}/K \times \frac{5}{9}$ = µin./in. × °F

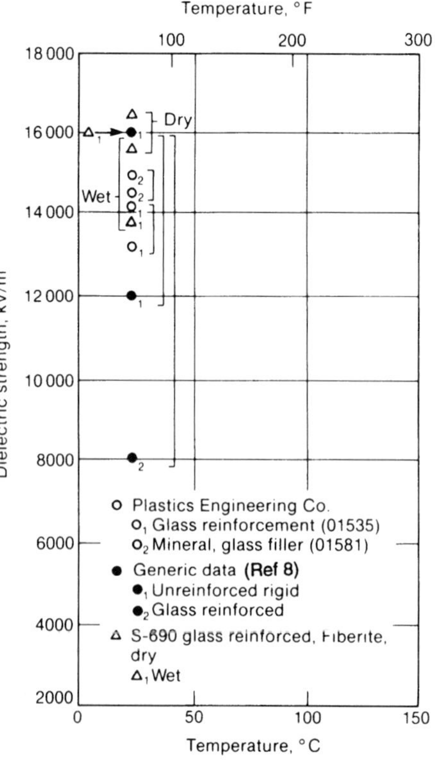

Fig. 44 Dielectric strength versus temperature for thermoset polyester resin and resin-matrix composites

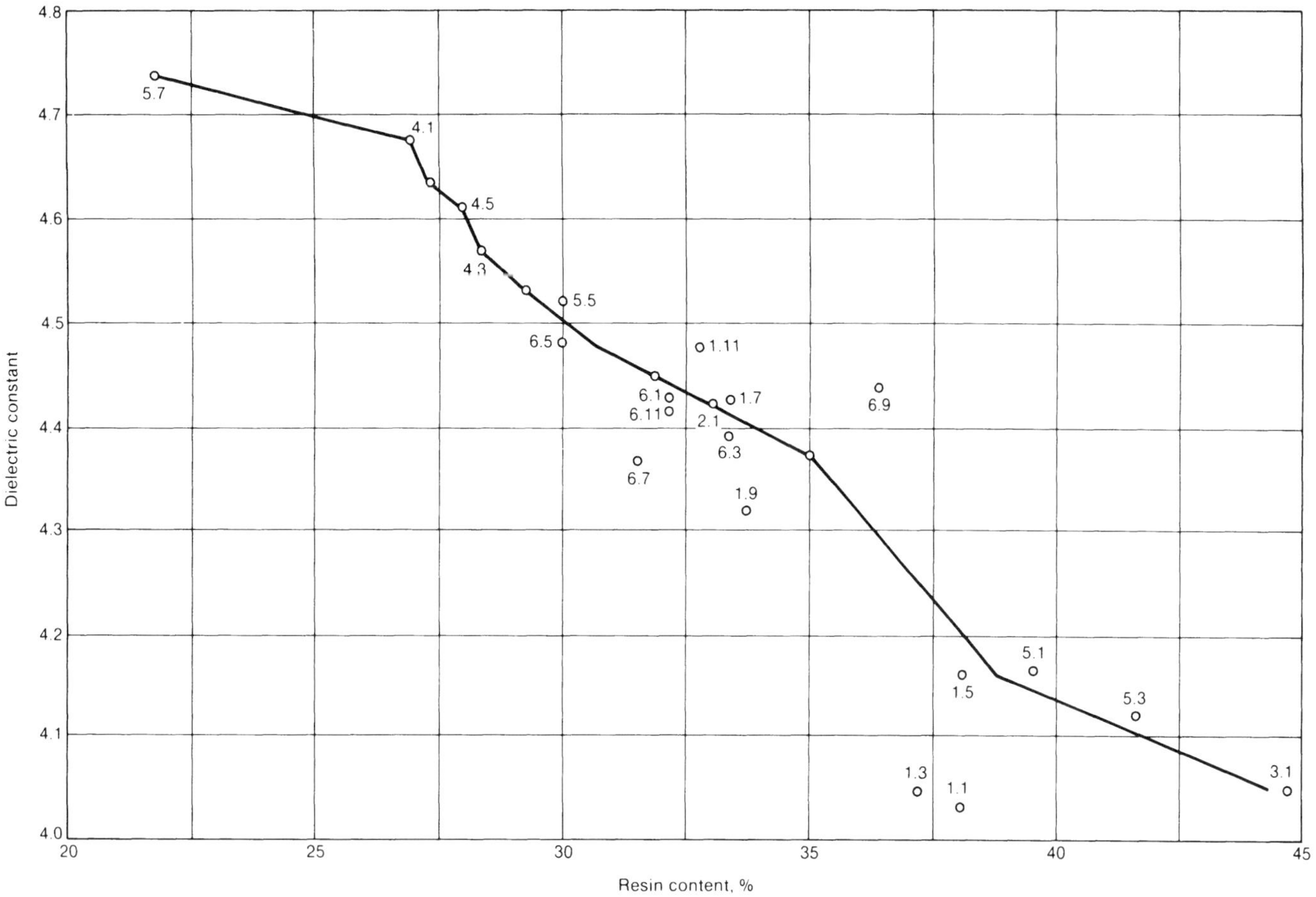

Fig. 45 Effect of resin content on dielectric constant for thermoset polyester-matrix composites. Glass fabric, all types. Numbers on field of figure are identification of data sets. Source: Ref 22

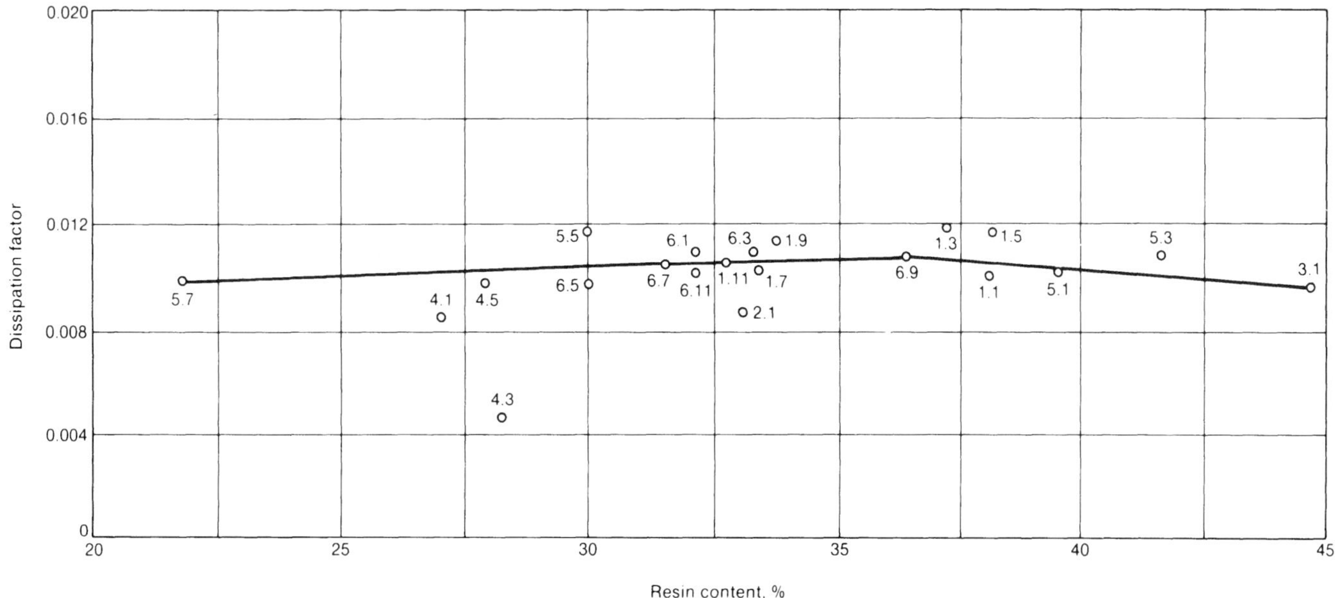

Fig. 46 Effect of resin content on dissipation factor (power factor) for thermoset polyester-matrix composites. Glass-fabric types of reinforcement. Numbers on field of figure are identification of data sets. Source: Ref 22

Table 7 Physical properties and service characteristics of thermoset phenolic resin and fiber-resin composites

Property	Phenolic resin	Fiber-resin composites: Molding compound (glass fiber)	Tape wrapping fabric composites: E-glass fabric	Carbon fabric	Graphite fabric
Specific gravity	1.28	1.95	1.90	1.45	1.42
Density, g/cm^3 (lb/in.^{3})	1.28 (0.046)	1.95 (0.070)	1.90 (0.069)	1.45 (0.052	1.42 (0.051)
Service temperature, °C (°F)	150–230 (300–450)	150 (300)	538 (1000)	3038 (5500)	3038 (5500)
Heat deflection temperature at 1820 kPa (264 psi), °C (°F)	120–315 (250–600)	...	...	...	...
UL flammability rating	94 V-1	94 V-0	94 V-0	...	...
Thermogravimetric analysis—stability temperature at 5–10% weight loss, °C (°F)	230 (450)	...	...	...	...
Reinforcement, wt%	...	35–45	63	55	55

UL, Underwriters' Laboratory

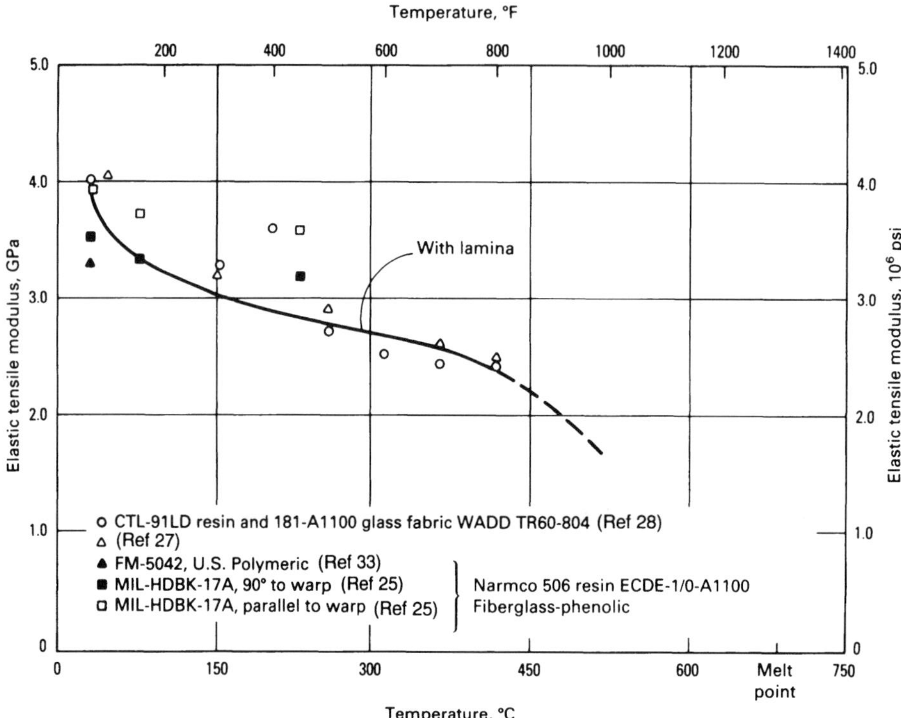

Fig. 47 Elastic tensile modulus versus temperature for thermoset phenolic resin-matrix composites with glass-cloth-fabric reinforcements

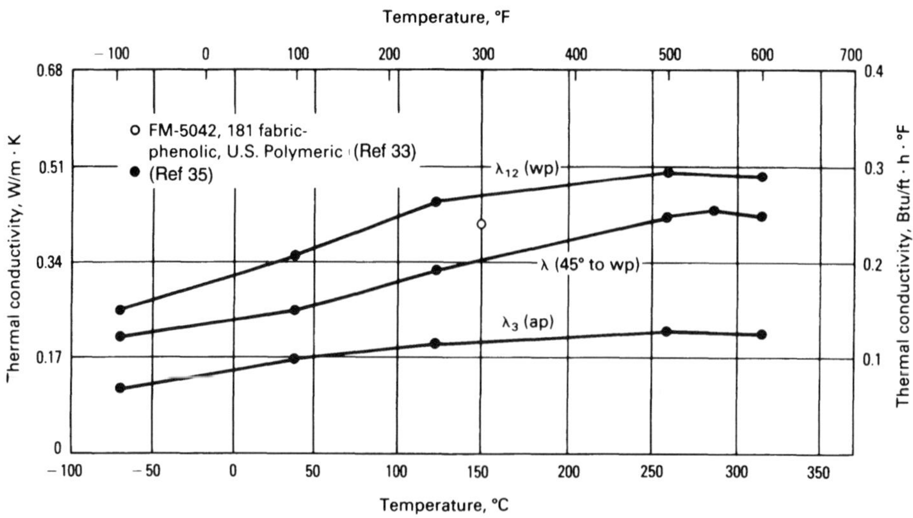

Fig. 48 Thermal conductivity versus temperature for thermoset phenolic resin-matrix composites with glass-cloth-fabric reinforcements

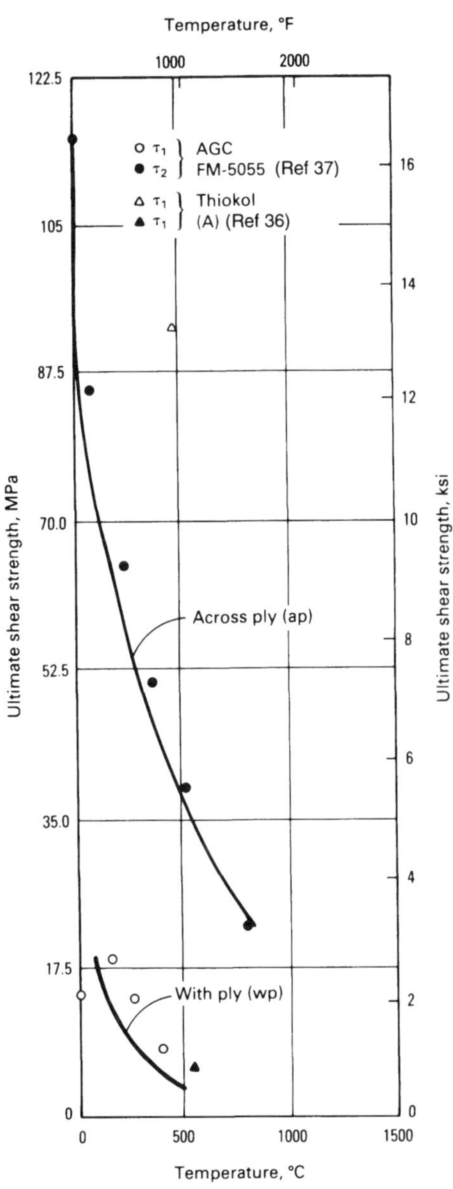

Fig. 49 Ultimate shear strength versus temperature for thermoset phenolic resin-matrix composites with carbon-fabric reinforcements

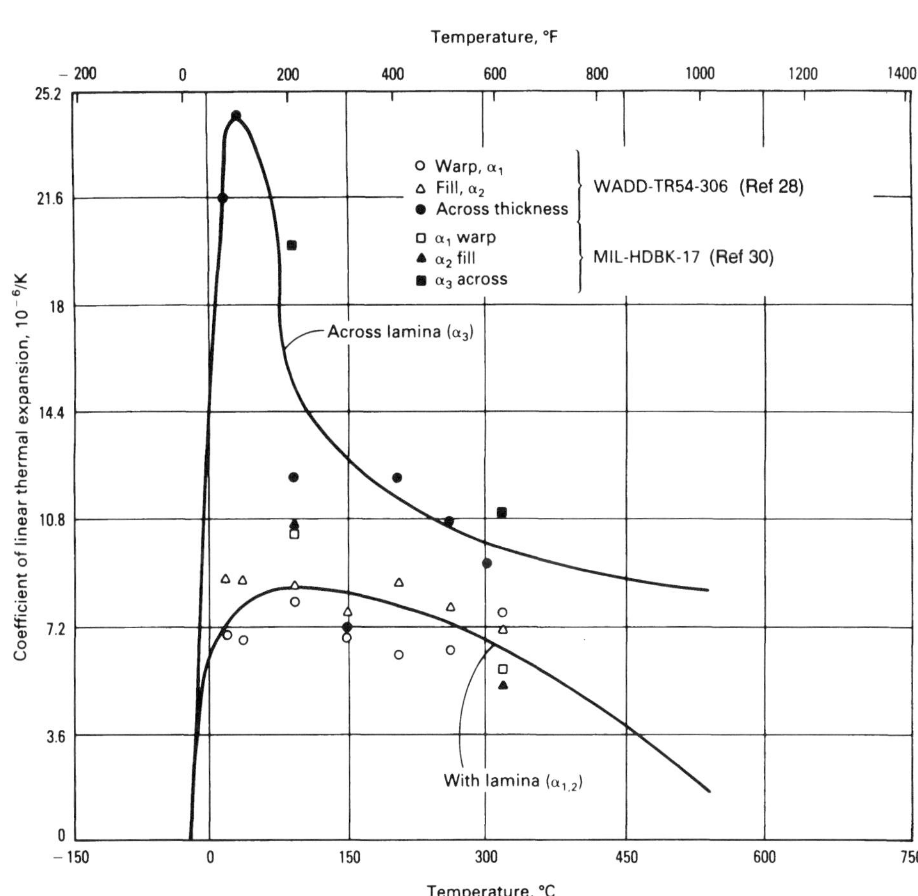

Fig. 50 Coefficient of thermal expansion versus temperature for thermoset phenolic resin-matrix composites with glass-cloth–fabric reinforcements. 10^{-6}/K × $\frac{5}{9}$ = μin./in. × °F

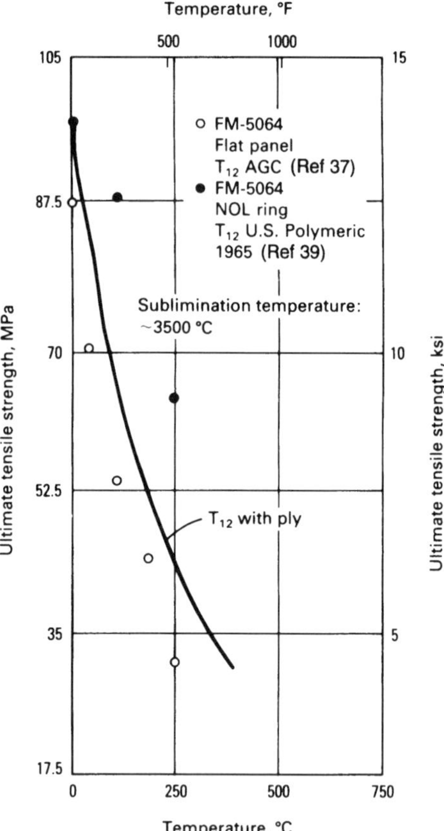

Fig. 51 Ultimate tensile strength versus temperature for thermoset phenolic resin-matrix composites with graphite-fabric reinforcements

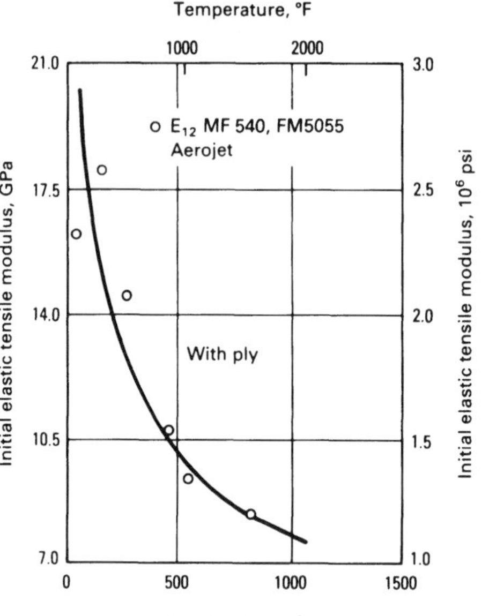

Fig. 52 Initial elastic tensile modulus versus temperature for thermoset phenolic resin-matrix composites with carbon-fabric reinforcements. Source: Ref 37

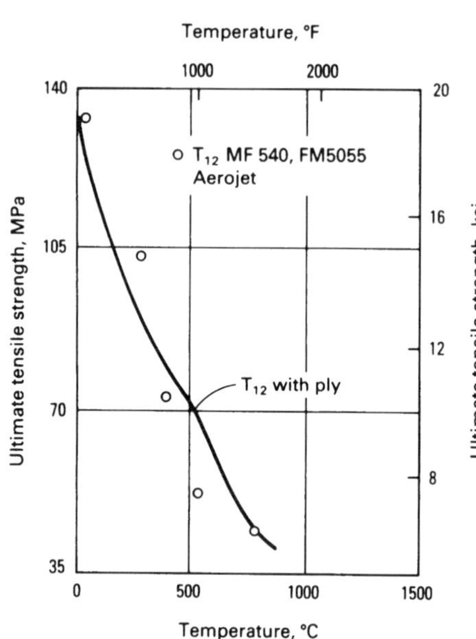

Fig. 53 Ultimate tensile strength versus temperature for thermoset phenolic resin-matrix composites with carbon-fabric reinforcements. Source: Ref 37

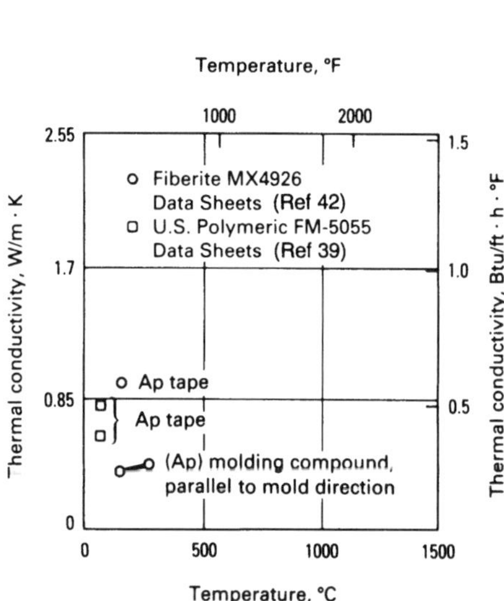

Fig. 54 Thermal conductivity versus temperature for thermoset phenolic resin-matrix composites with carbon-fabric reinforcements

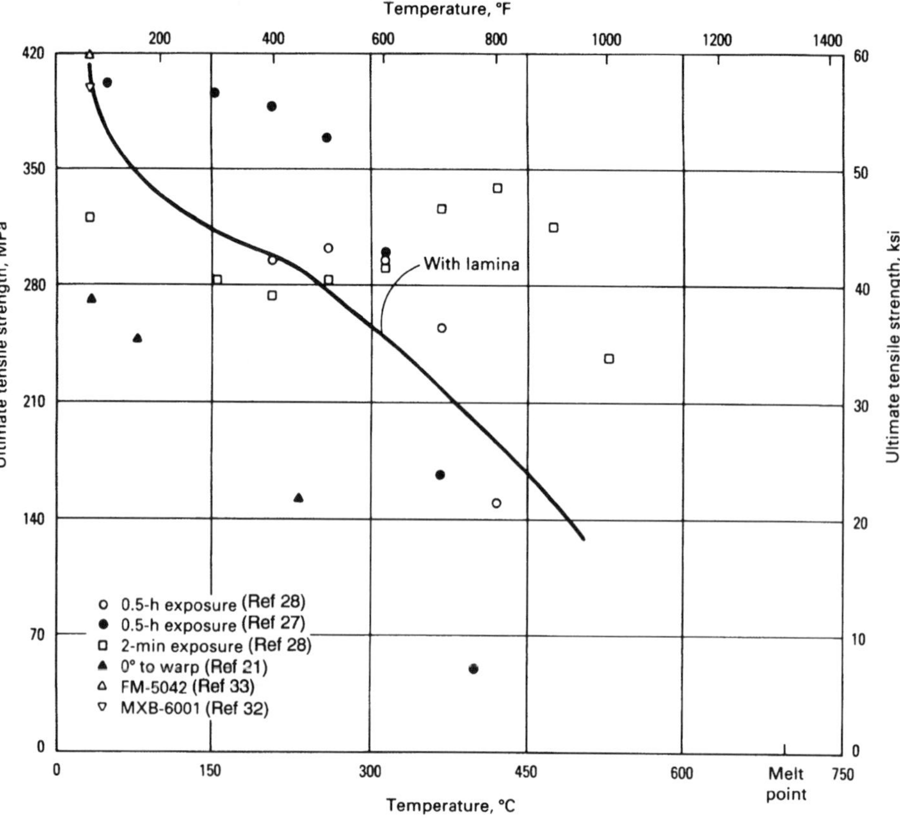

Fig. 55 Ultimate tensile strength versus temperature for thermoset phenolic resin-matrix composites with glass-cloth–fabric reinforcements

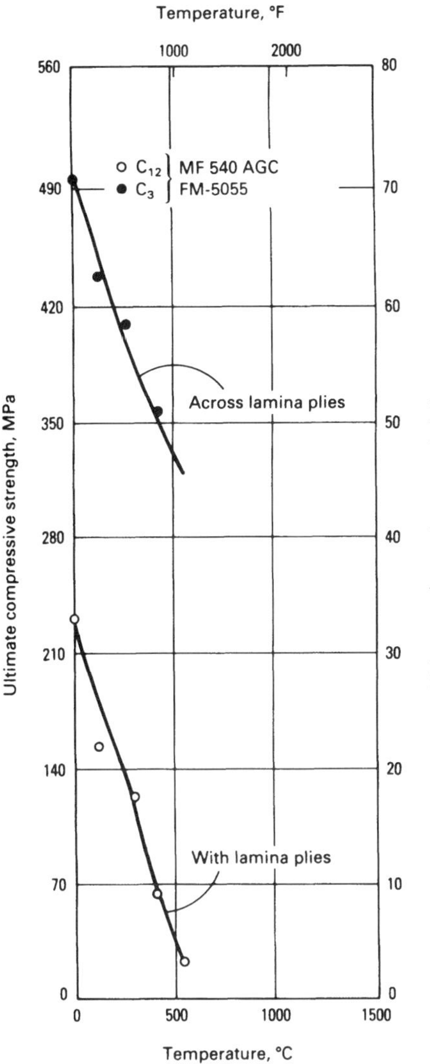

Fig. 56 Ultimate compressive strength versus temperature for thermoset phenolic resin-matrix composites with carbon-fabric reinforcements. Source Ref 37

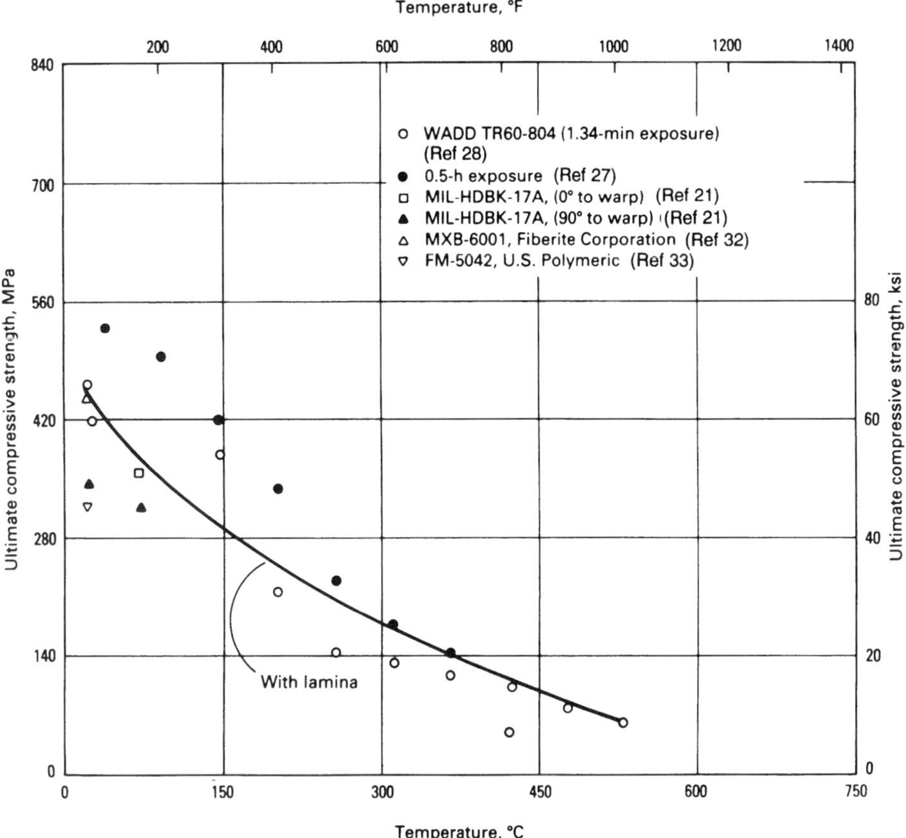

Fig. 57 Ultimate compressive strength versus temperature for thermoset phenolic resin-matrix composites with glass-cloth–fabric reinforcements

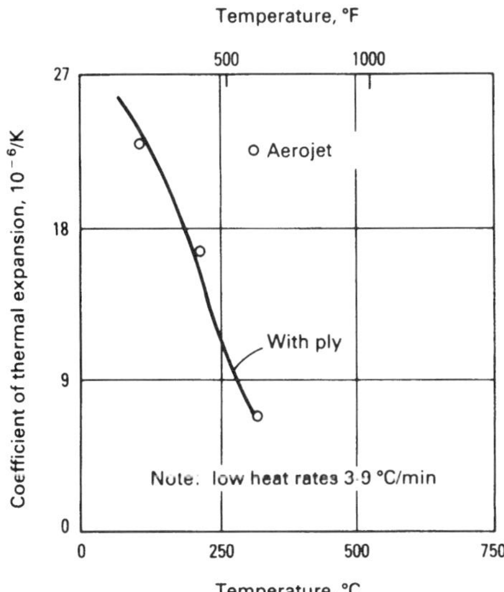

Fig. 58 Coefficient of thermal expansion versus temperature with ply for thermoset phenolic resin-matrix composites with graphite-fabric reinforcements. 10^{-6}/K × 5/9 = µin./in. × °F. Source: Ref 37

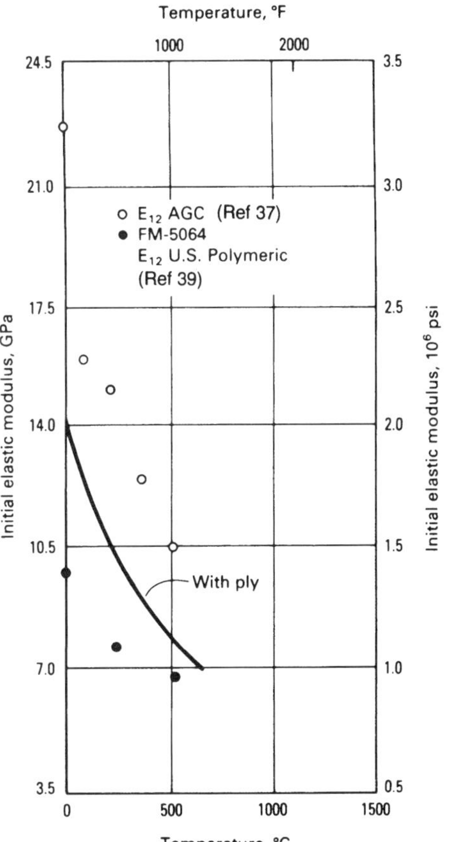

Fig. 59 Initial elastic tensile modulus versus temperature for thermoset phenolic resin-matrix composites with graphite-fabric reinforcements

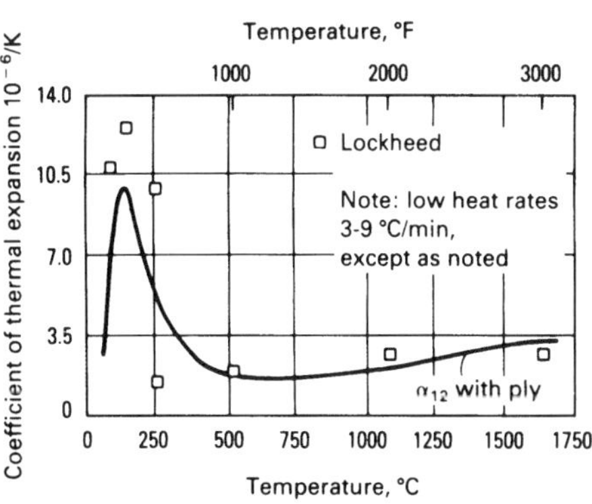

Fig. 60 Coefficient of thermal expansion versus temperature with ply—low heating rates for thermoset phenolic resin-matrix composites with carbon-fabric reinforcements. 10^{-6}/K × 5/9 = µin./in. × °F. Source: Ref 38

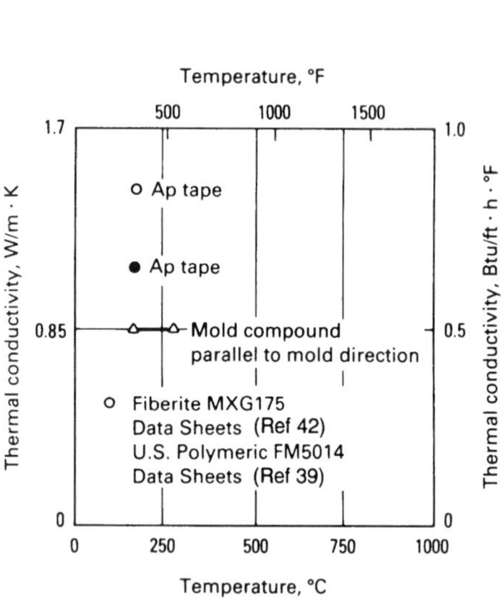

Fig. 61 Thermal conductivity versus temperature for thermoset phenolic resin-matrix composites with graphite-fabric reinforcements

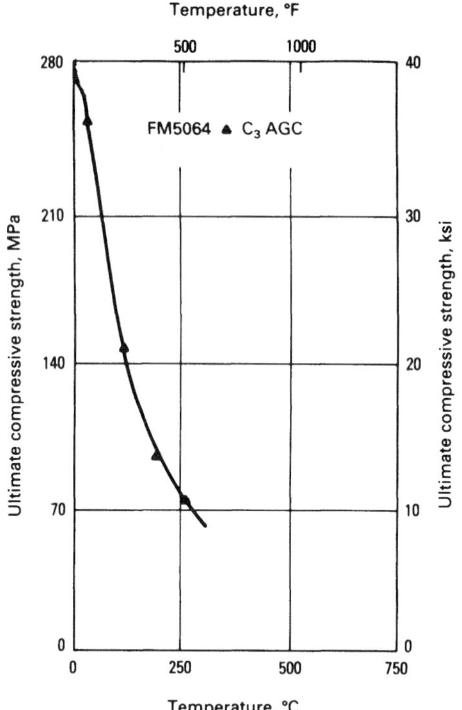

Fig. 62 Ultimate compressive strength versus temperature for thermoset phenolic resin-matrix composites with graphite-fabric reinforcements. Source: Ref 37

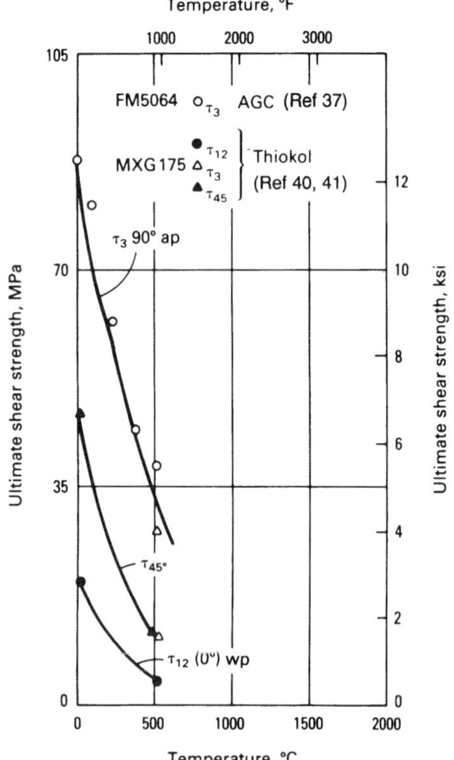

Fig. 63 Ultimate shear strength versus temperature for thermoset phenolic resin-matrix composites with graphite-fabric reinforcements

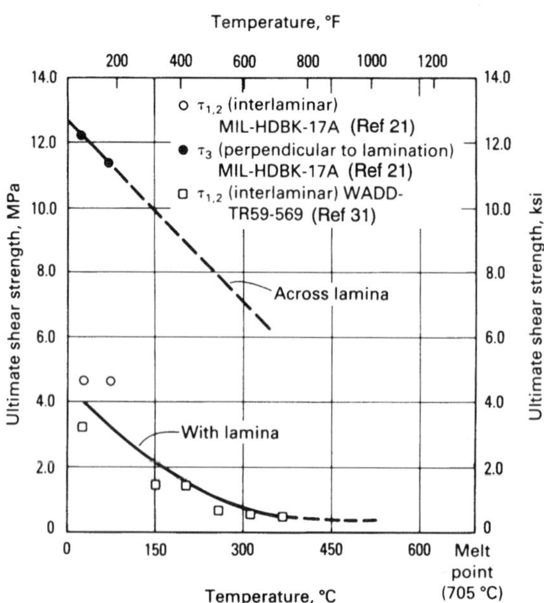

Fig. 64 Ultimate shear strength versus temperature for thermoset phenolic resin-matrix composites with glass-cloth–fabric reinforcements

Table 8 Physical properties and service characteristics of thermoset epoxy resin-matrix fiber- and fabric-reinforced composites

Properties	S-2 filament winding glass fiber composite	Kevlar composite	Carbon composite	Graphite fiber composite	Layup quartz fabric composite
Specific gravity	1.86	1.25	1.46	1.58	1.75
Density, g/cm^3 (lb/in.^{3})	1.86 (0.067)	1.25 (0.045)	1.46 (0.053)	1.58 (0.057)	1.75 (0.063)
Service temperature, °C (°F)	150 (300)	150 (300) for 1 to 2 min	150 (300)	150 (300)	150 (300)
Reinforcement volume, wt%	60	62.9	56	54	65

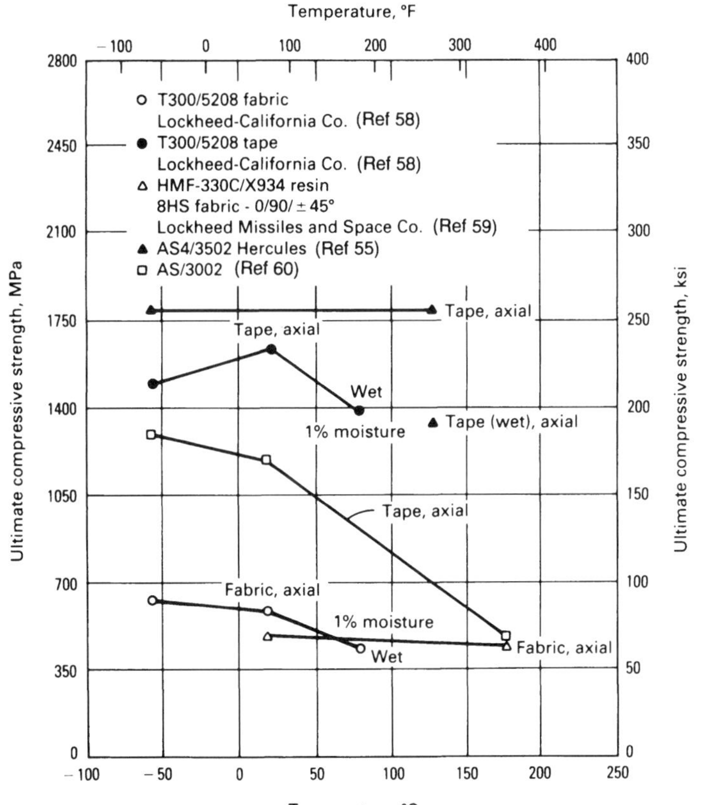

Fig. 65 Ultimate compressive strength versus temperature for thermoset epoxy resin-matrix composites with carbon reinforcements

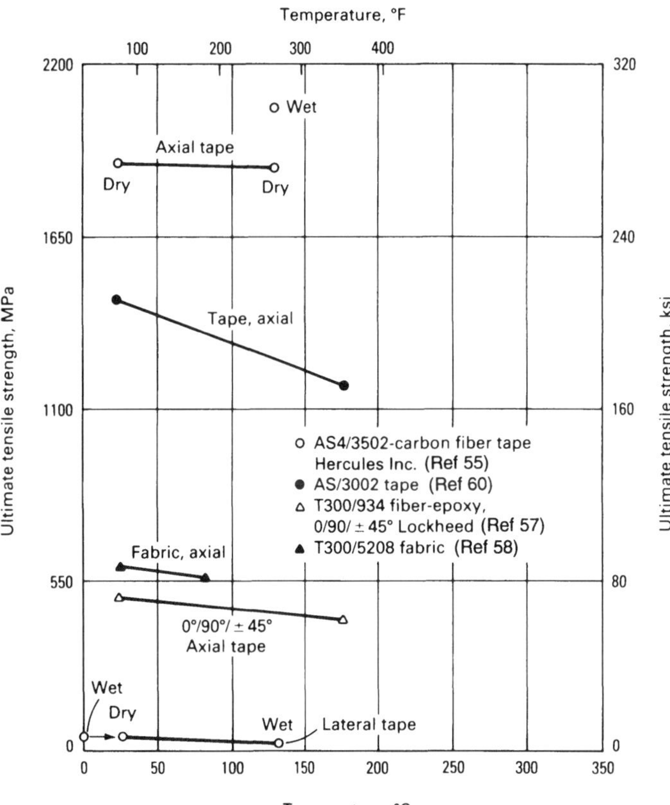

Fig. 66 Ultimate tensile strength versus temperature for thermoset epoxy resin-matrix composites with carbon reinforcements

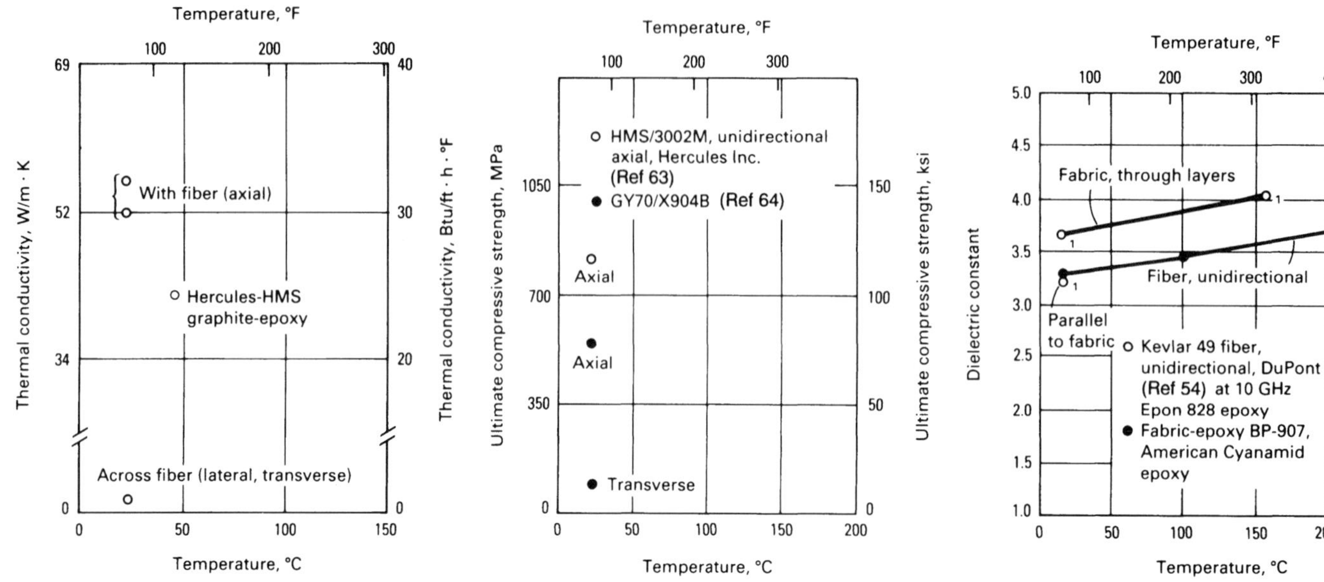

Fig. 67 Thermal conductivity versus temperature for thermoset epoxy resin-matrix composites with graphite-fiber reinforcements

Fig. 68 Ultimate compressive strength versus temperature for thermoset epoxy resin-matrix composites with graphite-fiber reinforcements

Fig. 69 Dielectric constant versus temperature for thermoset epoxy resin-matrix composites with Kevlar reinforcements

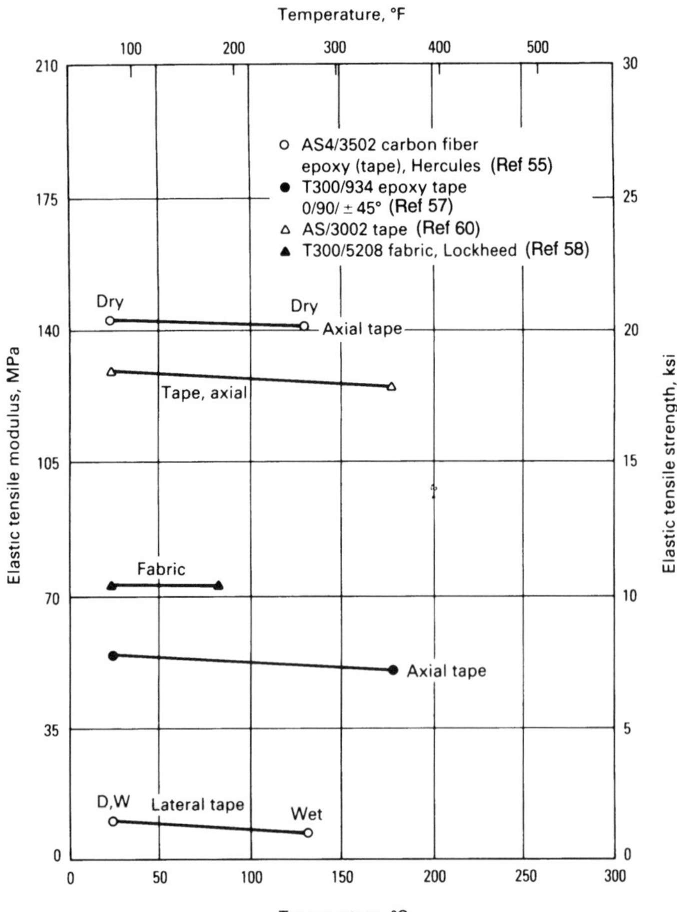

Fig. 70 Elastic tensile modulus versus temperature for thermoset epoxy resin-matrix composites with carbon reinforcements

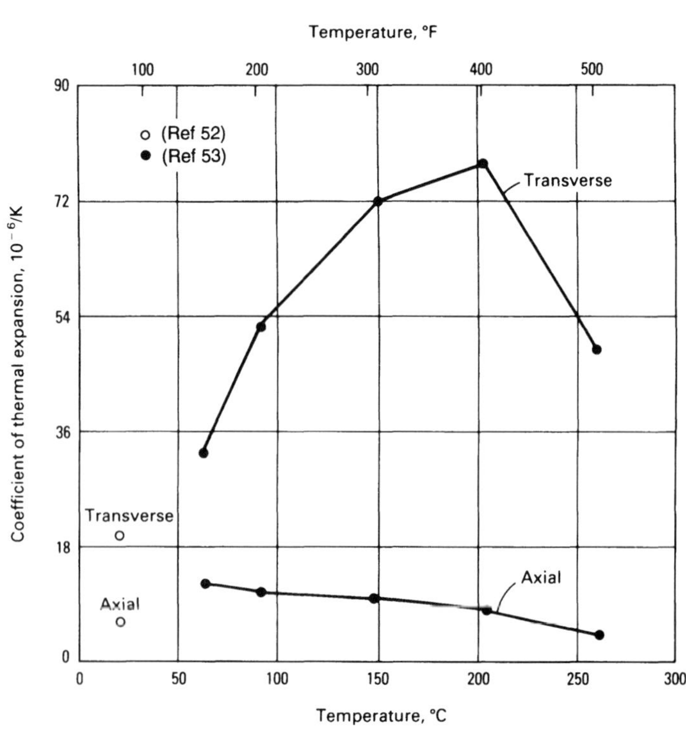

Fig. 71 Coefficient of thermal expansion versus temperature for thermoset phenolic resin-matrix composites with S-glass fabric reinforcements. $10^{-6}/K \times 5/9 =$ µin./in. × °F

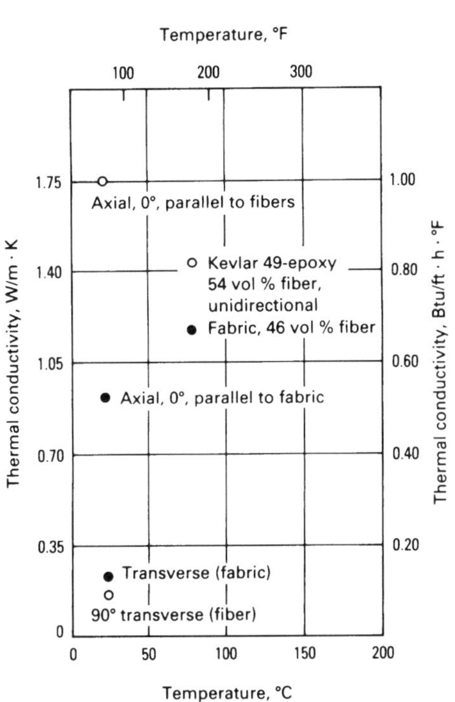

Fig. 72 Thermal conductivity versus temperature for thermoset epoxy resin-matrix composites with Kevlar reinforcements. Source: Ref 54

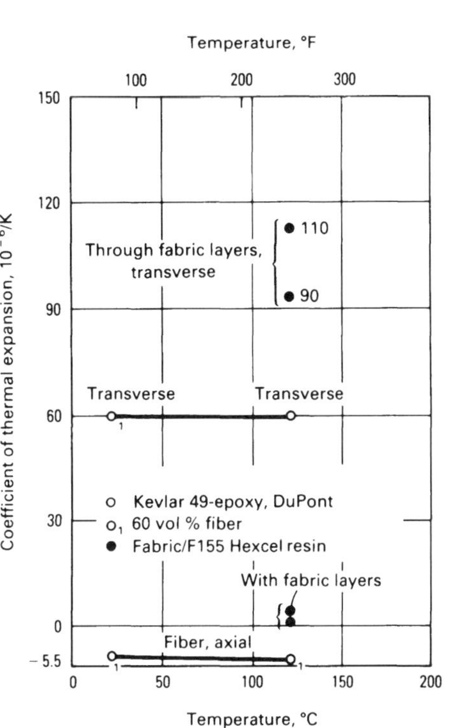

Fig. 73 Coefficient of thermal expansion versus temperature for thermoset epoxy resin-matrix composites with Kevlar reinforcements. 10^{-6}/K × $\frac{5}{9}$ = μin./in. × °F

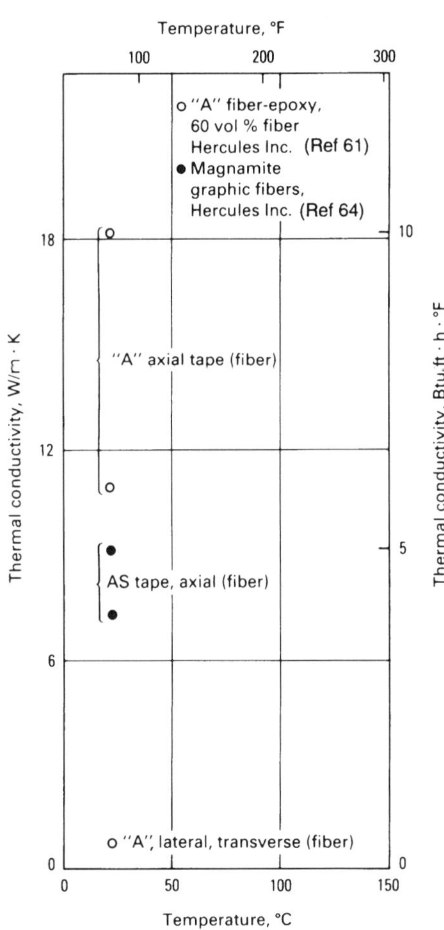

Fig. 74 Thermal conductivity versus temperature for thermoset epoxy resin-matrix composites with carbon reinforcements

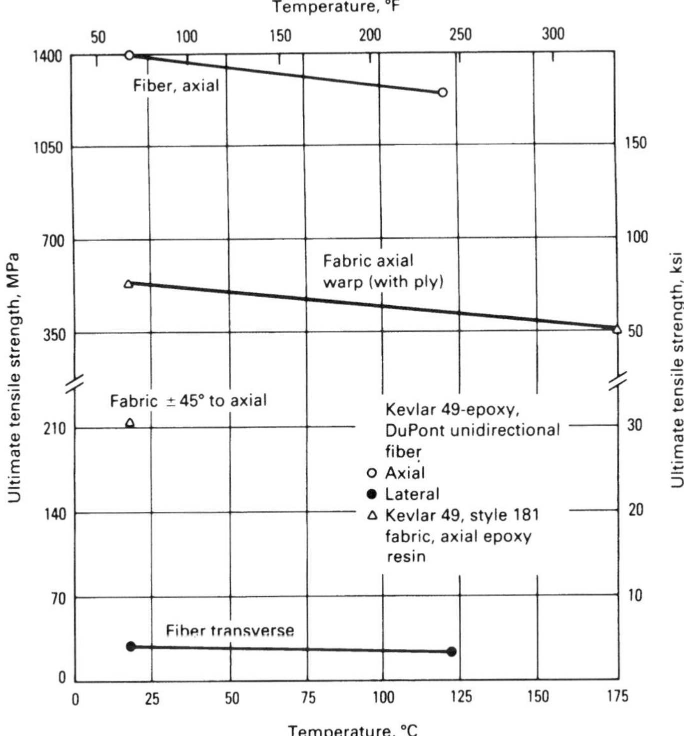

Fig. 75 Ultimate tensile strength versus temperature for thermoset epoxy resin-matrix composites with Kevlar reinforcements. Room-temperature tensile elongation: axial fiber, 1.85%; axial fabric, 1.78%; transverse lateral fiber, 0.58%. Source: Ref 54

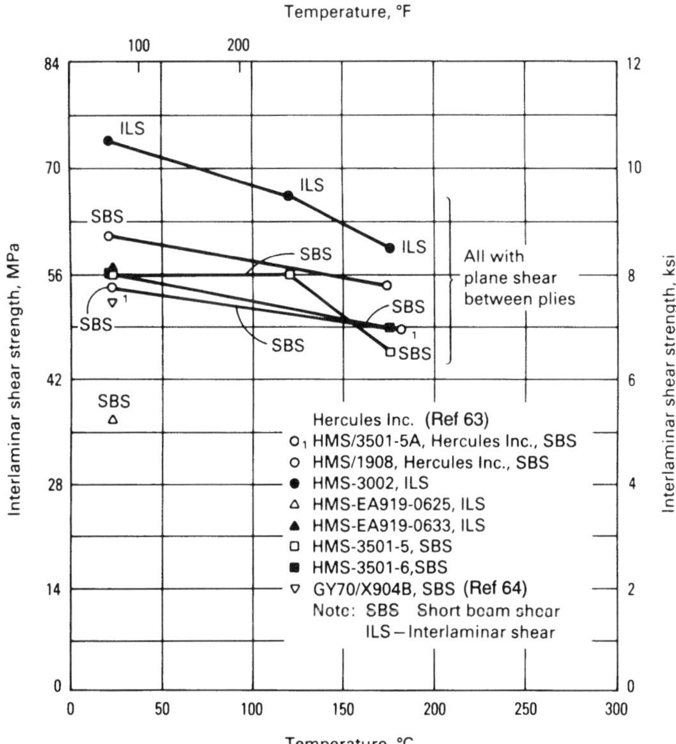

Fig. 76 Interlaminar shear versus temperature for thermoset epoxy resin-matrix composites with graphite-fiber reinforcements

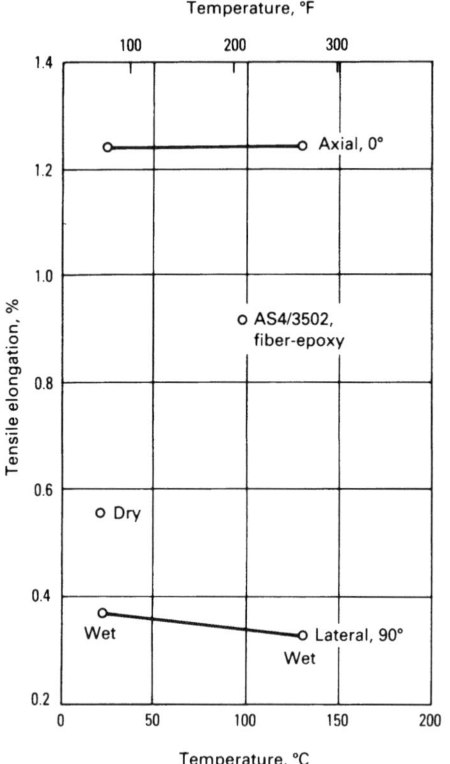

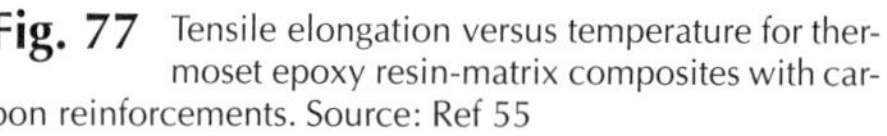

Fig. 77 Tensile elongation versus temperature for thermoset epoxy resin-matrix composites with carbon reinforcements. Source: Ref 55

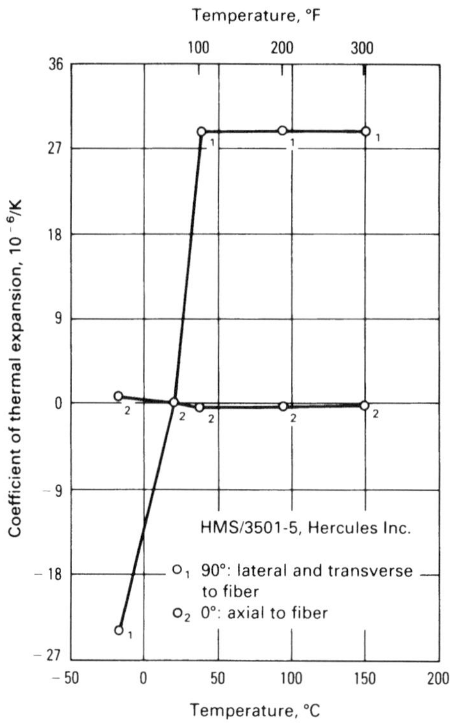

Fig. 78 Coefficient of thermal expansion versus temperature for thermoset epoxy resin-matrix composites with graphite-fiber reinforcements. 10^{-6}/K × $5/9$ = μin./in. × °F

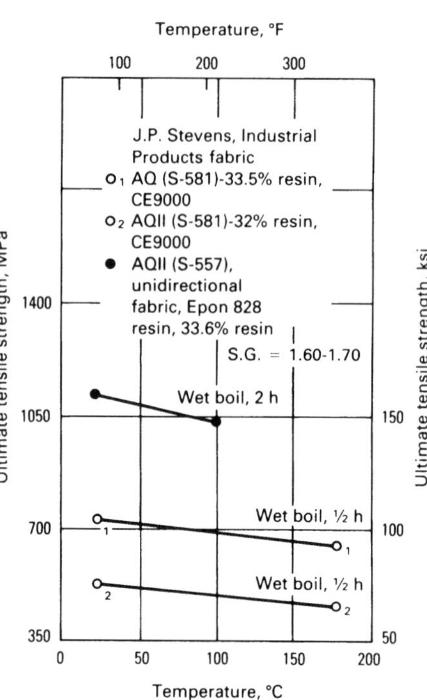

Fig. 79 Ultimate tensile strength versus temperature for thermoset epoxy resin-matrix composites with quartz-fabric reinforcements. S.G., specific gravity. Source Ref 65

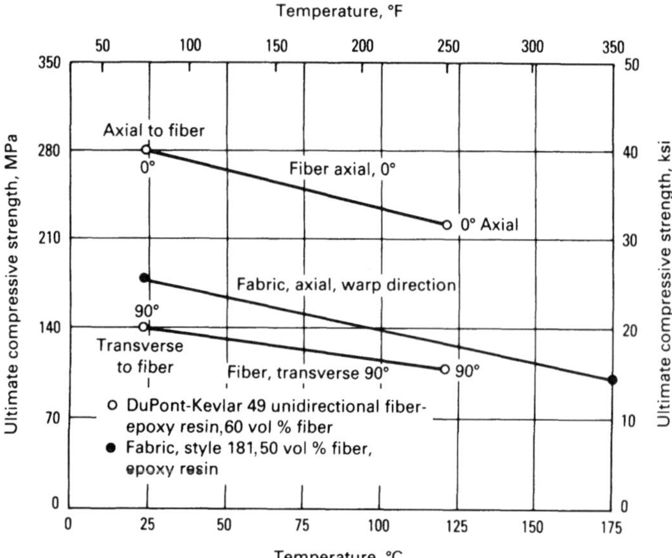

Fig. 80 Ultimate compressive strength versus temperature for thermoset epoxy resin-matrix composites with Kevlar reinforcements. Room-temperature tensile elongation: axial fiber, 1.85%; axial fabric, 1.78%; transverse lateral fiber, 0.58%. Source: Ref 54

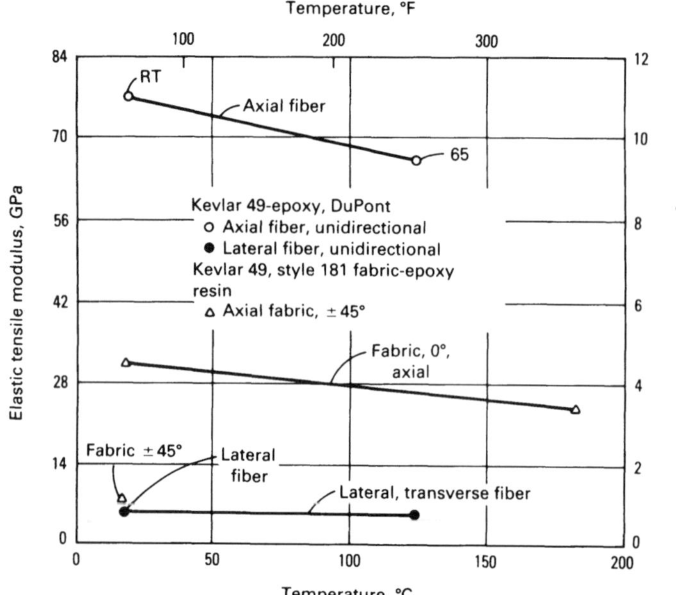

Fig. 81 Elastic tensile modulus versus temperature for thermoset epoxy resin-matrix composites with Kevlar reinforcements. Room-temperature (RT) tensile elongation: axial fiber, 1.85%; axial fabric, 1,78%; transverse lateral fiber, 0.58%. Source: Ref 54

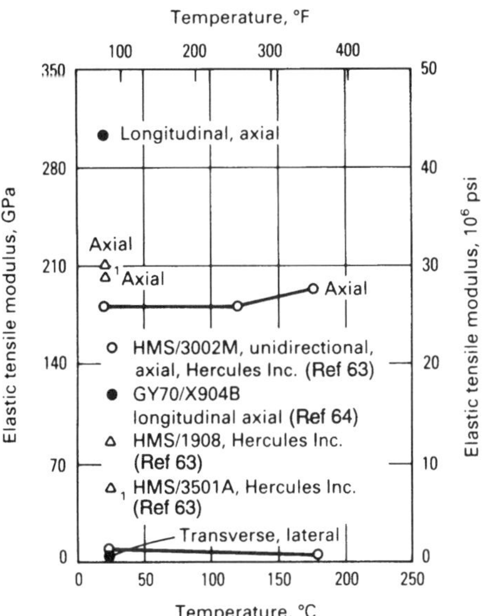

Fig. 82 Elastic tensile modulus versus temperature for thermoset epoxy resin-matrix composites with graphite-fiber reinforcements

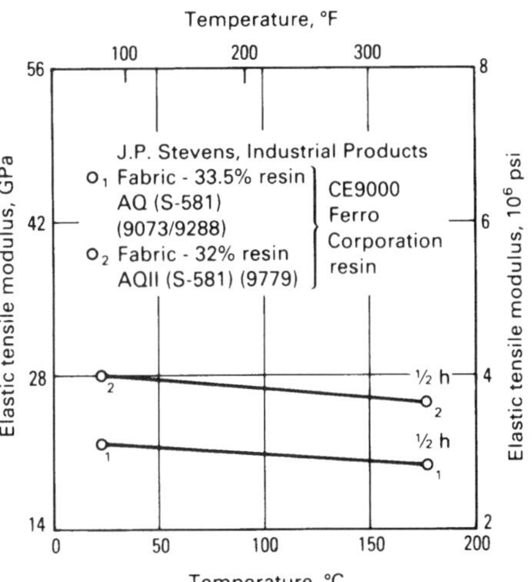

Fig. 83 Elastic tensile modulus versus temperature for thermoset epoxy resin-matrix composites with quartz-fabric reinforcements. Source: Ref 65

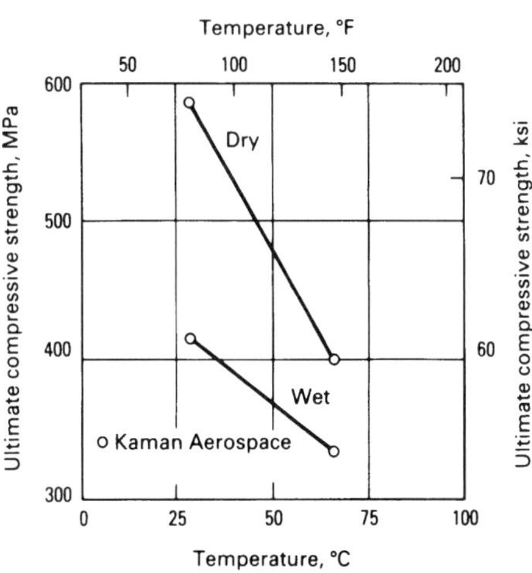

Fig. 84 Ultimate compressive strength versus temperature for thermoset phenolic resin-matrix composites with S-glass fabric reinforcements. Source: Ref 51

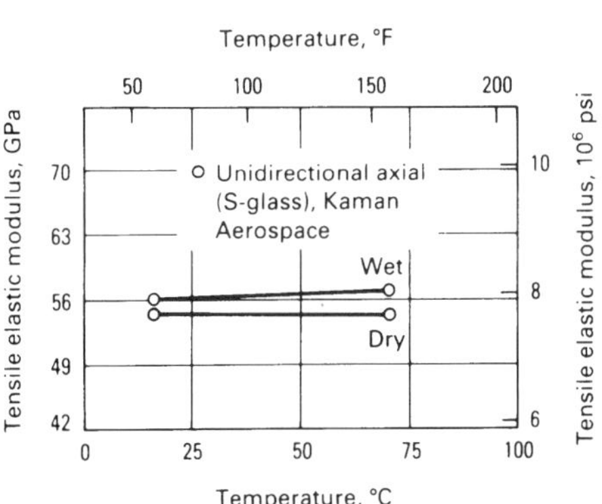

Fig. 85 Tensile elastic modulus versus temperature for thermoset phenolic resin-matrix composites with S-glass fabric reinforcements. Source: Ref 51

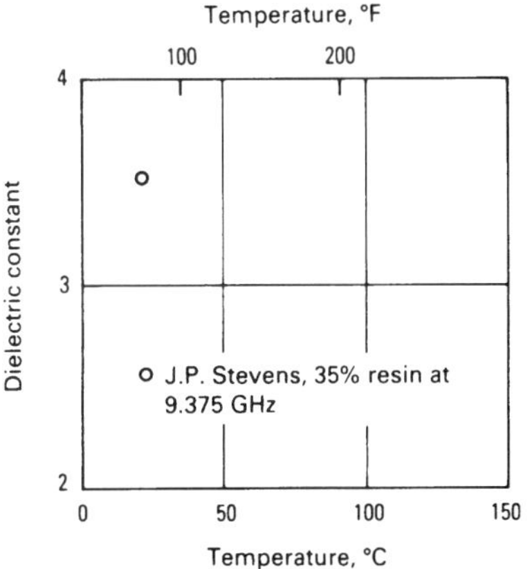

Fig. 86 Dielectric constant versus temperature for thermoset epoxy resin-matrix composites with quartz-fabric reinforcements. Source: Ref 65

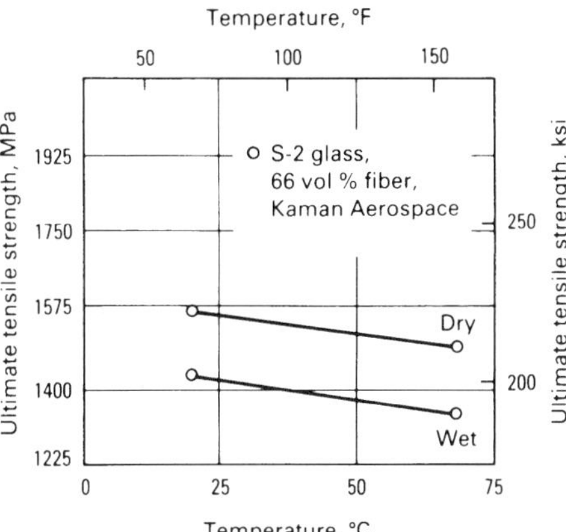

Fig. 87 Ultimate tensile strength versus temperature for thermoset phenolic resin-matrix composites with S-glass fabric reinforcements. Source: Ref 51

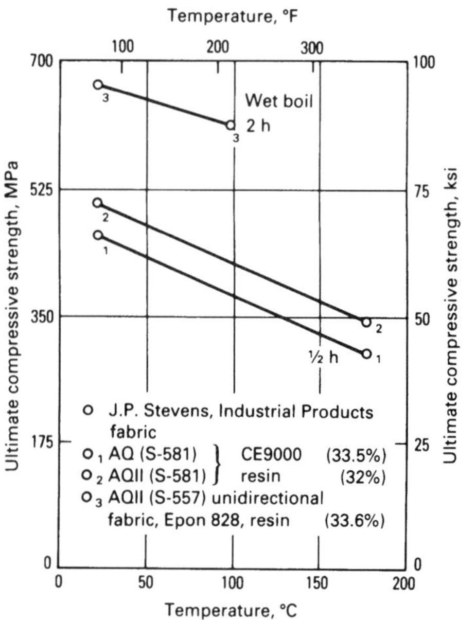

Fig. 88 Ultimate compressive strength versus temperature for thermoset epoxy resin-matrix composites with quartz-fabric reinforcements. Source: Ref 65

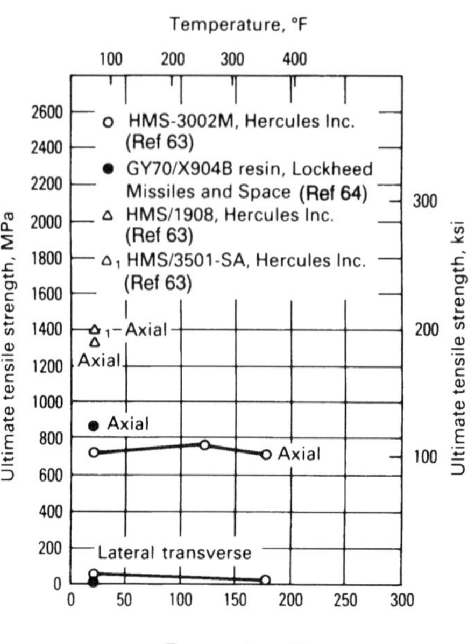

Fig. 89 Ultimate tensile strength versus temperature for thermoset epoxy resin-matrix composites with graphite-fiber reinforcements

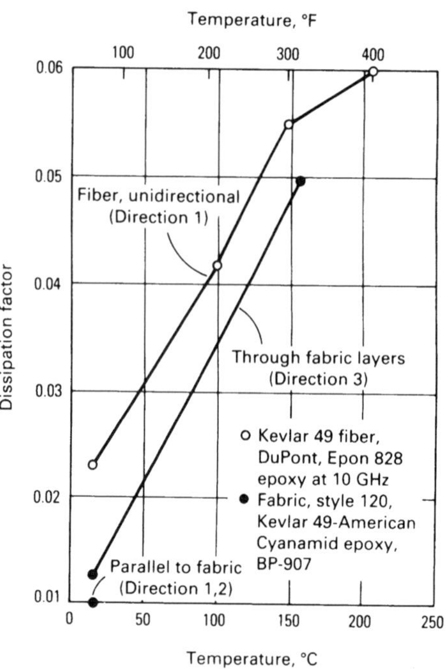

Fig. 90 Dissipation factor versus temperature for thermoset epoxy resin-matrix composites with Kevlar reinforcements

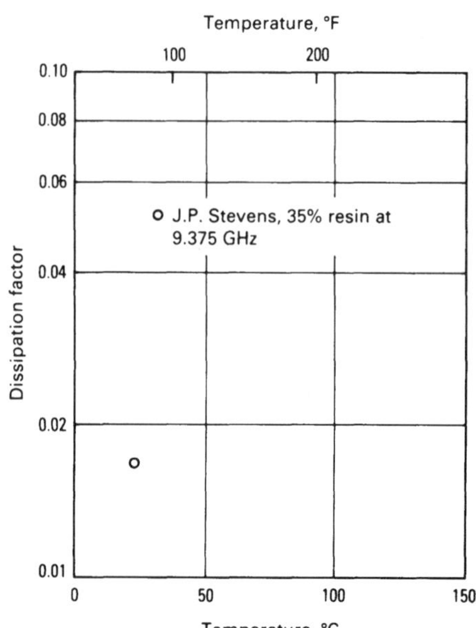

Fig. 91 Dissipation factor versus temperature for thermoset epoxy resin-matrix composites with quartz-fabric reinforcements. Source: Ref 65

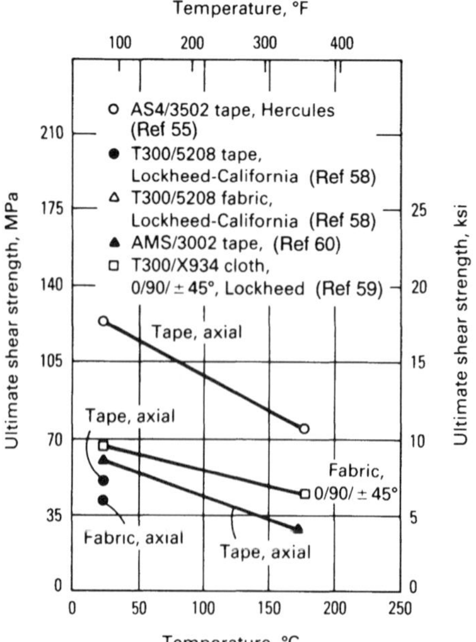

Fig. 92 Ultimate shear strength versus temperature for thermoset epoxy resin-matrix composites with carbon reinforcements

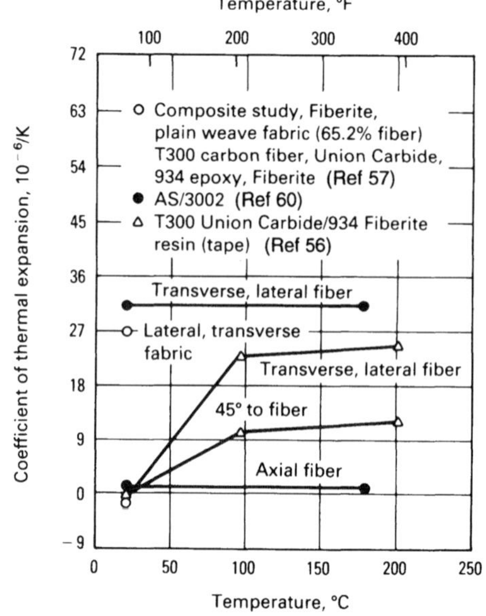

Fig. 93 Coefficient of thermal expansion versus temperature for thermoset epoxy resin-matrix composites with carbon reinforcements. $10^{-6}/K \times 5/9 = \mu in./in. \times °F$

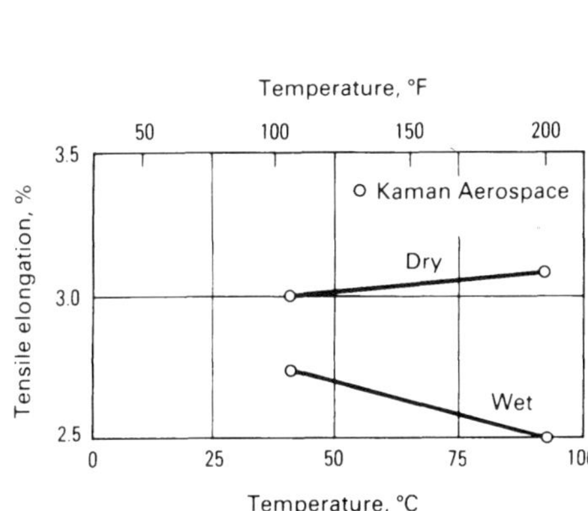

Fig. 94 Tensile elongation percent versus temperature for thermoset phenolic resin-matrix composites with S-glass reinforcements. Source: Ref 51

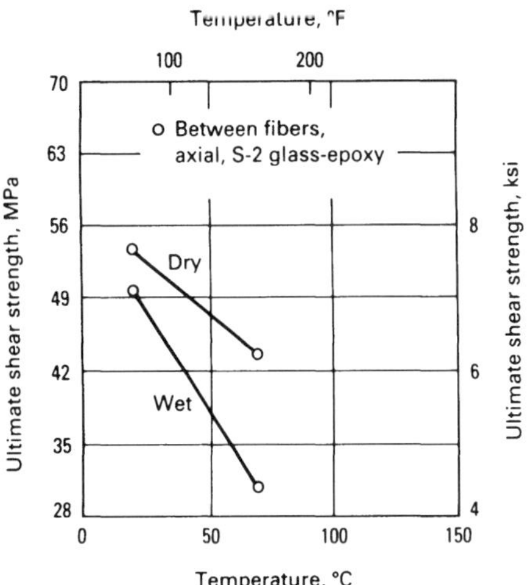

Fig. 95 Ultimate shear strength versus temperature for thermoset phenolic resin-matrix composites with S-glass fabric reinforcements. Source: Ref 51

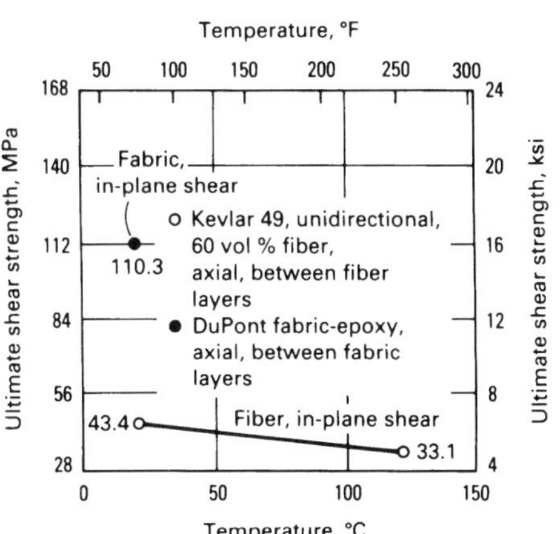

Fig. 96 Ultimate shear strength versus temperature for thermoset epoxy resin-matrix composites with Kevlar reinforcements. Room-temperature tensile elongation: axial fiber, 1.85%; axial fabric, 1.78%. Source: Ref 54

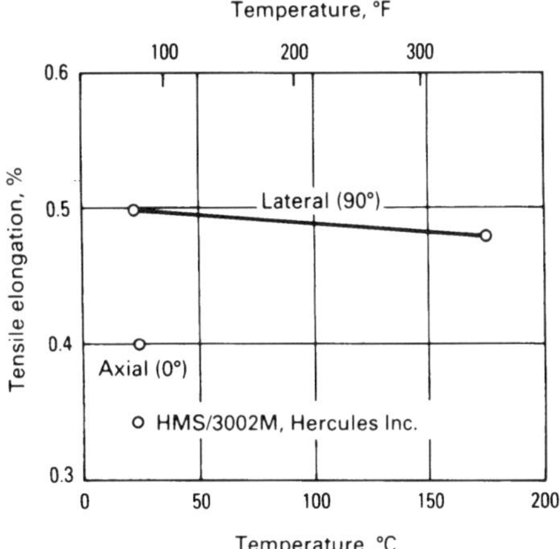

Fig. 97 Tensile elongation versus temperature for thermoset epoxy resin-matrix composites with graphite-fiber reinforcements. Source: Ref 63

Table 9 Physical properties and service characteristics of thermoset polyimide resin and fiber-resin composites

Properties	Resin	50% glass fiber composite
Heat deflection temperature at 1820 kPa (264 psi), °C (°F)	305–360 (582–680)	350 (660)
In-service temperature, °C (°F)	260–370 (500–700)	260 (500)
Specific gravity	1.43	1.65
Density, g/cm^3 (lb/in.^{3})	1.43 (0.052)	1.65 (0.060)

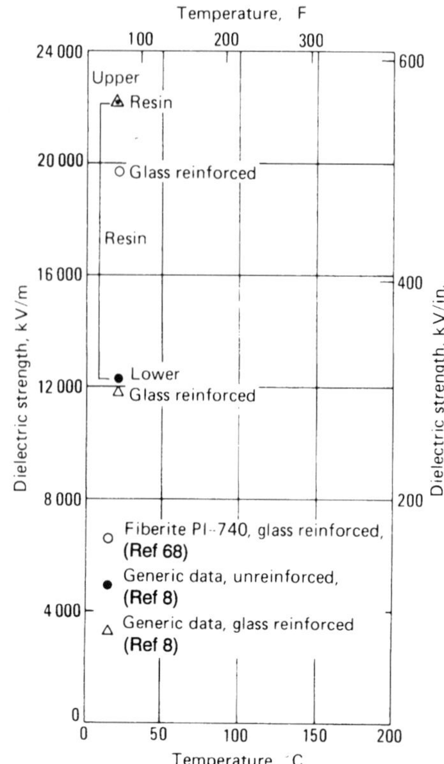

Fig. 98 Dielectric strength versus temperature for thermoset polyimide resin and resin-matrix composites

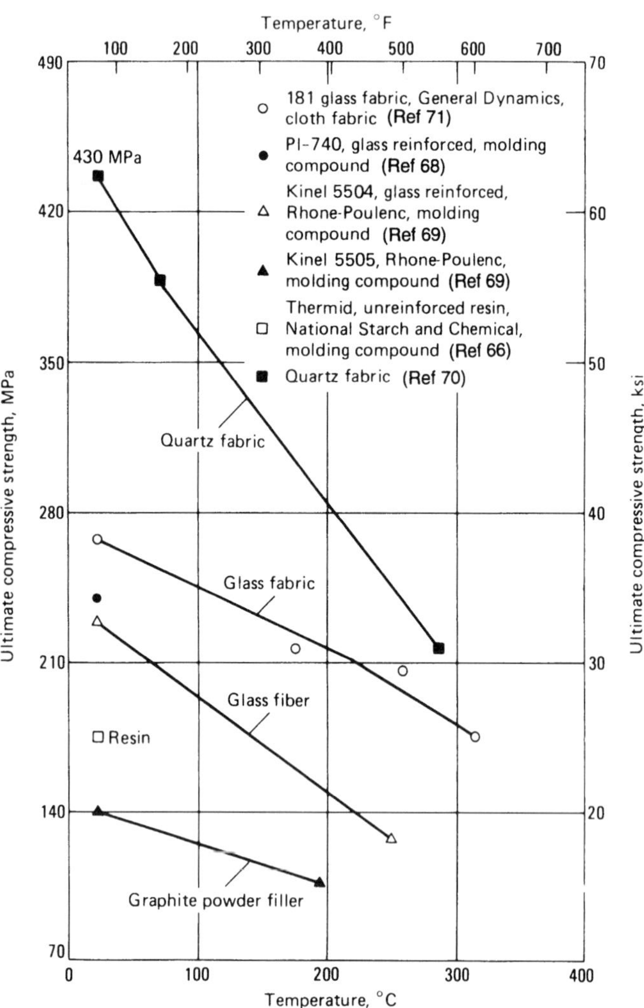

Fig. 99 Ultimate compressive strength versus temperature for thermoset polyimide resin and resin-matrix composites

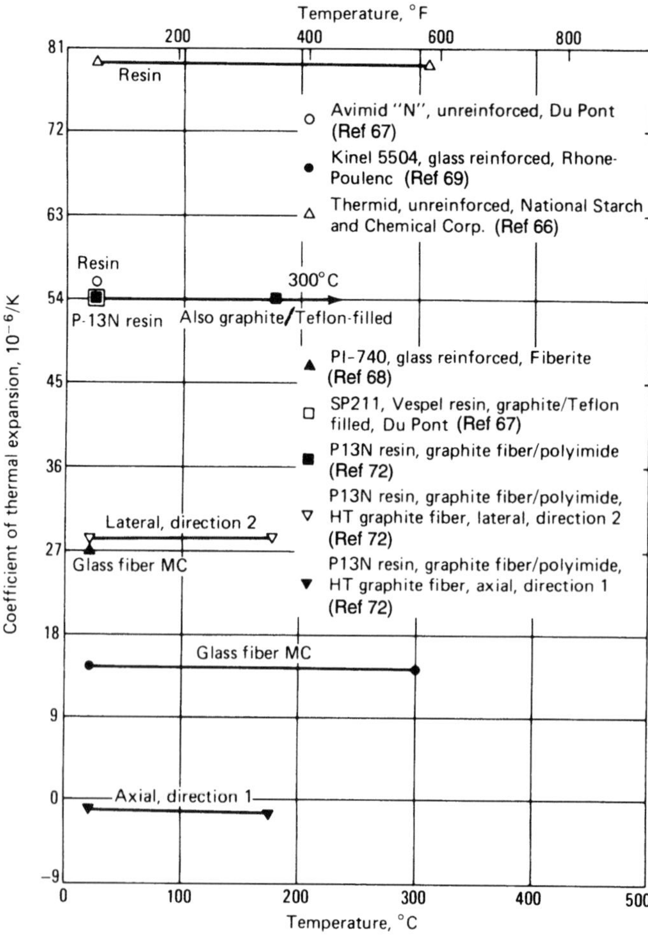

Fig. 100 Coefficient of thermal expansion versus temperature for thermoset polyimide resin and resin-matrix composites. 10^{-6}/K × $\frac{5}{9}$ = μin./in. × °F

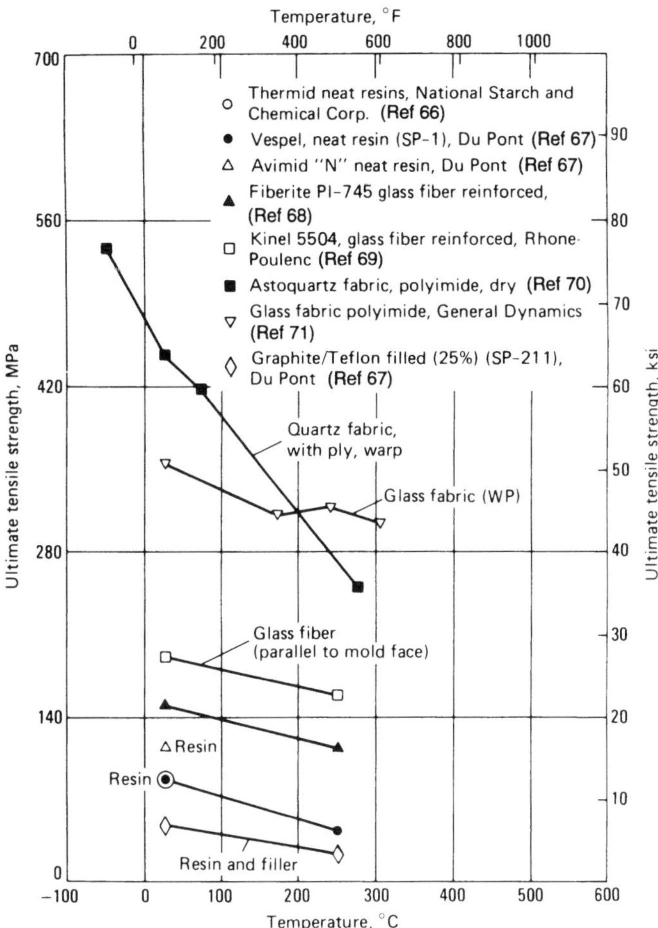

Fig. 101 Ultimate tensile strength versus temperature for thermoset polyimide resin and resin-matrix composites

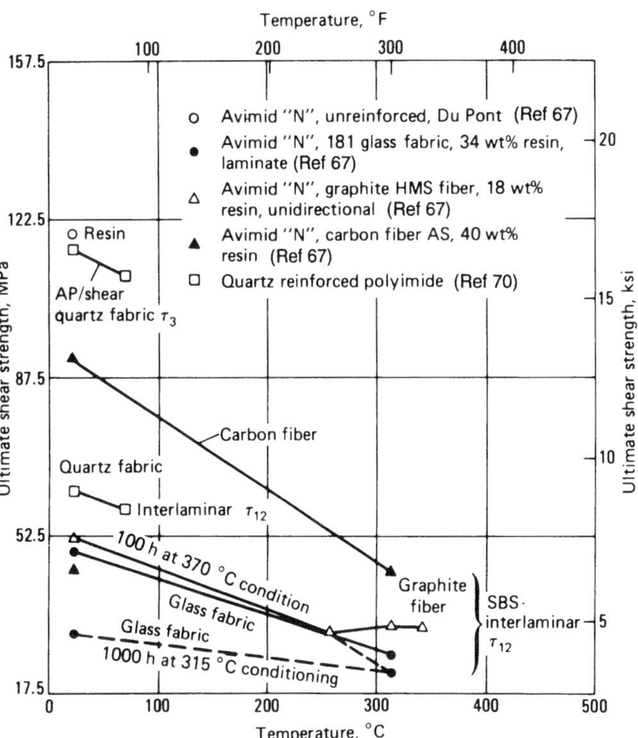

Fig. 102 Ultimate shear strength versus temperature for thermoset polyimide resin and resin-matrix composites

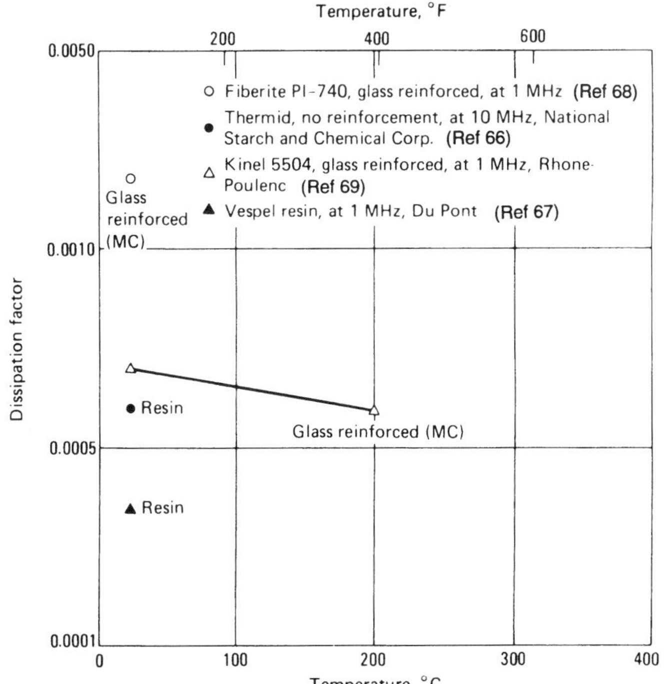

Fig. 103 Dissipation factor versus temperature for thermoset polyimide resin and resin-matrix composites. MC, molding compound

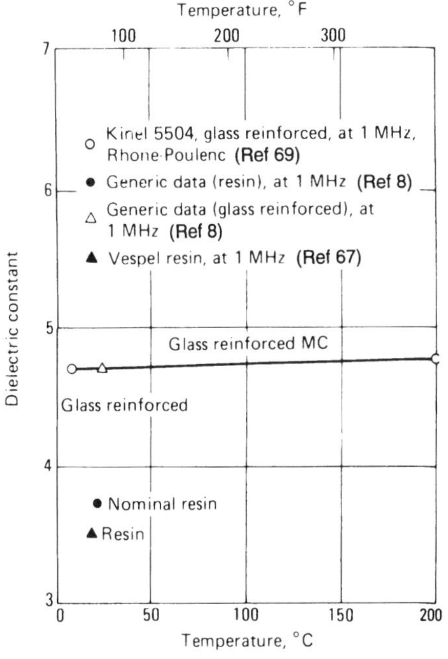

Fig. 104 Dielectric constant versus temperature for thermoset polyimide resin and resin-matrix composites

Table 10 Physical properties and characteristics of thermoset bismaleimide resin and resin-matrix composites

Properties	Neat resin	68.3 vol% T300 carbon fiber composite	57.7 vol% E-glass fiber fabric composite
Specific gravity	1.23	1.60	2.0
Density, g/cm^3 (lb/in.^{3})	1.23 (0.044)	1.60 (0.058)	2.0 (0.072)
In-service temperature			
Short-term, °C (°F)	315 (600)	315 (600)	315 (600)
Long-term, °C (°F)	230 (450)	230 (450)	230 (450)

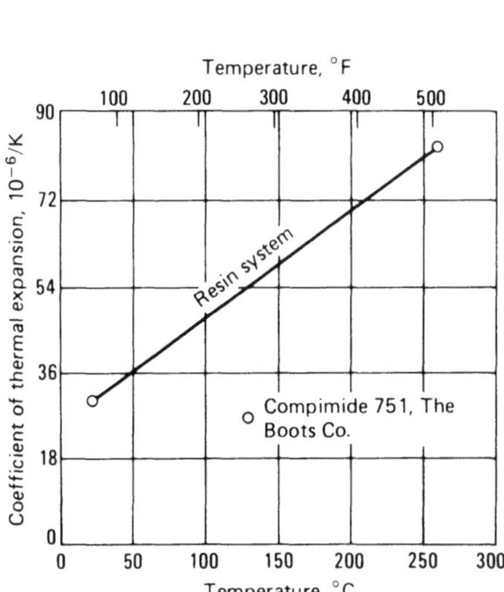

Fig. 105 Coefficient of thermal expansion versus temperature for thermoset bismaleimide resin. 10^{-6}/K × 5/9 = μin./in. × °F. Source: Ref 73

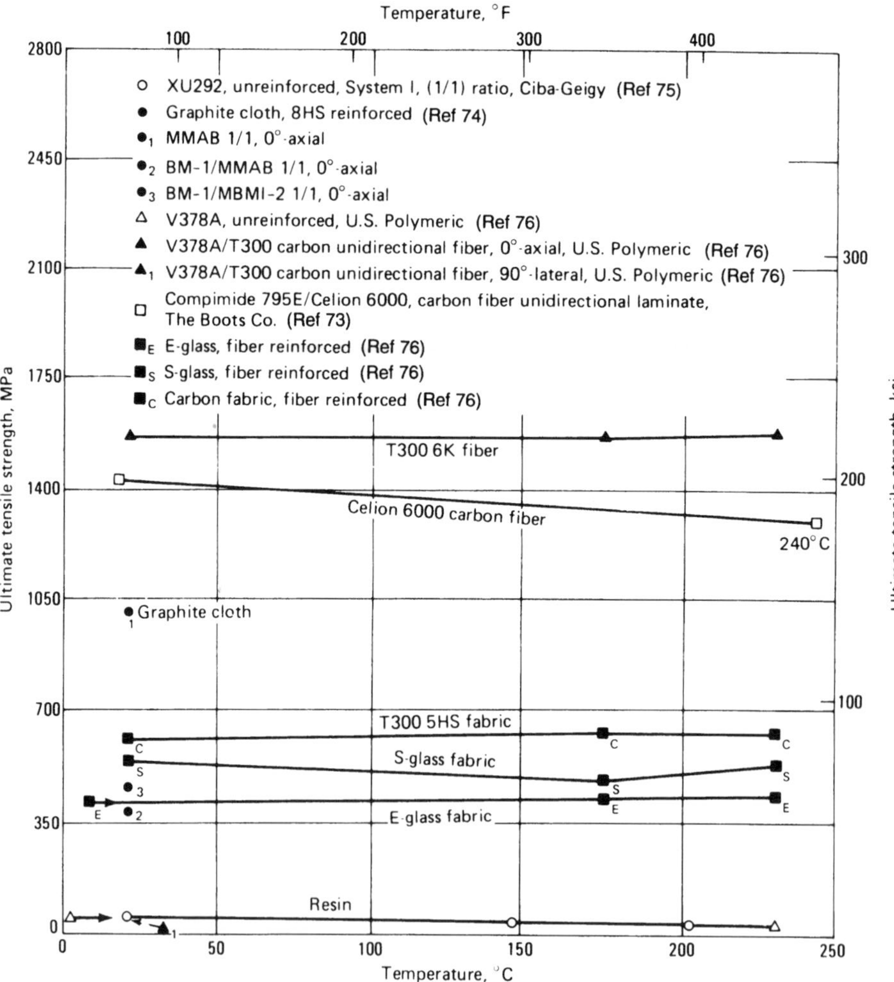

Fig. 106 Ultimate tensile strength versus temperature for thermoset bismaleimide resin and resin-matrix composites

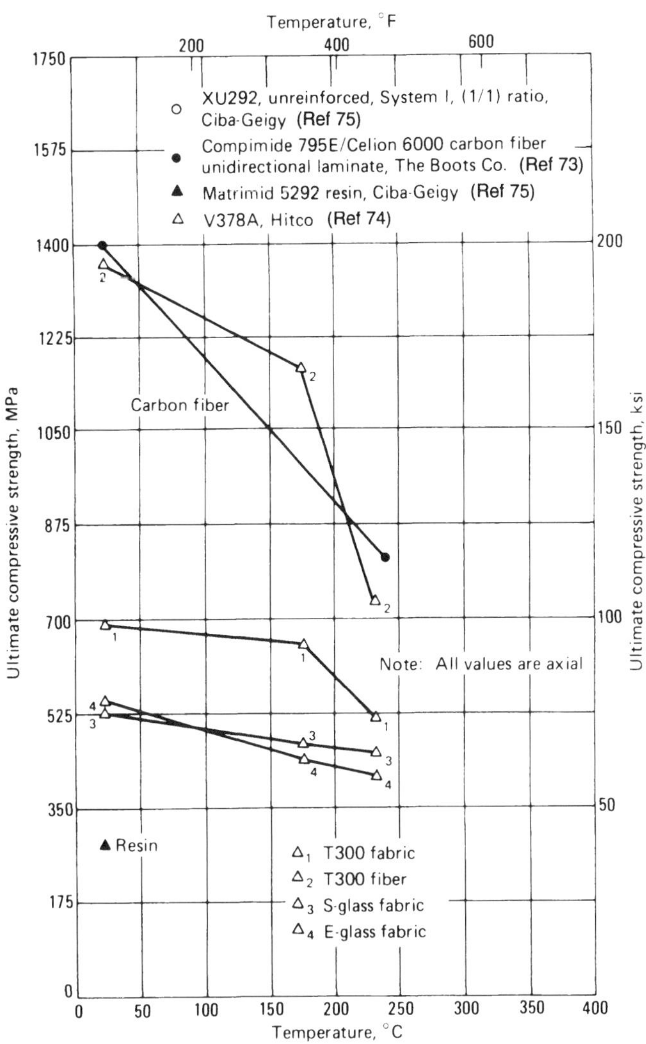

Fig. 107 Ultimate compressive strength versus temperature for thermoset bismaleimide resin and resin-matrix composites

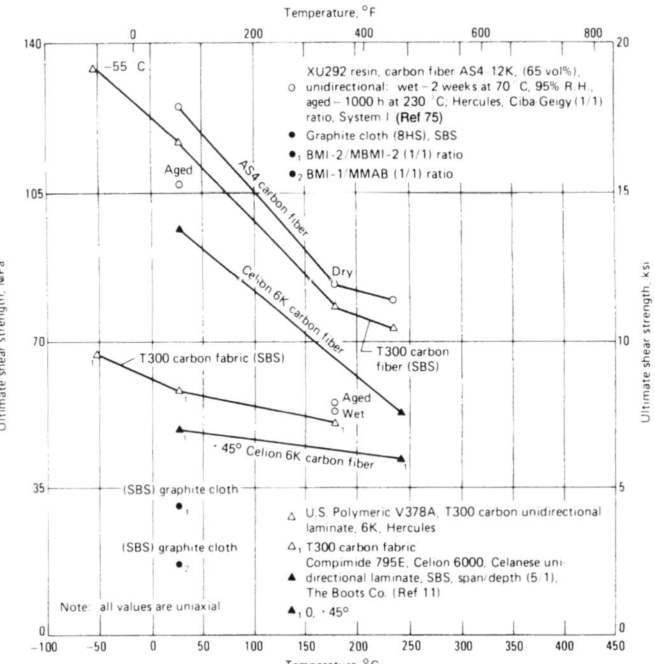

Fig. 108 Ultimate shear strength versus temperature for thermoset bismaleimide resin and resin-matrix composites

Properties of Metal-Matrix Composites

David E. Alman, U.S. Department of Energy, Albany Research Center

METAL-MATRIX COMPOSITES (MMCs) are a diverse class of materials that consist of a metallic alloy matrix typically reinforced with a ceramic phase in the form of particles, platelets, whiskers, short fibers, and continuously aligned fibers (Ref 1–3). Metal-matrix composites are used in structural applications, and in applications requiring wear resistance, thermal management, and weight savings. By far the most common commercial MMCs are based on aluminum, magnesium, and titanium alloys reinforced with either silicon carbide (SiC), alumina (Al_2O_3), carbon, or graphite.

Both continuously and discontinuously reinforced MMCs are used in structural applications. The incorporation of the reinforcement increases the stiffness and strength of the matrix. Figure 1 shows a comparison of the specific strength versus temperature for MMCs, conventional alloys, and other composites (Ref 4). However, the improvements in stiffness and strength generally come at the expense of ductility and fracture resistance. Hybrid laminated metallic (or ductile phase-toughened) composites combine strong materials with tough materials; they can offer an attractive combination of both strength and toughness.

Two types of MMCs are used in wear applications: composites with graphitic-type reinforcements and those with hard ceramic reinforcements. The addition of graphite to the matrix alloys alters the coefficient of friction between the composite and counterface, leading to prolonged wear life during sliding. The addition of hard ceramic particles increases the hardness of the composite, which enhances the resistance of the matrix to the penetration and reduces subsequent removal of material by wear debris and other third-body particles found in the wear environment. It should be emphasized that wear resistance is not a material property, but is a system response dependent on intrinsic materials properties and extrinsic factors related to the wear environment. Unlike mechanical properties, no single definable material parameter exists to universally quantify wear behavior.

Advancements in casting technologies have resulted in methods of manufacturing reinforced Al-MMCs containing high volume fractions (>40 vol%) of reinforcements. These composites have a coefficient of thermal expansion (CTE) similar to those of integrated circuit materials. Consequently, these types of composites are used as thermal management and support structures for electronic packages (Ref 1–3).

This article summarizes the properties of discontinuously reinforced MMCs, laminated metallic composites, and continuously aligned fiber reinforced MMCs.

Discontinuously Reinforced MMCs

Discontinuously reinforced MMCs are much less expensive to fabricate than continuously reinforced composites. Consequently, performance enhancement of the matrix comes at lower additional costs with discontinuous reinforcements compared with aligned reinforcements. Furthermore, the properties of discontinuously reinforced composites are nearly isotropic, whereas the properties of composites with continuous aligned reinforcements are highly anisotropic. Thus, in applications requiring isotropic properties, less expensive, discontinuously reinforced composites can outperform continuous fiber reinforced composites.

Typically, ceramics and graphitic materials are used as reinforcement phases in discontinuously reinforced MMCs. The properties of selected phases used as discontinuous reinforcements for MMCs are listed in Table 1 (Ref 5, 6). Silicon carbide, Al_2O_3, boron carbide (B_4C), and graphite are common reinforcements for aluminum matrices. Titanium carbide (TiC) and titanium boride (TiB) are common reinforcements for titanium alloys. Magnesium matrices are commonly reinforced with SiC, Al_2O_3, and graphite.

Properties of Discontinuously Reinforced Aluminum Composites

Discontinuously reinforced Al-MMCs, or DRAs, are the most widely applied commercial MMCs. The incorporation of hard particles strengthens (Fig. 2a) and stiffens (Fig. 2b) the aluminum matrix, but at the expense of ductility (Fig. 2a). The addition of softer graphitic particles decreases both strength and ductility. Al-

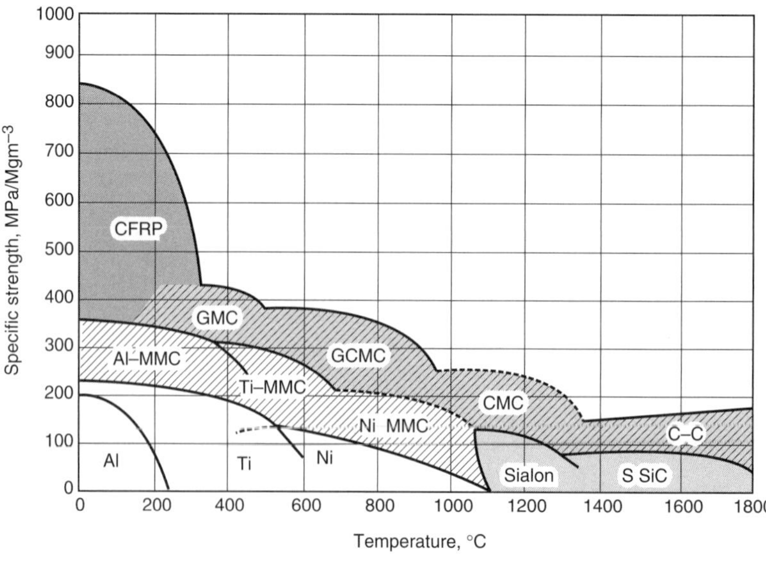

Fig. 1 Specific strength versus temperature. CFRP, carbon fiber reinforced polymers; GMC, glass-matrix composites; GCMC, glass-ceramic-matrix composites; CMC, ceramic-matrix composite; C-C, carbon-carbon composites; MMC, metal-matrix composites

MMCs components are manufactured using both cast and wrought metallurgical methods.

Cast Composites. Al-MMCs are melted and investment cast into near-net shapes in a manner similar to the techniques used for unreinforced aluminum alloys (Ref 7, 8). Due to the density difference between the reinforcement phase (Table 1) and the aluminum alloy (~2.7 g/cm^3), ceramic particles tend to sink and graphite tends to float in the molten metal. Stirring the melt can prevent separation of the matrix and reinforcement. However, investment-cast composites are limited to about 30 vol% reinforcement without phase segregation. Adding nickel-coated graphite particles can prevent segregation of ceramic phases in the molten aluminum, such as in GrA-Ni alloys developed by Inco Limited (Ref 9). During casting, the Al_2O_3 or SiC reinforcements form clusters with the graphite particles. The more dense ceramic particles prevent the lighter graphite particles from floating in the molten aluminum, and vice versa, the graphite particles prevent the ceramic particles from sinking in the molten aluminum. The result is a uniform mixture of particles in the aluminum matrix. The XD process developed by Martin Marietta (now Lockheed Martin) produces composites having a uniform dispersion of fine reinforcements in situ during melting (Ref 10, 11). In this process, compounding elements (such as titanium and carbon or titanium and boron) are mixed with a solvent metal (Al). During heating of the mixture, the compounding elements exothermically react to form an in situ composite (e.g., Al + TiC or Al + TiB_2). This precursor composite is remelted with pure aluminum or an alloy to form a composite containing the desired volume fraction of reinforcement.

Other casting methods, such as semisolid casting and liquid metal infiltration are also used to produce Al-MMCs (Ref 6–8). Semisolid casting methods, such as rheocasting, involve adding the reinforcement to the alloy in a semisolid state. Liquid metal infiltration involves infiltrating a porous preform (the reinforcement) with the molten matrix alloy. The preform can consist of either discontinuous (powders, whiskers, etc.) or continuous (aligned fibers) reinforcements. In processes such as squeeze casting, pressure is applied to the melt to force the liquid into the preform during solidification. Pressureless infiltration of the preform can also be accomplished in vacuum or in a gaseous environment, such as the Primex method developed by Lanxide Corporation. In this process, a ceramic preform (or a mixture of the ceramic with magnesium chips) is infiltrated by an aluminum-magnesium (or aluminum) alloy in a nitrogen (N_2) atmosphere (Ref 11). The magnesium reacts with the N_2 to form magnesium nitride (Mg_3N_2). The formation of these particles enhances the infiltration process, with the particles subsequently reduced by the aluminum to form aluminum nitride (AlN) in the final composite. Composites containing larger volume fractions of reinforcements can be produced more easily using molten-metal infiltration than by using investment casting.

Typical tensile properties for selected cast Al-MMCs are listed in Table 2. Gravity-fed investment-cast composites are commonly used in automotive (e.g., brake rotors, brake calipers, and materials for moving parts in engines) and recreational (e.g., sporting goods) applications. Al-MMCs are particularly attractive materials for use in automotive brake applications because they are lighter and conduct heat three times more efficiently than cast iron (Table 3).

Figure 2(c) illustrates the CTE as a function of volume fraction for the Al-SiC and Al-Al_2O_3 systems. The CTEs of several Al-SiC composites are similar to those of integrated circuit and

Table 1 Properties of selected discontinuous reinforcement materials used for MMCs

Reinforcement	Modulus of elasticity, GPa	Modulus of elasticity, 10^6 psi	Fracture toughness, MPa $\sqrt{m}$	Fracture toughness, ksi $\sqrt{in.}$	Poisson's ratio	Specific heat, J/g · °C	Thermal conductivity, W/m · K	Coefficient of thermal expansion, 10^{-6}/K	Density, g/cm^3
SiC	400	58	4.6	4.2	0.20	0.67	52	4.3	3.20
Al_2O_3	393	57	4.0	3.7	0.25	0.71	30	7.0	3.96
B_4C	445	64.5	3.3	3.02	0.21	0.84	26	4.78	2.51
TiC	451	65.5	...	...	0.185	0.50	35	7.7	4.94
Graphite(a)	8–15	55–103	...	...	...	0.71–0.83	25–450	1.2–8.2	2.24–2.26(b)

(a) The properties of graphite are dependent on the grade (e.g., impurity, ash content, etc.). (b) Theoretical value for graphite; density values for bulk graphite range from 1.3–1.9 g/cm^3. Source: Ref 5, 6

Table 2 Room-temperature tensile properties of selected discontinuously reinforced cast Al-MMCs

Material	Modulus, GPa	Modulus, 10^6 psi	Yield strength, MPa	Yield strength, ksi	Ultimate tensile strength, MPa	Ultimate tensile strength, ksi	Ductility, %
Al (99%) + SiC_w pressure infiltration of preform (Ref 7)							
Al	...	...	127	18.4	225	32.6	4
Al + 20 vol% SiC	...	...	207	30.0	260	37.7	4
Al + 23 vol% SiC	...	...	190	27.5	250	36.2	4
Al + 28 vol% SiC	...	...	200	29.0	270	39.1	3.5
Al + 32 vol% SiC	...	...	260	37.7	312	42.5	2.8
Al + 40 vol% SiC	...	...	340	49.3	390	56.5	0.8
A356Al + SiC gravity cast into sand mold (Ref 8)							
A356Al	75.2	10.9	200	29.0	255	36.9	4
A356 + 10 vol% SiC	77.2	11.2	262	37.9	276	40.0	0.7
A356 + 15 vol% SiC	92.4	13.4	296	42.9	303	43.9	0.4
A356 + 20 vol% SiC	95.8	13.9	296	42.9	317	45.9	0.5
Al-8Si + SiC-graphite (nickel coated)-gravity cast (Ref 9)							
Al-8Si + 10 vol% SiC-4 vol% graphite	...	...	260	37.7	275	39.8	0.6
A359 (Al-9Si) + 20SiC	...	...	310	44.9	317	45.9	0.5
F3S/F3K(a) (Al-Si-Mg) + SiC—gravity cast into permanent mold T6 condition (Ref 8, 12)							
A356	75.2	10.9	200	29.0	276	40.0	6
F3K + 10 vol% SiC	87.6	12.7	359	52.0	372	53.9	0.3
F3K + 20 vol% SiC	101	14.6	372	53.9	372	53.9	<0.1
F3S + 10 vol% SiC	86.2	12.5	303	43.9	338	49.0	1.2
F3S + 20 vol% SiC	98.6	14.3	338	49.0	359	52.0	0.4
F3D/F3N(b) (Al-Si-Cu-Mg-Fe-Ni) + SiC—pressure die cast (Ref 8, 12)							
A380	71	10.3	159	23.0	317	45.9	3.5
A390	81.4	11.8	241	34.9	283	41.0	1.0
F3N + 10 vol% SiC	91	13.2	221	32.0	310	44.9	0.9
F3N + 20 vol% SiC	108.2	15.7	248	35.9	303	43.9	0.5
F3D + 10 vol% SiC	93.8	13.6	241	34.9	345	50.0	1.2
F3D + 20 vol% SiC	113.8	16.5	303	43.9	352	51.0	0.4
206 (Al-Cu) + TiC-XD processes (Ref 11)							
206	70	10.2	345	50.0	434	62.9	12
206 + 20 vol% TiC	96	13.9	358	51.9	400	58.0	1.2
306 + 35 vol% TiC	138	20.0	372	53.9	407	59.0	1.2
A380Al + fly ash gravity cast (Ref 13)							
A380	...	...	165	23.9	331	48.0	3
A380 + 18.9 vol% fly ash	...	...	139	20.1	242	35.0	2.9
A380 + 21.8 vol% fly ash	...	...	118	17.1	228	33.0	3.2
A380 + 27.6 vol% fly ash	...	...	121	17.5	210	30.4	2.7
A380 + 32.8 vol% fly ash	...	...	135	19.5	203	29.4	2.1

(a) F3S = Al + 9Si-0.2Fe-0.2Cu-0.55Mg-0.2Ti; F3K = Al + 10Si-0.3Fe-3Cu-1Mg-1.25Ni-0.2Ti. (b) F3N = Al + 10Si-1Fe-0.2Cu-0.65Mn-0.4Mg; F3D = Al + 10Si-1Fe-3.25Cu-0.65Mn-0.4Mg-1.25Ni

Table 3 Properties of selected Al-MMC used for thermal management applications

Material	Density, g/cm^3	Tensile strength		Modulus		Fracture toughness		Poisson's ratio	Coefficient of thermal expansion, 10^{-6}/K	Heat capacity, J/g · °C	Thermal conductivity, W/m · K	Process
		MPa	ksi	GPa	10^6 psi	MPa $\sqrt{m}$	ksi $\sqrt{in.}$					
Reinforcement, vol%												
54% SiC_p	2.96	...	...	167	24	...	...	0.251	9.5	0.768	180	Infiltration(a)
64% SiC_p	3.01	...	...	192	28	11.3	10.3	0.242	7.5	0.741	180	Infiltration(a)
70% SiC_p	2.99	...	...	217	31	11.7	10.7	0.154	6.6	0.741	180	Infiltration(a)
63% SiC_p	3.01	253	37	220	32	...	...	...	7.9	...	175	Pressure infiltration(b)
68% SiC_p	3.03	207	30	255	37	...	...	...	7.3	...	175	Pressure infiltration(b)
55–70% SiC_p	2.90	225–250	33–36	220–250	32–36	9–10	8.2–9.1	0.23	6.5–7.3	0.72–0.76	160–180	Primex(c)
18–40% SiC_p	2.77–2.87	...	...	108–151	16–22	...	...	...	11.9–16	...	132–183	Primex(c)
Al alloys												
A356	2.69	172	25	72.4	10.5	17.4	15.8	0.33	21.5	0.963	167	...
6061	2.68	290	42	70.3	10.2	29.7	...	0.34	23.5	...	171	...
Structural, cast												
55 vol% Al_2O_3	3.40	380	55	167	24	18.5	27.0	...	13.2	0.831	88.5	Vacuum infiltration(d)
10 vol% SiC	2.71	303	44	86.2	12.5	17.4	15.8	...	20.7	0.879	151	F3S.10S(e)
20 vol% SiC	2.77	338	49	98.6	14.3	15.9	14.5	...	17.5	0.837	185	F3S.20S(e)
Structural, wrought												
6061-10 vol% Al_2O_3	2.81	352	51	81.4	11.8	24.1	21.9	...	20.9	...	156	W6A.10A-T6(e)
6061-15 vol% Al_2O_3	2.86	365	53	88.9	12.9	22.0	20.0	...	19.8	...	144	W6A.15A-T6(e)
6092-15 vol% SiC	2.78	468	68	91.6	13.3	...	...	...	19.1	...	185	HS-series(f)
6092-40 vol% SiC	2.92	544	79	135.8	119.7	...	...	...	13.6	...	190	HS-series(f)
Related materials												
Gray cast iron	7.2	300–400	44–58	99–119	90–108	...	...	...	...	0.402	47	...
GaAs	...	...	...	...	...	...	...	...	5.8	...	...	...
Al_2O_3	3.9	...	...	...	...	...	...	...	6.7	...	20	...
Silicon	2.3	...	...	...	...	...	...	...	4.1	...	150	...
Copper	8.9	...	...	...	...	...	...	...	17	...	400	...
Kovar (Ni-Fe)	8.3	...	...	...	...	...	...	...	5.9	...	17	...
W-10Cu	16.6	...	...	...	...	...	...	...	6.5	...	167	...

(a) Ceramics Process Systems (Ref 14). (b) PCC-Advanced Forming Technology (Ref 15). (c) Lanxide (Ref 16). (d) MMCC, Inc. (Ref 17). (e) Duralcan (Ref 12). (f) Alyn Corp. (Ref 18)

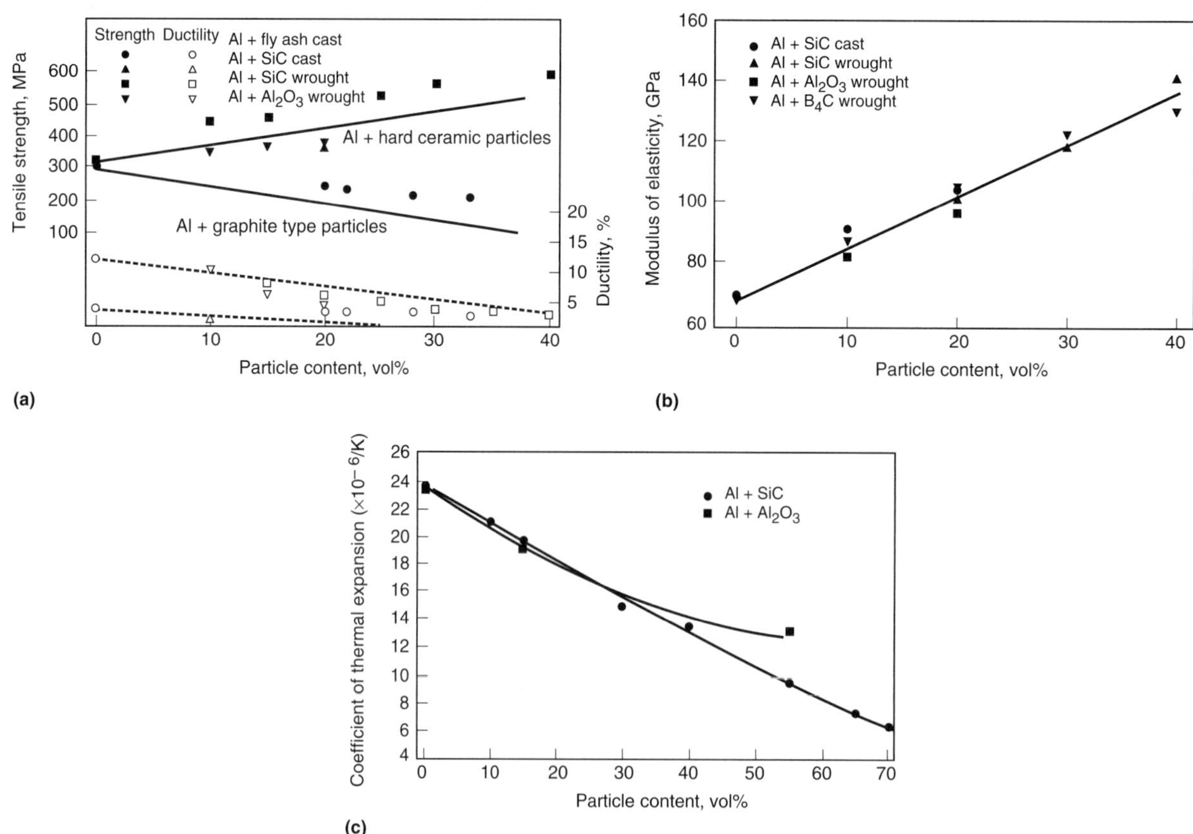

Fig. 2 The effect of particulate concentration on the properties of Al-MMCs. (a) Strength and ductility. (b) Modulus. (c) Coefficient of thermal expansion

electronic packaging materials, so these composites are used as heat sinks and structural supports for electronic packages. Al-MMCs are less dense than traditional heat-sink materials, Kovar (Fe-Ni) alloys, for example, which is advantageous in weight-sensitive applications such as avionics. Table 3 lists the mechanical and thermal properties for selected Al-MMCs, as well as properties for several related materials.

The influence of SiC particle size on the tensile properties of squeezed-cast Al-4Mg + 50 vol% silicon carbide particulate (SiC_p) composites is shown in Fig. 3 (Ref 19). Particle size has a strong effect on the failure mode, strength, and ductility of the composite; both strength and ductility decrease with increasing particle size. The fracture process is dominated by metal failure (e.g., few broken SiC particles, Fig. 3b) in composites having small reinforcements (<6.5 μm) and by particle breakage for large reinforcements (>23 μm). The optimal combination of properties occurs in the intermediate-size regime where neither mode of primary failure predominates. A similar trend has been noted for the tensile strength of aluminum alloy 2014-55 vol% Al_2O_3 composites produced via pressure infiltration (Ref 20). The tensile strength decreases with increasing Al_2O_3 particle size (ultimate tensile strengths of 440, 360, and 300 MPa for composites having 5, 12.85, and 29.2 μm Al_2O_3 particles, respectively). The influence of particle size on strength can be rationalized by considering that the strength distribution of the ceramic particle population in the composite follows Weibull statistics. Therefore, larger particles are detrimental to strength as they are more likely to contain flaws and thus fail at a lower stress levels, which reduces the overall strength of the composite.

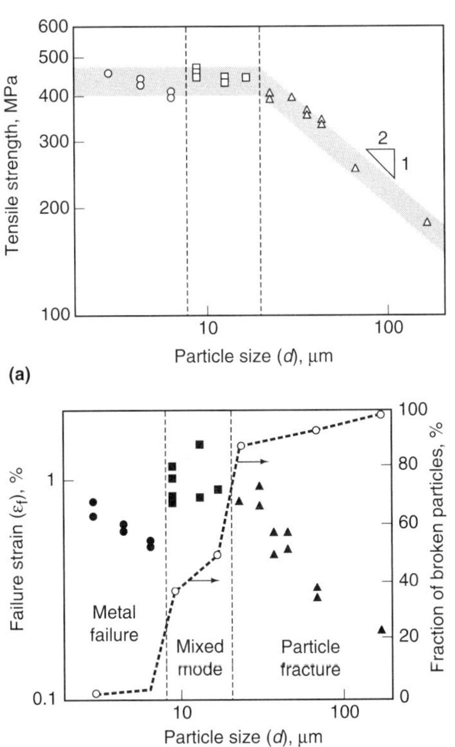

Fig. 3 Influence of SiC particle size on (a) strength and (b) failure properties of Al-4Mg + 50 vol% (nominal) SiC_p composites. Source: Ref 20

Wrought Composites. Wrought Al-MMCs typically contain less than 40 vol% reinforcement. These composites are manufactured by preparing a billet or an ingot, which is subsequently forged, rolled, or extruded. The billet can be produced using casting, spray forming, or powder metallurgy (P/M) methods. Extrusions are used as bicycle frames, automotive shafts, and fan exit guide vanes for gas turbines (Ref 21, 22). Sheet products are used in aerospace applications, such as fuel access cover panels and ventral fins for the F16 fighter aircraft (Ref 22). Forgings find applications as chip carriers for electronic packages (Ref 21). Table 4 lists typical properties for selected wrought aluminum alloys reinforced with SiC, B_4C, or Al_2O_3 particles.

Deformation processing breaks the reinforcement into smaller particles, enhances the bond strength between the particle and matrix, and aligns the reinforcement parallel to the direction of material flow. Reinforcement alignment imparts composite texture with respect to the orientation of the reinforcement phase, especially for composites reinforced with whiskers. Table 5 lists the influence of orientation on the properties of several deformation-processed Al-SiC composites. The properties of composites having SiC whiskers are more anisotropic than composites produced with particles. This is due in part

Table 4 Room-temperature tensile properties of selected wrought particulate reinforced Al-MMCs (T6 condition)

	Modulus		Yield strength		Tensile strength		
Particle content, vol%	GPa	10^6 psi	MPa	ksi	MPa	ksi	Ductility, %
6061 (Al-Mg-Si)-SiC							
0	68.9	10.0	275.8	40.0	310.3	45.0	12
15	95.5	13.8	400	58	455.1	66.0	7.5
20	103.4	15.0	413.7	60.0	496.4	72.0	5.5
25	113.8	16.5	427.5	62.0	517.1	75.0	4.5
30	120.7	17.5	434.3	63.0	551.6	80.0	3.0
35	134.5	19.5	455.1	66.0	551.6	80.0	2.7
40	144.8	21.0	448.2	65.0	586.1	85.0	2.0
6092 (Al-Mg-Si)-SiC							
0	68.9	10.0	379	55	447.8	64.9	11
5	75.8	11.0	385.8	55.9	440.9	63.9	8
10	84.1	12.2	399.6	57.9	454.7	65.9	6
15	91.6	13.3	413.4	59.9	468.5	67.9	5
20	100	14.5	427.2	61.9	482.3	69.9	4.5
25	108.2	15.7	447.9	64.9	503.0	72.9	3
30	119.9	17.4	461.6	66.9	516.8	74.9	1.5
35	124.0	18.0	475.4	68.9	537.4	77.9	1.0
40	131.6	19.1	482.3	69.9	544.3	78.9	0.8
2124 (Al-Cu-Mg)-SiC							
0	71	10.3	420.6	61.0	455.1	66.0	9
10	93.8	13.6	437	63	484	70.2	7
20	103.4	15.0	400	58	555.6	80.6	7
25	113.8	16.5	413.7	60.0	565.4	82.0	5.6
30	120.7	17.5	441.3	64.0	593.0	86.0	4.5
40	151.7	22.0	517.1	75.0	689.5	100.0	1.1
6092 (Al-Mg-Si)-B_4C							
0	68.9	10.0	379	55	447.8	64.9	11
5	77.9	11.3	358.3	52.0	427.2	61.9	12
10	86.8	12.6	372.1	54.0	454.7	65.9	6
15	95.7	13.9	365.2	53.0	447.8	64.9	6
20	104.7	15.2	258.3	37.4	427.2	61.9	3
25	113.7	16.5	379	55	461.6	66.9	3
30	122.6	17.8	365.2	53.0	447.9	64.9	1
35	131.6	19.1	258.3	37.4	441	63.9	0.8
6061 (Al-Mg-Si)-Al_2O_3							
0	68.9	10.0	275	40	310.3	45.0	12
10	81.4	11.8	295	43	350	50.8	10
15	89	12.9	325	47	365	52.9	6
20	97.2	14.1	350	51	370	53.7	4
2014 (Al-Cu-Mg)-Al_2O_3							
0	73.1	10.6	475	69	525	76.1	13
10	84.1	12.2	495	72	530	76.9	3
15	93.8	13.6	505	73	530	76.9	2
20	101	14.6	505	73	515	74.7	1

Source: Ref 7, 18, 21

to the texture effect, that is, composites having whiskers tend to be stronger than similar matrix composites reinforced with particles. However, this phenomenon is also related to the relative diameters of the whiskers and particles. The diameter of available whiskers are an order of magnitude smaller than the diameter of available SiC particles. Experimental composites produced using either particles or whiskers of similar diameters have nearly identical tensile properties; yield strength (σ_{YS}) is 167 MPa (24 ksi) and ultimate tensile strength (σ_{UTS}) is 299 MPa (43 ksi) for an Al + 20 vol% SiC composite containing 0.5 μm diameter and 2 to 3μm long whiskers compared with σ_{YS} of 172 MPa (25 ksi) and σ_{UTS} of 250 MPa (36 ksi) for an Al + 20 vol% SiC composite containing 0.5 μm diameter spherical particles (Ref 23). The amount of deformation (extrusion reduction ratio) can influence the properties of the composites. Figure 4 illustrates the influence of extrusion ratio on the properties of 6061/Al_2O_3 particulate composite (Ref 24). Larger extrusion ratios result in stronger composites. This is attributed to the effect that extrusion has on reinforcement particle size (larger reductions result in composites with smaller reinforcements).

Age-Hardened Composites. The properties of any MMC that utilizes a matrix that can be age hardened (e.g., 2*xxx*, 6*xxx*, and 7*xxx* series alloys) will be influenced by subsequent heat treatment (Fig. 5) (Ref 1). The addition of reinforcement particles to aluminum alloy matrix may accelerate aging kinetics as illustrated in Fig. 6 and has been observed to occur in alloys reinforced with SiC, Al_2O_3, and B_4C particles and whiskers (Ref 25). Accelerated aging is due in part to the mismatch between the CTE of the matrix and reinforcement. During cooling, the strain field generated by the CTE mismatch is relaxed in the matrix through the generation of dislocations. These serve as nucleation sites for matrix-strengthening precipitates, and as a consequence the aging process is accelerated compared with unreinforced alloys.

Elevated-Temperature and Creep Properties. Elevated-temperature tensile properties for selected Al-MMC s are listed in Table 6. There have been numerous studies on the creep behavior of Al-SiC, Al-Al_2O_3, Al-TiC, and Al-TiB_2 composites reported in the literature (Ref 27–43). As with elevated-temperature strength, the addition of the reinforcement enhances creep life of the composite.

Early onset of tertiary creep occurs during creep testing of Al-MMC in tension and at high stress levels. Little deformation occurs in the composite until severe localized deformation (cavitation) initiates around the reinforcement. Consequently, the minimum strain rate determined in tension at high stress levels does not always correspond to the steady-state secondary strain rate. Tests performed in compression or shear delay the onset of tertiary creep, and thus may provide more accurate values for the steady-state creep parameters.

Powder-processed composites tend to have better creep resistance than cast composites due to the oxides associated with powder matrices (e.g., oxides on the surfaces of the starting aluminum powder), which inhibit dislocation motion (Ref 39). The size of the reinforcement is an important factor in determining creep resistance (Ref 39). Smaller, more numerous reinforcements are more effective in enhancing creep resistance via impeding matrix dislocation motion, stabilizing grain growth, and so forth. The distribution of the reinforcement has a critical effect on creep damage. Clustering of the reinforcement results in severe cavitation near the reinforcement and concomitant rapid failure of the composite. For isolated reinforcements, damage occurs at reinforcement angularities.

Creep in Al-MMCs is unique in several aspects. First, the dependency of the steady-state secondary creep rate on the applied stress, measured by the power-law creep stress exponent, n, is high, ranging from 7 to 25. This compares with about 4 for aluminum alloys. Second, the temperature dependence of steady-state creep rate, measured by the creep activation energy, Q, is much larger than for self-diffusion in aluminum; Q varies from 200 to 500 kJ/mol compared with 146 kJ/mol for aluminum (Ref 27). In these aspects, the creep behavior of Al-MMC resembles that of dispersion-strengthened alloys, where the creep behavior can be explained in terms of a threshold stress (σ_0) for creep. Unlike dispersion-strengthened alloys, where the origin of the threshold stress arises from the interaction of dislocations with a fine dispersion of particles, the origin of the threshold stress for Al-MMCs is complex and is not fully understood. Furthermore, in composites the applied load will be carried by both the matrix and the reinforcement. A modified power-law creep equation for discontinuous composites that incorporates a stress-partition parameter has been proposed, as follows (Ref 36):

$$\dot{\varepsilon} \propto \{(1-\alpha_{LT})(\sigma-\sigma_0)\}^n \exp\left[-\frac{Q}{RT}\right] \quad \text{(Eq 1)}$$

Table 5 Influence of specimen orientation on the properties of wrought Al-MMCs

Orientation	Modulus, GPa	Modulus, 10^6 psi	Yield strength, MPa	Yield strength, ksi	Ultimate strength, MPa	Ultimate strength, ksi	Ductility, %	Coefficient of thermal expansion, 10^{-6}/K	Density, g/cm^3
6092 + 17.5 vol% SiC particles (T6) plate extrusions									
6.35 mm (0.25 in.) thick									
L	123	17.9	478	65	537	78	4	...	2.83
LT	119	17.3	427	62	517	75	3	...	2.83
12.7 mm (0.5 in.) thick									
L	122	17.7	429	61	516	75	5	15.3	2.82
LT	116	16.8	388	58	482	70	4	...	...
18.8 mm (0.75 in.) thick									
L	121	17.6	429	61	516	75	5	...	...
LT	114	16.6	388	58	482	70	4	...	...
6092 + 17.5 vol% SiC particles (T6) rolled sheet									
1.00 mm (0.03 in.) thick									
L	100	14.6	400	58	475	69	7	16.7	2.80
LT	98	14.2	372	54	454	66	7	16.4	...
2.00 mm (0.07 in.) thick									
L	101	14.7	386	56	455	66	8	16.7	2.80
LT	101	14.7	385	52	448	65	8	16.6	...
2.50 mm (0.10 in.) thick									
L	101	14.7	393	57	461	67	8	17.5	2.80
LT	101	14.7	365	53	455	66	7	16.9	...
3.17 mm (0.12 in.) thick									
L	101	14.7	393	57	461	67	8	16.7	2.80
LT	101	14.7	365	53	455	66	8	16.4	...
2024Al + 20 vol% SiC whiskers (T6), cylindrical billet (305 mm, or 12 in., diam)									
L			351	50.9	496	71.9	...	16.1	2.86
2024Al + 20 vol% SiC whiskers, 13 × 125 mm (0.5 × 5 in.) plate extrusion									
L			448	64.9	731	107	...	13.1	2.86
LT			379	54.9	426	67	...	19.6	...
2124Al + 15 vol% SiC whiskers (T6) rolled sheet 2.54 mm, or 0.1 in. thick									
L	114	16.5	573	83.1	718	104	5.3	...	...
LT	95	14	386	56.4	559	81	8.5	...	...
2009Al + 15 vol% SiC whiskers sheet (T8)									
L	106	15.3	483	70	634	92	6.4	...	...
LT	98	14.2	400	58	552	80	8.4	...	...
2009Al + 20 vol% SiC particles sheet (T8)									
L	109	15.8	462	67	593	86	5.2	...	...
LT	109	15.8	421	61	672	97.5	5.3	...	...

Source: Ref 3, 7, 22

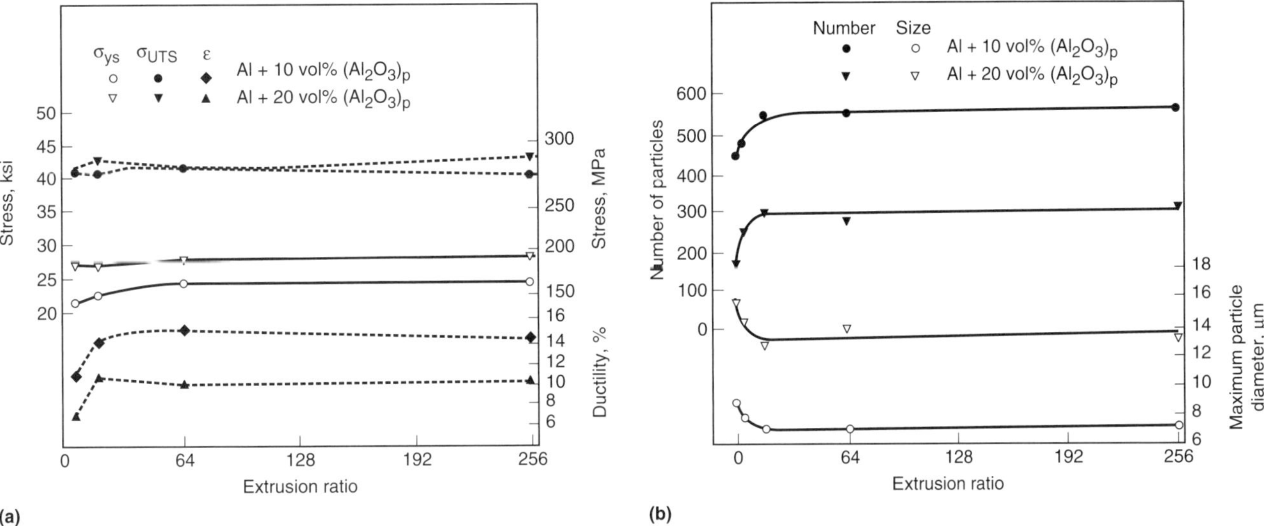

Fig. 4 Effect of extrusion ratio on (a) tensile properties (T4-condition) and (b) microstructural features of 6061Al-Al_2O_{3p} composite. After Ref 24

where $\dot{\varepsilon}$ is the minimum creep rate, σ is the applied stress, α_{LT} is a stress partition function (experimentally determined for a 6061Al-30 vol% SiC_p as 0.55, 0.48, and 0.45 at 618, 648, and 678 K, respectively, Ref 36), T is the temperature, and R is the gas constant. (Note: in the original publication, Park and Mohamed (Ref 36) related minimum creep rate in shear strain rate, $\dot{\gamma}$, to shear stress, τ.)

Power-law creep analyses primarily account for deformation occurring through dislocation climb in the matrix. As previously mentioned, damage during creep initiates near the particles. Wakashima et al. (Ref 43) defined a micromechanics-based constitutive equation that incorporates this effect. They describe two components for creep: creep in the matrix and viscous (or diffusional) creep occurring at the matrix-reinforcement interface. The matrix creep rate is given in terms similar to Eq 1, incorporating parameters such as the actual stress carried by the matrix, the threshold stress for power-law creep, volume diffusivity, and matrix dislocation properties (e.g., Burgers vector). The diffusional flow rate is similar in nature to Nabarro-Herring creep and is associated with atomic transport in the matrix around the reinforcement phase, incorporating the stress carried by the reinforcement phase, size of the reinforcement, and parameters related to the mass transport in the vicinity of the interface (e.g., boundary-diffusion coefficient, the effective thickness of the boundary through which diffusive transport occurs, and the volume of diffusing matter). Steady-state creep is established when both components are balanced.

Fracture and Fatigue. The incorporation of discontinuous reinforcements generally decreases the fracture toughness of the matrix (Table 7). Generally, there is a slight tendency for fracture toughness to increase with increasing particle size (Table 8). This can be explained by considering that interparticle spacing increases with particle size and a greater volume of matrix material is available for unconstrained plastic flow in the wake of the propagating crack, resulting in the higher fracture toughness. Improvements in toughness of Al-MMC can be accomplished by producing hybrid laminated metal composites consisting of Al-MMCs and tougher unreinforced alloys (discussed later in this article).

Fatigue and fatigue crack growth studies have been performed on Al-MMCs (Ref 45–55). The fatigue life of the matrix can be either improved (Fig. 7) or degraded by the addition of the reinforcement phase, depending on the loading and type of fatigue test (Ref 45–47). For stress-controlled fatigue, the composite exhibits a much lower total strain during a fatigue cycle than the unreinforced alloys (Fig. 8a). This is a result of the higher modulus and work-hardening rates of the composite compared with the monolithic matrix, and therefore fatigue life is improved with the incorporation of the reinforcement. Following the same reasoning, under strain-controlled conditions (Fig. 8b), the composite experiences a higher level of stress per cycle than the unreinforced alloy to accumulate a comparable strain level. This accelerates the formation of fatigue damage in the composite, and this degrades fatigue life.

Under stress-controlled fatigue, increasing the volume fraction of the discontinuous phase will increase fatigue life, due to increases in modulus and work-hardening rates. Composites having smaller reinforcements tend to have longer fatigue lives (the fatigue strength at 10^7 cycles (R = 1) decreased from about 240 to 200 and 150 MPa (35 to 29, and 22 ksi) for a 2124 Al + 20 vol% SiC particulate composite, as the particle size increased from 2.5, 17.5, and 35 μm) (Ref 45). This behavior has been attributed to the interparticle spacing and fracture behavior of the particles. As mentioned previously, due to the statistical nature of the fracture of the ceramics,

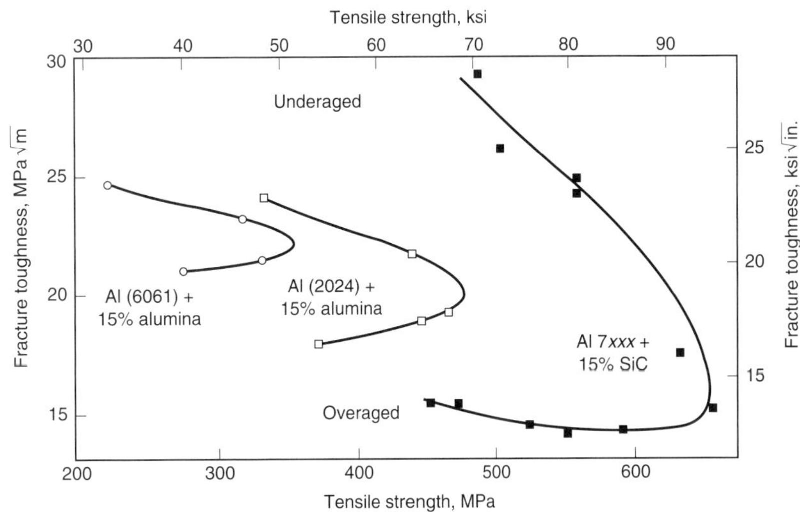

Fig. 5 Variation in fracture toughness for selected Al-MMCs subjected to various heat treatments. Source: Ref 1

large particles have a greater propensity to crack than smaller particles. Thus, these particles are more easily fractured during fatigue, reducing fatigue life. Also for a constant volume fraction, the interparticle spacing decreases with decreasing particle size. Thus, the addition of smaller particles provides for a greater barrier to dislocation motion, which enhances fatigue life.

At low R values (under 0.3) Al-MMCs typically have a higher threshold stress intensity (ΔK_{th}) for fatigue crack growth initiation than the matrix alloys (Table 9) (Ref 48). Composites generally possess a steeper Paris region, and the transition to unstable fracture occurs at lower ΔK values (Fig. 9) (Ref 45, 46). This is a direct result of the lower fracture toughness of the composites. Particle morphology and distribution play an important role in fatigue crack growth (Ref 48). Fatigue cracks are attracted to stress concentrators, such as whisker ends, particle corners, and reinforcement clusters. ΔK_{th} tends to increase with increasing volume fraction, which is explained in terms of crack closure concepts. Closure levels appear to be determined by a crack path roughness mechanism, which is dependent on the size, distribution, and volume fraction of reinforcements. For wrought-processed, whisker-reinforced composites, ΔK_{th} is anisotropic, with higher values obtained in the L-T orientation than in T-L orientation. This is also explained in terms of crack closure and roughness mechanisms. A dependency on orientation, reinforcement morphology, and volume fraction of ΔK_{th} at higher R (0.7) is not observed due to the minimal effect of crack deflection and thus the ineffectiveness of closure mechanisms (Ref 48).

Wear and Corrosion. As previously mentioned, wear is not a materials property, but a systems response. Wear behavior is dependent on materials properties and the wear environment. Small changes in environmental conditions can dramatically alter wear behavior, as a result changing the relative ranking of different materials. Thus, interpretation and application of results of wear experiments are difficult and should be made with caution.

Sliding wear is a common form of wear experienced by various automotive engine components (cylinder blocks, pistons, piston insert rings, etc.) that are fabricated from Al-MMCs (Ref 56). Sliding or adhesive wear is defined as the transfer of material from one surface to another during the relative motion of contacting surfaces. The repeated contact of asperities on the surfaces may cause them to be detached from the parent body during sliding. The detached particles, or wear debris, are either temporarily or permanently attached to the other surface. Other wear mechanisms include plastic flow and fracture, both of which can result in excavation and detachment of material. Important parameters that affect wear behavior are the relative hardness of the surfaces and the coefficient of friction between the sliding surfaces. Therefore, wear resistance of an alloy can be improved through the addition of hard particles, which enhances surface hardness, or through addition of softer graphitic-type particles, which alter the coefficient of friction between the surfaces by providing a self-lubricant. Two reviews on sliding wear of Al-MMCs can be found in the literature (Ref 56, 57).

Figure 10(a) illustrates the influence of reinforcement volume fraction on the sliding wear rate (related to material loss) of an Al-SiC MMC worn against a steel counterface (Ref 56). The addition of a small volume fraction of hard particles can significantly reduce the wear rate of the unreinforced aluminum. However, a decrease in the wear rate of the composite can be accompanied by an increase in the wear rate of the counterface. The improvement in wear resistance can be attributed to the hard particles remaining intact when struck by asperities or abrading particles, under conditions such that material would be plowed from the surface of the unreinforced alloy. Thus, high reinforcement strength and strong interfacial bonding are factors that lead to improved wear resistance of MMCs.

The influence of temperature on the wear rate of an Al-15 vol% SiC composite worn against a

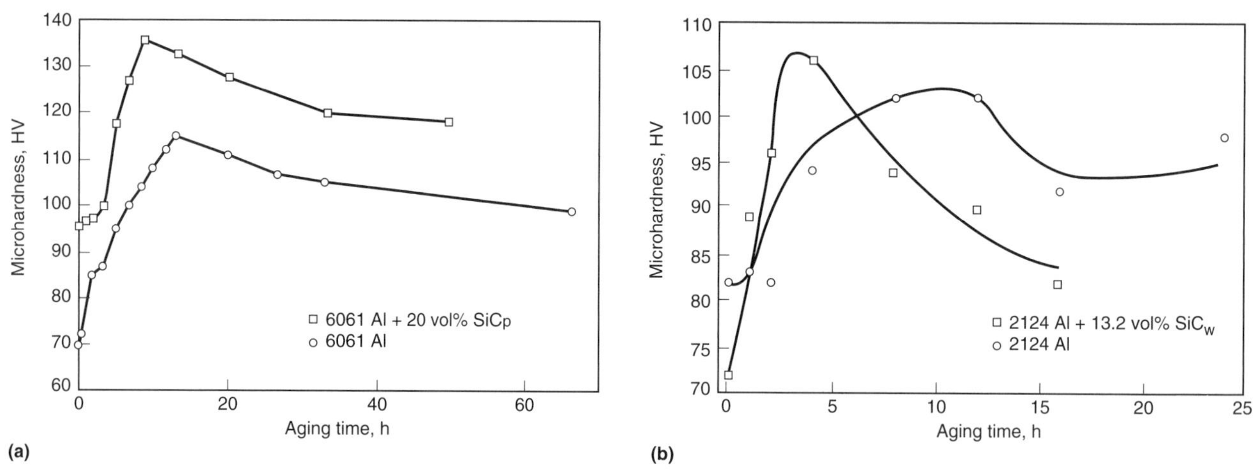

Fig. 6 Influence of particle additions on the matrix microhardness as a function of aging time. (a) 6061Al + SiC_p at 180 °C (360 °F) (after Ref 25). (b) 2124Al + SiC_w at 177 °C (350 °F) (after Ref 26)

Table 6 Elevated-temperature tensile properties of discontinuous reinforced Al-MMC

Temperature		Yield strength				Tensile strength				Yield strength				Tensile strength				Yield strength				Tensile strength			
		2014		$+15Al_2O_3$		2024		$+15Al_2O_3$		6061		$+15Al_2O_3$		6061		$+15Al_2O_3$		F3K + 10SiC		+20SiC		F3K + 10SiC		+20SiC	
°C	°F	MPa	ksi	MPa	ksi	MPa	ksi	MPa	ksi	MPa	ksi	MPa	ksi	MPa	ksi	MPa	ksi	MPa	ksi	MPa	ksi	MPa	ksi	MPa	ksi
22	72	524	76	531	77	476	69	503	73	276	40	324	47	310	45	365	53	179	26	214	31	255	37	262	38
93	200	434	63	490	71	393	57	393	57	262	38	290	42	283	41	331	48	...	...	...	...	...	...	...	...
149	300	379	55	434	63	352	51	352	51	248	36	269	39	262	38	303	44	...	...	...	...	...	...	...	...
204	400	310	45	338	49	283	41	283	41	221	32	241	35	228	33	262	38	145	21	165	24	179	26	186	27
260	500	172	25	214	31	159	23	159	23	165	24	172	25	172	25	179	26	90	13.0	117	17	124	18	145	21
316	600	76	11.0	110	16	62	9.0	62	9.0	90	13.0	110	16	97	14.0	117	17	62	9.0	83	12	83	12	110	16
371	700	41	5.9	55	8.0	34	4.9	34	4.9	55	8.0	62	9.0	59	8.6	69	10.0	41	5.9	62	9.0	55	8.0	76	11.0

2014 and 6061, wrought composites; F3K cast composite, nominal composition of F3K = Al-10Si-3Cu-1.25Ni-1Mg-0.3Fe-0.2Ti. Source: Ref 21

steel counterface is shown in Fig. 10(b) (Ref 58). The main effect of the SiC reinforcement on sliding wear at high temperatures is to delay the transition from mild to severe wear by about 50 °C (90 °F). This is attributed to the presence of the SiC particles improving the high-temperature strength of the matrix.

Increasing applied load tends to increase wear rates during sliding (Fig. 10c). At low applied loads (regime I), composites typically are more wear resistant than unreinforced matrix alloys, and material removal occurs through oxidative wear processes. In this wear mechanism, oxide layers form on both sliding surfaces, resulting from the frictional heating associated with sliding. Oxidized asperities become detached from the surface and can be compacted on the countersurface to form a wear film. Wear rates tend to be low, as material removal is confined to the thickness of the oxide reinforcement. At intermediate loads (regime II), the wear mechanism changes from oxidative wear to metallic wear. In this regime, significant subsurface plastic deformation occurs, and when strain exceeds the fracture strain, material is detached from the surface. In this regime, composites have similar wear rates to those of unreinforced alloys. At high loads (regime III), the wear rates of the composite are much lower (typically, two orders of magnitude) than those of the unreinforced matrix alloy. The unreinforced matrix alloy experiences severe wear associated with adhesion and seizure during sliding. Wear maps delineate material removal mechanisms, and thus wear rates, for the wear conditions (applied load and sliding speed) of a specific wear environment. Figure 10(d) shows a wear map for a 6061Al-20 vol% SiC_w composite worn against a steel counterface (Ref 56). It should be noted that while the emphasis of this section is on Al-SiC particles, incorporation of Al_2O_3, B_4C, TiC, and other hard particles into aluminum has similar effects on wear resistance (Ref 56, 59).

Superior sliding resistance is obtained through the addition of softer graphitic-type reinforcements, as illustrated in Fig. 11(a) and (b). During sliding, the graphite reinforcement can become smeared on the surface and function as a lubricant, which decreases the coefficient of friction between the surfaces and extends component life (Ref 1, 57). However, this effect is very sensitive to the ambient environment, as moisture content in the environment significantly affects the tribological properties of these types of composites.

Hybrid composites containing both hard and soft phases offer improved sliding resistance, particularly at high applied loads, as shown in Fig. 11(c) (Ref 9). Frictional heating decreases in the hybrid composites as a result of a lower coefficient of friction. This prevents the transition from mild to severe wear for the Al-SiC hybrid composite.

Corrosion of MMCs tends to center on localized corrosion, which arises from galvanic effects between the matrix and reinforcement,

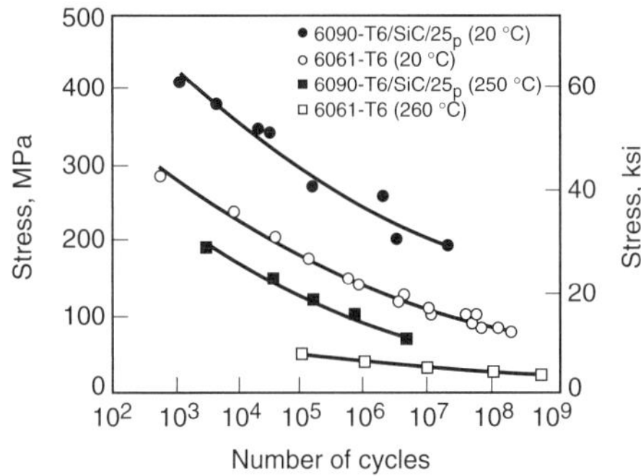

Fig. 7 Comparison of stress-life data for 6069Al and 6069Al + 25 vol% SiC_p. Source: Ref 47

Table 7 Influence of discontinuous reinforcement on the fracture toughness of Al-MMCs

Composite/vol% reinforcement	Fracture toughness, MPa $\sqrt{m}$	Fracture toughness, ksi $\sqrt{in.}$
6061Al-T6 (Ref 25)		
6061	29.7	27.0
+ 10 vol% $(Al_2O_3)_p$	24.1	21.9
+ 20 vol% $(Al_2O_3)_p$	21.5	19.6
+ 10 vol% SiC_p	24.7	22.5
+ 20 vol% SiC_p	20.5	18.7
2124Al-T6 (Ref 12)		
2124	29.7	27.0
+ 10 vol% $(Al_2O_3)_p$	24.1	21.9
+ 15 vol% $(Al_2O_3)_p$	22.0	20.0
+ 20 vol% $(Al_2O_3)_p$	21.5	4.1
2618Al (T651) (Ref 44)		
2618Al		
At 25 °C (77 °F)	22.7	20.7
At 200 °C (390 °F)	22.5	20.5
2618Al + 15 vol% SiC_p		
At –150 °C (–238 °F)	17.4	15.8
At –50 °C (–58 °F)	16.5	15.0
At –20 °C (–4 °F)	18	16.4
At 0 °C (30 °F)	17.5	15.9
At 25 °C (77 °F)	17.8	16.2
At 50 °C (122 °F)	18.5	16.8
At 100 °C (210 °F)	20.1	18.3
At 125 °C (260 °F)	17.4	15.8
At 150 °C (300 °F)	17.0	15.5
At 200 °C (390 °F)	16.8	15.3

Table 8 Influence of particle size on fracture toughness of Al-MMCs

Particle size, μm	Fracture toughness, MPa $\sqrt{m}$	Fracture toughness, ksi $\sqrt{in.}$
Al-SiC_p (Ref 1)		
5	14.5	13.2
7	16.5	15.0
16	16.8	15.3
21	18.7	17.0
Al + 55 vol% Al_2O_3 (Ref 21)		
5	18.0	16.4
12.8	19.5	17.7
29.2	24.0	21.8

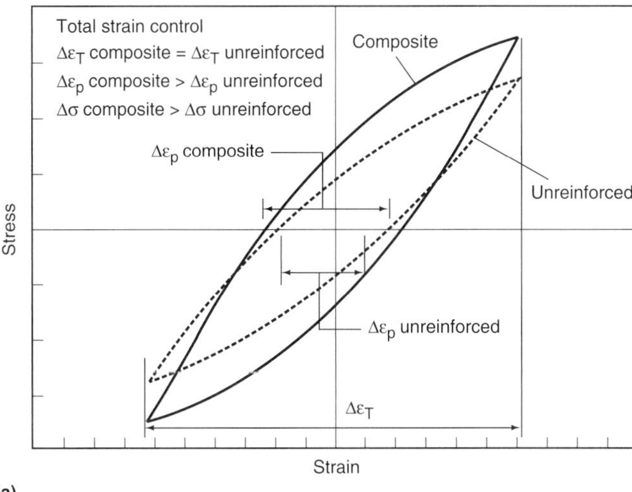

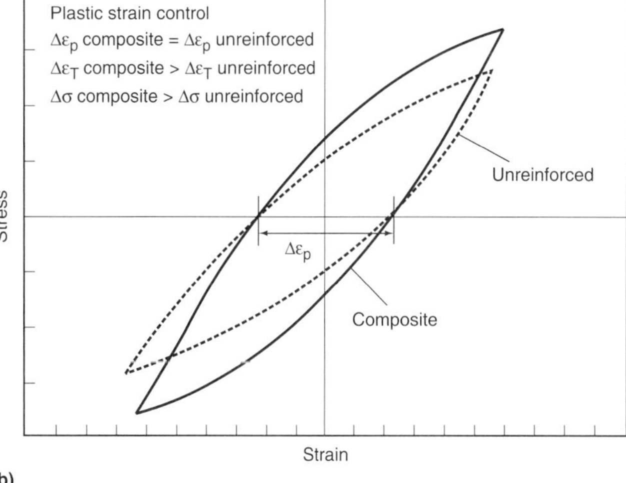

Fig. 8 Cyclic stress-strain loops for a discontinuously reinforced composite compared to unreinforced matrix alloy. (a) Stress-controlled conditions. (b) Strain-controlled conditions. Source: Ref 45

crevice corrosion at the interface between the matrix and reinforcement, and pitting reaction at interfacial reaction products (Ref 1). A brief summary of the corrosion behavior in MMCs follows, with more details found in Ref 60.

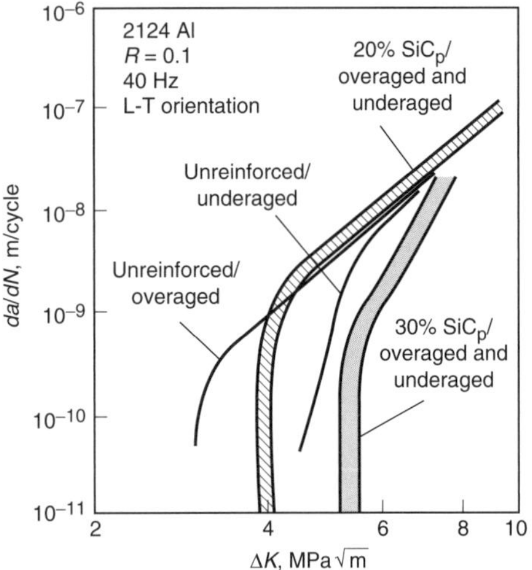

Fig. 9 Effect of volume fraction on fatigue crack growth rates in 2124Al + SiC_p composites. Source: Ref 46

Galvanic corrosion is driven by the electrode potential difference between the two constituent phases. For Al-MMCs, galvanic effects occur in Al-graphite composites in solutions containing sodium chloride (NaCl), such as seawater, causing severe corrosion. Electrochemical experiments conducted on Al + 3 wt% graphite particulate composites in seawater show that the cathodic curve (hydrogen evolution) is strongly polarized by the presence of graphite, more than doubling the corrosion current density for this reaction for the composite compared with unreinforced aluminum. The corresponding anodic reaction (dissolution of aluminum matrix) proceeds at a higher rate for the composite material compared with the unreinforced alloy (Ref 1).

Galvanic corrosion does not occur in aluminum composites containing Al_2O_3 or SiC particles or whiskers to the extent that it does in graphite reinforced composites (Ref 60). Electrochemical experiments reveal that the corrosion potential does not vary greatly with SiC content. Al-SiC composites, however, are susceptible to localized corrosion at the Al/SiC interface in NaCl and acidic environments. The degree of corrosion increases with increasing SiC content.

Properties of Other Discontinuously Reinforced Composites

Magnesium MMCs containing discontinuous reinforcements can be fabricated via the same methods as Al-MMCs. Magnesium materials are attractive based on density (1.8 g/cm^3) alone. In general, the behavior of Mg-MMCs is very similar to Al-MMCs; that is, the addition of the reinforcement increases the strength and modulus of the matrix. Tensile properties of some of these MMCs are listed in Tables 10 and 11. The same microstructural factors discussed for Al-MMCs also influence the properties of magnesium-based composites. Stress-controlled, high-cycle fatigue behavior of AZ1D-SiC_p composite has been studied (Ref 62), and the fatigue life was very dependent on the size of the SiC_p. The addition of smaller (15 μm) reinforcements provides improved fatigue performance with respect

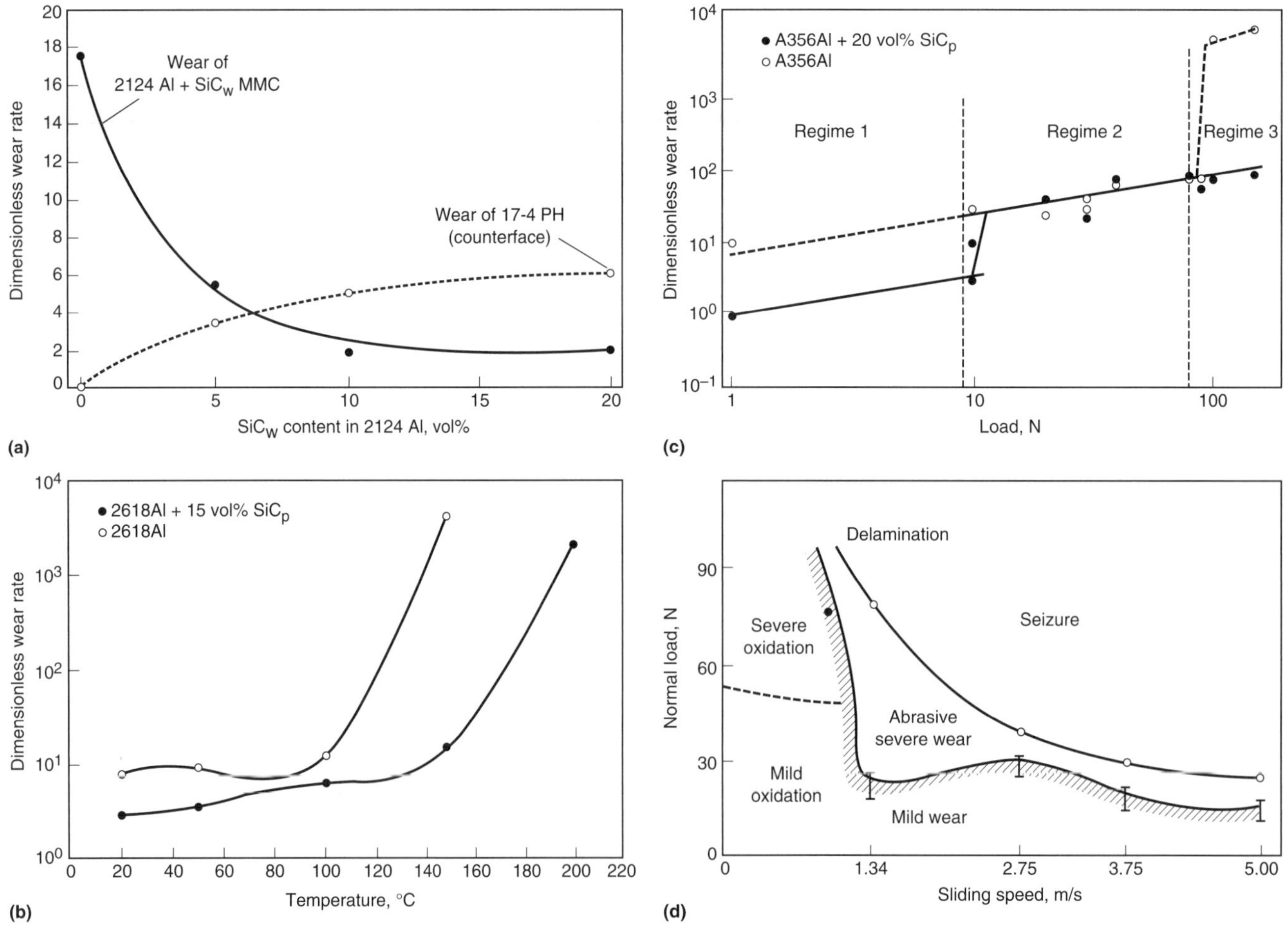

Fig. 10 Sliding wear behavior of Al-SiC MMCs. (a) Effect of SiC content on wear of composite and steel counterface. (b) Effect of temperature of wear rate. (c) Effect of applied load on wear rate. (d) A wear map for Al-SiC composite. After Ref 56, 58

Table 9 Tensile, fracture and fatigue crack growth threshold stress intensity data for 2124Al-SiC composites

Reinforcement content, vol%, and form	Rolling direction	Modulus of elasticity		Aging condition	Yield strength		Tensile strength		Elongation, %	ΔK_{th} threshold							
										K_{Ic}		$R = 0.1$		$R = 0.1$, ΔK_{th}^{eff}		R = 0.7	
		GPa	10^6 psi		MPa	ksi	MPa	ksi		MPa $\sqrt{m}$	ksi $\sqrt{in.}$	MPa $\sqrt{m}$	ksi $\sqrt{in.}$	MPa $\sqrt{m}$	ksi $\sqrt{in.}$	MPa $\sqrt{m}$	ksi $\sqrt{in.}$
0	L-T	7.25	10.5	OA	370	53.7	440	63.8	10.2	...	...	2.0	1.8	...	...	...	...
				PA	447	64.8	479	69.5	10.0	...	...	2.4	2.2	...	...	...	...
				UA	360	52.2	488	70.8	17.8	...	...	3.6	3.3	...	...	...	...
$15SiC_w$	L-T	94.3	13.7	OA	465	67.4	589	85.4	2.9	15.1	13.7	3.6	3.3	2.0	1.8	2.2	2.0
				PA	504	73.1	690	100.1	3.0	15.3	13.9	4.7	4.3	...	...	...	...
				UA	501	72.6	650	94.3	3.5	19.3	17.6	4.2	3.8	1.8	1.6	2.3	2.1
	T-L	83.3	12.0	OA	403	58.4	487	70.6	4.8	13.2	12.0	2.7	2.5	1.3	1.2	1.8	1.6
				UA	432	62.6	568	82.4	6.4	18.4	16.7	3.1	2.8	1.6	1.5	1.9	1.7
$20SiC_p$	L-T	108	15.7	OA	403	58.4	561	81.3	4.0	11.3	10.3	3.4	3.1	2.1	1.9	2.2	2.0
				PA	509	73.8	567	82.2	2.9	14.0	12.7	4.5	4.1	...	...	...	...
				UA	445	64.5	580	84.1	4.1	11.8	10.7	3.8	3.4	1.5	1.4	1.8	1.6
$30SiC_p$	L-T	127	18.4	OA	487	70.6	541	78.4	1.9	15.9	14.5	4.9	4.5	2.1	1.9	2.3	2.1
				PA	609	88.3	660	95.7	1.7	17.6	16.0	5.1	4.6	...	...	...	...
				UA	526	76.3	618	89.6	1.9	18.9	17.2	5.7	5.2	2.2	2.0	2.3	2.1
	T-L	125	18.1	OA	496	71.9	542	78.6	2.1	17.9	16.3	4.9	4.6	2.2	2.0	2.2	2.0
				UA	447	64.8	557	80.8	2.3	17.6	16.0	4.5	4.1	2.9	2.6	2.3	2.1

UA = 177 °C, 1 h; PA = 177 °C, 5 h; OA = 175 °C, 50 h. Source: Ref 48

to the unreinforced magnesium alloy. However, the fatigue life of composites containing larger particles (52 μm) is shorter than AZ91D. This behavior is attributed to a larger percentage of cracked SiC_p found both at and beneath the fracture surface of composites containing the larger-sized particles. Like aluminum-graphite composites, magnesium-graphite composites also undergo galvanic corrosion in NaCl solutions (Ref 60).

Table 10 Properties of discontinuously reinforced magnesium MMCs

Composite/vol% reinforcement	Yield stress		Tensile strength		Ductility, %	Modulus		Comments
	MPa	ksi	MPa	ksi		GPa	10^6 psi	
Pure Mg (Ref 61)								
Mg	135	19.6	196	28.4	12	38	5.5	P/M
+ 20 SiC_p	229	33.2	258	37.4	2	59	8.6	Cast
+ 10 SiC_p	222	32.2	280	40.6	1.2	57	8.3	P/M
+ 20 SiC_p	232	33.6	250	36.3	0.3	59	8.6	P/M
+ 30 SiC_p	217	31.5	217	31.5	0.1	77	11.2	P/M
AZ91D (Ref 62)								
AZ91D	204	29.6	360	52.2	9.9	42	6.1	Cast + extruded
+ 20 SiC_p (15 μm)	330	47.9	390	56.6	1.3	71	10.3	Cast + extruded
+ 20 SiC_p (52 μm)	270	39.2	320	46.4	1.1	72	10.4	Cast + extruded
+ 25 SiC_p (15 μm)	310	45.0	330	47.9	0.8	78	11.3	Cast + extruded
+ 25 SiC_p (52 μm)	290	42.1	340	49.3	1.1	79	11.5	Cast + extruded
ZK60A (Ref 2)								
ZK60A	193	28.0	310	45.0	...	45	6.5	Density = 1.8 g/cm^3
+ 20 SiC_w	454	65.8	578	83.8	1.58	96.5	14.0	P/M: density = 2.04 g/cm^3 Coefficient of thermal expansion = 11.7 × 10^{-6}/K
+ 30 B_4C_p	454	65.8	510	74.0	0.93	...	...	P/M

Titanium is another metal matrix commonly reinforced with discontinuous reinforcements to improve high-temperature strength and wear resistance (Ref 63). The most common reinforcements are TiB and TiC, and composites have been produced via ingot and powder metallurgical methods. Titanium boride particles and whiskers are formed in situ in the melt during alloy preparation (Ref 64–66). Titanium boride reinforced composites also are prepared via powder routes (Ref 67–70), in which TiB_2 is blended with the matrix powder, and the TiB_2 powder reacts with titanium to form TiB during processing. Titanium carbide reinforced composites are commonly produced via blending and consolidation of powders. Titanium carbide particles have also been formed in situ during gas atomization of carbon-modified Ti-6Al-4V alloys (Ref 66).

Room-temperature tensile properties of selected Ti-MMCs are listed in Table 12. As with the Al-MMCs, the incorporation of the ceramic phase increases both strength and modulus of the

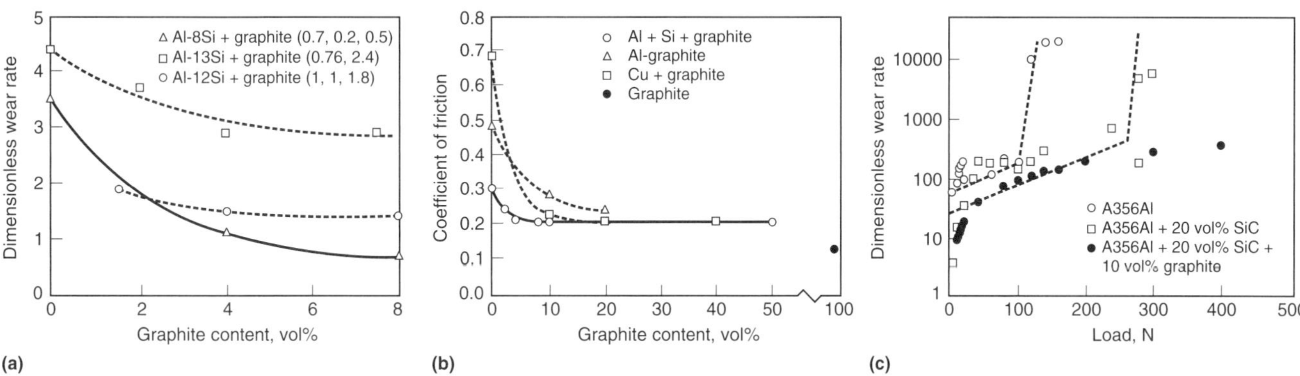

Fig. 11 Sliding wear of Al-graphite MMCs. (a) Wear rate versus graphite content (number in parenthesis in legend correspond to load, sliding speed, and sliding distance). (b) Measured coefficient of friction versus graphite content. (c) Comparison of wear behavior for unreinforced Al, Al + SiC_p, and Al + SiC + graphite composites. Source: Ref 1, 19, 57

matrix, but at the expense of ductility. The strengthening effect of the reinforcements is retained at elevated temperatures (Table 13). The addition of TiB particles improves creep resistance (Fig. 12), fatigue resistance (Fig. 13), and wear resistance of the matrix (Fig. 14). The incorporation of TiC also improves wear resistance. Table 14 shows the fracture toughness of a Ti-6Al-4V + 20 vol% TiC particle composite from liquid nitrogen temperature to 750 °C (1380 °F).

Intermetallics. Alloys based on intermetallic compounds are an emerging new class of materials. In general, intermetallic compounds are characterized by having high strengths, low densities, high melting points, and good resistance to oxidation and corrosion. Unfortunately, these compounds tend to be brittle because they possess ordered crystal structures, like ceramics, which hinders easy dislocation motion. This has limited the engineering application of these compounds as oxidation-resistant coatings. Like ferritic steels, these compounds undergo a brittle to ductile transition at elevated temperature, but tend to have poor creep resistance above this transition temperature. Composite strengthening has been used to improve both toughness and elevated-temperature strength of these alloys. Discontinuous reinforcements can be added to improve strength and creep resistance. Table 15 shows tensile properties for titanium aluminide (TiAl) and nickel aluminide (NiAl) matrices reinforced by TiB_2 particles (Ref 73–80). The addition of particles not only strengthens the matrices at room and elevated temperatures, but also improves creep resistance, as shown in Fig. 15 for NiAl + TiB_2 composites (Ref 75, 79). XD-TiAl reinforced with <1 vol% TiB_2 particles is of specific interest because the particles refine the grain size of the TiAl matrix, which is beneficial for a variety of TiAl mechanical properties (Ref 80). NiAl-base composites may find use in applications where wear resistance is required, such as barrels for extruders for the processing of food, plastics, chemicals, and pharmaceuticals (Ref 81). The addition of TiB_2 particles is effective in improving wear resistance, as shown in Fig. 16 (Ref 82). The particles can, however, have a detrimental effect on oxidation resistance of the matrix. Tests on NiAl-TiB_2 composites exposed to an oxidizing environment at between 800 and 1200 °C (1470 and 2190 °F), show that TiB_2 particles located on the surface tend to selectively oxidize, thereby reducing the oxidation resistance of the matrix. Composites with smaller TiB_2 particles are more oxidation resistant than similar composites containing larger particles (Ref 83).

Hybrid Laminated Metal and Ductile Phase Composites

Laminated metal composites (LMCs) consist of bonded alternating metal layers that have very distinct, or sharp, interfaces (Ref 84). The composites differ from functional gradient materials, which also can consist of alternating layers having less distinct, or diffuse, interfaces. Laminated metal-metal composites are produced via diffusion bonding or deformation bonding (roll bonding, coextrusion, etc.). A variety of layered composites have been produced including discontinuous reinforced aluminum (DRA) with unreinforced aluminum, ultrahigh-carbon steel (UHCS) with mild steel, and UHCS with brass (Ref 85–90). These types of composites are easily engineered by altering processing history and layer thickness to produce composites having prescribed properties (Ref 84).

Laminated metal composites can dramatically improve many properties including fracture toughness, fatigue, and impact behavior of an otherwise brittle material. As illustrated in Fig. 17(a), the Charpy-V notch behavior of UHCS/

Table 11 Properties of discontinuously reinforced magnesium MMCs at elevated temperatures

Temperature		Yield stress		Tensile strength			Modulus	
°C	°F	MPa	ksi	MPa	ksi	Ductility, %	GPa	10^6 psi
AZ31B (Ref 2)								
25	77	165	23.9	250	36.3	12	45	6.5
150	300	105	15.2	170	24.7	39	...	...
AZ31B + 20 vol% 600 grit SiC_p (Ref 2)								
25	77	251	36.4	330	47.9	5.7	79	11.5
150	300	154	22.3	215	31.2	10.4	56	8.1
AZ31B + 20 vol% 1000 grit SiC_p (Ref 2)								
25	77	341	49.4	270	39.2	4	79	11.5
150	300	215	31.2	167	24.2	9	68	9.9
Mg (Ref 61)								
25	77	135	19.6	196	28.4	12	...	...
250	480	47	6.8	66	9.6	48	...	...
300	570	33	4.8	42	6.1	63	...	...
350	660	15	2.2	22	3.2	43	...	...
Mg + 30 vol% SiC_p (Ref 61)								
25	77	229	33.2	258	37.4	2	...	...
250	480	68	9.9	91	13.2	20	...	...
300	570	42	6.1	57	8.3	22	...	...
350	660	31	4.5	42	6.1	16	...	...
400	750	24	3.5	26	3.8	19	...	...

Table 12 Room-temperature tensile properties of discontinuously reinforced Ti-MMC

	Yield stress		Tensile strength			Modulus	
Composite/alloy	MPa	ksi	MPa	ksi	Ductility, %	GPa	10^6 psi
Ti-6Al-4V + TiB (in situ during powder atomization, consolidation via powder extrusion) (Ref 66)							
Ti-6Al-4V-0.9B	1190	173	1312	190	5	127	18.4
Ti-6Al-4V-1.4B	1135	165	1297	188	6.7	140	20.3
Ti-6Al-4V-1.7B	1202	174	1359	197	3.3	136	19.7
Ti-6Al-4V-2.2B	1315	191	1470	213	3.1	144	20.9
Ti-6Al-4V-1.3B-0.5C	1424	207	1424	207	6.7	138	20.0
Ti-6Al-4V + TiC (in situ during powder atomization, consolidation via powder extrusion) (Ref 66)							
Ti-6Al-4V-0.5C	1183	172	1306	189	6.3	127	18.4
Ti-6Al-4V-0.9C	1124	163	1237	179	4.7	123	17.8
Ti-6Al-4V-1.8C	1329	193	1329	193	0	145	21.0
Ti-6Al-4V + TiB whiskers (during in situ induction skull melting followed by extrusion) (Ref 65)							
Ti-6.5Al-4.2V-0.48B	1041	151	1156	168	15	129	18.7
Ti-6Al-4V	986	143	1035	150	15	...	...
Ti-17Mo + TiB (in situ arc melted) (Ref 64)							
Ti-17Mo	640	92.8	...	...	...	96	13.9
Ti-17Mo + 14 vol% TiB	825	119.5	...	...	...	126	18.3
Ti-17Mo + 21 vol% TiB	840	121.8	...	...	...	155	22.5
Ti-6Al-2Sn-4Zr-2Mo + TiB (in situ reactive sintering Ti + TiB_2 powders) (Ref 71)							
Ti-6Al-2Sn-4Zr-2Mo	...	...	1039	151	15	...	...
Ti-6Al-2Sn-4Zr-2Mo + 8.2 vol% TiB	...	...	1228	178	2	...	...
Ti-6Al-4V + TiC (mixed powders cold and hot pressed) (Ref 63)							
Ti-6Al-4V + 10 vol% TiC	792	114.8	799	116	1.1	...	...
Ti-6Al-4V + 20 vol% TiC	943	136.7	959	139	0.3	139	20.2

mild steel laminate composite is superior to both constituent alloys. The composites were tested with the interface between the layers oriented perpendicular to the direction of crack propagation—in a crack arrester mode. Extensive delamination between the layers of the composite occurred during fracture. The added energy required for delamination results in the improvement in toughness. The strength of the interface is paramount in determining toughness of the composite. Sharp (chemically weak) interfaces promote toughness in these types of composites. When the UHCS/mild steel composite is heat treated to produce a stronger chemical bond between the layers, the impact properties of the composite are degraded (Fig. 17b). More detailed information regarding these composites can be found in Ref 84.

A variety of DRA-Al laminates have also been produced. Figure 18 illustrates the fracture toughness versus global SiC content of these composites (Ref 90). The laminate composites have higher fracture toughnesses than comparable base-particulate reinforced composites. The microstructure of these composites does not have to consist of laminates. For example, Microstructural Toughened composites (United Technologies) use tubular reinforcements instead of layers, and composites consisting of

Table 13 Elevated-temperature tensile properties of discontinuously reinforced Ti-MMC

Composite/alloy	Yield stress, MPa	Yield stress, ksi	Tensile strength, MPa	Tensile strength, ksi	Ductility, %	Modulus, GPa	Modulus, 10^6 psi
Ti-6Al-4V + TiB at 550 °C (1020 °F) (in situ during powder atomization, consolidation via powder extrusion) (Ref 66)							
Ti-6Al-4V-0.001B	500	72.5	620	89.9	22	80	11.6
Ti-6Al-4V-1.4B	700	101.5	850	123.3	8	110	16.0
Ti-6Al-4V-1.7B	760	110.2	875	126.9	8	118	17.1
Ti-6Al-4V-1.3B-0.5C	800	116.0	950	137.8	7	128	18.6
Ti-6Al-4V + TiB at 650 °C (1200 °F) (in situ during powder atomization, consolidation via powder extrusion) (Ref 66)							
Ti-6Al-4V-0.001B	325	47.1	450	65.3	29	72	10.4
Ti-6Al-4V-1.4B	425	61.6	675	97.9	14		
Ti-6Al-4V-1.7B	350	50.8	675	97.9	8	112	16.2
Ti-6Al-4V-1.3B-0.5C	375	54.4	675	97.9	20	72	10.4
Ti-6Al-4V + TiB whiskers at 200 °C (390 °F) (during in situ induction skull melting followed by extrusion) (Ref 65)							
Ti-6.5Al-4.2B-0.48B	721	104.5	725	105.1	19	125	18.1

Table 14 Effect of temperature on the fracture toughness of Ti-6Al-4V + 20 vol% TiC composite

Temperature, °C	Temperature, °F	Fracture toughness, MPa $\sqrt{m}$	Fracture toughness, ksi $\sqrt{in.}$
−173	−279	20	18.2
−73	−99	29	26.4
27	81	30	27.3
427	801	27	24.6
627	1161	23	20.9
727	1341	17	15.5

Source: Ref 72

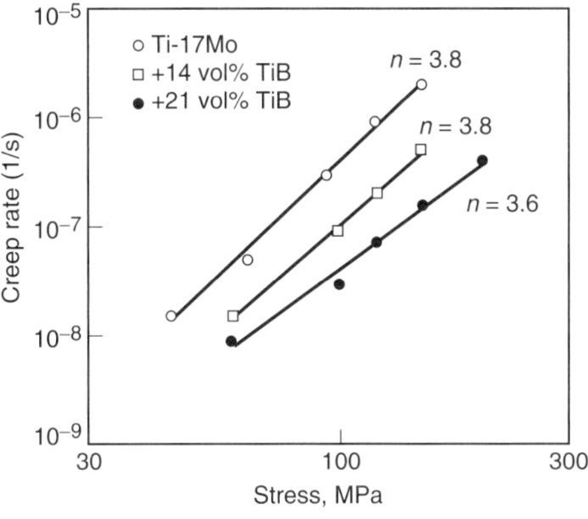

Fig. 12 Steady-state creep behavior of Ti-TiB composites tested at 600 °C (1100 °F). After Ref 64

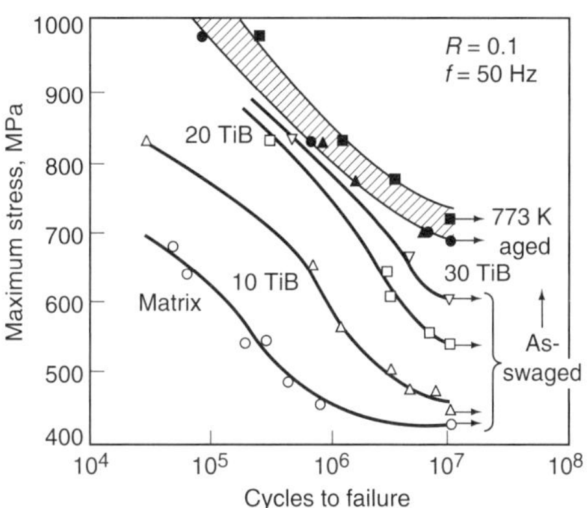

Fig. 13 S-N curves for Ti-TiB MMCs. Source: Ref 67

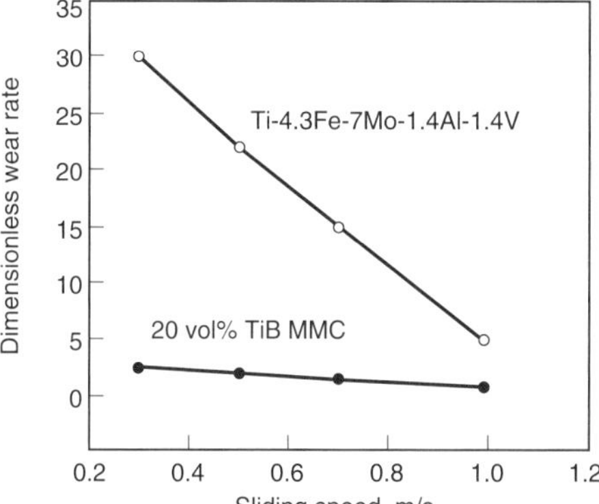

Fig. 14 Sliding wear behavior of Ti-TiB composite compared to the unreinforced alloy. After Ref 67

Table 15 Tensile properties of selected discontinuously reinforced intermetallic-matrix composites

Composite vol% reinforcement	Yield stress, MPa	Yield stress, ksi	Tensile strength, MPa	Tensile strength, ksi	Ductility, %	Modulus, GPa	Modulus, 10^6 psi	Fracture toughness, MPa $\sqrt{m}$	Fracture toughness, ksi $\sqrt{in.}$
TiAl (Ti-48Al-2Cr-2Nb) + TiB2, XD processed (Ref 73, 74); temperature = 25 °C									
0	275–380	39.9–55.1	360–500	52.2–72.5	1–3	160–175	23.2–25.4	22	20.0
0.8	400–600	58.0–87.0	485–720	70.3–104.4	0.5–1.5	160–175	23.2–25.4	17	15.5
7.5	793	115.0	862	125.0	0.5	...	...	...	...
NiAl + TiB_2 XD processed (Ref 75); temperature = 25 °C									
20	504	73.1	773	112.1	0.5	232	33.6	...	...
NiAl + TiB_2 powder processed (Ref 76); temperature = 700 °C									
0	173	25.1	191	27.7	3	...	...	...	...
20	344	49.9	344	50.0	0	...	...	...	...
Temperature = 800 °C									
0	135	19.6	154	22.3	14	...	...	...	...
20	310	45.0	360	52.2	6.5	...	...	...	...
NiAl + TiB_2 rapid solidified (Ref 77); temperature 760 °C									
2.7	209	30.3	251	36.4	64.7	...	...	...	...

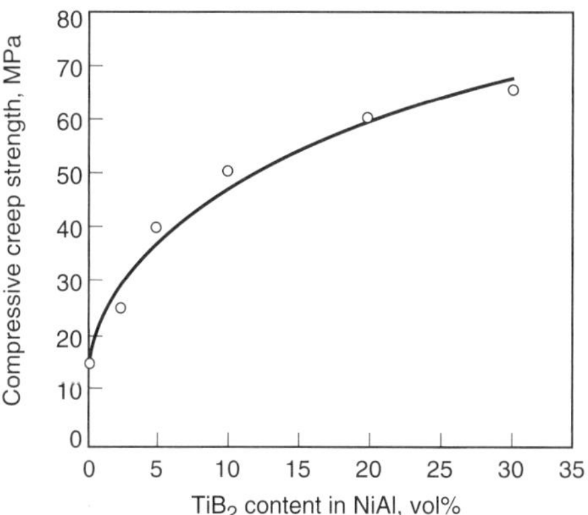

Fig. 15 Influence of TiB_2 particles on the creep strength of NiAl. Temperature, 1300 K (1027 °C); strain rate, 10^{-7} s^{-1}. After Ref 79

DRA with aluminum alloy tubes (Ref 86), DRA with commercially pure (CP) titanium tubes (Ref 86), and NiAl + B_4C with stainless steel tubes have been produced (Ref 87, 88). Another simpler method of producing these composites is by coextruding a mixture of the DRA powder blend with very large particles (e.g., 0.3 and 10 mm) of the unreinforced aluminum alloy. Note that the particle size of the unreinforced alloy is significantly larger than the size of powders that comprise the DRA blend (Ref 90). An advantage of this approach is that the properties of the composites are much more isotropic than those of laminate or Microstructural Toughened composites. These composites should also be less expensive to fabricate, as this method requires fewer manufacturing steps. The room-temperature tensile properties of these composites are listed in Table 16.

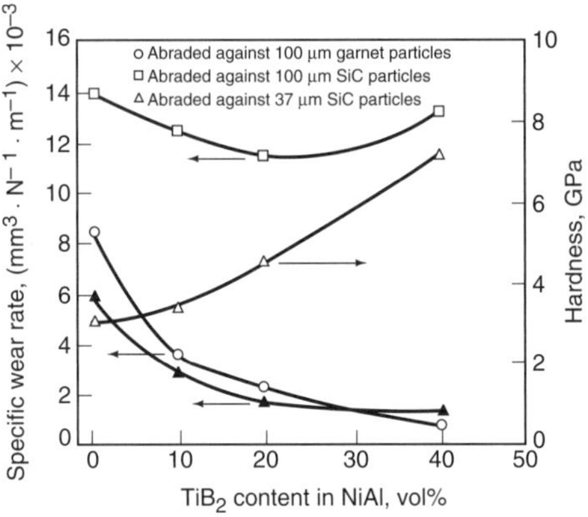

Fig. 16 Abrasive wear behavior of NiAl-TiB_2 composites compared to the unreinforced alloy. Source: Ref 83

Ductile phase-toughened intermetallics are closely related to laminated composites. These composites combine a brittle matrix, such as a ceramic or intermetallic compound, with a ductile metallic alloy in the form of particles, fibers (wires), or layers. The fracture resistance of the matrix is enhanced by:

- Ductile rupture of the metallic phase at the tip of a crack propagating through the matrix
- Bridging of the crack by the ductile phase
- Deflection of the crack by the ductile phase

The degree to which these mechanisms are operational is dependent on the morphology (particles, fibers, etc.) of the metallic phase and the bond strength between the phases incorporated into the matrix. Both artificial and in situ composites have been produced, and a compilation of fracture toughness values for numerous ductile phase-toughened composites can be found in Ref 91. The in situ eutectic composites are particularly attractive because they are more readily fabricated than artificial composites and the microstructure (e.g., volume fractions) can easily be modified through adjusting the alloy composition (Ref 92–96). Nb/Nb_5Si_3-type in situ composites based on Nb-Si-Ti alloys appear to be ideally suited for use in high-temperature applications, because they have both elevated-temperature oxidation resistance and low-tempera-

Table 16 Tensile properties of extruded DRA (7093Al + 15 vol% SiC_p) + Al particles

Composite	Modulus of elasticity		Yield stress		Tensile strength		Ductility, %	Initiation fracture toughness(a) $K_{(a\text{-}eq)}$		Steady-state fracture toughness(a) (K_{ss})	
	GPa	10^6 psi	MPa	ksi	MPa	ksi		MPa $\sqrt{m}$	ksi $\sqrt{in.}$	MPa $\sqrt{m}$	ksi $\sqrt{in.}$
Underaged heat treatment (400 °C/4 h/QQ + 125 °C/25 min)											
DRA	89.9	13.0	503	72.9	629	91.2	5.9	16.0	14.6	20	18.2
+ 10% large Al particles(b)	87.4	12.7	436	63.2	533	77.3	5.4	16.5	15.0	25.2	22.9
+ 25% large Al particles	91	13.2	466	67.6	546	79.2	2.2	20.5	18.7	33.8	30.8
+ 25% small Al particles	92	13.3	453	65.7	546	79.2	4.4	24.0	21.8	34.6	31.5
+ 10% large Cu-50Al particles	89	12.9	502	72.8	595	86.3	2.9	24.8	22.6	26.8	24.4
Overaged heat treatment (490 °C/4 h/QQ + 120 °C/24 h + 150 °C/8 h)											
DRA	91.5	13.3	591	85.7	642	93.1	2.4	19.6	17.8	...	...
+ 10% large Al particles(b)	99	14.4	611	88.6	652	94.5	4.4	19.3	17.6	22.3	20.3
+ 25% large Al particles	95	13.8	562	81.5	599	86.9	0.5	21	19.1	32.7	29.8
+ 25% small Al particles	89	12.9	469.1	68.0	562.7	81.6	1.3	19	17.3	21.1	19.2
+ 10% large Cu-50Al particles	96	13.9	618	89.6	652	94.5	1.5	16	14.6	18.5	16.8
Laminated DRA underaged								32.9	29.9	42.8	38.9

(a) See Ref 90 for definition. (b) Large particles = 10 mm in size; small particles = 0.3 mm in size. Source: Ref 90

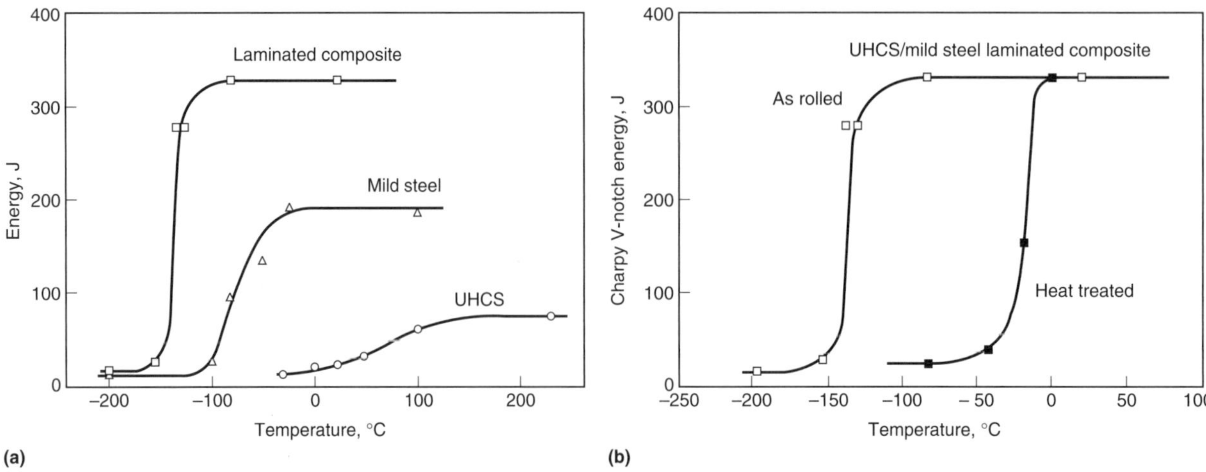

Fig. 17 Charpy V-notch impact energy versus test temperature. (a) Laminated ultrahigh carbon steel (UHCS)/mild steel composite compared to constituent alloys. (b) Effect of interface condition on impact behavior of UHCS/mild steel laminated composite (heat treating produced a strong interface between layer, as-rolled produced a weak interface between layers). Source: Ref 85

ture fracture toughness (Ref 95, 96), as illustrated in Fig. 19.

Metal-polymer composites, such as GLARE (Akzo) and ARALL (Alcoa), consist of alternating layers of high-strength aluminum and fiber reinforced epoxy adhesives (Ref 97). ARALL composites consist of adhesive prepregs of 50 vol% high-modulus aramid fibers. GLARE composites consist of an adhesive prepreg consisting of 60 vol% high strength glass fibers either uniaxially or biaxially oriented. Because the glass fiber is stronger than aramid fiber, GLARE laminates are stronger in a cross-ply lay-up in both L and LT orientation compared with ARALL laminates (Table 17). The principal benefit of these composites is the ability to impede and self-arrest fatigue cracks. In monolithic aluminum sheet, fatigue cracks can grow until the metal panel fails. In the layered composites, the fatigue crack only develops in the aluminum layer or layers. The fibers remain intact due to their high strength and toughness. As the crack grows, fibers bridging the crack carry an increasing portion of the load, decreasing the stress intensity at the crack tip and, consequently, arresting further crack growth. In addition to the superior crack growth properties, GLARE and ARALL composites are lighter and more damage tolerant than 2024-T3 Al sheet. A high-temperature version of these composites consists of titanium, carbon fibers, and a thermoplastic resin (Ref 98). More details on these composites can be found in Ref 97.

Continuous Fiber Reinforced Composites

Continuously aligned, fiber reinforced metal-matrix composites are used primarily in aerospace structural applications requiring high stiffness and strength (Ref 99). Common composite matrices reinforced with continuous fibers are aluminum, magnesium, copper, titanium and titanium aluminide (Ti_3Al-α_2 and Ti_2AlNb-orthorhombic) compounds. Common commercial fibers are SiC, Al_2O_3 and carbon, or graphite. Al_2O_3, SiC, carbon, or graphite fibers are used to reinforce aluminum matrices, Al_2O_3 and graphite are used in magnesium matrices, and SiC is used in titanium matrices. Potential aerospace applications for Ti-MMCs include compressor disks, blades, shafts, and casings. Weight savings of up to 40% are possible in using Ti-MMCs over conventional titanium alloys (Ref 99). Al-MMCs are being developed for use in two main aerospace applications, net-shaped castings, and simple shapes (such as I-beams and T-sections) for structural supports (Ref 99).

Emphasis in this article is on aluminum-, magnesium-, and titanium-matrix composites. Discussion of other aligned fibrous metal-matrix composites is not possible due to space limitations. However, other fiber reinforced metal-matrix composites systems that have been studied include intermetallics reinforced with Al_2O_3 fibers and superalloys with refractory metal wires. Detailed information regarding the properties of these other composites can be found in Ref 100 and 101, respectively.

Aligned fibrous composites are produced using solid-state methods; various fabrication methods have been developed with the objective of producing high-quality and cost-effective components. Titanium-matrix composites are commonly produced by diffusion bonding of matrix foils and fiber tapes (foil-fiber-foil method), plasma spraying fiber tapes with the matrix, and coating the fiber by physical vapor deposition (PVD) with the matrix.

The foil-fiber-foil method consists of the consolidation through diffusion bonding of alternately stacked layers of alloy foil (80–120 μm) and a fiber mat made of aligned monofilament. The fiber mat is produced by weaving the fibers together into a ribbon, or they are held in place using a fugitive organic binder that is outgassed in the final consolidation step. A major disad-

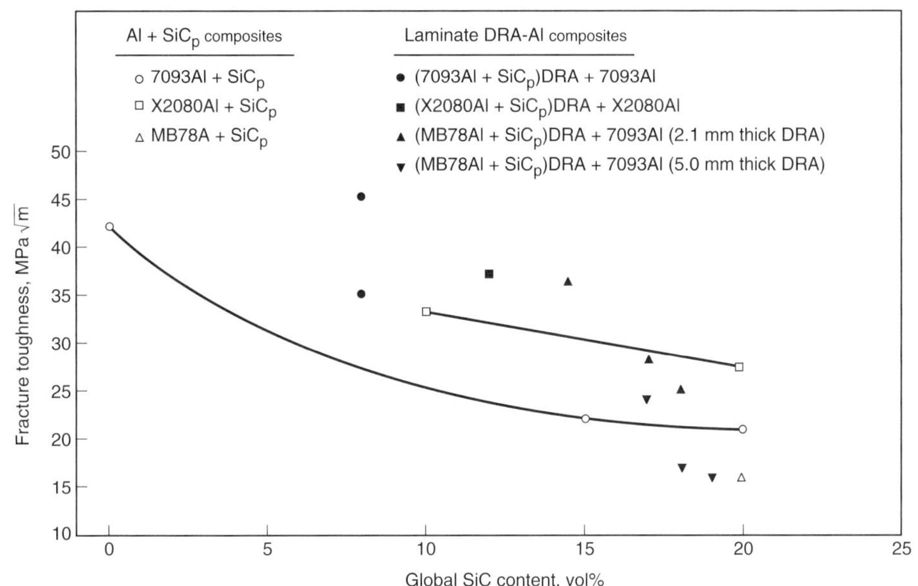

Fig. 18 Fracture toughness as a function of SiC_p concentration for particulate and laminated discontinuously reinforced aluminum (DRA) composites. After Ref 89

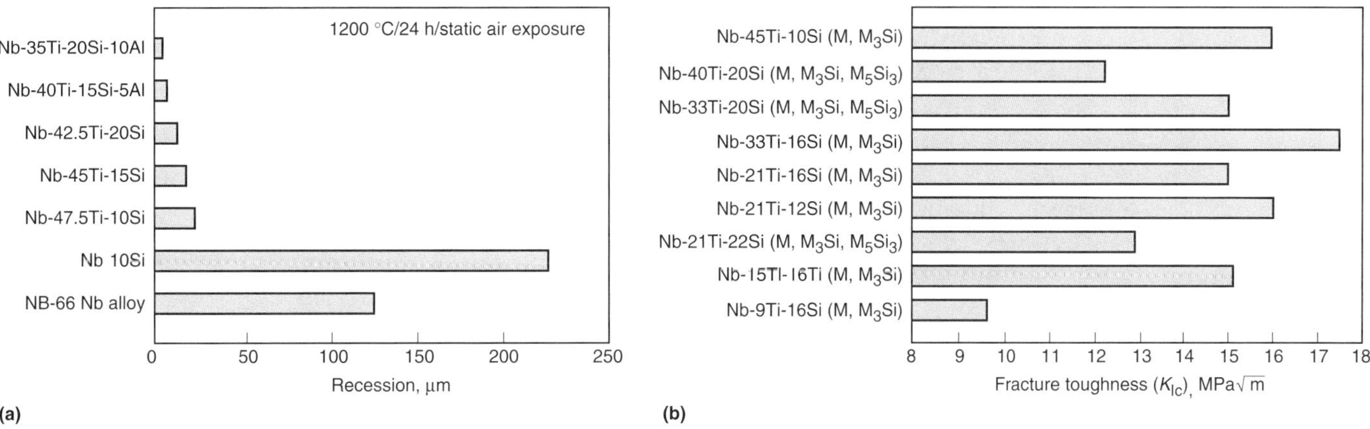

Fig. 19 (a) Oxidation and (b) fracture toughness of selected metal (M)-metal-silicide (M_3Si, M_5Si_3) in situ composites based on Nb-Ti-Si. After Ref 95, 96

vantage of this method is that the fibers tend to be poorly distributed, and they touch each other, both of which have a detrimental effect on mechanical properties. Also, this technique can only be applied to matrices that are easily formed into thin foils. Powder cloths can be used for matrices that are not readily formed into foils.

Vacuum plasma spray is used to manufacture Ti-MMCs monotapes. Metallic powders are introduced into a plasma where they are melted and propelled at high velocity onto a single layer of fibers wound on a drum. The monotapes are subsequently cut, stacked, and hot pressed to form the composite. Typically, fiber distribution is superior in plasma spray composites than in foil-fiber-foil composites. However, the quality of the monotapes depends on the impurities associated with the powders. The PVD process consists of coating the fiber with a thick layer of matrix material by means of sputtering or electron beam deposition. The volume fraction of fibers in the matrix is controlled through the thickness of matrix coating. The coated fibers are then laid up and hot pressed to produce the composite. The main advantage of this technique is achieving a very uniform fiber distribution with no touching fibers.

Aluminum and magnesium composites can be fabricated using the methods described above and through the molten-metal infiltration of fiber preforms, as previously described. Two major advantages of the infiltration method are that

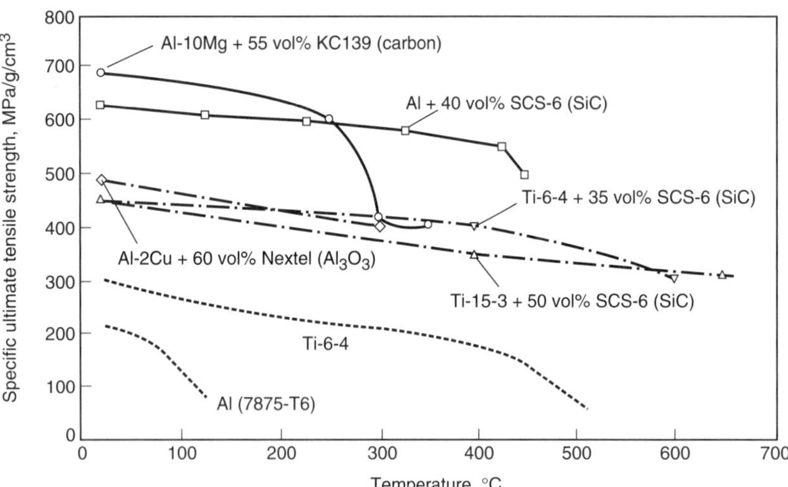

Fig. 20 Specific strength versus temperature for unidirectional fiber reinforced MMCs. After Ref 2 and 99

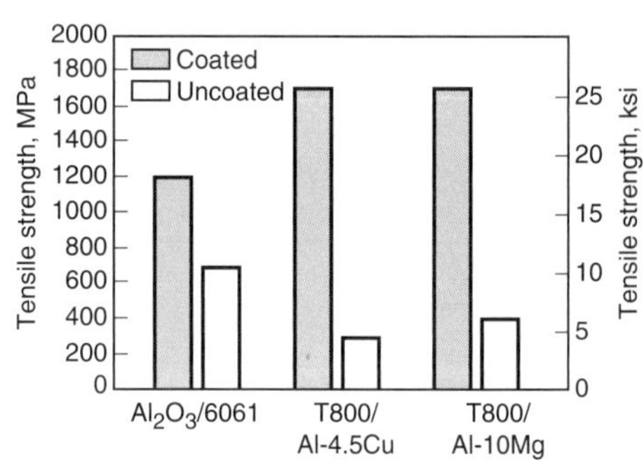

Fig. 21 Influence of fiber coatings on longitudinal tensile strengths of Al-MMCs at room temperature. C + TiB_2 coating on Al_2O_3 fiber, carbon coating on T800 carbon fiber. After Ref 99

Table 17 Properties of metal-polymer laminate composites

Mechanical properties (orientation)	Glare 2(a), 3/2(b)	Glare 3(a), 3/2(b)	ARALL 2(a), 3/2(b)	2024-T3
Tensile ultimate strength, MPa (ksi)				
L	1214 (176)	717 (104.0)	717 (104.0)	455 (66.0)
LT	317 (46.0)	716 (103.8)	317 (46.0)	448 (65.0)
Tensile yield strength, MPa (ksi)				
L	360 (52.2)	305 (44.2)	365 (52.9)	359 (52.1)
LT	228 (33.0)	283 (41.0)	228 (33.0)	324 (47.0)
Tensile modulus, GPa (10^6 psi)				
L	65 (9.4)	58 (8.4)	66 (9.6)	72 (10.4)
LT	50 (7.3)	58 (8.4)	53 (7.7)	72 (10.4)
Ultimate strain, %				
L	4.7	4.7	2.5	19
LT	10.8	4.7	12.7	19
Compressive yield strength, MPa (ksi)				
L	414 (60.0)	309 (44.8)	255 (37.0)	303 (43.9)
LT	236 (34.2)	306 (44.4)	234 (33.9)	345 (50.0)
Compressive modulus, GPa (10^6 psi)				
L	67 (9.7)	60 (8.7)	65 (9.4)	74 (10.7)
LT	52 (7.5)	60 (8.7)	53 (7.7)	74 (10.7)

(a) Glare 2: 2024-T3 Al with unidirectional glass prepregs. Glare 3: 2024-T3 Al with cross ply of 50/50 fibers in L direction and LT direction. ARALL 2: 2024-T3 Al with unidirectional aramid fibers. (b) Number of layers: 3, metal; 2, polymer. Source: Ref 97

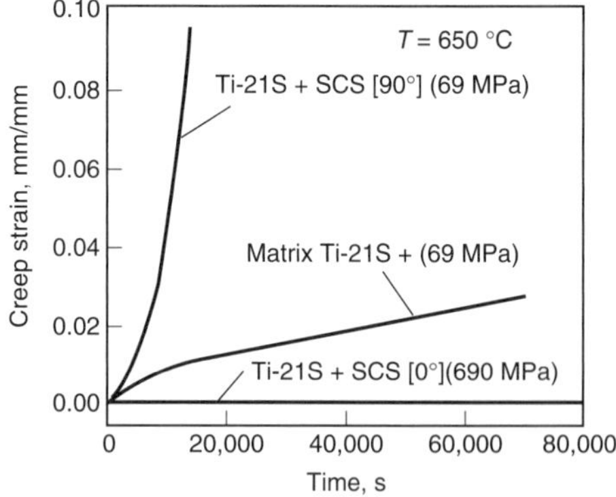

Fig. 22 Comparison of creep behavior of Ti-21S + SCS6 fibers loaded parallel [0°] and [90°] to fibers with unreinforced matrix. Temperature, 650 °C (1200 °F). After Ref 111

Table 18 Survey of reinforcement morphology on the properties of Al-MMCs

Composite	Tensile strength		Modulus of elasticity		Fracture toughness		Density, g/cm^3	Coefficient of thermal expansion, 10^{-6}K	Thermal conductivity, W/m · K
	MPa	ksi	GPa	10^6 psi	MPa $\sqrt{m}$	ksi $\sqrt{in.}$			
Al/Al_2O_3 continuous fiber	1300–1900	189–276	220–300	31.9–43.5			3.5	10–12	80
Al/Al_2O_3 short fibers	300–450	43.5–65.3	120–140	17.4–20.3	15–20	13.7–18.2	3.1	17	100
Al/Al_2O_3 particles	300–500	43.5–72.5	170–190	24.7–27.6	15–30	13.7–27.3	3.2	12–14	55
Al/Al_2O_3 particles 3D	300–500	43.5–72.5	120–140	17.4–20.3	15–30	13.7–27.3	3.1	14–16	60–90
Al/graphite 2D fabric	...	...	...	...	...	...	2.3	2.8	280
Al/graphite 3D fiber mat	...	...	...	...	...	...	2.3	5.5	226 (*x-y*) 178 (*z*)

Source: MMCC, Inc. (Ref 17)

near-net-shape components can be cast, and complex preforms (e.g., three-dimensional fiber weaves) can be used to produce composites having unique reinforcement architectures. Table 18 shows the influence of reinforcement architecture on the properties of selected Al-MMCs (Ref 17).

Properties of Continuous Fiber Reinforced Composites

Strength and Stiffness. Typical tensile properties (at room and elevated temperatures) for selected Al-, Mg-, and Ti-MMCs reinforced with continuous fibers are listed in Tables 19 to 24 (Ref 3, 17, 102–108).

The addition of fibers improves the axial, or longitudinal (0° orientation; fibers aligned parallel to the tensile axis), stiffness of the matrix by a factor of 3. In this orientation, the composites take on the properties of the reinforcement, and the composites are an order of magnitude stronger than the unreinforced matrix. The composites retain their strength and stiffness at elevated temperatures, relative to the unreinforced matrices, as illustrated in Fig. 20. As loads rotate off-axis, the properties fall quickly once the direction of the fibers and the direction of the loads differ. Typically, transverse strengths (90° orientation; fibers perpendicular to the tensile axis) are about 10% of the longitudinal strengths. Higher transverse strength can be obtained by the use of cross-ply laminates.

Interfacial properties have a pronounced effect on the mechanical behavior of the composites. Strong interfaces lead to moderate longitudinal strengths and good transverse strengths, while weak interfaces produce high longitudinal strengths, close to those predicted by the rule of mixtures, but with reduced transverse strengths. As discussed in the section "Creep and Fatigue," weak interfaces also improve fracture resistance and fatigue life.

Figure 21 illustrates the effect of fiber coatings on the longitudinal properties of Al-MMCs containing Al_2O_3 and carbon fibers. In the absence of a coating, both Al_2O_3 and carbon fibers form a strong bond with the matrix; carbon fibers react with aluminum to form an Al_4C_3 interfacial layer during molten metal processing. In principle, if the matrix yield stress is sufficiently low (e.g., such as for aluminum and Al-2Cu alloys), then shearing of the matrix in the vicinity of the fibers can occur, functioning as a weak interface. With stronger alloys, such as 6061, coatings can be applied to the surface of the fibers to promote a weak interface. For Al_2O_3 fibers, a C/TiB_2 duplex coating has been developed, and for carbon fibers, the deposition of a pyrolytic carbon coating can serve as a diffusion barrier (Ref 99, 109, 110).

For Ti-SiC composites, the longitudinal tensile properties are consistent with simple models in which the strength is dominated by the bundle properties of the fibers (Ref 111–113). All other properties are strongly dependent on interfacial properties of the composites. For composites having relatively weak interfaces (i.e, Ti-15-3 containing carbon-coated SCS-6 fibers), fiber debonding occurs readily via mode I and mode II fracture modes, and frictional sliding occurs at the debonded interface (Ref 111–113). The slid-

Table 19 Properties of selected Al- and Mg-MMC composites

Composite/vol% reinforcement	Orientation	Modulus of elasticity		Tensile strength		Poisson's ratio	Ductility, %	Coefficient of thermal expansion, 10^{-6}/K
		GPa	10^6 psi	MPa	ksi			
Al + 65% Al_2O_3 (3M-Nextel)(a)	0	262	38.0	1833	266	0.295	0.73	...
	90	123	17.8	178	25.8	...	1.16	...
Al + 2wt% Cu + 65% Al_2O_3 (3M-Nextel)(a)	0	267	38.7	1805	262	0.31	0.73	...
	90	173	25.1	318	46.1	...	0.55	...
Al + 60% Al_2O_3 (3M-Nextel)(a)	0	241	34.9	1653	240	...	...	7
	90	172	24.9	318	46.1	...	...	16
Al + 2wt% Cu + 60% Al_2O_3 (3M-Nextel)(a)	0	241	34.9	1515	220	...	...	9
	90	158	22.9	275	39.9	...	...	16
Al + 45% Al_2O_3 (3M-Nextel)(a)	0	165	23.9	1255	182	...	0.8	...
6061Al + 48% B (Textron)(b)	0	210	30.5	1520	220	...	...	5.8
	90	138	20.0	110	16.0	...	...	19.1
6061Al + 60% B (Textron)(b)	0	214	31.0	1490	216	...	...	...
	90	138	20.0	138	20.0	...	...	...
AZ31B Mg + 70% B(c)	0	285	41.3	2255	327	...	...	...
ZK Mg + 70% B(c)	0	296	42.9	1048	152	...	...	...
HZK Mg + 70% B(c)	0	300	43.5	1089	158	...	...	...
6061Al + 47% SiC (SCS-2 Textron)(b)	0	204	29.6	1462	212	0.27	0.89	6.6
	±45	95	13.8	309	44.8	0.395	10.6	...
	90	118	17.1	86	12.5	0.124	0.08	21.3
	Cross ply, 0/90/0/90	136	19.7	673	97.6	...	0.90	...
	Cross ply, 0/±45/0	146	21.2	800	116	...	0.86	...
	Cross ply, 0/±45/90	127	18.4	572	82.9	...	1.0	...
6061Al + 48% SiC (SCS-6 Textron)(b)	0	220	31.9	1750	254	...	...	...
	90	...	...	105	15.2	...	...	...
7075Al + 35% SiC (Nicalon)(b)	0	105	15.2	850	123.3	...	...	12
	90	...	...	90	13.0	...	...	25
6061Al + 47% graphite (P-100)(b)	0	301	43.6	543	78.7	...	...	...
	90	48	7.0	13	1.9	...	...	...
6061Al + 37.5% carbon (T-300)(b)	0	124	18.0	1100	160	...	...	...
Al-5Mg + 35% carbon (M40)(c)	0	180	26.1	728	105.6	...	...	...
Al-3Mg-2Zr + 35% carbon (M40)(c)	0	160	23.2	1110	161	...	...	...
Mg + 30% carbon (T-300)(c)	0	84	12.2	522	75.7	...	...	...
Mg + 35% carbon (T-300)(c)	0	80	11.6	498	72.2	...	...	...
Mg-4Al + 30% carbon (T-300)(c)	0	93	13.5	655	95.0	...	...	...
Mg-4Al + 35% carbon (T-300)(c)	0	76	11.0	638	92.5	...	...	...

(a) 3M Inc., Ref 102. (b) Ref 2. (c) Ref 8

Table 20 Elevated-temperature properties of Al-Al_2O_3 (Nextel) and Al-SiC (Nicalon) MMCs (longitudinal orientation)

Property	Property at indicated test temperature, °C (°F)				
	−50 (−58)	25 (77)	100 (210)	300 (570)	400 (750)
Al + 45 vol% Al_2O_3(a)					
Modulus of elasticity, GPa (10^6 psi)	165 (23.9)	165 (23.9)	133 (19.3)	133 (19.3)	133 (19.3)
Strength, MPa (ksi)	1220 (177)	1255 (178)	1247 (181)	1110 (161)	1061 (154)
Ductility, %	0.73	0.80	0.85	0.82	0.79
Al + 65 vol% Al_2O_3(a)					
Modulus of elasticity, GPa (10^6 psi)	...	261 (37.8)	...	200 (29.0)	...
Strength, MPa (ksi)	...	1833 (266)	...	1447 (210)	...
Ductility, %	...	0.73	...	0.850	...
Al + 30 vol% SiC(b)					
Strength, MPa (ksi)	...	610 (88.5)	...	650 (94.3)	550 (79.8)
Al + 35 vol% SiC					
Strength, MPa (ksi)	...	850 (123.3)	...	700 (101.5)	760 (110.2)

(a) Source: 3M, Inc. (Ref 102). (b) Source: Ref 2

Table 21 Typical longitudinal tensile properties of Ti-SiC composites containing nominally 35 vol% SCS-6 fibers

Matrix	Test temperature		Modulus		Strength		Ductility, %
	°C	°F	GPa	10^6 psi	MPa	ksi	
T-6Al-4V(a)	23	73	202	29.3	1932	280.1	1.09
	538	1000	183	26.5	1370	198.7	0.87
	650	1202	167	24.2	1221	177.0	0.86
Ti-1100 (Ti-6Al-2.75Sn-4Zr-0.4Mo-0.45SI)(a)	23	73	198	28.7	1219	176.8	0.73
	538	1000	178	25.8	1004	145.6	0.65
	650	1202	166	24.0	971	140.8	0.68
Ti-25Al-10Nb-3V-1Mo (Ti_3Al alloy)(a)	23	73	217	31.5	1517	220.0	0.79
	538	1000	200	29.0	1472	213.4	0.85
	650	1202	188	27.3	1360	197.2	0.82
Ti-24Al-11Nb (Ti_3Al alloy)(b)	23	73	205	29.7	1496	216.9	0.97
	650	1202	159	23.1	997	144.6	0.79
	815	1499	153	22.2	740	107.3	0.65
Ti-22Al-23Nb (Ti_2AlNb orthorhombic alloy)(c) (Ultra-SCS fibers)	23	73	202	29.3	2213	320.9	1.48
	650	1202	173	25.1	1820	263.9	1.35
	760	1400	135	19.6	1115–1318	161.7–191.1	1.22

(a) Ref 103. (b) Ref 104. (c) Ref 105, 106

Table 22 Longitudinal (0°) tensile properties of Ti-15-3 (Ti-15V-3Cr-3Al-3Sn) + SCS6 SiC composites

Fiber content, vol%	Ultimate tensile strength		Modulus of elasticity		Poisson's ratio	Ductility, %
	MPa	ksi	GPa	10^6 psi		
Test temperature, 25 °C (77 °F)						
0	850	123	85	12	...	19.3
15	1275	185	138	20	...	1.21
35	1380	200	183	27	0.28	0.84
41	1565	227	214	31	...	0.82
Test temperature, 425 °C (800 °F)						
15	945	137	131	19	0.38	0.81
25	1345	195	165	24	0.32	0.90
35	1560	226	186	27	...	0.95
45	1710	248	213	31	0.30	0.84

Source: Ref 107, 108

ing can be influenced by normal compression at the interface, suggestive of the Coulomb friction law (Ref 112). These interfacial features cause the composite flow strength in both transverse tension and shear to be appreciably lower than the matrix flow stress (Ref 112). Exposure at elevated temperatures can alter the interfacial properties and degrade the strength and stiffness of the composite (Ref 106, 111).

Thermal Properties. Graphite fibers have a negative coefficient of thermal expansion. Composites having unique thermal expansion and thermal conductivity properties (Table 25) can be produced by combining these fibers with aluminum and copper matrices (Ref 3). Composites can be designed to have a CTE of nearly zero, which is attractive for use in space applications in an environment where the temperature can vary by hundreds of degrees. These composites also have high thermal conductivities, and, as with particulate composites discussed previously, are being used in thermal management applications in electronic devices.

Creep and Fatigue. Creep rupture data for selected Ti-SCS-6 composites are listed in Table 26 (Ref 103, 114). Continuous fiber reinforced composites are expected to exhibit greater creep resistance than particulate or short fiber composites. However, as with strength and stiffness, the creep rate of a composite can be quite anisotropic (Fig. 22). Creep rates tend to be very low when loaded parallel to the fibers. Under transverse loadings, creep rates tend to be quite rapid, especially if the specimen is also exposed to thermal cycling. Research suggests that creep life is reduced when interfacial sliding occurs; thus, composites having strong fiber/matrix interfaces are desired for creep resistance (Ref 115, 116).

Under parallel loading conditions, the fibers carry most of the applied load; therefore, the creep rate of the composite is dependent on the creep characteristics of the fiber. In this case, the fiber deforms elastically, and the overall creep strain of the composite (ε_c) rises asymptotically (Fig. 22) from an instantaneous value ($\varepsilon_{t=0}$) to a maximum value (ε_{max}). The creep strain (ε_c) of the composite at any given time (t) can be given by a power law model (Ref 1):

$$\frac{1}{(\varepsilon_{max}-\varepsilon_c)^{n-1}} - \frac{1}{(\varepsilon_{max}-\varepsilon_{t=0})^{n-1}} = \frac{AE_M(1-f)}{E_c} \times \left(\frac{fE_f}{1-f}\right)^n t \quad \text{(Eq 2)}$$

where the matrix creep rate is given by $A\sigma^n$, $(\varepsilon_{t=0}) = \sigma/E_c$, and $\varepsilon_{max} = \sigma/E_f$. E_c, E_M, and E_f are the modulus of the composite, matrix, and fiber, respectively, f is the volume fraction, σ is the applied load, and A and n are constants.

Fatigue life and fracture resistance are important parameters when considering aerospace engine applications—even more important than strength and stiffness. Therefore, considerable effort has been devoted to understanding the fatigue behavior of MMCs, particularly for Ti-MMCs. The following summary attempts to highlight salient features of the fatigue behavior of MMCs. Considerably more detail can be found by examining Ref 117 to 133.

The mechanisms of fatigue failure have been summarized in Ref 120, 124, 127, and 131 to 135. The effect of both R ratio and volume fraction of fibers on fatigue behavior have been studied (Ref 128, 129), and the fatigue of Ti-SiC cross plies (Ref 126, 130) and hybrid Ti-SiC-TiAl composites have been evaluated (Ref 124).

Table 23 Transverse (90°) tensile properties of Ti-15-3 (Ti-15V-3Cr-3Al-3Sn) + SCS6 SiC composites

Fiber content, vol%	Ultimate tensile strength		Modulus of elasticity		Poisson's ratio	Ductility, %
	MPa	ksi	GPa	10^6 psi		
Test temperature, 25 °C (77 °F)						
0	850	123	85	12	...	19.3
15	661	96	124	18	...	1.91
35	420	61	124	18	0.12	1.41
41	192	28	124	18	...	0.61
Test temperature, 425 °C (800 °F)						
35	282	41	117	17	...	0.99

Source: Ref 107, 108

Table 24 Fiber orientation effects on tensile properties of Ti-15-3 (Ti-15V-3Cr-3Al-3Sn) + 35 vol% SCS6 SiC composites

Fiber orientation, degrees	Ultimate tensile strength		Modulus of elasticity		Poisson's ratio	Ductility, %
	MPa	ksi	GPa	10^6 psi		
Test temperature, 25 °C (77 °F)						
0	1380	200	183	27	0.28	0.84
30	965	140	153	22	...	1.24
45	530	77	117	17	...	>4
60	390	57	117	17	...	1.8
90	420	61	124	18	0.18	1.41
0/90 cross ply	1020	148	144	21	0.18	1.09
Test temperature, 425 °C (800 °F)						
0	1560	226	186	27	0.95	...
30	923	134	138	20	1.52	...
45	468	68	90	13	7.29	...
60	330	48	97	14	2.95	...
90	282	41	117	17	0.71	...

Source: Ref 107, 108

Table 25 Thermal properties of Al- and Cu-MMCs reinforced with graphite fibers

Composite	Fiber content, vol%	Density, g/cm^3	Axial thermal conductivity, W/m · K	Coefficient of thermal expansion, 10^{-6}/K
Al	0	2.70	170	23
Al/graphite	40	2.52	200	6.7
Al/graphite	60	2.41	419	−0.32
Al/SiC_p	40–70	2.91–3.03	160–180	12.6–6.5
Cu	0	8.94	400	17.6
Cu/graphite	40	6.86	300	7.4
Cu/graphite	60	4.90	522	−0.07

Source: Ref 2, 17

Fatigue life of unnotched MMCs laminates is a function of the stress/strain range in the 0° fibers. At high peak stress levels, the fibers fail ahead of the crack tip and fatigue life is relatively short. The growth of the fatigue crack is dominated by the properties of the matrix, with minimal contribution from fiber pullout. Prior to catastrophic failure, a plastic strip forms ahead of the crack, similar to what is observed in ductile metals. In this region, all of the fibers break prior to final fracture. Typically, under these conditions, referred to as regime 1, the fatigue life of the composite is lower than the fatigue life of the unreinforced matrix. At low peak stress levels (regime 3), fatigue life is long (i.e., near the endurance limit) and damage is initiated in the matrix. Matrix cracks can grow past the fibers, leaving the fibers intact in the wake of the crack. Continued cycling is accommodated by debonding and sliding along the fiber/matrix interface. The bridging fibers exert closing traction forces on the crack faces, reducing the crack tip stress intensity range and rate of fatigue crack growth. Below a threshold stress level, the stress borne by a bridging fiber is less than the strength of the fibers. Consequently the fibers never break, and a steady-state fatigue crack growth rate is reached and is independent of crack length. Under these loading conditions the fatigue life of the composite is relatively long and is superior compared with the unreinforced matrix. Above the threshold stress level (regime 2) at intermediate peak stress levels, the fibers begin to break when the crack reaches a critical length, which is dependent on fiber strength and crack dimensions. Subsequently, the composite fractures. In this regime, the composites have similar characteristics to monolithic materials in that there is a power-law-type relationship between the stress range and fatigue life.

Substantial crack growth in the matrix can occur without unstable failure, as the fibers bridge matrix cracks. The bridged fibers can drastically improve fatigue crack growth (FCG) properties and can even result in crack arrest. Because the crack propagates through the matrix, FCG rates of the composite correlate with FCG rates in the unreinforced matrix alloy, provided that the driving force for crack growth in the matrix is corrected for the reduced stress intensity at the crack tip due to the fibers bridging. Because fiber debonding plays an important role in FCG, the strength of the interface is an important parameter in governing FCG behavior (Ref 121, 125). Generally, composites having weaker interfaces can significantly enhance FCG behavior. However, substantial fatigue resistance can also be achieved with strong interfaces (Ref 125). This is important because use of Ti-MMCs in aeroengine applications will require improvements in transverse properties.

Typically, exposure to oxidizing environments tends to decrease fatigue life of Ti-SiC composites, under conditions in which matrix cracking is the dominant failure mode (regimes 2 and 3) (Ref 123, 132). For Ti_3Al-SiC, oxidizing atmospheres can reduce the fatigue life by an order of magnitude compared with that in inert environments (Ref 132). Likewise, for a Ti-SiC composites, samples tested in inert environments had twice the fatigue life compared with that of similar samples tested in oxidizing atmospheres (Ref 123). Under fatigue conditions in which the fatigue failure is dominated by fiber fracture (regime 1), environment has little effect on fatigue life.

Fatigue life in MMCs can be complicated by combining thermal cycling with mechanical fatigue (thermal mechanical fatigue, or TMF). Fatigue life is prolonged when the temperature cycling is in phase with the mechanical cycling (i.e., maximum temperature level coincides with the maximum stress level) as opposed to out of phase (i.e., maximum temperature level coincides with minimum stress level), as shown in Fig. 23 (Ref 121).

The corrosion resistance of fiber reinforced composites is different from that of particulate reinforced composites because of the interfacial

Table 26 Creep rupture data for Ti-SCS composites (nominally 35 vol%)

Matrix	Orientation	Temperature °C	Temperature °F	Stress MPa	Stress ksi	Rupture time, h	Larson-Miller parameter
Ti-6-4(a)	[0]	538	1008	965	139.9	932	...
				1103	160	252	...
	[0]	650	1202	758	109.9	>500	...
				827	119.9	392	...
Ti-1100(a)	[0]	538	1000	689	99.9	>500	...
				827	119.9	16	...
		650	1202	758	109.9	6	...
				827	119.9	0.7	...
Ti-25-10-3-1(a)	[0]	538	1000	689	99.9	>600	...
				827	119.9	>500	...
		650	1202	758	109.9	591	...
				827	119.9	54	...
Ti-21S(b)	[0]	650	1202	825	119.6	173.2	20.52
				862	125.0	6.9	19.23
		760	1400	621	90.0	161	22.93
				672	97.4	22.2	22.05
		815	1499	517.5	75.0	111.0	23.98
	[±45]	650	1202	69	10.0	122	20.38
				103	14.9	5.8	19.16
		760	1400	55.2	8.0	277.7	23.18
		815	1499	34.5	5.0	92.2	24.23
	[90]	650	1202	86.2	12.5	1.0	18.49
				69	10.0	3.9	19.00
				44.8	6.5	14.0	19.53
				41.4	6.0	44.3	19.98
				34.5	5.0	117.3	20.37
	[0/90] cross ply	650	1202	379.5	55.0	190	20.78
				400	58.0	93.8	20.02
				425	61.6	18	19.61
		815	1499	310	45.0	116.8	24.01
				345	50.0	9.0	22.79
	[0/±45/90] cross ply	650	1202	220	31.9	138	22.56
				241	34.9	121.6	21.78
		760	1400	200	29.0	194	23.02

(a) Ref 107. (b) Ref 109

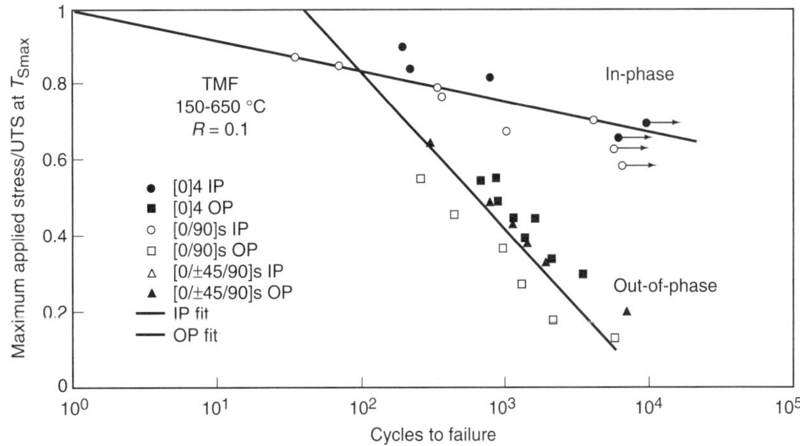

Fig. 23 Thermomechanical fatigue life for SCS-6/Ti-21S composites, normalized for maximum applied stress basis. Source: Ref 120

coating applied to many fibers. Also, many fibers are not pure materials. For instance, SCS-type SiC fibers are produced by depositing SiC around a carbon core. Also, these fibers commonly have carbon layer on their surfaces. The core and any interfacial coating alter the electrical properties relative to the pure phase. Thus, galvanic corrosion can occur in Al-SCS fibrous composites in environments where such corrosion does not normally occur in Al-SiC particulate composites. Furthermore, the interfacial region can become a region for localized corrosion. Similarly, with Al_2O_3 fibers, interfacial reaction phases can preferentially corrode.

As mentioned previously, Al-graphite particulate composites are susceptible to severe galvanic corrosion. The same is true for fibrous reinforced composites. Al-graphite fiber composites swell upon exposure to chloride-containing environments; corrosion products penetrate deep into the subcutaneous layers of the composite. Al-graphite fiber MMCs are also susceptible to exfoliation, with debonding along the fiber/matrix interface due to localized corrosion at the interface. Furthermore, aluminum and graphite can react during processing to form an Al_4C_3 reaction layer. In the presence of moist or humid environments, Al_4C_3 hydrolyzes, producing methane and aluminum hydroxide. Al-graphite composites readily decompose in water.

Methods evaluated to prevent the corrosion of Al-graphite composites include cathodic protection, use of protective coating, and electrical decoupling. Normal cathodic protection methods that are generally applied to prevent galvanic corrosion in unreinforced aluminum alloys are unsuitable for Al-graphite MMCs. Overprotection occurs, and corrosion rates actually increase because of alkalization of the cathode surface. The effectiveness of coatings on surfaces of the bulk composites is related to the integrity of the applied coatings. Corrosion rates follow the corrosion rate of the unreinforced alloy until the coating is breached, exposing the underlying Al-graphite MMC. Electrically decoupling of the graphite fiber from the aluminum matrix through the deposition of insulating coating of the fibers, as well as the deposition of metallic (nickel) interlayers to alter the coupling behavior have also been examined to improve the corrosion resistance of Al-graphite composites. Greater detail can be found in Ref 60.

ACKNOWLEDGMENT

The author would like to thank Jeffrey A. Hawk of the Albany Research Center for reviewing this article prior to submission.

REFERENCES

1. T.W. Clyne and P.J. Withers, *An Introduction to Metal Matrix Composites,* Cambridge University Press, Cambridge, U.K., 1993
2. M.M. Schwartz, *Properties, Nondestructive Testing, and Repair,* Vol 1, *Composite Materials,* Prentice Hall, 1997
3. S. Suresh, A. Mortensen, and A. Needleman, *Fundamentals of Metal Matrix Composites,* Butterworth-Heinmann, 1993
4. T.S. Srivatsan, T.S. Sudarshan, and E.J. Lavernia, *Prog. Mater. Sci.,* Vol 39, 1995, p 317
5. *Ceramics and Glasses,* Vol 4, *Engineered Materials Handbook,* ASM International, 1991
6. P.T.B. Schaffer, *ART-Handbook of Advanced Ceramic Materials,* Advanced Refractories Technologies, Inc., 1994
7. *ASM Specialty Handbook: Aluminum and Aluminum Alloys,* ASM International, 1993
8. R.B. Bhagat, *Metal Matrix Composites, Processing and Interfaces,* R.K. Everett and R. J. Arsenault, Ed., Academic Press, 1991, p 43
9. J.A.E. Bell, A.E.F Warner, and T.F. Stephenson, *Processing, Properties, and Applications of Cast Metal Matrix Composites,* P. Rohatgi, Ed., TMS, 1996, p 247
10. L. Christodoulou and J.M. Brupbacher, *Mater. Edge,* Nov/Dec 1990, p 29
11. D.L. Lewis III, Metal Matrix Composites: Processing and Interfaces, P.K. Everett and R.J. Arsenault, Ed., Academic Press, 1991, p 121
12. "Duralcan Aluminum Metal Matrix Composites," Duralcan, 1999
13. X. Liu and M. Nilmani, *Processing, Properties, and Applications of Cast Metal Matrix Composites,* P. Rohatgi, Ed., TMS, 1996, p 297
14. Materials Data, Ceramics Process Systems, Inc., 2000
15. Materials Data, PCC-Advanced Forming Technologies, Inc., 2000
16. "Property Data, Materials Selector & Recommended Applications," Lanxide Electronic Components, Inc., 2000
17. Materials Data, Metal Matrix Cast Composites, Inc., Waltham MA, 2000
18. Boralyn Properties, Ayln Corp., 2000
19. J.Y. Yang, F.W. Zok, and C.G. Levi, *Processing, Properties, and Applications of Cast Metal Matrix Composites,* P. Rohatgi, Ed., TMS, 1996, p 77
20. M.L. Seleznev, I.L. Selznev, J.A. Cornie, A.S. Argon, and R.P. Manson, Paper 980700, SAE International Congress and Exposition (Detroit, MI), 23–26 Feb 1998, Society of Automotive Engineers
21. "Duralcan Aluminum Metal Matrix Composites," Duralcan, 1999
22. DWA Aluminum Composites, DWA, Chatsworth, CA, 2000
23. R.J. Arsenault and S.B Wu, *Scr. Metall.,* Vol 22, 1998, p 767
24. W. Dixon and D.J. Lloyd, *Processing, Properties, and Applications of Cast Metal Matrix Composites,* P. Rohatgi, Ed., TMS, 1996, p 259
25. J.K. Park and J.P. Lucas, *Processing, Properties, and Applications of Cast Metal Matrix Composites,* P. Rohatgi, Ed., TMS, 1996, p 201
26. T. Christman and S. Suresh, *Acta Metall.,* Vol 36, 1998, p 1691
27. D.C. Dunand and B. Derby, *Fundamentals of Metal Matrix Composites,* S. Suresh, A. Mortensen, and A. Needleman, Ed., Butterworth-Heinemann, 1993, p 191
28. T.G. Nieh, *Metall. Trans.,* Vol 15A, 1985, p 139
29. V.C. Nardone and J.R. Strife, *Metall. Trans.,* Vol 18A, 1987, p 109
30. T. Morimoto, T. Yamaoka, H. Lilholt, and M. Taya, *J. Eng. Mater. Technol.,* Vol 110, 1988, p 77
31. E.T. Park, E.J. Lavernia, and F.A. Mohamad, *Acta Metall. Mater.,* Vol 38, 1990, p 2149
32. A.B. Pandey, R.S. Mishra, and Y.R. Mahajan, *Acta Metall. Mater.,* Vol 40, 1992, p 2045
33. T.L. Dragone and W.D. Nix, *Acta Metall. Mater.,* Vol 40, 1992, p 2781
34. G. Gonzalez-Doncel and O.D. Sherby, *Acta Metall. Mater.,* Vol 41, 1993, p 2797
35. A.B. Pandey, R.S. Mishra, and Y. Mahajan, *Mater. Sci. Eng. A,* Vol A189, 1994, p 95
36. K.T. Park and F.A. Mohamed, *Metall. Mater. Trans. A,* Vol 26A, 1995, p 3119
37. A.B. Pandey, R.S. Mishra, and Y. Mahajan, *Mater. Sci. Eng. A,* Vol A206, 1996, p 270
38. J. Cadek, M. Pahutova, and V. Sustek, *Mater. Sci. Eng. A,* Vol A246, 1998, p 252
39. A.F. Whitehouse, H.M.A. Winand, and T.W. Clyne, *Mater. Sci. Eng. A,* Vol A242, 1998, p 57
40. Y. Li and T.G. Langdon, *Metall. Mater. Trans. A,* Vol 30A, 1999, p 315
41. H.W. Nam and K.S. Ham, *Metall. Mater. Trans. A,* Vol 29A, 1998, p 1983
42. A.-B. El-Nasr, F.A. Mohamed, and J.C. Earthman, *Mater. Sci. Eng. A,* Vol A214, 1996, p 31
43. K. Wakashima, T. Moriyama, and T. Mori, *Acta Mater.,* Vol 48, 2000, p 891
44. J. Llorca and P. Poza, *Scr. Met. Mater.,* Vol 29, 1993, p 261
45. J.E. Allison and J.W. Jones, *Fundamentals of Metal Matrix Composites,* S. Suresh, A. Mortensen, and A. Needleman, Ed., Butterworth-Heinemann, 1993, p 269
46. J.J. Lewandowski and P.M. Singh, Fracture and Fatigue of DRA Composites, *Fatigue and Fracture,* Vol 19, *ASM Handbook,* ASM International, 1996, p 895–904
47. D. Lesuer, C.S. Syn, and T.G. Nieh, *Aluminum and Magnesium for Automotive Applications,* J.D. Bryant and D.R. White, Ed., TMS, 1996
48. J.J. Manson and R.O. Ritchie, *Mater. Sci. Eng. A,* Vol 231, 1997, p 170
49. D.M. Knowles, T.J. Downes, J.E. King, *Acta Metall. Mater.,* Vol 41, 1993, p 1189

50. V.K. Varma, S.V. Kamat, M.K. Jain, V.V. Bhanuprasad, and Y.R. Mahajan, *J. Mater. Sci.,* Vol 28, 1993, p 477
51. Y. Sugimura and S. Suresh, *Metall. Trans.,* Vol 23A, 1992, p 2231
52. D.L. Davidson, *Metall. Trans.,* Vol 22A, 1991, p 97
53. J.K. Shang and R.O. Ritchie, *Acta Metall.,* Vol 37, 1989, p 2267
54. D.M. Knowles and J.E. King, *Acta Metall.,* Vol 39, 1991, p 793
55. J.J. Bonnen, *Metall. Trans.,* Vol 22A, 1991, p 1007
56. R.L. Deuis, C. Subramanian, and J.M. Yellup, *Compos. Sci. Technol.,* Vol 57, 1997, p 415
57. P.K. Rohatgi, S. Ray, and Y. Liu, *Int. Mater. Rev.,* Vol 37, 1992, p 129
58. A. Martin, M.A. Martinez, and J.L. Lorca, *Wear,* Vol 193, 1996, p 169
59. M. Roy, B. Venkataraman, V.V. Bhanuprasad, Y.R. Mahajan, and G. Sundararjan, *Metall. Trans.,* Vol 23A, 1992, p 2833
60. L.H. Hihara and R.M. Laranision, *Int. Mater. Rev.,* Vol 39, 1994, p 245
61. R.A. Saravanan and M.K. Surppa, *Mater. Sci. Eng. A,* Vol A276, 2000, p 108
62. A.R. Vaidya and J.J. Lewandowski, *Mater. Sci. Eng. A,* Vol A220, 1996, p 85
63. S. Ranganth, *J. Mater. Sci.,* Vol 32, 1997, p 1
64. J.A. Philliber, F.C. Dary, F.W. Zok, and C.G. Levi, *Titanium'95 Science and Technology,* P.A. Blenkinsop, W.J. Evans, and H.M. Flower, Ed., The Institute of Metals, London, 1995, p 2714
65. T.S. Srivatsan, W.O. Soboyejo, and R.J. Lederich, *Composites Part A,* Vol 28A, 1997, p 356
66. C.F. Yolton and J.H. Moll, *Titanium'95 Science and Technology,* P.A. Blenkinsop, W.J. Evans, and H.M. Flower, Ed., The Institute of Metals, London, 1995, p 2755
67. T. Saito, H. Takamiya, and T. Furuta, *Titanium'95 Science and Technology,* P.A. Blenkinsop, W.J. Evans, and H.M. Flower, Ed., The Institute of Metals, London, 1995, p 2859
68. M. Kobayashi, K. Funami, S. Suzuki, and C. Ouchi, *Mater. Sci. Eng. A,* Vol A243, 1998, p 279
69. T. Saito, H, Takamiya, and T. Furuta, *Mater. Sci. Eng. A,* Vol A243, 1998, p 273
70. L. Wang, M. Niiomi, S. Takahashi, M. Hagiwara, S. Emura, Y. Kawabei, and S.-J. Kim, *Mater. Sci. Eng. A,* Vol A263, 1999, p 319
71. P. Wanjara, R.A.L. Drew, and S. Yue, *Titanium'95 Science and Technology,* P.A. Blenkinsop, W.J. Evans, and H.M. Flower, Ed., The Institute of Metals, London, 1995, p 2843
72. G. Lui, D. Zhu, and J.-K. Shang, *Scr. Met. Mater.,* Vol 28, 1993, p 729
73. P.A. Bartollotta and D.L. Krause, *Gamma Titanium Aluminides, 1999,* Y.-W. Kim, D.M. Dimiduk, and M.H. Loretto, Ed., TMS, 1999, p 3
74. L. Christodoulou, P.A. Parrish, and C.R. Crowe, *High Temperature. High Performance Composites,* F.D. Lemkey, S.G. Fishman, A.G. Evans, and J.R. Strife, Symp. Proc. 120, Materials Research Society, 1988, p 29
75. K.S. Kumar, R. Darolia, D.F. Lahrman, and S.K. Mannan, *Scr. Metall. Mater.,* Vol 26, 1992, p 1001
76. D.E. Alman and N.S. Stoloff, *Int. J. Powder Metall.,* Vol 27 (No. 1), 1991, p 29
77. S.C. Jha and R. Ray, *J. Mater. Sci., Lett.,* Vol 7, 1988, p 285
78. J.A. Christodoulou and H.M. Flower, *Gamma Titanium Aluminides, 1999,* Y.-W. Kim, D.M. Dimiduk, and M.H. Loretto, Ed., TMS, 1999, p 315
79. M.Y. Nazmy, *Physical Metallurgy and Processing of Intermetallic Compounds,* N.S. Stoloff and V.K. Sikka, Ed., Chapman and Hall, 1996, p 126
80. W. Voice, *Gamma Titanium Aluminides, 1999,* Y.-W. Kim, D.M. Dimiduk, and M.H. Loretto, Ed., TMS, 1999, p 3
81. J.-H. Jin and D.J. Stephenson, *Wear,* Vol 217, 1998, p 200
82. J.A. Hawk and D.E. Alman, *Mater. Sci. Eng. A,* Vol A329-240, 1997 p 889
83. P.S. Korinko, D.E. Alman, N.S. Stoloff, and D.J. Duquette, *Intermetallic Matrix Composites II,* D.B. Miracle, D.L. Anton, and J.A. Graves, Ed., Symp. Proc. 120, Material Research Society, 1992, p 183
84. D.R. Lesuer, C.K. Syn, O.D. Sherby, J. Wadsworth, J.J. Lewandowski, and W.H. Hunt, *Int. Mater. Rev.,* Vol 41, 1996, p 169
85. C.K. Syn, D.R. Lesuer, J. Wolfenstine, and O.D. Sherby, *Metall. Trans. A,* Vol 24A, 1993, p 1647
86. V.C. Nardone, J.R. Striffe, and K.M. Prewo, *Metall. Trans. A,* Vol 22A, 1991, p 17
87. V.C. Nardone and J.R. Striffe, *Metall. Trans. A,* Vol 22A, 1991, p 181
88. V.C. Nardone, *Metall. Trans. A,* Vol 23A, 1992, p 563
89. T.M. Osman, J.J. Lewandowski, and D.R. Lesuer, *Mater. Sci. Eng. A,* Vol A299, 1997, p 1
90. A.B. Pandey, B.S. Majumdar, and D.B. Miracle, *Mater. Sci. Eng. A,* Vol A259, 1999, p 296
91. K.S. Ravichandran, *Scr. Metall. Mater.,* Vol 26, 1992, p 1389
92. D.M. Shah, D.L. Anton, D.P. Pope, and S. Chin, *Mater. Sci. Eng. A,* Vol A192/193, 1995, p 658
93. M.G. Mendiratta, J.J. Lewandowski, and D.M. Dimiduk, *Metall. Trans. A,* Vol 22A, 1991, p 1573
94. G.A. Henshall, M.J. Strum, B.P. Bewlay, and J.A. Sutliff, *Metall. Mater. Trans. A,* Vol 28A, 1997, p. 2555
95. P.R. Subramanian, M.G. Mendiratta, and D.M. Dimiduk, *High Temperature Silicides and Refractory Alloys,* C.L. Briant, J.J. Petrovic, B.P. Bewlay, A.K. Vasudenvan, and H.A. Lipsitt, Ed., Symp. Proc., Vol 322, Materials Research Society, 1994, p 491
96. B.P. Bewlay, M.R. Jackson, and H.A. Lipsitt, *High Temperature Ordered Intermetallic Alloys VII,* C.C. Koch, C.T. Liu, N.S. Stoloff, and A. Wanner, Ed., Symp. Proc., Vol 460, Materials Research Society, 1997, p 491
97. G. Nordmark, *Fatigue and Fracture,* Vol 19, *ASM Handbook,* ASM International, 1996, p 910–913
98. J.L Miller, D.J. Progar, W.S. Johnson, and T.L. St. Clair, *J. Adhes.,* Vol 54, 1995, p 223
99. A. Vassel, *Mater. Sci. Eng.,* Vol A263, 1999, p 305
100. D.M. Shah and D.L. Anton, *Structural Intermetallics,* R. Darolia, J.J. Lewandowski, C.T. Liu, P.L. Martin, D.B. Miracle, and M.V. Nathal, Ed., TMS 1993, p 775
101. D.W. Petrasek and R.A Signirelli, *Superalloys and Supercomposites and Superceramics,* J.K. Tien and T. Caulfield, Ed., Academic Press, 1989, p 629
102. "Al Matrix Composites," Material Data Sheet, 3M, St. Paul, MN, 1999
103. S.W. Schwenker and D. Eylon, *Titanium'95 Science and Technology,* P.A. Blenkinsop, W.J. Evans, and H.M. Flower, Ed., The Institute of Metals, London, 1995, p 2787
104. P.K. Brindley, S.L. Draper, J.I. Eldridge, M.V. Nathal, and S.M. Arnold, *Metall. Trans. A,* Vol 23A, 1992, p 2527
105. D.B. Miracle, P.R. Smith, and J.A. Graves, *Intermetallic Matrix Composites III,* J.A Graves, R.R. Bowman, and J.J. Lewandowski, Symp. Proc. 350, Materials Research Society, 1994 p 133
106. P.R. Smith, J.A. Graves, and C.G. Rhodes, *Metall. Mater. Trans. A,* Vol 25A, 1994, p 1267
107. Metal Matrix Composites, *Composite Materials Handbook,* MIL-HDBK-17-4, U.S. Department of Defense, 21 Sept 1999
108. B.A. Lerch and J.F. Saltsman, *Composite Materials: Fatigue and Fracture,* Vol 4, STP 1156, W.W. Stinchomb and N.E. Ashbaugh, Ed., ASTM, 1993, p 161
109. M.H. Vidal-Setif, M. Lancin, C. Marhic, R. Valle, J.-L. Raviart, J.-C. Daux, and M. Rabinovitch, *Mater. Sci. Eng. A,* Vol A272, 1999, p 321
110. C. McCullough, H.E. Deve, and T.E. Channel, *Mater. Sci. Eng. A,* Vol A189, 1994, p 147
111. T.W. Clyne, P. Feillard, and A.F. Halyton, *Life Prediction Methodology for Titanium Matrix Composites,* STP 1253, W.S. Johnson, J.M. Larson, and B.N. Cox, Ed., ASTM, 1996, p 5
112. S. Jansson, H.E. Deve, and A.G. Evans, *Metall. Trans. A,* Vol 22A, 1991, p 2975

113. S.M. Jeng, J.-M. Yang, and C.J. Yang, *Mater. Sci. Eng. A,* Vol A138, 1991, p 169
114. M. Khobaid, R. John, and N.E. Ashbaugh, *Life Prediction Methodology for Titanium Matrix Composites,* STP 1253, W.S. Johnson, J.M. Larson, and B.N. Cox, Ed., ASTM, 1996, p 185
115. R. Nagarajan, I. Dutta, J.V. Funn, and M. Esmele, *Mater. Sci. Eng. A,* Vol A259, 1999, p 237
116. D.B. Miracle and B.S. Majumdar, *Metall. Mater. Trans. A,* Vol 30A, 1999, p 301
117. W.S. Johnson, *Fatigue and Fracture,* Vol 19, *ASM Handbook,* ASM International, 1996, p 914
118. W.S. Johnson, J.M. Larson, and B.N. Cox, Ed., *Life Prediction Methodology for Titanium Matrix Composites,* STP 1253, ASTM, 1996
119. W.S. Johnson, *Metal Matrix Composites: Testing, Analysis and Failure Modes,* STP 1032, W.S. Johnson, Ed., ASTM, 1989, p 194
120. T. Nicholas, *Mater. Sci. Eng. A,* Vol A200, 1995, p 29
121. J.M. Larsen, J.L. Moran, J.R. Jira, and D. Blatt, *Titanium'95 Science and Technology,* P.A. Blenkinsop, W.J. Evans, and H.M. Flower, Ed., The Institute of Metals, London, 1995, p 2803
122. J.L. Miller, M.A. Portanova, and W.S. Johnson, *Composite Materials: Fatigue and Fracture,* Vol 6, STP 1285, E.A. Armanios, Ed., ASTM, 1997, p 260
123. A.H. Rosenberger and T. Nicholas, *Composite Materials: Fatigue and Fracture,* Vol 6, STP 1285, E.A. Armanios, Ed., ASTM, 1997, p 394
124. P.C. Wang, Y.C. Her, and J.-M. Yang, *Mater. Sci. Eng. A,* Vol A245, 1998, p 100
125. S.G. Warrier, B. Maruyama, B.S. Majumdar, and D.B. Miracle, *Mater. Sci. Eng. A,* Vol A259, 1999, p 189
126. E.A. Boyum and S. Mall, *Mater. Sci. Eng. A,* Vol A200, 1995, p 1
127. B.S. Majumdar and G.M. Newaz, *Mater. Sci. Eng.,* Vol A200, 1995, p 114
128. S.J. Covey, B.A. Lerch, and N. Jayaraman, *Mater. Sci. Eng. A,* Vol A200, 1995, p 68
129. B. Lerch and G. Halford, *Mater. Sci. Eng. A,* Vol A200, 1995, p 47
130. W.O. Soboyejo and B. M. Rabeeh, *Mater. Sci. Eng. A,* Vol 2000, 1995, p 89
131. S.Q. Guo, Y. Kagawa, J.-L. Bobet, and C. Masuda, *Mater. Sci. Eng. A,* Vol A220, 1996, p 57
132. P.K. Brindley and P.A. Bartolotta, *Mater. Sci. Eng. A,* Vol A200 , 1995, p 55
133. F.W. Zok, Z.-Z. Du, and S.J. Connell, *Mater. Sci. Eng. A,* Vol A200, 1995, p 103
134. P.C. Wang, S.M. Jeng, and J.-M. Yang, *Mater. Sci. Eng. A,* Vol A200, 1995, p 173
135. Y.C. Her. J.-M. Yang, and Y. Kagawa, *Mater. Sci. Eng. A,* Vol A271, 1999, p 407

SELECTED REFERENCES

- T.W. Clyne and P.J. Withers, *An Introduction to Metal Matrix Composites,* Cambridge University Press, Cambridge, U.K., 1993
- R.L. Deuis, C. Subramanian, and J.M. Yellup, Dry Sliding Wear of Aluminum Composites—A Review, *Compos. Sci. Technol.,* Vol 57, 1997, p 415
- P.K. Everett and R.J. Arsenault, Ed., *Metal Matrix Composites: Processing and Interfaces* and *Metal Matrix Composites: Mechanisms and Properties,* Academic Press, Boston, 1991 (2 volumes)
- Z.X. Guo and B. Derby, Solid-State Fabrication and Interfaces of Fiber Reinforced Metal Matrix Composites, *Prog. Mater. Sci.,* Vol 39, 1995, p 411
- L.H. Higara and R.M. Katanision, Corrosion of Metal Matrix Composites, *Int. Mater. Rev.,* Vol 39, 1994, p 245
- W.S. Johnson, J.M. Larson, and B.N. Cox, *Life Prediction Methodology for Titanium Matrix Composites,* STP 1253, ASTM, 1996
- D.R. Lesuer, C.K. Syn, O.D. Sherby, J. Wadsworth, J.J. Lewandowski, and W.H. Hunt, Mechanical Behavior of Laminated Metal Composites, *Int. Mater. Rev.,* Vol 41, 1996, p 169
- D.J. Lloyd, Particulate Reinforced Aluminum and Magnesium Matrix Composites, *Int. Mater. Rev.,* Vol 39, 1994, p 1
- P.G. Partridge and C.M. Ward-Close, Processing of Advanced Continuous Fiber Composites: Current Practice and Potential Developments, *Int. Mater. Rev.,* Vol 38, 1993, p 1
- D.W. Petrasek and R.A Signirelli, Fiber Reinforced Superalloys, *Superalloys and Supercomposites and Superceramics,* J.K. Tien and T. Caulfield, Ed., Academic Press, 1989, p 629
- S. Ranganath, A Review on Particulate-Reinforced Titanium Matrix Composites, *J. Mater. Sci.,* Vol 32, 1997, p 1
- P.K. Rohatgi, S. Ray, and Y. Lui, Tribological Properties of Metal Matrix-Graphite Particulate Composites, *Int. Mater. Rev.,* Vol 37, 1992, p 129
- T.S. Srivatsan, T.S. Sudarshan, and E.J. Lavernia, Processing of Discontinuously Reinforced Metal Matrix Composites by Rapid Solidification, *Prog. Mater. Sci.,* Vol 39, 1995, p 317
- S. Suresh, A. Mortensen, and A. Needleman, *Fundamentals of Metal Matrix Composites,* Butterworth-Heinmann, 1993
- A. Vassel, Continuous Fiber Reinforced Titanium and Aluminum Composites: A Comparison, *Mater. Sci. Eng.,* Vol A263, 1999, p 305

Properties and Performance of Ceramic-Matrix and Carbon-Carbon Composites

Cynthia Powell Doğan, U.S. Department of Energy, Albany Research Center

TECHNOLOGY has made giant strides in recent decades so that when engineers today apply their ideas they frequently are limited only by the materials that are readily available at a reasonable cost. After centuries of wondering "What can I make with this kind of material?" scientists and engineers have reached the point of asking "What kind of materials need to be developed in order to advance this technology?" The answer to this question is often a composite material, in which the performance requirements of the specific application are engineered into the component by combining materials of different characteristics. Composites can be made of ceramics, metals, intermetallics, polymers, or some combination of these materials. For most ceramic-matrix composites (CMCs), the driving force for taking the composites approach is to enhance the mechanical reliability of a traditionally brittle material, while retaining such properties as low density, high hardness, high strength, high stiffness, thermal stability, corrosion resistance, and wear resistance.

The current interest in ceramic-matrix and carbon-carbon (C-C) composites derives primarily from the need for materials that can operate reliably at very high temperatures in harsh environments. The need for high-temperature materials spans the range of industries, from aerospace to pulp and paper, and is often driven by the desire to increase energy efficiency and/or reduce emissions. Current metals-based technology can produce materials that are stable to 1000 °C (1830 °F), and superalloys can be utilized to slightly higher temperatures if thermal barrier coatings and cooling systems are included. However, further technological advances in the high-temperature arena will probably not come from the use of metallic materials. Components produced from ceramic-based materials can operate at temperatures that are hundreds of degrees above the melting point of superalloys. Carbon-base components are stable to temperatures approaching 3000 °C (5430 °F). Clearly the next step is to fully exploit the high-temperature capabilities of these materials. Ceramic-matrix and carbon-carbon composite technology is one way to do so.

Ceramic-matrix composites can be broadly classified into three types: discontinuously reinforced ceramic-matrix composites (DR-CMCs), continuous fiber ceramic composites (CFCCs), and carbon-carbon composites. In the following sections, the mechanisms for enhancing the reliability of each type of composite is discussed, along with examples of the mechanical and physical properties, and the current limitations of the materials. Examples of the properties of commercially available materials are provided where available. Because the mechanisms of toughening are much the same, glass-matrix composites are not discussed here as a separate type of CMC, but are included in the general discussion of DR-CMCs and CFCCs.

Discontinuously Reinforced Ceramic-Matrix Composites

Discontinuously reinforced ceramic-matrix composites are a class of materials designed to retain the attractive properties of monolithic ceramics, while enhancing their reliability for structural applications. Although strictly speaking almost any multiphase ceramic can be classified as a DR-CMC, the materials referred to in this section are those in which discrete particles, platelets, whiskers, fibers, and so forth are incorporated into a ceramic or glass matrix in order to enhance composite performance. For the purposes of this discussion, transformation-toughened zirconia ceramics such as the partially stabilized zirconias (Ref 1–3) are not considered DR-CMCs, although ceramic matrices with added zirconia particles, such as the zirconia-toughened aluminas, are included.

In addition to the specific advantages of each composite system, DR-CMCs are characterized by the following:

- Their processing methodology is similar to that of monolithic ceramics, and therefore any increases in the cost of the composite relative to the monolithic should be small.
- Their mechanical and physical properties are approximately isotropic.
- Their fracture toughness is typically 25 to 100% higher than the corresponding monolithic ceramic (Ref 4, 5).

However, even though the possible increases in fracture toughness are relatively large with the addition of discontinuous reinforcement, DR-CMCs remain similar to monolithic ceramics in that they will fail catastrophically when a crack or flaw grows beyond a critical size.

Currently DR-CMCs are in the early stages of commercialization, with applications that include cutting tools, dies, advanced turbine engine components, heat exchangers, pressure seals, and wear-resistant parts. Although the principal driving force behind the addition of a discontinuous reinforcement to a ceramic matrix is most often the need to increase its structural reliability, it is important to remember that other properties of the material can also be enhanced, or tailored, by the composite approach (Ref 6).

Toughening Mechanisms. The magnitude of the change in the properties of a material that result from the addition of a discontinuous reinforcement phase can frequently be estimated by a rule of mixtures approximation. However, any changes in the toughness of the composite depend on the specific toughening mechanism(s) that are activated by the addition of the reinforcement, and the magnitude of the change can be difficult to predict. Possible toughening mechanisms for these materials include: crack deflection, crack bridging, pullout, microcracking, crack pinning, and phase transformation, as illustrated in Fig. 1. In most instances the toughening observed in a DR-CMC is the result of the combination of two or more of these toughening mechanisms. The effect of these mechanisms on

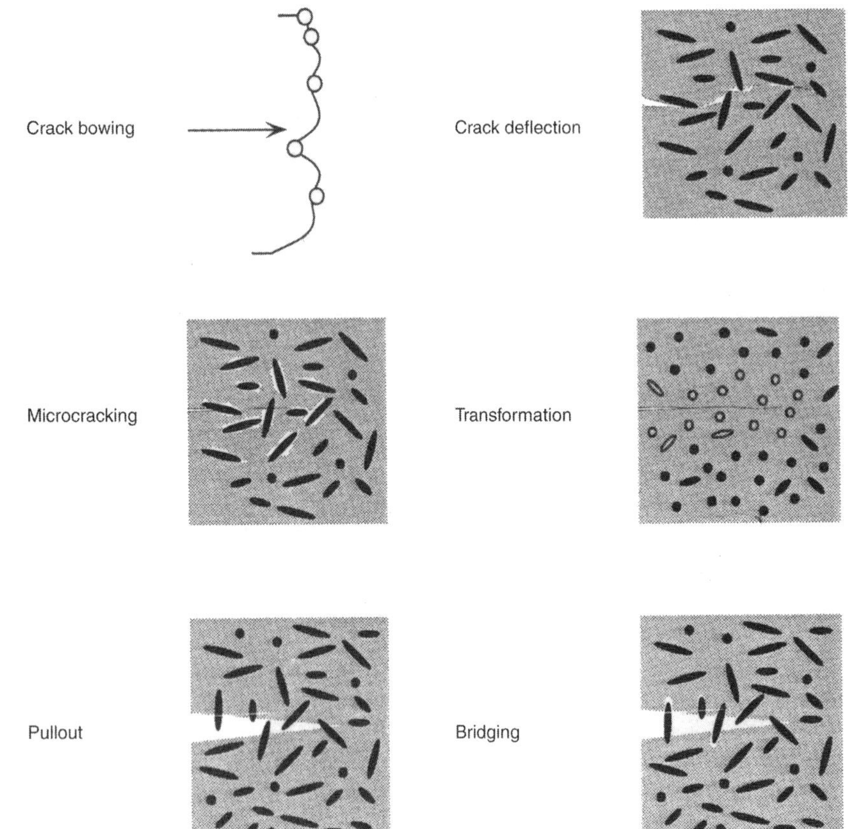

Fig. 1 Toughening mechanisms that can be activated in a discontinuously reinforced ceramic-matrix composite. Source: Ref 7

the room-temperature strength and fracture toughness of several DR-CMCs is presented in Table 1.

With crack deflection, a crack propagating through the matrix is deflected by the reinforcement phase, causing the crack to travel a longer distance and resulting in a corresponding decrease in the stress intensity at the crack tip (and thus an increase in the fracture toughness). Deflection results from the residual strain caused by the presence of the reinforcement phase and/or from the relatively weak reinforcement-matrix interfaces. This mechanism is operative in almost all DR-CMCs, although it may not be the dominant toughening mechanism. For most composite systems, the following generalities about toughening by crack deflection hold (Ref 8, 9): the increase in toughness depends on the reinforcement particle shape and volume fraction, but not on the reinforcement particle size; a rod shape is the most effective reinforcement morphology for increasing toughness; and the toughness increases with increased volume fraction of reinforcement particles up to a volume fraction of ~20%, but increases very little at higher volume fractions.

In crack bridging, the reinforcement phase does not fracture as the crack front passes by, creating "bridges" of material that remain intact behind the crack tip. The presence of these bridges limits the opening displacement of the crack, inhibiting further crack propagation, and thereby increasing fracture toughness. Whiskers, fibers, ductile metallic particles, or even large matrix grains can act as bridging elements in DR-CMCs. Typically, crack bridging is enhanced by an increase in the strength, diameter, and/or volume fraction of the ceramic reinforcement phase. With ductile reinforcement, on the other hand, toughness generally increases with volume fraction up to 15 vol% metal; however, composites containing greater than 5 vol% metal particles typically experience some degradation in strength and hardness.

When the shear strength of the reinforcement-matrix interfaces is less than the strength of the reinforcement phase, fracture along these interfaces will occur, leading to pullout of the reinforcement phase. Pullout increases the work of fracture of the composite and therefore increases its fracture toughness. Both fibers and whiskers can enhance the pullout toughness of a DR-CMC, although the pullout lengths of whiskers are relatively small, and thus their toughening effects are correspondingly less. When pullout is the dominant toughening mechanism, a balance between composite strength and fracture toughness must be achieved by carefully engineering the reinforcement-matrix interfaces so that they are sufficiently weak to maximize the number of pullouts that will occur, but not so weak as to compromise the integrity of the composite. Interfacial strength is governed by both the chemical reactions that occur at the interface and the degree of mechanical bonding.

A misfit in the coefficients of thermal expansion between the matrix and reinforcement phases can produce stresses in the composite that, if sufficiently high, will result in the spontaneous microcracking of the material. Composite toughening can occur if these microcracks are not initiated until an external stress is applied to the system. In this case, microcracks form only at the tip of the primary crack, reducing the stress intensity and therefore increasing fracture toughness. However, increases in the composite toughness as a result of this mechanism are generally not greater than 10%, and if not carefully controlled, excessive microcracking can lead to a decrease in the fracture toughness and strength of the material.

With crack pinning, the crack is pinned by the reinforcement phase, causing an increase in the fracture energy (toughness) as the crack front bows out between the pinning points. Effective crack pinning requires both a strong reinforcement-matrix interface and a strong reinforcement phase. In addition, the spacing between the individual pinning points (reinforcement particles) must be small relative to the crack size.

Transformation toughening occurs in DR-CMCs primarily through the addition of tetragonal zirconia particles to the ceramic matrix. Toughening occurs when these particles undergo a martensitic transformation to monoclinic symmetry in the presence of an external stress, resulting in a volume expansion that exerts closure stresses on the crack tip (Ref 1–3). Transformation toughening is maximized when the tetragonal zirconia particles are below a critical size, typically 0.5 to 0.8 μm in alumina-base materials. Microcracking, which may also occur during the tetragonal-to-monoclinic phase transformation, can also impact composite fracture toughness.

Table 1 General trends in room-temperature strength and toughness for ceramic-matrix composites with the addition of a discontinuous reinforcement phase

Composite	Fracture strength	Fracture toughness
Particulate Reinforced CMC		
Glass + Al_2O_3 (p)	Increase	Increase
Al_2O_3 + ZrO_2 (p)	Increase	Increase
Al_2O_3 + Ni (p)	Decrease	Increase
Platelet Reinforced CMC		
Al_2O_3 + SiC (pl)	Decrease	Increase
Whisker Reinforced CMC		
Glass + SiC (w)	Increase	Increase
Al_2O_3 + SiC (w)	Increase	Increase
Si_3N_4 + SiC (w)	Increase	Increase
ZrO_2 + SiC (w)	Decrease	Increase

Reinforcement: p, particulate; pl, platelet; w, whisker. Source: Ref 7

Optimal toughness in DR-CMCs is typically achieved by first determining which toughening mechanisms are possible within a particular composite system and then selecting the reinforcement particle type, shape, size, and volume fraction that maximize each of them. Because strength is typically a secondary concern in these materials, most DR-CMCs are designed for enhanced toughness, with little change in strength relative to the monolithic ceramic. In addition, it is important to recognize that while these various toughening mechanisms are active at low to intermediate temperatures, almost all of them can be predicted to degrade during prolonged exposure to temperatures above ~1100 °C (~2010 °F) (Ref 10). To date little experimental work has focused on the high-temperature stability of DR-CMCs; however, toughening mechanisms that rely on mismatches in thermal expansion or phase transformations will certainly not have the same influence at elevated temperatures. Long-term exposure to high temperatures is also likely to change reinforcement particle size and morphology and to influence the chemical nature of the matrix-reinforcement interfaces, potentially reducing the contributions of mechanisms such as pullout, bridging, and deflection to the overall toughness of the composite. Finally, characteristics of the composite unrelated to the reinforcement can also influence the high-temperature performance of the material, such as the presence of an amorphous grain-boundary phase within the matrix.

A list of the effect of the various types of ceramic reinforcement on the room-temperature strength and toughness of several ceramic and glass matrices can be found in Table 2.

Composite Architecture. The ceramic matrix in a DR-CMC may either be an oxide or nonoxide material and, depending on the processing techniques employed, may also contain some residual metal. The more common oxide matrices include polycrystalline alumina (Al_2O_3), silica (SiO_2), and mullite ($3Al_2O_3$-$2SiO_2$), and barium-aluminosilicate, calcium-aluminosilicate, and lithium-aluminosilicate glasses. However, alumina and mullite are by far the most common oxide-matrix materials because of their thermal and chemical stability and their compatibility with most of the common reinforcement materials. Nonoxide-matrix materials tend to have superior structural properties to their oxide counterparts, and they have better corrosion resistance in some environments. However, they are sensitive to oxidizing environments at elevated temperatures. The more common nonoxide matrices are silicon carbide (SiC), aluminum nitride (AlN), silicon nitride (Si_3N_4), and boron carbide (B_4C). Of these SiC is the more widely used, although AlN may be employed when high conductivity is a requirement, and Si_3N_4 may be selected when higher strength is needed.

The reinforcement phase in a DR-CMC can have a variety of morphologies and is typically composed of one of the following: SiC, Si_3N_4, AlN, TiC, TiB_2, BN, or B_4C. Because of its stability in a wide variety of ceramic matrices, and because of its commercial availability in a variety of morphologies, SiC is the most widely used reinforcement phase. However, for applications that require long-term exposure to high temperatures, an oxide reinforcement may be a better choice. Silicon carbide is susceptible to degradation in oxygen-containing environments at temperatures above 1200 °C (2190 °F), and even when used as a reinforcement at these temperatures, it must be protected by some sort of coating system to ensure reliable service.

Particulate Reinforced CMCs. The technique of adding a distribution of particles to a ceramic or glass matrix in order to enhance its properties is well known, and a wide variety of particle-matrix systems have been explored over the years. The particle reinforcements added may either be ceramic or metallic, with their effectiveness generally determined by their chemical compatibility with the ceramic matrix and other factors such as thermal expansion and elastic mismatch. The toughening mechanisms that are activated in these types of composites may include crack deflection, crack pinning, microcracking, and transformation toughening in zirconia-containing composites; however, crack deflection is most often the primary toughening mechanism in ceramic-ceramic systems. In these cases, the degree of chemical interaction between matrix and particle is important in determining the ease of debonding at the matrix-reinforcement interface and therefore the level of toughening that can be achieved by crack deflection. In addition, for maximum toughness it is important that the reinforcement particles remain as a discrete phase within the matrix; in other words, it is important that chemical reactions between particles and matrix are not so extensive that a variety of second phases are formed at the expense of the reinforcement. The level of thermal expansion mismatch between matrix and reinforcement phases is also important in defining composite reliability. When there is a mismatch in thermal expansion, stresses form within and around the particles that can lead to spontaneous microcracking of the material. This may either enhance or degrade the toughness of the composite, as described previously. When microcracking does not occur,

Table 2 Room-temperature strength and fracture toughness of selected discontinuously reinforced ceramic-matrix composites

Composite system	Vol % reinforcement	Fracture strength		Fracture toughness		Reference
		MPa	ksi	MPa $\sqrt{m}$	ksi $\sqrt{in.}$	
Alumina matrix						
99.5% Al_2O_3	0	375	54.4	4–5	3.6–4.5	11
Al_2O_3 + ZrO_2 (p)	20	450	65.2	5–6	4.5–5.4	11
Al_2O_3 + ZrO_2 (p)	15	480–940	69.6–136.3	9	8.2	14
Al_2O_3 + TiC (p)	30	700	101.5	3.2	2.9	15
Al_2O_3 + SiC (p)	20	520	75.4	4–5	3.6–4.5	16
Al_2O_3 + SiC (pl)	30	480	69.6	7.1	6.5	17
Al_2O_3 + SiC (w)	30	700	101.5	8.7	7.9	18
Al_2O_3 + SiC (w)	20	620	89.9	7–8	6.4–7.3	13
Al_2O_3 + TiC (p) + SiC(w)	10 TiC (p) 20 SiC (w)	690	100	9.6	8.7	13
Silicon carbide matrix						
SiC	0	480	69.6	4–5	3.6–4.5	11
SiC + TiB_2 (p)	16	480	69.6	8.9	8.1	19
SiC + TiC (p)	15	680	98.6	5.1	4.6	19
Silicon nitride matrix						
Si_3N_4	0	800	116	7	6.4	12
Si_3N_4 + TiC (p)	30	800	116	4.3	3.9	15
Si_3N_4 + SiC (p)	20	600	87	7	6.4	20
Si_3N_4 + SiC (pl)	30	503	72.9	4.9	4.4	21
Si_3N_4 + SiC (w)	30	994	144	8.0	7.3	22
Si_3N_4 + SiC (w) + SiC (p)	10 SiC (p) 20 SiC (w)	550	79.7	10.5	9.5	5
Si_3N_4 + β-Si_3N_4	30	680	98.6	8.6	7.8	23
Mullite matrix						
Mullite	0	170	24.6	2	1.8	11
Mullite + SiC (p)	10	240	34.8	2.2	2.0	24
Mullite + SiC (pl)	10	163	23.6	3.0	2.7	25
Mullite + SiC (w)	10	422	61.2	3.6	3.3	26
Borosilicate glass matrix						
Borosilicate glass	0	77	11.1	1	0.9	27
Borosilicate glass + SiC (w)	20	136	19.7	5.5	5.0	27
Aluminosilicate glass matrix						
Aluminosilicate glass + SiC (w)	30	338	49.0	3.4	3.1	28

Reinforcement: p, particulate; pl, platelet; w, whisker

stress fields around the reinforcement particles may activate a crack deflection mechanism, enhancing composite toughness.

In metal particle reinforced CMCs, optimal toughness occurs when the particles can deform in the wake of the crack, bridging the crack and thereby reducing the crack opening displacement. Very high toughnesses can be achieved in these composites by this mechanism, with reports of room-temperature toughness values as high as 35 MPa$\sqrt{m}$ (31.8 ksi$\sqrt{in.}$) for an aluminum reinforced alumina (Ref 29). However, use of metal particle reinforced CMCs is severely hampered by the temperature and oxidation limits of the metal reinforcement.

Platelet Reinforced CMCs. Ceramic particles in the shape of platelets have only recently become widely available, and therefore the number of studies on the physical properties of platelet reinforced CMCs is relatively small. Work to date suggests that ceramic matrices reinforced with platelets will not be as tough as whisker reinforced CMCs, although they can be as tough, or tougher than particle reinforced CMCs (Table 2). However, composite strengths are frequently reduced by the addition of platelet reinforcements, either because of excessive microcracking in the case of larger platelets, or because they can act as strength-limiting flaws in the case of smaller platelets (Ref 5). Crack deflection and platelet crack bridging appear to be the primary toughening mechanisms in these materials (Ref 30).

Whisker Reinforced CMCs. The addition of ceramic whiskers (defined here as rod or needle-shaped single crystals) to ceramic matrices results in composites that are stronger and tougher than similar materials with particulate or platelet reinforcement (Table 2). This increase in material reliability results from the combination of superior reinforcement properties and the wide range of toughening mechanisms that are invoked by the presence of the whiskers. Silicon carbide whiskers, with a tensile strength approaching 7 GPa (1×10^6 psi) and a high elastic modulus of 550 GPa (79.8×10^6 psi), are the most commonly used whisker reinforcement, although a variety of other ceramic whiskers are also available. The presence of these whiskers can activate as many as five different toughening mechanisms, including crack bridging, whisker pullout, crack deflection, crack pinning, and microcracking. Which of these mechanisms will be activated at any given time depends on the local stress state and the orientation of the whiskers at the crack tip. However, in general each of these toughening mechanisms leads to increasing composite toughness with an increase in whisker content (Ref 31, 32).

Whisker-toughened CMCs typically retain their high toughness to temperatures of approximately 1100 °C (2010 °F). At higher temperatures, the apparent toughness will increase due in part to longer pullout and bridging lengths and the nucleation of creep cracks; however, this increase in toughness is typically offset by the onset of creep, which occurs at around 1200 °C (2190 °F). In addition, nonoxide whiskers are reactive at elevated temperatures, which affects their usefulness as structural components in severe environments. Both SiC and Si_3N_4 decompose to gaseous by-products in the presence of oxygen at temperatures as low as 1200 °C (2190 °F), and they will react with most matrix materials at high temperatures to form compounds such as SiO_2 and mullite, which will further reduce composite toughness.

In addition to toughness, the incorporation of ceramic whiskers into a ceramic matrix can result in an improvement of other material properties such as hardness and thermal conductivity. Increases in hardness translate to better wear resistance, although this can be tempered by a localized decrease in the fracture toughness at the microscale (Ref 33). Increases in thermal conductivity, combined with toughening mechanisms that resist the coalescence of thermal-shock-induced cracks into critical flaws, result in enhanced thermal shock resistance relative to the monolithic ceramic.

Because of their superior properties and their relative ease of manufacture, whisker-toughened CMCs have enjoyed more commercial success to date than any of the other ceramic-based composite systems. Alumina toughened by SiC whiskers (Al_2O_3/SiC_w) is used with considerable success as a cutting tool for nickel-base superalloys. The advantages of these CMCs in this application include: increased tool lifetimes, reduced downtime, improved surface finish, lower maintenance costs, and increased production rates. Although the Al_2O_3/SiC_w composites cost more to manufacture than the more traditional carbide tools, their increased cost is more than compensated for by their superior performance.

Hybrid DR-CMCs. Reinforcements of several morphologies and/or compositions can also be added to a ceramic matrix to produce hybrid DR-CMCs. In many cases, this can lead to an enhancement in the mechanical properties of the composite, as indicated for several systems in Table 2. However, it cannot be assumed that all material properties will benefit from this combination. For example, the combination of SiC whiskers and tetragonal ZrO_2 particles in an alumina matrix results in an increase in composite toughness relative to either a whisker-toughened alumina or a zirconia-transformation-toughened alumina. However, when this hybrid composite is exposed to an oxygen-containing atmosphere at elevated temperatures, the oxidation of the SiC whiskers is enhanced by the presence of zirconia, resulting in severe degradation in composite properties in a relatively short time (Ref 34).

Continuous Fiber Ceramic Composites

Continuous fiber ceramic composites represent the ceramic industry's best success thus far in overcoming the inherent brittleness characteristic of most ceramic materials, while retaining many of their attractive qualities. As a result, CFCCs can be produced that have the high hardness, high strength, high melting point, chemical inertness, good wear resistance, and low density common to monolithic ceramics. However, unlike monolithic ceramics, CFCCs can be designed to be strain tolerant and therefore to have a much lower probability of failing catastrophically in a high stress environment. The development of CFCCs for application at high temperatures is not without its challenges, however. Because the fibers and fiber-matrix interfacial regions of the most successful CFCCs tend to be either carbides or nitrides, they can exhibit poor stability at elevated temperatures when exposed to oxygen-containing environments. The performance of CFCCs depends critically on the integrity of these regions, and thus their degradation can be catastrophic. In addition, because they require specialized materials and processing techniques, CFCCs are expensive to produce relative to either monolithic ceramics or DR-CMCs.

Most CFCCs are currently in the precommercial/demonstration stage of development, with the best of the current generation CFCCs considered to be competitive with the best metallic materials for specific niche applications. However, once problems with poor creep resistance are resolved, oxide-oxide CFCCs are predicted to be the ultimate materials solution for many high-temperature structural applications in the military, power-generating, and transportation industries.

Composite Architecture. Continuous fiber ceramic composites consist of a continuous network of ceramic or carbon fibers in a ceramic or glass matrix. A wide variety of ceramics have potential as matrix materials for CFCCs, including SiC, Si_3N_4, $MoSi_2$, Al_2O_3, mullite, yttrium-aluminum-garnet (YAG), and spinel. However, SiC and Al_2O_3 are currently the most commonly used matrix materials. Silicon-carbide-matrix CFCCs are designed for applications where high thermal conductivity, low thermal expansion, light weight, and good corrosion and wear resistance are desired. Alumina-matrix CFCCs are better in applications where a high tolerance to salt corrosion, molten glass, or oxidation is required in combination with light weight and high thermal shock resistance. In addition, a variety of glass and glass-ceramic matrices can be used in applications that do not require structural stability above the softening temperature of the glass (for example, ~600 °C, or 1100 °F, for a borosilicate glass or ~1150 °C, or 2100 °F, for a high silica glass). For such applications, the relative ease of processing glass-matrix CFCCs can result in a significant cost savings.

The fiber reinforcement within a CFCC is typically either SiC or carbon, although a number of other oxide and nonoxide fibers are currently under development and several are commercially available. The properties of several ceramic- and carbon-base fibers can be found in Tables 3 and 4. In order to act as a reinforcement, the fibers must have the following characteristics: high strength, environmental stability (particularly in oxygen-containing environments), creep resistance, and a coefficient of thermal expansion that is close to that of the matrix. In addition, the ideal fibers must be processible with a small enough diameter to allow weaving, and their production should be relatively inexpensive. Currently, it is oxidation and creep resistance that are the limiting factors for most fiber reinforcement. In the absence of oxygen, carbon is the choice fiber for most applications. However, carbon fibers can suffer from oxidation at temperatures as low as 350 °C (660 °F). Silicon carbide fibers have good strength up to 1000 °C (1832 °F), but begin to creep at higher temperatures. In addition, all SiC fibers will suffer from oxidation at temperatures greater than 1200 °C (2190 °F) and have a maximum-use temperature of not more than 1400 °C (2550 °F). Current-generation oxide fibers, such as Al_2O_3, are polycrystalline materials with silica at their grain boundaries. As a result, alumina-base fibers begin to creep at temperatures as low as 900 °C (1650 °F) and retain almost no strength at temperatures above 1150 °C (2100 °F). Thus, although alumina and other oxide fibers have considerable potential as CFCC reinforcement because of their oxidative stability, their poor high-temperature mechanical properties currently limit their usefulness. The application of single-crystal oxide fibers, currently under development, may be the solution to this problem of high-temperature stability.

The fibers within a CFCC can be oriented in a variety of ways, depending on the performance requirements of the specific application. A unidirectional (0°) alignment of fibers results in the highest level of property translation efficiency, but at the expense of intralaminar and interlaminar strength. A two-dimensional, planar interlaced fiber architecture results in better intralaminar properties; however, the interlaminar strength is limited by the properties of the matrix due to the lack of through-thickness reinforcement. A three-dimensional, integrated, fiber architecture results in enhanced interlaminar properties by providing reinforcement in the through-thickness direction. The type of fiber architecture that is best suited for a particular application will depend on the performance requirements of that application.

Mechanical Behavior. The mechanical behavior of a CFCC is determined to a large degree by three factors: the strength of the reinforcing fibers, the characteristics of the fiber-matrix interface, and the residual stress present in the composite due to thermal expansion mismatch between fibers and matrix. High-strength fibers are important because once a matrix crack is initiated and extended, load is transferred from the matrix to the fibers in the wake of the crack. As a result, the ultimate load-bearing capability of the composite is determined by the load-bearing characteristics of the fibers. The level of toughening imparted by the fibers depends on how well the interface between matrix and fibers is engineered. In an ideal composite, the interface will be strong enough to transfer load from the matrix to the fiber, yet weak enough to allow debonding of the fiber in the path of a crack. Actual composite toughening then occurs by the mechanisms of crack deflection, crack bridging, and fiber pullout when the fibers finally do fail, as shown in Fig. 2. In addition to the chemical bonding at the interface, residual stresses from thermal expansion mismatch between the matrix and fibers can contribute to the mechanical strength of the fiber-matrix interface and thus influence composite toughness.

The ways in which fiber-matrix interface strength influences the toughness of a CFCC is illustrated by the four stress-strain curves in Fig. 3. The first curve, labeled BSG, is that of an unreinforced glass in which the stress-strain behavior is purely elastic and failure is brittle. Curve A illustrates the stress-strain behavior of a fiber reinforced glass with a strong fiber matrix interface. Because the elastic modulus of the fibers is higher than that of the matrix, some strengthening of the composite is observed. However, because the fiber-matrix interface does not allow for debonding in the presence of a matrix crack, the potential toughening mechanisms of crack deflection and crack bridging are not activated, and both matrix and fibers fail in a brittle manner. The CFCC represented by curve B has a fiber-matrix interface that is engineered such that debonding occurs as the crack passes by the fiber, leaving the fiber intact in the wake of the crack to continue to bear load and to toughen the composite by crack bridging. Curve C represents the stress-strain behavior of a CFCC in which fiber pullout has been added as a toughening mechanism, in addition to crack deflection and crack bridging. Thus, through the addition of a continuous network of strong fibers, and well-engineered fiber-matrix inter-

Table 3 Physical properties of selected commercially available ceramic fibers

Trade name	Composition, wt%	Fiber diameter, μm	Density, g/cm^3	Strength, GPa	Strength, ksi	Modulus, GPa	Modulus, 10^6 psi	Strain to failure, %
α-Al_2O_3 fiber								
Almax	99.9% Al_2O_3	10	3.60	1.0	145	344	49.9	0.30
Nextel-610	99% Al_2O_3	10–12	3.75	1.9	275.5	370	53.7	0.5
Nextel-440	70% Al_2O_3 28% SiO_2 2% B_2O_3	10–12	3.05	2.1	304.5	190	27.6	1.11
SiC fiber								
Nicalon	56.6% Si 31.7% C 11.7% O	14	2.55	2.0	290	190	29.6	1.05
Hi-Nicalon	62.4% Si 37.1% C 0.5% O	14	2.74	2.6	377	263	38.1	1.0
Tyranno Lox-M	54% Si 31.6% C 12.4% O	8.5	2.37	2.5	362.5	180	26.1	1.4
Tyranno Lox-E	54.8% Si 37.5% C 5.8% O 1.9% Ti	11	2.39	2.9	420.5	199	28.8	1.45
Tyranno ZMI	56.6% Si 34.8% C 7.6% O 1.0% Zr	11	2.48	3.4	493	200	29.0	1.7
Tyranno ZE	58.6% Si 38.4% C 1.7% O 1.0% Zr	11	2.55	3.5	507	233	35.8	1.5

Source: Ref 35

Table 4 Properties of selected commercially available polyacrylonitrile-based carbon fibers

Trade name	Grade	Density, g/cm^3	Stiffness, GPa	Stiffness, 10^6 psi	Strength, GPa	Strength, ksi	Strain at failure, (%)
Celion	G30	1.78	234	33.9	3.8	551	1.6
	G40	1.77	300	43.5	5.0	725	1.7
	G50	1.78	358	51.9	2.5	362.5	0.7
Magnamite	AS4	1.8	235	34.1	3.8	551	1.5
	IM6	1.73	276	40.0	4.4	638	1.5
	HMU	1.84	380	55.1	2.8	406	0.7
Thornel	T-650/35	1.77	241	34.9	4.6	671.6	1.8
	T-650/42	1.78	290	42.0	5.0	725	1.7
	T-50	1.81	390	56.5	2.4	348	0.7

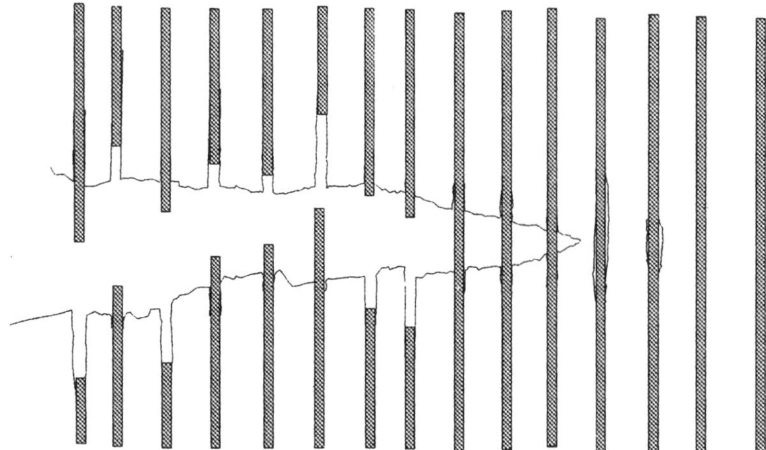

Fig. 2 Mechanisms of fiber debonding, crack bridging, and fiber pullout as a result of crack propagation within a continuous fiber ceramic composite. Source: Ref 35

faces, a normally brittle material can be designed to have improved tolerance to strain and reduced probability of catastrophic failure. The mechanics of fracture initiation and propagation is detailed and modeled in "Fracture Analysis of Fiber-Reinforced Ceramic-Matrix Composites" in this Volume.

Interface bonding is controlled either by selecting fiber and matrix materials that are thermodynamically stable at both the processing and the service temperatures, or by applying coatings that act as diffusion barriers and therefore prevent a strong bond between fiber and matrix. Currently, carbon and boron nitride are the coating materials most often used to control the interfacial properties of the CFCC because of their weak crystallographic orientations, which can preferentially delaminate. These coatings also serve to prevent mechanical damage to the fibers during processing. However, both carbon and boron nitride are susceptible to environmental degradation at elevated temperatures. As a result, a variety of alternative multilayer and oxide-base coatings are in the design/feasibility stage.

Mechanical and Physical Properties. In CFCCs, the principal driving force in adding a continuous distribution of fibers is to mitigate against the inherent brittleness of the ceramic matrix. Enhancement of other physical properties, such as strength, hardness, or conductivity, may be the result of the addition of reinforcement to the CFCC, but it is rarely the objective of their production. Table 5 provides a list of the room-temperature mechanical properties of several commercially available CFCCs, and Table 6 lists the thermal properties of the same suite of composites.

Limitations to Current Technology. Although ceramic materials are noted for their high-temperature stability, characteristics of a polycrystalline ceramic microstructure make the current generation of materials susceptible to deformation and creep at temperatures as low as 900 °C (1650 °F). This is true both for the matrices and for the fibers that are used to produce CFCCs. This susceptibility results from the presence of grain boundaries and the tendency for relatively low-melting phases, which may be introduced either intentionally or unintentionally during processing, to reside there. When these grain-boundary phases begin to soften, the grains can slide relative to one another, resulting in the initiation of creep cracks and the deformation of the bulk material at temperatures much lower than the softening point of the matrix. Because of grain-boundary creep, current generation oxide fibers have a maximum-use temperature of approximately 1000 °C (1830 °F), rendering them unsuitable for many CFCC applications. Depending on the amount of oxygen present in the material, SiC fibers can also exhibit significant creep in the same temperature range. As a result, poor fiber stability is considered one of the major barriers to the high-temperature application of CFCCs, and research emphasis is now focusing on the potential of single-crystal oxide fibers as a possible reinforcement material.

In addition to high-temperature deformation, environmental susceptibility is a problem for many of the nonoxide matrix and reinforcement materials used in CFCCs. Both SiC and Si_3N_4 form a SiO_2 surface layer upon exposure to an oxidizing environment, which is protective to temperatures approaching 1200 °C (2190 °F). However, decomposition reactions at higher temperatures render the oxide coating nonprotective, and volatilization of the material can be problematic. This high-temperature decomposition occurs even in nonoxide fibers embedded within the composite matrix. In the case of fibers, cracks in the matrix can expose the reinforcement to an oxygen-containing environment. Alternatively, fast diffusion of oxygen along grain boundaries, or along interfaces, can cause internal volatilization of the reinforcement, resulting in cavitation, bloating, and/or blistering. Finally, oxidation of the protective boron nitride or carbon coating typically applied to fibers can result in the formation of a strong interfacial bond that will embrittle the composite.

As a result of these limitations, it appears that oxide-oxide CFCCs, which include single-crystal reinforcement, have the highest potential for

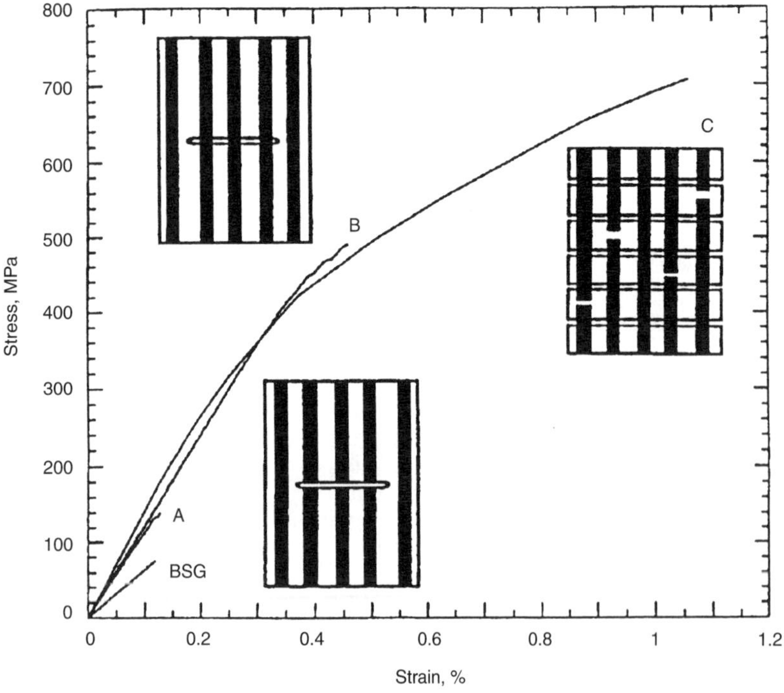

Fig. 3 Stress-strain curves for (a) unreinforced glass (BSG), fiber reinforced glass with a strong fiber matrix interface, (b) fiber reinforced glass with a relatively weak fiber matrix interface in which toughening by fiber debonding and bridging can occur, and (c) fiber reinforced glass in which the toughening mechanisms of debonding, bridging, and pullout are active. Source: Ref 36

Table 5 Room-temperature mechanical properties of several commercially available CFCCs

Fiber matrix system	Fiber architecture	Volume fraction fibers, %	Tensile strength				Tensile modulus				Compressive strength				Compressive modulus				Shear strength	
			x-y		z		x-y		z		x-y		z		x-y		z			
			MPa	ksi	MPa	ksi	GPa	10^6 psi	GPa	10^6 psi	MPa	ksi	MPa	ksi	GPa	10^6 psi	GPa	10^6 psi	MPa	ksi
C/SiC	3D	...	69	10	48	7	83	12	48	6.9	503	72.9	73	10.6	110	16	16	2.3	103	14.9
SiC/Al_2O_3	2D	37.5	246	35.7	...	...	144	21	...	...	550	79.7	...	...	84	12.2	...	...	63	9.1
SiC/SiC	2D	31.2	215	31.2	...	...	140	20.3	...	...	502	72.8	...	...	145	21	...	...	30	4.3

3D, three-directional; 2D, two-directional. Source: Ref 36

structural applications at temperatures greater than 1400 °C (2550 °F). However, issues with grain-boundary creep of the matrix and thermal shock resistance have yet to be resolved, and thus it will be several years before these materials can be developed and commercialized.

Carbon-Carbon Composites

A number of advantages—including stable mechanical properties to temperatures greater than 2000 °C (3630 °F), high strength-to-weight ratio, high thermal conductivity, good thermal shock resistance, good abrasion resistance, and good corrosion resistance—make C-C composites a candidate material for virtually any application requiring structural integrity at very high temperature. In addition, C-C composites are biocompatible, and this characteristic, combined with the ability to tailor the directional properties of these materials, makes them attractive for use in various load-bearing prosthetic devices. However, C-C composites have at least two drawbacks that prevent their widespread application. The first is that C-C composites are extremely susceptible to degradation by oxidation at temperatures as low as 350 °C (660 °F). As a result, the long-term use of these materials as structural components at high temperature in oxygen-containing environments is impossible without some form of protective coating. The second drawback is that production costs can be quite high, making C-C composites a prohibitively expensive solution for many applications. Because of these drawbacks, use of C-C composites to date has been limited primarily to military and space applications. However, C-C composites have also been successfully utilized as commercial aircraft brakes, where their superior performance outweighs their increased costs.

Carbon-carbon Composite Architecture. Carbon-carbon composites are composed of carbon fibers embedded in a carbon matrix. The microstructural characteristics, and therefore the physical properties, of the carbon matrix can vary widely depending on the starting materials used and methods of composite fabrication. For example, the matrix carbon can be approximately isotropic, composed of small, randomly oriented crystallites of poorly graphitic or turbostratic carbon. The matrix can also be strongly anisotropic, consisting of relatively large crystallites of highly graphitized carbon. More often, however, the matrix microstructure is a combination of these two extremes and includes some porosity and microcracking. The level of porosity is determined by the methods of manufacture, whereas the matrix microcracking most often results from the strong anisotropy of carbon in thermal expansion.

The carbon fibers within a C-C composite are most often continuous, with a variety of orientations. Available fiber architectures include unidirectional, bidirectional (two-dimensional) laminates, three-directional (three-dimensional) orthogonal weaves, or multidirectional weaves and braids. The fiber architecture selected depends on the properties desired in the composite. Multidirectional C-C composites containing reinforcing fibers in three or more directions are advantageous because their fiber architecture can be designed to accommodate the specific requirements of the final component. Unidirectionally reinforced C-C composites, on the other hand, tend to have very high on-axis strength and fracture toughness, but at the expense of their off-axis mechanical properties. In addition to fiber architecture, C-C performance also depends on the physical properties of the fibers themselves, as well as on the characteristics of the interface between fibers and matrix. The carbon fibers used in C-C composites range from the isotropic variety, with low elastic moduli and modest strengths, to highly oriented, high-performance fibers, with high elastic moduli and strengths between 3 and 5 GPa (0.4 and 0.7 × 10^6 psi). Most of these fibers are derived from polyacrylonitrile (PAN) resin, although petroleum pitch or rayon may also be used as fiber precursors. Table 4 lists the mechanical properties of several commercially available PAN-based carbon fibers.

In C-C composites, the strain-to-failure of the carbon matrix is typically much lower than that of the reinforcing fibers, and as noted earlier the matrix is frequently microcracked as a result of thermal expansion mismatch stresses created during processing. As a result, it is frequently the characteristics of the interfacial bonding between matrix and fiber that govern the mechanical properties of the C-C composite. When the bonding between fibers and matrix is strong, cracks that form in the matrix are propagated across the fiber-matrix interface, resulting in fiber failure. Brittle failure of the composite results, with the ultimate strength of the composite governed by the strain-to-failure of the matrix, as illustrated in the stress-strain curve of Fig. 4(a). Weak interfaces between fibers and matrix, on the other hand, allow matrix cracking to occur without crack propagation through the fibers. Intact fibers bridge the matrix cracks and maintain load-bearing capability until increasing load finally initiates fiber fracture and failure. This process results in a much tougher composite, as illustrated in the stress-strain curve of Fig. 4(b). A more complete discussion of the effect of interfacial strength on the mechanical properties of C-C composites can be found in the work of Fitzer and Hüttner (Ref 38) and Thomas and Walker (Ref 39).

Although top mechanical performance depends on weak fiber-matrix interfaces, other physical properties are enhanced by strong fiber-matrix interfaces. As a result, fiber treatments and fabrication methods are varied to tailor the interfacial characteristics of the C-C composite to match the requirements of the specific application (Ref 40, 41). A number of theoretical models are available to predict composite behavior based on variables such as fiber volume fraction, fiber properties, matrix properties, porosity, degree of microcracking, and so forth (Ref 42–48).

Thermal and Mechanical Properties. Fiber architecture, fiber type, matrix precursor, and processing methodology will all contribute to determine the physical properties of C-C composites. As a result of the large number of variables involved, C-C composites can be produced with a wide range of properties. Nonetheless, all C-C composites have the following basic char-

Table 6 Thermal properties of selected commercially available CFCCs

Fiber matrix system	Fiber architecture	Volume fraction fibers, %	Thermal expansion (a), 10^{-6}/K		Thermal diffusivity(b), 10^{-6} m^2/s		Thermal conductivity(b), 10^2 W/m · K		Specific heat(b), J/kg · K
			x-y	z	x-y	z	x-y	z	
C-SiC	3D	...	4.27	3.10	6.4	5.8	11.6	10.5	1351
SiC-Al_2O_3	2D	37.5	5.8	...	...	...	5.7	...	...
SiC-SiC	2D	35	5.2	...	1.7	...	...	...	1500

3D, three-directional; 2D, two-directional. (a) From 20–1500 °C (68–2730 °F). (b) Measured at 1000 °C (1830 °F). Source: Ref 37

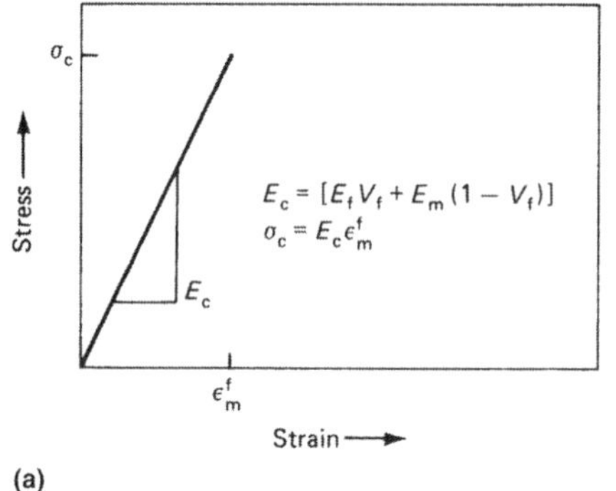

(a)

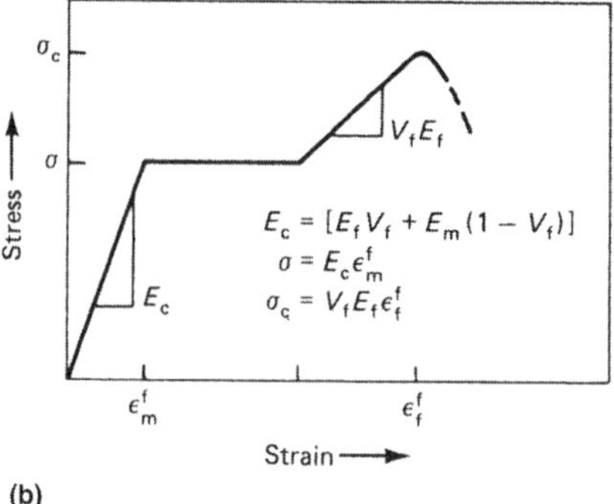

(b)

Fig. 4 Stress-strain curves for C-C composites. (a) Strong bonding between fibers and matrix and therefore little toughening of the composite. (b) Well-engineered fiber matrix interface in which significant toughening occurs

Table 7 Room-temperature mechanical properties of graphite and C-C composites

Material	Elastic modulus		Tensile strength		Compressive strength		Fracture energy, kJ/m^2
	GPa	10^6 psi	MPa	ksi	MPa	ksi	
Graphite	10–15	1.46–2.17	40–60	5.8–8.7	110–200	16–29	0.01
Unidirectional C-C composite	120–150	17.4–21.7	600–700	87–101	500–800	72.5–116	1.4–2.0
Three-directional C-C composite	40–100	5.8–14.5	200–350	29–50.7	150–200	21.7–29	5–10

Source: Ref 49

acteristics in common: low thermal expansion that increases with temperature, good strength that increases with temperature in inert environments, and thermal conductivity that decreases with temperature. To illustrate the influence of carbon fibers and their architecture on the properties of the composite, Table 7 compares the room-temperature mechanical properties of a fine-grained monolithic graphite with unidirectional and three-directional C-C composites (Ref 49). Tables 8 and 9 list the mechanical and thermal properties of several C-C composites with different fiber architectures (Ref 50).

A comparison of the data in Table 7 clearly indicates the benefits of adding carbon fibers to the carbon matrix. All room-temperature mechanical properties are improved in the composites to a level that depends on fiber architecture. Unidirectional fibers provide dramatic increases in the strength of the material in the principal fiber direction. The addition of a three-dimensional network of fibers results in more modest increases in room-temperature strength, but a tremendous increase in fracture toughness. Tables 8 and 9 illustrate the directional nature of the mechanical and thermal properties. Room-temperature mechanical properties are many times higher when measured in the principal axis directions of both the unidirectional and fabric laminate composites. The woven orthogonal (three-dimensional) composite, on the other hand, has more isotropic mechanical properties.

Generally, the elastic modulus that is measured in the principal fiber direction of C-C composites reflects the fiber modulus according to the law of mixtures. Strength utilization of the fibers is typically between 25 and 50%, depending on how the composite is processed (Ref 50). However, as is common with fiber reinforced composites, the shear properties of the C-C composites tend to be relatively low and therefore will usually have a strong influence on materials selection and design. The same is true for the tensile properties of one- and two-dimensional composites in directions normal to the principal fiber directions. These low properties are the direct result of the weak fiber-matrix interfaces that are designed to prevent composite brittleness and low fracture strengths parallel to the fiber directions.

Carbon-carbon composites are unique in that their mechanical properties do not degrade with increasing temperature until 2200 °C (3990 °F). Increases in the tensile strength and decreases in the elastic modulus of the composites (measured in the principal fiber directions) as the temperature increases are typical of carbon fibers (Ref 51). However, it is the properties of the matrix, and of the matrix-fiber interface, that dictate the effect of temperature on the shear, cross-fiber tensile, and compressive strengths of the composites (Ref 50). Generally, these properties also improve with increase in temperature, a phenomenon that is attributed to the closing of matrix microcracks as the temperature is increased. Creep behavior has received only minimal attention to date; however, the steady-state creep rates of most C-C composites are predicted to be at least four orders of magnitude lower than that of most technical grade ceramics (Ref 52).

As with the mechanical properties in C-C composites, the bulk thermal expansion and thermal conductivity can be highly anisotropic in the unidirectional composite (reflecting the large anisotropy in these properties in single-crystal graphite), but approximately isotropic in the three-dimensional composite (Table 9). The thermal expansion of C-C composites tends to increase with increasing temperature, although the value remains low relative to other ionic and covalently bonded materials. The thermal conductivity, on the other hand, tends to decrease with increasing temperature. The combination of good strength, relatively high thermal conductivity, and low thermal expansion makes C-C composites very resistant to thermal shock.

Oxidation Resistance. The retention of mechanical properties to high temperature, combined with a resistance to damage by thermal shock, makes C-C composites an ideal candidate for many high-temperature structural applications. However, the lack of reliable oxidation protection for these materials has been, and continues to be, a serious limitation to their widespread application.

Depending on its crystal structure, carbon can become susceptible to oxidation at temperatures as low as 350 °C (660 °F), especially when the environment contains atomic oxygen. This susceptibility to oxidation increases with increase in temperature until approximately 800 °C (1470 °F), where the rate of oxidation is limited only by the diffusion rate of oxygen to the carbon surface. Because the oxides of carbon are gaseous, oxidation results in significant material loss and serious degradation in material performance. As a result, some form of oxidation protection is essential to the long-term reliable use of C-C composites at all but the lowest temperatures.

Table 8 Room-temperature mechanical properties of selected C-C composites

Construction	Fiber volume fraction			Tensile strength				Tensile elastic modulus				Compressive strength				Compressive elastic modulus			
				x		z		x		z		x		z		x		z	
	x	y	z	MPa	ksi	MPa	ksi	GPa	10^6 psi	GPa	10^6psi	MPa	ksi	MPa	ksi	GPa	10^6 psi	GPa	10^6 psi
Unidirectional (one-dimensional)	0.65	0	0	1000	145	2.0	0.29	260	37.7	3.4	0.5	620	89.9	...	...	250	36.2	...	...
Fabric laminate (two-dimensional)	0.31	0.30	0	350	50.7	5.0	0.72	115	16.7	4.1	1.59	150	21.7	...	...	100	14.5	...	...
Woven orthogonal (three-dimensional)	0.13	0.13	0.21	170	24.6	300	43.5	55	7.97	96	13.9	...	...	140	20.3	...	...	90	13.0

Source: Ref 50

Table 9 Thermal properties of selected C-C composites

Construction	Fiber volume fraction			Coefficient of thermal expansion(a), 10^{-6}/K		Thermal conductivity(b), W/m · K	
	x	y	z	x	z	x	z
Unidirectional (one-dimensional)	0.65	0	0	1.1	10.1	125	10
Fabric laminate (two-dimensional)	0.31	0.30	0	1.3	6.1	95	4
Woven orthogonal (three-dimensional)	0.13	0.13	0.21	1.3	1.3	57	80

(a) Thermal expansion measured from room temperature to 1650 °C (3000 °F). (b) Thermal conductivity measured at 800 °C (1470 °F). Source: Ref 50

External coatings are the most direct, and to date the most effective, method of oxidation protection for these materials. However, the thermal expansion characteristics of C-C composites make establishing and maintaining coherent and adherent coatings extremely difficult. In addition, coating defects are unavoidable with current coating technology, and thus the addition of some mechanism for coating self-healing and/or internal oxidation protection is an absolute necessity for these materials.

The primary coating candidate for oxidation protection at temperatures below 1200 °C (2190 °F) is SiC, because it forms a surface layer of SiO_2 that is highly oxidation resistant, it is chemically compatible with carbon, and it has a relatively low coefficient of thermal expansion. The temperature limitation for SiC in oxidizing environments results from a reaction between SiC and SiO_2 that renders the SiO_2 nonprotective, and this leads to the rapid erosion of the SiC coating (Ref 53). Coatings of Si_3N_4 can also be used, but have essentially the same temperature limitations as SiC. Silicon carbide and Si_3N_4 are usually applied to the C-C composite surface in combination with a boron-containing inner coating to protect the carbon from the inevitable formation of coating cracks. Oxidation of this inner coating through the cracks results in the formation of a sealant glass that flows into and closes the cracks (Ref 54) and thus prevents the oxidation of the underlying composite.

Oxidation protection for C-C composites above ~1500 °C (2730 °F) requires the use of either a noble metal or a highly refractory ceramic coating as a primary oxygen barrier. The most attractive noble metal for carbon protection at high temperatures is iridium, which has a melting point of 2440 °C (4425 °F). In addition, iridium has a very low oxygen permeability to 2100 °C (3810 °F), is nonreactive with carbon below 2280 °C (4135 °F), and is an effective carbon diffusion barrier (Ref 55). However, there are also disadvantages to iridium, including a susceptibility to erosion by volatile oxide formation, a lack of adherence to carbon, and a thermal expansion incompatibility with C-C composites. The use of refractory ceramic coatings for high-temperature oxidation protection, on the other hand, is limited by the high oxygen permeabilities of the refractory oxides. All of the refractory carbides, nitrides, borides, and silicides oxidize rapidly at temperatures above 1750 °C (3180 °F), and most oxidize at significantly lower temperatures. As a result, refractory ceramic coatings cannot provide long-term oxidation protection to C-C composites without the identification of effective additives that can act as oxygen barriers. Problems such as chemical compatibility with carbon at high temperature and thermal expansion mismatch will also have to be solved.

REFERENCES

1. Science and Technology of Zirconia, *Advances in Ceramics,* Vol 3, A.H. Heuer and L.W. Hobbs, Ed., American Ceramic Society, 1981
2. Science and Technology of Zirconia II, *Advances in Ceramics,* Vol 12, N. Claussen, M. Rühle, and A.H. Heuer, Ed., American Ceramic Society, 1984
3. Science and Technology of Zirconia III, *Advances in Ceramics,* Vol 24, S. Somiya, N. Yamamoto, and H. Yanagida, Ed., American Ceramic Society, 1988
4. R. Warren and V.K. Sarin, Particulate Ceramic-Matrix Composites, *Ceramic Matrix Composites,* R. Warren, Ed., Chapman and Hall, 1992, 146–166
5. T.N. Tiegs, Structural and Physical Properties of Ceramic Matrix Composites, *Handbook on Discontinuously Reinforced Ceramic Matrix Composites*, K.J. Bowman, S.K. El-Rahaiby, and J.B. Wachtman, Jr., Ed., Purdue University and American Ceramic Society, 1995, p 225–273
6. Company literature from Ceradyne, Inc., Costa Mesa, CA, July 2000
7. R.N. Katz and K.J. Bowman, Introduction and Overview, *Handbook on Discontinuously Reinforced Ceramic Matrix Composites*, K.J. Bowman, S.K. El-Rahaiby, and J.B. Wachtman, Jr., Ed., Purdue University, West and American Ceramic Society, 1995, p 1–30
8. K.T. Faber and A.G. Evans, Crack Deflection Processes I. Theory, *Acta Metall.*, Vol 31, 1983, p 565–576
9. K.T. Faber and A.G. Evans, Crack Deflection Processes II. Experiment, *Acta Metall.*, Vol 31, 1983, p 577–584
10. R. Raj, Fundamental Research in Structural Ceramics for Service near 2000 °C, *J. Am. Ceram. Soc.*, Vol 76, 1993, p 2147–2174
11. Material Properties Standard 2000, CoorsTek, Golden, CO, July 2000
12. Silicon Nitride Data Sheet, Rauschert Industries, Inc., Madisonville, TN, July 2000
13. Crystaloy Ceramic Composites Data Sheet, Industrial Ceramic Technology, Inc., Ann Arbor, MI, July 2000
14. D.W. Shin, K.K. Orr, and H. Schubert, *J. Am. Ceram. Soc.*, Vol 73, 1990, p 1181
15. J.G. Baldoni and S.T. Buljan, Ceramics for Machining, *Am. Ceram. Soc. Bull.*, Vol 67, 1988, p 381–387
16. K. Niihara, A. Nakahira, T. Uchiyama, and T. Hirai, High-Temperature Mechanical Properties of Al_2O_3-SiC Composites, *Fracture Mechanics of Ceramics,* Vol 7, Plenum Press, 1986, p 103–116
17. Y. Chou and D.J. Green, Silicon Carbide Platelet/Alumina Composites: II., Mechanical Properties, *J. Am. Ceram. Soc.,* Vol 76, 1993, 1452–1458
18. P.F. Becher, T.N. Tiegs, J.C. Ogle, and W.H. Warwick, Toughening of Ceramics by Whisker Reinforcement, *Fracture Mechanics of Ceramics,* Vol 7, Plenum Press, 1986, p 61–73
19. G.C. Wei and P.F. Becher, Improvements in Mechanical Properties in SiC by the Addition of TiC Particles, *J. Am. Ceram. Soc.,* Vol 76, 1984, p 571–574
20. F.F. Lange, Effect of Microstructure on Strength of Si_3N_4-SiC Composite System, *J. Am. Ceram. Soc.,* Vol 56, 1973, p 445–450
21. G. Pezzoti, Si_3N_4/SiC Platelet Composite without Sintering Aids: A Candidate for Gas Turbine Engines, *J. Am. Ceram. Soc.,* Vol 76, 1993, p 1313–1320
22. S.T. Buljan, J.G. Buldoni, M.L. Huckabee, J. Neil, and J. Hefter, "Development of Ceramic Matrix Composites for Application in Technology for Advanced Engines Program," ORNL/Sub/85-22011/2, Oak Ridge National Laboratory, 1992
23. J. Homeny and L.J. Neergard, Mechanical Properties of β-Si_3N_4-Whiskers/ Si_3N_4-Matrix Composites, *J. Am. Ceram. Soc.,* Vol 73, 1990, p 3493–3496
24. R. Warren and V.K. Sarin, Particulate Ceramic-Matrix Composites, *Ceramic Matrix Composites,* R. Warren, Ed., Chapman and Hall, 1992, p 146–166
25. C. Nischik, M.M. Seibold, N.A. Travitzky, and N. Claussen, Effect of Processing on Mechanical Properties of Platelet-Reinforced Mullite Composites, *J. Am. Ceram. Soc.,* Vol 74, 1991, p 2464–2468
26. T.N. Tiegs, P.F. Becher, and P. Angelini, Microstructures and Properties of SiC Whisker Reinforced Mullite Composites, *Mullite and Mullite Matrix Composites*, Vol 6, Ceramic Transactions, American Ceramic Society, 1990, p 463–472
27. F.D. Gac, J.J. Petrovic, J.V. Milevski, and P.D. Shalek, *Ceram. Eng. Sci. Proc.,* Vol 7, 1986, p 978–982
28. K.P. Gadjaree and K. Chyung, Silicon Carbide Whisker Reinforced Glass and Glass-Ceramic Composites, *Am. Ceram. Soc. Bull.,* Vol 65, 1986, p 370–376
29. B.D. Flinn, C.S. Lo, F.W. Zok, and A.G. Evans, Fracture Resistance Characteristics

of a Metal-Toughened Ceramic, *J. Am. Ceram. Soc.,* Vol 76, 1993, p 369–375
30. Y.S. Chou and D.J. Green, Silicon Carbide Platelet/Alumina Composites: III., Toughening Mechanisms, *J. Am. Ceram. Soc.,* Vol 76, 1993, p 1985–1992
31. P.F. Becher, C.H, Hsueh, P. Angelini, and T.N. Tiegs, Toughening Behavior of Whisker-Reinforced Ceramic Matrix Composites, *J. Am. Ceram. Soc.,* Vol 71, 1988, p 1050–1061
32. M. Bengisu and O.T. Inal, Whisker Toughening of Ceramics: Toughening Mechanisms, Fabrication, and Composite Properties, *Ann. Rev. Mater. Sci.,* Vol 24, 1983, p 83–124
33. C.P. Dogan and J.A. Hawk, Influence of Whisker Toughening and Microstructure on the Wear Behavior of Si_3N_4- and Al_2O_3-Matrix Composites Reinforced with SiC, *J. Mat. Sci.,* Vol 35, 2000, p 5793–5807
34. M. Backhaus-Ricoult, Oxidation Behavior of SiC Whisker Reinforced Alumina Zirconia Composites, *J. Am. Ceram. Soc.,*
35. A.R. Bunsell, M-H Berger, and A. Kelly, Fine Ceramic Fibers, *Fine Ceramic Fibers*, A.R. Bunsell and M-H Berger, Ed., Marcel-Dekker, 1999, p 1–62
36. P.G. Karandi-Kar, T.W. Chou, and A. Parvizi-Majidi, Mechanical Properties, *Handbook on Continuous Fiber Reinforced Ceramic Matrix Composites,* R.L. Lehman, S.K. El-Rahiaby, and J.B. Wachtman, Ed., Purdue University and American Ceramic Society, 1996, p 62–95
37. Material Data Sheets, Honeywell Advanced Composites, July 2000
38. E. Fitzer and W. Hüttner, Structure and Strength of Carbon/Carbon Composites, *J. Phys. D., Appl. Phys.*, Vol 14, 1981, p 347
39. C.R. Thomas and E.J. Walker, Carbon-Carbon Composites as High Strength Refractories, *High Temp. High Press.*, Vol 10, 1979, p 79
40. E. Fitzer, K.H. Geigl, and W. Hüttner, *Carbon,* Vol 18, 1980, p 265
41. P.K. Jain, O.P. Bahl, and L.M. Manocha, *SAMPE Q.*, Vol 23, 1992, p 43
42. J.J. Kibler, *Carbon-Carbon Materials and Composites*, J.D. Buckley and D.D. Edie, Noyes, 1993, p 169–195
43. B.W. Rosen and C. Zweben, *CR-2057,* National Aeronautic Space Administration, 1972
44. B.W. Rosen, *Fiber Composite Materials*, ASM, 1965
45. Z. Hashin, *J. Appl. Mech.,* Vol 46, 1979, p 543–550
46. R.M. Jones, *Mechanics of Composite Materials*, McGraw-Hill, 1975
47. B.W. Rosen, S.N. Chatterjee, and J.J. Kibler, *Composite Materials: Testing and Design, STP 617*, ASTM, 1977, p 243–257
48. N.J. Pagano and G.P. Tandon, *Comp. Sci. Technol.,* Vol 31, 1988, p 273–293
49. T. Windhorst and G. Blount, Carbon-Carbon Composites: A Summary of Recent Developments and Applications, *Mater. & Des.,* Vol 18, 1997, p 11–15
50. J.E. Sheehan, K.W. Buesking, and B.J. Sullivan, Carbon-Carbon Composites, *Ann. Rev. Mater. Sci.,* Vol 24, 1994, p 19–44
51. C.R. Rowe and D.L. Lowe, *Carbon,* Vol 13, 1983, p 170–171
52. M.S. Dresselhaus, G. Dresselhaus, K. Sugihara, and I.L. Spain, *Graphite Fibers and Filaments*, Springer-Verlag, 1988, p 382
53. G.H. Schiroky, J.L. Kaae, and J.E. Sheehan, "High Temperature Oxidation of CVD Silicon Carbide," presented at the 87th Annual Meeting, American Ceramic Society, May 1985
54. J.R. Strife and J.E. Sheehan, *Am. Ceram. Soc. Bull.,* Vol 67, 1988, p 368–374
55. "High Temperature Oxidation Resistant Coatings," ISBM 0-309-01769-6, National Academy of Sciences and Engineering, 1970

SELECTED REFERENCES

- K.J. Bowman, S.K. El-Rahaiby, and J.B. Wachtman Jr., Ed., *Handbook on Discontinuously Reinforced Ceramic Matrix Composites*, Purdue University and American Ceramic Society, 1995
- A.R. Bunsell, Ed., *Fibre Reinforcements for Composite Materials*, Elsevier, Amsterdam, 1988
- A.R. Bunsell and M-H Berger, Ed., *Fine Ceramic Fibers*, Marcel-Dekker, 1999
- K.K. Chawla, *Ceramic Matrix Composites*, Chapman & Hall, London, 1993
- R.R. Lehman, S.K. El-Rahaiby, and J.B. Wachtman Jr., Ed., *Handbook on Continuous Fiber-Reinforced Ceramic Matrix Composites*, Purdue University and American Ceramic Society, 1995
- G. Savage, *Carbon-Carbon Composites*, Chapman & Hall, London, 1993

Product Reliability, Maintainability, and Repair

Chairpersons: Michael J. Hoke, Abaris Training Resources, Inc.
Richard B. Heslehurst, Australian Defence Force Academy

Introduction to Product Reliability, Maintainability, and Repair

Michael J. Hoke, Abaris Training Inc.
Rikard B. Heslehurst, Australian Defence Force Academy

THE RANGE OF APPLICATIONS of advanced composite structures is very broad. Operators of equipment that use structural composites must be well aware of the in-service implications with respect to maintenance, reliability, and repairs. These implications require a fresh approach to in-service operations and maintenance activities. Knowledge of the composite system is essential to provide adequate and effective in-service support of composite structures.

Facilitating Effective Repair of Composite Structures

This Section covers a range of topics that first include the general issues for reliability, maintenance, and repair of composite structures. Specific structural applications are also discussed, including marine, infrastructure, and aircraft related issues. The first article, "Designing for Repairability," discusses the need to begin by designing repairable structures. At the preliminary and detailed design stages, composite structures must be developed with the aim of reparability. Replacement of composite components is costly, particularly with the design requirements attempting to reduce parts by having large one-piece sections. The article "Repair Engineering and Design Considerations" provides comment and direction on designing simple repairs to composite structures. This article is aimed at the design of simple and effective repairs. Fabrication and application issues with respect to the repair scheme must be addressed for long-term justification of any maintenance activity. The quality-control and quality-assurance inspection requirements and their implementation provide for this reassurance. Practical methods in achieving quality repair schemes are provided in the article "Repair Applications, Quality Control, and Inspection."

Repair Issues for Specific Applications

The next three articles provide detailed discussions on the repair issues and practices for marine vessels, civil infrastructure, and aircraft. While there are many common elements across all applications of composite structural repair, each application discusses in their respective articles the unique requirements of repair.

Composite materials are also a medium to achieve effective and structurally efficient repairs to existing structures. Using a composite repair patch to overcome structural deficiencies has been proven for many years. But the details of engineering design and practical application of composite repair patches are still considered a unique field of engineering. The article "Bonded Repair of Metal Structures Using Composites" discusses the composite repair scheme as applied to metal structures, such as that found on aging aircraft. Civil infrastructure issues with respect to repairing concrete and steel-based constructions are covered in the article "Rehabilitation of Reinforced Concrete Structures Using Fiber-Reinforced Polymer Composites." Repairs of marine craft are addressed in the article "Ship Structure Repairs." Issues related to in-service maintainability of aircraft are discussed in the article "Maintainability Issues."

Repair Standardization and Reliability Considerations

In today's climate of structural repair validation and verification, there is a need for the standardization of repair design, applications, and materials. The article "Worldwide Repair Standardization" provides an overview of these requirements and then discusses several of the key issues in detail. The final article, "Product Reliability, In-Service Experience, and Lessons Learned" looks at overall product reliability and the specific aspects that pertain to composite structures. A significant part of understanding the reliability of the composite components of today is based on the lessons learned for several aging composite structure applications.

Composite structures are here to stay! Their applications and general uses are growing steadily. Operators of equipment employing composite structures in primary load applications must understand the issues with respect to maintenance and repair action. This Section looks at a significant portion of these requirements. The authors have provided the current state-of-the-art in composite structure reliability, maintenance, and repair. However, this area is a very dynamic engineering system. New materials, fabrication methods, and design and analysis approaches are being developed. It is imperative that the in-service equipment operators keep up-to-date with the latest trends and maintain their own skills and those of their employees.

Designing for Repairability

L.J. Hart-Smith, The Boeing Company
R.B. Heslehurst, Australian Defence Force Academy

DESIGN is typically a compromise of conflicting requirements. This is particularly so with the design of composite structures. On one hand, there is the ability to produce very efficient structures that are lightweight and cost-effective with respect to manufacture. On the other hand, in-service maintenance and repair often require a structure that does not have the best strength-to-weight ratio or stiffness-to-weight ratio and could be more complex and costly to fabricate. The final structure needs to be both production and structurally efficient and simple to maintain and repair. This article discusses the requirement for designing repairable composite structures by providing general and specific design guidelines. Several examples are used to illustrate how this can be achieved. This article is largely based on the content of Ref 1–4. While these reports may seem dated, the content is still regarded as significant in the design of composite joints.

Introduction to Designing for Repairability

The de Havilland DH-98 Mosquito "Wooden Wonder" or "Mossie" fighter-bomber of World War II is an excellent example and source of very valuable information about the design of composite aircraft structures, in particular, the principles of structural joints in composite materials. The most important lesson for designers today is that the wood (a natural composite) in the Mosquito was used only to carry in-plane loads. Metal fittings were used for all triaxially loaded components—the landing gear, engine mounts, control surface mounting brackets, wing-to-fuselage junction, and so on. Such a policy of avoiding triaxial or interlaminar loads on composite structures makes even more sense today, because the resin matrix is far weaker compared to graphite fibers, for example, than the cellulose was compared to the wood fibers.

Another key feature of the Mosquito was the extensive use of adhesive bonding throughout the primary and secondary structures, even though the early casein adhesives used survived only in the cold environment of Europe and not in the tropical environment of the Far East. Later production models used formaldehyde adhesives instead. The extensive use of adhesive bonding on the Mosquito is in sharp contrast to the widespread malpractice today of bolting together thin, lightly loaded composite components that would be far better suited to bonding. Bolting should be reserved for thicker, more heavily loaded composite structures, as it was on the Mosquito. This reluctance to make greater use of adhesively bonded advanced composite structures is particularly difficult to fathom, because the adhesives of today are much stronger than the resin matrices that hold the fibers together.

The BAe/Boeing AV-8B Harrier II uses approximately 25% composite materials in its structural weight. The distribution of composite materials includes wing, empennage and fuselage skins, and the substructure of the forward fuselage and wing. Figure 1 illustrates the material use. The all-composite wing on the AV-8B Harrier is an excellent example of composite structure where repair and maintenance were considered during the initial design phase rather than as the more customary afterthought. The fiber pattern is near quasi-isotropic throughout. The strain levels are sufficiently low to permit U.S. Marines to perform quick bolted repairs anywhere without first having each specific repair reviewed by the manufacturer. A slightly orthotropic fiber pattern would have been more appropriate for some other wings with higher aspect ratios, but the structural efficiencies would not have been much greater than with the quasi-isotropic pattern.

On the other hand, in the Bell/Boeing V-22 Osprey (Fig. 2), which has a more orthotropic fiber pattern for strength-to-weight and stiffness-to-weight advantages, bolt holes and cutout develop a higher stress concentration. Because the Harrier wing contains no major splices, being continuous from tip to tip, the design of the bolted joints could be performed according to a simple design procedure.

Review of Joining Methods. The choice between mechanical or bonded repair of advanced composites is often dictated by the nature of the component. For instance, minimum gage control surfaces are lighter if bonded than bolted, because there is no need for locally thickened seams to allow for countersunk fastener heads. Very thick primary structures, on the other hand, are best made by bolting or riveting together simple details that do not have the critical weaknesses due to laminate wrinkling that seems to

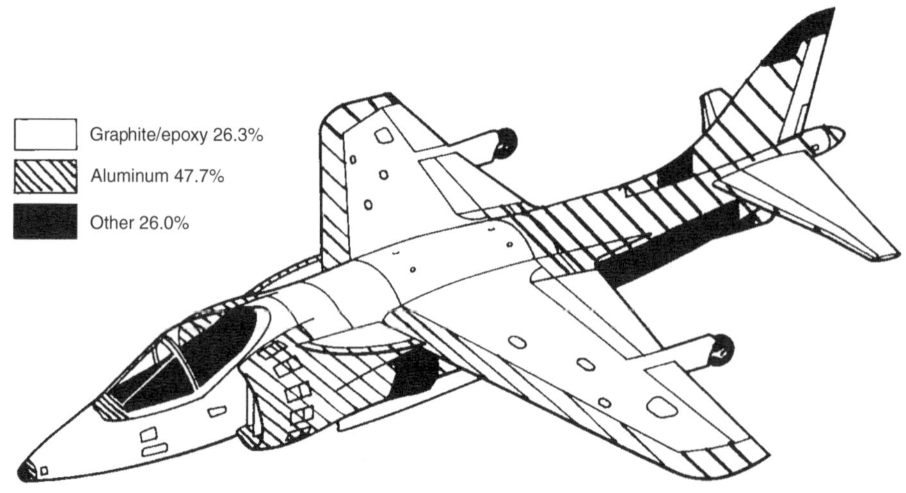

Fig. 1 AV-8B material breakdown. Courtesy of Boeing

be inherent in many integrally stiffened co-cured panels (Fig. 3).

Bolted or riveted composite repairs may be preferred to bonded repairs, because they take less time, can be done with fewer skills and special equipment, and because some structures lend themselves to mechanical repairs with no loss of static strength. In any event, it is important to plan and to use a laminate pattern that is compatible with bolted holes.

Bolted Joint Failure Modes. The failure modes of mechanically fastened joints are illustrated in Fig. 4. The individual mode of failure is dependent upon the joint geometry as well as the lay-up pattern. The strongest joint usually fails by tension through the hole at a particular width-to-diameter (*w*/*d*) ratio. The width is the strip width or bolt pitch distance, and the diameter is that of the hole or fastener. Bearing failures occur at lower total loads per unit width and at greater *w*/*d* ratios, where the bolts are further apart. Shear-out failure is controlled by near quasi-isotropic laminate patterns and sufficient edge distances; whereas fastener-type failure is restricted by appropriate fastener diameter-to-component thickness ratios. It suffices here to state that in both original structure and repairs, the strongest joints are developed only by keeping the fastener loads low in comparison with both the rated shear strength and the laminate bearing allowable.

Adhesively bonded repairs are needed for advanced composite structures that have already been manufactured and were not designed for bolted repairs. They are also needed for the very thin skins used on fairings and control surfaces. However, despite the need, many of today's composite designs contain areas in which no structural repair at all is possible.

The understanding of what can be adhesively bonded and what cannot starts with an assessment of the relative strengths of the bonded joints themselves and the laminates that are to be bonded together. That assessment is best performed in terms of the local load intensity (load per unit width) rather than of the stresses (load per unit area) in either the adherends or adhesive. As a rule, light loads are resisted by thin structure and heavy loads by thick structure, so the thickness of the laminate is the most appropriate independent variable here. For thin laminate, it is always possible to design an adhesively bonded joint that is inherently stronger than the adherends being bonded together (see Fig. 3 in

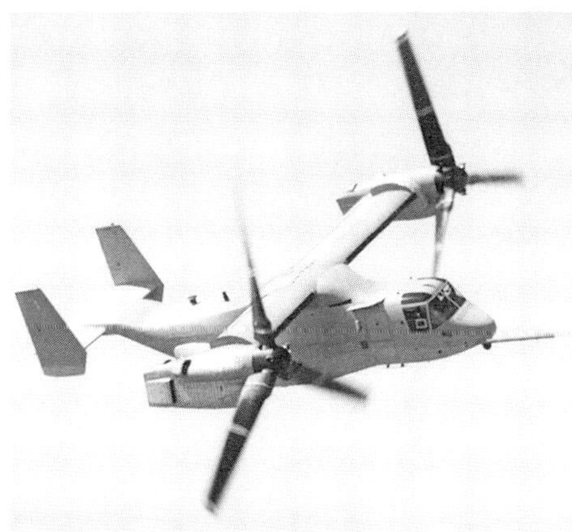

Fig. 2 V-22 Osprey. Courtesy of Boeing

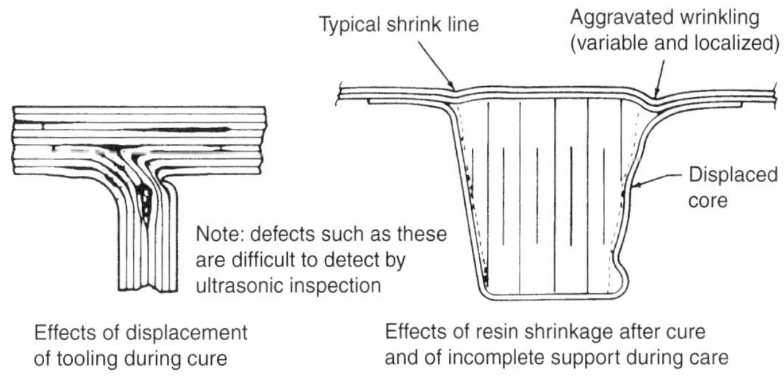

Fig. 3 Internal wrinkling of co-cured composite structures

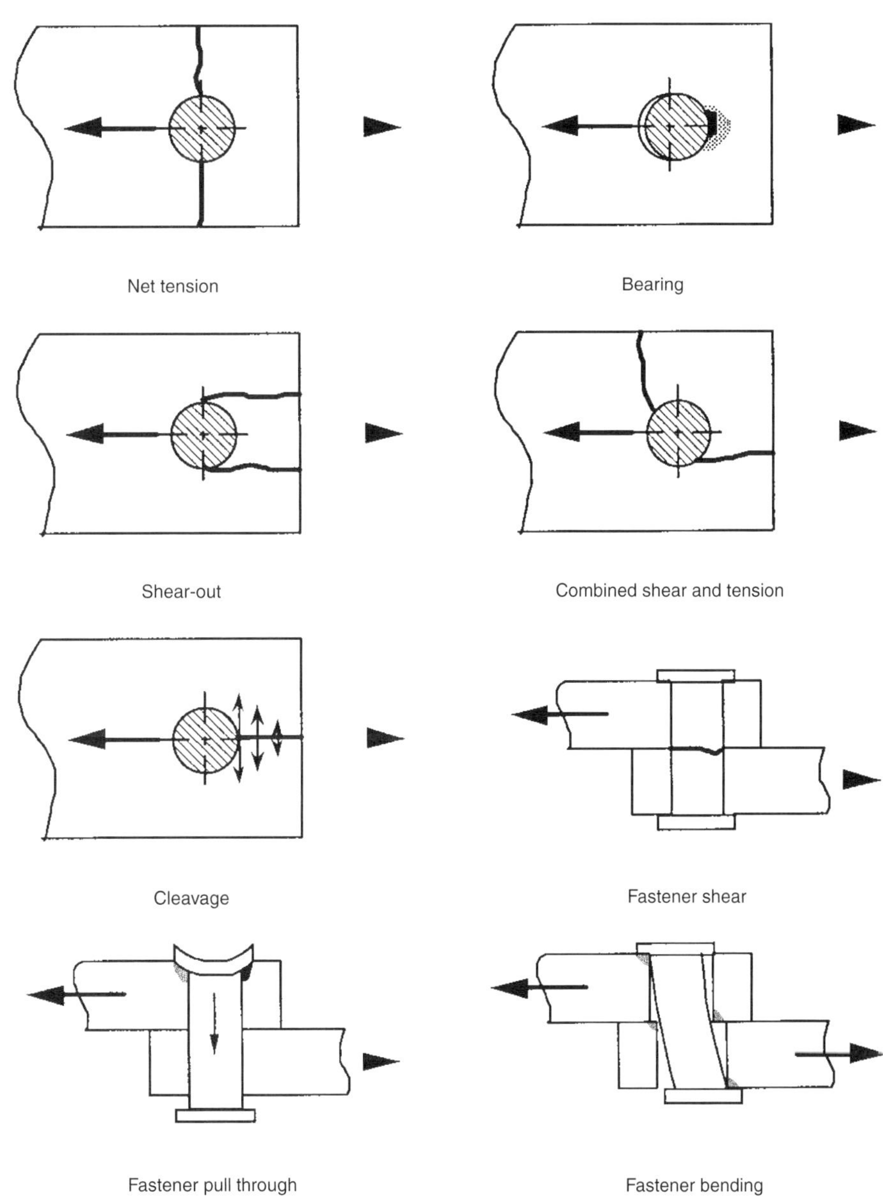

Fig. 4 Failure modes of mechanically fastened joints

the article "Bolted and Bonded Joints" in this Volume). For this discussion, it is sufficient to recognize that the simplest joint configurations are applicable to thin bonded structures, while thick structures need more complex joints, as shown in Fig. 5.

Adhesively Bonded Joint Failure Modes. The failure modes of adhesively bonded joints are illustrated in Fig. 6. Adherend failure is the preferred failure mode, and the strength of the adhesive in cohesive shear must be designed to be at least half as much stronger than the adherends. Adherend and cohesive peel failure mode are controlled by detailed joint end design. Adhesive failure is excluded by specific and detailed attention to surface preparation.

Design Guidelines

Some proponents of advanced composite structures claim that the main weight savings are attained because fiber patterns can be tailored to be orthotropic, thereby uncoupling the materials needed for the bending and torsion requirements of wings, for example. Actually, the converse is closer to the truth. Composite monolayers have so little strength in the transverse fiber direction that it is necessary to include fibers in every direction for which some load condition exists. In contrast, for adhesively bonded laminated metal alloy structures, each laminate can perform double or triple duties, because the same layers can react to different loads that do not occur simultaneously.

The need for fibers in every direction in a composite laminate is most pronounced around bolt holes. (The distribution of hoop and bearing stresses is shown in Fig. 24 in the article "Bolted and Bonded Joints" in this Volume.) It is not surprising that the quasi-isotropic pattern (0°, ±45°, 90°) with one quarter of the layers in each of the four directions lies in the middle of a plateau (of bolt bearing strength) on the plane of varying fiber patterns. Excessive deviation from that pattern involves substantial loss of bolted joint strength. The preferred fiber patterns for bolted or riveted composite structures are shown in Fig. 7 for the family of laminates based on the 0°, ±45°, 90° directions.

It should be noted that there is a minimum requirement for about 12.5% of the fibers in each of the four directions. In addition, a good balance of strength around the circumference of the bolt bearing area is achieved with a maximum 37.5% of the fibers in any one direction. Figure 8 shows a larger regime than Fig. 7, limited by no more than 50% of the fibers in any one of the four directions, that is suitable for the mechanical repair of lightly loaded, minimum gage composite structures. Those laminates will not split longitudinally provided that the applied loads are re-

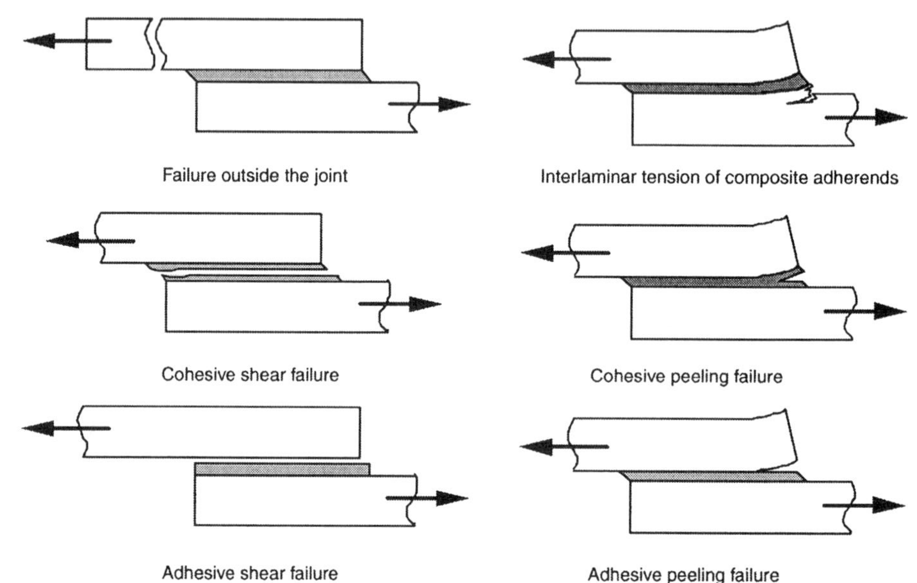

Fig. 6 Failure modes of adhesively bonded joints

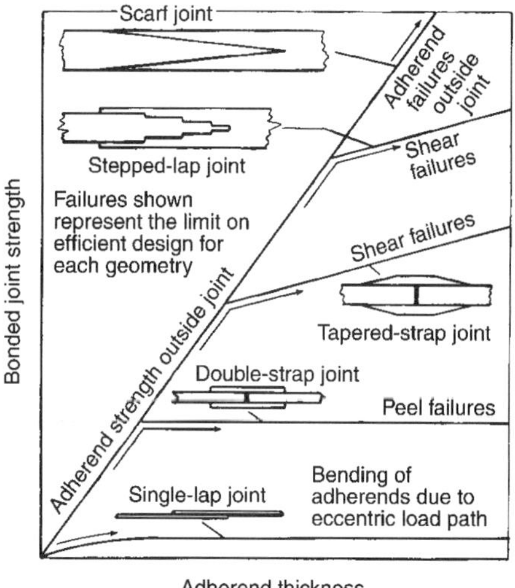

Fig. 5 Relative uses of different bonded joint types

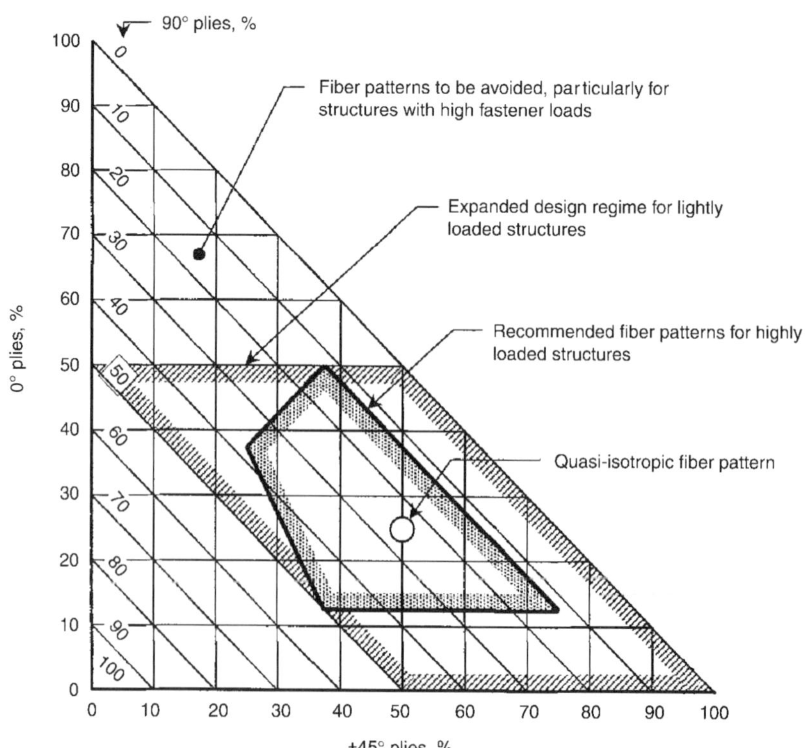

Fig. 7 Selection of lay-up pattern for carbon-fiber-reinforced composite laminates

stricted. However, for the heavily loaded primary composite structures, the fiber patterns should be confined within the area shown in Fig. 7, not Fig. 8.

Adhesively bonded repairs are most suitable for thin, lightly loaded structures for two reasons. The first reason is the complexity of the joints needed for the transfer of large bond loads. The titanium-to-composite stepped-lap joints are difficult enough to make as original structure, let alone as an after-the-fact repair. Second, an adhesively bonded joint must never be allowed to be weaker than the members it is joining; otherwise, it does not tolerate damage and could act as a weak link fuse. Another powerful reason for not using bonded repair of a small hole in thick laminates is the large amount of undamaged material that is removed for a scarf repair. For the majority of structural adhesives used, the scarf angle is limited to 3°.

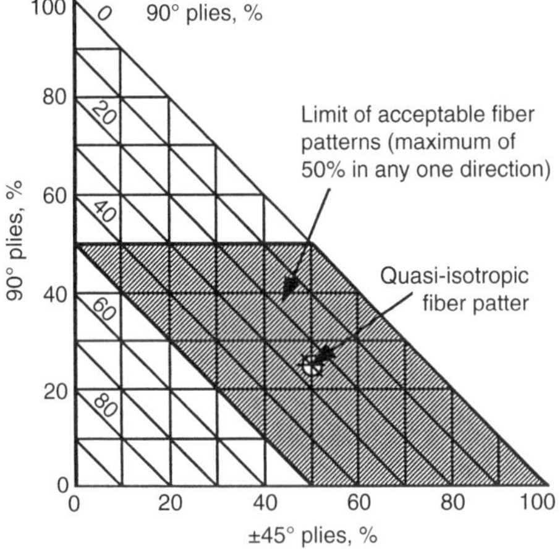

Fig. 8 Selection of lay-up pattern for bolted repair of lightly loaded fibrous composite laminates

Bolted or Riveted Repairs. The few keys to successful bolted or riveted repairs of advanced composite structures can be expressed as follows:

- The original laminate must have no location where the stresses are so high that drilling repair holes will result in an unacceptable loss of ultimate strength. Typical stress limits are given in Fig. 9; they indicate a need to design to no more than about 50% of the unnotched material allowable strengths. More such design information is given in Fig. 10, in terms of the more customary design strain levels. It should be noted, however, that these strains are not as independent of fiber pattern as was once believed.
- The bearing stresses must be kept much lower than the single-hole bearing allowables, if efficient bolted joints are to be designed. The need to restrict the design bearing stress is indicated in Fig. 10, which relates the interaction between bearing and bypass stresses to the strengths of the laminate. These load increments also apply at each bolt in a multirow joint.
- The original laminates must not be excessively orthotropic. A minimum of 12.5% of the fibers in each of the 0°, ±45°, and 90° directions is desirable, along with a maximum

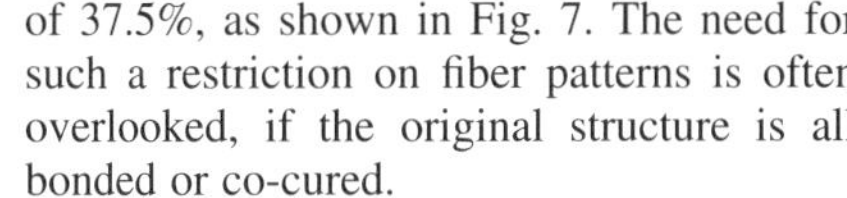

of 37.5%, as shown in Fig. 7. The need for such a restriction on fiber patterns is often overlooked, if the original structure is all bonded or co-cured.
- Optimal bolted joint geometries can be computed, as in Ref 5 and 6. Nonoptimal geometries can easily result in joints far weaker than anticipated.
- Neither fully plastic nor perfectly elastic bolted joint analyses are suitable for advanced composites. This is evident from Fig. 11, which shows that the two-straight-line designs, akin to typical metal structural analysis, are inappropriate and often dangerous for composites. That two-straight-line method is based on a uniform bearing allowable applied to the hole and a fictitious universal tensile strength applied to the net section. Linear finite-element analysis of bolted composite joints is unduly conservative, unless some fudge factor is used. Actually, designing bolted composite joints is not very difficult, as explained in Ref 6 and 7, unless one seeks the maximum efficiency for a splice.
- The need for repair should be recognized at the time of the design, and the use of laminate

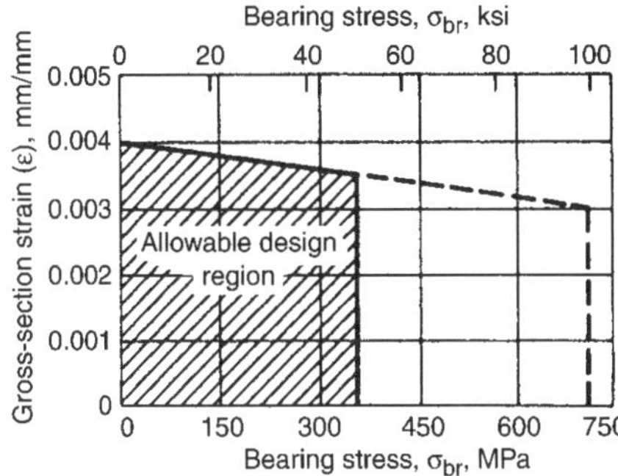

Fig. 10 Design strain levels for bolted graphite/epoxy structures

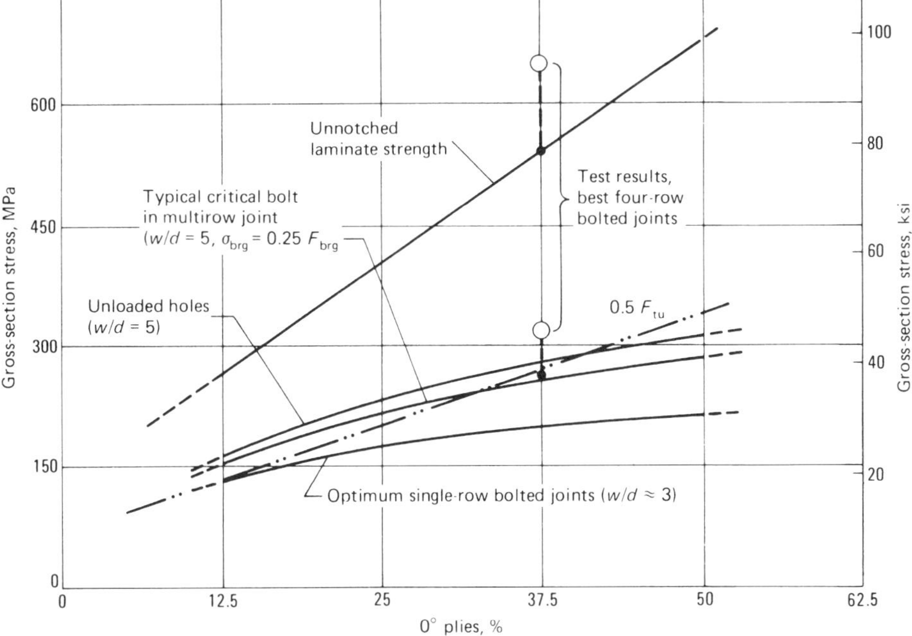

Fig. 9 Gross-section design stresses (*B*-basis allowables) for bolted composite structures (graphite/epoxy laminates). Chart is applicable for bolts up to 9.5 mm (0.375 in.) in diameter. Larger bolts are associated with progressively lower laminate stresses. σ_{brg}, bearing stress ($\sigma_{brg} = P/dt$, where P is the load, d is the bolt diameter, and t is laminate thickness), F_{brg}, composite ultimate bearing strength; F_{tu}, composite ultimate tensile strength parallel to the applied loads.

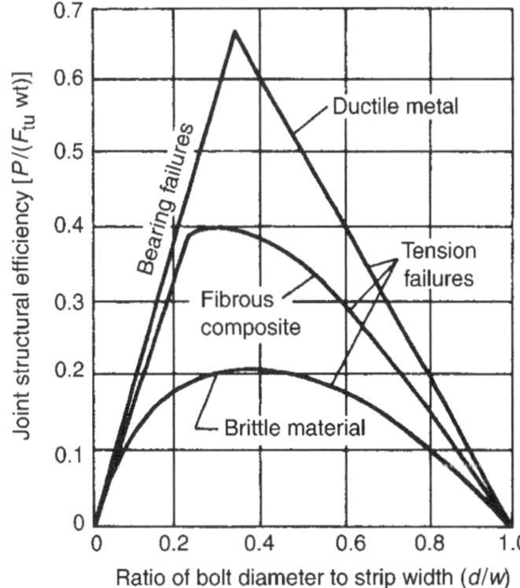

Fig. 11 Relationship between strengths of bolted joints in ductile, fibrous composite and brittle materials

optimization programs that ignore such practical considerations as repair should be resisted, even if doing so results in a reduction in the weight saved.

Adhesively Bonded Repairs. The few keys to successful adhesively bonded repairs of advanced composite structures are as follows (but are based on good initial design):

- Only lightly loaded structures are considered practical for bonded repairs. The limits are the equivalent of 3.2 mm (0.125 in.) thick aluminum alloy for a two-side bond or 1.6 mm (0.063 in.) if only a one-side bond can be accomplished.
- An effective surface preparation technique is of paramount importance, especially if a metallic adherend is involved (in which case a chemical surface treatment may be essential).
- Patches should be precured wherever possible to avoid overheating the basic structure or joggling the fibers in the patch, even though such precured patches would usually not permit flush repairs to be made.
- Particularly for a co-cured repair, it is imperative to slowly and carefully dry out any absorbed moisture in the laminate or free water in honeycomb cells. Some honeycomb parts have been known to have so much water in the cells that the weight of the parts has been increased to as much as three times the dry structural weight. More closely monitored inspection of this past problem in sandwich panels limits this occurrence today. However, moisture ingress into honeycomb cells through thin porous (usually co-cured) face sheets remains a potentially serious problem with many such structures in service today. When the resin was not subject to autoclave pressure during the cure cycle, but to the vent pressure (i.e. atmospheric pressure at the most, or some level of vacuum at the least) higher than usual levels of porosity exist in such structures. Consequently, it is imperative not to use bare aluminum cores in such structures, but to use phosphoric acid anodized (PAA) cores instead. Even Nomex cores soften appreciably when immersed in standing water. For this reason, more recent structures have included surfacing layers of adhesive film (akin to gel coating on marine vessels) to minimize the occurrence of pin holes in the outer face sheets. Many have impervious Tedlar sheets cured on the inside of the parts to act as a barrier there, where the skins are often even thinner. (Some such structures now use pre-cured outer face sheets, cured at autoclave pressure, before the remainder of the structure is co-bonded to them.) The added structural weight is far less than that of the water that would otherwise have been absorbed which has, on occasions been far greater than the original structural weight. Nevertheless, when this additional weight needed to keep the water out is accounted for properly in the initial design trade-off studies, it is usually found that the multirib postbuckled thin-skin design, such as the DC-10 composite upper aft rudder, is lighter. Such designs can also be less expensive to build as well as easier to maintain than equivalent honeycomb designs. The same cannot be said for designs involving a combination of honeycomb sandwich cores, in which water collects, and ultrathin composite facesheets, through which it passes.
- The design of bonded repair splices is straightforward—unless one has to adhesively bond a thick, damaged laminate that had been designed to a high strain level that will not permit the use of a bolted or riveted repair.

Honeycomb Sandwich Panel Construction. Honeycomb sandwich constructions have been used extensively for lightly loaded control surfaces, access doors, and fairings on large commercial transport aircraft; however, it is questionable whether this represents an improvement over the sheet metal components they replaced. Paradoxically, there has been a dearth of honeycomb composite structures in applications where slightly greater load intensities would make them more appealing. This is explained at length in Ref 3.

Leaving aside the difficulties associated with manufacturing fibrous composite honeycomb panels, there are service problems that become acute when the facesheets contain less than three layers of woven fabric. Because of high tensile residual thermal stresses in the resin matrix for autoclave-cured graphite/epoxies and aramid/epoxies, through-cracks grow easily in the middle of each bundle of fibers, and the components fill up rapidly with water. While actually a design problem, this situation is often misinterpreted as a Kevlar/Nomex (DuPont) material problem. (With graphite/epoxy, so far the cracks have not penetrated right through the facesheets; there is not any sign of water accumulation, mainly because most graphite fabrics have a finer weave than is customarily used with Kevlar.) There was no counterpart to these problems with the earlier oven-cured fiberglass/epoxy components because the residual stresses were lower and the resins were tougher. (Curiously, 20 years of satisfactory service with resins cured at 120 °C, or 250 °F, has been overridden by laboratory test-coupon results showing that 175 °C, or 350 °F, cures are needed to ensure durability in the service environment.)

The obvious solution to the moisture-ingress problem is to add more layers of composites to the facesheets, because the locally thickened areas where the fastener seams are located do not develop through-cracks. Weaves with smaller fiber bundles would also help. However, adding extra plies creates an apparent weight problem. The water absorbed through the minimum-gage facesheets is only in the part and not called out on the drawing; whereas the added plies would be counted as part of the weight even though they would weigh less than the water eventually transmitted through thinner and lighter facesheets.

Perfectly satisfactory metal control surface skins can be made from 0.4 mm (0.016 in.) thick aluminum alloy sheet, with adhesively bonded metal doublers to thicken the skin locally where the rivets are installed and to enhance the resistance to sonic fatigue. A structurally equivalent postbuckled design was used in the DC-10 graphite/epoxy rudders made at Douglas Aircraft Company under contract to National Aeronautics and Space Administration (NASA)-Langley. The composite skin was only 0.76 mm (0.030 in.) thick, and the entire structural box weighed only about two-thirds as much as the highly efficient metal design, even though during both initial testing and retesting of a composite rudder examined for possible deterioration in service, the rudder withstood 400% of design limit load without failure.

Despite concerns in some quarters about delaminations in postbuckled skins, more than 10 years of flight service on about 15 rudders has not revealed any such problems, mainly because the thin skins were not reinforced to delay the onset of buckling. Instead, they were allowed to deflect out of the way to relieve themselves of as much load as possible. Highlights of this technically very successful DC-10 composite rudder program are recorded in Ref 8.

This good application of composites to lightweight aircraft structures has not often been emulated, perhaps because most of the research into postbuckled composite structures has concerned thicker structures. In those cases, there is a very real possibility that any skin wrinkling would delaminate the structure at the stiffeners. The induced peel stresses are proportional to the fourth power of the thickness of the members being bonded together. Consequently, excessively thick postbuckled co-cured or bonded composite structures will delaminate, and moderately thick structures will need to be stitched together to prevent such delaminations. Another result of that same power law is that very thin composite structures can be allowed to buckle with impunity, because the induced peel stresses will be trivial, if the flange widths are adequate.

Honeycomb sandwich designs simply cannot compete with postbuckled designs of composites or metal. The 0.76 mm (0.030 in.) of graphite/epoxy, which alone is structurally adequate when bonded to stable rib caps and spar caps, can be compared with the combination of a typical (nonbuckling) minimum gage exterior facesheet 0.63 mm (0.025 in.) thick, an interior facesheet 0.43 mm (0.017 in.) thick, a honeycomb core of 12.7 mm (0.5 in.), and four layers of film adhesive, each 0.125 mm (0.005 in.) thick. The smaller number of ribs in the honeycomb designs does not make up for the heavier skins. Worse, that sandwich skin is very prone to impact damage by debris thrown up from the runway and by hailstorms. The authors are concerned that the high incidence of minor damage to thin-skinned honeycomb structures in service will become a black mark against all composite structures. They fear that people might change back to metal structures, rather than admit that the problem was really caused by an inappropriate design concept. Such a reaction has already occurred in relation to Kevlar/Nomex construction, with a reversion to heavier fiberglass/epoxy facings to solve the problem of entrapment of water in the honeycomb core. An alternative solution of retaining the Kevlar skin because of its high impact resistance and eliminating the honeycomb has not been adopted, presumably because doing so would have added to the redesign and tooling costs. Yet, the microcracks in the Kevlar would never have been of concern if there had not been cavities in which water could collect.

A further undesirable feature common to many advanced composite control surfaces is the use of mechanical fasteners instead of adhesive bonding. This practice is particularly undesirable for mass-balanced control surfaces. There is a widespread irrational aversion to the use of secondary adhesive bonding with advanced composites. Because the fasteners must be countersunk and the minimum-size threaded fastener used is 4.76 mm ($\frac{3}{16}$ in.) in diameter, whereas 3.2 mm ($\frac{1}{8}$ in.) diameter rivets are permitted in the metal structure, the composite panels include thickened seams over all rib caps and spar caps that are not needed for structural reasons, but merely accommodate the greater countersunk head size. That weight penalty is compounded by replacing 3.2 mm ($\frac{1}{8}$ in.) diameter rivets with 4.76 mm ($\frac{3}{16}$ in.) diameter threaded fasteners on an almost one-for-one basis and by the need for additional balance weights.

In the DC-10 rudder design philosophy, the unreinforced skins would be bonded directly to the rib caps and rear spar caps in the future. The 20 rudders made under the flight service evaluation program were co-cured as complete boxes in a single operation, but because the design remains an object lesson for the future, the manufacturing method used needs to be improved. Hart-Smith first saw such work in Europe early in the 1980s, by which time it had already been developed to include preheating both the flat layups and the rubber bag to enable even thicker sections to be flanged. Suggested design and manufacturing improvements for subsequent work on lightly loaded composite structures are given in Ref 8. Any such future designs would be bonded together from individual, uniformly thick details. The only thickening for fasteners would be along a removable front spar, where the moment arm with respect to the hinge line is small and so is the effect on the balance weights.

It is noteworthy that the key to the considerable excess strength of the DC-10 composite rudders was between 0.11 and 0.23 kg ($\frac{1}{4}$ and $\frac{1}{2}$ lb) of conservatism at the bolted joints attaching the hinge and actuator fittings to the composite structure; the remainder of the structure was almost all of minimum gage. The judicious decision to not seek the last possible ounce of weight saving was directly responsible for an uneventful and quick series of certification tests.

The use of honeycomb construction for fairings, such as at the wing roots, is also not an optimal solution. Unfortunately, it has been used extensively, because it is the quickest to draw and the cheapest to tool, due to the small number of parts. Consequently, such designs can also maximize the return on investment for subcontractors by minimizing their up-front costs. The higher recurring costs are passed on to the customer.

Apart from the weight and moisture absorption problems discussed earlier, honeycomb panels present one other serious potential problem. If they warp out of shape during manufacture, they require tremendous force to make them fit on assembly to the basic structure or line up properly with similar adjacent panels. Such problems were not as severe with the older fiberglass panels, because of the low modulus of those facesheets. When co-cured as a single assembly, the panels also tend to suffer from pinholes on the surface, and these must be filled and glazed before the panels can be painted. An alternative design concept that is torsionally soft and easy to assemble is a hollow-hat stiffened single-skin arrangement, as shown in Fig. 12. If a secondary adhesive bonding process were used instead of co-curing, spare parts would be available to facilitate repairs. In addition, repairs would not often be needed, because the single solid skin would be less prone to impact damage than today's minimum-gage skins on each side of a honeycomb or foam core.

Skin tools for such fairings can easily be made by stretch forming a metal sheet over a numerically machined wooden master model. Such woodwork is common for automobile prototyping. The Lear Fan spar masters were made from wood in a most successful subcontract. Stiffener tools can be made by draping long sections of flexible rubber mandrels (made in simple straight tools) inside the skin tool, if only a few panels are needed. Machined metal tools would be preferable, if many components are needed.

Designs of the type shown in Fig. 12 are easily adaptable to low-cost manufacture using thermoplastics by designing components, such as the trailing-edge panel in Fig. 13, as two uniformly thick panels subsequently glued or fused together. One panel defines the exterior shape, while the other provides the stiffening elements and local doublers. Each component is formed from a fully cross-plied flat pattern to avoid the internal bridging and wrinkles associated with a layer-by-layer hand lay-up directly on the tool.

It is noteworthy that the skin and stiffener tools are each complete in a single component, without any removable details of the type needed to co-cure integral blade stiffeners, for example. The design concept in Fig. 13 is actually a development of an earlier idea for making such panels out of thermoset resins in a single operation. Figure 14 shows the arrangement of the first such panel built.

The rational use of honeycomb sandwich construction with fibrous composites requires that applications with higher load intensities be found to justify the necessarily thicker facings than have been used on aircraft control surfaces and fairings. Figure 15 shows how the optimal structural geometry varies with load intensity; honeycomb is best only for a limited range between thin postbuckled single-skin structures and thick discretely stiffened structures that are resistant to buckling without the need for a continuous second skin. Alternatively, as on the wing of the round-the-world Voyager and modern composite sailplanes, sandwich construction can be justified by the greatly improved control of the wing section profile, leading to a dramatic reduction in drag. Similar special cases include the passenger floors of large aircraft; it would be virtually impossible to wheel the food and drink carts around on a spongy, discretely stiffened single-skin floor.

Integrally Stiffened Co-cured Composite Structures. Many of today's advanced composite structures contain integrally stiffened co-cured panels or assemblies. These are used to save on tooling costs, but there is also a desire to strengthen composites by eliminating bolt holes. This improves the fracture toughness by

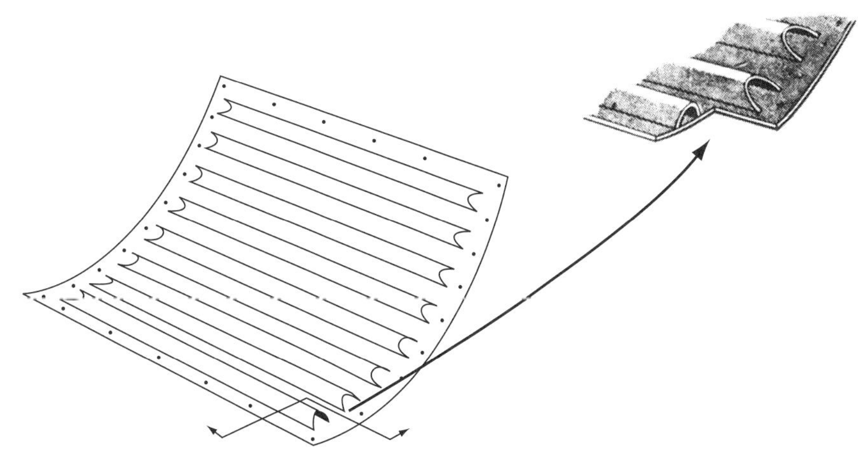

Fig. 12 Hollow-hat stiffened composite panel

alternating hard and soft areas to prevent any initial damage from spreading catastrophically under subsequent loads. The reason for this latter technique is that basic uniformly patterned composites have specific fracture toughness only about half as high as that of today's pressurized metal fuselages. By alternating stiff and soft strips, where the stiff strips are stronger than the soft strips, damage to either is confined or will not spread beyond the adjacent strips. While that technique has been shown by test to control the spread of damage, neither the stiff nor the soft areas lend themselves to bolted or riveted repairs. The stiff areas, being rich in 0° fibers, tend to split or delaminate longitudinally. Indeed, that is how the spread of damage is confined. The soft areas, having very few 0° fibers, cannot develop substantial strength, because the strains there are limited by the bolt holes in the adjacent stiff areas. These different strains-to-failure for each fiber pattern are explained in Ref 5.

This technique of attaining damage tolerance at the cost of repairability is obviously unsatisfactory. A careful study of the manner in which damage tolerance is achieved in metal aircraft structures and an appreciation of the behavior of bolted joints in different composite fiber patterns indicate that other approaches could achieve both goals simultaneously. Integrally stiffened machined metal planks are known to provide the least damage tolerance of all, in the sense that a crack, once started, will continue to grow across skin area and stiffener alike. In built-up metal structures, on the other hand, neither a slow-growing fatigue crack nor a fast fracture needs transfer from one member into another. In thin adhesively bonded structure, the glue layer provides the flexibility and the unbroken member the alternate load path to arrest the crack. The rivets or bolts in light or heavy built-up metal structures achieve the same purpose.

In short, damage tolerance in metal structures relies upon the absence of one-piece integrally stiffened structures, which are used mainly in the compression skins of wings, which are not fatigue-critical, and on horizontal tails, where the normal operating stresses are only a small fraction of those experienced with an extreme design load.

There is no reason to expect that the use of discrete members in fibrous composite structures would be any less effective in providing damage tolerance than in metal aircraft structures. Likewise, depending on the thickness of the members involved, adhesive bonding, rivets, or bolts should be used, as appropriate, for joining. For example, consider a composite wing skin. Determinable amounts of spanwise bending and torsion material are needed, along with a compatible amount of chordwise material. All of this material could be co-cured together in the scheme at the left of Fig. 16. Alternatively, the structure could be created by bolting together the elements shown at the right, where the skin would typically be of a quasi-isotropic (25, 50, 25) pattern to provide the torsional material. The stiffeners and doubler would be made from the (50, 37.5, 12.5) pattern and would provide the bulk of the bending material. All of these patterns could be bolted together, or, if the structure were thin enough, they could be adhesively bonded.

Now, this built-up composite structure obviously has good damage tolerance as well as inherent repairability. Moreover, it also has some very powerful manufacturing advantages. The difficulty in manufacturing parts is roughly proportional to the maximum thickness of the parts. It is not at all unusual to have to consolidate complex lay-ups every 0.76 mm (0.030 in.) or so during the lay-up to eliminate trapped voids and to minimize wrinkling of the plies. The three simple detail parts to the right of Fig. 16 are far easier to lay-up than the complex assemblies on the left and involve far fewer bagging cycles. The reason for the doubler, rather than a thicker stiffener, is that the two individually thinner parts are easier to lay-up and to fit together for

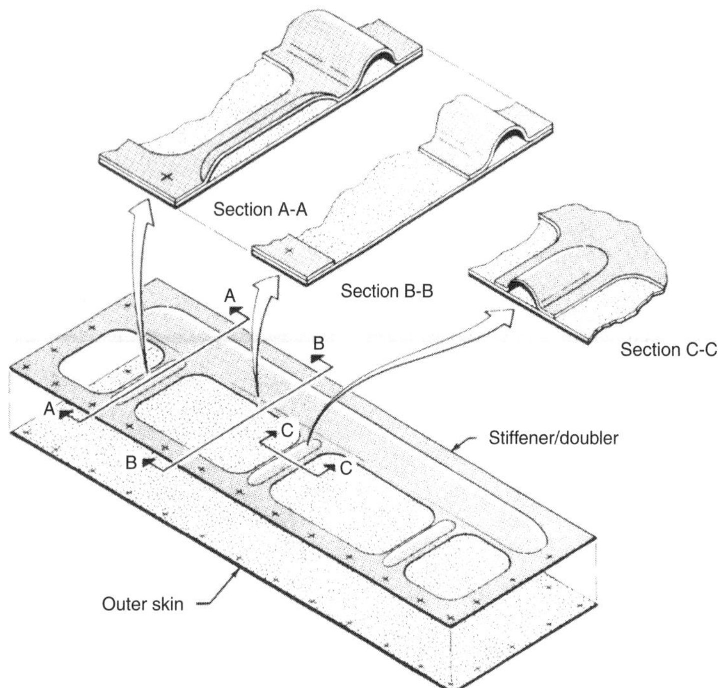

Fig. 13 Construction of two-piece thermoplastic composite access panels. Exploded views (not to scale). Section views show outer skin bonded to reinforcement.

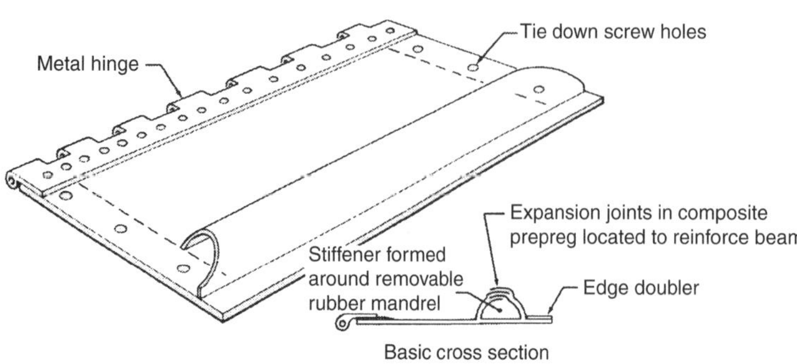

Fig. 14 Integrally stiffened co-cured composite trailing-edge panel

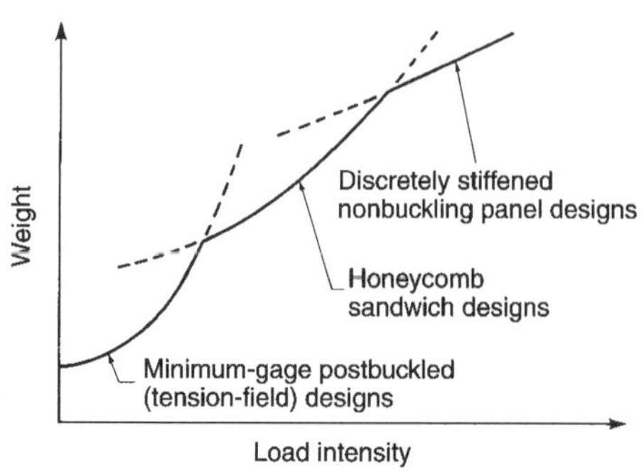

Fig. 15 Relative weights of different structural configurations

final assembly. The choice of a hat stiffener is based on three considerations: its structural efficiency, the ease of forming it from a flat layup, and the way it can be flattened out for easy splicing at manufacturing breaks in the wing skins. The integrally stiffened constructions need not have any advantage in terms of compressive allowables; the built-up assemblies can be bonded and bolted just as easily as they can be bolted and sealed.

The price paid for these superior laminates is having a large number of fasteners. However, those fasteners may be needed anyway to arrest the spread of delamination. They can be looked upon as giant stitches, performing the same role that fiber stitches do in thin composite structures. The effectiveness of such fasteners in controlling the spread of delaminations in thick composite structures is analyzed in Ref 9 and 10.

There is another often-overlooked reason for avoiding highly loaded, integrally stiffened composite structures. Were a designer to advocate adhesive bonding the stringers to the wing skins in a C-5, 747, DC-10, or L-1011 instead of drivematic riveting, he would be quickly reassigned to another task. The same fate would befall him, and deservedly so, were he to advocate adhesive bonding alone for a large all-composite wing. Thin layers of structural adhesives are simply not strong enough to provide damage tolerance in such cases, even if they could transfer the running shear loads in a carefully designed structure with no discontinuities. Yet when some other designer advocates leaving that layer of adhesive out of such a composite wing structure and relying instead on a single layer of resin to connect the skin and stiffeners together, few people understand that such an integrally stiffened structure is weaker than an equivalent adhesively bonded one. (Actually, the adjacent layers of resin would fail prematurely and prevent the development of the full strength of such an adhesive layer.)

Unfortunately, integrally stiffened laminated designs are usually perceived as equivalent to integrally stiffened isotropic metal structures, with total disregard of the weak interlaminar strength of the composite. A more appropriate comparison would be with adhesively bonded metal structures in which someone replaced the layer of adhesive with a layer of wet paint primer.

To be fair, it should be acknowledged that a few of the integrally stiffened composite panels have been designed in such a way that the fibers, rather than the resin, transfer most of the load between the stiffeners and the skin. The criticism in the preceding paragraph was not intended to refer to these design concepts. The following comments, however, do refer to all integrally stiffened panels.

Perhaps the greatest difficulty associated with integral stringers on large composite wing structures is in transferring massive loads into or out of the stringers at manufacturing breaks. For typical average wing skin load intensities of 207 MPa (30 ksi), it is usual to have individual stiffener loads of 220 to 440 kN (50 to 100 kips) at the nacelle or the side of the fuselage. In most panels tested thus far, such loads have been applied with block compression into potted ends of the composite structure. Transferring such loads through a bolted or adhesively bonded splice is no easy task. Most major aerospace manufacturers in the United States and abroad have experienced catastrophic failures of large composite structures that resulted from single overloaded bolt holes. This was true for the A-4 horizontal stabilizer failure from the front spar fitting and the Falcon 10 lower wing skin near the landing gear cutout. The DC-10 vertical tail failed through a rear spar access hole, because of insufficient structural deformation for bolts in clearance holes to pick up load. Each component was redesigned and retested before being shown to have adequate strength.

One is reminded of the difficulties encountered when trying to use 7079 aluminum alloys that were once supposed to be superior to 7075 material for aircraft structures. They presented so many problems that they are no longer used. Highly orthotropic composite laminates present much the same kind of problem, both in the original designs and for repairs—it is very difficult to design reliably for very high loads in any very brittle material, and the material is very unforgiving of any error in design or analysis.

There is another powerful reason for preferring to secondarily bond precured composite skins and stiffeners instead of co-curing them together. The bonding approach avoids the highly visible exterior mark-off associated with co-curing. As shown in Fig. 3, the locally excessive resin buildups in the co-cured structures contract during the cool-down period after cure. That mark-off even occurs around the perimeters of honeycomb panels at the edge of the core. Because the remainder of such co-cured panels is usually visually perfect, the mark-off needs subsequent filling and sanding before painting to enhance the cosmetic appearance of the panels.

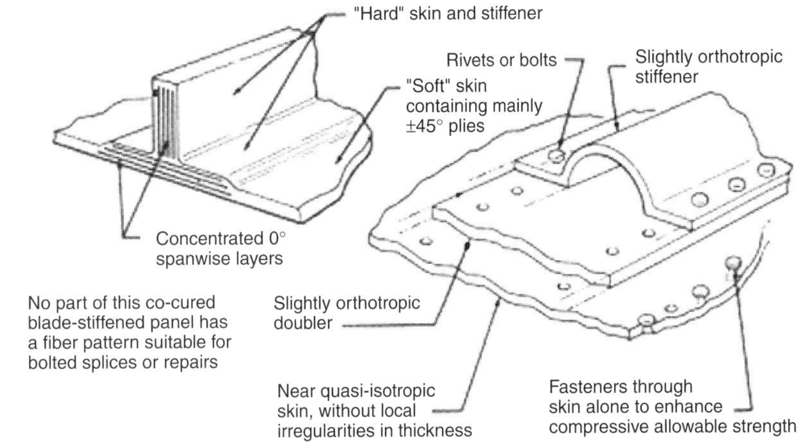

Fig. 16 Merits of not co-curing primary composite structure

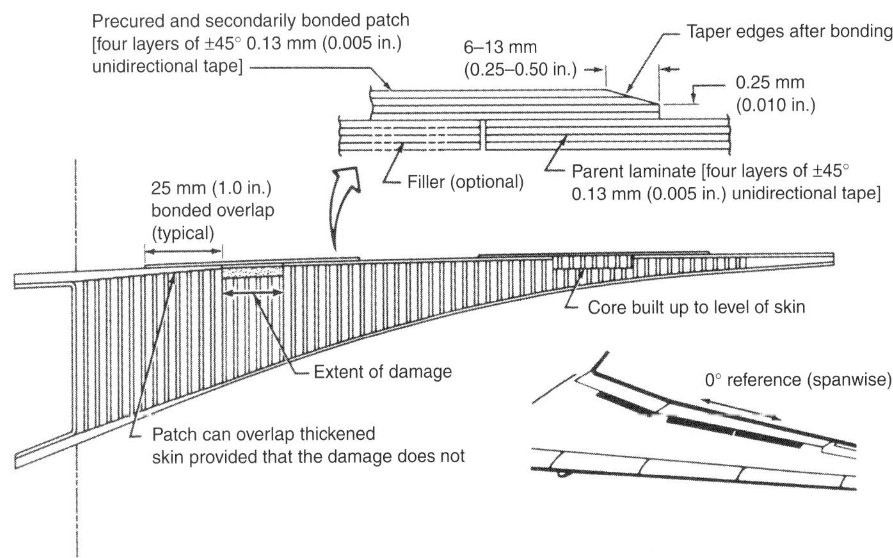

Fig. 17 Precured composite skin repair for MD-80 spoiler

Those subsequent operations tend to negate the original savings from co-curing.

In summary, it can be stated that experience has shown that the manufacturing economies sought by co-cured integrally stiffened constructions are often illusory for large panels. More importantly, the co-curing has frequently led to designs that cannot be repaired. The authors suggest other ways of achieving desirable goals in terms of manufacturing costs and damage tolerance without sacrificing repairability, such as bonding or mechanically fastening separate precured details.

Design for Supportability

It is possible to extract valuable lessons about what to do and what not to do in the future from the many composite aircraft components that have been built since the 1980s. Perhaps the most valuable conclusion is that it is vital to start with a well-conceived plan that coordinates the concurrent activities of various participating groups, rather than allowing work to pass from group to group sequentially. Success can be achieved only when good use is made of the preliminary design phase to uncover and solve potential problems before the majority of the budget has been committed. Failure to confirm that the tooling and manufacturing approaches will work before the formal design commences is an invitation to disaster. Experience has also taught that success is unlikely if the assigned personnel do not include a core of proficient experts; composites are too unforgiving for learning on the job. Perhaps the greatest trap is a feeling of complacency that composites are such wondrous materials that nothing can go wrong.

The Dos and Don'ts of Composites Structural Design.

Some technical and managerial lessons learned include the following:

- Don't design for primary loads being transferred by interlaminar shear; also, avoid secondary induced interlaminar loads.
- Do plan the tooling and manufacturing approach during the preliminary design phase to ensure that all three are compatible. Don't complete the design in isolation and then worry afterward about how to build it at a specified production rate.
- Don't begin the formal design drawings until after the first part has been completed. Do the drawings last to ensure that they are in conformity with the part.
- Don't design integral co-cured stiffening without expecting to pay for the more-expensive tooling needed to avoid hidden internal wrinkles. While seeming to be rather expensive, the metal-block tooling techniques developed at Messerschmitt-Bolkow-Blohm for Airbus tail surfaces and spoilers are appropriate for such components.
- Do thoroughly intersperse the different fiber directions and avoid having more than two 0.125 mm (0.005 in.) thick unidirectional plies adjacent when the angle change to the next direction is 90°, or more than four such plies when the angle change is 45°. (It should be noted that this imposes a limit on the maximum permissible percentage of fibers in any one direction.)
- Do require a minimum content of about 12.5% of the fibers in each of the four standard directions, 0°, +45°, 90°, and –45° (see Fig. 7).
- Don't permit in excess of 37.5% of the fibers to be oriented in any one direction, if the structure is mechanically fastened.
- Do be aware of abrupt internal ply drop-offs. Drop off plies in small increments, not all together; otherwise, the transitions in thickness will cause wrinkling of the fibers and possibly delaminations under load.
- Don't trust computer strength analysis or optimization programs that advocate the use of highly orthotropic fiber patterns.
- Don't design the basic structure first and the joints last—design the joints first, to maximize the structural efficiency, and fill in the gaps in between afterward.
- Do allow for the presence of loaded bolt holes, cutouts, or both in establishing the design strain levels that will be, in nearly all cases, appreciably less than those of unnotched laminates.
- Do not adhere blindly to original plans when difficulties arise. If three cure cycles are

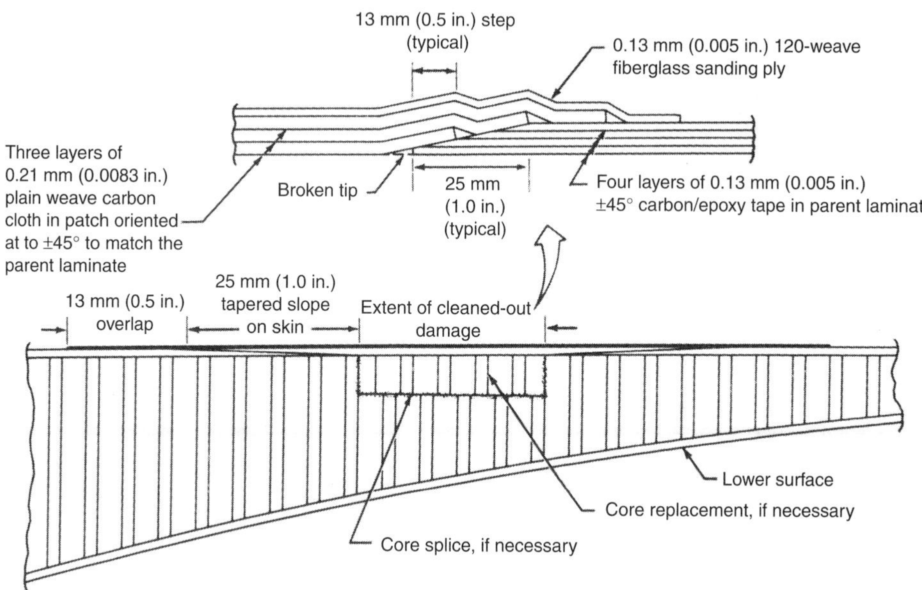

Fig. 18 Co-cured composite skin repair for MD-80 spoiler

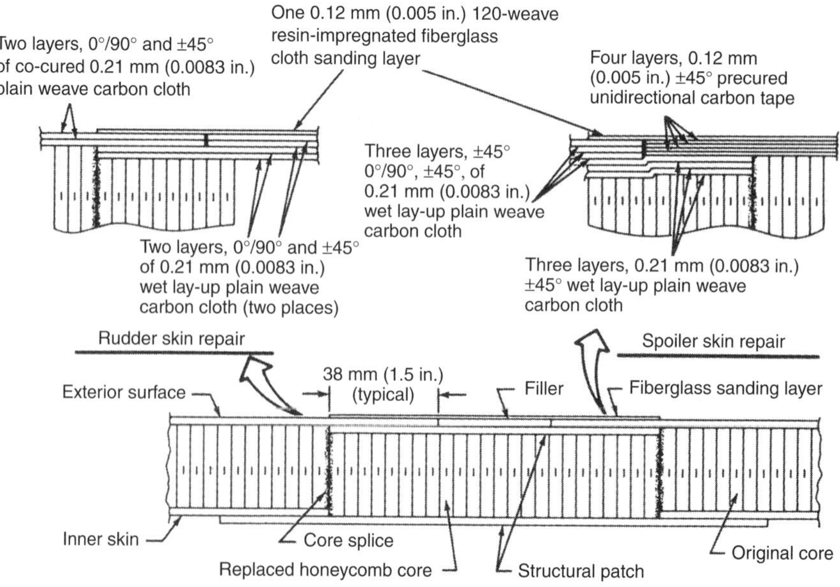

Fig. 19 Flush co-cured repairs for MD-80 spoilers and rudder

needed to manufacture a design that was supposed to be made in one shot, it is time to change to a different optimal design for two-stage manufacture.

- Do beware of subscale testing and proof-of-tool demonstrations. Many effects can be simulated only in actual size.
- Do understand the reasons behind historical precedents before following them in the future. What is optimal for one set of circumstances is often quite unsuitable for others.
- Do use secondary adhesive bonding extensively for thin, lightly loaded composite structures, restricting the use of mechanical fastening mainly to thicker, more heavily loaded structures.
- Don't be afraid to let thin composite skins wrinkle or buckle, but beware of allowing thick structure to do the same. It is wrong to add reinforcement to a structure merely to delay the onset of buckling; doing so just reduces the ultimate strength.
- Do consider the required production rate when deciding between a subassembly approach and fabrication of an essentially complete co-cured structure in one tool. The latter is best only for very low production rates, because, otherwise, it requires more replicates of the largest and most-costly tools.
- Don't be a slave to fashion. Understand the merits and limitations of past design and manufacturing techniques thoroughly before deciding on an approach for some given application.
- Don't repudiate 50 years of experience in designing metal aircraft structures as being of no value in composite construction. There is no real reason why composite structural arrangements should be fundamentally different from equivalent metal ones.
- Do take advantage of the greater dimensional control of composite detail parts made on metal tooling to integrate into one simple component what would normally have been made from several adjustable pieces in pressed or bent metal.
- Do understand that optimal design solutions are not generic. They vary, in particular, with load level, with the production rate, and with the need, or otherwise, for repair.
- Don't treat repairability and damage tolerance as afterthoughts once the static ultimate-strength design has been accomplished. All conditions need to be treated simultaneously.
- Don't complicate designs by seeking the last ounce of weight saving. Doing so will add unreasonably to the design and manufacturing costs.
- Don't be reluctant to design conservatively in local critical areas. The weight penalty for doing so is insignificant, while the savings in time during the development program can be enormous. Don't design to excessive bolt bearing stresses; doing so reduces the structural efficiency of the composite laminate.
- Don't ever design an adhesive bond to be the weak link in a structure. The bonds should always be stronger than the members being joined.
- Do be wary of induced peel stresses, both in adhesive layers and in the composite laminates.
- Don't be blind to the possibility that, for some structures, metals may be better or more cost-effective than fibrous composites.
- Don't standardize by using only one fiber and one resin for all applications. Follow metal practice that uses different alloys and heat treatments, as appropriate.
- Do remember the need to put fibers in every direction for which there is some significant load. When there are multiple load conditions, it is not permissible to optimize for only the most severe load on its own.
- Do remember to allow for expansion and contraction of the tools and composite material at different times during the cure cycle.
- Do be wary of unacceptably slow heat-up rates whenever the tooling (particularly rubber) has an excessive heat sink.
- Do be cautious about oversimplified cure cycles with no feedback control. Quality is often improved and inspection and rework costs reduced by extended consolidation periods prior to cure, by relating the pressure profile in the autoclave to the thermal profile and by temperature dwells within the cure cycles.
- Do provide slip joints within complicated lay-ups to ensure proper compaction and to ensure that there are no voids, bridges, or resin-rich buildups in the finished article. The same

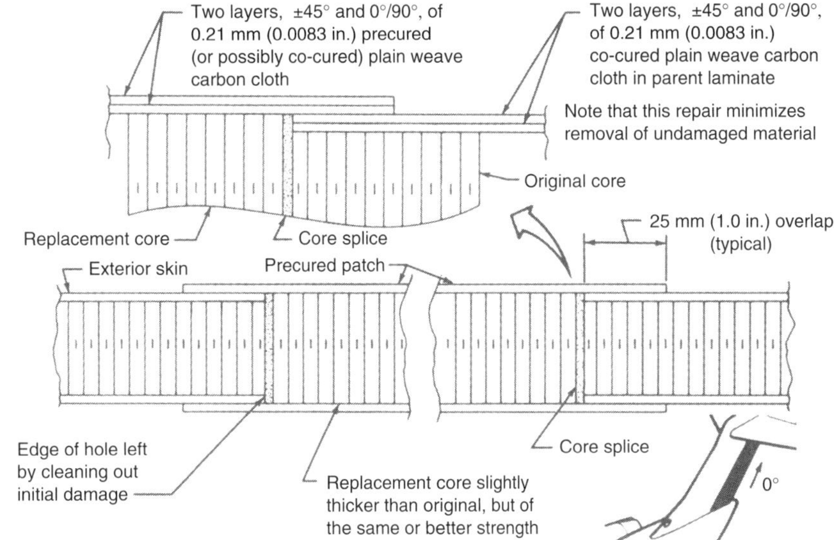

Fig. 20 Precured patch repair of MD-80 rudder skins

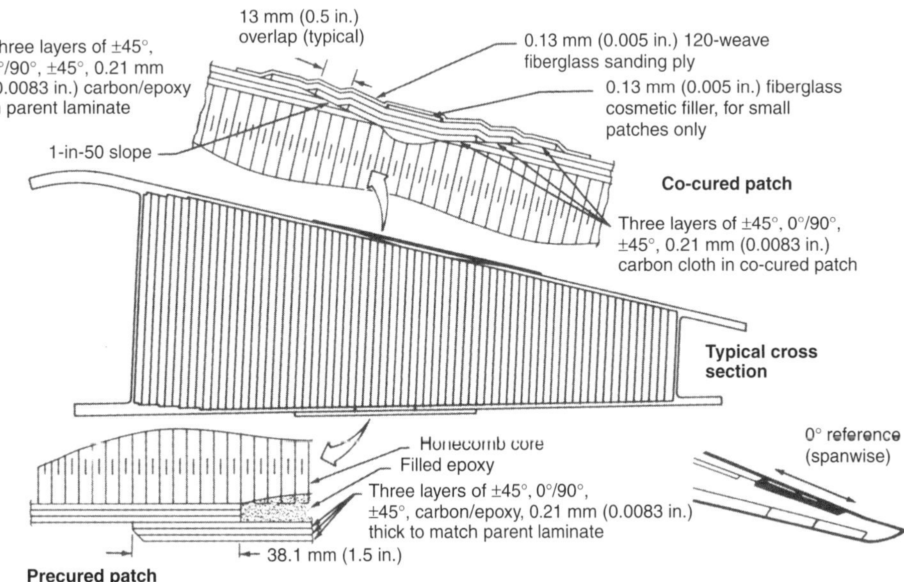

Fig. 21 Repair of MD-80 aileron skins

is true for the installation of bagging and breather material. Once verified by initial production, such details should be included in the drawings. Reference axes at one location of a compound-curved panel are not sufficient to define the lay-up.

- Do remember that composites are very brittle. There is no yielding to provide forgiveness for mistakes about internal load distributions or underestimated stress concentrations.
- Don't be overawed by the mystique of the composites. With well-thought-out load paths and a sensible manufacturing plan, good composite structures are not difficult to design.

Specific Examples

Several typical skin repairs for the graphite/ and Kevlar/epoxy components on the MD-80 are described in this section. The same techniques can be applied to the Kevlar/ and fiberglass/epoxy fairings on this and other aircraft. The techniques are applicable to such components on virtually all subsonic aircraft, except for those in proximity to the engines.

Consider the MD-80 composite spoiler. The basic exterior skin consists of four layers of unidirectional AS4/3501-6 tape aligned in the $\pm 45°$ directions with respect to the 0° reference of the leading and trailing edges of the spoiler. It has a full-depth honeycomb core of 4.8 mm ($\frac{3}{16}$ in.) hexagonal cell size. Most of the in-service damage is expected to consist of small punctures to the 0.51 mm (0.020 in.) facings or dings in the trailing edge that will cause local delaminations. There also might be some surface bruising that crushes the honeycomb core without damaging the facesheets. If any damage is not too close to the fitting or front spar, there is no limit to the size of the damaged area that may be repaired structurally.

Co-cured repairs using the original composite material are not encouraged, because of the high probability that the 450 K (350 °F) cure would react adversely with any moisture that may have been absorbed by the laminate or collected in the cells. No repairs should be performed above 394 K (250 °F), and the range of 355 to 366 K (180 to 200 °F) is preferred.Those restrictions leave the options of repairing by using either a patch of precured tape made to the original specifications or a wet lay-up with three layers of 0.21 mm (0.0083 in.) thick 3PW AS4 woven graphite fabric impregnated with a resin (e.g., EA-956 or Ciba-Geigy 1300) that cures at room temperature, but is usually postcured at 355 to 366 K (180 to 200 °F). The initial cure may also be accelerated at the same temperature to reduce the elapsed time for repair. These repairs are illustrated in Fig. 17 and 18.

The precured patch could be used for any size damage; whereas the wet lay-up patch would be preferred only when cosmetic considerations are important. Large co-cured patches tend to be very heavy, particularly if potting compound is used to fill the core cells. The compound would not be necessary, however, if the spoiler was removed from the aircraft and the patch cured with the repaired skin facing down. The mechanical properties of co-cured composite facesheets are inherently inferior to those of precured facesheets, even on a per-ply basis that allows for the additional resin needed to prevent pinholes; therefore, two layers of 0.25 mm (0.010 in.) graphite cloth would not suffice in this case. Naturally, the repair fibers would be oriented in the same $\pm 45°$ directions as in the parent laminate. The technique of using a thin 0.13 mm (0.005 in.) 120-weave glass surfacing ply to facilitate sanding and painting is shown in Fig. 18.

While on the subject of sanding, it is appropriate to remind the reader of the difficulties associated with sanding Kevlar fibers. Kevlar tends to break up into fuzzy balls, rather than break off smoothly the way glass and graphite fibers do. For that reason, and because of the difficulty of impregnating Kevlar fabric, it is customary to use fiberglass repairs for Kevlar panels.

The execution of a structurally adequate, perfectly flush repair for honeycomb skins is shown in Fig. 19. With the appropriate overlaps, this repair would work for either the MD-80 spoilers or the MD-80 rudder skins. Obviously, such a repair would be used infrequently, because of the

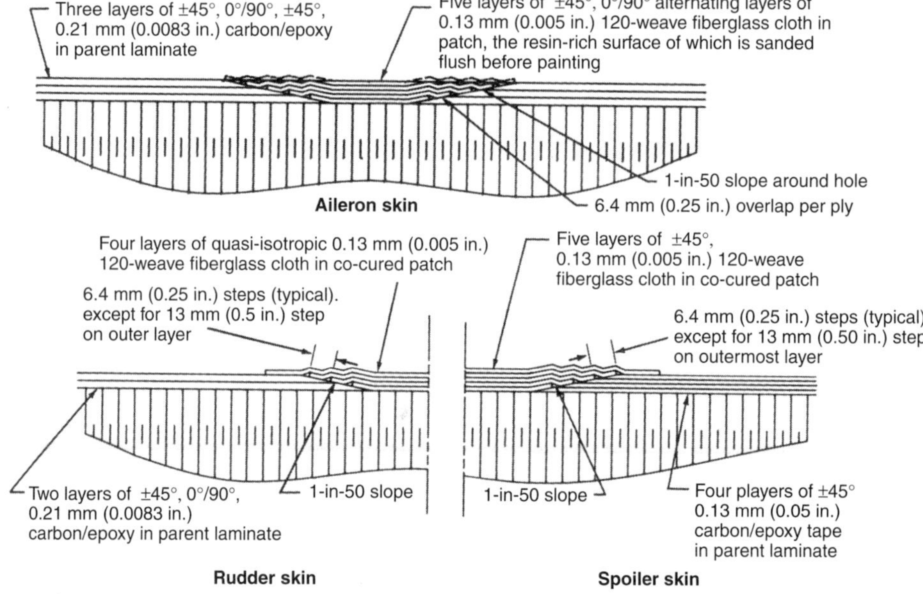

Fig. 22 Cosmetic repairs of minor damage to MD-80 composite control surfaces

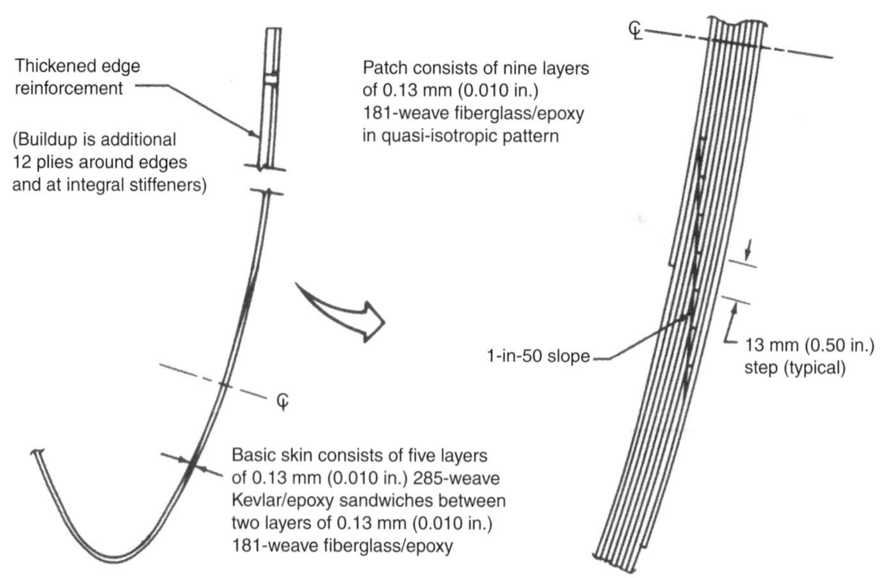

Fig. 23 Repair of MD-80 extended flap hinge fairings

complexity, and would not be used at all on the (full-depth honeycomb) aileron for which there is no unexposed surface on which to conceal the buildup on the other skin. Its greatest applicability would seem to be for the repair of large-area damage suffered by a compound-curved wing/fuselage fillet, tail cone, or radome for which no reference shape is available other than a plaster splash taken from a spare part. Even for those shapes, if the inner skin is undamaged, it is common for airlines to reconstruct the damaged part from the inside out and to tolerate the substantial additional finishing required, rather than create an exterior mold surface.

The skin of the MD-80 graphite/epoxy rudder is a double-skin, Nomex-honeycomb-cored panel having two layers of 0.21 mm (0.0083 in.) thick plain-weave AS4/3501-6 graphite/epoxy woven fabric on each side. One layer has a 0°/90° orientation, and the other is at ±45° to the 0° spanwise reference axis. The composite skins are thus quasi-isotropic, and a repair of the same kind could be oriented in any direction, provided that the two individual layers are rotated 45° with respect to each other. Nevertheless, it is customary to match the original fiber orientations, particularly for large repairs.

There is a possibility that the outside skin will be covered by a thin fiberglass layer, as part of a flame sprayed lightning-strike protection system. This is not shown here, because it would not be considered structural.

Because the sides of the MD-80 rudder are essentially flat, it would also be possible to perform repairs using two-ply (0°/90° and ±45°) precured skins bonded with a room-temperature curing adhesive that would subsequently be postcured. The details of such a repair are shown in Fig. 20. Even though the panel appears to be thermally unbalanced, it will not warp, because each cloth layer is symmetric about its midplane, and the thermal characteristics are identical in all in-plane directions. Figure 20 shows repairs performed to both skins, not because it is mandatory for precured repairs, but because precured repairs are more likely to be used for large areas of damage, and they, in turn, are likely to be associated with the puncture of both thin and thick skins.

The extent of such precured patch repair work is limited only by the possibility of its intruding into the reinforced areas around the spars and rib caps. Were a relatively large area (more than about 0.3 m, or 12 in., in diameter) to be repaired using the wet lay-up technique, it would be prudent to add one additional layer of graphite fabric—in the ±45° direction, because the primary load is in torsion due to the fact that the mechanical properties of such laminates will be inferior to those of the original laminate manufactured in an autoclave. The extra layer could be omitted, if justified by an examination of the stress levels in any area of specific concern, with a stronger case for doing so existing near the top of the rudder rather than near the bottom where it is actuated.

The composite ailerons on the MD-80 are of full-depth honeycomb construction, except for the inboard end that is unreinforced skin in the area through which the push-rods pass to the inboard tab. (The push-rods to the outboard tab are contained in hollow external fairings.) The facings on the skin consist of three layers of AS4/3501-6 graphite/epoxy 0.21 mm (0.0083 in.) thick plain weave cloth in the (±45°, 0°/90°, ±45°) directions, with the 0° reference being spanwise. Both wet lay-up and precured patches could be used to repair these skins, with typical dimensions shown in Fig. 21. Note that in this case, the skin facings are not quasi-isotropic, and it is important that the patch fiber orientations match those in the parent material. Perfectly flush repairs are not desirable, except possibly for small cosmetic fiberglass repairs of the form shown in Fig. 22. The corresponding cosmetic (and waterproofing) repairs on the thinner facings of the rudder and spoiler should have one 0.13 mm (0.005 in.) layer of fiberglass outside the loft surface to ensure adequate bonding. Even for the aileron skin, the semiflush nonstructural repair is structurally preferable.

If a composite elevator is produced for the MD-80, it will have much the same multirib, postbuckled (tension-field) skin design that has given such trouble-free service on about a dozen DC-10 rudders in flight-service evaluation. With tail-mounted engines, it is very important to maximize the weight savings associated with any redesign of the elevator. In addition, nonhoneycomb designs are preferred for mass-balanced control surfaces, because they preclude water from collecting in undrainable cavities. The ribs would be located on a 125 to 150 mm (5 to 6 in.) pitch, and the skin would be made of seven layers of 0.13 mm (0.005 in.) graphite/epoxy unidirectional tape in a [0°, +45°, –45°,

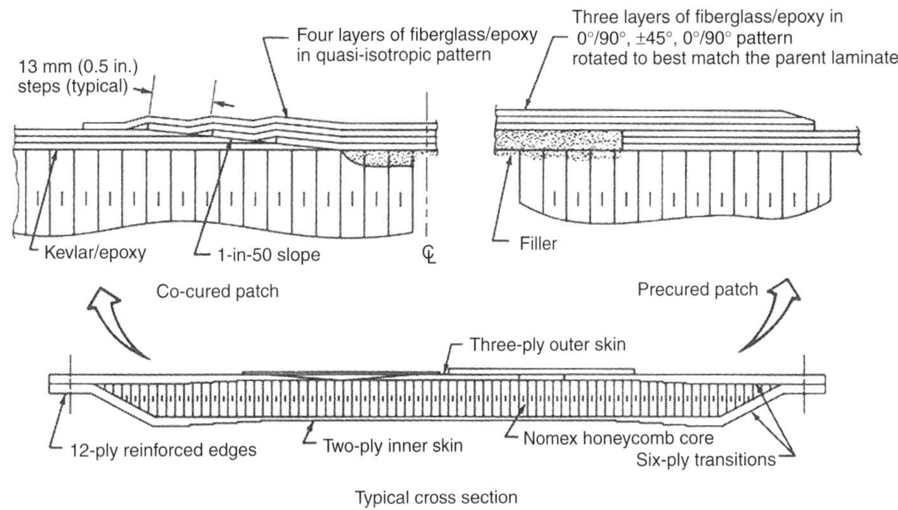

Fig. 24 Repair of MD-80 Kevlar/epoxy wing trailing-edge panels

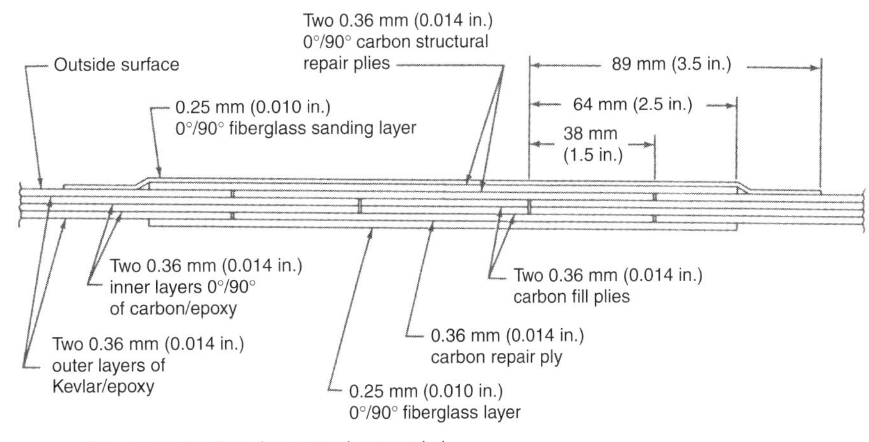

Fig. 25 Repair of Kevlar-graphite/epoxy MD-80 engine cowl

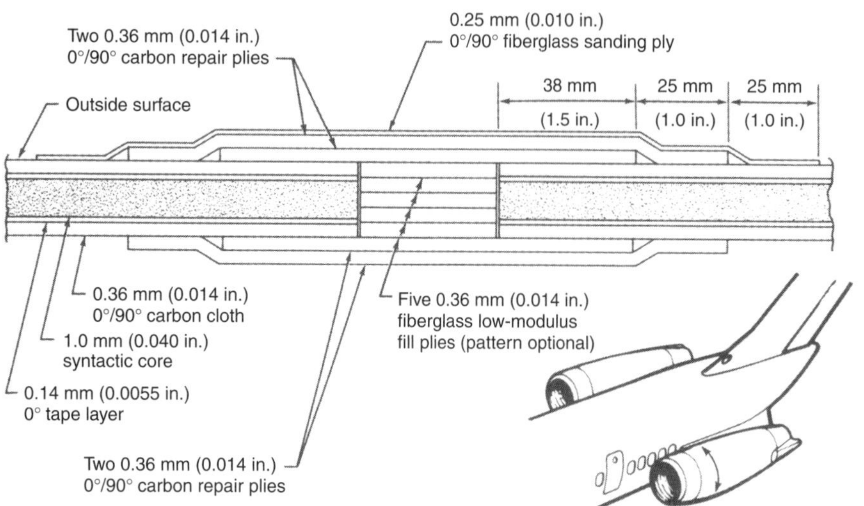

Fig. 26 Repair of syntactic-core graphite/epoxy MD-80 engine cowl

90°, –45°, +45°, 0°] pattern, with the 0° reference again being spanwise. The DC-10 upper-aft-rudder skins are the same, except that the chordwise (90°) layer is not distributed uniformly, but concentrated in a narrow double layer as part of each rib cap.

The relatively few repairs actually performed on the DC-10 rudder skins have been made with slightly thicker patches of quasi-isotropic wet lay-up graphite fabric, using a semi-flush exterior patch over a 1-in-50 scarf slope. A steeper-than-normal slope could be justified by the proximity of a spar cap containing bolt holes and, therefore, operating at a reduced strain level. Test samples proved satisfactory at a slope of 1-in-50, as reported in Ref 11, but similar trials with a 1-in-30 slope failed unacceptably in the bonded joint. Larger damage could easily be repaired by using a properly oriented precured patch made from unidirectional tape and having a uniform bonded overlap of 38 mm (1.5 in.) all around.

The low-drag extended flap hinge fairings for the MD-80 are simple solid laminates made from basically five layers of Kevlar/epoxy cloth sandwiched between fiberglass/epoxy outer and inner faces. The fairings have co-cured local buildups serving as edge reinforcements and transverse stiffeners; all attachments pass through locally reinforced areas. The compound-curved shape renders the use of precured patches impractical, although both scarfed and uniform co-cured patches could be suitable. A repair concept for the unreinforced skin areas of this component is shown in Fig. 23. It should be noted that not only should the outer surface be smooth for low drag, there are some areas on the inner surface that cannot be built up excessively, because they would interfere with the metallic flap support structure.

The more-recently delivered MD-80s have had many of the older fiberglass/epoxy fairings replaced by Kevlar/epoxy ones, particularly on the wing trailing edges and the wing root fillets. The typical wing trailing-edge panel construction consists of three layers of 0.25 mm (0.010 in.) 285-weave (4-harness) Kevlar cloth on the outside and two layers on the inside of the Nomex honeycomb cells. Because the direction of the fibers is not controlled on the drawings for these lightly loaded covers, reference must be made to the actual part in the area surrounding the damage. Typical basic repairs for such components are shown in Fig. 24. The greatest problem with repairing in this manner is in sanding the scarf angle accurately. A simple exterior three-ply patch, while not as aesthetically pleasing, may be considered far more practical.

In an attempt to avoid the problem of sanding Kevlar, the original MD-80 composite engine cowl repair uses a stepped-lap patch of the type shown in Fig. 25. This requires that the parent material be peeled apart and cut back ply-by-ply, without ever cutting into the underlying layer(s). Such an operation is felt to be risky for normal use, and the second nacelle design (with syntactic core) is to be repaired using the simpler double-lap patch shown in Fig. 26. This also permits the repair of larger skin damage than would the more restrictive method shown in Fig. 25 which requires the removal of a considerable amount of previously undamaged material without the patch spreading too close to hinge or latch areas. Unfortunately, because of regulations requiring that engine cowls withstand specific burn tests, it is not possible to authorize the structurally improved repairs retroactively without first verifying that they meet other requirements also.

REFERENCES

1. L.J. Hart-Smith, "The Design of Repairable Advanced Composite Structures," Douglas Aircraft Company Paper 7550, presented at Society of Automotive Engineers Aerospace Technology Conf., 14–17 Oct 1985 (Long Beach, CA)
2. L.J. Hart-Smith, "Design Details for Adhesively Bonded Repairs of Fibrous Composite Structures," Douglas Aircraft Company Paper 7637, presented at 31st National Society for the Advancement of Material & Process Engineering Symposium and Exhibition, 8–10 April 1986 (Las Vegas, NV)
3. L.J. Hart-Smith, "Designing with Advanced Fibrous Composites," Douglas Aircraft Company Paper 8011, presented at the Australian Bicentennial International Congress in Mechanical Engineering, 8–13 May 1988 (Brisbane)
4. L.J. Hart-Smith, "Innovative Concepts for the Design and Manufacture of Secondary Composite Aircraft Structures," Douglas Aircraft Company Paper MDC 93K0081, presented at the Fifth Australian Aeronautical Conf., 13–15 Sept 1993 (Melbourne)
5. M. Klotzsche et al., "ACEE Composite Structures Technology," papers by Douglas Aircraft Company, NASA Contractor Report 172359, presented to NASA Oral Review on ACEE Composites Programs, Aug 1984 (Seattle, WA)
6. W.D. Nelson, B.L. Bunin, and L.J. Hart-Smith, "Critical Joints in Large Composite Aircraft Structure," Douglas Aircraft Company Paper 7266, presented to Sixth Conf. on Fibrous Composites in Structural Design, Jan 1983 (New Orleans, LA)
7. L.J. Hart-Smith, "Design and Analysis of Bolted and Riveted Joints in Fibrous Composite Structures," Douglas Aircraft Company Paper 7475, to be published in *Joining Fiber Reinforced Plastics*, F.L. Matthews, Ed., Elsevier Applied Science, Essex, England
8. L.J. Hart-Smith, "Lessons Learned from the DC-10 Graphite/Epoxy Rudder Program," Society of Automotive Engineers, Trans. 861675, 1986
9. L.J. Hart-Smith, "Design Methodology for Bonded-Bolted Composite Joints," Air Force Wright Aeronautical Laboratories TR-81-3154, Feb 1982
10. L.J. Hart-Smith, "Bonded-Bolted Composite Joints," Douglas Aircraft Company Paper 7398, presented to American Institute of Aeronautics and Astronautics/American Society of Mechanical Engineers/American Society of Civil Engineers/American Helicopter Society 25th Structures, Structural Dynamics and Materials Conference, May 1984 (Palm Springs, CA)
11. B.R. Fox, "Flight Service Program for Advanced Composite Rudders on Transport Aircraft," Douglas Aircraft Company Ninth Annual Summary Report to NASA Langley Research Center, Contract NASI-12954, Sept 1985

Repair Engineering and Design Considerations

Rikard B. Heslehurst, Australian Defence Force Academy
Mark S. Forte, U.S. Air Force Research Laboratory

Repair of advanced composite structures is a relatively new area of engineering design and analysis. Repair engineering requires a thorough understanding of composite structural mechanics and structural joining of composites and metal structures. These two aspects, in combination with other considerations, such as damage removal, surface preparation, and repair fabrication, require a clearly defined engineering process. The level of repair will be determined by such factors as damage criticality, operational requirements, and repair station capabilities. All of these add up to a unique repair for most composite structural damage restoration.

Figure 1 illustrates an example of the repair application steps for a composite sandwich structure. The damaged region is mapped out in Fig. 1(a). Then the damage is removed and the surface is prepared for a scarf repair scheme; Fig. 1(b) shows the removed core plug and scarfed skin. The replacement core plug is installed (Fig. 1c) and the repair plies are cured in place (Fig. 1d).

Types of Repairs to Composite Structures

There are three typical repair types for composite structures. The first is a temporary repair that essentially maintains aerodynamic smoothness or prevents the damaging environment from entering the damaged site. For relatively thin structures, adhesively bonded repair patches are likely to be used because they are structurally efficient. Where thick, primary structures are to be repaired, bolted repair patches are likely choices. Although they are not necessarily structurally efficient, bolted joints are economical for repair over all size constraints. An example of each repair type is shown in Fig. 2, 3, and 4.

Repair design in each of the three design schemes is based on the specific requirements of the repair medium. The fundamental analysis for each type is summarized as follows:

Temporary Repairs. Temporary repairs do not specifically require substantial analysis. The design requirements are based on minor structural damage. The temporary repair should be designed so that it does not attract load into itself; therefore, it should be made from a material with a relatively low stiffness.

Adhesively Bonded Repairs. Adhesively bonded repairs are designed so the adhesive shear and peeling strengths and interlaminar strengths of the composite are not critical. Special attention is directed to surface preparation in the design application. However, for the design analysis of adhesively bonded repairs, complete adhesive material properties are required.

Bolted Repairs. The analysis of mechanically fastened repairs in composite structures will require specific information on the composite laminate material structural or orthotropic properties for both on-axes and off-axes. The need to develop bearing-strength properties for the composite laminate is of particular interest.

Repair Requirements

Table 1 lists general design requirements and considerations for the repair of composite struc-

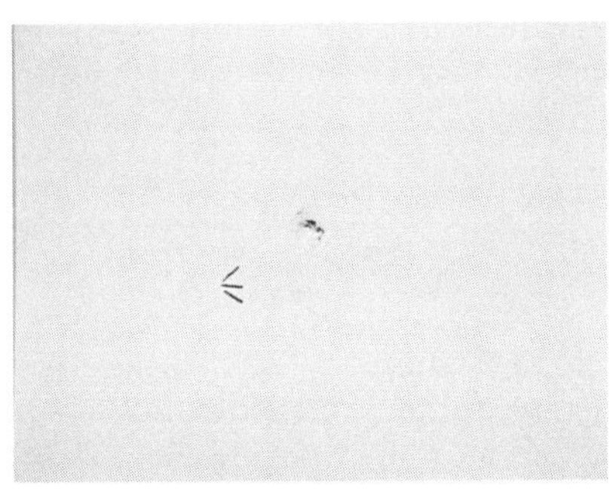

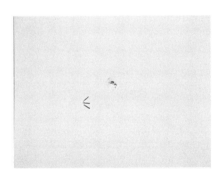

(a) Damaged region

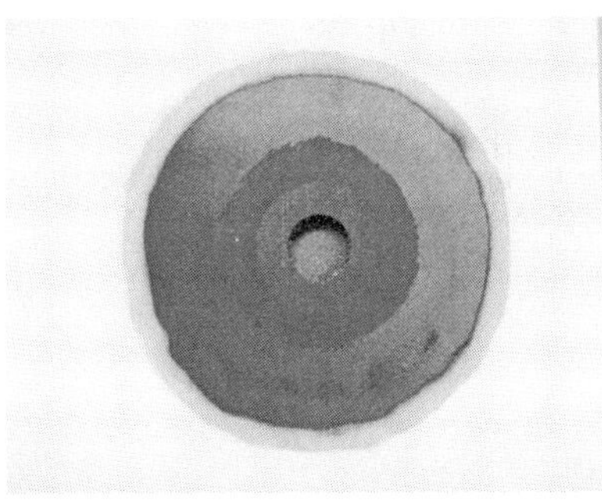

(b) Damaged removed

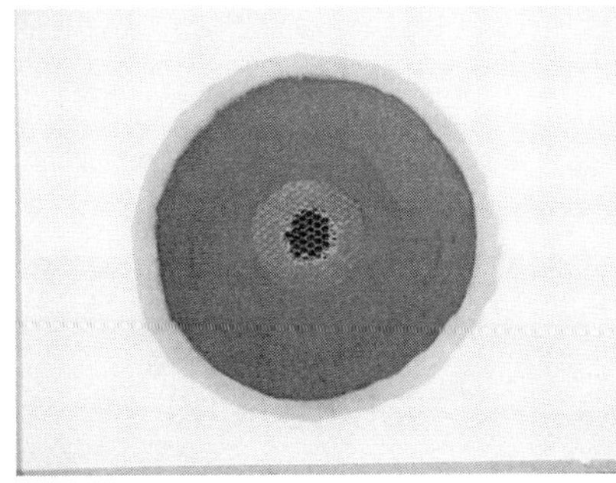

(c) Replacement core plug

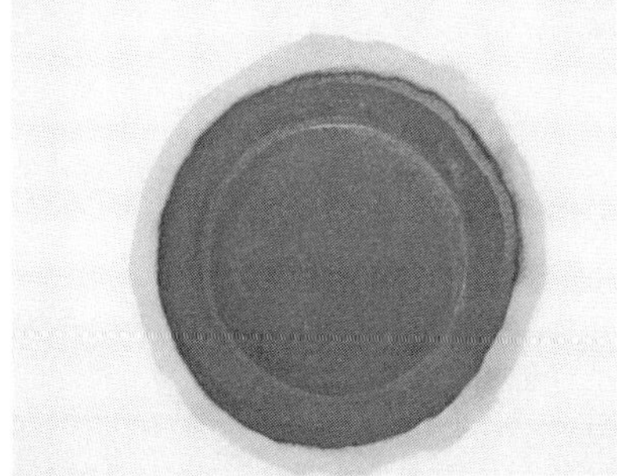

(d) Repair plies

Fig. 1 Example of a repair to a sandwich structure. See text for discussion.

tures. Several of these are described subsequently in greater detail.

Static Strength and Stability. Any repair must be capable of supporting the design loads applied to the original structure. There are two major aspects:

- *Strength Restoration:* The first question to ask is if full strength restoration is required. The answer is determined from the results of damage stress analysis.
- *Stability Requirements*: The greatest concerns in many of the damaged structures are instability under compressive loading and restoration of structural stiffness. The damage analysis will indicate where structural instability exists. The repair design is then focused on how to overcome this instability.

Repair Durability. Any repair designed to restore aircraft to flying condition is generally expected to remain an integral part of the airframe for the remaining service life of the craft (exceptions are rapid-action or battle-damage type repairs). Durability of the repair scheme must consider the following in its design phase:

- Fatigue loading of the structure and its effects on bolted and bonded joints, damage growth, and monitoring for airworthiness
- Corrosion of components where dissimilar materials have been used in the repair and maintenance of corrosion protection precautions
- Environmental degradation of resin-system-based repairs, particularly via moisture absorption and hot or wet environments.

Stiffness Requirements. In aircraft where lightweight structures are an essential design requirement, stiffness is often more critical than strength. Likewise, repaired structures must maintain the integrity of structural stiffness. The following requirements must be considered in a stiffness-critical repair design:

- Deflection limitations of flying surfaces, such as wings and flight controls, are based on aerodynamic and performance requirements of the aircraft, repair should not unduly alter the flying characteristics of the aircraft.
- Flutter and other aeroelasticity effects limit the design of a repair so that the repair scheme stiffness should be essentially equal to that of the parent structure.
- Load path variations are undesirable in any structure. As a general rule, the repair area stiffness should match that of the parent structure, so as not to change the load path significantly.

Aerodynamic Smoothness. Aerodynamic smoothness is an important consideration when maximum speed or fuel efficiency is required. Those parts of the aircraft that require good aerodynamic smoothness, that is, leading edges and locations where the boundary layer is laminar, must have flush or very thin external patch repair schemes. These repair types are based on local capabilities in manufacturing techniques, the effects of performance degradation, repair size, and the possible effects of multiple damage sites.

Weight and Balance. The size of the repair and the local changes in weight can be insignificant to the total component weight, but in weight-sensitive structures such as flight controls, the effect on the mass balance can be highly significant. The effective change in local weight must be controlled and kept within defined limits; in some cases, component rebalancing may be necessary.

Operational Temperature. The operating temperature influences the selection of repair materials, particularly adhesives and composite resins. Materials that maintain adequate properties within the required operational temperature range must be selected. The combination of extreme temperatures with environmental exposure, the hot and wet condition, is the critical design condition for the repair.

Environmental Effects. Composite and adhesively bonded joints are prone to property degradation when exposed to various environments, in particular, to fluids and to thermal cycling. Absorbed moisture is known to have major long-term concerns. Durability of the repair design must consider environmental aging.

Related On-Board Aircraft Systems. The repair design must also be compatible with onboard aircraft systems. Such onboard aircraft systems include the following:

- *Fuel System*: In many aircraft, the fuel is carried within the wing structure as a "wet wing." Therefore, any repair to wing skins, which are in direct contact with the fuel system, must seal the fuel tank, cater for out-of-plane fuel pressure forces, and not contaminate the fuel system during the repair process.
- *Lightning Protection*: If electrical conductivity of the parent structure is required for lightning protection, then the repair must also incorporate the same degree of electrical conductivity.
- *Mechanical System Operation*: Any component that is required to move during aircraft operations or is in close proximity to a moving component that is subsequently repaired must not impede component operation; for example, repair of a retracting flap must provide adequate retraction clearance.

Table 1 Requirements and considerations for repair of composites

Repair requirement or consideration	Important factors
Static strength and stability	Full versus partial strength restoration
	Stability requirements
Repair durability	Fatigue loading
	Corrosion
	Environmental degradation
Stiffness requirements	Deflection limitations
	Flutter and other aeroelasticity effects
	Load path variations
Aerodynamic smoothness	Manufacturing techniques
	Performance degradation
Weight and balance	Size of the repair
	Mass balance effect
Operational temperature	Low and high temperature requirements
	Temperature effects
Environmental effects	Types of exposure
	Effects to epoxy resins
Related on-board aircraft systems	Fuel system sealing
	Lightning protection
	Mechanical system operation
Costs and scheduling	Downtime
	Facilities, equipment and materials
	Personnel skill levels
	Materials handling
Low observable characteristics	Radar cross section
	Laser cross section

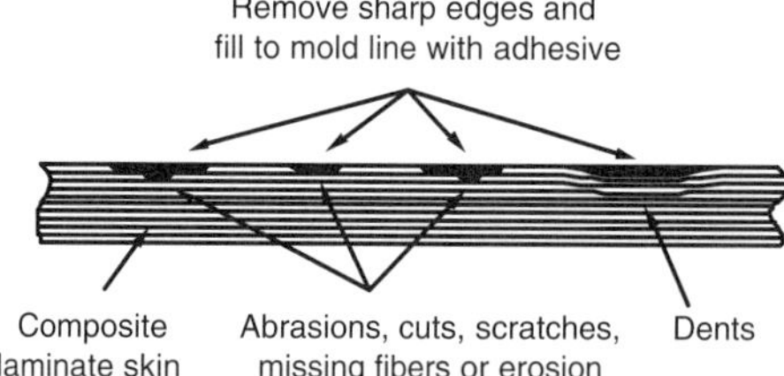

Fig. 2 Temporary or minor repair to a composite laminate

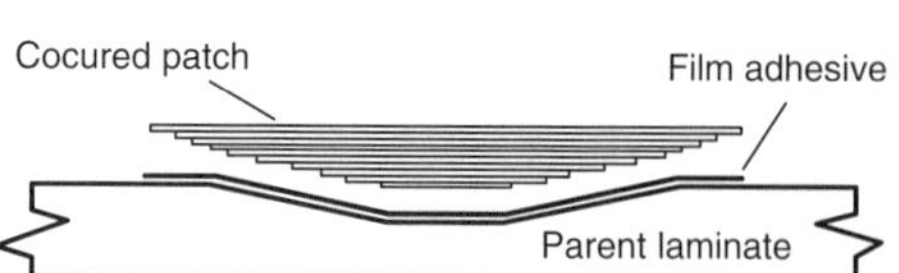

Fig. 3 Adhesively bonded repair to a composite laminate

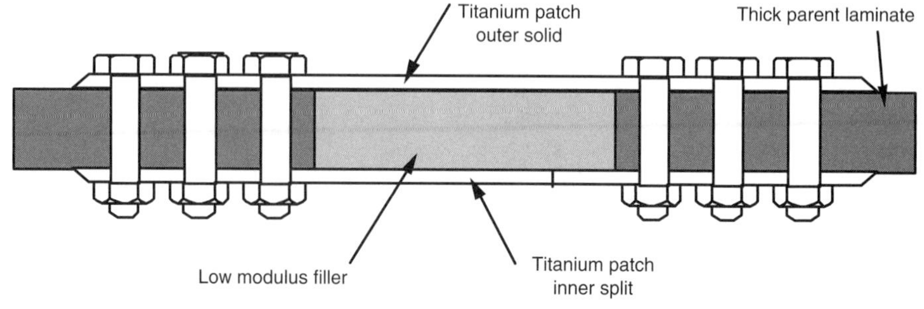

Fig. 4 Bolted repair to a composite laminate

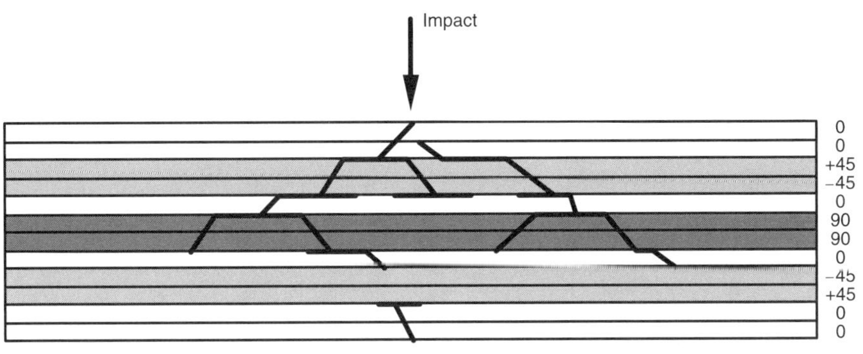

Fig. 5 Impact damage barely visible on the surface but showing extensive subsurface delaminations

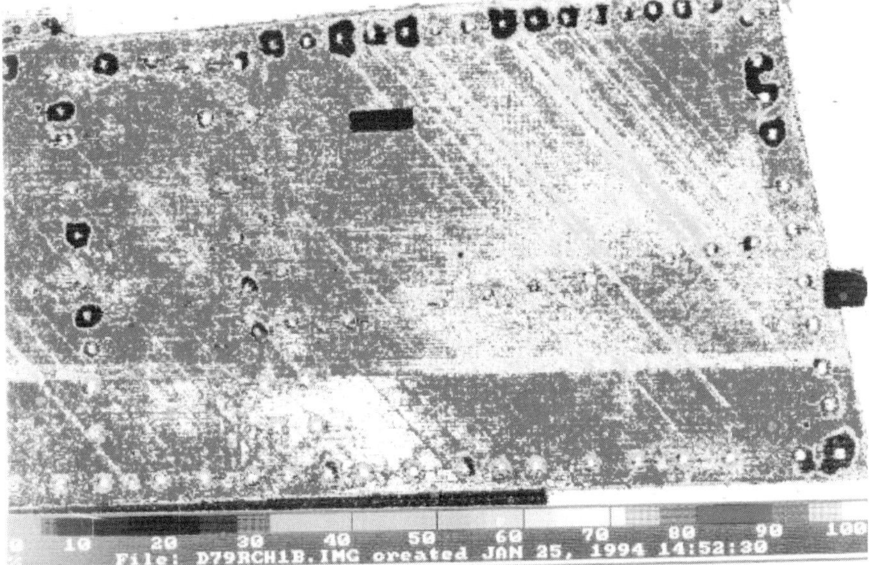

Fig. 6 C-scan of a composite panel with fastener hole delaminations

Costs and Scheduling. Repair and repair design result in aircraft downtime and increased operating expenses. However, experience has shown that it is less expensive to repair than replace, given that appropriate facilities and adequate personnel skilled to do the repair.

Low Observable Characteristics. An important attribute for military aircraft is reduced radar cross section (RCS), which is a major contributor to low observable characteristics of the aircraft. If the aircraft is a stealth type by design, then repairs must be designed to maintain the mold line and not have reflective corners.

Considerations Prior to, During, and After Repair Action

The recommended engineering approach to more effectively restore structural integrity to damaged composite components entails a ten-step methodology. This methodology is based on the current level of damage stress and the damage tolerance required in structural strength and stiffness restoration of a repair scheme. The ten steps are described below.

Step 1: Find the Damage. The location of the composite structure damage is found by either a visual inspection of the external surface of the component or through the inadequate performance or structural behavior. This step has significant implications for the damage tolerance of the composite structure. Internally hidden damage to a composite structure does not show itself readily on the surface (Fig. 5). Nonvisible or barely visible impact damage can result in little evidence on the structural surface but significant internal damage in the form of delaminations. A good understanding of the likely sites of potential damage is essential in locating such damage. The common tap hammer test provides an acceptable method for finding near-surface damage.

Step 2: Assess the Extent of Damage. Following the visual inspection or observation, a more sophisticated nondestructive inspection (NDI) technique is used to determine the physical geometry of the damage state (see the article "Nondestructive Testing" in this Volume). The appropriately selected NDI technique will determine the size, shape, and depth of damage. Because composite laminates are known to have damage hidden beneath the surface, the NDI techniques applied will exhibit the true extent of the damage. A typical C-scan result is shown in Fig. 6. In this figure, the details of delaminations around fastener holes can be scrutinized.

Step 3: Analyze the Damage Stress State. Before the most effective repair scheme can be designed, the damage stress state must be evaluated. This analysis will determine the type of repair scheme to be designed for the damage. From the calculated stress state, the residual structural strength can be compared against the design allowable or ultimate strength. Hence, the structural integrity or the loss of damage tolerance can be ascertained. The details of the damage stress analysis are discussed in Ref 1–4. A brief summary is provided later in this article.

Step 4: Design the Repair Scheme. The repair-scheme design is typically one of three generic repair design categories. The generic repair categories are non-structural, semi-structural, or full-strength repair schemes. Each of these three generic repair schemes is illustrated in Fig. 7, 8, and 9, respectively. The various repair designs are generically the same, but each design should be analyzed to determine its adequacy. The de-

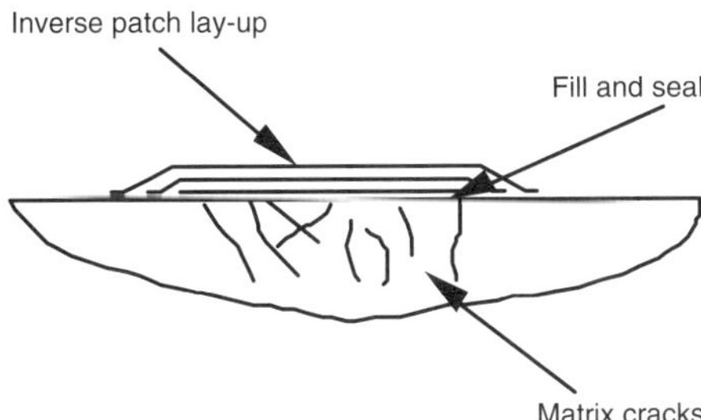

Fig. 7 Doubler patch installation over matrix cracking for non-structural repairs

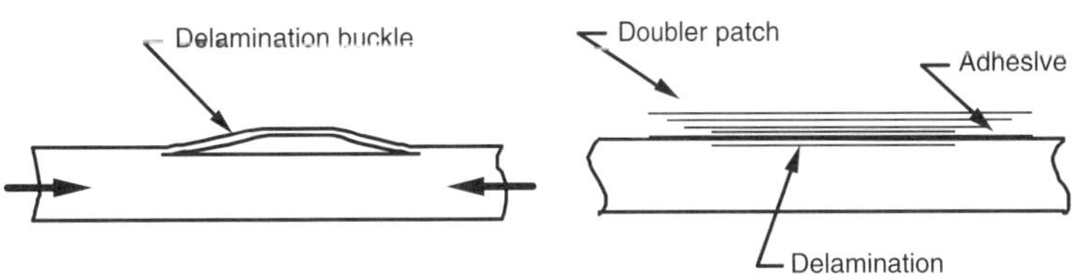

Fig. 8 Doubler patch installation over delamination for semistructural repairs

sign variables are the repair-ply configuration and thickness and the overlap length. Simple repair design techniques are discussed in Ref 5–9.

Step 5: Remove the Damage and Prepare the Component for Repair. Using standard composite machining techniques, the damage is removed (Fig. 1b). If a hole is produced, then simple geometric shapes should be used, such as holes or rounded rectangles. The preparation of the structure for repair application involves moisture removal and surface preparation for repair patch bonding. Both of these steps are crucial to ensure complete repair scheme structural integrity.

Step 6: Fabricate the Repair Scheme. To ensure that the repair patch meets material property specifications, the materials and fabrication process used must be to the appropriate engineering standards. Precured autoclave patches are preferred; however, if a vacuum bagging technique without positive pressure cures the patches, strength properties must be reduced accordingly.

Step 7: Apply the Repair Scheme. Whether the repair scheme is cured in place (co-bonded) or secondarily bonded, three aspects are critical. First, surface preparation is most important for bondline structural integrity; also, cure temperature and time of cure must be within specified limits. The cure profile requires careful understanding, as improper curing can have major consequences.

Step 8: Conduct a Post-Repair Inspection of the Repair Scheme. A quality assurance check by an appropriate NDI method will identify any apparent repair scheme deficiencies. At the least, a visual inspection of adhesive fillet flow and an acoustic-hammer tap test should be done to indicate gross defects.

Step 9: Document the Repair Scheme. Repair documentation is required of repair management and design-certification procedures. Flight-critical structural repairs must have supportive documentation to verify repair structural integrity and mass-balance effects. Multisite-damage concerns necessitate engineering management of the component repair history.

Step 10: Monitor the Repair Zone. Due to material and fabrication anomalies and/or unknown stress states around the repaired region, the repair scheme and parent structure should be regularly monitored for ongoing validation.

Validation and Certification of Repairs

The relative infancy of composite-material application in aircraft structures and the growing use of adhesive bonding in primary structures have caught most aircraft operators by surprise. Design and manufacturing techniques for advanced composite structures have advanced by leaps and bounds, but, unfortunately, corresponding repair and maintenance techniques have lagged behind.

Because of this sudden increase and the importance of the maintenance and integrity of composite structure repair, management activities have to take a new thrust. All areas of the repair activity need detailed managing. This is particularly true with a developing composite structural repair capability. However, because of rapidly growing technology, ongoing attention for the improvement of current capabilities needs a concerted management effort.

Certification and structural worthiness of composite structures in the manufacturing area is still developing, and only a few rules have been formulated by the structural-worthiness authorities. In the repair and maintenance fields, there are no defined requirements to certify repairs or define what constitutes structural worthiness. The following discussion is a general review of certification and structural worthiness requirements for manufacture and design of composite structures. These requirements are directly related to the repair and maintenance of composite structures.

Management

Requirements for an Effective Repair Capability. The development of an effective composite structural repair capability needs to address the following requirements:

- Engineering damage assessment, analysis, and repair design skills
- Engineer and repair technician training, which includes maintaining learned skills
- Repair station quality control and assurance
- Repair station facilities
- Repair management and certification procedures
- Personal safety and environmental health policy

Some of these requirements are discussed in more detail in the following paragraphs. The article "Maintainability Issues" in the Section "Product Reliability, Maintainability, and Repair" of this Handbook also discusses these repair requirements.

Engineer and Technician Training. The training of engineers and technicians in repair of composite structures is of the utmost importance. Both engineers and technicians must understand the issues in the structural mechanics, limitations and influencing factors of composite materials. They are also required to have a very thorough appreciation of the repair process issues discussed earlier. Other issues that are necessary for engineers and technicians to understand are as follows:

- Materials handling
- Damage removal and surface pretreatment requirements and methods
- Repair fabrication requirements
- Repair application methods
- Quality control and assurance of the repair process and finished product
- Continuation training to keep pace with the rapidly changing technology
- Regular work in the repair procedures to maintain learned skills

Repair Station Facilities. The requirements of any composite structure repair station depend on the level of repair to be undertaken. The three typical levels of repair activity, operation-level maintenance (OLM), intermediate-level maintenance (ILM), and depot or deeper-level maintenance (DLM), have different composite-structure repair requirements, outlined as follows:

Operation-Level Maintenance. Limited repair action is typically undertaken at the OLM facility. Such activities would include preliminary NDI and simple cosmetic repairs. Minimal equipment, material storage, and infrastructure facilities are required.

Intermediate-Level Maintenance. A significantly greater level of repair activity is expected at ILM. Vacuum sources for full-flow and local-vacuum extraction of contaminants and air supply for tools and breathing equipment are required in the damage removal process. In a separate clean room with temperature and humidity controls as well as positive pressure, vacuum bag/heater blanket curing equipment are required. Cold-storage facilities for prepreg and adhesive materials are essential. Prior to repair, some composite structures may need to have absorbed moisture removed; a drying room may be required. More sophisticated NDI equipment is required for ILM than for OLM.

Depot Level Maintenance. In addition to the requirements of an ILM facility, DLM facilities also require autoclaves and/or heated platen

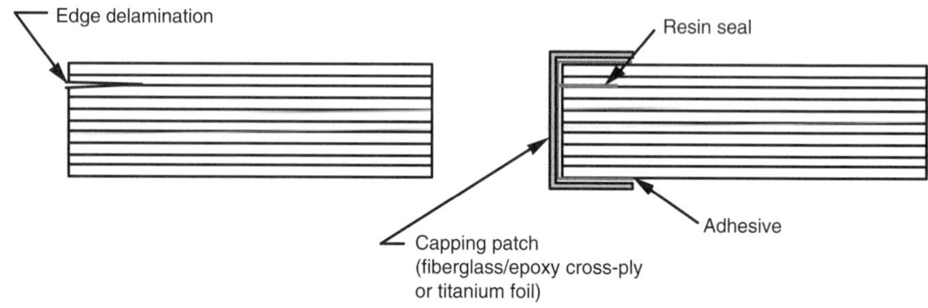

Fig. 9 Out-of-plane reinforcing capping patch over edge delamination

pressing, honeycomb profilers, prepreg cutters, anodizing process tanks, and C-scan facilities.

Repair Validation

To ensure that the repaired composite components are structurally sound, repair validation is required. The driving needs for repair validation are the rapid technological changes that occur in composite structure design, design capabilities, and new materials substantiation. Furthermore, composite components in primary loaded structures have only had a limited life cycle, so repair tracking is critical in the ongoing validation of repair methods and techniques. Finally, multisite damage is only beginning to be understood in metal structures; in composite structures, the interaction with neighboring repairs is not yet well understood. The monitoring of damage growth will also provide a better understanding of repair limits and damage criticality.

Certification

Structural Design Certification. The issues in structural design certification are static loads and margins of factors, static-strength substantiation, cyclic loading, impact resistance and damage development, repair design and strength restoration, erosion resistance, stiffness variations, and damage-inspection capabilities.

Elements of Certification for Composite Structures. The elements for certifying composite structures and their subsequent repairs are as follows:

- Design criteria (stiffness, strength, or other)
- Analysis requirements and capabilities
- Design allowables, including static, fatigue, and damage tolerance with environment and scatter factors
- Design/configuration development
- Quality control and quality assurance from receipt of materials through to completed task
- Verification testing for static, fatigue, and damage tolerance properties
- Other considerations, including lightning, flammability, individual component tracking, inspection, and repair

Structural Worthiness Considerations

The main concerns here are the proper allowance for environmental effects (moisture and temperature) on the static and fatigue properties of composite structures and their repair, and the data scatter, which is greater than that of metals (improving for static properties). The use of A-allowable or B-allowable properties is defined for a limited number of structural composites in MIL-HDBK-17. A significantly extensive testing program is called for to allow for new structural composites to become structurally certified. Included in the certification requirements are the curing conditions and other process variables.

Design Guidelines

Designing a repair first requires analyzing the damage and then analyzing possible strategies for making a repair.

Damage Analysis

The repair scheme developed for a damage-stress state can be based on the loss of structural integrity. The damage-stress state can be examined by generalizing the damage into one of four categories. Table 2 provides a summary of these generalized damage types and how they typically affect the structural integrity of the composite component. The size of the damage does play a key role in the degree of degradation.

Core Damage. Damage to the core material must be very substantial to result in a significant loss of structural integrity. The skin material is usually damaged with fiber fracture. The fiber fracture will become the dominant damage type. Core-to-skin separation can be more common. The resulting disbond will cause concern under compression or in-plane shear loading. Loss of stiffness integrity due to a disbond can be analyzed by the same method as that used for delaminations.

Intralaminar Matrix Cracks. Intralaminar matrix cracks in composite structures are confined to those cracks within a ply or lamina. These intralaminar cracks tend to be transverse to the fiber direction and terminate at the ply boundaries. Crazing and heat damage are examples of matrix cracks. Local stiffness loss is attributed to intralaminar matrix cracks. Local loss of stiffness can easily be evaluated by using a degraded value of the matrix stiffness and strength properties of the individual ply effect. This value, generally about a 60 to 80% reduction, can be applied directly to the ply transverse properties or used in micromechanics analysis and then used in any of the structural analysis techniques. If the effect of stiffness reduction is severe, particularly under compressive loads and fatigue cycling, then delaminations may be initiated. If matrix cracks are present with delaminations or fractured fibers, their influence becomes insignificant. Repair of matrix cracks is done by using a low-viscosity resin to fill the surface cracks and then applying a surface patch to prevent moisture absorption and restore any loss of local stiffness (Fig. 7). Always ensure that the repair patch has a stiffness that is less than or equal to that of the parent laminate. A stiffer patch will attract load to the damaged area. The repair region should be inspected at each major service or at regular intervals to determine if the crack density has grown and/or delaminations have been initiated. Removing the matrix cracks by cutting out the damage and therefore removing the fibers will do more damage and can cause more degradation to the repaired structural integrity.

Delaminations. Delaminations are also a form of matrix cracking, but they lie in the plane of the laminate and between plies. The delaminations typically grow from transverse intralaminar matrix cracks. Structural instability under compressive loading is of greatest concern in the presence of delaminations. Linear elastic fracture mechanics (LEFM) has been used to determine the delamination propagation. However, LEFM methods require determination of basic material property values relating to each method. These material properties have been difficult to obtain for composite structures. Under compressive loading, the delamination generally grows after sublaminate buckling. After an initial estimate of potential delamination crack growth, the stability of the sublaminate under design loading conditions can be determined. Several methods of determining the loss of buckling stiffness are found in the literature. A modification to laminated plate theory for a sublaminate (the delamination) allows for evaluation of the critical buckling load. This critical buckling load is then compared to the design loads in the laminate. Repair of delamination damage (Ref 10) can be accomplished by four principal methods:

- *Resin Injection*: The injection of a low-viscosity resin into the laminate has been a commonly used delamination repair method for many years. However, there are several concerns about the effectiveness of the repair method, such as complete infusion of resin and the cut fibers, which result from drilling the holes. The method is best used on lightly loaded structures.
- *Doubler Patch*: The bonding of a doubler patch over the delaminated region, as shown in Fig. 8, to increase the critical buckling loads has been suggested in several reports. This allows the delamination to remain in the structure but restores the structural integrity of the damaged region. The repair region should be monitored at regular intervals to ensure that the delamination does not grow. The basic principle behind this method is the same as that for the crack patching technology used to restore metal-structure fatigue in-

Table 2 Effect of local damage on residual strength and stiffness

Damage type	Production error	Low-energy impact	Puncture	Effect on: Residual strength	Effect on: Residual stiffness
Core damage	Minimal	Moderate	Significant	Limited	Small
Cut fibers	Few	Minimal	Significant	Significant	Significant
Matrix cracks	Few	Many	Many	Limited	Small
Delaminations	Minimal	Significant	Moderate	Moderate	Significant

tegrity. The structural stiffness of the doubler must be matched to that of the parent laminate, so that it will not attract additional load to the damaged region.

- *Damaged Removal*: Removing the delaminations by cutting out the material results in a partial through-the-thickness hole, which can be treated as a fiber-fracture (hole) damage type.
- *Edge Delaminations*: Edge delaminations require special attention, as it is very difficult to restore out-of-plane structural integrity without cutting out the damage. Another suggested repair method is to fill the edge damage with a low-viscosity resin and support the out-of-plane properties with a wrap-around patch (Fig. 9).

Fiber Fracture (Holes). In the event that fibers are fractured, the damage removal process will result in the drilling of a hole with circular ends. The stress state can be determined by calculating the stress concentration factor for the hole. The stress state is then evaluated against the structural design allowables.

There are several methods of calculating the stress concentration factor for a hole in a composite structure. The most common methods are the point stress failure criteria (Ref 11) and a stress-field model (Ref 12); a more detailed method exists where the hole is elliptical in shape and the far-field in-plane loads are complex (Ref 13). Generally, there are only two methods of restoring the structural integrity in the presence of a hole. The repair scheme will either be an adhesively bonded patch or a mechanically fastened patch.

Repair Design Analysis

When developing the repair scheme, the stress analysis will be based on whether the repair is a core replacement, an adhesively bonded patch, or a mechanically fastened patch. These three repair schemes are discussed briefly.

Core Replacement. The replacement of the core material (Fig. 1b) is relatively straightforward. There are a few simple rules:

- The replacement core ribbon direction should match so that the core stiffness/strength properties remain directionally consistent, and the cell densities are the same.
- When bonding the replacement core to an existing lower skin, the adhesive should fillet to the core cell walls (Fig. 10).
- Use a foaming adhesive to lock the replacement core to the existing core.
- Ensure that the top of the replacement core allows the replacement skin to lie flat.

Adhesively Bonded Joints. There are two methods of adhesively bonding repair patches: doubler repair patches and scarf, or stepped, repairs.

Doubler Repair Patch. This is the simplest of the adhesively bonded repair patch schemes (Fig. 10). However, the bonded-joint overlap length here must be sufficient to allow for an elastic-load trough to develop in the adhesive. Also, the ends of the repair must be checked for peel stresses. Tapering the joint ends will reduce peel stresses substantially. Standard practice is to taper the repair laminate, with the largest ply placed last (Fig. 11). Based on the idealized adhesive stress/strain curve (Fig. 12), the load carrying capacity of the joint (P) is as follows:

$$P = 2\sqrt{\eta\tau_p\left(\frac{\gamma_e}{2}+\gamma_p\right)Et}$$

where η is the adhesive thickness (nominally 0.13 mm, or 0.005 in.), τ_p is the peak adhesive shear stress, γ_e and γ_p are the adhesive elastic and plastic shear strains, respectively, and Et is the effective stiffness of the patch or parent laminate. The allowable load per unit width of the patch is given by:

$$P_{all} = E\varepsilon_{all}t$$

where nominally ε_{all} = 4000 microstrain. (Microstrain is the strain over a gage length comparable to the material's interatomic distance.)

The patch overlap length is:

$$l_{overlap} = \left[\frac{P}{\tau_p}+\frac{2}{\lambda}\right]FS$$

where $\lambda = \sqrt{2G/\eta Et}, G = \tau_p/\gamma_e$, and FS is the factor of safety.

Scarf or Stepped Repair. When higher loads are to be transferred through the repair region or a smooth surface contour needs to be maintained, an adhesively bonded scarf repair is recommended (Fig. 1). A flush repair to a thin laminated section will be either a scarf joint or stepped-lap joint. Generally the damage removed results in a scarfed section, and the replacement plies are stepped (Fig. 13). For preliminary design purposes, a scarf joint analysis is used. In the simple analysis, try to maintain stiffness and thermal coefficient of expansion balance; therefore, if the load is acting over a scarf angle of 0°, the shear and normal stresses (Fig. 14) are:

$$\tau = \frac{P\sin(2\theta)}{2t}$$

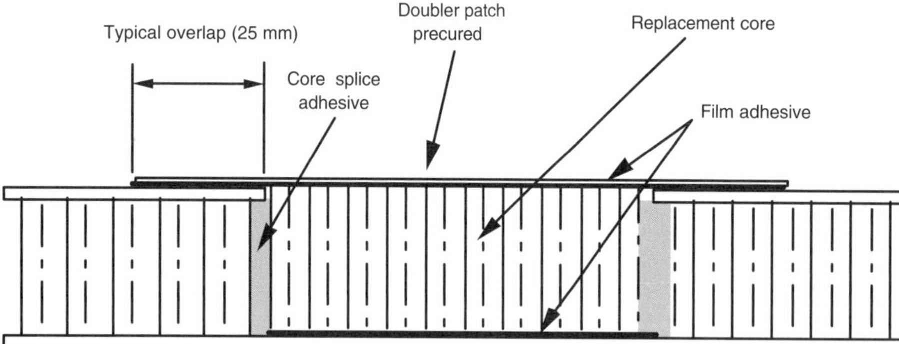

Fig. 10 Structural doubler and plug repair

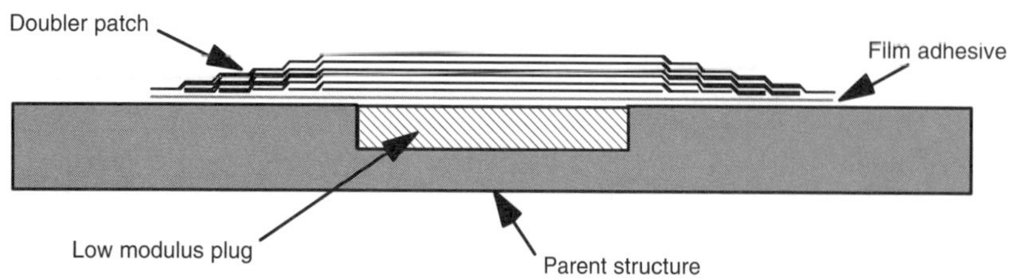

Fig. 11 Inverted doubler and plug repair

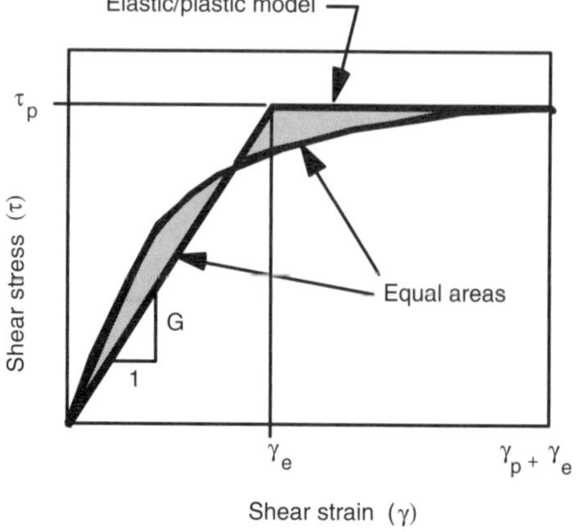

Fig. 12 Idealized adhesive stress-strain curve

and

$$\sigma = \frac{P \sin^2 \theta}{t}$$

As θ gets smaller, the normal stress will approach zero. By letting $\tau = \tau_p$, the allowable load carrying capacity of the joint is:

$$P = E\varepsilon_{ult} t = \frac{2\tau_p t}{\sin(2\theta)}$$

where E_{ult} = nominally 4000 microstrain. Therefore, the scarfing angle is given as:

$$\theta = \frac{\tau_p}{E\varepsilon_{ult}} \text{ (in radians)}$$

For the majority of structural adhesives and adherends, the scarf angle θ is limited to 3°. This gives a repair scheme length expression of:

$$l_{patch} = \frac{2t}{\tan\theta} + D_{hole}$$

where t is laminate thickness and D_{hole} is the hole diameter. As a function of the laminate thickness for a hole size of 50 mm (2 in.), Table 3 indicates the increasing patch size if a 3° scarf joint is used and clearly shows that this repair design is limited to thinner structures.

Additional information on adhesive bonding is provided in the articles "Bolted and Bonded Joints" and "Secondary Adhesive Bonding of Polymer-Matrix Composites" in this Volume and in Ref 14 and 15.

Mechanically Fastened Joints. As the skin thickness increases, scarf repairs become impractical in terms of repair design. At this stage, a bolted repair is more practical. The analysis of a bolted repair follows the methodology of a mechanically fastened joint using the allowable load per unit width of:

$$P_{all} = E\varepsilon_{all} t$$

The following design points are recommended for a bolted repair design:

- Attempt to use a low-modulus plug that restricts the load into the filled hole. A loaded hole (inclusion) can have a greater strength reduction than an open hole.
- Where a patch is relatively thick, taper the patch edges or use a stepped-lap configuration; this will reduce the load on the first row of fasteners, which are typically critically loaded.
- Seal the patch to the parent laminate and install the fasteners with sealant in the wet condition.
- Bearing/bypass loads require specific design attention, noting that the bearing strength of composite structures is often low and significantly affected by environmental conditions.

Additional information on mechanical fastening of composites is provided in the articles "Bolted and Bonded Joints" and "Mechanical Fastener Selection" in this Volume.

Pitfalls and Problems

Repair design for composite structures assumes several factors. The first assumption is that the repair patch materials properties are the same as those of the parent structure. This assumption is acceptable if the repair patch is autoclave precured. However, most adhesively bonded composite repair patches are co-bonding to the parent structures. This raises a number of problems:

- Repair patch material properties will not be the same as those of the parent structure. Several factors influence this property variation, particularly when using the vacuum bag and heater-blanket curing process. The inability to achieve high consolidation pressure will result in a lower fiber-volume ratio. Due to thermal variations across the heater blanket and heat sinks from local substructure changes, the cure rheology will be different.
- When doing heat-cured repairs, the level of absorbed moisture in the parent laminate can result in poor repair and bondline properties, due to the formation of voids. Only through drying out the parent laminate prior to repair can this be overcome. Significant levels of absorbed moisture can result in extensive damage to the structure, such as blown skins.
- The choice of either doing the repair in the field or removing the structural component to be repaired and doing the work in a workshop also results in structural property variability. Repairing the composite structure in a workshop where the environment is controlled will provide a better repair. This is particularly true for moisture removal and surface preparation when doing adhesively bonded repairs.

A second potential pitfall is the adequacy of the repair analysis. In the repair design analysis for both adhesively bonded and mechanically fastened repairs, the material properties are typically assumed from vendor data, with ample margins of safety applied to cover environmental conditions. This is particularly true for bearing strength of composite materials. However, the complex interaction of stress transfer is usually not applied, even if understood. The removed damage does not result in geometrically perfect interfaces; however, the analysis assumes this to be so. The skill of the technician thus plays a critical role in the development of uniform load transfer into the repair patch. The preparation of the surface for adhesively bonded repair schemes is also critical and depends on the skill and thoroughness of the technician. Surface preparation to composite structures is not as critical as in metallic structures, but the effect of poor surface preparation is the same: the repair patch will eventually fail at the bondline interface (adhesive failure mode) due to bondline degradation.

Corrosion is always a problem in repair design application and durability. The selection of repair materials must be consistent with the parent structure. The situation is more critical in mechanically fastened repair schemes, where the composite repair scheme can be bolted to a metallic substructure. Adhesively bonded repair schemes have several concerns. The bondline, if broken, can allow moisture to enter, resulting in substructure corrosion. This is a real concern with metallic honeycomb core structures.

Table 3 Relationship between scarf patch size and laminate thickness for a hole size of 50 mm (2 in.)

No. of plies	Laminate(a)		Scarf length		Patch length		Ratio of patch length to hole diameter
	mm	in.	mm	in.	mm	in.	
8	1.0	0.04	19.1	0.75	88.2	3.47	1.8
12	1.5	0.06	28.6	1.13	107.2	4.22	2.2
16	2.0	0.08	38.2	1.50	126.4	4.98	2.5
24	3.0	0.12	57.2	2.25	164.4	6.47	3.3
36	4.5	0.18	85.9	3.39	221.8	8.73	4.4
52	6.5	0.26	124.0	4.89	298.0	11.73	6.0

(a) Based on a ply thickness of 0.125 mm (0.005 in.)

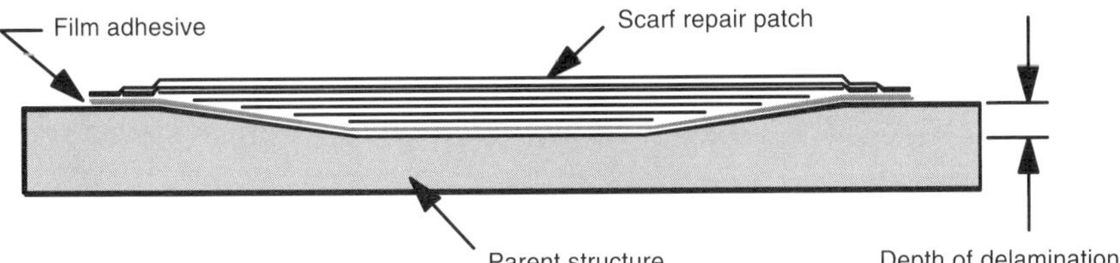

Fig. 13 Stepped-lap/scarf repair scheme

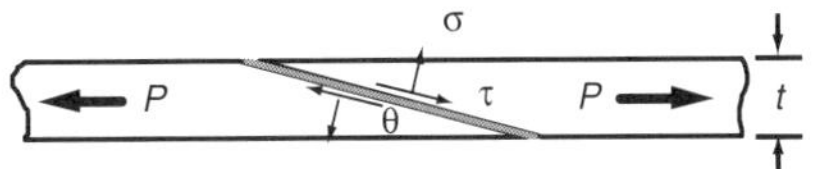

Fig. 14 Scarf joint analysis geometry

Finally, the stress state in the structure and the repair scheme is typically considered uniform. However, the stress state is often complex and includes some degree of out-of-plane loading. Careful design of the repair scheme is required in order to either eliminate the severity of the complex three-dimensional stress state or to allow the repair scheme to accommodate such a stress state. The first option is typically preferred but not always easy to do.

REFERENCES

1. R.B. Heslehurst, The Accuracy of Simple Damage Analysis Methods in Composite Structures, *Proc. of 37th International SAMPE Symposium and Exhibition* (Anaheim), Society for the Advancement of Material and Process Engineering, March 1992, p 321–332
2. R.B Heslehurst, Analysis and Modelling of Damage and Repair of Composite Materials in Aerospace, *Numerical Analysis and Modelling of Composite Materials*, J.W. Bull, Ed., Blackie Academic & Professional Publishing, Glasgow, 1996
3. R.B. Heslehurst, "Evaluation of Damage Analysis Techniques for Composite Aircraft Structures–Executive Summary," Defence Fellowship Report, Australian Defence Department, Feb 1990
4. R.B. Heslehurst, The Accuracy of Simple Damage Analysis Methods in Composite Structures, *Proc. of 37th International SAMPE Symposium* (Anaheim), March 1992, p 321–332
5. A.A. Baker and R. Jones, *Bonded Repair of Aircraft Structures,* Martinus Nijhoff Publishing, Dordrecht, 1988
6. B.C. Hoskin and A.A. Baker, Ed., *Composite Materials for Aircraft Structures, AIAA Education Series,* AIAA, 1986
7. L.J. Hart-Smith, "Design Methodology for Bonded-Bolted Composite Joints," AFWAL-TR-81-3154, Feb 1982
8. L.J. Hart-Smith, Design Details for Adhesively Bonded Repairs of Fibrous Composite Structures, Douglas Paper 7637, presented at 31st National SAMPE Symposium and Exhibition (Las Vegas, NV), Society for the Advancement of Material and Process Engineering, 8–10 April 1986
9. R.B. Heslehurst, Composite Structural Repairs–An Engineering Approach, *Proc. of the 39th SAMPE International Symposium and Exhibition* (Anaheim), Society for the Advancement of Material and Process Engineering, 11–14 April 1994, p 602–609
10. R.B. Heslehurst, Repair of Delamination Damage—A Simplified Approach, *Proc. of the 41st SAMPE International Symposium and Exhibition* (Anaheim), Society for the Advancement of Material and Process Engineering, 25–28 March 1996, p 915–924
11. J.M. Whitney and R.J. Nuismer, Stress Fracture Criteria for Laminated Composites Containing Stress Concentrations, *J. Compos. Mater.,* Vol 8, July 1974, p 253–265
12. L.B. Greszczuk, Stress Concentration and Failure Criteria for Orthotropic and Anisotropic Plates with Circular Openings, *Composite Materials: Testing and Design, Second Conf.,* STP 497, ASTM, 1971, p 363
13. S.W. Tsai, *Composite Design*, 4th ed., Think Composites, 1988
14. M.J. Davis, "A Workshop on the Practical Adhesive Bonding Performance and Durability: Standards and Standardization," a workshop presented during ICCM-11, International Conference on Composite Materials (Brisbane, Australia), 11 July 1997
15. L.J. Hart-Smith, "Adhesive-Bonded Double-Lap Joints," NASA Contractual Report, NASA CR-112235, Jan 1973

SELECTED REFERENCES

- "Advanced Composite Repair Guide," Northrop Corporation Report NOR 82-60, Hawthorne, 1982
- "Advanced Composite Structures: Fabrication and Damage Repair," Abaris Training, Reno NV, 1998
- The Composite Materials Handbook—MIL-HDBK-17, Technomic Publishing, 1999. Also available on the Web at www.mil17.org
- K.B. Armstrong and R.T. Barrett, *Care and Repair of Advanced Composites*, Society of Automotive Engineers, 1997

Repair Applications, Quality Control, and Inspection

Michael J. Hoke, Abaris Training Resources Inc.

REPAIR OF DAMAGED ADVANCED COMPOSITE COMPONENTS often is more economical than replacing them. Many thousands of composite structural repairs have been made over the years, so they obviously can be done well. For lightly loaded nonstructural parts, such repairs may sometimes be only cosmetic. For loaded structures, however, repairs must be more than cosmetic and are generally intended to restore the ability of the component to carry design loads. These types of repairs are discussed in this article, together with other issues surrounding advanced composite repair technology.

Composite repairs can be complex, with many possible variations and differences of opinion as to how they are best performed. They are not necessarily more difficult than metallic structural repairs, but they are different. The major difference is that in repairing a composite, one is not only accomplishing the repair, but also "creating" the strength of the materials as the repair plies are laid up and the resin is cured. This additional level of complexity, and the difficulty of inspecting composites after cure, leads to many of the quality- and process-control considerations that are so important to achieving reliable repairs. New skills are required of not only repair technicians, but also of the engineers who are designing repairs for composite structures.

As structural design engineers become more comfortable with using composites in heavily loaded structures, the design allowables are creeping ever upward, and the materials are being used at higher microstrain levels, closer to their true limits. While this is necessary to achieve efficient structures, it makes the job of the repair design engineer and repair technicians more difficult. With overdesigned composite structures, there is some leeway for understrength repairs to work successfully. This may not be so in more efficiently designed structures. So repair personnel have to be careful in assuming that what they "got away with" in the past will work in the future. As always, a true understanding of the detailed complexities of these structures is what is needed to repair them safely and economically.

In a theoretically ideal repair, one is trying to match, not exceed, the strength, stiffness, and weight of the original structure. A "perfect" repair would be to replace the damaged component with a new one. Then those three parameters would be matched exactly. In an actual repair, it is not possible to match all three simultaneously. To achieve the original strength, the repaired part will be stiffer and heavier than the original. To match the original stiffness, the repaired part would be weaker and slightly heavier than the original, and so on.

Therefore, repair design involves evaluating trade-offs among these parameters, especially with stiffness-critical structures, such as helicopter rotor blades. Other considerations also come into play, such as the physical practicality of performing the repair successfully, the time involved, inspection and substantiation of the quality of the repair, cosmetic appearance, cost, and so on.

In type-certified civilian aircraft, one is obligated to follow the repair procedures outlined in the aircraft structural repair manual (SRM). If the damage is outside the allowable limits defined in the SRM, then the repair will require specific engineering support from an authorized source, and a specific repair designed for that particular damage case will be required. If the engineering support is not available, then the part must be replaced. Military organizations have their own similar procedures.

Durability and inspectability of repairs are also a concern. Since a large percentage of composite repairs are bonded rather than bolted, the long-term durability of the adhesive bond is important. Small details in the repair process, especially regarding surface preparation, are vital in determining the quality of the repair. Control of the repair materials and processes is therefore crucial.

Types of Damage

Various types of damage can occur in a fiber reinforced polymer-matrix composite as a result of impact severity, as shown in Fig. 1. Damage includes holes and punctures, delaminations, disbonds, core and resin damage, and water intrusion.

Holes and punctures usually are caused by high- or medium-level impact. Damage can be severe, but usually is easily detected and generally is localized near the point of impact.

Delaminations, perhaps the most common of all types of damage, often are caused by low-energy impacts, such as a tool drop or a glancing bird strike on an aircraft. They sometimes are visible if near the surface, but the full extent of damage is often not readily detectable.

Disbonds indicate an adhesive bond failure between joined structures. They usually are observed with a face sheet disbonding from an underlying sandwich core material.

Core damage can occur with any type of core. Causes of core damage include handling damage in manufacturing, impact, improper vacuum bagging, and fluid ingress.

Resin damage can be caused by many factors including fire or excessive heat, ultraviolet (UV) rays, paint stripper, and impacts. It may be hard to detect, and it is especially difficult to quantify the effects of such damage on the structural integrity of the part. As a general rule, resin damage leads to a greater loss in compressive strength than in tensile strength.

Water intrusion is especially a problem with honeycomb cores, resulting in weight gain, corrosion in aluminum honeycomb, and core cell ruptures and disbonds if water freezes and expands. A very common problem in high-temperature repairs is that the heat of curing the repair causes the trapped water to turn to steam, disbonding face sheets around the repair; this is an excellent way to inadvertently convert a small area of damage into a large one. Water intrusion also softens the cured matrix, reducing compressive properties, particularly bearing strength.

Damage Detection in Field Conditions

Visual inspection can be a quite effective and often underrated technique for detecting damaged composite structures. Even low-energy impacts may leave a slight marring, paint scrape, or faint surface blemish on a part. A slight wave or ripple on the surface may indicate an underlying delamination or disbond. A light spot or "whitish" area on a fiberglass part may indicate trapped air, a resin-lean area, or a delamination.

However, one of the common problems with composites is "hidden damage." Often, low-energy impacts will leave no visible marks on the surface, but underlying delaminations can be extensive, spreading out in a cone-shape from the impact point. Often plies on the back side will be visibly delaminated, but this is not visible from the front. Some, but not all, hidden damage can be detected using the methods discussed in this section.

Tap testing probably is the most common inspection technique used other than visual examination. By tapping gently on the surface of a composite part, often it is possible to hear a change in sound from a clear sharp tone to a dull thud. By tapping back and forth over the area in question, and making a small mark at the point where the tone just begins to change, it is possible to outline large, irregularly shaped areas of delaminations or disbonds.

However, there are many limitations to tap testing. For example, it does not work well through a core material; that is, it is difficult to detect damage on the back side of a sandwich structure without access to both sides. It does not work well on deep damage in thick laminates—a reasonable limit typically is about 4 to 6 plies deep, depending on the type of composite material being inspected.

In addition, when performed correctly, one is listening for very small changes in tone. This means tap testing has to be done in a quiet area by a person who has good hearing. As with all nondestructive inspection techniques, the inspector has to have a good knowledge of the underlying structure. Internal doublers, bonded stiffeners, core potting compound, and the like will change the tone and could lead to false interpretations.

A digital tap tester can help overcome some of these limitations. It reads the bounce time of a small plastic tap hammer in microseconds and can give better resolution and read deeper damage than can manual tapping. It also is unaffected by external noise and so is especially good for tap testing on an aircraft ramp with jet engines running nearby.

Ultrasonic inspection consists of two main methods: pulse-echo and through-transmission. Both methods can detect many types of hidden defects, but not all defects.

Pulse-echo requires rather expensive portable equipment and a very well-trained inspector, and it can be performed with access from one side only—on a part still mounted on an aircraft, for example. It is more suitable for small-area inspections because it is difficult to cover large areas using typical portable equipment in a reasonable time. Delaminations and disbonds can be detected deeper down inside the structure than those detectable using tap testing. The method provides information about the depth of the defect, down to the particular ply level in many cases. Pulse-echo primarily is used at repair facilities or at manufacturing facilities to give more detailed information about a defect uncovered by another method. It does not work well through a core material to detect problems on the back-side skin.

Through-transmission requires access to both sides of a part and often is performed using rather expensive fixed equipment. It can be automated and can cover large areas fairly quickly and may or may not give depth information. It is most commonly used in manufacturing and large repair stations.

X-radiography requires expensive equipment and well-trained inspectors. It is an excellent method for detecting metallic inclusions and for inspecting aluminum honeycomb—it is relatively good at finding water trapped in honeycomb—but is not good for detecting delaminations parallel to the plane of the x-ray image.

Thermography uses an infrared camera to videotape parts as they are heated or cooled and uses the visible thermal differences to extract information about the part. It is useful in bondline inspection, detection of inclusions, and in some cases detecting water trapped in honeycomb.

Component Identification

Ideally, fiber reinforced composite components should be fully identified before a repair is performed. Such details as material specifications, ply numbers and ply orientations, core ribbon direction, ply buildups and drop-offs, and numerous other details need to be understood before a repair commences.

For aircraft, this type of information usually is available in the SRM, design drawings, or equivalent documents. In repairs of nonaerospace components, an SRM or equivalent often is not available. However, the types of information described previously are still needed for proper repairs and should be obtained by the repair technician. Determination of these details can often be made by careful taper sanding through a scrap of material and reading the information directly

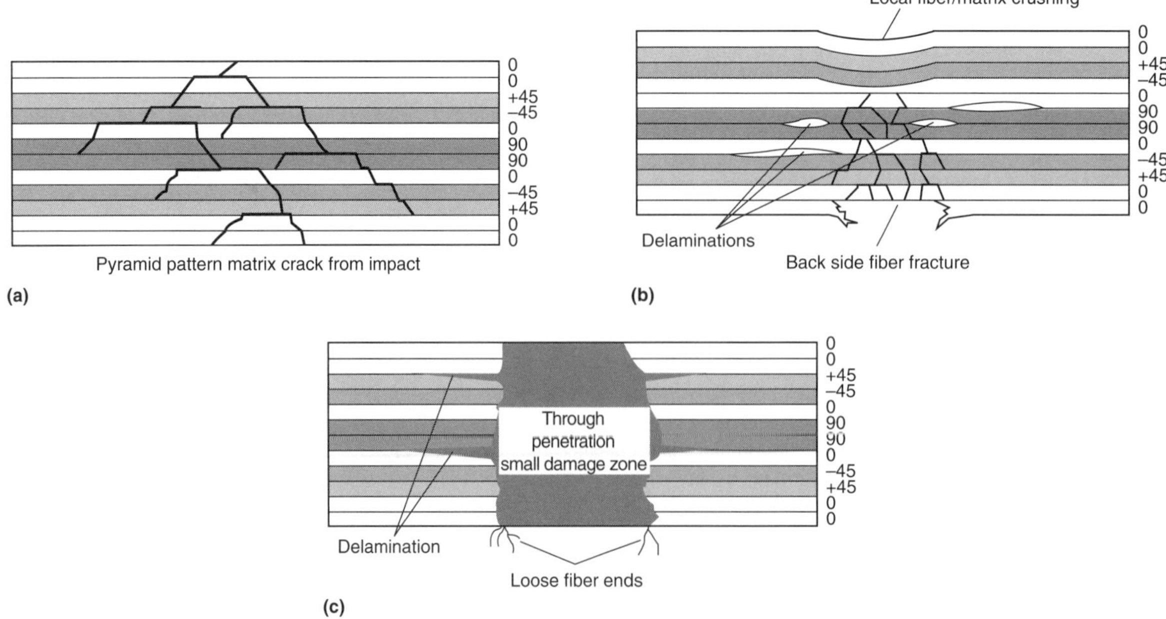

Fig. 1 Damage to fiber reinforced polymer-matrix composites resulting from different impact severity. (a) Low-energy impact. (b) Medium-energy impact. (c) High-energy impact

from the composite itself. A thorough understanding of composite materials, weave patterns, ply orientation concepts such as balance, symmetry, nesting, and so forth, is mandatory for this type of analysis to be meaningful.

Paint Removal

Chemical Stripping. Most paint strippers (solvents) are methylene-chloride based, which will attack cured epoxy resin, and, therefore, are not recommended for use on composite structures. Alternatives include hand sanding and various particulate-blasting methods.

Hand sanding is widely used as a paint-removal method for composites. No expensive equipment is needed, and the sanding pressure can easily be controlled to avoid laminate damage. Hand sanding is recommended for paint removal in a small area (in an area to be repaired, for example). One must be careful not to damage fibers in the surface ply, unless a specific "sanding ply" has been included on the surface of the component. The obvious disadvantage is the high labor cost, especially on large parts. However, this is by far the most common paint-removal method in preparation for repair.

Blasting involves the use of various types of blasting media including sand, aluminum oxide, plastic particles, wheat starch, and others.

Sandblasting is possible, but must be done very carefully, as it is extremely likely that fibers on the top ply would be damaged.

Aluminum oxide blasting is similar to sandblasting, and the same precautions apply.

Plastic media blasting is less aggressive than sand or aluminum oxide blasting and is used quite a bit on composites. While effective, this technique has shown some difficulties in the field. The plastic media most often are cleaned and reused in such systems, which can lead to the following problems:

- The cleaning process is largely designed to remove paint chips and solid matter. If the plastic media become contaminated with oil, grease, fuel, and so forth, these contaminates can be driven back into the composite surface, causing paint adhesion problems.
- The plastic particles become dull with reuse, and a poorly trained operator may turn up the air pressure to compensate. This can lead to damage of the composite surface or even blowing a hole through these rather brittle materials.

Wheat starch blasting is a fairly new method used to blast paint off parts. Boeing has approved this method for paint removal from composites. Corn-hybrid polymer blasting is an even newer but similar method. There is no chemical attack to worry about; wheat starch and corn-hybrid polymers are environmentally benign, biodegradable material that can easily be disposed of.

Other Methods. There are many other methods, such as dry ice blasting, Xenon flash lamps, baking-soda blasting, and so forth. Work in this field is continuing, and better methods are being sought by many organizations.

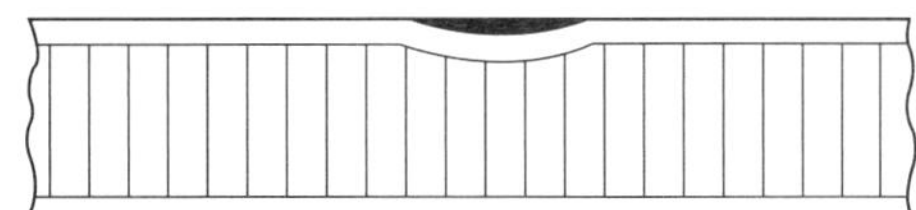

Fig. 2 Cosmetic repair using superficial nonstructural filler

Repair Design

Designing for repair involves various considerations including structure types and repair types.

Structure types include:

Type	Criteria	Example
Primary	Heavily loaded or safety-of-flight structures	Helicopter blade
Secondary	Intermediate loading and safety structures	Aerodynamic fairing
Tertiary	Lightly loaded or noncritical structures	Interior sidewall panel

Note that in some cases, a structure is designated as secondary or tertiary from a design load point of view, but it may be treated as primary structure regarding the critical nature and location of the component. An example would be a lightly loaded fairing located in front of the intake of a jet engine. Failure of the fairing itself would not be structurally critical. However, if it gets sucked into the engine, the resulting engine failure could cause more interesting problems.

Repair types include cosmetic, semistructural, structural, and temporary.

A cosmetic repair is a superficial nonstructural filler as shown in Fig. 2. This type of repair will not regain any strength and must be used only where strength is unimportant. However, it can serve to keep water out of a hole until a more permanent repair is made. Due to high shrinkage with some fillers, these types of cosmetic repairs often will start to crack after a relatively short time in service.

Semistructural repairs include a plug-and-patch repair (Fig. 3) and resin-injection repair (Fig. 4). These types of repairs can regain some strength. The mechanically fastened plug-and-patch repair can be especially effective where thick solid laminates are used because they withstand bolt loads well. Resin injection can be effective in limited instances, where the delamination is restricted to one ply. However, not much strength is regained, and the primary benefit of this type of repair is that it is quick and inexpensive. At best, one can hope to slow the spread of a delamination with this type of repair, and it is generally considered a temporary measure.

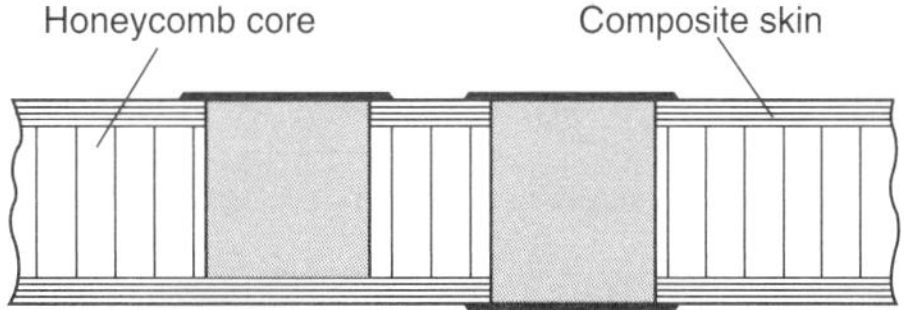

Fig. 3 Semistructural plug-and-patch repair

Structural repairs include mechanically fastened doublers (metallic or precured composite), bonded external doublers, and flush (aerodynamic) patches.

Full structural repairs using bolted doublers (Fig. 5) can be used in heavily loaded solid laminates and are often the only practical means of repairing such structures. However, such repairs are not aerodynamically smooth and may cause "signature" problems in structures where low observability is a design criteria.

Bolted repairs are used in repairing structures such as F-18 wing skins, Boeing 777 horizontal and vertical stabilizers, AV-8B Harrier wing skins, and other similar items. It is important to note that the original design must allow for the use of bolted repairs, otherwise a significant reduction in design load allowables will result.

Bonded (as opposed to bolted) doublers often are used, especially with wet lay-up materials, to perform repairs to lightly loaded, thin laminate structures. They may be either room- or high-temperature cured, depending on the repair matrix system. They can regain a significant portion of the original strength of the structure, or even full strength, although with a significant stiffness and weight penalty in many cases. They are generally easy and relatively quick and do not require the highly developed skills of the flush repairs described below.

Flush (aerodynamic) patches, called "taper sanded" or "scarfed" repairs, are most commonly applied to thin solid laminates or sandwich structures. They require careful (smooth, flat) removal of material at a precise angle, all around the cleaned-up damaged area (Fig. 6). This is usually accomplished by hand using a compressed-air-powered high-speed grinder. Significant skill and practice on the part of the repair technician are mandatory.

These repairs currently are considered the best in terms of the strength, stiffness, and weight trade-offs discussed previously and are very commonly called out in aircraft SRMs. They can be almost perfectly flush with the surface if performed very carefully. Typical scarf distances are from 20 to 120 times the thickness of the laminate being scarfed.

Stepped repairs are similar in geometry to scarfed repairs, but the plies are cut back one by one in a terraced pattern (Fig. 7). The resulting plateaus are then filled in with new plies. Many of the same advantages as scarfed repairs are obtained. However, it can be very difficult in many laminates to cut cleanly through a ply without damaging any fibers in the ply below. The sharp

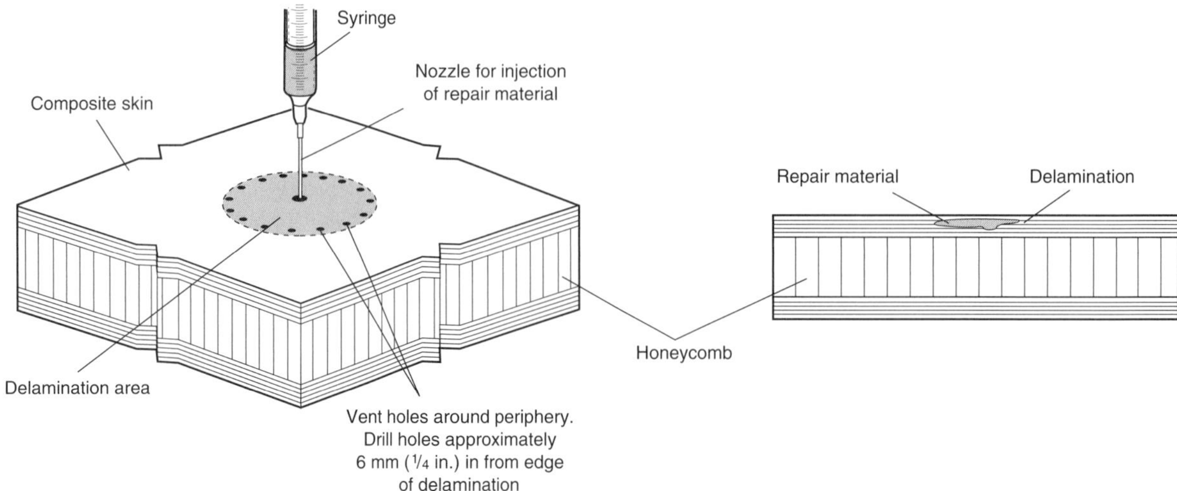

Fig. 4 Semistructural resin-injection repair

edges of the steps also can lead to abrupt stress concentrations in the repaired laminate. While theoretically all of the repair plies in a stepped repair can lay perfectly flat, which is not possible at the very edges of a scarfed repair, the practical difficulties of performing a stepped repair without damaging underlying plies have led to a reduction in use in recent years.

Temporary repairs commonly are used in cases of battle damage and limited service (ferry flight, etc.). Temporary repairs often are performed to return an aircraft to a location where a permanent repair can be performed. Structural repair manuals spell out the limits of such repairs. They often are performed using materials such as speed tape, potting compound, or other such materials. The primary purpose is to limit the further spread of damage—and to keep water, airflow, and so forth out of the damaged area—until a permanent repair can be made. If a temporary repair is desired that falls outside the allowable SRM limits for such repairs, then engineering approval is needed, and for U.S.-certified civilian aircraft a "ferry permit" might be required to allow a one-time flight to a station that can perform a permanent repair.

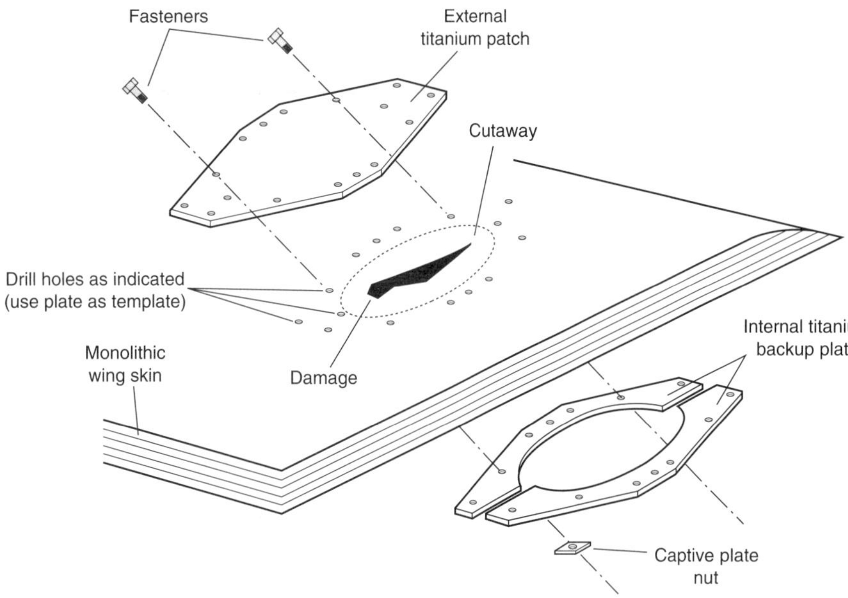

Fig. 5 Mechanically fastened doubler (bolted patch repair) on thick skin composite

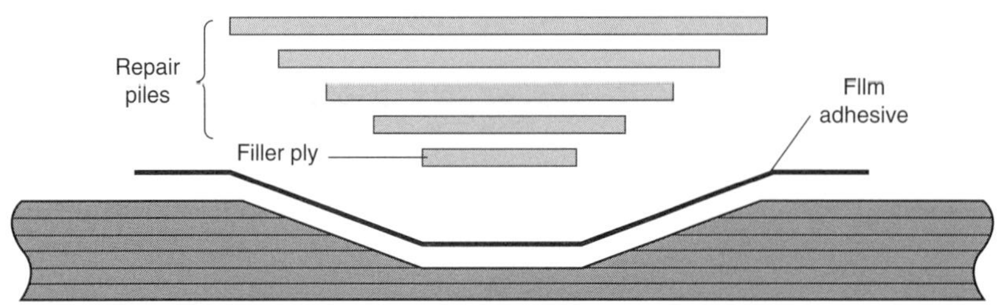

Fig. 6 Scarf removal for flush (aerodynamic) repair

Repair Design Considerations

Stiffness Discontinuities. Repairs should not have high stiffness near edges. This leads to peel mode failures in adhesive bonded repairs. In addition, an abrupt change in stiffness at the edge of a repair can lead to failure of the underlying part during structural loading at the edge of the repair. This failure can occur at a lower load than that at which the unrepaired part would have failed, due to the high concentration of load at the edges of the stiff repair. This is why gently tapered repairs are often performed. Softening of the edge of the repair is often performed by ply drop-offs and/or "pinking" the edges of the outermost repair plies.

Available Equipment. Often the equipment and materials available determine to a large extent the repair scheme. For example, SRMs frequently offer several different repair schemes, such as wet lay-up room-temperature cure, generally with a higher-temperature postcure; prepreg 121 °C (250 °F) cure; or prepreg 177 °C (350 °F) cure. As a general rule, the higher the temperature, the larger the allowable repair. However, in some cases, such as a honeycomb core structure having possible water contamination, a lower-temperature repair often is preferable to avoid further damage. As a general

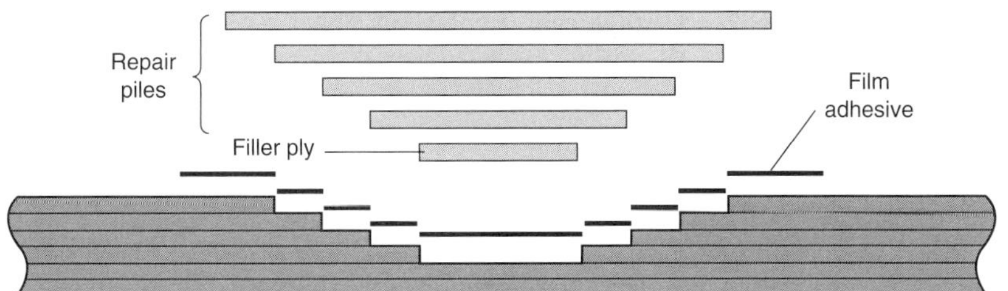

Fig. 7 Step removal for flush (aerodynamic) repair

guideline, if multiple repair methods are authorized for a given area of damage, choose the lowest-temperature approved method. The lower the temperature, the fewer the problems, and the lower the chances of moisture turning to steam and disbonding a sandwich skin or creating excessive porosity in a bondline.

An additional important equipment consideration concerns availability of vacuum bagging and curing equipment. These items are discussed in the following paragraphs.

Lightning-Strike Considerations. Occasionally, the surface of an external composite component will be a ply or layer of conductive material. In addition to a normal structural repair, one must also recreate the electrical conductivity designed into such a part. These conductive materials are of many different types, ranging from nickel-coated graphite cloth to metal meshes to aluminized fiberglass to conductive paints. These types of repairs generally require a conductivity test be performed with an ohmmeter to verify minimum electrical resistance across the structure. It is extremely important in repairing these types of structures to use only the approved materials from the specific vendors authorized, including such items as potting compounds, sealants, adhesives, and so forth.

Available Quality-Assurance Methods. It is important to consider whether the quality of the repair is inspectable. How does one know, for example, that a bonded repair will not fall off in the short term (the next day or week) or the long term (the next year)? This is a difficult problem. As of 2000, there is no known commercially available method to nondestructively measure the strength of an adhesive bond. One can destructively test them, carefully control the process of making the actual bonded joints, and get a good, but not perfect, degree of confidence in the strength of a bond.

However, some things can be inspected. If there are delaminations in a repair, this can usually be detected by tap testing or ultrasonic inspection. Obvious resin starvation, ply wrinkles, and so forth also can be observed. If a faulty repair is suspected, then the usual course of action is to remove and replace it.

Training of Repair Personnel. As composite structural repairs become more common on heavily loaded primary structures, the quality of the repairs becomes more critical. In years past, composite components often were so overdesigned that they could tolerate poor repairs and still perform adequately at their design loads.

As engineers become more confident at designing structures to be operated at higher loads, more near the true limits of the materials, understrength repairs are becoming more of a problem. Repair techniques that are acceptable on a lightly loaded structure may be truly dangerous on a heavily loaded structure. The job of the repair specialist is becoming more difficult as composites become more commonplace.

Therefore, training is becoming more important. Development of more standardized materials, processes, and training for repairs is proceeding slowly but steadily. Because a fundamental issue with composite repairs is their limited inspectability, the quality of the repair is very much dependent on the training and integrity of the repair specialist.

Repair Instructions

Manufacturer's Repair Instructions. In military or type-certified-civilian aircraft, repairs must be performed in accordance with approved repair instructions issued by the aircraft manufacturer or military organization responsible. In the airline world, these instructions are located in SRMs. For military aircraft, these are in Technical Orders, Technical Manuals, or the equivalent.

Classification Criteria. Typically, these repair instructions have limits on the size and location of repairable damage. These limits vary considerably from part to part, depending on such things as location of the damage, size and severity of the damage, adjacent damage, part construction details, criticality of the structure, ease of subsequent inspection, temperature requirements, and so forth.

Engineered Repairs and Instructions. If the damage falls outside the allowable repair criteria, then either the part must be replaced, or a specific repair must be designed for that particular component and damage level by an engineer specifically trained and qualified to design composite repairs. This type of engineered repair design is very often done with the close cooperation of the aircraft manufacturer or may be done by engineers from the manufacturer.

Repair Materials

When performing a permanent repair, the most common repair techniques involve using the same materials used to manufacture the original structure to try to recreate the original structural properties as closely as possible. However, this is not feasible in some cases, especially when the original structure was manufactured with a fiber/resin system that required an autoclave cure, and the repair is being performed without using an autoclave. Therefore, material substitutions may be allowed or even required by the SRM. In battle damage or temporary repairs, often more flexibility in material substitution is allowed than would be normal for permanent repairs.

In any composite repair, the repair materials must be considered and evaluated before the repair is begun to ensure that the repair is structurally sound. Types of repair materials are shown in Table 1.

Curing Methods

Portable repair systems are suitcase-sized or smaller units designed to allow for the accurate application of controlled heat and vacuum to a composite repair. They are especially useful for field repairs, in situations where it is not possible to remove the damaged part for repair. Portable systems offer programmable cure cycles, with hard-copy documentation of the actual temperatures and vacuum achieved during the repair.

Table 1 Types of repair materials for making fiber reinforced polymer-matrix composites repairs

Matrix resin systems(a)
Wet lay-up
Prepreg
Low temperature
High temperature
Reinforcement fibers and fabrics
Fiberglass
Aramid
Carbon
Boron
Others
Reinforcement form
Unidirectional tape
Woven cloth
Weave style
Core materials
Honeycomb
Foam
Balsa wood
Potting compounds
Others
Lightning-strike materials
Aluminum mesh
Copper mesh
Conductive fibers
Nickel coating
Conductive paints
Flame spray coatings

(a) Also must consider cure cycle requirements and available equipment

They are most commonly used to control heat blankets, but can also be used to control heat lamps, hot air guns, and even ovens. An electrical power source and a clean compressed air source are required, and the system relies on accurate thermocouple readings. Thermocouple features for "J"-type wire and plugs, accurate to 370 °C (700 °F), are:

Grade	Accuracy	Cost
Standard grade	±0.75% or ±2 °C (4 °F); two can vary 4.5 °C (8 °F)	\$1–2/m (\$0.30–0.60/ft)
Special grade	±0.40% or ±1 °C (2 °F); two can vary 2 °C (4 °F)	\$12–20/m (\$3.60–6.00/ft)

Wires (24 or 28 gage) are insulated with Kapton coating. Calibration is not a function of length. 0.5 °C (1 °F) temperature change per 38 m (125 ft)

Vacuum bags always are used with prepreg materials and often are used with wet lay-up materials.

Ovens and autoclaves offer the capability to use original molds (if available) and require that panels be removed from the structure. The size of the repaired panel is limited by the size of the available equipment.

SELECTED REFERENCES

- *Advances in Aircraft Composite Repair Symposium* (Farnborough, England), 5–7 Sept 1994, Society of Automotive Engineers, 1994
- *Advances in Composite Repair,* SAE TOPTEC (Seattle, WA), 1–2 Nov 1993, Society of Automotive Engineers, 1993
- K.B. Armstrong and R.T. Barrett, *Care and Repair of Advanced Composites,* Society of Automotive Engineers, 1997
- A.J. Baker and R. Jones, Ed., *Bonded Repair of Aircraft Structures,* Martinus Nijhoff Publishers, 1988
- Commercial Aircraft Repair Committee, Repair Design Task Group, "Design of Durable, Repairable, and Maintainable Aircraft Composites," Document Reference AE-27, Society of Automotive Engineers, 1997
- J.W. Deaton, Repair of Advanced Composite Commercial Aircraft Structures, *Adhesives and Sealants,* Vol 3, *Engineered Materials Handbook,* ASM International, 1990, p 829–839
- S.H. Myhre and C.E. Beck, Repair Concepts for Advanced Composites Structures, *Adhesives and Sealants,* Vol 3, *Engineered Materials Handbook,* ASM International, 1990, p 821–828

Ship Structure Repairs

A.P. Mouritz, RMIT University, Australia
R.S. Trask, DERA Farnborough, United Kingdom
A.J. Russell, Dockyard Laboratory Pacific, DRDC, Canada

A WIDE VARIETY of marine craft, boats, and ships can be made of fiber-reinforced polymer composites, including yachts, fishing trawlers, naval patrol boats, minehunting ships, and corvettes. Composites are also being used increasingly in the superstructures of ferries and naval frigates, funnels of cruise liners, and antenna masts of large warships. Future applications for composites include rudders, propellers, and propeller shafts for naval ships and propulsors and control surfaces for submarines. Most composite ship structures are made of thick-section glass-reinforced polyester (GRP) laminate or a sandwich material consisting of GRP face skins covering a balsa or polymer foam core (Ref 1).

There are many ways that a composite component can be damaged in service, but in general it is due to mechanical loading or environmental conditions that are either unexpected or of low probability, and hence were not allowed for in the original design. A description of the various damage mechanisms to GRP marine composites is given in Table 1. The most common types of damage to GRP vessels are gouges and delamination cracks at the outer hull surface caused by impact with debris in the water and repeated sliding against a wharf in heavy seas. Mechanical damage can include surface scratches, matrix cracking, delamination cracking, fiber failure, and, in severe cases, rupture and penetration of the composite hull. The significance of these damage types will depend upon the particular ship structure. Table 2 gives descriptions and illustrations of the different types of damage. Other types of damage commonly experienced by sandwich composites is disbonding of skins from the core, which is normally caused by poor design or fabrication, and core crushing caused by impact or excessive overloading.

The repair of minor surface damage, such as to gel coats, is not necessary unless the appearance of the ship is important or the long-term properties of the composite will be degraded. The repair of damage consisting of delaminations, broken fibers, and joint failures is essential when the structural integrity or watertightness of the vessel is compromised. Currently, there are no clear guidelines for determining whether damage has weakened a vessel. However, the hulls of most composite ships have good damage tolerance because of the high safety factors used in design. For example, the design safety factors for minehunting ships are typically between 3 and 6, and this allows the hull to contain a delamination at least 0.3 m (1 ft) long without the stiffness, strength, or fatigue performance being notably affected (Ref 2). Fracture mechanics techniques and finite element analysis tools are being developed to estimate the loss in mechanical performance of composite ship structures due to damage (e.g., Ref 2), although the models are usually simplistic in that only single cracks and simple load conditions are considered. Despite these developments, the amount of damage needed to degrade the structural integrity of a composite ship structure is extremely difficult to specify accurately using modeling techniques. As a result, it is recommended that repairs be made whenever damage consists of delamination cracks or broken fibers.

The aircraft industry has undertaken most of the research, development, and certification of repair techniques for composite structures (e.g., Ref 3–5). Some repair methods that were originally developed for aircraft composite structures, such as adhesive patching and scarf repairs, were adapted later for composite ship structures (e.g., Ref 6–8). With some repair methods, such adaptation has been fraught with danger, because the composite structures for aircraft are different from composite ship structures. Furthermore, some boat builders are using in-house repair methods that have not been scientifically evaluated for structural efficiency or durability. Navies and coast guards are alleviating the problem to some extent by the introduction of repair standards that have been certified for composite vessels (Ref 9–11). The methods outlined in this article, which covers gel coat repairs, patching, scarfing, and step repairs, have undergone extensive development and rigorous testing for use on composite ship structures. Resin infusion repair, which is a relatively new method for repairing marine composites, is also briefly described, even though it has not been completely assessed for ship structures.

Repair Classification, Characterization, and Cycle

The objective of any repair is to return the ship structure as far as practical to its undamaged condition, such that it can support all design loads for the intended service life. Clearly, the objective of the repair will vary on the specific circumstances, but it is likely to include:

- Restoration of static strength, stiffness, and/or elastic stability of the structure
- Restoration of fatigue performance and long-term durability of the structure
- Restoration of surface profile (e.g., clearances or appearance unaffected)

Table 1 Common damage mechanisms of marine composite structures

Damage mechanism	Description
Impact damage	This is the main cause of damage in composite structures. It occurs most often from low-velocity impacts, either locally, such as a tool being dropped onto a surface, or from a more general collision between moving objects. Abrasion of the surface can occur by the vessel rubbing against the wharf.
Overload	The design loads may be exceeded by unexpected loading conditions. (This could be due to inferior design or poor-quality fabrication.)
Fatigue	Composite materials are usually highly fatigue resistant to fatigue loading, but damage may still occur at high strains, usually initiating at notches and fastener holes.
Environment	If the maximum operating temperature of the material is exceeded, or if it is exposed to fire or chemicals (for example, fuel or paint stripping fluid), then damage such as decomposition of the resin matrix may occur. The properties of the matrix material and fiber-matrix interface can also degrade due to weathering (e.g., moisture, ultraviolet radiation).
Wartime environment	Small-arms fire, missile strikes, air blasts, and underwater explosions can also damage naval ships.

In addition to achieving the structural requirements, the repair will also be designed to meet additional factors:

- Minimum weight increase (if applicable)
- Simple procedures for implementation
- Accessibility to the damage
- Minimum downtime of equipment and minimum total cost

Emphasis on each of the previous factors will depend on the type of structure, the repair environment, and whether the repair is nonstructural or structural. For example, a structural repair to a composite hull will be more lengthy, compared with the repair of an internal bulkhead. For repairs carried out in-service and away from the dedicated repair yards, the need to use simple procedures takes a higher priority than it might for repairs carried out at a specialized maintenance facility.

When considering bonded composite repairs, it is important to correctly characterize the severity of the damage and the implications on the operational capability of the structure. For the purpose of simplicity, the different repair types can be classified as nonstructural or structural methods. A description of these repair types is provided in Table 3. Nonstructural damage can be defined as any form of damage contained within the surface layers of the composite, or areas of damage penetrating the composite that are of little structural significance. Typical approaches for this type of damage include:

- Mark and monitor over time
- Cosmetic repair
- Temporary repair

Structural damage can be defined as any form of damage that affects the stiffness or strength of the vessel, that is, damage occurring in areas of the vessel that have structural significance. Typical repair methods for this type of damage include:

- Minor repair (restoration to full serviceability)
- Major repair (restoration to original integrity)

A typical repair cycle for a composite structure is summarized in Fig. 1. The repair cycle itself contains a number of distinct levels: the survey of the damage and defect identification; making the repair decision; fabricating the repair; and then monitoring its performance throughout the life of the structure. Although all stages are important, a critical stage of the cycle concerns the defect identification phase, when it is essential to gather as much information as possible to help make an informed decision. Furthermore, a diligent approach at this stage will help eliminate the necessity of requesting any additional structural surveying, which only serves to delay the repair process. The second area that requires close control concerns the fabrication of the repair. In some cases, a repair might involve simple filling of cosmetic damage. However, at the other extreme, a badly damaged hull laminate may well necessitate major reconstruction.

Repair to Gel Coats

Gel coats on marine composites can experience hairline cracking, blistering, and abrasion that can be unsightly and may, over a long period, affect the mechanical performance of the underlying laminate (Ref 12, 13). Gel coat cracks are caused by many factors, including inadequate design, poor application of the gel coat, impact loading, stress concentrations around drilled holes, thermal expansion, and thermal fatigue effects. Blisters usually occur because of poor adhesion between the gel coat and the com-

Table 2 Types of damage to marine composites

Defect type	Defect description	Illustration of defect
Surface impact damage or gouge	Extended surface indentation, often approximately linear in form, on the laminate surface. Often associated with witness marks from the impactor and delamination damage. Direction of impact event can be inferred from the gouge orientation.	
Abrasion damage	The wearing away of a portion of the GRP laminate by either natural (rain, wind, etc.) or man-made (overblasting, collision) events. Confined to the laminate surface	Minor; Shallow; Deep; Gelcoat/resin rich layer; Chopped strand mat; Woven roving laminate
Delamination damage	Single plane or multiplane separation of adjacent layers within a multilayer component. In GRP laminates, it can be associated with a lightening of the damaged region. Often has a curved boundary	
Fracture	Through-thickness discontinuity or separation of the GRP laminate. Defined both as surface rupture (partial separation) of the laminate and as complete separation due to external or internal forces	Broken fibers; Crack penetrates depth of laminate

Table 3 Description of damage types

Damage type	Repair classification	Description
Nonstructural	Mark and monitor	This approach is undertaken when the nature of the damage does not warrant any form of repair. With this technique, it is necessary to record all information about the nature of the damage in order to be able to compare any worsening of the defect while the structure is subjected to operational loading.
	Cosmetic	Cosmetic repairs are designed to repair localized surface defects to the original profile and to prevent moisture ingress.
	Temporary	Temporary repairs are only to be conducted when there are operational reasons that prevent the recommended repair approach. These types of repairs must be made permanent at the next designated maintenance period.
Structural	Minor	Restoration of the structure to full serviceability, but requiring increased inspection frequencies to ensure that the repair remains effective
	Major	Restoration of the composite structure to its original integrity

posite, or by hydrolysis of the gel coat and subsequent ingress of moisture by osmosis. Most blisters are 2 to 50 mm (0.08 to 2.0 in.) in diameter and raised about 1 to 3 mm (0.04 to 0.12 in.) above the surrounding laminate. Blisters usually occur within the gel coat or at the bond line with the laminate, but occasionally blistering occurs beneath the first or several ply layers in the composite (Fig. 2). Gouges in gel coats occur mostly by the repeated action of the hull sliding against the dock, and severe abrasion marks can be several meters long. Removal of antifouling coatings by scraping can also cause mechanical damage, while the use of chemical paint strippers may degrade the gel coat properties. Some solvent-based paint strippers may impair the abrasion resistance by causing a permanent loss in hardness, while alkaline formulations may increase the likelihood of cracking.

The cracks, blisters, and abrasions to gel coats are usually cosmetic when they first develop and do not affect the structural integrity of the vessel. Blisters less than 5 mm (0.2 in.) in diameter, small cracks, and abrasion marks need not be repaired, although it is recommended they be regularly monitored, because over time the damage may spread. Larger damaged areas may be repaired using the following process:

1. Cracks, blisters, or gouges should be removed by light sanding. The gel coat can be removed until the laminate surface is exposed. Sanding of the laminate must be avoided, unless dry fibers are exposed or the damage occurs immediately beneath the laminate surface.
2. The sanded area should be thoroughly cleaned and dried.
3. The affected area should be filled with an epoxy, vinyl ester, or polyester resin. Care must be taken to ensure that the filler resin is compatible with follow-on gel-coating materials to ensure long-term adhesion and durability. For example, most common marine gel coats are compatible with polyester and vinyl ester commonly used as the matrix resin in many marine composites, but the gel coats may not adhere strongly to epoxy resin.
4. In repairs that require the removal of a small amount of laminate, the cavity should be filled with chopped strand mat wetted with resin or a filler compound consisting of resin and milled glass fibers. The resin used should be the same matrix resin of the composite, or a toughened resin that is compatible with the composite.
5. After curing, the repaired area can be painted, if necessary.

Composite Patch Repairs

Composite patching is one of the most common techniques for repairing minor structural damage to small marine craft with hulls thinner than about 8 to 10 mm (0.31 to 0.40 in.), such as canoes, powerboats, and small yachts. Patching can also be used to repair secondary structures to large composite ships, such as decks and superstructure, when a scarf repair is not possible or necessary. Composite patches can be easily and quickly applied while the boat is dockside.

A schematic diagram of a bonded composite patch is shown in Fig. 3. With a patch repair, the sound material surrounding the damaged area is first sanded and cleaned of dust. Because relatively little material is removed by sanding, it is important to then clean the prepared surface with a nonreactive solvent to remove any contamination. Several layers of glass-reinforced polyester are applied over the damaged area and then cured. A distinct feature of the repair is the offsetting of the ply drop-offs around the edges of the patch. This is done to minimize the localization of edge peel strains that can occur with this type of repair. The consolidation of the repair is improved if the patch is compacted during curing by a vacuum bagging process, although this may not always be practical, particularly when performed as a field repair. Patches rarely recover more than 70% of the original strength, due to the uneven shear stress distribution along the adhesive layer. Bolting can be used to more firmly secure an adhesively bonded patch to the composite substrate and support out-of-plane loads, although drilling the bolt holes can introduce further damage and create stress concentrations.

Scarf Repairs

The most common technique for repairing damaged composite ship structures is the scarf repair. Scarf repairs are popular with many boat builders because they can be applied to almost all types of craft, are durable and watertight, and usually restore an acceptable degree of structural integrity. The repairs restore between 50 and 90% of the original stiffness and strength of the composite structure, depending upon the quality of the repair and whether it is loaded in bending, compression, or tension. Disadvantages of scarf repairs are: they must be performed at a dockyard by skilled workers; they are time-consuming; and they may require the removal of a large amount of undamaged material to form the required taper angle. Scarf repairs can be made on both single-skin laminates and sandwich composites.

Laminates. Three types of scarf repairs that can be used to repair single-skin laminates are commonly known as single-scarf, double-scarf, and partial-thickness scarf (Fig. 4). Single-scarf repair is generally used when access to both sides of the damaged structure is not possible, or on composite structures thinner than several millimeters. Double-scarf repair should be used whenever practical, and is strongly recommended for the repair of damage that severely degrades the mechanical properties of the composite structure, such as a hole through the hull

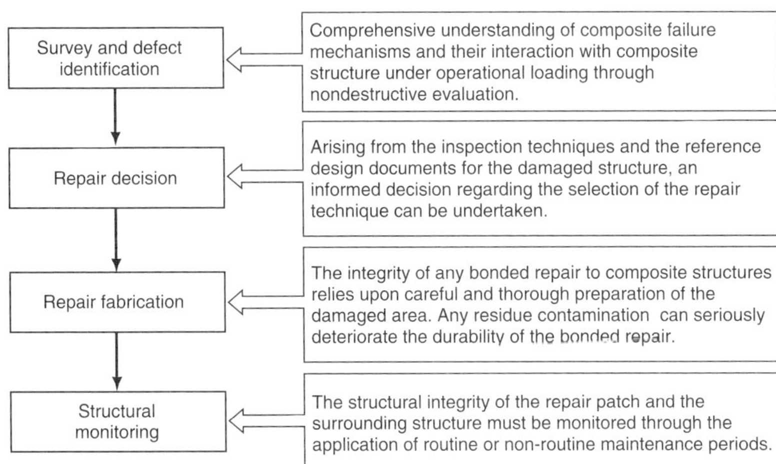

Fig. 1 A typical repair cycle for a composite structure

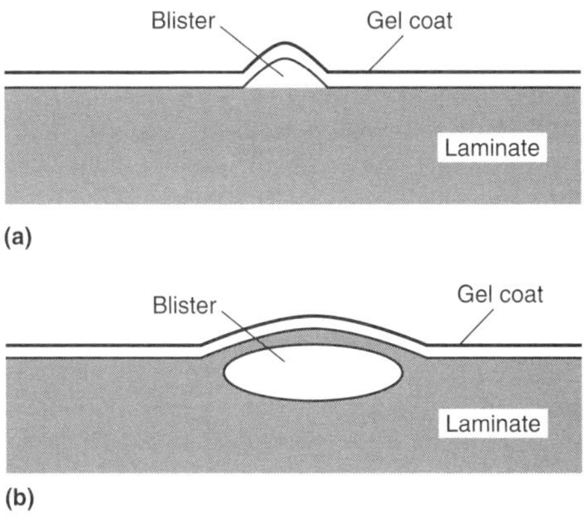

Fig. 2 Blistering. (a) Blistering of a gel coat. (b) Blistering beneath a gel coat

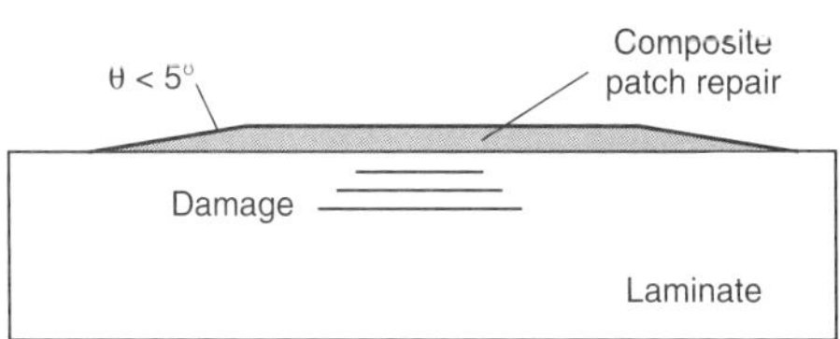

Fig. 3 Configuration of a composite patch repair

near or below the waterline. Partial-thickness repair is applied to thick composite structures that have damage confined to a region close to the surface, such as near-surface delaminations or gouges that penetrate only partway through the laminate.

Scarf Repair Steps. Scarf repairs are performed in the sequence of steps described below.

Step 1: Inspection and Mapping of Damage. The size and depth of damage to be repaired must be accurately surveyed using appropriate nondestructive evaluation (NDE) techniques. A variety of NDE techniques can be used to inspect for damage in composite ship structures, and these are reviewed by Bar-Cohen (Ref 14). The simplest technique is visual inspection, where "whitening" due to delamination and/or resin cracking can be used to indicate the damage area in semitransparent composites such as glass/polyester and glass/vinyl ester laminates. Visual inspection is not an accurate technique because not all damage is detectable to the eye, particularly damage hidden by paint, damage located deep below the surface, and damage in nontransparent composites such as carbon and aramid laminates. A popular technique is tap testing, where a lightweight object such as a coin or hammer is used to softly tap the composite surface. A change in the frequency of the tapping sound is used to indicate the presence of damage. The main benefits of tap testing are that it is simple and can be used to rapidly inspect large areas. Tap testing can usually be used to detect delamination damage close to the surface, but becomes increasingly less reliable the deeper the delamination is located below the surface. Tap testing is not useful for detecting other types of damage, such as resin cracks and broken fibers. More advanced NDE techniques for inspecting composite ships are impedance testing, x-ray radiography, thermography, and ultrasonics (see the article "Nondestructive Testing" in this Volume). Of these techniques, ultrasonics are arguably the most accurate and practical, and are often used for surveying damage. Ultrasonics can be used to detect small delaminations located deep below the surface, unlike visual inspection and tap testing.

Step 2: Removal of Damaged Material. The damaged laminate must be removed and the edges of the sound laminate tapered back to a shallow angle. The taper slope ratio, also known as the scarf angle, should be less than 12 to 1 ($\theta < 5°$) to minimize the shear strains along the bond line after the repair patch is applied. The shallow angle also compensates for some errors in workmanship and other shop variables that might diminish patch adhesion.

Step 3: Surface Preparation. The laminate close to the scarf zone should be lightly abraded with sandpaper, followed by the removal of dust and contaminates. It is recommended that if the scarf zone has been exposed to the environment for any considerable period of time, it should be cleaned with a solvent to remove contamination.

Step 4: Molding. A rigid backing plate having the original profile of the composite ship structure is needed to ensure the repair has the same geometry as the surrounding structure.

Step 5: Laminating. Laminated repairs are usually done using the smallest-ply-first taper sequence that is illustrated in Fig. 5(a). While this repair is acceptable, it produces relatively weak, resin-rich areas at each ply edge at the repair interface. A better alternative is the largest-ply-first laminate sequence, where the first layer of reinforcing fabric completely covers the work area, followed by successively smaller layers, and then finished with an extra outer layer or two extending over the patch and onto the sound laminate for some distance, as shown in Fig. 5(b).

Selection of the reinforcing material is critical to ensuring the repair has acceptable mechanical performance. The reinforcing fabric or mat should be identical to the reinforcement material used in the original composite. Also, the fiber orientations to the reinforcing layers within the repair laminate should match those of the original hull laminate, so that the mechanical properties of the repair will be as close to original as possible. Resin selection is another important factor in repair. Isophthalic laminating-grade polyester resins are generally acceptable in most marine repairs, although vinyl esters are recommended for hull repairs below the waterline to achieve superior adhesion, better durability, and higher mechanical properties.

The laminating process used in the repair should be similar to that used for original construction of the ship laminate to ensure the repair material has the same fiber-to-resin ratio as the original structure. In other words, a ship laminate originally made using vacuum bagging or resin infusion should not be repaired with an open hand lay-up process, because this will result in a repair with a much lower fiber-to-resin ratio than the base material.

Step 6: Finishing. After the patch has cured, a gel coat and/or paint should be applied.

Properties and Durability of Scarf Repairs to Laminates. Scarf repairs to marine craft should ideally have similar mechanical properties and durability to that of the original composite. Unfortunately, this is not always the case, with the efficiency of a scarf repair being affected by factors such as matching plies, quality of adhesive, scarf angle, and the general quality of workmanship. Most scarf repairs restore up to 80 to 90% of the original stiffness, strength, and fatigue life, and this is considered adequate for a permanent repair. However, the restoration of properties may be much lower than this in some cases. In other cases the stiffness and strength of the repair may be greater than the original mechanical properties of the laminate. This situation is to be avoided because it creates a "hard" spot that may affect the long-term fatigue performance of the structure. Scarf repairs have good long-term durability in the marine environment, and are affected no more than the original structure by contaminates such as oil and fuel.

Sandwich Composites. Sandwich composites used in marine craft can experience three classes of damage, known as type A, B, or C, as illustrated in Fig. 6, 7, and 8. Type A damage is confined to one skin, and is usually produced by gouging or a low-speed impact that creates matrix cracks, fiber breaks, and delaminations in one of the skins. Type A damage can also include disbonding of one skin from the core. Type B involves damage to one skin and the core, where the core may be crushed or cracked. Type C is damage to both skins and the core, and can be complete rupture of the sandwich structure.

The first step in the scarf repair of a sandwich composite is to inspect and map the damage. The detection of core failures for types B and C damage is difficult using most conventional nondestructive inspection techniques, such as tap testing and ultrasonics. Nondestructive evaluation techniques that may be used to detect damage are impedance testing, thermography, and, possibly, microwave. The repair of type A damage is similar to a single-scarf repair of a single-skin laminate (Fig. 6). The damaged skin is removed, the surrounding sound material is tapered to a scarf angle of about 5°, and then the skin is replaced, often with an extra lay of GRP to ensure high stiffness and strength. Afterwards, the repaired area can be gel coated and painted. The reinforcement and resin should be the same as

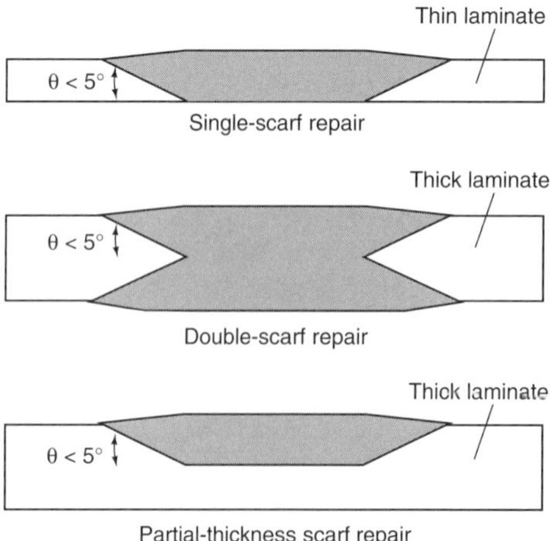

Fig. 4 Illustrations of different types of scarf repairs for single-skin composites

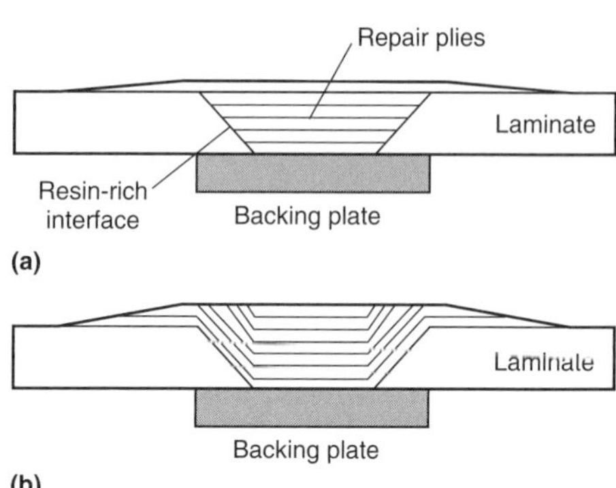

Fig. 5 Illustrations of (a) conventional and (b) improved scarf repair techniques

those of the original skin. It is also suitable in some cases to use resins with higher elongation properties than the original resin, provided both resins are compatible. In addition, the plies must be laminated in the same stacking sequence as the reinforcement in the original skin to achieve optimal structural efficiency. A major problem with scarf repairs of sandwich composites is the entrapment of air at the bond line between the new skin and core, which can result in lower mechanical properties. This problem can be overcome by good workmanship to establish an acceptable bond between the lowest repair ply and the core. The removal of air from along the bond line can also be achieved by vacuum bagging of the wet lay-up repair or by using prepreg repairs.

Different techniques are available for repairing type B damage, with one such technique shown schematically in Fig. 7 (Ref 11, 16, 17). The main differences between type B repair techniques are the geometry of the replacement core and the taper angle to the core. When the core has been slightly damaged, it is possible to apply a foaming adhesive or a laminate as a replacement. When the core has been extensively damaged, it must be cut out and replaced with the original core material. Some methods recommend replacing the damaged core with square or rectangular blocks with a scarf angle of 90° (Fig. 7). Other methods recommend using triangular wedges with a scarf taper of 45°. Accurately machining a 45° taper through the core of a damaged boat can be difficult, and therefore most boat builders prefer a scarf angle of 90°, however the repairs are more prone to shear core failure along the bond line.

The replacement core is bonded into place using a polyester resin, syntactic foam putty, or rubber-toughened vinyl-ester-based putty and, if necessary, fastened with small screws or pins (Ref 16). Extreme care is needed when inserting the replacement core sections so that air does not become trapped along the bond line with the undamaged skin. Entrapped air usually occurs during hand lay-up repairs, and the problem can be prevented using vacuum-bagging methods to consolidate the repair. After the replacement core has been inserted, the skin is replaced using the same method as for the type A repair. Type B repairs usually recover about 80% of the structural properties, although repairs having strength and fatigue properties as low as 50% of the original material have been reported (Ref 17, 18).

Various techniques are available for repairing type C damage. A type C repair method is illustrated in Fig. 8, which is an extension of the type B repair shown in Fig. 7. The steps involved in a type C repair are similar to those for a type B repair, with the only obvious difference being the need to replace the second damaged skin. Supplemental "doubler" laminates, larger in area than the repair itself, are commonly applied to the interior laminates in this type of repair, where facing or cosmetic considerations make oversized repair plies impractical for the outer skin. The mechanical properties of sandwich composites repaired by a type C technique are generally similar to those of the original material (Ref 17).

Step Repairs

Typical sea-loading conditions on a GRP ship induce cyclic horizontal bending of the hull and shear and torsion of the hull girder, together with static and wave-induced pressures on the hull surface (Ref 1). Due to the bending nature of these loading situations, a step repair profile should be selected in preference to the scarf profile. A schematic illustration showing the basic stages of the step repair technique is given in Fig. 9. As with the other repair techniques, the first stage involves accurately surveying the extent of damage using NDE techniques. After this, the area immediately surrounding a damaged section of hull is removed using a cut and peel-back method, as shown in Fig. 10. A rectangular stepped surface is created by cutting into the hull to a set depth and peeling out material within this area along the level of the laminate. This process is repeated within the peeled out area down to the depth of the damage/delamination, as shown in Fig. 9. The step lengths and step depths are determined depending on the structural criticality of the damaged site.

Producing a stepped profile can be difficult, particularly when performed at sea or in bilges, and it is common to experience problems with the repair. Figure 11 highlights the most common problem with the repair step, namely, the problem of excessive undercutting. When the step into the parent material is made, it is necessary to cut slightly deeper (1–2 mm, or 0.04–0.08 in.) than the nominal step depth. This is so the repair area can be peeled out of the bulk material without delamination extending into the remaining material. Due to the waviness in the ply layers of a composite made by the hand lay-up process, the temptation (on the part of the person cutting out the damage) is to always cut slightly deeper than necessary to prevent this peel-back into the parent laminate. Although it may be expected that the undercut would pose a structural weakness in the repair site, this generally does not appear to be the case. For example, in the Royal Navy composite minehunting vessels, where this technique is used for the repair of all

Type A damage

Core

Taper skin

Apply replacement skin

Fig. 6 Schematic of basic steps in the scarf repair to a sandwich composite with type A damage. (Adapted from Ref 15)

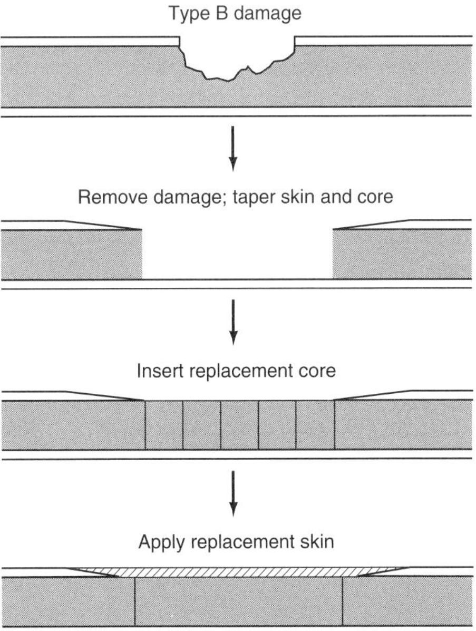

Fig. 7 Schematic of steps in the repair to a sandwich composite with type B damage. (Adapted from Ref 16)

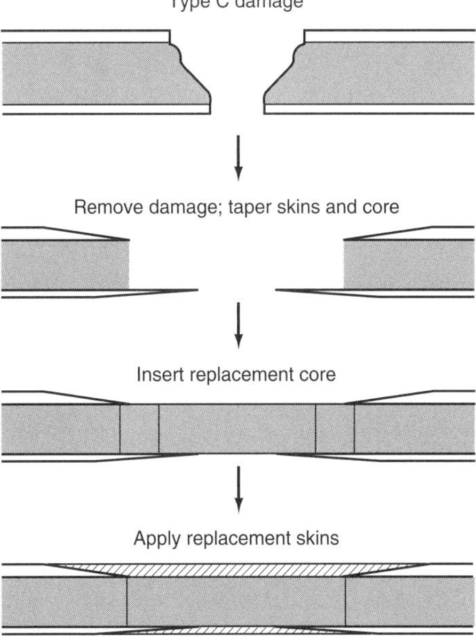

Fig. 8 Schematic of steps in the repair to a sandwich composite with type C damage. (Adapted from Ref 16)

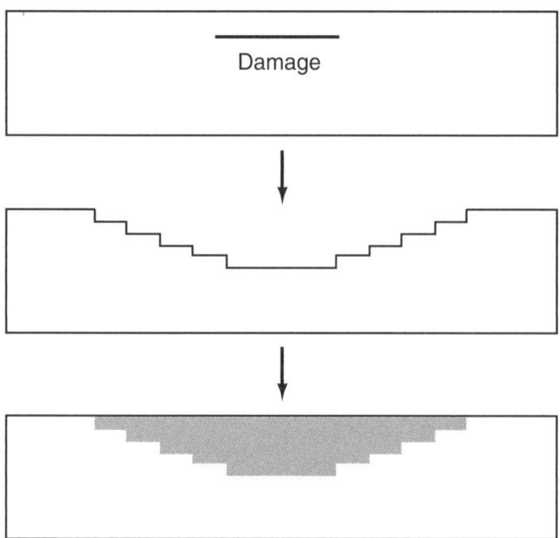

Fig. 9 Schematic of the stages in the step repair of a single-skin composite

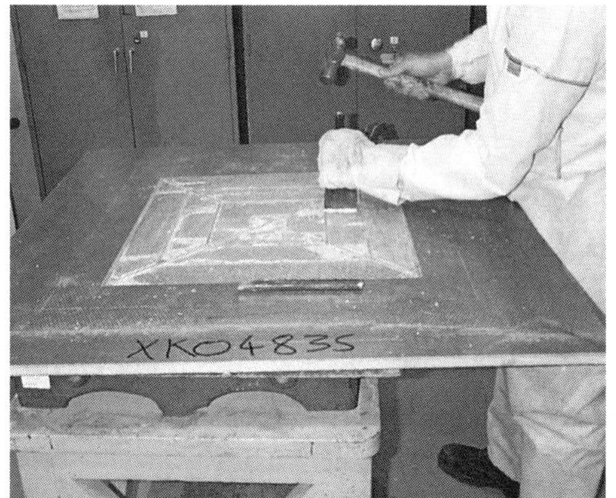

Fig. 10 Mechanical extraction of damage to form a step profile

structural damage, there has been no indicated in-service failure of this type of repair.

After the damaged material is removed and the step profile is complete, the hollowed-out area is given a standard surface preparation, and the repair material is laid up into it with only manual consolidation and cured in situ at ambient temperature.

Resin-Infusion Repairs

Resin-infusion repair methods are relatively new techniques being developed to restore minor structural damage to single-skin laminates and to repair disbonds between the skin and core of sandwich composites (Ref 19). As with any repair technique, the first step in a resin-infusion repair is to survey and map the extent of damage. Narrow holes are then drilled through the damaged material at several locations, with the holes usually spaced 5 to 30 cm (2 to 12 in.) apart. Plastic hoses are connected from the holes to a vacuum pump, which extracts any moisture that may have seeped into the crack. Following this, some of the hoses are connected to a resin source. Resin is then drawn under vacuum into the crack, until filled. The hoses are disconnected, the resin cured within the defect, and the repair is complete. A resin-infusion repair to a composite ship is shown in Fig. 12.

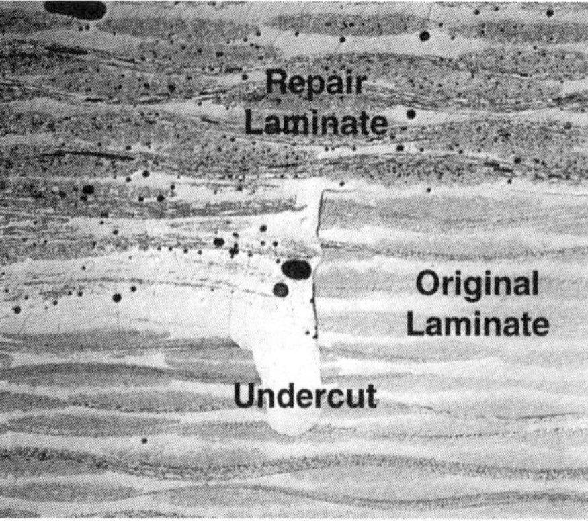

Fig. 11 Micrograph showing a typical undercut in a GRP step repair

The resin-infusion method has not been thoroughly tested on a wide range of marine craft, although in the future the method may be used increasingly instead of scarf or step repairs because it is cheaper, simpler, and does not require removing a large amount of undamaged material. However, there are several factors that are likely to limit the severity of damage that can be repaired in this way. These include the difficulty of removing contaminants, such as salts and oily residues, from the fracture surfaces prior to rebonding, the inability to mend broken fibers, and problems establishing the effectiveness of a given repair.

An alternate to resin infusion is a resin-injection repair, where resin is forced into the cracks and disbonds under an externally applied pressure. The advantage over resin infusion is that it has a greater potential for infiltrating most of the damage, and can be implemented with some flow-through of the resin in order to flush contaminants from the disbonded surfaces. However, it is difficult to fill the crack front with resin because of entrapped air, and the externally applied pressure may cause further growth of the cracks. Resin-injection repairs have been developed for use on aircraft composite structures, but have not yet been widely adapted for composite ship repairs. While both resin-infusion and resin-injection repairs can be remarkably successful in restoring stiffness and strength, validating the structural efficiency of a specific repair is likely to remain a problem.

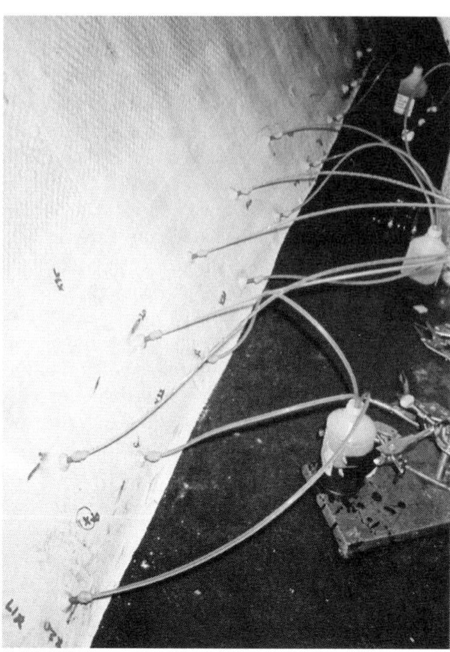

Fig. 12 Resin-infusion repair of a composite ship structure

REFERENCES

1. C.S. Smith, *Design of Marine Structures in Composite Materials,* Elsevier Applied Science, London, 1990
2. J.D.G. Sumpter, A.C. Swift, D.M. Elliott, D. Faulke, R. Court, and P.W. Lay, "Defect Tolerance of GRP Ships," Proc. Advances in Marine Structures III, 20–23 May 1997 (Dunfermline, Scotland)
3. R.W. Kiger and C.E. Beck, "Large Area Composite Structure Repair," Paper 17-D, Proc. 33rd Annual Conf. Reinforced Plastics/Composites Institute, 1978
4. S.H. Myhre, Advanced Composite Repair—Recent Developments and Some Problems, *Proc. 26th National SAMPE Symposium,* 28–30 April 1981, p 716–727
5. A.A. Baker, Repair Techniques for Composite Structures, *Composite Materials in Aircraft Structures,* D.H. Middleton, Ed., Longman Scientific and Technical, United Kingdom, 1990, p 207–227
6. P.J. Petrick, *Fiberglass Repairs,* Cormell Maritime Inc., Cambridge, MD, 1976
7. Owens-Corning Fiberglass, "Fiberglass Repairability: a Guide and Directory to the Repair of Fiberglass Commercial Fishing Boats," 5-BO-12657, Toledo, OH, 1985
8. B. Pfund, "Fiber in the Hole," *Professional Boatbuilder,* Aug/Sept 1995, p 34–39
9. "GRP Ships and Boats Maintenance Survey and Repair: Maintenance and Repair Requirements for GRP Surface Ships, Boats and Craft (Single Skin)," Naval Engineering Standard 752, Part 2 (Issue 2), MoD, Bath, 1981
10. "Notes on Design, Construction, Inspection and Repair of Fibre Reinforced Plastic (FRP) Vessels," USCG NVIG 8-87, 1987
11. "Bay Class Minehunter Inshore Glass Reinforced Plastic Repair Manual," Defence Instruction (Navy) ABR 5803, Royal Australian Navy, July 1992
12. L. Whitfield et al., *Repairs to Blisters in Glass Fibre Hulls,* The British Plastics Federation, 1979

13. E. Greene, "Marine Composites: Investigation of Fiberglass Reinforced Plastics in Marine Structures," Ship Structure Committee Report SSC-360, National Technical Information Service, VA, 1990
14. Y. Bar-Cohen, "Nondestructive Evaluation (NDE) of Fibreglass Marine Structures: State-of-the-Art Review," Report c\CG-D-02-91, McDonnell Douglas Corporation, 1991
15. S. Martinsen and C. Madsen, "Production, Research and Development in GRP Materials," Paper 8-F, Proc. of the 46th Annual Conference of the Composites Institute, 18–21 February 1991
16. J. Sjogren, C.G. Celsing, K.A. Olsson, C.G. Levan, and S.E. Hellbrat, "Swedish Development of MCMV-Hull Design and Production," RINA Symposium, June 1984 (London)
17. R. Thomson, R. Luescher, and I. Grabovac, "Repair of Damage to Marine Sandwich Structures: Part I—Static Testing," DSTO Technical Report DSTO-TR-0736, 1998
18. S.D. Clark, R.A. Shenoi, and H.G. Allen, Influence of Impact Damage and Repair Schemes on the Strength of Foam-Cored Sandwich Beams, *Proc. 11th International Conf. Composite Materials,* 14–18 July 1997 (Gold Coast, Australia), p VI-385 to VI-394
19. N.A. St. John, G.J. Simpson, and K.E. Challis, Resin Infusion Repair of Delaminated GRP Structures, *Proc. ACUN-3,* 6–9 Feb 2001 (Sydney, Australia), p 482–487

Rehabilitation of Reinforced Concrete Structures Using Fiber-Reinforced Polymer Composites

A. Zureick and L. Kahn, Georgia Institute of Technology

FIBER-REINFORCED POLYMER (FRP) COMPOSITE MATERIALS provide an outstanding means for rehabilitating and strengthening existing reinforced and prestressed concrete bridges, buildings and other structures. Whether a structure has been damaged due to overload, earthquake or materials deterioration, or whether the structure requires strengthening to resist increased future live loads, wind, or seismic forces, FRPs provide an efficient, cost-effective, and easy-to-construct means or reinforcing concrete members. These advanced composites may be designed to act as flexural, shear, and confinement reinforcement. Use of these composites requires less disturbance to building occupancy, bridge traffic, and other functions than rehabilitation that uses additional steel reinforcement.

The concept of strengthening with FRP was pioneered by Professor U. Meier at the Swiss Federal Laboratories for Materials Testing and Research Institute in the early 1980s. His extensive research activities led to the first-time field implementation of FRP rehabilitation for both bridge and building applications. Both the Ibach bridge near Lucerne, Switzerland and the City Hall of Gossau, St. Gall in northeastern Switzerland were strengthened in 1991 by bonding pultruded carbon-fiber polymer plates to the exterior surfaces of the concrete structures. Details on some of these and other early applications are described in Ref 1. Since then, there has been keen worldwide interest not only to use polymeric materials in strengthening structures, but also to examine their structural behavior under a variety of loading and environmental conditions. Reference 2 is a review highlighting some fundamental concepts pertaining to the use of FRP materials in structural rehabilitation; comprehensive expositions of past research activities, test results, and case studies on the same subject are given in a monograph (Ref 3).

To effectively design and execute a rehabilitation scheme using FRPs, the engineer must fully understand the condition of the existing structure, the properties and characteristics of the composite materials, the interaction between the FRP and concrete, and construction methodology.

The terms rehabilitation, repair, and strengthening are defined as follows:

- Rehabilitation: the process of repairing or modifying a structure to a desired useful condition
- Repair: the process of replacing or correcting deteriorated, damaged, or faulty materials, components, or elements of a structure
- Strengthening: the process of increasing the load-carrying capacity of a structure or portion thereof

Structural Assessment

The structure must be evaluated prior to application of FRPs, so that the actual load-carrying capacity may be determined and the causes for prior deterioration or damage may be identified and eliminated. Cracked, chipped, and deteriorated concrete must be repaired; corroded steel reinforcement must be cleaned and evaluated prior to further rehabilitation.

The first step of the structural assessment should be a review of the plans, specifications, and construction records of the structure. These documents provide the minimum strength of the concrete and reinforcement, the size of the members, and the size and location of all reinforcement. An analysis based upon these plans gives an estimate of the anticipated strength of the structure, provided no deterioration has occurred.

The second step, site observation, includes measurement of the geometry of the structure and determination of cracks and other deterioration or damage. The geometry is compared with the plans to assure the correctness of the documentation. The presence of cracks and damage provides a basis for the design of repairs needed prior to rehabilitation.

Provided that cracking and deterioration are not extensive, nondestructive testing of the structure is used to verify the strength of the concrete and the location of the reinforcement. The quality of the concrete can be investigated using acoustic impact (e.g., chain dragging), rebound hammers (Schmidt Hammer shown in Fig. 1), and penetration resistance (Windsor Probe). Magnetic detection devices (pachometers) may be used to measure the extent and location of reinforcement. If the quality of the concrete appears poor, destructive tests are necessary. Cores are taken; cutting of reinforcement is avoided. Compression testing of the cores provides an acceptable determination of compressive strength (f_c'). Petrographic analysis is required if the suspected cause of deterioration is alkali-silica reaction.

Cracking and/or pop-outs in the vicinity of reinforcement indicate potential corrosion of the reinforcement. In those locations, the concrete should be removed and the reinforcement in-

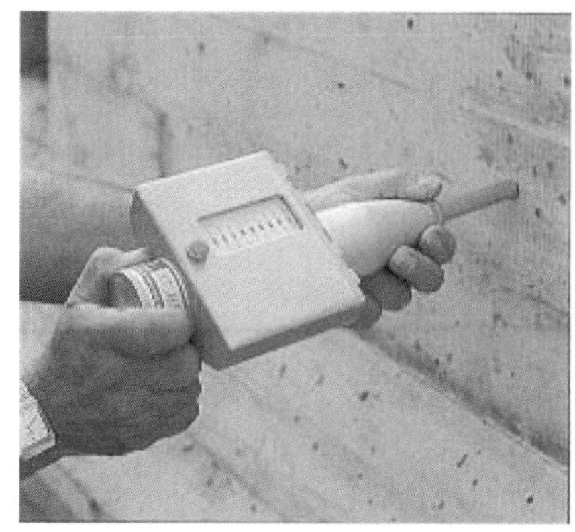

Fig. 1 Schmidt Hammer for evaluating concrete quality. Courtesy of PROCEQ SA

spected. If the reinforcement is rusted such that loose rust is noted, the concrete must be removed from around the corroded reinforcing bars, and the bars must be cleaned of rust. The actual cross-sectional area of the bars should be determined and used in subsequent analysis. Further, the chloride content of the concrete should be determined, along with its electrical potential, so that the probability of continued active corrosion is determined. Permitting active corrosion of the reinforcement to continue after FRP rehabilitation will limit the life of the rehabilitation system.

With the previously mentioned assessment complete, areas of damaged and deteriorated concrete should be repaired prior to placement of FRP materials. Areas where concrete has been removed and corroded reinforcement cleaned should be patched with compatible materials. In general, Portland cement mortar patches provide good bond and compatibility with the existing concrete substrate. Polymer concretes are preferred for small patches (less than 20 mm, or 0.79 in. thick).

Where damage has occurred due to overload, differential settlement, or restraint of shrinkage and creep of the concrete, cracks may be large. An assessment of those cracks may indicate that the concrete cannot transmit shear or compressive forces. In such cases, cracks with widths between 0.3 and 3.0 mm (0.012 and 0.12 in.) should be filled by injection with a low viscosity epoxy; cracks wider than 3.0 mm (0.12 in.) should be injected with either a polymer or cement grout. Wherever cracks are injected and patches are placed, the surface of the resulting structure should be smooth and even for optimal application of the FRP.

Finally, the strength of the existing structure should be assessed, based on the actual condition of the structure.

Composite Materials Reinforcing Systems for Concrete Strengthening

Fiber-reinforced polymer composites used for strengthening reinforced concrete structures are made of aramid, carbon, or glass fibers with an epoxy thermoset-resin matrix to bind them together. They can be classified into two systems: shop-manufactured and field-manufactured.

Shop-manufactured composites are premanufactured in the form of plates, shells, or other shapes and are bonded in the field to the surface of the concrete member using structural adhesives. These composites are manufactured by a variety of techniques, such as pultrusion, filament winding, and resin transfer molding. Some of the common commercially available shop-manufactured composite systems are briefly described below:

- CarboDur (Sika Corporation, Lyndhurst, NJ) composites are 1.2 mm (0.05 in.) thick carbon-epoxy pultruded unidirectional plates that can be bonded to the concrete surface with an epoxy-based adhesive. The fiber volume in this system is approximately 68% (Fig. 2).
- SNAP-Tite (ISCO Industries LLC, Louisville, KY) a 3 mm (1/8 in.) thick prefabricated E-glass/isophthalic polyester shell that can be bonded to a round concrete column using polyurethene adhesive. Additional shells can be bonded over the first bonded shell to achieve the desired thickness.
- Hardshell structures are prefabricated E-glass/vinyl ester shells manufactured by the vacuum-assisted resin transfer molding process with a fiber volume of about 60%. The shells can be bonded to round concrete columns using an adhesive system.

Field-manufactured composites are fibers in the form of tows or fabrics and are impregnated in the field before being placed on the surface of the structure requiring strengthening. Impregnation can be accomplished manually (hand lay-up), by a portable impregnator machine, or by infusion under vacuum. The composite is bonded to the concrete and left to cure under ambient or elevated temperature.

Commercially available field-manufactured composite systems include, but are not limited to, the following:

- MBrace (Master Builders, Inc., Cleveland, OH) and Replark (Mitsubishi Chemical Corp., Tokyo) are similar systems that include a primer, putty, epoxy-resin matrix, and dry unidirectional carbon-fiber sheets weighing approximately 300 g/m^2 (8.8 oz/yd^2). The composite reinforcing system is manufactured by the hand lay-up technique.
- SikaWrap Hex (Sika Corporation, Lyndhurst, NJ) and Tyfo Fiberwrap Systems (Fyfe Co. LLC, San Diego, CA) are unidirectional fabrics weighing approximately 612 g/m^2 (18 oz/yd^2). The fabrics are impregnated with epoxy resin using a portable impregnator machine, as illustrated in Fig. 3.
- XXsys Technologies, Inc. system is one in which columns are wound with prepreg carbon tows using a Robo-Wrapper (XXsys Technologies, Inc., San Diego) winding machine as shown in Fig. 4. The resin is cured at elevated temperature, using a portable oven known as Robo-Curing System shown in Fig. 5.

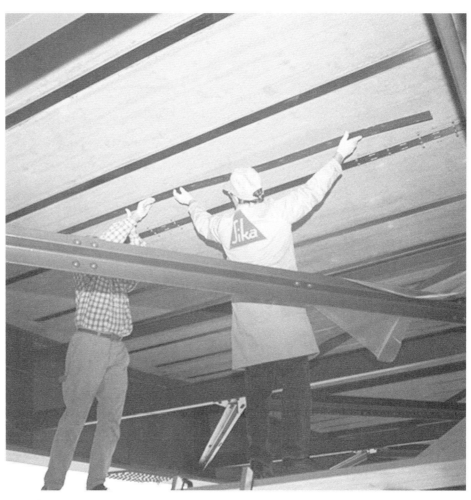

Fig. 2 Application of shop-manufactured carbon composite plates to the underside of a bridge deck

An advantage of the shop-manufactured composites over the field-manufactured composites is the ability to control the quality and uniformity in the composite reinforcing systems. An advantage of the field-manufactured composites is their ability to conform to nonuniform concrete surfaces.

Properties of Polymer Composite Reinforcing Systems

Because of the absence of national codes and standards, manufacturers report their data in a variety of ways. This variation presents both the engineer and the owner with a dilemma for properly comparing different systems and for assessing the benefit of using such materials in construction projects. Reported data should include the method of testing used to obtain such data, the number of tested specimens, the number of batches from which test specimens were drawn, the mean value, the minimum and maximum values, and the coefficient of variation. Manufacturers also may elect to provide the minimum guaranteed property values, along with the methods by which such values are obtained. As a minimum, the contractor should furnish the owner the following information pertaining to the matrix (binding resin or adhesive):

- For the matrix material and any of its components, the commercial designation, name of manufacturer, and materials safety data sheet, prepared in compliance with the Federal Occupational Safety and Health Administration (OSHA) Hazard Communication Standard 29 CFR 1910.1200
- The density of the matrix material and any of its components, determined according to ASTM D 792, "Test Methods for Specific Gravity and Density of Plastics by Displacement"
- The gel time, determined according to ASTM D 2472, "Standard Test Method for Gel Time and Peak Exothermic Temperature of Reacting Thermosetting Resins"
- The curing behavior, determined according to ASTM D 4473, "Standard Practice for Measuring the Cure Behavior of Thermosetting Resins Using Dynamic Mechanical Procedures"
- The water absorption, determined according to ASTM D 570, "Standard Test Method for Water Absorption of Plastics"
- The glass transition temperature, according to ASTM D 3418, "Standard Test Method for Temperatures of Polymers by Differential Scanning Calorimetry"
- The tensile properties, according to ASTM D 638, "Standard Test Method for Tensile Properties of Plastics"
- The compressive properties, according to ASTM D 695, "Standard Test Method for Compressive Properties of Rigid Plastics"
- The flexural properties, according to ASTM D 790, "Standard Test Method for Flexural Properties of Unreinforced and Reinforced Plastics and Electrical Insulating Materials"

The contractor should furnish the following information about the reinforcement materials:

- The commercial designation, name of manufacturer, fiber form (e.g., yarns, strands, tows, fabric, and prepreg), fiber orientation, fiber dimensions, and fiber surface treatments
- The density of the fiber, according to ASTM D 3800, "Standard Test Method for Density of High-Modulus Fibers"
- For prepregs, the matrix solid content and matrix content, determined according to ASTM D 3529, "Standard Test Method for Matrix Solids Content and Matrix Content of Composite Prepreg"
- For epoxy-carbon fiber-based prepreg, the volatiles content, reported according to ASTM D 3530, "Volatiles Content of Carbon-Fiber Prepreg"

For a composite system, cured under specified conditions approximating the conditions of the actual use, the following materials properties determined experimentally should be provided:

- The density, according to ASTM D 792, "Test Methods for Specific Gravity and Density of Plastics by Displacements"
- The tensile properties (ultimate strength, ultimate strain, and modulus) of the composite

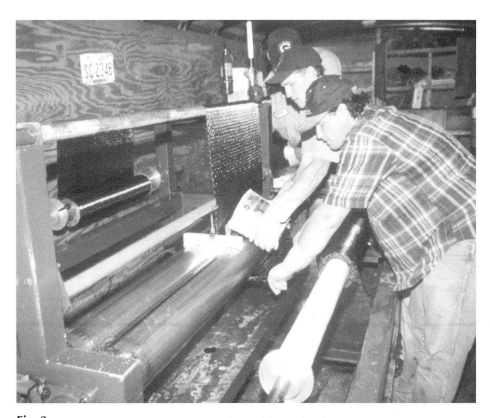

Fig. 3 Portable impregnator machine for field manufacture of fiber-reinforced composites

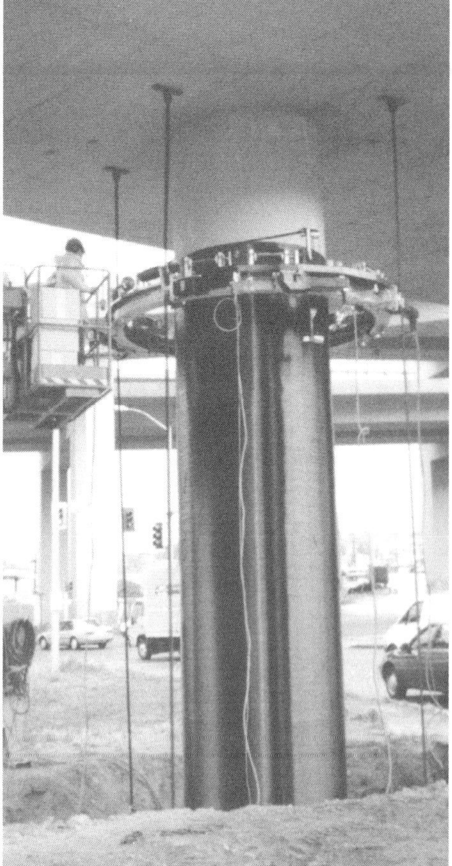

Fig. 4 Robo-Wrapper machine for winding columns with prepreg carbon tows. Courtesy of XXsys Technologies, Inc.

materials, according to ASTM D 3039, "Test Method for Tensile Properties of Polymer Matrix Composite Materials"

- The fiber volume, according to ASTM D 2584, "Test Method for Ignition Loss of Cured Reinforced Resins," or D 3171, "Test Method for Fiber Content of Resin-Matrix Composites by Matrix Digestion"
- The void volume, according to ASTM D 2734, "Test Method for Void Content of Reinforced Plastics"
- Moisture diffusivity and absorption or desorption properties, according to ASTM D 5229, "Test Method for Moisture Absorption Properties and Equilibrium Conditioning of Polymer Matrix Composite Materials"

The wealth of information gained from over 30 years of composite applications for aerospace use makes the task of reporting properties straightforward in the case of shop-manufactured composites. However, difficulties arise when composites are manufactured in the field, especially with the hand lay-up technique, where both geometrical (e.g., thickness) and materials properties (e.g., mechanical) are strongly influenced, not only by the operator fabricating the composites but also by climate curing conditions, dust from occasional wind, and other environmental factors.

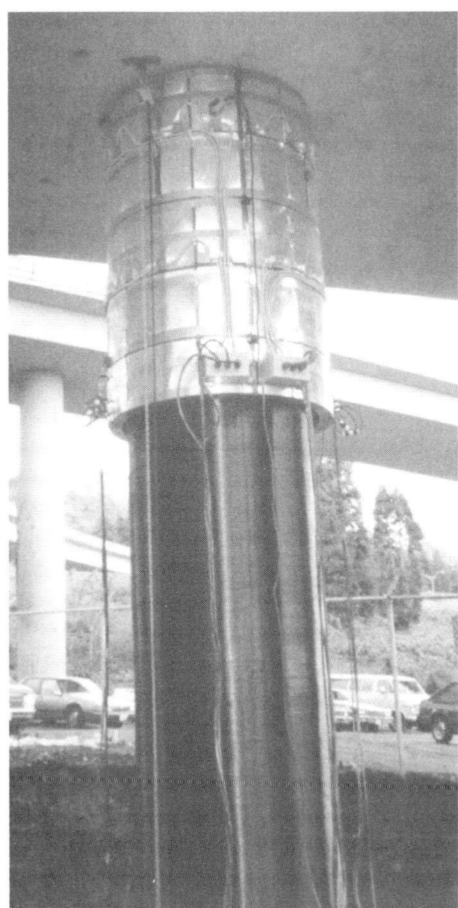

Fig. 5 Portable oven (Robo-Curing System) for curing columns wound from prepreg carbon tows. Courtesy of XXsys Technologies, Inc.

Materials Property Requirements for Design

When used to strengthen concrete structures, polymeric composite reinforcing systems will virtually always be subjected to not only various combinations of loads (e.g., dead loads, live loads, wind loads, and earthquake loads) but also to complicated environmental exposures (ambient temperature, solar radiation, humidity, organic growth, chemicals, etc.) that change continually. Therefore, the composite properties need to be stable or undergo insignificant changes during the lifetime of the strucuture.

Temperature is of particular importance. Defining the operating temperature range requires a proper examination of the climatological data for the location in which the structure is to be built. The data can be statistically analyzed for trends and variations (see Ref 4), so that high and low temperature values can be estimated for a given region and time interval; these values have a specified annual probability of being within the admissible range. Temperature records in the United States are readily available through the National Climatic Data Center. We define the operating temperatures as the range bounded by the overall temperature maximum and minimum recorded daily in a given location from the observed climate. Figures 6 and 7 show these extreme values for each state individually.

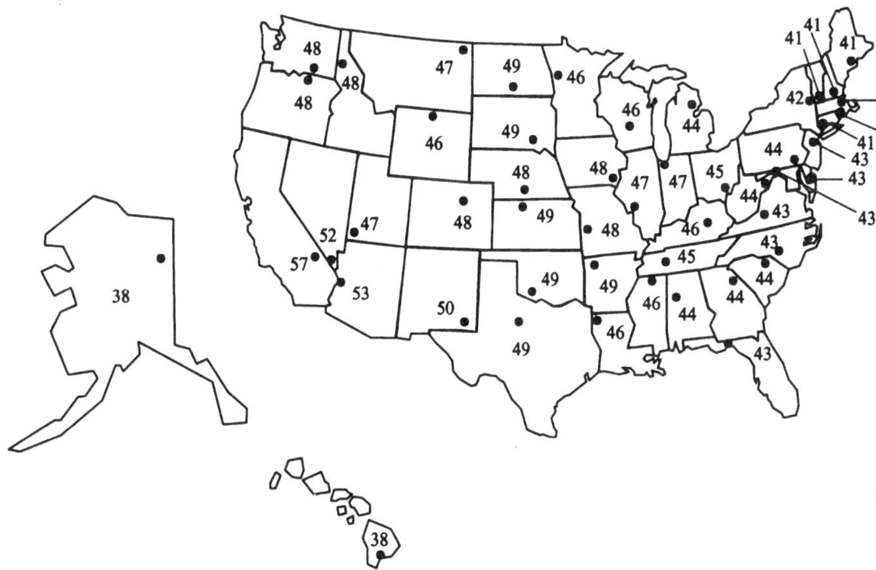

Fig. 6 Record highest temperature (°C) by states through 1998. Source: National Climatic Data Center

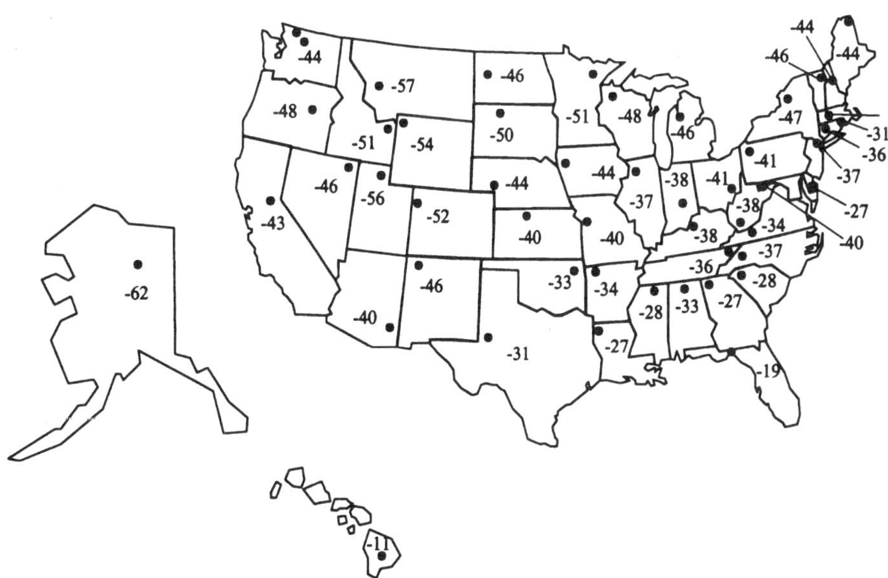

Fig. 7 Record lowest temperature (°C) by states through 1998. Source: National Climatic Data Center

To appropriately select the polymeric composite most suitable for strengthening purposes, the designer relies upon the dimensional stability, strength, and stiffness properties of the materials for which the main determinant is their glass transition temperature, (T_g). The T_g is defined as the approximate temperature value or temperature range at which the matrix changes from a glassy to a rubbery state. Above T_g, the composite softens and its mechanical properties are degraded, as illustrated in Fig. 8. In addition, it is to be noted that T_g decreases as the moisture content in the composite increases. The T_g of the resin, when cured in a manner recommended for rehabilitation, should be at least 30 °C (86 °F) above the operating temperature. Note that measurements on actual structures strengthened with carbon-fiber composites showed that the composite surface temperature was approximately 15 to 20 °C (59 to 68 °F) higher than the air temperature. Polymers with a T_g of less than 55 °C (131 °F) must be avoided when rehabilitating civil engineering structures, because their mechanical properties degrade under various service environmental conditions. Polymers demonstrate significantly greater creep above T_g than at the operating temperature. For example, the bond strength in a concrete beam reinforced externally with carbon/epoxy composites having T_g of 50 °C (122 °F) is reduced by almost 40% when the temperature rises from 20 °C (68 °F) to 60 °C (140 °F).

FRP-Reinforced Concrete Behavior

The failure mode of a FRP-rehabilitated reinforced concrete member depends on whether the failure is flexural, shear, or axial and on the ratio of steel and FRP reinforcement. In flexure, the failure of the member may be determined by either the maximum compressive strain in the concrete (assumed as 0.003), the effective ultimate strain in the FRP, or the FRP-to-concrete bond. In shear, the failure is typically controlled by the strain in the FRP or by the FRP-to-concrete bond. Finally, when a composite is used to confine an axial load-resisting member, the ultimate failure of the member is controlled by concrete axial strain or by tensile strain in the composite. Experiments by the authors and others (see Ref 2) have shown that the ultimate flexural response of FRP-strengthened concrete beams is generally controlled by the delamination of the FRP from the tension side of the beam. This delamination is different from a bond failure, in that the delamination results from a tensile-shear failure in the concrete at a level adjacent to the FRP; a bond failure results from either an inadequate length of FRP needed to develop the strength of the FRP or from a failure of the adhesive, as evidenced by a separation of the adhesive from the FRP. The tension-shear failure in the concrete is a consequence of the tensile strength of the cement paste and local stress risers. Flexural cracks in the concrete, large pieces of aggregate near the surface, and deviations in field construction of the FRP are causes of these stress risers.

The values of FRP strain at which concrete tensile-shear delamination occurs vary widely, especially between shop- and field-manufactured composites. The strain is almost never as high as the breaking strain of the FRP; that is, the breaking stress of a composite is generally not the cause of failure.

Based on the evidence to date, the authors recommend a value of 0.004 as the effective ultimate strain (ε_{max}) in the FRP for flexural rehabilitation. While the strain at concrete tensile-shear delamination may be less than this, it is generally significantly greater. The 0.004 value provides for the uncertainties associated with field construction and the misalignment of fibers, and it gives reasonable stresses in the composite for flexural design.

Flexure. Figures 9 and 10 illustrate a beam in flexure, where a composite is bonded to the bottom tension surface. It is assumed that the reinforced concrete member carries the dead load of the structure and that the rehabilitated beam carries the total factored load. Under an ultimate moment, either strain condition in Fig. 9 or in Fig. 10 exists; Fig. 9 defines failure as crushing of the concrete with a compression strain ε_c of 0.003, while Fig. 10 defines failure as a maximum, effective ultimate strain in the composite, which is taken as 0.004, as discussed previously. Under the condition of Fig. 9, the full capacity of the concrete in compression is developed, and an equivalent rectangular stress block analysis may be used. The steel reinforcement may or may not be yielding (in the figure it is assumed to yield); the composite is elastic. Under the condition of Fig. 10, a parabolic stress distribution is assumed for the concrete, such as the Todeschini model (Ref 5); the composite has reached its maximum, effective ultimate strain. The steel reinforcement is typically yielding. In the rectangular stress block model (Fig. 9):

$$a = \beta c$$

where c is the distance between the neutral axis and the compressive face of the section, and

$$\beta = 0.85 \text{ for } f_c' \leq 28 \text{ MPa (4000 psi)}$$

$$\beta = 1.05 - 0.05\frac{f'c}{1000} \text{ for } f'c \text{ in units of psi}$$

$$\text{when } 4000 \text{ psi} < f'c < 8000 \text{ psi}$$

$$\beta = 1.05 - \frac{f'c}{6.9} \text{ for } f'c \text{ in units of MPa}$$

$$\text{when } 28 \text{ MPa} < 56 \text{ MPa}$$

and

$$\beta = 0.65 \text{ for } f_c' \geq 56 \text{ MPa (8000 psi)}$$

Further:

$$\alpha = \frac{A_s f_y + T_{FRP}}{0.85 f_c' b}$$

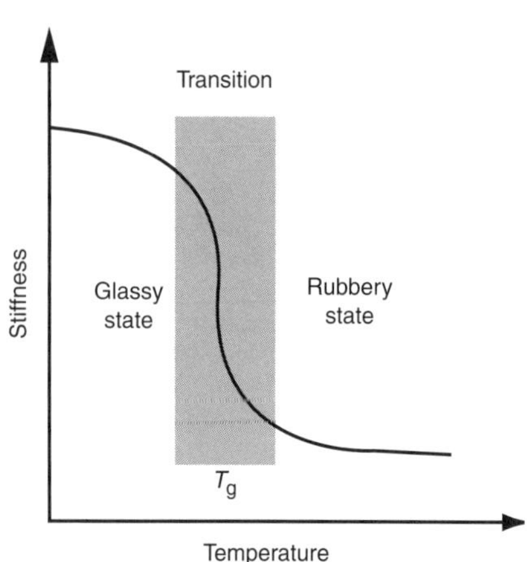

Fig. 8 Effect of temperature on the stiffness of composites. Above the glass transition temperature, T_g, the composite softens.

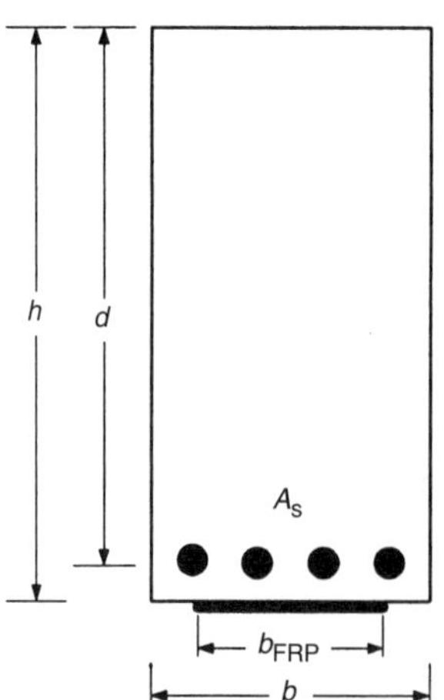

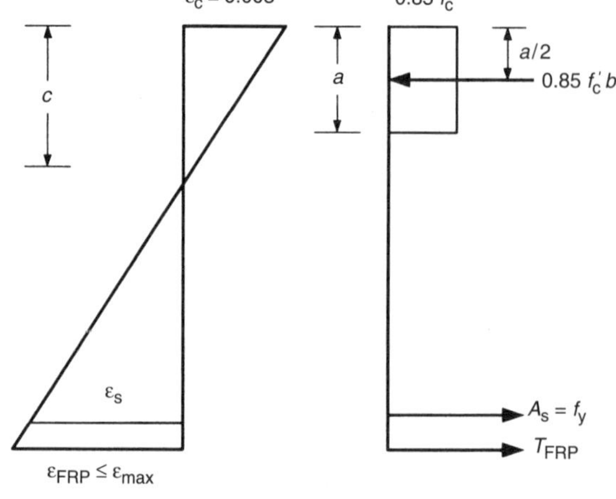

Fig. 9 Flexural condition based upon ultimate compressive strain of the concrete ε_C. b_{FRP} = width of composite. The other terms are defined in the text.

where b is the width of the concrete under compression, A_s the area of steel reinforcement, f_y is the yield stress of the steel, and T_{FRP} is the tensile force in the composite. The nominal moment capacity M_n is:

$$M_n = A_s f_y \left(d - \frac{a}{2}\right) + T_{FRP}\left(h - \frac{a}{2}\right) \quad \text{(Eq 1)}$$

where d is the distance from the compression face to the centroid of steel reinforcement and h is the depth of the section. In the Todeschini model, the concrete compressive stress-strain distribution is assumed parabolic according to the following equation:

$$f_c = \frac{2(0.9f_c')(\varepsilon_c/\varepsilon_o)}{1+(\varepsilon_c/\varepsilon_o)^2} \quad \text{(Eq 2)}$$

where f_c and ε_c are the maximum compressive stress and strain in the concrete, respectively. f_c' is the compressive strength of the concrete and ε_o is the strain, corresponding to the maximum stress, computed from the following equation:

$$\varepsilon_o = 1.71\frac{f_c'}{E_c} \quad \text{(Eq 3)}$$

The modulus of elasticity, E_c, for normal-weight concrete can be computed from:

$$E_c = 57{,}000\sqrt{f_c'} \quad \text{(Eq 4)}$$

where the unit for f_c' is in psi and

$$E_c = 4{,}730\sqrt{f_c'} \quad \text{(Eq 5)}$$

where the unit for f_c' is in MPa.

Based upon Eq 2–5, the compressive force in the concrete may be computed from an assumed rectangular stress block having a depth of "c" and an average stress $\beta_1(0.9f_c')$ as illustrated in Fig. 10, where β_1 is a factor computed from the following equation:

$$\beta_1 = \frac{\ln\left[1+\left(\frac{\varepsilon_c}{\varepsilon_o}\right)^2\right]}{\left(\frac{\varepsilon_c}{\varepsilon_o}\right)} \quad \text{(Eq 6)}$$

The center of gravity of the compression zone is k_2c from the compression surface, where:

$$k_2 = 1 - \frac{2\left[\left(\frac{\varepsilon_c}{\varepsilon_o}\right) - \tan^{-1}\left(\frac{\varepsilon_c}{\varepsilon_o}\right)\right]}{\left(\frac{\varepsilon_c}{\varepsilon_o}\right)^2 \beta_1} \quad \text{(Eq 7)}$$

Assuming yielding of the steel reinforcement, the nominal moment resistance is then given as

$$M_n = A_s f_y (d - k_2c) + T_{FRP}(h - k_2c) \quad \text{(Eq 8)}$$

Figure 11 illustrates a failure of a slab in flexure where the concrete in compression crushed prior to the delamination of the composite reinforcement. Figure 12 shows a delamination type of failure.

Shear. FRPs are applied to the side faces of a beam in order to improve the shear strength of the member, as shown in Fig. 13. The effective ultimate strain for the FRP in this shear condition is 0.004. This effective ultimate strain is used for shear conditions to assure aggregate interlock shear in the concrete and to compensate for the lack of adequate bond development length in the FRP reinforcement. The diagonal shear-tension cracks formed in the concrete must be kept small, to allow for shear transfer across the crack for full development of the concrete shear strength, V_c. On the sides of beams and columns, the transverse FRP reinforcement generally has about 25 mm (1 in.) to develop its effective strength, so that it can participate in shear strengthening. This short length is insufficient to develop the same strength in the FRP as found for flexural strengthening. When the ultimate strain is limited to this 0.004 strain value, it may be assumed that the concrete, V_c, transverse steel shear reinforcement, V_s and FRP materials V_{FRP}, act together to provide shear strength, V_n, as given by:

$$V_n = V_c + V_s + V_{FRP} \quad \text{(Eq 9)}$$

At that effective ultimate strain, the steel stirrups are yielding and the concrete strength may be taken as:

$$V_c = \frac{\sqrt{f_c'}}{6} b_w d \quad \text{(Eq 10)}$$

where b_w is the width of the web and the unit of f_c' is in MPa or

$$V_c = 2\sqrt{f_c'} b_w d \quad \text{(Eq 11)}$$

where f_c' is in psi. The steel strength is:

$$V_s = \frac{A_v f_y d}{s} \quad \text{(Eq 12)}$$

where s is the stirrup spacing, A_v is the area of the stirrups crossing one diagonal crack, and the FRP strength is:

$$V_{FRP} = \frac{T_{FRP} d_{FRP}}{S_{FRP}} \quad \text{(Eq 13)}$$

where T_{FRP} is the strength at a strain of 0.4%, S_{FRP} is the center-to-center spacing of FRP strips, and d_{FRP} is the length of the FRP strips.

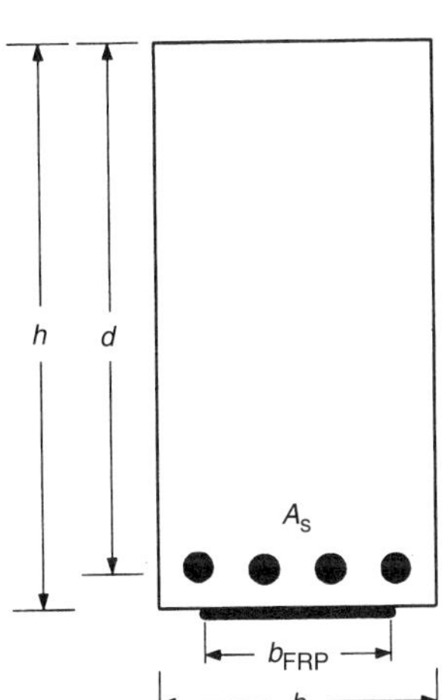

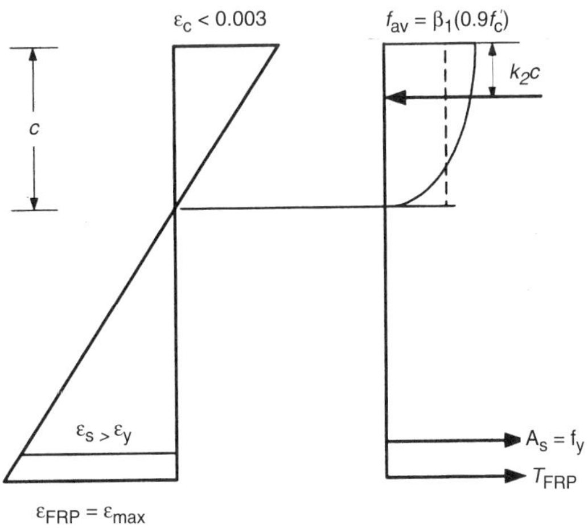

Fig. 10 Flexural condition based upon maximum, effective ultimate strain in the composite $\varepsilon_{FRP} = \varepsilon_{max}$. The terms are defined in the text.

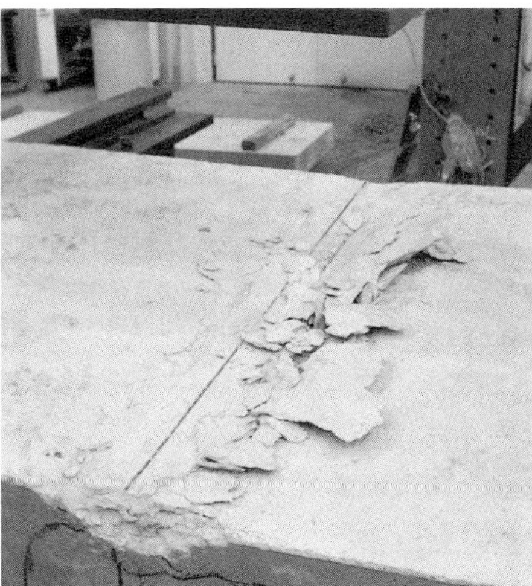

Fig. 11 Crushing of concrete deck in flexural failure. The fiber-reinforced polymer tensile reinforcement remained elastic while the steel reinforcement yielded.

The strips should be wrapped under the bottom of the section. While it would be most desirable to wrap the FRP over the top of the beam, it is generally impossible to do so. Most beams have a slab cast atop the beam. Slots could be drilled through the slab for wrapping the FRP around the beam, but such construction is expensive. Adequate shear strengthening results when the FRP strips are placed immediately below the slab and wrapped around the bottom edge of the beam. The d_{FRP} is then the distance from the bottom layer of steel reinforcing to the bottom of the slab. Additional guidelines on the subject are presented in Ref 6 and 7.

Surface Preparation

Effective rehabilitation techniques using bonded fiber-reinforced polymeric materials depend strongly upon the condition of the substrate to which composite materials will be bonded. To maximize this bond, it is recommended that at least the following surface preparation procedure be followed:

1. Remove all loose and damaged concrete material by mechanical means. Saw cutting, water blasting, and air hammers are effective, as long as 'bruising' (added cracking) of surrounding sound concrete is avoided.
2. Repair the corroded reinforcing steel or prestress tendons by mechanically cleaning the rust; high-pressure washing is effective.
3. Restore the shape of the structure with a new structural concrete or mortar system.
4. Round all corner edges of the rehabilitated elements to a minimum radius of 25 mm (1 in.) to permit effective bends in the composite reinforcement.
5. Inject all cracks that are wider than 0.25 mm (0.01 in.) with structural resin.
6. Remove deleterious materials such as laitance, dust, oil, and so on by means of abrasive blasting. All residue from blasting should be removed with compressed air. When abrasive blasting is not an option due to environmental restrictions, grit blasting, where grits and debris are collected by a vacuum system, can also be used. Hydroblasting is an effective surface cleaning technique; when used, the concrete surface shall be allowed to dry prior to any subsequent repair step.
7. Remove all protrusions higher than 1.5 mm (1/16 in.) and fill all holes and depressions greater than 3 mm (1/8 in.) in diameter with structural mortar.
8. Apply a penetrating epoxy primer to the clean, dry concrete surface. Apply only when the ambient temperature is between 5 and 32 °C (40 and 90 °F), the relative humidity is less than 90%, the concrete surface temperature is more than 2 °C (5 °F) above the dew point, and the concrete moisture content is no greater than 4%.

Composite Materials Applications

After allowing the epoxy primer to dry for a period of time as specified by the manufacturer, the rehabilitation procedure may continue, provided that the ambient temperature is between 5 and 32 °C (40 and 90 °F), the relative humidity is less than 90%, the concrete surface temperature is more than 2 °C (5 °F) above the dew point, and the concrete moisture content is dry (moisture content is less than 4%). Elapsed time between mixing and application of the first ply and also between any two successive plies shall be within a time period not exceeding the gel time of the resin.

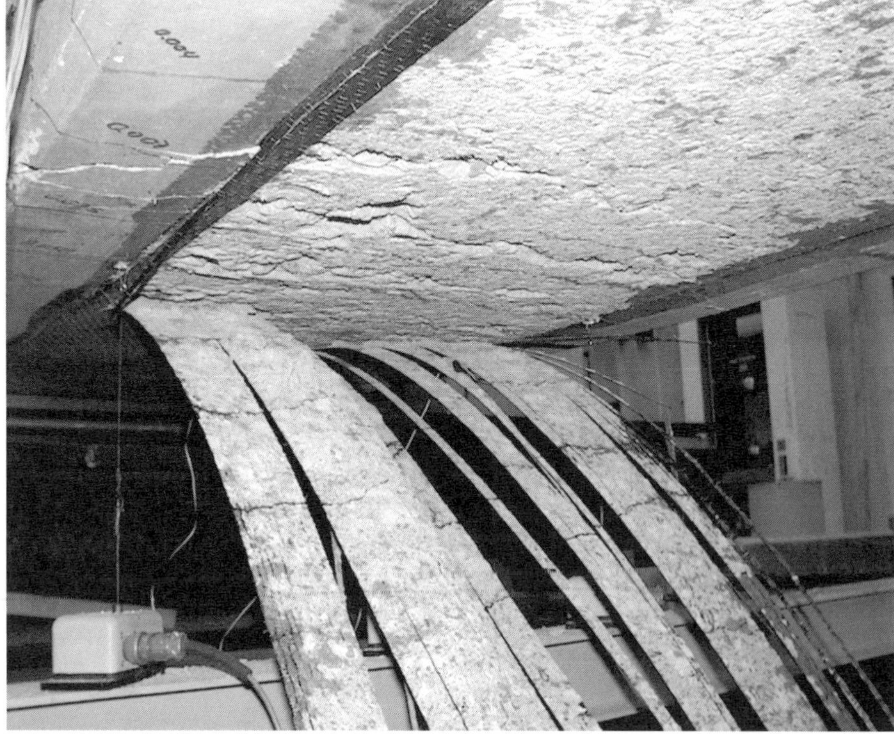

Fig. 12 Delamination of fiber-reinforced polymer composite from concrete slab in flexural failure. The concrete remaining on the composite indicates good bond.

Records

During the rehabilitation of concrete structures with composite materials, records of key data should be kept. The following is an example of the types of information that should be recorded:

- Name of the project
- Date of strengthening
- Ambient air temperature and relative air humidity measured in the shade
- Concrete surface temperature and relative humidity at the time of rehabilitation
- The compressive strength of the concrete to be strengthened
- The commercial designation, name of manufacturer, date of manufacturing, and the manufacturer lot number, as shown on the shipping label for each component used to form the binding resin matrix
- The commercial designation, name of manufacturer, date of manufacturing, and the manufacturer lot number, as shown on the shipping label for the reinforcing fibers, fabric, or prepreg, as applicable

Acceptance Criteria

A few days after the rehabilitation, the structure should be inspected visually and also by per-

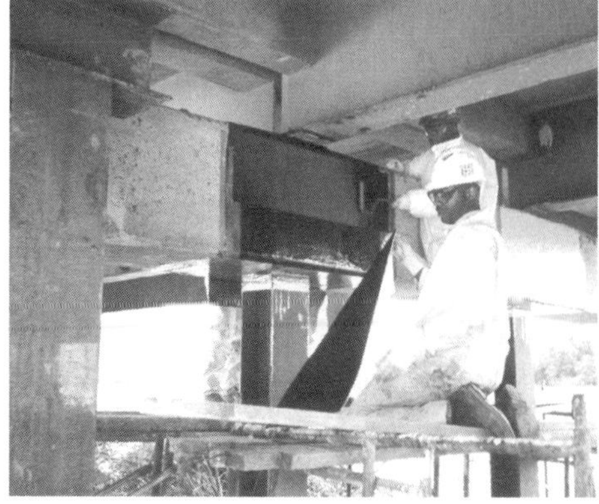

Fig. 13 Fiber-reinforced polymer sheet applied to the side of a beam to increase the shear strength of the beam

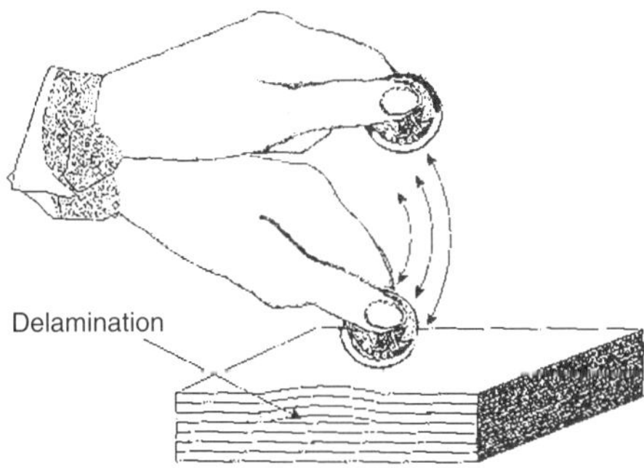

Fig. 14 Tap test for detecting delaminations between the composite layers or between the composite and concrete. Courtesy of Abaris Training

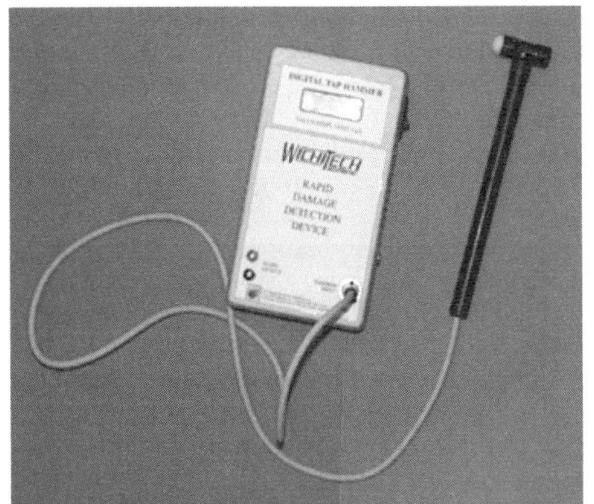

Fig. 15 Automated tap hammer for detecting voids and delaminations

forming a tap test with a coin or a small piece of metal, as shown in Fig. 14. An automated version of this test can be performed with the instrument shown in Fig. 15. The structure also can be inspected much more accurately using thermography (Fig. 16). The strengthened structure should be free of any defects (e.g., voids, bubbles, and delamination). In the presence of such defects, a repair of the composite should be done. A valuable destructive test to measure bond strength is the direct composite pull-out test, conducted on an area adjacent to the actual rehabilitated area and performed after the manufacturer's recommended curing time period (Fig. 17). The test area should have the same number of plies and/or ply orientations as those of the rehabilitated areas, and should not affect the rehabilitation in any manner. The recommended number of composite pull-off tests is 3 for every 23 m^2 (250 ft^2) of rehabilitated area. These tests should demonstrate that failure always occurs in either the substrate or along the bond line with a minimum average tensile stress

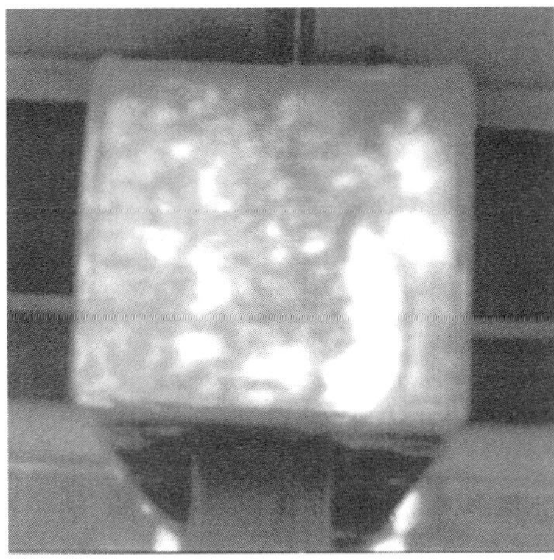

Fig. 16 Thermographic image showing delamination

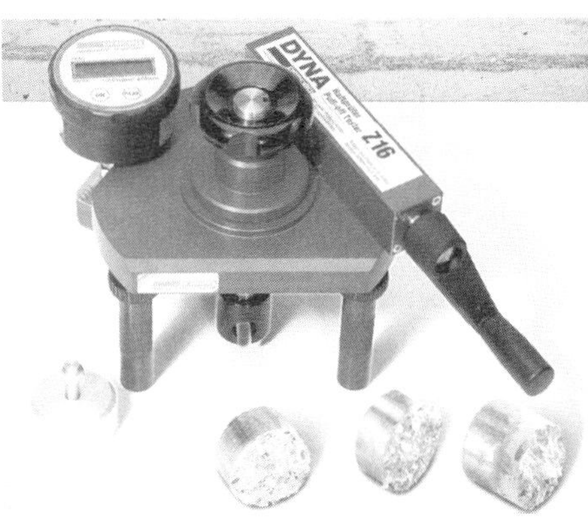

Fig. 17 Pull-off tester for measuring bond strength. Courtesy of PROCEQ SA

of 1380 kPa (200 psi). In addition, it is necessary to conduct tests for verifying the glass transition temperature and the tensile properties in the direction of interest. This can be done on field-prepared panels (Fig. 18) that have the same number of plies and fiber orientations and the same curing condition as those of the rehabilitated areas.

ACKNOWLEDGMENTS

This work was supported in part by the Earthquake Engineering Research Centers Program of the National Science Foundation under Award Number EEC-9701785. Additional support was provided by the Georgia Department of Transportation and the Federal Highway Administration under GDOT Project NO 9606 and GDOT R. P. 9702. The subject presented herein represents the views and opinions of the writers only.

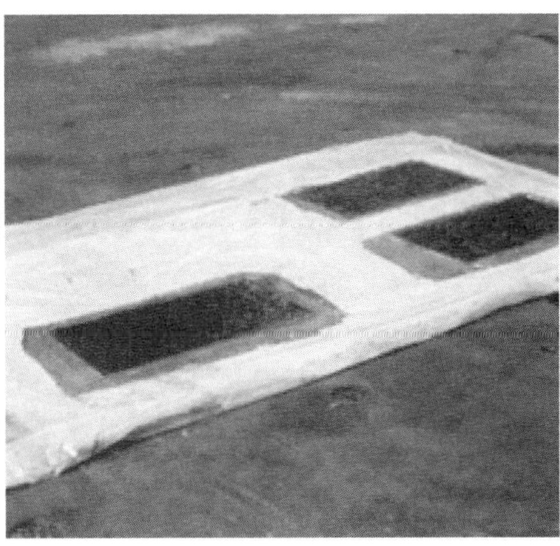

Fig. 18 Field-prepared composite panels for materials property verifications

SELECTED REFERENCES

- "Guide for Evaluation of Concrete Structures Prior to Rehabilitation," ACI 364.1-94, American Concrete Institute, 1994, p 22
- "Concrete Repair Guide," ACI 546R-96, American Concrete Institute, 1996, p 41

REFERENCES

1. U. Meier, M. Deuring, H. Meier, and G. Schwegler, Strengthening of Structures with Advanced Composites, *Alternative Materials for the Reinforcement and Prestressing of Concrete,* J.L. Clarke, Ed., Blackie Academic and Professional, Glasgow, 1993, p 153–171
2. T.C. Triantafillou, Strengthening of Structures with Advanced FRPs, *Prog. Struct. Eng. Mater.,* Vol 1 (No. 2), 1998, p 126–134
3. L.C. Hollaway and M.B. Leeming, *Strengthening of Reinforced Concrete Structures,* Woodhead Publishing Limited, Cambridge, England, 1999
4. Hans Von Storch and Francis W. Zwiers, *Statistical Analysis in Climate Research,* Cambridge University Press, Cambridge, United Kingdom, 1999
5. Claudio Todeschini, Albert Bianchini, and Clyde Kesler, Behavior of Concrete Columns Reinforced with High Strength Steels, *ACI Mater. J.,* Vol 61 (No. 6), June 1964, p 701–716
6. Ahmad Kahlifa, William J. Gold, Antonio Nanni, and M.I. Abdel Aziz, Contribution of Externally Bonded FRP to Shear Capacity of RC Flexural Members, *J. Compos. Constr.,* ASCE, Nov 1988, p 195–203
7. T.C. Triantafillou and Costas P. Antonopoulos, Design of Concrete Flexural Members Strengthened in Shear with FRP, *J. Compos. Constr.,* Vol 4 (No. 4), Nov 2000, p 198–205

Maintainability Issues

William F. Cole II, United Airlines
Mark S. Forte, Air Force Research Laboratory
Rikard B. Heslehurst, Australian Defence Force Academy

IN-SERVICE MAINTAINABILITY is a primary ongoing issue associated with composite aircraft structures. The increase in use of composite materials in aviation has been accompanied by more complicated designs and significantly loaded structures. Damage types experienced by composite structures, the methods of inspecting for damage, and the techniques for repair typically are more complex compared with those involving aluminum structures. As a result, performance and weight benefits inherent to composite materials can be reduced or lost if the cost associated with maintaining these structures is too high. This cost is directly related to the durability, damage tolerance, and repairability built in during the design process. There are a range of issues that need to be addressed in maintaining composite structures. A better understanding of, as well as improvement of, maintenance procedures will go a long way in maintaining composite structures more cost effectively.

Composite materials, mostly reinforced with glass fiber, began to replace aluminum secondary structure on aircraft in the early 1960s. Those first introduced were typically aerodynamic fairings and wing leading edges. As the potential benefits of composites were realized, other polymer composites reinforced with advanced fibers offering increased specific stiffness and strength, reduced weight, and improved corrosion and fatigue resistance over aluminum were successfully introduced. The most common base materials for these advanced fibers were graphite (carbon) and aramid. These materials were used in structures such as flight controls and engine cowlings.

These designs were lighter, thin-skinned sandwich structures that proved to be less damage resistant than those made of aluminum and introduced new damage phenomena that were complex by comparison. This complicated the maintenance actions of damage assessment, inspection, and repair. These problems, not foreseen at the design stage, made in-service damage a frequent occurrence, which was further aggravated by the lack of experience and materials needed to carry out corrective action. Out-of-service aircraft, expensive spare components, training liability for technicians, and expensive materials and facilities reduce or eliminate the cost benefits that composites are intended to provide through increased performance.

The most recent aircraft designs include graphite/epoxy solid composite laminates in primary structures such as floor beams and other critical substructures. These uses demonstrate continued confidence in the capabilities of composite materials. However, the effort needed to maintain composite components must be reduced to realize the complete life-cycle cost potential.

Maintainability is a function of the durability, damage tolerance, and repairability of the structure. Durability is the ability of the structure to maintain its strength and stiffness throughout its service life. Damage tolerance is the capability of the structure to sustain a level of damage and yet safely perform its intended operational functions. The initial design phase of these parameters has the greatest influence for maintainability and reliability.

Types of Composite Structures

Over the past several years, advanced fiber reinforced polymer-matrix composites (PMCs) have emerged as a structural material to replace aluminum and titanium alloys. Composites, which were initially used as a direct replacement of metallic structures, have been utilized for many types of increasingly complex components. Advanced composites have been constructed with boron, Kevlar, and graphite fibers, with the predominant fiber of choice being graphite. Resins used in composite construction include epoxy, bismaleimide (BMI), and polyimide (PI), with epoxy resin used most exclusively.

Several configurations of composite structures are being used in military and commercial aviation applications. The three main configurations used in commercial aircraft composites are sandwich, stiffened-skin, and monolithic structures.

Sandwich Structure. Two forms of sandwich structures are found in aircraft applications: honeycomb panels and sandwich panels. Sandwich structures are the result of the bonding of thin face sheets separated by a low-density core (Fig. 1). This type of structure results in an efficient and light structure of high flexural stiffness. The face sheets are laminates of glass, graphite, aramid, or a combination of these materials in an epoxy matrix. The core is typically an aramid or fiberglass paper honeycomb, aluminum honeycomb, foam, or balsa wood material. Sandwich structures composed of a solid laminate plus an equivalent core thickness will be seven times the stiffness and almost four times the strength of the monolithic skin alone. However, thin-skinned sandwich structure is highly prone to impact damage and fluid ingression contamination. Aircraft components using sandwich core include control surface fairings, access doors, fuselage, and flooring.

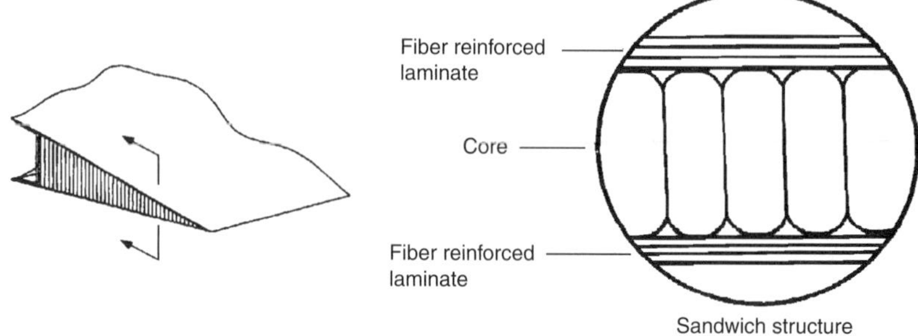

Fig. 1 Sandwich structure

Stiffened structure (Fig. 2), can be either strength or stiffness critical. This type of construction utilizes advanced composites as the skin material ranging from 8 to 20 plies. The stiffeners are typically constructed of composites and are either fabricated as integral to the skin or secondarily bonded, although mechanical fastening of the stiffeners is also used. The stiffeners currently utilized include hat, bead, and I-beam designs. The stiffeners range from 8 to 30 plies. Stiffened-skin structure is significantly more durable than sandwich structure and can approach the same stiffness, but will generally be slightly heavier. A well-designed stiffened-skin structure, designed with repair in mind, will typically provide superior maintainability compared with a sandwich structure. Aircraft components using stiffeners include fuselage, control surfaces, tail skins, wing panels, and wing skins.

Monolithic structure can be either strength or stiffness critical and are a form of stiffened structure. This type of construction utilizes advanced composites as the skin material and can be more than 100 plies. The monolithic skin panels are typically bolted to a composite or metallic substructure. Aircraft components using monolithic panels include main torque box, wing, and vertical tail.

Designing for Maintainability

The conceptual design phase is a time of greatest influence on maintainability. It is likely that a high level of maintainability will be achieved if a designer of a composite structure takes the following into consideration during the conceptual design phase:

- Understand that all composite structures will experience significant damage while in service.
- Understand all damage sources for the structure and design to minimize their effects.
- Understand the operating environment for the structure and design to accommodate this.
- Define the repair philosophy for this structure and develop all interim and permanent repairs simultaneously with the original design. If certain areas of the design do not lend themselves easily to repair, strongly consider an alternate configuration.
- Test candidate repairs during original development test programs. This will establish their effectiveness and provide a basis for maximum allowable and repairable damage limits.
- Consider only standardized repair techniques.
- Provide sufficient access to properly inspect and prepare the damaged area, fit and install repair parts, and use repair tools and bonding equipment. If adequate access is not possible, design for ease of removal and/or disassembly.
- Minimize the variety and amount of materials necessary to meet the requirements of both interim and permanent repairs.
- Establish minimum levels of damage resistance based on the type of structure, expected type of impact, and the level of impact energy.
- Design to reestablish the balance moment of flight controls by allowing for the increase in weight due to repair. Electrically servocontrolled flight controls do not have this requirement.
- Establish and verify level of nondetectable damage by test that will not endanger the normal operation of the aircraft structure for two lifetimes.
- Assess, based on the structure and its configurations, which methods of inspection are practical and usable to detect potential damage. No single nondestructive inspection method can locate and isolate all defects.
- Take into account material fatigue behavior, even though it is far superior to that of metallic structures.

Sources of Defects and Damage

Advanced composites can be damaged from several manufacturing or in-service sources. The vulnerability of a particular composite structure depends on factors including type of construction, function, and location on the aircraft.

Manufacturing defects include voids, delaminations, surface damage, and misdrilled holes.

Void-type defects can occur in a laminate or the bondline of adhesively bonded structure, (Fig. 3). The most common cause of this defect is poor process control during fabrication. In the case of a composite laminate, voids can result from lack of pressure during the curing operation or using incorrect cure cycle. Bonded structure can have excessive voids due to inadequate pressure during cure, lack of adhesive in the bondline, or improper fit with tooling or adjacent surfaces.

Delaminations are separations between laminate plies and can occur in any composite structure. The most common causes of this defect are poor process control, poor dimensional tolerance, faulty hole-drilling procedures, and inclusion of release film during fabrication. A majority of delaminations occur because the laminate is subjected to out-of-plane loading.

Surface damage can occur in a laminate or bonded structure, especially at an exposed edge. The most common causes of this type of defect are poor process control or incorrect handling of the composite. An example of surface damage due to poor process control is a structure not releasing from a tool in which prying for removal results in laminate or edge damage. Thin composite laminates are vulnerable to impact damage from dropped tools or from contact with heavy objects.

Misdrilled holes are typically the result of incorrect drilling procedures or faulty fixturing prior to the drilling operation. This type of damage can result in a repair of the hole or scrapping of the entire laminate.

In-service defects include cuts and scratches, penetration damage, abrasion and erosion, delaminations and disbonds, hole elongation, dents and crushed core, core corrosion, edge damage, and overheat damage.

Cuts and scratches can range from gouging of the resin to breaking of fibers, which can reduce the laminate structural strength. They typically occur as a result of impact or handling damage while the aircraft is on the ground.

Penetration damage is an extension of the previous category, with complete penetration of the skin and corresponding resin and fiber breakage (Fig. 4). This damage is likely to cause a reduction in load-carrying capability. This damage can occur as a result of severe impact or handling while the aircraft is on the ground, or in the case of military aircraft, ballistic impact.

Abrasion and erosion typically affect leading-edge components that are exposed to airflow (Fig. 5). The damage occurs in flight as a result of air, rain, and/or grit impingement on the surface. Damage levels range from removal of coating to stripping of complete laminate surface plies.

Delaminations and disbonds can occur in any laminate or bondline of a bonded structure. The causes of this defect are low-velocity impact (dropped tools), high-velocity impact (hailstones, runway debris), overload, and freeze/thaw expansion. A majority of delaminations and disbonds occur because the laminate is min-

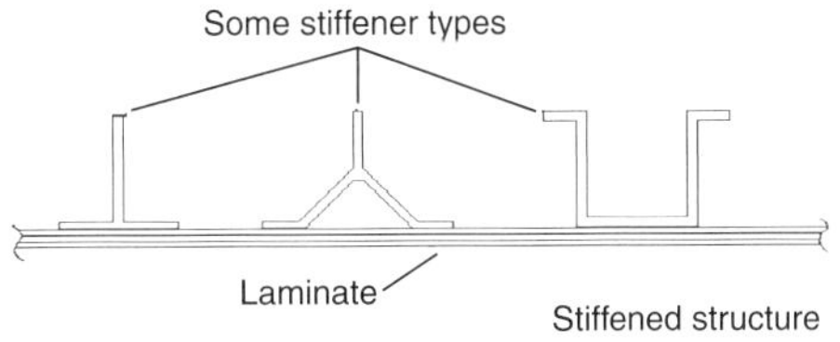

Fig. 2 Stiffened panels

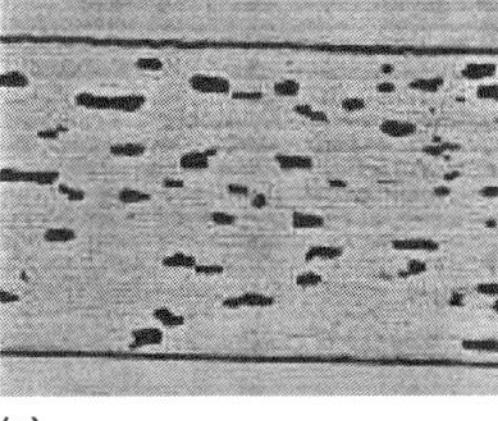

(a)

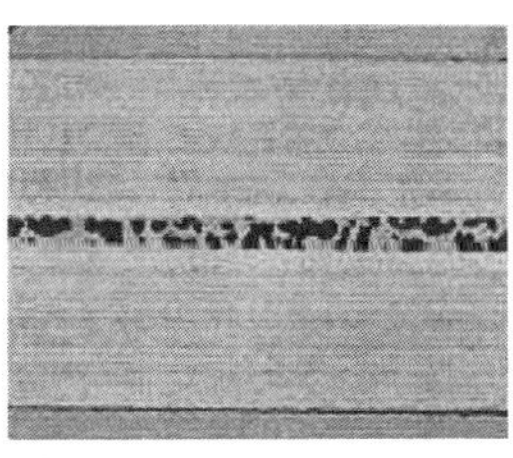

(b)

Fig. 3 Typical void defects in (a) laminates and (b) at the bondline

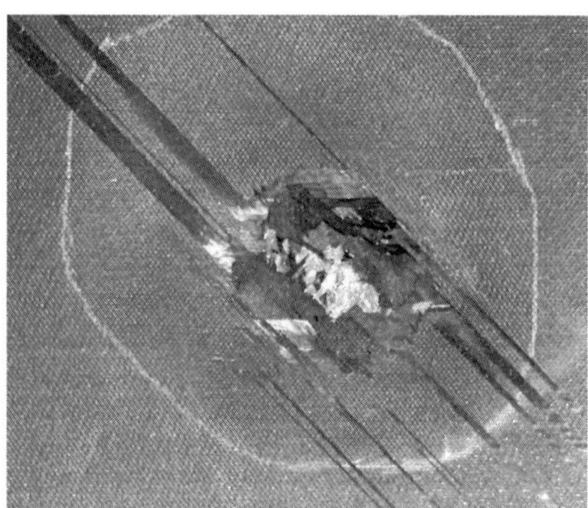

Fig. 4 Penetration damage

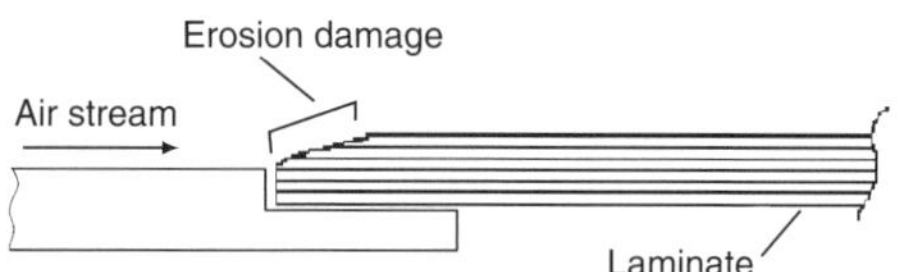

Fig. 5 Laminate edge erosion

imum thickness and subjected to out-of-plane loading.

Hole elongation can occur in laminates with mechanical fasteners that have seen extended removal and reinstallation use. Other causes of damage include inadequate shimming and overtorqued fasteners.

Dents and crushed core can occur in sandwich structures. The causes of this defect are low-velocity impact (dropped tools) or high-velocity impact (hailstones, runway debris). A majority of dents and crushed cores occur because the laminate is minimum thickness and subjected to out-of-plane loading.

Core degradation is a result of cumulative effects on honeycomb substructure being exposed to standing water over a period of time (Fig. 6). The water typically enters the core through the face sheet or an edge member, often due to fiber breakage from impact damage, sealant loss, or missing surface finish. The aluminum honeycomb corrodes, while paper-type and resin-type honeycomb disbonds or loses material properties.

Edge damage can result in disbonding, delamination, and fiber breakage. The most common cause of this type of defect is incorrect handling of the composite. Cured composite thin structures (laminates, edges, or corners) prove to be fragile and susceptible to impact damage from dropped tools or other heavy objects.

Overheat damage can occur in a laminate or bonded structure. The causes for overheat damage are hot gas impingement, fire, repair over temperature (Fig. 7), lightning strikes (Fig. 8), and battle damage that heat the composite over the intended use temperature, resulting in reduced mechanical properties.

Nondestructive Inspection Requirements

Nondestructive Inspection (NDI) methods are used in the repair of composite structures to locate damage, characterize the extent of damage, and ensure post-repair quality. The first and most important activity in a repair process is to identify the region of the defect or damage. Initial assessment of the damage is usually achieved by visual inspection. Visual inspection localizes the damaged area external surface. This is followed by a more sensitive NDI method that maps the extent of any internal damage. Detailed NDI is very important when dealing with composite structures because of the ease with which damage is hidden.

Nondestructive inspection methods currently available include:

- Visual, which includes optical magnification and defect enhancement
- Acoustic methods, which identify changes in sound emission
- Ultrasonic methods, such as A-scan and C-scan and also Lamb waves
- Thermography
- Interferometry
- Radiography
- Microwave
- Material property changes, that is, stiffness and dielectric strength

A detailed discussion of the various NDI methods can be found in the Selected References at the end of this article and in the article "Nondestructive Testing" in this Volume.

For the successful application of any NDI method, a selection process to identify the most suitable method must be in place with personnel trained and qualified in that method. The NDI selection process is based on configuration of the component and its construction materials, type and size of defects to be inspected, accessibility to the assessment area, and availability of both equipment and skilled operators. Table 1 lists the ability of selected NDI methods to find various defects in composite structures.

The NDI operator and assessor must be familiar with several different inspection techniques and be able to set up equipment and effectively modify the standard diagnostic arrangements to suit the part being evaluated. Other requirements include having the skill to interpret the resulting NDI information, a knowledge of safety standards and procedures, and the ability to comply with MIL-STD-410 or its equivalent.

Three requirements for NDI to be successful in detecting the extent of damage in composite structures and components are:

- Suitable NDI equipment (calibrated and in good working order) and facilities, including personnel safety and environmental health procedures
- Adequately trained and experienced operators of NDI equipment to ensure that the results from any damage assessment survey are both accurate and reliable

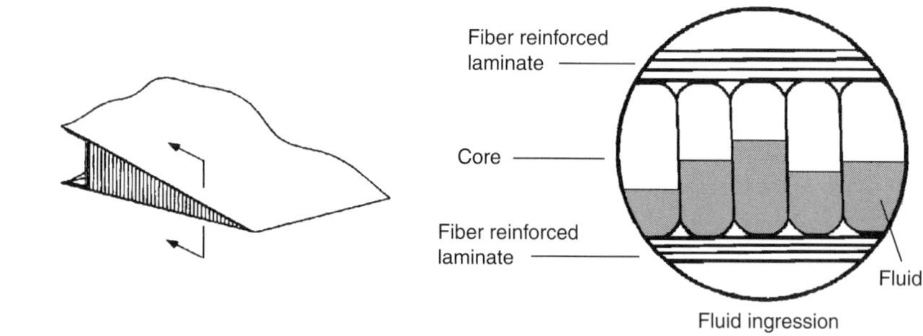

Fig. 6 Fluid ingression in honeycomb structure

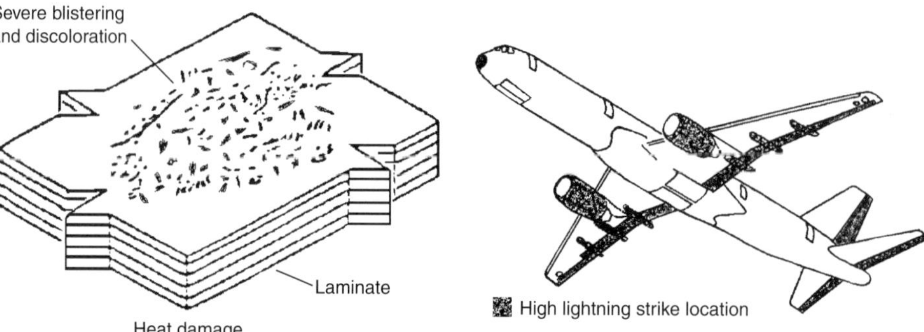

Fig. 7 Heat damage in laminate

Fig. 8 Locations subject to high number of lightning strikes

- Available comparative specimens, because any NDI technique is comparative in nature, and results of an assessment usually are compared with a good or similarly damaged specimen. This is particularly important when calibrating NDI equipment.

Design Recommendations

This section lists suggestions that can be used as guidelines when designing for the durability of a composite structure. Many of the suggestions provided would minimize the effects of the damage sources discussed in the previous section.

Adhesive bonding design guidelines include:

- Do not bond parts having significantly different coefficients of thermal expansion to avoid thermally induced residual bond stresses.
- Apply film adhesive at stiffener to skin interfaces to improve peel strength.
- Make bonded stiffener flanges wide enough to accommodate a row of structural fasteners that may be needed in making future repairs.
- Do not use sealants that become strong adhesives over time on joints that require separation for repair.
- Avoid structural eccentricities that can cause stress risers and lead to repair joint deterioration and failure.
- Confirm that any state-of-the-art automated processing methods used to manufacture a part lend themselves to in-service repair. Filament winding, for example, is not easily repaired using standard processes.
- Do not design components prone to mechanical impact damage (such as nacelles, flaps, and service doors) with thin face sheets.
- Reinforce and protect latch, corner, and edge areas from mishandling damage.

General composite structure design guidelines include:

- Consider breaking down complicated components into simpler subassemblies to make disassembly for repair and the repairs themselves easier. This will be a trade-off because structural efficiency and manufacturing part-count costs are both optimized by larger composite structures.
- Do not require the removal of components from the aircraft to gain access to equipment.
- Provide the maximum possible access for internal inspection and repair for hollow components.
- Provide adequate space for removal of hinge or actuator pins when using standard tools.
- Provide easy removal and replacement of access panels covering hinges, actuators, and ports.
- Design laminates having a fabric outer ply (particularly at fastener locations) to resist the cracking, splitting, and peeling often experienced with unidirectional outer plies.
- Accurately trim panel edges and locate holes using fixtures.
- Locate ground-handling fitting attachments to facilitate attachment of hoist fixtures during component change.
- Design robust attachments.
- Provide hole protection in access panels requiring frequent removal.
- Use galvanic compatible barrier plies when installing metallic hardware such as fasteners, fittings, metal-filled adhesives, and metallic core against graphite-based structures.
- Develop repair designs that do not degrade the design fatigue life of the structure.

Sandwich structure design guidelines include:

- Establish minimum face sheet thickness criteria based on realistic impact energy criteria and handling criteria.

Table 1 Defects detectable by means of selected nondestructive inspection methods

	Detection method												
Defect type	Visual	DP	Tap test	Bond tester	UP	TT	X-ray	Dielectric	Thermography	Interferometry	Microwave	NR	MI
Laminate defects													
Delaminations	1, 2	1	X	X	X	X	3		X	X			X
Macrocracks	1, 2	2	X	X			3		X	X			
Fiber fracture							X		2, 3	2, 3			
Interfacial cracks									2, 3	X			
Microcracks		1	2	2					X	X			
Porosity	1		2	2	X	X	X		2	X			
Inclusions	1			2	2	2	X		X	X			X
Heat damage	1		2	2				2		2			
Moisture							2	X		2	X	X	
Voids				2	X	X	X		X	X			
Surface protrusions	X								X	X			
Wrinkles	X								v	X			
Improper cure								X	2	2		X	
Bondline defects													
Debonds	1, 2	1	X	X	X	X	X		X	X			X
Weak bonds									2	X			
Cracks	1, 2	1	2	2	2	2	3		X	X			
Voids			X	X	X	X	X		X	X			X
Moisture							X	X		2	X	X	
Inclusions			2	2	2	2	X		X	X			X
Porosity				2	X	X	X		X	X			
Lack of adhesive			X	X	X	X	X		X	X			
Sandwich panel defects													
Blown core			X	X	X	X	X					X	X
Condensed core			2	2		2	X					X	
Crushed cure			2	2		2	X					X	
Distorted core							X					X	
Cut core			X	X		X	X					X	
Missing core			2	2	2	2	X					X	X
Node debond							X		2	X			
Water in core			2	2		2	X				X	X	
Debonds			X	X	X	X	X		X	X			X
Voids			2	2	X	X	X		X	X			
Core filler cracks			2		2	X	3		2	2			
Lack of filler			2	2	2	X	X		2	2		X	

1, Must be open to the surface; 2, unreliable detection; 3, dependent on defect orientation. DP, dye penetrant; UP, ultrasonic pulse echo; TT, through transmission; NR, neutron radiography; MI, mechanical impedance

- Protect the inner face sheet from damage by establishing a minimum core thickness and density consistent with the outer face sheet damage threshold. The core should be able to absorb the impact energy passing through the outer face sheet without the inner face sheet being damaged.
- Avoid the use of honeycomb core septums, because it is very difficult to remove all moisture with access to only one side during repair.
- Avoid the use of fasteners or tooling holes that penetrate into the core area to avoid creating fluid leak paths. If fasteners must be used, pot hole with filler material that will not crack over time.
- Use ramped core closeouts instead of square-edged core closeouts to avoid fluid leak paths. If this is not possible, seal the edge with a closure rib, composite wrap, or flexible sealant.
- Avoid low-pressure core-to-skin bonding processes to avoid fluid leak paths due to a porous bondline. This is a consideration for the processing of secondarily bonded precured skins.
- Provide adequate sealing to prevent moisture ingression.

Material selection guidelines include:

- Strive for commonality of materials; the use of exotic, high-performance materials may prove impractical or unacceptable for repair.
- Select a small number of repair materials that will be compatible with those used in manufacture. A lower-temperature cure repair material is preferable for repair.
- Choose materials and processing that result in low porosity when cured to reduce fluid ingression.
- Use higher-resin-content plies on the outer surface to reduce laminate porosity.
- Avoid the use of aramid materials in areas where moisture exists. Components with aramid plies are known to have problems with microcracking and moisture absorption.
- Use thicker laminates and, for sandwich applications, denser core materials to improve damage resistance.

Erosion and abrasion design guidelines include:

- Provide erosion protection on forward edges and avoid the possibility of positive steps in the air stream. This protection should be easily replaceable.
- Provide easily replaceable, sacrificial materials or coatings on wear areas to protect from abrasion.

Fasteners. Design considerations when using fasteners include:

- Use readily available, easily removed, standard fastener types and lengths.
- Use fasteners that are compatible in the galvanic series with the material of the contacting structure to prevent corrosion. Titanium and Monel (nickel-copper alloy), fasteners are used most often to join carbon fiber/epoxy-based structures.
- Use fastener systems that do not initiate damage to the structure upon removal and replacement.
- Drill fastener holes precisely so that they align when alternate parts are installed. Automated drilling or the use of drilling fixtures can ensure this.
- Use nut plates and reusable screws for panel attachment or where access to the far side is restricted.
- Do not cover fasteners with filler compound.
- Consider that blind fasteners will often require that stems be punched through for removal. If this is in a cavity where removal is not possible, these stems will move around in service, potentially damaging the composite structure.

Lightning-strike protection guidelines include:

- Avoid the use of aluminum honeycomb combined with graphite fiber face sheets due to the higher risk of lightning-strike damage.
- Provide easily replaceable conductive material with adequate conductive area at critical lightning-zone locations.
- Make all conductive path attachments easily accessible.
- Ensure that lightning-protection schemes, such as flame spray or metallic mesh, are easily restored during repair. If this is not possible for a particular protection scheme, consider using alternate protection options.

Thermal Degradation. Provide adequate materials or improved thermal insulation, such as heat blankets, for components used in environments of 120 °C (250 °F) or higher.

Personnel, Facilities, and Equipment

Training/Skill Level Required. Trained personnel in a composite workshop are of the utmost necessity, particularly in the aviation industry where cured composite and bonded metallic patches require high levels of engineering design development and technician skills. Once the repair has been completed, any nonconformity in material and component properties are hidden until loaded. Furthermore, errors can be expensive to fix. All personnel must be qualified in the preparation and handling of repair materials and repair methods. Inspectors must have the same qualifications, as well as significant work experience. The quality of the repair, to maintain structural integrity throughout the life of the structure, is directly dependent on the design talents and workmanship employed.

Materials Storage and Handling. All incoming materials need to be handled and stored in accordance with the vendor's Materials Safety Data Sheet (MSDS) instructions. This is most necessary for hazardous and shelf-life materials, which are common in the composite and adhesive-bonding materials. The cold storage of shelf-life materials—in particular the composite prepregs, film adhesives, and two-part adhesives—is essential in order to maintain material property standards. The time duration that the material is out of cold storage must be well documented, and the appropriate reduction in remaining life made.

The thaw time of any materials held in cold storage is most important. When a material is taken from the freezer, it should not be removed from its protective sealed wrapping until all of it has reached room temperature. Otherwise, water vapor will condense onto the surface and be absorbed into the resin materials. This moisture degradation will have the same effect as using overaged materials, that is, reduced mechanical properties. However, the degree to which moisture continues to condense on the sealing package can give a ready indication of the "ready-to-use" status of the material. If water vapor no longer condenses on the bag, it is near enough to room temperature to open it.

When the materials are returned to cold storage, ensure that the packaging is airtight, even to the point of removing the air from the package. This again will stop moisture absorption. In general, storage temperatures of –18 °C (0 °F), will provide the full storage life that is guaranteed by the materials supplier. Temperatures of –40 °C (–40 °F) will provide an indefinite life, but this is not guaranteed by the material suppliers. Finally, complete appropriate material storage documentation.

Repair Fabrication Rooms and Equipment. The two major processes in the repair of composite structures are damage removal and repair patch fabrication and application. Each of these processes must be done in separate rooms and with dedicated tooling to prevent contamination.

Environmental Controls for Work Areas. In a composite and adhesive-bonding workshop, the materials used are temperature and moisture sensitive. They are temperature sensitive because the material processing requires a time duration at elevated temperature to produce the finished product. High working temperatures can prematurely begin the curing process of resins and adhesives, thus shortening their working life. Humidity control is important as polymeric materials absorb moisture readily from the atmosphere, contaminating the material and possibly reducing the mechanical properties. Excessively low humidity and temperature will make the prepregs and film adhesive stiff and difficult to work with due to lack of tackiness. In the repair of flight critical structures, environmental controls must not be waived. If, however, field repairs are necessary, then the repair scheme is fabricated in a controlled environment (precured patch), sealed, and shipped to the field where it is attached as quickly as possible.

Access Control. Damage removal and clean rooms both are hazardous to personnel and have the potential to contaminate components. Access to these rooms should be restricted to personnel trained in health and safety procedures and composite processing.

Repair Documentation. From a quality-control perspective, four levels of repair documentation are required to ensure that the repair will be of the highest standard:

1. Equipment operations
2. Component tracking, including: initial NDI survey, damage details, repair action and scheme, moisture-removal requirements and method, damage removal action, repair fabrication details (including materials used), repair application procedure, cure details, and post-repair NDI action and results
3. Shelf-life materials tracking
4. Cure documentation (see Ref 1)

Health and Safety. Three main issues to be addressed in the environmental health and safety for composite structural repairs are:

Common Sense Approach: In all aspects of working with damaged composite structures and their repair, a common-sense approach to health and safety is expected. If there is the slightest concern, then appropriate safeguards and protective systems must be put in place. A good record-keeping is very important. This includes the availability of up-to-date Material Safety Data Sheets, (MSDS), suitable storage requirements and facilities for toxic and harmful materials, appropriate relabeling (particularly when batches of materials are broken down into more usable sizes), and material disposal.

Protect the Worker: At all times the worker, that is, the person directly involved in damaged-component removal, composite structure machining and grinding, and the preparation of repair schemes and their application needs to be protected. This means that engineering management must ensure that the worker has a safe environment within which to work and is encouraged to follow safe work practices stringently.

Local, State, and Federal Legislation: Government legislation must be strictly observed at all times. Disposal action is steadily becoming a legislated requirement. Reference 1 details the specifics of the disposal requirements for toxic and hazardous composite materials. The details of legislation vary from one location or country to another. The appropriate authorities must be contacted for specific guidelines.

Sharp needlelike fibers are exposed when composite components are damaged. The needlelike spikes are a result of resin-stiffened fibers, and they easily protrude into skin or soft body tissues. Of particular threat are the fingers, hands, and eyes. The precautionary personal safety equipment required includes at least: disposable coveralls, face shields or goggles, and heavy rubber or canvas gloves.

There are a number of environmental and safety concerns when machining and/or grinding composite components. Fiber dust could be potentially hazardous to human health, both physically and chemically. Free-floating composite fibers are not seen as a particular carcinogenic concern (as opposed to asbestos) due to their fiber diameter to length ratio. However, workers should avoid breathing them. The microfibrils of aramid fibers are an unresolved concern. Therefore, the minimal safety equipment to be used includes: high-efficiency particulate respirators, local vacuum or dust extractors, face shields and/or goggles, appropriate gloves, and disposable coveralls.

Safety protection when working with uncured adhesives and resins, solvent cleaning, acid etching prior to bonding, and during the cure process include: disposable coveralls; gloves—surgical, cotton, or rubber depending on the application; vacuum hood or air extraction system; and face shields or goggles, if liquid resins and solvents are used. The major concerns are splashing of liquids and the absorption of vapors through the skin and other orifices of the body. The MSDS will specify the requirements for each material type. All of the processes that emit vapors should be performed with extraction systems outside the working space, in fume cupboards or in well-ventilated rooms. Note that many of these vapors are flammable. A further concern when working with uncured two-part resin systems is exothermic reactions. The mixing of two-part resin systems produces heat in the reaction. If this heat production (exothermic reaction) is not controlled, the resin mix may exotherm uncontrollably. This can lead to an explosive reaction or fire hazard. Follow the MSDS requirements and be observant to any heat buildup or unusual color changes. The hazards associated with the various types of adhesives and composite resins are provided in Table 2.

Quality Control and Quality Assurance. In any composite-structures workshop, whether components are being manufactured or repaired, one of the most important process requirements, and usually the one most often neglected, is quality control. In terms of both manufacture and repair facilities, quality control is the process that provides the customer's full acceptance of the integrity of the product, its technology, and the producer.

The material and process quality-control aspects in a composite and bonded structure workshop deal principally with the actual materials used in the fabrication of the component or repair scheme and the process by which the fabrication takes place. This particular component of quality control covers the entire product or service process. In addition, the level of skill in the work force, both technician and engineer, is a fundamental part of material and process quality control.

To ensure that repair materials are of the highest quality and that the repair station is set up to maintain an appropriate working environment, certain quality-control procedures or guidelines should be in place. As a minimum, such guidelines would include:

- Supplied material quality checks and receiving inspections
- Materials handling procedures and storage facilities for shelf-life materials
- Clean room for patch repair fabrication and application
- Damage removal area with suitable dust-extraction equipment
- Humidity and temperature controls in the clean room, including positive pressure for dust control
- Controlled access to the clean room
- Consumables, environmental controls, and repair procedure documentation
- Appropriately trained technical staff, with skill levels set and ongoing training programs

Quality-assurance testing is the physical testing of a product to show or demonstrate that it meets its acceptance standards. That is, the product achieves the desired mechanical strength, stiffness, and durability properties, for which it is designed. Quality-assurance testing is the final proof of successful quality-control implementation. The types of quality-assurance tests required fall under three main areas:

- Material quality assurance
- Process quality assurance
- Component quality assurance

Material quality assurance is in effect prefabrication testing of constituent materials. Such testing is used to screen incoming materials to ensure that they conform to the manufacturer's documented standards, and that lifetime-expired materials can also be checked against that standard. Tests that can be used on prepreg composites and adhesives (or any resin material) include: composite prepreg tack test, adhesive flow tests (Ref 3), and other test methods provided in

Table 2 Hazards associated with selected adhesives

Adhesive type	Causes burns	Flammability	Explosion	Harmful vapors	Harmful to skin and eyes
Solvent-borne		X	X	X	X
Water-borne				X maybe	X
Hot melts	X			X maybe	X
Powder form			X		
Curing rubber	X			X	
Epoxies		X		X maybe	X
Polyesters					X
Phenolics		X		X	X
Polyurethanes		X		X	X
Acrylics				X	X
Cyanoacrylates				X	X

X, Hazardous. Source: Ref 2

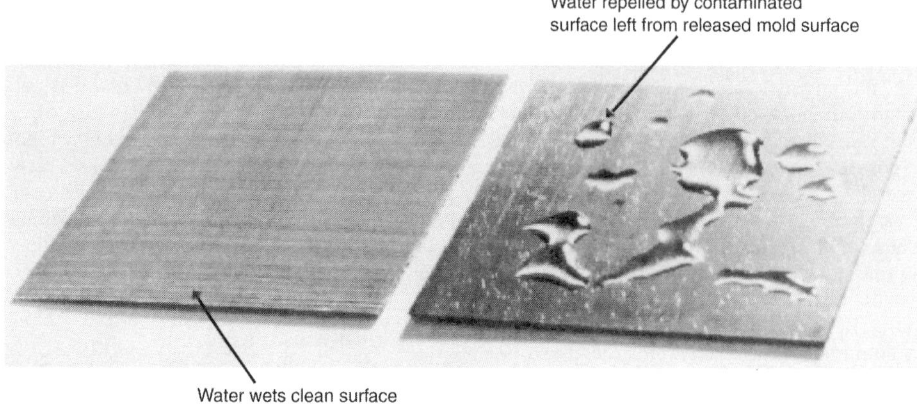
Water repelled by contaminated
surface left from released mold surface
Water wets clean surface

Fig. 9 Good (left) and poor (right) water break test results. Source: Ref 4

ASTM standards and Suppliers of Advanced Composite Materials Association (SACMA) test methods.

Cofabrication quality-assurance testing takes place during the actual fabrication of the repair scheme and its placement on the damaged area. The testing in effect is simple in that little expense and time is required, but such tests have a large impact on the structural integrity of the final repair. The testing procedure also ensures that all repair steps are completed and that critical steps are independently inspected prior to continuing with the repair. The testing process (both physical test and procedural checks) include backing ply count, water break test (Fig. 9), repair procedure checklist, and independent inspector's check.

Finished-component quality-assurance testing is a postfabrication test procedure, which is either a mechanical test on the completed component for adequate material properties, (a proof-load test or comparative coupon test) and/or a nondestructive test.

Mechanical property testing includes (for composites):

- Short-beam shear test—(ASTM D 2344 (Ref 5) or SRM 8-88 (Ref 6)
- Iosipescu shear test (Ref 7)
- Tension and compression tests—ASTM D 3039 (Ref 8), ASTM D 3410 (Ref 9), SRM 1-88 (Ref 10), and SRM 4-88 (Ref 11).

and (for bonded joints):

- Lap-shear test—ASTM D 3165 (Ref 12)
- Boeing wedge test—ASTM D 3762 (Ref 13)
- Postrepair NDI

REFERENCES

1. K.B. Armstrong and R.T. Barrett, *Care and Repair of Advanced Composites,* SAE International, 1997
2. K. Armstrong and R. Barrett, *Care and Repair of Advanced Composites*, Society of Automotive Engineers, 1998, p 193
3. "Standard Test Method for Flow Properties of Adhesives," D 2183, *Annual Book of ASTM Standards,* ASTM
4. L.J. Hart-Smith, R.W. Ochsner, and R.L. Radecky, "Surface Preparation of Fibrous Composites for Adhesive Bonding or Painting," Douglas Service Paper, First Quarter, 1984
5. "Standard Test Method for Apparent Interlaminar Shear Strength of Parallel Fiber Composites by Short-Beam Method," D 2344, *Annual Book of ASTM Standards,* ASTM
6. "SACMA Recommended Test Method for Apparent Interlaminar Shear Strength of Oriented Fiber-Resin Composites by the Short-Beam Method," SRM 8-88, Suppliers of Advanced Composite Materials Association
7. D.F. Adams and D.E. Walrath, Iosipescu Shear Properties of Composite Materials, *Composite Materials: Testing and Design* (Sixth Conference), STP 787, ASTM, 1982, p 19–33
8. "Standard Test Method for Tensile Properties of Fiber-Resin Composites," D 3039, *Annual Book of ASTM Standards,* ASTM
9. "Standard Test Method for Compressive Properties of Unidirectional or Crossply Fiber-Resin Composites," D 3410, *Annual Book of ASTM Standards,* ASTM
10. "SACMA Recommended Test Method for Compressive Properties of Oriented Fiber-Resin Composites, SRM 1-88, Suppliers of Advanced Composite Materials Association
11. "SACMA Recommended Test Method for Tensile Properties of Oriented Fiber-Resin Composites," SRM 4-88, Suppliers of Advanced Composite Materials Association
12. "Standard Test Method for Strength Properties of Laminated Assemblies Adhesives in Shear by Tension Loading," D 3165, *Annual Book of ASTM Standards,* ASTM
13. "Standard Test Method for Adhesive-Bonded Surface Durability of Aluminum (Wedge Test)," D 3762, *Annual Book of ASTM Standards,* ASTM

SELECTED REFERENCES

- *Adhesives and Sealants,* Vol 3, *Engineered Materials Handbook,* ASM International, 1990
- "Advanced Composite Repair Guide," NOR 82-60, Northrop Corp., Hawthorne, CA, March 1982
- "Advanced Composite Structures: Fabrication and Damage Repair," Abaris Training, Reno, NV, 1998
- *Aircraft Bonded Structure,* Training Manual, IAP Inc., Casper, WY, 1985
- *Airframe Section Textbook,* EA-ITP-AB, IAP Inc., Casper WY, 1985
- *ASTM Standards and Literature References for Composite Materials,* 2nd ed., ASTM, 1990
- A.A. Baker and R. Jones, *Bonded Repair of Aircraft Structures,* Martinus Nijhoff, Dordrecht, Netherlands, 1988
- C.E. Bakis and K.L. Reifsnider, Adiabatic Thermoelastic Measurements, *Manual on Experimental Methods for Mechanical Testing of Composites,* R.L. Pendleton and M.E. Tuttle, Ed., Elsevier Applied Science, 1989
- Y. Bar-Cohen, Nondestructive Inspection and Quality Control—Introduction, Section 9, *Adhesives and Sealants,* Vol 3, *Engineered Materials Handbook,* ASM International, 1990, p 727–728
- T. Bitzer, *Honeycomb Technology,* Chapman & Hall, London, 1997
- W. Cole, Commercial Aircraft Composite Repair Committee, Repair Design Task Group, *Design of Durable, Repairable, and Maintainable Aircraft Composites,* Society for the Advancement of Material and Process Engineering, 1997
- *Design of Durable, Repairable, and Maintainable Aircraft Composites,* Document Reference AE-27, Society of Automotive Engineers, 1997
- *Handling Precautions for Araldite Epoxy Resin Materials,* Safety Manual No. 37m, Ciba-Geigy Plastics, Duxford, England, May 1989
- R.B. Heslehurst, Observations in the Structural Response of Adhesive Bondline Defects, *Int. J. Adhes. Adhes.,* Vol 19, 1999, p 133–154
- R.B. Heslehurst, "Application and Interpretation of Holographic Interferometry Techniques in the Detection of Damage to Structural Materials," Ph.D. Dissertation, School of Aerospace and Mechanical Engineering, University College, University of New South Wales, Canberra, 1998
- R.B. Heslehurst, J.P. Baird, H.M. Williamson, and R.K. Clark, Can Aging Adhesively Bonded Joints Be Found?, *Proc. 41st SAMPE International Symposium and Exhibition* (Anaheim CA), 25–28 March 1996, Society for the Advancement of Material and Process Engineering, 1996, p 925–935
- R.B. Heslehurst, J.P. Baird, and H.M. Williamson, The Effect on Adhesion Stiffness

Due to Bonded Surface Contamination, *SAMPE J.,* Vol 26 (No. 3), April 1995, p 11–15

- B.C. Hoskin and A.A. Baker, Ed., *Composite Materials for Aircraft Structures,* AIAA Education Series, American Institute of Aeronautics and Astronautics, 1986
- A.J. Kinloch, *Adhesion and Adhesives—Science and Technology,* Chapman and Hall, London, 1987
- M.J. Kroes, W.A. Watkins, and F. Delp, *Aircraft Maintenance & Repair,* 6th ed., Macmillan/McGraw-Hill, 1993
- A.H. Landrock, *Adhesives Technology Handbook,* Noyes Publications, 1985
- M.C.Y. Niu, *Composite Airframe Structures: Practical Design Information and Data,* Conmilit Press Ltd., Hong Kong, 1992
- D. Perl, "Depot Repairs of F/A-18 Composite Aircraft Structures," Naval Aviation Depot Report, July 1983
- P. Peters, *Maintenance of Fibre Reinforced Plastics on Aircraft,* Department of Aviation, Aircraft Maintenance—Text 5, AGPS, Canberra, 1986
- "Safe Handling of Advanced Composite Materials Components: Health Information," Suppliers of Advanced Composite Materials Association, 1989
- Save Your Skin! A Guide to the Prevention of Dermatitis, Suppliers of Advanced Composite Materials Association, Arlington VA.
- "Standard Test Method for Flow Properties of Adhesives," D 2183, *Annual Book of ASTM Standards,* ASTM
- J. Summerscales, Ed., *Non-Destructive Testing of Fibre-Reinforced Plastics Composites,* Vol 1, Elsevier Applied Science, London, 1987
- *Utilization of Data,* Vol III, *Polymer Matrix Composites,* MIL-HDBK-17-3D, Department of Defense, 1994
- L.F. Vosteen and R.N. Hadcock, "Composite Chronicles: A Study of the Lessons Learned in the Development, Production, and Service of Composite Structures," NASA Contractor Report 4620, Langley Research Center, National Aeronautics and Space Administration, Nov 1994
- R.F. Wegman and T.R. Tullos, Nondestructive Inspection, *Handbook of Adhesive Bonded Structural Repair,* Noyes, 1992, Chapter 11

Bonded Repair of Metal Structures Using Composites

Richard J. Chester, Aeronautical and Maritime Research Laboratory, Australia
James J. Mazza, Air Force Research Laboratory

MODERN AIRCRAFT are becoming increasingly sophisticated and therefore more expensive to purchase. For this reason, aircraft are remaining in service for lengthy periods that, in some cases, exceed their original design lives. Some military aircraft are now expected to remain in service for 50 years or more; this would have been unthinkable when they were designed. To achieve such life extension, careful attention must be paid to managing both corrosion and fatigue, because they are the main problems associated with aging aircraft structure.

Composite bonded repair technology (Ref 1) enables cost-effective and durable repairs to be made to damaged or defective aircraft structure. This technology was developed in the early 1970s and is now routinely used for repairs to tertiary and secondary structure and noncritical repairs to primary structure (Ref 2). Some structurally significant repairs have also been made to primary structure (Ref 3, 4). Composite bonded repair technology is based on the use of advanced composite repairs or reinforcements that are adhesively bonded to the damaged structure. This contrasts with conventional repairs that are usually made from the same material as the parent structure (normally aluminum) and mechanically fastened to transfer the load into the repair material. The lack of conventional fasteners in a composite bonded repair is one of the main advantages. Fastener holes are points of stress concentration in a structure and may cause the initiation of new fatigue cracks. Adhesively bonded repairs have a much more uniform stress transfer mechanism, resulting in a stiffer joint, because the load is not transferred only at a few discrete locations, as is the case for fasteners. Composite bonded repairs are typically thinner, weigh less, and can be applied more rapidly than conventional repairs. They also do not suffer from subsequent corrosion during service, because the patch is immune to corrosion and the adhesive effectively seals the repair interface.

Because composite bonded repairs provide greater reinforcing efficiency than a mechanically fastened joint, it is often possible to leave the defect in the structure. Simple nondestructive inspection (NDI) methods can subsequently be used to confirm the effectiveness of the repair in service. Not having to remove the defect is one of the ways in which significant savings in repair time can be achieved. A major difference between mechanically fastened and adhesively bonded joints is that there is no NDI technique currently available that can provide a measure of the adhesively bonded joint strength or durability after the joint has been made. For this reason, it is essential that all adhesively bonded repairs be undertaken using quality management principles.

As well as repairing damaged structure, adhesively bonded composite materials can also be used to reinforce structure to reduce excessive deflection or stress and prevent the initiation of a defect. It is important that the details of the structure and nature of loading be understood to ensure that an effective reinforcement can be designed.

Due to the research carried out since the 1970s, the technology is now mature for relatively straightforward repairs. Research is continuing into its use on thicker structures that are highly loaded, highly curved structure and safety-of-flight-critical structure, where the defect has reduced the load capacity of the structure below design ultimate load.

This article aims to introduce the reader to the technology and explain some of the key steps that are normally encountered in the design, certification, and application of an adhesively bonded repair. In the space available, it is not possible to completely describe all aspects of this technology; readers interested in designing and applying such repairs are referred to the references for more complete details. Some examples are given of successful repairs to military aircraft, and finally, future trends and developments in this area are forecast.

Damage Assessment

An important precursor to the design phase is a careful assessment of the damage to establish if the repair design will be effective. Cracking, in particular, should be carefully inspected to determine the nature of the loads that are responsible. In many cases, tensile loads are involved; however, in some cases, shear or bending stresses may be present, and a repair may need to be specifically designed for these loads. Cracks should be inspected to determine if they are fatigue cracks, acoustically generated fatigue cracks, or stress corrosion cracks. Different design approaches will be required in each case.

The nature of the damaged structure is important. Considerations include material type and thickness, the nature of the loading, environmental conditions present, and local geometry, including curvature. The degree of support to the structure in the repair area is also important, together with the available length of the load transfer zone. If the structure is well supported or is sufficiently thick, a repair to only one side of the damage may be appropriate. For thin, poorly supported structure, a one-sided repair may induce bending, due to the shift of the neutral axis of the repaired structure, so a double-sided repair may need to be considered.

Accurate NDI is desirable to ensure the full extent and nature of the damage is known. If the defect is to be left in the structure, this information will be used during subsequent inspections to check for any defect growth during service.

Repair Design

Following a thorough assessment of the nature of the damage, an appropriate repair can be designed. In some cases, the designs of bonded composite repairs are deceptively simple, but some understanding of the technology is required if the repair is to perform its required function. Although strength and stiffness will be primary considerations during the design process, many other issues need to be considered to ensure that the repair is effective. Some of these are listed in Table 1. For any bonded repair, the designer must also recognize the crucial importance of correct manufacture and application procedures (covered in the section "Repair Application" in this article).

Materials Selection and Engineering. There is no single repair material that will be optimal for every repair situation, and so the designer needs to select the best material for the situation (Ref 5). Materials that have been used effectively include boron/epoxy and graphite/epoxy composites (fiber-reinforced plastics, FRP), GLARE (a laminated metallic material reinforced with glass fibers in an adhesive layer), and conventional metallic materials. Fiber-reinforced plastic materials are most commonly used, because they are relatively resistant to fatigue damage and impervious to corrosion (Ref 1). Their high specific stiffness allows repairs to be made thin and with low weight, they can usually be molded readily to complex aerodynamic curvatures, and they can be readily made with tapered ends to reduce peel stresses. Potential FRP disadvantages include cost, availability, and the need to carefully insulate graphite/epoxy repairs to avoid galvanic corrosion of aluminum substrates. Boron/epoxy repairs do not cause galvanic corrosion and also readily permit the use of NDI methods, such as eddy current inspection, to check for growth of the defect underneath the installed repair material. As a result of thermal expansion mismatch between the composite and metal (Table 2), residual stresses are generated when composites are bonded to a metallic substrate with an elevated-temperature-curing adhesive. Boron/epoxy is often preferred to graphite/epoxy as a repair material, because it gives rise to lower residual stresses. Note that thermally induced residual stresses do not normally compromise the design of a composite bonded repair; however, it is important that they be considered during the design phase.

GLARE has been demonstrated by the United States Air Force (USAF) for fuselage repairs and appears to have greatest advantage for applications where the operating temperature is normally low (high-altitude cruise conditions) (Ref 6). This is because at low temperatures, the residual stresses caused by composites are enhanced, while GLARE produces minimal residual stress. Disadvantages of GLARE include relatively low stiffness that results in comparatively thick and heavy repairs, difficulty in molding the patch to complex curves, and difficulty in performing NDI to check on growth of any underlying damage. These same disadvantages apply to the use of conventional metals for repair materials, but metals are more susceptible to fatigue and corrosion than GLARE.

The operating temperature is an important design consideration that can influence the choice of repair material. Apart from the low-temperature condition described previously, many high-temperature locations are present around engines, bleed air (de-icing) locations, and on leading edges of military aircraft. The glass transition temperature of composite materials and the composite interlayers in GLARE need to be carefully checked to ensure that an adequate margin is allowed for safe operation under worst-case hot/wet conditions.

Adhesives used for bonded composite repairs are often structural film adhesives (epoxies, phenolics); however, some paste adhesives, such as epoxies and modified acrylics, have also been used successfully. The designer needs to consider whether the mechanical properties of the adhesive (shear modulus, shear yield strength, and strain-to-failure) are adequate for the repair application. Note that the lap/shear strength data usually provided by adhesive manufacturers are convenient for comparison purposes but are not pure shear (rather, mixed peel and shear) and, therefore, should not be used for design. The correct design value is the shear strain at yield, measured by the thick-adherend shear test (for example, ASTM D 3983 and D 5656). Good repair design will have the adhesive being stressed in shear with low peel stresses at the ends of the joint. Designs in which high levels of peel stress are present should not be considered; however, it is important to recognize that some adhesives are much better able to withstand peel stress than others. High-temperature adhesives (phenolics, polyimides), in general, are essentially brittle and so are much more likely to fail due to peel stresses than lower-temperature, toughened adhesives (modified acrylics and toughened epoxies). It should be noted that failure of a composite bonded repair may not be within the adhesive layer, but rather within the relatively more-brittle matrix resin of the composite repair material. Designing only to the adhesive strength may be unconservative, if actual repair failure occurs within the composite repair material.

The cure temperature is usually an important factor to be considered, because this directly affects the ability of the adhesive to function satisfactorily under the operating temperature. Cure temperature is also the critical consideration if residual stresses are deemed to be important, and cure time can sometimes be important where the repair must be completed quickly, due to operational requirements.

Stress Analysis. Bonded composite repairs are normally intended to restore the load path that the damage/defect has removed from the structure. For this reason, the design is typically undertaken so that the repair restores the lost stiffness, and checks are made to confirm that adequate strength levels have been achieved. Designing to restore strength with composite materials could result in the structure being overstiffened, which will result in extra load being attracted to the region. In practice, it is found that most simple repairs can be modeled approximately as a representative bonded joint, the solutions for which have previously been published (Ref 7, 8). The shear stress distribution in a typical repair is shown in Fig. 1.

At the ends of the repair, the adhesive shear stress (τ_p) is high and may reach the yield stress at high loads. As the longitudinal strains in the repair and substrate adherends become equal, the adhesive shear stress reduces. A sensible design

Table 1 Partial list of issues to be considered during repair design

Static strength
Fatigue strength
Weight
Stiffness
Aerodynamic smoothness
Cost
Operating temperature
Repair interactions
Nondestructive inspection
Stress intensity following repair
Post-repair inspections
Durability under operating environment

Table 2 Coefficients of thermal expansion of substrates and repair materials

Material	Coefficient of thermal expansion 10^{-6}/°C	Coefficient of thermal expansion 10^{-6}/°F
Boron/epoxy (unidirectional)	4.5	2.5
Graphite/epoxy (unidirectional)	–0.3	–0.16
GLARE-3 3/2, 0.2 (longitudinal)	16.3	9.1
Aluminum (typical)	23(a)	12.8(a)

(a) In typical aircraft structure, the aluminum component is constrained by the relatively cool surrounding structure, and so the actual expansion is usually significantly lower than would be the case for free expansion.

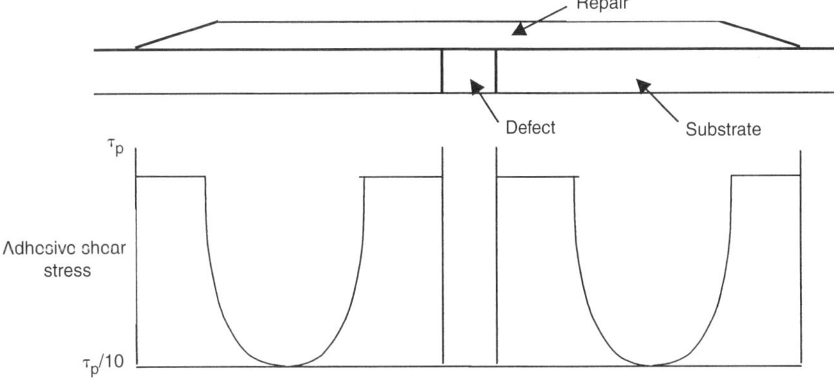

Fig. 1 Example of the shear stress distribution in a bonded repair where the defect remains in the structure and the substrate is restrained from bending

approach is to adjust the length of the repair to allow this stress to reduce to less than one-tenth of the plastic shear stress value. This provides necessary damage tolerance with respect to voids or other defects in the adhesive bondline and against failure by creep rupture.

The design should be checked for static strength using the maximum load the structure is expected to see in service (for aircraft this is the design ultimate load). Checks need to be made of the stress intensity at the defect after repair to confirm that the repaired structure has an adequate margin of static strength. The maximum strain in the repair material needs to be less than the design allowable for the material, and a check must be made of the load-carrying capability of the adhesive in the joint. The maximum load to be transmitted by the joint is checked to confirm that it is less than the load-carrying capacity of the adhesive. This is related to the strain energy capacity of the adhesive (area under the stress-strain curve) and the influence of residual stresses in the joint. Where the repair will operate at low or elevated temperatures, these strength checks need to be made using the appropriate adhesive properties. As noted in the section "Materials Selection and Engineering" in this article, if the adhesive strength does not determine the joint strength, as may occur with composite adherends, this design strategy may be unconservative.

If the repair demonstrates adequate static strength, it should not be the weak link in the structure if maximum load is applied. Checks should also be made on the expected crack growth of the defect, using the postrepair stress-intensity factor and the fatigue load spectrum. Due to the efficiency of bonded repairs, it is usual to find zero or very low crack-growth rates following the application of a bonded composite repair. Using the fatigue spectrum, checks can then also be made to ensure that the adhesive is not likely to suffer fatigue damage and that the repair material is operating below the fatigue threshold. Simple repairs can be designed using this analytical approach, while more complex repairs (to thick structure or complex geometries) are likely to require the use of finite-element analysis (Ref 1).

Repair Application

Successful application of a bonded repair design is not necessarily difficult, but requires proper execution of a number of processing steps, including surface preparation for both the aircraft structure and the composite repair material, as well as heating and pressurization. Other considerations include the nature of the repair installation environment, handling of repair materials, health and safety issues, training of repair installers, and postbond operations. In all cases, it is important that installation procedures be considered during repair design and validation, because they directly influence the final properties of the adhesively bonded joint.

Surface Preparation. Preparation of adherend surfaces prior to bonding is the single most-important application process step for ensuring a successful repair (Ref 9). Surface preparation is necessary for the attainment of adequate initial bond strength and long-term durability in the service environment. Although the environment includes temperature extremes and exposure to many aircraft fluids and maintenance chemicals, moisture tends to be the biggest impediment to long-term durability, particularly for aluminum bonded joints. Nearly all failures in aluminum adhesive joints on aircraft have been initiated by moisture (Ref 10).

In the broadest sense, prebond surface preparation encompasses several steps required to provide a durable interface between the substrate and adhesive (or primer). These can include cleaning, deoxidizing, chemical and/or physical modification of the surface, and application of adhesive bond primer. Prior to surface preparation, existing inorganic and organic coatings or surface layers must be removed from the surface via locally approved processes. Cleaning, typically solvent degreasing, is required to remove oils, greases, hydraulic fluids, jet fuel, and other gross organic contaminants. This should be accomplished prior to and subsequent to coatings removal. Care must be taken to use degreasing solvents that can remove the likely contaminants.

After cleaning, metals are usually abraded, grit-blasted, or etched to remove loosely adhered oxides, to prepare a contaminant-free surface, and to generate a rough surface topography. Abrasion can be accomplished by a variety of means, including sandpaper and nylon abrasive pads, such as Scotch-Brite (3M Corporation). Grit-blasting, typically with fine alumina, is a good method for roughening surfaces and removing existing oxide layers. Care must be taken not to damage aircraft structure, with particular caution for fatigue-critical components, and removal of abrasive media and debris must be done in such a way that the clean surface is not contaminated. Etching with a strong acid or base can also be used to deoxidize, clean, and roughen metal components. After degreasing and roughening, the water break test (Ref 11) is often used to assess the cleanliness of the surface, although it does not guarantee that the surface is free of contaminants.

Adhesive bonding is sometimes conducted on surfaces that have simply been cleaned and roughened. However, this is not recommended, particularly for critical components or those intended for a long service life, because a clean, rough surface does not guarantee adequate initial bond strength and does very little toward providing a metal-polymer interface that can resist long-term moisture attack. Additional surface modification is necessary to create a robust interface capable of resisting moisture for extended periods of service. This modification is often referred to as the surface treatment step, whereas the precursor cleaning and roughening steps are often designated the pretreatment. The actual surface treatment can be accomplished via anodizing, etching, or application of a coupling agent. Many anodizing and etching processes are available for metal alloys (Ref 12). The anodizing processes grow a fairly stable, microrough oxide layer on the metal surface that allows for mechanical interlocking with an adhesive or primer. Etching treatments produce less microroughness, but also provide bond strength and durability via mechanical interlocking (Ref 13). The use of coupling agents is intended to produce adhesion via strong chemical bonds. Coupling agents, most often silanes with appropriate organic functionalities, are formulated to bond two dissimilar materials, such as a metal oxide surface and a polymer (primer or adhesive). This approach eliminates problems associated with acid use on aircraft, such as embrittlement of certain high-strength steels (Ref 14), health/safety issues, and possible corrosion if not properly rinsed away. Variants of the grit-blast/silane (GBS) approach have been used successfully by a number of organizations (Ref 15, 16). Silane coupling agent application is shown in Fig. 2 for a F-16 aircraft repair. A similar but improved approach based on sol-gel technology has been developed and is now beginning to see application (Ref 17, 18). Application of a corrosion-inhibiting adhesive primer is also required to maximize long-term moisture durability for all of the surface treatments, and its use is recommended in most cases. Primers, though, can be difficult to properly apply on aircraft, and they can present health/safety concerns. Environmental durability data for several surface preparations, as measured by the ASTM D 3762 wedge test, are presented in Table 3.

Table 3 Wedge test data (ASTM D 3762) for several surface preparations

Surface preparation	Initial crack, mm (in.)	Cumulative crack growth, mm (in.) 1 h	8 h	24 h	7 days	28 days	Failure mode(a)
Abrade/solvent wipe	40.1 (1.58)	82.3 (3.24)	85.1 (3.35)	Removed due to gross failure			0% co
Grit-blast only	30.7 (1.21)	4.1 (0.16)	9.1 (0.36)	12.2 (0.48)	16.6 (0.65)	23.1 (0.91)	0% co
Grit-blast/silane-no primer	30.5 (1.20)	1.8 (0.07)	2.3 (0.09)	2.5 (0.10)	3.3 (0.13)	4.3 (0.17)	80% co
Grit-blast/silane-BR 127(b)	30.7 (1.21)	1.8 (0.07)	1.8 (0.07)	2.5 (0.10)	3.3 (0.13)	3.8 (0.15)	100% co
Grit-blast/sol-gel-BR 6747-1(c)	29.7 (1.17)	0.8 (0.03)	1.3 (0.05)	2.3 (0.09)	2.3 (0.09)	3.8 (0.15)	100% co
PAA-BR 127(b)	32.0 (1.26)	0.3 (0.01)	0.8 (0.03)	0.8 (0.03)	0.8 (0.03)	1.0 (0.04)	100% co

U.S. Air Force Research Laboratory Materials Directorate data on aluminum 2024-T3 bonded with AF 163-2M (3M Corporation, St. Paul, MN) adhesive and conditioned at 49 °C (120 °F) and 95–100% relative humidity. Data represent the average of 5–10 specimens from one or two panels and typify data routinely obtained by the Air Force Research Laboratory for the represented surface preparations. (a) co, cohesive failure within the adhesive layer; remaining failure was interfacial between metal and primer or adhesive. (b) BR 127, Cytec Fiberite chromated solvent-based bond primer. (c) BR 6747-1, Cytec Fiberite chromated waterborne bond primer

Repair materials such as metals, GLARE, and precured FRPs must also be treated prior to bonding. Because the outer surface of the GLARE laminate is anodized and primed, it must only be degreased with a suitable solvent prior to bonding. Precured FRP materials must also be prepared by cleaning and roughening prior to bonding; however, because they do not have an oxide layer, there is no need for a chemical modification or treatment step to ensure a strong and durable bond, as is the case for metals. The primary function of the surface preparation is to remove contaminants, such as oils, mold lubricants, or general dirt. There are two main techniques used to accomplish this: the peel ply method and solvent cleaning and abrasion, often conducted after a peel ply surface has been exposed (Ref 19). Solvent cleaning to remove gross organic contaminants is conducted with the same type of solvents used to degrease metals. Abrasion can be accomplished using a variety of media, including abrasive papers and nylon pads. A grit-blast with aluminum oxide is the best surface preparation known for composites. This method is preferred, if at all practical for a given application, and its superiority has been confirmed by a series of tests at a number of companies. It results in optimal bond strengths with a minimum of scatter (Ref 20).

A peel ply can be incorporated, during manufacture, as the outer layer on the bonding surface of a composite laminate to be removed just prior to bonding (Fig. 3). In principle, a clean surface is exposed that is ready for immediate bonding. However, it is difficult to ensure that the peel ply has not left behind sufficient contamination to reduce the bond strength and increase the coefficient of variation considerably (Ref 21). The choice of peel ply material is important as well as controversial (Ref 22). The safest approach is to abrade or grit-blast after peel ply removal. The peel ply then prevents contamination of the bond surface until its removal just prior to bonding, and the abrasion ensures the peel ply itself does not contaminate the surface. The cleanliness of the prepared FRP surface can be checked using the standard water break test (Ref 23). The FRP should then be thoroughly dried prior to adhesive application. Primers are not typically used on FRP materials.

After the aircraft repair area and repair material surfaces are prepared for bonding, adhesive is applied, and the repair material is mated to the aircraft within a predetermined time interval. Film adhesives are usually applied to the repair material, which is then taped in place on the aircraft. If paste adhesives are used, they are applied to both mating surfaces. Some means of bondline thickness control is required for pastes, such as glass beads or a scrim cloth, whereas most film adhesives used for repair already contain a carrier cloth. In all cases, the procedure used should be validated prior to the actual repair. Handling and application of adhesives should be done in such a way as to avoid contamination and minimize air entrapment.

Heating and Pressurization. If surface preparation is the single most important bonded repair application process, heating and pressurization are likely next. In fact, heat application is an essential part of many surface preparations. For instance, the GBS process requires controlled elevated-temperature drying of the silane immediately after its application to the metal surface. Heating may also be used to dry surfaces after rinsing acids or conducting water break tests. Controlled heating is also required to cure adhesive primers, and elevated temperatures are often used to dry structure prior to repair. Of course, heating is required to cure many repair adhesives, and elevated temperatures are often used to accelerate the cure of ambient-curable adhesives. Many adhesives can cure over a range of temperatures, provided they exceed a minimum temperature for a specified time. It is often desirable to cure for longer times at lower temperatures to reduce the effect of coefficient of thermal expansion mismatch between aircraft structure and repair material (see the section "Materials Selection and Engineering" in this article). The actual cure cycle to be used should be validated with the design, because adhesive properties can vary for differing cures.

Pressure application is necessary to mate the repair material to the aircraft structure. Although pressure is not required to actually cure the adhesive, sufficient pressure is required to achieve desired bond strength and durability. Pressure causes the adhesive to flow and properly "wet" the bond surfaces; it ensures proper bondline thickness, and it helps reduce the extent of bondline voids and porosity.

Heating may be conducted by any of a number of methods, provided they are able to safely control the temperature in the repair area within prescribed tolerances for the time required, without contaminating the repair. Typical on-aircraft heating methods include electric-resistance heat blankets, infrared heat lamps, and hot air devices. Application specifics determine the method best suited to a given repair. Heat blankets are typically used to cure adhesives, whereas heat lamps are usually the choice for silane drying and precuring primers. All heating devices must be controlled by some means so that heat can be applied when and to the levels required. This is particularly important for adhesive cure, because controlled heat-up and cooling rates are usually prescribed. "Hot bonders" that automatically control heating based on temperature feedback from the repair area are

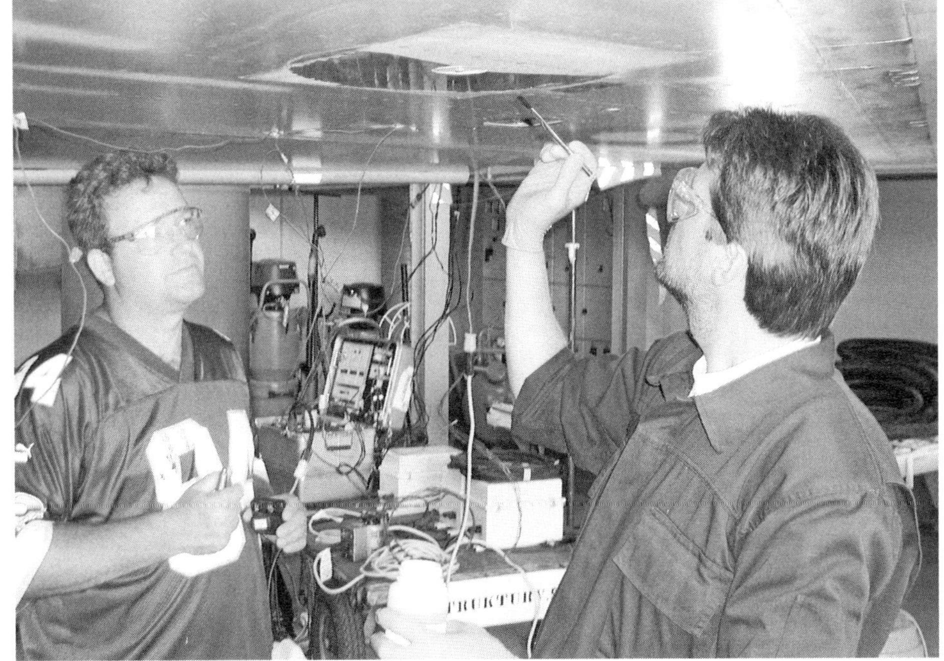

Fig. 2 Application of silane coupling agent (GBS surface preparation) during a F-16 aircraft repair

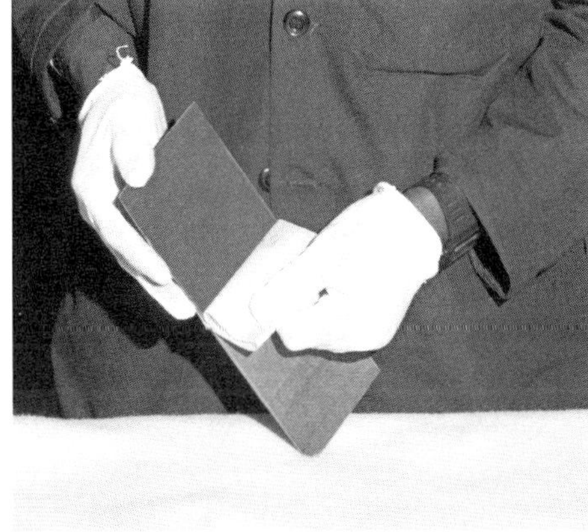

Fig. 3 Peel ply removal from composite doubler

normally used with heat blankets. These units or similar means can be employed to control heat lamps and hot air devices.

Achieving prescribed repair temperatures within desired tolerances can often be difficult on aircraft, because portions of the structure can act as "heat sinks." These regions conduct heat away from the repair site and become locally cooler regions where there is a danger that the adhesive may not fully cure. Thermal surveys of the repair area are important to ensure proper heating will be attainable. The surveys should be conducted on the actual repair area, using the equipment to be employed during the repair. They can determine the placement of insulation materials or the locations needed for supplemental heating to overcome "heat sinks," and they will reveal the required temperature readings for surrounding "monitoring" locations that can be used to determine the temperature in the repair area. The goal is to reduce the temperature delta in the repair area to an acceptable value considered during the repair design. In complex situations where large heat sinks exist, a sound philosophy is to monitor and control the hottest point, so as to avoid any damage to the structure, and then use the coldest point as the basis for ensuring complete cure of the adhesive.

Pressure application on aircraft may also be achieved by a variety of means. These include vacuum bag, inflated bladder, or various forms of mechanical pressure. The use of a vacuum bag is the most common, because it is almost always the most convenient. Vacuum bags are light, conform to almost any surface, apply uniform pressure, can remove volatiles from the repair area, and can hold a heat blanket in place (Fig. 4). To apply pressure this way, a bag is built over the repair area and air is extracted, allowing atmospheric pressure to be applied. In most cases, it is not desirable to achieve a full vacuum throughout the cure cycle, because the vacuum allows volatiles in the adhesive, such as moisture or solvents, to boil more readily, and it allows entrapped air to expand more easily. Often, high vacuum levels are applied initially to remove volatiles from the repair, then vacuum levels are reduced before the adhesive gels, in order to minimize porosity in the bondline. Levels corresponding to 34 to 69 kPa (5 to 10 psi) pressure are common. The process decision is influenced by the particular repair adhesive and should be considered during repair design. A common problem with the use of vacuum bags is that they also tend to draw air and contaminants into the repair area through leakage points in the structure, for example, from around and under fastener heads or from around intersecting ribs that cannot be completely sealed.

Bladders inflated with air can be used to apply positive pressure (as opposed to vacuum) on a repair area. This may be desirable to minimize void formation due to the evolution of volatiles. However, this approach is not usually convenient, because bladders must be held against the structure in some way, and they require a frame or fixture to react against. If this fixture is fastened to the structure, pressure is limited to prevent damage. Mechanical pressure may also be applied by clamping or other means. Again, these forces must be reacted, and it is difficult to apply uniform pressure over a large area via clamps.

Precured FRP repair materials should be cured via positive pressure in accordance with manufacturer's recommendations. This is normally done in an autoclave to minimize porosity and achieve the per-ply thickness value envisioned by the design. Fiber-reinforced plastic materials can also be cocured with the adhesive during repair installation. This can be a convenient method for ensuring the repair material matches surface contours.

After the repair material is bonded in place, the edges of the repair should be sealed to slow moisture ingress. Adhesive "flash" that has squeezed out onto the prepared surface during bonding should be left in place around the periphery of the repair, with only excessive squeezeout carefully removed. The metal corrosion protection scheme should then be reestablished in the area surrounding the repair, and the edge of the repair should also be coated with sealant, such as Aerospace Materials Specification (AMS) S 8802 (Ref 24).

Repair Certification

A number of design, installation, and in-service inspection issues must be addressed in order to certify a bonded repair. Unfortunately, there is no widely accepted standard for certification. The problem that sets bonded repair apart is the concern over long-term bond durability in the service environment, particularly moisture, and the current inability to satisfactorily predict or nondestructively measure this durability. This is less important for repair of structure that is not flight-critical, because risks are lower, and these types of repairs are becoming accepted. However, a fail-safe approach is often taken for safety-of-flight-critical structure. This does not allow full credit to be given to the repair for restoring residual strength and reducing the fatigue crack growth rate. In other words, it is assumed the repair can fail at any time. To receive full credit, there must be assurances that the risk of losing repair effectiveness is acceptably low, or a technique must be available to detect significant loss before it is a problem (Ref 25).

Certification Guidelines. Aside from the critical environmental durability issue, repairs can be designed on the basis that patch efficiency can be predicted, and they should be designed conservatively, with respect to the possible failure modes, to include the surrounding structure. In this regard, an approach similar to the one outlined by the USAF Structural Integrity Program identified in MIL-HDBK-1530 (Ref 26) can be used as the basis for certification. The environmental durability issue greatly increases the significance of quality control and associated testing, because quality is assured by complying with approved and validated process specifications. Validation of surface preparation procedures is particularly difficult, due to the current lack of a definitive test to accelerate the effects of service environment in a way that is quantifiable. Although not as complex as the issue of adhesive bond durability, validation of all the other aspects of repair implementation is also required to enable certification. This includes repair design methods, processes, and software and repair application methods and processes.

Nondestructive Inspection and Quality Control. Nondestructive inspection plays a role in determining whether a repair has been successfully installed and is performing as expected in service. Several different NDI techniques can be used to inspect bonded composite repairs. Ultrasonics can be used to readily detect disbonds between the repair and the parent structure, and defects within the adhesive bondline, such as large voids or delaminations within a composite patch or reinforcement. Ultrasonic bond testers using a low-frequency impedance technique can also detect disbonds and voids within a repair joint. Thermography is gaining increased acceptance as a rapid way of detecting the presence of disbonds and larger voids within bondlines. Also, simple tap tests can normally be used to provide a quick indication of the presence of a disbond under a repair, and inspection of the squeezeout after bonding can give an indication as to proper pressure application and bondline porosity. Eddy current methods are particularly useful for determining the length of cracks in metallic substructure under a composite repair and are most efficient for repair materials, such as boron/epoxy, that are electrically nonconductive. Further details of these and other NDI methods can be found in Ref 27 and 28.

Even with the large number of techniques available, NDI plays a supporting role that is necessary but not sufficient for assuring bondline integrity. This is because there is no NDI technique currently available that can measure the strength of a bond and therefore provide evidence of gradual adhesive bond degradation. When such a technique becomes available, it will be possible to confirm that the surface treatment procedures have produced a bond with the required level of strength, and then, while in ser-

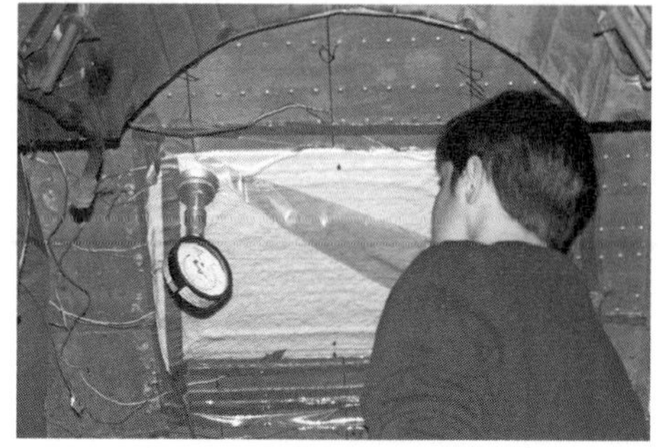

Fig. 4 Installation of vacuum bag containing heat blanket and thermocouples

vice, the technique can be periodically used to confirm that no deterioration of the joint strength has occurred. The only way in which such assurance can currently be obtained is by quality management of the repair application. Critical aspects of quality management include:

- Effective training of design and technical staff
- The use of in-life materials that have been qualified and properly handled
- The use of validated design and application procedures (in particular, surface treatment procedures)
- Control of the repair environment and the use of validated procedures to ensure full cure of the adhesive and the absence of defects after the repair has been applied

The previously mentioned process, coupled with NDI and the judicious use of process control (witness) coupons, is the best method currently available to assure a successful repair that has long-term durability. This process has been applied successfully in the repairs described subsequently.

Repair Examples

Thousands of bonded repairs have been made to metallic aircraft structures using composite materials. Most have been applied to instances of metal fatigue cracking, although bonded repairs have been used to address damage caused by corrosion, stress corrosion, and other types of damage. The Royal Australian Air Force (RAAF) was the first to routinely use bonded composites to repair metal structure, and they have applied a large number of these repairs, including applications on several aircraft types (Ref 25). In particular, thousands of repairs have been installed on RAAF C-130 aircraft, saving nearly $100 million (Ref 2), with a successful history of over 25 years of service. The USAF has installed bonded composite repairs on a number of aircraft types, including C-141, C-130, C-5, B-52, and F-16. The most notable application is the "weep hole" crack repair for the C-141 aircraft wings. This application and an example of the repair of a crack beyond critical length on an RAAF F-111 aircraft are discussed subsequently.

Example 1: USAF C-141 Weep Hole Repair. The C-141 aircraft lower wing skins are constructed of extruded 7075-T6 aluminum panels stiffened by integral risers containing weep holes to prevent fuel entrapment in the wings. In 1993, fatigue cracks were discovered at a large number of inner-wing weep holes, causing 45 of the approximately 250 aircraft in the fleet to be grounded and others to be restricted. All of the nearly 1500 inner-wing weep holes per aircraft were inspected using the bolt-hole eddy current NDI method, and more than 13,000 cracks were discovered. Oversizing holes eliminated over 80% of the cracks. In cases where a significant quantity or cluster of holes could not be cleaned up by oversizing, wing panels were replaced. In other cases, on about 170 aircraft where the maximum allowable oversize could not eliminate cracks, bonded composite repairs were accomplished.

A durability and damage tolerance analysis completed in the 1980s identified the wing weep holes as a potential concern. The C-141 manufacturer, Lockheed Martin, designed an initial bonded composite repair and accomplished a finite-element analysis (FEA). When cracking became a problem, Warner Robins Air Logistics Center (WR-ALC) built from these early efforts to produce a final repair design. A conservative approach was taken, assuming the riser was totally severed, and a coarse shell element analysis was used to evaluate the effect of several repairs in close proximity. The original 5-doubler Lockheed design was simplified to three, one on either side of the affected riser (inside the wing) and one on the wing skin below the riser (on the outer moldline). Figure 5 illustrates the wing configuration and 3-doubler repair. The outer doubler was later split into two for repairs over splice joints between wing panels, creating a 4-doubler repair in these cases.

Warner Robins Air Logistics Center's experience with composite repair of composite structure and various literature sources were used to size and shape doublers and determine ply stacking and stepoff. A detailed two-dimensional (2-D) shell element analysis of an assumed standard repair was accomplished to look at ply stresses and optimize doubler configuration, location, and quantity. The 3-doubler approach was verified at this time, and boron/epoxy was selected as the repair material. Although graphite/epoxy was considered viable, boron/epoxy was chosen, due to the desire to avoid galvanic corrosion issues in the event fasteners had to be put through the doublers. A considerable amount of detailed three-dimensional (3-D) FEA was conducted to further optimize the doubler and evaluate its impact on the surrounding structure. A segment of actual wing plank was repaired to identically match the 3-D model, instrumented and statically tested. Correlation was very good and even allowed reduction of spacing between repairs. Based on the detailed FEA, a damage tolerance assessment was performed. This was validated by fatigue testing to a critical flight spectrum of the area, indicating that the desired 15,000 flight hours could be achieved by repaired wing panels. Fatigue testing was conducted at ambient temperature and at –54 °C (–65 °F). Thermal shock and salt fog testing were also conducted on freestanding repaired specimens, with no negative effects.

Installation procedures for the precured doublers were developed in collaboration between WR-ALC and the Air Force Research Laboratory (AFRL). As expected, the key issue was metal surface preparation. Warner Robins Air Logistics Center's requirement for nonacid surface preparation was accommodated by selection of the GBS process developed by AFRL and based on a similar procedure used in Australia (Ref 15). The GBS procedure included the ap-

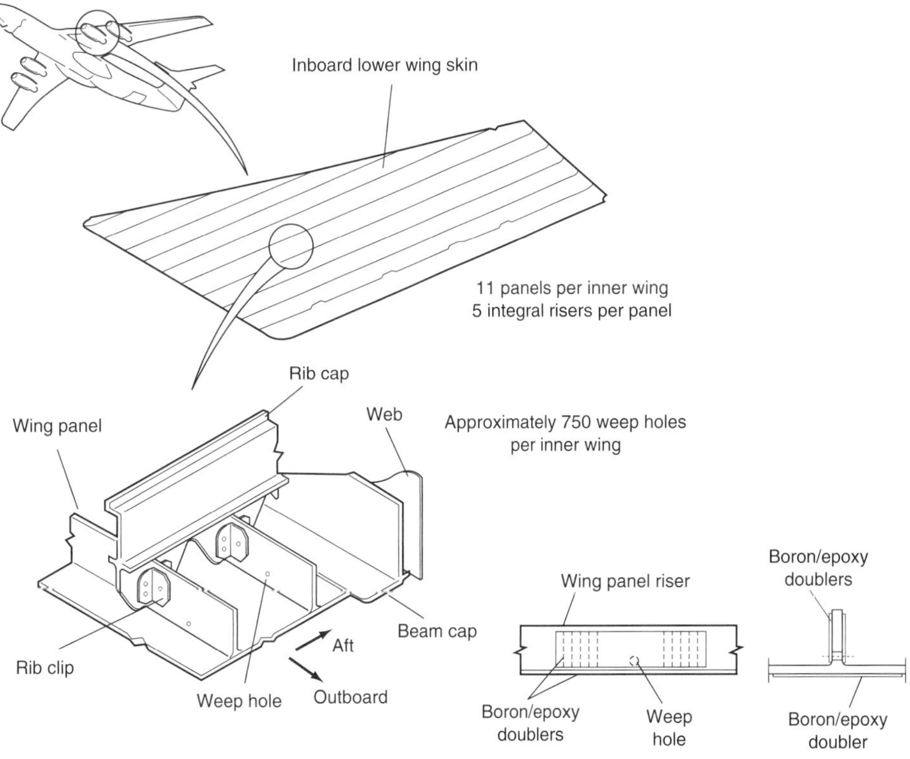

Fig. 5 C-141 wing configuration with weep holes; 3-doubler repair

plication of BR 127 (Cytec Fiberite, Inc.) adhesive primer. Although time-consuming, the GBS/primer approach proved to be very successful when implemented with strict quality control measures. The precured boron/epoxy doublers contained an untreated resin-rich nylon peel ply outer layer that was removed just prior to bonding. In most cases, no further treatment was provided. Silane was dried and primer was cured on the risers using a heat blanket placed on the outside moldline, whereas silane and primer applied to the moldline were heated by means of heat lamps. Doublers were installed using one of three 120 °C (250 °F) curing modified epoxy film adhesives. Pressure was applied by vacuum bag at about 381 mm Hg. In most cases, heat was provided to all three bondlines simultaneously via a heat blanket located on the bottom of the wing skin in the vacuum bag over the outer moldline doubler. The ability to heat in this way had been previously established during thermal surveys on an actual C-141 wing.

The first repairs were made in August 1993. In less than two years, over 800 bonded composite repairs (representing over 2400 doublers) were installed by several organizations. In total, over 900 repairs have now been installed, over half by WR-ALC. Routine inspections are conducted using thermography, and none of the repairs installed using the GBS surface preparation have failed. Cost savings for the WR-ALC effort alone are estimated at approximately $40 million, based on avoiding the replacement of over 250 wing panels. This success has led to expanded applications on other C-141 primary structure. External doublers for weep hole repairs are shown in Fig. 6.

Example 2: RAAF F-111 Lower Wing Skin Repair. F-111 aircraft in service with the RAAF have recently been found to suffer from fatigue cracking in the outboard section of the lower wing skin (Ref 3). The cracking is caused by a stress concentration from a runout in the forward auxiliary spar to create a fuel flow passage. When the first crack was discovered, fracture mechanics calculations indicated that it was beyond critical length at design limit load. A conventional, mechanically fastened metallic repair was considered, but this was unattractive from an aerodynamic standpoint (excessive thickness). New fastener holes would not have been acceptable in this highly stressed primary structure, and the crack would have been uninspectable beneath such a repair. A bonded composite repair was the only alternative to scrapping the wing. It must be emphasized that because of its criticality this repair is not a typical example, but rather represents the limit of what bonded repair technology can achieve. Because of certification concerns (Ref 25), repairs to critical defects in primary aircraft structure are unlikely to become commonplace in the near future, and in this case, an extensive program was required to certify this repair.

Extensive and detailed 2-D and 3-D finite-element analyses were conducted, so that the stress distribution around the defect could be quantified. This revealed that the wing skin at this location was subject to secondary bending, and this was the explanation for the observation that the crack had initiated on the inside surface of the wing skin. The model was validated with strain measurements from a full-scale wing test undertaken at the Aeronautical and Maritime Research Laboratory. In addition, three levels of specimen testing were undertaken:

- Small, inexpensive coupon-sized specimens were used to investigate the effects of impact damage, temperature, and moisture and load spectrum truncation effects.
- Panel specimens with a full-scale representation of the local wing geometry were used as structural details in a fatigue and environmental study.
- Large box specimens were used to represent the wing as a quasi-full-scale test article in testing static and fatigue strength and an examination of thermal residual stresses.

A repair was designed using boron/epoxy as the repair material, because this provides lower levels of thermally induced residual stress compared with graphite/epoxy and enables the ready use of eddy current NDI methods to confirm the length of the crack that was left in the wing. Cytec Fiberite FM 73 epoxy adhesive was selected and cured at the comparatively low temperature of 80 °C (180 °F) to minimize the thermally induced residual stresses (Ref 29). This cure cycle had previously been carefully validated for another complex repair (Ref 5). The surface treatment used was the GBS process described previously. Advantage was taken of nearby hard-points on the wing to make use of positive pressure during the cure. An inflated bladder was used to apply pressure to the repair, and the pressurization loads were reacted out via a rigid plate to the hard-points. A similar system was used in the earlier application of doublers to the upper surface of F-111 wing pivot fittings (Ref 5).

This lower wing skin repair was predicted, and subsequently proven in service, to substantially reduce the crack growth rate of the defect. Because most wings in the RAAF fleet have not yet developed cracks, these repairs are currently being applied to the fleet as preventative reinforcements to prevent the initiation of cracks in the future. This is an excellent example of how the technology can be used to extend the life of airframes. The repair to the wing is shown in Fig. 7.

Future Trends

The greatest future advance affecting the application of bonded composite repairs will arguably be the development of an NDI technique that can reliably and accurately measure the level of adhesive bond strength and long-term environmental durability. As mentioned in the section "Repair Certification," such a method will enable the management of repairs using risk analysis where the risk can be readily quantified by the NDI method. Unfortunately, due to the considerable technical complexity of this task, a practical NDI technique is unlikely to be available for many years. A more achievable goal is the development of a low-cost, accelerated test method that can be shown to accurately predict the long-term behavior of adhesively bonded joints. In the past, the Boeing wedge test (ASTM D 3762) has been proposed as such a test, after wedge specimens cut from the structure of aged airframes were found to correlate well with the observed behavior of the bonded sections of the structure. More work, possibly based on existing

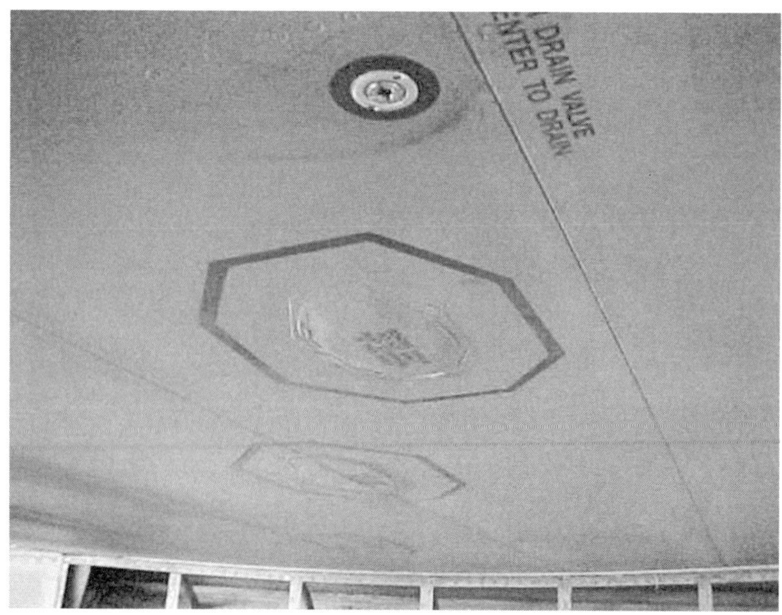

Fig. 6 Doublers installed on C-141 for "weep hole" repair

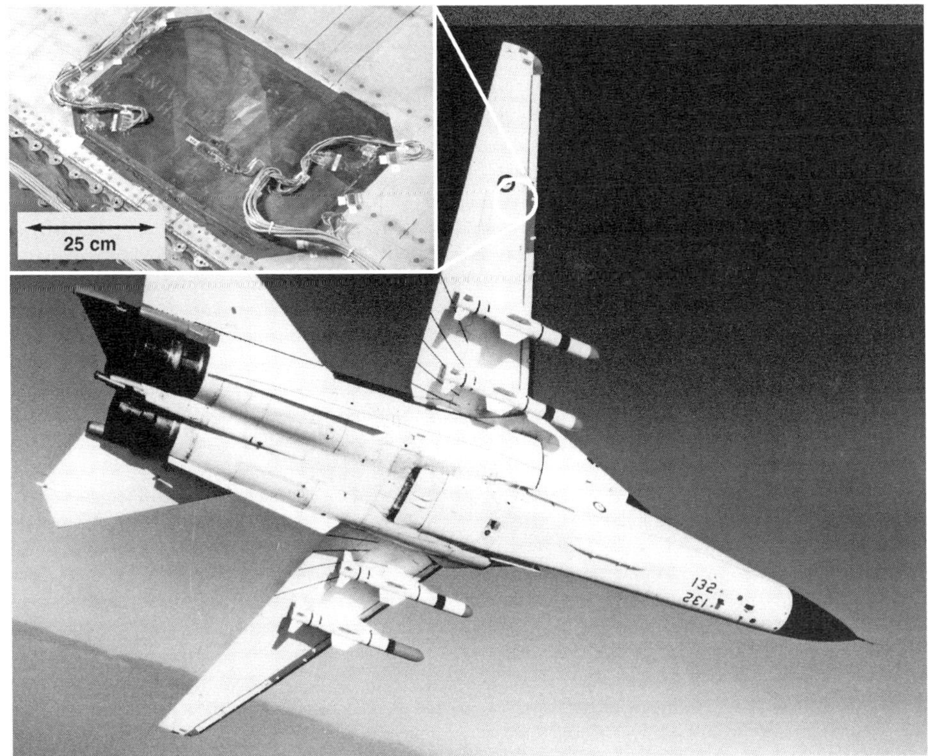

Fig. 7 Bonded composite repair to F-111 lower wing skin

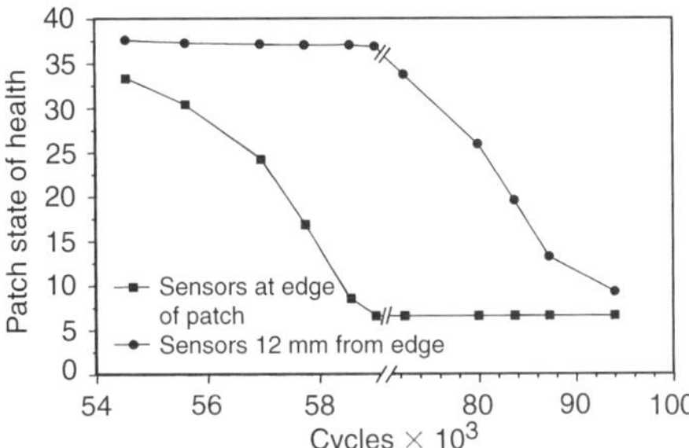

Fig. 8 Results from a demonstration "smart patch" showing a reduction in strain ratio ("patch state of health," the ratio of strains in the patch to those in the parent structure) as a function of fatigue cycles due to disbond growth under the patch. Source: Ref 30

service durability data, is required to confirm that this method is able to reliably predict the long-term behavior of adhesively bonded joints made with a range of adhesives and processes.

Improvements are also possible in the development of adhesives and surface treatment processes. Adhesively bonded repairs can be produced with levels of durability approaching the best factory treatments; however, because of the greater difficulty of controlling the repair environment, very high levels of quality control are required for repairs when compared with the manufacturing situation. New adhesives that are significantly more tolerant of poor surface treatment could, for example, reduce the level of quality control that is currently required.

Another approach to the problem of long-term bond degradation is to assume that a small risk exists that a disbond may occur in the future and to construct a repair/reinforcement that is able to sense any such damage. This so-called "smart patch" concept (Ref 30) makes use of modern electronic and sensor technology. It is envisaged that the sensors and electronics could be fully embedded within the patch. Piezoelectric films could be used to "harvest" power from the usual fatigue stresses in the structure, avoiding the need for a separate power supply. One approach is to compare the strains present in the patch to those in the parent structure, as a ratio describing the "patch state of health." If this ratio decreases (Fig. 8), it is an indication that a disbond may be growing under the patch. A single value representing this ratio could be stored in memory within the patch and then downloaded by means of a wireless technique to technical staff at a convenient time. Another concept being considered is to have embedded actuators inside the patch that would be capable of applying load to the bondline (without the aircraft being flown) to measure the load transfer into the repair. In all these concepts, it will of course be necessary to show that the smart systems themselves are highly reliable and have excellent long-term durability.

REFERENCES

1. A.A. Baker and R. Jones, *Bonded Repair of Aircraft Structures*, Martinus Nijhoff Publishers, Dordrecht, 1988
2. A.A. Baker, Bonded Composite Repair of Metallic Aircraft Components—Overview of Australian Activities, *Proc. 79th Meeting of the AGARD Structures and Materials Panel on Composite Repair of Military Aircraft Structures*, AGARD CP 550, Advisory Group for Aerospace Research and Development (NATO), Jan 1995, p 1-1 to 1-14
3. R.J. Chester, P.D. Chalkley, and K.F. Walker, Adhesively Bonded Repairs to Primary Aircraft Structure, *Int. J. Adhes. Adhes.*, Vol 19, 1999, p 1–8
4. A.A. Baker, Bonded Composite Repair of Fatigue-Cracked Primary Aircraft Structure, *Compos. Struct.*, Vol 47, 1999, p 431–443
5. A.A. Baker, R.J. Chester, M.J. Davis, J.D. Roberts, and J.A. Retchford, Reinforcement of the F-111 Wing Pivot Fitting with a Boron/Epoxy Doubler System—Materials Engineering Aspects, *Composites*, Vol 24, 1993, p 511–521
6. R. Fredell, C. Guyt, J. Mazza, S. Knighton, and E. Collas, Repair of C-5 Fuselage Cracking with Bonded GLARE Patches, *Proc. 41st Society for the Advancement of Material and Process Engineering International Conf.*, Spring 1996 (Anaheim, CA), p 962–974
7. A.A. Baker, Joining and Repair of Aircraft Composite Structures, *Composites Engineering Handbook*, P.K. Mallick, Ed., Marcel Dekker, New York, 1997
8. F.E. Penado and R.K. Dropek, Numerical Design and Analysis, *Adhesives and Sealants*, Vol 3, *Engineered Materials Handbook*, H.F. Brinson, technical chairman, ASM International, 1990, p 476–500
9. *Adhesive Bonded Aerospace Structures Standardized Repair Handbook*, AFML-TR-77-206, final report for U.S. Air Force Contract F33615-73-C-5171, Dec 1977, p 5-1
10. H.M. Clearfield, D.K. McNamara, and G.D. Davis, Surface Preparation of Metals, *Adhesives and Sealants*, Vol 3, *Engineered Materials Handbook*, H.F. Brinson, technical chairman, ASM International, 1990, p 261
11. "Standard Guide for Preparation of Metal Surfaces for Adhesive Bonding," ASTM D 2651, *Annual Book of ASTM Standards*, ASTM
12. H.M. Clearfield, D.K. McNamara, and G.D. Davis, Surface Preparation of Metals, *Adhesives and Sealants*, Vol 3, *Engineered Materials Handbook*, H.F. Brinson, technical chairman, ASM International, 1990, p 259–275
13. H.M. Clearfield, D.K. McNamara, and G.D. Davis, Surface Preparation of Metals, *Adhesives and Sealants*, Vol 3, *Engineered Materials Handbook*, H.F. Brinson, technical chairman, ASM International, 1990, p 260–261
14. W.B. Pinnell, "Hydrogen Embrittlement of Metal Fasteners due to PACS Exposure," AFRL-ML-WP-TR-2000-4153, report for Delivery Order 0004, Task 2 of U.S. Air

Force Contract F33615-95-D-5616, University of Dayton Research Institute, Aug 1999
15. A.A. Baker and R.J. Chester, Minimum Surface Treatments for Adhesively Bonded Repairs, *Int. J. Adhes. Adhes.*, Vol 12, 1992, p 73–78
16. J.J. Mazza, J.B. Avram, and R.J. Kuhbander, "Grit Blast/Silane (GBS) Aluminum Surface Preparation for Structural Adhesive Bonding," WL-TR-94-4111, interim report under U.S. Air Force Contracts F33615-89-C-5643 and F33615-95-D-5617
17. D.B. McCray and J.J Mazza, Optimization of Sol-Gel Surface Preparations for Repair Bonding of Aluminum Alloys, *Proc. 45th International Society for the Advancement of Material and Process Engineering Symposium*, Vol 45, May 2000 (Long Beach, CA), p 53–54
18. J. Mazza, G. Gaskin, W. DePiero, and K. Blohowiak, Faster Durable Bonded Repairs Using Sol-Gel Surface Treatment, *Proc. Fourth Joint Department of Defense/Federal Aviation Administration/National Aeronautics and Space Administration*, Conf. on Aging Aircraft, May 2000 (St. Louis, MO)
19. A.J. Kinloch, *Adhesion and Adhesives Science and Technology*, Chapman and Hall, London, 1987, p 123
20. L.J. Hart-Smith, R.W. Ochsner, and R.L. Radecky, Surface Preparation of Composties for Adhesive-Bonded Repair, *Adhesives and Sealants*, Vol 3, *Engineered Materials Handbook*, H.F. Brinson, technical chairman, ASM International, 1990, p 841
21. A.J. Kinloch, *Adhesion and Adhesives Science and Technology*, Chapman and Hall, London, 1987, p 124
22. L.J. Hart-Smith, G. Redmond, and M.J. Davis, The Curse of the Nylon Peel Ply, *Proc. 41st International Society for the Advancement of Material and Process Engineering Symposium*, Vol 41, March 1996 (Anaheim, CA)
23. L.J. Hart-Smith, R.W. Ochsner, and R.L. Radecky, Surface Preparation of Composties for Adhesive-Bonded Repair, *Adhesives and Sealants*, Vol 3, *Engineered Materials Handbook*, H. F. Brinson, technical chairman, ASM International, 1990, p 840–844
24. "Sealing Compound, Temperature Resistant, Integral Fuel Tanks and Fuel Cell Cavities, High Adhesion," Aerospace Materials Specification Society of Automotive Engineers, Inc., May 1999
25. A. Baker, Issues in the Certification of Bonded Composite Patch Repairs for Cracked Metallic Aircraft Structures, *Proc. 20th Symposium of the International Committee on Aeronautical Fatigue*, June 1999 (Seattle), p 312–313
26. "General Guidelines for Aircraft Structural Integrity Program," MIL-HDBK-1530, 31 Oct 1996
27. D.J. Hagemaier, End-Product Nondestructive Evaluation of Adhesive-Bonded Metal Joints, *Adhesives and Sealants*, Vol 3, *Engineered Materials Handbook*, H.F. Brinson, technical chairman, ASM International, 1990, p 743–776
28. Y. Bar-Cohen and A.K. Mal, End-Product Nondestructive Evaluation of Adhesive-Bonded Composite Joints, *Adhesives and Sealants*, Vol 3, *Engineered Materials Handbook*, H.F Brinson, technical chairman, ASM International, 1990, p 777–784
29. M.J. Davis, K.J. Kearns, and M.O. Wilkin, Bonded Repair Cracking to Primary Structure: A Case Study, *Proc. Sixth Australian Aeronautical Conf.*, 20–23 March 1995 (Melbourne), p 323–329
30. S.C. Galea and A.A. Baker, "Smart Structures Approaches for Health Monitoring of Aircraft Structures," Paper 4235-39, Proc. SPIE 2000 Symposium on Smart Materials and MEMS: Smart Structures and Devices Conf., 13–15 Dec 2000 (Melbourne, Australia), SPIE–The International Society for Optical Engineering.

Worldwide Repair Standardization

K.B. Armstrong, Consultant

COMPARED WITH METALS, which have specified alloy content and which are covered by standard test methods, composites comprise a range of different fibers and resins, and the resins are of undisclosed formulations having a wide range of mechanical and other properties. Likewise, the test methods for composites are in the process of standardization with the International Standards Organization (ISO), but at present there are still some differences between the methods used by the fiber and prepreg producers and those used by the aircraft manufacturers. Efforts to introduce some degree of standardization are described in this article together with an indication of progress at the time of this writing. This work has been done by the Commercial Aircraft Composite Repair Committee (CACRC), a combination of previous Air Transport Association of America (ATA), International Air Transport Association (IATA), and Society of Automotive Engineers (SAE) committees with the support of the Federal Aviation Administration (FAA), SAE, and Airlines and Airframe and Engine Manufacturers. It is hoped that the standardization efforts of the aerospace industry may be of benefit in other areas and that other industries may make standardization efforts of their own.

In May 1988, IATA formed a Composite Repair Task Force (CRTF) at its Engineering and Maintenance Advisory Committee (EMAC) meeting in Geneva, Switzerland, with the aim of standardizing composite repairs as much as possible. The Society of Automotive Engineers (SAE) and ATA had similar committees at the time.

The first document resulting from CRTF was IATA DOC: GEN: 3043, "Guidance Material for the Design, Maintenance, Inspection, and Repair of Thermosetting Epoxy Matrix Composite Aircraft Structures," in 1990. Only epoxy systems were covered by this document because it was impossible in the short time allowed to include other matrix systems. Similar documents could be produced for other resin systems as required. The IATA CRTF was disbanded on completion of the document, and the original intention was that airlines should use it when purchasing aircraft so that manufacturers would know the requirements of airlines regarding design, maintainability, inspectability, and repairability of future composite structures and components. It was considered that a further effort should be made to standardize repair materials and techniques and training and inspection methods throughout the world and that the findings of the IATA CRTF needed to be implemented in a positive manner. The current airline practice of outsourcing maintenance made this even more important. At this stage, the ATA, IATA, and SAE Task Forces were combined to form the CACRC. The Society of Automotive Engineers provided the administrative support for the CACRC and have published all the documents it has produced. Many of these documents will be incorporated into Original Equipment Manufacturer (OEM) repair instructions as alternative means of compliance with FAA, Joint Aviation Authorities (JAA), and other regulatory requirements. This will help to standardize procedures around the world.

Repair Types and Materials

There is a need to recognize repair as a separate subject, needing different materials and techniques from manufacture, if operational delays and maintenance costs are to be kept to a minimum. It should be borne in mind that composites are now being considered more from a life-cycle cost point of view rather than pure weight savings. Manufacturing cost and repair cost of a composite item throughout its service life will both need to be reduced. Manufacturers offer various repair techniques of different permitted sizes depending on the method, materials, and cure temperature used.

One of the problems of repair is that often it cannot be done by repeating procedures used in manufacture. Repair almost always needs to be carried out quickly with the minimum of equipment and often without tooling. Ideally, it also needs to be done without major disassembly of components such as rudders, flaps, and so forth. Experience has shown that if moisture is present in a honeycomb core, then heating to 180 °C (355 °F) can produce an internal steam pressure of about 1.2 MPa (180 psi). At this temperature the strength of the adhesive is seriously reduced, and disbonding between skin and core often takes place. In solid laminates, overheating can cause delamination between the plies. This means that repair needs to be performed at a lower temperature than manufacture (25–50 °C, or 45–90 °F lower), to avoid further damage, while retaining the resin glass transition temperature needed to meet design requirements.

It is essential during repair procedures to avoid causing further damage to a structure or component for several reasons:

- The permitted size of each type of repair is limited, and if the damage size is increased a more complex, expensive, and time-consuming repair may be necessary.
- The larger a repair becomes, the more likely it will be that some form of tooling will be required to maintain the shape.
- If the damage becomes too large, the part may be beyond economical repair.
- The larger the repair, the longer the delay that will be incurred in completing it.

The types of repair include:

- Wet lay-up liquid resins (cold or warm-cured) are available.
- Hot-cured, preimpregnated fabrics or tapes (prepreg repairs), which can take the form of precured or cocured patches. The precured patches have to be bonded with a suitable adhesive after they have been cured. A hot-curing film adhesive is usually used for this purpose, but a cold- or warm-curing adhesive can be used depending on the service temperature required from the repair. Bonded repairs (hot or cold cured) may be made with overlap joints, stepped lap joints, or scarf joints. All of these must be made strictly to the OEM repair instructions using only the specified type.
- Bolted repairs to solid laminate structures can be used with either titanium plates (in the case of the Harrier) or bolted precured composite sections. Bonded repairs are not often done on laminates more than 2 or 3 mm (0.078 or 0.12 in.) thick as overlaps are large and the weight of bolted joints is actually lower. However, there may be other reasons that require a bonded repair to be used. The OEM repair instructions must be complied with in each individual case.

- Bolted repairs to solid laminates are similar in appearance and concept to metal repairs, but their execution requires the use of the correct and special fasteners. These special fasteners require the use of the correct drill types and shapes and also the use of controlled feed drills and special lubricants (Boelube) to avoid overheating and backing plates to avoid breakout of the back skin as the drill goes through. Drills need to be sharpened frequently and reground accurately to achieve the close tolerance hole sizes required, especially when slight interference fits are specified. Bolt fitting must be done with great care to avoid delamination.

Special fasteners are needed to give an adequate clamping area and washers may have to be used to avoid scoring of laminates and to give clamping area to avoid crushing by nuts during torque tightening. Torque values for bolts need to be checked with the OEM instructions, as composites sometimes require slightly lower torque values. It is essential to avoid using higher torque values than those specified. As more solid laminate composite structure is used in fins, tailplanes, and wing structures, the use of bolted repairs will increase and special training will become necessary to ensure adequate quality. Original Equipment Manufacturer instructions give the information required on fastener type, drill type, and drilling procedures. It is usual to bond these parts with an adhesive in addition to bolting.

Training

The increasing number of applications of composite materials means that more and more people will become involved in their maintenance and repair, and the need for good training can only increase. It may be worth mentioning that experienced technicians are becoming difficult to find, and it may soon be necessary to look outside the aircraft industry for new people. This means two problems instead of one. Firstly, there is a need to find enough mechanically inclined people. Secondly, if they come from outside the aircraft industry and from outside the world of composites they will need to be trained, not only technically but also to accept the high standards of workmanship that will be expected of them. These high standards are also necessary in other industries using composites such as automobiles, boat building, railway carriages, space vehicles, and sporting equipment. Composites are also being used to build and to repair bridges, and these applications also need good quality, long-life repairs.

Table 1 Aerospace Material Specifications for repair of polymer matrix composites

Specification No.	Title
Issued	
AMS 2980	Carbon Fiber Fabric and Epoxy Resin, Wet Lay-up Repair Material
Work in progress	
AMS 2960	Glass Fabric with Epoxy Resin, Wet Lay-up Repair Material
AMS 3970	CFRP Repair Prepreg 125 °C Vacuum Curing

Major Standardization Issues

While a number of individual issues are involved, a review of the CACRC Task Group assignments gives an excellent overview of the major areas of concern in composite repair standardization. Each of these Task Groups has prepared recommended standard procedures and/or highlighted problem areas that need to be addressed. Topics of current work are given below, with some future needs.

Design. This group has produced AE-27 (Aerospace Information Report AIR 4928) Guide for the Design of Durable and Maintainable Composites and is working on a Life-Cycle Cost Model (Aerospace Information Report 5416) because there is a need to develop composite components with a lower life-cycle cost than metallic parts. Many small detail design changes can greatly increase the service life of composite parts, and this book should help designers avoid previous mistakes. AEs are automotive or aerospace engineering design manuals, handbooks, or guidebooks developed by SAE technical committees.

Repair Materials. The CACRC Task Group on Repair materials has issued one standard and is working on several others, as shown in Table 1. There is a need for a greater understanding of the importance of resin and adhesive mechanical and other properties to make the choice of alternatives easier when this is necessary.

Table 2 Aerospace Recommended Practices for polymer matrix composites repair techniques

Standard No.	Title
Issued	
ARP 4916	Masking and Cleaning of Epoxy and Polyester Matrix Thermosetting Composite Materials
ARP 4977	Drying of Thermosetting Composite Materials
ARP 4991	Core Restoration of Thermosetting Composite Materials
ARP 5144	Heat Application for Thermosetting Composite Repairs
ARP 5256	Resin Mixing
Work in progress	
ARP 5143	Vacuum Bagging of Thermosetting Composite Repairs
ARP 5319	Impregnation of Dry Fabric and Ply Lay-up
AIR 5367	Machining of Epoxy and Polyester Matrix Thermosetting Composite Structures
AIR 5416	Maintenance Life Cycle Cost Equations and Definition of Variables
AIR 5431	Tooling for Composite Repair

One material combination is in the process of qualification to AMS 2980 (Carbon Fiber Fabric and Epoxy Resins, Wet Lay-Up Repair Material), and it is hoped that other materials will be qualified. Qualification to AMS 2960 (Glass Fabric with Epoxy Resin, Wet Lay-Up Repair Material) and AMS 3970 (CFRP Repair Prepreg 125 °C Vacuum Curing) will follow later, and it is hoped that more than one material combination will be qualified to these specifications. The fiber type is expected to remain the same in each case, but could come from a different source. The most likely difference will be the use of different resin systems, although with very similar mechanical and other properties.

Repair Techniques. The CACRC Task Group on Repair Techniques has issued several recommended repair practices and is working on others, as shown in Table 2. The group also is working on a technique for the repair of lightning strike protection systems. Work also is needed on techniques for the repair of thermoplastic composites and another for the preparation of bolted repairs.

Inspection. The task group on inspection issued ARP 5089: Composite Repair NDT/NDI) Handbook to address nondestructive testing techniques and is working on a generic set of Composite Reference Standards for use on all types of aircraft. It is intended to produce design drawings and manufacturing procedures for test blocks for honeycomb panels and solid laminates. A phenolic-based set of standard blocks is considered acceptable as representative of carbon, glass, and aramid composites. The group also is responsible for investigating improved NDI techniques.

Training. The task group on training has issued the following documents:

AIR 4844C	Composite and Metal Bonding Glossary (updated annually)
AIR 4938	Composite and Bonded Structure Technician/ Specialist Training Document
AIR 5278	Composite and Bonded Structure Engineers: Training Document
AIR 5279	Composite and Bonded Structure Inspector: Training Document

There is a need in the training area to update existing documents to include repair techniques for thermoplastics and the preparation of bolted repairs to solid laminates.

Analytical Repair Techniques. This is a new group making good progress on its first document to provide a theoretical basis for the design of composite repairs. It would be helpful if this work included the design of bolted joints.

Future projects. There is a need for a nondestructive method of measuring adhesive bond strength and also a method of measuring the "bondability" of a surface, perhaps a measure of surface energy, after the surface preparation process has been performed. This could replace the "water break test" if found to be superior. At this point, these topics have not been allocated to any Task Group.

ACKNOWLEDGMENT

All documents mentioned in this article written in the CACRC Task Groups are published and available from SAE, Warrendale, PA, USA. Advisory Circular Number 145-6: Repair Station for Composite and Bonded Aircraft Structures is published as a collaborative effort between IATA, ATA, and SAE.

SELECTED REFERENCES

- *Advances in Aircraft Composite Repair Symposium,* 5–7 Sept 1994 (Farnborough, U.K.), Society of Automotive Engineers
- *Advances in Composite Repair,* SAE TOPTEC, 1–2 Nov 1993, (Seattle,WA), Society for Automotive Engineers
- K.B. Armstrong, Repairing the Damage, *Conference Bonding and Repair of Composites,* 14 July 1989 (Birmingham, UK), Butterworth, p 93–99
- K.B. Armstrong, Ph.D. thesis, "The Selection of Adhesives and Composite Matrix Resins for Aircraft Repairs," The City University, London, U.K, 1990
- K.B. Armstrong, "Care and Repair of Advanced Composites," paper presented at *Meeting Today's Maintenance Challenges,* 21 April 1998 (London)
- K.B. Armstrong, Eleven Years of Work to Standardise Aerospace Composite Repairs 1988–1999, *International Conference on Joining and Repair of Plastics and Composites,* 16–17 March 1999 (London, UK), Professional Engineering Publishing Ltd
- K.B. Armstrong, Ed., *Int. J. Adhes. Adhes.* Vol 19 (No. 2, 3), 1999. Special double issue entitled *Aircraft Repairs.*
- K.B. Armstrong and R.T. Barrett, "Care and Repair of Advanced Composites", presented at Meeting Today's Maintenance Challenges, 21 April 1998 (London, UK), Society of Automotive Engineers, 1997
- A.A. Baker and R. Jones, Ed., *Bonded Repair of Aircraft Structures,* Martinus Nijhoff 1988
- *Composite Structures Awareness,* video tape, Boeing and CACRC, available from Society of Automotive Engineers
- M.H. Datoo, Mechanics of Fibrous Composites, Elsevier, 1991
- "Guidance Material for the Design, Maintenance, Inspection, and Repair of Thermosetting Epoxy Matrix Composite Aircraft Structures," DOC:GEN: 3043, International Air Transport Association, 1st ed., May 1991
- D. Hull, *An Introduction to Composite Materials,* Cambridge Solid State Science Series, Cambridge University Press, 1993
- A. Kelly, Ed., *Concise Encyclopaedia of Composite Materials,* Pergamon, 1995
- I.H. Marshall, Ed., *Composite Structures,* Vol 10 (No. 1), 1988 Special Issue, *Supportability of Composite Airframes,* F. Demuts, Guest Editor
- D.H. Middleton, Ed., *Composite Materials in Aircraft Structures,* Longman Scientific and Technical, 1990
- J. Murphy, *The Reinforced Plastics Handbook,* 2nd ed., Elsevier, 1988
- M.C. Niu, *Composite Airframe Structures—Practical Design Information and Data,* Conmilit Press Ltd, Hong Kong, Technical Book Co., 1992
- R.J. Palmer, "Investigation of the Effect of Resin Material on Impact Damage to Graphite/Epoxy Composites," NASA Contractor Report 165677, McDonnell-Douglas Corp., Long Beach, CA
- L.N. Phillips, Ed., *Design with Advanced Composite Material,* The Design Council/Springer Verlag, 1989

Product Reliability, In-Service Experience, and Lessons Learned

Eric Chesmar, United Airlines

SERVICE EXPERIENCE AND PRODUCT RELIABILITY have become increasingly important over time. When the use of composites has been compared to other materials, they are evaluated not just for weight savings and original cost, but for overall life cycle performance, including in-service reliability, maintainability, reparability, and durability. The value of reliability has risen as aircraft operators demand greater return on the large investment in aircraft, including lower maintenance costs.

The scope of this article is limited to nonproprietary and noncompetition-sensitive information related to aircraft applications. Those interested in specific aircraft or manufacturer data should contact the companies directly. In spite of these limitations, the experiences from past reliability and in-service problems can be found in various sources, such as publications by industry associations, textbooks, and symposiums. Although the specific design of any part determines the part's performance, the published literature contains consistently recurring failure modes, which will be presented as general types, and then specific component examples.

The following presents an overview of reliability and commonly used measurements. More importantly, the many failure modes that cause the negative performance are discussed. This catalog of failure modes is compiled from many types of sources: manufacturer service bulletins, reliability and customer service departments, literature reviews, demonstration programs, in-service evaluations, design guides, and surveys of commercial and military aircraft maintenance organizations. Lessons learned will also be described, while attempting to avoid overlapping the many other related topics in this Volume, such as maintainability, reparability, and materials choice.

Reliability

The importance of operational (or in-service) reliability has been increased over the years as the use of composites has been compared to other materials choices, and the materials are evaluated not just for weight savings or original cost, but for reliability in service. Data on actual operational reliability is used to identify areas for improvements on existing aircraft and to identify design improvements for future aircraft. Reliability analysis at commercial airlines and airframe manufactures is required by Federal Aviation Administration (FAA) regulations for continued airworthiness. In addition to regulatory reasons, aircraft operators perform reliability analysis in order to optimize aircraft utilization and reduce costs and improve safety, and the aircraft original equipment manufacturers (OEMs) as a service to their customers to solve problems beyond their own capabilities and improve their product.

Reliability can be measured in many ways, but all result in performance that is less than trouble-free or maintenance-free. The trouble ranges from routine maintenance and servicing that ensures performance (such as lubrication), to active monitoring, to instrumented inspections at various intervals, to required overhauls at defined intervals, to mandatory scrapping of life-limited parts. Formal maintenance programs, as required by regulatory agencies, are specific to each model and can include any one of these tasks.

A general definition of *reliability* is the probability that a system or product will perform in a satisfactory manner for a given period of time when used under specified operating conditions (Ref 1). The elements of this definition are worthy of further examination for how they apply to composite structures as opposed to system components and line replaceable units, which account for most of the reliability studies. To be judged "satisfactory," structures made of composites are expected by the aircraft operator to be equivalent to or better than the previous aircraft models or better than the same structure made in metallic materials; preferably they will require no routine maintenance. The "period of time" for structures is usually the life of the aircraft, or at least the interval between heavy-maintenance visits. The "specified operating conditions" for structures is usually the entire life cycle, including the aircraft's flying envelope, maintenance visits, and a component's time during maintenance, storage, and shipping. The elements of this definition are determined and specified in more detail during the design phase, together with concepts for maintenance, servicing, and repairs. These factors all influence the inherent reliability. The composite designer has the responsibility to translate the failure modes learned from past experience to a risk probability with associated inspectability and maintenance program, as well as to determine loads and design a part accordingly. One example of such a design process was that for Aerospatiale's ATR72 outer wing, certified in 1989 (Ref 2).

The field of reliability engineering has developed many measurements for reliability to describe the different impacts. In reviewing the total life cycle of an aircraft structure, measurements of "satisfactory performance" can be made at many different levels and different aspects, which reflect the repercussion of failure, such as a flight cancellation, delay, replacement, repair, servicing, repetitive inspection, or other maintenance action. At the highest level (the aircraft as a whole), reliability can be defined as the ability to complete the aircraft's mission, either a military sortie or a flight segment for commercial passenger or freight (e.g., 87% completed flights). Each type of event can be expressed as a percent (such as 97% on-time arrivals), frequency (e.g., 5 cancellations per year), or rate that normalizes based on use of the system, part, or aircraft (e.g., 0.0001 in-flight shutdowns per flying hour). For components, the most commonly used expression is the mean time between unscheduled removal (MTBUR), expressed in flight hours. Mean time to failure in flight hours is the removals without the no-fault-found. The units of measurements can also be calendar time, but in order to compare between different operators, they can be normalized for amount of use by dividing by flight hours or flight cycles.

One of the roles played by airline engineering and OEM customer service representatives is to identify and report the reasons for removal and failure modes. These reports form the basis for design changes, modifications, and improvements embodied in service bulletins, service letters, and production changes. To widen the experience base and increase the validity of these reports, the airline industry has worked together with aircraft manufacturers to establish standardized formats and variables for reliability reports (via the Air Transport Association and OEM reliability departments).

Additional information on reliability concepts is provided in the article "Reliability in Design" in *Materials Selection and Design,* Volume 20 of *ASM Handbook.*

Context of In-Service Experiences within Aircraft Operations

Many of the failure modes may seem insignificant, but for a variety of reasons can result in delays, cancellations, or other significant operational impact. This kind of operational impact is similar to that seen when any new technology or change is introduced, for example, lack of repair instructions, reliance on OEM advice, requirements for nonstandardized materials, tooling, testing, or skills. More details on these are covered in other articles, but they are significant in that they are usually a new failure mode compared to previous metallic designs. Furthermore, even though maintenance actions may be routine, they add up to significant resources, such as for paint, erosion, sealant, or minor wet layup repairs. The total maintenance life cycle includes not only the scheduled maintenance and inspection cycles, but also the daily walkarounds, the shop repairs, repairs on-wing, and unscheduled inspections after damage. Failures or damage may occur at all times, but all may not be reported. Without reports on all the phases of the aircraft operation, the exact reliability and total life-cycle cost is incomplete. One should recognize this fact and understand the source of the reports and the missing data. Therefore, a review of published studies follows.

Don Joynes at Boeing made a study on the composite control surfaces (aileron, elevator, and rudder) on the Boeing 737-300, 757, and 767, which were introduced to service in 1982, 1982, and 1986, respectively (Ref 3). The study involved analyzing reported incident data for these components. The sample included about 1400 aircraft (7000 components), which had accumulated in excess of 15 million hours and 10 million flight cycles since they entered service, through July 1990. Figures 1, 2, and 3 show the incidents per airplane per year, major causes, and the zones affected. The category "Design and Wear," was defined to include general nonstructural items such as wear, panel-edge erosion and paint condition, peeling, and so on. It is important to note that even though these were considered "nonstructural" by the design engineers at the OEM, the impact on the operator can be the same as a "structural" damage if documentation inadequately describes the allowable damage. The reduction in incidents reported is not due to reliability improvements, but Joynes attributed it "to the airlines becoming familiar with the com-

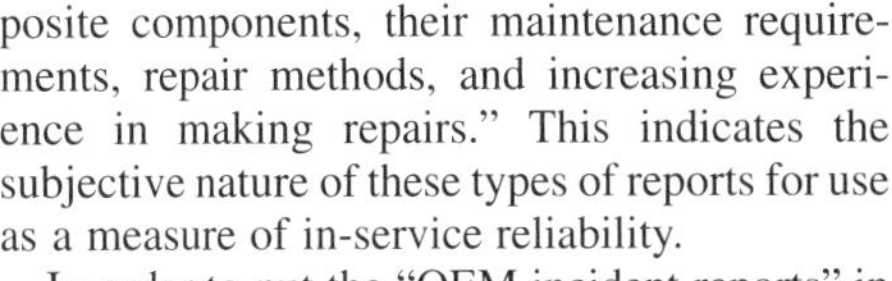

posite components, their maintenance requirements, repair methods, and increasing experience in making repairs." This indicates the subjective nature of these types of reports for use as a measure of in-service reliability.

In order to put the "OEM incident reports" in perspective with overall aircraft maintenance and to collect cost of all maintenance, a study was performed by British Aerospace (BA) at United Airlines (UAL) in 1998 by Dunkley (Ref 4). This study attempted to record all the maintenance actions at all levels of maintenance for the entire wing (BA's design responsibility in the Airbus partnership) and horizontal stabilizer. British Aerospace gathered data from UAL's records from all maintenance locations, including 4 years of line maintenance, 53 airframe annual visits (C-checks), and 5 each airframe heavy visits (or D-checks, approximately every 5 years). Based on the sample of 639 findings, the following causes were found: a large percentage of write-ups were due to paint erosion, numerous dents of unknown source, numerous cracks, few hail (six each) and bird strikes (three each), and no significant repairs or flight delays due to composites. None of the write-ups resulted in a query or report to the OEM, but were corrected using existing maintenance documents or the support of airline engineering. The study also noted the distribution of write-ups against the structure by material type (see Fig. 4).

Furthermore, even though maintenance actions may be routine, they add up to significant resources and costs, such as for paint or for minor wet lay-up repairs. Although some may be preventable with better designs, these repairs become an accepted and institutionalized "cost of doing business" for airlines. Customer service and engineering departments respond to problems brought to them, but the cost impact may be just as great for the "institutionalized" maintenance. Airline requests account for less than five percent of all the repairs.

Failure Modes

Some efforts have been made by industry groups to identify commonly occurring failures.

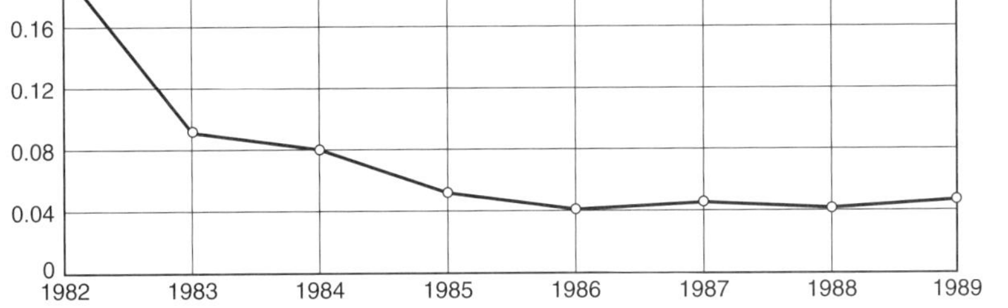

Fig. 1 Incidents reported per airplane per year for 737, 757, 767 control surfaces (aileron, elevator, and rudder). Source: Ref 3

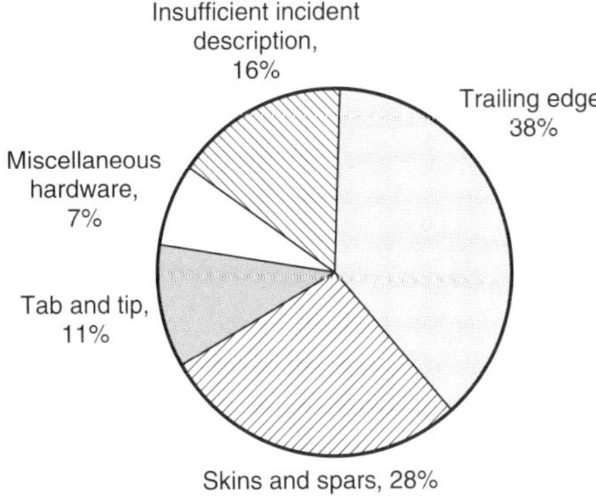

Fig. 2 Damage by zone for 737, 757, 767 control surfaces. Source: Ref 3

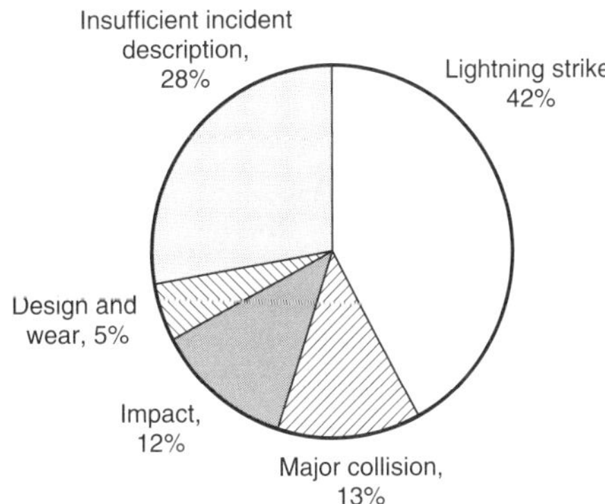

Fig. 3 Cause of major damage to 737, 757, 767 control surfaces. Source: Ref 3

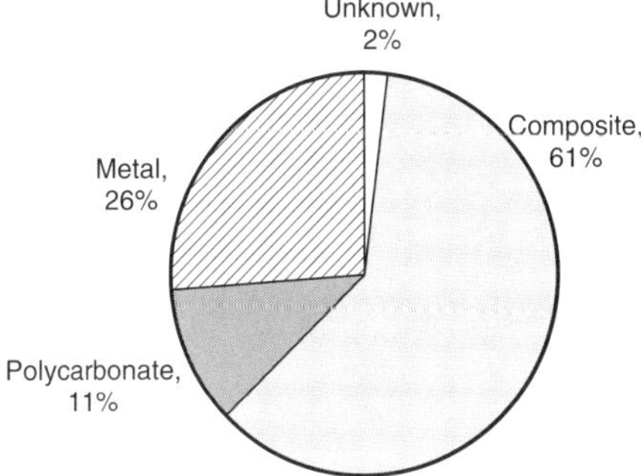

Fig. 4 Distribution of maintenance record write-ups (639 records total) by material type for A320 wings and stabilizer

Examples include the Commercial Aircraft Composite Repair Committee (CACRC), National Aeronautics and Space Administration (NASA), National Research Council, the International Air Transport Association (IATA) in 1991 (and detailed in Ref 5), and the MIL-HDBK-17 Committee.

In 1998, the CACRC published the guide "Design of Repairable, Maintainable, and Durable Composite Structure" (Ref 6), which contains a compilation of failure modes based on survey observations and in-service experiences of airlines, OEMs, and repair stations (Table 1). The failure modes are organized by type and then the general zones, specific components, or structures they affect. One unique feature of this publication is the illustrations of design details and suggested solutions. This list of failure modes is reinforced by other surveys of operators, such as by National Research Council, NASA, and most comprehensively in the MIL-HDBK-17.

In reviewing studies of in-service damage, the term "failure mode" is subjective. Hence, some studies may not report minor, easily repaired or common wear, damage such as wear and tear, paint, and so on, although they are included in comprehensive lists. Major failure modes, which result in the component removal and repair or scrapping, are all that is reported in some studies, with no minor damage and wear and tear, which may be an error of omission. A review of shop findings reveals that nearly all removed components have many other minor defects that are corrected during overhaul. In the subsequent review of many past studies, usually only the major failure modes are discussed to highlight their severity and the need to improve future designs based on experiences. Although the specific construction of each part is not always possible to disclose, by focusing on the failure mode and source, the lessons for the future can still be identified.

Ground Handling Damage. In all major studies and reports of production aircraft, ground handling damage is ranked as the largest cause of damage. In the early 1990s, Boeing investigated in order to understand the sources of damage and determine the extent of ground handling equipment damage. Eleven operators were asked about ground damage incidents during the period from 1990 to 1993 (Ref 8). The types of equipment that induced the 1,894 reported incidents are detailed in Table 2. The large number of "unknown" causes is a good indication of why it is so difficult for airline support operations to reduce these incidents—many of the people "at the wheel" in those incidents either fear retribution if they are reported or are unaware of the damage caused to composites. In addition, ramp employees are often driven to increase productivity through faster aircraft turn-arounds.

The CACRC recognized the need to reduce ground equipment damage and sponsored a video (produced by Boeing) aimed at ramp personnel to increase awareness of consequences and appropriate actions. No one realistically expects that this damage can be totally eliminated by improved design; however, it must be recognized as the largest source of damage and taken into account when considering allowable damage, dispatch limits, battle damage repairs, repairability, ease of removing and installing parts, interchangeability, spare availability, and so on. The life-cycle cost associated with this fact of life has already motivated one airline launch customer to demand commonly damaged parts be made of aluminum to decrease flight delays and cancellations and to reduce life-cycle cost.

Moisture Ingression. The second major failure mode is moisture ingression, which primarily affects sandwich structure as opposed to monolithic (i.e., solid laminate) construction. Moisture absorption even at the equilibrium levels, in a laminate over sandwich or in monolithic, complicates the repair and is discussed widely in industry literature (see the other articles in this Section, Ref 9, etc.). This discussion concentrates on ingression that causes removal of the component. The problem is widespread due to the many sources of ingression and the many ways it affects the composite component. Water has been reported to ingress via the following means: cracked end potting, cracked paint, failed/cracked sealant, through fasteners, porosity in the skins of cloth or thin unidirectional

Table 1 Damage sources and areas affected

General category	Specific source	Aircraft parts affected
Foreign object damage in flight	Hail damage	Radome, engine inlet cowls and interior engine components, wing leading edges, horizontal and vertical leading edges
	Bird strike damage	Radomes, engine inlet cowls, fan blades, leading edges
	Engine failure or foreign object damage	Nacelles, acoustic liners
	Engine uncontained failure damage	Fuselage, body fairing, lower wing panels, horizontal stabilizer leading edge
	Tire separation	Trailing edge flaps, lower wing to body fairings, landing gear doors, fixed wing panels
Foreign object damage on ground	Hail damage	Radome, engine inlet cowls and interior engine components, wing leading edges, horizontal and vertical leading edges
	Runway debris	Trailing-edge flap lower surface, environmental control system inlet, wing upper fixed trailing-edge panels, engine inlet cowls, lower fuselage aft of landing gear
	Ground handling equipment damage	Engine cowling outer surfaces, leading and trailing edges of wings and stabilizer, wing-to-body fairings, flap track fairings, radomes
	Personnel mishandling	Engine cowling near latches, access doors. Areas surrounding all latches should resist prying.
	Shipping and transportation damage	All removable components, especially without well-designed containers
Environmental damage in flight	Lightning strikes	Affected zones as specified by regulations; generally near attachment and detachment areas, such as radomes, engine cowlings, outer 18 in. of ailerons and elevators, rudder
		Designs frequently sustain a strike that results in damage greater than allowable without repair.
		Avoid use of aluminum honeycomb with carbon facesheets.
	Overheat	Engine cowling, parts near high-temperature ducts or borescope plugs, aft of air-conditioning exhaust
	Moisture ingression	Honeycomb parts, laminates during repair or high heat exposure
	Erosion	Radome, engine inlet cowl, leading-edge fairing
Overstress	Overactuation due to system failure	Actuated components such as flaps, powered doors
	Buffeting, sonic fatigue, vibration	High sonic areas such as near engines, i.e., flap track fairings, pylon panels
Chemical contamination	Hydraulic fluid leakage	Actuated components, fairings under hydraulic systems such as belly fairing, engine cowling
	Jet fuel	Components under fuel system, i.e., engine cowling, pylon
	Paint stripper	All painted surfaces, especially adjacent to metallic parts being stripped
	Corrosion	Improperly isolated aluminum attaching hardware, aluminum honeycomb with fluid ingression

Source: Ref 6, 7

Table 2 Sources of ground equipment damage

Cause of damage	Percentage of incidents
Unknown	41
Jetway	13
Baggage cart	7
Catering	7
Belt loader	6
Tug/towbar/taxi	6
Loader	5
Maintenance	5
Cargo loading	3
Lavatory and water service	3
Container	2
Fueling	2

Source: Ref 8

skins, porous adhesive in lap joints, wicking through aramid fibers, and wicking along foaming adhesive and along metallic doublers. Once inside the sandwich, the fluid causes failures via various mechanisms. Water absorbed in the epoxy matrix or adhesive lowers its glass transition temperature and significantly degrades mechanical properties. Fluid also degrades the honeycomb cell wall, which increases the ease of water migration. Eventually, when a honeycomb cell is full of water, the expansion during freezing is strong enough to cause the skin to delaminate from the core. During repairs, water must be removed for any epoxy repairs to cure and bond properly, even at room temperature. Drying of water adds time to repairs. If water is not detected and sufficiently dried, the following elevated temperature cure generates steam that often causes delaminations, both in sandwich structures and in solid laminates (Ref 10).

Honeycomb sandwich structures have the potential to carry much more water weight than fibers and matrix. The empty space that makes honeycomb such an efficient structural element (by weight) also acts as a holding tank for water. Most honeycomb thickness ranges from 10 mm (0.4 in.) for typical panels (rudders or fixed skins), to 25 mm (1 in.) for wing-to-body fairings, to 150 mm (6 in.) for full-depth core such as ailerons and flap wedges. An estimate for the weight of the 757 spoilers was made during their overhaul at UAL. Two hundred and fifty spoilers were x-rayed to find detectable amounts and weighed before and after replacement of one skin and honeycomb core. The average water weight per spoiler was 1.6 kg (3.5 lb).

To determine the extent of honeycomb parts with water, a joint study was made by UAL, University of Washington, Boeing, and Hexcel. Using infrared thermography, thirty-six UAL aircraft were surveyed from the ground, covering about 60% of the composite structures. Of the fifteen 767-200 aircraft between 12 and 15 years old, water was detected in an average of 15 parts. Closer analysis of the water patterns to find ingression point and an analysis of the design, materials, and processes used on the parts revealed there was no single mode on any one part, and all were types seen previously. These included: fastener penetration, cracking/wicking through potting around fastener, wicking through expanding foam core splice adhesive, porous prepreg skins, cracked sealant on honeycomb closeouts, and so on (Ref 11).

The U.S. Navy and U.S. Air Force have both reported that "honeycomb sandwich structures have had the most disbond problems in service." The root cause for these military aircraft parts is suspected to be foreign object damage (FOD) or maintenance-induced damage, which produced a site for water to ingress (Ref 12). Use of aluminum for the type of honeycomb further exacerbates the problem due to the fast rate of corrosion. "Aluminum honeycomb sandwich structures caused major problems on Air Force and Navy aircraft because of moisture ingress, core corrosion, and for supersonic aircraft, debonding of skin to core adhesive due to pressure buildup in the core after moisture ingression."

Manufacturing Defects. Although manufacturing of composites is discussed in more detail elsewhere, manufacturing defects are sometimes detected during in-service operations. Although these are not considered to be "failure modes" unless the defects are specifically documented as allowable damage/defects in the Structural Repair Manual, operators must treat them as any other damage discovered during inspections. Therefore, if not allowed, the defects have the same effect on an airline operation as damage. Furthermore, some defects will propagate, or affect long-term durability, such as peel ply not removed or resin-rich areas resulting in cracking and moisture ingression. Table 3 lists some of the manufacturing defects (Ref 9).

Part-Specific In-Service Experiences

Documentation of experiences with composite structural parts comes from many sources: demonstration programs, limited use research and development parts, reliability reports service, bulletins or service letters, surveys of maintenance organizations, telexes to the original manufacturer's customer service organization (usually from maintenance engineers for repairs), and anecdotal stories. Some examples are listed subsequently. Although the different sources and reports may be written for various purposes and emphasize different aspects, they all contain valid feedback on failure modes of composite structures. The author has gathered previously published reports, starting with the NASA Advanced Composite Energy Efficiency (ACEE) program, and then grouped by the specific components. Much more information can be found in each OEM's model-specific service bulletins and service letters.

NASA ACEE Program

Beginning in 1973, the ACEE program, the largest in-service evaluation program, was conducted by NASA Langley Research Center. The program's end goal was to reduce aircraft fuel consumption via the use of weight-saving advanced composite materials and to encourage the use and acceptance of composites in the aircraft industry. Other specific objectives were: "to establish confidence in the long-term durability of advanced composites through flight experience of numerous composite components on transport aircraft," "to evaluate the effects of realistic flight environments on composite components," and to allow "airlines to develop inspection and repair procedures prior to making production commitments."

In 1979, NASA Langley and the U.S. Army initiated joint programs to evaluate composite components on commercial and military helicopters. Although helicopters accumulate fewer flight hours than do transport aircraft, the environments and fatigue loading are sometimes more severe for the helicopter components. The helicopters in which composite components were tested included the Bell 206L and the Sikorsky S-76 and CH-53. They were flown in Canada, Alaska, and the northeast, southwest, and gulf coast of the United States, with selected components removed periodically from service for residual strength testing. However, emphasis was on commercial aircraft because of their high utilization rates, exposure to worldwide environmental conditions, and systematic maintenance procedures. The ACEE program contracted many aerospace companies to produce composite versions of aircraft components already in production, put them in service with the modified inspection and maintenance program, periodically remove some of them either at planned or unplanned times for an in-depth inspection, and sometimes test them for residual strength. The in-service experience is summarized in Table 4. The discussion that follows is adapted from the previous edition of this Volume, which has more photos (Ref 13, 14, 15).

L-1011 Kevlar 49-Epoxy Fairings. The L-1011 fairings were fabricated with Kevlar 49 fibers (in fabric form), F-155 and F-161 epoxy resins, and Nomex (E.I. DuPont de Nemours & Co., Wilmington, DE) honeycomb. The configurations of the center-engine fairing, under-wing fillet, and wing-to-body fairing are shown in Fig. 5, along with the various types of damage incurred. During the ten-year service evaluation period, the Kevlar 49-epoxy fairings installed on L-1011 aircraft were inspected annually. Minor impact damage from equipment and foreign objects was noted on several fairings, primarily the honeycomb sandwich wing-to-body fairings.

Table 3 Manufacturing defects in fiber composite laminates

Structure	Defect
Solid laminates	Voids Delaminations Disbonds Foreign body inclusions (e.g., release film) Resin-starved areas Resin-rich area (leading to cracks) Incomplete resin cure Incorrect fiber orientation (including wavy fibers) Incorrect ply sequence Fiber gaps Wrinkled layers Poor surface condition (i.e., poor release from mold) Tolerance errors (including mis-shimming) Misdrilled holes Surface damage Voids
Sandwich panels (in addition to the above)	Poor core splice Disbonds form skins Crushed core Core gaps Excessive thickness of polymeric surfaces and paint, leading to cracking and moisture ingress through surface laminate

Surface cracks and indentations were repaired with filler epoxy and, in general, the cracks did not propagate with continued service. Paint adherence was a minor problem, particularly with parts in contact with hydraulic fluid. Fastener holes in several fairings were frayed, primarily because of nonoptimal drilling procedures and improper fit. Elongated holes were also noted, primarily caused by improper fit and nonuniform fastener load distribution. There were no moisture intrusion problems with the Kevlar 49-epoxy fairings, and they performed similarly to production fiberglass-epoxy fairings. Additional details on the design, fabrication, and service evaluation of the Kevlar 49-epoxy fairings are presented in Ref 16 and 17.

B-737 Graphite-Epoxy Spoilers. The B-737 spoilers used three different graphite-epoxy unidirectional tape systems: T300-5209, T300-2544, and AS-3501. The spoilers were fabricated with upper and lower graphite-epoxy skins, aluminum fittings, spar, and honeycomb core, and fiberglass-epoxy ribs (Fig. 6). During the 13-year service evaluation period, several types of damage were encountered, with over 75% of the damage incidents being related to design details. Damage was most often due to actuator rod interference with the graphite-epoxy skin, which was resolved by redesigning the actuator rod ends. The second most frequent cause of damage was moisture intrusion and corrosion at the spar-to-center hinge fitting splice, which could be resolved by redesigning the splice to prevent disbonds between the skin and spar cap. Miscellaneous cuts and dents related to airline use were also encountered. Damage from hailstones, bird strikes, and ground handling equipment occurred on several spoilers.

A typical corrosion damage scenario occurs at the spar-to-center hinge fitting splice (see Fig. 6). The corrosion damage can be characterized by three phases of development. Phase 1 involves corrosion initiation at an aluminum fitting or at the aluminum spar splice. The corrosion is initiated by moisture intrusion through cracked paint and sealant material. If the corrosion products are not removed and new sealant applied, the damage progresses to phase 2, where moisture penetrates under the graphite-epoxy skin along the aluminum C-channel front spar. Normal service loads combined with moisture contribute to crack growth and subsequent corrosion. If the phase 2 corrosion is not repaired, the damage progresses to phase 3, where extensive skin-to-spar separation takes place. Phase 3 corrosion can result in significant loss of strength and stiffness. Uninterrupted flight service of two to three years is required before phase 3 separation becomes significant. Residual strength tests were conducted annually to establish the effects of service environments on the graphite-epoxy spoilers. The spoilers were tested with compression load pads on the upper surface to simulate airloads. Trailing-edge tip deflection was measured as a function of applied load for each spoiler tested. The test results were compared with the strength and stiffness of 16 new spoilers. The strength for each spoiler through 12 years of service generally fell within the strength scatter band for the baseline spoilers. However, spoilers with significant corrosion damage that were tested after seven to eight years of service, respectively, indicated a strength reduction of up to 35%. The load deflection response of the spoilers, compared with that of the baseline spoilers, followed similar trends.

In addition to structural tests of the spoilers, measurements were made to determine absorbed moisture content of the graphite-epoxy skins. The moisture content was determined from plugs cut near the trailing edge. The plugs consisted of aluminum honeycomb core, two graphite-epoxy face sheets, two layers of epoxy film adhesive, and two exterior coats of polyurethane paint. About 90% of the plug mass was in the composite facesheets, including the paint and adhesive. The moisture content was determined by drying the plugs and recording the mass change.

The data for plugs removed from spoilers after nine years of service indicated moisture levels in the graphite-epoxy skins ranging from 0.59 to 0.90%. The moisture levels for the T300-5209 and AS-3501 systems were similar to those for unpainted material coupons exposed to worldwide outdoor environments. However, the moisture content of 0.90% for the T300-2544 plugs was only about half that of the unpainted outdoor-exposure material coupons. Extensive ultraviolet radiation degradation of the T300-2544 unpainted specimens may partially explain the higher moisture absorption. Additional details on the design, fabrication, testing, and service evaluation of the B-737 graphite-epoxy spoilers are presented in Ref 18 and 19.

C-130 Boron-Epoxy-Reinforced Center-Wing Boxes. The design of the boron-epoxy-reinforced aluminum center-wing boxes installed on the two C-130 aircraft in 1974 included uniaxial strips of boron-epoxy bonded to the aluminum alloy skin panels and to the hat section stringer crown. The objective of this program was to compare the strength and fatigue endurance of the boron-epoxy-reinforced boxes and equivalent all-aluminum wing boxes.

The boron-epoxy-reinforced aluminum wing boxes performed excellently in service, with no damage or defects reported. No maintenance actions were required during a 12-year service evaluation period. On the basis of results of ground tests on a third wing box, the boron-epoxy-reinforced wing boxes are expected to have greater fatigue endurance than the baseline aluminum boxes. Additional details on the design, fabrication, and ground tests of the boron-epoxy-reinforced wing boxes can be found in Ref 20–22.

DC-10 Boron-Aluminum Aft-Pylon Skins. The boron-aluminum skin panels installed on the three DC-10 aircraft in 1975 were located above the aft-engine and encountered high acoustic fatigue loading and moderate thermal loads. Two of the skin panels were still in service after 11 years. However, one panel was removed from service after seven years because of corrosion damage (see Fig. 7); the outer layer of boron filaments on the inside of the panel was almost completely exposed. The panel contained a light residue of ester oil similar to turbine engine oil; however, the specific corrodent was not identified. A second panel also had some corrosion damage and a small crack, but was monitored closely during service to check for crack growth and further corrosion damage. The crack in the panel was probably caused by exterior mechanical damage during removal and reinstallation of the adjacent engine cowling.

It was concluded that the method of corrosion protection used was inadequate. In general, the boron-aluminum panels did not perform as well as similar production titanium panels. Additional details on the DC-10 boron-aluminum skin panels are presented in Ref 23.

DC-10 Graphite-Epoxy Rudders. The configuration of the fifteen T300-5208 graphite-epoxy upper aft rudders installed on DC-10 aircraft in 1976 is shown in Fig. 8. The entire structure was co-cured in an oven at the materials supplier's recommended cure cycle for T300-5208.

Table 4 NASA ACEE composite structures flight service summary

Aircraft	Component	Components in service: Originally	Components in service: As of June 1991	Start of service
L-1011	Fairing panels	18	15	January 1973
	Aileron	8	8	
B-737	Spoilers	108	33	July 1973
	Horizontal stabilizer	10	8	
C-130	Center wing box	2	2	October 1974
DC-10	Aft pylon skin	3	2	August 1975
	Upper rudder	15	10	April 1976
	Vertical stabilizer	1	1	January 1987
B-727	Elevator	10	8	March 1980
L-1011	Aileron	8	8	<March 1982
B-737	Horizontal stabilizer	10	8	March 1984
S-76	Tail rotors and horizontal stabilizer	14	0	February 1979
206L	Fairing, doors, and vertical fin	160	51	March 1981
CH-53	Cargo ramp skin	1	1	May 1981
Total		**350**	**139**	

Source: Ref 15

Expandable rubber was used inside the rudder to apply pressure against an outside steel tool.

There were seven incidents that required rudder repairs, including three minor disbonds, rib damage due to ground handling, and damage due to lightning. Minor lightning strike damage to the trailing edge of a rudder and rib damage occurred while the rudder was off the aircraft for other maintenance. The lightning strike damage was limited to the outer four layers of graphite-epoxy, and a room-temperature repair was performed in accordance with procedures established when the rudders were certified by the FAA. The rib damage was more extensive, and a portion of a rib was removed and rebuilt (see Ref 24 for more details).

More extensive lightning damage was sustained on another graphite-epoxy rudder. Inspection of the rudder revealed that the lightning protection strap had been inadvertently left off after the previous maintenance check. The skin in the damaged area was eight-plies thick over an eight-ply spar cap. Fiber damage and resin vaporization extended through the skin forward of the spar, and the skin and spar cap aft of the rear spar were completely destroyed. Details of the repair procedures are given in Ref 25.

A graphite-epoxy rudder was removed from service for residual strength testing after 5.7 years and 22,265 flight hours on Air New Zealand aircraft. The load-deflection response indicated that this rudder had an initial stiffness higher than that of the baseline rudder, but a similar overall response. The baseline and the 5.7-year tests were stopped at approximately 400% limit load because of instability of the loading apparatus. Although the rudders were designed by stiffness considerations and only one residual strength test was conducted, the overall response of the rudder indicated that no degradation had occurred after 22,265 flight hours.

B-727 Graphite-Epoxy Elevators. The T300-5208 graphite-epoxy elevator was constructed with Nomex honeycomb sandwich skins and ribs, and laminated spars (see the article "Aircraft Applications" in this Volume). Following initiation of flight service of ten elevators in 1980, three B-727 graphite-epoxy elevators were damaged by minor lightning strikes and two elevators were damaged during ground handling. The most severe damage occurred when the static discharge of one B-727 penetrated the elevator of another B-727 during ground handling. Skin panels were punctured, resulting in four holes in the lower surface and one hole in the upper surface, and the lower horizontal flange at the front spar was cut inboard of the outboard hinge. Figure 9 shows typical lightning damage to the trailing edge of an elevator and trailing-edge fracture of another elevator caused by impact from a deicing apparatus. Damage from lightning strikes ranged in severity from scorched paint to skin delamination. All of the elevator repairs were performed by airline maintenance personnel.

The lightning damage was repaired with epoxy filler and milled glass fibers. The skin punctures were repaired with T300-5208 prepreg fabric and Nomex honeycomb core plugs. The front spar was repaired with a machined titanium doubler, which was mechanically fastened to the lower skin flange of the spar chord. The repaired graphite-epoxy elevators were reinstalled on aircraft for continued commercial service. Details of the design and fabrication of the graphite-epoxy elevators are given in Ref 26.

L-1011 Graphite-Epoxy Ailerons. After four shipsets of T300-5208 graphite-epoxy inboard ailerons (Fig. 10) were installed on L-1011 commercial aircraft in 1982, an additional shipset was installed on the L-1011 flight-test aircraft.

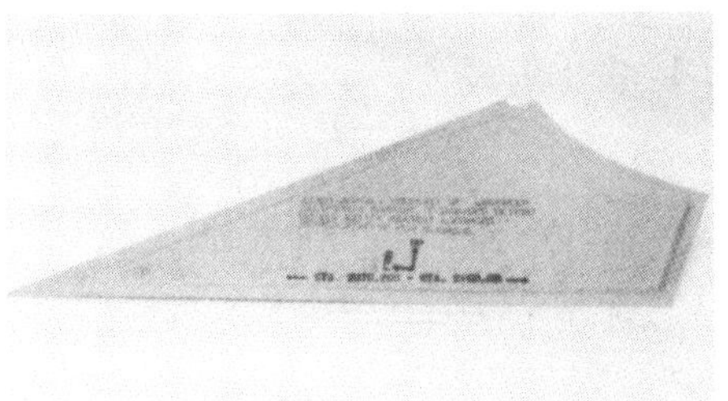

Center-engine fairing

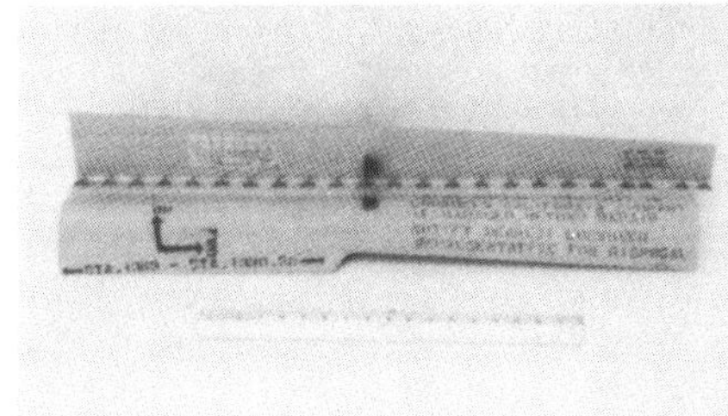

Under-wing fillet

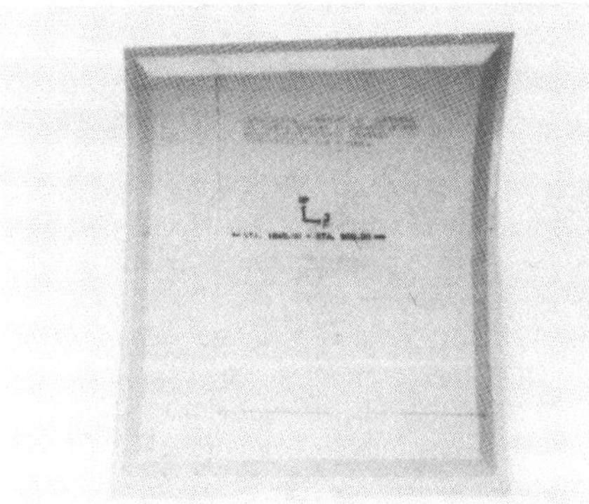

Wing-to-body fairing

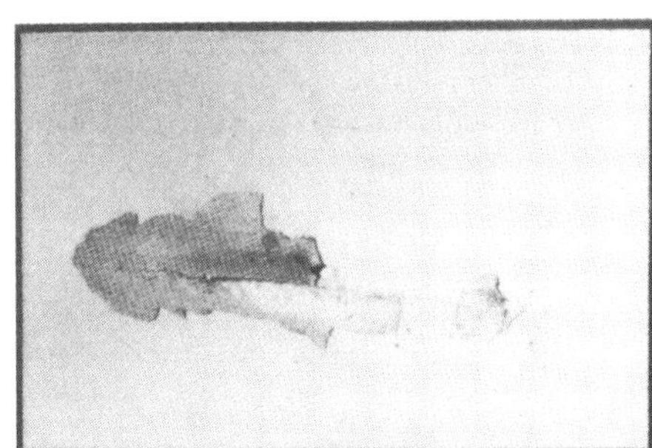

External surface crack

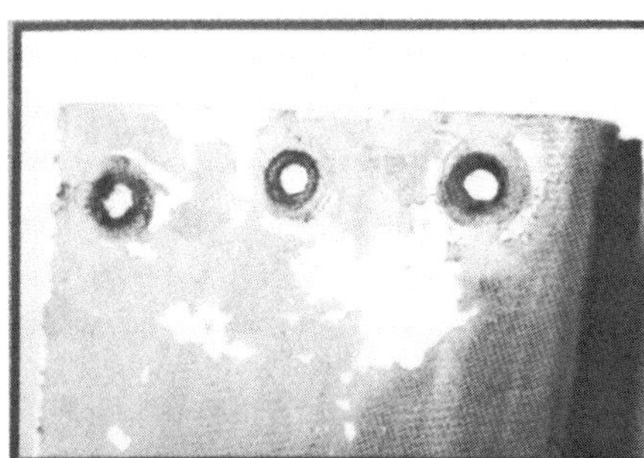

Lack of paint adherence

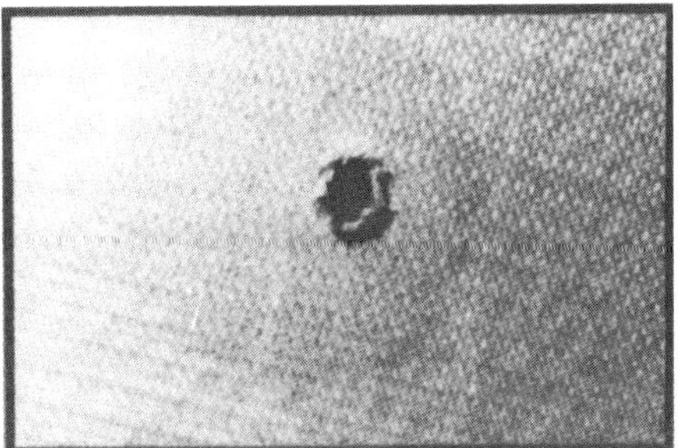

Frayed fastener hole

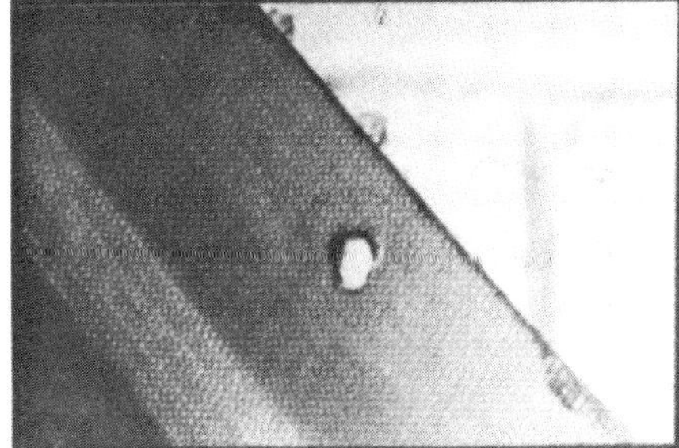

Elongated fastener hole

Fig. 5 Configurations of L-1011 Kevlar 49-epoxy fairings (top) and typical in-service conditions (below)

During the four-year service evaluation period, no damage incidents occurred and no major maintenance actions were required. Minor paint touch-up was performed periodically, and loose fibers around one fastener hole on the flight-test aircraft were rebonded with epoxy. Details on the development of the graphite-epoxy ailerons are reported in Ref 27.

B-737 Graphite-Epoxy Horizontal Stabilizers. The configuration of the five shipsets of T300-5208 graphite-epoxy horizontal stabilizers installed on B-737 aircraft beginning in 1984 is shown in Fig. 11. The graphite-epoxy stabilizer features stringer-reinforced skins, laminated spars, and Nomex honeycomb-reinforced ribs. This structure was the first certified primary structure for commercial airplanes. No damage incidents occurred and no maintenance actions were required on any of the stabilizers. Details on the development of the graphite-epoxy stabilizers are reported in Ref 28.

Helicopter (Bell 206L) Components. The four composite components evaluated on the 206L are shown in Fig. 12. Installation of the 40 shipsets of composite components was initiated in March 1981. Design-related and normal-use problems were encountered with some of the components, but service experience with the forward fairing and the vertical fin was excellent. Two graphite-epoxy vertical fins were struck by lightning. One fin was repaired and returned to service; the second fin was returned to the manufacturer for residual-strength testing. Service experience with the Kevlar 49-epoxy litter door was good, but underdesigned metal hinges caused problems. New hinges were installed on all the litter doors. A design-related thermal distortion problem occurred with Plexiglas (Rohm & Haas Company, Philadelphia, PA) windows in the litter doors, necessitating redesign of the window attachment to the door. The baggage doors had the poorest service record; the major problem was disbanding of the outer Kevlar 49-epoxy skin from the Nomex honeycomb core, to which the outer skin had been co-cured with no additional adhesive. Poor resin filleting was the primary cause of the skin-to-core disbonds, which could probably be prevented by using a film adhesive between the skin and core.

Residual-strength tests were conducted on 24 components removed from service in the Gulf of Mexico, eastern Canada, Alaska, and the northeastern United States. The service times ranged from 12 to 34 months, and flight times ranged from 668 to 3387 h. All the flight-service components, except two baggage doors with disbonds, failed at loads higher than the design requirements. Additional details on flight-service performance of the 206L components are reported in Ref 29.

S-76 Components. The two composite components evaluated on the S-76 were tail rotors (graphite-epoxy spar, glass-epoxy skin) and horizontal stabilizers (Kevlar 49-epoxy torque tube reinforced with full-depth aluminum honeycomb and graphite-epoxy spar caps, Kevlar 49-epoxy skin, Nomex honeycomb sandwich core). These were baseline designs for the S-76 and went into commercial production.

Three horizontal stabilizers removed from service for residual-strength testing met baseline proof load requirements. Seven tail rotor spars were removed from service for either static or fatigue testing, and test results were compared to the baseline room-temperature dry strength of ten spars tested for FAA certification. These components exhibited minimum strength retention of 93% of FAA certification values, which compares well with strength retention factors projected from laboratory-conditioned specimens.

Coupons cut from spars were tested in short-beam shear, and the results were compared with those from coupons cut from panels exposed in an outdoor exposure rack in Stratford, Connecticut. The average short-beam shear strength of the spar coupons was 5% lower than that of the coupons machined from the outdoor ground-exposure panels. The spar coupons had service times ranging from 37 to 51 months, and the panel coupons had exposure times ranging from 35 to 49 months. The foregoing results indicate excellent in-service performance for all the S-76 composite components. Additional details on the evaluation program are reported in Ref 30.

CH-53D Cargo-Ramp Skin. A ±45° Kevlar 49 fabric-5143 epoxy composite skin was installed on the aft end of a CH-53D cargo ramp for U.S. Marine Corps service evaluation in 1981 to assess the wear, impact, and damage resistance of Kevlar 49-epoxy in an environment where ground impact occurs frequently. The skin panel was 508 × 2032 mm (20 × 80 in.) and ranged in thickness from 1.0 to 2.0 mm (0.04 to 0.08 in.). Because of the location and thinness of the panel, the potential for damage was significant. However, no damage or service-related problems were reported following annual inspections.

Other Part-Specific In-Service Experiences

Elevators and Ailerons. In Joynes' 1990 study of the 737-300, 757, and 767 models, the aileron and elevator control surfaces had the most reported incidents. "Being closest to the ground, they present the greatest opportunity for collisions with ground equipment, stands, and so on, and also the greatest area for falling-object damage. The elevators are particularly susceptible to damage from runway debris," sometimes disturbed by engine exhaust and tires. "Lightning strike damage also occurs more frequently to the elevators because they are subjected to both direct strikes and to the attachment of swept strikes off the wing, engine nacelles, or fuselage that stream aft over the horizontal stabilizer" (Ref 3). Elevators have suffered from a moisture ingression problem due to the thin skins they are often designed with, such as on the 737 and A320, as stated in Airbus Service Bulletin.

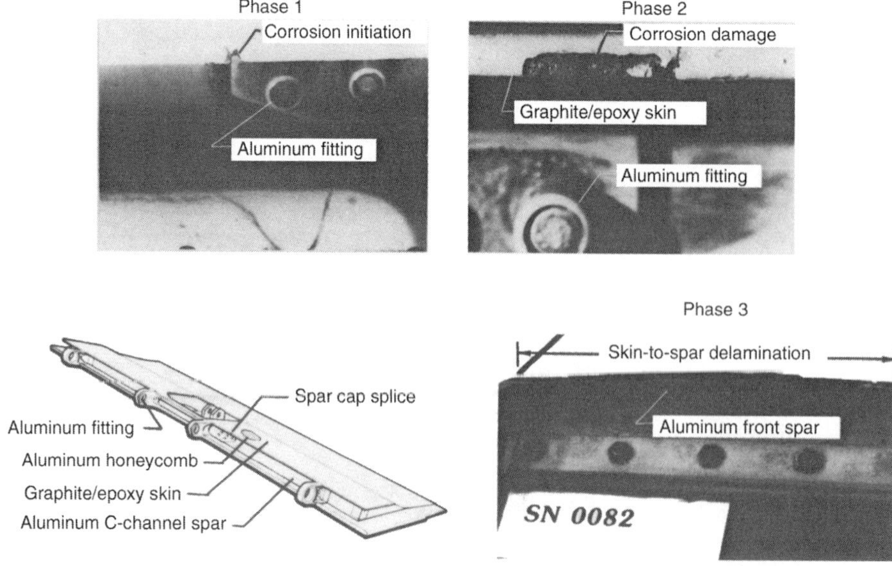

Fig. 6 Corrosion damage to B-737 graphite-epoxy spoiler

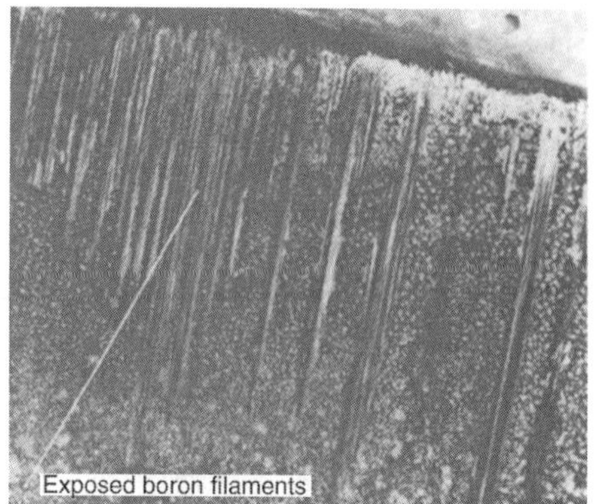

Fig. 7 Interior corrosion damage to DC-10 boron-aluminum aft-pylon skin panel

Rudders. Joynes reports that the majority of the rudder damage on 737-300s, 757s, and 767s was due to lightning strikes, impacts due to collisions with other aircraft or hangers, or uncoordinated surface movements while the aircraft was near workstands (Ref 3).

Nacelles. Nacelles, in general, due to their location, suffer from several frequent damage modes: damage by ground vehicles, erosion, lightning strike, heat damage on inner and outer skins, and fluid ingression (Ref 6).

Engine inlet cowls are a structure complicated by the need to incorporate noise attenuation to meet lower engine noise requirements. These acoustic panels have a perforated outer skin that necessarily allows water in the honeycomb and must use materials very resistant to water. If drainage is not designed or manufactured properly, water will accumulate to cause other damage (such as service bulletins for the CF6-6 and CFM56). On some designs, the acoustic panels use materials that are difficult to bond or not durable under impact, such as stainless steel mesh or coarse weave graphite cloth. Due to their low bond strength, these materials delaminate easily after impact or under environment stress or corrosion (Ref 6).

Fan Cowls. One early service demonstration study was conducted by Rolls-Royce on an RB211-524 engine (Ref 31). A substitute was designed for the aluminum-skinned unit using skins of T300 graphite. A left-hand and right-hand fan cowl were installed on a commercial turbine engine and examined after 5795 hours and 2663 cycles. Visual inspection found paint erosion, disbond of edge erosion protection, disbonding of door lands, fiber splintering at leading edge, damaged connecting plates, and dents on the outer skins. The "majority of the damage sustained was . . . of a minor nature." X-ray inspection revealed honeycomb cell wall buckling near the dents and fluid ingress near the visible skin damage. Testing on sections cut from the cowls showed no change in four-point bending, flatwise tensile strength, thermal analysis, and a moisture content of 1.2% by weight. Rolls Royce concluded, "In view of the many small areas of local impact damage, the absence of delamination and . . . unbond gives confidence that composite components and bonded assemblies of this type can withstand normal environmental condition."

Thermal degradation of nacelles is quite common in nacelle composite due to failures of other components, such as bleed valves, anti-ice systems, high-pressure bleed air ducts, and unplugged borescope ports. Normal operation of various exhausts, such as from the engine inlet anti-ice system, can result in hot air flowing over the fan cowl or reverser and leading to delamination. A polyimide demonstration fan cowl was evaluated in service by Lufthansa. The cowl was found to have a large amount of hydraulic fluid that diffused through the skin. The root cause of the damage was identified as thermal degradation and matrix cracking. During an effort to investigate nacelle temperatures, Lufthansa ran a short monitoring program on an A300-600 aircraft with CF6-80-C2 engines. Temperatures recorded on the inner surface of the fan cowl were found to be much higher than the manufacturer's designed continuous service temperature (Ref 32).

Other failure modes identified that are specific to fan cowls include: mishandling damage around the latch cutouts, erosion, punctures of the inner skin by clamps on engine accessories, and ingression of oil/hydraulic fluid. Use of aluminum honeycomb with graphite skins seems to increase the lightning damage (Ref 6).

Fuselage Fairings. Many aircraft models are reported to require many repairs and maintenance to the belly fairings, due to the high ex-

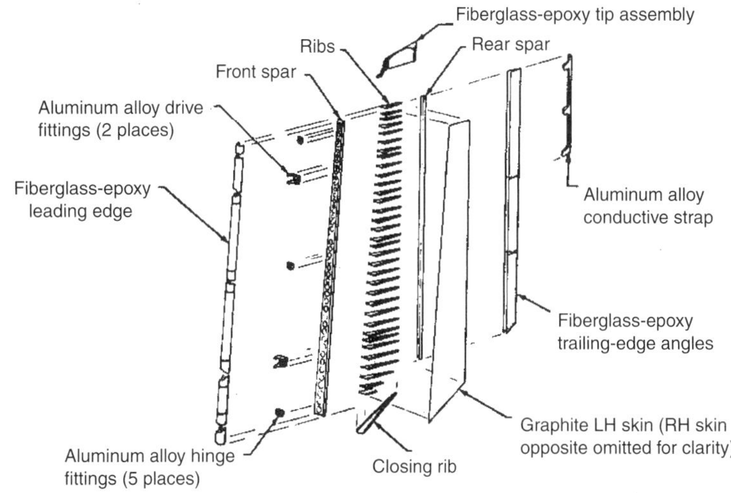

Fig. 8 Configuration of DC-10 graphite-epoxy upper aft rudder

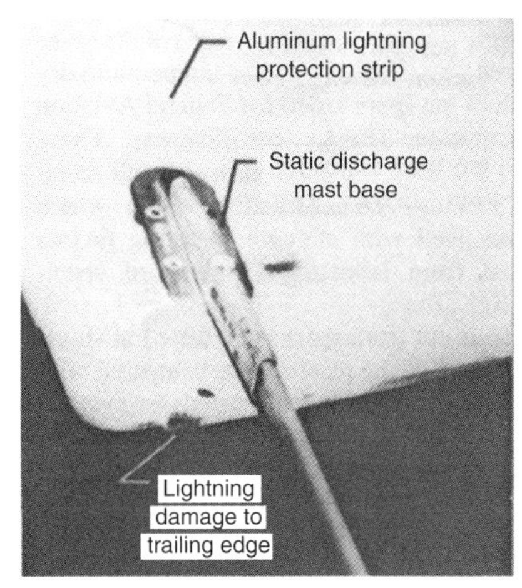

Lightning damage

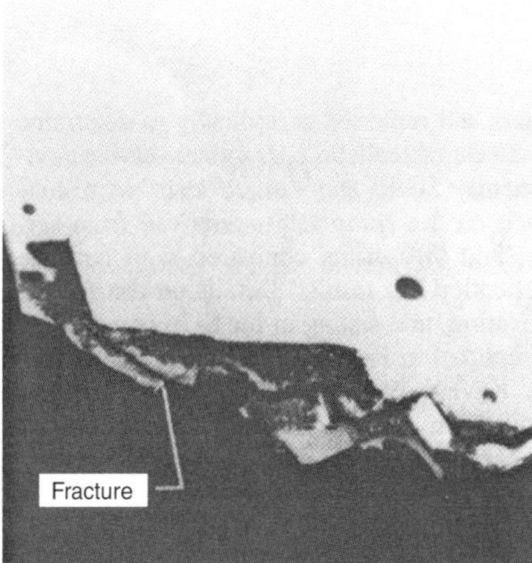

Ground handling damage

Fig. 9 B-727 graphite-epoxy elevator damage

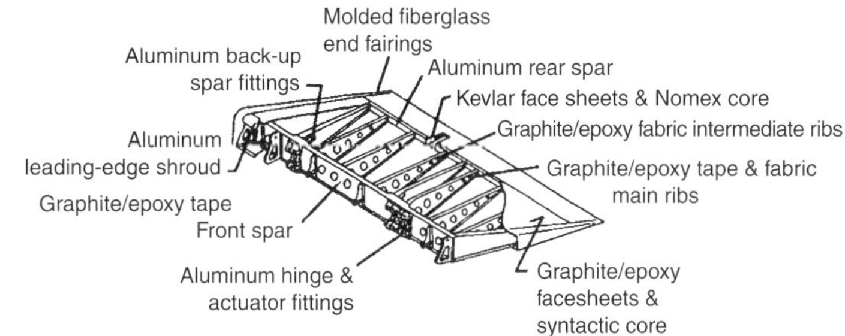

Fig. 10 Configuration of L-1011 graphite-epoxy aileron

posure to vehicle damage or runway FOD, and due to lightweight designs. However, one failure that is easier to prevent is fluid ingression, especially from leaky hydraulic components mounted above the panels. Armstrong reported early in the B-747 service that some of the fairings collect moisture (Ref 31). One specific case was described in AE-27 and the Airbus Service Bulletin A320-53-1116. The belly panels were constructed of honeycomb sandwich with one ply aramid cloth on the inside skin. The inner skin was not protected by any fluid barrier, such as a polyvinyl fluoride film or paint, and allowed the ingress of hydraulic fluid, fuel, and water. This is a common failure mode with honeycomb panels on many aircraft models, even with protection schemes, which will degrade with time, allowing ingression into thin permeable skins.

Radomes. Radomes have been cited in many studies as a troublesome part, because they are in a vulnerable location on the nose of the aircraft, and there is the additional complication that they must have transparency to radar waves. The MTBUR reported by various sources ranges from 1,000 to 40,000 flight hours. Keith Armstrong reported that radomes needed repair after . . ."rain and hail erosion and penetration, overshoe deterioration, lightning strike, and impact with ground service vehicles." (Ref 31). At UAL, an internal study on removal reasons from line aircraft found similar failures, as shown in Table 5. This study was based on almost 400 radomes removed during three years of non-maintenance visits on UAL's DC10, A320, 727, 737, 757, and 767 fleets. At UAL, of all the composite removable components in all fleets, radomes are the worst in causing delays and cancellations, in removal rate, and in the number of spares.

Spoilers. Slightly predating the ACEE, Vought established a program for a four-year study with 28 composite spoilers on the S-3A. The objective of the program was to establish the practicality of advanced composite materials. Flight-service test complements laboratory test result and serves to validate the long-term structural integrity of the material design and manufacturing process. They also recognized the necessity to obtain management approval from both the manufacturer and the airline user for production and fleet usage. The 41 incidents of in-service damage are summarized in Table 6 (Ref 33).

By far the worst failure mode has been due to moisture intrusion in the honeycomb. In the NASA ACEE program, the B-737 Spoiler, made of graphite skins with aluminum honeycomb and fittings, was reported to have a design flaw where moisture and corrosion entered the overlap between the spar and the hinge fitting after sealing protection (paint and a fillet sealant) failed in places. After 15 years in service, types of damage found included (in order of frequency): dents from actuator, moisture intrusion with corrosion where the skin and spar overlap, miscellaneous cuts and dents, hailstones, bird strikes, and ground handling equipment. Even though "design changes and improved sealing methods could prevent corrosion damage," the "im-

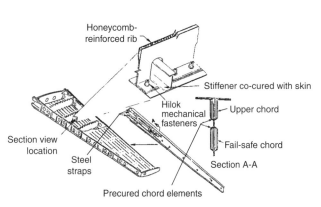

Fig. 11 Configuration of B-737 graphite-epoxy horizontal stabilizer

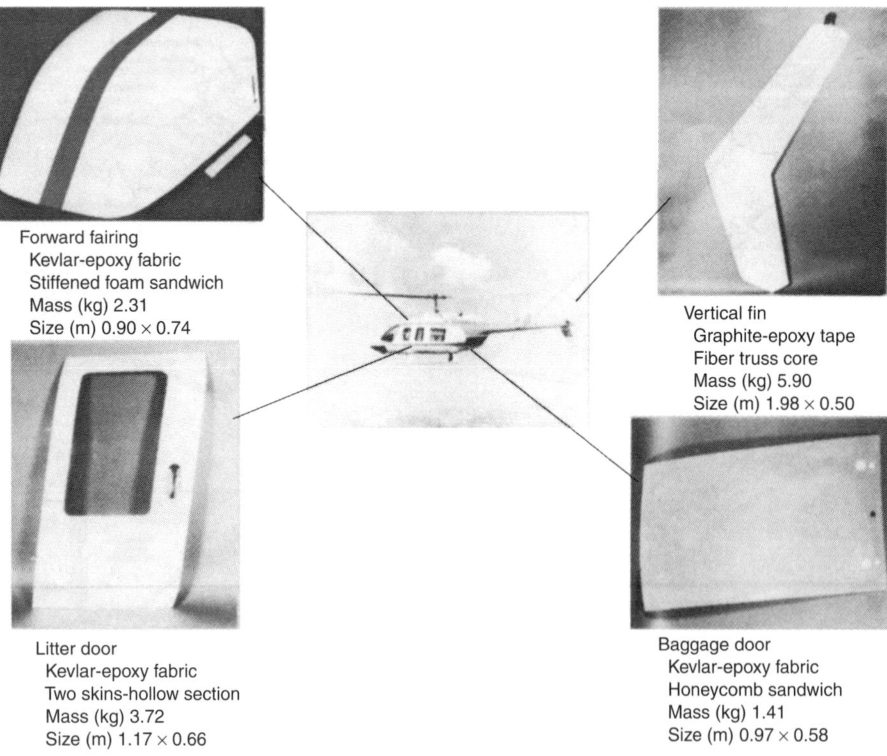

Fig. 12 Composite components in 206L helicopter

Table 5 United Airlines radome removal reasons, three year

Reason for Removal	Number	Percent
Bird	14	3.5
Boot	18	4.5
Color scheme wrong	22	5.5
Cracked	3	0.8
Damage found	26	6.5
Delamination/hail/soft	28	7.0
Fibers exposed	15	3.8
Hole	31	7.8
Lightning strike	86	21.6
Moisture	16	4.0
Paint chips	63	15.8
Pinhole	40	10.1
Radome noise	2	0.5
Static burn	34	8.5
Total	**398**	**100.0**

Table 6 S-3A composite spoilers in-service damage

Problem	Number of incidents	Percent of total	Cause
Blister above center hinge fitting	24	58	Design
Spar exfoliation corrosion	9	22	Manufacturing
Miscellaneous cuts and dents	6	15	Airline use
Trailing-edge delamination	2	5	Environment
Total	**41**	**100**	

Source: Ref 33

proved" sealing methods have never materialized (Ref 15). Reliance on sealant or paint to never crack has been demonstrated to eventually have some percentage of failures, which are sometimes as small as pinholes. Additionally, the water intrusion can lead to failure of the skin-to-core bondline.

757 Spoilers have also been a recent example of moisture intrusion. Although the root cause was identified as manufacturing noncompliance with sealing in accordance with the drawing, disassembly also revealed water ingression at tooling holes and hinge fittings. The water propagated rapidly through porous foaming adhesive and along the fiberglass septum (Boeing Service Bulletin 757-57-0047).

Table 7 Lessons learned for in-flight durability

Design aspect affected	Lesson
Solid laminate	Avoid abrupt termination of bonded solid laminate stiffeners; design flanges of stiffeners wide enough to accommodate bearing loads for fasteners; avoid bonding materials with different coefficients of thermal expansion.
Honeycomb sandwich	Establish minimum skin thickness criteria based on realistic impact energy levels; avoid self-adhesive prepregs when bonding to sandwich core; avoid fasteners penetrating into the core; potting around fasteners sufficient diameter; potting susceptible to cracking over time, or to moisture absorption; avoid square-edge honeycomb; avoid geometry and tools with local areas of low pressure, leading to porous bondline.
Materials selection	Avoid prepregs with high porosity when cured, such as solvated impregnation, and especially when cured only with vacuum pressure; take care with aramid fibers, especially in thin skins that are more susceptible to microcracking and moisture absorption; avoid surface finishes that can crack after subjected to combined stress of thermal, aging, and cyclic fatigue, or reduce the amount used.
Erosion	Provide erosion protection on leading edge and forward facing, such as radomes; erosion protection on forward edges with positive step; use easily replaceable, sacrificial materials or coatings.
Lightning strikes	Affect zones as specified by FARs, generally near attachment and detachment areas, such as radomes, engine cowlings, outer 18 in. of ailerons and elevators, rudder; allow for easy access to bonding jumpers and attachments; designs frequently do not sustain a strike without damage greater than allowable. Use sacrificial protection instead of sacrificing laminate; avoid use of aluminum honeycomb with carbon facesheets.
Thermal durability	Aircraft systems, especially powerplants, experience increase in operation temperatures with age. Do not underestimate temperature margins near engines; provide materials with adequate temperature capability; use insulation blankets, which have superior durability and repairability, instead of insulating/fire resistant coatings.

Source: Ref 6

Empennage and Primary Structure. Most operators report relatively few problems with composite fixed horizontal stabilizers and vertical stabilizer. The primary airframe structures have had very few occurrences of damage (Ref 34). The CACRC "Guide for Design . . ." has described the A320 vertical stabilizer as a "success story" for composites, saving weight and requiring little unforeseen maintenance (Ref 6). Service bulletins written against the tail have been minor.

Metallic alloy structures make up the vast majority of the airframes in the Air Force aging aircraft. However, more-recent aircraft have significant quantities of primary flight controls (C-17) and primary airframe structures (B-2, F-22) constructed from carbon-fiber-reinforced polymeric composites. Limited Navy and commercial aircraft service experience with composite laminate primary structures has indicated very few occurrences of damage in primary structures. The committee recommends that the Air Force undertake long-term research to monitor potential deterioration of composite structures, including the development of improved nondestructive evaluation methods, and to develop or improve maintenance and repair technologies, especially for composite primary structures.

In addition to the ACEE program, a paper was published in 1980, early in the life of the eight A-7 composite wings (Ref 35). After only 2.2 years and an average of 682 flight hours, no major problems were found. The following "minor" effects were reported, and the associated corrective actions:

- Small delamination. Injected with paste adhesive
- Suspected crack along rear spar. Paint sanded down, and crack found only in the aerodynamic filler material
- Blind fasteners installed with wrong grip length
- 13 mm (0.5 in.) crack in the upper cover at the access door support structure
- "Herringbone" cracks were detected in the upper and lower surfaces. Paint sanded down, and cracks found only in the aerodynamic filler material
- Delamination in leading edge of the lower skin. Repair with bolted doubler picking up nearby fastener

Lessons Learned

With any maturing technology, dispersal of the technology is related to the comfort level and acceptance. "Lessons learned" is an effort to document and pass on to future users of the technology the experiences and mistakes of the past, and therefore encourage the use of and reduce the risk of the technology. These lessons are often learned by the users while the aircraft are in service, but need to be absorbed by the designers and decision-makers at the OEMs, and then implemented whenever possible on production aircraft or new aircraft. The CACRC compiled some lessons oriented toward increasing durability, which have been summarized in Table 7 (Ref 6). The most comprehensive compilation of lessons for all stages of the lifecycle is found in *Composite Materials,* MIL-HDBK-17, Volume 3, Chapter 9 (Ref 36).

Materials. Even though the materials and process used in composite structures are still evolving, many of the failure modes can be attributed to materials or their inappropriate processing and design. However, these materials are still in use due to the economics of their continued use, which is often driven by the expense of changing or qualifying a new material. The two most obvious examples include: high-porosity prepreg cloths (Ref 37), and surface finishes that crack and chip (Ref 6).

Furthermore, the failure modes observed in service do correlate to degradation mechanisms for the materials. In a report on "Accelerated Aging of Materials and Structures," the National Research Council identified the four most significant degradation mechanisms: matrix cracking, thermal degradation and oxidation, hygrothermal degradation, and phase separation or macrostructural changes (see Table 8). The root cause of many of the current failure modes is in those areas identified in the column "missing information," which is a fruitful area for future materials research. The National Research Council summarized nicely: "The principal barriers to increased use for new high-performance materials are acquisition, manufacturing, certification, life-cycle cost, and incomplete understanding of failure mechanisms and the interactions" (Ref 39).

In the military aircraft, lessons for materials are embodied formally in aircraft specifications. For example, the U.S. Navy currently prohibits the use of honeycomb sandwich structure and aramid/epoxy. The Navy also has prohibited the use of polyimide and bismaleimide resins, because of potential for corrosion in the presence of jet fuel and salt (Ref 12). In a 1997 study, the Committee on Aging of U.S. Air Force Aircraft reported on the need " . . .to continue to monitor the performance of their composite components." Potential degradation mechanisms to monitor for future composite structural applications include (Ref 34):

- The development of transverse matrix cracking resulting from mechanical, thermal, or hygrothermal stresses
- The growth of impact damage under fatigue loading
- The growth of manufacturing-induced damage, especially from fastener installation
- The development of corrosion in adjacent metal structures

Design Opportunities and Documentation. Although such lessons learned have been documented for many years in various places, they have been difficult to implement, and known mistakes are often repeated by copying

Table 8 Aging materials lessons learned

Degradation mechanism	Most important variables	Modeling approach	Ways to accelerate tests	Missing information
Matrix cracking	Processing parameters Temperature cycle range Static and fatigue loading Moisture/thermal cycle Number of cycles Ply thickness Residual stresses	Damage accumulation models	Increase temperature cycle range Increase applied stress Increase frequency	Effects of moisture Rate effects
Thermal degradation and oxidation	Temperature Oxygen concentration Exposure time Mass-transfer models	Reaction kinetics models	Increase temperature Increase oxygen concentration	Chemical degradation models Effect of matrix cracking
Hygrothermal degradation	Exposure temperature Moisture concentration Heating rate	Moisture diffusion models	Increase exposure temperature Increase moisture content Cycle moisture sorption	Effect of moisture on residual stresses Description effects Moisture gradient effects Effect of matrix cracking Effect of imposed stress
Phase separation/ microstructural changes	Exposure time Exposure temperature Moisture content	None	Increase temperature Increase moisture content	Microstructural characterization methods Solubility methods

Source: Ref 38

previous designs. One obvious opportunity to take advantage of the lessons learned from past experience is during the design process for new aircraft models or redesign for a new fleet. Recently, aircraft manufacturers have attempted to use a team approach to design, involving designers, production, and the airline customers. If given the opportunity, this is the time during the aircraft life cycle when the airline customer can most easily influence the design and therefore, the maintenance and airline operating costs.

The OEM can incorporate lessons into general design guidelines, new test requirements, or materials specifications. Boeing uses documents called Design Requirements and Objectives (DR&O), which translate both mandatory Federal Aviation Regulations (FARs) and nonmandatory targets into specifics. One change for these DR&O for composites was an increase in the hail resistance, specifically the minimum thickness for the sandwich skins. Don Joynes stated in 1990, "To reduce time-consuming replacement of the fixed upper panels, a new hail and impact damage criteria was established that increased the thickness of the outer upper skin for production airplanes" (Ref 3). An example of new and revised specifications and design guidelines was presented by R. Thevénin in response to airline requests for more durable composites. Several specifications were described: EN2563 for testing for mechanical degradation from fluids, AITM 2-0037 for fluid tightness of the completed structure, AITM 1-0029 for resistance against erosion, improved potting compounds, and larger area of potting around fasteners, ABD0076 for elimination of a layer of pore filler, and AIMS 10-01-000 for material qualification for surfacers (Ref 40).

Another method of capturing the lessons of the past is to create a living document containing a generic, state-of-the-art design. The B.F. Goodrich-Aerostructures company has incorporated all the lessons they have learned from their hardware in a "best practices" nacelle design (Ref 41). The advantage with this approach is that there is continual feedback from customer service groups, continual updating of the design, and the design is not associated only with specific engines or aircraft models. This type of document also avoids the pitfalls of relying on existing designs or copying the experience of individuals.

ACKNOWLEDGMENTS

The author thanks those who have contributed to his understanding of composite aircraft structures, including Murray Kuperman, John Player, and the technicians at United Airlines. He also thanks Jahan Shafizadeh, who assisted with a much-appreciated literary search.

REFERENCES

1. B. Blanchard and W. Fabrycky, *Systems Engineering and Analysis,* 2nd ed., Prentice Hall, Englewood Cliffs, NJ, 1990
2. A. Tropis, Determination of Maintenance Program, Design and Justification of Repairs for Primary Composite Structures, *Proc. Flight Safety Foundation 48th International Air Safety Seminar,* Nov 1995, p 391–410
3. D. Joynes, Inservice Experience and Maintenance of Advanced Composite Structures In Airline Service, *22nd National SAMPE Technical Conf.,* Nov 1990, p 1131–1145
4. M. Dunkley, "British Aerospace Report on Inservice A320 Maintenance," Minutes of Commercial Aircraft Composite Repair Committee, SAE, Nov 1997
5. K.B. Armstrong and R. Barrett, "Care and Repair of Advanced Composites," SAE, 1998
6. Commercial Aircraft Composite Repair Committee, "Design of Durable, Repairable, and Maintainable Aircraft Composites," SAE AE-27, 1997
7. C. Blohm, "Advanced Composite Structures: In-Service Experience in the View of a Carrier," paper presented at the Workshop on Long-Term Aging of Materials and Structures, National Materials Advisory Board, National Research Council, Washington, D.C., 10–12 Aug 1994
8. *Ramp Rash,* Boeing Airliner magazine, April-June 1994
9. B.C. Hoskins and A.A. Baker, *Composite Materials for Aircraft Structures,* American Institute of Aeronautics and Astronautics, New York, 1986, p 85
10. J. Shafizadeh and J. Seferis, Ed., "Perceptions of Technological Innovation, Development, and Transfer; via an In-Service Evaluation of Moisture Migration Through Honeycomb Sandwich Structures," team certificate program final report, University of Washington, 1997
11. J. Shafizadeh, J. Seferis, E. Chesmar, and B. Geyer, Evaluation of the In-Service Behavior of Honeycomb Composite Sandwich Structures, *J. Mater. Eng. Perform.,* Vol 8 (No. 6), Dec 1999, p 661–668
12. L.F. Vosteen and R.N. Hadcock, "Composite Chronicles: A Study of the Lessons Learned in the Development, Production, and Service of Composite Structures," NASA contractor report, NASA CR-4620 4004995481, 1994
13. H.B. Dexter, "Long-Term Environmental Effects and Flight Service Evaluation of Composite Materials," NASA TM-89067, National Aeronautics and Space Administration, Jan 1987
14. H.B. Dexter, Long-Term Environmental Effects and Flight Service Evaluation, *Composites,* Vol 1, *Engineered Materials Handbook,* ASM International, 1987, p 823–831
15. H.B. Dexter and D.J. Benson, *Flight Service Environmental Effects on Composite Materials and Structures,* Kluwer Academic Publishers, 1994, p 51–85
16. J.H. Wooley, D.R. Paschal, and E.R. Crilly, "Flight Service Evaluation of PRD-49/Epoxy Composite Panels in Wide-Bodied Commercial Transport Aircraft," NASA CR-112250, National Aeronautics and Space Administration, March 1973
17. R.H. Stone, "Flight Service Evaluation of Kevlar 49/Epoxy Composite Panels in Wide-Bodied Commercial Transport Aircraft—Tenth and Final Annual Flight Service Report," NASA CR-172344, National Aeronautics and Space Administration, June 1984
18. R.L. Stoecklin, "A Study of the Effects of Long-Term Ground and Flight Environment Exposure on the Behavior of Graphite/Epoxy Spoilers—Manufacturing and Test," NASA CR-132682, National Aeronautics and Space Administration, June 1975

19. R.L. Coggeshall, "737 Graphite Composite Flight-Spoiler Flight Service Evaluation, Eighth Report," NASA CR-172600, National Aeronautics and Space Administration, May 1985
20. W.E. Harvill, J.J. Duhig, and B.R. Spencer, "Program for Establishing Long-Time Flight Service Performance of Composite Materials in Center Wing Structure of C-130 Aircraft. Phase II–Detailed Design," NASA CR-112272, National Aeronautics and Space Administration, April 1973
21. W.E. Harvill and A.O. Kays, "Program for Establishing Long-Time Flight Service Performance of Composite Materials Center Wing Structure of C-130 Aircraft. Phase III–Fabrication," NASA CR-132495, National Aeronautics and Space Administration, Sept 1974
22. W.E. Harvill and J.-A. Kizer, " Program for Establishing Long-Time Flight Service Performance of Composite Materials in Center Wing Structure of C-130 Aircraft. Phase IV–Ground/Flight Acceptance Tests," NASA CR-145043, National Aeronautics and Space Administration, Sept 1976
23. B.R. Fox, "Flight Service Evaluation of Advanced Metal Matrix Aircraft Structural Component–Flight Service Final Report," MDC Report J3827, McDonnell Douglas Corporation, Aug 1985
24. G.M. Lehman, "Flight-Service Program for Advanced Composite Rudders on Transport Aircraft–Sixth Annual Summary Report," MDC Report J6574, McDonnell Douglas Corporation, Aug 1982
25. B.R. Fox, "Flight-Service Program for Advanced Composite Rudders on Transport Aircraft–Ninth Annual Summary Report," MDC Report J-3871, McDonnell Douglas Corporation, Sept 1985
26. D.V. Chovil et al., "Advanced Composite Elevator for Boeing 727 Aircraft—Volume 2 Final Report," NASA CR-15958, National Aeronautics and Space Administration, Nov 1980
27. C.F. Griffin and E.G. Dunning, "Development of an Advanced Composite Aileron for L-1011 Transport Aircraft," NASA CR-3517, National Aeronautics and Space Administration, Feb 1982
28. J.E. McCarty and D.R. Wilson, "Advanced Composite Stabilizer for Boeing 737 Aircraft," *Proc. Sixth Conference on Fibrous Composites in Structural Design,* AMMRC MS83-2, Army Materials and Mechanics Research Center, Nov 1983
29. H. Zinberg, "Flight Service Evaluation of Composite Components on Bell Model 206L—First Annual Flight Service Report," NASA CR-172296, National Aeronautics and Space Administration, March 1984
30. M.J. Rich and D.W. Lowry, "Flight Service Evaluation of Composite Components. Second Annual Report. May 1982 through September 1983," NASA CR-172562, National Aeronautics and Space Administration, April 1985
31. D. Middleton, Ed., *Composite Materials in Aircraft Structures,* Longman Scientific & Technical, Essex, England, 1990, p 341–389
32. R. Gaag, R. Grove, W. Paplham, B. Smith, J. Sonnett, T. Streyczek, M. Tanikella, and C. Velisaris, "Risk Assessment for New Technology: A Study on the In-Service Evaluation of High Temperature Composite Materials in an Engine Environment," team certificate program final report, University of Washington, 1999
33. R.C. Knight and E.L. Rosenweig, "S-3A Composite Spoilers Service Experience," 12th National SAMPE Technical Conf., 1980
34. Committee on Aging of U.S. Air Force Aircraft, *Aging of U.S. Air Force Aircraft,* National Academy of Science Press, Washington, D.C., 1997
35. J.H. Pimm and F.J. Fechek, "A-7 Composite Outer Wing Service Experience," 12th National SAMPE Technical Conf., 1980
36. *The Composite Materials Handbook,* MIL-17, Materials Sciences Corporation, University of Delaware, Army Research Laboratory. Available in print from Technomic Inc. Available on the Web at http://www.materials-sciences.com/mil17/
37. F. Buehler, C. Martin, J. Seferis, and S. Zeng, "Evaluation of Secondary Airplane Structure Prepreg Systems," *Proc. 13th Annual Technical Conference on Composite Materials,* American Society of Composites, 1998
38. Committee on Evaluation of Long-Term Aging of Materials and Structures Using Accelerated Test Methods, Ed., *Accelerated Aging of Materials and Structures,* National Academy Press, 1996
39. National Research Council et al., "Report on Materials for Next-Generation Commercial Transport," National Academy Press, Washington, D.C., 1996
40. R. Thevénin, "Airbus Implementation of CACRC AE-27," Minutes of Commercial Aircraft Composite Repair Committee, SAE, May 1999
41. C. English, B.F. Goodrich-Aerostructures, private conversation, 2000

SELECTED REFERENCES

- K.B. Armstrong, "Guidance Material for the Design, Maintenance, Inspection and Repair of Thermosetting Epoxy Matrix Composite Aircraft Structures," 1991 National Conference Publication, Institution of Engineers, Number 91 Part 17, Australia, 1991, p 64–75
- J. Ayling, C-130 Hercules Composite Flaps Fatigue Test Program, *Proc. 44th International SAMPE Symposium,* 23-27 May 1999
- L.S. Blue, "Composite Materials in the Civilian Aerospace Industry: Composites in the 80's in Civil Aviation," *Second Annual Materials Technology Conf.,* Southern Illinois University, April 1985
- B. Cole, "Presentation of CACRC Survey," Minutes of Commercial Aircraft Composite Repair Committee, SAE, May 1999
- B. Geyer and J. Thompson, "Water In Airplane Honeycomb Sandwich Structures; Where Is It?," *44th International SAMPE Symposium,* May 1999
- "Guidance Material for Design, Maintenance, Inspection, and Repair of Thermosetting Epoxy Matrix Composite Aircraft Structures," International Air Transport Association, Montreal/Geneva, 1991
- International Air Transport Association (IATA), "Conclusions of IATA Questionnaire on Composite Structures Maintenance," Montreal, Canada, 1991
- MIL-HDBK-470A, "Designing and Developing Maintainable Products and Systems," Dept. of Defense, Aug 1997
- MIL-STD-721, "Reliability and Maintainability Definitions," Dept. of Defense
- R.L. Stoecklin, "Commercial Composite Component Service Experience," *12th National SAMPE Technical Conf.,* 1980

Failure Analysis

Chairperson: Patricia L. Stumpff, Hartzell Propeller, Inc.

Introduction to Failure Analysis

Patricia L. Stumpff, Hartzell Propeller, Inc.

ADVANCED COMPOSITES are being used as structural materials in automotive, recreational, aerospace, and other industries due to their low weight and inherent structural stiffness. As these materials continue to be used, it is inevitable for premature failures to occur as a result of manufacturing defects, unexpected loads, environmental exposure, and in-service damage. The need to understand and analyze these failures has led to an increased interest in determining whether the techniques and procedures used for failure analysis of metallic materials can be applied to composite materials as well. Analysts have been trying to establish, modify, and amend metallic failure analysis procedures to fit the procedures required for conducting failure analysis investigations of composite materials. This work has resulted in significant strides in this area since the 1980s. While failure analysis of composite materials is similar to that of metallic materials, the anisotropy of composites, the frequent use of adhesive bonding for joining dissimilar materials and structures, as well as the potential for composites to fracture in different and multiple failure modes, sometimes make their analysis much more complex. Therefore, while much has been accomplished in this regard, there is still much that needs to be done.

Overview of Failure Analysis

Any failure investigation begins with obtaining background information about the manufacture of the part and its service history. Part manufacturing information includes things such as part drawings, materials, manufacturing process specifications utilized, and any materials and/or manufacturing changes. Service history includes information regarding part usage, service time prior to failure, the number of failures, changes in the number of failures as a function of time, expected loading, and service environment.

After the background information has been obtained, the laboratory investigation can proceed. The purposes of the laboratory investigation are to determine if the material was manufactured according to the specifications and to identify any potential problems that may have played a role in the failure of the part. The laboratory investigation begins by conducting a thorough visual analysis of the failed parts to verify the type and location of the damage and to initiate ideas as to how the failure may have occurred. Appropriate nondestructive evaluation should also be conducted in order to verify all visual determinations of damage and to find other damage that may or may not be visible. It is necessary that all damage to the component be found and evaluated, in order to understand the failure mode and sequence. The next step in the investigation is verification of the materials and processes. This includes taking measurements, wherever possible, to ensure that the part exhibited dimensional conformance. Next, sections should be removed to verify material chemistry. Cross sections are extracted and mounted to evaluate ply type, count, and orientation. Glass transition temperature and degree of resin cure should be determined using thermal analysis techniques to ensure that the part was processed as required. Fracture surfaces should be removed and analyzed using both optical and scanning electron microscopy in order to determine failure initiation sites, crack growth directions, environmental influences, defects, and failure modes. Chemical analyses of potential foreign materials or contaminants may also be conducted.

If the laboratory investigation up to this point does not yet adequately explain the failure, additional testing can be conducted to further define the failure cause. Additional testing could include such things as mechanical testing to verify material strength and modulus, and/or stress analysis to determine the maximum failure stresses and potential sequence of fracture. The failure analysis is concluded when the cause of the failure has been adequately explained.

The sequence of conducting these investigative efforts is as important as the information actually obtained. This is because there can be a loss of relevant information that cannot be obtained later, once sectioning of the part has begun. Additionally, the information obtained from the previous analyses may be needed or useful in conducting subsequent analyses. The investigative sequence for conducting a failure investigation has been identified as the failure analysis logic network (FALN), and is shown in Fig. 1.

Coverage of this Section

This Section has been significantly overhauled since the last edition, mainly because of a significant increase in the understanding and actual use of the analytical procedures and techniques developed in prior years. Although it is not possible to describe in detail all the analytical procedures and techniques that might be useful in any investigation, it is hoped that this

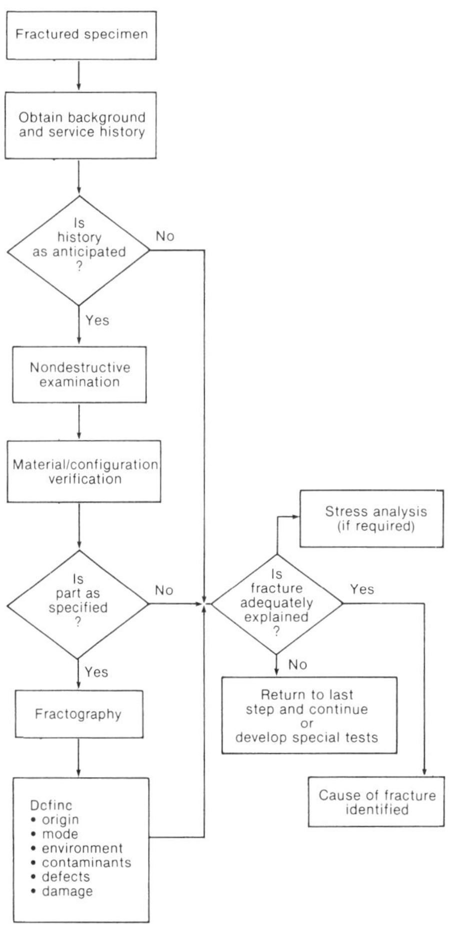

Fig. 1 Failure analysis logic network (FALN) for determining sources of failure in composite parts. Original FALN was developed by Boeing.

Section will at least provide the analyst with some general guidelines for conducting an investigation.

Most of the information in this Section is geared toward organic-matrix composites, although there is some information on failure analysis and fractography of ceramic- and metal-matrix composites (CMCs and MMCs). It is hoped that many, or at least some, of these procedures and techniques, which were originally developed for organic-matrix composites, can be applied to CMC and MMC materials as well.

The remainder of this Section is divided into nine articles. The first article, "Failure Causes," details the types of failures in composites, including those due to material and manufacturing defects, mechanical, thermal, and residual stresses, and environmental exposure.

The second article, "Failure Analysis Procedures," gives a general overview of the investigative sequence, as well as many of the specific techniques that can be used in an investigation. These techniques include both nondestructive techniques, such as x-ray and ultrasonics, and destructive techniques, such as cross-sectioning, thermal analysis, fractography, and mechanical testing. In addition to defining the technique, the article gives numerous examples of the types of data obtained and how those data can be used in a composite failure investigation.

The third article, "Visual Analysis, Nondestructive Testing, and Destructive Testing," is devoted to obtaining information relative to the current damage state of the component. Nondestructive analysis techniques, including visual examination, ultrasonics, x-radiography, and tape replicas, are discussed in relation to their usefulness in determining the location and severity of all damage.

The fourth article, "Microscopy," details the procedures for obtaining part cross sections. Cross sections are necessary in order to determine the material and processing conditions used to manufacture the part, including fiber, resins, and adhesives; ply type, count, and orientation; fiber, matrix, and void-volume fractions; fiber/matrix adhesion; material crystallinity; and material defects such as porosity, delaminations, and microcracking. The article also details several different techniques used for sample preparation of different materials, including information regarding thin section preparation. It describes the use of reflected bright-field, dark-field, polarized, and transmitted light, as well as phase contrast, differential interference contrast, modulation contrast, and optical staining in the analysis of material microstructure.

The fifth article, "Thermal Analysis," is devoted to detailing specific thermal analysis techniques utilized in composite failure analysis. Thermal analysis techniques, such as differential scanning calorimetry, thermomechanical analyses, dynamic mechanical analysis, and dielectric analysis, are generally used for determining the prior processing history, thermal exposure, and environmental service history. These analyses are used to help define the time/temperature exposures experienced by the composite either during manufacture or in service.

The sixth article, "Fractography," provides fractographs that help define the specific features used to determine the crack initiation site, crack growth direction, fracture mode, material/manufacturing defects, and environmental conditions at the time of failure. This article gives just a glimpse of the numerous fractographic features encountered when working with composite materials, although features from a broad range of materials and failure modes are provided. There is also a short discussion provided with each fractographic feature to describe what the feature tells an analyst about the failure.

The seventh article, "Case Histories," is devoted to describing three composite failure investigations. The purpose of this section is to provide the analyst with a description of how the procedural sequence and specific techniques were used in conducting several specific composite failure investigations.

The eighth article, "Fatigue Properties and Quantitative Fractography of Metal-Matrix Composites" is devoted to fatigue testing and the fractography associated with metal-matrix composites.

The ninth and final article, "Failure Analysis of Ceramic-Matrix Composites," is devoted to the fractographic analysis of ceramic-matrix composites, including characteristic failure modes, fractography, and failure mechanisms.

It is hoped that the information presented in this Section will be useful to the composite failure analyst and encourage future work in these areas. There is still a significant amount of research that needs to be conducted in the areas of visual, metallographic, and fractographic analyses before the analyses of composite materials and structures are as routine as the analysis of metals.

Failure Causes

John E. Moalli, Exponent Failure Analysis Associates

AS WITH MOST ENGINEERING MATERIALS, the failure of composite materials, no matter how complex, can be divided into three discrete arenas: improper design, improper manufacturing, and improper use of the end product. Each of these categories can be further subdivided, but it is rare that a failure cannot be assigned to one or more of them. This article looks at these failure causes from a broad perspective so that the composites designer, manufacturer, and user can readily see some of the more common issues associated with these unique materials.

Design

Design is sometimes described as a circular process that involves conceptualization of a product, construction of a prototype, evaluation and testing of the prototype, and return to the conceptualization/design phase to correct any deficiencies discovered during testing. Clearly, this is a great simplification, with each of these phases representing multiple steps. For example, in order to design and build a prototype, one must come up with dimensions that satisfy the relevant design criteria (Ref 1).

In composite materials, sizing the part based on its ability to support loads can be a challenging process, as stress analysis in composite materials is complicated by the inherent anisotropy of the material. In certain nonsymmetric laminated structures, it is possible to require 21 independent elastic constants to describe fully the component of interest, that number being reduced to 9 and 4 constants for three- and two-dimensional orthotropy, respectively (Ref 2). This is not to say that anisotropy should be avoided. In fact, it is anisotropy that allows composite structures to be designed so efficiently; the structure can be tailored to have different strengths in different directions to effectively handle directionally dependent loads and stresses.

It is important to note that not only are composite materials anisotropic because of the macrostructures (fiber orientation and laminate sequence), but also because of the anisotropy in the materials from which they are made. For example, many synthetic polymeric fibers have different moduli in tension and compression. Failure to consider this can lead to failures if one assumes that composites made from these materials will behave identically in push/pull situations. Even a unidirectional laminate in flexure will require special analytical consideration with different tensile and compressive moduli, as the neutral axis will no longer be coincident with the centroidal one. Equally important is the fact that the compressive and tensile strengths may be different, and the associated failure criteria may have to be examined separately.

Anisotropy is not limited to mechanical properties; composites often have directionally dependent thermal characteristics as well. It is not uncommon to have a factor of 10 difference in longitudinal and transverse thermal expansion coefficients (Ref 3), a variation dominated by the thermal characteristics of the constituent materials. Some graphite fibers, in fact, have negative longitudinal thermal expansion coefficients; they actually shrink when they are heated (Ref 4).

When considering internal thermal (often called residual) stresses from a design standpoint, it is critical to remember that the reference, zero-strain temperature is the curing temperature, not the ambient one. In laminated composites, the variation in ply orientation can cause thermally induced internal stresses to be quite large; ignoring these stresses and considering applied stresses only can promote overloading and resultant failure. Thermal stresses resulting from external conditions should use a different, appropriate reference temperature. For example, attaching a composite structure to a material of different composition can lead to applied stresses from differential thermal expansion and should use the attachment temperature as the reference condition.

Analysis of composite materials also needs proper consideration of product-dependent inhomogeneities including holes and notches, the presence of which can lead to structural failure at stresses well below nominal ultimate strength. Even the edges of composite plates with plies oriented at significant angles to each other need to be considered; the large ply stress gradients are not always considered and sometimes lead to premature failure.

Finally, analysis can be further complicated by selection of appropriate failure criteria. Those familiar with design based on load-limit-type analyses may find that, in many occasions with composites, strain limits are a more appropriate selection. For example, in composite pipes carrying aggressive media it may be important for the resin not to crack as the fibers will no longer be protected; this will likely occur at a strain level much lower than ultimate. If the pipe is designed solely from a strength standpoint, premature cracking of the resin may result.

As part of the design process described previously, prototype components should be fabricated and tested in actual end-use conditions. All expected load conditions should be evaluated, including transient or impact loads; it is well known that in certain composite structures, compressive strength after impact can be substantially reduced. Cyclic loads can also have detrimental effects, and fatigue damage created by them should be tested for and examined carefully. Carbon fiber reinforced composites generally display better fatigue resistance than glass reinforced ones; this is often attributed to the lower matrix strains in the higher-modulus carbon fiber reinforced material at a given stress level (Ref 5).

The time-dependent nature of extended loads must also be considered, as composites can be susceptible to both creep and stress relaxation. Finally, it is important to evaluate prototypes under representative environmental conditions (temperature, chemical, and ultraviolet exposure). For example, exposure of composite pressure vessels to acidic conditions has led to premature failure from environmental stress corrosion of the glass reinforcement (Ref 6).

Manufacturing

Manufacturing processes for composite materials are quite varied, from hand lay-up of laminated structures to computer-controlled processing of sheet molding compound, and failures can and do result from manufacturing errors. In the context of this discussion, manufacturing includes both processing of the composite and assembly of final components.

Typical processing-related failures include improper mixing and curing of matrix resins, which can have a number of effects on composite properties. An overcured resin can become embrittled, crack prematurely, and expose the reinforcement to environmental conditions it might not otherwise be exposed to. An undercured resin may be too soft and not transmit loads efficiently to fibers. Improper resin curing and mixing can also affect the chemical and thermal resistance of the matrix material.

If the composite is manufactured in such a way as to induce substantial voids in the resin, the flexural, transverse tensile, compressive, and interlaminar shear strength can all be negatively affected. Excessive voids can also reduce the environmental resistance of the composite. Because the end-use requirements of composite structures are so different, allowable void contents vary as well. Applications that demand minimal voids are usually autoclaved or vacuum bagged.

Since the strength and stiffness of composites is mostly governed by the reinforcing fibers, placement of them within the composite can be critical. In a thin, unidirectional laminate, for example, a variation in fiber orientation as small as 15° can reduce the laminate strength by a factor of 2. In some cases, random fiber placement is desired to produce a more isotropic structure. Flow-induced fiber orientation from processing can reduce isotropy, increasing strength and stiffness along the flow direction and reducing them transverse to the flow direction.

Errors related to assembly and fabrication of composites can also lead to failure. Composite materials are often bonded together with adhesives, the curing of which can affect strength and ultimate performance. Proper curing, as well as minimization of voids and contaminants, are important items to monitor during adhesive bonding.

Other types of mechanical joints also need to be monitored carefully during assembly. For example, excessive applied torque in bolted joints not only can cause visible bearing failures, but subsurface interlaminar failures can also be induced. Because these failures are not readily observed, they tend to be more insidious as they can propagate without notice.

As mentioned previously, the temperature at which a bonded or adhesive joint is made can also be a factor in composite failure. If the joint connects materials with dissimilar thermal expansion coefficients and is made at a temperature significantly different than the service temperature, significant stresses can be induced from differential thermal expansion.

Improper Use

Although the incidence of misuse in composite materials should be similar to conventional ones, the results can be quite different. An impact, not expected in typical service conditions, may dent a metallic component that can be used thereafter without consequence. The same impact in a composite structure can cause an internal delamination that can propagate unseen and contribute to subsequent premature failure. For example, application of force with blunt objects to composite pressure vessels may leave little visible sign of external damage, but can cause subsequent failure of the vessel after filling to service pressures. For this reason, it is often necessary to inspect critical parts for nonvisible damage and also to make composite designs more robust than their traditional counterparts.

Failures from misuse can also be caused by not following specific instructions associated with the composite component. For example, buried composite tanks need to be installed in the ground in a very specific way, as they rely on the surrounding soil for support and stiffness. If they are not properly installed (misused), they tend to fail prematurely. For products such as these, designers and manufacturers should ensure that use instructions are clear and simple to comprehend.

REFERENCES

1. J.E. Moalli, Translating Failure into Success—Lessons Learned from Product Failure Analysis, *Proc., ANTEC 1999*, May 1999
2. L.R. Calcote, *The Analysis of Laminated Composite Structures*, Van Nostrand Reinhold, 1969
3. G. Lubin, *Handbook of Composites*, Van Nostrand Reinhold, 1982
4. W. Watt and B.V. Perov, *Strong Fibers*, Elsevier Science, 1985
5. R.W. Hertzberg and J.A. Manson, *Fatigue of Engineering Plastics*, Academic Press, 1980
6. Federal Register 63 FR 68819, 14 Dec 1998

Failure Analysis Procedures

Patricia L. Stumpff, Hartzell Propeller, Inc.

FAILURE ANALYSIS procedures for composites are generally similar to those used for other material systems. As with any thorough analysis, the investigation should follow a series of chronological steps that includes at least:

1. A review of available in-service records
2. A review of required materials and processing methods, print requirements, and manufacturing records
3. Visual analysis, documentation of damage and any other nondestructive part evaluation
4. Verification of materials, including the fiber/resin/adhesive systems
5. Determination of fiber, matrix, and void volume fractions and verification of the lay-up, ply type, and orientation
6. A review of the processing parameters used to manufacture the component, including the type of equipment, pressure, times, and temperatures used to effect the proper cure
7. Fractographic analysis, including failure origin, crack growth direction, environmental influences, and failure mode
8. Mechanical testing and stress analysis as warranted to adequately determine failure cause

The purpose in following a specific test sequence is to try to avoid the loss of necessary evidence that may come about during the destructive evaluation of the component. The techniques to be used in these analyses are described in more detail in this article.

Review of Available In-Service Records, Materials and Processing Methods, Print Requirements, and Manufacturing Records

Available service records are a good source of information to determine:

- How long the fractured component has been in service
- Whether or not the component was properly maintained during its service history
- If and when the component had ever been repaired or overhauled
- The types and magnitudes of the loads the component experienced at the time of failure, and whether or not those loads were typical or atypical for that part
- The environment experienced in service, and whether or not that environment was as initially anticipated during the design phase
- Whether or not there have been any other failures similar to the current failure of this particular component

A review of the materials and processing methods, print requirements, and manufacturing methods will entail a determination of the fiber/resin/adhesive systems, the type and number of plies and their orientation, the dimensional requirements and tolerances of the part, and the pressures, temperatures, times, and cure cycles used to process the materials into the finished component. A review of this information should provide answers to questions regarding whether the design, materials, manufacturing or processing methods, loads, environment, maintenance, or repair procedures might have been implicated in the failure event.

Visual Analysis and Nondestructive Examination

Visual analysis is usually the first step in the nondestructive evaluation process. The purpose of a visual examination is to document all damage and to determine how the component may have separated, and from this information, to try to discern which specific fracture or fractures initiated the failure event. The purpose in defining the initiating fractures from subsequent ones is to reduce the number of surfaces needing further evaluation in order to determine failure cause. Figure 1 depicts the three different stages in the failure of a helicopter rotor. The area labeled "A" depicts a fatigue initiation region; the area labeled "B" depicts a region of translaminar bending failure; and the area labeled "C" depicts an area of fiber crushing during final fracture. These three distinct regions are visually apparent on the fracture surface and are indicative of the different types of loading on the part during the failure event.

Although most translaminar fractures are visually apparent, composites, because of their laminated construction, will also exhibit interlaminar fractures that may be hidden from view. As a result, nondestructive evaluation of the component to find these interlaminar fractures often represents a particularly critical step in the analysis of composite structures.

The most successful nondestructive inspection methods for composite materials include through-transmission ultrasonics (TTU), pulse-echo ultrasonics, and dye-penetrant enhanced x-radiography. In the first two methods, internal damage is detected by placing an ultrasonic transducer on either one (pulse echo) or both sides (TTU) of the component and measuring the attenuation of 1 to 25 MHz acoustic waves transmitted into it. Signal attenuation levels are then measured, grouped together, and assigned different gray levels or colors on the scale of the chart recorder. The greater the level of signal attenuation, the more internal damage in the component. Figure 2 depicts an ultrasonic inspection record from a section of a damaged radome. In this case, the signal is highly attenuated in the dark, damaged region, identified as section A, where a delamination has occurred. No signal attenuation, however, was noted in the light-colored area shown in the center of section B, meaning no damage exists in that region. Moderate attenuation of the signal can be noted in the darker areas surrounding the undamaged area in section B. Moderate attenuation of the signal is probably indicative of some minor form of damage to the composite, such as resin micro-cracking or fiber-matrix separation.

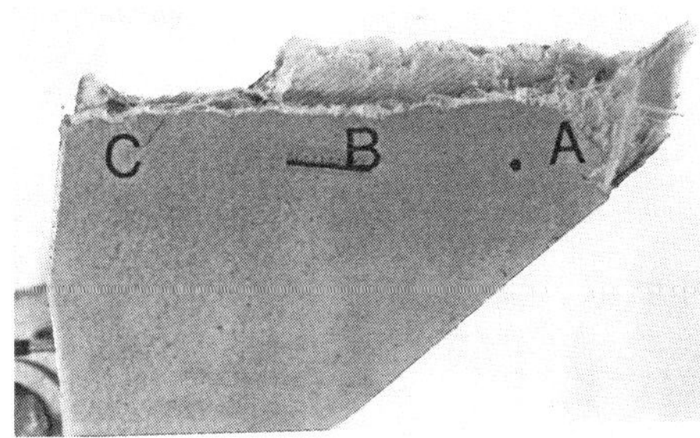

Fig. 1 Three different failure modes exhibited on the surface of a fractured, translaminar helicopter rotor. A, fatigue initiation; B, translaminar bending; C, fiber crushing during final fracture

The detection of damage in composites using x-radiography is carried out in the same basic manner as it is for metals, except that prior to the x-ray inspection, a radiopaque penetrant is wetted into the open surface cracks to enhance damage visibility. In general, x-ray equipment operable in the 10 to 50 kV, 5 mA range with diiodobutane penetrant yields the best results. Figure 3 details the damage evident in the 45° plies of a composite specimen following tensile loading in a mechanical test frame. The radiograph was taken following the addition and penetration of the radiopaque penetrant from the edges toward the center of the specimen. The use of penetrant to enhance this type of damage is often important in defining the depth of the interlaminar damage in a specimen prior to ultimate failure.

In addition to dye-penetrant-aided x-radiography, standard x-ray analysis can provide information regarding ply counts, ply orientations, and ply drop-offs. Foaming of resins or adhesives will also be apparent, as will water ingression into core details. The orientation, cell size, and web materials of honeycomb cores (particularly nonmetallic cores) can often be determined with x-ray inspection.

The use of any of these nondestructive evaluation techniques requires that some forethought be given to the type of failure likely to be encountered. With both ultrasonic methods, as well as with x-radiography with radiopaque penetrant, liquids will penetrate into the fracture surfaces. These liquids may alter the chemical nature of the fracture surfaces that may have initiated and/or propagated the failure. In those cases where surface-analysis techniques, such as x-ray photoelectron spectroscopy (XPS), are to be used later on to define the type of contamination on the fracture surface, the water or penetrant should be prevented from entering the fracture surfaces by sealing the exposed ends of the fracture with a water-resistant tape.

Verification of Materials and Processing Methods

The first step in the destructive portion of the investigation is to verify that the correct materials and processing methods were used in the manufacture of the component. These analyses include verification of:

- The fiber, resin, and adhesive systems
- The size, type, number, location, and orientation of all plies and adhesive layers
- The cure cycle used to cure the component

Verification of the resin and adhesive systems is usually conducted using a technique known as Fourier transform infrared (FTIR) spectroscopy. Each resin or adhesive used in the composite exhibits a unique infrared spectrum, as depicted in Fig. 4. The spectrum obtained for the resin or adhesive in the component is then compared to reference spectra in a materials database. This analysis generally reveals the specific material type and delineates materials such as epoxies from bismaleimides. Additionally, if enough database profiles are available for comparison, the uniqueness of the FTIR trace may even be able to verify a specific resin and its manufacturer, for example, Cytec FM 73 epoxy. The spectrum obtained during this analysis may also exhibit peaks that are not indicative of the material being analyzed; peaks that may be indicative of a potential contaminant that may be related to failure cause. The FTIR technique is also used to verify the fiber type as well, although visual analysis is often all that is required to identify fiber systems such as carbon, glass, boron, and aramid.

Following verification of the material, the next step in the investigative process is to determine glass transition temperatures and degrees of cure for all resin and adhesive systems. The assurance of a full cure is generally obtained by measuring both the glass transition temperature (T_g) and the residual heat of reaction (ΔH). These measurements are conducted using thermomechanical analysis (TMA) and differential scanning calorimetry (DSC), both standard thermodynamic instruments.

The T_g is defined as the temperature at which the matrix undergoes a transition from a glassy to a rubbery state. It is measured by inputting heat into the test sample and monitoring the rate of change of one of several materials properties, such as thermal expansion or stiffness, as a function of increasing temperature (see Fig. 5). The T_g can also be defined as the temperature at which the tangents to the curve, before and after

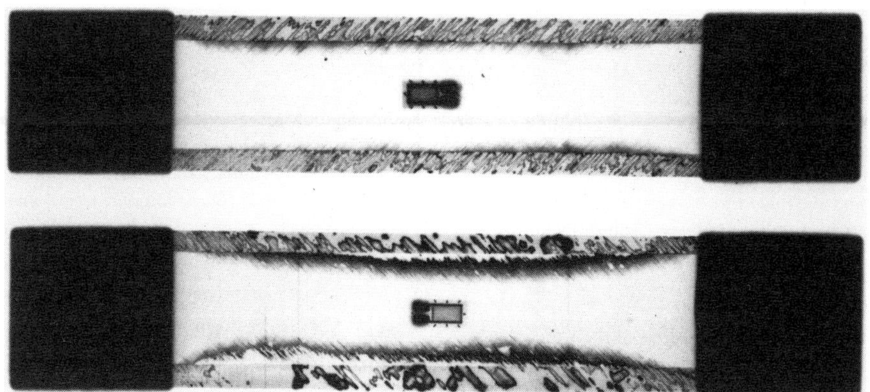

Fig. 3 Penetrant-enhanced radiograph revealing the microcracking and edge delaminations in a tensile test specimen

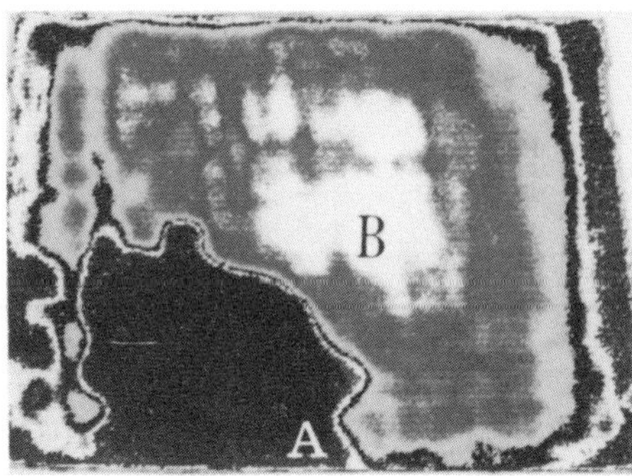

Fig. 2 Ultrasonic C-scan evaluation of a delaminated section of an aramid/epoxy radome. A, damaged region; B, undamaged region

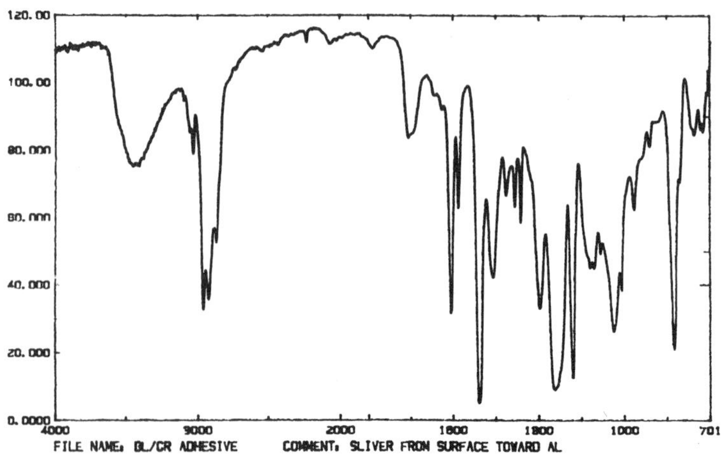

Fig. 4 Fourier transform infrared (FTIR) spectroscopy trace of an adhesive from a composite component

the transition, intersect. The specimens used for determining the T_g of the material, however, must be completely dry prior to the start of the test. This is because any moisture in the composite will generally lower the T_g and give a false reading. Specimens can generally be dried out by placing them in a vacuum oven set at 60 to 95 °C (140 to 200 °F), depending on the T_g of the material, until no weight loss is noted. (It should be noted, though, that predrying TMA samples prior to T_g determination may raise the T_g of the sample over the level seen at the time of the failure. In this case, the T_g may not be representative of the in-service condition of the failed part.)

If the T_g is still lower than expected after the specimen has been fully dried, then a DSC test should be conducted by inputting heat into the sample and measuring ΔH. The ΔH is basically the area under the curve on the thermogram in Fig. 6. A test specimen that has a thermogram with ΔH indicates that the specimen was not fully cured. Further analysis of the area under the curve reveals the degree of undercure in the specimen. This is done by comparing the ΔH for the test sample against that required to cure a similar amount of the original prepreg material. The two samples are each individually heated and the ΔH calculated. The ratio of the two ΔH values per gram of material is then used for determining the ratio or percentage of cure in the test sample. (It should be noted that using DSC to determine the extent of cure [and the completeness of the cure] will work well only for systems with well-defined reaction endpoints. Other systems are more difficult to characterize by this method.)

Determination of Fiber, Matrix, and Void Volume Fractions and Verification of Ply Lay-Up and Orientation

Composite failures can also be the result of improper fiber, matrix, and void volume fractions or incorrect ply lay-up and orientation. For determination of the fiber, matrix, and void volume fractions, two techniques are often used: the chemical matrix digestion method, and the microstructural analysis method. In the chemical matrix digestion method, the composite is first weighed in air and water to determine the density, using the Archimedean principle (that is, that a body immersed in fluid undergoes an apparent loss in weight equal to the weight of the fluid it displaces). The composite is then put into hot nitric acid until the resin is gone and nothing remains but the fibers. The fibers are then weighed, and a calculation is made to determine the volume percentages of the fibers and the resin, using standard density measurements. Fiber, resin, and void volume percentages can be determined as follows:

$$V_f = 100\frac{W_f/\rho_f}{W_c/\rho_c}$$

$$V_r = 100\frac{W_r/\rho_r}{W_c/\rho_c}$$

$$V_v = 100 - \left(100\frac{(W_r/\rho_r)+(W_f/\rho_f)}{W_c/\rho_c}\right)$$

where V is volume percent, W is weight, ρ is density, and subscripts f, r, v, and c are fiber, resin, void, and composite, respectively.

Fiber, matrix, and void volume fractions can also be determined by metallographic means, by taking several cross-sectional samples (Fig. 7) both near and away from the fracture surfaces and using image analysis techniques to determine average percentages of each constituent.

Improper ply lay-up and orientation can also be the cause of failure in composite materials. The number and orientation of plies can be examined through simple metallographic cross-sectioning procedures. The metallographic sections are cut so that they are perpendicular to the 0° or 90° plies, in order to enable relatively easy identification of the ply orientation and lay-up. Sections are then mounted using a cold mounting epoxy resin, so as not to expose the matrix material to the high temperatures used in hot presses. Mounting may not be necessary for laminate samples or for sandwich constructions if the skins are of interest. However, the examination of the core requires mounting for best results. Grinding of the samples is accomplished using standard metallographic techniques similar to that used for metallic specimens. Polishing is best accomplished with wheels covered with cloths without appreciable nap, such as nylon or silk. Diamond lapping films (9 μm) provide a good rough polish in advance of the final steps.

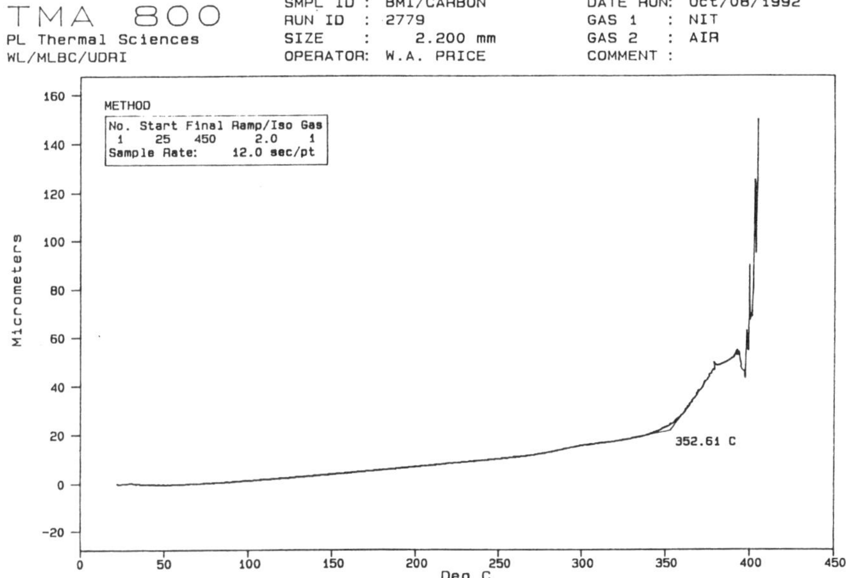

Fig. 5 Thermomechanical analysis (TMA) trace of a carbon/bismaleimide composite

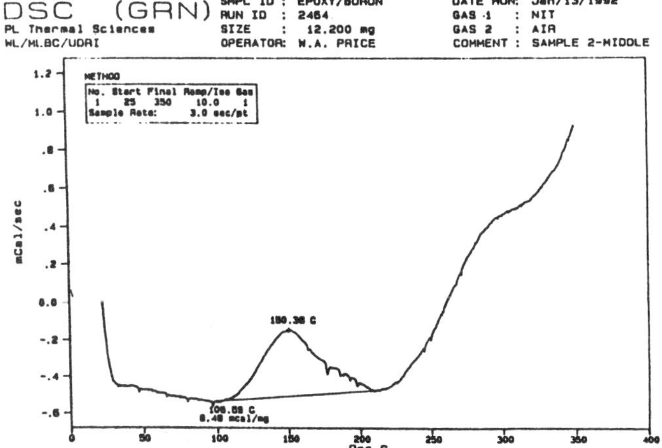

Fig. 6 Differential scanning calorimetry (DSC) trace of an undercured boron/epoxy laminate

Polymer-coated wheels can be used in lieu of cloths with alumina suspensions for final polishing steps. Etching is generally not required, because of the distinct optical differences that exist between most fiber-matrix systems. An exception to this, however, is fiberglass, for which a dilute hydrofluoric acid etch may be necessary to enhance fiber visibility.

The resin-rich regions between the plies often help in the identification of ply lay-up. Additionally, because the fibers in each of the different angular plies exhibit a different profile (round, elliptical, and so on), the orientation of the plies is also usually determined using a simple formula. Known as the fiber ellipse aspect ratio, the angles of the fiber and hence, the plies are determined from the equation:

$$\sin\theta = \frac{2b}{2a}$$

where b is the short transverse radius of the ellipse and a is the long transverse radius of the ellipse. Using cross-sectional metallography for ply orientation verification does not distinguish ± 45 plies, unless the cross section is taken at a 45° angle from the normal direction of the laminate surface.

Review of Composites Processing Parameters

Knowing the exact processing methods used in the manufacture of the component is also useful when evaluating failure cause. Knowing whether the part was manufactured using vacuum bag, press, or autoclave techniques enables the analyst to better understand how the microstructural characteristics of the composite may have affected the overall mechanical properties of the component. For example, autoclaved components generally exhibit better fiber, resin, and void contents and have better consolidation and higher mechanical properties than either press-molded or vacuum-bagged components. In addition to knowing what type of temperature/pressure system was used, the actual cure cycle for the component should be examined to ensure that proper pressures, ramp rate, times at temperature, and cool-down cycles were as specified by the materials supplier.

Fractography and Surface Analysis

Fractography. Composites can exhibit either relatively simple or extremely complex failure modes. Complex failures may include one or more interlaminar, intralaminar, or translaminar fractures, and hence, many fracture surfaces may need to be examined. To reduce the number of surfaces for examination, a decision must be made as to which surfaces are likely to give the most useful information. This decision often represents one of the most difficult tasks involved in composite failure analysis. Generally, the selection of which surfaces to examine depends first upon the predominant failure mode exhibited by the component and second, the necessity to examine the secondary fractures in order to explain the primary fracture.

In general, fractography is used to determine failure mode, initiation site, crack growth direction, and all environmental influences on the failure. For now, it is sufficient to say that translaminar fractures can exhibit tensile, compressive, shear, flexural, or fatigue failure modes, while intra- and interlaminar fractures can exhibit both overload and fatigue in mode I tension, mode II shear, and mixed-mode failure. Additional information regarding features associated with specific loading conditions, as well as crack initiation and propagation direction and features related to environmental exposure, can be found in the article "Fractography" in this Section.

Surface Analysis Techniques. A number of chemical techniques can also be used to define surface contaminants noted during the fractographic evaluation. Some of these techniques include XPS, FTIR spectroscopy, secondary ion mass spectroscopy (SIMS), and Auger electron spectroscopy (AES).

In XPS, a sample is irradiated with x-rays, causing each element to emit photoelectrons at specific energies, thus identifying the elements present. All elements, except hydrogen and helium, can be detected by this method. Fourier transform infrared spectroscopy is a technique for identifying the basic compound or chemical family in which a foreign contaminant might belong. The technique uses a mechanism whereby infrared radiation is absorbed by the material at distinct frequencies associated with characteristic molecular vibrations in the molecules. The result is an infrared spectrum that reveals the characteristic infrared radiation frequencies that relate to the specific chemical bonds. Secondary ion mass spectroscopy is based on energetic ion beam impact of the contaminant, with subsequent ionization and removal of the surface atoms that are then detected with a mass spectrometer. A plot of intensity versus atomic mass units is generated. This technique is used when XPS cannot provide sufficient sensitivity or chemical information regarding the contaminant, but does not work very well on nonconducting composite surfaces. Auger electron spectroscopy is a technique based on the induced Auger electron emission characteristic energy for each element. Many instruments are capable of performing both AES and XPS, but because AES requires a conductive specimen, its application is limited in composites.

Mechanical Testing and Stress Analysis

Mechanical testing is often used in an investigation to determine the effect of various defects or environmental influences on the material. For example, mechanical testing may be required to determine the reduction in compressive properties of a skin or spar that exhibited excessive fiber waviness, high levels of porosity, weak fiber-matrix interfaces, or impact damage that resulted in an undetected delamination. Similarly, tensile or fatigue testing might be required if it is determined that the maximum or minimum loads experienced by the component were more than expected, if the number and/or ori-

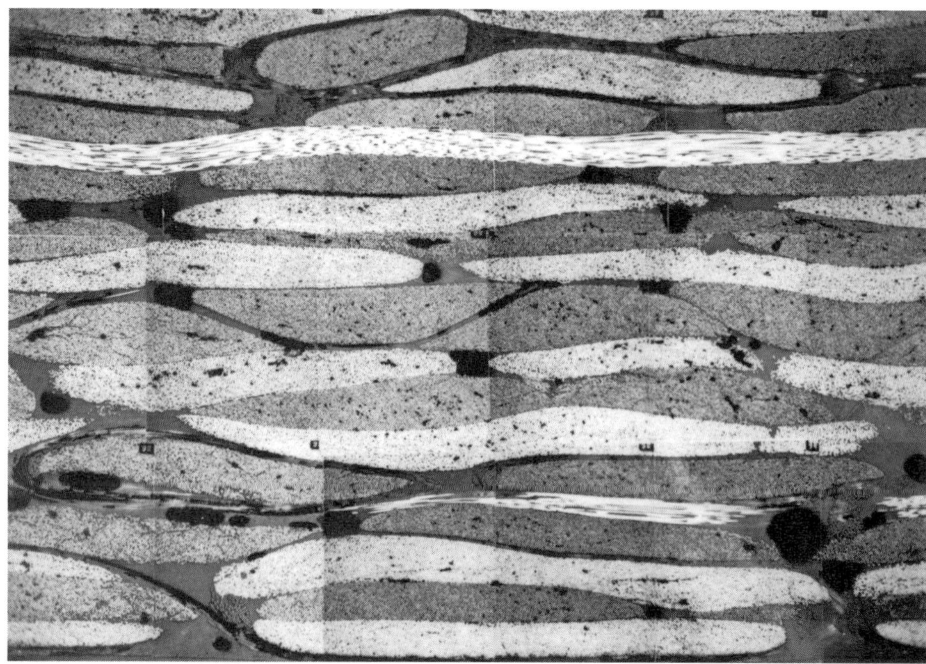

Fig. 7 Micrograph of a cross section obtained from a carbon/epoxy, resin transfer molded component

entation of the plies was different in the part than specified in the design, or if there was an undetected fatigue load noted on the part. Mechanical testing of composite materials is generally conducted using typical ASTM standards. Some of the more common test methods for composites include:

ASTM No.	Title
D 790	Standard Test Methods for Flexural Properties of Unreinforced and Reinforced Plastics and Electrical Insulating Materials
D 2344/D 2344M	Standard Test Method for Short-Beam Shear Strength of Polymer-Matrix Composite Materials and Their Laminates
D 3039/D 3039M	Standard Test Method for Tensile Properties of Polymer-Matrix Composite Materials
D 3410/D 3410M	Standard Test Method for Compressive Properties of Polymer-Matrix Composite Materials with Unsupported Gage Section by Shear Loading
D 3479/D 3479M	Standard Test Method for Tension-Tension Fatigue of Polymer-Matrix Composite Materials
D 4255/D 4255M	Standard Guide for Testing In-Plane Shear Properties of Composite Laminates

Further information regarding mechanical test methods can be found in other Sections in this Volume.

Stress Analysis. In most cases, an accurate understanding of the loads and stress levels in component operation is one of the critical ingredients involved in defining the source of failure. Although fractographic and visual methods of analysis may identify the origin, direction, and mode of crack propagation, stress analysis is the technique that most often provides the quantitative explanation for the failure cause. Through this analysis step, engineers involved in future or corrective redesigns are provided with direct feedback regarding the actual loads experienced by the component, poor design practices and configurations, and the effectiveness of the analysis methods used in the design.

Stress analysis procedures for composite materials can be relatively complex, and because they are fabricated by the lamination of highly anisotropic plies, a nearly infinite variety of directional moduli and strengths can be achieved. Because of this tailorability, a different set of materials properties must be considered for each failure examined. As a further complication, because of their laminated and anisotropic construction, significant variations in stress can exist within the laminate itself. As a result, consideration must be given to failure at the microstructural, or individual ply, as well as the gross, or overall, laminate levels.

Typically, analyses at the individual ply level provide the greatest level of detailed information. This method basically predicts materials properties by modeling the composite as a plate built up from individual plies. The calculated properties may include the effect of hygrothermal expansion, moisture diffusivity, and density of the composite, but are, in general, estimated from individual fiber and resin properties using micromechanics equations. Through this method, the stiffness characteristics of the overall laminate can be determined for the general case of in-plane and/or flexural loads. Based upon this stiffness, the gross stress generated for any given load can be calculated.

However, as noted previously, consideration must also be given to the stresses carried by each individual ply. These stresses depend on the modulus and orientation of each ply and can be determined using basic lamination theory. One of the chief advantages of lamination theory is its ability to quantify these stresses and to examine them on an individual ply level. Although lamination theory provides a powerful tool with which to examine the stress state operating within a composite, there are several disadvantages. The most notable of these is in its application in predicting the onset of failure. Such predictions are achieved by evaluating the stress within each individual ply against semiempirical models that define the maximum stress envelope to which a ply can be exposed without failure. However, predictions of the onset of interlaminar and intralaminar failure using such criteria have not been entirely successful. One of the reasons for this lack of success centers around the fact that standard lamination theory is unable to predict the three-dimensional state of stress that exists in laminates near free edges and other discontinuities, such as holes, cut-outs, and ply drop-offs.

Various approaches can be used, however, to predict the three-dimensional state of stress within a laminate. Typically, these methods, including finite-element analysis, generalized plane strain, three-dimensional elements, and approximate strength-of-materials methods (Ref 1), are relatively specific. Using these methods, failure criteria based on principles of fracture mechanics (Ref 2) have been somewhat successful in predicting the onset and growth of interlaminar and intralaminar matrix damage, including fatigue effects.

The prediction of catastrophic failure at the laminate level has followed two distinctly different approaches. The first, which may be referred to as a statistical approach, uses coupon test data to determine the maximum allowable strains for each laminate design. From this, traditional methods of stress analysis can be applied, load versus area, to determine the occurrence of failure, without regard to individual ply or interlaminar stresses. In this case, failure occurs when the statistically determined maximum allowable strain is exceeded. The second approach to predicting translaminar failure involves a more mechanistic approach in which the load redistribution due to intralaminar and interlaminar matrix damage is taken into account. In its simplest form, this approach can be applied directly with lamination theory and has been referred to as the global ply discount method (Ref 3). Applications of this method rely on a predetermined definition of characteristic intralaminar and interlaminar damage. Using the lamination theory, the state of stress surrounding this damage is defined, and the magnitude of the applied load necessary to create failure is determined.

Conclusions

This section was aimed at describing some of the numerous techniques used in the analysis of failed composite structure. Although the techniques described are not all-inclusive by any means, it is hoped that the number and variety of techniques outlined in this section are adequate for an investigator to begin his analyses. Further information regarding composite failure analysis techniques, fractographic data, and case history studies can be found in Ref 4. More detailed information on failure analysis in general can be found in *Failure Analysis and Prevention*, Volume 11 of *ASM Handbook*.

ACKNOWLEDGMENTS

This article was adapted from B.W. Smith, Failure Analysis Procedures, *Composites*, Vol 1, *Engineered Materials Handbook*, ASM International, 1987, p 770–778.

REFERENCES

1. W.S. Johnson, Ed., *Delamination and Debonding of Materials,* STP 876, American Society for Testing and Materials, 1985
2. A.S.D. Wang, "Fracture Mechanics of Sub-Laminate Cracks in Composite Laminates in AGARD, Conf. Characterization Analysis and Significance of Defects in Composite Materials AGARD CP-355," Advisory Group for Aerospace Research and Development, 1983
3. K.L. Reifsnider, K. Schultz, and J.C. Duke, Long-Term Fatigue Behavior of Composite Materials, *Long-Term Behavior of Composites,* T.K. O'Brien, Ed., STP 813, American Society for Testing and Materials, 1983, p 136–159
4. *Composite Failure Analysis Handbook,* distributed by CINDAS/USAF CRDA Handbooks Operation, Purdue University, Lafayette, IN, Feb 1992

Visual Analysis, Nondestructive Testing, and Destructive Testing

Patricia L. Stumpff, Hartzell Propeller, Inc.

MECHANICAL AND ENVIRONMENTAL LOADINGS cause a variety of failure modes in composites, including matrix cracking, fiber-matrix debonding, delamination between plies, and fiber breakage. A cumulative state of damage for a composite includes a percentage of each of these loading-related failure modes as well as materials defects originating from processing, which include voids, fiber-rich or matrix-rich regions, fiber misalignment, and laminate stacking errors. The integrated effect of the cumulative damage state of the composite results in the final failure mode. Therefore, to analyze and understand a composite failure, one must recognize the complexity and extent of damage that might have been present before final failure.

Visual analysis, nondestructive testing, and destructive testing are all important techniques in failure analysis of composites. Visual analysis usually is the first and perhaps most important step in failure analysis. In many cases, the diagnosis can be made by visual examination, and testing is performed to confirm or contradict it. Many experimental nondestructive and destructive test techniques have been developed to measure damage levels in composites. Nondestructive testing (NDT) techniques may be categorized as field (bulk) methods or detail (micro) methods, depending on the type of information they yield. Field methods provide test parameters that are a function of the volume of material interrogated by the NDT technique, but do not provide microscopic information on the actual type of damage present. Detail methods provide information on the microscopic damage state. As a general rule, two or more NDT methods should be used to provide complementary information on the state of damage to composites. This article summarizes useful NDT methods for failure analysis; more detail on NDT techniques is provided in the article "Nondestructive Testing" in this Volume. Destructive techniques are quite useful in the laboratory for evaluating materials response, but obviously have limited use for in-service applications.

Visual Analysis

Visual analysis of failed polymer-matrix composites can provide a significant amount of information regarding failure cause. In particular, examination of a composite fracture can be useful in determining the crack initiation site, crack growth direction, fracture sequence, and failure mode.

Crack Initiation, Growth Direction, and Failure Mode. For transverse fractures, initiation site and crack growth direction can often be ascertained by an analysis of the crack pattern. Transverse cracks in a laminate can exhibit the feature known as crack branching, with increases in the number of the branches generally indicative of increasing crack propagation direction. In Fig. 1, the branched crack in the graphite-epoxy wing box is indicative of crack growth in the component from right to left. Other features visually apparent on the fracture surfaces are indicative of failure mode. Figure 2 reveals a transverse fracture of a graphite-epoxy composite wing section, which failed in bending. The upper

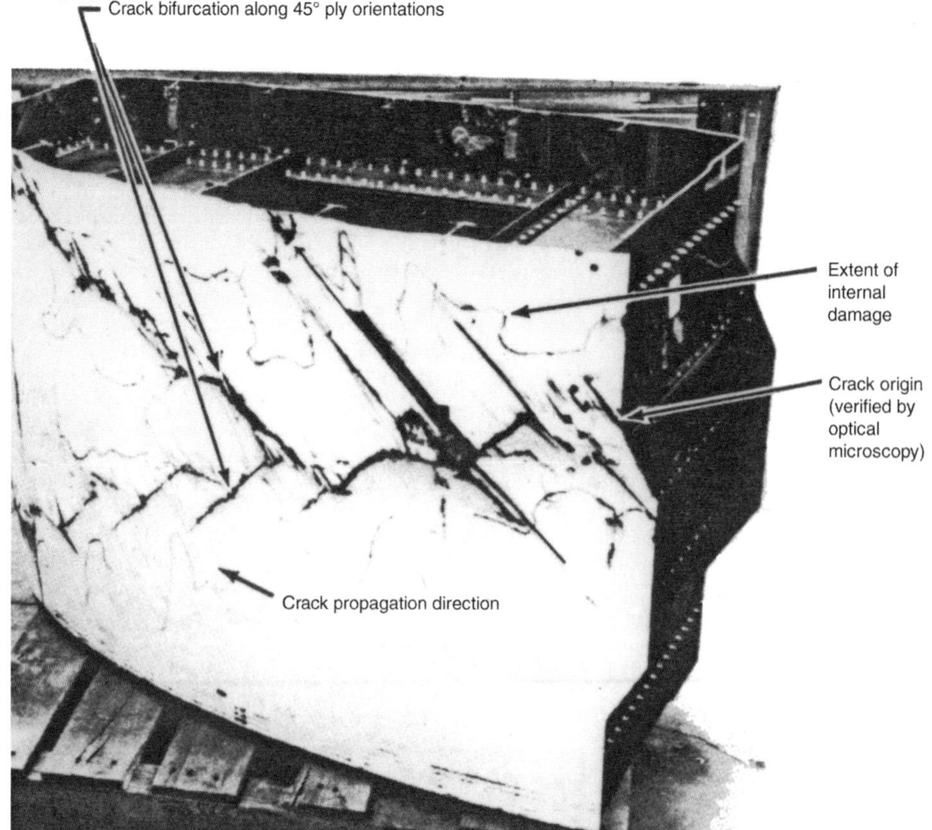

Fig. 1 Crack branching indicative of crack growth direction in transverse fractures. ~0.02×

skin surface exhibits a relatively flat fracture surface with minimal fiber pullout, indicative of a compressive failure, whereas the lower skin surface exhibits a roughened fracture surface with extensive fiber pullout, indicative of tensile failure.

For delaminated fracture surfaces, crack initiation and crack growth direction may be ascertained using the fracture feature known as banding. Banding, identified by the white arrows in Fig. 3, often appears on delaminated surfaces formed following a Mode I tensile or mixed-mode failure of the specimen. Banding generally indicates crack growth direction from the convex to the concave side of the bands, with the banding in Fig. 3 depicting crack growth from left to right.

Other features on the delaminated surfaces are indicative of failure mode. In graphite-epoxy materials, Mode II shear failures are generally less reflective than Mode I tensile failures. Mode II shear failures generally exhibit a dull, "whitish" appearance, whereas Mode I tensile failures generally exhibit a shiny, black surface appearance. The difference in reflectivity between these two failure modes is thought to be due to the difference in actual fracture features, with hackles formed on surfaces failed in shear, and river patterns formed on the surfaces failed in tension. The differences in reflectivity not only help in the interpretation of Mode I tension versus Mode II shear failure, but can also help in the identification of prior impact damage in a laminate. A graphite-epoxy laminate with internal delaminations due to impact damage was opened at a delaminated surface by Mode I tensile loading. One side of the partially delaminated, and now fully separated, surface is shown in Fig. 4. The internal delamination (area surrounded by arrows in the figure) resulting from the impact damage exhibits a whitish appearance, whereas the newly separated, Mode I tensile failure had a dark, reflective surface appearance. The differences in reflectivity are thought to be the result of the differences in failure modes, with the impact region in this specimen more representative of a combination of compression and Mode II shear failure, and the separated region more indicative of Mode I tensile failure.

Other fracture features can also be indicative of crack growth direction and failure mode. Figure 5 is a photo depicting numerous small cracks found in the resin of a fractured, graphite-epoxy wing spar. These cracks were visually evident and progressed along the length of the delaminated spar interfaces. Further investigation into the cause of the spar failure revealed that it failed as a result of the wings going into a flutter-failure mode, which then resulted in the extensive, progressive cracking noted along the length of the spar. Further evidence of a dynamic failure such as flutter was found on the transverse fracture surfaces of the spar. The transverse fractures exhibited extensive smearing of the entire fracture surface, a feature not generally found in overload failures of a component.

Fracture Sequence. In addition to crack growth direction and failure mode, however, composite materials often require the determination of fracture sequence in order to identify an initiation site. Fracture initiation and sequence in composite materials can sometimes be difficult to determine, although detailed fractographic analyses of the fracture surfaces can help. Figure 6 depicts a cross section of a composite specimen that was overheated on one side of the sample and then failed in compression. The failed specimen contains both delaminated and transverse fractures. To determine whether the delamination(s) occurred prior to the transverse fracture, the following techniques can be employed. Figure 7 depicts mating fracture surfaces of a delamination obtained from a complex specimen failed in compression. The failed specimen itself exhibited numerous transverse fractures and delaminations, but not all the plies exhibited transverse failure. In this case, only one of the two neighboring plies exhibited a full transverse fracture. Upon examination of the ply without the complete transverse fracture, evidence of the transverse cracking and damage of the opposite ply (reference the damage between the two arrows) can be seen. The fact that the transverse fracture of one ply is evident on the surface of the delaminated ply most probably indicates that the two plies were not delaminated or separated prior to the transverse fracture of the first ply. It is also possible, however, that the two plies were initially delaminated, but not actually separated, when the transverse fracture occurred.

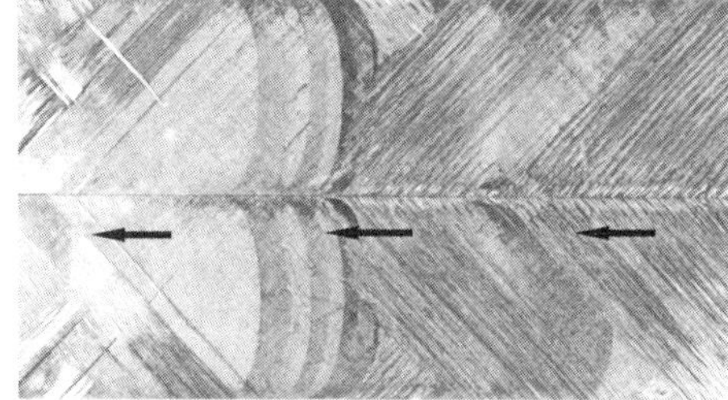

Fig. 3 Delaminated surface revealing beach marks (arrow) indicative of mixed-mode failure in a graphite-epoxy laminate. ~0.7×

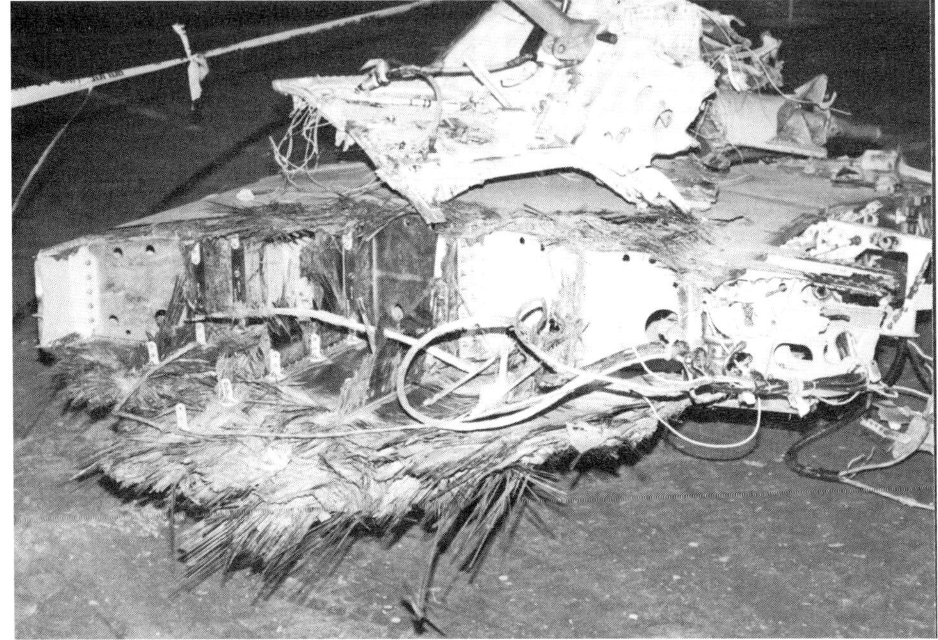

Fig. 2 Flexural failure of a graphite-epoxy wing box. ~0.03×

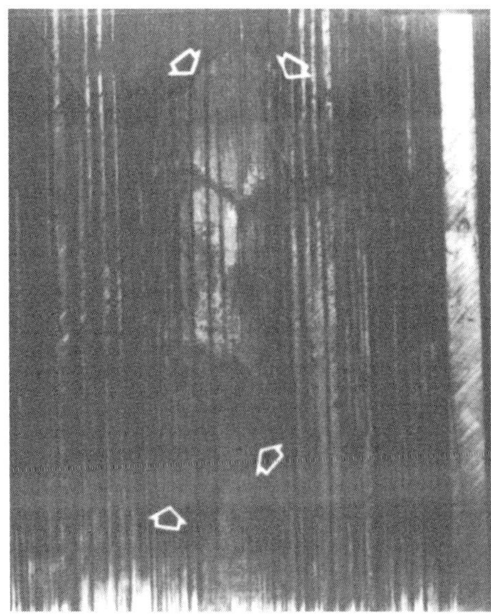

Fig. 4 Reflectivity differences on a delaminated fracture surface indicative of impact damage. ~0.5×

Figure 8 also depicts how fracture sequence information can be gleaned from visual examination of the fracture surfaces. In this figure, numerous transverse cracks are evident in the thick adhesive layer between the wing skin and its mating spar. The cracks in the adhesive are curved, with the convex surface toward the inboard side of the wing, and the spacing between the cracks increasing as the cracks move outboard. This curvature and increased spacing of the transverse fractures in the adhesive indicate that the fracture initiated at inboard section of the wing and progressed outboard. Additionally, because the transverse cracking in the adhesive is evident on the surfaces of both the wing spar and the wing skin, it is believed that this transverse cracking in the adhesive is the cause of the skin/spar separations. Had there been any separation of the skin or the spar from the adhesive prior to the transverse cracking, no evidence of adhesive cracking would have been found on the separated surface. Evidence of the transverse cracks in the adhesive, however, was noted on both skin and spar surfaces throughout the failure location.

Other Information from Visual Analysis. Other information about the failure can be obtained from a visual analysis of the variations in the color of the resin and/or the adhesive. Variations from the original resin/adhesive color can be indicative of moisture absorption, undercure, overheat exposure, or the actual amount of resin or adhesive on the surface or within the plies.

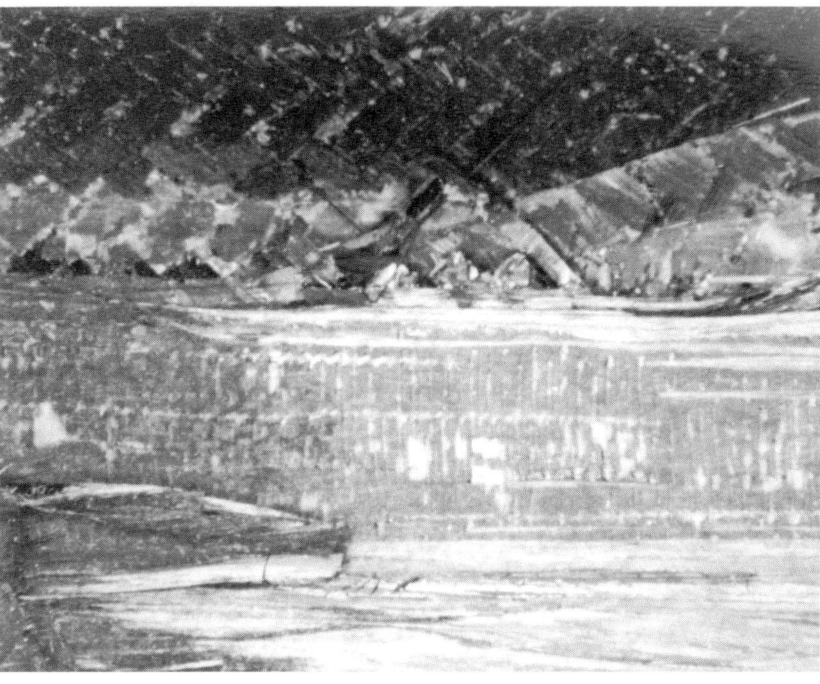

Fig. 5 Longitudinal cracks on a delaminated fracture surface indicative of progressive fracture. ~5×

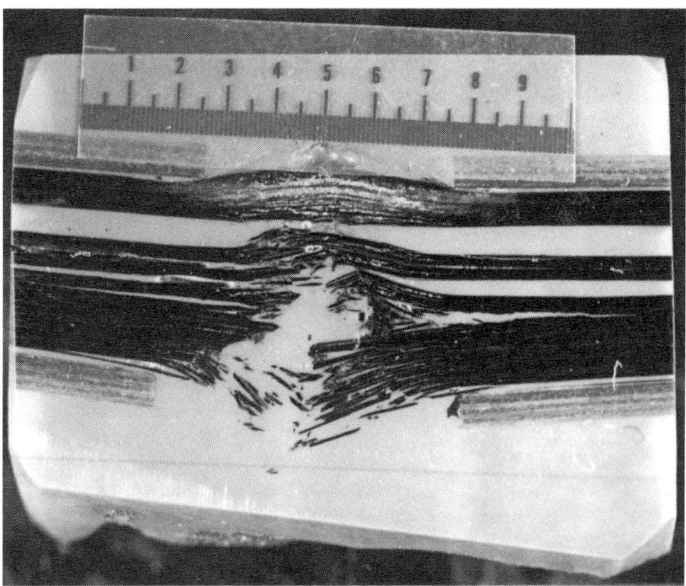

Fig. 6 Cross section of a composite laminate, which failed in compression, containing both delaminations and transverse fractures for examination of fracture sequence. ~2×

Nondestructive Test Techniques

Determining failure modes in a composite is often better performed before final catastrophic failure. Incrementally studying the mechanical state of the composite that is a result of previous loading is useful even though no definitive knowledge exists as to how the final failure event itself would have been related to the damage state prior to failure. Nondestructive tests are performed prior to final failure either in real time—by continuously monitoring the composite during service (or testing in the laboratory)—or at selected service intervals by removing the composite from the load environment to perform the tests. Nondestructive testing is also performed on components after failure, but just prior to destructive analysis.

The lack of definition as to what constitutes "important" damage necessitates searching for all indications of damage. Because NDT methods have different sensitivities to different types of damage, it is usually necessary to apply several NDT techniques to the same specimen to obtain complementary information on the damage state. In addition to matrix cracking, fiber-matrix debonding, delamination between plies, and fiber breakage, all of which are loading-related damages, other important types of damage resulting from the manufacturing process are

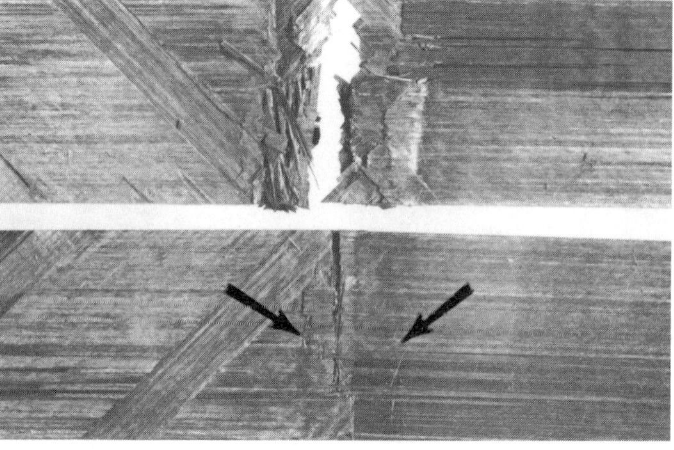

Fig. 7 Examination of separated plies in a graphite-epoxy laminate to determine sequence of fracture. ~0.8×

voids, foreign objects, misalignment of fibers, and either bunching or lack of fibers.

To monitor damage progression in composites, a number of NDT methods used with homogeneous materials have been modified and adapted. These techniques include edge replication, stiffness measurement, radiography, ultrasonics, acoustic emission, and thermography.

Surface or edge replication is a technique that has found wide application by materials scientists studying surface topography. Because replication tape is typically used to record the surface topography along the edge of a composite laminate, the method is known as edge replication. The technique only requires application of: cellulose-acetate tape (or solution) to the surface, a solvent such as acetone to one side of the tape to soften and partially dissolve it, and a small amount of pressure to the back side of the softened tape so that it will conform to the surface of the material. When the tape hardens, it can be removed from the surface and will carry with it a record of the surface topography at the time the replica was made (Fig. 9).

This technique was first applied by D.O. Stalnaker and W.W. Stinchcomb (Ref 1) to the study of composites. Since their early work, edge replication has been used by a large number of investigators and is currently recognized as a standard technique for following the development of damage in composites. J.E. Masters and K.L. Reifsnider (Ref 2) applied the technique extensively to composite laminates and found that it provided a very good record of damage progression. Information on damage at the specimen edge provides an accurate record of the transverse cracks occurring in the specimen. Evidence suggests that, at least for laboratory-sized specimens, the cracks observable along the edge run through the entire width of the specimen.

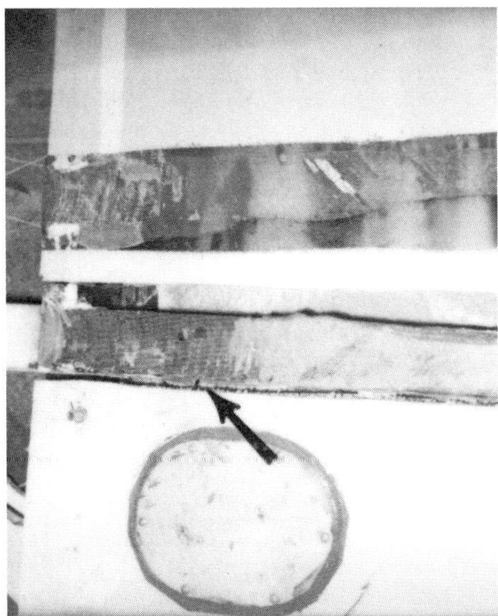

Fig. 8 Mating fracture surfaces of an adhesively bonded wing skin and wing spar. ~0.2×

Edge replication can be used to ascertain the degree to which the "characteristic damage state" has been achieved. This concept, developed by K.L. Reifsnider et al. (Ref 3), describes the state at which a saturated number of transverse cracks develop in each off-axis ply of a composite laminate as a result of tensile loading. Attaining the characteristic damage state corresponds to the knee of the bilinear stress-strain curve in a number of laminates (Ref 3).

Stiffness. The elastic modulus of a composite laminate can be predicted using classical laminate theory (Ref 4) based on the concept of ideal laminate behavior; that is, it assumes that each lamina has its respective elastic properties and is bonded to its neighbor without delaminations, and that no damage exists in the laminae to affect their individual elastic properties. As a laminate is quasi-statically loaded to high stress levels or fatigue loaded, damage (such as transverse cracking) develops in the plies. This damage affects laminae stiffnesses and results in as much as 20 to 30% stiffness degradation of the entire laminate, depending on the laminate stacking sequence.

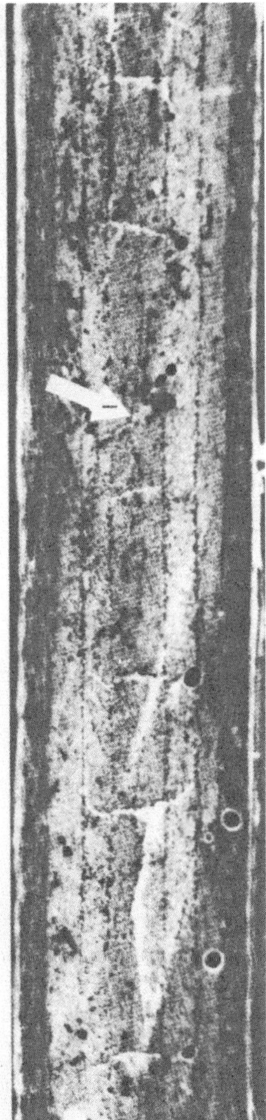

Fig. 9 Edge replica of graphite-epoxy specimen

Stiffness degradation in a graphite-epoxy laminate resulting from fatigue loading is shown in Fig. 10. Each of the tensorial stiffness components is affected to some degree (Ref 5). Therefore, stiffness measurement is an acceptable technique for monitoring the degree of damage development in a material. Following the work of T.K. O'Brien and K.L. Reifsnider (Ref 5), stiffness measurements can be made for each of the in-plane tensor elastic moduli. In general, a better correlation between stiffness degradation and damage development is obtained when measurements are made over a relatively large specimen length. For example, when using extensometers, a 5 cm (2 in.) gage length will give better results than a 2.5 cm (1 in.) gage length because the greater the length integrated, the more inhomogeneities in the damage state can be averaged out.

Radiography is an NDT technique that can provide extensive and detailed information on the state of damage. A variety of penetrating particles and rays, including neutron, gamma, and x-ray, are used to study composites. Detailed information on radiography techniques is provided in the article "Nondestructive Testing" in this Volume.

Ultrasonic techniques are most frequently used for nondestructive inspection of composites. Various materials properties, including stiffness (through the measurement of elastic wave speeds), volume fraction of voids, and attenuation, in addition to various damage modes, including delamination and matrix cracking, are monitored by different ultrasonic methods. Velocity measurement, attenuation measurement, C-scan, and acousto-ultrasonics are ultrasonic techniques that are related, but are distinguished differently, depending on how the data are obtained, analyzed, and presented. Detailed information on ultrasonic testing techniques is provided in the article "Nondestructive Testing" in this Volume.

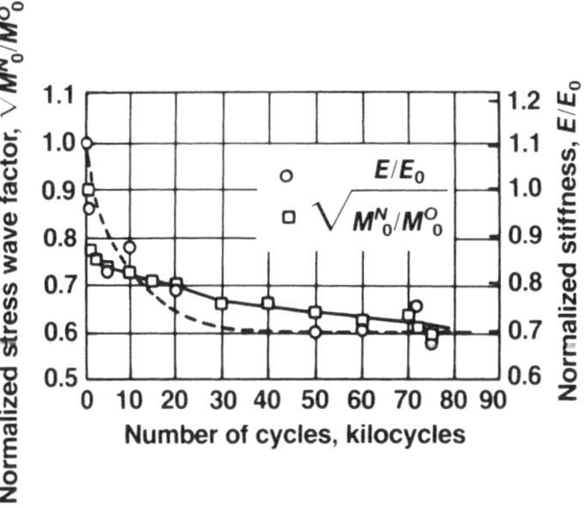

Fig. 10 Change in acousto-ultrasonic stress wave parameter during fatigue test of graphite-epoxy specimen

Acoustic emission (AE) is a phenomenon familiar to metallurgists; mechanical twinning in tin and tin alloys is known as "tin cry." Composite materials are equally noisy under load, particularly during quasi-static tension testing; therefore, AE has received significant attention as a technique for monitoring damage development in composites. An article by M.A. Hamstad (Ref 6) reviews use of AE as a tool for composite material studies, including the following studies, which are pertinent to damage analysis: time-dependent composite properties, impact, relationship of AE-detected damage to other measures of damage, interface, and environmental effects.

Many researchers have attempted to develop AE testing to the point that different failure modes could be distinguished by their respective acoustic emissions. However, no definitive conclusions can be made at present. Several authors have suggested that failure modes might be distinguished by grouping received signals according to energy levels; Ref 7 indicates that there are three distinct energy-level groupings that indicate the differing amounts of energy emitted from fiber breakage, matrix cracking, and delamination. Additional studies of AE in composites need to be performed.

Thermography, or surface mapping of isothermal contour lines, can be performed through a variety of techniques, but use of a video-thermographic camera is the most efficient and offers the highest resolution.

Because matter emits infrared radiation with an intensity dependent upon its absolute temperature and surface emissivity, infrared energy-sensitive sensors can be used indirectly to measure the temperature of the emitting surface. Other materials parameters, specifically surface emissivity, affect the intensity of the emitted radiation and thus the value of the measured temperature. However, as the only concern is relative temperature differences (as in nondestructive inspection for damage), this is of minor concern as long as care is taken to condition the examined surface to ensure that the emissivity is as uniform as possible across the entire surface.

Thermography has been used by a number of investigators to detect and analyze damage in composites (Ref 7–12). Thermal gradients are generated using either a passive or active method to delineate defects or damage. In the passive method, an external heat source is applied to the material. Heat may be conducted either into or away from the examined object by an external heat source of either higher or lower temperature. In the active method, energy is applied in a form other than thermal, such as electrical or mechanical energy. Heat is generated by internal mechanisms that transform the applied energy into thermal energy. In either method, differences in the local properties of the material affect heat conduction or heat generation through the region surrounding the damage, thus delineating areas of damage. Both the passive and active methods have been used to examine composites (Ref 11, 12).

Additional information on thermography is provided in the article "Nondestructive Testing" in this Volume.

Destructive Test Techniques

Destructive test techniques are also useful for studying damage in composite materials whether the objective is to develop fundamental knowledge of materials response in the research laboratory, or to analyze a materials failure. Most of these techniques are similar to those used to evaluate homogeneous metal and alloy systems. Therefore, only those two methods peculiar to studying composite failures are described here.

Matrix digestion techniques are used to determine fiber and void-volume fractions in both metallic- and organic-matrix composites. The volume fraction of the fiber present is an important aspect of failure analysis because it is used to determine the apparent strength and modulus of the reinforcing fibers in the composite. Void content is one indication of the quality of the fabrication process and resulting material.

Standard test methods (Ref 13, 14) have been established for both metallic- and organic-matrix composites. The test procedure requires a sample of the material to be weighed and its volume determined by a fluid displacement technique so that the density of the composite can be calculated. The sample is then placed in a hot, liquid medium that can specifically digest the matrix. The mixture is filtered, and the residue is dried and weighed to determine the amount of fiber present. If the density of the fiber is known, the volume fraction of fiber, V_f, present in the composite sample is:

$$V_f = \frac{(W_f / \rho_f)}{(W_c / \rho_c)} \quad \text{(Eq 1)}$$

where W_f is the fiber weight, W_c is the composite weight, ρ_f is the fiber density, and ρ_c is the composite density. If, in addition, the matrix density, ρ_m, is also known, the same measurements can be used to calculate the volume fraction of void content, V_v, present in the sample:

$$V_v = 1 - \left\{ \frac{\left[W_f/\rho_f + (W_c - W_f)/\rho_m \right]}{(W_c/\rho_c)} \right\} \quad \text{(Eq 2)}$$

It is sometimes necessary to make corrections for loss of fiber material during the digestion process if the fiber material has some degree of solubility in or reactivity to the digestion mixture.

The deply technique developed by S.M. Freeman (Ref 15) provides information on the discrete nature of fiber fracture in the interior of a layered composite and is presently used with organic-matrix composites. A sample is heated for a predetermined time period at a temperature sufficient to partially pyrolyze the resin matrix. This process diminishes the interlaminar bond strength to the point that the individual plies can be easily separated by simply applying a piece of adhesive tape to the top lamina, peeling it off, and continuing in the same manner through the laminate, ply by ply. Each lamina can then be examined in an optical or scanning electron microscope (in the latter case, after applying a graphitic or metallic surface coat using a sputtering technique, if fibers are electrically nonconducting). Individual broken fibers can then be easily detected.

Freeman also observed that an image-enhancing agent could be used to delineate in each ply the regions adjacent to delaminations or matrix cracks. This is accomplished by applying a gold chloride solution to the composite before pyrolysis to penetrate cracks and delaminations. During pyrolysis, the solution breaks down and leaves a residue of gold, which demarcates any crack or delamination. When viewed under the microscope, the relationship between broken fibers and cracking/delamination is easily deduced (Ref 16).

Additional information about destructive tests for composites is provided in the Sections "Quality Assurance" and "Testing and Certification" in this Volume.

ACKNOWLEDGMENT

Portions of this article are adapted from E.G. Henneke, Destructive and Nondestructive Tests, *Composites,* Volume 1, *Engineered Materials Handbook,* ASM International, 1987, p 774–778.

REFERENCES

1. D.O. Stalnaker and W.W. Stinchcomb, Load History—Edge Damage Studies in Two Quasi-Isotropic Graphite Epoxy Laminates, *Composite Materials: Testing and Design (Fifth Conference)*, STP 674, S.W. Tsai, Ed., American Society for Testing and Materials, 1979, p 620–641
2. J.E. Masters and K.L. Reifsnider, An Investigation of Cumulative Damage Development in Quasi-Isotropic Graphite/Epoxy Laminates, *Damage in Composite Materials*, STP 775, K.L. Reifsnider, Ed., American Society for Testing and Materials, 1982, p 40–62
3. K.L. Reifsnider, E.G. Henneke, and W.W. Stinchcomb, "Defect-Property Relationships in Composite Laminate," AFML Final Report 76-81, Air Force Materials Laboratory, June 1979
4. R.M. Jones, *Mechanics of Composite Materials*, McGraw-Hill, 1975
5. T.K. O'Brien and K.L. Reifsnider, Fatigue Damage: Stiffness/Strength Comparisons for Composite Materials, *J. Test. Eval.*, Vol 5 (No. 5), 1977, p 384–393

6. M.A. Hamstad, A Review: Acoustic Emission, a Tool for Composite Materials Studies, *Exp. Mech*., Vol 26 (No. 1), March 1986, p 7–13
7. J. Awerbuch, M.R. Gorman, and M. Madhudar, Monitoring Acoustic Emission During Quasi-Static Loading-Unloading Cycles of Filament-Wound Graphite-Epoxy Laminate Coupons, *Mater. Eval*., Vol 43 (No. 6), 1985, p 754–764
8. R.T. Schaum, "Development of a Nondestructive Inspection Technique for Advanced Composite Materials Using Cholesteric Liquid Crystals," AD-A032322, National Technical Information Service, Sept 1976
9. J.D. Whitcomb, Thermographic Measurement of Fatigue Damage, *Composite Materials: Testing and Design,* STP 674, S.W. Tsai, Ed., American Society for Testing and Materials, 1979, p 502–516
10. E.G. Henneke and T.S. Jones, Detection of Damage in Composite Materials by Vibrothermography, *Nondestructive Evaluation Flaw Criticality*, STP 696, R.B. Pipes, Ed., American Society for Testing and Materials, 1979, p 83–95
11. S.S. Russell and E.G. Henneke, Dynamic Effects During Vibrothermographic NDE of Composites, *NDT Int*., Vol 17 (No. 1), Feb 1984, p 19–25
12. P.V. McLaughlin, E.V. McAssey, and R.C. Deitrich, Nondestructive Examination of Fiber Composite Structures by Thermal Field Techniques, *NDT Int*., Vol 13 (No. 2), p 56–62
13. "Standard Test Method for Fiber Content of Resin-Matrix Composites by Matrix Digestion," D 3171, *Annual Book of ASTM Standards*, American Society for Testing and Materials
14. "Standard Test Method for Fiber Content by Digestion of Reinforced Metal Matrix Composites," D 3553, *Annual Book of ASTM Standards*, American Society for Testing and Materials
15. S.M. Freeman, Characterization of Lamina and Interlaminar Damage in Graphite-Epoxy Composites by the Deply Technique, *Composite Materials: Testing and Design (Sixth Conference)*, STP 787, I.M. Daniel, Ed., American Society for Testing and Materials, 1982, p 50–62
16. R.D. Jamison, "Advanced Fatigue Damage Development in Graphite Epoxy Laminates," Ph.D. thesis, Virginia Polytechnic Institute and State University, 1982

Microscopy

Brian S. Hayes, University of Washington
Luther M. Gammon, The Boeing Company

MICROSCOPY is a valuable tool in materials investigations related to problem solving, failure analysis, advanced materials development, and quality control. Microscopy has been used for many decades to provide insight into the microstructure and macrostructure of fiber reinforced composites (FRC). The most widespread use of microscopy for composites is determining void content, ply counts, and fiber orientations. While this makes up the majority of analysis, the investigation of failure mechanisms and microstructural analysis is also common. Furthermore, insight into fiber morphology, matrix modifiers, fillers, and process parameters of composite materials are also elucidated using microscopy techniques.

For most cases, standard reflected light microscopy provides most of the necessary information one would desire. In some cases however, etchants, stains, or dyes may be required for further clarification of the morphology or crack identification. If reflected light techniques do not yield the required information, transmitted-light optical microscopy can provide insights into the microstructures of materials that would otherwise remain hidden when using standard bulk metallographic preparation techniques and reflected illumination. Because most polymeric materials are inert to metallographic etchants, they can be best observed with transmitted polarized light and various contrast media to enhance the differences in refractive index of discrete phases in the composite.

Although an array of different types of composite materials are in use today, the utilization of both thermosetting and thermoplastic (polymer) matrix fiber reinforced composites (PMC) continues to dominate the field in terms of both volume and applications (Ref 1). This is due to easy processing, a wide range of materials and properties, and a much lower cost than that of other composite materials, such as metal matrix (MMC) and ceramic matrix composites (CMC). While not to discount the limited use of other types of composites, all of these heterogeneous and anisotropic materials have unique properties and characteristics lending their use in specific applications.

Throughout this article, the easiest, most cost-effective, and reproducible techniques the authors have found for sample preparation, polishing, and analysis are emphasized. The most common types of composite materials, PMC, are the primary focus, but preparation methods for other composite materials are also discussed.

Sample Preparation

Sectioning. The first question to ask when analyzing a composite material with light microscopy is what type of information is desired. Once this is determined, the part or sample must be systematically and meticulously documented and labeled. After labeling the samples, the composite part typically needs to be sectioned so that it is manageable for polishing. It is important in this stage that no damage is done to the specimen so that artifacts are not introduced. Therefore, when sectioning the part, never use a band saw with a tooth blade, because it may damage the specimen. Instead, use an abrasive band saw to cut large parts down to a manageable size. Rough cutting may be performed without lubrication or cutting fluids; however, a vacuum apparatus should be used to minimize dust. For final composite specimen cutting, an abrasive cut-off saw with coolant should be used to minimize damage to the specimen. The use of coolant is necessary since increases in temperature during cutting can alter the microstructure of polymer matrices. In general, thin blades reduce damage and material loss; however, thin blades may bend, resulting in a nonplanar surface. Additionally, thin blades are more likely to break during cutting that can be quite costly.

In some cases, if the sample is small enough or after rough cutting, it can be ground down to the required size with the use of 60 or 120 grit silicon carbide (SiC) paper. It is important to realize that the use of 60 grit paper can damage the specimen, so care must be taken when using it for grinding. To use this technique, the ground edge of the sample must be stout enough so that it is not destroyed during the removal process or distorted. For thin materials, the specimen must be mounted first to resist deformation and then ground down to size. This grinding operation should also be done with ample cooling water so that the temperature is not increased.

Before mounting the specimens, thoroughly cleaning the samples to remove any particulates from the cutting or sectioning process is necessary. Also, at this point, any greases or oils (e.g., kerosene from cutting) that may have come in contact with the specimens must be removed. This will enable optimum adhesion of the specimens to the mounting resin during the mounting procedure. Specimen preparation is a key aspect that determines the quality of the microstructural information that can be obtained.

Mounting the Sample. The best mount is no mount, meaning that the specimen is prepared and polished without the use of a permanent mounting resin or material. Automated polishers have holders that allow easy mounting of the specimens by mechanical clamping or grips. The benefit is that after polishing, the specimens may be removed and directly viewed. Likewise, the original sample identifications are easier to discern. A rectangular holder with a 35 by 76 mm (1.4 by 3.0 in.) opening works very well for both laminate and honeycomb composite materials. With this type of mount it is necessary to use scrap backup pieces to protect the edges. After polishing, these scrap pieces can be easily removed. For carbon fiber reinforced polymer (CFRP) samples, CFRP backup pieces are recommended, as the material removal rates will be well matched. The same is true with other composite materials: backup pieces of similar materials and hardness provide superior results. Using this method, void analysis and ply-count specimens may be prepared quickly with excellent results.

Hand-polishing unmounted specimens is possible but often difficult. The long and narrow nature of most composite samples makes it difficult to maintain a high-quality flat surface free of artifacts. Additionally, the edges are prone to tearing the polishing cloth. With special exceptions, this is the least favorable specimen preparation method.

Fragile materials, multiple samples, or samples with surface features require support to ensure a flat planar surface. The use of a mounting medium such as epoxy, polyester, or acrylic resin is necessary. Of these resins, epoxy is preferred, since it has the least shrinkage during cure. Room temperature curing resins are often ideal;

however, they frequently need to be cured at least 8 h at 20 °C (68 °F), as oven curing may increase shrinkage. To ensure full impregnation of the specimens, the mold can be placed in a vacuum impregnation chamber while infusing the resin. The use of moderate vacuum to remove entrapped air, followed by applying pressure during cure, is highly effective for sample preparation and creating good adhesion.

The following steps are recommended to achieve a good mounted specimen without voids or specimen pull-out:

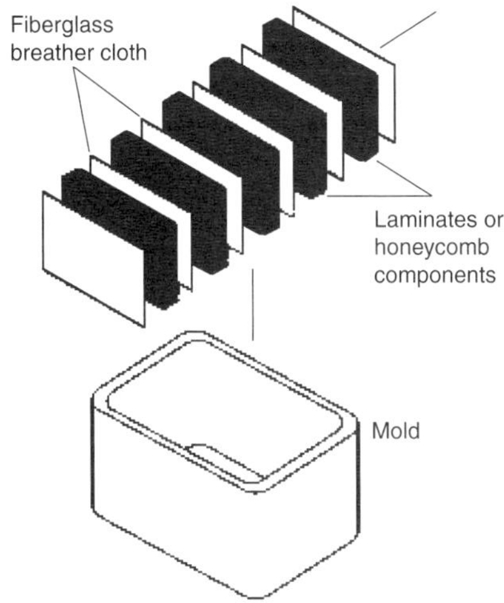

Fig. 1 Schematic showing the mounting of composite specimens in a rubber mold. Note the glass breather cloth used for separation of the samples.

1. Select a mold to hold the specimens and rinse with mold release agent. Silicone rubber molds are the most convenient and can be used repeatedly. A convenient size mold for composite specimens is 57 by 25 by 25 mm (2.2 by 1.0 by 1.0 in.). The resulting samples may be used in automated polishers, hand-polishing applications, and thin sections. Circular plastic molds can also be used for these applications but are not as convenient for mounting or for polishing later.
2. Wash and degrease the samples to create a clean interface to bond to the mounting resin.
3. Completely dry all the components of the sample before mounting. A vacuum desiccator or low-temperature, 40 to 50 °C (105 to 120 °F), drying oven should be considered for at least 12 h.
4. Place dry specimens in the mold and position a strip of loosely woven glass cloth between the flat adjacent surfaces of the sample. This will ensure sufficient wetting with the resin (Fig. 1). The glass fabric allows the resin to impregnate (wick) between the specimens, no matter how tightly they are packed together. This provides the best possible bonding of the specimens so that the mounted sample does not come apart during the grinding and polishing stages.
5. When possible, excess specimens should be used for backup material within the mount to aid in polishing. As a general rule, use materials with the same mechanical properties for the best support.
6. Vacuum impregnate the specimens in the mold with epoxy resin. After the impregnation step, it is recommended that the mount be pressure cured using at least 400 kPa (58 psi) for 12 h at 21 °C (70 °F). The time depends on the epoxy mounting resin selected since curing times may vary.

While the previous mounting directions focused on filling specimens in a preset-sized mold, followed by impregnation, another type of mounting is also beneficial for manual or hand polishing. This type mounting is quite fast and economical. Samples can be mounted, polished, and viewed within 20 min. The mount for manual polishing can be prepared as follows (Fig. 2):

1. Cut samples of the laminate or honeycomb specimen into strips that are 25 to 65 mm (1.0 to 2.6 in.) long by 12 to 25 mm (0.5 to 1.0 in.) high (Fig. 2a).
2. Cut sacrificial side panels that are 12 mm (0.5 in.) longer than the subject specimens, using scrap laminates of a similar material to create a custom mold (Fig. 2b).
3. Tightly hold and bind the sample together on five sides with gray vinyl electrical tape or an equivalent product. The open side should be opposite the side to be polished (Fig. 2c).
4. Fill the custom mold with 5 min epoxy. The result is a mount that can be handled easily and maximizes the surface area of the sample. After the specimen is cured, the gray vinyl tape can be easily peeled off, leaving the specimen ready to polish (Fig. 2d).

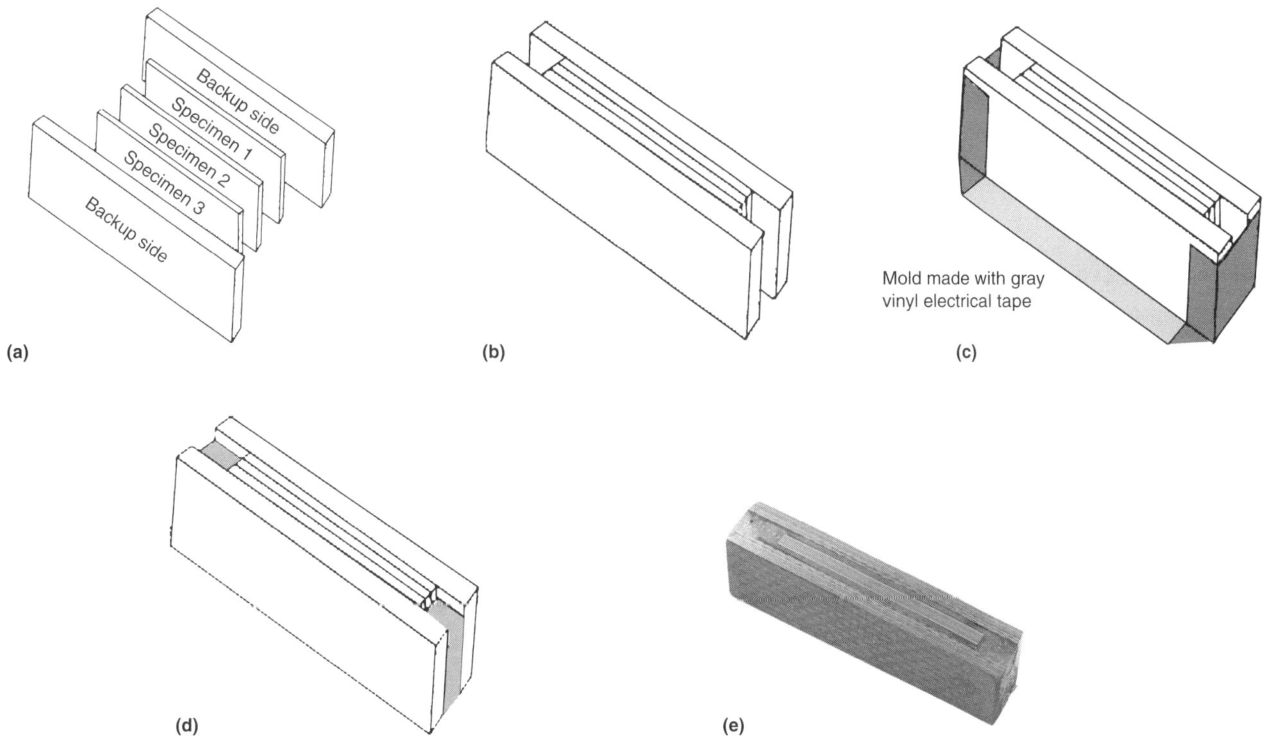

Fig. 2 Preparation steps for the development of a manual polishing mount. (a) Backup sides and three specimens. (b) The mount before bonding with epoxy. (c) Mold with taped ends for retaining mounting resin and holding samples while curing. (d) Mounted specimens ready to polish. (e) Manual mount after final polish

A photograph of a mounted and polished specimen is shown in Fig. 2e. Notice that the backup pieces are of the same type of material, carbon fiber composite laminates, as the sample to be viewed in the middle of the mount, providing similar sample removal rates.

Rough Grinding and Polishing

Sample Removal (Rough Grinding). The first stage of grinding should be aggressive enough to remove the material quickly and easily, but not so aggressive as to induce damage. Sixty-grit paper, like the band saw, can induce significant damage and may leave the sample in worse condition than it was before grinding. Wet-grinding with silicon carbide (SiC) paper will not introduce damage that cannot be removed easily if 120, 320, and 600 grit papers are used sequentially. However, because of their short useful life, SiC papers are one of the most expensive options for rough and fine sanding (each sheet will not last much beyond three CFRP specimens). Do not use dual papers, the removal rate is decreased and may introduce damage.

Rough and fine grinding using water-lubricated, diamond-impregnated discs remains one of the most efficient means of preparing specimens for final polishing. If used only for composites, a single diamond disc can last for years. A high-quality diamond disc can remove material at a continuous rate with less damage than SiC papers for a given grit size (e.g.,70 μm or 120 grit platen), making it possible to move to the next step (9 μm diamond lapping film, 15 μm or 1200 grit platen). A noncontinuous diamond pattern or a low-density distribution is recommended, as the water and removed material are easily sluiced away, ultimately increasing material removal rate.

The two methods for grinding described previously can be summarized as follows:

- *Method 1:* 120, 320, and 600 grit SiC paper
- *Method 2:* 70 and 15 μm diamond platens or 120 and then 1200 grit diamond platens

Rough Polishing. For automated polishing, a 1200 grit diamond disc or 9 μm diamond lapping film provides excellent results. Likewise, as one sheet is capable of polishing up to 1000 specimens, it is also highly economical. For hand preparation, however, 15 μm aluminum oxide (Al_2O_3 alumina) is recommended.

Polishing (micromachining) with levigated Al_2O_3 is inexpensive and effective if used correctly. Al_2O_3 alumina may be used on most composites with fiber hardness less than that of Al_2O_3. The rough polish Al_2O_3 comes in three sizes: 15.0, 5.0, and 0.3 μm. A fine balance of Al_2O_3 concentration in the lubricant (distilled water) and its proper application is necessary for efficient and quality micromachining as is the cloth type, revolutions per minute of the platen, and applied pressure. Achieving this balance will lock the cutting material into the cloth, resulting in a clean cut across both the soft resin and hard fibers. The Al_2O_3 distribution can be best controlled by adding it to the cloth in a premixed colloidal solution. *Never apply dry aluminum oxide to the cloth.* After the 0.3 μm step, the surface will be nearly free of artifacts that can be seen at 100× magnification. It should be noted that although diamond abrasives can also be used effectively, they are not recommended since the cost is much more significant.

The right concentration of Al_2O_3 is critical. There is a tendency to over concentrate the mixture. In this case, the Al_2O_3 will roll, becoming an ineffective cutting material. In addition, the rolling action will erode the resin from around the fibers leaving the fibers rounded and the surrounding resin undercut. This condition ultimately destroys the surface plane. For this reason, it is better to use a less concentrated Al_2O_3 solution to accomplish the micromachining polishing. A ratio of 5 g of 0.3 μm Al_2O_3 to 1 L of distilled water and 12 g of 15 μm Al_2O_3 to 1 L of distilled water has been found to be optimum.

The purpose of a lubricant is to dissipate the heat from polishing and to act as a carrier for the abrasive material, such as Al_2O_3. The lubricant needs to have a low viscosity to prevent hydroplaning during polishing. Usually, the lubricant consists of distilled water. Any contaminant in the lubricant can cause deep gouges, so avoid using tap water as it often contains abrasive particles.

Although there are many types of cloths promoted for polishing, such as Dacron (E.I. DuPont de Nemours & Co.) and nylon, cloths made from silk are recommended. Silk cloths come in a variety of different types and allow the fastest removal rates.

The speed of the platen is best kept high–typically 300 to 1000 rpm for a 200 to 300 mm (8 to 12 in.) platen. Although this may by limited by the type of equipment, the higher surface speed/pressure helps lock the Al_2O_3 into the cloth without excess buildup of Al_2O_3 on the cloth. Higher sample surface speed, whether increased through wheel speed, wheel diameter, or counter specimen rotation, will increase removal rates.

The pressure needs to be high enough to eliminate hydroplaning, but it is often limited by the capacity of the equipment. A fully loaded automatic head can have as much as 80 cm^2 (12 $in.^2$) of contact area with the platen. It may not be possible to apply sufficient pressure without overloading the equipment. For hand polishing, the pressure is limited by the ability of the operator to hold the specimen under control.

The right application of all the components may be accomplished in several ways. The key is the introduction of the colloidal Al_2O_3 mixture at the right rate: 1 to 2 drops per s will cool the sample and supply an ample amount of abrasive. Since silk cloth has no nap to retain lubricant, caution must be exercised. Damage to the samples may occur in 4 to 10 s if the platen is allowed to run dry.

Final Polishing. The final polish step transitions from micromachining using napless cloths and high pressure to one of lapping with low speed and low pressure. The most efficient process involves using a premixed 0.05 or 0.06 μm colloidal Al_2O_3 suspension diluted with distilled water in conjunction with a napless cloth. The critical parameters of fine polishing are very low vertical force, complementary rotation of the sample relative to the platen rotation, and a low platen speed. If the vertical force is too high, the fiber-resin interface will display cupping. In addition, if the platen speed is too high, the sample will become difficult to control if it is being hand-polished, and the sample will want to stick to the platen. It should be noted that it is hard to control the sample when hand polishing in a counter direction during this step. When hand polishing or automated polishing is done, platen speeds <120 rpm with a complementary sample rotation give $\frac{1}{4}$ μm (or better) surfaces in 30 to 180 s. This should be performed using a neoprene cloth (pad). Figure 3 shows how a polished surface of a composite material should look after this final step.

A vibratory polisher can also be used for the final polish. Silk or synthetic silk cloth is recommended, with a diluted premixed 0.05 or 0.06 μm colloidal Al_2O_3 suspension and low applied pressure. There are prestretched synthetic cloths on metallic plates that work very well and are tough. Silk can be used, but it is difficult to stretch over the platen. The vibratory polisher is slower than other automated polishing techniques and is easily contaminated but gives the best possible final surface. This process extends the micromachining with lapping.

The more traditional technique of final polishing with either a high- or low-nap cloth is not recommended. After as little as 20 s, rounding on the fiber-resin interface can be greater than 1 μm. This effect can be seen in Fig. 4 when compared to Fig. 3.

The following steps summarize the rough and fine polishing steps for both hand and automated techniques:

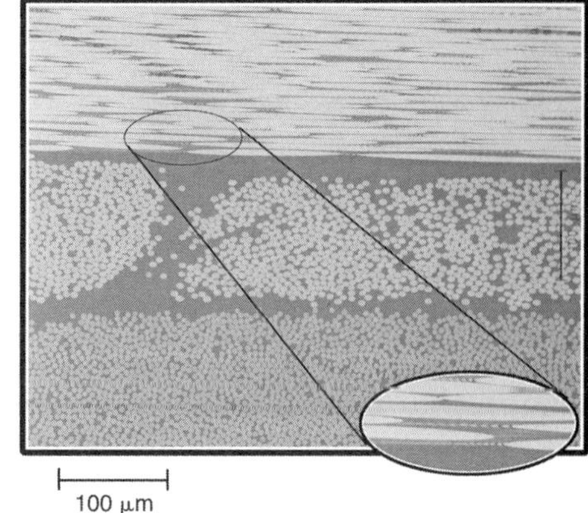

Fig. 3 Bright-field illumination (200×) of a composite specimen after alumina polish. Note the interferometer bands on the longitudinal fibers. This is one way to check the flatness of the polish.

Method 1. Hand polishing

1. 15 μm levigated alumina slurry (12 g Al_2O_3 to 1 L distilled water), silk cloth, 1000 rpm
2. 0.3 μm levigated alumina slurry (5 g Al_2O_3 to 1 L distilled water), silk cloth, 1000 rpm
3. Finish with a premixed solution of 0.05 or 0.06 μm levigated Al_2O_3 diluted with distilled water, neoprene cloth (pad).

Method 2. Automated polishing

1. 9 μm lapping film or 1200 grit diamond platen (note: use a high-quality diamond platen; not all are the same.)
2. 0.3 μm levigated alumina slurry (5 g Al_2O_3 to 1 L distilled water) with silk cloth
3. Finish with a premixed solution of 0.05 or 0.06 μm levigated Al_2O_3 diluted with distilled water on a neoprene cloth or silk cloth with vibratory polisher.

Preparation and Polishing Boron Fiber Composites. Polishing boron fiber composites is very difficult. The fibers are extremely brittle and the critical crack length is sufficiently short that any stress riser or abrasion may result in the fiber shattering. Given this, trying to cross-section and polish boron fiber composites with conventional techniques can be frustrating, as the boron particles break loose and gouge the polishing surface, frequently inflicting damage faster than it can be removed (Fig. 5). Although diamond is more expensive than Al_2O_3, it is necessary for polishing the harder, brittle fibers such as boron nitride.

Most of the problems associated with cutting and polishing boron fiber composites can be averted by combining sawing and polishing into a single step. Using a diamond wafering saw, cut the mounted specimen in half. This will result in a specimen that is ready for final polish. Likewise, this process will bypass the steps that cause the majority of the damage. After being sawed with the wafering saw, the sample is ready for a 1 μm polish (micromachining). Use a 1 μm polydiamond abrasive and a stainless steel mesh cloth or phenolic pad platen. Of these two polishing surfaces, the phenolic pad platen works the best; however, both result in a slow process. The vertical force should be high with a platen speed of 150 rpm and the head rotating counter to the platen. The polishing surface must be kept wet with a diluted solution of the diamond abrasive and ethanol. If the polishing plane is allowed to dry, the fibers can overheat and protrude from the surface of the sample. Destruction of the sample will follow. With its high vapor pressure, ethanol evaporates quickly, helping to cool the specimen-polishing plane. It is therefore imperative that the ethanol be applied at a rate that keeps the wheel wet. A small automatic atomizer works well. This step will take some time, as the hardness of the fiber approaches that of the diamond. Properly performed, this methodology will prepare specimens with no visible artifacts and with less than one-quarter interface edge rounding. To this point in the preparation procedure using hand polishing is not really recommended, as the brittle fibers will fracture.

Because the fibers do not allow the diamond abrasive to penetrate very deeply into the sample, a final polish is not required. However, a neoprene cloth with a premixed solution of 0.05 or 0.06 μm levigated Al_2O_3 diluted with distilled water and light pressure can clean up the last of the artifacts if so desired (Fig. 6).

The polishing of other types of composites, such as MMCs is not nearly as difficult as the boron fiber-polymer matrix composite. Most MMCs can be prepared by grinding with 70 μm diamond platen to a 9 μm lapping film, followed by 1 μm diamond abrasive polishing using the same technique as previously discussed for boron fiber composites. An example of a polished metal matrix composite is shown in Fig. 7.

Thin-Section Preparation

Ultrathin sections are typically used as a research tool rather than a production tool. At the ultrathin level, even opaque materials become optically transparent. This preparation is needed in order to resolve and analyze microstructural features at the theoretical limit for optical microscopy. Thin sections allow the use of several types of transmitted-light microscopy on materials normally considered opaque. Transmitted-light methods reveal more details of the morphology of polymers and similar materials than any other microscopy techniques available (Ref 2).

Ultrathin-section transmitted-light microscopy is time and labor intensive, and its use typically can only be justified when required data cannot be obtained by an alternative method. An ideal thin section is one where the only residual stress and strain that should be seen is that from the original specimen rather than due to the preparation (Ref 3, 4). Polymeric materials cannot be microtomed (which induces stress and strain as artifacts) to obtain the high resolution or detail that can be achieved with a polished ultrathin section. The following sections detail the various aspects relating to the selection and preparation of ultrathin section specimens of polymeric composites and other materials and their examination by transmitted-light microscopy techniques.

Procedure and Selection of Rough Section. The selection of the area of interest for thin-section examination and the procedure for the preparation of the rough section will depend on the nature of the starting bulk material from which the specimen is to be extracted and the type of information sought. When preparing thin sections, the orientation of the section relative to the fiber alignment is a major consideration for fiber-reinforced composites (FRCs). The angle at which the section is taken is important when quantifying anomalies such as voids and microcracks. If extensive microcracking of the resin matrix has occurred, thin sections normal to the fibers would be extremely fragile, and the specimen may tend to fall apart. In this situation, a section parallel to the longitudinal fibers is beneficial because the fibers provide support to hold

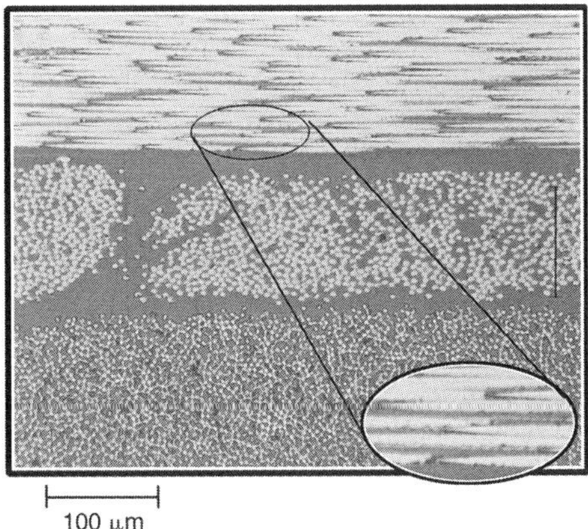

Fig. 4 Same specimen as in Fig. 3, repolished with 6 and 1 μm diamond on a nap cloth. Note the rounded fiber interface and the lack of interferometer bands on the longitudinal fibers.

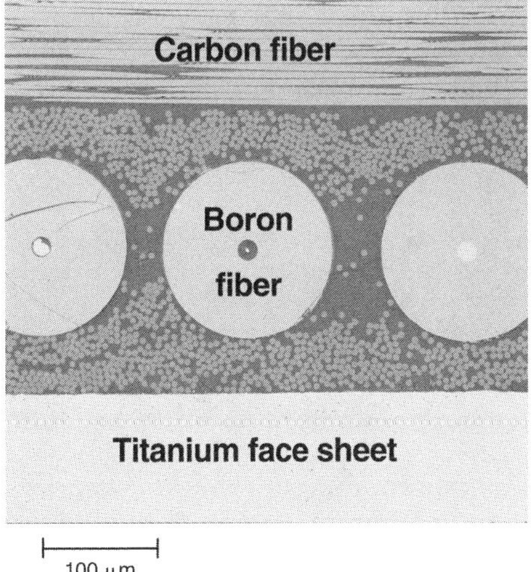

Fig. 5 Results of a diamond saw cut and the effect on the brittle boron fibers. 200×

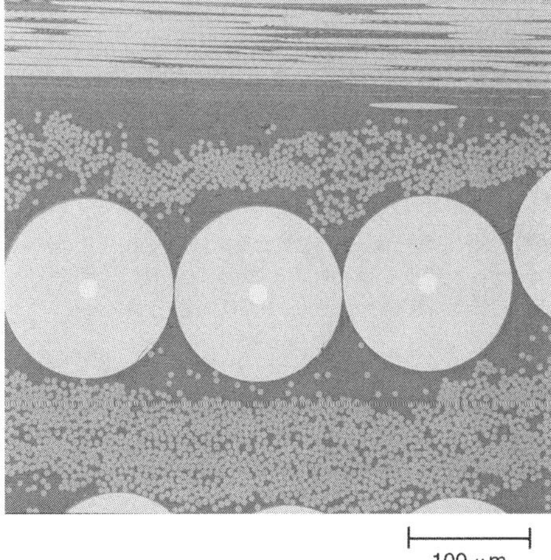

Fig. 6 Boron fiber composite cross section after final polish. 200×

the cracked matrix together. Here, a section along the longitudinal fibers on a heavily microcracked area can be used to hold the sample together.

Thin-section transmitted light microscopy has been successfully used for the following types of investigations:

- A single small area, such as the fracture origin in a laminate or honeycomb composite part. The feature can be a small zone that requires several sections for broader sampling.
- Finely dispersed particles or chopped fibers imbedded in resin
- Large, complex structures such as honeycomb composites with an array of materials. Frequently, there are zones with intermingled phases between components that need to be documented.
- Surfaces where oxidation or contamination is to be observed and documented.

The mounting of the specimens in a rubber mold can be done as previously described. In all cases, the final mount should be centered to feature the portion of interest. It is easier to control the removal of the material from the center than the edges.

It is better to make an initial slab of the rough cut larger than the final 46 by 27 mm (1.8 by 1.1 in.) petrographic glass slide so that the excess can later be trimmed, thereby eliminating artifacts on the edge of the final product. The "first surface" will become the surface glued to the glass slide. Be careful when preparing the first surface; any artifacts created at this point will affect the optical light path on the final section. Flatness of the surface is also critical, not only on the section plane, but also on the structure interface of different components (e.g., carbon fiber and thermoplastic resin). Polishing this face is performed the same as previously described for the reflected light specimens.

Mounting the First Surface on a Glass Slide. Once the first face is polished, mounting this surface to a glass slide is the next step in the process. The lack of a homogeneous adhesive bond between the sample and the glass slide will decrease the quality of the thin section. Trapped air and contaminants can cause the sample to separate from the slide during final polish, resulting in the self-destruction of the thin section. The following steps should be used to mount the sample onto a glass slide:

1. Clean a standard 46 by 27 mm (1.8 by 1.1 in.) petrographic glass slide with an appropriate solvent.
2. Clean and dry the sample.
3. Vacuum impregnate the polished surface and bond to the glass slide with low-viscosity, highly adhesive epoxy resin to ensure that any cavities opened by the polishing are filled and sealed.
4. Clamp sample to slide and allow to completely cure. The easiest way to bond the sample to the slide is to place a 1 kg (2.2 lb) weight on top of the sample.

Preparing the Second Surface (Top Surface). The second surface is prepared by grinding and polishing down the section from 1 mm (rough cut) to a nominal 1 to 7 μm-thick surface, parallel to the first surface. Like the first surface, this needs to be artifact-free. Any artifact, especially on the top surface, will show up in the microscope optical path. With epi-illumination, scratches can be a problem. When using transmitted light microscopy, the residual stress and strain associated with scratches affect the optical path and interfere with the microscopic analysis. The following sequence of steps is recommended for the preparation of the second surface after mounting the first surface to the glass slide.

Step 1: Trimming the Rough Sample. Trim the flashing from around the slide so it will fit into the vacuum chuck. The excess flashing has to be trimmed to match the slide (Fig. 8).

Step 2: Wafering the Sample.

1. Place the primary mount and glass slide in a vacuum chuck.
2. Mount the glass slide, with the primary mount bonded to it, in the wafering saw in preparation for the 1 mm (0.04 in.) cut.
3. Use the wafering saw to cut off a nominal 1 mm (0.04 in.) thick sample bonded to glass. The manufacturer's recommendation for speed and pressure should be followed because these parameters will vary with the resins used and the materials that are cut. The remaining rough-cut specimen may be reprocessed from the primary mount to obtain a series of thin sections.

If a wafering saw is not available, sample removal can also be done by grinding the mounted specimen, using 120 grit SiC paper, to a final thickness of 1 mm (0.04 in.). This is often time-consuming, depending on the original specimen thickness.

Step 3: Mounting the Wafer in the Vice for Grinding the Second Surface. Coarse and fine grinding are performed with the aid of a sacrificial hand vice:

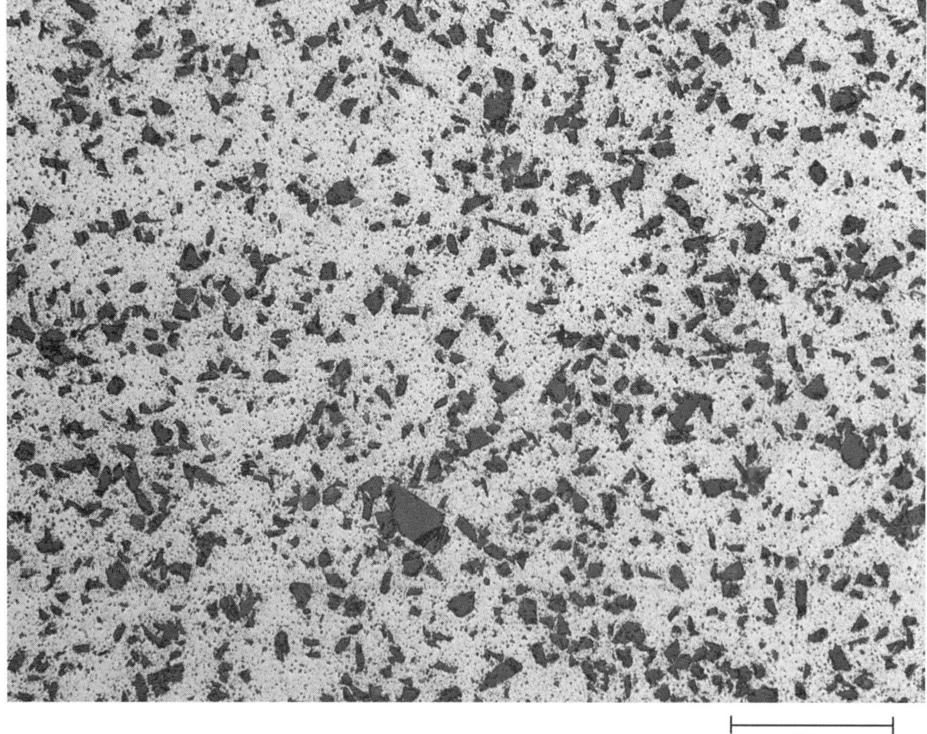

Fig. 7 Polished metal matrix composite made of 6061 aluminum and silicon carbide aggregate. 250×

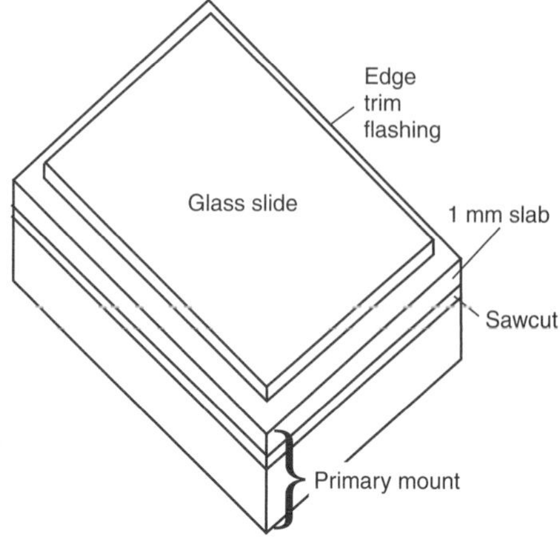

Fig. 8 Schematic of primary mount and area of saw cut

1. Mount the sample in a sacrificial hand vice using glycerin (Fig. 9). The purpose of this type of vice is to increase the surface area of the specimen and provide a holder. The sacrificial hand vice is an aluminum cylinder with a 46 by 27 mm (1.8 by 1.1 in.) removable rectangular piston.
2. The surface of the piston and the surface of the hand vice must be synchronized on the same plane for each use, which is accomplished by grinding them to a common plane. After the piston and the hand vice have been "planed," the piston should be reset to 375 μm, plus the thickness of the glass slide, into the cylinder. The easiest way to set the standoff distance is to use a blank slide and 375 μm of shim material.
3. At this point, a few drops of glycerin are placed on the recessed piston, and the glass-bonded 1 mm wafer is inserted into the cylinder. The sacrificial hand vice with the glass-bonded 1 mm wafer is now ready for the grinding process (Fig. 10).

Step 4: Grinding the Second Surface:

1. Grind the excess material with 120 grit SiC paper until the excess sample is removed so that it is flush to the aluminum vice surface. Do not use coarse paper because damage and deep scratches may result. Use reflection off surface to identify high spots where additional grinding is required.
2. Continue the grinding process in the vice with 320 grit SiC paper down to a level of roughly 50 μm above the first surface.
3. Finish the grinding process in a vice with 600 grit SiC paper down to approximately 25 μm. This completes the grinding process, and now the polishing process can begin. The sacrificial hand vice is no longer needed.

Step 5: Polishing the Second Surface. Mount the specimen in a hand vice. The purpose of the hand vice is to serve as a handle to hold the slide while polishing. A few drops of glycerin should be applied to the well to hold the specimen. The specimen can be removed at any time for a microscopic evaluation and reinstalled in this vice holder for further preparation. The polish action is hand pressure on a polish wheel. The direction of rotation is critical to follow. As previously described, the polishing can be done by hand. However, the 15 μm polishing step should be stopped when the thin section is within 1 to 3 μm of the final thickness. Shaping is done by center-weighting or off-center-weighting to control the final plane of the thin section so that it is parallel to the first surface or is a wedge to a very thin edge (Fig. 11). This is the last opportunity to do any major shaping of this plane.

The second polishing step uses a 0.3 μm alumina slurry on a silk cloth. This step removes the last 1 to 2 μm and will achieve the final plane, leaving the surface at a point where it can be examined. It is important to maintain center-weighting. Overpolishing can cause the sample to disbond. This step will test the effectiveness of the adhesive. The last polishing step can be accomplished as previously mentioned using a diluted 0.05 or 0.06 μm levigated alumina suspension either by hand or with automated vibratory polishing.

General Considerations for Thin-Section Sample Preparation. It is important to pay attention to all aspects of polishing (e.g., center-weighting, hand pressure, and cutting rate). Even the sounds of the sandpaper and the polishing cloth as the specimen is prepared can help guide the microscopist to maintain the desired plane. Going through the steps involved in preparing a specimen, a good microscopist continuously checks the specimen by viewing the light refracting off the surface. This technique saves time and is an excellent tool. Knowing when to stop and when to continue to the next step is critical and usually done by feel and experience. Each step leaves damage of decreasing magnitude. When too much material is removed at any given step, the sample in most cases is either lost or distorted. If not enough of the sample is ground down at any given step, it becomes difficult and sometimes impossible to reach ultrathin dimensions.

Feathering out is defined as the process of creating a slight wedge that is spread across the entire sample thickness varying from 0 to 5 μm. The advantage of feathering is that it allows the entire thickness range to be scanned utilizing the thickness effect on the optical contrast, refractive indices, and resolution. This allows the microscopist to obtain the maximum information and photographic detail. The biggest advantage of this is that the different optical contrast modes can be utilized for different portions or thicknesses of the sample. By carefully controlling the weighting of the sample during polishing, the specimen can be tuned to any shape or thickness needed. It is possible to obtain a near parallel surface; however, most polymeric composite materials have an optimal thickness that corresponds to differences in contrast. Therefore, tapering the surface of the specimens may offer more information while also providing easier identification of sample removal.

Viewing the Specimen

Reflected Light Microscopy. There are many factors to consider when viewing a specimen. The first is what type of specimen: what are the fibers and what is the matrix? What are the capabilities of the microscope? Viewing samples with the light microscope is the preferred start. In most cases, relevant detail may be resolved from 5 to 100× magnification. An understanding of the microscope is helpful in order to fully use its capabilities (Ref 5–12).

Epi-bright-field illumination (reflected bright field) is used in most cases. Bright field is used >90% of the time and on all types of composites. This method is particularly useful for imaging samples for void studies, fiber-orientation verification, resin-to-fiber ratio determination, and most microcrack studies. In general, it is advisable to observe all polished specimens with bright field before continuing with other illumination methods. Macro bright field (<30× magnification) can be difficult to achieve. The 6 to 10× range is where a large portion of documenting porosity in composites falls. Most microscopes are not set up for this range, and those that are have difficulty achieving the quality of a dedicated macroscope.

Void analysis of composite specimens can be performed using low-magnification bright-field illumination of the cross section (6 to 50×). An example of a unidirectional-fiber polymer composite material containing a significant number of voids is shown (Fig. 12). The voids show up as dark holes on the surface.

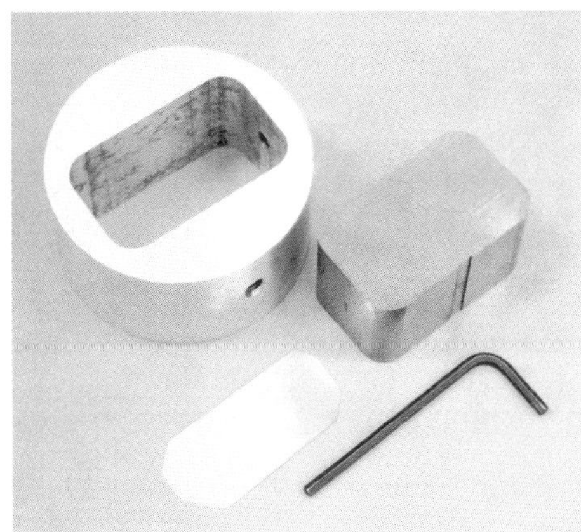

Fig. 9 Sacrificial hand vice with 375 μm shim material

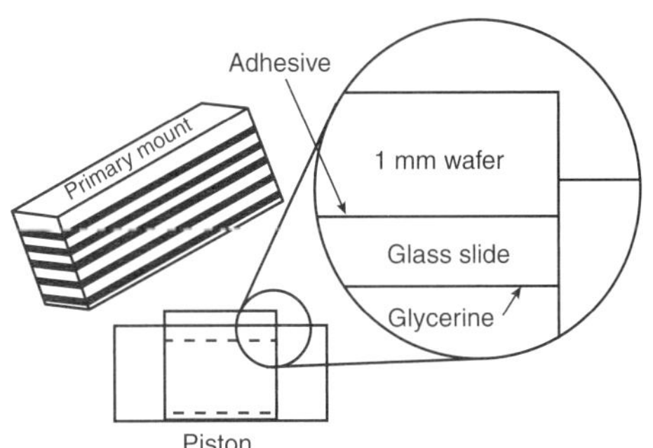

Fig. 10 Sacrificial hand vice with wafer assembly

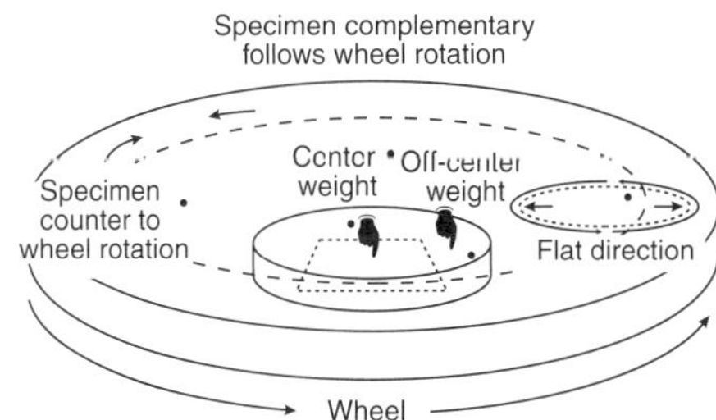

Fig. 11 Polishing wheel and specimen movement

Ply counts on unidirectional carbon fiber composite laminates can be accomplished by mounting and polishing the specimen at 45° to the plane view. This is the easiest way to sort the ply angles with only bright field (Fig. 13). Likewise, ply counts can best be performed on carbon fiber fabric composites using low magnification bright-field illumination of the cross section (30 to 80×). 90° tows can hide in the node zone. It is important to use a large field of view because of the structure of the weave. Figure 14 shows a montage of a chamfer area of a honeycomb composite structure where the 3K-70 plain-weave carbon-fabric plies are easily observed, as are voids in the structure.

Different composites present different types of resoluble features, depending on the reflectivity of the individual components present. The carbon fibers tend to be very reflective (or to show a high degree of contrast) and are easily resolved in thermoset resins. By comparison, glass fiber composites tend to absorb light equally across the spectrum, making it difficult to resolve the individual components (Fig. 15). Note the bright-field image of the glass fabric on the edge (top) and the carbon fiber plies.

Epi-dark-field illumination (dark field) is used to bring out subsurface features such as microcracks. With dark field, the light path is blocked from the objective center and is directed to the specimen at an oblique angle. This eliminates the reflected image in favor of the image formed as light passes through the sample subsurface. Using bright field, microcracks in CFRP composites are easily resolved. Similarly, samples with low surface contrast, such as glass fiber composites, are often visualized using dark field. However, there may be cases where subsurface features remain indistinct. The use of penetrant dyes or a red permanent ink felt-tip pen is often effective in highlighting these features (Fig. 16).

Epi-polarized light (polarized light) is similar to dark field, except that there is a polarizing element at the light source and an analyzer-polarizer between the sample and the eye. These additional elements allow the visualization of contrast created as light to be both reflected and polarized by the sample surface. An advantage of polarized light is best exemplified with fiber-orientation studies of CFRP composites (Fig. 15). The carbon fibers on the transverse (0°) axis are "blacked out" using polarized light, while the

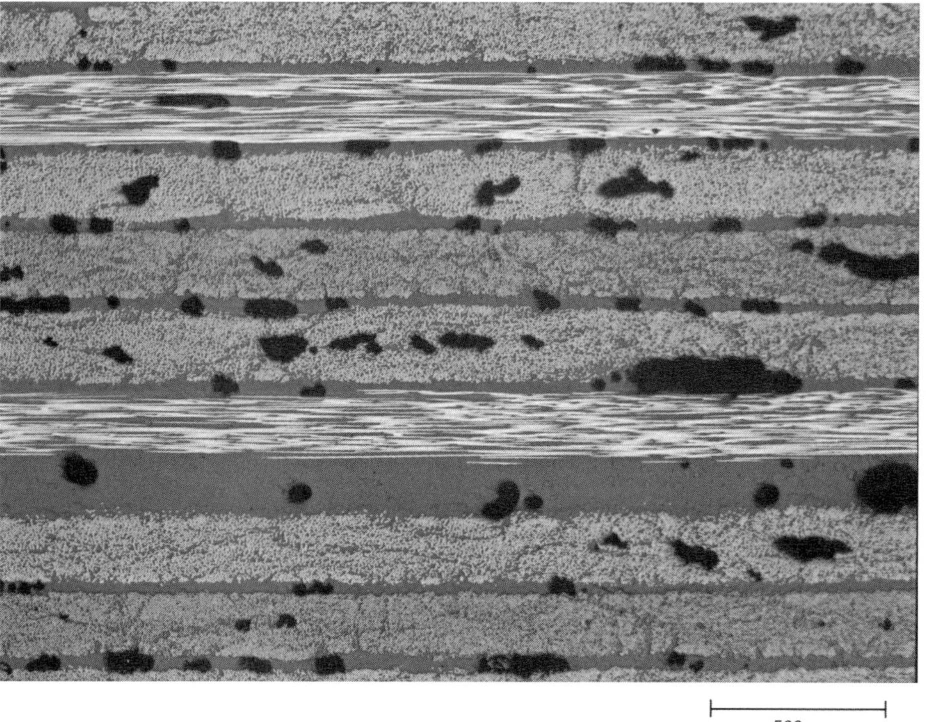

Fig. 12 Unidirectional composite specimen showing voids in the cured structure. 50×

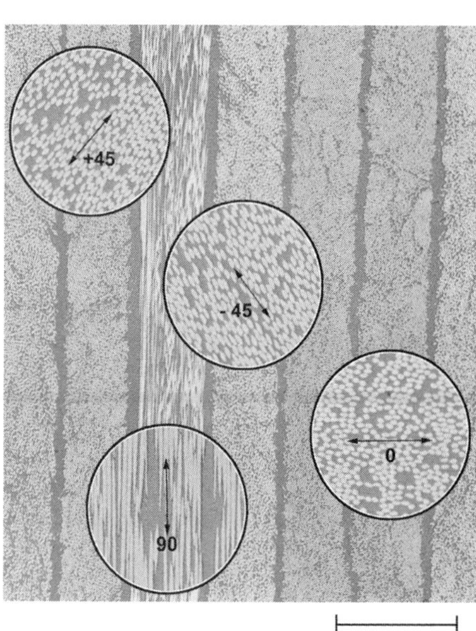

Fig. 13 Bright-field illumination of a unidirectional carbon fiber composite specimen showing the ply angles. 80 to 200×

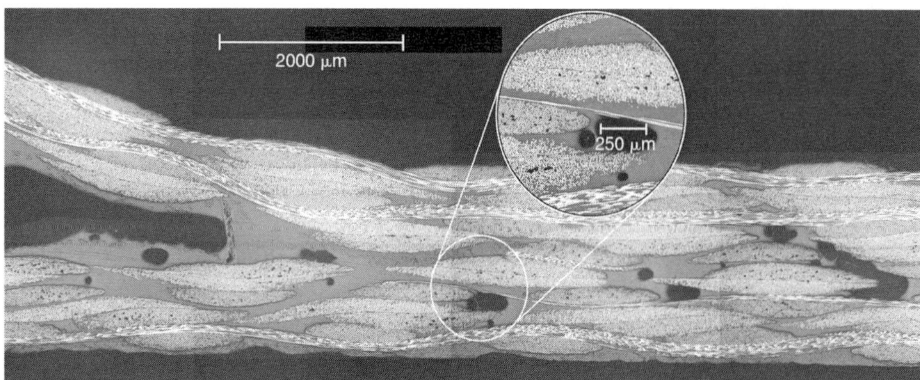

Fig. 14 A montage of a chamfer area of a honeycomb composite part made with carbon fabric skins. A highlighted area of a void in the structure is also shown.

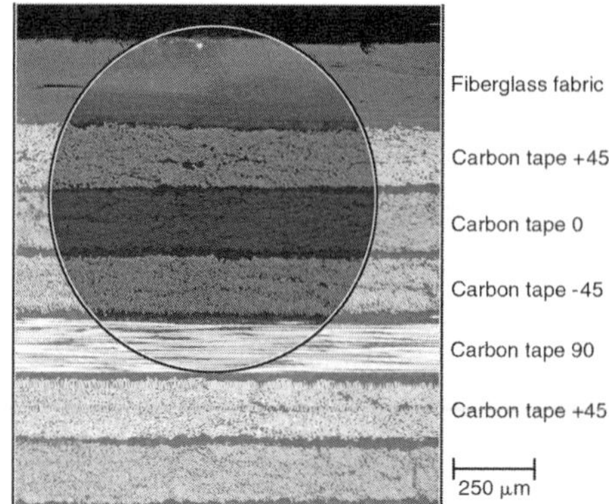

Fig. 15 Ply-count image showing bright-field background and polarized light center. A cross section of a glass fabric/unidirectional carbon fiber composite (80×). Note the lack of contrast of the glass fabric when compared to the carbon fibers.

longitudinal (90°) fibers depolarize the light and, as a result, are seen as bright features. With a 540 nm wave shift, the transverse fibers appear as first-order magenta; the longitudinal fibers appear white. While these two orientations appear in this manner with any type of illumination, the real advantage of polarized light is the ability to discern other orientations (e.g., ±45). Using polarized light, the ±45 fibers appear pink. Those closer to 0° will turn progressively more first-order magenta, while those that are closer to 90° will fade, eventually becoming white (Fig. 15).

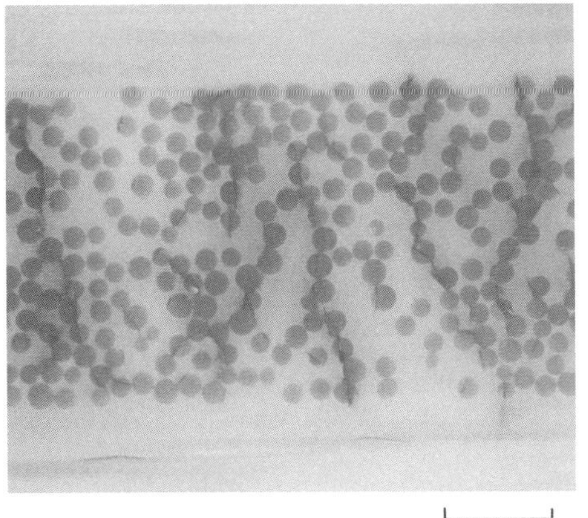

Fig. 16 Dark-field image (200×) of a nylon fiber composite with Magnaflux Spotcheck Penetrant SKL-H (Magnaflux, Glenview, IL). The transverse fibers and microcracks appear red. This technique works well for most translucent fibers.

Epi-fluorescence uses an ultraviolet light source (mercury or xenon) for illumination. Light is transmitted though an excitation filter that blocks all but a narrow bandwidth of the light spectrum. The narrow bandwidth of light strikes the sample surface, which is mostly reflected. However, some of the light is absorbed and reemitted, causing a lengthening of selected light bands. The image is passed through a dichroic mirror that filters some of the spectrum that then passes through a barrier filter. The filter removes all light except that which was emitted (fluoresced) from the sample.

It is important to note that with fluorescence microscopy, one does not see detail but sees only the fluorescing illumination. The selection of appropriate light source and filters is critical. All microscope manufacturers offer a wide range of filter combinations for this purpose. One of the most useful combinations is the following: 390 to 440 nm light, a 460 nm dichroic mirror, and a 475 nm barrier filter. Although some polymeric resins naturally fluoresce, most do not. In some multiphase resins, it is possible to selectively dye certain phases with laser dye for increased contrast. Dyeing the specimen is accomplished by first dissolving the laser dye in methanol and then adding it to three parts methylene chloride and a few drops of a wetting agent (Tergitol 15 S-7 surfactant, Union Carbide Corp., Danbury, CT). The specimen can then be immersed in the solution. The dyes can be absorbed through the skin and are extremely toxic. The most common application of fluorescence is observing microcracks that remain obscure with any other type of microscopy. Some carbon fiber composites and thermoplastics can have microcracks that will be invisible with bright field, dark field, and circularly polarized light (Fig. 17a). These microcracks can be easily observed with MagnaFlux Zyglo Penetrant ZKL-H (Magnaflux, Glenview, IL), a commercially available laser dye solution, wicked into the microcracks (Fig. 17b).

Use of Dyes and Etchants. For the majority of specimens, the microstructure is readily visible after polishing, though some features may need to be etched or dyed to be fully visible (Ref 13). The features of a multiphase polymer matrix, such as a thermoset containing a second phase thermoplastic or elastomer, are usually not resolved using bright-field microscopy. Although some phases may be observable with dark-field techniques, most multiphase polymer matrices require additional sample preparation after polishing. One option is the ultrathin section, but other methods such as etching and staining (dyeing) are less time consuming and work well for elastomers and thermoplastics. Some recommended etchants include: tetrahydrofuran

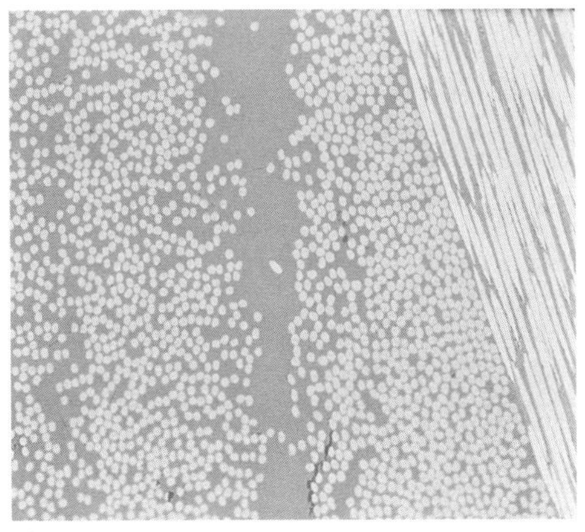

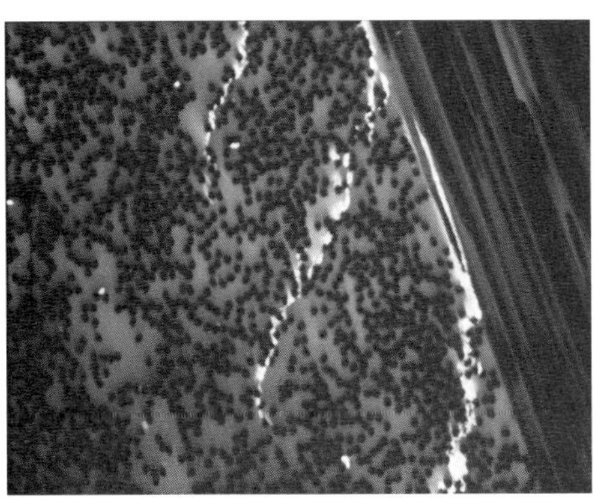

Fig. 17 A composite specimen containing a crack. (a) Bright-field illumination. (b) Same location with the use of fluorescence 390 to 440 nm and Zyglo Penetrant (Magnaflux, Glenview, IL). Both 200×

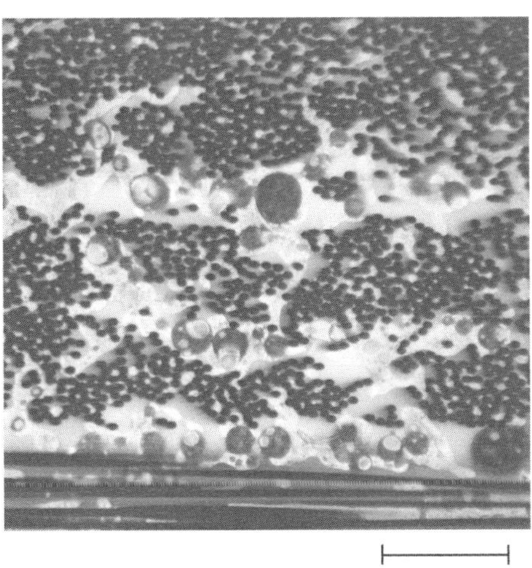

Fig. 18 Image of a composite cross section dyed with rhodamine-B and viewed at 390 to 440 nm. The use of dye was necessary to distinguish the dispersed second phase in the matrix.

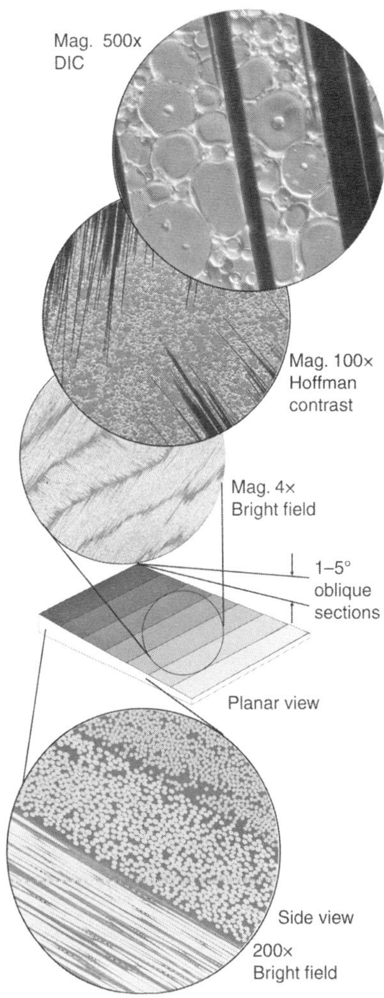

Fig. 19 Examples of laminate micrographs showing a side view and planar views of a thin section using different contrast modes and magnifications.

(THF), etch time 16 to 48 h; formic acid, etch time 20 to 120 s; a solution of CrO_3 12.5 g, HNO_3 50 mL, and 50 mL water, etch time 10 to 120 s. If the second phase material is known, it can be etched from within the thermosetting matrix with a suitable solvent for that material (e.g., a second phase consisting of polyetherimide in a thermosetting matrix can be etched with methylene chloride). An example of a carbon-fiber composite with a dyed multiphase epoxy matrix that contains a second phase thermoplastic and elastomer is shown in Fig. 18. This specimen was dyed with rhodamine B and viewed at 390 to 440 nm using fluorescence microscopy (1 g of rhodamine/25 ml of methanol/75 g methylene chloride; soak for 30 s).

Transmitted light microscopy methods use several contrast-enhancement methods that are not commonly used in metallurgical reflective microscopy. These methods include bright field; polarized light; phase contrast; differential interference contrast (DIC), also known as Nomarski; modulation contrast, also known as Hoffman contrast; epi-illumination; and optical staining. The methods of transmitted optical microscopy are to enhance or selectively detect changes in light intensity or color. The human eye and photodetectors are sensitive to differences in light intensity or wave amplitude and changes in color indicating changes in frequency of light. An example of several contrast methods applied to one material is shown in Fig. 19. At low magnification, bright-field microscopy shows the composite with good contrast. Modulation contrast at 100× and DIC at 200× are used to bring out the features at higher magnification.

Color and/or light intensity effects shown in the image are related to the rate of changes in refractive index (RI) and the thickness of the specimen or both. Use RI oils with a cover slide to increase relief and contrast of the specimen (Ref 5, 6). This requires a basic knowledge of the RI of the composite or polymer components in order to select appropriate oils. Optical path differences are sometimes referred to as optical thickness or optical color staining (Ref 5).

REFERENCES

1. P.K. Mallick, Fiber-Reinforced Composites, Materials, Manufacturing, and Design, 2nd ed., Dekker, NY, 1993
2. L.M. Gammon and D.J. Ray, "Preparation of Ultra-Thin Sections for Fiber-Reinforced Polymer Composites and Similar Materials," paper A-21, presented at 30th Annual IMS Convention, International Metallographic Society, July, , 1997
3. N.T. Saenz, Ultrathinning Section Techniques for the Characterization of Brittle Materials, Microstructural Science, Vol 18, 1991, p 147–159
4. L.M. Gammon, Optical Techniques for Microstructural Characterization of Fiber-Reinforced Polymers, Microstructural Science, Vol 19, 1992, p 653–657
5. M. Abromowitz, "Contrast Methods in Microscopy: Transmitted Light, Basics and Beyond," Olympus Corp., Lake Success, NY, 1987
6. F.D. Bloss, An Introduction to the Methods of Optical Crystallography, Saunders College Publishers, Philadelphia, 1989
7. P.F. Kerr, Optical Mineralogy, McGraw-Hill Co., 1977
8. C.W. Mason, Handbook of Chemical Microscopy, Vol 4, John Wiley & Sons, 1983
9. W.C. McCrone and J.G. Delly, The Particle Atlas Principles and Techniques, Vol 2, Ann Arbor Science Publishers, Ann Arbor, MI, 1973
10. L.C. Sawyer and D.T. Grubb, Polymer Microscopy, Vol 2, Chapman & Hall, 1996
11. D. Shelley, Optical Microscopy, Vol 2, Elsevier Science Inc., 1985
12. C. Viney, Transmitted Polarized Light Microscopy, McCrone Research Institute, 1990
13. L.M. Gammon and B.S. Hayes, Microscopy of Fiber-Reinforced Polymer Composites (workshop handbook), International Metallographic Society, October 1999

Thermal Analysis

George Dallas, TA Instruments

FAILURE OF A COMPOSITE STRUCTURE can be caused by several factors, such as tensile failure (dominated by fiber properties) and fiber/resin interface or interphase problems (e.g., failures in 90° plies). Thermal analysis is of limited use for such failures. However, in failure modes sensitive to the properties of the matrix resin, thermal analysis can help determine whether the matrix resin of a failed composite has the appropriate glass transition temperature (T_g). Some thermal analysis techniques, especially dynamic mechanical analysis (DMA), can also be used to "fingerprint" resins by determining properties over a wide temperature range.

Composite Failure Modes Affected by Matrix Resin

If failure occurs under high-temperature conditions, then the T_g of the resin should be checked using a thermal analysis technique. Even if failure occurs at low temperatures, T_g should be checked for indications of overcure, because an excessively high T_g can lead to microcracking. In addition, for a multiphase resin (for example, elastomeric or thermoplastic modified), thermal analysis can determine the T_g of the modifying second phase. If such a fingerprint differs to a significant degree from a control sample, there may be a problem with the composition of the modifier, the resin preparation (for example, improper prereaction), the formulation (too little or too much modifier), or the cure cycle. For example, such changes in fingerprint could indicate that the modifiers are not acting to toughen the resin effectively, which could lead to low interlaminar toughness.

Testing Approach

Usually, it is neither possible nor informative to compare the T_g of a laminate to a literature or brochure value. It is therefore necessary to run a control specimen with a test specimen from the failed laminate. Ideally, the control laminate should be made from a batch of prepreg that is within composition specifications for which quality control data are available from both the manufacturer and the end user. The control laminate lay-up should be of the same configuration as the failed laminate and should be done under controlled, or at least monitored, humidity. Also, it should then be cured under the same cycle as was the test specimen. Then a thermal analysis can be performed, and the T_g and other transitions for both specimens can be compared.

Reasons for Variations in T_g. There are several reasons that T_g may be lower in the test laminate than in the control laminate. The test laminate may have been undercured because an incorrect cure cycle was used. This sometimes occurs if the cure cycle is controlled using tool temperature rather than part temperature when the specified cycle is based on part temperature. The T_g also can be lower if the prepreg were cut and laid up under high relative humidity (RH). For example, T_g can be lowered by as much as 20 °C (36 °F) if it is exposed to 80% RH at 30 °C (85 °F) for 4 h (compared with dry prepreg). Incorrect formulation can also lead to a low T_g.

The T_g of the failed laminate could be higher than the control laminate if an incorrect cure or postcure were used. In addition, if temperatures higher than cure or postcure were experienced in service, T_g could be increased. Incorrect formulation can also raise T_g.

Thermal Analysis Techniques

Several thermal analysis techniques can be used to verify the cure of a polymer composite and to determine if the polymer had other associated thermal history that might have resulted from aging or faulty processing.

Thermal analysis is a family of techniques used for studying the thermophysical and kinetic properties of materials. Uses for polymers include monitoring the cure of thermosetting resins, measuring the degree of cure of the final product, studying crystallinity in thermoplastics, studying the compatibility of multiphase sys-

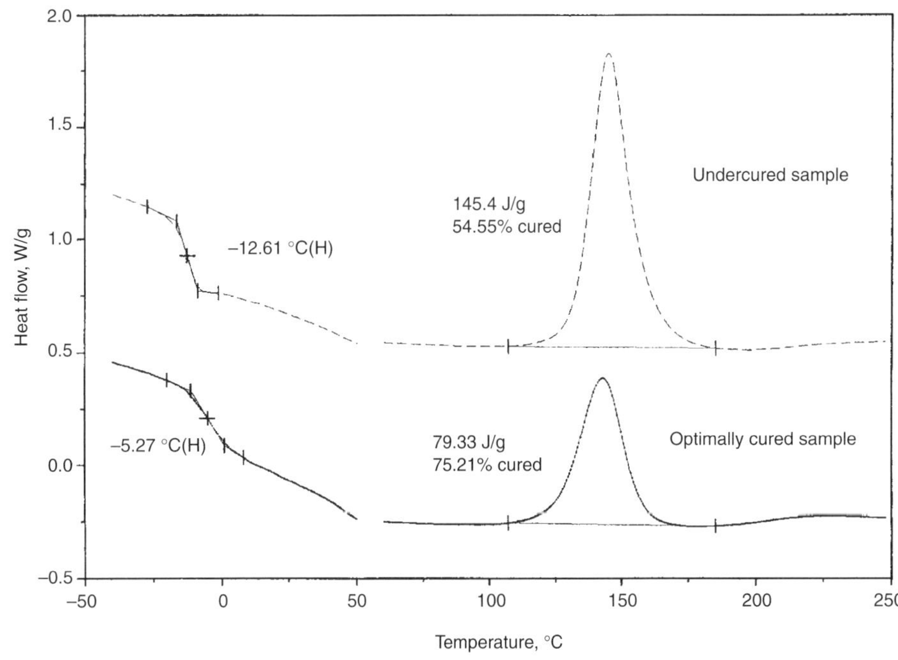

Fig. 1 Degree of cure determined using DSC. Graph shows advancement in T_g and measurement of heat of reaction. Heating rate: 10 °C/min; nitrogen gas purge (50 mL/min). Curves rescaled and shifted for readability

tems (Ref 1, 2), and identifying transitions imposed upon the polymer by faulty processing or aging (Ref 1). The techniques include differential scanning calorimetry (DSC); its advanced analog, modulated DSC (MDSC) (TA Instruments, New Castle, DE); thermomechanical analysis (TMA); DMA; and dielectric analysis (DEA). Differential scanning calorimetry and TMA are simpler, lower-cost methods compared with the others.

These techniques monitor the resin-curing process or determine the degree of cure of the finished product either by measuring the increase in T_g as cure advances, or by a technique-specific measurement of the curing reaction itself (e.g., increase in modulus by DMA). However, the low-energy T_g signal that is easily observed by DSC or TMA in a polymer-matrix, laminate, or a lightly filled composite may be difficult or impossible to detect in conditions of high humidity or in a highly filled composite of the same polymer due to the damping effect of the fillers. Dynamic mechanical analysis, however, should easily detect the same T_g, since it offers nearly two orders of magnitude of additional sensitivity over DSC to this measurement.

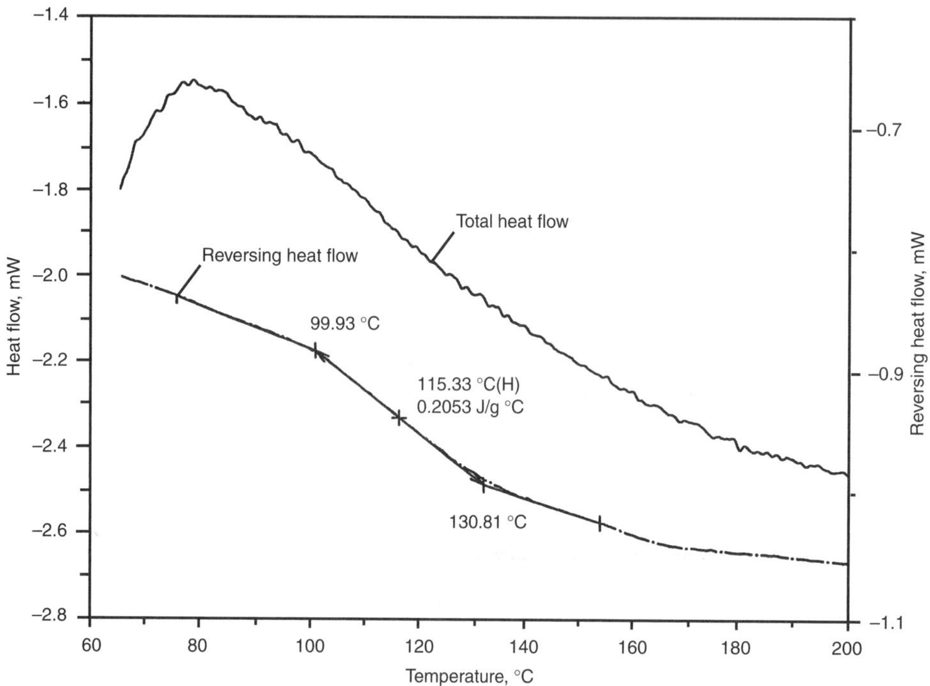

Fig. 2 High-sensitivity T_g detection using MDSC. Sample: glass fiber reinforced epoxy-Kevlar/polyimide; sample size: 32.9 mg; method: MDSC 2.5/60 at 1 °C/min; crimped pan; nitrogen gas purge

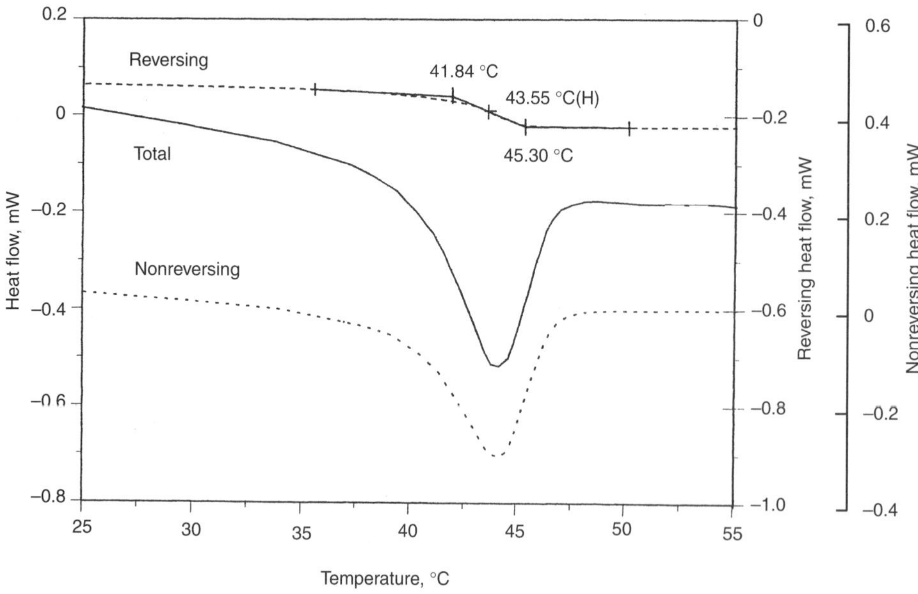

Fig. 3 MDSC separation of T_g from enthalpic relaxation. Upper curve: T_g; lower curve: enthalpic relaxation

Differential scanning calorimetry is the most popular thermal technique for polymer characterization. It is easy to use, requires small samples (~20 mg), operates from –180 to 725 °C (–290 to 1335 °F) and measures heat flow associated with sample transitions as a function of temperature (or time) under controlled-atmospheric conditions. Differential scanning calorimetry has been used to study thermodynamic processes (glass transition, heat capacity) and kinetic events such as cure and enthalpic relaxations associated with physical aging or stress (Ref 1).

Differential scanning calorimetry is commonly used to measure the T_g of uncured prepregs and cured laminates, advancement in cured laminates, and also the degree of cure of the final product, the heat of reaction during prepreg processing, and relative resin reactivity. The degree of cure is determined either by the increase in the T_g with cure, or by measurement of the heat evolved from the curing reaction. Figure 1 shows an example of both techniques in a comparison of an undercured and an optimally cured epoxy resin system for a given end use. The T_g shift with advance in cure is evident, while the residual cure is directly quantified. If the heat of reaction of a 100% unreacted resin is known, the degree of cure of each sample can be computed. If not, relative degrees of cure can also be assessed. If the material was 100% cured, upon reanalysis the exothermic heat of reaction peak would be absent.

As mentioned previously, detection of the T_g by DSC may prove difficult or impossible in highly filled composites or where moisture is present. In filled composites with reactive resin matrices (epoxy), the heat of reaction is usually sufficient for comparisons to be made of degree of cure. However, quantitative accuracy can be affected by variability of fiber (and filler) content in the small samples used.

Modulated DSC, a high-performance version of DSC, improves the possibility for T_g detection because it can offer a fivefold increase in sensitivity over DSC and with no loss in signal resolution (Ref 3). Figure 2 shows MDSC detection of a broad T_g in a complex glass fiber reinforced epoxy-Kevlar/polyimide composite that was unobservable using DSC even at highest sensitivity. Modulated DSC can also resolve the total heat flow signal into its thermodynamic (heat capacity related) and kinetic (temperature/time related) components. This allows direct analysis of the effects of aging or process-induced stresses, which appear as an enthalpic relaxation that can mask the T_g, with the net result being a signal that looks like an endothermic melt. The total heat flow signal is shown in Fig. 3. Modulated DSC can resolve these overlapping events; the actual T_g of the epoxy composite appears in the

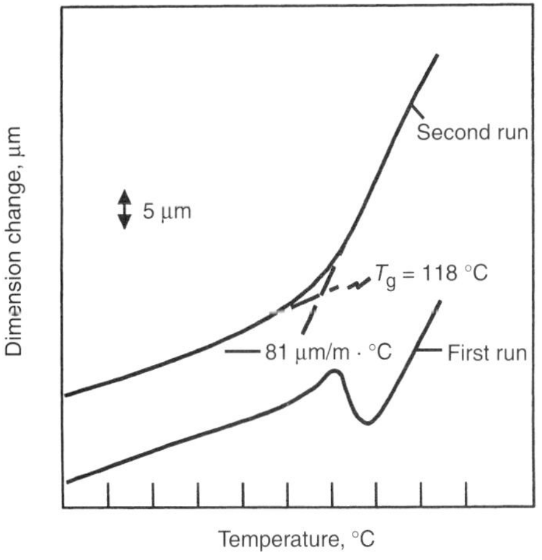

Fig. 4 TMA analysis of a PCB laminate

upper curve in Fig. 3, while the relaxation is resolved into a second kinetic-related signal (nonreversing).

Thermomechanical analysis determines dimensional changes in a material as a function of temperature (or time) under a controlled atmosphere. It is easy to use, has a wide temperature range (–150 to 1000 °C, or –240 to 1830 °F), and its multiple measurement modes (penetration, expansion, flexure, compression, tension, stress relaxation) permit analyses of a wide variety of materials. The primary applications of TMA to thermosets are the measurement of both T_g and the changes in its coefficient of linear thermal expansion (CTE) with cure.

In TMA, the T_g is measured as the intersection of the expansion curves in the glassy and rubbery states of the polymer matrix, possible for most polymers because there is a threefold difference in CTE at this point in the TMA curve (Ref 1).

Figure 4 shows measurement of the expansion coefficient and the T_g in a printed circuit board (PCB) laminate, where the signal is affected by an enthalpic relaxation effect due to stress induced by processing (lower curve). Annealing the sample removes the relaxation and allows clear detection of the glass transition upon reanalysis (upper curve).

As with DSC, the success of a glass transition measurement using TMA may be compromised by effects of moisture, fiber orientation with respect to the probe, and the presence of filling materials.

Dynamic mechanical analysis measures the stiffness (modulus) and damping of a material as a function of temperature, time, and frequency under a controlled atmosphere. Operational from –150 to 600 °C (–240 to 1110 °F) and over a wide frequency range, DMA is used to probe material structure by measuring mechanical, flow, and viscoelastic properties (E', E'', G', G'', tan δ, η^*). Multiple clamping systems allow operation in a variety of measurement modes (single and dual cantilever, three-point bending, shear, compression, and tension) on a range of samples. Its high sensitivity makes DMA an ideal tool for following the course and kinetics of the cure process and for analyzing the viscoelastic properties of the final product. Dynamic mechanical analysis can detect some or all of the events in a thermoset curing cycle, including initial T_g of the uncured resin, the temperature of minimum viscosity, the onset of gelation, the cross-linking reaction, the cure completion, and the modulus of the fully cured material. The sharp increase in the shear modulus with cure in Fig. 5 shows the high sensitivity of DMA to the cross-linking reaction even with complex materials such as a highly filled sheet molding composite.

Dynamic mechanical analysis is also used to measure the T_g of a cured material versus a target value and in relative-cure comparisons. Its very high sensitivity to T_g detection is valuable in samples where the T_g is inherently weak or reduced by the presence of moisture or fillers. Absolute modulus numbers both below and above the T_g can easily be obtained. The higher the modulus above the T_g, the higher is the degree of cure, while in comparative situations, the higher the T_g, the greater is the degree of cure. In analyzing composites by DMA, the sample should be loaded in a resin-dominated direction. In fiber-dominated orientations, the superior fiber stiffness controls the composite stiffness and masks the effect of the resin.

Dielectric analysis measures dielectric properties of a material as a function of temperature, time, and frequency under a controlled atmosphere. Ceramic parallel plate and ceramic single-surface sensors permit analysis of powders, liquids, pastes, and films from –150 to 500 °C (–240 to 930 °F) and over a wide frequency range (0.003 to >100 kHz). Measured properties are dielectric permittivity (ε') and loss factor (ε''), from which other useful parameters (tan δ, ionic conductivity, complex permittivity) can be automatically computed. Permittivity (dielectric constant) is related to the ability of a material to store energy, while loss factor describes its conductive nature and is composed of two factors: energy loss associated with time-dependent polarization and bulk conduction. The former dominates below the T_g, and the latter above it, due to ionic mobility (Ref 4). Dielectric analysis is useful in resin-curing studies because it readily detects the T_g, minimum viscosity (seen as maximum ionic mobility), resin cure, and vitrification. It is very sensitive to the last stages of the curing reaction (Ref 5). Dielectric analysis is at least an order of magnitude better than DSC or TMA in detection of the T_g and can also measure lower energy β and γ transitions.

Figure 6 shows a DEA curing study on an Epon 828/DDS system, where the T_g, flow, minimum viscosity, and cure portions of the curve are readily apparent. Dielectric analysis is also

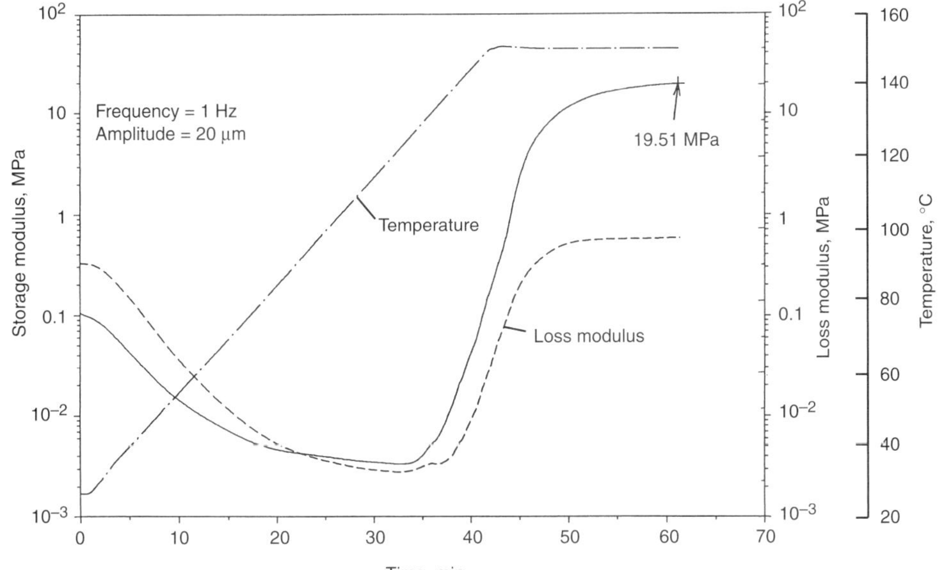

Fig. 5 Cure of sheet molding compound in shear sandwich mode. Cross-linking reaction indicated by sharp increase in shear modulus. Frequency: 1 Hz; amplitude: 20 µm

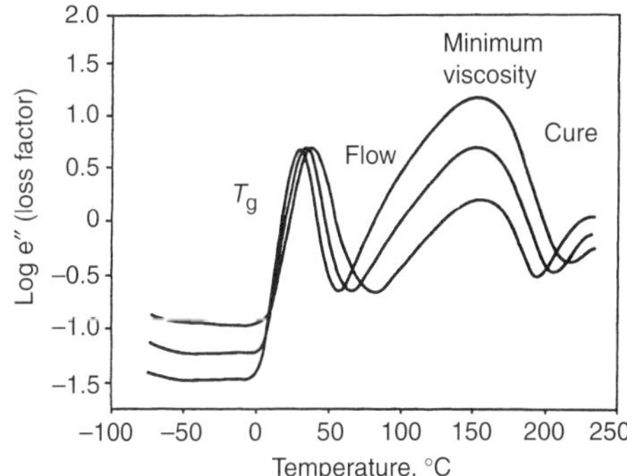

Fig. 6 Epoxy resin cure determined using DEA with a single-surface sensor. Sample: Epon 828/DDS; heating rate: 3 °C/min; frequency: 10, 30, 100 kHz

useful for evaluating cure in solvent-based urethane/isocyanate systems, which pose problems for DSC and DMA due to the low viscosity of the initial resin, the small heat of reaction, and solvent volatilization.

Dielectric analysis may have limited utility in analysis of highly filled composites, since the filler material can reduce signal sensitivity by restricting dipolar alignment with the electric field (permittivity) and also impede ionic mobility. Dielectric analysis is impractical if electrically conductive fillers or supporting fibers are present, because these would short the electrodes.

REFERENCES

1. R.B. Prime, *Thermal Characterization of Polymeric Materials,* 2nd ed., Vol 2, E.A. Turi, Ed., Academic Press, 1997, Chap. 6
2. R.J. Morgan, *Thermal Characterization of Polymeric Materials,* 2nd ed., Vol 2, E.A. Turi, Ed., Academic Press, 1997, Chap. 9
3. L.C. Thomas, "Modulated DSC Theory," Technical Publication, TA 211, TA Instruments, 1993
4. T. Grenntzer and J. Leckenby, *Am. Lab.,* Jan 1989
5. T. Grenntzer, "Characterization of Cure of High Temperature Urethane Resins by Dielectric Analysis" Application Brief, TA 103, TA Instruments, 1989

Fractography

Patricia L. Stumpff, Hartzell Propeller, Inc.

FRACTURE SURFACES are examined during most investigations of failed structural components because these surfaces provide an actual physical record of the events at the time of failure. Fractographic analyses of the surfaces of metallic components reveal useful information about the cause and sequence of failure. Those surfaces reveal features that identify the crack origin, crack propagation direction, failure mode, load, and environmental conditions at the time of failure. This information is extremely useful in the determination of failure cause. Hence, as composites developed into structural materials, a similar need arose to understand the fractographic evidence that these materials can provide.

The best method of developing an understanding of the fractographic evidence provided by those failures is to obtain pedigreed, fractographic data. These data are obtained by documenting the fractographic characteristics of specimens manufactured from different composite materials under different processes and exposed to different environmental and load conditions. The fracture surfaces of the pedigreed test specimens are examined, documented, and analyzed to determine which features are specific to a particular material, process, load, and/or environmental condition. The fractographs can then be used in the analysis of component failures.

This article depicts typical fractographic features for a number of different composite materials. Although not all-inclusive by any means, the fractographs depict a range of different, yet typical, fractographic features obtained from various composite materials that were manufactured and tested under different load and environmental conditions. It is hoped the fractographic data provided are useful for comparison with actual fractured surfaces to help determine the cause of component failures.

Material systems examined include epoxy resins with different fibers, such as carbon/epoxy (AS4/3501-6), fiberglass/epoxy (Hexcel E-glass/F155) and aramid/epoxy (Kevlar 49/3501-6), as well as fibers with different thermosetting resins, including carbon/bismaleimide (AS4/5250-3) and glass/polyimide (Celion 3K/PMR-15). Carbon fiber and thermoplastic resin composite systems are also highlighted, mainly for comparison purposes, and include carbon/thermoplastic (AS4/APC-2) and (AS4/KIII).

The specimens used for the fractographs depicted in this section were generally manufactured according to material supplier recommendations. Those specimens that were not manufactured according to manufacturer recommendations were processed with changes made solely to examine the effect of different material processing conditions. Material processing variations included changes in cure cycle, such as overcure or undercure conditions, surface contamination, and reduced resin content.

Environmental conditioning of the test specimens was conducted as noted in the fractographs provided. Environmental conditions examined included the effect of moisture in the laminate, moisture saturation followed by elevated temperature exposure (i.e., hot/wet conditions), and elevated temperature exposure without prior moisture conditioning.

Loading on the specimens was conducted using a variety of test specimens and load conditions. Mode I tension and tension fatigue failures were obtained using double cantilever beam (DCB) specimens; mode II shear and shear fatigue failures were obtained using end-notched flexural (ENF) specimens. Translaminar tension and compression specimens used either the notched bend bar specimens with four-point loading or the specimen configurations defined in ASTM D 3039, "Tensile Properties of Fiber-Resin Composites" and ASTM D 3410, "Compressive Properties of Unidirectional or Cross-Ply Fiber Resin Composites."

Following manufacture, environmental conditioning, and testing to failure, the fracture surfaces of the test specimens were examined in the scanning electron microscope (SEM). Typical fractographic features of each test specimen

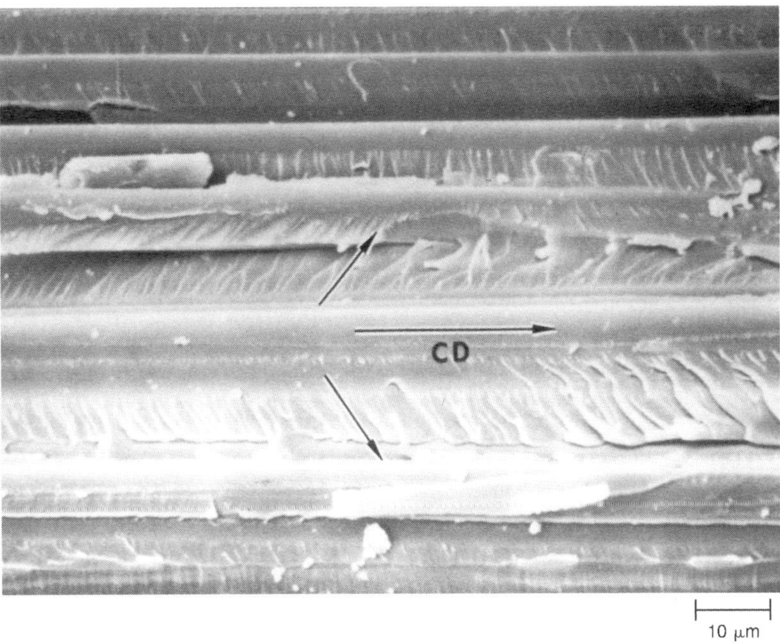

Fig. 1 River patterns on the surface of a mode I tensile failure in a carbon/epoxy (AS4/3501-6) composite laminate. Overall crack growth direction is from left to right. 1000×

were then identified and documented. Further examination and analysis of the fractographs were then conducted in order to define the specific fractographic features that were indicative of a specific material, processing, environmental, or load condition at failure.

Interlaminar Fracture Features

An interlaminar fracture occurs when the load is applied perpendicular to the composite laminate and failure occurs in the plane of the reinforcement. Interlaminar fractures occur following mode I tension or fatigue loading, mode II shear or fatigue loading, flexural loading, and impact loading on the surface of the laminate.

Interlaminar Fracture of Composites with Brittle, Thermoset Matrices. Most of the fractographic evidence in interlaminar fractures that would be indicative of the material, processing, load, and/or environmental conditions at failure are found in the matrix materials, rather than the fibers, of the composite. Analysis has shown that the fractographic features associated with these brittle thermoset matrices, including the epoxies, bismaleimides, and polyimides, are similar in nature. Because of this, most of the fractographic data presented in this section were obtained from epoxy matrix materials; minimal fractographic data from the other brittle thermoset resin systems are presented.

Differences in Fracture Characteristics Due to Different Loading Conditions. In general, brittle matrix composite materials tested under interlaminar, mode I tension loads fail in the plane of the reinforcement. Visually, these surfaces exhibit a glossy appearance, with some banding and resin covering most of the fibers on the fracture surfaces. On a microscopic level, the fractographic features evident in this failure mode consist mainly of river patterns on the surface of the matrix, as shown in Fig. 1 and 2, and matrix feathering, as shown in Fig. 3. River patterns are basically created by cleavage of the matrix on different levels, resulting in what appear to be branches or small tributaries of a river. They can be found emanating from the resin at the surface of the fibers or fiber imprints, as shown in Fig. 2(b), or in the matrix between fibers. Matrix feathering, on the other hand, consists of small flow lines in the matrix that emanate from an imaginary centerline as the crack moves forward. Feathering is particularly evident in large, flat, resin-rich regions, where river patterns are not usually noted. Both river patterns and matrix feathering are not only indicative of mode I tension loading in brittle composite materials, but have also been noted to be indicative of crack growth direction. Crack growth direction can be ascertained by noting the direction in which the smaller rivers combine into the one large river, as shown in Fig. 1. In this figure, the crack-growth direction is from left to right. It has also been noted during fractographic examination that larger river patterns tend to give a better indication of the overall direction of crack growth in the specimen, as the larger river patterns are less influenced by the fibers themselves. In general, however, river patterns are indicative of mode I tensile loading and must be vectorially added across the majority of the fracture surface in order to obtain a definitive crack initiation site and crack-growth direction. Flow lines are also indicative of crack growth direction, as shown in Fig. 3, where they are indicative of crack-growth direction from right to left.

Composites with brittle matrices tested under interlaminar mode II shear loading exhibit different fractographic features than those tested under interlaminar mode I tension loading. Visually, these surfaces exhibit milky white, dull fracture surfaces. Again, failure of the laminate generally occurs in the plane of the reinforce-

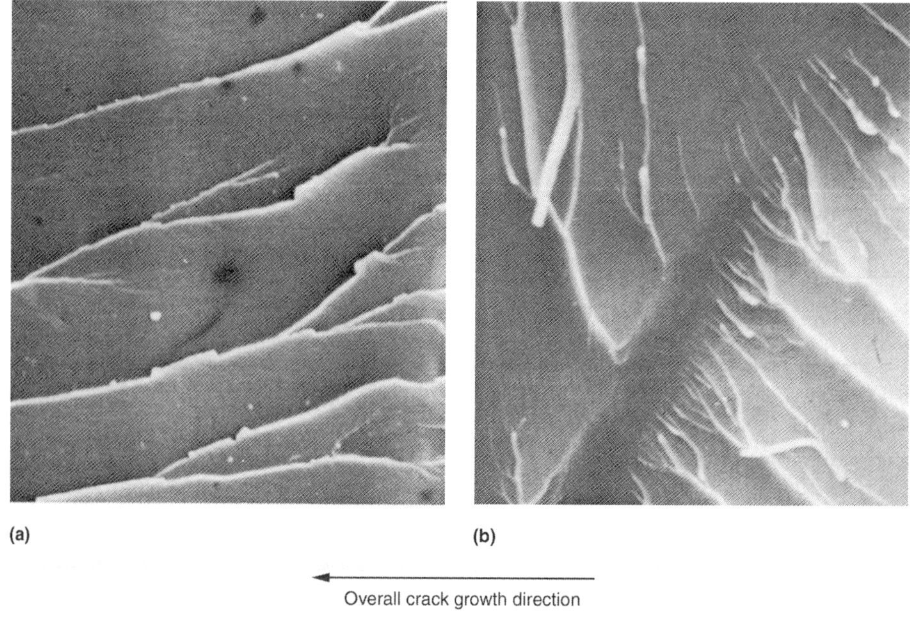

Fig. 2 Mode I tension interlaminar fractures that propagated at various angles to the direction of fiber reinforcement. (a) Fracture between adjacent 0° and 90° plies. (b) Fracture between 45° and –45° plies. 2000×. Source: Ref 1

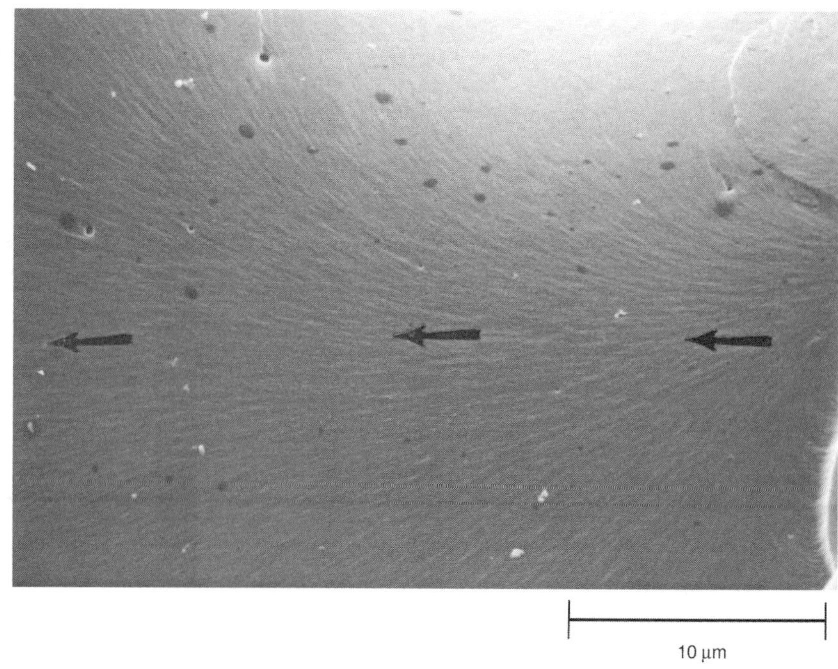

Fig. 3 Matrix feathering produced under interlaminar mode I tension. 3600×. Source: Ref 1

ment, and SEM analysis reveals distinctive fractographic features. On these fracture surfaces, the appearance of the feature known as *hackles* becomes evident, as shown in Fig. 4 and 5. Hackles appear to form by the coalescence of numerous, small, 45°, tensile micro cracks that form between the fibers under shear loading, as illustrated in Fig. 6 and 7. The size, shape, and form of the hackles are quite varied over the fracture surface, and the variation appears to be related to the actual percentage of mode I versus mode II loading, the amount of resin between the fibers, and the orientation of the fibers to the applied load. Under some mode II shear or mixed mode load conditions, small river patterns are sometimes evident at the base of the hackle or on the surface of the hackle as depicted in Fig. 5. These river marks can sometimes be used to help in determining the crack-growth direction.

Specimens tested under mode I tension and mode II shear fatigue loading generally result in fracture surfaces that contain fatigue striations. Fatigue striations, however, are not easily found in composite materials. This is partly because there may be little difference macroscopically between specimens that failed in fatigue and those that failed in overload by tension or shear. Unlike metallic materials, in which beach marks can often be found radiating outward from a visual fatigue initiation site, composite materials lack an apparent visual fatigue initiation site, which makes the diagnosis of fatigue failures at the macroscopic level somewhat more difficult. Additionally, fatigue failures can also be difficult to diagnose on the microscopic level. There are usually relatively few areas on the fracture surface that contain the fatigue striations. This lack of a significant number of striations on a fatigue fracture surface and the large separation between areas containing fatigue striations make locating them somewhat difficult and more time-consuming than in metals. The difficulty in finding these features is also enhanced by the fact that a certain amount of specimen tilt is often required in order to make them visible in the SEM. The amount of specimen tilt is of utmost importance in detecting the striations; higher tilt angles (>30°) often are required to find them. However, when fatigue striations are found, they can be found either in the matrix between two fibers, as shown in Fig. 7 and 8, or in the matrix itself, as shown in Fig. 9.

Impact damage is another form of loading that can result in specific interlaminar fracture characteristics in composite materials. In general, a delamination resulting from an impact load can often be ascertained by opening up the laminate in the plane of the delamination under mode I tension or mixed-mode loading. Visually, the delamination will generally exhibit a whitish, damaged surface, as compared to the darker, smoother, reflective surface of the manually fractured region. The delamination due to impact will also exhibit more evidence of shear (i.e., hackle formation in the damaged region) as compared to the surrounding area, which will generally have more river patterns indicative of the manually applied, mixed mode, or mode I tensile loading. The impact damaged region will also exhibit considerable matrix debris on the surface of the laminate, as compared to the surrounding area. For woven Kevlar/epoxy laminates, the fractographic evidence of impact damage can be found in both the matrix and in the fibers. Figures 10 and 11 depict the difference between an interlaminar fracture due to impact damage and an interlaminar fracture due to mode I tension loading for this particular material system. In addition to the visual differences noted above, the microscopic features in the impact damaged region (Fig. 10) include hackles, matrix debris, and significant fiber fibrillation and damage. The microscopic features in the mode I tensile region (Fig. 11) include the formation of river patterns, minimal matrix debris, and significantly less fiber fibrillation than in the impact-damaged zone.

Differences in Fracture Characteristics Due to Different Material Processing Conditions. Composite materials were then manu-

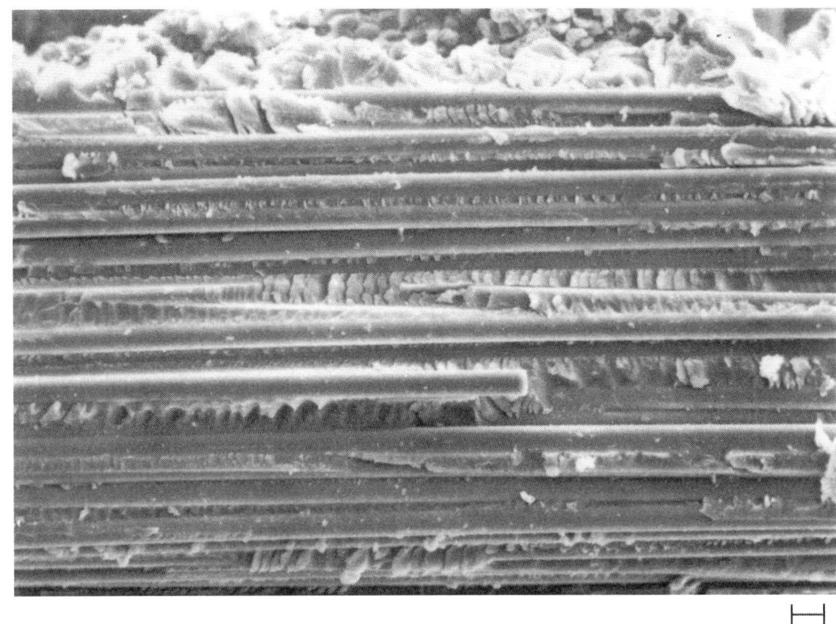

Fig. 4 Hackles in the resin of a carbon/epoxy (AS4/3501-6) laminate, indicative of mode II shear failure. 480×

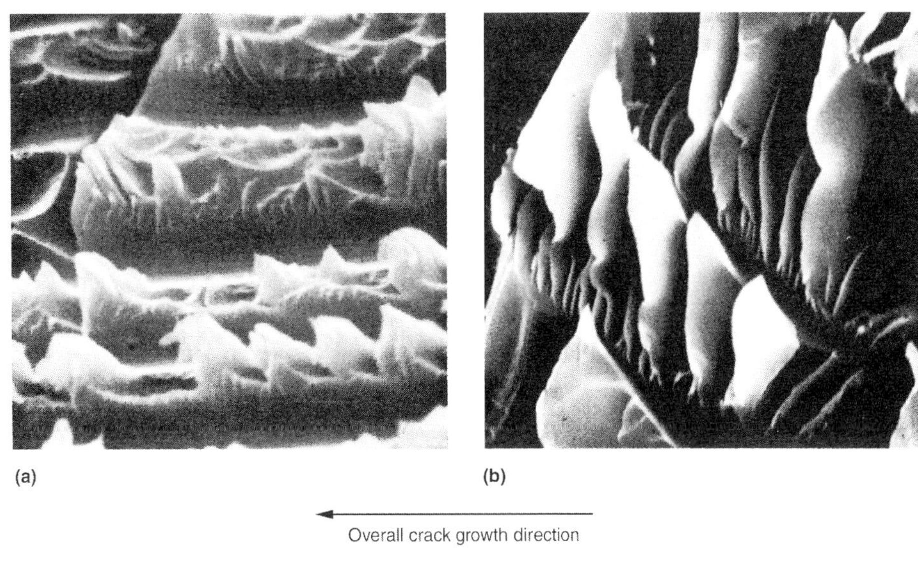

Fig. 5 Interlaminar mode II shear fractures that propagated at an angle to the direction of fiber reinforcement. (a) Delamination between 0° and 90° plies. 5000×. (b) Fracture between 45° and –45° plies. 2000×. Source: Ref 1

factured using material processing conditions other than those recommended by the manufacturer. The purpose of manufacturing and testing these specimens was to determine if material processing defects could be identified in the fracture characteristics of the laminates. Brittle thermoset-matrix composite test specimens were either overcured or undercured during the processing of the laminates and then tested to failure under mode I tension loading. The fracture surfaces of these specimens exhibit variations in the fractographic features that appeared to coincide with the variations in processing conditions. In specimens that were undercured and then tested to failure under mode I tension, the river patterns generally exhibited a more feathery appearance than the specimens that had received a normal cure cycle. Specimens that were overcured and then tested to failure under mode I tension generally exhibited more brittle-looking and distinct river patterns in the matrix. Other material processing variations, including the use of materials with inadequate resin content, generally resulted in interlaminar fracture surfaces with fewer matrix-rich regions and, hence, fewer fracture features, such as river marks, matrix feathering, hackles, and fatigue striations. Inadequate resin content in laminates also generally reveals the fracture characteristic known as fiber splinters. Fiber splinters are fibers that separate readily from the fracture surface because insufficient adherent-matrix cannot keep them attached to the rest of the specimen under mode I tension loading. These splinters are shown in Fig. 12 for a woven, glass/polyimide composite laminate. Other processing defects, such as contamination of an internal ply of the composite laminate with a release agent such as Frekote (Dexter Adhesive & Coating Systems) can also be found on the delaminated fracture surface during routine examination, as shown in Fig. 13.

Differences in Fracture Characteristics Due to Different Environmental Conditions. Environmental exposure of the test specimens

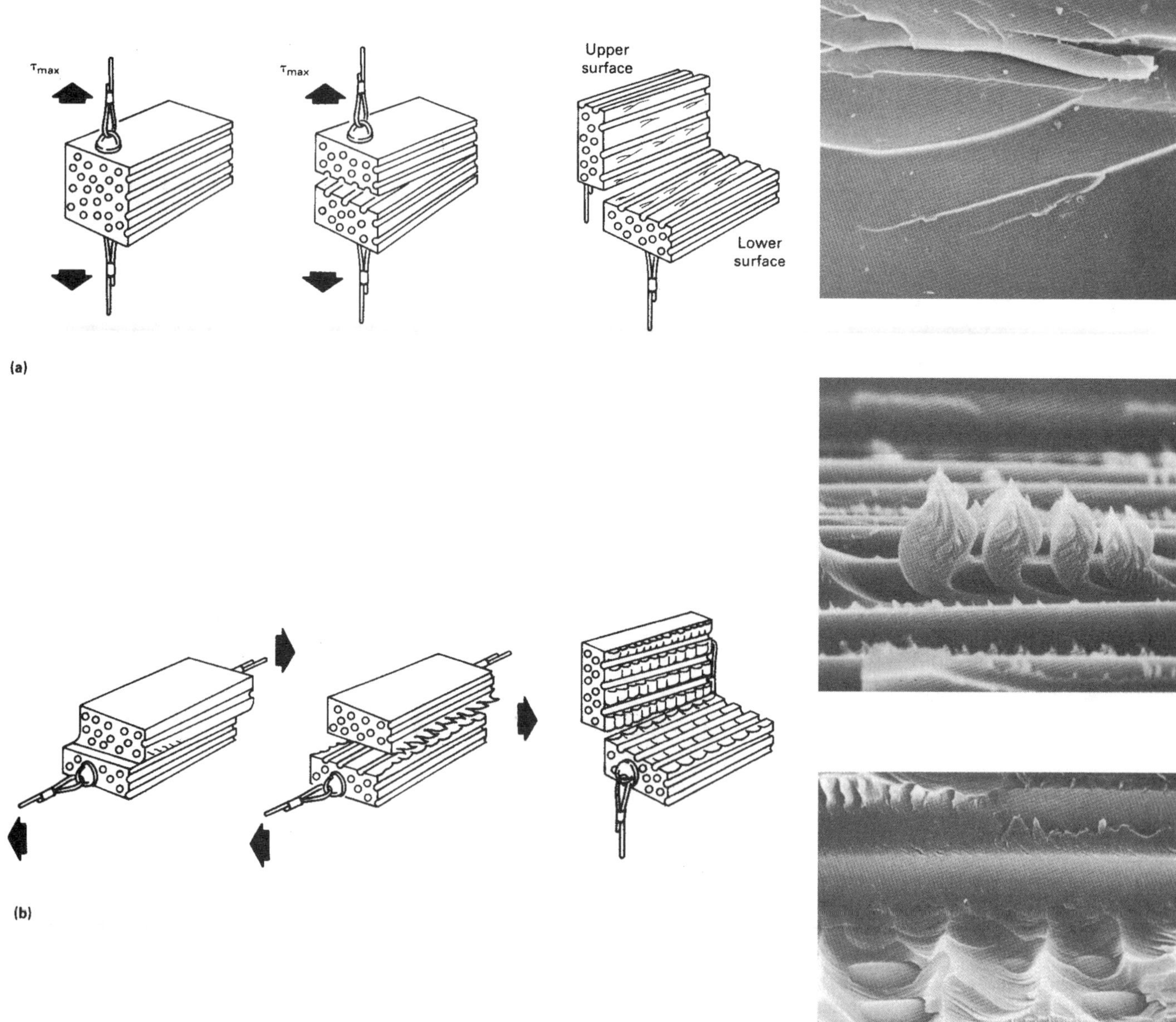

Fig. 6 Schematic of mode II interlaminar shear failure

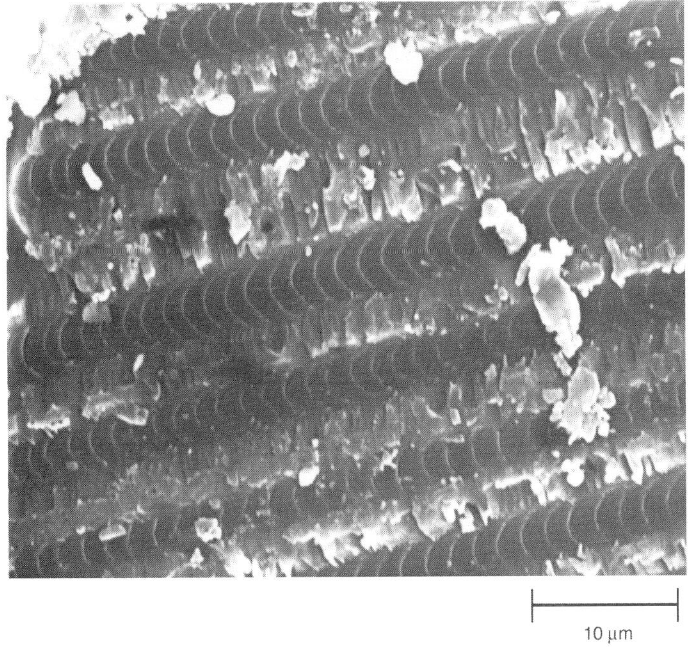

Fig. 7 Fatigue striations in a carbon fiber composite. 2000×

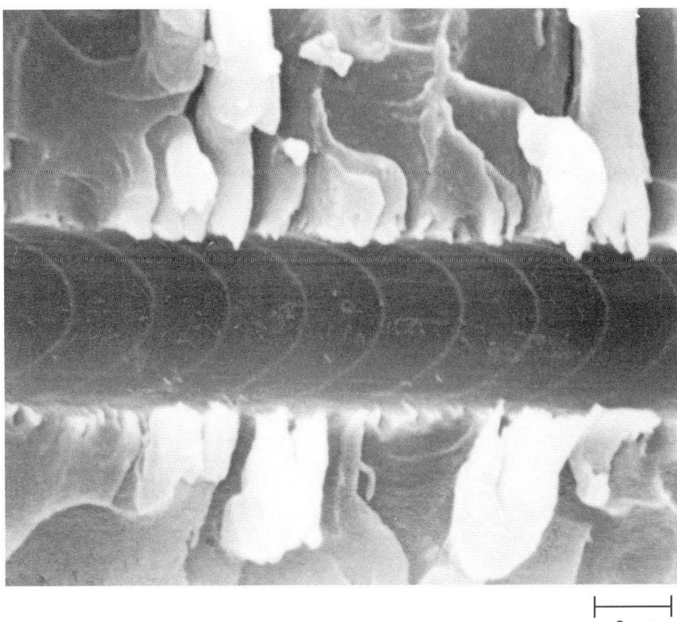

Fig. 8 Fatigue striations in the resin beneath a carbon fiber that was pulled out of a carbon/epoxy (AS4/3501-6) laminate following mode I fatigue loading. 5000×

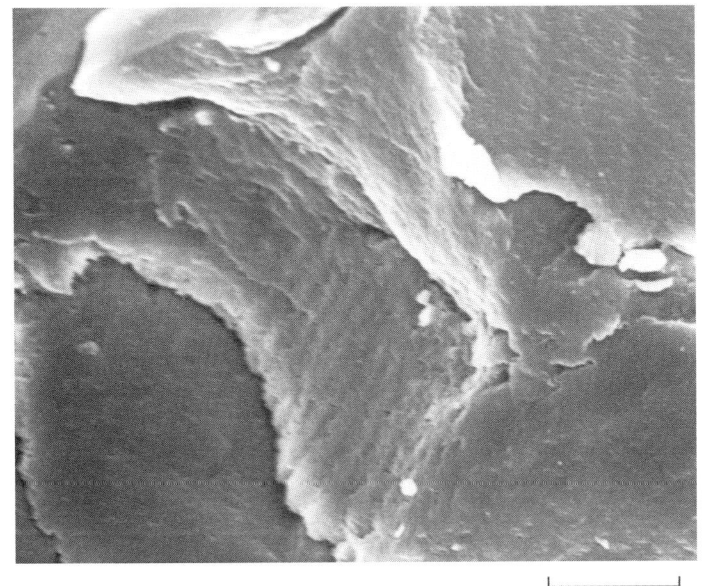

Fig. 9 Fatigue striations in the resin of a carbon/fiber composite laminate that failed in mode I fatigue loading. Striations cover the surfaces of several fibers. 1000×

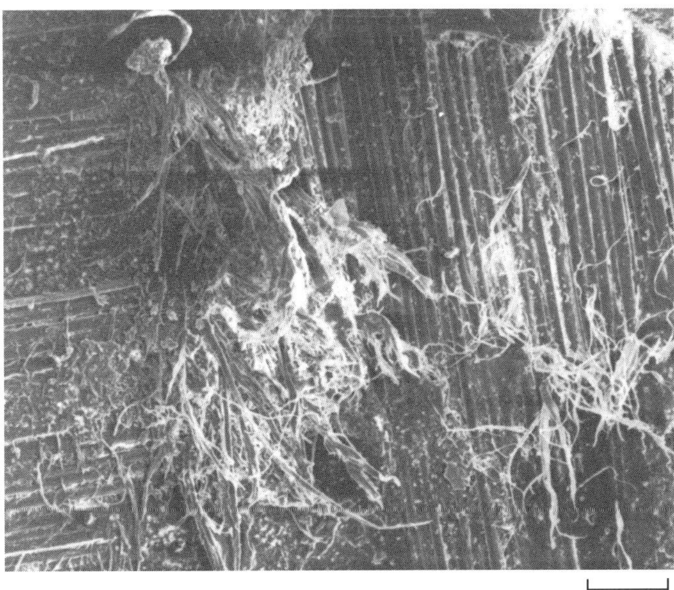

Fig. 10 Impact damage in a Kevlar/epoxy composite laminate depicting hackle formation indicative of shear loading; resin debris indicative of impact loading and fiber fibrillation. 120×

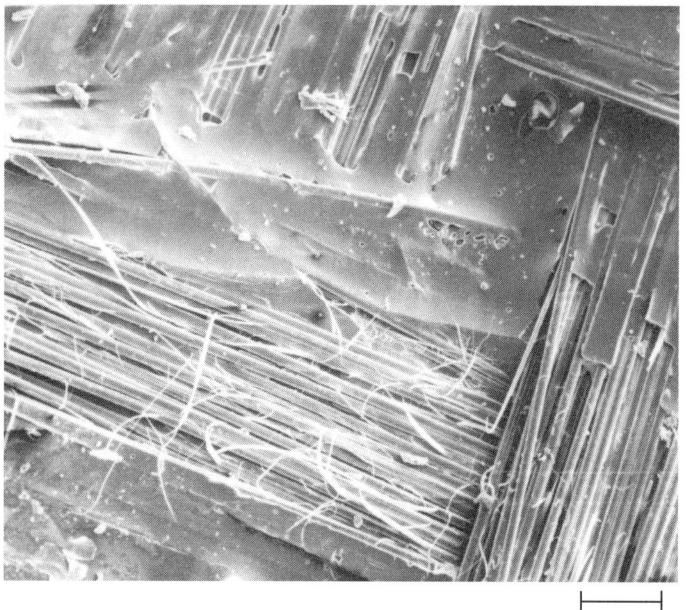

Fig. 11 River patterns and fiber fibrillation in a Kevlar/epoxy laminate in the region surrounding the impact damage, following peel failure of the laminate. 120×

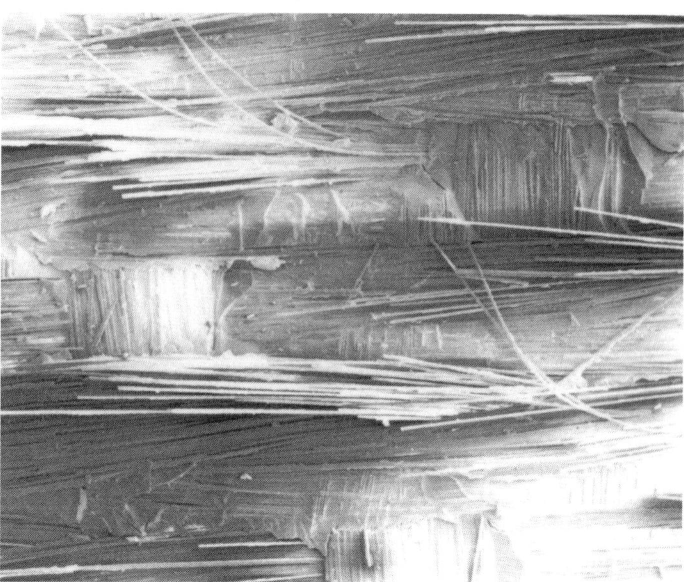

Fig. 12 Exposure of fiber splinters in a glass/polyimide laminate having inadequate resin content, following mode I tension loading of the specimen. 40×

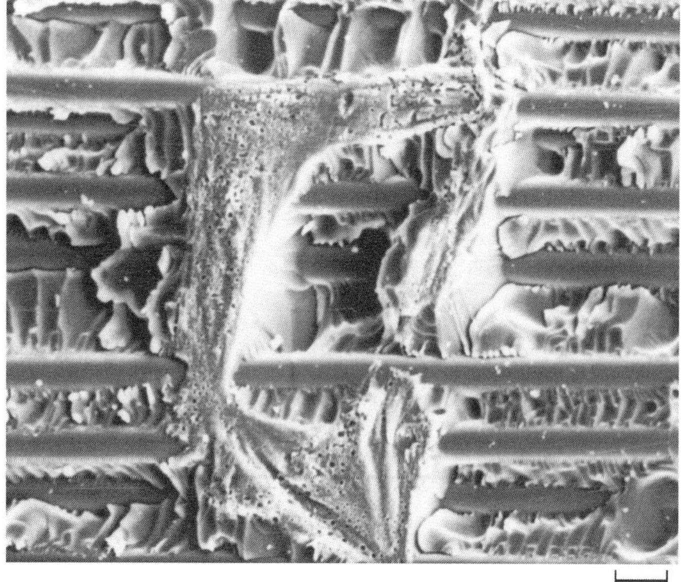

Fig. 13 Frekote contamination on the center portion of the fracture surface of a carbon/epoxy specimen, following mode II shear loading. 780×

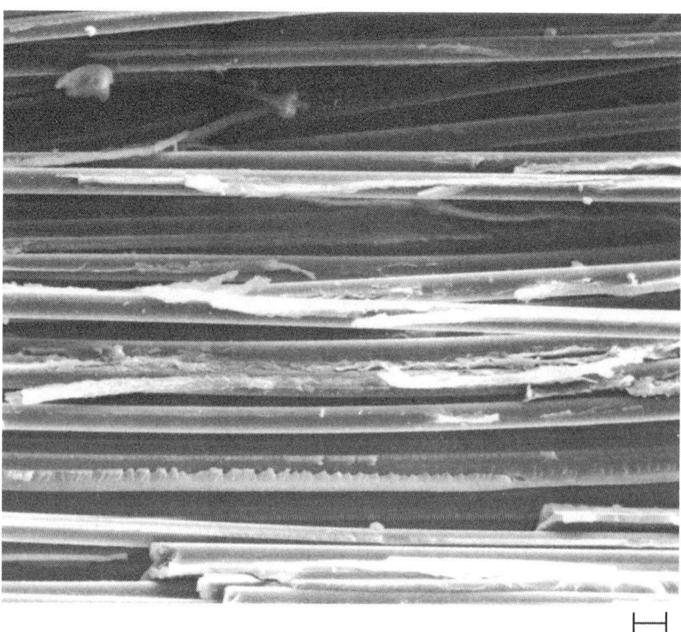

Fig. 14 Fiber/matrix interfacial failure in a carbon/epoxy (AS4/3501-6) test specimen after full moisture saturation and mode I tension loading at 130 °C (270 °F). 480×

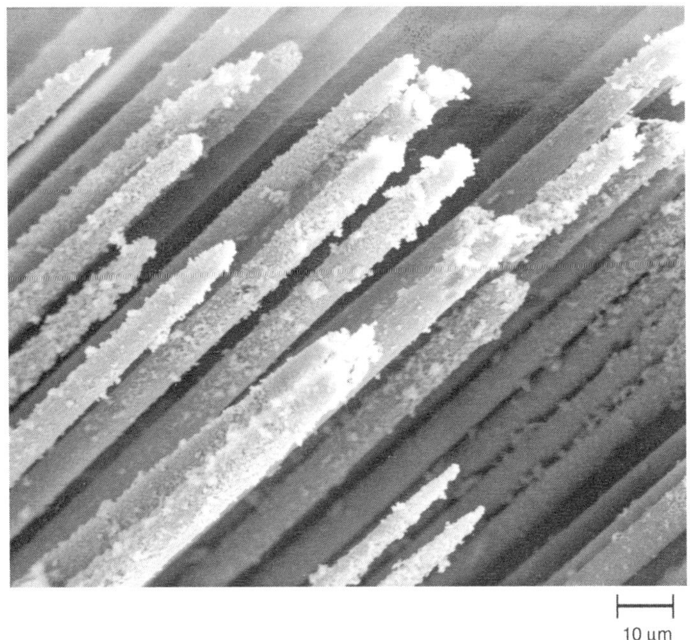

Fig. 15 Carbon fibers in a carbon/epoxy (AS4/3501-6) laminate, following exposure to fire for an unknown time period. 780×

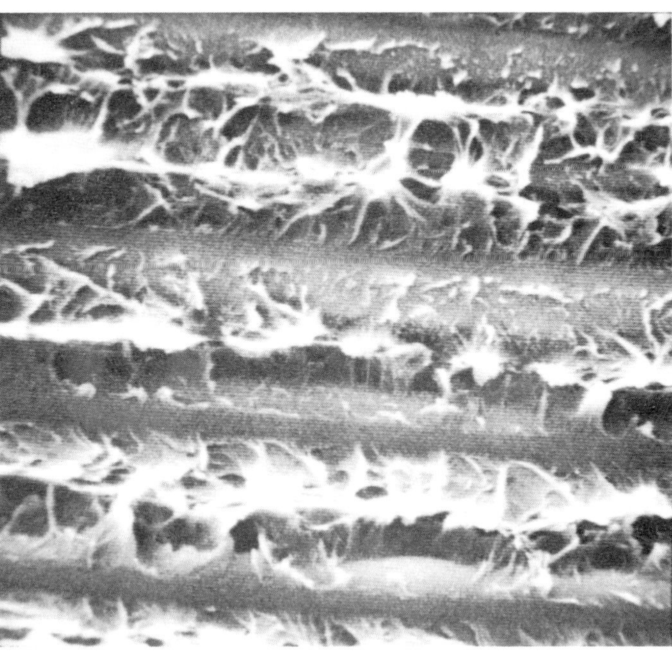

Fig. 16 Surface features of carbon/polyetheretherketone (AS4/APC-2), following mode I tensile fracture. 1500×

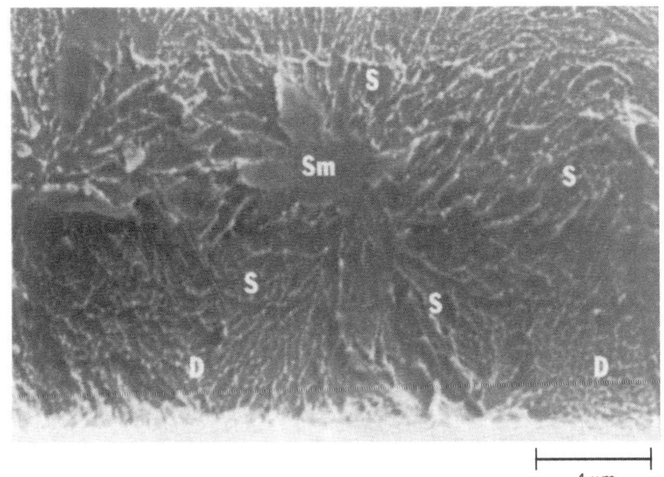

Fig. 17 Radial features thought to be crystallites in the matrix of the APC-2 material, indicative of the crystalline nature of the carbon/thermoplastic (AS4/APC2) resin system, following failure due to mode I tension loading. 5000×

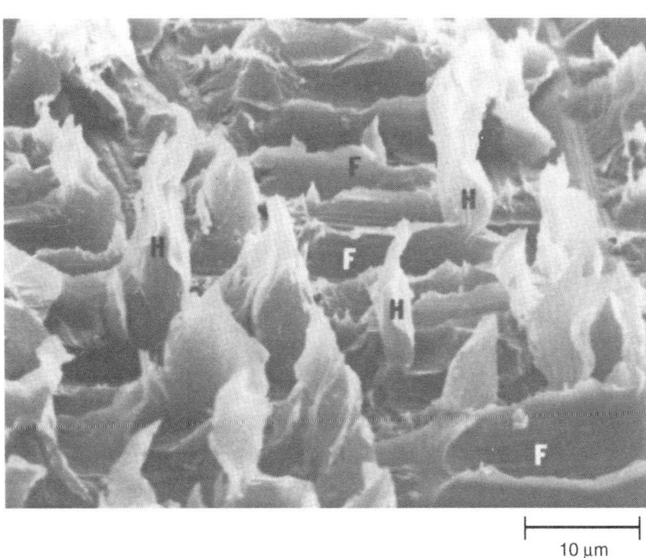

Fig. 18 The formation of the feature known as *spikes* in a mode II shear fracture surface of a carbon/PEEK composite laminate. 1700×

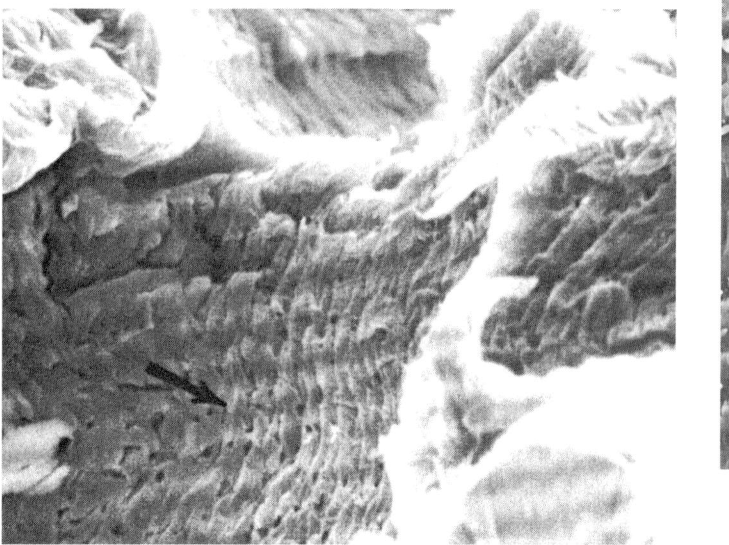

Fig. 19 Fatigue striations in the resin of an interlaminar failure, following mode I loading of a carbon/PEEK composite laminate. 900×

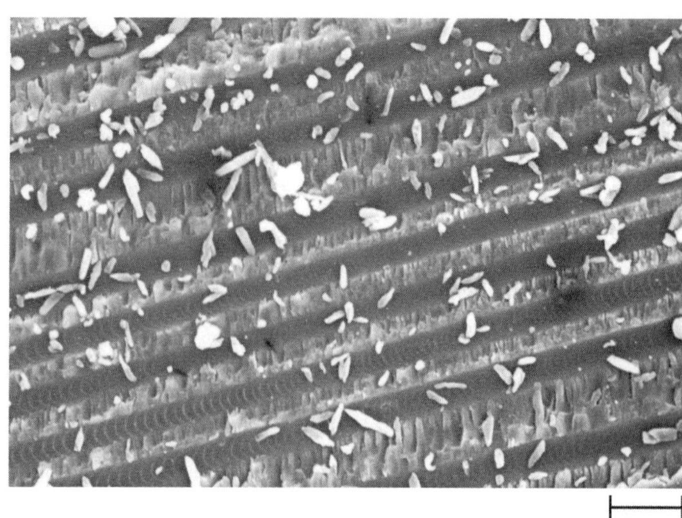

Fig. 20 Fracture feature known as *matrix rollers* on the surface of a carbon/KIII thermoplastic composite, following failure under mode II shear loading conditions. 1000×

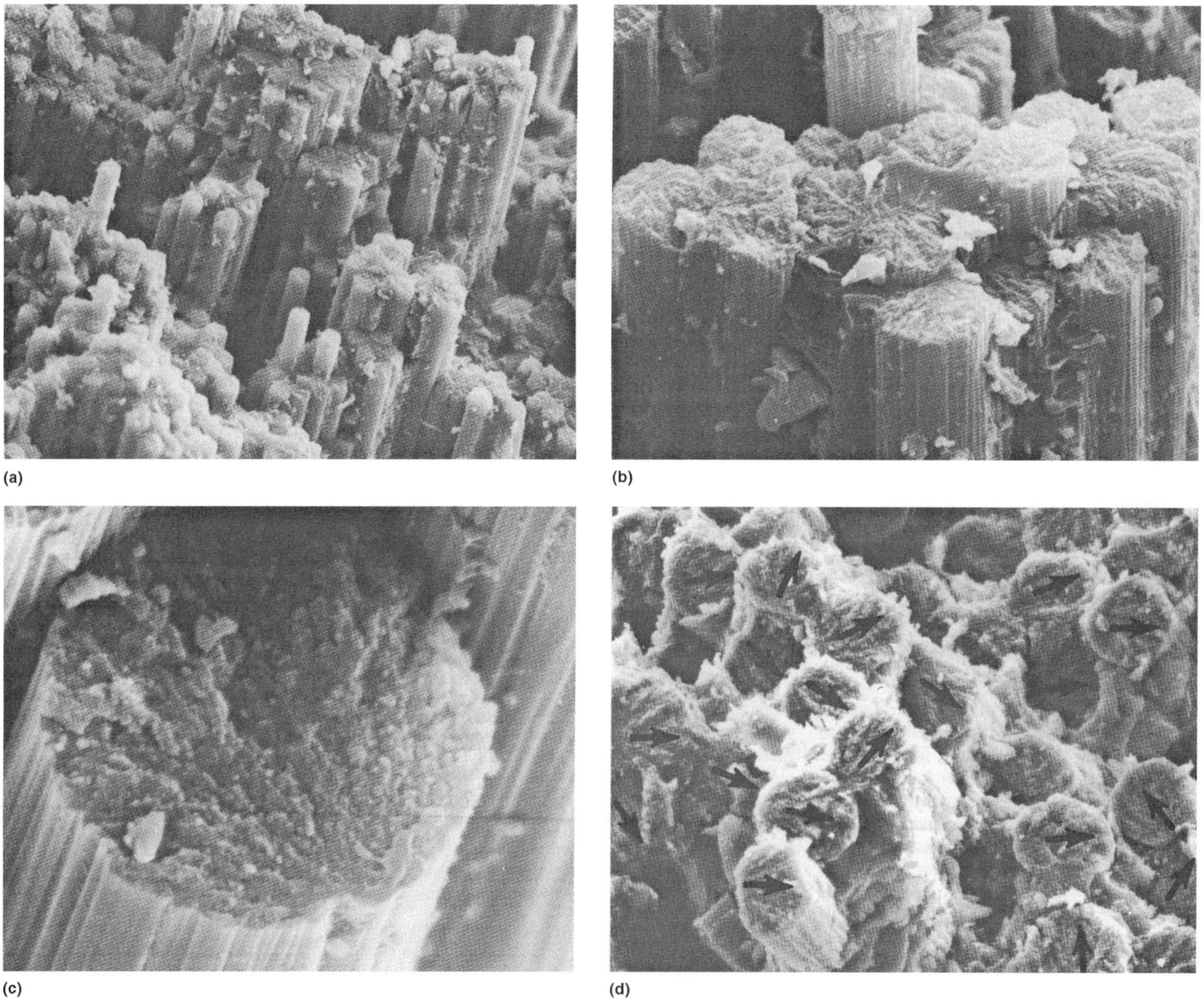

(a)

(b)

(c)

(d)

Fig. 21 Examples of translaminar tension fractures. (a) Translaminar tension fracture in a graphite/epoxy composite. Note fiber bundles and individual fiber pullout. 400×. Source: Ref 2. (b) Translaminar tension failure with localized area of flat fracture. 2000×. Source: Ref 2. (c) Radial fracture topography of an individual graphite-fiber failure under translaminar tension. 10,000×. Source: Ref 2. (d) Variations in fiber fracture mapped to determine overall crack growth direction. 2000×. Source: Ref 3

either before, during, or after loading also influences the fractographic features of brittle matrix composite materials. Specimens first exposed to moisture and then tested at room temperature or specimens exposed to moisture and then tested at elevated temperature revealed specific, identifiable fracture characteristics. Composites that were moisture-saturated and then tested at room temperature generally revealed more plasticity in their fracture characteristics than those specimens that were not moisture-conditioned. This effect, however, is very subtle and may or may not be evident, unless a similarly manufactured and tested dry specimen is available for comparison. For specimens that were moisture-conditioned and then exposed to elevated temperature, however, the fracture characteristics include not only an increase in matrix plasticity, but also an increase in the amount of fiber/matrix interfacial failure in the composite, as shown in Fig. 14. Although an increase in the amount of fiber/matrix interfacial failure may also be somewhat subjective in nature and difficult to discern, this effect is usually more significant, particularly at high moisture contents and temperatures near the wet, glass transition temperature of the resin. Environmental exposure of an organic, composite laminate to high heat or fire, without prior moisture exposure, may also be determined from the fractographic evidence. Following exposure to elevated temperatures, the resin itself is often degraded or pyrolized. The carbon fibers themselves tend to become thinner and more distorted; they have a loss of fiber end fracture features and decomposition products appear on the surface, as shown in Fig. 15. The amount of degradation will depend upon the glass transition and oxidation temperatures of the particular resin system used in the composite, as well as the time and temperature of the exposure. The result can be a partial or total loss of matrix fracture features, including river patterns, hackles and striations, which makes analysis of composites exposed to high temperatures or fire significantly more difficult.

Interlaminar Fracture of Composites with Ductile Thermoplastic Matrices. In ductile thermoplastic resin systems, the interlaminar mode I and mode II fracture characteristics of composite materials are significantly different than for the brittle, thermoset resin systems. In the case of carbon/thermoplastic (AS4/APC-2), the mode I tension fracture surfaces do not exhibit river patterns. These surfaces exhibit small matrix peaks, as shown in Fig. 16, or small flat, radiating, crystallite formations on the fiber surfaces, as shown in Fig. 17. Both of these formations are indicative of the semicrystalline nature of the polyetheretherketone (PEEK) resin system.

For thermoplastic composite laminates such as AS4/APC-2, tested under mode II shear, the fracture features are again unique and unlike the brittle thermoset matrices in which hackles are formed. However, in this case, a similar, repetitive formation of the resin occurs on the surface of the fibers, as shown in Fig. 18. These formations have been termed "spikes." The tilt of the spikes and the flow of the material from the base to the tip can again be used as an indication of crack-growth direction.

Thermoplastic composite specimens, tested under mode I tension and mode II shear fatigue loading conditions, were also examined and fractographically documented. The fracture surfaces of these specimens also exhibit fatigue striations. These striations are similar to those formed in brittle thermoset-matrix composite systems but seemed to exhibit considerably more matrix plasticity, as shown in Fig. 19. The striations in these thermoplastic materials also tend to take on a somewhat irregular shape, often following the ductile matrix material; in brittle thermoset composites, the striations are generally sharp and regular and follow a relatively flat fracture path. Additionally, another feature indicative of fatigue has been noted on the fracture surface of other thermoplastic composite materials, including the carbon/KIII thermoplastic system; when tested under mode II shear fatigue loading conditions, the fracture surfaces of this material exhibit the feature known as *matrix rollers*. This feature consists of resin that tends to roll up upon itself, as shown in Fig. 20. The appearance of these rollers, either between two fibers and/or on the top of the fracture surface, also indicates fatigue failure of the part.

Minimal changes in the manufacturing processes were explored and minimal environmental exposure was conducted for the thermoplastic composite systems. Moisture conditioning of the thermoplastic composite with room temperature testing, however, did not appear to significantly alter fracture features of the carbon/PEEK material.

Translaminar Fracture Features

Translaminar fractures occur when loading of the composite specimen causes fracture perpendicular to the plane of fiber reinforcement. Unlike interlaminar failures, where most of the fractographic information is in the matrix material, translaminar fractures have the majority of the fractographic information in the fiber ends. Visually, translaminar fractures that fail under tensile loads, particularly those with some zero-degree or other off-axis plies, will exhibit considerable fiber pullout and have very irregular fracture surfaces. Scanning electron microscopic examination of the fiber end fractures of carbon and glass fibers will often depict the feature known as *fiber radials*, as shown in Fig. 21 and 22. These fiber radial patterns can often be found in groups, particularly if failure occurred directionally across the laminate, as in the four-point, notched-bend specimens. In these directionally failed test specimens, the fiber radials can be used to determine the direction of the crack propagation. To do this, the direction of each fiber fracture must first be determined. The direction of fiber fracture is determined by creating a vector from the initiation point of the fiber, where the lines on the fiber ends radiate outward, to a point 180° across the fiber surface. Crack growth direction in the laminate can then be determined from addition of these vectors on each fiber across the entire fracture surface.

For composites loaded under translaminar compression, the fracture surfaces are straighter and less jagged than those that failed under translaminar tension. The fracture surface of a com-

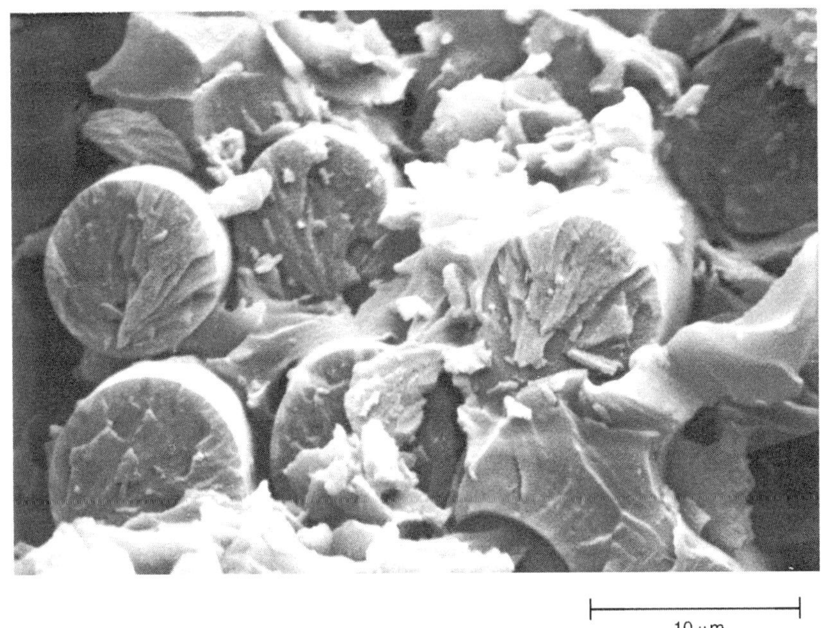

Fig. 22 Radial marks on the surfaces of glass fibers indicative of tensile failure in a glass/polyimide composite following failure of a notched four-point bend specimen. 3000×

posite failed in compression exhibits several different fracture layers, secondary cracking and minimal fiber pullout. They often exhibit shear crippling due to microbuckling of the fibers, which occurs when the fibers kink under compressive loads (Fig. 23a, b). This shear crippling then results in the fracture feature known as *chop marks,* along with pieces of matrix debris on the surface, as shown for carbon fibers in Fig. 23(c) and (d) and for glass fibers in Fig. 24. Chop marks generally have three specific regions on the fiber ends: a tensile region, indicated by fiber radials, a compressive region, indicated by a flat, often angled, fracture surface, and a neutral axis or line separating the two regions.

Translaminar flexural failure of composite laminates generally exhibits both tensile and compressive failure regions on the fracture surface. The amount of each depends upon the loading conditions and the differences between the tensile and compressive strengths of the fibers. The differences between the two regions are generally quite visible, and the location of the neutral axis line can be easily identified from the differences in the fiber end fractures.

Conclusion

In conclusion, the fracture surfaces of a number of composite test specimens have been ex-

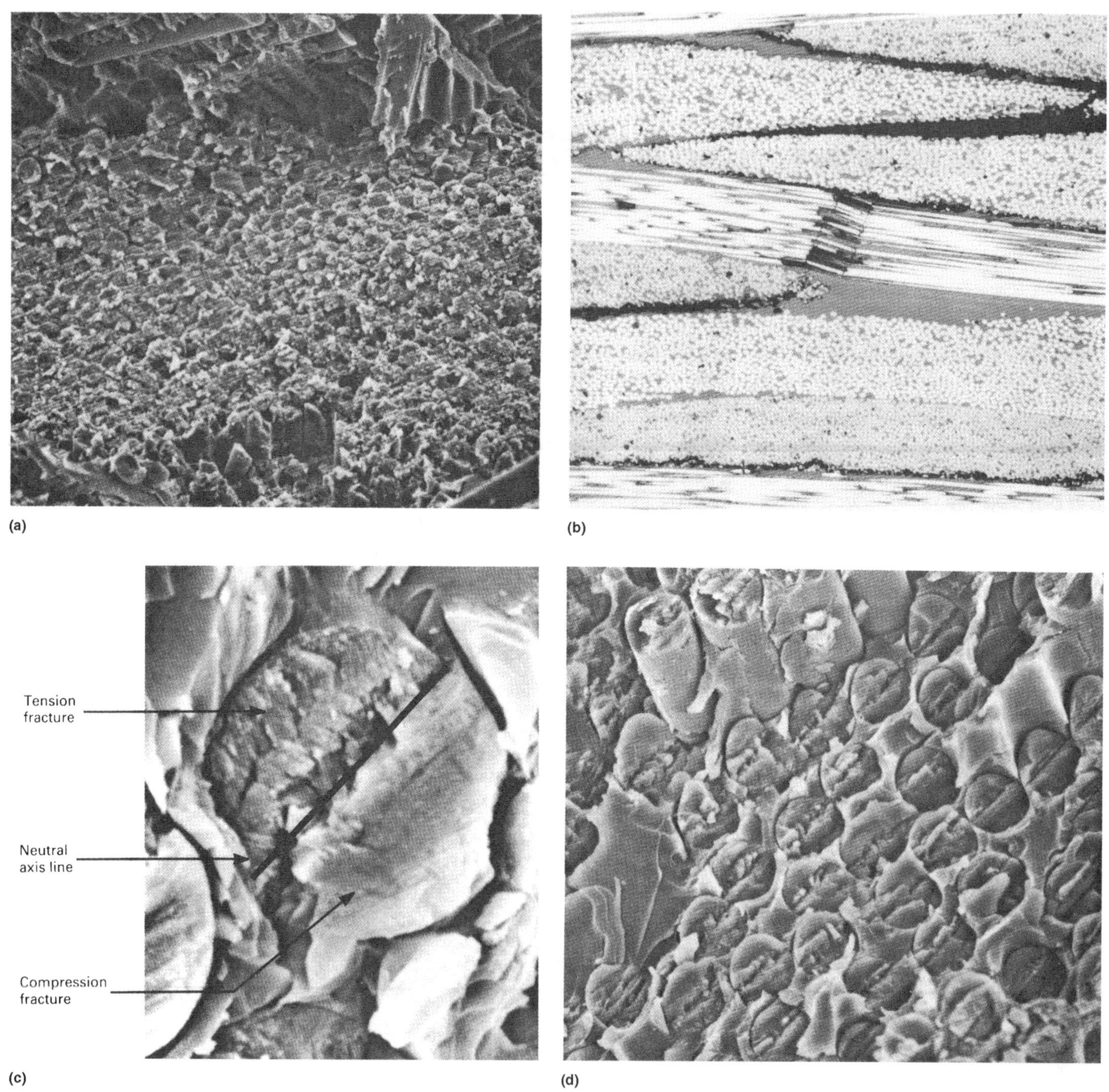

Fig. 23 Examples of translaminar compression fractures. (a) Translaminar compression fracture with extensive post-failure damage to fiber ends. 750×. (b) Translaminar compression-generated fiber kink in graphite/epoxy fabric. 100×. (c) Flexural fracture characteristics on fiber ends of a compression specimen. 10,000×. (d) Translaminar compression fracture illustrating parallel neutral axis lines representative of unified crack growth. 2000×

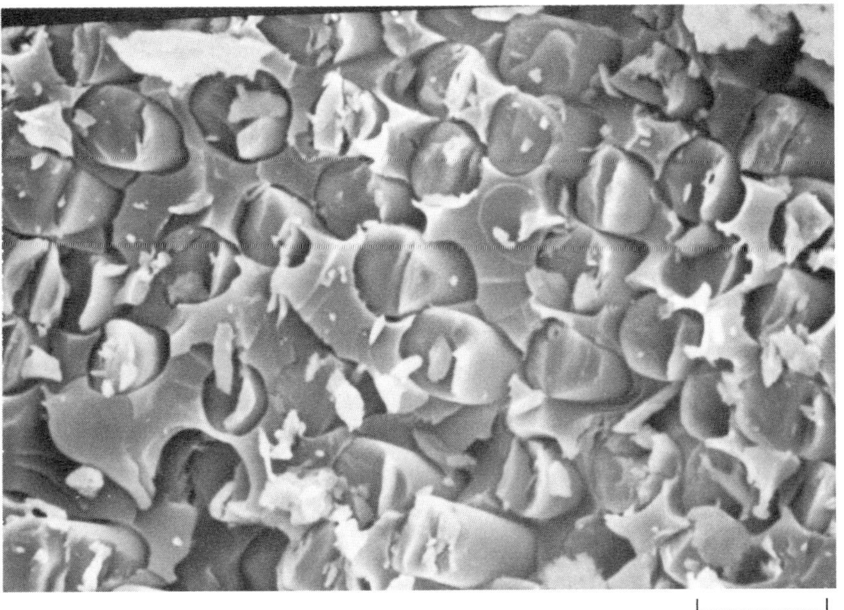

Fig. 24 "Chop marks" on the fracture surface of the glass fibers in a glass/polyimide composite tested as a notched four-point bend specimen that failed in compression. 1800×

amined and fractographically documented. It appears that, similar to metallic materials, composite materials have unique fractographic features that can be related to specific materials, processing methods, environmental exposures, and load conditions. These features have been catalogued by a number of researchers over the years and have been evaluated, based on the type of information they are able to provide about the fracture. The features can be used for determining information about component failures, particularly, information regarding crack initiation site, crack-growth direction, environmental conditioning, and failure mode. It should be noted, however, that even with the large amount of fractographic data that have become available in recent years, it still may not be possible to always determine the failure cause. This is because some of the fractographic information may have been obliterated, lost, or destroyed by some postfailure condition. Additionally, there are limitations as to the amount and type of information that can be obtained from a fractographic analysis, and additional techniques, such as mechanical testing and stress analysis, may be required to determine failure cause in some instances.

ACKNOWLEDGMENTS

The author would like to recognize the assistance of Boeing Military Airplane Company and Northrop Grumman, who provided some of the test specimens and fractographs for this work under Air Force Contracts F33615-84-C-5010 and F33615-87-C-5212.

REFERENCES

1. B.W. Smith et al., Fractographic Analysis of Interlaminar Fractures in Graphite-Epoxy Material Structures, *International Conference: Post Failure Analysis Techniques for Fiber Reinforced Composites*, Air Force Wright Aeronautical Laboratories, MLSE, July 1985
2. A.G. Miller et al., "Fracture Surface Characterization of Commercial Graphite/Epoxy Systems," *Nondestructive Evaluation and Flaw Criticality for Composite Materials,* STP 696, American Society for Testing and Materials, 1979, p 223–273
3. S.W. Tsai and H.T. Hahn, *Introduction to Composite Materials,* Technomic Publishing, 1980

Case Histories

Patricia L. Stumpff, Hartzell Propeller Inc.

THIS ARTICLE describes the results of several case history studies of the failure of polymer-matrix composite (PMC) components to provide not only some representative types of failures one can encounter, but also to provide some insight into the investigative process. These case histories deal mainly with structures that exhibit an initial material and/or manufacturing defect or anomaly—failures that are most prevalent and most easily solved. Component failures traced to some initial material- and/or manufacturing-related defects seem to have fewer fracture surfaces compared with those that do not have any initial defects. In addition, more complex failures (those without defects and those having transverse fractures) often require the use of stress analysis in addition to fractographic analysis.

In the investigations presented here, final analysis often was considerably more involved than is possible to describe in a brief summary. However, the results of these investigations hopefully will enable the reader to understand the need not only for careful technical analyses, but also the need for insight, patience, persistence, and experience to solve the myriad types of problems related to the failure analysis of composite structures.

Helicopter Rotor Blade Failure

Circumstances Leading to Failure. A helicopter rotor blade failed after a minimal number of flight hours. The blade failure consisted of a complete separation of the outer carbon/epoxy sleeve from the internal Kevlar/epoxy paddle, as well as complete transverse failure of the paddle and the sleeve (Fig. 1). The outer sleeve and the paddle are manufactured separately and then adhesively bonded together during final assembly of the blade. The Kevlar/epoxy paddles are machine sanded after molding to remove any traces of silicon that may have adhered to the surface of the paddle during the molding process. The paddle itself has a convex curvature across its width, with foam inserts bonded to the underside of the paddle to fill in the concave area. The woven carbon/epoxy plies of the outer sleeve, the Kevlar/epoxy paddle, and the foam inserts are bonded together during final assembly of the blade.

Test Procedures and Results. Visual analysis of the failed blade revealed that the top surface of the paddle had a smooth, glossy surface, except for two strips along the length of the paddle, which exhibited duller fracture features. Examination of the glossy areas on the surface of the paddle at low magnification revealed relatively featureless fracture surfaces (Fig. 2). By comparison, the dull areas had a number of areas with resin fracture as indicated by the arrows in Fig. 3. Examination of the glossy surface at higher magnification revealed small rounded globules (Fig. 4), while the dull surfaces at higher magnification revealed considerable plastic deformation (Fig. 5).

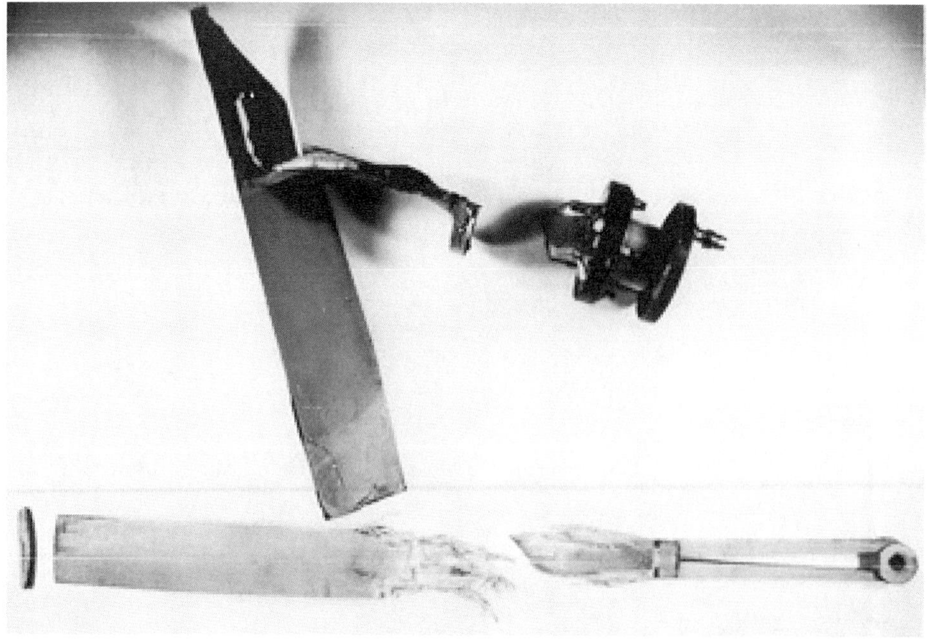

Fig. 1 Separation and fracture of internal Kevlar/epoxy paddle and external carbon/epoxy sleeve of failed helicopter blade

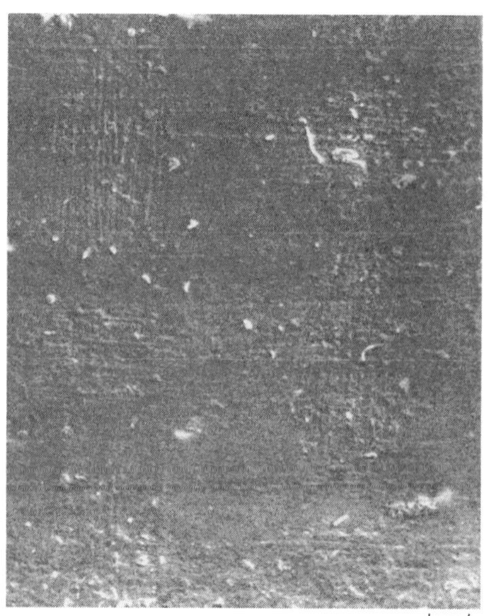

Fig. 2 Low magnification SEM view of shiny areas on Kevlar/epoxy paddle surface. 48×

Fourier transform infrared (FTIR) analysis of the paddle surface showed that the spectrum is typical of that for an epoxy resin, but also contains an additional peak at 1741 cm^{-1}, which is indicative of a carbonyl band (Fig. 6). Electron spectroscopy for chemical analysis (ESCA) of the surface of the paddle revealed unexplained silicon peaks as shown by the small peaks to the right in Fig. 7.

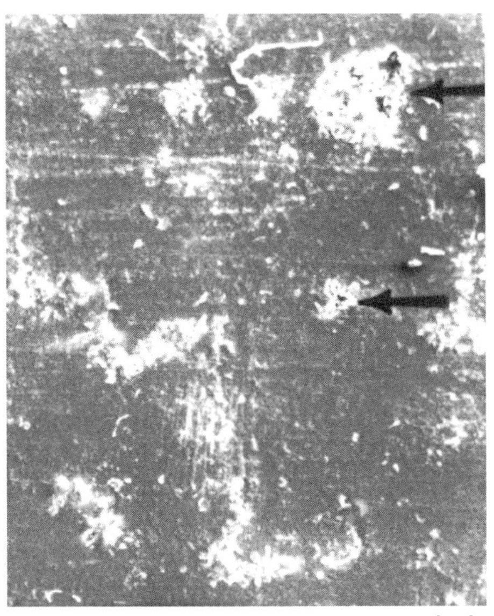

Fig. 3 Low magnification SEM view of dull areas on Kevlar/epoxy paddle surface. 48×

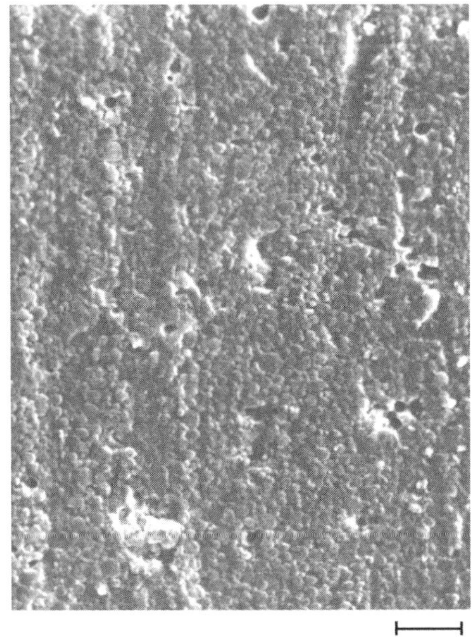

Fig. 4 Higher magnification SEM view shiny surface of Kevlar/epoxy paddle showing resin swelling and no resin fracture. 720×

Evaluation and Conclusions. Both the glossy surface appearance and the presence of silicon indicated the possibility of inadequate sanding of the paddles prior to the adhesive-bond operation. Additional paddles from the manufacturer (both before and after the sanding operation) were evaluated to verify or disprove this hypothesis. Paddle surfaces prior to the sanding operation exhibited smooth, glossy surfaces, intact fibers, and silicon contamination, as well as rounded globules indicative of resin swelling. By comparison, sanded paddles exhibited a dull, whitish surface finish, fiber damage, resin deformation, and no evidence of silicon contamination.

Further analyses of the other fractures were limited. In addition to the debonding of the paddle from the sleeve, the paddle and sleeve also exhibited transverse fractures. These fractures occurred at approximately the same lengthwise location, but investigators were unable to determine the mode of fracture. The fact that the sleeve failed in the same location as the paddle appears to indicate that these two transverse fractures were related or occurred at nearly the same time and/or under the same loading conditions.

Overall visual evaluation of the fractured components appears to indicate that the paddle debonded from the sleeve prior to the transverse fracture of either subassembly. Transverse fracture of either portion of the blade prior to a debond most probably would have revealed some damage, such as markings on either the inside surface of the sleeve or on the outer surface of the paddle, which is not the case. If the transverse fracture occurred first in both the sleeve

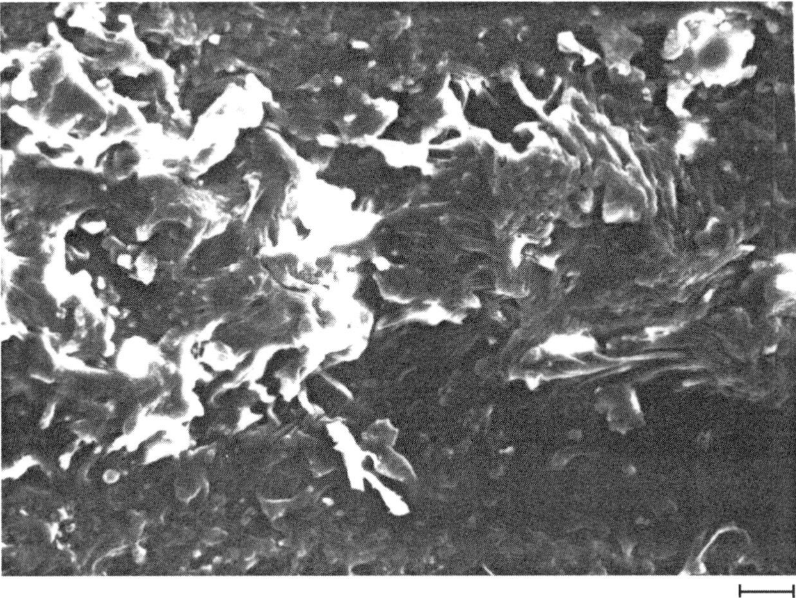

Fig. 5 Higher magnification SEM view of dull surface of Kevlar/epoxy paddle showing significant resin deformation and fracture. 720×

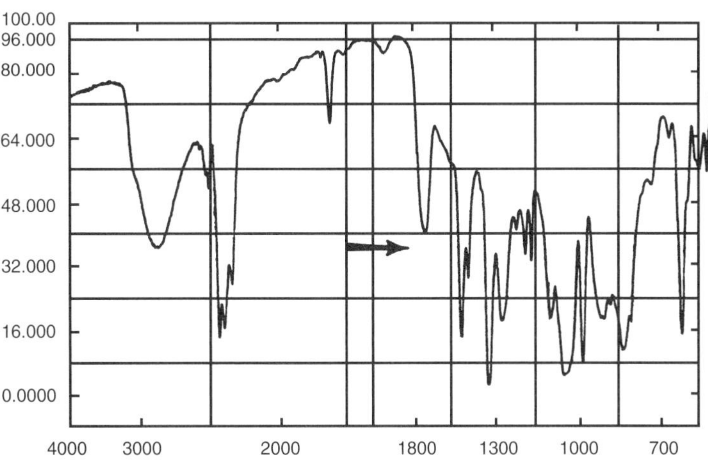

Fig. 6 FTIR spectrum of Kevlar/epoxy paddle surface showing additional carbonyl peak (arrow) at 1741 cm^{-1}

and the paddle together, there would have been no reason for a disbond to occur at all. Therefore, the most likely scenario is that the disbond occurred prior to any transverse fracture. Debonding between the paddle and the sleeve would significantly reduce the stiffness of the blade; reduced stiffness in both the paddle and the sleeve may have resulted in the transverse failure of the paddle and the sleeve under normal loads. It is believed that premature debonding occurred as a result of either inadequate or incomplete sanding of the paddles prior to the bond operation. Inadequate sanding resulted in a contaminated surface having a slick, glossy finish, which is unsuitable for subsequent bonding of the paddle to the sleeve.

Composite Wing Spar Failure

Circumstances Leading to Failure. A wing spar on a small aircraft failed prematurely; the aircraft reportedly had some flight time prior to failure, but no overloads on the wing were believed to have occurred. The spar section is shown in Fig. 8; the leading edge of the wing is at the bottom and the aft edge at the top of the photo. The wing spar is in the shape of a box spar with upper and lower carbon/epoxy and glass/epoxy caps and shear webs made of Nomex honeycomb core and glass/epoxy skins.

Test Procedures and Results. Further examination of the spar revealed a flexural failure, with the lower cap exhibiting tensile failure and fibers bent aft (Fig. 9) and the upper cap exhibiting compressive failure with the fibers bent forward (Fig. 10). This analysis is consistent with a wing bending upward and twisting forward.

Nondestructive evaluation of the wing spar using x-radiography did not reveal any evidence of damage in the component except for the visually apparent fracture. Following visual and nondestructive evaluation, fracture surfaces were removed for examination using scanning electron microscopy (SEM). Scanning electron microscopy evaluation revealed fiber radials, which are indicative of tensile failure in the lower cap, and fiber chop marks and debris, which are indicative of a compressive failure of the upper cap; these results further support the occurrence of a bending failure of the spar.

A cross section of the spar near the fracture revealed that the upper and lower caps were manufactured using unidirectional carbon/epoxy prepreg, with several glass/epoxy plies on either side. The number of plies, their orientation and layup were as specified by the manufacturer. The shear webs were manufactured using Nomex honeycomb core with glass/epoxy skins, which are subsequently bonded to the upper and lower caps. The cross sections of the upper and lower caps reveal several significant manufacturing anomalies including a large amount of fiber waviness (Fig. 11), a 12% void content (Fig. 12), and an abnormally low fiber volume fraction of only 45%.

Thermal-mechanical analysis of the carbon/epoxy cap indicated a glass transition temperature of 115 °C (239 °F), which is slightly on the low side for a 120 °C (250 °F) carbon/epoxy system. Differential scanning calorimetry did not reveal any exothermic reactions, indicating a full cure of the composite spar.

Further fractographic examination of several interlaminar fracture surfaces revealed evidence of striations, which are indicative of fatigue (Fig. 13). Most of the striations are found in the upper cap, but some also are present in the lower cap.

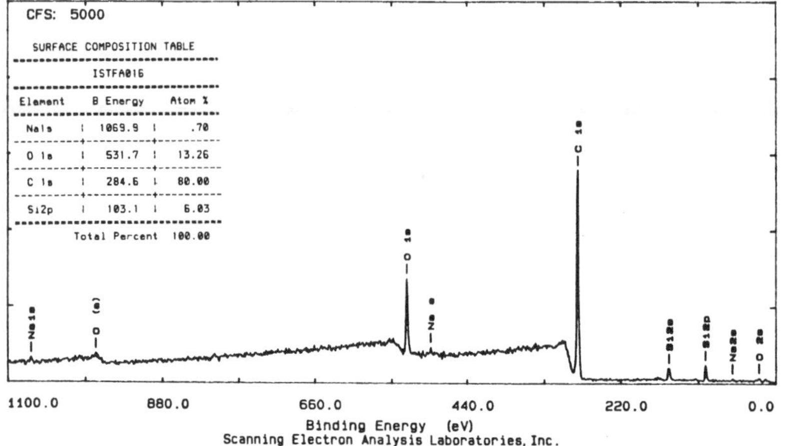

Fig. 7 ESCA analysis of Kevlar/epoxy paddle surface showing silicon peaks (small peaks on the right)

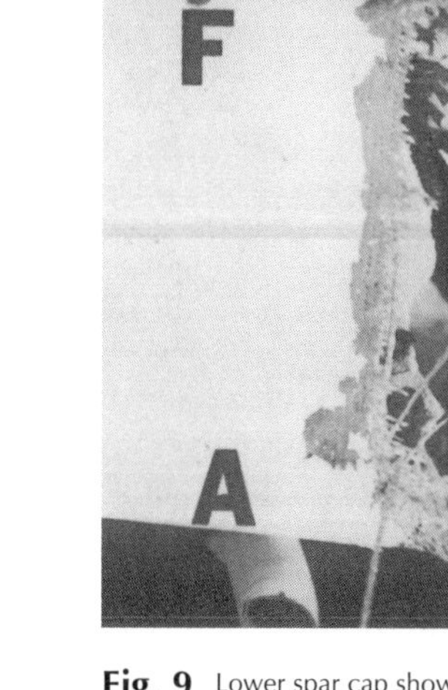

Fig. 9 Lower spar cap showing tensile failure and fiber distortion aft (arrow). F: forward, or leading edge; A: aft, or trailing edge

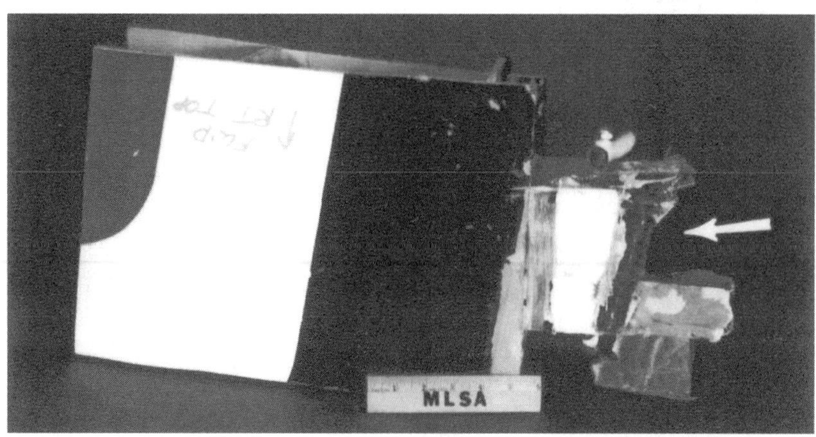

Fig. 8 Section of failed wing spar

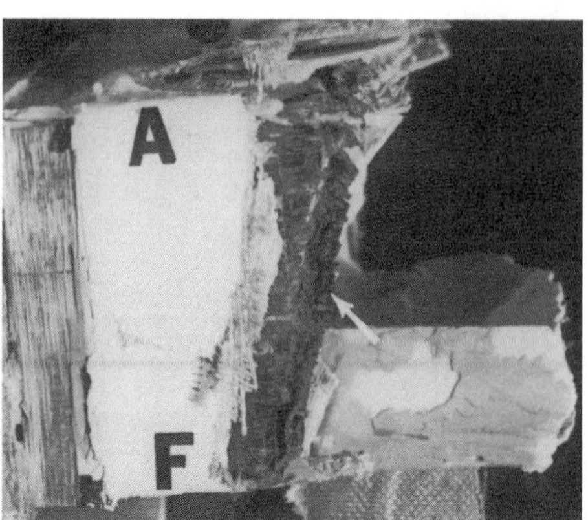

Fig. 10 Upper spar showing compressive failure and fiber distortion forward (arrow). F: forward, or leading edge; A: aft, or trailing edge

Test specimens were sectioned from the spar to determine mechanical property data. Five 0° tensile (ASTM D 3039-76) and five 0° compressive (ASTM D 3420-87) specimens were machined from the carbon/epoxy portions of the upper and lower caps, respectively. Average tensile and compressive strengths of the test specimens were determined to be only 670 and 267 MPa (97.3 and 38.7 ksi), respectively. These values are significantly lower than the 0° tensile strength of 1585 to 1792 MPa (230–260 ksi) and 0° compressive strength of 1516 to 1723 MPa (220–250 ksi) reported by the materials supplier.

A compression-compression fatigue test (R = 0.1) was conducted by loading the specimen at 80% of the average ultimate compression strength determined from the prior compression test. Ultimate failure occurred after only a few cycles. A second compression-compression fatigue test was conducted at a maximum compression load of only 192 MPa (27.8 ksi), or 72% of the ultimate compression strength of the spar cap. In this case, failure occurred after approximately 156,619 cycles.

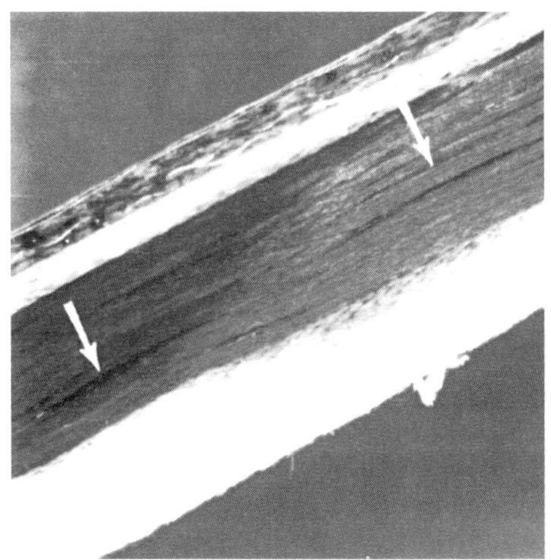

Fig. 11 Wing spar cross section showing delaminations (arrows) and excessive fiber waviness. 3.5×

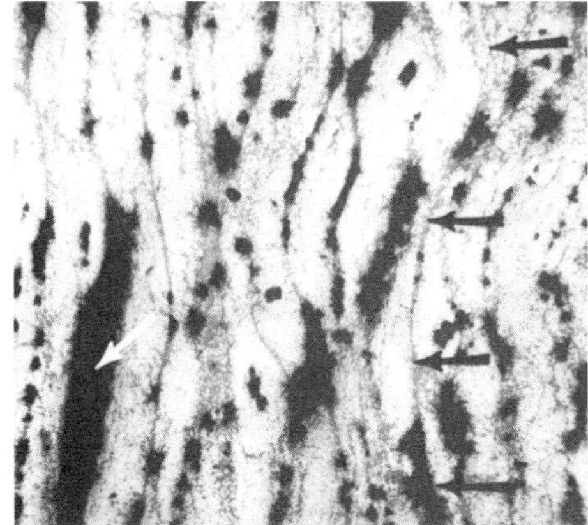

Fig. 12 Higher magnification of spar cap cross section showing excessive fiber waviness (black arrows) and high void content (white arrow). 40×

Evaluation and Conclusions. The fractographic evidence indicates that the failure of the spar is consistent with bending fatigue, with evidence of compressive failure on the upper cap of the spar and tensile failure on the lower cap. The bending fatigue in the spar may have initiated and propagated due to either higher than anticipated fatigue loads on the spar or to anticipated fatigue loads in conjunction with a reduction in the fatigue strength resulting from a number of manufacturing anomalies.

Manufacturing anomalies in the spar noted during the investigation include significant fiber waviness, high porosity, and low fiber volume fraction. According to the materials supplier, resins used in the manufacture of this particular spar generally were formulated for use in autoclave or press molding. However, the manufacturer noted that composites were successfully processed using this resin and vacuum bag molding techniques, stressing that the component must be debulked regularly to extract trapped air from the layers.

Whatever method was used in the manufacture of this spar, it resulted in manufacturing anomalies and relatively low mechanical properties, which may have contributed to the premature fatigue failure of the spar.

Aircraft Rudder Failure

Circumstances Leading to Failure. The skin from a composite rudder assembly separated from the core. Visual analysis revealed that the right side of the rudder (Fig. 14) had undergone almost complete skin/core separation; only a small piece of composite skin remained attached to the rudder at the trailing edge. The separated skin was lost and not available for evaluation. The adhesive, still attached to the aluminum core, did not exhibit any visible fracture features, although porosity is evident throughout. The adhesive itself is a consistent shade of light gold over most of the fracture surface, except under the remaining section of skin, where the adhesive is white in color.

The left side of the rudder was intact. Markings found on the leading edge of the intact left side of the rudder are believed to be indicative of a disbond/delaminated area previously detected by nondestructive evaluation. Examination of adhesive on the left side of the rudder after removing a small section of skin revealed characteristics similar to those on the right side, that is, porosity with no visible fracture features. This adhesive also is white in color, similar to the adhesive under the remaining skin on the right side of the rudder.

Test Procedures and Results. Background information on this particular rudder revealed that nondestructive evaluation after manufacture showed no evidence of any skin/core disbond or skin delamination. Rudders manufactured after the one being evaluated exhibited some small disbonds/delaminations on their leading edges following manufacture. Other rudders exhibited some small disbonds/delaminations after some time in service. However, the rudder under investigation was said to be the first to undergo a complete, in-flight skin/core separation.

Rudder construction consists of an aluminum frame and honeycomb core with carbon/epoxy face sheets containing a single glass/epoxy fabric ply on the either side of the carbon/epoxy skin. The skins are precured and then subsequently

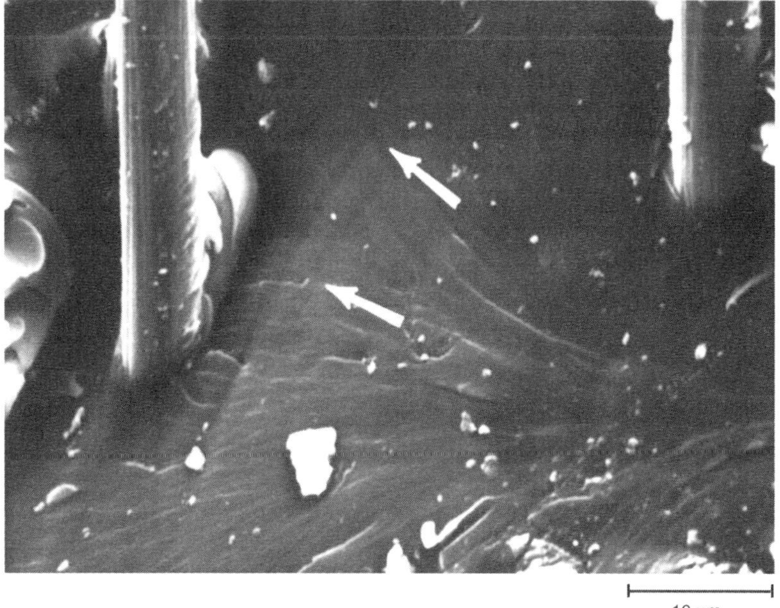

Fig. 13 Striations (arrows) in resin of fractured surfaces, indicative of fatigue failure. 2000×

bonded to the aluminum substructure. During manufacture of the skins, polyester peel plies are added to the exterior skin surfaces and are removed just prior to bonding the skins to the aluminum frame and honeycomb core. The removal of a peel ply generally results in clean, roughened, fractured surfaces, immediately suitable for bonding. The precured composite skins are then bonded to the aluminum substructure using a typical aircraft adhesive manufactured for composite and aluminum bonding.

Pulse-echo ultrasonics was used to verify whether there was any damage actually present on the leading edge on the left side of the rudder. The test revealed a disbond/delamination in the marked area and a small delamination at the other end on the leading edge of the rudder, but no other damage.

A portion of the remaining glass/epoxy composite skin and its mating adhesive on the right side of the rudder was removed and examined using SEM. For comparison, a small piece of skin and its mating adhesive surface from the left side of the rudder also were examined following separation by peel forces. Similar fracture characteristics were identified at both interfaces on both sides of the rudder. Figure 15 depicts the adhesive surface characteristics on the right side of the rudder. The adhesive takes on the shape of the peel ply imprints that were left on the skin surface upon removal of the peel ply. Examination of the adhesive surface at higher magnification reveals some evidence of epoxy from the composite skin surface (the short, wide arrow in Fig. 16) adhering to the adhesive at the interstices of the peel ply imprints. Mating fracture characteristics were found on the surface of the composite skin samples that were originally attached to the adhesives.

Although the adhesive itself does not exhibit any features indicative of fracture mode or direction, river patterns—indicative of peel forces—were evident in the epoxy matrix that remained attached to the adhesive. The river patterns, often located in the epoxy at the interstices of the peel ply imprints, were used to determine the direction of skin separation and indicated that the origin of the failure on the right side of the rudder is at the lower leading edge, or forward corner. Crack growth proceeded from the lower forward leading edge corner toward the top and trailing edge of the rudder, as identified in the schematic, in Fig. 17. Crack growth direction in the crosshatched area of the schematic could not be determined because fracture at this location occurred at the interface of two adhesive layers. Two layers of adhesive are used in this location of the rudder, and because fracture of this particular adhesive does not exhibit river patterns, no crack growth direction could be determined in this area.

Fourier transform infrared spectroscopy was used to identify the adhesive system. Although no exact match could be found in the reference database, the spectra obtained bore some similarity to modified, inorganic, filled epoxies. Differential scanning calorimetry tests conducted on the adhesive showed no significant exothermic reactions, indicating the adhesive samples were fully cured.

Electron spectroscopy for chemical analysis (ESCA) was used to analyze the glass/epoxy skin and adhesive surfaces from both sides of the rudder to determine if there was any contamination present on the right side of the rudder that might have contributed to the failure. The spectra for the adhesive/glass interface on the right side of the rudder showed 70% C and 30% O. Similar results were obtained on the left side of the rudder (following peel fracture), indicating surface contamination did not contribute to the separation of the skin from the rudder.

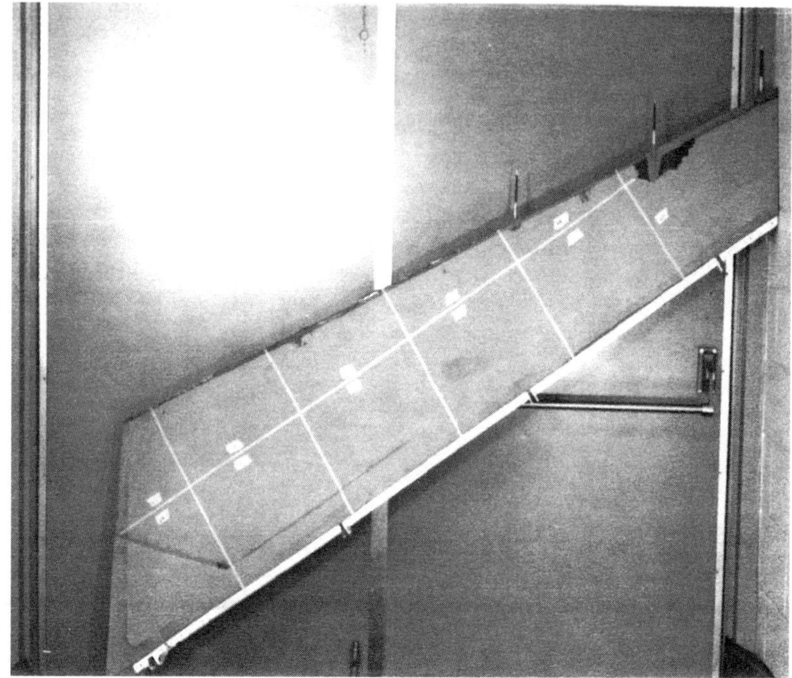

Fig. 14 Loss of the outer skin (except small section near the antennae at the top of the photograph) on right side of composite rudder

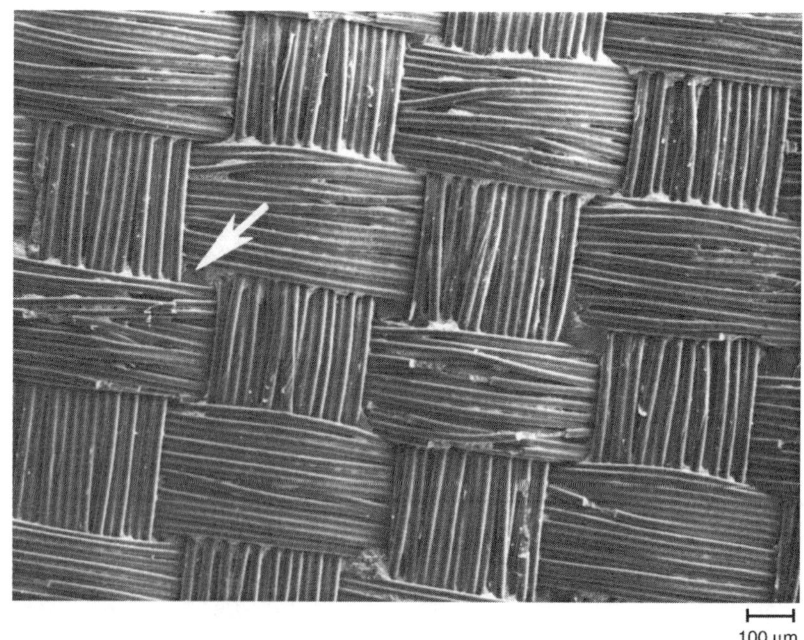

Fig. 15 Adhesive surface showing mirror image of peel ply imprints on glass/epoxy skin surface (river patterns at interstitial areas of weave indicated by white arrow). 66×

Investigation of the color variation in the adhesive showed that humidity aged an adhesive sample at a slightly elevated temperature; the white adhesive turned to a light golden yellow, similar to the color of the adhesive on the right side of the rudder.

Evaluation and Conclusions. The almost complete separation of the skin of the rudder from the core is believed to be the result of inadequate adhesive bonding of the skin to the aluminum core and possible moisture intrusion into the bondline. Inadequate bonding of the skin to the core was evident particularly at the lower forward leading edge corner of the rudder where the fracture initiated. The two layers of adhesive noted in this location, a history of delaminations in this area in manufactured rudders, and evidence of a delamination in this same location on the opposite side of the rudder support this conclusion. Poor bonding is also suspected because the majority of the failure was interfacial in nature; only about 5% of the adhesive fracture surface had epoxy on it. Additionally, it was noted that the bonded side of the skin surfaces exhibited smooth, mirror images of the peel plies that were not removed prior to the adhesive-bonding operation. Bonds that are manufactured using laminates that have smooth, reflective surfaces following peel-ply removal generally have poorer mechanical properties than bonds manufactured using laminates that have roughened fracture surfaces following peel-ply removal.

There is also evidence of possible moisture intrusion into the bondline. Moisture intrusion is suspected because the adhesive on the delaminated surface changed color from white to light gold, similar to the color change experienced by adhesive specimens upon exposure to moisture and temperature in the humidity chamber. It is suspected that the moisture entered the bond at the delamination at the leading edge and helped propagate the failure over time, mainly because the color change was evident only on the delaminated portion of the fracture.

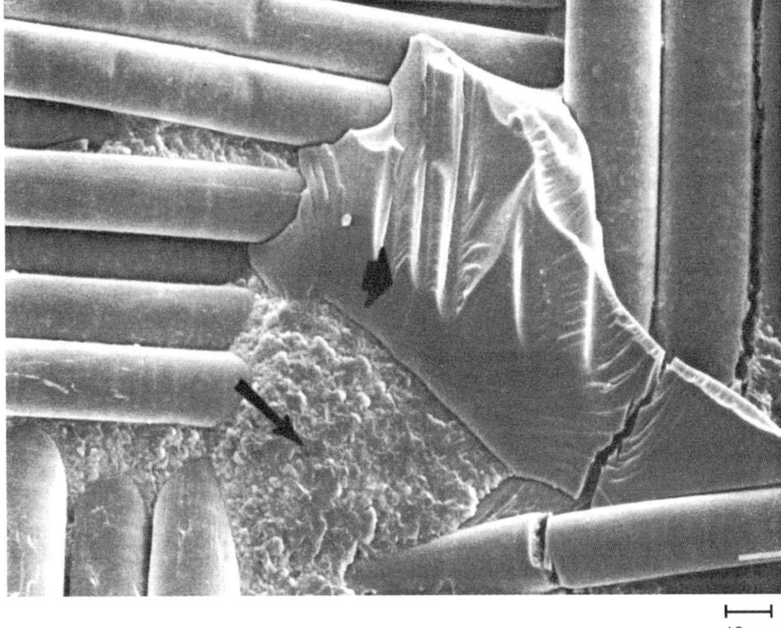

Fig. 16 Higher magnification view showing river patterns in epoxy resin at interstitial areas (short arrow) and fracture of the adhesive (long, thin arrow). 600×

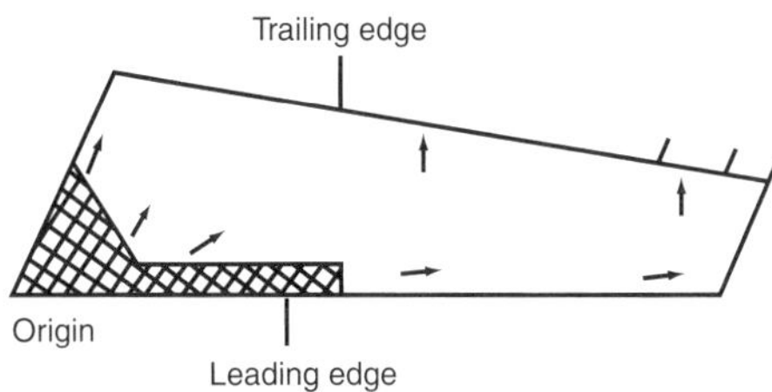

Fig. 17 Schematic of direction of skin separation (small arrows) on horizontal stabilizer from lower leading edge to upper trailing edges

Fatigue Properties and Quantitative Fractography of Metal-Matrix Composites

Bruce Crawford, Deakin University, Australia

FATIGUE PROPERTIES of particle-reinforced metal-matrix composites (PR-MMCs) and the quantitative examination of their fracture surfaces are the principal concerns of this article. The general properties of MMCs are not described here. A full review of these can be found in Ref 1 and in the article "Properties of Metal-Matrix Composites" in this Volume. The experimental and fractographic techniques described here resemble those used with unreinforced metallic alloys, but the fracture surfaces of MMCs contain features, such as fractured and decohered reinforcement particles, that distinguish them from those of unreinforced materials.

Fatigue Properties of Metal-Matrix Composites

This section reviews the fatigue properties of MMCs in terms of mechanisms of crack initiation, fatigue life, and fatigue crack growth.

Mechanisms of Crack Initiation

The initiation of cracks in SiC and Al_2O_3 reinforced MMCs has been extensively studied. Most of these studies have concentrated on MMCs with aluminum alloy matrices. Four major sources of crack initiation have been identified. These are:

- *Fracture of the reinforcement particles (Fig. 1a):* Reinforcement particles are typically very brittle. They fracture in the initial stages of fatigue, sometimes in the first loading cycle, and rapidly initiate microcracks in the surrounding matrix. This is due to the high strain concentration produced by the intersection of microcracks in reinforcement particles with the surrounding matrix. This mechanism is most commonly observed in composites reinforced with Al_2O_3 particles or fibers (Ref 2–4).
- *Decohesion of the reinforcement from the matrix:* This can occur either at the interface between the reinforcement and the matrix or in the matrix near the reinforcement-matrix interface. It is most common in SiC-reinforced composites (Ref 5–11), but it has also been observed in alumina-reinforced composites (Ref 12). In many cases, cracks are initiated from particle clusters (Ref 5, 7, 8, 10). These typically act as a single, large particle as plastic flow of the matrix material within the cluster is heavily constrained. Also, in MMCs prepared using liquid metallurgy techniques, poor penetration of the matrix material into particle clusters can lead to poor particle-matrix bonding within the cluster, which increases the likelihood of decohesion (Ref 13).
- *Fracture of large particles,* other than reinforcement particles: Examples of such particles include large inclusions and intermetallics. These are very prone to fracture because of their large size relative to the reinforcement particles (20 to 100 μm) and brittle nature. This mechanism is common in composites with Al-Cu-Zn (2*xxx*) matrices because of the high alloy content of these materials (Ref 9, 12). In general, these particles fracture in the early stages of fatigue and rapidly initiate cracks.
- *Porosity* (Fig. 1b): Fatigue cracks can initiate from porosity in composites (Ref 4, 8) just as they do in unreinforced metals (Ref 14). As the size of the pores increases, so does their effectiveness in initiating cracks relative to the other mechanisms described here. An MMC containing large pores will typically fail due to a fatigue crack initiated from one of these pores (Ref 4). For liquid metallurgy MMCs, pores typically arise from incomplete penetration of the matrix material into particle clusters.

Fatigue crack initiation typically occurs at or near the surface of a material (Ref 10, 11), regardless of the nature of the initiating defect. This is because surface defects are exposed to higher cyclic plastic strains and, once fractured, to higher stress-intensity factors (K) than defects located within the bulk of the material. As a consequence, cracks will initiate far earlier from surface defects than from bulk defects and will grow faster once initiated.

Fatigue Life

The increased stiffness and strength of MMCs increase their fatigue life under the load-control conditions of a typical fatigue life test (Ref 10). This increased life is most pronounced under high cycle conditions. In contrast, under strain-control conditions, the fatigue life of MMCs is often worse than that of the corresponding matrix alloy (Ref 10). The reason for this change is the higher elastic modulus of MMCs compared to their base alloys. Under load-controlled conditions, the higher modulus of the MMC means that the strain imposed on the matrix is reduced. This increases the fatigue life. The opposite occurs under strain control. In this case, the strain is the same in both materials, but the stress is higher in the MMC. This increases the probability of reinforcement fracture or decohesion, which, in turn, encourages the initiation and growth of fatigue cracks that reduce the fatigue life of the composite.

Fatigue Crack Growth

The interaction between reinforcement particles and the fatigue crack controls the local direction of crack growth in MMCs. This is because reinforcement particles modify the stress field surrounding the crack tip. The exact nature of this modification depends on whether the particles fracture, decohere, or remain intact during fatigue. The main factors controlling the fatigue of MMCs are therefore:

- Reinforcement type (composition and shape)
- Reinforcement volume fraction and size
- Matrix aging condition

The residual stresses produced by thermomechanical treatment also influence the fatigue of MMCs. The effects of residual stresses are discussed in the section "Long Fatigue Crack Growth" in this article.

Reinforcement Type. It is difficult to find any direct comparisons between the fatigue behavior of similar alloys reinforced with different types of reinforcement particle. This is principally due to the pre-eminence of SiC as a reinforcing particle for MMCs. A similar problem exists for the effect of particle shape, as SiC particles are significantly larger than SiC whiskers. In general, however, elongated particles (such as SiC whiskers) will inhibit crack growth when the crack is growing perpendicular to the particles and accelerate growth when the crack is parallel (Ref 5, 15).

Reinforcement Volume Fraction and Size. The effect of reinforcement volume fraction varies with the mean size of the reinforcement. An increase in volume fraction decreases fatigue crack growth rate in composites reinforced with large (>10 μm) particles (Ref 16–18) and increases the fatigue crack growth rate in composites reinforced with very small (<3 μm) particles (Ref 19, 20). The difference arises from the way in which reinforcement particles of differing size react to an approaching fatigue crack. Fine particles are resistant to fracture, which tends to constrain the crack path. This produces a flat fracture path, low levels of roughness-induced closure, and faster fatigue crack growth. At a given reinforcement volume fraction, larger reinforcement particles are spaced further apart and are, by virtue of their larger size, more prone to fracture. Fractured particles attract the fatigue crack, which, when combined with the increased particle spacing, produces a rougher fracture surface and higher levels of roughness-induced crack closure. This effect is, therefore, most pronounced near the fatigue threshold, and so MMCs containing fine particles tend to have lower fatigue thresholds than those containing coarser particles.

Matrix Aging Condition. In unreinforced aluminum alloys, the fatigue threshold decreases with increased aging (Ref 21). This is because aging alters the slip character of the matrix. Reinforcement particles suppress this effect in MMCs (Ref 22). This occurs because fatigue cracks avoid uncracked particles while seeking out cracked particles. Therefore, the crack path is controlled by the size, spacing, and fracture behavior of the reinforcement particles. As aging treatments cannot alter these parameters, fatigue properties of the MMCs remain unchanged.

Fatigue Testing of MMCs

Specimen Preparation

As described previously, the fatigue life of MMCs and the initiation of cracks in them during fatigue have been extensively studied. The techniques, samples, and equipment used for this work resemble those used with unreinforced metallic alloys. However, the reinforcement particles in MMCs mean that tungsten carbide or diamond-coated tooling is required for specimen machining. In addition, the difference in hardness between the matrix and reinforcement can cause surface relief to develop during polishing. This surface relief should be avoided as it can decrease the fatigue endurance of MMCs. This can be achieved by using polishing cloths with a low nap during polishing.

Microscopy

Fatigue crack initiation and short crack growth in MMCs can be readily studied using an optical microscope. Detailed methodology is found in the article "Microscopy" in this Volume. The use of Normarski interference contrast greatly aids the identification of fractured reinforcement particles and fatigue microcracks in polished initiation samples of MMC. This is due to the distortion of the surface of the sample by the plastic zones surrounding these fatigue microcracks. The resultant surface relief is quite obvious under Normarski interference contrast conditions (see Fig. 1a). Crack initiation and growth can also be studied using acetate or rubber molding compound replicas. These have the advantage of providing a more complete record of the surface of the specimen than optical microscopy can.

Another method of studying crack initiation and short crack growth in MMCs is using a scanning electron microscope (SEM) equipped with a cyclic loading stage. This allows very detailed study of the interaction between reinforcement particles and fatigue cracks. However, the rarity of the cyclic loading stages makes this method unavailable to most researchers.

Long Fatigue Crack Growth

The long fatigue crack growth behavior of MMCs can be evaluated using the test methods

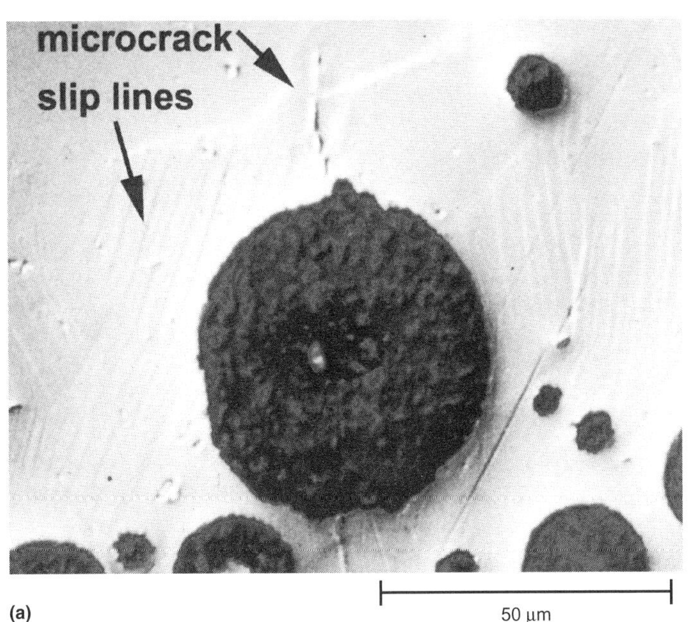

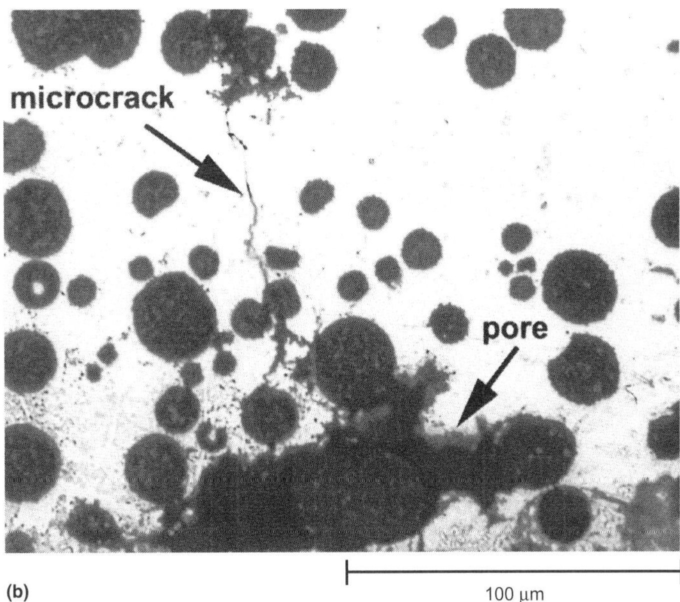

Fig. 1 Initiation of fatigue microcracks in metal-matrix composites. (a) A fatigue microcrack initiated from a fractured Micral-20 (mullite-alumina) reinforcement particle in Comral-85 (6061-20% Micral-20). Note that the reinforcement particle has fractured across its vertical equatorial plane, perpendicular to the applied load. (b) Initiation of a fatigue microcrack from a large pore in Comral-85

and specimens used for unreinforced metallic alloys. Most of the published fatigue crack growth data for MMCs has been obtained using either compact tension or tensile single-edge notch specimens as described in ASTM E 647 (Ref 23). However, MMCs have several features that must be accounted for if they are to be tested successfully. The most important of these are described subsequently.

Macroscopic Residual Stresses and Consequent Crack Bowing Induced by Heat Treatment. Macroscopic residual stresses are significantly higher in MMCs than in unreinforced alloys (Ref 24). As a result, MMCs are prone to increased crack-front bowing. The edges of the crack can grow unevenly, with one side being a millimeter or so ahead of the other (in a crack of between approximately 10 and 50 mm, or 0.4 and 2.0 in., in length). In extreme cases, the center of the crack can grow several millimeters ahead of its edges. This contravenes the requirements of ASTM E 647 (Ref 23) and should be minimized. This can be achieved, with various degrees of success, by prestraining after either solution treatment or aging, annealing out the residual stresses in the MMC, reducing their effect during testing, or by compensating for the resultant crack bowing during analysis after testing is complete. Prestraining the MMC before testing can reduce residual stresses (Ref 25, 26). This, however, increases the yield stress of the MMC and decreases its ductility, which will bias the collected fatigue results. Despite this, prestraining is widely used. It is less problematic if performed after solution treatment, where the low strength of the matrix reduces damage to the reinforcement particles. Annealing to remove the residual stresses is impractical, because the temperatures required exceed those used in artificial aging in aluminum alloys. The effect of residual stresses during testing can be minimized by using high load ratios ($R \geq 0.4$, where R is P_{min}/P_{max}, the ratio of minimum load to maximum load in cyclic loading) (Ref 24). This increases the crack-opening displacement, which reduces crack closure and crack-front bowing. This approach, however, does not allow the fatigue properties of the MMC to be fully evaluated. Finally, the effect of crack bowing can be compensated by recalculating K based upon measurements of crack-front curvature collected after the completion of testing. This approach has been successful in reducing the scatter in fracture toughness results for an aluminum alloy and for an alumina-reinforced MMC (Ref 27, 28). The use of this method with fatigue cracks and MMCs, however, has not been validated.

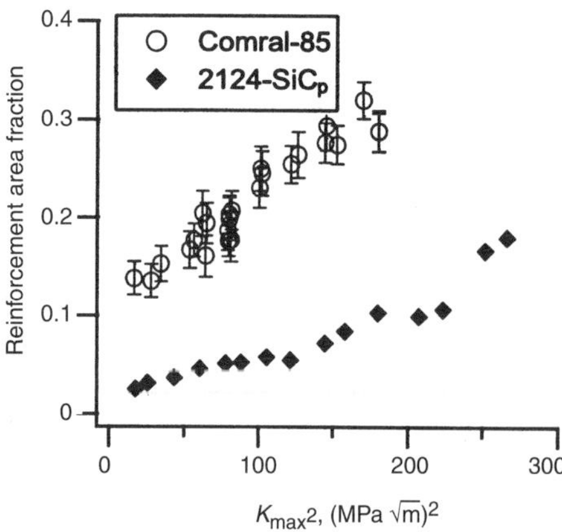

Fig. 2 Area fraction of reinforcement on the fatigue fracture surface of a SiC-reinforced MMC (Ref 11) and Comral-85, a Micral-20- (mullite-alumina) (Ref 25) reinforced MMC as a function of K_{max}^2

Increased Electrical Resistance and Decreased Compliance Compared to Unreinforced Materials. Automatic crack-length measurement methods use either the electrical resistance or compliance of the specimen to estimate the length of the fatigue crack. Therefore, changes in these values due to reinforcement must be accounted for if these methods are to be used successfully. Additionally, the compliance of MMCs can change due to damage in the process zone ahead of the crack tip. This will cause compliance methods to overestimate the true crack length. The magnitude of this error increases with increasing K_{max} due to the fracture of reinforcement particles ahead of the crack tip. For this reason, automatic crack-length measurements should be supplemented with visual measurements to confirm their accuracy.

Fractography of MMCs under Plane-Strain Conditions

Observed Features of MMC Fatigue Fracture Surfaces

A major feature of the fatigue fracture surfaces of MMCs produced under plane-strain conditions is that the area fraction of reinforcement particles on the fracture surface (A_f) is proportional to K_{max}^2 (Fig. 2) (Ref 11, 26). This suggests that A_f is controlled by the size of a process zone preceding the fatigue crack (Ref 10, 11, 26). Fractographic evidence (Fig. 3) from Comral-85, an MMC consisting of a 6061 matrix reinforced with mullite-alumina microspheres, supports this supposition (Ref 26). Note that several of the reinforcement particles visible in Fig. 3(a) are surrounded by plateaus, which are microcracks initiated by the reinforcement particle during fatigue. These plateaus are characterized by river lines radiating from the perimeter of the reinforcement particle. Closer examination shows that these lines initiate from surface features of the reinforcement particle at the center of the plateau. These lines, and the plateaus on which they appear, indicate that the reinforcing particles fractured ahead of the main crack tip. Figure 4 shows the effect of a change in K_{max} on the fracture surface of a MMC reinforced with SiC particles (Ref 29). These fracture surfaces are similar to those of Comral-85 except that there is no SiC visible on the fracture surface at low (< 8 MPa $\sqrt{m}$, or 7 ksi $\sqrt{in.}$) stress-intensity factors (Fig. 4a).

In addition to K_{max}, the type, size, shape, and volume fraction of reinforcement, the aging state of the matrix material, and the stress state under which fatigue crack propagation occurred influence A_f (Ref 11, 26). A_f also depends on K_{Ic} because this is the highest value of K_{max} possible for a given material. In contrast, A_f is independent of ΔK and R, as shown in Fig. 5 for Comral-85 (Ref 26). Similar results for SiC-reinforced composite are currently unavailable.

Using four variants of a 2124 Al/20 vol% SiC$_p$ composite, Hall et al. (Ref 11) demonstrated that A_f increases with the mean size of the reinforcement particles. This increase is most likely due to the decreased resistance to fracture of larger particles. Hall et al. (Ref 11) also observed that A_f increased as the reinforcement volume fraction increased. This increase in A_f, however, was not proportional to the increase in V_f and is therefore not merely a result of the increased amount of reinforcement in the composite. Instead, the proportion of A_f as a function of the reinforcement volume fraction of the composite decreased as the volume fraction increased.

The appearance of the fracture surface around the reinforcement particles changes dramatically between threshold and fast fracture (Ref 11, 26). (Compare Fig. 3a with 3b and Fig. 4a with 4b.) Near the fatigue threshold the fracture surface is quite flat, with the exception of river marks growing from those reinforcement particles that are visible on the fracture surface. The regions between the plateaus are characterized by shear steps. Striations are visible on the fracture surface of the SiC-reinforced composite (Fig. 4a). As ΔK increases into the Paris Law region*, the plateaus around the particles shrink and the steps between the plateaus become rougher and more distinct. Toward the upper end of the Paris Law region, the plateau boundaries take on the appearance of ductile knife edges. By this stage, however, the plateaus are very small, because the spacing between the reinforcement particles has dropped dramatically. Eventually, the plateaus disappear, leaving a fracture surface consisting entirely of fractured or decohered reinforcement particles surrounded by ductile knife edges. This occurs at K_{max} values approaching K_{Ic}. At this stage, the fracture surface can no longer be distinguished from that produced by fast fracture.

The presence of reinforcement particles in MMCs prevents the formation of the regular striations observed in some aluminum alloys (Ref 26). However, some irregular striations may be observed in areas free of reinforcement particles (Ref 26, 28). Striations can be seen in the center of Fig. 4(a). The lack of regular striations indicates that the crack front in MMCs is highly irregular. This is consistent with the plateaus described previously. Together these features

*The Paris Law region is the central portion of the da/dN versus ΔK curve where the curve can be modeled as $da/dN = C(\Delta K)^m$, where da/dN is the crack growth rate, ΔK is the stress-intensity factor range, and C and m are constants.

indicate the initiation of microcracks ahead of the main crack front.

Method of Observation

The fracture surfaces of MMCs are most efficiently examined by studying areas of the surface produced under known loading conditions. This is best achieved by determining the areas of interest using an initial visual examination followed by examination under a microscope. After this, the fracture surface can be examined in the SEM. In general, MMCs should be considered to be nonconductive. Therefore, they should be carbon coated prior to SEM examination and examined at accelerating voltages between 5 and 10 kV to minimize beam charging.

Location of Specific Points and Calculation of K_{max}. In examining the fracture surfaces of MMCs, it is vital that the loading conditions at the point being examined are known or can be confidently estimated. The method used to achieve this varies with the type of specimen being examined. If the specimen is a fatigue life specimen, then the methods used in Ref 10 and 11, which are based on a *K*-calibration developed by Raju and Newman (Ref 30), are appropriate. For fatigue crack growth specimens, the loading conditions at a specific point can be determined from the records of fatigue testing. Automated crack-length measurements should be backed up with visual crack-length measurements (if available) so that the extent of crack-front curvature is known.

The typical examination method for fatigue life samples is to record a sequence of overlapping fractographs from the crack origin in a straight line to the boundary of the fatigue region and beyond (Ref 10, 11). The distance between the crack-initiation site and any point of interest can be measured directly from this sequence, and *K* can be determined from standard calibrations (Ref 30). It should be noted that valid values of *K* can only be determined when linear elastic fracture mechanics apply, and prior to fast frac-

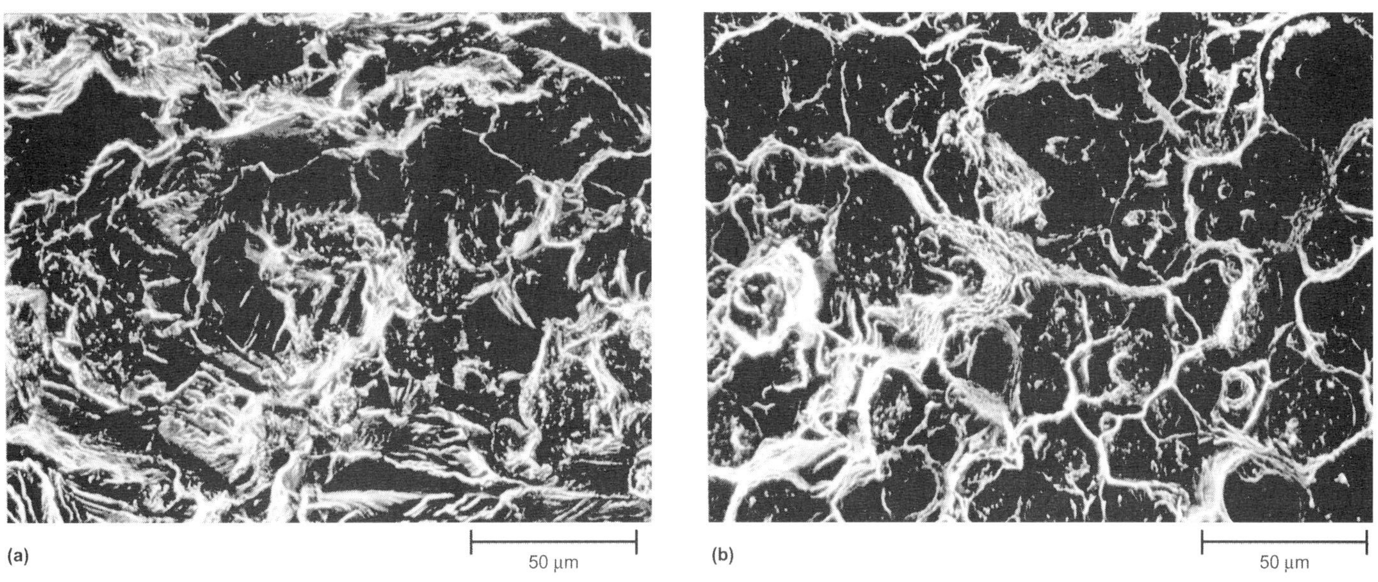

Fig. 3 Comparison of fatigue fracture surfaces for (a) low (K_{max} = 4.04 MPa$\sqrt{m}$, or 3.68 ksi$\sqrt{in.}$) and (b) high (K_{max} = 13.0 MPa$\sqrt{m}$, or 11.8 ksi$\sqrt{in.}$) values of K_{max} in Comral-85, a 6061-T6 wrought aluminium alloy reinforced with 20 vol% Micral-20 particles. Source: Ref 26

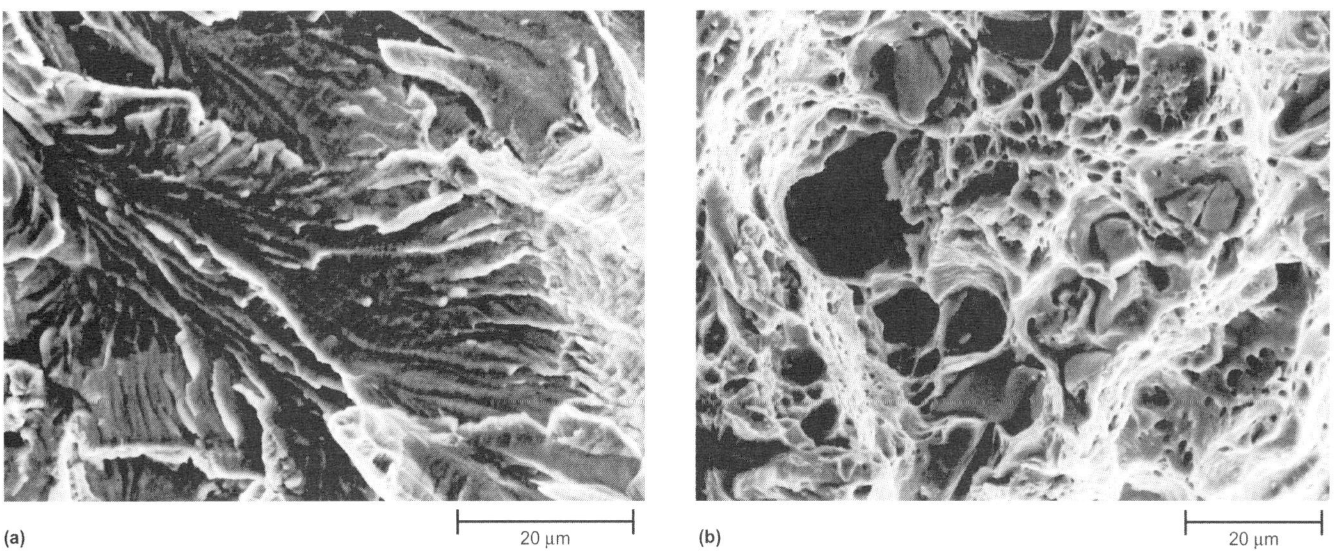

Fig. 4 Comparison of fatigue fracture surfaces for (a) low ($\Delta K < 8$ MPa $\sqrt{m}$, or 7 ksi $\sqrt{in.}$) and (b) high ($\Delta K > 11$ MPa$\sqrt{m}$, or 10 ksi$\sqrt{in.}$) values of ΔK in Duralcan F3A.20S, an Al-7%Si cast alloy reinforced with 20 vol% SiC particles. Courtesy of J. Baïlon. Source: Ref 28

ture. The first of these conditions means that K is undefined near the initiating defect due to short crack effects. The second condition arises simply because K_{Ic} is the maximum stress-intensity factor that a material can withstand under plane-strain conditions. K is also undefined if gross section yield occurs in the remaining ligament of the specimen.

The examination method for fatigue crack growth (FCG) specimens is somewhat more involved. The fracture surface of a FCG sample often consists of multiple regions, each of which was produced at different values of ΔK and/or R. It is therefore necessary to have a method of locating required points on fracture surfaces. A suitable method, which is based on a coordinate transformation between FCG specimen and SEM stage position coordinates, is described in Ref 31. The advantage of using FCG specimens is that they provide a much larger fracture surface than fatigue life samples. As a result, the data obtained from their fracture surfaces can be much more reliable than those from fatigue life specimens. In addition, in FCG testing it is possible to produce a region of fracture surface of constant loading (ΔK and R) conditions. This increases the accuracy of the K_{max} value of the fracture surface being examined and reduces transient effects.

It should be noted that there has been no direct comparison of fractographic data obtained from fatigue life and fatigue crack growth samples. This may be a significant oversight, given that stress state is known to influence A_f (Ref 26).

Measurement of Reinforcement Area Fraction. The area fraction of reinforcement particles appearing on a fracture surface of an MMC can be estimated using techniques similar to those used on plane-polished sections (Ref 11, 26). The point-counting method outlined in ASTM E 562 is suitable in this case (Ref 32). It allows both the area fraction of reinforcement and the error in these estimates to be determined with statistical reliability. This has been a weakness of previous research into the relationship between area fraction and loading conditions. This weakness is a result of the limited fracture surface area available on fatigue life samples that have been used in most of the fractographic studies of metal-matrix composites (Ref 10, 11).

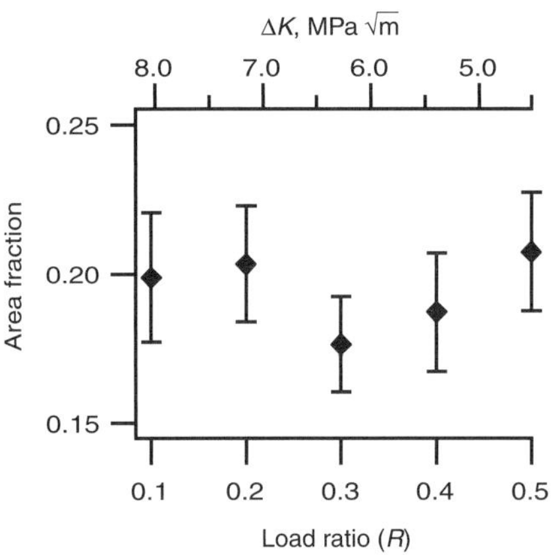

Fig. 5 Area fraction of reinforcement on the fracture surface of Comral-85 as a function of load ratio at constant K_{max} = 8.9 MPa$\sqrt{m}$, or 8.1 ksi$\sqrt{in.}$

An appealing alternative to visual examination is to analyze the x-ray emissions from fracture surfaces. Such a method was used by Baïlon and Tong (Ref 29), who found that the intensity (I) of an x-ray peak due to SiC increased as a function of crack growth rate in an MMC reinforced with SiC_p. This indicates an increase in the amount of SiC on the fracture surface. At this stage, no conversion between I and A_f is available, other than a comparison with the I-value obtained from a plane-polished surface. When such a conversion becomes available, this method is likely to significantly increase the speed with which MMC fracture surfaces can be quantitatively examined.

ACKNOWLEDGMENTS

The author would like to acknowledge Jeremy Leggoe of Texas Tech University (USA) and Jean-Paul Baïlon of École Polytechnique de Montreal (Canada) for providing several of the micrographs included in this article.

REFERENCES

1. T.W. Clyne and P.J. Withers, *An Introduction to Metal Matrix Composites*, Cambridge University Press, Cambridge, United Kingdom, 1993
2. S.J. Harris and G. Yi, "Fatigue Behaviour of Short-Fibre and Particle-Reinforced Metal Matrix Composites," *Proc., Seventh International Conf. on Composite Materials (ICCM-7)*, Beijing, People's Republic of China, 1989, p 659–668
3. A. Melander, M. Rolfson, S. Savage, and S. Preston, Fatigue Crack Growth Behaviour of a α-alumina Short Fibre Reinforced Al-2Mg Alloy – Part I: Short Cracks, *Proc., Fatigue '90: Fourth International Conf. on Fatigue and Fatigue Thresholds*, July 1990, p 905–910
4. B.R. Crawford and J.R. Griffiths, Initiation and Growth of Short Cracks in an Alumina Reinforced Metal Matrix Composite, *Proc., Materials Research Forum 1997: Materials Conservation*, Nov 1997, Monash University, Australia, p 105–108
5. K. Ishii, K. Tohgo, H. Araki, and K. Oshima, Fatigue Behaviour of SiC/Al Composite Materials, *Proc., Sixth International Conf. on Mechanical Behaviour of Materials (ICM-6)*, July-Aug, 1991, Kyoto, Japan, p 421–426
6. G.M. Vyletel, J.E. Allison, and D.C. Van Aken, The Influence of Matrix Microstructure and TiC Reinforcement on the Cyclic Response and Fatigue Behaviour of 2219 Al, *Metal. Trans. A*, Vol 26A, 1993 p 2545–2557
7. K. Komai, K. Minoshima, and H. Ryoson, Tensile and Fatigue Fracture Behaviour and Water-Environment in SiC-Whisker/7075 Composite, *Proc., Sixth International Conf. on Mechanical Behaviour of Materials (ICM-6)*, July-Aug 1991, Kyoto, Japan, p 404–408
8. P.K. Sharp, B.A. Parker, and J.R. Griffiths, The Fatigue of SiC-Reinforced Aluminium Alloys, *Proc., Fatigue '90: Fourth International Conf. on Fatigue and Fatigue Thresholds*, July 1990, p 875–880
9. S. Kumai, J.E. King, and J.F. Knott, Fatigue Crack Growth Behaviour in Molten-Metal Processed SiC Particle-Reinforced Aluminium Alloys, *Fatigue Frac. Eng. Mater. Struct.*, Vol 15 (No. 1), 1992, p 1–11
10. J.J. Bonnen, J.E. Allison, and J.W. Jones, Fatigue Behaviour of a 2*xxx* Series Aluminum Alloy Reinforced with 15% v/o SiC_p, *Metall. Trans. A*, Vol 23A, 1991, p 1007–1019
11. J.N. Hall, J.W. Jones, and A.K. Sachdev, Particle Size, Volume Fraction and Matrix Strength Effects on Fatigue Behaviour and Particle Fracture in 2124 Aluminum-SiC_p Composites, *Mater. Sci. Eng.*, Vol A183, 1994, p 69–80
12. N.J. Hurd, Fatigue Performance of Alumina Reinforced Metal Matrix Composites, *Mater. Sci. Technol.*, Vol 4, 1988, p 513–517
13. A. Martin and J. Llorca, Mechanical Behaviour and Failure Mechanisms of a Binary Mg-6%Zn Alloy Reinforced with SiC Particulates, *Mater. Sci. Eng.*, A201, 1995, p 77–87
14. M.J. Couper, A.E. Neeson, and J.R. Griffiths, Casting Defects and the Fatigue Behaviour of an Aluminium Casting Alloy, *Fatigue Frac. Eng. Mater. Struct.*, Vol 15, 1990, p 213–227
15. K. Tanaka, M. Kinefuchi, and Y. Akinawa, Fatigue Crack Propagation in SiC Whisker Reinforced Aluminum Alloys, *Proc., Fatigue '90: Fourth International Conf. on Fatigue and Fatigue Thresholds*, July 1990, p 857–862
16. T. Christman and S. Suresh, Effects of SiC Reinforcement and Aging Treatments on Fatigue Crack Growth in an Al-SiC Composite, *Mat. Sci. Eng. A*, Vol 102, 1988, p 211–216
17. D.L. Davidson, The Growth of Fatigue Cracks through Particulate SiC Reinforced Aluminum Alloys, *Eng. Fract. Mech.*, Vol 33, 1989, p 965–975
18. J.-K. Shang and R.O. Ritchie, On the Particle-Size Dependence of Fatigue-Crack Propagation Thresholds in SiC-Particulate Reinforced Aluminum-Alloy Composites: Role of Crack Closure and Crack Trapping, *Acta Metall.*, Vol. 37, 1989, p 2267–2278
19. S. Kumai, J.E. King, and J.F. Knott, Fatigue Crack Growth in SiC Particulate-Reinforced Aluminium Alloys, *Proc., Fatigue '90: Fourth International Conf. on Fatigue and Fatigue Thresholds*, July 1990, p 869–874

20. Y. Sugimura and S. Suresh, Effect of SiC Content on Fatigue Crack Growth in Aluminum Alloys Reinforced with SiC Particles, *Metal. Trans. A,* Vol 23A, 1992, p 2231–2242
21. S. Suresh, *Fatigue of Materials*, Cambridge University Press, 1991, p 209–211
22. T. J. Downes, D.M. Knowles, and J.E. King, Effect of Particle Size and Ageing on the Fatigue Behaviour of an Aluminum Based Metal Matrix Composite, *Proc., 8th Biennial Conf. on Fracture (ECF-8)*, Oct 1990, Turin, p 296–302
23. "Standard Test Method for Measurement of Fatigue Crack Growth Rates", E 647, *Annual Book of ASTM Standards*, ASTM
24. D.M. Knowles and J.E. King, Influence of Macroscopic Residual Stress Fields on Fatigue Crack Growth Measurement in SiC Particulate Reinforced 8090 Aluminium Alloys, *Mater. Sci. Technol.*, Vol 7, 1991, p 1015–1020
25. M. Levin and B. Karlsson, Influence of SiC Particle Distribution and Prestraining on Fatigue Crack Growth Rates in AA 6061-SiC Composite Material, *Mater. Sci. and Technol.*, Vol 7, 1991, p 596–607
26. B.R. Crawford and J.R. Griffiths, The Role of Reinforcement Particles during Fatigue Cracking of a Micral-20-Reinforced 6061 Alloy, *Fatigue Fract. Eng. Mater. Struct.*, Vol 22, 1999, p 811–819
27. B. Roebuck, Parabolic Curve Crack Fronts in Fracture Toughness Specimens of Particulate Reinforced Aluminum Alloy Metal Matrix Composite, *Fatigue Fract. Eng. Mater. Struct.*, Vol 15, 1992, p 13–22
28. J.W. Leggoe, X.Z. Hu, and M.B. Bush, Crack Tip Damage Development and Crack Growth Resistance in Particulate Reinforced Metal Matrix Composites, *Eng. Fract. Mech.*, Vol 53 (No. 6), 1996, p 873–895
29. J.P. Baïlon and Z.-X. Tong, Mechanics of Fatigue Crack Propagation in an Aluminum Matrix Composite, *Proc., Fatigue 99: 7th International Fatigue Congress*, Vol 3, (Beijing, People's Republic of China), 1999, p 1457–1464
30. I.S. Raju and J.C. Newman, "Stress-Intensity Factors for Circumferential Surface Cracks in Pipes and Rods under Tension and Bending Loads," NASA TM 87594, National Aeronautics and Space Administration, Aug 1985
31. B. Crawford, A Method for the Location of Specific Points on Surfaces in the SEM, *J. Micros.*, Vol 181 (No. 1), 1996, p 18–22
32. "Standard Test Method for Determining Volume Fraction by Systematic Manual Point Count," E 562, *Annual Book of ASTM Standards*, ASTM

Failure Analysis of Ceramic-Matrix Composites

Michael G. Jenkins, University of Washington—Seattle
Raj N. Singh, University of Cincinnati

INTERPRETATION OF FAILURES of ceramic-matrix composites (CMCs), and in particular continuous fiber reinforced ceramic-matrix composites (CFCCs) is complicated by the complex structure of the composite material. To perform successfully (that is, to exhibit damage tolerance without undergoing catastrophic brittle failure), CFCCs often must incorporate three constituents (fiber, matrix, interphase between the fiber and matrix) for use in room-temperature applications and up to four constituents (fiber, matrix, interphase between the fiber and matrix, and an environmental and/or thermal barrier coating over the entire composite) for use in high-temperature applications. In addition to the thermomechanical performance of the composite and each of its constituents, attention must be paid to the chemical compatibility of the constituents. The complex composite structure of a CFCC is necessary, because without a debonding interphase between the brittle ceramic matrix and the brittle ceramic fiber, brittle fracture of the CFCC would result with none of the nonlinear behavior and inherent damage tolerance. An example of this composite structure is shown in Fig. 1 (Ref 1).

Although CMCs and CFCCs can exhibit many of the basic failure modes of other composite laminates: in-plane and out-of-plane failures (Ref 2), this article concentrates on those failure mechanisms unique to CMCs, in particular those involving interaction of the constituents.

Characteristic Failure

Continuous fiber reinforced ceramic-matrix composites retain many of the characteristics of monolithic advanced ceramics (for example, erosion and corrosion resistance, stiffness, and high-temperature properties) while avoiding the main drawback of monolithic ceramics (that is, brittleness) by exhibiting increased toughness

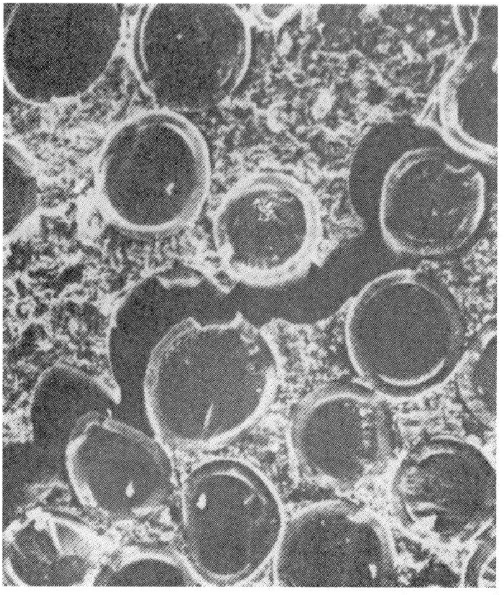

Fig. 1 Scanning electron micrograph of a CMC with a thick interphase (Nicalon fibers, SiC-BN-SiC interphase, and $ZrTiO_4$ matrix). Source: Ref 1

Monolith
(greater strength, lower toughness)
Composite
(lower strength, greater toughness)
Tensile stress, σ
Longitudinal strain, ε

Fig. 2 Tensile stress-strain curves for a monolithic ceramic and a ceramic-matrix composite. Source: Ref 3

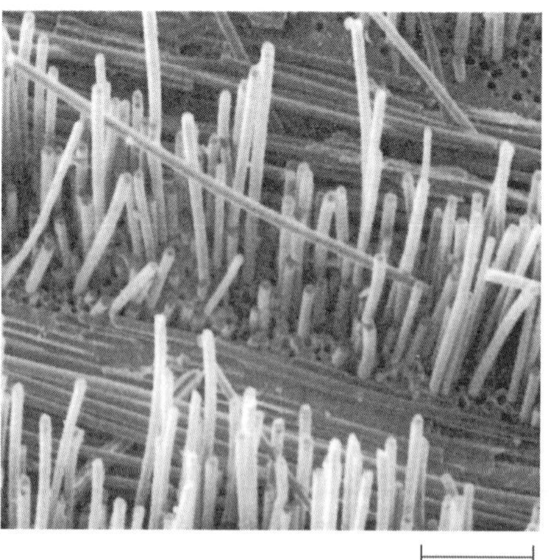

Fig. 3 Brushy fracture surface indicative of nonlinear, energy-absorbing stress-strain behavior (good toughening behavior of CMCs); 0°/90° laminate Nicalon fiber reinforced calcium aluminosilicate (CAS) glass-matrix composite. Source: Ref 4

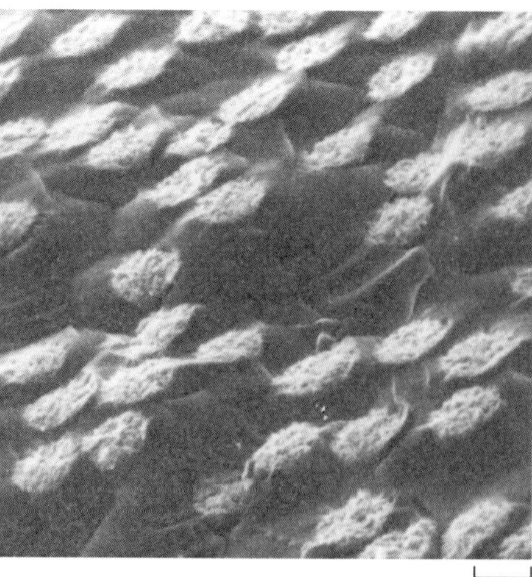

Fig. 4 Flat, nearly featureless fracture surface indicative of linear-elastic, very low energy absorbing stress-strain behavior (poor toughening behavior of CMCs); alumina (PRD-166) fiber reinforced glass-matrix composite. Source: Ref 5

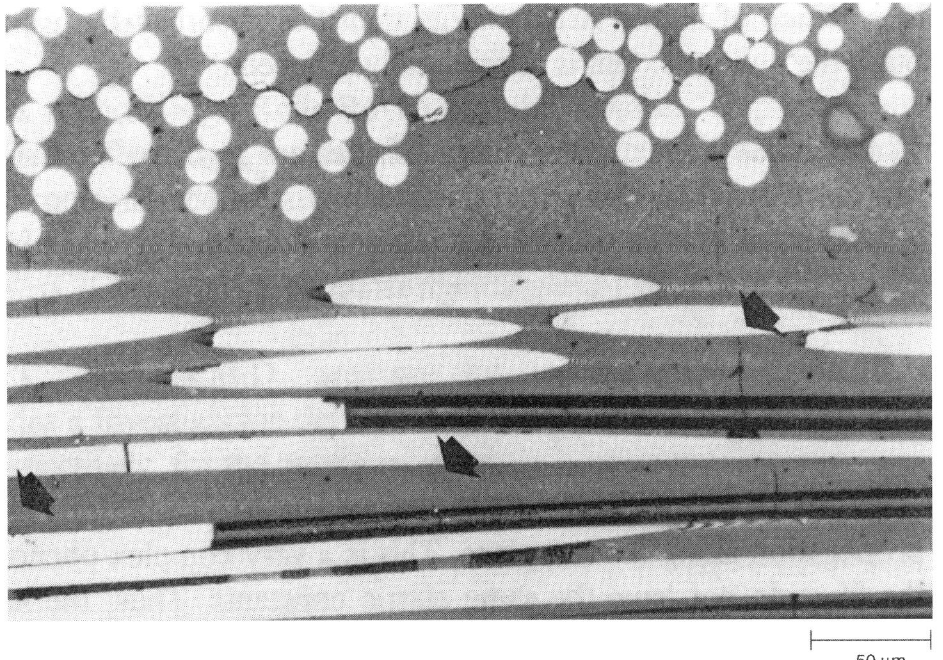

Fig. 5 Matrix cracks related to the proportional limit stress and onset of nonlinearity of the stress-strain curve; arrows indicate matrix cracks in 0°/90° laminate Nicalon fiber reinforced CAS glass-matrix composite. Source: Ref 4

and, therefore, increased reliability. Figure 2 illustrates this increased toughness, contrasting the lower strength but nonlinear energy-absorbing quasi-ductile behavior of ceramic composites with the linear-elastic but brittle behavior of monolithic ceramics.

A key characteristic feature of the fracture surfaces of the energy-absorbing nonlinear stress-strain behavior is a "brushy" appearance with many pulled-out fibers as shown in Fig. 3. Note in Fig. 3 that not only are long fiber lengths apparent, but also many holes are visible from which fibers have been pulled out. It is important to note that the nonlinear stress-strain behavior occurs because of debonding of the fiber/matrix interface and subsequent fiber pullout due to fracture of the interphase and fibers. If a strong or highly fracture-resistant interphase is present, or if no interphase is present, such that the fiber is tightly bonded to the matrix, then the composite will behave in a brittle manner similar to the monolithic ceramic shown in Fig. 2. The resulting fracture surface will show little or no fiber pullout; the nearly featureless fracture surface is shown in Fig. 4.

Evidence of Failure Mechanisms

Fractography can reveal evidence of individual fracture mechanisms, as well as the overall fracture behavior shown in Fig. 3 and 4. For example, the onset of nonlinearity (proportional limit stress) indicated in the stress-strain curve for the ceramic composite shown in Fig. 2 is often equated to a matrix cracking stress. Figure 5 shows evidence of matrix cracking, often first occurring around the fibers oriented 90° to the loading direction (Ref 4). The nature of fracture surface appearance of individual fibers can also be related to fiber strength, fiber fracture resistance and fiber degradation (for example, surface defects) as shown in Fig. 6 (Ref 6). Degradation of fibers at elevated temperatures is indicated by changes of the fracture mirrors and fracture origins (surface or volume). These changes in fracture surface appearances are consistent with changes in fracture strength for fibers.

Changes in macroscopic fracture features can often be related to environmental degradation of the composite. For example, in Fig. 7 low-magnification scanning electron microscopy (SEM) reveals changes in fiber-dominated fracture (Fig. 7a) at room temperature to matrix-dominated transverse fracture at elevated temperatures (Fig. 7b and c). Such overall changes in fracture features often cannot be discerned at high magnification. Figure 8 indicates that fatigue loading results in multiple cracks in the matrix, spaced about 300 μm apart. Such microcracking can eventually lead to environmental degradation and possible brittle fracture of the composite.

REFERENCES

1. B.A. Bender, T.L. Jessen, and D. Lewis III, Electron Microscopy of the Interfacial Regions in Various SiC Fiber/$ZrTiO_4$ Composites, *Ceram. Eng. Sci. Proc.,* Vol 12 (No. 9–10), 1991, p 2262–2274
2. J.E. Masters, Basic Failure Modes of Continuous Fiber Composites, *Composites,* Vol 1, *Engineered Materials Handbook,* 1987, p 781–785

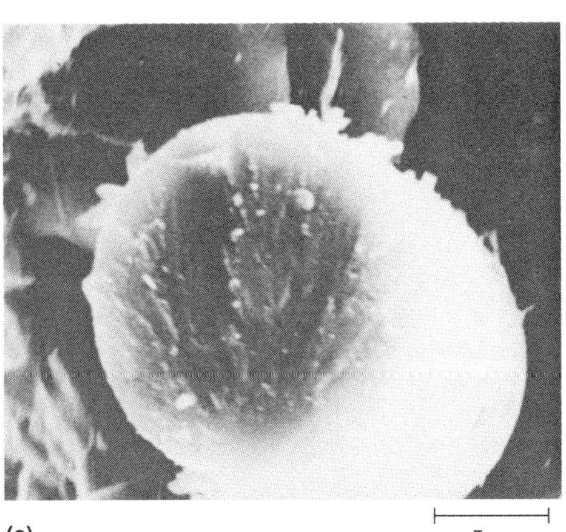

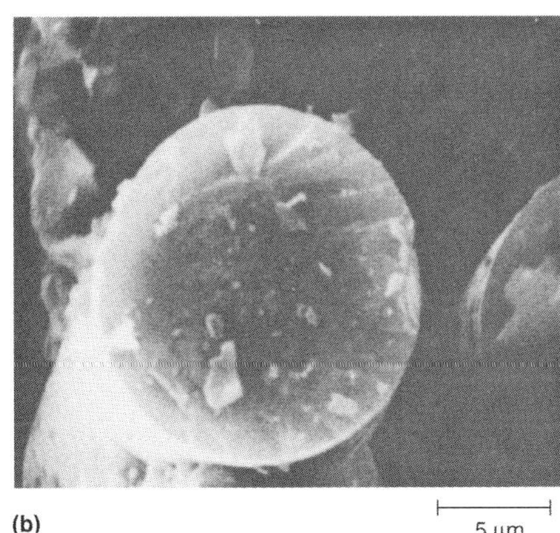

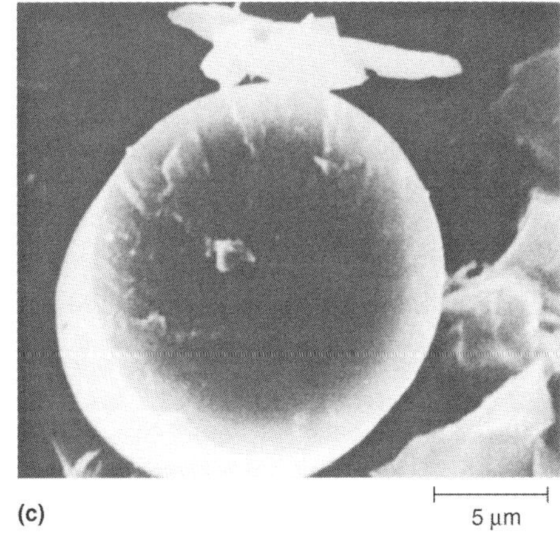

Fig. 6 Fracture mirrors on pulled-out fiber fracture surfaces of Nicalon fiber reinforced SiC-matrix composites with carbide interphase. (a) 298 K. (b) 800 K. (c) 1200 K. Source: Ref 6

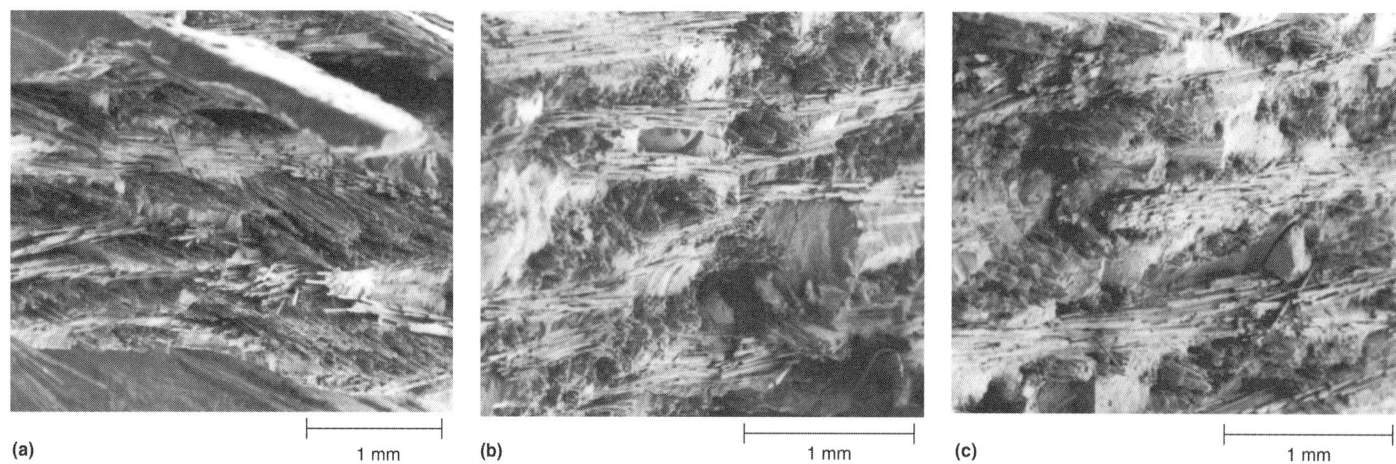

Fig. 7 Changes in macroscopic fracture with increasing temperatures. Fracture mirrors on pulled-out fiber fracture surfaces of Nicalon fiber reinforced Al_2O_3-matrix composites with boron nitride interphase. (a) 293 K. (b) 1073 K. (c) 1273 K. Source: Ref 7

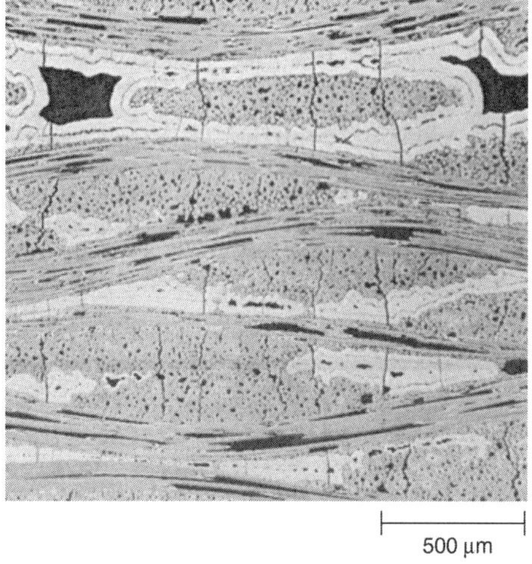

Fig. 8 Matrix microcracking due to cyclic fatigue loading of Nicalon fiber reinforced SiC-matrix composites with carbide interphase. Source: Ref 8

3. K.L. Munson and M.G. Jenkins, Retained Tensile Properties and Performance of an Oxide Matrix Continuous Fiber Ceramic Composite after Elevated Temperature Exposure in Ambient Air, *Thermal and Mechanical Test Methods and Behavior of Continuous Fiber Ceramic Composites,* STP 1309, M.G. Jenkins, S.T. Gonczy, E. Lara-Curzio, N.E. Ashbaugh, and L.P. Zawada, Ed., ASTM, 1997, p 176–189
4. J.M. Sanchez, I. Putente, R. Elizalde, A. Martin, J.M. Martinez, A.M. Daniel, M. Fuentes, and C.P. Beesely, Effect of High Strain Rate on the Tensile Behavior of Nicalon/CAS Continuous, Fiber Ceramic Composites, *Thermal and Mechanical Test Methods and Behavior of Continuous Fiber Ceramic Composites,* STP 1309, M.G. Jenkins, S. T. Gonczy, E. Lara-Curzio, N.E. Ashbaugh, and L.P. Zawada, Ed., ASTM, 1997
5. K.K. Chawla, *Ceramic Matrix Composites,* Chapman-Hall, 1993
6. S. Guo and Y. Kagawa, Temperature Dependence of In Situ Constituent Properties of Polymer Infiltration Pyrolysis Processed Nicalon SiC Fiber-Reinforced SiC Matrix Composite, *J. Mater. Res.,* Vol 15 (No. 4), 2000, p 951–960
7. K.R. Fehlmann, "Effects of Material Removal Processes and Elevated Temperature Exposure on Properties of Continuous Fiber Ceramic Composites," M.S. Thesis, University of Washington, Seattle, WA, 1996
8. Ö. Ünal, Tensile and Fatigue Behavior of a Silicon Carbide/Silicon Carbide Composite at 1300 °C, *Thermal and Mechanical Test Methods and Behavior of Continuous Fiber Ceramic Composites,* STP 1309, M.G. Jenkins, S.T. Gonczy, E. Lara-Curzio, N.E. Ashbaugh, and L.P. Zawada, Ed., ASTM, 1997

Recycling and Disposal

Chairperson: Nicholas J. Gianaris, Visteon Corporation

Introduction to Recycling and Disposal of Composites

Nicholas J. Gianaris, Visteon Corporation

THE RECYCLABILITY of all materials, components, and systems has gained increased international emphasis, and this is certainly true of structural materials including composites. Composite materials have traditionally been selected for increased performance, mass reduction, safety, and ease of manufacturing for all applications including transportation, civil, as well as military. However, with the recently increased regulatory and ecological emphasis on recycling, composite materials must now be examined for their potential as recyclable and reusable materials.

Many drivers, including energy usage, greenhouse gas minimization, cost, and waste stream management, have escalated the emphasis on recycling. The Kyoto Protocol to the 1992 Climate Change Treaty has placed the responsibility on the United States, Japan, and the European Union to create open- and closed-loop material recycling schemes that decrease greenhouse gas emissions from 1990 levels to lower levels by 2008 to 2012. Additionally, the European Union passed a directive in 2000 for member nations to adopt by 2002 that requires all used automobiles to be 100% reusable or recyclable by 2007, with all costs borne by the automotive manufacturers. This also includes having vehicles manufactured with reusable or recyclable components that constitute 85% of the mass of the vehicle by 2006, and 95% of the mass of the vehicle by 2015. This directive is intended to force automotive manufacturers to use ecologically friendly materials and design schemes. As one can observe, regulatory and environmental factors will more greatly influence the decision of material use for all applications.

The choice of low-density and high-strength materials such as composites has always been viewed as the ultimate solution for mass reduction and increased fuel economy of automotive as well as aerospace vehicles. If, however, the recyclability of composite materials is not well understood and advantageously demonstrated, then the use of composites for all applications can be limited by the regulatory and ecological drivers, as stated previously. It is important, therefore, that the scientist and engineer be presented with the most comprehensive and timely information on the recycling and disposal of composite materials.

The articles presented in this Section give the reader the most recent developments in the open- and closed-loop recycling of polymer and metal matrix composites. Much of the innovation presented is based on developing processes that take existing materials and reuse them at equivalent or less value than the previous loop in which they were used. There also are material innovations presented that allow the engineer to use high-quality structural composites that are easily processed at high production volumes and can be closed-loop recycled for equivalent or even higher value new applications. Such developments are exciting and are featured in this Section.

The automotive industry is the focus of recycling efforts due to high-volume production, and this will be emphasized most heavily in this Section. This information is also designed so that it may be applicable to the use of composites in any area.

Recycling and Disposal of Polymer-Matrix Composites

John M. Henshaw, The University of Tulsa

RECYCLING AND REUSE of fiber-reinforced polymer-matrix composite materials can be difficult, although much progress has been made. These materials obtain their useful and unusual blend of properties from their constituent phases: fibers, organic resins, and fillers. That these disparate phases are so finely interspersed in composites accounts for some of the difficulties in recycling postconsumer and factory-generated scrap. Nonetheless, many researchers have attempted to develop technically feasible, economically viable, and environmentally acceptable recycling processes for polymer-matrix composites. This article reviews those processes after first discussing the driving forces for composites recycling.

Driving Forces for Recycling of Composites

Why recycle composites? The answers are much the same as for other commodity materials, such as aluminum and glass, for which recycling processes are older, better established, and more successful. Some of these reasons include: to conserve non-renewable natural resources (both materials and energy), to reduce solid wastes (in particular, to reduce landfill volumes), to reduce hazardous wastes, to make money, and to comply with governmental regulations. Each of these driving forces for the recycling of composites is briefly discussed subsequently.

Composites Contribution to Solid Waste. Where do polymer composites fit into the total plastics picture? The data in Fig. 1 show that while total plastics production in the United States exceeds 35×10^9 kg (77×10^9 lb) and is increasing, the total for polymer composites is only about 1.4×10^9 kg (3.1×10^9 lb), or about 4% of the total plastics mass (Ref 1). A breakdown of the polymer composites fraction is included in Fig. 2.

It is also important to consider the uses and types of composites currently being produced. Figure 2 shows the total weight of composites produced along with the weight of sheet molding compound (SMC) and advanced composites prepreg for comparison (Ref 1). The figure shows that disposal issues for prepreg (traditionally an aerospace material) are not driven by production volume. In other words, it may be important to

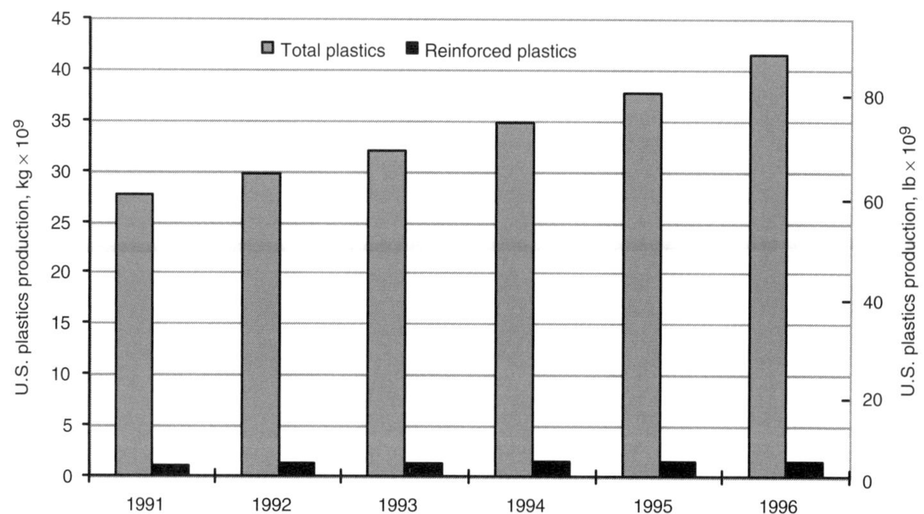

Fig. 1 Comparison of reinforced plastics production to total plastics production in the United States

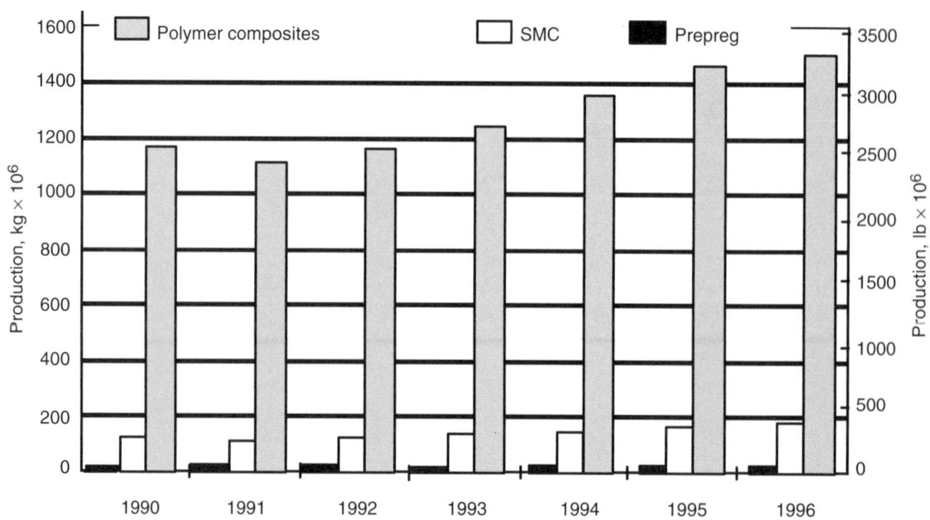

Fig. 2 Sheet molding compound and prepreg production versus total reinforced plastics production in the United States

recycle prepreg composites, perhaps because of their value, but not because their sheer mass or volume are creating societal problems.

More surprising, perhaps, than the low fraction of prepreg in the total composites stream shown in Fig. 2 is the relatively low fraction of total composites production made up of SMC. Even within the automotive industry, SMC comprises only about 50% of total composites use.

The totals for composites production, shown in Fig. 2, may also be broken down by industry, as shown in Fig. 3. The data in Fig. 2 and 3 are presented to show that polymer composites represent a broad class of materials employed in a wide range of applications. This can make recycling more difficult, because it complicates the collection and separation of composites scrap and can result in recycling feedstock of widely varying composition.

Composites Contribution to Conservation of Nonrenewable Resources. Reprocessing polymer composites into usable products represents the reuse of a non-renewable natural resource, namely hydrocarbons. In the hydrocarbon life cycle, non-renewable resources are extracted and refined into fuels and nonfuels. The fuel stream accounts for 86% of hydrocarbon production (Fig. 4). Nonfuels or petrochemicals represent only 14% of the hydrocarbon stream. Petrochemicals include plastics, synthetic fibers, solvents, lubricants, detergents, paints, and other products. Petrochemicals can be disposed of by burning, burying, or reusing them (Ref 2). Just as composites represent a small fraction of the total plastics stream, plastics represent a small fraction of the hydrocarbon stream. In terms of resource conservation, then, the recycling of reinforced plastics has extremely limited utility compared to reduction of fuels usage or the recycling of unreinforced plastics. Figure 4 also shows why the burning of waste plastics and composites for energy recovery is so appealing to some, because that is what society does with the vast majority of hydrocarbon products in the first place.

Hazardous Waste Reduction. There are some cases in which composites waste material can be considered as hazardous waste. Automobile shredder residue (ASR), the fraction of materials left over from the automated shredding and recovery of materials (mostly metals) from cars, is considered as hazardous waste by some European countries (Ref 3). The same is true of uncured composite scrap, such as SMC or prepreg.

Economic Incentives. Recycling is traditionally an economic activity. Historically, environmental pressures to recycle materials are relatively recent. Most successful recycling efforts, such as that involving aluminum cans, are also successful economically. Composites recycling efforts will eventually have to show acceptable economic returns, particularly in the absence of strict governmental regulations mandating recycling.

Governmental Regulations. Governmental regulations have influenced the development of composites recycling. For example, as noted previously, ASR is considered as hazardous waste in some European countries.

Disposing of Composite Scrap

Having described some of the driving forces for recycling composites, it is appropriate to briefly consider the options for dealing with solid waste in general. According to William Rathje, all options for handling solid wastes can be divided into four categories: burying, burning, reusing, or using less in the first place (Ref 2). Burying generally refers to landfilling methods. Landfilling is under pressure due to shortages of landfill space in some areas and to environmental problems, particularly with older landfills. Burning refers to combustion processes used to dispose of solid wastes, often accompanied by energy recovery. Reuse refers to the direct reuse of a discarded item or to the reprocessing of the material into raw materials for use in a manufacturing process. The fourth option listed, using less of a material, is of particular interest for composites. This option is sometimes referred to as "source reduction." Composites are frequently employed because they save weight over other materials that could be specified. If by saving weight in an automobile, for example, a composite component can be shown to improve fuel economy, that component has source-reduced the use of fuel in that car. Considered from a life cycle perspective, this type of source reduction is important for polymer composites. If polymer composites can reduce the overall amount of hydrocarbons consumed during the life cycle of the product they are a part of, then, in life cycle terms, the composite part may have an advantage over a heavier (metal) component that is more readily recycled. The evaluation of the life cycle merits of saving fuel versus ease of reuse fall under the category of "life cycle analysis," which is somewhat beyond the scope of this article; an overview of life cycle concepts is available in the article "Life Cycle Engineering and Design" in *Materials Selection and Design,* Volume 20 of *ASM Handbook.*

The Recycling Chain. Having briefly considered the generic ways in which scrap composites can be handled, the remainder of this article focuses on techniques for the reuse/reprocessing of polymer composites. A number of technologies have been or are in the process of being devel-

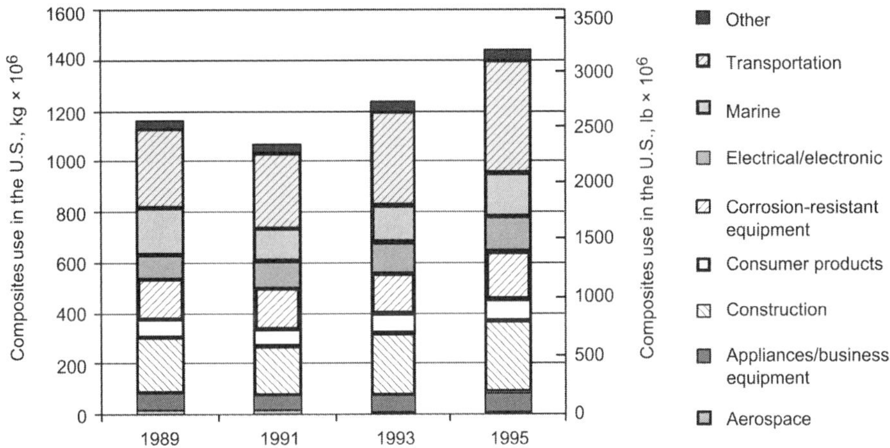

Fig. 3 Composites use by industry in the United States

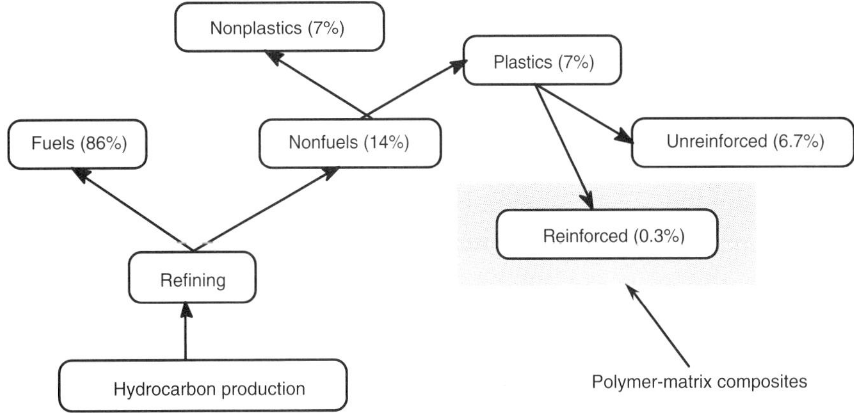

Fig. 4 Relation of polymer-matrix composites to the overall use of hydrocarbons

Table 1 Thermoset composites recycling processes

Process	Feedstock	Products/wastes
Pyrolysis (Ref 12)	In-house or postconsumer SMC	Fuel gas, oil, inorganic solid
Pyrolysis and milling (Ref 8)	SMC	Fuel gas, oil, inorganic solid
Pyrolysis (Ref 14)	Polyurethane foams, ASR	Gas, oil, solid waste
Hydrolysis (Ref 10, 11)	Foams, RIM resin, and elastomers	Monomers of the input material
Fluidized bed combustion (Ref 14)	RIM	Energy recovery, solid and gaseous wastes
Rotary kiln combustion (Ref 13)	RIM	Energy recovery, solid and gaseous wastes
Incineration (Ref 11, 15)	ASR "pellets," mixed polymer waste, fuel supplement	Energy recovery, solid and gaseous wastes
Incineration in pure O_2 (Ref 11)	Auto battery plastics scrap, ASR	Energy recovery, solid and gaseous wastes
RIM regrind (Ref 4, 5)	In-house or postconsumer RIM polyurethane	Ground particles for use as filler
Phenolic regrind (Ref 1)	Phenolic scrap parts, other thermosets	Ground phenolic for use as filler
SMC regrind (Ref 6, 7)	In-house (cured) or postconsumer SMC	Ground particles for use as filler
Vitrification/energy recovery (Ref 1)	ASR	Glassy solids for use in asphalt/concrete, energy
Fluidized bed and separation (Ref 9)	SMC, filament-wound pipe, or glass-reinforced sandwich panels	Short fibers, fillers, and energy

ASR, automobile shredder residue; RIM, reaction injection molding; SMC, sheet molding compound

oped. These processes use scrap composites as feedstock for the production of a variety of useful materials. Whatever the merits of these particular processes, they are only one element in an overall recycling system for composites.

The successful recycling of composites depends on a sequence of events, each of which is crucial to the overall success of the system. Reprocessing techniques are an important part, but only a part, of that system. The recycling chain is shown schematically in Fig. 5. There are five necessary elements in a recycling system for composites, or indeed for any recycling system: (1) a source of materials to be recycled, (2) a means to collect those materials and (3) deliver them to a reprocessor, (4) efficient means to reprocess those materials, and (5) economical markets for the reprocessed materials. If any one of those elements is missing, economically nonviable, or otherwise unsuitable, the entire recycling system will fail. In this respect, composite materials are no different from aluminum beverage cans or other materials. While most of the research and development efforts for composites have focused on the reprocessing techniques themselves (as does the remainder of this article), it must be recognized that those techniques by themselves do not constitute "recycling."

The reprocessing of thermoset- and thermoplastic-matrix polymer composites are considered in the sections that follow.

Recycling of Thermoset-Matrix Composites

Figure 6 shows an overview of some of the main options for recycling thermoset-matrix composites. Table 1 summarizes specific recycling technologies for these composites. The first column in the table lists the process name and associated literature references. The second column lists the feedstocks to the recycling process, while the third shows the major products produced by the process.

The processes for recycling of thermoset-matrix composites listed in Table 1 fit into several broad categories. These include regrind processes, chemical processes, energy recovery processes, and other thermal processes for fiber and filler recovery. As is seen, some overlap exists among categories. These categories are discussed subsequently.

Regrind Processes for Recycling of Thermoset Composites. A great deal of research, development, and commercial activity has revolved around the shredding and regrinding of thermosetting composites, particularly SMC, into particles suitable for use as filler in materials such as SMC and bulk molding compound (BMC). A number of investigations has shown this type of process to have technical merit. At least one commercial enterprise in North America, Phoenix Fibreglass of Canada, was able to commercialize a process of this type, although the company closed its operations in 1996.

In general, regrind processes for thermosetting composites begin with "shredded" composite components—the pieces of which have dimensions on the order of 100 mm (4 in.). To date, most of this type of recycling has been done on postindustrial (cured) scrap and not on postconsumer scrap. Such materials may contain molded-in metallic components, but are typically free of adhesives and coatings. Magnets separate out ferromagnetic materials at several stages in the process. The shredded feedstock is further shredded into smaller pieces and passed through several more metal-separation processes. In the next step, the material is shattered in a process that allows much of the fiber content of the material to be separated from the fillers and polymer matrix. At the former Phoenix Fi-

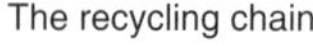

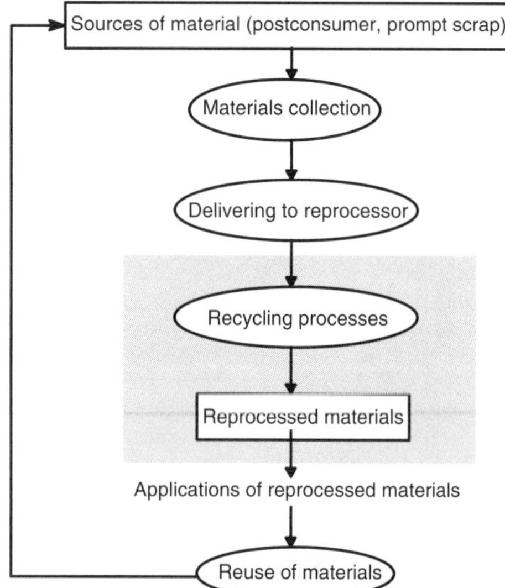

Fig. 5 Flow chart for the recycling and reuse of materials

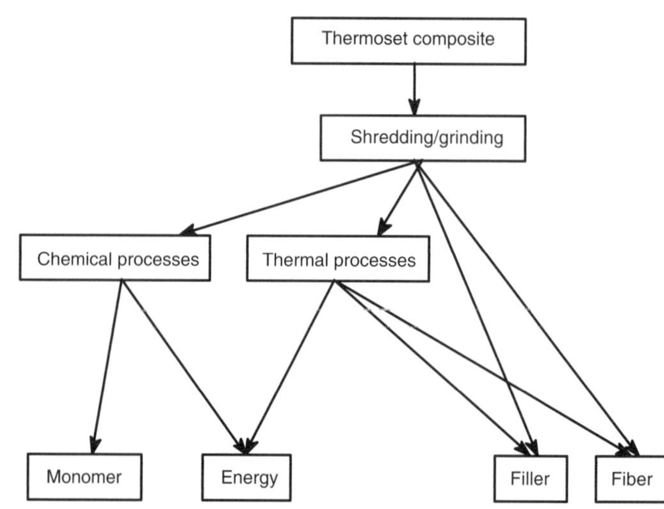

Fig. 6 Thermoset composites recycling

breglass operation, separation was accomplished through proprietary screening processes that allowed Phoenix to market products consisting of filler (pulverized polymer and calcium carbonate), chopped-strand glass fiber, and discrete fibers in several length categories. The recycled filler product was milled down to an average particle size, as specified by the customer. In a process such as this, the finer the particle size, the more expensive the product, but the more suitable it will be for recycling as filler for "class A" automotive components. (Class A components require a very smooth surface finish and thus, a finer particle size for their filler component.)

Recycled filler has been used in a number of production SMC and BMC automotive applications. Recycled content of 5 to 15% by weight has been achieved, with up to 25% believed to be possible. (Virgin SMC contains up to 40% filler by weight.) The recycled material has the added bonus of weight savings, because a blend of powdered polymer and calcium carbonate is less dense than 100% calcium carbonate. Recycled content of 25% in an SMC component is said to yield a weight savings of almost 10% over virgin SMC.

Recycling of other composites has been investigated, using related regrind-to-filler technology. Developmental work on recycling reaction injection molded (RIM) polyurethane automotive scrap is ongoing. One technique involves regrinding RIM scrap and then using approximately 10% of the regrind as filler in other molding processes (Ref 4).

Compression molding of these materials is limited to simple shapes and requires very high pressures. The Polyurethanes Recycle and Recovery Council announced plans to establish pilot facilities to develop similar recycling processes. Phenolic scrap containing glass fibers or carbon fibers has been shown, by phenolic suppliers, to be capable of being pulverized into suitably sized particles and then used as fillers and extender in molding compounds (Ref 5). Rogers Corporation has shown that it is possible for cured phenolic compounds to be ground and reformulated into other phenolic-based compounds. The properties of the compounds containing recycled phenolics are similar to virgin materials. Besides structural reaction injection molded (SRIM) and RIM materials, regrinds of thermoplastics such as acrylonitrile-butadiene-styrene (ABS) and polypropylene have also been used as fillers. Test results show a significant increase in modulus of elasticity. Researchers claim that the cost of the final part may be reduced because of the substitution of recycled RIM or SRIM into the virgin material (Ref 5). Union Carbide Chemicals and Plastics Company has results showing that the properties of the thermoplastic-matrix composites containing recycled SMC as fillers can be as good as or better than those containing virgin materials (Ref 6). Owens-Corning Fiberglass Corporation has reported that fully cured SMC scrap can be shredded, ground, and milled into powder and then used directly as a filler and reinforcement in BMC and thermoplastic polyolefin molding compounds (Ref 7).

Chemical Processes for Recycling of Thermoset Composites. Included in this category of recycling processes for thermoset-matrix composites are processes such as pyrolysis and hydrolysis that result in the chemical and thermomechanical decomposition of composites into gases, liquids, and solids. Some of these decomposition products have economic value, while others must be disposed of as waste.

Pyrolysis. Pyrolysis of polymers and their composites involves thermal decomposition of organic materials at high temperature in the absence of oxygen. Typical pyrolysis processes involve melting vessels, blast furnaces, autoclaves, tube reactors, rotary kilns, and fluidized bed reactors. Rotary kilns and fluidized beds are among the most widely used pyrolysis processes for use in recycling. The reaction products of the pyrolysis of polymers include various hydrocarbons that can often be used as fuels or as feedstocks for petrochemicals. Pyrolysis processes may eventually become a feasible alternative in the market for recycling thermosetting composites, if the waste composites can be collected in large quantities. Attempts to pyrolyze cured and uncured SMC in-house manufacturing scrap have been carried out. Three trial SMC pyrolysis runs were completed at a converted tire pyrolysis facility (Ref 16). Based on a pyrolysis project sponsored by the SMC Automotive Alliance, the pyrolysis yielded about 30% by weight gas and oil and 70% solid by-product. The solid residue was milled to a particle size suitable for use as filler. The mechanical property data for SMC using pyrolyzed and milled SMC have demonstrated that pyrolysis followed by milling is a technically feasible recycling technology (Ref 8).

A difficulty with pyrolysis of glass-reinforced composites such as SMC is the large inorganic fraction (mainly glass and calcium carbonate) that must be dealt with following pyrolysis. The SMC Automotive Alliance concluded that recycling of cured in-house SMC scrap by pyrolysis is less cost-effective than simply grinding scrap SMC to a powder and using it as filler (Ref 8). Uncured prompt scrap seems to be a better candidate for pyrolysis. It is possible that post-consumer SMC will be a better candidate for the direct regrind and milling process than for pyrolysis, or perhaps for the thermal process for fiber and filler process (Ref 9) described subsequently.

Some research has been done on pyrolysis of ASR. Auto shredder residue is what remains after automobiles have passed through the shredding process and after a variety of metals have been separated out. Auto shredder residue contains an increasing fraction of polymer composites as composites use in cars becomes more common. One major difficulty with the pyrolysis of ASR is the variability of the feedstock. Unlike pyrolyzing SMC prompt scrap, pyrolyzing ASR requires dealing with a constantly varying mix of polymers and other materials, making the process difficult to control.

Hydrolysis. Recycling through hydrolysis can be used for recovering the monomers of materials manufactured by various polymerization reactions. Polymers capable of recycling through hydrolysis include polyesters, polyethylene, polyurethanes, polyamides (Ref 10), and the composites of these polymers—for both thermosets and thermoplastics. The polyester polyethylene terephthalate can be hydrolyzed using water and an acid or base catalyst, producing terephthalic acid and ethylene glycol. Success of this type of process requires the scrap materials to be separated by polymer type, and is thus not applicable to ASR (unless the ASR can be separated by polymer type—a difficult proposition) (Ref 11). In the 1970s, General Motors Corporation and Ford Motor Company extensively investigated hydrolysis of polyurethane foams. General Motors found that flexible polyurethane foam was hydrolyzed to a diamine, a polyol, and CO_2, and discovered that high-pressure steam would hydrolyze flexible foam rapidly at temperatures of 232 to 316 °C (450 to 600 °F). The diamines could be distilled and extracted from the steam and the reclaimed polyols recovered from the hydrolysis residue. Ford explored the hydrolysis of polyurethane flexible foam seat cushion material at a lower temperature than that of General Motors. Bayer AG patented a continuous hydrolysis process using a specially designed extruder (Ref 12).

Most hydrolysis research on recycling has been directed toward unreinforced polymers. Extension to composites should be possible, although the presence of the inorganic phases (fibers and fillers) complicates the process.

Energy Recovery Processes for Recycling of Thermoset Composites. Like unreinforced plastics, composites have an appreciable energy content (although the frequently inorganic reinforcement phase significantly lowers the specific heat content). For example, it was estimated that the energy equivalent of the 1990 RIM production in North America alone would be 30 to 35 million liters (8 to 9 million gallons) of crude oil (Ref 13). The potential for energy recoverable from waste plastics is thus significant. The most common energy recovery methods are fluidized bed, rotary kiln, and mass burn. Dow Chemical Company conducted a study of the combustion of RIM materials. The Dow facility included a rotary kiln with a burner operating temperature of 870 to 1200 °C (1600 to 2200 °F). A multipass boiler was used to recover heat from the gases from the incinerator. The gases then went through a quench chamber and scrubber to remove acid gases and particulates (Ref 13). The Miles, New Martinsville WV plant used a waste-energy fluidized bed combustor to burn RIM. The facility operated at 900 °C (1650 °F). The unit used 12,700 kg (28,000 lb) of silica sand, which provided very high combustion efficiency. A three-stage boiler was used to recover the heat. The cooled gases were then led to an electrostatic precipitator and a two-stage scrubber to remove particulate and acid gas (Ref 14).

Auto shredder residue can be used as a substitute or supplement for fossil fuel, because its heat value is typically equivalent to that of a low-grade coal. EnerGroup has reported that ASR, for 12 samples used, has an average heat value of 12.6 MJ/kg. The mass of ASR may be reduced 50% by incineration—thus reducing disposal costs and landfill volumes (Ref 15). Japanese researchers have suggested separating the combustible portion of ASR, mixing with resin, and compressing the mixture into briquettes (Ref 11). Others proposed a similar process that would generate steam from the incineration of ASR in pure oxygen as an energy source for the shredder mill itself (Ref 3). While the use of pure oxygen instead of air for combustion is more expensive, it is compensated for by a reduction in reactor size and reduced emissions. For most ASR incineration schemes, a flue gas scrubber is still necessary due to the concentration of chlorine and sulfur. The solid wastes from such a process (with ASR as a feedstock) are said to consist of an inert slag that has applications as a building material.

Some investigators believe that incineration processes are the only practical solution for the disposition of certain types of mixed plastic/nonplastic wastes (Ref 3). Composites are an important component in many such types of waste, including ASR. In fact, it is possible that separating such mixed wastes and employing a recycling process designed to reuse the material (rather than just capturing its energy content) is more costly in energy terms than simply producing more of the material in virgin form (Ref 3). If that is true, then incineration processes for recycling of composites-rich mixed plastics do represent an important option, provided the incineration processes themselves are environmentally acceptable.

Thermal Processes for Fiber and Filler Recovery. A recently developed thermal process shows promise for the recovery of both fibers and fillers from thermoset-matrix glass-fiber composites (Ref 9). This process, shown schematically in Fig. 7, uses a low-temperature (450 °C, or 840 °F) fluidized bed reactor to separate fibers and fillers from the resin-matrix materials in shredded composite feedstock. The organic matrix is volatilized in this process. Novel separation techniques are then used to separate fibers from fillers, while a second, higher-temperature (1000 °C, or 1830 °F) reactor combusts the volatilized organic materials. Heat is then recovered from this last reaction and the resulting gaseous emissions are scrubbed and released.

This process has been tested separately on feedstocks of SMC (25% polyester, 22% E-glass, 35% calcium carbonate, and 15% aluminum hydroxide), filament wound pipe (35% polyester, 34% E-glass, and 31% silica filler), and on an E-glass/polyester automobile body sandwich panel (polyurethane foam core with about 15% E-glass and 15% calcium carbonate as a weight percent of the total panel weight). The sandwich panels also contained some molded-in aluminum inserts and were also primed and painted.

Initial experimental results for this process are promising. Fiber yields for the three feedstocks (SMC, pipe, and sandwich panel) were from 40 to 46% of the fiber content of the feedstock. The organic content of separated fiber and filler recyclates varied from 3 to 10%. This was due to incomplete volatilization of the feedstock in the first reactor.

Fibers recovered from this process were recycled into two different kinds of products to investigate the quality of recycled material. Molded components containing 50% recycled fiber content showed no significant change in molding characteristics or mechanical or electrical properties. Incorporation of recycled fibers into veil products resulted in significant reduction in veil strengths. In addition, recycled fibers were incompatible with virgin fibers due to the difference in surface chemistry of the two types of fibers.

An economic analysis of this recycling process showed that, within the assumptions of the model, revenues could exceed expenses for throughputs in excess of 8×10^6 kg (18×10^6 lb) per year. Assumptions included that all scrap would be collected within 80 km (50 miles) of the plant at a cost equivalent to landfill charges in the United Kingdom. Recovered fiber was assumed to retail at 80% of the price of virgin chopped-glass strand, and recovered filler at the same price as calcium carbonate.

Recycling of Thermoplastic-Matrix Composites

Thermoplastic-matrix fiber-reinforced composites have several potential advantages over thermoset-matrix composites. Toughness and damage resistance are among these properties. Because of the fundamental ability of thermoplastics to be reshaped upon heating, there are, at least potentially, some recycling advantages as well.

A schematic overview of recycling of thermoplastic composites is shown in Fig. 8. Specific processes and references are shown in Table 2. Because of the nature of thermoplastic polymers, several processes exist for the recycling of thermoplastic-matrix composites that do not exist for thermoset composites. However, it should not be assumed that all the thermoset-matrix recycling processes listed in Table 1 are also feasible options for thermoplastics.

Most thermoplastic composite material recycling investigations have involved variations on the following processing sequence. First, a virgin

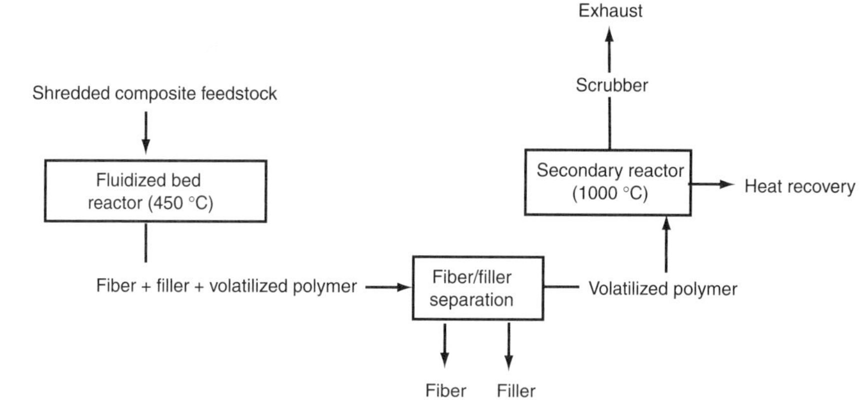

Fig. 7 Schematic of thermal recycling process for thermoset composites. Source: Ref 9

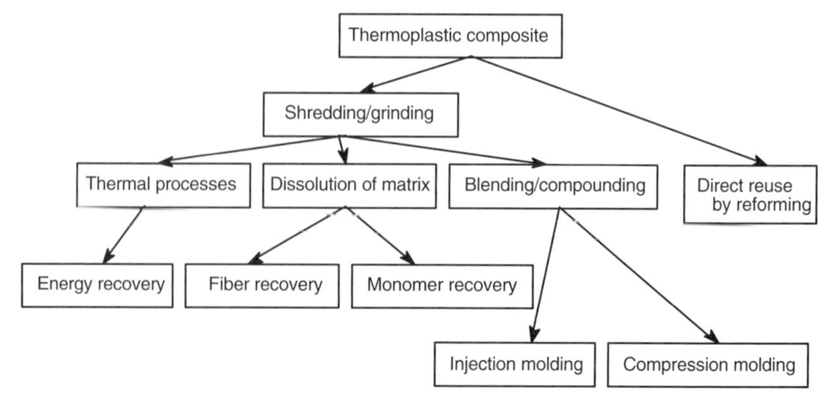

Fig. 8 Thermoplastic composite recycling

composite, either short- or continuous-fiber-reinforced, is shredded, cut, and/or ground into relatively small pieces. This regrind is then compounded with virgin unreinforced thermoplastic. The thus-reformulated material is then extruded into either injection or compression molding pellets. Injection or compression molded parts are then produced and their properties compared to virgin composites of similar composition.

Regrinding Thermoplastic Composites. The regrinding process has been investigated by many researchers. Schinner and coworkers compared hammer mills to knife-like cutters for reducing continuous-carbon-fiber-reinforced polyetheretherketone (PEEK) laminates to pieces small enough for recompounding and recycling (Ref 17). Before entering the hammer or cutter mills, large laminates had to be shredded to thumb-size pieces. Analysis of the resulting ground composites showed that the cutter mills resulted in a more uniform distribution of fiber lengths, with over 60% of the fibers being 0.5 mm (0.02 in.) or longer. Hammer milling resulted in over 80% of the fibers being shorter than 0.5 mm (0.02 in.). The researchers noted a high wear rate on the cutter blades as a result of chopping the carbon fibers. Hammer mill components seemed to hold up better.

Compounding/Blending and Reprocessing. Schinner and coworkers blended reground PEEK with virgin PEEK resin to produce injection molding pellets. This technique was found to be satisfactory for fiber contents from 30 to 50 wt%. Tensile strength, tensile modulus, and elongation at break were found to compare favorably with virgin PEEK/carbon injection molding materials with similar fiber contents.

Table 2 Thermoplastic composites recycling processes

Process	Feedstock	Recycled products
Regrind/compression molding (Ref 17–22)	Short- or long-fiber thermoplastic composites	Flake for use in compression molding
Regrind/extrusion-injection molding (Ref 17–22)	Short- or long-fiber thermoplastic composites	Injection molding pellets
Regrind followed by extrusion-compression molding (Ref 19)	Short- or long-fiber thermoplastic composites	Pellets for use in compression molding

Cutter-mill reground PEEK was also reprocessed directly by press molding, thus avoiding the recompounding step. As expected, properties were reduced from those of the continuous-fiber-reinforced virgin PEEK laminates. However, the mechanical properties of the press-molded recycled laminates were both consistent and useful and exceeded the properties of comparable virgin injection molded materials.

Other researchers have considered the effects of service life on the properties of recycled thermoplastic composites. Van Lochem and coworkers investigated various types of artificial aging designed to simulate ten years service life (Ref 18). The materials evaluated were injection molded polyphenylene sulfide (PPS) and polybutylene terephthalate (PBT) reinforced with 30 or 40 wt% glass fibers. Tensile bars of virgin material were injection molded and then aged in a variety of environments, including elevated temperatures, high humidity, and high and low pH. Aged materials were physically and mechanically characterized, and then the composites were reground, blended with varying amounts of virgin material, and remolded.

The results of this research were mixed. The aged-then-recycled PPS composites generally performed better than the PBT composites, particularly when a fiber-matrix coupling agent was blended with the material during compounding. The PBT composites were deemed unsuitable for use in applications for which the virgin material was intended.

Chu and Sullivan investigated the recyclability of several different glass-reinforced thermoplastic-matrix composites (Ref 19, 20). The composites investigated included a woven glass fabric-reinforced polycarbonate and a continuous strand mat glass-reinforced PBT. The virgin materials were ground in a cutting-type granulator and prepared for recycling. Some of the reground materials were treated with various types of silane coupling agents to assess the need to improve fiber-matrix interface in the recycled materials. Reprocessing was then accomplished using either injection molding, compression molding, or a hybrid process called extrusion-compression molding. This latter process was developed to improve the homogeneity of the final compression molded product, but without the attendant reduction in molecular weight and fiber length associated with injection molding. Results showed that the silane coupling agents improved the properties of the recycled materials. The properties of the recycled PBT composite were generally better than that of a virgin 35 wt% Valox (General Electric Company) reference material, as shown in Table 3, but inferior to those of the continuous-fiber virgin material.

Steenkamer and Sullivan investigated the recyclability of a liquid molded cyclic thermoplastic composite (Ref 21). The material investigated was a novel cyclic PBT. This polymer may be prepared as a low-molecular-weight, relatively low-viscosity liquid that can be processed by one of the liquid molding processes (resin transfer molding, etc.). Once inside the mold, the resin polymerizes into PBT in a proprietary process. Recyclability was one of the strong driving forces behind the development of this material by General Electric Company and Ford. Liquid molded panels with glass-fabric reinforcement were prepared and then reprocessed by grinding/compounding/injection molding. The properties of the recycled material compared very favorably to those of a virgin commercial PBT injection molding material with the same glass content.

Ramakrishna and coworkers also recycled continuous-fiber carbon/PEEK composites by shredding, grinding in a cutting mill, and then compression molding the resulting ground composite. The mechanical properties of the recycled moldings were once again found to be greatly reduced from those of the virgin continuous-fiber laminates, but were nonetheless considered to be useful (Ref 22).

Properties of Recycled Composite Fibers

Allred and coworkers investigated the properties of carbon fibers reclaimed from a chemical recycling process that had been applied to uncured, out-of-date carbon/epoxy unidirectional prepreg and cured carbon fabric/epoxy factory scrap (Ref 23). Single-fiber mechanical tests were performed on fibers reclaimed from the cured scrap and compared to virgin fibers of the same type. The reclaimed fibers showed about a 10% reduction in tensile load capacity, with a similar Weibull statistical distribution as the virgin fibers. The investigators attribute most of the fiber degradation to other factors in the life cycle of the fiber-weaving, molding, part fabrication, and shredding prior to the reclaiming process—

Table 3 Comparison of properties of recycled PBT composites to virgin materials

Material	Reprocessing technique	Tensile strength		Tensile modulus		Maximum elongation, %	Notched Izod impact strength	
		MPa	ksi	GPa	10^6 psi		J/m	ft · lbf/ft
Virgin continuous swirl mat (35 wt% glass)	. . .	103	15	9.0	1.3	2.1	700	159
Virgin Valox (35 wt %)	Injection molded	126.4 ± 2.6	18.3 ± 0.4	10.2 ± 0.8	1.5 ± 0.12	3.5 ± 0.4	86.1 ± 5.2	19.6 ± 1.2
Recycled with silane(a)	. . .	131.9 ± 2.3	19.1 ± 0.3	10.2 ± 0.9	1.5 ± 0.13	1.8 ± 0.1	115.2 ± 9.0	26.2 ± 2.0
Recycled with silane(a)	Extrusion-compression molded	97.2 ± 6.5	14.1 ± 0.9	12.0 ± 1.9	1.7 ± 0.28	1.3 ± 0.2	105.9 ± 5.4	24.1 ± 1.2
Recycled with silane(a)	Compression molded	57.4 ± 3.9	8.3 ± 0.6	6.3 ± 1.06	0.9 ± 0.15	1.2 ± 0.1	298.3 ± 32.2	67.8 ± 7.3

(a) Dow Corning Z-6040. Source: Ref 20

and not to the reclaiming process itself. For example, they cite a typical 5 to 10% strength reduction due to weaving alone.

The same investigators also analyzed the surface chemistry of reclaimed AS4 carbon fibers and compared it to virgin AS4. No significant differences in surface chemistry were noted. This is important if the fibers are to be reused in composites applications, where fiber/matrix adhesion is critical.

Kennerley and coworkers (Ref 24) investigated the properties of glass fibers reclaimed through the use of thermal processes for fiber and filler recovery similar to those described earlier (Ref 9). They found that the strength of single glass fibers subjected to 450 °C (840 °F) was only 44% of that of untreated fibers. Treatment at 650 °C (1200 °F) reduced residual strength to only 5% of the untreated value. Longer times at the various temperatures resulted in greater strength loss. Fiber modulus was relatively unaffected by the various treatments. Reclaimed glass fibers were successfully used in semistructural molded products and veils (Ref 24).

Finally, Steenkamer and Sullivan investigated the substitution of recycled A-glass fibers for E-glass in composite applications (Ref 25). A-glass in the form of bulk glass cullet (predominately broken bottles, jars, and car windows) is an industrial commodity. These researchers investigated the use of fiber spun from A-glass and then incorporated in polymer-matrix composites. A-glass has inferior mechanical properties compared to E-glass. For example, the elastic modulus of A-glass is 66 $\pm$ 0.5 GPa (9.6 $\pm$ 0.007 $\times$ 10^6 psi), while that of E-glass is 78 $\pm$ 0.8 GPa (11.3 $\pm$ 0.12 $\times$ 10^6 psi). The strength of A-glass is 863 $\pm$ 301 MPa (125 $\pm$ 44 ksi), while that of E-glass is 1261 $\pm$ 517 MPa (183 $\pm$ 75 ksi) . These property differences are reflected in the composites that are produced from the two types of fibers. The study concluded that A-glass fibers produced from recycled material are capable of producing acceptable composites with a predictable and somewhat lower performance than their E-glass counterparts. It was further concluded that the use of recycled A-glass fibers could thus increase "recycled content" in products, such as automobiles. Recycled content can be an important marketing factor for environmentally conscious consumers and could potentially be the subject of governmental regulation.

REFERENCES

1. J.M. Henshaw, W. Han, and A.D. Owens, An Overview of Recycling Issues for Composite Materials, *J. Thermoplast. Compos. Mater.*, Vol 9, Jan 1996, p 4–20
2. W. Rathje and C. Murphy, *Rubbish!*, Harper Collins, 1992
3. G. Menges, Chemical Recycling as a Sink for Problematic Waste from Fiber-Reinforced Plastics, *J. Thermoplast. Compos. Mater.*, Vol 7, Jan 1994, p 65–73
4. S.A. Wood, *Mod. Plast.*, June 1988, p 62
5. C. Bambrick, D. Babbington, and D. Waszeciak, Recycling Options for SRIM Composites, *Advanced Composites: Design, Materials and Processing Technologies*, 2–5 Nov 1992 (Chicago, IL), ASM International, p 231–237
6. R. Godlewski and W. Herdle, Recycling of Ground SMC into Polypropylene and Recovery of Scrap Azdel to Produce Quality Molded Parts, *Advanced Composites: Design, Materials and Processing Technologies*, 2–5 Nov 1992 (Chicago IL), ASM International, p 239–246
7. R.B. Jutte and W.D. Graham, Recycling SMC Scrap as a Reinforcement, *Plast. Eng.*, May 1991, p 13–16
8. A.J. Stanley, Recycling SMC, *Plastics Recycling as a Future Business Opportunity*, 22–23 May 1991 (Washington DC), Plastics Institute of America, p 2–12
9. S.J. Pickering, R.M. Kelly, J.R. Kennerley, C.D. Rudd, and N.J. Fenwick, A Fluidised-Bed Process for the Recovery of Glass Fibers from Scrap Thermoset Composites," *Compos. Sci. Technol.*, Vol 60, 2000, p 509–523
10. A. Weber, "Aspects on Recycling Plastics Engineering Parts," BASF, Ludwigshafen, Germany
11. G. Menges et al., *Kunstst. Ger. Plast.*, Vol 78 (No. 7), 1988
12. W.J. Farrissey, Thermosets, *Plastics Recycling: Products and Processes*, R.J. Ehrig, Ed., Hanser Publishers, 1992, p 231–262
13. G.F. Baumann, W.J. Farrissey, and J.I. Myers, Energy Recovery From Automotive RIM Parts, *Polyurethanes World Congress 1991: The Voice of Advancement*, 24–26 Sept 1991 (Nice, France), p 355–360
14. W.J. Farrissey, Recycle of Thermoset Polyurethanes, *Plastics Recycling as a Future Business Opportunity*, 22–23 May 1991 (Washington DC), Plastics Institute of America, p 15–22
15. E.J. Daniels, B.J. Jody, and P.V. Bonsignore, Alternatives for Recycling of Auto Shredder Residue, *J. Resour. Manage. Technol.*, Vol 20 (No. 1), 1992, p 14–25
16. D.R. Norris, *Proc. ASM/ESD Advanced Composites Conf.*, Vol 6, ASM International and the Engineering Society of Detroit, 1990, p 277–283
17. G. Schinner, J. Brandt, and H. Richter, Recycling Carbon-Fiber-Reinforced Thermoplastic Composites, *J. Thermoplast. Compos. Mater.*, Vol 9, July 1996, p 239–245
18. J.H. van Lochem, C. Henriksen, and H.H. Lund, Recycling Concepts for Thermoplastic Composites, *J. Reinf. Plast. Compos.*, Vol 15, Sept 1996, p 865–876
19. J. Chu and J.L. Sullivan, Recyclability of a Continuous E-Glass Fiber Reinforced Polycarbonate Composite, *Polym. Compos.*, Vol 17 (No. 4), Aug 1996, p 556–567
20. J. Chu and J.L. Sullivan, Recyclability of a Glass Fiber Poly(Butylene Terephthalate) Composite, *Polym. Compos.*, Vol 17 (No. 3), June 1996, p 523–531
21. D.A. Steenkamer and J.L. Sullivan, On the Recyclability of a Cyclic Thermoplastic Composite Material, *Compos. B*, Vol 29B, 1998, p 745-752
22. S. Ramakrishna, W.K. Tan, S.H. Teoh, and M.O. Lai, Recycling of Carbon Fiber/PEEK Composites, *Key Eng. Mater.*, Vol 137, 1998, p 1–8
23. R.E. Allred, A.B. Coons, and R.J. Simonson, Properties of Carbon Fibers Reclaimed from Composite Manufacturing Scrap by Tertiary Recycling, *28th International SAMPE Technical Conf.*, Nov 1996, p 139–150
24. J.R. Kennerley, N.J. Fenwick, S.J. Pickering, and C.D. Rudd, The Properties of Glass Fibres Recycled from the Thermal Processing of Scrap Thermoset Composites, *Proc. ANTEC '96*, Society of Plastics Engineers, p 890–894
25. D.A. Steenkamer and J.L. Sullivan, Recycled Content in Polymer Matrix Composites through the Use of A-Glass Fibers, *Polym. Compos.*, Vol 18 (No. 3), June 1997, p 300–312

Recycling and Disposal of Metal-Matrix Composites

David Weiss, Eck Industries Inc.

THE NEED TO RECYCLE metal-matrix composites (MMCs) to reduce cost and meet environmental goals becomes more important as these materials are used increasingly in higher-volume applications, including the automobile industry. The worldwide market of MMCs reached 2.5 million kg in 1999 (Ref 1). Metal matrix materials can have an initial cost of two to more than 100 times the cost of the base alloy. The ability to recycle into a usable metal matrix composite therefore becomes a significant overall cost driver for their use. Most of the significant tonnage in metal matrix composites is done in aluminum-base materials, and the most progress in recycling and recovery has been done in the aluminum matrix composites as well.

Recycling of Aluminum MMCs

Aluminum matrix composites typically consist of an aluminum matrix and a high-performance second phase. In the most common production alloys, a hard second phase such as silicon carbide (SiC) or aluminum oxide (Al_2O_3) is used. Other reinforcements include graphite, boron, boron carbide, fly ash, and titanium carbide. The alloys can be discontinuously reinforced with particles and whiskers or continuously reinforced with fibers and filaments or compacted preforms. The type and method of reinforcement influences the ability of the alloys to be recycled for reuse. The manufacturing methods used to produce the composite shape and subsequent use and environmental exposure also impact recyclability. Since the cost of metal matrix composites is greater than that of the matrix alloy, it is desirable to recycle for direct reuse whenever possible. In most cases it is possible to recover at minimum the matrix alloy for reuse or sale.

Discontinuous SiC Reinforced Aluminum MMCs. Recycling procedures will vary with product form and manufacturing methods. The efficiency of the recycling effort in terms of product loss and quality of the final product can be quite variable. This variability impacts final product cost through material and quality costs. Manufacturing with recycling in mind reduces that variability.

Die-cast scrap that is produced as a by-product of the casting process is usually remelted directly without further processing. Experiments (Ref 2) have shown that the type and quantity of die and plunger lubrication affect the recovery rates of die-cast remelt. Heavy, oil-based lubricants that are trapped on or in the castings can reduce recovery rates to 80%. Castings made with water-based graphite lubricants have recovery rates in excess of 95%. Castings that show signs of surface grease or lubricant can be degreased by heating to 540 °C (1000 °F) for 6 h prior to remelting.

Foundry Scrap. The amount of work required to yield fully reusable material depends on the type and condition of the scrap. Foundry scrap, gates, risers, and clean, uncoated parts can be grit or shot blasted, blown clean, and melted with new ingot. Since the production of castings often creates some oxides in the finished product, excessive amounts of recycled materials may contribute to excessive oxides in the melt, reducing fluidity and part integrity. Good casting techniques direct oxides into the gate and riser system. Therefore, a more conservative approach would be to process gating separately with the fluxing procedure outlined below. Extra cleaning is required as the level of SiC in the alloy increases, since even low levels of oxides in alloys containing 20% or more volume content of SiC significantly reduces the ability to cast the product successfully (Fig. 1). Critical castings requiring very good mechanical properties; thin wall parts and parts cast with 30% SiC require the use of either all new material or material processed using dry argon cleaning.

Dirty Scrap, Gates, and Risers. Dirty scrap can be recovered using a fluxing and degassing procedure originally developed by Duralcan USA (Ref 3). This procedure uses a diffuser wand to introduce dry argon into the bath of molten metal (Fig. 2). The detailed procedure is as follows:

1. Mix the composite for approximately 20 min at a temperature of 700 ° C (1290 °F).
2. Preheat the end of the diffuser wand to ensure that it is dry. Diffuser wands are typically graphite or silica.
3. Begin a flow of dry argon (less than 3 ppm water) through the diffuser wand at approximately 0.14 m^3/h (5 ft^3/h). With the mixing impeller off, slowly immerse the diffuser wand in the composite bath to a level at or slightly below the end of the impeller, letting the argon bubble through the composite (Fig. 3).
4. Restart the mixing impeller and increase the argon flow rate through the wand to the flow rate of the degassing curve shown in Fig. 4. During the degassing the dross should be skimmed and discarded.
5. When dross formation ceases, remove the wand and stop the gas flow.
6. Allow the molten composite to sit for 40 to 60 min without mixing to allow any remaining entrapped gas to rise to the surface.
7. Manually stir the SiC from the bottom of the furnace, start the stirrer, and mix for at least 10 min before casting.

Very dirty scrap, scrap containing ceramic filters, or scrap that no longer contains the proper

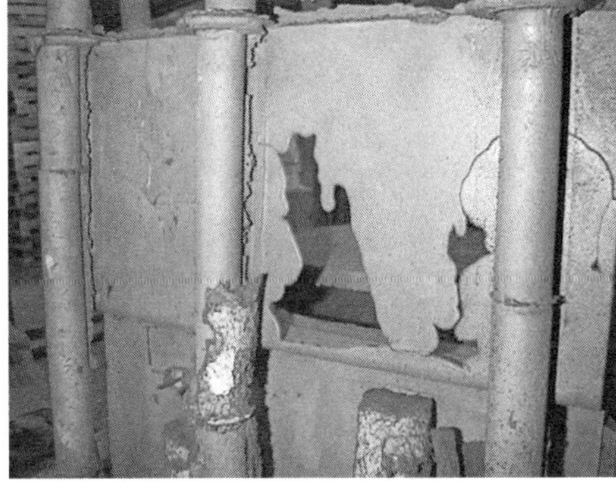

Fig. 1 Casting misrun due to low fluidity caused by presence of oxides in SiC/Al matrix MMC

amount of reinforcement can be recovered for its aluminum content in the foundry or scrap yard. Specific procedures for aluminum recovery are discussed in the section "Continuous Reinforced Aluminum MMCs" in this article.

The techniques described here for discontinuous SiC-reinforced aluminum MMCs are generally useful for most gravity and die-castable particulate reinforced aluminum-matrix composites. Alumina foundry composites may experience dewetting during the recycling procedure and are generally recycled to recover the aluminum alloy only.

Continuous Reinforced Aluminum MMCs

Aluminum alloys can be continuously reinforced with fibers or filaments of graphite, boron, SiC, and Al_2O_3. In order to separate these reinforcements from the matrix aluminum, a material must be used that has a smaller free energy than that of the matrix material when the material contacts the reinforcement (Ref 4). In the molten state, this material infiltrates into the interface and if the material is not soluble in the matrix metal, separation of the reinforcement from the matrix metal will begin. Various salts and salt combinations that are typically used for removing oxides from molten aluminum have lower surface energies than aluminum:

Material	Surface energy, mJ/m^{-2}
Aluminum (Al)	860–900
Sodium chloride (NaCl)	190.8
Potassium chloride (KCl)	155.2
Barium chloride ($BaCl_2$)	162.6
Sodium (Na)	151
Potassium (K)	86

Experiments conducted by Nishida et al. (Ref 5) using a $NaCl{\cdot}KCl{\cdot}Na_2SiF_6$ (ratio 40:40:20) showed separation rates of matrix material from alumina short fibers of 50 to 60% by adding flux during agitation of the molten metal. Separation rates of only 20% were found when recovering aluminum from 0.6 μm SiC whiskers. This type of flux gives off chlorine and fluorine gas as the flux decomposes in molten aluminum. These gases serve an important role in pushing the molten matrix from the composite. It has long been recognized that fluxing with chlorine gas will effectively strip the SiC from particulate reinforced composite. Other gases have been used with mixed effectiveness to remove particulate reinforcements, although their uses for recycling continuous reinforced aluminum MMCs have not been documented.

Aluminum that has had the reinforcement phase removed is generally filtered to remove oxides and traces of reinforcement, checked for chemistry, and recovered in ingot form. Reinforcement phases are generally not reused, but are benign waste products that can be disposed of in a landfill.

Aluminum MMCs Containing Preforms. Preforms can be considered a special type of continuous reinforcement. One of the advantages to the use of preforms is the possibility of selective reinforcement of a component. Preforms are primarily ceramic, but may contain metallic reinforcement separately or in combination with the ceramic. Recycling can be done in two stages, with the reinforcement area sawed or otherwise removed from the component followed by recovery of the aluminum trapped in the preform. If the area of the reinforcement cannot be determined precisely, it may be possible to melt the surrounding product from it using a dry-hearth-type furnace (Fig. 5). A dry hearth furnace has a separate melting chamber connected to the bath by a slanted channel. The aluminum will melt and run down the channel, leaving the preform in the melting chamber. The preforms can later be removed by using a tool to pull them from the chamber or waiting to remove them until after the furnace cools.

Quality Issues

Most recycling of metal matrix composites occurs during manufacture of the products, typically as a way to recover gates, risers, stubs, or scrap. Material control at the point of manufacturing makes alloy identification and separation easy to maintain. However, repeated melting of MMCs or repeated melting of aluminum recovered from MMCs can change the chemistry of the base alloy as well as the amount and distribution of reinforcement.

Base alloy chemistry should be checked using optical emission spectroscopy or similar tech-

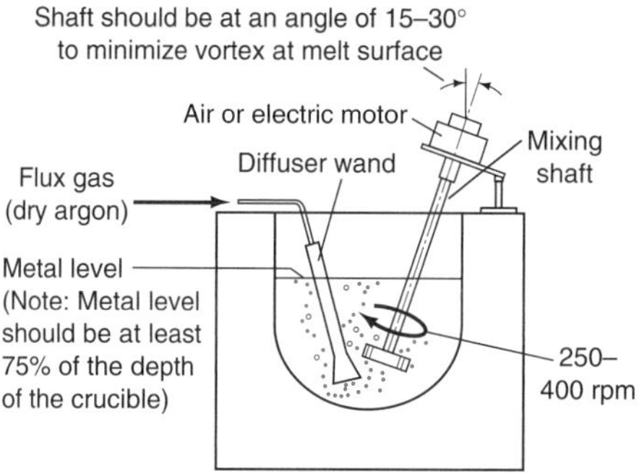

Fig. 3 Orientation of mechanical stirring device and degassing tube for crucible-style furnace

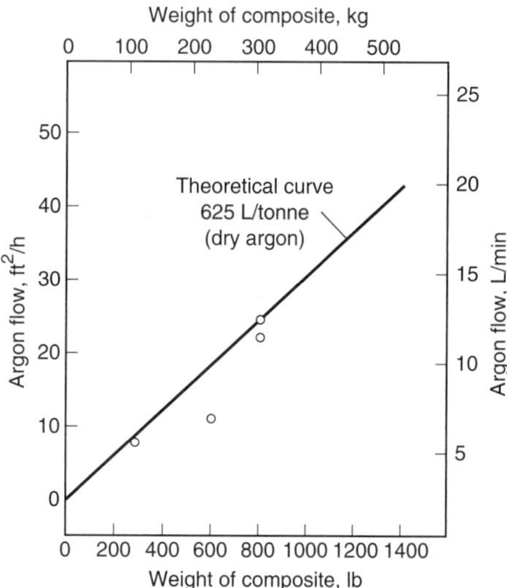

Fig. 4 Degassing curve based on degassing for 20 min

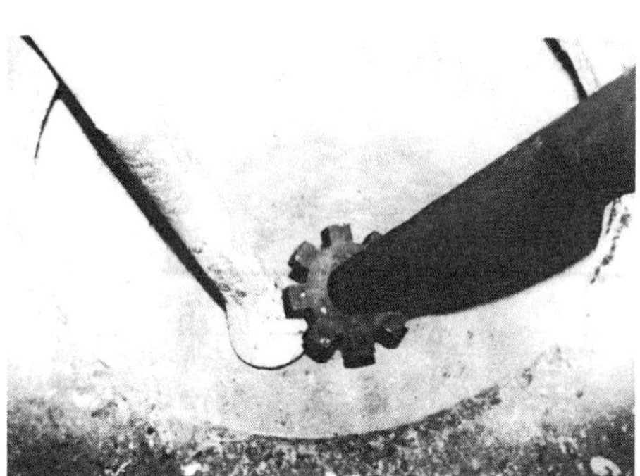

Fig. 2 Molten SiC/Al-matrix MMC fluxed and degassed by introducing dry argon gas via diffuser wand

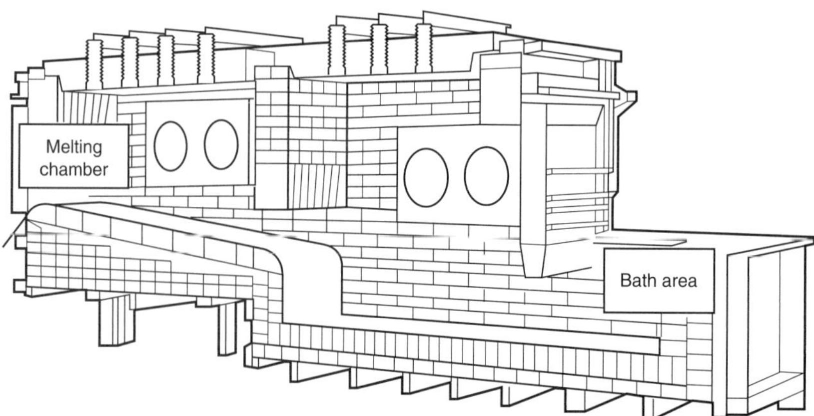

Fig. 5 Dry hearth furnace for recovering aluminum from preform reinforced aluminum-matrix MMC

Table 1 Property comparison for castings made of virgin and recycled material

Al MMC type F3S.20S-T71	Tensile strength MPa	Tensile strength ksi	Yield strength MPa	Yield strength ksi	Elongation, %
100% virgin ingot	241–262	35–38	200–214	29–31	1–2
100% remelt castings	220–241	32–35	200–214	29–31	1–2

nique. Magnesium, an important alloying element in aluminum casting alloys, is lost through successive remeltings and alloy cleaning procedures. Iron may be picked up through repeated contact with skimming and stirring devices and furnace cleaning tools. Materials may be inadvertently mixed that will cause the alloys to be out of specification.

When recycling composite alloys for direct reuse, sampling of the base alloy can be done in a number of different ways. The reinforcement phase can be allowed to settle or float, and a base alloy sample can be pulled from the segregated melt, which is then checked using spectrographic techniques. For the SiC reinforced composites, techniques have been developed (Ref 3) to check both particle loading and elemental chemistry using optical emission spectroscopy with a spectrometer equipped with a carbon line.

Repeated remelting of particulate reinforced composites can lead to gradual loss of particles from particle settling or particle removal by melt cleaning methods. Particle loading can be determined through wet chemistry, optical emission spectroscopy for some alloys, or ultrasonic testing.

Properties of Recycled Aluminum MMCs

The recycling techniques developed for aluminum MMCs are meant to ensure adequate mechanical properties for recycled materials. However, repeated recycling using the best techniques can eventually add dispersed oxides that may affect the tensile properties of the materials. Weiss et al. (Ref 6) have demonstrated the correlation between oxides in the microstructure and mechanical properties. Mechanical properties of permanent mold test bars produced from virgin material versus a melt prepared from 100% recycled scrap castings (Ref 7) are shown in Table 1. Generally, a mixture of 50% new ingot and 50% recycled materials will yield acceptable mechanical properties under most conditions.

Disposal of Aluminum MMCs

Good particulate reinforced composite material or aluminum recovered from composite materials is often directly reused. Aluminum that has been stripped from the reinforcement can also be sold to secondary aluminum processors for alloying and subsequent resale. Particulate, continuous reinforcements and preforms removed from the aluminum are not generally reused and are typically sent to a landfill. Commonly used reinforcements do not present an environmental hazard. Often these reinforcements are mixed with other rich dross and sent to secondary reprocessors for further removal and recovery of the aluminum.

Recycling Other MMCs

Other ferrous and nonferrous metals have been used as matrix materials for a wide range of metal matrix composite materials. A partial list of these materials includes:

Reinforcement	Matrix alloys
Boron fiber	Aluminum, titanium
Silicon carbide fiber	Aluminum, titanium, magnesium, copper
Graphite Fiber	Aluminum, magnesium
Aluminum oxide fiber	Aluminum, magnesium
Tungsten fiber	Nickel, cobalt, iron

Generally, recycling of these materials is based on recovery of the matrix materials and disposal of the reinforcement. Little information has been documented on the particular techniques used with titanium, magnesium, copper, superalloy, and iron-base composites. Filtering, exploitation of density differences, and chemical separation techniques have been discussed as possible techniques. Chemical composition of the base alloy needs to be verified since some reinforcements and reinforcement coating can cause a change to base alloy chemistry.

REFERENCES

1. "Metal Matrix Composites in the 21st Century: Markets and Opportunities," Business Communications Co., Inc., Norwalk, CT, 1999
2. Recycling studies done at Eck Industries, Manitowoc, WI, Dec 1996 to March 1998
3. Duralcan Composites Casting Guidelines, April 1993
4. Y. Nishida, N. Izawa, and Y. Kuramasu, *Metall. Mater. Trans.A*, Vol 30, March 1999, p 839–844
5. Y. Nishida, N. Izawa, and Y. Kuramasu, *Metall. Mater. Trans. A*, Vol 30, March 1999, p 840–842
6. D. Weiss, P. Rohatgi, Q. Liu, "Correlation Between Structure and Mechanical Properties of Cast SiC Particulate Reinforced Al-Alloy Matrix Composites," Paper 00–073, 2000 AFS Casting Congress, American Foundrymen's Society
7. Properties Database, Eck Industries, Manitowoc, WI

Applications and Experience

Chairpersons: Tia Benson Tolle, Air Force Research Laboratory
Warren H. Hunt, Jr., Aluminum Consultants Group Inc.

Introduction to Applications

Tia Benson Tolle, Materials and Manufacturing Directorate, Air Force Research Laboratory
Warren H. Hunt, Jr., Aluminum Consultants Group, Inc.

APPLICATIONS of advanced composite materials have demonstrated significant system-level benefits over conventional materials to a point where they are now accepted engineering materials. This Section highlights selected applications of polymer-matrix composites (PMCs), metal-matrix composites (MMCs), and ceramic-matrix composites (CMCs). The focus is on important applications that are representative of the current state of practice.

Advanced Polymer-Matrix Composites

Although the basic concepts of composite materials were understood from a technical sense early on, it was in the 1940s that glass-reinforced plastics came into existence as an industrial material. Their potential benefits for structural applications were recognized in 1941 when the first task force was initiated at Wright-Patterson Air Force Base to examine fiber-reinforced plastics for aircraft applications. In 1943, the first reinforced composite airframe structures were demonstrated at the Wright-Patterson Air Force Base Structures and Materials Laboratory, where the aft fuselage of the Vultee BT-15 trainer aircraft was designed and fabricated in composites, based on development and analysis. Testing proved the composite structure to be approximately 50% stronger than a metallic or wooden construction. Since then, advanced composite materials have found many applications in aeronautical and spacecraft structures. Their inherent characteristics offered new capabilities and dramatic improvements to many aerospace structures and ensured their widespread application in performance-driven systems. Sports and recreation equipment also exploited the characteristics of composites. Glass-reinforced PMCs have found wide use in marine applications since the late 1940s and have begun to migrate into automotive applications.

Today, advanced composites continue to be extensively used in aerospace applications and are becoming increasingly utilized in non-aerospace applications such as infrastructure and automotive structures. Although advanced composites are not yet a commodity material, they have reached the level of an accepted specialty engineering material. New application areas such as infrastructure offer the opportunity for composites to become more of a commodity material with widespread and diverse usage. These applications are based on a foundation of research, development, and experience that spans over 50 years. Advanced composite technologies continue to be developed, and new and significant applications can be envisioned for the future, based not only on new markets, but also on the continual understanding of new materials and processes and associated capabilities.

Metal-Matrix Composites

Advanced composites based on metallic matrices have a somewhat more recent history than PMCs, yet the opportunities look no less promising. The first MMCs were developed in the 1970s for high-performance applications using continuous fibers and whiskers for reinforcement. Specialty applications in the space shuttle, Hubble telescope, and other systems have been seen. Increasing emphasis on lower-cost composite systems was driven by the interest of the automotive industry in cost-effective performance. Aluminum-matrix composites employing ceramic-particle reinforcement and amenable to inexpensive net shape processes such as casting and extrusion have led to the application of these materials in automotive brakes, drive shafts, and cylinder liners. The recent recognition that additions of ceramic reinforcement enable tailoring of physical as well as mechanical properties of MMCs has led to increasingly widespread use of these materials in electronic-packaging and thermal-management applications. Recent market forecasts for MMC use suggest the prospect for accelerating growth as the materials are more widely understood and costs decrease, suggesting a bright future for this class of materials.

Ceramic-Matrix Composites

Current applications for CMCs include cutting tool inserts and other wear-resistant parts, aerospace and military applications, and various industrial applications, including engines and energy-related applications. Advanced continuous-fiber CMCs are now emerging from laboratories and show potential for high-performance applications. Currently these materials are considered to be expensive. However, their high-temperature stability, corrosion resistance, and toughness make continuous-fiber CMCs attractive for a wide range of potential applications in both the aerospace and industrial sectors.

Automotive Applications

Nicholas J. Gianaris, Visteon Corporation

COMPOSITE MATERIALS have a history that parallels that of the automotive industry since the 1940s. Henry Ford first demonstrated the "soybean" car in 1941 when he swung an axe against it during a media demonstration (Fig. 1). The body panels were constructed of cellulose-fiber reinforcement in a soybean-resin matrix. The ability for composites to withstand impact loads was confirmed, curb weight was reduced by 900 kg (2000 lb), and the opportunity to use environmentally friendly natural fiber technologies was shown (Ref 1). The ingenious design and manufacture of composites in automotive and aerospace in parallel was shown when Convair built the Flying Car in 1946 (Fig. 2). Six of these auto-aerospace vehicles were manufactured with a glass-epoxy structural composite body and chassis (Ref 1). Composites were subsequently used for various prototype automotive vehicles. Perhaps the most famous use of composites in the automotive industry was the use of fiberglass reinforced composites for the body panels of the Chevrolet Corvette, starting in 1953 (Fig. 3).

Today, structural polymer-matrix composites (PMCs) are seen as a material critical to achieving the goals of an optimally designed car that uses a systems engineering approach in a simultaneous engineering environment. The energy crises of the 1970s and 1980s, the implementation of corporate average fuel economy regulations in the United States for domestically produced vehicles, and the high rate of taxation on automotive fuels in most countries has resulted in a focus on fuel economy. Improvements in fuel economy are most drastically realized through improvements in the efficiency of the automotive engine and powertrain reduction in weight, and through increased aerodynamic efficiency. This has resulted in an extensive use of emission control systems and the now-familiar look of aerodynamically sleek automobiles. Recently published reports by the United States Cooperative Automotive Research (USCAR) alliance have shown that a 30% mass reduction in the automobile can potentially increase fuel economy by 30%. The ripest areas for mass reduction have been shown to be the chassis

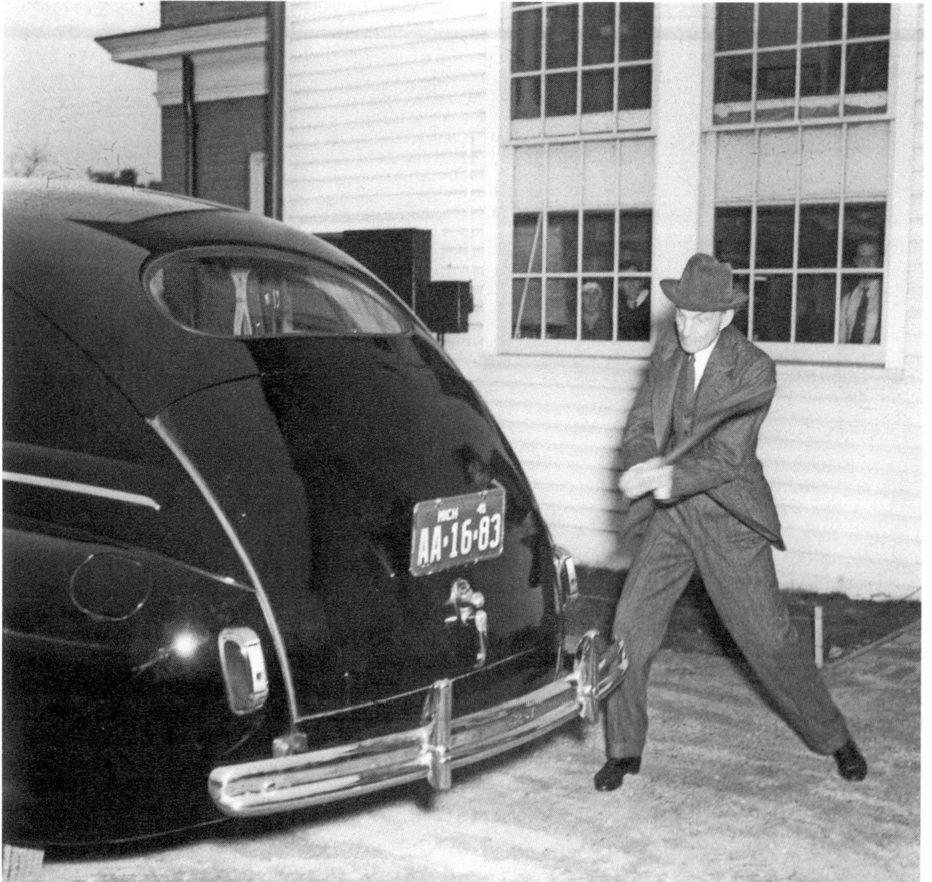

Fig. 1 Henry Ford demonstrating the durability of the "soybean" composites car. Courtesy of Ford Motor Company

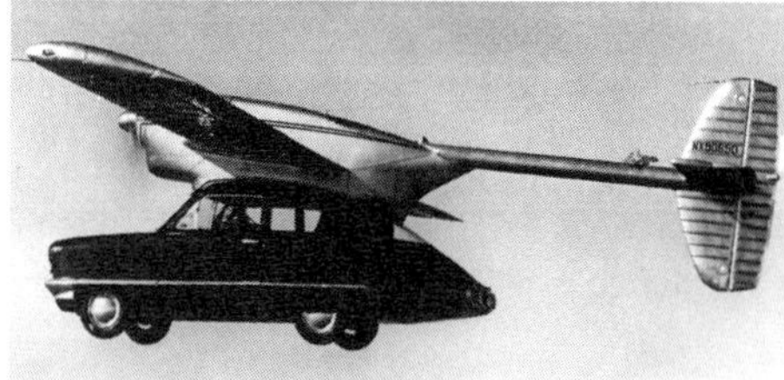

Fig. 2 Convair Flying Car. Courtesy of W. Brandt Goldsworthy & Associates

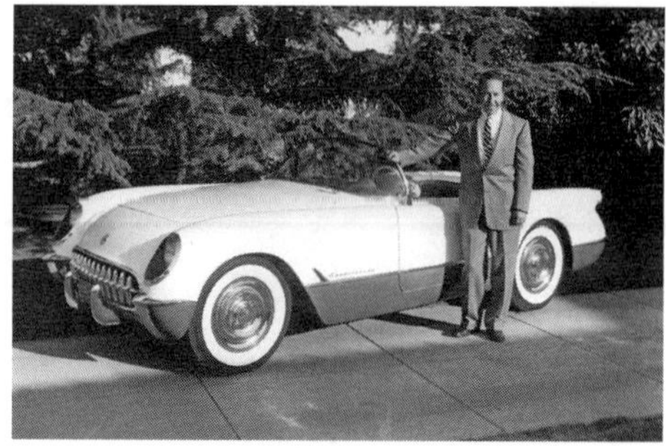

Fig. 3 Chevrolet Corvette. Courtesy of W. Brandt Goldsworthy & Associates

area—which includes the suspension, driveline, braking, and steering components—and the body and underbody structural systems. The high strength-to-mass ratio of composite materials makes them a candidate materials system for successfully achieving mass reduction in the automobile. Because composite materials have different inherent properties and different manufacturing methods than the traditional materials used for automotive applications, pure materials substitution into metal-based designs will not allow an automotive engineer to realize the advantages of the high strength-to-mass ratio of composites. A cost penalty also may be incurred, which is one principal reason why composites have not yet become a dominant material in the automotive industry. Hence, design practices that focus on optimization of the material and the system design will allow structural composites to be successfully and cost-effectively implemented on automobiles, pick-up trucks, and sport utility vehicles.

Automotive Composites

Composite materials are those with any two or more distinct and identifiable constituent materials that differ in form or composition and whose combination results in properties that are superior to those of the constituent materials. When the composite material is engineered and optimized for structural applications, the constituent materials are typically a high-strength and an intermediate-to-high apparent modulus, high aspect ratio fiber that is combined with a semicoherent or coherent matrix that usually serves as a binder. Typically, composites are engineered to withstand primary static and dynamic structural requirements and environmental factors. However, in automotive applications, composites are also engineered to satisfy appearance requirements, secondary structural needs (i.e., reduction of noise, vibration for harshness for structures such as body panels and hoods), high- or low-volume manufacturing and process drivers, cost, and crash safety. Secondary structural applications in many cases tend to trade off structural properties for appearance or high-volume, low-cycle manufacturing. Hence, these types of composites are considered as semistructural. The general properties of thermoplastic and thermoset composites are listed in Table 1. Multifunctional composites are those which take advantage of other nonstructural properties, such as conductivity, health monitoring, and sensing materials. These properties are underused in today's automobile, but will be important for future applications. The design and manufacture issues that are associated with PMCs are addressed subsequently.

Design Drivers

Composites are generally regarded as structural materials that are suitable for stiffness-critical designs and have a great potential for automotive applications. One design driver for which PMCs are useful is mass reduction and distribution. Mass reduction of the total vehicle system helps to increase fuel economy. This is especially true of rotating unsprung mass at the hub, wheel, and brake system. The structural parts of the automobile, the body and the chassis, are also mass sensitive for vehicle dynamics and performance. The reduction of unsprung mass, or the mass that is not carried by the suspension system, improves vehicle performance much more than when mass is reduced for sprung, or suspended, mass. Hence, mass reduction of the chassis, especially the braking, and suspension systems, affects vehicle dynamics more favorably than the reduction of body mass. Additionally, the mass distribution from front to rear and side to side also greatly affects vehicle dynamics. If mass reduction results in an unbalanced chassis, then the performance and the feel of the vehicle are affected, despite any overall reduction of vehicle mass. Hence, fuel economy and vehicle dynamics are the critical drivers for lean mass automotive designs.

Noise, Vibration, and Harshness (NVH). Polymer-matrix composites also have the inherent advantage of increasing the natural frequencies of NVH produced in a vehicle while it is being driven. The high stiffness-to-mass ratios and damping characteristics of PMCs raise these frequencies to levels that are indistinguishable to the driver and passenger, hence increasing customer satisfaction. The use of PMCs eliminates the need for the addition of bushings, other damping materials, and spot welds that are added solely to increase structural stiffness and reduce noise transmission. Hence, total vehicle mass and cost is reduced.

Body and Chassis. Structural PMCs are applied mainly to the body and chassis areas. These areas of the automobile must carry internal and external static and dynamic loads. Hence, PMC designs based on rules of mixture and generalized Hooke's law can be used to provide globally—and locally—optimized strength and stiffness properties for the structural needs of the body and chassis. This design tailorability is one of the greatest advantages for the use of PMCs with automotive applications, but also is one of the greatest challenges.

Process and Materials Property Constraints. The advantages of structural composites can only be realized if process limitations are understood and if materials properties and differing design principles receive proper attention. Engineers who have designed applications using traditional linear, elastic, homogeneous, and isotropic materials must remember that simple materials substitution is not sufficient to ensure a successful product. Systems engineering principles and discipline must be followed in a simultaneous engineering environment. The specific needs of an individual design should drive the selection of the optimal material and process, as opposed to using a specific materials system to meet all design requirements. A decision flow chart that shows this is in Fig. 4.

Safety and Reliability. Automobiles are consumer products that are regulated for safety and fuel economy. One of the most critical design safety drivers is the performance of the vehicle during a crash. The automobile must meet vehicle dynamic and performance expectations that differentiate it from its competition. The reliability and service costs associated with a particular automotive product are also quite important.

Design Optimization. The automotive industry must also develop optimized designs that push the processing technology envelope, as opposed to process-driven designs for which only semistructural materials may be used. The automotive industry has already successfully implemented the use of computer-aided design (CAD) and computer-aided engineering (CAE) tools for design and process optimization. Design CAE tools have been limited to linear, elastic, homogeneous, and isotropic materials assumptions. These tools have been quite effective in design optimization and finite-element analysis (FEA) studies, but the more complex models that are required for composite material design and optimization are just now becoming commercially available. Even more critical are the safety aspects of automotive designs. Crash computer simulation models have successfully been implemented in the automotive design community for metal designs, but are still in development for composites. The Automotive Composites Consortium group of USCAR has been making significant progress in this area.

Previous materials substitution successes and failures must be documented to lay the foundation for product improvements. Sometimes, structurally optimized properties typically require trade-offs with appearance requirements.

Design Challenges and Constraints

Polymer-matrix composites have been shown to have great potential for use in automotive applications; but their full range of potential advantages is not well understood in the automo-

Table 1 General characteristics of thermoplastic and thermoset composites

Property	Thermoplastic composites	Thermoset composites
Fiber content	Low to medium	Medium to high
Fiber type	Continuous and discontinuous	Continuous and discontinuous
Solvent resistance	Low	High
Heat resistance	Low to medium	Low to high
Molding time	Fast (<5 min)	Slow (typically $\frac{1}{2}$ to 4 h)
Molding pressure	High (>14 bar, or 1400 kPa)	Low (1 bar–7 bar, or 100–700 kPa)
Material cost	Low to medium	Low to high
Safety/handling	Excellent	Good
Storage life	Indefinite	Good (6–24 months with refrigeration)

Source: Ref 2

tive design community. One of the most common mistakes made is *direct materials substitution*, where a component that was originally designed for another materials system (i.e., steel, cast iron) is manufactured with PMCs without any changes. This is a poor approach because the design advantages of the PMC are underutilized, thus increasing the cost of a part that is using an already costly material. PMCs permit the designer to consolidate parts.

Structural and Appearance Requirements. Automotive applications have both structural and appearance requirements that have tended to change with time. High quality surface appearance on secondary structures, such as hoods and body panels, is required.

Automotive applications have stringent design and appearance requirements that are, at times, in conflict with each other. Fenders and fascias are primarily appearance parts, with only local strength and stiffness requirements for attachments and oil-canning resistance. Load floors and floor pans are structural, with only minor appearance needs. Hoods, roofs, and doors, however, contribute in varying degrees to the overall vehicle structure and must provide the same quality appearance as fenders and fascias.

Structural requirements can be subdivided into primary and secondary requirements. The primary structure reacts to major loads, such as static and dynamic external loads and component loads, while the secondary structure supplements the primary one by addressing local requirements, such as surface appearance, sealing, and carrying minor components. The secondary structure can act to stabilize the primary structure for an optimized overall design. Hence, if the load paths of the body and chassis structure are modeled with FEA and well understood, the anisotropic properties of continuous or long fiber PMCs can be used to optimize strength and modulus of the PMC material design.

In the automotive industry, the application of structural composites has been mostly limited to secondary structures and appearance panels. For example, doors contribute to crashworthiness, but are largely secondary structures. Aerospace and aircraft applications are often considerably different from automotive applications in that the exterior surfaces are often an integral part of the primary structure of the product. The fact that structural composites have been used extensively for both primary and secondary structures in aerospace applications is due to the low production rates and an emphasis on the reduction of weight as opposed to cost.

Computer Aided Engineering. Another area in which automotive design with PMCs has great emphasis is in the use of CAE. As previously stated, CAE models are used extensively for designing with linear, elastic, homogeneous, and isotropic materials, such as most metal materials. These computer tools are valuable in design optimization and simulation. Areas in which CAE tools have become invaluable include vehicle dynamics and crashworthiness simulations. Crash safety is driven by engineering standards and government regulations internationally and is expensive to validate due to the number of vehicles that must be tested for crash safety certification. Computer-aided engineering tools provide a significant potential for the digital validation of crashworthiness, but are limited mainly to linear, elastic, homogeneous, and isotropic materials systems. Automotive companies, including the USCAR consortium, are concentrating resources in order to develop CAE models for PMCs.

Recyclability. Recyclability of composites is also of concern to the international automotive community. In response to the Kyoto Summit and the European Economic Community, PMCs must be able to demonstrate closed-loop recycling. Other parts of this Volume are more specific on this area, but a great challenge exists in being able to use PMCs to their advantage while also being recyclable.

Life Cycle Assessment. Polymer-matrix composites have been compared with other materials to estimate the environmental burdens in

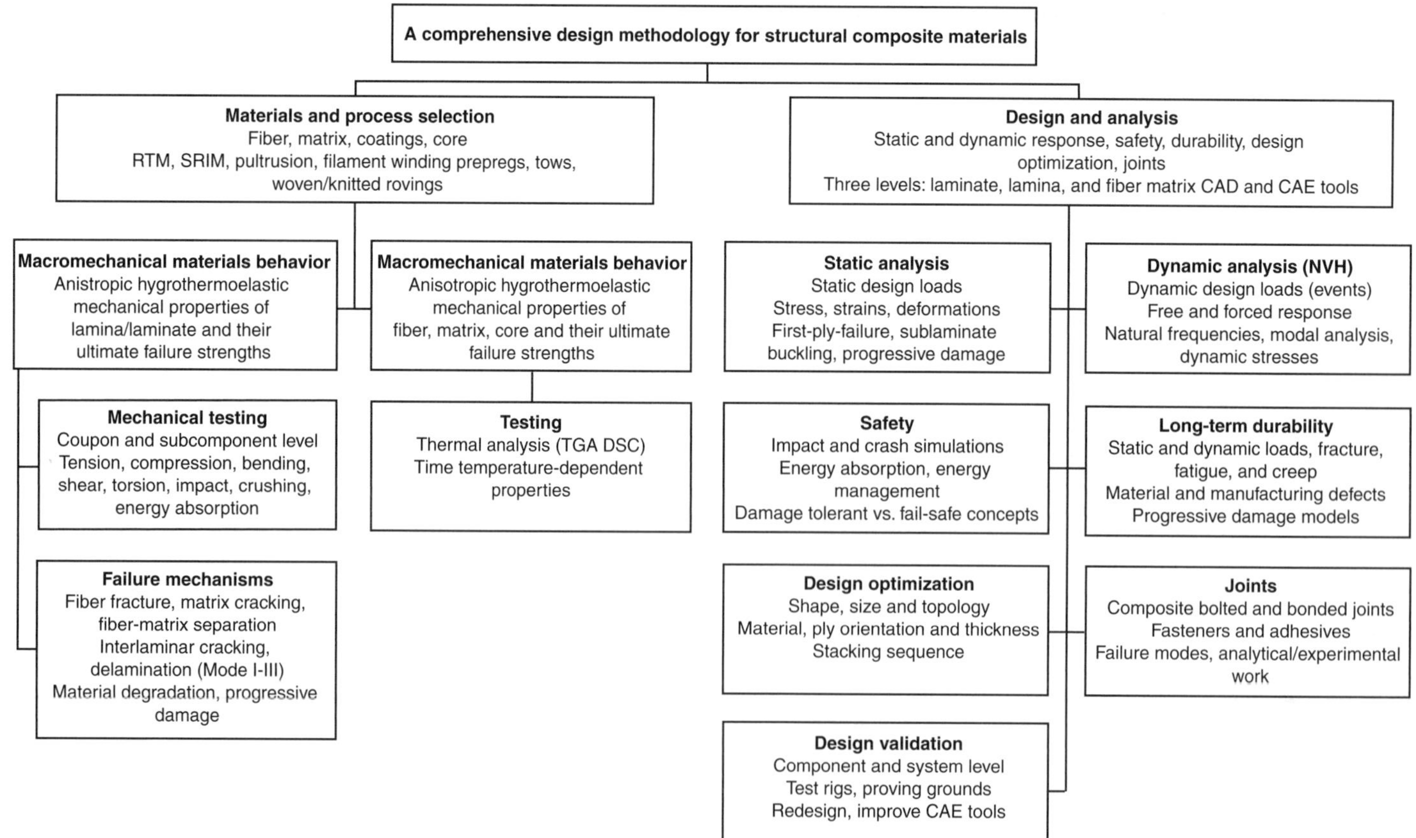

Fig. 4 Design methodology for automotive composite structures. RTM, resin transfer molding; SRIM, structural reaction injection molding; CAD, computer-aided design; CAE, computer-aided engineering; TGA, thermogravimetric analysis; DSC, differential scanning calorimetry

automobile applications over the entire product life cycle. It was found that carbon- or glass-fiber-reinforced thermoplastic-matrix PMC had the lowest total life cycle environmental burden compared to steel, aluminum, or magnesium. This was despite the fact that carbon-fiber PMC has higher initial costs and energy burdens to produce the material. But, when taking into account life cycle energy use, greenhouse gas emissions, water emissions, solid waste, and hydrogen fluoride emissions, PMC imposed the lowest environmental life cycle burden (Ref 3).

Repair and Maintainability. Similar to the challenges with the use of composites in the aerospace area, the repair and the maintainability of automotive PMCs is a significant design as well as infrastructure challenge. Unlike other transportation applications, automotive maintenance is not limited strictly to certified mechanics. Most repairs are geared to steel-based procedures. However, with the evolution of the use of aluminum and modular electronics in automobiles, mechanics are becoming more versed in the special procedures that must be followed to service automobiles. This may provide promise for the servicing of technologically advanced automotive vehicles, but still entails the challenge of designing PMC automotive systems with servicing in mind. An excellent example of this is the LiteCast control link (National Composite Center), which provides a simple mechanism to indicate damage to the composite portion of the component (Fig 5). This mechanism is a stress concentrator at the end of the control link that induces failure at the composite-to-aluminum interface.

Processability. Processing of composites has been a constraint in being able to use fully optimized composite designs for automotive applications. Hand lay-up of composite structures is used to process racing vehicles, and this is still a primary process in aerospace manufacturing. Such a process that is touch-labor intensive and also wastes more than 1% of PMC material during production is quite prohibitive for automotive applications because of the cost involved. Thus, either highly automated processes or cost-effective labor-intensive processes must be used today to be able to produce design- and cost-optimized automotive vehicles. Examples of such processes are listed in Table 2. One step toward this goal is an automated process developed by the Automotive Composites Consortium (ACC) called P4 (which stands for programmable powder preforming process). This process has the potential for low-cost, high-volume production of optimized-design automotive PMC, due to its highly automated and low-waste method of applying chopped fiber to contoured surfaces. The fiber length and direction can be controlled, thus allowing for the design advantages of PMCs to be exploited (Fig 6). The P4 process is an example of how processes must be adapted to accommodate the design advantages of PMCs, instead of limiting the implementation of PMCs in automotive applications to existing high-volume processes.

An example of PMCs used to achieve low materials cost, short process cycle time, and part consolidation is DaimlerChrysler's composites vehicle (Fig 7). This vehicle was designed to use fiber-reinforced thermoplastic PMC and adhesives to achieve structural and surface finish requirements at a reasonable cost, due to part consolidation and process time reduction (Ref 6).

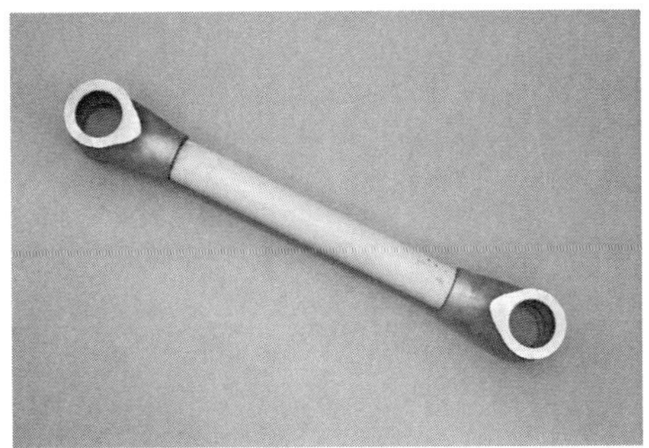

Fig. 5 LiteCast control link. Courtesy of National Composite Center

Design Environments

The design environment for automotive PMCs is still in the emerging technology stage for most applications that involve primary structure. Secondary structural applications are dominated by the use of sheet molding compounds (SMCs) and reinforced reaction injection molding (RRIM). Applications tend to emphasize body panel consolidation and the inclusion of special cosmetic design features, such as an integral step pad in a pick-up truck fender or header ports in a hood. Additionally, the design and processing knowledge and expertise lies mainly at the original equipment manufacturer (OEM) level, hence limiting "black box" designs at the tier one supplier level. Therefore, the design environment today is appearance dominated, with primary design responsibility at the OEM level. However, great potential exists for the PMC design environment to mature as primary structural and multifunctional applications are developed. A successful and proven design strategy will be one that used systems engineering principles and disciplines in a simultaneous engineering environment.

Application Drivers and Constraints

Production, Regulatory, and Consumer Attributes. The automotive industry sells vehicles that range from the utilitarian vehicles, such as pick-up trucks, to sports and sports-luxury vehicles. In all parts of this spectrum, the design advantages of PMCs lend themselves to fuel economy and vehicle dynamics and performance. Applications are differentiated by passenger and load capacity, in addition to regulatory classifications of vehicles. Today, PMCs tend to be used mostly in niche vehicle applications where production volumes are low and premium prices are charged per vehicle. This is because in the existing automotive design and assembly paradigm, the cost of PMC generally is not cost-effective over 50,000 units per year, despite lower tooling costs than those associated with metal material forming and processing. Sport utility and pick-up vehicles are obvious applications in which PMCs may be used, especially because fuel economy, vehicle dynamics, and NVH are more critical in these markets than they used to be. For example, SMCs are

Table 2 Characteristics of common processes for manufacturing polymer-based composites

Method	Fiber content, %	Resin content, %	Fiber geometry	Resins	Comments
Filament winding	60–70	30–40	Continuous, geodesic paths	Highly developed for thermosets, recently thermoplastics	Body revolves
Pultrusion	60 (varies)	40	Continuous, +90 an issue	Polyesters, others, some epoxy, recently thermoplastics	Constant cross section
Hand lay-ups	60	40	Continuous aligned and woven	Epoxy and thermoplastics	Airplane parts, surfboards
Hand lay-ups	40	60	Strand mat	Polyester	Boat hulls
Spray-up	30	70	Random chopped	Polyester, others	Fast, fumes
RTM and SRIM	20–50	50–80	Fiber preforms	Polyester, others	Low pressure, tooling issue
Compression molding (sheet molding compound)	20–50	50–80	Long, random	Polyester, others	Fiber orientation, surface finish issues
Stamping	20–60	40–80	Random coiled, continuous aligned	Thermoplastic	New developments
Injection molding	10–20	80–90	Short, random	Thermoplastic, polyester, polyurethane, others	Fast, RRIM, BMC, new developments

RTM, resin transfer molding; SRIM, structural reaction injection molding; RRIM, reinforced reaction injection molding; BMC, bulk molding compound. Source: Ref 2

used in cross truck beams. Implementation of PMCs in today's automotive environment has been mostly limited to areas such as the pick-up box area, although U.S. automakers recognize the need to increase the use of composites in order to meet fuel economy and safety goals for these vehicles. This can be accomplished at high-volume automotive line production rates if the total cost equation of material, tooling, design optimization, and ownership costs are addressed in order to take full advantage of the benefits of composites.

Cost. A consumer product, such as the automobile or the pick-up truck, can inspire endless application ideas, but the primary constraint of any application is cost. Materials cost is a significant constraint for PMCs in the automotive industry. With optimized design tools and practices, materials cost can be counterbalanced by reduced design and development cost, reduced capital investment and tooling cost, and enhanced value of the vehicle to the consumer. Thus, the total cost to the consumer becomes much more advantageous.

High-Volume Composite Descriptions, Properties, and Processes

Over 50% of automotive composites used in today's production vehicles consist of SMC and reaction injection molded (RIM) composites. Information is presented subsequently on the properties and processes of these automotive composite materials systems.

Sheet Molding Compounds. Sheet molding compounds are fiber-reinforced plastics that are fabricated in sheets and compression molded to final shape. They are reinforced in the plane of the sheet, but are not significantly reinforced in the through-thickness direction. The reinforcement may consist of continuous fibers (SMC-C), randomly chopped fibers (SMC-R), or a blend of both (SMC-C/R). The weight percent of fiber is generally indicated after the "C" or "R".* Continuous fibers can be placed parallel to get maximum stiffness and strength in one direction, but at the price of very low properties in the direction normal to the fibers. A wide range of intermediate properties can be obtained by combining continuous and random fibers or by laying continuous fibers in an "X" pattern, oriented at a specific angle to get the desired directional properties (XMC). Of these types, SMC-R materials are the most widely used for automotive applications.

Properties of typical appearance-grade (SMC-R25), structural-grade (SMC-R50), mixed continuous/random (SMC-C20/R30), and $\pm 7.5°$ X-pattern continuous (XMC-3) SMC compounds are given in Table 3. These properties are from compounds made from typical polyester resins with calcium carbonate filler and glass fibers.

*Weight percent is used for SMC instead of volume percent because of the traditional practice of the automotive plastics industry, which has served as the main supplier of SMC to the automotive industry. The amount of fiber reinforcement is measured by weight percent to describe the plastics-oriented manufacturing process of SMC. This is in contrast to the customary use of volume percent by manufacturers of primary structural composites. Volume percent is more useful in describing the design and the mechanics of structural composites.

The SMC molding process involves placing an SMC charge in a heated mold and compressing the material at pressures of roughly 5.5 to 6.9 MPa (0.80 to 1.0 ksi). Polymerization of the partially reacted matrix is completed in the molding process. Faster dual-acting presses with accurately controlled parallelism, closing speed, and pressing force are also used in production. These presses have the potential to reduce press cycle time to less than 1 min. Molded coating can be applied during the molding cycle to fill surface porosity and to uniformly coat the surface for optimal surface appearance and quality.

Complex shapes and refined details that may be impractical with sheet metal are often easy to achieve with SMC. Parts may also be molded with varying thicknesses for local stiffness requirements. The design must be planned, however, so that all shape and detail is formed in a one-step molding process. While this can be an advantage over the multiple press-forming operations found in sheet metal fabrication, it must be understood that a molded SMC part cannot be reformed or flanged by a restrike operation, as is common with sheet metal parts.

It is critical that SMC parts be designed with sufficient draft to allow easy removal from the mold. Unlike parts made of more flexible polymeric materials, SMC parts cannot be designed with features that require parts to be snapped or peeled out of the mold. The use of lifters and slides to achieve features that are common in injection molded parts is more limited in SMC parts, because of the requirement for placing the uncured SMC material into the mold before it is closed.

Reaction Injection Molding. Reaction injection molding materials are prepared by polymerizing monomers or prepolymers during the process of molding finished parts. Milled glass fiber can be added to obtain reinforced RIM (RRIM). Milled glass RRIM tends to have directional properties due to fiber orientation during injection. Substituting glass flakes for the milled fibers can greatly reduce directional differences. As in SMC materials, reinforcement is primarily in the local plane of the material and

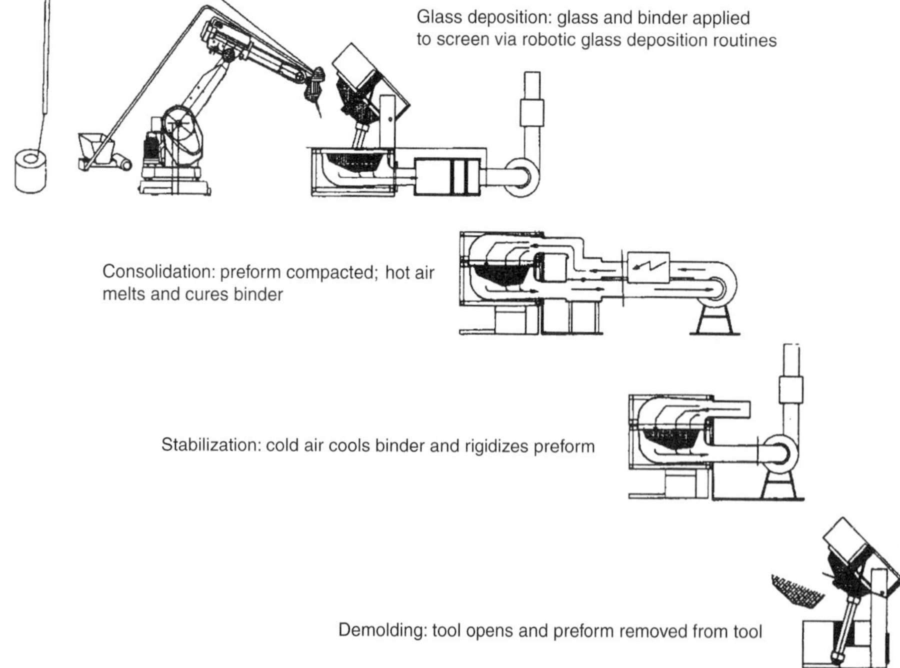
Glass deposition: glass and binder applied to screen via robotic glass deposition routines
Consolidation: preform compacted; hot air melts and cures binder
Stabilization: cold air cools binder and rigidizes preform
Demolding: tool opens and preform removed from tool

Fig. 6 Programmable powder preforming process (P4) composites manufacturing technology. Source: Ref 4. Courtesy of N.G. Chavka, Ford Motor Company

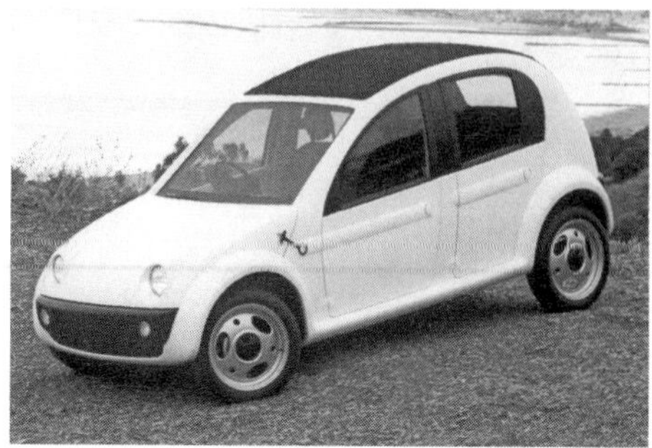

Fig. 7 Chrysler composite vehicle. Source: Ref 5. Courtesy of G.B. Chapman II, DaimlerChrysler Corporation

not through the thickness. The RIM and RRIM materials described previously do not have significant structural applications, because their strength and stiffness properties are relatively low compared to those of SMC. Strength and stiffness properties similar to those of SMC can be obtained by placing fiber preforms in the mold before injecting and reacting the RIM matrix. This material is referred to as structural RRIM, sometimes called SRRIM or SRIM. Properties of typical RRIM and structural RRIM materials—commercial polyurethane and polyurea resins—are given in Table 4.

The RIM process involves mixing the matrix reactants and injecting them into the mold. The reinforcing material can be injected with the reactants or can be placed in the mold as preformed mat before injection. Mold pressures are about 0.7 to 1.0 MPa (0.1 to 0.15 ksi) for RIM and RRIM, increasing to 1.4 to 2.0 MPa (0.20 to 0.30 ksi) for structural RRIM. Fast-acting polyurea and prepolymer chemicals are available that shorten reaction times to less than 10 s. New developments include equipment that provides precise temperature control, mixing ratios, and injection of filled and reinforced material.

As with SMC, the RIM processes permit complex shapes, refined details, and variations in thickness that would be impractical in sheet metal. Again, this is a one-step process, and secondary or restrike operations are not possible. An advantage of the RIM process is that it can use lifters and slides to achieve features common on other injection molding processes. The lower stiffness of RIM and RRIM permit some degree of snapping or peeling the parts out of the mold. On the other hand, the lower stiffness reduces the applicability of these materials to meet many structural requirements, unless the operation of fabricating a preform mat is added. Newer mat-making processes include the use of ultraviolet light-activated powder binder and woven composites with *z*-axis fibers.

Processes for Directed and Oriented Fiber. Specific fiber orientation often is required for structural composites. Other sections of this article describe the need for design optimization and its relation to fiber orientation in primary structural composites. The typical properties of oriented fiber composites are given in Table 5, although more specific properties are given elsewhere in this Volume. Though there are new processes, such as the P4 process described earlier in this article, other processes that have been used for commercial automotive application include filament winding, tape laying, and braiding.

In general, the filament winding and tape laying processes for each technique are similar in that fibers are precoated with resin by the fiber manufacturer or are coated in the fabrication process just before the fiber-placement operation. The parts are then cured, either in a mold or on a supporting surface. The fiber-placement techniques have evolved to high-volume processes. Examples of this include high-volume automated filament winding of composite driveshafts, where several driveshafts can be wound at a time on removable mandrels.

Complex shapes and varying thicknesses can be obtained with these processes. However, the design must be planned so that any supporting surface for the fibers can be removed after curing or can remain as a part of the product.

Resin Transfer Molding and Squeeze Molding. Resin transfer molding and squeeze molding are low-pressure, long cycle time processes that are generally used for low-volume commercial products, such as class eight trucks. They can be thought of as low-productivity, low-pressure versions of the SMC and structural RIM processes. They have the capacity for producing parts that approximate the properties of the higher-productivity processes and, as such, are useful for producing prototype parts for evaluation.

Design Guidelines for Body and Secondary Structural Panels. Although the multitude of composite materials and processes available today for high-volume automotive applications makes design and process decisions difficult, most major automobile companies have developed materials selection and design criteria based on previous experience and through the efforts of the ACC. This section features those points that must be considered when determining which materials are best-suited for automotive body panels.

In general, the structural qualities of panels can be categorized by stiffness and strength requirements. The stiffness requirements provide the rigidity necessary to resist deflection, oil canning, and buckling and to ensure the desired vibration response. The strength requirements provide the needed failure resistance under service loading. In addition, certain panels contribute to crash resistance and energy management when a vehicle is tested under safety loading conditions.

Table 3 Typical properties of sheet molding compounds

Type	Specific gravity	Glass, wt%	Filler, wt%	Resin, wt%	Tensile strength MPa	Tensile strength ksi	Elongation, %	Flexural modulus GPa	Flexural modulus 10^6 psi	Coefficient of linear thermal expansion, 10^{-6}/K
SMC-R25	1.83	25	46	29	82.4	12.0	1.34	11.7	1.70	23.2
SMC-R50	1.87	50	16	34	164	23.8	1.73	15.9	2.30	14.8
SMC-C20/R30	1.81	50	16	34	...	...	...	...	...	...
Longitudinal	...	...	...	...	289	41.9	1.73	25.7	3.73	11.3
Lateral	...	...	...	...	84.0	12.2	1.58	5.9	0.86	24.6
XMC-3 ± 7.5° X-pattern	1.97	75	...	25	...	...	...	...	...	...
Longitudinal	...	...	...	...	561	81.4	1.66	34.1	4.95	8.7
Lateral	...	...	...	...	69.9	10.1	1.54	6.8	0.99	28.6

Table 4 Typical properties of reinforced reaction injection molding materials

Type	Specific gravity	Glass, wt%	Resin, wt%	Tensile strength MPa	Tensile strength ksi	Elongation, %	Flexural modulus GPa	Flexural modulus 10^6 psi	Coefficient of linear thermal expansion, 10^{-6}/K
Polyurethane reinforced with milled glass	1.08	15	85	...	...	...	...	...	...
Longitudinal	...	...	...	19.3	2.80	110	0.538	0.0780	90
Lateral	...	...	...	17.9	2.60	140	0.331	0.0480	135
Polyurethane reinforced with flake glass	1.15	20	80	...		...	...	...	...
Longitudinal	...	...	...	24.1	3.50	25	1.34	0.194	54
Lateral	...	...	...	25.2	3.65	25	1.24	0.180	58
Polyurea reinforced with flake glass	1.18	20	80	...	...	...	...	...	...
Longitudinal	...	...	...	33.3	4.83	31	1.68	0.244	50
Lateral	...	...	...	30.5	4.42	31	1.72	0.250	53
Structural RRIM	1.5	37	63	172	24.9	4.2	12.4	1.80	12

Table 5 Typical properties of oriented fiber composites

Type	Specific gravity	Fiber, wt%	Resin, wt%	Tensile strength MPa	Tensile strength ksi	Flexural modulus GPa	Flexural modulus 10^6	Coefficient of linear thermal expansion, 10^{-6}/K
Epoxy 0° S-glass	1.80	70	30	...	...	...	...	...
Longitudinal	...	...	...	849	123	40	5.8	...
Lateral	...	...	...	47.0	6.82	11	1.6	...
Epoxy 0° AS carbon	1.26	70	30	...	...	...	...	...
Longitudinal	...	...	...	966	140	138	20.0	–0.2
Lateral	...	...	...	37.3	5.41	9.7	1.4	13.0
Epoxy ± 45° AS carbon	1.26	70	30	...	...	...	...	...
Longitudinal	...	...	...	89.7	13.0	15.9	2.31	0.8
Lateral	...	...	...	89.7	13.0	15.9	2.31	0.8

AS, designation for surface-treated fiber

In the case of body panels, the stiffness requirement is selected as the primary performance constraint. This can be justified for preliminary design evaluation, because experience has shown that stiffness requirements are usually the most restrictive. A structural panel can be evaluated for strength after it has been designed for stiffness, and modifications for strength can be added.

Other experience has shown that the secondary structural panels contribute somewhat to the global stiffness of a vehicle, but that local stiffness requirements predominate. The local stiffness is defined as the stiffness of a support-free region of the panel bounded by stiffeners or edge beams. Therefore, a typical body panel assembly could have one or more support-free regions. In the case of uniform-thickness design, the region with the lowest stiffness is used to determine the panel thickness for the entire panel assembly.

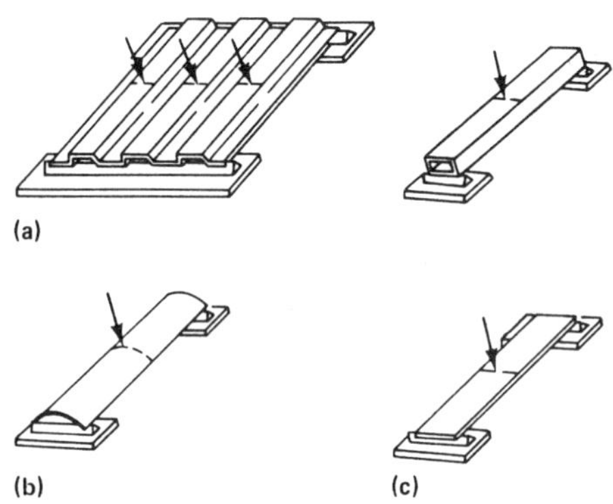

Fig. 8 Panel stiffness criteria. (a) $\alpha = 1$, pure membrane resistance. (b) $\alpha = 2$, oil-canning resistance. (c) $\alpha = 3$, flat panel bending

Panel stiffness is proportional to the modulus of elasticity (E) of the material under consideration and can be approximated as:

$$D \propto E \cdot t^{\alpha}$$

where D is panel stiffness, t is the panel thickness, and α is the stiffness parameter, which is a function of panel curvature and of the loading and boundary conditions imposed on the panel. The value of α for laterally loaded panels can range from $\alpha = 1$ for closed-box sections and corrugated panels governed by membrane stiffness, to $\alpha = 3$ for flat panels governed by pure bending stiffness. In general, all secondary structural applications have an α value between 1 and 3, because they have a combination of bending and membrane requirements. Figure 8 depicts the general conditions found in body panels.

Table 6 lists the relative thickness, weight, and materials cost for several materials, based on the three general stiffness schemes shown previously. In this example, the thickness and weight calculations have been normalized to SMC. Approximate material costs (not processing costs) and properties are listed in Table 7. Costs and materials properties are approximate and will change with economic, process, and materials developments.

To relate the above information to actual applications, Table 8 lists values for typical panel applications. The values can change with size and curvature as well as boundary and loading conditions. It should be noted that using a smaller α value results in a conservative materials substitution design that may be more costly and not take advantage of the composite materials properties in an optimized manner.

Preliminary evaluation of alternative materials can be made by comparing Table 6 with Table 8. After identifying the most likely materials, an in-depth investigation of processing and tooling costs and assembly alternatives should be conducted before finalizing the design, process, and manufacturing scheme. In this context, manufacturing includes all postprocessing steps as well, including corrosion protection, joining techniques, and final appearance coating.

Table 6 Relative thickness, weight, and cost of materials used for automobile body panels

	Pure membrane resistance ($\alpha = 1, t^1$)			Oil-canning resistance ($\alpha = 2, t^2$)			Flat panel bending ($\alpha = 3, t^3$)		
Material	t	wt	Cost	t	wt	Cost	t	wt	Cost
Appearance SMC	1.0	1.0	1.0	1.0	1.0	1.0	1.0	1.0	1.0
Structural SMC	0.73	0.77	0.62	0.86	0.91	0.72	0.90	0.95	0.76
RRIM (flake glass)	6.8	4.5	6.0	2.6	1.7	2.3	1.9	1.3	1.8
Structural RRIM	0.94	0.78	0.78	0.97	0.81	0.81	0.98	0.82	0.82
Amorphous nylon	5.6	3.4	9.2	2.4	1.4	3.9	1.8	1.1	2.9
Nonappearance engineering thermoplastic	2.1	1.3	1.9	1.5	0.89	1.3	1.3	0.78	1.2
Glass-filled (30%) thermoplastic	1.7	1.3	3.0	1.3	1.0	2.3	1.2	0.92	2.1
Steel	0.06	0.25	0.12	0.24	1.0	0.51	0.38	1.7	0.82
Aluminum	0.17	0.22	0.49	0.41	0.62	1.3	0.55	0.83	1.6

Table 7 Properties and costs for materials listed in Table 6

	Modulus				Cost	
Material	MPa	ksi	Specific gravity	Specific modulus(a)	\$/lb	\$/kg
Appearance SMC	11.7	1.70	1.8	6.5	0.75	0.34
Structural SMC	15.9	2.31	1.9	8.4	0.60	0.27
RRIM	1.72	0.249	1.2	1.4	1.00	0.454
Structural RRIM	12.4	1.80	1.5	8.3	0.75	0.34
Amorphous nylon	2.07	0.300	1.1	1.9	2.00	0.907
Engineering thermoplastic	5.52	0.801	1.1	5.0	1.10	0.499
Glass-filled thermoplastic	6.90	1.00	1.4	4.9	1.70	0.771
Steel	207	30.0	7.8	26.5	0.38	0.17
Aluminum	69	10.0	2.7	25.6	1.44	0.653

(a) Modulus (in MPa) divided by specific gravity

State-of-the-Art and Developing Technologies

Composite-intensive automotive designs have been demonstrated with aerospace design principles as a basis, but have not been shown to be manufacturable for the automotive industry environment. A concentration by the automotive industry on high-volume processes, such as sheet-molded compound PMCs, has shown limited results. Three technologies under development for potential automotive applications are the P4 process, low-cost carbon fiber, and cyclic thermoplastic polymer systems. The P4 process is described earlier and shows the best potential for cost-effective manufacture of structural and optimized automotive PMC systems and components (Fig 6). Derivatives of this process have been implemented for the pick-up box of the General Motors Silverado and Sierra pick-up trucks and for structural systems on the Aston Martin Vanquish 2001 vehicle.

Designs Incorporating Composites. The ACC Partnership for a New Generation of Vehicles (PNGV) has also worked with MultiMatic to design and prototype a hybrid material automotive body that was based on the Chrysler Cirrus body in white. The goal of the project was to see if a vehicle could be designed to save 70% of the mass versus a traditional steel body. It uses woven glass, aramid, and carbon-fiber thermo-

Table 8 Typical stiffness parameter (α) values for automotive body panels

Panel	α
Floor pan	1.0
Rear compartment pan	2.5
Motor compartment front panel	3.0
Dash panel	3.0
Roof panel	2.0
Rear end panel	2.0
Quarter inner panel	3.0
Quarter outer panel	2.0
Trunk lid inner panel	1.0
Trunk lid outer panel	2.5
Front fenders	2.5
Hood assembly	2.5

set-matrix PMC that also achieves class "A" surfaces. Aluminum honeycomb sandwich composites were also used. Basic modeling techniques were used to determine proper composite laminate design for structural and crash safety requirements. (Fig 9). This vehicle was tested recently in a controlled standard crash test with reasonable results (Ref 7). This vehicle did not, however, meet the PNGV goals for high-volume manufacturability and lower cost.

Similarly, a composite vehicle that takes advantage of optimized design for braided and woven composites is the Solectria Sunrise electric vehicle (Fig. 10). The automobile is manufactured using stitched woven and braided composite fibers. The entire structure for the body and chassis consists of six separate sections and are assembled at a cost that may be comparable to those for high-volume manufacturing of traditional automotive structures.

Composite Fuel Storage Tanks. Another area that has received much attention is the fuel storage tank (Fig. 11). The automotive industry has implemented the use of natural gas-powered vehicles. Composite storage tanks have been shown to be advantageous as a lightweight and durable storage alternative to the more traditional tank storage media (Ref 9, 10). With the further development of hydrogen fuel-based powertrains, the need for hydrogen storage may increase in the future until fuel-cell technology is perfected.

Lower-Cost Carbon Fibers. The composite materials supply base has taken initiatives to produce good-quality carbon fiber at attractive prices, and this has become a catalyst for the automotive design community to further investigate its use. As stated earlier, the need for high stiffness in the automotive structure can be fulfilled by the use of carbon fiber.

Composite driveshafts have enjoyed limited success in the automotive market since the 1980s. In the past, these applications have been driven by the weight savings, natural frequency, and energy management opportunities this technology can provide.

Cost competitiveness with metal (steel, aluminum) and high-temperature performance have impeded broad market penetration. Cost is primarily driven by the cost of carbon fibers, although glass fiber has been used to dilute cost if the application requirements allow. Volume production of standardized low-modulus carbon fibers has had a significant impact on the cost reduction of a carbon composite materials system. Advancements in resin-matrix chemistry have provided much-improved high-temperature strength and stiffness without significant economic penalty.

Automotive OEMs have come under increased market and regulatory pressure to reduce weight and improve NVH characteristics. Many rear-wheel drive and all-wheel drive applications have been driven to two-piece metal driveshaft architectures for improved NVH and vehicle speed requirements. Composite driveshafts can meet many of these application requirements in a one-piece architecture.

There are several performance characteristics that an optimized composite driveshaft can provide. The weight savings and higher natural frequency (critical speed) capability of composite driveshaft technology have been well documented in the industry. The NVH response has generally been acceptable, due to the inherent superior damping qualities of the composite materials system. Design optimization may provide improved NVH response by also tuning the higher-order breathing modes through three-dimensional modeling. The stiffness-to-weight ratio allows smaller shaft diameters to meet application natural frequency requirements, providing increased package space to the OEM. Torsional stiffness may be tuned for drivetrain shock load management. Crush initiators and optimized bias plies may be used to attain an optimal energy management profile. Reduced rotating inertia reduces drivetrain losses in vehicle acceleration.

The reduced pricing of carbon fiber and the increased capability of modeling tools to optimize and enhance other performance characteristics of composite technology has motivated OEM and suppliers to reevaluate composite driveshaft technology. While many challenges remain in system drivetrain simulation and volume composite production methods, the cost-benefit ratio of composite driveshaft technology is stronger than ever.

Natural Fibers. An alternative and ecologically friendly fiber system that has seen use in secondary automotive interior structures is natural fiber. These fibers are found in common organic biological structures, such as flax, leaf, and seeds. These fibers have the advantage of low mass, renewability and recyclability, low cost, and good thermal and acoustic properties. The disadvantages include lower strength properties, variable quality, moisture absorption, limited processing temperatures, poor fire resistance, and variable prices (Ref 11). Much work is being performed with natural fibers that may result in further use for automotive applications.

Cyclic Thermoplastic Composites. Lastly, the development of cyclic thermoplastic polymer systems for the matrix of structural composites

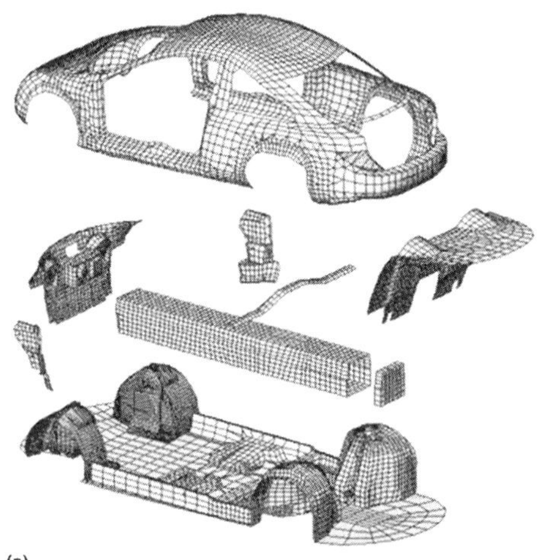

(a)

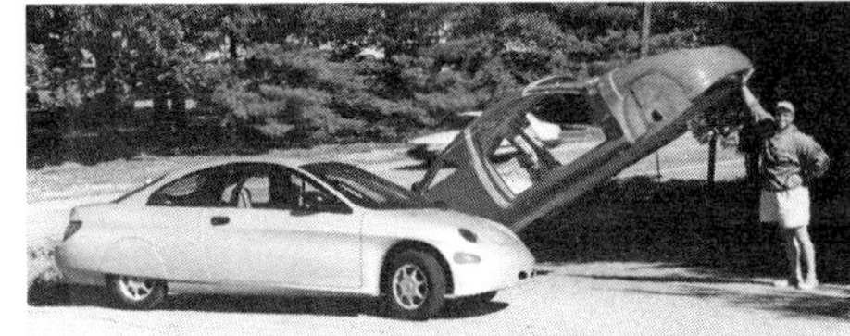

(b)

Fig. 10 Solectria Sunrise composite electric vehicle. (a) Assembly view. (b) View showing lightweight body. Source: Ref 8. Courtesy of V. Brachos, Solectria

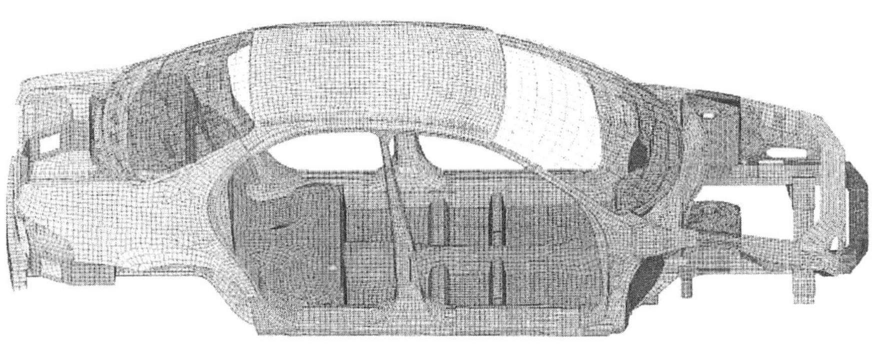

Fig. 9 MultiMatic PNGV hybrid material body in white finite-element model. Source: Ref 7

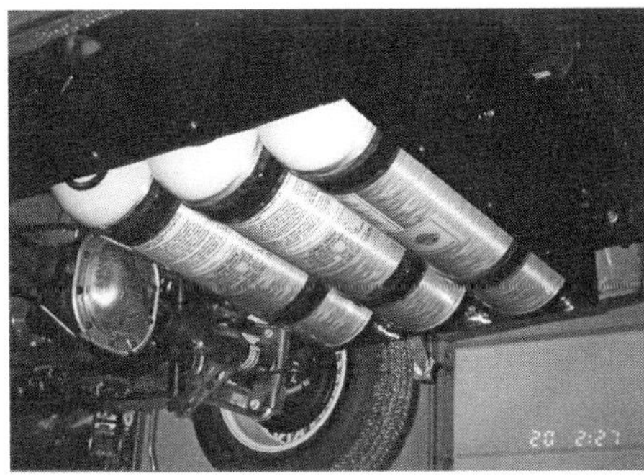

Fig. 11 Composite fuel storage tank. Reprinted by permission from the Society for the Advancement of Material and Process Engineering (SAMPE)

holds promise for high-volume production of automotive composite systems that are recyclable as well. This polymer system has the design and processability attributes of thermoset PMCs. This polymer also has the recyclability attributes of thermoplastic PMCs. Hence, one this polymer system is proven out for its properties for automotive applications, it holds the promise of low-cost structural PMCs that are closed-loop recyclable.

REFERENCES

1. *Automotive Composites: A Design and Manufacturing Guide,* Ray Publishing, Wheat Ridge, Colorado, 1997
2. D. Haygood, G. Lallas, and J.H. Porter, Technical Paper Series Report 960240, Society of Automotive Engineers, 1996
3. T.L. Gibson, Technical Paper Series Report 2000-01-1486, Society of Automotive Engineers, 2000
4. N.G. Chavka and J.S. Dahl, "P4 Preforming Technology: Development of a High Volume Manufacturing Method for Fiber Preforms," presented at the 13th Annual Engineering Society of Detroit Advanced Composites Conference and Exposition (Detroit), 1998
5. J.G. Argeropoulos, R.C. Fielding, and L.J. Oswald, Technical Paper Series Report 1999-01-3244, Society of Automotive Engineers, 1999
6. G.B. Chapman II, Technical Paper Series Report 1999-01-3222, Society of Automotive Engineers, 1999
7. J. Prsa, PNGV Hybrid Material Automotive Body Structure Development, Technical Paper Series Report 1999-01-3224, Society of Automotive Engineers, 1999
8. V. Brachos, G.A. Rossi, and W. Kirk, "Design of an All Composite Vehicle Platform–Solectria's Sunrise EV," presented at the 13th Annual Engineering Society of Detroit Advanced Composites Conference and Exposition (Detroit) 1998
9. J.B. Carrigan, L.W. Smith, N.J.H. Holroyd, et al., CNG Fuel Container Systems for Maximum Payload Space and Vehicle Range, *SAMPE J.,* Vol 36 (No. 6), 2000, p 26–33
10. J.-J. Koppert and A. Beukers, Full Composite Isotensoid Pressure Vessels or How Composites Can Compete with Steel, *SAMPE J.,* Vol 36 (No. 6), 2000, p 8–15
11. W.D. Brouwer, Natural Fibre Composites: Where Can Flax Compete with Glass? *SAMPE J.,* Vol 36 (No 6), 2000, p 18–23

Automotive Applications of Metal-Matrix Composites

Warren H. Hunt, Jr., Aluminum Consultants Group, Inc.
Daniel B. Miracle, Air Force Research Laboratory

METAL-MATRIX COMPOSITES (MMCs) have been used commercially in the automotive market for nearly 20 years. Properties of interest to the automotive engineer include increased specific stiffness, wear resistance, and improved high-cycle fatigue resistance (Ref 1). While weight savings is also important in automotive applications, the need for achieving performance improvements with much lower-cost premiums than tolerated by aerospace applications drives attention toward low-cost materials and processes. The raw material cost of cast iron or steel is less than $0.60/kg ($0.25/lb), and discontinuously reinforced aluminum (DRA) cast ingot currently costs about $3.30 to 4.40/kg ($1.50 to 2.00/lb) for large-scale production, so that the raw material cost of MMCs is higher than that of the material typically replaced. However, the DRA component would weigh 45% less than steel, significantly improving the cost comparison. Nevertheless, wider application of this technology will require performance improvements coupled with novel or innovative process improvements to drastically lower overall cost.

There has been successful application in several automotive applications in which the combination of properties and cost satisfied a particular need. As a result of these successful applications, the 1999 total world market of MMCs for ground transportation (automotive and rail) amounted to 1566 metric tonnes, valued at over $7 million (Ref 2). Some of these applications are described subsequently, emphasizing the innovations that have led to MMC insertion and the system-level benefits that have been obtained.

Engine Applications

Pistons. The piston is subjected to a severe dynamic thermal and mechanical environment. It must support cyclic mechanical loads at frequencies approaching 100 Hz, so excellent fatigue response is a primary requirement. The piston must also maintain a tight tolerance with the cylinder to retain maximum combustion pressure and withstand ring groove pounding. Dynamic strength, excellent wear resistance and a coefficient of thermal expansion (CTE) that matches the cylinder are the desired attributes. The temperature can be as high as 300 °C (570 °F) on the piston dome, so high-temperature properties are important. Finally, thermal gradients and thermal cycling are present, so that a high thermal conductivity is desired to reduce overall temperature and thermal stresses. Prior to 1983, a cast iron insert was often used for the piston top plate and ring groove area for direct-injection diesel engines (Ref 3).

A watershed application for aluminum MMC was the Toyota Motor Manufacturing piston for diesel engines (Ref 4). These pistons were placed into commercial production in Japan in 1983. The part consists of selective reinforcement of the aluminum alloy by a chopped fiber preform in the ring groove area, to provide improved wear and thermal fatigue resistance. The porous ceramic preform is placed in a permanent die mold, and complete infiltration by the molten metal matrix is accomplished by rapid pressurization. This squeeze casting process provides a high-quality component with low cost and very high production rates, as high as 100,000 per month (Ref 3).

The selectively reinforced piston provides significant improvement in wear resistance. As important, the low CTE has allowed redesign of the piston, using tighter tolerances and resulting in higher pressure and improved heat transfer properties (Ref 2). The lower reciprocating mass also adds to improved performance. Finally, the squeeze casting process, which integrates the reinforced top plate and ring groove material with the casting in a single step, resulted in an overall cost reduction compared to the previous design. Thus, although the aluminum MMC is more expensive on a raw material per unit mass basis, the selective reinforcement and simplified process result in a cost reduction at the component level. The performance improvements are added benefits in the use of the MMC.

To date, the selectively reinforced MMC piston has not been strongly considered in the U.S. market, because diesel engines in North America tend to be larger and operate at lower rotational speeds (rotations per minute, or rpm). As a result, the wear and fatigue requirements are not as stringent, and so the benefits are not as compelling. Nonetheless, MMC pistons provide a strong advantage in Asian and Western European designs, and continued growth is expected in this area. For example, Mazda Ford Motor Company introduced a selectively reinforced piston produced by a low-pressure die casting process in 1998 (Ref 2).

Other piston applications have included the use of SiC particulate- and whisker-reinforced aluminum forgings in racing applications. Due to the lower CTE of the MMC, reduced clearances between the piston and cylinder wall are possible. In some cases, an order of magnitude reduction in the specified clearance is possible (Ref 2). Based on trials of MMC pistons in drag racing bikes, improved performance compared to conventional hypereutectic aluminum-silicon alloys can result (Ref. 5).

Cylinder Liners. Widespread use of aluminum engine blocks has led to the need for protective cylinder liners for many of the same reasons discussed previously for pistons. Historically, the first and still the most widespread approach has been to use cast iron inserts as a result of the successful performance of cast iron engine blocks. Good wear resistance has been the primary consideration, even though the cast iron has a high density and relatively poor thermal conductivity.

Aluminum MMC cylinder liners have been in mass production since 1990 in the Honda Prelude 2.3 liter engine (Ref 6). In this case, hybrid preforms consisting of carbon and alumina (Al_2O_3) fibers are infiltrated by molten aluminum to form the cylinder liners during the medium-pressure squeeze casting process for the engine block. This innovative process eliminates the need for separate cast liners to be placed into a die cast machine or pressed into a pre-machined engine block. This reduces the number of parts previously required, and eliminates the assembly step that was required to place the cast iron liners into the engine block. This engine is shown in Fig. 1.

The wear resistance of the aluminum MMC is better than that of cast iron. The overall weight reduction of the aluminum engine block is 20% with the MMC inserts (Ref 3)—a dramatic improvement. In addition, the aluminum MMC has a higher thermal conductivity, so that the operating temperature is lower, thus further extending the life of the engine. Finally, the MMC liner is thinner than the previous cast iron, so that an increase in engine displacement has been achieved without redesign of the engine. Over 300,000 of these engines have now been produced. In addition to the Honda Prelude, MMC cylinder liners are now used in the Honda S2000 sports car, a premium version of the Acura NSX, and in the Porsche Boxter engine (Ref 2). The engine for the 2000 Toyota Celica also incorporates MMC piston liners, and 25,000 units were produced in the first model year. Finally, an aluminum MMC cylinder liner is used in high performance Honda motorcycles, using a powder metallurgy (P/M) process (Ref 3).

Valves. Intake and exhaust valves coordinate the transportation of the air-fuel mixture for combustion and the exhaust gases in automotive engines. Both intake and exhaust valves are subjected to cyclic mechanical loading at frequencies as high as 50 Hz, so fatigue properties are of primary importance. The valves must also possess good resistance to sliding wear in the valve guide. The exhaust valve operates in gas temperatures as high as 900 °C (1650 °F), so good creep resistance is required at the neck, where the maximum stress occurs. The atmosphere of exhaust gases changes, depending on acceleration, but the average gas composition is oxidizing, so that the exhaust valve material must have good oxidation resistance. Finally, the valve is subjected to high-frequency hammering forces, and good resistance to galling adhesion on the valve seat is required. Automotive valves are typically produced from austenitic steel. While the cost is low, these parts have relatively high mass. In addition, high spring forces are required to maintain continuous contact between the valve lifter (follower) and the camshaft lobe at higher rpm, so that a higher spring mass is required. This higher spring force increases frictional forces on the cam, the tensile stress at the neck, and the contact forces with the cylinder head. Finally, the energy required to compress the springs is lost to the cycle and decreases the overall fuel efficiency.

Discontinuously reinforced titanium (DRTi) MMCs have been used as automotive valves since 1998 in the Toyota Altezza 2.0 liter L-4 engine (Ref 7). The DRTi is made by a P/M process using low-cost titanium hydride powder, powders of the appropriate master alloys, and TiB_2 (Ref 8). The powders are mixed in an attritor, then metal-die pressed and sintered. The sintering step provides homogenization, densification, and allows the TiB_2 to react and form the stable titanium monoboride (TiB) reinforcements. Sintered billets can be processed into valves by an intermediate extrusion step followed by upset forging. The matrix alloys for intake valves is Ti-6Al-4V, and for exhaust valves is Ti-6.5Al-4.6Sn-4.6Zr-1Nb-1Mo-0.3Si (Ref 7, 8). Rigorous certification testing included endurance testing at 10,500 rpm (87 Hz).

Since the introduction of the Altezza, over 500,000 DRTi valves have been produced, representing a mass of about 13 metric tonnes. No defective units have been reported. A set of 16 DRTi valves weighs 408 g (14 oz), relative to 677 g (24 oz) for a full steel valveset, for a direct weight savings of 269 g (10 oz) per engine (Ref 7). In addition, the valve spring mass has been reduced by 7 g (0.2 oz) each, so that the total engine weight reduction is 381 g (13 oz). In addition to the reduced mass, the cam contact frictional forces and the energy required to compress the springs are reduced. The cost of the DRTi valves is currently about twice as high as for steel, due to the relatively low volume of production. However, the cost has been projected to be comparable to steel for full-scale production. Yamaha Motor Corporation, an affiliate company of Toyota Motor Manufacturing, announced that DRTi valves will be used in two of their motorcycles introduced in 2001. An annual production volume of 500,000 units is expected. Figure 2 shows an intake and exhaust valveset used in the Toyota Altezza.

Pushrods. Cylindrical pushrods translate motion from the cam to the valve train in overhead valve (OHV) engines. A typical 8-cylinder OHV engine has 16 ultrahigh-strength steel pushrods. It is vital that the pushrod faithfully reproduces the desired motion from the cam to the valves. Limiting behavior at high engine rpm includes pushrod flexure, "valve toss" or "lofting" caused by loss of contact past the nose of the cam, "valve bounce" associated with lofting, and vibrations induced throughout the valve train caused by exciting a natural frequency of the pushrods. Flexure, lofting, and valve bounce limit engine performance, and excessive vibrations severely limit the lifetime of valvetrain components, especially springs. A high pushrod stiffness is required to control bending, a low mass is needed to reduce lofting, and good damping is essential to limiting vibration.

A fiber-reinforced aluminum MMC is now used in pushrods for high-performance OHV racing engines. The 3M Corporation produces the material by infiltrating 60% of Nextel 610 Al_2O_3 fibers with an aluminum matrix. Hollow pushrods of several diameters are made, where the fibers are axially aligned along the pushrod length. Hardened steel end caps are bonded to the ends of the MMC tubes. The aluminum MMC pushrods provide 25% higher bending stiffness and twice the damping capacity relative to 4340 steel pushrods (Ref 9). The MMC density is less than half that of steel, so that engine speed can be increased by an average of 250 to 400 rpm before valve bounce begins. In addition, it has been projected that the use of aluminum MMC pushrods could provide an extension in spring life of up to 600% as a result of the improved damping characteristics of the MMC (Ref 9). Because valvetrain springsets are generally a significant expense, this benefit provides a value far in excess of the initial acquisition cost. Further benefits of the 3M Corporation MMC pushrods may be achieved through optimization of cam design.

Connecting Rods. Other drivetrain components, and particularly the connecting rod, have been a focus of development (Ref 5). By reducing the mass of the connecting rod/piston assembly, the objectionable secondary shaking forces that can develop, particularly in smaller engines, can be reduced. In addition, lower reciprocating loads should lead to lower loads on the crankshaft and lower friction losses, and increased fuel

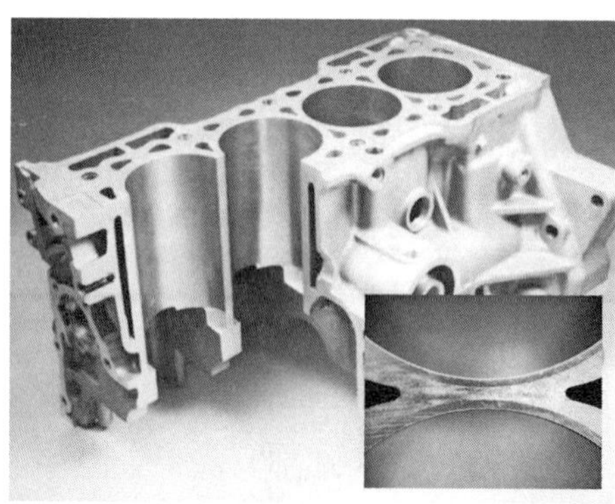

Fig. 1 Engine with integrally cast aluminum MMC cylinder liners

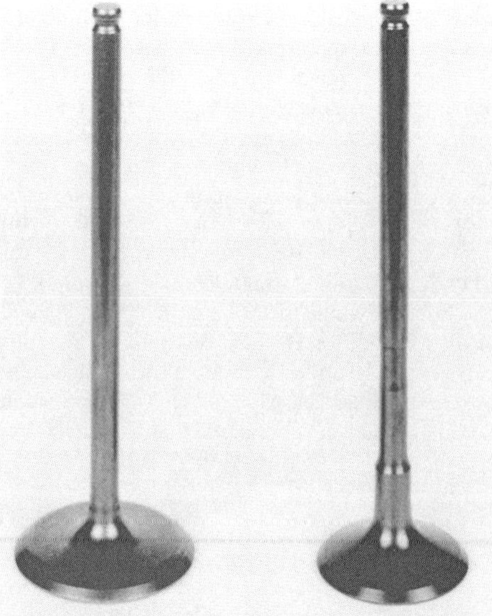

Fig. 2 Discontinuously reinforced titanium (DRTi) automotive valves for the Toyota Altezza. The valve on the left is an intake valve, and on the right is an exhaust valve. Courtesy of Toyota Central Research and Development Laboratories

economy or performance can be realized (Ref 1). In fact, it has been stated that for every 1 kg (2 lb) of weight removed from the connecting rods, 7 kg (15 lb) of weight required by steel connecting rods for support and counterbalance can be removed (Ref 2).

Commercial applications of MMC connecting rods in high-volume vehicles have not yet been achieved, largely because of the difficulty in obtaining a material with the necessary high cycle fatigue performance and low-cost combination. While prototype connecting rods from hot-forged aluminum MMC have successfully been produced and tested, further cost reduction is required. A prototype connecting rod is shown in Fig. 3.

Brake System Applications

Aluminum-based MMCs offer a very useful combination of properties for brake system applications in replacement of cast iron. Specifically, the wear resistance and high thermal conductivity of aluminum MMCs enable substitution in disk brake rotors and brake drums, with an attendant weight savings on the order of 50 to 60%. Because the weight reduction is unsprung, it also reduces inertial forces, providing an additional benefit in fuel economy. In addition, lightweight MMC rotors provide increased acceleration and reduced braking distance. It is reported that, based on brake dynamometer testing, MMC rotors reduce brake noise and wear, and have more uniform friction over the entire testing sequence compared to cast iron rotors (Ref 1).

Metal-matrix composite brake rotors and drums are typically produced by casting processes such as semipermanent gravity casting. Aluminum-magnesium and aluminum-silicon-matrix alloys and both SiC and Al_2O_3 particle reinforcements have been used, typically of at least 20% by volume. A number of automobiles now use MMC brake components. The Lotus Elise used four DRA brake rotors per vehicle from 1996 to 1998, and the specialty Plymouth Prowler has used DRA in the rear wheels since production started in 1997. Discontinuously reinforced aluminum rotors are particularly attractive in lightweight automobiles and are featured in the Volkswagen Lupo 3L and the Audi A2. In addition, a number of electric and hybrid vehicles, such as the Toyota RAV4, Ford Prodigy, and the General Motors Precept, are reported to use MMC brake components (Ref 2). Figure 4 shows a selection of DRA brake rotors.

Discontinuously reinforced aluminum brake rotors are now being used on the InterCity Express (ICE), the German high-speed trains. Metal-matrix composite brake discs are now used on the ICE-1 and ICE-2, representing over 100 trainsets. Application of aluminum MMC in automotive racing applications, where higher-priced material is acceptable for improved performance, has been reported. Brake calipers for Formula 1 racecars produced from a 2124/SiC/25p MMC provide less displacement, more leverage, and quicker stops, due to the increased material stiffness (Ref 10). Metal-matrix composites are also reportedly being used as brake pads in conjunction with the Porsche 911 ceramic-matrix composite brake rotors.

Driveshaft Applications

Use of aluminum MMCs in the driveshaft takes advantage of the increased specific stiffness obtained in these materials. Current driveshafts, whether aluminum or steel, are constrained by the speed at which the shaft becomes dynamically unstable. The critical speed of the driveshaft is a function of the length, inner and outer radius, and specific stiffness. In vehicles with packaging constraints that do not allow increased driveshaft diameter, MMCs offer a desirable solution. Use of MMCs enables longer driveshaft lengths at a given diameter, or smaller diameter shafts at a given length. This is important in trucks and large passenger vehicles, where a two-piece driveshaft is sometimes used because of length restrictions. Substitution of a two-piece aluminum or steel driveshaft with a single-piece DRA driveshaft provides a direct weight savings, eliminates the weight and cost associated with the center support structure for the two-piece driveshaft, and reduces the mass required for corrective counterweights and balancing. As much as 9 kg (20 lb) can be saved (Ref 2).

As a result of these benefits, driveshafts comprised of 6061/Al_2O_3 materials produced by stir casting and subsequent extrusion into tube have been applied. In 1996, DRA driveshafts were introduced in the Chevrolet S-10 and GMC Sonomo pickup trucks. The following year, DRA driveshafts became standard equipment on the Chevrolet Corvette. An MMC driveshaft is now also used in the Ford "Police Interceptor" version of the Crown Victoria. Figure 5 shows the driveshaft used in the Chevrolet Corvette.

Other Applications

Metal-matrix composites, specifically those based on aluminum matrices, are candidates for application in brake calipers, pump housings, gears, valves, brackets, pulleys, turbocharger and supercharger compressors, and suspension components (Ref 1). In addition, they have been cited for clutch parts, suspension pushrods and rock-

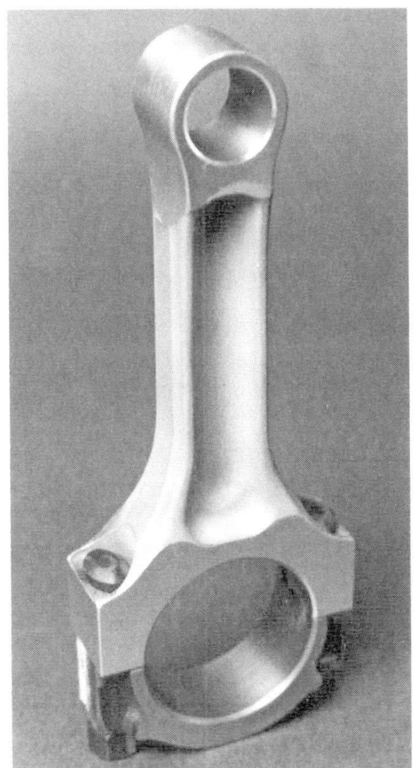

Fig. 3 Prototype aluminum MMC connecting rod

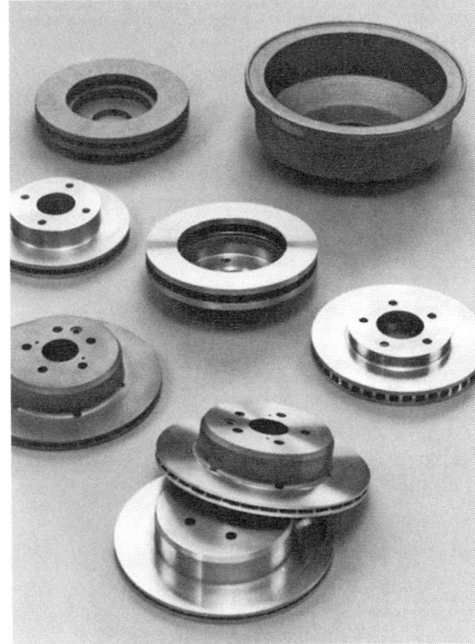

Fig. 4 Aluminum MMC brake rotors

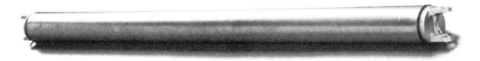

Fig. 5 Aluminum MMC driveshaft

ers, as well as other gearbox and engine parts (Ref 10). Discontinuously reinforced titanium is also under consideration for some of these components.

Snow tire studs have been manufactured from 6061/Al_2O_3 drawn wire. In Finland, where steel tire stud jackets have been outlawed and unreinforced aluminum has insufficient wear resistance, the MMC tire stud jackets have been successfully applied since the mid-1990s (Ref 11), and represent an annual market of about 150 metric tonnes (Ref 2).

Conclusions

A growing market has been established for MMCs in the automotive industry. Important applications have resulted when performance and weight benefits overcome the added component cost. Performance benefits have been obtained from reduced weight, improved wear resistance, low coefficient of thermal expansion, and good thermal properties. However, high volume process and material innovations are needed before MMCs are widely applied to the automobile across all product offerings. Continued pressure in the ground transportation industry for lower weight to improve environmental emissons and fuel efficiency is expected to generate growth in the existing application areas, as well as new opportunities for MMCs.

REFERENCES

1. J.E. Allison and G.S. Cole, *JOM*, Vol 45, 1993, p 19–24
2. M.N. Rittner, in "Metal Matrix Composites in the 21st Century: Markets and Opportunities," Report GB-108R, Business Communications Co., Inc., Norwalk, CT, 2000
3. V.M. Kevorkijan, *JOM*, Vol 51 (No. 11), 1999, p 54–58
4. T. Donomoto et al., SAE Paper 830252, Society of Automotive Engineers, 1983
5. W.C. Harrigan, in *Handbook of Metallic Composites,* S. Ochiai, Ed., Marcel Dekker, Inc., New York, 1994, p 759–773
6. K. Hamajima, A. Tanaka, and T. Suganama, *JSAE*, Vol 11, 1990, p 80–84
7. F.H. Froes and R.H. Jones, *Light Met. Age*, Vol 57 (No 1, 2), 1999, p 117–121
8. T. Saito, *Adv. Perform. Mater.*, Vol 2, 1995, p 121–144
9. G. Mendelson, *Trackside*, Vol 7 (No. 23), 1996, p 82–88
10. S. Hurley, *MBM*, 1995, p 54–55
11. A.I. Nussbaum, *Light Met. Age*, Vol 55 (No. 1, 2), 1997

Space Applications

Suraj P. Rawal, Lockheed Martin Astronautics
John W. Goodman, Material Technologies, Inc.

TYPICAL SPACE STRUCTURES require high stiffness, low coefficient of thermal expansion, and dimensional stability during the operational lifetime. High-performance composites do satisfy these requirements, and also offer the minimum weight material solution for space applications. Composites have been used in space applications almost from the start of the space program in the 1950s. Building upon the first successful use of composite for solid-fuel rocket motor cases in the 1950s, composites have been continually developed for the aircraft, launch vehicles, missiles, and spacecraft structures.

Elastic response, strength, failure mode, and damage tolerance characteristics of fiber-reinforced laminated composites are quite different from metals. More specifically, polymer-matrix composites are also different from metals in terms of the sensitivity to temperature, moisture, and the space environment. Recognizing these differences, specific design methods, materials, manufacturing processes, and test techniques are used for composite structures. In the last two decades, significant advances have been made in the areas of fibers, matrix materials, design and analysis methods, and composite manufacturing technology. As a result, composite materials have been increasingly used for both structural and nonstructural applications on spacecraft (Ref 1–15). These applications include truss structure, equipment-panel structure, optical benches, radiators, solar array support structures, antenna reflectors, antenna masts, electronic enclosures, and engine shields. In space launch vehicles and missiles, composites have been increasingly used for rocket motor cases, nozzles, payload fairings, payload support structures, igniters, and the interstage structures.

This article is primarily directed to address composites for unmanned space vehicles. More specifically, a brief overview of the key design drivers, challenges, and environment for use of composites in spacecraft, launch vehicles, and missiles is presented here.

Design Drivers and Challenges

The primary design drivers with respect to selecting composites for space applications typically are reduced weight, reduced part count and structural complexity, improved structural/thermal performance (e.g., specific strength and stiffness, dimensional stability, high thermal conductivity), and potentially lower cost than conventional metallic materials.

When using composites for space applications, major challenges are in the areas of design allowables, cost of manufacturing and test, and perceived risk. For example, there is ongoing need to perform materials characterization testing due to a lack of applicable industry data with respect to mechanical properties of materials, impact resistance, and damage protection. Usually, recurring process control verification testing is expensive. Driven by cost, schedule, and risk-avoidance guidelines, some program managers may not evaluate composites for use despite their benefits in terms of mass/cost savings and significant improvements in performance. While composites do provide the improved performance because of high stiffness, dimensional stability, and low density, they complicate several system-level design issues. These issues include grounding, shielding, handling damage, shelf life, variability in raw materials properties, environmental interactions, adaptability to post-build design modifications, nondestructive inspection, full-scale test requirements, fracture control, compatible interfaces and attachments, and so on. To address these issues, there is a critical need for interactions among designers, analysts, and materials scientists with extensive composite experience.

Environments

Spacecraft are subjected to various environments during fabrication, transportation, handling, testing, and service life. Design of most structures in a spacecraft is driven by environment on earth, during launch, and in space. In each program, a structural environment definition document is prepared, including specific values of the structural design environment. Key spacecraft environments include transient/steady state, vibration (random and sine), acoustic, pyroshock, pressure, thermal, handling, and transport. In addition, structural design may be affected by other environmental considerations, such as salt-fog, humidity, ambient temperature, and space environment.

The space environment (Ref 14–21) includes naturally occurring phenomena such as atomic oxygen (AO), very low-density atmosphere (near vacuum), ionizing radiation, plasma, charged-particle plasma, neutral atomic and molecular particles, micrometeoroids, and man-made debris. Vacuum describing the low pressure in space varies significantly with altitude, being about 10^{-15} torr (1.3×10^{-13} Pa) for geosynchronous spacecraft, compared to atmospheric pressure of 760 torr (101, 325 Pa, exact) at sea level. When exposed to space vacuum, including temperatures experienced, polymer-based composites release substances in the form of gas. This outgassing can lead to two potentially undesirable effects: degradation of key mechanical properties and condensation of gasses on critical surfaces of lenses, mirrors, and sensors, which influences optical performance (Ref 8, 16, 19, 20).

Design Processes and Trade-Offs

While composites do offer significant performance improvements, one of the key drivers for the use of composites on spacecraft has always been the payoff in terms of reduced mass and, consequently, reduced launch cost. An industry-accepted figure for satellite payload mass savings varies from $20,000 to 100,000 per kilogram (kg). According to these figures, a 25 kg savings in mass reflects a projected cost reduction of at least $500,000. Lack of attention to spacecraft weight might result in a payload too heavy to be boosted into orbit by the launch vehicle originally scheduled for the spacecraft. This would be a calamity in virtually any program. Not only would the use of a larger vehicle cost substantially more due to the increase in unplanned expense, but such vehicles are most often difficult to schedule. Delay in the launch date in turn extends the cost of the development period. For a scientific payload, delay may eliminate the usefulness of the payload altogether. For a government utility satellite such as a weather monitor, the functional loss would be noticeable and embarrassing to the government, and costly to the public relying on accurate prediction of weather patterns.

Reduction in structural mass can also be converted into obtaining greater functionality by using upgraded instruments or electronic components for longer life, higher reliability, or additional capability. Even very late in the program, a weight savings in one area can be used to store additional fuel or compressed gas for longer life with attitude control on orbit.

Design, Analysis, and Tests for Composites. Any design process begins with the mission/system/subsystem requirements as they are reduced to structural design criteria, such as weight, launch acceleration, and minimum acceptable natural vibration frequency. Stiffness and stability constraints are imposed on the structure to minimize distortion and maintain alignment and stability for payload sensors during operational environment. Primary strength and stiffness of the composites are in-plane, and the composite parts are designed, exploiting the anisotropy features and tailorability of materials to satisfy the specific requirements. Basic considerations of fabrication and producibility aspects of composites are also included in the design of each part. Accessibility of components and subsystems is very important, and therefore a modular approach is followed when possible. Scientific instruments must have obstruction-free view angles. Instruments, like magnetometers, may have to be isolated from the satellite with long booms. Some subsystems need quantitatively specified surface areas, while others need 4π steradians of solid-angle field of view. This may necessitate using deployable appendages, such as booms, panels, antennas, and so on. The structure must be electrically conductive to act as a common ground plane for all equipment. The thermal loads typically involve temperatures in the range from –157 to 121 °C (–250 to 250 °F). The structure must provide a minimum mass heat path for the dissipation of excess thermal energy in order to remove all the heat generated inside the spacecraft. For construction and support of optical and antenna components, the acceptable limits on thermal distortion are specified. For unique components, design of the manufacturing tools and fixtures may be a key part of the process. Structural analyses are generally similar to aircraft practice also, but with a stronger reliance on vibration analysis to predict natural frequencies. Additional special analyses include thermal cycling associated with the periodic passage through the earth shadow in orbit, and thermoelastic calculation of the displacements of optical supports.

Structural testing usually does not include building a full-scale structural model for destructive testing; instead, full-scale articles are tested with limited loads and eventually prepared for launch. Subscale or partial components known as "pathfinders" are fabricated and tested to validate new designs and new fabrication procedures. For a typical value, low-production (one to three of a kind) spacecraft, coupons of scraps/edges cut from production parts are tested routinely to ensure that the materials properties are consistent with the design values. In the large production programs, critical design, production, inspection, and tests are established in the first 4 to 6 units, thus minimizing the testing of subsequent units. Additional information is provided in the articles "Element and Subcomponent Testing" and "Full-Scale Structural Testing" in this Volume.

Materials and Process Trade-Offs. Materials trade-off studies at the beginning of the design phase often involve a design iteration process to arrive at alternative concepts incorporating material capable of meeting design requirements. Trade-off study parameters include structural configurations, materials (fibers and resin matrices), manufacturing methods, and joining and assembly processes. An accurate and reliable database is needed to obtain a legitimate comparison of materials; typical materials properties used for materials trades can be obtained from the materials manufacturer. Figure 1 shows a typical trade-off study to identify the composite material and attachment methodology for hardware and bus structure. For example, a miniature spacecraft bus (primary support structure) could be a truss structure or a skin frame structure. Usually, if a monocoque structure has to be fabricated, then the selected fiber should exhibit ease of handling and adequate strain to failure. There are several options for an epoxy or cyanate-ester matrix system. A cyanate matrix with a desired cure temperature of 121 or 177 °C (250 or 350 °F) is often used, because it exhibits good microcracking resistance and low outgassing characteristics compared to conventional epoxies. Figure 1 also includes the design criteria for each parameter, thus providing a basis for down-selection of specific composite design. Based on this preliminary evaluation, M55J/cyanate-ester composite is an optimal materials option to satisfy performance requirements and provide a cost-effective honeycomb panel structure for a specific application.

Lamination theory is often used to predict laminate properties for use in materials selection and the fiber orientation required to meet performance requirements. In general, the fiber directions are oriented parallel to the major loading directions of the component. For components that are stiffness or coefficient of thermal expansion (CTE) driven, the fiber orientation and stacking sequence of each lamina are selected to achieve composite laminates that meet specific stiffness and dimensional stability requirements. Several lay-up or materials combinations may meet the required performance parameters; selection of the final lay-up and materials combinations finally depends on variables such as cost, availability, fabrication experience, available database, and risk toleration.

If high-heat load components are mounted on the bus walls or deck panels, then the composite facesheet material should have high-conductivity fibers. The high-conductivity composite substrates help to spread heat efficiently, thus keeping the components within acceptable temperature limits.

Joining and assembly of composite hardware is accomplished by adhesive bonding and mechanical fastening methods. The lack of a plastic region in the material stress-strain response makes a joint in a composite part less tolerant of misalignment, fabrication tolerances, and damage from flaws or fatigue than similar joints in metallic materials. Proper consideration of critical composite joints includes basic understanding of load transfer function and detailed analysis that is complemented by elemental and component tests. In general, bonded joints are most suitable for thin members, and mechanical fasteners are used for thicker members. Bonded joints are designed such that the residual stress is minimized at the bond line and adhesive is stressed in the direction of shear, the direction of its maximum strength. Bonded joints are readily used in dimensionally stable composite structures. In recent years, the use of bonded joining techniques, such as mortise and tenon and corner blocks, has increased significantly. Mechanically fastened joints require no surface preparation and offer ease of inspection and disassembly, compared to bonded joints. Mechanically fastened joints are designed so that bearing is the critical failure mode. Typical quasi-isotropic composite laminate provides optimal bearing strength.

Fabrication and Acceptance of Composite Components for Spacecraft. Spacecraft laminates are usually thin, and most components are, in fact, sandwich structures with composite facesheets. Some sandwich panels consist of precured facesheets adhesively bonded to the aluminum honeycomb core. The "cocured" sandwich, in which the facesheet and the adhesive are cured simultaneously, is becoming common. The cure temperature varies from 121 to 177 °C (250 to 350 °F), depending on the laminating resin and adhesive selected. The pressure during cure is typically 207 kPa (30 psi), rather than the 689 kPa (100 psi) employed for solid laminates.

A general principle of manufacturing composite components holds that costs are reduced by reducing the number of individual operations and the number of individual parts. Cocuring of large components achieves such savings. Other methods to reduce fabrication cost include processing resin-transfer-molded composite shapes, which superficially resemble the metal extrusions in aircraft. Such parts can be processed for significantly less cost than the cost of hand lay-up of complex shapes. Some bolted joints must be provided to permit separation (or rework and repair) during assembly and test to permit equipment installation. Composite fasteners are becoming available but are not yet widespread.

Typical design verification testing of composite components for spacecraft includes the following four types of tests: (a) development, (b) qualification, (c) protoflight, and (d) acceptance. Development tests are conducted as necessary (on simulated components) to provide engineering design and test information to validate analytical techniques, evaluate optimal designs, and test procedures. Qualification tests are performed to provide verification that the flight-quality component, subsystem, or an entire vehicle has met its full performance/design requirements. Test levels and duration normally exceed the expected flight limits to ensure that the specified design safety margins are available. Often, prototype hardware, a nonflight hardware, is built to flight hardware requirements and then subjected to qualification-level test environments. In the protoflight-level tests, the test article (flight hardware) is subjected to the qualification environment-reduced (acceptance) duration. Protoflight testing of the first flight unit qualifies the flight hardware so that subsequent flight hardware need undergo acceptance-level testing only. Acceptance tests are conducted primarily to detect latent material and workmanship defects by performing tests at levels equal to or greater than the limit levels predicted for flight.

Composite Materials Properties

Design allowable properties are the numerical values of mechanical and physical properties used in structural analysis for preliminary design and subsequent design verification. These properties are generally based on tests of unidirectional [0], simple cross-plied $[0/90]_s$, or quasi-isotropic $[0/+45°/-45°/90°]_s$ laminates. In contrast, aircraft and automotive industries generate design allowables by testing a statistically significant number of specimens of every laminate lay-up and local structural configuration. Design allowable properties for actual spacecraft laminates, however, are implicitly calculated by anisotropic computer laminate analysis programs for stiffness and failure criteria for strength in the prescribed stress state. With so many potential combinations of fibers and lay-ups, it is impractical and cost-prohibitive to test the hundreds of specimens to rigorously establish A-basis allowables for all spacecraft composites. More specifically, MIL-HDBK-17 recommends that five prepreg batches of the composite material need to be tested so that materials properties data can be included in the handbook. Based on this recommendation, thirty tests per data point (six tests per batch) provide the basis to determine the B-basis properties.

Tests for both the physical and mechanical properties of cured lamina are performed in accordance with the American Society for Testing and Materials (ASTM) recommended test methods. Physical property tests include density, fiber, volume, resin volume, ply thickness, and glass transition temperature. The mechanical property tests include 0° and 90° tension, 0° and 90° compression, and in-plane shear tests. Short beam shear tests are required for determining process control test minimum values. Most often, a limited number (average ten) of coupon specimens are tested to generate a limited database, and small sample statistical analysis is employed to estimate minimum design allowables for strength and average values for stiffness and other parameters. The designers use structural allowables that are a combination of vendor and test data, with appropriate knockdown factor, if needed.

Manufacturers of composite structures for spacecraft generate materials property databases, often proprietary, on composite materials. The MIL-HDBK-17 committee on spacecraft composites has documented the available data from open literature, vendors, and spacecraft manufacturers. For preliminary design use, typical property data are available for nearly all spacecraft composite materials from the fiber and prepreg manufacturers. Typical fibers used in the spacecraft composite structures include a variety of fibers, such as S-glass, high silica, quartz, aramid, boron, and carbon. Carbon fibers are dominant for spacecraft bus structure, including, in the manufacturer's nomenclature, T300, M46J, M55J, XN50, M60J, P75, XN70, P120, K13C2U, and K1100. While a significant amount of test data is available in MIL-HDBK-17 and other sources, Tables 1 to 3 list the typical properties (Ref 22–26) of different carbon-fiber-reinforced organic-matrix composites used in spacecraft applications. Tables 1 to 3 include the test data of unidirectional carbon-fiber/cyanate-resin laminates, carbon-fiber/epoxy-resin laminates, and high-thermal conductivity carbon-fiber laminates.

Effect of the Space Environment on Composite Materials. Many materials used on

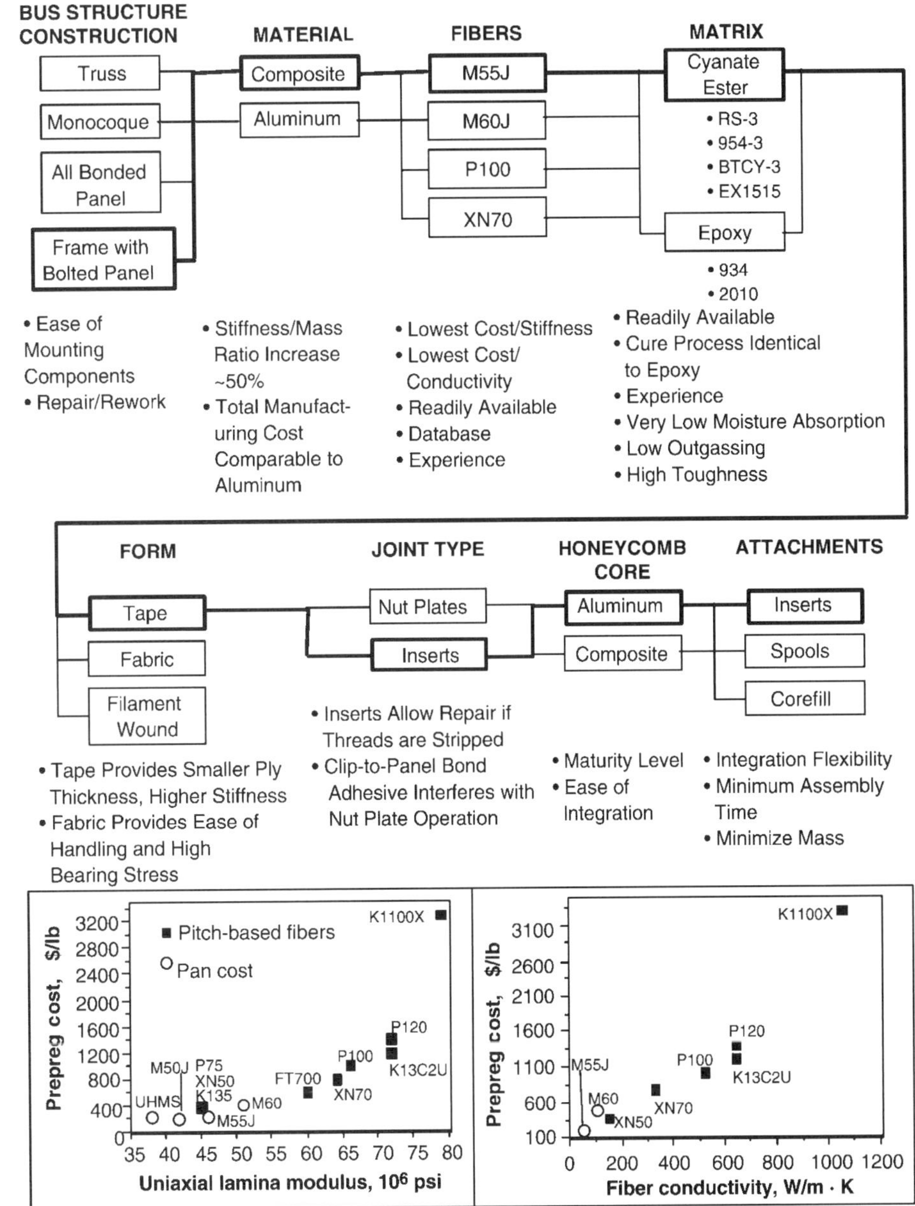

Fig. 1 Example of a design trade-off study used to select optimal composite materials and processes

spacecraft surfaces are susceptible to attack by nascent atomic oxygen (AO), a major atmospheric constituent in the low earth orbit (LEO) region (Ref 16–19, 26). The harsh environment of LEO includes not only AO erosion, but also solar ultraviolet radiation, temperature cycling in orbit, vacuum, condensates of volatile organic substances evaporated from spacecraft surfaces, micrometeoroid and man-made debris impacts, and high-energy radiation. The combined effects of the space environment can lead to serious deterioration of mechanical, optical, and thermal properties of some material surfaces. Optical properties (solar absorptivity and thermal emissivity) may change due to AO bleaching or ultraviolet (UV) radiation darkening. Polymeric films may peel due to thermal cycling. In turn, this opens new surfaces that can be attacked by AO or AO and UV. The electrical conductivity of a material may be affected by AO, resulting in spacecraft charging. The strength and stiffness of composite structures may degrade due to AO erosion of resin binders, although the strength is rarely needed after reaching orbit and completing deployment. However, degradation of stiffness of an optical bench or main support structure for a typical optical system will compromise system performance. Temperature cycling, as experienced by any orbiting system, must be controlled or compensated to maintain optical alignment. Based on the testing of composite specimens exposed to LEO environment, there is very limited degradation in the fiber-dominated properties. Also, the measured CTE values exhibit no substantial degradation other than that associated with outgassing. Careful selection of materials can ensure satisfactory performance over the design life of the system. Absolute protection from AO erosion is not realistic, but specific spacecraft are provided with AO protection optimized for the planned mission life, plus an operating margin to allow for variations in orbital conditions or for reasonable mission extensions. Spacecraft operating for short periods in LEO and spacecraft bound for high orbits or interplanetary trajectories require far less AO protection than spacecraft designed to operate for several years at intermediate Earth orbits. Geostationary, deep-space, and planetary spacecraft structures do not require AO protection, because the oxygen population in those environments is negligible.

State-of-the-Art Applications

General discussion of specific applications of composites is often limited by the information available in the open literature. Tables 4 and 5 provide brief lists of composite applications in spacecraft and rocket-motor cases, respectively. In each of the structural and non-structural applications, composites do offer unique performance characteristics and the ability to realize weight savings. The following sections describe the specific state-of-the-art applications of composite materials for spacecraft missiles and launch vehicles.

Spacecraft Applications

A spacecraft consists of a "payload," which is the mission-specific equipment, and a "bus" structure, which includes components of different subsystems. Table 6 lists the spacecraft subsystems, functions, and its major components.

The bus is the body of the spacecraft that attaches to the expendable booster vehicle at an interface, including a separation device. The bus, as the primary structure, is the major load path between the spacecraft components and the launch vehicle. Electrical, optical, and other instruments are mounted within the bus. While primary structure is loaded mainly by steady state and transient loads, secondary and tertiary structures are loaded mainly by vibroacoustic loads. Secondary structures, such as antennas and solar arrays, are folded up and stowed during launch and deployed from the bus after orbit is reached. The electronic boxes and brackets that support cables are tertiary structures.

Antennas may be parabolic shells or more (electrically and geometrically) complex components. Solar arrays include interconnected solar cells on composite sandwich panels, or sometimes planar frames supporting membranes that in turn support the solar cells. The propulsion system on some spacecraft has included carbon-carbon composite nozzle/exit cone parts. Carbon-fiber wrapping of high-pressure gas storage tanks is becoming more and more the norm. The bus also provides attachment points that allow handling of spacecraft during assembly, testing, transportation, and launch.

Minimum weight is achieved with composites if the (compressive) strength-to-density ratio and the modulus-to-density ratio are tailored for spe-

Table 1 Properties of a carbon/cyanate ester unidirectional laminate

Property	UHMS	M55J	M60J	XN70
Design strength (typical)				
Ultimate longitudinal tensile strength, MPa (ksi)	1171 (170)	1826 (265)	1723 (250)	1550 (225)
Ultimate longitudinal compressive strength, MPa (ksi)	689 (100)	758 (110)	655 (95)	275 (40)
Elastic properties (typical)				
Longitudinal tensile modulus, GPa (10^6 psi)	234 (34)	296 (43)	330 (48)	400 (58)
Transverse tensile modulus, GPa (10^6 psi)	8.3 (1.2)	6.9 (1.0)	6.9 (1.0)	6.9 (1.0)
In-plane shear modulus, GPa (10^6 psi)	4.1 (0.6)	4.1 (0.6)	4.1 (0.6)	4.1 (0.6)
Longitudinal Poisson's ratio	0.27	0.25	0.28	0.3
Physical constants (typical)				
Density, g/cm^3	1.6714	1.6988	1.6988	1.781
Coefficient of thermal expansion, 10^{-6}/°C				
Longitudinal	−0.22	−0.22	−0.22	−0.33
Transverse	8.89	8.89	8.89	8.89
Thermal conductivity (longitudinal), W/m · K	51.9	69.2	86.5	155.7

Fiber volume percentage (V_f), 60%

Table 2 Typical properties of different composite laminates used in spacecraft applications

Property	P75/1962 graphite/epoxy $[\pm 30/0_4]_s$	P75/1962 graphite/expoxy $[0/\pm 45/90]_s$	IM7/epoxy $[\pm 30/0_4]_s$	IM7/epoxy $[0/\pm 45/90]_s$	AS4/3501-5 [0/90]
Density, g/cm^3	1.73	1.73	1.58	1.58	0.058
Modulus of elasticity (E), GPa (10^6 psi)					
Longitudinal (E_x)	225 (33)	105 (15)	125 (18)	50.3 (7.3)	58.6 (8.5)
Transverse (E_y)	12.3 (1.8)	105 (15)	11.3 (1.6)	53.1 (7.7)	58.6 (8.5)
Poisson's ratio	1.21	0.31	1.02	0.291	. . .
Ultimate tensile strength (F_{tu}), MPa (ksi)					
Longitudinal (F_{tux})	589 (85)	308 (45)	2050 (297)	896 (130)	600 (87)
Transverse (F_{tuy})	30.3 (4.4)	345 (50)	101 (15)	929 (135)	600 (87)
Ultimate compressive (crushing) strength (F_{cu}), MPa (ksi)					
Longitudinal (F_{cux})	374 (54)	183 (27)	880 (128)	467 (68)	758 (110)
Transversel (F_{cuy})	122 (18)	190 (28)	159 (23)	338 (49)	758 (110)
Shear strength (F_{su}), MPa (ksi)	44.0 (6.4)	34.7 (5.0)	250 (36)	312 (45)	. . .
Thermal conductivity (k) at room temperature, W/m · K					
Longitudinal (k_x)	83	44	5	3	. . .
Transverse (k_y)	8	44	1.2	3	. . .
Through thickness k_z	1.5	1.5	0.6	0.6	. . .
Coefficient of thermal expansion (α) at room temperature, 10^{-6}/K					
Longitudinal (α_x)	−1.02	−0.454	−0.62	1.37	. . .
Transverse (α_y)	5.83	−0.14	12.56	1.16	. . .
Reference	22	22	22	22	23

Fiber volume fraction (V_f), 62%

cific applications. Composites with the highest stiffness currently available contain carbon/graphite fibers derived from pitch, with elastic modulus about 900 GPa (130 × 10^6 psi). For components that require moderate strength to withstand the launch acceleration and vibration, slightly lower modulus fibers, about 500 GPa (73 × 10^6 psi), are appropriate. For small clips and brackets, stiffness properties are not critical, and lower modulus carbon fibers about 225 GPa (33 × 10^6 psi) in fabric form are sufficient. Fibers with very high thermal conductivity, which are also very stiff and exhibit relatively low compressive strength and low strain to failure, are used in both structural and nonstructural thermal management applications. Glass and aramid fibers are rarely used on spacecraft, but quartz fibers are sometimes employed for their dielectric properties.

The structural components of spacecraft are in the forms of trusses, platforms, pressure vessels, and shells. A brief description of the key applications, such as spacecraft bus module, optical bench, solar array, and reflector structure, is presented here.

Spacecraft Bus Module. Composites provide low mass, high stiffness, and thermal stability for the spacecraft bus modules. The platform structures use the two most common forms of construction: sandwich construction and isogrid. Both of these constructions offer high stiffness and high buckling strength relative to their mass. A sandwich structure consists of two thin facesheets separated by and adhesively bonded to a lightweight aluminum honeycomb core. Most often, the facesheets are composite laminates with quasi-isotropic lay-up (e.g., $[0/\pm45/90]_s$ or $[0/\pm60]_s$). The facesheets carry the axial loads, bending moments, and in-plane shear loads acting on the panel, and the core carries out-of-plane flexure shear loads. Bus modules using panel structure have been used in several spacecraft, including Mars Global Surveyor (Fig. 2). Composite grid (including isogrid) stiffened structures have also been fabricated using a mortise-and-tenon-based flat laminate fabrication technology (Fig. 3). Using simple molded tubes, angles, and cylinders, the composite bus structures would ideally be designed such that the bonds are not in the load paths. Lay-ups are tailored to increase the structure stiffness without adding weight. While most spacecraft bus structure panels are fabricated using graphite/epoxy or graphite/cyanate composite, carbon-carbon (C-C) composite has also been used to fabricate

Table 3 Candidate thermal-structural polymer-matrix composites

Material	Tensile strength (0°) MPa	Tensile strength (0°) ksi	Tensile modulus (0°) GPa	Tensile modulus (0°) 10^6 psi	In-plane shear strength MPa	In-plane shear strength ksi	Compressive strength (0°) MPa	Compressive strength (0°) ksi	Compressive modulus (0°) GPa	Compressive modulus (0°) 10^6 psi
P100XHT/EX515	1798	261	469	68	. . .	. . .	379	55	517	75
XN70/RS3	1667	242	427	62	48	7	331	48	420	61
P120/934	958	139	475	69	41	6	276	40	441	64
K13C2U/EX1515	2005	291	48	7	41	6	386	56	524	76
XN80/RS3	1488	216	441	64	. . .	. . .	227	33	482	70
K1100X/1939-3	1461	212	558	81	34	5	248	36	565	82

Material	Compressive strength (90°) MPa	Compressive strength (90°) ksi	Compressive modulus (90°) GPa	Compressive modulus (90°) 10^6 psi	Coefficient of thermal expansion (longitudinal), 10^{-6}/K	Thermal conductivity, W/m · K	Density, g/cm^3
P100XHT/EX515	96	14	5.5	0.8	−0.7	. . .	1.8
XN70/RS3	. . .	. . .	. . .	. . .	. . .	. . .	1.8
P120/934	103	15	4.8	0.7	−0.7	380	1.8
K13C2u/EX1515	145	21	5.5	0.8	−0.7	366	1.8
XN80/RS3	. . .	. . .	. . .	. . .	−1.4	. . .	1.8
K1100X/1939-3	. . .	. . .	. . .	. . .	−1.2	540	1.9

90° is in-plane perpendicular to the 0° unidirectional fiber. Source: Ref 23

Table 4 Application of advanced composites on spacecraft

Spacecraft (S/C)	Launch year	Composite hardware
Intelsat IV (10 S/C)	1971–1979	Hybrid boron and fiberglass-epoxy aluminum foil waveguide; carbon-epoxy (C-epoxy) stiffeners on supporting structure for Earth coverage horn antennas
Apollo (3 S/C)	1971–1972	Boron-epoxy lunar surface drill
Anik B 1, 2, 3	1972, 1973, 1974	C-epoxy mesh grid offset parabolic antenna reflector
Explorer 49	1973	Boron-epoxy booms
ATS-6 (F/G)	1974	C-epoxy antenna feeds support truss
SATCOM	1974–1975	Aramid/epoxy antenna reflector assemblies
HEAO 2	1978	C-epoxy x-ray telescope optical bench
FLTSATCOM 1–7	1978–1986	C-epoxy tubular boom for helical receiver antenna deployment; aramid ground plane support
Intelsat V (8 S/C)	1980–1985	Aramid/epoxy and GY-70/epoxy on Nomex H/C for 4 and 6 GHz reflectors; 51 and 25 mm (2.0 and 1.0 in.) diam GY-70/epoxy tube truss for antenna feed structure; copper-coated T300/epoxy waveguides; T300/epoxy feed arrays (copper clad); P75/epoxy Al honeycomb solar panel; T300/epoxy solar array yoke
TDRSS 1-8	1980s–1990s	2 m (8 ft) length carbon/epoxy antenna ribs (18 tapered tubes (41–25 mm, or 1.6–1.0 in.); quartz fiber/epoxy radome; 1.9 m (6.5 ft) diam carbon/epoxy-aluminum honeycomb ground link antenna; aramid/epoxy substrate for the antenna; C-epoxy tubes for solar array frame
Hubble space telescope	1990	Carbon/aluminum high-gain antenna mast; 4.8 m (16 ft) carbon/epoxy metering truss structure; C-epoxy truss tube focal plane array; C-epoxy optical bench for camera assembly
Milstar LDR for flights 1, 2	1994	Spot beam antennas: • GY-70/epoxy with Al H/C reflectors (990 and 635 mm, or 39 and 25 in. diam) • GY-70 epoxy with Al H/C feed support tower • GY-70 epoxy with Al H/C upper platform UHF antenna: T300/epoxy tubular boom Agile beam antenna: • Aramid/epoxy with Al H/C lens support structure • T300/epoxy corner fittings
Intelsat VII (4 S/C)	1994–1995	Numerous composite parts, including K1100/PC; central cylinder; solar array substrates; carbon/PC thrust tube
AXAF "Chandra"	1999	M55J/PC with Al H/C solar array substrates; M60J/PC for optical bench and ISIM module
Mars mission spacecraft and Stardust	1996–1999	M55J/PC for bus structure; carbon-carbon for engine shield; low-modulus carbon-carbon thermal doublers; K13C2U/PC for battery support and radiator

H/C, honeycomb; PC, polycyanate

Table 5 Rocket motor cases manufactured with filament-wound composites since the 1950s

Missile category	Solid rocket motor name	Missile stage application	Composite fiber
Space launch vehicles	Altair	4	Glass
	Antares	3	Glass
	BE-3	(Various)	Glass
	S/SRM-1	(Various)	Aramid
	S/SRM-2	(Various)	Aramid
	Space shuttle FWC	1	Graphite
Strategic	Polaris A-2	2	Glass
	Minuteman	3	Glass
	Polaris A-3	1, 2	Glass
	Poseidon	1, 2	Aramid
	Trident 1	1, 2, 3	Aramid
	Peacekeeper	1, 2, 3	Aramid
	Trident 2	1, 2, 3	Graphite
Defense	Sprint	1, 2	Glass
Tactical	Viper	1	Glass
	ADATS	1	Glass
	ASW/SOW	1	Aramid
	Pershing	1, 2	Aramid
	Hypervelocity missile	1	Graphite

Source: Ref 3

some structural panels for high-temperature applications. A flat C-C composite panel, using aluminum honeycomb core, provided higher stiffness and thermal conductivity than a baseline aluminum panel. This C-C panel was successfully flown as a structural radiator on an operational spacecraft (Ref 27).

Truss structures usually consist of an assemblage of tubes. The tubes are designed to have high axial and bending stiffness and low CTE. Tube-to-end fitting (generally titanium) joints are designed to withstand thermal stresses caused by temperature cycling, and also to provide stiffness compatibility to minimize the stresses caused by any imposed loads. The application technology satellite was one of the first satellites (in 1974) to use composite truss structure that provided 50% weight savings over a similar metallic design.

Small spacecraft bus structures (octagon or hexagon shapes) usually have separation interfaces with launch vehicles that also provide the main supports for the bus structures. It is desirable to have load paths directly connected to the supports, such as the corners of the bus frame. The frames are assembled from pieces that are cut from quasi-isotropic flat laminates. Frames and panels may be fabricated in parallel and then integrated together using simple assembly fixtures.

Conventional aluminum structures inherently satisfy other system-level concerns, such as grounding and shielding requirements of the spacecraft bus module, but for composite laminates, a thin aluminum or copper foil is co-cured with the laminates to satisfy electron-magnetic interference shielding requirements. If needed, nickel powder is added to the adhesive to meet the electrical conductivity requirement. Furthermore, to minimize thermal stresses at the composite/metallic fitting interface, titanium is usually used for fittings due to its low CTE, low density, and high strength.

Optical benches are structural platforms with mounting interfaces for the attachment of optics, telescopes, interferometers, and other precision instruments. Key requirements for optical bench structures are high stiffness, thermal and mechanical stability, high strength, and light weight. Critical design considerations for an optical bench are near-zero CTE and coefficient of moisture expansion (CME) for the final assembly (Ref 28–30). Sandwich panels and trusses are conventionally employed. High- or ultrahigh-modulus graphite fibers impregnated with epoxy or cyanate-ester resin are normally used to fabricate the laminates or tubes. In a quasi-isotropic laminate configuration with a 60% fiber volume fraction, these materials systems can offer: a near-zero CTE ($\sim 0.0 \pm 0.1$ ppm/°C), a low coefficient of moisture expansion (80–160 ppm/%M), an in-plane tensile modulus of up to 147 GPa (21×10^6 psi), tensile strength as high as 450 MPa (65 ksi), and densities of approximately 1.7 g/cm^3. For example, the optical bench structure for the Hubble space telescope (Fig. 4)

Table 6 Spacecraft systems

Subsystem	Functions	Key components
Attitude control subsystem	Determines and controls the spacecraft's attitude (orientation) and orbital position	Sensors for determination; actuators for control (components that introduce forces or moments)
Propulsion subsystem	Changes the spacecraft's orbit	Propellant, storage tanks, pipes, and thrusters
Communications subsystems	Communicates directly or indirectly with ground control personnel and enables spacecraft tracking	Receiver, transmitter, and antenna
Command and data handling subsystem	Processes and distributes commands; stores, encrypts, and decrypts data	Data recorder and computer
Electrical power subsystem	Generates, stores, regulates, and distributes electrical power	Solar arrays, batteries, electronics, and cables
Thermal control subsystem	Monitors and controls temperatures	Heaters, radiators, heat pipes, louvers, insulation, and coatings
Structures and mechanisms subsystem	Physically supports spacecraft components, moves them as necessary, and protects them from dynamic loading	Primary, secondary, and tertiary structures; mechanisms

Subsystem makeup varies from one spacecraft to the next. Some spacecraft may not need all of these subsystems. Source: Ref. 8

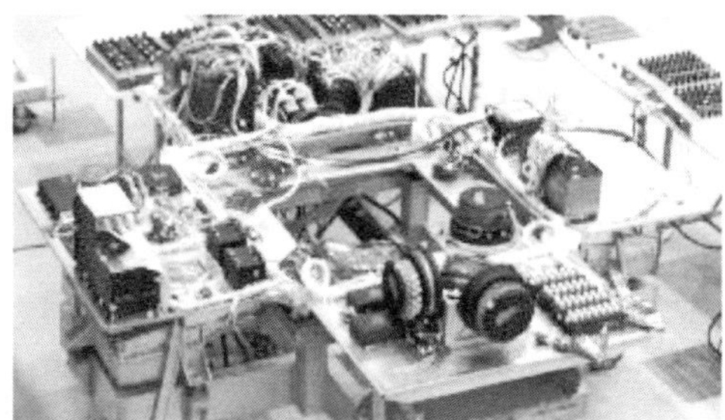

(a)

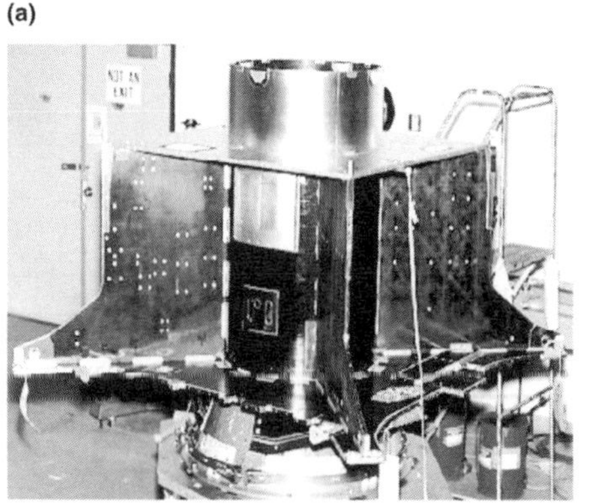

(b)

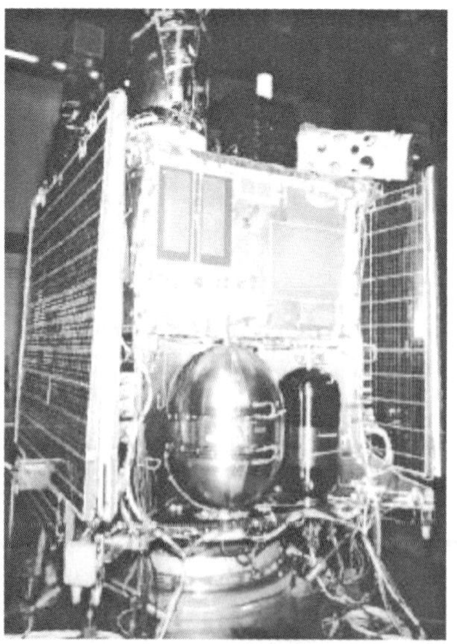

(c)

Fig. 2 Mars Global Surveyor. (a) The equipment module with M55J/CE panels in the unfolded state. After the subsystems were tested, it was folded up into a box placed on top of the propulsion module. (b) A view of the composite propulsion module with the hydrazine tank (left) and the helium pressurant tank (right). (c) The nearly complete spacecraft with solar array panels

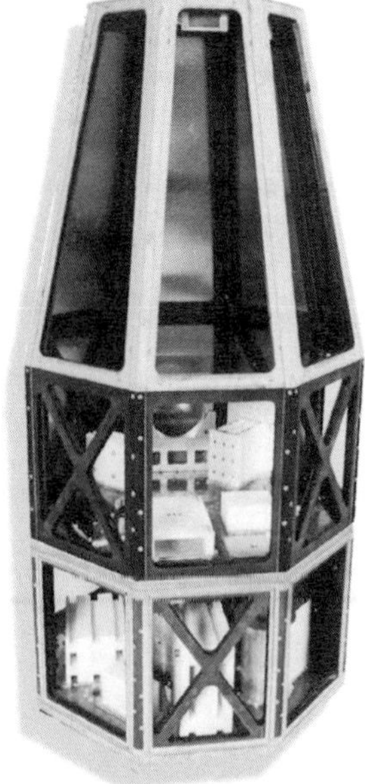

Fig. 3 Composite grid structure for the fast orbit-recording transient events spacecraft. Courtesy of Composite Optics Inc./Los Alamos National Laboratory

satisfies the CTE requirement of 0.0 ± 0.1 ppm/°C. Figure 5 shows a composite truss-type optical bench structure, consisting of tubes with plates and a thick honeycomb sandwich panel. Optical benches have also been designed with facesheets and internal egg-crated ribs. Ribs are made from thin laminates and slotted half-height to allow crossing through. The slots cause change of CTE from one side of the rib to the other; counter slots sometimes are required to balance the CTE. Ribs may also have tabs to engage with the slots in the facesheets. This configuration can include mortise-and-tenon joints in which the bond line is in shear and therefore able to take higher load than a tensile bond. Average bond-line thickness needs to be uniform, because inconsistent thickness may cause unpredictable thermal distortions due to varying CTE. Most fittings used in optical bench assemblies are Invar, possessing both low CTE and high modulus.

Solar arrays are usually categorized as rigid or flexible structures. Flexible arrays demonstrate their best performance advantages for large applications and unique launch envelope requirements. The rigid solar arrays are predominately used in the small-to-medium size applications and even into the large applications. The state-of-the-art rigid solar array substrate (SAS) that supports the solar cell population is a relatively large panel that is required to be flat, lightweight, thermally conductive through the panel, electrically nonconductive in-plane at the cell interface, and structurally capable of surviving launch conditions.

The rigid SAS is manufactured from the smallest sizes up to approximately 4 × 3 m (13 × 10 ft). Overall panel flatness usually is maintained at 1 mm/m (0.01 in./ft), but can be tightened up to approximately 30 to 50% of that value if required. The state-of-the-art SAS is a honeycomb sandwich construction with discrete hinge and/or snubber attachment fittings around the perimeter, and shear tie fittings nested in the interior of the panel. Usually, aluminum honeycomb core is used because of cost and thermal conductivity considerations. Often, the reticulated adhesive film (which cures at 122 or 177 °C, or 250 or 350 °F) is used to bond the skin to the core. Local doublers are incorporated in high shear areas and as strongbacks to maintain overall panel stiffness and local skin strength. These doublers can be embedded within the panel skins or bonded to the panel skin exterior.

Candidate materials for rigid SAS panels can be aluminum, aramid (unidirectional tape or woven fabric), high-modulus graphite/epoxy or cyanate ester (350 to 525 GPa, or 50 to 75 × 10^6 psi, unidirectional tape), ultrahigh-modulus graphite/epoxy or cyanate ester (560 to 910 GPa, or 80 to 130 × 10^6 psi, unidirectional tape), or conductive K1100 graphite/epoxy or cyanate ester unidirectional tape. Hybrid combinations of these materials for skins and doublers are common. Composite skins offer 30 to 40% mass savings and ease of bonding surface preparation compared to the aluminum skins. Because the composite-graphite fibers in the skins are electrically conductive in-plane, the panel skins are insulated from the solar cell population by using a nonconductive film, such as aramid/epoxy skin, which can be co-cured with the composite skin or secondarily bonded.

Reflectors. Two common reflector designs include composite honeycomb sandwich and isogrid structure. Most reflectors with a surface accuracy requirement of 0.100 mm (0.004 in.) root mean square (rms) or greater are honeycomb sandwich designs. The isogrid ribbed design requires more labor than the sandwich design, but it has been fabricated to satisfy the requirements of a few micron RMS surface roughness. Composite materials used to manufacture some reflectors are aramid and graphite/cyanate ester. These materials offer high stiffness-to-weight ratio and nearly zero CTE. Figure 6 shows an antenna reflector assembly, consisting of a 1 m (3 ft) dish fabricated by using advanced co-cured sandwich structure. However, laminates and sandwiches made from these materials have high CTE through the thickness and high CME. Determination of the CTE and CME is very crucial in order to predict and control the surface accuracy during manufacturing as well as on orbit.

In addition to reflector and solar array support structures, polymer-matrix composites have been used to fabricate attachment fittings, avionics boxes/enclosures, thermal planes (i.e., heat sinks for circuit cards), thermal doublers (i.e., heat sinks under high-heat-generating components), radiator fins, and antenna elements (including waveguides, feed horns, and integrated feed towers).

Metal-Matrix Composite Parts. While polymer-matrix composites have been used for most of the primary and secondary structure applications, there have been a few applications where metal-matrix composites and C-C composites have also been successfully used. The space shuttle is one of the first production applications of metal-matrix composites. Unidirectional boron-aluminum structural tubular struts have been used as the frame and rib truss members in the midfuselage section and as the landing gear drag link of the space shuttle orbiter. The 242 boron-aluminum tubes construction weighing 150 kg (330 lb) resulted in nearly 44% weight savings over baseline aluminum extrusions design. Driven by the high stiffness and low CTE requirements, diffusion-bonded graphite-fiber-reinforced aluminum composite has been used as the high-gain antenna boom for the Hubble space telescope. The structure is 3–6 m (10–20 ft) long, with internal dimensional tolerances of 0 ± 0.15 mm (0 ± 0.006 in.) along the entire length so that the tube can act as a wave guide.

Carbon-Carbon Composite Parts. Carbon-carbon composites have also been used in spacecraft applications for both structural (e.g., radiator [Ref 25]) and nonstructural (e.g., engine shield, thermal planes, and thermal doublers [Ref 29]) applications. For example, if the ther-

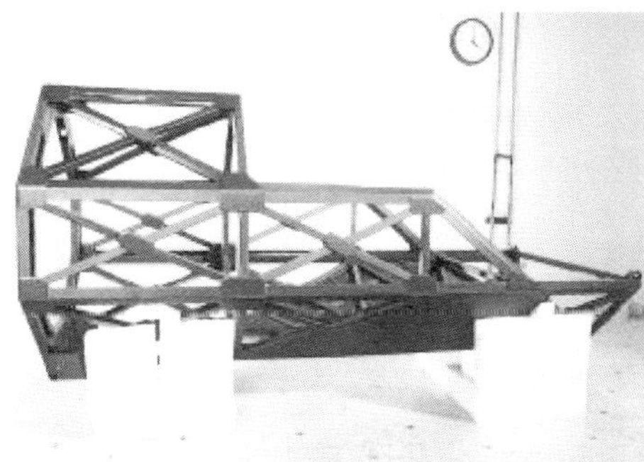

Fig. 4 Dimensionally stable optical bench for the near-infrared camera and multi-object spectrometer on the Hubble space telescope. Courtesy of NASA/Ball Aerospace/Alliant Techsystems

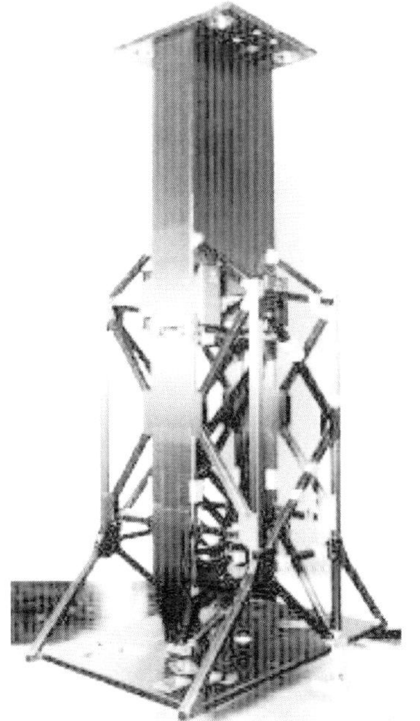

Fig. 5 Thermally stable bench for the far-ultraviolet spectroscopic Explorer spacecraft. Courtesy of NASA/Swales/Alliant Techsystems

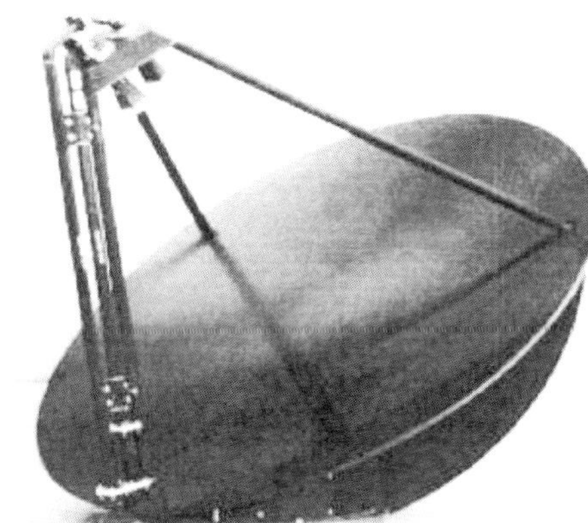

Fig. 6 Antenna assembly for the Seawinds spacecraft. Courtesy of Composite Optics, Inc./JPL

mal management needs of the electronic box necessitates the use of a thermal doubler, then the spacecraft designer needs a composite material that has high thermal conductivity, low CTE (equivalent to the facesheet), and low elastic modulus (compared to the facesheet). Conventional aluminum thermal doublers do not satisfy these requirements, because the combination of its high CTE and stiffness nearly equivalent to the facesheet could induce structural damage in the composite facesheet. A low-modulus two-dimensional and three-dimensional C-C for thermal doublers for composite structures provides the best combination of low density, low elastic modulus, low CTE, and high thermal conductivity (K). More specifically, a two-dimensional C-C doubler, processed at high graphitization temperatures, exhibits in-plane thermal conductivity of 130 to 160 W/m · K, and through-the-thickness conductivity of ≈40 W/m · K, whereas a three-dimensional C-C thermal doubler, heat treated at high temperature, exhibits in-plane conductivity ≥200 W/m · K, and through-the-thickness conductivity of 170 W/m · K, nearly equivalent to the thermal properties of an aluminum thermal doubler at lower weight.

Space Launch Vehicle and Missile Applications

Composites are used in a large number of space launch vehicle and missile components, such as rocket motor cases, nozzles, control surfaces, aerodynamic fairings, and launch canisters. Since the early days of lunar missions, filament-wound composite tanks have been used for the storage of fuels and pressurized gases on launch vehicle upper stages and satellites. A brief description of key applications, including solid rocket motor casings, payload fairings, and payload support (adapter) structures, is presented subsequently.

Solid Rocket Motors. Space motor components must be highly reliable and lightweight structures. Building upon the early successful use of composites for Altair, Antares, and BE-3 motor cases (in the 1950s) for the Vanguard and Scout launch vehicle programs, composites have been used in solid rocket motors of nearly all expendable launch vehicles. In the solid-propellant-type motor, fuel burns inside the case, generating moderately high pressures, which are contained by the large case wall. Composites with high tensile strength and low density offer an excellent materials solution. These families of expendable launch vehicles include Delta, Titan IV, Pegasus, and Ariane, each designed with capability to launch payloads of different weights to the desired altitude. For example, Delta II comprises a large family of expendable rockets that can be configured as two- or three-stage vehicles, depending on mission needs. The first stage of Delta II is powered by Boeing Rocketdyne-built RS-27A main engine, and by solid rocket strap-on graphite/epoxy motors (GEMs) (Fig. 7) for added boost during lift-off. The use of solid rocket motor upgrade system provided 25% increased performance and heavier lift capability than the boosters of the previous design of Titan IV launch vehicles. In particular, Titan IV-B rocket motor cases use high-strength IM7 fiber and durable HBRF-55B epoxy-resin composites. These cases are filament wound and produced by state-of-the-art automation, robotics, and process controls.

Filament-wound solid rocket motor casings have been extensively used in almost all missile systems, including strategic ballistic and defensive missile systems. For example, three filament-wound composite motor cases form the primary structure of the Trident I solid propellant missile system. These cases use Kevlar-49 (DuPont) aramid-fiber/epoxy composite in the pressure vessel section of the case and standard-modulus carbon-fiber/epoxy composite in the highly loaded, integrally wound thrust skirts. The Trident II (D5) missile is a three-stage, solid propellant missile that makes extensive use of composite structures. Major composite components of the missile include first-, second-, and third-stage rocket motors, igniters, the interstage structure, and equipment section. For example, the first-stage motor structure consists of a 2.1 m (6.9 ft) diameter by 7.3 m (24.0 ft) long standard-modulus carbon/epoxy filament-wound motor case (Fig. 8) with integral forward and aft skirts, aluminum attach rings, and aluminum port adapters that are integrally wound into the dome sections of the composite case.

Payload Fairings and Adapters. The payload fairings constitute a critical element of payload accommodation, because they protect the spacecraft/payload during the launch and ascent phases of flight. With respect to payload fairings, composite structures, and adapters, the current state-of-the-art is exemplified by the products being used by the European Space Agency and on the Atlas V program. For example, Arian 5 and Atlas V launch vehicles typically use 5.4 m (17.7 ft) diameter composite payload fairings. The payload fairings are constructed using vented aluminum honeycomb core co-cured to self-adhesive graphite/epoxy facesheets and cork thermal protection. They are fabricated in sections using hand lay-up of the facesheets. The Delta II and Delta III use 3 and 4 m (10 and 13 ft) diameter composite fairings, respectively, that separate into halves in flight to permit payload deployment. These composite fairing designs also incorporate acoustic blankets to protect payloads from noise and vibration at lift-off. In addition to honeycomb sandwich structures, composite payload shrouds have also been constructed using an advanced grid-stiffened (AGS) structure, a rib-skin configuration. A conical AGS shroud fabricated by Air Force Research Laboratory, New Mexico, was successfully flown in 1997. Advanced grid-stiffened

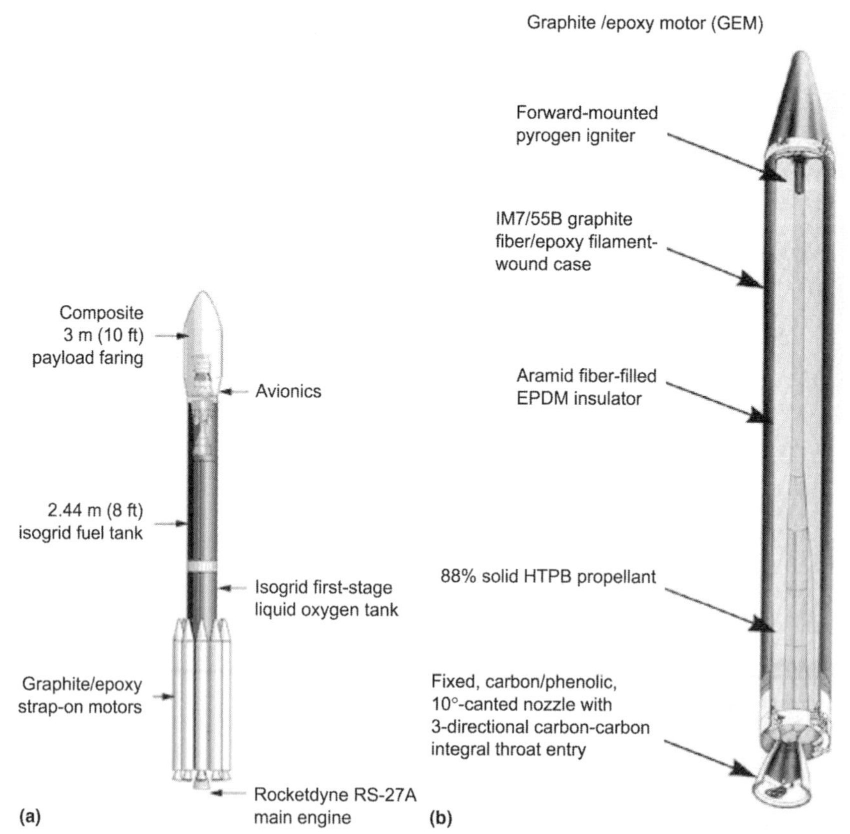

Fig. 7 Delta II launch vehicle. (a) View showing solid rocket strap-on graphite/epoxy motors (GEMS). (b) 3 m (10 ft) composite payload fairing

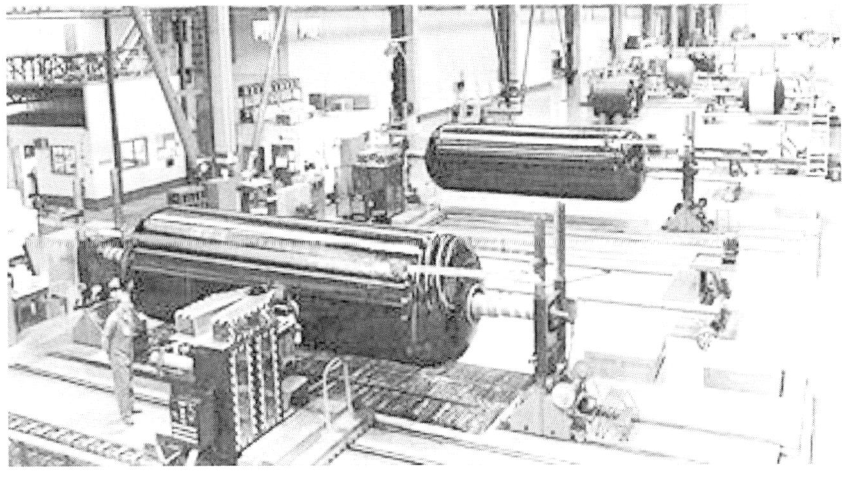

Fig. 8 High-performance graphite/epoxy motor chambers fabricated using computerized filament winding. Courtesy of Alliant Aerospace Company

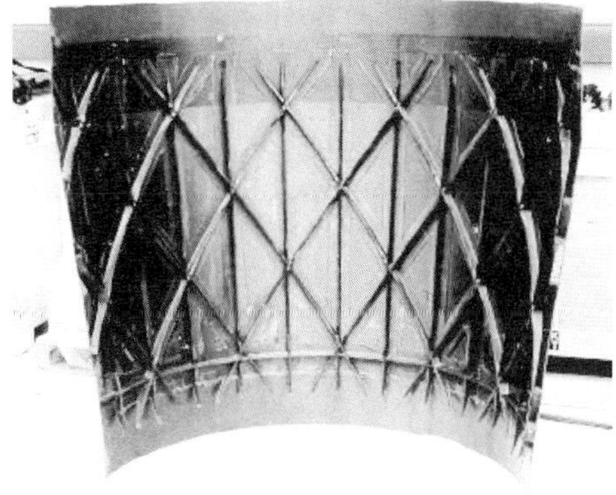

Fig. 9 Advanced grid-stiffened structure for launch veicle systems. Courtesy of Air Force Research Laboratory, Kirtland Air Force Base

structures are composed of composite shells supported by a "grid pattern" of composite stiffeners (Fig. 9). These structures are of interest due to their structural efficiency, high damage tolerance, suitability for propensity toward automated manufacture, and environmental robustness.

The interstate adapters used on the Atlas V program are constructed with similar materials, but are fabricated using automated fiber placement, which reduces touch labor, minimizes material scrap, and improves process control and repeatability. Graphite/epoxy facesheets are used based upon exhibiting good strength and stiffness, reasonable cost, good elevated temperature (i.e., up to about 150 °C, or 300 °F) capability, and fairly extensive heritage in space applications. Aluminum honeycomb is preferred over structural foam and on metallic cores due to its superior compression and shear strength properties, lighter weight, and reduced cost. Cork is still generally less expensive and more effective than spray-on insulations and ablatives for exterior thermal protection. Spray-ons are used, and do work, but they rarely fully deliver on their promises. Bismaleimides and polyimides are frequently studied and sometimes used to improve facesheet performance at higher temperatures. With the proper postcure processing, the materials can be used at temperatures up to 188 and 233 °C (370 and 450 °F), respectively, without the need for ancillary thermal treatments. However, they are quite expensive, generally more difficult to process, and sometimes exhibit problems resisting launch vehicle environments, such as moisture absorption.

New Developments and Future Needs

For several years, the trend in composite materials for spacecraft has been regular introduction of new fibers and new composite product forms; it is likely to continue. In particular, fibers with still-higher thermal conductivity are anticipated, and the use of carbon-carbon for thermal conductance will increase. In the long run, a locally leak-free (nonpermeable) composite will be developed, capable of containing a fluid and leading to wholly composite heat pipes embedded in composite laminates and sandwich panels.

For low-cost small satellites, such as those produced by the dozens for LEO telephone communications, composite designs and procedures will evolve to still-simpler shapes and methods. For these satellites, redundancy of systems on orbit will permit acceptance of risk of structural/functional failure of composite components. The motivation, of course, is cost reduction by eliminating expensive inspection and quality control procedures.

For unique high-value spacecraft, such as the next-generation (optical) space telescope, more and more adaptive structures with embedded piezoelectric or magnetostrictive elements will be employed to obtain precise dimensional control.

In processing, resin transfer molded and pultruded parts will be available in sufficient variety to replace most hand lay-up long, straight shapes for frames and stiffeners in bus structure.

In design of solar arrays and other secondary structures, the trend will continue to lighter composite sheets. Already, honeycomb core sandwich structure employs ultralight carbon-fiber facesheets that may be a single ply of a triaxial weave fabric, a single ply of conventional square weave fabric, or even two crossed plies of unidirectional prepreg tape. An additional weight reduction is likely from ultrathin prepregs, thinner than 0.1mm (0.004 in.). Composite truss tubes will routinely contain integrally formed composite end fittings.

The impact of composite advances on evolving ultrasmall micro- (10 kg, or 22 lb) and nano- (1 kg, or 2 lb) satellites is still unclear; if huge weight savings are accomplished with the functional components, the savings available from structural composite materials may be less attractive. On the other hand, advances in carbon nanotube based composites should offer multifunctional structure design solutions for the fabrication of micro- and nano-satellites.

Composite users for reusable launch vehicles require an extensive database containing mechanical properties of common graphite/epoxy systems, which would be most useful. These data should be based on lamina, common laminates, and honeycomb sandwich specimens tested in sufficient quantities to yield A-basis allowables at room temperature dry and wet, elevated-temperature dry and wet, and reduced temperature (cryogenic) dry and wet. More work needs to be done to characterize the effects of compression after barely visible impact and standard repair techniques. Lower-cost materials and processes and more-consistent process repeatability will also help the future of composites. Also, more work needs to be performed to improve cost and weight effectiveness of acoustic transmission loss characteristics without the need for heavy ancillary treatments. The inherent advantages of graphite/epoxy honeycomb sandwich structures in terms of improved specific stiffness make them ideal transmitters of acoustic noise. Frequently, the treatments applied to mitigate acoustic transmission severely penalize the performance of composite structures.

REFERENCES

1. "Advanced Composite Design Guide," 3rd ed., 2nd revision, Air Force Flight Dynamics Laboratory (FBC), Wright-Patterson Air Force Base, Dayton, OH, 1976
2. G. Lubin, Ed., *Handbook of Composites*, Van Nostrand Reinhold Company, New York, NY, 1982, p 197 271
3. F.J. Policelli and A.A. Vicario, Space and Missile Systems, *Composites*, Vol 1, *Engineered Materials Handbook*, ASM International, 1987, p 816–822
4. Michael D. Griffin and James R. French, "Space Vehicle Design," American Institute of Aeronautics and Astronautics, Washington, D.C.

5. Wiley J. Larson and James R. Wertz, Ed., *Space Mission Analysis and Design*, Kluwer Academic Publishers and Microcosm, Inc., 1992
6. J.B. Rittenhouse and J.B. Singletary, "Space Materials Handbook," Technical Report AFML-TR-68-205, Defense Technical Information Center, Cameron Station, Alexandria, VA, 1968
7. Carl Zweben, Advanced Composites in Spacecraft and Launch Vehicles, *Launchspace*, June/July 1998, p 55–58
8. Thomas P. Sarafin, Ed., and Wiley J. Larson, Managing Ed., *Spacecraft Structures and Mechanisms—From Concept to Launch*, Microcosm, Inc. and Kluwer Academic Publishers, 1995
9. D. Schmidt, K. Davidson, and L. Theibert, Unique Applications of Carbon-Carbon Composite Materials (Part Two), *SAMPE J.*, Vol 35 (No. 4), July/Aug 1999, p 51–63
10. Brent Strong, *Fundamentals of Composite Manufacturing: Materials, Methods and Applications*, Society of Manufacturing Engineers, 1989
11. Edward Silverman, Composite Isogrid Structures for Spacecraft Components, *SAMPE J.*, Vol 35 (No. 1), Jan/Feb 1999, p 51–58
12. J.E. Rule, *Thermal Stability and Surface Accuracy Considerations for Space-Based Single- and Dual-Shell Antenna Reflectors*, San Diego, CA, 1990
13. K. Dodson and J. Rule, Thermal Stability Considerations for Space Flight Optical Benches, *34th International SAMPE Symposium*, Vol 34, (Reno, NV), 1989, p 1578–1589
14. A.A. Vicario, Composites in Missiles and Launch Vehicles, *Comprehensive Composite Materials*, A. Kelly and C. Zweben, Ed., Vol 6, *Design and Applications*, Elsevier, 2000, p 317–340
15. S.P. Rawal and J.W. Goodman, Composites for Spacecraft, *Comprehensive Composite Materials*, A. Kelly and C. Zweben, Ed., Vol 6, *Design and Applications*, Elsevier, 2000, p 279–316
16. F. James, O.W. Norton, and M.B. Alexander, "The Natural Space Environment: Effects on Spacecraft," NASA Reference Publication 1350, Nov 1994
17. C.A. Belk, J.H. Robinson, M.B. Alexander, W.J. Cooke, and S.D. Pavelitz, "Meteoroids and Orbital Debris: Effects on Spacecraft," NASA Reference Publication 1408, Aug 1997
18. B.J. Anderson and R.E. Smith, "Natural Orbital Environment Guidelines for Use in Aerospace Vehicle Development," NASA Technical Memorandum 4527, June 1994
19. D. Dooling and M.M. Kinckenor, "Material Selection Guidelines to Limit Atomic Oxygen Effects on Spacecraft Surfaces," NASA/TP-1999-209260, June 1999
20. J.H. Adams, R. Silberg, and C.H. Tszo, "Cosmic Ray Effects on Microelectronics, Part 1: The Near-Earth Particle Environment," NRL-MR-4506-1, Naval Research Laboratory, Washington, D.C.
21. G. C. Messenger and M.S. Ash, *The Effects of Radiation on Electronic Systems*, Van Nostrand Reinhold, 1986
22. Compiled data from several vendors, including Hercules, Amoco/BP, Toray, Mitsubishi
23. Compiled from data provided by vendors, such as Hexcel/Fiberite, YLA Inc., and Bryte Industries
24. S.P. Rawal, M.S. Misra, and R.G. Wendt, "Composite Materials for Space Applications," NASA Contractor Report 187472, Contract NAS1-18230, Aug 1990
25. "DoD/NASA Advanced Composite" Guide, Rockwell International, AFWAL/FDL, Chapter 4.2, July 1983
26. Edward M. Silverman, "Composite Spacecraft Structures Design Guide," NASA Contractor Report 4708, Part 1, Contract NAS1-19319, March 1996
27. W. Vaughn, E. Shinn, S. Rawal, and J. Wright, "Carbon-Carbon Composite Radiator Development for the EO-1 Spacecraft," Paper 30-3, Proc. 13th Annual Conf. American Society for Composites, 21–23 Sept, 1998 (Baltimore, MD)
28. M.P. Campbell, J.H. Hoste, K.T. Kedward, and G.C. Krumweide, "Designing Composite Structures for Thermally Stable Applications," Fifth DoD/NASA Conf. Fibrous Composites in Structural Design, Jan 1981, (New Orleans)
29. G.C. Krumweide, and D.N. Chamberlain, "Adaption and Innovation in High-Modulus Graphite/Epoxy Composite Design: Notes on Recent Developments," S.P.I.E. O-E LASIE 1988, (Los Angeles, CA), Jan 1988
30. C. Blair, and J. Zakreewski, Coefficient of Thermal and Moisture Expansions and Moisture Absorption for Dimensionally Stable Quasi-Isotropic High Modulus Graphite/Epoxy Composites, *S.P.I.E. Proc., Advances in Optical Structural Systems*, Vol 1303, (Orlando, FL), April 1990

Aeronautical Applications of Metal-Matrix Composites

Daniel B. Miracle, Air Force Research Laboratory

METAL-MATRIX COMPOSITES (MMCs) could claim only a few significant applications as recently as the 1980s. None of these were aeronautical applications. Since that time, however, dramatic advancements have been made in the areas of material and process development, design, manufacturing scale-up, and certification of MMCs. As a result, a number of significant MMC applications are now in service in the aeronautical field. Metal-matrix composites are used in both military and commercial aeronautical systems. Major applications exist for aerostructural components and parts in aeropropulsion systems, and a growing number of uses in aeronautical subsystems is evident. The current generation of MMC applications largely includes structural components and applications for thermal management, but important applications for wear resistance have also been considered.

The primary motivation for the insertion of MMCs into aeronautical systems is the excellent balance of specific strength and stiffness offered by MMCs relative to competing structural materials. As shown in Fig. 1, fiber-reinforced MMCs offer specific strengths and stiffnesses significantly higher than those of aerospace metal alloys. However, their properties are highly anisotropic, limiting potential applications, as discussed in more detail subsequently. Further, their specific properties are still inferior to those of organic-matrix composites, such as graphite/epoxy, in the uniaxial orientation. Discontinuously reinforced aluminum (DRA) MMCs have isotropic properties and provide specific stiffness values that are higher than those of aerospace metal alloys by as much as 100%. While the highest levels of specific stiffness are obtained by using higher volume fractions of particulate reinforcement, good fracture properties (ductility, toughness, and fatigue) can only be obtained with current technology for volume fractions of 25% or less.

Data points for the most widely used DRA aerospace materials are labeled in Fig. 1 and have volume fractions that range from 15 to 25% of SiC particles. These materials have isotropic specific stiffnesses up to 50% higher than those of metal alloys and isotropic specific strengths that are equivalent to those of the best commonly-used aerospace metal alloys, such as Ti-6Al-4V and 7075-T6 aluminum. These MMCs also provide specific stiffnesses equivalent to those of the best graphite/epoxy cross-plied material and have specific strengths in the midrange of cross-plied organic composites. The structural properties of discontinuously reinforced titanium (DRTi) are shown in Fig. 1 to illustrate the potential of this class of MMCs. Although less mature than DRA, these materials already have important applications, including intake and exhaust valves in production automobiles (see the article "Automotive Applications of Metal-Matrix Composites" in this Section). The labeled bubble illustrates the current range of specific properties of DRTi for reinforcement volume fractions to 20%, and the larger bubble outlines the projected range of properties that may be achieved with higher volume fractions.

A great deal of effort has been undertaken to develop fiber-reinforced MMCs for aerospace applications. Early success was achieved with aluminum alloys reinforced with boron monofilaments or graphite fibers, resulting in spacecraft applications (see the article "Space Applications" in this Section). However, no applications in aeronautical systems resulted from fiber-reinforced aluminum MMCs. Additional matrix alloys based on copper, magnesium, nickel, and niobium have been studied, but by far the largest effort has focused on fiber-reinforced titanium alloys. The motivation for this research and development activity was to obtain exceptional specific strength and stiffness for high-temperature applications in systems such as the National Aerospace Plane (NASP) in the United States and in advanced gas turbine engines. Candidate matrix alloys included α-titanium alloys, α + β-titanium alloys, β-titanium alloys, and titanium-aluminide alloys. Alumina was sometimes considered as a reinforcing fiber, but SiC monofilaments were most commonly used. A number of innovative processes were explored and developed. Although the required material properties goals were largely achieved in these research and development efforts, the high raw material cost associated with the SiC monofilament and difficulty in processing and machining provided critical barriers to insertion.

Significant resources have been applied to develop these materials for critical components in gas turbine compressors of advanced gas turbine engines. In one case, such efforts are still underway, and it is not certain whether a successful insertion will result. Nonetheless, fiber-reinforced titanium has been specified as bill of material in an actuator piston rod for a nozzle actuator in the F119 engine for the F-22 aircraft and for use as an actuator linkage in the F110 engine for the F-16 aircraft. These parts provide a simple component shape, easing manufacturing concerns. The loading is purely axial, which takes best advantage of material properties. Finally, the part is not fracture-critical, providing

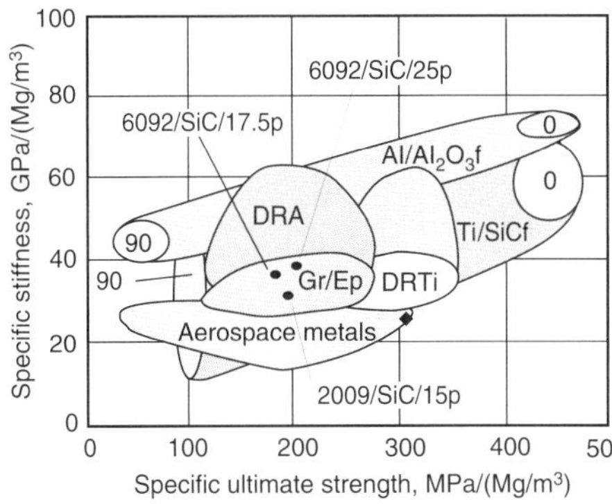

Fig. 1 Specific strength and specific stiffness of existing aerospace structural materials with isotropic properties, including metal alloys, discontinuously reinforced aluminum (DRA), discontinuously reinforced titanium (DRTi), and cross-plied graphite/epoxy (Gr/Ep). Graphite/epoxy/overlaps the lower-stiffness region of DRA. Three data points for particular aerospace-qualified DRA materials are labeled. Fiber-reinforced MMCs (Al/Al_2O_3f and Ti/SiCf, or TMC) are also shown. Data for DRTi are available only for reinforcement volume fractions of ≤20%, as represented by the labeled oval, and the larger oval suggests the potential properties that may be achieved with higher volume fractions of reinforcement. The diamond represents data for high strength specialty steel.

a low-risk component for first insertion. These components are discussed later in this article.

An equally large, though more diffuse, activity on discontinuously reinforced metals has been undertaken in the past 20 years. Many international efforts have explored MMCs based on alloys of magnesium, copper, iron, and titanium. A number of important applications have been developed for discontinuously reinforced Fe, including hard, wear-resistant parts such as industrial rollers and extrusion dies. Discontinuously reinforced titanium has been successfully developed for a few significant applications, including intake and exhaust valves in the automotive industry (Ref 1). Clearly, however, the most significant success over this time period has been the development and commercialization of DRA. Self-sustaining industries are now established in Great Britain, Canada, and the United States, satisfying demands from the automotive, aerospace, thermal management, tribology, and recreation industries. Applications of DRA range from sophisticated, high-technology components such as net shape, integrally processed multifunctional parts to simple commodities such as automotive-cylinder liners and snow tire studs. By far the widest range of applications exists in the automotive, space, thermal management, and aeronautical fields. The current aerospace powder metallurgy (P/M) market in the United States alone amounts to 50 tonnes per year, and the automotive market represents a volume over an order of magnitude larger.

The DRA materials constitute an extremely broad and flexible material system. Matrix alloys can be based on either cast or wrought compositions, and a full range of microstructural modifications from thermal and mechanical treatment is available. SiC, Al_2O_3, B_4C, and graphite are commonly used as reinforcements. Reinforcements may be particulate or whiskers and may comprise a volume fraction from 10 to 70% by volume. A significant degree of control can be exercised over the size and distribution of reinforcing particles. A number of commercial primary and secondary processes have been established for DRA, and the interested reader is referred to other articles within this Volume for a detailed description.

A convenient standardized nomenclature, ANSI H35.5-1997, has been established for aluminum MMCs and is illustrated here: 2009/SiC/15p-T4. The four-digit Aluminum Association alloy designation, which specifies the matrix alloy composition, is followed by the reinforcement composition. This is followed by the reinforcement volume fraction (in volume percent), and a single letter that signifies the morphology of the reinforcements (p = particle, w = whisker, and f = fiber). The standard Aluminum Association temper designation (T4 in the example) is used at the end of the MMC designation, as appropriate.

The following briefly describes the most significant aeronautical applications of MMCs. With only one exception (the hydraulic manifold for the V-22), the components described are now in production—the remaining component had been selected as bill of material and was awaiting certification testing at the time of publication. Each description includes discussion of the main features and requirements of the particular application, including service requirements and deficiencies of previous materials. Design considerations and trade-off studies that led to the selection of the MMC are highlighted. The MMC material and process as it applies to the specific component is then described. Finally, the benefits that have resulted from the use of MMCs are highlighted. In this article, a distinction is drawn between applications for aeronautical systems, which are covered here, and space systems, which are covered elsewhere in this Section. Many important applications of DRA are established in aeronautical systems for thermal management and electronic packaging, but these are covered elsewhere in this Section (in the article "Thermal Management and Electronic Packaging Applications"). Automotive uses of MMCs are described in the article "Automotive Applications of Metal-Matrix Composites" in this Section.

Aerostructural Applications

Ventral Fin. The F-16 aircraft has two ventral fins on the lower half of the fuselage just aft of (behind) the wings (Fig. 2). In a number of operational regimes, including those with high angles of attack, the horizontal stabilizers become less effective due to turbulence from the wings. The purpose of the ventral fins is to provide additional flight stability to the aircraft under such conditions. The ventral fins are subjected to aerodynamic loading and require high strength and stiffness. The ventral fins, however, were experiencing a higher than expected rate of failure. The failure mode was dramatic and resulted in complete destruction of the component. The cause of these failures was identified as unanticipated loading from aerodynamic turbulence (that occurred during certain flight maneuvers), such as a rapid decrease in power to the engines (a "throttle chop"). This causes a wave of highly turbulent air, originating at the front of the engine intake, to propagate along the fuselage. The ventral fins were subjected to a rolling moment and a first mode torsion, which twisted the fin along the fuselage axis. Measurements on operational aircraft during such maneuvers showed that the peak-to-peak amplitude of the ventral fin oscillation at the tip, resulting from the rolling moment, was as much as 10 cm (4 in.). These bending moments produced elongation of the bolt holes and eventual failure. While pilot and aircraft were not seriously endangered, the frequent failures led to high downtime and significant repair costs.

The original ventral fins were made of a built-up structure consisting of a 2024-T4 aluminum alloy sheet over an internal structure. This internal structure consists of a central root rib that projects normal to the fuselage skin, and a front and rear spar, which are parallel to the fuselage skin. The sheet is attached to these structures, and a honeycomb core completes the assembly. The assembly is attached to an engine access panel, which is, in turn, attached to the fuselage. Design trade studies were conducted to identify the best solution to the ventral fin failure problem described. Critical design properties included high stiffness and good high cycle fatigue strength. Preferred solutions that would provide the same form, fit, and function of the original design were sought, so that additional certification of significantly different materials or component configurations would not be required. As an example, a preferred solution would allow stripping, painting, and repair of battle damage (bullet holes) by techniques that had already been specified and standardized for the existing aluminum part. In addition, the preferred solution should be affordable. Candidate solutions included a graphite/epoxy skin over the existing spar structure, regions of increased thickness of the original 2024-T4 aluminum alloy, and a DRA sheet over the aluminum alloy spar. Graphite/epoxy was eliminated because of the difficulties of support and cost, and the modified aluminum alloy and DRA approaches underwent testing.

The DRA material selected for study was 6092/SiC/17.5p. The 6092 aluminum matrix alloy is a modified 6*xxx* age-hardenable aluminum alloy that was optimized to be used as a matrix alloy for DRA. This alloy has been approved by the Aluminum Association and is the DRA matrix analog to 6013. Design trade studies and material and process development were undertaken as a collaborative effort between Lockheed-Martin, the U.S. Air Force Air Logistics Center at

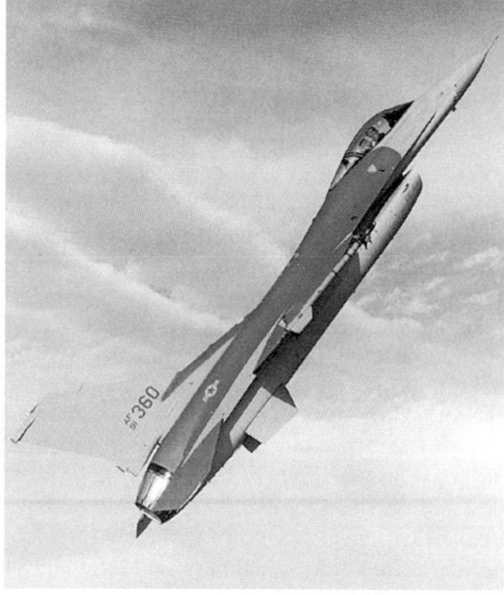

Fig. 2 An F-16 aircraft, illustrating the ventral fins, which are located on the bottom of the fuselage just aft of (behind) the wings. The ventral fins are now assembled from 6092/SiC/17.5p discontinuously-reinforced aluminum sheet material produced via a powder metallurgy process.

Ogden, UT, DWA Aluminum Composites, and the U.S. Air Force Materials and Manufacturing Directorate. Material and process development and process scale-up were conducted by DWA Aluminum Composites Specialties, Inc. under a contract with the U.S. Air Force. In this work, powder handling, mixing, outgassing, and consolidation were established. Sheet rolling of consolidated powder was also established. Initial billets 51 cm (20 in.) in diameter were extruded to 7.5 × 36 cm (3 × 14 in.) rolling stock. This was cut to 66 cm (26 in.) lengths, then cross-rolled from 36 cm to 76 cm. The material was then rotated 90° and rolled to final thickness (3.18 and 1.02 mm, or 0.125 and 0.040 in.). The material was sheared to length, heat treated, and quenched. Flatness was obtained by stretching (3.18 mm) or offset rolling (1.02 mm). The DRA sheet was then inserted into the existing repair line established for the original aluminum fins. The only modifications required were the use of polycrystalline diamond tooling and a new chemical masking agent. The standard chemical milling process established for the original aluminum component was used for surface activation required for adhesive bonding to the honeycomb core.

In addition to establishing the commercial processes required to produce the DRA material in sufficient quantity and of quality, the DRA material satisfactorily completed the rigorous testing schedule required for MIL-HDBK-5 certification testing, providing design-allowables properties for the 6092/SiC/17.5p material. Data obtained from this study are shown in Table 1. The design trade studies showed DRA to be the preferred solution. Extensive flight testing was conducted in collaboration between the U.S. Air Force, Lockheed Martin, the Royal Netherlands Air Force, and the National Aerospace Laboratory of the Netherlands (NLR). The flight testing was fully successful, and the DRA ventral fin has been established as the preferred spare.

The DRA sheet provided a 40% increase in specific stiffness over the baseline design. This increased stiffness nearly eliminated the first mode torsional loads on the fin, providing a solution to the bolt hole elongation. Instrumented flight testing showed that the peak tip deflections of the ventral fin were reduced by 50%. As a result of this effort, replacement of the original ventral fins is now in progress with the 6092/SiC/17.5p DRA ventral fins. A projected improvement in service life of 400% is expected for the new ventral fins, and flight experience over the past several years now bears this number out. The reduced maintenance, inspection, and downtime costs associated with the DRA ventral fins have resulted in a life-cycle cost savings to the Air Force of over $26 million.

Fuel Access Door Covers. During high-G maneuvers, the fuselage of the F-16 aircraft is subjected to bending stresses, which produce significant axial stresses in the skin. The upper fuselage skin is perforated by many fuel access doors (Fig. 3). In the original aircraft design, these doors did not carry any of the load in the fuselage skin, and so the corners of the door openings act as stress concentrators. As a result, the F-16 fuselage skin was cracking near the vertical tail root. As a solution to this problem, special door fasteners were designed that allowed the doors to carry some of the load, thus reducing the stress at the door openings. These new fasteners required a redesign of the doors, since the original doors were not designed to support a load. Several design options were considered, including 2024 Al doors of double thickness and 6092/SiC/17.5p DRA doors. Critical design properties for the new doors included high strength and stiffness, high bearing strength, good high-cycle fatigue resistance, and compatibility with jet fuel equivalent to aluminum alloys.

The doors are made of 6092/SiC/17.5p wrought P/M material in sheet form. The process is identical to that described for the F-16 ventral fins, with the exception that the final sheet thickness is 2.54 mm (0.10 in.) for most doors, with a few at 2.03 mm (0.08 in.). After producing the sheet, the doors are shipped to the fabricator. The final dimensions are obtained with a high-speed routing operation followed by finish machining. Holes are pre-punched and then drilled. Routing and drilling are done with diamond tooling, and the punching operation is done using standard equipment. The DRA punches much better than standard aluminum alloys do, due to the higher modulus. The punched surface is much cleaner, with no edge rollover. The door is roll-formed to the final contour and given the final aging heat treatment. Since the upper fuselage skin is a fuel-cell wall, the door material must be compatible with JP-4 jet fuel. Exposure studies established that the DRA response is equivalent to that of the unreinforced metal alloy. The part is cleaned and painted in a final operation.

In combination with the improved door fasteners, the 6092/SiC/17.5p DRA doors provided the best solution to the cracking problem because of the combination of higher specific strength and stiffness compared to that of 2024 aluminum. The DRA was also able to satisfy a higher bearing allowable, which was required by the new door fasteners. Doors of DRA have been inserted in 23 of the 26 fuel access doors on the F-16 aircraft in an active retrofitting program called Falcon Up. This is the first military retrofit application for a MMC. As a result of the new doors and fasteners, the peak skin stresses have been reduced by 38% and the average skin stresses have been lowered by 10%. This has fully eliminated the cracking previously observed in the F-16 upper fuselage skins and has extended the durability life calculation for the F-16 fuselage to over 8000 flight hours.

Helicopter Blade Sleeve. The Eurocopter France EC120 and N4 helicopters are used for civilian law enforcement and search and rescue in Europe, the United States, and in many other countries. The large centrifugal loads of each rotor blade (the N4 has five blades) are supported by a blade sleeve, which holds the rotor blade to the drive shaft (Fig. 4). This component requires an infinite fatigue life, excellent fretting fatigue resistance, high specific strength, and good fracture toughness. The blade sleeve is designated as a Class I vital critical rotating part, since component failure results in total loss of the craft and its inhabitants. Helicopter performance and durability are linked very strongly to rotating mass, and the principle motivation for consideration of DRA in this application is the reduction in rotating mass and the high cost associated with titanium alloy, which has now been replaced by DRA.

Forged 2009/SiC/15p-T4 DRA has replaced the wrought titanium alloy component originally specified. Extrusion of a 36 cm (14 in.) P/M billet, which weighs 95 kg (210 lb), provides a 95 mm (3.7 in.) diameter preform. After cutting to length, each piece is blocker forged, followed by

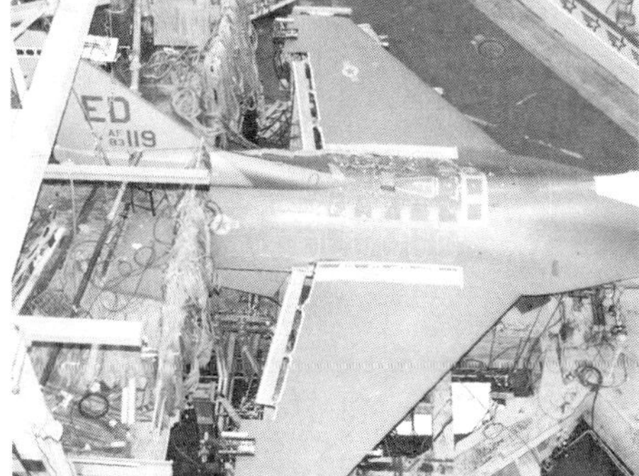

Fig. 3 An F-16 center fuselage, illustrating the size and location of fuel access door covers, which are located between the wings. Of the 26 doors on each F-16, 23 are now made from 6092/SiC/17.5p discontinuously-reinforced aluminum.

Table 1 Properties of 6092/SiC/17.5p and 2009/SiC/15p-T4 MMCs

Property	6092/SiC/17.5p	2009/SiC/15p-T4
Tensile yield strength, MPa (ksi)	434 (63)	343 (54)
Ultimate tensile strength ± 1 standard deviation, MPa (ksi)	490 (71)	498 ± 4.5 (72 ± 0.7)
Tensile modulus, GPa (10^6 psi)	107 (15.5)	93 (13.5)
Strain to failure, %	6	6.2
Fracture toughness, MPa $\sqrt{m}$ (ksi $\sqrt{in.}$)	Not measured	25 (23)
High cycle fatigue strength at 10^7 cycles	Not measured	270 (39)
Bearing ultimate strength (*e*/*D* 2.0), MPa (ksi)	924 (134)	Not measured
Shear strength (longitudinal), MPa (ksi)	296 (43)	Not measured
Density, g/cm^3 (lb/in.^{3})	2.80 (0.101)	2.83 (0.102)

closed-die forging to a sonic inspection envelope. The sonic envelope is also the final component shape, and less than 1% of material is discarded as scrap after drilling and final machining. As a result of the criticality of this component, extensive testing and certification are conducted. Twenty-five-year traceability is provided for raw materials and finished goods via archived documentation of processing and inspection. In addition to measuring minimum mechanical properties in the transverse orientation on each billet, the electrical conductivity (as a quality check for microstructural uniformity), chemistry, reinforcement volume fraction, and density are also documented for each billet. Inspection is performed via a macroetch and ultrasonic inspection using MIL-STD 2154 Class AA (no defect ≥1.2 mm, or $\frac{3}{64}$ in., is allowed). The primary requirement is for infinite fatigue life. The 2009/SiC/15p-T4 material has a fatigue strength of 270 MPa (39 ksi) at 10^7 cycles, compared to 155 and 180 MPa (22 and 26 ksi) for 2024-T4 and 7075-T6, respectively. This excellent fatigue performance allows DRA to compete successfully with wrought titanium. The fracture toughness of this DRA material is 25 MPa $\sqrt{m}$ (23 ksi $\sqrt{in.}$), and the specific strength is comparable to the displaced titanium alloy. Other properties for the 2009/SiC/15p-T4 DRA material are provided in Table 1.

Nearly 14 kg (over 30 lb) of rotating mass have been saved by the use of 2009/SiC/15p-T4 DRA, which is a dramatic reduction for helicopter rotors. In addition to reduced weight, the DRA blade sleeves are less costly to produce, providing a saving in acquisition cost. This is the first aerospace application of DRA in a fracture-critical component.

Aeropropulsion Applications

Fan Exit Guide Vane. The fan exit guide vane (FEGV) of high-bypass gas turbine engines removes the "swirl" component of bypass air, so that maximum thrust can be obtained from the redirected air flow. In commercial engines, primary design requirements include high specific stiffness, excellent erosion and ballistic response, and low acquisition and support costs. Recent engines have specified graphite/epoxy for this application. However, poor ballistic performance and susceptibility to erosion from airborne particulates and rain have led to high in-service costs and concerns regarding flight safety. An interim solution, bonding a titanium-alloy foil over the graphite/epoxy leading edge, provided improvement in the erosion response (but no improvement in ballistic performance) and increased the cost significantly.

Between 1996 and 1998, 6092/SiC/17.5p DRA has entered service in the Pratt & Whitney 4084, 4090 and 4098 engines, replacing graphite/epoxy. The DRA material is a P/M product that is consolidated into billets. A large reduction ratio during extrusion provides improved particulate distribution, which enhances the fracture properties of the material. A high-tolerance extrusion produces the net shape airfoil contour of the component, and a double-hollow internal configuration is produced to remove unnecessary mass (Fig. 5). The bridge between the two hollow cavities is both formed and joined during the extrusion process, and this bridge improves the structural performance of the airfoil. The resulting DRA component weight is equivalent to the solid graphite/epoxy unit initially specified. Extrusion of this part utilizes existing metalworking infrastructure with only minor modifications. The extrusion die is a standard tool steel die, with a Ferro-TiC die insert. (Ferro-TiC, a trademark of Alloy Technology International Inc., is a discontinuously reinforced iron alloy that uses TiC particulates as reinforcement; it is used in the tool and die industry, and for high wear applications such as industrial rollers.) Current FEGV dimensions include a chord width of 14 cm (5.5 in.) or 19 cm (7.5 in.) and a length of 61 cm (24 in.). After cutting to length, each part is coined to provide a slight camber and is then embedded in thermoplastic end fittings with an elastomeric coupling agent. Over 10,000 piece parts have been manufactured to date.

This component, used in engines that power the Boeing 777 aircraft, was the first commercial aerospace production application of DRA. The DRA components have demonstrated a sevenfold reduction in erosion rate and significant increase in resistance to ballistic damage from foreign objects, such as hailstones. A dramatic reduction in the unit acquisition cost was realized at the time of introduction. In addition, an overall increase in service life of 300% and reduced maintenance and repair costs also increase the life-cycle cost savings. The total realized savings since introduction has been well in excess of $100 million.

TMC Nozzle Actuator Piston Rod. Turbine-engine nozzle flaps increase the efficiency of gas turbine engines by controlling the velocity and, in some cases, the direction of the exhaust gas. This is accomplished by controlling the nozzle flap position via actuator and linkage devices. A pair of divergent nozzle flaps are used on each of the two Pratt & Whitney F119 engines used on the F-22 aircraft. Each divergent nozzle flap is driven by an actuator assembly consisting of a hydraulic cylinder and a metallic piston, which is connected, in turn, to a linkage mechanism. The piston must support large axial loads and must also possess high stiffness. Weight is a primary concern in the F-22 aircraft, so specific strength and stiffness are the primary selection criteria. The piston rod is subjected to fatigue loading, and the maximum operating temperature is 450 °C (850 °F). The initial material specified for the piston actuator was a solid rod of 13-8 Cr-Ni precipitation hardened stainless steel, which has now been replaced by a SiC fiber-reinforced titanium alloy MMC. This MMC is often referred to as a titanium-matrix composite (TMC), and it is inferred that the reinforcement is continuous when this acronym is used.

The TMC actuator piston rod is manufactured by a novel metal wire process. A Ti-6Al-2Sn-4Zr-2Mo (Ti-6242) alloy is hot-drawn in a conventional wire drawing process to a diameter of 178 μm (0.007 in.). The Trimarc-1 SiC monofil-

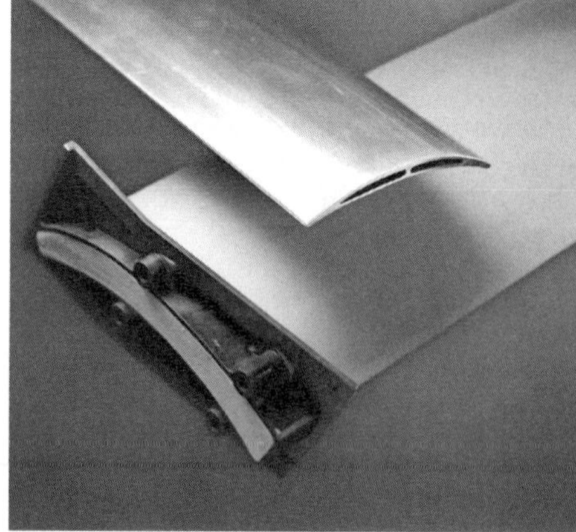

Fig. 5 Fan exit guide vane blank (top), showing the high quality of the as-extruded product and the double-hollow construction. Below is an assembled fan exit guide vane mounted in the endcap. This component is used in Pratt & Whitney 4084, 4090, and 4098 gas turbine engines. Component dimensions are provided in the text. Courtesy of DWA Aluminum Composites, Inc.

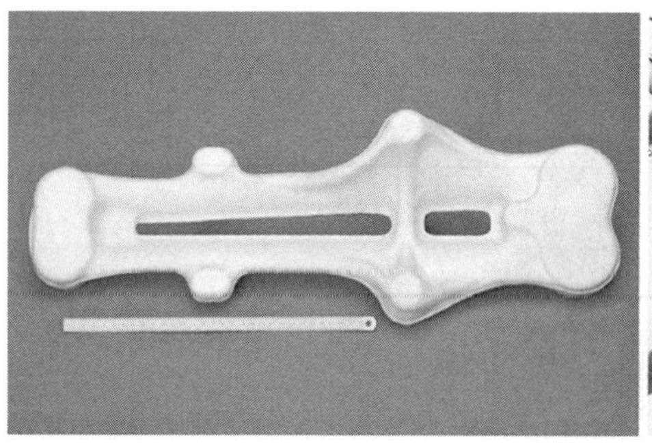

(a)

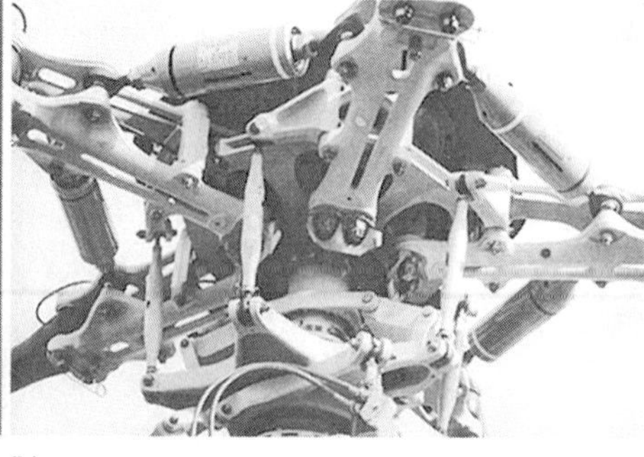

(b)

Fig. 4 EC-120 helicopter rotor application. (a) Rotor blade sleeve. The part is made of forged 2009/SiC/15p discontinuously reinforced aluminum (DRA). The scale below the part is 30 cm long. (b) Rotor assembly showing the DRA blade sleeves. Photos courtesy of DWA Aluminum Composites, Inc.

ament reinforcement is 129 μm (5.07 × 10–3 in.) in diameter, and is produced by a chemical vapor deposition process on a tungsten wire core. An outer C-based coating protects the fiber from chemical interaction with the matrix during consolidation and service. The Ti-6242 metal wire is combined with 34 vol% of the SiC monofilament by wrapping on a rotating drum. The wires are held together with an organic binder and are then cut and removed from the drum to make a preform "cloth." This cloth is wrapped around a solid titanium mandrel, so that the SiC and Ti-6242 wires are parallel to the long axis of the mandrel. A short Ti-6242 cylinder, with an outer diameter of 10 cm (4 in.) and 5 cm (2 in.) high, is placed around one end of the cloth-wrapped mandrel, from which the piston head will be formed. After hot isostatic pressing consolidation, the piston head is machined from the stocky cylinder at one end of the piston, and a threaded connection is machined from the titanium mandrel at the other end. The remainder of the mandrel is removed by gun drilling. The final component is 30.5 cm (12 in.) long, and the shaft is 3.79 cm (1.49 in.) in diameter (Fig. 6a). The excellent fiber spacing is shown in the figure inset.

The use of a TMC in the actuator piston is a landmark application and represents the first aerospace application of TMCs. In addition to providing significant improvement in the specific strength and stiffness over steel (compare steel properties, indicated by the diamond data point, with Ti/SiCf in Fig. 1), the TMC material passed fatigue properties certification by a very wide margin. Certification of the TMC actuator piston rods has resulted in a direct weight savings of 3.4 kg (7.4 lb) per aircraft. The F-22 is an extremely weight-sensitive aircraft, so this weight savings is considered significant. Further, since the weight removed is in the aft end of the aircraft, counterweights added in the fore section of the aircraft to shift the aircraft center of gravity forward can also be removed, providing additional weight savings. At the time of publication, the first orders of the TMC actuator pistons had been shipped for the initial production phase of F-22 aircraft.

TMC Nozzle Actuator Links. Based on the experience gained from the success of the TMC actuator piston rod, TMCs have now been certified as nozzle links on the General Electric F110 engine, used for F-16 aircraft. The nozzle of the F110 engine consists of 24 nozzle flaps arranged symmetrically around the exhaust periphery in a "turkey feather" configuration. Every second nozzle flap is driven by an actuator via a nozzle link, so that 12 TMC nozzle link actuators are now specified for each engine. The original link was produced from a square tube of Inconel 718, which was formed from sheet and welded along its length.

The manufacturing process begins by winding Trimarc-2 SiC monofilament, which is similar to Trimarc-1 but is produced on a carbon core, on a drum as for the piston rod. Rather than using metal wire, Ti-6242 powder is sprayed with an organic binder over the wound SiC fibers to produce a preform cloth. This cloth is then cut and removed from the drum as before, and wrapped around a mandrel. Added at each end are Ti-6242 fittings for a clevis attachment and a threaded end, and the entire assembly is consolidated via HIP. After machining the clevis and the threaded end, the mandrel is removed. A finished part is shown in Fig. 6(b).

The new TMC links have been certified for F110 engine rebuilds in the F-16. The TMC links provide a 50% increase in buckling resistance relative to the Inconel 718 component. Insertion of the TMC links have provided a direct weight savings of over 2 kg (4.5 lb) per shipset. This application provides a low-risk first insertion of TMCs for the F110 engine. From this, the end-user will gain critical field experience in the application and support of TMCs, and the manufacturer (Atlantic Research Corporation) will be able to identify and implement important process improvements anticipated to improve material quality and reduce costs.

Aeronautical Subsystem Applications

T-1 Racks. The first flight application of DRA in a military aircraft occurred as avionics support racks for the Lockheed-Martin U2/TR-1 Spy Plane. The material used was 6091/SiC/25p DRA. The matrix alloy is the DRA analog to 6061. The principal requirements for the racks are isotropic stiffness, good bearing strength, and high electrical conductivity, necessary for a high-quality grounding plane for the avionics. The original structure was an aluminum alloy, but this was replaced by graphite/epoxy in order to save weight. However, the need for isotropic stiffness required a quasi-isotropic lay-up, which produced section channels that were thicker than necessary to support the primary loads. The poor bearing strength of the graphite/epoxy also added weight to the structure, since local reinforcement was required. Finally, the high-quality grounding plane was provided by bonding aluminum foil to the structure. This added both weight and cost, and introduced significant support issues when the aluminum foil was damaged as avionics racks were slid across the surface.

The rack section channels were the first successful attempt to produce precision mill shapes of DRA from multiple-holed extrusion dies. Straight tubing was produced with a minimum gage thickness. The reduced mass allowed by the minimum gage, along with the high intrinsic electrical conductivity and good bearing strength, allowed the DRA rack to save 20% in weight over the graphite/epoxy design and 34% relative to the original aluminum design. Reduced material costs improved manufacturability, and improved supportability led to reduced component cost. This part was first introduced in 1988.

Hydraulic Manifold in V-22 Osprey Tiltrotor and F-18 E/F. Materials of DRA are being used to produce hydraulic manifolds for the Navy Osprey V-22 Tiltrotor aircraft. The manifolds redistribute high-pressure hydraulic fluid (up to 70 MPa) to flight control surfaces. In addition to high mean pressures, the manifold is subjected to impulse loading during flight. The operating temperature is up to 100 °C (210 °F). Selection criteria include affordable near net shape processing, high specific strength to support the high hydraulic pressures, and good resistance to high-cycle fatigue from the impulse loading. Two manifolds are used for each V-22 aircraft.

The initial design specified 7050 aluminum, but the hydraulic manifold failed in burst tests, so a whisker-reinforced 2009/SiC/15w DRA is now being used. Components are manufactured by a P/M process, whereby a solid block is produced, and the manifold is machined from this solid block of DRA. This material satisfies the service requirements, but the material cost is high due to the whisker reinforcements used. The component cost is high due to the significant machining required.

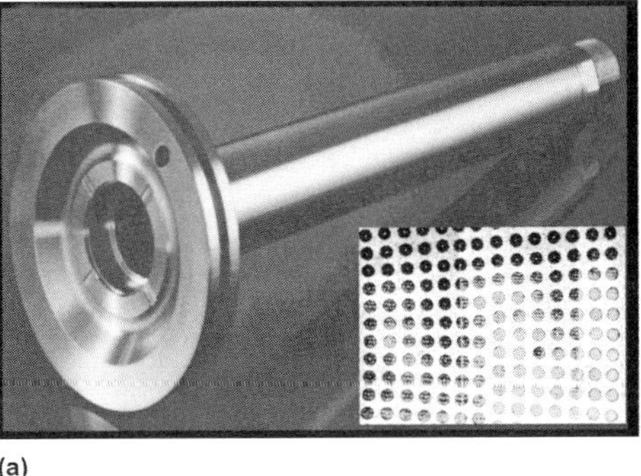

(a)

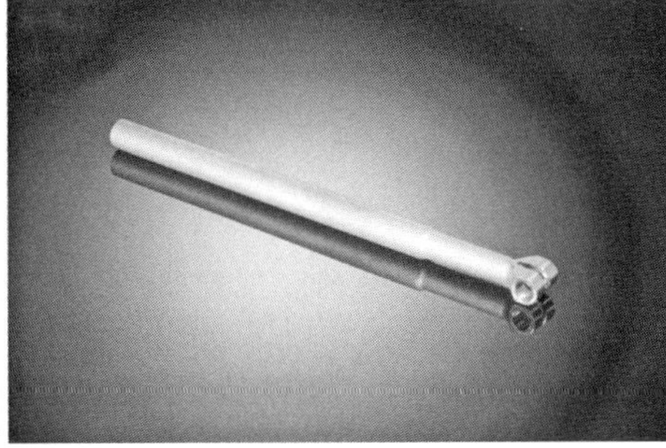

(b)

Fig. 6 Jet engine applications of titanium-matrix composites. (a) A nozzle actuator piston rod used on the Pratt & Whitney F119 engine for F-22 aircraft. The part is made of a Ti-6Al-2Sn-4Zr-2Mo alloy reinforced with SiC monofilaments that are 129 μm in diameter. The inset shows the typical distribution of the SiC reinforcements (inside diameter of the rod is to the left in this inset micrograph). (b) A nozzle actuator link from the General Electric F110 engine, made of a similar metal-matrix composite, used for F-16 aircraft. Component dimensions are provided in the text. Courtesy of Atlantic Research Corporation.

An alternate DRA material, A206/SiC/40p DRA, produced by pressure infiltration casting of a molten aluminum alloy into a particulate ceramic preform, is now being pursued. Preform manufacture is simplified by a unique castable process, providing a preform that is near net shape. Controlled reinforcement volume fractions from 30 to 70% can be achieved. A clean preform that is free of organic material is produced, and a uniform particle distribution is achieved. This process uses low-cost SiC particulates, which significantly reduces the cost of producing a manifold. The near net shape processing requires only finish machining, further reducing component cost. Full-scale components have passed proof, impulse, and burst testing. This component was awaiting certification testing by Bell Helicopter at the time of publication. An image of this component is provided in Fig. 7.

A DRA fluid manifold end gland is currently in production for the F-18 E/F. This component is part of the subsystem that controls the rudder and aileron. The end gland is 7.5 cm (3 in.) in diameter and is less than 7.5 cm (3 in.) in length. There are two fittings per aircraft. The operational conditions are similar to those described for the V-22 manifold. In addition, this component requires good wear resistance. The original component was made from an aluminum bronze. While this performed well, the high density of this material led to an excessive part weight. The DRA component is made from 2009/SiC/15p, which is machined from an extrusion. This is precisely the same material and process as described above for the helicopter blade sleeve, and so certification requirements were minimal. The DRA component provides reduced weight, and has a lower coefficient of thermal expansion, a higher wear resistance, and a fatigue limit that is twice that of the initial component. This last property is notable, since standard high-strength aluminum alloys typically possess poor fatigue response in hydraulic fluid when the pressure is greater than about 34 MPa (5 ksi). As a result, titanium is often specified for these applications. However, the DRA component performed very well in fatigue testing in high-pressure hydraulic fluid, so that DRA can now be considered a replacement for titanium alloys in similar applications.

Implementation Strategy

Critical evaluation of the case histories above provide useful guidance for future successful efforts to apply MMCs in new applications. Since technical considerations for the selection of an MMC are reviewed earlier in this article and elsewhere in this Volume, discussion here emphasizes nontechnical approaches. Experience has shown that the nontechnical factors are often at least as important as are the technical details in selecting materials to meet specific application requirements.

In every single component described above, the MMC displaced some other material that had been initially specified. This reflects the embryonic familiarity and confidence with which the design community views MMCs. This poor familiarity is manifested as a perceived high initial cost, concern about availability and depth of supply chain, lack of field experience, questions on reparability, and knowledge base and analysis tools available to design engineers that address MMCs. It is therefore essential that an internal advocate exists within the organization considering the use of an MMC. This advocacy function must be knowledgeable in MMC capabilities and limitations and should also possess some contact within the design function for the organization. Previous examples described herein also strongly support the importance of a close collaboration between the system manufacturer, the materials and component suppliers, and the end-use customer. The customer (or user) provides system requirements and constraints. When a solution to an existing problem is sought, the customer can provide information relating to causes and modes of failure; the customer establishes the value of the proposed improvement and also may provide insights into possible solutions. The manufacturer typically provides the design function. Internal testing and certification by the manufacturer is also critical, since data generated in house is often considered more relevant and reliable. Finally, the supply chain provides detailed information regarding the material capability and processing options and limitations. Such partnerships divide the risk and combine expertise to achieve an optimum solution. Many of the successes described resulted from such teamwork.

Another important point is that MMCs nearly always solved an existing operational problem or deficiency in the previous examples. Very infrequently are new materials such as MMCs selected simply because they provide a benefit over an existing system if that system is not currently deficient in some operational consideration. This follows from the high cost of certifying a new material and from the conservative design philosophy typically followed in the aeronautical industry.

The approach of developing a single MMC material that can satisfy the requirements for a range of applications is an effective strategy for reducing certification costs. Thus, certification costs for a particular material can be shared by several business units within a given company. Multiple applications provide an expanded payoff, thus providing a better return on investment for certification costs. In two cases above, a second application of an MMC within an organization followed a successful first insertion. A related approach is to form cross-industry teams (such as aeropropulsion and rocket propulsion, or aerostructures and automotive), which can share ideas and resources while minimizing issues of competition. Thus, a useful materials development strategy is to achieve a balance of properties that are acceptable for several requirements, rather than tailoring an MMC to achieve an optimum set of properties for a single application. Again, this approach shares the risk and expands the impact.

With regard to fiber-reinforced MMCs, the conservative approach of focusing on applications with simple geometric shapes and relatively low risk for failure is proposed until the technology matures and designer familiarity and confidence increases. Components with nearly axial loading are also suggested, since the technology for producing isotropy via cross-plied architectures is expected to remain difficult in the coming years.

View of the Future

While the emphasis of this Volume is as a practical guide for existing technologies, a brief

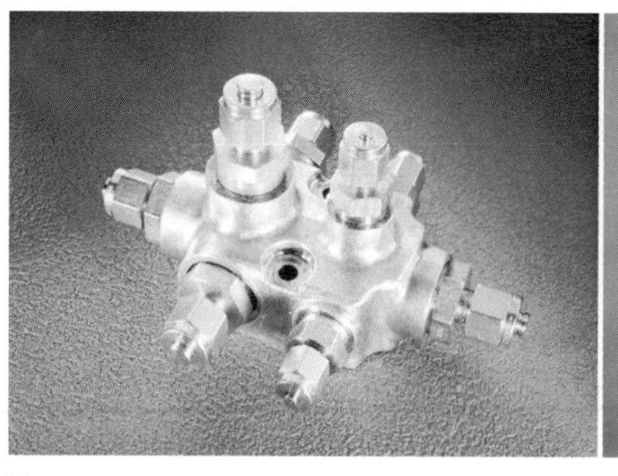

(a)

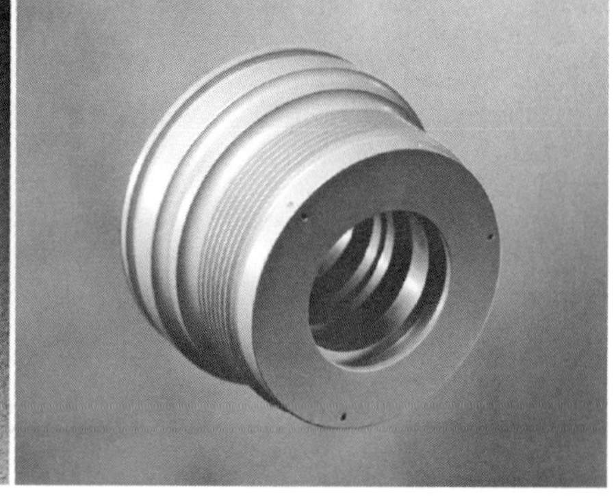

(b)

Fig. 7 Manifold applications. (a) A manifold used to redistribute high-pressure hydraulic fluid to flight control surfaces in V-22 Osprey Tiltrotor aircraft. This component is made by infiltration casting of A206/SiC/40p discontinuously reinforced aluminum. Courtesy of Triton Systems, Inc. (b) A fluid manifold end gland currently used in F-18 E/F aircraft as part of the subsystem that controls the rudder and aileron. The material is a powder metallurgy discontinuously reinforced aluminum, 2009/SiC/15p. Dimensions for the end gland are provided in the text. Courtesy of DWA Aluminum Composites, Inc.

look forward may be helpful to anticipate and benefit from major advancements as they develop.

The use of DRA is almost certain to continue the current trend of increasing application. The existing stable, production-oriented supplier base has brought costs down significantly, so that cast DRA can compete on a cost basis in some applications even with steel, and P/M DRA competes very favorably with titanium alloys. Subsystem uses provide the lowest risk of insertion, but aerostructural applications are expected to provide a strong market. Cast DRA is the standard MMC material and process for the automotive industry, and steady progress in this technology, especially infiltration casting, for high-quality aerospace applications is expected to produce initial applications in coming years. This near net shape process will improve the overall affordability of this material. Efforts to produce uniform ceramic preforms at reinforcement volume fractions below 30% is important to ensure that infiltration cast DRA components retain adequate fracture properties.

A great deal of progress has been achieved in producing affordable aluminum MMCs reinforced with alumina fiber tows. This is now a commercial product, and markets include high-performance automotive and mechanical subsystems. Power transmission cables are likely to enter first service within a few years. Many aerospace applications have largely axial loading and simple component shape, and so are candidates for this material. Candidate components include cases, shrouds, struts, rods, and shafts. In many cases these have requirements that eliminate organic-matrix composites from consideration, and so significant benefit over existing metal materials are expected. The processing technology has been well established for a simple unit product shape.

Two remaining MMC technologies with significant potential in the next ten years include DRA for application at temperatures up to about 200 °C (400 °F), and DRTi. High-temperature DRA is a prime candidate for replacing many titanium components that are specified because the use temperature is just a little higher than the full-life capability of aluminum alloys (about 150 °C, or 300 °F). Examples include engine pylon structures for transport aircraft and aft fuselage structure for fighter aircraft where the engine is embedded in the fuselage. In both cases, conduction and radiation from the engine heats the surrounding structures. Titanium provides a significant cost and weight penalty, and so is an important target for these applications. The DRTi materials may provide the highest level of isotropic strength and stiffness of any common structural material and so have a very broad range of possible applications. The DRTi materials may be produced by cast, wrought, or P/M technology, providing flexible processing and forming options.

REFERENCE

1. F.H. Froes, "Fourteenth International Titanium Application Conference and Exhibition," *Light Met. Age,* Vol 57 (No. 1, 2), 1999, p 117–121

High-Temperature Applications

Tito T. Serafini
Stephen C. Mitchell, General Electric Aircraft Engines

HIGH-TEMPERATURE-RESISTANT POLYMERS are used in aerospace, electronic, and other applications that demand outstanding elevated-temperature physical and mechanical properties. Major product forms of these polymers include adhesives, coatings, fibers, film, foam, insulation paper laminating resin solutions, molding powders, and wire enamels. A wide range of literature is available on their chemistry, processing characteristics, properties, and applications.

Early applications of high-temperature polymers as matrix resins in fiber-reinforced composites were limited to nonstructural (nonload-bearing) components. However, following the development of in situ polymerization of monomer reactants (PMR) polyimides at the National Aeronautics and Space Administration (NASA) Lewis (now NASA Glenn) Research Center (Ref 1–3) and their commercialization by prepreg suppliers, the fiber-reinforced PMR polyimide based on PMR-15 has found increased acceptance as an engineering material for high-performance structural applications. Because it has become the most widely used high-temperature polymer, most of the applications discussed in this article are representative examples of the use of fiber-reinforced PMR-15 polyimide. In addition, resin systems that compete with and, in some cases, extend the temperature range of PMR-15 are BMI, AFR700C, Avimid RB, PETI, PMR-II, Avimid N, AFR700B, and phthalonitriles. Other resins that have found use in composites for high-temperature applications include phenolics and bismaleimides; applications for these materials are described in the articles "Phenolic Resins" and "Bismaleimide Resins" in this Volume.

General Characteristics

For a material to function as a viable matrix in a fiber-reinforced composite, the matrix must bind the constituents, transfer loads, provide environmental stability, and perhaps most important, provide processibility. Most organic polymers soften or melt below 204 °C (400 °F). The key to preparing high-temperature polymers is to incorporate highly stable structural units in the polymer chain, such as aromatic and/or heterocyclic rings. These structural units are able to absorb thermal energy and contain a minimum of oxidizable hydrogen atoms.

In addition to being resistant to elevated temperatures, many high-temperature polymers are also resistant to being processed into useful structural components. The poor processing characteristics of early high-temperature polymers prevented them from performing the necessary functions of a matrix material. Composites fabricated with these polymers exhibited high void contents, poor fiber translation efficiencies, inferior elevated-temperature mechanical properties, and inferior thermooxidative stabilities. Little progress was made in developing polymers with improved processibility, because the major thrust of polymer synthesis research up until 1970 was in the area of improved thermal stability, without any concern for processibility.

Condensation-Type Polyimides

High-temperature laminating resins of the class known as condensation-type polyimides were first commercialized in 1962 and 1965 and emerged as the sole contenders for resin-matrix applications. Although these materials presented processing difficulties, they had good high-temperature properties along with cost and availability advantages. Because polyimide laminating resins generally used the same monomers as those used in versions for other product forms, such as film and wire enamels, it was a relatively easy matter to make the laminating resins commercially available at a reasonable cost.

The major problems in processing condensation-type polyimide prepreg materials can be attributed both to the inherent nature of condensation reactions (by-product evolution) and to the use of high boiling point aprotic solvents, leading to void content problems. During thermal processing of the prepreg to effect chain growth and solvent/by-product removal, appreciable imidization also occurs, converting the resin to an intractable state. Reduced resin flow prevents the removal of the last traces of solvent and by-products. The entrapment of these volatile materials results in composites having void contents in the range of 5 to 10 vol%, particularly for thick sections (>1 mm, or 0.04 in.). The presence of these voids adversely affects mechanical and thermooxidative stabilities of the composite.

Applications of Condensation-Type Polyimides. The earliest applications for fiber-reinforced condensation-type polyimides, in 1972, were for radomes on advanced aircraft (Ref 4) and for sound-suppression panels in the engine nacelles of subsonic commercial transports. Both applications can be considered secondary structural applications. In fact, the high void content of condensation polyimides is desirable for the sound-suppression panels. The formidable processing problems of these materials were solved by using dynamic dielectric analysis. More than 200 fiberglass-polyimide radomes measuring 4.6 × 0.5 × 0.6 m (15 × 1.6 × 2.0 ft) have been produced for EA-6B aircraft.

PMR Polyimides

A major advance in high-temperature resins was the development of polyimides that cured by an addition reaction (Ref 5 and 6). Low-molecular-weight amide-acid prepolymers whose chain ends were terminated, or end-capped, were synthesized. In the early 1970s, attempts to commercialize a resin, designated P13N, met with limited success because of several shortcomings. It was to circumvent the shortcomings of condensation-type and addition-type prepolymer polyimides that investigators at NASA Lewis developed the novel PMR polyimides. In the PMR approach, the reinforcing fibers are impregnated with a monomer reactant mixture dissolved in a low-boiling-point alkyl alcohol, such as methanol or ethanol. In situ polymerization of the monomer reactants occurs when the impregnated fibers are heated, followed by final polymerization to a void-free composite. Further details on the polymer reactions are available in Ref 1 and Ref 7 to 10. Prepreg materials based on PMR-15 are commercially available in the United States from the major prepreg suppliers. The structures of the monomers used in PMR-15 are shown in Fig. 1. Additional information on resin chemistry is provided in the article "Polyimide Resins" in this Volume.

The early studies (Ref 1, 7) conducted at NASA Lewis also clearly demonstrated the efficacy and versatility of the PMR approach. By varying the chemical nature of either the dialkyl ester acid or the aromatic diamine, or both, and the monomer reactant stoichiometry, PMR matrices having a broad range of processing characteristics and properties could easily be synthesized. Figure 2 shows that significantly higher resin flow for high tensile strength (HTS) graphite-PMR composites can be achieved by reducing the formulated molecular weight. However, the PMR compositions that exhibited increased resin flow were found to be less thermooxidatively stable at 288 °C (550 °F). The lower resin flow and increased thermooxidative stability in going from PMR-10 to PMR-15 clearly show the sensitivity of these properties to imide ring and alicyclic contents. The reduction in resin flow with increased formulated molecular weight also serves to account qualitatively for the intractable nature of condensation-type polyimides at an early stage of their process cycle.

High-pressure (compression) and low-pressure (autoclave) molding cycles have been developed for fabrication of fiber-reinforced PMR composites. Although the thermally induced addition cure reaction of the norbornenyl group occurs at temperatures in the range of 275 to 350 °C (527 to 662 °F), nearly all the processes developed use a maximum cure temperature of 316 °C (600 °F). Cure times of 1 to 2 h followed by a free-standing postcure in air at 316 °C (600 °F) for 4 to 16 h are also normally used. Compression molding cycles generally use high heating rates (5 to 10 °C/min, or 9 to 18 °F/min) and pressures in the range of 3.5 to 6.9 MPa (0.5 to 1.0 ksi). Vacuum bag autoclave processes at low heating rates (2 to 4 °C/min, or 3.6 to 7.2 °F/min) and pressures of 1.38 MPa (0.200 ksi) or less have been used successfully to fabricate void-free composites. Autoclave processing methodology can be successfully applied to PMR polyimides, because of the presence of a thermal transition, termed melt flow, which occurs over a fairly broad temperature range (Ref 11). The lower limit of the melt-flow temperature range depends on a number of factors, including the chemical nature and stoichiometry of the monomer reactant mixture and the thermal history of the PMR prepreg.

Differential scanning calorimetry analysis has shown that four thermal transitions occur during the overall cure of a PMR polyimide. During the first and second thermal transitions, solvent and condensation by-products can be volatilized without converting the polymer to an intractable state. During the third thermal transition, and with the application of pressure, fusion occurs. At still higher temperatures, and while maintaining the applied pressure, the addition cure reaction occurs. The high-temperature postcure mentioned previously must be used to obtain optimal thermooxidative stability and mechanical properties retention at elevated temperatures. The cure temperature requirements of PMR polyimides exceed the capabilities of many existing autoclave facilities and impose a severe strain on the temperature capabilities of current bagging and sealant materials (Ref 12–14). It should be noted that the increase in production applications of high-temperature composites has increased the availability of appropriate high-temperature autoclaves and the ruggedness of bagging materials.

Many investigations have been conducted to determine the effects of various hostile environments on the physical and mechanical properties of PMR-15 composites. The thermooxidative stability and retention of mechanical properties at elevated temperatures have been found to be far in excess of what would be predicted on the basis of polymer molecular structure criteria for polymer thermal stability. Graphite-PMR-15 composites have been reported (Ref 15) to be suitable for use in air at 288 °C (550 °F) for at least 5000 h. At 316 °C (600 °F), the useful life of graphite-PMR-15 composites is in the range of 1200 to 1400 h.

Fiber-reinforced PMR-15 polyimide composites are finding increased acceptance as engineering materials for the design and fabrication of aerospace structural components, particularly in aeropropulsion. Components being fabricated range from small, compression-molded bearings to large, autoclave-molded aircraft engine cowls and ducts. Processing technology and baseline materials data are also being developed for the application of PMR-15 composites in weapon systems. Firms involved in manufacturing small, compression-molded bearings made from particulate or chopped-fiber PMR molding compounds have found it convenient to become captive producers of PMR-15 resin. In contrast, firms involved in fabricating larger components made from tape or fabric materials rely on traditional sources of composite materials for PMR-15 prepreg. Materials based on PMR-15 are commercially available from the major suppliers of composite materials in the form of solutions, molding compounds, prepregs, and adhesives.

The presence of methylene dianiline (MDA) in the PMR-15 polyimide resin requires individuals to comply with the Occupational Safety and Health Administration (OSHA) Standard 29 CFR 1910.1050 document entitled "Occupational Exposure to 4,4′methylenedianiline (MDA)." This document applies when a material contains greater than 0.1% MDA by weight or volume. Because MDA is a suspected carcinogen, much effort has been put into developing alternatives to PMR-15. Other high-temperature polyimides, such as PMR-II, Avimid N, and AFR700B, do not use MDA. Additional information is provided in the article "Polyimide Resins" in this Volume.

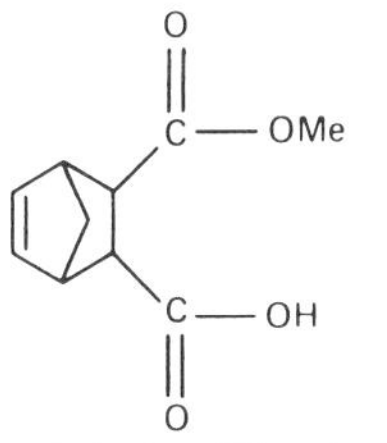

Monomethyl ester of 5-norbornene-2,3-dicarboxylic acid (NE)

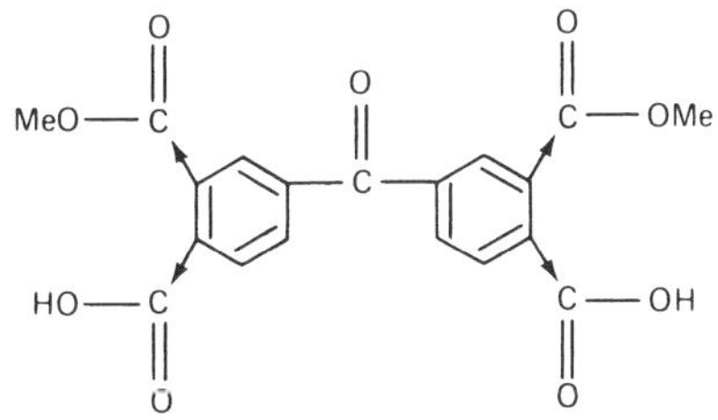

Dimethyl ester of 3,3′,4,4′-benzophenonetetracarboxylic acid (BTDE)

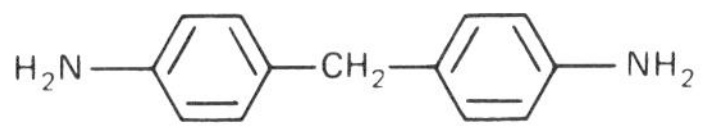

4,4′-methylenedianiline (MDA)

Fig. 1 Structures of monomers used in PMR-15

Applications of PMR-15

The development of PMR-15 resin as a viable, high-temperature composite system had a profound effect on increasing the number of applications of composite components. Prior resin systems placed significant size and thickness constraints on potential applications; however, the advent of PMR-15 allowed engineers to design large, complex components with thick sections. PMR-15 produced significant interest within the military propulsion community, due to the high operating temperatures within the low-pressure system. In addition, the high weight savings of composite rotor components saw the initial PMR-15 applications occur in both rotors (blades) and stators (vanes).

The blade illustrated in Fig. 3 was the first structural airfoil component fabricated with a PMR-15 resin and reinforced with HTS graphite fiber. The blade was designed and fabricated for an ultrahigh-speed fan stage (Ref 16, 17). The blade span is 28 cm (11 in.), the chord is 20 cm (8 in.), and the thickness ranges from about 13

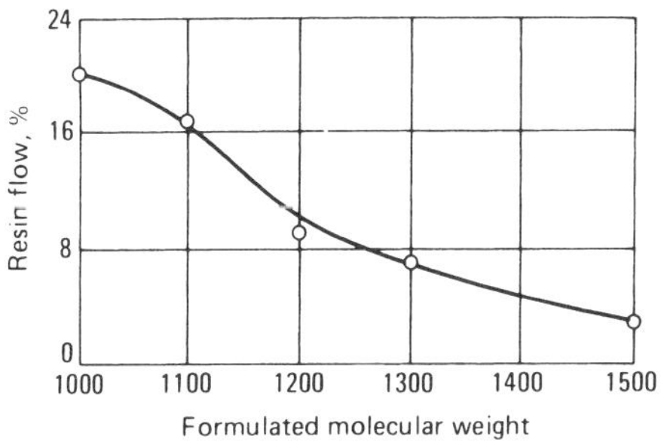

Fig. 2 Effect of formulated molecular weight on resin flow of HTS graphite fiber-PMR

mm (0.5 in.) in the dovetail to about 0.5 mm (0.020 in.) at the leading edge. At the thickest section, the composite structure consists of 77 plies of material arranged in varying fiber orientations. The airfoil surface line visible at approximately one-third the height from the blade tip resulted from a change in fiber orientation from 40° in the lower region to 75° in the upper region, in order to meet torsional stiffness requirements. Although some minor internal defects were induced in the blade during low-cycle and high-cycle fatigue testing, the successful fabrication of these highly complex blades established PMR-15 as a processible matrix resin.

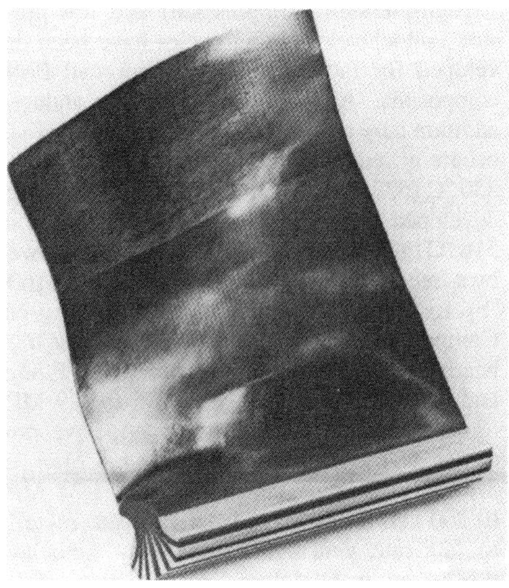

Fig. 3 Graphite fiber-PMR-15 fan blade

Another early application of PMR-15 composites in rotating components was the fourth-stage compressor blade shells and spacers (Fig. 4) in a supersonic wind tunnel. More than 24,000 pounds of fiberglass-PMR-15 were processed for this application (Ref 18). The total quantity of material was equally divided between 360 blade shells and 600 blade spacers.

The success with small airfoil components developed the interest in applying PMR-15 to large static structures. In 1975, NASA and General Electric Aircraft Engines (GEAE) launched the most aggressive use of composite components in a propulsion system. Figure 5 shows a cross section of this quiet, clean, short-haul experimental engine commonly known as the quiet, clean, short-haul, experimental engine (QCSEE) propulsion system. To meet the program goals for low weight, low noise, clean emissions, and improved efficiency, composites were used extensively in the fan blades, vane frame, containment, integrated nacelle, inlet, external flaps, and inner core cowl (Ref 19). The blades, frame, and nacelle components were fabricated with carbon-epoxy tape and fabric; the containment was fabricated with aramid fabric; and the inner core cowl was fabricated with graphite-PMR-15 fabric. The high-temperature environment of the core cowl was not the result of any operating condition, but rather the product of radiant heating at shutdown. The absence of any airflow at shutdown raised the temperature of the core cowl to approximately 315 °C (600 °F).

Figure 6 shows the inner core cowl installed on the QCSEE occupying the region below the pylon and aft of the vane frame. The core cowl was a honeycomb sandwich structure with a maximum diameter of 90 cm (35 in.) and a length of 165 cm (65 in.). Fiberglass-polyimide honeycomb was used as the core material that was bonded to the inner surface of the premolded, perforated outer skin. The inner skin was then cocured to the honeycomb core. In an effort to reduce acoustic emissions, the entire flowpath surface of the core cowl was perforated with 0.5 mm (0.020 in.) holes to a 10% porosity level. In addition, the size limitations of the autoclave forced the core cowl to be a bonded assembly of four sectors. Today's large autoclaves would allow the fabrication of a unitized cowl without any bonded sectors. Complete details of the core cowl fabrication are provided in Ref 20. The cowl did not exhibit any degradation after 300 hours of engine ground testing (Ref 21). The successful autoclave fabrication and ground engine testing of the QCSEE core cowl established the feasibility of using graphite-PMR-15 composite materials for large static structures.

In the late 1970s, the U.S. Navy and NASA jointly sponsored a program (NAS3-21854) to replace the F404 titanium bypass duct with the world's first, large primary production engine structure fabricated with graphite-PMR-15. Studies conducted by GEAE indicated weight savings in excess of 4.5 kg (10 lb) (Ref 22). The duct shown in Fig. 7 is about 75 cm (30 in.) in diameter, 100 cm (40 in.) long, 2.3 mm (0.090 in.) thick, and sized from large loads attempting to compress and buckle the shell. The titanium outer bypass duct is a sophisticated casing located between the engine mounts and fabricated by forming, welding, machining, and chemical milling. Difficulties in the bonding and inspection operations of the QCSEE core cowl dictated

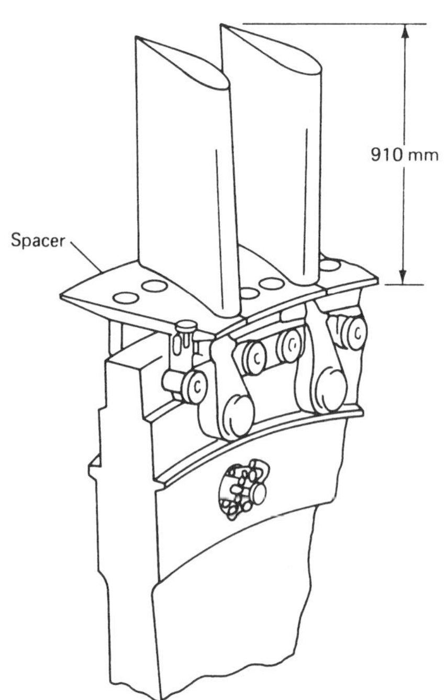

Fig. 4 Application of PMR-15 in supersonic wind tunnel

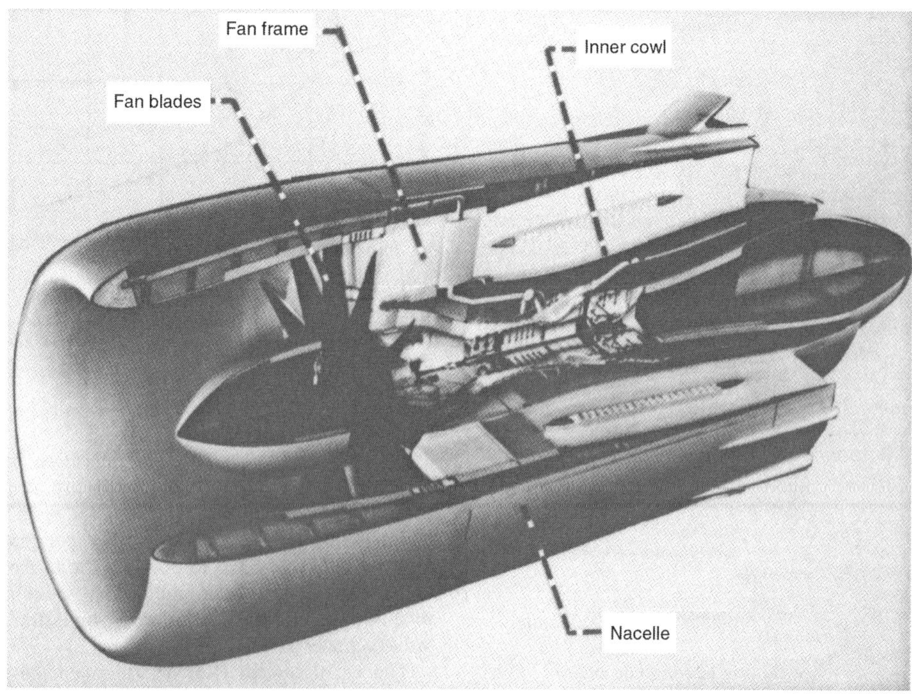

Fig. 5 Application of composites on QCSEE

that the F404 bypass duct would be a solid monolithic shell. The initial prototype F404 composite ducts contained titanium flanges bonded and riveted to a composite shell; however, within six months, the production duct of the F404 contained integral composite flanges. Another feature of the duct was the use of metal grommets needed for the attachment of approximately 100 configuration components. The top and bottom duct halves are fabricated by hand lay-up of T300 carbon-PMR-15 preimidized fabric into external molds. The parts are then bagged and autoclave cured. Prior to production, the duct successfully underwent 2500 hours of ground testing and 700 hours of flight testing. By 2000, over 1000 composite ducts had accumulated over 1.4 million flight hours on F-18 aircraft.

The success of the F404 carbon-PMR-15 bypass duct resulted in a carbon-PMR duct as the prime production "bill of materials" for the F414 in the early 1990s. The F414 duct shown in Fig. 8 became a second-generation component by incorporating several significant improvements in material, manufacturing, and design. To improve thermal oxidation resistance, the carbon-fiber fabric was changed from T300 to T650-35. The lay-up fabrication was improved by changing from two external molds for the top and bottom to one single internal mandrel. The axial flange design was improved by replacing the upright bolted flange used in the F404 with a bolted double-splice joint. These three changes significantly improved the quality and producibility of the F414 duct. The duct was introduced into production in 1997.

The success of the F404 bypass duct led to the 1984 production introduction of the carbon-PMR F110 fan frame splitter panels and forward inner duct shown in Fig. 9. Although these components are secondary structures, they provide important flowpath performance benefits. The inner duct has a 100 cm (40 in.) diameter, 40 cm (15 in.) length, and 1.5 mm (0.060 in.) thick shell, and is fabricated with T300-PMR-15 fabric. The frame splitter panels (Ref 23) are eight separate curved panels approximately 25 cm (10 in.) long and 15 cm (6 in.) wide. In 1986, the metal outer exhaust nozzle flap on the F110-400 was replaced with the hand lay-up carbon-PMR fabric design shown in Fig. 10. This 1.4 kg (3 lb) rib-stiffened part is 70 cm (27 in.) long, 30 cm (12 in.) wide, and varies in thickness from 1.8 to 13 mm (0.07 to 0.50 in.) at the stiffeners.

The success of the F404 carbon-PMR bypass duct also generated interest in swirl frame struc-

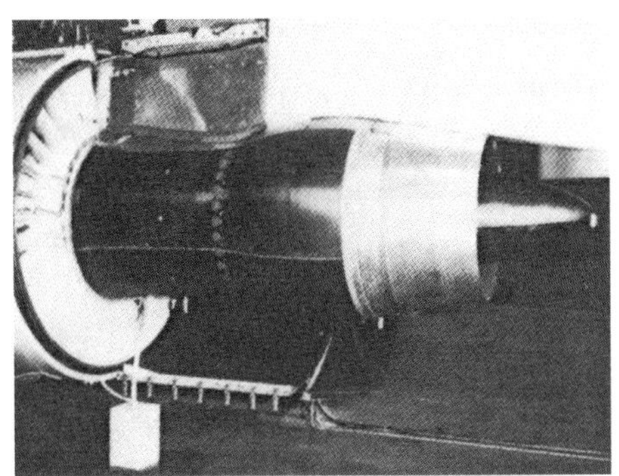

Fig. 6 Carbon fiber-PMR-15 polyimide QCSEE inner cowl

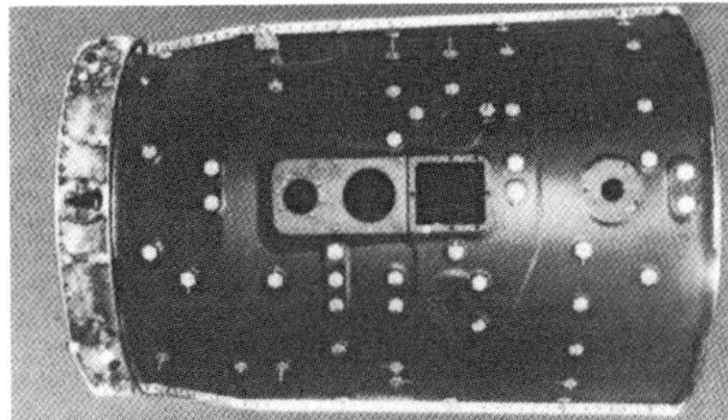

Fig. 7 Carbon fiber-PMR-15 polyimide F404 outer duct

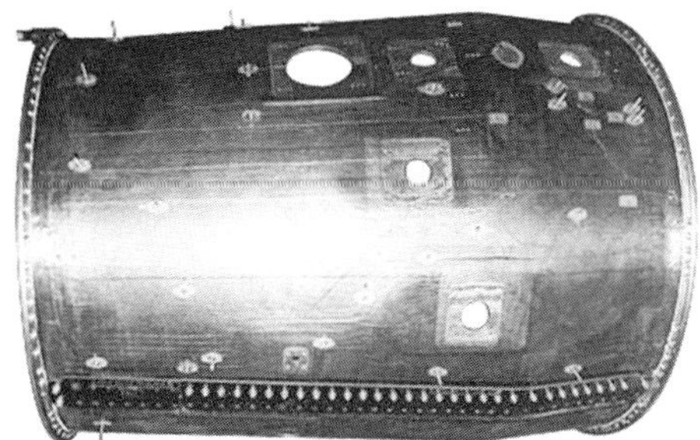

Fig. 8 Carbon-PMR-15 F414 outer duct

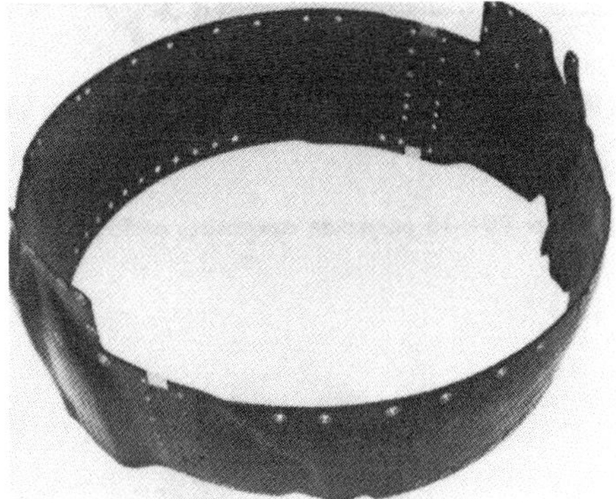

Fig. 9 Carbon fiber-PMR-15 polyimide F110 inner duct

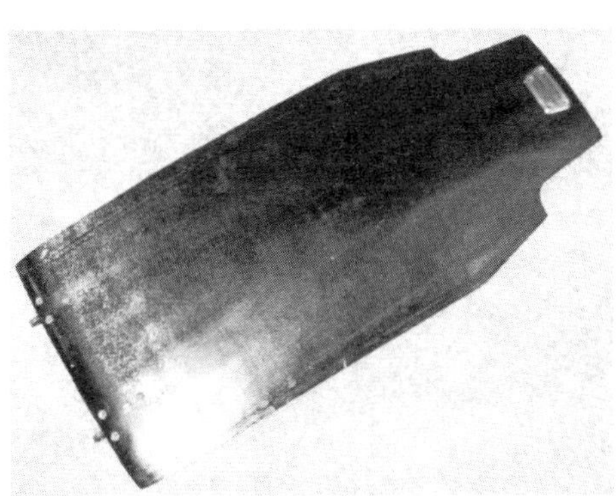

Fig. 10 Carbon-PMR General Electric (GE) F110-400 exhaust nozzle flap

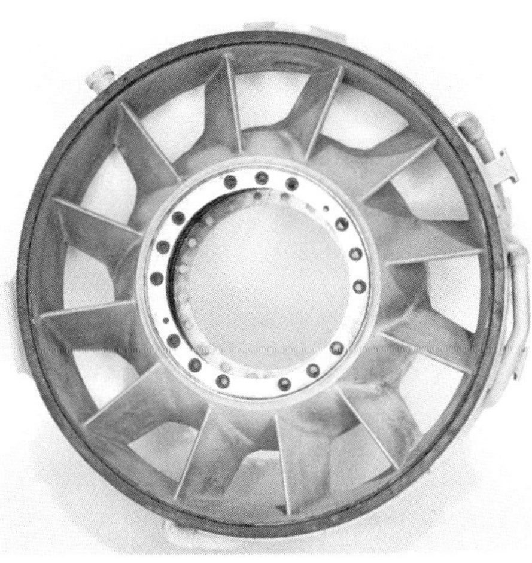

Fig. 11 Composite PMR hybrid swirl frame

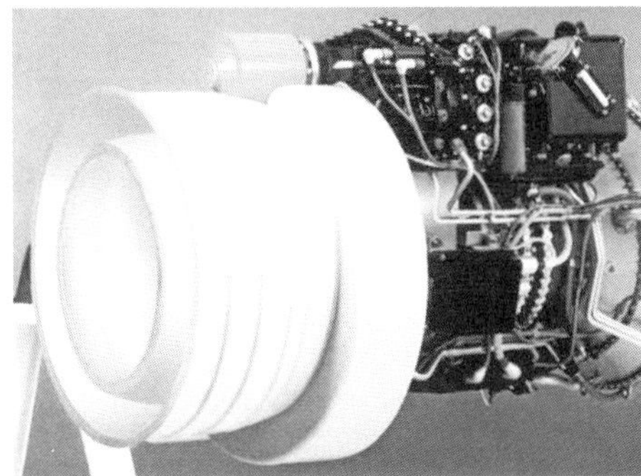

Fig. 12 GE27 engine with carbon-PMR inlet particle separator

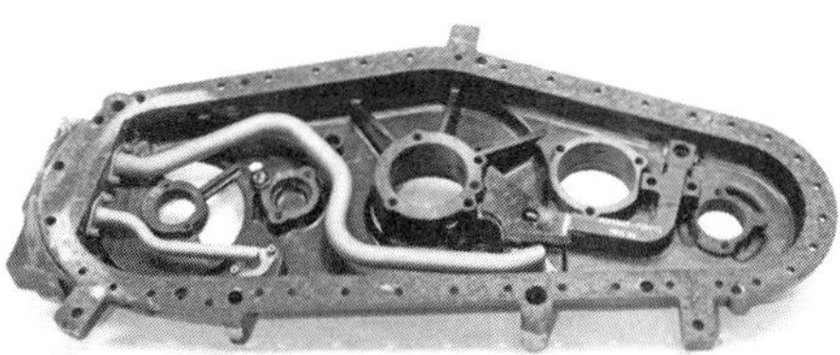

Fig. 13 GE27 carbon-PMR accessory gearbox

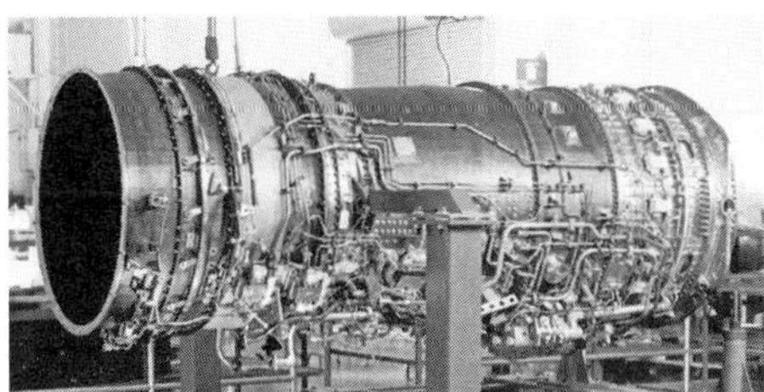

Fig. 14 GE YF120 engine with carbon-PMR parts

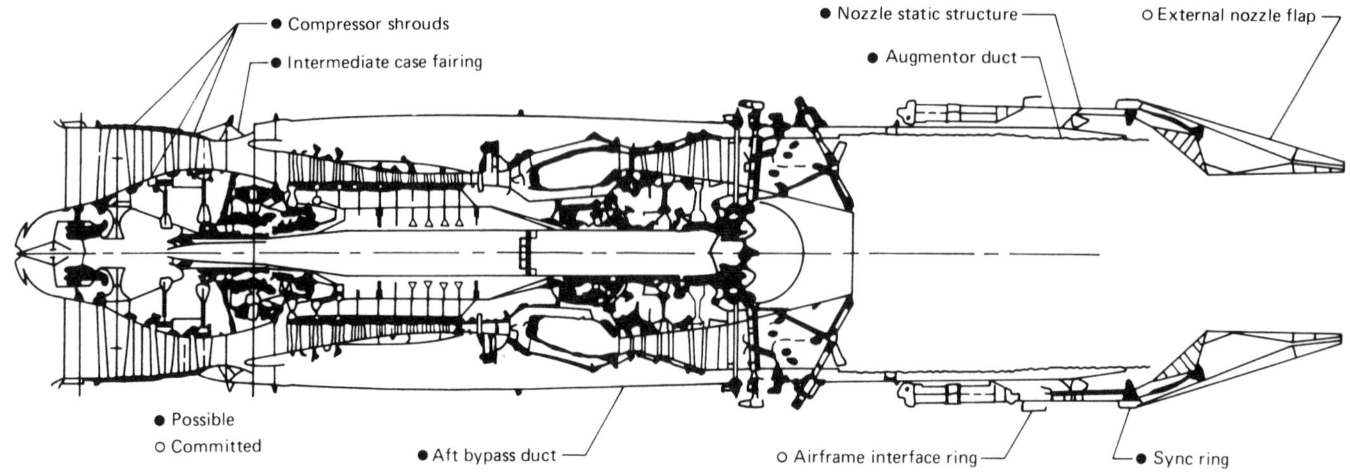

Fig. 15 Possible and committed applications of graphite fiber-PMR-15 polyimide components on PW1120 engine

tures. In late 1978, GEAE conducted design studies that indicated a 30% cost and weight savings of a hybrid composite swirl frame versus a brazed metal frame. In 1979, GEAE was awarded an Army contract (DDAK51-79-C0018) to fabricate and test three composite metal hybrid swirl frames for the T700 engine (Ref 24). The frames had an outside diameter of 50 cm (20 in.) and an axial length of 20 cm (8 in.). Figure 11 shows a section of the hybrid frame fabricated from a brazed cage of 410 stainless steel hollow struts and rings and bonded with various types of PMR-15 materials. The low transverse thermal conductivity of carbon-PMR material forced the struts to be steel. The antiiced hub and outer flowpath were fabricated from aluminized glass-PMR-15, due to improved thermal conductivity and superior erosion resistance. The structural flanged aft portion of the outer case was fabricated as a manifold from carbon-PMR fabric with laser-drilled holes on the inside surface. The manifold was used to distribute water for washing the inside of the swirl frame. The forward portion of the outer case contained an air manifold used to distribute hot air into struts for antiicing. Hot air exited the bottom of the struts and entered the hub flowpath. After bonding, the entire inside flowpath was coated with an aluminum oxide coating to provide erosion resistance. All three frames were subjected to a series of tests. The first and second frames successfully passed all iceball impact, sand erosion, static load, and fire tests. The third frame successfully ran on the T700 engine for over 100 hours. This program proved the structural viability of a hybrid frame, and in 1985 the GE27 engine (Fig. 12) incorporated a hybrid carbon-PMR composite inlet particle separator.

The GE27 engine provided an opportunity to explore another carbon-PMR composite component, but with a molding compound form of material. In 1983, GEAE was awarded an Army contract to fabricate an engine accessory gearbox. A considerable series of trial fabrications were conducted to identify the proper fiber length needed to successfully fill the complicated press mold, plus provide adequate strength. The final design, shown in Fig. 13, was a press-molded shell with rib-stiffened integral flanges and separately bonded metal tubes for bearing lubrication. After two years, four forward portions of the accessory gearbox were fabricated and successfully tested. Testing consisted of static, bench, ballistic, and fire tests. The final

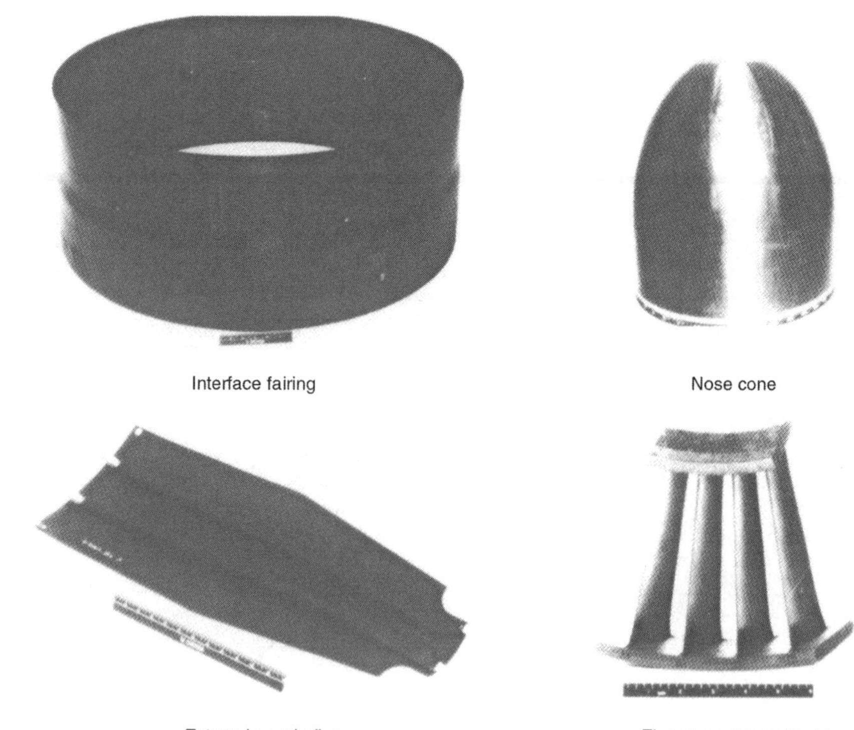

Fig. 16 Graphite fiber-PMR-15 composites on PW1120 and 1130 engines

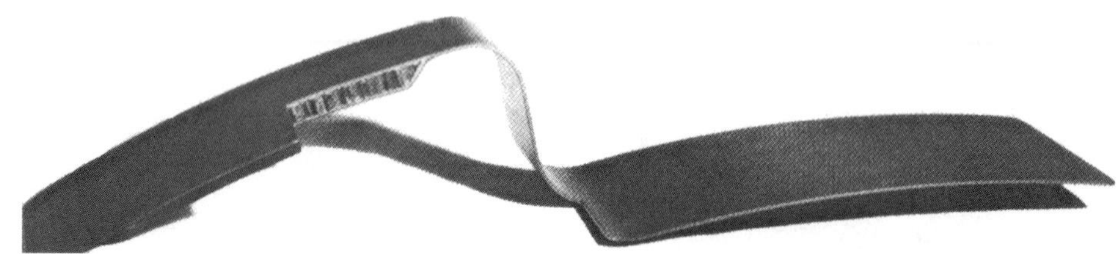

Fig. 17 Graphite fiber-PMR-15 sandwich structure

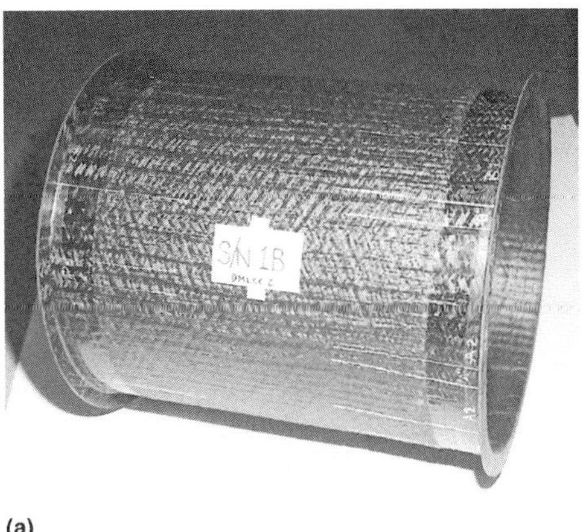

(a)

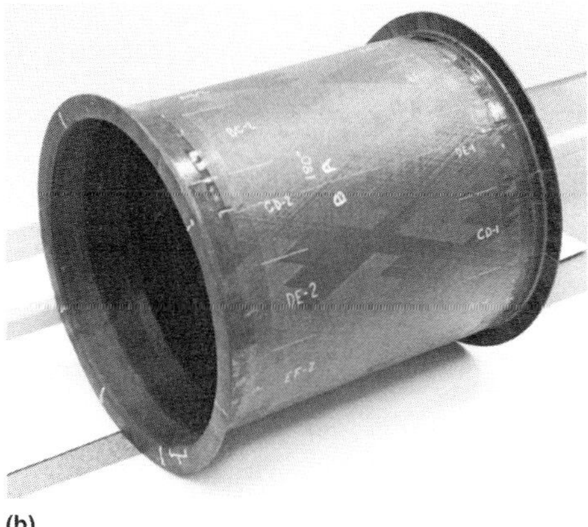
(b)

Fig. 18 DMLCC,E subscale ducts. (a) Carbon-PMR braided duct. (b) Carbon-PMR filament-wound duct

design demonstrated a 10% weight savings over the metal baseline.

Perhaps the largest single application of carbon-PMR structures occurred in the 1982 to 1989 time frame when the General Electric (GE) YF120 engine, shown in Fig. 14, incorporated a carbon-PMR front frame, fan case, stator vanes, and bypass ducts. All of these components were successfully static, engine, and flight tested. The front frame struts were hollow for air antiicing requirements, and the frame casing supported the variable flaps. The fan case bolted to the front and fan frames and supported the outer ends of the fan stator vanes. The bypass duct consisted of two structures. The forward duct was split into a top and bottom half, whereas the aft duct was a complete continuous casing.

Figure 15 shows "committed" and "potential" applications of graphite-PMR-15 composite materials on the PW1120 turbojet under development. A committed application is one for which a metal backup component is not being developed. The only committed applications for graphite-PMR-15 composites are the external nozzle flaps and the airframe interface ring. Graphite-PMR-15 external nozzle flaps are on the PW1130 turbofan engine. Figure 16 shows different components fabricated from graphite-PMR-15 for both the PW1120 and PW1130 engines (Ref 25).

Figure 17 shows a PMR-15 sandwich structure for which the skins were procured and then bonded to a glass-polyimide honeycomb using a commercially available adhesive based on PMR-15 (Ref 26). Interest has also been shown in applying PMR-15 composites to filament-wound structures. In 1985, a small, integrally flanged carbon-PMR conical shell was wet wound on a filament winder by Brunswick Corporation. Although this component lacked numerous details, it showed promise for future filament winding.

In 1990, GEAE was awarded an Air Force Manufacturing Technology program (F33615-91-C-5719) to significantly reduce the cost of high-temperature engine structures. The goal of the Design and Manufacturing of Low-Cost Composites for Engines (DMLCC,E) program was to reduce the cost of hand lay-up carbon-PMR bypass ducts by 50%. The program examined every aspect of duct design and incorporated numerous changes to reduce cost. The basic changes involved a new form of carbon-PMR material, automation, and a new axial flange design. In order to incorporate automation, the prepreg fabric had to be replaced with a new form of tow material. A preimidized tow was developed that allowed the material to be used on filament winders, braiders and tape placement machines. In order to satisfy all of the equipment requirements, 3 K, 6 K, and 12 K prepreg tows were manufactured and evaluated. The evaluation consisted of fabricating by filament winding, braiding, and tape placement on both cylindrical shells and integrally flanged subscale ducts, shown in Fig. 18. The shells were 50 cm (20 in.) in diameter and 90 cm (36 in.) long, and the subscale ducts were 50 cm (20 in.) in diameter and 75 cm (30 in.) long. Over 50 subcomponent shells and ducts were fabricated and tested. Testing consisted of buckling tests, flange subelement tests, and material property tests. Results of a down selection showed filament winding and braiding as viable alternatives. Tape placement results indicated continued development needs in manufacturing methods. In 1996, an Industry and Government team was formed to move the technology from subscale to a full-scale F110 production design. General Electric Aircraft Engines and Lincoln Composites teamed with the U.S. Air Force Manufac-

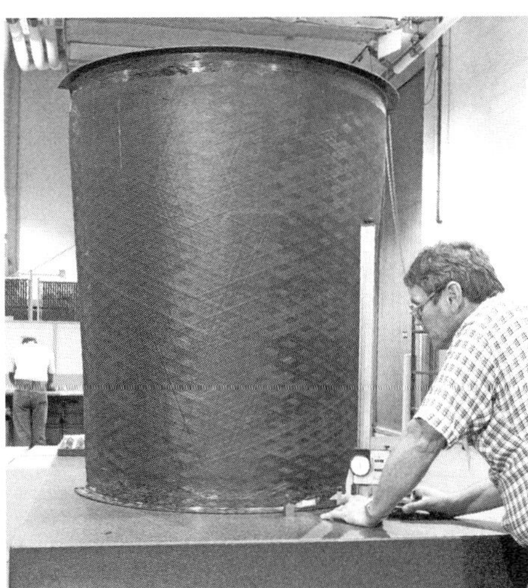

Fig. 19 F110 carbon-PMR filament-wound duct

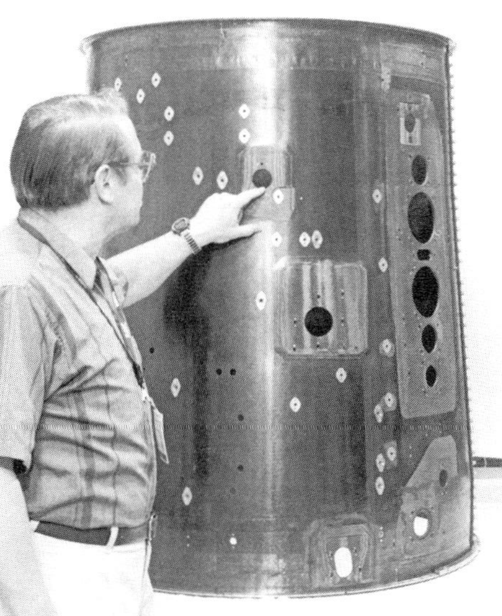

Fig. 20 F110 carbon-PMR hand lay-up fabric duct

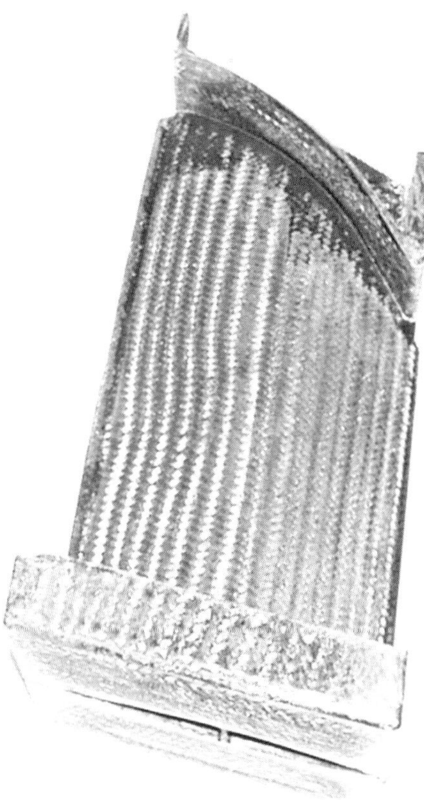

Fig. 21 Braided hollow fan frame strut

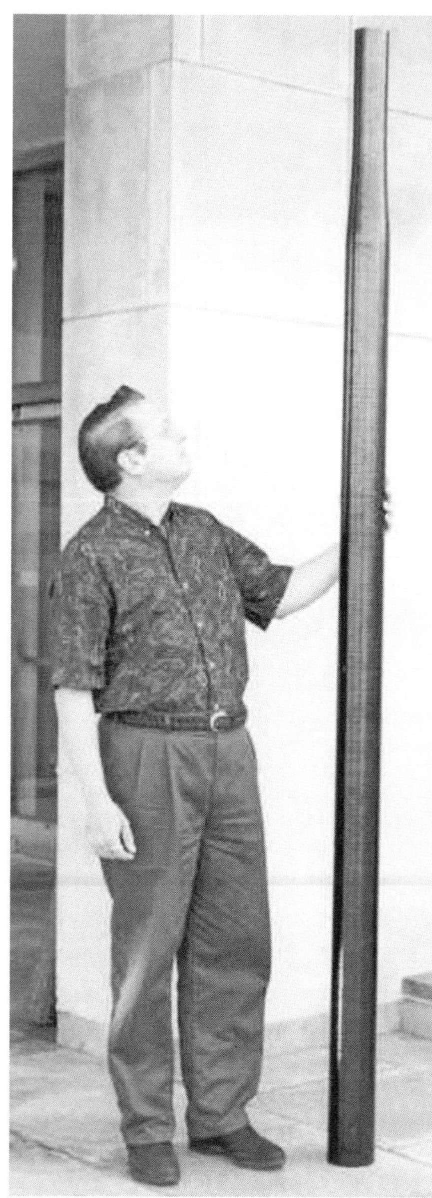

Fig. 22 Braided GE90 carbon-PMR vent tube

turing and Propulsion Directorates to design, fabricate, and test a full-scale bypass duct. Numerous towpreg production adjustments and filament-winding trials were conducted on subscale ducts and full-scale prototype tools. In late 2000, the first filament-wound, carbon-PMR, integrally flanged duct was fabricated, as shown in Fig. 19. In a parallel effort, GE also developed the hand lay-up carbon-PMR bypass duct, shown in Fig. 20. Both ducts are approximately 15% lighter than the current titanium duct. Structural and engine testing is ongoing for planned production in 2002. Results of this program can be found in Ref 27.

In 1996, the DMLCC,E program also explored solvent-assisted resin transfer molding (SaRTM) of braided preforms as a low-cost manufacturing method for carbon-PMR. Subcomponent frame struts shown in Fig. 21 were fabricated to assess manufacturability and structural viability. These struts demonstrated braided-SaRTM of carbon-PMR as a viable system for low-cost manufacturing. This success prompted a NASA Glenn-funded development program for an engine thrust link using the braided-SaRTM process. Under an internally funded program, GE investigated replacing the production hand lay-up GE90 center vent tube with the braided carbon-PMR tube, shown in Fig. 22.

ACKNOWLEDGMENT

This article is updated from T.T. Serafini, High-Temperature Applications, *Composites,* Volume 1, *Engineered Materials Handbook,* ASM International, 1987, p 810–815

REFERENCES

1. T.T. Serafini, P. Delvigs, and G.R. Lightsey, *J. Appl. Polm. Sci.,* Vol 16, 1972, p 905
2. T.T. Serafini, P. Delvigs, and G.R. Lightsey, U.S. Patent 3,745,149, 1973
3. T.T. Serafini, in *International Conference on Composite Materials,* E. Scala, Ed., Vol 1, American Institute of Mining, Metallurgical, and Petroleum Engineers, 1976, p 202
4. L.M. Poveromo, in *High Temperature Polymer Matrix Composites,* NASA CP2385, National Aeronautics and Space Administration, 1983, p 339
5. H.R. Lubowitz, Polyimide Polymers, U.S. Patent 3,528,950, Sept 1970
6. E.A. Burns, H.R. Lubowitz, and J.F. Jones. “Investigation of Resin Systems for Improved Ablative Materials,” NASA CR-72460, TRW-05937-6019-RO-00, TRW Systems Group, Oct 1968
7. P. Delvigs, T.T. Serafini, and G.R. Lightsey, NASA TN D-6877, National Aeronautics and Space Administration, 1972
8. F.I. Hurwitz, NASA TM-8 1580, National Aeronautics and Space Administration, 1980
9. R.J. Jones, R.W. Vaughan, and E.A. Burns. “Thermally Stable Laminating Resins,” NASA CR-72984, TRW-16402-6012-RO-00, TRW Systems Group, Feb 1972
10. A.C. Wong and W.M. Ritchey, *Macromolecules,* Vol 14 (No. 3), 1981, p 825
11. R.D. Vannucci, in *Materials and Processes—In-Service Performance,* Society for the Advancement of Material and Process Engineering, 1977, p 171
12. T.T. Serafini, P. Delvigs, and R.D. Vannucci, NASA TMX-8 1705, National Aeronautics and Space Administration, 1981
13. P. Delvigs, NASA TM-82958, National Aeronautics and Space Administration, 1982
14. R.H. Pater, NASA TM-82733, National Aeronautics and Space Administration, 1981
15. C.H. Sheppard and D. McLaren, in *High Temperature Polymer Matrix Composites,* NASA CP 2385, National Aeronautics and Space Administration, p 329
16. J.E. Halle, E.D. Burger, and R.E. Dundas, NASA CR-135 122, PWA-5487, Pratt and Whitney Aircraft, 1977
17. P.J. Cavano, NASA CR-134727, TRW-ER-7677-F, TRW Equipment Laboratories, 1974
18. L.A. Lottridge, Hamilton Standard Division, United Technologies, private communication
19. A.P. Adamson, in *Quiet Powered-Lift Propulsion,* NASA CP-2077, National Aeronautics and Space Administration, 1979, p 17
20. C.L. Ruggles, NASA CR-135279, R78AEG206, General Electric Company, 1978
21. C.L. Stotler, in *Quiet Powered-Lift Propulsion,* NASA CP-2077, National Aeronautics and Space Administration, 1979, p 83
22. C.L. Stotler, The 1980’s—Payoff Decade for Advanced Materials, *SAMPE Proc.,* 1980, p 176
23. A.J. Wilson, Aircraft Engine Business Group, General Electric Company, private communication
24. S.C. Harrier, S. Mitchell, and J.A. Saunders, USAAVRADCOM-TR-83-D20A and 20B, U.S. Army, 1983
25. T.E. Schmid, Pratt and Whitney Aircraft Group, private communication
26. R.A. Buchanan, Brunswick Corporation, Defense Division, private communication
27. S. Gowda and S. Mitchell, DMLCC,E Presentation, *SAMPE Proc.,* Society for the Advancement of Material and Process Engineering, 2000

Aircraft Applications

Mark Wilhelm, Boeing Commercial Airplane Company

FIBER-REINFORCED COMPOSITES have become an increasingly attractive alternative to metal for many aircraft components. Composites are strong, fatigue resistant, damage tolerant, and have been shown to be very durable when the design of the component includes proper consideration for the operating environment common to the component. They meet design and certification requirements and offer significant weight advantages. Composites also can provide significant cost reductions, especially when viewed in terms of aircraft life-cycle costs.

The composite materials used in the aircraft industry are generally reinforcing fibers or filaments embedded in a resin matrix. The most common fibers are carbon, aramid, and fiberglass, used alone or in hybrid combinations. Carbon fiber is replacing fiberglass as the most widely used reinforcement. The resin matrix is usually an epoxy-based system requiring curing temperatures between 120 and 180 °C (250 and 350 °F). Both past and current applications of fiber-reinforced composites in commercial and military aircraft are described in this article.

Early Commercial Applications

Contracts awarded in the early 1970s by the U.S. Air Force and the National Aeronautics and Space Administration (NASA) to investigate and encourage the use of composites resulted in the design, test, certification, and in-service use of a large number of composite components on commercial aircraft. Building on the contract and military experience, composites were incorporated into civil aircraft, such as the 757, 767, and 777. Table 1 summarizes these applications.

One example of these government-sponsored programs, the composite spoiler for the Boeing 737, was funded by the NASA Langley Research Center. Its design featured carbon-fiber-reinforced skins and end-closure ribs made of fiberglass. The other components of the spoiler, including the center hinge fitting, front spar sections, and honeycomb core, were existing aluminum parts. The composite spoiler was completely interchangeable with the standard aluminum version. By July 1973, the Boeing Commercial Airplane Company had placed 111 composite spoilers in regular airline service for evaluation; these were periodically removed and tested in laboratories. Construction details of the part are illuminated in Fig. 1.

Under a NASA contract, Lockheed-California Company manufactured three advanced composite fins for the L-1011 airliner. Shown in Fig.

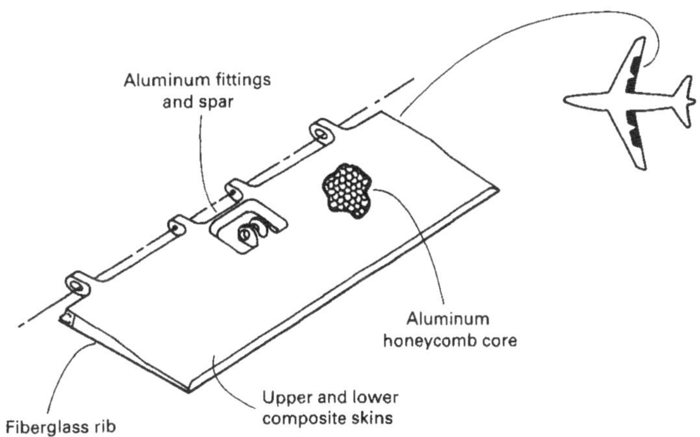

Fig. 1 Construction of Boeing 737/NASA composite spoiler. Length, 130 cm (52 in.); width, 56 cm (22 in.); surface area, 1.5 m^2 (15.8 ft^2); weight, 5 kg (12 lb)

Table 1 Composite components in various types of aircraft

Composite component	F-14	F-15	F-16	F-18	B-1	AV-8B	A340-500/600	ATR 72	757	767-400	777	Lear Fan
Doors	x	...	...	x	x	x	x	x	x	x	x	x
Rudder	...	x	...	...	...	x	x	x	x	x	x	x
Elevator	...	...	...	...	...	...	x	x	x	x	x	x
Vertical tail	...	x	x	x	x	x	x	x	...	...	x	x
Horizontal tail	x	x	x	x	x	x	x	x	...	...	x	x
Aileron	...	...	...	...	...	x	x	x	x	x	x	...
Spoiler	...	...	...	...	...	...	x	x	x	x	x	...
Flap	...	...	...	...	x	x	x	x	x	x	x	x
Wing box	...	...	...	x	...	x	...	x	...	...	...	x
Body	...	...	...	...	...	x	...	...	...	...	...	x
Fairings	x	...	...	x	...	x	x	x	x	x	x	x
Miscellaneous	...	Speed brake	...	Speed brake	Slats, inlet	...	Keel beam, aft pressure bulkhead, fan cowl doors	Nacelle components	Nacelle components	Raked wing tip, nacelle components	Floor beams, nacelle components	Propeller blades

2, the fin box configuration had a span of 760 cm (300 in.), a root chord of 270 cm (107 in.), and a tip chord of 120 cm (46 in.), for a surface area of 15 m^2 (150 ft^2). The box had 2 covers, 2 spars, and 11 ribs. The skins were co-cured in a single piece from a 180 °C (350 °F) curing tape material.

In the late 1970s, in reaction to the oil crisis, NASA created the Aircraft Energy Efficiency (ACEE) program. The NASA-ACEE funded a program for the McDonnell Douglas DC-10 upper aft rudder that resulted in the fabrication of 20 carbon-fiber-reinforced components for flight service evaluation. Furthermore, NASA-ACEE sponsored the design and fabrication of elevators and horizontal stabilizer boxes for the empennage of Boeing 727 and 737 jetliners. The 727 elevator shown in Fig. 3 is composed of one-piece upper and lower honeycomb skin panels, laminated front and rear spars, and honeycomb ribs. The program provided for fabrication of five slip sets for flight service evaluation, all of which were certified December 1979 and continue to be deployed on commercial aircraft. The composite components resulted in a weight reduction of 68 kg (150 lb), or 26%. The 737 horizontal stabilizer box shown in Fig. 4 was the first application of a composite primary structure on a Boeing commercial airplane. Five and one-half ship sets of stabilizer boxes were fabricated. All components were certified May 1981 and are still in commercial service. The stabilizer box shown in Fig. 5 consists of I-stiffened, laminated lower and upper skins mechanically fastened to laminated front and rear spin. The ribs are of a honeycomb sandwich-type construction and are very similar to those fabricated for the 727 carbon-fiber-reinforced epoxy elevator. A 22% weight savings (55 kg, or 116 lb) was achieved on the stabilizer box.

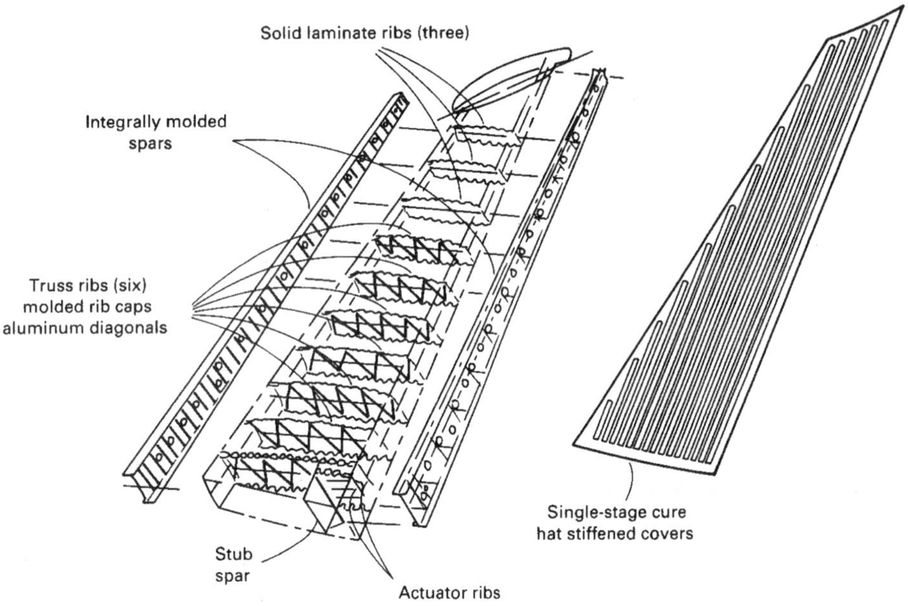

Fig. 2 L-1011 advanced composite vertical fin configuration

Current Production Aircraft

Composite components are used extensively on current commercial production aircraft such as the Boeing 757 and 767 and the Airbus A310, which employ about 1500 kg (3300 lb) each, while smaller planes such as the 737-300 use approximately 680 kg (1500 lb). Composite utilization on selected Boeing aircraft is listed in Table 2. While composite primary structure for the 737 horizontal stabilizer was certified in 1982, a follow-on production commitment was not made. In contrast, the vertical fin of the Airbus A310 was produced from carbon-reinforced epoxy as a production commitment and certified in 1985. In fact, the empennage primary structure for all Airbus models beginning with the A320 have been made from carbon/epoxy materials. Boeing's reentry into primary composite structure occurred on the 777 empennage (Fig. 6 and 7). To support the certification process, a total of 8059 material coupon and element tests were conducted. The 777-200 was certified jointly by United States and European regulatory

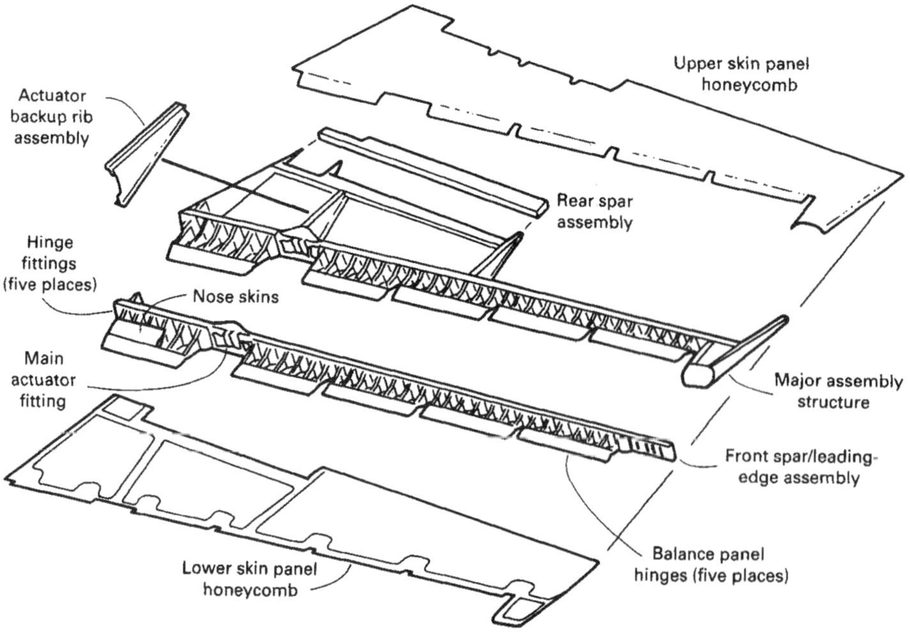

Fig. 3 Boeing 727 elevator structural arrangement

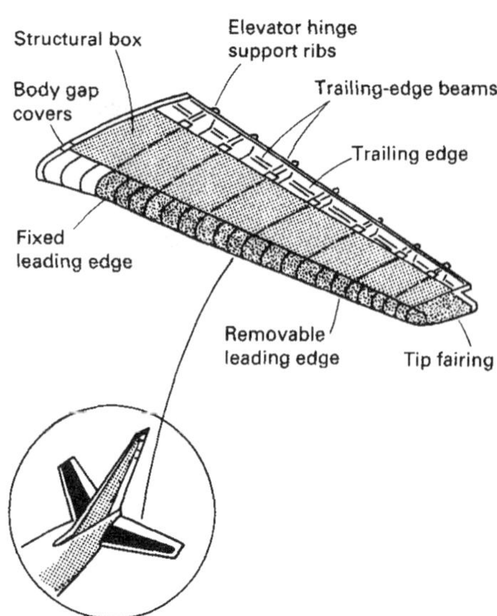

Fig. 4 Boeing 737 composite stabilizer box

agencies in April 1995. This aircraft was the first to enter commercial service with approval for extended range twin engine operations. The composite utilization for the 777-200 is shown in Fig. 8. Excluding the payload (interiors), each aircraft contains approximately 7450 kg (16,400 lb) of carbon- and fiberglass-composite material; 71% of this amount is carbon reinforced. The majority of the carbon/epoxy quantity is an intermediate modulus fiber impregnated with a toughened epoxy-based matrix used in floor beams, the horizontal stabilizer, and the vertical fin.

On the 737, composites are used for control surfaces, fairings, and nacelle components for about 3% of the total structural weight of the aircraft. Individual composite parts are 20 to 30% lighter than their metallic counterparts.

Small, general aviation airplanes make extensive use of advanced composites. The Lear Fan 2100 uses carbon-, glass-, and aramid-fiber materials totaling approximately 820 kg (1800 lb) per aircraft. The Beech Starship I includes approximately 1360 kg (3000 lb) of composites.

With the exception of small detail parts, empennage primary structure spars, and skin panels, most composite components for commercial airplanes are of honeycomb sandwich construction. These may be either full-depth designs, such as the 767 outboard aileron shown in Fig. 9, or structures built of separate panels, such as the 767 rudder in Fig. 10. The 767 rudder is approximately 11 m (36 ft) long and 3 m (8 ft) in chord width at the root. Both examples use 177 °C (350 °F) curing materials. This elevated-temperature cure provides the most environmentally durable composite, particularly in its strength and modulus retention after moisture and thermal exposure.

Figure 11 shows a Boeing 757 as a typical example of composites used for an engine nacelle. Because the structure is in close proximity to the power plant, 177 °C (350 °F) curing materials are generally employed.

Structures such as fairings, fixed wing, and empennage trailing-edge panels are generally fabricated as a sandwich. Facesheets for these panels are made of carbon fiber or carbon fiber combined with aramid or fiberglass fabric. Such panels most often employ self-adhesive 120 °C (250 °F) curing systems. Phenolic-coated fiberglass or Nomex (DuPont) honeycomb core is used. The panels are fabricated in a single-stage curing process that provides significant cost advantages in addition to weight savings as a result of the use of self-adhesive prepregs.

Table 2 Examples of advanced composites use and associated weight savings in commercial aircraft

Model	Total advanced composites		Weight savings	
	kg	lb	kg	lb
737-300	681	1500	272	600
757	1516	3340	676	1490
767	1535	3380	636	1400

Composites are also widely used in the interiors of commercial aircraft. In addition to meeting mechanical property and processibility requirements, all materials used within the pressurized portion of the aircraft must meet both the flammability-resistance requirements defined by regulatory agencies and, if applicable, smoke and toxic-gas emission guidelines of the airframe manufacturers. Additionally, visible portions of interior components must meet stringent aesthetic requirements to satisfy the airlines and their customers.

Interior parts, such as overhead luggage compartments, sidewalls, ceilings, floors, galleys, lavatories, partitions, cargo liners, and bulkheads are routinely made of composite components. In general, these are fiber-reinforced epoxy or phenolic resin honeycomb sandwich constructions. The phenolic resin system is used because of its excellent fire-resistant properties, including low flammability and low smoke and toxic gas emissions. The predominant design considerations for interior components are impact resistance, stiffness, and surface smoothness.

The choice of fiber depends not only on structural requirements, but on part contour and fabrication method. For relatively flat parts, unidirectional or woven fabrics can be used. For compound contours, stretchable, knitted fabrics are often necessary. The predominant fiber used in interior composites is fiberglass; however, carbon fiber use is increasing as structural applications increase. For example, a filament-wound door spring is employed on the 767. Using unidirectional carbon fibers in an epoxy matrix, the springs are only one-third as heavy as comparable steel springs and only half the weight of state-of-the art titanium springs.

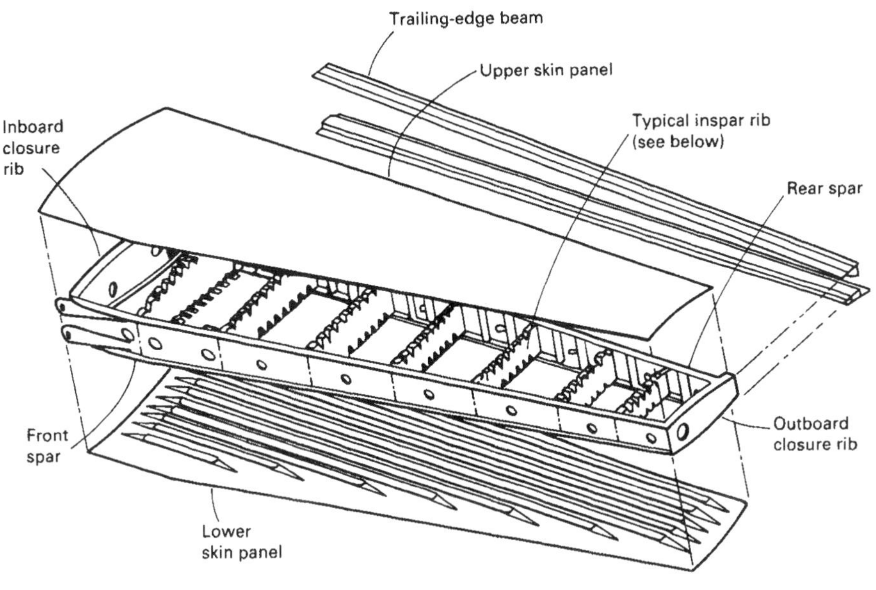

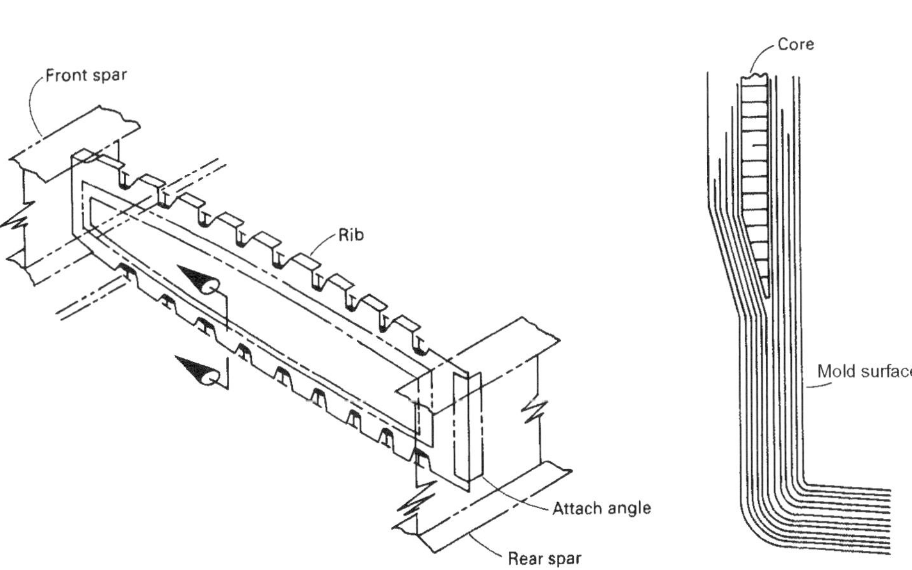

Fig. 5 Boeing 737 horizontal stabilizer assembly

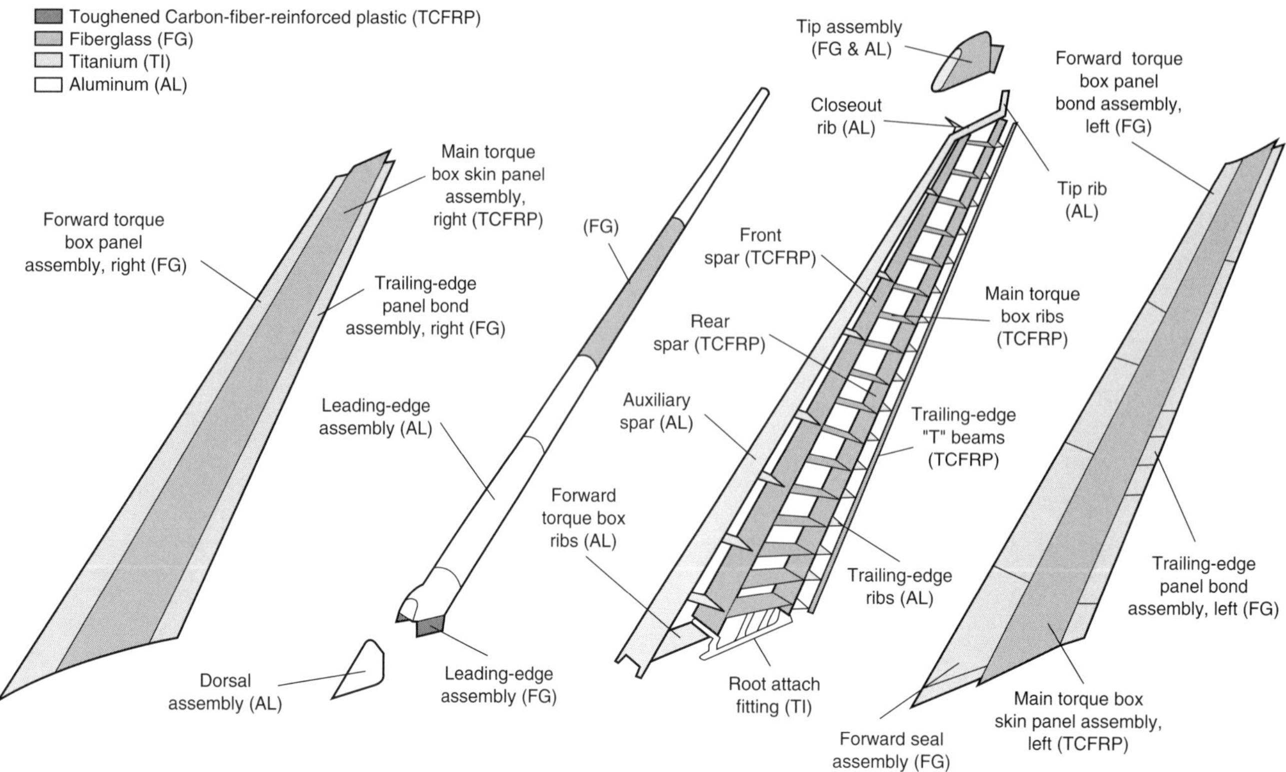

Fig. 6 Boeing 777 vertical fin

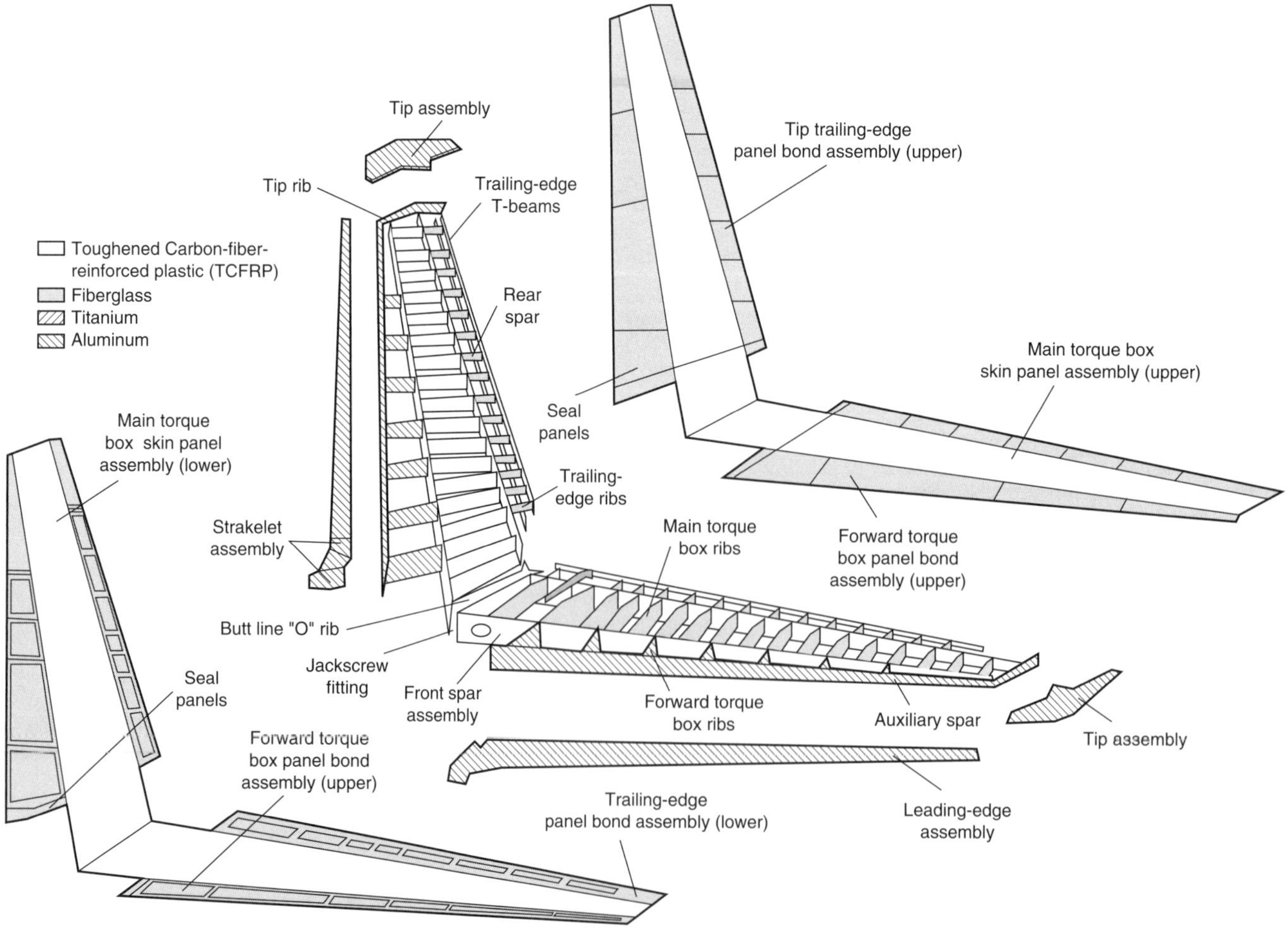

Fig. 7 Boeing 777 horizontal stabilizer

Military Applications

U.S. Military Applications. In the United States, the largest application by far of composite material is for military programs, which constitute more than 40% of the aerospace total. Most military aircraft applications use carbon-fiber-reinforced epoxy composites.

About 26% of the structural weight of the U.S. Navy's AV-8B is carbon-fiber-reinforced composites. Components include the wing box, forward fuselage, horizontal stabilizer, elevators, rudder and other control surfaces, and over-wing fairings. The wing skins are one piece tip-to-tip laminate, mechanically fastened to a multispar composite substructure; the design of the horizontal stabilizer is similar to that of the wing. Approximately 590 kg (1300 lb) of carbon-fiber epoxy is used on the AV-8B, providing a weight reduction of almost 225 kg (500 lb).

On the F-18 aircraft, carbon-fiber-reinforced composites make up approximately 10% of the structural weight and more than 50% of the surface area, as illustrated in Fig. 12. They are used in the wing skins, the horizontal and vertical tail boxes, the wing and tail control surfaces, the speed brake, the leading-edge extension, and various doors. The F-18 composite wing skins are solid laminate; their thickness varies from root to tip, with a minimum thickness of about 2 mm (0.08 in.). The tail primary structure is similar in construction.

The B-1B bomber employs a number of composite structural components. Shown in Fig. 13, these include the dorsal longeron, weapons bay doors, aft equipment bay doors, and flaps. All of the materials, including adhesives, are 180 °C (350 °F) curing systems. The structures include laminate, full-depth honeycomb-reinforced panels, and composite facesheets bonded to aluminum core. The weapons bay doors shown in Fig. 14 employ carbon-fiber-reinforced tape facesheets, aluminum honeycomb core, and titanium fittings. Because the doors are in a position that is particularly vulnerable to foreign object damage, an aramid-fiber-reinforced phenolic outer layer provides penetration resistance. At a production rate of four aircraft per month, the B-1B uses 127,000 kg (280,000 lb) per year of composite structure—3040 kg (6700 lb) per aircraft—resulting in weight savings of approximately 1360 kg (3000 lb) on each bomber.

Grumman Aerospace Corporation fabricates F-14A horizontal stabilizers from a boron-fiber-reinforced composite material. The stabilizers are moving surfaces that pivot about shafts that protrude from the fuselage; each has an area of 6.5 m^2 (70 ft^2), with a thickness chord ratio of 5% at the root and 3% at the tip. The stabilizer consists of the main structural box, leading- and trailing-edge sections, and tip. The latter three components have conventional aluminum skins over a full-depth aluminum honeycomb core. The main box is a boron-fiber-reinforced composite structure consisting of the root rib, two intercostals, outer bearing, outboard rib, front and rear beams, tip rib, honeycomb core, and two covers. Figure 15 shows the front and rear beams and the root tip, which are of fiberglass construction. The stabilizer was designed so that there are no mechanical fasteners through the boron. In regions of high shear transfer between the substructure and cover, titanium is carried over the areas to distribute load, and the stabilizer is mechanically fastened. In regions of reduced loads, bonded joints are employed. A unique feature of this structure is a bonded splice at the pivot region (Fig. 16). The total weight of the stabilizer is 350 kg (778 lb), a savings of approximately 20%.

The F-16 employs a carbon-fiber-reinforced epoxy horizontal stabilizer, vertical stabilizer, leading-edge, and rudder in the empennage of the fighter. The vertical stabilizer structural box is a multispar, multirib, laminate skin design. The horizontal stabilizer (Fig. 17) has composite skins with aluminum honeycomb core.

Another program that employed a considerable amount of composite material is the A-6 wing replacement program. In the A-6 program, high-flight-time metal wings were being replaced by lighter composite wings with improved fatigue characteristics and much greater resistance to corrosion. The A-6 wing was being

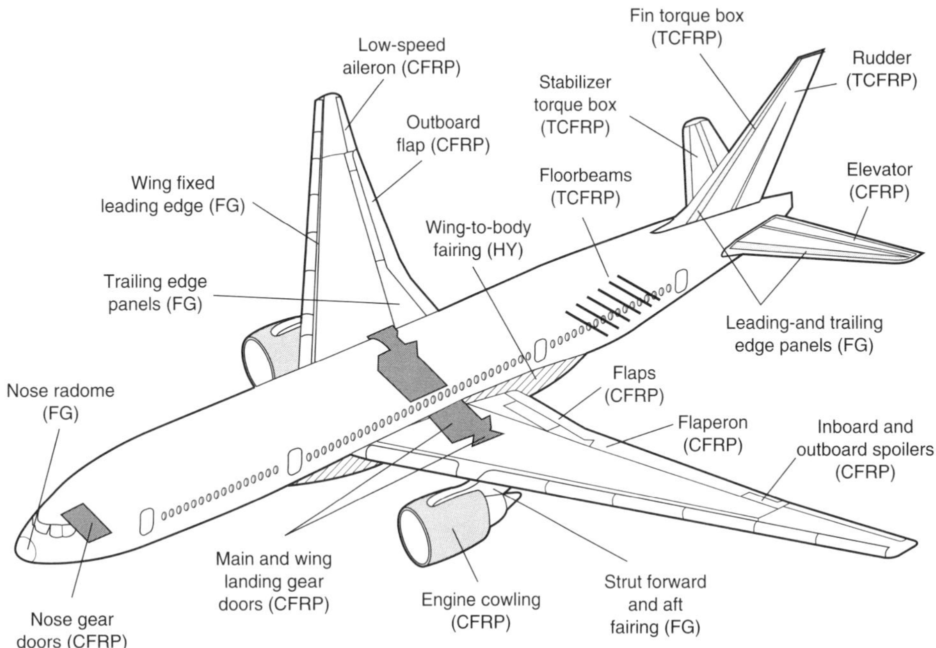

Fig. 8 Composites use on the Boeing 777-200. CFRP, carbon fiber reinforced plastic; TCFRP, toughened CFRP; FG, fiberglass; HY, hybrid

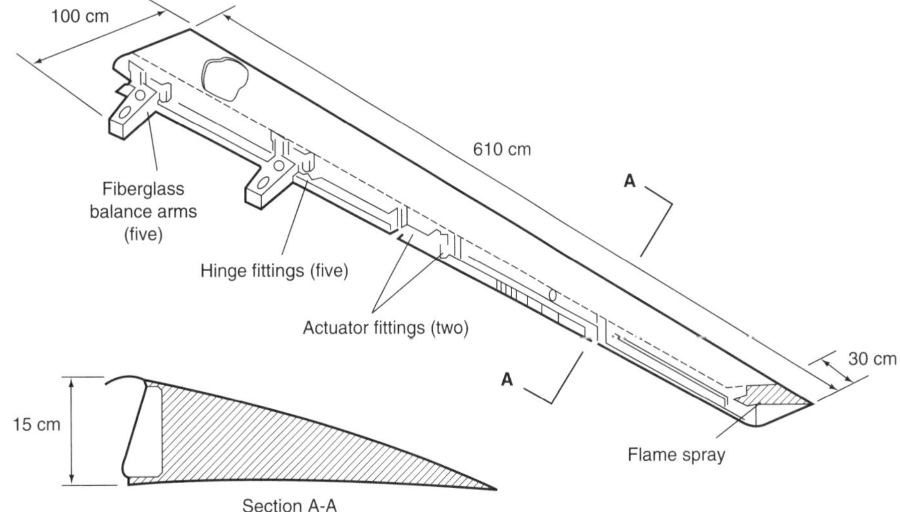

Fig. 9 Boeing 767 outboard aileron

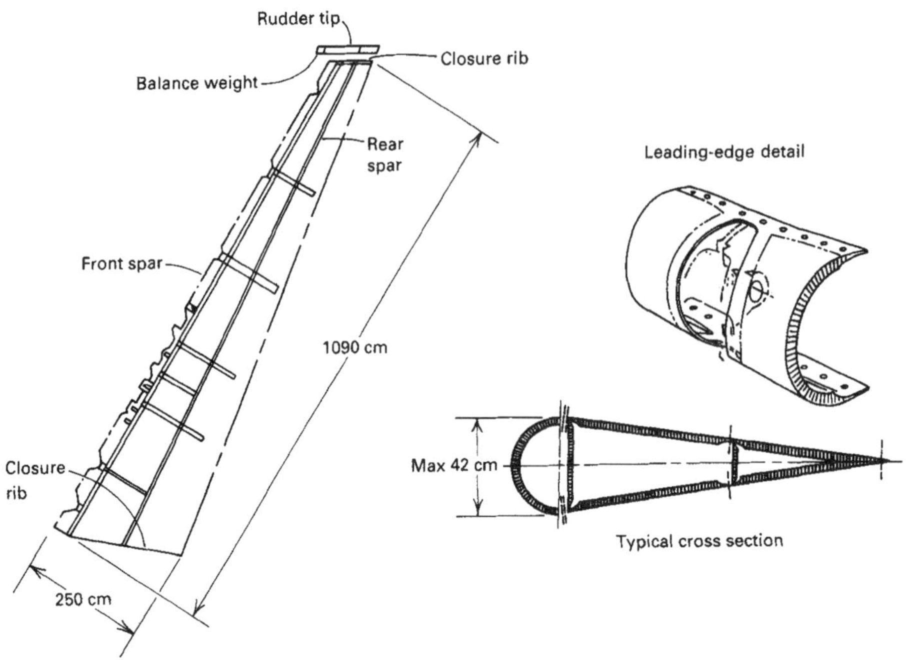

Fig. 10 767 carbon-fiber-reinforced epoxy rudder

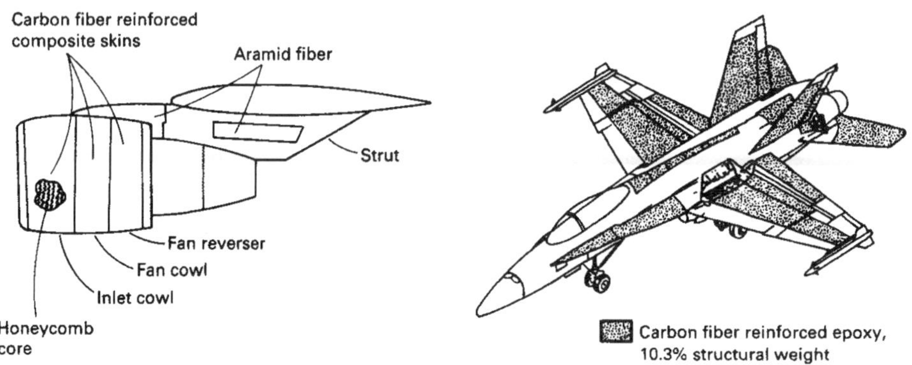

Fig. 11 757 engine strut applications

Fig. 12 F-18 composites applications

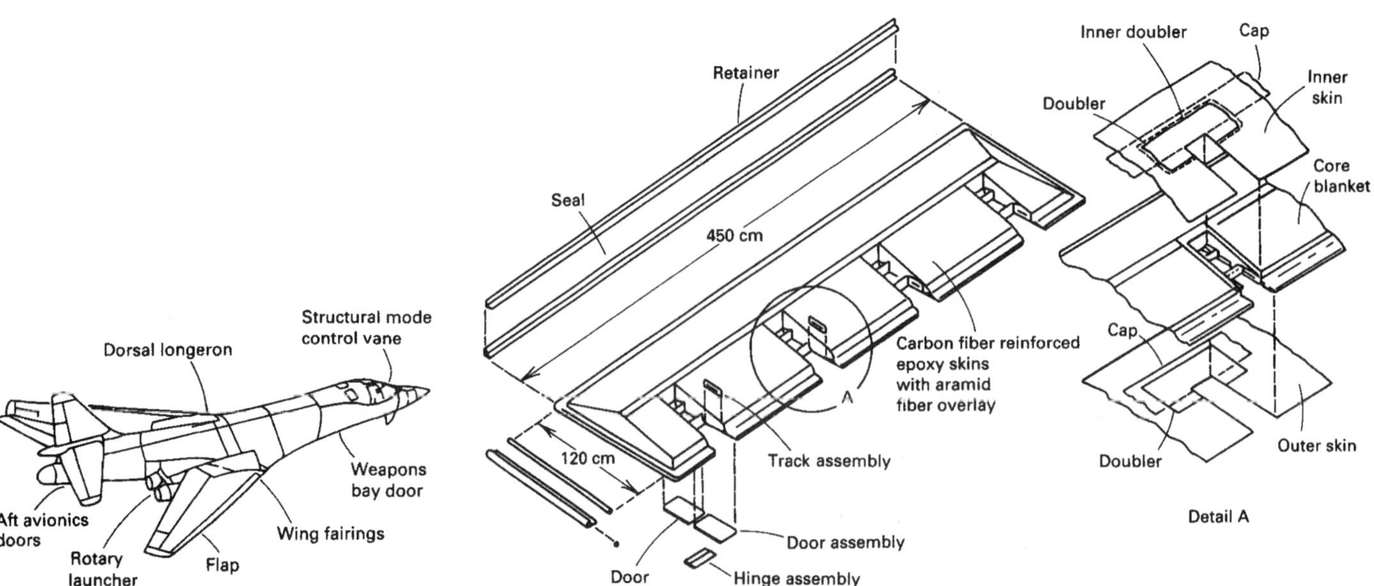

Fig. 13 B-1B composite applications

Fig. 14 B-1B weapons bay door

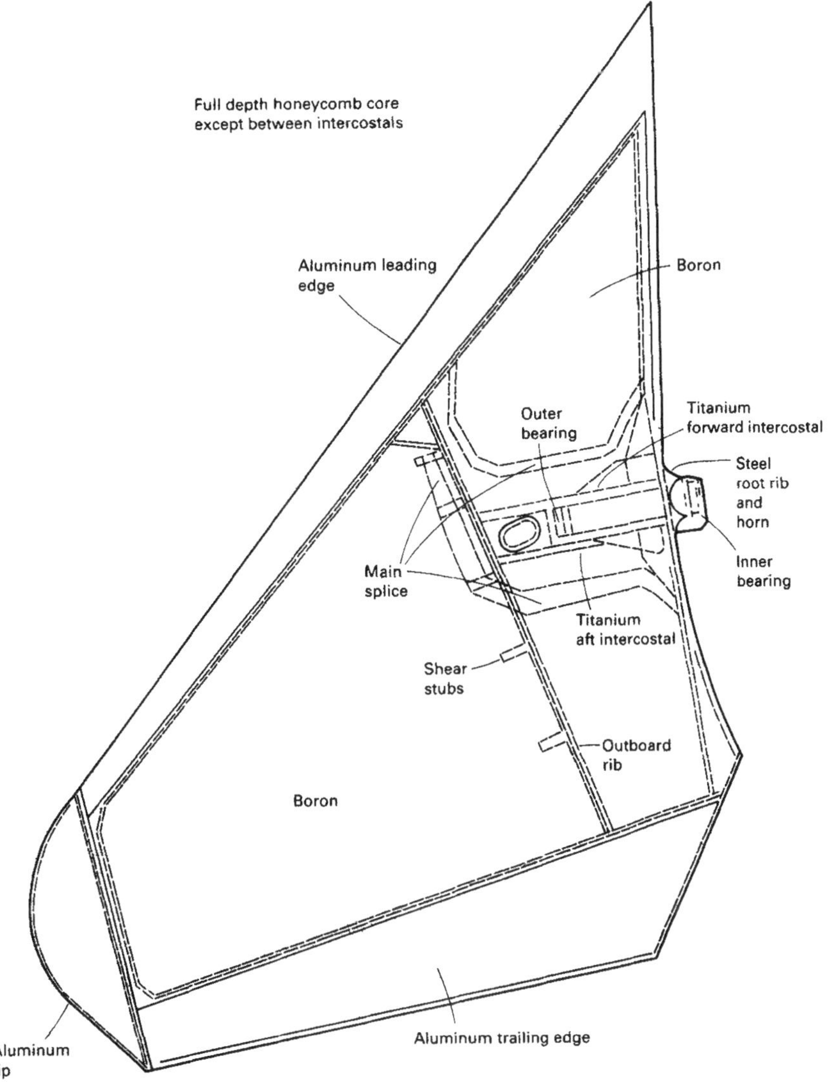

Fig. 15 F-14A boron-epoxy stabilizer, plan view

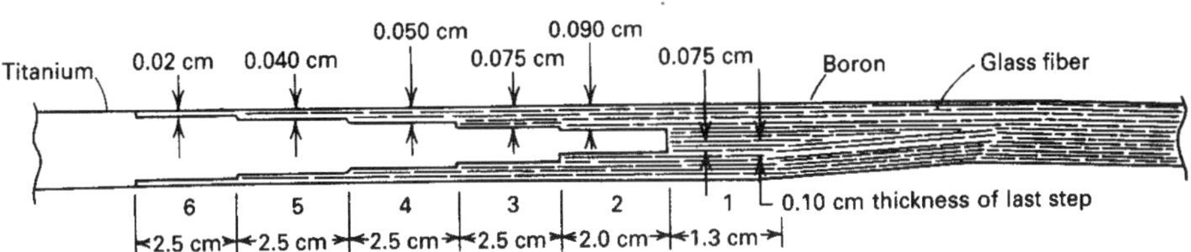

Fig. 16 Section through main splice of the F-14A stabilizer

designed and built by Boeing Military Airplane Company. The A-6 replacement program requires a wing structural box made of carbon-fiber-reinforced epoxy. Figure 18 shows the design configuration of laminate skin fastened to composite intermediate ribs and spars, with titanium front and rear spars, and inboard and outboard lank end ribs. The skin panels were manufactured in a single piece using a 180 °C (350 °F) curing tape material.

The V-22 Osprey aircraft is an innovative design that combines the advantages of the vertical takeoff and landing of a helicopter with the smooth, high-speed cruise and extended range of a fixed-wing airplane. The V-22 engines and propellers are vertically oriented for takeoff and landing, then pivot forward for cruise, with conventional wing surfaces providing aerodynamic lift. The V-22 wing panels have integrally stiffened laminate skins. The fuselage of the V-22 (Fig. 19) is also made of composite materials that make up 50% of its structural weight.

European Military Application (the Eurofighter). On the Typhoon (Eurofighter) aircraft, carbon-fiber-reinforced composites make up approximately 30% of the structural weight and more than 70% of the surface area, as illustrated in Fig. 20. Almost all components are made of a 185 °C (365 °F) curing system (Hexcel 8552 toughened epoxy, Hexcel Corp.). Primary structures are made from unidirectional prepregs. Secondary structures may have portions of fabric prepregs.

The skins of the wing (Fig. 21) are solid laminate, with thicknesses varying from root to tip between about 20 and 4 mm (0.8 and 0.16 in.). They are laminated by automated tape laying. During manufacturing, the wing skins are cured first. Afterwards, the solid laminate spars are cured and simultaneously bonded to the already cured lower skin in a second autoclave cycle (co-bonding process).

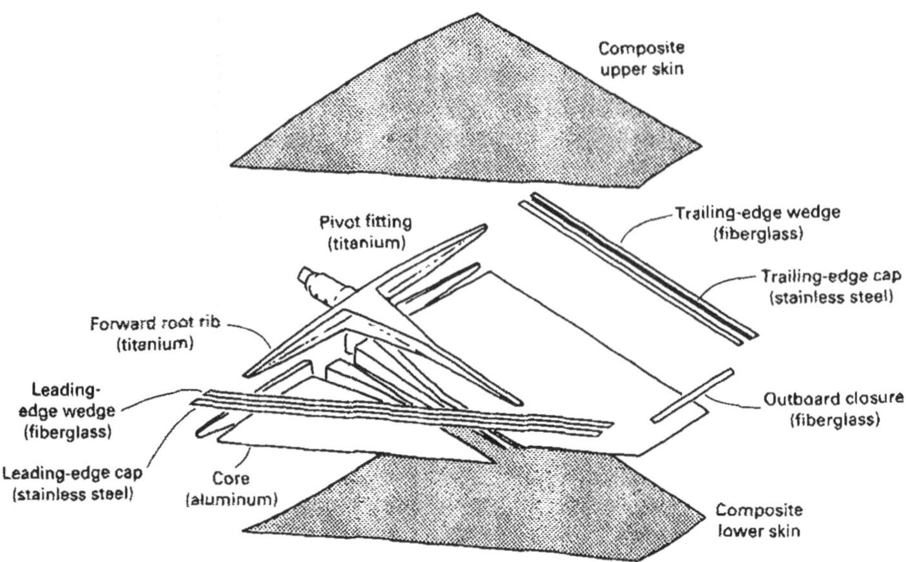

Fig. 17 F-16 composite horizontal stabilizer

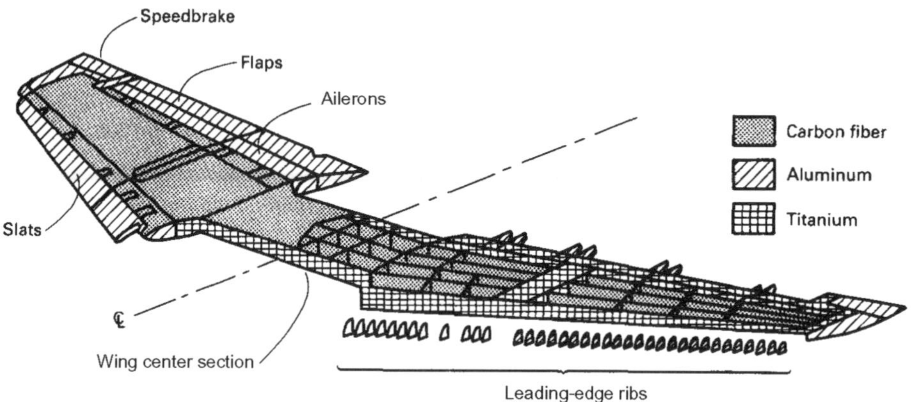

Fig. 18 A-6 composite wing

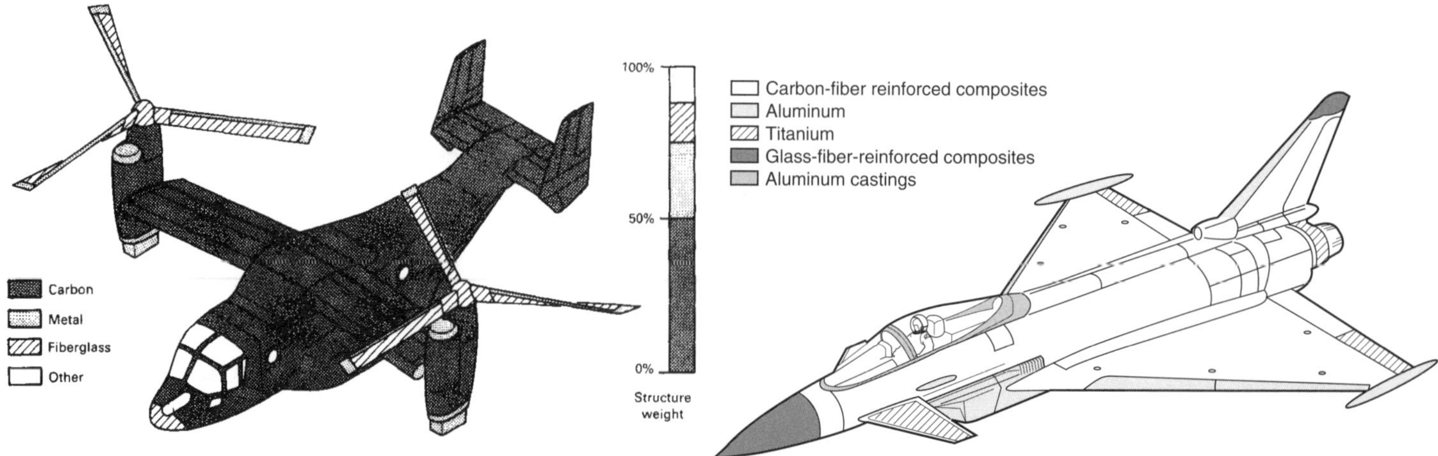

Fig. 19 V-22 material applications. Structure (wing, fuselage, empennage, nacelle, rotor): 6120 kg (13,496 lb). Carbon epoxy: 3100 kg (6856 lb)

Fig. 20 Materials use in the Typhoon (Eurofighter) airplane

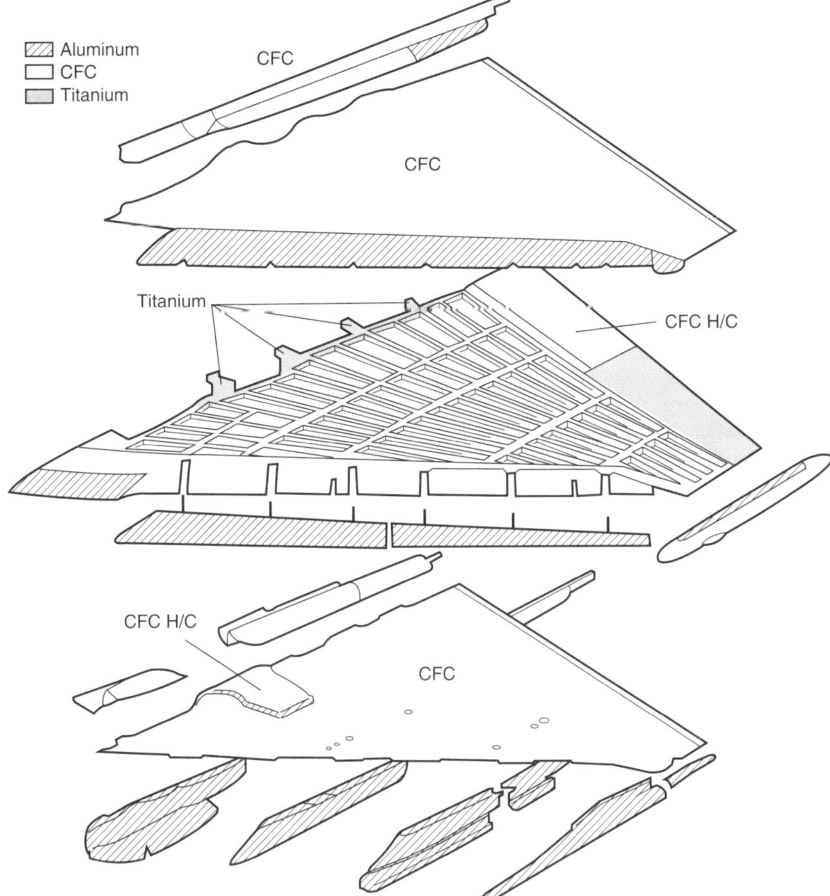

Fig. 21 Typhoon wing. CFC, carbon-fiber composite; H/C, honeycomb

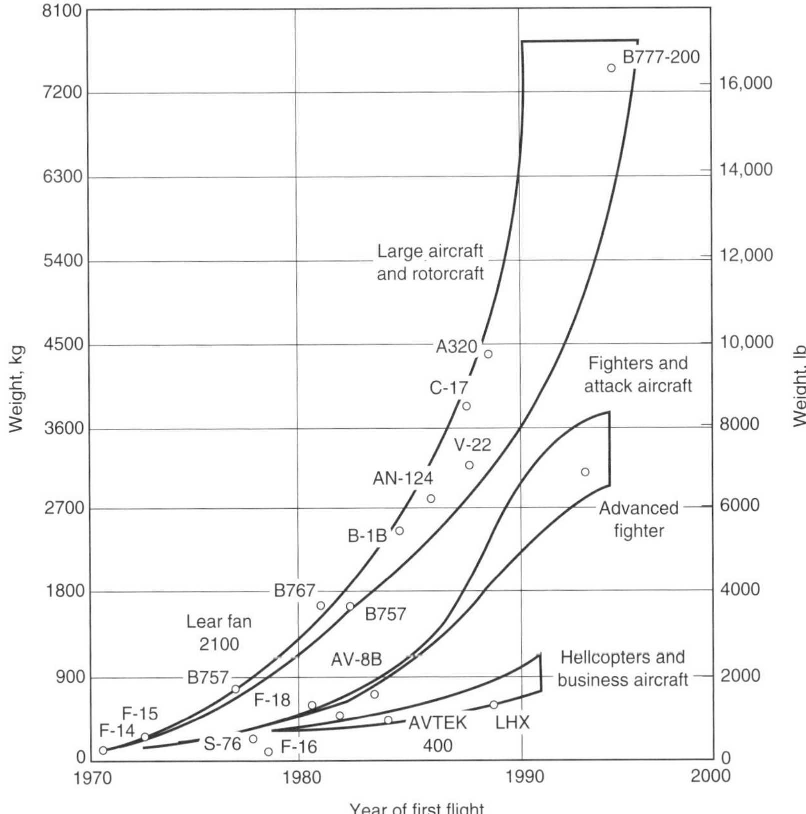

Fig. 23 Composite aircraft structure by weight

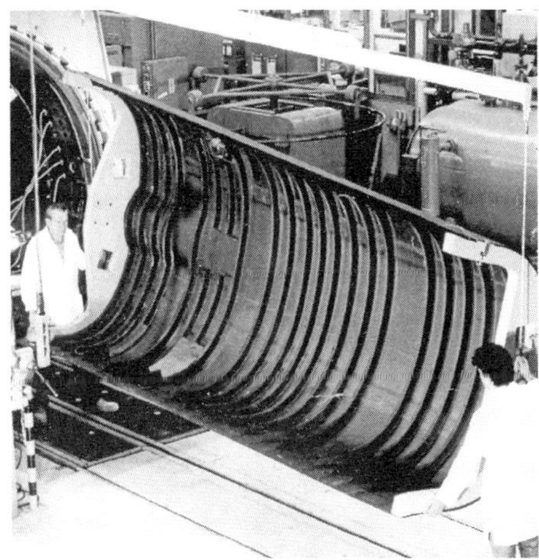

Fig. 22 Typhoon center fuselage skin with J-stiffeners

The center fuselage skin (Fig. 22) is integrally J-stiffened solid laminate, with thicknesses varying between 11 and 3.5 mm (0.43 and 0.14 in.). During manufacturing, the skin and the stiffeners are jointly cured in one autoclave cycle (co-curing process).

Fin, rudder, in-board aileron, and airbrake have skins of solid laminate. For rudder and in-board aileron, the substructure also is solid laminate. Sandwich panels are used for the side skins of the forward fuselage, the upper and side skins of the rear fuselage, the landing gear doors and for load-carrying covers of the center fuselage.

Outlook

Trends clearly indicate that the use of composite structures will continue to grow in both commercial and military aircraft. New materials, with both improved properties and increased suitability to new automated processes, will result in weight savings and cost competitiveness with traditional metal structures. Figure 23 depicts the rapid increase of composites in aircraft and an implied projection of increase in use.

However, factors that may inhibit wider use of composites include cost, schedule, capital investment, and inspectability. Furthermore, unexpected variations in raw materials and poorly defined cost data, as well as a lack of uniform, industry-wide specifications, test techniques, environmental conditioning, standards, and design allowables all combine to create a degree of conservatism at this time. Because of these factors, a detailed business case must be prepared and analyzed in order to ensure selection of composites for applications for which they are technically and economically most appropriate.

From a commercial aircraft manufacturing perspective, the change in approach from the 1960s (technology rules) to the early 1970s (oil crisis) to the present (focus on shareholder and customer value) has been monumental. Technology for technology's sake and designs that consider only minimizing component weight are not relevant in the marketplace of 2001. The emergence of business-case analysis applied to potential projects has interjected needed discipline into the technology development process. Likewise, knowledge of the composite value chain enables analysis of new technology and its potential to reduce cost and create value along the chain. Early involvement of existing and potential customers has been shown to be an effective tool to define composite utilization opportunities as well as to bring needed lessons learned from customer experiences.

The need to predict and understand design and fabrication costs continues to be important. It is apparent that currently employed cost collection systems do not adequately capture costs at a low enough level. As a result, this situation is responsible for data being suboptimal when used for value chain or business-cases development. Additionally, cost data is typically treated as proprietary information—not only outside, but also often within organizations. Lack of detailed cost information complicates the analysis and identification of cost-reduction opportunities. It is imperative that these obstacles be eliminated in order to make meaningful inroads in the quest for cost reduction.

For commercial aircraft, a critical success factor is to ensure that certification via the appropriate regulatory agency is an integral part of any development program. The certification requirement forces the program structure to think of the big picture in terms of developing the necessary engineering and manufacturing data. An example of how this was successfully accomplished was demonstrated during the Boeing/NASA-ACEE program described in this article.

ACKNOWLEDGMENTS

Portions of this article have been adapted from J.M. Anglin, Aircraft Applications, *Composites,* Volume 1, *Engineered Materials Handbook,* ASM International, 1987, p 801–809. ASM International wishes to thank Hans-Wolfgang Schröder, EADS Deutschland GmbH, for providing information about the Typhoon (Eurofighter) aircraft.

SELECTED REFERENCES

- *DOD/NASA Advanced Composites Design Guide,* Volume III, U.S. Air Force Flight Dynamics Laboratory, July 1983
- A. Fawcett, J. Trostle, and S. Ward, "777 Empennage Certification Approach," Boeing internal documentation 130344, Boeing Commercial Airplane Group, Seattle, WA
- R.N. Hadcock, "Status and Viability of Composite Materials in Structures of High Performance Aircraft," paper presented to the National Research Council Aeronautics and Space Engineering Board, Naval Postgraduate School, Monterey, CA, Feb 1986
- L.G. Hansen, D. Lossee, and W.L. O'Brien, Advanced Composites Applications for the B-1B Bomber—An Overview, *Proc. 31st International SAMPE Symposium,* Society for the Advancement of Material and Process Engineering, 1986
- J.K. Kuno, Growth of the Advanced Composites Industry in the 1980s, *Proc. 31st International SAMPE Symposium,* Society for the Advancement of Material and Process Engineering, 1986
- J.E. McCarty, R.W. Johnson, and D.R. Wilson, "737 Graphite-Epoxy Horizontal Stabilizer Certification," AIAA 82-0745, American Institute of Aeronautics and Astronautics
- J.C. McMillan and J.T. Quinlivan, Commercial Aircraft Applications, *Advanced Thermosets Composites,* J.M. Margolis, Ed., Van Nostrand Reinhold, 1986
- M.M. Schwartz, *Composite Materials,* Volume II, *Processing, Fabrication, and Applications,* Prentice-Hall, 1997
- S.A. Zervas-Berg, Composites for Applications in Aircraft, *Chem. Eng. Prog.,* June 1986

Applications of Carbon-Carbon Composites

Kristen M. Kearns, Materials and Manufacturing Directorate, Air Force Research Laboratory

CARBON-CARBON COMPOSITES have historically been utilized for applications requiring ablation and high-temperature stability (i.e., rocket nozzles and exit cones) or wear resistance at moderate temperatures (i.e., aircraft brakes). These applications utilize thicker materials with moderate mechanical-performance requirements. The processes that have been developed for these thick material applications are tailored to produce a dense material with the required properties. The processes typically include fabricating some type of organic composite preform, heating that preform to high temperature to decompose the organic material to carbon (referred to as carbonization), and then infiltrating the composite to fill the gaps left after decomposition (referred to as densification). The carbonization and densification processes can be repeated as many times as needed until the materials reach the desired density.

Beginning in the mid-1980s, carbon-carbon was considered for applications requiring a stiff, structural material with very thin walls. This interest has led to the investigation into other properties of carbon that could be exploited in a carbon-carbon composite. One area that has been explored is carbon-carbon for thermal management. Many systems require heat control, either by rejecting or by absorbing "waste heat energy." This has led to much interest in carbon-carbon for such applications as electronic thermal planes; spacecraft thermal doublers, radiators, and thermal and shields; and aircraft heat exchangers.

Material Properties

Carbon has many characteristics that are appealing for many different thermal management applications. Carbon has a very low density, a tailorable thermal conductivity, and very low thermal expansion with acceptable mechanical properties. This means a carbon composite can be fabricated with high specific thermal conductivity and low thermal expansion. These properties are very desirable for many different thermal management applications.

Typical mechanical properties of carbon-carbon are shown in Fig. 1. These plots show the range of specific strength and modulus (actual modulus divided by the density) of a variety of carbon-carbon materials. Due to the fibers used in carbon-carbon composites used for thermal management applications, typical tensile strengths are approximately 70 to 280 MPa (10–40 ksi) and moduli are about 70 to 175 GPa (10 to 25 $\times 10^6$ psi) for two-dimensional isotropic (0/90/$\pm$45), woven composites.

For many thermal management applications it is desirable to have a material that has a very low thermal expansion or a thermal expansion close to the material to which it is bonding or attaching. Figure 2 shows how the thermal expansion of carbon compares to other metallic materials. Notice there is a range of values for carbon because it is not isotropic like the other materials.

Another important material property for thermal management is the thermal conductivity. Most applications need a material with good thermal conductivity and low mass; thus the specific thermal conductivity (conductivity/density) of various materials is shown in Fig. 3 below. It can be seen that metallic materials are isotropic, while the composite materials are directionally conductive. Composite thermal conductivity is achieved primarily from fiber contribution. An organic-matrix composite is essentially a thermal insulator through the thickness. The difference in the through-thickness and fiber direction (in-plane) conductivity of the carbon-carbon composite is due to the alignment of the carbon planes within the matrix versus the fiber. Typical pitch-derived fibers, such as P100 and K1100, possess well-aligned carbon/graphite planes within their microstructure (the greater the alignment the higher the thermal conductivity). Because the carbon/graphite planes are deposited semirandomly during processing, the matrix has no orderly alignment. This lack of alignment results in reduced thermal conductivity in the carbon matrix compared to the carbon fibers.

Applications

Electronic Thermal Planes. One of the first thermal management applications investigated for carbon-carbon was thermal planes for electronics. A thermal plane dissipates the heat from the electronic board to keep the chips at a temperature at which they can properly operate. The thermal plane also must not expand too much under heat loads so that it does not induce loads

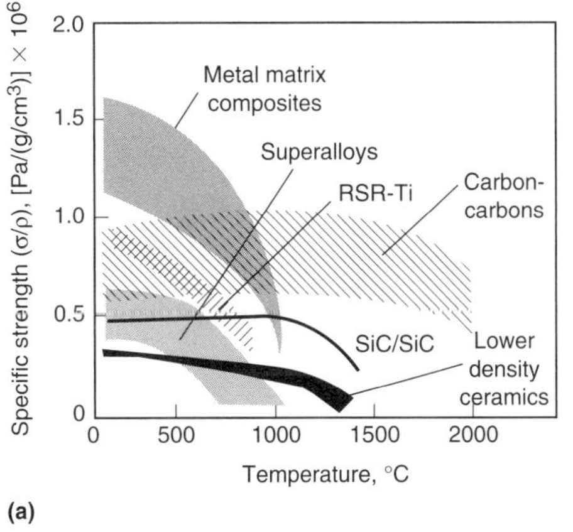

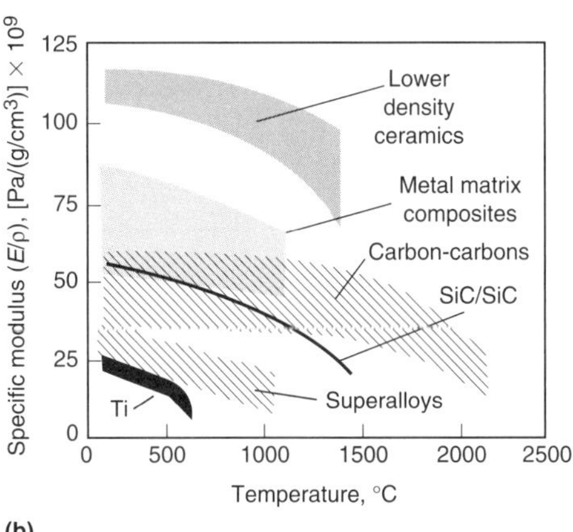

Fig. 1 Specific strength (a) and modulus (b) of carbon-carbon composites

that wear the joints that attach the chips to the electronic board. Therefore, the thermal plane material must have high thermal conductivity as well as low thermal expansion. In addition, high stiffness material results in less vibration transmitted to the electronic board and thus a reduction in fatigue on the joints as well as reduced deflections. If the electronic boards do not deflect under loading, they can be packed together more closely without risk of impact. This allows a designer to get more electronic capability into a smaller volume.

From the application requirements it can be seen that carbon-carbon possesses many of the needed properties. Carbon-carbon has a low thermal expansion, thus reducing the thermal fatigue of the chip soldering. The high thermal conductivity allows the thermal plane to keep the electronics from overheating. Testing has shown that a carbon-carbon thermal plane reduces the electronic packaging temperature by 4 to 16 °C (7–29 °F), depending on the input power level, over the conventional aluminum thermal plane. This temperature reduction translates to increased reliability of the electronic package. Carbon-carbon also has a high stiffness that reduces deflections during vibrational loading. These properties combined with its low density make carbon-carbon composites an ideal material for electronic thermal planes. Figure 4 shows electronic modules utilizing carbon-carbon thermal planes.

Two major concerns, which have delayed the utilization of carbon-carbon, are electrical insulation from the electronics and cost of the composite. Carbon is a good thermal and electrical conductor and must be insulated from any electronics. This includes preventing any carbon on the surface from "dusting" and depositing carbon on the electronic modules or their solder joints. The coatings must be thin to minimize the effect on the thermal conductivity and must adhere well to the carbon surface. Efforts are underway to develop a coating and application technique. Current progress has shown various materials are capable of encapsulating carbon-carbon and allowing the composite properties to dominate performance. Cost of carbon-carbon must be reduced for it to be used in many systems. The costs associated with the long densification times and high costs prevent the composite from being regularly used.

Spacecraft thermal doublers perform a similar thermal function as thermal planes, but the mechanical requirements are different. The thermal doubler is typically used to remove heat from part of a spacecraft and then radiate that heat to space. Therefore, a high thermal conductivity material is needed. The components to which the thermal doubler attaches require the material to have a fairly low stiffness to reduce vibration (as opposed to the electronic thermal plane, which utilizes a high stiffness material). The final and very critical requirement for a thermal doubler material is it must be lightweight. The cost of launching a spacecraft is significant, and weight can considerably affect launch costs. Therefore, designers desire the lowest-density material that can meet the performance requirements.

Carbon-carbon can be fabricated for all of the required thermal doubler properties. It has a high thermal conductivity and a low density. By choosing a lower-modulus fiber with good conductivity and arranging it in the appropriate architecture, carbon-carbon can be made into a fairly low-modulus material. Carbon-carbon thermal doublers have been fabricated (Fig. 5) and used on some spacecraft.

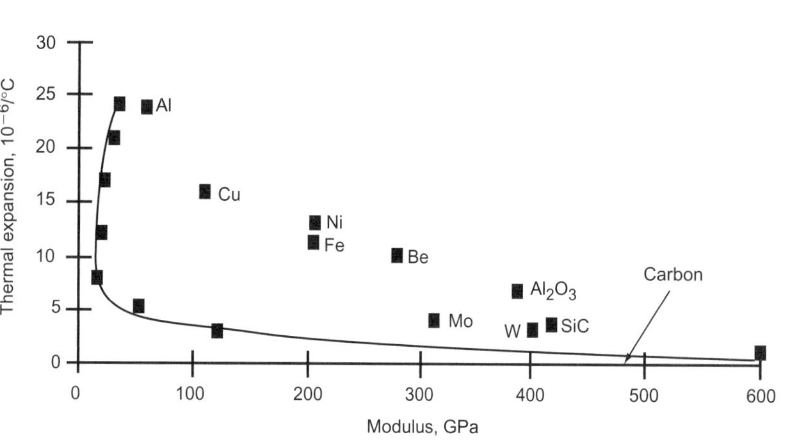

Fig. 2 Comparison of thermal expansion of various materials

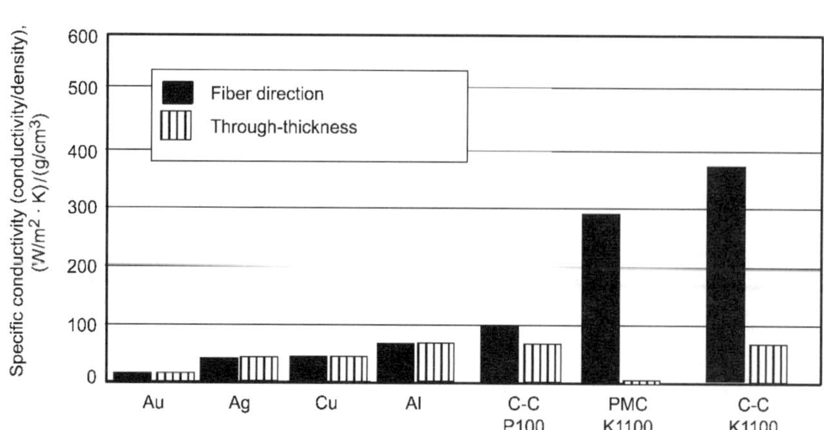

Fig. 3 Specific thermal conductivity comparison of carbon-carbon (C-C) composites, polymer-matrix composite (PMC) and high-conductivity metals. For composites, the fiber type is indicated under C-C or PMC.

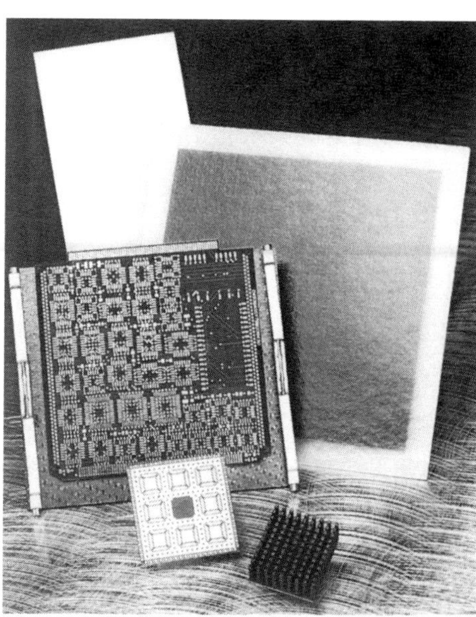

Fig. 4 Electronics with carbon-carbon thermal planes

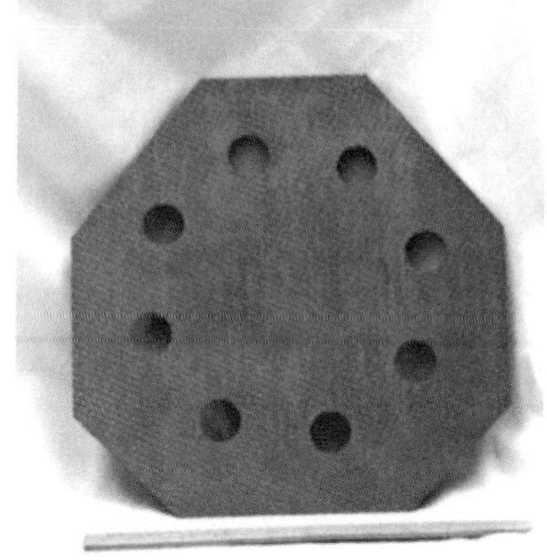

Fig. 5 Typical carbon-carbon space radiator. Courtesy of B.F. Goodrich

While procurement costs for space components are not the dominant issue, the fabrication time is significant. The average time to deliver a finished component from the time it is ordered is approximately three months due to the densification iteration. This required lead time is typically too long for users. Thus, producers have been working to significantly decrease the typical process time.

Spacecraft thermal shields represent a different type of thermal management application. The role of this component is to shield the remaining spacecraft system from the waste heat of the propulsion system. The material requirements include high-temperature stability and high stiffness at a low density. The high-temperature stability requirement is due to the amount of heat generated by the propulsion system. The material must be able to withstand this heat and still maintain mechanical integrity. The vibrational loading contributes the requirement for a material with high stiffness. The material must be able to survive under fairly high vibrational loading from the acoustics. A critical requirement for a thermal shield material is it must be lightweight, and therefore the most important advantage of a carbon-carbon thermal shield is the low density of the material. Carbon-carbon thermal shields have been shown to provide an approximately 50% weight reduction over metallic ones. The temperature stability and stiffness have been proven to be acceptable, as carbon-carbon thermal shields have performed successfully. Figure 6 shows a carbon-carbon thermal shield with Fig. 7 providing a concept of how it could be arranged in a spacecraft system.

Overall, the cost savings due to the weight savings overshadows any additional material costs. While procurement costs are not a significant issue, the time for composite fabrication is important, as it can be longer than desired by the customer.

Spacecraft radiators are another application in which the material must conduct "waste heat" from a source and radiate it to space. Its function is to keep whatever it attaches to cool enough to operate properly. Therefore, the material requirements include high thermal conductivity, reasonable strength and stiffness, and especially low density. A material with high thermal conductivity keeps the components from overheating. The material must have reasonable mechanical properties to support the components attached to it as well as survive any launch loads. Once again density is a critical material property.

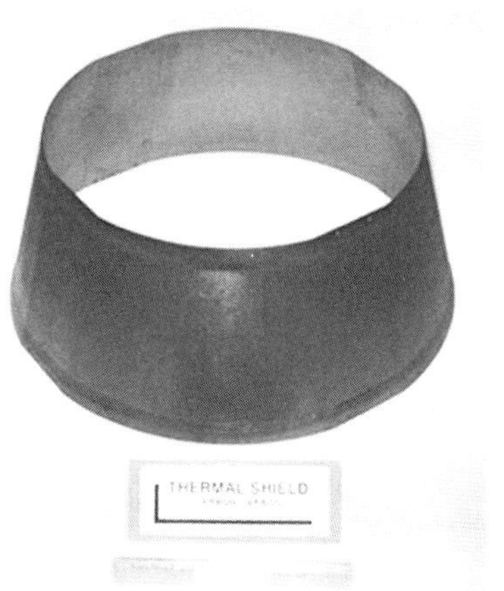

Fig. 6 Uncoated, as-fabricated carbon-carbon thermal shield. Courtesy of Lockheed Martin Astronautics

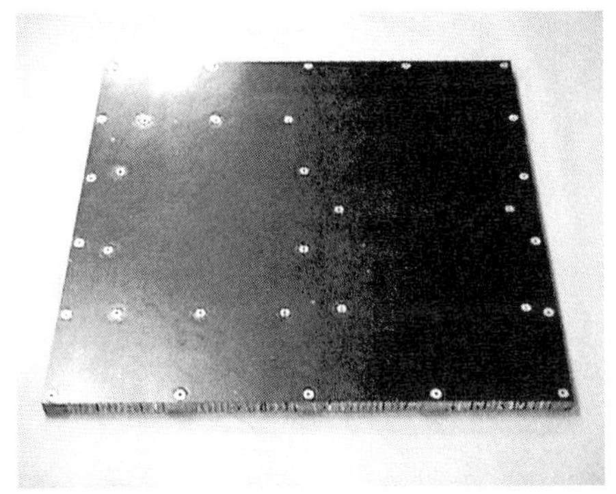

Fig. 8 Carbon-carbon space radiator with attachments. Courtesy of Lockheed Martin Astronautics

From the application requirements it can be seen that carbon-carbon possesses many of the needed properties. The high thermal conductivity allows the radiator to provide the needed cooling capabilities. Carbon-carbon also has a high stiffness that reduces deflections during launch. These properties combined with its low density make carbon-carbon composites an ideal material for spacecraft radiators. Figure 8 shows an assembled carbon-carbon radiator with an aluminum honeycomb core and the attachments included.

Attaching or bonding to a carbon-carbon radiator has not been an area of emphasis. Techniques have been tried, but have not been thoroughly tested. The radiator shown in Fig. 8 is based on the design required for an aluminum or polymeric-matrix composite radiator. There has not been enough work to determine the best design for carbon-carbon. Finally, the cost of carbon-carbon must be reduced for it to be used as a radiator material, and the fabrication time must be decreased. The current materials (aluminum or polymeric-matrix composites) are providing adequate performance at lower acquisition cost and time. Without the demonstration of significantly improved performance, it will be hard to justify carbon-carbon radiators over current materials.

Aircraft Heat Exchangers. Many different heat exchangers are used on many different systems all over an aircraft. Figure 9 shows a metallic heat exchanger, housing, and core. The operating conditions can range from room temperature to as high as 650 °C (1200 °F) with low to fairly high fluid pressures. The specific conditions depend on where in the aircraft the heat-exchanger is located and its function. The role of the heat-exchanger material is basically to conduct heat from the hot fluid to the cold. The material requirements are high thermal conductivity, corrosion resistance, strength, stiffness, low permeability, and moderate temperature capability (depending on the specific heat exchanger). Corrosion resistance is required because of the composition of some of the fluids flowing through the heat-exchanger channels. For instance, an aircraft flying over the ocean

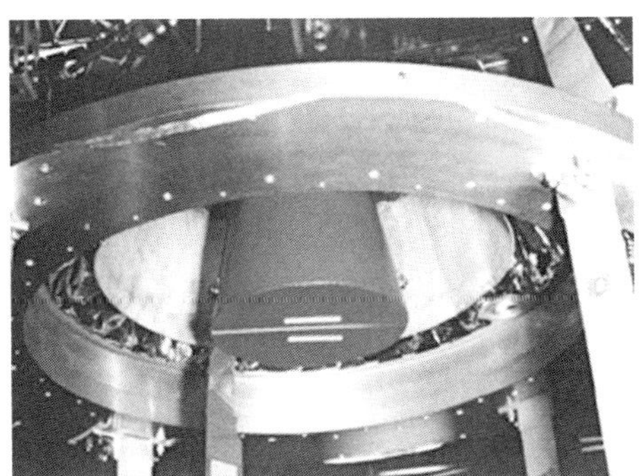

Fig. 7 Coated carbon-carbon thermal shield shown in spacecraft. Courtesy of Lockheed Martin Astronautics

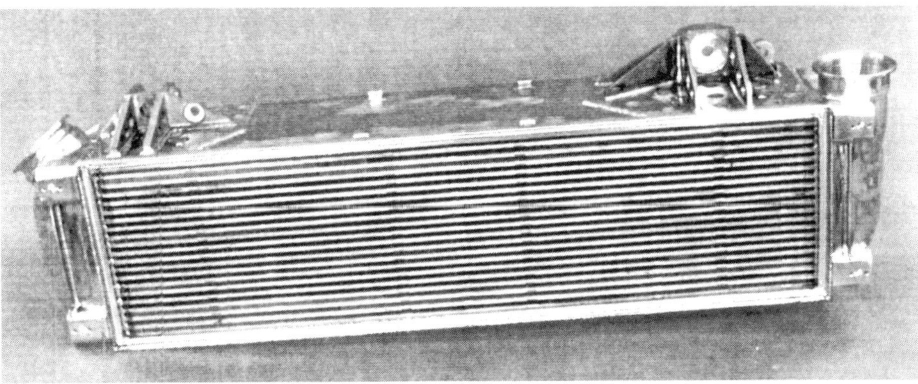

Fig. 9 Typical aircraft plate fin heat exchanger. Courtesy of SPARTA/Hamilton Standard

will ingest salt spray as part of the cooling or heating fluid. So the heat-exchanger material must be resistant to saltwater corrosion or maintenance costs will be high.

For the lower-temperature heat exchangers with air fluids, carbon-carbon may be the ideal material. It has a high thermal conductivity, reasonable strength and stiffness, and low density. Corrosion is not a concern at temperatures below 370 °C (700 °F). The higher-temperature heat exchangers are typically fabricated from very heavy metallic materials. The weight savings and high thermal conductivity of carbon-carbon offers the payoff of a higher-performance heat exchanger or a reduced-volume heat exchanger.

Many issues need to be resolved in fabricating a carbon-carbon heat exchanger. The structure of the core consists of parting plates and fins that are very delicate designs for any composite material. The core structure has been demonstrated with carbon-carbon, but must be more automated for better reproducibility and quality and lower costs. The higher-temperature heat exchangers require operating temperatures up to 650 °C (1200 °F). Above 370°C (700 °F), carbon begins to oxidize in the presence of oxygen (the higher the temperature the faster the oxidation rate). Oxidation protection schemes are being developed and tested to determine their capabilities.

Conclusions

The many properties of carbon have just begun to be exploited in carbon-carbon composites. Thermal management has become a logical application to explore with the composite material. Its tailorable thermal conductivity, stiffness, and strength in combination with its inherent low density make it an ideal replacement for some of the applications currently using a heavier metallic material. The applications discussed in this article are being investigated with the potential payoff being more efficient heat dissipation and/or lighter-weight components. However, research and demonstration efforts are required before carbon-carbon can be considered the "baseline" material for any of the applications. The applications that are being investigated represent only a few of the many that could benefit from carbon-carbon.

REFERENCES

1. D.L. Schmidt, K.E. Davidson, and L.S. Theibert, *SAMPE J.*, Vol 32 (No. 4), 1996, p 44
2. W.T. Shih, F.H. Ho, and B.B. Burkett, *7th Int. SAMPE Electronic Conference,* Society for the Advancement of Materials and Processing Engineering, 1994, p 296
3. R. Watts, Air Force Research Laboratory, personal communications, Dec 1997
4. S. Rawal, Lockheed Martin Astronautics, personal communications, Oct 1997
5. W.T. Shih, B.F. Goodrich, personal communications, Dec 1997

Sports and Recreation Equipment Applications

THE ADVANTAGES of composite construction have been applied to equipment for a wide range of sports and recreation activities. These advantages include strength, ductility, stiffness (modulus), and low density. This article opens with some historical background and then describes several examples of current composites applications for a variety of sports and recreation activities. A general overview of advanced materials for sports equipment is provided in Ref 1.

Historical Background

Modern composite construction in recreational equipment and sporting goods has been used for over 100 years. The paper canoe manufactured in 1874 by E. Waters & Sons of Troy, New York, probably the first one ever built, was a very early example of modern composite structure in recreational equipment.

Construction proceeded over a wooden mold that was rabbeted to accept internal framing. Two kinds of paper were used: that made from Manila and that prepared from pure unbleached linen stock. Several sheets were laid on the mold, wetted, and then glued together. An analogy can be drawn directly to modern fiber-glass cloth-resin construction. After drying, the hull was removed from the mold, waterproofed, and the woodwork finished. The thickness of the paper layers was controlled to provide adequate strength at various positions on the hull; this was done to make the canoe as light and as strong as possible. This variable-strength feature of composite manufacture provides a unique design freedom that is still used in modern composites.

Unfortunately, Waters & Sons burned down for the last time in 1901. The first paper canoe, the *Maria Theresa,* perished in a 1920 fire at the New York Canoe Club. It had been made famous by Nathaniel Bishop, who paddled it from Troy, New York, to Cedar Keys, Florida. The entire matter is an amazing testimony to the soundness of composite construction in recreational equipment, even with materials that would now be considered inadequate.

Laminated wood construction, or plywood, was later used in various forms for sport and pleasure boating, as well as in such items as tennis rackets and the delicate, glued flyrods constructed of tapered bamboo sections. More recently, the term composite has been associated with such materials as fiberglass, carbon fibers, silicon carbide platelets and whiskers, and aramid fibers. These materials have greatly broadened composite use in sport and recreational equipment by introducing filamentary materials with tensile strength versus weight and stiffness versus weight properties that greatly exceed those of wood, steel, and other more common materials. All of these new materials are embedded in a resin matrix, such as an epoxy or polyester, for fiber alignment and stable form.

Composite construction permits a designer to vary the mechanical properties almost microscopically in any section of the composite. This is done by controlling the amount of fiber reinforcement inserted, as well as its direction, and by combining layers of different reinforcing fibers of varying elasticity and strength. The end result is a macroscopic body that can have nearly ideal stress-strain and strength properties for the application. This application-efficient construction, along with modern fiber reinforcements, markedly minimizes overall weight in recreational equipment.

The common component of these composites is the resin that binds the mass together. The early nonwaterproofed glues were a severe constraint on paper canoes. With the availability of waterproof adhesives, the use of plywood in recreational equipment increased greatly. However, the same development problems remain true today. One of the most recent discoveries is the long-term failure of certain polyester resins used in pleasure craft, which led to severe blistering of the hull surface due to water absorption. The story of composite development in recreational equipment could also be expressed in terms of resin and adhesive development. The combination of modern resins with advanced filaments of great strength and stiffness has created new opportunities for composites in recreational and sporting goods, as well as other applications.

Bats, Rackets, and Clubs

Baseball Bats. Many softball teams and college baseball teams are now using composite bats. The bats are made of a graphite-reinforced polycarbonate (PC) blend. The graphite-reinforced bat is light and durable like aluminum, with the sound of wood. The bat is highly resistant to impact. It is tested against an air cannon that rockets balls in at 290 km/h (180 mph), nearly twice as fast as a major league fastball.

Both baseball and softball bats are formed by molding the graphite-PC blend around a steel core pin. A hollow shell is produced, which can be selectively filled with cellular urethane foam. The foam provides a center of gravity for the "sweet spot" of the bat, the area from which the ball travels farthest.

The graphite-reinforced resin shell is lightweight, strong, and stiff, allowing minimum material to achieve high strength. The weight savings allows greater options in the placement of the urethane filler. The sweet spot can be made larger. Graphite also reduces vibration and the sting of ball shock, the tingling feeling sent to the hands usually when a batter misses hitting the ball in the sweet spot of the bat.

The center of gravity of the bat also can be moved down the handle, permitting the hitter to generate more bat speed. With a larger sweet spot and greater bat speed, a batter can hit the ball farther.

Tennis Rackets. With many professional players smashing tennis balls at over 160 km/h (100 mph), tennis is a game of speed and control. Trying to hit the ball at high speeds and return it in-bounds requires concentration and a great degree of racket control. Rackets made from graphite-fiber composites give the player better ball control without increasing physical energy. The graphite rackets are stronger and stiffer than metal or wood and have a reduced head torque that provides a solid feel over a larger area of the racket head.

A graphite racket dissipates less energy, allowing the player to hit the ball with greater velocity. Manufacturers also can tailor the weight and balance the racket to a player's individual needs. The endurance life of a graphite racket is longer than that of conventional rackets.

Composite rackets are also being made with a combination of braided and unidirectional carbon fibers. Braided carbon fibers help prevent the racket from twisting. Rackets are made with 65% carbon, 30% glass, and 5% aramid. Graphite is stiffer, but more brittle; fiberglass is more flexible, but tougher.

Another racket is made with 84% carbon, 12% aramid, and 4% alumina fibers. The racket combines the performance of carbon with the comfort of a ceramic racket. Carbon adds stiffness and strength, resulting in controllable power. Aramid damps vibration, preventing "tennis elbow." Alumina has a higher modulus and damps vibration better than silicon carbide, which is commonly used in ceramic rackets. The net result: the racket delivers power, stroking control, and a soft but solid feel that is easy on the arm.

Golf Clubs. One of the greatest professional golf players, Jack Nicklaus, once said, "To play strategic and tactical golf, you have to be able to hit the ball more or less in a predictable direction a good part of the time." Thus, the key to better golf scores is not just strength but control. Composite golf shafts, reinforced with graphite fibers, give the golfer more control. They are 40% lighter than metal shafts, allowing weight to be added to the club head, while still reducing the overall club weight. With more weight in the head area, a golfer can drive the ball farther. The lighter club helps the golfer to improve the accuracy with his shots.

Composite golf shafts are usually made by either roll wrapping or filament winding. Filament winding, because it is an automated process, tends to maintain lower shaft frequency variations, often to ±1 cycle per minute (cpm) compared to ±4 cpm for roll-wrapped shafts (see the article "Filament Winding" in this Volume).

Golf club shafts are also being made of a combination of carbon- and boron-reinforcing fibers. Many Professional Golf Association (PGA) players prefer the carbon-boron club. Boron has much higher stiffness and fiber diameter than carbon, so it may serve better when used longitudinally. Compression-molded carbon cores serve to increase strength and power, while damping vibration.

To combat crushing loads, the manufacturing process begins with a close spiral wrap (to prevent the collapsing-straw effect), followed by a second spiral wrap that places the fibers at a lesser angle relative to the shaft axis. These layers form the effective core that handles torsional and radial impact loads. Here, the material of the wrap and the number of filaments in it control the off-center, springlike response of the golf club head to impact with the ball. The head should return to an appropriately neutral position when the ball leaves contact with the club in order to maintain optimal directional control. The inner windings, with resin applied, are enveloped by a layer of parallel fibers running along the axis of the shaft, which respond to flexural loads along the axis of the golf club. Using this method of construction, adjusting the thicknesses of the helical and parallel fibers, and using a predetermined inside and outside diameter for the shaft, the designer has enough variables under his control to construct the most efficient golf shaft available.

Even golf heads are being made of graphite-reinforced epoxy. The graphite heads are stronger, stiffer, and lighter, leading to more head speed and greater control. Golf club faces are being made by a combination of quartz yarn and carbon-fiber/epoxy composite, which compresses the ball more, leading to longer drives.

Bicycling

Bicycle races often end in sprints, with the cyclist achieving speeds of 80 km/h (50 mph). Cycling requires training, endurance, strategy, and equipment. Bike racing demands a high level of concentration. No energy is wasted in unnecessary movements. While pedaling, power should be applied all the way around, and the lighter the bike, the faster it can go.

Carbon-fiber-reinforced bicycle frames are stiffer than steel and lighter than aluminum. Hubs and wheels are being fabricated with glass-fiber-reinforced nylon. Drive plates are being made of polyethylene terephthalate reinforced with glass fibers. Even the drive chains are being replaced with polymer composites.

Bicycle Frames. Graphite/epoxy composite frames allow more flexibility in design, permitting designs that reduce drag. They also provide vibration damping. The Softride suspension system from Allsop, Inc. employs a graphite and glass, cantilevered seat beam to reduce shock.

Bicycle frames are being braided with graphite prepreg. Braiding provides high strength and resistance to torsion, or twisting.

In a Kestrel design, the carbon/epoxy frame has no seat tube (Fig. 1). The one-piece frame has integrally molded tubes and junctures and eliminates the seat tube by using a passive suspension system for a smoother, more aerodynamic ride.

In another one-piece design, the frame is molded with true airfoils to reduce drag. It is reinforced with a hybrid of carbon and polyethylene (PE) fibers. Carbon fibers supply stiffness, while PE fibers provide lightweight strength. Polyethylene fibers also damp shock and resist fatigue. The frame has no bonded joints, which are regions of stress concentration. The frame is very stiff in-plane, so energy goes to driving the bike forward. Unlike metal, the composite frame is more flexible out-of-plane, so it is easier on bumps, especially important in long races. Further, the composite frame can withstand fatigue and crushing three to four times better than steel.

Air resistance accounts for up to 90% of the total force slowing a cyclist down. The U.S. Olympic team used carbon composite tubes in the bicycle frame. Each tube is shaped like an airfoil to reduce drag, yet it is stiffer and lighter than steel. Olympic cyclists also used an aerodynamic bicycle frame that is laid up with carbon-fiber/epoxy prepreg and glass-fiber prepreg sandwiched around a closed-cell foam core. Spoke and disc wheels are also composite.

Bicycle frames are being fabricated with boron-reinforced aluminum. Boron-reinforced aluminum is lighter, stronger, and stiffer than pure aluminum, yet it retains much of the toughness of aluminum. Hybrid frames, such as carbon-fiber-reinforced polymer composites combined with titanium, have been provided.

Bicycle Wheels. The SPIN bicycle wheel from Innovations in Composites is made with a long carbon-fiber-reinforced nylon blend. The long fiber compounds are prepared in a pultrusion process that permits a high level of fiber impregnation. The three-spoke 1 kg (2.2 lb) SPIN wheel is a one-piece hollow construction made by a lost-core injection molded process. An aluminum rim is bonded to the wheel. The result is a strong and lightweight composite wheel at half the cost of a traditional carbon/epoxy hand-laid-up wheel.

Aramid-fiber composites are being made into disc wheels. The aramid wheels cut the wind resistance of a normal bicycle wheel in half. The spokeless wheels knife through the air, eliminating the drag of numerous spokes. Aramid-reinforced tires weigh less than 0.1 kg (¼ lb) each. The feather-light wheels and tires reduce rolling friction.

A one-piece bicycle wheel rim is being formed with braided carbon-fiber/epoxy prepreg. The braided prepreg permits closer tolerances—down to 0.05 mm (0.002 in.)—so less energy is lost to sideways motion.

Winter Sports

Hockey sticks must be light and stiff like golf clubs. However, hockey sticks take a beating from slapping against the ice, crashing into the boards, and swinging at other players. The average hockey stick lasts only 5 to 15 games.

Hockey stick handles from Sherwood Products are made with a core of aspen wood surrounded by layers of fiberglass. Fiberglass lowers the weight while adding stiffness and durability. The critical region of the blade consists of 80% fiberglass and 20% graphite fibers for increased stiffness. Aramid is sometimes added to the heel of the blade for impact.

Hockey sticks are also being fabricated by Easton Aluminum Inc. with an aluminum tube overwrapped by layers of bonded high-modulus

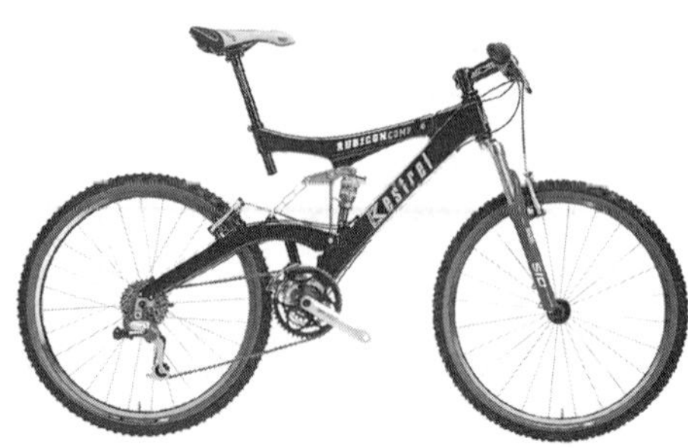

Fig. 1 One-piece carbon/epoxy bicycle frame. Courtesy of Kestrel

carbon-fiber/epoxy. The hockey stick is said to be the lightest and stiffest made.

Sleds. Olympic bobsleds race at speeds up to 90 mph, rounding a turn at five times the force of gravity. A composite monocoque replaces previous steel sleds. The composite sled is four times stronger than steel. It is also safer; the driver's body is protected during a crash by the composite monocoque. In a steel sled, the driver bangs into the steel rods; in the composite sled, there are no protrusions to bang into.

The composite sled is comprised of Nomex (DuPont) honeycomb, sandwiched between layers of aramid and graphite-fiber-reinforced epoxy. The epoxy withstands subzero temperatures without losing its adhesive properties. The composite sled allows greater freedom in aerodynamic design, reducing drag by 40%. The sled weighs only 45 kg (100 lb), a fifth as much as a metal sled. The result: greater speed and greater control.

Luge sleds are also made of composites. They are composed of a carbon-fiber/vinyl ester resin that withstands the subzero temperatures without a loss in properties. The sled is highly resistant to impact, which is important in a sled that can tip over at speeds up to 130 km/h (80 mph).

Snowboards. A composite snowboard is constructed by Hexcel Corporation. The board consists of a thermoplastic cap or top layer, a layer of glass, carbon, or hybrid prepreg, a polyurethane honeycomb core, another layer of glass, carbon or hybrid prepreg, and a PE running surface. Prepregs are used, because they provide easier handling and a better working environment than wet lay-up. They also are lighter than wet lay-up, because they have a lower resin content. Further, they are easier to mass produce to an exact specification (thickness and weight).

The composite board has a polyurethane (PUR) honeycomb core, because it provides significant weight savings over a wood core, with no loss of stiffness. Polyurethane reduces production times (less than 10 min from mold preparation to demolding) and reduces the number of components. Polyurethane provides excellent adhesive properties and an ideal balance of flexibility and stiffness when combined with laminates. The use of PUR reaction injection molding material makes production extremely quick and provides excellent adhesive properties. Honeycombs combine very low weight with excellent stiffness.

A snowboard from Morrow Snowboards has a Baydur polyurethane foam core from Bayer Corporation (Fig. 2). Polyurethane is poured into a clamshell mold to form the composite core. The mold is heated to 55 to 60 °C (130 to 140 °F), with pressure reaching 240 kPa (35 psi). After 10 to 12 min, the foam core is demolded. Thicknesses range from 9 mm (0.35 in.) in the center, tapering down to 2 mm (0.08 in.) at the front and back. The foam core is covered with fiberglass that has been impregnated with epoxy resin. A decorated top layer is applied last.

Snow Skis. The world's record for downhill racing is nearly 210 km/h (130 mph). To reach these speeds, high-strength, lightweight materials are essential. Snow skis are made out of graphite-reinforced epoxy. The high stiffness and reduced damping of graphite permit sharper, faster turns.

Some skis are made with glass-fiber-reinforced epoxy. The fiberglass/epoxy skis do not break as easily as wood. Aramid fibers are also reinforcing skis. The aramid fibers dampen vibration for smoother, more comfortable skiing. The fibers resist abrasion and lessen fatigue, so skiers can ski faster and longer, while retaining control.

Snow skis have been made with braided composites. Braiding is an automated process that ensures uniformity, while it eliminates seams and overlaps. Braided skis resist torsion better and weigh 0.45 kg (1 lb) less than hand lay-up skis—due to closer tolerances and less excess resin.

Hexcel Corporation is manufacturing Alpine and cross-country skis using honeycomb cores. The skis have a layered structure, consisting of an aluminum/epoxy/fiberglass top layer, a rigid foam/wood/honeycomb core, a reformed thermoplastic cap, a layer of epoxy/fiberglass prepreg, a polyurethane rigid foam core, another epoxy/fiberglass bottom laminate, and a PE running surface. The multilayered skis have the toughness and durability to resist the stresses and strains of Alpine and cross-country skiing, yet the skis are ultralight and comfortable to use.

Ski poles are manufactured by pultruding glass fibers. Ski poles are also made out of graphite-reinforced epoxy. Both woven and unidirectional graphite fibers are used. In a ski pole, swing weight is critical. Composites allow the center of gravity to be moved closer to the handle, reducing the swing weight. In a 15 km (9 mile) cross-country ski race, the poles swing 5,000 times, so carbon-fiber shafts, which weigh only 100 g (3.4 oz), can save 3400 J (2,500 ft · lbf) of energy during a race. Ski poles also need compressive strength, with the carbon/epoxy pole at 860 MPa (125 ksi) compared to 550 MPa (80 ksi) for aluminum.

Ice skates and boots, from K2 Exotech have long fiber-glass-reinforced nylon with chopped carbon fibers injection molded into the ice skate frames, boot base, and heel counters. K2 also produces 4-wheel and 5-wheel cross-training skates, made from fiberglass/epoxy prepreg and graphite/epoxy prepreg continuous woven fabric.

Merlin Technologies developed a low-cost/high-production system for hybrid glass-carbon composite structures used in lightweight skating boots. The composite components replace 90% of the structural leather in traditional boots, reducing the overall weight while improving control response for ice, roller, and blade skaters. In figure skating, the reduced weight means higher leaps and a greater chance of completing multiple-spin movements, while increased stiffness allows better blade control at landing impact. Reebok makes a fiberglass/carbon-fiber hybrid arch support in their athletic footwear.

Aquatic Sports

Water Skis. Like snow skiing, water skiing is a sport that relies heavily upon balance and coordination. Skiing slalom, on just one ski, requires an even greater degree of control. Composite slalom skis are reinforced with PE fibers. The PE fibers are 10 times stronger than steel for the same weight. The stronger, lighter PE-fiber reinforced skis help the skier to regain speed after turns and jumps and to accelerate faster. The ski is more stable in rough water and provides the skier with greater control. The impact resistance and toughness are improved, giving the skier a competitive edge.

Slalom water skis are also being made of a hybrid of glass and carbon fibers to achieve the desired combination of flex and performance. The skis are constructed by wrapping fiberglass and carbon-fiber-reinforced epoxy prepreg around a high-density PUR foam core that has been premolded, sanded, and cured so that shrinkage takes place before the ski is fabricated. Skis are typically cured by compression molding at around 95 °C (200 °F). Trick skis and jump skis are constructed from carbon-fiber prepreg with aluminum honeycomb cores.

Another water ski from Connelly Skis, Inc. has Baydur PUR foam core surrounded by a graphite-fiberglass composite, with an acrylic top shell and acrylam (acrylic) base. The PUR foam core gives the basic shape to the ski, has a high strength-to-weight ratio and provides structural stability and torsional control. It helps

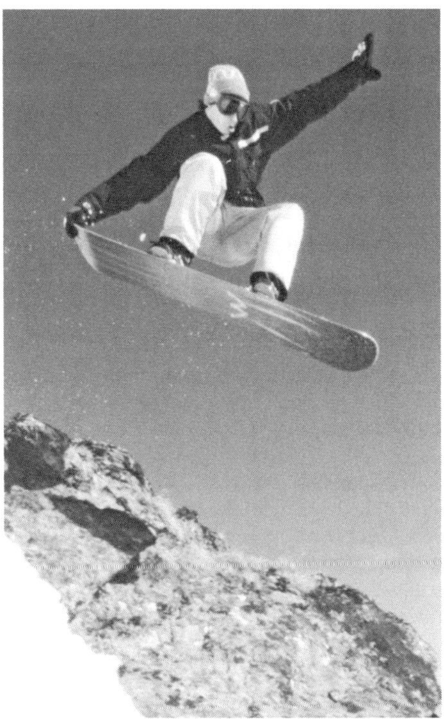

Fig. 2 Fiberglass/epoxy snowboard with a polyurethane foam core. Courtesy of Bayer Corp.

skiers maintain control—providing the right amount of acceleration and deceleration and enabling them to carve smooth turns without losing edge.

A hybrid composite containing aramid and boron fibers is being fabricated into water skis. Aramid provides lightweight tensile strength and toughness. Boron offers stiffness and strength in both compression and bending.

A wake board, or surfboard, from Connelly Skis, Inc. (Fig. 3) is compression molded with a core of Baydur PUR. The core is then wrapped with a graphite-fiberglass composite. This in turn is sandwiched between the top and bottom layers of the board. The top layer is an acrylic material. The bottom of the board is made with acrylam (acrylic). The wake board is stiff, light, and strong.

Windsurfers. Windsurfing boards are constructed of high-density 6 mm (0.25 in.) polyvinyl chloride foam sandwiched between layers of high-strength, epoxy-impregnated fiberglass. This sandwich construction is then wrapped around an expanded polystyrene foam core. The board lay-up is placed in die molds and cured under heat and pressure. The resulting board is light and very strong. Carbon strips are used for strategic placement, such as in the area under the feet of the sailor, which can see high stress from landing jumps from up to 6 m (20 ft) high, typical when sailing in ocean waves.

Another design of windsurfing board is started from the inside out. The dry laminate (roving, mat, and carbon) is stapled with plastic stitches to the foam blank, coated with acrylonitrile-butadiene-styrene (25 to 50 μm, or 1 to 2 mil, thick), and thermoformed in an injection press.

Windsurfer masts (Fig. 4) are braided with carbon and glass fibers by Fiberspar. The masts are 5 m (16 ft) long with a base diameter of 48 cm (19 in.) and a tip diameter of 25 cm (10 in.). The masts weigh only 2.3 kg (4.7 lb) and must endure considerable torsional forces, because bend in the mast is critical for speed. Braiding the masts helps control the torsion within the design limits. The lighter masts are easier to hang on to, manipulate, and lift out of the water.

A case history in materials selection for a windsurfer mast is provided in the article "Performance Indices" in *Materials Selection and Design,* Volume 20 of *ASM Handbook.*

Canoes, kayaks, and racing hulls are being made with carbon-fiber/epoxy as well as aramid and glass fibers. The lighter-weight boats travel faster in competition. Canoes are being built with carbon fibers, aramid fibers, and a core material called Spheretex (Spheretex GmbH), a woven fabric with high silica glass. These boats provide greater tensile strength and abrasion resistance.

Composite canoes from We-No-Nah Canoe, Inc. are manufactured using Tuf-Weave fiberglass-orthopolyester 0.3 kg (10 oz) fabric blend, with a small amount of aramid for stiffening in the bow and stern. They also make vinyl ester/aramid canoes. Both are thin-skin laminates formulated with a high fiber-resin ratio and cured under vacuum bag pressure to provide good flexibility and resilience.

Personal watercraft, such as the JetSki from Kawasaki Motors Corporation, are being manufactured with sheet molding compound, which uses half-inch chopped glass and precision-matched steel dies. Personal watercraft are also being made by hand lay-up fiberglass and resin transfer molding with glass reinforcement for structural parts, such as hulls and decks.

A composite kayak is reinforced with PE fibers. The high strength-weight ratio of the PE fibers causes the ends of the boat to be lighter, allowing it to go over waves more easily. The composite kayak sustains travel over rocks without damage. The kayak is 4 kg (9 lb) lighter than comparable carbon or aramid kayaks, leading to faster acceleration.

Canoe paddles are made out of a hybrid composite. The paddle has a rigid polyimide foam core covered with a layer of unidirectional graphite/epoxy tape. On top of that is a hybrid braid of aramid, fiberglass, and selectively placed graphite wraps, with twice the amount of graphite on the compression side as the tension side. The compression side of the paddle blade is comprised of unidirectional graphite/woven fiberglass hybrid cloth. The tension side of the paddle blade is comprised of unidirectional aramid/woven fiberglass hybrid cloth.

The overall result of this bent-shape canoe paddle is high strength and ultralightweight. The paddle is tough, yet provides smooth and efficient propulsion.

A Big Blade oar from Concept II is combining graphite/epoxy with glass fibers for durability and light weight. The short, fat, meat-cleaver-shaped oar has 15% more surface area on the blade, leading to more force on the water per stroke with less effort than longer conventional-shaped oars.

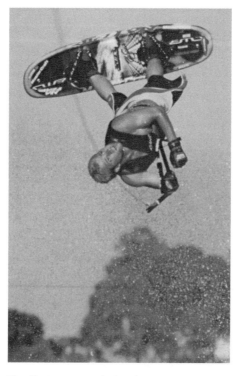

Fig. 3 Composite wake board. Courtesy of Connelly Skis Inc.

Use of composites in larger watercraft is addressed in the article "Marine Applications" in this Volume.

Fishing Gear. To catch a large number of fish, a fisherman needs a lightweight rod that requires minimum casting energy. Fishing rods, with glass-fiber-reinforced epoxy wound around a mandrel, are lightweight and flexible. The rods are made by a combination of pultrusion and modified filament winding.

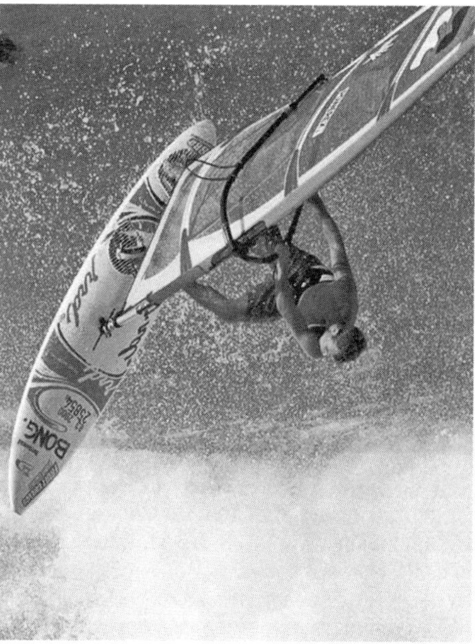

(a)

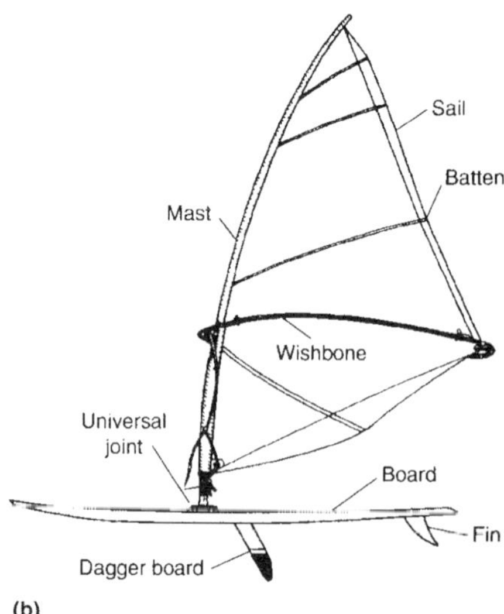

(b)

Fig. 4 Windsurfers. (a) Windsurfer with a braided composite mast. Courtesy of Fiberspan. (b) General design of a windsurfer. The flexure of the mast controls the shape of the sail; its pivoting about the universal joint controls the response of the craft.

Graphite-reinforced rods are even lighter, typically weighing 38 g (1.3 oz). Lighter weight rods increase the response and "handfeel." When casting, vibrations in a graphite rod dampen more rapidly than other rods, minimizing the line drag. The reduced drag helps the fisherman to cast a greater distance and more accurately. Graphite rods vibrate less than bamboo, wasting less energy and allowing 20% greater casting distance.

A hybrid graphite/glass/epoxy fishing pole made by Shakespeare Products is ultralight, allowing a fisherman to cast farther and make more casts without tiring out his arm, yet the rod is strong enough to pull in a large bass. The rod can actually be bent 360° without breaking. These rods use a hollow tubular structure to minimize weight and to optimize the strength and sensitivity of the rod in sport fishing. All such tubular fishing rods are created around a removable metal mandrel, which forms the tapered inner diameter of the finished product. The taper and diameter of this cylindrical cone constitute the starting point of the design. On this inner mandrel are placed the various fibers that provide the strength of the fishing rod and the resin that bonds the fibrous structure together.

One particular construction (Fig. 5) begins with an inner layer of carbon fiber, wound spirally around the mandrel from the butt end to the tip of the rod. This continuous spiral of fibers dramatically improves the radial integrity, or hoop strength, of the rod blank by distributing pressure over a larger area. It virtually eliminates the collapsing-straw effect that can plague hollow rods constructed with a fiber direction (for example, rolled woven fibers) that does not take into account the actual stress distribution in a bending tube. A second layer of fiberglass fibers is then placed over the initial graphite layer and oriented longitudinally along the axis of the rod, which increases the sensitivity of the rod, because the vibrations of the fish are readily transmitted in the direction of the fiber. The final function of these fibers is to increase the overall bending strength of the fishing rod. In a premium rod, a third layer of longitudinal carbon fiber is added to the blank for further strength and controlled stiffness. The small, solid tip on such a rod becomes a light, very strong section of 100% carbon fiber embedded in resin.

The end result is a piece of recreational equipment in which material choice, material configuration, and overall shape maximize the strength and sensitivity of the rod at minimum weight, illustrating how modern composite materials and design permit optimization to suit the final purpose of the application. Such design freedom is simply not available with metal or wood.

Figure 6 shows the equipment used to produce high-quality composite rods. The machine starts at the butt of a rod mandrel and uses the maximum number of fiberglass or graphite rovings required by the design. These are then cut out or reduced in number in a preset manner as the rod blank is formed from butt to tip. Consequently, some of the fiber filaments run the full length of the mandrel, and others run only a partial length. Impregnation with resin, usually an epoxy, is carried out simultaneously. By altering the mandrel and changing the amount and locations of the fibers used in construction, fishing rods of different characteristics can be made for all segments of the market on a few basic pieces of manufacturing equipment.

The spool of a bait-casting fishing reel should be light to start rotating quickly and stop quickly with a minimum inertia. A heavy spool is hard to start or stop. A glass-fiber-reinforced polybutylene terephthalate (PBT) reel is significantly lighter than its metal counterparts.

The PBT reel costs less to manufacture than a metal reel. By means of part consolidation, the PBT reel has only 47 parts compared to 58 parts for metal reels, while eliminating many assembly and finishing steps. It also resists corrosion better.

A trolling motor shaft from Strongwell Company is being manufactured from a 29 mm (1.125 in.) diam by 760 mm (30 in.) long pultruded tube, threaded to fit into a steel housing and given a black satin finish. The fiberglass-polyester shaft does not transmit motor sound waves, a big advantage to a fisherman. For fishing underwater, Bedford Reinforced Plastics Inc. pultrudes fiberglass-isopolyester rods and tubes that are used for diving spears, diver's flag floats, and tickle sticks for poking lobster out of holes.

Track and Field Equipment

Pole-Vaulting Poles. Pole vaulting as a sport has never imposed any particular constraints on the construction or design of the pole. However, there was little change in the design or materials of construction until the advent of fiberglass composites. The poles had been made of bamboo, steel, or wood, but in the 1950s, fiberglass-resin poles were successfully introduced. These poles copied the earlier wood or metal poles

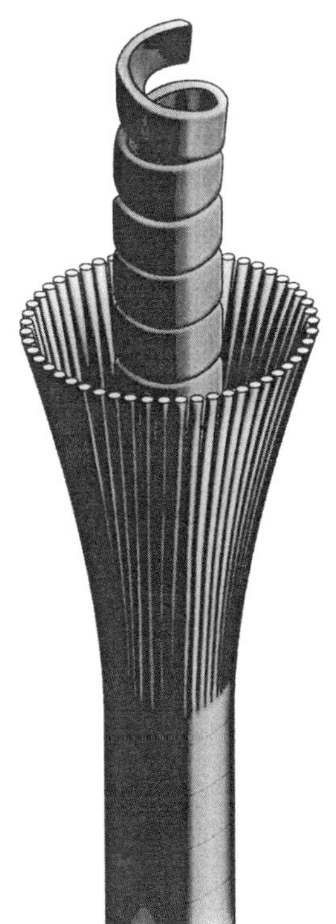

Fig. 5 Composite fishing rod construction. Courtesy of Shakespeare Products

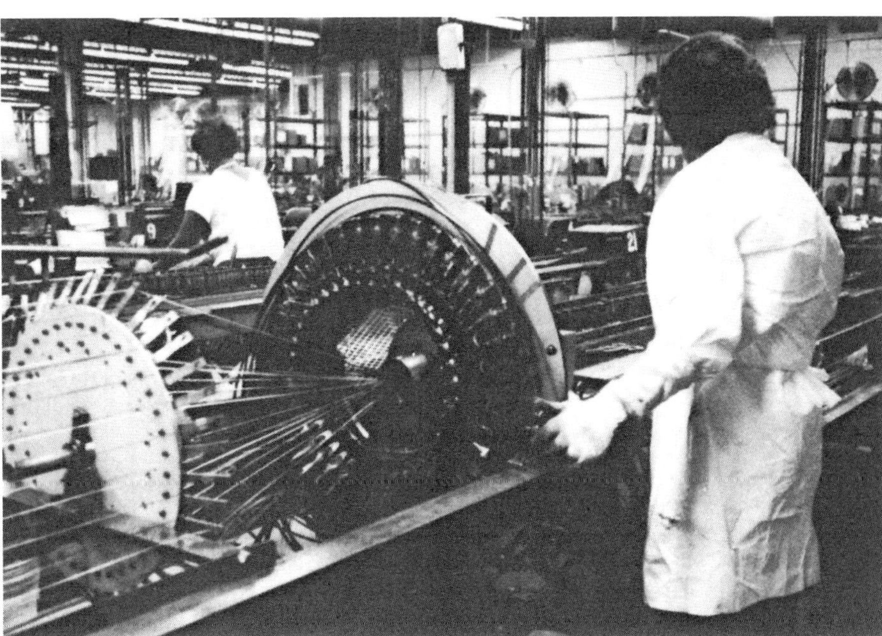

Fig. 6 An inner layer of spiral wrapping of carbon filaments being applied to a carbon-fiberglass fishing rod. Courtesy of Shakespeare Products

without any pronounced use of empty cores or changing of diameters or fiber concentrations to improve the pole in a way comparable to that described for fishing rods or golf clubs.

The engineering problem involves the design of a very light, highly efficient tubular spring that is loaded by impact when the running vaulter places one end of the pole in the planting box beneath the vertical bars of the vault. The kinetic energy of running must be converted into a rotational energy that is sufficient to carry the vaulter to a vertical position and over the measuring rod. The basic vibrational period required for the pole to straighten from its initial loading must equal the time it takes for this quarter revolution of the vaulter to occur. The spring constant must therefore be designed to take the weight of the vaulter into account. Because the vaulter tries to maximize the kinetic energy by sprinting toward the vault, the pole needs to be as light as possible. Above all, it should not break.

This is the type of problem that, once thoroughly understood in engineering terms, makes it impossible to become a successful vaulter. This point may seem facetious, but the customer for recreational equipment must be approached with this matter in mind. The acceptance of an innovative piece of sports equipment is often achieved through performance factors recognizable by the athlete in a framework entirely different from that used by the engineer.

The strength of the composite fiberglass poles per unit weight was greater than earlier materials. Therefore, the poles were made lighter and were more flexible. This required vaulters to develop new techniques for their successful use. The early fiberglass poles were not yet designed for all the desirable requirements from the viewpoint of the vaulter, and this probably slowed their initial acceptance.

The requirements of the vaulting pole have led to a specialized form of fishing rod, rather than a pole that bends uniformly from end to end. The major manufacturers have recently redesigned the poles to be nonlinear springs, which are stiffer at the butt end than at the other. Carbon fiber has also been introduced in an attempt to reduce weight while improving stiffness. Fiberglass, with about five times the strength-to-weight ratio of steel, is roughly equal to steel in specific stiffness. Carbon fibers have about five times the specific strength and about five times the specific stiffness of steel. The resultant optimal pole is therefore likely to be a combination of these two fibrous materials in a suitable resin matrix.

The pole design consists of two layers of fiberglass tape spiral wrapped to the outside of a hollow aluminum mandrel. Next, unidirectional fiberglass/epoxy prepreg is ironed to the spiral wrap. Carbon fiber is added in the inner wrap. A "sail piece" of the same prepreg material is cut to a taper and wrapped around the pole. The pole is put into a silicone bag, air pressure is applied to the outside of the bag, and steam heat is directed into the aluminum mandrel, curing the part from the inside.

Sports wheelchairs used for racing and sports such as basketball, use graphite/epoxy frames, weighing only 1 kg (2.3), integrally laid-up lugs, and elliptically shaped tubes that are 29% stronger than round tubing across major load planes. Composites allow varied wall thickness to build in stress reinforcement. They also dampen shock. The Power Bar, a T-shaped graphite/epoxy wheelchair frame, has a wall thickness of 2.54 mm (0.10 in.). The Power Bar also has a braided prepreg sock. Composites in the frame have four times the longitudinal stiffness as aluminum.

Sprinters' Prostheses. Springlite manufactures a one-piece graphite-fiber/epoxy sprinter foot prosthesis that features a radial shape and high strength and stiffness, allowing sprinters to run on their toes without fear of the prosthesis breaking. The Flex Sprint from Flex Foot has graphite-fiber/epoxy pylons that allow length variation and a balance of strength and flexural properties that vary with a runner's weight and speed (Fig. 7). Composite plantar flexes are designed to angle forward and down, striking first in the toe, thus storing and returning more energy to the runner.

For above-knee runners' prosthetics, the Endolite Sports Limb (Chas. A. Blatchford & Sons Ltd) contains a graphite/epoxy knee. The Sports Limb features a lightweight composite cradle able to withstand loads generated during running, which can be four times the athlete's body weight.

Archery Equipment

In competition, an arrow must be shot usually 55 m (180 ft), but it must be shot right on target. Both distance and precision depend upon arrow speed. Compounded bows formed of pultruded fiberglass produce greater arrow velocity than bows of laminated wood.

Fiberglass archery limbs have a higher strength than wood and superior resistance to fatigue. They can endure higher stresses when flexed and still return to their original shape. Labor costs are up to 50% less in production. Laminated wood limbs are produced by hand, requiring time-consuming spraying, finishing, and sanding operations.

Graphite fibers also are reinforcing bows. The high strength of graphite fibers helps to shoot the arrow farther and faster. The high modulus of graphite helps give the archer bull's-eye accuracy. Another bow has a syntactic foam core sandwiched between unidirectional glass and graphite fibers. The design is strong, light, and stable, allowing the archer to shoot an arrow at high speed. The bow accelerates the arrow to a velocity of over 67 m/s (220 ft/s), with forces that cause the arrow to buckle and vibrate all the way to the target.

Arrows are also being made of composites. One arrow shaft is made from a carbon composite. Through a special wrapping process, the several layers of carbon are combined as one super-strong and extremely smooth arrow. The arrow resists bending and shattering better than aluminum arrows.

Composites are being pultruded into arrow shafts. Each Carbon Tech arrow shaft starts as 348,000 separate carbon fibers. Through a pultrusion process, they are bonded together with a matrix resin, producing a seamless shaft with an extremely smooth surface. The lighter, smoother arrows travel swiftly and accurately to their target.

In Olympic competition, a hybrid composite arrow has won gold and bronze medals. The arrow, manufactured by Easton Aluminum Inc., is fabricated with an aluminum tube overwrapped by layers of bonded, high-modulus carbon-fiber/epoxy. The arrow shaft is said to be the lightest and stiffest made. Because the arrow is stiffer, it oscillates at higher frequencies. The higher-frequency oscillation increases velocity. The shafts travel at up to 8 m/s (25 ft/s) faster than pure aluminum arrows. Because the flight time is shortened, it lessens the effect of wind and weather on the arrow, thereby increasing accuracy.

Conclusions

Modern composite construction has been applied in some degree to almost every modern sport. The design flexibility and, in some cases, lower production costs are used to build equipment that provides superior performance. For example, few people who have used a light, well-designed carbon-fiberglass fishing rod would return to an older steel or bamboo version. The

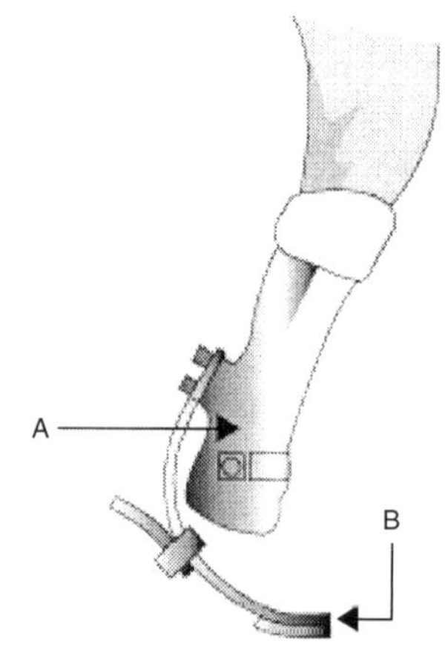

Fig. 7 Schematic of a sprinter's prosthesis, used by Tony Volpentest at the 1992 Barcelona Paralympics. Born without feet, Volpentest won gold metals in Barcelona in the 100 meter (11.63 s) and 200 meter (23.07 s). The socket of the prosthesis (A) is flexible, allowing for various muscles, tendons, and bones to function inside. It also features a flexed toe (B) that ensures landing on the forward 5 cm (2 in.) of the toe—the normal gait for sprinting. Source: Ref 2

penetration has been so complete that the revolution is almost over in the sport and recreational markets. What remains, however, is continuous improvement within the general fiber-resin composite concept as designers learn how to optimize the use of these materials to fit the distinct mechanical loads applied to various parts of sporting equipment.

ACKNOWLEDGMENTS

Portions of this article were adapted from W.J. Spry, Sports and Recreation Equipment, *Composites*, Vol 1, *Engineered Materials Handbook,* ASM International, 1987, p 845–847. Additional information was prepared for this edition by Allen Klein.

REFERENCES

1. K.E. Easterling, *Advanced Materials for Sports Equipment,* Chapman and Hall, 1993
2. F.H. Froes, Is the Use of Advanced Materials in Sports Equipment Unethical?, *JOM,* Vol 49 (No. 2), 1997, p 15–19

Thermal Management and Electronic Packaging Applications

Carl Zweben, Composites Consultant

A VARIETY of new advanced composite materials that provide great advantages over conventional materials for thermal management and electronic (also called microelectronic) packaging are available now. Their advantages include:

- Extremely high thermal conductivities (over twice that of copper)
- Low, tailorable coefficients of thermal expansion (CTE)
- Weight savings up to 80%
- Size reductions up to 65%
- Extremely high strength and stiffness
- Reduced thermal stresses
- Increased reliability
- Simplified thermal design
- Potential elimination of heat pipes
- Low cost, net-shape fabrication processes
- Potential cost reductions

Composites are in a state of continual development that undoubtedly will result in improved and new materials providing even greater benefits. The number of production applications is increasing rapidly, and composites are well on their way to becoming the twenty-first century materials of choice for thermal management and electronic packaging. This article provides an overview of advanced composites used in thermal management and electronic packaging, including properties, applications, and future trends. The focus is on materials having thermal conductivities at least as high as those of aluminum alloys. Future trends in thermal management materials and the potential for composites in other aspects of the electronics industry, such as high-speed assembly machine materials of construction, are also examined.

Application Requirements and Candidate Materials

In the *Electronic Materials Handbook,* Volume 1 (Ref 1), published in 1989, an overview of composites developed for use in electronic packaging and thermal management was presented. This article presents an update on that work, expanding the topic to include other types of composites and advanced materials. Electronics packaging is an important industry with worldwide sales of $100 billion; sales are expected to double by 2005 or 2010.

Although this article deals with composites developed for thermal management aspects of electronic packaging, the use of and potential for composites in packaging is much broader. Combining two or more constituents makes possible the creation of materials with unique combinations of properties that cannot be achieved any other way. Perhaps the best example is printed circuit boards (PCBs) for which dielectric properties are critical. The most common PCB material, E-glass fiber-reinforced epoxy, was first developed over a half century ago.

In addition to microelectronic packaging, composites are well suited for other packaging applications, such as optoelectronic components and microelectromechanical systems (MEMS). Both are important growth areas.

Application Requirements. Electronic packaging provides a number of primary functions: it provides power, transfers signals in and out, provides mechanical support and protection to the components it houses, and dissipates heat generated in the package. In addition, electronic packaging may have to be hermetic and provide electromagnetic interference (EMI) shielding.

The continuing increase in packaging density has resulted in a need for materials with high thermal conductivities. In addition, to minimize thermal stresses that can cause component or solder-joint failure, packaging materials must have CTEs matching those of the materials to which they are attached, especially ceramic substrates and semiconductors, which are weak, brittle materials. Further, low density is desirable in many applications, including portable systems such as laptops, handheld telephones, and avionics. Reducing weight also minimizes potentially damaging stresses resulting from shock loads that can occur during shipping and other activities. Of course, low cost is also a key consideration. Traditional materials used in electronic packaging do not meet all of these requirements. In response to this need, new composite materials have been and continue to be developed.

Improved materials are also needed in other thermal management applications. One of the best examples is spacecraft, for which mass and thermal management are critical issues.

Candidate Composite Materials. A composite material can be defined as two or more materials bonded together (Ref 2). Composites are nothing new in electronic packaging. For example, polymer-matrix composites (PMCs) in the form of E-glass fiber-reinforced polymer (GFRP) PCBs are well-established packaging materials. Similarly, a variety of particles are added to polymers to reduce CTE and increase thermal conductivity, electrical conductivity, or both. These materials are particle-reinforced PMCs. New composites have been developed in recent years that provide unique combinations of properties that make them outstanding candidates for packaging applications.

The four key classes of composite materials are PMCs, metal-matrix composites (MMCs), ceramic-matrix composites (CMCs), and carbon-matrix composites, which encompasses carbon-carbon composites (CCCs). At this time, PMCs, MMCs, and CCCs are the key composites of interest for thermal management, the focus of this article.

Figure 1, which plots thermal conductivity as a function of CTE for a variety of materials used in electronics, illustrates the limitations of traditional packaging materials. In order to minimize thermal stresses in many packaging designs, it is necessary to match the CTEs of semiconductors like silicon and gallium arsenide and ceramics used for substrates, such as alumina, beryllia, and aluminum nitride. These materials have CTEs in the range of about 4 to 7 ppm/K (shaded area). As the figure shows, aluminum and copper have good thermal conductivities but CTEs that are much higher than desired.

Traditional microelectronic packaging materials used to achieve low CTEs include Kovar, a nickel-iron alloy, and blends of copper and tungsten (Cu-W) or copper and molybdenum (Cu-Mo). Kovar has a low thermal conductivity and a density much higher than that of aluminum. Low-CTE materials with higher thermal conductivities than Kovar are obtained by blending copper with tungsten or molybdenum. As the two constituents are not alloyed, these materials can be considered composites; that is, they satisfy our definition of a composite material as two or more materials bonded together. For clarity in this article, materials consisting of two distinct metals bonded together are referred to as metal-metal composites. The term metal-matrix composite is reserved for metals reinforced with fibers or particles. Table 1 presents more detail about the properties of many of the materials in Fig. 1.

Although the thermal conductivities of Cu-W and Cu-Mo are much greater than that of Kovar, they are in the range of aluminum alloys. Higher values, along with low CTE and density, are desired.

There are several composite materials in Fig. 1 that have CTEs in the desired range and significantly higher thermal conductivities than traditional materials. These materials include silicon carbide particle-reinforced aluminum ($[SiC]_p/Al$), carbon fiber-reinforced copper (C/Cu), carbon fiber-reinforced aluminum (C/Al), diamond particle-reinforced copper ($[diamond]_p/Cu$), and beryllia particle-reinforced beryllium ($[BeO]_p/Be$). A number of other materials are seen to have high thermal conductivities, but these materials lie outside the shaded area. In addition to silver, aluminum, and copper, such materials include pyrolitic graphite, CCCs, carbon fiber-reinforced epoxy (C/Ep) and, of course, diamond.

The CTE of E-glass fiber-reinforced epoxy (E-glass/Ep), the most widely used PCB material, is much higher than that of silicon. Coefficients of thermal expansion range between 12 and 18 ppm/K. This can give rise to warpage and high thermal stresses in solder joints when integrated circuits (ICs, or chips) made from silicon and other semiconductors are directly attached to PCBs. To reduce stresses in the solder joints and ICs, which can cause premature failure, adhesive called an underfill is commonly introduced between the chip and PCB. However, this is a relatively slow, costly step, which does not necessarily eliminate undesirable warpage.

In some designs, lids used to remove heat from chips are bonded to the PCB, and a compliant thermal grease, gel, or other interface material is used between the chip and lid. In this case, it is desirable to have the CTE of the lid match that of the PCB. One of the big advantages of composites is that it is possible to tailor properties like CTE over a wide range. For example, we find commercial metal-metal and metal-matrix composite formulations with CTEs similar to those of both silicon and E-glass/Ep.

To compare packaging materials in applications for which both thermal conductivity and density are important, a useful figure of merit is specific thermal conductivity, defined as thermal conductivity divided by density (for simplicity, specific gravity, which is dimensionless, is used). Materials with high specific thermal conductivities are desirable in weight critical applications. Figure 2 presents specific thermal conductivity as a function of CTE for packaging materials. The specific thermal conductivities of traditional low-CTE packaging materials like Kovar, Cu-W,

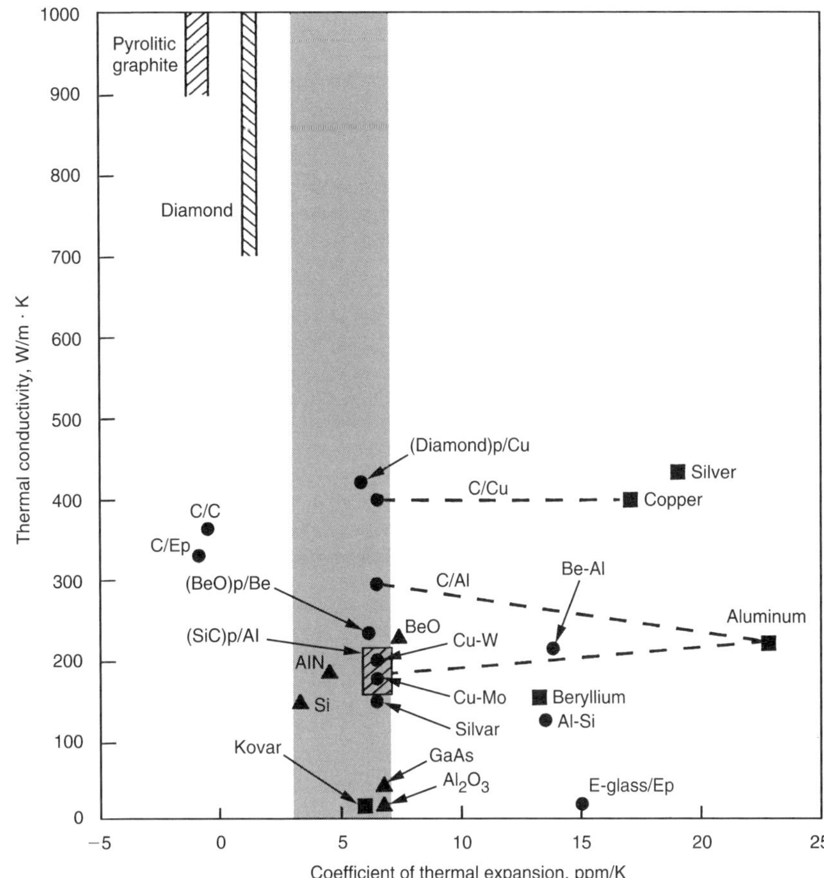

Fig. 1 Thermal conductivity as a function of coefficient of thermal expansion for materials used in electronic packaging

Table 1 Properties of selected electronic packaging materials

Reinforcement	Matrix	Thermal conductivity, W/m · K	Coefficient of thermal expansion, ppm/K	Modulus of elasticity GPa	Modulus of elasticity 10^6 psi	Specific gravity
Unreinforced	Silicon	150	4.1	. . .	. . .	2.3
	Alumina	20	6.7	380	55	3.9
	Aluminum	120	23	69	10	2.7
	Copper	400	17	117	17	8.9
	Epoxy	1.7	54	3	0	1.2
	Kovar	17	5.9	131	19	8.3
	Pyrolitic graphite	1600–1700	–1.0	. . .	. . .	2.3
Copper	Tungsten	167	6.5	248	36	16.6
	Molybdenum	184	7.0	282	41	10.0
Beryllium	Aluminum	210	13.9	179	26	2.1
E-glass fibers	Epoxy	0.16–0.26	11–16	16–19	2–3	2.1
Invar	Silver	153	6.5	110	16	8.8
Continuous carbon fibers	Epoxy	300	–1.1	186	27	1.8
	Copper	400	6.5	158	23	7.2
	Aluminum	290	6.5	131	19	2.5
Discontinuous carbon fibers	Aluminum	185	6.0	14	2	2.5
	Polymer	20	4–7	30 50	4–7	1.6
	Carbon	400	–1.0	255	37	1.9
Silicon	Aluminum	126–160	6.5–13.5	100–130	15–19	2.5–2.6
SiC particles	Aluminum	170–220	6.2–7.3	225–265	33–38	3.0
Discontinuous carbon-graphite	Aluminum	400–600	4.5–5.0	90–100	13–15	2.3
Diamond particles	Aluminum	550–600	7.0–7.5	. . .	. . .	3.1
Beryllia particles	Beryllium	240	6.1	330	48	2.6

Coefficients of thermal expansion, thermal conductivities, and elastic moduli for composites reinforced with continuous fibers are in-plane isotropic values. Fiber volume fractions for metal-matrix composites reinforced with continuous fibers are selected to achieve an in-plane coefficient of thermal expansion of 6.5 ppm/K.

and Cu-Mo are very low. However, the low density of many composites combined with their high thermal conductivities enhances their relative position. In fact, the specific thermal conductivities of some composites are more than an order of magnitude greater than those of traditional materials like Kovar, Cu-W, and Cu-Mo.

A rule of thumb states that improving a critical property by an order of magnitude produces revolutionary change in a technology. It is not surprising, therefore, that composites are making significant inroads in thermal management and electronic packaging.

A key advantage of some of composites is that they can be used with processes that produce parts having the final desired shape (net-shape processes) or that require only a small amount of machining (near-net shape processes). Minimizing machining enhances the cost effectiveness of these materials. This is particularly true for silicon carbide particle-reinforced aluminum (often called Al/SiC in the electronic packaging industry and discontinuously reinforced aluminum, or DRA, in the aerospace industry), which is one of the most important of the new composite packaging materials.

In the following sections, the key types of reinforcements and composites used for microelectronic packaging and thermal management, significant applications, and future directions are considered.

Important issues must be taken into account when considering properties of composites and ceramics. First, there are a large and increasing number of materials in these categories, all of which are proprietary. In addition, there are a variety of test methods used to measure properties. As a consequence, reported properties may vary significantly. For example, reported properties of aluminum oxide from one manufacturer may differ significantly from a nominally identical material made by another manufacturer. This is particularly true for composites, for which reinforcements, reinforcement volume fractions, reinforcement geometry, matrix materials, and processes may differ significantly. The properties of composites are very process sensitive. Another consideration is that many properties, including CTE and thermal conductivity, are often strongly temperature dependent. Room temperature values are presented in this article. A fundamental issue is that, especially in the early stages of development, the only source of material properties may be the manufacturer rather than an independent source.

For the reasons cited, properties presented in this article should be considered representative values. They are intended to be used for comparative purposes, not design allowables. It is always good practice to verify material properties used for design.

Reinforcements

Several types of reinforcements are used in composite materials: continuous fibers, discontinuous fibers, whiskers (elongated single crystals), and particles. Flakes are included in the last category. At this time, the most important reinforcements for obtaining high thermal conductivity are pitch-based carbon (also called graphite) fibers, which are used in continuous and discontinuous forms, and two types of ceramic particles, silicon carbide (SiC) and beryllia (beryllium oxide, BeO). As a rule, continuous fibers are much more efficient than discontinuous fibers and particles for achieving high thermal conductivity, stiffness, and strength. An increasing number of reinforcements are of interest.

Composites reinforced with discontinuous fibers or particles may have processing advantages in some instances. A key characteristic of materials reinforced with equiaxed (roughly spherical, sandlike) particles is that they tend to be isotropic. That is, their properties are similar in all directions. This is not true of materials reinforced with continuous fibers or platelike flake particles, which are almost always anisotropic, which means that their properties vary with direction.

If a composite is reinforced with discontinuous fibers that are truly randomly oriented, its properties are statistically isotropic. However, virtually all processes produce some degree of preferred fiber orientation, and there are no strictly isotropic random-fiber composites. It is possible and quite common to make fiber reinforced materials with properties that are approximately isotropic in a plane. These materials are called quasi-isotropic or pseudoisotropic materials.

A major advantage of using continuous fibers is that it is possible to vary directional properties significantly. For example, it is possible to produce composites with very high thermal conductivities, stiffnesses, and strengths in particular directions by orienting a high percentage of fibers along these axes. In some instances, this can make fiberreinforced composites more efficient than heat pipes in transporting heat over relatively short distances. An additional benefit is that solid-state methods of heat transfer are more reliable.

Carbon Fibers. The most important types of commercial carbon fibers at this time are made from polyacrylonitrile (PAN) and pitches derived from petroleum and coal. Figure 3, which is adapted from one developed by Amoco Performance Products (now BP-Amoco), shows how thermal conductivity varies with electrical resistivity for selected metals and carbon fibers. There are commercial pitch-based carbon fibers with thermal conductivities almost three times that of copper. At the upper end of the spectrum

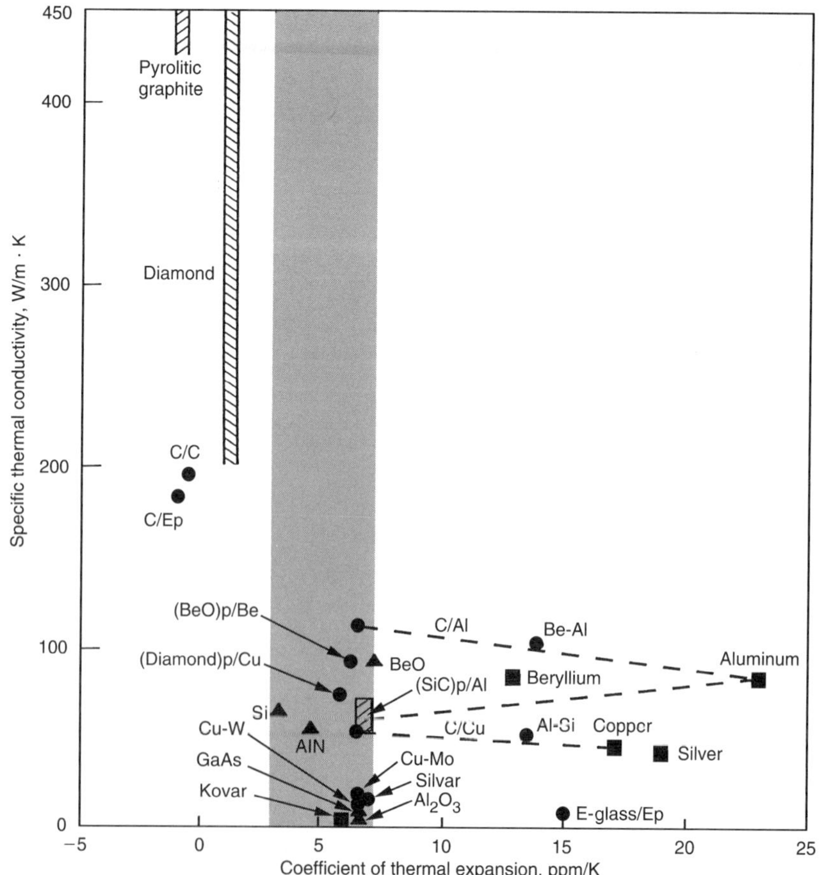

Fig. 2 Specific thermal conductivity (thermal conductivity divided by specific gravity) as a function of thermal expansion for materials used in electronic packaging

are experimental fibers made by chemical vapor deposition (CVD) that have thermal conductivities in the range of 2000 W/m · K, five times that of copper. These reinforcements are also called vapor-grown carbon fibers.

At the time of publication, the commercial fiber with the highest thermal conductivity was K1100, manufactured by BP-Amoco (Chicago, IL), which has a nominal axial thermal conductivity of 1100 W/m · K. Other companies also produce pitch-based carbon fibers with high thermal conductivities.

Note that carbon fibers are generally strongly anisotropic. For example, the radial thermal conductivity of K1100 carbon fibers is at least an order of magnitude lower than the axial value.

In addition to their high thermal conductivities, pitch-based carbon fibers have other attractive attributes for packaging and structural applications: elastic moduli as high as 965 GPa (140×10^6 psi), more than an order of magnitude greater than that of aluminum, and very low densities. These reinforcements are being used with polymer, metal, and carbon matrices to create light, stiff composites with extremely high thermal conductivities and low, tailorable CTEs.

Additional information is available in the article "Carbon Fibers" in this Volume.

Ceramic Particles. As previously noted, ceramic particles have been used to increase the thermal conductivity and reduce the CTE of polymers for some time. Although these particulate PMCs are significantly more thermally conductive than monolithic (unreinforced) resins, their thermal conductivities are still an order of magnitude lower than that of aluminum. Since the 1980s, however, ceramic particles have been added to metals to achieve the same objectives as for polymers, high thermal conductivity and low CTE, creating MMCs that are now used in significant production applications. These composites also have much lower densities than traditional low-CTE metallic materials used in packaging.

As mentioned earlier, the two key materials currently used as particulate reinforcements are silicon carbide and beryllia. Diamond particles also have been used to reinforce metals on an experimental basis. Because of the difficulty of measuring the thermal conductivity of particles, it is common to assume that they have values similar to those of bulk materials. However, there are considerable differences in published thermal conductivities for ceramics. In general, transport properties like thermal conductivity are more difficult to measure than bulk properties such as modulus.

Additional information is available in the article "Ceramic Fibers" in this Volume.

Thermal Management Composites and Other Advanced Materials

In this section, the three key classes of composite materials used in thermal management and electronic packaging at this time, PMCs, MMCs, and CCCs, are considered. Pyrolitic graphite, a monolithic material, some forms of which have very high in-plane thermal conductivity, is also discussed.

Polymer-Matrix Composites. Polymers reinforced with continuous K1100 carbon fiber offer the highest thermal conductivity of all commercial PMCs. Table 1 shows the in-plane properties of quasi-isotropic epoxy-matrix composites reinforced with continuous K1100 fibers. Composite properties depend strongly on reinforcement content; the fiber volume fraction of the composites listed in Table 1 is 0.60. The in-plane thermal conductivity and elastic modulus of this composite are much higher than the corresponding properties of aluminum, and its density is much lower. The specific thermal conductivities of these composites are greater than that of copper. Note that the in-plane CTE is negative. This is not an error; carbon fibers generally have negative CTEs. Although the CTE of this composite does not fall in the desired range of 4 to 7 ppm/K, it is much closer to it than those of aluminum and copper.

Note that a K1100 carbon-fiber-reinforced PMC with a fiber volume fraction of 0.60 having all fibers oriented in the same direction, which is called a unidirectional composite, would have a nominal axial thermal conductivity of 660 W/m · K, over 150% greater than that of copper (approximately 400 W/m · K).

Although continuous fibers offer the best properties, PMCs reinforced with discontinuous fibers can be used with relatively inexpensive net-shape processes such as injection molding. Table 1 shows representative properties of a composite with discontinuous K1100 fibers. Note that both thermal conductivity and elastic modulus are much lower than those for composites reinforced with continuous fibers. Despite these limitations, the manufacturing advantages of discontinuous fiber PMCs have led to some very high production volumes.

Metal-Matrix Composites. At this time, the key electronic-packaging MMCs are:

- Silicon carbide particle-reinforced aluminum (Al/SiC, also known as discontinuously reinforced aluminum, or DRA)
- Beryllia particle-reinforced beryllium
- Carbon fiber-reinforced aluminum
- Aluminum-silicon, a metal-metal composite

Table 1 presents properties of these materials.

In recent years, a number of new metal-metal composites also have been developed, including beryllium-aluminum, Invar-silver (Silvar) and Invar-copper (Cuvar). An Al-Si composite consisting of 60% aluminum and 40% silicon that has been commercially available for many years also has been used for packaging. It is interesting that one manufacturer of this material, who for many years called it an aluminum-silicon alloy, now refers to it as a metal-metal composite. Because the solubility of aluminum and silicon at room temperature is relatively low, the material consists of an interpenetrating network of aluminum and silicon. Recently, a new family of Al-Si materials with higher levels of silicon has been made by a powder spray process. One formulation has a CTE in the range of ceramic substrates and semiconductors and another a CTE similar to that of E-glass/epoxy (Ref 3). A key advantage of Al-Si is that it is much easier to machine than Al/SiC. Table 1 presents properties of these materials.

The most successful of the newer MMCs presently is silicon-carbide particle-reinforced aluminum (Al/SiC), which was first discussed as a packaging material in Ref 4 to 10. Figure 4 shows how the CTE of Al/SiC varies with particle content. For particle volume fractions in the range of 0.7, it is possible to match the CTE of silicon. That, and its low density and net-shape-fabrication capability, have led to rapidly increasing use of this material. As discussed earlier, Al/SiC formulations with CTEs matching that of E-glass/epoxy PCBs are being used in IC lids. The particle volume fraction of these MMCs is in the range of 20%. They are relatively ductile and can be formed by stamping, a low-cost process. Lids made of this material are cost competitive with the machined-copper parts they are replacing.

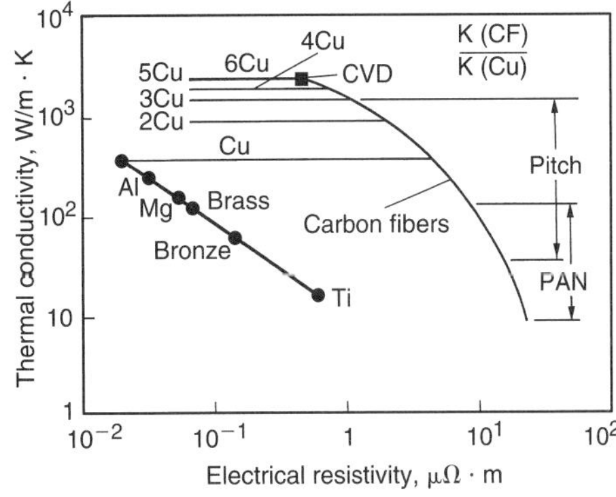

Fig. 3 Thermal conductivity as a function of electrical resistivity for metals and carbon fibers

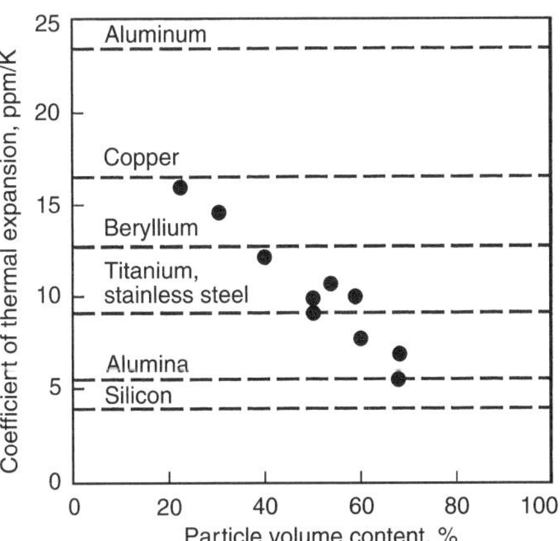

Fig. 4 Coefficient of thermal expansion as a function of particle content for silicon carbide particle-reinforced aluminum

Beryllia-particle-reinforced beryllium also has been used in production applications, although not as widely as Al/SiC because of higher cost.

Metal-matrix composites consisting of continuous and discontinuous thermally conductive carbon fibers are also being employed in packaging and thermal management applications. Materials made with continuous fibers are relatively expensive, and there have been relatively few applications to date. However, recent developments have resulted in significant cost reductions for discontinuous-fiber MMCs, and these materials are now entering production systems. It should be noted that, like common laminated metals used in electronic packaging such as copper-Invar-Copper and copper-molybdenum-copper, MMCs reinforced with continuous fibers may display significant hysteresis when subjected to large thermal excursions or mechanical stresses (Ref 1).

Other MMCs with high thermal conductivities are made by infiltrating porous carbon/carbon composites and fibrous carbon-fiber preforms or felts with aluminum or copper. For materials with highly oriented fibers such as ThermalGraph, axial thermal conductivities as high as 890 W/m · K have been reported (Ref 11). Another MMC infiltrated with copper has reported in-plane and through-thickness thermal conductivities of 700 W/m · K and 250 W/m · K, respectively.

A recently developed MMC consists of aluminum reinforced with nonfibrous discontinuous carbon graphite. The reported in-plane and through-thickness thermal conductivities are 420 to 600 W/m · K and 100 to 150 W/m · K, respectively.

The thermal conductivity of particle-reinforced MMCs depends greatly on the thermal properties of the interface. Early experimental diamond-particle-reinforced aluminum composites had thermal conductivities in the range of aluminum alloys, perhaps because of nonoptimum heat transfer across particle-matrix interfaces. Recent improvements have resulted in materials with a reported isotropic thermal conductivity in the range of 550 to 600 W/m · K and a CTE of 7 to 7.5 ppm/K.

Carbon-Carbon Composites and Pyrolitic Graphite. There are a large number of materials that fall in the category of CCCs, including ThermalGraph, which was discussed in the previous section. Carbon-carbon composites made from P120 carbon fibers, which have a nominal axial thermal conductivity of about 600 W/m · K, are reported to have an in-plane isotropic thermal conductivity of 250 W/m · K (Ref 11). This attribute, combined with a specific gravity of only 1.85, makes CCCs very attractive thermal-control materials for weight-sensitive applications (Ref 12). These materials are highly anisotropic, and through-thickness thermal conductivities are much lower.

CCCs with in-plane thermal conductivities as high as 400 to 450 W/m · K have been reported. Through-thickness values are in the range of 40 to 50 W/m · K.

There are other characteristics of CCCs worth noting. For one, they have relatively low strengths perpendicular to fiber directions. In addition, as discussed earlier, their in-plane CTEs are usually small, negative values. This is a characteristic they share with many PMCs reinforced with continuous fibers.

As shown in Fig. 1 and 2, pyrolitic graphite, a monolithic material, has very high in-plane thermal conductivity combined with a relatively low specific gravity of 2.5 (Ref 13). In-plane thermal conductivities as high as 1600 to 1700 W/m · K are reported. This material is highly anisotropic, and the through-thickness conductivity is only 25 W/m · K. One of the deficiencies of pyrolitic graphite is that, like other forms of monolithic graphite, it is relatively weak and brittle. To overcome this problem, pyrolitic graphite is being used as a laminate in which it is encapsulated with structural materials such as aluminum, copper, beryllium, Kovar, and two composites, Al/SiC and carbon/epoxy.

Applications

Composites are now being used in important commercial and aerospace thermal management and microelectronic packaging applications. Annual production for some packaging parts is in the hundreds of thousands. At this time, the most widely used composites are Cu-Mo, Cu-W, Al/SiC, and discontinuous thermally conductive carbon-fiber-reinforced polymers.

Microelectronic packaging components include carriers, complex hermetic microwave packages (modules), power semiconductor packages, solid and flow-through liquid-cooled PCB cold plates (thermal planes), heat sinks for integrated circuit packages, including pin-fin heat sinks, thermal straps, enclosures, and support structures (Ref 3–8, 10–18, 19–24).

Spacecraft applications, in addition to electronic packaging, include radiators, radiator panel thermal doublers, and battery sleeves (Ref 25–30). Additional information is provided in the article "Space Applications" in this Volume.

The composite electronic packaging components cited in the previous paragraph are being used in numerous commercial and aerospace products, including electric vehicles, motor controllers, cellular telephone ground stations, laptop computers, and aircraft and spacecraft microwave and power supply subsystems. In addition, composites are key materials in developmental integrated multifunctional structural/electronic systems (Ref 30).

Future Trends

Virtually all of the experts predict that packaging density will continue to increase, and, with it, the need for continuing improvements in thermal management. This will require a variety of new solutions including use of heat pipes and active fluid cooling. However, it is unlikely that the latter two approaches will solve all thermal management problems. Further, a passive solution, such as use of materials with improved thermal conductivities, simplifies thermal management and improves reliability. In addition, use of active cooling and heat pipes does not eliminate the issue of thermal stresses resulting from thermal-expansion mismatch.

Another important trend is the continuing competition to reduce the weight of portable systems, such as laptop computers and handheld cellular telephones. In addition to these commercial products, the drive to reduce weight in electronics and thermal management systems used in aircraft, spacecraft, and even shipboard applications will continue.

Based on these facts, it is concluded that there will continue to be a need for improved materials that have high thermal conductivities and low, tailorable CTEs. In addition, there is a need for low-density materials in many applications. Cost will continue to be a critical issue in both the aerospace and commercial industries.

It is clear that the early stages of an important new materials technology are underway. The future will undoubtedly see development of improved and new reinforcements, matrix materials, material systems, and manufacturing processes. Increasing material production volumes and improved processes will reduce costs, making composites even more competitive.

As a historical point of reference, carbon fibers sold for $500/kg ($225/lb) when they were first introduced commercially in the early 1970s. It is now possible to buy commercial structural grade fibers for as little as $4/kg ($2/lb). Further price reductions appear likely as volume builds. In particular, the following trends in reinforcements appear likely:

- Silicon carbide particles with much higher thermal conductivities (over 400 W/m · K has been measured for high-purity single crystals)
- Use of diamond, aluminum nitride, and cubic boron nitride particles
- Commercial pitch-based and vapor-grown carbon fibers with higher thermal conductivities, perhaps approaching 2000 W/m · K
- Commercial diamond and diamond-coated carbon fibers with thermal conductivities also approaching 2000 W/m · K
- Reinforcement coatings to promote adhesion, reduce reinforcement-matrix reactions, and improve thermal conductivity
- Use of carbon nanotubes, which have very high thermal conductivities

Based on experience in the field of structural composites, expecting the development of polymer, metal, and carbon-matrix material systems, which are tailored for use in thermal management and packaging applications with the reinforcements listed previously, is also reasonable. In addition, use of inherently electronically conductive polymers could be advantageous in providing EMI shielding.

The field of nanocomposites, which includes the carbon nanotubes cited previously, is likely to contribute some interesting new materials. For example, incorporation of ceramic nanoparticles could be useful in tailoring CTE and increasing thermal conductivity.

Current development efforts are likely to result in improved processes for production of net-shape components. This will eliminate machining costs and make composites more competitive with traditional materials.

In summary, the need for improved thermal management and microelectronic packaging materials will continue for the foreseeable future. The present infancy of an important materials technology will continue to produce new and improved composite materials and manufacturing processes. Advances will make composites more technically attractive and also reduce costs. The result will be increasing use of composites in many thermal-control and electronic-packaging applications.

Beyond the thermal management materials discussed in this article, major opportunities for composites in other areas of electronic packaging exist. For example, there are great needs for new materials with improved dielectric properties and high thermal conductivities for use in PCBs and electrically insulating substrates. Materials of interest here include ceramic fibers and particles in ceramic and polymeric matrices. Because the requirements of packaging materials for optoelectronics and MEMS are similar to those of microelectronics, composites also have great potential in these important and rapidly growing applications.

Extending to other aspects of the electronics industry, great potential also exists for composites in high-speed, precise manufacturing and assembly machinery, such as pick-and-place machines. Lasky dramatically points out the inefficiency inherent in current equipment (Ref 31). He observes that gantries used to place a 1 mg component may weigh 100 kg, or 100,000,000 times as much.

When components of current electronic-industry assembly machines are examined, the materials of construction, that is, steel, cast iron, aluminum, and granite, are found to have been developed in previous centuries. There is little doubt that in the twenty-first century, composites will be the materials of choice in high-performance machinery because of their unmatched properties. Benefits of composites in machinery include:

- Order of magnitude improvements in specific stiffness (stiffness divided by density)
- Outstanding fatigue resistance
- Excellent corrosion resistance
- Low CTEs (some nearly zero)

Other applications of composites in the electronics industry include photolithography equipment and wafer-handling devices.

As a result of their unique attributes, all four classes of composites, PMCs, MMCs, CMCs and CCCs, are now being used in countless commercial-production applications including automobile engine blocks, automobile and truck diesel engine pistons, automobile and pickup truck-brake rotors and drive shafts, rollers used in printing presses, audio- and videotape production machines, coordinate-measuring machines, automated ultrasonic inspection equipment, cutting tools, and equipment used in the manufacture of optical fibers and glass products (Ref 19, 20). In short, the limitless potential for composites has barely been explored, not only in electronics packaging, but also throughout the electronics industry.

ACKNOWLEDGMENT

Figures 1 to 4 and some of the data in this article were taken from Ref 19 and appear courtesy of John Wiley & Sons, Inc.

REFERENCES

1. K.A. Schmidt and C. Zweben, Section Editors and Authors, "Advanced Composite Packaging Materials," *Electronic Materials Handbook*, Vol 1, *Packaging*, ASM International, 1989, p 1117–1131
2. A. Kelly, *Concise Encyclopedia of Composite Materials*, Pergamon Press, Oxford, 1988
3. S.P.S. Sangha et al., Novel Aluminum-Silicon Alloys for Electronics Packaging, *Eng. Sci. Edu. J.*, Oct 1997, p 195–201
4. C. Thaw, J. Zemany, and C. Zweben, Metal Matrix Composite Microwave Packaging Components, *SAMPE J.*, Vol 23 (No. 6), 1987
5. C. Thaw, J. Zemany, and C. Zweben, Metal Matrix Composites for Microwave Packaging Components, *Electronic Packaging and Production*, Aug 1987, p 27–29
6. C. Thaw, J. Zemany, and C. Zweben, "Metal Matrix Composite Hybrid Microelectronic Package Components," presented at National Electronic Packaging Conf., - NEPCON East '87 (Boston), Reed Exhibition Companies, June 1987
7. C. Zweben, Lightweight, Low-Thermal-Expansion Composite Heat Sink, *Proc. National Electronic Packaging and Production Conf.*, presented at NEPCON East '88 (Boston), Reed Exhibition Companies, June 1988
8. K.A. Schmidt and C. Zweben, "Advanced Composite Materials for Microelectronic, Power Semiconductor, Microwave and Laser Diode Packaging," presented at Metal Matrix Composites - 88 (Philadelphia), Society of Manufacturing Engineers, Sept 1988
9. C. Zweben, Mechanical and Thermal Properties of Silicon Carbide Particle-Reinforced Aluminum, *Thermal and Mechanical Behavior of Metal Matrix and Ceramic Matrix Composites*, STP 1080, L.M. Kennedy, H.H. Moeller and W.S. Johnson, Ed. American Society for Testing and Materials, Philadelphia, 1989
10. C. Zweben, Overview of Metal Matrix Composites for Electronic Packaging and Thermal Management, *JOM*, July 1992
11. J. Miller, "ThermalGraph Product Forms for Use in Space, Electronics and Satellite Applications," seminar on Pitch Fiber Composites for Space Structures (Long Beach, CA), Oct 1995
12. W.T. Shih, Carbon-Carbon (C-C) Composites for Thermal Plane Applications, *Proc. Seventh International SAMPE Electronics Conf.*, June 1994
13. M.J. Montesano, New Material for Thermal Management Has Four Times Thermal Conductivity of Copper, *Mat. Technol.*, 1996, Vol 11 (No. 3), 1996, p 87–91
14. M. DiNardo, J. Kreitz, and C. Zweben, Lightweight Composite Electronics Enclosure for High Stress and Temperature Environments, *Proc. 35th International SAMPE Symposium and Exhibition* (Anaheim), April 1990
15. C. Zweben, The Future of Advanced Composite Electronic Packaging, *Materials for Electronic Packaging,* D.D.L. Chung, Ed., Butterworth-Heinemann, Oxford, 1995
16. T.F. Fleming, C.D. Levan, and W.C. Riley, Applications for Ultra-High Thermal Conductivity Fibers, *Proc. of the International Electronic Packaging Conf.* (Wheaton, IL), International Electronic Packaging Society, 1995, p 493–503
17. D.D.L. Chung, Overview of Materials for Electronic Packaging, *Materials for Electronic Packaging.*, D.D.L. Chung, Ed. Butterworth-Heinemann, Oxford, 1995
18. C. Zweben, course notes, workshop on Cost Effective, High Performance Composite Materials for Electronic Packaging and Thermal Control, National Electronic Packaging and Production Conf., NEPCON West '98, (Anaheim), March 1998
19. C. Zweben, Composite Materials and Mechanical Design, *Mechanical Engineers' Handbook,* 2nd ed., M. Kutz, Ed., John Wiley & Sons, Inc., New York, 1998
20. C. Zweben, "Advanced Composite Materials for Mechanical Engineering Applications," American Society of Mechanical Engineers Distinguished Lecture Program, 1998
21. C. Zweben, Advances in Thermal Management Materials for Electronic Applications, *JOM Special Topics Series*, June 1998
22. D.D.L. Chung and C. Zweben, Composites for Electronic Packaging and Thermal Management, *Comprehensive Composite Materials*, Vol 6, *Design and Applications*, A. Kelly and C. Zweben, Ed., Pergamon Press, Oxford, 2000
23. C. Zweben, High Performance Thermal Management Materials, *Electron. Cool.*, Vol 5 (No. 3), Sept 1999, p 36–42
24. C. Zweben, Heat Sink Materials for Electronic Packaging, *Encyclopedia of Materials: Science and Technology*, K.H.J. Buschow et al., Ed., Pergamon Press, Oxford, in press
25. J.L. Kuhn, S.M. Benner, C. D. Butler, and

E.A. Silk, Thermal and Mechanical Performance of a Carbon-Carbon Composite Spacecraft Radiator, *Proc. Conf. on Composite Materials and Applications*, SPIE International Symposium on Optical Science, Engineering and Instrumentation (Denver), Society of Photo-Optical Instrumentation Engineers, July 1999

26. C. Zweben, Overview of Composite Materials for Optomechanical, Data storage and Thermal Management System Applications, *Proc. Conf. on Composite Materials and Applications*, SPIE International Symposium on Optical Science, Engineering and Instrumentation (Denver), Society of Photo-Optical Instrumentation Engineers, July 1999
27. C. Zweben, Advanced Composites in Spacecraft and Launch Vehicles, *Launchspace*, June/July 1998, p 55–58
28. C. Zweben, "Material Selection and Manufacturing for Spacecraft and Launch Vehicles," state-of-the-art report, Advanced Materials and Processes Technology Information Analysis Center (AMPTIAC), Rome, New York, in press
29. S.P. Rawal and J.W. Goodman, Composites for Spacecraft, *Comprehensive Composite Materials*, Vol 6, *Design and Applications*, A. Kelly and C. Zweben, Ed., Pergamon Press, Oxford, 2000
30. S.P. Rawal, Multifunctional Composite Materials and Structures, *Comprehensive Composite Materials*, Vol 6, *Design and Applications*, A. Kelly and C. Zweben, Ed., Pergamon Press, Oxford, 2000
31. R. Lasky, Software and Assembly Line Integration, *Electr. Packag. Prod.*, Jan 1998, p 64–66

Marine Applications

A.P. Mouritz, RMIT University, Australia
C.P. Gardiner, Defence Science & Technology Organisation, Australia

THE FIRST MARINE APPLICATION of fiber-reinforced polymer (FRP) composite materials was in the construction of boats shortly after World War II. This was about the time that composites were first used for other applications, such as in aircraft, electrical devices, and building materials. Boat builders began to use FRP composites instead of timber, which was traditionally used in small maritime craft, because wood was becoming increasingly scarce and expensive. Timber was also losing favor with many boat builders and owners, because wooden boat hulls are degraded by seawater and marine organisms and therefore require ongoing maintenance and repairs that can be expensive. The earliest attempt to fabricate boat hulls with FRP composites was in 1947 when twelve small surfboats were made for the United States Navy. At the time, little was known about the design and construction of composite boats, the fabrication technologies were underdeveloped, and the materials had low strength and poor durability in seawater. This combination of factors led to the construction of composite boats that were not seaworthy, and many had to be scrapped. The early history of the development and application of composites to marine craft has been reported (Ref 1–3).

The design techniques, processing technology, fiber reinforcements, and resins improved rapidly after the early problems, and composites were used successfully during the 1950s in small leisure craft, yachts, and naval boats as well as in ship and submarine structures, such as radomes, sonar domes, and casings. Knowledge and confidence in composites grew with these applications, and this further expanded the number and types of maritime craft made of composites. For example, by the mid-1960s, over 3000 boats had been built of composite materials for the United States Navy, including over 800 motor whaleboats, 330 utility boats, 250 landing craft, 220 personnel boats, and 120 patrol boats. Since the 1970s, composites have also been used in niche applications on offshore oil drilling platforms and, as with maritime craft, the use of FRP materials is expanding into new platform applications.

Most maritime craft are built using glass-reinforced polyester (GRP) composites, although sandwich composites and advanced FRP materials containing carbon or aramid fibers with vinyl ester or epoxy-resin matrices are commonly used for high-performance structural applications. Composites are now used in a wide variety of craft, ranging in size from canoes, dinghies, and yachts to racing maxis, hovercraft, patrol boats, naval minehunting ships, and corvettes. Composites are also used in lightweight structures on warships, such as advanced mast systems and superstructure sections. The application of composites to leisure craft, yachts, boats, ships, submarines, and offshore structures has been extensively reviewed (e.g., Ref 4–10). The purpose of this article is to briefly outline current and potential applications of composites for maritime craft and offshore drilling platforms. The key benefits gained from using FRP materials together with an examination of the drawbacks and major issues impeding the more widespread use of composites in marine structures are given.

Naval Applications of FRP Composites

The application of FRP composites to maritime craft was initially driven by a need for lightweight, strong, corrosion resistant, and durable naval boats (Ref 1–3). The United States Navy sponsored most of the early design, research, and development work that led to the production of composite boats. Initially, the navy funded the production of small personnel boats, although this was followed in the 1950s by support for a variety of other craft, including patrol boats, landing craft, and minesweeping boats. The United States Navy was also the first to use composites on large ships for deckhouses, pipes, and fuel and water tanks, as well as on submarines for fairwaters and mast shrouds (Ref 1–3). From the 1950s, other navies, most notably the British, French, and Swedish Navies, began to use composites on their vessels, which further expanded the marine applications of FRP materials (Ref 11, 12). The expansion in the use of composites on naval ships and submarines during the 1950s and 1960s was dramatic, and by the mid-1960s the number of applications was extremely diverse, as shown in Table 1. Most of these early applications were driven by the need to overcome corrosion problems experienced with steel or aluminum alloys or environmental degradation suffered by wood. Another reason for using composites was to reduce weight, particularly the topside weight of ships. The high acoustic transparency of composites also resulted in their use in radomes on ships and sonar domes on submarines.

Up to the 1960s, however, the only naval boats built entirely of composites were under 20 m (66 ft) in length. It was not safe to build larger warships with composites, because they would not have adequate hull girder stiffness due to the low Young's modulus of FRP materials. Low hull girder stiffness would cause excessive hogging and sagging of a composite ship in heavy seas. Such large hull deflections cause fatigue-induced failures of the hull, bulkheads, and joints and also cause serviceability problems, such as shaft misalignment and loss of sealing to watertight hatches. The problem of low hull girder stiffness for small warships (less than ~50 m, or 165 ft, long) was overcome in the early 1970s with the construction of the Royal Navy

Table 1 Early naval applications of FRP composites (1945–1965)

Minesweeper (15.5 m, or 51 ft, long)
Landing craft (15.2 m, or 50 ft)
Personnel boat (7.9 m, or 26 ft)
Sheathing of wood hulls
Submarine sonar dome
Submarine fins
Masts and mast shrouds
Rudders
Tanks (fuel, lube oil, water)
Torpedo tubes
Hatch covers
Landing craft reconnaissance (15.8 m, or 52 ft)
River patrol boat (9.5m, or 31 ft)
Pilot boat
Submarine fairwater
Submarine nonpressure hull casing
Deckhouses for small ships
Radomes
Antenna trunks
Piping
Crew shelters
Rope guards

minesweeper HMS *Wilton* (Ref 13, 14). This ship was 46.6 m (153 ft) long with a full-load displacement of 450 tons, making it the largest all-composite ship at the time. High hull girder stiffness was achieved by building the ship with an innovative composite hull known as the framed single-skin design. The hull basically consisted of a thin FRP laminate shell stiffened with longitudinal and transverse frames, mostly of "top hat" cross-section sandwich composite construction. Not only did the hull have adequate stiffness, but it also had excellent impact and underwater blast damage resistance that is essential for naval ships.

Since the mid-1970s, hundreds of patrol boats and minehunter ships in the 50 to 60 m (165 to 200 ft) length range have been built using composites (Ref 8). While the framed single-skin hull remains popular, two other hull forms have been developed for composite ships up to about 70 m (230 ft). These forms are monocoque construction, which basically consists of the thick laminate hull, and sandwich construction, which consists of thin FRP face skins over a thick core of medium-density polyvinyl chloride foam or polyurethane foam or end-grain balsa (Ref 5). Figure 1 shows examples of naval ships with the framed single-skin, monocoque, and sandwich hull types.

Increasingly, naval patrol boats are being built with an all-composite design or a composite hull fitted with an aluminum superstructure (Ref 8). The growing popularity of FRP patrol boats is due mainly to their excellent corrosion resistance, which reduces maintenance costs, and light weight, which can result in higher speeds and better fuel economy. It is estimated that composite patrol boats are usually approximately 10% lighter than an aluminum boat and over 35% lighter than a steel boat of the same size (Ref 15). However, the fabrication cost of a composite patrol boat is estimated to be about 30% higher than for a steel boat, which is a major impediment to their construction. An example of a modern composite patrol boat is the Skjøld class operated by the Royal Norwegian Navy, as shown in Fig. 2. The Skjøld is 46.8 m (154 ft) long with a full-load displacement of 270 tons and is made of a sandwich composite material (Ref 16). The core of the sandwich composite is polyvinyl chloride foam, and the face skins consist of glass- and carbon-fiber polymer laminates. Carbon-fiber composites are rarely used on naval vessels because of their high cost, however it is used in the Skjøld for structures requiring high stiffness, such as the mast, beam frames, and the support base to the gun.

The other type of naval vessel that is commonly built of composites is minehunting ships. Nearly 250 minehunter ships have been built since the mid-1970s using composite materials. A wide variety of minehunter ships made of single-skin or sandwich composites are in service, and three types are shown in Fig. 1. The main reasons for building minehunting ships with composite are they are nonmagnetic and corrosion resistant (Ref 5, 8, 17).

As a general design rule, the structural performance of ships less than approximately 50 to 60 m (165 to 200 ft) long, such as patrol boats and minehunters, is determined by the response of local structures, such as bulkheads and decks. On the other hand, the performance of ships longer than about 60 m (200 ft) is dominated by the hull girder stiffness. Because of the relatively low stiffness of most glass-reinforced polymer materials, almost all composite ships are under 60 m (200 ft) long. The only composite naval vessel built to date above this size is the 72 m (236 ft) long Visby class corvette for the Royal Swedish Navy (Ref 18), which is shown in Fig. 3. The Visby uses a sandwich composite incorporating a polyvinyl chloride foam core and carbon-fiber/vinyl ester laminate skins manufactured using a resin-infusion laminating method. The use of carbon-fiber composite reflects the

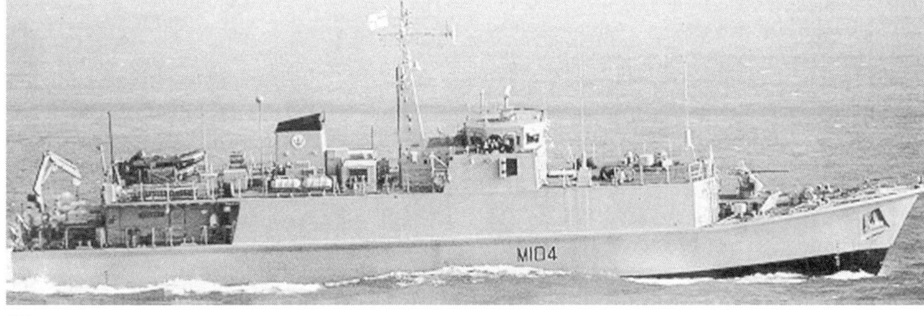

(a)

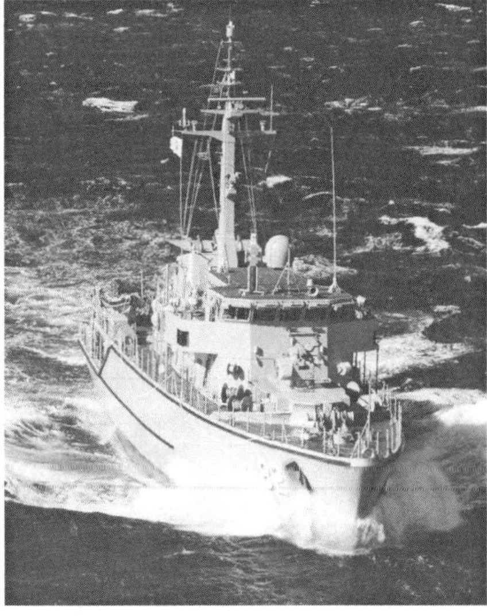

(b)

(c)

Fig. 1 Composite naval ships. (a) Sandown class minehunter ship with a framed single-skin hull form. (b) Huon class minehunter ship with a monocoque hull form. (c) Bay class minehunter ship with a sandwich composite hull form

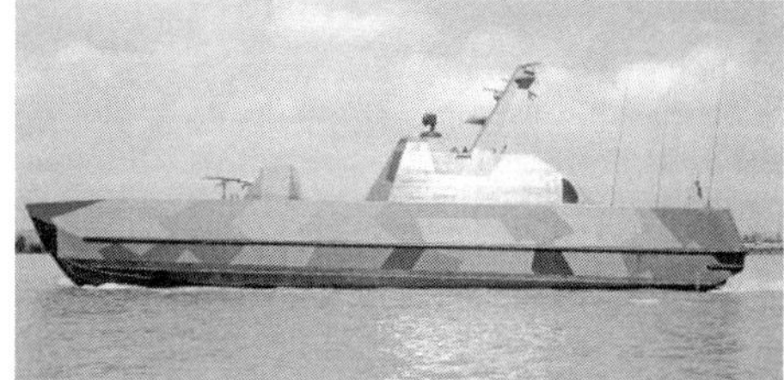

Fig. 2 The Skjøld class patrol boat

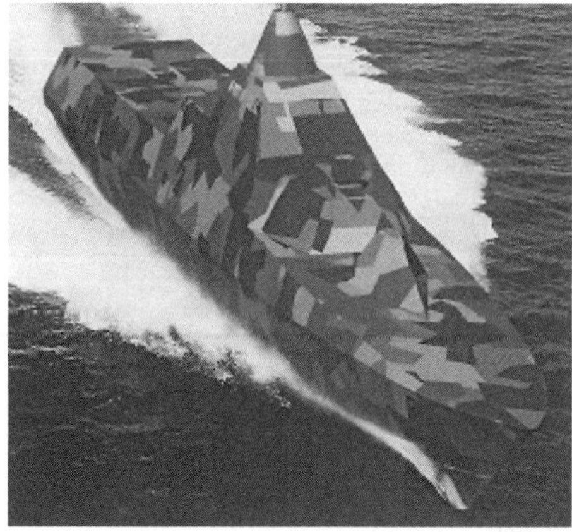

Fig. 3 Artist drawing of the all-composite Visby class corvette

increased demand on hull girder stiffness from a vessel of this length. The composite design also affords a high level of strength and durability, good shock resistance, a low magnetic signature, and a lightweight structure, as necessary for a ship designed for a multimission capability. The ship is undergoing sea trials and evaluation, and five more corvettes will be built.

An all-composite patrol boat/corvette, known as the NGPV class, is being designed for the Royal Singapore Navy and is expected to be 80 m (260 ft) long with a full-load displacement of 1016 tons. The United States Navy is also considering building their next-generation corvettes with composite materials (Ref 19). Navy ships longer than about 100 m (330 ft), such as frigates, destroyers, and aircraft carriers, are not likely to be constructed entirely with composites because it is much cheaper to build large ships with welded steel construction. At this stage in the development of large composite ships, it is glass-fiber-reinforced structures that have the longest service history. However, as carbon-reinforced ships, such as the Visby corvette, enter service and as the price of carbon-fiber material continues to drop, larger carbon-reinforced ship structures may become practical.

While it is not feasible to build large naval ships using composites, these materials are now used in a wide variety of topside structures and internal equipment on frigates, destroyers, and aircraft carriers. Composites are used in the superstructures on some naval ships to eliminate corrosion and fatigue cracking, lower topside weight, and reduce the radar cross section (Ref 20–22). The first large naval ship built with a composite superstructure was the La Fayette class frigate (Ref 23), which is shown in Fig. 4. Sandwich composite is used in the aft section of the superstructure, which includes a helicopter hangar and funnels. The aft section is 38 m (125 ft) long, 15 m (50 ft) wide, 6.5 to 8.5 m (21 to 28 ft) high from the main deck, and weighs 85 tons, which makes it the largest and heaviest composite superstructure on a naval ship. The forward section of the superstructure, which includes the bridge and combat and telecommunications centers, is built of steel because it was considered that a composite structure would not provide adequate protection against a high-pressure air blast. It is estimated that composite superstructures are 30 to 40% lighter than a steel structure, which results in better ship stability and fuel savings (Ref 21, 22, 24, 25). Composite superstructures are also more resistant to corrosion and fatigue, and therefore require less maintenance and fewer repairs. However, composite superstructures are estimated to be 35 to 50% more expensive to build (Ref 24, 25), and for this reason, most naval ships will continue to be built with steel or aluminum superstructures for at least the next ten years. However, the United States, British, and Norwegian Navies are considering fitting composite superstructure sections and helicopter hangars to some of their next-generation warships (Ref 24, 25).

Another major composite topside structure being developed for future use on large naval ships is masts. The feasibility of fabricating advanced communication and surveillance masts using composites is being explored because of numerous problems with conventional steel truss masts. The major problems with steel masts are that they corrode, increase the radar signature of the ship, and interfere with the ships own radar and communications systems because of their open structure. In 1997, the advanced enclosed mast/sensor (AEM/S) system was installed on the Spruance class destroyer USS *Arthur W. Radford* as a technology demonstrator (Ref 26). The entire mast is made of sandwich composite material and is 28 m (92 ft) tall and up to 10.7 m (35 ft) wide, as shown in Fig. 5. A major reason for building the AEM/S system with composites is that these materials enable the passage of radar and communications signals with very little interference or attenuation, unlike metals. This, then, allows all the antennas, sensors, and other sensitive electronic equipment to be enclosed within the mast structure and thereby protected from the weather. Other benefits of the AEM/S system are that it is lighter and more corrosion resistant than steel truss masts; however, composite masts are much more expensive to build. The AEM/S system has performed beyond the expectations of the United States Navy, and consideration is currently being given to installing advanced composite masts on future amphibious ships, destroyers, and sea-lift vessels (Ref 26). A composite mast structure similar to the AEM/S system is also being developed in the United Kingdom for next-generation warships (Ref 27). Smaller composite masts have been fitted to some naval submarines to lower weight, reduce corrosion, and dampen vibrations (Ref 28).

The feasibility of using composites in a wide variety of secondary structures and equipment on warships and submarines is under investigation. For example, a major effort is being given to the development of composite propellers, propulsors, and propulsion shafts (Ref 29–36). Composites are expected to offer a number of important benefits over metals when used in propulsion systems, including lower costs, reduced weight, lower magnetic signature, better noise-damping properties, and superior corrosion resistance (Ref 29–36). It is anticipated that propulsion shafts made of composites will be 25 to 80% lighter than a steel shaft of the same size and will reduce life-cycle costs by at least 25% because of fewer problems associated with corrosion and fatigue (Ref 33, 35, 36). Despite the projected benefits, the use of composites in propulsion systems has been limited. Composite propellers have only been used on torpedoes and one minehunter ship (Ref 33), composite propeller shafts have only been installed on a small number of patrol boats, including the Skjøld (Ref 16), whereas composite propulsors have not yet been used. However, within the next ten years the use of composites in these applications is expected to increase, albeit at a slow rate.

Composites are also being evaluated for use in rudders for ships and control surfaces for submarines (Ref 22, 37, 38). Other potential applications include funnels, bulkheads, decks, watertight doors, machinery foundations, pipes, ventilation ducts, and components for diesel en-

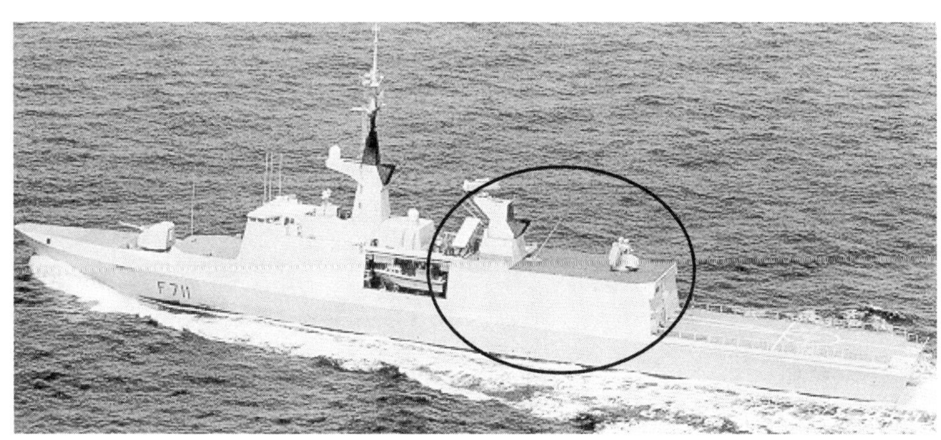

Fig. 4 La Fayette frigate with the composite superstructure section shown within the circled region

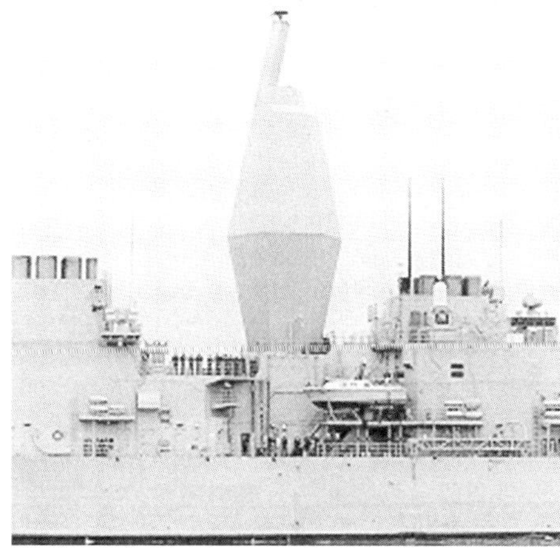

Fig. 5 Advanced enclosed mast/sensor (AEM/S) composite mast on the USS *Arthur W. Radford*

gines, pumps, and heat exchangers on large warships (Ref 8, 22, 36, 39–41).

Leisure, Sporting, and Commercial FRP Composite Craft

The diverse application of composite materials to naval vessels is matched by their wide-ranging use in leisure, sporting, and commercial vessels and small submersibles. Composites were first used in leisure craft and yachts in the 1950s and in commercial craft, such as fishing trawlers and pilot boats as well as submersibles, in the late 1960s (Ref 4, 5, 42). The use of composites in these vessels was due to the successful application of FRP materials to naval boats during the 1950s and 1960s. It is interesting to note, however, that the experience and knowledge gained from using composites in leisure and commercial craft later facilitated the wider use of these materials in naval ships.

Since the 1970s, the use of composites in the hulls of marine craft has increased dramatically, and currently most vessels under a length of 15 to 20 m (50 to 65 ft) are built with FRP materials. The types of craft in this size range that are made of composites include kayaks, canoes, dinghies, jet skis, lifeboats, yachts, and powerboats (Ref 4, 5). Vessels longer than approximately 20 m (50 ft) are usually made of steel or aluminum alloy, although the use of composites is increasing as their fabrication cost continues to fall and as boat operators become aware of the reduced through-life costs. Among the largest commercial vessels that are built using composites are luxury cruisers, passenger ferries, hovercraft, and fishing trawlers. Several years ago, between 50 and 60% of all fishing boats under 60 m (200 ft) were made of GRP, and the proportion of trawlers built of composites is expected to continue to rise (Ref 5). Composites are often used because the lightweight construction allows a heavier fishing haul to be carried, the fish holds are easier to clean than wooden holds, and the hulls are easier to maintain and repair. Composites have also been used in propellers of fishing trawlers as well as powerboats to overcome corrosion and noise problems that can be experienced with metal propellers (Ref 35, 43). Composites are also being used increasingly in high-speed ferries capable of carrying 350 to 400 passengers. The ferries are usually built with a composite hull and an aluminum superstructure. Ferries are rarely built with a composite superstructure because of the poor fire resistance. The hoisting decks and bow gates on car ferries have also been made of sandwich composite material.

As with naval ships, the composite material most commonly used in leisure and commercial craft is GRP in the form of a thick laminate or a sandwich composite. Over 95% of all composite marine craft are built with GRP because of its low cost, which is similar to the cost of steel and aluminum alloy. There are, however, a number of other reasons for the popularity of GRP composites in marine craft, and these include:

- Ability to easily and inexpensively mold GRP to the near-net shape, even for marine structures with a complex shape, such as boat hulls, thus making it suitable for mass production
- Excellent corrosion resistance
- Light weight, resulting in reduced fuel consumption
- Simple to repair
- Good ability to absorb noise and dampen vibrations, which makes for a more comfortable ride on motor-powered boats

High-performance yachts competing in the world's most prestigious races, such as the America's Cup and Admiral's Cup, are built with aerospace-quality composite materials rather than GRP (Ref 44–47). Advanced composites are also used in the construction of racing powerboats and skiff sailing hulls (Ref 44, 45). A state-of-the-art International America's Cup Class (IACC) yacht and a racing powerboat that have been built using advanced composites are shown in Fig. 6. Racing yachts and boats such as these are built using ultralight sandwich composite materials that have thin laminate skins containing carbon, glass and/or aramid (Kevlar, DuPont) fibers and a core of polyvinyl chloride foam or Kevlar honeycomb. Advanced fabrication processes, such as resin transfer molding, resin film infusion, or autoclaving, are used in the construction of the hull and decks to produce composites that are defect-free, excellent dimensional tolerance, and a high fiber content for maximum stiffness, strength, and fatigue resistance (Ref 48).

The main advantages of using advanced composites are optimal weight distribution, good fatigue resistance, vibration damping, and most importantly, high stiffness-to-weight and strength-to-weight ratios. The use of advanced composites with high stiffness- and strength-to-weight ratios allows lighter hull structures to be built with stiffness and strength equivalent to much thicker GRP hulls. This is desirable for planing craft, such as powerboats and sailing hulls, for reducing hydrodynamic resistance. Similarly, for displacement craft such as yachts,

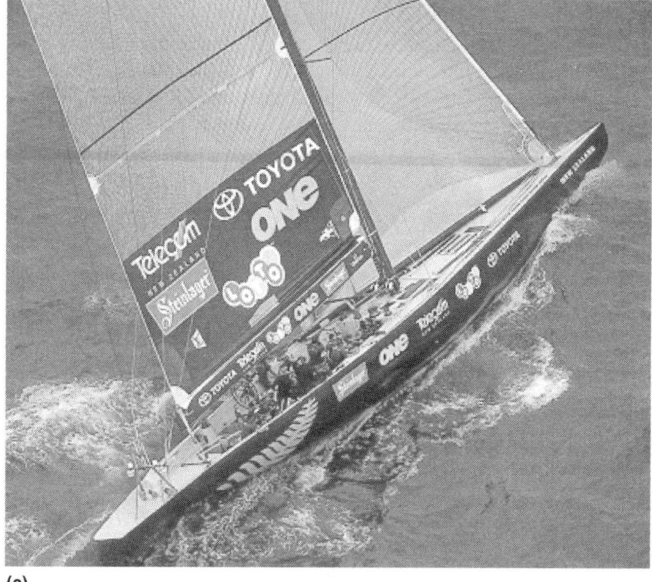

(a)

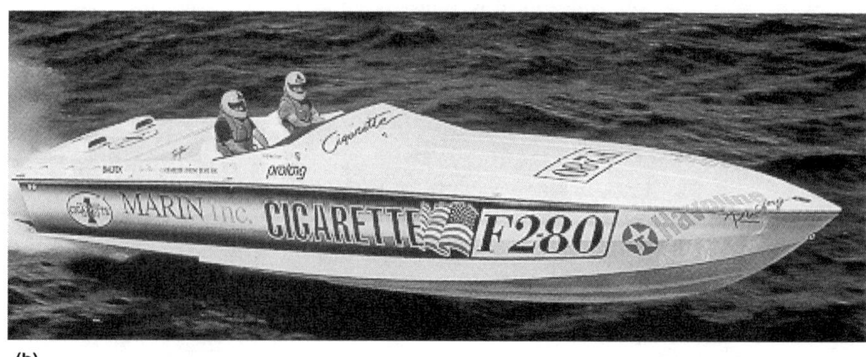

(b)

Fig. 6 Boats built almost entirely from aerospace-grade composite materials. (a) 2000 Team New Zealand IACC yacht. (b) F-2 series race boat

a reduction in hull structure weight allows increased ballast to be used for a given displacement. Appendages such as centreboards and rudders on high-performance sailing hulls, trim tabs on powerboats, and rudders on high-performance yachts are also commonly constructed using advanced sandwich materials. This is beneficial for hydrodynamic performance because the overall weight is minimized, higher appendage stiffness is obtained, and a reduction in the weight of the rudder contributes to lower hull-pitching moments.

Composites are also commonly used for spars (mast, boom, and spinnaker poles), fittings, and fitting reinforcements on sailing boats and yachts (Ref 49). Mast tips, which are about the top one-third of the mast, on sailing boats are made of glass- or carbon-reinforced composite to obtain desired flexibility for optimal gust response (Ref 50). Carbon-fiber composite is also used in masts for IACC and other high-performance-class yachts. Composite masts are 40 to 50% lighter than similar masts made of aluminum alloy, which results in a reduced heeling moment and therefore, improved performance. The high stiffness obtained with carbon-fiber composite spars is also beneficial for maintaining sail shape under high rig loads. Similarly, the use of high-performance composites in hull structures is beneficial for maintaining high rig loads with minimal hull distortion and added hydrodynamic resistance.

Offshore Applications of FRP Composites

FRP composites have been used in offshore drilling platforms for many years, although the oil industry has only used these materials in niche applications and not in major structural elements. Steel is the primary structural material used in drilling platforms and is expected to remain so for the foreseeable future, because it has many benefits that other materials, including composites, cannot match. The benefits include low materials cost, the ability to fabricate large structures at low cost, good flame resistance, well-established design rules, and a long service history for using steel in offshore platforms. However, steel has a number of drawbacks that have allowed composites to be used to a limited extent.

The greatest problem with using steel in an offshore structure is the poor corrosion resistance against seawater and other highly corrosive agents, such as hydrogen sulfide and hydrogen chloride, that occur during drilling. It is estimated that the oil industry spends several billion dollars each year in maintaining, repairing, and replacing corroded steel structures (Ref 51). Composites offer the potential to reduce these costs because of their outstanding corrosion resistance against most types of chemicals.

Composites also offer the possibility of reducing the topside weight of offshore platforms when used in such applications as accommodation modules, helicopter landing pads, and decks. It is estimated that composites provide a weight saving of 30 to 50% compared to steel for many non-structural components (Ref 52). The increased use of composites in topside structures is expected to make the transportation and installation of platforms easier, reduce the weight of tethers, foundations, and piles needed to anchor platforms, and allow drilling in deeper waters than is currently possible with heavier steel platforms.

Composites are used in a variety of structures and components on offshore platforms because of their better corrosion resistance and lighter weight compared with steel. The most common types of composites used are GRP and phenolic composites, with the latter being used because of good fire resistance. Advanced composites containing carbon fibers, Kevlar fibers, or epoxy resins are used sparingly because of their high cost. Some of the current applications of FRP materials are (Ref 7, 10, 51–56):

- Low pressure pipes
- Diesel storage tanks, lube tanks, and utility tanks
- Walkway gratings, stair steps, and handrails
- Cable ladders and trays
- Fire protection panels and sections of accommodation modules
- Buoys and floats
- Strengthening of primary steel structures
- Helicopter landing decks

It is worth noting that not all offshore platforms use composites, and in most applications, composite components have been used to replace corroded steel sections. New platforms are rarely built with significant amounts of composite, although this may change as the oil industry assesses the feasibility of using FRP materials for new applications. Potential applications include (Ref 51, 52):

- High-pressure (firewater) pipes
- Drill pipes, tubing, and risers
- Mooring tendons for tension leg platforms and semisubmersible platforms
- Walls and floors to provide protection against blast and fire

The use of composites is expected to grow as some of these new applications are realized, however, there remain many economic and technical issues that must be resolved before FRP materials are more widely used in offshore platforms (Ref 10, 52). The higher cost of fabricating offshore structures with composites compared with welded steel is a concern to the oil industry. However, there is growing recognition that significant through-life cost savings can be gained with composites due to reduced maintenance and replacement of corroded structures. There is also concern about the lack of design codes and well-established oilfield standards in the use of composites. An important safety concern is that most FRP materials have poor fire-resistant properties, such as short ignition times and high rates of heat release, smoke production, and flame spread. While it is generally recognized that composites have much lower thermal conductivity than metallic materials, these factors make it difficult for composites to meet the stringent fire safety requirements applied to offshore oil and gas platforms.

REFERENCES

1. T.M. Buermann, and R.J. Della Rocca, Fibreglass Reinforced Plastics for Marine Applications, *Proc. of the Spring Meeting of the Society of Naval Architects and Marine Engineers*, 26–28 June 1960, p 138–192
2. K.B. Spaulding, A History of the Construction of Fibreglass Boats for the Navy, *Bur. Ships J.*, March 1966, p 2–11
3. S.R. Heller, ‘The Use of Composite Materials in Naval Ships, *Mechanics of Composite Materials: Proc. of the Fifth Symposium on Structural Mechanics*, 8–10 May 1967, Pergamon Press, Oxford, p 69–111
4. W.R. Graner, Marine Applications, *Handbook of Composites*, G. Lubin, Ed., Van Nostrand Reinhold, New York, 1982, p 699–721
5. C.S. Smith, *Design of Marine Structures in Composite Materials*, Elsevier Applied Science, London, 1990
6. “Use of Fibre Reinforced Plastics in the Marine Industry,” Ship Structure Committee Report SSC-360, National Technical Information Service, Springfield, VA, 1990
7. Sea Duty for Composites?, *Adv. Mater. Process.*, Vol 142 (No. 2), 1992, p 16–20
8. A.P. Mouritz, E. Gellert, P. Burchill, and K. Challis, Review of Advanced Composite Structures for Naval Ships and Submarines, *J. Compos. Struct.*, Vol 53 (No. 1), 2001, p 21–44
9. S.W. Beckwith and C.R. Hyland, FRP and Advanced Composites in the Oilfield, *Compos. Fabr.*, Aug 1998, p 37–48
10. J.F. Wellicome, Composites in Offshore Structures, in *Composite Materials in Marine Structures*, Vol 2, R.A. Shenoi and J.F. Wellicome, Ed., Cambridge University Press, Cambridge, p 199–228
11. D. Henton, Glass Reinforced Plastics in the Royal Navy, *Trans. Royal Inst. Nav. Archit.*, Vol 109, 1967, p 487–501
12. K. Mäkinen, S.-E. Hellbrat, and K.-A. Olsson, The Development of Sandwich Structures for Naval Vessels during 25 Years, *Mechanics of Sandwich Structures*, A. Vautrin, Ed., Kluwer Academic Publishers, Netherlands, 1998, p 13–28
13. R.H. Dixon, B.W. Ramsey, and P.J. Usher, Design and Build of the GRP Hull of HMS *Wilton*, *Royal Institution of Naval Architects Symposium on GRP Ship Construction* (London), 1972, p 1–32
14. D.W. Chalmers, R.J. Osburn, and A. Bunney, “Hull Construction of MCMVs in the

United Kingdom," Paper 13, Proceedings of the International Symposium on Mine Warfare Vessels and Systems, Royal Institution of Naval Architects (London), 12–15 June 1984

15. P. Goubalt and S. Mayes, Comparative Analysis of Metal and Composite Materials for the Primary Structure of a Patrol Boat, *Nav. Eng. J.*, Vol 108 (No. 3), 1996, p 387–397
16. D. Foxwell, 'Skjøld Class Comes in from the Cold, *Jane's Navy Int.*, Vol 104 (No. 6), 1999, p 14–20
17. H. Schultz, "Aspects of Materials Selection for MCMVs Hulls," Paper 14, Proc. of the International Symposium on Mine Warfare Vessels and Systems, Royal Institution of Naval Architects (London), 12–15 June 1984
18. A. Lönnö, "The Visby Class Corvette: The World's Biggest CFRP-Sandwich Ship," Proc. of the Conf. on Offshore and Marine Composites, 5–6 April 2000, University of Newcastle-upon-Tyne (Newcastle, UK)
19. S. Mayes and B. Scott, Advanced All-Composite Surface Combatant, *Proc. of the American Society of Naval Engineers (ASNE) Symposium*, Feb 1995 (Biloxi, Mississippi), Vol 1, p 16–17 & Vol 2, p 73–112
20. P. Cahill, Composite Materials and Naval Surface Combatants: The Integrated Technology Deckhouse Project, *J. Ship Prod.*, Vol 8, 1992, p 1–7
21. M.O. Critchfield, T.D. Judy, and A.D. Kurzweil, Low-Cost Design and Fabrication of Composite Ship Structures, *Mar. Struct.*, Vol 7, 1994, p 475–494
22. A.W. Horsman, Composites for Large Ships, *J. Ship Prod.*, Vol 10, 1994, p 274–280
23. J. Janssen, The Shape of Ships to Come, Jane's World of Defence 1995, *Jane's Def. Wkly.*, London, 1995, p 123–128
24. B. Høyning and J. Taby, "Warship Design: the Potential for Composites in Frigate Superstructures," Paper Number 6, *Proc. of the International Conf. on Lightweight Construction—Latest Developments*, 24–25 Feb 2000
25. A.R. Dodkins and T.J. Williams, "Sandwich Structures for Naval Vessels," Proc. of the International Conf. on Offshore and Marine Composites, 5–6 April 2000, University of Newcastle-upon-Tyne (Newcastle, UK)
26. J.L. Benson, The AEM/S System, A Paradigm-Breaking Mast, Goes to Sea, *Nav. Eng. J.*, Vol 110 (No. 4), 1998, p 99–103
27. R. Scott, DERA Puts Integrated Mast Concept to the Test, *Jane's Def. Wkly.*, Vol 31 (No. 18), 1999, p 35–37
28. M.R. Newan, "Development of Non Hull Penetrating Masts and Periscopes," Paper No. 6, Proc. Warship '99: The International Symposium on Naval Structures 6, Royal Institution of Naval Architects (London), 14–16 June 1999
29. C. Kane and R. Dow, Marine Propulsors—Design in Fibre Reinforced Plastics, *J. Def. Sci.*, Vol 4, 1994, p 301–308
30 A. Macander, An X-D Braided Composite Marine Propeller, *Proc. of the Tenth DOD/NASA/FAA Conf. on Fibrous Composites in Structural Design*, April 1994, Vol 2, p VII–19 to VII–34.
31. Deformation-Controlled Composite CP Propeller Blades, *Maritime Def.*, Vol 16 (No. 2), 1991, p 42–43
32. S. Womack, Carbon Propeller Allows Ships to Go Softly Softly, *Engineer*, Vol 276, 1993, p. 30
33. R.L. Pegg and H. Reyes, Progress in Naval Composites, *Adv. Mat. & Process.*, Vol 131 (No. 3), 1987, p 35–39
34. T. Searle and D. Shot, Are Composite Propellers the Way Forward for Small Boats?, *Mater. World*, Vol 2 (No. 2), 1994, p 69–70
35. G.F. Wilhelmi, W.M. Appleman, and F.T.C. Loo, Composite Shafting for Naval Propulsion Systems, *Nav. Eng. J.*, Vol 98 (No. 4), 1986, p 129–136
36. J.E. Gagorik, J.A. Corrado, and R.W. Kornbau, An Overview of Composite Developments for Naval Surface Combatants, *Proc. of the 36th International SAMPE Symposium*, 15–18 April 1991, p 1855–1867
37. P. Lazarus, Revisiting RIRM, *Professional Boatbuilder*, Aug/Sept 1997, p 48
38. R. Phelan, Design, Analysis, Fabrication and Testing of a Composite Control Surface, *Nav. Eng. J.*, Vol 107 (No. 2), 1995, p 41–55
39. V. Bhasin, D. Conroy, and J. Reid, Development of a Family of Commercial Marine Composite Ball Valves', *Nav. Eng. J.*, Vol 110 (No. 4), 1998, p 51–65
40. D. Suitt and F. Girona, Development of a Standard Family of Composite Material Centrifugal Pumps for Naval Surface Ships, *Nav. Eng. J.*, Vol 105 (No. 4), 1993, p 167–180
41. G.F. Wilhelmi and W.H. Schab, Glass Reinforced Plastic (GRP) Piping for Shipboard Applications, *Nav. Eng. J.*, Vol 89 (No. 2), 1977, p 139–160
42. H.R. Hallet and J.H. Simpson, Fabrication of Large RP Trawlers, *Reinf. Plast.*, Vol 12 (No. 6), June 1968
43. Y.Z. Ashkenazi, I.B. Gol'fman, L.P. Rezhkov, and N.P. Sidorov, *Glass-Fiber-Reinforced Plastic Parts in Ship Machinery*, Sudostroyeniye Publishing House, Leningard, 1974
44. B. Pfund, Working with Carbon Fiber, *Professional Boatbuilder*, Oct/Nov 1999, p 34–50
45. P. Lazarus, The Near Future of Marine Composites, *Professional Boatbuilder,* April/May 1999, p 36–52
46. B. Pfund, Designing and Building with Kevlar, *Professional Boatbuilder*, Dec/Jan 1999, p 61–73
47. Q. Warren, A Builder's Designer, *Professional Boatbuilder*, Oct/Nov 1999, p 66–80
48. P. Lazarus, Reporting on the Resin Infusion Front, *Professional Boatbuilder*, Dec/Jan 1997, p 30–34
49. N. Calder, Carbon Fiber Spars, *Professional Boatbuilder*, June/July 1997, p 44–55
50. F. Bethwaite, *High Performance Sailing*, Shrewsbury, England, 1993
51. J.G. Williams, Opportunities for Composites in the Offshore Oil Iindustry, *Proc. of the Conf. on the Use of Composite Materials in Load-Bearing Marine Structures*, Vol 2, 25–26 Sept 1990 (Arlington, VA), p 41–65
52. F.J. Barnes, Composite Materials in the UK Offshore Oil and Gas Industry, *SAMPE J.*, Vol 32 (No. 2), 1996, p 12–17
53. S.W. Beckwith and C.R. Hyland, FRP and Advanced Composites in the Oilfield, *Compos. Fabr.*, Aug 1988, p 36–48
54. V.P. McConnell, Fibreglass Goes Offshore, *Composites Technology Magazine*, Jan/Feb 1996, p 48–50
55. W.B. Goldsworthy and C.J. Wiernicki, Logical vs. Traditional: The Use of Composites in Offshore Industry, *Proc. of the Ninth International Conf. on Offshore Mechanics and Arctic Engineering*, 18–23 Feb 1990 (Houston, TX), Vol III, Part A, American Society of Mechanical Engineers International, p 29–36
56. P.R. Godfrey and A.G. Davis, The Use of GRP Materials in Platform Topside Construction and the Regulatory Implications, *Proc. of the Ninth International Conference on Offshore Mechanics and Arctic Engineering*, 18–23 Feb 1990 (Houston, TX), Vol III, Part A, American Society of Mechanical Engineers International, p 15–20

Civil Infrastructure Applications

Vistasp M. Karbhari, University of California, San Diego

CIVIL INFRASTRUCTURE, such as bridges, buildings, waterfront structures, waste treatment facilities, and facilities for transmission and transport of utilities, represents an investment of trillions of dollars worldwide. Increasingly the security of this investment is being questioned. The infrastructure of constructed facilities for the transportation and housing of people, goods, and services, which was developed and rapidly expanded in the middle of the last century, is now reaching a critical age, with widespread signs of deterioration and inadequate functionality. Composites—particularly fiber-reinforced polymer (FRP) materials—are increasingly being adopted or considered as alternatives to conventional materials for infrastructure applications. Within the vast applications area in civil infrastructure, this article concentrates on a few specific examples related to the use of composites in seismic retrofit, component strengthening and repair, and in new structural systems. Reviews of the state-of-the-art as practiced in various regions of the world have been recently published (Ref 1–6) and readers are referred to them for further detailed information.

The Need for Infrastructure Renewal

The existing infrastructure is in critical need of renewal. For example, deficiencies in the existing bridge inventory include those related to wear, environmental deterioration, and aging of structural components, increased traffic demands and changing traffic patterns, insufficient detailing at the time of original design, the use of substandard materials in initial construction, and inadequate maintenance and rehabilitation measures taken through the life of the structure. In the United States, an estimated 35% of all bridges on the federal inventory are judged to be structurally deficient or functionally obsolete and require repair, strengthening, widening, or replacement. In addition to increasing or changing traffic demands, common deficiencies include:

- Deck deterioration due to wear, deicing salts, temperature gradients, freeze-thaw cycles, and other environmental factors
- Scour at bridge substructures in flowing water
- Corrosion of structural steel members and steel reinforcement in structural concrete
- Problems associated with dynamic response under wind or earthquake conditions
- Physical and chemical aging and deterioration of materials

These deficiencies are not isolated to bridges and other transportation-related structures alone, but are endemic to the built environment, including residential housing, pipelines used for the distribution of water, and industrial structures. This deterioration and inability to provide required services has a tremendous impact on society in terms of socioeconomic losses resulting from delays, accidents, and irregularity in supply.

Within the scope of rehabilitation of civil infrastructure, it is essential to differentiate among *repair, strengthening,* and *retrofit.* These terms often are used interchangeably, but in fact should be used to refer to three different structural conditions (Fig. 1). In "repairing" a structure, the composite material is used to fix a structural or functional deficiency, such as a crack or a severely degraded structural component. In contrast, the strengthening of structures is specific to those situations where the addition or application of the composite would enhance the existing designed performance level, as would be the case in attempting to increase the load rating (or capacity) of a bridge deck through the application of composites to the deck soffit. The term retrofit, although often used as a generic term for rehabilitation, is increasingly being specifically used in relation to the seismic upgrade of facilities, such as in the use of composite jackets for the confinement of columns. The differentiation is important not just on the basis of structural functionality, but also because the specifics related to the use of the material in conjunction with existing conventional materials and its expected life have a significant effect on the selection (or rejection) of fiber-resin combinations from a variety of alternatives.

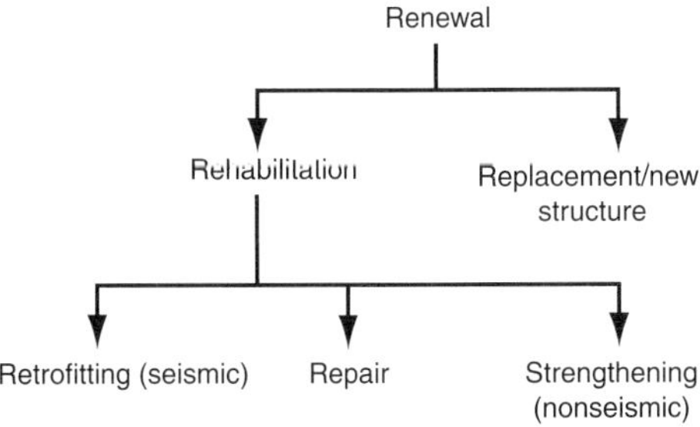

Fig. 1 Types of renewal strategies for civil infrastructure

Conventional Materials versus Composites

Conventional materials, such as steel, concrete, and wood, have a number of advantages, not the least of which is the relatively low cost of materials and construction. However, it is clear that conventional materials and technologies, although suitable in many situations and with a history of good applicability, lack in longevity in some cases and, in others, are susceptible to rapid deterioration, emphasizing the need for better grades of these materials or newer technologies to supplement the conventional ones used. Also note that design alternatives may be constrained by the current limitations of materials used, for example, in the length of the clear span of a bridge due to weight constraints, or the size of a column due to restrictions on design and minimum dimensions needed. In a similar manner, the use of conventional materials is often not possible in cases of retrofit, or may be deemed as ineffective in terms of functionality. In other situations, restraints such as dead load restrict the widening of current structures or the carriage of higher amounts of traffic over existing lifelines. In all such (and other) cases, there is a critical need for the use of new and emerging materials and technologies, with the end goal of facilitating functionality and greater structural and life-cycle efficiency.

The human race has a long history of attempts to create new materials with enhanced properties for the construction of structural systems. The use of combinations of materials to provide both ease of use and enhanced performance, as in the use of straw reinforcement in mud by the ancient Israelites (800 B.C.), or in the combination of different orientations of veneers of wood, as in plywood, has a long history. The concept of combining materials to create a new system having some of the advantages of each of the constituents can be seen in reinforced concrete (steel, aggregate, sand, and cement) and, to an extent, in the use of special compounds and chemicals in alloys of steel. Fiber-reinforced composites take this concept one step further in civil infrastructure, potentially giving the designer a wide palette of materials choices to fit the specific requirements of the structure and showing immense potential to add to the current range of materials being used. The tailorability of these materials, derived from the inherent anisotropy predicated by the arrangement of the fiber reinforcement in the polymer matrix, as well as the corrosion resistance, light weight, high strength, and stiffness-to-weight ratios permit their use in ways that are not available to conventional materials. These unique characteristics provide significant impetus for their use in rehabilitation and restoration of historic structures without causing significant changes to the aesthetic features or geometric configurations of the original structures. Similarly, the performance attributes, in conjunction with their light weight, enable their use in strengthening severely degraded structural elements, as well as in the modification of existing structures without egress on available headroom or open space. Further, when used in new structural systems, they provide the designer with the ability to truly blend form and function.

Although this article focuses on aspects related to rehabilitation through external application of FRP composites and the development of new structural systems, it needs to be emphasized that composites are also being used in the form of internal reinforcement in structural concrete, as tendons/cables for internal and external prestressing, and as cable stays. In these areas, the primary drivers for the use of composites as replacements for conventional steel members have been corrosion resistance, light weight, and performance attributes. Composite rebar, used for the reinforcement of concrete, is already commercially available in a variety of configurations using carbon, glass, and aramid fibers, and has found application primarily in corrosive regimes, such as coastal and marine structures, and in structures where the magnetic and conductive transparency of composites is advantageous. Design guidelines and specifications for the use of composite rebar have already been developed by associations such as the American Concrete Institute and the Japan Society of Civil Engineers. They have also been included to a level in the Canadian Highway Bridge Design Code. The use of cables and tendons, primarily of carbon and aramid fibers, has been demonstrated on a number of bridges in Europe and Japan. Their application appears to have significant merit, as long as issues related to cost and anchorages can be resolved.

Seismic Retrofit Applications

Recent earthquakes, such as those in Whittier, CA (1987), Loma Prieta, CA (1989), Northridge, CA (1994), and Kobe, Japan (1995), have repeatedly shown the vulnerability of existing bridge columns built before the 1971 San Fernando, CA, earthquake. For reinforced concrete columns, conventional retrofit measures include the external confinement of the core by heavily reinforced external concrete sections; the use of steel cables wound helically around the existing column at close spacing, which are then covered by concrete; and the use of steel shells or casings that are welded together in the field, confining the existing columns. Although some of these methods are very effective, they are time-consuming, needing days for installation; can cause significant traffic disruption due to access and space requirements for heavy equipment; rely on field welding, the quality and uniformity of which are often suspect; and are susceptible to degradation due to corrosion. Also, due to the isotropic nature of the material in steel casings or jackets, the jacket not only provides the needed confinement, but also causes an increase in stiffness and strength capacity of the retrofitted column. Both of these attributes are not desirable, because higher seismic force levels are typically transmitted to adjacent structural elements. The use of fiber-reinforced composites not only provides a means for confinement without the attendant increase in stiffness (through the use of hoop reinforcement only, i.e., no axial reinforcement), but also enables the rapid fabrication of cost-effective and durable jackets, with little to no traffic disruption in a large number of cases.

Numerous methods (based on the form of jacketing material or fabrication process) have been tested at large- or full-scale, many of which are now used commercially in Japan and the United States. Generically, fiber-reinforced composite wraps (or jackets) can be classified into six basic categories, as a function of process and/or materials form, as shown in Fig. 2. In the wet lay-up process, fabric is impregnated on-site and wrapped around a column, with cure generally taking place under ambient conditions. In wet winding, the process of fabrication is automated, but essentially follows the same schema, with the difference being that the ensuing jacket has a nominal prestress due to the use of winding tension. The use of prepreg tow presents the opportunity not only for elevated-temperature cure (with the consequent advantages of higher degree of cure, higher glass transition temperature, and greater overall durability associated with moisture and humidity resistance), but also the use of standardized and uniform materials that are easy for the structural designer to specify. In the case of adhesively bonded shells, the concept of uniformity and standardization is carried even further, through the use of prefabricated single- or dual-section jackets that can be assembled in the field through bonding and layering. This process affords a high level of materials quality control due to prefabrication of the elements under factory conditions, but, as in the case of external strengthening, relies on the integrity of the adhesive bond.

The structural effectiveness of composite jackets has been demonstrated through an ample

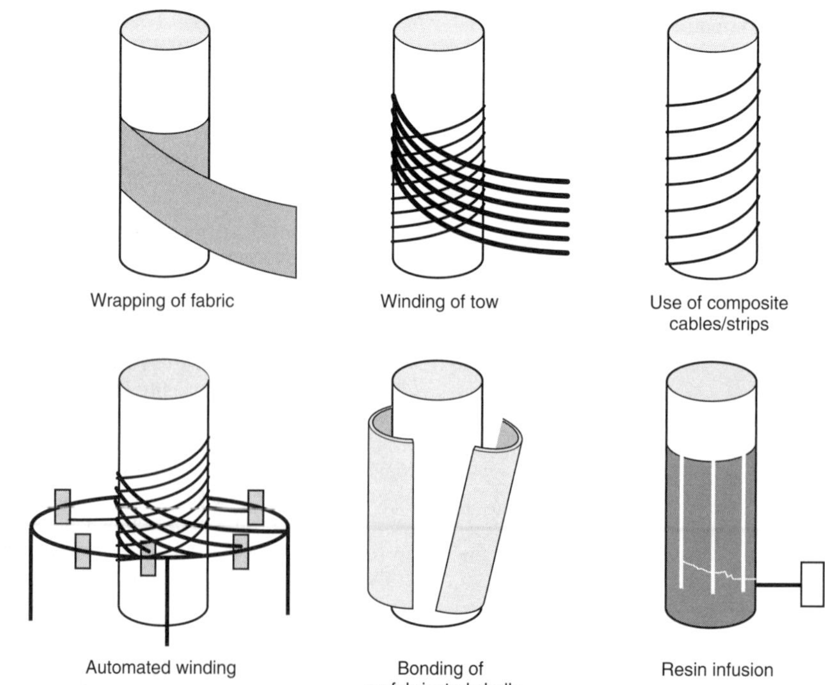

Fig. 2 Schematic of methods of seismic retrofit of columns using composites

number of large- and full-scale tests (Ref 7, 8), and through demonstration projects in Japan (Ref 5) and the United States (Fig. 3, for example). One of the largest applications of composites in seismic retrofit was conducted using the adhesively bonded shells technique on columns of the Yolo causeway west of Sacramento, California.

The use of composites for seismic retrofit is fairly well developed, with established principles for design and analysis of standard column configurations. Design examples and methodology are detailed in Ref 7 and 9. In most cases, the use of composites results in a cost-effective and structurally efficient retrofit scheme that significantly increases structural ductility and, thereby, seismic resistance.

The determination of thickness of the composite retrofit depends on the requirements to correct the failure modes expected under seismic load/deformation, which can be differentiated into four general classes: shear strengthening, plastic hinge confinement, bar-buckling restraint, and lap-splice clamping. A comparison of jacket thicknesses for three typical systems is shown in Table 1, where system A is representative of a tow-preg-based graphite/epoxy composite similar to that used in automated winding, system B is representative of an aramid/epoxy system similar to that used in Japan using wet lay-up, and system C is representative of an E-glass/vinylester similar to that used in prefabricated, adhesively bonded shells. All values in Table 1 are normalized to the thickness values determined for system A. It can be seen that jacket thicknesses for shear, bar-buckling restraint, and lap-splice clamping are driven by the modulus of the jacket in the hoop direction that favors the selection of higher modulus materials (carbon, aramid), whereas the requirements for flexural hinge confinement can be efficiently achieved with a lower modulus, but high-strength and higher strain-capacity material (e.g., E-glass).

Beyond the flexibility afforded by composites for the rapid and cost-effective retrofit of circular and rectangular columns/piers, composites are also invaluable for seismic retrofit of historical structures, such as arch bridges with spandrel columns. (An example is shown in Fig. 4.) Because of historical considerations, the rectangular columns cannot be retrofit using steel jackets without significant changes in the original shape and other architectural considerations. Further, location considerations also make the use of the steel option difficult, in this case emphasizing the overall effectiveness of composites in providing a solution where conventional materials and methods cannot be used easily.

It should be noted that in a number of situations, the method of wrapping has also been used to protect and retard corrosion of steel reinforcement. In addition to the protection afforded by the composites as a barrier to moisture diffusion and penetration, the added confinement also assists in resisting cracking of concrete. Although questions still remain regarding the efficacy of FRP jackets in reducing corrosion in reinforcing steel through encapsulation of the structure after treatment of the concrete, the method has been used in the field to potentially extend the life of bridge columns.

Repair and Strengthening of Beams and Slabs

Degradation due to corrosion of steel reinforcement, spalling of concrete cover, extensive cracking of concrete due to excessive carbonation and/or freeze thaw action, effects of alkali-silica reaction, and rapidly changing traffic needs (both in terms of number of vehicles and load levels) have created a critical need for methods of repair and strengthening of beams and girders, as well as deck soffits and bridge deck slabs. The need for increasing load capacity/rating of bridges due to requirements for uniform postings over a region, such as in Europe, or the need to enhance capacity to ensure safe carriage of increased truck axle weights, as in Australia and Japan, provide significant impetus for the adoption of technology that is capable of achieving this in both a cost-effective manner and without significant distress to traffic. In buildings, materials degradation, changing needs of building occupancy (e.g., residential to office), and upgrades to facilities (e.g., cutting of floor slabs in older buildings to facilitate the construction of shafts for elevator installation) necessitate the strengthening of existing slabs and beams.

Conventional methods for external strengthening range from the use of external post-tensioning to the addition of epoxy-bonded steel

Table 1 Comparison of hypothetical jacket thicknesses

Property	Proportionality relationship	System A	System B	System C
Mechanical characteristics of composite jacket in the hoop direction				
Modulus of elasticity (E_j), GPa (10^6 psi)	...	124 (18)	76 (11)	21 (3)
Ultimate tensile strength (f_{ju}), MPa (ksi)	...	1380 (200)	1380 (200)	655 (95)
Ultimate strain at failure (ε_{ju}), %	...	1	1.5	2.5
Normalized jacket thickness				
Shear strength	$t_j^v \sim \frac{1}{E_j D} \times C_v$	1	1.6	6.0
Plastic hinge confinement	$t_j^c \sim \frac{D}{f_{ju}\varepsilon_{ju}} \times C_c$	1	0.7	0.9
Bar-buckling restraint	$t_j^b \sim \frac{D}{E_j} \times C_b$	1	1.6	6.0
Lap-splice clamping	$t_j^s \sim \frac{D}{E_j} \times C_s$	1	1.6	6.0

D, diameter of column; t_j, minimum required jacket thickness for indicated parameter; C_v, parameter for shear strength; C_c, parameter for plastic hinge confinement; C_b, parameter for bar buckling restraint; C_s, parameter for lap-splice clamping

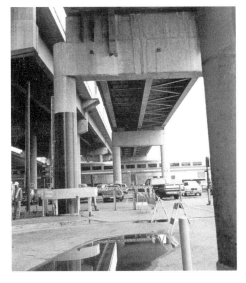

Fig. 3 Columns on the Santa Monica viaduct wrapped with carbon/epoxy prepreg

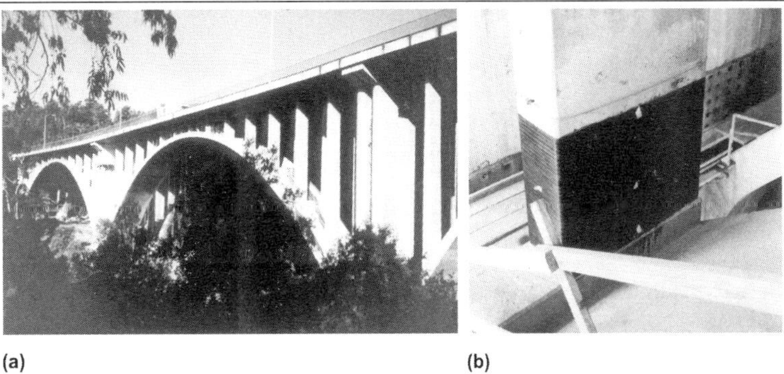

(a) (b)

Fig. 4 Seismic retrofit of bridges with spandrel columns. (a) Arch bridge showing spandrel column. (b) Composite jacket on the lower third of a spandrel column

plates to the soffit of the deck superstructure. Although the latter technique is simple and has been used in Europe and the United States in the past, it suffers from a number of disadvantages, ranging from difficulty in placement to concerns related to overall durability and corrosion resistance. Steel plates are heavy and unwieldy and thus difficult to handle during erection. At the minimum, jacks, extensive scaffolding, and winches or cranes are needed. The length of individual plates is restricted to a maximum of 6 to 10 m (20 to 30 ft) to facilitate handling, and even at these lengths, it may be difficult to erect them due to preexisting service facilities below the deck slab. Composites fabricated either through wet processes on-site or prefabricated in strips and then adhesively bonded to the concrete surface provide an efficient and easy means of strengthening that can be carried out with no interruptions in traffic flow.

In general, composites can be applied in three ways (as described in Table 2), of which the first two are the most widely used. It should be noted that although the wet lay-up process affords significant flexibility for work on-site, there may be important, technical and psychological advantages in the use of prefabricated, and thus standardized, strips and plates, which are adhesively bonded to the concrete substrate. Regardless of the method of application, it is important to note that the efficacy of the method depends primarily on the appropriate selection of the composite material, based on stiffness and strength requirements, and the efficiency and integrity of the bond between the concrete surface and the composite. The bond between the composite and concrete, whether established through the use of an adhesive or through the use of the same resin system used in the wet lay-up of the composite itself, must be capable of performing under ambient conditions. It must also be capable of providing the required response under extremes of temperature (including temperature gradients between the top and bottom surfaces of concrete), the resulting stress and strain conditions, and in the presence of moisture (which may be absorbed not only from the atmosphere, but could also gather at the adhesive-concrete interface due to moisture collection and ingress through concrete, which itself is a porous material).

Regardless of the method used, the external application of composites to concrete beams and slabs, if conducted in an appropriate manner, can result in the significant enhancement of load carrying capacity and flexural and shear strength of the original structural element. Test results show that the use of external composite reinforcement (fabric placed using wet lay-up and pultruded strips that were adhesively bonded to the surface), dramatically increase the load-carrying capacity of the slabs, whereas the ductility (or deformation capacity) at initial failure (though at a significantly higher load than possible with a typical reinforced concrete slab) is drastically reduced. Although the procedure provides an efficient means of strengthening, care must be taken to ensure that the rehabilitation design addresses the possibility of elastic failure of the system, with a sudden drop in strength when the composite fails through catastrophic fracture, failure of the composite-concrete bond interphase, limits on capacity increase related to yielding of steel reinforcement, or the use of an appropriately factored, equivalent-energy-based design approach.

Significant research related to the strengthening of beams has already been conducted (Ref 10–12) and is being used extensively in the field. The method has found the most applicability in the flexural strengthening of beams and girders through the addition of composite reinforcing strips/plates to the lower surface of beams, or around the entire web area to provide shear strengthening. A carbon-fiber-based strengthening system, consisting of stabilized unidirectional fabric impregnated in the field with an epoxy resin using the wet lay-up process, was used recently for the repair and enhancement of shear capacity of precast, prestressed double-T beam stems at the Pittsburgh airport parking complex. The project consumed over 3400 m^2 (36,600 ft^2) of the fabric, representing one of the largest uses of this material in the United States. It was completed in less than four months, with minimal closure of the garage. In another application, 3000 m (9800 ft) of pultruded carbon/epoxy strips were used at LaGuardia Airport to strengthen runway slabs over Flushing Bay in Queens, NY. The strips were used to restore the ultimate capacity of the slabs and to stiffen them to prevent localized surface cracking and failure initiation from holes that had been cut in the slabs for the installation of additional piling.

The strengthening or repair of slabs is being increasingly considered, but it should be kept in mind that, due to differences in conventional steel reinforcement detailing and structural response between beams and slabs, results derived from the application of composites to beams cannot be directly extrapolated to application of slabs, especially as related to the selection of form and positioning of the external reinforcement (Ref 13). This application is considered to be of significant importance for the future, in terms of buildings, highway infrastructure, piers and waterfront structures, and even tarmacs, not just for purposes of strengthening and increase in load capacity, but also for the repair of deficient structures, such as those where local punching shear failures are seen in bridge decks between longitudinal girders.

Figure 5 shows an area of extensive cracking and punching shear failure in the deck of a bridge (Ref 14). Cracking was initiated in transverse spanning decks in longitudinal bending due to lack of flexural capacity. Subsequently, the effective width in the transverse direction was limited to the spacing between the transverse cracks, resulting in significant flexure and shear overloads. As a consequence, longitudinal cracks develop that spread over the entire deck length due to the moving nature of wheel loads, resulting in the local shear capacity being exceeded over a shear area limited by existing flexural cracks in both directions.

A common conventional recourse is the complete reconstruction of the area, often at significant cost and with protracted distress to traffic. In comparison, fiber-reinforced composites can easily be applied without any disruption of traffic. If the repair scheme is designed properly, the external composite reinforcement will not only repair the area that was damaged by punching shear, but will also ensure that existing cracks do not open, causing further deterioration. The repair of this deficiency through the use of adhesively bonded pultruded composite strips and through wet lay-up of unidirectional fabric is shown in Fig. 6. The rehabilitation was conducted under traffic conditions without blocking or otherwise contaminating the aqueduct that carried water underneath it, again exemplifying the significant potential of composites for rehabilitation (Ref 15).

Similar schemes can be applied, not just in bridges, but also for the strengthening and repair of floor slabs of parking garages, which often suffer rapid deterioration due to salt-induced cracking, efflorescence of concrete, and corrosion of steel reinforcement. Further, the use of composite strips/bands provides an efficient mechanism for repair where the installation of liftwells and shafts in buildings results in cutting through existing steel reinforcement to form a cutout. Composite strips or bands can be easily applied externally to make up the lost reinforcing capacity, as well as to provide the means for redistribution of loads and resulting stresses. Where preexisting slabs have to be cut for the installation of a liftwell during changes in building use, conventional methods would result in

Table 2 Methods of application of external composite reinforcement for strengthening

Procedure	Description	Time
Adhesive bonding	Composite strip/panel/plate is prefabricated and cured (using wet lay-up, pultrusion, or autoclave cure) and then bonded onto the concrete substrate using an adhesive under pressure	Very quick application
Wet lay-up	Resin is applied to the concrete substrate and layers of fabric are then impregnated in place using rollers and/or squeegees. The composite and bond are formed at the same time.	Slower and needs more set-up
Vacuum infusion	Reinforcing fabric is placed over the area under consideration and the entire area is encapsulated in a vacuum bag. Resin is infused into the assembly under vacuum with compaction taking place under vacuum pressure. Unlike the wet lay-up process this is a closed process. In a variant the outer layer of fabric in contact with the vacuum bag is partially cured prior to placement in order to assure a good surface.	Far slower with significant setup time needed

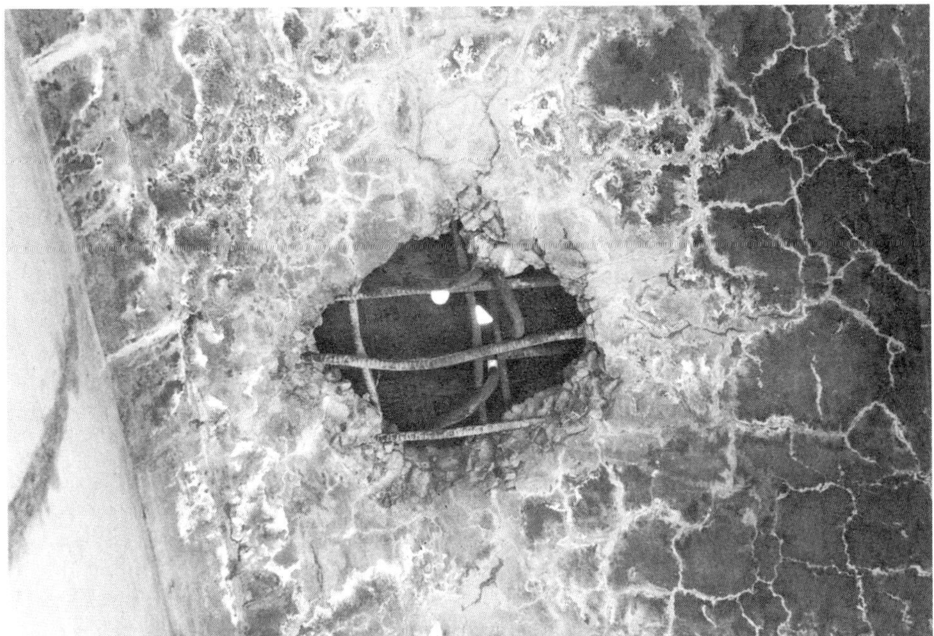

Fig. 5 Extensive cracking and punching shear damage to a bridge deck

the construction of deep supporting beams, enclosure walls, or columns to support the resulting weaker structure. Not only would all of these alternatives cause valuable space to be used, but significant cost and extended inconvenience to the inhabitants would also result. Composites, as shown in the example in Fig. 7 (Ref 15), thus provide a means not just for strengthening and repair, but also for effecting change in occupancy or use of structures while allowing rapid and nonintrusive reconstruction. Appropriate design can assure that failure is through delamination at the level of cover concrete, with load level decreasing to that of the yield response of the slab with a cutout, thereby ensuring gradual rather than catastrophic failure.

In addition to the uses described previously, FRP composites have also been used for the repair and strengthening of historical structures or those with local community value, due to the ease of application without causing changes in the overall aesthetics and geometry of the structural components under consideration. In an interesting application in this area, three 65 m (215 ft) tall concrete smoke stacks of a cement plant in San Antonio, TX, were strengthened in 1998 using glass-fiber-reinforced polymer composites over the full height of the stacks to repair them from a structural aspect, while improving the aesthetics of a local landmark. The entire plant, with the smoke stacks as the signature elements, was renovated and converted into a shopping and entertainment complex.

Repair of Large-Diameter Pipes

Prestressed concrete cylinder pipe (PCCP) is widely used for the transportation and distribution of water in municipal, industrial, and agricultural irrigation systems. Pipe diameters range from 1.5 to 6 m (5 to 20 ft), and pressure heads range in height from 15 to 300 m (50 to 1000 ft). Recently, there has been an increasing fear of pipeline ruptures caused by:

- Cracking of the mortar coating or concrete cover, resulting in inadequate protection over a localized portion of prestressing wire, which can then corrode over time and lead to loss of section and ultimate loss in prestress of the pipe
- Defects in the original manufacturing process that could lead to water ingress into the pipe structure, leading to corrosion of the prestressing strands and ultimate loss of prestress
- Defects in the prestressing wire material, leading to accelerated pitting and corrosion

A number of sections have recently failed, with bursts leading to severe structural failure and damage to the surrounding area through cratering (Fig. 8). A number of these pipelines are below roads and in urban areas, leading to realistic fears of severe damage in case of failure, and necessitating the development of in situ repair methods that can be conducted without having to excavate the ground to replace pipe sections.

Although repair can be conducted through the use of conventional materials, such as installing

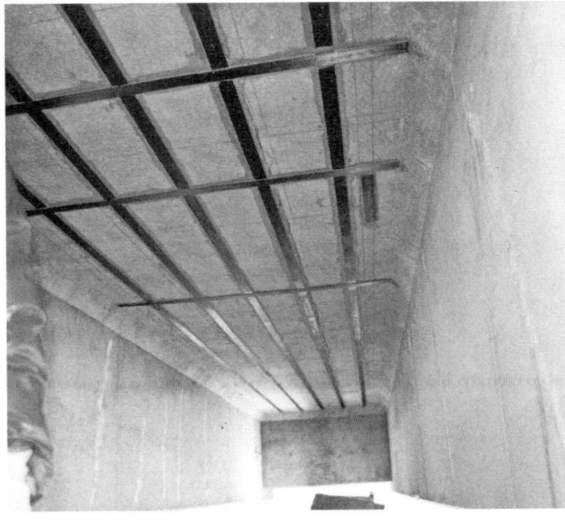

(a)

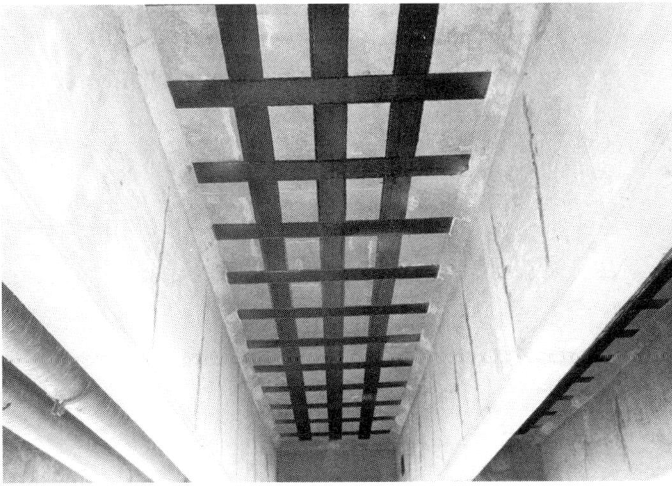

(b)

Fig. 6 Repair/strengthening of deck using (a) pultruded strips adhesively bonded to the concrete substrate, and (b) unidirectional fabric placed using wet lay-up

an inner steel liner, installation is problematic due to the lack of clear access and the need for welding on-site inside the pipe. Moreover, the use of this method results in significant decreases in pipe cross section, leading to loss in flow. Further, the use of metallic liners necessitates the use of expensive corrosion protection schemes. Taking advantage of the high strength and stiffness of thin cross sections of composite materials, the use of a thin composite liner bonded to the inner surface of the concrete lining (Fig. 9) presents an attractive means to counteract the loss in prestressing due to corrosion of the outer prestressing wire. Recent tests have shown that the use of appropriately designed composite liners having predominant hoop reinforcement can ensure that the full capacity of the pipe can be achieved with very small reduction in inner diameter, thus using composites to effect a rapid and significantly lower cost repair. Similar to the methods of external strengthening described in the previous section, these structural liners can be installed using the wet lay-up process or through the adhesive bonding of prefabricated strips in spiral or hoop fashion. Because the primary need for reinforcement is in a specific direction (along the circumference), materials use can also be optimized in a composite through implementation of predominantly unidirectional (hoop oriented) layers. This method has already been demonstrated in the field as an efficient means of both repair and life-extension, as well as a cost-efficient means of preventive maintenance. Although the application was developed for purposes of repair and strengthening, it could also be used in the fabrication of new large-diameter pipelines to enhance pressure capacity and overall durability.

Replacement Bridge Decks

Of all elements in a bridge superstructure, bridge decks may require the maximum maintenance, for reasons ranging from the deterioration of the wearing surface to the degradation of the deck system itself. Added to the problems of deterioration are issues related to the need for higher load ratings and increased number of lanes on existing bridges to accommodate the constantly increasing traffic flow on major arteries. Beyond the costs and visible consequences associated with continuous retrofit, repair, and upgrade of such structural components are the intangible, but nonetheless important, consequences related to losses in productivity and overall economies related to losses of time and resources caused by delays and detours. Reasons such as those listed previously provide significant impetus for the development of new bridge decks out of materials that are durable, light, and easy to install. Besides the potential savings in life-cycle costs due to increased durability, decks fabricated from composites would be significantly lighter, thereby affecting savings in substructure costs, enabling the use of higher live-load levels by offsetting the higher dead weight of existing conventional decks, and giving designers the potential of longer unsupported spans and enhanced seismic resistance. These deck structures can either be used as replacements for existing, but deteriorated or substandard concrete/conventional decks, or used as new structural components on conventional or new supporting structural elements.

For use as replacement decks, FRP composite decks have to be designed with four criteria in mind:

- Stiffness developed in the composite deck system (usually through the combination of a core and facesheets) must fall in the range between that of an equivalent uncracked and a cracked concrete deck, and the resulting response must have deformations not exceeding those of the conventional systems.
- Methods of attachment must match those useable on the existing girders and superstructure.
- Factors of safety must be designed in through the use of an appropriately factored equivalent energy approach, so as to offset the initial linear response followed by irreversible cracking/delamination/separation of fabric layers in composite decks.
- Processing methods must enable uniformity at costs comparable with the in-place costs of existing deck systems.

It should be noted that enhanced durability and the consequent lower life-cycle cost, although important, might not be an overriding factor in systems selection at the acquisition stage if cost differences are too high. Thus, it is important that savings arising from faster erection, need for less installation equipment, savings in supporting/foundation structure costs, and significantly reduced disruption of traffic be factored into the systems-level cost.

Fiber-reinforced polymer composite decks have been fabricated using a number of processes, such as wet lay-up (with one of the first vehicular demonstrations being the Miyun Bridge in China, Ref 16), resin-infusion-based processes (Ref 17, 18), pultrusion (Ref 18–21), or a combination thereof. The use of modular sections that can "snap" together in the field provide flexibility while satisfying the civil engineer's desire to use standardized sections. Large-scale tests on deck subelements and the use of these in a number of projects in the field have demonstrated that adequate performance levels can be easily achieved at significantly lower weights. It should be noted that because designs are primarily driven by deflection (i.e., stiffness-related) constraints, materials and structural configurations are selected to optimize stiffness, and therefore stress levels in the composite are extremely low under service conditions (generically in the range of 10–15% of ultimate). Although the typical response envelope is linear to failure, it is possible to design for a failure envelope that mimics the overall structural ductility of reinforced concrete by allowing failures at nodes within the composite through mechanisms of delamination and layer separation. Although these modes are irreversible, they do provide a slow degradation of performance with substantial "pseudoductility." Fiber-reinforced polymer bridge decks have already been installed as replacements for existing concrete, steel, and timber decks in a number of cases, and in others have been used

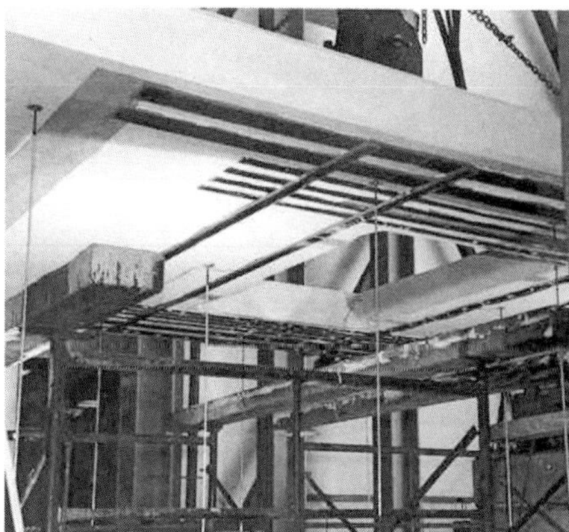

Fig. 7 Placement of composites around cutout in slab to provide external reinforcement for stress redistribution

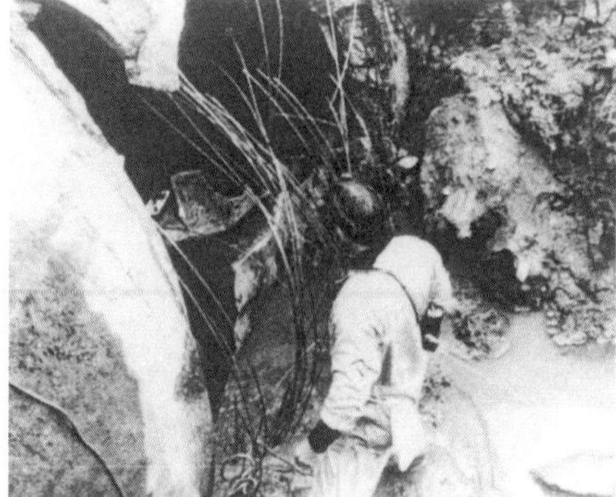

Fig. 8 Damage due to prestressed concrete cylinder pipe burst (Mojave Desert)

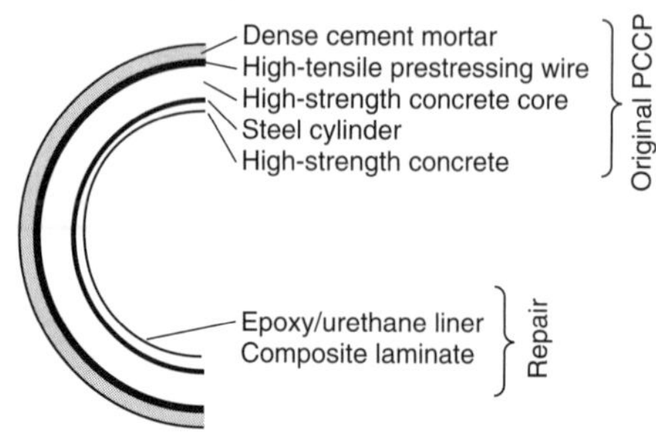

Fig. 9 Schematic for placement of composite structural liner for preventive maintenance of large-diameter water pipes. PCCP, prestressed concrete cylinder pipe

as complete replacements for existing superstructure between abutments.

New Structural Systems

The current emphasis on the use of composites in the areas of rehabilitation and replacement can be traced to the greater ease of its introduction in this area due to urgent needs for methods and greater flexibility in accepting technologies without the establishment of standards. However, there is significant long-term potential for the development of new infrastructure systems, using either composites by themselves or in conjunction with existing materials, such as timber, steel, and concrete. The intrinsic light weight and tailorability of composites enable the integration of form and function into civil engineering designs without constraints previously in place due to limitations of conventional materials. Building ecosystems having large, unsupported domes, such as those needed for artificial desert and undersea habitats, long span bridges, such as between Italy and Sicily, or bridges that meld in with environments without upsetting the fragile surrounding ecosystems could all be possible in the 21st century using large and long unsupported prefabricated composite systems, either as full structural elements or as the primary reinforcement. Applications such as floor panels and gratings on offshore platforms are already being used as part of primary structure, both decreasing topside weight (which generically results in a minimum of three times the savings below the waterline) and increasing occupant safety in cases of fire, due to decreased levels of heat conduction as compared with steel and aluminum. Electrical transmission towers fabricated using specially designed interlocking pultruded elements (Ref 22) are already providing immense advantages over metallic incumbent structures due to increased durability and ease of installation, especially in areas that are difficult to access.

The development of new structural concepts and systems that combine the superior mechanical characteristics of directional strength in tension in the direction of the fiber with the dominant characteristics of conventional materials, such as compression in concrete, show great potential for development of new advances in the design and construction of civil infrastructure systems. The concept of using composite tubes as both the formwork and the primary tension reinforcement for columns (Ref 23) provides an efficient means of replacing the reinforcing steel (and the attendant problems related with assemblage in the field and deterioration due to corrosion) while providing a prefabricated reinforcing formwork into which lower strength concrete could be easily and rapidly poured. This provides better seismic response and overall durability, coupled with greater speed of erection. This concept is currently being studied not just for the fabrication of new columns using "stay-in-place" formwork, but also as a framing system for large industrial facilities.

An extension of these concepts is possible for complete bridge systems where both columns and supporting girders for superstructure are prefabricated from hollow shells, assembled on site, and then filled with lightweight, high-flowable concrete under pressure for rapid modular construction. Both composite and reinforced concrete (precast or cast-in-place) decks could be used in this scheme. Prototype systems for slab and girder bridge systems have already been tested (Ref 24) at levels of individual components and large-scale structural subsystems and have shown that performance (both static and fatigue) criteria can readily be reached, with ultimate capacities being significantly in excess of required shear and moment demand for full vehicular operation. A prototype 20.1 m (66 ft) span bridge (Fig. 10) has recently been completed in Palm Desert, CA, using this concept for full vehicular traffic (Ref 25).

The use of rectangular and "conrec" shell configurations, such as described in (Ref 26), in place of circular cross sections permits greater optimization of materials usage through hybridization, using both carbon- and glass-fiber reinforcements, while simultaneously enabling greater ease of construction/assembly using tension-tie-plates to position and hold the assembly

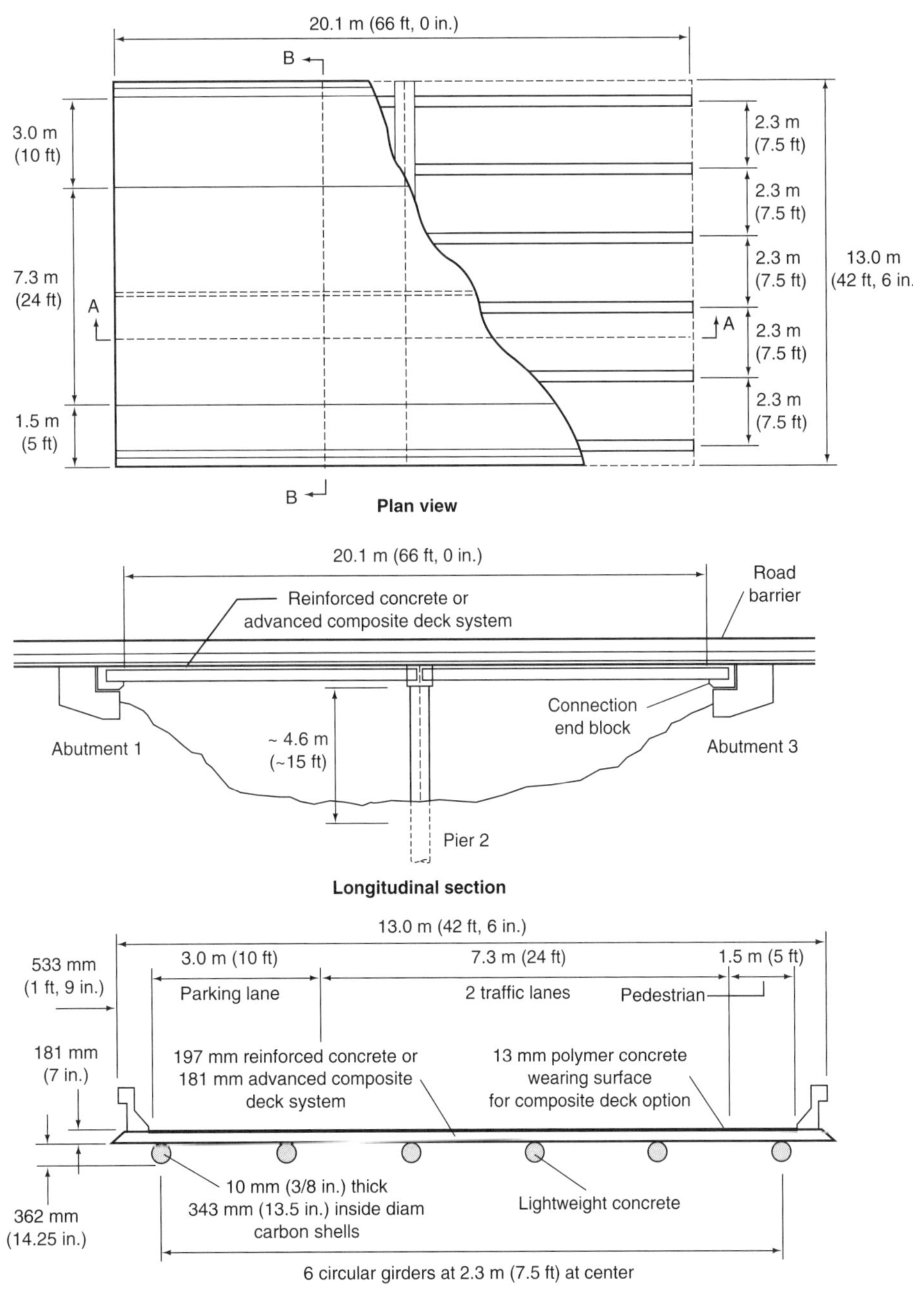

Fig. 10 Geometry of the Kings stormwater channel bridge (Palm Desert, CA)

together (Fig. 11). Such systems, comprised of composite tube and plate assemblies used synergistically with concrete infill and selective use of conventional embedded connection details, can provide design enhancements that were envisioned earlier with the use of concrete-filled steel tubes, but did not find widespread use due to difficulties associated with steel yielding, corrosion-related degradation, and weight. Such concepts could also conceivably be extended for use in rapid fabrication of large industrial facilities without the use of heavy equipment in areas where labor is either unskilled or not readily available.

A number of other systems using combinations of deck systems and pultruded beams as girders have already been erected in the field over short spans and are being monitored for performance (Ref 27–29). Further developments, such as the envisioned construction of the Interstate 5/Gilman Drive bridge (San Diego, CA) (Fig. 12), which uses concrete-filled carbon/epoxy tubes as the longitudinal girders, E-glass/vinylester hollow rectangular box-type transverse girders, and a set of structural stiffened deck panel overlaid with fiber–reinforced concrete with steel rebar spanning between the transverse girders (Ref 25, 26), provide additional impetus for the rapid acceptance of composites in civil construction.

Outlook

Although the use of polymer-matrix composites is increasing in the area of civil infrastructure, it must be noted that, except in the areas of seismic retrofit and strengthening, most of the other applications are in the realm of demonstrations, rather than in the commercial area. There is no doubt, however, that the intrinsic tailorability and performance attributes of both glass- and carbon-fiber reinforced composites make these materials very attractive for use in civil infrastructure applications, and a welcome addition to the current palette of construction materials. Due to the large volume of material needed, even for niche applications, the civil infrastructure market is expected to provide a significant impetus for further development of new composite material systems (primarily in the area of hybrids and textile structural composites) and new or modified processes capable of fabricating large structural components in a cost-efficient manner.

These developments are likely to range from the production of cheaper carbon fibers and E-glass fibers with greater alkaline resistance, to the greater use of hybrid composites, with hybridization taking place at the level of the tow as well as in textile preform structures. Needs for greater resistance to fires have already spurred the renewed development of phenolic resins with greater flexibility in processing. In an environmentally conscious industry, requirements for the fabrication of large structural components using low-cost processes, such as pultrusion, resin infusion, and resin transfer molding, have lead to the development of low-viscosity, lower-styrene- and volatile-content vinylesters, and phase-transforming resin systems. Field conditions and the intrinsic need for composites that must be able to perform under wide ranges of temperature and humidity levels is leading to intense research in areas related to alternate cure mechanisms capable of achieving rapid cure and higher-than-ambient glass transition temperatures without the use of external heat.

By their very nature, most composite components used in civil infrastructure have to be cost-competitive on an acquisition cost basis, if not at the component level, then at least at the systems level, with incumbents made of conventional materials. Further, the very nature of the applications set almost assures that significant fabrication will be conducted in the field or in partially controlled, but changing environments. The exigencies of size also dictate that, in general, traditional autoclave-based fabrication will not be used widely. The emphasis is increasingly being placed on processes such as wet lay-up, pultrusion, winding, and resin transfer molding, and in the development of newer processes, such as injection pultrusion and resin infusion. It should be noted that these and other developments brought about by the needs of civil infrastructure will not only provide solutions specific to civil infrastructure requirements, but will also have a positive influence on other applications of composites.

In spite of the high level of current interest in this area, the extent and nature of the future use of composites in civil infrastructure will depend on a number of factors, including:

- Resolution of outstanding issues related to durability, fire resistance, and reparability, to the extent of having a good determination of the level of knowledge and assurance of each of these factors
- Development of manufacturing processes and schemes that are amenable to the high-quality, repeatable, and uniform production of primary structural elements in a cost-effective (as related to civil infrastructure economics) manner, both in controlled factory conditions (for prefabricated elements) and in the field (for in situ fabrication)
- Development of validated codes, standards, and guidelines for the use of these materials by the civil engineering community
- Development of low-cost, in situ health-monitoring devices and schemes, especially to provide a level of comfort about the safety of using structures/components fabricated from composites, until a time when an appropriate history of in-field use has been attained
- The synergistic education of both the civil engineering/construction and the composites communities about the needs and methods of development in both areas

Recent advances in materials, manufacturing, mechanics, and design point to the continued development of innovative materials and structural systems that will enable:

- Synthesis of form and function
- Greater emphasis to be paid to aesthetics and blending of the structure into the environment
- Construction of true long-span bridges
- Use of intelligent, self-monitoring structural systems
- Development of very large-scale structural systems, such as large integrated city-structural complexes, built as independent envi-

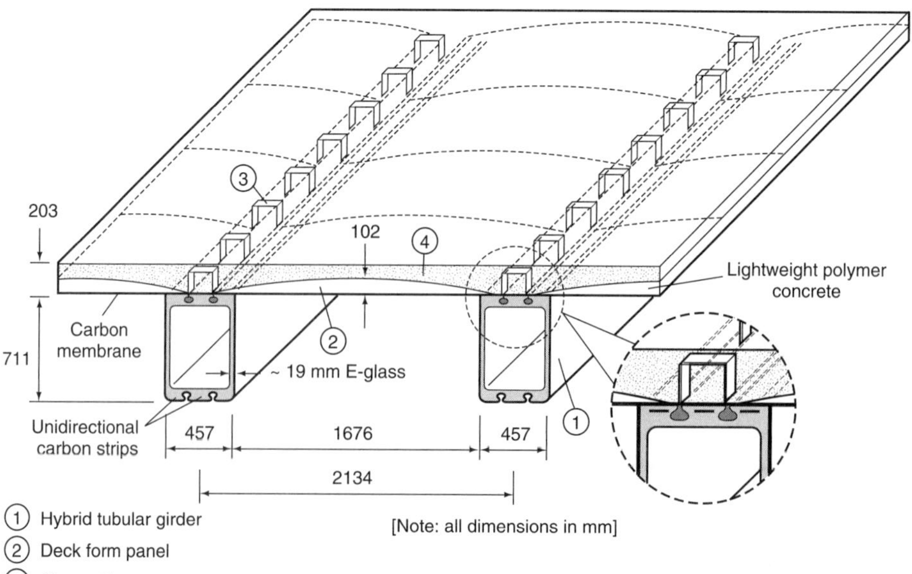

Fig. 11 Modular "snap-in" bridge system

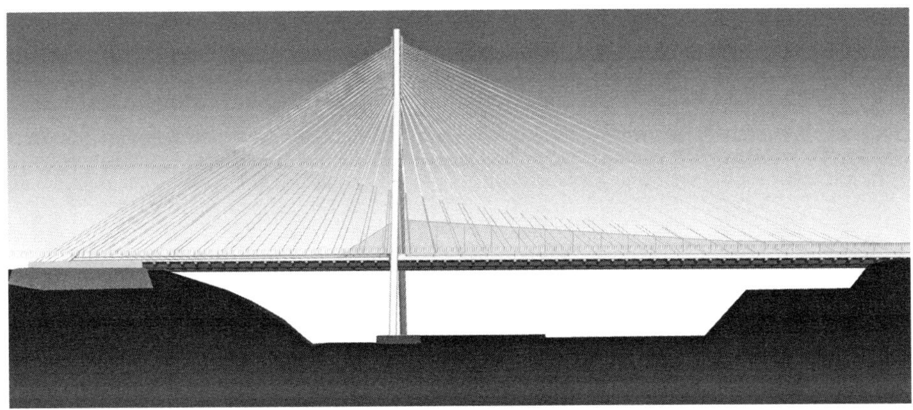

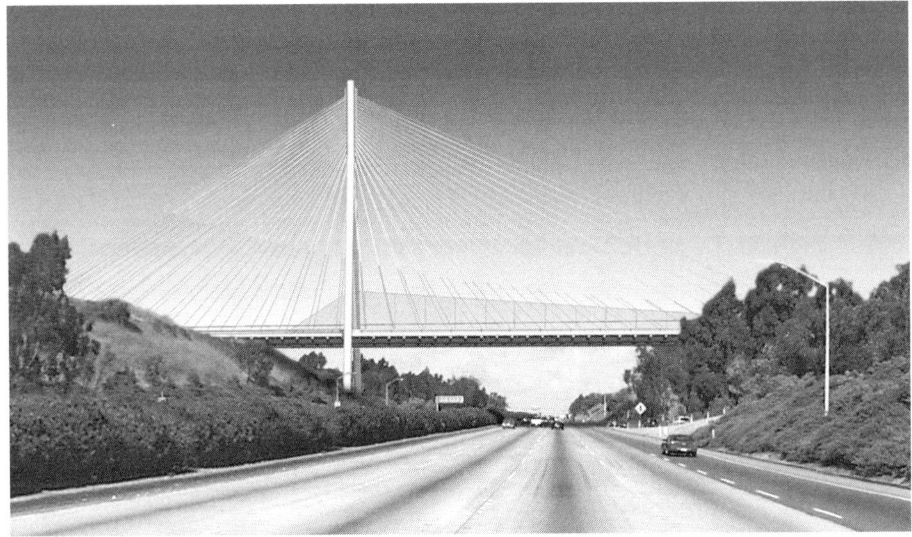

Fig. 12 Artist's rendition of the Interstate 5/Gilman Drive cable-stayed bridge

ronments on land, in the air/space, or underground

Perhaps in civil infrastructure applications, fiber-reinforced polymer-matrix composites will finally demonstrate their potential as true structural materials and become not just "materials of the future," but "materials for everyday construction."

REFERENCES

1. F.S. Rostasy, FRP: The European Perspective, *Proc. ICCI '96*, (Arizona), 1996, p 12–20
2. F. Seible and V. Karbhari, Advanced Composites for Civil Engineering Applications in the United States, *Proc. ICCI '96*, (Arizona), 1996, p 21–40
3. K.W. Neale and P. Labossiere, State-of-the-Art Report of Retrofitting and Strengthening by Continuous Fibre in Canada, *Proc. Third International Symposium on Non-Metallic (FRP) Reinforcement for Concrete Structures*, (Japan), 1997, p 25–39
4. U. Meier, Post Strengthening by Continuous Fiber Laminates in Europe, *Proc. Third International Symposium on Non-Metallic (FRP) Reinforcement for Concrete Structures*, (Japan), 1997, p 41–56
5. V.M. Karbhari, "Use of Composite Materials in Civil Infrastructure in Japan," WTEC report, National Science Foundation, 1998
6. *Structural Engineering International, Special Issue on Advanced Materials*, Vol 9 (No. 4), 1999
7. F. Seible, M.J.N. Priestley, G.A. Hegemier, and D. Innamorato, Seismic Retrofit of RC Columns with Continuous Carbon Fiber Jackets, *ASCE J. Compos. Constr.*, Vol 1 (No. 2), 1997, p 40–52
8. M.J.N. Priestley and F. Seible, Design of Seismic Retrofit Measures for Concrete and Masonry Structures, *Constr. Build. Mater.*, Vol 9 (No. 6), 1995, p 365 377
9. F. Seible and V.M. Karbhari, "Seismic Retrofit of Bridge Columns Using Advanced Composite Materials," The National Seminar on Advanced Composite Materials Bridges (Washington, D.C.), May 1997
10. B. Taljsten, "Plate Bonding," doctoral thesis, Lulea University of Technology, Sweden, 1994
11. H. Saadatmanesh and M.R. Ehsani, RC Beams Strengthened with FRP Plates I: Experimental Study, *ASCE J. Struct. Eng.*, Vol 117 (No. 11), 1991, p 3417–3433.
12. U. Meier, M Deuring, M. Meier, and G. Schwegler, Strengthening of Structures with Advanced Composites, *Alternative Materials for Reinforcement and Prestressing of Concrete*, Blackie Academic & Professional, 1993, p 153–171
13. V.M. Karbhari and F. Seible, Design Considerations for FRP Rehabilitation of Concrete Structures, *Proc. First International Conf. on the Behavior of Damaged Structures, Damstruc '98*, May 1998
14. F. Seible and V.M. Karbhari, "Byron Road Bridge Rehabilitation Project, Structural Systems Research Project," SSRP–98/10, University of California, San Diego, Aug 1998
15. V.M. Karbhari, Renewal of Civil Infrastructure Using FRP Composites—Efficient Use of Materials and Processes for Rehabilitation, *Proc. Second International Conf. on the Behavior of Damaged Structures*, June 2000 (Rio de Janeiro, Brazil)
16. F. Seible, Z. Sun, and G. Ma, "Glass Fiber Composite Bridges in China," ACTT—93/01,University of California, San Diego, 1993
17. M. Chajes, J. Gillespie, D. Mertz, and H. Shenton, Advanced Composite Bridges in Delaware, *Proc. ICCI '98*, Vol 1, 1998, p 645–650
18. V.M. Karbhari, F. Seible, G. Hegemier, and L. Zhao, Fiber Reinforced Composite Decks for Infrastructure Renewal—Results and Issues, *Proc. 1997 International Composites Expo*, 1997, p 3C/1–3C/6
19. R. Lopez-Anido, H.V.S. GangaRao, D. Troutman, and D. Williams, Design and Construction of Short-Span Bridges with Modular FRP Composite Decks, *Proc. ICCI '98*, Vol 1, 1998, p 705–714
20. P.R. Head, Advanced Composites in Civil Engineering—A Critical Overview at This High Interest, Low Use Stage of Development, *Proc. ICCI '98*, Vol 1, 1998, p 3–15
21. V.M. Karbhari, Fiber Reinforced Composite Decks for Infrastructure Renewal, *Proc. Second International Conf. on Advanced Composites in Bridges and Structures*, 1996, p 759–766
22. W.B. Goldsworthy and C. Hiel, Composite Structures are a Snap, *Second International Conf. Composites in Infrastructure*, Vol 2, 1998, p 382–396
23. F. Seible, R. Burgueno, M.G. Abdallah, and R. Nuismer, "Advanced Composite Carbon Shell Systems for Bridge Columns Under Seismic Loads," *National Seismic Conf. Bridges and Highways*, (San Diego) Dec 1995
24. V.M. Karbhari, F. Seible, R. Burgueno, A. Davol, M. Wernli, and L. Zhao, Structural Characterization of Fiber Reinforced Composite Short- and Medium-Span Bridge Sys-

tems, *Appl. Compos. Mater.*, Vol 7, 2000, p 151–182
25. F. Seible, V.M. Karbhari, and R. Burgueno, Kings Stormwater Channel and I-5/Gilman Bridges, USA, *Struct. Eng. Int.*, Vol 9 (No. 4), Nov 1999, p 250–253
26. F. Seible, V.M. Karbhari, R. Burgueno, and E. Seaberg, "A Modular Advanced Composite Bridge System for Short and Medium Span Bridges," Fifth International Conf. Short and Medium Span Bridges, (Calgary, Canada), July 1998
27. A.B. Temeles, T.E. Cousins, and J.J. Lesko, Composite Plate and Tube Bridge Deck Design: Evaluation in the Troutville, Virginia Weigh Station Test Bed, *Proc. ACMBS-III*, Aug 2000, (Ottawa), p 801–808
28. D. Richards, and G. Solomon, Review of Field Data on the All-Composite Highway Bridge, Tech-21, *Proc. 1999 International Composites Exposition*, May 1999, (Cincinnati, Ohio), p 25B/1–25B/6
29. M.D. Hayes, J.J. Lesko, J. Haramis, T.E. Cousins, J. Gomez, and P. Masarelli, Laboratory and Field Testing of Composite Bridge Superstructure, *ASCE J. Compos. Constr.*, Vol 4 (No. 3), 2000, p 120–128

Applications of Ceramic-Matrix Composites

J.R. Davis, Davis & Associates

APPLICATIONS for ceramic-matrix composites (CMCs) fall into four major categories:

- Cutting tool inserts
- Wear-resistant parts
- Aerospace and military applications
- Other industrial applications, including engines and energy-related applications

This article reviews application examples in each of these four categories, with emphasis placed on those applications/materials that have achieved commercial viability. Advanced CMCs that are now emerging from laboratories and that show potential for high-performance applications or that are in the prototype stage are also surveyed. An in-depth economic analysis on CMCs, including their processing, new applications, current markets and trends, and U.S. and international companies and institutions involved in CMCs, can be found in Ref 1.

Applications for Discontinuously Reinforced CMCs

Discontinuous reinforcement involves the addition of particles, platelets, whiskers, or chopped fibers, typically to a polycrystalline ceramic, glass, or glass-ceramic matrix. From an application viewpoint, the most important matrix material is alumina (Al_2O_3), although discontinuously reinforced CMCs have also been produced from silicon carbide (SiC), silicon nitride (Si_3N_4), mullite ($3Al_2O_32SiO_2$), and aluminosilicate matrices. Important reinforcements include SiC, zirconia (ZrO_2), and titanium carbide (TiC). Additional information on discontinuously reinforced CMCs, including their toughening mechanisms and properties, can be found

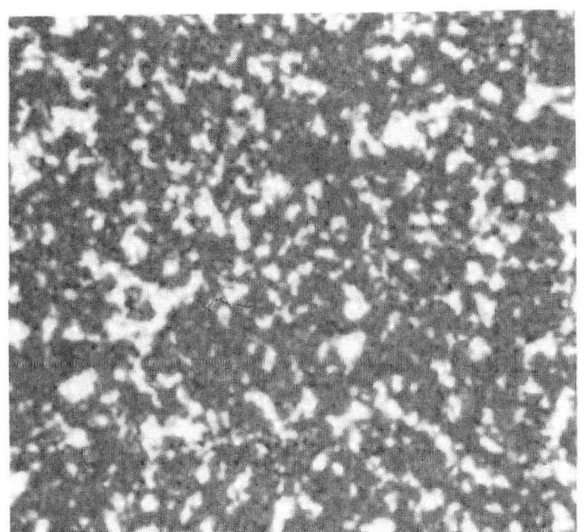

Fig. 1 Microstructure of a hot-pressed Al_2O_3-TiC ceramic tool material. 1500×

Table 1 Typical property values for cutting tool materials, including discontinuously reinforced CMCs

Tool material	Transverse rupture strength		Hardness, HRA	Fracture toughness	
	MPa	ksi		MPa $\sqrt{m}$	ksi $\sqrt{in.}$
Al_2O_3	500–700	70–100	93–94	3.5–4.5	3.2–4.1
Al_2O_3-ZrO_2	700–900	100–130	93–94	5.0–8.0	4.5–7.3
Al_2O_3-TiC	600–850	90–120	94–95	3.5–4.5	3.2–4.1
Al_2O_3-SiC_w	550–750	80–110	94–95	4.5–8.0	4.1–7.3
Si_3N_4	700–1050	100–150	92–94	6.0–8.5	5.5–7.7
SiAlON	700–900	100–125	93–95	4.5–6.0	4.1–5.5
WC-Co alloys	1250–2100	180–300	91–93	10.0–13.5	9.1–11.4

Source: Ref 2

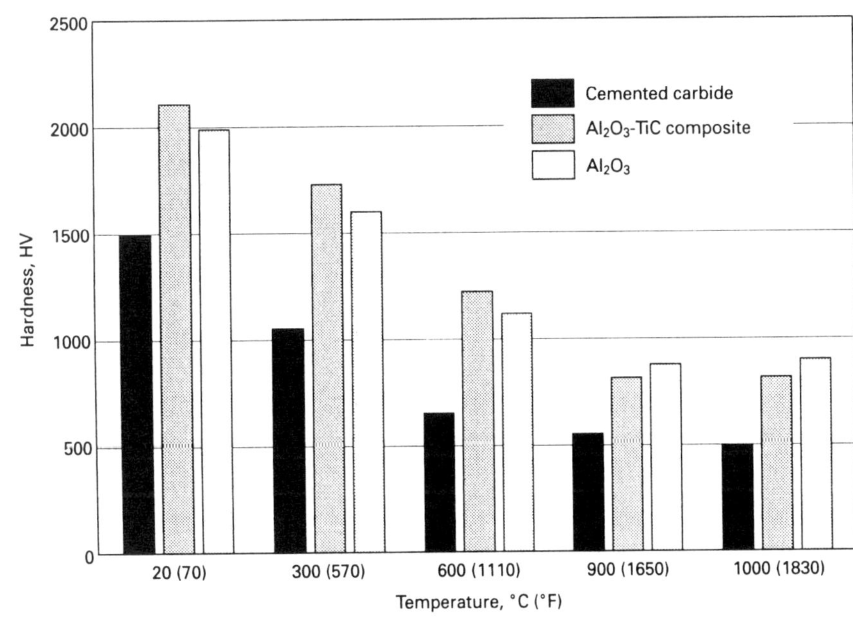

Fig. 2 Hot hardness comparison of monolithic Al_2O_3, Al_2O_3-TiC, and cemented carbide tool materials. Source: Ref 3

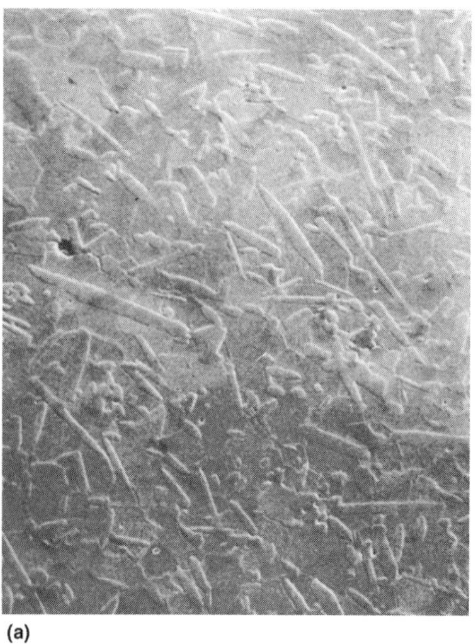

(a)

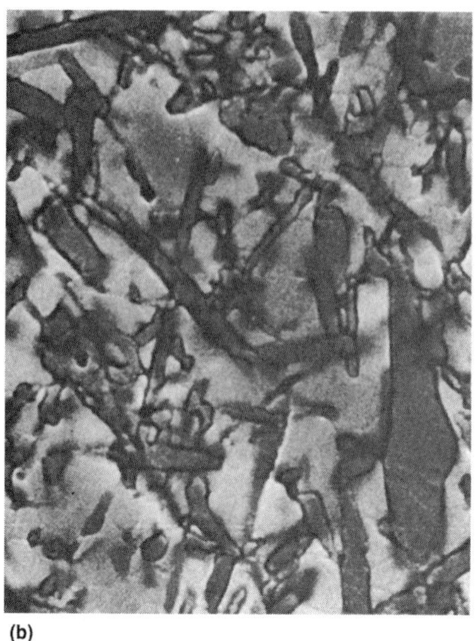

(b)

Fig. 3 Microstructure of SiC whisker-reinforced Al_2O_3 composite. (a) 2100×. (b) 5000×

Fig. 4 Fracture surface of a SiC whisker-reinforced Al_2O_3 ceramic. Note hexagonal voids or holes due to whisker pull-out upon fracture. 950×

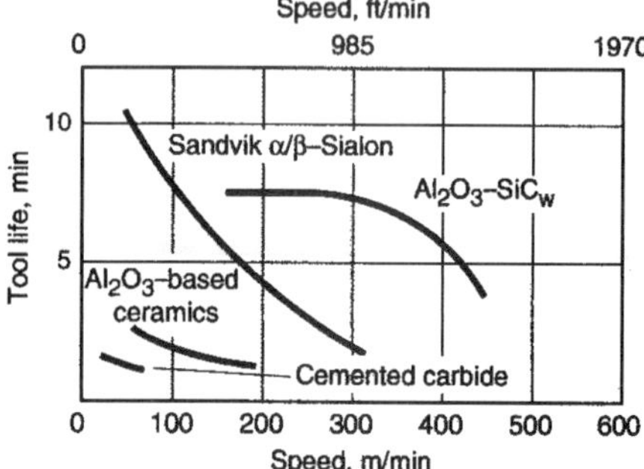

Fig. 5 Tool life of ceramic, CMC, and cemented carbide materials when machining Inconel 718 (feed of 0.2 mm/rev; depth-of-cut of 2 mm). Source: Ref 8

in the article "Properties and Performance of Ceramic-Matrix and Carbon-Carbon Composites" in this Volume.

Cutting Tools

Both particulate-reinforced and whisker-reinforced Al_2O_3 have found use as cutting tool inserts. The development of these composite tool materials was partially based on the advances in high-temperature monolithic ceramic materials and processing technology developed for automotive gas turbine and other high-temperature structural applications. Table 1 compares the room-temperature properties of ceramic and cemented carbide tool materials, including several of the CMCs discussed subsequently.

Al_2O_3-TiC Composites. In the early 1970s, it was discovered that Al_2O_3 admixed with a refractory metal particulate (for example, titanium carbide) could produce a cutting tool with superior hardness and fracture resistance. These hot-pressed or hot isostatically pressed (HIPed) composites consist of approximately 70% Al_2O_3 with 30% TiC particulate. Such composites are referred to as black ceramics due to their color,

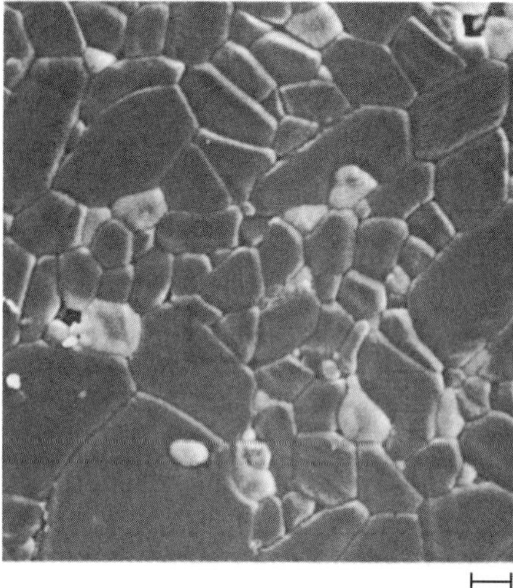

Fig. 6 Scanning electron micrograph of high-purity zirconia-toughened alumina (ZTA) showing dispersed ZrO_2 phase (white) within an Al_2O_3 matrix

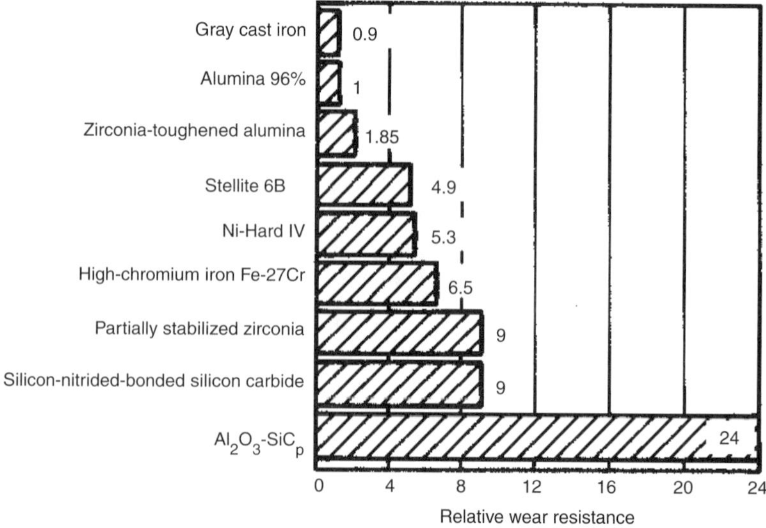

Fig. 7 Relative slurry erosion wear performance of metallic, ceramic, and CMC (Al_2O_3-SiC_p) materials. This evaluation compared measured material losses in a slurry pot test in which 14 mm (0.54 in.) diam by 60 mm (2.4 in.) long test pins were rotated at 10 m/s (33 ft/s) for 20 h in a slurry of 40 wt% 300 to 600 μm SiO_2 particles in neutral water. Source: Ref 18

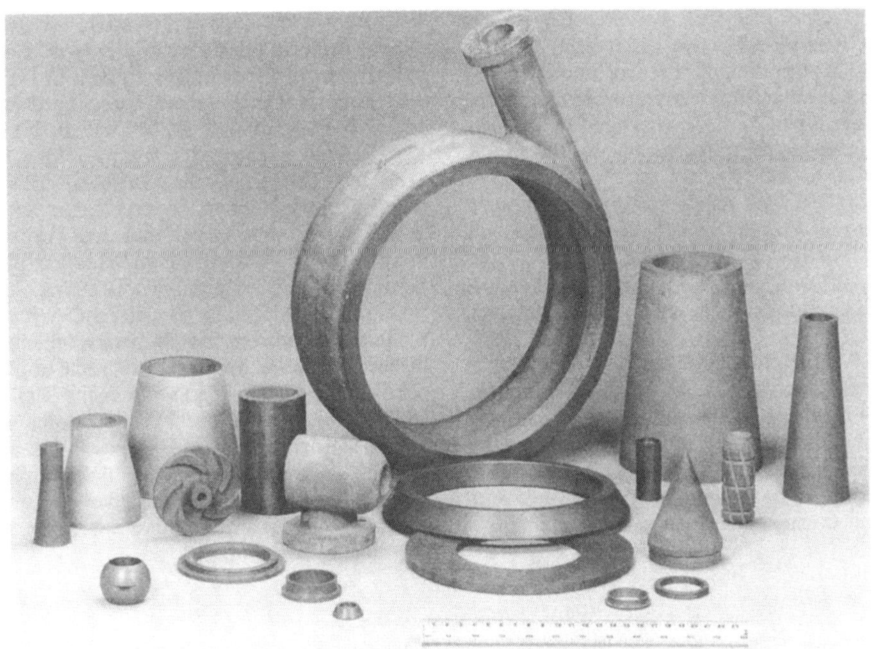

Fig. 8 Examples of wear-resistant Al_2O_3-SiC_p components produced for use in applications requiring resistance to slurry erosion. The pump housing is approximately 640 mm (25 in.) in diameter. Large wear rings are produced up to 1.2 m (48 in.) in diameter.

which results from the presence of TiC. The typical microstructure of an Al_2O_3-TiC composite is shown in Fig. 1.

The dispersion of hard refractory particles increases the hardness of these composites at temperatures up to 800 °C (1470 °F) when compared to monolithic oxide ceramics (Fig. 2). Simultaneously, the fracture toughness and bending strength is improved through crack impediment, crack deflection, or crack branching caused by the dispersed hard particles. The higher hardness in combination with the higher toughness increases the resistance to abrasive and erosive wear considerably. The lower thermal expansion and higher thermal conductivity of the composites improve thermal-shock resistance when compared to monolithic oxide ceramics. At temperatures exceeding 800 °C (1470 °F), however, the TiC particles oxidize and begin to lose their reinforcing properties and the composite weakens. Thus, this phenomenon must be taken into consideration when selecting cutting conditions such as cutting speed, depth of cut, and feed rate.

The HIPed Al_2O_3-TiC composite tool grades are used for interrupted cuts, and for roughing and finishing of high-temperature superalloys, hardened steels (30 to 50 HRC), chilled irons (50 to 60 HRC), and gray and ductile cast irons with hardnesses ranging from 140 to 300 HB. Additional information on machining of these materials with Al_2O_3-TiC composite tool inserts can be found in Ref 4.

Silicon carbide whisker-reinforced alumina (Al_2O_3-SiC_w) is the newest Al_2O_3-base tool material. The incorporation of SiC whiskers (20 to 45 vol%) into an Al_2O_3 matrix with subsequent hot pressing results in a composite with significantly improved toughness. Figure 3 shows the microstructure of SiC whisker-reinforced Al_2O_3.

The whiskers, which are small fibers of single-crystal SiC about 0.5 to 1 μm in diameter and 10 to 125 μm long, have a higher thermal conductivity and a lower coefficient of thermal expansion than Al_2O_3. This improves thermal-shock resistance.

The SiC whiskers in the Al_2O_3 matrix also produce a twofold increase in fracture toughness (Table 1). The fracture toughness is enhanced by the occurrence of whisker "pull-out." A close examination of the fracture surface at high magnification will reveal not only a clear indication of the whiskers randomly dispersed throughout the matrix, but also the obvious hexagonal voids where whiskers have actually been pulled out during the fracture process (Fig. 4). A large amount of energy is required to pull the whiskers out, and this greatly inhibits crack propagation. More detailed information on the fracture toughness of Al_2O_3-SiC_w composites can be found in Ref 5 to 7.

The Al_2O_3-SiC_w composite tool grades are used for rough turning of alloy and hardened steels (32 to 65 HRC), ductile irons (150 to 300 HB), and chilled irons (50 to 65 HRC). Their primary application area, however, is for roughing, finishing, and milling of difficult-to-machine age-hardenable nickel-base superalloys. Much higher cutting speeds and longer tool life can be achieved when machining these materials with whisker-reinforced Al_2O_3 (Fig. 5). Additional information on the use of Al_2O_3-SiC_w ceramic tooling for machining of superalloys can be found in Ref 9.

Si_3N_4-Base Composites. A number of particle-reinforced and whisker-reinforced Si_3N_4 composites have also been evaluated as cutting tool materials (Ref 10–14). The addition of dispersed phases such as TiC, titanium nitride (TiN), and hafnium carbide (HfC) to a Si_3N_4 matrix results in an increase in hardness. Hot-pressed whisker-reinforced composites, containing from 10 to 30 vol% SiC, exhibit higher fracture toughness values than do their unreinforced counterparts. Despite these advantages, Si_3N_4-base composite tool materials have not reached commercial viability as have monolithic Si_3N_4 and SiAlON cutting tools.

Wear-Resistant Materials/Applications

Zirconia-Toughened Ceramics. Particulate-toughened ceramics, such as the zirconia-toughened ceramics, are filling applications such as bearings, bushings, precision balls, valve seats, and die inserts where their friction and wear characteristics have improved both performance and cost. One example is zirconia-toughened alumina, or ZTA (Al_2O_3-ZrO_2), where Al_2O_3 is considered the primary or continuous (70 to 95%) phase. Zirconia particulate additions from 5 to 30% (either as pure ZrO_2 or stabilized ZrO_2) represent the second phase (Fig. 6). The ZrO_2 is present either in the tetragonal or monoclinic symmetry. Zirconia-toughened Al_2O_3 is a mate-

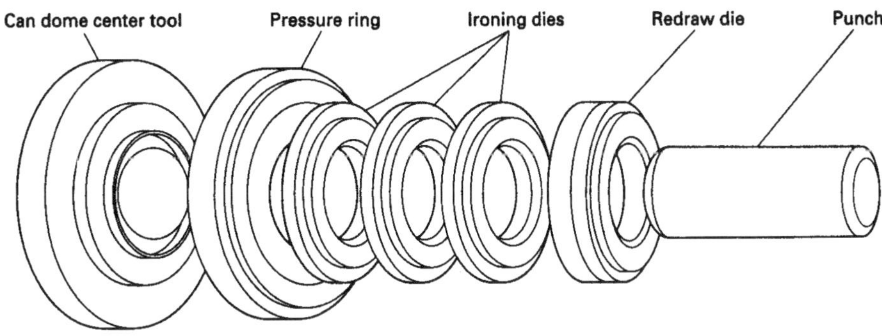

Fig. 9 Exploded view of a Si_3N_4-SiC_w can-making tooling assembly. Source: Ref 19

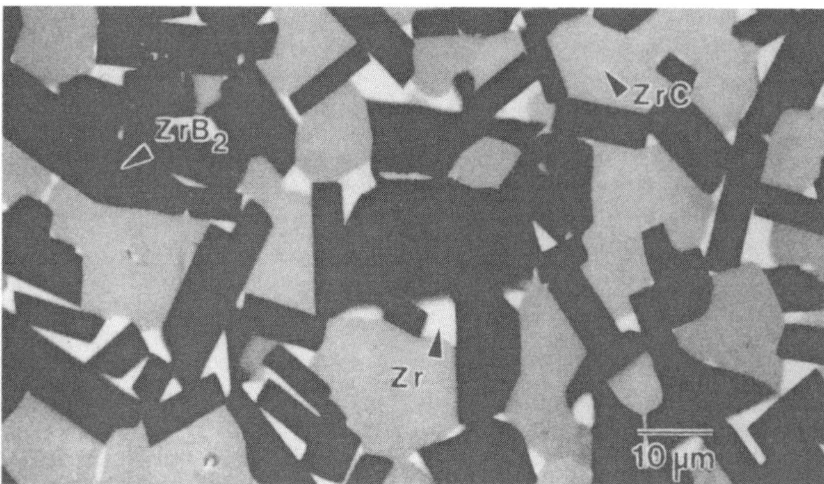

Fig. 10 Microstructure of a ZrB_2 platelet-reinforced composite with a ZrC matrix that also contains controlled amounts of zirconium metal. Source: Ref 18

rial of interest primarily because it has a significantly higher strength and fracture toughness than monolithic Al_2O_3 (Table 1).

The microstructure and subsequent mechanical properties can be tailored to specific applications. Higher ZrO_2 contents lead to increased fracture toughness and strength values, with little reduction in hardness and elastic modulus, provided most of the ZrO_2 can be retained in the tetragonal phase. Strengths up to 1050 MPa (152 ksi) and fracture toughness values as high as 8.0 MPa $\sqrt{m}$ (7.3 ksi $\sqrt{in.}$) have been measured (Table 1). Wear properties in some applications may also improve due to mechanical property enhancement compared to alumina. These types of ZTA compositions have been used in transportation equipment where they need to withstand corrosion, erosion, abrasion, and thermal shock (see subsequent discussion). Other applications for ZTA include cutting tool inserts and its use as an abrasive grinding medium.

Zirconia-toughened alumina has also seen some use in thermal shock applications. Extensive use of monoclinic ZrO_2 can result in a severely microcracked ceramic body. This microstructure allows thermal stresses to be distributed throughout a network of microcracks where energy is expended opening and/or extending microcracks, leaving the bulk ceramic body intact (Ref 15).

SiC Particle-Reinforced Al_2O_3 Matrix Composites. An Al_2O_3 matrix composite reinforced with coarse SiC particles has been optimized for applications requiring slurry erosion resistance (Ref 16, 17). Processing was carried out by directed metal oxidation (see the article "Processing of Ceramic-Matrix Composites" in this Volume for details). Wear test data for the Al_2O_3-SiC_p composite and other ceramic and metallic materials are compared in Fig. 7. Silicon carbide particle-reinforced Al_2O_3 composites of this type are being used successfully in a range of applications including slurry pump components, hydrocyclone liners, chute liners, and materials handling systems. Figure 8 shows several examples of wear components that are available commercially. A similar composite has been commercialized for armor applications.

Another variant of a SiC particle-filled Al_2O_3 matrix composite has been optimized for resistance to sliding and rolling contact wear (Ref 18). This composite uses fine SiC particles with modifications to the residual metal in the Al_2O_3 ceramic matrix. Successful prototype test results have been obtained for piston engine cam follower rollers made of this material.

CMCs for Can-Making Tooling. Ceramic-matrix composites have gained acceptance in aluminum can-making equipment and associated tooling. Products made from CMCs include (Ref 19):

- Punches
- Bodymaker toolpack (redraw dies, ironing dies, pressure rings)
- Domer tooling
- Cupper tooling
- Stripper tooling
- Necker tooling
- Trimmer blades

Materials used for these applications include transformation-toughened zirconia, Al_2O_3-SiC_w, and Si_3N_4-SiC_w. The latter material has the least affinity for aluminum metal pickup during two-piece can-making operations. Figure 9 shows an exploded view of a ceramic can-making tool assembly. Such assemblies are generally made from the same material, with Si_3N_4-SiC_w the most commonly used.

Aerospace Applications

Although most CMCs under development for aerospace structural applications are the continuous fiber CMCs discussed later in this article, there have been attempts to develop discontinuously reinforced CMCs for such applications. One example is the zirconium diboride (ZrB_2) platelet-reinforced zirconium carbide (ZrC) composite described subsequently. This is another example of CMC processing by direct metal oxidation.

ZrB_2 Platelet-Reinforced ZrC Composites. To form this composite, molten zirconium is di-

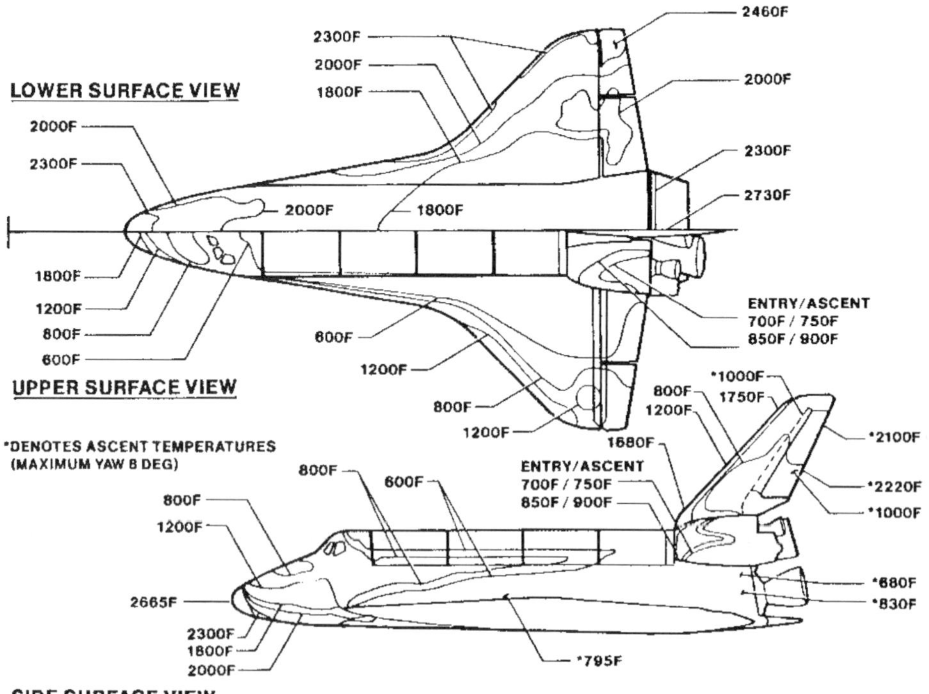

Fig. 11 Space shuttle orbiter isotherms for a typical trajectory. Source: Ref 22

rectionally reacted with B_4C powder in a graphite mold at temperatures of about 1850 to 2000 °C (3350 to 3630 °F) (Ref 20). The B_4C is completely reacted to form the two ceramic phases ZrB_2 and ZrC. The ZrB_2 takes the form of hexagonal platelets in a ZrC matrix containing controlled amounts of free zirconium, as illustrated by the microstructure shown in Fig. 10.

Typical room-temperature mechanical properties for composites in the 3 to 12 vol% Zr range include flexural strengths of 800 to 900 MPa (116 to 130 ksi), Weibull moduli of 20 to 30, and fracture toughnesses (chevron notch method) of 12 to 15 MPa$\sqrt{m}$ (11 to 14 ksi$\sqrt{in.}$) (Ref 21). The fracture toughness values depend on the metal content. Toughness values of 10 to 12 MPa$\sqrt{m}$ (9 to 11 ksi$\sqrt{in.}$) at very low metal contents result from platelet toughening mechanisms (that is, crack deflection and crack bridging/platelet pull-out). As the metal content increases, the toughness increases due to an additional contribution from ductile rupturing of metal ligaments during crack propagation.

This composite has been successfully tested in very high temperature (> 2700 °C, or 4900 °F), short time applications in rocket engines. These results derive from the highly refractory nature of the ZrB_2 and ZrC phases and the excellent thermal shock resistance of the composite. Longer-term structural applications at high temperatures may not be possible, because of the limited resistance of these materials to high-temperature oxidation and creep.

This composite is also being evaluated for applications in prosthetic devices based on its strength, fracture toughness, wear resistance, and biocompatibility. Mechanical seals and other special wear parts are additional promising application areas for these materials.

Space Shuttle Thermal Protection System

A key to the success of the space shuttle orbiter is the development of a fully reusable thermal protection system (TPS) capable of being used for up to 100 missions. The key element of the TPS is the thousands of ceramic tiles that protect the shuttle during reentry. Figure 11 shows the orbiter and the temperatures reached during reentry in a typical trajectory. During reentry of the shuttle into the earth's atmosphere, its surface reaches 1260 °C (2300 °F) where the ceramic tiles are used. Even hotter regions (up to 1650 °C, or 3000 °F) occur at the nose tip and the wing leading edges, where reinforced carbon-carbon (RCC) composites must be employed. Figure 12 indicates the materials chosen for various areas of the TPS.

The basic tile system is composed of four key elements: a ceramic tile, a nylon felt mounting pad, a filler bar, and a room-temperature vulcanizing (RTV) silicone adhesive. The tile, coated with a high emittance layer of glass, functions as both radiator (to dissipate heat) and insulator (to block heating to the structure). The felt mounting pad, called a strain isolator pad (SIP), isolates the tile from the thermal and mechanical strains of the substructure. The filler bar, also a nylon felt material coated with silicone rubber, protects the structure under the tile-to-tile gap from overheating. The RTV adhesive bonds the tile to the SIP and the SIP and filler bar to the substructure (Fig. 13). The substructure (tile substrate) consists of aluminum alloys or graphite-epoxy composites. More detailed information on the tile system can be found in Ref 22.

The ceramic tiles are made from very-high-purity amorphous silica fibers ~1.2 to 4 μm in diameter and 0.32 cm (0.125 in.) long, which are felted from a slurry and pressed and sintered at ~1370 °C (2500 °F) into blocks. Two tile densities are used: 144 kg/m^3 (9 lb/ft^3) (LI-900) and 352 kg/m^3 (22 lb/ft^3) (LI-2200). The LI-900 depends on a colloidal silica binder to achieve a fiber-to-fiber bond, whereas LI-2200 depends entirely on fiber-to-fiber sintering.

Most of the tiles are made from LI-900; however, in areas where higher strength is required, LI-2200 is used. All tiles have a borosilicate glass coating on five sides to provide the proper thermal properties. Those on the underside of the vehicle appear black because of the addition of silicon tetraboride for high emittance at high temperatures, whereas those on upper surfaces generally are white to limit on-orbit system temperature. The black tiles are usually a 15.2 by 15.2 cm (6 by 6 in.) square planform and typically 1.3 to 8.9 cm (0.5 to 3.5 in.) thick, as required. White tiles are generally a 20.3 by 20.3 cm (8 by 8 in.) square planform, 0.5 (0.2) to ~2.5 cm (1 in.) thick. There are special shapes or sizes—as small as ~4.4 cm (1.75 in.) square—as vehicle geometry dictates in some areas.

The silica tiles offer many advantages. The tile is 93% void; thus, it is an excellent insulator, having conductivities (through the thickness) as low as 0.017 to 0.052 W/m · K (0.01 to 0.03 Btu · ft/h · ft^2 · °F). The low coefficient of expansion of amorphous silica, as well as the low modulus of the tile, eliminates thermal-stress and thermal-shock problems. Because of the very high purity (99.62%), devitrification is limited, avoiding the high stresses associated with the expansion or contraction of the crystalline phase (cristobalite). Silica has high temperature resistance; it is capable of exposure above 1480 °C (2700 °F) for a limited time. Since it is an oxide, further protection is unnecessary, whereas RCC and refractory metals must have oxidation-protective coat-

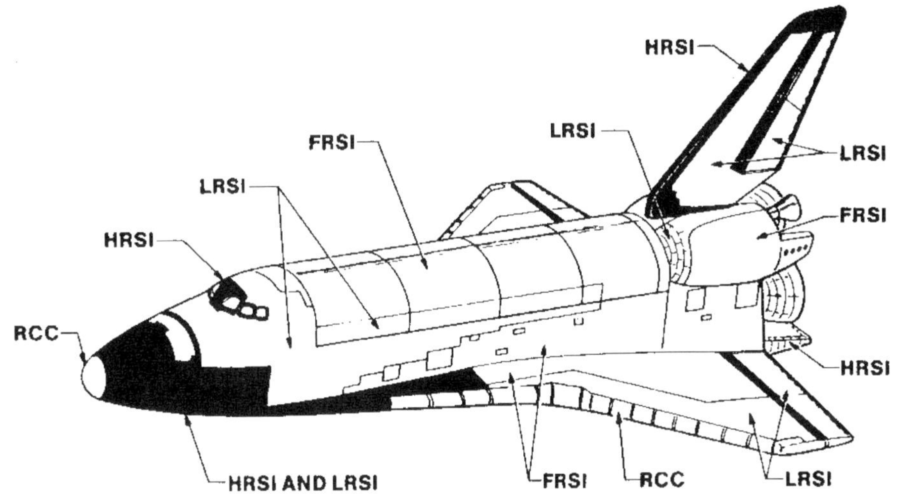

Material generic name	Material temperature capability, °C (°F)(a)	Material composition	Areas of orbiter
Reinforced carbon-carbon (RCC)	to 1650 (3000)	Pyrolized carbon-carbon, coated with SiC	Nose cone, wing leading edges, forward external tank separation panel
High-temperature reusable surface insulation (HRSI)	650–1260 (1200–2300)	SiO^2 tiles, borosilicate glass coating with SiB^4 added	Lower surfaces and sides, tail leading and trailing edges, tiles behind RCC
Low-temperature reusable surface insulation (LRSI)	400–650 (750–1200)	SiO^2 tiles, borosilicate glass coating	Upper wing surfaces, tail surfaces, upper vehicle sides, OMS(b) pods
Felt reusable surface insulation (FRSI)	to 400 (750)	Nylon felt, silicone rubber coating	Wing upper surface, upper sides, cargo bay doors, sides of OMS(b) pods

(a) 100 missions; higher temperatures are acceptable for a single mission. (b) Orbital maneuvering system (OMS) engines

Fig. 12 Thermal protection system materials for the U.S. space shuttle. More than 30,000 ceramic tiles are included in the system. Other materials making up the system are reinforced carbon-carbon composites (44 panels and the nose cap) and 333 m^2 (3581 ft^2) of felt reusable surface insulation. Source: Ref 22

ings. Oxidation of the silicon tetraboride in the coating results in boria and silica, the basic ingredients of the glass itself.

Heat-Resistant Industrial Applications

Another CMC processed by directed metal oxidation also using SiC particles in an Al_2O_3 matrix has been developed for high-temperature applications, such as furnace and heat exchanger components. These composites use very fine SiC particles (<10 μm), and the parent metal and processing conditions are selected to optimize high-temperature stability and mechanical characteristics. Elevated-temperature flexural strengths for three such composites are given in Fig. 14. Tests on similar composites have shown that these high-temperature strengths are unaffected by holding at temperatures at least up to 1500 °C (2730 °F) for a thousand hours or more. Prototype heat exchanger tubes and furnace components have been tested successfully, including a rig test of a burner tube involving temperature cycling to 1530 °C (2790 °F). Figure 15 shows examples of heat exchanger and furnace components made of this composite.

Biomedical Applications

A number of ceramics have found use as a biomaterial for surgical implants. For example, monolithic Al_2O_3 is widely used in hip and dental implants, and calcium hydroxyapatite is applied as a coating for orthopedic prostheses. In terms of biocomposites, a number of polymer matrices reinforced with carbon fibers, glass fibers, or tricalcium phosphate particulate have been studied. One example of a CMC biomedical application is the use of a polymer-reinforced glass-ceramic composite for use as a new bone substitute (Ref 23). Other ceramic-polymer combinations are also under consideration.

Applications for Continuous Fiber Ceramic Composites

Continuous fiber ceramic composites (CFCCs) are the most recently developed advanced ceramic. The continuous fibers in CFCCs overcome the brittle fracture problem associated with ceramics by providing increased fracture toughness (Fig. 16). The principal mechanisms that toughen CFCC components are:

- Deflection and bridging of cracks by the ceramic fibers
- Fiber pull-out from the ceramic matrix (Fiber pull-out is achieved by applying a coating to the fiber, allowing the fiber to be pulled out under stress.)

As the matrix cracks, the fibers continue to carry the load, thus avoiding the catastrophic behavior that is familiar in ceramic materials. Figure 17 compares the stress-strain behavior of monolithic ceramics and CFCCs.

Processing. As shown in Table 2, CFCCs are processed by various methods, including chemical vapor infiltration (CVI), polymer impregnation pyrolysis (PIP), melt infiltration, reaction bonding (also referred to as "nitride bonding"), sol gel infiltration, slurry infiltration, directed metal oxidation, and a combination of cold isostatic pressing and hot isostatic pressing (CIP/HIP). More detailed information on these methods can be found in the article "Processing of Ceramic-Matrix Composites" in this Volume.

Matrix-Reinforcement Materials. The most common matrix materials for CFCCs are SiC, Al_2O_3, Si_3N_4, mullite, and aluminosilicates (see Table 2). The predominant fiber material is SiC, although Al_2O_3 and carbon fibers are also used. Fiber loadings are often high, on the order of 35 to 50 vol%.

Property ranges typical for CFCCs are listed in Table 3. Additional property data can be found in the article "Properties and Performance of Ceramic-Matrix and Carbon-Carbon Composites" in this Volume.

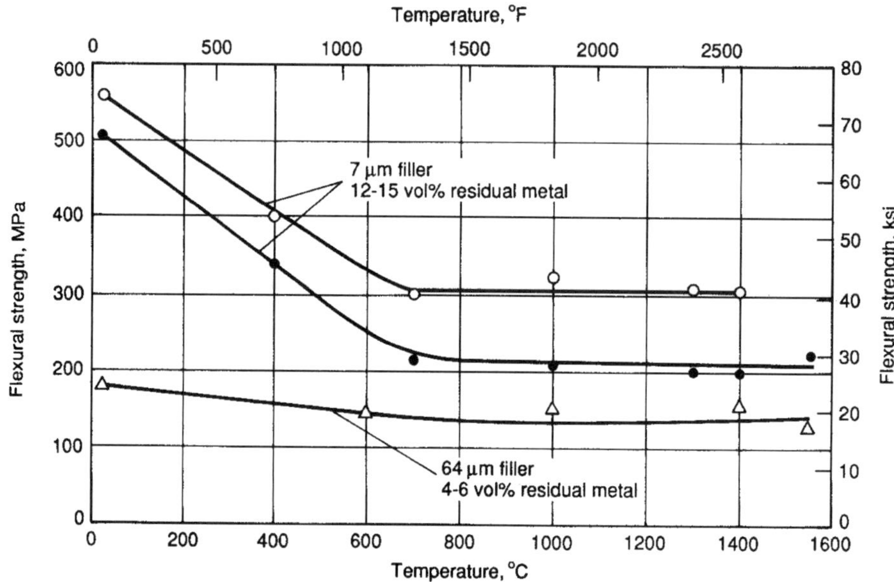

Fig. 14 Four-point flexural strengths of three SiC particle-filled Al_2O_3 matrix composites over a range of temperatures. The upper two curves represent processing differences using the same nominal filler particle size. Source: Ref 18

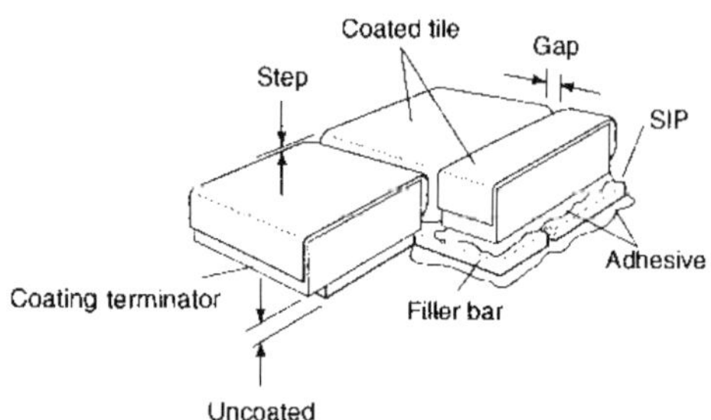

Fig. 13 The silica-silica tile thermal protection system configuration. SIP, strain isolator pad. Source: Ref 22

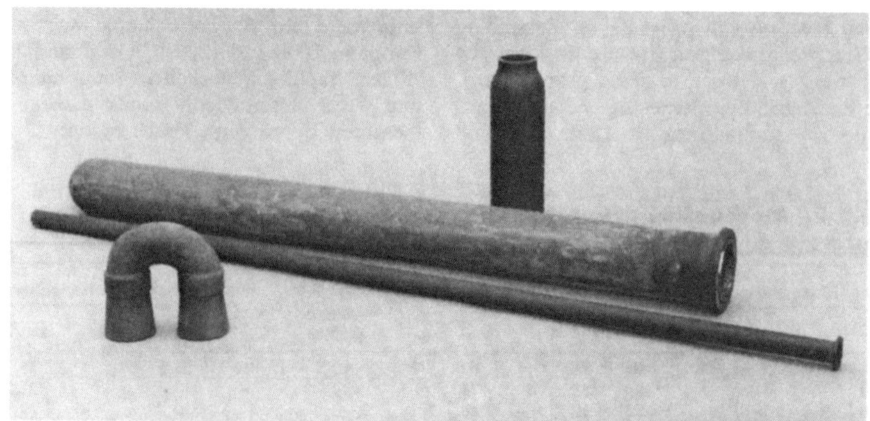

Fig. 15 Heat exchanger and furnace components made from an Al_2O_3-SiC_p composite. Source: Ref 18

Application Examples. The high-temperature stability, corrosion resistance, and toughness of CFCCs make them suitable for a wide range of applications in both the aerospace and industrial sectors. Many of the subsequent applications surveyed were brought about by The Continuous Fiber Ceramic Composite (CFCC) Program supported by the Department of Energy (DOE) Office of Industrial Technologies (OIT). This was a collaborative effort between industry, national laboratories, universities, and the U.S. government. A summary of this program can be found on the internet at http://www.oit.doe.gov/cfcc/. Examples of potential applications for CMCs include (Ref 25–27):

- *Turbine engine components:* combustor liners, shrouds, seals, vanes, blades, and other parts used in gas turbines, including utility, industrial, and aeronautical engine applications. Both SiC-SiC and Al_2O_3-SiC composites are under development for such applications. Various processing methods, including melt infiltration, CVI, PIP, and directed metal oxidation, are used to produce these components.
- *Radiant burner screens:* SiC-SiC reverberatory screens for natural gas burners are being produced by CVI. These burners are used in industrial applications, such as paper or paint drying, chemical processing, metal treating, and glass forming. The single-layer porous mesh screen is mounted directly above the burner surface.

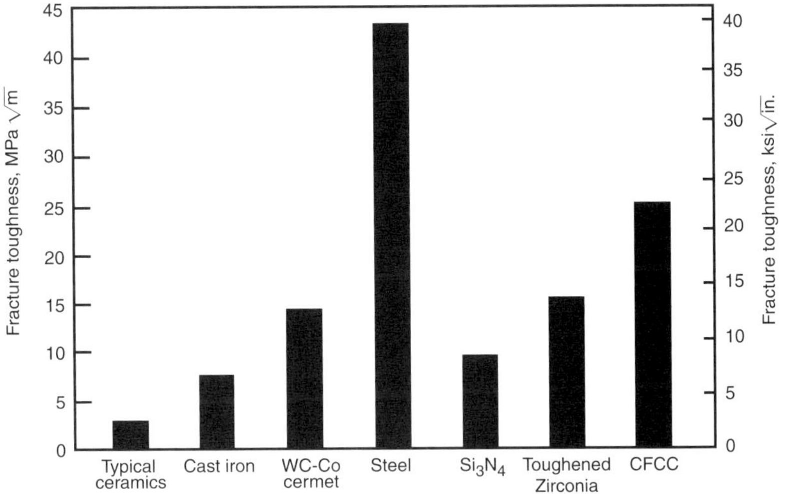

Fig. 16 Fracture toughness comparison for various materials, including CFCCs. Source: Ref 24

Table 2 Examples of various CFCC materials and processes

Process	Matrix	Fiber
Chemical vapor infiltration (CVI)	SiC	SiC, carbon
Polymer impregnation pyrolysis (PIP)	SiC, SiOC, SiNC	SiC
Melt infiltration	SiC-Si	SiC
Reaction bonding	Nitride-bonded SiC	SiC
Sol gel	Mullite, Al_2O_3	SiC, Al_2O_3
Slurry infiltration	Aluminosilicates	Al_2O_3
Directed metal oxidation	Al_2O_3	SiC, Al_2O_3
CIP/HIP	Si_3N_4	Carbon

Source: Ref 25, 26

Table 3 Property ranges typical of CFCCs

Property	Range
Density, g/cm^3	2.1–3.1
Open porosity, %	0–20
Tensile properties	
Strength, MPa (ksi)	250–400 (35–60)
Modulus, GPa (10^6 psi)	90–250 (13–36)
Strain-to-failure, %	0.4–0.8
Flexure properties	
Strength, MPa (ksi)	200–480 (29–70)
Modulus, GPa (10^6 psi)	83–240 (12–35)
Compressive strength, MPa (ksi)	450–1100 (65–160)
Shear strength, MPa (ksi)	28–68 (4–10)
Room-temperature thermal conductivity, W/m · K	1–40

Source: Ref 26

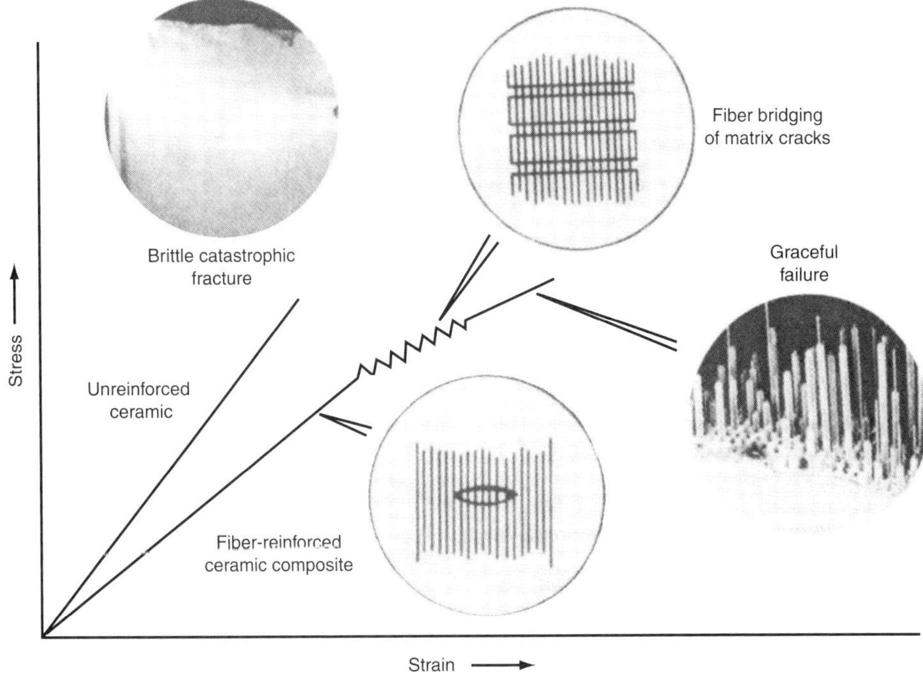

Fig. 17 Stress-strain behavior of reinforced and unreinforced ceramics. Fiber reinforcement of CMCs avoids the brittle catastrophic fracture characteristic of monolithic materials.

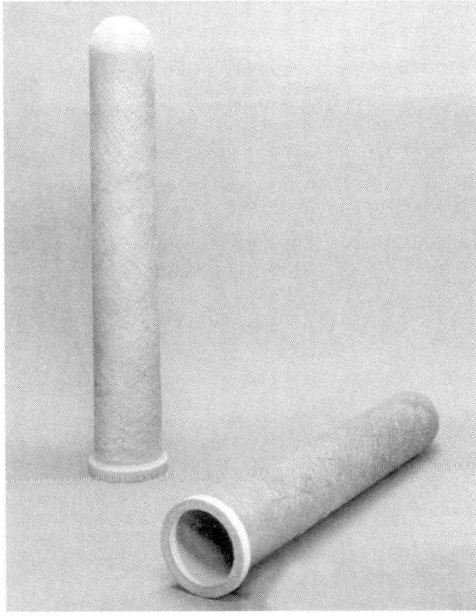

Fig. 18 Immersion tubes for molten aluminum holding furnaces made from a filament-wound CFCC. Courtesy of Textron Systems

- *Immersion heater tubes:* SiC-SiC composite burner tubes (Fig. 18) have been developed for melting aluminum in casting foundries. The CFCC is not wetted or chemically attacked by the molten aluminum. The processing approach involves the application of a water-based ceramic slurry onto a mandrel that is filament wound with SiC fiber. The green preform is nitride bonded (thermally treated in a nitrogen atmosphere), which results in a material composed of SiC fibers in a matrix of SiC and Si_3N_4.
- *Hot gas filters:* Al_2O_3-Al_2O_3 composites are being evaluated for use as hot gas filters in advanced coal-fired energy applications. Removing coal-ash particles from the exhaust gas of a coal-fired pressurized fluidized-bed combustor protects the downstream equipment, such as gas turbine engines, from damage, enabling the generation of energy with reduced emissions and with higher efficiency. Sol gel and slurry infiltration methods are used to produce these filters.
- *Turbine disks for rocket engines:* Integrally bladed disks ("blisks") for rocket engine turbopumps have been produced from carbon-fiber-reinforced SiC. Figure 19 shows the Fastrac engine developed by the National Aeronautics and Space Administration (NASA) and the locations of the turbopump and blisk. The blisks were produced by CVI of a woven preform, which was subsequently machined and thermally treated to complete densification. Figure 20 shows the final turbopump assembly.

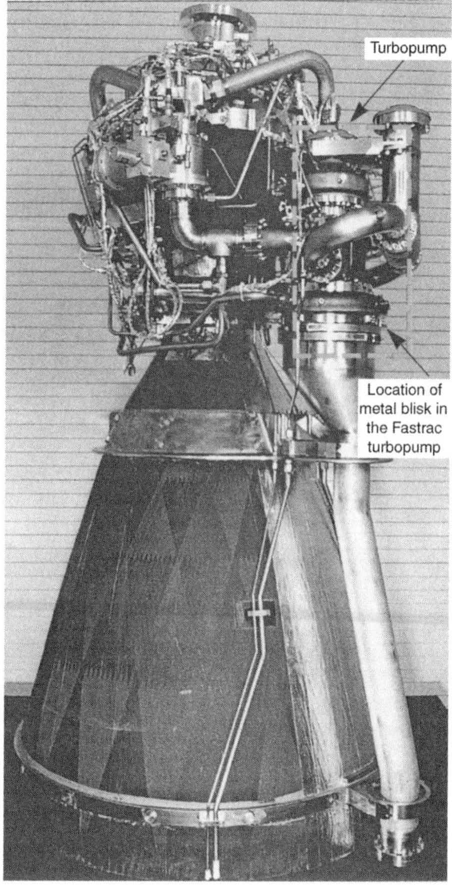

Fig. 19 Fastrac rocket engine showing the location of the turbopump that contains the CFCC blisk shown in Fig. 20. Source: Ref 27

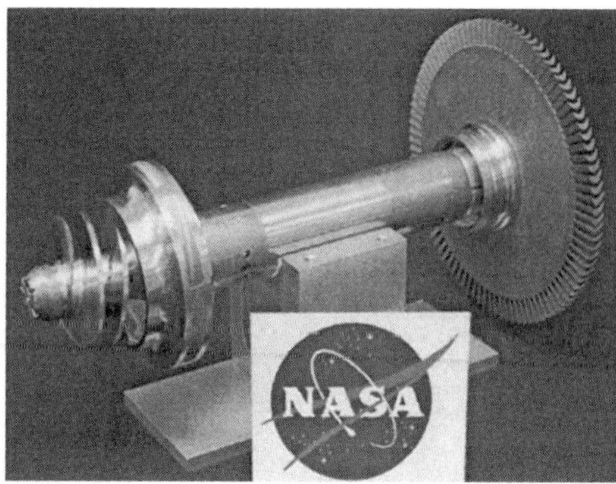

Fig. 20 Turbopump assembly showing the carbon-fiber-reinforced SiC blisk (right) and a metal inducer and impeller mounted on its shaft. The use of CFCCs for this application increases the temperature capability up to 1370 °C (2500 °F). Source: Ref 27

Other potential applications for CFCCs include heat exchanger tubes, armor, pipe hangers for petroleum refining, submersible pump housings for chemical processing, parts for ethylene cracking reformers, parts exposed to methyl chloride and dimethylchlorosilane, heat treating furnace fans, hot particle separators in municipal waste incinerators, and low-heat-rejection diesel engine exhaust valve guides that are self-lubricating.

REFERENCES

1. T. Abraham, "Ceramic Matrix Composites," Report GB-110R, Business Communications Company Inc. (Norwalk, CT), 2000
2. S.J. Burden et al., Comparison of Hot-Isostatically-Pressed and Uniaxially Hot Pressed Alumina-Titanium Carbide Cutting Tools, *Ceram. Bull.,* Vol 67 (No. 6), 1988, p 1003
3. W.W. Gruss and K.M. Friedrich, Aluminum Oxide/Titanium Carbide Composite Cutting Tools, *Ceramic Cutting Tools,* E.D. Whitney, Ed., Noyes Publications, 1994, p 48–62
4. Ceramics, in *ASM Specialty Handbook: Tool Materials,* J.R. Davis, Ed., ASM International, 1995, p 67–76
5. G.C. Wei and P.F. Becher, Development of SiC-Whisker-Reinforced Ceramic Composite, *Am. Ceram. Soc. Bull.,* Vol 64 (No. 2), 1985, 296–304
6. T.N. Tiegs and P.F. Becher, Whisker-Reinforced Ceramic Composites, *Tailoring Multiphase and Composite Ceramics,* Plenum Press, 1986, p 639–647
7. C.K. Jun and K.H. Smith, Alumina-Silicon Carbide Whisker Composite Tools, *Ceramic Cutting Tools,* E.D. Whitney, Ed., Noyes Publications, 1994, p 86-111
8. G. Brandt, Ceramic Cutting Tools, *Ceramic Technology International,* I. Birkby, Ed., Sterling Publications Ltd., 1995, p 77–80
9. Machining of Nickel Alloys, in *ASM Specialty Handbook: Nickel, Cobalt, and Their Alloys,* J.R. Davis, Ed., ASM International, 2000, p 235–244
10. S.-T. Buljan and V.K. Sarin, Machining Performance of Ceramic Tools, *Cutting Tool Materials,* F.W. Gorsler, Ed., American Society for Metals, 1981, p 335–348
11. V.K. Sarin and S.-T. Buljan, "Advanced Silicon Nitride-Based Ceramic Cutting Tools," SME paper MR83-189, Society of Manufacturing Engineers, 1983
12. S.-T. Buljan and V.K. Sarin, Improved Productivity Through Application of Silicon Nitride Cutting Tools, *Carbide Tool J.,* Vol 14 (No. 3), 1982, p 40–46
13. J.G. Baldoni and S.-T. Buljan, "Silicon Nitride-Based Ceramic Cutting Tools," SME paper MR86-913, Society of Manufacturing Engineers, 1986
14. S. Hampshire, Engineering Properties of Nitrides, *Ceramics and Glasses,* Vol 4, *Engineered Materials Handbook,* ASM International, 1991, p 812–820
15. G.L. DePoorter, T.K. Brog, and M.J. Readey, Structural Ceramics, *Properties and Selection: Nonferrous Alloys and Special-Purpose Materials,* Vol 2, *ASM Handbook,* ASM International, 1990, p 1019–1029
16. J. Weinstein and B.R. Rossing, Application of a New Ceramic/Metal Composite Technology to Form Net Shape Wear Resistant Composites, *Proc. TMS Sixth Northeast Regional Symposium on High Performance Composites for the 1990s,* TMS/American Institute of Mining, Metallurgical and Petroleum Engineers, 1990, p 339–360
17. B.R. Rossing and M.A. Rocazella, Slurry Erosion of Silicon Carbide Particulate Reinforced Alumina Composites, *Proc. Fourth Berkeley Conference on Corrosion-Erosion-Wear of Materials at Elevated Temperatures,* National Association of Corrosion Engineers, to be published
18. A.W. Urquhart, Directed Metal Oxidation, *Ceramics and Glasses,* Vol 4, *Engineered Materials Handbook,* ASM International, 1991, p 232–235
19. C.J. Dziedzic and J.J. Parson, "Ceramics for the Canmaking Industry," Process Forming Systems, Golden, CO
20. W.B. Johnson, T.D. Claar, and G.H. Schiroky, Preparation and Processing of Platelet Reinforced Ceramics by the Directed Reaction of Zirconium with Boron Carbide, *Ceram. Eng. Sci. Proc.,* Vol 10 (No. 7–8), 1989, p 588–598
21. T.D. Claar, W.B. Johnson, C.A. Andersson, and G.H. Schiroky, Microstructure and Properties of Platelet Reinforced Ceramics Formed by the Directed Reaction of Zirco-

nium with Boron Carbide, *Ceram. Eng. Sci. Proc.,* Vol 10 (No 7–8), 1989, p 599–609
22. L.J. Korb, C.A. Morant, R.M. Calland, and C.S. Thatcher, The Shuttle Orbiter Thermal Protection System, *Ceram. Bull.,* Vol 60 (No. 11), 1981, p 1188–1193
23. L. Claes, S. Wolf, A. Ignatius, and D. Reif, "Glass-Ceramic-Composites Show Adequate Mechanical Properties for Use as New Bone Substitute Materials," paper presented at the Society for Biomaterials 25th Annual Meeting, 28 April to 2 May 1999 (Providence, RI); also published in the *Trans. Soc. Biomater.,* Vol XXII, May 1999
24. D.W. Richerson and D.A. Haught, "Advanced Ceramics for High-Temperature Service," Paper 273, *Corrosion 99,* National Association of Corrosion Engineers International, 1999
25. P.A. Craig, "Continuous Fiber Ceramic Composites—A New Generation of Materials for Industrial and Corrosive Applications," Paper 268, *Corrosion 99,* National Association of Corrosion Engineers International, 1999
26. J.K. Wessel and W.G. Long, "Applications of Continuous-Fiber-Reinforced Ceramic Composites (CFCC) in Corrosive/Erosive Environments," Paper 00563, *Corrosion 2000,* National Association of Corrosion Engineers International, 2000
27. M.R. Effinger, G.G. Genge, and J.D. Kiser, Ceramic Composite Turbine Disks for Rocket Engines, *Adv. Mater. Process.,* June 2000, p 69–73

Reference Information

Glossary of Terms

A

A-basis. The "A" mechanical property value is the value above which at least 99% of the population of values is expected to fall, with a confidence of 95%. Also called A-allowable. See also *B-basis, S-basis,* and *typical-basis.*

abhesive. A material that resists adhesion. A film or coating applied to surfaces to prevent sticking, heat sealing, and so on, such as a parting agent or mold release agent.

ablation. The degradation, decomposition, and erosion of a material caused by high temperature, pressure, time, percent oxidizing species, and velocity of gas flow. A controlled loss of material to protect the underlying structure.

ablative plastic. A material that absorbs heat (with a low material loss and char rate) through a decomposition process (pyrolysis) that takes place at or near the surface exposed to the heat.

abrasive waterjet. Similar to a conventional water jet except that a fine grit (usually garnet) is mixed into the high-pressure water stream. Useful for cutting cured organic-matrix and metal-matrix composite materials. The main cutting action is an accelerated erosion process.

absorption. (1) The penetration into the mass of one substance by another. (2) The process whereby energy is dissipated within a specimen placed in a field of radiant energy. (3) The capillary or cellular attraction of adherend surfaces to draw off the liquid adhesive film into the substrate.

accelerated test. A test procedure in which conditions are increased in magnitude to reduce the time required to obtain a result. To reproduce in a short time the deteriorating effect obtained under normal service conditions.

accelerator. A material that, when mixed with a catalyst or a resin, speeds up the chemical reaction between the catalyst and the resin (either in the polymerizing of resins or vulcanization of rubbers). Also called promoter.

accuracy. The agreement of an experimental or calculated value to an accepted recognized standard or specified value. Compare with *precision.*

acoustic emission. A measure of integrity of a material, as determined by sound emission when a material is stressed. Ideally, emissions can be correlated with defects and/or incipient failure.

acrylic plastic. A thermoplastic polymer made by the polymerization of esters of acrylic acid and its derivatives. Its full name is polymethyl methacrylate. See also *polymethyl methacrylate.*

activation. The (usually) chemical process of making a surface more receptive to bonding to a coating or an encapsulating material.

activator. See *accelerator.*

addition polymerization. A chemical reaction in which simple molecules (monomers) are added to each other to form long-chain molecules (polymers) without forming by-products.

additive. Any substance added to another substance, usually to improve properties, such as plasticizers, initiators, light stabilizers, and flame retardants. See also *filler.*

adherend. A body that is held to another body, usually by an adhesive. A detail or part prepared for bonding.

adhesion. The state in which two surfaces are held together at an interface by mechanical or chemical forces, interlocking action, or both.

adhesion, mechanical. See *mechanical adhesion.*

adhesion promoter. A coating applied to a substrate, before it is coated with an adhesive, to improve the adhesion of the plastic. Also called primer.

adhesive. A substance capable of holding two materials together by surface attachment. Adhesive can be in film, liquid, or paste form.

adhesive, anaerobic. See *anaerobic adhesive.*

adhesive assembly. A group of materials or parts, including adhesive, that are placed together for bonding or that have been bonded together.

adhesive bonding. A materials joining process in which an adhesive, placed between facing surfaces, solidifies to bond the surfaces together.

adhesive, cold-setting. See *cold-setting adhesive.*

adhesive, contact. See *contact adhesive.*

adhesive failure. Rupture of an adhesive bond such that the separation appears to be at the adhesive-adherend interface.

adhesive film. A synthetic resin adhesive, with or without a film carrier fabric, usually of the thermosetting type, in the form of a thin film of resin, used under heat and pressure as an interleaf in the production of bonded structures.

adhesive, gap-filling. See *gap-filling adhesive.*

adhesive, heat-activated. See *heat-activated adhesive.*

adhesive, heat-sealing. See *heat-sealing adhesive.*

adhesive, hot-melt. See *hot-melt adhesive.*

adhesive, hot-setting. See *hot-setting adhesive.*

adhesive, intermediate temperature setting. See *intermediate temperature setting adhesive.*

adhesive joint. The location at which two adherends or substrates are held together with a layer of adhesive. The general area of contact for a bonded structure.

adhesive, pressure-sensitive. See *pressure-sensitive adhesive.*

adhesive strength. Strength of the bond between an adhesive and an adherend.

adhesive, structural. See *structural adhesive.*

admixture. The addition and homogeneous dispersion of discrete components, before cure.

adsorption. (1) The adhesion of the molecules of gases, dissolved substances, or liquids in more or less concentrated form, to the surfaces of solids or liquids with which they are in contact. (2) A concentration of a substance at a surface or interface of another substance.

advanced ceramics. Ceramic materials that exhibit superior mechanical properties, corrosion/oxidation resistance, or electrical, optical, and/or magnetic properties. This term includes many monolithic ceramics as well as particulate-, whisker-, and fiber-reinforced glass, glass-ceramics, and ceramic-matrix composites. Also known as engineering, fine, or technical ceramics.

advanced composites. Composite materials that are reinforced with continuous fibers having a modulus higher than that of fiberglass fibers. The term includes metal-matrix and ceramic-matrix composites, as well as carbon-carbon composites.

afterbrake. See *postcure.*

aggregate. A hard, coarse material usually of mineral origin used with an epoxy binder (or other resin) in plastic tools. Also used in flooring or as a surface medium.

aging. (1) The effect on materials of exposure to an environment for an interval of time. (2) The process of exposing materials to an environment for an interval of time.

air-bubble void. Air entrapment within and between the plies of reinforcement or within a bondline or encapsulated area; localized, noninterconnected, spherical in shape.

air vent. Small outlet to prevent entrapment of gases in a molding or tooling fixture.

alkyd plastic. Thermoset plastic based on resins composed principally of polymeric esters, in which the recurring ester groups are an integral part of the main polymer chain, and in which ester groups occur in most cross links that may be present between chains.

allotropy. The existence of a substance, especially an element, in two or more forms (for example, crystals). See also *graphite.*

alloy. (1) In plastics, a blend of polymers or copolymers with other polymers or elastomers under selected conditions; for example, styrene-acrylonitrile. Also called polymer blend. (2) In metals, a substance having metallic properties and being composed of two or more chemical elements of which at least one is a metal.

allyl plastic. A thermoset plastic based on resins made by addition polymerization of monomers containing allyl groups; for example, diallyl phthalate (DAP).

alternating stress. A stress varying between two maximum values that are equal but with opposite signs, according to a law determined in terms of the time.

alternating stress amplitude. A test parameter of a dynamic fatigue test; one-half the algebraic difference between the maximum and minimum stress in one cycle.

ambient. The surrounding environmental conditions, such as pressure, temperature, or relative humidity.

amorphous plastic (amorphous phase). A plastic that has no crystalline component. There is no order or pattern to the distribution of the molecules.

anaerobic adhesive. An adhesive that cures only in the absence of air after being confined between assembled parts.

anelasticity. A characteristic exhibited by certain materials in which strain is a function of both stress and time, such that while no permanent deformations are involved, a finite time is required to establish equilibrium between stress and strain in both the loading and unloading directions.

angle-ply laminate. A laminate having fibers of adjacent plies, oriented at alternating angles.

angle wrap. Tape fabric wrapped on a starter dam mandrel at an angle to the centerline.

anisotropic. Not isotropic. Exhibiting different properties when tested along axes in different directions. See also *anisotropy of laminates.*

anisotropic laminate. One in which the properties are different in different directions.

anisotropy of laminates. The difference of the properties along the directions parallel to the length or width of the lamination planes and perpendicular to the lamination.

annealing. In plastics, heating to a temperature at which the molecules have significant mobility, permitting them to reorient to a configuration having less residual stress.

antioxidant. A substance that, when added in small quantities to the resin during mixing, prevents its oxidative degradation and contributes to the maintenance of its properties.

antistatic agents. Agents that, when added to a molding material or applied to the surface of the molded object, make it less conductive, thus hindering the fixation of dust or the buildup of electrical charge.

aramid. A type of highly oriented organic material derived from polyamide (nylon) but incorporating aromatic ring structure. Used primarily as a high-strength, high-modulus fiber. Kevlar and Nomex (E.I. DuPont de Nemours & Co., Inc., Wilmington, DE) are examples of aramids.

arc resistance. Ability to withstand exposure to an electric voltage. The total time in seconds that an intermittent arc may play across a plastic surface without rendering the surface conductive.

areal weight. The weight of fiber per unit area (width × length) of tape or fabric.

aromatic. Unsaturated hydrocarbon with one or more benzene ring structures in the molecule.

artificial weathering. The exposure of plastics to cyclic laboratory conditions, consisting of high and low temperatures, high and low relative humidities, and ultraviolet radiant energy, with or without direct water spray and moving air (wind), in an attempt to produce changes in their properties similar to those observed in long-term continuous exposure outdoors. The laboratory exposure conditions are usually intensified beyond those encountered in actual outdoor exposure in an attempt to achieve an accelerated effect. Also called accelerated aging.

ash content. Proportion of the solid residue remaining after a reinforcing substance has been incinerated (charred or intensely heated).

aspect ratio. (1) In essentially two-dimensional rectangular structures such as panels, the ratio of the long dimension to the short dimension. (2) In compressive loading, the ratio of the dimension in the load direction to the dimension in the transverse direction. (3) In fiber micromechanics, the ratio of length to diameter.

assembly time. The time interval between the spreading of the adhesive on the adherend and the application of pressure and/or heat to the assembly.

A-stage. An early stage in the preparation of certain thermosetting resins in which the material is still soluble in certain liquids, and may be liquid or capable of becoming liquid upon heating. See also *B-stage* and *C-stage.*

attenuation. The diminution of vibrations or energy over time or distance. The process of making thin and slender, as applied to the formation of fiber from molten glass.

autoclave. A closed vessel for conducting and completing a chemical reaction or other operation, such as cooling, under pressure and with or without heat.

autoclave molding. A process in which, after lay-up, winding, or wrapping, an entire assembly is placed in a heated autoclave, usually at 340 to 1380 kPa (50 to 200 psi). Additional pressure permits higher density and improved removal of volatiles from the resin. Lay-up is usually vacuum bagged with a bleeder and release cloth.

automated tape laying. A fabrication process in which prepreg material, typically unidirectional tape, is laid across the surface of a mold in multiple layers and directions by an automated tape-application machine to form a structure.

automatic mold. A mold for injection or compression molding that repeatedly goes through the entire cycle, including ejection, without human assistance.

automatic press. A hydraulic press for compression molding or an injection machine that operates continuously, being controlled mechanically, electrically, hydraulically, or by a combination of any of these methods.

axial strain. The linear strain in a plane parallel to the longitudinal axis of the specimen.

axial winding. In filament-wound reinforced plastics, a winding with the filaments parallel to, or at a small angle to, the axis (0° helix angle). See also *polar winding.*

B

back pressure. Resistance of a material, because of its viscosity, to continued flow when mold is closing.

bagging. Applying an impermeable layer of film over an uncured part and sealing the edges so that a vacuum can be drawn.

bag molding. A method of molding or laminating that involves the application of fluid pressure, usually by means of air, steam, water, or vacuum, to a flexible barrier material that transmits the pressure to the material being molded or bonded.

bag side. The side of the part that is cured against the vacuum bag.

balanced construction. Equal parts of warp and fill in fiber fabric. Construction in which reactions to tension and compression loads result in extension or compression deformations only and in which flexural loads produce pure bending of equal magnitude in axial and lateral directions.

balanced design. In filament-wound reinforced plastics, a winding pattern so designed that the stresses in all filaments are equal.

balanced in-plane contour. In a filament-wound part, a head contour in which the filaments are oriented within a plane and the radii of curvature are adjusted to balance the stresses along the filaments with the pressure loading.

balanced laminate. A composite laminate in which all laminae at angles other than 0° and 90° occur only in ± pairs (not necessarily adjacent). See also *symmetrical laminate.*

balanced twist. An arrangement of twists in a combination of two or more strands that does not cause kinking or twisting on themselves when the yarn produced is held in the form of an open loop.

band density. In filament winding, the quantity of fiberglass reinforcement per inch of band width, expressed as strands (or filaments) per inch.

band thickness. In filament winding, the thickness of the reinforcement as it is applied to the mandrel.

band width. In filament winding, the width of the reinforcement as it is applied to the mandrel.

Barcol hardness. A hardness value obtained by measuring the resistance to penetration of a sharp steel point under a spring load. The instrument, called the Barcol impressor, gives a direct reading on a 0 to 100 scale. The hardness value is often used as a measure of the degree of cure of a plastic.

bare glass. Glass, such as yarns, rovings, and fabrics, from which the sizing or finish has been removed. Also, such glass before the application of sizing or finish.

barrier coat. An exterior coating applied to a composite wound structure to provide protection.

barrier film. The layer of film used during cure to permit removal of air and volatiles from a composite lay-up while minimizing resin loss.

barrier plastics. A general term applied to a group of lightweight, transparent, impact-resistant plastics, usually rigid copolymers of high acrylonitrile content. Barrier plastics are generally characterized by gas, aroma, and flavor barrier characteristics approaching those of metal and glass.

batch. In general, a quantity of materials formed during the same process or in one continuous process and having identical characteristics throughout. Also called a lot.

batt. Felted fabrics. Structures built by the interlocking action of compressing fibers, without spinning, weaving, or knitting.

B-basis. The "B" mechanical property value is the value above which at least 90% of the population of values is expected to fall, with a confidence of 95%. See also *A-basis, S-basis,* and *typical-basis.*

bearing area. The diameter of the hole times the thickness of the material. The cross-section area of the bearing load member on the sample.

bearing strain. The ratio of the deformation of the bearing hole, in the direction of the applied force, to the pin diameter. Also, the stretch or deformation strain for a sample under bearing load.

bearing strength. The maximum bearing stress that can be sustained. Also, the bearing stress at that point on the stress-strain curve where the tangent is equal to the bearing stress divided by *n*% of the bearing hole diameter.

bearing stress. The applied load in pounds divided by the bearing area. Maximum bearing stress is the maximum load in pounds sustained by the specimen during the test, divided by the original bearing area.

bending-twisting coupling. A property of certain classes of laminates that exhibit twisting curvatures when subjected to bending moments.

bias fabric. Warp and fill fibers at an angle to the length of the fabric.

biaxial load. A loading condition in which a laminate is stressed in two different directions in its plane. A loading condition of a pressure vessel under internal pressure and with unrestrained ends.

biaxial winding. In filament winding, a type of winding in which the helical band is laid in sequence, side by side, with crossover of the fibers eliminated.

bidirectional laminate. A reinforced plastic laminate with the fibers oriented in two directions in its plane. A cross laminate. See also *unidirectional laminate.*

binder. The resin or cementing constituent (of a plastic compound) that holds the other components together. The agent applied to fiber mat or preforms to bond the fibers before laminating or molding.

bismaleimide (BMI). A type of polyimide that cures by an addition rather than a condensation reaction, thus avoiding problems with volatiles formation, and which is produced by a vinyl-type polymerization of a prepolymer terminated with two maleimide groups. Intermediate in temperature capability between epoxy and polyimide.

bisphenol "A." A condensation product formed by the reaction of two molecules of phenol with acetone. This polyhydric phenol is the standard intermediate resin that is reacted with epichlorohydrin in the production of epoxy resins.

bladder. An elastomeric lining for the containment of hydroproof or hydroburst pressurization medium in filament-wound structures.

blanket. Fiber or fabric plies that have been laid up in a complete assembly and placed on or in the mold all at one time (flexible bag process). Also, the type of bag in which the edges are sealed against the mold.

bleeder cloth. A woven or nonwoven layer of material used in the manufacture of composite parts to allow the escape of excess gas and resin during cure. The bleeder cloth is removed after the curing process and is not part of the final composite.

bleeding. The removal of excess resin from a laminate during cure. The diffusion of color out of a plastic part into the surrounding surface or part.

bleedout. The excess liquid resin that migrates to the surface of a winding. Primarily occurs in filament winding.

blister. An imperfection, a rounded elevation of the surface of a plastic, with boundaries that may be more or less sharply defined, somewhat resembling in shape a blister on the human skin.

bloom. A visible local exudation or finish change on the surface of a plastic. Bloom can be caused by a lubricant or plasticizer or by atmospheric contamination.

BMC. See *bulk molding compound.*

BMI. See *bismaleimide.*

body putty. A pastelike mixture of plastic resin (polyester or epoxy) and talc used in repair of metal surfaces, such as auto bodies.

bond. To unite materials by means of an adhesive.

bond line. The layer of adhesive that attaches two adherends.

bond strength. The unit load applied to tension, compression, flexure, peel, impact, cleavage, or shear required to break an adhesive assembly with failure occurring in or near the plane of the bond.

boron fiber. A fiber produced by vapor deposition of elemental boron, usually onto a tungsten filament core, to impart strength and stiffness.

boss. See *polar boss.*

braid. A system of three or more yarns that are interwoven in such a way that no two yarns are twisted around each other.

braiding. (1) Weaving of fibers into a tubular shape instead of a flat fabric, as for graphite-fiber-reinforced golf club shafts. (2) Textile process where two or more strands, yarns, or tapes are intertwined in the bias direction to form an integral structure.

branched polymer. In molecular structure of polymers, a main chain with attached side chains, in contrast to a linear polymer.

breaking extension. The elongation necessary to cause rupture of a test specimen. The tensile strain at the moment of rupture.

breaking factor. The breaking load divided by the original width of a test specimen, expressed in lb/in.

breaking length. A measure of the breaking strength of yarn. The length of a specimen whose weight is equal to the breaking load.

breakout. Fiber separation or break on surface plies at drilled or machined edges.

breather. A loosely woven material that serves as a continuous vacuum path over a part but is not in contact with the resin.

breathing. The opening and closing of a mold to allow gas to escape early in the molding cycle. Also called degassing; sometimes called bumping, in phenolic molding.

bridging. (1) Condition in which fibers do not move into or conform to radii and corners during molding, resulting in voids and dimensional control problems. (2) In the fracture mechanics of composites, the toughening mechanism of the reinforcing fibers behind the crack tip, before these fibers fail.

broad goods. Fiber woven to form fabric up to 1270 mm (50 in.) wide. It may or may not be impregnated with resin and is usually furnished in rolls of 25 to 140 kg (50 to 300 lb).

B-stage. An intermediate stage in the reaction of certain thermosetting resins in which the material softens when heated and is plastic and fusible but may not entirely dissolve or fuse. Also called resistol. The resin in an uncured prepreg or premix is usually in this stage. See also *A-stage* and *C-stage.*

buckling (composite). A mode of failure generally characterized by an unstable lateral material deflection due to compressive action on the structural element involved.

bulk density. The density of a molding material in loose form (granular, nodular, and so forth), expressed as a ratio of weight to volume.

bulk factor. The ratio of the volume of a raw molding compound or powdered plastic to the volume of the finished solid piece produced therefrom. The ratio of the density of the solid plastic object to the apparent or bulk density of the loose molding powder.

bulk modulus. The ratio of the hydrostatic pressure to the volume strain.

bulk molding compound (BMC). Thermosetting resin mixed with strand reinforcement, fillers, and so on, into a viscous compound for compression or injection molding. See also *premix* and *sheet molding compound.*

bundle. A general term for a collection of essentially parallel filaments or fibers.

burned. Showing evidence of thermal decomposition or charring through some discoloration, distortion, destruction, or conversion of the surface of the plastic, sometimes to a carbonaceous char.

burst strength (bursting strength). Measure of the ability of a material to withstand internal hydrostatic or gas dynamic pressure without rupture. Hydraulic pressure required to burst a vessel of given thickness.

bushing. (1) An electrically heated alloy container encased in insulating material, used for melting and feeding glass in the forming of individual fibers or filaments. (2) A special extraheavy load-carrying short cylinder inserted in bolt or pin holes.

butt joint. A type of edge joint in which the edge faces of the two adherends are at right angles to the other faces of the adherends.

C

calender. To produce a smooth finish and a desired dimensional thickness for sheet material by passing it between sets of pressure rollers.

carbon. The element that provides the backbone for all organic polymers. Graphite is a more ordered form of carbon. Diamond is the densest crystalline form of carbon.

carbon-carbon. A composite material consisting of carbon or graphite fibers in a carbon or graphite matrix.

carbon fiber. Fiber produced by the pyrolysis of organic precursor fibers, such as rayon, polyacrylonitrile (PAN), and pitch, in an inert environment. The term is often used interchangeably with the term graphite; however, carbon fibers and graphite fibers differ. The basic differences lie in the temperature at which the fibers are made and heat treated, and in the amount of elemental carbon produced. Carbon fibers typically are carbonized in the region of 1315 °C (2400 °F) and assay at 93 to 95% carbon, while graphite fibers are graphitized at 1900 to 2480 °C (3450 to 4500 °F) and assay at more than 99% elemental carbon. See also *pyrolysis (of fibers).*

carbonization. The process of pyrolyzation in an inert atmosphere at temperatures ranging from 800 to 1600 °C (1470 to 2910 °F) and higher, usually at about 1315 °C (2400 °F). Range is influenced by precursor, individual manufacturer's process, and properties desired.

catalyst. (1) A substance that changes the rate of a chemical reaction without itself undergoing permanent change in composition or becoming a part of the molecular structure of the product. (2) A substance that markedly speeds up the cure of a compound when added in minor quantity, compared to the amounts of primary reactants. See also *accelerator, curing agent, hardener, inhibitor,* and *promoter.*

catastrophic failures. Totally unpredictable failures of a mechanical, thermal, or electrical nature.

catenary. (1) A measure of the difference in length of the strands in a specified length of roving as a result of unequal tension. (2) The tendency of some strands in a taut, horizontal roving to sag more than the others.

caul plates. Smooth metal plates, free of surface defects, the same size and shape as a composite lay-up, used immediately in contact with the lay-up during the curing process to transmit normal pressure and temperature, and to provide a smooth surface on the finished laminate.

cavity. (1) The space inside a mold in which a resin or molding compound is poured or injected. (2) The female portion of a mold. (3) That portion of the mold that encloses the molded article (often referred to as the die). Depending on the number of such depressions, molds are designated as single cavity or multiple cavity.

cell. In honeycomb core, a cell is a single honeycomb unit, usually in a hexagonal shape.

cell size. The diameter of an inscribed circle within a cell of honeycomb core.

cellular plastic. A plastic containing numerous cells, interconnecting or not, distributed throughout the mass. Also called expanded plastic or foamed plastic.

ceramic. A rigid, frequently brittle material made from clay and other inorganic, nonmetallic substances and fabricated into articles by sintering, that is, cold molding followed by fusion of the part at high temperature.

ceramic-matrix composites. Advanced composites that consist of fibers or whiskers in a ceramic matrix. Typical reinforcing materials include carbon fibers and silicon carbide fibers or whiskers. Matrix materials commonly used are glass, glass-ceramics, alumina, and silicon nitride. Ceramic-matrix composites are resistant to both oxidation and wear. See also *continuous fiber ceramic composite, discontinuous fiber-reinforced composite,* and *particulate reinforced ceramic-matrix composite.*

cermet. Composite materials consisting of two constituents, one being either an oxide, carbide, boride, or similar inorganic compound, and the other a metallic binder.

CFCC. See *continuous fiber ceramic composite.*

C-glass. A glass with a soda-lime-borosilicate composition that is used for its chemical stability in corrosive environments.

chain length. The length of the stretched linear macromolecule, most often expressed by the number of identical links.

chalking. Dry, chalklike appearance of deposit on the surface of a plastic.

Charpy impact test. A test for shock loading in which a centrally notched sample bar is held at both ends and broken by striking the back face in the same plane as the notch.

charring. The heating of a composite in air to reduce the polymer matrix to ash, allowing the fiber content to be determined by weight.

chemical vapor deposited (CVD) carbon. Carbon deposited on a substrate by pyrolysis of a hydrocarbon, such as methane.

chemical vapor deposition (CVD). Process used in manufacture of several composite reinforcements, especially boron and silicon carbide, in which desired reinforcement material is deposited from vapor phase onto a continuous core, for example, boron on tungsten wire (core).

chopped strand mat. A mat formed of strands cut to a short length, randomly distributed, without intentional orientation, and held together by a binder.

chopped strands. Short strands cut from continuous filament strands, not held together by any means.

circuit. In filament winding, one complete traverse of a winding band from one arbitrary point along the winding path to another point on a plane through the starting point and perpendicular to the axis.

circumferential ("circ") winding. In filament-wound reinforced plastics, a winding with the filaments essentially perpendicular to the axis (90° or level winding).

clamping pressure. In injection molding and transfer molding, the pressure that is applied to the mold to keep it closed in opposition to the fluid pressure of the compressed molding material.

closure. The complete coverage of a mandrel with one layer (two plies) of fiber. When the last tape circuit that completes mandrel coverage lays down adjacent to the first without gaps or overlaps, the wind pattern is said to have "closed."

cloth. See *woven fabric* and *nonwoven fabric.*

co-curing. The act of curing a composite laminate and simultaneously bonding it to some other prepared surface, or curing together an inner and outer tube of similar or dissimilar fiber-resin combination after each has been wound or wrapped separately. See also *secondary bonding.*

coefficient of elasticity. The reciprocal of Young's modulus in a tension test. See also *compliance.*

coefficient of expansion. A measure of the change in length or volume of an object, specifically measured by the increase in length or volume of an object per unit length or volume.

coefficient of friction. A measure of the resistance to sliding of one surface in contact with another surface.

coefficient of thermal expansion (CTE). The change in length or volume per unit length or volume produced by a 1° change in temperature.

cohesion. (1) The propensity of a single substance to adhere to itself. (2) The internal attraction of molecular particles toward each other. (3) The ability to resist partition of itself. (4) The force holding a single substance together.

cohesive failure. Failure of an adhesive joint occurring primarily in an adhesive layer.

cohesive strength. Intrinsic strength of an adhesive.

coin test. Using a coin to tap a laminate in different spots, listening for a change in sound, which would indicate the presence of a defect. A surprisingly accurate test in the hands of experienced personnel.

coke. Carbonaceous residue resulting from the pyrolysis of pitch.

cold flow. The distortion that takes place in materials under continuous load at temperatures within the working range of the material without a phase or chemical change. See also *creep.*

cold-setting adhesive. A synthetic resin adhesive capable of hardening at normal room temperature in the presence of a hardener.

collet. A rigid, lateral container for the mold-forming material. A dam, a restriction box. The drive wheel that pulls glass fibers from the bushing. A forming tube is placed on the collet, and a package of strand is wound up on the tube. A metal band, ferrule, collar, or flange, often used to hold a tool or workpiece.

collimated. Rendered parallel.

collimated roving. Roving that has been made using a special process (usually parallel wound), so that the strands are more parallel than in standard roving.

colloidal. A state of suspension in a liquid medium in which extremely small particles are suspended and dispersed but not dissolved.

compaction. The application of a temporary vacuum bag and vacuum to remove trapped air and compact the lay-up.

compatibility. The ability of two or more substances combined with one another to form a homogeneous composition of useful plastic properties; for example, the suitability of a sizing or finish for use with certain general resin types. Nonreactivity or negligible reactivity between materials in contact.

complex dielectric constant. The vectorial sum of the dielectric constant and the loss factor.

complex shear modulus. The vectorial sum of the shear modulus and the loss modulus.

complex Young's modulus. The vectorial sum of Young's modulus and the loss modulus. Analogous to the complex dielectric constant.

compliance. Tensile compliance: the reciprocal of Young's modulus. Shear compliance: the reciprocal of shear modulus. Also, a term used in the evaluation of stiffness and deflection.

composite material. A combination of two or more materials (reinforcing elements, fillers, and composite matrix binder), differing in form or composition on a macroscale. The constituents retain their identities; that is, they do not dissolve or merge completely into one another although they act in concert. Normally, the components can be physically identified and exhibit an interface between one another. Composite materials are usually man-made and created to obtain properties that cannot be achieved by any of the components acting alone.

compound. The intimate admixture of a polymer with other ingredients, such as fillers, softeners, plasticizers, reinforcement, catalysts, pigments, or dyes. A thermoset compound usually contains all the ingredients necessary for the finished product, while a thermoplastic compound may require subsequent addition of pigments, blowing agents, and so forth.

compression molding. Technique for molding in which a part is shaped by placing the fiber and resin into an open mold cavity, closing the mold, and applying heat and pressure until the material has cured or achieved its final form. Compression molding can be used for making parts from glass mat thermoplastics, long-fiber thermoplastics, and short-fiber reinforced sheet molding compounds (thermosets).

compressive modulus. Ratio of compressive stress to compressive strain below the proportional limit. Theoretically equal to Young's modulus determined from tensile experiments.

compressive strength. The ability of a material to resist a force that tends to crush or buckle. The maximum compressive load sustained by a specimen divided by the original cross-sectional area of the specimen.

compressive stress. The normal stress caused by forces directed toward the plane on which they act.

condensation polymerization. A chemical reaction in which two or more molecules combine, with the separation of water or some other simple substance. If a polymer is formed, the process is called polycondensation. See also *polymerization.*

conditioning. Subjecting a material to a prescribed environmental and/or stress history before testing.

conductivity. Reciprocal of volume resistivity. The measure of the ability of a material to transfer heat or electric current from one face of a unit cube to the opposite face (conductivity per unit volume).

consolidation. In metal-matrix or thermoplastic composites, a processing step in which fiber and matrix are compressed by one of several methods to reduce voids and achieve desired density.

constituent. In general, an element of a larger grouping. In advanced composites, the principal constituents are the fibers and the matrix.

contact adhesive. An adhesive that is apparently dry to the touch and that will adhere to itself simultaneously upon contact. An adhesive applied to both adherends and allowed to become dry, which develops a bond when the adherends are brought together without sustained pressure.

contact molding. A process for molding reinforced plastics in which reinforcement and resin are placed on a mold. Cure is either at room temperature using a catalyst-promoter system or by heating in an oven, without additional pressure.

contact pressure molding. A method of molding or laminating in which the pressure, usually less than 70 kPa (10 psi), is only slightly more than necessary to hold the materials together during the molding operation.

contact pressure resins. Liquid resins that thicken or polymerize on heating, and, when used for bonding laminates, require little or no pressure.

contaminant. An impurity or foreign substance present in a material or environment that affects one or more properties of the material, particularly adhesion.

continuous fiber ceramic composite (CFCC). A ceramic-matrix composite in which the reinforcing phase(s) consists of continuous filaments, fibers, yarn, or knitted or woven fabrics.

continuous filament yarn. Yarn formed by twisting two or more continuous filaments into a single, continuous strand.

copolymer. A long-chain molecule formed by the reaction of two or more dissimilar monomers. See also *polymer.*

core. (1) The central member, usually foam or honeycomb, of a sandwich construction to which the faces of the sandwich are attached or bonded. (2) The central member of a plywood assembly. (3) A channel in a mold for circulation of heat transfer media. (4) A device on which prepreg is wound.

core crush. A collapse, distortion, or compression of the core.

core depression. A localized indentation or gouge in the core.

cored mold. A mold incorporating passages for electrical heating elements, steam, or water.

core separation. A partial or complete breaking of the core node bond.

core splicing. The joining of segments of a core by bonding, or by overlapping each segment and then driving them together.

corrosion resistance. The ability of a material to withstand contact with ambient natural factors or those of a particular, artificially created atmosphere, without degradation or change in properties. For metals, this could be pitting or rusting; for organic materials, it could be crazing.

count. For fabric, number of warp and filling yarns per inch in woven cloth. For yarn, size based on relation of length and weight.

coupling agent. Any chemical substance designed to react with both the reinforcement and matrix phases of a composite material to form or promote a stronger bond at the interface.

coupon. Usually, a specimen for a specific test, such as a tensile coupon.

crack. An actual separation of material, visible on opposite surfaces of the part, and extending through the thickness. A fracture.

crack growth. Rate of propagation of a crack through a material due to a static or dynamic applied load.

crazing. Region of ultrafine cracks, which may extend in a network on or under the surface of a resin or plastic material. May appear as a white band. Often found in a filament-wound pressure vessel or bottle.

creel. A device for holding the required number of roving balls (spools) or supply packages in desired position for unwinding onto the next processing step, that is, weaving, braiding, or filament winding.

creep. (1) The change in dimension of a material under load over a period of time, not including the initial instantaneous elastic deformation. (Creep at room temperature is called cold flow.) (2) The time-dependent part of strain resulting from an applied stress.

creep, rate of. The slope of the creep-time curve at a given time. Deflection with time under a given static load.

crimp. The waviness of a fiber or fabric, which determines the capacity of fibers to cohere under light pressure. Measured by the number of crimps or waves per unit length.

critical length. The minimum fiber length required for shear loading to its ultimate strength by the matrix.

critical longitudinal stress. (1) Applied to fibers, the longitudinal stress necessary to cause internal slippage and separation of a spun yarn. (2) The stress necessary to overcome the interfiber friction developed as a result of twist.

critical strain. The strain at the yield point.

cross laminate. A laminate in which some of the layers of material are oriented approximately at right angles to the remaining layers with respect to the grain, or strongest direction in tension. See also *parallel laminate.*

cross-linking. Applied to polymer molecules, the setting-up of chemical links between the molecular chains. When extensive, as in most thermosetting resins, cross-linking makes one infusible supermolecule of all the chains.

cross-linking, degree of. The fraction of cross-linked polymeric units in the entire system.

cross-ply laminate. (1) A laminate with plies usually oriented at 0° and 90° only. (2) Any filamentary laminate that is not uniaxial.

crosswise direction. Crosswise refers to the cutting of specimens and to the application of load. For rods and tubes, crosswise is any direction perpendicular to the long axis. For other shapes or materials that are stronger in one direction than in another, crosswise is the direction that is weaker. For materials that are equally strong in both directions, crosswise is an arbitrarily designated direction at right angles to the lengthwise direction.

crystalline plastic. A polymeric material having an internal structure in which the atoms are arranged in an orderly three-dimensional configuration.

C-scan. The back-and-forth scanning of a specimen with ultrasonics. A nondestructive testing technique for finding voids, delaminations, defects in fiber distribution, and so forth.

C-stage. The final stage in the reaction of certain thermosetting resins in which the material is practically insoluble and infusible. Sometimes referred to as resite. The resin in a fully cured thermoset molding is in this stage. See also *A-stage* and *B-stage.*

cure. To irreversibly change the properties of a thermosetting resin by chemical reaction, that is, condensation, ring closure, or addition. Cure may be accomplished by addition of curing (cross linking) agents, with or without heat and pressure.

cure cycle. The time/temperature/pressure cycle used to cure a thermosetting resin system or prepreg.

cure monitoring, electrical. Use of electrical techniques to detect changes in the electrical properties and/or mobility of the resin molecules during cure. A measuring of resin cure.

cure stress. A residual internal stress produced during the curing cycle of composite structures. Normally, these stresses originate when different components of a wet lay-up have different thermal coefficients of expansion.

curing agent. A catalytic or reactive agent that, when added to a resin, causes polymerization. Also called hardener.

CVD carbon. See *chemical vapor deposited (CVD) carbon.*

cyanate ester resins. Thermosetting resins that are derived from bisphenols or polyphenols, and are available as monomers, oligomers, blends, and solutions.

cycle time. In molding, the total time used to carry out a complete sequence of operations making up the molding cycle.

D

dam. Boundary support or ridge used to prevent excessive edge bleeding or resin runout of a laminate and to prevent crowning of the bag during cure.

damage tolerance. A design measure of crack growth rate. Cracks in damage tolerant designed structures are not permitted to grow to critical size during expected service life.

damping. The decay, with time, of the amplitude of free vibrations of a specimen. See also *hysteresis* and *attenuation.*

daylight. The distance, in the open position, between the moving and fixed tables or the platens of a hydraulic press. In the case of a multiplaten press, daylight is the distance between adjacent platens. Daylight provides space for removal of the molded part from the mold.

debond. (1) A deliberate separation of a bonded joint or interface, usually for repair or rework purposes. (2) An unbonded or nonadhered region; a separation at the fiber-matrix interface due to strain incompatibility. See also *disbond* and *delamination.*

debulking. Compacting of a thick laminate under moderate heat and pressure and/or vacuum to remove most of the air, to ensure seating on the tool, and to prevent wrinkles.

deep-draw mold. A mold having a core that is long in relation to the wall thickness.

deflashing. A finishing technique used to remove the flash (excess, unwanted material) on a plastic molding.

deflection temperature under load. The temperature at which a simple cantilever beam deflects a given amount under load. Formerly called heat distortion temperature.

deformation under load. The dimensional change of a material under load for a specified time following the instantaneous elastic deformation caused by the initial application of the load. See also *cold flow* and *creep.*

degassing. See *breathing.*

degradation. A deleterious change in the chemical structure, physical properties, or appearance of a plastic.

degree of polymerization. Number of structural units, or mers, in the average polymer molecule in a sample measure of molecular weight.

delamination. Separation of the layers of material in a laminate, either local or covering a wide area. Can occur in the cure or subsequent life.

denier. A yarn and filament numbering system in which the yarn number is numerically equal to the weight in grams of 9000 meters. Used for continuous filaments. The lower the denier, the finer the yarn.

densification process. Consolidation of a loose or bulky material.

density, apparent. The weight in air of a unit volume of a material.

density, bulk. The weight per unit volume of a material, including voids inherent in material as tested.

deposition. The process of applying a material to a base by means of vacuum, electrical, chemical, screening, or vapor methods, often with the assistance of a temperature and pressure container.

design allowables. Statistically defined (by a test program) material property allowable strengths, usually referring to stress or strain. See also *A-basis, B-basis, S-basis,* and *typical basis.*

desizing. (1) The process of eliminating sizing, which is generally starch, from gray (also greige) goods before applying special finishes or bleaches (for yarn such as glass or cotton). (2) Removing lubricant size following weaving of a cloth.

desorption. A process in which an absorbed material is released from another material. Desorption is the reverse of absorption, adsorption, or both.

devitrification. The formation of crystals (seeds) in a glass melt, usually occurring when the melt is too cold. These crystals can appear as defects in glass fibers.

D-glass. A high boron content glass made especially for laminates requiring a precisely controlled dielectric constant.

diaphragm forming. A method of simultaneously consolidating and forming thermoplastic composites in which the lay-up is sandwiched between two heat-formable sheets (often superplastic aluminum sheets) and placed under gas pressure in a press to form and consolidate the desired shape.

dielectric. (1) A nonconductor of electricity. (2) The ability of a material to resist the flow of an electrical current.

dielectric constant. The ratio of the capacitance of an assembly of two electrodes separated solely by a plastic insulating material to its capacitance when the electrodes are separated by air. See also *complex dielectric constant.*

dielectric curing. The curing of a synthetic thermosetting resin by the passage of an electric charge (produced from a high-frequency generator) through the resin.

dielectric heating. The heating of materials by dielectric loss in a high-frequency electrostatic field.

dielectric loss. A loss of energy evidenced by the rise in heat of a dielectric placed in an alternating electric field.

dielectric monitoring. A means of tracking the cure of thermosets by changes in their electrical properties during material processing.

dielectric strength. (1) The property of an insulating material that enables it to withstand electric stress. (2) The average potential per unit thickness at which failure of the dielectric material occurs.

dielectrometry. Use of electrical techniques to measure the changes in loss factor (dissipation) and in capacitance during cure of the resin in a laminate.

differential scanning calorimetry (DSC). Measurement of the energy absorbed (endotherm) or produced (exotherm) as a resin system is cured. Also detects loss of solvents and other volatiles.

differential thermal analysis (DTA). An experimental analysis technique in which a specimen and a control are heated simultaneously and the difference in their temperatures is monitored. The difference in temperature provides information on relative heat capacities, presence of solvents, changes in structure (that is, phase changes, such as melting of one component in a resin system), and chemical reactions. See also *differential scanning calorimetry.*

diluent. An ingredient added to an adhesive, usually to reduce the concentration of bonding materials.

dimensional stability. Ability of a plastic part to retain the precise shape to which it was molded, cast, or otherwise fabricated.

disbond. (1) An area within a bonded interface between two adherends in which an adhesion failure or separation has occurred. (2) An area of separation between two laminae in the finished laminate (in this case, the term delamination is normally preferred). See also *debond.*

discontinuous fiber-reinforced composite. A ceramic-matrix composite material reinforced by chopped fibers.

displacement angle. In filament winding, the advancement distance of the winding ribbon on the equator after one complete circuit.

dissipation factor, electrical. See *electrical dissipation factor.*

distortion. (1) In fabric, the displacement of fill fiber from the 90° angle (right angle) relative to the warp fiber. (2) In a laminate, the displacement of the fibers (especially at radii), relative to their idealized location, due to motion during lay-up and cure.

doctor blade or bar. A straight piece of material used to spread resin, as in application of a thin film of resin for use in hot melt prepregging or for use as an adhesive film. Also called paste metering blade.

dolly. In filament winding, the planar reinforcement applied to a local area between windings to provide extra strength in an area where a cut-out is to be made, for example, port openings. Usually placed at the knuckle joints of cylinder to dome.

dome. In filament winding, the portion of a cylindrical container that forms the spherical or elliptical shell ends of the container.

doubler. Localized areas of extra layers of reinforcement, usually to provide stiffness or strength for fastening or other abrupt load transfer. See also *tabs.*

draft. The taper or slope of the vertical surfaces of a mold designed to facilitate removal of molded parts.

draft angle. The angle of a taper on a mandrel or mold that facilitates removal of the finished part.

drape. The ability of a fabric or prepreg to conform to a contoured surface.

drawn fiber. Fiber with a certain amount of orientation imparted by the drawing process by which it was formed.

dry laminate. A laminate containing insufficient resin for complete bonding of the reinforcement. See also *resin-starved area.*

dry lay-up. Construction of a laminate by the layering of preimpregnated reinforcement (partly cured resin) in a female mold or on a male mold, usually followed by bag molding or autoclave molding.

dry winding. A term used to describe filament winding using preimpregnated roving, as differentiated from wet winding, where unimpregnated roving is pulled through a resin bath just before being wound onto a mandrel. See also *wet winding.*

DSC. See *differential scanning calorimetry.*

DTA. See *differential thermal analysis.*

ductility. The amount of plastic strain that a material can withstand before fracture. Also, the ability of a material to deform plastically before fracturing.

dwell. (1) A pause in the application of pressure or temperature to a mold, made just before it is completely closed, to allow the escape of gas from the molding material. In filament winding, the time that the traverse mechanism is stationary while the mandrel continues to rotate to the appropriate point for the traverse to begin a new pass. (2) In a standard autoclave cure cycle, an intermediate step in which the resin matrix is held at a temperature below the cure temperature for a specified period of time sufficient to produce a desired degree of staging. Used primarily to control resin flow.

dynamic modulus. The ratio of stress to strain under vibratory conditions (calculated from data obtained from either free or forced vibration tests, in shear, compression, or elongation).

E

edge distance ratio. The distance from the center of the bearing hole to the edge of the specimen in the direction of the principal stress, divided by the diameter of the hole.

edge joint. A joint made by bonding the edge faces of two adherends.

EEW. See *epoxide equivalent weight.*

E-glass. A family of glasses with a calcium aluminoborosilicate composition and a maximum alkali content of 2.0%. A general-purpose fiber that is most often used in reinforced plastics, and is suitable for electrical laminates because of its high resistivity. Also called electric glass.

elastic deformation. The part of the total strain in a stressed body that disappears upon removal of the stress.

elasticity. That property of materials by virtue of which they tend to recover their original size and shape after removal of a force causing deformation. See also *viscoelasticity.*

elastic limit. The greatest stress a material is capable of sustaining without permanent strain remaining after the complete release of the stress. A material is said to have passed its elastic limit when the load is sufficient to initiate plastic, or nonrecoverable, deformation.

elastic recovery. The fraction of a given deformation that behaves elastically. A perfectly elastic material has an elastic recovery of 1; a perfectly plastic material has an elastic recovery of 0.

elastomer. A material that substantially recovers its original shape and size at room temperature after removal of a deforming force.

elastomeric tooling. A tooling system that uses the thermal expansion of rubber materials to form composite parts during cure.

electrical dissipation factor. The ratio of the power loss in a dielectric material to the total power transmitted through it; thus, the imperfection of the dielectric. Equal to the tangent of the loss angle.

electric glass. See *E-glass.*

electroformed molds. A mold made by electroplating metal on the reverse pattern of the cavity. Molten steel may then be sprayed on the back of the mold to increase its strength.

elongation. Deformation caused by stretching. The fractional increase in length of a material stressed in tension. (When expressed as percentage of the original gage length, it is called percentage elongation.)

elongation at break. Elongation recorded at the moment of rupture of the specimen, often expressed as a percentage of the original length.

encapsulation. The enclosure of an item in plastic. Sometimes used specifically in reference to the enclosure of capacitors or circuit board modules.

end. A strand of roving consisting of a given number of filaments gathered together. The group of filaments is considered an "end" or strand before twisting, a "yarn" after twist has been applied. An individual warp yarn, thread, fiber, or roving.

end count. An exact number of ends supplied on a ball of roving.

endurance limit. See *fatigue limit.*

engineered plastic. A material that has been made by specific design and through use of particular monomers and monomer sequences to produce a plastic with desired properties, possibly for a specific application.

engineering plastics. Those plastics and polymeric compositions for which well-defined properties are available such that engineering rather than empirical methods can be used for the design and manufacture of products that require definite and predictable performance in structural applications over a substantial temperature range.

environment. The aggregate of all conditions (such as contamination, temperature, humidity, radiation, magnetic and electric fields, shock, and vibration) that externally influence the performance of an item.

environmental stress cracking. The susceptibility of a thermoplastic resin to crack or craze when in the presence of surface-active agents or other environments.

epichlorohydrin. The basic epoxidizing resin intermediate in the production of epoxy resins. It contains an epoxy group and is highly reactive with polyhydric phenols such as bisphenol A.

epoxide. Compound containing the oxirane structure, a three-member ring containing two carbon atoms and one oxygen atom. The most important members are ethylene oxide and propylene oxide.

epoxide equivalent weight (EEW). The weight of a resin (in grams) that contains one gram equivalent of epoxy.

epoxy plastic. A polymerizable thermoset polymer containing one or more epoxide groups and curable by reaction with amines, alcohols, phenols, carboxylic acids, acid anhydrides, and mercaptans. An important matrix resin in composites and structural adhesive.

equator. In filament winding, the line in a pressure vessel described by the junction of the cylindrical portion and the end dome. Also called tangent line or point.

even tension. The process whereby each end of roving is kept in the same degree of tension as the other ends making up that ball of roving. See also *catenary.*

exotherm. The liberation or evolution of heat during the curing of a plastic product.

expanded plastic. See *cellular plastic.*

extend. To add fillers or low-cost materials in an economy-producing endeavor. To add inert materials to improve void-filling characteristics and reduce crazing.

extenders. Low-cost materials used to dilute or extend high-cost resins without extensive lessening of properties. See also *filler.*

extensibility. The ability of a material to extend or elongate upon application of sufficient force, expressed as percent of the original length.

extensional-bending coupling. A property of certain classes of laminates that exhibit bending curvatures when subjected to extensional loading.

extensional-shear coupling. A property of certain classes of laminates that exhibit shear strains when subjected to extensional loading.

extensometer. A mechanical or optical device for measuring linear strain due to mechanical stress.

F

fabric (1) A material made of woven fibers or filaments. (2) A planar textile also known as cloth.

fabricating (fabrication). The manufacture of products from molded parts, rods, tubes, sheeting, extrusions, or other form by appropriate operations, such as punching, cutting, drilling, and tapping. Fabrication includes fastening parts together or to other parts by mechanical devices, adhesives, heat sealing, welding, or other means.

fabric fill face. That side of the woven fabric where the greatest number of the yarns are perpendicular to the selvage.

fabric, nonwoven. See *nonwoven fabric.*

fabric prepreg batch. Prepreg containing fabric from one fabric batch, impregnated with one batch of resin in one continuous operation.

fabric warp face. That side of the woven fabric where the greatest number of the yarns are parallel to the selvage.

fabric, woven. See *woven fabric.*

facings. (1) Skins and doublers in any lay-up. (2) The outermost layer or composite component of a sandwich construction, generally thin and of high density, which resists most of the edgewise loads and flatwise bending moments, synonymous with face, skin, and facesheet.

fairing. A member or structure, the primary function of which is to streamline the flow of a fluid by producing a smooth outline and to reduce drag, as in aircraft frames and boat hulls.

fatigue. The failure or decay of mechanical properties after repeated applications of stress. Fatigue tests give information on the ability of a material to resist the development of cracks, which eventually bring about failure as a result of a large number of cycles.

fatigue life. The number of cycles of deformation required to bring about failures of the test specimen under a given set of oscillating conditions (stresses or strains). Also known as safe life.

fatigue limit. The stress level below which a material can be stressed cyclically for an infinite number of times without failure.

fatigue ratio. The ratio of fatigue strength to tensile strength. Mean stress and alternating stress must be stated.

fatigue strength. The maximum cyclical stress a material can withstand for a given number of cycles before failure occurs. The residual strength after being subjected to fatigue.

faying surface. The surfaces of materials in contact with each other and joined or about to be joined together.

felt. A fibrous material made up of interlocked fibers by mechanical or chemical action, moisture, or heat. Made from fibers such as asbestos, cotton, glass, and so forth. See also *batt.*

fiber. A general term used to refer to filamentary materials. Often, fiber is used synonymously with filament. It is a general term for a filament with a finite length that is at least 100 times its diameter, which is typically 0.10 to 0.13 mm (0.004 to 0.005 in.). In most cases it is prepared by drawing from a molten bath, spinning, or deposition on a substrate. A whisker, on the other hand, is a short, single-crystal fiber or filament made from a wide variety of materials, with diameters ranging from 1 to 25 μm (40 to 1400 μin.) and aspect ratios (a measure of length) between 100 and 15,000. Fibers can be continuous or specific short lengths (discontinuous), normally no less than 3.2 mm (1/8 in.).

fiber content. The amount of fiber present in a composite. This is usually expressed as a percentage volume fraction or weight fraction of the composite.

fiber count. The number of fibers per unit width of ply present in a specified section of a composite.

fiber diameter. The measurement (expressed in hundred thousandths) of the diameter of individual filaments.

fiber direction. The orientation or alignment of the longitudinal axis of the fiber with respect to a stated reference axis.

fiberglass. An individual filament made by drawing molten glass. A continuous filament is a glass fiber of great or indefinite length. A staple fiber is a glass fiber of relatively short length, generally less than 430 mm (17 in.), the length related to the forming or spinning process used.

fiberglass reinforcement. Major material used to reinforce plastic. Available as mat, roving, fabric, and so forth, it is incorporated into both thermosets and thermoplastics.

fiber pattern. Visible fibers on the surface of laminates or molding. The thread size and weave of glass cloth.

fiber placement. Continuous process for fabricating composite shapes with complex contours and/or cutouts by means of a device that lays preimpregnated fibers (in tow form) onto a nonuniform mandrel or tool. Differs from filament winding in several ways. There is no limit on fiber angles; compaction takes place on-line via heat, pressure, or both; and fibers can be added and dropped as necessary. The process produces more complex shapes and permits a faster put-down rate than filament winding.

fiber-reinforced plastic (FRP). A general term for a composite that is reinforced with cloth, mat, strands, or any other fiber form.

fiber show. Strands or bundles of fibers that are not covered by plastic and that are at or above the surface of a composite.

fiber wash. Splaying out of woven or nonwoven fibers from the general reinforcement direction. Fibers are carried along with bleeding resin during cure.

filament. The smallest unit of a fibrous material. The basic units formed during drawing and spinning, which are gathered into strands of fiber for use in composites. Filaments usually are of extreme length and very small diameter, usually less than 25 μm (1 mil). Normally, filaments are not used individually. Some textile filaments can function as a yarn when they are of sufficient strength and flexibility.

filamentary composite. A major form of advanced composite in which the fiber constituent consists of continuous filaments. Specifically, a filamentary composite is a laminate comprised of a number of laminae, each of which consists of a nonwoven, parallel, uniaxial, planar array of filaments (or filament yarns) embedded in the selected matrix material. Individual laminae are directionally oriented and combined into specific multiaxial laminates for application to specific envelopes of strength and stiffness requirements.

filament winding. A process for fabricating a composite structure in which continuous reinforcements (filament, wire, yarn, tape, or other), either previously impregnated with a matrix material or impregnated during the winding, are placed over a rotating and removable form or mandrel in a prescribed way to meet certain stress conditions. Generally the shape is a surface of revolution and may or may not include end closures. When the required number of layers is applied, the wound form is cured and the mandrel removed.

fill. Yarn oriented at right angles to the warp in a woven fabric.

filler. A relatively inert substance added to a material to alter its physical, mechanical, thermal, electrical, and other properties, or to lower cost or density. Sometimes the term is used specifically to mean particulate additives. See also *inert filler.*

fillet. A rounded filling or adhesive that fills the corner or angle where two adherends are joined.

filling yarn. The transverse threads or fibers in a woven fabric. Those fibers running perpendicular to the warp. Also called weft.

film adhesive. A synthetic resin adhesive, usually of the thermosetting type, in the form of a thin, dry film of resin with or without a paper or glass carrier.

finish. Chemical finish applied to glass and other fibers, after sizing has been removed, to facilitate resin wetting, resin bonding, and good environmental performance of the cured laminate. See also *size.*

first-order transition. A change of state associated with crystallization or melting in a polymer.

flame resistance. Ability of a material to extinguish flame once the source of heat is removed. See also *self-extinguishing resin.*

flame retardants. Certain chemicals that are used to reduce or eliminate the tendency of a resin to burn.

flammability. Measure of the extent to which a material will support combustion.

flash. That portion of the charge that flows from or is extruded from the mold cavity during the molding. Extra plastic attached to a molding along the parting line, which must be removed before the part is considered finished.

flexibilizer. An additive that makes a finished plastic more flexible or tough. See also *plasticizer.*

flexible molds. Molds made of rubber or elastomeric plastics, used for casting plastics. They can be stretched to remove cured pieces with undercuts.

flexural modulus. The ratio, within the elastic limit, of the applied stress on a test specimen in flexure to the corresponding strain in the outermost fibers of the specimen.

flexural strength. The maximum stress that can be borne by the surface fibers in a beam in bending. The flexural strength is the unit resistance to the maximum load before failure by bending, usually expressed in force per unit area.

flow. (1) The movement of resin under pressure, allowing it to fill all parts of a mold. (2) The gradual but continuous distortion of a material under continued load, usually at high temperatures; also called creep.

flow line. A mark on a molded piece made by the meeting of two flow fronts during molding. Also called striae, weld mark, or weld line.

flow marks. Wavy surface appearance of an object molded from thermoplastic resins, caused by improper flow of the resin into the mold.

fluoroplastic. A plastic based on polymers made from monomers containing one or more atoms of fluorine, or copolymers of such monomers with other monomers, the fluorine-containing monomer(s) being in greatest amount by mass.

fluted core. An integrally woven reinforcement material consisting of ribs between two skins in a unitized sandwich construction.

foamed plastics. (1) Resins in sponge form, flexible or rigid, with cells closed or interconnected and density over a range from that of the solid parent resin to 0.030 g/cm^3. Compressive strength of rigid foams is fair, making them useful as core materials for sandwich constructions. (2) A chemical cellular plastic, the structure of which is produced by gases generated from the chemical interaction of its constituents.

foaming agent. Chemicals added to plastics and rubbers that generate inert gases on heating, causing the resin to assume a cellular structure.

foam-in-place. Refers to the deposition of foams when the foaming machine must be brought to the work that is "in place," as opposed to bringing the work to the foaming machine. Also, foam mixed in a container and poured into a mold, where it rises to fill the cavity.

force. The male half of the mold that enters the cavity, exerting pressure on the resin and causing it to flow. Also called punch.

FP fiber. Polycrystalline alumina fiber (Al_2O_3). A ceramic fiber useful for high-temperature (1370 to 1650 °C, or 2500 to 3000 °F) composites.

fracture. The separation of a body. Defined both as rupture of the surface without complete separation of laminate and as complete separation of a body because of external or internal forces.

fracture stress. The true, normal stress on the minimum cross-sectional area at the beginning of fracture.

fracture toughness. A measure of the damage tolerance of a material containing initial flaws or cracks. Used in aircraft structural design and analysis.

free-radical polymerization. A type of polymerization in which the propagating species is a long-chain free radical initiated by the introduction of free radicals from thermal or photochemical decomposition.

free wall. The portion of a honeycomb cell wall that is not connected to another cell.

friction, coefficient of. See *coefficient of friction.*

FRP. See *fiber-reinforced plastic.*
fungus resistance. The resistance of a material to attack by fungi in conditions promoting their growth.
fuzz. Accumulation of short, broken filaments after passing glass strands, yarns, or rovings over a contact point. Often, weighted and used as an inverse measure of abrasion resistance.

G

gage length. Length over which deformation is measured, for a tensile or compressive test specimen. The deformation over the gage length divided by the gage length determines the strain.
gap. (1) In filament winding, the space between successive windings in which windings are usually intended to lay next to each other. (2) Separations between fibers within a filament winding band. (3) The distance between adjacent plies in a lay-up of unidirectional tape materials.
gap-filling adhesive. An adhesive subject to low shrinkage in setting, used as sealant.
gel. The initial jellylike solid phase that develops during the formation of a resin from a liquid. A semisolid system consisting of a network of solid aggregates in which liquid is held.
gelation. The point in a resin cure when the resin viscosity has increased to a point such that it barely moves when probed with a sharp instrument.
gelation time. (1) That interval of time, in connection with the use of synthetic thermosetting resins, extending from the introduction of a catalyst into a liquid adhesive system until the start of gel formation. (2) The time under application of load for a resin to reach a solid state.
gel coat. A quick-setting resin applied to the surface of a mold and gelled before lay-up. The gel coat becomes an integral part of the finished laminate, and is usually used to improve surface appearance and bonding.
gel permeation chromatography (GPC). A form of liquid chromatography in which the polymer molecules are separated by their ability or inability to penetrate the material in the separation column.
gel point. The stage at which a liquid begins to exhibit pseudoelastic properties. This stage may be conveniently observed from the inflection point on a viscosity time plot.
geodesic. The shortest distance between two points on a surface.
geodesic isotensoid. Constant stress level in any given filament at all points in its path.
geodesic-isotensoid contour. In filament-wound reinforced plastic pressure vessels, a dome contour in which the filaments are placed on geodesic paths so that the filaments will exhibit uniform tensions throughout their length under pressure loading.
geodesic ovaloid. A contour for end domes, the fibers forming a geodesic line: the shortest distance between two points on a surface of revolution. The forces exerted by the filaments are proportioned to meet hoop and meridional stresses at any point.
glass. An inorganic product of fusion that has cooled to a rigid condition without crystallizing. Glass is typically hard and relatively brittle, and has a conchoidal fracture.
glass cloth. Conventionally woven glass fiber material. See also *scrim.*
glass fiber. A fiber spun from an inorganic product of fusion that has cooled to a rigid condition without crystallizing.
glass filament. A form of glass that has been drawn to a small diameter and extreme length. Most filaments are less than 0.15 mm (0.005 in.) in diameter.
glass filament bushing. The unit through which molten glass is drawn in making glass filaments.
glass finish. A material applied to the surface of a glass reinforcement to improve the bond between the glass and the plastic resin matrix.
glass flake. Thin, irregularly shaped flakes of glass, typically made by shattering a thin-walled tube of glass.
glass former. An oxide that forms a glass easily. Also, one which contributes to the network of silica glass when added to it.
glass mat thermoplastic (GMT). A semifinished resin-fiber combination supplied as blanks for compression molding.
glass, percent by volume. The product of the specific gravity of a laminate and the percent glass by weight, divided by the specific gravity of the glass.
glass stress. In a filament-wound part, usually a pressure vessel, the stress calculated using the load and the cross-sectional area of the reinforcement only.
glass transition. The reversible change in an amorphous polymer or in amorphous regions of a partially crystalline polymer from, or to, a viscous or rubbery condition to, or from, a hard and relatively brittle one.
glass-transition temperature (T_g). (1) The approximate midpoint of the temperature range over which the glass transition takes place; glass and silica fiber exhibit a phase change at approximately 955 °C (1750 °F) and carbon/graphite fibers at 2205 to 2760 °C (4000 to 5000 °F). (2) The temperature at which increased molecular mobility results in significant changes in the properties of a cured resin system. (3) The inflection point on a plot of modulus versus temperature. The measured value of T_g depends to some extent on the method of test.
GMT. See *glass mat thermoplastic.*
graphite. The crystalline allotropic form of carbon.
graphite fiber. A fiber made from a precursor by an oxidation, carbonization, and graphitization process (which provides a graphitic structure). See also *carbon fiber.*
graphitization. The process of pyrolyzation in an inert atmosphere at temperatures in excess of 1925 °C (3500 °F), usually as high as 2480 °C (4500 °F), and sometimes as high as 9750 °C (5400 °F), converting carbon to its crystalline allotropic form. Temperature depends on precursor and properties desired.
green strength. The ability of the material (such as urethane elastomer), while not completely cured, to undergo removal from the mold and handling without tearing or permanent distortion.
greige, gray goods. Any fabric before finishing, as well as any yarn or fiber before bleaching or dyeing; therefore, fabric with no finish or size.

H

hand. The softness of a piece of fabric, as determined by the touch (individual judgment).
hand lay-up. The process of placing (and working) successive plies of reinforcing material or resin-impregnated reinforcement in position on a mold by hand.
handling life. The out-of-refrigeration time over which a material retains its handleability.
hardener. A substance or mixture added to a plastic composition to promote or control the curing action by taking part in it.
hardness. The resistance to surface indentation usually measured by the depth of penetration (or arbitrary units related to the depth of penetration) of a blunt point under a given load using a particular instrument according to a prescribed procedure. See also *Barcol hardness, Mohs hardness, Rockwell hardness,* and *Shore hardness.*
harness satin. Weaving pattern producing a satin appearance. "Eight-harness" means the warp tow crosses over seven fill tows and under the eighth (repeatedly).
heat-activated adhesive. A dry adhesive that is rendered tacky or fluid by application of heat, or heat and pressure, to the assembly.
heat buildup. The rise in temperature in a part resulting from the dissipation of applied strain energy as heat or from applied mold cure heat. See also *hysteresis.*
heat cleaned. A condition in which glass or other fibers are exposed to elevated temperatures to remove preliminary sizings or binders not compatible with the resin system to be applied.
heat distortion temperature. The temperature at which a standard test bar deflects a specified amount under a stated load.
heat resistance. The property or ability of plastics and elastomers to resist the deteriorating effects of elevated temperatures.
heat sealing. A method of joining plastic films by simultaneous application of heat and pressure to areas in contact.
heat-sealing adhesive. A thermoplastic film adhesive that is melted between the adherend surfaces by heat application to one or both of the adjacent adherend surfaces.

heat sink. A contrivance for the absorption or transfer of heat away from a critical element or part. Bulk graphite is often used as a heat sink.

heat treating. Term used to cover annealing, hardening, tempering, and so on.

helical winding. In filament-wound items, a winding in which a filament band advances along a helical path, not necessarily at a constant angle, except in the case of a cylinder.

heterogeneous. (1) Descriptive term for a material consisting of dissimilar constituents separately identifiable. (2) A medium consisting of regions of unlike properties separated by internal boundaries. Note that not all nonhomogeneous materials are necessarily heterogeneous.

hexa. Shortened form of hexamethylenetetramine, a source of reactive methylene for curing novolacs.

high-frequency heating. The heating of materials by dielectric loss in a high-frequency electrostatic field. The material is exposed between electrodes and is heated quickly and uniformly by absorption of energy from the electrical field.

high-pressure laminates. Laminates molded and cured at pressures not lower than 6.9 MPa (1.0 ksi), and more commonly in the range of 8.3 to 13.8 MPa (1.2 to 2.0 ksi).

high-pressure spot. See *resin-starved area.*

HIP. See *hot isostatic pressing.*

homogeneous. (1) Descriptive term for a material of uniform composition throughout. (2) A medium that has no internal physical boundaries. (3) A material whose properties are constant at every point, that is, constant with respect to spatial coordinates (but not necessarily with respect to directional coordinates).

honeycomb. Manufactured product of resin-impregnated sheet material (paper, glass fabric, and so on) or metal foil, formed into hexagonal-shaped cells. Used as a core material in sandwich construction. See also *sandwich construction.*

hoop. Ply laid onto a mandrel at a 90° angle. Primarily used in reference to filament winding of cylindrically shaped objects.

hoop stress. The circumferential stress in a material of cylindrical form subjected to internal or external pressure.

hot isostatic pressing. A process for fabricating certain metal-matrix composites. A preform is consolidated under fluid pressure (usually an inert gas) at high temperature and pressure in a pressure vessel.

hot-melt adhesive. An adhesive that is applied in a molten state and forms a bond after cooling to a solid state. A bonding agent that achieves a solid state and resultant strength by cooling, as contrasted with other adhesives that achieve the solid state through evaporation of solvents or chemical cure. A thermoplastic resin that functions as an adhesive when melted between substrates and cooled.

hot-setting adhesive. An adhesive that requires a temperature at or above 100 °C (212 °F) to set.

hot working. Any form of mechanical deformation processing carried out on a metal or alloy above its recrystallization temperature but below its melting point.

hybrid. A composite laminate consisting of at least two distinct types of matrix or reinforcement. Each matrix or reinforcement type can be distinct because of its (1) physical and/or mechanical properties, (2) material form, and (3) chemical composition. See also *interply hybrid* and *intraply hybrid.*

hydraulic press. A press in which the molding force is created by the pressure exerted by a fluid.

hydromechanical press. A press in which the molding forces are created partly by a mechanical system and partly by an hydraulic system.

hydrophilic. Capable of absorbing water; easily wetted by water.

hydrophobic. Capable of repelling water; poorly wetted by water.

hygroscopic. Capable of absorbing and retaining atmospheric moisture.

hygrothermal effect. Change in properties due to moisture absorption and temperature change.

hysteresis. The energy absorbed in a complete cycle of loading and unloading. This energy is converted from mechanical to frictional energy (heat).

I

ignition loss. The difference in weight before and after burning. As with glass, the burning off of the binder or size.

impact strength. The ability of a material to withstand shock loading. The work done in fracturing a test specimen in a specified manner under shock loading.

impact test. Measure of the energy necessary to fracture a standard notched bar by an impulse load. See also *Izod impact test, reverse impact test,* and *Charpy impact test.*

impregnate. In reinforced plastics, to saturate the reinforcement with a resin.

impregnated fabric. A fabric impregnated with a synthetic resin. See also *prepreg.*

inclusion. A physical and mechanical discontinuity occurring within a material or part, usually consisting of solid, encapsulated foreign material. Inclusions are often capable of transmitting some structural stresses and energy fields, but in a noticeably different degree from the parent material. See also *voids.*

induction bonding. A secondary joining process for thermoplastic composite parts in which a metallic susceptor is placed in the bondline and an induction coil is used to heat the joint above the melt temperature of the thermoplastic matrix.

inert filler. A material added to a plastic to alter the end-item properties through physical rather than chemical means.

infrared. Part of the electromagnetic spectrum between the visible light range and the radar range. Radiant heat is in this range, and infrared heaters are frequently used in the thermoforming and curing of plastics and composites. Infrared analysis is used for identification of polymer constituents.

inhibitor. A substance that retards a chemical reaction. Also used in certain types of monomers and resins to prolong storage life.

initial modulus. The slope of the initial straight portion of a stress-strain or load-elongation curve. See also *Young's modulus.*

initial strain. The strain produced in a specimen by given loading conditions before creep occurs.

initial (instantaneous) stress. The stress produced by force in a specimen before stress relaxation occurs.

initiator. Peroxides used as sources of free radicals. They are used in free-radical polymerizations, for curing thermosetting resins, as cross-linking agents for elastomers and polyethylene, and for polymer modification.

injection molding. Method of forming a plastic to the desired shape by forcing the heat-softened plastic into a relatively cool cavity under pressure.

inorganic. Designating or pertaining to the chemistry of all elements and compounds not classified as organic. Matter other than animal or vegetable, such as earthy or mineral matter. Applies to the chemistry of all elements and compounds not classified as organic.

inorganic pigments. Natural or synthetic metallic oxides, sulfides, and other salts that impart heat and light stability, weathering resistance, color, and migration resistance to plastics.

insert. An integral part of a plastic molding consisting of metal or other material that may be molded or pressed into position after the molding is completed.

insulation resistance. (1) The electrical resistance between two conductors or systems of conductors separated only by insulating material. (2) The ratio of the applied voltage to the total current between two electrodes in contact with a specified insulator. (3) The electrical resistance of an insulating material to a direct voltage.

insulator. A material of such low electrical conductivity that the flow of current through it can usually be neglected. Similarly, a material of low thermal conductivity, such as that used to insulate structural shells.

integral composite structure. Composite structure in which several structural elements, which would conventionally be assembled together by bonding or mechanical fasteners after separate fabrication, are instead laid up and cured as a single, complex, continuous structure, for example, spars, ribs, and one stiffened cover of a wing box fabricated as a single integral part. The term is sometimes applied more loosely to any composite structure not assembled by mechanical fasteners. All or some parts of the assembly may be co-cured.

integrally heated. A term referring to tooling that is self-heating, through use of electrical heaters such as cal rods. Most hydroclave tooling is integrally heated. Some autoclave tooling is integrally heated to compensate for thick sections, to provide high heat-up rates, or to permit processing at a higher temperature than is otherwise possible with the autoclave.

integral skin foam. Urethane foam with a cellular core structure and a relatively nonporous skin.

interface. (1) The boundary or surface between two different, physically distinguishable media. (2) On fibers, the contact area between fibers and sizing or finish. (3) In a laminate, the contact area between the reinforcement and the laminating resin.

interference fits. A joint or mating of two parts in which the male part has an external dimension larger than the internal dimension of the mating female part. Distension of the female by the male creates a stress, which supplies the bonding force for the joint.

interlaminar. Descriptive term pertaining to an object (for example, voids), event (for example, fracture), or potential field (for example, shear stress) referenced as existing or occurring between two or more adjacent laminae.

interlaminar shear. Shearing force tending to produce a relative displacement between two laminae in a laminate along the plane of their interface.

intermediate temperature setting adhesive. An adhesive that sets in the temperature range from 30 to 100 °C (87 to 211 °F).

interpenetrating polymer network. A combination of two polymers in a network in which at least one (or both) is crosslinked around the other. Interpenetrating polymer networks are frequently used to toughen epoxy matrices where the epoxy is continuous and a thermoplastic polymer is discontinuous.

interphase. The boundary region between a bulk resin or polymer and an adherend in which the polymer has a high degree of orientation to the adherend on a molecular basis. It plays a major role in the load transfer process between the bulk of the adhesive and the adherend or the fiber and the laminate matrix resin.

interply cracks. Through-cracking of individual layers within a composite lay-up, perpendicular to the ply interfaces.

interply hybrid. A composite in which adjacent laminae are composed of different materials.

intralaminar. Descriptive term pertaining to an object (for example, voids), event (for example, fracture), or potential field (for example, temperature gradient) existing entirely within a single lamina without reference to any adjacent laminae.

intraply hybrid. A composite in which different materials are used within a specific layer or band.

irradiation. As applied to plastics, the bombardment with a variety of subatomic particles, usually alpha-, beta-, or gamma-rays. Used to initiate polymerization and copolymerization of plastics and in some cases to bring about changes in the physical properties of a plastic.

irreversible. Not capable of redissolving or remelting. Chemical reactions that proceed in a single direction and are not capable of reversal (as applied to thermosetting resins).

isocyanate plastics. Plastics based on resins made by the condensation of organic isocyanates with other compounds. Generally reacted with polyols on a polyester or polyether backbone molecule, with the reactants being joined through the formation of the urethane linkage. See also *polyurethane* and *urethane plastics.*

isostatic pressing. Pressing powder under a gas or liquid so that pressure is transmitted equally in all directions, for example, in sintering.

isotropic. Having uniform properties in all directions. The measured properties of an isotropic material are independent of the axis of testing.

Izod impact test. A test for shock loading in which a notched specimen bar is held at one end and broken by striking, and the energy absorbed is measured.

J

joint, adhesive. See *adhesive joint.*
joint, butt. See *butt joint.*
joint, edge. See *edge joint.*
joint, lap. See *lap joint.*
joint, scarf. See *scarf joint.*

K

Kapton. Trade name (E.I. DuPont de Nemours & Co., Inc., Wilmington, DE) for a polyimide film that emits low smoke and flame, resists hydraulic fluids, and has good low- and elevated-temperature performance.

kerf. The width of a cut made by a saw blade, torch, waterjet, laser beam, and so forth.

Kevlar. Trade name (E.I. DuPont de Nemours & Co., Inc., Wilmington, DE) for an organic polymer composed of aromatic polyamides having a para-type orientation (parallel chain extending bonds from each aromatic nucleus).

***K*-factor.** The coefficient of thermal conductivity. The amount of heat that passes through a unit cube of material in a given time when the difference in temperature of two opposite faces is 1°.

knitted fabrics. Fabrics produced by interlooping chains of yarn.

knuckle area. The area of transition between sections of different geometry in a filament-wound part, for example, where the skirt joins the cylinder of the pressure vessel. Also called Y-joint.

L

lamina. A single ply or layer in a laminate made up of a series of layers (organic composite). A flat or curved surface containing unidirectional fibers or woven fibers embedded in a matrix (metal-matrix composite).

laminae. Plural of lamina.

laminate. (1) To unite laminae with a bonding material, usually with pressure and heat (normally used with reference to flat sheets, but also rods and tubes). (2) A product made by such bonding. See also *bidirectional laminate* and *unidirectional laminate.*

laminate coordinates. A reference coordinate system (used to describe the properties of a laminate), generally in the direction of principal axes, when they exist.

laminate orientation. The configuration of a cross-plied composite laminate with regard to the angles of cross-plying, the number of laminae at each angle, and the exact sequence of the lamina lay-up.

laminate ply. One fabric-resin or fiber-resin layer of a product that is bonded to adjacent layers in the curing process.

lap. In filament winding, the amount of overlay between successive windings, usually intended to minimize gapping. In bonding, the distance one adherend covers another adherend.

lap joint. A joint made by placing one adherend partly over another and bonding the overlapped portions.

lattice pattern. A pattern of filament winding with a fixed arrangement of open voids.

lay-up. (1) The reinforcing material placed in position in the mold. (2) The process of placing the reinforcing material in position in the mold. (3) The resin-impregnated reinforcement. (4) A description of the component materials, geometry, and so on, of a laminate. (5) A fabrication process involving the assembly of successive layers of resin-impregnated material.

***L*-direction.** The ribbon direction, that is, the direction of the continuous sheets of honeycomb.

level winding. See *circumferential winding.*

linear expansion. The increase of a given dimension, measured by the expansion or contraction of a specimen or component subject to a thermal gradient or changing temperature. See also *coefficient of thermal expansion.*

liner. In a filament-wound pressure vessel, the continuous, usually flexible coating on the inside surface of the vessel, used to protect the laminate from chemical attack or to prevent leakage under stress.

liquid crystal polymer. A thermoplastic polymer that is melt processable and develops high orientation in molding, with resultant tensile strength and high-temperature capability that is notably improved. First commercial availability was as an aromatic polyester. With or without fiber reinforcement.

liquid metal infiltration. Process for immersion of metal fibers in a molten metal bath to achieve a metal-matrix composite; for example, graphite fibers in molten aluminum.

liquid shim. Material used to position components in an assembly where dimensional alignment is critical. For example, epoxy adhesive is introduced into gaps after the assembly is placed in the desired configuration.

load-deflection curve. A curve in which the increasing tension, compression, or flexural loads are plotted on the ordinate axis and the deflections caused by those loads are plotted on the abscissa axis.

longos. Low-angle helical or longitudinal windings.

loop tenacity. The tenacity or strength value obtained by pulling two loops, as two links in a chain, against each other in order to demonstrate the susceptibility that a fibrous material has for cutting or crushing itself; loop strength.

loss factor. The product of the dissipation factor and the dielectric constant of a dielectric material.

loss modulus. A damping term describing the dissipation of energy into heat when a material is deformed.

loss on ignition. Weight loss, usually expressed as percent of total, after burning off an organic sizing from glass fibers, or an organic resin from a glass fiber laminate.

loss tangent. See *electrical dissipation factor.*

lot. A specific amount of material produced at one time using the same process and the same conditions of manufacture, and offered for sale as a unit quantity.

low-pressure laminates. In general, laminates molded and cured in the range of pressures from 2760 kPa (400 psi) down to and including pressure obtained by the mere contact of the plies.

lubricant. A material added to most sizings to improve the handling and processing properties of textile strands, especially during weaving.

M

macerate. To chop or shred fabric for use as a filler for a molding resin.

macro. In relation to composites, denotes the gross properties of a composite as a structural element but does not consider the individual properties or identity of the constituents.

mandrel. The core tool around which resin-impregnated paper, fabric, or fiber is wound to form pipes, tubes, or structural shell shapes.

mat. (1) A fibrous material for reinforced plastic consisting of randomly oriented chopped filaments, short fibers (with or without a carrier fabric), or swirled filaments loosely held together with a binder. Available in blankets of various widths, weights, and lengths. (2) A sheet formed by filament winding a single-hoop ply of fiber on a mandrel, cutting across its width and laying out a flat sheet.

matched metal molding. A reinforced plastics manufacturing process in which matching male and female metal molds are used (similar to compression molding) to form the part, with time, pressure, and heat.

matrix. The essentially homogeneous material in which the fiber system or reinforcing particles of a composite are embedded. Both thermoplastic and thermoset resins may be used, as well as metals, ceramics, and glasses.

mechanical adhesion. Adhesion between surfaces in which the adhesive holds the parts together by interlocking action.

mechanical properties. (1) The properties of a material, such as compressive and tensile strengths and modulus, that are associated with elastic and inelastic reaction when force is applied. (2) The individual relationship between stress and strain.

melt. A charge of molten metal or plastic. See also *liquid metal infiltration.*

mer. The repeating structural unit of any polymer.

mesophase. An intermediate phase in the formation of carbon from a pitch precursor. This is a liquid crystal phase in the form of microspheres, which, upon prolonged heating above 400 °C (750 °F), coalesce, solidify, and form regions of extended order. Heating to above 2000 °C (3630 °F) leads to the formation of graphite structure.

mesoscopic. Pertaining to the size range between microscopic and macroscopic.

metallic fiber. Manufactured fiber composed of metal, plastic-coated metal, metal-coated plastic, or a core completely covered by metal.

metal-matrix composites. Advanced composites that consist of a nonmetallic reinforcement incorporated into a metallic matrix. Reinforcements may constitute from 10 to 60 vol% of the composite. Continuous fiber or filament reinforcements include graphite, silicon carbide, boron, alumina, and refractory metals. Matrix materials include aluminum (the most common), titanium, magnesium, copper, and ordered intermetallic compounds (NiAl and Ti_3Al).

M-glass. A high beryllia (BeO_2) content glass designed especially for high modulus of elasticity.

micro. In relation to composites, denotes the properties of the constituents, that is, matrix, reinforcement, and interface only, and their effects on the composite properties.

microcracking. Cracks formed in composites when thermal stresses locally exceed the strength of the matrix. Since most microcracks do not penetrate the reinforcing fibers, microcracks in a cross-plied tape laminate or in a laminate made from cloth prepreg are usually limited to the thickness of a single ply.

micromechanics. Analysis of the structural behavior of composites on a constituent (matrix, reinforcement, interface) level.

microstructure. A structure with heterogeneities that can be seen through a microscope.

mil. A unit of length used in measuring the diameter of glass fiber strands, wire, and so on (1 mil = 0.001 in., or 0.0254 mm).

milled fiber. Continuous glass strands hammer milled into very short glass fibers. Useful as inexpensive filler or anticrazing reinforcing fillers for adhesives.

modulus, initial. See *initial modulus.*

modulus of elasticity. The ratio of the stress or load applied to the strain or deformation produced in a material that is elastically deformed. If a tensile strength of 13.8 MPa (2.0 ksi) results in an elongation of 1%, the modulus of elasticity is 13.8 MPa (2.0 ksi) divided by 0.01, or 1380 MPa (200 ksi). Also called Young's modulus. See also *offset modulus* and *secant modulus.*

modulus, offset. See *offset modulus.*

modulus of resilience. The energy that can be absorbed per unit volume without creating a permanent distortion. Calculated by integrating the stress-strain curve from zero to the elastic limit and dividing by the original volume of the specimen.

modulus of rigidity. The ratio of stress to strain within the elastic region for shear or torsional stress. Also called shear modulus or torsional modulus.

modulus of rupture, in bending. The maximum tensile or compressive stress value (whichever causes failure) in the extreme fiber of a beam loaded to failure in bending.

modulus of rupture, in torsion. The maximum shear stress in the extreme fiber of a member of circular cross section loaded to failure in torsion.

modulus, secant. See *secant modulus.*

modulus, tangent. See *tangent modulus.*

Mohs hardness. A measure of the scratch resistance of a material. The higher the number, the greater the scratch resistance (No. 10 being termed diamond).

moisture absorption. The pickup of water vapor from air by a material. It relates only to vapor withdrawn from the air by a material and must be distinguished from water absorption, which is the gain in weight due to the take-up of water by immersion.

moisture content. The amount of moisture in a material determined under prescribed conditions and expressed as a percentage of the mass of the moist specimen, that is, the mass of the dry substance plus the moisture present.

moisture equilibrium. The condition reached by a sample when it no longer takes up moisture from, or gives up moisture to, the surrounding environment.

moisture vapor transmission. A rate at which water vapor passes through a material at a specified temperature and relative humidity (g/mil/24 h/100 in.^{2}).

mold. (1) The cavity or matrix into or on which the plastic composition is placed and from which it takes form. (2) To shape plastic parts or finished articles by heat and pressure. (3)

The assembly of all the parts that function collectively in the molding process.

molded edge. An edge that is not physically altered after molding for use in final form, and particularly one that does not have fiber ends along its length.

molded net. Description of a molded part that requires no additional processing to meet dimensional requirements.

molding. The forming of a polymer or composite into a solid mass of prescribed shape and size by the application of pressure and heat for given times. Sometimes used to denote the finished part.

molding cycle. (1) The period of time required for the complete sequence of operations on a molding press to produce one set of moldings. (2) The operations necessary to produce a set of moldings without reference to the total time taken.

molding powder or compound. Plastic material in varying stages of pellets or granulation, and consisting of resin, filler, pigments, reinforcements, plasticizers, and other ingredients, ready for use in the molding operation.

molding pressure. The pressure applied to the ram of an injection machine, compression press, or transfer press to force the softened plastic to fill the mold cavities completely.

mold-release agent. A lubricant, liquid, or powder (often silicone oils and waxes) used to prevent sticking of molded articles in the cavity.

mold shrinkage. (1) The immediate shrinkage that a molded part undergoes when it is removed from a mold and cooled to room temperature. (2) The difference in dimensions, expressed in inches per inch, between a molding and the mold cavity in which it was molded (at normal-temperature measurement). (3) The incremental difference between the dimensions of the molding and the mold from which it was made, expressed as a percentage of the mold dimensions.

mold surface. The side of a laminate that faced the mold (tool) during cure in an autoclave or hydroclave.

molecular weight. The sum of the atomic weights of all the atoms in a molecule. A measure of the chain length for the molecules that make up the polymer.

monofilament. A single fiber or filament of indefinite length, strong enough to function as a yarn in commercial textile operations.

monolayer. The basic laminate unit from which cross-plied or other laminate types are constructed. Also, a "single" layer of atoms or molecules adsorbed on or applied to a surface.

monomer. A single molecule that can react with like or unlike molecules to form a polymer. The smallest repeating structure of a polymer (mer). For addition polymers, this represents the original unpolymerized compound.

morphology. The overall form of a polymer structure, that is, crystallinity, branching, molecular weight, and so on.

multicircuit winding. In filament winding, a winding that requires more than one circuit before the band repeats by laying adjacent to the first band.

multifilament yarn. A large number (500 to 2000) of fine, continuous filaments (often 5 to 100 individual filaments), usually with some twist in the yarn to facilitate handling.

MVT. See *moisture vapor transmission.*

Mylar. A trade name (E.I. DuPont de Nemours & Co., Inc., Wilmington, DE) for a polyester film used as a release sheet in adhesive and composite bonding. Also used as food packaging.

N

NDE. See *nondestructive evaluation.*

NDI. See *nondestructive inspection.*

NDT. See *nondestructive testing.*

neat resin. Resin to which nothing (additives, reinforcements, and so on) has been added.

necking. The localized reduction in cross section that may occur in a material under tensile stress.

needled mat. A mat formed of strands cut to a short length, then felted together in a needle loom with or without a carrier.

nesting. In reinforced plastics, the placing of plies of fabric so that the yarns of one ply lie in the valleys between the yarns of the adjacent ply (nested cloth).

net resin content prepreg. A prepreg product form that contains the final desired resin content and does not require resin bleeding (removal) during the cure process.

netting analysis. The analysis of filament-wound structures that assumes the stresses induced in the structure are carried entirely by the filaments, and the strength of the resin is neglected, and assumes also that the filaments possess no bending or shearing stiffness and carry only the axial tensile loads.

node. The connected portion of adjacent ribbons of honeycomb.

NOL ring. A parallel filament- or tape-wound hoop test specimen developed by the Naval Ordnance Laboratory (NOL) (now the Naval Surface Weapons Laboratory) for measuring various mechanical strength properties of the material, such as tension and compression, by testing the entire ring or segments of it. Also known as a parallel fiber reinforced ring.

Nomex. A trade name (E.I. DuPont de Nemours & Co., Inc., Wilmington, DE) for an aramid fiber or paper used for honeycomb construction.

nominal stress. The stress at a point calculated on the net cross section without taking into consideration the effect on stress of geometric discontinuities, such as holes, grooves, fillets, and so on. The calculation is made by simple elastic theory.

nominal value. A value assigned for the purpose of a convenient designation. A nominal value exists in name only. It is often an average number with a tolerance so as to fit together with adjacent parts.

nondestructive evaluation (NDE). Broadly considered synonymous with nondestructive inspection (NDI). More specifically, the analysis of NDI findings to determine whether the material will be acceptable for its function.

nondestructive inspection (NDI). A process or procedure, such as ultrasonic or radiographic inspection, for determining the quality or characteristics of a material, part, or assembly, without permanently altering the subject or its properties. Used to find internal anomalies in a structure without degrading its properties.

nondestructive testing (NDT). Broadly considered synonymous with nondestructive inspection (NDI).

nonhygroscopic. Lacking the property of absorbing and retaining an appreciable quantity of moisture (water vapor) from the air.

nonwoven fabric. A planar textile structure produced by loosely compressing together fibers, yarns, rovings, and so on, with or without a scrim cloth carrier. Accomplished by mechanical, chemical, thermal, or solvent means, and combinations thereof.

normal stress. The stress component that is perpendicular to the plane on which the forces act.

notched specimen. A test specimen that has been deliberately cut or notched, usually in a V-shape, to induce and locate point of failure.

notch factor. Ratio of the resilience determined on a plain specimen to the resilience determined on a notched specimen.

notch sensitivity. The extent to which the sensitivity of a material to fracture is increased by the presence of a surface nonhomogeneity, such as a notch, a sudden change in section, a crack, or a scratch. Low notch sensitivity is usually associated with ductile materials, and high notch sensitivity is usually associated with brittle materials.

novolac. A linear, thermoplastic, B-staged phenolic resin, which, in the presence of methylene or other cross-linking groups, reacts to form a thermoset phenolic.

nylon. The generic name for all synthetic polyamides.

nylon plastics. Plastics based on a resin composed principally of a long-chain synthetic polymeric amide that has recurring amide groups as an integral part of the main polymer chain. Numerical designations (nylon 6, nylon 6/6, and so on) refer to the monomeric amides of which they are made. Characterized by great toughness and elasticity.

O

off-axis laminate. A laminate whose principal axis is oriented at an angle (θ) other than 0 or 90° with respect to a reference direction, usually related to principal load or stress direction.

offset modulus. The ratio of the offset yield stress to the extension at the offset point.

offset yield strength. The stress at which the strain exceeds by a specific amount (the offset) an extension of the initial, approximately linear, proportional portion of the stress-strain curve. It is expressed in force per unit area.

olefin. A group of unsaturated hydrocarbons of the general formula C_nH_{2n} named after the corresponding paraffins by the addition of "-ene" or "-ylene" to the root, for example, ethylene, propylene, and pentene.

open-cell foam. Foamed or cellular material with cells that are generally interconnected. Closed cell refers to cells that are not interconnected.

orange peel. An uneven surface somewhat resembling that of an orange peel; said of injection moldings that have unintentionally ragged surfaces.

organic. Matter originating in plant or animal life, or composed of chemicals of hydrocarbon origin, either natural or synthetic.

orientation. The alignment of the crystalline structure in polymeric materials in order to produce a highly aligned structure. Orientation can be accomplished by cold drawing or stretching in fabrication.

oriented materials. Materials, particularly amorphous polymers and composites, whose molecules and/or macroconstituents are aligned in a specific way. Oriented materials are anisotropic. Orientation can generally be divided into two classes, uniaxial and biaxial.

orthotropic. Having three mutually perpendicular planes of elastic symmetry.

outgassing. Release of solvents and moisture from composite parts under vacuum. Also occurs during the normal curing process under vacuum.

out time. The time a prepreg is exposed to ambient temperature, namely, the total amount of time the prepreg is out of the freezer. The primary effects of out time are to decrease the drape and tack of the prepreg while also allowing it to absorb moisture from the air.

ovaloid. A surface of revolution symmetrical about the polar axis that forms the end closure for a filament-wound cylinder.

oven dry. The condition of a material that has been heated under prescribed conditions of temperature and humidity until there is no further significant change in its mass.

overlay sheet. A nonwoven fibrous mat (of glass, synthetic fiber, and so on) used as the top layer in a cloth or mat lay-up to provide a smoother finish, minimize the appearance of the fibrous pattern, or permit machining or grinding to a precise dimension. Also called surfacing mat.

oxidation. (1) In carbon/graphite fiber processing, the step of reacting the precursor polymer (rayon, PAN, or pitch) with oxygen, resulting in stabilization of the structure for the hot stretching operation. (2) In general use, oxidation refers to any chemical reaction in which electrons are transferred.

P

package. Yarn, roving, and so on in the form of units capable of being unwound and suitable for handling, storing, shipping, and use.

PAN. See *polyacrylonitrile*.

parallel laminate. (1) A laminate of woven fabric in which the plies are aligned in the same position as originally aligned in the fabric roll. (2) A series of flat or curved cloth-resin layers stacked uniformly on top of each other.

particulate composite. Material consisting of one or more constituents suspended in a matrix of another material. These particles are either metallic or nonmetallic.

particulate reinforced ceramic-matrix composite. A ceramic-matrix composite in which the reinforcing components are particles of equiaxed or platelet geometry (in contrast to whiskers or short fibers).

parting agent. See *mold-release agent*.

parting line. A mark on a molded piece where the sections of a mold have met in closing.

PAS. See *polyarylsulfone*.

PBI. See *polybenzimidazole*.

PC. See *polycarbonate*.

PEEK. See *polyether etherketone*.

peel ply. A layer of open-weave material, usually fiberglass or heat-set nylon, applied directly to the surface of a prepreg lay-up. The peel ply is removed from the cured laminate immediately before bonding operations, leaving a clean, resin-rich surface that needs no further preparation for bonding, other than application of a primer where one is required.

peel strength. Adhesive bond strength, as in pounds per inch of width, obtained by a stress applied in a peeling mode.

penetration. The entering of an adhesive into an adherend.

permanence. The property of a plastic that describes its resistance to appreciable changes in characteristics with time and environment.

permanent set. (1) The deformation remaining after a specimen has been stressed a prescribed amount in tension, compression, or shear for a definite time period and released for a definite time period. (2) For creep tests, the residual unrecoverable deformation after the load causing the creep has been removed for a substantial and definite period of time. (3) The increase in length, expressed as a percentage of the original length, by which an elastic material fails to return to original length after being stressed for a standard period of time.

permeability. The passage or diffusion (or rate of passage) of a gas, vapor, liquid, or solid through a barrier without physically or chemically affecting it.

pH. The measure of the acidity or alkalinity of a substance, neutrality being at pH 7. Acid solutions are less than 7, alkaline solutions are more than 7.

phenolic (phenolic resin). A thermosetting resin produced by the condensation of an aromatic alcohol with an aldehyde, particularly of phenol with formaldehyde. Used in high-temperature applications with various fillers and reinforcements.

phenylsilane resins. Thermosetting copolymers of silicone and phenolic resins. Furnished in solution form.

physical catalyst. Radiant energy capable of promoting or modifying a chemical reaction.

PI. See *polyimide*.

PIC. See *pressure-impregnation-carbonization*.

pick. An individual filling yarn, running the width of a woven fabric at right angles to the warp. Also called fill, woof, and weft.

pick count. The number of filling yarns per inch of woven fabric.

pin holes. Small cavities that penetrate the surface of a cured part.

pit. A small, regular or irregular crater in the surface of a plastic, usually of a width approximately the same order of magnitude as its depth.

pitch. A high molecular weight material left as a residue from the destructive distillation of coal and petroleum products. Pitches are used as base materials for the manufacture of certain high-modulus carbon fibers and as matrix precursors for carbon-carbon composites.

plain weave. A weaving pattern in which the warp and fill fibers alternate; that is, the repeat pattern is warp/fill/warp/fill, and so on. Both faces of a plain weave are identical. Properties are significantly reduced relative to a weaving pattern with fewer crossovers.

planar. Lying essentially in a single plane.

planar helix winding. A winding in which the filament path on each dome lies on a plane that intersects the dome, while a helical path over the cylindrical section is connected to the dome paths.

planar winding. A winding in which the filament path lies on a plane that intersects the winding surface. See also *polar winding*.

plastic. (1) A material that contains as an essential ingredient an organic polymer of large molecular weight, hardeners, fillers, reinforcements, and so on; is solid in its finished state; and, at some stage in its manufacture or its processing into finished articles, can be shaped by flow. (2) Made of plastic. A plastic may be either thermoplastic or thermoset.

plastic deformation. Change in dimensions of an object under load that is not recovered when the load is removed, as opposed to elastic deformation.

plastic flow. Deformation under the action of a sustained hot or cold force. Flow of semisolids in the molding of plastics.

plasticizer. (1) A material incorporated in a plastic to increase its workability and flexibility or distensibility. Normally used in thermoplastics. (2) A lower molecular weight material added to an epoxy to reduce stiffness and brittleness, thereby resulting in a lower glass transition temperature for the polymer.

plastic memory. The tendency of a thermoplastic material that has been stretched while hot to return to its unstretched shape upon being reheated.

platens. The mounting plates of a press, to which the entire mold assembly is bolted.

plied yarn. Yarn made by collecting two or more single yarns. Normally, the yarns are twisted together, though sometimes they are collected without twist.

ply. (1) In general, fabrics or felts consisting of one or more layers (laminates, and so on). (2) The layers that make up a stack. (3) Yarn resulting from twisting operations (three-ply yarn, and so on). (4) A single layer of prepreg. (5) A single pass in filament winding (two plies forming one layer).

PMMA. See *polymethyl methacrylate.*

PMR polyimides. A novel class of high-temperature-resistant polymers. PMR represents in situ polymerization of monomer reactants.

Poisson's ratio. (1) The ratio of the change in lateral width per unit width to change in axial length per unit length caused by the axial stretching or stressing of a material. (2) The ratio of transverse strain to the corresponding axial strain below the proportional limit.

polar boss. In filament winding, a metal end fitting located in the center of each dome that describes the pole about which winding bands are wrapped.

polar winding. A winding in which the filament path passes tangent to the polar opening at one end of the chamber and tangent to the opposite side of the polar opening at the other end. A one-circuit pattern is inherent in the system.

polyacrylonitrile (PAN). Used as a base material or precursor in the manufacture of certain carbon fibers.

polyamide. A thermoplastic polymer in which the structural units are linked by amide or thio-amide groupings (repeated nitrogen and hydrogen groupings). Many polyamides are fiber-forming.

polyamideimide. A polymer containing both amide (nylon) and imide (as in polyimide) groups; properties combine the benefits and disadvantages of both.

polyamide plastic. See *nylon plastics.*

polyarylsulfone (PAS). A high-temperature-resistant thermoplastic with T_g values ranging from 190 to 275 °C (375 to 525 °F). The term is also occasionally used to describe the family of resins that includes polysulfone and polyethersulfone.

polybenzimidazole (PBI). A condensation polymer of diphenyl isophthalate and 3,3′-diaminobenzidine. Extremely high-temperature resistant. Available as adhesive and fiber.

polycarbonate (PC). A thermoplastic polymer derived from the direct reaction between aromatic and aliphatic dihydroxy compounds with phosgene, or by the ester exchange reaction with appropriate phosgene-derived precursors. Highest impact resistance of any transparent plastic.

polycondensation. See *condensation polymerization.*

polyesters, thermoplastic. See *thermoplastic polyesters.*

polyesters, thermosetting. See *thermosetting polyesters.*

polyether etherketone (PEEK). A linear aromatic crystalline thermoplastic. A composite with a PEEK matrix may have a continuous-use temperature as high as 250 °C (480 °F).

polyetherimide. An amorphous polymer with good thermal properties, for a thermoplastic. Reported T_g of 215 °C (419 °F) and continuous-use temperature of about 170 °C (338 °F).

polyimide (PI). A polymer produced by reacting an aromatic dianhydride with an aromatic diamine. It is a highly heat-resistant resin ≥ 315 °C (600 °F). Similar to a polyamide, differing only in the number of hydrogen molecules contained in the groupings. Suitable for use as a binder or adhesive. May be either thermoplastic or thermoset.

polymer. A high molecular weight organic compound, natural or synthetic, whose structure can be represented by a repeated small unit, the mer, for example, polyethylene, rubber, and cellulose. Synthetic polymers are formed by addition or condensation polymerization of monomers. Some polymers are elastomers, some are plastics, and some are fibers. When two or more dissimilar monomers are involved, the product is called a copolymer. The chain lengths of commercial thermoplastics vary from near a thousand to over one hundred thousand repeating units. Thermosetting polymers approach infinity after curing, but their resin precursors, often called prepolymers, may be relatively short—6 to 100 repeating units—before curing. The lengths of polymer chains, usually measured by molecular weight, have very significant effects on the performance properties of plastics and profound effects on processibility.

polymerization. A chemical reaction in which the molecules of a monomer are linked together to form large molecules whose molecular weight is a multiple of that of the original substance. When two or more monomers are involved, the process is called copolymerization.

polymer matrix. The resin portion of a reinforced or filled plastic.

polymethyl methacrylate (PMMA). A thermoplastic polymer synthesized from methyl methacrylate. It is a transparent solid with exceptional optical properties; available in the form of sheets, granules, solutions, and emulsions. Used as facing material in certain composite constructions. See also *acrylic plastic.*

polyphenylene sulfide (PPS). A high temperature thermoplastic useful primarily as a molding compound. Optimal properties depend on slightly cross-linking the resin. Known for chemical resistance.

polypropylene. A tough, lightweight thermoplastic made by the polymerization of high-purity propylene gas in the presence of an organometallic catalyst at relatively low pressures and temperatures.

polysulfide. A synthetic polymer containing sulfur and carbon linkages, produced from organic dihalides and sodium polysulfide. Material is elastomeric in nature, resistant to light, oil, and solvents, and impermeable to gases.

polysulfone. A high-temperature-resistant thermoplastic polymer with the sulfone linkage, with a T_g of 190 °C (375 °F).

polyurethane. A thermosetting resin prepared by the reaction of diisocyanates with polyols, polyamides, alkyd polymers, and polyether polymers. See also *isocyanate plastics* and *urethane plastics.*

porosity. A condition of trapped pockets of air, gas, or vacuum within a solid material. Usually expressed as a percentage of the total nonsolid volume to the total volume (solid plus nonsolid) of a unit quantity of material.

postcure. Additional elevated-temperature cure, usually without pressure, to improve final properties and/or complete the cure, or decrease the percentage of volatiles in the compound. In certain resins, complete cure and ultimate mechanical properties are attained only by exposure of the cured resin to higher temperatures than those of curing.

postforming. The forming, bending, or shaping of fully cured, C-staged thermoset laminates that have been heated to make them flexible. On cooling, the formed laminate retains the contours and shape of the mold over which it has been formed.

pot life. The length of time that a catalyzed thermosetting resin system retains a viscosity low enough to be used in processing. Also called working life.

PPS. See *polyphenylene sulfide.*

precision. The closeness of agreement between the results of individual replicated measurements or tests. Precision may be expressed as the standard deviation of the data. Compare with *accuracy.*

precure. The full or partial setting of a synthetic resin or adhesive in a joint before the clamping operation is complete or before pressure is applied.

precursor. For carbon or graphite fiber, the rayon, PAN, or pitch fibers from which carbon and graphite fibers are derived.

prefit. A process for checking the fit of mating detail parts in an assembly prior to adhesive bonding, to ensure proper bond lines. Mechanically fastened structures are sometimes prefitted to establish shimming requirements.

preform. (1) A preshaped fibrous reinforcement formed by distribution of chopped fibers or cloth by air, water flotation, or vacuum over the surface of a perforated screen to the approximate contour and thickness desired in the finished part. (2) A preshaped fibrous reinforcement of mat or cloth formed to the desired shape on a mandrel or mock-up before being placed in a mold press.

preform binder. A resin applied to the chopped strands of a preform, usually during its formation, and cured so that the preform will retain its shape and can be handled.

pregel. An unintentional, extra layer of cured resin on part of the surface of a reinforced plastic. Not related to gel coat.

preheating. The heating of a compound before molding or casting, to facilitate the operation or reduce the molding cycle.

preimpregnation. The practice of mixing resin and reinforcement and effecting partial cure before use or shipment to the user. See also *prepreg.*

premix. A molding compound prepared prior to and apart from the molding operations and containing all components required for molding: Resin, reinforcement, fillers, catalysts, release agents, and other ingredients.

premolding. The lay-up and partial cure at an intermediate cure temperature of a laminated or chopped-fiber detail part to stabilize its configuration for handling and assembly with other parts for final cure.

preply. A composite material lamina in the raw-material stage, ready to be fabricated into a finished laminate. The lamina is usually combined with other raw laminae before fabrication. A preply includes a fiber system that is placed in position relative to all or part of the required matrix material to constitute the finished lamina. An organic matrix preply is called a prepreg. Metal-matrix preplies include green tape, flame-sprayed tape, and consolidated monolayers.

prepolymer. A chemical intermediate whose molecular weight is between that of the monomer or monomers and the final polymer or resin.

prepreg. Either ready-to-mold material in sheet form or ready-to-wind material in roving form, which may be cloth, mat, unidirectional fiber, or paper impregnated with resin and stored for use. The resin is partially cured to a B-stage and supplied to the fabricator, who lays up the finished shape and completes the cure with heat and pressure. The two distinct types of prepreg available are (1) commercial prepregs, where the roving is coated with a hot melt or solvent system to produce a specific product to meet specific customer requirements; and (2) wet prepreg, where the basic resin is installed without solvents or preservatives but has limited room-temperature shelf life.

press clave. A simulated autoclave made by using the platens of a press to seal the ends of an open chamber, providing both the force required to prevent loss of the pressurizing medium and the heat required to cure the laminate inside.

pressure bag molding. A process for molding reinforced plastics in which a tailored, flexible bag is placed over the contact lay-up on the mold, sealed, and clamped in place. Fluid pressure, usually provided by compressed air or water, is placed against the bag, and the part is cured.

pressure-impregnation-carbonization (PIC). A densification process for carbon-carbon composites involving pitch impregnation and carbonization under high temperature and isostatic pressure conditions. This process is carried out in hot isostatic press (HIP) equipment.

pressure intensifier. A layer of flexible material (usually a high-temperature rubber) used to ensure the application of sufficient pressure to a location, such as a radius, in a lay-up being cured.

pressure-sensitive adhesive. A viscoelastic material that, in solvent-free form, remains permanently tacky. Such material will adhere instantaneously to most solid surfaces with the application of very light pressure.

primer. A coating applied to a surface, before the application of an adhesive, lacquer, enamel, and so on, to improve the adhesion performance or load-carrying ability of the bond.

processing window. The range of processing conditions, such as stock (melt) temperature, pressure, shear rate, and so on, within which a particular grade of plastic can be fabricated with optimal or acceptable properties by a particular fabricating process, such as extrusion, injection molding, sheet molding, and so on. The processing window for a particular plastic can vary significantly with design of the part and the mold, with the fabricating machinery used, and with the severity of the end-use stresses.

promoter. A chemical, itself a feeble catalyst, that greatly increases the activity of a given catalyst. See also *accelerator.*

proof. To test a component or system at its peak operating load or pressure.

proof pressure. The test pressure that pressurized components shall sustain without detrimental deformation or damage. The proof pressure test is used to give evidence of satisfactory workmanship and material quality.

proportional limit. The maximum stress that a material is capable of sustaining without deviation from proportionality of stress and strain (Hooke's law). It is expressed in force per unit area. See also *elastic limit.*

prototype. A model suitable for use in complete evaluation of form, design, performance, and material processing.

puckers. Areas on prepreg materials where material has locally blistered from the separator film or release paper.

pulp molding. The process by which a resin-impregnated pulp material is preformed by application of a vacuum and subsequently is oven cured or molded.

pultrusion. A continuous process for manufacturing composites that have a constant cross-sectional shape. The process consists of pulling a fiber-reinforcing material through a resin impregnation bath and through a shaping die, where the resin is subsequently cured.

pyrolysis. With respect to fibers, the thermal process by which organic precursor fiber materials, such as rayon, polyacrylonitrile (PAN), and pitch, are chemically changed into carbon fiber by the action of heat in an inert atmosphere. Pyrolysis temperatures can range from 800 to 2800 °C (1470 to 5070 °F), depending on the precursor. Higher processing graphitization temperatures of 1900 to 3000 °C (3450 to 5430 °F) generally lead to higher modulus carbon fibers, usually referred to as graphite fibers. During the pyrolysis process, molecules containing oxygen, hydrogen, and nitrogen are driven from the precursor fiber, leaving continuous chains of carbon.

Q

quasi-isotropic laminate. A laminate approximating isotropy by orientation of plies in several or more directions.

R

random pattern. A winding with no fixed pattern. If a large number of circuits is required for the pattern to repeat, a random pattern is approached. A winding in which the filaments do not lie in an even pattern.

reaction injection molding (RIM). A process for molding polyurethane, epoxy, and other liquid chemical systems. Mixing of two to four components in the proper chemical ratio is accomplished by a high-pressure impingement-type mixing head, from which the mixed material is delivered into the mold at low pressure, where it reacts (cures). Also known as structural reaction injection molding.

reinforced plastics. Molded, formed, filament-wound, tape-wrapped, or shaped plastic parts consisting of resins to which reinforcing fibers, mats, fabrics, and so on, have been added before the forming operation to provide some strength properties greatly superior to those of the base resin.

reinforced reaction injection molding (RRIM). A reaction injection molding with a reinforcement added. See also *reaction injection molding.*

reinforcement. A strong material bonded into a matrix to improve its mechanical properties. Reinforcements are usually long fibers, chopped fibers, whiskers, particulates, and so on. The term should not be used synonymously with filler.

relaxation time. The time required for a stress under a sustained constant strain to diminish by a stated fraction of its initial value.

relaxed stress. The initial stress minus the remaining stress at a given time during a stress-relaxation test.

release agent. A material that is applied in a thin film to the surface of a mold to keep the resin from bonding to the mold. Also called parting agent. See also *mold-release agent.*

release film. An impermeable layer of film that does not bond to the resin being cured. See also *separator.*

release paper. A sheet, serving as a protectant or carrier, or both, for an adhesive film or mass, which is easily removed from the film or mass prior to use.
residual strain. The strain associated with residual stress.
residual stress. The stress existing in a body at rest, in equilibrium, at uniform temperature, and not subjected to external forces. Often caused by the forming and curing process.
resilience. (1) The ratio of energy returned, on recovery from deformation, to the work input required to produce the deformation (usually expressed as a percentage). (2) The ability to regain an original shape quickly after being strained or distorted.
resin. A solid or pseudosolid organic material, usually of high molecular weight, that exhibits a tendency to flow when subjected to stress. It usually has a softening or melting range, and fractures conchoidally. Most resins are polymers. In reinforced plastics, the material used to bind together the reinforcement material; the matrix. See also *polymer.*
resin content. The amount of resin in a laminate expressed as either a percentage of total weight or total volume.
resin film infusion (RFI). A variant of the resin transfer molding process in which a layer of solid resin film is placed along with a dry preform in a matched die. During the autoclave cure cycle, the resin film melts and flows to impregnate the dry preform.
resinoid. Any class of thermosetting synthetic resins, either in their initial temporarily fusible state or in their final infusible state.
resin pocket. An apparent accumulation of excess resin in a small, localized section visible on cut edges of molded surfaces, or internal to the structure and nonvisible. See also *resin-rich area.*
resin-rich area. Localized area filled with resin and lacking reinforcing material. See also *resin pocket.*
resin-starved area. Localized area of insufficient resin, usually identified by low gloss, dry spots, or fiber showing on the surface.
resin system. A mixture of resin and ingredients such as catalyst, initiator, diluents, and so on, required for the intended processing and final product.
resin transfer molding (RTM). A process whereby catalyzed resin is transferred or injected into an enclosed mold in which the fiberglass reinforcement has been placed. See also *resin film infusion* and *vacuum-assisted resin transfer molding.*
resistivity. The ability of a material to resist passage of electrical current either through its bulk or on a surface.
resite. See preferred term *C-stage.*
resitol. See preferred term *B-stage.*
resole. See preferred term *A-stage.*
reverse helical winding. In filament winding, as the fiber delivery arm traverses one circuit, a continuous helix is laid down, reversing direction at the polar ends, in contrast to biaxial, compact, or sequential winding. The fibers cross each other at definite equators, the number depending on the helix. The minimum region of crossover is three.
reverse impact test. A test in which one side of a sheet of material is struck by a pendulum or falling object, and the reverse side is inspected for damage.
RFI. See *resin film infusion.*
rheology. The study of the flow of materials, particularly plastic flow of solids and the flow of non-Newtonian liquids. The science treating the deformation and flow of matter.
rib. A reinforcing member designed into a plastic part to provide lateral, horizontal, hoop, or other structural support.
RIM. See *reaction injection molding.*
rise time. In urethane foam molding, the time between the pouring of the urethane mix and the completion of foaming.
Rockwell hardness. A value derived from the increase in depth of an impression as the load on an indenter is increased from a fixed minimum value to a higher value and then returned to the minimum value. Indenters for the Rockwell test include steel balls of several specific diameters and a diamond cone penetrator having an included angle of 120° with a spherical tip having a radius of 0.2 mm (0.0070 in.). Rockwell hardness numbers are always quoted with a prefix representing the Rockwell scale corresponding to a given combination of load and indenter, for example, HRC 30.
room-temperature curing adhesive. An adhesive that sets (to handling strength) within an hour at temperatures from 20 to 30 °C (68 to 86 °F) and later reaches full strength without heating.
room-temperature vulcanizing (RTV). Vulcanization or curing at room temperature by chemical reaction; usually applies to silicones and other rubbers.
roving. A number of yarns, strands, tows, or ends collected into a parallel bundle with little or no twist.
roving ball. The supply package offered to the winder, consisting of a number of ends or strands wound to a given outside diameter onto a length of cardboard tube. Usually designated by either fiber weight or length in yards.
roving cloth. A textile fabric, coarse in nature, woven from rovings.
***R*-ratio (*R*-factor).** In cyclic fatigue testing, the ratio of applied minimum stress to maximum stress. When $R = -1$, the cycle is equally compressive and tensile.
RRIM. See *reinforced reaction injection molding.*
RTM. See *resin transfer molding.*
RTV. See *room-temperature vulcanizing.*
rubber. Cross-linked polymers having glass transition temperature below room temperature that exhibit highly elastic deformation and have high elongation.
rule of mixtures. When two materials are mixed together, it is normally the case that the properties of the mixture are an average of the properties of the constituents according to the proportion of each in the mixture. This applies, for example, to particulate reinforced composites and fillers in resins.
rupture. (1) A cleavage or break resulting from physical stress. (2) Work of rupture. (3) The integral of the stress-strain curve between the origin and the point of rupture.

S

safe life. See *fatigue life.*
sandwich construction. Panels composed of a lightweight core material, such as honeycomb, foamed plastic, and so on, to which two relatively thin, dense, high-strength or high-stiffness faces or skins are adhered.
satin. A type of finish having a satin or velvety appearance, specified for plastics or composites.
satin weave. See *harness satin.*
S-basis. The S-basis property allowable is the minimum value specified by the appropriate federal, military, SAE, ASTM, or other recognized and approved specifications for the material.
SBS. See *short beam shear.*
scarf joint. A joint made by cutting away similar angular segments on two adherends and bonding the adherends with the cut areas fitted together. See also *lap joint.*
scrim. A low-cost reinforcing fabric made from continuous filament yarn in an open-mesh construction. Used in the processing of tape or other B-stage material to facilitate handling. Also used as a carrier of adhesive, to be used in secondary bonding.
sealant. A material applied to a joint in paste or liquid form that hardens or cures in place, forming a seal against gas or liquid entry.
secant modulus. Idealized Young's modulus derived from a secant drawn between the origin and any point on a nonlinear stress-strain curve. On materials whose modulus changes with stress, the secant modulus is the average of the zero applied stress point and the maximum stress point being considered. See also *tangent modulus.*
secondary bonding. The joining together, by the process of adhesive bonding, of two or more already cured composite parts, during which the only chemical or thermal reaction occurring is the curing of the adhesive itself.
secondary structure. In aircraft and aerospace applications, a structure that is not critical to flight safety.
self-extinguishing resin. A resin formulation that will burn in the presence of a flame but will extinguish itself within a specified time after the flame is removed.
self-skinning foam. A urethane foam that produces a tough outer surface over a foam core upon curing.

selvage. The woven-edge portion of a fabric parallel to the warp.

semicrystalline. In plastics, materials that exhibit localized crystallinity. See also *crystalline plastic.*

separator. A permeable layer that also acts as a release film. Porous Teflon-coated fiberglass is an example. Often placed between lay-up and bleeder to facilitate bleeder system removal from laminate after cure.

set. (1) The irrecoverable or permanent deformation or creep after complete release of the force producing the deformation. (2) To convert an adhesive into a fixed or hardened state by chemical or physical action, such as condensation, polymerization, oxidation, vulcanization, gelation, hydration, or evaporation of volatile constituents.

set up. To harden, as in curing of a polymer resin.

S-glass. A magnesium aluminosilicate composition that is especially designed to provide very high tensile strength glass filaments. S-glass and S-2 glass fibers have the same glass composition but different finishes (coatings). S-glass is made to more demanding specifications, and S-2 is considered the commercial grade.

shear. (1) An action or stress resulting from applied forces that causes or tends to cause two contiguous parts of a body to slide relative to each other in a direction parallel to their plane of contact. (2) In interlaminar shear, the plane of contact is composed primarily of resin. See also *shear strength* and *shear stress.*

shear compliance. See *compliance.*

shear edge. The cutoff edge of the mold.

shear modulus. The ratio of shearing stress to shearing strain within the proportional limit of the material.

shear strain. The tangent of the angular change, caused by a force between two lines originally perpendicular to each other through a point in a body. Also called angular strain.

shear strength. The maximum shear stress that a material is capable of sustaining. Shear strength is calculated from the maximum load during a shear or torsion test and is based on the original cross-sectional area of the specimen.

shear stress. The component of stress tangent to the plane on which the forces act.

sheet molding compound (SMC). A composite of fibers, usually a polyester resin, and pigments, fillers, and other additives that have been compounded and processed into sheet form to facilitate handling in the molding operation.

shelf life. The length of time a material, substance, product, or reagent can be stored under specified environmental conditions and continue to meet all applicable specification requirements and/or remain suitable for its intended function.

shell tooling. A mold or bonding fixture consisting of a contoured surface shell supported by a substructure to provide dimensional stability.

shoe. A device for gathering filaments into a strand, in glass fiber forming.

Shore hardness. A measure of the resistance of material to indentation by a spring-loaded indenter. The higher the number, the greater the resistance. Normally used for rubber materials.

short beam shear (SBS). A flexural test of a specimen having a low test span-to-thickness ratio (for example, 4:1), such that failure is primarily in shear.

short shot. Injection of insufficient material to fill the mold.

shot capacity. The maximum weight of material an injection machine can provide from one forward motion of the ram, screw, or plunger.

shrinkage. The relative change in dimension from the length measured on the mold when it is cold to the length of the molded object 24 h after it has been taken out of the mold.

silicon carbide. Reinforcement, in whisker, particulate, and fine or large fiber, that has application as metal-matrix reinforcement because of its high strength and modulus, density equal to that of aluminum, and comparatively low cost. As a whisker or particulate, it gives the composite isotropic properties.

silicone plastics. Plastics based on resins in which the main polymer chain consists of alternating silicon and oxygen atoms, with carbon-containing side groups. Derived from silica (sand) and methyl chlorides and furnished in different molecular weights, including liquids and solid resins and elastomers.

single-circuit winding. A winding in which the filament path makes a complete traverse of the chamber, after which the following traverse lies immediately adjacent to the previous one.

sink mark. A shallow depression or dimple on the surface of an injection-molded part due to collapsing of the surface following local internal shrinkage after the gate seals. An incipient short shot.

sintering. The bonding of powders by solid-state diffusion, resulting in the absence of a separate bonding phase. The process is generally accompanied by an increase in strength, ductility, and, occasionally, density.

size. Any treatment consisting of starch, gelatin, oil, wax, or other suitable ingredient applied to yarn or fibers at the time of formation to protect the surface and aid the process of handling and fabrication or to control the fiber characteristics. The treatment contains ingredients that provide surface lubricity and binding action, but unlike a finish, contains no coupling agent. Before final fabrication into a composite, the size is usually removed by heat cleaning, and a finish is applied.

sizing content. The percent of the total strand weight made up by the sizing; usually determined by burning off or dissolving the organic sizing; known as *loss on ignition.*

skein. A continuous filament, strand, yarn, or roving, wound up to some measurable length and usually used to measure various physical properties.

skin. The relatively dense material that may form the surface of a cellular plastic or of a sandwich.

skirt. The extension of a motorcase from the tangency plane, used for interstage connections, usually wound or laid up as an integral part of the case.

slenderness ratio. The unsupported effective length of a uniform column divided by the least radius of gyration of the cross-sectional area.

slip. The relative collinear displacement of the adherends on either side of the adhesive layer in the direction of the applied load.

slip angle. The angle at which a tensioned fiber will slide off a filament-wound dome. If the difference between the wind angle and the geodesic angle is less than the slip angle, fiber will not slide off the dome. Slip angles for different fiber-resin systems vary and must be determined experimentally.

slippage. Undesired movement of the adherends with respect to one another during the bonding process.

sliver. A number of staple or continuous-filament fibers aligned in a continuous strand without twist. Pronounced "slyver." See also *strand.*

slurry preforming. Method of preparing reinforced plastic preforms by wet processing techniques similar to those used in the pulp molding industry. For example, glass fibers suspended in water are passed through a screen that passes the water but retains the fibers in the form of a mat.

SMC. See *sheet molding compound.*

***S-N* diagram.** (1) A plot of stress (*S*) against the number of cycles to failure (*N*) in fatigue testing. A log scale is normally used for *N*. For *S*, a linear scale is often used, but sometimes a log scale is used here, too. (2) A representation of the number of alternating stress cycles a material can sustain without failure at various maximum stresses.

softening range. The range of temperatures in which a plastic changes from a rigid to a soft state. Actual values will depend on the test method. Sometimes erroneously referred to as softening point.

solvation. The process of swelling, gelling, or dissolving a resin by a solvent or plasticizer.

specific gravity. The density (mass per unit volume) of any material divided by that of water at a standard temperature.

specific heat. The quantity of heat required to raise the temperature of a unit mass of a substance 1° under specified conditions.

specific properties. Material properties divided by the material density.

SPF. See *superplastic forming.*

splay. A fanlike surface defect near the gate on a part.

splice. The joining of two ends of glass fiber yarn or strand, usually by means of an air-drying adhesive.

sprayed-metal molds. Molds made by spraying molten metal onto a master until a shell of predetermined thickness is achieved. The shell is then removed and backed up with plaster, cement, casting resin, or other suitable material. Used primarily as a mold in the sheet-forming process.

spray-up. Technique in which a spray gun is used as an applicator tool. In reinforced plastics, for example, fibrous glass and resin can be simultaneously deposited in a mold. In essence, roving is fed through a chopper and ejected into a resin stream that is directed at the mold by either of two spray systems. In foamed plastics, fast-reacting urethane foams or epoxy foams are fed in liquid streams to the gun and sprayed on the surface. On contact, the liquid starts to foam.

spread. The quantity of adhesive per unit joint area applied to an adherend, usually expressed in pounds of adhesive per thousand square feet of joint area.

spring constant. The number of pounds required to compress a spring or specimen 25 mm (1 in.) in a prescribed test procedure.

sprue. A single hole through which thermoset molding compounds are injected directly into the mold cavity.

spun roving. A heavy, low-cost glass or aramid fiber strand consisting of filaments that are continuous but doubled back on themselves.

stabilization. In carbon fiber forming, the process used to render the carbon fiber precursor infusible prior to carbonization.

stabilized core. Honeycomb cores in which the cells have been filled with a specified reinforcing material.

stacking sequence. A description of a laminate that details the ply orientations and their sequence in the laminate.

staging. Heating a premixed resin system, such as in a prepreg, until the chemical reaction (curing) starts, but stopping the reaction before the gel point is reached. Staging is often used to reduce resin flow in subsequent press molding operations.

staple fibers. Fibers of spinnable length manufactured directly or by cutting continuous filaments to short lengths (usually 12.7 to 50 mm, or 1/2 to 2 in. long; 1 to 5 denier).

starved area. An area in a plastic part that has an insufficient amount of resin to wet out the reinforcement completely. This condition may be due to improper wetting, impregnation, or resin flow; excessive molding pressure; or improper bleeder cloth thickness.

starved joint. An adhesive joint that has been deprived of the proper film thickness of adhesive due to insufficient adhesive spreading or to the application of excessive pressure during the lamination process.

static fatigue. Failure of a part under continued static load. Analogous to creep rupture failure in metals testing, but often the result of aging accelerated by stress.

static modulus. The ratio of stress to strain under static conditions. It is calculated from static stress-strain tests, in shear, compression, or tension. Expressed in force per unit area.

static stress. A stress in which the force is constant or slowly increasing with time, for example, test to failure without shock.

stiffness. (1) A measure of modulus. (2) The relationship of load and deformation. (3) The ratio between the applied stress and resulting strain. (4) A term often used when the relationship of stress to strain does not conform to the definition of Young's modulus. See also *stress-strain.*

stitching. A method of three-dimensional (translaminar) reinforcement in which a needle is used to insert a reinforcing thread (usually aramid or glass) through a two-dimensional laminate. Both dry preforms and prepreg laminates have been stitched.

stops. Metal pieces inserted between die halves. Used to control the thickness of a press-molded part. Not a recommended practice, because the resin will receive less pressure, which can result in voids.

storage life. The period of time during which a liquid resin, packaged adhesive, or prepreg can be stored under specified temperature conditions and remain suitable for use. Also called shelf life.

storage modulus. A quantitative measure of elastic properties in polymers, defined as the ratio of the stress, in phase with the strain, to the magnitude of the strain. The storage modulus may be measured in tension, flexure, compression, or shear.

strain. Elastic deformation due to stress. Measured as the change in length per unit of length in a given direction, and expressed in percentage or mm/mm (in./in.).

strain, axial. See *axial strain.*

strain gage. Device to measure strain in a stressed material based on the change in electrical resistance.

strain, initial. See *initial strain.*

strain relaxation. Reduction in internal strain over time. Similar molecular processes occur as in creep, except that the body is constrained.

strain, residual. See *residual strain.*

strain, shear. See *shear strain.*

strain, transverse. See *transverse strain.*

strain, true. See *true strain.*

strand. Normally an untwisted bundle or assembly of continuous filaments used as a unit, including slivers, tows, ends, yarn, and so on. Sometimes a single fiber or filament is called a strand.

strand count. The number of strands in a plied yarn. The number of strands in a roving.

strand integrity. The degree to which the individual filaments making up the strand or end are held together by the applied sizing.

strand tensile test. A tensile test of a single resin-impregnated strand of any fiber.

strength, compressive. See *compressive strength.*

strength, flexural. See *flexural strength.*

strength, shear. See *shear strength.*

strength, tensile. See *tensile strength.*

strength, wet. See *wet strength.*

strength, yield. See *yield strength.*

stress. The internal force per unit area that resists a change in size or shape of a body. Expressed in force per unit area.

stress concentration. On a macromechanical level, the magnification of the level of an applied stress in the region of a notch, void, hole, or inclusion.

stress-concentration factor. The ratio of the maximum stress in the region of a stress concentrator, such as a hole, to the stress in a similar strained area without a stress concentrator.

stress corrosion. Preferential attack of areas under stress in a corrosive environment, where such an environment alone would not have caused corrosion.

stress crack. External or internal cracks in a plastic caused by tensile stresses less than that of its short-time mechanical strength, frequently accelerated by the environment to which the plastic is exposed. The stresses that cause cracking may be present internally or externally or may be combinations of these stresses. See also *crazing.*

stress cracking. The failure of a material by cracking or crazing some time after it has been placed under load. Time-to-failure may range from minutes to years. Causes include molded-in stresses, postfabrication shrinkage or warpage, and hostile environment.

stress, fracture. See *fracture stress.*

stress, initial (instantaneous). See *initial (instantaneous) stress.*

stress, nominal. See *nominal stress.*

stress, normal. See *normal stress.*

stress relaxation. The decrease in stress under sustained, constant strain. Also called stress decay.

stress, relaxed. See *relaxed stress.*

stress, residual. See *residual stress.*

stress, shear. See *shear stress.*

stress-strain. Stiffness at a given strain.

stress-strain curve. Simultaneous readings of load and deformation, converted to stress and strain, plotted as ordinates and abscissae, respectively, to obtain a stress-strain diagram.

stress, tensile. See *tensile stress.*

stress, torsional. See *torsional stress.*

stress, true. See *true stress.*

structural adhesive. Adhesive used for transferring required loads between adherends exposed to service environments typical for the structure involved.

structural bond. A bond that joins basic load-bearing parts of an assembly. The load may be either static or dynamic.

structural reaction injection molding. See *reaction injection molding.*

structural sandwich construction. A laminar construction comprising a combination of alternating dissimilar simple or composite materials assembled and intimately fixed in relation to each other so as to use the properties of each to attain specific structural advantages for the whole assembly.

superplastic forming (SPF). A strain rate sensitive metal forming process that uses characteristics of materials exhibiting high elongation-to-failure.

surface preparation. Physical and/or chemical preparation of an adherend to make it suitable for adhesive bonding.

surface treatment. A material (size or finish) applied to fibrous material during the forming operation or in subsequent processes. For carbon fiber surface treatment, the process used to enhance bonding capability of fiber to resin.

surfacing mat. A very thin mat, usually 180 to 510 μm (7 to 20 mil) thick, of highly filamentized fiberglass, used primarily to produce a smooth surface on a reinforced plastic laminate, or for precise machining or grinding.

symmetrical laminate. A composite laminate in which the sequence of plies below the laminate midplane is a mirror image of the stacking sequence above the midplane.

syntactic foams. Composites made by mixing hollow microspheres of glass, epoxy, phenolic, and so on, into fluid resins (with additives and curing agents) to form a moldable, curable, lightweight, fluid mass, as opposed to foamed plastic, in which the cells are formed by gas bubbles released in the liquid plastic by either chemical or mechanical action.

synthetic resin. A complex, substantially amorphous, organic semisolid or solid material (usually a mixture) built up by chemical reaction of comparatively simple compounds, approximating the natural resins in luster, fracture, comparative brittleness, insolubility in water, fusibility or plasticity, and some degree of rubberlike extensibility, but commonly deviating widely from natural resins in chemical constitution and behavior with reagents.

T

tabs. Extra lengths of composite or other material at the ends of a tensile specimen to promote failure away from the grips.

tack. Stickiness of an adhesive or filament-reinforced resin prepreg material.

tack range. The period of time in which an adhesive will remain in the tacky-dry condition after application to the adherend, and under specified conditions of temperature and humidity.

tangent modulus. The slope of the line at a predefined point on a static stress-strain curve, expressed in force per unit area per unit strain. This is the tangent modulus at that point in shear, tension, or compression, as the case may be. See also *secant modulus.*

tape. Unidirectional prepreg fabricated in widths up to 305 mm (12 in.) for carbon and 75 mm (3 in.) for boron. Woven broad goods carbon and glass tapes up to 1250 or 1500 mm (50 or 60 in.) wide are available commercially.

tape wrapped. Fabric tape is heated and wrapped onto a rotating mandrel and subsequently cooled to firm the surface for the next tape layer application.

Tedlar. Trade name (E.I. DuPont de Nemours & Co., Inc., Wilmington, DE) for polyvinylfluoride (PVF) used as a waterproof film on some composites.

template. A pattern used as a guide for cutting and laying plies.

tenacity. The term generally used in yarn manufacture and textile engineering to denote the strength of a yarn or of a filament of a given size. Numerically, it is the grams of breaking force per denier unit of yarn or filament size. Grams per denier is expressed as gpd.

tensile compliance. See *compliance.*

tensile modulus. See *Young's modulus.*

tensile strength. The maximum load or force per unit cross-sectional area, within the gage length, of the specimen. The pulling stress required to break a given specimen.

tensile strength, ultimate. See *ultimate tensile strength.*

tensile stress. The normal stress caused by forces directed away from the plane on which they act.

tenth-scale vessel. A filament-wound material test vessel based on a one-tenth subscale of the prototype.

terpolymer. A polymeric system that contains three monomeric units.

tex. A unit for expressing linear density equal to the mass or weight in grams of 1000 meters of filament, fiber, yarn, or other textile strand.

textile fibers. Fibers or filaments that can be processed into yarn or made into a fabric by interlacing in a variety of methods, including weaving, knitting, and braiding.

T_g. See *glass transition temperature.*

TGA. See *thermogravimetric analysis.*

thermal conductivity. (1) Ability of a material to conduct heat. (2) The physical constant for the quantity of heat that passes through a unit cube of a substance in unit time when the difference in temperature of two faces is 1°.

thermal endurance. The time at a selected temperature for a material or system of materials to deteriorate to some predetermined level of electrical, mechanical, or chemical performance under prescribed conditions of test.

thermal expansion molding. A process in which elastomeric tooling details are constrained within a rigid frame to generate consolidation pressure by thermal expansion during the curing cycle of the autoclave molding process.

thermal stress cracking. Crazing and cracking of some thermoplastic resins, resulting from overexposure to elevated temperatures. See also *stress cracking.*

thermoforming. Forming a thermoplastic material after heating it to the point where it is soft enough to be formed without cracking or breaking reinforcing fibers.

thermogravimetric analysis (TGA). The study of the mass of a material under various conditions of temperature and pressure.

thermoplastic. Capable of being repeatedly softened by an increase of temperature and hardened by a decrease in temperature. Applicable to those materials whose change upon heating is substantially physical rather than chemical and that in the softened stage can be shaped by flow into articles by molding or extrusion.

thermoplastic polyesters. A class of thermoplastic polymers in which the repeating units are joined by ester groups. The two important types are (1) polyethylene terephthalate (PET), which is widely used as film, fiber, and soda bottles; and (2) polybutylene terephthalate (PBT), primarily a molding compound.

thermoset. A plastic that, when cured by application of heat or chemical means, changes into a substantially infusible and insoluble material.

thermosetting polyesters. A class of resins produced by dissolving unsaturated, generally linear, alkyd resins in a vinyl-type active monomer such as styrene, methyl styrene, or diallyl phthalate. Cure is effected through vinyl polymerization using peroxide catalysts and promoters or heat to accelerate the reaction. The two important commercial types are (1) liquid resins that are cross linked with styrene and used either as impregnants for glass or carbon-fiber reinforcements in laminates, filament-wound structures, and other built-up constructions, or as binders for chopped-fiber reinforcements in molding compounds, such as sheet molding compound (SMC), bulk molding compound (BMC), and thick molding compound (TMC); and (2) liquid or solid resins cross linked with other esters in chopped-fiber and mineral-filled molding compounds, for example, alkyd and diallyl phthalate.

thick adherend test. A test method for film adhesives using thick metallic adherends that allows the true shear stress, strain, and modulus of the adhesive to be determined for stress analysis of bonded joints.

thixotropic (thixotropy). Concerning materials that are gel-like at rest but fluid when agitated. Having high static shear strength and low dynamic shear strength at the same time. To lose viscosity under stress.

thread. See *fiber.*

thread count. The number of yarns (threads) per inch in either the lengthwise (warp) or crosswise (fill or weft) direction of woven fabrics.

tolerance. The specified permissible deviation from the specified nominal value of a component characteristic at standard or stated environmental conditions.

tooling resin. Resins that have applications as tooling aids, coreboxes, prototypes, hammer forms, stretch forms, foundry patterns, and so on. Epoxy and silicone are common examples.

tool side. The side of the part that is cured against the tool (mold or mandrel).

torsion. Twisting stress.

torsional stress. The shear stress on a transverse cross section caused by a twisting action.

toughness. A measure of the ability of a material to absorb work, or the actual work per unit volume or unit mass of material that is required to rupture it. Toughness is proportional to the area under the load-elongation curve from the origin to the breaking point.

tow. An untwisted bundle of continuous filaments. Commonly used in referring to man-made fibers, particularly carbon and graphite, but also glass and aramid. A tow designated at 140K has 140,000 filaments.

towpreg. A tow of fibers that has been preimpregnated with a resin and is typically used in either filament winding or fiber placement operations.

TPI. See *turns per inch.*

tracer. A fiber, tow, or yarn added to a prepreg for verifying fiber alignment and, in the case of woven materials, for distinguishing warp fibers from fill fibers.

transfer molding. Method of molding thermosetting materials in which the plastic is first softened by heat and pressure in a transfer chamber and then forced by high pressure through suitable sprues, runners, and gates into the closed mold for final shaping and curing.

transition, first order. See *first-order transition.*

transition temperature. The temperature at which the properties of a material change. Depending on the material, the transition change may or may not be reversible.

transversely isotropic. Term describing a material exhibiting a special case of orthotropy in which properties are identical in two orthotropic dimensions but not the third. Having identical properties in both transverse directions but not in the longitudinal direction.

transverse strain. The linear strain in a plane perpendicular to the loading axis of a specimen.

true strain. The natural logarithm of the ratio of gage length at the moment of observation to the original gage length for a body subjected to an axial force.

true stress. The stress along the axis calculated on the actual cross section at the time of observation instead of the original cross-sectional area. Applicable to tension and compression testing.

turns per inch (TPI). A measure of the amount of twist produced in a yarn, tow, or roving during its processing history. Also, the lead rate of a hoop layer at a specified band width. See also *twist.*

twist. The spiral turns about its axis per unit of length in a yarn or other textile strand. Twist may be expressed as turns per inch (TPI), and so forth. *S* and *Z* refer to direction of twist, in reference to whether the twist direction conforms to the middle-section slope of the particular letter.

twist, balanced. See *balanced twist.*

typical-basis. The typical property value is an average value. No statistical assurance is associated with this basis.

U

ultimate elongation. The elongation at rupture.

ultimate tensile strength. The ultimate or final (highest) stress sustained by a specimen in a tension test. Rupture and ultimate stress may or may not be the same.

ultrasonic testing. A nondestructive test applied to materials for the purpose of locating internal flaws or structural discontinuities by the use of high-frequency reflection or attenuation (ultrasonic beam).

ultraviolet (UV). Zone of invisible radiations beyond the violet end of the spectrum of visible radiations. Since UV wavelengths are shorter than visible wavelengths, their photons have more energy, enough to initiate some chemical reactions and to degrade most plastics, particularly aramids.

ultraviolet (UV) stabilizer. Any chemical compound that, when admixed with a thermoplastic resin, selectively absorbs UV rays.

unbond. An area within a bonded interface between two adherends in which the intended bonding action failed to take place, or where two layers of prepreg in a cured component do not adhere to each other. Also used to denote specific areas deliberately prevented from bonding in order to simulate a defective bond, such as in the generation of quality standards specimens.

undercure. A condition of the molded article resulting from the allowance of too little time and/or temperature or pressure for adequate hardening of the molding.

undercut. A protuberance or indentation that impedes the withdrawal of a molded part from a two-piece, rigid mold. Any such protuberance or indentation, depending on the design of the mold.

uniaxial load. A condition whereby a material is stressed in only one direction along the axis or centerline of component parts.

unidirectional laminate. A reinforced plastic laminate in which substantially all of the fibers are oriented in the same direction.

unsaturated compounds. Any compound having more than one bond between two adjacent atoms, usually carbon atoms, and capable of adding other atoms at that point to reduce it to a single bond.

unsymmetric laminate. A laminate having an arbitrary stacking sequence without midplane symmetry.

urethane plastics. Plastics based on resins made by condensation of organic isocyanates with compounds or resins that contain hydroxyl groups. The resin is furnished as two component liquid monomers or prepolymers that are mixed in the field immediately before application. A great variety of materials are available, depending upon the monomers used in the prepolymers, polyols, and the type of diisocyanate employed. Extremely abrasion and impact resistant. See also *isocyanate plastics* and *polyurethane.*

UV. See *ultraviolet.*

V

vacuum-assisted resin transfer molding (VARTM). A variant of the resin transfer molding process that uses only vacuum pressure to impregnate the dry preform during cure. The advantages of this process are that because only vacuum pressure is used, the tooling does not have to withstand high pressures, and only single-sided tooling is required because a vacuum bag arrangement is used on the top side.

vacuum bag molding. A process in which a sheet of flexible transparent material plus bleeder cloth and release film are placed over the lay-up on the mold and sealed at the edges. A vacuum is applied between the sheet and the lay-up. The entrapped air is mechanically worked out of the lay-up and removed by the vacuum, and the part is cured with temperature, pressure, and time. Also called bag molding.

vacuum hot pressing (VHP). A method of processing materials (especially powders) at elevated temperatures and consolidation pressures, and low atmospheric pressures.

vacuum infusion. A resin injection technique, derived from *resin transfer molding,* in which the resin injection tank and inlet port are at ambient pressure and the pressure gradient is created by vacuum on the outlet port.

vapor-liquid-solid (VLS) process. A process using vapor feed gases and a liquid catalyst, and producing solid crystalline whisker growth. Used to produce silicon carbide whiskers.

VARTM. See *vacuum-assisted resin transfer molding.*

veil. An ultrathin mat similar to a surface mat, often composed of organic fibers as well as glass fibers.

vent. A small hole or shallow channel in a mold that allows air or gas to exit as the molding material enters.

vent cloth. A layer or layers of open-weave cloth used to provide a path for vacuum to "reach" the area over a laminate being cured, such that volatiles and air can be removed. Also causes the pressure differential that results in application of pressure to the part being cured. Also called breather cloth.

venting. In autoclave curing of a part or assembly, turning off the vacuum source and venting the vacuum bag to the atmosphere. The pressure on the part is then the difference between pressure in the autoclave and atmospheric pressure.

vermiculite. A granular material mixed with resin to form a filler of relatively high compressive strength.

VHP. See *vacuum hot pressing.*

vinyl esters. A class of thermosetting resins containing esters of acrylic and/or methacrylic acids, many of which have been made from epoxy resin. Cure is accomplished, as with unsaturated polyesters, by copolymerization with other vinyl monomers, such as styrene.

virgin filament. An individual filament that has not been in contact with any other fiber or any other hard material.

viscoelasticity. (1) A property involving a combination of elastic and viscous behavior in the application of which a material is considered to combine the features of a perfectly elastic solid and a perfect fluid. (2) Phenomenon of time-dependent, in addition to elastic, deformation (or recovery) in response to load.

viscosity. The property of resistance to flow exhibited within the body of a material, expressed in terms of relationship between applied shearing stress and resulting rate of strain in shear. Viscosity is usually taken to mean Newtonian viscosity, in which case the ratio of shearing stress to the rate of shearing strain is constant. In non-Newtonian behavior, which is the usual case with plastics, the ratio varies with the shearing stress. Such ratios are often called the apparent viscosities at the corresponding shearing stresses. Viscosity is measured in terms of flow in Pa · s (P), with water as the base standard (value of 1.0). The higher the number, the less flow.

VLS process. See *vapor-liquid-solid process.*

void content. Volume percentage of voids, usually less than 1% in a properly cured composite. The experimental determination is indirect, that is, calculated from the measured density of a cured laminate and the "theoretical" density of the starting material.

voids. Air or gas that has been trapped and cured into a laminate. Porosity is an aggregation of microvoids. Voids are essentially incapable of transmitting structural stresses or nonradiative energy fields.

volatile content. The percent of volatiles that are driven off as a vapor from a plastic or an impregnated reinforcement.

volatiles. Materials, such as water and alcohol, in a sizing or a resin formulation, that are capable of being driven off as a vapor at room temperature or at a slightly elevated temperature.

volume fraction. Fraction of a constituent material based on its volume.

volume resistance. (1) The volume resistance between two electrodes in contact with or embedded in a specimen is the ratio between the direct voltage applied to them and that portion of the current between them that is distributed through the volume of the specimen. (2) The electrical resistance between opposite faces of a 1 cm (0.40 in.) cube of insulating material. Also called specific insulation resistance.

vulcanization. A chemical reaction in which a rubber is cured by reaction with sulfur or other suitable agents.

W

wafer. A reinforcement for motorcase port openings.

warp. The yarn running lengthwise in a woven fabric. A group of yarns in long lengths and approximately parallel. A change in dimension of a cured laminate from its original molded shape.

warpage. Dimensional distortion in a composite part.

water absorption. Ratio of the weight of water absorbed by a material to the weight of the dry material.

water break. The appearance of a discontinuous film of water on a surface signifying nonuniform wetting and usually associated with a surface contamination.

water break test. A test to determine if a surface is chemically clean by the use of a drop of water, preferably distilled water. If the surface is clean, the water will break and spread; a contaminated surface will cause the water to bead.

waterjet. Water emitted from a nozzle under high pressure (70 to 410 MPa, or 10 to 60 ksi or higher). Useful for cutting organic materials. See also *abrasive waterjet.*

weathering. Exposure of plastics to the outdoor environment.

weathering, artificial. See *artificial weathering.*

weave. The particular manner in which a fabric is formed by interlacing yarns. Usually assigned a style number.

weeping. Slow leakage manifested by the appearance of water on a surface.

weft. The transverse threads or fibers in a woven fabric. Those fibers running perpendicular to the warp. Also called fill, filling yarn, or woof.

Weibull modulus (β). A statistical constant that relates strength to survival probability. The smaller the value of β, the greater the range of strength values for a material.

weld line. The mark visible on a finished part made by the meeting of two flow fronts of plastic material during molding. Also called weld mark or flow line.

weld mark. See *flow line.*

wet installation. A bolted joint in which sealant is applied to the head and shank of the fastener so that after assembly a seal is provided between the fastener and the elements being joined.

wet lay-up. A method of making a reinforced product by applying the resin system as a liquid when the reinforcement is put in place.

wet-out. The condition of an impregnated roving or yarn in which substantially all voids between the sized strands and filaments are filled with resin.

wet strength. (1) The strength of an organic matrix composite when the matrix resin is saturated with absorbed moisture, or is at a defined percentage of absorbed moisture less than saturation. (Saturation is an equilibrium condition in which the net rate of absorption under prescribed conditions falls essentially to zero). (2) The strength of an adhesive joint determined immediately after removal from a liquid in which it has been immersed under specified conditions of time, temperature, and pressure.

wetting. The spreading, and sometimes absorption, of a fluid on or into a surface.

wet winding. In filament winding, the process of winding glass on a mandrel in which the strand is impregnated with resin just before contact with the mandrel. See also *dry winding.*

whisker. A short single crystal fiber or filament used as a reinforcement in a matrix. Whisker diameters range from 1 to 25 μm (40 to 980 μin.), with aspect ratios between 100 and 15,000.

wind angle. The angular measure in degrees between the direction parallel to the filaments and an established reference. In filament-wound structures it is the convention to measure the wind angle with reference to the centerline through the polar bosses, that is, the axis of rotation.

winding pattern. (1) The total number of individual circuits required for a winding path to begin repeating by laying down immediately adjacent to the initial circuit. (2) A regularly recurring pattern of the filament path after a certain number of mandrel revolutions, leading eventually to the complete coverage of the mandrel.

winding tension. In filament winding or tape wrapping, the amount of tension on the reinforcement as it makes contact with the mandrel.

woof. See *weft.*

work hardening. (1) Increase in resistance to further deformation with continuing distortion. (2) Hardening and strengthening of a metal or alloy caused by the strain energy absorbed from prior deformation.

working life. The period of time during which a liquid resin or adhesive, after mixing with catalyst, solvent, or other compounding ingredients, remains usable. See also *gelation time* and *pot life.*

woven fabric. A material (usually a planar structure) constructed by interlacing yarns, fibers, or filaments to form such fabric patterns as plain, harness satin, or leno weaves.

woven fabric composite. A major form of advanced composite in which the fiber constituent consists of woven fabric. A woven fabric composite normally is a laminate comprised of a number of laminae, each of which consists of one layer of fabric embedded in the selected matrix material. Individual fabric laminae are directionally oriented and combined into specific multiaxial laminates for application to specific strength and stiffness requirements.

woven roving. A heavy glass fiber fabric made by weaving roving or yarn bundles.

wrinkle. A surface imperfection in laminated plastics that has the appearance of a crease or fold in one or more outer sheets of the paper, fabric, or other base, which has been pressed in. Also occurs in vacuum bag molding when the bag is improperly placed, causing a crease.

X

***x*-axis.** In composite laminates, an axis in the plane of the laminate that is used as the 0° reference for designating the angle of a lamina.

***xy*-plane.** In composite laminates, the reference plane parallel to the plane of the laminate.

Y

yarn. An assemblage of twisted filaments, fibers, or strands, either natural or manufactured, to form a continuous length that is suitable for use in weaving or interweaving into textile materials.

yarn bundle. See *bundle.*

yarn, plied. See *plied yarn.*

***y*-axis.** In composite laminates, the axis in the plane of the laminate that is perpendicular to the *x*-axis. Contrast with *x*-axis.

yield point. (1) The first stress in a material, less than the maximum attainable stress, at which the strain increases at a higher rate than the stress. (2) The point at which permanent deformation of a stressed specimen begins to take place. Only materials that exhibit yielding have a yield point.

yield strength. (1) The stress at the yield point. (2) The stress at which a material exhibits a specified limiting deviation from the proportionality of stress to strain. (3) The lowest stress at which a material undergoes plastic deformation. Below this stress, the material is elastic; above it, the material is viscous. Often defined as the stress needed to produce a specified amount of plastic deformation (usually a 0.2% change in length).

Young's modulus. The ratio of normal stress to corresponding strain for tensile or compressive stresses less than the proportional limit of the material. See also *modulus of elasticity.*

Z

***z*-axis.** In composite laminates, the reference axis normal to the plane of the laminate.

zero bleed. A laminate fabrication procedure that does not allow loss of resin during cure. Also describes prepreg made with the amount of resin desired in the final part, such that no resin has to be removed during cure.

ACKNOWLEDGMENTS

This glossary has been adapted from H.E. Pebly, Glossary of Terms, *Composites,* Volume 1, *Engineered Materials Handbook,* ASM International, 1987, p 3–26. The updates and revisions were compiled for this edition by Joseph R. Davis, Davis & Associates. ASM International would like to thank Flake C. Campbell, Jr., The Boeing Company, and Michael J. Hoke, Abaris Training Inc., for supplying new terms and definitions.

SELECTED REFERENCES

- Glossary of Terms, *Adhesives and Sealants,* Vol 3, *Engineered Materials Handbook,* ASM International, 1990, p 3–31
- Glossary of Terms, *Engineered Plastics,* Vol 2, *Engineered Materials Handbook,* ASM International, 1988, p 2–47
- Glossary of Terms, *Engineered Materials Handbook Desk Edition,* ASM International, 1995, p 3–72
- "Standard Terminology for Composite Materials," ASTM D 3878, *Annual Book of ASTM Standards,* Vol 15.03
- "Standard Terminology of Adhesives," ASTM D 907, *Annual Book of ASTM Standards,* Vol 15.06
- "Standard Terminology of Advanced Ceramics," ASTM C 1145, *Annual Book of ASTM Standards,* Vol 15.01
- "Standard Terminology of Structural Sandwich Constructions," ASTM C 274, *Annual Book of ASTM Standards,* Vol 15.03
- "Standard Terminology Relating to Manufactured Carbon and Graphite," ASTM C 709, *Annual Book of ASTM Standards,* Vol 15.01
- "Standard Terminology Relating to Plastics," ASTM D 883, *Annual Book of ASTM Standards,* Vol 08.01
- "Standard Terminology Relating to Textiles," ASTM D 123, *Annual Book of ASTM Standards,* Vol 07.01
- S.W. Horstman, "Composites and Metal Bonding Glossary," Aerospace Information Report (AIR) 4844, SAE International, 2000
- *The Composite Materials Handbook,* MIL-HDBK-17, Department of Defense (DoD) release: Vol 1E, Materials Sciences Corporation, University of Delaware, and Army Research Laboratory, 2000

Metric Conversion Guide

This Section is intended as a guide for expressing weights and measures in the Système International d'Unités (SI). The purpose of SI units, developed and maintained by the General Conference of Weights and Measures, is to provide a basis for worldwide standardization of units and measure. For more information on metric conversions, the reader should consult the following references:

- *The International System of Units,* SP 330, 1991, National Institute of Standards and Technology. Order from Superintendent of Documents, U.S. Government Printing Office, Washington, DC 20402-9325
- *Metric Editorial Guide,* 5th ed. (revised), 1993, American National Metric Council, 4340 East West Highway, Suite 401, Bethesda, MD 20814-4411
- ''Standard for Use of the International System of Units (SI): The Modern Metric System,'' IEEE/ASTM SI 10-1997, Institute of Electrical and Electronics Engineers, 345 East 47th Street, New York, NY 10017, USA
- *Guide for the Use of the International System of Units (SI),* SP 811, 1995, National Institute of Standards and Technology, U.S. Government Printing Office, Washington, DC 20402

Base, supplementary, and derived SI units

Measure	Unit	Symbol
Base units		
Amount of substance	mole	mol
Electric current	ampere	A
Length	meter	m
Luminous intensity	candela	cd
Mass	kilogram	kg
Thermodynamic temperature	kelvin	K
Time	second	s
Supplementary units		
Plane angle	radian	rad
Solid angle	steradian	sr
Derived units		
Absorbed dose	gray	Gy
Acceleration	meter per second squared	m/s^2
Activity (of radionuclides)	becquerel	Bq
Angular acceleration	radian per second squared	rad/s^2
Angular velocity	radian per second	rad/s
Area	square meter	m^2
Capacitance	farad	F
Concentration (of amount of substance)	mole per cubic meter	mol/m^3
Current density	ampere per square meter	A/m^2
Density, mass	kilogram per cubic meter	kg/m^3
Dose equivalent, dose equivalent index	sievert	Sv
Electric charge density	coulomb per cubic meter	C/m^3
Electric conductance	siemens	S
Electric field strength	volt per meter	V/m
Electric flux density	coulomb per square meter	C/m^2
Electric potential, potential difference, electromotive force	volt	V
Electric resistance	ohm	Ω
Energy, work, quantity of heat	joule	J
Energy density	joule per cubic meter	J/m^3
Entropy	joule per kelvin	J/K
Force	newton	N
Frequency	hertz	Hz
Heat capacity	joule per kelvin	J/K
Heat flux density	wa per square meter	W/m^2
Illuminance	lux	lx
Inductance	henry	H
Irradiance	wa per square meter	W/m^2
Luminance	candela per square meter	cd/m^2
Luminous flux	lumen	lm
Magnetic field strength	ampere per meter	A/m
Magnetic flux	weber	Wb
Magnetic flux density	tesla	T
Molar energy	joule per mole	J/mol
Molar entropy	joule per mole kelvin	J/mol · K
Molar heat capacity	joule per mole kelvin	J/mol · K
Moment of force	newton meter	N · m
Permeability	henry per meter	H/m
Permiivity	farad per meter	F/m
Power, radiant flux	wa	W
Pressure, stress	pascal	Pa
Quantity of electricity, electric charge	coulomb	C
Radiance	wa per square meter steradian	$W/m^2 \cdot sr$
Radiant intensity	wa per steradian	W/sr
Specific heat capacity	joule per kilogram kelvin	J/kg · K
Specific energy	joule per kilogram	J/kg
Specific entropy	joule per kilogram kelvin	J/kg · K
Specific volume	cubic meter per kilogram	m^3/kg
Surface tension	newton per meter	N/m
Thermal conductivity	wa per meter kelvin	W/m · K
Velocity	meter per second	m/s
Viscosity, dynamic	pascal second	Pa · s
Viscosity, kinematic	square meter per second	m^2/s
Volume	cubic meter	m^3
Wavenumber	1 per meter	1/m

Conversion factors

To convert from	to	multiply by
Angle		
degree	rad	1.745 329 E−02
Area		
in.^{2}	mm^2	6.451 600 E+02
in.^{2}	cm^2	6.451 600 E+00
in.^{2}	m^2	6.451 600 E−04
ft^2	m^2	9.290 304 E−02
Bending moment or torque		
lbf · in.	N · m	1.129 848 E−01
lbf · ft	N · m	1.355 818 E+00
kgf · m	N · m	9.806 650 E+00
ozf · in.	N · m	7.061 552 E−03
Bending moment or torque per unit length		
lbf · in./in.	N · m/m	4.448 222 E+00
lbf · ft/in.	N · m/m	5.337 866 E+01
Current density		
A/in.^{2}	A/cm^2	1.550 003 E−01
A/in.^{2}	A/mm^2	1.550 003 E−03
A/ft^2	A/m^2	1.076 400 E+01
Electricity and magnetism		
gauss	T	1.000 000 E−04
maxwell	μWb	1.000 000 E−02
mho	S	1.000 000 E+00
Oersted	A/m	7.957 700 E+01
Ω · cm	Ω · m	1.000 000 E−02
Ω circular-mil/ft	μΩ · m	1.662 426 E−03
Energy (impact, other)		
ft · lbf	J	1.355 818 E+00
Btu (thermochemical)	J	1.054 350 E+03
cal (thermochemical)	J	4.184 000 E+00
Cal (nutritional)	J	4.184 000 E+03
kW · h	J	3.600 000 E+06
W · h	J	3.600 000 E+03
Flow rate		
ft^3/h	L/min	4.719 475 E−01
ft^3/min	L/min	2.831 000 E+01
gal/h	L/min	6.309 020 E−02
gal/min	L/min	3.785 412 E+00
Force		
lbf	N	4.448 222 E+00
kip (1000 lbf)	N	4.448 222 E+03
onf	kN	8.896 443 E+00
kgf	N	9.806 650 E+00
Force per unit length		
lbf/ft	N/m	1.459 390 E+01
lbf/in.	N/m	1.751 268 E+02
Fracture toughness		
ksi $\sqrt{in.}$	MPa $\sqrt{m}$	1.098 800 E+00
Heat content		
Btu/lb	kJ/kg	2.326 000 E+00
cal/g	kJ/kg	4.186 800 E+00
Heat input		
J/in.	J/m	3.937 008 E+01
kJ/in.	kJ/m	3.937 008 E+01
Impact energy per unit area		
ft · lbf/ft^2	J/m^2	1.459 002 E+01
Length		
Å	nm	1.000 000 E−01
μin.	μm	2.540 000 E−02
mil	μm	2.540 000 E+01
in.	mm	2.540 000 E+01
in.	cm	2.540 000 E+00
ft	m	3.048 000 E−01
yd	m	9.144 000 E−01
mile, international	km	1.609 344 E+00
mile, nautical	km	1.852 000 E+00
mile, U.S. statute	km	1.609 347 E+00
Mass		
oz	kg	2.834 952 E−02
lb	kg	4.535 924 E−01
ton (short, 2000 lb)	kg	9.071 847 E+02
ton (short, 2000 lb)	kg × 10^3(a)	9.071 847 E−01
ton (long, 2240 lb)	kg	1.016 047 E+03
Mass per unit area		
oz/in.^{2}	kg/m^2	4.395 000 E+01
oz/ft^2	kg/m^2	3.051 517 E−01
oz/yd^2	kg/m^2	3.390 575 E−02
lb/ft^2	kg/m^2	4.882 428 E+00
Mass per unit length		
lb/ft	kg/m	1.488 164 E+00
lb/in.	kg/m	1.785 797 E+01
Mass per unit time		
lb/h	kg/s	1.259 979 E−04
lb/min	kg/s	7.559 873 E−03
lb/s	kg/s	4.535 924 E−01
Mass per unit volume (includes density)		
g/cm^3	kg/m^3	1.000 000 E+03
lb/ft^3	g/cm^3	1.601 846 E−02
lb/ft^3	kg/m^3	1.601 846 E+01
lb/in.^{3}	g/cm^3	2.767 990 E+01
lb/in.^{3}	kg/m^3	2.767 990 E+04
Power		
Btu/s	kW	1.055 056 E+00
Btu/min	kW	1.758 426 E−02
Btu/h	W	2.928 751 E−01
erg/s	W	1.000 000 E−07
ft · lbf/s	W	1.355 818 E+00
ft · lbf/min	W	2.259 697 E−02
ft · lbf/h	W	3.766 161 E−04
hp (550 ft · lbf/s)	kW	7.456 999 E−01
hp (electric)	kW	7.460 000 E−01
Power density		
W/in.^{2}	W/m^2	1.550 003 E+03
Pressure (fluid)		
atm (standard)	Pa	1.013 250 E+05
bar	Pa	1.000 000 E+05
in. Hg (32 °F)	Pa	3.386 380 E+03
in. Hg (60 °F)	Pa	3.376 850 E+03
lbf/in.^{2} (psi)	Pa	6.894 757 E+03
torr (mm Hg, 0 °C)	Pa	1.333 220 E+02
Specific heat		
Btu/lb · °F	J/kg · K	4.186 800 E+03
cal/g · °C	J/kg · K	4.186 800 E+03
Stress (force per unit area)		
tonf/in.^{2} (tsi)	MPa	1.378 951 E+01
kgf/mm^2	MPa	9.806 650 E+00
ksi	MPa	6.894 757 E+00
lbf/in.^{2} (psi)	MPa	6.894 757 E−03
MN/m^2	MPa	1.000 000 E+00
Temperature		
°F	°C	5/9 · (°F − 32)
°R	K	5/9
K	°C	K − 273.15
Temperature interval		
°F	°C	5/9
Thermal conductivity		
Btu · in./s · ft^2 · °F	W/m · K	5.192 204 E+02
Btu/ft · h · °F	W/m · K	1.730 735 E+00
Btu · in./h · ft^2 · °F	W/m · K	1.442 279 E−01
cal/cm · s · °C	W/m · K	4.184 000 E+02
Thermal expansion		
in./in. · °C	m/m · K	1.000 000 E+00
in./in. · °F	m/m · K	1.800 000 E+00
Velocity		
ft/h	m/s	8.466 667 E−05
ft/min	m/s	5.080 000 E−03
ft/s	m/s	3.048 000 E−01
in./s	m/s	2.540 000 E−02
km/h	m/s	2.777 778 E−01
mph	km/h	1.609 344 E+00
Velocity of rotation		
rev/min (rpm)	rad/s	1.047 164 E−01
rev/s	rad/s	6.283 185 E+00
Viscosity		
poise	Pa · s	1.000 000 E−01
stokes	m^2/s	1.000 000 E−04
ft^2/s	m^2/s	9.290 304 E−02
in.^{2}/s	mm^2/s	6.451 600 E+02
Volume		
in.^{3}	m^3	1.638 706 E−05
ft^3	m^3	2.831 685 E−02
fluid oz	m^3	2.957 353 E−05
gal (U.S. liquid)	m^3	3.785 412 E−03
Volume per unit time		
ft^3/min	m^3/s	4.719 474 E−04
ft^3/s	m^3/s	2.831 685 E−02
in.^{3}/min	m^3/s	2.731 177 E−07

(a) kg × 10^3 = 1 metric ton or 1 megagram (Mg)

SI prefixes—names and symbols

Exponential expression	Multiplication factor	Prefix	Symbol
10^{24}	1 000 000 000 000 000 000 000 000	yotta	Y
10^{21}	1 000 000 000 000 000 000 000	zetta	Z
10^{18}	1 000 000 000 000 000 000	exa	E
10^{15}	1 000 000 000 000 000	peta	P
10^{12}	1 000 000 000 000	tera	T
10^{9}	1 000 000 000	giga	G
10^{6}	1 000 000	mega	M
10^{3}	1 000	kilo	k
10^{2}	100	hecto(a)	h
10^{1}	10	deka(a)	da
10^{0}	1	BASE UNIT	
10^{-1}	0.1	deci(a)	d
10^{-2}	0.01	centi(a)	c
10^{-3}	0.001	milli	m
10^{-6}	0.000 001	micro	µ
10^{-9}	0.000 000 001	nano	n
10^{-12}	0.000 000 000 001	pico	p
10^{-15}	0.000 000 000 000 001	femto	f
10^{-18}	0.000 000 000 000 000 001	atto	a
10^{-21}	0.000 000 000 000 000 000 001	zepto	z
10^{-24}	0.000 000 000 000 000 000 000 001	yocto	y

(a) Nonpreferred. Prefixes should be selected in steps of 10^3 so that the resultant number before the prefix is between 0.1 and 1000. These prefixes should not be used for units of linear measurement, but may be used for higher order units. For example, the linear measurement, decimeter, is nonpreferred, but square decimeter is acceptable.

Abbreviations and Symbols

a crack length
A ampere; alkali (glass fiber designator)
A area; ratio of the alternating stress amplitude to the mean stress
Å angstrom
ABS acrylonitrile-butadiene-styrene
ac alternating current
AE acoustic emission
AES Auger electron spectroscopy
AESO acrylated epoxidized soybean oil
AFRL Air Force Research Laboratory
AGATE Advanced General Aviation Transport Experiments
AMS Aerospace Materials Specification
ANOVA analysis of variance
ANSI American National Standards Institute
AO atomic oxygen
APB aminophenoxy benzene
ARC accelerated rate calorimeter
AS designation for surface-treated fiber
ASR automobile
ASTM American Society for Testing and Materials
at.% atomic percent
ATL automated tape layer
atm atmosphere (pressure)
AU designation for untreated fiber
B width of faces; test section length and width
BET Brunauer-Emmett-Teller
BF_3 boron trifluoride
BJSFM bolted-joint stress field model
BMC bulk molding compound
BMI bismaleimide (resin)
BPA bisphenol A
Btu British thermal unit
BVID barely visible impact damage
C Kozeny constant
c composite specific heat (c_p = constant pressure, c_v = constant volume)
CACRC Commercial Aircraft Composite Repair Committee
CAD/CAM computer-aided design/computer-aided manufacturing
CAE computer aided engineering
CAI compression after impact
CAS calcium aluminosilicate
CAT computer-aided tomography
C-C carbon-carbon
CDCA cyclohexane dicarboxylic anhydride
CFCC continuous fiber ceramic composite
CFRC carbon fiber reinforced composite
CFRM continuous filament random mat
CFRP carbon fiber reinforced plastic
CIP cold isostatic pressing
cm centimeter
CMC ceramic-matrix composite
CME coefficient of moisture expansion
CMM coordinate measuring machine
CMOD crack mouth opening displacement
CNC computer numeric control
CP commercially pure
cpm cycles per minute
cps cycles per second
CSAI compression strength after impact
CSM chopped-strand mat
CTE coefficient of thermal expansion
CV coefficient of variation PENDING AQ confirmation
CVD chemical vapor deposition
CVI chemical vapor infiltration
CVN Charpy V-notch (impact test or specimen)
d an operator used in mathematical expressions involving a derivative (denotes rate of change)
d depth; diameter
da/dn crack growth rate
dB decibel
DABA diallylbisphenol A
DAP diallyl phthalate
DBTT ductile-brittle transition temperature
dc direct current
DCB double-cantilever beam
DCPD dicyclopentadiene
DDA dynamic dielectric analysis
DEA dielectric analysis
DERA Defence Evaluation and Research Agency (United Kingdom)
DETA diethylene triamine
DFMA design for manufacture and assembly
DGEBA diglycidyl ether of bisphenol A
DGEBF diglycidyl ether of bisphenol F
diam diameter
DIC differential interference contrast
DMA dynamic mechanical analysis
DMAC dimethylacetamide
DMF dimethylformamide
DMLCC,E design and manufacturing of low-cost composites for engines
DoD Department of Defense
DOE Department of Energy
DOF degrees of freedom
DRA discontinuously reinforced aluminum
DRTi discontinuously reinforced titanium
DSC differential scanning calorimetry
DTA differential thermal analysis
DTUL deflection temperature under load
e natural log base, 2.71828
E electrical (designator for glass)
E modulus of elasticity; Young's modulus
EB electron beam
EC eddy current
ECR special-purpose glass fiber characterized by high corrosion resistance
EEW epoxy per equivalent weight
EMI/RFI electromagnetic interference/radio-frequency interference
ENF end-notched flexure
Eq equation
et al. and others
ESCA electron spectroscopy for chemical analysis
ESD electrostatic discharge
ETD elevated temperature, dry
ETW elevated temperature, wet
f fiber
F force; strength
FAA Federal Aviation Administration
FALN failure analysis logic network
FE finite element
FEM finite element model
FAW fiber areal weight
FCG fatigue crack growth
FEA finite element analysis
FEP fluorinated ethylene propylene
FG fiberglass
FOD foreign object damage
FOS factor of safety
FP polycrystalline alumina fiber
FPL Forest Products Laboratory
FRC fiber reinforced composites
FRP fiber-reinforced plastic
ft foot
FTIR Fourier transform infrared
g gram
G shear modulus
G′ storage modulus
G″ loss modulus
G_{Ic} interlaminar fracture toughness (mode I, peel; mode II, shear; mode III, scissor shear)
gal gallon
GFRP glass-fiber-reinforced plastic
GMT glass mat thermoplastics
GL/EP glass/epoxy
GPa gigapascal

GPC gel permeation chromatography
gpd grams per denier
gr grain
GRP glass reinforced plastic
h hour
h height
H height
HAZ heat-affected zone
HDT heat-deflection temperature
HEPA high-efficiency particulate air
HERF high-energy-rate forging
HEXA hexamethylenetetramine
HIP hot isostatic pressing
HLU hand lay-up
HM high modulus
HO/MA hydroxylated oil, maleinized
HPC high-performance compound
HPLC high-performance liquid chromatography
HS high-strength
HSO/MA hydroxylated soybean oil, maleinated
HT high tensile
Hz hertz
I moment of inertia
ICP inductively coupled plasma
ID inside diameter
IFT interlaminar fracture toughness
IM intermediate modulus
IMC in-mold coating
IMC intermetallic-matrix composite
IR infrared (radiation)
ISO International Standards Organization
ISS interlaminar shear strength
J joule
k notch sensitivity factor; thermal conductivity
K Kelvin
K coefficient of thermal conductivity; bulk modulus of elasticity
K_c plane-stress fracture toughness
K_I stress-intensity factor
K_{Ic} plane-strain fracture toughness; mode I critical stress-intensity factor
K_{Id} dynamic fracture toughness
K_{Iscc} threshold stress intensity for stress-corrosion cracking
K_t stress-concentration factor
K_{th} threshold crack tip stress-intensity factor
kg kilogram
km kilometer
kPa kilopascal
ksi kips (1000 lb) per square inch
kV kilovolt
l length
L liter; longitudinal direction
L length
lb pound
LCF low cycle fatigue
LEFM linear-elastic fracture mechanics
LEO low earth orbit
LFG long fiber granulate
LFT long fiber thermoplastics
LM low modulus
LMC laminated metal composite
ln natural logarithm (base ***e***)
LOM laminated object manufacture
LS low shrink
LSE low-styrene emission
LVID low velocity impact damage
m matrix
M modulus (glass fiber designator)
M moment
MAS magnesium aluminosilicate
MDA methylenedianiline
MEK methyl ethyl ketone
Mg megagram
min minute; minimum
MJ megajoule
mL milliliter
mm millimeter
MMA methyl methacrylate
MMC metal-matrix composite
MOL material operational limit
mol% mole percent
MPa megapascal
mph miles per hour
MSDS materials safety data sheet
MTE medium-toughness epoxy
MVT moisture vapor transmission
N Newton
N fatigue life (number of cycles)
NA not applicable
NASA National Aeronautics and Space Administration
NC numerical control
NDE nondestructive evaluation
NDI nondestructive inspection
NDT nondestructive testing
NGV natural gas vehicle
nm nanometer
NMP N-methyl pyrrolidinone
NMR nuclear magnetic resonance
NOL Naval Ordnance Laboratory
No. number
NPG neopentyl glycol
OD outside diameter
OEM original equipment manufacturer
OHC open-hole compression
OHV overhead valve
OMC organic-matrix composite
OMS orbital maneuvering system
OSHA Occupational Safety and Health Administration
oz ounce
p particulate
P applied load; pressure
Pa pascal
PA polyamide
PAI polyamide-imide
PAN polyacrylonitrile
PAS polyarylsulfone
PBI polybenzimidazole
PBT polybutylene terephthalate
PC polycarbonate
PCB printed circuit board
PEI polyetherimide
PEEK polyetheretherketone
PES polyether sulfone
PET polyethylene terephthalate
PF phenol formaldehyde
phr parts per hundred parts resin
PI polyimide
PIC pressure-impregnation-carbonization
PIP polymer infiltration and pyrolysis
pl platelet
P/M powder metallurgy
PMC polymer-matrix composite
PMMA polymethyl methacrylate
PMR in situ polymerization of monomer reactants
PP polypropylene
ppb parts per billion
PPE polyphenylene ether
ppm parts per million
PPS polyphenylene sulfide
Pr Prandtl number
PRF phenol resorcinal formaldehyde
PR-MMC particle-reinforced metal-matrix composites
PS polysulfone
psi pounds per square inch
psia pounds per square inch absolute
psid pounds per square inch differential
psig pounds per square inch gage
PTFE polytetrafluoroethylene
PUR polyurethane
PVA polyvinyl alcohol
PVAC polyvinyl acetate
PVC polyvinyl chloride
PVD physical vapor deposition
PVDF polyvinylidene fluoride
PVF polyvinyl fluoride
PZT lead-zirconium titanate
r radius; rate of reaction
R radius; ratio of the minimum stress to the maximum stress; load ratio
RA reduction of area
Ref reference
RFI resin-film infusion
RGA residual gas analysis
RH relative humidity
RI refractive index
RIM reaction injection molding
RMS root mean square
ROM rule of mixtures; rough order of magnitude
RP rapid prototyping
rpm revolutions per minute
RRIM reinforced reaction injection molding
RT room temperature
RTD room temperature, dry
RTM resin transfer molding
RTW room temperature, wet
RTV room temperature, vulcanizing
RVE representative volume element
s second
s symmetry of stacking about the midplane
S strength (glass fiber designator)
SACMA Suppliers of Advanced Composite Materials Association
SAE Society of Automotive Engineers
SaRTM solvent-assisted resin transfer molding
SAVE structural analysis using variable-order elements
SBS short beam shear
SCRIMP Seeman composite resin infusion molding process
SD standard deviation
SEM scanning electron microscope or microscopy

SHS self-propagating high-temperature synthesis
SI Systeme International d'Unites
SIMS secondary ion mass spectroscopy
SLA stereolithography
SLS selective laser sintering
SM standard modulus
SMC sheet molding compound
SMC-C sheet molding compound-continuous
SMC-R sheet molding compound-random
S-N stress-number of cycles
SOMG/MA soybean oil monoglyceride, maleinated
SPC statistical process control
SPF superplastic forming
sp gr specific gravity
SRIM structural reaction injection molding
SSB small-scale bridging
SSY small-scale yielding
t thickness; time
T transverse direction
T temperature; tenacity
tan equal to ratio of the loss modulus to the storage modulus
TEM transmission electron microscope or microscopy
TFE tetrafluoroethylene
T_g glass transition temperature
TGA thermogravimetric analysis
TLC thin-layer chromatography
T_m melting temperature
TMA thermomechanical analysis
TMC thick molding compound; titanium-matrix composite
TMF thermal mechanical fatigue
TPI turns per inch
TS thermoset
TTU through-transmission ultrasonics
U velocity
UD unidirectional
UDC unidirectional composite
UHM ultrahigh modulus
UL Underwriters' Laboratory
UP, UPE unsaturated polyester
USAF United States Air Force
UTS ultimate tensile strength
UV ultraviolet
VARI vacuum-assisted resin injection
VARTM vacuum-assisted resin transfer molding
v viscosity; void
V velocity; volume fraction
VCXPS voltage contrast x-ray photoelectron spectroscopy
V_f volume fraction of fiber
VHP vacuum hot pressing
VLS vapor-liquid-solid
V_m volume fraction of matrix
VOC volatile organic compound
vol volume
vol% volume percent
V_v volume fraction of void content
w whisker
W watt
W width
WPE weight per epoxide
WR woven roving
wt% weight percent
XPS x-ray photoelectron spectroscopy
YAG yttrium-aluminum-garnet
yr year
ZTA zirconia-toughened alumina
1-D one dimensional
2-D two dimensional
3-D three dimensional
3DP three-dimensional printing
° angular measure; degree
°C degree Celsius (centigrade)
°F degree Fahrenheit
0° fiber direction
90° perpendicular to fiber direction
α angle; coefficient of thermal expansion
Δ change in quantity; an increment; a range
η viscosity
ε strain
$\dot{\varepsilon}$ strain rate
ε-N strain life, strain-number of cycles
γ shear strain; surface tension; surface energy
$\dot{\gamma}$ shear strain rate
μin. microinch
μm micrometer (micron)
ν Poisson's ratio
π pi (3.141592)
ω excitation frequency
ψ damping
ρ density
σ tensile stress
τ shear stress
θ angle
$\pm\theta$ angle plies
ϕ porosity
⇔ direction of reaction
÷ divided by
= equals
^ circumflex
≈ approximately equals
≠ not equal to
≡ identical with
> greater than
≫ much greater than
≥ greater than or equal to
∞ infinity
∝ is proportional to; varies as
∫ integral of
< less than
≪ much less than
≤ less than or equal to
± maximum deviation
− minus; negative ion charge
× diameters (magnification); multiplied by
· multiplied by
Ω ohm
/ per
% percent
\+ plus; positive ion charge
√ square root of
~ approximately; similar to

Greek Alphabet

Α, α alpha
Β, β beta
Γ, γ gamma
Δ, δ delta
Ε, ε epsilon
Ζ, ζ zeta
Η, η eta
Θ, θ theta
Ι, ι iota
Κ, κ kappa
Λ, λ lambda
Μ, μ mu
Ν, ν nu
Ξ, ξ xi
Ο, ο omicron
Π, π pi
Ρ, ρ rho
Σ, σ sigma
Τ, τ tau
Υ, υ upsilon
Φ, φ phi
Χ, χ chi
Ψ, ψ psi
Ω, ω omega

Index

A

B

C

D

E

F

G

H

I

J

K

L

M

N

O

Q

R

T

U

V

W

X

Y

Z